Appendices

KIRK'S
CURRENT VETERINARY THERAPY
XIII
SMALL ANIMAL PRACTICE

Consulting Editors

CARL A. OSBORNE
Special Therapy

NISHI DHUPA and ROBERT J. MURTAUGH
Critical Care

MICHAEL J. MURPHY
Toxicologic Disorders

EDWARD B. BREITSCHWERDT
Infectious Diseases

MARK E. PETERSON
Endocrine and Metabolic Disorders

BRUCE R. MADEWELL
Hematology, Oncology, and Immunology

CRAIG E. GRIFFIN and WAYNE S. ROSENKRANTZ
Dermatologic Diseases

DAVID C. TWEDT
Gastrointestinal Disorders

BRUCE W. KEENE and LINDA B. LEHMKUHL
Cardiopulmonary Diseases

JEANNE A. BARSANTI
Urinary Disorders

VICKI N. MEYERS-WALLEN
Reproductive Disorders

STEVEN C. SCHRADER and KYLE G. BRAUND
Neurologic and Musculoskeletal Disorders

THOMAS J. KERN and MARK P. NASISSE
Ophthalmologic Diseases

NANCY L. ANDERSON and R. ERIC MILLER
Diseases of Birds and Exotic Pets

ROBERT M. JACOBS and MARK G. PAPICH
Appendices

KIRK'S CURRENT VETERINARY THERAPY

XIII
SMALL ANIMAL PRACTICE

Edited by

JOHN D. BONAGURA, D.V.M., M.S.

Dipl. A.C.V.I.M. (Cardiology, Internal Medicine)
Gilbreath-McLorn Professor of Veterinary Cardiology
Department of Veterinary Medicine and Surgery
University of Missouri Veterinary Medical Teaching Hospital
Columbia, Missouri

W.B. SAUNDERS COMPANY
A Harcourt Health Sciences Company
Philadelphia   London   New York   St. Louis   Sydney   Toronto

W.B. SAUNDERS COMPANY
A Harcourt Health Sciences Company

The Curtis Center
Independence Square West
Philadelphia, Pennsylvania 19106

Library of Congress Cataloging-in-Publication Data

Current veterinary therapy. 1964/65—Philadelphia, W. B. Saunders "Small animal practice." Editor: 1964/65- R. W. Kirk. Key title: Current Veterinary Therapy

v. 26 cm.

1. Veterinary medicine—Periodicals.   2. Pets—Diseases—Periodicals.   I. Kirk, Robert Warren, ed. [DNLM: W1 CU823]

SF 745,C8   636.0896   64—10489
                            MARC-S

Library of Congress   [8308]

KIRK'S CURRENT VETERINARY THERAPY XIII   ISBN 0–7216–5523–8

Last digit is the print number: 9   8   7   6   5   4   3

To my parents,
Peter J. Bonagura and Hazel Young Bonagura

JDB

CONTRIBUTORS

Noha Abou-Madi, D.V.M., M.Sc.
Post-Doctorate Associate, College of Veterinary Medicine, Cornell University, Ithaca, New York
Dysecdysis (Abnormal Skin Shedding) in Reptiles

Anthony C. G. Abrams-Ogg, D.V.M., D.V.Sc., Dipl. A.C.V.I.M.
Associate Professor, Department of Clinical Studies, Ontario Veterinary College, University of Guelph, Guelph, Ontario, Canada
Antimicrobial Therapy for the Neutropenic Dog and Cat

Janette Ackerman, D.V.M.
Director of Veterinary Services, American Wildlife Foundation, Molalla, Oregon
Care of Orphan Birds

Verena K. Affolter, D.V.M., F.V.H. Pathology
Dermatopathologist, Department of Veterinary Pathology, Microbiology and Immunology, School of Veterinary Medicine, University of California, Davis, California
Immunophenotyping in the Dog; Canine Cutaneous Histiocytic Diseases

Gustavo D. Aguirre, V.M.D., Ph.D., Ph.D. (hc), Dipl. A.C.V.O.
Alfred H. Caspary Professor of Ophthalmology, James A. Baker Institute for Animal Health, College of Veterinary Medicine, Cornell University, Ithaca, New York
DNA Testing for Inherited Canine Diseases

F. J. Allan, B.V.Sc., M.V.Sc.
Lecturer, Companion Animal Medicine, Centre for Companion Animal Health, Institute of Veterinary, Animal and Biomedical Sciences, Massey University, Palmerston North, New Zealand
Assessment of Gastrointestinal Motility

Nancy L. Anderson, D.V.M., Dipl. A.B.V.P. (Avian)
Graduate Teaching Associate, Department of Evolution, Ecology, and Organismal Biology, College of Veterinary Medicine, The Ohio State University, Columbus, Ohio
Section 14, Consulting Editor; Appendices

Tammy E. Anderson, D.V.M.
Veterinary Internal Medicine Resident, Small Animal Teaching Hospital, College of Veterinary Medicine, University of Tennessee, Knoxville, Tennessee
Tumors of the Respiratory Tract

Natalie Antinoff, D.V.M., Dipl. A.B.V.P. (Avian)
Staff Veterinarian, Gulf Coast Avian and Exotics, Gulf Coast Veterinary Specialists, Houston, Texas
Neoplasia in Ferrets

Max J. G. Appel, D.V.M., Ph.D.
Professor of Virology, James A. Baker Institute for Animal Health, College of Veterinary Medicine, Cornell University, Ithaca, New York
Lyme Disease Vaccination

P. Jane Armstrong, D.V.M., M.S., Dipl. A.C.V.I.M.
Professor, Internal Medicine/Clinical Nutrition, College of Veterinary Medicine, University of Minnesota, St. Paul, Minnesota
Mechanical Devices for Percutaneous Placement of Gastrostomy Tubes: Use of Eld Applicator; Feline Cholangiohepatitis

Susi Arnold, PhD, Dr. Med. Vet.
Privatdozentin, Department of Reproduction, Veterinary Faculty, University of Zurich, Zurich, Switzerland
Urethral Sphincter Mechanism Incompetence in Male Dogs

Clarke E. Atkins, D.V.M., Dipl. A.C.V.I.M. (Internal Medicine and Cardiology)
Professor of Medicine and Cardiology, College of Veterinary Medicine, North Carolina State University, Raleigh, North Carolina
CVT Update: Diagnosis and Prevention of Heartworm Disease in Cats

Glenn W. Austin
President, Louis C. Herring & Company, Orlando, Florida
Adverse Effects of Drugs on Formation of Canine and Feline Crystalluria and Uroliths

Helio Silva Autran de Morais, D.V.M., Ph.D., Dipl. A.C.V.I.M. (Internal Medicine and Cardiology)
Associate Professor and Department Chair, Departamento de Clínicas Veterinárias; Internist/ Cardiologist, Hospital Veterinário, Universidade Estadual de Londrina, Londrina, Paraná, Brazil
Routes of Fluid Administration: Indications, Contraindications, Techniques, and Complications; Feline Congenital Heart Disease

Rodney S. Bagley, D.V.M., Dipl. A.C.V.I.M.

Associate Professor, Neurology and Neurosurgery, College of Veterinary Medicine, Washington State University, Pullman, Washington

Vestibular Disease of Dogs and Cats

A. Catherine Barr, Ph.D. (Toxicology)

Adjunct Assistant Professor, Department of Veterinary Anatomy and Public Health, College of Veterinary Medicine, Texas A&M University; Assistant Toxicologist, Texas Veterinary Medical Diagnostic Laboratory, College Station, Texas

Grass, Poinsettias, and Nontoxic Plants

Jeanne A. Barsanti, D.V.M., M.S., Dipl. A.C.V.I.M.

Professor, Department of Small Animal Medicine, College of Veterinary Medicine, University of Georgia; Internist Chief, Small Animal Medical Section, University of Georgia Veterinary Teaching Hospital, Athens, Georgia

Section 10, Consulting Editor; Diagnostic Approach to Polyuria and Polydipsia; Recent Developments in the Management of Progressive Renal Failure; Bacterial Urinary Tract Infection in Cats

Stephen L. Barten, D.V.M.

Partner, Vernon Hills Animal Hospital, Mundelein, Illinois

Egg Laying Problems in Green Iguanas, Iguana iguana

Joseph W. Bartges, D.V.M., Ph.D., Dipl. A.C.V.I.M., A.C.V.N.

Associate Professor of Medicine and Nutrition, Department of Small Animal Clinical Sciences, College of Veterinary Medicine; Internist and Clinical Nutritionist, Veterinary Teaching Hospitals, University of Tennessee, Knoxville, Tennessee

Management of Anorexia; Parenteral Nutrition Products; Refeeding Syndrome; CVT Update: Therapy for Hepatic Lipidosis; Summary of Dietary Recommendations in Urinary Diseases; Recent Developments in the Management of Progressive Renal Failure; Ammonium Urate Uroliths in Dogs With Portosystemic Shunts; Bacterial Urinary Tract Infection in Cats

Linda Barton, D.V.M., Dipl. A.C.V.E.C.C.

Staff Veterinarian, Emergency Critical Care, The Animal Medical Center, New York, New York

Open Chest Cardiopulmonary Resuscitation

Neal Bataller, M.E., D.V.M.

Coordinator, FDA/CVM Adverse Drug Experience Reporting System, Center for Veterinary Medicine, U.S. Food and Drug Administration, Rockville, Maryland

Adverse Drug Reactions

Karin M. Beale, D.V.M., Dipl. A.C.V.D.

Staff Dermatologist, Dermatology & Allergy, Gulf Coast Veterinary Specialists, Houston, Texas

Feline Demodicosis

Stephanie L. Beardsley, D.V.M., Dipl. A.C.V.S.

Chief of Staff, Central Texas Veterinary Surgery, P.C., Austin, Texas

Shearing and Degloving Wounds on the Extremities of Dogs and Cats

Ellen N. Behrend, V.M.D., M.S., Dipl. A.C.V.I.M.

Fellow in Endocrinology, Department of Anatomy, Physiology, and Pharmacology, College of Veterinary Medicine, Auburn University, Auburn, Alabama

CVT Update: Interpretation of Endocrine Diagnostic Test Results for Adrenal and Thyroid Disease

Anna-Lena Berg, D.V.M., Ph.D.

Senior Researcher, Department of Pathology, Swedish University of Agricultural Sciences, Uppsala, Sweden

Borna Disease in Cats

Philip J. Bergman, D.V.M., M.S., Dipl. A.C.V.I.M. (Oncology)

American Cancer Society PRTA Fellow, M.D. Anderson Cancer Center, Department of Cell Biology, Houston, Texas

Multidrug Resistance

Sonya V. Bettenay, M.A.C.V.Sc., Fellow A.C.V.Sc.

Australian College of Veterinary Sciences (Dermatology), Animal Skin & Allergy Clinic, Mount Waverly, Australia

Feline Atopy

G. Daniel Boon, D.V.M., M.S., Dipl. A.C.V.P.

President and Director of Pathology, United Veterinary Laboratories, Garden Grove, California

Interpretation of Cytograms and Histograms of Erythrocytes, Leukocytes, and Platelets

Mona J. Boord, D.V.M., Dipl. A.C.V.D.

Dermatologist Veterinarian Consultant, Animal Dermatology Clinic, Animal Allergy Specialists, San Diego, California

In Vitro Assays in the Diagnosis and Treatment of Atopic Disease

Rosemary J. Booth, B.V.Sc.

Senior Veterinarian, Healesville Sanctuary, Healesville, Victoria, Australia

General Husbandry and Medical Care of Sugar Gliders

Dawn Merton Boothe, D.V.M., M.S., Ph.D., Dipl. A.C.V.I.M., A.C.V.C.P.

Associate Professor, Department of Veterinary Physiology and Pharmacology, College of Veterinary Medicine, Texas A&M University; Director, Clinical

Pharmacology Laboratory; Clinician, Veterinary Medical Teaching Hospital, Texas Veterinary Medical Center, College Station, Texas

Therapeutic Drug Monitoring; Do's and Don'ts of Antimicrobial Therapy; Fluorinated Quinolones: Use and Misuses

Dino Bradley, D.V.M., M.S.

Research Associate, Scott-Ritchey Research Center, College of Veterinary Medicine, Auburn University, Auburn, Alabama

Acral Lick Dermatitis

Kyle G. Braund, B.V.Sc., M.V.Sc., Ph.D., F.R.C.V.S., Dipl. A.C.V.I.M. (Neurology)

Professor, Small Animal Medicine and Surgery, College of Veterinary Medicine, Auburn University; Director, Neuromuscular Diagnostic Laboratory, Scott-Ritchey Research Center, Auburn, Alabama

Section 12, Consulting Editor; Chronic Inflammatory Demyelinating Polyneuropathy in Dogs

Edward B. Breitschwerdt, D.V.M., B.S., Dipl. A.C.V.I.M.

Professor of Medicine and Infectious Diseases, College of Veterinary Medicine, North Carolina State University, Raleigh; Adjunct Assistant Professor of Medicine, Duke University Medical Center, Durham, North Carolina

Section 4, Consulting Editor; Why Are Infectious Diseases Emerging?; Bartonella vinsonii Infection in Dogs; Bartonella Infections in Domestic Cats

Marjory Brooks, D.V.M., Dipl. A.C.V.I.M.

Associate Director, Comparative Coagulation Laboratory, Department of Population Medicine and Diagnostic Sciences, College of Veterinary Medicine, Cornell University, Ithaca, New York

Platelet Dysfunction

Michael C. Brown, Ph.D.

International Canine Genetics, Malvern, Pennsylvania

Use of Serum Relaxin for Pregnancy Diagnosis in the Bitch

Scott A. Brown, V.M.D., Ph.D., Dipl. A.C.V.I.M.

Associate Professor, Department of Physiology and Pharmacology, College of Veterinary Medicine, University of Georgia; Associate Professor, Department of Small Animal Medicine, University of Georgia Veterinary Medical Teaching Hospital, Athens, Georgia

The Kidney and Hyperthyroidism; Diagnosis of Systemic Hypertension in Dogs and Cats; Therapy for Systemic Hypertension in Dogs and Cats; Summary of Dietary Recommendations in Urinary Diseases; Recent Developments in the Management of Progressive Renal Failure

Susan A. Brown, D.V.M.

Partner, Midwest Bird & Exotic Animal Hospital, Westchester, Illinois

Neutering of Rabbits and Rodents

David S. Bruyette, D.V.M., Dipl. A.C.V.I.M.

Medical Director, VCA West Los Angeles Animal Hospital, Los Angeles, California

L-Deprenyl Therapy for Canine Cognitive Dysfunction; CVT Update: L-Deprenyl in the Treatment of Canine Pituitary-Dependent Hyperadrenocorticism

Steven C. Budsberg, D.V.M., M.S., Dipl. A.C.V.S.

Professor of Surgery, Department of Small Animal Medicine, College of Veterinary Medicine, University of Georgia, Athens, Georgia

Use of Chondromodulating Drugs and Substances in the Prevention and Treatment of Osteoarthritis in Dogs

C. A. Tony Buffington, D.V.M., Ph.D., Dipl. A.C.V.N.

Department of Veterinary Clinical Sciences, College of Veterinary Medicine, The Ohio State University, Columbus, Ohio

CVT Update: Idiopathic (Interstitial) Cystitis in Cats

Susan E. Bunch, D.V.M., Ph.D., Dipl. A.C.V.I.M.

Professor of Medicine, and Internist, Veterinary Teaching Hospital, College of Veterinary Medicine, North Carolina State University, Raleigh, North Carolina

Diagnostic Approach to Hepatobiliary Disease

Janice L. Cain, D.V.M., Dipl. A.C.V.I.M.

Internist, Specialty Practice, Norris Canyon Veterinary Medical Center, San Ramon, California

CVT Update: Infertility in the Bitch

Marco Caldin, Dr. Med. Vet.

Senior Lecturer in Veterinary Medical Pathology, Faculty of Veterinary Medicine, University of Padua; Director of Medicine, Chief of Service, Veterinary Clinic San Marco, Padua, Italy

Recognition and Treatment of Disseminated Intravascular Coagulation

Clay A. Calvert, D.V.M., Dipl. A.C.V.I.M.

Professor, Department of Small Animal Medicine, College of Veterinary Medicine, University of Georgia, Athens, Georgia

CVT Update: Doberman Pinscher Occult Cardiomyopathy

Richard C. Cambre, B.S., D.V.M.

Head, Department of Animal Health, National Zoological Park, Smithsonian Institution, Washington, District of Columbia

Salmonella in Reptiles

Elaine R. Caplan, D.V.M., Dipl. A.B.V.P.

Surgery Instructor, Veterinary Teaching Hospital, Iowa State University, Ames, Iowa

Treatment of Insulinoma in the Dog, Cat, and Ferret

James W. Carpenter, M.S., D.V.M., Dipl. A.C.Z.M.

Professor, Exotic Animal, Wildlife, and Zoo Animal Medicine Service, Department of Clinical Sciences, College of Veterinary Medicine, Kansas State University, Manhattan, Kansas

Trichobezoars and Gastric Stasis in Rabbits

Anthony P. Carr, Dr. Med. Vet., Dipl. A.C.V.I.M.

Staff Internist, Emergency Clinic for Animals, Madison, Wisconsin

Von Willebrand's Disease and Other Hereditary Coagulopathies

James L. Catalfamo, M.S., Ph.D.

Director, Comparative Coagulation Laboratory, Department of Population Medicine and Diagnostic Sciences, College of Veterinary Medicine, Cornell University, Ithaca, New York

Platelet Dysfunction

Sharon A. Center, D.V.M., Dipl. A.C.V.I.M.

Professor, Internal Medicine, College of Veterinary Medicine, Cornell University, Ithaca, New York

Hepatoportal Microvascular Dysplasia

Erin S. Champagne, D.V.M., Dipl. A.C.V.O.

Visiting Clinical Assistant Professor, Department of Veterinary Medicine and Surgery, College of Veterinary Medicine, University of Missouri, Columbia, Missouri

Eyelid Diseases

Dennis J. Chew, D.V.M., Dipl. A.C.V.I.M.

Professor, Department of Clinical Sciences, College of Veterinary Medicine, The Ohio State University; Attending Clinician, The Ohio State University Veterinary Medical Teaching Hospital, Columbus, Ohio

Treatment of Hypoparathyroidism; CVT Update: Idiopathic (Interstitial) Cystitis in Cats

Mary M. Christopher, D.V.M., Ph.D., Dipl. A.C.V.P.

Department of Pathology, Microbiology and Immunology, School of Veterinary Medicine; Clinician, Veterinary Medical Teaching Hospital, University of California, Davis, California

Disorders of Feline Red Blood Cells

Jane Owens Clark, D.V.M., Ph.D.

Senior Research Scientist, Animal Health Product Development, Safety and Metabolism, Pfizer Central Research, Groton, Connecticut

Common Household Chemical Hazards; Toxicities From Newer Over-the-Counter Drugs

Victoria L. Clyde, D.V.M.

Staff Veterinarian, Milwaukee County Zoo, Milwaukee, Wisconsin

Avian Analgesia

Leah A. Cohn, D.V.M., Ph.D., Dipl. A.C.V.I.M.

Assistant Professor of Veterinary Medicine, College of Veterinary Medicine, University of Missouri, Columbia, Missouri

CVT Update: Diagnosis and Treatment of Parvovirus

Patrick W. Concannon, M.S., Ph.D., A.C.T. (Hon.)

Senior Research Associate, Department of Biomedical Sciences, College of Veterinary Medicine, Cornell University, Ithaca, New York

Pregnancy Diagnosis in the Bitch

Gheorghe M. Constantinescu, D.V.M., Ph.D., Dr.h.c.

Professor of Veterinary Anatomy, College of Veterinary Medicine, University of Missouri, Columbia, Missouri

Feline Respiratory Tract Polyps

Larry M. Cornelius, D.V.M., Dipl. A.C.V.I.M.

Professor of Small Animal Medicine, College of Veterinary Medicine; Small Animal Internist, Veterinary Teaching Hospital, University of Georgia, Athens, Georgia

CVT Update: Therapy for Hepatic Lipidosis; Ammonium Urate Uroliths in Dogs With Portosystemic Shunts

Nancy B. Cottrill, D.V.M., M.S., Dipl. A.C.V.O.

Staff Ophthalmologist, Animal Eye Clinic, Metairie, Louisiana

Differential Diagnosis of Anisocoria

Laine A. Cowan, D.V.M., Dipl. A.C.V.I.M.

Associate Professor, Department of Clinical Sciences, College of Veterinary Medicine, Kansas State University, Manhattan, Kansas

Cutaneous and Renal Glomerulopathy of Greyhound Dogs

Larry D. Cowgill, D.V.M., Ph.D., Dipl. A.C.V.I.M.

Associate Professor, Department of Medicine and Epidemiology, School of Veterinary Medicine; Director, Companion Animal Hemodialysis Unit, Veterinary Medical Teaching Hospital, University of California, Davis, California

Acute Renal Failure

Michael R. Cranfield, D.V.M.

Faculty, Division of Comparative Medicine, School of Medicine, Johns Hopkins University; Head Veterinarian, Baltimore Zoo Medical Department, Baltimore, Maryland

Cryptosporidia in Reptiles

Carolyn Cray, Ph.D.

Research Assistant Professor, College of Veterinary Medicine, University of Miami, Miami, Florida

Diagnostic Use of Protein Electrophoresis in Birds

Kathy L. Crenshaw, D.V.M., Dipl. A.C.V.I.M.

Staff Veterinarian, The Rogosia Institute, New York, New York

CVT Update: Monitoring Treatment of Diabetes Mellitus in Dogs and Cats

David A. Crossley, B. Vet. Med.

Head of Dentistry, Animal Medical Centre, Manchester, United Kingdom

Dental Disease in Lagomorphs and Rodents

Dennis T. Crowe, D.V.M., Dipl. A.C.V.S., A.C.V.E.C.C.

Chief of Emergency and Critical Care Services and Staff Surgeon, Georgia Veterinary Specialists, Alpharetta, Georgia; Staff Surgeon and Emergency and Critical Care Specialist, Carson Tahoe Veterinary Hospital, Carson City, Nevada

Microenteral Nutrition; Open Chest Cardiopulmonary Resuscitation

Deborah J. Davenport, D.V.M., M.S., Dipl. A.C.V.I.M.

Director, Extramural Research, Hill's Science and Technology Center; Associate in Clinical Nutrition, Mark Morris Institute; Adjunct Professor, Department of Clinical Sciences, College of Veterinary Medicine, Kansas State University, Manhattan, Kansas

Small Intestinal Bacterial Overgrowth

Autumn P. Davidson, B.S., D.V.M., Dipl. A.C.V.I.M.

Associate Clinical Professor, School of Veterinary Medicine; Staff, Small Animal Clinic, Veterinary Medical Teaching Hospital, University of California, Davis; Staff Internist, Encina Veterinary Hospital, Walnut Creek; Staff, Guide Dogs for the Blind, San Rafael, California

CVT Update: Therapy for Nasal Aspergillosis; CVT Update: Infertility in the Queen

Thomas K. Day, D.V.M., M.S., Dipl. A.C.V.A.

Emergency and Critical Care Veterinarian, Kentucky Veterinary Specialists Emergency Services, Inc., Louisville, Kentucky

Intravenous Anesthetic Techniques for Emergency and Critical Care Procedures

Linda J. DeBowes, D.V.M., Dipl. A.C.V.I.M. (Internal Medicine), A.V.D.C.

Associate Professor, Department of Clinical Sciences, College of Veterinary Medicine, Kansas State University, Manhattan, Kansas

Feline Stomatitis and Faucitis

Teresa C. DeFrancesco, D.V.M., Dipl. A.C.V.I.M. (Cardiology)

Clinical Assistant Professor, Department of Companion and Special Species Medicine, College of Veterinary Medicine, North Carolina State University, Raleigh, North Carolina

CVT Update: Infectious Endocarditis

Robert C. DeNovo, D.V.M., M.S., Dipl. A.C.V.I.M.

Associate Professor of Medicine, College of Veterinary Medicine, University of Tennessee, Knoxville, Tennessee

Canine Megaesophagus

Avi Deshmukh, B.V.Sc., Ph.D.

Ralston Purina Company, St. Louis, Missouri

Nutritional Assessment of Pet Food Labels

Jennifer J. Devey, D.V.M., Dipl. A.C.V.E.C.C.

Director of Intensive Care Unit and Emergency Service, South Paws Veterinary Referral Center, Springfield, Virginia

Microenteral Nutrition

Chad M. Devitt, D.V.M.

Veterinary Teaching Hospital, Colorado State University, Fort Collins, Colorado

Esophageal Feeding Tubes

Mark W. Dewhirst, D.V.M., Ph.D.

Professor, Department of Radiation Oncology, Duke University Medical Center, Durham; Adjunct Professor, College of Veterinary Medicine, North Carolina State University, Raleigh, North Carolina

Hyperthermia

Ravinder S. Dhaliwal, D.V.M., M.S., Dipl. A.C.V.I.M.

Resident in Oncology, College of Veterinary Medicine, University of Illinois, Urbana, Illinois; Staff Oncologist, All Care Animal Referral Center, Fountain Valley, California

CVT Update: Anticancer Drugs and Protocols: Using Traditional Drugs

Nishi Dhupa, B.V.M., Cert. S.A.C., M.R.C.V.S., Dipl. A.C.V.I.M., A.C.V.E.C.C.

Clinical Assistant Professor, Tufts University School of Veterinary Medicine, North Grafton, Massachusetts

Section 2, Consulting Editor; Sodium Nitroprusside: Uses and Precautions

Stephen P. DiBartola, D.V.M., Dipl. A.C.V.I.M.

Professor of Medicine, Department of Veterinary Clinical Sciences, College of Veterinary Medicine; Clinician, Small Animal Medicine, Veterinary Medical Teaching Hospital, The Ohio State University, Columbus, Ohio

The Kidney and Hyperthyroidism; Diagnostic Approach to Polyuria and Polydipsia

David C. Dorman, D.V.M., Ph.D., Dipl. A.B.V.T.

Scientist II (Neurotoxicologist), Chemical Industry Institute of Toxicology, Research Triangle Park, North Carolina

Common Household Chemical Hazards; Toxicities from Newer Over-the-Counter Drugs

Steven W. Dow, D.V.M., Ph.D., Dipl. A.C.V.I.M.

Instructor, National Jewish Medical and Research Center; Instructor, Department of Dermatology, University of Colorado Health Sciences Center, Denver, Colorado

Why Are Infectious Diseases Emerging?; Gene Therapy for Cancer

Cherie L. Drenzek, M.S., D.V.M.

Assistant Professor, Department of Medical Microbiology and Parasitology, College of Veterinary Medicine, University of Georgia, Athens, Georgia

The Rabies Pandemic

Kenneth J. Drobatz, D.V.M., Dipl. A.C.V.I.M., A.C.V.E.C.C.

Associate Professor, Department of Clinical Studies; Director, Emergency Service, Veterinary Hospital, School of Veterinary Medicine, University of Pennsylvania, Philadelphia, Pennsylvania

Differential Diagnosis of Laboratory Abnormalities in Critical Care Settings; Noncardiogenic Pulmonary Edema

David A. Dzanis, D.V.M., Ph.D., Dipl. A.C.V.N.

Owner, Dzanis Consulting and Collaborations, Santa Clarita, California

Appendices

Lisa Ann Dzyban, D.V.M., B.S., Dipl. A.C.V.I.M.

Staff, Companion Animal Hospital, San Carlos, California

CVT Update: Peritoneal Dialysis

Denise A. Elliott, B.V.Sc. (Hons), Dipl. A.C.V.I.M.

Department of Molecular Biosciences, School of Veterinary Medicine; Nutrition Support Service, Veterinary Medical Teaching Hospital, University of California, Davis, California

Acute Renal Failure

Robyn E. Elmslie, D.V.M., Dipl. A.C.V.I.M.

Clinical Oncologist, Veterinary Referral Center of Colorado, Veterinary Cancer Specialists, Denver, Colorado

Gene Therapy for Cancer

Theresa L. Entriken, D.V.M.

Clinical Trials Coordinator, Deprenyl Animal Health, Inc., Overland Park, Kansas

L-Deprenyl Therapy for Canine Cognitive Dysfunction

S. A. Ewing, D.V.M., M.S., Ph.D.

Wendell H. and Nellie G. Krull Professor of Veterinary Parasitology, College of Veterinary Medicine, Oklahoma State University, Stillwater, Oklahoma

Ticks as Vectors of Companion Animal Diseases

Andrea J. Fascetti, V.M.D., Dipl. A.C.V.N.

Hill's Fellow in Clinical Nutrition, School of Veterinary Medicine, University of California, Davis, California

Nutritional Management of Diarrheal Diseases

Leah S. Faudskar, B.S., D.V.M., Dipl. A.C.V.E.C.C.

Staff Veterinarian, Affiliated Veterinary Emergency Service, Golden Valley, Minnesota

Routes of Fluid Administration: Indications, Contraindications, Techniques, and Complications; Point-of-Care Laboratory Testing in the Intensive Care Unit

Bernard F. Feldman, D.V.M., Ph.D.

Professor of Veterinary Clinical Hematology and Biochemistry, and Chief of Laboratory Diagnostic Services, Virginia-Maryland Regional College of Veterinary Medicine, Veterinary Medical Teaching Hospital, Virginia Polytechnic Institute and State University, Blacksburg, Virginia

Recognition and Treatment of Disseminated Intravascular Coagulation; Blood Transfusion Guidelines

Edward C. Feldman, D.V.M., Dipl. A.C.V.I.M.

Professor, Small Animal Internal Medicine, Department of Medicine and Epidemiology, School of Veterinary Medicine, University of California, Davis, California

Hypercalcemia and Primary Hyperparathyroidism in Dogs; Complications Associated With Insulin Treatment of Diabetes Mellitus; Diagnosis and Management of Large Pituitary Tumors in Dogs With Pituitary-Dependent Hyperadrenocorticism

Peter J. Felsburg, V.M.D., Ph.D.

Trustee Professor of Clinical Immunology and Chairman, Department of Clinical Studies, School of Veterinary Medicine, University of Pennsylvania, Philadelphia, Pennsylvania

Hereditary and Acquired Immunodeficiency Diseases

Delmar R. Finco, D.V.M., Ph.D., Dipl. A.C.V.I.M. (Internal Medicine)

Professor, Department of Physiology and Pharmacology, College of Veterinary Medicine, University of Georgia, Athens, Georgia

Diagnostic Approach to Polyuria and Polydipsia; Diagnosis of Systemic Hypertension in Dogs and Cats; Recent Developments in the Management of Progressive Renal Failure

Ava Firth, D.V.M., M.V.S., M.A.C.V.Sc., Dipl. A.C.V.E.C.C.

Assistant Clinical Specialist, Department of Small Animal Clinical Sciences, Veterinary Teaching Hospital, University of Minnesota, St. Paul, Minnesota

Treatments Used in Small Animal Toxicoses

James A. Flanders, B.S., D.V.M., Dipl. A.C.V.S.

Associate Professor, Department of Clinical Sciences, College of Veterinary Medicine, Cornell University, Ithaca, New York

Diseases of the Canine Testes

Richard B. Ford, D.V.M., M.S., Dipl. A.C.V.I.M.

Professor of Medicine, College of Veterinary Medicine, North Carolina State University, Raleigh, North Carolina

Vaccines and Vaccinations: Issues for the 21st Century; Bacterial Pneumonia

S. Dru Forrester, D.V.M., M.S., Dipl. A.C.V.I.M. (Internal Medicine)

Associate Professor, Director of Student Affairs, Department of Small Animal Clinical Sciences, Virginia-Maryland Regional College of Veterinary Medicine; Small Animal Internist, Veterinary Medical Teaching Hospital, Virginia Polytechnic Institute and State University, Blacksburg, Virginia

Urinary Tract Infections Associated With Endocrine Disorders in Dogs

Theresa W. Fossum, D.V.M., Dipl. A.C.V.S.

Associate Professor and Chief of Surgery, Department of Small Animal Medicine and Surgery, College of Veterinary Medicine, Texas A&M University, College Station, Texas

Medical and Surgical Management of Pleural Effusion

Philip R. Fox, D.V.M., M.Sc., Dipl. A.C.V.I.M., A.C.V.E.C.C.

Cardiologist, Bobst Hospital of the Animal Medical Center; Director, Caspary Research Institute, The Animal Medical Center, New York, New York

CVT Update: Therapy for Feline Myocardial Diseases

Linda A. Frank, M.S., D.V.M., Dipl. A.C.V.D.

Associate Professor of Dermatology, College of Veterinary Medicine, University of Tennessee, Knoxville, Tennessee

Dermatophytosis

Lisa M. Freeman, D.V.M., Ph.D., Dipl. A.C.V.N.

Assistant Professor, Tufts University School of Veterinary Medicine, North Grafton; Scientist, Jean Mayer USDA Human Nutrition Research Center on Aging at Tufts University, Boston, Massachusetts

Nutritional Management of Heart Disease

Joni L. Freshman, D.V.M., M.S., Dipl. A.C.V.I.M.

Staff Internist, East Springs Animal Hospital, Colorado Springs, Colorado

Current Therapeutic Recommendations for Pregnant Dogs

Angela E. Frimberger, V.M.D., Dipl. A.C.V.I.M.

Research Fellow, University of Massachusetts Memorial Cancer Center, Worcester, Massachusetts

Anticancer Drugs: New Drugs or Applications for Veterinary Medicine

James Gaarder, D.V.M., Dipl. A.C.V.O.

Resident in Ophthalmology, Veterinary Medical Teaching Hospital, College of Veterinary Medicine, Cornell University, Ithaca, New York

Canine Glaucoma

Josanne M. Gagne, D.V.M.

Veterinarian, Inver Grove Heights Animal Hospital, Inver Grove Heights, Minnesota

Feline Cholangiohepatitis

Lee Garrod, D.V.M.

Consultant, New England Veterinary Specialists, Brentwood, New Hampsire

Transvenous Pacing

Urs Giger, Dr. Med. Vet., M.S., F.V.H, Dipl. A.C.V.I.M., E.C.V.I.M.

Charlotte Newton Sheppard Professor of Medicine, and Chief, Section of Medical Genetics, School of Veterinary Medicine, University of Pennsylvania, Philadelphia, Pennsylvania

Blood Typing and Crossmatching to Ensure Compatible Transfusions; Hereditary Erythrocyte Disorders

Brian C. Gilger, D.V.M., M.S., Dipl. A.C.V.O.

Associate Professor, Department of Ophthalmology, College of Veterinary Medicine; Ophthalmology Clinical Director, Veterinary Teaching Hospital, North Carolina State University, Raleigh, North Carolina

Ocular Manifestations of Systemic Infectious Diseases; Diagnosis and Treatment of Canine Conjunctivitis

Tony Glover, M.S., D.V.M., A.C.V.O.

Clinical Ophthalmologist, Veterinary Eye Specialist, Carolina Veterinary Specialists, Charlotte, North Carolina

Ocular Emergencies

Laura T. Goldsmith, Ph.D.

Department of Obstetrics and Gynecology, University of Medicine and Dentistry of New Jersey, Newark, New Jersey

Use of Serum Relaxin for Pregnancy Diagnosis in the Bitch

Jody Gookin, D.V.M., Dipl. A.C.V.I.M.

Graduate Student, Department of Anatomy, Physiology, and Radiology, College of Veterinary Medicine, North Carolina State University, Raleigh, North Carolina

Indications for Nephrectomy and Nephrotomy

Marielle Goossens, D.V.M., Dipl. A.C.V.M.

The Encina Veterinary Hospital, Walnut Greek, California

Diagnosis and Management of Large Pituitary Tumors in Dogs With Pituitary-Dependent Hyperadrenocorticism

Thaddeus K. Graczyk, M.Sc., Ph.D.
Associate Scientist, Lecturer, Course Director,
Department of Molecular Microbiology and
Immunology, School of Hygiene and Public Health,
Johns Hopkins University, Baltimore, Maryland
Cryptosporidia in Reptiles

Carlos M. Gradil, L.M.V., M.Sc., Ph.D.
Resident, Theriogenology Section, Veterinary Medical
Teaching Hospital, College of Veterinary Medicine,
Cornell University, Ithaca, New York
Pregnancy Diagnosis in the Bitch

Gregory F. Grauer, D.V.M., M.S., Dipl. A.C.V.I.M.
Professor and Section Chief, Small Animal Medicine,
Department of Clinical Sciences; Staff Internist,
Veterinary Teaching Hospital, College of Veterinary
Medicine and Biomedical Sciences, Fort Collins,
Colorado
CVT Update: Canine Glomerulonephritis

Deborah S. Greco, D.V.M., Ph.D., Dipl. A.C.V.I.M.
Associate Professor, Small Animal Medicine, Veterinary
Teaching Hospital, Colorado State University, Fort
Collins, Colorado
*Use of Endogenous Thyrotropin and Free Thyroxine
Determinations for Monitoring Thyroid Replacement
Treatment in Dogs With Hypothyroidism; Treatment
of Non–Insulin-Dependent Diabetes Mellitus in Cats
Using Oral Hypoglycemic Agents*

Clare R. Gregory, D.V.M., Dipl. A.C.V.S.
Professor, Department of Surgical and Radiological
Sciences; Director, Comparative Transplantation
Laboratory, School of Veterinary Medicine, University
of California, Davis, California
Immunosuppressive Agents

Barbara Greig, B.S., D.V.M., Dipl. A.C.V.P.
Veterinary Clinical Pathologist, Clin Path Veterinary
Specialty, Eden Prairie, Minnesota
Granulocytic Ehrlichioses

Victoria L. Grevan, D.V.M., M.S., Dipl. A.C.V.O.
Veterinary Ophthalmologist, Animal Eye Specialty
Clinic, West Palm Beach, Florida
Nonulcerative Corneal Disease

Stephen M. Griffey, D.V.M., Ph.D.
Senior Veterinarian and Director, Comparative Pathology
Laboratory, School of Veterinary Medicine, University
of California, Davis, California
*Modern Diagnostic Strategies for Cancer: Sampling
Guidelines*

Craig E. Griffin, D.V.M., Dipl. A.C.V.D.
Clinician and Partner, Animal Dermatology Clinics, San
Diego and Garden Grove, California
Section 7, Consulting Editor; Pseudomonas *Otitis
Therapy*

Carol B. Grindem, D.V.M., Ph.D., Dipl. A.C.V.P.
Professor, Clinical Pathology, Department of
Microbiology, Pathology, and Parasitology, College of
Veterinary Medicine, North Carolina State University,
Raleigh, North Carolina
Infectious and Immune-Mediated Thrombocytopenia

W. G. Guilford, B.V.Sc., Ph.D., Dipl. A.C.V.I.M.
Associate Professor, and Head, Institute of Veterinary,
Animal and Biomedical Sciences, Massey University,
Palmerston North, New Zealand
Assessment of Gastrointestinal Motility

Timothy B. Hackett, D.V.M., M.S., Dipl. A.C.V.E.C.C.
Assistant Professor, Emergency Medicine and Critical
Care, Veterinary Teaching Hospital, Colorado State
University, Fort Collins, Colorado
Thoracoscopy

Kevin A. Hahn, D.V.M., Ph.D.
Associate Professor of Oncology, and Director, Tumor
Biology Laboratory, Department of Comparative
Medicine, College of Veterinary Medicine, University of
Tennessee, Knoxville, Tennessee
Tumors of the Respiratory Tract

Edward J. Hall, M.A., Vet. M.B., Ph.D.
Lecturer in Small Animal Internal Medicine, Department
of Clinical Veterinary Science, Division of Companion
Animals, University of Bristol, Bristol, United Kingdom
Dietary Sensitivity

Jean A. Hall, D.V.M., M.S., Ph.D., Dipl. A.C.V.I.M.
Assistant Professor, Department of Biomedical Sciences,
College of Veterinary Medicine, Oregon State
University, Corvallis, Oregon
Gastric Prokinetic Agents

Holly L. Hamilton, D.V.M., M.S., Dipl. A.C.V.O.
Assistant Professor, Veterinary Clinical Sciences,
Louisiana State University, Baton Rouge, Louisiana
Diagnosis of Blindness

Ralph E. Hamor, D.V.M., M.S., Dipl. A.C.V.O.
Assistant Professor, Comparative Ophthalmology
Service, Department of Veterinary Clinical Medicine,
College of Veterinary Medicine, University of Illinois at
Urbana-Champaign, Urbana, Illinois
Ocular Neoplasia

**Bernie Hansen, D.V.M., M.S., Dipl. A.C.V.I.M.,
A.C.V.E.C.C.**
Assistant Professor, College of Veterinary Medicine,
North Carolina State University, Raleigh, North Carolina
Acute Pain Management; Epidural Analgesia

Elizabeth M. Hardie, Ph.D., D.V.M., Dipl. A.C.V.S.
Associate Professor, College of Veterinary Medicine,
North Carolina State University, Raleigh, North Carolina
Therapeutic Management of Sepsis

Benjamin L. Hart, D.V.M., Ph.D., Dipl. A.C.V.B.

Professor, and Chief, Behavior Service, Veterinary Medical Teaching Hospital, School of Veterinary Medicine, University of California, Davis, California

L-Deprenyl Therapy for Canine Cognitive Dysfunction

Richard G. Harvey, B.V.Sc., Dipl. E.C.V.D., M.R.C.V.S.

Partner, Godiva Referrals, Coventry, United Kingdom

Essential Fatty Acids

Steve C. Haskins, D.V.M., M.S., Dipl. A.C.V.E.C.C.

Professor, Department of Surgical and Radiological Sciences; Director, Small Animal Intensive Care Unit, Veterinary Medical Teaching Hospital, University of California, Davis, California

Therapy for Shock

Eleanor C. Hawkins, D.V.M., Dipl. A.C.V.I.M.

Associate Professor, Internal Medicine, Department of Companion Animal and Special Species Medicine, College of Veterinary Medicine; Internist, Veterinary Teaching Hospital, North Carolina State University, Raleigh, North Carolina

Medical and Surgical Management of Pleural Effusion

Pilar M. Hayes, D.V.M.

Resident in Zoological Medicine, Oklahoma City Zoo and Oklahoma State University, Oklahoma City, Oklahoma

Diseases of Chinchillas

Stuart C. Helfand, D.V.M., Dipl. A.C.V.I.M. (Oncology and Internal Medicine)

Associate Professor, Oncology and Internal Medicine, Department of Medical Sciences, School of Veterinary Medicine, University of Wisconsin-Madison; Member, University of Wisconsin Comprehensive Cancer Center, Madison, Wisconsin

Hematopoietic Cytokines: The Interleukin Array

Mattie J. Hendrick, V.M.D., Dipl. A.C.V.P.

Associate Professor and Head, Laboratory of Pathology and Toxicology, Department of Pathobiology, School of Veterinary Medicine, University of Pennsylvania, Philadelphia, Pennsylvania

Feline Fibrosarcoma: Vaccine Associated

Joan C. Hendricks, V.M.D., Ph.D., Dipl. A.C.V.I.M.

Professor, Department of Clinical Studies, School of Veterinary Medicine, University of Pennsylvania, Philadelphia, Pennsylvania

Airway Management

Diane V. H. Hendrix, D.V.M., Dipl. A.C.V.O.

Assistant Professor of Veterinary Ophthalmology, Department of Small Animal Clinical Sciences, College of Veterinary Medicine, University of Tennessee, Knoxville, Tennessee

Differential Diagnosis of the Red Eye

Paula K. Hendrix, D.V.M., Ph.D., Dipl. A.C.V.A.

Associate Clinical Specialist, Department of Small Animal Clinical Sciences, College of Veterinary Medicine, University of Minnesota, St. Paul, Minnesota

Acute Pain Management

Rosemary A. Henik, D.V.M., M.S., Dipl. A.C.V.I.M.

Clinical Associate Professor, Small Animal Internal Medicine, Department of Medical Sciences, School of Veterinary Medicine, University of Wisconsin-Madison, Madison, Wisconsin

Diagnosis of Systemic Hypertension in Dogs and Cats; Therapy for Systemic Hypertension in Dogs and Cats

Carolyn J. Henry, D.V.M., M.S., Dipl. A.C.V.I.M. (Oncology)

Assistant Professor of Oncology, Department of Veterinary Medicine and Surgery, College of Veterinary Medicine, University of Missouri-Columbia, Columbia, Missouri

CVT Update: Diagnosis and Treatment of Systemic Lupus Erythematosus

Michael E. Herrtage, M.A., B.V.Sc., D.V.R., D.V.D., D.S.A.M., M.R.C.V.S., Dipl. E.C.V.I.M., Dipl. E.C.V.D.I.

Lecturer in Small Animal Medicine, The Queens Veterinary School Hospital, Department of Clinical Veterinary Medicine, University of Cambridge, Cambridge, United Kingdom

Management of Tracheal Collapse

Donna M. Hertzke, D.V.M., Ph.D.

Pathologist, Veterinary Division, Marshfield Laboratories, Marshfield, Wisconsin

Cutaneous and Renal Glomerulopathy of Greyhound Dogs

Paul R. Hess, D.V.M., Dipl. A.C.V.I.M.

Graduate Student, Center for Genetic and Cellular Therapies, Duke University Medical Center, Durham; and College of Veterinary Medicine, North Carolina State University, Raleigh, North Carolina

Diagnostic Approach to Hepatobiliary Disease

Fiona H. Hickford, B.V.Sc., M.A.C.V.Sc.

Assistant Lecturer, Department of Veterinary Clinical Sciences, Institute of Veterinary, Animal and Biomedical Sciences, Massey University, Palmerston North, New Zealand

Congenital Myotonia in the Cat

Karin M. Hinkle, D.V.M.

Intern, Department of Veterinary Clinical Medicine, College of Veterinary Medicine, University of Illinois at Urbana-Champaign, Urbana, Illinois

Ocular Neoplasia

Dwight C. Hirsh, D.V.M., Ph.D.
Professor of Microbiology, Department of Pathology, Microbiology and Immunology, School of Veterinary Medicine; Chief, Microbiology Service, Veterinary Medical Teaching Hospital, University of California, Davis, California
Disinfectant and Antiseptic Use in Small Animal Practice

Heidi L. Hoefer, D.V.M., Dipl. A.B.V.P.
Staff Veterinarian, Animal Medical Center, New York; Exotics Consultant, Long Island Veterinary Specialists, Plainview, New York
Heart Disease in Ferrets

David Holt, B.V.Sc., Dipl. A.C.V.S.
Assistant Professor of Surgery, Department of Clinical Sciences, School of Veterinary Medicine, University of Pennsylvania, Philadelphia, Pennsylvania
Feline Constipation and Idiopathic Megacolon

Stephen B. Hooser, D.V.M., Ph.D., Dipl. A.B.V.T.
Assistant Professor, Department of Veterinary Pathobiology, School of Veterinary Medicine; Chief, Toxicology Section, Animal Disease Diagnostic Laboratory, Purdue University, West Lafayette, Indiana
Hepatotoxins

Carl S. Hornfeldt, M.S., Dipl. A.B.A.T.
Clinical Assistant Professor, College of Pharmacy, University of Minnesota; Veterinary Service Coordinator, Hennepin Regional Poison Center, Hennepin County Medical Center, Minneapolis, Minnesota
Summary of Small Animal Poison Exposures in a Major Metropolitan Area

Johnny D. Hoskins, D.V.M., Ph.D., Dipl. A.C.V.I.M.
Professor Emeritus, Department of Veterinary Clinical Sciences, School of Veterinary Medicine, Louisiana State University, Baton Rouge, Louisiana
Neonatal Diarrhea in Puppies and Kittens

Dez Hughes, B.V.Sc., M.R.C.V.S., Dipl. A.C.V.E.C.C.
Senior Lecturer, Section of Critical Care, Department of Clinical Studies, School of Veterinary Medicine, University of Pennsylvania, Philadelphia, Pennsylvania
Lactate Measurement: Diagnostic, Therapeutic, and Prognostic Implications

Walt Ingwersen, D.V.M., D.V.Sc., Dipl. A.C.V.I.M.
Hospital Director, MacKay Animal Clinic, Whitby, Ontario, Canada
Electronic Pet Identification and Retrieval Systems

Robert M. Jacobs, D.V.M., Ph.D., Dipl. A.C.V.P.
Professor, Department of Pathobiology, Ontario Veterinary College, University of Guelph, Guelph, Ontario, Canada
Appendices, Consulting Editor

Elliott Jacobson, D.V.M., Ph.D., Dipl. A.C.Z.M.
Wildlife and Zoological Medicine, Department of Small Animal Clinical Sciences, College of Veterinary Medicine; Service Chief, Wildlife and Zoological Medicine, Veterinary Medical Teaching Hospital, University of Florida, Gainesville, Florida
Antibiotic Therapy for Reptiles

André Jaggy, P.D., Ph.D.
Associate Professor, Institute of Animal Neurology, University of Bern, Bern, Switzerland
Neurologic Manifestations of Canine Hypothyroidism

Cheri A. Johnson, D.V.M., M.S., Dipl. A.C.V.I.M.
Professor, Department of Small Animal Clinical Sciences, College of Veterinary Medicine, Michigan State University, East Lansing, Michigan
Effects of Hypothyroidism on Canine Male Infertility

Justine A. Johnson, D.V.M., Dipl. A.C.V.E.C.C.
Warwick Animal Hospital, Warwick, Rhode Island
Craniocerebral Trauma

Lynelle Johnson, D.V.M., M.S., Dipl. A.C.V.I.M.
Research Assistant Professor, University of Missouri, Columbia, Missouri
CVT Update: Canine Chronic Bronchitis

Shirley D. Johnston, D.V.M., Ph.D., Dipl. A.C.T.
Dean, College of Veterinary Medicine, Western University, Pomona, California
Use of Serum Progesterone for Ovulation Timing in the Bitch; Artificial Insemination in the Bitch

Boyd R. Jones, B.V.Sc., F.A.C.V.Sc., M.R.C.V.S.
Department of Small Animal Clinical Studies, Faculty of Veterinary Medicine, University College Dublin, Dublin, Ireland
Hypokalemic Myopathy in Cats; Congenital Myotonia in the Cat

Andrew J. Kaplan, D.V.M., Dipl. A.C.V.I.M.
Veterinarian, Greenbrae Pet Hospital, Greenbrae, California
Effects of Nonadrenal Disease on Adrenal Function Tests in Dogs

Richard D. Kealy, Ph.D.
Ralston Purina Company, St. Louis, Missouri
Nutritional Assessment of Pet Food Labels

Bruce W. Keene, D.V.M., M.S., Dipl. A.C.V.I.M. (Cardiology)
Associate Professor, Department of Clinical Sciences, College of Veterinary Medicine, North Carolina State University, Raleigh, North Carolina
Section 9, Consulting Editor; Outpatient Management of Chronic Heart Failure

Charlotte B. Keller, Dr. Med. Vet., Dipl. A.C.V.O., Dipl. E.C.V.O.

Assistant Professor, Department of Clinical Studies, Ontario Veterinary College, University of Guelph, Guelph, Ontario, Canada

Epiphora

William C. Keller, D.V.M., M.S.

Director, Division of Epidemiology and Surveillance, Center for Veterinary Medicine, U.S. Food and Drug Administration, Rockville, Maryland

Adverse Drug Reactions

Robert J. Kemppainen, D.V.M., Ph.D.

Professor and Director of the Endocrine Diagnostic Laboratory, Department of Anatomy, Physiology, and Pharmacology, College of Veterinary Medicine, Auburn University, Auburn, Alabama

CVT Update: Interpretation of Endocrine Diagnostic Test Results for Adrenal and Thyroid Disease

Thomas J. Kern, D.V.M., Dipl. A.C.V.O.

Associate Professor of Ophthalmology, College of Veterinary Medicine, Cornell University, Ithaca, New York

Section 13, Consulting Editor

Lesley G. King, M.V.B., M.R.C.V.S., Dipl. A.C.V.E.C.C., A.C.V.I.M.

Associate Professor, Section of Critical Care, Department of Clinical Studies, School of Veterinary Medicine, University of Pennsylvania, Philadelphia, Pennsylvania

Colloid Osmometry; Airway Management

Peter P. Kintzer, D.V.M., Dipl. A.C.V.I.M.

Clinical Assistant Professor, Department of Clinical Sciences, School of Veterinary Medicine, Tufts University, North Grafton; Staff Internist, Boston Road Animal Hospital, Springfield, Massachusetts

Differential Diagnosis of Hyperkalemia and Hyponatremia in Dogs and Cats

Rebecca Kirby, D.V.M., Dipl. A.C.V.I.M., A.C.V.E.C.C.

Director of Medicine and President, Animal Emergency Center and Referral Services, Milwaukee, Wisconsin

Cats Are Not Dogs in Critical Care; Colloids: Current Recommendations; Recognition and Treatment of Disseminated Intravascular Coagulation

Barbara E. Kitchell, D.V.M., Ph.D., Dipl. A.C.V.I.M.

Assistant Professor of Medicine, College of Veterinary Medicine, University of Illinois at Urbana-Champaign, Urbana, Illinois

CVT Update: Anticancer Drugs and Protocols: Using Traditional Drugs

Mark D. Kittleson, D.V.M., Ph.D., Dipl. A.C.V.I.M.

Professor, Department of Medicine and Epidemiology, School of Veterinary Medicine; Associate Director and Staff Cardiologist, Veterinary Medical Teaching Hospital, University of California, Davis, California

Taurine- and Carnitine-Responsive Dilated Cardiomyopathy in American Cocker Spaniels

Jeffrey Klausner, D.V.M., M.S., Dipl. A.C.V.I.M. (Internal Medicine, Oncology)

Professor and Chair, Department of Small Animal Clinical Sciences, College of Veterinary Medicine, University of Minnesota, St. Paul, Minnesota

From Journal to Patient: Evidence-Based Medicine

David H. Knight, D.V.M., M. Med. Sc., Dipl. A.C.V.I.M. (Cardiology)

Professor of Cardiology, School of Veterinary Medicine; Chief, Section of Cardiology, Veterinary Hospital, University of Pennsylvania, Philadelphia, Pennsylvania

Reason Must Supersede Dogma in the Management of Ventricular Arrhythmias; CVT Update: Heartworm Testing and Prevention in Dogs

Kim Knowles, D.V.M., M.S., Dipl. A.C.V.I.M.

Assistant Professor of Medicine, Clinical Neurologist, Tufts University School of Veterinary Medicine, North Grafton, Massachusetts

CVT Update: Deafness in Dogs and Cats

Dorsey L. Kordick, Ph.D.

Department of Companion Animal and Special Species Medicine, College of Veterinary Medicine, North Carolina State University, Raleigh, North Carolina

Bartonella Infections in Domestic Cats

Susan A. Kraegel, D.V.M., Dipl. A.C.V.I.M. (Oncology)

Lecturer, Surgical and Radiological Sciences, Veterinary Medical Teaching Hospital, University of California, Davis, California

Practical Mechanics of Drug Delivery

Karl H. Kraus, D.V.M., M.S., Dipl. A.C.V.S.

Department of Clinical Sciences, Tufts University School of Veterinary Medicine, North Grafton; Instructor in Anaesthesia, Brigham and Women's Hospital, Harvard University Medical School, Boston, Massachusetts

Medical Management of Acute Spinal Cord Disease

Donald R. Krawiec, D.V.M., Ph.D., Dipl. A.C.V.I.M.

North County Specialty Animal Hospital, San Marcos, California

Urologic Emergencies; Gastrointestinal Complications of Uremia

John M. Kruger, D.V.M., Ph.D., Dipl. A.C.V.I.M.

Associate Professor, Department of Small Animal Clinical Sciences, College of Veterinary Medicine, Michigan State University, East Lansing, Michigan

Nonobstructive Idiopathic Feline Lower Urinary Tract Disease: Therapeutic Rights and Wrongs

Stephen A. Kruth, D.V.M., Dipl. A.C.V.I.M.

Professor, Department of Clinical Studies, Ontario Veterinary College, University of Guelph, Guelph, Ontario, Canada

Antimicrobial Therapy for the Neutropenic Dog and Cat

Charles A. Kuntz, D.V.M., Dipl. A.C.V.S.

Fellow, Surgical Oncology, Department of Clinical Sciences, College of Veterinary Medicine and Biomedical Sciences, Colorado State University, Fort Collins, Colorado

Sacral Fractures and Sacrococcygeal Injuries in Dogs and Cats

Andrew E. Kyles, B.V.M.S., Ph.D., Dipl. A.C.V.S.

Assistant Professor, Department of Surgical and Radiological Sciences, School of Veterinary Medicine, University of California, Davis, California

Diagnosis and Management of Ureteral Obstruction

Mary Anna Labato, D.V.M., Dipl. A.C.V.I.M.

Clinical Associate Professor, Department of Clinical Sciences, Tufts University School of Veterinary Medicine; Staff Veterinarian, Foster Hospital for Small Animals, North Grafton, Massachusetts

CVT Update: Peritoneal Dialysis

Dorothy P. Laflamme, M.S., D.V.M., Ph.D., Dipl. A.C.V.N.

Research Fellow, Research and Development, Ralston Purina Company, St. Louis, Missouri

Nutritional Management of Liver Disease

Michael Lagutchik, D.V.M.

Resident, Emergency and Critical Care Medicine, Veterinary Teaching Hospital, College of Veterinary Medicine and Biomedical Sciences, Colorado State University, Fort Collins, Colorado

Defibrillation

Nadine Lamberski, D.V.M.

Staff Veterinarian, Riverbanks Zoological Park and Botanical Garden, Columbia, South Carolina

Salmonellosis in Birds

India F. Lane, D.V.M., M.S., Dipl. A.C.V.I.M.

Assistant Professor, Department of Small Animal Clinical Sciences, College of Veterinary Medicine, University of Tennessee, Knoxville, Tennessee

Use of Anticholinergic Agents in Lower Urinary Tract Disease

Michael R. Lappin, D.V.M., Ph.D., Dipl. A.C.V.I.M.

Associate Professor, Department of Clinical Sciences, College of Veterinary Medicine and Biomedical Sciences, Colorado State University, Fort Collins, Colorado

ELISA Tests: Methods and Interpretation

Kenneth S. Latimer, D.V.M., Ph.D., Dipl. A.C.V.P.

Professor, Department of Pathology, College of Veterinary Medicine, University of Georgia, Athens, Georgia

Overview of Neutrophil Dysfunction in Dogs and Cats

Alfred M. Legendre, D.V.M., M.S., Dipl. A.C.V.I.M.

Professor of Medicine, Department of Small Animal Clinical Sciences, College of Veterinary Medicine, University of Tennessee, Knoxville, Tennessee

Diagnosis and Prevention of Feline Infectious Peritonitis; Diagnosis and Treatment of Fungal Diseases of the Respiratory System

Linda B. Lehmkuhl, D.V.M., M.S., Dipl. A.C.V.I.M.

Assistant Professor, Department of Veterinary Clinical Sciences; Cardiologist, Veterinary Teaching Hospital, The Ohio State University, Columbus, Ohio

Section 9, Consulting Editor

Michael S. Leib, D.V.M., M.S., Dipl. A.C.V.I.M.

Professor, Small Animal Medicine, Virginia-Maryland Regional College of Veterinary Medicine; Staff Internist, Veterinary Medical Teaching Hospital, Virginia Polytechnic Institute and State University, Blacksburg, Virginia

Chronic Colitis in Dogs

Cynthia R. Leveille-Webster, D.V.M., Dipl. A.C.V.I.M.

Assistant Professor, Tufts University School of Veterinary Medicine, North Grafton, Massachusetts

Ursodeoxycholic Acid Therapy

Julie K. Levy, D.V.M., Ph.D., Dipl. A.C.V.I.M.

Assistant Professor, Small Animal Internal Medicine, College of Veterinary Medicine, University of Florida, Gainesville, Florida

CVT Update: Feline Immunodeficiency Virus

Gregory A. Lewbart, M.S., V.M.D.

Assistant Professor of Aquatic Medicine, College of Veterinary Medicine, North Carolina State University, Raleigh, North Carolina; Adjunct Assistant Professor, School of Veterinary Medicine, University of Pennsylvania, Philadelphia, Pennsylvania

CVT Update: Antibiotic Treatment of Aquarium Fish

Daniel Dean Lewis, D.V.M., Dipl. A.C.V.S.

Associate Professor, Small Animal Surgery, Department of Small Animal Clinical Sciences; Interim Director of

Center for Veterinary Sports Medicine, College of Veterinary Medicine, University of Florida, Gainesville, Florida

Gracilis-Semitendinosus Myopathy

Scott W. Line, D.V.M., Ph.D.

Associate Clinical Specialist, College of Veterinary Medicine, University of Minnesota, St. Paul, Minnesota

Sensory Mutilation and Related Behavioral Syndromes

Dawn Logas, D.V.M., Dipl. A.C.V.D.

Owner and Staff Dermatologist, Veterinary Dermatology Center, Winter Park, Florida

Ear Flushing Techniques and Therapeutic Importance; Appropriate Use of Glucocorticoids in Otitis Externa

Cheryl London, D.V.M., Dipl. A.C.V.I.M.

Postdoctoral Research Fellow, Brigham and Women's Hospital, Division of Immunology, Department of Pathology, Harvard University Medical School, Boston, Massachusetts

Hematopoietic Cytokines: The Myelopoietic Factors

Randall C. Longshore, D.V.M., Dipl. A.C.V.I.M.

Veterinary Neurologist, Veterinary Neurological Center, Phoenix, Arizona

Diagnosis and Management of Dysautonomia in Dogs

Brenda C. Love, D.V.M., Ph.D.

Adjunct Instructor, School of Veterinary Medicine, The Ohio State University, Columbus; Veterinary Microbiologist, Animal Disease Diagnostic Laboratory, Ohio Department of Agriculture, Reynoldsburg, Ohio

Disinfectant and Antiseptic Use in Small Animal Practice

Richard T. Lovell, M.S., Ph.D.

Distinguished University Professor, College of Veterinary Medicine, Auburn University, Auburn, Alabama

Nutrition of Ornamental Fish

Chris L. Ludlow, D.V.M., M.S., Dipl. A.C.V.I.M.

Staff Veterinarian, Veterinary Internal Medicine Specialists of Kansas City, Overland Park, Kansas

Small Intestinal Bacterial Overgrowth

Jody P. Lulich, D.V.M., Ph.D., Dipl. A.C.V.I.M.

Assistant Professor, Department of Small Animal Clinical Sciences, College of Veterinary Medicine, University of Minnesota, St. Paul, Minnesota

Quantitative Urine Collection as an Aid to Diagnosis and Therapy; Alternatives to Exploratory Celiotomies: First Do No Harm; Adverse Effects of Drugs on Formation of Canine and Feline

Crystalluria and Uroliths; Compound Uroliths: Treatment and Prevention; Forceps Biopsy of the Lower Urinary Tract; Nonobstructive Feline Lower Urinary Tract Disease: Therapeutic Rights and Wrongs

John H. Lumsden, D.V.M., M.Sc., Dipl. A.C.V.P.

Professor, Department of Pathobiology, Ontario Veterinary College, University of Guelph, Guelph, Ontario, Canada

Appendices

Elizabeth Lund, D.V.M., M.P.H., Ph.D.

President and CEO, Epi Center, Inc., Lake Elmo, Minnesota

From Journal to Patient: Evidence-Based Medicine

George Lust, Ph.D.

Professor of Physiological Chemistry, James A. Baker Institute for Animal Health, College of Veterinary Medicine, Cornell University, Ithaca, New York

Use of Serum Relaxin for Pregnancy Diagnosis in the Bitch

Ronald Lyman, D.V.M., Dipl. A.C.V.I.M.

President, Animal Emergency and Referral Center, Fort Pierce, Florida

Hepatoportal Microvascular Dysplasia

John M. MacDonald, D.V.M., Dipl. A.C.V.D.

Associate Professor, Department of Surgery and Medicine, College of Veterinary Medicine, Auburn University, Alabama

Acral Lick Dermatitis

Douglass K. Macintire, D.V.M., M.S., Dipl. A.C.V.I.M., A.C.V.E.C.C.

Associate Professor, Department of Small Animal Surgery and Medicine, College of Veterinary Medicine, Auburn University, Auburn, Alabama

Bacterial Translocation: Clinical Implications and Prevention; Canine Hepatozoonosis

Douglas R. Mader, D.V.M., Dipl. A.B.V.P. (C.A.)

Staff, Marathon Veterinary Hospital, and Marathon Sea Turtle Hospital, Marathon; Staff, Key West Aquarium, Key West, Florida

Nutritional Secondary Hyperparathyroidism in Green Iguanas

Bruce R. Madewell, V.M.D., M.S., Dipl. A.C.V.I.M.

Professor, Department of Surgical and Radiological Sciences; Chief, Oncology Service, Veterinary Medical Teaching Hospital, University of California, Davis, California

Section 6, Consulting Editor; Modern Diagnostic Strategies for Cancer: Sampling Guidelines

Michael L. Magne, D.V.M., M.S., Dipl. A.C.V.I.M.

Staff Internist, Animal Care Center, Rohnert Park, California

Gastrointestinal Neoplasia

Deborah C. Mandell, V.M.D., Dipl. A.C.V.E.C.C.

Lecturer, Emergency Medicine, Section of Critical Care, Department of Clinical Studies, School of Veterinary Medicine, University of Pennsylvania, Philadelphia, Pennsylvania

Differential Diagnosis of Laboratory Abnormalities in Critical Care Settings

F. A. Mann, D.V.M., M.S., Dipl. A.C.V.S., A.C.V.E.C.C.

Associate Professor, Veterinary Medical Teaching Hospital, University of Missouri-Columbia, Columbia, Missouri

Acute Abdomen: Evaluation and Emergency Treatment

Ann Marie Manning, D.V.M., Dipl. A.C.V.E.C.C.

Staff Veterinarian, Emergency and Critical Care Medicine, Angell Memorial Animal Hospital, Boston, Massachusetts

Alpha- and Beta-Adrenergic Agonist Intoxications

Denis J. Marcellin-Little, D.E.D.V., Dipl. A.C.V.S., E.C.V.S.

Assistant Professor, Orthopedic Surgery, College of Veterinary Medicine, North Carolina State University, Raleigh, North Carolina

Incomplete Ossification of the Humeral Condyle in Dogs

Dominic J. Marino, D.V.M., Dipl. A.C.V.S.

President, and Chairman, Department of Surgery, Long Island Veterinary Specialists, Plainview, New York

Diseases of the Spleen

Stanley L. Marks, B.V.Sc., Ph.D., Dipl. A.C.V.I.M. (Internal Medicine, Oncology), A.C.V.N.

Assistant Professor, Department of Medicine and Epidemiology; Chief, Nutrition Support Service, School of Veterinary Medicine, University of California, Davis, California

Nutritional Management of Diarrheal Diseases

Steven L. Marks, B.V.Sc., M.S., M.R.C.V.S., Dipl. A.C.V.I.M.

Assistant Professor of Internal Medicine, Department of Veterinary Clinical Sciences, School of Veterinary Medicine, Louisiana State University, Baton Rouge, Louisiana

CVT Update: Diagnosis and Treatment of Systemic Lupus Erythematosus

Ruth M. Marrion Malenda, D.V.M., Ph.D.

Staff Ophthalmologist, Essex County Veterinary Specialists, North Andover, Massachusetts

Ulcerative Keratitis

Kenneth V. Mason, B.Sc., M.V.Sc., F.A.C.V.Sc.

Dermatologist, Albert Animal Hospital, Springwood, Queensland, Australia

Therapy for Drug Eruptions

Karol A. Mathews, D.V.M., D.V.Sc., Dipl. A.C.V.E.C.C.

Staff Veterinarian, Service Chief, Emergency and Critical Care, Ontario Veterinary College, University of Guelph, Guelph, Ontario, Canada

Gastric Dilatation-Volvulus

Kyle G. Mathews, D.V.M., M.S., Dipl. A.C.V.S.

Assistant Professor, Department of Companion Animal and Special Species Medicine, College of Veterinary Medicine, North Carolina State University, Raleigh, North Carolina

CVT Update: Therapy for Nasal Aspergillosis

Glenna E. Mauldin, D.V.M., M.S., Dipl. A.C.V.I.M.

Assistant Professor of Veterinary Oncology and Companion Animal Medicine, School of Veterinary Medicine, Louisiana State University, Baton Rouge, Louisiana

Nutritional Support of the Cancer Patient

John W. McCall, M.S., Ph.D.

Professor of Parasitology, Department of Medical Microbiology and Parasitology, College of Veterinary Medicine, University of Georgia, Athens, Georgia

Current Uses and Hazards of Melarsomine

Robert J. McCarthy, D.V.M., M.S., Dipl. A.C.V.S.

Clinical Assistant Professor, Tufts University School of Veterinary Medicine, Foster Hospital for Small Animals, North Grafton, Massachusetts

Emergency Management of Open Fractures

Margaret C. McEntee, D.V.M., Dipl. A.C.V.I.M. (Medical Oncology), A.C.V.R. (Radiation Oncology)

Assistant Clinical Professor, Radiation Oncology, College of Veterinary Medicine, University of California, Davis, California

Radiation Therapy: Systems of Application and Eligible Patients

Michael W. McGuill, D.V.M., M.P.H.

Adjunct Faculty, Center for Animals and Public Policy, Tufts University School of Veterinary Medicine, North Grafton; State Public Health Veterinarian, Massachusetts Department of Public Health, Boston, Massachusetts

Salmonella in Reptiles

Susan A. McLaughlin, D.V.M., M.S., Dipl. A.C.V.O.

Associate Professor, Department of Small Animal Surgery and Medicine, College of Veterinary Medicine, Auburn University, Auburn, Alabama

Diagnosis of Blindness

Paul S. McNamara, Jr., D.V.M.
Capital District Veterinary Surgical Associates, Pattersonville, New York
Use of Chondromodulating Drugs and Substances in the Prevention and Treatment of Osteoarthritis in Dogs

Erick A. Mears, D.V.M., Dipl. A.C.V.I.M.
Staff Internist, Florida Veterinary Specialists, Tampa, Florida
Canine Megaesophagus

Karelle A. Meleo, D.V.M., Dipl. A.C.V.I.M.
Senior Oncologist, Veterinary Oncology Services, Redmond, Washington
Treatment of Insulinoma in the Dog, Cat, and Ferret

Carlos Melián, D.V.M., Ph.D.
Director, Clinica Veterinaria Atlantico, Las Palmas de Gran Canaria, Spain
The Incidentally Discovered Adrenal Mass

Lindsay K. Merkel, D.V.M.
Assistant Clinical Specialist, Internal Medicine, Veterinary Teaching Hospital, College of Veterinary Medicine, University of Minnesota, St. Paul, Minnesota
Mechanical Devices for Percutaneous Placement of Gastrostomy Tubes: Use of Eld Applicator

Linda M. Messinger, D.V.M., Dipl. A.C.V.D.
Head Dermatologist, Veterinary Skin and Allergy Specialists, P.C., Veterinary Referral Center of Colorado, Denver, Colorado
Pruritus Therapy in the Cat

Kathryn M. Meurs, D.V.M., Ph.D., Dipl. A.C.V.I.M.
Assistant Professor, Department of Veterinary Clinical Sciences, College of Veterinary Medicine, The Ohio State University, Columbus, Ohio
CVT Update: Doberman Pinscher Occult Cardiomyopathy

Denny J. Meyer, D.V.M., Dipl. A.C.V.I.M., A.C.V.P.
Clinical Pathologist, Research Fellow, Nexstar Pharmaceuticals, Boulder, Colorado; Adjunct Professor, Department of Small Animal Clinical Sciences, College of Veterinary Medicine, University of Florida, Gainesville, Florida
Effect of Extrahepatic Disease on the Liver

Vicki N. Meyers-Wallen, B.S., V.M.D., Ph.D., Dipl. A.C.T.
Associate Professor, James A. Baker Institute for Animal Health, College of Veterinary Medicine; Chief-of-Service, Small Animal Fertility and Infertility Service, Cornell University, Ithaca, New York
Section 11, Consulting Editor; CVT Update: Inherited Disorders of the Reproductive Tract in Dogs and Cats; Medical Management of Dystocia and Indications for Cesarean Section in the Bitch

Cheryl C. Miller, D.V.M., M.S.
Department of Physiology and Pharmacology, College of Veterinary Medicine, University of Georgia, Athens, Georgia
Parenteral Nutrition Products; Refeeding Syndrome; CVT Update: Therapy for Hepatic Lipidosis

Ellen Miller, D.V.M., M.S., Dipl. A.C.V.I.M.
Columbine Veterinary Medical Referral Services, Fort Collins, Colorado
CVT Update: Diagnosis and Treatment of Immune-Mediated Hemolytic Anemia

E. Phillip Miller, D.V.M., M.S., Dipl. A.B.V.T, A.B.T.
Director of Product Safety and Efficacy, Hill's Pet Nutrition, Inc., Topeka, Kansas
Pet Food Safety

Matthew W. Miller, D.V.M., M.S., Dipl. A.C.V.I.M. (Cardiology)
Associate Professor, Department of Small Animal Medicine and Surgery, College of Veterinary Medicine; Staff Cardiologist, Veterinary Medical Teaching Hospital, Texas Veterinary Medical Center, Texas A&M University, College Station, Texas
Interventional Cardiology: Catheter Occlusion of Patent Ductus Arteriosus in Dogs

R. Eric Miller, B.S., D.V.M., Dipl. A.C.Z.M.
Adjunct Assistant Professor in Medicine and Surgery, College of Veterinary Medicine, University of Missouri, Columbia; Director of Animal Health and Conservation, St. Louis Zoological Park, St. Louis, Missouri
Section 14, Consulting Editor; Appendices

Barry T. Mitzner, D.V.M.
Southeast Vetlab, Inc., Miami, Florida
Hematology Instrumentation for the In-House Laboratory

N. Sydney Moïse, D.V.M., M.S., Dipl. A.C.V.I.M. (Internal Medicine, Cardiclogy)
Professor of Medicine, College of Veterinary Medicine, Cornell University, Ithaca, New York
CVT Update: Ventricular Arrhythmias

Carmel T. Mooney, M.V.B., M.Phil., Ph.D., M.R.C.V.S., R.W.S. Specialist in Small Animal Medicine (Endocrinology)
College Lecturer in Small Animal Medicine, Department of Small Animal Clinical Studies, Faculty of Veterinary Medicine, University College Dublin, Dublin, Ireland
CVT Update: Medical Treatment for Hyperthyroidism in Cats

Cecil P. Moore, D.V.M., M.S., Dipl. A.C.V.O.
Professor of Veterinary Ophthalmology, Department of Veterinary Medicine and Surgery, College of Veterinary Medicine; Acting Chairman and Hospital Director, Veterinary Medicine and Surgery and Veterinary Medical Teaching Hospital, University of Missouri, Columbia, Missouri
  Keratoconjunctivitis Sicca

Lisa Erin Moore, D.V.M., Dipl. A.C.V.I.M.
Assistant Professor, Department of Clinical Sciences, College of Veterinary Medicine, Kansas State University, Manhattan, Kansas
  Protein-Losing Enteropathies

Peter F. Moore, B.V.Sc., Ph.D.
Professor, Veterinary Medicine Pathology, Microbiology and Immunology, School of Veterinary Medicine, University of California, Davis, California
  Immunophenotyping in the Dog; Canine Cutaneous Histiocytic Diseases

Daniel O. Morris, D.V.M.
Assistant Professor and Chief, Dermatology, Veterinary Hospital of the University of Pennsylvania, Philadelphia, Pennsylvania
  Feline Demodicosis

Patrick J. Morris, D.V.M., Dipl. A.C.Z.M., Dipl. A.C.V.D.
Senior Veterinarian, Department of Veterinary Services, San Diego Zoo, San Diego, California
  Zoonotic Diseases of Pet Birds

Michael J. Murphy, D.V.M., Ph.D., Dipl. A.C.T.
Veterinary Diagnostic Laboratory, St. Paul, Minnesota
  Section 3, Consulting Editor; Summary of Small Animal Poison Exposures in a Major Metropolitan Area; CVT Update: Rodenticide Toxicosis

Robert J. Murtaugh, D.V.M., M.S., Dipl. A.C.V.I.M., A.C.V.E.C.C.
Director of Critical Care, Dove Lewis Emergency Animal Hospital, Portland, Oregon
  Section 2, Consulting Editor; Craniocerebral Trauma

Russell Muse, D.V.M., Dipl. A.C.V.D.
Clinician/Partner, Animal Dermatology Clinic, Garden Grove, California
  Malassezia Dermatitis

Masahiko Nagata, D.V.M., M.S.
Dermatologist, Animal Dermatology Center, ASC, Tokyo, Japan
  Canine Papillomaviruses

Larry A. Nagode, D.V.M., M.S., Ph.D.
Associate Professor, Veterinary Pathology, Department of Veterinary Biosciences, College of Veterinary Medicine, The Ohio State University, Columbus, Ohio
  Treatment of Hypoparathyroidism

Mark P. Nasisse, D.V.M., Dipl. A.C.V.O.
Carolina Veterinary Specialists, Greensboro, North Carolina
  Section 13, Consulting Editor; Ocular Feline Herpesvirus-1 Infection

Richard W. Nelson, D.V.M., Dipl. A.C.V.I.M.
Professor, Department of Medicine and Epidemiology, School of Veterinary Medicine, University of California, Davis, California
  Hypercalcemia and Primary Hyperparathyroidism in Dogs; Complications Associated With Insulin Treatment of Diabetes Mellitus

Rhett Nichols, D.V.M., Dipl. A.C.V.I.M.
Internal Medicine Consultant, Antech Diagnostics, Farmingdale, New York
  Clinical Use of the Vasopressin Analogue DDAVP for the Diagnosis and Treatment of Diabetes Insipidus

Chiara Noli, D.V.M., Dipl. E.C.V.D.
Veterinary Dermatology Consulting Service, Milan, Italy
  Practical Laboratory Methods for the Diagnosis of Dermatologic Diseases

Dennis P. O'Brien, D.V.M., Ph.D., Dipl. A.C.V.I.M.
Associate Professor, Veterinary Neurology, College of Veterinary Medicine, University of Missouri, Columbia, Missouri
  Diagnosis and Management of Dysautonomia in Dogs

Barbara Oglesbee, D.V.M., Dipl. A.V.B.P. (Avian)
Associate Clinical Professor, College of Veterinary Medicine, The Ohio State University, Columbus, Ohio
  Psittacine Behavior and Training

E. Christopher Orton, D.V.M., Ph.D., Dipl. A.C.V.S.
Professor, Department of Clinical Sciences; Veterinary Teaching Hospital, Colorado State University, Fort Collins, Colorado
  Current Indications for Cardiac Surgery

Carl A. Osborne, D.V.M., Ph.D., Dipl. A.C.V.I.M.
Professor, Department of Small Animal Clinical Sciences, College of Veterinary Medicine, University of Minnesota, St. Paul, Minnesota
  Section 1, Consulting Editor; Quantitative Urine Collection as an Aid to Diagnosis and Therapy; Alternatives to Exploratory Celiotomies: First Do No Harm; Enhancing Compliance with Treatment Recommendations; Adverse Effects of Drugs on Formation of Canine and Feline Crystalluria and Uroliths; Ammonium Urate Uroliths in Dogs With Portosystemic Shunts; Compound Uroliths: Treatment and Prevention; Forceps Biopsy of the Lower Urinary Tract; Nonobstructive Feline Lower Urinary Tract Disease: Therapeutic Rights and Wrongs

Philip Padrid, R.N., D.V.M.

Associate Professor of Medicine and Committee on Immunology; Chief, Academic Programs, Committee on Comparative Medicine and Pathology, University of Chicago, Chicago, Illinois

CVT Update: Feline Asthma

David L. Panciera, D.V.M., M.S., Dipl. A.C.V.I.M.

Associate Professor, Department of Small Animal Clinical Sciences, Virginia-Maryland Regional College of Veterinary Medicine, Virginia Polytechnic Institute and State University, Blacksburg, Virginia

Complications and Concurrent Conditions Associated With Hypothyroidism in Dogs; Von Willebrand's Disease and Other Hereditary Coagulopathies; Cardiovascular Complications of Thyroid Disease

Mark G. Papich, D.V.M., M.S., Dipl. A.C.V.C.P.

Associate Professor of Clinical Pharmacology, and Supervisor of the Clinical Pharmacology Laboratory, College of Veterinary Medicine; Clinical Pharmacologist, Veterinary Teaching Hospital, North Carolina State University, Raleigh, North Carolina

Appendices, Consulting Editor; Antihistamines: Current Therapeutic Use; Bacterial Resistance

Brandee L. Pappalardo, B.S.

College of Veterinary Medicine, North Carolina State University, Raleigh, North Carolina

Bartonella vinsonii Infection in Dogs

Manon Paradis, D.V.M., M.V.Sc., Dipl. A.C.V.D.

Professor in Veterinary Dermatology, Faculté de Médecine Vétérinaire, Université de Montreal, Montreal, Québec, Canada

Melatonin Therapy in Canine Alopecia

Joanne Paul-Murphy, D.V.M., Dipl. A.C.Z.M.

Assistant Professor, School of Veterinary Medicine, University of Wisconsin, Madison, Wisconsin

Avian Analgesia

Mark E. Peterson, D.V.M., Dipl. A.C.V.I.M.

Head, Division of Endocrinology, Department of Medicine, and Associate Director, Caspary Research Institute, The Animal Medical Center, New York, New York

Section 5, Consulting Editor; Effects of Nonadrenal Disease on Adrenal Function Tests in Dogs; The Incidentally Discovered Adrenal Mass; Hyperadrenocorticism in the Ferret; Growth Hormone Therapy in the Dog

David N. Phalen, D.V.M., Ph.D., Dipl. A.B.V.P. (Avian)

Assistant Professor, College of Veterinary Medicine, Texas A&M University, College Station, Texas

Avian Mycobacteriosis

Lesley Phillips, D.V.M.

Staff Surgeon, Animal Emergency and Referral Center, Fort Pierce, Florida

Hepatoportal Microvascular Dysplasia

Michael Podell, M.Sc., D.V.M., Dipl. A.C.V.I.M.

Associate Professor, Department of Veterinary Clinical Sciences, College of Veterinary Medicine; Adjunct Associate Professor, Department of Otolaryngology; Member, Comprehensive Cancer Center, Arthur G. James Cancer Hospital; Member, Neuroscience Graduate Studies Program, College of Medicine, The Ohio State University, Columbus, Ohio

Seizure Management in Dogs

David J. Polzin, D.V.M., Ph.D., Dipl. A.C.V.I.M.

Professor, Department of Small Animal Clinical Sciences, College of Veterinary Medicine, University of Minnesota, St. Paul, Minnesota

From Journal to Patient: Evidence-Based Medicine

Eric R. Pope, D.V.M., M.S., Dipl. A.C.V.S.

Associate Professor of Surgery, College of Veterinary Medicine, University of Missouri, Columbia, Missouri

Feline Respiratory Tract Polyps

Lauren C. Prause, M.S., D.V.M., Dipl. A.C.V.I.M.

Staff Internist, Alameda East Veterinary Hospital, Denver, Colorado

Hepatic Nodular Hyperplasia

Jeffrey Proulx, D.V.M.

Resident in Emergency and Critical Care, Tufts University School of Veterinary Medicine, North Grafton, Massachusetts

Sodium Nitroprusside: Uses and Precautions

Marc Raffe, D.V.M., M.S., Dipl. A.C.V.A., A.C.V.E.C.C.

Professor of Anesthesia and Critical Care, Department of Small Animal Clinical Sciences, College of Veterinary Medicine, University of Minnesota, St. Paul, Minnesota

Medical Use of Colloids; Point-of-Care Laboratory Testing in the Intensive Care Unit

David T. Ramsey, D.V.M., Dipl. A.C.V.O.

Assistant Professor, Comparative Ophthalmology, College of Veterinary Medicine, Michigan State University, East Lansing, Michigan

Exophthalmos

John F. Randolph, D.V.M., Dipl. A.C.V.I.M.

Associate Professor, Department of Clinical Sciences, College of Veterinary Medicine; Small Animal Internist, Companion Animal Hospital, Cornell University, Ithaca, New York

Growth Hormone Therapy in the Dog

Clarence A. Rawlings, D.V.M., Ph.D., Dipl. A.C.V.S.

Professor and Head, Department of Small Animal Medicine, College of Veterinary Medicine, University of Georgia, Athens, Georgia

Current Uses and Hazards of Melarsomine

Renate Reimschuessel, V.M.D., Ph.D.

Associate Professor, School of Veterinary Medicine, University of Maryland, Baltimore, Maryland

Necropsy Techniques in Aquarium Fish

Craig R. Reinemeyer, D.V.M., Ph.D.

Executive Officer, East Tennessee Clinical Research, Inc., Knoxville, Tennessee

Appendices

Virginia Rentko, V.M.D., Dipl. A.C.V.I.M.

Clinical Assistant, Tufts University School of Veterinary Medicine, North Grafton; Director, Veterinary Medicine, Biopure Corporation, Cambridge, Massachusetts

Leptospirosis; Practical Use of a Blood Substitute

Jennifer M. Rewerts, D.V.M., Dipl. A.C.V.I.M.

Internist and Owner, Veterinary Specialties of Omaha, Omaha, Nebraska

CVT Update: Diagnosis and Treatment of Parvovirus

Mark Rishniw, B.V.Sc., M.S., Dipl. A.C.V.I.M.

Lecturer in Cardiology, College of Veterinary Medicine, Cornell University, Ithaca, New York

Bradyarrhythmias

Margaret V. Root Kustritz, D.V.M., Ph.D., Dipl. A.C.T.

Associate Clinical Specialist, Small Animal Reproduction, College of Veterinary Medicine, University of Minnesota, St. Paul, Minnesota

Use of Serum Progesterone for Ovulation Timing in the Bitch; Artificial Insemination in the Bitch

Wayne S. Rosenkrantz, D.V.M., Dipl. A.C.V.D.

Owner and Partner, Animal Dermatology Clinics of Garden Grove and San Diego, Garden Grove and San Diego, California

Section 7, Consulting Editor; Pyotraumatic Dermatitis ("Hot Spots")

Karen L. Rosenthal, D.V.M., M.S., Dipl. A.B.V.P.

Director of Avian and Exotic Animal Services, Antech Diagnostics, Farmingdale, New York

Hyperadrenocorticism in the Ferret

Linda A. Ross, D.V.M., M.S., Dipl. A.C.V.I.M.

Associate Dean for Clinical Programs, Hospital Director, Tufts University School of Veterinary Medicine, North Grafton, Massachusetts

Leptospirosis; CVT Update: Peritoneal Dialysis

Edmund J. Rosser, Jr., D.V.M., Dipl. A.C.V.D.

Professor of Dermatology, Department of Small Animal Clinical Sciences, College of Veterinary Medicine, Michigan State University, East Lansing, Michigan

Therapy for Sebaceous Adenitis

Philip Roudebush, D.V.M., Dipl. A.C.V.I.M.

Adjunct Professor, College of Veterinary Medicine, Kansas State University, Manhattan; Veterinary Fellow, Hill's Science and Technology Center, Topeka, Kansas

Hypoallergenic Diets for Dogs and Cats; Nutritional Management of Heart Disease

Elke Rudloff, D.V.M., Dipl. A.C.V.E.C.C.

Director of Medical Services, Animal Emergency Center and Referral Services, Milwaukee, Wisconsin

Cats Are Not Dogs in Critical Care; Colloids: Current Recommendations

William W. Ruehl, V.M.D., Ph.D., Dipl. A.C.V.P. (Clinical Pathology)

Vice President, Scientific Affairs, Deprenyl Animal Health, Inc., Overland Park, Kansas

L-Deprenyl Therapy for Canine Cognitive Dysfunction; CVT Update: L-Deprenyl in the Treatment of Canine Pituitary-Dependent Hyperadrenocorticism

Wilson K. Rumbeiha, D.V.M., Dipl. A.B.V.T.

Assistant Professor of Clinical Toxicology, College of Veterinary Medicine, Michigan State University, East Lansing, Michigan

Nephrotoxins

Charles E. Rupprecht, V.M.D., M.S., Ph.D.

Chief, Rabies Section, Centers for Disease Control and Prevention, Atlanta, Georgia

The Rabies Pandemic

John E. Rush, D.V.M., M.S., Dipl. A.C.V.I.M. (Cardiology), A.C.V.E.C.C.

Associate Professor and Associate Chair, Department of Clinical Sciences, Section Head, Emergency and Critical Care Medicine, Tufts University School of Veterinary Medicine, North Grafton; Medical Director, Veterinary Emergency Treatment Services of Walpole, Walpole, Massachusetts

Transvenous Pacing; Diagnosis and Treatment of Pericardial Effusion

H. Carolien Rutgers, D.V.M., M.S., M.R.C.V.S., D.S.A.M., Dipl. A.C.V.I.M.

Senior Lecturer, Department of Small Animal Medicine and Surgery, Royal Veterinary College, Hatfield, Hertfordshire, United Kingdom

Hepatic Fibrosis in the Dog

William G. Ryan, M.B.A., B.V.Sc.
Senior Director, Technical Services, Merial Limited, Iselin, New Jersey
CVT Update: Diagnosis and Prevention of Heartworm Disease in Cats

Sherry Sanderson, D.V.M., B.S., Dipl. A.C.V.I.M.
Veterinary Medical Associate, Department of Small Animal Clinical Sciences, College of Veterinary Medicine; Resident/Graduate Student in Small Animal Internal Medicine and Clinical Nutrition, Veterinary Teaching Hospital, University of Minnesota, St. Paul, Minnesota
Management of Anorexia

H. Mark Saunders, V.M.D., M.S., Dipl. A.C.V.R.
Associate Professor and Chief, Section of Radiology, Department of Clinical Studies, School of Veterinary Medicine, University of Pennsylvania, Philadelphia, Pennsylvania
Noncardiogenic Pulmonary Edema

Thomas Schermerhorn, V.M.D., Dipl. A.C.V.I.M.
Graduate Research Associate, Department of Molecular Medicine, College of Veterinary Medicine, Cornell University, Ithaca, New York
Hepatoportal Microvascular Dysplasia

Donald H. Schlafer, D.V.M., M.S., Ph.D., A.C.V.P., A.C.V.M., A.C.T.
Professor of Comparative Reproductive Pathology, Department of Biomedical Sciences, Section of Pathology, College of Veterinary Medicine, Cornell University, Ithaca, New York
Diseases of the Canine Testes

Steven C. Schrader, D.V.M., Dipl. A.C.V.S.
Associate Professor, College of Veterinary Medicine, The Ohio State University, Columbus, Ohio
Section 12, Consulting Editor; Diagnosis and Management of Pelvic Fractures and Dislocation of the Sacroiliac Joint

Rhonda L. Schulman, D.V.M.
Mesa Veterinary Hospital, Mesa, Arizona
Gastrointestinal Complications of Uremia

Ronald D. Schultz, Ph.D., Dipl. A.C.V.I.M. (Hon.)
Professor and Chair, Department of Pathobiological Sciences, School of Veterinary Medicine, University of Wisconsin-Madison, Madison, Wisconsin
Vaccines and Vaccinations: Issues for the 21st Century

Juergen Schumacher, Dr. Med. Vet.
Assistant Professor in Avian and Zoological Medicine, Department of Comparative Medicine, College of Veterinary Medicine, University of Tennessee, Knoxville, Tennessee
Fluid Therapy in Reptiles; Viral Diseases of Reptiles

Peter D. Schwarz, D.V.M., Dipl. A.C.V.S.
Staff Surgeon and Owner, Veterinary Surgical Specialists of New Mexico, PC, Albuquerque, New Mexico
Canine Elbow Dysplasia

Christine M. Schweizer, B.S., D.V.M., Dipl. A.C.T.
Lecturer, Theriogenology, and Chief of Service, Large Animal Theriogenology, College of Veterinary Medicine, Cornell University, Ithaca, New York
Medical Management of Dystocia and Indications for Cesarean Section in the Bitch

Michael Scott, D.V.M., Ph.D., Dipl. A.C.V.P.
Assistant Professor, College of Veterinary Medicine, University of Missouri-Columbia, Columbia, Missouri
Interpretation of Cytograms and Histograms of Erythrocytes, Leukocytes, and Platelets

Howard B. Seim, III, D.V.M., Dipl. A.C.V.S.
Professor and Chief, Small Animal Surgery Section, Veterinary Medical Teaching Hospital, Colorado State University, Fort Collins, Colorado
Esophageal Feeding Tubes; Diagnosis and Treatment of Cervical Vertebral Instability-Malformation Syndromes

Rance K. Sellon, D.V.M., Ph.D., Dipl. A.C.V.I.M.
Assistant Professor, Department of Veterinary Clinical Sciences, College of Veterinary Medicine, Washington State University, Pullman, Washington
Vaccination of the Immunocompromised Animal

David F. Senior, B.V.Sc., Dipl. A.C.V.I.M.
Professor and Head, Veterinary Clinical Sciences, School of Veterinary Medicine, Louisiana State University, Baton Rouge, Louisiana
Management of Difficult Urinary Tract Infections

Nicholas J. H. Sharp, B.V.M., Ph.D.
Assistant Professor of Neurology, Department of Companion Animal and Special Species Medicine, College of Veterinary Medicine, North Carolina State University, Raleigh, North Carolina
Molecular Biology of Infectious Disease

Linda G. Shell, D.V.M., Dipl. A.C.V.I.M.
Professor, Virginia-Maryland Regional College of Veterinary Medicine, Virginia Polytechnic Institute and State University, Blacksburg, Virginia
Feline Seizure Disorders

Eric R. Simonson, A.S., R.L.A.T.
Co-Clinical Instructor, Medical Oncology, Veterinary Medical Teaching Hospital, University of California, Davis, California
Practical Mechanics of Drug Delivery

Kenneth W. Simpson, B.V.M.t.S., Ph.D., Dipl. A.C.V.I.M.
Assistant Professor of Medicine, Department of Clinical Sciences, College of Veterinary Medicine, Cornell University, Ithaca, New York
Gastrinoma in Dogs

David Sisson, D.V.M., Dipl. A.C.V.I.M.
Associate Professor, and Director, Cardiology Service, Veterinary Medical Teaching Hospital, University of Illinois at Urbana-Champaign, Urbana, Illinois
Medical Management of Refractory Congestive Heart Failure in Dogs

Daniel Smeak, D.V.M., Dipl. A.C.V.S.
Professor and Head of Small Animal Surgery, College of Veterinary Medicine, The Ohio State University, Columbus, Ohio
Pneumothorax in the Dog

Anthony J. Smith, D.V.M.
Principal, Canis Consulting, Alameda, California
General Husbandry and Medical Care of Hedgehogs

Francis W. K. Smith, Jr., D.V.M., Dipl. A.C.V.I.M. (Internal Medicine, Cardiology)
Clinical Assistant Professor, Tufts University School of Veterinary Medicine, North Grafton, Massachusetts; Chief of Medicine, Cardiopet, Little Falls, New Jersey
Diagnosis and Treatment of Pericardial Effusion

Patricia J. Smith, M.S., D.V.M., Ph.D., Dipl. A.C.V.O.
Adjunct Assistant Professor, College of Veterinary Medicine, University of Florida, Gainesville, Florida; Ophthalmologist, Animal Eye Care, Fremont, California
Hypertensive Retinopathy

Brian L. Speer, D.V.M., Dipl. A.B.V.P. (Avian)
Owner, The Medical Center for Birds, Oakley, California
Egg Laying Problems in Caged Birds

Gary J. Spodnick, D.V.M., Dipl. A.C.V.S.
Head, Department of Surgery, Veterinary Specialty Hospital of the Carolinas, Cary, North Carolina
Canine Cutaneous Pythiosis

Jörg M. Steiner, Dr. Med. Vet.
Clinical Investigator, Gastrointestinal Laboratory, Department of Small Animal Medicine and Surgery, College of Veterinary Medicine, Texas A&M University, College Station, Texas
Canine Pancreatitis; Feline Exocrine Pancreatic Disease

Bernard G. Steinetz, Ph.D.
Professor, Nelson Institute for Environmental Medicine, New York University Medical Center, Tuxedo, New York
Use of Serum Relaxin for Pregnancy Diagnosis in the Bitch

Lani A. Steinohrt, D.V.M.
Clinical Assistant Professor, College of Veterinary Medicine, Ohio State University; General Practice, Avian and Exotics, Columbus, Ohio
Diagnosis and Treatment of Common Diseases of Finches

Rebecca L. Stepien, D.V.M., M.S., Dipl. A.C.V.I.M. (Cardiology)
Clinical Assistant Professor of Cardiology, Department of Medical Sciences, School of Veterinary Medicine; Staff Cardiologist, Veterinary Medical Teaching Hospital, University of Wisconsin-Madison, Madison, Wisconsin
Feline Congenital Heart Disease

Mark D. Stetter, D.V.M., Dipl. A.C.Z.M.
Staff Veterinarian, Disney's Animal Kingdom, Lake Buena Vista, Florida
Diagnostic Imaging of Reptiles

Phillip F. Steyn, B.Sc., B.V.Sc., M.S., Dipl. A.C.V.R.
Associate Professor, Radiology, Veterinary Teaching Hospital, Colorado State University, Fort Collins, Colorado
Radiographic Diagnosis of Portosystemic Anomalies

Daniel Stobie, D.V.M., M.S., Dipl. A.C.V.S.
Staff Surgeon, Garden State Veterinary Specialists, Tinton Falls, New Jersey
Bicipital Tenosynovitis in Dogs

Elizabeth Arnold Stone, D.V.M., M.S., Dipl. A.C.V.S.
Professor and Head, Department of Companion Animal and Special Species Medicine, College of Veterinary Medicine, North Carolina State University, Raleigh, North Carolina
Indications for Nephrectomy and Nephrotomy; Diagnosis and Management of Ureteral Obstruction

Sara Z. Sudo, D.V.M., Ph.D.
Research Scientist, Urolith, Nephrology, Urology Center, Department of Small Animal Clinical Sciences, College of Veterinary Medicine, University of Minnesota, St. Paul, Minnesota
Enhancing Compliance with Treatment Recommendations

Patricia Talcott, M.S., D.V.M., Ph.D., Dipl. A.B.V.T.
Assistant Professor, Department of Food Science & Toxicology, Holm Research Center, University of Idaho, Moscow, Idaho; Adjunct Assistant Professor, VCAPP, School of Veterinary Medicine, Washington State University, Pullman, Washington
Toxicity of Flea and Tick Products

Judith A. Taylor, D.V.M., D.V.Sc.
Staff Pathologist, Department of Pathobiology, Ontario Veterinary College, University of Guelph, Guelph, Ontario, Canada
Appendices

Alain Théon, Dr. Med. Vet., M.S., Dipl. A.C.V.R.

Associate Professor, Department of Veterinary Medicine: Surgery and Radiological Science, School of Veterinary Medicine, University of California, Davis, California

Diagnosis and Management of Large Pituitary Tumors in Dogs With Pituitary-Dependent Hyperadrenocorticism

Keith L. Thoday, B. Vet. Med., Ph.D., D.V.D., Dipl. E.C.V.D., M.R.C.V.S.

Senior Lecturer in Veterinary Medicine, Head of Small Animal Teaching Hospital, Head of Dermatology Service, Department of Veterinary Clinical Studies, The Royal (Dick) School of Veterinary Studies, The University of Edinburgh, Edinburgh, Scotland

CVT Update: Medical Treatment for Hyperthyroidism in Cats

William P. Thomas, D.V.M., Dipl. A.C.V.I.M.

Professor, Medicine and Epidemiology, School of Veterinary Medicine; Chief, Cardiology Service, Veterinary Medical Teaching Hospital, University of California, Davis, California

Bradyarrhythmias

Mark S. Thompson, D.V.M., Dipl. A.B.V.P.

Staff Veterinarian, Brevard Animal Hospital, Brevard, North Carolina

Diseases of the Anal Sacs

Amy S. Tidwell, D.V.M., Dipl. A.C.V.R.

Associate Professor, Department of Clinical Sciences, Tufts University School of Veterinary Medicine, North Grafton, Massachusetts

Use of Computed Tomography in Cardiopulmonary Disease

Andrea Tipold, P.D., D.V.M., Dipl. E.C.V.N.

Associate Professor, Institutes of Animal Neurology and Veterinary Virology, University of Bern, Bern, Switzerland

Steroid-Responsive Meningitis-Arteritis in Dogs

Robert L. Toal, D.V.M., M.S., Dipl. A.C.V.R.

Associate Professor of Radiology, Department of Large Animal Clinical Sciences, College of Veterinary Medicine, University of Tennessee, Knoxville, Tennessee

Diagnosis and Treatment of Fungal Diseases of the Respiratory System

Rory J. Todhunter, B.V.Sc., M.S., Ph.D., Dipl. A.C.V.S.

Assistant Professor, College of Veterinary Medicine, Cornell University, Ithaca, New York

Use of Chondromodulating Drugs and Substances in the Prevention and Treatment of Osteoarthritis in Dogs

Gregory C. Troy, D.V.M., M.S., Dipl. A.C.V.I.M.

Professor, Department of Small Animal Clinical Sciences, and Chief, Animal Medicine, Virginia-Maryland Regional College of Veterinary Medicine, Virginia Polytechnic Institute and State University, Blacksburg, Virginia

Urinary Tract Infections Associated With Endocrine Disorders in Dogs

Harold Tvedten, D.V.M., M.S., Ph.D., Dipl. A.C.V.P.

Professor of Pathology, and Chief of Veterinary Clinical Pathology Section, Veterinary Teaching Hospital, Michigan State University, East Lansing, Michigan

Interpretation of Cytograms and Histograms of Erythrocytes, Leukocytes, and Platelets

David C. Twedt, D.V.M., Dipl. A.C.V.I.M.

Professor, Department of Clinical Sciences, College of Veterinary Medicine and Biomedical Sciences, Colorado State University Fort Collins, Colorado

Section 8, Consulting Editor; Effect of Extrahepatic Disease on the Liver; Hepatic Nodular Hyperplasia

Lisa K. Ulrich, Certified Veterinary Technician

Principal Veterinary Technician, Department of Small Animal Clinical Sciences, College of Veterinary Medicine, University of Minnesota, St. Paul, Minnesota

Adverse Effects of Drugs on Formation of Canine and Feline Crystalluria and Uroliths

Shelly L. Vaden, D.V.M., Ph.D., Dipl. A.C.V.I.M.

Associate Professor, Internal Medicine, College of Veterinary Medicine, North Carolina State University, Raleigh, North Carolina

Differentiation of Acute From Chronic Renal Failure

Amy K. Valentine, M.S., D.V.M.

Surgeon, Small Animal, Oregon Veterinary Referral Associates, PC, Springfield, Oregon

Pneumothorax in the Dog

William Vernau, B.Sc., B.V.M.S., D.V.Sc., Dipl. A.C.V.P.

Clinical Pathologist, Veterinary Medicine Pathology, Microbiology and Immunology, School of Veterinary Medicine, University of California, Davis, California

Immunophenotyping in the Dog

John Paul L. Verstegen, D.V.M., M.Sc., Ph.D.

Professor, and Head of the Small Animal Theriogenology Group of the Veterinary College of the University of Liege, Department of Small Animal Clinical Sciences, Veterinary College, University of Liege; President of the European Veterinary Society for Small Animal Reproduction, Liege, Belgium

Overview of Mismating Regimens for the Bitch

Nancy Vincent-Johnson, D.V.M., M.S., Dipl. A.C.V.I.M.

Major, U.S. Army Veterinary Command, 94th Medical Detachment (VM), Fort Sam Houston, San Antonio, Texas

Canine Hepatozoonosis

Don R. Waldron, B.S., D.V.M., Dipl. A.C.V.S.

Professor of Surgery, Section Chief Small Animal Surgery and Anesthesiology, Virginia-Maryland Regional College of Veterinary Medicine, Virginia Polytechnic Institute and State University, Blacksburg, Virginia

Urine Diversion by Tube Cystostomy

Patricia Walter, D.V.M., M.S., Dipl. A.C.V.R.

Associate Professor, College of Veterinary Medicine, University of Minnesota; Staff Radiologist, Lewis Hospital For Companion Animals, St. Paul, Minnesota

From Journal to Patient: Evidence-Based Medicine

Ronald S. Walton, D.V.M., M.S., Dipl. A.C.V.I.M., A.C.V.E.C.C.

Major, U.S. Army, Deputy Commander, 51st Medical Detachment, Kaiserslautern, Germany

Thoracoscopy

Wendy A. Ware, D.V.M., M.S., Dipl. A.C.V.I.M.

Associate Professor, Departments of Veterinary Clinical Sciences and Biomedical Sciences, College of Veterinary Medicine; Staff Cardiologist, Veterinary Teaching Hospital, Iowa State University, Ames, Iowa

Outpatient Management of Chronic Heart Failure

Robert J. Washabau, V.M.D., Ph.D., Dipl. A.C.V.I.M.

Associate Professor and Section Chief of Medicine, Department of Clinical Studies, School of Veterinary Medicine, University of Pennsylvania, Philadelphia, Pennsylvania

Gastric Prokinetic Agents; Feline Constipation and Idiopathic Megacolon

Urs Weber, Dr. Med. Vet., D.E.C.V.S.

Owner of a private referral clinic, Tennikon, Switzerland

Urethral Sphincter Mechanism Incompetence in Male Dogs

Douglas J. Weiss, D.V.M., Ph.D., Dipl. A.C.V.P.

Professor of Pathology, College of Veterinary Medicine, University of Minnesota, St. Paul, Minnesota

Feline Cholangiohepatitis

Elizabeth A. Weyrauch, D.V.M.

Lecturer (Clinical Nutrition), College of Veterinary Medicine, Texas A&M University, College Station, Texas

Esophagitis

Richard A. S. White, B. Vet. Med., Ph.D., D.S.A.S., D.V.R., Dipl. A.C.V.S., E.C.V.S.

Lecturer in Small Animal Soft Tissue Surgery, Department of Clinical Veterinary Medicine, The Queens Veterinary School Hospital, University of Cambridge, Cambridge, United Kingdom

Management of Tracheal Collapse

Stephen D. White, D.V.M., Dipl. A.C.V.D.

Professor, Department of Medicine and Epidemiology, School of Veterinary Medicine, University of California, Davis, California

Nonsteroidal Immunosuppressive Therapy

Michael D. Willard, D.V.M., M.S., Dipl. A.C.V.I.M.

Professor of Small Animal Medicine and Surgery, College of Veterinary Medicine, Texas A&M University, College Station, Texas

Esophagitis

David A. Williams, M.A., Vet. M.B., Ph.D., M.R.C.V.S., Dipl. A.C.V.I.M.

Professor and Head, Department of Small Animal Medicine and Surgery, College of Veterinary Medicine, Texas A&M University, College Station, Texas

Treatment of Canine Pancreatitis; Feline Exocrine Pancreatic Disease

Wanda Wilson, B.S., D.V.M.

Senior Resident, Emergency and Critical Care, Animal Emergency Center and Referral Center, Milwaukee, Wisconsin

Cats Are Not Dogs in Critical Care

Wayne E. Wingfield, M.S., D.V.M., Dipl. A.C.V.E.C.C.

Department of Clinical Sciences and Veterinary Teaching Hospital, College of Veterinary Medicine and Biomedical Sciences, Colorado State University, Fort Collins, Colorado

Defibrillation

James S. Wohl, D.V.M., Dipl. A.C.V.I.M., A.C.V.E.C.C.

Assistant Professor and Co-Director, Intensive Care Unit, College of Veterinary Medicine, Auburn University, Auburn, Alabama

Vascular Access Techniques

Alice M. Wolf, D.V.M., Dipl. A.C.V.I.M., A.B.V.P.

Professor, Small Animal Medicine and Surgery, College of Veterinary Medicine, Texas A&M University, College Station, Texas

CVT Update: Feline Leukemia Virus

Kathy N. Wright, D.V.M., Dipl. A.C.V.I.M.

Research Assistant Professor, Children's Hospital Medical Center, Division of Cardiology, Cincinnati, Ohio

Assessment and Treatment of Supraventricular Tachyarrhythmias

Amy E. Yeager, D.V.M., Dipl. A.C.V.R.

Staff Veterinarian, Radiology Section, Teaching Hospital, College of Veterinary Medicine, Cornell University, Ithaca, New York

Pregnancy Diagnosis in the Bitch; Diseases of the Canine Testes

Roger A. Yeary, D.V.M., Dipl. A.B.V.T.

Emeritus Professor, College of Veterinary Medicine, The Ohio State University, Columbus; Vice President, Health, Safety, and Environmental Stewardship, Trugreen Chemlawn, Delaware, Ohio

Lawn Care Products

Elisabeth Zenger, D.V.M., Ph.D., Dipl. A.C.V.I.M.

AIDS Program at San Francisco General Hospital, University of California, San Francisco, San Francisco, California

Retroviral Infection of the Nervous System

PREFACE

The organization of the 13th edition of *Kirk's Current Veterinary Therapy* will be familiar to long-time users of *"CVT."* This volume is divided into 14 sections that embrace a wide range of medical disorders of companion animals. Twenty veterinarians renowned for their clinical expertise serve as Consulting Editors for these sections and the accompanying Appendices. Current topics in small animal practice are detailed within 310 individual chapters contributed by nearly 400 authors. The initial sections of *Kirk's Current Veterinary Therapy* consider topics in special therapy, critical care, toxicology, and infectious disease. Next are nine sections that address important disorders of companion animals based on an organ-systems approach. The final section describes diseases of birds and exotic pets. *Current Veterinary Therapy* concludes with in-depth appendices and an updated Table of Common Drugs. We have tried to maintain the chapters in an easy-to-read format that considers the salient clinical features of a disorder, the basis for rational therapy, and clear and practical pointers for treatment. Most chapters are directed toward the management of a specific condition. Other chapters concentrate on important principles of therapy or general management approaches to diseases of small animals or exotic pets.

We continue our policy of integrating the previous edition of *Current Veterinary Therapy* with the current one. The first page of each section of *CVT XIII* lists the chapters from *CVT XII* that are considered "still current." These chapters and topics can also be found by consulting the index of the current edition. While this approach may require a reader to pull the previous edition from the bookshelf, I believe that it is preferable to duplicating chapters unnecessarily when the management of a disorder has not changed significantly since the last edition. When used together, *CVT XIII* and *CVT XII* provide a relatively comprehensive review of current therapy in small animal practice. I am hopeful that the student or first-time reader of *"CVT"* who holds only this current edition will find the information so useful as to forgive the occasional omission of a topic.

The fastest way of finding information in *Current Veterinary Therapy* is through the cumulative index. The index has been reorganized to emphasize diseases based on anatomic and physiologic disorders, and is extensively cross-referenced. Using the index, the reader should be able to locate a concise chapter detailing most clinical problems. Of course, many readers familiar with the *CVT* format will head straight for the individual tables of contents that appear on each section opening page. Since many subjects "overlap" individual sections, we have made every attempt to cross-index information in chapters throughout the book.

I am most thankful to the veterinarians and scientists who have contributed chapters to this edition and for the expertise and guidance of our Consulting Editors. The staff at W.B. Saunders Company also deserve mention. I am especially appreciative of Dolores Meloni, Senior Developmental Editor, for her organizational skills and supervision of manuscripts. My deepest appreciation is directed to Gina Scala for her expert editing and her patience. Linda R. Garber and Natalie Ware have combined to supervise production of *CVT XIII*. Ray Kersey, Senior Acquisitions Editor, has provided general supervision for this edition. A special thanks is extended to Dr. Debra Primovic for indexing this volume.

Current Veterinary Therapy is written for the veterinary practitioner and for the veterinary student. I am always grateful to receive comments from our readership, including any concerns about possible errors or omissions. Ideas designed to improve this textbook are most welcome. I have tried to maintain *Current Veterinary Therapy* on the course first set by Dr. Robert W. Kirk, and I am most appreciative of the acceptance of previous volumes and this new edition.

JOHN D. BONAGURA, D.V.M.
Columbia, Missouri

CONTENTS

Section 3
Toxicologic Disorders
Michael J. Murphy, *Consulting Editor*

Section 4
Infectious Diseases
Edward B. Breitschwerdt, *Consulting Editor*

Section 5
Endocrine and Metabolic Disorders
Mark E. Peterson, *Consulting Editor*

Section 6

Hematology, Oncology, and Immunology

Bruce R. Madewell, *Consulting Editor*

Section 7

Dermatologic Diseases

Craig E. Griffin and Wayne S. Rosenkrantz, *Consulting Editors*

Section 8
Gastrointestinal Disorders
David C. Twedt, *Consulting Editor*

Section 9

Cardiopulmonary Diseases

Bruce W. Keene and Linda B. Lehmkuhl, *Consulting Editors*

Section 10

Urinary Disorders

Jeanne A. Barsanti, *Consulting Editor*

Section 11
Reproductive Disorders
Vicki N. Meyers-Wallen, *Consulting Editor*

Section 12
Neurologic and Musculoskeletal Disorders
Steven C. Schrader and Kyle G. Braund, *Consulting Editors*

Section 13
Ophthalmologic Diseases
Thomas J. Kern and Mark P. Nasisse, *Consulting Editors*

Section 14
Diseases of Birds and Exotic Pets
Nancy L. Anderson and R. Eric Miller, *Consulting Editors*

Appendices 1205
Robert M. Jacobs and Mark G. Papich

Special Therapy

CARL A. OSBORNE

Consulting Editor

From Journal to Patient: Evidence-Based Medicine

David J. Polzin

Elizabeth Lund

Patricia Walter

Jeffrey Klausner

St. Paul, Minnesota

CONCEPTS OF EVIDENCE-BASED MEDICINE

Overview

Rapid advances in medical knowledge constantly challenge our ability to provide the best and most current clinical information for our patients. When faced by uncertainty as to the best or most current approach to a clinical problem, we can choose among several options: (1) when possible, we can rely on traditional tried-and-true protocols and resort to established habits to justify our decisions and give us confidence to proceed down a particular path of diagnosis and treatment; (2) we can proceed on the basis of our personal experiences or clinical intuition; (3) we can seek the advice of an expert in the field; or (4) we can rely on scientific evidence. Evidence-based medicine (EBM) is an approach to solving patient problems and providing better clinical care through the use of scientific evidence available in the medical literature. EBM is accomplished by systematically searching the medical literature for applicable studies, critically evaluating the selected study or studies, and determining the applicability of evidence to the patient or patients.

Origins

Pioneered by a group of physicians at McMasters University in Hamilton, Ontario, EBM is a specific approach to clinical decision-making. Although the name has undergone transformation over the years—from clinical epidemiology to critical appraisal of the literature to EBM—the basic premise and orientation have remained constant. EBM involves the application of population or epidemiologic research to individual patient care. This process objectifies the science of the art of medicine and stresses rational clinical practice.

Premise

In EBM, the medical literature is thoughtfully evaluated and applied to enhance medical decision-making. For some, this approach is in conflict with existing clinical paradigms. Existing paradigms may suggest that (1) clinical experience is a valid way of gaining understanding about a diagnosis, prognosis, or treatment; (2) physiologic rationale is a valid way of guiding treatment; (3) common sense and solid medical training are the only qualities needed to evaluate the medical literature; and (4) expertise is highly valued—the expert is always correct. The EBM paradigm suggests that (1) personal experience may be misleading and is therefore potentially of less value; (2) randomized trials are required to validate results because predictions about patient response based on physiology may be wrong; (3) reading the literature requires more than common sense—certain evidence must be available; and (4) experts can be wrong, and so they need to justify and defend their opinions.

OVERVIEW OF METHODS USED IN EVIDENCE-BASED MEDICINE

From Patient to Literature

The evidence-based approach to problem solving begins with a clinical question generated as a result of a patient encounter. Although every clinical question need not be addressed by reference to the literature, when legitimate options exist, the most relevant current published information should be sought. Clinicians should begin by formulating *answerable* clinical questions. Questions should be clinically relevant and as specific as possible with the goal of focusing on patient outcomes of importance to the patient or owner, or both.

The clinician then searches the literature via computer to identify relevant published clinical studies that may serve as the basis for an informed clinical decision. The search can be conducted by breaking down the question into concepts that are combined with the Boolean operators, AND, OR, and AND NOT. Ideally, randomized, prospective clinical trials should be sought because, when properly performed, they typically provide the most reliable data concerning clinical problems. Unfortunately, few randomized clinical trials have been published in the veterinary literature. If they cannot be found, it may be necessary to rely on *potentially* less valid or applicable resources such as experimental studies, uncontrolled clinical trials, case series and reports, or observational studies.

Options for Searching the Veterinary Literature

A variety of electronic options are available to search and access medical literature (Table 1). The choice of a particular source depends on factors such as cost, type of computer, need for other services, and areas of clinical

TABLE 1. **Sources for Searching the Veterinary Medical Literature**

Diskette-Based Bibliographic Databases

FOCUS ON: Veterinary Science and Medicine (800-336-4474)
FOCUS ON includes references from over 160 core veterinary journals and also features selected veterinary-related references from nonveterinary publications. FOCUS ON is a product of the Institute for Scientific Information (ISI) and is a veterinary subset of their Current Contents databases with practitioner-oriented journals added. The content pages of journal issues can be browsed and specific topics across all issues can be searched. FOCUS ON also features document ordering through ISI's "Request a Print" and "The Genuine Article." Updates are monthly and the price is $225 per year.* It is available for both Macintosh and DOS operating systems (with or without Windows). The URL for contacting FOCUS ON is http://www.isinet.com.

CD-ROM–Based Bibliographic Databases

VET CD (800-343-0064, ext. 744)
The VET CD database is a subset of the CAB ABSTRACT database. VET CD includes all information from the printed Index Veterinarius and Veterinary Bulletin as well as other indices. The focus of VET CD is on animal disease of all origins as well as public health. Animal species coverage is broad, from domestic species to zoo, wildlife, laboratory, and aquatic species. Updates are distributed quarterly. SilverPlatter is the vendor that packages this database as well as MEDLINE (discussed further on). SilverPlatter allows flexible searching on keywords as well as a number of other field types. Cost for a yearly subscription to VET CD covering 1973 to 1997 is $2,995. Quarterly updates are free. The programs are available for both Macintosh and DOS operating systems (with or without Windows).

Current Contents—Agriculture, Biology & Environmental Sciences (800-336-4474)
Current Contents—Agriculture, Biology & Environmental Sciences is a multidisciplinary database that includes more than 1,350 life science journals from around the world. A subscription consists of 51 weekly discs (or CDs) for updating the database and an annual archival disc. There are three other editions also available on CD-ROM: Clinical Medicine; Life Sciences; and Physical, Chemical & Earth Sciences. The cost of a 1-year subscription (including the weekly updates) varies from $600 to $2,930. Current Contents is for use on IBM-compatible (MS-DOS with or without Windows and Macintosh computers). The URL is http://www.isinet.com.

Medline (MEDLARS onLINE)
MEDLINE is one of the bibliographic databases of the National Library of Medicine MEDLARS (MEDical Literature Analysis and Retrieval System) that contains all the references that appear in the Index Medicus, Index to the Dental Literature, and the International Nursing Index. More than 3,800 journals (68 in veterinary medicine) from 75 countries are currently indexed; about 70% of the records include abstracts. Although CD-ROM access to MEDLINE is available for a fee through SilverPlatter and other vendors, on-line options discussed below are more cost-effective for practitioners.

On-Line Bibliographic Databases and Other Information Sources

Internet Grateful Med and PubMed (888-346-3656)
Internet Grateful Med (IGM) and PubMed are two free (Internet service provider charges still apply) WWW-based search interfaces offered by the National Library of Medicine. IGM provides free access to MEDLINE (1966 to present) as well as 9 other MEDLARS databases (AIDSLINE, HealthSTAR, AIDSDRUGS, AIDSTRIALS, DIRLINE, HISTLINE, HSRPROJ, OLDMEDLINE, SDILINE). Using pull-down menus, the user can search for bibliographic citations by

language, publication type, and so forth. PubMed provides free access to MEDLINE only with a range of choices for searching from simple keywords to Boolean expressions. As part of PubMed, the user can create a clinical query form with built-in search filters for diagnosis, etiology, therapy, and prognosis. PubMed also has embedded links to publishers' Web sites for access to full-text articles for approximately 100 journals (some are subscription only). A document-ordering service called Loansome Doc is available with either IGM or PubMed and allows the user to order full-text articles from local medical libraries (local charges may apply). The URL for IGM and PubMed is http://www.nlm.nih.gov/databases/freemedl.html.

Network of Animal Health (NOAH) (800-248-2862, ext. 297)
Although the American Veterinary Medical Association (AVMA) launched NOAH through the commercial network CompuServe in 1994, it is currently accessible directly through the World Wide Web. NOAH has four resource areas: discussion groups, databases, a NOAH forum library, and NOAH conferences. Through NOAH, abstracts from three veterinary journals can be searched (*American Journal of Veterinary Research, Journal of the American Veterinary Medical Association,* and the *Canadian Veterinary Journal*). Other databases on-line through NOAH include the Veterinary Drug Handbook and the AVMA Membership directory (read-only). These are five "forums," including Clinical Medicine, Specialty Medicine, and Professional Issues. The ISI/NOAH World Veterinary Index is also available to subscribers and contains abstracts from 85 journals from the past 5 years (updated quarterly). ISI's document ordering service can also be utilized as part of this Index ("The Genuine Article"). The subscription rate for NOAH is $120/year for AVMA members and $175/year for non-AVMA members. NOAH is available for both DOS, Windows, and Macintosh operating systems. NOAH may be accessed through the AVMA web site: http://www.avma.org/.

Veterinary Information Network (VIN) (800-700-4636)
VIN was initiated in 1990 and runs on the commercial network America Online (AOL). VIN provides access to discussion groups by topic (e.g., Clinical Pathology, Internal Medicine); questions can be posted to be answered by VIN consultants. Also included are weekly rounds-type discussions and access to VIN libraries (logs of on-line discussions, conference logs, and Association and Foundations [e.g., Association Newsletters]). VIN offers on-line continuing education courses for credit. A searchable database provides access to 8 years of interpretative summaries from the Quarterly Index; 20 professional journals, a Veterinary Drug Handbook and indexed transcripts of discussions that have taken place on the network. Subscription costs $37 per month. AOL connect charges are additional. VIN is available for DOS, Windows, and Macintosh operating systems. A VIN demonstration site can be found at http://www.mother.com/~vin/.

CONSULTANT (607-253-3419)
CONSULTANT is a veterinary diagnostic support system developed and maintained by Dr. Maurice E. White and Mr. John Lewkowicz at the College of Veterinary Medicine at Cornell University. Among the many features of CONSULTANT are its 4,000 disease descriptions that include one or more journal article citations and links to other World Wide Web sites. It is estimated that the database includes upward of 10,000 citations to the current literature in veterinary medicine. These citations are reviewed and selected by Dr. White, who monitors the literature and adds or replaces references as needed; he also incorporates links to other World Wide Web sites or home pages that may have useful information. It is currently available on the World Wide Web free of charge. The URL is http://www.vet.cornell.edu/consultant/consult.asp.

---

*All prices were accurate at the time of this writing.

practice and interest. Factors influencing the selection of a bibliographic database include (1) specific journals contained in the database, (2) currentness of the information, that is, how often the database is updated, (3) cost of the application, (4) kind of computer system that will be used to access the database (operating system, memory, and so on), and (5) the need for other information services. Although all these factors influence decisions, the most critical factor is selection of journals included in the database.

Another feature to consider is the method used in accessing the database. Three basic methods are diskette, compact disc–read only memory (CD-ROM), and on-line access. Diskette and CD-ROM packages create a bibliographic database on a local computer, whereas the on-line option uses a database at a distant site, connecting through a modem and phone line. Diskette or CD-ROM options require an initial investment and subscription fee for updates. The majority of cost for on-line searches is associated with contact time with the database through the phone and modem. In general, diskette or CD-ROM databases are updated less often than the on-line databases. In contrasting diskette and CD-ROM based products, the extent and comprehensiveness of CD-ROMs are impressive; however, purchase and update costs for CD-ROMs may be substantial. Many databases are now accessible through the Internet using the Worldwide Web (WWW). A compilation of many of these resources can be seen at http://www.nnlm.nlm.nih.-gov/pnr/etc/vetmed.html (the Veterinary Medicine Resource sampler).

From Literature to Patient—Studies on Effectiveness of Treatments

EBM is not simply the application of published treatment recommendations to patient care. It involves critically appraising clinical studies to establish the accuracy, clinical usefulness, and applicability of reported findings. According to the principles of EBM (Guyatt et al, 1993), clinicians should address three concerns before applying results contained in an article about treatment:

1. Are the results of the study valid?
2. How useful is the treatment likely to be?
3. Will the results of this article help me in managing my patients?

Are the Study Results Valid?

Before considering the results of a study, it is important to assess whether the results are valid. Do the results indicate the true direction and magnitude of the treatment effect? To answer this question, the study design and analysis should be examined with the goal of establishing whether the researchers have taken appropriate steps to minimize bias. Guyatt and colleagues suggest that clinicians assess the validity of clinical studies on the basis of a limited number of primary and secondary guidelines (Guyatt et al, 1993). Primary guidelines allow rapid assessment of validity "on the clinic floor." Secondary guidelines, although important, may be reserved for articles deserving more in-depth review. The two primary and three secondary guidelines, applied in sequence, will help readers establish whether results of an article are worthy of further consideration.

Primary Guides to Validity

Was assignment of patients to treatments randomized? Randomized trials provide the strongest evidence for or against treatment effects. The "materials and methods" section should state whether subjects were randomly assigned to treatment and control groups. Ideally, the method of randomization should also be described.

Randomization is important because treatment is only one of the factors that may affect clinical outcome. Many other prognostic factors may bias the treatment effect being studied. Some prognostic factors are obvious and may be addressed by the researchers (e.g., severity of illness, comorbid conditions). Unfortunately, not all important prognostic factors can be accounted for or are known. These factors may also influence decisions concerning inclusion of study subjects or assignment of treatments. Randomization overcomes many of these concerns because when sample size is large enough, it assures that both known and unknown determinants of outcome are allocated evenly between treatment and control groups. It is important to recognize that nonrandomized trials provide weaker evidence than do randomized trials.

Were all patients entering into the study accounted for and evaluated at its conclusion? Answering this question involves assuring that follow-up evaluations were complete for all subjects and that subjects were analyzed in the groups to which they were assigned. Every subject should be accounted for at the conclusion of a study. Because subjects lost during study may have different prognoses than subjects that are retained, failure to account for subject losses may bias results. In clinical studies, subjects may fail to complete treatment protocols because their clinical signs worsen or because they are doing so well that owners neglect to return for follow-up. In experimental (induced-disease) studies, subjects suffering adverse consequences may be withdrawn from study. These losses may or may not be consequences of the treatments studied. The validity of the study is open to question when authors fail to account for all subjects or when substantial numbers are reported as lost during the study.

Treatment plans may change after group assignment because of factors related to prognosis. Therefore, analyzing patients according to treatment administered rather than by assigned treatment may bias the outcome. Analyzing subjects according to the group to which they were assigned preserves randomization and is referred to as an intention-to-treat analysis.

Secondary Guides to Validity

Were study participants "blind" to the assigned treatments? Owners and personnel involved in studies often have expectations concerning the outcome of a study. These expectations can influence measures of outcome and distort results. Ideally all participants in a study would be unaware of which subjects received which treatments during the study (double-blinding). However, when double-blinding is not possible, it is wise to note whether efforts were made to "blind" those individuals responsible for assessing clinical outcomes.

Were groups similar at the start of the study? It is reassuring to learn that control and study groups differ only in the treatments received. If randomization has resulted in groups balanced with regard to known prognostic factors, unknown prognostic factors are also likely balanced. However, randomization does not always produce groups balanced for known prognostic factors, especially when group sizes are small, which is typical of many veterinary trials.

Aside from the treatment studied, were the groups treated equally? Because clinical trials are performed on patients that need individual management, it is often necessary to allow clinicians judgment to influence the management of study participants. However, individual management of patients may lead to differences between treatment groups. Even in laboratory-based animal studies, unequally applied interventions may distort the results. For example, in a study of the impact of dietary protein intake on dogs with chronic renal failure, a large percentage of the dogs fed the higher protein diet were also given an alkalinizing agent to alleviate metabolic acidosis. Alkalinizing agents have been hypothesized to influence prognosis in renal failure. Thus, administering this drug to only one treatment group reduces confidence in the findings of this study.

Interventions other than the treatment under study, when differentially applied to treatment and control groups, are called *cointerventions*. Such interventions may refer to medications or differences in patient management, such as frequency of follow-up examinations. The prognostic effect of unequally applied cointerventions is often unknown. Cointerventions and their frequency should be explicitly documented in the "methods" section of the study. Clinicians can be most confident in the results when cointerventions are shown to be infrequent.

How Useful Is the Treatment?

In managing a patient, it is helpful to know the magnitude of benefit likely to accrue from the therapy being considered. Randomized clinical trials often monitor the frequency of adverse events or outcomes. The magnitude of the effect of therapy for dichotomous outcomes (outcomes that either do or do not happen such as death, recurrence of neoplasia, or resolution of disease) may be reported in several ways: (1) absolute risk reduction, (2) relative risk, or (3) relative risk reduction. Absolute risk reduction $(X - Y)$ is the difference between the proportion with adverse outcomes in the control group (X) and the proportion with adverse outcomes in the treatment group (Y). The impact of this therapy could also be expressed as the relative risk (RR): the risk of adverse outcomes among treated patients relative to that among the controls (i.e., RR $= Y/X$). Another useful means of expressing the magnitude of effect (and the most commonly reported measure in human randomized clinical trials) is the relative risk reduction (RRR):

Relative risk reduction =
$$[1 - (Y/X)] \times 100\% \text{ or } [(X - Y)/X] \times 100$$

The RRR provides a measure (expressed as a percentage) of the extent to which the treatment studied will reduce the incidence of the defined adverse outcome.

Results of a study should provide a "point estimate" of the effect of a treatment. The *true* effect may be greater or less than the estimate. Investigators should provide an estimate of the range around the point estimate by providing 95% confidence intervals (CI). The true value for treatment effect will extend to greater than or less than the 95% CI extremes only 5% of the time.

Providing CIs around the RRR is useful in that it allows the reader to examine the extreme values that could represent the true treatment effect and determine if the reported treatment effect is *clinically* significant, as opposed to just statistically significant. For a positive study (i.e., a study that concludes a statistically significant effect occurs), the lower end of the 95% CI should be examined to determine whether the value of such a benefit would likely be considered clinically important (because the true effect may be this small). Thus, a statistically important effect may not be a clinically important effect. In contrast, for a negative study (i.e., a study that fails to detect a statistically significant effect), the upper boundary of the 95% CI should be examined to determine if the study has failed to exclude a potentially important clinical effect. Small sample sizes can influence these assessments because the significant differences may not be measured (low statistical power); in addition, CI increases with smaller sample size.

Unfortunately, 95% CI around the RRR is not always reported. If the P-value reported for the statistic is exactly 0.05, the lower limit for the 95% CI is 0 and the possibility that the treatment has no effect cannot be excluded. As the P-value declines to less than 0.05, the lower boundary of the 95% CI rises to greater than 0. When the standard error (SE) of the RRR or RR is reported, the 95% CI can be established by adding and subtracting twice the SE to the point estimate for the RRR.

Will These Results Help Me in Caring for My Patients?

When evaluating a clinical study, ask yourself whether the results can be applied to your patients. Stated another way, do the subjects studied in this report differ in any important way from your patients? The specific criteria to apply in deciding whether your patients are similar will vary depending on the conditions and treatments studied. In most instances, this question can be answered by asking whether there is a compelling reason why the results should not be applied to your patients. A consideration that may be unique to veterinary medicine is the application of findings from studies of induced disease. Consider how well the disease model replicates the spontaneous disease. How do the circumstances under which the experiment was performed compare to the clinical setting? The more closely the conditions of the study compare to those of your patients, the more confident you can be in applying the findings.

It is also important to decide whether all clinically important outcomes were considered. The critical concern here is whether the study provides evidence that the treatment improves outcomes important to the patient. For example, if you are attempting to decide whether to use an antihypertensive medication in a cat with chronic renal failure, you want to know whether administering the drug reduces the incidence of death or adverse outcomes (e.g., retinal detachment, neurologic disease). Data indicating that the drug effectively reduces blood pressure in this setting does not directly address the clinical question at hand because your therapeutic goal is to reduce the incidence of adverse outcomes, not simply to reduce blood pressure. Some studies focus on effects that have little or no impact on quality of life or survival while overlooking more important clinical effects. Even when a favorable clinically relevant outcome is reported, it is important to consider any deleterious effects of treatment.

Finally, it is important to decide whether the likely benefits of treatment are worth the potential harms and costs to the patient and owner. To put the value of treatment in perspective, it is possible to calculate the "number needed to be treated" to prevent one event (Guyatt et al, 1994). This calculation takes into account the RRR of the treatment as well as the risk of the adverse outcome it is designed to prevent. For example, in a study on dietary phosphorus restriction in dogs with induced renal failure, phosphorus restriction had an RRR (using death as the end point) of 63% (Brown et al, 1991). This RRR suggests that phosphorus restriction has a profound beneficial effect in enhancing survival in dogs with renal failure. However, when applied to different patient populations, the conclusion may be different. Consider two dogs with chronic renal failure. Dog A is a 2-year-old Shih Tzu with congenital renal dysplasia and a serum creatinine concentration of 1.8 mg/dl. Dog B is a 9-year-old Labrador retriever with chronic renal failure of undetermined causes and a serum creatinine concentration of 3.5 mg/dl. Table 2 compares the effects of phosphorus restriction on each of these patients.

These calculations suggest that dietary phosphorus intake would have to be restricted in 27 dogs similar to the Shih Tzu to prevent a single death in this group. In contrast, by treating fewer than four dogs similar to the Labrador retriever, one would expect to prevent one death over the 2-year period. These calculations do not clearly indicate that one should or should not intervene with such therapy in an individual patient, but they do put the benefits of therapy in a perspective that allows owners and veterinarians to make informed choices. Similar methods can be used to incorporate side effects into these calculations (Guyatt et al, 1994).

From Literature to Patient—Studies of Diagnostic Tests

Application of EBM involves critical appraisal of clinical studies to establish the accuracy, clinical usefulness, and applicability of reported findings. Clinicians should ask three questions when attempting to apply the results of an article about a diagnostic test (Jaeschke et al, 1994):

1. Are the results of the study valid?
2. What is the accuracy of the diagnostic test?
3. Will the results presented in this article help me in caring for my patients?

Are the Study Results Valid?

Valid studies concerning diagnostic tests have at least the following two characteristics: (1) there is an independent, blind comparison of the diagnostic test with a reference "gold" standard, and (2) the sample of patients tested includes a spectrum of patients similar to those in which the test will be applied in clinical practice. Studies that fail to meet these basic standards may not provide reliable results.

The accuracy of a diagnostic test is determined by comparing the test to a reference standard. For example, depending on the type of diagnostic test being evaluated, biopsy, long-term follow-up, or necropsy, or a combination, and results of other tests can provide "gold" standards for comparison. If one does not accept the reference standard (this is relative), the paper is unlikely to provide valid results. If the reference standard is acceptable, the next question to ask is whether or not test results and the reference standard were compared without knowledge of or independently of each other (blinded). Interpretation of a new test can be biased by knowledge of the reference standard (or vice versa).

Tests should be evaluated in a spectrum of patients similar to those in which the test would be performed in clinical practice. If the test is only evaluated in severely affected patients, the test results may appear to have more power to discriminate normal from abnormal than is truly present. This is a frequent problem when only populations of referred patients are considered.

Although less critical, it is also desirable that (1) the results of the test being performed did not influence the decision to perform the reference standard and (2) the methods used in performing the test are described in sufficient detail to permit replication. Performance of a reference standard should not be influenced by the result of the test being evaluated. Work-up bias occurs when clinicians are reluctant to subject patients with a low probability of disease to an invasive procedure for definitive diagnosis.

What Is the Accuracy of the Diagnostic Test?

Pretest Probability

The probability of a given disorder prior to performing a diagnostic test is termed *pretest probability*. Ideally, the

TABLE 2. Comparison of the Effects of Phosphorus Restriction on Two Patients

Risk Calculation	Patient A	Patient B
Estimated risk of death at 2 years without therapy:*	0.10	0.75
(X)	(10%)	(75%)
Relative risk reduction with phosphate restriction:	0.63	0.63
(Y)	63%	63%
Risk of death with treatment:	0.063	0.47
(Y = X × 0.63)	6.3%	47%
Absolute risk reduction:	0.037	0.28
(X − Y)	3.7%	28%
Number needed to treat to prevent one event:	27	3.6
[1/(X − Y)]		

*The estimate used here is not based on published or unpublished data.

pretest probability should be obtained from reports in the veterinary literature, but this type of information is not readily available. Clinicians must rely on their own clinical experience or the clinical experience of others to estimate the pretest probability.

Consider the following two patients: patient 1 is an 8-year-old spayed female Norwegian elkhound with a history of vomiting of 24 hours' duration. The owners report that the dog was not eating and seemed depressed. Physical examination revealed that the dog was depressed and dehydrated. Pain in the anterior abdomen, generalized lymphadenopathy, and a temperature of 103°F (39.44°C) were also noted. Patient 2 is a 3-year-old female poodle with a history of vomiting of 2 weeks' duration. The vomiting was intermittent and the dog had a good appetite. Physical examination did not reveal abnormalities. Because of the vomiting, you are considering the possibility of acute pancreatitis in both dogs. Obviously, the probability of pancreatitis is significantly different in the two dogs.

Each item in the history and physical examination can be considered as a test that either increases or decreases the probability of a particular disorder. In patient 1, the history of short-duration vomiting, lethargy, pyrexia, and anorexia increases the probability of pancreatitis, whereas lymphadenopathy reduces the probability of pancreatitis. In patient 2, the dog's age, 2-week duration of vomiting, and a good appetite all decrease the probability of acute pancreatitis. If one knew the probability of each historical and physical examination finding, one would be able to sequentially calculate and recalculate the probability of pancreatitis as each of the findings is considered. Although the exact probabilities may be unknown, clinicians intuitively use this process when ranking differential diagnoses and when making decisions on which test or tests to perform.

In this example, consider the estimated pretest probability of pancreatitis to be 85% in patient 1 and 15% in patient 2. How might the finding of serum amylase activity that is three times greater than normal influence diagnoses in these patients?

Likelihood Ratios

The usefulness of a diagnostic test is determined by the ability of the test to identify a specific disorder (test accuracy). Perhaps the most useful measure of the clinical usefulness of a diagnostic test is the likelihood ratio (LR). These ratios are estimates of the ability of a diagnostic test to raise or lower the pretest probability of the disease in question and allow calculation of the post-test probability of disease. An LR is calculated as:

$$\frac{\text{(Proportion of subjects testing positive that do have the specific condition)}}{\text{(Proportion of subjects testing positive that do not have the specific condition)}}$$

An LR of X is interpreted as meaning that a positive test is X times more likely to occur in a patient with the specific condition than in a patient that does not have this condition. An LR of 1 indicates that the test has not altered

the pretest probability of disease. Ratios greater than 1 increase the probability of disease, whereas ratios less than 1 decrease the probability of disease. LRs greater than 10 and less than 0.1 are likely to have a major impact on post-test probability. LRs of 5 to 10 and 0.2 to 0.1 generate moderate shifts in post-test probability, whereas those between 2 and 5 and 0.5 and 0.2 generate small, but sometimes important, changes in probability. LRs of 1 to 2 and 0.5 to 1 have only a small, and rarely important, effect on post-test probability.

To calculate the post-test probability of disease, one must convert the pretest probability to odds, then multiply the pretest odds by the LR and convert the post-test odds back to probability:

$$(\text{Pretest probability}) \times (\text{LR}) = \text{Post-test probability}$$

The formula to convert probabilities into odds is:

$$\text{Odds} = \text{Probability}/(1 - \text{probability})$$

In the previous examples, patient 1 with a pretest probability of pancreatitis of 85% would have pretest odds of 5.66 $(0.85/1 - 0.85)$. If the amylase test result was three times the normal value and the LR for this finding were 11 (Lund et al, 1995), the post-test odds would be 11.0×5.66 or 62.2. The formula: probability = odds/(odds + 1) can be used to calculate the post-test probability from the post-test odds—$(62.2/\{62.2 + 1\}) = 0.98$ or 98%. Thus, we are virtually assured of the diagnosis of acute pancreatitis in this dog. Patient 2, with a pretest probability of pancreatitis of 15%, would have pretest odds of 0.17. Finding an amylase value that was three times normal would increase the probability of pancreatitis in this patient to 66%. In this case, the probability of pancreatitis has greatly increased, but the diagnosis remains far from conclusive. A detailed description of the calculation and application of LR has been published (Jaeschke et al, 1994).

Will These Results Help Me in Caring for My Patients?

Factors to consider when deciding to use a diagnostic test include (1) reproducibility of the test, (2) applicability of study results to your patients, and (3) whether the test result will provide sufficient power to influence your case management. Reproducibility of the test is an important consideration. Poor reproducibility can result from the test itself (e.g., variations in test kits to measure amylase) or variation in a test because interpretation is required (presence of nodules on a thoracic radiograph). If interpretation is required, the authors should describe the diagnostic criteria used and the level of agreement among observers.

Will the test have the same accuracy in your patients as those described in the study? In considering whether reported results are applicable to your patients, compare the population studied to the patients typically seen in your practice. Test properties often change substantially with severity of disease. When the severity of disease in the population increases, LRs increasingly become greater than 1.

The ultimate value of a diagnostic test is its ability to

influence the management of the case. Will the results of this test change patient management? For any disease, there is a post-test probability at which one would feel confident in establishing a diagnosis and a post-test probability at which one would feel confident in dismissing a diagnosis (thresholds). When the test result falls between these two thresholds, additional, different tests are warranted. Setting threshold values is a matter of judgment based on the potential "costs" of missing a diagnosis and the potential "costs" of treating a patient who does not have the disease. The most useful tests are those with very high or very low LRs because these tests (or levels within a test) are most likely to move the probability of disease across a threshold value.

References and Suggested Reading

Brown SA, Crowell WA, Barsanti JA, et al: Beneficial effects of dietary mineral restriction in dogs with marked reduction of functional renal mass. J Am Soc Nephrol 1:1169, 1991.

Department of Clinical Epidemiology and Biostatistics, McMaster University, Hamilton, Ontario: Clinical disagreement: I. How it occurs and why. Can Med Assoc J 123:499, 1980.

Department of Clinical Epidemiology and Biostatistics, McMaster University, Hamilton, Ontario: Clinical disagreement: II. How to avoid it and how to learn from one's mistakes. Can Med Assoc J 123:613, 1980.

Department of Clinical Epidemiology and Biostatistics, McMaster University, Hamilton, Ontario: How to read clinical journals: III. To learn the clinical course and prognosis of disease. Can Med Assoc J 124:869, 1981.

Evidence-Based Medicine Working Group: Evidence-based medicine: A new approach to teaching the practice of medicine. JAMA 268:2420, 1992.

Guyatt GH, Sackett DL, Cook DJ: Users guide to the medical literature: II. How to use an article about therapy or prevention. A. Are the results of the study valid? JAMA 270:2598, 1993.

Guyatt GH, Sackett DL, Cook DJ: Users guide to the medical literature: II. How to use an article about therapy or prevention. B. What were the results and will they help me in caring for my patients? JAMA 271:59, 1994.

Jaeschke R, Guyatt GH, Sackett DL: Users' guide to the medical literature: III. How to use an article about a diagnostic test. A. Are the results of the study valid? JAMA 271:389, 1994.

Jaeschke R, Guyatt GH, Sackett DL: Users' guide to the medical literature: III. How to use an article about a diagnostic test. B. What are the results and will they help me in caring for my patients? JAMA 271:703, 1994.

Lund L, Klausner JK, Polzin DJ, et al: Bridging the gap from paper to patient. Proceedings of the 13th annual Veterinary Medical Forum. Orlando, FL, 1995.

McKibbon KA, Walker-Dilks CJ: Beyond ACP Journal Club: How to Harness MEDLINE for Therapy Problems. Ann Intern Med 121(suppl 1):A-10, 1994.

Oxman A, Sackett DL, Guyatt GH: Users' guide to the medical literature: I. How to get started. JAMA 270:2093, 1993.

Sackett DL, Hayes RB, Guyatt GH, et al: Clinical Epidemiology, 2nd ed. Boston: Little, Brown, 1991.
A comprehensive guide to understanding and applying evidence-based medicine.

ELISA Tests: Methods and Interpretation

MICHAEL R. LAPPIN
Fort Collins, Colorado

Immunoassays are procedures that use antibody-antigen interactions to qualitatively or quantitatively detect substances. Enzyme-linked immunosorbent assays (ELISAs) are immunoassays in which the measurable signal is generated by an enzyme and its reaction with a reporter substance (substrate). Enzyme immunoassay (EIA) is generally used interchangeably with ELISA (Table 1). ELISAs are frequently used to detect antigen, antibodies, or antibody-antigen complexes associated with infectious agents. However, an ELISA can be developed to detect any substance against which a specific antibody can be generated.

Depending on the specific substance (analyte) to be measured and the type of ELISA, either antigen or antibody is bound to a solid phase. In general, the solid phase is either plastic wells of a microtiter ELISA plate (usually polystyrene) or a membrane (usually nitrocellulose). The material that potentially contains the analyte in question is added to the solid phase to allow the primary antigen-antibody reaction to occur. The conjugate (enzyme-linked detection system) is then added to detect the primary antigen-antibody reaction; if the conjugate is bound, indicating that the primary antigen-antibody reaction has occurred, a color reaction will develop when the reporter substance is added (Fig. 1).

Antibodies used in the detection systems of ELISA can be monoclonal or polyclonal, and can be heterogeneous (different species) or homogeneous. Multiple enzymes and substrates are used. There are numerous potential derivations of ELISA, including direct ELISA, indirect ELISA, sandwich ELISA (Fig. 2), and competitive ELISA (Fig. 3). ELISA results can be interpreted visually by comparing the color reaction of the suspect samples with that of controls, or by determining the absorbance values with a spectrophotometer. When a spectrophotometer is used, results can be calculated by measuring the reaction several times (kinetic) or at one individual time (end point). Results can be reported as a titer or other units, including %ELISA, enzyme activity, antibody activity, or specific concentrations of the substance measured. A titer is the reciprocal of the highest dilution of sample giving a predefined positive reaction in an immunoassay. In general, titers cannot be directly compared between assays or laboratories.

It is impossible to make generic statements concerning the sensitivity, specificity, predictive values, and precision of ELISA, in general, compared with other types of assays or even with other ELISAs that detect the same substance. Use of different antibodies, buffers, solid-phase materials,

TABLE 1. Definition of Terms Commonly Used With ELISA

Term	Definition
Affinity	The intrinsic attractiveness of one substance for another (antibody for an antigen).
Analyte	The antigen or antibody to be measured.
Antiglobulin	An antibody that detects another antibody.
Antibody binding site	The site of the variable region of antibodies that binds to the antigen epitope.
Antigen	Substances specifically recognized by the immune system (antibody in immunoassays).
Avidity	The property of a molecular dissociation that inhibits disassociation. Usually the combination of affinity and the interaction of reagents with the solid phase.
Blocking	Protein or detergent used to block nonspecific reactions between reagents of an ELISA or between reagents and the solid phase.
Capture antibody	Immobilized antibody used to capture the antigen of interest from the sample.
Competitive ELISA	An ELISA in which the detection of the analyte is based on its ability to quantitatively inhibit the binding of a known amount of a standard analyte to a limiting amount of antibody.
Conjugate	A covalent complex of two biomolecules. In ELISA, the conjugate is an antibody or antigen bound to enzyme.
Direct ELISA	An ELISA in which the primary antigen-antibody interaction is directly measured, since the enzyme is directly labeled to one or the other.
Epitope	The portion of a biomolecule (antigen) that is specifically recognized by the antibody binding site. Antigenic determinant is synonymous.
Immunoblot	An immunoassay in which the immunochemical reaction between antigen and antibody occurs on a blotting membrane.
Indirect ELISA	An ELISA in which the primary antigen-antibody reaction is detected with the use of an enzyme-labeled antiglobulin.
Nitrocellulose	The most common membrane used for immunoblot.
Nonspecific binding	Binding of the conjugate in a nonimmune/nonspecific fashion, possibly resulting in a high signal and false-positive reactions.
Precision	Agreement of replicate measurements within an assay or between assays; a measure of reproducibility.
Reporter substance	A biomolecule that generates a signal as indication of its presence. In ELISA, the substrate is often the reporter substance.
Sandwich ELISA	A type of ELISA in which the analyte is captured by one antibody and detected by another enzyme-linked antibody.
Titer	The reciprocal of the highest dilution of sample giving a predefined positive reaction in an immunoassay.
Western blot	A method by which molecules are electrophoretically separated on a gel, transferred to a blotting membrane, and then detected by antibodies or special stains.

substrates, and incubation periods dramatically changes results of ELISA. Each individual assay must be validated (Jacobson and Romatowski, 1996). When new ELISA or other immunoassays become available, the veterinary health care worker should critically evaluate the assay prior to use.

When evaluating the ELISA itself, the *analytical sensitivity* defines the minimum detectable amount of the substance in question that can be accurately measured; the *analytical specificity* defines whether the substance detected cross-reacts with other substances. The *diagnostic sensitivity* is the proportion of positive test results from known infected animals; the *diagnostic specificity* is the proportion of negative test results from known uninfected animals. The *predictive value* of a positive test is the probability that a test-positive animal is diseased; the predictive value of a negative test is the probability that a test-negative animal is normal. The lower the prevalence of disease, the lower the predictive value of a positive test (Jacobson, 1991). This concept is important to clinicians, as the number of false-positive results increase when tests are applied to populations at low risk for the tested disease. Disease prevalence has little effect on negative predictive values.

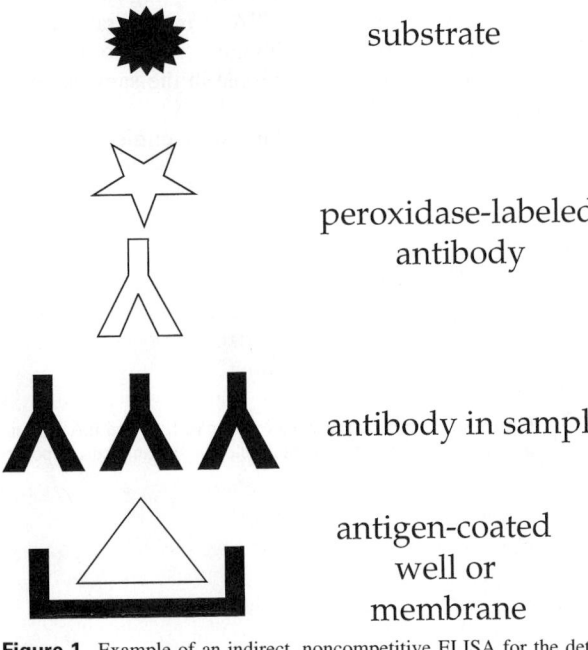

Figure 1. Example of an indirect, noncompetitive ELISA for the detection of specific antibody.

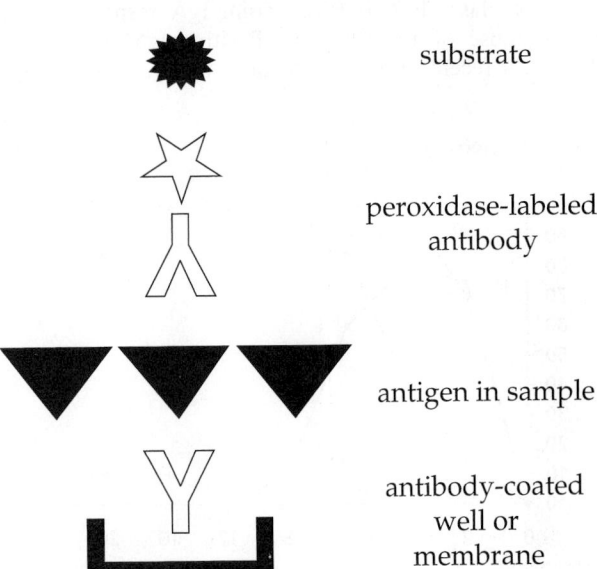

Figure 2. Example of a sandwich ELISA for the detection of antigen.

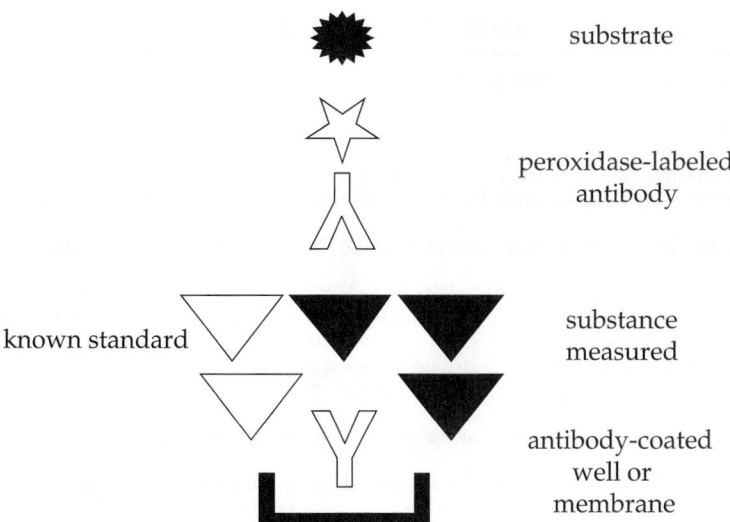

substrate

peroxidase-labeled
antibody

known standard

substance
measured

antibody-coated
well or
membrane

Figure 3. Example of a competitive ELISA. The known concentration of standard competes with the unknown concentration of substance for antibody binding sites.

The following is a brief discussion of the ELISA-based antibody and antigen detection systems utilized in small animal veterinary practice.

ANTIBODY DETECTION

Serum

ELISAs are used commonly to detect antibodies in serum and can be adapted to detect specific antibody classes. Complement fixation, hemagglutination inhibition, serum neutralization, and agglutination assays generally detect all antibody classes in serum samples. When one interprets results of a serologic test, it is important to know whether the assay is specific for one or more immunoglobulins. Once exposed to foreign antigens, the immune system generates serum antibodies (humoral immune response). Specific antibodies commonly assayed include immunoglobulin M (IgM), immunoglobulin G (IgG), immunoglobulin A (IgA), and immunoglobulin E (IgE). Dogs and cats generally produce IgM first, followed by rapid antibody class shift to IgG. Serum IgA responses often mirror those of IgG (Fig. 4). Positive IgM titers often document recent or active infection, whereas positive IgG

titers often indicate more chronic exposure to the specific antigen.

Individual animals vary in their humoral responses against specific antigens. Some animals are high responders and produce large concentrations of specific antibody; whereas others do not. Thus, the magnitude of an antibody titer does not definitely document that an antigenic exposure was or was not recent. This is particularly true for the IgG class of antibody and for agents resulting in persistent infections. For example, many healthy cats experimentally inoculated with *Toxoplasma gondii* have IgG antibody titers greater than 10,000 6 years after the last inoculation.

Documentation of increasing antibody titers suggests recent exposure to an antigen. However, the time interval between the first positive result and maximal antibody titers can be very short; for example, antibodies in cats inoculated with *Bartonella henselae* can be detected by day 14 after inoculation, and maximal titers are usually detected by day 21 after inoculation. If you are attempting to document increasing antibody titers by ELISA, it is preferable to use the same assay and the same laboratory, and to assay the acute and convalescent serum sample in the same assay to minimize interassay variation.

Some infectious diseases can cause clinical signs of

Percent positive

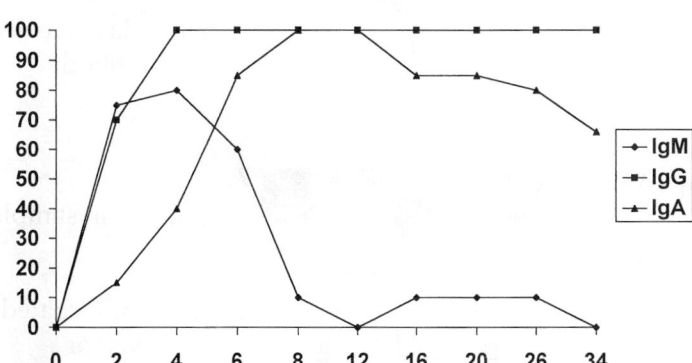

Figure 4. Graphic representation of IgM, IgG, and IgA immune responses characteristic for cats following an antigenic exposure on week 0.

Weeks after inoculation

disease prior to the development of positive antibody titer, particularly if the antibody class measured is IgG. Examples include *Ehrlichia canis,* feline immunodeficiency virus, and *Rickettsia rickettsii.* If negative serologic results are found in animals with acute disease that could be referable to the tested agents, serologic evaluation should be repeated in 2 to 3 weeks.

The timing of antibody testing is very important in kittens because of the potential to detect antibodies, derived from the queen, which are transmitted in the colostrum. In general, positive serum antibody tests cannot be interpreted as kitten-derived until kittens are at least 8 to 12 weeks of age.

Many of the infectious agents encountered in small animal practice infect a large percentage of the population, resulting in serum antibody production but induce disease in only a small number of the infected group. Examples include coronaviruses, canine distemper virus, herpesvirus 1, calicivirus, *Toxoplasma gondii, Borrelia burgdorferi,* and *Rickettsia rickettsii.* Assays with good analytical sensitivity and specificity for detection of serum antibodies against these pathogens are available; however, the predictive value of a positive test for disease is extremely low, since antibodies are commonly detected in healthy animals. The diagnostic utility of some serologic tests are also limited, owing to antibodies induced by vaccination. Examples include feline coronaviruses, *Borrelia burgdorferi,* feline herpesvirus 1, calicivirus, and canine distemper virus. Since there is no serologic test that correlates to clinical illness with many infectious diseases, clinicians must be careful not to overdiagnose these diseases based on just a positive serologic result. A positive diagnosis should be based on the combination of serologic findings, typical historical findings, characteristic clinical and laboratory evidence of disease, exclusion of other likely etiologies, demonstration of the organism, and/or response to appropriate management.

Body Fluids

Documentation of agent-specific antibodies in aqueous humor, vitreous humor, or cerebrospinal fluid (CSF) can be used to support the diagnosis of infection of these tissues; the ELISA is a good methodology for this type of testing, since results can be easily quantified. Measurement of ocular and CSF antibodies is difficult to interpret if serum antibodies and inflammatory disease are present because serum antibodies leak into ocular fluids and CSF in the setting of inflammation. The following is a method for proving local antibody production by the eye or central nervous system.

$$\frac{\text{Aqueous humor or CSF specific antibody}}{\text{Serum specific antibody}} \times$$

$$\frac{\text{Serum total antibody}}{\text{Aqueous humor or CSF total antibody}}$$

If this ratio is greater than 1, it suggests that the antibody in the aqueous humor or CSF was produced locally and is consistent with infection of the eye or central nervous system.

ANTIGEN DETECTION

ELISA can be used to measure any substance against which an antibody can be generated. Examples include antigens of infectious agents, cell-associated antigens (including tumors), receptors, hormones, and drugs. In general, any substance that can be measured by radioimmunoassay could potentially be measured by ELISA.

Antigens of some infectious agents can be detected in body fluids or feces with the use of ELISA. Commercially available ELISA for the detection of antigens in serum or plasma are available for *Dirofilaria immitis* and feline leukemia virus. ELISAs for measurement of feline leukemia virus antigen in saliva and tears have also been developed. In general, the sensitivities and specificities of these assays are good. *Dirofilaria immitis* antigen tests can yield false-negative results in some animals with low worm burdens or single sex (male) infections; this is particularly true for cats. Feline leukemia virus antigen test results can be falsely negative in cats with localized or sequestered viral infection (latent). Serum- or plasma-based feline leukemia virus antigen test results can also be transiently positive in cats that are limiting infection; thus, positive ELISA test results in healthy cats should always be confirmed by repeat ELISA testing in 3 to 4 weeks or by immunofluorescent antibody testing. Since clinically normal animals can be antigen positive by ELISA, the positive predictive value for disease is not 100%, particularly if the prevalence of disease is low. Positive feline leukemia antigen test results also do not prove immunodeficiency.

ELISAs for detection of parvovirus, *Cryptosporidium parvum,* and *Giardia* spp. in feces are available. The parvovirus assay detects both canine and feline parvovirus antigens. Minimal sensitivity and specificity results for the *C. parvum* and *Giardia* spp. assays, when used with feces from small animals, are currently available. If these assays are used, the results should be interpreted with results from fecal examination techniques for oocysts (*Cryptosporidium*) or cysts (*Giardia*).

References and Suggested Reading

Butler JE: Perspectives, configurations, and principles. In: Butler JE, ed: Immunochemistry of Solid-Phase Immunoassay. Boca Raton, FL: CRC Press, 1991, pp 3–26.

Butler JE, Hamilton RG: Quantitation of specific antibodies: Methods of expression, standards, solid-phase considerations and specific applications. In: Butler JE, ed: Immunochemistry of Solid-Phase Immunoassay. Boca Raton, FL: CRC Press, 1991, pp 173–198.

Hamilton RG: Antigen quantification: Measurement of multivalent antigens by solid-phase immunoassay. In: Butler JE, ed: Immunochemistry of Solid-Phase Immunoassay. Boca Raton, FL: CRC Press, 1991, pp 139–150.

Jacobson RH: How well do serodiagnostic tests predict the infection or disease status of cats? J Am Vet Med Assoc 199:1343–1347, 1991.

Jacobson RH, Romatowski J: Assessing the validity of serodiagnostic test results. Semin Vet Med Surg 11:135–143, 1996.

Lappin MR: Feline toxoplasmosis: Interpretation of diagnostic test results. Semin Vet Med Surg 11:154–160, 1996.

Ngo TT: Enzyme systems and enzyme conjugates for solid-phase ELISA. In: Butler JE, ed: Immunochemistry of Solid-Phase Immunoassay. Boca Raton, FL: CRC Press, 1991, pp 85–102.

Tyler JW, Cullor JS: Titers, tests, and truisms: Rational interpretation of diagnostic serology testing. J Am Vet Med Assoc 194:1550–1558, 1989.

Quantitative Urine Collection as an Aid to Diagnosis and Therapy

JODY P. LULICH
CARL A. OSBORNE
St. Paul, Minnesota

In health, the composition of urine reflects the ability of normal kidneys to retain and reabsorb substances essential to basic metabolism and homeostasis and to excrete excess materials from the diet together with end-products of metabolism. This is accomplished through glomerular filtration of blood, selective resorption of useful components from glomerular filtrate, and tubular secretion of unwanted metabolites. Constant adjustment of these renal functions maintains the composition of all intracellular and extracellular compartments within narrow limits. However, pathologic or pharmacologic conditions affecting many body systems may alter the normal formation of urine so that unwanted substances are conserved or wanted substances are unavoidably lost, or both. Evaluation of timed urine samples can provide useful information about (1) altered mechanisms of urine excretion, (2) excretion of excess metabolites associated with disorders of other systems and organs, and (3) effects and side effects of therapy (Table 1).

RATIONALE FOR EVALUATING TIMED URINE COLLECTIONS

Measuring urinary excretion of amino acids is of greater clinical value than measuring their plasma concentrations for the detection of many inherited errors of metabolism (Woo and Henry, 1996). Typically, amino acid disorders are related to the absence of an enzyme involved in their conversion to other metabolites. Without this enzyme, amino acids that would normally serve as substrate for the enzyme accumulate in the plasma or urine, or both. Increased urinary excretion of amino acids can be categorized as either overflow or renal. Overflow aminoacidurias occur when the concentrations of amino acids in plasma, and subsequently in glomerular filtrate, greatly exceed the reabsorptive capacity of normally functioning renal tubules. Renal aminoacidurias are associated with defects in renal tubular transport mechanisms that result in decreased reabsorption of amino acids from the glomerular filtrate; plasma concentrations of amino acids are usually normal. Cystinuria is an excellent example of renal aminoaciduria that occurs in dogs and cats.

Improvement of nitrogen balance is the nutritional parameter most consistently associated with improved outcomes in critically ill patients (Konstantinides, 1992). Protein turnover is assessed by measuring the daily intake and excretion of nitrogen. Collection of timed urine samples and feces is essential for determining the daily quantity of nitrogen eliminated.

Measuring the urine volume of timed urine collections provides a basis for calculating fluid excesses and deficits in animals with polyuria or oliguria. For example, without considering the rate of urine production, a patient with oliguric renal failure could become overhydrated if repeated administration of fluids was calculated on the basis of normal maintenance requirements (Table 2). In contrast, polyuric patients would become dehydrated if they were provided with only normal maintenance fluid volumes without considering coexisting losses in urine.

Circadian release of hormones altering plasma concentrations of metabolites promotes short-term variations in the quantity of metabolites in urine. Postprandial variations in urine volume and composition also occur. Therefore, the volume and quantity of various metabolites in randomly collected urine samples from the same patient vary significantly throughout the day. Timed urine samples minimize diagnostic and therapeutic errors inherent to interpretation of values determined from random urine samples. The specific time intervals during which urine is collected may vary but should be long enough to minimize the influence of short-term biologic variations. We routinely collect 24-hour urine samples to assess urinary excretion of most minerals, electrolytes, and hormones. In contrast, we typically assess fluid balance in oliguric or polyuric patients every 2 to 6 hours to facilitate rapid assessment and replacement of needed fluid.

TECHNIQUE

Urine Collection

1. Because urinary excretion of minerals and electrolytes varies during fasting and postprandial states and with different types of diets, optimal results are most likely to be obtained when animals are evaluated under conditions similar to those used when normal values were established. To meaningfully assess the effects of therapy, samples collected during treatment should be compared with baseline values collected prior to treatment.
2. To facilitate acclimation of patients to hospital environments, house and feed patients in collection cages for at least 1 day prior to urine collection. As dogs and cats become acclimated to new environments, they are more likely to consume quantities of food and water similar to those consumed in their home environment.
3. Begin each timed urine collection by removing all urine from the urinary bladder. Transurethral catheterization provides the most reliable method of urine removal; however, other methods may also be considered (Table 3). Urine removed at the beginning of the timed sample collection may be discarded or submitted

TABLE 1. Indications for Timed Urine Collections

Indication	Test	Technical Consideration	Interpretation
Diagnosis of mild renal failure	Endogenous creatinine clearance	24-hr urine sample is best; shorter time intervals have also been performed. A midpoint serum sample is required for creatinine concentration.	Values less than normal (2–4 ml/min/kg in the dog, 1.6–3.8 ml/min/kg in the cat) are indicative of a decreased glomerular filtration rate and may explain clinical signs of urinary incontinence, nocturia, or polyuria in nonazotemic patients. In these patients, water restriction is not advised to control increased urine volume.
Diagnosis and management of oliguric renal failure	Monitor successive urine volumes every 2 to 4 hr	Serum biochemical analyses are needed to adjust for imbalances in serum electrolyte concentrations appropriately.	Hydrated dogs and cats forming urine in quantities less than 0.5 to 1 ml/kg/hr are considered oliguric. A brisk diuresis should be noticed following appropriate fluid therapy in nonliguric patients. With pathologic oliguria, fluid therapy should be adjusted so that volumes administered during the subsequent intervals are equal to urine volumes lost in the previous period, plus approximately 1 ml/kg/hr to account for insensible losses. In patients with no urine production, consider urinary tract obstruction as the underlying cause.
Maintain area of fluid balance in polyuric renal failure patients	Monitor successive urine volumes every 4 to 6 hr	Serum biochemical analyses are needed to adjust for deficits and excesses in serum electrolyte concentrations appropriately.	The amount of fluid replaced over that next time period is equal to the quantity lost in urine plus approximately an additional 1 ml/kg/hr to account for insensible evaporative losses. Alternatively, fluid can be replaced to maintain body weight: 1 ml for every gram of weight loss by the patient. Once the patient is drinking, oral administration can gradually replace parenteral administration.
Diagnosis and evaluation of therapy for protein-losing glomerulonephropathy	24-hr urine protein excretion	Alternatively, calculation of a urine protein-urine creatinine ratio from a random urine sample can be used.	Urine protein excretion greater than 20 mg/kg/day is consistent with glomerular disease in patients without evidence of preglomerular (e.g., increased small molecular weight plasma proteins) or postglomerular (e.g., hematuria) protein loss.
Monitoring urine mineral excretion in patients with urolithiasis	24-hr urine sample	Pretreatment samples are helpful for comparison. Activity products can be calculated with the aid of computer programs.	Concentrations of calculogenic minerals should become reduced and activity product ratios should be less than 1.
Identification of cystinuric patients	24-hr amino acid excretion	During urine collection, the sample is kept cold.	Cystine excretion is usually greater than 220 mg/gm of creatinine; clinically healthy dogs excrete approximately 70 mg/gm of creatinine. Quantities of ornithine, lysine, and arginine may also be increased.
Prevention of urate urolith recurrence in Dalmatians and other breeds	24-hr uric acid excretion	The aliquot submitted for analysis is diluted 1:20 with deionized water (1 ml urine to 19 ml water) to minimize precipitation of urate following collection.	A 24-hr uric acid excretion of 275 to 325 mg has been suggested as sufficient allopurinal therapy to prevent urate urolith recurrence and minimize allopurinol-induced xanthine urolith formation.
Diagnosis of Fanconi's syndrome	24-hr amino acid excretion	During urine collection, the sample is kept cold.	Affected dogs excrete higher levels of a variety of amino acids, glucose, and phosphorus.
Diagnosis of pheochromocytoma	24-hr urine catecholamine excretion	Urine is assayed for epinephrine, norepinephrine, vanillylmandelic acid, metanephrine, and normetanephrine. To prevent chemical degradation of catecholamines during urine collection, the sample is kept cold and acidified (pH <3).	Normal values have not been determined; compare with a clinically healthy dog of similar age and breed. Catecholamine values should be higher in dogs with pheochromocytomas.
Confirm polyuria	24-hr urine volume	Average 24-hr urine volume determined over several days.	Values in excess of 50 ml/kg/day warrant investigation as to the physiologic or pathologic causes of disease.
Nitrogen balance studies	24-hr urine nitrogen	Feces are also collected and analyzed for their nitrogen content.	Nitrogen balance is equal to nitrogen output subtracted from nitrogen input. A negative nitrogen balance indicates that the rate of protein catabolism exceeds the rate of protein anabolism, indicating the need for additional nutritional support.

TABLE 2. Definition and Quantification of Related Terms

Polyuria means excessive excretion of urine and may be physiologic, pharmacologic, or pathologic. Normal dogs housed in metabolism cages excrete 10.5 to 17.9 ml/kg/day of urine. Urine excretion in excess of 50 ml/kg is polyuric for dogs. Polyuria is an appropriate physiologic response to polydipsia or increased sodium consumption. Polyuria is an inappropriate response in dehydrated patients.

Oliguria may be physiologic or pathologic. Dogs and cats forming inappropriately concentrated urine in quantities less than 0.5 to 1 ml/kg/hr are considered to have pathologic oliguria. Prompt recognition of pathologic oliguria is important because affected patients are unable to compensate for parenteral administration of excessive quantities of fluid. Oliguria and appropriate urine concentration are normal physiologic responses to dehydration. This situation will occur following adequate fluid replacement. If oliguria is not reversed with fluid administration, further fluid must be carefully monitored to prevent iatrogenic overhydration.

Anuria connotes almost total suppression of urine formation and usually occurs as a result of total obstruction of urine outflow. Infrequent causes of anuria include processes that severely curtail renal blood flow (e.g., bilateral renal artery thrombosis) and possibly bilateral severe acute tubular necrosis.

Pollakiuria connotes abnormally frequent urination. Owners often confuse pollakiuria and polyuria. Pollakiuria is an indication of lower urinary tract inflammation; polyuria suggests renal involvement. Although polyuric animals also may urinate more frequently, they are not considered pollakiuric because the amount voided is normal or larger.

Normal daily maintenance fluid requirements represent physiologic losses of water via urine, feces, and respiration. Maintenance fluid volumes are closely linked to daily caloric requirements; however, the relationship between water requirements and body weight is not linear. Small patients require more water per unit of body weight; large patients require less. Formulas are available to calculate daily maintenance water requirements for dogs (140 × [body weight in kg]$^{0.73}$) and cats 80 × [body weight in kg]$^{0.75}$). Because increases in body temperature increase metabolic rate, water requirements also increase during elevations in body temperature. It has been suggested that maintenance fluid volumes increase 10% for every 1.8°F (−16.77°C) rise in body temperature above normal.

Sensible water losses are those that can be easily measured and predominantly consist of urinary and digestive losses.

Insensible water losses are those that are not easily quantified and primarily represent losses from the respiratory tract. Insensible losses account for approximately one third of maintenance fluid needs; the volume is lower for animals at rest and higher for animals with increased respiratory rate.

Polydipsia is defined as fluid intake greater than 50 ml/kg/day in either dogs or cats. Polydipsia is typically a normal physiologic compensatory response to replenish excessive fluid loss.

---

for baseline urinalysis or bacterial culture. When the bladder has been completely emptied, record the exact time that quantitative urine collection is initiated.

4. Accurately weigh the patient.
5. Feed patients their usual diet and provide unlimited amounts of water, unless test protocols specify modifications of diet and water. For example, it is essential to withhold water and food during water deprivation tests to assess urine concentrating capacity.
6. During urine collection, keep the patient in the collection cage. When animals void in cages designed for urine collection, periodic evacuation of the urinary bladder is not needed except at the end of the collection period. However, some house-trained dogs will not voluntary void urine while confined to metabolism cages. For these dogs, we periodically remove urine

by catheterization to keep them comfortable (typically every 6 to 8 hours). Urine collected in this manner is added to the collection container.

7. At the end of the specified collection period (usually 24 hours), the urinary bladder should be completely emptied, preferably by transurethral catheterization. This urine is added to the collection container (see Table 3).
8. The exact time that urine collection is completed should be recorded.
9. All urine collected during the allotted period should be pooled in a single container and its volume measured.
10. Pooled urine should be thoroughly mixed prior to removing aliquots for analysis or storage.
11. Urine volume can be approximated in sick animals by weighing absorbent bedding following voiding (remember to weigh the bedding before placing it in the cage). Urine volume in cats can be approximated by weighing pans containing litter. When voided urine is to be analyzed for its various constituents, we use nonabsorbable litter or litter pans that funnel urine into a collection vial.

Urine Preservation

1. Urine preservatives have different roles, but most are used to minimize bacterial growth, reduce chemical decomposition, and/or solubilize constituents that might otherwise precipitate or decrease atmospheric oxidation of unstable compounds.
2. For some tests, preservatives should not be added to urine specimens because they interfere with analytic methods.
3. Methods of preservation vary according to the substances being measured and the tests used to measure them. Consult with the staff at the laboratory performing the analysis of the specimen for recommended methods of preservation.
4. Refrigeration is a common method for preserving substances excreted in urine. Urine removed from the bladder by intermittent catheterization can be refrigerated in clean containers with screw top lids. Containers used to collect urine voided by patients in metabolism cages can be surrounded by ice packs and then insulated. Immediately following collection of all urine, the composite sample is mixed, and preservatives are added to aliquots, which are then stored until analysis. Remember that refrigeration can cause some minerals in solution to precipitate, leading to errors in measurement of their excretion in urine.
5. Acidification (10 ml of 1N HCl/L to achieve a pH of 3 or less) is commonly used to preserve urine specimens collected for analysis of oxalate and calcium. However, acidified urine is unsuitable for preservation of samples for measuring uric acid analysis because urates precipitate in acidic solutions.

Additional Considerations

1. *Midpoint blood samples.* Evaluation of blood during the midpoint of timed urine collections may help to deter-

TABLE 3. Methods of Emptying the Bladder

Method	Advantages	Disadvantages
Transurethral catheterization	With the opening "eye" of the catheter in the region of the trigone of the urinary blader, the bladder is effectively emptied	Catheterization of the female urethra requires experience Potential to induce iatrogenic bacterial infection
Palpation-induced voiding	Applying steady digital pressure to the urinary bladder is a noninvasive method to induce voiding	Some may resist bladder compression Unsure of degree of complete bladder evacuation Hematuria Microbes from urinary blader may reflux into ureters and kidneys
Urecholine-induced micturition	A subcutaneous injection of 0.1 to 0.2 mg/kg is a noninvasive method to induce voiding	May induce salivation and abdominal pain Profuse salivation may affect urine volume and composition
Voluntary voiding	No risk of iatrogenic injury to the patient	May not void unless bladder is at least moderately filled Unsure of degree of complete bladder evacuation Lower urogenital contaminants may modify urine composition
Transabdominal cystocentesis	Provides a relatively clean urine sample free of lower urogenital contaminants	Complete urinary evacuation is not possible because needle will traumatize mucosal surface and perhaps other portions of the bladder wall

mine if changes in urine concentrations of various metabolites reflect changes in their serum or plasma concentration. This information can assist in detection of underlying causes and mechanisms of abnormal analyte excretion. Likewise, evaluation of blood concentrations of some hormones (e.g., parathyroid hormone, calcitriol, and so on) may be helpful in determining the role of hormones in the regulation of mineral excretion. A midpoint blood sample is also required for calculating renal clearance of endogenous substances such as creatinine.

2. *Antimicrobial agents.* Antimicrobial drugs are commonly administered to patients to prevent iatrogenic urinary tract infection during catheterization of the urinary bladder. The dosage, dosing interval, and route should be based on the recommendations of the manufacturer. If antimicrobial drugs are known to interfere with the volume or composition of urine, they should be given following completion of urine collection. For patients with normal urinary tracts, antimicrobial agents are usually continued for 3 to 5 days after urine collection. We estimate that this represents the approximate time required for normal urothelial repair of catheter-induced trauma to the urethra and bladder mucosa.

We select antimicrobials that are primarily excreted in urine and that minimally affect urine concentrations of minerals, proteins (promoters and inhibitors associated with urolith formation), and amino acids. Some antimicrobials are formulated as salts of sodium or potassium, resulting in correspondingly high concentrations of sodium or potassium in urine. We routinely use cephalosporins when collecting urine for evaluation of amino acids, and ampicillin when collecting urine for evaluation of calcium, oxalate, or uric acid.

3. *Fasting urine collections.* Evaluation of timed urine collections during periods of food fasting has been used to characterize pathophysiologic mechanisms of some disorders. One representative example is hypercalciuria in dogs with calcium oxalate uroliths (Lulich et al,

1991). We usually collect fasting urine collections immediately after urine collections during standard feeding. Dogs that absorb excessive amounts of calcium from their diet and subsequently excrete high quantities of calcium in their urine have intestinal hypercalciuria. In dogs with intestinal (or absorptive) hypercalciuria, the hypercalciuria primarily occurs during food consumption; normocalciuria or hypocalciuria occurs when food is withheld. In addition, intestinal hypercalciuria is associated with normal serum concentrations of calcium and normal or low serum concentrations of parathyroid hormone. In contrast, hypercalciuria occurs during feeding and fasting in dogs with primary hyperparathyroidism (resorptive hypercalciuria) or impaired renal tubular absorption of calcium (renal leak hypercalciuria).

4. *Urine pH.* The solubility of many mineral salts is influenced by urine pH. Determination of the pH of timed urine samples may be helpful in evaluating crystal formation and diagnosing various forms of renal tubular acidosis. Urine pH values are required to calculate activity products for several mineral salts commonly found in uroliths. An ion selective electrode and pH meter should be used to measure urine pH accurately.

CALCULATIONS

24-Hour Urine Volume

Although 24-hour urine specimens are recommended to minimize the effects of short-term biologic variations in mineral excretion, completion of urine collection in exactly 24 hours is often impractical. To adjust collected urine volume to a 24-hour period, use the following formula:

1440 (number of minutes in 24 hours)/actual collection time interval (minutes) × urine volume

Example:
A 24-hour urine collection was started at 9:30 AM and ended the following day at 8:30 AM. During this period, 350 ml of urine was collected. What is the 24-hour urine volume?

$$(1440/1380) \times 350 = 356.2 \text{ ml}$$

Conversion of mmol/L to mg/dl

In order to standardize measurements, the scientific community is promoting adoption of a uniform system of measurement known as the *System International d'Unites*. In this system, concentration is often expressed as molarity (moles or millimoles of a substance per liter of fluid). However, in the United States, most values are expressed as milligrams per deciliter. The following formula can be used to convert millimoles per liter to milligrams per deciliter:

$$\text{mmol/L} \times \text{gram atomic weight of substance}/10$$

The formula is divided by 10 because there are 10 dl in a liter. The gram atomic weights of elements can be found in the periodic table of general chemistry textbooks.

Example:
The concentration of calcium from a 24-hour urine sample was 1.35 mmol/L. To convert this value to milligrams per deciliter for comparison with normal values, multiply 1.35 mmol/L × the gram atomic weight of calcium (40.08); 1.35 mmol/L × 40.08/10 = 5.4 mg/dl.

Expressing Excretion of a Substance in mg/kg Per 24 Hours or mEq/kg Per 24 Hours

Excretion of metabolites is often expressed on a per kilogram body weight basis to standardize excretion for different sized animals. The following formula can be used:

$$\text{Concentration of substance} \times 24 \text{ hour urine}$$
$$\text{volume/body weight (kg)}$$

Units used to express the volume of urine, and the concentration of the substance measured in urine must be the same.

Example:
The concentration of calcium in a 24-hour urine sample is 5.4 mg/dl. In 24 hours, 356.2 ml of urine was collected. The dog weighed 10 kg. What is the daily calcium excretion on a kilogram body weight basis?
First, express the volume of urine collected in the same units as the urine concentration of the substance measured; 356.2 ml per 24 hours is equal to 3.562 dl per 24 hours.
Substituting variables in the formula results in (5.4 mg/dl × 3.562 dl per 24 hours)/10kg = 1.92 mg/kg per 24 hours.

Endogenous Creatinine Clearance

Serum concentrations of urea nitrogen and creatinine are not sensitive tests to detect mild renal failure because values usually remain within the range for normal dogs until three quarters of the nephrons of both kidneys become nonfunctional. In chronic progressive diseases, impaired urine concentration typically occurs prior to azotemia. Thus, early clinical signs of chronic progressive renal failure include polyuria, nocturia, and sometimes urinary incontinence. To rule out early renal failure as a cause of these urinary signs, endogenous creatinine clearance may be used to evaluate kidney function. Endogenous creatinine

clearance can also be used to monitor progression of renal failure more accurately.

After all urine is removed from the bladder at the beginning of the study, a 24-hour urine sample is collected and assayed for creatinine excretion. At the midpoint of the urine collection, a blood sample is obtained for determination of serum creatinine concentration. Using the weight of the dog, urine volume, and serum and urine concentrations of creatinine, the glomerular filtration rate is calculated as follows:

$$\text{(Urine creatinine concentration in mg/dl)} \times \text{(urine}$$
$$\text{volume)} \div \text{(serum creatinine concentration in}$$
$$\text{mg/dl} \times \text{time of collection} \times \text{body weight in kg)}$$

Normal values are 2.0 to 4.0 ml/min/kg for dogs and 1.6 to 3.8 ml/min/kg for cats (Ross, 1986). Abnormally low values are consistent with impaired renal function.

Example:
The owner of a 5-year-old, female, well-hydrated, nonazotemic Golden retriever with nephrogenic diabetes insipidus wanted to restrict the dog's water availability at night to prevent nocturia. However, water should not be restricted in patients with obligatory polyuria associated with renal failure. Before agreeing with the owner's request, a 24-hour endogenous creatinine clearance test was performed to determine whether or not this nonazotemic patient had early renal failure. Midpoint serum creatinine was 1.2 mg/dl; urine creatinine was 54 mg/dl, 24-hour urine volume was 1550 ml, and the dog's weight was 30 kg. Endogenous creatinine clearance is (184 mg/dl × 1550 ml)/(1.2mg/dl × 30 kg × 1440 min) = 1.6 ml/min/kg. Although this patient is not azotemic, the abnormally low endogenous creatinine clearance value indicates that early renal failure is present. Therefore, water should not be restricted. As an alternative, feeding diets restricted in protein and minerals may help reduce urine volume by minimizing solute diuresis.

Fractional Excretion of Electrolytes

Urinary fractional excretion of a substance represents the portion (or fraction) of the substance that is filtered by the kidneys but not reabsorbed by renal tubules (the fraction of glomerular filtrate that is ultimately excreted). Determining fractional excretion traditionally requires collection of a timed urine sample. Because the variables of time and urine volume can be factored out of the fractional excretion equation, fractional excretions may be calculated from nontimed spot urine samples using the following formula:

$$\frac{\text{Concentration of substance in urine/}}{\text{concentration of substance in serum}}$$
$$\overline{\text{Urine creatinine concentration/}}$$
$$\text{serum creatinine concentration}$$

Example:
In order to evaluate the effects of dietary phosphorus restriction in a dog with renal failure, measure the fractional excretion of phosphorus during consumption of a phosphorus-restricted renal failure diet and compare this value with the fractional excretion of phosphorus during consumption of a standard maintenance diet (baseline fractional excretion of

phosphorus was 0.56). Blood and urine should be obtained concurrently and evaluated for their phosphorus concentrations (serum = 5.3 mg/dl, urine = 38.4mg/dl) and creatinine concentrations (serum = 3.6mg/dl, urine = 102 mg/dl). The fractional excretion of phosphorus is (38.4/5.3)/(102/3.6) = 0.26. This lower value indicates a favorable response to dietary phosphorus reduction.

Approximating Urine Volume by Weighing Absorbent Material

One gram of water equals 1 ml of water. Since the weight of water is similar to the weight of urine, 1 gm of urine is approximately equal to 1 ml of urine. The difference in the weight of absorbent material before placing patients in cages and after patients have urinated on the absorbent material can be used to estimate the volume of urine voided.

Example:
What is the volume of urine voided by a cat whose litter pan weighs 1.5 pounds (original weight = 0.8 pounds)? The weight of urine = 1.5 pounds − 0.8 pounds = 0.7 pounds; 0.7 pounds × 454 gm/pound = 317.8 gm. Therefore, this patient urinated approximately 320 ml of urine. Remember that urine spread over a large surface area, such as litter or a towel, has a tendency to evaporate at a faster rate than urine in the bladder or urine that is collected in a container.

Urine Analyte:Creatinine Ratios

To minimize technical difficulties with collection of timed urine samples, the magnitude of excretion of various substances in urine is sometimes assessed by determining the concentration of the substance in urine from a random urine sample and then dividing it by the creatinine concentration in the same urine sample. Accuracy of urine analyte:creatinine ratios are based on the assumptions that (1) the glomerular filtration rate is constant, (2) the quantity of the substance lost in the urine is constant during a 24-hour period, and (3) glomerular filtration and tubular concentration of urine affect both the substance measured and creatinine similarly. Although this method is reliable for assessment of 24-hour urine protein excretion, it has not been reliable in estimating 24-hour urinary excretion of many minerals (e.g., potassium, urate, calcium, phosphorus).

Example:
Proteinuria designated as 2+ was identified by a qualitative reagent strip test in a 5-year-old Labrador retriever with weight loss. To quantitate protein loss more accurately, a 5-ml urine sample was removed from the bladder by cystocentesis and analyzed. The protein concentration was 1105 mg/dl and the creatinine concentration was 184 mg/dl. What is the patient's urine protein:creatinine ratio? 1105/184 = 6. Normal urine protein:creatinine ratio values are less than 1 (which equals approximately 20 mg/kg per day). A value of 6 supports a diagnosis of glomerular disease provided that the patient does not have evidence of preglomerular or postglomerular protein loss.

References and Suggested Reading

Konstantinides FN: Nitrogen balance studies in clinical nutrition. Nutr Clin Pract 7:231, 1992.
Human reference for performing nitrogen balance studies.
Lulich JP, Osborne CA, Nagode LA, et al: Evaluation of urine and serum analytes in miniature schnauzers with calcium oxalate urolithiasis. J Am Vet Res 52:1583, 1991.
Effects of fasting on some urine values.
Ross LA: Assessment of renal function in the dogs and cat. In: Kirk RW, ed: Current Veterinary Therapy IX: Small Animal Practice. Philadelphia: WB Saunders, 1986, pp 1103–1107.
Procedure for endogenous creatinine clearance.
Woo J, Henry JB: Metabolic intermediates and inorganic ions. In: Henry JB, ed. Clinical Diagnosis and Management by Laboratory Methods. Philadelphia: WB Saunders, 1996, pp 169–170.
Diagnosis and localization of aminoacidurias.

Alternatives to Exploratory Celiotomies: First Do No Harm

CARL A. OSBORNE
JODY P. LULICH
St. Paul, Minnesota

ARE YOU A CUTTING SURGEON OR A THINKING SURGEON?

With the development and widespread availability of excellent surgical equipment, safe and effective methods of anesthesia, intraoperative monitoring devices, and surgical support therapy, most veterinarians feel very confident about their ability to perform celiotomies. Unfortunately, knowing how to perform celiotomies is not synonymous with knowing why and when to perform them. Why should celiotomies be performed? When should they be performed? How often have exploratory celiotomies been without benefit or even detrimental to the patient? One clinician provided an indirect answer to these questions by stating, "A negative laparotomy is disappointing. However, it is more disappointing to delay the operation, have the patient die, and find a correctable lesion on postmortem examination. If an error in judgment is to be made, it is better to be too aggressive than not aggressive enough." Another clinician provided this perspective, "Far more patients have died because an exploratory celiotomy was delayed than because the procedure was performed without finding significant lesions." These recommendations appear to be based on the premise that many patients will die if exploratory celiotomies are not performed. However, is this premise valid? Are there data to support these generalities? Could the same generalities be applied to exploratory thoracotomies? Utilizing a computerized search, we could not find controlled retrospective or prospective studies in the veterinary literature designed to provide quantitative information about risk/benefit ratios of exploratory celiotomies. Why is this situation of concern? Because in the absence of acceptable evidence of therapeutic efficacy, the occasional dramatic result is often vividly remembered, the failures are often forgotten, and unquestioned therapeutic dogma becomes established.

The authors recognize that most exploratory celiotomies are performed with good intent. However, as experience has taught us all, good intent does not always result in a beneficial outcome. As internists in a referral hospital, the author's experience has been that too many exploratory celiotomies are performed without the operators giving balanced thought to probable risks and benefits to the patients. Because of what we will symbolically describe as a "cutting surgeon mentality," it is the author's opinion that records will confirm that the abdomens of too many patients with undiagnosed abdominal disease have been "opened up." When we view outcomes through our "retrospectoscopes," it becomes apparent that some exploratory celiotomies did not always benefit the patients. Yet despite some negative outcomes clearly recognized in hindsight, the vision of those with a "cutting surgeon" philosophy does not always improve. Instead of becoming 20/20, it remains at 60/80. Why so? Could it be because veterinarians as a group have been reluctant to criticize seemingly logical diagnostic and/or therapeutic intervention that resulted in an unfavorable outcome as long as there was some faith that some good might be achieved? Have we as a profession promulgated an unrealistic concept about the efficacy of exploratory surgery? Is it not true that many clients have blind faith that many diseases can be resolved or helped by surgery? How often have we heard clients say, "Will you have to do surgery, Doctor?" And what is our response if following surgery the patient is not helped? Often we excuse ourselves by saying, "Well, at least we tried."

What is the point? When clearly defined objectives for exploratory celiotomies have not been considered in light of the probable risks and benefits to the patient, the outcome is often disappointing from a diagnostic and therapeutic perspective.

The purpose of this essay is not to create disunity between literal surgeons and literal internists. Rather, the author's desire is to promote high-quality patient care by fostering a thinking surgeon mentality, rather than a cutting surgeon mentality, in all of us. Whereas the motto of the cutting surgeon mentality is "a chance to cut is chance to cure," the paradigm of the thinking surgeon mentality is to minimize the philosophy of "chance" in terms of cure. The precept of thinking surgeons is that although there are some patients we cannot help, there are none we cannot harm. They clearly recognize the difference between activity (performing an exploratory celiotomy) and accomplishment (performing an exploratory celiotomy when the probable benefit to the patient outweighs the risks). Isn't it true that no patient should be worse for having seen the doctor? Ethics demand that we not let poorly conceived choices to perform technically sound exploratory celiotomies jeopardize the welfare of our patients. With high-quality patient care in mind, let us consider why and when exploratory celiotomies should be performed, some risks and benefits of exploratory celiotomies, and also some alternatives to exploratory celiotomies.

EXPLORATORY CELIOTOMY VERSUS EXPLORATORY LAPAROTOMY

The term laparotomy is sometimes used as a synonym for the term celiotomy. However, the term laparotomy is derived from the Greek words "laparo" meaning flank (the part of the body below the ribs and above the ilium), and "tome" meaning to cut. Laparotomy is defined as a surgical incision through the flank.

The term celiotomy is derived from the Greek words "celio" meaning abdomen, and "tome." Thus, a celiotomy is a surgical incision into the abdominal cavity. The term abdomen is derived from the Latin root word "abdere," meaning "to hide away." Thus an exploratory celiotomy is a surgical incision into the abdominal cavity performed to facilitate examination of the structural and functional integrity of various "hidden" abdominal organs, and/or with the intent of restoring adequate function and structure to various abdominal organs.

EXPLORATORY CELIOTOMY

Objectives

There are at least four basic objectives of exploratory celiotomies, including: (1) restoration of hemostasis, (2) control of contamination (e.g., by utilizing noncrushing intestinal clamps to prevent further loss of ingesta from a rent in the intestines), (3) localization and identification of the cause or causes of injury or disease, and (4) repair of abnormal tissues and restoration of lost function.

One additional objective may become important. If an exploratory celiotomy does not result in diagnosis of the underlying cause of abdominal disease, before the abdominal wall is closed it is wise to consider whether or not appropriate biopsy specimens should be taken from organs or tissues thought to be involved with the disease process. On occasions too numerous to count, the authors have consulted with colleagues about persistent signs of disease of various abdominal structures following negative exploratory celiotomies. Procurement of biopsy samples from appropriate structures at this opportune time was frequently overlooked. The impact of this oversight becomes magnified if additional anesthesia and/or surgery is subsequently needed to obtain biopsy samples from abdominal structures.

Potential Benefits and Risks

The practice of veterinary medicine is often difficult, because it requires judgment in the absence of certainty (see *CVT XII*, p. 11). This statement is especially applicable to patients with undiagnosed illness, especially with acute diseases of the abdomen. Experience has taught us all that there are avoidable and unavoidable risks associated with general anesthesia and exploratory abdominal surgery. What can be done to recognize and minimize these risks? What can be done to enhance the benefits to the patient as a result of this procedure?

When considering exploratory celiotomy as a diagnostic and/or therapeutic option, what "operative" and "nonoperative" risks should be evaluated? Operative risks encompass (1) the availability, sensitivity, and specificity of nonsurgical techniques to evaluate and/or treat the patient (Table 1), (2) the level of diagnostic refinement of the abdominal disorder and concomitant unrelated disorders (Table 2), (3) the status of the patient (e.g., age, functional status of body systems and organs), (4) the technical skills and experiences of the anesthesia and/or surgical team, (5) the technical difficulty of anticipated diagnostic or corrective surgical procedures (e.g., splenectomy, intestinal anastomosis, ureteral anastomosis), (6) the need for and availability of postoperative supportive care, (7) risks associated with anesthetic "stress," and (8) potential sequela to the

TABLE 2. Four Conceptual Diagnostic Levels of Problem Refinement

Problem(s)	Level of Refinement
1. Subjective history or physical examination findings	Lowest
a. Vomiting	
b. Diarrhea	
c. Painful abdomen	
d. Abdominal distention	
e. Other	
2. Objective reproducible diagnostic findings	Low
a. Laboratory data	
b. Radiographic or ultrasonographic data	
c. Microscopy of biopsy samples	
d. Results of endoscopy or laparoscopy	
e. Other	
3. Pathophysiologic syndrome	Higher
a. Shock due to unexplained rupture of the kidney	
b. Intestinal malabsorption syndrome	
c. Postrenal uremia and uroperitoneum due to unexplained rupture of the urinary bladder	
d. Other	
4. Specific diagnosis	Highest
a. Transudative ascites and portal hypertension due to hepatic cirrhosis	
b. Hemoperitoneum and hemodynamic instability due to rupture of splenic hemangiosarcoma	
c. Septic bacterial peritonitis due to perforation of the ileum by a foreign body	
d. Other	

TABLE 1. Diagnostic Procedures That May Help Determine Patient Risk/Benefit Ratios of Exploratory Celiotomies

Diagnostic Procedure	Reference

1. Problem-specific database including
  a. Predetermined questions about patient's history
  b. Predetermined physical examination protocol
  c. Predetermined laboratory tests
  d. Other diagnostic tests relevant to specific problem(s)
	Osborne, 1983

2. Paracentesis of abdominal fluid
  a. Cytology
  b. Bacterial culture
  c. Biochemical tests (e.g., protein, amylase, urea nitrogen, creatinine, bilirubin)
	Birchard & Fingland, 1986; Ellison, 1986

3. Diagnostic peritoneal lavage
  a. A rapid and sensitive but nonspecific method to confirm intraperitoneal bleeding*
  b. Especially helpful in assessing whether hemoperitoneum exists in a patient with progressive hemodynamic instability
	Birchard & Fingland, 1986; Ellison, 1986

4. Imaging techniques
  a. Survey radiography
  b. Contrast radiography
  c. Ultrasonography; ultrasound-guided biopsy
  d. Fluoroscopy
  e. Angiography
  f. Computed tomography
	Burk & Ackerman, 1996; Feeney et al, 1991; O'Brien et al, 1981

5. Endoscopy and laparoscopy	Tams, 1996
6. Specialist consultation	
7. Referral	

*See *CVT XII*, p. 766.

surgery itself (e.g., postsplenectomy sepsis, organ loss or dysfunction). Nonoperative risks encompass (1) the biologic behavior of the underlying cause or causes of the abdominal disorders, and (2) the probable morbidity and mortality associated with nonsurgical treatment of the disorder or disorders, especially compared with accepted protocols for surgical treatment of the abnormality. For example, if a patient known to have marginal renal function subsequently develops hemoperitoneum as a consequence of severe trauma following needle biopsy of the kidney, what are the short- and long-term benefits and risks of conservative treatment by blood transfusion versus exploratory celiotomy and partial or total nephrectomy? This question becomes especially relevant in light of the undesirable immunosuppressive effects of blood transfusions.

A major decision that often influences patient risk/benefit ratios is whether exploratory celiotomies are required on an emergency basis, or whether there is time for additional diagnostic investigation (see Table 1). Understandably, it is not possible to develop "always" or "never" criteria to answer this question. However, it is important to consider whether direct visualization of abdominal structures by means of exploratory celiotomy would be of probable benefit to the patient by (1) permitting verification and/or localization of the site or sites and/or cause or causes of abdominal signs, (2) facilitating aspiration, needle, or wedge biopsies of abnormal structures, and/or (3) surgically restoring normal structure and function of abdominal organs.

Diagnostic information that will most effectively allow assessment of probable patient risk/benefit ratios of exploratory celiotomies has not been determined. This is not surprising since selection of the appropriate diagnostic protocol would be influenced by (1) the mechanism or mechanisms of injury or disease, (2) the hemodynamic or homeostatic stability of the patient, (3) the level of problem refinement (see Table 2) and the need for additional diagnostic or prognostic tests (see Table 1), (4) the availability of needed diagnostic tests or procedures, and (5) the estimated cost of desired diagnostic tests and procedures.

Whether or not exploratory celiotomies are performed on an emergency basis, it is important to collect appropriate samples of blood, serum, plasma, urine, and material for bacterial culture and/or exfoliative cytology before any diagnostic, preanesthetic, anesthetic, or therapeutic agents are given to the patient. If subsequent developments preclude the need for these samples, they may be discarded. More often, they may be submitted at the time of, or following, surgery. Even though the results of laboratory tests may not become available until after an "emergency" exploratory celiotomy is performed, they represent pretreatment results unaltered by diagnostic or therapeutic agents. Thus, they can be used to help retrospectively evaluate the benefit of the choice to perform an exploratory celiotomy. They may also be used as baseline data with which to compare results of serially collected laboratory data obtained following celiotomy to monitor the rate of remission or progression of the problem.

TABLE 3. Probable Patient Risk/Benefit Outcomes Associated With Management of Some Abdominal Diseases by Exploratory Celiotomy

1. Some abdominal diseases for which benefits of exploratory celiotomy probably outweigh risks
   a. Penetrating gunshot wounds of the abdomen, even if signs secondary to organ injury have not yet developed
   b. Sudden unexplained blood loss associated with overt hemoperitoneum in a hemodynamically unstable patient
   c. Overt diffuse septic peritonitis
   d. Evisceration of abdominal contents
   e. Obstructive uropathy of the ureter or renal pelvis associated with concomitant bacterial urinary tract infection
   f. Intestinal obstruction
   g. Rupture of the renal pelvis, ureter, or urinary bladder associated with uroperitoneum
   h. Bile peritonitis
2. Some abdominal diseases for which the risk/benefit ratio of exploratory celiotomy often requires further study
   a. Abdominal stab wounds unassociated with hemodynamically unstable hemoperitoneum or diffuse septic peritonitis
   b. Hemoperitoneum in a hemodynamically stable patient, especially as a result of low-pressure traumatic bleeding from the liver or spleen
   c. Rupture of the urinary bladder unassociated with uroperitoneum or septic peritonitis
   d. Intra-abdominal malignancy
3. Some abdominal diseases for which risks of exploratory celiotomy are likely to outweigh benefits
   a. Exploratory cystotomy of cats with idiopathic feline lower urinary tract disease
   b. Persistent or intermittent vomiting that has not been localized and evaluated with conventional nonsurgical diagnostic methods
   c. Persistent or intermittent diarrhea that has not been localized and evaluated with conventional nonsurgical diagnostic methods
   d. Ascites that has not been evaluated by conventional nonsurgical diagnostic methods
   e. Renoliths and/or ureteroliths that are not obstructing outflow of urine

Alternatives

Unquestionably, there are many circumstances in which exploratory celiotomies are of great benefit to the patient; often they are life-saving. However, a positive outcome is more likely to be linked to informed choice rather than chance.

Development of and experience with nonsurgical methods of visualizing intra-abdominal structures and evaluating the function of abdominal organs has reduced the frequency of unnecessary exploratory celiotomies in human patients. Our experience has been that a similar trend is occurring in veterinary medicine (Table 3). In addition, better understanding of the biologic behavior of traumatic and nontraumatic abdominal disorders has revealed that exploratory celiotomies are frequently unnecessary and, sometimes, contraindicated.

There remain a substantial number of patients with abdominal disorders for which the risk/benefit ratio of exploratory celiotomy cannot be clearly forecast. When uncertainty exists as to whether an exploratory celiotomy is, or is not, in the best interests of the patient, the authors try to assess the following questions. Based on all available information, would I elect to have an exploratory celiotomy if I were this patient? Based on knowledge of my own skill and experience, and the availability of support staff and equipment, would I consent to the proposed plan of diagnostic and therapeutic action if I were in this patient's exact situation? What diagnostic and/or therapeutic goals are likely to be achieved? If an exploratory celiotomy is or is not performed, in all probability will the overall benefits of this plan of action justify the associated risks and costs.

References and Suggested Reading

Birchard SJ, Fingland RB: Abdominal trauma. In: Bright RM, ed: Surgical Emergencies (Contemporary Issues in Small Animal Practice). New York: Churchill Livingstone, 1986, pp 111–125.
  This chapter provides details about diagnostic peritoneal lavage.
Bordin JO, Blajchman MA: Transfusion-associated immunosuppression. In: Simon TL (Rossi EC, et al, eds): Principles of Transfusion Medicine, 2nd ed. Baltimore: Williams & Wilkins, 1996, pp 803–812.
  This chapter summarizes evidence about the consequences of the immunosuppressive effects of blood transfusions.
Burk RL, Ackerman N: Small Animal Radiology and Ultrasonography, 2nd ed. Philadelphia: WB Saunders, 1996.
Crowe DT, Jr: The abdominal cavity: Peritoneum, retroperitoneum, abdominal hernias, and adrenal glands. In: Harvey CE, Newton CD, Schwartz A, eds: Small Animal Surgery. Philadelphia: JB Lippincott, 1990, pp 279–322.
  This chapter provides details about abdominal surgery.
Ellison GW: Nontraumatic surgical emergencies of the abdomen. In: Bright RM, ed: Surgical Emergencies (Contemporary Issues in Small Animal Practice). New York: Churchill Livingstone, 1986, pp 127–172.
  This chapter provides information about diagnostic peritoneal lavage.
Fabian TC, Croce MA: Abdominal trauma including indications for celiotomy. In: Feliciano DV, Moore EE, Mattox KL, eds: Trauma, 3rd ed. Stamford, CT: Appleton & Lange, 1996, pp 441–459.
  An up-to-date review about the diagnosis and treatment of abdominal trauma in humans.
Feeney DA, Fletcher TF, Hardy RM: Atlas of Correlative Imaging Anatomy of the Normal Dog: Ultrasound and Computed Tomography. Philadelphia: WB Saunders, 1991.
O'Brien TR, Biery DN, Park RD, et al: Radiographic Diagnosis of Abdominal Disorders in the Dog and Cat. Philadelphia: WB Saunders, 1981.
Osborne CA: The problem-oriented medical system: Improved knowl-

edge, wisdom, and understanding of patient care. Vet Clin North Am Small Anim Pract 13:745, 1983.
This article provides guidelines about the development of problem-specific databases.
Osborne CA, Sanderson SL, Lulich JP, et al: Medical management of iatrogenic rents in the wall of the feline urinary bladder. Vet Clin North Am Small Anim Pract 23:551, 1996.
Rozycki GS: Abdominal ultrasonography in trauma. Surg Clin North Am 75:175, 1995.
Shackford SR: The evolution of modern trauma care. Surg Clin North Am 75:147, 1995.

A review emphasizing the need for a systematized or organized approach to trauma care.
Simon RJ, Ivatury RR: Current concepts in the use of cavitary endoscopy in the evaluation and treatment of blunt and penetrating truncal injuries. Surg Clin North Am 75:157, 1995.
A review of the indications, contraindications, techniques, and pitfalls of laparoscopy and thoracoscopy as they apply to humans.
Tams TR: Handbook of Small Animal Gastroenterology. Philadelphia: WB Saunders, 1996.
This book provides details about laparoscopy.

Enhancing Compliance With Treatment Recommendations

SARA Z. SUDO

CARL A. OSBORNE

St. Paul, Minnesota

The best practitioners strive to give their patients the least medications.

Do Your Clients Comply With Your Recommendations? The overall rate of compliance with physician instructions, based on a review of a large number of articles, is approximately 50% (Sackett, 1976). If this rate reflects the situation in veterinary medicine, then the effect of noncompliance on therapeutic outcomes is greater than most veterinarians realize. In our experience, veterinarians and their staff typically overestimate rates of compliance among their clients. In addition, veterinarians are often unable to identify noncompliant individuals. However, it is certain that veterinarians may have a positive or negative effect on many variables that influence compliance. The following comments are based on our own experiences and information extrapolated from studies of human patients.

Roles of Doctors, Clients, and Patients. In terms of compliance, who is most important: the doctor, the client, or the patient? A common assumption is that it is the doctor's role to order medications, whereas the proper role of the client and the patient is to comply with the doctor's orders. Recent studies indicate that this type of relationship is not optimal in achieving compliance with treatment recommendations (Weinstein, 1995; Tebbi, 1993). Specifying whether the doctor, the client, or the patient is most important in achieving compliance is comparable to asking which leg is most important on a three-legged stool. The interaction among the three frequently determines the effectiveness of a therapeutic regimen. Each must contribute to the effort for a successful outcome. The veterinarian must provide or validate the correct diagnosis, and then must educate the client about the consequences of the disease

with or without therapy. Following a review of therapeutic options, the doctor and the client together should select a mutually agreeable plan. The client must be committed to implementing the therapeutic plan, and to providing follow-up information to the veterinary health care team. But are treatment plans selected by veterinarians always conducive to compliance? Furthermore, do clients carry out the plans, and can our patients cooperate with them? The following discussion highlights some problems commonly encountered and provides our suggestions about improving client and patient compliance.

Defining Problems and Selecting Therapeutic Options. There is a difference between doing things right (e.g., devising the right components and sequence of treatments) and doing the right things (giving the properly devised treatments to the right patients at the right times to help eliminate or control the right diseases). For example, on several occasions we have evaluated patients who have not responded to technically correct therapeutic techniques (the treatment plan was right) because of a misdiagnosis (thus, the therapy was not appropriate to manage that disorder). Correct assessment of the patient's problems is a basic requirement for consistently successful therapy. In fact, a well-defined problem is usually half-solved! Once the disease is properly defined, current treatments can often be found in journals or textbooks or by consulting with colleagues via telephone, fax, or computer (see p. 2).

Yet an accurate assessment of the illness, coupled with accurate formulation of a therapeutic plan, may not result in cure or control of the problem. The most advanced diagnostic and therapeutic techniques are useless if they cannot be transformed into therapeutic action that can be consistently implemented by the client.

CLIENT EDUCATION

Client education requires that providers of veterinary care make judgments about what clients need to know and do, what they are capable of learning and willing to learn, how they can best be taught, and how to assess what they have learned. Interactive learning is often more effective than traditional instructor-oriented monologues. Clients, like students, usually learn best by actively participating in the learning process.

Understanding Disease Processes. Facts and concepts about various diseases are best explained with the use of clear, nontechnical language, whether it be in the spoken or written word. However, to be most effective, the approach used to facilitate learning should be adapted to the client. For example, consider a scenario of three clients—a retired physician, an accountant, and a carpenter—each with the same level of innate intelligence but possessing acquired knowledge and wisdom that are quite different. In this situation, their understanding of clinical problems will be enhanced if explanations are adapted to the knowledge base of each individual. This requires assessment of the client's concept of illness, which then becomes a starting point from which to build understanding. It is also best to keep the conversation simple and focused. Overloading the client with too much data may have the same effect as giving them too little information. Use of relevant illustrations that clients can readily understand and remember is an extremely powerful method of communication. Likewise, viewpoint questions that avoid simple "yes" and "no" responses are also powerful learning tools. For example, instead of asking the client, "Do you know what kidney failure is?", the client might be asked, "What is your understanding about the effects of kidney failure?" In turn, the client must also be given the opportunity to ask questions.

Discussion of complicated diseases is facilitated by the use of illustrated brochures or printed fact-sheets. We find that commercially produced client handouts and videotapes designed to explain and illustrate specific problems are very helpful. We also compose our own information sheets about common problems, and print the material as needed using a word processor. In addition, we distribute information sheets or brochures about common problems (heartworms, flea infestation, obesity, urolithiasis, chronic renal failure, etc.) supplied by corporations. At the time that brochures are given to clients, we direct their attention to major points in the material, highlighting information that is specifically relevant to the patient. We encourage them to read short passages of relevant information to us, and then ask them for their interpretation of the information using their own words. This technique allows us to immediately assess their understanding, and may arouse their interest, leading to additional review of the material at home. If the recommended therapy is to be prolonged, complicated, or expensive, compliance is usually enhanced if the client conceptually understands why the problems have occurred, the anticipated biological behavior, and the expectations of treatment. Our goal is to provide clients with a foundation that will help them conceptually understand the benefits of recommended therapy.

Understanding Therapeutic Benefits and Risks. After the client has a conceptual understanding of the biologic behavior of the disease, therapeutic options should be discussed. Clients are more likely to properly use medications if they understand why they are beneficial. Most forms of therapy can be classified as (1) specific, (2) supportive, (3) symptomatic, or (4) palliative. Suggestion is a powerful therapeutic tool that often influences the client's expectations about the value of each of these forms of therapy. If a veterinarian communicates optimism about the benefits of a particular mode of therapy, it will often have a more positive effect compared with a neutral suggestion about the same form of therapy. Of course, all recommendations should be based on proper ethical principles.

For most diseases, it is usually best to review "tried and true" protocols associated with well-established outcomes. The client should understand what is to be done and why, and should be asked if they are able to perform the necessary treatments. Therapeutic pros and cons, costs in terms of time and money, availability of medications, and the short-term and long-term prognoses associated with each option should be discussed. The client and the veterinarian should discuss, and when possible jointly negotiate, the type of management that best fits the client's circumstances. Better treatment outcomes can be expected if there is agreement between the veterinarian and the client about the importance of problems and methods for their management. Veterinarians must also remember that all clients do not desire the same level of patient care, a point illustrated by the familiar question "Does my client want a dog—or this dog?" The negotiated approach also facilitates a shared responsibility for therapy and minimizes unrealistic expectations by either client or veterinarian.

The client must develop a conceptual knowledge of the desired effect of each medication, how much medication to give, and when to give it. Clients must also be informed of potential side effects. Undesirable effects are often associated with less frustration if clients can anticipate them and have been taught how to deal with them (Short, 1993; Tebbi, 1993). We also predict the probable time required for expected improvement to occur, and emphasize the importance of consultation if there are significant deviations from these expectations. We reassure clients that if objective improvement does not occur within a reasonable period, treatment will be re-evaluated.

Clients often require instruction to properly administer oral and parenteral medications. The size, shape, taste, and physical form of oral medications may profoundly influence client and patient compliance. Logically, the first step is a demonstration of how we administer medications. Next, we give the client an opportunity to administer the medication under our supervision. Occasionally, owners cannot give needed medications to their pets. Solutions to this predicament include short-term hospitalization of the patient or having the owner and patient come to the hospital for help. Alternatively, we discuss whether family, friends, or neighbors can assist. If there is uncertainty about the client's physical ability to perform the desired treatment, we discuss this problem to devise a practical solution. When we view these difficulties as "our problems" rather

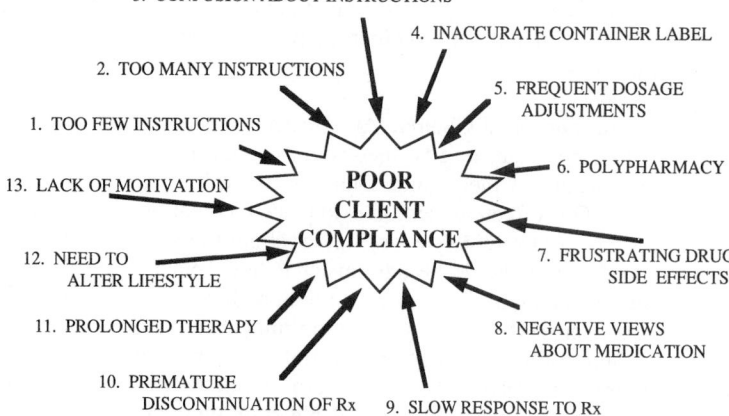

Figure 1. Factors that contribute to poor client compliance.

than "their problems," we can expect a higher rate of compliance and therapeutic benefit.

APPLYING PRINCIPLES THAT ENHANCE COMPLIANCE

Common reasons for client noncompliance and suggestions for correcting them are summarized in Figures 1 and 2. In many situations, the expectation of full compliance may be unrealistic. Less than full compliance is often acceptable to us, as long as the desired therapeutic result can safely be achieved over an appropriate time.

Recognizing Inconveniences. Studies of human patients reveal that their compliance with directions to take medications once or twice per day is significantly higher than their compliance with directions to take medications three or more times daily (Haynes, 1976; Eisen et al, 1990). Results of human studies also indicate that when medications are prescribed twice a day, the evening dose is more frequently omitted than the morning dose. If the medication schedule can be altered to accommodate the client's convenience, compliance is likely to improve. The use of slow-release drugs may also be of value. However, skipping a dose of some long-acting drugs may result in an increased interval of suboptimal blood, tissue, or urine concentrations of the drug. Therefore, the client should be educated about the importance of complying with instructions when utilizing sustained-release medications, and also should be informed about what adjustment is recommended in the event a dosing interval is missed (Waeber et al, 1994).

Disregard for the client's time can also lead to noncompliance. Long waiting times on the phone, at re-evaluation, or at the hospital pharmacy are frustrating and may contribute to noncompliance.

Encouragement When Prolonged Therapy Is Needed. While some medical problems often resolve in a week or less, others require prolonged treatment. Unfortunately, when longer periods of therapy are needed, compliance with administration of medications tends to decrease. In fact, some studies revealed that compliance decreased after only 4 or 5 days of therapy (Ellerbeck et al, 1995; Tebbi, 1993; Sackett, 1976).

When therapy must be given for longer periods, compliance is often enhanced if clients are given positive motivation at appropriate intervals. Scheduled re-evaluations and consultations typically enhance compliance. As the patient is being re-examined, we ask the client whether there have been difficulties associated with providing the needed medication. If problems have occurred, we seek the client's input about how to make adjustments. If a recheck visit is unnecessary, we have a staff member periodically call the

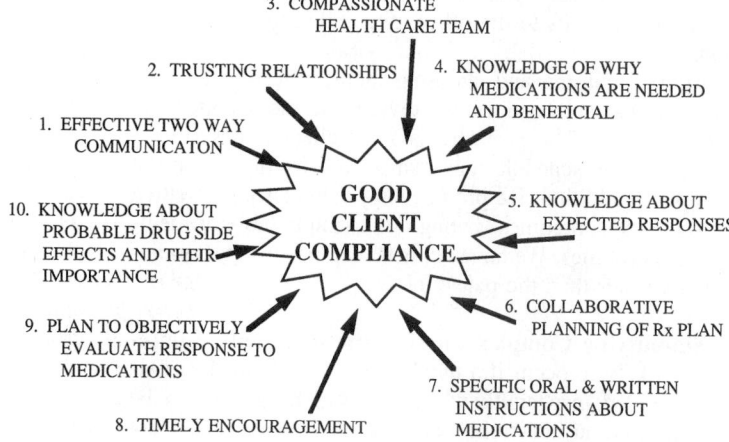

Figure 2. Factors that contribute to improved client compliance.

client to ask whether the patient is making progress as expected, and to determine whether there are problems with medications.

Reminding Forgetful Clients. An effective remedy for some clients who forget to give medications at the proper times is to customize the dosing intervals to conform to their lifestyle. One effective method is to place medications next to objects used routinely every day at about the same time the medication should be administered (e.g., placing the evening medication vial next to a toothbrush after the morning dose, or next to car keys or a morning coffee cup after the evening dose). Timely administration of medications that must be given on a long-term basis will be facilitated by the use of pill trays available from pharmacies. Once each week, the client can distribute the proper medication into each of seven daily compartments. If the patient is medicated with pills contained in the proper compartment, it is possible to quickly ascertain whether a dose has been removed or whether one has been missed. If three or more daily medications are involved, we find it easier to use trays with 28 compartments (four compartments for each day).

Understanding Misunderstandings. A significant degree of noncompliance is related to client misunderstanding of ambiguous instructions given by doctors (Elliot, 1994). Such misunderstandings often occur because different people attach different definitions or meanings to what might appear to be universally accepted terms. For example, what is your interpretation of a label that states that four capsules are to be given, divided four times per day? Are four capsules to be given every 6 hours, or is one capsule to be given every 6 hours? Is it necessary to interrupt work or sleep to adhere to a rigid 6-hour dosage interval? If medication is to be given three times per day, are the intervals to be spaced at exactly 8 hours, or can the medication also be given in the morning, afternoon, and evening? What are the advantages and disadvantages of customizing dosing regimens according to convenience compared with ideal dosage regimens based on the pharmacodynamics of the drug?

Some misunderstandings can be attributed to events that distract the client or the veterinarian. Misconceptions are especially common when a hospitalized patient is reunited with its owner before discharge instructions are discussed. It frequently occurs when young children, while accompanying their parents to the office, need attention or supervision.

After discussing and choosing therapeutic maintenance intervals that are feasible, we review the therapeutic plan with the client. Then we often ask the client to describe to us the specific schedule they plan to use to implement the therapy. In addition, we provide simple but specific written instructions, sometimes writing out a simple table of medications and times. We have learned that the strongest memory is weaker than the palest ink.

Simplifying Complex Therapeutic Regimens. Confusion is likely to occur if a number of different medications are provided, especially when different drugs are to be administered at different intervals, and when there are frequent changes in drugs or dosages. Giving drugs at multiple intervals tends to compound the problem and the likelihood of side effects. To enhance compliance, we strive to (1) use the least number of drugs; (2) select the lowest effective dosages; and (3) give the drugs the fewest number of times necessary. When several drugs must be given, we use a medication chart (Table 1). Discharge sheets incorporating the medication chart can be generated with the use of computer spreadsheets or word processors. After medications are labeled, we fill in the blanks on the chart for each medication while explaining the protocol to the client. We also add additional instructions or reminders at that time. The next appointment may be established at this time, or at the time the client pays the hospital fee.

Coping With Medication Side Effects. As veterinarians, we have a tendency to overstate the benefits and understate the risks of drugs that we prescribe. When unexplained clinical signs occur following initiation of new treatments, clients may choose not to comply with further needed treatment if they perceive that there are side effects associated with the medication (Short, 1993; Ellerbeck et al, 1995). An effective way of minimizing this problem is to list major side effects, the likelihood of their occurrence, and the recommended action should they occur. We have found it beneficial to distinguish between "nuisance" side effects and those likely to be harmful. It is best to avoid discussion of every potential side effect, as this may heighten the client's anxiety. Computer software packages can be used to generate a notation about side effects of drugs that appears on the invoice each time a specific drug is entered. The key point is that clients are more likely to be satisfied and compliant if educated about what to expect and how to proceed when the unexpected occurs.

Evaluating Apparent Cures and Apparent Nonresponses. If rapid improvement is likely, but will be sustained only if medication is continuously provided (e.g., insulin for diabetes mellius), this situation should be emphasized to the client. We also recommend that this information be provided with the written or printed notes dispensed with the drugs. If detection of a beneficial response to the medication by the client is unlikely, we advise them about how the beneficial response will be verified (e.g., repeat complete blood count [CBC], urinalysis, urine culture, blood glucose).

Making Unaffordable Care Affordable. Lack of compliance related to the high cost of drug and prescription therapy is a frustrating problem. It is essential that veterinarians understand the cost to the client of care and of medications. The more refined, or specific, the diagnosis, the greater the likelihood of choosing cost-effective medications. For example, selection of an inexpensive but effective antibiotic for long-term treatment of bacterial pyelonephritis may be possible if one can base the selection on the results of bacterial culture and antimicrobial tests. Without appropriate testing, and because of uncertainty about microbial susceptibility, the alternative may be the selection of an expensive, broad-spectrum antimicrobic.

In cases in which the preferred brand of drug is too expensive, less expensive generic forms should be consid-

TABLE 1. Therapy Chart Containing Therapeutic Recommendations for a Geriatric Cat With Moderate Chronic Polyuric Renal Failure Caused or Complicated by *Escherichia coli* Pyelonephritis

Daily Medication	6 to 9 AM	11 to 1 PM	4 to 7 PM	9 to 11 PM
Prescription Diet Feline k/d (canned)	½ can		½ can	
Calcium acetate	150 mg mixed with food		150 mg mixed with food	
Potassium citrate	200 mg oral		200 mg oral	
Enrofloxacin				12.5 mg oral
Amlodipine	3 mg oral			

ADDITIONAL THERAPY
Erythropoietin—inject 500 U under the skin twice a week.
Lactated Ringer's solution—inject 150 ml under the skin once a week.
Re-evaluation on June 6 at 10:00 AM

ered, provided that they are known to be effective. If cost considerations are a high priority, less convenient but less expensive, rapid-release drugs may be used instead of more expensive extended-release forms. These decisions can create ethical dilemmas for veterinarians. Should one prescribe the veterinary drug or the (extra-label) human preparation if the latter is significantly cheaper? Should medications be dispensed by the veterinary hospital or discount, chain-store pharmacy? These issues are complex and impact patient, client, and veterinarian.

Keeping Appointments. When the patient's progress must be monitored at the hospital, clients are more likely to return on schedule if appointments are made before they leave the hospital (Murray, 1996). One strategy is to make the appointment with the client at the time of payment of the invoice and also to include an appointment reminder with the discharge sheet. If the follow-up consists of laboratory tests on samples submitted by clients, reminders can be entered into the hospital's computer system at the time of invoicing. Most software systems can be programed to generate phone call or card reminders at the time the invoice is generated. A simple calendar and note card system can also be used to organize follow-up care.

Helping Uncooperative Patients to be Cooperative. Refusal by companion animals to cooperate with administration of medications by clients is a major reason for involuntary compliance. Clients should receive a full demonstration of how to administer medication. Such demonstration is especially important when one deals with cats (especially those with front claws) or potentially aggressive dogs. Specific devices used to prepare medication (pill cutters, droppers) or to administer treatment may need to be discussed. Clients may also be taught techniques that will help avoid future problems. For instance, some clients may not realize that some eyedrops placed directly on the cornea are painful, especially if the eye is inflamed. Natu-

rally, the animal learns to anticipate the discomfort and becomes progressively more uncooperative. In this situation, demonstrating placement of the medication in the lower cul-de-sac or on the dorsal sclera, before the patient acquires distrust, is often beneficial. In addition, a treat or some other form of reward can be provided immediately after the medication is given. Minimizing pain and offering positive reinforcement are likely to enhance cooperation.

Refusal to take oral medication is a common problem. The size, shape, taste, and physical form of oral medications may have a profound influence on client and patient compliance. Pills can be hidden in food to overcome this problem, but some pets have an uncanny ability to find the medication and eject it. To minimize this behavior, a "shell game" may be effective. Prepare about five bite-sized pieces of food that the animal is known to relish. Give one piece. After it is eaten, give another (if possible, encourage the animal to earn it by obeying a command). The goal is to reduce the pet's suspicion so that it will carelessly eat the treat. Place the tablet or capsule in the third treat to be given. After offering the third piece, immediately offer the fourth treat. Most animals will quickly swallow the third treat in order to get the fourth. Finally, give one more treat while praising the pet.

References and Suggested Reading

Eisen SA, Miller DK, Woodward RS, et al: The effect of prescribed daily dose frequency on patient medication compliance. Arch Intern Med 150:1881, 1990.

Ellerbeck E, Khallaf N, El Ansary KS, et al: Caretaker compliance with different antibiotic formulations for treatment of childhood pneumonia. J Trop Pediatr 41:103, 1995.

Elliott WJ: Compliance strategies. Curr Opin Nephrol Hypertens 3:271, 1994.

Haynes RB: A critical review of the determinants of patient compliance with therapeutic regimens. In: Sackett D, Haynes RB, eds: Compliance with therapeutic regimens. Baltimore: Hohns Hopkins Press, 1976, p 26.

Hungerbuhler P, Bovet P, Shamlaye C, et al: Compliance with medication among outpatients with uncontrolled hypertension in the Seychelles. Bull World Health Organ 73:437, 1995.

Murray MJ, LeBlanc CH: Clinic follow-up from the emergency department: Do patients show up? Ann Emerg Med 27:56, 1996.

Sackett DL: The magnitude of compliance and non-compliance. In: Sackett DL, Haynes RB, eds: Compliance with therapeutic regimens. Baltimore: Johns Hopkins Press, 1976, p 9.

Short D: The art of good prescribing. Br J Hosp Med 50:609, 1993.

Tebbi CK: Treatment compliance in childhood and adolescence. Cancer suppl 71:3441, 1993.

Waeber B, Erne P, Saxenhofer H, et al: Use of drugs with more than a twenty-four-hour duration of action. J Hypertens 12(suppl 8):S67, 1994.

Weinstein AG: Clinical management strategies to maintain drug compliance in asthmatic children. Ann Allergy Asthma Immunol 74:304, 1995.

Therapeutic Drug Monitoring

DAWN MERTON BOOTHE

College Station, Texas

The success of fixed dosing regimens (e.g., the labeled dose of a drug) is most often based on the patient's clinical response to the drug. Fixed dosing regimens are designed to generate plasma drug concentrations (PDC) within a therapeutic range, that is, to achieve the desired effect while avoiding toxicity. Recommended dosing regimens have proved most successful when based on scientific pharmacokinetic studies performed in a population of normal mature animals of the species intended to receive the drug. However, marked interindividual variability (within a species) has been confirmed for many drugs. Of greater importance is the fact that the veterinary patient receiving the drug rarely meets the above criteria. Rather, the patient usually is sick and is often being treated with more than one drug. All the factors that determine drug disposition are amenable to change in the unhealthy patient. Physiologic, pathologic, and pharmacologic factors can so profoundly alter the disposition of a drug that therapeutic failure or adverse reactions occur. Changes in drug metabolism and excretion induced by age, sex, disease, or drug interactions are important factors causing PDC to be higher or lower than expected. Sometimes, recommended dosing regimens are designed to compensate for the impact of some of these factors. Examples include many feline dosing regimens (e.g., aspirin, some selected antimicrobials) and the use of body surface area, rather than body weight, for drugs with a high potential of toxicity (e.g., anticancer drugs). Unfortunately, the factors and their impact on drug disposition often are unpredictable and cannot be anticipated or avoided in the individual patient, despite innovative dosing calculations.

If the patient's response to a drug is perceived as inappropriate owing to failure or toxicity, a trial-and-error approach generally is used for modifying the dose. Although this approach is adequate when clinical efficacy is easy to detect (e.g., anesthetics) or when the drug is very safe (e.g., most antibiotics), it is inefficient and potentially dangerous when (1) the drug response cannot be easily measured (most drugs), (2) the drug has a narrow margin of safety (e.g., digoxin), (3) or the patient's condition is life-threatening (e.g., convulsions or septicemia). Therapeutic drug monitoring (TDM) provides a guide to effective and safe drug therapy for individual patients. Monitoring can be used to determine whether plasma drug concentrations are above or below the therapeutic range, thus enhancing timely corrective measures.

INDICATIONS FOR THERAPEUTIC DRUG MONITORING

Clinical Indications

Therapeutic drug monitoring (TDM) is indicated when the expected therapeutic effect of a drug (1) has not been observed (e.g., the heart rate has not slowed sufficiently in a patient receiving digoxin; an epileptic patient on anticonvulsant therapy continues to have seizures) or (2) is difficult to observe (e.g., reduction in seizures in a patient with a long seizure interval, or correction of a hypothyroid or hyperthyroid state), or (3) if an adverse reaction (for which toxicity is due to high PDC) is suspected (e.g., a patient receiving digoxin is anorectic, or a patient receiving anticonvulsants is groggy). In addition, TDM can be used to establish whether optimum therapeutic concentrations have been achieved for drugs used to treat life-threatening diseases and when the trial-and-error approach to dose modification is unacceptable (e.g., the use of anticonvulsants in a patient prone to status epilepticus, or administration of aminoglycosides in a patient suffering from septicemia). When chronic drug administration is likely, TDM can be used to define the effective target plasma drug concentration in the patient. The target PDC can then be used if pharmacokinetics change in the patient over the course of chronic drug administration, owing to progression of disease or successful treatment of the disease, environmental changes, age-related changes, or drug interactions (e.g., phenobarbital, thyroid supplementation). Unexpected toxicity due to drug interactions can also be detected with TDM, as with enrofloxacin-induced theophylline toxicity or chloramphenicol-induced phenobarbital toxicity. Drug monitoring is also useful in identifying owner noncompliance as a cause of therapeutic failure or adverse reactions.

Characteristics of Drugs To Be Monitored

Drugs for which TDM is most useful are characterized by one or more of the following: (1) serious toxicity coupled with a poorly defined or difficult to detect clinical endpoint (e.g., anticonvulsants); (2) a steep dose-response curve for which a small increase in dose can result in a marked increase in desired or undesired response (e.g., theophylline); (3) nonlinear pharmacokinetics that may lead to rapid accumulation of drugs to toxic concentrations; (4) a narrow therapeutic range (e.g., digoxin); (5) marked interindividual pharmacokinetic variability, which increases the variability in the relationship between dose and PDC (e.g., phenobarbital); and (6) a drug whose disposition has not been determined in the species of interest (e.g., phenobarbital in a ferret). Not all drugs can be monitored by TDM, and specific criteria must be met. First, patient response to the drug must correlate with PDC. Second, drugs with active metabolites that constitute a large proportion of the desired pharmacologic response must have all active metabolites and the parent drug measured. Third, an effective drug therapeutic or toxic range must have been identified for the species and disease under treatment. Controlled clinical trials that establish therapeutic ranges for various diseases generally have not been performed in animals, and most recommended therapeutic ranges have simply been extrapolated from those used in human patients. Fourth, the pharmacokinetics of the drug must be established in a large population of animals intended to receive the drug so that normal ranges are available for the predictive pharmacokinetic parameters. Fifth, the drug must be detectable in a relatively small serum sample, and analytical methods must be available to rapidly and accurately detect the drug in plasma. The methods must be specific for the drug and must be able to differentiate it from other compounds of interest, including inactive metabolites. Sixth, the drug assay must be validated in the species of interest (or control sera containing no drug from the same species of animal should be provided with the sample containing the drug of interest). Seventh, the cost of the analytical method must be reasonable.

Drugs that meet the above criteria and for which TDM has proved useful in veterinary medicine include some anticonvulsants (phenobarbital, primidone, potassium bromide, selected benzodiazepines), antimicrobials (e.g., aminoglycosides, gentamicin, amikacin), cardioactive drugs (digoxin, procainamide, lidocaine, quinidine), and theophylline (Table 1). Although thyroid hormones are endogenous in origin, exogenous manipulation of their concentrations renders them subject to therapeutic drug monitoring.

IMPLEMENTING THERAPEUTIC DRUG MONITORING

Impact of Drug Elimination Half-life on TDM

Following the decision to monitor a drug, certain questions must be answered: Once therapy with the drug has begun, how long must one wait before monitoring the drug? Is one plasma sample sufficient, or should two samples be collected? At what time or times after the drug is administered should the sample be collected? In what should the sample be collected? The first three answers are primarily dependent on the relationship of the elimination half-life of the drug to the dosing interval. Two scenarios

illustrate the extreme situations: a drug with a long elimination half-life compared to the dosing interval, and a drug with a short elimination half-life compared to the dosing interval.

Drugs With a Long Elimination Half-Life Compared to the Dosing Interval

In general, TDM should not be performed until PDC has reached steady state in the patient. Steady-state PDC occurs at the time when drug input and drug elimination are equal. The steady state is important for drugs that accumulate with repetitive dosing because the peak PDC during the steady state is higher than concentrations following the first dose. The drug accumulates in plasma if the half-life is longer than the dosing interval. For example, in many animals phenobarbital has an elimination half-life of approximately 72 hours. If the drug is given every 12 hours, 6 doses (6 $\times$ 12 hours) will be given before 50% of the first dose has been eliminated and the drug will accumulate. Comparison of steady-state PDC with that after the first dose is referred to as the accumulation ratio. The magnitude of accumulated drug depends on how much longer its half-life is than the dosing interval. A drug whose half-life is equal to its dosing interval will accumulate two fold (i.e., at steady state, peak PDC will be twice what it was following the first dose). A drug administered at intervals equal to half the drug half-life will accumulate three fold; at one third the drug half-life, accumulation will be four fold, and so on. With multiple drug dosing, PDC will reach 50% of the steady-state concentration at one half-life, 75% by two half-lives, 87.5% at three half-lives, and so on. Thus, regardless of the drug, steady-state concentrations are attained only after four to five elimination half-lives have elapsed once fixed-dosing drug administration has begun. If any portion of the original dosing regimen (i.e., dose, frequency, or route) is changed, the same time period (i.e., four to five drug half-lives) must elapse for steady-state PDCs to be re-established. Evaluation of a drug's efficacy is often inappropriate until steady state has been reached because it is only then that maximum peak and trough drug concentrations and, thus, maximal response will have been achieved. The magnitude of peak and trough drug concentrations at steady state is also dependent on the elimination half-life. For a drug whose elimination half-life is much longer than the dosing interval, peak and trough concentrations are not likely to differ much (e.g., with a 72-hour half-life, little phenobarbital will be eliminated during a 12-hour dosing interval). Although PDC changes to some degree during the dosing interval at steady state, the peak and trough concentrations remain constant between intervals at steady state (Fig. 1).

Often, it is desirable to proactively monitor drug concentrations to ensure that safe yet effective concentrations will be reached at steady state. This monitoring is particularly important for patients experiencing seizures and that are receiving a drug with a long elimination half-life. It may be more effective to predict where concentrations will be at steady state for bromide (steady state at 2 to 3 months) to prevent seizures during that time period. In such instances, PDC can be measured at approximately one drug half-life as reported for the population. The PDC at that

TABLE 1.

Drug	Usual Dosage	Interval (hr)	Therapeutic Range	Volume of Distribution (L/kg)	Elimination Half-Life	Time to Steady State	Sample No.
Amikacin (dog)	7–20	12–24	2–25	0.25	1–2 hr	1 day	2 (plastic only)
Aspirin (dog) (cat)	10 mg/kg 10 mg/kg	8–12 72	50–100 μg/ml	0.19 0.19	8 hr 38 hr	40 hr 8 days	1
Benzodiazepines (dog)	1–2 mg/kg		100–200 ng/ml*		<8 hr	1 day	2
Digoxin (dog) (cat)	.011 mg/kg .008 mg/kg	12 12–24	0.9–3.0 ng/ml 0.9–2.0 ng/ml	19 14.5	31.3 hr 33.5 hr	7 days 7 days	1–2† (glass only)
Gentamicin (dog)	2–8 mg/kg	12–24	0.5–1.5 μg/ml t	0.3–0.4	0.9–1.3 hr	6.5 hr	1–2
Phenobarbital (dog)	2 mg/kg	12	14–45 μg/ml	0.7	32–75 hr	14–16 days	1–2‡
KBr (dog)	15–20 mg/kg	12–24	1.0–3.5 mg/ml	—	24 days	2–3 months	1
Primidone§ (dog) (cat)	11–25 mg/kg 11–20 mg/kg	12–24	Based on phenobarbital‡	0.7	6.1 hr	14–16 days	1–2
Procainamide (dog)	15 mg/kg	12		1.4–2.1	2.9 hr	15 hr	1–2
Quinidine (dog) (cat)	6–20 mg/kg Not recommended		2.5–5.0 μg/ml	2.9 2.2	5.6 hr 1.9 hr	28 hr 10 hr	1–2
Theophylline (dog)	7–11 mg/kg 4 mg/kg		10–20 μg/ml	0.82 0.46	5.7 hr 7.9 hr	29 hr 40 hr	1–2‖

p, peak; tr, trough.

*600 ng/ml listed in humans. Assay measures all benzodiazepines (parent and metabolites) relative to dosing interval. For drugs with very short half-life, trough sample may no longer have detectable drug. Wait 1 or 2 predicted elimination drug half-lives between peak and trough sample collections.

†Both peak and trough recommended for short half-life.

‡Peak and trough recommended if seizures are difficult to control.

§Based on phenobarbital concentrations.

‖For slow-release preparations, one sample may be sufficient.

time should be about 50% of steady-state concentrations. In either case, one can modify the dose early, rather than waiting for steady-state PDC. This approach might be beneficial for the evaluation of phenobarbital (half-life up to 5 days; steady state occurring at 2 to 3 weeks) and especially for bromide (half-life 24 days; steady state occurring at 2 to 3 months). A proactive approach can also be taken when steady-state PDCs must be reached immediately. A loading dose can be administered to rapidly achieve therapeutic PDC (see Fig. 1B). The loading dose needed to achieve a known therapeutic concentration of a drug depends on the volume of distribution (V_d) of that drug in the patient (Table 2) and the target concentration (see Table 1). Although a loading dose can decrease the time required for maximum response to occur, the hazards of adverse reaction to the drug are greater because the body has no time to accommodate to the drug. Thus, loading doses generally are not advised for drugs, such as digoxin, with a narrow therapeutic index. However, for safer drugs (e.g., bromide, phenobarbital), a loading dose can be administered if deemed appropriate. If a loading dose is given, maintenance doses may be too high or too low. However, the need for maintenance dose modification may not become evident until steady state occurs (i.e., three to five drug half-lives). When giving loading doses, TDM should be performed after the loading dose is complete to establish a baseline, and again one drug half-life later (e.g., for bromide at 24 to 30 days), to ensure that the maintenance dose is able to maintain the plasma concentrations achieved by loading. If the second sample (collected at one half-life) does not approximate the first (collected after loading), one can modify the maintenance dose at that

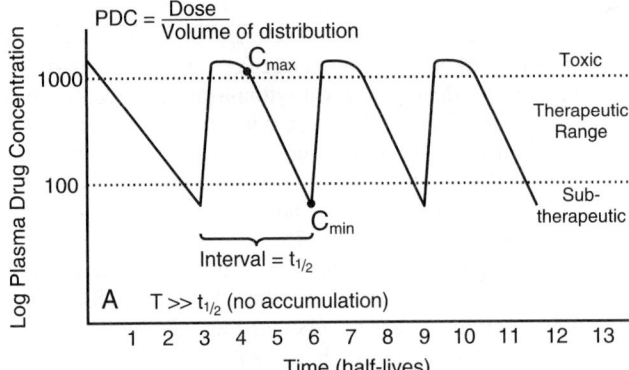

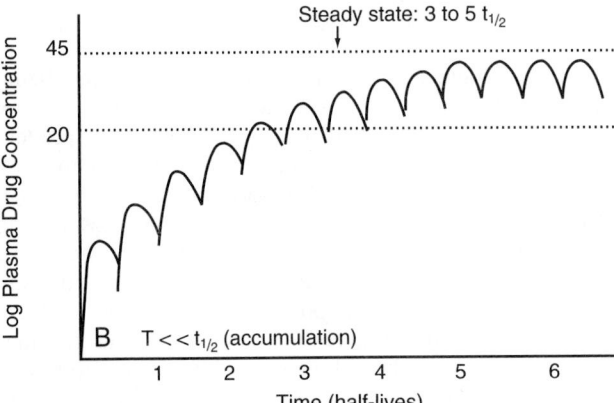

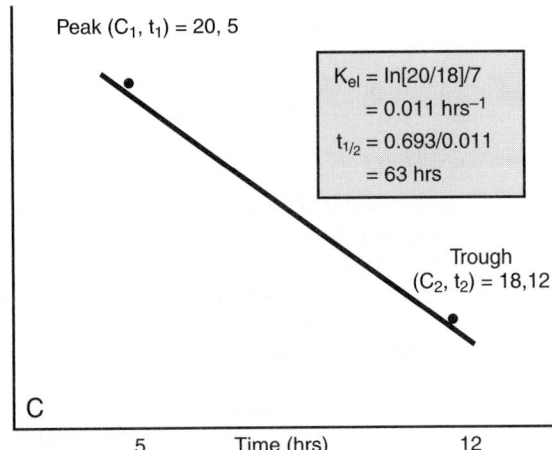

Figure 1. Plasma drug concentration–versus–time curves following multiple extravascular dosing. The therapeutic range of a drug is defined by a maximum concentration (C_{max}) above which toxicity is more likely, and a minimum concentration (C_{min}) below which therapeutic failure is more likely. The amount of accumulation determines the drug concentration at steady state. The relationship between dosing interval T and drug half-life ($t_{1/2}$) determines the amount of drug accumulation. A drug whose dosing interval is longer than its half-life *(A)* is not likely to accumulate, since most of the drug will be eliminated during a dosing interval. In contrast, a drug administered at an interval shorter than its half-life *(B)* will accumulate because most of the drug remains in the body by the next dose. Steady state occurs at five drug half-lives, when the amount of drug eliminated during a dosing interval equals the amount of the dose reaching systemic circulation. Drug half-life can be determined from peak (C_{max}) and trough (C_{min}) plasma drug concentrations *(C)*.

time, rather than waiting for steady state and the potential advent of adverse drug reactions.

Drugs With a Short Elimination Half-Life Compared to the Dosing Interval

Many drugs are characterized by half-lives that are much shorter than the dosing interval. For these drugs, little or no accumulation occurs and the concept of *steady state* is perhaps irrelevant. When the elimination half-life is shorter than the dosing interval, the response to the drug can often be evaluated with the first dose (or as soon as the disease or body has had time to respond). For example, many antimicrobials (e.g., aminoglycosides) characterized by a half-life that is less than 2 hours (e.g., amikacin in dogs) are given at a dosing interval of 8 to 12 hours. Thus, four to six drug half-lives will have elapsed and less than 5% of the dose will remain in the body by the next dose. With this dosing regimen, amikacin will not accumulate in the plasma and a steady-state equilibrium will not be reached. Therapeutic drug monitoring is useful with these drugs to ensure that therapeutic concentrations are achieved and sufficiently maintained, and to avoid toxic concentrations during each dosing interval. For drugs with short elimination half-lives, the PDC may fluctuate dramatically during a dosing interval. The magnitude of the fluctuation will be greater for drugs with shorter half-lives. A PDC may reach the toxic concentration after each dose, only to drop below the minimum effective concentration before the next dose. Increasing the dose will increase the risk of toxicity after dosing; decreasing the dose will increase the risk of therapeutic failure. In such cases, the dosing interval must be modified to minimize these fluctuations. The new dosing interval should be decided not only on the basis of drug elimination half-life but also with consideration of other drug effects. For some drugs, dosing intervals can be longer than expected, based on their elimination half-lives. For drugs (aminoglycosides and many other antibiotics) whose effects are manifested even in the absence of the drug in plasma, the interval need not be modified even if the dose drops below the therapeutic range during the dosing interval. Aminoglycosides will be undetectable in

TABLE 2. Formulas for Calculating Dosing Regimens

Elimination rate constant	$k_{el} = \ln (C_1/C_2)/(t_2 - t_1)$
Drug elimination half-life	$t_{1/2} = 0.693/k_{el}$
Maximum time that can lapse between doses	$T_{max} = \ln(C_{max}/C_{min})/K$
Amount of drug to be administered during a dosing interval	$D_{M,max} = (V_d/F)*(C_{max} - C_{min})$
Dose per unit time	$D_{M,max}/T_{max}$
Dose each interval	$\dfrac{D_{M,max} * \text{Interval}}{T_{max}}$
Loading dose	$D_L = (V_d/F)*C_{ss,max}$
Accumulation ratio	$1/(1 - [1/2]^Z)$

C_{max}, maximum PDC (peak); C_{min}, minimum PDC (trough); $C_{ss,max}$, maximum (target) PDC at steady state (mg/ml); V_d, volume of distribution (L/kg); F, bioavailability (100% if IV); Z, $T/t_{1/2}$ (interval/half-life).

normal animals if a 12-hour, or perhaps more appropriately, 24-hour dosing interval is used. However, the drugs are still effective because their postantibiotic effect allows a relatively long (and convenient) dosing interval to be used despite the short drug half-life.

For some drugs, the therapeutic drug concentration should not be monitored immediately at steady state. Drugs that target the endocrine system can be used as an example. Even though the elimination half-life of thyroid hormones is less than 12 hours in dogs and cats, the physiologic response to their effects may take several weeks. Thus, the duration of time before steady state is achieved (which includes physiologic equilibration to the hormone) is longer than five elimination half-lives of the drug.

One Versus Two Sample Collections

The number of plasma samples collected for TDM depends on the half-life of the drug and the purpose of monitoring. For most drugs, PDCs are likely to continue to fluctuate during a fixed dosing interval unless drug half-life is much longer than the dosing interval (e.g., bromide). The trough PDC, or the lowest drug concentration (C_{min}) during a dosing interval (see Fig. 1), occurs just prior to administration of the next dose and represents the maximum effects of drug elimination (i.e., metabolism and excretion) that occur between doses. The time of the peak PDC, or maximum concentration (C_{max}), after a dose is administered is less predictable than the trough concentration. Peak PDC depends on the route of administration, the rate of absorption (if not administered intravenously), and the rate of distribution into peripheral tissues. The peak concentration of interest is usually that which occurs after the drug has been distributed to the site of action. For intravenous drugs, the magnitude of C_{max} is based on the volume of distribution of the drugs; for oral drugs, its magnitude is also dependent on the rate and extent of drug absorption.

For drugs with a long elimination half-life compared with the dosing interval, peak and trough concentrations will not differ substantially during the dosing interval. For such drugs, a single sample is generally sufficient to guide drug dose modification. For the sake of consistency in sample collection across time in the same patient, the author recommends collecting a trough sample (just before the next dose), since there is no doubt about the timing (i.e., C_{min} will occur just before the next dose). Single samples might also be indicated for slow-release products (e.g., theophylline) because constant drug absorption mitigates a detectable difference between peak and trough concentrations regardless of elimination half-life. Single samples can also be collected following a loading dose (i.e., bromide), as the question to be answered is the magnitude of the PDC following loading.

The relationship between peak and trough PDCs is determined by drug elimination half-life. Drugs with a short half-life compared to the dosing interval have different peak and trough concentrations. For such drugs, both a peak and a trough sample should be collected, since a single sample collected at any time during the dosing interval provides no information regarding the other times

of the dosing interval. Thus, an advantage of collecting both peak and trough drug samples is confirmation of achievement of a minimum effective concentration (C_{min}) throughout the dosing interval without drug concentrations above the maximum (C_{max}). Collection of at least two samples during a single dosing interval is particularly important for drugs characterized by a short elimination half-life (compared to the dosing interval) and a narrow therapeutic range (e.g., digoxin). Because effective and toxic drug concentrations of these drugs are not widely separated, they are more likely to cause adverse reactions.

Often, determination of whether the half-life is short or long requires collection of both peak and trough samples. For phenobarbital, the elimination half-life may initially be much longer (e.g., greater than 48 hours) than the dosing interval. However, following several months of therapy, the half-life may be shorter (e.g., even less than 12 hours) in the same patient owing to induction of drug-metabolizing enzymes. The need for peak and trough samples may not be evident if a long half-life is anticipated. A prudent approach for patients beginning phenobarbital therapy would be to collect peak and trough samples as a baseline, but single samples for rechecks if the patient is responding to therapy. Peak and trough plasma samples should be collected from patients that are not responding to therapy in order to rule out the possibility of a short half-life and subtherapeutic drug concentrations. Digoxin provides a good example of the risk associated with collecting only a single sample. Toxicity can be confirmed by evaluating a single sample collected at the time clinical signs of toxicity occur. However, neither toxicity nor efficacy can be confirmed throughout the dosing interval, unless two samples (peak and trough) are collected. Digoxin is characterized by a half-life that ranges from less than 12 hours (for which a 12-hour dosing interval is indicated) to more than 36 hours (for which a 24-hour dosing interval may be most appropriate). The latter is more likely to occur in patients with renal disease. The elimination half-life generally becomes shorter if renal perfusion and digoxin clearance increase in response to therapy for cardiac failure.

If TDM is performed to evaluate a kinetic profile of a patient, at least two samples must be collected to establish a PDC-versus-time curve. The samples preferentially are collected at peak and trough times unless the interval is so long that the drug may not be detectable at the trough time. For example, the elimination half-life of aminoglycosides is generally about 2 hours, yet these drugs are administered at 12- or 24-hour dosing intervals. If a trough sample is collected prior to the next dose, at least six elimination half-lives will have elapsed and drug concentrations are likely to be undetectable. Because data will be available only for one time point, a kinetic profile cannot be generated (i.e., volume of distribution and elimination half-life). In such cases, the trough sample should be collected at one to two drug elimination half-lives (with the use of values reported in the literature for normal animals). The most accurate kinetic information is generated from patients receiving an intravenous dose, since the volume of distribution can be estimated (see Table 2) along with drug elimination half-life. For oral doses, only the rate of elimination and drug half-life can be obtained.

Timing of Sample Collection

If single samples are to be collected, trough samples are recommended for consistency across time. Trough samples should be collected as close to, but before giving, the next dose. Time of peak PDC is more difficult to predict because peak PDC should be determined after drug absorption and distribution are complete. The route of drug administration can influence the times at which peak PDC occurs. For orally administered drugs, absorption is slower (1 to 2 hours) and distribution is often complete by the time peak PDCs have been achieved. However, absorption rates can vary widely owing to product preparation, the effect of eating, and individual patient variability. Obviously, a drug prepared as an elixir will be absorbed more rapidly than the same drug prepared as a capsule or tablet. Because food can slow the absorption of many drugs, fasting is generally indicated (if safe) prior to therapeutic drug monitoring. Generally, peak PDC occurs 2 to 4 hours after oral administration. Some drugs (e.g., phenobarbital) are simply absorbed more slowly than others, and the time of peak PDC sample collection is longer (e.g., 2 to 5 hours for phenobarbital). For drugs administered intravenously, distribution rather than absorption is a concern. For some intramuscular and subcutaneous administrations, absorption occurs rapidly (i.e., 30 to 60 minutes), but drug distribution may take longer. Thus, PDCs generally are measured 1 to 2 hours after parenteral drug administration, regardless of the route. Exceptions occur for slowly absorbed drugs.

INTERPRETING RESULTS OF THERAPEUTIC DRUG MONITORING

Information Needed for TDM

The minimum information necessary for interpretation of PDC includes the following:

1. The total daily dose (mg/kg) of drug that will be correlated with the patient's measured PDC. The patient's PDC will then be compared to the target concentration, and the dose modified proportionately.
2. Time of drug administration and sample collection (for each dose if two samples are collected), which is particularly important for drugs with short half-lives (e.g., aminoglycosides). From these data, a drug half-life can be calculated and a proper dosing interval can be determined.
3. The patient's clinical status, because both acute and chronic diseases can dramatically alter drug disposition patterns. Such alterations are particularly marked in patients with renal, liver, or cardiac disease. If this information is lacking, disease-induced changes in drug disposition cannot be distinguished from other causes, such as noncompliance or drug interactions.
4. Knowledge of concurrently administered drugs, since they may alter drug disposition patterns and thus contribute to individual differences in drug disposition.
5. Physiologic characteristics, such as patient species, breed, and age, that may influence drug disposition or pharmacodynamic responses. For intravenous drugs, weight must be provided to determine the volume of distribution.

6. The reason for evaluating TDM (i.e., has the patient failed therapy or is the patient exhibiting signs of toxicity?).

Kinetic Calculations

At least two data points are needed to develop a pharmacokinetic profile. Generally for TDM, these consist of the peak and trough sampler (see Fig. 1) collected during a single dosing interval. For convenience, a trough sample can be collected just prior to a dose, and the peak sample collected 2 to 5 hours following dosing. This protocol is based on the assumption that the drug is handled consistently by the body during both dosing intervals. Often, the dose is not the same for both morning and evening. Regardless of when the samples are collected (assuming they are collected after absorption and distribution are complete), when plotted on semilogarithmic graph paper, the slope between these two points reflects K_{el} (see Fig. 1), which is used to determine drug half-life in the patient. Half-life can be either calculated or estimated from the PDC-versus-time curve drawn on semilogarithmic graph paper. On the plot, the two points are connected, and the resultant line is extrapolated to both the x and y axis. Elimination half-life can then be estimated by determining the time that elapses (i.e., the x axis) between any two concentrations (the y axis) as long as one concentration is twice the second. Alternatively, one can calculate the half-life from the slope of the line (rise over run), which is also the elimination rate constant ($t_{1/2} = 0.693/K_{el}$), using the two points. For the calculation, the peak = C_1,t_1 and the trough = C_2,t_2. Thus, K_{el} = natural log [ln] of the rise or [$C_1 - C_2$] over the run [$t_2 - t_1$]; $K_{el} = \ln[C_1/C_2]/t_2 - t_1$ (see Table 2).

Once the elimination half-life is determined, a proper dosing interval can be determined. The interval is based on the maximum time that can elapse between doses in the patient before PDC does fall below the recommended minimum effective concentration during the dosing interval (T_{max}) (see Table 2). The V_d of drugs administered intravenously can be calculated from the peak PDC and dose (see Table 2). From these data, a proper dose can be calculated. If the drug is 100% bioavailable following oral, subcutaneous, or intramuscular administration, V_d can also be estimated from these data. If the bioavailability of orally administered drugs is not known, a population V_d measured in normal animals must be used. However, the individual patient V_d may not be accurately estimated by population V_d. Changes in patient V_d compared to normal animals can be best interpreted if information regarding patient factors that influence V_d (e.g., obesity, edema, ascites, dehydration, serum protein concentrations) are known. The V_d is used to calculate the amount of drug that must be administered to achieve C_{max}, the target (generally maximum) effective drug concentration (loading dose D_L), and the amount of drug necessary to replace drug eliminated during the dosing interval (maintenance dose, D_{max}) (see Table 2). Once D_{max} and T_{max} have been established, dosing regimens can be appropriately altered to ensure that PDC falls within a recommended therapeutic range (see Table 2).

Not all modifications in dosing regimens require pharmacokinetic calculations. Generally, a dose can be modified with the use of the following equation, as long as concentrations were measured at steady state:

$$\text{New dose} = \text{Old dose} \times \frac{\text{Measured PDC}}{\text{Observed PDC}}$$

or

$$\text{New interval} = \text{Old interval} \times \frac{\text{Observed PDC}}{\text{Measured PDC}}$$

The decision as to whether to change the dose or the interval depends on the drug itself, its therapeutic index, and the need to maintain PDC within the therapeutic range throughout a dosing interval. Even if TDM is used to ensure that PDC remains within a therapeutic range during a dosing interval, a patient may react adversely (including failure to respond therapeutically). Recommended therapeutic ranges generally reflect the range in which a certain percentage (i.e., 95%) of patients are expected to respond. Some patients will respond at the low end of the range; some will not respond until the maximum is reached; and a smaller percentage of the population will respond at concentrations outside the recommended range. Disease, age, and other factors may play a role in the minimum effective concentration necessary for each patient. Therefore, it is imperative that PDCs be interpreted in conjunction with the desired therapeutic end point (i.e., complete eradication of seizures versus a decrease in the severity and frequency) as well as the clinical status of the patient.

WHERE IS TDM OFFERED?

Currently, TDM is being offered as an aid to rational drug therapy at several veterinary academic institutions and veterinary diagnostic laboratories throughout North America. The availability of TDM for specific drugs varies with the laboratory. In addition, TDM has received wide acceptance in the human medical field. Clinical laboratories providing TDM services to human patients may also be amenable to provision of the same services to veterinary practitioners. Some laboratories have contracts with overnight delivery services allowing sample pick up and overnight delivery to the laboratory for a reduced fee. Each laboratory should be contacted regarding its pick-up services.

Therapeutic ranges may differ between animals and people. Examples include clorazepate and bromide. Regardless of the type of laboratory (i.e., human and medical), veterinarians should use laboratories that offer a good qual-ity control program. Under such a program, assays that detect drugs have been validated in the species of interest, and controls are used daily or with each test to make sure that the assay is valid. Many veterinary laboratories use automated assays designed to measure drugs in humans. To assume that the assays will detect the drug in animals is incorrect because the constituents in plasma differ substantially between species, and these constituents can interfere with the methodology of some assays. Laboratories should be contacted prior to use to ensure that quality control procedures are followed, and that assays used in animals have been validated at concentrations commonly found in animal patients.

Attention should be given as to how the sample is handled following collection. Some drugs may require refrigeration or freezing. Sample size may vary for each drug or even for the same drug, depending on the methodology used. Drugs can interact with containers in which they are collected or mailed. In general, serum separator tubes should not be used to collect or mail samples containing drugs because drugs can bind to the silicon gel, which will decrease the concentrations measured in blood. Because aminoglycosides can bind to glass, samples should be collected and submitted in plastic tubes. The effects of hemolysis and hyperlipidemia on drug assays vary; however, it is wise to avoid either factor in sample collection. The laboratory to which the sample will be submitted should be contacted about idiosyncrasies regarding timing of sample, collection, and storage apparatus (i.e., tubes and anticoagulants) and mailing instructions (including conditions) and cost.

References and Selected Reading

Abbott Laboratories: Therapeutic Drug Monitoring, Clinical Guide. Dallas, TX: Diagnostic Division, 1984.

Atkins CE, Snyder PS, Keene BW, et al: Effects of compensated heart failure on digoxin pharmacokinetics in cats. J Am Vet Med Assoc 195:945, 1989.

Bundtzen RW, Gerber AU, Cohn DL, et al: Postantibiotic suppression of bacterial growth. Rev Infect Dis 3:28, 1981.

Drayer DE: Review problems in therapeutic drug monitoring: The dilemma of enantiomeric drugs in man. Ther Drug Monit 10:1, 1988.

Neff-Davis CA: Therapeutic drug monitoring in veterinary medicine. Vet Clin North Am Small Anim Pract 18:1287, 1988.

Pippenger CF, Massoud N: Therapeutic Drug Monitoring. In: Benet LZ, ed: Pharmacokinetic Basis for Drug Therapy. New York: Raven Press, 1984, p 367.

Price CP: Analytical techniques for therapeutic drug monitoring. Clin Biochem 17:52, 1984.

Ravis WR, Nachreiner RF, Pedersoli WM, et al: Pharmacokinetics of phenobarbital in dogs after multiple oral administration. Am J Vet Res 45:1283, 1984.

Wilson RC: Therapeutic drug monitoring. Auburn Vet 42:20, 1987.

Do's and Don'ts of Antimicrobial Therapy

DAWN MERTON BOOTHE
College Station, Texas

INTRODUCTION

The goal of antimicrobial therapy is to achieve effective concentrations of an appropriate drug at the site of infection while avoiding toxic concentrations of drug. Antimicrobial treatment of an infected patient involves several decisions (Table 1). Each decision must account for microbial, drug, and patient factors (Table 2).

Don't Use Antimicrobial Therapy Indiscriminately

A common "mistake" of antimicrobial therapy is the use of an antimicrobial in the absence of an infection. Indiscriminate use of antimicrobials is discouraged for many reasons, including the risk of superinfection, development of resistant organisms, cost, inconvenience, and increased host toxicity. The patient should be carefully evaluated to detect the source of infection. Although oral, respiratory, skin, and urinary tract infections may be identified easily, bacteremia and gastrointestinal infections are more insidious. Fever, inflammation, clinical signs or clinical pathology indicative of organ dysfunction, or structural changes indicated by radiography or other imaging techniques may support but do not conclusively prove infection. Gram-staining, cytology, and cultures can be used to document that bacteria are present, but a diagnosis of infection generally must be based on supporting data (see *CVT XII,* p. 137).

Do Target a Specific Microorganism

Selection of antimicrobial drugs, even for simple or uncomplicated infections, should be based on the antici-

pated or known identity of infectious organisms. Although a drug with a broad spectrum may be selected empirically (see *CVT XII,* p. 276), the drug should be selected for its anticipated efficacy against the presumed infecting organism. The need for more exact bacterial identification becomes important as infections become chronic, recurrent, or associated with a high risk of morbidity or mortality. The source of infection is often a useful guide for empirical selection of antimicrobial therapy, since some bacteria are more commonly found in some body systems than others. For example, genitourinary tracts are often infected with gram-negative aerobes, while abdominal infections generally are caused by gram-negative aerobes initially, then by anaerobes. Granulocytopenic or immunocompromised patients are more likely to be infected by aerobic gram-negative organisms. Bacterial pathogens often reflect the normal bacterial flora of the infected sites, as with *Escherichia coli, Pseudomonas aeruginosa, Klebsiella pneumoniae,* or *Staphylococcus aureus.* In particularly critical patients, organisms from the alimentary canal or nosocomial organisms may be involved, often with resistant patterns that require more expensive and potentially toxic drugs for effective therapy.

Properly collected tissue specimens that have been gram-stained are often of value in the selection of antimicrobial therapy. Whereas a single species of bacteria often indicates the need for antibiotic therapy, isolation of multi-

TABLE 1. Decisions To Be Made About Antimicrobial Therapy

The need for antimicrobial therapy
The source of infection and target organism
  Culture and susceptibility
  Empirical therapy
Assessment of clinical status
  Immune status
  Physiologic status
Determining host factors detrimental to drug efficacy
Selecting the antimicrobial
  Single versus combination therapy
  Drug pharmacokinetics
Determining the dosing regimen
Assessing response
  Efficacy
  Toxicity
Re-evaluating antimicrobial protocol
Discontinuing therapy

TABLE 2. General Criteria for Antimicrobial Selection

Microbial Factors
  Target organism
  Susceptibility pattern
  Bactericidal vs. static needs
  Presence of LPS covering (gram-negative bacteria)
  Aerobic vs. anaerobic
Host Factors
  Effects of disease on drug disposition
  Effects of disease on drug toxicity
  Severity of illness
  Target site
    accessibility
    environmental effects
  Immunocompetence
Drug Factors
  Mechanism:
    of action
    of toxicity
    of resistance
  Disposition characteristics
    distribution
    route of elimination
    convenience of administration
  Toxicity
  Availability
  Cost

ple species of bacteria may represent either contamination of the sample, colonizing flora, or a polymicrobial infection. The distinction between gram-negative and gram-positive bacteria is important. The lipopolysaccharide (LPS) covering gram-negative bacteria may protect them from host defenses, can act as a barrier to movement of drugs into the organism, and represents the source of endotoxin responsible for the morbidity and mortality associated with gram-negative infections. If the specific identity of bacterial pathogens is unknown, broad-spectrum or combination antimicrobials, with a low incidence of resistance and toxicity, should be selected for empirical therapy. Discriminating between aerobic and anaerobic bacteria is also important because anaerobes are inherently resistant to a number of antimicrobial drugs. In addition, an anaerobic environment may impair antimicrobial efficacy and host immune response particularly for bacteriostatic drugs.

Don't Neglect Bacterial Culture and Antimicrobial Susceptibility Data in Complicated Infections

Bacterial culture and antimicrobial susceptibility tests are especially beneficial when the infecting microorganism is resistant to the antimicrobials being used, when the dose of the drug requires modification, or when an equally effective but less expensive drug is available. Culture and susceptibility tests are particularly critical for patients recently treated with antimicrobials. Even if antimicrobial therapy is immediately initiated, culture and susceptibility data may still be critical to therapeutic success. For example, initial antimicrobial treatment of critically ill patients is changed as frequently as 35% of the time following evaluation of culture and susceptibility data.

Not only do culture and susceptibility tests identify the infecting organism or organisms, but also they provide specific data regarding drug efficacy. Two methods of bacterial culture, disc diffusion and tube dilution, are commonly used (see *CVT XII*, p. 261). Each type provides different information. The disc diffusion technique is a semiquantitative method of identifying susceptibility patterns. Drug concentrations in the agar surrounding the disc are roughly proportional to drug concentrations in the patient's serum when the drug is given at recommended (labeled) doses. However, the relative susceptibility of the bacteria to drugs cannot be determined with this method. In contrast, the tube dilution method provides quantitative data regarding the amount of drug necessary to inhibit bacterial growth. Evaluation of the ability of bacteria to grow in media containing decreasing concentrations of drug allows the minimum inhibitory concentration (MIC) of the drug to be determined (Table 3). The in vitro MIC of the drug guides selection of drugs that can reach similar concentrations in vivo and provides a basis for comparing the relative susceptibility of the organism to other drugs. Drug concentrations at the site of infection presumably must at least equal the MIC to be effective. In turn, PDCs usually must be higher to ensure adequate tissue concentrations of the drug. However, indiscriminate increases in antimicrobial doses to achieve the MIC for a particular bacterium can result in host toxicity. The "breakpoint MIC" of a drug is the highest drug concentration that can be reasonably achieved safely with the use of the clinically accepted dose and route of administration of the drug (see Table 3). Whereas the MIC is specific to the bacteria cultured and a specific drug, the breakpoint MIC is specific to the host and drug. Thus, the breakpoint MIC of a drug will be the same for any organism (see Table 3). The breakpoint for a specific organism may vary among animal species (because of differences in drug susceptibility or disposition) and laboratories. The laboratory providing culture and susceptibility data should be contacted regarding the breakpoint values used in their tests. With the use of tube dilution data, bacteria are considered susceptible (S) to the drug if the MIC is well below the breakpoint MIC. Bacterial pathogens with medium susceptibility (MS) or intermediate susceptibility (I) are inhibited by drug concentrations that approach the breakpoint MIC and may or may not cause adverse reactions in the patient. The MIC for resistant (R) bacteria will surpass the breakpoint. It is unlikely that effective concentrations of that drug against the target organism will be reached in the patient. In such cases, the risk of toxicity may also outweigh the potential benefits of therapy. The breakpoint of newer antimicrobials may be less clear with the advent of professional flexible labeling of dosage ranges.

Drugs should be selected so that the nontoxic dosing regimen will result in PDCs that sufficiently surpass the MIC. Many bacteria will be susceptible to a drug at concentrations well below the breakpoint. The difference between the breakpoint and the MIC can be used to compare relative efficacy among antimicrobials. For example, based on the breakpoint of 32 μg/ml for amikacin, an *E. coli* with an MIC of 2 μg/ml is relatively more sensitive to amikacin than is an *E. coli* with an MIC of 16 μg/ml. Both might be considered susceptible (although the latter might be given a medium susceptibility), but the former should be easier to inhibit. If the same *E. coli* with an MIC of 2 μg/ml exhibited an MIC of 16 μg/ml to amoxicillin (with a breakpoint of 32 μg/ml), presumably, the organism would be easier to inhibit with amikacin than with amoxicillin because the MIC of amikacin is further from its breakpoint MIC than is the MIC of amoxicillin from its breakpoint MIC. Although the difference of an MIC of 16 versus 32 for a particular bacterium and drug may seem quite large (particularly in the context of PDCs), it represents a difference of only one tube dilution. This observation exemplifies one of the hazards of overinterpreting susceptibility data. If the MIC of an organism is close to the breakpoint, variability in interpretation may result in an "S" or "MS" designation by one laboratory, but an "R" by another. This variability is one reason why, with one exception, drugs to which an organism is MS (or where the MIC is close to the breakpoint) should be avoided. The exception occurs if the drug can be concentrated at the site of infection well beyond the MIC measured in the in vitro test. Good examples of this situation would be the use of drugs eliminated by the kidneys to treat a urinary tract infection, or the use of drugs eliminated in the bile to treat a biliary infection. Concentration of selected drugs by white blood cells (i.e., fluorinated quinolones, macrolides) may also result in drug concentrations that markedly surpass the MIC (or breakpoint MIC) at the tissue site despite lower concentrations in plasma.

TABLE 3. Minimum Inhibitory Concentrations (MIC$_{90}$ [μg/ml]) of Selected Antimicrobials for Common Bacterial Pathogens[1]

Drug	Breakpoint	Staphylococcus aureus	E. coli	Klebsiella sp.	Proteus sp.	Serratia sp.	Pseudomonas aureus
Amikacin	≥32	2–≥64	1–2	1–2	2–4	4–16	2–64
Amoxicillin (alone) with clavulanic acid	≥32 / ≥16	4–64 / 0.25–≥16	≥8–2048 / 8–16	≥16–1024 / 8–32	≥0.5–≥128 / 1–8	≥32–512 / ≥16–256	2048 / 32–512
Ampicillin	≥32	0.125–64	8–512	≥512[2]	≥2	≥512[2]	—
Cefazolin	≥32	4–32	2–≥128	4–32	8–16	512	—
Cefotaxime	≥32	2–64	0.06–16	0.125	0.03–≤0.125	4–32	≥32–64
Cefoxitin	≥32	≥16	4	8	4	64	—
Ceftiofur	≥32						
Cephalexin	≥32	4–≥128	8–32	8–32	8–64	≥32–256	≥128–≥2048
Cephalothin	≥32	32	8	16	—	≥256	—
Chloramphenicol	≥32	8	128	512	64	512	
Ciprofloxacin	≥32	0.25–4	≥.0075–.25	.03–0.25	0.03–0.25	0.125–8	0.012–1
Clindamycin	≥32	25–≥128	—				
Doxycycline	≥32	8	64	32	32	32	32
Enrofloxacin	≥32	—	—	—	—	—	—
Gentamicin	≥32	—	0.5–16	0.05–≥16	0.5–4	8–32	1–≥32
Imipenem/cilastin	≥32	0.06–≥16	0.125–0.5	0.25–0.5	1–4	2	2–8
Kanamycin	≥32	2	16	32	8	128	
Penicillin G	≥32	0.5–32	—	—	—	—	—
Piperacillin	≥32	4–1024	1–≥1024	16–128	2–≥1024	8–256	16–512
Ticarcillin (alone) with clavulanic acid	≥32 / ≥32	–2 /	512 / 32	512 / 32	8 / 0.5	512 / 128	100–512 / 512
Tobramycin	≥32	0.25	0.5	1	0.5	32	4–6
Trimethoprim-sulfonamide	≥32						
Vancomycin	≥32	1–2	—	—	—	—	—

[1]MIC information extrapolated from human literature. MIC$_{90}$ is the MIC necessary to inhibit 90% of the organisms tested. Ranges reflect different MICs from the various reports. Data can be compared to organisms cultured from patients to order to evaluate the relative susceptibility of those organisms to organisms reported in the literature (Lorian, 1996).
[2]Klebsiella sp. or Serratia sp.
[3]Reported as MIC only.
[4]The dose of an antimicrobial necessary to achieve PDCs that are 4 to 10 times the MIC of a microbe can be calculated using the volume of distribution (V$_d$) of the drug: Dose (mg/kg) = $4 \cdot \text{MIC} \cdot V_d$. For example, for an MIC of 2 μg/ml for gentamicin and a therapeutic factor of 4, the dose would be $4 \cdot (2 \text{ mg/L}) \cdot 0.25$ L/kg, or 2 mg/kg. This assumes normal disposition of the drug in the patient.

The MIC of a bacterium may differ with subsequent infections by the same bacterium. The MIC may also change during the course of an infection. An increase in the MIC may simply represent a difference in interpretation (especially if the difference is only a tube dilution) but might also be interpreted as the development of resistance against a drug. In such instances, antimicrobial therapy could be altered by adding an additional drug or changing to a more effective drug. For polymicrobial infections, the MIC of a drug is likely to be different for each infecting bacterium. A bacterium with a lower MIC for a given drug should be easier to inhibit than an organism with a higher MIC for the same drug.

Do Localize the Site of Infection

The elimination half-life of many antimicrobials is much shorter than the dosing interval (e.g., 2-hour half-life for aminoglycosides given at 12- to 24-hour intervals). As a result, concentrations in plasma or at the site of infection may be well below the MIC, and undetectable for some portion of the dosing interval. Fortunately, this nadir in drug concentration may not impair antimicrobial efficacy. Persistence of antimicrobial effect after brief exposure to (or the lack of detectable concentrations of) an antimicrobial has been termed the postantibiotic effect (PAE). The PAE is therapeutically important for some antimicrobials against some organisms. The duration of the PAE differs among bacteria for each drug. For some bacteria, the duration of the PAE is dependent on the relationship between PDCs and MIC. For example, the PAE for aminoglycosides is maximized by a large inhibitory quotient (perhaps best defined by the ratio of PDC:MIC) and then a drug-free period (i.e., a long interval between doses). In contrast, the efficacy of many beta-lactam antimicrobial agents is enhanced by continuous drug administration or shorter dosing intervals that result in PDCs above the MIC for much of the dosing interval. The PAE can impact the dosing interval for some antimicrobials. Presumably, the dosing interval should equal the time for which PDCs are above the MIC, plus the duration of the PAE. The PAE may be absent for some drugs, some bacteria, or some patients (e.g., perhaps immunocompromised patients).

The relationship among PDC, MIC, and therapeutic efficacy (and the PAE) varies with the drug, as exemplified by comparing beta-lactam with aminoglycoside antimicrobials. Although the efficacy of aminoglycosides is dose dependent (i.e., efficacy is enhanced with maximization of the inhibitory quotient), the efficacy of beta-lactam antimicrobials is time dependent, (i.e., efficacy is enhanced if the PDC remains above the MIC for the majority of the dosing interval). Thus, using a dose that is too low is particularly detrimental with aminoglycoside therapy, but prolonging the dosing interval should be avoided for beta-lactams. The optimal relationship between PDC and MIC and the parameter that best predicts antimicrobial efficacy (e.g., peak PDC; area under the drug concentration versus time curve; duration of PDC above MIC) have not been established definitively for all antimicrobials. The efficacy of fluorinated quinolones appears to be dose related but may also be time related (see p. 41).

The relationship between MIC and PDC can also provide a basis for understanding the difference between bacteriostatic and bactericidal drugs. Organisms whose growth is merely inhibited by bacteriostatic drugs must be killed by host defenses. In contrast, organisms subjected to bactericidal drugs are killed by the drug. Patients that are immunodeficient and, in particular, granulocytopenic are dependent on bactericidal drugs for eradication of infection. Effective treatment of infections in immunocompromised patients is also dependent on bactericidal antimicrobial activity, as may occur with septicemia, meningitis, valvular endocarditis, and osteomyelitis. For a bactericidal drug, the MIC is very close to the concentration necessary to kill the organism. However, the distinction between a bactericidal and a bacteriostatic drug depends on the concentration to which bacteria are exposed. A bactericidal drug can be easily rendered nonbactericidal if concentrations sufficient to kill the bacteria are not reached at the site of infection. In contrast, when drugs are concentrated in tissues (e.g.,

urinary tract and prostate gland), even a static drug might become bactericidal in selected instances.

Consideration must be given to factors that reduce concentrations of active drug at the site of infection. In general, the target PDC of a drug is the MIC of the drug multiplied by a "therapeutic factor" of 4 to 10. Higher factors should be used for especially virulent organisms, immunocompromised patients, serious infections, or infections associated with host factors that preclude penetration of or efficacy at the site of infection. Higher factors should also be used for infections in tissues that are normally difficult to penetrate (i.e., the ratio of drug in tissues compared to that in plasma is less than 0.75). In general, the MIC times the therapeutic factor should result in a PDC below the breakpoint MIC for that bacterium to avoid drug toxicity. Thus, the closer the MIC of a bacterium is to the breakpoint MIC for the drug, the narrower is the margin of error. As MICs approach breakpoints, the recommended dose of a drug must be increased to maintain a therapeutic factor. Fortunately, most antimicrobial drugs are sufficiently safe that doses can be increased to levels beyond the breakpoint (i.e., beyond the labeled dose) for infections caused by organisms with high MICs.

Therapeutic failure may occur despite the achievement of targeted PDC if host factors decrease the concentration of active drug at the infection site. Changes in the patient can lead to changes in drug disposition, resulting in lower than anticipated PDCs. The volume to which drugs are distributed is affected by fluid compartments that vary with age, species, and hydration status. Distribution to target organs can be affected profoundly by cardiovascular responses, particularly as a result of shock or retention of salt and water (i.e., edema). Factors that affect elimination of antimicrobials must be considered when one treats critical patients. Changes in glomerular filtration cause parallel changes in renal excretion of drugs. In patients with renal dysfunction, serum creatinine concentrations should be used to reduce doses, or to prolong the dosing intervals of potentially toxic drugs. Likewise, severe changes in hepatic function may indicate selection of antimicrobial drugs that are not dependent on hepatic function for activation or excretion.

Other host factors may also alter drug efficacy at sites of infection. Deposition of fibrous tissue at the infected site reduces drug penetration. The microenvironment can profoundly impair antimicrobial activity (Table 4). For example, purulent exudate, which is typically acidic, hyperosmolar, and hypoxic, impairs the efficacy of many antimicrobials. The hypoxic environment may also impair host phagocytic defenses. Hemoglobin and products of inflammation can bind antimicrobials. Some antimicrobials inhibit neutrophil function. Antimicrobials can also be impaired by host factors that alter the mechanism of action of the drug. For example, beta-lactam antimicrobial agents become less effective in a hypertonic environment, might be found in the renal medullary interstitium or in inflammatory debris.

Not all host factors negatively impact antimicrobial efficacy. For example, leukocytes at the site of inflammation may actively concentrate some antimicrobials (including macrolides, lincosamides, and fluorinated quinolones) more than 20 times that of the plasma or surrounding fluids.

TABLE 4. Effects of the Microenvironment on Antimicrobial Efficacy

Factor	Effect
Acidic pH	Penicillins inactivated at pH <6.0
	Aminoglycosides and enrofloxacin more effective in alkaline pH
Hypertonicity, hyperosmolarity	Impaired efficacy of beta-lactam antibiotics
Pus	Acidic pH
	Hypertonic
	Hyperosmolar
	Protein binding of selected drugs
	Binding to sediment (aminoglycosides)
Low O₂ tension	Aminoglycosides inactive
	Growth of organisms slowed → decreased efficacy of bactericidal drugs
	Impaired phagocytic activity of leukocytes
Large inoculum	Greater concentration of antimicrobial inactivating enzymes
	Greater concentration of drug molecules required
Leukocyte effects	Impaired chemotaxis, phagocytosis, metabolism

Thus, drugs that achieve only bacteriostatic concentrations in plasma may become bactericidal inside cells and particularly against intracellular pathogens, unless the drug is sequestered in subcellular organelles.

Don't Neglect Differences in Drug Distribution as the Antimicrobial Is Selected

Most antimicrobials become well distributed in extracellular fluids. Notable exceptions are the brain, prostate, and eye. Water-soluble drugs (whose volume of distribution is generally less than 0.3 L/kg) tend to distribute only in extracellular fluid; whereas lipid-soluble drugs (whose volume of distribution is generally equal to or greater than 0.6 L/kg) penetrate lipid membranes and are thus more likely to distribute throughout total body water. The male genitourinary tract offers two extremes in this regard. Urine is an easy target as long as the drug is eliminated in the urine in an active form. However, the kidney and prostate are more difficult to penetrate. Lipid-soluble antimicrobials should be used for infections of the tissues as well as infections associated with marked tissue reaction or by intracellular organisms. The distribution of aminoglycosides and most beta-lactam antimicrobials is limited to the extracellular fluid. In contrast, fluorinated quinolones and trimethoprim-sulfonamide combinations are distributed to all body tissues, including prostate and eye. The blood-brain barrier represents a particularly challenging site for drug distribution, since it prevents movement of antimicrobials into the central nervous system and also actively removes or destroys some drugs (some cephalosporins). Imipenem, trimethoprim-sulfonamide combinations, and fluorinated quinolones can achieve bactericidal concentrations against some central nervous system infections, while chloramphenicol may achieve bacteriostatic concentrations against

others. Drug movement into bacteria must also be considered. Gram-negative organisms are protected beneath several layers of structures in cell walls. Proteins embedded in the outermost membrane—known as porins or outer membrane proteins—form channels through which small molecules (including drugs) can penetrate. Lipid-soluble drugs are generally able to passively diffuse to varying degrees through cell walls, but water-soluble drugs (e.g., beta-lactams and aminoglycosides) predominantly pass these microbes through porins. The variable size of porins help contribute to the differences in antimicrobial drug resistance. For example, *Pseudomonas* spp. have very small porins, which exclude penetration of many drugs.

Finally, drug binding to proteins can be an issue. Protein-bound drugs are not distributed into tissues, and once at the site of infection these drugs can again become bound to inflammatory proteins.

Do Avoid Antimicrobial Resistance

Bacterial resistance to antimicrobials is a common cause of therapeutic failure. The ability of bacteria to develop resistance to antimicrobial agents varies with the species and strain. Resistance may be inherent or acquired. The lack of efficacy of aminoglycosides against anaerobic organisms occurs because the drugs must be actively transported into the cell (an oxygen-dependent process). Acquired resistance often occurs during the course of therapy and can be caused by a chance mutation or the transfer of genetic material between organisms, usually via plasmids. Mutational resistance typically develops slowly and often is accompanied by other changes that render the organism less viable and thus more likely to be destroyed by other drugs. Plasmid-mediated resistance, on the other hand, is of great clinical significance. Plasmid-mediated resistance in gram-negative bacteria is common, can develop rapidly, and can be transmitted between species. A single transfer of plasmid genetic material can result in antimicrobial resistance against as many as seven antimicrobials.

The mechanisms of bacterial resistance vary and may involve the following: (1) changes in cell wall structures, proteins (i.e., penicillin-binding proteins), or enzymes; (2) development of enzymes that destroy antimicrobials (i.e., (beta-lactamases destroy penicillins); or (3) changes in intracellular transport proteins (tetracyclines), metabolic pathways (sulfonamides), or binding sites (i.e., on ribosomes as for aminoglycosides) for antibiotics. Bacteria often respond to the antimicrobial agent through one or more of these mechanisms. The recent recognition of decreased efficacy of antimicrobial agents that have traditionally been very effective for the treatment of bacterial infections underscores the significance of antimicrobial resistance. Plasmid-mediated resistance is of particular concern because of its rapid onset and potential for transmission among species of microbes.

Proper procedures should be followed to minimize antimicrobial resistance for the benefit of the patient, hospital, and community. Even if an antimicrobial (e.g., enrofloxacin) has a low incidence of plasmid-mediated resistance, resistance may develop over several decades. Whether antimicrobials have been recently used in the patient should be considered. Development of infection, during recent or ongoing antimicrobial therapy, suggests that the infecting organism is resistant to the antibiotics being given. Previous antimicrobial therapy can change the resistance pattern of a group of organisms to a number of drugs, even if the drugs have not been previously administered. Basing drug selection on bacterial culture and antimicrobial susceptibility information is probably the best method for reducing the risk of resistance. However, secondary resistance can also occur during antimicrobial therapy; subsequent bacterial culture and antimicrobial susceptibility can help detect resistance in patients receiving long-term antibiotic therapy. In complicated infections, clinicians should take advantage of manipulations by pharmaceutical manufacturers designed to minimize resistance. For example, bacterial resistance to antimicrobial agents has been decreased by (1) synthesizing smaller molecules that can penetrate smaller porins (e.g., the extended spectrum penicillins, ticarcillin, and piperacillin); (2) "protecting" the antibiotic from beta-lactamases (e.g., addition of clavulanic acid); (3) modifying the compound so that it is more difficult to destroy by bacterial enzymes (e.g., amikacin, which is larger than gentamicin); and (4) development of lipid-soluble compounds better able to achieve effective concentrations in various tissues (e.g., doxycycline compared to other tetracyclines).

Ensuring that adequate drug concentrations are present at the site of infection is probably the single most important action in reducing the incidence of resistance. Development of bacterial resistance to antimicrobials can be minimized in critical or chronic situations by ensuring that organisms are exposed to maximum drug concentrations for a sufficient period. Therefore, intravenous administration should be considered in life-threatening conditions or prophylactic therapy, or for treatment of tissues that are difficult for antimicrobials to penetrate. Doses should be maximized and based on MIC or therapeutic drug monitoring whenever possible, and the proper dosing interval should be used. Patient factors should be considered when one designs the dosing regimen. Drugs inherently more resistant to bacterial inactivation should be selected (i.e., amikacin rather than gentamicin). Combination antimicrobial therapy (e.g., beta-lactamase protected antimicrobial combinations; combination of beta-lactams with aminoglycosides) can also be expected to reduce the incidence of antimicrobial resistance.

Don't Harm the Patient

Because host cells are eukaryotic, while the targets of most antibiotics are prokaryotic bacterial cells, the toxicity of antibiotics frequently is not related to their mechanisms of antimicrobial action. In general, antimicrobials tend to be very safe drugs; however, notable problems include immune-mediated diseases associated with trimethoprim-sulfonamide combinations, cartilage defects in large-breed growing dogs receiving enrofloxacin, and nephrotoxicity induced by aminoglycosides (which can be largely avoided with once-daily therapy). Also, drugs that target cell membranes (colistin, polymixin B) are so nephrotoxic that they can only be administered topically. Endotoxin release following antimicrobial therapy may result in toxicity. Release of endotoxin may influence antimicrobial selection in the patient infected with large numbers of gram-negative organisms. Endotoxins initiate the release of cytokines and other mediators of septic shock (see *CVT XII,* pp. 139 and 547). Among the drugs traditionally used to treat septicemia, aminoglycoside therapy has been associated with the least endotoxin release, whereas beta-lactams (with the notable exception of imipenem) have been associated with the greatest release. Quinolones are associated with release of variable amounts of endotoxin.

Don't Indiscriminately Extrapolate Drug Dosing Regimens But Modify the Dose and Route When Indicated

Adequate concentrations of drug at sites of infection are obviously required for effective therapy. Dosing recommendations printed on product labels are based on studies of healthy members of the target species. The use of a nonscientifically based dose of a drug approved in one species in an unhealthy member of another species may result in therapeutic failure, resistance, or toxicity. Drugs approved for use in human patients should be evaluated before they are used in infected animals.

Antimicrobial therapy must be implemented in a timely fashion. A dose of antimicrobials administered at the first appearance of a clinical infection will have a much greater therapeutic effect. Although label dosing recommendations should be followed, exceptions have become recognized. Product labels may not reflect new findings regarding antimicrobial efficacy. Modifications beyond label dosage should be based on current literature and logic. Therapeutic drug monitoring (see p. 26) can be used to establish a drug dose or maintenance interval in individual patients and is the optimum basis for dose modification in critical patients. Unfortunately, few drugs can be rapidly and accurately measured at a reasonable cost. If sufficient knowledge is known about the antimicrobial, the dose can be calculated from MIC data (dose is equal to MIC times a therapeutic factor of 4 to 10 times the volume of distribution). Alternatively, if the volume of distribution of the drug is unknown, the labeled dose of an antimicrobial can be increased based on the magnitude of separation of the MIC from the breakpoint MIC, and the likelihood that drug will reach the site of infection. Doubling the dose is indicated for drugs whose efficacy is determined primarily on the basis of the ratio of MIC to PDC (e.g., fluorinated quinolones, aminoglycosides, metronidazole); decreasing the interval is indicated for drugs whose efficacy depends on PDC surpassing the MIC during most of the interval (e.g., beta-lactam and "bacteriostatic" antibiotics). Parenteral, and particularly intravenous administration, are indicated for life-threatening infections or any time tissue concentrations need to be maximized.

Don't Combine Antimicrobials Indiscriminately

The indications for combination therapy include the following: (1) achieving a broad antimicrobial spectrum for empirical therapy; (2) treatment of a polymicrobial infection involving organisms not susceptible to the same drugs; (3) reducing the likelihood of antimicrobial resistance; and (4) reducing the risk of adverse drug reactions by minimizing doses of potentially toxic antimicrobials. The rational use of combinations of antimicrobials is often an effective method of enhancing antimicrobial efficacy in critically ill patients. The primary reasons for avoiding combination therapy include increased risk of suprainfections, risk of toxicity if both drugs are potentially toxic, cost, and inconvenience. Combinations of antimicrobials should be selected on the basis of target organisms as well as mechanisms of action (Fig. 1).

Antimicrobial combinations may result in either antagonistic, additive, or synergistic antimicrobial effects. Antimicrobic *antagonism* must be avoided, particularly in patients with impaired host defenses. In general, drugs that inhibit ribosomes and thus microbial growth (e.g., chloramphenicol, tetracyclines, and erythromycin) should not be combined with drugs whose mechanism of action is dependent on protein synthesis and growth of the organism (i.e., beta-lactams) or formation of a target protein (e.g., fluorinated quinolones). Antagonism between beta-lactams and bacteriostatic ribosomal inhibitors has been well documented. Antagonism between ribosomal inhibitors and fluorinated quinolones is less clear, although antagonism of chloramphenicol with ciprofloxacin has been documented. Chemical antagonism between two or more antimicrobials is also possible. Aminoglycosides are chemically inactivated by sufficient concentrations of penicillins. However, chemical antagonism between these agents is an unlikely event in most clinical settings. An exception would be simultaneous intravenous use of high doses of both drugs. In general, drugs that have the same mechanism of action have additive actions. Additive effects are also likely when active metabolites are produced from an active parent compound, such as metabolism of enrofloxacin to ciprofloxacin. However, antagonistic effects might occur if the drugs compete for a limited number of target sites (i.e., chloramphenicol

and erythromycin). Synergism between antimicrobials is most likely to occur if two antimicrobial agents kill bacteria by independent mechanisms or by acting in sequence to interrupt a metabolic pathway. Combinations of trimethoprim and a sulfonamide or amoxicillin and clavulanic acid exemplify synergism due to sequential inhibition of pathways. Synergism between beta-lactams and aminoglycosides exemplifies synergism due to killing by independent pathways. Not only do their mechanisms of action complement one another, but also efficacy is enhanced because aminoglycoside movement into bacteria is enhanced by beta-lactam–induced increases in cell wall permeability. Other synergistic combinations include beta-lactams with fluorinated quinolones; this combination may render a *Pseudomonas* sp. that was not susceptible to the fluorinated quinolone as susceptible. Aminoglycosides act synergistically with potentiated sulfonamide combinations against *Nocardia* and *Actinomyces* sp. Beta-lactams and, specifically, penicillins also act synergistically against *Nocardia* and *Actinomyces*.

Combination antimicrobial therapy may be selected because of a polymicrobial infection. Aminoglycosides or fluorinated quinolones are often combined with beta-lactams, metronidazole, or clindamycin to target both aerobic gram-positive and gram-negative infections, or infections caused by both aerobes and anaerobes.

Don't Treat When the Intent Is To Prevent

The use of antibiotics for treatment must be distinguished from their use for prevention. Bacterial infection, or anticipated infection, following bacterial contamination (i.e., a compound fracture; contamination of abdominal contents with intestinal fluid) indicates the need for antimicrobial treatment, rather than antimicrobial prophylaxis. If antimicrobial *prophylaxis* is to be implemented in association with an invasive procedure (i.e., surgery), the follow-

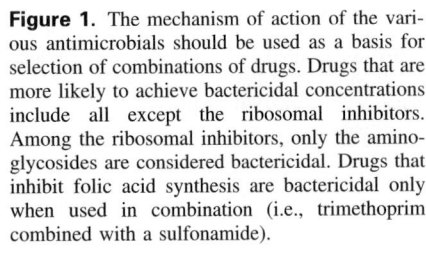

Figure 1. The mechanism of action of the various antimicrobials should be used as a basis for selection of combinations of drugs. Drugs that are more likely to achieve bactericidal concentrations include all except the ribosomal inhibitors. Among the ribosomal inhibitors, only the aminoglycosides are considered bactericidal. Drugs that inhibit folic acid synthesis are bactericidal only when used in combination (i.e., trimethoprim combined with a sulfonamide).

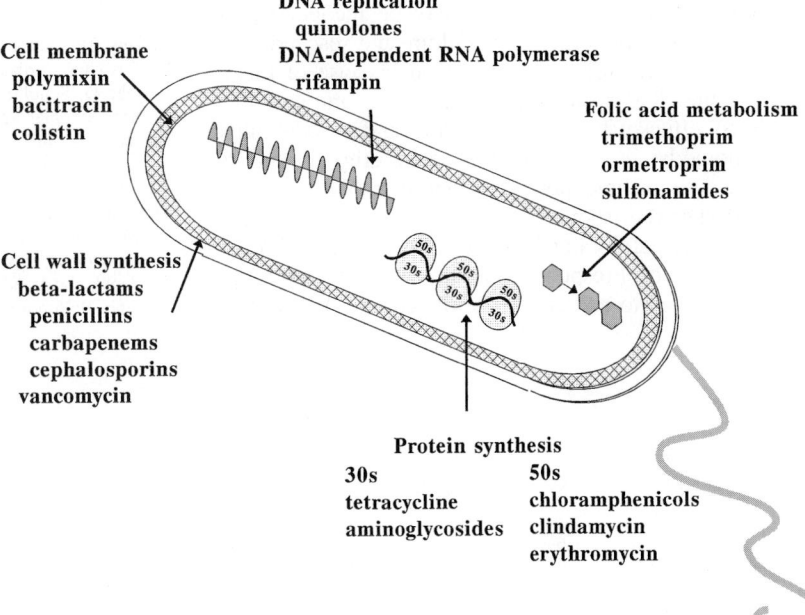

ing should serve as a basis for selection: (1) the antimicrobial should target the most likely pathogenic organism (i.e., *Staphylococcus* or gram-negative coliforms for many surgical procedures, or anaerobes for dental procedures); (2) adequate concentrations of drug should be at the site of invasion prior to potential contamination; (3) the antimicrobial should either have a long elimination half-life or should be redosed during lengthy procedures; (4) the least toxic drug should be selected; and (5) the duration of therapy should be as short as possible. Generally, a single dose should be given so that peak tissue drug concentrations occur at the time of bacterial exposure. For surgical cases, a second dose might be given intraoperatively or postoperatively. For dental prophylaxis, several doses might be given prior to the dental procedure to decrease the bacterial load in the oral cavity.

Don't Risk Inappropriate Therapy in the Interest of Cost or Convenience

Convenience of administration for outpatient therapy may profoundly alter drug efficacy simply because of owner compliance. A drug that can be given twice daily is more likely to be effective than a drug given every 8 hours. The cost of antimicrobials certainly has an impact on antibiotic selection but should be considered only after other factors have been considered. The cost of an excellent but expensive antimicrobial can be easily surpassed by the selection and use of several cheaper, but less effective antimicrobials.

Evidence of improvement in clinical status is expected 48 to 72 hours following the start of antimicrobial therapy. Although fever and leukocytosis have been hallmarks indicating the need for antimicrobial therapy, there are noninfectious causes of inflammation and fever. In addition, leukocytosis may be absent in the immune-compromised patient. Therapeutic failure may be associated with inappropriate antimicrobial use or selection, improper dose or maintenance interval, or a number of host factors. The first two causes of therapeutic failure may be recognized by therapeutic drug monitoring or by culture and susceptibility tests. When antimicrobials are changed because of therapeutic failure, the cheapest and least toxic antimicrobial that shows efficacy by in vitro culture and susceptibility results should be chosen as long as active drug is likely to reach the site of infection. The antimicrobial with the narrowest spectrum should also be used to minimize suppression of normal flora and the risk of antimicrobial resistance. An equivocal response to antimicrobial therapy may indicate the need to add another antimicrobial to eradicate potentially resistant organisms. Therapy should be given for a sufficient period to allow complete resolution of infection, yet the duration should be short enough to avoid toxicity, development of resistance, and suprainfection. The duration of antimicrobial therapy often varies with the severity of illness; 10 to 14 days is generally recommended for granulocytopenic, septicemic, or seriously ill patients, whereas 7 to 10 days of therapy may be sufficient in patients with less severe infections. Febrile patients should be treated until they have been afebrile for 4 to 5 days.

References and Suggested Reading

Acar JR, Goldstein FW: Disk susceptibility testing. In: Lorian V, ed: Antibiotics in Laboratory Medicine. Baltimore: Williams & Wilkins, 1991, p 17.

Amsterdam D: Susceptibility testing of antimicrobials in liquid media. In: Lorian V, ed: Antibiotics in Laboratory Medicine. Baltimore: Williams & Wilkins, 1991, p 53.

Bergan T: Pharmacokinetics of tissue penetration of antibiotics. Rev Infect Dis 3:45, 1981.

Blaser J: Efficacy of once- and thrice-daily dosing of aminoglycosides in in-vitro models of infection. J Antimicrob Chemother 27(Suppl C):21, 1991.

Boothe DM: Principles of pharmacology for the practicing veterinarian. In: Current Veterinary Therapy XII, Small Animal Practice. Philadelphia: WB Saunders, 1995, p 339.

Brown SA: Minimum inhibitory concentrations and postantimicrobial effects as factors in dosage of antimicrobial drugs. J Am Vet Med Assoc 191:871, 1987.

Brumbaugh G: Antimicrobial susceptibility and therapy: Concepts and controversies. Parts I and II. Proc Am Coll Vet Intern Med 8:525, 1990.

Craig WA, Gudmundsson S: Postantibiotic effect. In: Lorian V, ed: Antibiotics in Laboratory Medicine. Baltimore: Williams & Wilkins, 1996, p 403.

Eliopoulos GM, Moellering RC: Antimicrobial combinations. In: Lorian V, ed: Antibiotics in Laboratory Medicine. Baltimore: Williams & Wilkins, 1991, p 432.

LeFrock JL, Prince RA, Richards ML: Penetration of antimicrobials into the cerebrospinal fluid and brain. In: Ristuccia AM, Cuhna BA, eds: Antimicrobial Therapy. New York: Raven Press, 1984, p 397.

Lesar TS, Zaske DE: Modifying dosage regimens in renal and hepatic failure. In: Ristuccia AM, ed: Antimicrobial Therapy. New York: Raven Press, 1984, p 95.

Lorian V, ed: Antibiotics in Laboratory Medicine. Baltimore: Williams & Wilkins, 1996.

Murray BE: Problems and mechanisms of antimicrobial resistance. Infect Dis Clin North Am 3:423, 1989.

Nitsche D, Schulze C, Oesser S, et al: The effects of different types of antimicrobial agents on plasma endotoxin activity in Gram-negative bacterial infections. In: Garrard C, ed: Ciprofloxacin I.V.: Defining Its Role in Serious Infections. International Symposium, Salzburg, September 1993. Berlin: Springer-Verlag, 1994, pp 21–38.

Tomasz A: Multiple antibiotic resistant pathogenic bacteria. N Engl J Med 330:1247, 1994.

Wiedemann B, Atkinson BA: Susceptibility to antibiotics: Species incidence and trends. In: Lorian V, ed: Antibiotics in Laboratory Medicine. Baltimore: Williams & Wilkins, 1991, p 962.

Fluorinated Quinolones: Use and Misuses

DAWN MERTON BOOTHE

College Station, Texas

Fluorinated quinolones are a relatively new class of minimally toxic synthetic antimicrobials effective against gram-negative and selected gram-positive organisms. Drugs of this class used in veterinary medicine in the United States include the veterinary products enrofloxacin, difloxacin, and orbifloxacin and the human products ciprofloxacin and norfloxacin. Other fluorinated quinolones are under evaluation for use in people or animals. Included in this group are danofloxacin and marbofloxacin, intended for use in animals, and sparfloxacin, for use in human patients. The primary focus of this article is the approved veterinary fluorinated quinolone products in the United States. Enrofloxacin will serve as the prototypic veterinary fluorinated quinolone product. However, much of the discussion applies to fluorinated quinolones as a class of drugs.

CLINICAL PHARMACOLOGY

Structure-Activity Relationship

Nalidixic acid is the progenitor of the fluorinated 4-quinolones. The addition of the fluorine atom and other synthetic changes in nalidixic acid resulted in a broader antibacterial spectrum, better tissue distribution, and fewer side effects. All the fluorinated quinolones contain a carboxylic acid group that is necessary for antibacterial action, the fluorine atom, and many also contain a piperazine ring. Much of the information regarding enrofloxacin has been extrapolated from studies of the human drug ciprofloxacin. The two compounds are very similar in structure, as enrofloxacin is an ethylated version of ciprofloxacin, and their spectrum of antimicrobial activity and tissue distribution are similar. In addition, since enrofloxacin is at least partially metabolized to ciprofloxacin in many species, information about ciprofloxacin is pertinent to enrofloxacin. Less information is available about orbifloxacin and difloxacin. They are approved strictly for animal use; thus, the reliability of information extrapolated from other fluorinated quinolones as it pertains to orbifloxacin is less clear.

Mechanism of Action

Fluorinated quinolones inhibit DNA gyrase (DNA topoisomerase), a topoisomerase enzyme responsible for supercoiling of DNA during bacterial division (Fig. 1). Bacterial DNA must separate prior to replication, but separation is preceded by an excessive (positive) supercoiling of DNA. Bacterial DNA gyrase, an ATP-dependent enzyme, causes negative supercoils in DNA and supports the separated strands of DNA as each strand passes through the break and then is resealed. Bacterial DNA gyrase is composed of two alpha and two beta subunits. The alpha subunits carry out the strand-cutting function, whereas the beta subunits cause the ATP hydrolysis necessary for gyrase supercoiling. The actions of alpha subunits, the target of quinolone antimicrobials, are inhibited by concentrations of enrofloxacin of 0.1 to 10 μg/ml.

The concentration of enrofloxacin (and ciprofloxacin) necessary for inhibition of the growth of susceptible organisms (i.e., the minimum inhibitory concentration, or MIC) is very close to the concentration necessary to kill the organisms (the minimum bactericidal concentration). The unique mechanism of antimicrobial action of the fluorinated quinolones results in rapid bactericidal activity, with minimal detrimental effects to the patient. Eukaryote cells do not contain DNA gyrase, although they do contain type II DNA topoisomerase. However, the affinity of eukaryote topoisomerases for fluorinated quinolones is less than 0.001 that of bacterial DNA gyrase.

Spectrum of Activity

The spectrum of activity of the fluorinated quinolones as a class might be considered broad; however, the term does not apply universally to all members of the class. For example, although the spectrum of activity of enrofloxacin against gram-negative organisms is broad, its activity against gram-positive bacteria is less so, and enrofloxacin is not effective against anaerobic organisms. Gram-positive organisms predictably susceptible to enrofloxacin include *Staphylococcus* sp. and some species of *Corynebacterium*. Most gram-negative organisms are susceptible to enrofloxacin. Common bacterial pathogens in small animals particularly susceptible to enrofloxacin include *Escherichia coli, Klebsiella* sp., *Enterobacter cloacae, Proteus mirabilis, Citrobacter freundii, Serratia marcescens*, and *Pseudomonas aeruginosa*. Various species of *Salmonella, Shigella*, and *Campylobacter* are also susceptible. Other susceptible organisms include *Yersinia*. Enrofloxacin has variable efficacy against *Streptococcus* spp. and *Enterococcus faecalis*. (The concentration of antibiotic at which 90% of all bacterial isolates investigated showed inhibition of growth.) The MIC_{90} of enrofloxacin for most susceptible gram-negative organisms is 0.25 μg/ml or less. An exception is *P. aeruginosa*, whose MIC often approaches the breakpoint MIC of enrofloxacin (i.e., 1 μg/ml; Table 1). For example, in one study, the MIC of 97% of isolates of *Staphylococcus intermedius* was reported as 0.25μg/ml or less (Stegemann et al, 1996). For enrofloxacin, organisms with an MIC of as much as 2 μg/ml are considered susceptible to enrofloxacin, whereas organisms with an MIC of more than 4 μg/ml are considered resistant. However, this is based on a dose of 2.5 mg/kg (oral).

Veterinarians who submit samples for culture and susceptibility testing to human laboratories are likely to re-

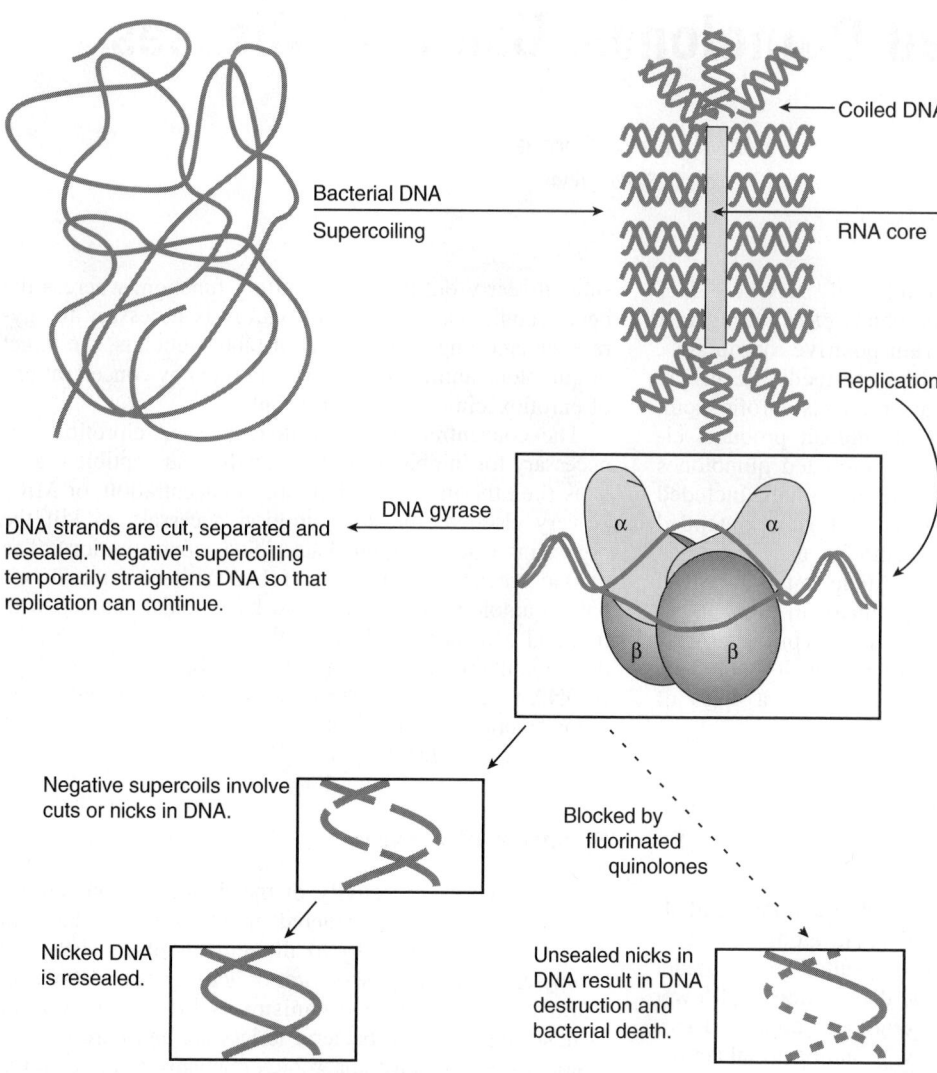

Coiled DNA

Bacterial DNA
Supercoiling

RNA core

Replication

Figure 1. The fluorinated quinolones act by impairing DNA supercoiling during bacterial replication. The alpha subunit of the enzyme is the target of fluorinated quinolone activity.

DNA strands are cut, separated and resealed. "Negative" supercoiling temporarily straightens DNA so that replication can continue.

DNA gyrase

Negative supercoils involve cuts or nicks in DNA.

Blocked by fluorinated quinolones

Nicked DNA is resealed.

Unsealed nicks in DNA result in DNA destruction and bacterial death.

ceive data regarding ciprofloxacin, rather than enrofloxacin. The spectrum of activity of ciprofloxacin is similar to that of enrofloxacin. The breakpoint MIC for ciprofloxacin is ≤ 2 μg/ml for susceptible bacteria; bacteria with an MIC of 8 μg/ml or more are considered resistant to ciprofloxa-

cin. For norfloxacin, susceptibility data apply only to bacteria infecting the urinary tract; bacteria with an MIC of 2 μg/ml or less are considered susceptible.

The spectrum of activity of orbifloxacin is similar to that of enrofloxacin. The drug is new, and so a consensus

TABLE 1. Plasma MIC_{50} and MIC_{90} (μg/ml) of Selected Antimicrobials for Selected Organisms

	Ciprofloxacin ($\leq$2)[a]		Enrofloxacin (1.3)[b]		Orbifloxacin (2.3)[b]		Difloxacin (1.8)[c]	
	MIC_{50}	MIC_{90}	MIC_{50}	MIC_{90}	MIC_{50}	MIC_{90}	MIC_{50}	MIC_{90}
Staphylococcus sp.	0.125–1	0.25–4	0.3–1	0.25	—	—	0.23	0.46
Escherichia coli	0.0075–0.06	$\geq$0.075–0.25	<0.01–0.5	0.125	0.0975	0.39	0.05	0.11
Klebsiella pneumoniae	$\geq$0.0075–0.03	0.03–0.25	0.03–0.5	0.25	—	—	Y 0.11	0.11
Proteus sp.	$\geq$0.004–0.125	0.03–0.25	0.03–0.5[b]	—	0.78	1.56	Y 0.11	1.83
Serratia marcescens	0.03–0.125	0.125–8	0.01–1	—	—	—	—	—
Pseudomonas aeruginosa	$\geq$0.0075–12.5	0.012–1	0.25–2	2.0	3.12	12.5	0.11	0.92

[a]Breakpoint MIC (μg/ml)

[b]Peak serum concentration following administration of 2.5 mg/kg orally (μg/ml).

[c]Peak serum concentration following administration of 10 mg/kg orally (μg/ml).

Adapted from Wiedemann B, Atkinson BA: Susceptibility to antibiotics Species incidence and trends. In: Lorian V, ed: Antibiotics in Laboratory Medicine. Baltimore: Williams & Wilkins, 1996, p 962; and Aucoin D: Target. The Antimicrobial Reference Guide to Effective Treatment. Port Huron, MI: North American Compendiums, Inc., 1993, with permission and package inserts (orbifloxacin and difloxacin).

has not been reached on breakpoint MIC data. However, the manufacturer's recommendations suggest that organisms with an MIC of as much as 1 μg/ml be considered susceptible; those with an MIC between 1 to 4 μg/ml be considered moderately susceptible; and those with an MIC of 8 μg/ml or more be considered resistant. Among susceptible gram-positive organisms are *Staphylococcus intermedius* and *aureus* and *Streptococcus* spp. (MIC_{90} = 0.39 μg/ml). The gram-negative spectrum is broad and includes *Pasteurella* spp. (MIC range of 0.003 to 0.78), *E. coli* (MIC_{90} = 0.39 μg/ml), and *Klebsiella* sp. (MIC range of 0.0975 to 0.195 μg/ml). Less susceptible gram-negative organisms include *Bordetella bronchiseptica* (MIC_{90} = 2) and selected *Proteus* (MIC_{90} ranges from 0.048 to 1.56 for *P. mirabilis*). Susceptibility of *Pseudomonas aeruginosa* is questionable, since MIC_{90} is above the breakpoint (12.5 μg/ml).

A number of intracellular organisms are also susceptible to enrofloxacin, including *Brucella, Chlamydia, Mycoplasma*, and several species of *Mycobacterium* (including *M. tuberculosis*). Rickettsial organisms also are susceptible in vitro, and the clinical efficacy of enrofloxacin in the treatment of ehrlichiosis and Rocky Mountain spotted fever is just being reported in animals. As is the case with the aminoglycosides, anaerobic organisms are generally resistant to the fluorinated quinolones. Sparfloxacin, a product currently not approved for animal use in the United States, is an exception. However, in contrast to the aminoglycosides, the fluorinated quinolones are effective against susceptible facultative anaerobic organisms located in an anaerobic environment. Newer fluorinated quinolones are likely to have a different spectrum of antimicrobial activity; this spectrum should be reviewed prior to the use of the new drugs. Generally, a difference in spectrum among the fluorinated quinolones approved for veterinary use has not been established. However, differences in efficacy should be compared based on differences in tissue concentrations at the site of infection compared to the MIC_{90} of the target organism or, ideally, the MIC of the organism cultured from the patient (see Tables 1 and 2). Care should be taken that equivalent doses are compared.

Resistance

A major advantage of the fluorinated quinolones compared with many other antimicrobials has been the lack of plasma-mediated resistance in clinical cases. Resistance occurs as a result of mutational changes in DNA gyrase or changes in the size of porins located in the outer lipopolysaccharide covering of gram-negative organisms. Increased movement of the drug out of the organism has also been documented for *S. aureus*. Changes in DNA gyrase occur only in the alpha subunit, the portion of the enzyme responsible for bacterial DNA cutting. Resistance of this nature has been documented for *E. coli, P. aeruginosa, C. freundii*, and *S. marcescens*. Changes in the bacterial outer lipopolysaccharide layer of gram-negative organisms impairs drug transport into the organism. Resistance to fluorinated quinolones exhibited by *Pseudomonas* often reflects changes in the size or an absence of porins in the outer membrane. Even though resistance is mutational, it can occur rapidly during the course of therapy. However, resistance induced

by mutational changes in bacterial DNA may cause changes in other coding, rendering the bacterial offspring less viable and thus more susceptible to destruction by other drugs or host defenses. Although not documented, cross-resistance between ciprofloxacin and enrofloxacin should be expected because of similarities in structure. Culture and susceptibility data that indicates resistance to enrofloxacin but susceptibility to ciprofloxacin should be interpreted with caution.

Compared with plasmid-mediated resistance, mutational resistance develops more slowly. Yet, even though the therapeutic use of the quinolones does not appear to be limited by the development of plasmid-mediated resistance, caution is recommended with continued and indiscriminant use of this class of antimicrobials. Development of plasmid-mediated resistance may take several decades of intense antibiotic use, suggesting that like other antimicrobials the use of fluorinated quinolones ultimately may be limited by plasmid-mediated resistance. Concern about the development of resistance to fluoroquinolones by human bacteria has led to a ban on the use of fluorinated quinolones in food animals (with the exception of poultry), including food additives (i.e., growth promoters). Already an increasing pattern of clinical resistance has been noted for both ciprofloxacin (in humans) and enrofloxacin (in veterinary medicine) against several bacteria, including *S. aureus, P. aeruginosa*, and other gram-negative organisms. Prudent use of these drugs (i.e., limiting their use to critical or chronic, nonresponsive infections) may limit the development of resistance. The author encourages the use of drugs other than fluorinated quinolones for simple, uncomplicated infections. Whenever possible, the use of enrofloxacin should be based on culture and susceptibility data to ensure susceptibility.

Pharmacokinetics

Enrofloxacin is partially metabolized to ciprofloxacin by many animals. Different methodologies may be used to determine enrofloxacin concentrations in animal tissues. The type of methodology used can profoundly influence the results. For example, bioassay measures active metabolites (ciprofloxacin) of enrofloxacin as well as enrofloxacin. In contrast, high-performance liquid chromatography (HPLC) detects only the parent drug (enrofloxacin). Thus, concentrations of enrofloxacin in animals as measured by bioassay are often higher than concentrations of enrofloxacin measured by HPLC. In vitro data from MIC determination are not influenced by these differences in methodology, since drug enrofloxacin is not metabolized to ciprofloxacin. The metabolites of orbifloxacin and difloxacin apparently are not active.

Following oral administration, enrofloxacin, orbifloxacin and difloxacin are rapidly and nearly completely (>80%) absorbed from the gastrointestinal tract. Magnesium and aluminum decrease oral absorption. Following oral administration to dogs, both norfloxacin and ciprofloxacin are characterized by substantially less oral bioavailability. Oral bioavailability of ciprofloxacin is as little as 30% in the dog. Following the administration of similar doses, the area under the concentration curve for ciprofloxacin equals less than 35% of that for enrofloxacin. The differences in oral bioavailability among animals result in plasma drug concentrations (PDCs) that are less predictable for ciprofloxacin than for enrofloxacin. This unpredictability is an undesirable characteristic for a fluorinated quinolone antibiotic because efficacy is likely to be maximized by high plasma drug concentrations. Following oral administration of enrofloxacin, peak serum concentrations occur between 1 and 2.5 hours. Plasma drug concentrations of enrofloxacin increase proportionately with the dose. Based on a bioassay that measures total microbiologic activity, in dogs peak concentrations of enrofloxacin (and of active metabolites) following intravenous administration at 2.5, 5.5, and 11 mg/kg twice daily for 4 days are 1.0, 2.45, and 4.56 μg/ml, respectively (Walker et al, 1992). These data can be compared to MIC data from the target organism. In contrast to total microbiologic activity, following a single dose of enrofloxacin of 5 mg/kg, peak concentrations as measured by HPLC are 1.3 μg/ml (Kung et al, 1993). Peak concentrations following oral administration are approximately 80% less, although bioavailability approaches 100%. Peak serum concentrations following subcutaneous administration are higher than those after oral administration of the same dose.

An intravenous preparation of enrofloxacin is not available. A parenteral preparation is available for use in animals that cannot be given oral medications, or in animals in which peak serum and tissue concentrations have to be maximized. This preparation is intended for intramuscular or subcutaneous administration, but it can also be used intravenously if administered cautiously. Rapid intravenous administration may cause nausea and vomiting. An anaphylactoid reaction has occurred in some animals. The solution should be diluted at least 1:1 in saline and administered slowly (over 20 to 30 minutes) to minimize these adverse reactions.

The fluorinated quinolones are not substantially bound to serum or tissue proteins. As lipid-soluble drugs, they are well distributed to most body tissues, including bone and prostate, and to bile and urine. The volume of distribution for enrofloxacin in normal adult dogs is 2.7 L/kg. Higher enrofloxacin concentrations can be achieved in many tissues, including lung, liver, kidney, spleen, and muscle and in urine and bile (Table 2). Concentrations that are effective against many bacteria can be achieved in the prostate and central nervous system, although combination therapy or increased doses will probably be necessary for organisms with an MIC that approaches breakpoint. Maximum tissue concentrations are not likely to be achieved as rapidly as maximum plasma concentrations, but the tissue half-life of the drug is likely to be longer (i.e., 5 to 6 hours).

Both enrofloxacin and ciprofloxacin are eliminated principally unchanged in the urine. However, a small proportion of enrofloxacin is metabolized (presumably by liver, but potentially by other tissues) to microbiologically active metabolites, including ciprofloxacin. Both dogs and cats metabolize enrofloxacin to ciprofloxacin. Data in the author's laboratory indicate that the breakpoint MIC of ciprofloxacin ($\leq$2 μg/ml) will be reached in both species receiving 5 mg/kg PO twice daily. Metabolism of the drug to an active metabolite not only increases the antimicrobial efficacy of enrofloxacin but also prolongs antimicrobial actions. Alkaline urine increases the proportion of diffusible drug in the urine, thus increasing resorption of both enrofloxacin and ciprofloxacin, and prolonging the elimination half-life. In dogs, the elimination half-life of enrofloxacin and its active metabolites ranges from 6.5 hours (2.75 mg/kg) to 4.0 hours (5.5 mg/kg twice daily for 4 days; Walker et al, 1992; Stegemann et al, 1996). In contrast, the elimination half-life of enrofloxacin itself (5 mg/kg IV) is 2.5 hours (Cester et al, 1996) to 3.9 hours (Kung et al, 1993). The half-life of marbofloxacin is approximately 10 hours (Cester et al, 1996). Based on differences in data provided by studies that measure enrofloxacin alone (HPLC) versus studies that measure enrofloxacin and its active metabolites (microbiologic assay), it can be assumed that an additive antimicrobial effect is associated with ciprofloxacin in patients receiving enrofloxacin. This fact, the reduced oral bioavailability of ciprofloxacin, similarities in the antibacterial spectrum of ciprofloxacin and enrofloxacin and the illegalities associated with extralabel use of a human drug for which a veterinary product is available make the use of ciprofloxacin in lieu of enrofloxacin in animals questionable. The current labeled dose of enrofloxacin may not achieve therapeutic concentrations for organisms with higher, yet susceptible MIC values. Higher doses (5 to 20 mg/kg) may be necessary, particularly for *Pseudomonas* sp. causing infections in difficult-to-penetrate tissues. These tissues include prostate, eye or central nervous system, and tissues associated with marked inflammatory debris. The efficacy of the quinolones appears to correlate more closely with peak concentrations than with the duration of the PDC above the MIC; thus, care must be taken not to underdose the patient.

Orbifloxacin is distributed to a volume that is smaller (1.3 L/kg) than that of enrofloxacin but, nonetheless, indicative of its lipophilic nature. The smaller volume suggests that tissue distribution may not be as large as that of enrofloxacin or difloxacin. It is eliminated primarily by the kidneys, resulting in an elimination half-life of 5.6 hours. Maximum serum concentrations following oral administration of 2.5 mg/kg (the low end of the recommended dose spectrum) should approximate 2.3 μg/ml, whereas concentrations achieved after administration of 7.5 mg/kg (the high end of the dose) should approximate 5.5 to 6 μg/ml. Although drug concentrations of orbifloxacin approximate or slightly exceed those of enrofloxacin when the same dose is given, the breakpoint MIC of orbifloxacin is higher than that of enrofloxacin, suggesting that plasma concentrations should be higher for the two drugs to be equally effective against a susceptible organism. Although orbifloxacin is widely distributed in tissues, specific concentration data in tissues are not available on the package insert at the time of the publication of this article (see Table 2). No studies have yet documented the accumulation of orbifloxacin or difloxacin in white blood cells.

Difloxacin is the newest fluorinated quinolone approved for use in dogs. Following administration of 5 mg/kg, peak concentrations are 1.8 μg/ml, which presumably is the breakpoint at that dose. Difloxacin's spectrum of activity is similar to orbifloxacin and enrofloxacin. The ranges of MIC for *Escherichia coli* are less than 0.05 to 3.66 μg/ml and 0.05 to 1.83 for *Staphylococcus* spp. Like orbifloxacin and enrofloxicin, difloxacin is labeled for once-daily use. Differences compared with orbifloxacin and enrofloxacin include elimination via the bile, a larger volume of

TABLE 2. Concentrations of Active Ingredients in Tissues of Dogs After a Single Oral Dose of a Fluorinated Quinolone[a]

Tissue	Enrofloxacin (5 mg/kg)[b]	Orbifloxacin (5 mg/kg)[c]	Difloxacin (10 mg/kg)[c]
Serum	0.9	1.56	1.2
Urine	>30	—	21
Bile	>30	280	—
Cerebrospinal fluid	0.9	0.548	—
Brain	0.4	0.66	—
Lung	2.5	1.81	0.9
Kidney	3.5	4.28	2.8
Liver	5.8	3.30	7.8
Spleen	2.8	—	1.1
Skin	0.97	1.57	—
Fat	1.4	—	0.8
Muscle	2.3	2.21	1.2
Bone	0.97	0.152	7.2
Rib	0.7	—	—
Heart	3.1	—	1.6
Adrenal	2.1	—	—
Uterus	0.3	—	—
Prostate	2.20[d]	1.35	1.5
Small intestine	1.11[d]	6.91	38.7[e]
Aqueous humor	0.66[d]	0.526	—

[a]Data from this table can be used to compare drug concentrations in tissues among the fluorinated quinolones. Care should be taken to compare equivalent times and doses. Concentrations in tissues also should be compared to the MIC of the organism.

[b]8 hours after dosing, from Sheer M: Concentrations of active ingredient in serum and tissue after oral and parenteral administration of Baytril. Vet Med Res 2:104–118, 1987.

[c]6 hours after dosing, personal communication, Gerryll Gae, Schering-Plough (orbifloxacin) and package insert (difloxacin).

[d]8 hours after dosing of 2.5 mg/kg.

[e]Reflects enterohepatic circulation.

distribution (3.8 L/kg), and a longer half-life (9.3 hours). Although a larger VD suggests improved tissue distribution compared with enrofloxacin, comparison of tissue to serum concentrations between the two drugs reveals that the ratios for enrofloxacin are equal to or exceed the ratios for difloxacin in most tissues. The larger volume of distribution is likely to reflect, in part, elimination and accumulation in the bile. The longer elimination half-life for difloxacin compared with enrofloxacin and orbifloxacin probably reflects enterohepatic circulation. The importance of a longer half-life is not clear, inasmuch as these drugs are concentration dependent, rather than time dependent. It is probable that the susceptibility of an organism to any one of these drugs, including ciprofloxacin, will be the same. However, caution is recommended in interpreting culture and susceptibility data until it is clear that comparable doses have been used to generate the breakpoint drug concentration on which the susceptibility to each drug is based. For example, if the disk for enrofloxacin is based on a dose of 2.5 mg/ kg and the disk for orbifloxacin is based on a dose of 7.5 mg/kg, differences in susceptibility may simply reflect differences in dosing. Currently, no veterinary labeled flourinated quinolone appears to have a clinically significant advantage over others.

THERAPEUTIC USE

Selection of antimicrobial drugs should be based on knowledge of the (1) susceptibility of the microorganism, either anticipated or based on culture and susceptibility data; (2) the disposition of the drug, with an emphasis on distribution to the site of infection and host safety; and (3) the effect of host factors on drug efficacy and safety.

Effect of Host Factors on Efficacy of Fluorinated Quinolones

The bactericidal effects of the fluorinated quinolones are both time dependent and, especially, concentration dependent. The postantibiotic effect—the duration of inhibition after only brief exposure to the drug—of these drugs can be long (up to 8 hours), but it is also concentration dependent. For many bacteria, the postantibiotic effect is not evident until concentrations have reached 10 to 20 times the MIC. At this concentration of drugs, not only is the postantibiotic effect longer, but also a second bactericidal effect occurs and the emergence of resistant organisms decreases. For organisms with a high MIC, such as *Pseudomonas aeruginosa*, a postantibiotic effect may not occur because drug concentrations are too low, particularly in tissues. However, exposure of such organisms to sub-MIC drug concentrations may render the bacteria more susceptible to destruction by host white blood cells. For example, when *Pseudomonas aeruginosa* is exposed to sub-MIC concentrations of ciprofloxacin, it is less able to express exotoxins and thus becomes more susceptible to phagocytosis.

The size of the bacterial inoculum should have minimal effect on fluorinated quinolone efficacy, since bacteria do not produce enzymes capable of destroying these drugs. However, higher drug concentrations are necessary for the eradication of larger inocula of bacteria. Growing cells are more likely to be susceptible to the killing effects of fluorinated quinolones compared with nongrowing cells. Thus, drugs that inhibit the growth of organisms (i.e., ribosomal inhibitors), inflammatory environments, or anaerobic environments may decrease the efficacy of fluorinated quinolones. White blood cell activity (i.e., phagocytosis and intracellular killing mechanisms) may also be impaired in anaerobic conditions, reducing the host's ability to kill bacteria. Recognizing anaerobic conditions at the site of infection can be important in antimicrobial selection because with the exception of *Pseudomonas* sp. many gram-negative and gram-positive organisms are facultative anaerobes (i.e., can survive in anaerobic conditions). Aerobic cultures of material obtained from these sites yield growth, leading the clinician to believe that the site of infection is aerobic, rather than anaerobic. However, proof of the efficacy of fluorinated quinolones, in the treatment of anaerobic conditions is controversial. Enrofloxacin appears effective against gram-negative organisms under anaerobic conditions but may be less effective against *Staphylococcus*.

Inflammatory debris may be a mechanical barrier to impair passive drug diffusion. However, the lipid solubility of the fluorinated quinolones renders them less susceptible to such detrimental effects on passive diffusion compared with water-soluble drugs, such as beta-lactams and aminoglycosides. In fact, inflammatory debris may actually increase the concentrations of fluorinated quinolones at the site of infection. Fluorinated quinolones accumulate in white blood cells. Intracellular concentrations can exceed those of plasma, or surrounding fluid, by 10 to 20 fold. High intracellular concentrations of fluorinated quinolones may account for the clinical efficacy that occurs when culture and susceptibility data indicate microbial resistance. The release of drug from white blood cells that migrate to drug-free infection sites also may increase the extracellular concentrations of drugs. Fluorinated quinolones do not bind to inflammatory proteins or other debris.

The efficacy of the fluorinated quinolones is pH dependent. The pH of inflamed tissues, particularly abscesses, and inside phagocytic cells is acidic. As a result, not only will white blood cell activity be reduced, but also the proportion of non-ionized, and thus diffusible, fluorinated quinolone will decrease logarithmically as pH decreases from 8.0 to 6.3. Changes in pH are accompanied by decreased concentrations of active drug that reaches the bacterial target. However, in acidic tissue, white blood cells containing fluorinated quinolones increase. Thus, although the in vitro efficacy of fluorinated quinolones may be decreased in acidic conditions, in vivo they remain effective for the treatment of infections associated with inflammatory debris. Evidence of inflammation should be considered when formulating the dose of enrofloxacin.

Dosing Regimen

The time to effect for fluorinated quinolones, and specifically for enrofloxacin, is a half hour. The postantibiotic effect may persist for as long as 8 hours after drug exposure. Like the efficacy of the aminoglycosides, that of the fluorinated quinolones appears to be more closely correlated with the ratio of peak PDCs compared to MIC than it is to the duration of the dosing interval that the PDC is above the MIC. Thus, once-daily dosing, rather than twice-daily dosing, may and perhaps should become the accepted normal interval. Orbifloxacin and difloxacin are dosed according to a flexible label, and a similar label has been approved for enrofloxacin. However, the efficacy of once-daily dosing should be based on the results of clinical trials. It is the author's recommendation to encourage clinical trials as the basis of efficacy for once-daily dosing. Doses should be increased up to 4 fold when indicated by MIC data. This recommendation is particularly important for infections of tissues that are difficult to penetrate, including those with marked inflammation, and also when the MIC of bacteria approaches breakpoint. An exception is for bacterial urinary tract infections, for which once-daily dosing may prove effective.

The MIC of fluorinated quinolones for susceptible organisms is often low compared with most other antimicrobial drugs, and high inhibitory quotients (i.e., PDC:MIC ratios > 10) are easy to achieve. *Pseudomonas aeruginosa* may be an exception to this generality because the MIC often approaches the breakpoint MIC for enrofloxacin and more so for orbifloxacin. When possible, differences in the efficacy of fluorinated quinolones against susceptible organisms should be based on MIC data, and the dose should be modified accordingly. For example, based on a peak plasma concentration of 1.3 μg/ml, for organisms with an MIC of 0.1 μg/ml or less, at least 10 times the MIC will be reached in plasma, although a lower ratio may be achieved in the target tissue. However, for *Pseudomonas* whose MIC is 1 μg/ml, the MIC will just be reached in plasma and may not be reached in tissues. Because infections are in tissues and often are accompanied by inflammatory debris that may decrease drug distribution to the site of infection, it is likely that the MIC will not be reached in tissues for susceptible organisms with relatively high MICs. Doses should be increased accordingly. The failure to adjust doses increases the risk of therapeutic failure and increases the risk of antimicrobial resistance.

Combination Therapy

Combination antimicrobial therapy with fluorinated quinolones may be indicated (1) for polymicrobial infections caused by anaerobes or other bacteria resistant to fluorinated quinolones; (2) to enhance efficacy, targeting a synergistic effect, against a susceptible organism (usually associated with life-threatening disease or difficult-to-penetrate tissues); (3) to enhance the safety of an otherwise toxic drug; or (4) to reduce the risk of bacterial resistance. The selection of antimicrobials to be used in combination therapy should be based on their spectrum of antibacterial action and mechanism of action.

In general, drugs that impair the growth of bacteria (i.e., ribosomal inhibitors) should not be used in combination with drugs whose action is dependent on the rapid growth of bacteria. A few drugs have antagonized the actions of the fluorinated quinolones. For example, chloramphenicol, a ribosomal inhibitor, antagonizes the actions of fluorinated quinolones (ciprofloxacin) in vitro. One could speculate that the reason the drug is antagonistic is that less target enzyme (i.e., DNA gyrase) is synthesized in organisms that are not growing. Drugs that target DNA gyrase (e.g., novobiocin) also antagonize the actions of fluorinated quinolones. Rifampin appears to reduce the bactericidal actions of ciprofloxacin against *Staphylococcus* sp.

While antagonism of fluorinated quinolones with other

antibiotics is rare, synergism has been documented when a fluorinated quinolone (usually ciprofloxacin) is combined with other antibiotics. Although infrequent, synergism occurs in vitro against selected strains of Enterobacteriaceae when ciprofloxacin is combined with aminoglycosides. Synergism occurs in as many as one third of *Pseudomonas* sp. isolates when ciprofloxacin is combined with enrofloxacin. However, synergism occurs more commonly when ciprofloxacin is combined with a beta-lactam (e.g., imipenem); synergism may occur even against *Pseudomonas aureus*, which is otherwise resistant to fluorinated quinolones. Synergistic activities between fluorinated quinolones and other antimicrobials may reflect, in part, the reduced emergence of resistance. As with aminoglycosides, synergism between fluorinated quinolones and beta-lactams also may reflect, in part, increased movement of the quinolone into the cell. Even though combination therapy is likely to enhance the efficacy of either drug used in combination, the doses of either drug used in combination should not be reduced. Rather, the recommended dose, or a dose calculated from MIC data (for both drugs), should be used to ensure effective concentrations at the site of infection.

When one treats polymicrobial infections, one should select drugs that target anaerobic organisms or improve the gram-positive activity spectrum of the fluorinated quinolones. Beta-lactams—and specifically penicillins or cefoxitin—and clindamycin accomplish both of these goals simultaneously. Metronidazole can be used in combination for its anaerobic spectrum, but it offers no additional actions against aerobic gram-positive organisms.

Adverse Reactions

Adverse reactions to the fluorinated quinolones are limited. Cartilage deformities and joint growth disorders have been documented in young dogs following treatment with enrofloxacin and orbifloxacin. All fluorinated quinolones are likely to cause cartilage degeneration and should be avoided in animals 12 (large) to 18 (giant) months of age and in pregnant animals. The use of chondroprotectants (i.e., polysulfated glycosaminoglycans) might be considered if fluorinated quinolone therapy must be used to treat growing dogs. The mechanism of chondrodestruction by the fluorinated quinolones may be related to the loss of magnesium in cartilage. Quinolones appear to accumulate in cartilage and are potent chelators of magnesium. The chelation of magnesium in cartilage may affect selected proteins in the cartilage; damage may be exacerbated with malnourishment (Stahlman et al, 1995).

Intramuscular injection of enrofloxacin frequently causes pain. Gastrointestinal upset evidenced by nausea, vomiting, and possibly diarrhea may occur following administration of enrofloxacin by any route, but particularly oral administration. Seizures have been precipitated in human and veterinary patients. Predisposing factors include a pre-epileptic state, high doses (resulting in high plasma drug concentrations), and concurrent use of nonsteroidal anti-inflammatory drugs. Adverse reactions including nausea and vomiting have been reported when the intramuscular enrofloxacin solution is given intravenously. The intramuscular solution is alkaline (pH = 10); diluting the drug in saline and administering it over a 30-minute period may reduce the nausea. Crystalluria is a rare complication that reportedly may occur if hydration is not maintained.

In patients infected with large numbers of gram-negative organisms (Nitsche, 1994), the potential for release of endotoxins may influence antimicrobial selection. Endotoxins cause the release of cytokines and other mediators of septic shock. Most of these effects are mediated by the inner lipid A component of lipopolysaccharide molecules, which becomes exposed following antimicrobial therapy. In human patients experiencing endotoxic shock, the outcome of antimicrobial therapy has been related to plasma endotoxin levels. Quinolones (ciprofloxacin) release variable amounts of endotoxin, depending on the study. The magnitude of endotoxin release varies with the specific type of drug. For example, in a study of mouse *E. coli* peritonitis, imipenem and ciprofloxacin caused less endotoxin release than did cefotaxime (Nitsche, 1994). The release of endotoxin may also be dose dependent. For example, endotoxin release is greater at half the recommended dose of ciprofloxacin (3 mg/kg versus 7 mg/kg) using the previously described model (Nitsche, 1994). Actions that may minimize the sequelae of endotoxin release after antimicrobial therapy have not been established. Presumably, administering a dose more slowly would decrease the rate of endotoxin release. Binding and subsequent inactivation of endotoxin by antimicrobials has been documented and may occur with the quinolones, as it does with other cationic antimicrobials (e.g., aminoglycosides and polymyxin; Nitsche, 1994). The binding effect, at least for ciprofloxacin, appears to be concentration dependent, albeit at supratherapeutic concentrations. The clinical relevancy of endotoxin binding by antimicrobials, including the fluorinated quinolones, has yet to be established.

Drug Interactions

Fluorinated quinolones have few drug interactions. This lack of interaction probably reflects, in part, the fact that the drugs are minimally metabolized by the liver. A notable exception occurs, however, with methylxanthine derivatives, including theophylline. Either ciprofloxacin or enrofloxacin will increase plasma concentrations of theophylline in patients receiving both theophylline and a fluorinated quinolone after several doses of the combined therapy. The concentrations of theophylline may become toxic. Reduction of the theophylline dose by 25% may avoid toxicity. Alternatively, theophylline concentrations should be monitored during and after combined therapy, and the doses of theophylline modified accordingly. The combination of fluorinated quinolones with nonsteroidal anti-inflammatory drugs increases the potential of fluorinated quinolones to lower seizure threshold. Orally administered fluorinated quinolones can complex with food or drugs that contain aluminum and magnesium, reducing the bioavailability of the drug.

References and Suggested Reading

Aucoin D: Target. The Antimicrobial Reference Guide to Effective Treatment. Port Huron, MI: North American Compendiums, Inc., 1993.

Aucoin DP: Intracellular-intraphagocytic dynamics of fluoroquinolone antibiotics: A comparative review. Suppl Compend Contin Educ Pract Vet 18:9, 1996.

Boothe DM: Antimicrobial therapy in the critically ill patient. Suppl Compend Contin Educ Pract Vet 18:66, 1996.

Cester CC, Schneider M, Toutain PL: Comparative kinetics of two orally administered fluoroquinolones in dog: Enrofloxacin versus marbofloxacin. Rev Med Vet 147:703, 1996.

Kung K, Riond JL, Wanner M: Pharmacokinetics of enrofloxacin and its metabolite ciprofloxacin after intravenous and oral administration of enrofloxacin in dogs. J Vet Pharmacol Ther 16:462, 1993.

McKellar QA: Clinical relevance of the pharmacologic properties of fluoroquinolones. Suppl Compend Contin Educ Pract Vet 18:14, 1996.

Nitsche D: The effects of different types of antimicrobial agents on plasma endotoxin activity in gram-negative bacterial infections. In: Garrard C, ed: Ciprofloxacin IV: Defining its Role in Serious Infections. International Symposium, Salzburg, September 1993. New York: Springer-Verlag, 1994, pp 21–38.

Stahlman R, Forster C, Shakibaier M, et al: Magnesium deficiency induces joint cartilage lesions in juvenile rats which are identical to quinolone-induced arthropathy. Antimicrob Agents Chemother 39:2013, 1995.

Stegemann M, Keukamp U, Scheer M: Kinetics of antibacterial activity after administration of enrofloxacin in dog serum and skin: In vitro susceptibility of field isolates. Suppl Compend Contin Educ Pract Vet 18:30, 1996.

Walker RD, Stein GE, Hauptman JG, et al: Pharmacokinetic evaluation of enrofloxacin administered orally to dogs. Am J Vet Res 53:2315, 1992.

Wetzstein H-G, de Jong A: In vitro bactericidal activity and postantibiotic effect of fluoroquinolones used in veterinary medicine. Suppl Compend Contin Educ Pract Vet 18:22, 1996.

Wiedemann B, Atkinson BA: Susceptibility to antibiotics: Species incidence and trends. In: Lorian V, ed: Antibiotics in Laboratory Medicine. Baltimore: Williams & Wilkins, 1996, p 962.

Antihistamines: Current Therapeutic Use

MARK G. PAPICH

Raleigh, North Carolina

Antihistamine drugs have been classified as H_1 and H_2 receptor antagonists. An H_3 histamine receptor has been identified that serves as a feedback inhibitor, but at this time there is no reported veterinary use of an H_3 antagonist. The H_1 antagonists are divided into first-generation antihistamines (e.g., chlorpheniramine, diphenhydramine, and hydroxyzine) and second-generation antihistamines (e.g., terfenadine, astemizole, and loratadine). First-generation antihistamines are generally older, familiar drugs developed before 1982 (Table 1). Second-generation antihistamines are newer, nonsedating drugs (Table 2). The H_2 receptor antagonists are antisecretory drugs that include cimetidine, ranitidine, and famotidine and are used to suppress gastric acidity. The H_2 antagonists attenuate histamine effects on blood vessels to some degree, but this is not a primary use of these drugs. In this article, *antihistamine* refers to blockers of the H_1 receptor, whether they are of the first-generation or second-generation type.

The primary difference between the first- and second-generation antihistamines is that second-generation antihistamines do not easily cross the blood-brain barrier. Therefore, they lack central nervous system side effects, particularly sedation, common to first-generation antihistamines. Second-generation antihistamines also do not have antimuscarinic properties (atropine-like effects) associated with first-generation antihistamines.

ACTION OF HISTAMINE

Histamine is released from mast cells and basophils. Mast cells are the predominant tissue source of histamine; basophils are the predominant source in circulating blood. Tissues such as the skin, bronchial mucosa, and gastrointestinal mucosa that contain a high population of mast cells have the highest concentration of histamine.

Histamine is released from storage granules when IgE antibodies on the surface of mast cells are cross-linked by antigen. The antibody may be a specific subclass of IgG (IgGd) in atopic individuals. Other inflammatory mediators released from activated mast cells include leukotrienes, prostaglandins, heparin, and cytokines. Other compounds can trigger release of mediators from mast cells without activation by antibodies. Compounds known to activate mast cells in this manner include concanavalin A (Con A), compound 48/80, calcium ionophores, and radiographic contrast material. Therapeutic agents such as amphotericin B, morphine, and doxorubicin also can degranulate mast cells and induce a systemic reaction that has been mistaken for drug allergy.

Histamine produces multiple effects throughout the body. Primarily, it acts as an inflammatory mediator to produce local edema and erythema. Histamine stimulates H_1 receptors in the respiratory tract and causes contraction of bronchial smooth muscle. This contraction produces severe bronchoconstriction in some species (e.g., Guinea pig) during an anaphylactic reaction. In the gastrointestinal tract, activation of H_1 receptors causes muscle contraction.

Vascular Effects

Stimulation of H_1 and H_2 receptors on blood vessels causes vasodilation. H_1 receptors produce a more rapid and short-lived vasodilation, whereas H_2 receptors produce vasodilation that develops more slowly and is longer-lasting. Vascular H_1 receptors reside on the endothelial cells. When stimulated, the endothelial cells retract, creating larger openings in vessels resulting in leakage of fluid, cells, and proteins. The result is local edema, erythema, and inflammation from activated leukocytes. Stimulation of local nerve endings in these tissues produces the familiar pain and itch associated with histamine release.

TABLE 1. First-Generation Antihistamines

Drug Class	Generic Name	Common Brand	Formulation	Approximate Dose
Alkylamine	Chlorpheniramine maleate	Chlor-Trimeton (Schering-Plough), and various other brands	4-, 8-, 12-mg tablets; 1 or 2 mg/5 ml syrup; 10 or 100 mg/ml injection	Dog: 4–8 mg/dog to a maximum of 0.5 mg/kg q8–12hr PO Cat: 2–4 mg/cat q12hr PO
	Brompheniramine maleate	Dimetane (Robins)	4-, 8-mg tablets; 2 mg/5 ml elixir; 10 mg/ml injection	No dose established for animals Dose for people is 4 mg q4–6hr PO
Ethanolamine	Diphenhydramine HCL	Benadryl (Parke-Davis)	25-, 50-mg capsules; 12.5 mg/5 ml elixir; 6.35 mg/5ml syrup; 50 mg/ml injection	2–4 mg/kg q8–12hr PO 1 mg/kg q8–12hr IM, SC, IV (do not exceed 40 mg total dose)
	Dimenhydrinate	Dramamine (Pharmacia & Upjohn), and other brands	50-mg capsules; 50-mg tablets; 12.5 mg/5 ml elixir; 12.5 mg/4 ml syrup; 50 mg/ml injection	4–8 mg/kg q8–12 hr
	Clemastine fumarate	Tavist (Sandoz) and generic	Tavist-1 is 1.34-mg tablets Tavist-2 is 2.68-mg tablets 0.67 mg/5 ml syrup	Dog: 0.05–0.1 mg/kg q12hr PO Cat: 0.67 mg/cat q12hr PO
Piperazine	Hydroxyzine	Atarax (Roerig)	10-, 25-, 50-mg capsules; 10-, 25-, 50-, 100-mg tablets 10 mg/5 ml syrup; 25 or 50 mg/ml injection	0.5–2 mg/kg q6–8hr PO (for pruritus 2.2 mg/kg has been used)
Phenothiazine	Trimeprazine	Temaril-P (Pfizer), and Temaril	Temaril contains 2.5 mg/tablet, or 2.5 mg/5 ml syrup Each tablet of Temaril-P contains trimeprazine tartrate (5 mg) and prednisolone (2 mg)	0.5 mg/kg q12hr PO (of the trimeprazine)
	Promethazine	Phenergan (Wyeth-Ayerst) and generic	6.25 mg/5 ml syrup; 12.5-, 25-, 50-mg tablets; 25 mg/ml injection	0.2–0.4 mg/kg IM or PO q8hr (or every 4 hr as needed for vomiting)
	Chlorpromazine	Thorazine (SmithKline Beecham) and generic	10-, 25-, 50-, 100-, 200-mg tablets; 10 mg/5 ml syrup; 25 mg/ml injection	Antiemetic dose: 0.5 mg/kg q6–8hr IM or SC
	Prochlorperazine	Compazine (SmithKline Beecham)	5-, 10-, 25-mg tablets; 5 mg/ml injection	0.1–0.5 mg/kg q6–8hr IM, SC, or PO
Ethylenediamine	Tripelennamine HCL	PBZ (Geigy)	25-, 50-mg tablets	No dose established for animals Dose for humans is 25–50 mg q4–6hr PO
Tricyclic (tricyclic antidepressant with antihistamine activity)	Doxepin	Sinequan (Roerig)		Dose not established

Histamine produces a wide range of responses in other tissues. Histamine stimulates the stomach to secrete gastric acid by binding to specific H_2-receptors of the gastric parietal cell. Histamine (H_1) receptors in the central nervous system may play a part in wakefulness, explaining the somnolence associated with administration of some antihistamines.

EFFECTS OF ANTIHISTAMINE DRUGS

Competitive Antagonism

The benefit from antihistamines lies in their ability to block the inflammatory effects of histamine. The antagonism is competitive, which implies that blockade of the receptor is dose-dependent. If the drug concentration at the

TABLE 2. Second-Generation Antihistamines*

Drug Class	Generic Name	Common Brand Name
Piperidines	Terfenadine	Seldane (Hoechst Marion Roussel)
	Fexofenadine	Allegra (Hoechst Marion Roussel)
	Astemizole	Hismanal (Janssen Pharmaceutical)
	Loratadine	Claritin (Schering-Plough)
	Levocabastine	Livostin
Piperazines	Cetirizine	Reactine (Pfizer)

*Doses are not listed for these drugs because effective doses have yet to be established.

receptor site (which should correlate with dose) is not sufficiently high, released histamine can overwhelm the effects of a histamine blocker. Therefore, in some patients, doses may need to be escalated to match the degree of histamine liberated from mast cells. Because antagonism is competitive, antihistamines are most effective when administered *before* histamine binds to receptor sites.

Other Receptors Affected

First-generation antihistamines may also block muscarinic cholinergic receptors, serotonin (5-HT) receptors, and alpha-adrenergic receptors. The drugs vary in their affinity for these receptors, which will be discussed with the specific drug groups. Cyproheptadine (Periactin [Merck]) also blocks $5-HT_{2A}$ (serotonin) receptors. The therapeutic significance of this effect in veterinary patients is not well established. Antihistamines have some local anesthetic effects, but the concentration required for this effect is higher than that usually achieved with doses used clinically. The local anesthetic effect probably does not have any clinical benefit.

Anti-inflammatory Effects

In addition to blockade of the histamine receptor, some antihistamines decrease the release of inflammatory mediators from mast cells by inhibiting increases in intracellular calcium that trigger mast cell degranulation (Simons, 1992). The clinical importance of this effect has been debated. In vitro studies have shown that concentrations of antihistamine drugs necessary to inhibit mast cell degranulation are higher than achieved with usual "antiallergy" doses. The second-generation antihistamines terfenadine and loratadine induce a dose-dependent inhibition of canine mast cell release (Garcia et al, 1997). But in clinical trials terfenadine was ineffective for suppressing pruritus in dogs (Scott et al, 1994).

Antiemetic Effects

Antihistamines have been used to treat motion sickness and vestibulitis and vomiting caused by drugs and toxins. Drugs and toxins stimulate vomiting via their effect on the chemoreceptor trigger zone (CRTZ), where histamine is an important neurotransmitter in dogs, but not cats (Washabau

and Elie, 1995). Antihistamines alone may not block vomiting induced via the CRTZ because muscarinic stimulation, as well as the neurotransmitters dopamine, serotonin, and norepinephrine, also stimulate vomiting at this site.

CHARACTERISTICS OF H₁ RECEPTOR ANTAGONISTS

The H_2 antagonists are primarily used to treat gastritis and disorders associated with gastric hyperacidity; information on their use can be found in more specific articles (Papich, 1993).

All of the antihistamines have a tertiary amino group linked to two or three carbons and two aromatic groups. Antihistamines are weak bases that are cationic at physiologic pH. They have been grouped into chemical classes that predict to some degree the action of each drug (see Table 1). Examples of each class are in parentheses. The *ethanolamines* (diphenhydramine) have the greatest antiemetic activity but also produce the greatest degree of sedation. The *alkylamines* (chlorpheniramine) include some of the most potent antihistamines. A comparison of the relative potency is demonstrated in the dose rates in Table 1. These drugs are not as likely to produce sedation; in some patients, they may cause paradoxical stimulation and excitement. *Piperazines* (hydroxyzine) may cause considerable central nervous system depression. Cetirizine is an active metabolite of hydroxyzine but does not cross the blood-brain barrier. *Phenothiazines* (promethazine) have both H_1 blocking and antimuscarinic activity. They have prominent sedative effects and can be effective antiemetics. *Piperidines* (terfenadine) are highly selective for H_1 receptors; they do not cross the blood-brain barrier. They are virtually free from antimuscarinic side effects.

Pharmacokinetic Properties

Except for a few isolated studies, the pharmacokinetics of the antihistamines have not been reported in domestic animals. Most of the information about them comprises assumptions extrapolated from human studies. Antihistamines all appear to be well absorbed after oral administration, but there may be high presystemic metabolism by the liver (high first-pass effect). Antihistamines all appear to be highly metabolized, with only a small percentage of the intact drug eliminated in urine. Some metabolites are active. For example, the new drug cetirizine is an active metabolite of hydroxyzine. In humans, antihistamines have half-lives of 12 to 24 hours. In dogs, chlorpheniramine has an elimination half-life of 24 hours. Because antihistamines are metabolized by the liver, veterinarians should consider whether hepatic disorders and drug interactions will affect hepatic metabolism.

Duration of Effect

The clinical effects persist longer than what one would expect from the plasma half-life (Simons and Simons, 1994). In people, clinical effects have persisted for 7 days after a course of treatment. In dogs, 3 mg/kg of hydroxyzine inhibited skin test reactivity for 3 to 5 days after treatment was discontinued (Barbet and Halliwell, 1989). An explanation for the long duration of effect is persistence of antihistamines in tissues despite elimination from the blood. In the skin, for example, antihistamines reach high concentrations that may exceed plasma concentrations. For some drugs, the active metabolites may have a longer half-life than the parent drug.

Adverse Effects and Side Effects

Side effects are undesirable but unavoidable consequences from drug therapy usually attributed to the drug's mechanism of action. Secondary adverse effects are usually more serious, often requiring discontinuation of therapy. Although several adverse effects and side effects may occur, in case studies of animals, it has been unusual to discontinue medication because of side effects or adverse effects alone.

Central Nervous System. First-generation antihistamines produce sedation and can inhibit appetite. However, in some people, there has been an increase in appetite and weight gain. The appetite stimulation caused by cyproheptadine in some patients is probably caused by the serotonin receptor effects and is not related to the antihistamine properties. Sedation is usually the predominant central nervous system effect. For example, antihistamines are the active ingredient in over-the-counter sleeping aids. But, paradoxical stimulation from antihistamines can occur in some individuals or species. This may lead to restlessness and excitement. Chlorpheniramine and diphenhydramine, for example, may cause excitement in cats. In people, dizziness, incoordination, and impaired cognitive function have been reported; the incidence of these effects in animals is not known.

Antimuscarinic Effects. Antimuscarinic anticholinergic (atropine-like) effects can be significant. A dry mouth can contribute to dental disease and can cause some dogs to drink more water. Drying of the respiratory passages may stimulate coughing. Antimuscarinic effects can also account for constipation, loss of appetite, and intestinal problems. Either diarrhea or constipation may occur. Decreased stomach emptying and a bloating sensation have been reported in people. The antimuscarinic effect is a contraindication in patients with glaucoma or disorders of urine retention. Tachycardia may occur, but whether or not these drugs are contraindicated in patients with heart disease is not established.

Adverse Effects Unique to Second-Generation Antihistamines. Although considered to lack most of the side effects produced from first-generation antihistamines, adverse effects from second-generation antihistamines have received recent attention. High concentrations of terfenadine (Seldane [Marion Merrell Dow]) and astemizole (Hismanal [Janssen Pharmaceutical]) have caused near-fatal cardiac events. This has been caused by overdoses (Otto and Greentree, 1994), or drug interactions. Drug interactions in people known to increase concentrations of these drugs include ingestion of ketoconazole, itraconazole,

erythromycin, or other drugs that may inhibit hepatic metabolizing enzymes.

CLINICAL USE

Acute Allergic Reactions

An acute allergic reaction, especially one that may be life-threatening such as anaphylaxis, should be treated with epinephrine (5 µg/kg IV or IM), *not* antihistamines. Antihistamines are not as likely to be beneficial once histamine has been released.

Antihistamines may be beneficial as a so-called pretreatment to prevent histamine reactions because they can block receptors before histamine has been released. They are administered prior to treatments that may induce an allergic response, such as blood transfusions, cancer treatment with asparaginase (Elspar) or doxorubicin (Adriamycin), or administration of radiographic contrast agents. In the author's experience, clinicians prefer diphenhydramine (Benadryl [Parke-Davis]) for this purpose. However, there are no comparative studies of the effects of other antihistamines, and there is no reason to suspect that other antihistamines would not be efficacious for this use. The commonly used dose of diphenhydramine is 1 mg/kg IM or IV, immediately prior to administration of the drug or treatment that may induce a histamine reaction. Diphenhydramine has the additional benefit of producing an antiemetic effect, which may be of benefit for some treatments. In the case of cancer chemotherapeutic agents, dexamethasone is often administered, which has an antiemetic effect in addition to decreasing the effects of histamine on blood vessels.

When chemotherapy is used to treat mast cell tumors, degranulation of mast cells may induce a histamine reaction. Both H_1 type and H_2 type antihistamines have been administered to patients during this treatment. In the author's experience, clinicians prefer chlorpheniramine at a dose of 4 to 8 mg/dog or 2 mg/cat up to a maximum of 0.5 mg/kg PO every 8 to 12 hours for this use.

Allergic Skin Disease

Antihistamines have been used in an attempt to control pruritus and skin inflammation in animals, but the success has not been consistent. Efficacy rates reported by dermatologists have been mixed (Scott et al, 1995). But these drugs can be considered for the short-term treatment of pruritus in patients who do not tolerate corticosteroids. The exact mechanism by which they act is not certain. Presumably, they block the action of histamine on the H_1 receptor. But histamine may not be an important mediator of pruritus in dogs; thus, these drugs may also exert their effects by inhibiting mast cell degranulation. The side effect of sedation may also play a role by decreasing the animal's urge to scratch.

Clemastine (Tavist), an ethanolamine antihistamine, may be the most effective antihistamine in dogs, with 30% of the dogs responding to treatment in one study (Paradis et al, 1991b). Chlorpheniramine reduces pruritus in cats with a 73% reported success rate (see Section 7). Clemastine is also effective in cats with a reported 50% success rate. Chlorpheniramine, diphenhydramine, and hydroxyzine appear to be somewhat effective in dogs with success rates from 10 to 20% of patients treated (Scott and Buerger, 1988). Trimeprazine (Panectyl [May & Baker, Canada]) alone has not been effective.

Second-generation antihistamines, astemizole, loratadine (Claritin [Schering-Plough]), and terfenadine (when administered at 5 mg/kg every 12 hours) do not appear to be effective in dogs and cats. Doxepin (Sinequan [Roerig]), a tricyclic antidepressant with antihistamine effects, and cyproheptadine, an antihistamine with antiserotonin effects, are ineffective in dogs.

Combinations With Other Drugs

There may be a synergistic effect of antihistamines in combination with omega-3/omega-6 fatty acids or corticosteroids. Trimeprazine, a phenothiazine derivative with antihistamine effects, has little effect alone but is an effective drug when combined with a corticosteroid (Temaril-P [Pfizer]) (Paradis et al, 1991a). When antihistamines are combined with corticosteroids, the dose of prednisone can be lowered (30% reduction) (Paradis et al, 1991a). In a study in dogs, a combination of a fatty acid product plus clemastine was more effective (43% response) than either drug used alone (Paradis et al, 1991b). In cats, chlorpheniramine plus fatty acids (see p. 538) are more effective than either drug used alone (Scott and Miller, 1995).

Allergic Respiratory Disease

Antihistamines have been considered for treatment of allergic airway disease and allergic rhinitis in dogs and cats, but there is no evidence to support this use. In people, allergic airway disease or asthma is not managed with antihistamines because histamine is not an important mediator of the disease. Inflammatory airway diseases in dogs and cats are most often managed with environmental control, corticosteroids, or bronchodilator drugs (methylxanthines or beta-agonists). There is some experimental evidence that a serotonin antagonist (cyproheptadine) may be helpful for feline asthma, but clinical trials have not yet confirmed this benefit (see p. 538).

Antihistamines that produce marked anticholinergic effects may affect respiratory passages. This drying effect may temporarily alleviate some signs of respiratory disease, but the chronic effects on respiratory passages are uncertain. Other antimuscarinic drugs have been beneficial for treatment of asthma in human patients and chronic obstructive pulmonary disease in horses, because acetylcholine may stimulate bronchoconstriction in these species. However, benefit from treatment with these drugs in dogs and cats has not been demonstrated.

Antiemetic Therapy

Antihistamines are often administered to control nausea and vomiting. Although there are no controlled studies to demonstrate the effectiveness of antihistamines for this use—nor are there any reports of comparisons among the antihistamines—there is a general consensus among veterinarians that these drugs are helpful. Drugs administered

most often include the ethanolamines, diphenhydramine and dimenhydrinate (Dramamine [Pharmacia & Upjohn]). Diphenhydramine is the active part of dimenhydrinate. Phenothiazines with H_1-blocking effects, promethazine (Phenergan [Wyeth-Ayerst]) and cyclizine, also have been used (Washabau and Elie, 1995). Antihistamines are more likely to be beneficial for dogs than cats. Motion sickness in cats should be treated with a drug that has more specific antimuscarinic effects. Promethazine, chlorpromazine (Thorazine [SmithKline Beecham]), or prochlorperazine (Compazine [SmithKline Beecham]) have been used for this purpose and as general antiemetics in cats. None of the second-generation antihistamines have these antimuscarinic properties.

H_2-Receptor Antagonists

The H_2-receptor antagonists include cimetidine, ranitidine, and famotidine. Antisecretory effects of these drugs are beneficial in treating gastric ulcers and gastric hypersecretory disease. There is also some evidence that these drugs may be effective for some dermatologic diseases. In human patients with urticaria refractory to treatment of H_1-receptor antagonists alone, cimetidine or ranitidine enhanced relief of pruritus and wheal formation. However, one study showed only a minimal response when cimetidine was used alone for treatment of pruritus in animals. These drugs are probably more effective when combined with H_1-receptor antagonists.

The H_2-receptor antagonists can inhibit metabolism of other drugs. They have been reported to inhibit metabolism of H_1-receptor antagonists if they are co-administered, thus increasing plasma levels of the H_1-receptor antagonist.

References and Suggested Reading

Barbet JL, Halliwell REW: Duration of inhibition of immediate skin test reactivity by hydroxyzine hydrochloride in dogs. J Am Vet Med Assoc 194:1565, 1989.
Describes the duration of antihistamine activity.

Garcia G, DeMora F, Ferrer L, et al: Effect of H_1-antihistamines on histamine release from dispersed canine cutaneous mast cells. Am J Vet Res 58:293, 1997.
Recent report that describes the effect of antihistamine on in vitro canine mast cells.

Otto CM, Greentree WF: Terfenadine toxicosis in dogs. J Am Vet Med Assoc 205:1004, 1994.
Case report of antihistamine toxicosis.

Papich MG: Antiulcer therapy. Vet Clin North Am (Small Anim Pract) 23:497, 1993.
Thorough reference that describes the use of histamine H_2 receptor antagonists.

Paradis M, Scott DW, Giroux D: Further investigations on the use of nonsteroidal and steroidal antiinflammatory agents in the management of canine pruritus. J Am Anim Hosp Assoc 27:44, 1991a.
The most comparative reference on antihistamines and other drugs for treatment of pruritus in dogs.

Paradis M, Lemay S, Scott DW: The efficacy of clemastine (Tavist), a fatty acid-containing product (Derm Caps) and the combination of both products in the management of canine pruritus. Vet Dermatol 2:17, 1991b.
This reference demonstrates the efficacy of clemastine and combination therapy for treatment of pruritus.

Scott DW, Buerger RG: Nonsteroidal antiinflammatory agents in the management of canine pruritus. J Am Anim Hosp Assoc 24:425, 1988.
This is the first reference that compared the efficacy of several drugs, including antihistamines, for treatment of pruritus in dogs.

Scott DW, Cayette SM, Decker GA: Failure of terfenadine (Seldane) as an antipruritic agent in atopic dogs: Results of an open trial. Can Vet J 35:286, 1994.

This reference demonstrates the failure of second-generation antihistamines for treating skin disease in dogs.

Scott DW, Miller WH: The combination of an antihistamine (chlorpheniramine) and an omega-3/omega-6 fatty acid–containing product for the management of pruritic cats: Results of an open clinical trial. N Z Vet J 43:29, 1995.

This reference demonstrates the efficacy of chlorpheniramine and combinations for treatment of pruritus in cats.

Scott DW, Miller WH, Griffen CE: Immunologic skin disease. In: Scott DW, Miller WH Jr, Griffin CE, eds: Muller & Kirk's Small Animal Dermatology, 5th ed. Philadelphia: WB Saunders, 1995, p 484.

This is a thorough, current reference that summarizes all of the antihistamines used to treat skin disease in animals.

Simons FER: The antiallergic effects of antihistamines (H$_1$-receptor antagonists). J Allergy Clin Immunol 90:705, 1992.

This is a good, current, summary of the effects of antihistamines for treating allergy in people.

Simons FER, Simons KJ: The pharmacology and use of H$_1$-receptor-antagonist drugs. N Engl J Med 330:1663, 1994.

This is a recent thorough summary of all antihistamines and their uses in people.

Washabau RJ, Elie MS: Antiemetic therapy. In: Bonagura JD, ed: Current Veterinary Therapy XII. Philadelphia: WB Saunders, 1995, p 679.

This is a complete, detailed summary of antiemetic drugs for small animals.

L-Deprenyl Therapy for Canine Cognitive Dysfunction

WILLIAM W. RUEHL
Overland Park, Kansas

BENJAMIN L. HART
Davis, California

THERESA L. ENTRIKEN
Overland Park, Kansas

DAVID S. BRUYETTE
West Los Angeles, California

Thanks to improvements in medical care, many dogs, like people, are living longer. Currently in the United States, more than 7.3 million pet dogs are 10 years of age or older. A substantial number of elderly pet dogs are at risk for developing age-related medical and behavioral disorders. The occurrence of geriatric behavioral problems in pet dogs is usually referred to by pet owners and veterinarians as part of the "old dog syndrome" or as "senility." Pet owners commonly and often incorrectly attribute all these problems to "simple aging" or "normal aging." They are frustrated by a perceived deterioration in the quality of their pet's life as well as by sequelae such as housesoiling and nocturnal anxiety. The purpose of this article is to provide pragmatic guidelines to help veterinarians diagnose and pharmacologically manage patients with cognitive dysfunction (CD).

Cognitive dysfunction refers to the geriatric onset of multiple behavioral problems that cannot be wholly attributed to medical problems, such as neoplasia, infection, and organ failure. Dogs with severe CD may fulfill the diagnostic criteria for dementia (Ruehl et al, 1995). As currently used in animal behavior, cognition refers to mental processes such as memory, learning, awareness, and perception. Behaviors involving spatial orientation, memory, learning, housetraining, and recognizing and reacting to human family members are examples of external manifestations of cognition.

CLINICAL ONSET AND BIOLOGIC BEHAVIOR

Although the history and clinical onset of CD is unique for each dog, as it is for humans with dementia, a consistent set of behavioral patterns have been identified from recent studies. Some signs commonly observed in geriatric dogs include decreased activity and attention, apparent hearing impairment, loss of housetraining, changes in the sleep-wake cycle, altered or diminished interaction with family members, disorientation, and reduced ability to navigate stairs unrelated to musculoskeletal or visual impairment (Ruehl et al, 1995.) These CD behavioral changes can be categorized as (1) disorientation, (2) decreased or altered social interactions or responsiveness to family members, (3) loss of prior housetraining, (4) disturbances in the sleep-wake cycle, and (5) decreased activity (Ruehl and Hart, 1998).

From the time that signs of CD are first observed, many dogs survive an average of 18 to 24 months. Typically, linear or stepwise deterioration of function occurs during this period. Affected dogs are ultimately euthanatized because of clinical manifestations of CD, such as wandering and loss of housetraining, or owing to unrelated general medical problems.

PREVALENCE OF COGNITIVE DYSFUNCTION IN PET DOGS

The prevalence of dementia in humans markedly increases with age, ranging from 1 to 3% of people 65 to 70 years of age to as high as 47% in people 85 years of age or older. A study of the prevalence of CD signs in dogs is underway. To date, 139 dogs, 11 to 16 years of age, have been studied at the Veterinary Medical Teaching Hospital of the University of California, Davis (Nielson et al, cited in Hart and Hart, 1997). Included in the study were dogs without major debilitating medical conditions or a history of drug therapy that might explain the behavioral problems. Owners who had been questioned specifically about the occurrence of signs of CD in their pets stated that signs in at least one of the CD behavioral categories (described earlier) were observed in 62% of the dogs. Within each age group, the prevalence of CD signs in spayed females was similar to that observed in castrated males. Insufficient numbers of sexually intact subjects made meaningful comparisons impossible. It was evident that the prevalence of CD signs increased with advancing years, similar to the age-related increase in prevalence of CD signs observed in elderly people. In the 11- to 12-year-old age group, 47% of dogs exhibited changes in at least one behavioral category, compared with 86% of dogs in the 15- to 16-year-old age group.

In contrast, a survey of 250 veterinarians throughout the United States and Canada revealed that only 7% of clients seeking routine examinations for their elderly, otherwise healthy dogs reported (without prompting) that their older pets had one or more behavioral problems typical of CD. This low percentage may be related, in part, to the owner's incorrect perception that the problems are due to "normal aging" and that "nothing can be done." Thus, veterinarians should specifically question owners regarding the occurrence of behavioral changes in elderly pets to minimize the likelihood that owners will underreport the signs.

DIAGNOSIS

The diagnosis of CD in dogs (and the diagnosis of dementia in people) is often based primarily on thorough behavioral and medical histories, in conjunction with adequate medical evaluation and other testing as needed. Since pet owners may underreport the occurrence of these signs unless specifically queried by the veterinarian or staff, the first step is to ask the owner of each dog 7 years of age or older whether the dog has specific behavioral changes or problems. To facilitate early recognition of geriatric behavioral problems and the diagnosis of CD, veterinarians may encourage owners to address a checklist of common CD signs, the results of which are incorporated into the medical record. If the owner notes one or more problems, additional history is obtained to characterize the behavioral problems with respect to onset, severity, duration, frequency of occurrence, and impact on the lifestyle and quality of life of both the pet and the owner.

It is also important to perform a medical work-up, since many patients with CD have concurrent unrelated general medical conditions (neoplasia, infection, organ failure) or develop them within 1 week to 1 year of the time of diagnosis of CD. Alternatively, the medical condition may contribute to the behavioral problems, in which instance treatment of the former may mitigate or eliminate the latter. The medical evaluation of dogs with geriatric behavioral problems often includes physical examination, neurologic examination focusing on cranial nerve function and evaluation of the perineal reflex (especially in housesoiling dogs), and routine laboratory procedures such as a complete blood count (CBC), biochemistry profile, and urinalysis. Urine culture and endocrine tests may also be indicated. Some patients may require evaluation by electrocardiography, radiology, ultrasound, magnetic resonance imaging (MRI) or computed tomography (CT).

Brain imaging studies of humans with dementia help rule out vascular and neoplastic causes of cognitive deterioration. However, these studies cannot establish a diagnosis of Alzheimer's disease (AD), which can be confirmed only with light microscope examination of brain tissue obtained by biopsy (rarely) or autopsy (Morris, 1996). Thus, therapy for AD in human patients is instituted without a diagnosis confirmed by light microscopy.

ETIOLOGY AND PATHOGENESIS

There are more than 60 recognized causes of dementia in humans. Alzheimer's disease is the most common, followed by vascular disease. The etiologies of these disorders and other age-related brain changes are unknown. Recent findings emphasize remarkable similarities between the brains of elderly dogs with CD and people with AD (Cummings et al, 1996). The Alzheimer's neuropathology in dogs occurs primarily in the cerebral cortex and hippocampus, the same regions affected in humans with AD. Perhaps the most significant light microscopic findings in old dog brains pertain to accumulations of beta-amyloid and formation of plaques. The results of additional studies in dogs have revealed that an impaired ability to perform some neuropsychological tasks correlates strongly with the amount of beta-amyloid in their brains. In people, a similar correlation exists between the quantity of brain amyloid and cognitive test scores (Cummings et al, 1996). An additional age-related decline in the various aspects of cognition has been documented in dogs and other species. Since an increased accumulation of beta-amyloid is associated with increased severity of cognitive impairment in dogs and humans, studies are in progress to investigate how beta-amyloid might affect cognition. Beta-amyloid identified in brains differs from various types of amyloid associated with diseases of other organs, such as the kidneys, liver, and pancreas. The amino acid sequences of beta-amyloid proteins found in dogs, cats, and humans are identical. Beta-amyloid is neurotoxic and can disrupt neuronal function.

Neurotransmitter Dysfunction

A variety of neurotransmitter abnormalities have been described in patients with AD. They include depletion or imbalances of acetylcholine, serotonin, norepinephrine, and dopamine, which contributes to cognitive deficits associated with degenerative changes of late-stage AD. Monoamine oxidase B (MAOB) is an enzyme that catalyzes the breakdown of dopamine, leading to the production of free radicals. In a variety of mammalian species, brain MAOB activity is higher in the aged than in the young. MAOB activities can be extremely high in patients with neurodegenerative disorders, such as Parkinson's syndrome and AD (Tariot et al, 1993). These observations suggest that some cases of CD may be treated with drugs that inhibit MAOB, facilitate dopaminergic tone, and/or decrease free radical production.

Endocrine Dysfunction

Endocrine and metabolic disorders may cause dementia in people. For example, 27 to 52% of people with Alzheimer-type dementia also exhibit hypothalamic-pituitary-adrenal (HPA) axis dysregulation, characterized by a lack of suppression following administration of dexamethasone (Jenike and Albert, 1984). In a recent prospective study in people with mild cognitive dysfunction, patients with a "subclinical" imbalance of the HPA axis were at high risk for further deterioration of cognitive ability (Lupien et al, 1994). While recruiting geriatric dogs for a chemotherapeutic clinical trial, the authors encountered numerous dogs with signs of cognitive dysfunction and dysregulation of the HPA axis. Elevated urinary cortisol/creatinine ratios were observed in 86% of the dogs. Lack of suppression of plasma cortisol concentration subsequent to intravenous administration of dexamethasone, 0.01 mg/kg (low-dose dexamethasone suppression [LDDS] test) occurred in 31% (Ruehl et al, 1997). These dogs did *not* exhibit signs typical of Cushing's syndrome, such as polyuria, polydipsia, polyphagia, alopecia, and changes in body conformation. Behavioral manifestations have been described in humans with Cushing's syndrome (Nieman and Cutler, 1995) and in dogs with pituitary-dependent hyperadrenocorticism.

STRATEGIES FOR DRUG THERAPY

Few articles have been devoted to the treatment of behavioral problems in geriatric pet dogs. For dogs with behavioral signs related, at least in part, to an identifiable underlying cause or that display problematic but normal behavior, treatment is directed toward the specific cause, often in conjunction with symptomatic therapy, as will be discussed. In dogs with signs typical of CD unrelated to an identifiable underlying cause, Alzheimer-like pathology may be present (Cummings et al, 1996). Symptomatic or preventive drug therapy, or both, may be used to treat these dogs (Shihabuddin and Davis, 1996). One goal of symptomatic therapy is to replace depleted neurotransmitters or prolong their effect. Neurotransmitter function can be enhanced by increasing synthesis, inhibiting degradation, promoting release, decreasing reuptake after nerve firing, or replacing them with agonists.

Another goal of therapy is to slow or reverse the progression of the disease by modulating inflammatory or immune responses. Another approach is to alter amyloidogenesis by reducing the toxicity of beta-amyloid, inhibiting synthesis, altering its processing, or promoting its removal. In addition toxic free radical burden can be decreased.

PHARMACOTHERAPY WITH L-DEPRENYL

Overview

L-Deprenyl (Anipryl, Pfizer Animal Health) has been approved by the Canadian Bureau of Veterinary Drugs for the treatment of both canine pituitary-dependent hyperadrenocorticism (PDH) and cognitive dysfunction. The United States Food and Drug Administration (FDA) has approved L-deprenyl for the control of clinical signs of canine PDH, as well as for the control of clinical signs associated with canine cognitive dysfunction. Anipryl tablets are supplied in strengths of 2 mg, 5 mg, 10 mg, 15 mg, and 30 mg.

L-Deprenyl may reduce the severity of CD symptoms and/or slow neurodegenerative disease progression. First, it enhances brain dopamine concentrations and metabolism by irreversible inhibition of MAOB and perhaps other mechanisms. Second, L-deprenyl enhances the neuronal impulse-mediated release of catecholamines in the brain. Third, L-deprenyl decreases free radical production and increases free radical removal. These effects are clinically relevant, since L-deprenyl (selegiline) may slow the progression of Parkinson's disease in some human patients, rather than merely provide symptomatic relief (Olanow et al, 1995).

Safety and Efficacy

The safety of L-deprenyl (Anipryl) has been evaluated in normal dogs and by clinical evaluation of pet dogs with CD and Cushing's disease (see p. 364). The drug has been demonstrated to be generally well tolerated in controlled clinical laboratory trials that involved more than 400 dogs. A 6-month placebo-controlled safety study in laboratory Beagles demonstrated that L-deprenyl was safe when administered at doses of no more than 2.0 mg/kg PO every 24 hours. At daily doses of at least 3.0 mg/kg, salivation, decreased pupillary response, and decreased body weight occurred; at 6.0 mg/kg PO every 24 hours, panting, decreased skin elasticity, and transient stereotypies (e.g., weaving) were noted. No changes were noted in blood pressure, heart rate, and electrocardiographic parameters, nor were there any ophthalmic changes. During a placebo-controlled cognitive dysfunction clinical trial (see below), the overall incidence of adverse events was similar in dogs treated with L-deprenyl and in placebo-treated control subjects.

The results of a double-blind, placebo-controlled trial demonstrated that L-deprenyl improved the cognitive performance of dogs (Head et al, 1996). In a prospective, open-label clinical trial designed to evaluate L-deprenyl for the treatment of CD in pet dogs, improvement was observed in 77% of cases after 1 month of therapy, and benefits were generally maintained in a high percentage (78%) of patients after 3 months of therapy (Ruehl et al, 1995).

In a placebo-controlled, fully blinded trial, 199 client-owned dogs with cognitive dysfunction were studied. During the first treatment phase, each dog was randomly assigned to one of three treatment groups: placebo; L-deprenyl, 0.2 mg/kg; or L-deprenyl, 1.0 mg/kg PO given every 24 hours in the morning. Dogs completing the first 4 weeks received 1.0 mg/kg L-deprenyl in open-label fashion for an additional 8 weeks. After 4 weeks of treatment, behavior was significantly improved in L-deprenyl–treated dogs compared with placebo-treated control subjects. L-Deprenyl therapy at 1.0 mg/kg every 24 hours was superior to 0.2 mg/kg, with 69% of dogs improved in the 1.0 mg/kg dose group. This 69% response rate was maintained after 12 weeks (Ruehl et al, 1998).

Indications and Precautions

L-Deprenyl is indicated for the control of clinical signs associated with canine cognitive dysfunction. Concurrent medical problems should also be treated. L-Deprenyl is not recommended for other behavioral problems, such as aggression. Some patients might also benefit from advice provided by veterinary behavioral specialists. Patients who do not adequately respond or who relapse after initial improvement should be re-evaluated for concurrent medical or behavioral problems. L-Deprenyl should not be administered at doses exceeding those recommended. In humans, severe central nervous system toxicity, including death, has been reported with the combination of L-deprenyl and tricyclic antidepressants, and L-deprenyl and selective serotonin reuptake inhibitors. Although no adverse drug interactions were reported in the field trials in dogs, it seems prudent to avoid the combination of L-deprenyl and tricyclic antidepressants, and L-deprenyl and selective serotonin reuptake inhibitors. This warning is extended to include tetracyclic antidepressants and other antidepressants, including amoxapine, protriptyline HCl, trimipramine maleate, and venlafaxine HCl. At least 14 days should elapse between discontinuation of L-deprenyl and initiation of treatment with a tricyclic antidepressant or selective serotonin reuptake inhibitor. Because of the long half-life of fluoxetine HCl (Prozac, Dista) and its metabolites, at least 5 weeks should elapse between discontinuation of fluoxetine and initiation of treatment with L-deprenyl. The concurrent use of L-deprenyl with ephedrine or potential MAO inhibitors, such as amitraz, is not recommended.

Although L-deprenyl has been used in cats with geriatric behavioral problems (housesoiling, inappropriate vocalization), clinical trials have not been performed. When L-deprenyl was given at typical canine doses, no adverse events attributable to the drug were observed in a pilot study in cats (Ruehl et al, 1996); however, at higher doses (6 to 10 mg/kg PO every 24 hours), vomiting and excessive salivation occurred.

Dosage and Administration of L-Deprenyl

L-Deprenyl therapy is initiated at a dose of 0.5 to 1.0 mg/kg PO every 24 hours (Ruehl et al, 1995; Ruehl and Hart, 1998). Morning administration is preferable, especially in dogs with sleep-wake cycle disturbances. After oral administration, L-deprenyl is readily absorbed; tablets can be administered with or without food. It is metabolized by the liver; metabolites are excreted in the urine.

Owners typically report improvements in behavior within the first 2 to 4 weeks of therapy; some have observed that improvement begins within the first few days. Improvement can be expected in approximately 69 to 77% of patients by the end of the first month. In some dogs, improvement has been first observed during the second month of therapy. Further improvement may occur during the second and third months of therapy.

The rate of response and the magnitude and duration of benefit vary from patient to patient, possibly because of differences in the severity and duration of the brain pathology prior to treatment, variability in concurrent medical conditions, environmental factors, and the pet's behavioral repertoire prior to the onset of CD. Learning or memory may be impaired as a result of pathology in the central nervous system. Therefore, behavioral modification (e.g., rehousetraining), environmental changes (e.g., dog door, fence), client education, and supportive care should be instituted as necessary.

Periodically during the first 3 months of treatment, patients should be re-evaluated by interviewing the owner via telephone or, if warranted, by personal interview of the owner and physical examination of the patient. If behavioral improvement is not evident after 3 months of treatment, or if at any time behavioral problems progress during drug treatment, the patient should be re-evaluated for concurrent disorders. If CD signs are stable or improved in otherwise healthy patients, the authors recommend re-examination every 3 to 6 months, since elderly dogs often manifest new medical problems in that time period.

References and Suggested Reading

Cummings BJ, Head E, Ruehl WW, et al: The canine as an animal model of human aging and dementia. Neurobiol Aging 17:259, 1996.
   A review of the evidence supporting the use of the aged canine as a model of human aging, including neuropathology, clinical aspects, and response to L-deprenyl therapy.
Hart BL, Hart LA: Selecting, raising, and caring for dogs to avoid problem aggression. J Am Vet Med Assoc 210:1129, 1997.
   Data are presented from a study on age-related behavioral changes in elderly dogs.
Head E, Hartley J, Kameka AM, et al: The effects of L-deprenyl on spatial short-term memory in young and aged dogs. Prog Neuropsychopharmacol Biol Psychiatry 20:515, 1996.
   Prospective study of spatial memory task performance in young and aged dogs given L-deprenyl or placebo, showing that L-deprenyl improved spatial memory in aged dogs.
Jenike MA, Albert MS: The dexamethasone suppression test in patients with presenile and senile dementia of the Alzheimer's type. J Am Geriatr Soc 32:441, 1984.
   Documents inadequate dexamethasone suppression in people with severe cognitive dysfunction or dementia.
Lupien S, LeCours A, Lussier I, et al: Basal cortisol levels and cognitive deficits in human aging. J Neurosci 14:2893, 1994.
   Documents that altered cortisol levels precede and predict the development of cognitive dysfunction.
Morris JC: Diagnosis of Alzheimer's disease. In: Khachaturian ZS, Radebaugh TS, eds: Alzheimer's Disease: Cause(s), Diagnosis, Treatment, and Care. Boca Raton, FL: CRC Press, 1996, p 76.
   Discusses differentiating dementia from normal aging, the criteria for the clinical diagnosis of dementia of the Alzheimer's type and for definite histopathologic diagnosis of Alzheimer's disease.
Nieman LK, Cutler GB: Cushing's syndrome. In: DeGroot LJ, ed: Endocrinology, 3rd ed. Philadelphia: WB Saunders, 1995, p 1741.
   Discusses human Cushing's syndrome, including behavioral signs.
Olanow CW, Hauser RA, Gauger L, et al: The effect of deprenyl and levodopa on the progression of Parkinson's disease. Ann Neurol 38:771, 1995.
   This clinical trial confirms that L-deprenyl slows the clinical progression of neurodegenerative disease.
Pfizer Animal Health: Anipryl tablets package insert. Exton, PA: Pfizer Animal Health, 1997.
   Package insert for the veterinary formulation of L-deprenyl.
Ruehl WW, Hart BL: Canine cognitive dysfunction. In: Dodman NH, Shuster L, eds: Psychopharmacology of Animal Behavior Disorders. Malden, MA: Blackwell Science, 1998, pp 283–304.
   Reviews recent studies in both dogs and human patients pertaining to

age-related behavior changes, including prevalence, etiopathogenesis, results from neuropsychological laboratory studies, pharmacotherapy clinical trials, diagnosis, and management.

Ruehl WW, Bruyette DS, DePaoli A, et al: Canine cognitive dysfunction as a model for human age-related cognitive decline, dementia and Alzheimer's disease: Clinical presentation, cognitive testing, pathology and response to L-deprenyl therapy. Prog Brain Res 106:217, 1995.
Discusses similarities of cognitive dysfunction between dogs and people and presents findings of a prospective clinical trial of L-deprenyl therapy in dogs with cognitive dysfunction.

Ruehl WW, Bruyette DS, Entriken TL, et al: Adrenal axis dysregulation in geriatric dogs with cognitive dysfunction. J Vet Intern Med 11:119, 1997 (abstract).
Results of endocrine function tests from 249 geriatric dogs with cognitive dysfunction confirm that hypothalamic-pituitary-adrenal (HPA) axis dysregulation occurs in the absence of typical physical signs of Cushing's syndrome or medical problems expected to activate the HPA axis.

Ruehl WW, Griffin D, Bouchard G, et al: Effects of L-deprenyl in cats in a one-month dose escalation study. Vet Pathol 33:621, 1996 (abstract).
Results of a dose-escalation study to assess the toxicity of L-deprenyl in four cats.

Ruehl W, Hart B, Reisner I, et al: L-Deprenyl therapy for geriatric dogs with cognitive dysfunction (Abstract). J Vet Intern Med 12:206, 1998.
Results of a clinical trial to assess the efficacy and safety of L-deprenyl in management of geriatric behavioral problems associated with cognitive function.

Shihabuddin L, Davis KL: Treatment of Alzheimer's disease. In: Khachaturian ZS, Radebaugh TS, eds: Alzheimer's disease: Causes(s), Diagnosis, Treatment and Care. Boca Raton, FL: CRC Press, 1996, p 258.
Discusses rationales and drugs for the treatment of dementia of the Alzheimer's type.

Tariot PN, Schneider LS, Patel SV, et al: Alzheimer's disease and L-deprenyl: Rationales and findings. In: Szelenyi I, ed: Inhibitors of Monoamine Oxidase B. Basel: Birkhauser Verlag, 1993, p 301.
Summarizes rationales and clinical trial results of L-deprenyl treatment for dementia of the Alzheimer's type.

Acute Pain Management

PAULA K. HENDRIX
St. Paul, Minnesota

BERNIE HANSEN
Raleigh, North Carolina

Pain management in veterinary medicine has improved significantly since cage confinement alone was an accepted method of pain control. Recent advances in the understanding of the pathophysiology, recognition, and management of pain have underscored the importance of providing adequate pain relief in veterinary patients. It is no longer acceptable to leave a painful animal untreated on the premise that the discomfort will prevent excessive movement and additional injury. Appropriate pain control has become an integral and rewarding aspect of medical and surgical case management in veterinary medicine.

PATHOPHYSIOLOGY AND RECOGNITION OF PAIN

Traditionally, pain has been considered as merely a protective mechanism designed to guard against further tissue or bodily damage; however, recent research has shown that pain syndromes incorporate pathophysiologic responses that are themselves damaging to the body (Sinatra, 1992). Peripheral responses to tissue injury include local release of algogeneic substances, including histamine, prostaglandins, substance P, serotonin, bradykinin, and hydrogen and potassium ions. In addition to causing or contributing to the local inflammatory response, these chemicals mediate transmission of nociceptive signals to the central nervous system (CNS) (Woolf, 1993). Persistent stimulation from inflamed tissue sensitizes the CNS, eliciting functional changes in the spinal cord and brain accompanied by biochemical alterations in substrate concerned

with nociception. This process, also called "wind-up," amplifies central responses to subsequent stimulation and may intensify pain. The process of sensitization may explain such common findings as tenderness following injury and phantom pain after limb amputation.

The pathologic consequences of peripheral and central sensitization include enhanced sympathetic output and alterations in neurohumoral balance. Elevated plasma epinephrine and norepinephrine concentrations increase heart rate, blood pressure, and systemic vascular resistance. Sympathetic nervous system activation increases plasma cortisol, glucagon, adrenocorticotropic hormone (ACTH), lactate, and ketone concentrations. Pain-induced chest wall muscle spasms reduce pulmonary compliance and tidal volume. Pain management is therefore necessary from both the humane and the medical standpoint.

Determining the existence and severity of pain is the first step in providing appropriate pain management. Recognition of animal pain is particularly challenging when one deals with species that display only subtle behavioral responses to injury. Individuals of many species hide physical evidence of pain because animals that draw attention to themselves may become favored prey. This strategy, so advantageous to species in the wild, guarantees veterinarians great difficulty in recognizing and treating pain. Even domesticated animals, long selected for human interaction, may not display signs of pain when our intuition suggests that they should. This difficulty is compounded by often dramatic and unpredictable individual variation of response.

The signs of pain common to companion animals include avoidance, inappetence, tachycardia, rapid shallow respirations, and vocalization. Significant species differences exist among companion animals. For example, cats that are experiencing pain may favor avoidance behavior such as hiding in the back of the cage, whereas dogs that are experiencing pain may solicit human interaction and may be more likely to vocalize.

Heavy reliance on observations of pain-induced behaviors may be a mistake. The absence of behaviors suggesting distressing pain can lead the care provider to the incorrect assumption that pain is not present or not severe enough to warrant treatment, even when severe injuries have occurred. Furthermore, abnormal behavior may prompt a diagnosis of pain when, in fact, the behavior may have been a response to some other stimulus. For example, vocalization prompted by fear and anxiety in dogs may be indistinguishable from pain-induced vocalization. Obvious distress behaviors should never be ignored, even when the stimulus appears trivial. However, in the absence of such behavior, the decision to treat pain is often best made by consideration of the *severity of injury instead of relying solely on physical signs*. Pain threshold and pathophysiologic responses to tissue injury are similar between animals and humans (Haskins, 1992). It is therefore likely that conditions painful enough to warrant treatment in humans are also painful enough to warrant treatment in animals.

Examples of conditions that produce mild pain include localized soft tissue injury such as an abscess or a sprained limb, a superficial laceration, and placement of large-bore intravenous catheters or chest tubes. Soothing nursing care and administration of a local anestheia or a short-acting systemic analgesic are adequate to control mild pain in most cases. Conditions producing moderate to severe pain include invasive orthopedic or soft tissue surgical procedures such as cat declawings, fracture repairs, cruciate ligament repairs, pelvic procedures, ovariohysterectomies, abdominal and thoracic exploration, ear resection, and enucleation of the eye. Traumatized animals who have sustained extensive soft tissue or orthopedic injuries should be given appropriate analgesics, as should those with painful gastrointestinal conditions such as gastric–dilatation volvulus syndrome, pancreatitis, or peritonitis. Frequently, the sicker the animal, the more likely the need for analgesic therapy. Unfortunately, some traumatized and sick animals who are in enough pain to warrant judicious treatment with analgesics do not receive them because of unfounded fear of worsening their condition.

MANAGEMENT OF PAIN

Simple but essential means of relieving pain include provision of comfort, warmth, and a quiet stress-free environment. Appropriate padding, stabilization of the injured area, exercise restriction, and assistance in moving also help minimize pain. However, pharmacologic intervention is necessary for animals with significant acute pain.

Principles of Pain Management

Treatment with local, regional, or systemic analgesia immediately preoperatively or intraoperatively reduces CNS sensitization in human and animal patients maintained under general anesthesia with isoflurane or halothane and reduces postoperative analgesic requirements in humans (Abram and Yaksh, 1993; Dickenson and Sullivan, 1987; Tverskoy et al, 1990). These observations support the concept of *preemptive analgesia* (Woolf, 1993). Opioids and/or local anesthetics given preoperatively may reduce inflammatory response and decrease the need for postoperative analgesics compared with analgesia initiated after the onset of pain. Therefore, preoperative administration of analgesics such as an opioid alone or in conjunction with an applicable local or regional block should be considered.

For many patients, administration of one dose of an analgesic preoperatively or intraoperatively will minimize postoperative pain following minor surgical procedures. If postoperative analgesics are required, drugs should be administered according to dosing intervals determined by the duration of action of the chosen drug, rather than on an "as-needed" basis. Dosing on an as-needed basis requires the animal to show obvious behavioral signs of pain before analgesics are given. This method of pain management is *inappropriate* for several reasons. Once the animal shows physical signs of pain, the pain is often severe enough to have already triggered pathophysiologic responses. As previously mentioned, many animals who are experiencing pain do not show behavioral signs of distress. Finally, the dosages of analgesics necessary to control recurrent pain are higher than those necessary to preempt pain. Higher dosages of drugs are associated with higher incidences of adverse drug effects.

Opioids

The authors recommend opioids for relief of moderate to severe acute pain (Table 1). Opioids bind reversibly to specific opiate receptors in the CNS to inhibit nociception. Activation of opiate receptors is responsible for both the analgesic and the adverse effects associated with opioid administration. Mu receptor activation produces excellent dose-dependent analgesia but also causes respiratory depression. However, respiratory depression after opioid administration is rarely life-threatening and therefore should not be used as a contraindication to administering opioids. Respiratory depression is undesirable in animals with severe head injuries, metabolic acidosis, or decreased central respiratory drive. Opioids also alter awareness. Sedation is common after opioid administration and is often desirable during the initial postoperative hours. Most dogs become sedate after receiving mu-agonists; however, some dogs and cats become dysphoric, especially if the opioid is rapidly administered intravenously. Concomitant low-dose administration of acepromazine (0.01 to 0.03 mg/kg IM or IV) to young, healthy animals, or administration of a benzodiazepine to geriatric or debilitated animals, may reduce the incidence of opioid-induced dysphoria. Intramuscular or very slow (over 2 to 3 minutes) intravenous administration of the opioid may also prevent dysphoria.

Most opioids reduce the heart rate of companion animals, especially during general anesthesia. Administration of an anticholinergic agent such as glycopyrrolate or atropine may be indicated if opioid treatment results in signs of inadequate cardiac output due to bradycardia. The gas-

TABLE 1. **Dosage Guidelines for Systemic Opioid Administration in Cats and Dogs**

Cats				Dogs			
Drug	Dosage (mg/kg)	Dosing Interval (hr)	Comments	Drug	Dosage (mg/kg)	Dosing Interval (hr)	Comments
Mu Agonists			Moderate to profound analgesia	*Mu Agonists*			Moderate to profound analgesia
Morphine	0.1–0.4 IM, SC	3–6	Concomitant tranquilization recommended	Morphine	0.5–2.0 IM, SC	3–4	For SLOW IV administration, use 10% of recommended IM dosage
Oxymorphone	0.05–0.1 IM, IV, SC	1–3	Concomitant tranquilization recommended	Oxymorphone	0.1–0.2 IM, IV, SC	1–3	
Buprenorphine	0.005–0.01 IM, IV, SC	6–12		Buprenorphine	0.005–0.02 IM, IV, SC	6–12	
Kappa Agonists			Mild to moderate analgesia	*Kappa Agonists*			Mild to moderate analgesia
Butorphanol	0.1–1.0 IM, IV, SC	1–3		Butorphanol	0.1–1.0 IM, IV, SC	1–3	
Nalbuphine	0.1 IM, IV, SC	1–3		Nalbuphine	0.1–0.5 IM, IV, SC	1–3	
				Pentazocine	1.0–6.0 IM, SC	1–3	

trointestinal effects of mu-agonist administration include nausea, vomiting, and defecation. Although vomiting is often observed in healthy dogs treated with opioids as anesthetic premedication, vomiting is much less common following opioid treatment of animals in pain from surgery or disease. The authors have observed that animals already experiencing gastrointestinal discomfort and vomiting do not tend to vomit more after receiving an opioid.

Drugs acting as full agonists at mu opiate receptors include morphine, oxymorphone, and fentanyl. These drugs are recommended for the prevention or treatment of moderate to severe pain. The choice of a specific mu-agonist is dependent on the desired duration of effect and route of administration. Meperidine has a very limited role in companion animal practice because of a very short duration of action and profound cardiovascular side effects in unstable patients. Morphine is the gold standard by which all other opioids are compared; it is inexpensive and provides 3 to 4 hours of profound analgesia after systemic administration. Morphine can cause histamine release with associated hypotension when administered intravenously. Therefore, the authors recommend intramuscular or very slow intravenous administration of reduced dosages when morphine is administered to dogs under general anesthesia. Development of arterial hypotension following administration of morphine to an awake animal usually indicates previously undetected hypovolemia. This problem is prevented and treated with proper fluid therapy. Indications for the use of systemic morphine include preoperative administration to provide preemptive analgesia, postoperative administration, and relief of pain in traumatized animals. Administration of morphine immediately after the induction of general anesthesia and intubation will prevent problems with vomiting in healthy dogs and will reduce the amount (and cost) of inhalant anesthesia required. A combination of morphine and low dosages of acepromazine provides excellent analgesia and long-lasting tranquilization in hemodynamically stable animals who are experiencing pain.

Oxymorphone is the only mu-agonist approved for use as a sole agent in dogs and cats. It can be administered either intramuscularly or intravenously and provides 1 to 3 hours of excellent pain relief. Oxymorphone is very useful when immediate pain relief is necessary in hypovolemic animals or those under general anesthesia because it can be given intravenously without causing histamine release. Oxymorphone is also useful as a preanesthetic medication for preemptive analgesia, and at recommended dosing intervals for analgesia in high-risk patients requiring close monitoring. A combination of oxymorphone and low dosages of either diazepam or the water-soluble benzodiazepine midazolam is a good analgesic choice for geriatric or debilitated dogs or cats.

Fentanyl is a very potent mu-agonist most commonly administered intravenously to provide intraoperative analgesia in high-risk animals. Fentanyl can cause profound bradycardia; therefore, heart rate should be monitored closely during intravenous administration. The duration of action of intravenous fentanyl is only 20 minutes. Therefore, unless administered continuously in intravenous fluids, it is a poor choice if a long duration of analgesia is desired.

Fentanyl has become available recently as a transdermal patch (Duragesic, Janssen Pharmaceutical) designed to provide continuous analgesia for up to 3 days in human patients experiencing chronic pain. It has become popular in veterinary medicine for control of traumatic, surgical, and cancer pain in small animal patients (Hardie, 1995). The self-adhesive patch is applied to a clean, clipped area of skin. Adequate plasma fentanyl concentrations are not achieved for 6 to 48 hours after patch application, and the patch may never provide adequate analgesia for some patients. Therefore, other mu-agonists or nonopioid analgesics should be provided to animals that continue to experience pain following treatment with fentanyl patches.

Buprenorphine is a partial mu-agonist; it binds to mu opiate receptors but does not provide the same degree of pain relief or sedation as full mu-agonists, such as morphine. It has a long duration of action, providing 4 to 8 hours of relief from pain. Buprenorphine is useful for relief of moderate pain, but because it is only a partial agonist, it may be unsuitable for treatment of severe pain. Additionally, it binds avidly to mu receptors and may be difficult to displace with the use of an antagonist or another mu-agonist.

Activation of kappa opiate receptors also produces analgesia, but not as profound as that following mu receptor activation. Administration of kappa-agonists produces mild analgesia, minimal to no sedation, and mild respiratory depression, and rarely causes vomiting. These drugs are indicated for the treatment of mild pain when minimal sedative or respiratory depressant effects are desired. Kappa receptor agonists include butorphanol, nalbuphine, and pentazocine. Butorphanol is reported to increase the pain threshold up to 6 hours in cats, and up to 4 hours in dogs. However, its analgesic effects rarely last longer than 1 to 2 hours when it is used to treat acute pain. Frequent dosing is required to maintain analgesia. Additionally, because it is a kappa-agonist, the pain relief afforded by butorphanol is inadequate for the treatment of moderate to severe pain. Nalbuphine and pentazocine are kappa-agonist analgesics with durations of action similar to butorphanol. Kappa-agonists may also act as antagonists at mu opiate receptors; therefore, they are useful for antagonism of the sedative effects of mu-agonists with maintenance of mild analgesia via kappa receptor activation. The effects of both kappa and mu opiate receptor agonists can be antagonized by naloxone.

Local Anesthetic Drugs and Techniques

Local anesthetic (LA) techniques are often overlooked yet are a readily available, effective, and inexpensive means of providing surgical anesthesia and analgesia. The LA agents reversibly block nerve conduction by inactivating sodium channels. Lidocaine is the most widely used local anesthetic in veterinary medicine. When combined with 1:200,000 dilution of epinephrine, it provides 1 to 2 hours of surgical anesthesia after local infiltration, and up to 3 hours of pain relief after epidural administration. Bupivacaine (Marcaine, Winthrop Pharmaceuticals) is a more potent and longer lasting local anesthetic than is lidocaine. It has a 3- to 6-hour duration after local infiltration and up to 6 to 8 hours after epidural administration. It is preferred over lidocaine when long-lasting local or regional anesthesia is desired. Mepivacaine (Carbocaine, Upjohn Co.) is similar in potency to lidocaine but has a slightly longer duration of action, lasting up to 3 hours after local infiltration.

Toxicity associated with the use of LA agents occurs primarily as a result of inadvertent intravenous administration or after intravenous absorption of a toxic dose. The signs of toxicity include neurotoxicity, seizures, coma, and cardiovascular collapse. To minimize the risk of LA toxicity, avoid lidocaine and mepivacaine dosages exceeding 8 mg/kg in dogs and 4 mg/kg in cats. Avoid bupivacaine dosages exceeding 4 mg/kg in dogs and 2 mg/kg in cats. Additionally, use care to prevent inadvertent intravenous administration.

A variety of simple techniques using local anesthesia provide excellent pain relief. Subcutaneous infiltration of LA agents along the site of surgical incision will provide surgical anesthesia and postoperative analgesia for hours. Injection of LA into the exposed ends of nerves during limb amputation or ear resections and into declawing sites after claw removal may provide some postoperative analgesia. A brachial plexus block provides analgesia distal to the elbow (Skarda, 1996). Intercostal infiltration of 0.25 to 0.5 ml of LA immediately dorsal to, and one to two intercostal spaces immediately cranial and caudal to, a fractured rib or intercostal incision site provides excellent analgesia. Interpleural analgesia can be used to provide pain relief to animals experiencing thoracic wall pain too widespread to block with selective intercostal nerve blocks. Interpleural analgesia can be provided by carefully administering 0.5% bupivacaine through an existing chest tube or injecting it into the thoracic cavity via a butterfly needle or small-bore catheter. The dosage is 1.0 mg/kg (cats) to 2.0 mg/kg (dogs) diluted with sterile isotonic saline or water to a volume between 5 ml (animals <10 kg) and 20 ml (animals >25 kg). Placing the animal in dorsal recumbency for 5 to 10 minutes after administering the solution may improve the effect by blocking the intercostal nerves as they exit the spinal cord. In dogs with a chest tube positioned immediately adjacent to the injured area, undiluted 0.25% bupivacaine may be administered at a dosage of 1 mg/kg every 6 hours. The injured site should be positioned down during, and for 10 minutes after, injection. Intra-articular administration of 0.5% bupivacaine, 0.5 ml/kg, provides analgesia following stifle arthrotomies in dogs (Sammarco et al, 1996).

Local anesthetics and opioids can also be administered epidurally in dogs and cats to provide surgical anesthesia or analgesia. The technique of performing lumbosacral epidural puncture and recommended dosages of LA agents and opioids in dogs and cats have been described (Pascoe, 1997).

Nonopioid Analgesic Agents

Alpha₂-Adrenergic Agonists

Alpha₂-adrenergic agonists produce analgesia and sedation by inhibiting the release of the excitatory neurotransmitter norepinephrine. Alpha₂-agonists provide excellent pain relief, especially for visceral pain. However, adverse effects limit their usefulness. These effects include sedation, vomiting, profound bradycardia, second degree atrioventricular block, widespread vasoconstriction, reduced cardiac output, hypertension followed by hypotension, and inhibition of anti-diuretic hormone and insulin secretion. Because of the numerous side effects, alpha₂-agonists should be considered only for use in young, healthy animals. Alpha₂-adrenergic agonists may have a role in veterinary pain management if used in low dosages combined with opioids for the treatment of acute pain.

Nonsteroidal Anti-inflammatory Drugs

Nonsteroidal anti-inflammatory drugs (NSAIDs) provide analgesia primarily by modification of local inflammation; however, recent findings suggest that NSAIDs also have central analgesic properties. The principal mechanism of action of NSAIDs is inhibition of the inducible form of cyclooxygenase necessary for the production of algogeneic prostaglandins. Many NSAIDs currently available are of limited usefulness for the management of acute severe pain because they produce inadequate analgesia or because they produce serious adverse effects by potently inhibiting the constitutive form of cyclooxygenase. Signs of gastrointestinal irritation, manifested as vomiting, diarrhea, and ulceration, are common side effects following repeated administration. Acute renal failure is a more serious sequela to NSAID administration. Both of these organ effects are more likely to occur in hemodynamically unstable animals or animals given NSAIDs more than once. One new oral agent approved for the treatment of canine osteoarthritis, carprofen (Rimadyl, Pfizer Animal Health), is a weak peripheral cyclooxygenase inhibitor and yet is an effective analgesic. It has low gastrointestinal toxicity, except for occasional liver toxicity, and may prove to be safe for perioperative administration to dogs. Another potentially useful agent is ketorolac (Toradol, Roche Laboratories). Ketorolac is available in injectable form labeled for human use. A *single dose* of 0.3 to 0.5 mg/kg IV or IM provides significant postoperative analgesia with minimal side effects in hemodynamically stable dogs (Mathews, 1996).

References and Suggested Reading

Abram SE, Yaksh TL: Morphine, but not inhalation anesthesia, blocks post-injury facilitation: The role of preemptive suppression of afferent transmission. Anesthesiology 78:713, 1993.
Demonstration of the inability of inhalation anesthesia to block spinal cord sensitization.

Clark GN: Epidural analgesia. In: Kirk RW, ed: Current Veterinary Therapy XI. Philadelphia: WB Saunders, 1992, p 96.
Review of pharmacology and technique of epidural analgesia.

Dickenson AH, Sullivan AF: Evidence for a role of the NMDA receptor in the frequency dependent potentiation of deep rat dorsal horn nociceptive neurones following C fibre stimulation. Neuropharmacology 26:1235, 1987.
Demonstration of spinal cord dorsal horn windup in response to peripheral stimulation in rats under 1 MAC general anesthesia.

Hardie EM: New horizons in pain management: Transdermal fentanyl patches. Perspectives, Jan/Feb 1995, p 35.
Review of fentanyl patch use in dogs.

Haskins SC: Postoperative analgesia. Vet Clin North Am Small Anim Pract 22:353, 1992.
Review of pain pathophysiology, assessment, and treatment in small animals.

Mathews KA: Nonsteroidal anti-inflammatory analgesics in pain management in dogs and cats. Can Vet J 37:539–545, 1996.
Indications and adverse effects of nonsteroidal anti-inflammatory drugs in dogs and cats.

Pascoe P: Local and regional anesthesia and analgesia. Semin Vet Med Surg (Small Anim) 12:94, 1997.

Sammarco JL, Conzemius MG, Perkowski SZ, et al: Postoperative analgesia for stifle surgery: A comparison of intra-articular bupivacaine, morphine, or saline. Vet Surg 25:59, 1996.
Prospective clinical analysis of intra-articular analgesics in dogs.

Sinatra RS: Acute Pain: Mechanisms and Management. St. Louis: Mosby-Year Book, 1992.
Comprehensive review of pain pathophysiology, anatomy, and management in humans.

Skarda RT: Local and regional anesthesia and analgesia techniques: Dogs. In: Thurman JC, Tranquilli WJ, Benson GJ, eds: Lumb and Jones' Veterinary Anesthesia, 3rd ed. Baltimore: Williams & Wilkins, 1996, p 432.
Review of local anesthetic techniques in dogs.

Tverskoy M, Cozacoy C, Avache M, et al: Postoperative pain after inguinal herniorrhaphy with different types of anesthesia. Anesth Analg 70:29, 1990.
Demonstration of the efficacy of preoperative local and regional anesthesia to limit postoperative pain for days in adult humans.

Woolf CJ: Preemptive analgesia—treating postoperative pain by preventing the establishment of central sensitization. Anesth Analg 77:362, 1993.
Review of peripheral and central pain mechanisms, and benefit of preemptive analgesia.

Routes of Fluid Administration: Indications, Contraindications, Techniques, and Complications

LEAH S. FAUDSKAR
Golden Valley, Minnesota

HELIO SILVA AUTRAN DE MORAIS
Londrina, Paraná, Brazil

Five routes of fluid administration are commonly used: oral, subcutaneous (SC), intraperitoneal (IP), intravenous (IV), and intraosseous (IO). Several factors influence the choice of route of administration of fluids, including (1) severity and duration of the underlying disease processes, (2) type of fluid administered, (3) cost of equipment and supplies, and (4) technical skills of personnel. The goal of fluid therapy may also significantly influence the route selected for administration. The goals of fluid therapy include correcting dehydration, restoring vascular volume, supporting the vascular system during anesthesia, improving delivery of oxygen to tissues, providing nutritional support, correcting anemia, correcting acid-base abnormalities, delivering drugs or additives, or correcting electrolyte abnormalities.

ORAL ROUTE

Indications and Contraindications

The oral route of administration of replacement and maintenance fluids is often overlooked and underutilized. The oral route of therapy is safe and economical and allows both caloric and fluid needs to be replaced and maintained. Modern oral replacement therapy began in human medicine in the 1940s when pediatricians used electrolyte solutions as maintenance therapy in children with mild diarrhea (Ferreira and Cash, 1990). Conditions that have been successfully treated with oral administration of fluids in veterinary patients include parasitic, viral, bacterial, and dietary causes of diarrhea (Zenger and Willard, 1989). Oral rehydration therapy is used less frequently in patients with metabolic problems, such as pancreatitis and renal disease (Zenger and Willard, 1989).

Fluid Composition

Early oral rehydrating solutions contained water and electrolytes. A carbohydrate source was added later when research in the 1950s and 1960s demonstrated that sodium and organic solutes (sugars and amino acids) were cotransported across the small intestinal mucosa (Ferreira and Cash, 1990). Extensive research over the last 35 years has led to the development of several oral rehydrating solutions. Their electrolyte content is designed to replace deficits in major ion species, including sodium, potassium, chloride, and bicarbonate. Even though the quantity of sodium in oral rehydrating solutions has been studied extensively, controversy still exists over the optimum sodium concentration. Ideal solutions contain 60 to 90 mmol/L of sodium and 60 to 110 mmol/L of glucose (Zenger and Willard, 1989). Whether a base should be added to these solutions also remains controversial. Cost and palatability also influence components contained in oral rehydrating solutions.

Technique

When parenteral fluid therapy is not possible, oral rehydration therapy can be considered. A variety of solutions may be taken voluntarily or administered via a nasogastric tube. The most successful treatment protocols in humans utilize oral rehydrating solutions at a rate sufficient to replace fluids lost in feces, and vomitus and insensible losses. Hydration, serum electrolyte status, and urine specific gravity should be monitored during oral rehydration. Water should be available at free choice.

When vomiting occurs, oral rehydration therapy is usually more successful when limited to small volumes or given as a continuous infusion through a nasogastric (NG) tube. It may be necessary to periodically remove residual fluids in the stomach lumen by suctioning through the NG tube. A promotility drug may enhance emptying of fluids from the stomach. An antiemetic given as a continuous-rate infusion may help control vomiting (see Section 8).

Complications

Electrolytes and hydration status should be monitored serially to prevent worsening of dehydration or development of hypernatremia. The complications associated with home feeding through an NG tube can be minimized with proper client training. Patients with active pancreatitis, persistent vomiting, or severe fluid losses require parenteral fluid therapy.

SUBCUTANEOUS ROUTE

Indications and Contraindications

The subcutaneous route of administration of fluids is practical and inexpensive, especially for small dogs and cats. It is an excellent choice for many patients that are not severely dehydrated. Subcutaneous administration of fluids may also be used to prevent dehydration in anorectic animals, or as a transition to oral intake in patients receiving intravenous fluids. Subcutaneous fluids should not be used in patients with marked peripheral vasoconstriction because of delayed absorption of the infused fluid. Hypothermic patients, patients that are severely dehydrated, and patients with acute and severe loss of fluids are not candidates for SC fluid replacement. As a rule of thumb, if the fluids given remain in the SC space 6 hours after administration, the patient requires fluids administered by another route (e.g., intravenously or intraosseously).

Fluid Composition

Only isotonic or mildly hypotonic fluids should be given subcutaneouly. As much as 35 mEq/L of potassium can be safely given by this route. Solutions without electrolytes (e.g., 5% dextrose in water) should not be routinely administered subcutaneously because electrolytes in the extracellular fluid will move into the hypotonic fluid in the SC space before absorption of this fluid can occur.

Technique

Fluids can be given subcutaneously with a large syringe or an IV fluid administration set. The skin should be gently pulled away from the body to allow atraumatic insertion of a 22- to 18-gauge hypodermic needle. Fluid warmed to body temperature should be infused slowly. Several different SC sites should be used when substantial quantities of fluids are given to avoid the discomfort associated with overdistention of the skin. Gently massaging the area where the fluid is being infused also helps decrease the occurrence of pain during administration. The volume of fluid that can be administered subcutaneously is limited by the animal's skin elasticity and may range from 10 to 100 ml per site. Animals differ in their ability to tolerate the infused load comfortably. Maintenance doses of fluids (40 to 60 ml/kg per day) can be infused in most patients. Some animals can even tolerate larger doses of fluids subcutaneously.

Complications

Cellulitis and infection leading to SC abscesses may occur as a complication of SC fluid therapy. An effort to maintain sterile technique is a standard of practice.

INTRAPERITONEAL ROUTE

Indications and Contraindications

Fluids administered by the IP route are affected by many of the same factors that affect subcutaneously administered fluid. In addition to the use of fluids at proper temperatures and osmolality, one must use caution to avoid injury to abdominal organs when placing needles or catheters into the peritoneal cavity. Absorption of fluid from the peritoneal cavity is normally slower than that of fluids given by the IV route and may be delayed even further by hypotension and hypothermia. Although IP fluid administration is not advocated for routine use, it provides an option for bolus fluid administration to patients with systemic hypoperfusion and thus may facilitate the establishment of vascular access.

Intraperitoneal fluid absorption is ineffective in the treatment of hemorrhagic shock. Solute and fluid in the peritoneal cavity move through a large network of pores on the mesothelial surface into the interstitial space surrounding the peritoneum (McNamara et al, 1993). Absorption of solute and fluid from the peritoneal interstitium is dependent on the availability of capillary pores. The availability of these capillary pores is directly related to the amount of vasoconstriction. It is probable that mesenteric capillary constriction associated with shock states results in poor absorption.

Intraperitoneal infusion of red blood cells (RBCs) has been advocated as a method of blood administration when vascular overload is of concern (Aba et al, 1991). Pediatric dogs and cats that are anemic because of severe parasitism, for example, often need RBCs even though their vascular volume is normal. In one study in dogs, RBCs labeled with radioactive iron (^{59}Fe) were injected into the abdominal cavity equivalent to 50% of the estimated total RBC volume. Maximum absorption of approximately 90% of the RBCs occurred by 96 hours. Random destruction of the cells occurred, and the estimated half-life of the administered cells was 66 days. At necropsy, only minor serosal reactions attributed to the infusion of RBCs were seen in the peritoneal cavity.

Other indications for infusion of solutions into the intraperitoneal cavity include peritoneal dialysis and intraperitoneal antineoplastic therapy.

Fluid Composition

Only isotonic and nonirritating fluids should be administered by this route. Hypotonic fluids, such as 5% dextrose in water, are not routinely recommended, particularly if the patient is severely dehydrated, because electrolytes diffuse into the peritoneal cavity until they have equilibrated with the fluid; this may further contract the extracellular volume.

Technique

In a study of children with more than 10% loss of body weight due to fluid loss, IP fluid resuscitation was utilized as an alternative method of fluid administration because of adverse conditions (Tighe et al, 1993). Intraperitoneal needles were inserted into the linea alba midway between the pubic symphysis and the umbilicus and attached to a container of warmed lactated Ringer's solution (LRS). The needle was advanced with the flow control half open until a loss of resistance was felt and, as the needle entered the peritoneal cavity, free fluid flow was observed. Aseptic technique must be observed. Fluid may be administered as rapidly as tolerated by the patient.

Complications

Complications from IP administration of fluids include failure to restore vascular volume, infection, trauma to abdominal viscera, inflammation, and leakage of fluid into the subcutaneous tissue adjacent to the abdomen.

INTRAVENOUS ROUTE

Indications and Contraindications

The IV route of fluid administration is recommended for treatment of severe dehydration (shock) and for acute fluid loss (see *CVT XII,* p. 34). Provided that patients do not have underlying cardiac dysfunction, large fluid volumes may be rapidly infused intravenously. The IV route should also be used when accurate delivery of fluid is necessary, or when precise infusion rates of drugs are required (see *CVT XII,* pp. 184 and 188).

Fluids are usually intravenously infused with wing-tip (butterfly), over-the-needle, or through-the-needle catheters. The use of smaller catheters made of soft materials is less traumatic to the veins.

Wing-tip catheters are useful for short-term fluid therapy or short-term drug administration. They are easy to place. However, the sharp needle bevel remains exposed inside the vein; thus, the risks of puncturing the far vessel wall and fluid extravasation are increased. Because wing-tip catheters are short, they are easily displaced if left inside the vessel for more than a few hours.

Over-the-needle catheters are often used in peripheral vessels. They can be used for short-term drug administration or for IV fluid administration. They are commonly utilized for small animal patients. Typically used catheter sizes range from 24 to 14 gauge. Over-the-needle catheters are readily available, inexpensive, and easy to place and to secure. The primary disadvantage of the catheters in peripheral veins is that flow may be affected by limb position. Conversely, shorter catheters offer less resistance to flow than an IV catheter of similar caliber but longer length. This difference can be an issue when fluids must be bolused, as in shock.

Through-the-needle catheters are frequently used in central lines, although they can be placed in peripheral veins (with flow impacted by limb position). These catheters are substantially more expensive than over-the-needle catheters.

A central line is a relatively wide-bore, long catheter placed so that the tip is positioned in the cranial or caudal vena cava. The length of the catheter needed to enter the vena cava is determined by the distance of the access vein from the vena cava. Some of the indications for central lines include (1) patients needing large amounts of rapidly infused fluids, (2) patients requiring frequent blood sampling (e.g., patients with diabetic ketoacidosis), or (3) patients receiving hypertonic or viscous solutions. Large volumes of fluids can often be infused at high speeds through these catheters, making them useful for emergency fluid administration. Through-the-needle catheters also allow withdrawal of blood. Central lines allow measurement of central venous pressure, which can help the clinician optimize right ventricular filling in hypotensive patients.

The site of venipuncture used for IV fluid therapy depends primarily on individual clinician preference. The jugular and cephalic veins are most commonly chosen for IV catheterization; however, the lateral saphenous and medial saphenous veins are also used. The advantages of the jugular venous route include the ability to measure central venous pressure and obtain serial blood samples. The jugular vein also allows the use of large-bore catheters for rapid infusions, administration of hypertonic or viscous solutions, and dilution of irritating drugs (Table 1). Blood flow to the region should be considered before one places the catheter (hindlimb veins are not options in dogs with gastric dilatation–volvulus or cats with aortic thromboembolism). The possibility of contamination should also be considered. Avoid areas with skin lesions. Use veins on the forelimbs or the jugular veins in patients with polyuria or diarrhea; use hindlimb veins in vomiting patients.

Intravenous fluid therapy is more expensive than the SC route of fluid therapy because of increased cost of supplies and the increased personnel time required for catheter care (e.g., bandaging, adjusting drip, flushing).

Fluid Composition

Fluids suitable for intravenous administration include all isotonic crystalloids (for example, 0.9% NaCl, lactated Ringer's solution), synthetic colloids (for example, dextrans, hetastarch, pentastarch), plasma, blood, hypotonic crystalloids (for example, 0.45% NaCl, 5% dextrose in water), hypertonic crystalloids (for example, 7% NaCl, 50% dextrose in water), and viscous solutions (for example,

lipid solutions). Specific fluid therapy regimens for renal failure are described in *CVT XII* (p. 951).

Technique

The technique for IV catheter placement has been described in detail (Hansen, 1992). Catheters should always be placed aseptically. Aseptic technique includes clipping a wide margin of hair in the area of the vein and completing a standard surgical scrub of the site. An antimicrobial cream should be placed at the catheter-skin interface of the puncture site. To minimize problems with catheters, sterile technique should always be followed. Catheters should remain in a vein no longer than 72 hours.

Patients with indwelling IV catheters should be monitored for fever and leukocytosis. If fever develops after placement of the catheter, the catheter should be assumed to be the source until proved otherwise. The catheter should be promptly removed, and the tip cultured. If bacterial growth is detected by culture, appropriate therapy, based on antimicrobial susceptibility tests, should be started. Catheter sites should always be clean and dry. Vascular catheters not in use can be flushed with heparinized saline (0.9% saline with 5 U of heparin/ml) every 6 hours to minimize formation of blood clots in the catheter lumen.

Complications

Complications of IV fluid therapy include extravasation of fluid into perivascular tissue, thrombosis, thrombophlebitis, infections, air embolism or embolism caused by catheter fragments, and bleeding. Thrombosis is more likely to occur when catheters are placed in small peripheral veins, or when the catheters are placed in veins that traverse a mobile joint. The use of IV catheters in animals with immune-mediated hemolytic anemia or vasculitis is associated with a high incidence of thrombosis. Peripheral veins are preferred in these patients because thrombosis of central veins is associated with greater morbidity (e.g., chylothorax) than thrombosis of peripheral veins.

To decrease the prevalence of infection at the site of entry of the catheter through the skin, standard surgical preparation of the site is recommended. These sites should be inspected once or twice daily. Bandages should be changed every other day or when they become wet or dirty. To decrease the risk of thrombophlebitis and infection, catheters should be removed after 72 hours.

INTRAOSSEOUS ROUTE

Indications and Contraindications

The IO route of fluid administration is reserved exclusively for resuscitation when vascular access is difficult to obtain. Patients in which IO fluid administration is most often used include neonates (see *CVT XII*, p. 34), exotic animals (see CVT XII, p. 1331), and patients with severe cardiac dysfunction. When vascular access cannot be obtained, or when time is a factor, intraosseous infusion is an acceptable temporary alternative.

Uptake and distribution from bone marrow occurs via medullary sinuses that drain into nutrient veins leading to

TABLE 1. Recommended Veins for Intravenous Fluid Therapy

Viscous or hypertonic solutions → central vein
Large volumes of fluids at high speed → central vein
Vomiting → central or hindlimb veins
Polyuria → central or forelimb veins
Diarrhea → central or forelimb veins
Aortic thromboembolism → central or forelimb veins
Immune-mediated hemolytic anemia → peripheral veins
Gastric dilatation–volvulus → central and forelimb veins

the general circulation. Uptake of fluid has been demonstrated to occur within 9.9 seconds in normal dogs and within 12.8 seconds in hypovolemic dogs with the use of technetium-labeled albumin (Cameron et al, 1989).

Intraosseous administration provides a quick and reliable method for resuscitation until a vascular access can be established. Intraosseous needles should be removed as soon as intravascular access is obtained to minimize the risk of osteomyelitis.

Fluid Composition

Most solutions that are satisfactory for IV administration may also be administered intraosseously. Drugs that have been administered intraosseously include antibiotics, atropine, dexamethasone sodium phosphate, diazepam, digoxin, dobutamine, dopamine, epinephrine, heparin, insulin, lidocaine, morphine, dextran 70, plasma, dextrose up to 50%, lactated Ringer's solution, sodium bicarbonate, normal and hypertonic saline, and whole blood (Cameron et al, 1989; Driggers et al, 1991).

Technique

Clip and aseptically prepare healthy skin. Local anesthesia is recommended for conscious patients. A 2- to 3-mm skin incision facilitates penetration of the IO or bone marrow biopsy needle through the skin. The needle is held against the bony cortex at a 45- to 90-degree angle to the long axis of the bone and inserted with a twisting motion. Typically, a change in resistance can be felt when the needle passes through the bony cortex and enters the marrow cavity. This positioning may be confirmed by aspirating marrow or venous blood, or by noting little resistance during the injection of normal saline. The needle may be sutured to the skin or protected by a padded bandage. The site of insertion must be maintained aseptically. If repeated attempts are needed to place an IO needle, a second site should be utilized because solutions will leak from earlier entry sites into the bony cortex.

Intraosseous needles and bone marrow biopsy needles may be used for IO fluid administration. In smaller patients, spinal needles may be used. Needles without stylets may also be utilized for IO fluid administration but may become plugged with a core of cortical bone.

The sites for IO needle placement in mammals include the iliac crest, the anterior tibia, the trochanteric fossa of the femur, and the head of the humerus. The ulna is commonly used in birds.

For routine administration of fluids, gravity-dependent flow rates are satisfactory. However, gravity flow and flow from pressurized fluid bags may not deliver volumes of crystalloids adequate for shock resuscitation. A study of IO infusions of hypertonic saline and dextrans was shown to improve cardiac output and mean arterial pressure in a canine model of hemorrhagic shock (Okrasinski et al, 1992).

Complications

Complications associated with IO fluid administration include osteomyelitis, loss of fluid from the administration site with local swelling or edema, and embolization (Driggers et al, 1991). Microscopic changes associated with administration of fluid through a needle placed in the bone marrow cavity are characterized by cellular displacement and disruption as well as migration of inflammatory cells into the area. Changes do not include the physis; however, the needle is generally directed away from areas of bone growth in immature animals.

References and Suggested Reading

Aba MA, Pissani AA, Alzola RH, et al: Evaluation of the intraperitoneal route for the transfusion of erythrocytes using rats and dogs. Acta Physiol Pharmacol Ther Latinoam 41:387, 1991.
Measurements of uptake and survivability of RBCs transfused via the peritoneal cavity.

Cameron JL, Fontanarosa PB, Passalaqua AM: A comparative study of peripheral to central circulation delivery times between intraosseous and intravenous injection using a radionuclide technique in normovolemic and hypovolemic canines. J Emerg Med 7:123, 1988.
A study demonstrating no difference between intravenous and intraosseous delivery times.

Driggers DA, Johnson R, Steiner JF, et al: Emergency resuscitation in children: The role of intraosseous infusion. Emerg Res 89:129, 1991.
A description of the indications, technique, and pharmacokinetics of intraosseous infusions.

Ferreira RM, Cash RA: History of the development of oral rehydration therapy. Clin Ther 12(suppl A):2, 1990.
A history of the research into and use of oral rehydration therapy.

Hansen BD: Technical aspects of fluid therapy: Catheters and monitoring of fluid therapy. In: DiBartola SP, ed: Fluid Therapy in Small Animal Practice. Philadelphia: WB Saunders, 1992, pp 341–370.
A description of catheters, complications, and monitoring of fluid therapy.

McNamara RM, Schoffstall JM, Fuerst RS: Inefficacy of intraperitoneal fluid administration in a shock model. Pediatr Emerg Care 9:77, 1993.
A study of the response to intraperitoneal fluid resuscitation in hemorrhaged immature swine.

Okrasinski EB, Krahwinkle DJ, Sanders WL: Treatment of dogs in hemorrhagic shock by intraosseous infusion of hypertonic saline and dextran. Vet Surg 21:20, 1992.
Hemodynamic monitoring during shock resuscitation utilizing hypertonic saline and dextrans administered intraosseously.

Schedl HP: Scientific rationale for oral rehydration therapy. Clin Ther 12(suppl A):14, 1990.
A discussion of the physiology and pathophysiology of intestinal mucosal function as related to the development of oral rehydration solutions.

Tighe SQM, Rudland PM, Kershaw CR: Paediatric resuscitation in adverse circumstances: A comparison of three routes of systemic access. J R Nav Med Serv 79:75, 1993.
A comparison of IV, IO, and IP routes of fluid administration in dehydrated Kurdish children.

Zenger E, Willard MD: Oral rehydration therapy in companion animals. Comp Anim Pract 19(4 and 5):6, 1989.
Indications and clinical use of oral rehydration therapy in companion animals.

Medical Use of Colloids

MARC RAFFE

St. Paul, Minnesota

Successful management of fluid and electrolyte balance in critically ill patients is often a challenge. In recent years, macromolecular solutions (colloids) have been successfully used to maintain intravascular fluid balance, and for shock resuscitation. A growing body of evidence indicates the value of colloids in supporting intravascular fluid retention and reducing transcompartmental fluid shifts associated with acute and chronic diseases. This article provides an overview of the role of colloids in achieving these goals and compares their efficacy to saline-based fluids commonly used in clinical practice. Measuring the effective colloid osmotic pressure is described on page 112. Additional therapeutic guidelines are found on page 131.

FUNCTION OF COLLOIDS

Intercompartmental fluid balance is highly dependent on the concentrations of sodium and plasma proteins. When sodium or protein depletion occurs, significant "shifts" in water volume occur at the expense of intravascular and interstitial fluid spaces. Redistribution of water away from these compartments results in reduced intravascular fluid volume and contributes to hypotension and shock.

Colloids are "active" molecules that "draw" water across permeable membranes into the fluid compartment where the colloids are located, a physiologic process known as "osmosis." Colloids dynamically contribute to transcompartmental fluid balance by regulating water distribution among vascular, extravascular, and intracellular fluid spaces. The dynamic relationship between osmotic activity and local capillary perfusion pressure is termed the Starling law of the capillary. The role of colloids in Starling forces is to prevent or minimize abnormal fluid redistribution (edema) from the intravascular space into interstitial and intracellular fluid spaces. Colloids are not the only therapeutic solutions that exert an in vivo osmotic effect; hypertonic saline (3 to 10%) and sugar solutions (10% dextrose, 20% mannitol) also share the ability to shift water between fluid compartments. However, when compared with colloids, these actions are transient (1 to 3 hours) and may not achieve the desired clinical response under all circumstances.

COLLOID SOLUTIONS

Colloids are pharmacologically classified, on the basis of their origin, as endogenously synthesized (albumin, plasma protein) or artificially manufactured (dextrans, hetastarch, pentastarch, gelatins). Table 1 summarizes the main characteristics.

Plasma Protein (Albumin). Albumin is the major protein produced in the liver. It has a molecular weight of approximately 69,000 daltons (D). Albumin accounts for approximately 80% of the intravascular colloid osmotic pressure provided by protein molecules. Each gram of albumin has the capacity to retain 18 ml of fluid in the vascular space.

Albumin synthesis is governed by osmoreceptors in the hepatic interstitium. The rate of biosynthesis is correlated with several factors, including nutritional level and stress response. Albumin biosynthesis is unaffected by other plasma proteins. Following synthesis and release, approximately 40% of albumin remains in the intravascular space, while 60% is distributed into the interstitial and intracellular spaces. Interstitial albumin can be returned to the systemic circulation by lymphatic drainage. Approximately 10% of interstitial albumin remains tissue bound and unavailable for mobilization. Approximately 8% of albumin is metabolized daily.

Albumin has several functions unrelated to its colloid activity. Albumin binds and contributes to intravascular transport of many substances, including drugs, hormones, metals, and enzymes. Albumin also acts as a free radical scavenger and binds inflammatory mediators that are potentially injurious to tissues and organs.

Albumin is found in the plasma protein fraction following separation of blood components. Following intravenous administration, peak oncotic action occurs within 30 to 60 minutes and produces interstitial fluid translocation into the intravascular space. In severely dehydrated patients, administration of supplemental saline-based fluid is indicated to prevent intravascular hyperoncotic syndrome. The half-life of albumin is approximately 16 hours following intravenous administration.

Several *complications* have been associated with albumin administration. Pulmonary edema is a concern; however, many studies refute this theoretical consideration. Hypocalcemia has been reported following albumin administration and may be a reflection of the properties of commonly used anticoagulant agents that act to bind calcium. Changes in coagulation have been reported following administration, which may reflect intravascular dilution of coagulation factors associated with intravascular volume expansion. Allergic reactions characterized by hypotension and prekallikrein activation may infrequently occur.

Economics and shelf life of plasma proteins are also considerations inasmuch as the expense associated with harvesting and processing blood products may be significant. Storage times in excess of 6 months are not recommended for processed plasma components.

Dextran (Gentran 70). Dextrans are produced by the bacterium *Leuconostoc mesenteroides* grown in sucrose. Dextran solutions contain a range of molecular-weight polymers that reflect bacterial biosynthesis and subsequent purification processes. Dextran 70 is currently the most

TABLE 1. **Colloid Solutions**

Colloid	Average Mol. Wt. (Daltons)	Colloid Oncotic Pressure (mm Hg)	Plasma Half-Life (hr)	Route of Elimination	Side Effects	Usual Dose (ml/kg)
Albumin	69,000	18–20	18	Hepatic metabolism	Anaphylactoid Hypocalcemia	10–20 ml/kg
Hydroxyethyl starch (HES; hetastarch)	69,000	30	36–48	Mixed Renal Hepatic storage	Coagulopathy Hyperamylasemia Anaphylaxis	20 ml/kg/day
Dextran 70 (Gentran; Rheomacrodex)	70,000	30	25	Mixed Renal Hepatic metabolism	Coagulopathy Anaphylaxis	20–30 ml/kg/day
Modified fluid gelatin (Plasmagel)	35,000	38	2.5–4	Renal GI	Anaphylaxis	10–20 ml/kg
Urea-linked gelatin (Haemaccel)	35,000	39	2.5–4	Renal GI	Coagulopathy	10–20 ml/kg
Succinylated gelatin (Gelofusine)	35,000		2–4	Renal GI	Coagulopathy	10–20 ml/kg
Polyoxygelatin (Vetaplasma)	30,000	45–47	4–8	Renal GI	Coagulopathy	5 ml/kg q1hr × 2

commonly used dextran solution. Dextran 70 solution has dextran polymers with a mean molecular weight of 70,000 D. It is commercially prepared as a 6% solution in a 0.9% saline base fluid. The osmotic pressure of the solution is 30 mm Hg; it has an osmolality of 308 mOsm/L when compounded as a 6% solution in normal saline. Dextrans are removed from the vascular space by several mechanisms. Small dextran molecules are directly filtered by the kidneys. Larger molecules are stored in hepatocytes and reticuloendothelial cells until metabolized into carbon dioxide and water.

Infusion of dextran 70 results in plasma volume expansion and enhanced hemodynamic performance. Each gram of infused dextran 70 can retain up to 30 ml of water in the vascular compartment. Three hours following dextran 70 infusion, approximately 70% of the administered dose is retained in the vascular space. In comparison, approximately 15% of a saline-based fluid solution, such as lactated Ringer's solution, is retained in the intravascular space 3 hours following intravenous infusion. Approximately one third of the administered dose of dextran 70 is present 24 hours following infusion. The hemodynamic improvement noted following dextran administration is partly attributed to improved microcirculatory blood flow. The rheologic (viscosity) effects of dextran include decreased interaction of cellular blood elements with the endothelium. Decreased platelet adhesiveness, red blood cell aggregation, and platelet aggregation have also been associated with dextran administration (see p. 131).

Dextran administration may be associated with several side effects. Acute renal failure has been reported with lower-molecular-weight dextran preparations (dextran 40). However, in human and animal studies, dextran 70 has rarely been associated with this complication. Anaphylactoid reactions have been reported in humans and sporadically noted in dogs. Severe reactions can occur; the incidence varies between 0.03 and 0.5%. The source of the reaction is dextran-producing bacteria in the gastrointestinal tract.

The major side effect associated with administration of dextrans is increased bleeding tendency. It vitro studies have revealed a multifactorial dose-related hemostatic defect, primarily associated with reduced platelet adhesion and aggregation mediated through factor VIII antigen activity. Dextrans also (1) lower all clotting factor levels by hemodilution; (2) coat blood vessel walls and cellular elements, impairing initial clot development; and (3) impair the elasticity and tensile strength of fibrin clot aggregates. Bleeding may occur more readily in patients with coagulation abnormalities, such as thrombocytopenia. If patients have pre-existing renal failure, uremic platelet dysfunction may occur. Interference with crossmatching blood may also occur, owing to delayed development of antigen-antibody complexes. Interference with certain serum glucose assays has also been reported. However, when dextran infusion does not exceed 20 ml/kg/day, these side effects are uncommon.

Hydroxyethyl Starch, Hetastarch (Hespan). Hydroxyethyl starch (HES) is synthesized by enzymatic cleavage of a base amylopectin (starch) molecule. HES, like dextrans, contains a heterogeneous mixture of molecular weights ranging from 10,000 to one million, with a mean molecular weight of 69,000 D. When compounded as a 6% solution in normal saline, the osmotic pressure of the solution is 30 mm Hg and has an osmolality of 310 mOsm/L. Molecules less than 50,000 D are cleared by the kidneys; larger molecules are trapped in the liver, spleen, and reticuloendothelial system and metabolized to glucose.

HES is an effective volume expander. Each gram of HES has the capacity to retain 30 ml of water in the intravascular fluid space. Three hours following administration, the effective intravascular fluid volume is greater than the infused HES volume, and this effect may persist as long as 24 hours. Fifty percent of the original HES dose is retained within the vessels 48 hours following administration; one third the administered dose is present in the intravascular space 8 days following administration. The intravascular retention time following HES administration is equivalent to plasma protein administration.

An increased bleeding tendency may occur following HES administration. Studies of humans indicate that HES infusion causes a dilutional effect on plasma fibrinogen and antithrombin III levels. Increased partial thromboplastin times and decreased factor VIII activity also occur. In humans, a single case of a subclinical von Willebrand's carrier demonstrating increased bleeding tendencies following HES administration has been reported. Corollary studies are not available in companion animal species.

Serum amylase concentrations increase following HES administration in humans. Resolution of HES-associated hyperamylasemia without clinical complications occurs within 72 hours following administration. Anaphylactoid reactions following HES administration have been infrequently noted. The overall incidence of side effects following HES administration in humans is 0.085%. Dosing is discussed on page 131.

Gelatins. Gelatin origin colloid solutions are available throughout the world and have recently been introduced in the United States. Gelatins are modification of animal collagen (cattle bone). Medically available solutions include modified fluid gelatin, urea-linked gelatin, succinylated gelatin, and oxypolygelatin. Currently, only oxypolygelatin is available for veterinary medical use in the United States.

Gelatin-based colloids have a molecular weight of 30,000 to 35,000 D with a colloid content of 3.5 to 5.5 gm/dl. Because of their lower mean molecular weight, they differ from dextrans and HES in several important ways. The "denser" concentration of molecules per unit volume produces greater osmotic action. Gelatin-based colloids have the ability to retain 45 to 47 ml of water/gm of colloid in the intravascular space. However, the smaller molecular weight is also a liability in that intravascular retention times following administration average only about 2 hours. Elimination is by direct renal filtration; however, extrarenal mechanisms, including gastrointestinal excretion and metabolism, also occur. The clinical characteristics of gelatin-based colloids are different from those of dextrans or hydroxystarch. A large volume is required to achieve therapeutic effect compared with other colloids. Approximately two times the estimated blood loss is required to achieve an equivalent resuscitation end point. This dose must be repeated approximately every 2 hours to maintain colloid oncotic pressure activity.

The side effects associated with gelatin administration include complement-mediated anaphylaxis resulting in hypotension, urticaria, pulmonary edema, and gastrointestinal disturbances. Dilutional coagulopathies may occur following large volume administration. Acute pulmonary edema has been reported following overadministration; however, no specific literature supports this reported side effect. Renal complications following gelatin administration have not been reported.

MEDICAL INDICATIONS FOR COLLOIDS

Colloids have been used in a variety of medical and surgical conditions in human and veterinary medicine. One principal indication for colloids is shock resuscitation. Research studies indicate that colloids provide effective resuscitation in acute hypovolemia. Colloids are valuable in providing vascular volume support both in the initial resuscitation period and for an extended time following administration. These characteristics are important in the initial management and stabilization of the clinical shock (see p. 140). Studies support the inclusion of colloids in resuscitation and indicate no difference in adverse clinical outcomes when colloids are compared with saline-based fluid resuscitation. A major concern associated with aggressive crystalloid administration for shock resuscitation is the hemodilution effect of acellular fluids on plasma proteins. A balanced approach is to combine both fluid bases in a resuscitation protocol. The rationale for this protocol is that the crystalloid solutions will provide immediate intravascular volume expansion, while colloids will increase the time of crystalloid retention in the intravascular compartment. The optimal "ratio" of infused volume to achieve a resuscitation end point remains unresolved. Most reports support reducing the crystalloid infusion by 33 to 50% if colloids are coadministered at standard dose rates.

Colloids are also used for replacement of perioperative blood loss. They provide excellent intravascular volume support that extends into the postoperative period. Colloids are selected for human use to replace lost blood volume and also to reduce the risk of infectious disease transmission associated with transfusion.

Colloids have also been advocated for use in hypoproteinemic patients to re-establish and maintain intercompartmental water balance. Natural colloids such as albumin or plasma protein fraction are preferred because of their increased intravascular retention time. Recent studies in hypoproteinemic patients indicate that HES may provide a similar result. A significant clinical response can occur within 12 hours following colloid administration and may be noted as reduced peripheral edema, increased urine production, decreased extravascular lung water (noted radiographically as interstitial edema), and reduced "gelatinous" consistency to the subcuticular tissue.

Additional indications for colloids have been cited in the clinical literature. Colloids are protective against edema formation in "leaky" capillary syndromes associated with sepsis or other pansystemic inflammatory diseases. They prevent water shifts from the vascular to interstitial and extracellular spaces, thereby reducing edema formation and preserving hemodynamic function. Colloids have also been useful in the treatment of acute head injury characterized by impaired regulation of transcompartmental fluid balance. Finally, the addition of colloids to readministered red blood cell products following plasmapheresis reduces the incidence of complications associated with this procedure.

References and Suggested Reading

Concannon KT: Colloid oncotic pressure and the clinical use of colloidal solutions. J Vet Emerg Crit Care Med 3:49, 1993.
  An excellent review of the principles and use of colloids in clinical practice.
Griffel MI, Kaufman BS: Pharmacology of colloids and crystalloids. Crit Care Clin 8:235, 1992.
  An overview of the comparative pharmacology of synthetic colloids available in clinical practice.
Mishler JW: Synthetic plasma volume expanders: Their pharmacology, safety, and clinical efficacy. Clin Haematol 13:75, 1983.
  An overview of the comparative pharmacology of synthetic colloids available in clinical practice.

Prough DS: Crystalloids versus colloids in the perioperative period. Anesthesiol Clin North Am 14:341, 1996.
An overview of the comparative role of crystalloids and colloids in surgical patients.

Smiley LE, Garvey MS: The use of hetastarch as adjunct therapy in 26 dogs with hypoalbuminemia. J Vet Intern Med 8:195, 1994.
A clinical study evaluating hydroxyethyl starch in a population of hypoalbuminemic dogs.

Management of Anorexia

SHERRY SANDERSON
St. Paul, Minnesota

JOSEPH W. BARTGES
Knoxville, Tennessee

CLINICAL IMPORTANCE

Anorexia is an abnormality characterized by partial or complete loss of appetite or aversion to food. Anorexia differs from satiety, which is a physiologic state produced by having a *specific need fulfilled,* in this instance hunger. Hunger, or the desire for food, is the opposite of satiety.

Anorexia is a frequently recognized, but all too often-ignored symptom. In people, rapid unintentional weight loss and low body weight are associated with increased morbidity and mortality. Many of the complications of anorexia that occur in human patients also occur in veterinary patients; thus, it is logical to postulate that ignoring anorexia in animals will have the same outcome. The point is that managing anorexia early during the course of various diseases often results in clinical improvement and shorter hospital stays.

Some clinicians choose to ignore anorexia in overweight patients because of an erroneous assumption that weight loss will benefit the patient. Ignoring anorexia in overweight patients is not advisable because obese patients, as well as thin ones, can become malnourished, lose lean body mass, and suffer deleterious results.

For many patients, anorexia may need to be addressed before the underlying cause can be detected and treated. In some patients, ignoring anorexia may be more detrimental to the patient than ignoring other manifestations of the underlying disorder. A conceptual understanding of the mechanisms and consequences of anorexia will enhance patient care and increase the likelihood of a successful outcome.

MECHANISMS

Voluntary consumption of food is controlled, in part, by centers in the central nervous system. Eating also involves an interplay of other mechanisms, including neurologic, hormonal, gastrointestinal, environmental, and sensory factors. Therefore, mechanisms that trigger the onset of anorexia may be complex. The numerous potential underlying causes of anorexia include psychological causes (e.g., stress, fear, or pain), and pathophysiologic causes such as degenerative, anatomic (oropharyngeal lesions and obstructions, etc.) metabolic, neurologic, neoplastic, infectious, inflammatory, and traumatic disorders. Anorexia can also be caused by drugs that cause nausea, delay gastric emptying, or alter the sense of smell and taste.

Influence of Neurotransmitters. Stimulation of the lateral hypothalamus causes hunger, whereas stimulation of the "satiety" center in the medial hypothalamus results in a diminished appetite (Morley, 1980). Disorders that reduce arousal of the "hunger" center or stimulate the "satiety" center may result in decreased food intake. For example, neurotransmitters, such as serotonin, inhibit appetite. Therefore, serotonin antagonists, such as cyproheptadine, are sometimes used to stimulate appetite. Other neurotransmitters, such as gamma-aminobutyric acid (GABA), also stimulate the hunger center or inhibit the satiety center. As a result, drugs that facilitate GABA activity and inhibit serotonin release, such as benzodiazepines, are sometimes used as appetite stimulants.

Influence of Hormones. Hormones often play a role in anorexia. For example, insulin has a negative effect on appetite. That is why insulin-deficient patients, such as diabetics, often have voracious appetites. In contrast, patients with too much insulin, such as those with insulinomas, may have suppressed appetites. Cortisol and thyroid hormones tend to stimulate appetite, providing a logical explanation of why dogs with hyperadrenocorticism and cats with hyperthyroidism often have voracious appetites.

Gastrointestinal Factors. Gastrointestinal (GI) stimulation may affect appetite by several hormonal and neural mechanisms. Nutrients in the GI tract stimulate vagal nerves, which in turn stimulate the satiety center. Nutrients in the GI tract also cause release of hormones, such as cholecystokinin, a strong inhibitor of appetite. In addition, gastric distention and rate of gastric emptying, as well as the nutrient content of the diet, all can influence appetite. For instance, in dogs, dietary fat, in addition to causing release of cholecystokinin, slows the rate of gastric emptying to a greater degree than does dietary protein or carbohydrate. This decreased gastric emptying often results in reduced food intake during a subsequent meal.

Environmental and Sensory Factors. Appetite is influenced by environmental and sensory factors, such as the texture, shape, and smell of food. Flavor preferences and nutrient preferences are also important and often vary between species. For example, dogs often like sweet flavors, but cats usually do not. Dogs also readily accept diets high in carbohydrates, whereas cats may not.

The appetite levels of dogs and cats may also be influenced by acquired behaviors. For instance, a dog that has been fed primarily human food may not readily accept dog food. Likewise, a cat given primarily dry food its entire life may be reluctant to eat canned food.

Food Aversion. Force-feeding diets to nauseated animals may lead to food aversions, which can create problems, especially if there are only a limited number of therapeutic diets available for treatment of the associated disorders. Even if a diet is not force-fed, occasionally the smell of food placed in front of a nauseated patient may contribute to food aversion. Therefore, withhold the diet designed for long-term use until the patient's appetite improves. Consider feeding the patient an alterative diet until the nausea is controlled.

EFFECTS OF ANOREXIA

Protein-energy malnutrition occurs in 25 to 60% of hospitalized human patients and is associated with increased morbidity and mortality. However, despite improvements in the recognition and treatment of malnutrition, protein-energy malnutrition often persists. In veterinary medicine, the malnourished patient often goes untreated because the signs of malnutrition are overlooked, and guidelines for nutritional support have not been stan-

dardized. For example, in one study, approximately 10% of dogs admitted to a teaching hospital were considered to have less than optimum body condition (Kronfeld et al, 1991).

Nutritional deprivation has adverse effects on the structure and function of nearly all the organs and systems of the body (Table 1). These changes may produce clinical disease or have a detrimental effect on concurrent illness (Remillard and Martin, 1990). For example, metabolic rate is increased and protein conservation is impaired. Increased metabolic rate and protein catabolism are approximately proportional to the severity of the insult. The neuroendocrine changes that occur include sympathetic nervous system activation; increased production of catecholamines, glucagon, and glucocorticoids; increased production of antidiuretic hormone; and activation of the renin-angiotensin-aldosterone system. These neuroendocrine changes can result in increased cardiac output, increased peripheral vascular resistance, relative insulin resistance, increased protein catabolism and nitrogen loss, increases in the mediators of inflammation, increased metabolic rate, and rapid development of malnutrition (see Table 1). The adverse consequences of protein-energy malnutrition include impaired cell-mediated and humoral immunity (Burkholder and Swecker, 1990); increased susceptibility to infection and shock; delayed wound and fracture healing (Remillard and Martin, 1990); increased wound dehiscence; poor tolerance to chemotherapy and radiation therapy; cardiac, skeletal, and smooth muscle weakness; and organ failure and death.

TREATMENT AND PREVENTION
Selection of Patients for Nutritional Support

Nutritional support should be initiated early during the management of anorexic patients to prevent malnutrition,

---

TABLE 1. Potential Adverse Effects of Inadequate Food Intake

Cardiac
 Decreased cardiac output
 Decreased ability to metabolize lactic acid
 Decreased heart weight
 Myofibrillar atrophy
 Electrophysiologic changes
  Sinus bradycardia
  Increased QT interval
  Decreased voltage of waves
Drug metabolism—altered:
 Drug absorption
 Protein binding
 Pharmacodynamics
 Metabolism
 Clearance
Gastrointestinal tract
 Prolonged gastric emptying
 Prolonged transit time
 Decreased gastric acid secretion
 Flattening of villi
 Decreased epithelial cell renewal
 Reduced absorptive area
 Inflammatory infiltration in wall
 Mucosal congestion and edema
 Carbohydrate and fat maldigestion
 Ileus

Hematologic
 Anemia
 Thrombocytopenia
 Leukopenia
Host defenses
 Impaired antibody synthesis
 Impaired interferon synthesis
 Low T-cell lymphocyte counts
 Decreased inflammatory response
 Decreased leukocyte function
 Decreased acute-phase proteins
 Decreased complement
 Inability to contain localized infections
Kidney
 Becomes a gluconeogenic organ
 Impaired response to acid-base changes
 Decreased glomerular filtration rate
 Decreased plasma flow rate
 Altered regulation of electrolytes
 Altered regulation of minerals
 Polyuria
Liver
 Lipid deposition
 Increased bromosulfophthalein
  retention time

Pancreas
 Atrophy and fibrosis
 Exocrine insufficiency
Pulmonary
 Reduced lung elasticity
 Decreased amount of secretions
 Increased viscosity of secretions
 Decreased respiratory rate
 Decreased tidal volume
 Susceptible to pneumonia
Skeletal muscle
 Decreased synthesis
 Increased degradation
 Increased fatiguability
Bone
 Osteoporosis
 Spontaneous fractures
Wound healing
 Decreased neovascularization
 Decreased collagen synthesis
 Decreased wound remodeling
 Decreased healing with edema

Modified and reprinted with permission from Bartges J: Nutritional support. In: Lipowitz AJ, Caywood DD, Newton CD, et al, eds: Complications in Small Animal Surgery. Baltimore: Williams & Wilkins, 1996, pp 35–72.

especially protein malnutrition. Unfortunately, there are no specific tests available that will consistently identify patients likely to benefit from nutritional supplementation. However, patients with any one or a combination of the following abnormalities should be considered for nutritional support (Carnevale et al, 1991).

Anorexia or Decreased Food Intake for at Least 3 Days. Many patients have been anorectic for at least 3 days at the time of their initial evaluation. In this situation, nutritional support should be considered even before the underlying cause of anorexia is ascertained. When possible, blood and urine samples for diagnostic tests should be collected prior to any form of therapy.

Loss of at Least 10% of Body Weight. Accurate body weights recorded during routine examination of patients serve as baseline data with which to compare weight loss during illness. If an accurate body weight prior to illness is not available, it is safer to assume that significant weight loss has occurred and to initiate nutritional support rather than to wait until a 10% weight loss can be verified. Weight and hydration status should also be monitored at least daily while the patient is hospitalized.

Decreased Serum Albumin Concentration. Serum proteins reflect the functional mass of internal organs. The evaluation of multiple serum proteins, including albumin, transferrin, prealbumin, and retinol-binding protein, provides the most accurate assessment of the patient's protein nutritional status. Unfortunately, with the exception of albumin, methods for measuring these other proteins are usually not readily available. Therefore, veterinarians must usually rely on serum albumin concentrations. Because serum albumin has a half-life of approximately 8 days in dogs, decreases in serum albumin concentration usually reflect chronic states of protein deficiency. Albumin concentrations of less than 2.5 g/dl in cats and less than 2.1 g/dl in dogs may indicate protein malnutrition (Carnevale et al, 1991). However, protein malnutrition may not be the only cause of hypoalbuminemia. Hypoalbuminemia can also occur as a result of hepatic diseases associated with impaired albumin synthesis, or protein-losing glomerulonephropathies and enteropathies associated with increased albumin loss.

Inadequate Muscle Mass or Diseases Associated With High Metabolic Demands. Inadequate muscle mass may result from inadequate caloric intake, or from diseases that impair protein synthesis, increase protein loss, or increase protein requirements. Some diseases, such as cancer or sepsis, are often associated with rapid loss of muscle mass and cachexia. Even if patients with these diseases are not anorectic, they often are unable to keep up with increased metabolic demands. Such patients often benefit from nutritional supplementation. Recording of body condition score as well as body weight during routine examination provides useful information.

Routes of Nutritional Support

The generally accepted rule to follow when one chooses between enteral and parenteral nutritional support is that *"if the gut works, use it."* Enterocytes rely on luminal substrates for at least 40% of their nutrition and rapidly atrophy when nutrition is supplied solely by the parenteral route. Enteral nutrition helps maintain the integrity of enterocytes and is physiologically superior to parenteral nutrition.

Appetite Stimulants. Pharmacologic appetite stimulants may be of value in partially anorectic patients for short periods. However, in our experience, pharmacologic appetite stimulants rarely are of long-term benefit. In addition, many appetite stimulants, such as glucocorticoids and benzodiazepines, have undesirable side effects. Although glucocorticoids may stimulate appetite, catabolic and immunosuppressive side effects may offset any benefits gained from their use. Benzodiazepines often cause drowsiness, making clinical evaluation of the patient's attitude difficult. In addition, diazepam has been associated with hepatitis in some cats. Although appetite stimulants may occasionally "jump-start" the appetite of anorectic patients, it is not advisable to depend solely on this type of therapy. If the patient does not respond to one appetite stimulant, we recommend the use of involuntary feeding methods, such as feeding tubes, for nutritional support.

Enteral Nutrition. Enteral nutrition is the cornerstone of nutritional support for most anorectic patients. Exceptions where parenteral nutritional support may be a better choice include patients with frequent vomiting, those lacking a gag reflex, or those which are comatose. The following sections summarize the available types of enteral feeding methods. Tables 2 to 4 summarize advantages, indications, contraindications, and complications. Numerous articles describe techniques of placing an indwelling

TABLE 2. Advantages of Different Types of Enteral Feeding Methods

Feeding Method	Invasive Procedure	Anesthesia or Sedation Required	Inexpensive	Type of Diets Used	Additional Advantages
Nasoesophageal or nasogastric tubes	No	No (a)	Yes	Liquid only	(b)
Esophagostomy tubes	Yes	Yes	Yes	Liquid or gruel	(b)
Gastrostomy tubes	Yes	Yes	No	Liquid or gruel	(b), (c), (d), (e)
Jejunostomy tubes	Yes	Yes	No	Liquid only	(b), (f)

(a), advantageous in patients that are high anesthetic risks or in critically ill patients prior to more invasive procedures; (b), can be used to administer liquid medications; (c), can be used to administer ground-up tablet medications; (d), can be kept in place for up to a year without the need for replacement; (e), advantageous in patients where head needs to be bypassed (e.g., facial trauma); (f), advantageous in patients where stomach lacks persistaltic activity.

TABLE 3. Indications and Contraindications for Use of Different Enteral Feeding Methods

Feeding Method	Frequent Vomiting	Lack of Gag Reflex	Esophageal Motility Disorders	Comatose Patients	Additional Contraindications
Nasoesophageal or nasogastric tubes	Avoid	Avoid	Avoid	Avoid	(a)
Esophagostomy tubes	Avoid	Avoid	Avoid	Avoid	(b)
Gastrostomy tubes	Avoid	Avoid	OK (f)	Avoid	(b), (c)
Jejunostomy tubes	OK	OK	OK	OK	(b), (d), (e)

(a), severe facial or head trauma; (b), patients that are poor anesthestic risks; (c), animals with ascites or peritonitis (nonsurgical); (d), caution should be used in patients with peritonitis (closed abdomen) or ascites; (e), contraindicated in patients with severe underlying intestinal pathology and impaired intestinal healing; (f), occasionally dogs with megaesophagus will continue to regurgitate with gastrostomy tubes.

feeding tube (Crowe, 1990; Bright, 1992; Fulton and Dennis, 1992).

Repeated Orogastric Intubation. Repeated intubation of patients for feeding is often associated with significant stress to the patient, and increased chances of complications, such as incorrect tube placement, esophageal trauma, and aspiration pneumonia. Superior and less stressful methods for enteral feeding are available; thus, we do not recommend intubation for long-term management of anorexia. Providing nutrition to orphaned neonates is an exception to this generality.

Nasoesophageal or Nasogastric Tubes. Nasoesophageal and nasogastric tubes do not require sophisticated equipment. They are easy to place and well tolerated by most patients. We prefer to keep the far end of the tube in the distal esophagus, rather than in the stomach. Occasionally when the tube passes through the esphagogastric junction, gastric reflux along the tube causes esophagitis.

Esophagostomy Tubes. Placement of esophagostomy tubes is slightly more invasive and difficult than that of nasoesophageal or nasogastric tubes. However, in circumstances when a gastrostomy tube is not an option, such as in patients with facial trauma, esophagostomy tubes are a good alternative.

Gastrostomy Tubes. The ease of placing gastrostomy tubes has improved dramatically in the last decade. Originally, placement of gastrostomy tubes required a celiotomy. Subsequently, an endoscopic technique for the placement of percutaneous gastrostomy tubes was developed, eliminating the need for surgery. Recently, a comparatively inexpensive Eld gastrostomy tube applicator (Jorgensen Laboratories, Inc., 1-800-525-5614) has been developed that allows percutaneous gastrostomy tube placement without the need for endoscopy (see Section 8).

Once a gastrostomy tube is in place, even if the patient begins to voluntarily eat, it should not be removed for a minimum of 7 to 10 days to allow sufficient time for a fibrin seal to form between the stomach and the abdominal wall. Removing a tube prematurely may allow gastric contents to leak into the abdomen.

Jejunostomy Tubes. Jejunostomy tubes are used primarily to bypass the upper portion of the intestinal tract. Indications include poor stomach motility accompanied by satisfactory small intestinal function, such as occurs following surgical correction of gastric dilatation and volvulus. These tubes can also be used in patients with high intestinal resections, esophageal strictures, pancreatic abscesses, and peritonitis (open abdomen). We have also used jejunostomy tubes in patients with megaesophagus that continue to regurgitate frequently with gastrostomy tube feeding.

Because jejunostomy tubes bypass the stomach, small, frequent feedings or continuous slow feedings are needed to meet caloric requirements. In addition, only liquid diets can be used through the tube. Like gastrostomy tubes, enteral feeding tubes should not be removed for a minimum of 7 to 10 days.

Parenteral Nutrition. In patients in which enteral nutrition is not an option, parenteral nutrition should be considered for nutritional support. Indications for parenteral nutrition include (1) protracted vomiting or diarrhea, such as in puppies with parvoviral enteritis, and (2) pancreatitis. Parenteral nutrition is also useful in patients with intestinal ileus, those with massive bowel resection, and those that are comatose. Parenteral nutrition is useful in patients

TABLE 4. Complications Associated With Different Types of Enteral Feeding Methods

Feeding Method	Aspiration Pneumonia	Esophagitis or Stricture	Vomiting	Tube Extraction or Migration	Additional Complications
Nasoesophageal or nasogastric tubes	Yes	Yes	Yes	Yes	(a), (b), (c)
Esophagostomy tubes	Yes	Yes	Yes	Yes	(b), (d)
Gastrostomy tubes	Uncommon	Uncommon	Yes	Yes	(d), (e), (f), (g)
Jejunostomy tubes	Uncommon	Unlikely	Unlikely	Yes	(b), (d), (h), (i), (j), (k), (l)

(a), dacryocystitis; (b), tube clogging; (c), epistaxis; (d), peristomal infections; (e), splenic laceration (percutaneously placed); (f), pneumoperitoneum; (g), gastric hemorrhage; (h), diarrhea and vomiting from feeding too rapidly or using feeding formulas that are too concentrated; (i), hyperglycemia and electrolyte disturbances; (j), hypoglycemia if feedings are discontinued too rapidly; (k), tip of tube can perforate small intestine; (l), leakage of intestinal fluid into peritoneum.

maintained on artificial ventilation where the seriousness of the underlying disease prohibits anesthesia, or lack of sufficient esophageal and intestinal motility increases the risk of aspiration pneumonia with enteral nutrition support.

Total Parenteral Nutrition. The prototypical total parenteral nutrition (TPN) solution consists of 50% dextrose, 8.5 to 10% amino acids combined with electrolytes, 20% lipid, and vitamins and minerals. The amount of each component selected for use depends on the patient's underlying disease and nutritional status. (For specific TPN solutions used, see page 80).

Asepsis is essential when one prepares TPN solutions. The lipid emulsion should not be mixed directly with the dextrose solution because precipitation may occur. An effective memory aid for the order in which TPN components should be added is to add and mix them alphabetically. Mix the Amino acid solution with the Dextrose first, and then add the Lipid solution to this mixture.

All TPN solutions containing dextrose are hypertonic and must be administered through a central venous catheter. Administering TPN solutions through peripheral catheters is not advised because of the risk of phlebitis and thrombosis. The central venous catheter used for TPN administration should be dedicated only to that purpose. Drawing blood samples or administering medications concurrently through a catheter used for TPN increases the risk of bacterial contamination or thrombosis. TPN requires close monitoring; thus, it should be limited to clinics where 24-hour care is available.

If TPN solutions do not meet the patient's fluid requirements, they should be supplemented with parenteral fluids. TPN is usually started at 50% of the total calculated caloric rate for the first 12 hours. During this time, the patient should be monitored for hyperglycemia, hyperlipidemia, and azotemia. If these abnormalities do not develop, TPN can be administered at the full calculated rate. If hyperlipidemia occurs, reduce the amount of lipid solution in the formulation.

TPN solutions containing dextrose increase endogenous insulin production; however, if hyperglycemia occurs, low doses of insulin may be necessary to control blood sugar. When TPN is no longer required, stop insulin and gradually decrease the rate of administration over 12 hours. Rebound hypoglycemia may occur if TPN is discontinued abruptly.

Body weight, packed cell volume, total plasma protein, and blood glucose concentrations should be evaluated daily during TPN. The concentrations of serum electrolytes, blood urea nitrogen, and creatinine should be monitored at least every 48 hours, and a complete serum chemistry profile and complete blood cell count should be evaluated every 1 to 2 weeks.

Partial Parenteral Nutrition. We occasionally use partial parenteral solutions containing only amino acid solutions with electrolytes in puppies with parvoviral enteritis which are too small to readily accept a jugular catheter or other central line. Administering amino acid solutions to such patients helps minimize protein malnutrition. The amino acid solutions with electrolytes are usually isotonic or only slightly hyperosmotic and therefore can be administered through a peripheral vein. Partial parenteral nutrition may also be used temporarily in patients with severe intestinal malabsorption as a supplement to enteral nutrition.

CALCULATION OF NUTRIENT REQUIREMENTS

Fluid Requirements. For enteral nutrition, fluid is provided as premade liquid diets or added to canned pet foods to make a gruel. During parenteral nutrition, supplemental fluids are usually given intravenously. Dogs and cats require approximately 50 to 100 ml of water/kg body weight for daily maintenance. The daily fluid requirement is influenced by body surface area, environmental temperature, type of food, renal function, and level of activity. Normal daily fluid requirements are approximately equal to daily caloric requirements. The fluid intake of animals affected with diseases associated with polyuria or excessive blood loss into body cavities or through wounds is greater than what would be normally calculated. Abrupt changes in body weight usually reflect hydration status.

Energy Requirements. At a minimum, patients should receive sufficient calories to meet resting energy requirements (RER). This value may be calculated from the following equations: (1) $RER = 70(BWkg)^{0.75}$; or (2) $RER = 30(BWkg) + 70$, where BWkg is the body weight in kilograms. The expression $(Bwkg)^{0.75}$ may be readily calculated by using the Yx function key on most calculators.

During convalescence from illness or injury, the patient's energy requirement for maintenance of body weight is calculated from the RER. Numerous reports of critically ill human beings indicate that resting metabolic rates are higher than RER. For example, RER increases by 25 to 35% following surgery; 35 to 50% with trauma or cancer; 50 to 70% with sepsis; and 70 to 100% or more with major burns or head trauma.

The energy requirements of critically ill humans rarely approach normal maintenance energy requirements. Evidently, a reduction in physical activity due to illness or injury partially offsets the associated hypermetabolism. Based on data derived from human patients, various factors have been suggested for estimating the energy requirements of ill or injured animals (Lewis et al, 1987). A practical alternative to the use of complex factoring systems is to multiply the RER by a factor of 1.5 for dogs and 1.4 or 1.5 for cats for most situations.

Protein Requirements. Protein requirements during illness and injury vary. The variables include dietary energy content, dietary protein quantity and quality, species differences, individual patient differences, life stage, and type, degree, and stage of injury or illness. Unless renal or hepatic function is compromised, the levels of dietary protein should meet or exceed maintenance protein requirements. For maintenance, diets should provide a minimum of 4 gm of protein/100 kcal of metabolizable energy for dogs, and 6 gm of protein/100 kcal of metabolizable energy for cats. Protein sources of high biologic value should be used so that smaller quantities may be fed to an anorectic patient.

Special importance has been ascribed to the metabolism of specific amino acids in nutritional support. Arginine, an essential amino acid for dogs and cats, promotes wound healing, immune function, and a positive nitrogen balance. Glutamine is a principal nutrient for enterocytes and is important in nitrogen metabolism. Branched-chain amino acids (valine, leucine, and isoleucine) decrease trauma- and sepsis-induced muscle catabolism and improve nitrogen retention. Taurine, an essential sulfur-containing beta-amino acid for cats, helps maintain cardiac function. Carnitine plays an essential role in fatty acid metabolism.

Other Nutrient Requirements. The vitamin and mineral status of critically ill patients has not been extensively evaluated in animals, although deficiencies have been observed. One study of humans with a variety of illnesses revealed that micronutrient deficiency occurred in 64% of patients (Mobarhan et al, 1984). The use of balanced pet foods should provide adequate levels of micronutrients (see page 136). However, human enteral products may not provide adequate levels of nutrients for different species of animals. They should be supplemented with specific nutrients if a deficiency is present (e.g., taurine supplementation in cats, potassium supplementation if hypokalemia is present, iron supplementation if iron deficiency is present).

References and Suggested Reading

Bright RM: Percutaneous endoscopic gastrostomy (PEG) for nutritional support of the small animal patient. Waltham Int Focus 2:2, 1992.
Burkholder WJ, Swecker WS: Nutritional influences on immunity. Semin Vet Med Surg (Small Anim) 5:154, 1990.
Carnevale JM, Kallfelz FA, Chapman G, et al: Nutritional assessment: Guidelines to selecting patients for nutritional support. Compendium 13:255, 1991.
A practical guide for selecting patients that will benefit from nutritional support.
Crowe DT: Nutritional support for the hospitalized patient: An introduction to tube feeding. Compendium 12:1711, 1990.
Fulton RB Jr, Dennis JS: Blind percutaneous placement of a gastrostomy tube for nutritional support in dogs and cats. JAVMA 201:697, 1992.
Discusses percutaneous placement of gastrotomy tubes without the need for an endoscope.
Kronfeld DS, Donoghue S, Glickman LT: Body condition and energy intakes of dogs in a referral teaching hospital. J Nutr 121:S157, 1991.
Lewis LD, Morris MD Jr, Hand MS: Small Animal Clinical Nutrition III. Topeka, KS: Mark Morris Associates, 1987, pp 5-1 to 5-43.
Macy DW, Ralston SL: Cause and control of decreased appetite. In: Kirk RW, ed: Current Veterinary Therapy X. Philadelphia: WB Saunders, 1989, p 18.
Mobarhan S, Maiani G, Gerro-Luzzi A: Determinants of nutritional status in hospital patients in Italy. J Parenter Enter Nutr 11:122S, 1984.
Morley JE: The neuroendocrine control of appetite: The role of the endogenous opiates, cholecystokinin, TRH, gamma-amino-butyric-acid and the diazepam receptor. Life Sci 27:355, 1980.
A concise overview of appetite regulation by the hypothalamus and the interrelationships of the monoamines and peptides.
Remillard RL, Martin RA: Nutritional support in the surgical patient. Semin Vet Med Surg (Small Anim) 5:197, 1990.

Nutritional Assessment of Pet Food Labels

RICHARD D. KEALY

AVI DESHMUKH

St. Louis, Missouri

The label on a pet food product contains valuable information that helps the buyer assess its nutritional quality. In the following discussion, pet food label requirements and their relation to nutrition are categorized as follows: guaranteed analyses, ingredient statements, nutritional adequacy, feeding guidelines, calorie statement, and product names.

GUARANTEED ANALYSES

Regulations established by the Association of American Feed Control Officials (AAFCO) require that a pet food label contain guarantees for crude protein% (minimum), crude fat% (minimum), crude fiber% (maximum), and moisture% (maximum). Other nutrients included in AAFCO's nutrient profile may be added at the manufacturer's discretion and should follow the moisture guarantee. All chemical analysis procedures used to document nutrient levels can be found in the Association of Official Analytical Chemists handbook.

The moisture guarantee on the pet food label provides an upper limit for percentage of water in a product. Dry, extruded pet foods contain less than 20% moisture; semi-moist pet foods contain 20 to 50% moisture; canned pet foods contain 50% moisture or more. Most moisture analyses utilize oven drying techniques. However, sometimes oven drying volatiles are released, resulting in erroneously high moisture measurements. When this phenomenon occurs, a titration method may be used to obtain more accurate results. Any product containing in excess of 12% moisture is vulnerable to microbial degradation. Preservatives or special packaging must be used for products containing in excess of 12% moisture.

To compare nutrient levels in different types of diets, it is necessary to standardize the base of comparison. One method is to use dry matter conversion. The formula for converting nutrients in a pet food diet to dry matter (DM) equivalence is as follows:

$$\text{DM basis} = \frac{\% \text{ Nutrient}}{\% \text{ Dry matter}} \times 100$$

TABLE 1. Comparing Nutrients on a Dry Matter (DM) and an Energy Basis

Nutrient	Guaranteed Analysis on Label (as fed basis)	Moisture Adjusted Guarantees (DM basis)	Energy Adjusted Guarantees (DM)	AAFCO Profile (DM)	Energy Adjusted Guarantees vs. AAFCO
Crude protein	8%	32%	26%	22%	OK
Moisture	75%	—	—	—	—
Calcium	0.25%	0.8%	0.65%	1.0%	Low
ME (kcal/kg)	1,070	4,300	3,500	3,500	—

Since the direct measurement of protein in pet foods is impractical, nitrogen is measured and the result is referred to as "crude protein." The amount of nitrogen is multiplied by a factor of 6.25 to obtain "percent crude protein." Proteins found in foodstuffs contain approximately 16% nitrogen, which, divided into 100, yields the factor of 6.25. Since many foodstuff proteins vary from 15 to 19% nitrogen, this factor represents only an estimate of the protein present and assumes that all nitrogen present is proteinaceous.

Among others, crude protein is used as a commodity trading index and is also used by state feed control officials in feed law compliance control. Crude protein is not a reliable measure of protein quality in pet food. The best assessment of protein quality is obtained by relating the quantities of dietary essential amino acids in the specific pet food to the pet's requirement for those amino acids. Most reliable pet food companies provide essential amino acid values for the various pet foods they manufacture. Nutrient profiles of canine and feline foods, including amino acids, can be found in the AAFCO Handbook (1996) and in the Appendix.

Crude fat includes all lipid material in a foodstuff. It is measured by a quantitative procedure that gives no information as to the types of lipids or fatty acids present. The ether extraction method and the acid hydrolysis method are two recognized methods for determining crude fat content. The ether extract method uses petroleum ether to extract fats and oils from the foodstuff. The acid hydrolysis procedure involves hydrolysis of the food sample with dilute hydrochloric acid to free bound fats and oils and then extracts the sample with ether to remove lipid. Neither method gives an estimate of nutritionally essential fatty acids. However, this information is made available by most pet food companies.

Crude fiber includes cellulose and other complex polysaccharides. It is determined by an acid-alkali extraction procedure that removes protein, sugars, and starch (moisture and minerals are removed in separate steps). The

procedure was developed primarily for roughages and probably is not a good estimate of the quality of the fibrous material in a pet food.

The label of a dog or cat food may bear a statement about calorie content. Calories are listed separately from the guaranteed analyses and must be listed in kilocalories of metabolizable energy (ME) per kilogram of diet. Expression in other units is an option. Calorie content may be determined by calculation or by an official animal testing procedure. Determination of the calories in pet foods will be discussed below.

Many canned products are high in energy and fat content. As the guaranteed analysis on the label is provided on an "as fed" basis, the values for crude protein, crude fat, crude fiber, and energy do not look very high because of the high moisture content (about 75%). Therefore, it becomes important to convert these values to DM and energy (3,500 kcal/kg for dogs and 4,000 kcal/kg for cats) bases and compare them to the AAFCO's nutrient profile. The AAFCO's nutrient profile for dogs is based on ME of 3,500 kcal/kg of food and for cats is 4,000 kcal/kg of food.

This conversion based on DM and ME becomes more important when products of different moisture and energy levels are compared. Table 1 illustrates the importance of such conversions.

If the benefits of nutrients are illustrated on the label, those nutrients must be guaranteed in the guaranteed analysis. Figure 1 illustrates the concept.

INGREDIENT STATEMENT

The ingredient list on a pet food provides an indication of ingredient quantity and, in some cases, an estimate of ingredient quality. All ingredients are required to be listed on the pet food package in descending order of their contribution by weight. A manufacturer must list an ingredient even if is not added directly but comes as a part of another ingredient; for example, animal fat preserved with BHA (butylated hydroxyanisole). Specific nomenclature for

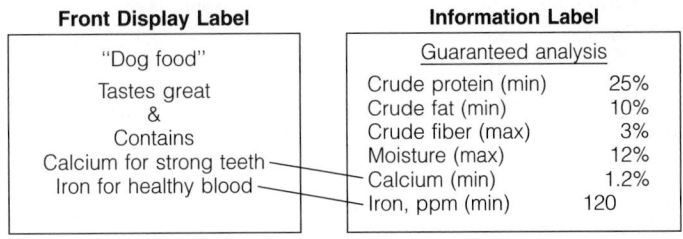

Figure 1. Nutrient benefits and guaranteed analysis relationship.

TABLE 2. Ingredient Comparison

This Ingredient*	Is Not the Same As	This Ingredient
Chicken	is not same as	Chicken meal
Chicken	is not same as	Chicken by-products meal
Chicken	is not same as	Chicken by-products
Chicken meal	is not same as	Chicken by-products meal
Chicken by-products	is not same as	Chicken by-products meal

*This concept also applies for other products of animal origin, such as beef, lamb, poultry, and fish.

pet food ingredients is defined by AAFCO regulations and the terms are listed in the AAFCO Handbook. For example poultry by-product meal and poultry by-products have specific definitions that dictate their usage on a pet food label. No reference to the *quality* of an ingredient is allowed in the ingredient list (e.g., chicken instead of pure chicken). When water is an integral part of the pet food formula, as in canned or semimoist foods, it must be listed as "water sufficient for processing." The first 5 to 10 ingredients in the list usually indicate the ingredients that constitute the greatest percentage of pet food formulas. The last 5 to 10 ingredients in the list generally represent micronutrients in the formula at levels of parts per million.

PRODUCT NAMES

The names of ingredients contained in the ingredient list become more critical when the product names are derived from the ingredients (Table 2). The names of the ingredients in the product name also tell the approximate percentage of the ingredient or ingredients in the product (Fig. 2).

NUTRITIONAL ADEQUACY

The Nutritional Adequacy Statement (NAS) informs consumers of the appropriateness of the product for a pet's life stage; for example, a "Complete and Balanced" pet food, without a specific life-stage qualifier, is assumed to be appropriate for growth, gestation and lactation, and adult maintenance (i.e., all life stages). A food that is "100% Complete and Balanced for Adult Dogs" conveys a message that the food is suitable for adult dogs; it may *not* be suitable for puppies and gestating or lactating females.

Nutritional Adequacy Statements

A product claiming to be complete and balanced for a pet's life stage is required to provide a nutritional adequacy statement. Pet food products that claim to be snacks or treats, those intended to be fed intermittently, or veterinary

---

All Beef Food for Dogs
Complete & Balanced
Tastes great

This product should contain *only* beef, preservatives, vitamins and minerals, etc. (Such names are found in canned products only)

Beef & Chicken for Cats
Complete & balanced
for adult cats
No artificial preservatives

This product should contain 95% beef & chicken. The chicken part should contain at least 3%; other ingredients are vitamins, minerals, etc. (Such names are found in canned products only)

Chicken & Rice Formula
Dog food
Delicious food
Complete & Balanced

This product contains a minimum of 25% chicken and rice. Rice makes up at least 3%. Other descriptors are dinner, supper, etc.

"With Beef"
Puppy food
Complete & balanced for puppies

This product contains a minimum of 3% beef.

Gourmet Cat Food
With Fish & Cheese
Complete & balanced
Eye-pleasing colors

This food contains a minimum of 3% fish and 3% cheese.

Cat Treats
Beef Flavored
Give to your cats as reward
Fun-shaped pieces

This food has to have a source of beef present. There is no requirement for minimum percentage of beef.

Figure 2. Approximate percentages of ingredients relative to product name.

medical foods need not bear such a nutrition adequacy statement on the label. However, some companies substantiate the nutritional adequacy of the veterinary medical foods by feeding trials. Therefore, they prefer to put the appropriate nutritional adequacy statements on the labels.

A nutrition adequacy statement on a complete and balanced dog food is often found (1) in an abbreviated form on the front display panel of the package (as shown in Figure 2), and (2) on the information portion (usually the side or back panel). The nutritional adequacy statement is generally presented in one of two different formats. The first format involves a statement that does not require animal testing: (1) "Barkies Dog Food" is formulated to meet the nutritional needs established by AAFCO dog food profiles for growth, gestation and lactation, maintenance, or "all life stages." This type of statement indicates that the stated product meets the minimum AAFCO nutrient profile by calculation, and that no animal studies were performed. The second format is a statement that does require animal testing: (2) Animal feeding tests using AAFCO procedures substantiate that "Barkies Dog Food" provides complete and balanced nutrition for growth, gestation and lactation, maintenance, or "all life stages." This type of statement indicates that the product's nutritional adequacy was established by animal studies according to AAFCO feeding trial protocols.

Manufacturers may conduct feeding studies according to the AAFCO protocol and apply claims, as mentioned in point 2 above, to products that are nutritionally similar or higher in nutrient levels, digestibility, and so forth.

Calorie Statement

Animals tend to eat to satisfy their energy needs. It is important for veterinarians and consumers to know the energy density of the diet because in balanced diets all required nutrients are usually based on the energy density of the diet. For example, AAFCO's nutrient profiles of dog foods are based on an energy density of 3,500 kcal ME/kg. If the energy density of the dog food exceeds 4,000 kcal/kg, the nutrients in the diet must be increased accordingly. However, if the diets are formulated to an energy density lower than 3,500 kcal ME/kg, nutrient levels in the diet should *not* be adjusted. Overfeeding of energy-dense diets may result in obesity. Information about the energy density of products helps veterinarians recommend diets and daily food amounts based on the specific caloric needs of the animals and thus helps avoid problems like obesity or undernutrition.

The energy on pet food labels is expressed as metabolizable energy (ME) and can be determined either by calculation or by conducting metabolic trials. Calculation of ME based on the "modified Atwater" formula is as follows:

$$ME \text{ (kcal/kg)} = 10[(3.5 \times \% \text{ Crude protein as fed}) + (8.5 \times \% \text{ Crude fat as fed}) + (3.5 \times \% \text{ Nitrogen free extract as fed})]$$

$$(\text{where } \% \text{ Nitrogen free extract} = 100 - [\% \text{ Crude protein} + \% \text{ Crude fat} + \% \text{ Crude fiber} + \% \text{ Ash} + \% \text{ Moisture}])$$

The percentages of crude protein and crude fat are arithmetic averages from proximate analyses of at least four production batches (AAFCO, 1995). Calculation of ME based on metabolic trials is described in detail on page 139 in AAFCO's 1996 publication.

ME Information on the Label

Listing the ME value of the product on the label is *voluntary*; a manufacturer is not legally required to provide the ME value on the label except for products that are "light" or "reduced calories" in nature. If the ME is determined by the calculation method, it must be declared as "Calculated Metabolizable Energy." If the ME is determined by metabolic trial, no such designation is needed. However, if the ME is determined by metabolic trial, it must not exceed or understate the calculated ME by more than 15%.

If the ME value of the product is included as part of the label, it must not be part of the guaranteed analysis (Fig. 3). There is no fixed place on the label where you can locate the ME value. However, if the ME information is given on the label, it must be under the heading of "Calorie Content." It is required that the ME value must be given as "ME: Kcal/kg." ME in other units, such as kcal/pound or kcal/cup, may follow.

DESCRIPTIVE TERMS

Reduced Calorie Diets

In August 1996, AAFCO approved the adoption of terms such "Lite or Light," "Lean or Low Fat," and "Reduced Fat or Reduced Calories." These terms are comparative in nature and carry a specific message to consumers (Table 3 and Fig. 4). Absolute values in calories for

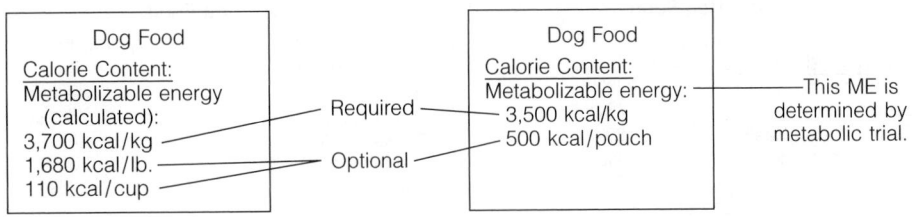

Figure 3. Examples of how ME values appear on labels.

TABLE 3. **Calories and Fat Levels in "Light or Lite" and "Lean" Dog and Cat Food Products**

	% Moisture (in Food)		
	20 or Less (Dry)	20–65 (Soft-Moist)	65 or More (Canned)
Light/lite (kcal/kg)			
Dog food	3,100	2,500	900
Cat food	3,250	2,650	950
(The label must bear "calorie content" statement)			
Lean/low fat (% fat)			
Dog food	9.0	7.0	4.0
Cat food	10.0	8.0	5.0
(The label must bear a guarantee for "maximum fat%" in guaranteed analysis)			

terms like "Light/Lite" reflect approximate percentage (15% for dogs and 10% for cats) reduction in calories relative to the average calories found for the products on the market under each category. Products bearing these claims should state the percentage reduction and the product of comparison. On adoption by the individual states, these regulations will assure consumers that a dry "Light Dog Food" will contain no more than 3,100 kcal ME/kg, rather than some arbitrary reduction from a product containing higher calories.

Feeding directions in "Light and Reduced Calorie" or similar products should reflect a reduction in calorie intake consistent with the intended use; that is, by feeding the recommended amount, animals should either lose or maintain body weight.

Natural Pet Foods

Often, pet foods come with the descriptor "Natural." The word "Natural" on the pet food label indicates that it does not contain synthetic or chemically altered ingredients (except vitamins or minerals) and chemical preservatives. The term "Natural" does not mean that the ingredients used in the product are of better quality or organically grown or have a special nutritional value.

When the descriptor "Natural" is used on a pet food label, it must be juxtaposed with words like "Fortified with Vitamins and Minerals." See Figure 5.

Feeding Directions

AAFCO regulations require that the product label of a complete and balanced dog or cat food must provide feeding directions. These instructions should be expressed in common terms such as weight or units of food per unit of body weight per day (e.g., 3 cups per 50 lb. body weight per day). Feeding directions are an important part of the information that instructs the veterinarians and consumers about daily food intake. Feeding directions on the label should be viewed *only* as guidelines and not as *absolute* directions.

Food intake is dependent on environment, breed, age, reproductive status, temperament, activity, and other factors. The recommended amount of food should be adjusted to these factors. Manufacturers generally tend to *overestimate* the recommended amount of food to avoid undernutrition and to cover individual animal variations.

Calorie statements on pet food labels serve as good information to determine the amount of food needed based on energy needs. Frequently pet food manufacturers will provide calorie charts upon request to help in proper feeding of dogs and cats.

Products such as dog and cat treats to be fed intermittently, and veterinary medical foods need not have feeding directions. However, for veterinary medical foods, veterinarians must be provided with information about intended use, indications, contra-indications, amount to be fed, and so forth.

Health Claims

Pet food labels also contain various claims including health claims. Claims pertaining to nutrients like "Contains Calcium and Phosphorus for strong bones and teeth," "Iron for healthy blood" are considered to be functional claims, and not health claims. A pet food claiming to be "Health Food" has no special significance. Any pet food which is

---

XYZ Light Dry Dog Food
Calorie Content: 3,100 kcal ME/kg

ABC Dry Dog Food
25% less calories than ABC Original Dry Dog Food
Calorie Content: 3,300 kcal ME/kg

XYZ Lean Dry Dog Food	
Guaranteed Analysis	
Crude protein (min)	22%
Crude fat (min)	7%
Crude fat% (max)	**8%**
Crude fiber (max)	3%
Moisture (max)	12%

ABC Dry Dog Food	
25% less fat than ABC Original Dry Dog Food	
Guaranteed Analysis	
Crude protein (min)	22%
Crude fat (min)	8%
Crude fat (max)	**9%**
Crude fiber (max)	3%
Moisture (max)	12%

Figure 4. Examples of pet food labels with descriptive terms.

Front Display Panel

Lamb & Rice Formula
(product names, indicates that lamb & rice make up as much as 25% of product, and
rice makes up at least 3%)

NATURAL
Fortified with Vitamins & Minerals
(indicates that chemically altered/synthesized ingredients
[except vitamins and minerals], and chemical preservatives are <u>not</u> used in the product)

Light Dry Dog Food
(indicates that the food contains ME less than 3,150 kcal/kg)

Complete & Balanced
(indicates that it is appropriate for growth,
gestation and lactation, and adult maintenance)

Helps Maintain Urinary Tract Health by:—
(health claim)

Figure 5. Important information on the front display panel of pet food labels from which the nutritional assessment of the pet food can be made.

Information Panel

Feeding Guidelines:
Recommended daily feeding amounts (8 oz cup) for adult dogs

Body Wt (lb)	3–12	13–20	21–50	51–100	Over 100
Cups	⅓–	1¼–	1¾–	3½–	6 plus ⅔
	1¼	1¾	3½	6	cup for each 10 lb
					over 100 lb

Puppy feeding instructions: Feed pups moistened food, all they can consume. As
puppies grow older offer them dry food. Avoid overweight problems in puppies.
Gestating and lactating females: This products provides all the nutrition needed by
gestating and lactating females. Food intake may double or quadruple during lactation.

Guaranteed Analysis:
Crude protein (min)   22%
Crude fat (min)   10%
Crude fiber (max)   3%
Moisture (max)   12%
Calcium (Ca) (min)   1.2%
Linoleic acid (min)   1.5%

Ingredient Statement
Lamb, rice, corn, wheat flour, poultry byproducts, ... vitamins and minerals

Nutritional Adequacy Statement:
Animal feeding tests using the AAFCO procedures substantiate that this product
provides complete and balanced nutrition for all life stages.

Caloric Statement (optional):
  Calorie Content:
  Metabolizable energy
  (calculated):
  3,700 kcal/kg
  1,680 kcal/lb
  110 kcal/cup

Figure 6. Important information on the information panel of pet food labels from which the nutritional assessment of the pet food can be made.

complete and balanced is a "Health Food." However, claims about maintaining urinary tract health or urine pH in cat foods are considered to be health claims and need prior review by the FDA-Center of Veterinary Medicine (CVM). Health claims are more commonly found in advertisements and brochures, but less commonly on pet food labels. When in doubt, check the validity of such claims with the State's Agriculture Department, or State Chemist's office, or the FDA-CVM.

Label Panels

Pet food labels contain significant nutritional information that is based on government and industry standards.

Information provided by the front display and the information panels can be useful in evaluating pet foods. A summary of the information printed on pet food labels from which a nutritional assessment can be made is presented in Figures 5 and 6.

References and Suggested Reading

Official Methods of Analysis of the AOAC, 16th ed. AOAC International, Gathersburg, MD: 1995.
Official Publication of Association of American Feed Control Officials. (Treasurer, Charles Frank). Atlanta: Georgia Department of Agriculture, 1996. (This publication can be purchased at this address.)

Parenteral Nutrition Products

CHERYL C. MILLER
Athens, Georgia

JOSEPH W. BARTGES
Knoxville, Tennessee

The decision whether to administer nutritional support orally, enterally, or parenterally to a patient is typically based on gastrointestinal tract function, as described in the previous article. In cases where the gastrointestinal tract is dysfunctional or oral nutrition is either impractical or insufficient, parenteral nutrients should be given. Supplying calories and amino acids through parenteral nutrition can correct malnourishment (Shizgal, 1993). However, parenteral nutritional support is labor intensive and time consuming and requires a strong commitment from both the veterinarian and the owner. Mechanical and metabolic complications are frequent (Bartges, 1996) and patients must be monitored closely while receiving nutritional support.

Once a decision has been made to utilize parenteral nutrition, nutrient requirements must be determined and product choices made. It is often advisable to begin with products from one manufacturer, because of incompatibility between products from different manufacturers (Bartges, 1996). Commercially available products include dextrose (glucose) solutions, crystalline amino acid solutions (with or without electrolytes), lipid emulsions, multivitamin supplements, and mineral supplements. Parenteral solutions, available in varying concentrations, should be individualized to the specific needs of each patient. Because dextrose solutions having concentrations greater than 7.7% (Table 1) and amino acid solutions having concentrations greater than 4.25% (Table 2) are hyperosmotic, they should be administered via a central vein, such as the cranial or caudal vena cava. Amino acid solutions range in concentration from 3.5 to 10% and are considered to be completely bioavailable. They are supplied with electrolytes, may be

compounded with crystalloid solutions (Table 3), or may be mixed with potassium, phosphorus, calcium, or sodium bicarbonate. Specialized amino acid formulations are also available for patients with renal dysfunction or hepatic dysfunction or that have sustained severe trauma.

Lipid emulsions (Table 4) are iso-osmotic and may be delivered via peripheral or central veins. They are available in 10 and 20% concentrations and provide energy along with dextrose solutions. Lipid emulsions prepared from soybean or safflower oil provide a mixture of neutral triglycerides, which are mainly unsaturated fatty acids. When hyperosmolar syndrome or glycosuria occurs as a result of rapid administration of hyperosmolar dextrose solutions, the lipid-to-dextrose ratio may be increased. Thus, energy requirements may be met, and hyperosmolar complications associated with altered dextrose metabolism can be mini-

TABLE 1. Parenteral Glucose Solutions

Glucose Concentration (%)	Caloric Content (kcal/L)	Osmolarity (mOsm/L)
5.0	170	253
7.7	262	388
10.0	340	505
20.0	680	1,010
30.0	1,020	1,515
40.0	1,360	2,020
50.0	1,700	2,525
60.0	2,040	3,030
70.0	2,380	3,535
100.0	3,400	5,050

TABLE 2. **Composition of Selected Parenteral Crystalline Amino Acid Solutions**

Product	Manufacturer	Total AA (gm/100 mL)	BCAA (% of total)	Osmolarity (mOsm/L)	Sodium (mEq/L)	Chloride (mEq/L)	Acetate (mEq/L)
Aminosyn	Abbott	3.5%	24.8	357	7.0	0	46.0
Aminosyn II	Abbott	3.5%	21.5	308	16.3	0	25.2
Aminosyn M	Abbott	3.5%	24.8	477	47.0	40.0	58.0
Aminosyn IIM	Abbott	3.5%	21.5	425	36.0	37.0	25.0
Travasol with Electrolytes	Clintec	3.5%	15.5	450	25.0	25.0	52.0
Aminosyn II in 5% Dextrose	Abbott	3.5%	21.5	585	18.0	0	25.2
Aminosyn II in 25% Dextrose	Abbott	3.5%	21.6	1,515	18	0	25.2
Aminosyn IIM in 5% Dextrose	Abbott	3.5%	21.5	616	41	36.5	25.1
Aminosyn II	Abbott	8.5%	21.5	742	33.3	0	61.1
Travasol without Electrolytes	Abbott	8.5%	15.5	890	0	34.0	73.0
FreAmine III	Abbott	8.5%	23.3	810	10.0	<3.0	72.0
Aminosyn with Electrolytes	Abbott	8.5%	24.7	1,160	70.0	98.0	142
Aminosyn II with Electrolytes	Abbott	8.5%	21.5	999	80.0	86.0	61.0
FreAmine III with Electrolytes	Abbott	8.5%	23.3	1,045	60.0	60.0	125
Travasol	Clintec	8.5%	15.5	1,160	70.0	70.0	141
Aminosyn	Abbott	8.5%	24.7	850	0	35.0	90.0
Aminosyn	Abbott	10%	24.9	1,000	0	0	148
TrophAmine	McGaw	10%	30.0	875	5.0	<3.0	97
Aminosyn-PF	Abbott	10%	26.9	829	3.4	0	46.3
Aminosyn II	Abbott	10%	21.5	873	45.3	0	71.8
Aminosyn (pH 6)	Abbott	10%	24.9	993	0	0	111
Travasol	Clintec	10%	19.1	1,000	40.0	0	87
FreAmine III	McGaw	10%	23.3	950	10.0	<3.0	89
Aminosyn II with Electrolytes	Abbott	10%	21.5	1,130	87.0	86.0	72

AA, amino acids; BCAA, branched-chain amino acids.

TABLE 3. **Composition of Selected Crystalloid Solutions**

Product	Manufacturer	Na (mEq/L)	K (mEq/L)	Ca (mEq/L)	Mg (mEq/L)	Cl (mEq/L)	Osmolarity (mOsm/L)
Plasma-Lyte 56	Baxter	40	13	0	3	40	111
Ringer's injection	Abbott Baxter McGaw	147	4	4	0	156	310
Lactated Ringer's injection	Abbott Baxter McGaw	130	4	3	0	109	273
Plasma-Lyte R	Baxter	140	10	5	3	103	312
Isolyte S (pH 6.7)	McGaw	140	5	0	3	98	295
Isolyte S (pH 7.4)	McGaw	141	5	0	3	98	295
Normosol-R	Abbott	140	5	0	3	98	295
Normosol-R (pH 7.4)	Abbott	140	5	0	3	98	295
Plasma-Lyte 148	Baxter	140	5	0	3	98	294
Plasma-Lyte A (pH 7.4)	Baxter	140	5	0	3	98	294
Isolyte E (pH 6.0)	McGaw	140	10	5	3	103	310
Hyperlyte	McGaw	25	40	5	8	33	6,015
Lypholyte	Lyphomed	25	40	5	8	33	7,562
Multilyte-40	Lyphomed	25	40	5	8	33	6,015
Nutrilyte	American Reagent	25	40	5	8	33	7,562
Lypholyte II	Lyphomed	35	20	4.5	5	35	6,200
TPN Electrolytes	Abbott	35	20	4.5	5	35	6,200
Nutrilyte II	American Reagent	35	20	4.5	5	35	6,212
TPN Electrolytes II	Abbott	18	18	4.5	5	35	4,320
TPN Electrolytes III	Abbott	25	40.6	5	8	33.5	7,520
Hyperlyte CR	McGaw	25	20	5	5	30	5,500
Hyperlyte R	McGaw	25	20	5	5	30	4,205
Multilyte-20	Lyphomed	25	20	5	5	30	4,205
0.9% Saline	Many	154	20–40	0	0	147–194	350–390

TABLE 4. **Composition of Selected Parenteral Fat Emulsions**

Product	Manufacturer	Triglyceride Source (wt/vol)	Triglyceride Distribution	Calories (kcal/ml)	Osmolarity (mOsm/L)
Intralipid 10%	Clintec	Soybean oil (10%)	100% LCT	1.1	260
Intralipid 20%	Clintec	Soybean oil (20%)	100% LCT	2.0	260
Liposyn II 10%	Abbott	Soybean oil (5%) Safflower oil (5%)	100% LCT	1.1	276
Liposyn II 20%	Abbott	Soybean oil (10%) Safflower oil (10%)	100% LCT	2.0	258
Liposyn III 10%	Abbott	Soybean oil (10%)	100% LCT	1.1	284
Liposyn III 20%	Abbott	Soybean oil (20%)	100% LCT	2.0	292

LCT, long-chain triglyceride.

TABLE 5. **Composition of Selected Parenteral Multiple Trace Element Preparations**

Product	Manufacturer	Cr (µg)	Cu (mg)	I (µg)	Mn (mg)	Se (µg)	Zn (mg)
Pedtrace-4	Lyphomed	0.85	0.10	0	0.025	0	0.50
Multiple Trace Element Neonatal	American Reagent	0.85	0.10	0	0.025	0	1.50
Neotrace-4	Lyphomed	0.85	0.10	0	0.025	0	1.50
PedTE-Pak-4	S&NSoloPak	1.00	0.10	0	0.025	0	1.00
P.T.E.-4	Lyphomed	1.00	0.10	0	0.025	0	1.00
Multiple Trace Element Pediatric	American Reagent	1.00	0.10	0	0.030	0	0.50
Trace Metals Additive in 0.9% NaCl	Abbott	2.00	0.20	0	0.16	0	0.80
M.T.E.-4	Lyphomed	4.00	0.40	0	0.10	0	1.00
MulTE-Pak-4	S&NSoloPak	4.00	0.40	0	0.10	0	1.00
Multiple Trace Element	American Reagent	4.00	0.40	0	0.10	0	1.00
Multiple Trace Element Concentrated	American Reagent	10.0	1.00	0	0.50	0	5.00
ConTE-Pak-4	S&NSoloPak	10.0	1.00	0	0.50	0	5.00
M.T.E.-4 Concentrated	Lyphomed	10.0	1.00	0	0.50	0	5.00
P.T.E.-5	Lyphomed	1.00	0.10	0	0.025	15.0	1.00
M.T.E.-5	Lyphomed	4.00	0.40	0	0.10	20.0	1.00
MulTE-Pak-5	S&NSoloPak	4.00	0.40	0	0.10	20.0	1.00
Multiple Trace Element with Selenium	American Reagent	4.00	0.40	0	0.10	20.0	1.00
M.T.E.-6	Lyphomed	4.00	0.40	25.0	0.10	20.0	1.00
M.T.E.-7	Lyphomed	4.00	0.40	25.0	0.10	20.0	1.00
M.T.E.-6 Concentrated	Lyphomed	10.0	1.00	75.0	0.50	60.0	5.00
Tracelyte Electrolyte Combination	Lyphomed	0.60	0.06	0	0.015	0	0.15
Tracelyte with Double Electrolytes	Lyphomed	0.30	0.03	0	0.0075	0	0.075
Tracelyte II Electrolyte Combination	Lyphomed	0.60	0.06	0	0.015	0	0.15
Tracelyte II with Double Electrolytes	Lyphomed	0.30	0.03	0	0.0075	0	0.075

TABLE 6. **Composition of Parenteral Vitamin Supplements**

Product	Manufacturer	Vitamins										
		A (IU)	D (IU)	E* (IU)	B_1 (mg)	B_2 (mg)	B_3 (mg)	B_5 (mg)	B_6 (mg)	B_{12} (µg)	C (mg)	Biotin (mg)
Berocca Parenteral Nutrition	Roche	3,300	200	10	3	3.6	40	15	4	5	100	60
M.V.I.-12 Injection	Astra	3,300	200	10	3	3.6	40	15	4	5	100	60
M.V.I.-12 Unit Vial	Astra	3,300	200	10	3	3.6	40	15	4	5	100	60
M.V.I. Pediatric	Astra	2,300	400	7	1.2	1.4	17	5	1	1	80	20
Multi Vitamin Concentrate Injection	Lyphomed	10,000	1,000	5	50	10	100	25	15	0	500	0
B-Complex with C & B_{12} Injection	Goldline	0	0	0	50	5	125	6	5	1,000	50	0

*Vitamin E as *dl*-alpha-tocopheryl acetate.

mized. Fatty acid composition must also be considered in terms of species requirements. Most lipid emulsions contain linoleic acid, but not the arachidonic acid that is essential for cats.

Vitamin and trace mineral preparations (Tables 5 and 6) are also available and are typically added to parenteral nutrition solutions on a daily basis. Single-entity vitamin-mineral products are also commercially available. Vitamin solutions contain both water- and fat-soluble vitamins and may be administered with or without trace minerals. Multiple-entity formulations typically contain 12 vitamins. Single-entity formulations are available for vitamins A, D, E, K, thiamine (B_1), riboflavin (B_2), niacin (B_3), pyridoxine (B_6), folic acid (B_9), cyanocobalamin (B_{12}), and ascorbic acid (C).

References and Suggested Reading

Bartges JW: Nutritional support. In: Caywood DD, Lipowitz AJ, Newton CD, et al, eds: Complications in Small Animal Surgery. Baltimore: Williams & Wilkins, 1996, p 58.
Brown RO, Dickerson RN, White KG: Parenteral nutrition solutions. In: Calwell MD, Rombeau JL, eds: Parenteral Nutrition, 2nd ed. Philadelphia: WB Saunders, 1993, p 310.
Fulton RB, Lippert AC, Parr AM: A retrospective study of the use of total parenteral nutrition in dogs and cats. J Vet Intern Med 7:52, 1993.
Shizgal HM: Anabolic steroids and total parenteral nutrition. Wien Med Wochenschr 143:375, 1993.

Mechanical Devices for Percutaneous Placement of Gastrostomy Tubes: Use of Eld Applicator

P. JANE ARMSTRONG
LINDSAY K. MERKEL
St. Paul, Minnesota

Percutaneous placement of gastrostomy tubes with the use of an endoscope is commonly performed in practices where endoscopic equipment is available. The wide application, safety, and client acceptance of the endoscopic procedure led to the development of innovative mechanical devices and techniques for nonendoscopic placement of these tubes. These devices have made the use of gastrostomy feeding tubes feasible in almost any practice.

GUIDELINES FOR THE USE OF GASTROSTOMY TUBES

Indications

Percutaneously placed gastrostomy tubes offer a practical method of providing nutritional support to cats and dogs when it is anticipated that the animal will be anorectic or unable to eat for at least 1 week or when more proximal access to the gastrointestinal tract (e.g., a nasoesophageal tube) cannot be used. Gastrostomy tubes are especially useful when the animal is to be fed on a long-term basis in the home environment.

Contraindications

Most of the contraindications for percutaneous placement of a gastrostomy tube parallel those for one placed endoscopically. Gastrostomy tubes are not recommended for animals that have primary gastric disease, gastric outflow obstruction, or gastric paresis. Animals with megaesophagus should be fed below the pylorus to lessen the risk of aspiration pneumonia (see p. 136). In some patients with esophageal motility disorders, however, this risk is accepted over the risks and costs involved in surgical placement of a jejunostomy tube. Two other relative contraindications to gastrostomy tube placement are clinically evident ascites and immunosuppression. In particular, problems with dehiscence at the tube exit site and subsequent peritonitis may be encountered in feline leukemia virus–positive cats. A specific contraindication to the nonendoscopic percutaneous placement of a gastrostomy tube is esophageal trauma or stricture that may predispose to esophageal perforation during passage of the placement device.

DEVICES AVAILABLE FOR PERCUTANEOUS PLACEMENT OF GASTROSTOMY TUBES

Three methods are available for placement of a gastrostomy tube: percutaneous, endoscopic, and surgical (see *CVT XII,* p. 669). In this review, only the percutaneous method is discussed. Several methods have been described or are available for percutaneous placement. All rely on some device to carry a piece of suture from the lateral body wall out through the mouth or vice versa. The use of large-bore vinyl tubing is effective, and the materials are inexpensive (Fulton and Dennis, 1992). This method, however, is technically more difficult than using an insertion instrument, such as the Eld applicator. The insertion device described by Mauterer is not commercially available, but a patent was issued for its use. The device could be constructed from the information given in the manuscript (Mauterer et al, 1994). Cook Veterinary Products Inc. (P.O. Box 2327, Bloomington, Indiana 47402; 1-800-826-2380) introduced a nonendoscopic gastrostomy tube insertion set in 1996 in 40-cm ($195.00) and 80-cm ($205.00) lengths. Either set accepts a 16- or 20-French (F) mushroom-tipped Cook silicone gastrostomy tube. These tubes cost $11.50 and $14.50, respectively. This insertion set differs from the Eld applicator (described below) in that a needle is passed percutaneously into a hollow tube through the body wall and the tube is used without an internal flange. Comparative safety data between the Cook and the Eld devices are not available. The remainder of this discussion is confined to use of the Eld gastrostomy tube applicator developed by Larry Eld, D.V.M., of Boise, Idaho.

GASTROSTOMY TUBE PLACEMENT USING THE ELD APPLICATOR

Materials Needed

The special materials needed for percutaneous placement of a gastrostomy tube using the Eld applicator are listed below in order of their use during tube insertion.

- The Eld gastrostomy tube applicator (Jorgensen Laboratories Inc., 1450 N. Van Buren Avenue, Loveland, CO 80538; 1-800-525-5614). The device is available in two sizes ($144.00 and $150.00, respectively). Use an applicator with a 45-cm shaft for all cats and dogs less than approximately 15 kg; use an applicator with an 80-cm shaft for larger dogs. In the authors' experience, the shorter applicator is used in more than 90% of cases. A tube can consistently be placed in less than 10 minutes in dogs and cats weighing less than 15 kg. Tube placement in larger dogs requires experience.
- Two lengths of 17-pound test fishing line, each approximately 80 cm. Zero (0) diameter monofilament nylon or similar large-diameter suture material can be used but is much less economical, and sterility is not required.
- A 200-μL MLA disposable pipette tip (Medical Laboratory Automation, Inc., 270 Marble Ave., Pleasantville, NY; 914-747-3020) to serve as a guide as the catheter exits the stomach and body wall. A 3½-F tomcat catheter (cut about 1 cm off the narrow end and discard) or the plastic guard from a 16-gauge over-the-needle type intravenous catheter can also be used. A pipette tip is an economical substitute for the tomcat catheter recommended in the directions accompanying the Eld applicator (cost is approximately $55.00 for 1,000 pipette tips).
- A Pezzer-type, mushroom-tip catheter (Bard Urological Catheter, Bard Urological Division of C.R. Bard Inc., 8195 Industrial Blvd., Covington, GA 30209; 800-526-4455). These catheters come in a wide variety of sizes. A syringeable diet can be fed through a 16-F catheter, so this standard size can be used in virtually all canine and feline cases (current cost of $11.80 per catheter). A 20- or 22-F catheter can be used in dogs weighing more than 15 kg (see *CVT XII*, p. 673). Some clinicians prefer these larger-bore catheters for all patients.

The type of catheter the authors recommend here differs from that described in the product literature that accompanies the Eld applicator. Experience with the use of the Pezzer-type urologic catheter has demonstrated that it is a robust tube suitable for long-term feeding (Armstrong and Hardie, 1990). The authors recommend adding an internal flange, as described below. Information is available about tube removal for this modified tube (DeBowes et al, 1993). Other authors prefer larger-diameter Pezzer tubes (18-F or larger) without an internal flange (Mauterer et al, 1994). Durability of a modified rubber or vinyl tube, as described in the product literature, has not been documented.

Other items required for tube placement are surgical scrub, three nonsterile hemostats, nonsterile scissors, a No. 11 scalpel blade, 2.5-cm white tape, a centimeter ruler, an indelible marker, water-soluble lubricant, a 20-gauge needle, an intravenous injection cap, antimicrobial ointment, a 10-cm gauze square, bandage material or 10-cm stockinette, and an Elizabethan collar.

Tube Assembly

The gastrostomy tube should be prepared in the following manner before the patient is anesthetized. Cut the flared proximal end off the mushroom-tip catheter (feeding tube) and discard. Cut two 2-cm pieces of tubing off the tube at the cut end. These pieces will serve as bumpers or flanges. With a No. 11 scalpel blade, make a stab incision in the center of each flange. Push a mosquito forcep through the slit in one flange and grasp the cut end of the feeding tube. Pull the feeding tube through the slit and push the flange down the tube until it rests adjacent to the mushroom tip. The other 2-cm piece of tubing will be used later as an external flange. Cut the nipple tip off the mushroom, to facilitate food delivery. Make several marks with an indelible marker at 1-cm intervals from the flange on the mushroom end of the tube. These marks will allow assessment of how much of the tube is in the stomach following placement. Lastly, the proximal end of the tube is cut at a sharp angle.

Anesthesia

Prior to gastrostomy tube placement, the animal should be fasted for 12 hours. Injectable anesthetic agents, such as propofol or ketamine with diazepam, or inhalant anesthesia, are satisfactory for tube insertion. The choice of anesthetic protocol is determined by evaluation of the individual patient. An endotracheal tube is recommended, particularly in cats, as pharyngeal manipulation may result in laryngospasm. The anesthetized patient is placed in *right lateral recumbency* and an area on the left flank extending approximately 10 cm behind the last rib is clipped and a surgical scrub performed.

Instructions for Tube Placement

- With the animal's neck extended, measure the distance from the nose to the last rib and mark this distance on the Eld applicator with a piece of tape. It is useful to note the direction of the curve of the Eld applicator tip on the piece of tape, to allow this orientation to be maintained during the procedure.

- With the Eld applicator tip oriented ventrally or slightly toward the animal's left side, introduce the lubricated tip into the mouth and pass it until the tape marker contacts the nose. To ensure that the trocar is not advanced inadvertently during passage, the authors recommend that the operator "guard" the trocar by wrapping the middle, ring, and baby fingers around the spring on the handle of the device. Smooth passage of the applicator is facilitated by extending the head and neck. Difficulty is occasionally encountered passing the tip of the applicator through the lower esophageal sphincter. Resistance here is best overcome by withdrawing the device a few centimeters and rotating the device 45 to 90 degrees before attempting passage. Gentle manipulation rather than force must be used to overcome any resistance. Another useful technique is to bring the animal's head to the end of the table, thereby allowing the applicator to be manipulated vertically as well as from side to side.
- Position the curved tip of the applicator so that it can be palpated in the stomach through the lateral abdominal wall. Palpation of the tip may be facilitated by bringing the animal's head to the end of the table, so that the handle of the applicator can be lowered. The location at which the tip is palpated must be *behind the last rib*, and preferably in the dorsal two thirds of the flank.
- With a gloved hand, apply digital pressure on both sides of the palpated tip to isolate it from any adjacent structures, and push the plunger, causing the trocar needle to advance from inside the stomach out through the body wall. *Take care to keep fingers clear of the advancing trocar.* Maintain pressure on the plunger to keep the trocar in the advanced position.
- Thread about 10 cm of fishing line through the trocar needle and tie it securely. Relax the pressure on the plunger, allowing the trocar to retract into the stomach. Slowly withdraw the applicator out through the mouth with the fishing line attached. Clamp a hemostat onto each end of the fishing line (one end is exiting the mouth and the opposite end is exiting the body wall) to maintain control of both ends, and cut the fishing line free of the applicator's trocar needle.
- Releasing the hemostat from the line exiting the mouth, thread the pipette tip (or alternative) onto the line, narrow end first. Attach the line securely to the cut proximal end of the stomach tube, using a 20-gauge needle or suture needle. Draw the end of the tube snugly into the pipette tip.
- Loop the second length of fishing line through the eyelets of the mushroom tip. Do not tie this line, but clamp the two ends together with a hemostat. If any difficulty is encountered during tube placement, traction on this safety loop will extract the tube.
- Lubricate the mushroom tip of the tube. Using steady traction, pull on the end of the line exiting the body wall, so that the tube advances through the mouth and out through the stomach and body wall. Guide the tube so that all obstructions in the mouth are avoided. Resistance encountered when the pipette tip contacts the body wall is overcome by steady traction and firm application of counterpressure to the body wall. As the pipette tip

emerges through the skin, grasp it with a hemostat to continue pulling. It is usually unnecessary to nick the exit site with a scalpel to enlarge it unless a large-diameter tube is selected. The safety loop through the mushroom tip is removed by releasing the hemostat and pulling on *one* end of the line.

- The stomach and body wall are brought into loose contact as the mushroom tip reaches the stomach wall. The remaining flange is fitted down the feeding tube by inserting a hemostat through the slit in the flange, grasping the end of the tube, and withdrawing the hemostat. Slide the flange down until it contacts, but does not create tension against, the body wall. Attach a piece of tape to the tube about 2 cm above the skin (or use superglue) to prevent flange slippage. Suturing the tube to the skin is not recommended. Cap the tube with an intravenous catheter cap or three-way stopcock.

TUBE USE AND MAINTENANCE

Antimicrobial ointment on a gauze square is fitted between the skin and the external flange at the exit site. Bandage material may be used to protect the tube and bring the end of the tube to a convenient point for feeding. The authors have found that a "sweater" fashioned out of 10-cm stockinette or a tube sock makes a very convenient alternative, especially in cats. For a cat, cut 45 cm of stockinette, and roll the sweater over the cat's head, inserting the forelegs into precut holes. Although the temperament of some dogs requires placement of an Elizabethan collar, most cats tolerate the tube without one. The tube exit site should be checked daily by rolling the caudal edge of the bandage or sweater forward. The tube covering need only be replaced if it becomes dislodged or soiled. The authors do not routinely use prophylactic antibiotics.

Feeding may begin 12 hours after tube placement. Tube location can be verified prior to each use by aspiration of a small quantity of gastric juice. If further confirmation of the location of the tube is required at any time, such as if the patient interferes with the tube, contrast radiography using a water-soluble contrast agent is readily accomplished. Commercially available syringeable diets, such as Hill's Prescription Diet a/d or Eukanuba Veterinary Diet Nutritional Recovery Formula (canned), may be used. Blenderized diets and commercially available liquid diets may also be fed via gastrostomy tube. The tube should always be flushed after feeding with a small volume of water (5 ml is adequate) to prevent tube clogging.

Pezzer-type gastrostomy tubes have been used without replacement for a year or more (Armstrong and Hardie, 1990). Use of a low-profile device to replace the standard tube has been described for long-term maintenance in dogs (Bright et al, 1995).

Tube Removal

Gastrostomy tubes are generally left in place a minimum of 5 to 7 days before removal, both to ensure that the tube is no longer required and to allow healing to occur at the tube exit site. Withhold food for 8 to 12 hours prior to tube removal. Anesthesia or tranquilization is not required. To remove the tube, the animal is usually restrained in right lateral recumbency. Exert firm traction on the tube, while applying counterpressure to the skin around the exit site. The mushroom tip will collapse as it pulls through the internal flange. The internal flange will pass in the feces. An alternative method of tube removal has been described for large-diameter tubes (see *CVT XII,* p. 673). Although, in the authors' experience, surgical intervention to retrieve the internal flange has never been needed, use of a large-diameter Pezzer tube without an internal flange eliminates any risk of intestinal obstruction following tube removal. Food is withheld for 12 hours after tube removal. The small gastrocutaneous fistula resulting from tube removal heals rapidly and thus requires no special care.

References and Suggested Reading

Armstrong PJ, Hardie EM: Percutaneous endoscopic gastrostomy: A retrospective study of clinical cases in dogs and cats. J Vet Intern Med 4:202, 1990.

Typical patient profiles, indications, and complications that may be encountered with gastrostomy tubes.
Bright RM, DeNovo RC, Jones JB: Use of a low-profile gastrostomy device for administering nutrients in two dogs. J Am Vet Med Assoc 207:1184, 1995.
A guide to insertion of the low-profile device with results of its use in two dogs.
DeBowes LJ, Coyne B, Layton CE: Comparison of French-Pezzer and Malecot catheters for percutaneously placed gastrostomy tubes in cats. J Am Vet Med Assoc 202:1963, 1993.
A study comparing the robustness of two types of gastrostomy tubes (placed endoscopically) and two methods of tube removal.
Fulton RB, Dennis JS: Blind percutaneous placement of a gastrostomy tube for nutritional support in dogs and cats. J Am Vet Med Assoc 201:697, 1992.
A guide to using large-diameter vinyl tubing for non-endoscopic gastrostomy tube placement.
Mauterer JV, Abood SK, Buffington CA, et al: New technique and management guidelines for percutaneous nonendoscopic tube gastrostomy. J Am Vet Med Assoc 205:574, 1994.
A description of an alternative device for nonendoscopic tube placement with results of its use in colony and client-owned animals.

Refeeding Syndrome

CHERYL C. MILLER
Athens, Georgia

JOSEPH W. BARTGES
Knoxville, Tennessee

Refeeding syndrome encompasses metabolic and functional abnormalities associated with providing nutrition to an anorectic and malnourished patient. The classic refeeding syndrome consists of severe hypophosphatemia that occurs in underfed patients who are refed with total parenteral nutrition (TPN). However, refeeding syndrome may also include other abnormalities, such as hypokalemia, hypomagnesemia, vitamin deficiencies, fluid intolerance, and glucose intolerance. Abnormalities have been observed in patients given enteral and parenteral nutrition after severe weight loss. The common cardiac, hematologic, respiratory, and neuromuscular abnormalities that may occur during refeeding syndrome strongly indicate that the disorder is a complication of a series of metabolic disorders (Brooks and Melnik, 1995; Havala and Shronts, 1990).

The exact prevalence of refeeding syndrome is unknown because it frequently is not recognized. However, ignorance about refeeding syndrome has caused death in underfed, yet otherwise healthy, human beings. Thus, recognition of metabolic changes associated with starvation (see *CVT XII,* p. 53), and the body's adaptation to starvation, is important in the prevention and management of refeeding syndrome. Exactly why the syndrome occurs in some patients and not others remains elusive. Therefore, nutritional support personnel must be aware of the potential for development of this syndrome and must be prepared to manage the metabolic complications.

METABOLIC CHANGES ASSOCIATED WITH STARVATION

During starvation, metabolic changes occur in the patient that allow adaptation to a calorie-deprived condition. During nonstressed starvation, total liver gluconeogenesis declines. Protein mobilization to provide amino acids for gluconeogenesis decreases, and protein sources are spared until fat stores are depleted. Other survival mechanisms include a reduction in basal metabolic rate, decreased insulin secretion, and the use of less glucose and some fatty acids by the brain for energy (Brooks and Melnik, 1995). Although the body strives to maintain serum electrolyte concentrations, total body potassium, magnesium, and phosphate are depleted as starvation persists. Serum concentrations of these metabolites are not indicative of total body stores. Additionally, starvation induces a catabolic response causing release of intracellular phosphate, which is lost from the body. Significant decreases in organ size occur during starvation. For example, cardiac contractility and ventricular mass are decreased. Changes in the gastrointestinal tract develop, including decreased absorptive surface area and villous atrophy (Brooks and Melnik, 1995).

HYPOPHOSPHATEMIA

Phosphorus is the major intracellular anion and exists as inorganic phosphate and as organic phosphate esters.

Organic phosphate (mainly intracellular) is present in many compounds, including phospholipids, phosphoproteins, nucleic acids, enzymes, and cofactors. These compounds represent important parts of plasma membranes, the electron transport chain, ATP, cAMP, and 2,3-diphosphoglycerate (2,3-DPG) and help maintain cell integrity. Inorganic phosphate is present mainly in the extracellular fluid. Approximately 10% is protein bound, and the remainder exists as monohydrogen phosphate and dihydrogen phosphate. Inorganic phosphate is an important substrate for many vital body functions, including glycogenolysis, 2,3-DPG production, and oxidative phosphorylation. Phosphates are also important buffers in maintaining acid-base balance (Forrester and Moreland, 1989).

The classic description of refeeding syndrome consists of *hypophosphatemia* resulting from decreased dietary intake, ineffective gastrointestinal absorption, increased nonrenal losses, and transcellular shifts. Nonrenal losses stem from disorders such as chronic diarrhea and vomiting. Renal losses of phosphorus are not significant, since urinary phosphorus concentrations approach zero during starvation as tubular resorption increases to approximately 100%. Transcellular shifts of phosphate from the extracellular to the intracellular compartment occur, and intensify the problem. Administration of carbohydrates, insulin, or amino acids promotes anabolism and glycolysis, thereby inducing cellular uptake of phosphate. Disturbances in acid-base balance also promote hypophosphatemia. Respiratory alkalosis is thought to increase intracellular pH, thus inducing glycolysis and the transcellular shift of phosphorus. Although dietary insufficiency or malnutrition alone will not lead to hypophosphatemia in a normal animal, a starved patient is particularly at risk because of inadequate nutritional intake and depleted phosphorus stores (Forrester and Moreland, 1989).

Calcium may also play a role in phosphate losses in animals during the early stages of starvation, and in association with TPN. Increasing calcium levels in TPN solutions lowered urine phosphate losses and the degree of hypophosphatemia in 3-day fasted rats (Al-Jurf and Chapmann-Furr, 1986).

The systemic abnormalities that may be caused by hypophosphatemia include cardiac dysfunction, hemolytic anemia, muscle weakness, ventilatory failure, ataxia, seizures, coma, metabolic encephalopathy, and renal, endocrine, and gastrointestinal disorders. These impairments specifically appear to be the result of decreased levels of ATP and 2,3-DPG associated with hypophosphatemia (Forrester and Moreland, 1989).

HYPOMAGNESEMIA AND HYPOKALEMIA

Hypomagnesemia and hypophosphatemia often coexist in patients at risk for developing refeeding syndrome. Both conditions lead to cardiac arrhythmias and neuromuscular signs (muscular weakness, seizures, confusion, and ataxia), making it difficult to determine which electrolyte disturbance is responsible (see *CVT XII,* p. 128). The dosage for repletion of either mineral that can be expected to result in incremental increases in serum concentrations is unknown. Therefore, it is recommended that phosphorus and magnesium (see *CVT XII,* p. 132) be repleted simultaneously. It is also recommended that repletion of both minerals be completed prior to the continuation of nutritional support, because continuation of nutritional support during electrolyte repletion creates an anabolic environment that exacerbates the problem.

The clinical signs of hypokalemia also overlap those of hypomagnesemia and hypophosphatemia (see *CVT XI,* p. 297). The effects of neither hypomagnesemia nor hypokalemia were recognized in early reports of refeeding syndrome. It is feasible that both conditions were present and acted synergistically to exacerbate the described hypophosphatemic disorder. Other factors that predispose to hypokalemia include insulin therapy (see *CVT XII,* p. 385), diuretic therapy, metabolic alkalosis, diarrhea, vomiting, and rapid glucose infusion (Havala and Shronts, 1990). Presumably, refeeding syndrome–induced hypokalemia develops because of a transcellular shift similar to development of hypophosphatemia. Supplemental potassium administration (see *CVT XII,* p. 954) prior to resuming nutritional support is recommended (Brooks and Melnik, 1995).

VITAMIN DEFICIENCIES

Several reports suggest that vitamin deficiencies, mainly thiamine, play a role in refeeding syndrome (Brooks and Melnik, 1995; Havala and Shronts, 1990). Thiamine (B_1), a water-soluble vitamin, is an important coenzyme for carbohydrate metabolism. Thiamine deficiency can develop in patients because of inadequate intake or prolonged intravenous hydration. The relationship between refeeding syndrome and severe vitamin deficiency is not yet clear. There is evidence that thiamine-deficient people developed carbohydrate loading–induced Wernicke's encephalopathy. Wernicke's encephalopathy can mimic hypophosphatemia; encephalopathy includes signs such as ataxia, vestibular dysfunction, confusion, and coma. Death has been reported in humans given thiamine-deficient TPN solutions. Therefore, even without direct scientific evidence of thiamine's contribution to refeeding syndrome in animals, the potential severity of the syndrome warrants consideration and probable supplementation. Thiamine can be supplemented as a component of B-vitamin complex at 1 ml/L of parenteral fluids.

GLUCOSE INTOLERANCE

Caution must be used when one administers exogenous glucose as nutritional support for underfed patients. In addition to inducing electrolyte and mineral imbalances (hypophosphatemia, hypomagnesemia, hypokalemia), exceeding optimal rates of glucose administration may result in hyperglycemia and may cause metabolic acidosis, osmotic diuresis, dehydration, or hypertension. Excessive calories may have other deleterious effects, such as conversion of excess carbohydrates to fat, predisposing to fatty liver. Insulin concentrations are depressed in starved patients; thus, abrupt refeeding with glucose may induce hyperinsulinemia. For unknown reasons, starvation induces fluid and sodium retention, leading to hypertension. Exogenous administration of excessive calories and fluid in parenteral glucose solutions stresses the atrophied heart and may predispose the patient to cardiac failure (Brooks and Melnik, 1995; Havala and Shronts, 1990; Solomon and Kirby, 1990).

REFEEDING SYNDROME IN VETERINARY MEDICINE

Of what significance is refeeding syndrome in veterinary medicine? Reports of refeeding syndrome in small animal medicine are rare, unlike the situation in human medicine. Electrolyte abnormalities occur in as many as 59% of human patients receiving TPN. In one study of TPN in dogs and cats, metabolic complications that developed included glucose intolerance, hypoglycemia, electrolyte abnormalities, and acid-base abnormalities. However, fewer than half of all animals developed these electrolyte abnormalities. More than 70% of animals receiving TPN survived and were discharged, and more than half of all animals receiving TPN gained weight (Lippert et al, 1993). The highest incidence of hypophosphatemia (the typical finding of refeeding syndrome) at any time period was only 8%, and the highest incidence of hypokalemia was 11%.

In a study of nondiabetic cats, only 2% of cats developed hypophosphatemia with enteral alimentation (Justin and Hohenhaus, 1995). Of these cats, four recovered, two died, and three were euthanized. All cats were thought to have been depleted of phosphate as a result of chronic malnutrition and anorexia. The authors postulated that the pathophysiology of hypophosphatemia in these cats was similar to that observed in human beings. Phosphorus abnormalities are reportedly as high as 57% in people receiving TPN; potassium abnormalities were recognized in as many as 36% of the patients. Thus, disorders often encountered in human patients receiving TPN appear far less common in small animals.

Unpublished data from the authors' hospital indicate that cats and dogs with feeding tubes did not readily develop refeeding syndrome. During a 2-year period, 17% of animals developed hypophosphatemia and 27% developed hypokalemia. However, both of these deficiencies resolved rapidly with tube feeding, and none of the animals died from electrolyte or mineral complications involving the tube feeding.

RECOMMENDATIONS

Published guidelines for providing enteral and parenteral nutritional support to small animals include calculating the basal energy requirement in kilocalories with the use of the following linear equation:

Basal energy requirement = 30 × (body weight [kg]) + 70

The basal energy requirement is then multiplied by an illness factor to correct for the illness energy requirement. The authors routinely use an illness factor of 1.5 for most dogs and cats. For enteral nutrition, tube feeding should be initiated at maintenance energy levels administered over several feedings (six to eight) on the first day. The amount of feed per meal is increased and the frequency of meals should be decreased over the next 2 to 3 days. For parenteral nutrition, half of the calculated rate for parenteral fluids should be administered for the first 12 hours; the full calculated rate should then be given if problems such as hyperglycemia, hyperlipidemia, azotemia, metabolic acidosis, or electrolyte imbalances do not develop (see p. 80).

If an animal given nutritional support develops hypophosphatemia, nutritional support should be discontinued until the electrolyte disorder is stabilized. At that time, nutritional support may be continued. Hypophosphatemia may be treated either orally or parenterally. The oral route is preferable; however, this route may not be feasible. If replacement phosphorus is given parenterally, serum phosphorus concentrations should be evaluated every 6 to 12 hours. Parenteral dosages of phosphate vary from 0.003 mmol/kg per hour for 24 hours to 0.03 mmol/kg per hour for 6 hours (Adams et al, 1993). Supplementation of potassium phosphate based on serum potassium levels, without regard to phosphate dose, has also been recommended (Adams et al, 1993). However, this method may be unsatisfactory because potassium deficits can greatly exceed phosphorus deficits. In this circumstance, severe iatrogenic hyperphosphatemia may develop. Treatment of hypophosphatemia with parenteral potassium phosphate is recommended, unless the animal becomes hyperkalemic. If hyperkalemia occurs, treatment with sodium phosphate is recommended (Adams et al, 1993).

References and Suggested Reading

Adams LG, Hardy RM, Weiss DJ, et al: Hypophosphatemia and hemolytic anemia associated with diabetes mellitus in hepatic lipidosis in cats. J Vet Intern Med 7:266, 1993.

Al-Jurf AS, Chapmann-Furr F: Phosphate balance and distribution during total parenteral nutrition: Effect of calcium and phosphate additives. J Parenteral Enteral Nutr 10:508, 1986.

Brooks MJ, Melnik G: The refeeding syndrome: An approach to understanding its complications and preventing its occurrence. Pharmacotherapy 15:713, 1995.

Forrester SD, Moreland KJ: Hypophosphatemia causes and clinical management. J Vet Intern Med 3:149, 1989.

Havala T, Shronts E: Managing the complications associated with refeeding. Nutr Clin Pract 5:23, 1990.

Justin RB, Hohenhaus AE: Hypophosphatemia associated with enteral alimentation in cats. J Vet Intern Med 9:228, 1995.

Lippert AC, Fulton RB, Parr AM: A retrospective study of the use of total parenteral nutrition in dogs and cats. J Vet Intern Med 7:52, 1993.

Solomon SM, Kirby DF: The refeeding syndrome: A review. J Parenteral Enteral Nutr 14:90, 1990.

Sensory Mutilation and Related Behavioral Syndromes

SCOTT W. LINE

St. Paul, Minnesota

Sensory mutilation, or self-mutilation, syndromes in dogs and cats are associated with a variety of behavioral patterns and may be considered stereotypic or compulsive. Stereotypic behaviors are generally defined as repetitive actions that have no apparent purpose or function yet have been observed in a wide variety of animal species. Included are normal behaviors performed with excessive frequency or duration, or truly abnormal idiosyncratic patterns.

Compulsions and obsessions are terms used to describe human behavioral disorders. Compulsions are behaviors that the patient is highly motivated to perform; they may experience high levels of anxiety if the behavior cannot be executed. The behaviors are often performed in a relatively fixed sequence and are repeated, frequently enough to interfere with the normal patterns of daily life. Obsessions are intrusive thoughts that cannot be ignored and, in some cases, can be relieved only through performance of a compulsive behavior. Since compulsions are observable behaviors and obsessions are cognitive by nature, I support the approach described by Hewson and Luescher (1996) and will refer to these behaviors in dogs and cats as compulsions rather than obsessions.

DIFFERENTIAL DIAGNOSIS

There are several potential causes of self-mutilation in dogs and cats, including attention getting, truly compulsive behavior, seizure-related disorders, and dermatologic conditions.

Attention getting is the appropriate diagnosis if the pet is performing the stereotypic pattern because it results in a reaction from the owner. In many cases, both positive and negative forms of attention are rewarding from the pet's perspective. Attention getting will occur mainly when a family member is present, but not when the pet is alone.

Truly compulsive self-mutilation occurs regardless of whether anyone is present and may occupy a large proportion of the pet's waking hours. In cats, self-mutilation often results from excessive grooming. While the original etiology may not be readily apparent, anxiety resulting from social stress can lead to grooming as a displacement behavior. Over time, physical lesions develop and they stimulate continued grooming. Eventually, the behavior may become compulsive. In dogs, compulsive self-mutilation also may begin in response to anxiety or in response to a lack of environmental stimulation. Other cases may occur spontaneously, without identifiable cause. The behavior gradually may become independent of the original cause and develop into a self-reinforcing habit.

In some cases, self-mutilation or other compulsive behaviors may be a form of seizure disorder. Abnormal activity in the temporal lobe has been associated with behavioral changes, including self-mutilation. Abnormal findings on electroencephalographic recordings, brain scans such as positron emission tomography (PET) or magnetic resonance imaging (MRI), or positive response to treatment with anticonvulsants can be used to diagnose seizure-related self-mutilation.

It is important to rule out primary dermatologic diseases as a cause of self-mutilation. Allergic, parasitic, and other infectious and inflammatory diseases may lead to pruritis, which results in self-mutilation. Successful treatment will require resolution of the primary condition.

Breed Predilections

In dogs, there are several breed predilections for self-mutilation: (1) flank sucking occurs in Doberman pinschers; (2) acral lick dermatitis (also known as lick granuloma or neurodermatitis) has been reported in some of the working and sporting breeds, including Golden retrievers, Labrador retrievers, Doberman pinschers, and German shepherds; (3) tail chasing and biting is seen in Bull terriers, Fox terriers, and German shepherds. Compulsive patterns similar to self-mutilation, including licking objects such as stoves or vacuum cleaners, have been seen in Miniature schnauzers. Fly snapping (lunging at imaginary objects) and other idiosyncratic patterns also occur in Bull terriers and other breeds. In Siamese cats, sucking and eating wool or similar cloth items also have been observed. These latter behaviors are not diagnosed as self-mutilation but *can be treated with the use of similar approaches.*

TREATMENT

Many cases of self-mutilation or compulsive behavior are difficult to treat. Historically, treatments have included making the area inaccessible through the use of restraining collars and bandaging, coating the affected area with foul-tasting lotions or sprays, or amputation of affected regions, such as the tip of the tail. However, reduction of the self-mutilating behavior itself was often not accomplished. Multiple approaches may be required for successful long-term management. These approaches may include behavior modification techniques, medication, and other supplemental tecnhiques.

Behavior Modification

If the primary motivation for the behavior is attention getting, removing all forms of attention to the pet from the

90

owner may help reduce self-mutilation. For some pets, all forms of attention are reinforcing, including looking at them, talking to them, or yelling at them. Removing the reinforcement by having owners ignore the pet will help extinguish the pattern. Actively ignoring the pet (turning away from the animal so there is no chance of eye contact or leaving the room) can speed up this process.

If an underlying source of anxiety can be identified, counter-conditioning the pet to that event or situation can help resolve self-mutilation. For example, a cat that is fearful of another cat in the household and subsequently licks and pulls out hair on the back may stop licking excessively if conditioned to tolerate the second cat. The first step would be to identify a suitable food (canned cat food, canned tuna, or canned salmon are often successful) that can be given to reward the patient for showing quiet, relaxed behavior. Starting in a quiet location in the house, the cat would be rewarded with attention, petting, and food for coming and responding to the owner. Several short repetitions per day of the training sessions should be done over 3 to 5 days to develop a positive association between the location in the house and the rewards. The second cat would then be added, but restrained in a carrier or held by another person and kept at a distance great enough to avoid provoking any fearful or anxious responses from the patient. Signs that the patient is not ready to proceed include growling, hissing, dilating pupils, or attempting to escape. The second cat should be present only for brief periods initially (1 to 2 minutes). Over time, the second cat should be brought closer, kept nearby for longer periods, and eventually given more freedom. The goal is to teach the patient to associate pleasant events with the second cat. It is important to progress only as fast as the patient can tolerate.

In cases of compulsive self-mutilation, counter-conditioning can also help reduce the frequency or duration of compulsive behavior. For example, sit-stay or down-stay activity can be taught to compete with tail chasing or biting. Because it is easier to interrupt a behavioral sequence in the early stages, to be most effective the command for the competing behavior should be given as soon as the pet shows signs of turning to bite or chew the affected area. For dogs, headcollars can also be used to interrupt licking or chewing.

Owners should be discouraged from using punishment to control self-mutilation. This approach is unlikely to be helpful for several reasons. First, pets that use self-licking as a means of getting attention may interpret any form of interaction (even reprimands) as reinforcing. Second, self-mutilation is often a result of anxiety, and punishment will generally increase anxiety. Finally, truly compulsive behavior is highly motivated, by definition, and punishment is unlikely to interrupt the behavior for very long.

In chronic cases, behavioral modification alone is usually unsuccessful but, when combined with anticompulsive medication, may greatly reduce the self-mutilation and enable the owner to gradually withdraw medication without leading to a relapse.

Medication

In recent years, antidepressant medications that inhibit reuptake of the neurotransmitter serotonin have proved highly effective in treating human obsessive-compulsive disorder. This syndrome is frequently characterized by excessive washing and grooming and may be similar to compulsive self-mutilation in dogs and cats. There are several anecdotal reports and two controlled studies (Goldberger and Rapoport, 1991; Rapoport et al, 1992) demonstrating that the tricyclic antidepressant clomipramine (Anafranil, Basel Pharmaceuticals) reduces acral lick dermatitis in dogs. The antidepressant fluoxetine (Prozac, Eli Lilly) is also effective in some patients (Rapoport et al, 1992). Other controlled studies designed to assess the effectiveness of other medications in animals are currently being conducted. Although published reports on efficacy are not available, other serotonin reuptake inhibitors such as sertraline (Zoloft, Roerig), fluvoxamine (Luvox, Solvay Pharmaceuticals), and paroxetine (Paxil, Smithkline Beecham Pharmaceuticals) may help control compulsive behaviors in animals.

Narcotic antagonists such as naloxone and naltrexone have been effective in reducing self-mutilation and other compulsive behaviors in some cases (Dodman et al, 1988). Naltrexone (ReVia, Dupont Merck Pharmaceuticals) is a useful drug for clinical treatment owing to its longer duration of action and oral dosing. However, naltrexone has recently been reformulated following approval of its use in treating alcoholism, and the cost has increased substantially. It is likely to be too expensive for most clients.

A syndrome has been described in Bull terriers that includes a range of abnormal behaviors, including severe aggression, fly snapping, tail chasing, and biting (Dodman et al, 1996a). Abnormal electroencephalographs were found in all affected dogs. One dog responded to treatment with clomipramine, and five of seven responded to treatment with phenobarbital. Although long-term treatment may lead to hepatotoxicity, anticonvulsants are likely to be much less expensive than clomipramine, fluoxetine, or other antidepressants and therefore may warrant consideration for treatment of self-mutilation in this syndrome.

Table 1 lists formulation, recommended dosage, dosing interval, and major side effects of medications used in treating self-mutilation and other compulsive behaviors in dogs and cats. The doses and dosing frequencies of many medications listed are based on extrapolation from human doses and anecdotal reports of use in dogs and cats, rather than controlled studies. The time to produce a reduction in self-mutilation may be up to 4 to 5 weeks in many cases. Individual animals may vary in their response to medication, so it is generally recommended that patients be started with a low dose, which is increased only if no positive response is observed after several weeks. The total duration of treatment is difficult to predict. In some cases treatment can be withdrawn after several months; however, in many cases long-term treatment (6 months to 1 year or longer) is needed to keep self-mutilation from recurring. When treatment is being stopped, the dose should be reduced over a 3- to 4-week period to reduce the chance that self-mutilation will recur.

Newer antidepressants are relatively safe, but they may be associated with adverse drug interactions. The main caution is that the tricyclic antidepressants (clomipramine and amitriptyline) and serotonin reuptake inhibitors (fluoxetine and similar drugs) should not be given at the

TABLE 1. Medications Used to Treat Self-Mutilation and Compulsive Behavior in Dogs and Cats

Medication	Formulation	Dosage (mg/kg)	Dosing Interval	Potential Side Effects
Primary Medications for Treating Compulsive Behavior				
Clomipramine (Anafranil) $	25-, 50-, 75-mg capsules	0.5–3	q12–24hr	Seizures, anticholinergic effects, hepatotoxicity, cardiac arrhythmias, sedation, vomiting, anorexia, diarrhea
Fluoxetine (Prozac) $$	10-, 20-mg capsules; 4 mg/ml solution	0.5–1	q24hr	Seizures, hepatotoxicity, anorexia, nausea, diarrhea, anxiety, rash, lethargy
Naltrexone (ReVia) $$$	50-mg tablets	2–5	q24hr	Sedation, diarrhea, hepatotoxicity, anxiety, pruritus
Phenobarbital $	8-, 16-, 32-, 62.5-, 100-mg tablets	2–20	q12–24hr	Hepatotoxicity, sedation
Additional Medications for Treating Anxiety				
Amitriptyline (Elavil)	10-, 25-, 50-, 75-, 100-, 150-mg tablets	1–2	q12hr	Seizures, anticholinergic effects, cardiac arrhythmias
Buspirone (BuSpar) $	5-, 10-mg tablets	1–2	q12hr	Dizziness, nausea, drowsiness, increased aggression, increased affection (cats)

$ indicates relative cost.

same time as monoamine oxidase inhibitors. In veterinary medicine, the most commonly used monoamine oxidase inhibitor is the acaricidal compound amitraz. A dog treated with a tricyclic antidepressant developed acute toxicity when an antitick collar with amitraz was used (Simpson and Davidson, 1996).

Since medication prescribed for behavioral problems *constitutes an extralabel use*, and since the possible adverse effects may not be well known in dogs and cats, a thorough pretreatment evaluation should be performed. At a minimum, a complete physical examination and blood chemistry profile should be performed. Most psychotropic medications are metabolized by conjugation in the liver and excretion in urine. Evaluation of liver and kidney function is important, particularly in older patients or those with a history of hepatic or renal impairment. Follow-up sampling should be repeated at regular intervals as long as treatment continues.

If fear or anxiety is identified as part of the underlying cause of self-mutilation, treatment with antianxiety medication can be a useful supplement to a behavioral modification program designed to reduce the fearful response. The anticompulsive medications listed in Table 1 generally also have anxiolytic effects. Additional medications that are used primarily to treat anxiety are also listed.

Although medication can be helpful in treating self-mutilation, medication alone will not completely eliminate the behavior in most pets. To be most successful, medication should be combined with the behavioral modification techniques outlined earlier. This approach will also reduce the chances of recurrence when medication is withdrawn, as well as decrease both the cost to the client and the chance of adverse side effects.

Supplemental Treatment Methods

Self-mutilation in some dogs will respond to radiation therapy (Rivers et al, 1993). Following treatment with orthovoltage or ^{60}Co radiation, approximately one third of patients, with a duration of symptoms ranging from 3 weeks to 2 years prior to treatment, showed no recurrence for periods ranging from 2 to 12 years. Another quarter showed temporary improvement, with lesions recurring 6 weeks to 1 year later. No improvement was observed in the remaining dogs.

Antibiotics and anti-inflammatory medication are useful as supplemental therapy for self-mutilation. Local infection and inflammation that occurs secondary to excessive licking or scratching may cause pruritus and increase the tendency to continue licking.

Physical methods of preventing self-mutilation are generally necessary to allow physical lesions to heal. While waiting for medication to take effect, the pet may need to wear a plastic Elizabethan collar whenever not directly supervised. A new stiff cylinder collar that fits between the skull and the shoulders prevents the animal from turning the neck (Bite Not collar, Bite Not Products). It may be more comfortable for some pets. Direct bandaging of the affected site may also be needed in some cases.

Diet and exercise are two other factors that may potentially play a role in reducing compulsive behavior. Many dogs who develop compulsive self-mutilation are terriers or sporting breeds that generally have a high level of activity. Providing regular aerobic exercise may help expend energy that would otherwise be directed at self-licking or self-chewing. It has been theorized that decreasing the amount of protein in the diet has the potential to decrease the motivation for self-mutilation, possibly through alteration of central neurotransmitter levels (Dodman et al, 1996b). At present, there is limited evidence to support this theory. In one published report, high levels of activity were not changed by decreasing dietary protein intake, but the duration of treatment was only 2 weeks (Dodman et al, 1996b). Fear-motivated territorial aggression was decreased by the low-protein diet, suggesting that self-mutilation that is motivated by anxiety may also be helped by a low-protein diet.

References and Suggested Readings

Dodman NH, Knowles KE, Shuster L, et al: Behavioral changes associated with suspected complex partial seizures in Bull Terriers. J Am Vet Med Assoc 208:688, 1996a.
A description of tail chasing and other compulsive behaviors in 8 Bull terriers, most of whom responded to treatment with phenobarbital.

Dodman NH, Reisner I, Shuster L, et al: Effect of dietary protein content on behavior in dogs. J Am Vet Med Assoc 208:376, 1996b.
Short-term feeding of a low-protein diet reduced fear-related territorial aggression in dogs, but had no effect on dominance aggression or high activity levels.

Dodman NH, Shuster L, White SD, et al: Use of narcotic antagonists to modify stereotypic self-licking, self-chewing, and scratching in dogs. J Am Vet Med Assoc 193:815, 1988.
Injection of nalmefene or naltrexone decreased self-mutilation in 10 of 11 dogs.

Goldberger E, Rapoport JL: Canine acral lick dermatitis: Response to the antiobsessional drug clomipramine. J Am Anim Hosp Assoc 27:179, 1991.
A single-blind, controlled study showing that treatment with clomipramine significantly reduced licking compared with treatment with desipramine.

Hewson CJ, Luescher UA: Compulsive disorder in dogs. In: Voith VL, Borchelt PL, eds: Readings in Companion Animal Behavior. Trenton: Veterinary Learning Systems, 1996, p 153.
An outline of the clinical presentation and history of compulsive behaviors in dogs, as well as general treatment recommendations.

Rapoport JL, Ryland DH, Kriete M: Drug treatment of canine acral lick: An animal model of obsessive-compulsive disorder. Arch Gen Psychiatry 49:517, 1992.
A series of double-blind crossover studies comparing clomipramine, fluoxetine, sertraline, desipramine, and fenfluramine for treatment of acral lick dermatitis. The first three medications all decreased licking significantly.

Rivers B, Walter PA, McKeever PJ: Treatment of canine acral lick dermatitis with radiation therapy: 17 cases (1979–1991). J Am Anim Hosp Assoc 29:541, 1993.
Permanent (6/17 cases) or temporary (4/17) resolution of lesions was noted following orthovoltage or ⁶⁰Co teletherapy.

Simpson BS, Davidson G: Concerns about possible drug interactions. J Am Vet Med Assoc 209:1380, 1996.
A letter describing an adverse reaction in a dog being treated with a tricyclic antidepressant (imipramine) and an antitick collar containing amitraz.

Simpson BS, Simpson DM: Behavioral pharmacotherapy. In: Voith VL, Borchelt PL, eds: Readings in Companion Animal Behavior. Trenton: Veterinary Learning Systems, 1996, p 100.
A description of the major classes of psychoactive medication used to treat pet behavioral problems, including common side effects and specific applications.

Electronic Pet Identification and Retrieval Systems

WALT INGWERSEN

Whitby, Ontario, Canada

The use of electronic means to identify animals is a relatively recent phenomenon that is quickly gaining widespread attention for companion animal application. It has evolved through necessity in the quest for a more effective means of animal identification to both better support animal control endeavors and fulfill owner expectations. Original identification methods, such as the collar tag and tattoo, stemmed from licensing and pedigree initiatives, respectively. Although they still have merit, and are in use today, tags and tattoos are limited in effectiveness because of their potential for loss, removal, and illegibility. The advent of electronic identification has provided a reliable, easy-to-implement method of identification that has overcome these limitations. Electronic identification was first utilized in the agricultural sector for identification of livestock, allowing for automation of data and herd management protocols. Initial implementation was in the format of an ear tag or other externally applied device. Similar systems were introduced for companion animals but did not generate widespread interest owing to their size and manner of implementation. Because of advancements in miniaturization and bar-coding technology, electronic identification has evolved into small, injectable microchips with a subsequent broader acceptance and application.

All electronic identification systems, also termed radio frequency identification (RFID) systems, are composed of the same three integrated components: a microchip, a reader, and an associated database.

MICROCHIP

The microchip, technically referred to as a transponder, has one main function: to store and, when prompted, to transmit its unique identification message. The microchip is composed of a silicon chip, which stores the identification code, that is connected to a wire coil antenna that both receives the energy necessary to power the microchip and transmits the radio signal containing the identification code. These two components are hermetically sealed within a biologically inert glass capsule with the overall size (approximately 2 mm by 12 mm) being comparable to a grain of rice. The structure and sequence of the information contained within the microchip has been standardized through the International Standards Organization (ISO) and allows for approximately 275 billion unique, 10-digit alphanumeric code combinations. The microchip has an exceptionally long life span, far exceeding that of the animal into which it is implanted, because it does not contain an internal power source. Rather, microchips are passive systems powered through the principle of electromagnetic

TABLE 1. Manufacturers of Microchips for Companion Animal Application

American Veterinary Identification Devices (AVID)
3179 Hamner Avenue
Norco, California, USA 91760
Phone: 909-371-7505 or 800-336-2843
Fax: 909-737-8967

Allflex SA
3300 Arapahoe, Suite 213
Boulder, Colorado, USA 80303
Phone: 303-449-9665
Fax: 303-440-0281

Datamars
Datamars SA—via Ponteggia
CH-6814 Cadempino-Lugano
Switzerland
Phone: (41) 91 968 2701
Fax: (41) 91 968 2741

Destron-Fearing Corporation*
490 Villaume Avenue
South St. Paul, Minnesota, USA 55075-2445
Phone: 612-455-1621
Fax: 612-455-0413

EID Electronic Identification Devices, Ltd. (Trovan)†
P.O. Box 40227
Santa Barbara, California, USA 93140
Phone: 805-565-1288
Fax: 805-565-1127

*Distributed by Schering-Plough Animal Health (800-341-5785) within the USA

†Distributed by InfoPET (612-890-2080) within the USA. A United States district court in Denver, Colorado, ruled in April 1996 that EID/Trovan microchip violated patents held by Destron-Fearing and enjoined InfoPET, as well as EID/Trovan, from further sales of their ID 100 injectable microchip within the US. This ruling was upheld on appeal in November 1997.

induction (see following section). Most current manufacturers (Table 1) also employ an external design or chemical coating that promotes the attachment of the microchip at the site of implantation, thereby greatly reducing the potential for migration. The microchip is supplied to the user in a preloaded device, much like a hypodermic needle, for easy subcutaneous implantation in a process very similar to vaccination. Therefore, no sedation is required and the procedure can be done in the veterinarian's office while the owner waits. In North America, as well as most user regions, implantation sites have been standardized based on the species involved (Table 2). Current research, development, and global standardization efforts are focusing on more complex microchip systems. Future applications, therefore, may include microchips designed as physiologic

TABLE 2. Standardized Microchip Implantation Sites Based on Species

Species	Site
Canine and feline*	The microchip is implanted subcutaneously on the dorsal midline, just cranial to the shoulder blades or scapula
Avian	The microchip is implanted intramuscularly within the pectoral muscles
Equine	The microchip is implanted within the nuchal ligament at the halfway point between the ears and the withers.

*In Europe, another common implantation site in the canine and feline is subcutaneously in the middle of the left side of the neck.

sensors potentially allowing for a noninvasive manner of providing information on body temperature, glucose, and hormonal measurements, among other factors.

READER

The microchip reader, also referred to as a scanner or transceiver, has two main functions. The first is to power the microchip, enabling it to transmit its message. The second is to receive and subsequently display the unique identification code transmitted. The energy necessary to power the microchip is derived through electromagnetic induction. This process is initiated when an alternating electrical current is passed through the excitation coil, or antenna, located within the reader. This produces a magnetic field in the space surrounding the reader. When the microchip is placed within this magnetic field, an alternating electrical current is induced within its own internal wire coil antenna. This electrical current ultimately gives the microchip the power to transmit the identification message. Although all electronic identification systems are based on the principle of electromagnetic induction, the specific manner and radio frequency in which a microchip and reader interact is called a communication protocol. Protocols currently vary between manufacturers. Despite the technical feasibility of reading any of the various protocols, there are compatibility problems between products because individual protocols are legally restricted from general use through patent protection laws. In markets with competing products, this lack of compatibility has resulted in a fragmentation rather than a coalescence of the recovery network, and has been the single most important impediment to the broad implementation of this technology. Fortunately, this is being addressed, both nationally and internationally, through standardization efforts. Globally, the ISO has facilitated the cooperative adoption of a single communication protocol that will overcome this concern and ensure the future compatibility of products. Published in October of 1996, the standard protects backward compatibility to pre-existing products by mandating the production and use of universal readers. A universal reader bridges the compatibility gap by providing a single reader that can identify the specific alphanumeric code of any microchip present, regardless of manufacturer.

The scanning protocol and reader maintenance should follow the manufacturer's recommendations to ensure optimal reader performance. It is strongly advised that the microchip implanted be scanned prior to and following implantation, as well as yearly, to verify proper function and location.

DATABASE

Most manufacturers, distributors, and users participate in, or offer their own, database registry where the unique identification code, as well as information pertaining to that microchip (i.e., animal name, owner, and contact phone number), is stored. Most databases offer accessibility to this information 24 hours per day, 7 days per week, often through internet linkup. Many databases are also protected through various veterinary medical associations or humane-shelter groups, ensuring that users can be guaranteed access to current information regardless of any eventuality. Also, most distributors and manufacturers have implemented sophisticated tracking systems to trace the microchip code to the ultimate user in the event the database information is incomplete. Both the database and the supporting tracking system are essential to the overall performance and integrity of electronic identification, and the user must ensure their existence when implementing this technology. The database is only as good as the information it contains. Owners of pets implanted with microchips should be counseled yearly to ensure that the pertinent information is current.

The distinct advantages of electronic identification and retrieval systems are their unalterable, unique identification, their permanence, and their long life span. They have greatly enhanced animal recovery programs where implemented, especially when done with municipal, shelter, and veterinary cooperation, and are currently being integrated into the licensing programs of many municipalities. However, they are not a panacea, because they require special equipment for implementation and they lack immediate visibility. These concerns have been partially dealt with through the use of external tags, supplied by the manufacturer, indicating that an animal has had a microchip implanted. It is also important not to rely on any single manner of pet identification, as no individual system is infallible. The likelihood of a lost pet's being returned to its rightful owner is greatly increased when electronic identification systems are combined with other methods of animal identification.

References and Supplemental Reading

Ingwersen W: To chip or not to chip. TRENDS Magazine (American Animal Hospital Association) February/March 12:6, 1996.
A review of the evolution of microchip technology, its implementation and standardization efforts, concentrating on companion animals in North America.

Olson P: Microchip technology: Coming of age. SHOPTALK (American Humane Association) 14:1, 1996.
A review of the implementation of microchip technology in the context of issues specific to the shelter environment.

Critical Care

Nishi Dhupa

Robert J. Murtaugh

Consulting Editors

Cats Are Not Dogs in Critical Care

REBECCA KIRBY
ELKE RUDLOFF
WANDA WILSON
Milwaukee, Wisconsin

Affectionate, independent, aloof, mysterious, unpredictable . . . the cat. Throughout the ages, the cat has mystified mankind. In the days of ancient Egypt, the cat was viewed as a domestic pet as well as a symbol of deity. Over time, artists, including Rembrandt, Renoir, and Picasso, have immortalized the personalities of the cat. Today, not only is the personality of the cat recognized as unequal and unpredictable, but also their responses to disease and therapy present constant challenges to the veterinarian. The cat is not a dog in critical care.

Cats and dogs in crisis share many of the same diseases, but they may not show the same clinical signs. Pancreatitis in the cat may cause anorexia and severe hypotension and hypothermia, without the vomiting or obvious abdominal pain typically seen in the dog. Heart disease in the cat may be evidenced by hindlimb paralysis, rather than respiratory distress. Common naturally occurring endocrine diseases in the dog, such as hyperadrenocorticism and hypoadrenocorticism, are rare in the cat. Cats have diseases and viruses almost unique to the species, such as hyperthyroidism, asthma, feline lower urinary tract disease, and feline leukemia virus and immunodeficiency virus–related diseases.

Many aspects of critical care are unique for the cat. The physiologic response to shock, procedures required for resuscitation, and the methods used in patient monitoring present specific challenges. It is often necessary to resuscitate, support, and stabilize the cat for extended periods of time prior to or throughout the course of definitive therapy. Struggling or aggressive manipulation can be debilitating or life-threatening. Optimal care requires a thorough and methodical approach to diagnostics, monitoring, therapeutics, and supportive care. By following the *Rule of 20* (Table 1), the major concerns in case management will be addressed (Kirby, 1995).

MANAGING THE CRITICALLY ILL CAT

Shock and Perfusion

Cats are difficult to resuscitate from hypotensive episodes. The heart rate is most often normal or slow with hypotension, instead of the typical tachycardia demonstrated by other species. In a series of hypotensive cats evaluated at the authors' center (systolic blood pressure by Doppler ultrasound was less than 90 mm Hg), most cats were found to have normal or slow heart rates. The heart rates of normotensive cats presented for emergency examination were 165 to 240 beats/min. Cardiac output is a function of myocardial contractility and heart rate; thus, the compensatory response to shock is blunted. Hyperdynamic, sympathomimetic signs of shock seen in other species are not typically observed in the cat. Shock in the cat is most commonly manifested by a normal or slow heart rate, severe hypothermia (≤98°F), weak or nonpalpable peripheral pulses, and profound mental depression. The mucous membranes are gray or white, and capillary refill time ranges from markedly delayed to absent. Bradycardia and low cardiac output contribute to hypothermia, and hypothermia accentuates the bradycardia by depressing the sinus node.

Vascular Access

In the authors' experience, long-term vascular access is best obtained from a medial saphenous vein. Long, flexible intravenous catheters are threaded cranially until the tip of the catheter is resting in the abdominal vena cava. Central venous pressure (CVP) estimates from this location are found to adequately reflect those of the thoracic vena cava. In addition, blood samples can be taken from the catheter, a procedure that avoids the stress of restraint for multiple venipunctures.

Fluid Balance and Colloid Oncotic Pressure

The blood volume in the cat is 66 ml/kg, in contrast to 90 ml/kg in the dog (Kohn, 1992). When intravascular volume deficits result in poor perfusion, crystalloids can be administered as fast as 45 to 66 ml/kg per hour. However, resuscitation with crystalloids alone frequently results in significant pulmonary and pleural fluid accumulations. The resultant hypoxemia contributes to the pathophysiology of shock.

TABLE 1. **Rule of 20 Checklist for Cats**

Fluid balance
Oncotic pull
Glucose
Electrolytes
Oxygenation/ventilation
Level of consciousness/mentation
Blood pressure
Heart rate/rhythm/contractility
Albumin
Coagulation
Red blood cells/hemoglobin
Renal function
Immune status/antibiotic dosages/WBCs
GI motility and mucosal integrity
Drug dosages and metabolism
Nutrition
Pain control
Nursing care/temperature control
Wound care/bandage change
Tender loving care

From Purvis D, Kirby R: Systemic inflammatory response syndrome: Septic shock. Vet Clin North Am Small Anim Pract 24:1225, 1994.

Resuscitation from hypovolemic shock in the cat is best accomplished with a combination of crystalloids and colloids. A rapid infusion of isotonic crystalloids is administered at 10 to 20 ml/kg. Since rapid intravenous infusion of hetastarch results in vomiting and hypotension in the cat, hetastarch (Hespan, DuPont) is administered at 5 ml/kg over 5 to 10 minutes. This amount is repeated at 5- to 10-minute intervals until the mean systemic arterial blood pressure is at least 60 to 80 mm Hg and the CVP is 6 to 8 cm H_2O (ensuring adequate cardiac and renal function). The cat is then maintained on a constant-rate intravenous infusion (CRI) at 10 to 40 ml/kg per day of hetastarch. Crystalloids are administered at the minimum amount required to maintain systemic arterial blood pressure and circulating blood volume.

The large fluid volumes typically required to initially resuscitate and maintain blood volume and pressure can lead to sudden intravascular volume overload and pulmonary edema. This situation can be avoided by titrating downward the amount of fluid being infused as soon as the CVP and systemic arterial blood pressure are stable for 1 to 2 hours with the volume infused. Should volume overload occur, decreasing the rate of crystalloid infusion, stopping colloid infusion, and administering furosemide (Lasix, Hoechst) at 2 to 4 mg/kg IV can help eliminate clinical signs.

Cats with systemic inflammatory response syndrome (SIRS) commonly develop intravascular fluid depletion with loss of albumin molecules through capillaries (see *CVT XII*, p. 139). During maintenance fluid therapy, when the albumin is less than 2.0 g/dl, fresh-frozen plasma (at 10 to 15 ml/kg) becomes the colloid of choice.

Glucose

The stress response in the cat frequently results in a transient hyperglycemia, requiring re-evaluation to exclude diabetes mellitus. The blood glucose concentration should be maintained between 100 and 200 mg/dl, and dextrose-containing fluids should not be administered. Conversely, hypotensive cats must be closely monitored for hypoglycemia, and glucose replacement can be accomplished by giving 0.25 to 0.5 gm/kg IV of a 50% dextrose solution, followed by a 2.5% concentration in the maintenance fluid.

Electrolytes

Alterations in potassium concentrations are common in critically ill cats. Cats with renal failure fed acidifying diets, high in protein and low in magnesium, can be presented with hypokalemic polymyopathy (Chew, 1994). Some cats with chronic renal failure can have profound potassium wasting and require long-term oral potassium supplementation. Although ventroflexion of the neck and generalized weakness can occur with hypokalemia, these signs are inconsistent. This consideration requires that serum potassium concentration be measured and that maintenance intravenous fluids be supplemented with potassium chloride (5 to 20 mEq KCl/250 ml of fluids) as needed.

Hyperkalemia can also be observed. Heart rate is not a reliable predictor of hyperkalemia in the cat. Normal and rapid heart rates have been seen in male cats with obstruction of urinary tract outflow and serum potassium concentrations greater than 10 mEq/L. When a cat has bradycardia (≤120 beats/min) due to hyperkalemia, there may be only minutes to respond before circulatory collapse and death. The administration of regular insulin (Humulin-R, Lilly), 0.2 to 0.4 U/kg IV accompanied by 2 gm of glucose IV/U of insulin, sodium bicarbonate, 0.5 to 1 mEq/kg IV, or calcium gluconate (Fujisawa), 0.2 to 1.5 ml/kg of 10% solution IV slowly, can be life-saving.

Hypophosphatemia, which can lead to red blood cell hemolysis and energy depletion, is most commonly seen in the anorectic cat beginning to receive nutritional supplementation. Careful monitoring of packed cell volume and serum color is required. Replacement therapy is administered as required (potassium or sodium phosphate, 0.01 to 0.06 mmol/kg per hour IV).

Oxygen and Ventilation

Oxygen supplementation is needed when perfusion or ventilation problems exist and is best supplied by nasal cannula or hood in the cat. Observation of the patient's breathing pattern can help determine the location of the problem and permit intervention often without stressful diagnostics (Table 2). Administration of a mild sedative such as butorphanol (Torbugesic, Fort Dodge) at a dosage of 0.2 to 0.4mg/kg IV or IM may be required while oxygen support is being given.

Cats with significant work of breathing must have the airway and ventilation controlled by intubation and positive-pressure ventilation with 100% oxygen early in the disease process. Do not wait until these animals are agonal! Cats with subclinical bronchial hypersensitivity can develop clinical signs of asthma with the stress of illness or from compounding cardiac and respiratory diseases.

TABLE 2. Breathing Patterns in Cats

Pattern	Location
Loud breathing (heard without stethoscope)	Large airway
Inspiratory stridor	Pharyngeal or laryngeal
Expiratory stridor	Intrathoracic trachea or bronchi
Rapid, shallow, smooth breathing	Parenchymal disease
Breathing with abdomen and chest moving in same direction at the same time; in and out motion of the cupula	
Short, choppy breathing	Pleural space disease
Breathing with abdomen and chest moving in opposite direction; inspiratory and expiratory times are short; no movement of the cupula	
Short inspiration, prolonged expiration with abdominal push	Small airway disease
Chest and abdomen moving in same direction at same time; expiratory push with the diaphragm*	

* May be combined with rapid, shallow, smooth breathing in cases of severe pulmonary edema with congestion of the small airways. The chest and abdomen move together, in the same direction, during each phase of respiration.

Cats with SIRS can develop pulmonary edema and pleural effusion due to capillary leakage and decreased myocardial performance. There are no obvious clinical signs until the edema is advanced. Initially, the cat has an increase in respiratory rate and poor mucous membrane color. Thoracic auscultation reveals louder than normal lung sounds and occasionally a pleural friction rub. When crackles are ausculted, pulmonary edema is severe.

Declining Level of Consciousness

A decline in the level of consciousness or mentation of the cat warrants immediate investigation for hypotension, hyperammonemia, and hypoglycemia. Other problems such as hyperosmolar syndromes, hypoxemia, thiamine deficiency, hypokalemia, and metabolic toxins from liver or renal failure should be considered. The inciting cause is treated, and the cat closely monitored. Vomiting and silent aspiration can cause a vasovagal-induced respiratory or cardiac arrest.

Blood Pressure

A comparison of indirect blood pressure measurement techniques in the cat (see *CVT XII,* p. 110 and p. 113) has found that Doppler techniques provide the most accurate information (McLeish, 1977). Hypotension or poor perfusion that is nonresponsive to intravascular volume resuscitation necessitates a search for ongoing fluid loss, hypoglycemia, hypoxemia, cardiac dysfunction, prolonged hypothermia and bradycardia, cardiac arrhythmias, electrolyte imbalances, cardiac tamponade, and brain stem disease. Persistent hypotension, not attributable to these complications, requires assessment of circulating blood volume, oxygen supplementation, pain control, evaluation of cardiac function, and treatment as indicated (e.g., vasopressor therapy).

Serial echocardiograms done by the authors in cats with persistent hypotension and SIRS demonstrate dilation of the left ventricle and decreased contractility during severe hypotensive stages of the syndrome. Although cardiac function improves as the disease resolves, positive inotropic support (dobutamine, 1.0 to 5.0 μg/kg per minute IV) can be required in the interim. A side effect of dobutamine in cats after approximately 24 hours of infusion is the development of seizures. Diazepam administration can be used to control the seizures until the dobutamine infusion is no longer required. It is ideal to monitor these patients by arterial blood pressure (ABP) measurement and even serial echocardiograms. Blindly placing a hypotensive cat on dobutamine may be a fatal mistake if the cat has underlying hypertrophic cardiomyopathy.

When intravascular volume and cardiac contractility are adequate and hypotension persists, dopamine (Abbott Labs), 5 to 15 μg/kg per minute IV, is infused for its vasopressor effects. The dosage is initially 5 μg/kg per minute and can be increased by increments of 2 μg/kg per minute (up to 15 μg/kg per minute) until the desired effect is seen. When systemic arterial blood pressure appears stable for 2 to 4 hours, the pressor drugs are gradually weaned to prevent ischemic renal damage.

Hypertension in the cat is suspected when systolic/diastolic systemic arterial blood pressures are repeatedly at least 160/100 mm Hg (Kobayashi et al, 1990). Pulse quality is not a reliable indicator. Severe hypertension can lead to poor peripheral perfusion, retinal hemorrhage and detachment, renal damage, and myocardial wall thickening. The underlying cause is identified, and a vasodilator chosen based on the cause (see pp. 835 and 838). In urgent situations (e.g., retinal detachment), initial therapy can be begun with amlodipine (Norvasc, Pfizer) at 0.625 mg every 24 hours.

Heart Rate, Rhythm, and Contractility

Careful auscultation of the heart is required to detect murmurs and gallops suggestive of underlying cardiac disease. Murmurs are most often heard in one location in the cat, just left of the sternum near the apical impulse. The gallop or murmur may be intermittent and very localized, requiring patience and concentration during auscultation.

Underlying cardiomyopathy can interfere with cardiovascular stabilization of other conditions. The authors follow a "Rule of 4" for cardiomyopathy in the cat. Cardiomyopathy can exist in different forms, including dilated, hypertrophic, or left ventricular endocardial fibrosis (also called restrictive or intermediate). The cardiac dynamics and therapeutics are different for each, and definitive therapy requires careful diagnostics (see Section 9). When any one of the following four clinical signs is present, cardiomyopathy must be excluded: (1) murmur or gallop, (2) unexplained hypothermia, (3) unexplained bradycardia, or (4) louder than normal or "moist" lung sounds (crackles). Frequently, a gallop or murmur becomes noticeable on day 2 or 3 of hospitalization, after volume resuscitation has occurred.

Fatal congestive heart failure has developed in cats with a heart murmur or gallop after they have received ketamine at sedative or anesthetic doses. Ketamine administration can increase systemic arterial blood pressure and myocardial oxygen consumption. These observations are relevant to cases of dyspnea following administration of ketamine. The drug should be used cautiously—if at all—in cats with unexplained murmurs or gallops.

Cardiac arrhythmias in cats most often have a definable and treatable underlying cause, such as hyperkalemia, hypokalemia, hypoxemia, hypercapnia, hypercalcemia, hypocalcemia, acidosis, hypomagnesemia, cardiomyopathy, or endogenous toxins from organ failure, including the liver or kidneys. It is always best to treat the underlying problem, rather than to administer palliative treatment with antiarrhythmic drugs alone. Oxygen supplementation and administration of potassium chloride are often appropriate initial steps. Infrequently, antiarrhythmic agents can be required for sustained ventricular tachycardia, with careful attention given to drug dosages in the cat (lidocaine, 0.25 to 1 mg/kg IV over 5 minutes; procainamide, 2 mg/kg IV over 5 minutes to 8 mg/kg).

Critically ill cats can express an increased vagal tone, making these cats highly susceptible to vagal-induced respiratory and cardiac arrest. This problem can occur with vomiting and straining to defecate or urinate. Recognition and prearrest interventions such as control of emesis and close monitoring of heart rate are recommended before cardiopulmonary resuscitation becomes necessary.

Coagulation

Coagulation times—activated clotting time (ACT), prothrombin time (PT), and activated partial thromboplastin time (aPTT)—in the cat are normally shorter than those observed in the dog, requiring a separate set of normal coagulation values. Cats can become hypercoagulable with low-flow states and SIRS, requiring careful monitoring of critically ill cats for declining platelet numbers and antithrombin (AT) levels. The authors have found AT activity higher than 90% to be normal in the cat. When AT levels fall below 60%, replacement of AT is required by administering plasma.

Profound hypothermia, as well as the administration of particular drugs (e.g., nonsteroidal anti-inflammatory medications or cephalosporins), can interfere with platelet function. The most common physical evidence of disseminated intravascular coagulation (DIC) is failure to form a solid clot in a clot tube. Occasionally, petechiae, ecchymoses, and subcutaneous hemorrhages are detectable. Transfusions of plasma or whole blood for replacement of coagulation factors and AT, along with administration of heparin (100 U/kg SC first dose, then 50 U/kg SC every 8 hours), treats DIC while the inciting cause is corrected. Fresh-frozen plasma and fresh whole blood are required for replacement of factors VIII and V. Fresh whole blood or platelet-rich plasma is required for replacement of platelets.

Cats with cardiomyopathy are prone to thrombus formation in the left atrium or thromboembolism to peripheral arterial vessels. Echocardiographic evidence of echogenic "smoke" thrombus in the left atrium or the presence of a peripheral thromboembolus is indication for anticoagulant therapy. Warfarin (Coumadin, DuPont), 0.5 mg/cat PO every 24 hours, is instituted, and heparin, 100 IU/kg IV every 8 hours, is administered for the initial 72 hours of warfarin therapy. The end point of the anticoagulant therapy is when the PT is prolonged 1.5 to 2 times normal. Thrombolytic therapy (streptokinase) has demonstrated mixed results.

Red Blood Cell/Hemoglobin Concentration

Frequent blood sampling of critically ill cats can cause iatrogenic anemia sufficient to require blood transfusion by day 3 or 4 of hospitalization. The use of blood collection and blood culture tubes designed for infants and babies minimizes the quantities of blood drawn. Microhematocrit tubes can be used to harvest small aliquots of serum for in-house biochemical testing.

Cats have three major blood types: A, B, and AB (see p. 115). Cats with type B erythrocytes have strong, naturally occurring anti-A antibody. Fewer than 30% of type-A cats have anti-B antibodies, and type AB cats have no preformed antibodies to blood types. A strong possibility of a significant transfusion reaction exists in type-B cats receiving type-A blood; thus, a crossmatch is always recommended prior to blood transfusion.

Other inherent differences in feline red blood cells exist. Feline erythrocytes have a life span of 72 days. Rouleaux formation is common and can be confused with red cell agglutination when viewed macroscopically. The two types of reticulocytes are punctate and aggregate. Aggregate (coarse clumping of ribosomes) reticulocytes mature into punctate (small individual inclusions) reticulocytes. Punctate reticulocytes have a relatively longer life span than aggregate reticulocytes (10 to 12 days versus 12 hours). Both the aggregate and punctate reticulocytes must be considered in the calculation of the corrected reticulocyte percentage. Large numbers of aggregate cells represent active regeneration, while punctate cells represent cumulative regeneration (Tvedten, 1989). A previously regenerative anemia that becomes nonregenerative can demonstrate a large number of punctate reticulocytes without aggregate reticulocytes. This finding requires repeated evaluation of reticulocyte morphology and indices.

Feline red blood cells often have Heinz bodies owing to physiologic oxidative stresses. These red blood cells are very sensitive to oxidation of hemoglobin by diseases and drugs such as methylene blue, acetaminophen, benzocaine, and propylthiouracil (see *CVT XII*, p. 443). Macrocytic-normochromic red blood cells, without reticulocytosis, are most common in feline leukemia virus–related myeloproliferative disorders. *Hemobartonella felis* can recrudesce in cats stressed by illness and cause hemolytic anemia. Normocytic-normochromic anemia commonly develops in critically ill cats. When a significant anemia is due to chronic renal failure, treatment with human recombinant erythropoietin (Epogen; Amgen: 100 U/kg SC or IV every 48 hours until packed cell volume reaches 30%, then 100 U/kg every 7 days) is indicated (see *CVT XII*, p. 961). In general, 4 to 12 weeks is required before maintenance (weekly) treatments are instituted. Serum iron-binding capacity must be adequate for production of new red blood cells, and supplemental iron administration may be required.

Renal Function

Geriatric cats have a high prevalence of chronic renal insufficiency. The inability to concentrate urine promotes volume depletion and potassium wasting. Hyperphosphatemia can cause hyperparathyroidism and hypocalcemia. Anorexia and chronic anemia are common clinical findings. Renal hypertension can complicate resuscitation procedures.

Prolonged hypertension, hypotension, or prolonged resuscitation with high-dosage vasopressor administration can lead to renal ischemia and acute renal failure. These factors necessitate rapid volume replacement in hypotensive episodes, monitoring and control of hypertension, and careful attention to weaning from vasopressors as soon as possible. Mannitol (0.1 gm/kg IV), furosemide (1 to 2 mg/kg per hour for 4 hours IV), and dopamine (1 to 3 µg/kg per minute IV) CRI administration can be used to support glomerular filtration and renal function.

Immune Status

Viral (feline leukemia virus, feline immunodeficiency virus, feline panleukopenia), protozoal (toxoplasmosis), and overwhelming bacterial (gram-positive and gram-negative) infections are common causes of immunosuppression (see p. 280). Feline leukemia virus can cause immunodeficiency by affecting lymphocyte function (Olsen and Krakowka, 1984). Feline immunodeficiency virus generally requires the presence of intercurrent bacterial or other infectious agents to induce immunosuppressive clinical syndromes. Testing for these viruses should occur when there are opportunistic infections or persistent or recurring diseases in the cat. When these viruses are discovered in the critically ill cat, treatment can be difficult and prolonged.

Chronic illness associated with fevers and neutropenia may also be due to toxoplasmosis infection. Serum IgM titers may suggest active infection. A response is generally seen with administration of clindamycin HCl (Antirobe, Upjohn) at 25 mg/kg PO every 12 hours for 2 to 3 weeks.

For bacterial infections, antibiotic selection is best when confirmed by the results of microbiologic culture and antibiotic sensitivity. In addition, the capability of the critically ill cat to metabolize and eliminate the antibiotic, and potential untoward side effects of the drug, are considered in the antibiotic selection process. In general, for empirical treatment pending culture results, a broad-spectrum intravenously administered antibiotic is selected (see pp. 267 and 272). Intravenous injections are administered slowly. In seemingly resistant bacterial infections, the considerations of *Mycobacterium* (see *CVT XII*, p. 622), *Mycoplasma* (see *CVT XII*, p. 301), and L-form bacteria should be investigated.

Bacterial L-forms and *Mycoplasma* are cell wall–deficient forms of bacteria. Penetrating bite wounds or surgical incisions are common locations of L-form infection, often manifesting with dermal abscesses, cellulitis, and polyarthritis. *Mycoplasma* is commonly associated with the development of secondary respiratory infections, which are not responsive to typical antibiotics, including cephalosporins. The diagnosis of infections with L-forms and *Mycoplasma* organisms is difficult because of the problems in isolating or identifying these bacteria by microbiologic culture techniques and light microscopy. The treatment of these infections consists of administration of oral doxycycline at 5 mg/kg PO every 12 hours until the discharges or respiratory signs have resolved for a week.

With geriatric cats, one must also consider concomitant chronic diseases that may contribute to immunosuppression and longer recovery periods in the intensive care unit. Other than chronic infectious diseases, hyperthyroidism, inflammatory bowel disease, renal insufficiency, diabetes mellitus, and dental disease need to be considered.

DRUG DOSES AND METABOLISM

Many drug dosages in the cat have been extrapolated from studies done in dogs. The cat's body surface area per unit of body weight is greater than that of the dog, and dosage extrapolation between these species can be inaccurate.

The liver plays a key role in the unique metabolism of many drugs in the cat. Lipid-soluble drugs (e.g., morphine, chloramphenicol, aspirin, primidone, acetaminophen, phenols, barbiturates, benzodiazepines, propofol) must be converted to water-soluble by-products before excretion. Cats lack many of the hepatic glucuronyl transferases that normally enable conjugation and excretion of these drugs. Toxic levels of these drugs or metabolites can accumulate. Enterohepatic recycling can also occur in cats, and this recycling can affect cumulative plasma concentrations of certain drugs, such as digoxin. Hepatic acetylation is well developed in the cat, causing faster clearance of drugs such as hydralazine and diltiazem.

Many of the published dosage recommendations are based on drug blood levels and clinical signs of toxicity. Unfortunately, there is scant information on the metabolic responses required for drug conversion and elimination by cats. The dosage recommendations for cats in the veterinary medical literature are often based on clinical experience and anecdotal information. When giving *any* drug to the cat, the proper dosage, route of administration, and dosing interval should be confirmed as safe and effective for cats.

NUTRITION

Being carnivores by nature, cats require no carbohydrates but need high levels of meat-based protein. The cat's protein requirement is 50% higher for growth and over 100% for maintenance compared with the dog.

Cats require dietary sources of arginine. Arginine is required for normal protein synthesis and ammonia detoxification. Domestic cats lack intestinal pyrroline-5-carboxylate synthase, which is required for the production of an arginine precursor, ornithine. A urea cycle intermediate, arginine enables conversion of ammonia to urea. Cats can develop severe hyperammonemia from anorexia or ingestion of an arginine-free meal (Morris and Rogers, 1978). Arginine has other important roles that include increasing endocrine secretagogue activity, improving nitrogen retention, acting as a substrate for nitric oxide production, reducing nitrogen loss in postoperative patients, enhancing collagen deposition in wounds, enhancing T-cell function, and the growth of lymphocytes (Babul and Hurson, 1994).

Cats also require a dietary source of taurine. Cats cannot synthesize enough taurine from dietary precursors to meet obligate intestinal loss. The cat uses only taurine for bile salt synthesis (in comparison to dogs, that can substitute glycine), causing an ongoing obligate loss of taurine with excreted bile salts. Taurine deficiency has been proved to cause dilated cardiomyopathy and retinal degeneration.

Cats do not have the ability to convert beta-carotene to active vitamin A (retinol). Cats lack dioxygenase enzymes in the intestinal mucosa that split the beta-carotene molecule to vitamin A aldehyde (retinal). Preformed vitamin A must be ingested or administered, as neither dietary nor intravenous beta-carotene can prevent the development of vitamin A deficiency and its consequence of blindness.

Since the cat cannot convert tryptophan to niacin, the niacin requirement of the cat is about four times that of the dog. Animal tissue is high in niacin, and this requirement is normally met by ingestion of a high-meat diet.

Arachidonic acid is needed in the feline diet, since cats cannot synthesize it from linoleic acid, in contrast to the dog. Arachidonic acid is an essential fatty acid required for maintenance of cell wall integrity and can be found in diets containing fats of animal source. Essential fatty acids should constitute 1% of the diet dry matter. Fatty acid deficiency results in poor quality of the hair coat and poor tissue integrity.

The nutritional requirements of the critically ill cat should be addressed early to minimize tissue catabolism and the development of hepatic lipidosis. Meat-based diets should be selected that provide a good-quality protein, vitamin A, thiamine, and niacin. The diet should be adequately supplemented with taurine and arginine. When the food is warmed prior to feeding or highly aromatic foods are fed, the palatability of the food offered to stressed and ill cats is often increased.

PAIN CONTROL

Pain can be manifested in the cat by mental depression, tachycardia (rare), anorexia, restlessness, or an irritable attitude. It is vital to the maintenance of cardiovascular function and the mental well-being of the cat to control pain. In the critically ill cat, it is best to titrate analgesics and sedatives to effect, as responses are variable and can be affected by underlying renal and hepatic dysfunction.

For mild to moderate pain control, butorphanol, 0.2 to 0.8 mg/kg IV every 2 to 6 hours, is given initially. For control of severe pain, the combination of injectable opioids—oxymorphone, (DuPont) 0.05 to 0.1 mg/kg IV, or morphine, 0.1 mg/kg IM—with diazepam, 0.2 mg/kg IV, is effective and reversible. In the hemodynamically stable feline, acepromazine, 0.02 to 0.1 mg/kg IV or IM, can be combined with the opioids. Fentanyl patches (Duragesic, Janssen), 25 μg/hr patch per cat, provide therapeutic blood levels after approximately 12 hours, and the effect lasts up to 72 hours.

Alternative approaches that can be used alone or in combination are regional anesthesia (nerve blocks or infusion in body cavities), epidural analgesia, and pre-emptive analgesia with administration of injectable opioids given prior to surgical intervention. Lidocaine administered subcutaneously or intravenously can cause methemoglobinemia and Heinz body anemia in the cat, and careful dosing is required.

NURSING CARE

The nursing staff should use minimal restraint to accomplish any task involving the manipulation of the critically ill cat. The cat must be removed from the cage and thoroughly examined at least twice daily. Any changes in the physical condition of the patient, including pulmonary function, may initially be very subtle and progress rapidly.

Hypothermia is a component of most diseases involving critically ill cats. These cats should initially be warmed passively. Warm fluids can be administered intravenously, and the cat can be wrapped in towels or blankets or placed in a warm incubator. Once intravascular volume replacement has been ensured, warm water–circulating blankets can be used. The cat must be mobile enough to move off of the heating blanket to minimize the risk of thermal injury. Geriatric cats especially can suffer impaired thermoregulation, and these patients should be monitored very closely.

TENDER LOVING CARE

Attention to the mental health of the cat is often as important as attention to the physical health of the patient. Visits by the owners are encouraged and having familiar items in the cage may minimize stress. It is important for cats to have fresh litter and a separate place for food within the confines of the cage. Blankets or bedding can be used to increase patient comfort. Providing a box for the cat to hide in or the use of other techniques for obstructing the view of strange animals (when the patient's condition allows) reduces the level of fear and stress.

References and Suggested Reading

Babul A, Hurson M: Arginine. In: Gay S, ed: Nutrition in Critical Care. St. Louis: Mosby–Year Book, 1994, p 107.

Chew D: Disorders of calcium and magnesium. In: Rush JE, ed: IVECCS Proceedings 1994, p 175.

Kirby R: Septic shock. In: Bonagura J, ed: Kirk's Current Veterinary Therapy XII. Philadelphia: WB Saunders, 1995, p 139.

Kobayashi DL, Peterson ME, Graves TK, et al: Hypertension in cats with chronic renal failure or hyperthyroidism. J Vet Intern Med 4:58, 1990.

Kohn CW, DiBartola SP: Composition and distribution of body fluids in dogs and cats. In: DiBartola SP, ed: Fluid Therapy In Small Animal Practice. Philadelphia: WB Saunders, 1992, p 1.

McLeish I: Doppler ultrasonic arterial pressure measurement in the cat. Vet Rec 100:290, 1977.

Morris JG, Rogers QR: Ammonia intoxication in the near adult cat as a result of dietary deficiency of arginine. Science 199:431, 1978.

Olsen RG, Krakowka S: Immune dysfunction associated with viral infections. Compen Cont Educ Pract Vet 6:422, 1984.

Rogers QR, Morris JR, Freedland RA: Lack of hepatic enzymatic adaption at low and high levels of dietary protein in the adult cat. Enzyme 22:348, 1977.

Tvedten H: Erythrocyte disorders. In: Willard MD, Tvedten H, Turnwald GH, eds: Small Animal Clinical Diagnosis By Laboratory Methods. Philadelphia: WB Saunders, 1989, p 36.

Differential Diagnosis of Laboratory Abnormalities in Critical Care Settings

Kenneth J. Drobatz
Deborah C. Mandell
Philadelphia, Pennsylvania

The measurement of clinical laboratory parameters is integral to the successful management of critically ill patients. The multitude of clinical laboratory abnormalities that occur in critically ill patients can be challenging to decipher. This article tabulates a variety of clinical laboratory abnormalities and the differential diagnoses associated with them (Tables 1 to 4). Also included are some major physiologic and clinical comments associated with each parameter and the most common causes, designated by an asterisk (*), of each laboratory abnormality observed at the authors' hospital. For selected clinical laboratory abnormalities, the authors have identified certain critical, or "panic," values, noting these in parentheses next to the stated abnormality in the accompanying tables. These values represent

Text continued on page 109

TABLE 1. Hematologic Studies

PCV	Total Solids	Differential Diagnosis
I. PACKED CELL VOLUME (PCV) AND TOTAL PLASMA SOLIDS		
Increased (>60%)	Increased (>9.5 g/dl)	Dehydration
	Normal	Splenic contraction (dog)
		Primary or secondary polycythemia
Normal	Normal	Dehydration with hypoproteinemia
		Anemia and hypoproteinemia with dehydration
	Decreased (<3.5 g/dl)	Decreased protein production (liver disease)
		Increased protein loss (gastrointestinal tract, kidney, third space)
	Increased	Anemia with dehydration
		Increased globulin production
Decreased	Normal	Increased red blood cell destruction
(Dogs <30%)		Decreased red blood cell production
(Cats <20%)		Chronic blood loss
	Decreased	Overhydration
		Blood loss

II. THROMBOCYTOPENIA (Critical value: <50,000/μl)
- A. Differential Diagnoses
  - 1. Decreased production
    - a. Immune mediated
    - b. Infections
    - c. Drugs
    - d. Neoplasms
  - 2. Sequestration
    - a. Hepatomegaly
    - b. Splenomegaly
    - c. Lungs (endotoxemia)
  - 3. Destruction
    - a. Primary immune-mediated thrombocytopenia (secondary causes have been ruled out)
    - b. Secondary immune-mediated thrombocytopenia (look for underlying cause, such as infectious agents, drugs, neoplasia, or systemic lupus erythematosus)

  - 4. Consumption or loss
    - a. Disseminated intravascular coagulation
    - b. Blood loss (usually causes only mild thrombocytopenia)
- B. Major Points
  - 1. Decreased platelet counts may be due to decreased production, increased consumption, destruction, or sequestration.
  - 2. Bleeding due to thrombocytopenia usually does not occur until the platelet count is less than 50,000/μl.
  - 3. Immune-mediated thrombocytopenias tend to cause the lowest platelet counts (<20,000/μl), although consumptive processes may rarely cause extremely low counts.

III. NEUTROPENIA (Critical value: <2500/μl)
- A. Differential Diagnosis
  - 1. Increased sequestration or consumption
    - a. Overwhelming bacterial infection
    - b. Endotoxemia
    - c. Viral infections
    - d. Anaphylaxis
  - 2. Decreased production
    - a. Viral infections (canine parvovirus, feline panleukopenia virus, feline leukemia virus)
    - b. Drugs (particularly chemotherapeutic agents)
    - c. Estrogen
- B. Major Points
  - 1. The major causes of neutropenia include decreased production, sequestration, or consumption.
  - 2. The major concern with neutropenia is immune compromise

IV. NEUTROPHILIA (Critical value: >35,000/μl)
- A. Differential Diagnosis
  - 1. Inflammation
  - 2. Infection
  - 3. Physiologic stress response
  - 4. Hypoxia
  - 5. Increased glucocorticoids (exogenous or endogenous)
  - 6. Neoplasia
  - 7. Regenerative anemia
- B. Major Points
  - 1. The major concern for an increased neutrophil count is infection, whether systemic or localized.

TABLE 2. Serum Electrolytes

I. HYPONATREMIA (Critical value: <125 mmol/L)
 A. Differential Diagnoses
  1. Diarrhea*
  2. Hypoadrenocorticism*
  3. Renal failure
  4. Potassium depletion
  5. Nephrotic syndrome
  6. Syndrome of inappropriate antidiuretic hormone (ADH) secretion
  7. Hypothyroidism
  8. Primary polydipsia
  9. Volume depletion (vomiting, diarrhea, polyuria)*
  10. Heart failure*
  11. Hypervolemia (fluid overinfusion)
  12. Metabolic acidosis
  13. Ketonuria
  14. Hyperglycemia*
  15. Pseudohypoadrenocorticism (whipworm [Trichuris trichiura] infection)
  16. Hyperosmotic agent administration (mannitol)
  17. Hyperlipidemia (pseudohyponatremia)*
  18. Hyperproteinemia (pseudohyponatremia)
 B. Major Points
  1. Changes in sodium concentration are due primarily to changes in free water distribution, loss, or gain.
  2. The common denominator in almost all hyponatremia states is an excess of water retention in relation to sodium.
  3. The clinical signs are dependent on the rate of development and degree of hyponatremia.
  4. The primary system affected is the central nervous system (CNS), owing to cerebral edema (CNS signs ranging from mild depression to stupor, coma, or seizures).
  5. Rapid correction of hyponatremia can result in CNS dehydration and central pontine myelinolysis.

II. HYPERNATREMIA (Critical value: >160 mmol/L)
 A. Differential Diagnoses
  1. Relatively sodium-free water loss
   a. Respiratory evaporation (hyperthermia, respiratory conditions)
   b. Renal loss (central diabetes insipidus, nephrogenic diabetes insipidus, osmotic diuresis)*
   c. Gastrointestinal loss (osmotic diarrhea)*
   d. Central nervous system disorders (primary hypodipsia, reset osmostat, essential hypernatremia)
  2. Intracellular free water shift
   a. Seizures or severe exercise
   b. Rhabdomyolysis
  3. Sodium retention
   a. Administration of fluids with a high concentration of sodium or sodium bicarbonate*
 B. Major Points
  1. Changes in sodium concentration are due primarily to changes in free water distribution, loss, or gain.
  2. Hypernatremia can result from sodium retention in excess of water, or water loss in excess of sodium, with the latter being the most common cause.
  3. Hypernatremia should not occur in patients that have constant access to free water and can drink.
  4. The clinical signs are dependent on the rate of development and degree of hypernatremia.
  5. The major organ system affected is the CNS, with signs ranging from mild depression to stupor, coma, or seizures.
  6. Rapid correction of chronic hypernatremia may result in cerebral edema.

III. HYPERKALEMIA (Critical value: >6 mmol/L)
 A. Differential Diagnoses
  1. Increased intake
   a. Oral
   b. Intravenous
  2. Shift of potassium from intracellular to extracellular space
   a. Pseudohyperkalemia (thrombocytosis, leukocytosis, hemolysis [Akitas])
   b. Metabolic acidosis (inorganic acids not organic acids such as lactic acidosis or ketoacidosis)
   c. Insulin deficiency (uncontrolled diabetes mellitus)
   d. Tissue catabolism or damage (rhabdomyolysis, tumor lysis syndrome, ischemia followed by reperfusion)
   e. Beta-adrenergic blockade
   f. Digitalis overdose
   g. Neuromuscular blockade (succinylcholine)
  3. Decreased urinary excretion
   a. Renal failure*
   b. Urinary obstruction*
   c. Ruptured urinary tract with urine retention*
   d. Effective volume depletion
   e. Hypoadrenocorticism*
   f. Pseudohypoadrenocorticism (whipworm infection—primary pathophysiologic cause unknown)*
 B. Major Points
  1. Hyperkalemia results from three major causes: increased intake, movement of potassium from the intracellular space to the extracellular space, and decreased urinary excretion.
  2. Cardiac electrophysiologic effects include tented T wave, widened QRS complex, prolonged PR interval, diminished or absent P wave, and merging of QRS complex and T wave.
  3. Muscle weakness and paralysis are other concerns with hyperkalemia.

IV. HYPOKALEMIA (Critical value: <3.0 mmol/L)
 A. Differential Diagnoses
  1. Decreased intake
   a. Anorexia*
   b. Administration of low potassium–containing fluids*
  2. Translocation of potassium into cells
   a. Alkalemia
   b. Hyperinsulinemia
   c. Beta-adrenergic agonist administration
   d. Hypothermia
  3. Increased gastrointestinal losses
   a. Vomiting*
   b. Diarrhea*
  4. Increased urinary losses
   a. Diuretic administration*
   b. Excessive administration of mineralocorticoids
   c. Cushing's disease (hyperadrenocorticism)
   d. Metabolic acidosis
   e. Penicillin administration
   f. Renal disease*
   g. Postobstructive diuresis*
   h. Polyuria*
   i. Vomiting, hypochloremia, and hypovolemia*
   j. Hypomagnesemia (may cause a severe and persistent hypokalemia until magnesium is replaced)
 B. Major Points
  1. The major categories of causes of hypokalemia include decreased intake, translocation of potassium into cells, increased gastrointestinal and/or renal losses, and hypomagnesemia.
  2. Muscle weakness and respiratory muscle dysfunction are the major consequences of hypokalemia.

TABLE 2. **Serum Electrolytes** *Continued*

V. INCREASED PHOSPHORUS (Critical value: >10 mg/dl)
  A. Differential Diagnoses
    1. Delayed separation of red blood cells and serum* (artifactual)
    2. Young animals*
    3. Vitamin D intoxication
    4. Cholecalciferol intoxication
    5. Tumor lysis syndrome
    6. Crush injury
    7. Tissue necrosis
    8. Decreased renal excretion (prerenal, renal, and postrenal causes)*
    9. Bone osteolysis
    10. Feline hyperthyroidism
    11. Administration of phosphate-containing enemas (especially cats)
  B. Major Points
    1. Hyperphosphatemia may cause ionized hypocalcemia resulting in neuromuscular and cardiovascular dysfunction.

VI. HYPOPHOSPHATEMIA (Critical value: <2.0 mg/dl)
  A. Differential Diagnoses
    1. Decreased intestinal absorption
      a. Decreased intake
      b. Malabsorption
      c. Vomiting or diarrhea
      d. Administration of oral phosphate binders
      e. Vitamin D deficiency
    2. Increased urinary excretion
      a. Primary hyperparathyroidism
      b. Diabetes mellitus*
      c. Hyperadrenocorticism
      d. Renal tubular defects
      e. Diuretics
      f. Administration of sodium bicarbonate
      g. Fluid diuresis
    3. Shift to the intracellular space
      a. Insulin therapy*
      b. Intravenous glucose administration
      c. Parenteral nutrition*
    4. Respiratory alkalosis
  B. Major Points
    1. The causes of hypophosphatemia are due primarily to three major problems: decreased intestinal absorption, increased urinary excretion, or a shift of phosphorus into the cell.
    2. Severe hypophosphatemia may cause red blood cell hemolysis and CNS dysfunction.
    3. Severe hypophosphatemia may cause thrombocytopenia.

VII. HYPOCALCEMIA (Critical value: <8 mg/dl)
  A. Differential Diagnoses
    1. Primary hypoparathyroidism*
    2. Chronic or acute renal failure*
    3. Hypoalbuminemia
    4. Acute pancreatitis*
    5. Eclampsia*
    6. Intestinal malabsorption
    7. Ethylene glycol intoxication
    8. Phosphate-containing enema administration (especially cats)
    9. Blood transfusion (citrated blood)
    10. Vitamin D deficiency
    11. Tumor lysis syndrome
    12. Massive soft tissue trauma
    13. Rhabdomyolysis
    14. Hyperphosphatemia*
    15. Hypomagnesemia
    16. Intravenous phosphate administration
  B. Major Points
    1. Calcium is integral to cardiovascular and neuromuscular function.
    2. Twitching, ataxia, and seizures are the major consequences of hypocalcemia.

VIII. HYPOMAGNESEMIA (Critical value: <1.5 mmol/L)
  A. Differential Diagnoses
    1. Administration of intravenous fluids lacking magnesium*
    2. Diarrhea*
    3. Osmotic diarrhea*
    4. Diuretics (furosemide, thiazides, osmotic)*
    5. Aminoglycoside therapy
    6. Ticarcillin therapy
  B. Major Points
    1. Magnesium is the second most abundant intracellular cation (potassium is the most abundant).
    2. Magnesium is a cofactor for all enzyme reactions that involve ATP.
    3. Magnesium is part of the membrane pump that maintains electrical excitability in nerve and muscle cells.
    4. Hypomagnesemia can be a cause of refractory hypokalemia.
    5. Hypomagnesemia can cause hypocalcemia, owing to reduced parathyroid hormone (PTH) secretion.
    6. Other clinical manifestations of hypomagnesemia include cardiac arrhythmias and muscle weakness.

*Most common causes.

TABLE 3. Acid-Base Disorders

I. METABOLIC ACIDOSIS (Critical value: HCO_3 <10 mmol/L)
  A. Differential Diagnoses
    1. Normal anion gap
      a. Diarrhea*
      b. Renal insufficiency*
      c. High chloride containing fluid administration
      d. Compensation for respiratory alkalosis
      e. Renal tubular acidosis
    2. High anion gap
      a. Lactic acidosis*
      b. Ketoacidosis*
      c. Renal failure*
      d. Toxins (ethylene glycol, salicylates)
  B. Major Points
    1. The four major causes of metabolic acidoses are renal failure, ketoacidosis, lactic acidosis, and toxin ingestion.
    2. Cardiac arrhythmias may occur secondary to severe metabolic acidosis.
    3. Cardiac contractility and responsiveness to catecholamines may be compromised with severe metabolic acidosis.

II. RESPIRATORY ACIDOSIS (Critical value: PA_{CO_2} >50 mm Hg)
  A. Differential Diagnoses
    1. Drug-induced respiratory center depression (anesthetics)*
    2. Central nervous system lesions*
    3. Peripheral neuromuscular diseases (myasthenia gravis, polyradiculoneuritis, botulism, tick paralysis)*
    4. Electrolyte disorders causing muscle weakness (severe hypokalemia or hypophosphatemia)
    5. Upper airway obstruction*
    6. Intrinsic lung disease*
    7. Severe pleural space disease*
    8. Inadequate mechanical ventilation*
  B. Major Points
    1. Carbon dioxide is normally the major stimulus for respiration.
    2. Hypercapnia and respiratory acidosis are almost always due to a reduction in effective alveolar ventilation, rather than an increase in carbon dioxide production.
    3. Hypercapnia with intrinsic lung disease is thought to be due primarily to a ventilation-perfusion imbalance (perfused areas are underventilated).
    4. CNS effects (range from restlessness, anxiety, and tremors to delirium or somnolence) are mediated partly by acidemia-induced increases in cerebral blood flow and increased intracranial pressure.
    5. Cardiac arrhythmias may result from respiratory acidosis.
    6. Respiratory acidosis can cause peripheral vasodilation and hypotension.

*Most common causes.

TABLE 4. Serum Biochemical Abnormalities

I. INCREASED CREATININE (Critical value: >4.0 mg/dl)
  A. Differential Diagnoses
    1. Prerenal
      a. Dehydration*
      b. Cardiac insufficiency*
      c. Hypovolemia*
      d. Septic shock*
      e. Traumatic shock*
    2. Renal
      a. Pyelonephritis*
      b. Leptospirosis*
      c. Toxin (ethylene glycol, nonsteroidal anti-inflammatory medications, aminoglycosides)
      d. Neoplasia
      e. Congenital*
      f. Trauma
      g. Ischemia
    3. Postrenal
      a. Urethral obstruction*
      b. Ureter obstruction
      c. Urinary tract rupture*
  B. Major Points
    1. Creatinine concentration is not significantly affected by diet and catabolic factors.
    2. An increase in serum creatinine concentration above normal implies that at least 75% of the nephrons are not functioning when nonrenal variables have been eliminated as the cause of the increased creatinine.
    3. An increased creatinine level may be the result of prerenal, renal, or postrenal causes.

II. HYPOGLYCEMIA (Critical value: <60 mg/dl)
  A. Differential Diagnoses
    1. Sepsis*
    2. Neoplasia (insulin-secreting tumor, extrapancreatic tumors)*
    3. Insulin overdose*
    4. Oral hypoglycemia drugs
    5. Neonatal hypoglycemia*
    6. Severe and prolonged seizures
    7. Liver failure (end-stage)
    8. Artifactual (left in contact with red blood cells for too long)*
    9. Toy breed hypoglycemia*
    10. Hunting dog hypoglycemia
    11. Hypoadrenocorticism
    12. Glycogen storage disease
    13. Starvation combined with systemic illness (mild)*
    14. Heatstroke
  B. Major Points
    1. Glucose is the major source of energy for the brain under normal conditions.
    2. Blood glucose concentration is determined by the amount of glucose entering and leaving the blood stream. The principal determinants are dietary intake, the rate of entry into the cells, and the glucostatic activity of the liver.
    3. The major hormones involved in glucose homeostasis are insulin and the counterregulatory hormones glucagon, catecholamines, growth hormone, and cortisol.
    4. The brain is the primary organ affected by hypoglycemia. Signs may range from mild depression to stupor, coma, or seizures.
    5. In the critically ill patient, even mild hypoglycemia warrants an investigation for a septic process as the cause of the hypoglycemia.

TABLE 4. **Serum Biochemical Abnormalities** *Continued*

III. HYPERGLYCEMIA (Critical value: >300 mg/dl)
   A. Differential Diagnoses
      1. Stress (cats)*—usually <400 mg/dl
      2. Diabetes mellitus*
      3. Corticosteroid administration or hyperadrenocorticism*
      4. Acute pancreatitis
      5. Head trauma
      6. Severe hypothermia
      7. Administration of glucose-containing fluids*
   B. Major Points
      1. Persistent, fasting hyperglycemia occurs as the result of relative insulin deficiency or insulin resistance.
      2. Extreme hyperglycemia causes an increase in serum osmolality and potential central nervous system effects.
      3. Glucosuria results in polyuria and energy losses through the urine.
      4. Polyuria resulting in dehydration can occur in animals that are unable to drink enough to keep up with the urinary fluid losses.
      5. Transient hyperglycemia can be seen with severe head trauma or other severe central nervous system insults.
      6. Hyperglycemia can be detrimental to the brain in patients with poor cerebral perfusion.

IV. HYPERBILIRUBINEMIA (Critical value: >4 mg/dl)
   A. Differential Diagnoses
      1. Prehepatic
         a. Hemolysis*
      2. Hepatic
         a. Bacterial infections of the liver
         b. Neoplasia*
         c. Chronic active hepatitis
         d. Hepatic lipidosis*
         e. Hepatic necrosis
         f. Sepsis*
      3. Posthepatic
         a. Pancreatitis*
         b. Cholecystitis
         c. Cholelithiasis
         d. Ruptured biliary tract (bile peritonitis)
         e. Neoplasia
   B. Major Points
      1. Increased bilirubin is due to one or a combination of three major causes: prehepatic, hepatic, and posthepatic.

V. HYPOCHOLESTEROLEMIA
   A. Differential Diagnoses
      1. Liver failure*
      2. Anorexia*
      3. Malabsorption*
      4. Maldigestion*
      5. Lymphangiectasia or lymphatic disorders
      6. Heatstroke*
   B. Major Points
      1. Fifty percent of cholesterol is synthesized in the liver.
      2. Cholesterol is required for the synthesis of bile acids, steroid hormones, and vitamin D.

VI. HYPERCHOLESTEROLEMIA
   A. Differential Diagnoses
      1. Diabetes mellitus*
      2. Pancreatitis
      3. Extrahepatic biliary obstruction
      4. Hyperadrenocorticism*
      5. Hypothyroidism*
      6. Primary hyperlipidemia
      7. Glomerulonephritis or protein-losing nephropathy
      8. Postprandial
   B. Major Points
      1. Chronic hypercholesterolemia with hypothyroidism may lead to atherosclerosis and thromboembolism.
      2. Hyperlipidemia may interfere with measurements of sodium, potassium, bilirubin, alkaline phosphatase, calcium, phosphorus, amylase, lipase, and albumin.

VII. INCREASED ALANINE AMINOTRANSFERASE (ALT)
   A. Differential Diagnoses
      1. Toxin-induced hepatocellular necrosis
      2. Liver hypoxia*
      3. Trauma*
      4. Infection
      5. Inflammation
   B. Major Points
      1. Increased serum ALT occurs when there is leakage from hepatocytes (increased cell membrane permeability or damage).

VIII. INCREASED ALKALINE PHOSPHATASE
   A. Differential Diagnoses
      1. Glucocorticoid administration or Cushing's syndrome* in dogs
      2. Phenobarbital administration*
      3. Bone growth or remodeling*
      4. Hyperparathyroidism
      5. Panosteitis
      6. Osteomyelitis
      7. Neoplasia
      8. Biliary obstruction
      9. Intrahepatic cholestasis*
   B. Major Points
      1. Major sources of increased serum alkaline phosphatase include drug induction of isoenzymes, bone, and liver.

*Most common cause.

a critical concentration when action should be quickly taken to correct the abnormality.

These numbers and values should be taken as guidelines, and the clinician should assess the findings in the context of the patient's physiologic status or the trend of change of the parameter. For example, a change in creatinine level from 1.0 mg/dl to 3.5 mg/dl should alert the clinician that the patient's renal function is deteriorating and rapid action should be taken despite the fact that the value falls below the panic value of 4.0 mg/dl.

References and Selected Reading

Marino PL: The ICU Book. Philadelphia: Lea & Febiger, 1991.
   A practical yet comprehensive book addressing all aspects of critical care medicine.
Rich LJ, Coles EH: Textbook of Veterinary Internal Medicine. Philadelphia: WB Saunders, 1995, pp 11–16.
   A comprehensive list of differential diagnoses for a variety of laboratory abnormalities.
Rose BD: Clinical Physiology of Acid-Base and Electrolyte Disorders. New York: McGraw-Hill, 1994.
   A clinical and practical book reviewing electrolyte and acid-base abnormalities.

Point-of-Care Laboratory Testing in the Intensive Care Unit

Marc R. Raffe

St. Paul, Minnesota

Leah S. Faudskar

Golden Valley, Minnesota

The complexity and demands of medical practice have dramatically increased in the past decade. The introduction of advanced technologies has provided the clinician with an array of diagnostic and therapeutic capabilities that were unheard of until a few years ago. A feature common to many of the diagnostic and therapeutic advances is the reduced time required between the test evaluation and availability of results. Centralized facilities for laboratory services have been the standard for several decades. Time requirements for processing patient samples and reporting results have been long because of complex technology and methods, the characteristics of chemical reagents used for analysis, and the need for dedicated personnel to manage the equipment and perform the assays. Recently, advances in laboratory testing technology have permitted relocating elements of the central laboratory facility to sites closer to the patient. This is an exciting development that promises to address concerns and limitations associated with centralized laboratory facilities. Accurate laboratory information is now available to the clinician in time frames that were not previously possible. This advance has significant implications in the diagnosis and therapy of the critically ill patient. Time savings in diagnosis and therapy may be lifesaving in emergency or critically ill patients. Monitoring therapeutic response is also easier and faster in many cases. The goal of this chapter is to introduce this exciting new concept and provide insights into the current status and future direction of this emerging area.

WHAT IS POINT-OF-CARE TESTING?

By definition, point-of-care testing (POCT) is testing performed anywhere medically indicated. In the context of this review, it will be limited to clinical laboratory tests and testing procedures that are performed in proximity to the patient. Synonyms for POCT include bedside testing, near bedside testing, and decentralized laboratory testing.

POCT is feasible because of the design and production of biosensors that measure established laboratory parameters using unseparated whole blood. A unique feature of these biosensors is that they do not require chemical reagents to perform an analysis. Only physical contact between the blood sample and biosensor is necessary for measurement. The development of this technology has simplified testing methodologies and has resulted in the capability of gaining more analytic information from a smaller blood volume.

Coupled with biosensor development are significant advances in electronic design and rechargeable power sources that have resulted in transportable laboratory instruments. Many POCT devices are in the size range of a personal stereo system. Several devices are the size of a cellular telephone. The overall instrument size and weight of POCT devices have contributed to the ease of transporting the POCT instrument to the patient rather than the patient or sample to the instrument.

WHAT ARE ADVANTAGES OF POINT-OF-CARE TESTING?

Several advantages are apparent when comparing POCT with central laboratory methods. Many POCT devices are "self-contained" and require no external connections for operation. They have a modular design in that a test cartridge is inserted in the analyzer base for sample analysis. The blood sample size required to perform a test is small compared with traditional laboratory requirements, thus minimizing the physiologic impact associated with withdrawing large volume blood samples. The cartridge is discarded following analysis, thereby minimizing contamination and refreshing the biosensors for each test sample. Most analyzers have reagent standards incorporated into the test cartridge that confirm instrument calibration and provide quality control prior to patient sample testing. Calibration reagents and accessories are periodically used to confirm calibration in accordance with human hospital laboratory standards for quality assurance. Finally, POCT is user-friendly and may be successfully operated by individuals with diverse training backgrounds. In our experience, mastery is quickly achieved by support staff who assume an active role in performing POCT evaluation.

WHAT LABORATORY TESTS ARE AVAILABLE USING POINT-OF-CARE TESTING?

The range of laboratory tests available varies by device manufacturer. Biochemical tests available in at least one POCT analyzer system include hemoglobin, glucose, blood gas analysis (pH, P_{O_2}, P_{CO_2}, T_{CO_2}, HCO_3, base excess, calculated hemoglobin saturation), electrolyte profile (Na, K, Cl, Ca^{2+}), and blood urea nitrogen. Coagulation monitoring including activated clotting time, activated partial thromboplastin time, prothrombin time, and thrombin time is available with dedicated devices. Glucose monitoring may also be performed using POCT analyzers or glucometers. However, these are well-established devices that will not be specifically discussed other than to recognize that they conform to the definition of POCT devices. Specific capabilities of POCT devices are compared in Table 1.

HOW ACCURATE ARE POINT-OF-CARE TESTING DEVICES COMPARED WITH TRADITIONAL LABORATORY ANALYZERS?

Several human studies have compared the accuracy of POCT devices with standard laboratory methods. Excellent correlation has been reported between POCT analyzers and standard methods. Correlation coefficients for pH, Po_2, Pco_2, blood urea nitrogen, potassium, calcium, and hematocrit have exceeded 95% in one or more studies. Correlation between POCT analyzers and standard methods for chloride ranged from 85 to 94% in several studies. Correlation between POCT analyzers and standard methods for sodium and glucose is less than 85%. Studies in dogs parallel the human results except for a lower potassium correlation with central laboratory facilities. Bias and precision studies comparing methods indicate similar results between human and canine studies completed to date.

Based on these results, it appears that POCT devices compare favorably with most standard laboratory methods. Further evaluation is indicated to determine if consistency can be achieved in larger population studies and across species lines. The reasons that specific analytes have lower correlations also needs to be further defined.

WHAT FACTORS INFLUENCE POINT-OF-CARE TESTING RESULTS?

Laboratory results obtained by POCT methods are susceptible to errors that are common to other laboratory testing methodologies. Some manufacturers require biosensor cartridges to be stored at 4°C and require a minimum warming period at room temperature prior to use. Failure to warm the cartridge to room temperature has been shown to affect results. Appropriate sample handling is a main factor in accuracy of results. For example, failure to use an anticoagulant in blood gas samples may cause sample clotting and invalidate results. Failure to inject an appropriate sample volume into the POCT cartridge is another major error. However, clear instructions for filling volumes or procedures are displayed on each cartridge unit. Failure to adhere to time requirements following cartridge calibration may render the test invalid. The time window from calibration to sample analysis varies with manufacturer but is approximately 2 to 4 minutes following completion of the quality control check. Quality control failure invalidates the individual cartridge and the blood sample used to fill the cartridge.

HOW DOES THE PRICE STRUCTURE OF POINT-OF-CARE ANALYZERS COMPARE WITH CENTRAL LABORATORY COSTS?

The price structure of POCT analyzers varies with the cartridge configuration and test profile. In general, the cost of multiple test cartridges is equivalent to a central laboratory analyzer on a per test basis. Single test cartridges—for example, a glucose test—are more expensive compared with standard portable or central laboratory analyzers. The cartridge cost for blood gas analysis is approximately equal to central laboratory fees on a per test basis.

The current price structure reflects two advantages of POCT analyzers compared with central laboratory facilities. One advantage is timely access to laboratory information at sites remote from the central laboratory facility. This helps in rapid, accurate diagnosis and therapeutic planning, thus providing a cost saving based on time saved. A second advantage is the immediate access to updated laboratory information that is essential for monitoring therapy in the critically ill patient. This "convenience" and rapid information access 24 hours a day contributes to

TABLE 1. Point-of-Care Testing Devices and Current Capabilities

Device	Manufacturer or Distributor	Patient Tests per Cartridge	Hematocrit-Hemoglobin	Blood Gas	Electrolytes	Glucose	Other	Coagulation
i-STAT	SDI Corp	1	Y	Y	Na, K, Cl, Ca	Y	BUN	N
IRMA	Diametrics Inc.	1/Multiple	Y	Y	Na, K, Cl, Ca	Y		N
Stat-Pal II	PPG Industries	Up to 30	N	Y	N	N		N
AVL	AVL Scientific	1	N	Y	Na, K, Ca	N		N
NOVASTAT Profile 5,7	Nova	Multiple	Y	Y	Na, K, Cl, Ca	Y	Lactate	
GEM-STAT	Mallinckrodt systems	1	Y	Y	Na, K, Ca			
Sendx 100	Sendx Medical Inc.	Multiple	Y	Y	Na, K, Ca	N		N
Hemochrom 401	International Technidyne Corp.	1	N	N	N	N		ACT, PT, aPTT, TT
Hemochrom Jr.	International Technidyne Corp.	1	N	N	N	N		ACT, PT, aPTT, TT
TAS	Cardiovascular Diagnostics Inc.	1	N	N	N	N		PT, aPTT, TT

Y, yes; N, no; ACT, activated clotting time; aPTT, activated partial thromboplastin time; PT, prothrombin time; TT, thrombin time.

improved quality and timeliness of patient care. These advantages are significant in critical or intensive care unit environments and outweigh cost penalties that may be present with POCT analyzers.

WHAT IS THE FUTURE IN POINT-OF-CARE TESTING?

The future of POCT is exciting. Over the next several years, an expanded spectrum of devices and testing capabilities will be introduced into the marketplace. Additional test "batteries" will become available that will permit use of the same POCT analyzer for several different testing profiles. POCT devices may expand to include designs that will measure specific parameters by automated sample withdrawal from the catheter site (ex vivo analysis). First-generation devices using these technologies are commercially available on the human medical market and may soon be evaluated in veterinary medicine.

Adaptation of POCT devices to areas of clinical practice beyond emergency and critical care medicine will likely occur. Use of POCT analysis in practice locations outside a hospital setting is feasible. POCT technology may prove ideal for use in species with limited blood volumes because of the small sample size requirement for testing. Additional uses not currently considered will be discovered and adapted as POCT evolves and is accepted in clinical practice.

The technology and approach to POCT is an exciting field that will address limitations previously associated with laboratory support. This technology will complement central laboratory facilities and permit further sophistication in diagnostic capability for the clinical veterinarian.

References and Suggested Reading

Castro HJ, Oropello JM, Halpern N: Point-of-care testing in the intensive care unit. Am J Clin Pathol 104:S95, 1995.
Provides an overview of the advantages of point-of-care testing in a clinical setting.
Gault HM, Harding CE: Evaluation of i-STAT portable clinical analyzer in a hemodialysis unit. Clin Biochem 29:117, 1996.
Compares the i-STAT POCT device with several testing modules to a central laboratory analyzer in a defined patient population.
Jacobs E, Nowakowski M, Colman N: Performance of Gem Premier blood gas/electrolyte analyzer evaluated. Clin Chem 39:1890, 1993.
Compares the Gem Premier POCT device with a central laboratory blood gas analyzer and a portable multichannel analyzer in a defined patient population.
Kost GJ, Hague C: The current future status of critical care testing and patient monitoring. Am J Clin Pathol 104:S2, 1995.
Provides an overview of POCT and defines future directions and technologies associated with POCT.
Mock T, Morrison D, Yatscoff R: Evaluation of the i-STAT system: A portable chemistry analyzer for the measurement of sodium, potassium chloride, urea, glucose, and hematocrit. Clin Biochem 28:187, 1995.
Compares the i-STAT POCT device with a Kodak Ektachem 700XR dry reagent chemistry analyzer in a defined patient population.
Oberhardt BJ: Thrombosis and hemostatasis testing at the point of care. Am J Clin Pathol 104:S72, 1995.
Reviews POCT devices available for coagulation monitoring.
Oyer D, Devey J, Crowe DT, et al: Instrument correlation study between the i-STAT and the Stat 5 profile in an emergency setting. Proceedings of the International Veterinary Emergency and Critical Care Symposium V. San Antonio, TX, 1996, p 881.
Comparison study of i-STAT and Nova Stat 5 analyzer in an emergency setting.
Raffe MR, Randall D, Kulas C, et al: Validation of a point of care chemistry and blood gas analyzer in dogs. Proceedings of the International Veterinary Emergency and Critical Care Symposium V. San Antonio, TX, 1996, p 879.
Comparison study of i-STAT and central laboratory analyzers for blood gas and electrolyte evaluation in a normal dog population.
Salem M, Chernow B, Burke R, et al: Bedside diagnostic blood testing. JAMA 266:382, 1990.
Comparison of a NovaStat 5 portable analyzer with a central laboratory analyzer in a critical care setting.
Zaloga GP, Roberts PR, Black K, et al: Hand-held blood gas analyzer is accurate in the critical care setting. Crit Care Med 24:957, 1996.
Comparison of an IRMA portable analyzer with a central laboratory analyzer in a critical care setting.

Lactate Measurement: Diagnostic, Therapeutic, and Prognostic Implications

DEZ HUGHES
Philadelphia, Pennsylvania

The clinical value of measuring lactate concentrations in blood and other tissue fluids has been recognized for more than 40 years. Lactate determination offers the clinician a unique means by which to detect and monitor anaerobic tissue metabolism. Although lactate measurement has been shown to be particularly useful for the detection and monitoring of systemic and local tissue hypoperfusion, it also serves as an accurate prognostic indicator in many critically ill patients. Lactate quantitation may also prove a useful diagnostic adjunct (e.g., in the detection of bacterial infections of body cavities such as peritonitis, meningitis, and bacterial arthritis). Because of the relatively rapid changes seen in lactate levels, its clinical use has been limited by slow or complicated assay methods; however, with the advent of simple, rapid, and readily available methods of quantitation, the full potential of lactate analysis should soon be realized in veterinary medicine.

BIOCHEMISTRY

Cellular metabolic energy, in the form of high-energy phosphate compounds, is generated via three major processes: glycolysis, the citric acid cycle, and the electron transport chain–oxidative phosphorylation. Glycolysis occurs in the cytosol, whereas the necessary enzymes and cofactors for the citric acid cycle and the electron transport chain–oxidative phosphorylation are located in mitochondria. In contrast to the latter two processes, which require aerobic conditions, glycolysis does not require oxygen, thereby allowing energy production to continue in conditions of relative or absolute cellular hypoxia. The energy generating capacity of glycolysis is much less than that of aerobic metabolism on a molar basis. Only 2 mol of adenosine triphosphate (ATP) are produced per mole of glucose converted to lactate, compared with 36 mol of ATP generated when glucose is fully oxidized to carbon dioxide and water. Glycolysis can, however, proceed at a much faster rate than the aerobic components of cellular energy production. In addition to high-energy phosphate, glycolysis produces pyruvate and consumes nicotinamide adenine dinucleotide (NAD^+). To enable anaerobic energy production to continue, the cell disposes of excess pyruvate and regenerates NAD^+ by converting pyruvate to lactate. The disadvantage of lactate production is that it indirectly results in the production of H^+ ions and acidosis. Lactate can either be converted back to pyruvate and oxidized via the citric acid cycle in the presence of adequate tissue oxygen supplies or used for gluconeogenesis in the liver and kidney. Metabolism of lactate consumes H^+ ions and, after oxidation, generates carbon dioxide, which is in equilibrium with bicarbonate. It can be seen, therefore, that once tissue hypoxia is reversed, lactic acidosis should be self-correcting.

BLOOD LACTATE CONCENTRATION

Lactate produced by cellular metabolism is primarily the levorotatory isomer, or L-lactate. Lactate and lactic acid are not synonymous: lactic acid, $CH_3CH(OH)COOH$, is a strong acid that is almost completely ionized to lactate, $CH_3CH(OH)COO^-$, and H^+ at physiologic pH. An elevated blood lactate concentration is termed *hyperlactatemia*; however, depending on buffer reserves and concurrent acid-base disturbances, hyperlactatemia may or may not be associated with *acidemia* (a blood pH lower than 7.35). *Lactic acidosis* should be used to denote a situation in which lactate production exceeds lactate clearance, that is, a state in which lactic acid tends to cause a fall in pH. *Lactic acidemia* refers to an acidemic blood pH and hyperlactatemia. Plasma lactate levels greater than 5 mmol/L are usually associated with acidemia. Because both the anion gap and base excess are insensitive and nonspecific indicators of plasma lactate concentration, lactate concentrations must be measured directly rather than estimated.

Although lactate is a charged molecule, it equilibrates rapidly across cell membranes via the action of a bidirectional membrane transport system in which lactate (or other monocarboxylates) are carried across the membrane in conjunction with free H^+. Increased cellular lactate production therefore elevates the interstitial and blood lactate concen-

tration. Although all tissues have the capacity to produce lactate, basal lactate production is highest in skin, red blood cells (which lack mitochondria), brain, and muscle, whereas basal lactate utilization is highest in liver and kidney. In keeping with the role of lactate as an important metabolic energy fuel, the kidney does not excrete significant quantities of lactate until a moderate degree of hyperlactatemia is present. Plasma lactate concentration is therefore determined by the balance between the relative rates of lactate production and lactate extraction from the blood. Red blood cell lactate concentration equilibrates with, but lags behind, acute changes in plasma lactate concentration, so the lactate concentration in plasma, rather than that in whole blood, should be used in the clinical setting. The reference range for plasma lactate concentration in normal dogs in the author's hospital (by direct amperometry) is less than 2.5 mmol/L.

ETIOLOGY OF DISORDERED LACTATE METABOLISM

Hyperlactatemia occurs whenever the rate of lactate production exceeds that of lactate extraction. Because glycolysis can proceed more rapidly than can the oxidation of pyruvate, hyperlactatemia can occur with increased lactate production in the absence of tissue hypoxia in conditions that speed glycolysis, such as alkalosis, glucose infusion, and sepsis without hypoperfusion. Hyperlactatemia can also occur from relative, rather than absolute, tissue hypoxia when energy requirements exceed the capacity of aerobic metabolism, as in exercise, trembling, and seizures. The hyperlactatemia observed with increased muscular activity is significantly different from that seen in other causes in that resolution is much more rapid with a half-life on the order of 2 hours. Extreme exercise in greyhounds can generate lactate concentrations greater than 30 mmol/L, whereas seizures tend to cause elevations in the 6 to 10 mmol/L range. Hyperlactatemia due to tissue hypoxia can result from hypoperfusion or severe reductions in arterial oxygen content in the absence of hypoperfusion, or rarely from an inability of the cells to utilize oxygen. By far the most common and clinically significant cause of hyperlactatemia (and usually the most severe) is systemic or local tissue hypoperfusion. Hyperlactatemia should always prompt an aggressive search for tissue hypoperfusion regardless of concurrent conditions. The main causes of hyperlactatemia with potential relevance to veterinary medicine are shown in Table 1 and are categorized according to the most widely used scheme (Cohen and Woods, 1976). Not all these potential causes have been definitively documented in veterinary practice. Since this classification scheme was developed, many of the causes of hyperlactatemia have been shown to include some component of tissue hypoperfusion.

CLINICAL USE OF PLASMA LACTATE QUANTITATION

Technical Concerns

The effects of blood sampling and sample handling are important. In an ongoing study by the author, restraint

TABLE 1. **Major Causes of Hyperlactatemia Relevant to Veterinary Medicine**

Type A (clinical evidence of absolute or relative tissue hypoxia)
  Shock (systemic hypoperfusion)
    Hypovolemic
    Cardiogenic
    Septic
  Local hypoperfusion
    Gastric necrosis and other causes of splanchnic ischemia
    Aortic thromboembolism
  Severe hypoxemia (Pao_2 <30–40 mm Hg)
  Severe anemia (packed cell volume <15%)
  Carbon monoxide toxicity
  Excessive muscular activity
    Exercise
    Trembling
    Seizures
Type B (no clinical evidence of tissue hypoxia)
  Type B_1 (in association with an underlying disease)
    Diabetes mellitus
    Severe liver disease
    Malignancy
    Sepsis
    Pheochromocytoma
    Thiamine deficiency
  Type B_2 (due to drugs or toxins)
    Acetaminophen
    Cyanide
    Epinephrine
    Ethanol
    Ethylene glycol
    Insulin
    Methanol
    Morphine
    Nitroprusside
    Propylene glycol
    Salicylates
    Terbutaline
  Type B_3 (due to inborn metabolic defects)
    Mitochondrial myopathy
  Miscellaneous
    Alkalosis-hyperventilation
    Hypoglycemia

per se and prolonged venous occlusion caused only mild elevations of plasma lactate concentration (2.5 to 3.5 mmol/L). It appears that the degree of muscular activity during sampling is more important, with elevations of the magnitude of 6 to 7 mmol/L seen in normal dogs that tremble during venipuncture. Although the vast majority of studies have used arterial blood samples, clinical evidence supporting the use of arterial samples is largely lacking. In normal dogs, the differences among arterial, central venous (jugular), and cephalic samples are minimal (Hughes and Drobatz, 1996). Clinical experience and data from human patients suggest that this premise also holds true in hypoperfused patients. Consequently, an inability to obtain arterial blood samples should not preclude lactate analysis.

Blood samples should be held on ice or the plasma or serum sample promptly separated from red blood cells and kept at room temperature. There is no elevation of lactate concentration if such samples are analyzed within 30 minutes. The lactate concentration in whole blood samples held at room temperature rises by approximately 0.2 mmol/L in 30 minutes because of glycolytic activity in red blood cells.

Tissue Perfusion

Several authors have demonstrated that for severe lactic acidosis to ensue, increased lactate production must be associated with a reduction in net lactate clearance from the body. The major determinant of the relative contribution to lactate production or extraction by different tissues in hypoperfused states appears to be the blood flow to that tissue. For example, in mild to moderate hemorrhagic shock in dogs, blood flow to the gut is greatly reduced, whereas blood supply to the liver is preserved. Accordingly, intestinal lactate production is high, and the liver actually extracts lactate, albeit at a reduced rate. Only in late and severe hemorrhagic shock does the liver begin to produce lactate. Experimental evidence has shown a correlation between the magnitude of hyperlactatemia and the reduction in oxygen supply to the tissues. Clinical experience suggests that mild systemic hypoperfusion is associated with lactate levels of 3 to 5 mmol/L, moderate hypoperfusion yields lactate concentrations of 5 to 10 mmol/L, and in severe hypoperfusion lactate concentrations exceed 10 mmol/L. More importantly, plasma lactate concentrations almost invariably fall with successful fluid resuscitation and can be used to guide fluid therapy in the treatment of hypoperfusion. Failure of the lactate concentration to normalize following appropriate fluid resuscitation suggests ongoing systemic hypoperfusion or an occult local source of lactate production.

Prognosis

The prognostic significance of lactate quantitation in critically ill humans has been extensively documented. It should be intuitive that the cause of hyperlactatemia influences the respective cutoff values, for example, survival for a given lactate concentration is better in hemorrhagic than in septic shock. In one landmark human study (Weil and Afifi, 1970), as lactate concentration increased from 2.1 to 8.0 mmol/L, survival decreased from 90 to 10%. Clinical experience suggests that similar results will be obtained in canine patients. If plasma lactate concentrations fail to fall to less than 10 mmol/L following appropriate fluid challenge, or if a significant rise in plasma lactate concentration occurs, the prognosis appears to be poor regardless of the underlying cause of the hyperlactatemia.

In an ongoing study, currently composed of 43 dogs with gastric dilatation volvulus, we have demonstrated that plasma lactate concentration is a useful indicator of gastric necrosis. A cutoff value of 6.0 mmol/L yields a sensitivity of 63% and a specificity of 85% for the presence of gastric necrosis. Seventy-one percent of dogs with a lactate concentration greater than 6.0 mmol/L had gastric necrosis, whereas only 21% of dogs with a lactate concentration less than 6.0 mmol/L had gastric necrosis. Because gastric necrosis is one of the main determinants of mortality in this patient population, these types of data should facilitate more accurate prognostication. In our study group, a plasma lactate concentration of less than 5.0 mmol/L was associated with a survival rate of 96%, whereas a plasma lactate concentration of greater than 5.0 mmol/L was associated with a survival rate of 71%. Another interesting and potentially useful application of lactate concentration in veterinary patients may be its use to predict survival or the likelihood of limb salvage in cases of feline aortic thromboembolism, using both jugular venous samples and venous samples obtained from the ischemic limbs. Serum lactate concentration has also been shown to be predictive of survival in dogs in a veterinary intensive care unit (Lagutchik et al, 1996), in dogs with heartworm caval syndrome, and in horses with acute abdominal crises.

Other Causes of Hyperlactatemia

Hyperlactatemia in association with underlying disease processes in the absence of hypoperfusion and drug-induced causes remains largely undocumented in clinical veterinary medicine. It is particularly important to note that hypoxemia alone in veterinary patients should not cause hyperlactatemia. Severe anemia, conversely, may result in hyperlactatemia in the absence of hypoperfusion. Lymphoma in dogs has been shown to be associated with elevated resting lactate levels and a greater degree of hyperlactatemia following glucose challenge. The elevations in lactate concentrations were minimal, however, and perfusion parameters were not reported. An increased susceptibility to the development of hyperlactatemia following intravenous fluid therapy with lactate-containing crystalloids has also been reported in dogs with lymphoma. Although the elevations were also relatively minor, and no dogs experienced acidemia, it would seem wise to choose a crystalloid without lactate in this patient population.

LACTATE ANALYSIS IN OTHER BODY FLUIDS

The use of lactate quantitation in fluids other than blood has been investigated as a predictor of bacterial infection, an indicator of a successful response to antibiotic therapy, and an objective means of assessing the degree of tissue injury and therefore prognosis. Lactate levels in abdominal effusions, cerebrospinal fluid, and synovial fluid may have clinical application. Lactate concentration in abdominal fluid in patients with ascites may be helpful in the diagnosis of bacterial peritonitis (Swann et al, 1996). Abdominal fluid lactate concentration in the presence of bacterial peritonitis was 8.4 ± 4.2 mmol/L (mean $\pm$ standard deviation) compared with 4.2 ± 2.9 mmol/L ($P < 0.001$) in nonbacterial causes of abdominal effusion. The gradient between venous and abdominal fluid lactate concentration appears to be a more accurate predictor of bacterial peritonitis than is the absolute concentration. An effusion-to-venous lactate gradient of greater than 4.6 mmol/L yielded a specificity of 100% and a sensitivity of 55% for the presence of bacterial peritonitis. The best predictor of bacterial peritonitis in this study was an effusion glucose concentration of less than 55 mg/dl or the presence of intracellular bacteria identified on effusion cytologic studies. Quantitation of lactate concentration in cerebrospinal fluid has been correlated with the presence of bacterial meningitis and the severity of central nervous system damage and prognosis in many human clinical and animal experimental studies. Evidence for the use of lactate as a diagnostic adjunct and prognostic indicator in brain disease, ischemic spinal cord injury, and intervertebral disc prolapse suggests that these areas are especially worthy of investigation in veterinary medicine. Synovial fluid lactate concentration may also be helpful in the diagnosis of bacterial arthritis.

TREATMENT

Lactic acidosis is usually a manifestation of an underlying disease process rather than a primary diagnosis; therefore, treatment for lactic acidosis is almost entirely directed toward the diagnosis and correction of the underlying problem. Although it would seem cautious to avoid lactate-containing fluids in this patient population, the majority of available experimental evidence does not support this premise. *Correction of hypoperfusion* should be paramount in the patient with hyperlactatemia. Aggressive intravenous fluid therapy using crystalloids, colloids, or blood products is usually necessary for the patient with lactic acidosis caused by hypovolemia provided that cardiac disease is absent. Maintaining a packed cell volume of greater than 20% would seem wise with respect to the effects of anemia on arterial oxygen content and hyperlactatemia. The use of intravenous bicarbonate infusions in the treatment of lactic acidosis is controversial; however, the benefits of intravenous bicarbonate therapy appear to outweigh the risks in patients with severe hemodynamic compromise and acidosis (pH <7.1) refractory to intravenous volume loading provided that pulmonary ventilation is adequate. Cautious bicarbonate therapy (1 mEq/kg IV) may be used in refractory lactic acidosis but should never supplant the administration of adequate volumes of intravenous fluids.

Studies investigating the use of buffers that do not generate carbon dioxide, such as Carbicarb (a mixture of sodium bicarbonate and sodium carbonate), have yielded equivocal results. Specific therapy aimed at correcting hyperlactatemia per se has centered on the use of dichloroacetate, which decreases blood lactate levels and increases systemic pH through stimulation of pyruvate dehydrogenase, increased myocardial ATP content, improved cardiac contractility, and peripheral vasodilatation. Concerns regarding neurotoxicity with chronic administration have largely restricted its use. As thiamine is an essential cofactor in the oxidation of pyruvate, and this vitamin has a high therapeutic index, thiamine treatment has been advocated in lactic acidosis. Recommended doses of thiamine vary widely, but an empirical dosage of 1 to 2 mg/kg IM would seem appropriate.

References and Suggested Reading

Cohen RD, Woods RF: Clinical and Biochemical Aspects of Lactic Acidosis. Boston: Blackwell Scientific, 1976, p 42.
    Although some chapters are somewhat outdated, this is still one of the landmark publications dealing with lactic acidosis.
Hindman BJ: Sodium bicarbonate in the treatment of subtypes of acute lactic acidosis: Physiological considerations. Anesthesiology 72:1064, 1990.
Hughes D, Drobatz KJ: Comparison of plasma lactate concentration from cephalic, jugular, and femoral arterial blood samples in normal dogs. J Vet Emerg Crit Care 6:115, 1996.
    Provides reference range for plasma lactate in normal dogs by direct amperometry.

Lagutchik MS, Ogilvie GK, Wingfield WE: Lactate levels in critically ill and injured dogs. J Vet Emerg Crit Care 6:119, 1996.

Mizock BA, Falk JL: Lactic acidosis in critical illness. Crit Care Med 20:80, 1993.
   Clinically oriented review of lactic acidosis in human critical care medicine.

Swann H, Hughes D, Drobatz KJ: Use of abdominal fluid pH, PO_2, PCO_2, [glucose], and [lactate] to differentiate bacterial peritonitis from non-bacterial causes of abdominal effusion in dogs and cats. J Vet Emerg Crit Care 6:114, 1996.

Toffaletti JG: Blood lactate: Biochemistry, laboratory methods, and clinical interpretation. Crit Rev Clin Lab Sci 28:253, 1991.
   Good review of lactate biochemistry and overview of laboratory methods of lactate quantitation.

Weil MH, Afifi AA: Experimental and clinical studies on lactate and pyruvate as indicators of the severity of acute circulatory failure (shock). Circulation 41:989, 1970.
   One of the landmark studies documenting the prognostic significance of hyperlactatemia in circulatory shock.

Colloid Osmometry

LESLEY G. KING

Philadelphia, Pennsylvania

The emergency database—including determination of packed cell volume, total plasma solids (TS), blood glucose, and blood urea estimation—is an integral part of the initial assessment and management of critically ill patients. The TS is easily measured with a refractometer and provides the clinician with an estimate of plasma total protein (TP) concentration. For stabilization of critical patients (rather than from a diagnostic perspective), the most important reason for measuring TS is to obtain a general indication of the colloid osmotic pressure (COP) of the blood. If the TS (and therefore COP) is low, edema is possible, which may be exacerbated by the administration of crystalloid fluids. The clinician faced with this situation often reaches for plasma or synthetic colloids as resuscitation fluids.

With increased use of synthetic colloids in critical patients, using TS or TP as an estimate of COP becomes problematic. Following the administration of these solutions to patients, any correlation between TP and COP is lost. The TP and TS may be low, but COP may be within the normal range because of the presence of the synthetic colloid molecules. Without the ability to measure COP directly, the only way of monitoring synthetic colloid therapy is by the use of clinical signs. This is analogous to the situation that would occur if we gave blood transfusions without monitoring the results by sequentially measuring hematocrit or packed cell volume. Therefore, colloid osmometry is one of the most important monitoring tools available to the critical care clinician who uses synthetic colloid therapy.

WHAT IS COLLOID OSMOTIC PRESSURE?

The *osmolality* of a solution is defined as the total concentration of dissolved solute particles (in millimoles per kilogram of solvent). Osmolality is independent of particle size and electrical charge and is measured by freezing point depression. In physiologic terms, the solute particles in plasma can be divided into crystalloids (mainly electrolytes) that have molecular weights less than 30,000

dalton (D), and colloids (mainly plasma proteins) that weigh more than 30,000 D.

The vascular endothelium acts as a semipermeable membrane that does not usually allow passage of colloids into the interstitium but allows free passage of crystalloid particles. If one solution (plasma) contains more colloid particles and therefore less solvent than the other solution (interstitial fluid), solvent will gradually diffuse through the pores of the semipermeable membrane into the area where its concentration is lower. *Colloid osmotic pressure*, therefore, is a relative characteristic of one colloid solution compared with another colloid solution from which it is separated by a semipermeable membrane.

The presence of protein in plasma promotes the maintenance of intravascular volume by retention of water and crystalloids in the intravascular compartment. The colloid osmotic pressure of blood is therefore one important characteristic that determines fluid flux among the various body fluid compartments.

Osmotic pressure depends on the fundamental properties of both solutions, as well as on the pore characteristics of the semipermeable membrane. When synthetic membranes are used for colloid osmometry, the ideal membrane should have a narrow distribution of pore sizes and should reject any solute with a molecular weight greater than 30,000 D. In plasma, both the colloid and crystalloid particles carry electrical charges, which can greatly affect COP via the Gibbs-Donnan effect. At normal blood pH, the plasma proteins carry a net negative charge. Since electroneutrality must be maintained on both sides of the membrane, positively charged ions are retained to balance the negative charge on the plasma proteins. The net COP in physiologic solutions, therefore, is a nonlinear summation of the effect of both the colloid particles and the positive ions.

THE COLLOID OSMOMETER

The colloid osmometer (Wescor 4400 Colloid Osmometer, Wescor Inc, Logan, Utah) (Fig. 1) basically consists of two chambers, a semipermeable membrane, and a sensitive pressure transducer. The reference chamber is filled with normal saline to approximate the Gibbs-Donnan effect of interstitial fluid. Heparinized whole blood, plasma, or serum is slowly injected into the test chamber, which is separated from the reference chamber by the semipermeable membrane. Accurate results require a test sample volume of 0.5 ml. Water molecules migrate into the test chamber, resulting in a negative pressure gradient in the reference chamber. Equilibration across the membrane usually takes 30 to 90 seconds. The negative pressure gradient is measured by the sensing diaphragm of the pressure transducer. Minute pressure changes cause changes in electrical impedance and are displayed in digital form as COP (millimeters of mercury) on the instrument display.

The colloid osmometer must be carefully maintained to ensure the accuracy of the results. The instrument should be calibrated daily, with the use of commercially available test solutions of albumin of known standard COP (Osmocoll II Standard/Control, Wescor Inc, Logan, Utah). Additionally, both the upper and lower chambers must be flushed with saline daily, and the instrument should be carefully zeroed with saline before and after each use. Saline and sample solutions must be injected carefully to avoid the introduction of air bubbles. If properly maintained, the semipermeable membrane should have a long life of several thousand samples. The most common problem recognized during use of the instrument is failure to reach a plateau pressure, which can often be corrected by tightening the upper chamber or replacing the semipermeable membrane. Detailed trouble-shooting instructions are available in the instruction and service manual. The approximate cost of the instruments is $5,000.

NORMAL VALUES FOR COLLOID OSMOTIC PRESSURE

We established normal values using the Wescor Colloid Osmometer with 2 ml whole blood collected in lyophilized

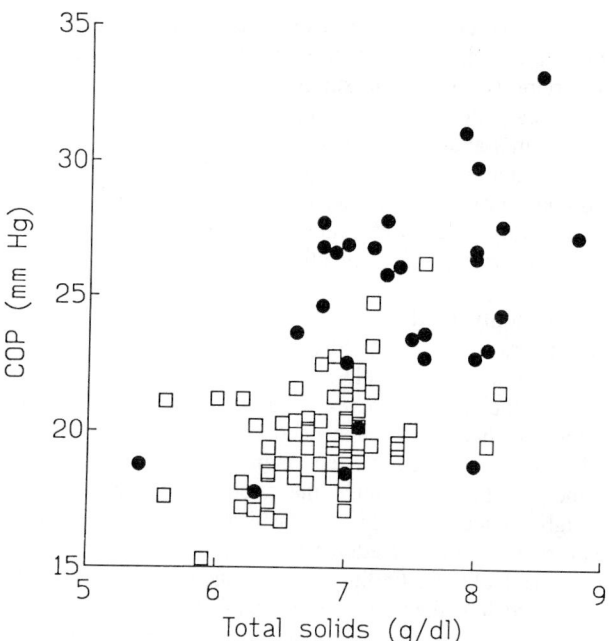

Figure 2. Relationship between colloid osmotic pressure and total solids in normal dogs (n = 63) and normal cats (n = 31). Cats tended to have higher values for COP and for total plasma solids (TS) than did dogs. Notice the poor correlation between TS and COP, as a TS of 7 g/dl might produce a COP ranging from 17 to 26 mm Hg in different individuals.

heparin tubes (Fig. 2). In 63 normal dogs, the mean COP of whole blood was of 19.95 ± 2.1 (range 15.3 to 26.3) mm Hg (Culp et al, 1994). In 31 normal cats, the COP of whole blood was significantly different ($P < .0001$), with a mean of 24.7 ± 3.7 (range 17.6 to 33.1) mm Hg (Culp et al, 1994).

The effects of sample handling were studied in six normal dogs. We found that the results were not affected when the standard 3-ml lyophilized heparin tubes were underfilled. Samples anticoagulated with ethylenediamine tetra-acetic acid, citrate, and liquid heparin provided significantly lower results than the standard, presumably because of dilution. When COP was determined with the use of plasma or serum, the values were significantly higher than those of whole blood. For ease of clinical utility in cage-side monitoring, samples are usually run using whole blood. As a research tool, plasma or serum can be used. Freezing and thawing appears to have minimal effect on COP.

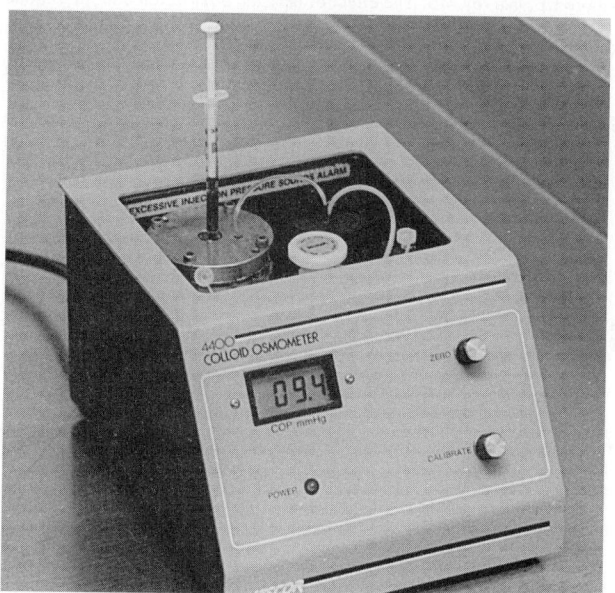

Figure 1. The Wescor 4400 colloid osmometer. Heparinized whole blood is injected into the test chamber, and the colloid osmotic pressure (COP) is determined by equilibration of the sample with saline across a semipermeable membrane.

RELATIONSHIPS AMONG COLLOID OSMOTIC PRESSURE, TOTAL PROTEIN, AND SYNTHETIC COLLOIDS

Studies have evaluated the relationship between COP and TP and have suggested equations for prediction of COP from the plasma protein concentration. These nonlinear equations showed high correlation between COP and TP (Thomas and Brown, 1992).

Unfortunately, TP is not the only factor that affects COP. A great deal of variability exists among individual animals, which is probably related to several factors, including the ratio of albumin to globulin, the plasma pH, and the ionic composition of the plasma due to the Gibbs-Donnan effect. Since even more factors can contribute to variability of TS measurements, there is even greater discrepancy in the relationship between TS and COP in both normal and ill patients (see Fig. 2). Unfortunately, the experimentally developed equations, derived by dilution and concentration of plasma samples from individual dogs, do not provide accurate enough estimates of COP to be useful in widely differing clinical patients (Brown et al, 1994).

Commonly used synthetic colloids such as hetastarch and dextrans do not predictably change the TP or TS measurements. Nevertheless, these solutions can effectively increase the COP, with resolution of effusions or edema, despite unchanged or even decreased TS. When synthetic colloids are used for patient management, it can be extremely difficult to gauge the adequacy of therapy. Although clinical findings such as improved hemodynamic state or resolution of edema may provide useful information, these clinical findings are dependent on a variety of factors, such as the presence of sepsis or vasculitis, not just COP. Additionally, synthetic colloids do not predictably increase the COP in a dose-related manner (Smiley and Garvey, 1994). Ongoing losses of colloids resulting from vasculitis, effusions, or gastrointestinal tract loss may result in a minimal increase in COP despite apparently adequate dosing. Direct measurement of COP is therefore the only way of monitoring synthetic colloid therapy effectively.

USING COLLOID OSMOMETRY IN CLINICAL PATIENTS

In a sample of 100 critically ill dogs and cats admitted to the intensive care unit at the Veterinary Hospital of the University of Pennsylvania, the mean COP prior to synthetic colloid therapy was 13.9 ± 3.1 (range 7.6 to 23.8) mm Hg (King et al, 1994). In this sample, we found no direct relationship between COP and the presence of peripheral edema, presumably because of concurrent vasculitis in many of our patients. It is the author's impression that COP values less than 14 mm Hg are clinically significant in the dog and cat; however, the decision to administer plasma or synthetic colloids should be based on the clinical status of the patient rather than simply on the TP or COP value. Intervention may not be required in a patient recovering uneventfully from abdominal surgery who is beginning to eat, with no vomiting, and has a COP of 13 mm Hg. Conversely, a vomiting postoperative septic peritonitis patient with an open abdomen and a COP of 14 mm Hg should be aggressively supported with colloid therapy.

We often measure COP several times daily as a routine part of cage-side monitoring of patients receiving synthetic colloids. Since this tool has become available, we have found that the volume of synthetic colloids administered to individual patients has increased, whereas the incidence of peripheral edema has decreased. When 24 dogs were treated with hetastarch at varying rates, the COP increased significantly from 11.5 ± 3.0 (range 4.4 to 20.2) mm Hg to 19.3 ± 4.4 (range 11.5 to 31) mm Hg (King et al, 1994). Most of our patients require hetastarch at dosage rates of 20 to 40 ml/kg per day to achieve and maintain effective elevations of their COP values. Depending on the needs of the individual patient, we aim to increase the COP to a value greater than 15 mm Hg. We and others (Moore and Garvey, 1996) have found that single doses of hetastarch result in transient increases of COP and that multiple doses or continuous administration is necessary to maintain the COP within optimal ranges.

References and Suggested Reading

Brown SA, Dusza K, Boehmer J: Comparison of measured and calculated values for colloid osmotic pressure in hospitalized animals. Am J Vet Res 5:910, 1994.

Culp AM, Clay ME, Baylor IA, et al: Colloid osmotic pressure (COP) and total solids (TS) measurement in normal dogs and cats. Fourth International Veterinary Emergency and Critical Care Symposium. San Antonio, TX: Omnipress, 1994, p 705(abstract).

King LG, Culp AM, Clay ME, et al: Measurement of colloid osmotic pressure (COP) in a small animal intensive care unit. (Abstract) Fourth International Veterinary Emergency and Critical Care Symposium, San Antonio, TX: Omnipress, 1994, p 701.

Moore LE, Garvey MS: The effect of hetastarch on serum colloid osmotic pressure in hypoalbuminemic dogs. J Vet Intern Med 10:300, 1996.

Smiley LE, Garvey MS: The use of hetastarch as adjunct therapy in 26 dogs with hypoalbuminemia: A phase two clinical trial. J Vet Intern Med 8:195, 1994.

Thomas LA, Brown SA: Relationship between colloid osmotic pressure and plasma protein concentration in cattle, horses, dogs and cats. Am J Vet Res 53:2241, 1992.

Vascular Access Techniques

JAMES S. WOHL
Auburn, Alabama

Percutaneous placement of intravascular catheters is the most common method for achieving access to the vasculature for fluid therapy, frequent blood collection, and physiologic monitoring. In emergency patients, percutaneous venous catheterization can be problematic because of hypotension, hypovolemia, vascular collapse, trauma, and skin stiffness. Percutaneous arterial catheterization is technically difficult because arteries are surrounded by a dense adventitia, are located deeper in fascial tissues than are veins, and are not visible through the skin. Arterial catheterization can be further complicated by hypotension or hypovolemia. Intraosseous cannulation (see *CVT XI*, p. 107) provides a route for fluid and drug administration but is inadequate for blood collection and cardiovascular monitoring. In some instances, emergency venous or arterial access requires a cutdown procedure. Knowledge of reliable anatomic landmarks and proper surgical technique facilitates successful placement of vascular catheters in the critically ill patient.

PATIENT PREPARATION

Except in the most emergent situations, aseptic technique should be maintained during catheter placement. Clipping and surgical preparation of the skin 180 degrees around the cutdown site allows aseptic handling of a limb. Infusion of lidocaine into the skin and subcutis of the proposed cutdown site facilitates placement in awake patients. Final preparation includes a last surgical scrub and the maintenance of a sterile field containing the necessary instruments, catheters, syringes filled with heparinized saline, injection plugs, stopcocks, and fluid tubing. Sterile latex gloves should be worn when one attempts invasive vascular access techniques. Since the focus of the surgeon will be on the cutdown site, it is essential that nongloved assistants be present to monitor the patient's vital signs during the procedure.

VENOUS CUTDOWN TECHNIQUES

Mini Cutdown

The mini cutdown technique is used for gaining access to the cephalic and lateral saphenous veins. With the bevel facing the operator, a sterile 20- or 22-gauge hypodermic needle is scraped across the skin directly over and parallel to the underlying vein in a proximal to distal direction. Tearing of the skin in this fashion will release skin tension without damaging the underlying vessel. Alternatively, a small incision can be made over the vein with a scalpel blade. Although an incision will cause a less traumatic defect to the skin, care must be taken to avoid incising the vessel and subcutaneous tissue. A mini cutdown can be used to visualize a collapsed vein but is more commonly used to avoid tissue drag during catheter placement. This technique is most useful in cats with thick skin or when burring of an over-the-needle catheter is prohibiting percutaneous placement. Infusion of lidocaine prior to mini cutdown is rarely needed, especially in very sick patients.

Surgical Cutdown

Surgical cutdowns can be used over the external jugular, maxillary, cephalic, or lateral saphenous veins. Cutdown incisions should be made in the middle to cranial portion of the jugular groove when one attempts to catheterize the external jugular vein. The maxillary vein is a branch of the external jugular vein and is located half the distance between the wing of the atlas and the mandibular salivary gland. For cephalic and lateral saphenous vein cutdowns, incisions are made over their expected locations on the dorsal antebrachium and lateral aspect of the distal tibia, respectively.

The surgical technique is similar for all venous sites. A scalpel blade is used to incise the skin directly over or adjacent to the vein. Either a transverse or a parallel skin incision can be made. Care should be taken to incise only the full thickness of the skin. Blunt dissection (e.g., with mosquito forceps) may be required to visualize the vein as a blue to purple tubular structure within the subcutaneous tissue. Minimal dissection is usually required for the placement of an over-the-needle or through-the-needle catheter.

In some instances, it may be necessary to isolate the vein. Isolation is accomplished by blunt dissection parallel to the vein. Subcutaneous or adventitial tissue adjacent to the vein is retracted with atraumatic thumb forceps, exposing the vessel. Dissection with the use of sharp-ended scissors is then performed dorsally and ventrally to the vein. Dissecting in a parallel fashion minimizes the chances of rupturing or traumatizing the vessel. After freeing the vein from the subcutaneous tissue, a hemostat is advanced beneath the vein. A silk suture is then clasped by the hemostat and drawn beneath the vessel (Fig. 1). The vein can be briefly occluded proximally to enhance filling. The suture can then be used to retract the vein distally and provide adequate tension for the catheterization of the vessel (Fig. 2). Alternatively, the vessel may be sacrificed by ligating the vein distally and using the ligature to retract the vessel. A second suture is placed beneath the vessel proximally. The vein is then cannulated through a venotomy (or by venipuncture) between the two ligatures. Following catheterization, the proximal suture is ligated, securing the catheter in the vein.

ARTERIAL CUTDOWN TECHNIQUES

Percutaneous placement of arterial catheters (see *CVT XII*, p. 110) is indicated in patients requiring repeated

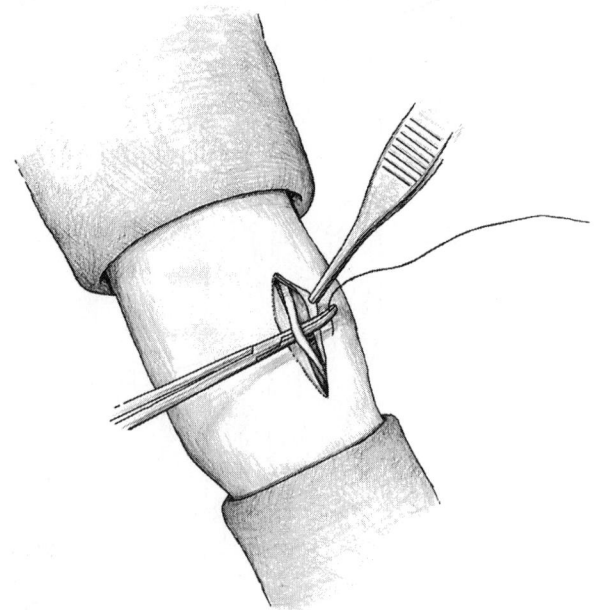

Figure 1. Following isolation of the blood vessel, a hemostat is used to pass a silk suture beneath the vessel. (Art by Lisa Makarchuk.)

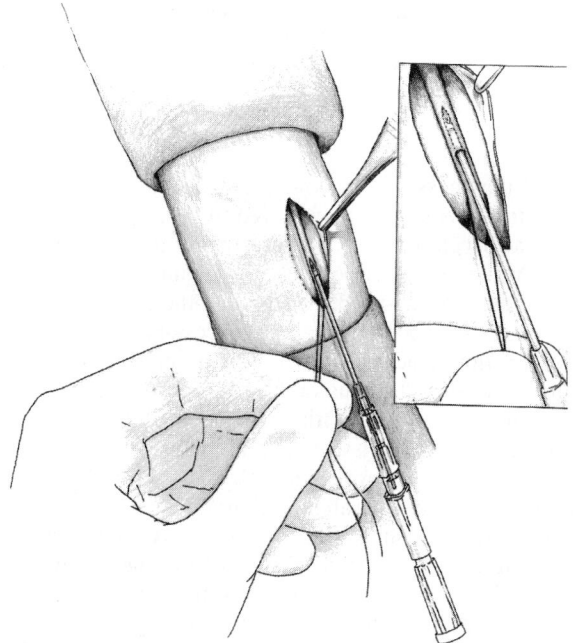

Figure 2. Retraction of the vessel with a suture applies tension to the vessel, allowing introduction of an over-the-needle catheter. (Art by Lisa Makarchuk.)

arterial blood gas analysis or direct arterial blood pressure measurement. The most common site for arterial catheterization is the dorsal metatarsal artery (Fig. 3). This artery is most superficial in the proximal metatarsus, medial to the

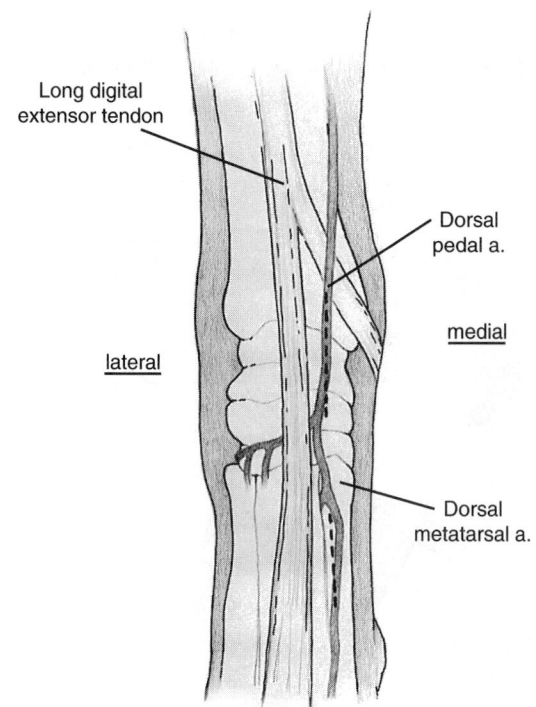

Long digital extensor tendon

lateral

Dorsal pedal a.

medial

Dorsal metatarsal a.

Figure 3. Location of dorsal metatarsal artery and dorsal pedal artery in the dog. Hashed lines depict location of cutdown sites. (Art by Lisa Makarchuk.)

extensor tendons, between the second and third metatarsal bones. A second arterial site is the dorsal pedal artery, which courses medial to the long digital extensor tendon at the level of the proximal tarsus (see Fig. 3). The femoral artery is less commonly used because of its location and the risk of hemorrhage, the potential danger of puncturing the external iliac artery, and retroperitoneal bleeding.

When a surgical cutdown is performed for arterial catheterization, a technique should be used that preserves vascular sufficiency. An incision is made over the pulsation of the dorsal metatarsal artery in the proximal metatarsus. When isolating the dorsal pedal artery, the incision is made medial and parallel to the long digital extensor in the proximal tarsus. Dissection is performed parallel to the direction of the artery, as described earlier for isolating a vein. The artery is identified as a white tubular structure. A pulse may be palpated, which will distinguish the artery from a nerve or tendon. A silk suture is placed beneath the artery and is retracted distally to expose and place tension on the vessel (see Fig. 2).

An over-the-needle catheter, primed with heparinized saline, is recommended for arterial cannulation. Through-the-needle catheters have a smaller diameter than the penetrating needle and puncture wound; consequently, leakage of blood can result at the catheter insertion site. A more expensive alternative to an over-the-needle catheter is to use the modified Seldinger technique. This method employs a guide wire over which the catheter is advanced into the artery. A vessel dilator is sometimes used prior to introducing the catheter. Although the Seldinger technique is thought to be the least traumatic method of catheter placement, arterial cannulation can usually be achieved with over-the-needle catheters.

Topical administration of a few drops of 2% lidocaine onto the artery may prevent arterial spasm and facilitate cannulation. Retracting the artery with silk suture, the needle catheter assembly is inserted into the artery until rapid flow of red arterial blood fills the needle hub. The assembly is then repositioned in line with the artery and advanced an additional few millimeters. The catheter is then advanced off the needle and into the artery. The needle is discarded, and a sterile Luer-Lok injection plug is attached to the catheter. The catheter is flushed with a small volume of heparinized saline. Aspiration of arterial blood through the plugged catheter with a needle and syringe confirms the appropriate placement within the artery. It is important to keep the artery retracted during this procedure to prevent slippage of the artery off the unsecured catheter. In anesthetized patients, venous blood may be superoxygenated and have the appearance of arterial blood. Observing pulsatile, rapid blood flow through the open catheter prior to the insertion of an injection cap indicates the cannulated vessel is an artery. Blood gas analysis revealing an oxygen tension compatible with arterial blood, or connection to a pressure-monitoring system, will further confirm proper placement.

Securing the Catheter Without Sacrificing the Artery

The silk retraction suture is removed from beneath the artery. A silk suture with a swaged-on needle is placed above the artery but beneath the hub of the catheter. A

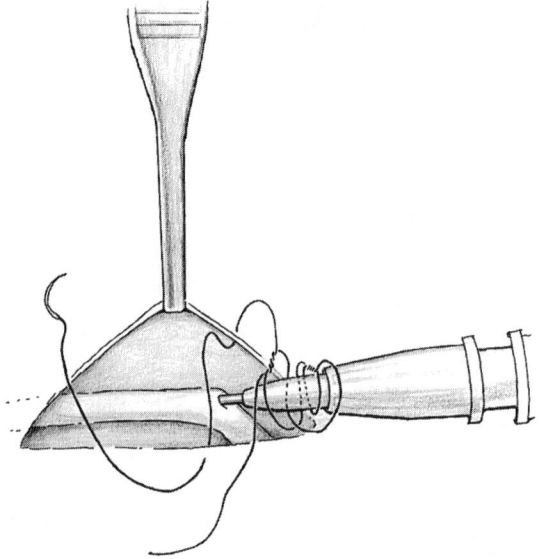

Figure 4. A finger trap suture is placed around the catheter hub only. An interrupted skin suture is then placed anchoring the catheter in place. (Art by Lisa Makarchuk.)

finger trap suture is tied around the catheter hub, leaving excess suture on both ends of the second knot (Fig. 4). The catheter is allowed to lie in a stationary position, and the remaining length of suture is used to anchor the catheter through the skin, placing minimal tension on the catheter. This method secures the catheter in place without sacrificing the artery and allows withdrawal of the catheter after cutting the anchoring skin suture. One or two interrupted skin sutures may be required proximal to the anchor suture to close the incision site.

MAINTENANCE OF ARTERIAL CATHETERS

Following suturing of the catheter and the incision site, a sterile dressing is applied, and the catheter is bandaged routinely. In awake patients, a soft padded bandage can be used to inhibit movement of the tarsus. Patency of the catheter is maintained by periodic flushing with small volumes (1 to 2 ml) of heparinized saline injected through the injection cap with a 25-gauge needle. Manual flushing of larger volumes of fluid with a syringe can cause retrograde blood flow and embolization of particulate matter or air. Most transducer systems used for direct blood pressure monitoring employ a squeeze clamp or pigtail flushing device. Attaching a multiport stopcock to the catheter allows connections to a blood pressure monitor and a flushing system and provides an additional site for blood collection. When not in use, stopcock ports should be attached to sterile injection plugs.

Blood Collection

With the stopcock turned off to the designated collection port, the sterile injection plug is removed and protected from contamination by placing it on a sterile gauze square or other sterile field. A sterile 3-ml syringe containing 1 ml of heparinized saline is then attached to the collection

TABLE 1. Hazards and Complications of Arterial Catheters

Arterial embolization of fibrin, air, or particulate matter
Hemorrhage and hematoma formation
Vascular insufficiency
Ischemic necrosis of the overlying skin
Infection
Accidental intra-arterial drug injection

port. The stopcock is then turned off to the flushing system and 1 ml of blood is drawn into the flush syringe. The stopcock is turned off to the patient and sample port and the flush syringe is discarded. The flushed blood mixture should *not* be reinfused following arterial blood collection. A new sterile syringe that has been purged with heparin (if obtaining a blood gas sample) is then attached. The stopcock is then turned off to the flushing system, and the desired amount of blood is drawn *slowly* into the syringe. Rapid, forced withdrawal may injure the artery. After sample collection, the stopcock is turned off to the sample port, the sample syringe is removed, and the system is flushed for 1 second via the flushing system. To minimize thrombus formation and bacterial contamination, the sample stopcock should be flushed following blood collection. This is achieved by turning the stopcock off to the patient and allowing irrigation solution to flow through the open sample port. Sterile gauze can be used to collect the expelled solution. Following this procedure, the sterile injection plug is returned to the sample port.

Complications and Removal of Arterial Catheters

An arterial catheter should be removed as soon as it is no longer essential for proper patient management. Table 1 lists hazards and complications of arterial catheterization. In human patients, arterial catheters are associated with a higher rate of thrombus formation after a 3- or 4-day dwell time. Evidence of vasculitis, skin discoloration, hemorrhage, or an unexplained fever should prompt evaluation of the catheter site. Cooler than normal skin temperature distal to the catheter insertion site may be indicative of developing catheter-related insufficiency in blood supply and impending ischemic necrosis.

When one removes an arterial catheter, all bandage and dressing material should be removed. The anchoring suture is then cut. Firm pressure is applied proximal and distal to the insertion site while the catheter is removed with mild continuous suction applied by a syringe. This method facilitates aspiration of clots surrounding and within the catheter. On catheter removal, firm manual pressure is applied over the insertion site for 5 to 10 minutes. After the application of manual pressure, a pressure dressing is applied for several hours. The insertion site is monitored periodically for internal or external hemorrhage.

Acknowledgment
The author acknowledges the medical illustrations of Lisa Makarchuk.

Intravenous Anesthetic Techniques for Emergency and Critical Care Procedures

THOMAS K. DAY

Louisville, Kentucky

Chemical restraint is often required to perform medical and minor surgical procedures in critically ill or injured veterinary patients. Most chemical restraint techniques require a combination of anesthetic drugs because single-agent therapy offering adequate chemical restraint with minimal cardiopulmonary side effects is currently unavailable. Application of local anesthesia in combination with chemical restraint can also be helpful in providing adequate time to perform procedures.

Several excellent reviews of general anesthesia for the critically ill or traumatized veterinary patient address the physiology and clinical pharmacology of anesthetic drugs used for premedication, induction, and maintenance of anesthesia for major surgical intervention (Bednarski, 1989; Faggella, 1992). This article concentrates specifically on intravenous injectable anesthetic techniques using combinations of drugs that provide chemical restraint for procedures other than major surgery. The following discussion can be applied to both dogs and cats; any differences between dogs and cats concerning the use of the recommended intravenous injectable anesthetics will be noted in the text.

INJECTABLE ANESTHETIC DRUGS CONTRAINDICATED IN THE CRITICALLY ILL PATIENT

Alpha₂-Agonists

Xylazine (Rompun, Miles, Inc.) and medetomidine (Domitor, Pfizer) provide dose-dependent sedation, muscle relaxation, and analgesia, all of which are desirable qualities for performing most procedures. In addition, specific antagonists are available for xylazine (yohimbine [Yobine, Lloyd Laboratories]) and medetomidine (atipamezole [Antesedan, Pfizer]) that will reverse all of the effects, including side effects. However, both drugs produce a degree of cardiopulmonary depression that is not acceptable in critically ill animals. Therefore, xylazine and medetomidine are not indicated for chemical restraint in the critically ill veterinary patient.

Phenothiazine Tranquilizers

Acepromazine (ProMACE, Fort Dodge) is the most commonly used phenothiazine tranquilizer in veterinary anesthesia. Acepromazine produces reliable mental calming and potentiates the analgesic and sedative properties of opioids. The cardiovascular effects include dose-dependent peripheral vasodilation with the potential for hypotension. There is no antagonist for acepromazine, and the duration of action can be as long as 4 to 6 hours. Most critically ill animals are unable to tolerate or provide adequate compensation to the effects of acepromazine. Acepromazine should

be considered an anesthetic drug that is contraindicated in critically ill veterinary patients.

USEFUL INJECTABLE ANESTHETIC TECHNIQUES

Neuroleptanalgesia

Neuroleptanalgesia is the effect produced by the combination of a tranquilizer and an opioid. The most commonly used tranquilizer in a neuroleptanalgesic combination is acepromazine, which is generally contraindicated in the critically ill animal. Xylazine and medetomidine can be used as the tranquilizer portion of a neuroleptanalgesic, but both are also considered to be contraindicated in most patients. Therefore, the class of drugs used most often as the tranquilizer in a neuroleptanalgesic combination for critically ill animals is the benzodiazepines—diazepam and midazolam.

The benzodiazepines are considered minor tranquilizers in normal animals. Minimal sedation and paradoxical excitement or aggression can occur after intravenous or intramuscular administration of a benzodiazepine to a normal animal. In critically ill animals, however, the benzodiazepines can have a profound sedative effect when administered alone. The patient with severely depressed mentation may appear to be anesthetized following administration of benzodiazepines, whereas the somewhat alert patient can appear minimally affected. Most clinical situations require that benzodiazepines be administered in combination with opioids to produce adequate chemical restraint (see discussion further on). The benzodiazepines minimally depress the cardiovascular and respiratory systems and are generally considered safe in critically ill animals.

Diazepam (Elkins-Sinn, Inc.) and midazolam (Versed, Roche Pharma, Inc.) are two commercially available benzodiazepine tranquilizers. Diazepam is formulated in a propylene glycol base, whereas midazolam is water-soluble. Diazepam should not be mixed with other drugs (with the exception of ketamine) to prevent the formation of precipitates. In human patients, midazolam induces sedation and heavy hypnosis (sleep) at subanesthetic doses, is approximately three times more potent than diazepam, and has a shorter duration of action. These effects are not as evident in dogs and cats, in which time to complete recovery is similar to diazepam (Thurmon et al, 1996). Midazolam is approximately 10 times more expensive than diazepam. Therefore, diazepam is generally the benzodiazepine of choice.

The central nervous system effects of diazepam and midazolam can be effectively reversed by the administration of the benzodiazepine antagonist flumazenil (Romazicon, Roche Pharma, Inc.). However, with the minimal cardiopulmonary depression produced by the benzodiazepines, there is rarely a need to administer flumazenil. Animals with severe liver disease that have been sedated with a benzodiazepine neuroleptanalgesic may require flumazenil administration because of the possibility of the benzodiazepine exacerbating clinical signs of hepatic encephalopathy. The cost of flumazenil may currently be prohibitive for routine use in veterinary practice.

The second class of drugs used to produce neuroleptanalgesia is the opioids. In normal animals, opioids provide analgesia and possibly some degree of sedation, but this effect is not consistent among opioids. Once again, however, the compromised animal may exhibit a profound sedative effect following administration of an opioid that seemingly exerts no effect in a normal animal.

The physiologic effect of the opioids is determined by the opioid receptor activated (Thurmon et al, 1996). The primary effect on the cardiovascular system following opioid administration is a bradyarrhythmia resulting from the parasympathomimetic effects of opioids. Bradyarrhythmias are more likely to occur with opioid agonists than with agonist-antagonists and rarely occur when appropriate dosages are administered. Bradyarrhythmias can be treated with the anticholinergic atropine (Butler Co.) or glycopyrrolate (Robinul, Elkins-Sinn, Inc.). Opioids do not decrease myocardial contractility and have no effect on the peripheral vasculature. Opioid agonists produce dose-dependent respiratory depression, but this effect is minimized with the use of opioid agonist-antagonists. Panting can be a prominent side effect of opioid administration.

Opioid agonists are more likely to produce sedation than are opioid agonist-antagonists in normal animals. Both opioid agonists and agonist-antagonists are likely to produce sedation when combined with a tranquilizer, with acepromazine combinations producing more profound effects than benzodiazepine combinations. In contrast to effects in normal animals, opioid agonists are likely to produce very profound sedation, whereas opioid agonist-antagonists are likely to produce reliable sedation in compromised animals, especially when combined with a benzodiazepine tranquilizer.

The opioids that are recommended for neuroleptanalgesic combinations with benzodiazepines include the opioid agonist oxymorphone (Numorphan, DuPont Pharma), the opioid agonist-antagonist butorphanol (Torbugesic, Fort Dodge), and the partial opioid agonist buprenorphine (Buprenex, Reckitt & Colman). Oxymorphone causes the most profound sedation and is more likely to produce respiratory depression and bradycardia. Butorphanol produces minimal respiratory depression and rarely produces bradycardia. Both oxymorphone and butorphanol, when combined with a benzodiazepine, produce sedation within 1 to 2 minutes in a compromised patient for a total duration of reliable sedation of approximately 15 to 20 minutes. Buprenorphine is similar to butorphanol in producing minimal respiratory depression and rarely producing bradycardia. Buprenorphine differs from oxymorphone and butorphanol in that it has a relatively longer onset of action (5 to 10 minutes) and a longer duration of reliable sedation (20 to 30 minutes).

The effects produced by opioids can be reversed by the administration of the opioid antagonist naloxone (Astra Pharmaceutical Products, Inc.). The duration of action of naloxone is short (15 to 20 minutes), and administration of a second or third dose may be necessary when used to reverse the effects of oxymorphone or buprenorphine, respectively. If oxymorphone was administered as the opioid to provide analgesia, the sedative effects can be reversed by administration of butorphanol without reversing the analgesic effects (partial opioid reversal).

Adjuncts to Neuroleptanalgesia

Intravenous Induction Agents

There may be techniques or procedures that require more time than the neuroleptanalgesic combination offers. Administration of an intravenous anesthetic induction agent, at doses less than those required for intubation, is an effective technique to prolong the effects of neuroleptanalgesia. The criteria for choosing an induction agent would include one that has a rapid onset of action, short duration, rapid redistribution, and minimal cardiopulmonary depression. The most important aspect of choosing an induction agent is to consider each patient individually. The anesthesia induction agents that are most commonly used in conjunction with neuroleptanalgesia are ketamine (Ketaset, Fort Dodge), propofol (Diprivan; Zeneca), etomidate (Amidate, Abbott), and in some instances, thiopental (Pentothal; Abbott).

Ketamine can be used alone or in combination with diazepam. Ketamine can cause seizures and muscle rigidity in dogs and cats if administered alone. The diazepam used in the neuroleptanalgesic combination usually suffices to prevent seizures and provides adequate muscle relaxation if the animal is adequately sedated. Ketamine produces minimal cardiovascular depression when administered to animals with adequate intravascular volume. Blood pressure can decrease in dogs and cats heavily sedated prior to ketamine administration, but the effect is transient. Ketamine produces minimal respiratory depression, but this effect can be exacerbated when the drug is combined with oxymorphone.

Propofol is an induction agent with a short duration of action and noncumulative effects (see *CVT XII*, p. 77). The cardiopulmonary properties of propofol are reportedly similar to those of thiopental, including transient decreases in arterial blood pressure and profound respiratory depression. Apnea produced by propofol can be more profound than that observed with thiopental. However, the dose of propofol used for neuroleptanalgesia is lower than the dose needed for induction of anesthesia. Very slow administration of propofol results in a less profound and shorter duration of apnea, even when propofol is used with oxymorphone. Propofol is the induction agent of choice if repeated boluses or a constant rate infusion (CRI) is required in addition to neuroleptanalgesia. Propofol is rapidly redistributed and metabolized in the liver by glucuronidation. The recovery from propofol in cats does not seem to be prolonged unless the CRI used is longer than 30 minutes (Ilkiw, 1992) or multiple boluses are administered over a period of 30 minutes. The use of propofol on consecutive days is not recommended in cats because of the development of Heinz bodies on feline red blood cells (Andress and Day, 1995).

Etomidate is an induction agent with a short duration of action and minimal cardiopulmonary effects; heart rate, heart rhythm, arterial blood pressure, myocardial contractility along with respiratory rate and rhythm are maintained. Side effects (myoclonus, pain on injection) rarely occur when etomidate is administered following neuroleptanalgesia. Repeated intravenous boluses of etomidate are not recommended. Etomidate is a hypertonic solution and can produce hemolysis of red blood cells if more than two boluses are administered or if etomidate is administered as a CRI.

Thiopental has limited use in the critically ill animal. Administration of thiopental following neuroleptanalgesia should be limited to younger animals with no cardiopulmonary compromise. Repeated boluses of thiopental are not recommended because of the cumulative effects. The availability of induction agents with less adverse cardiopulmonary effects (ketamine) and the development of newer induction agents (propofol and etomidate) preclude the use of thiopental in most instances.

Local Anesthesia

Local anesthesia can provide additional analgesia to prolong the effective sedation time of neuroleptanalgesics administered with or without an intravenous induction agent. The most commonly used techniques are infiltrative, epidural, and intravenous regional local anesthesia (Skarda, 1996). Infiltrative local anesthesia involves placing local anesthetic in or surrounding a specific site and can be used anywhere on the body. Epidural anesthesia (see the next article) is usually reserved to provide anesthesia to the caudal half of the body. Application of epidural local anesthesia is difficult in cats. Intravenous regional anesthesia is a technique that is limited to the distal limb, either distal to the elbow or the hock, using the cephalic and saphenous veins, respectively.

Lidocaine (Lidoject, Vetus) and bupivacaine (Sensorcaine-MPF, Astra) are used most commonly. The choice of a local anesthetic will be determined by the desired duration of analgesia. The duration of lidocaine is approximately 60 to 90 minutes, and the duration of bupivacaine is approximately 4 to 6 hours. Local anesthesia techniques should be used with caution in patients that are severely compromised. Vasodilation can occur with epidural local anesthesia techniques, which could exacerbate or produce hypotension. Cardiovascular and neurotoxicity can occur at lower dosages in animals (especially in cats) with altered intravascular blood volumes. Lidocaine also has central nervous system depressant effects that are not reversible.

CLINICAL EXAMPLES

The following case scenarios are designed to give clinicians a basis for determining the intravenous injectable anesthesia techniques and dosages to provide adequate sedation and analgesia with minimal adverse cardiopulmonary effects. A range of dosages is presented in Table 1. In general, animals that are minimally depressed require higher dosages. Cats generally appear to require the higher dosage range for neuroleptanalgesia when a benzodiazepine is used as the tranquilizer.

Neuroleptanalgesia

A 14-year-old poodle presents with a history of anorexia, depression, and weight loss. Clinical signs include icterus and moderate abdominal distention resulting from ascites. Hypoproteinemia is the most important laboratory result. Primary liver disease is suspected and an ultrasound-guided liver biopsy is required. Adequate hydration status is obtained within 24 hours. A combination of diazepam (0.2 mg/kg IV) and butorphanol (0.2 mg/kg IV) should be adequate to perform this procedure. Oxymorphone (0.05 mg/kg IV) could be used, but butorphanol should be adequate based on the patient's signalment and mental status. Oxymorphone will likely result in panting, which could interfere with biopsy procedure, and bradycardia, which may require therapy with an anticholinergic agent. Low doses of diazepam and butorphanol were chosen for this dog because hypoproteinemia will result in a greater amount of free drug available to produce the desired clinical effects. The effects of both diazepam and butorphanol can be reversed, if necessary.

A 10-year-old cat presents with a 5-day history of anorexia and depression. Diabetic ketoacidosis is diagnosed, and fluid support is administered through a cephalic vein catheter for rehydration. Sedation will be required in this cat so that a catheter can be placed in the jugular vein. A combination of diazepam (0.3 mg/kg IV) and oxymorphone (0.1 mg/kg IV) could be administered. Panting does not seem to be a prominent feature when opioids and neuroleptanalgesics are administered to cats. The duration of effective sedation (IV, 5 to 10 minutes; IM, 10 to 15 minutes; a slightly longer duration in older cats) with this combination seems to be less in cats than in dogs. Recovery from anesthesia after diazepam and oxymorphone use in critically ill cats is usually smooth and uncomplicated when compared with recovery from ketamine-diazepam combinations.

A 4-year-old dog presents after being hit by a car. Intravascular volume resuscitation is established and maintained. The dog is alert and in pain, with normal cardiovascular parameters. The dog remains somewhat tachypneic. The dog requires thoracic and abdominal radiography, and there is a large area of soft tissue damage to the thorax and abdomen. A combination of diazepam (0.4 mg/kg IV) and buprenorphine (0.02 mg/kg IV) can be administered to obtain radiographs. Buprenorphine takes a little longer to produce sedation but provides minimal respiratory depression when compared with oxymorphone. The latter agent also causes panting that can make obtaining a thoracic radiograph more difficult. Buprenorphine also provides analgesia for 4 to 6 hours.

Neuroleptanalgesia and Intravenous Induction

A 10-year-old female Boxer presents with anorexia, lethargy, depression, anemia, and generalized lymphadenopathy. The diagnostic plan includes a bone marrow biopsy, but the dog will not allow manual restraint so that the procedure can be performed. A combination of diazepam (0.4 mg/kg IV) and oxymorphone (0.1 mg/kg IV) is administered, but the dog responds when the procedure

TABLE 1. Recommended Anesthetic Drugs Used for Emergency and Critical Care Procedures

Drug (mg/ml)	Intravenous Dose (mg/kg)	Approximate Cost ($/ml)	Comments
		Neuroleptanalgesia	
Tranquilizers			
Diazepam or midazolam (5 mg/ml)	0.2–0.4	Diazepam ($1.10) Midazolam ($8.00)	Hemodynamic stability, minimal respiratory depression; should not mix diazepam with other drugs (except ketamine)
Opioids			
Oxymorphone (1.5 mg/ml)	0.05–0.1	$4.00	Opioid agonist, respiratory depression
Butorphanol (10 mg/ml)	0.2–0.4	$3.30	Opioid agonist-antagonist, minimal respiratory depression
Buprenorphine (0.3 mg/ml)	0.005–0.02	$2.80	Partial opioid agonist, minimal respiratory depression, difficult to reverse
		Induction Agents	
Propofol (10 mg/ml)	1–2 mg/kg	$0.75	Transient decrease in blood pressure, respiratory depression, apnea, rapid redistribution, rapid recovery
Etomidate (2 mg/ml)	0.5–1.0	$1.40	Minimal cardiorespiratory depression, repeat boluses or CRI not recommended
Ketamine (100 mg/ml)	2–4	$0.80	May require diazepam concurrently, respiratory depression possible
Thiopental (25 mg/ml)	2–6	$0.08	Transient decrease in blood pressure, respiratory depression, apnea, cumulative
		Antagonists	
Naloxone (0.4 mg/ml)	0.01–0.04	$1.15	Opioid antagonists, may need repeat administration for oxymorphone and buprenorphine
Flumazenil (0.1 mg/ml)	0.05–0.1	$6.00	Benzodiazepine antagonist, may be cost-prohibitive
		Anticholinergics	
Atropine (0.54 mg/ml)	0.01–0.04	$0.03	Administer lower dose first
Glycopyrrolate (0.2 mg/ml)	0.025–0.05	$0.60	Administer lower dose first

CRI, continuous rate infusion.

begins. One bolus of ketamine (4 mg/kg IV), propofol (2 mg/kg IV) or thiopental (4 mg/kg IV) could be administered to complete the sedation and analgesia required to perform this procedure.

A 4-year-old male Doberman pinscher with a 6-month history of dilated cardiomyopathy that is responding to medication presents with an ulcerated mass on the lateral canthus of the left eye. The diagnostic plan includes a punch biopsy of the mass. The dog will not allow manipulation of the mass. A combination of diazepam (0.4 mg/kg IV) and butorphanol (0.3 mg/kg IV) can be administered for sedation. One bolus of etomidate (0.5 mg/kg IV) should allow the procedure to be completed without cardiopulmonary depression. Butorphanol can be reversed with naloxone (0.04 mg/kg IV) at the completion of the procedure.

Neuroleptanalgesia and Intravenous Induction and Local Anesthetic

A 2-year-old dog is presented following trauma produced by a lawn mower. The dog has a degloving injury to the distal portion of the left rear leg from the hock to the digits, which is immediately bandaged. The dog is in the compensatory stage of shock and adequate intravascular volume is established with crystalloid fluid therapy. The leg requires radiography and the wound requires cleaning and debridement. A combination of diazepam (0.4 mg/kg IV) and oxymorphone (0.1 mg/kg IV) can be administered so that radiography can be performed. Ketamine (3 mg/kg IV) could then be administered to allow bandage removal. An intravenous regional anesthesia technique with lidocaine or a lumbosacral epidural using lidocaine or bupivacaine can provide adequate analgesia to clean and debride

the wound without the need to administer additional anesthetic drugs.

A 6-year-old Dalmatian presents for urethral obstruction and uroabdomen. Fluid and electrolyte balance is addressed prior to attempting urethral catheterization and placement of a peritoneal drain. A combination of diazepam (0.3 mg/kg IV) and buprenorphine (0.02 mg/kg IV) could be administered to provide initial sedation. Oxymorphone (0.05 mg/kg IV) could be used in place of buprenorphine if the dog seems alert. If attempts to place a urethral catheter are not successful because of the animal's pain and discomfort, a bolus of ketamine (4 mg/kg IV) or propofol (2 mg/kg IV) could be administered. If repeated boluses are anticipated, propofol is the preferred choice of induction agents. A lumbosacral epidural using lidocaine or bupivacaine could be applied to allow placement of a peritoneal drain. An infiltration technique for the lidocaine could also be used. The epidural technique would also allow prolonged analgesia (urethral and peritoneal pain), especially if bupivacaine is used.

References and Suggested Reading

Andress JL, Day TK: The effects of consecutive day propofol anesthesia on feline red blood cells. Vet Surg 24:277, 1995.
Study that demonstrated the production of Heinz bodies on feline red bloods cells after administration of propofol over a period of 3 consecutive days.
Bednarski RM: Anesthesia and pain control. Vet Clin North Am Small Anim Pract 1989, p 1223.
Excellent overview of anesthesia for the critically ill veterinary patient including tables with drug dosages.
Faggella AM: Anesthesia for the critical or trauma patient. In: Kirk RW, Bonagura JD, eds: Kirk's Current Veterinary Therapy XI, Small Animal Practice. Philadelphia: WB Saunders, 1992, p 88.

Excellent overview of the approach to critically ill or trauma patients with recommendations of anesthetic techniques for specific disorders. It is another good source for anesthetic drug dosages.

Ilkiw JE: Other potentially useful new injectable anesthetic agents. In: Haskins SC, Klide AM, eds: The Veterinary Clinics of North America, Small Animal Practice, Opinions in Small Animal Anesthesia. Philadelphia: WB Saunders, 1992, p 281.
This entire volume is dedicated to specialists' views on anesthesia. A great source for current information.

Skarda RT: Local and regional anesthetic and analgesic techniques. In: Thurmon JC, Tranquilli WJ, Benson GJ: Lumb and Jones' Veterinary Anesthesia, 3rd ed. Baltimore: Williams & Wilkins, 1996, p 426.
Simple, detailed pictorial and written explanation on the various local anesthesia techniques in dogs.

Thurmon JC, Tranquilli WJ, Benson GJ: Lumb and Jones' Veterinary Anesthesia, 3rd ed. Baltimore: Williams & Wilkins, 1996, p 183.
Comprehensive source of current information on tranquilizers and opioids in veterinary anesthesia.

Epidural Analgesia

BERNIE HANSEN
Raleigh, North Carolina

Seventy years ago, E.R. Frank described a technique of epidural procaine anesthesia in dogs and cats as a practical alternative to hazardous contemporary anesthetics (Frank, 1927). Interest in this technique was sustained during the next two decades but waned following the widespread introduction of more convenient inhalation anesthesia. However, the discovery 20 years ago that intrathecal injection of opioids induces profound analgesia in animals has renewed interest in epidural techniques in human and veterinary patients. Although many different classes of drugs have been evaluated for epidural injection, only local anesthetic agents, opioids, and alpha₂-agonists are currently administered by epidural or intrathecal (subarachnoid) injection to companion animals. As intrathecal administration offers few advantages over epidural injection and may increase the risk of complications, only the epidural administration of agents are reviewed here.

INDICATIONS, PRECAUTIONS, AND CONTRAINDICATIONS FOR EPIDURAL ANALGESIA

Although epidural anesthesia and analgesia are widely used in companion animals, clear indications for these techniques remain to be fully defined. Nevertheless, it appears that these methods can provide effective analgesia in animals undergoing surgery caudal to the umbilicus (or up to and including the thoracic limbs if using morphine). Other potential indications include peritonitis, severe pancreatitis, and caudal trauma. The drug therapy options most widely used at present include single injections of opioids or local anesthetics, or combinations of the two.

Relative or absolute *contraindications* to spinal analgesia include coagulopathies, bacteremia, severe systemic infection, infection at the site of needle placement, thoracolumbar neurologic deficits, lumbosacral fractures or dislocations, uncorrected hypovolemia, and lack of operator experience. Potential complications of epidural drug administration include infection, epidural or intrathecal hemorrhage, spinal or nerve root trauma, and persistent weakness or ataxia. Motor blockade or central effects may be

undesirable side effects of some agents. Serious complications appear rare when the technique is performed by experienced clinicians.

Drug formulation should be evaluated prior to use. Most local anesthetics and opioids sold in multiple-dose vials contain one or more preservatives, some of which have been shown to be neurotoxic in animals. Nevertheless, these products have been successfully used epidurally in many patients, and there have been no reports of neurotoxicity attributable to preservative agents following single injections of these drugs. However, it would be prudent to avoid using preserved drugs whenever possible and to avoid intrathecal injections and repeated epidural administration of those agents. The antioxidant sodium metabisulfite is added to local anesthetics that contain epinephrine. This compound, although not a preservative, should not be administered intrathecally.

EPIDURAL LOCAL ANESTHETICS

Epidural administration of local anesthetics is perhaps most often used to provide regional anesthesia during surgery. These agents reversibly bind to neuronal voltage-gated sodium channels and block nerve impulse conduction. When applied to the epidural space, they effect anesthesia at segmental nerve roots. When administered into the cerebrospinal fluid (CSF) by subarachnoid injection, local anesthetics exert a direct spinal effect. The onset of action following either route is rapid, and analgesia or anesthesia begins within minutes of injection. The pharmacodynamics of individual agents is influenced by the drug's lipid solubility, dissociation constant, and protein-binding characteristics. In general, local anesthetics with high lipid solubility are more potent than are hydrophilic agents.

Two local anesthetics commonly used for epidural analgesia or anesthesia in companion animals are lidocaine and bupivacaine. The latter is perhaps the most useful agent for epidural use. Compared with lidocaine, bupivacaine is more potent with a slower onset and a longer duration of action (Table 1). The relatively high affinity of bupivacaine for sodium channels may be responsible for its increased

TABLE 1. Drugs Useful for Epidural Analgesia and Anesthesia

Drug	Dose (mg/kg)*	Duration Following Single Injection
Local Anesthetics		
Lidocaine for injection or preservative-free, 1.0–2.0%		
Single lumbosacral injection:	1 ml/5 kg lean BW for caudal procedures	1 hr
	1 ml/3.5 kg lean BW for abdominal procedures with epinephrine	(1.5 to 2 hr if combined)
Bupivacaine with epinephrine, 0.25–0.5%		
Single lumbosacral injection:	1 ml/5 kg lean BW for caudal procedures	6 hr
	1 ml/3.5 kg lean BW for abdominal procedures	
Bupivacaine preservative-free without epinephrine, 0.0625–0.125%		
For catheter delivery:	1 ml/3.5–5 kg lean BW, followed by 0.1–0.4 ml/kg/hr CRI; do not exceed 4 mg/kg/day (dog)	4–6 hr
Preservative-free 0.25% bupivacaine with 1 mg/ml preservative-free morphine, mixed in a 50:50 ratio by volume:	0.2–0.5 ml initial dose, followed by 0.1 ml/hr CRI (cat)	—
	0.2 ml/kg initial dose, then 0.025 ml/kg/hr CRI (dog)	—
Opioids		
Morphine for injection, 15 mg/ml		
Single epidural injection:	0.1–0.3 mg/kg	8 hr
(may be diluted in saline to 1–2 mg/ml)		
Morphine preservative-free, 1 mg/ml (Duramorph, Elkins-Sinn)		
Single injection:	0.1–0.3 mg/kg	8 hr
Catheter delivery:	0.1–0.2 mg/kg	8 hr
	0.3–0.5 mg/kg/day CRI	
Oxymorphone for injection, 1.0 mg/ml		
Single injection:	0.05–0.3 mg/kg	8 hr
Fentanyl, preservative-free, 50 μg/ml		
Single injection:	5–10 μg/kg (dogs)	
Catheter delivery:	1–5 μg/kg/hr CRI	
Buprenorphine, preservative-free, 300 μg/ml (Buprene)		
Single injection:	5–20 μg/kg (dog)	8 hr
	5–10 μg/kg (cat)	8 hr
Catheter delivery (dog):	5–20 μg/kg q 8 hr	
	15–60 μg/kg/day CRI	
Alpha₂-Agonists		
Medetomidine, single epidural injection, administered with morphine	2–5 μg/kg	13 hr

*Reduce dose to 30–50% of calculated for subarachnoid injection.
BW, body weight; CRI, continuous rate of infusion.

cardiotoxicity compared with other local anesthetics. Because of its relatively high lipid solubility, the drug must be administered in a reasonably large volume to affect upper lumbar spinal segments following injection at the lumbosacral (LS) space. Both bupivacaine and lidocaine gravitate to dependent areas of the spinal canal following epidural injection and will therefore have the greatest effect on nerve roots on the dependent side of an animal in lateral recumbency (Heath et al, 1989).

Local anesthetics in general, and bupivacaine in particular, may provide analgesia with minimal motor blockade when used in dilute concentrations. Bupivacaine 0.0625–0.125% may be used to provide analgesia with minimal motor blockade. This dilution may be achieved by mixing 1 part 0.25% bupivacaine with 1 to 3 parts sterile saline or an opioid by volume.

Advantages of local anesthetics include effective analgesia, the potential for complete regional anesthesia, and potentiation of epidurally administered opioids. In humans, postoperative neural blockade with local anesthetics attenu-

ates the stress response and improves respiratory function and hemodynamic stability. When included as part of a patient management strategy designed to provide early ambulation and self-sufficiency, these analgesic techniques may reduce morbidity and mortality (Kehlet, 1995). A practical advantage of local anesthetics over opioids is that the motor blockade achieved with higher concentrations provides vivid proof of correct injection. Disadvantages of local anesthetic agents include a relatively short duration of action following a single injection, the possibility of unwanted motor blockade, and potential for blockade of spinal sympathetic nerves, which could cause or aggravate hypotension.

EPIDURAL OPIOIDS

Morphine, oxymorphone, buprenorphine, and fentanyl have been administered epidurally to dogs and cats. The analgesic activity of opioids following epidural administration is attributed to binding at opioid receptors on interneurons of the superficial laminae of the dorsal horn of the spinal cord segments. Thus, epidurally administered opioids must cross the dura to gain access to the CSF and spinal cord. Analgesia is produced by modulation of spinal cord processing of nociceptive information and occurs without significant central effects or motor, sensory, or sympathetic blockade.

Morphine is the least lipid-soluble of the opioids. This characteristic slows spinal and systemic absorption of the drug. Consequently, the peak analgesic effect may not be reached for 90 minutes following injection, and analgesia may persist for up to 24 hours in some patients. In contrast to local anesthetics, the extent of cephalad migration of morphine appears to be relatively independent of the volume in which it is administered. When used for perioperative analgesia, it is important to administer morphine immediately after the induction of general anesthesia and prior to surgery because of the relatively long latency to peak effect. Oxymorphone is only slightly more lipophilic than morphine and has been used successfully for epidural analgesia. Fentanyl is very lipid soluble and rapidly absorbed into the blood, resulting in a short latency and rapid onset of central effects. When combined with morphine, epidural fentanyl reduces latency to analgesia, a feature that is useful for the management of intraoperative pain (Leighton et al, 1989). There appears to be little use for fentanyl as a single epidural agent. Buprenorphine is nearly as lipophilic as fentanyl, limiting its extent of analgesia to a short distance from the injection site. However, its longer duration of action renders it more useful than fentanyl.

The most common side effect of epidural opioids in human beings is pruritus at affected dermatomes (particularly following administration of morphine), and the most serious side effect is delayed respiratory depression. Some patients may experience respiratory depression up to 24 hours after the administration of epidural morphine. Although uncommon (<2% of patients), this delayed respiratory depression may be severe and is the principal reason human patients are routinely monitored following epidural opioid administration. Clinically significant respiratory depression following epidural opioids has not been reported in the companion animals.

Common side effects of epidural morphine or oxymorphone in dogs and cats include posterior ataxia and urine retention. The ataxia is subtle and usually goes unnoticed. Urine retention is due to detrusor muscle weakness and can be problematic in some animals, necessitating manual expression of the bladder or bladder catheterization for up to 24 hours after epidural opioid administration. Urine retention is less likely following administration of buprenorphine (Drenger and Magora, 1989). Although opioid-induced pruritus appears uncommon in dogs, the author has observed three dogs that developed marked *hyperesthesia* following intrathecal injections of morphine. It has been suggested that in humans, this rare side effect may be due to metabolites of morphine and may be controlled by administration of other opioids such as fentanyl (Sjogren et al, 1994).

Following administration of high doses of epidural morphine, or after inadvertent injection of an epidural dose into the subarachnoid space, significant central effects may be observed. Dogs may experience sedation and miosis,

and cats may experience agitation and mydriasis. Respiratory depression occurs but appears no more severe than that observed following parenteral administration of the agent.

EPIDURAL ALPHA$_2$-ADRENERGIC AGENTS

Alpha$_2$-adrenoceptors are present on the membrane of the same cells that contain opioid receptors. The natural ligand for these receptors is norepinephrine, and the cell response following activation is similar to that following binding of opioids to their receptors. Among the alpha$_2$-agonists evaluated in veterinary patients are xylazine and medetomidine. Although the use of epidural xylazine in the horse and ruminant has been standard practice, there has been comparatively little application of epidural alpha$_2$-agonist drugs in companion animals. Although epidural administration of low doses of these agents alone does provide measurable analgesia with minimal cardiovascular side effects, they may work best when low doses are combined with other agents such as morphine (Branson et al, 1993; Greene et al, 1995).

TECHNIQUES OF ADMINISTRATION

Single Injections

Single injections are most often administered to anesthetized animals during preparation for surgery. The LS space is the preferred location owing to the relatively large distance between vertebrae at that site; moreover, in most dogs, the dural sac terminates just cranial to that location, reducing the likelihood of subdural injections. Because the dural sac of many cats extends to the LS junction, attempts at epidural injection of the LS space in that species frequently results in subdural injections. Most subdural injections will also be subarachnoid, and injected medications immediately enter the CSF. Complications of subarachnoid injection include leakage of CSF (which causes "dural puncture headache" in humans), migration of the drug to the brain stem, and complete spinal blockade when using local anesthetics.

In preparation for an LS injection, an area of skin is clipped from the posterior sacrum caudally to L4 cranially and laterally past the wings of the ilea. The skin is aseptically prepared as for surgery. If the animal is awake, the skin, midline fibrous tissue, ligamentum flavum, and epidural space near the ligamentum flavum may be anesthetized with an injection of 1 to 2% lidocaine administered with a 1- to 1.5-inch, 22-gauge needle (or a longer spinal needle if needed). The lidocaine may be mixed with sodium bicarbonate solution at a ratio of 9 parts lidocaine to 1 part bicarbonate (by volume) to eliminate the "sting" of injected lidocaine. Materials needed for injection include sterile latex gloves, a 1- to 3-inch 20- to 22-gauge spinal needle (Monoject, Sherwood Medical, St. Louis, MO) or an 18- to 20-gauge Tuohy needle (Becton Dickinson and Company, Franklin Lakes, NJ), a 3-ml syringe, and a syringe containing the agent to be injected.

The animal may be positioned in lateral or sternal recumbency. If a unilateral surgical procedure is to be performed, the patient should be positioned in lateral recumbency with the surgical site down. The pelvic limbs should be drawn cranially to flex the spine at the LS junction. The most prominent aspects of the dorsal wings of the ilea are palpated, and an imaginary line connecting the two points is visualized. In most animals, the dorsal process of L6 lies near this line, usually just cranial to it. Because the dorsal process of L7 is substantially shorter than that of L6, it may be difficult to palpate in some animals. The sacrum is crowned with the closely spaced, indistinct dorsal processes of the fused sacral vertebrae. The LS space lies under a palpable depression just cranial to the first dorsal sacral process and a slightly greater distance caudal to the dorsal process of L7.

Plain injection needles (20- to 22-gauge, 1 to 1.5 inches in length) may be used in small dogs and cats, but the long sharp bevel and tip increase the risk of penetration of the dura. Spinal and Tuohy needles differ from regular injection needles because they have shorter bevels, include a steel stylet, and are available in longer lengths. Compared with spinal needles, Tuohy needles are larger in diameter, stiffer, and duller.

The needle is advanced transcutaneously perpendicular to the skin at the center of the LS depression, with the bevel oriented cranially. The needle is advanced to the LS space. During this time, the operator must keep the needle shaft oriented on the midline. If bone is encountered, positioning is reassessed by inspection and palpation, and the needle is withdrawn slightly and "walked" cranially or caudally to find the LS space. When misplaced, the needle tip is usually cranial to the LS space. The primary source of resistance to advancement of the needle at the LS space is the dorsal spinal ligament, or ligamentum flavum. When using sharp needles in small patients, the resistance offered by the ligamentum flavum is minimal. In larger and older animals, the ligamentum flavum is considerably more fibrous and offers more resistance. The "feel" of needle passage through the ligamentum is a valuable aid to determine that the needle has entered the proper location.

Once the needle has entered the ligamentum flavum, it is advanced 2 mm further until there is a loss of resistance. This usually indicates that the entire bevel surface has entered the spinal canal. At that time, the stylet is withdrawn and the hub of the needle is inspected for the presence of blood or CSF. If blood is encountered, this usually signifies deviation of the needle tip from the midline and penetration of an epidural vein. The needle should be partially withdrawn and redirected to the midline. If CSF is observed, the needle should be partially withdrawn and repositioned. If desired, preservative-free agents without epinephrine can be safely administered into the subarachnoid space, although the dose should be reduced to 30 to 50% of the epidural dose.

If no blood or CSF is encountered, an attempt should be made to confirm that the needle tip is located in the epidural space. The following sections discuss several methods to accomplish this.

Air Leakage

If the needle tip is located in the epidural space, an injection of 0.5 to 2.0 ml of air will proceed with no resistance and with no visible leakage into subcutaneous tissue. The observation of air bulging the skin around the needle shaft during injection signifies that the needle has not penetrated the ligamentum flavum. If the air is injected into the epidural space, one can often aspirate at least a portion of it back.

The "Whoosh" Test

In the "whoosh" test, the operator uses a stethoscope to auscultate directly over the spine just cranial to the needle during the injection of 0.5 to 2.0 ml of air (Lewis et al, 1992). Proper placement of the needle in the epidural space results in a "whoosh" sound during injection that is relatively free of crepitus. Injection of air into any extraspinal tissue produces loud crepitus.

Loss of Resistance

The loss of resistance technique works well only with Tuohy needles. A 3-ml syringe with 0.5 to 2.0 ml of air is attached to the hub of the needle, the needle-syringe assembly is bent caudally, and a test injection of air is carried out. This maneuver forces the beveled tip of the needle in a cranial direction. If the tip is within the epidural space, the ligamentum flavum serves as a fulcrum for the needle, and the bevel is forced cranially. The only tissue to come in direct contact with the needle bevel is spinal fat, and this tissue offers no resistance to injected air. If the needle tip lies in paraspinal tissue, the maneuver will force the bevel surface to compress the muscle and connective tissue in front of it, and these tissues significantly increase the resistance to injection.

Hanging Drop Technique

This technique is best performed with a Tuohy needle and is initiated prior to penetration of the ligamentum flavum. The needle is advanced to a point near the ligamentum flavum, the stylet is withdrawn, and the lumen of the needle is filled with some of the agent to be injected. The hub of the needle should be filled so that some of the liquid protrudes beyond the edge of the hub orifice. The needle is then advanced into the epidural space. When the needle bevel enters the epidural space, the normally negative pressure within the space will cause the drop of fluid to be aspirated down the needle shaft.

Once the needle is properly positioned, the injection may proceed. The operator should confirm that the bevel is directed cranially (the hubs of spinal and Tuohy needles are marked on the bevel side), and the agent should be injected slowly, over 10 to 20 seconds (longer, if possible, in awake animals). Rapid injection into conscious animals often provokes vomiting and may be painful.

Epidural Catheterization

There are several commercially available brands of epidural catheters approved for human use. All are inserted through a Tuohy (or similar) needle placed in the same manner as for single injections. Tuohy needles are characterized by having a 90-degree bend at the needle tip that produces a bevel orifice parallel to the long axis of the needle. This causes the catheter to exit the needle at a right angle to it, facilitating its advancement into the epidural space. Examples of kits successfully used in dogs include the Arrow Flex-Tip Plus catheter (Arrow Epidural Catheter Kit, product No. AM-05500, Arrow International, Reading, PA) and the Arrow Theracath (Arrow Epidural Catheter Kit, product No. AK-05000, Arrow International, Reading, PA).

Additional helpful supplies include an in-line bacterial filter (Sterile Acrodisc 0.2 micron syringe filter, Gelman Sciences, Ann Arbor, MI), a small-volume extension set (Medex Mini-Vol Extension Set, part No. 1855-00, Medex Inc., Duluth, GA), and an injection cap with Luer-Lok fitting. Using sterile technique, the gloved and masked operator connects the injection cap to the bacterial filter, which is, in turn, connected to the extension set. The entire system is purged of air using the desired analgesic agent and is laid on the sterile glove wrap until needed. The skin is prepared and anesthetized as for single-needle injections, and the area is covered with a sterile field drape.

In cats and small dogs, a long (8 to 12 inch) 22-gauge through-the-needle venous catheter may be used successfully. The catheter should be made of polyurethane (not Teflon) to limit kinking and should include a wire stylet and a clear plastic sheath over the catheter to maintain sterility. Because the bevel of IV catheter needles is not parallel to the needle, the needle should penetrate the skin somewhat more caudally than for a single injection, at a level approximately over the first dorsal process of the sacrum. The needle is then directed cranially and advanced just over the anterior-dorsal edge of the sacrum, into the ligamentum flavum and epidural space. The sterile plastic catheter sheath is left in place to cover the needle hub and catheter for the procedure. If the operator is not sure of proper placement, the plastic sleeve and catheter may be temporarily removed and the needle position tested with an injection of air as described earlier. The plastic sleeve and catheter are then carefully repositioned on the needle hub. The operator should ensure that the bevel of the needle is always directed cranially.

Once proper placement of either needle type is determined, the catheter is advanced through the needle. Lowering the hub of the needle to make the long axis of the needle more parallel to the spinal canal facilitates egress of the catheter from the needle tip and directs it up the spinal canal. The catheter should be advanced past the desired location (it will later be partially withdrawn back to that level). The catheter should advance with minimal resistance and must not be forced. The needle should then be withdrawn from the skin, taking care not to withdraw the catheter. The needle is then removed from the catheter (if using an epidural kit) or is split off the catheter or covered with a needle guard, depending on the product used (if using an IV catheter). The stylet is removed from the catheter and may be held along the side of the catheter and patient for use as a depth gauge to determine the position of the catheter tip. The catheter is then partially withdrawn to the desired level.

At this time, the primed extension set is connected to the catheter hub to maintain the sterility of the system. A small "butterfly" of 1-inch waterproof white tape is applied to the catheter at the exit site, and this may be

reinforced with more overlaid 1-inch tape. The proximal edge of the tape is then sutured to the skin 3 to 5 mm to either side of the catheter. The exit site is covered with antiseptic ointment and the 2-inch × 2-inch sponge and the entire IV catheter and a sufficient portion of the extension set is coiled and adhered to the body surface with overlapping strips of 2-inch white tape. Tape adherence to the skin may be improved by spraying the tape with medical adhesive or ether. All connections among injection cap, filter, extension set, and catheter are covered and reinforced with the waterproof tape to maintain the integrity of the system.

All subsequent injections should be made using a 22- to 25-gauge needle through the injection cap after first cleaning the cap with alcohol. Alternatively, a second extension set may be used to connect a syringe pump assembly directly to the proximal extension set to facilitate constant infusion of drug.

The sterility of the system must be carefully maintained, and any break in technique should prompt consideration of catheter removal. The insertion point should be inspected frequently for evidence of inflammation, and the patient should be evaluated for evidence of local pain or swelling, indicating infection. Epidural catheters have been left in human patients for many weeks at a time, and the author has successfully maintained them in dogs and cats for up to 2 weeks. The injection cap, filter, and extension set should be replaced at least every 2 to 4 days using aseptic technique.

References and Suggested Reading

Branson KR, Ko JCH, Tranquilli WJ, et al: Duration of analgesia induced by epidurally administered morphine and medetomidine in dogs. J Vet Pharmacol Ther 16:369, 1993.
A prospective study of the analgesia provided by epidural morphine, medetomidine, or a combination of the two in dogs subjected to experimental pain.

Drenger B, Magora F: Urodynamic studies after intrathecal fentanyl and buprenorphine in the dog. Anesth Analg 69:348, 1989.
A prospective study of detrusor function following intrathecal administration of fentanyl or buprenorphine to healthy dogs.

Frank ER: Regional anesthesia in the dog and cat. J Am Vet Med Assoc 72:336, 1927.
An early report of epidural anesthesia in the dog.

Greene SA, Keegan RD, Weil AB: Cardiovascular effects after epidural injection of xylazine in isoflurane-anesthetized dogs. Vet Surg 24:283, 1995.
A prospective study of the cardiovascular side effects of epidural xylazine in anesthetized dogs.

Heath RB, Broadstone RV, Wright M, et al: Using bupivacaine hydrochloride for lumbosacral epidural analgesia. Compend Contin Educ Pract Vet 11(1):50, 1989.
A review and retrospective analysis of clinical use of epidural bupivacaine in dogs.

Kehlet H: Does analgesia benefit postinjury outcome? In: Parker MM, Shapiro MJ, Porembka DT, eds: Critical Care: State of the Art, vol 15. Anaheim, CA: Society of Critical Care Medicine, 1995, p 213.
A review of the literature on the effects of epidural analgesia on morbidity and mortality in human surgery and trauma patients.

Leighton BL, DeSimone CA, Norris MC, et al: Intrathecal narcotics for labor revisited: The combination of fentanyl and morphine intrathecally provides rapid onset of profound, prolonged analgesia. Anesth Analg 69:122, 1989.
A prospective study of the effects of epidural combination fentanyl and morphine in humans.

Lewis MPN, Thomas P, Wilson LF, et al: The "whoosh" test. A clinical

test to confirm correct needle placement in caudal epidural injections. Anaesthesia 47:57, 1992.
A description of this technique in humans.
Sjogren P, Jensen N-H, Jensen TS: Disappearance of morphine-induced

hyperalgesia after discontinuing or substituting morphine with other opioid agonists. Pain 59:313, 1994.
Report of morphine-induced hyperalgesia and its reversal with fentanyl in humans.

Colloids: Current Recommendations

ELKE RUDLOFF

REBECCA KIRBY

Milwaukee, Wisconsin

Severe intravascular volume depletion, as may occur with hemorrhage, trauma, systemic inflammatory response syndrome, and other metabolic diseases, results in poor tissue perfusion, tissue hypoxia, and cellular energy depletion. Vascular tone and integrity become compromised, leading to maldistribution of fluid among the intravascular, interstitial, and intracellular compartments. Fluid replacement in the form of crystalloids and colloids is the foundation of treatment.

The goal of fluid resuscitation and maintenance in the critically ill animal is to restore perfusion and hydration and at the same time prevent volume overload and the attendant complications of pulmonary, peripheral, and brain edema. Determining ongoing fluid requirements can be challenging because of vascular leakage, vasodilation, excessive vasoconstriction, inadequate cardiac function, alterations in fluid composition, or ongoing fluid loss. Whether the fluid administered remains in the intravascular compartment, or moves into the interstitial or intracellular spaces, depends on fluid compartment and capillary dynamics and the composition of the fluid administered.

FLUID DYNAMICS

The body's fluid space is divided into three compartments (intracellular, interstitial, and intravascular), which are separated by a cellular and capillary membrane freely permeable to water, but not to most solutes. When "free water" (no osmotically active particles) is administered to the intravascular compartment, it is distributed to all fluid compartments. The water moves under the force of hydrostatic pressure and osmotic pull.

Starling's law defines the forces that determine the volume of fluid that remains within the intravascular compartment. Membrane pore size, and differences in colloid oncotic pressure (COP) and hydrostatic pressure between the interstitial and intravascular compartments, play the major role in determining intravascular volume. The size of the pore varies from tissue to tissue. The "filtration coefficient" has been found to be variable relative to the amount of albumin in the interstitial space.

The *cellular membrane* is impermeable to most ions. Intracellular ions keep water in the cell by osmotic action. The *capillary membrane* is permeable to electrolyte ions

in the plasma, but not the plasma protein anions. As electrolyte ions move out of the capillary, water follows. The intravascular retention of protein anion is largely responsible for the retention of water in the capillary. This mechanism is responsible for COP.

The dynamics of fluid movement across the capillary membrane can change with certain diseases. Whenever intravascular hydrostatic pressure increases over COP, membrane pore size becomes larger, or intravascular COP becomes lower than interstitial COP, the movement of fluid from the intravascular into the interstitial space is favored. Membrane pore size can increase with systemic inflammation, burns, or trauma. When the hole becomes larger than the plasma proteins, they pass into the interstitium, pulling water with them. Treatment of leaking capillary membranes is aimed at maintaining intravascular COP, with larger anions that will not pass through the holes.

The Landis-Pappenheimer equation, which calculates COP from total protein, fails to provide an accurate measurement of COP for dog plasma (see p. 112). Direct measurement of COP becomes more important. Colloid oncotic pressure in the normal dog is 17.5 mm Hg ± 3.04 with a normal protein concentration of 6.08 ± 0.83 g/dl. In the patient with acute volume depletion, this value can increase when there is water loss (hemoconcentration), remain the same as with hemorrhage, or decrease with protein loss.

In addition to capillary dynamics, the composition of a fluid administered determines how the administered fluid is distributed. The two major categories of administered fluids are crystalloids and colloids. A crystalloid is a water-based solution with electrolyte ions permeable to the capillary membrane. A colloid fluid is a water-based solution with both small molecules that are permeable to the capillary membrane as well as impermeable anions.

When large-volume fluid resuscitation and maintenance are required, crystalloids may fail to provide appropriate intravascular volume without also causing interstitial volume overload and edema. The treatment of critically ill animals requiring large-volume resuscitation or suffering from hypo-oncotic states is greatly facilitated by the administration of colloid fluids. The selection of a colloid or a combination of colloids is based on the pharmacology of the fluid and the disorder requiring treatment.

BASIC COLLOID PHARMACOLOGY

Whole blood, plasma products, and concentrated albumin contain natural colloids in the form of proteins, primarily albumin (Kaufman, 1992). Oxypolygelatin, dextrans 40 and 70, and hydroxyethyl starches (hetastarch and pentastarch) are synthetically derived colloids (Table 1 and Table 2). Synthetic colloids were developed to provide timely and convenient fluid resuscitation and to avoid the problems encountered with rapid, natural colloid infusions. Colloids provide an increase in COP beyond what is attainable with whole blood or plasma. These fluids are not, however, to be considered a substitute for blood products when albumin, red blood cells, antithrombin, or coagulation proteins are needed.

It is the difference in macromolecular structure and weight that dictates the oncotic effect, method of excretion, and half-life of the colloidal solution. The number-averaged molecular weight of a colloid is the arithmetic mean of the molecular weights of the polymers in solution. Weight-averaged molecular weight is the sum of the number of molecules at each number-averaged molecular weight divided by the total of all molecules. This weight is generally larger when larger polymers are present in solution. In general, the greater the number of small molecules that exist per unit volume, the greater the initial oncotic effect and plasma volume expansion. The greater the number of large molecules, the better the colloid is retained in the vascular space. The degree of molar substitution, the size of the molecule, and the enzymatic processes required for breakdown determine the half-life of the molecule in the body. Synthetic colloids are eliminated via the gastrointestinal system, uptake and storage in the tissues of major organs, and filtration at the glomerulus and subsequent appearance in urine.

Whether resuscitating with crystalloids, colloids, or a combination of both, large-volume resuscitation decreases the concentration of coagulation proteins in the plasma and can cause a dilution coagulopathy. In addition, dextrans and hetastarch, at recommended dosages, can have an effect on von Willebrand's factor concentration that is not explained by dilution alone. A notable prolongation in activated partial thromboplastin time occurs in human patients receiving hetastarch, which is attributed to its effects on factor VIII. Partial thromboplastin and prothrombin times were prolonged in dogs reported to have received therapeutic doses of dextran 70 (Concannon et al, 1992). The authors have experienced prolongation in activated clotting times (ACT; less than 50% above normal) without clinical evidence of bleeding in animals receiving hetastarch. However, elevation in ACT above 50% of the normal reference range warrants investigation for concurrent coagulation problems.

Surgeons have voiced concern about increased bleeding during surgical procedures if synthetic colloids are administered. A study of human patients requiring abdominal aortic aneurysm repair and infused with equal concentrations of either 5% albumin or hetastarch at 16 ml/kg showed no significant difference in coagulation times (Gold, 1990). Used at recommended dosages, dextran 70 and hetastarch do not appear to cause an increase in bleeding at surgical sites. However, there is an increase in microcirculatory flow, requiring careful and aggressive surgical hemostasis. When massive quantities of synthetic colloids are required for patient stabilization, the administration of plasma, albumin, and whole blood may be required to provide necessary coagulation proteins, albumin, or red blood cells.

Much of the basic pharmacology of colloids is similar between synthetic colloid groups. However, significant differences exist among groups and within each group. These differences make each colloid unique and form the basis for making an appropriate colloid selection for a specific patient (see Table 1).

TABLE 1. Natural and Synthetic Colloids: Pharmacologic Characteristics

Colloid	Number Avg. Mol. Weight (Daltons)	Avg. Mol. Weight (Daltons)	Mol. Weight Range (Daltons)	Half-Life	Solvent and Contents	Max. H₂O Binding (ml H₂O/g colloid)	COP (mm Hg)	% Concentration
Whole blood	69,000	69,000	69,000–320,000	35 days	Water Albumin Red blood cells White blood cells* Coagulation factors† Platelets‡ Antithrombin	18	20	3.5
Plasma	69,000	69,000	69,000–320,000	17–19 days	Water Albumin Coagulation factors† Antithrombin	18	20	3.5
Oxypolygelatin	23,000	30,000	5,600–100,000	2.5 hours	Electrolyte solution	39	46	5.6
Dextran 40	25,000	40,000	10,000–80,000	2.5 hours	0.9% NaCl or 5% Dextrose	37	40	10
Dextran 70	39,000	70,000	15,000–160,000	25 hours	0.9% NaCl or 5% Dextrose	29	—	6
Pentastarch	39,000	280,000	10,000–1 million	2.5 hours	0.9% NaCl	30	25	10
Hetastarch	70,000	450,000	10,000–3.4 million	25 hours	0.9% NaCl	20	30	6

*White blood cell concentration decreases with age of transfusion.
†Concentrations of factors V and VII decrease within 6 to 8 hours after donation and are not of significant levels in stored whole blood or frozen plasma.
‡Platelet function and numbers decrease significantly within 6 to 8 hours after donation.

TABLE 2. **Natural and Synthetic Colloids: Indications, Dosage, and Adverse Effects**

Colloid	Indication	Dosage: Acute Volume Resuscitation IV*	Dosage: Volume Maintenance IV†	Potential Adverse Effects‡
Whole blood	Severe, acute hemorrhage Anemia with low albumin Thrombocytopenia or coagulopathy from bleeding crisis§	*Dogs:* 20 ml/kg *Cats:* 10–20 ml/kg until PCV = 25–30%	*Dogs:* 20 ml/kg *Cats:* 10–20 ml/kg until PCV = 25–30% over 4–6 hours	Crossmatch and blood-typing recommended Transfusion reaction Blood-borne illnesses Hypocalcemia Expense Availability
Plasma	Coagulopathies Disseminated intravascular coagulation Low antithrombin Acute hypoalbuminemia¶	—	*Dogs:* 250 ml/10–20 kg *Cats:* 10 ml/kg until plasma albumin >2.0 g/dl over 4–6 hours	Need large volumes for COP effect Hypocalcemia Availability
Oxypolygelatin	Hypovolemic, traumatic, or hemorrhagic shock	5 ml/kg over 15 minutes This dose can be repeated twice	In dogs and cats in distributive shock due to SIRS, the initial bolus can be followed by a CRI of hetastarch‖	Anaphylaxis
Dextran 40	Hypovolemic or traumatic shock Prophylaxis of deep vein thrombosis and pulmonary emboli	*Dogs:* 10–20 ml/kg *Cats:* 5 ml/kg increments over 5–10 minutes	In dogs and cats in distributive shock due to SIRS, the initial bolus can be followed by a CRI of hetastarch‖	Acute renal failure Anaphylaxis Bleeding diathesis
Dextran 70	Hypovolemic shock Traumatic shock	*Dogs:* 10–40 ml/kg *Cats:* 5 ml/kg increments over 5–10 minutes	In dogs and cats in distributive shock due to SIRS, the initial bolus can be followed by a CRI of hetastarch‖	Allergic reaction Increases ACT Increased total solids by refractometry
Pentastarch	Hypovolemic shock Traumatic shock	*Dogs:* 10–40 ml/kg *Cats:* 5 ml/kg increments over 5–10 minutes	In dogs and cats in distributive shock due to SIRS, the initial bolus can be followed by a CRI of hetastarch‖	Allergic reaction Increases ACT
Hetastarch	Hypovolemic shock Traumatic shock Low-volume resuscitation COP maintenance	*Dogs:* 10–40 ml/kg *Cats:* 5 ml/kg increments over 5–10 minutes to total 10–40 ml/kg** Cardiogenic shock: 5 ml/kg increments to effect	Constant rate infusion *Dogs:* 10–20 ml/kg/day *Cats:* 10–40 ml/kg/day	Allergic reaction Increases ACT Volume overload Increased amylase

*Titrated to an intravascular volume and blood pressure that support perfusion without causing volume overload. This generally means a mean systemic arterial blood pressure of 80 mm Hg and a central venous pressure of 5 to 8 cm H_2O.

†Set at a rate that maintains perfusion and intravascular volume. The rate depends on the disease process and ongoing fluid losses.

‡At or exceeding recommended dosages.

§Stored blood has decreased concentrations of platelets, and factors V and VIII.

¶Replacement of albumin is important for its function as a carrier of drugs, hormones, and electrolytes.

‖Colloid oncotic pressure maintenance is more easily achieved with large-molecular-weight hydroxyethyl starch, especially in the setting of leaky capillary membranes caused by SIRS.

**It has been the authors' experience that if colloids are required to restore blood pressure and perfusion in the cat, a constant rate infusion of colloid should be immediately initiated.

Oxypolygelatin

Oxypolygelatin (SmithKline Beecham) is produced from cattle bone-marrow gelatin and prepared by gradual controlled heating and oxidation with hydrogen peroxide. Antibodies to raw unmodified gelatin can be found prior to administration of the gelatin products. There is a relevant risk of allergic reaction with oxypolygelatin, mediated by histamine and complement activation. The reported prevalence of anaphylactic reactions for gelatins is higher than that for other synthetic colloids (Kaufman, 1992).

Gelatins have been reported to significantly lower serum calcium concentration, initiating tetany. For this reason, the oxypolygelatin product for veterinary use is supplemented with calcium. The manufacturer of oxypolygelatin recommends extreme caution when it is used in animals with coagulation disorders, hypoproteinemia, cardiac or pulmonary insufficiency, and renal diseases.

Dextran

Dextrans are polysaccharides composed of linear glucose residues. These compounds are produced by the enzyme dextran sucrase during the growth of various strains of the bacterium *Leuconostoc* in media containing sucrose. Different molecular weight dextrans can be produced by acid hydrolysis of the parent macromolecule. Dextran 40 and dextran 70 (McGaw) are available for acute volume resuscitation, with a greater number of large molecules in the dextran 70 preparation.

Disease states that result in vascular subendothelial exposure or hemolytic anemia induce coagulation factor consumption and activation of platelets. During this hypercoagulable period, thromboemboli can develop, causing microcirculatory obstruction and ischemia. Dextran 40 administration decreases circulatory stasis by its effects of improved rheology, inducing temporary functional change in factor VIII:RAg (vWF:Ag), and decreasing platelet aggregability and thrombus stability. Dextran 40 is recommended for use in people as an antithromboembolic agent (Sewester, 1996).

Dextran 40 administration has been associated with development of acute renal failure, anaphylaxis, and bleeding diathesis. Significant amounts of dextran 40 are freely filtered by the glomerulus, entering the renal tubules. As tubular water is reabsorbed, a highly viscous urine is formed. The dextran may precipitate and irreversibly obstruct the tubules, causing acute renal failure. Renal problems are more likely to occur when there is underlying renal disease or pre-existing dehydration. Dextran 70 administration has rarely been associated with the development of acute renal failure.

Clinical and experimental experience with dextran 70 in the dog suggest moderate to life-threatening allergic reactions are rare. Blood glucose concentration may be elevated from dextran metabolism into its glucose residues. Serum bilirubin concentration can be falsely increased for unknown reasons. The presence of dextran 70 in the circulation may cause a change in the total solids value obtained via refractometry, not reflecting actual protein content (see p. 116). Additionally, red blood cell cross-linking occurs with dextran 70, and appears as rouleaux formation, potentially interfering with blood type crossmatching.

Hydroxyethyl Starch

Hydroxyethyl starch (HES; DuPont Pharma), the parent name of a polymeric molecule made from a waxy species of either maize or sorghum, is composed primarily of amylopectin (98%). It is a highly branched polysaccharide closely resembling glycogen, formed by the reaction between ethylene oxide and amylopectin in the presence of an alkaline catalyst. The molecular weight and molar substitution can be adjusted by acid hydrolysis of the parent amylopectin molecule. Two species of HES are currently commercially available for fluid resuscitation and maintenance, hetastarch and pentastarch. However, pentastarch is used only in Europe and Canada as a hemodiluting and volume-expanding agent. Hetastarch contains a greater concentration of large-molecular-weight particles compared with pentastarch. The greater concentration of large molecules in hetastarch and its specific stereochemistry make it superior at maintaining intravascular volume in animals with leaking capillaries or animals hypo-oncotic from low plasma albumin.

In addition to providing low-volume resuscitation, hydroxyethyl starch has been shown to reverse changes in microvascular permeability caused by oxygen free radicals during reperfusion injury (Zikria et al, 1989). It also decreases the plasma concentration of soluble adhesion molecules, decreasing leukocyte-endothelial adhesion and improving microcirculation (Boldt et al, 1996). Whether this is an effect of improved microvascular perfusion or an independent characteristic of its molecular architecture has yet to be determined.

Hetastarch is nontoxic and nonallergenic in doses up to 100 ml/kg in dogs (Ballinger et al, 1966). Hetastarch has been shown to cause complement activation. The authors have observed a moderate reaction to rapid intravenous infusion in the cat, with signs of nausea, occasional vom-

iting, and hypotension. The administration of hetastarch in small volume increments (5 ml/kg), given slowly over 5 to 15 minutes, has eliminated these side effects in cats.

CLINICAL USE

Synthetic colloids each have pharmacologic qualities, specific characteristics, and potential side effects that make each unique. Selection of a specific synthetic colloid is based on these individual traits (see Tables 1 and 2). Based on the disease process, colloids may be used alone or in combination for maximum benefit.

With the possible exception of oxypolygelatins, dogs can tolerate rapid intravenous boluses of synthetic colloids for immediate intravascular resuscitation. All synthetic colloids are given slowly, titrated to effect, in the cat. Colloids are *always* administered in conjunction with isotonic crystalloids; however, the crystalloid volume is decreased by 40 to 60% of the expected requirement.

Based on their experience, the authors recommend maintaining the plasma COP of the animal with systemic inflammatory response syndrome (SIRS) at 14 to 17 mm Hg with synthetic colloids to minimize edema formation and third-space fluid loss. Based on the disease process and resuscitation needs, a single colloid or a combination of colloids is selected to obtain the desired benefits. As colloids are dissolved in potassium-free crystalloids, the ongoing need for potassium supplementation must be carefully determined.

Hypovolemic and Traumatic Shock

Rapid Intravascular Volume Replacement

Indications. Rapid intravascular volume replacement is indicated when there is poor peripheral perfusion owing to intravascular fluid volume deficits, without evidence of ongoing hemorrhage or closed cavity bleeding.

Colloid Selection. Hetastarch, dextran 70, oxypolygelatin.

Dosage and Administration. In the dog, begin rapid intravenous infusion of isotonic crystalloids at 40 to 50 ml/kg per hour and administer 10 to 20 ml/kg of hetastarch or dextran 70 by rapid intravenous infusion.* Monitoring of the patient's perfusion parameters is important in administering colloid as needed to bring the mean systemic arterial blood pressure to 80 mm Hg or higher. Following resuscitation, reduce the crystalloid infusion rate to the minimal amount required to provide for maintenance fluid needs and replacement of ongoing losses. The patient should be monitored for volume overload and assessed for the need of natural colloid administration.

In the cat, begin rapid intravenous infusion of isotonic crystalloids at 10 to 30 ml/kg per hour and administer hetastarch or dextran 70 at a dosage of 5 ml/kg over 5 to 10 minutes. This bolus administration is repeated until the mean systemic arterial blood pressure is at least 60 to

---

*If oxypolygelatins are used, follow manufacturers' recommendations of administering 5 ml/kg IV slowly over 15 minutes.

80 mm Hg. Immediately following resuscitation, begin a constant rate of infusion (CRI) of hetastarch or dextran 70 at 10 to 40 ml/kg per day and reduce the crystalloid infusion rate to the minimum amount required to provide for maintenance fluid needs and replacement of ongoing losses. This volume of crystalloids will be lower than that normally calculated owing to the CRI of colloid. Monitor for volume overload.

Hypotensive Resuscitation

Indications. Hypotensive resuscitation is preferred when closed cavity (abdominal, thoracic, intrapulmonary, intracranial) hemorrhage is suspected. The patient is resuscitated to a blood pressure only adequate to ensure organ perfusion but low enough to preserve vascular clots that have formed.

Colloid Selection. Hetastarch, dextran 70, or oxypolygelatin.

Dosage and Administration. Begin rapid infusion of isotonic crystalloids (dog, 40 to 50 ml/kg per hour; cat, 10 to 30 ml/kg per hour). Administer hetastarch or dextran 70 by giving 5 ml/kg over 5 to 10 minutes.* This dosage is repeated until the mean arterial pressure is at least 60 to 80 mm Hg, infusing the minimum amount required to reach the perfusion end point. Reduce the crystalloid infusion rate to the minimum required to provide for maintenance and replacement of ongoing losses. Cats may require a CRI of the colloid to maintain an adequate blood pressure. Monitor for volume overload or ongoing fluid or blood loss.

Ongoing Hemorrhage

Indications. Animals that have experienced trauma may be hypotensive on presentation and have ongoing hemorrhage that is evident.

Colloid Selection. Hetastarch, dextran 70, oxypolygelatin, whole blood, packed red blood cells (PRBCs), plasma.

Dosage and Administration. The dog and cat are resuscitated as described for hypotensive resuscitation. The administration of natural colloids may be required, based on the packed cell volume (PCV), serum albumin concentration, and clotting ability of the patient. The administration of whole blood or packed red blood cells (PRBCs) with fresh or fresh-frozen plasma, hetastarch, or dextran. Hetastarch and dextran 70 can be mixed with PRBC. The combination of oxypolygelatin with PRBCs must be done with caution because of its low osmolarity and potential risk of RBC swelling. Fresh or fresh-frozen plasma may be required if there is prolongation of clotting times or decreased antithrombin concentrations. The dosages and administration rates of synthetic colloids are the same as for hypotensive resuscitation.

---

*If oxypolygelatins are used, follow manufacturers' recommendations of administering 5 ml/kg IV slowly over 15 minutes.

Small-Volume Resuscitation

Small-volume resuscitation is considered when there is a need to decrease the risk of volume overload and minimize the amount of fluid that can efflux from the intravascular to the interstitial spaces.

Indications. Clinical conditions such as trauma with hemorrhage or edema in the brain or lungs, hypovolemic heart failure in a critically hypotensive animal, or hypovolemia in the chronically hypoalbuminemic animal may require small-volume resuscitation. The goal is to administer the smallest volume of fluids necessary to restore general organ perfusion.

Colloid Selection. Hetastarch.

Dosage and Administration. Administer hetastarch by giving 5 ml/kg IV over 5 to 10 minutes. This dosage is repeated until the mean arterial pressure is at least 60 to 80 mm Hg, infusing the minimum amount required to reach the perfusion end point. Reduce the crystalloid infusion rate to the minimum required to provide for maintenance and ongoing losses. Cats may require a CRI of the colloid to maintain an adequate blood pressure. Monitor for volume overload or ongoing fluid or blood loss.

Systemic Inflammatory Response Syndrome (SIRS)

The systemic inflammatory response syndrome results in vasodilation of capillaries and postcapillary venules, along with increased permeability of the capillaries.

Indications. Initiators of SIRS include clinical conditions such as pancreatitis, pneumonia, peritonitis, pyometra, gastroenteritis, neoplasia, burns, hyperthermia, multiple trauma, systemic fungal, rickettsial, or viral diseases, immune-mediated diseases, cold exposure, and other causes of systemic inflammation. The common denominator is hypovolemia, capillary and postcapillary dilatation, and increased capillary permeability.

Colloid Selection. Hetastarch.

Dosage and Administration. Administer hetastarch as described earlier for rapid intravascular volume resuscitation. If perfusion is adequate, the initial dose of hetastarch (15 to 40 ml/kg in dogs and 10 to 15 ml/kg in cats) can be administered over 4 to 6 hours. Immediately begin a CRI of hetastarch (20 ml/kg per day in dogs and 10 to 40 ml/kg per day in cats) and maintain a plasma COP at 14 to 17 mm Hg. Reduce crystalloid infusion to the amount required to provide for maintenance and replacement of ongoing fluid or blood losses. Synthetic colloid administration is temporarily discontinued during blood product administration. Monitor for volume overload. Assess for natural colloid administration. Frozen plasma is administered to maintain a minimum plasma albumin level of 2.0 g/dl.

References and Suggested Reading

Ballinger WF II, Solanke TF, Thompson WL: Effect of hydroxyethyl starch upon survival of dogs subjected to hemorrhagic shock. Surg Gynecol Obstet 122:33, 1966.

When hetastarch was infused, percentage of dogs that survived was greater than when dextran was given as a volume replacement fluid.

Boldt J, Mueller M, Heesen M, et al: Influence of different volume therapies and pentoxifylline infusion on circulating soluble adhesion molecules in critically ill patients. Crit Care Med 24:385, 1996.
Long-term volume therapy with hydroxyethyl starch decreased plasma concentrations of soluble adhesion molecules, in contrast to albumin and pentoxifylline, which further increased their concentration.

Concannon KT, Haskins SC, Feldman BF: Hemostatic defects associated with two infusion rates of dextran 70 in dogs. Am J Vet Res 53:1369, 1992.
Measurements of coagulation parameters in normal dogs receiving dextran 70.

Dextran 40. In: Sewester CS, Olin BR, Hebel SK, et al, eds: Drug Facts and Comparisons. St. Louis: Wolters Kluwer, 1996, p 93g.
Pharmacology of dextran 40, its indications and uses.

Gold MS, Russo J, Tissot M, et al: Comparison of hetastarch to albumin for perioperative bleeding in patients undergoing abdominal aortic aneurysm repair: A prospective, randomized study. Ann Surg 211:482, 1990.

Kaufman BS: Fluid resuscitation of the critically ill. Crit Care Clin 8:235, 1992.
A practical guide to the use of various fluid types in critically ill people.

Zikria BA, Subbarao C, Oz MC, et al: Macromolecules reduce abnormal microvascular permeability in rat limb ischemia-reperfusion injury. Crit Care Med 17:1306, 1989.
Reduction of abnormally increased microvascular permeability may be accomplished by appropriately sized intravenous hydroxyethyl starch molecules.

Microenteral Nutrition

JENNIFER J. DEVEY
Springfield, Virginia

DENNIS T. CROWE
Alpharetta, Georgia

Anorexia in the acutely ill or injured patient can lead to a rapid loss of critical energy stores and compromise the immune system to the point that the stressed animal is at increased risk for the development of infections and organ dysfunction. The deleterious effects of anorexia in these patients may occur within as little as 24 to 96 hours (Moss et al, 1976). A continuous supply of energy in the form of glucose is required as a fuel source, not only for the brain and red blood cells but also for the functions of macrophages or leukocytes and for wound repair. Additionally, the delivery of enteral nutrients is required for the production of secretory IgA, which is vital to the gut mucosal defense system. Enteral nutrients also are essential in maintaining the integrity and function of the gut mucosal barrier. Breakdown of this gut barrier leads to translocation of bacteria and endotoxin, which is thought to play a major role in the development of the systemic inflammatory response syndrome and multiple organ failure in the critically ill or injured animal.

Anorexia leads to gastrointestinal (GI) mucosal atrophy, down-regulation of digestive enzyme systems, pancreatic atrophy, and cholestasis. As a result, the ability of the gut to digest and absorb nutrients is significantly decreased. Enteral nutrition, but not parenteral nutrition, prevents, alleviates, or reverses these conditions (Alverdy et al, 1988; Levine et al, 1974; Lippert et al, 1989; Hughes et al, 1978; Feldman et al, 1976).

Enteral nutrition should be considered an important form of therapy in every ill or injured patient, especially if the patient requires hospitalization. Voluntary oral intake, forced oral intake (syringe feeding) or the use of nasal feeding tubes that terminate in the esophagus or stomach are the three most common methods for providing enteral nutrition in veterinary medicine. However, not all patients tolerate this form of nutritional support. When enteral feeding is attempted in patients with a dysfunctional GI tract, nausea, vomiting, and diarrhea may result. The patient with an underlying disease that causes frequent vomiting or severe diarrhea often will not tolerate complete enteral nutrition. The delivery of a large volume of nutrients into the upper GI tract of the patient with a decreased level of consciousness may be hazardous because of the possibility of regurgitation and aspiration.

Microenteral nutrition was a term proposed in 1991 by Crowe to define the delivery of small amounts of water, electrolytes, and readily absorbed nutrients (glucose, amino acids, and small peptides) directly to the GI tract (Crowe, 1992). The solutions are delivered by either constant rate infusion or bolus infusion every 1 to 2 hours via an indwelling feeding tube. Typically the volumes delivered are less than 0.25 ml/kg per hour. The solution is usually delivered into the esophagus and stomach, although it can also be delivered directly into the duodenum or jejunum via a nasoenteral, duodenostomy, or jejunostomy tube. This chapter discusses the rationale behind the use of microenteral nutrition based on results from research involving animal models and clinical use in more than 1,000 small animal patients. The technique employed by the authors for the delivery of microenteral nutrition, the evolution of this technique as it has been used clinically, and our impressions of the clinical effects of this type of nutritional therapy in canine and feline patients are described.

GOALS

The goal of microenteral nutrition is not to meet protein or caloric needs but rather to improve GI blood flow, to help protect the upper GI mucosa from atrophy and mechanical dysfunction, to help prevent down-regulation of the gut mucosal enzyme system, and to help preserve gut immune function (Table 1). By using microenteral nutrition, it is hoped that patient morbidity will be decreased, that the patient will return more rapidly to full enteral nutrition, and that discharge from the hospital will be more rapid. Preliminary evidence in experimental studies on animals and in human patients supports these findings (Zaloga, 1997, personal communication).

BACKGROUND

Cortisol, catecholamines, and cytokines released during the response to an acute injury or illness lead to the development of a metabolic state characterized by an increase in protein catabolism, an increase in glucose production, and a dramatic increase in energy consumption at the cellular level. This catabolic state leads to a loss of skeletal and visceral muscle mass with secondary organ dysfunction, impaired wound healing, and an increased susceptibility to infection. Although the catabolic state cannot be wholly prevented through the use of nutritional support, the provision of nutrients may allow sparing of protein, which is a major goal of nutritional therapy in the acutely ill or injured patient. Protein substrates are essential for wound healing, acute-phase protein production, immune function, and providing substrates for gluconeogenesis. Early administration of enteral nutrition can decrease the hypermetabolic response associated with acute illness and injury (Wilmore, 1990).

A lack of nutritional substrates in the lumen of the intestine leads to increased absorption of bacteria and endotoxin from the bowel lumen into the bloodstream and lymphatics. The continued absorption of enterotoxin from the gut lumen promotes the inflammatory response through a variety of mechanisms including the production of cytokines (e.g. interleukin-6), which then act on the hypothalamus to perpetuate the hypermetabolic response. The provision of enteral nutrients has been shown to decrease intestinal permeability and to decrease adherence of bacteria to the microvilli (Zaloga, 1997).

Current research on enteral nutrition is examining the value of specific nutrients in modulating the immune response. For instance, cranberry juice appears to have properties that limit bacterial translocation from the gut and

supplementation of arginine and dietary nucleotides improves resistance to infection. Antibiotics administered to sick patients often alter the microbial population of the gut and the provision of specific nutrients such as fructo-oligosaccharides may help maintain more "stable" bacterial populations in the gut. The provision of omega-3 and omega-6 fatty acids in a ratio between 5:1 and 10:1 has been shown to have beneficial effects on regulating systemic inflammatory responses.

The stress response in the ill or injured patient initially creates a hyperglycemic response. Liver glycogen stores are often depleted within 6 hours in dogs. If the rate of catabolism cannot keep up with the cellular energy requirement, serum glucose levels may become subnormal. This is especially true in the hypothermic or the very young or very old patient. The provision of enteral glucose may help prevent hypoglycemic states, as the intestinal tract has an efficient system for the absorption of glucose (Jeevandam et al, 1992). Conversely, despite providing an exogenous source of energy, intravenous dextrose infusions (5% concentration) alone are not protein-sparing. Nitrogen balance only improves when amino acid solutions are added to the parenteral dextrose solutions, and this improvement steadily increases as the concentration of dextrose infusion is increased (Elwyn et al, 1978). Similar studies have not been performed using enteral solutions, but, since infusion of enteral nutrients utilizes a more physiologic route than parenteral infusion of nutrients, it would seem logical that the same benefits might result as long as the gut is functional.

STRESS MUCOSAL INJURY

Stress ulcers can develop in human patients within hours of entry into an intensive care unit (ICU). Gastric and duodenal ulceration is a significant problem in these human patients and may pose a similar problem in veterinary intensive care units. The underlying cause of the ulceration has not been clearly determined, but it is known to be associated with inadequate circulation to the GI mucosa. The delivery of glucose (isosomolar and hyperosmolar solutions) to the gastric mucosa helps prevent gastric ulcers (Ephgrave and Horton, 1985; Pingleton and Hadzima, 1983). The delivery of parenteral glucose, however, does not provide the same protection (Shorr et al, 1984). The exact mechanism for the mucosal protection observed with enteral glucose administration is unknown; however, it is thought to be related to a combination of stimulated neural and hormonal effects, an increase in gastric pH, and an increase in gastric volume (Ephgrave et al, 1990). The infusion of glucose into the lumen of the gut causes a "hyperemic response" substantially increasing GI blood flow in laboratory animals (Zaloga, 1997). This may be the major reason for the protective effect of luminal glucose because the development of stress ulcers and increased bacterial translocation are associated with low flow states.

INDICATIONS

Microenteral nutrition should be used whenever the clinician believes the patient is not ready for complete enteral

TABLE 1. Goals of Microenteral Nutrition

1. To preserve or increase blood flow to the GI tract
2. To prevent gastric and duodenal ulceration
3. To preserve secretory-IgA levels, other immune defense systems, and normal GI bacterial populations
4. To decrease bacterial adherence to the gut mucosa and decrease GI permeability
5. To increase GI mucus production
6. To prevent the down-regulation of GI brush border enzyme systems
7. To promote GI peristalsis
8. To help perserve intestinal function via provision of nutrients and humoral stimulation
9. To promote the continued presence of endogenous opioid receptors and opioid-like drug production in the GI tract
10. To promote more rapid return to full enteral feeding

GI; gastrointestinal.

TABLE 2. Indications for Microenteral Nutritional Support

Altered level of consciousness
Presence of NG tube for decompression
Transition phase to enteral nutrition
Recovery stage from GI disese
Patient at risk for stress ulcers and bacterial translocation
Gastric ulcerative disease
Immediate postoperative period (0–3 days)
Traumatic injury—from admission to full enteral nutrition
Acute renal failure
Acute hepatic failure
Gut protection during the provision of parenteral nutrition

NG; nasogastric; GI, gastrointestinal.

nutrition but that enteral nutritional support would be beneficial (Table 2). Research would also indicate that the effects of nutrient instillation into the gut early in the course of resuscitation of critically ill or injured animals may enhance regional GI blood flow and protect against bacterial and enterotoxin absorption (Zaloga, 1997). Additionally, canine and feline patients that have gastric motility disorders or persistent vomiting problems may benefit from gastric decompression using a nasogastric (NG) tube.

After decompressing the stomach by aspirating the NG tube, a small volume of microenteral nutrition can be infused through the tube (see the protocol section further on). This approach is especially effective in treating postoperative patients and patients recovering from severe GI diseases such as parvovirus enteritis. Microenteral nutrition should be used if the patient is at risk for stress ulceration or has confirmed gastric ulceration. Patients at increased risk for gastric ulceration include those suffering from severe trauma, shock, hypoxia, and systemic inflammatory response syndrome. Microenteral nutrition is useful in the anorectic patient or in the patient with substantial vomiting as a transition phase to complete enteral nutrition. Persistent vomiting while microenteral nutrition is being delivered is an indication to stop the treatment and evaluate the patient to ensure that the diagnosis is correct (i.e., a puppy with parvovirus enteritis that develops an intussusception). In our experience, microenteral nutrition rarely appears to contribute to the prevalence of vomiting. Gastric secretions increase in response to a number of stimuli, including hypoglycemia, protein, and hyperosmolality. Since microenteral nutritional formulas are generally isosmotic, these formulations should not substantially change the volume of gastric secretions produced, and the provision of glucose may help decrease acid secretion in the stomach. Microenteral nutrition does not provide sufficient protein or calories to meet systemic nutritional requirements; therefore, if the patient shows signs that the microenteral feeding will not be able to progress quickly to full enteral feeding, parenteral nutritional support should also be used (see p. 80).

CONTRAINDICATIONS

There are few contraindications to the use of microenteral nutrition. Controversy exists as to the effectiveness and indications for microenteral nutrition in the patient with severe, persistent, uncontrolled vomiting. Infusion of nutrients into the stomach, even in small volumes, stimulates the pancreas. However, the authors' clinical experience is that microenteral nutrition may not contribute to worsening of pancreatitis in all patients. One case recently reported in the human literature supports this finding (McClave et al, 1997). Providing microenteral nutrition via an NG tube and periodically aspirating to determine the amount of gastric residuals can be useful in determining whether GI peristalsis is recovering.

PROTOCOL

Gastric distention leads to stimulation of receptors in the pyloric antral region and vomiting. By delivering only small volumes of liquid, this stimulus to vomiting is not triggered. The stomach normally receives a fluid volume of approximately 1.5 ml/kg per hour, which is composed of saliva and gastric secretions. Microenteral nutrition is administered in small volumes at frequent intervals or as a constant rate infusion. Initially, constant rate infusions of 0.05 to 0.2 ml/kg per hour are "trickle fed." This approach adds little volume to that normally produced within the stomach and is one of the major reasons this form of nutritional support may be well tolerated, even in the vomiting patient. The volume infused can be increased gradually to a total of 1 to 2 ml/kg per hour over a 24- to 48-hour period based on patient tolerance. If the volume consists of undiluted enteral formulas, this approach will provide full enteral nutrition.

Microenteral nutrition should be started within 2 to 12 hours of admission into the hospital unless there are specific contraindications. It is currently believed by some nutritional experts that nutrition should be provided as soon after admission as possible (Zaloga, 1997, personal communication). The solution can be administered by feeding tubes or can be force-fed by syringe or offered to the animal to drink. If the patient is showing signs of nausea with oral intake, it has been our experience that infusing the solution through a feeding tube is required.

Microenteral solutions can either be purchased commercially or formulated (Table 3). The goal initially is to deliver a nearly isotonic, balanced electrolyte solution containing glucose. Commercial oral rehydrating solutions containing glucose are the simplest to use (Re-Sorb,

TABLE 3. Microenteral Nutrition Solutions and Infusion Protocol

Begin within 2 to 12 hours of admission
Start with force feeding (syringe), nasoesophageal, or NG tube
Formulated: water, glucose (5 to 25 g/L), quarter-strength lactated
  Ringer's solution
Commercial: Re-Sorb, Pedialyte
Consider adding 20 to 40 mEq/L potassium chloride or 3% amino acid
  solution (FreAmine, Travasol)
Start feeding at 0.05 to 0.2 ml/kg per hour constant rate infusion or 0.1
  to 0.4 ml/kg every 2 hours
Increase volume by 0.2 ml/kg every 8 to 12 hours if patient tolerant
Switch to polymeric or peptide-based commercial liquid diet if clear
  liquid diet tolerated after 8 to 12 hours

NG, nasogastric.

SmithKline Beecham; Pedialyte, Ross Laboratories). The use of glucose not only has important physiologic effects but also helps with palatability when administered orally. Glycine is frequently found in commercial rehydrating solutions. Glycine has been shown to hasten the resolution of diarrhea, improve intestinal mucosa morphologic characteristics in animals with diarrhea, and enhance the uptake of glucose (Naylor et al, 1997). Other sources of electrolyte solutions include crystalloid fluids designed for parenteral use. In formulated and commercial solutions, glucose is often added to make a 5 to 25% solution. Laboratory studies evaluating the protection of the GI mucosal barrier support the use of a solution with up to 20% glucose concentration, and even higher glucose concentrations may be increasingly beneficial.

A mixture of amino acids can be added to microenteral nutrition formulations. Several commercial solutions are available containing from 3% (FreAmine, McGaw Inc.) to 8.5% (Travasol, Baxter Healthcare Corp.) amino acid concentrations. The use of a 3% amino acid solution has been shown to be protein-sparing in the critically ill patient (Freeman, 1978). The 8.5% solutions should be diluted with a maintenance electrolyte solution or an oral rehydrating electrolyte solution, if used. If these amino acid solutions are selected, glucose needs to be added via an oral rehydrating or glucose solution.

Amino acid solutions designed for intravenous use do not contain certain amino acids such as glutamine. Glutamine supplementation may be important because it is the preferred energy source for rapidly dividing cells, including gut mucosal cells, lymphocytes, and fibroblasts (Souba et al, 1990). Glutamine has been shown to play a role in the maintenance of the integrity of the GI mucosal barrier and in preventing bacterial translocation (Li et al, 1994). Small peptides (di- and tripeptides) appear to be absorbed much more efficiently than amino acids. Since small peptides play an important role in improving the integrity of the gut barrier, optimizing blood flow to the mucosa, and decreasing bacterial adherence, the administration of peptide-based diets (Peptamen, Clintec Nutrition Co.) would appear to be ideal in the early nutritional support of the critical patient.

Once it has been determined that the patient is tolerating the initial microenteral solution, more concentrated or polymeric liquid enteral diets can be introduced at the same small-volume infusion rates and the patient gradually converted to full enteral feeding. The definition of tolerance to the increased enteral feedings is based on finding minimal gastric residuals and a low prevalence or absence of vomiting.

POTENTIAL COMPLICATIONS

The potential to stimulate vomiting by administering microenteral nutrition does exist; however, we have found this to be a rare problem in clinical situations. The patient with a decreased level of consciousness is always at risk for regurgitation and aspiration. The use of microenteral nutrition does not contribute significantly to the volume of gastric fluids; however, if the stomach is not emptying, fluid could accumulate over time and put the patient at increased risk for regurgitation and aspiration. If an NG tube is being used, the tube should be aspirated periodically

(every 4 hours). If residual volumes are increasing, a decision may be made to decrease the volume or temporarily discontinue the infusion.

Critically ill patients may be insulin-resistant and may show signs of hyperglycemia when dextrose supplementation is provided. If significant hyperglycemia (greater than 300 mg/dl) exists, insulin should be administered. The goal is not necessarily to produce euglycemia, but to maintain a serum glucose concentration greater than 100 mg/dl and less than 300 mg/dl. Most studies that suggest the use of insulin for hyperglycemia have evaluated the use of intravenous dextrose supplementation in laboratory animals or human patients. There are very few studies looking at the provision of glucose via enteral administration in the same manner. Although it is possible to encounter hyperglycemia with enteral glucose administration, the chance of hyperglycemia is much less likely because the glucose administered is transported directly to the liver via the portal vein. We have not seen hyperglycemia develop with the use of microenteral nutrition except in known diabetics.

APPLICATION

The ideal enteral solution in the critically ill or injured patient includes glucose, small peptides, bile acids, and short chain fatty acids (Zaloga, 1997). A commercially available solution composed of these components is not currently available. Therefore, the closest approximation should be used and the solution modified as nutritional technology improves.

We have used microenteral nutrition in more than 1,000 small animals with good patient tolerance. However, there have been no controlled studies in human or veterinary medical patients to determine if the use of microenteral nutrition has any impact on outcome. Based on laboratory studies in the shock model and limited clinical studies in critically ill humans, the early provision of microenteral nutrition has been shown to significantly improve GI blood flow. This aids the maintenance of a normal gut mucosa and reduces complications associated with bacterial and endotoxin absorption. Microenteral nutrition is generally well tolerated even in the face of diarrhea and pancreatitis. Although not well studied, microenteral nutrition should aid in the maintenance and improvement in the function of the GI tract, the pancreas, and the biliary tract, enabling the anorectic patient to adapt to full enteral nutrition more quickly. Its use encourages clinicians to think about, and provide, enteral nutritional support by promoting continued attention to the nutritional needs of the patient. This approach, in our experience, appears to promote an earlier return to oral intake and a shorter hospital stay for the patient. The use of microenteral nutrition has many potential benefits and its use *early* in the course of hospitalization of the seriously ill or injured patient, or in the patient recovering from extensive surgical intervention, is highly recommended.

References and Suggested Reading

Alverdy JC, Aoys E, Moss GS: Total parenteral nutrition promotes bacterial translocation from the gut. Surgery 104:185, 1988.

Compares bacterial translocation in rats fed enterally versus parenterally.
Crowe DT: Ways to administer fluids. Tijdschrift Voor Diergeneeskunde 117:195, 1992.
Discusses parenteral and enteral techniques for administering fluids.
Elwyn DH, Gump FE, Iles M, et al: Protein and energy sparing of glucose added in hypocaloric amounts to peripheral infusion of amino acids. Metabolism 27:325, 1978.
Discusses importance of glucose supplementation when amino acids are provided as the sole nutritional source.
Ephgrave KS, Kleiman-Wexler RL, Adair CG: Enteral nutrients prevent stress ulceration and increase intragastric volume. Crit Care Med 18:621, 1990.
Investigates theories to explain protective effects of enteral nutrients against stress ulcers.
Ephgrave KS, Horton JW: Gastric mucosal protection during confinement stress: The role of intragastric glucose. Curr Surg 42:375, 1985.
Comparison of the effectiveness of intragastric glucose and antacids in ulcer protection in rats.
Feldman EJ, Dowling RH, McNaughton J, et al: Effects of oral versus intravenous nutrition on intestinal adaptation after small bowel resection in the dog. Gastroenterology 70:712, 1976.
Study examining the importance of enteral nutrients in maintaining structure and function of the intestine.
Freeman JB: Peripheral parenteral nutrition. Can J Surg 21:489, 1978.
Discusses partial peripheral parenteral nutrition and protein-sparing effects of glucose.
Hughes CA, Bates T, Dowling H: Cholecystokinin and secretin prevent the intestinal mucosal hypoplasia of total parenteral nutrition in the dog. Gastroenterology 75:34, 1978.
Investigates the trophic effects of pancreaticobiliary secretions on the intestine of beagles.
Jeevandam M, Shamos RF, Petersen SR: Substrate efficacy in early nutrition support of critically ill multiple trauma victims. J Parenter Enter Nutr 16:511, 1992.
Reviews findings in trauma patients fed glucose, and glucose and amino acids during catabolic phase.
Levine GM, Deren JJ, Steiger E, et al: Role of oral intake on maintenance of gut mass and disaccharide activity. Gastroenterology 67:975, 1974.
Discusses importance of enteral nutrients in maintaining gut structure and function.
Li J, Langkamp-Henken B, Suzuki K, et al: Glutamine prevents parenteral nutrition-induced increases in intestinal permeability. J Parenter Enter Nutr 18:303, 1994.

Discusses role glutamine plays in decreasing intestinal atrophy and increased permeability seen with total parenteral nutrition.
Lippert AC, Faulkner JE, Evan AT, et al: Total parenteral nutrition in clinically normal cats. J Am Vet Med Assoc 194:669, 1989.
Study examining clinical, hematologic, and histopathologic findings in cats fed total parenteral nutrition for 2 weeks.
McClave SA, Greene LM, Snider HC, et al: Comparison of the safety of early enteral vs parenteral nutrition in mild acute pancreatitis. J Parenter Enter Nutr 21:14, 1997.
Pancreatitis patients who received early enteral nutrition had similar outcomes when compared with those receiving TPN.
Moss G, Bierenbaum A, Bova F, et al: Postoperative metabolic patterns following immediate total nutritional support: Hormone levels, DNA synthesis, nitrogen balance, and accelerated wound healing. J Surg Res 21:383, 1976.
Immediate feeding following intestinal resection increases protein and DNA synthesis and wound healing.
Naylor JM, Leibel T, Middleton DM: Effect of glutamine or glycine containing oral electrolyte solutions on mucosal morphology, clinical and biochemical findings, in calves with viral induced diarrhea. Can J Vet Res 61:43, 1997.
Glycine as effective as glutamine in healing intestinal mucosa and treatment of diarrhea in calves.
Pingleton SK, Hadzima SK: Enteral alimentation and gastrointestinal bleeding in mechanically ventilated patients. Crit Care Med 11:13, 1983.
Comparison of antacids, histamine blockers, and enteral nutrients in protecting against GI bleeding.
Shorr LD, Sirnek KR, Page CP, et al: The role of glucose in preventing stress gastric mucosal injury. J Surg Res 36:384, 1984.
Discusses role glucose plays in gastric cytoprotection.
Souba WW, Klimberg VS, Plumley DA, et al: The role of glutamine in maintaining a healthy gut and supporting the metabolic response to injury and infection. J Surg Res 48:383, 1990.
Review of role glutamine plays in maintaining metabolism and GI structure and function and in fighting infection.
Wilmore DW: Catabolic illness: Strategies for enhancing recovery. N Engl J Med 325:695, 1990.
Review of stress response and therapeutic interventions to decrease the catabolic state.
Zaloga GP: Nutritional modulation in critical illness: Where's the beef? In Proceedings of the Critical Care Symposium, San Diego, CA, Feb 6–10, 1997, Society of Critical Care Medicine, Anaheim, CA, p 275.
Discusses effects of different nutrients on immune function in experimental and clinical studies.

Therapy for Shock

STEVE C. HASKINS
Davis, California

Shock is a condition of severe hemodynamic and metabolic dysfunction characterized by reduced tissue perfusion, impaired oxygen delivery, and inadequate cellular energy production. Many common disorders lead to shock, including those associated with severe heart failure, hypovolemia, peripheral vasoconstriction (maldistribution), large vein or arterial vessel occlusion (external compression, thromboembolism), sepsis, hypoxia (anemia, hypoxemia, methemoglobinemia, carboxyhemoglobin), heat stroke, severe hypoglycemia, and cyanide poisoning.

The clinical signs of shock vary, depending in part on the underlying condition. Typical features of sympathomi-

metic activation are common to most cases of cardiogenic shock (as with dilated cardiomyopathy or pericardial tamponade), hypovolemic shock (as with trauma or consequent to profound vomiting and diarrhea), and obstructive shock (as with gastric compression of the caudal vena cava or consequent to a large pulmonary embolus). The neurohormonal compensations activated to maintain blood pressure lead to the typical clinical signs of tachycardia, peripheral arterial vasoconstriction, pallor, coldness of mucous membranes, and reduced organ perfusion. Shock caused by volume depletion or obstruction of large blood vessels is often associated with a weak arterial pulse, systemic hypotension, and normal or collapsed jugular veins. With cardiogenic shock there are similar clinical features, but also elevated venous pressures causing jugular venous distention or cardiogenic pulmonary edema. A significant contrast to these examples is found with septic shock, which causes vasomotor dysfunction (so-called "distributive shock"). Septic shock is often characterized by an early hyperdynamic state with peripheral vasodilation, high cardiac output, and erythema or plethora of the mucous membranes (what used to be called "warm shock"), as described below in greater detail.

Most forms of shock are complicated by dysfunction of multiple organ systems. A fundamental disorder in oxygen delivery has a negative impact on aerobic metabolism and cellular energy production and frequently leads to metabolic and lactic acidosis. A host of systemic and local inflammatory and vasoactive mediators are released in shock. These mediators may alter local blood flow, initiate clotting or inflammatory responses, and injure tissues. Immunologic mechanisms can be altered, quite notably in cases of anaphylactic and septic shock. The aforementioned abnormalities, as well as stasis of blood, can cause disseminated intravascular coagulation (DIC). Reduced perfusion of the pancreatic, renal, and splanchnic circulatory beds releases myocardial depressant factors, impairs kidney and liver function, and seriously compromises the intestinal barrier, which permits gram-negative bacteria to enter the circulation. There may be deterioration of respiratory function related to capillary injury with pulmonary edema ("shock lung"), intrapulmonary shunting away from alveoli, or impaired skeletal muscular function. These conditions contribute to the development of arterial hypoxemia. Heart function may be impaired by inadequate venous return or through direct depression of myocardial contractility. Although the brain is reasonably well protected in shock, marked reduction of blood pressure or hyperventilation with hypercapnia can reduce cerebral perfusion and lead to neurologic dysfunction.

One of our greatest challenges today is septic shock. Systemic sepsis, including endotoxemia, can activate one or more enzymatic cascades, which "autoperpetuate" the entire systemic inflammatory response syndrome (SIRS), with subsequent deleterious systemic effects (see *CVT XII*, p. 139). When SIRS becomes severe, organ function deteriorates, causing septic shock or septic multiple organ dysfunction syndrome (MODS).

The clinical manifestations of septic SIRS include mild to moderate mental depression; poor appetite; fever; hyperglycemia; leukocytosis, possibly following a transient leukopenia, with a left shift and mild toxic change; vasodilation (red mucous membranes, accelerated capillary refill time); "bounding" pulse quality; normal to high cardiac output; normal to low arterial and central venous blood pressure; tachycardia; tachypnea; hyperventilation; nonhemorrhagic diarrhea; heart murmur; normal to hyperactive coagulation; normal to mildly impaired organ function; nonspecific increase of liver enzymes (particularly alkaline phosphatase); and hypoalbuminemia.

The clinical manifestations of septic MODS include moderate to severe depression; anorexia; subnormal core temperature; hypoglycemia; leukopenia or a large, rapid decrease in leukocyte count with a marked left shift and toxic neutrophils; vasoconstriction; low cardiac output; low arterial and central venous blood pressure; tachycardia; high venous oxygen; tachypnea; hyperventilation; hemorrhagic diarrhea; heart murmur; hypoactive coagulation with clinical petechiae or bleeding; lactic or metabolic acidosis; moderate to severe impairment of organ function (heart, kidneys, gut, lungs); moderate increases of liver enzymes; and hypoalbuminemia.

THERAPY

Restoration of Effective Circulation

Restoration of an Effective Circulating Blood Volume

CRYSTALLOIDS. Lactated Ringer's solution, or an equivalent solution with approximate extracellular concentrations of sodium, potassium, chloride, and a "bicarbonate-like" anion (bicarbonate, lactate, gluconate, or acetate), is a good fluid with which to begin. Hypotonic fluids such as 5% dextrose in water and low-sodium maintenance solutions should not be used for blood volume restoration therapy, since these crystalloids contain excessive free water and are very poor blood volume–expanding agents. Hypertonic (7.5%) saline (4 to 6 ml/kg) as a single initial bolus may be effective for rapid augmentation of blood volume.

Isotonic crystalloids may need to be administered in quantities of 40 to 90 ml/kg, or more, in the dog (25 to 60 ml/kg in the cat) to achieve adequate blood volume restoration. Fluids should be administered in quantities sufficient to alleviate peripheral vasoconstriction and to restore an acceptable pulse quality and a return of urine output. Central venous pressure (CVP), restored to a high normal level (8 to 10 cm H_2O), can provide a useful assessment of the adequacy of blood volume restoration and of preload pressure.

Only about 25 to 30% of a crystalloid fluid remains in the vascular fluid compartment 30 minutes following administration. The remainder readily diffuses across the endothelial membrane and is redistributed into the interstitial fluid compartment. The volume restoration achieved by crystalloid fluids may be fleeting, and if hypotension or vasoconstriction recurs, further fluid administration, perhaps in the form of colloids or whole blood, is indicated. Excessive hemodilution is another limitation to crystalloid fluid administration. Crystalloids should not be given when packed cell volume is below 15 to 25% (depending on the systemic status of the patient) or total protein is below approximately 3.5 gm/dl.

COLLOIDS. Plasma or a plasma substitute, such as dextran 70 or hetastarch, is indicated if the total protein is below approximately 3.5 gm/dl, the albumin is below approximately 1.5 gm/dl, or the colloid oncotic pressure (COP) is below approximately 15 mm Hg (see p. 116) or is likely to be reduced below this level with crystalloid therapy (see pp. 66 and 131). Colloids are more effective blood volume expanders than are crystalloids and should be considered when the patient does not appear to be responding appropriately to the crystalloid fluid infusion or when edema develops prior to adequate blood volume restoration. The dosage of any colloid, including whole blood, usually ranges between 10 and 40 ml/kg for the dog (5 to 25 ml/kg for the cat).

Dextran. Dextrans are mixtures of polysaccharides produced by the bacteria *Leuconostoc mesenteroides* or lactobacilli grown on sucrose media. Different molecular weights can be produced by acid hydrolysis of macromolecules. Molecular weights (MW) of less than 50,000 daltons (D) are rapidly excreted in the urine and exhibit a short duration of action (2 to 4 hours). Molecular weights above 50,000 D are widely distributed in the body and are metabolized at the rate of about 70 mg/kg of body weight per day.

Dextran 70 has an average MW of 70,000 D but a number-averaged MW of only 41,000 D. Molecular weights below 36,000 D have a half-life of less than 30 minutes; sizes between 44 and 55 have a half-life of 7.5 hours (Derrick and Guest, 1968). Dextran 70 is iso-osmotic (osmolality, 310 mOsm/kg) and hyperoncotic (COP, 60 mm Hg). Dextran 40 is even more hyperoncotic than dextran 70 but has a number-averaged MW of only 26,000 D and a duration of action of only 1.5 to 3 hours. Dextran 40 is rapidly filtered by the glomerulus and may be associated with an osmotic diuresis. In states of active tubular reabsorption of sodium and water, the dextran 40 concentrates in the tubular lumen, increasing the viscosity of the filtrate and, perhaps, precipitating out and plugging the tubule, resulting in renal failure.

Dextrans produce a dose-related defect of primary hemostasis that is somewhat greater than that due to simple dilution (Concannon et al, 1992). When administered in large volumes, dextrans can reduce factor VIII:C (factor VIII) activity and decrease platelet adhesiveness. It is not expected that even large doses would induce bleeding in patients with reasonable hemostatic reserves. The author has only rarely attributed a coagulopathy in a clinical patient to the administration of dextran. However, dextrans should be used conservatively in patients with von Willebrand's disease or hemophilia. Their inhibition of coagulation and platelet cascades may make them logical choices for part of the treatment of DIC.

Hetastarch. Hetastarch is a modified amylopectin, a branched glucose polymer. Hydroxylation makes it more resistant to degradation by serum amylase. Commercial hetastarch has an average MW of 450 D and is 0.7% hydroxylated. Its number-averaged MW is 69 D, and its COP is approximately 30 mm Hg. Hetastarch's elimination kinetics are complex because of the heterogeneity of hetastarch solutions: 18% has a half-life of 2 hours, 17% of 8.5 hours, and 30% of 67 hours. Hetastarch is much more expensive than dextran 70 per 500-ml bottle. It should enjoy a longer duration of action than dextran 70, but comparative studies reveal a marked similarity between the two (Metcalf et al, 1970). Hetastarch also causes prolongation of coagulation tests in a manner that is comparable to, but perhaps slightly less than, dextran 70 (Gollub et al, 1967). Starches are metabolized by plasma and interstitial alpha-amylase. Pentastarch has a smaller, more homogeneous particle size (264 D) with less hydroxyethyl substitu-

tion (0.5%). Its number-averaged MW is only about 39 D, and it has a COP of about 40 mm Hg.

Plasma. Albumin constitutes about 50% of the total plasma protein and 80% of the plasma COP. There is approximately 5 gm of albumin per kilogram of body weight in the extracellular fluid compartment (ECF). Forty percent of the albumin is in the plasma; its concentration is about 2.5 to 3.5 gm/dl. Sixty percent of the albumin is in the interstitial fluid compartment; the concentration is about 40% that of plasma. Albumin is strongly negatively charged and is an important carrier of certain drugs, hormones, metals, and enzymes, and certain chemicals and toxins such as cations, anions, toxic oxygen radicals, and toxic inflammatory substances. From the standpoint of COP, much of the albumin can be replaced with the artificial colloids, dextran 70 and hetastarch. Albumin is, however, functionally much more than just a colloid; therefore, it cannot be completely replaced.

The other common reason for the administration of plasma is to replenish coagulation factors and platelets. How the plasma is processed can be important with regard to the therapeutic purposes. Fresh plasma, of course, has everything (it is good for treating DIC and thrombocytopenia as well as all other coagulopathies). Freezing destroys the platelets (still good for treating hemophilia A and von Willebrand's disease). Refrigerator storage destroys both the platelets and the labile coagulation factors (factors V and VIII von Willebrand's factor); the stabile factors (II, VII, IX, X) persist (still good for treating warfarin-related rodenticide poisoning).

Red Cells. If the packed cell volume is below 15 to 25%, or it is likely to be reduced to that level by crystalloid therapy, red blood cells should be administered. Dogs are blessed with a very low incidence of weakly reacting, naturally occurring alloantibodies. In the dog, it is most likely that a first-time red blood cell transfusion will not be associated with a reaction. Although all erythrocytic antigens incite an antibody response, clinically significant transfusion reactions are likely to occur only following the second transfusion of dog erythrocytic antigens (DEA) 1.1 and 1.2 and, to a lesser extent, DEA 7. Potential donors should be typed, and they should be negative for these antigens. In vitro crossmatching is highly recommended if the recipient has received a previous transfusion or if the recipient suffers immune-mediated hemolytic anemia (see Section 6).

In cats, blood transfusions are both simpler and more complicated. There are only two identified red cell antigens: A and B. Type-A cats have low titers of naturally occurring anti-B antibodies. Type-B cats have high titers of strong, naturally occurring anti-A antibodies. Matched transfusions are associated with a mean survival time of labeled red blood cells of 29 to 39 days. Multiple, matched transfusions in presumably type-A cats result in shortened mean red blood cell survival times (Marion and Smith, 1983). Transfusion of type-B blood into type-A cats was associated with a mean red blood cell survival time of 2 days and minor transfusion reactions, while transfusion of type-A blood into type-B cats was associated with a mean red blood cell survival time of 1 hour and severe transfusion reactions (Giger and Bucheler, 1991). Virtually all the domestic shorthair "mongrel" cats are type A (Giger et al, 1989). Type-B populations are more likely to occur in breeds such as Scottish Fold, Birman, Himalayan, Abyssinian, Somali, Persian, Cornish and Devon Rex, and British shorthair. In vitro crossmatching or typing (if you know the blood type of your donors) may be particularly important, even with the first transfusion, especially when these exotic breeds are involved. Immunologic transfusion reactions may be manifested by restlessness, acute collapse, hypotension, dyspnea, wheezing, urticaria, hemoglobinemia or hemoglobinuria, or fever. Other adverse effects of blood transfusion include hypothermia if cold blood is administered; hypocalcemia and acidosis if large quantities of citrate are administered; and heparinization if large quantities of heparin are administered (see p. 400).

Sympathomimetic Therapy

Sympathomimetic therapy is indicated when fluid therapy alone has failed to restore acceptable tissue perfusion, pulse quality, arterial blood pressure, or cardiac output in the setting of high preload pressures (central venous pressure or pulmonary occlusion pressure). The goal of sympathomimetic therapy is to improve cardiac output and tissue perfusion and at the same time maintain systemic arterial blood pressure (for cerebral and coronary perfusion) without excessive vasoconstriction (vasoconstriction enhances arterial pressure but impairs visceral tissue perfusion) or excessive vasodilation (vasodilation enhances tissue perfusion but induces hypotension). In general, isoproterenol causes too much vasodilation and tachyarrhythmias, while epinephrine, norepinephrine, and phenylephrine cause too much vasoconstriction and therefore are not commonly used (see *CVT XII*, p. 184 and p. 188).

Dobutamine is the drug of choice for the management of these patients. It improves cardiac output and oxygen delivery more reliably than does dopamine and tends to be a mild to moderate vasodilator. The usual dosage is 5 to 15 μg/kg per minute IV by constant rate infusion (CRI). Dobutamine is a potent beta$_1$- and beta$_2$-agonist with less alpha effects compared with dopamine. A major metabolite, 3-O-methyldobutamine, is a potent alpha$_1$ and alpha$_2$ inhibitor. Dobutamine administration is usually associated with a decrease in systemic vascular resistance, and preload parameters and further fluid administration is often required. Cardiac output characteristically improves markedly, while systemic arterial blood pressure changes minimally.

Dopamine exhibits both direct and indirect cardiovascular effects. Dopamine is a potent beta$_1$ and beta$_2$, alpha$_1$ and alpha$_2$, and dopaminergic$_1$ and dopaminergic$_2$ agonist. The dosage of 1 to 3 μg/kg per minute IV by CRI enhances renal and visceral perfusion and provides some cardiovascular support (van Kesteren et al, 1988). Higher dosages (3 to 10 μg/kg per minute) should be used if greater cardiotonic and blood pressure support are indicated. Dopamine administration constricts capacitance veins and may increase central venous and pulmonary occlusion pressures. Dopamine administration increases systemic arterial blood pressure more than does dobutamine administration. Higher doses of dopamine may cause excessive vasoconstriction

and no further increase in cardiac output. Dopamine also decreases aldosterone secretion.

Ephedrine is an indirect-acting sympathomimetic, causing the release of norepinephrine from the sympathetic nerve endings. Prolonged use can deplete the stores of norepinephrine neurotransmitter, resulting in tachyphylaxis. Ephedrine is a general cardiovascular stimulant. Ephedrine does cross the blood-brain barrier and has a mild analeptic effect. Ephedrine mimics the actions of dopamine and dobutamine, although it is not as potent or as effective; it is easier to administer and has a longer duration of action.

Dopexamine is predominantly a beta$_2$-agonist (with indirect beta$_1$ effects) and a dopaminergic agonist without alpha-agonist activity. In dosages of 5 to 20 μg/kg per minute IV by CRI, it has been shown to increase cardiac output and decrease peripheral vascular resistance; systemic arterial blood pressure generally decreases somewhat, visceral tissue perfusion is improved (Einstein et al, 1994). Dopexamine administration is not associated with the tachyarrhythmias sometimes associated with dobutamine, nor with the peripheral vasoconstriction associated with higher dosages of dopamine, and its use may be efficacious in the management of oxygen delivery in septic patients.

Organ-Specific Therapy

Heart Failure

Impaired myocardial contractility is a cause of cardiogenic shock and is an early consequence of septic shock. Direct sympathomimetic support of myocardial function is indicated when preload (venous) parameters are high and forward-flow parameters (blood pressure, tissue perfusion) are low.

Acute Renal Failure

Acute renal failure is an early consequence of septic shock. Urine output is used as an index of adequate renal (and, by extrapolation, visceral) perfusion. A urinary catheter should be aseptically placed to verify and quantify urine output. Fluid administration is the mainstay of therapy to support renal perfusion. If restoration of an effective circulating volume does not generate an acceptable urine flow, aggressive diuretic therapy should be instituted. Furosemide (5 mg/kg IV) promotes mild renal (and visceral) vasodilation and is a potent loop diuretic. If urine flow is not detected within 10 minutes, mannitol (0.5 gm/kg IV) should be administered to osmotically increase blood volume and renal perfusion and cause an osmotic diuresis. If urine flow is not detected within 10 minutes, dopamine (3 μg/kg per minute IV) should be administered. Simultaneous administration of all three diuretics may be effective if serial administration fails.

Gastrointestinal Tract Protection

Gastrointestinal tract (GIT) mucosal ulceration and sloughing are common consequences of shock (see *CVT XII*, p. 133). The mechanism of GIT damage may be related to tissue hypoxia and diminished organ perfusion, oxygen radical–induced lipid peroxidation, diffusion of luminal hydrogen ions into mucosal cells, deterioration of the effectiveness of the mucus barrier, destructive action of bile acids and pancreatic proteases, or some combination of these causes (Arvidsson et al, 1990). The mainstay of GIT protection is the restoration of an effective circulating blood volume, and the re-establishment of adequate perfusion and oxygenation of the viscera. Other treatments, such as those discussed below, may be useful, but require further study.

Sucralfate reacts with hydrochloric acid to form a complex that binds to proteinaceous exudates at ulcers and protects the site from further damage by pepsin, acid, or bile. It may also stimulate prostaglandin E_2 and I_2 activity and therefore have a cytoprotective effect similar to that of misoprostol. It does not alter secretion of acid, trypsin, or amylase. Sucralfate decreases the bioavailability and absorption of other drugs and may also cause constipation. The recommended dosage is 0.25 to 1 gm every 8 to 12 hours.

Cimetidine, ranitidine, and *famotidine* block the H_2 receptor on the basolateral membrane of the parietal cells of the stomach. These drugs decrease acid production; they do not alter gastric emptying time or lower esophageal or pyloric sphincter tone or pancreatic or biliary secretion. Cimetidine—but not ranitidine—inhibits cytochrome P-450 microsomal enzyme function in the liver and may alter the metabolic rate of other drugs (beta-blockers, calcium channel blockers, diazepam, metronidazole). When administered orally, H_2 blockers should be given remotely (2 hours apart) from other drugs (antacids, metoclopramide, sucralfate). Cimetidine—but not ranitidine—binds H_2 receptors on red blood cells and platelets and may be associated with anemia and thrombocytopenia. Cimetidine (ranitidine much less so) crosses the blood-brain barrier and may be associated with mental confusion or depression. These agents, by virtue of increasing gastric fluid pH, may allow repopulation of the stomach and mouth with potentially pathogenic organisms, which, in turn, predisposes to nosocomial pneumonia. The dosage of cimetidine is 5 to 10 mg/kg PO, IV, or IM every 6 to 8 hours; of ranitidine is 0.5 to 2 mg/kg PO, IV, or IM every 8 to 12 hours; and famotidine is 0.5 mg/kg IM, SC, or PO every 12 to 24 hours.

Omeprazole is a gastric acid proton pump inhibitor. In an acid environment, it is activated to a sulphenamide that binds irreversibly to the H^+, K^+-exchanging ATPase enzyme on the secretory surfaces of the parietal cells. Recovery from the drug's effects depends on the synthesis of new H^+, K^+-ATPase protein (3 days). The drug also inhibits the cytochrome P-450 mixed-function oxidase system in the liver and therefore inhibits metabolism of a variety of other drugs (sedatives and anesthetics). It may cause abdominal cramping, vomiting, or diarrhea. The recommended dosage is 0.5 to 1 mg/kg PO every 24 hours.

Misoprostol directly inhibits gastric acid secretion of parietal cells and is cytoprotective by increasing secretion of gastric mucus and bicarbonate. The drug also enhances mucosal defense mechanisms and healing of acid-induced injuries. It is specifically therapeutic for the GI complications of antiprostaglandin drugs but does not interfere with their anti-inflammatory or analgesic effects. Misoprostol enhances uterine contractions and specifically should not be used in the pregnant animal. It also enhances GI motility; cramps, diarrhea, or vomiting may be a problem. The recommended dosage is 1 to 5 µg/kg PO every 8 hours.

Diffuse Infiltrative Pulmonary Parenchymal Disease

A diffuse infiltrative pulmonary parenchymal disease, referred to as respiratory distress syndrome (RDS), is a late complication of the septic shock process. This syndrome is caused by increased pulmonary capillary permeability resulting from the systemic inflammatory reaction. This diffuse infiltrative process decreases lung compliance and increases the work of ventilation. As the process worsens, small airways and alveoli collapse, causing venous admixture and hypoxemia. Development of RDS in septic MODS is not a good prognostic sign.

Initially, oxygen therapy (*CVT XII,* p. 175) is palliative, but as the parenchymal involvement worsens, positive-pressure ventilation becomes necessary to re-expand small airways and alveoli. Aggressive ventilatory settings are often necessary, owing to the severely reduced compliance of the lungs.

Coagulopathies

Activation of the coagulation and platelet aggregation cascades is an early consequence of septic SIRS and may be observed in other forms of shock. Disseminated intravascular coagulation is composed of an early hypercoagulable state (miliary microthrombosis) and a later hypocoagulable state (hemorrhagic diathesis) induced by the depletion of platelets and coagulation precursors, and the accumulation of thrombin-inhibiting fibrin degradation products. Small vessel thrombosis may cause microangiopathic red blood cell fragmentation (schistocytes), and intravascular and extravascular hemolysis. Postmortem fibrinolysis may negate histologic demonstration of these microinfarctions. The hypocoagulable phase, which is associated with multifocal hemorrhage and prolongation of in vitro coagulation times, is a consequence of the primary activation of platelet and coagulation cascades.

Treatment of the hypercoagulable phase of documented DIC involves the administration of drugs that inhibit these cascades. Treatment of the hypocoagulable phase involves the administration of fresh plasma (platelets and all coagulation factors are needed) in addition to therapy for the cause of the hypercoagulable phase. Heparin inhibits coagulation by several mechanisms. It binds with, and enhances the potency of, plasma antithrombin III, which inhibits several coagulation factors (particularly thrombin, factor X, and factor XII). Heparin also inhibits prothrombin activation and platelet aggregation. Low-dose heparin therapy is generally recommended (100 U/kg SC every 6 hours) in DIC when critical monitoring of in vitro coagulation times is not possible. The low-dose therapy regimen seldom, if ever, causes bleeding and uncommonly causes measurable changes in in vitro coagulation. Prolonged heparin therapy (6 to 12 days) may cause thrombocytopenia (an immune-mediated idiosyncratic reaction in fewer than 6% of human patients). Antiprostaglandins (especially aspirin) inhibit thromboxane synthesis and in the author's opinion should be administered, if possible, to DIC patients. The administration of dextran 70 may also be therapeutic.

General Medical Therapy

Antibiotic Therapy

The range of organisms involved in sepsis is unpredictable, as are the antibiotic susceptibilities (*CVT XII*, p. 137). A total of 30 to 70% of bacteremias are gram-negative, 25 to 50% are gram-positive, and 10 to 30% are anaerobic; mixed infections occur approximately 10 to 50% of the time. The antibiotic plan must be broad-spectrum and highly likely to be effective (Table 1).

Glucocorticosteroids

Pharmacologic doses of corticosteroids have been shown to have "antishock" effects in many different shock models. The mechanisms of the beneficial effects were attributed to organelle- and cell-membrane stabilization, improved cellular metabolism and gluconeogenesis, improved microcirculation, decreased production of endogenous toxins such as myocardial depressant factor and decreased absorption of endotoxin, decreased leukocyte activation and degranulation, minimized reticuloendothelial depression and histologic organ damage, and improved survival in some studies (Schumer, 1976; Hoffman et al, 1984; White et al, 1982). The recommended corticosteroids are hydrocortisone (100 to 300 mg/kg), prednisolone or methylprednisolone (10 to 30 mg/kg), or dexamethasone (4 to 6 mg/kg).

Corticosteroid therapy is not currently in vogue because the administration of these drugs did not improve survival in several large prospective human studies (Hinshaw et al, 1987; Bone et al, 1987; Luce et al, 1988). Mortality may not be the best end point for establishing the efficacy of any single therapy, since many patients in these studies have lethal underlying disease processes that would not be

expected to be responsive to corticosteroids. Thus, the efficacy of treatment with corticosteroids is unresolved, but they are often administered.

Antiprostaglandins

Prostaglandins released into the systemic circulation during shock can cause marked hemodynamic changes, including decreased cardiac output, systemic hypotension, pulmonary hypertension, and increased vascular permeability. Treatment with antiprostaglandins may ameliorate these cardiovascular changes. The adverse effects of antiprostaglandins include GIT hemorrhage and ulceration, and renal afferent vasoconstriction (causing acute renal failure). The narrow spectrum of beneficial effects coupled with these common disadvantageous effects have limited the use of these drugs in shock and in sepsis; their use is not recommended.

Glucose

Severe hypoglycemia is common in septic MODS. It may be a manifestation of impaired hepatic gluconeogenesis and peripheral anaerobic metabolism. If blood glucose concentration is very low, a bolus of 20% glucose (0.25 gm/kg IV) should be administered. Blood glucose concentration is then maintained by an intravenous infusion of a 2.5 to 10% glucose solution.

Alkalization

Metabolic acidosis during septic MODS is attributed primarily to lactic acidosis secondary to impaired aerobic metabolism. Alkalizing therapy should be instituted when the metabolic acidosis becomes severe. Sodium bicarbonate has been the traditional alkalizing agent used; however, the administration of sodium bicarbonate can also be associated with a number of problems, and so its use has become rather controversial.

The administration of sodium bicarbonate generates car-

TABLE 1. General Spectrum of Antibiotic Activity

	Gram-Negative	Gram-Positive		Anaerobic
		Staph. sp	Strep. sp	
Penicillins				
Penicillin, ampicillin, amoxicillin	No	Often	Yes	Yes (except some *B.*
Oxacillin, methicillin, nafcillin, cloxacillin	No	Yes	No	*fragilis* and
Carbenicillin, ticarcillin, azlocillin, piperacillin, mezlocillin	Yes	Yes	Variable	*Actinomyces*)
Cephalosporins				
First-generation	Variable	Yes	Yes	No
Second-generation	Variable	Yes	Yes	Variable
Third-generation	Yes	Variable	Yes	Yes
Imipenem/Cilastin	Yes	Yes	Yes	Yes
Aminoglycosides	Yes	Yes	No	No
Fluoroquinolones	Yes	Yes	No	No
Aztreonam	Yes	No	No	No
Metronidazole	No	No	No	Yes
Clindamycin	No	Yes	Yes	Yes

B. fragilis, Bacteroides fragilis; Staph., Staphylococcus; Strep., Streptococcus.

bon dioxide (via carbonic acid), which will result in hypercapnia if the patient is not ventilating well. Carbon dioxide rapidly diffuses into the intracellular compartment and into the cerebrospinal fluid (CSF; Pavlin and Hornbein, 1975a and 1975b). Once inside, it re-equilibrates across the carbonic acid equilibrium, generating an excess of hydrogen ion. Intracellular acidosis may be associated with myocardial and central nervous system (CNS) depression (Sun et al, 1996). Animals with normal respiratory responsiveness and capability eliminate this carbon dioxide in very short order, and intracellular acidosis does not occur (Sanders et al, 1988; Pavlin and Hornbein, 1975b). Sodium bicarbonate administration increases plasma sodium concentration and osmolality. The increase is moderate and similar to that associated with the administration of hypertonic saline. The administration of hypertonic solutions also promotes systemic vasodilation.

There are alternative alkalizing agents. Tromethamine (Tham-E, Abbott) is an organic amine buffer that binds directly with hydrogen ion. Tromethamine thus diminishes carbon dioxide via the carbonic acid system. The un-ionized portion of tromethamine (about 30% of it) is freely diffusible into the cell and therefore produces a more rapid intracellular buffering effect than does sodium bicarbonate. Tromethamine is also an osmotic diuretic. Tromethamine is a very alkaline solution (a 0.3 M solution has a pH of 10.6) and is irritating to tissues and small veins. The dosage is calculated by the formula: Base deficit $\times$ 0.4 $\times$ body wt kg (see discussion below). Carbicarb is a combination of a 0.33 M solution of sodium carbonate and a 0.33 M solution of sodium bicarbonate (International Medications Systems Ltd., South El Monte, CA). Carbicarb is associated with less carbon dioxide production than is sodium bicarbonate. There may be some advantages to tromethamine and Carbicarb, but the wholesale abandonment of sodium bicarbonate seems unwarranted, since it has been demonstrated to be efficacious and these other agents have not been demonstrated to be superior (Beech et al, 1994).

The milliequivalents of bicarbonate to administer can be calculated by multiplying the patient's weight (kg) by 0.3 (a slight overestimate of the extracellular fluid volume and the early redistribution fluid space of the administered bicarbonate) times the difference between the measured base deficit of bicarbonate and the goal level. This calculation often equates to a dose of 1 to 5 mEq of sodium bicarbonate per kilogram of body weight. This dose must be administered slowly (20 to 30 minutes). If administered too rapidly, sodium bicarbonate can cause vascular compartment alkalosis, hypokalemia, low ionized calcium, hypotension, restlessness, vomiting, collapse, and even death.

Nutrition

Nutrition should be started within 24 to 48 hours of onset of any critical illness (see other articles in sections 1 and 2). Enteral feeding is preferable to intravenous feeding because it preserves gut mucosal mass, gut impermeability, and mucosal immunity (see p. 136); reduces infectious complications and release of cytokine inflammatory mediators associated with a critical illness; and improves survival compared to intravenous feeding (Minard and Kudsk, 1994). Intravenous feeding is highly beneficial in patients

that cannot be fed enterally, and combinations of enteral and intravenous feeding can be used. A nasogastric tube or gastrostomy tube is commonly used. Many critically ill patients develop a gastric stasis that limits the efficacy of feeding by this route. Prokinetic agents such as metoclopramide or cisapride may be useful. A jejunostomy tube could also be placed during laparotomy so that the stomach can be bypassed.

Other Potential Therapies

Antisera

Antiendotoxin, anti–tumor necrosis factor, and anti–platelet-activating factor antisera, while protecting against experimental challenge with the specific agonist, have been reported not to be particularly efficacious in the management of clinical septic SIRS or MODS syndromes.

Reactive Oxygen Radical Scavengers

Reactive oxygen radicals (superoxide, hydrogen peroxide, and hydroxyl anion) cause protein denaturation and cell wall lipoperoxidation. The efficacy of inhibitors of reactive oxygen radical production (allopurinol, superoxide dismutase, and catalase), of scavengers of hydroxyl anion (mannitol, alpha-tocopherol), and of protectors of their effects (corticosteroids, 21-aminosteroids) remains to be established.

References

Arvidsson S, Falt K, Haglund U: Feline *E. coli* bacteremia: Effects of misoprostol/scavengers or methylprednisolone on hemodynamic reactions and gastrointestinal mucosal injury. Acta Chir Scand 156:215, 1990.

Beech JS, Nolan KM, Iles RA, et al: The effects of sodium bicarbonate and a mixture of sodium bicarbonate and carbonate ("Carbicarb") on skeletal muscle pH and hemodynamic status in rats with hypovolemic shock. Metabolism 43:518, 1994.

Bone RC, Fisher CJ, Clemmer TP, et al: A controlled clinical trial of high-dose methylprednisolone in the treatment of severe sepsis and septic shock. N Engl J Med 317:653, 1987.

Concannon KT, Haskins SC, Feldman BF: Hemostatic defects associated with two infusion rates of dextran 70 in dogs. Am J Vet Res 53:1369, 1992.

Derrick JR, Guest MM: Dextrans: Current Concepts of Basic Actions and Clinical Applications. Springfield, IL: Charles C Thomas, 1968.

Einstein R, Abdul-Hussein N, Wong TW, et al: Cardiovascular actions of dopexamine in anaesthetized and conscious dogs. Br J Pharmacol 111:199, 1994.

Giger U, Bucheler J: Transfusion of type-A and type-B blood to cats. J Am Vet Med Assoc 198:411, 1991.

Giger U, Kilran CG, Filippich LJ, et al: Frequencies of feline blood groups in the United States. J Am Vet Med Assoc 195:1230, 1989.

Gollub S, Schaefer C, Squittieri A: The bleeding tendency associated with plasma expanders. Surg Gynecol Obstet 124:1203, 1967.

Hinshaw L, Peduzzi P, Young E, et al: Effect of high-dose glucocorticoid therapy on mortality in patients with clinical signs of systemic sepsis. N Engl J Med 317:659, 1987.

Hoffman SL, Punjabi NH, Kumala S, et al: Reduction of mortality in chloramphenicol-treated severe typhoid fever by high-dose dexamethasone. N Engl J Med 310:82, 1984.

Luce JM, Montgomery AB, Marks JD, et al: Ineffectiveness of high-dose methylprednisolone in preventing parenchymal lung injury and improving mortality in patients with septic shock. Am Rev Respir Dis 138:62, 1988.

Marion RS, Smith JE: Survival of erythrocytes after autologous and allogeneic transfusion in cats. J Am Vet Med Assoc 183:1437, 1983.

Metcalf W, Papdopoulos A, Tufaro R, et al: A clinical physiologic study of hydroxyethyl starch. Surg Gynecol Obstet 130:255, 1970.

Minard G, Kudsk KA: Is early feeding beneficial? How early is early? New Horizons 2:156, 1994.

Pavlin EG, Hornbein TF: Distribution of H$^+$ and HCO$_3$$^-$ between CSF and blood during respiratory acidosis in dogs. Am J Physiol 228:1145, 1975a.

Pavlin EG, Hornbein TF: Distribution of H$^+$ and HCO$_3$$^-$ between CSF and blood during metabolic alkalosis in dogs. Am J Physiol 228:1141, 1975b.

Sanders AB, Otto CW, Kern KB, et al: Acid-base balance in a canine model of cardiac arrest. Ann Emerg Med 17:667, 1988.

Schumer W: Steroids in the treatment of clinical septic shock. Ann Surg 184:333, 1976.

Sun S, Weil MH, Tang W, et al: Effects of buffer agents on postresuscitation myocardial dysfunction. Crit Care Med 24:2035, 1996.

van Kesteren RG, van Alphen MMA, Charbon GA: Effects of dopamine on intestinal vessels in anesthetized dogs. Circ Shock 25:41, 1988.

White GL, White GS, Kosanke SD, et al: Therapeutic effects of prednisolone sodium succinate vs. dexamethasone in dogs subjected to E. coli septic shock. J Am Anim Hosp Assoc 18:639, 1982.

Open Chest Cardiopulmonary Resuscitation

LINDA BARTON
New York, New York

DENNIS T. CROWE
Alpharetta, Georgia

ADVANTAGES

Open chest cardiopulmonary cerebral resuscitation (CPCR) is physiologically superior but logistically inferior to standard external CPCR (Bircher and Safer, 1984). In standard external CPCR, blood flow is generated by both thoracic pump and cardiac pump mechanisms. In the thoracic pump mechanism, chest compression generates a global increase in intrathoracic pressure that is transmitted to the intrathoracic vascular structures. This results in forward blood flow, but also an increase in venous pressure. The increased venous pressure adversely affects coronary and cerebral perfusion by increasing resistance to flow. The thoracic pump is the most important mechanism in dogs weighing more than 20 kg (Crowe, 1988). Squeezing of the cardiac chambers (the cardiac pump mechanism) either indirectly in external CPCR or directly in open chest CPCR produces forward blood flow with less elevation in venous pressure. The cardiac mechanism results in diastolic perfusion pressure for coronary blood flow and cerebral blood flow compatible with full neurologic recovery.

Because of the increased blood flow produced, open chest CPCR provides a better chance for sustaining cerebral and myocardial viability and restoring spontaneous circulation. In addition, the open chest method permits direct palpation and observation of the heart, which helps guide fluid and drug therapy. Also, internal defibrillation may be performed more effectively than external defibrillation, if needed. Finally, the open chest method permits direct compression of a bleeding site in intrathoracic exsanguination, and in cases of intra-abdominal hemorrhage, allows temporary compression or clamping of the descending aorta above the diaphragm (Safer et al, 1995).

INDICATIONS

It has not been fully defined which situations in veterinary medicine justify the increased morbidity associated with an invasive procedure to achieve the improved perfusion possible with open chest CPCR. Direct cardiac massage is recommended when cardiac arrest occurs during an operative procedure in which the thorax or abdomen is already opened. Open chest CPCR should be initiated in patients with conditions that interfere with the generation of intrathoracic pressure, as outlined in Table 1. It has also been recommended in hypothermic arrest so that direct warming of the heart can occur simultaneously with resuscitation (American Heart Association, 1992).

Experimental studies and clinical experience suggest that open chest CPCR should be considered in cardiac arrest resulting from severe hypovolemia, such as that occurring secondary to trauma and hemorrhage (Crowe, 1988; Safar and Bircher, 1992a). Direct cardiac compression maximizes perfusion while rapid fluid replacement is initiated. Opening the chest also provides a means to control hemorrhage in either the thoracic or abdominal cavities. It also allows cross-clamping of the descending aorta

TABLE 1. Indications for Open Chest Cardiac Massage

Intraoperative arrest
Hypothermic arrest
Inability to generate high intrathoracic pressure
  Pneumothorax
  Diaphragmatic hernia
  Flail chest
  Severe obesity
  Pericardial effusion
  Very large animals
Arrest secondary to severe hypotension
  Multiple trauma
  Exsanguination
Ineffective closed chest CPCR

CPCR, cardiopulmonary cerebral resuscitation.

to direct blood flow cranially and improve coronary and cerebral perfusion. Open chest CPCR should be performed if closed chest techniques are ineffective.

The effectiveness of closed chest compressions can be evaluated by palpating for femoral pulses or by a flow detection devise such as a Doppler ultrasound transducer applied to the cornea (Crowe, 1992). If no flow can be detected after 2 minutes of closed chest CPCR, a thoracotomy should be performed to allow direct cardiac massage. Also, if closed chest CPCR has not resulted in a return to spontaneous circulation after 10 minutes, open chest CPCR should be initiated. Although there have been reports of successful resuscitation after a prolonged period of unsuccessful CPCR (Kern et al, 1987) the rate of successful resuscitation decreases markedly if internal cardiac compression is delayed beyond 15 minutes. Thoracotomy is not a procedure to be used as a last resort after everything else has failed. Although it has been proved effective in improving hemodynamic responses, open chest massage is unlikely to improve survival if it is performed after significant coronary and cerebral hypoxic damage has occurred.

TECHNIQUE
Emergency Thoracotomy

The emergent thoracotomy necessary to perform open chest cardiac massage is an easily learned procedure. It can be performed safely and efficiently within 10 to 30 seconds in most animals. With the animal in right lateral recumbency, a skin incision is made over the left fifth or sixth intercostal space, extending dorsally from the origin of the ribs to ventrally near the sternum. A rapid clip in a long-haired dog may facilitate the skin incision. A curved Mayo scissors is used to complete the thoracotomy.

The tips of the closed scissors are thrust through the intercostal muscle and into the pleural space ventrally near the costochondral junction. The depth of penetration is controlled by grasping the shaft of the scissors so that the exposed portion of the scissors is equal to the estimated thickness of the chest wall. The scissors tips are spread to enlarge the opening into the pleural cavity and to allow air to enter the pleural space to collapse the lung. The scissors are used in a sliding fashion to open the intercostal space. The tips are held open approximately 1 inch; with the deep blade held close to the parietal pleural surface, the scissors are pushed first dorsally along the cranial edge of the caudal rib. The incision is then extended ventrally. Ventral to the costochondral junction, the scissors are centered between the ribs to avoid the intercostal vessels that lie on the cranial and caudal edges of the ribs. The incision should stop short of the sternum to avoid injury to the internal thoracic artery and vein, which course longitudinally approximately 1 cm from the sternum. Positive-pressure ventilation should be temporarily interrupted during penetration into the pleural space and opening of the intercostal space. A Balfour abdominal retractor or a Finochietto rib spreader can be used to improve visualization and access to the heart and pericardium. If additional exposure is required, the caudal rib can be cut at the costochondral junction. This allows the rib to "shingle" under the next rib caudally and increases exposure. The same technique can be performed for the rib cranial to the incision.

Pericardotomy

The pericardium should be opened immediately on opening the chest. The index finger of the right hand is hooked around the phrenicopericardial ligament ventral to the apex of the heart. The pericardium is cut with a Mayo scissors ventrally near the ligamentous attachment. The incision in the pericardium is extended dorsally after visualizing the phrenic nerve. Opening the pericardium allows for detection of fine fibrillation and monitoring of coronary vessels to determine the effectiveness of CPCR and has been shown to increase the effectiveness of cardiac massage (Crowe, 1989).

Direct Cardiac Massage

The heart should be compressed in a smooth rhythmic fashion from the apex toward the base of the heart. Massage is performed with one or two hands, depending on the size of the heart. The palmar surfaces of the fingers and thumb are used to avoid fingertip penetration of the atrial or ventricular wall. Care should be taken not to rotate or displace the heart. "Kinking" of the heart may occlude inflow or cause tearing at the junction of the vena cava and right atrium. The heart should be compressed as soon as the ventricles fill. If a target heart rate of 80 to 120 beats/min cannot be achieved because of slow ventricular filling, the rate should initially be decreased as required to achieve filling while therapy is instituted to improve venous return. Therapy to increase venous return could include IV administration of a fluid bolus (lactated Ringer's or other similar replacement crystalloid solution at 90 ml/kg per hour or a 20 ml/kg bolus of a colloid such as hetastarch) or epinephrine (0.2 mg/kg IV).

Aortic Cross-Clamping

The descending aorta can be cross-clamped as an adjunctive resuscitative maneuver. By directing blood flow cranially, aortic cross-clamping significantly improves coronary and cerebral perfusion regardless of the prearrest intravascular volume. The thoracic descending aorta should be occluded just caudal to the base of the heart. The duration of cross-clamping should be limited to less than 10 minutes, if possible, to prevent ischemic spinal cord damage. The aorta can be occluded with a cardiovascular forceps or with a "tourniquet" of a soft flexible material such as a small feeding tube (3.5F or 5F), umbilical tape, or a Penrose drain. A curved hemostat is used to dissect around the aorta and facilitate the passage of the material to be looped around the vessel. The hemostat is slid down on the loop to tighten it around the aorta (Crowe, 1989). After spontaneous circulation has returned, the tourniquet is removed gradually over 5 to 10 minutes to prevent hypotension and possible rearrest.

Closure

After successful resuscitation, the patient should be taken to the operating room for copious irrigation and routine closure. The hair on the chest wall should not be clipped except very near the skin incision in dogs with long hair. Only a solution of chlorhexidine (Nolvasan, Fort Dodge) or povidone-iodine (Betadine, Purdue Frederick) should be used to clean the skin. Broad-spectrum, bacteriocidal antibiotics such as cefazolin sodium (20 mg/kg IV every 6 to 8 hours) should be administered. Infection is not reported to be a major complication in either veterinary or human patients (Crowe, 1989; Safar and Bircher, 1992a).

READINESS

The rate of survival from cardiac arrest in veterinary patients has been reported to be from 0 to 22% (Hackett and VanPelt, 1995). The effectiveness of CPCR efforts in a given setting will be dependent, in part, on the training and readiness of the hospital and staff. There should be designated areas where CPCR is performed. Essential equipment and drugs should be readily available in this area (see *CVT XII,* p. 167). Protocols for CPCR should be reviewed and practiced as a team. Practicing the techniques on cadavers is helpful to decrease the time it takes to perform the procedure, and to prevent iatrogenic injury.

PATIENT SELECTION

It should also be remembered that the goal of CPCR is to save "hearts and brains too good to die" (Safar and Bircher, 1992b). Every death is associated with the cessation of effective ventilation and circulation; however, resuscitation efforts should be restricted to patients not expected to die and when the life-threatening process believed responsible for their arrest is potentially reversible. When caring for patients with insurmountable problems, the owner should be honestly informed about the futility of the situation and gently guided to choose a "do not resuscitate" status for their pet. Resuscitation should not be attempted if it can be accurately (often difficult to determine) estimated that the animal has been dead for 15 to 20 minutes. Although we have an obligation to maximize resuscitation efforts in "treatable" patients, (including open-chest techniques) to apply resuscitation without judgment and compassion is morally and economically unacceptable (Safar and Bircher, 1992a).

References and Suggested Reading

American Heart Association: Standards for cardiopulmonary resuscitation and emergency cardiac care. JAMA 268:2171, 1992.
The American Heart Association's recommended guidelines for Basic Life Support and Advanced Life Support.
Bircher N, Safer P: Open-chest CPR: An old method whose time has returned. Am J Emerg Med 2:568, 1984.
Review of open and closed chest CPR.
Crowe DT: Cardiopulmonary resuscitation in the dog: A review and proposed new guidelines: Parts I and II. Semin Vet Med Surg (Small Animal) 3:321, 1988.
Review of CPR and suggested CPR protocols in veterinary patients.
Crowe DT: Symposium on critical care. Vet Med 84:77, 1989.
Review of critical care techniques including emergency thoracotomy for direct cardiac compression.
Crowe DT: Triage and trauma management. In: Murtaugh RJ, ed: Veterinary Emergency and Critical Care Medicine. St Louis: Mosby-Year Book, 1992, p 77.
Review of facility, equipment, and personnel readiness for resuscitation.
Crowe DT: Evaluation of a Doppler flow detector and probe on the eye for determining the effectiveness of blood flow generation with cardiac massage in dogs. Third International Veterinary Emergency and Critical Care Symposium 3:839, 1992.
Abstract about the use of the Parks Doppler flow on the eye in CPR.
Hackett TB, VanPelt DR: Cardiopulmonary resuscitation. In: Bonagura JD, ed: Current Veterinary Therapy XII: Small Animal Practice. Philadelphia: WB Saunders, 1995, p 167.
Review of CPR technique and suggested algorithms.
Kern KB, Sanders AB, Badylak SF, et al: Long-term survival with open chest cardiac massage after ineffective closed-chest compression in a canine preparation. Circulation 75:498, 1987.
Experimental canine study of the outcome of open-chest cardiac massage when instituted after failure of standard closed-chest compression CPR.
Safar P, Bircher N: Cardiopulmonary cerebral resuscitation: Basic and advanced life support. In: Schwartz GR, Cayten CG, Mangelsen MA, et al, eds: Principles and Practice of Emergency Medicine, 3rd ed, vol 1. Philadelphia: Lea & Febiger, 1992a, p 89.
Review of current guidelines for basic and advanced cardiopulmonary-cerebral resuscitation.
Safar P, Bircher N: The pathophysiology of dying and reanimation. In: Schwartz GR, Cayten CG, Mangelsen MA, et al, eds: Principles and Practice of Emergency Medicine, 3rd ed, vol 1. Philadelphia: Lea & Febiger, 1992b, p 3.
Summary of the pathophysiologic events that occur during dying and resuscitation.
Safer P, Abramson S, Bircher N: Cardiopulmonary-cerebral resuscitation. In: Shoemaker WC, Ayres SM, Grenuik A, et al, eds: Textbook of Critical Care. Philadelphia: WB Saunders, 1995, p 16.
Review of current guidelines for basic and advanced cardiopulmonary-cerebral resuscitation.

Defibrillation

WAYNE E. WINGFIELD

MICHAEL LAGUTCHIK

Fort Collins, Colorado

Total electrical disorder of the ventricles of the heart, accompanied by incoordination of contraction, is known as ventricular fibrillation (VF). For centuries, VF was recognized as a terminal event from which there was no recovery. In 1899, Prevost and Battelli reported on investigations into electrical methods of treatment of fibrillation in dog hearts. They were able to show that powerful electrical shocks applied directly to the heart could convert VF into a sinus rhythm. No clinical application of this technique was reported until 1947, when Beck successfully resuscitated a 16-year-old boy from VF by applying alternating-current electrical shock directly to the heart. Following further investigations, directly applied cardiac electrical shock became commonplace in human operating rooms. The need for conversion of VF without opening the chest soon became obvious, and external electrical defibrillators were developed in the mid-1950s independently by Zoll and Kouwenhoven and have since then received wide clinical application.

A chemical means of conversion of VF to sinus rhythm has been sought for many decades, beginning with the investigations of Hooker in 1928. Even today, no consistently effective chemical methods of defibrillation have evolved.

ELECTRICAL DEFIBRILLATION

Underlying the rationale of electrical defibrillation is the fact that a massive electrical shock will cause complete depolarization of all individual myocardial fibers. VF is a form of disordered re-entry, which requires at all times that some portion of the ventricular myocardium not be depolarized so that these segments can be next in line to be activated. When all the cells within the re-entrant circuit are depolarized, a condition of electrical homogeneity is re-established, which is unfavorable to the development of re-entry. In order to be successful, an electrical shock must produce a period of electrical homogeneity that persists for a sufficient time (>130 msec) (Chen et al, 1986).

The minimal amount of energy required to defibrillate the heart is called the *defibrillation threshold*. This is not a single value but rather a sigmoidal dose-response relationship: The greater the energy in a shock, the more likely it is to defibrillate a given heart (Davy et al, 1987). There is marked variability from animal to animal in the energy threshold, mainly because of interanimal differences in *transthoracic impedance*. This impedance has several important determinants: the size of the animal, electrode size, electrode-thoracic wall contact pressure and couplant ("electrode paste"), and phase of the respiratory cycle. Increases in transthoracic impedance during lung expansion are especially important considerations in animals receiving mechanical ventilation and in those receiving basic life support.

Impedance declines with multiple shocks partly because of the edema and tissue hyperemia in the pathway of electrical current (Sirna et al, 1989). Since *current*, and not energy,* is the determinant of successful defibrillation, recently developed defibrillators automatically deliver more energy when impedance is found to be high. Current required for defibrillation increases with heart and body weight, but excessive current impairs the contractile force of the myocardium. Therefore, defibrillation with the minimal effective peak current is obviously desirable. Hypoxia, hypothermia, pH, and ionic and catecholamine levels in the circulation are known to affect the amount of current required for defibrillation (Geddes and Baker, 1971).

Other factors besides transthoracic impedance can influence the defibrillation threshold. Lidocaine reversibly increases the defibrillation threshold by as much as 50% (Guarnieri et al, 1987). Beta-agonists and aminophylline, in contrast, lower the defibrillation threshold (Ruffy et al, 1988). The incidence of defibrillation is inversely proportional to the duration of fibrillation (Yakaitis et al, 1980). In Figure 1, the duration of fibrillation is seen to be proportional to the maximal achievable success of defibrillation and up to a certain point is directly related to the energy requirement for conversion. Energy is defined as the ability to do work. In a practical sense, it is the power multiplied by the time it is delivered; the unit employed is the joule (J) or watt-second. This defibrillation energy requirement is approximately *4–5 J/kg* (Yakaitis et al, 1980).

Defibrillation Equipment

The electrical defibrillator includes a bank of capacitors that can be charged from a voltage source (either line current or a battery) via a step-up transformer. Up to 7,000 volts may be required to charge capacitors for delivery of 400 J direct current. Inductance is added to the circuit to dampen the rise and fall of the current and voltage waveforms that are produced when the capacitors are discharged. These dampened waveforms are safer and more effective than undampened capacitor discharges. The optimal duration of a defibrillator shock has been found to be 4 to 12 msec (Ewy, 1978).

Alternating current (60 Hz) is not recommended for defibrillation. It is a potent fibrillating agent and is more dangerous to the animal and veterinarian. Although it is possible to defibrillate with alternating current, it faces a greater impedance than does direct current, and more en-

---

*Energy = Power × Duration

Power = Potential (volts) × Current (amps)

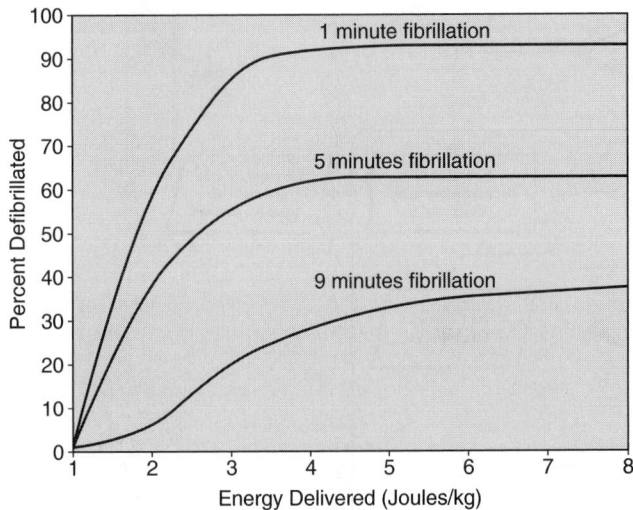

Figure 1. Curves showing estimated success of defibrillation versus delivered energy after 1, 5, and 9 minutes of fibrillation in dogs receiving closed-chest cardiac massage and artificial ventilation with epinephrine. (After Yakaitis RW, Ewy GA, Otto CW, et al: Influence of time and therapy on VF in dogs. Crit Care Med 8:157, 1980, with permission.)

ergy must be delivered to pass the same amount of current across the heart.

Electrode paddles are the key component to the defibrillation system. An optimal electrode size in humans is in the range of 8 to 12 cm. Smaller paddle electrodes (4.5 cm) are available for infants. For the veterinary patient, the 8-cm paddle should be used on any animal weighing more than 10 kg.

Emergency Defibrillation

Emergency defibrillation should be used to treat rhythms such as VF or rapid ventricular tachycardia that have caused the animal to be pulseless and unresponsive. In this situation, *speed* should be given the highest priority. The strongest determinant of survival is the interval between the onset of VF and the delivery of an effective electrical shock. If VF is witnessed in the electrocardiogram, defibrillation *precedes* basic life support techniques.

The electrode paddles should be coated well with gel, particularly around the edges. Although salt-containing electrode paste is typically used, ultrasound gel or surgical lubricant may also be used with equal success (Sirna et al, 1988). Alcohol-based solvents should *never* be used in proximity to the electrical defibrillator.

The paddles are applied firmly to the thoracic wall with about 25 pounds of pressure. This compresses the thorax, leading to a shorter electrode distance and lower thoracic impedance. Placement across the thorax likely makes little difference in the dog and cat. The paddle surface is generally as large as the heart, and only 28% of the fibrillating myocardial cells must be depolarized to cease fibrillation. In the larger dog, one may try to position the paddles so that defibrillation occurs from the base to the apex of the heart.

Extreme care must be taken to keep the paddles from touching each other and to prevent any bridging of the gap

TABLE 1. Confounding Variables Affecting Defibrillation

Body weight
Metabolic acidosis
Metabolic alkalosis
Hypoxia
Hyper- and hypokalemia
Hyper- and hypomagnesemia
Digitalis intoxication
Antiarrhythmic drugs
Acute reperfusion injury
Myocardial ischemia

between the electrodes by conductive gel. Once the paddles are in place, the defibrillator is charged. Prior to discharging the capacitors, the operator of the paddles *must* assure that no person is in contact with the animal, the table top, or a wet floor. Once a quick inspection has been made, the operator loudly announces *"ALL CLEAR."* After a second glance at the scene, the operator may discharge the defibrillator.

If the first attempt fails to convert the rhythm to a hemodynamically stable one, a second shock with nearly equal energy should be delivered. If the first two shocks fail to defibrillate the animal, a third shock with increased energy is immediately delivered. If all these attempts fail, the veterinarian should look for confounding factors such as inadequate electrode pressure, improper electrode positioning, and insufficient electrode-patient interface (i.e., inadequate gel amounts). Defibrillation may also fail when thoracic impedance is high because of pneumothorax. Table 1 lists other confounding variables that may interfere with defibrillation. Attempts should be made to correct these variables. Epinephrine can be used to lower the defibrillation threshold.

Efficacy of Defibrillation

No data are available from clinical experiences with defibrillation in the veterinary literature. In human patients, success rates are high for electrical conversion of ventricular dysrhythmias immediately after their onset. In experimental studies using the dog, 80% of induced ventricular tachycardia* and VF are converted with a single 200-J shock. Cumulative effectiveness is 95% after a second 200-J shock, and 99 to 100% after a third 300-J shock (Waldecker et al, 1986). Follow the algorithm in Figure 2 when defibrillating an animal. The amplitude of the fibrillation waveform has been shown to correlate with the time interval from initial cardiac arrest and to be a powerful predictor of outcome (Weaver et al, 1986). Human data indicate a fall in survival of 6% per minute in untreated VF so that no survival would be expected after 15 minutes (Larsen et al, 1993). Only 6% survival is seen in persons with very low amplitude ("fine") VF.

---

*The term *electrical cardioversion* is often used when converting supraventricular or ventricular tachyardias to sinus rhythm. Not synonymous with defibrillation, cardioversion uses a lower energy shock (e.g., 1J/kg) for a brief duration and is timed to the R wave of the electrocardiogram.

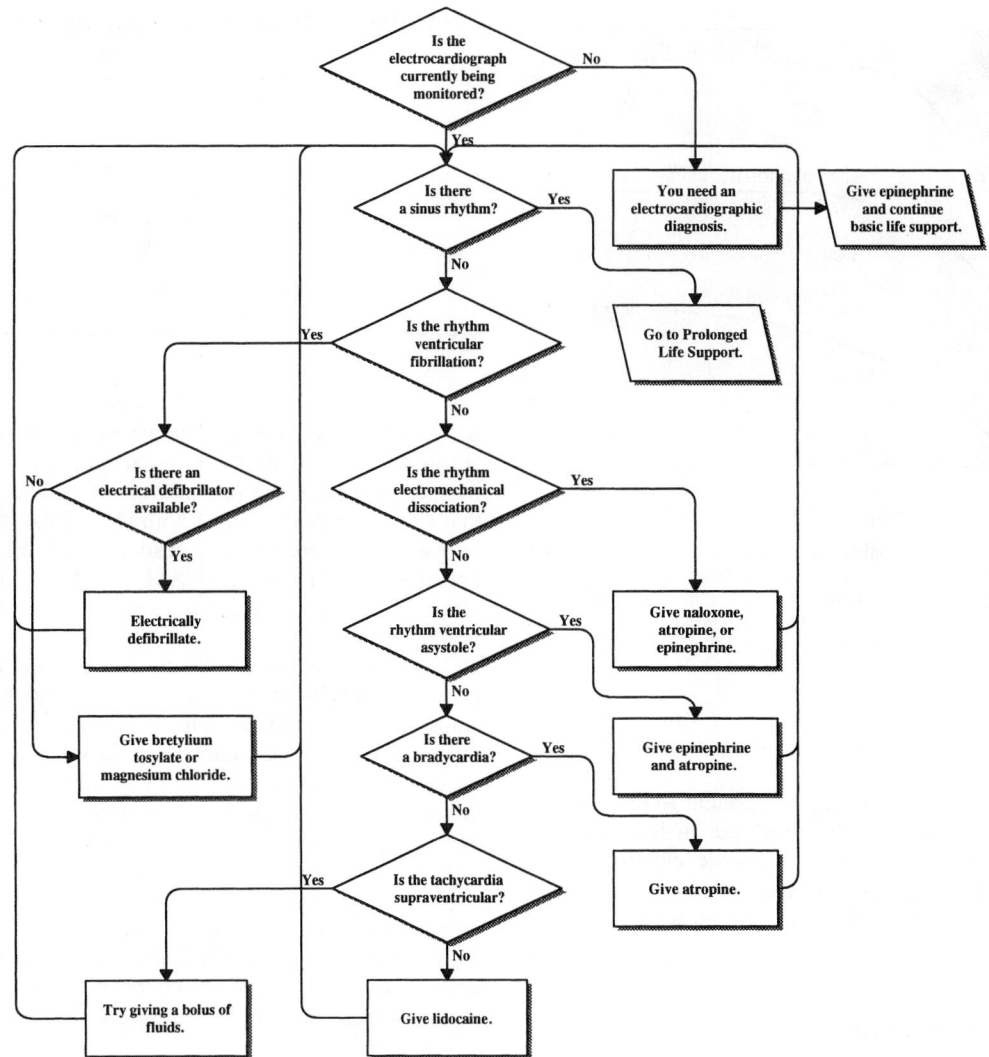

Figure 2. Algorithm for managing VF.

Open-Chest Defibrillation

Open-chest defibrillation involves direct application of the electrodes to the epicardium. The electrode paddles should be 6 to 8 cm in diameter and are covered with saline-soaked gauze. One paddle is applied on the base of the heart overlying the right atrium, whereas the second paddle is placed on the apex of the heart overlying the left ventricle. The electrical shock should not be administered in the presence of any explosive anesthetic agents. The shock is delivered under the control of the veterinarian holding the paddles and should follow the same safety guidelines outlined earlier for closed-chest defibrillation. Much less energy is required for open-chest defibrillation. Shocks varying from 10 to 60 J may be given. Epicardial burns may occur and may result in myocardial complications postresuscitation.

Spontaneous Defibrillation

Anecdotal reports persist regarding spontaneous defibrillation. These reports most frequently are associated with the cat and small dog. Although it is theoretically possible for spontaneous defibrillation to occur when a small heart is involved, the reason may well be good perfusion of the coronary arteries during cardiac compression (internal or external). This perfusion, the smallness of the heart, and the employment of myocardial stimulant drugs may be sufficient, in rare circumstances, to convert fibrillation to a sinus rhythm. Spontaneous defibrillation is rare and unpredictable and should play no role in the expectation of resuscitation.

CHEMICAL DEFIBRILLATION

Chemical defibrillating drugs have unproved efficacy in veterinary medicine. Unfortunately, many veterinarians do not have electrical defibrillators and thus chemical defibrillating drugs may be their only option. Several drugs are mentioned in the literature as useful for terminating VF. Although frequently mentioned, acetylcholine with potassium chloride is an unlikely choice for defibrillation because acetylcholine is not available as an injectable product. No clinical reports of successful chemical defibrillation using acetylcholine with potassium chloride are available in the veterinary literature.

Bretylium tosylate (10 mg/kg IV) is labeled for use in ventricular tachycardias and fibrillation. It will decrease the fibrillation threshold, but this must be balanced against the apparent loss of hemodynamic recovery. Bretylium possesses antiadrenergic and hypotensive actions associated with depletion of norepinephrine from peripheral adrenergic nerve endings. Thus, animals treated with bretylium may not be able to recover as well from fibrillation-defibrillation episodes because of less effective autonomic reflexes (Tacker et al, 1980).

Lidocaine has been offered as a possible chemical defibrillating agent in the past. Although lidocaine may possess an antifibrillatory effect under experimental conditions, the clinical relevance of such an effect is questionable. If cardiac arrest occurs, lidocaine has limited utility and may be deleterious secondary to diminished countershock efficacy or lidocaine-induced asystole (Wesley et al, 1991; Echt et al, 1994).

Magnesium is the most recently investigated chemical defibrillator drug. Hypomagnesemia is commonly seen in sick animals and is known to result in ventricular dysrhythmias (see *CVT XII*, p. 128). Most evidence points to a problem with potassium rather than magnesium as the cause, but magnesium infusion will occasionally convert ventricular dysrhythmias to normal sinus rhythms. Currently, the use of magnesium chloride (or sulfate) should be considered in the treatment of refractory VF. The dosage used is 0.15 to 0.3 mEq/kg infused intravenously over 2 minutes.

References and Suggested Reading

Chen PS, Shibata N, Dixon EG, et al: Activation during ventricular defibrillation in open-chest dogs. Evidence of complete cessation and regeneration of VF after unsuccessful shocks. J Clin Invest 77:810, 1986.

Davy J-M, Fain ES, Dorian P, et al: The relationship between successful defibrillation and delivered energy in open-chest dogs: Reappraisal of the "defibrillation threshold" concept. Am Heart J 113:77, 1987.

Echt DS, Gremillion ST, Lee JT, et al: Effects of procainamide and lidocaine on defibrillation energy requirements in patients receiving implantable cardioverter defibrillator devices. J Cardiovasc Electrophysiol 5:752, 1994.

Ewy GA: Cardiac arrest and resuscitation: Defibrillators and defibrillation. Curr Probl Cardiol 2:1, 1978.

Geddes LA, Baker LE: Response to passage of electric current through the body. J Assoc Advanc Med Instrument 5:13, 1971.

Guarnieri T, Levine JH, Veltri EP, et al: Success of chronic defibrillation and the role of antiarrhythmic drugs with the automatic implantable cardioverter/defibrillator. Am J Cardiol 60:1061, 1987.

Larsen MP, Eisenberg MS, Cummins RO, et al: Predicting survival from out-of-hospital cardiac arrest: A graphic model. Ann Emerg Med 22:1652, 1993.

Ruffy R, Monje E, Schechtman K: Facilitation of cardiac defibrillation by aminophylline in the conscious, closed-chest dog. J Electrophysiol 2:450, 1988.

Sirna SJ, Ferguson DW, Charbonnier F, et al: Electrical cardioversion in humans: Factors affecting transthoracic impedance. Am J Cardiol 62:1048, 1988.

Sirna SJ, Kieso RA, Fox-Eastham KJ, et al: Mechanisms responsible for the decline in thoracic impedance after direct current shock. Am J Physiol 257:H1180, 1989.

Tacker WA, Niebauer MJ, Babbs CF, et al: The effect of newer antiarrhythmic drugs on defibrillation threshold. Crit Care Med 8:107, 1980.

Waldecker B, Brugada P, Zehender M, et al: Dysrhythmias after direct-current cardioversion. Am J Cardiol 57:120, 1986.

Weaver WD, Cobb LA, Dennis D, et al: Factors influencing survival after out-of-hospital cardiac arrest. J Am Coll Cardiol 7:752, 1986.

Wesley RC Jr, Resh W, Zimmerman D: Reconsiderations of the routine and preferential use of lidocaine in the emergent treatment of ventricular arrhythmias [see comments]. Crit Care Med 21:305, 1991.

Yakaitis RW, Ewy GA, Otto CW, et al: Influence of time and therapy on VF in dogs. Crit Care Med 8:157, 1980.

Alpha- and Beta-Agonist Intoxications

ANN MARIE MANNING
Boston, Massachusetts

Alpha- and beta-agonist intoxicants encompass a group of drugs that elicit physiologic responses similar to those of endogenous catecholamines. These drugs are structurally similar to catecholamines and stimulate alpha- and beta-adrenergic receptors both directly and indirectly by causing the release of endogenous catecholamines. Toxicity is the result of excessive adrenergic stimulation.

Beta-agonists implicated in intoxication of animals include drugs used for the treatment of asthma in human patients. These drugs are usually in the form of an aerosol contained in a metered-dose inhaler, and intoxication occurs when the canister is punctured and the entire contents are delivered at one time. These drugs include epinephrine, albuterol, metaproterenol, terbutaline, and salmeterol.

Over-the-counter products that contain both beta- and alpha-agonists include nonprescription cold remedies, decongestants, stimulants, and appetite suppressants. These preparations are usually in the form of pills or liquids, and the active ingredients responsible include ephedrine, pseudoephedrine, and phenylpropanolamine. Similar preparations containing alpha-agonists as the prime ingredient are imidazolines and phenylephrine. Amitraz, a compound found in Preventic tick collars, and Mitaban, an acaricidal dip, are also alpha-agonists implicated in increasing numbers of intoxications.

BETA-AGONISTS

Inhaled beta-agonists are the most widely used drugs for the treatment of asthma in human patients. These are prescription drugs provided in the form of metered-dose inhalers, which are propellant-generated aerosols. Propellants contained within inhalers are chlorinated fluorocarbons (e.g., Freon 11 and Freon 12), which are relatively nontoxic with appropriate inhaler use but may be cardiotoxic at high doses, causing sinus bradycardia and asystole (Stiles and Plumb, 1993). Propellants have also been implicated in paradoxical bronchoconstriction and worsening of asthma in human asthma patients after the use of inhalers (Wilkinson et al, 1992). During normal inhaler use, a fixed amount of drug is delivered on activation. Approximately 12% of the drug is delivered to the airways, whereas the remainder is deposited in the mouth, pharynx, and larynx. The potential for poisoning exists when an animal punctures the canister and the entire contents are released into the oral cavity.

Metered-dose preparations of beta-agonists are classified as short-, intermediate-, or long-acting. Catecholamines comprise the group of short-acting beta-agonists. Epinephrine inhalers, which can be purchased over the counter, achieve instant bronchodilation (1 to 3 minutes), reach peak effect within 5 to 15 minutes, and effects wear off in 30 to 60 minutes. Epinephrine is a nonselective beta-agonist.

Intermediate-acting beta-agonists (albuterol, metaproterenol, terbutaline, bitolterol, and procaterol) have a slower onset of bronchodilation (3 to 6 minutes), a delayed peak (20 to 60 minutes) activity, and a sustained effect (4 to 6 hours). Intermediate-acting beta-agonists are the most commonly available. Each of the preceding products is $beta_2$-selective; however, selectivity is lost at higher concentrations, resulting in cardiac and central nervous system stimulation. The majority of these drugs are absorbed rapidly from the gastrointestinal (GI) tract, metabolized by the liver, and excreted by the kidneys. Although the effects from intoxication are similar for all, albuterol in particular is associated with a rapid, dose-related decrease in serum potassium concentrations (Vite and Gfeller, 1996).

Long-acting beta-agonists have prolonged receptor occupancy and persistent functional antagonism at $beta_2$-receptors. The onset of action may take up to 4 hours and effects last as long as 24 hours. Salmeterol is the most common long-acting beta-agonist in the United States. Table 1 lists the most common beta-agonists and the available drug on activation of metered inhalers (Nelson, 1995).

Toxicity and Clinical Signs

Signs of acute intoxication with beta-agonists are an extension of the pharmacologic effects and therefore are

TABLE 1. Common Beta-Agonists Used in Metered-Dose Inhalers*

Generic Name	Trade Name	Dose (per activation)
Intermediate-Acting (3–6 hr)		
Metaproterenol	Alupent, Metaprel	650 µg
Pirbuterol	Maxair	200 µg
Terbutaline	Brethaire	200 µg
Long-Acting (>12 hours)		
Salmeterol	Serevent	21 µg
Albuterol	Proventil, Ventolin	90 µg
Bitolterol	Tornalate	370 µg

*Dose equals the dose delivered per activation of inhaler.

predictable based on beta-agonist actions on adrenergic receptors in various organs. The cardiovascular, musculoskeletal, and central nervous systems are the main targets; however, most organ systems are affected in some manner.

Cardiovascular Effects

Clinical signs associated with the cardiovascular system include tachycardia, bounding femoral pulses, cardiac arrhythmias, and hypotension. Human patients complain of palpitations and angina. Cardiac effects can be explained by stimulation of both $beta_1$- and $beta_2$-adrenoreceptors by nonselective beta-agonists or by $beta_2$-specific agonists that lose selectivity as overdose occurs. Stimulation of $beta_1$- and $beta_2$-adrenoreceptors in the ventricular and atrial myocardium causes positive inotropic and chronotropic effects. Direct simulation of the sinoatrial node may also contribute to sinus tachycardia. Additionally, $beta_2$-selective agonists cause peripheral vasodilatation through stimulation of $beta_2$-receptors in the vascular smooth muscle endothelium, resulting in hypotension and reflex tachycardia (Reed, 1985). This hypotensive effect can create a substantial reduction in diastolic blood pressure, which may cause myocardial ischemia as cardiac perfusion pressure is decreased. Beta-agonists have opposing effects on coronary circulation. Beta-agonists enhance myocardial perfusion by a direct vasodilatory effect and diminish myocardial blood flow indirectly by causing systemic vasodilation. Reported cardiac arrhythmias include ventricular tachycardia, multifocal ventricular tachycardia, sinus tachycardia, and atrioventricular block. The development of cardiac arrhythmias may result from hypokalemia, hypomagnesemia, or myocardial damage from excessive sympathetic stimulation (reflected in increased aspartate aminotransferase and creatine phosphokinase levels). Sudden death is also possible.

Musculoskeletal Effects

Intoxicated animals may present with generalized muscle tremors due to direct stimulation of $beta_2$-receptors in skeletal muscle. All beta-agonists cause a dose-related decrease in serum potassium concentrations. Rapid transmembrane potassium shifts cause hyperpolarization of muscle tissue, increase the resting membrane potential of skeletal muscle, and result in muscular weakness and flaccid paralysis. Body temperature may also be elevated from excessive muscle activity.

Central Nervous System Effects

Beta-agonist intoxication causes stimulation of the central nervous system. Patients may exhibit anxiety, restlessness, hyperactivity, dizziness, prolapsed nictitating membranes, and dilated pupils.

Metabolic Effects

Hypokalemia, hypomagnesemia, hypophosphatemia, hyperglycemia, elevated free fatty acid levels, and increased plasma renin activity may result from beta-agonist intoxications. The serum potassium concentration initially increases as potassium is released from the liver, but levels drop within 30 minutes of intoxication as potassium accumulates in skeletal muscle. Serum potassium levels begin to rise 3 to 6 hours after the initial drop but often remain significantly lower than preintoxication values. Potassium shifts are explained by beta-agonist activation of the Na-K-ATPase pump and potassium accumulation in muscle cells (Clausen, 1983). It is important to note that actual body potassium stores remain normal despite low serum potassium concentrations. Hypokalemia contributes to weakness, dementia, and cardiac abnormalities. Decreased serum magnesium levels may also contribute to cardiac arrhythmias, and hypophosphatemia, in combination with hypokalemia, causes muscle weakness, respiratory muscle fatigue, and decreased tissue oxygen extraction (Bodenhamer et al, 1992). Hyperglycemia results from beta-agonist inhibition of insulin release, stimulation of glycogenolysis, and glucagon release. Increased free fatty acid levels have been incriminated in the development of myocardial necrosis in animals and result from beta-agonist–induced lipolysis.

Respiratory Effects

Tachypnea, dyspnea, and respiratory arrest secondary to severe bronchoconstriction may result from beta-agonist intoxication. Paradoxical bronchoconstriction may result from the propellants used in metered-dose inhalers and does not appear to be related to the beta-agonist (Nicklas, 1990).

Gastrointestinal Effects

Beta-agonist intoxications are associated with nausea, vomiting, and hypersalivation.

Diagnosis

The diagnosis of beta-agonist intoxication is based on a history of exposure and clinical signs. Laboratory findings may also be helpful in supporting a diagnosis. Such findings may include a transient hyperkalemia followed by hypokalemia, hyperglycemia, increased plasma free fatty acids, hypomagnesemia, hypophosphatemia, increased serum aspartate aminotransferase and creatine phosphokinase activities (indicating myocardial necrosis or skeletal muscle damage, or both) and a stress leukogram (mature neutrophilia, lymphopenia, monocytosis).

Treatment

Treatment should be directed at providing supportive and symptomatic care. Gastric lavage may be employed to decrease absorption of the drug if pills or liquids have been ingested; however, gastric lavage is of no value when intoxication is the result of punctured inhalers because the drug is rapidly absorbed from the GI tract. The administration of intravenous (IV) fluids can be used to increase intravascular volume and to enhance secretion of the drugs and metabolites. Potassium should be supplemented with IV fluids as needed. The administration of dextrose-containing fluids may contribute to decreases in serum potassium by stimulating insulin release and should be avoided.

The use of beta-blockers should be determined on a case-by-case basis. In general, the use of beta-blockers should be reserved for atrial tachycardia more than 250 beats per minute (beats/min), sustained ventricular tachycardia, intermittent ventricular tachycardia greater than 200 beats/min, multifocal ventricular tachycardia, ventricular depolarization associated with an R-on-T phenomenon, or clinical signs of decreased cardiac output (pale mucous membranes, weak pulses, cold extremities) (Stiles and Plumb, 1993). Propanolol, a nonselective beta-blocker, may be used at an initial dosage of 0.05 mg/kg of body weight IV. Propanolol is rapidly eliminated, and multiple dosages at 0.025 mg/kg IV may be required to control tachyarrhythmias. Propanolol should be administered cautiously because it may cause atrioventricular block and bronchoconstriction. Beta$_1$-selective blocking agents such as metoprolol (5 to 50 mg every 8 to 12 hours PO) and atenolol (6.25 to 12.5 mg every 12 hours PO) may be more beneficial, as these drugs help to decrease the heart rate but are less likely to cause bronchospasm that can be associated with nonselective beta blockade (Rush and Keene, 1990). Diazepam may be used as needed for sedation at a dosage of 0.5 mg/kg IV.

Monitoring

Continuous electrocardiographic monitoring is essential for cases of beta-agonist intoxication because cardiac arrhythmias are the most frequent manifestation of intoxication. Serial systemic arterial blood pressure measurements (see *CVT XII,* p. 110) and serum potassium, magnesium, and phosphorus levels should be monitored carefully during the initial 24 hours. The duration of toxicity is usually 24 to 36 hours.

ALPHA-AGONISTS

The effects of alpha-agonists vary depending on whether central or peripheral adrenoreceptors are affected preferentially. Stimulation of central alpha$_2$-adrenoreceptors in the ventrolateral medulla causes reduced sympathetic outflow, resulting in decreased systemic arterial blood pressure and bradycardia. Stimulation of central alpha$_2$-receptors can also enhance parasympathetic outflow, potentiating reflex bradycardia. The stimulation of peripheral alpha$_1$-receptors located on the postsynaptic membrane results in smooth muscle contraction, vasoconstriction, and increased systemic arterial blood pressure. A slow-onset, prolonged increase in cardiac contractility occurs when peripheral alpha$_1$-receptors, located on myocardial cells, are stimulated. Peripheral alpha$_2$-receptors are located on the presynaptic membrane of sympathetic nerves, and stimulation results in inhibition of norepinephrine release and local feedback regulation of activity at the sympathetic nerve terminus. The stimulation of alpha$_2$-receptors located on postsynaptic smooth muscle produces smooth muscle contraction (Ruffolo, 1994).

Imidazolines

Oxymetazoline, naphazoline, tetrahydrozoline, and xylometazoline are imidazolines used in topical nasal and ocular decongestants. These compounds are rapidly absorbed from the GI tract if ingested. The serum half-life is approximately 2 to 4 hours, and side effects disappear within 24 hours of exposure. The toxicity observed with these compounds is primarily due to central alpha$_2$-receptor activity. Cardiovascular parameters may vary markedly, ranging from hypotension and bradycardia due to central alpha$_2$-stimulation to hypertension and tachycardia due to peripheral alpha$_1$-stimulation (Certaruk and Aaron, 1994). Animals may alternate between central nervous system depression (lethargy, sedation, coma) and central nervous system excitation (nervousness, agitation, seizures). Intoxicated animals may also exhibit muscle tremors, nausea, and respiratory depression. Gastric lavage is of limited value because of rapid absorption; however, administration of activated charcoal (1 to 4 g/kg PO or 1 g/5 ml H_2O; 10 ml/kg) is indicated. Management of these patients is directed at maintaining stable hemodynamic and respiratory status.

Phenylephrine

Phenylephrine is a potent alpha-agonist found in nasal decongestants. It is erratically absorbed when ingested and undergoes first-pass metabolism by monoamine oxidase in the liver and gastrointestinal tract. The serum half-life is 2 to 3 hours and known side effects include hypertension and myocardial ischemia. Treatment of intoxication includes gastric lavage, administration of activated charcoal (1 to 4 g/kg PO or 1 g/5 ml H_2O; 10 ml/kg), and control of hypertension.

Amitraz

The ingestion of tick collars containing amitraz (Preventic 9% amitraz) is becoming more common in canine veterinary patients. The clinical signs associated with amitraz intoxication include bradycardia, hypotension, hypothermia (central alpha$_2$ effects), ileus, respiratory depression, vomiting, sedation, depression, disorientation, ataxia, hyperglycemia, and seizures. The clinical signs usually appear within hours of ingestion and persist as long as pieces of collar remain in the GI tract. The diagnosis of amitraz toxicity is based on a history of collar ingestion and the appearance of clinical signs. Abdominal radiographs can be taken to confirm pieces of collar in the GI tract. Treatment is aimed at removal of the collar pieces from the GI tract by induced vomiting or via endoscopic removal, followed by administration of activated charcoal as discussed earlier and a cathartic such as magnesium sulfate (5 gm PO). Intravenous fluids may be administered to provide intravascular volume expansion in hypotensive patients. Yohimbine is used to reverse the centrally mediated alpha effects of bradycardia and hypotension. The recommended dosage of yohimbine is 0.1 mg/kg of body weight IV, and repeated administration may be necessary. Serial systemic arterial blood pressure measurement and continuous monitoring of the patient for changes in mentation are necessary.

MIXED ALPHA- AND BETA-AGONISTS

Ephedrine and Pseudoephedrine

Ephedrine and pseudoephedrine are common ingredients of nonprescription cold remedies, decongestants, stimulants, and appetite depressants. These are usually oral preparations, which are metabolized slowly and have a prolonged duration of action. Pseudoephedrine is less potent than ephedrine, causing one-quarter the vasopressor effect and one-half the bronchodilator effect (Certaruk and Aaron, 1994). The clinical signs of toxicity include nausea, vomiting, agitation, tachycardia, hypertension, seizures, muscle tremors, and rhabdomyolysis. For treatment of intoxication, gastric lavage and activated charcoal (1 to 4 g/kg PO) are recommended, along with the administration of IV fluids to increase urine acidity and to hasten drug excretion. Hypertension can be controlled with enalapril (0.25 to 0.5 mg/kg every 12 hours PO) or direct-acting vasodilators such as sodium nitroprusside (see p. 194). Diazepam can be administered at a dose of 0.5 mg/kg IV to control seizures. Attempts to control tachyarrhythmias with propranolol should be avoided because this can worsen hypertension by causing unopposed alpha-mediated vasoconstriction. The duration of toxicity is usually 6 to 8 hours.

Phenylpropanolamine

Phenylpropanolamine is an indirect alpha-adrenergic receptor agonist that stimulates release of norepinephrine from postganglionic sympathetic nerve terminals. Phenylpropanolamine also has direct alpha-receptor agonist and weak beta-receptor agonist activity. The drug is rapidly absorbed from the GI tract and reaches peak plasma levels within 1.5 to 3 hours. The duration of action of phenylpropanolamine is 4 to 6 hours. The clinical signs of toxicity are manifested as hypertension and reflex bradycardia, cardiac arrhythmias, nausea, vomiting, lethargy, and rhabdomyolysis. The treatment of toxicity should include gastric lavage, administration of activated charcoal, and control of hypertension as for ephedrine and pseudoephedrine.

References and Suggested Reading

Bodenhamer J, Bergstrom R, Brown D, et al: Frequently nebulized beta-agonists for asthma: Effects on serum electrolytes. Ann Emerg Med 21:53, 1992.

Certaruk EW, Aaron CK: Hazards of non-prescription medications. Emerg Med Clin North Am 12:483, 1994.

Clausen T: Adrenergic control of Na^+ and K^+ homeostasis. Acta Med Scand 672(suppl):111, 1983.

Nelson HS: Beta-adrenergic bronchodilators. N Engl J Med 333:499, 1995.

Nicklas RA: Paradoxical bronchospasm associated with the use of inhaled beta agonists. J Allergy Clin Immunol 85:959, 1990.

Reed CR: Adrenergic bronchodilators: Pharmacology and toxicology. J Allergy Clin Immunol 76:335, 1985.

Ruffolo RR: Cardiovascular adrenoreceptors: Physiology and critical care implications. In: Chernow B, ed: The Pharmacologic Approach to the Critically Ill Patient, 3rd ed. Baltimore: Williams & Wilkins, 1994, p 168.

Rush JR, Keene BW: Metaproterenol intoxication in a dog. J Am Vet Med Assoc 197:1351, 1990.

Stiles J, Plumb DC: Toxicity associated with beta-agonist aerosol exposure in three dogs. J Am Anim Hosp Assoc 29:235, 1993.

Vite CH, Gfeller RW: Suspected albuterol intoxication in a dog. J Vet Emerg Crit Care 4:7, 1996.

Wilkinson JR, Roberts JA, Bradding P, et al: Paradoxical bronchoconstriction in asthmatic patients after salmeterol by metered dose inhaler. BMJ 305:931, 1992.

Zaritsky AL: Catecholamines, inotropic medications, and vasopressor agents. In: Chernow B, ed: The Pharmacologic Approach to the Critically Ill Patient. Baltimore: Williams & Wilkins, 1994, p 387.

Thoracoscopy

RONALD S. WALTON
Kaiserslautern, Germany

TIMOTHY B. HACKETT
Fort Collins, Colorado

Thoracoscopy is a minimally invasive operative procedure designed for visual inspection of the thoracic cavity and its organs. The techniques were first developed in the early 1900s using a simple cystoscope in an attempt to break down adhesive tuberculosis lesions in human patients. Thoracoscopy was in widespread use until the mid-1940s, when operative and anesthesia techniques as well as antibiotic therapy provided a successful avenue for the widespread use of operative thoracotomy techniques. Today, with expanded efforts to explore minimally invasive surgical techniques, there is a renewed interest in thoracoscopy in human thoracic medicine and surgery. With only a few isolated reports of thoracoscopy in the veterinary literature, its use has been limited to a few veterinary referral centers. Newer, more sophisticated, less expensive instrumentation makes this technique readily available to many veterinarians. Thoracoscopic techniques are in many ways easier to perform than is a standard laparoscopy. A knowledge of regional anatomy, appropriate preoperative staging, and a working knowledge of the equipment are required before beginning this diagnostic procedure. Many uses and techniques for thoracoscopy have recently been described in the human literature. The application of these techniques is limited only by the skill and imagination of the clinician.

INDICATIONS

Some of the indications for thoracoscopic exploration in humans include the following: general thoracoscopic exploration, management of malignant pleural effusion, staging of neoplasia, assessment of lesion resectability, implantation of epicardial pacemaker leads, and the correction of vascular anomalies. Thoracoscopy has been useful in veterinary medicine to biopsy hilar and mediastinal masses found during radiographic or ultrasonographic evaluation, when fluid loculation cannot be differentiated from solid masses, for treatment of malignant pleural effusions, and in pericardial disease. At our hospital, thoracoscopy has been used for staging neoplastic disease and preoperative evaluation of lesion resectability. Thoracoscopy is less invasive than is a traditional thoracotomy and is associated with lower morbidity and mortality. The view obtained with thoracoscopy is often superior to that obtained with a traditional thoracotomy because any structure within the thorax can be easily visualized in a magnified view. With the use of a small video camera, a well-illuminated view is displayed. *Surgical application* in the veterinary patient is largely undeveloped. The technology is available and the techniques of biopsy, partial lung lobectomies, partial pericardiectomies, and esophagomyotomies have been described.

EQUIPMENT

The basic instrumentation for thoracoscopy is the same as that needed for laparoscopy. One instrument set can be used for examination of both major body cavities. Traditionally, thoracoscopic instruments are shorter than are those commonly used in laparoscopy. The decreased length of the instruments and trocars makes them easier to maneuver in the limited confines of the thoracic cavity. Laparoscopic instruments, however, can easily be substituted in the veterinary patient. The basic set consists of a Hopkins rigid telescope (0 or 30 degree), introducing trocar-cannula apparatus, light source (xenon), and instrument set consisting of a palpation probe, grasping forceps, biopsy forceps, and scissors. A 4- to 5-mm set will accommodate the needs of most veterinary patients. A minor surgery set is required to place the trocars and to suture the sites closed at the completion of the procedure. Sufficient surgical instrumentation should be readily available in case conversion to a thoracotomy becomes necessary. A micro-video camera and monitor are highly recommended to enhance the view and ease of tissue manipulation. Electrocautery is also highly recommended but is not essential. Most of the available instrumentation is equipped for electrocautery attachment.

Video-assisted thoracoscopy is state of the art in human thoracic surgery and eliminates the need to use a small eyepiece with its limited visual field. Thoracoscopic instrumentation is a rapidly expanding field with many new innovations. One should refer to the References and Sug-

TABLE 1. Visualization of Thoracic Features by Trocar Insertion Site

	Trocar Insertion Site		
Anatomic Feature	*Paraxiphoid*	*Intercostal*	*Thoracic Inlet*
Diaphragm	+	+ + +	+ + +Ω
Pericardium	+ + +	+ +Ω	+Ω
Hilus of the lung	na	+ + +Ω	+ +Ω
Lung lobes	+ +	+ + +	+
Mediastinum	+ +	+ + +	+ + +Ω

na, nonvisualized structure; +, fair to poor visualization; + +, good visualization; + + +, excellent visualization. Ω indicates that manipulation of overlying structures was required by the use of additional trocars and a standard palpation probe to visualize certain structures.

gested Reading at the end of this chapter for descriptions of the advanced ligature, suturing, and stapling devices that are currently available for surgical and biopsy procedures.

PREOPERATIVE STAGING

It is important to plan thoracoscopic exploration. One should ask, "Why are you doing the procedure? What do you plan to do with the findings (open thoracotomy, biopsy, and so on)? Where is the lesion of interest? What approach or approaches will allow the best access to the lesion of interest? Which intercostal space do you plan to enter?"

Preoperative staging will help you avoid the common complications of thoracoscopy: spearing the lung with the trocar, entering the wrong side or location of the thorax, penetrating viscera through a large diaphragmatic hernia, or entering a clotted hemothorax. Limiting risk associated with thoracoscopy is necessary to complete an examination successfully. Patient evaluation, including thoracic radiographs within 24 hours of the procedure, limits costly mistakes.

TECHNIQUE

Anesthesia

Choice of anesthetic agent or agents is dictated by the patient's physical condition and is based on clinical judgment. General anesthesia with mechanical ventilation is recommended; however, we have performed this procedure repeatedly on spontaneous ventilating dogs without difficulty. A partial pneumothorax is induced when the pleural space is entered. The use of laparoscopic cannulas with one-way valves allows maintenance of a new airtight seal and precise regulation of the degree of pneumothorax induced. Free air can be added or removed by the insufflation port on the cannula. The use of nonvalved or open cannula ports makes mechanical ventilation mandatory, as the thorax is open to atmospheric pressure. As surgical procedures are developed and used, one-lung ventilation techniques will become necessary to provide complete visualization and precise manipulation of instrumentation and tissues. The full physiologic effects of one-lung ventilation techniques will allow greater exposure by collapsing the lung of interest while ventilating and maintaining respiratory function with the contralateral lung field. However, complete exploration of the thorax can be accomplished safely and easily without one-lung ventilation techniques. Based on prior research, it has been demonstrated that a large amount of air can be introduced into the thorax prior to any significant manifestation of respiratory or cardiovascular embarrassment.

There are three basic approaches to the thorax: the paraxiphoid transdiaphragmatic, intercostal, and thoracic inlet approaches. Each of the approaches has indications based on the anatomic features of interest. Table 1 lists several anatomic features accessible via thoracoscopy and the approaches that provide the best visibility. Figure 1 depicts the positions of trocar placement for the three basic approaches.

Paraxiphoid Transdiaphragmatic Approach

The paraxiphoid approach (see Fig. 1A) is useful for most applications. This allows excellent evaluation of the

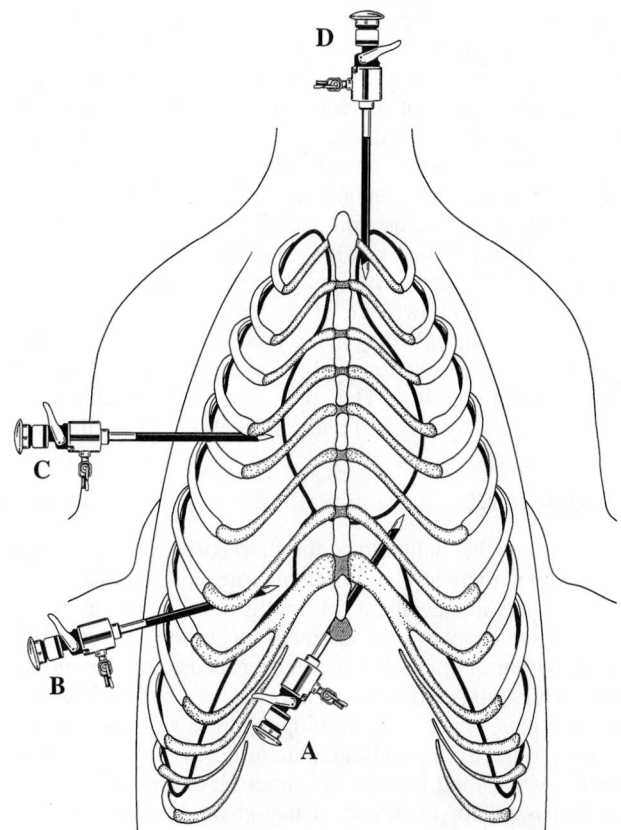

Figure 1. A dog in dorsal recumbency, with the various trocar insertion sites for thoracoscopic exploration. *A,* paraxiphoid transdiaphragmatic; *B,* caudal intercostal (7th ICS); *C,* cranial intercostal (4th ICS); *D,* thoracic inlet.

ventral aspects of both hemithoraces and requires less technical expertise. A typical laparoscopy (6 mm) multifunctional valve, or trumpet valve trocar is used for this insertion technique. The patient is positioned in dorsal recumbency and is clipped and prepared for a standard median sternotomy. The clinician should be prepared to convert to an open thoracic procedure if necessary. A small stab incision is made approximately 5 mm to the right or left of the xiphoid process. The trocar is grasped to control the penetration depth to just inside the thoracic cavity. On penetrating the ventral abdominal musculature and the abdominal surface of the ventromedial portion of the *pars sternalis*, the sharp tip of the trocar is directed in a cranial ventral direction (toward the sternum). When the pleural surface of the diaphragm is penetrated, the sharp trocar is withdrawn. The telescopic assembly is then inserted into the trocar valve and the scope is advanced until the ventral thoracic cavity is visualized. The thoracic cavity is examined by advancing the scope cranially.

Intercostal Approach

The intercostal approach is the most common approach described in the literature. The patient can be positioned in right or left lateral recumbency, in dorsal recumbency, or in an oblique fashion, depending on the structure or structures to be evaluated. The trocar is typically inserted at the seventh intercostal space (ICS) midway between the costochondral junction and ventral border of the epaxial muscles. Insertion caudally from the seventh ICS (see Fig. 1B) or craniad from the fourth ICS (see Fig. 1C) allows access to most anatomic features in each hemithorax. A short, rigid or flexible trocar cannula would typically be used for this location. A valve or nonvalved cannula can be used. Flexible cannulas such as the FLEXIPATH by Ethican Endo-Surgery can be cut to any length desired and allow introduction of standard operative instruments such as a right-angled forceps. Trocar insertion at the seventh ICS allows wide exploration and visualization of the entire lateral thorax. After making a small (6- to 7-mm) skin incision, blunt dissection of the subcutaneous tissue and underlying musculature with a hemostat will expose the pleura. Once atmospheric communication with the pleural space is achieved, the lung will fall away from the chest wall unless significant adhesions exist. The trocar can be gently and safely inserted with this technique. With placement of an additional trocar in the fourth ICS, a palpation probe will allow movement and examination of adjacent lung lobes and visualization of peribronchial tissues, pulmonary arteries and veins, hilar lymph nodes, and all aspects of the pleural surface of the diaphragm.

Thoracic Inlet Approach

Patients are positioned in dorsal recumbency. A small (6- to 7-mm) skin incision is made on the right or left side of the thoracic inlet between the cranial medial edge of the first rib and the lateral aspect of the trachea. The trocar is inserted under the skin and advanced in a caudal lateral direction toward the medial surface of the second rib. Both the right and left hemithoraces can be examined. The membranous nature of the cranial mediastinum makes anatomic orientation difficult with this approach. With patience, a cranial to caudal view of each hemithorax is possible. This technique carries more risk because blind trocar insertion is in close proximity to the internal thoracic artery and vein, brachycephalic trunk, subclavian artery and vein, common carotid artery, and vagus and phrenic nerves. There is little indication for this approach; most structures can be visualized with the safer cranial intercostal techniques.

POSTOPERATIVE CARE

After thoracoscopy, the air in the thoracic space should be withdrawn. Standard suction can be applied to the insufflation stopcock valve to evacuate the thorax. A thoracic drain should be placed after completion of the procedure and the patient should be monitored closely for signs of respiratory distress. Drain placement and function can be assessed thoracoscopically before the telescope trocar is removed. After removal of the cannulas, the wounds are sutured with a standard two-layer closure. Intermittent or continuous suction of the thoracic drain should be performed until the lungs are fully expanded. A postoperative thoracic radiograph may be used to confirm the resolution of the pneumothorax. In many patients, the thoracic drain can be removed in the early recovery period (within 4 to 6 hours); however, various pathologic processes may require long-term drainage. Systemic analgesics have rarely been necessary in the postoperative period when the trocar port sites are infused with local anesthetics at the conclusion of the procedure.

References and Suggested Reading

Allen MS, Deschamps C, Jones DM, et al: Video assisted thoracic surgical procedures: The Mayo experience. Mayo Clin Proc 71:351, 1996.

Bauer T, Thomas VP: Pulmonary diagnostic techniques. Vet Clin North Am Small Anim Pract 13:273, 1983.

Bennett RA, Orton EC, Tucker A, et al: Cardiopulmonary changes in conscious dogs with induced progressive pneumothorax. Am J Vet Res 50:280, 1989.

Braimbridge MV: The history of thoracoscopic surgery. Ann Thorac Surg 56:610, 1993.

Horswell JL: Anesthetic techniques for thoracoscopy. Ann Thorac Surg 56:624, 1993.

Kadukura M: Pathologic comparisons of video-assisted thoracoscopic lung biopsy with traditional lung biopsy. J Thor Cardiovasc Surg 109:494, 1995.

Kaiser LR, Vabaria JE: Complications of thoracoscopy. Ann Thorac Surg 56:796, 1993.

McCarthy TC, McDermaid SL: Thoracoscopy. Vet Clin North Am Small Anim Pract 20:1341, 1990.

Naruke T, Asamura H, Kondo H, et al: Thoracoscopy for staging of lung cancer. Ann Thorac Surg 56:661, 1993.

Potter LA: Video-assisted thoracic surgery (VATS). Am Coll Vet Surgeons Veterinary Symposium (Small Animal Proceedings) ACVS, Bethesda, 1996, pp 416–419.

Acute Abdomen: Evaluation and Emergency Treatment

F. A. MANN
Columbia, Missouri

Acute abdomen may be defined as the acute onset of abdominal pain necessitating prompt diagnosis and immediate medical or surgical intervention to prevent deterioration of the patient. Because many of the conditions responsible for acute abdomen may progress to a state of shock, abdominal pain may not be evident at the time the animal is presented for medical attention.

CLINICAL SIGNS

Abdominal pain may be manifested as peculiar posture, such as the praying position. In the praying position, the animal lies in sternal recumbency with the pelvic limbs in standing position to elevate the pelvis and caudal abdomen. Animals may also exhibit abdominal pain by a reluctance to move, by ambulating in a stilted gait, or by taking short, careful steps. Abdominal tenderness may be noted by an avoidance reaction, vocalization, or guarding ("splinting") when the abdomen is touched. Some animals with acute abdomen may become apprehensive in anticipation of abdominal contact. Nausea exhibited through hypersalivation may be apparent as a result of abdominal pain. Other clinical signs are related to the underlying cause of the acute abdomen, such as protracted vomiting from pancreatitis, fever due to septic peritonitis, hemorrhagic diarrhea resulting from canine parvoviral enteritis, and pale mucous membranes due to traumatic hemoabdomen.

DIFFERENTIAL DIAGNOSES

Differential diagnoses of disorders that may lead to the development of acute abdomen are listed in Table 1. Some of these causes have obvious surgical or medical indications, whereas others require some decision-making based on the individual situation. Many acute abdomen patients have serious diseases that require prompt attention to patient status and appropriate stabilization measures before a definitive diagnosis can be achieved and specific therapy implemented.

INITIAL PATIENT MANAGEMENT

On presentation, the patient with an acute abdomen should have a rapid primary survey to ascertain immediate needs and to determine priorities in diagnostics and therapeutics. The primary survey should include an abbreviated physical examination with emphasis on mental, respiratory, and cardiovascular status. Severely depressed animals with abnormal breathing and altered (weak or bounding) peripheral pulses should be interpreted to be in (or progressing toward) shock and should have appropriate resuscitative measures prior to detailed diagnostics and definitive therapy (see other chapters in this section). Immediately prior to emergency treatment procedures (such as shock doses of intravenous fluids), blood and urine samples should be obtained for a minimal database (see p. 140).

DIAGNOSTICS

Signalment and History

Signalment and history can be helpful in shortening the list of differential diagnoses and arranging those remaining according to likelihood. For example, a schnauzer with acute abdominal pain is more likely to have acute pancreatitis than gastric dilatation-volvulus. A history of dietary indiscretion in a well-vaccinated dog with no exposure to other dogs would prioritize garbage intoxication over parvoviral enteritis. A complete history should be taken, but certain questions should be emphasized in cases of acute abdomen as listed in Table 2.

Physical Examination

A complete body systems review is important for a full understanding of the patient's condition, but the patient's initial status may dictate that some aspects of the physical examination receive a low priority. Physical evaluation not directly related to the patient's immediate status can be postponed. The abdominal portion of the physical examination should be performed in each case of acute abdomen. However, the abdominal evaluation should be the last part of the physical examination for two reasons: (1) serious extra-abdominal abnormalities may be overlooked and (2) manipulation of a tender abdomen may elicit pain and apprehension that could interfere with further evaluation.

Physical examination of the abdomen should include visual inspection, auscultation, percussion, ballottement, superficial and deep palpation, and digital rectal palpation. The examination should proceed from the least to most likely technique to elicit a pain response. Abnormalities that may be detected on visual inspection include distention (such as with abdominal effusion), deformity (caused by a large abdominal mass or hernia), swelling (such as with cellulitis associated with urine leakage), and bruising (associated with coagulopathy or blunt trauma). Red discoloration around the umbilicus is indicative of intra-abdominal hemorrhage. Visual inspection may also reveal puncture wounds (associated with penetrating trauma such as animal bites or projectiles), but the wounds may not be evident without clipping of abdominal hair.

TABLE 1. Differential Diagnoses for the Acute Abdomen

Body System–Cause of Acute Abdomen	Treatment	Body System–Cause of Acute Abdomen	Treatment
Gastrointestinal Digestive System		**Reproductive System**	
Gastric dilatation	DS, PE	*Female*	
Gastric dilatation-volvulus	DS, DE	Acute metritis	PS, PE
Gastroduodenal ulceration	NS	Pyometra	DS, DE
Gastroduodenal perforation	DS, PE	Uterine torsion	DS, DE
Gastroduodenal rupture	DS, PE	Dystocia	PS, PE
Gastroduodenal dehiscence	DS, DE	Uterine rupture	DS, DE
Gastroenteritis (viral, bacterial, toxic, i.e., garbage)	NS	Ovarian cyst	PS, PE
Hemorrhagic gastroenteritis	NS	Ovarian neoplasia	DS, PE
Intestinal obstruction (foreign body, intussusception, neoplasia)	DS, PE	*Male*	
		Acute prostatitis	NS
Functional intestinal obstruction: ileus	NS	Prostatic abscess	DS, PE
Intestinal ulceration	NS	Prostatic cysts	DS, PE
Intestinal perforation	DS, DE	Prostatic neoplasia	DS, PE
Intestinal rupture	DS, DE	Testicular torsion	DS, DE
Intestinal dehiscence	DS, DE	**Hematopoietic System: Spleen**	
Intestinal volvulus	DS, DE	Splenic mass (hematoma, extramedullary hematopoiesis, neoplasia, nodular hyperplasia, abscess)	DS, PE
Cecal inversion	DS, PE		
Obstipation	NS		
Colitis	NS	Splenic rupture (mass)	DS, DE
Colonic ulceration	NS	Splenic rupture (trauma)	PS, PE
Colonic perforation	DS, DE	Splenic torsion	DS, DE
Colonic rupture	DS, DE	**Peritoneum and Mesentery**	
Colonic dehiscence	DS, DE	Peritonitis: septic	DS, DE
Hepatobiliary Digestive System		Peritonitis: chemical (bile, urine, pancreatic enzymes)	PS, PE
Acute hepatitis (toxic, infectious)	NS		
Hepatic abscess	DS, PE	Parietal peritoneal trauma: blunt	NS
Hepatic trauma	PS, PE	Parietal peritoneal trauma: penetrating	DS, DE
Hepatic rupture	PS, PE	Mesenteric traction–large masses	DS, PE
Hepato-biliary neoplasia	PS, PE	Mesenteric lymphadenopathy	PS, PE
Biliary obstruction (calculi, neoplasia, pancreatitis-abscess)	PS, PE	Mesenteric lymphadenitis	NS
		Mesenteric volvulus	DS, DE
Biliary rupture	DS, DE	Mesenteric avulsion	DS, DE
Cholecystitis	PS, PE	Mesenteric artery thrombosis	DS, DE
Cholangiohepatitis	NS	Adhesions with organ entrapment–internal hernias	DS, PE
Pancreatic Digestive System			
Acute pancreatitis	NS	**Abdominal Wall**	
Pancreatic abscess	DS, PE	Trauma	PS, PE
Pancreatic neoplasia	DS, PE	Abscess	DS, PE
Urinary System		Hematoma	PS, PE
Acute nephrosis (toxicosis)	NS	Strangulated hernias	DS, DE
Acute nephritis-pyelonephritis	NS	**Extra-abdominal**	
Urinary calculi: renal	PS, PE	Intervertebral disc disease	PS, PE
Urinary calculi: ureteral	PS, PE	Discospondylitis	PS, PE
Urinary calculi: cystic	PS, PE	Toxicities (heavy metal)	NS
Urinary calculi: urethral	PS, PE	Thoracic wall disease	PS, PE
Trauma-avulsion-rupture (renal, ureteral, cystic, urethral)	DS, PE	Steatitis	NS
		Myositis	NS
Obstruction (neoplasia, stricture): ureter	DS, PE	Hypoadrenocorticism	NS
Obstruction (neoplasia, stricture): urethra	DS, PE		
Renal artery thrombosis	PS, PE		
Renal neoplasia	PS, PE		

DS, definitely surgical; PS, potentially surgical; DE, definitely requires emergent surgery; PE, potentially requires emergent surgery (some conditions designated as PE may require surgery, although not on an emergent basis); NS, nonsurgical (the urgency of medical treatment depends on the specific problem and the condition of the animal; some nonsurgical acute abdomen cases may eventually require surgery on a nonemergent basis).

Abdominal auscultation is performed to characterize gut sounds. Increased gut sounds may be evident in acute cases of enteritis, intestinal obstruction, and toxin ingestion. Absence of gut sounds suggests ileus, chronic intestinal obstruction, peritonitis, or abdominal effusion. Anorexia causes decreased intestinal motility, necessitating a long period (2 to 3 minutes) of auscultation before ascertaining that gut sounds are absent. Failure to auscult abnormal (increased or absent) gut sounds does not mean that the abdomen is normal; normal gut motility may be maintained in the early post-traumatic period and in early peritoneal effusion.

Percussion can be performed with or without the aid of a stethoscope to detect hyperresonance (indicating intra-abdominal air, usually a gas-filled viscus) or hyporesonance (indicating intra-abdominal fluid). If the animal is standing, a fluid line may be percussed between areas of hyper- and hyporesonance. Ballottement can be performed in standing and in recumbent animals by tapping the abdomen and looking for a ripple effect to confirm the presence of intra-abdominal fluid. Animals with a large amount of intra- or extra-abdominal fat can appear to ripple on ballottement, yielding a false-positive diagnosis of abdominal effusion.

Palpation of the abdomen is performed to detect pain,

TABLE 2. Historical Information to be Included in Cases of Acute Abdomen

Diet
Appetite
Weight change
Water consumption
Urination: characterize—polyuria, anuria, pollakiuria
Defecation, Diarrhea: characterize—frequency, presence of blood, color, volume, relation to meals
Vomiting: characterize—frequency, presence of blood, color, volume, relation to meals
Exposure to toxins, trauma (blunt, penetrating), foreign body ingestion
Previous disease
Previous abdominal surgery
Length of illness
How quickly signs developed

masses, and enlargement, displacement, or other abnormalities of abdominal organs. Superficial palpation is used to detect, characterize, and potentially localize pain and should be performed prior to deep palpation. Reproducible abdominal guarding ("splinting") in response to superficial palpation is indicative of abdominal pain. Stimulation of irritated parietal peritoneum by superficial abdominal palpation is a major reason for the pain response. Another potential response to parietal peritoneum stimulation is nausea and vomiting. Deep palpation should be performed to characterize the structures and abnormal findings in each of three regions: cranial, middle, and caudal abdomen. The final evaluation of the caudal abdomen should include digital examination per rectum to assess the prostate, pelvis, pelvic urethra, sublumbar lymph nodes (if enlarged), and rectum, and to evaluate the character and color of the stool.

The physical examination will not necessarily provide a definitive diagnosis, nor will it necessarily dictate a particular therapeutic measure. However, it will help the clinician select the most appropriate diagnostic tests and, if performed serially, will keep the clinician abreast of changes in patient status.

Clinical Pathology

Laboratory testing of blood and urine is useful in providing confirmatory data, sometimes leading to a definitive diagnosis and, probably most important, providing a current picture of the patient's hematologic and metabolic status (see p. 110). A complete blood count provides information regarding anemia, platelet numbers, and hydration status (packed cell volume and total serum solids), which are important influences on treatment decisions. The leukogram provides information regarding the inflammatory status of the condition. A biochemistry profile may help localize the underlying disease to a specific organ and gives important information about the patient's acid-base balance and electrolyte status. Urinalysis, especially when interpreted in conjunction with biochemistry panels, provides essential information regarding renal function and other urinary tract abnormalities. In emergency situations, such as when contemplating emergent celiotomy, waiting for

laboratory test results can be detrimental to the patient's well-being. In such circumstances, an emergency minimal database should include determinations of packed cell volume, total serum solids, serum creatinine or blood urea nitrogen, serum glucose, serum electrolytes, and urine specific gravity as well as urine reagent strip test results. The remaining tests can be done later on pretreatment samples.

Diagnostic Imaging

Abdominal radiography, ultrasonography, and contrast studies may provide valuable directions to patient management. Abdominal radiographs should be taken as part of the standard evaluation in most cases of acute abdomen. Notable exceptions include (1) evisceration, (2) penetrating trauma, (3) postoperative abdomen with peritonitis confirmed on abdominocentesis, and (4) suspected cases of gastric dilatation-volvulus in which the patient is in respiratory distress. In the latter example, once the animal is stable and the stomach is decompressed, a right lateral abdominal radiograph may be obtained to confirm the diagnosis. Standing lateral views may be employed in cases of abdominal effusion that would otherwise have little abdominal detail. Notable positive radiographic findings in acute abdomen cases include the presence of fluid (abdominal effusion), gas-distended intestines (obstruction or ileus), free abdominal air (ruptured viscus), masses, organomegaly, foreign bodies, urinary calculi, and signs of pancreatitis (loss of detail in the right cranial quadrant and lateral displacement of a gas-filled descending duodenum).

Abdominal ultrasonography is helpful in defining masses and enlarged organs, especially when abdominal effusion causes loss of radiographic detail. Ultrasonography is particularly helpful in the identification of fluid-filled lesions (such as abscesses) and the characterization of abnormalities of the liver, spleen, prostate, and kidneys. Fine needle aspiration or needle biopsy of abnormal structures, or both, can be guided by ultrasonographic examination.

Contrast radiography of the gastrointestinal and urinary systems is sometimes necessary in acute abdomen if survey radiographs fail to define a suspected abnormality. Barium studies can be used to confirm and localize gastrointestinal obstruction. Water-soluble contrast agents should be used when gastrointestinal perforation is suspected. Intravenous urography and urethrocystography are used to confirm and localize discontinuity, obstruction, and other physical abnormalities of the urinary system. When diagnostic imaging fails to define the diagnosis and course of therapy clearly, sampling of abdominal fluid is necessary.

Abdominocentesis–Diagnostic Peritoneal Lavage

Sampling of abdominal fluid is most commonly performed to determine if the patient requires exploratory celiotomy, particularly emergent celiotomy. Abdominocentesis may result in a diagnostic sample if the abdominal fluid is of sufficient volume (approximately 20 ml/kg). Typically, each of four abdominal quadrants is aseptically tapped using a hypodermic needle or, preferably, a multiholed catheter. A standard over-the-needle intravenous catheter can be modified for abdominocentesis by making side holes with a scalpel blade. Care should be exercised to make the side holes small and smooth to prevent kinking and tearing of the catheter within the abdomen. The four-quadrant tap is performed with the animal in a standing position if he or she can stand voluntarily. If all four sites fail to yield fluid or are otherwise nondiagnostic, diagnostic peritoneal lavage is the next step.

Diagnostic peritoneal lavage is performed with a multiholed catheter. Commercially available dialysis catheters can be used, or standard intravenous catheters can be modified as described for abdominocentesis. The author prefers to use a commercially available thoracocentesis catheter (Argyle Turkel Safety Thoracentesis System, Sherwood Davis and Geck, St. Louis, MO) that has a protected needle-stylet and four offset side holes. Additional side holes can be made if desired. The ventral midline just caudal to the umbilicus has been recommended for diagnostic peritoneal lavage catheter placement (Crowe, 1988). However, the author prefers to enter the abdomen just to the right (2 to 3 cm in midsized dogs) of the umbilicus to avoid interference with the falciform ligament and median ligament of the bladder. The right side is used to minimize the chance of iatrogenic damage to the spleen and descending colon. A subcutaneous bleb of local anesthetic is placed at the proposed entry site, and a tiny stab incision is made in the skin with a No. 11 scalpel blade. The catheter is advanced through the skin stab and into the abdomen. Once the catheter is in the abdomen, a syringe is attached and gentle aspiration is applied. If a diagnostic sample is obtained, there is no need to progress with the lavage. In the absence of an adequate sample, 22 ml/kg of warmed, sterile isotonic saline is infused into the catheter via an intravenous infusion set with rapid gravity flow or by applying moderate pressure to the bag of saline. After completing the infusion, the patient is rolled gently from side to side and the abdomen is gently balloted to disperse the saline, taking care not to dislodge the catheter. Careful, slow aspiration of the catheter with a syringe is performed to collect a 10- to 20-ml sample. Ideally, all the infused fluid should be removed, but typically only a small portion is retrievable. The catheter can be retained temporarily for serial evaluation of abdominal fluid in some instances, such as for assessing whether hemoabdomen is ongoing.

Fluid from abdominocentesis–diagnostic peritoneal lavage should be evaluated for color, packed cell volume, white blood cell count, and cytologic features. Occasionally, bacterial cultures and chemistry panels should be performed. Red color suggests hemoabdomen. More definitively, a packed cell volume of diagnostic peritoneal lavage fluid that is 5% or greater indicates significant hemorrhage. Cloudiness suggests peritonitis. Cytologic features and white blood cell count are particularly useful in characterizing peritonitis. A normal white blood cell count in diagnostic peritoneal lavage is approximately 1,000 cells/mm^3. Local intra-abdominal infections may cause the white blood cell count to rise to greater than 4,000 cells/mm^3. Recent surgery will result in an elevated white blood cell count, but usually less than 10,000 cells/mm^3 (Crowe and Bjorling, 1993). Cytologic characteristics are more meaningful than are cell counts in differentiating septic from nonseptic peritonitis. Toxic changes in neutrophils and the presence of intra- or extracellular bacteria indicate septic peritonitis. In such cases, aerobic and anaerobic bacterial cultures are appropriate, particularly if antibiotic therapy is to be initiated before surgical samples can be obtained.

The most useful chemistry evaluation for abdominal fluid is creatinine in cases of suspected urinary system disruption. Urea nitrogen could also be used, but it is less desirable than creatinine because it is a smaller molecule and rapidly diffuses across the peritoneum and equilibrates with plasma. Diagnostic peritoneal lavage creatinine that is greater (usually two times greater) than serum creatinine indicates uroabdomen. Two other chemistry panels that are occasionally helpful are bilirubin and amylase measurements. Bilirubin test reagents can detect intraperitoneal bile, indicating disruption of the biliary system or duodenum. Elevated abdominal fluid amylase compared with serum amylase indicates pancreatitis or intestinal ischemia (Davenport and Martin, 1992).

Exploratory Celiotomy

When exploratory celiotomy is necessary in acute abdomen, the initial diagnostics should prepare the surgeon to anticipate certain findings. An acute abdomen condition for which surgery is indicated (see Table 1) should be on the differential diagnosis list for the patient in question. Exploratory celiotomy should be performed as soon as possible after the need for such is determined. A decision to delay surgery can be justified when the delay will decrease morbidity or the chance of mortality and when a delay is necessary for additional stabilization that will make the patient a better surgical candidate. Intraoperatively, the surgeon should perform a complete systematic exploratory celiotomy to detect and correct all significant abnormalities. Occasionally during emergent celiotomy, life-threatening problems (such as ongoing hemorrhage) will require immediate attention; systematic exploration can be performed later in the procedure. Only rarely should systematic exploration be abandoned altogether (for instance, in patients judged to be at risk of death or severe disability if recovery from anesthesia does not take place soon).

THERAPY

Specific medical and surgical therapeutic measures for animals experiencing acute abdomen are dictated by the clinical status of the patient and by the specific cause of the acute abdomen. Each patient should be considered at risk for deterioration; appropriate resuscitative measures are necessary in some cases before a definitive diagnosis can be achieved. Once the definitive cause is ascertained, specific medical or surgical treatments can be employed. It is difficult to identify any common therapy for all acute abdomen cases other than, perhaps, fluid therapy. However, there is one treatment that should not be overlooked—analgesic therapy.

If one considers that abdominal pain is present at some point in each case of acute abdomen and that definitive therapy is not necessarily going to immediately resolve the pain, analgesics become important. Analgesics should be administered to medical as well as surgical patients. Multiple analgesics are available, but most patients can be managed with either buprenorphine (dogs and cats) or morphine (dogs). Buprenorphine (0.005 to 0.02 mg/kg, every 6 hours or more frequently as needed, IV, IM, SC, or half IV and half IM or SC) is recommended if the major source of pain is thought to be visceral (such as a distended organ). Morphine (0.25 to 1.0 mg/kg, every 6 hours or more frequently as needed, IV, IM, SC, or half IV and half IM or SC) is recommended if the major source of pain is thought to be musculoskeletal (such as abdominal wall trauma). Although morphine would likely be effective for visceral pain, the potential side effects of nausea, emesis, urine retention, constipation, and a greater chance of respiratory depression than occurs with buprenorphine make morphine a less desirable analgesic for most acute abdomen cases (also see p. 57 for a more complete view of analgesics).

Analgesics should be given as early in the course of treatment as possible. In surgical patients, it is preferable to include analgesic administration as part of the preanesthetic medication and repeat administration as necessary before recovery from anesthesia. In nonsurgical patients and patients who undergo lengthy delays before surgery, analgesics are recommended as soon as it is ascertained that the drug effects will not interfere with the diagnostic evaluation. In most cases of acute abdomen, this means as soon

as the physical examination is complete. Withholding analgesics for fear of masking important clinical signs should be the exception rather than the rule. Analgesics are not administered immediately to animals who are presented in shock, but should be initiated soon after the shock state is reversed using the same guidelines discussed earlier. The duration of analgesic administration varies with the individual animal, but should be at least 24 hours in both postoperative and nonsurgical patients.

References and Suggested Reading

Crowe DT: The first steps in handling the acute abdomen patient. Vet Med 83:654, 1988.
Describes initial patient management, diagnostic techniques, and decision-making relevant to emergent surgery.
Crowe DT, Bjorling DE: Peritoneum and peritoneal cavity. In: Slatter DH, ed: Textbook of Small Animal Surgery, 2nd ed. Philadelphia: WB Saunders, 1993, p 407.
Describes anatomy, physiology, pathophysiology, and diseases of the peritoneal cavity and associated treatments, with particular emphasis on peritonitis.
Davenport DJ, Martin RA: Acute abdomen. In: Murtaugh RJ, Kaplan PM, eds: Veterinary Emergency and Critical Care Medicine. St. Louis: Mosby-Year Book, 1992, p 153.
Describes diagnostics for acute abdomen cases and exploratory surgery indications and methods.
Saxon WD: The acute abdomen. Vet Clin North Am Small Anim Pract 24:1207, 1994.
Discusses abdominal pain, diagnostics, exploratory surgery, and need for analgesia.

Gastric Dilatation-Volvulus

KAROL A. MATHEWS
Guelph, Ontario, Canada

Gastric dilatation-volvulus (GDV) is a complex medical and surgical emergency. Potentially, it can occur in any size or breed of dog, as well as in cats, but typically it is problematic in large and giant breeds of dogs. In smaller breeds, the dachshund is overrepresented. Deep-chested conformation may increase the susceptibility to GDV. The prevalence of GDV increases with increasing age, with the greatest occurrence between 7 and 10 years of age. The frequency of occurrence has been reported at 2.4 to 7.6 per 1,000 canine hospital admissions (Glickman et al, 1994). The cause of GDV has not been fully elucidated. Delayed gastric emptying, pyloric obstruction, aerophagia, and engorgement contribute to gastric dilatation (GD), with volvulus possibly occurring secondarily. Gastric volvulus can occur without prior dilatation. Exercise after consuming a large meal may predispose to GDV. Splenic torsion has also been causally implicated because malposition of the spleen frequently occurs with GDV; however, GDV can occur in splenectomized dogs. Inhibition of gastric motility by pharmacologic agents, blunt abdominal trauma, spinal cord injuries, prolonged surgical procedures, or prolonged

recumbency can predispose dogs to GD. Cereal diets have been suggested as a cause for GD; however, studies have not been able to confirm this finding.

This discussion focuses on the initial and postoperative treatment of the animal with GDV. A detailed description of the pathophysiology of GD and GDV is covered elsewhere (Leib, 1987) and is only briefly outlined here as a basis for treatment rationale. The various techniques used for surgical correction of GDV can be obtained from standard surgical texts.

As a consequence of GDV, local and systemic effects occur to varying degrees. Gastric ischemia results in gastritis progressing to necrosis, with possible perforation and peritonitis. Compression of the caudal vena cava and portal vein results in decreased venous return to the heart, with subsequent reduction in cardiac output, systemic arterial blood pressure, and perfusion of the myocardium and gastrointestinal tract. With gastrointestinal mucosal injury and subsequent translocation of bacteria and endotoxins, the patient is predisposed to sepsis and septic shock. Avulsion of the short gastric and right gastroepiploic vessels may occur, causing intra-abdominal hemorrhage. The splenic veins may also become thrombosed. The effect of these events is hypotension, hypovolemia (blood loss, plasma loss, increased production and sequestration of gastric secretions), hypoxemia, acid-base and electrolyte abnormalities, sepsis, myocardial dysfunction, and disseminated intravascular coagulation (DIC).

PRESENTATION

The clinical signs vary with the extent of GD or GDV and may not parallel the degree of gastric or splenic injury. Owners aware of the clinical signs associated with GDV may seek veterinary assistance at the onset of GD, whereas dogs left alone for several hours may present moribund. Typically dogs with GD or GDV have varying degrees of distention of the cranial abdomen with hypersalivation and unproductive retching. These animals are restless, dyspneic, or tachypneic and may or may not be depressed or moribund. In the early stages of GD, physical examination may reveal increased heart rate with strong pulses and normal capillary refill time, and mucous membrane color. In animals with advanced GDV, weak, rapid pulses—possibly associated with pulse deficits—are present; mucous membranes may be pale pink to pale gray with prolonged capillary refill time and the presence of petechiae, and the cranial abdomen may be tympanic with splenomegaly or free abdominal fluid present.

DIAGNOSIS

The diagnosis of GDV is often obvious from the presenting clinical signs. Radiographic examination is necessary and useful if the diagnosis is equivocal or, if after decompression, surgical management may not be an option (differentiation of dilatation from volvulus will direct further management). The ability to pass an orogastric tube does not rule out the presence of volvulus.

When necessary, abdominal radiographs with the dog in right lateral recumbency are usually diagnostic. Evaluation of this radiographic view initially may minimize the patient stress associated with obtaining multiple radiographic views. When volvulus is present, the pylorus is visualized on a right lateral survey radiograph as a gas-filled structure dorsal and cranial to the gastric fundus. A compartmentalization line is frequently observed between the pylorus and fundus. This line represents the pyloric antral wall folding back and contacting the fundic wall. The pylorus cannot be clearly identified in a left lateral projection. Free air within the abdomen may indicate gastric rupture or air leakage after gastrocentesis.

Electrocardiographic monitoring is essential in the patient with GDV and evidence of cardiac arrhythmias. Ventricular arrhythmias are the most common (Muir, 1982). Additionally, sinus tachycardia is almost always present in animals presenting with GDV.

Evaluation of systemic arterial blood pressure, packed cell volume (PCV), total plasma solids (TS), activated clotting time (ACT), platelet count, white blood cell count and differential, blood urea nitrogen and glucose concentrations, venous blood gases or total serum carbon dioxide

(these patients are frequently alkalemic in the early stage of GD but eventually become acidemic as the disease advances), and serum electrolytes are the minimal database required for assessing the patient and diagnosing complications associated with the GDV syndrome. This information is essential to manage the patient adequately and optimize outcome. A complete serum biochemical profile and complete hemostatic profile should be submitted to detect other potential organ dysfunction when appropriate and affordable.

INITIAL TREATMENT

Initial treatment should be considered in light of the presenting clinical signs and the consequences of the known pathophysiologic events. The primary objectives are to (1) prevent or reverse circulatory collapse (fluid and colloid resuscitation), (2) prevent or reduce the local and systemic events associated with GD or GDV by removing the inciting cause (gastric decompression and lavage), (3) treat associated complications (electrolyte and acid-base abnormalities, pain, cardiac arrhythmias, sepsis,) and (4) prepare the animal for surgical treatment. For the rare patient that presents with dilatation alone and without evidence of circulatory compromise, orogastric decompression is the initial treatment. For the typical patient with GDV, circulatory compromise or collapse is present, and reversal of the shock state should be addressed prior to gastric decompression. In seriously compromised patients, it may be necessary to partially decompress the stomach immediately to avoid impending respiratory or circulatory arrest. Gastrocentesis (see section on gastric decompression) is recommended in these situations to avoid the stress of orogastric intubation. In these patients, complete decompression should be avoided until rapid fluid resuscitation is well under way. All patients with GDV require surgical correction as soon as possible, as medical management alone results in a 75% recurrence rate.

Circulatory Resuscitation

A 14- or 16-gauge 2- to 4-inch catheter is placed into the jugular or cephalic vein or veins—not the saphenous vein. An alkalinizing (lactate or acetate) isotonic, balanced electrolyte solution (or acidifying if alkalemic; e.g., 0.9% NaCl solution) is administered at 90 ml/kg per hour initially, with continual monitoring and subsequent adjustment to effect. The crystalloid volume can be reduced by up to 40% if pentastarch (Pentaspan, DuPont Pharma Canada), hetastarch (Hespan, DuPont Pharma USA) or dextran-70 (Gentran, Baxter) is administered at 10–20 ml/kg over 15 to 30 minutes (see p. 131). If shock is severe, 4 ml/kg of 5% or 7.5% hypertonic saline is administered over 5 to 10 minutes, followed by the aforementioned infusions of isotonic crystalloid or synthetic colloid solution until clinical signs of shock are reversed (Table 1). TS and PCV should be measured every 30 minutes. If the PCV decreases to less than 25%, or the TS to less than 45 g/L, whole blood, packed red blood cell, or plasma transfusion should be considered. Blood or plasma is administered at a rate of 20 ml/kg over 1 to 2 hours depending on the resuscitative needs of the patient.

TABLE 1. Parameters to Assess and Goals to Achieve With Fluid and Colloid Resuscitation

Parameter	Goal
Mean arterial pressure (MAP)	70–80 mm Hg
Systolic blood pressure	100–120 mm Hg
Central venous pressure (CVP)	3–5 cm H₂O
Mucous membrane color	Pink
Capillary refill time	1–2 sec
Heart rate	120–140 bpm
Peripheral pulse (dorsal pedal) pressure	Moderate to normal strength
Mentation	Improved to normal for the situation
Urine output	1–2 ml/kg/hr

If hypotension persists, one should consider intravenous constant rate infusions (CRI) of dopamine (Intropin, DuPont Pharma) or dobutamine (Dobutrex, Eli Lilly) at 2 to 20 µg/kg per minute (see *CVT XII*, p. 184, for practical use of constant rate IV infusions). Adjustment in administration rates should be made as needed to achieve a satisfactory hemodynamic end point (see Table 1). Norepinephrine (Levophed, Sanofi Winthrop), 0.05 to 0.3 µg/kg per minute IV, or higher doses to effect, can be administered if dopamine or dobutamine infusions fail to achieve the desired effect.

The most common acid-base abnormality in animals with GDV is nonrespiratory (metabolic) acidosis. This abnormality is frequently corrected by treating the underlying cause (shock) with aggressive resuscitative fluid therapy and gastric decompression. Bicarbonate (HCO₃) administration is not routinely necessary but may be indicated if serum [HCO₃⁻] or total carbon dioxide is less than 12 mEq/L after fluid resuscitation. A suggested dose for HCO₃ administration (in milliequivalents) can be calculated using the following formula:

$$[body weight (kg) \times (12 - patient [HCO_3^-]) \times 0.3]$$

The calculated dose can be administered IV over 30 to 60 minutes. Occasionally, a patient may have a normal or increased blood pH, and empirical therapy with HCO₃⁻ may be deleterious.

Ventricular arrhythmias frequently improve after circulatory resuscitation and gastric decompression; however, treatment is advised by some (see p. 733) if the arrhythmia is sustained, paroxysmal, or polymorphic at an instantaneous rate greater than or equal to 170 beats/min (120 beats/min under general anesthesia), greater than or equal to 140 beats/min with mean arterial pressure (MAP) less than 70 mm Hg, when pre-existing cardiac disease is present, or when an R-on-T phenomenon or torsades de pointe is observed on the electrocardiogram. Initial treatment for ventricular tachyarrhythmias is lidocaine (Xylocaine, Astra) administration at 2 mg/kg IV. If the initial bolus is ineffective, one or two additional boluses can be administered within 5 to 10 minutes of the initial bolus. If the arrhythmia is lidocaine-responsive, an intravenous CRI of lidocaine at 30 to 80 µg/kg per minute is established. Failure of the rhythm to improve with lidocaine administration (reduction in rate to 120 to 140 beats/min and a

reduction in abnormal complex morphologic features) requires reassessment of the electrocardiographic diagnosis and overall status of the patient (electrolyte, acid-base, sepsis, pain, and so on) with consideration of alternative antiarrhythmic therapy. One should not expect to totally abolish the arrhythmia and should not feel compelled to treat those ventricular rhythms that are neither very fast nor causing hypotension. If there is uncertainty as to whether the arrhythmia is ventricular or supraventricular in origin, or the ventricular arrhythmia is not lidocaine-responsive, procainamide (Pronestyl, Squibb) is administered intravenously at 6 to 10 mg/kg (rarely up to 20 mg/kg) by 2 mg/kg increments every 5 minutes (to avoid hypotension). If procainamide administration is effective, it is continued at 6 to 10 mg/kg IM every 6 hours or as an IV CRI of 25 to 40 µg/kg per minute. The administration of 20% magnesium sulfate solution, at 0.15 to 0.3 mEq/kg (12.5 to 35 mg/kg) via 2- to 4-hour IV CRI three times in 24 hours, may abolish or enhance the treatment response of patients with ventricular arrhythmias. For life-threatening arrhythmia, a magnesium sulfate dose of 0.15 to 0.3 mEq/kg could be administered over 15 to 20 minutes. Caution must be used with magnesium sulfate administration in patients with renal insufficiency (see *CVT XII*, p. 132). Sinus tachycardia frequently resolves with resuscitative treatment and analgesic support. If sinus tachycardia persists, one should consider hypotension, hypovolemia (i.e., if not hypotensive, the possibility of maximal patient compensation requiring continuation of resuscitative treatment), hypoxemia, anemia, hypercarbia, inadequate control of pain, gastric perforation, splenic infarction, or other major organ complication that requires immediate exploratory celiotomy.

Potassium-supplemented fluids, delivered through an IV line separate from the rapid infusion of crystalloids, should be administered at a dosage of 30 to 80 mEq/L delivered at a maintenance fluid rate, when serum potassium concentrations are 3.5 mEq/L to less than 2.0 mEq/L, respectively. If the animal is acidemic, the serum potassium concentration may decrease during treatment with alkalinizing solutions. This possibility should be anticipated, assessed, and addressed by an increase in the rate of potassium infusion. Potassium infusions can be delivered at a maximal rate of 0.5 to 1.0 mEq/kg per hour when serum potassium levels are less than 3.0 mEq/L, ventricular arrhythmias are present, and continuous electrocardiography and serial serum potassium monitoring are possible every 2 hours.

Antibiotics with a spectrum of activity directed against gram-negative and anaerobic bacteria should be administered slowly intravenously during fluid resuscitation (cefoxitin, 20 mg/kg IV q6 hr, or ampicillin, 20 mg/kg IV q6 hr). Translocation of gut bacteria into the systemic circulation is a common complication of GDV and gastrointestinal hypoperfusion.

Administration of corticosteroids to patients with GDV is controversial. Some investigators have found no significant association between corticosteroid treatment and mortality of dogs with GDV (Brourman et al, 1996). The administration of prednisolone sodium succinate (Solu-Delta-Cortef, Upjohn), 10 mg/kg IV,, methylprednisolone (Solu-Medrol, Upjohn) at 10 mg/kg IV, or dexamethasone sodium-phosphate, 2 to 4 mg/kg IV over 20 minutes, has been suggested. Corticosteroids are not routinely administered to patients with GDV at our hospital. The administration of nonsteroidal anti-inflammatory analgesics is not recommended. Deferoxamine (Desferal, Ciba-Geigy Pharmaceutical Inc.), 50 mg/kg slowly IV,, administered 10 minutes before gastric decompression has shown promise in prevention of reperfusion injury when administered to dogs with experimentally induced GDV. However, this drug can cause significant hypotension when administered at 50 mg/kg; therefore, 20 to 25 mg/kg is suggested, given over 10 minutes to avoid hypotension. Clinical trials are needed to demonstrate its efficacy and limitations.

Gastric Decompression

After resuscitative fluid administration, gastric decompression is initiated. If the animal requires sedation, butorphanol (Torbugesic, Ayerst), 0.2 to 0.4 mg/kg IV, or oxymorphone (Numorphan, DuPont Pharma), 0.05 to 0.1 mg/kg IV, is administered. The addition of diazepam (Valium, Roche), 0.2 to 0.5 mg/kg IV, can be used concomitantly if needed in noncompliant dogs prior to decompression. If surgical correction is planned, oxymorphone administration is preferred, as this drug reduces the inhalant anesthetic requirements, has greater analgesic effect, and produces a better sedative effect that facilitates tracheal intubation.

To perform orogastric decompression, the dog is placed in sternal or lateral recumbency or in an upright sitting position. A large-bore tube is premeasured from the chin to the xiphoid, and the distance is marked on the tube with tape. The tube is lubricated with water-soluble jelly and passed carefully through an oral speculum (or 2-inch roll of tape) through the esophagus and into the stomach (the mark on the tube is at the level of the incisor teeth). Rupture of compromised areas of the lower esophagus or stomach can occur if excessive force is used in orogastric intubation. If resistance to passage of the orogastric tube is experienced, gently rotate the tube while reattempting passage or change the position of the dog to facilitate passage.

Gastrocentesis should be performed immediately in patients with severe gastric distention and incipient cardiopulmonary arrest or in patients in which attempts at orogastric intubation have been unsuccessful and delay in partial decompression with further repositioning will be detrimental to the patient. A 10 × 10 cm area is aseptically prepared caudal to the right costal arch. The area is percussed to identify the tympanic stomach and to avoid needle puncture of the spleen. An 18-gauge needle or needle-styleted catheter is placed through the abdominal wall into the lumen of the stomach to allow gas to escape. Orogastric decompression should be repeated after gastrocentesis because release of pressure on the cardia usually facilitates passage of the tube. After orogastric decompression, the stomach is lavaged with warm tap water to remove residual food. The absence of blood or coffee ground material in the lavage fluid does not rule out the presence of gastric necrosis.

If surgical correction cannot be performed immediately, decompression can be maintained by placement of a weighted nasogastric tube with stylet (EN-tube, Entech Inc. Lebanon, NJ), a temporary gastrostomy, or a pharyngostomy tube. Intermittent orogastric intubation is not recommended because this procedure is stressful and iatrogenic gastric rupture is a potential concern with repeated orogastric tube placement. The indications for maintaining temporary gastric decompression in these patients include (1) allowance of time to complete cardiovascular and metabolic stabilization in the more severely compromised patient unable to withstand general anesthesia, (2) maintenance of gastric decompression for patient transportation to a referral facility, and (3) unavailability of immediate surgical intervention. Rarely, a stabilization period of up to 12 hours may be indicated prior to definitive surgical intervention in dogs that are moribund and comatose with circulatory collapse.

Preparation for the placement of a temporary gastrostomy is as described for gastrocentesis. Anesthesia of the area to be incised can be obtained by infiltration of 4 to 6 ml of 1% lidocaine, through the skin and subcutaneous and muscle layers, including the peritoneum, in an inverted "L" pattern. A 6-cm incision is made through the skin and the approach to the peritoneum is made through muscle separation. The peritoneum is incised with caution, as the stomach is adjacent to it. A circumferential, simple continuous suture pattern is placed through the skin, abdominal wall, serosa, and muscles of the stomach. The stomach is then incised. Gastric emptying and lavage are then performed. Any temporary gastrostomy is closed and locally irrigated during the subsequent surgical approach for definitive surgical correction. In general, the recommendation would be for definitive surgical correction for GDV within 1 to 2 hours after presentation in the majority of cases. Early intervention, after an initial period of circulatory resuscitation, has been shown to reduce postoperative fatality rates (Brockman et al, 1995). The disadvantages of postponing surgical intervention are (1) the increased prevalence of cardiac arrhythmias by 12 to 72 hours, (2) an increased risk of splenic and gastric infarction resulting from continuing malposition, and (3) the increasing risk with time of gastric perforation, with consequent peritonitis (also see p. 764).

SURGICAL TREATMENT

Anesthesia regimens to be considered in patients with GDV include oxymorphone, 0.05 mg/kg, and mask administration of isoflurane (Forane, Ohmeda) for the severely compromised patient; ketamine (Ketaset, Ayerst), 2.0 to 5.0 mg/kg, combined with diazepam, 0.1 to 0.3 mg/kg, and isoflurane for the stable but moderately depressed patient; or oxymorphone, thiopental sodium (pentothal sodium, Abbott) and isoflurane for the hemodynamically stable patient with GDV. Crystalloid, colloid, blood, or blood component administration; antiarrhythmic and electrolyte therapy; and continuous electrocardiography, along with serial blood pressure monitoring, should continue throughout the intraoperative period.

The belt-loop gastropexy is the preferred technique for definitive correction of GDV in our hospital because of ease of performance and efficacy. The tube gastropexy was the preferred technique described in a recent report (Brockman et al, 1995). Regardless of the gastropexy used, during definitive surgical correction it is recommended that areas of gastric necrosis or questionably viable stomach be removed. Invagination into the gastric lumen of nonviable or potentially nonviable tissue, as suggested in some texts, can predispose to postoperative DIC. Similarly, if there are questionable areas of necrosis in the spleen or if the spleen does not return to a normal size after derotation (performed prior to gastropexy to allow time for venous drainage), the spleen should be removed. Unless pyloric outflow obstruction can be clearly demonstrated, pyloroplasty is not necessary, and the extended surgical time required to perform this procedure may contribute to patient morbidity. If there is a concern about pancreatitis, or if any extended ($>$24 hours) restriction of oral food intake is anticipated, a jejunostomy tube should be placed for nutritional support.

POSTOPERATIVE MANAGEMENT

Recent studies in patients with GDV and surgical intervention reported mortality rates as low as 15% (Brockman et al, 1995) to 18% (Brourman et al, 1996). Of the nonsurvivors, postoperative mortality associated with gastric resection was 28% (Brockman et al, 1995) to 35% (Brourman et al, 1996); with splenectomy, it was 32% (Brourman et al, 1996) to 38% (Brockman et al, 1995); and with cardiac arrhythmias that were present on admission, postoperative mortality was 38% (Brourman et al, 1996). Cardiac arrhythmias developing *postoperatively* did not influence outcome (Brourman et al, 1996; Brockman et al, 1995).

Complications to be anticipated in patients after surgical correction of GDV include cardiac arrhythmias; fluid overload; gastroparesis and ileus; vomiting; pancreatitis; DIC; gastric and incisional dehiscence; gastric ulceration; ischemic necrosis of stomach, spleen, or gallbladder with peritonitis; incarceration of small bowel dorsal to the gastropexy site; or the development of acute renal failure. The intensity of postoperative care will vary depending on the severity of illness and surgical intervention. To provide optimal care, the clinician should for the first 24 hours (1) continuously or serially observe the ECG and measure hemodynamics (goals are MAP $>$70 mm Hg, systolic pressure $>$110 mm Hg, CVP of 3 to 5 cm H_2O), provide pain assessment and treatment (oxymorphone 0.05 to 0.2 mg/kg every 4 hours or to effect), and measure urine output (1 to 2 ml/kg per hour); (2) assess at least every 8 hours serum electrolytes (goals are electrolytes within normal limits, with K^+ $>$4.5 mmol/L), nonrespiratory acid-base status (venous pH 7.28 to 7.4, [HCO_3^-] 16 to 24 mmol/L, base excess $\pm$5), PCV (25 to 45%), and TS (45 to 70 g/L); (3) measure every 12 hours ACT and blood glucose concentration; and (4) assess each day serum magnesium, creatinine, and albumin concentrations and CBC and antithrombin III levels (when DIC is suspected). Treatment approaches for abnormalities detected on serial postoperative testing need to be individualized to the patient.

The major electrolyte disturbance seen postoperatively in almost all patients with GDV is hypokalemia. Hypokalemia potentiates cardiac arrhythmias, and hypokalemia is potentiated by hypomagnesemia. In severely hypokalemic patients, potassium supplementation in intravenous fluids may exceed 80 mEq/L even though crystalloids are being delivered at twice to three times the normal requirement for maintenance. Magnesium sulfate 20% can be administered by intravenous CRI at 0.25 mEq/kg (30 mg/kg) di-

vided over 4 hours and repeated at 8-hour intervals for 24 hours or as an intravenous CRI of 1.0 mEq/kg per day (125 mg/kg per day). Serum potassium levels require frequent monitoring during potassium and magnesium infusions.

Sinus tachycardia should not be present postoperatively in patients without primary cardiac disease recovering from GDV. The presence of sinus tachycardia in these patients does not require antiarrhythmic therapy, as this rhythm often represents a physiologic response to heart failure, pain, hypoxia, anemia, hypotension, sepsis, and other potential problems previously mentioned. These primary abnormalities should be identified and treated. However, if a primary supraventricular tachyarrhythmia has been identified, appropriate antiarrhythmic therapy is administered based on the specific rhythm problem (see *CVT XII,* p. 164). Ventricular tachyarrhythmias are treated as described in the section on initial treatment (also see pp. 730 and 733).

In the postoperative GDV patient, isotonic crystalloid fluids and synthetic colloids are administered at a rate that maintains normal hydration, acid-base status, and urine output. Synthetic colloids, 20 to 30 ml/kg per day, should be administered when large-volume crystalloids are required to maintain the MAP at greater than 70 mm Hg, systolic arterial blood pressure at greater than 110 mm Hg, and urine output at greater than 1 ml/kg per hour or to prevent the development of interstitial or pulmonary edema in patients with decreased TS or colloidal oncotic pressure.

Antibiotic therapy, as recommended in the section on initial treatment, should be continued intravenously for 72 hours in patients requiring gastric resection or when gastric mucosal injury is highly suspect. Patients with simple GD or GDV without notable mucosal injury do not require antibiotic therapy postoperatively.

It is not uncommon for patients with GDV or GD to acquire gastric atony and ileus, postoperatively. This occurrence predisposes animals to recurrence of GD and vomiting. If a gastrostomy tube is not in place, maintenance of gastric decompression may require the placement of a nasogastric tube. Metoclopramide administration (Reglan, Wyeth-Ayerst), 0.2 to 0.5 mg/kg every 8 hours SC or 1 to 2 mg/kg per day by IV CRI, is recommended as a promotility drug to enhance gastric emptying and as an antiemetic. To enhance gastric mucosal healing, reduce the possibility of gastric ulceration with hemorrhage, and prevent esophageal stricture secondary to reflux esophagitis, ranitidine (Zantac, Glaxo), 0.5 to 1.0 mg/kg every 12 hours IV, and sucralfate (200 mg/ml suspension) (Sulcrate or Carafate, Nordic), 5 ml/dog every 8 hours PO, are recommended. Therapy may range from 2 to 5 days.

Gastric necrosis has been associated with abnormal hemostatic profiles (Millis et al, 1993). Therefore, when gastric or splenic necrosis is apparent at surgical correction, it should be assumed that DIC is present. These patients should receive at least one unit of fresh frozen plasma, preincubated with 75 U/kg heparin for 30 minutes prior to administration. A subsequent dose of heparin is administered SC at 16 hours and continued at 8-hour intervals thereafter. The continued "bedside" assessment of these patients includes serial assessment of ACT, TS, PCV, and platelet count and physical examination (incisional oozing, petechial hemorrhages, and deterioration in attitude). If further abnormalities develop in any of the assessed parameters, another unit of fresh frozen plasma or fresh whole blood (to raise the PCV to 25 to 30%) should be administered and consideration given to the possibility of an ongoing problem (progression of gastric or splenic necrosis) or another complication such as sepsis that may require further surgical treatment.

In most patients with uncomplicated surgical correction of GDV or GD, water should be offered at 12 hours postoperatively, and a low-fat, good-quality protein canned dog food slurry should be offered soon after if the patient is alert and not vomiting. Oral feeding to those patients with gastric resection should be started at the discretion of the surgeon based on the extent of, or surgical complications associated with, the resection and the presence or absence of a jejunostomy feeding tube.

If a jejunostomy feeding tube is in place, a CRI of an electrolyte solution with 5% dextrose (Plasma-Lyte, 56 with 5% dextrose, Baxter) is delivered at 0.5 ml/kg via the tube for the initial 12 hours postoperatively. If this is tolerated by the patient, the addition of a prepared liquid diet (Canine Clinicare, PetAg) at one half the daily, nonprotein, caloric requirements (see equation) diluted 50:50 with the aforementioned crystalloid solution is delivered at 0.5 ml/kg per hour for the subsequent 24 hours. If no signs of discomfort or nausea are noted after this 24-hour infusion, the infusion should be increased to meet full nutritional requirements. Peripheral intravenous fluid therapy should be reduced by the appropriate amount once oral intake occurs or enteral nutritional support is instituted. The duration of jejunostomy feeding is individualized to each patient.

$$1.5 \times [70 \text{ (body weight in kg}^{0.75})]$$

Parenteral nutritional support is recommended for patients unable to eat or drink or receive enteral nutrition for more than 36 hours postoperatively (also see p. 80). A common nutritional support technique used in our hospital is the administration of a partial parenteral nutritional (PPN) solution. In 1 L there is a 3.3% concentration of amino acids (Travasol, Baxter) and a 3.3% concentration of dextrose in an electrolyte solution (Plasma-Lyte 56 with 5% dextrose, Baxter). This can be prepared by removing 330 ml of the electrolyte solution from a 1-L bag and replacing it with 330 ml of Travasol, under sterile conditions. Lipids (20% Intralipid, Clintec) can be piggy-backed into the administration set and delivered at a volume up to 50% of the patient's nonprotein caloric requirements. Both can be delivered through a peripheral intravenous catheter. Although strict aseptic technique is used in preparing and delivering this solution, a dedicated peripheral line offers ease of PPN administration without compromising the patient through administration via a common central venous access that may be used for CVP monitoring, blood sampling, and delivery of crystalloid fluids or medications. The

amino acid–glucose solution is delivered as an IV CRI at a rate of 1 to 1½ normal daily fluid maintenance requirements. If further glucose supplementation appears necessary, it can be administered with the remaining replacement-maintenance crystalloid fluids. The hourly rate of administration for crystalloid fluid support should be reduced by an amount equal to that delivered via PPN to avoid overhydration. Guidelines for total parenteral nutritional support can be obtained elsewhere in *CVT XII* and *CVT XIII*.

The length of hospital stay will depend on the severity of illness but is expected to be 3 to 7 days. All dogs that have recovered from GDV or GD should be fed a good-quality canned dog food in small amounts (based on their normal daily nutritional requirements) four or five times daily initially, and no less than three times daily in the future to avoid engorgement. Exercise after eating should be avoided. Owners should be made aware that gastropexy is not a guarantee against future episodes of GD or GDV in the patient.

References and Suggested Reading

Brockman DJ, Washabau RJ, Drobatz KJ: Canine gastric dilation/volvulus syndrome in a veterinary critical care unit: 295 cases (1986–1992). J Am Vet Med Assoc 207:460, 1995.
A retrospective analysis of 295 medical records, with a description of a standardized protocol for the management of dogs with GDV, was undertaken to ascertain the efficacy of this protocol in reducing morbidity and mortality; risk factors associated with mortality are also presented.

Brourman JD, Schertel ER, Allen DA, et al: Factors associated with perioperative mortality in dogs with surgically managed gastric dilation-volvulus: 137 cases (1988–1993). J Am Vet Med Assoc 208:1855, 1996.
A retrospective analysis of the medical records of 137 dogs identifying factors associated with perioperative mortality in dogs with GDV and an evaluation of the differences in patient management and outcome between a university and a private specialty practice.

Glickman LT, Glickman NW, Perez CM, et al: Analysis of risk factors for gastric dilatation and dilatation-volvulus in dogs. J Am Vet Med Assoc 204:1465, 1994.
An epidemiologic study of GD and GDV using the Veterinary Medical Data Base to identify risk factors for GD and GDV and the frequency of occurrence in 12 institutions.

Leib MS: Therapy of gastric dilatation-volvulus in dogs. Compend Contin Educ Pract Vet 9:1155, 1987.
A good comprehensive review of GDV in dogs, including all aspects of management and personal experience; 63 references.

Matthiesen DT: Gastric dilation-volvulus syndrome. In: Slatter D, ed: Textbook of Small Animal Surgery, 2nd ed. Philadelphia: WB Saunders, 1993, p 580.
Detailed descriptions of current surgical techniques for GDV.

Millis DL, Hauptman JG, Fulton RB: Abnormal hemostatic profiles and gastric necrosis in canine gastric dilatation-volvulus. Vet Surg 22:93, 1993.
A prospective study using a preoperative hemostatic profile of 20 dogs with GDV to determine the correlation between abnormal tests and the presence of gastric necrosis.

Muir WW: Gastric dilatation-volvulus in the dog, with emphasis on cardiac arrhythmias. J Am Vet Med Assoc 180:739, 1982.
A retrospective study of the medical records of 156 dogs with GDV in which breed, age, sex, and prevalence of cardiac arrhythmias were identified and categorized.

Emergency Management of Open Fractures

ROBERT J. MCCARTHY

North Grafton, Massachusetts

Open fractures, defined as those in which fractured bone has been exposed to the external environment, represent between 5 and 10% of all fracture cases seen in small animal practice. Any open fracture must be considered contaminated and a source of potential infection. These fractures require immediate intervention and should be treated as surgical emergencies.

Open fractures have been classified into three types, based on the wounding mechanism and the degree of hard and soft tissue damage (Table 1). Type I open fractures are the result of the lowest energy trauma and are frequently associated with the sharp point of a fractured bone penetrating the skin from the inside. Wound size is generally less than 1 cm in length. There is little soft tissue injury, wounds are often relatively clean, and there is no crushing component. The bone end may remain exposed but more commonly returns to lie beneath the skin. Fractures are usually transverse or oblique, with minimal if any comminution. The tibia and radius are common sites of type I open fractures in small animals because of the close proximity of bone to the skin in the antebrachium and crus.

In a type II open fracture, an external force produces a penetrating wound that communicates with the fracture from the outside. Wounds are usually greater than 1 cm in length. These fractures have more severe soft tissue injury and contamination. There is a minimal to moderate crushing component to skin and musculature, and fractures may be comminuted. These fractures are about twice as likely to become infected as type I open fractures. Common examples include bite wounds and certain low-velocity gunshot fractures.

Type III open fractures are caused by high-energy trauma from an external source and are characterized by severe soft tissue damage and contamination. There is often soft tissue or bone loss, and bone may be stripped of soft tissue attachments. There is generally a severe crushing component. Fractures are usually highly comminuted, and repair may result in cortical defects. Risk of infection is considered about four times that in a type I open fracture.

Examples are degloving injuries with underlying fracture and high-velocity gunshot injuries.

INITIAL ASSESSMENT AND EMERGENCY MANAGEMENT

Treatment of an open fracture should be started at home. Owners are instructed to minimize all limb manipulation and to cover the wound and exposed bone with a sterile dressing if possible. A clean cloth or diaper are appropriate alternatives if bandage materials are not available. Owners should be warned that injured animals may bite, and they should consider placing a muzzle if necessary. Compression is usually sufficient to control hemorrhage during transport to the hospital. Initial veterinary management is directed toward evaluation and treatment of other potentially life-threatening injuries unless the wound is inadequately covered or is hemorrhaging profusely (Table 2). In this situation, a sterile dressing and pressure wrap should be applied. Ligation of actively bleeding vessels is occasionally required. Bone protruding from the wound should not be reduced into the wound at this time, as this allows additional contamination of the fracture site.

Evaluation of the stabilized patient is begun with a thorough case history. Owners are questioned regarding the cause of the injury and the environment in which the injury occurred. It is significant whether the animal was "run into" or "run over" because in the latter situation a significant crushing component is more likely. The environment where the injury occurred may help determine potential wound contaminants and dictate the choice of future antibiotic therapy.

Initial wound evaluation should be directed toward a careful assessment of the neurologic and vascular status of the limb, as they may alter treatment options. Simple diagnostic tests include clipping a toenail short to check for active bleeding, evaluation of extremity pulses distal to the wound, limb temperature assessment, and patient recognition of extremity sensation. Although the degree of

TABLE 1. Classification of Open Fractures

Classification	Wounding Mechanism	Soft Tissue and Bony Damage	Common Fracture Configuration	Relative Risk of Infection
Type I	Bone fragment protrudes outward from within	Minimal	Transverse, oblique	1
Type II	Penetrating external wound contacts bone	Moderate	Some comminution	2
Type III	Severe external force causes wound	Severe	Severe comminution	4

TABLE 2. Treatment Protocol for Management of Patients With Open Fracture

Evaluate patient status and treat life-threatening injuries
Control hemorrhage
Place sterile dressing and bandage during patient stabilization
Assess vascular and neurologic status of limb
Obtain preliminary deep wound culture
Start antibiotic therapy
Manage pain
Obtain radiographs
Perform definitive surgical debridement and fracture fixation within 6–8 hours if possible

wound contamination and apparent soft and bony tissue trauma should be determined, limb manipulation must be minimized and wound probing avoided, as they increase contamination, cause vascular damage, and result in pain. Potential problems associated with small puncture wounds should not be underestimated because debris may be under the skin, deep in the wound and medullary cavity. Preliminary deep wound cultures should be obtained at the time of initial wound evaluation. In humans, 50 to 70% of open fractures produce positive results when cultured at presentation, and in 66% of cases, the bacteria cultured at presentation are the same as those isolated later in infected wounds.

After the wound is assessed and cultured, radiographs are obtained, and a more functional immobilization dressing is applied. The purpose of this bandage is to prevent additional contamination, preserve vasculature, and decrease pain. Most organisms that are recovered from the wound after the development of an orthopedic infection can be traced to the hospital, so early protection of the wound is critical. Sterile dressings should be used in all cases and strict asepsis maintained. A splint is generally applied to support open fractures below the elbow or stifle, whereas a spica or Schroeder-Thomas bandage is required to immobilize fractures more proximal on the limb. Fractures proximal to the elbow or stifle are frequently difficult to immobilize properly, and in many cases it may be preferable simply to cover the wound and confine the animal to a small cage.

Antibiotics are always indicated for animals with open fractures because all wounds are contaminated, and wounds that occurred greater than 6 to 8 hours before definitive surgical debridement and lavage are infected. In humans, antibiotics administered within 3 hours of injury significantly decrease the rate of future wound infection. Risk of infection may be greater in animals with open fractures because of decreased host defense mechanisms caused by stress, high-dose corticosteroid use, or vascular compromise. Choice of antibiotic is based on the cause of injury, nature of the wound, likely bacterial contaminants, and knowledge of commonly isolated bacteria from patients with osteomyelitis. Staphylococcus spp. cause between 50 and 60% of bone infections in dogs, and many of these infections are monomicrobial. In general, concerns about penetration of antibiotics into bone interstitial fluid are unfounded.

First-generation cephalosporins such as cefazolin (Kefzol, Lilly; 20 mg/kg every 8 hours) are often the initial drugs of choice because they are broad spectrum, can be given intravenously, are usually effective against β-lactamase–producing Staphylococcus spp., and are relatively inexpensive. The intramuscular injection of a narrow-spectrum antibiotic (penicillin) is not an appropriate choice given the prevalence of β-lactamase–producing gram-positive and gram-negative bacteria in open fracture wounds. Anaerobic infections are more common than previously thought, and clindamycin (Antirobe, Upjohn; 5 to 10 mg/kg PO every 12 hours) or metronidazole (Flagyl, Searle; 25 to 40 mg/kg PO every 12 hours) should be considered in addition to first-generation cephalosporins in animals with severely necrotic, avascular wounds. The initial choice of antibiotic is altered when culture and sensitivity test results become available. In type I and II open fractures that are not infected, antibiotic use can be discontinued immediately after fracture repair. In any type III open fracture, or in type I or II open fractures that are infected, more prolonged use is indicated. In general, antibiotic therapy is continued for about 1 month in these cases. Antibiotics can be discontinued at that time if there is no clinical or radiographic evidence of infection.

Recognition of pain is difficult in dogs and cats because even animals with severe pain may show no overt clinical signs. Open fractures are associated with extensive pain and anxiety in humans, and a similar situation is expected in animals. Pain should be treated with narcotic analgesics. Butorphanol (Torbugesic, Fort Dodge; 0.2 to 0.4 mg/kg IV or IM), buprenorphine (Buprenex, Norwich Eaton; 0.01 mg/kg IV or IM), and oxymorphone (Numorphan, Dupont; 0.05 to 0.1 mg/kg IV or IM) all provide good analgesia, although oxymorphone may be better for severe pain. A dermal fentanyl patch is an excellent means for providing analgesia while avoiding the necessity of repeated injections.

SURGICAL DEBRIDEMENT

Patients with open fractures frequently require long hospitalization, multiple surgical procedures, and expensive medications, so before initiating definitive wound management and fracture repair, owners should be apprised carefully of the potential prognosis and cost. It is essential that the veterinarian communicate treatment options and prognosis in a manner that allows clients to understand the situation and then make rational, realistic decisions for themselves and their pets. An estimate in writing of the anticipated expense and treatment should be provided. Limb amputation may be a necessary alternative in some cases. Definitive surgical debridement of the open fracture wound should be performed as soon as safely possible, preferably within 6 to 8 hours after injury. This period is considered the "golden period" in which the wound is contaminated but bacteria have not had the opportunity to multiply and spread through adjacent tissues. If the patient is not yet stable for anesthesia, initial debridement can be attempted with a local anesthetic or a regional anesthesia technique such as an epidural. Neuroleptanalgesia can also be considered.

Surgical preparation and removal of gross debris may be performed in the surgical preparation area, but definitive debridement is performed in the operating room. Most orthopedic infections originate from hospital organisms, so strict aseptic technique is important. Sterile water-soluble gel can be placed in the wound to avoid contamination with hair while clipping. A water-impermeable barrier is placed between the limb and the rest of the body and surgery table during debridement, to prevent wicking of contaminated fluids from the environment into the operative field.

The goal of surgical debridement is to convert a contaminated wound to a clean one. All foreign material and contaminated or dead tissue is removed, but undermining of wound edges and extensive soft tissue dissection are avoided. Sharp dissection technique is preferred. Dependable features for predicting viability of muscle are ability to bleed, consistency, and contractility. Although commonly used, color is actually a relatively poor criterion because it depends greatly on the available light. If viability is questionable, it is better to leave tissue in place and remove it if necessary during a second procedure. As a guideline for debriding bone, if the bone has no soft tissue attachment, and is not critical for reconstruction of the fracture, it is excised. Bone that has no soft tissue attachment but is critical for fracture reconstruction should be saved. Any bone that has good soft tissue attachment is saved in the fracture site.

Wounds are irrigated with liters of isotonic saline or 0.05% chlorhexidine. Tap water has been used for wound irrigation but is not recommended because the hypotonicity of tap water may potentiate cellular damage. There is little evidence for incorporation of antibiotics into lavage fluids in dogs and cats. A pulsating irrigation delivery system is helpful, or lavage can be accomplished with a 35-ml syringe and an 18-gauge needle. Bullets retrieved from gunshot fracture wounds should be saved because of the potential for future litigation. A deep wound culture is obtained at the end rather than at the beginning of surgery, as this has been shown to correlate better with later infection.

FRACTURE REPAIR

Fracture fixation is performed as soon as safely possible, preferably during the initial wound debridement. If immediate fixation is planned, the operative field, the equipment, and the surgeon's gown and gloves should all be changed after the wound debridement. Rigid stabilization of the fracture increases patient comfort, improves blood supply to the tissues, facilitates wound healing, and promotes resistance to infection.

A number of techniques can be used for fracture repair. In general, after surgical debridement, type I open fractures can be treated in the same manner as a closed fracture. Higher grade open fractures require special consideration when planning repair. External coaptation with splints and casts is rarely appropriate, as wound care is difficult and stabilization is generally inadequate. Use of intramedullary pins is avoided, if possible, because they impede medullary circulation, may spread bacteria through the medullary cavity, and when used alone do not provide rigid stabilization. Bone screw and plate fixation can be used, but placement of a large metallic foreign body at the fracture site is a disadvantage. Implants potentiate bacterial proliferation

because the surfaces become covered with glycolipid, which allows *Staphylococcus* spp. and other gram-positive organisms to adhere. The extensive open surgical approach required for bone plating also further compromises vascularity. Despite these limitations, rigid fixation with a bone plate and screws is generally acceptable and usually results in uncomplicated healing.

External skeletal fixation is generally the fixation technique of choice, since fixation pins can be placed away from damaged tissue and rigid stabilization is possible. External skeletal fixation is economical, readily available, and does not require specialized equipment. The wound can be visualized and treated as needed. The Ilizarov ring external skeletal fixator has recently become available and may be particularly useful in these patients because very small fixation pins under tension are used.

Autogenous cancellous bone grafts are indicated in many open fractures, since cortical defects are common, and these fractures may heal slowly because of vascular and soft tissue damage. Transplanted cancellous bone facilitates bone healing by means of osteoconductive, osteoinductive, and osteogenic properties. Cancellous bone grafts rarely become infected, and when they do, they undergo harmless liquefactive necrosis. The graft should be collected with a separate set of equipment and gloves to avoid contamination of the graft site. In severely avascular wounds, bone grafting should be delayed 1 to 2 weeks, to allow sufficient proliferation of granulation tissue to provide vascular support for the graft. If delayed grafting is performed, the incision should be through previously undamaged tissue if possible. Although cortical allografts have been used successfully in open fractures, they are not recommended, because the risk of sequestration and resorption is high. Autogenous vascular bone grafts transplanted by microsurgery may prove beneficial in the future.

WOUND CLOSURE

Wound closure can be performed if debridement results in a surgically clean wound with adequate vascularity that can be closed without tension. Dead space drainage should be accomplished with aseptically placed closed suction drains. In general, more severe type II and all type III open fractures should be handled as open wounds, with delayed primary or secondary closure. If there is any doubt, it is always better to leave the wound open.

References and Suggested Reading

Anson LW: Emergency management of fractures. In: Slatter D, ed: Textbook of Small Animal Surgery. Philadelphia: WB Saunders, 1993, p 1603.
   A review of emergency management of both open and closed fractures.
Egger EL: Emergency treatment of musculoskeletal trauma. In: Bright RM, ed: Surgical Emergencies. New York: Churchill Livingstone, 1986, p 175.
   A review of emergency management of trauma to the musculoskeletal system, including bones, joints, muscle, and the central nervous system.
Tillson DM: Open fracture management. Vet Clin North Am Small Anim Pract 25:1093, 1995.
   A recent review of emergency management of open fractures.

Acute Renal Failure

DENISE A. ELLIOTT
LARRY D. COWGILL
Davis, California

CLASSIFICATION AND ETIOLOGY

Acute renal failure (ARF) is a clinical syndrome consequent to a sudden reduction of renal function or urine output with subsequent azotemia and failure to regulate fluid, electrolyte, and acid-base balance. The cause of ARF is multifactorial and is classified conventionally as *prerenal*, *intrinsic renal parenchymal*, and *postrenal* according to the anatomic target, extent, and duration of the inciting conditions promoting the syndrome (Table 1). Prerenal failure represents a functional (physiologic) decline in glomerular filtration secondary to deficiencies in renal blood flow or perfusion pressure or imbalances in renal vascular resistance. Prerenal failure is not associated initially with morphologic damage to the kidney and is fully reversible with correction of the underlying hemodynamic deficiencies. Prerenal failure frequently is a complication of other clinical conditions that disrupt extracellular volume or systemic hemodynamics. Intrinsic ARF occurs secondary to morphologic damage to the vasculature, glomeruli, tubular epithelium, or interstitium of the kidney. Intrinsic parenchymal damage can develop from prolongation of the hemodynamic deficiencies and ischemia causing prerenal ARF, systemic diseases with renal manifestations, infection, or exogenous causes (toxins) that target the kidneys. Postrenal ARF denotes obstruction or diversion of urine outflow and consequent accumulation of urinary excretory products within the body. Early recognition and correction of postrenal azotemia resolves the uremia quickly without permanent damage to the kidneys. Intrinsic ARF constitutes the most therapeutic challenge and constitutes the bulk of the remaining discussion.

PATHOPHYSIOLOGY

No single sequence of events can explain all manifestations of naturally occurring ARF or available ischemic and nephrotoxic models of this syndrome. However, an understanding of the prevailing pathophysiologic mechanisms is useful for prevention strategies and to guide the therapeutic intervention of intrinsic ARF. Following both ischemic and nephrotoxic insults to the kidney, afferent arteriolar vasoconstriction can be induced by increased adrenergic activity, release of vasoactive substances (thromboxane, endothelin, platelet-activating factor), endothelial or glomerular capillary cell damage and swelling, and intravascular coagulation. The resultant hypoperfusion causes cellular hypoxia, adenosine triphosphate depletion, and disruption of cellular transport and metabolism, resulting in membrane damage and death of the tubular epithelium. Conversely, intense vasodilation of the efferent arteriole reduces glomerular capillary hydrostatic pressure and glomerular filtration rate, decreasing urine production and regulation of solute and water reabsorption.

Either toxic or ischemic insults to the kidney can disrupt the integrity of the epithelial lining, permitting backleakage of filtrate into the interstitium and peritubular capillaries to perpetuate the initial reduction in urine formation. Further reduction of tubular fluid flow occurs by obstruction of

TABLE 1. Causes of Acute Renal Failure

Prerenal

Congestive heart failure	Trauma	Hypoalbuminemia	Dehydration
Hypoadrenocorticism	Surgery	Heat stroke	Anesthesia
Hypovolemic shock	Hemorrhagic shock	Hypotensive shock	Septic shock

Intrinsic Renal

Nephrotoxins

Ethylene glycol	Cisplatin	Nonsteroidal anti-inflammatory drugs	Hemoglobinuria
Aminoglycosides	Radiocontrast agents	Heavy metals	Myoglobinuria
Amphotericin B	Snake venom		

Hemodynamic

Hypovolemic shock	Cardiovascular shock	Hypotensive shock	Surgery
Hemorrhagic shock	Septic shock	Anesthesia	

Other Conditions

Hypercalcemia	Rickettsial infections	Lymphoma	Trauma
Leptospirosis	Pyelonephritis	Cardiovascular failure	Glomerulonephritis

Postrenal

Bilateral renal calculi	Urethral calculi	Extraluminal obstruction	Rupture of outflow tracts
Bilateral ureteral calculi	Urethral neoplasia	Prostatic disease	

the tubule with cellular debris and tubular casts. Tubular obstruction exacerbates increases in intratubular pressure associated with cellular swelling and interstitial edema, worsening the backleak and filtration failure. As these events resolve, tubular flow can be re-established, but the damaged tubular epithelium may be unable to regulate fluid and solute homeostasis, causing excessive fluid (polyuria) and electrolyte and acid-base abnormalities.

CLINICAL PRESENTATION

Acute renal failure is associated with a history of sudden onset (days) of anorexia, listlessness, vomiting, and diarrhea. Additional complaints of halitosis, ataxia, seizures, known toxin exposure, recent trauma, medical or surgical diseases (or medications), and observation of oliguria-anuria or polyuria are often reported. Lack of historical exposure to toxins does not exclude the potential of nephrotoxicosis, and the influence of concurrent therapeutic agents such as furosemide, angiotensin-converting enzyme (ACE) inhibitors, and antimicrobic and antineoplastic agents for pre-existing conditions should not be overlooked. Preenting clinical signs are nonspecific and include depression, lethargy, weakness, muscle tremors, stupor, or seizures. The presentation of animals with oliguria-anuria is roughly equal to those with nonoliguric presentations including polyuria.

Findings on initial physical examination may include dehydration, hypothermia, lingual or oral ulceration, necrosis of the margins of the tongue, scleral injection, tachypnea, and bradycardia. On abdominal palpation, the kidneys are usually large, swollen, and painful. Abdominal pain due to edema, swelling, and inflammation of the kidneys must be differentiated from other causes of acute abdomen, such as pancreatitis, peritonitis, and intestinal obstruction. The urinary bladder may be distended in animals with postrenal azotemia. Patients who have received fluid therapy prior to presentation may demonstrate chemosis, peripheral or pulmonary edema, and increased breath sounds on auscultation of the chest indicative of fluid overload. Animals with ARF and no other underlying medical conditions usually have normal body condition and healthy hair-coat and skin.

DIAGNOSTIC EVALUATION

Intrinsic ARF must be distinguished from prerenal and postrenal causes of ARF and from coexistent pre- and postrenal contributions. Similarly, concurrent prerenal azotemia and intrinsic ARF must be recognized in animals with acute exacerbations of underlying chronic renal disease. Azotemia and a concurrent urine specific gravity greater than 1.030 in dogs and 1.035 in cats is consistent with prerenal azotemia. Azotemia in the presence of inadequately concentrated urine (specific gravity 1.007 to 1.029 in dogs or 1.034 in cats) or isosthenuria supports a diagnosis of intrinsic ARF; however, renal concentrating ability may be impaired with some causes of *prerenal* azotemia such as hypoadrenocorticism or pre-existing renal disease or following diuretic administration. Prerenal azotemia resolves rapidly following correction of fluid volume deficits and restoration of blood pressure and renal perfusion. Prerenal azotemia can also be differentiated from intrinsic ARF by the demonstration of a fractional excretion of sodium less than or equal to 1%, but indices of sodium excretion are rarely used in veterinary practice and offer little advantage over careful clinical assessments. Postrenal azotemia is commonly associated with a history of stranguria, dysuria, or anuria and clinical evidence of a large distended bladder or hydroperitoneum. Hindrance or obstruction to passage of a urinary catheter suggests urethral outflow obstruction, and urine leakage may be associated with signs of hematuria, inguinal or perineal swelling and pain, or ascites. Abdominal fluid concentrations of potassium, creatinine, or urea greater than concurrent serum concentrations support the diagnosis of uroperitoneum. Ultrasonography (see *CVT XII*, p. 933) and plain and contrast radiographic studies (excretory urography, double-contrast cystography, or retrograde urethrography) are indicated for animals with postrenal azotemia to define the location and nature of the outflow failure.

Acute renal failure is associated with variable hyperkalemia and hypocalcemia, moderate to severe metabolic acidosis, and hyperphosphatemia in addition to azotemia. The anion gap is increased because of accumulation of phosphate, sulfates, and other organic acids. Urinalysis variably reveals proteinuria, glucosuria, and an active sediment including granular and cellular casts, red blood cells, white blood cells, epithelial cells, bacteria, or crystals, depending on the underlying cause of renal failure.

The kidneys of animals with ARF may appear of normal size or enlarged on survey radiographs, whereas small irregular kidneys are more indicative of chronic renal insufficiency. Radiographs should be inspected closely for calculi and prostatomegaly. Ultrasonography of the kidneys complements the physical and radiographic assessment of renal architecture. The kidneys commonly appear enlarged with good preservation of the corticomedullary junction. The cortex is typically thickened and relatively hyperechoic compared with liver, spleen, and renal medulla. Extremely hyperechoic (bright) renal cortices strongly suggest ethylene glycol toxicity as the cause. Dilated renal pelves may be seen with urinary tract obstruction or pyelonephritis or following fluid therapy.

Percutaneous renal biopsy will confirm the diagnosis of intrinsic ARF and help establish its cause, severity, and potential reversibility but is rarely indicated in the initial evaluation or management decisions. Percutaneous renal biopsy techniques are generally safe, but they may induce additional morbidity and delay definitive therapies like hemodialysis. Many animals with ARF will respond to supportive therapy and regain renal function whether or not a definitive diagnosis has been established. Percutaneous renal biopsy is indicated when a diagnosis other than toxic or ischemic renal disease is suspected to guide specific therapy, identify underlying chronic disease, or establish the reversibility of the renal lesions prior to discontinuing therapy.

Additional diagnostic tests to establish the cause include toxin analysis for ethylene glycol, glycolic acid, and gentamicin (see *CVT XII*, p. 943), and serologic tests for leptospirosis.

TREATMENT

The management of the acute uremia encompasses *reversing* the underlying cause or causes and ongoing risk factors (drugs, inadequate hemodynamics, concurrent diseases) for the renal injury; *correcting* the uremic intoxications and the fluid, electrolyte, and acid-base imbalances; *establishing* adequate urine production; and *providing* nutritional support until renal function has recovered. Delays in initiating appropriate treatments can prolong and worsen the renal damage, close finite windows of reversibility, and jeopardize a successful outcome. Identification and removal of the underlying cause or causes of ARF are not always possible. Induction of vomiting or gastric lavage should be performed shortly after presentation if a toxin has been ingested. Activated charcoal suspensions should be administered as an adjunct following gastric lavage to absorb residual toxin. Potentially nephrotoxic drugs should be discontinued and efforts made to prevent further or ongoing renal injury. Appropriate parenteral antibiotic therapy should be started if septicemia, pyelonephritis, or leptospirosis is suspected. The potential for exaggerated or toxic effects of drugs due to decreased renal clearance must be considered before they are administered routinely.

Correction of Fluid Imbalances

Animals with ARF typically are dehydrated and hypovolemic because of anorexia, vomiting, and diarrhea. An estimate of the initial fluid deficit should be made on the basis of body weight and skin turgor and determination of hematocrit, plasma proteins, capillary refill time, arterial blood pressure, pulse rate, and central venous pressure. The amount of replacement fluid to replete the deficit is calculated by multiplying the estimate of dehydration by the body weight in kilograms. The volume deficit should be corrected with normal saline or balanced polyionic solutions within 4 to 6 hours. Blood losses should be replaced with compatible blood transfusions to restore intravascular volume, blood pressure, and hematocrit. Further fluid administration should be provided to achieve mild (3 to 5% of body weight) volume expansion (balanced electrolyte solutions) and to replace insensible requirements (20 to 25 ml/kg per day 5% dextrose in water) and ongoing urinary and gastrointestinal losses (balanced electrolyte solutions). Maintenance solutions of 5% dextrose are generally inappropriate and ineffective to restore initial fluid deficits and initiate diuresis.

Fluid balance should be assessed regularly by changes in body weight and indices of hydration (see earlier) to direct ongoing fluid prescriptions. Oliguric or anuric animals are incapable of effectively excreting an excessive fluid load, so great care must be taken to avoid volume overload. Similar precautions should be taken in animals with cardiovascular insufficiency who are at risk for circulatory overload. Excessive fluid administration is associated with chemosis, serous nasal discharge, systemic hypertension, subcutaneous edema, ascites, pleural effusion, pulmonary edema, and elevated central venous pressure (>12 cm H_2O). Hypervolemia is a serious and potentially life-threatening complication of therapy that is difficult or impossible to correct. Further fluid administration is contraindicated, and diuretic administration or dialysis may be required to resolve the fluid burden. Maintenance fluid requirements are predicated on assessment of ongoing fluid losses (urinary, vomitus, fecal), which are replaced with isonatric solutions, and insensible fluid (free water) requirements, which must be supplied orally or by parenteral administration of 5% dextrose.

Correction of Acid-Base and Electrolyte Disorders

Severe metabolic acidosis and life-threatening hyperkalemia are common complications of ARF, but variable primary or mixed acid-base disturbances and potassium concentrations may develop depending on the underlying cause and extent of the vomiting, diarrhea, and respiratory components. Treatment decisions should be based on assessment of serum bicarbonate (or total carbon dioxide), blood gases, serum potassium, and an electrocardiogram. Metabolic acidosis should be treated with sodium bicarbonate if the serum bicarbonate is less than 15 mEq/L. The bicarbonate replacement (milliequivalents) equals the body weight (kilograms) $\times$ 0.3 $\times$ the bicarbonate deficit. One half of the calculated replacement is administered as a slow IV infusion over 20 to 30 minutes, and the remainder is provided with IV fluids over 4 to 6 hours. Serum bicarbonate or blood gases should be re-evaluated following the initial replacement to determine if the bicarbonate deficit is replete or if additional therapy is required. Most animals with oliguric or anuric ARF have an ongoing requirement for sodium bicarbonate at approximately 80 to 90 mg/kg per day to offset the production of metabolic acids. Administration of sodium bicarbonate can promote metabolic alkalosis and sodium excesses, potentiate a decrease in ionized calcium concentration, and induce paradoxical cerebral acidosis and cerebral edema (see *CVT XII*, p. 956).

Progressive electrocardiographic signs of hyperkalemia include bradycardia, decreased P wave amplitude, prolongation of the PR interval, peaking or biphasic T waves, and widening of QRS complexes. Severe hyperkalemia induces sine wave–appearing QRS complexes, idioventricular complexes, and ventricular escape complexes that may progress to ventricular fibrillation or asystole. These severe electrocardiographic signs require immediate intervention to counteract the cardiotoxicity and correct the hyperkalemia. Table 2 outlines conventional methods for managing hyperkalemia according to its severity and clinical effects. These treatments provide only transient protection from life-threatening arrhythmias until renal potassium excretion is restored or the potassium load is dissipated with dialysis.

Management of Oliguria-Anuria

Failure to induce an adequate diuresis by repletion of fluid deficits predicts severe renal parenchymal injury. A number of therapeutic agents have been advocated to attenuate the severity of the renal injury or induce urine formation in the initial oliguric or anuric phase of ARF. Despite demonstrated benefits in experimental forms of ischemic or toxic ARF, their efficacy remains controversial in clinical

TABLE 2. Management of Hyperkalemia in Acute Renal Failure

Therapy	Mechanism of Action
Mild Hyperkalemia (≤6.0 mEq/L)	
IV fluids (0.9% saline, lactated Ringer's)	Plasma volume expansion, dilutes K+, and increased glomerular filtration rate and renal potassium excretion
Moderate Hyperkalemia (6.0 to 8.0 mEq/L)	
Sodium bicarbonate 1–2 mEq/kg IV slowly over 20 min	Translocates potassium to intracellular space in exchange for hydrogen ions
Dextrose (20–50%) 1.5 gm/kg IV bolus	IV dextrose stimulates insulin release; insulin plus dextrose promotes transcellular entry of potassium into cells
Regular insulin and dextrose (20–50%) Insulin, 0.1–0.25 U/kg plus dextrose, 1–2 gm/U IV	Insulin plus dextrose promotes transcellular entry of potassium into cells
Severe Hyperkalemia (≥8.0 mEq/L)	
Calcium gluconate (10%) 0.5–1.0 ml/kg over 10–15 min; monitor the electrocardiogram during administration	Specific antagonist of the cardiotoxic effects of potassium

settings and should not supersede appropriate and timely administration of fluid therapy (Thadhani et al, 1996). The conversion of oliguric or anuric ARF to a nonoliguric state significantly facilitates the management of fluid, electrolyte, and acid-base disorders and has prompted the empirical use of diuretic agents such as mannitol and furosemide and the vasodilator dopamine, but induced changes in urine volume production may not be equated with improvements in renal function or recovery. Within judicious limits, however, these treatments pose minimal clinical risks and may facilitate the management.

Hypertonic mannitol (10 to 25%; Osmitrol, Baxter) can be given to fluid-replete animals as an initial slow bolus of 0.5 to 1.0 gm/kg IV to promote diuresis. Mannitol increases renal blood flow and tubular fluid flow, decreases epithelial swelling and intratubular obstruction, and scavenges oxygen free radicals. If significant diuresis is established within 30 minutes, mannitol can be continued as a constant rate infusion (CRI) at 1 to 2 mg/kg per minute IV or as intermittent boluses of 0.5 to 1.0 gm/kg every 4 to 6 hours IV for the next 24 to 48 hours. If adequate diuresis is not established, the initial dose may be repeated, but further administration is contraindicated if the animal is hypervolemic or has evidence of cardiac or pulmonary failure.

Furosemide (Lasix, Hoechst) is a powerful natriuretic agent with mild renal vasodilating effects and is used alone or in combination with mannitol or dopamine (Intropin, Du Pont; see further on) to promote urine formation. Furosemide is given initially at 2 to 6 mg/kg IV after correcting existing fluid deficits. If adequate diuresis is not evident

within 30 minutes, readministration at the initial or a higher dose is indicated, or the diuretic can be combined with dopamine. If diuresis is achieved, the dose is repeated every 8 hours to extend the diuresis for 24 to 48 hours, but fluid balance must be carefully monitored to prevent volume contraction and further compromise to renal hemodynamics.

Dopamine at 1 to 3 μg/kg per minute IV is a renal vasodilating agent with the potential to increase renal blood flow, glomerular filtration, and renal sodium excretion (Lindner et al, 1979; Flancbaum et al, 1994; Conger, 1995). Higher doses may cause renal vasoconstriction, tachycardia, and cardiac arrhythmias and are contraindicated in ARF unless required to maintain systemic blood pressure. Dopamine and furosemide are synergistic in their effects to increase urine production and generally are more effective when used in combination than when either agent is used alone. Once diuresis is established, strict attention to fluid and electrolyte balance is required.

With the onset of diuresis, some animals enter a polyuric phase that may signal recovery of renal function. During this state, fluid and electrolyte losses may exceed input, causing severe imbalances and recurrence of the uremia if the increased urine output is not accounted for in the assessment of maintenance and insensible losses (see *CVT XII*, p. 951). Hypokalemia may develop during the polyuric phase in response to diuretics, and supplemental potassium should be provided cautiously (not more than 0.5 mEq/kg per hour IV) to normalize serum potassium. Fluid therapy should continue until the azotemia has stabilized, electrolyte and acid-base abnormalities are corrected, and the animal is able to eat and drink. At this time, IV fluids can be withdrawn slowly or supplemented with subcutaneous fluids over 3 to 5 days.

If a diuretic response cannot be established or maintained within 4 to 6 hours following restoration of fluid deficits and administration of combined mannitol and furosemide or dopamine, or both, it is highly unlikely that additional administration of fluid or drugs will be safe or effective, and dialysis should be considered as an alternative. Peritoneal or hemodialysis is required when conservative medical management fails to increase urine production or the clinical complications associated with the azotemia, hyperkalemia, acid-base disturbances, and fluid overload cannot be controlled immediately (Cowgill, 1995; Cowgill and Langston, 1996). Dialysis can resolve the excretory complications of ARF and stabilize the animal until the renal injury is repaired and excretory function is regained. Without dialysis, most oliguric-anuric animals die before renal function is re-established. General indications for dialysis include severe oliguria or anuria, life-threatening fluid overload, electrolyte or acid-base disturbances, blood urea nitrogen levels greater than or equal to 100 mg/dl, serum creatinine levels greater than or equal to 10 mg/dl, or a clinical course refractory to medical therapy for more than 24 hours. Specific indications include acute poisoning with dialyzable toxins (ethylene glycol) or drugs that can be eliminated effectively from the body to prevent or minimize their toxicity. Peritoneal dialysis can be accomplished in private practice but is intensive and time-consuming and is complicated by catheter malfunction, dialysate leakage, fluid overload, and infection (see p. 859).

TABLE 3. Hemodialysis Centers in the United States

State	Institution or Center*	Phone Number
California	Veterinary Medical Teaching Hospital University of California at Davis Davis, CA 95616	916-752-1393
Maryland	Veterinary Referral Associates, Inc. 15021 Dufief Mill Road Gaithersburg, MD 20878	301-340-3224
Michigan	Veterinary Clinical Center Michigan State University East Lansing, MI 48824	517-347-5034
New York	The Animal Medical Center 510 East 62nd Street New York, NY 10021	212-838-8100

*Consult local specialists in your area for other possible sites.

Hemodialysis is effective and efficient in resolving the clinical complications of ARF (see *CVT XII,* p. 975) and is available on an emergency basis at regional centers throughout the United States for both dogs and cats (Table 3).

Nutritional Support

Recovery from ARF may require a prolonged convalescence during which animals are hypercatabolic, azotemic, hyperkalemic, acidotic, and hyperphosphatemic. Precise nutritional requirements for dogs and cats with ARF are unknown, but a high-energy, moderate-protein, potassium- and phosphate-containing diet comparable to those for chronic renal failure is a logical choice (see *CVT XII,* p. 971). Protein-calorie malnutrition is common, as dietary intake is compromised by anorexia, nausea, and vomiting and, initially, animals who can tolerate the additional fluid load benefit from parenteral nutrition until vomiting has ceased, at which time a commercial renal-failure diet can be substituted. Animals reluctant to eat appropriate amounts of food ad. lib. should have supplementation with enteral feeding via a nasogastric or gastrotomy tube. Enteral feeding to reach caloric and protein requirements can be achieved by blended commercial prescription diets (e.g., Prescription Diet Feline and Canine k/d, Hill's Pet Products; Canine Medium and Low Protein Diet or Feline Low Protein Diet, Waltham) or formulated liquid diets (Renal Care, Pet Ag).

Supportive Therapy

Antiemetics in combination with the restriction of all oral intake should be used to control protracted vomiting. Metoclopramide (Reglan, Robins), at 0.01 to 0.02 mg/kg per hour CRI or 0.1 to 0.5 mg/kg IM PO every 8 hours, or phenothiazine-derivative antiemetics (e.g., chlorpromazine [Thorazine, SK-Beecham; 0.5 mg/kg IM every 6 to 8 hours] or prochlorperazine [Darbazine, SK-Beecham; 0.1 to 0.5 mg/kg IM or SC every 12 hours]) suppress central vomiting centers. However, one must take into consideration the hypotensive potential of the phenothiazine derivatives. A histamine receptor–blocking drug such as cimeti-

dine (Tagamet, SK-Beecham; 5 to 10 mg/kg PO, IM, IV every 6 to 8 hours), ranitidine (Zantac, Glaxo; 2.0 mg/kg IV every 12 hours), or famotidine (Pepcid, Merck; 0.5 to 1.0 mg/kg PO or IV every 12 to 24 hours), in combination with a gastrointestinal protectant such as sucralfate (Carafate, Marion; 1 gm/30 kg PO every 6 to 8 hours in dogs; 0.25 to 0.5 gm PO every 6 to 8 hours in cats), may be used in the prevention of severe esophagitis and ulcerative gastritis during periods of severe azotemia and persistent vomiting.

Restriction of dietary phosphate is usually insufficient to prevent phosphate retention and hyperphosphatemia; therefore, phosphate binding products may need to be added to the therapeutic regimen. Phosphate binding agents combine with soluble phosphates derived from the diet and digestive secretions to form insoluble complexes that escape intestinal absorption and augment fecal phosphate excretion. Aluminum-based antacid compounds, such as aluminum hydroxide (Amphojel, Wyeth-Ayerst; ALterna-GEL, J&J-Merck) or aluminum carbonate (Basaljel, Wyeth-Ayerst) should be used at an empirical starting dosage of 30 to 90 mg/kg body weight per day divided with each feeding. To be effective, the binding agent must be administered simultaneously with the ingested meal. The dosage of phosphate binders must be adjusted appropriately until serum phosphate stabilizes.

Transfusion of compatible packed red blood cells or recombinant human erythropoietin (Epogen, Amgen) should be provided as needed for anemia associated with excessive blood sampling, gastrointestinal losses, decreased erythropoietin production, and decreased red blood cell survival. Other complications of severe uremia include stomatitis, enterocolitis, diarrhea, vasculitis, uremic encephalopathy and seizures, and uremic pneumonitis. Treatment for these disorders is empirical, and the conditions improve with resolution of the azotemia. Oral rinsing with 0.1% chlorhexidine solution is beneficial for uremic stomatitis and oral ulcerations. Systemic hypertension may require antihypertensive therapy to prevent retinal detachment and cerebral bleeding (see p. 838).

PREVENTION

Predisposition to the development of ARF includes preexisting renal disease, dehydration, concurrent cardiovascular or hepatic disease, sepsis, and use of diuretics or drugs with nephrotoxic potential (see *CVT XII,* p. 943). Clinical recognition of such predisposition is a major principle of prevention. Most preventable cases of ARF are caused by prolonged hypotension secondary to anesthesia or hemorrhage resulting from trauma or surgery. Anesthesia should be kept as brief as possible and mean blood pressure maintained at greater than 70 mm Hg to preserve renal perfusion. In addition, a mild solute diuresis should be maintained with a balanced electrolyte solution. The use of potentially nephrotoxic drugs such as aminoglycosides, cisplatin, or amphotericin B should be avoided or accompanied by brisk solute diuresis with 0.9% sodium chloride. Furosemide should not be used concurrently with gentamicin because it potentiates its nephrotoxicity. Prophylactic administration of mannitol with maintenance fluids may facilitate volume expansion and further protect animals at risk for the development of ischemic or nephrotoxic ARF.

EXPECTED OUTCOME AND PROGNOSIS

The potential for recovery is a fundamental difference between acute and chronic renal failure. Although some animals recover with no clinically apparent renal insufficiency, others have incomplete recoveries that require long-term management for chronic failure. The prognosis for recovery of renal function is good for pre- and postrenal causes of azotemia if the underlying conditions are identified and corrected. For mild forms of nonoliguric ARF, complete or partial recovery of renal function may be expected over 3 to 6 weeks, but the prognosis must remain guarded. Oliguric ARF has a guarded to poor prognosis for recovery. Recovery is often signaled by the onset of sudden diuresis and a gradual (usually partial) return of renal function over 4 to 12 weeks. Anuric ARF or conditions associated with multiple organ failure are generally fatal without dialysis support for extended periods to permit renal regeneration and repair. Renal transplantation is now a viable alternative for animals (especially cats) when kidney function remains compromised (Gregory and Gourley, 1992).

References and Suggested Reading

Conger JD: Interventions in clinical acute renal failure: What are the data? Am J Kidney Dis 26:565, 1995.
Cowgill LD: Application of peritoneal dialysis and hemodialysis in the management of renal failure. In: Osborne CA, Finco DR, eds: Canine and Feline Nephrology and Urology. Baltimore: Lea & Febiger, 1995, p 573.
  Discussion of the indications, applications, and complications of peritoneal and hemodialysis in dogs and cats.
Cowgill LD, Langston CE: Role of hemodialysis in the management of dogs and cats with renal failure. Vet Clin North Am 26:1347, 1996.
  Comprehensive discussion of the applications, benefits, and complications of hemodialysis in uremic animals.
Flancbaum L, Choban PS, Dasta FJ: Quantitative effects of low-dose dopamine on urine output in oliguric surgical intensive care unit patients. Crit Care Med 22:61, 1994.
Grauer GF, Lane IF: Acute renal failure. In: Ettinger SJ, Feldman EC, eds: Textbook of Veterinary Internal Medicine. Philadelphia: WB Saunders, 1995, p 1720.
  Comprehensive review of the etiology, diagnosis, and management of acute renal failure in dogs and cats.
Gregory CR, Gourley RM: Renal transplantation in clinical veterinary medicine. In: Kirk RW, Bonagura JD, eds: Current Veterinary Therapy XI. Philadelphia: WB Saunders, 1992, p 870.
  Provides a review of patient selection and procedure and complications of renal transplantation.
Lane IF, Graur GF, Fettman MJ: Acute renal failure: Part I. Risk factors, prevention, and strategies for protection. Compend Cont Ed Pract Vet 16:15, 1994.
  Reviews the pathophysiology, risk factors, early intervention, and prevention of acute renal failure.
Lane IF, Graur GF, Fettman MJ: Acute renal failure: Part II. Diagnosis, management, and prognosis. Compend Cont Ed Pract Vet 16:625, 1994.
  Review of the diagnosis and general management of patients with acute renal failure.
Lindner A, Cutler RE, Goodman G: Synergism of dopamine plus furosemide in preventing acute renal failure in the dog. Kidney Int 16:158, 1979.
Thadhani R, Pascual M, Bonventre JV: Acute renal failure. N Engl J Med 334:1448, 1996.
  Review of cause, pathogenesis, and management of acute renal failure in human patients.

Craniocerebral Trauma

JUSTINE A. JOHNSON
Warwick, Rhode Island

ROBERT J. MURTAUGH
North Grafton, Massachusetts

Primary injuries to the brain are a direct result of trauma, are completed at the time of the trauma, and do not lend themselves to reversal with medical therapy. Primary injuries include skull fractures, blood vessel disruption, and tearing or crushing of brain parenchyma. Although these injuries may be severe, most deaths occurring in patients surviving the initial trauma are attributed to secondary brain injury. Secondary injuries develop because of anatomic and physiologic changes that occur as a result of the primary injury and include hemorrhage, cerebral edema, increased intracranial pressure, and ischemia. These changes occur over hours to days after the traumatic event, and their control provides the principal opportunity for improvement of outcome through medical and surgical intervention.

PATHOPHYSIOLOGY

Intracranial pressure (ICP) increases as a result of intracranial mass lesions (tumors, edema, hematomas), increased intrathoracic or intra-abdominal pressure, or extracranial factors such as hypercarbia, hyperthermia, or fluid overload that cause increases in cerebral blood volume. The most detrimental effect of increased ICP is a reduction in cerebral blood flow (CBF). Adequate CBF is dependent on the pressure difference between arterial inflow and venous outflow. If ICP rises to the level of arterial blood pressure, or if parenchymal swelling occludes venous and ventricular outflow, blood flow across the brain may cease, leading to tissue ischemia and severe cellular injury.

The uninjured brain has several mechanisms to prevent

increases in ICP. Accommodation is the redistribution of blood and cerebrospinal fluid (CSF), which allows more room within the skull for swelling brain tissue. Capacitance vessels constrict, forcing blood into venous sinuses and jugular veins, and CSF is reabsorbed or displaced into the subarachnoid space and spinal canal.

Pressure autoregulation is the ability to maintain a constant CBF during periods of hypotension or hypertension by means of altered vascular diameter and cerebrovascular reactivity. In the uninjured brain, CBF remains stable across a wide range of systemic mean arterial blood pressure (MAP; 50 to 150 mm Hg). As the MAP decreases to less than 50 mm Hg, vasodilation progresses, but CBF decreases and becomes dependent on MAP. When MAP is maintained and cerebral perfusion pressure (CPP) increases, vasoconstriction of cerebral vessels serves to decrease overall cerebral blood volume and ICP (CPP = MAP − ICP).

Chemical autoregulation is the response of the cerebrovasculature to changes in $PaCO_2$, pH, and levels of oxygen, calcium, potassium, and arachidonic acid metabolites. Most significant is the effect of increased $PaCO_2$, which causes vasodilation and increased CBF. This "CO_2 reactivity" is preserved unless brain injury is severe. Vasodilation also occurs in response to hypoxemia (PaO_2 <50 mm Hg). In addition, cerebral ischemia, which occurs during periods of increased ICP or systemic hypotension, triggers an increase in systemic blood pressure (Cushing's reflex), thus potentially increasing CPP.

The development of cerebral edema is a significant contributor to increased brain volume and ICP. Cytotoxic edema is the result of abnormal cell metabolism and develops during periods of ischemia. In the absence of oxygen, there is a decrease in adenosine triphosphate synthesis and a decrease in the function of adenosine triphosphate–dependent membrane transport mechanisms. This leads to the accumulation of water and solutes within the neurons and glia. Cytotoxic edema is only minimally responsive to medical therapy. Vasogenic edema is more clinically significant and results from the disruption of the blood-brain barrier. Following periods of ischemia, reperfusion of ischemic tissues induces the production of free radicals and vasoactive substances (such as arachidonic acid metabolites). With iron as an important cofactor, free radicals react with polyunsaturated fatty acids in lipid membranes (including endothelial cell membranes and tight junctions), beginning a chain reaction of lipid peroxidation and membrane injury. This results in the leakage of proteins and small molecules into the interstitial space. The osmotic gradient produced by these solutes, as well as hydrostatic pressure from the circulating blood, drives water into the interstitium. Vasogenic edema is more responsive to therapy than is cytotoxic edema, but therapy for head trauma victims should be directed at preventing the degree and duration of cerebral ischemia to minimize the development of edema.

PATIENT EVALUATION

Neurologic Assessment

When an animal is presented with craniocerebral trauma, immediate evaluation for patency of the airway and stable vital signs is essential. Before neurologic injuries are assessed, the patient should be resuscitated from shock and evaluated for major body cavity injury. Significant body trauma can cause hemodynamic instability and lead to secondary brain injury. Initial neurologic assessment should include an evaluation of the state of consciousness, breathing pattern, size and responsiveness of pupils, ocular position and movements, and skeletal motor responses. Once the initial neurologic assessment is complete, the level of medical or surgical therapy can be selected (Fig. 1). Neurologic assessment should be repeated every 30 to 60 minutes (Table 1) in severely head-injured patients and therapies altered if changes in neurologic status occur.

A decreased level of consciousness is suggestive of injury to the cerebrum or the reticular activating system of the brain stem. Levels of consciousness range from normal, depressed, or delirious to stuporous or comatose. Patients presenting in a state of coma generally have bilateral or global cerebral abnormalities or severe brain stem injury and have a guarded prognosis.

Abnormalities or changes in respiratory pattern in the absence of significant thoracic or pulmonary trauma can signal severe brain injury or neurologic deterioration. Centrally mediated neurologic hyperventilation may occur as a result of cerebral acidosis or hypoxia, progressive damage to the mesencephalon, or transtentorial herniation secondary to increased ICP. Cheyne-Stokes respiration occurs as a cycle of hyperventilation followed by apnea. This pattern indicates a decreased responsiveness to increasing $PaCO_2$ and is most often associated with injury to the diencephalon. Ataxic respiration is characterized by irregularity in the rate, rhythm, and amplitude of respirations. The presence of this pattern usually indicates terminal brain stem damage. Concomitant bradycardia and hypertension are often present with this pattern and are associated with a grave prognosis.

Pupils that respond appropriately to light, even if miotic, indicate adequate function of the rostral brain stem, optic chiasm, optic nerves, and retinae. If there is no evidence of direct ocular trauma or Horner's syndrome from cervical injury, the presence of bilateral unresponsive, miotic pupils, mydriasis, or asymmetrical pupils suggests brain stem injury. Pupils that are initially miotic and that become mydriatic are indicative of a progressive brain stem lesion. Bilateral mydriasis with no response to light is usually indicative of irreversible midbrain damage or herniation of the cerebellum through the foramen magnum, or both. Unilateral mydriasis may indicate unilateral cerebellar herniation or brain stem hemorrhage. Oculocephalic reflexes (doll's eye) are abnormal with brain stem injury but may also be depressed by cerebral injury.

In cases of head trauma with no spinal involvement, segmental spinal reflexes are normal to exaggerated. Postural reflexes may be diminished. Extensor rigidity of the limbs may occur as a result of cerebral or cerebellar injury. Opisthotonos with hyperextension of all four limbs is suggestive of decerebrate rigidity, whereas variable flexion and extension of the hind limbs is seen in rigidity with cerebellar injury. Patients with decerebrate rigidity are semicomatose and have abnormal pupillary reactivity, whereas consciousness may be normal if the lesion is in the cerebellum. Other indicators of cerebellar injury are the presence of

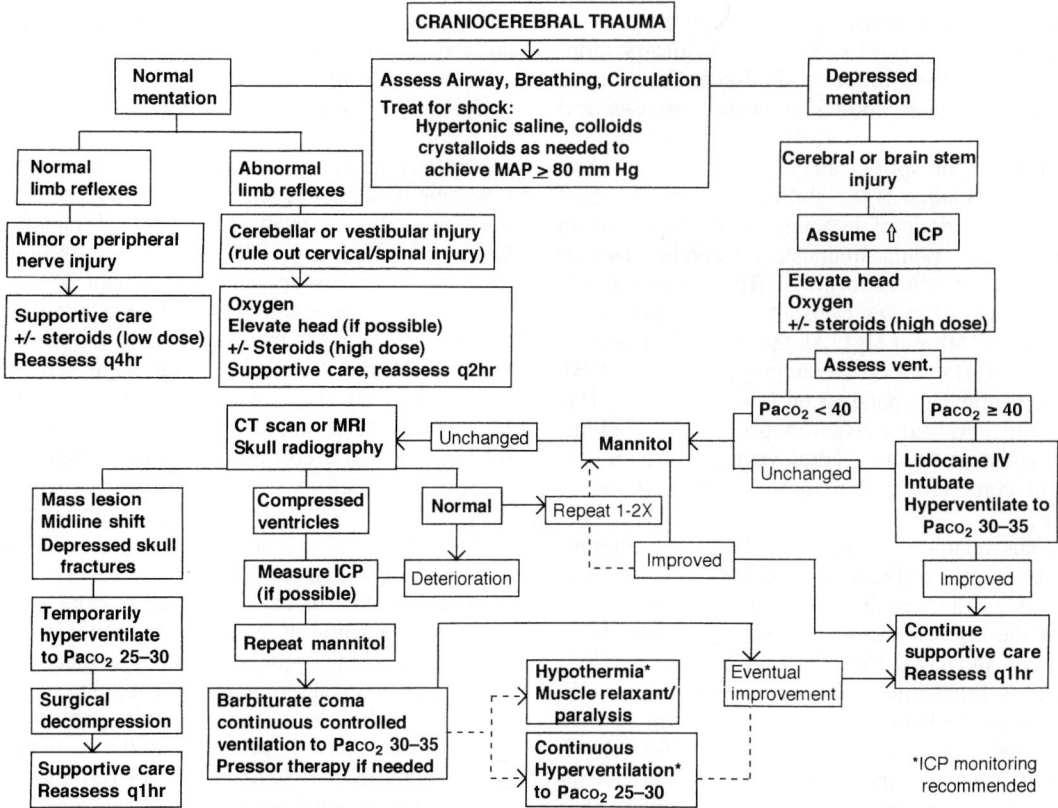

Figure 1. Algorithm for the treatment of craniocerebral trauma.

normal vision and palpebral reflexes, absent menace response, and intention tremors. Decerebrate rigidity is indicative of a loss of communication between the brain stem and cerebrum and carries a poor prognosis. The prognosis is better with cerebellar injury.

Clinical signs of increased ICP include papilledema, nausea, vomiting, decreased pupillary reactivity, decreased level of consciousness, altered gait, altered motor functions, and Cushing's reflex (increased blood pressure with bradycardia). Neurologic deterioration, as evidenced by progressive loss of consciousness, anisocoria or miosis progressing to fixed midrange or dilated pupils, the development of an abnormal respiratory pattern, or increased extensor tone in the limbs is strongly suggestive of progressively increasing ICP. If increased ICP is suspected, aggressive medical therapy should be instituted (Table 2). Neurologic deterioration despite aggressive medical management should prompt investigation (via diagnostic imaging) for compressive lesions such as depressed skull fractures or intracranial hematomas, which would necessitate surgical intervention.

Diagnostic Imaging

Radiographic evaluation of the skull is indicated for all cases of head trauma. Fractures of the cranium that are displaced more than the thickness of the calvarium should be repaired. Computed tomography (CT) and magnetic resonance imaging are useful in head trauma patients for the evaluation of skull fractures, bone fragments in the parenchyma, and intraparenchymal hemorrhage or extraparenchymal hematomas. In humans, CT is performed in all

cases of head injury because of the high prevalence of subdural hematomas. Subdural hematomas are considered rare in dogs and cats. However, one retrospective study in which the brains of traumatized dogs and cats were evaluated at surgery or necropsy revealed a high prevalence of intracranial hemorrhage. Ten of the 23 cases investigated had subdural hemorrhage, most of which could have been accessed with a lateral craniotomy (Dewey et al, 1993a). There have also been clinical reports of acute and delayed hematomas in dogs that were treated with surgical removal (Hopkins and Wheeler, 1991; Dewey et al, 1993b). If a subdural hematoma is apparent on CT or magnetic resonance imaging, craniotomy for decompression and evacuation of the hematoma is warranted. Increased ICP is evidenced on CT by compression of the ventricles and, if asymmetrical, may cause a shift of brain tissue away from midline. Intracranial hypertension is unlikely to develop in patients with no mass lesions or evidence of brain swelling on CT.

Intracranial Pressure Monitoring

Intracranial pressure monitoring is frequently employed in human hospitals and is being investigated for clinical use in dogs and cats. Methods for measuring ICP include the use of an intracranial (epidural, subarachnoid, or subdural) bolt or screw attached to a fluid-filled system with a pressure transducer or a fiberoptic transducer (Camino Laboratories) in the epidural, intraparenchymal, or intraventricular regions. The normal CSF pressure in dogs is 5 to 12 mm Hg, and the pressure in the brain parenchyma

TABLE 1. **Guidelines for Patient Monitoring Following Craniocerebral Trauma**

Monitoring Tools	Frequency	Goal	Action if Abnormal
Neurologic examination	30–60 min		If deteriorates, RESPOND with more aggressive medical therapy or surgery
Blood pressure	Continuous or q2hr	MAP 80–120 mm Hg	Fluid therapy $\pm$ pressor support if MAP <80 mm Hg
Central venous pressure	Continuous or q2hr	5–12 cm H_2O	Fluid therapy if CVP low
Blood gases	q.i.d., more often if hyperventilating	$Pao_2 \geq 80$ mm Hg $Paco_2 < 40$ mm Hg	Oxygen supplementation; intubate and ventilate if needed; to decrease ICP, ventilate 30 mm Hg < $Paco_2 < 35$ mm Hg
Pulse oximetry (SPO_2)	Continuous or q4–6hr	$SPO_2 \geq 95\%$	Oxygen supplementation; intubate; ventilate if $SPO_2 < 92\%$
Heart rate and rhythm	Continuous or q1hr	Normal rate varies by size and species	Treat arrhythmias; if tachycardic, evaluate for hypovolemia or pain and treat as indicated
Respiratory rate and rhythm	q1hr	10–25/min	Intubate and ventilate
Body temperature	q.i.d., more often if abnormal	100°–102.5°F	If febrile, evaluate for cause, treat with cool fluids, wet blanket, $\pm$ antibiotics, NSAIDs; for hypothermia therapy, maintain temperature between 31° and 34°C; warm slowly
Blood glucose	b.i.d., more often if abnormal or if during parenteral nutrition	80 < BG < 200 mg/dl	Add dextrose if BG <80 mg/dl; If hyperglycemic (BG >200 mg/dl), decrease parenteral dextrose, consider insulin
Electrolytes	b.i.d.	(See laboratory normals)	Alter fluid therapy as needed
Coagulation status	s.i.d.		If abnormal, administer fresh-frozen plasma
Hemoglobin	On presentation s.i.d. if abnormal, or if blood loss	Hb ≥ 7 gm/dl	Transfuse red blood cells if Hb <7 mg/dl
Intracranial pressure	q2hr	ICP 5–12 mm Hg	If ICP > 20 mm Hg, evaluate with CT or MRI. Decompress, evacuate hematomas; if not surgical, increase level of medical therapy

TABLE 2. **Therapeutic Agents Utilized in Patients With Craniocerebral Trauma**

Therapeutic	Beneficial Effects	Detrimental Effects
Hypertonic saline (7.5%) (3–5 ml/kg over 5 min)	Decreased ICP, increased CBF Induces vasomotor reflex to increase BP (small volume resuscitation of BP, CO) Improved rheology, oxygen delivery	Increased serum osmolality Hypernatremia (avoid if dehydration)
Colloids (Hetastarch, dextrans 20 ml/kg per 24 hr)	Decreased ICP	Coagulation abnormalities Anaphylactic reactions (dextrans)
Mannitol (0.25–1.0 gm/kg IV over 15 min)	Decreased brain density, water content Decreased ICP, increased CPP, CBF Decreased blood viscosity Free radical scavenging Decreased $CMRO_2$	Initial increase in ICP Hypernatremia, hyperkalemia Increased serum osmolality May accumulate in brain tissue and potentiate cerebral edema
Corticosteroids (Methylprednisolone sodium succinate, 30 mg/kg, then 15 mg/kg at 2 and 8 hr—high dose) (Dexamethasone, 2 mg/kg IV—low dose)	Decreased inflammatory response to necrosis Membrane stabilization via inhibition of lipid peroxidation	Perpetuates neuronal damage during periods of ischemia Promotes increases in blood glucose, metabolic acidosis, lactic acidosis
Hyperventilation (to $Paco_2$ 30–35 mm Hg)	Vasoconstriction causes decreased ICP	Decreased CBF may cause ischemia Shunting of blood to severely damaged areas Decreased cerebral O_2 delivery
Barbiturates (Pentobarbital 5–15 mg/kg to effect then 0.2–1 mg/kg/hr infusion)	Decreased $CMRO_2$ Decreased ICP Increased intracellular pH	Respiratory, myocardial depression Decreased vascular resistance $\rightarrow$ hypotension Vasoconstriction, shunting of blood to most damaged areas
Head elevation (30 degrees)	Decreased ICP (promotes venous and CSF drainage)	Decreased CPP (minimal if $\leq$30 degrees)
Hypothermia (to 31°–34°C)	Decreased $CMRO_2$ Decreased brain necrosis Decreased ICP	Herniation of brain during rewarming Coagulation abnormalities Cardiac arrhythmias Increased ICP with shivering (consider neuromuscular blockade)

ICP, intracranial pressure; CBF, cerebral blood flow; CPP, cerebral perfusion pressure (CPP = MAP − ICP); MAP, mean arterial pressure; $CMRO_2$, cerebral metabolic rate of oxygen consumption; CSF, cerebrospinal fluid; CO, cardiac output.

is slightly higher (Bagley, 1996). In humans, neurologic outcome is related to the amount of time the patient spends with an ICP greater than 20 mm Hg (Saul and Ducker, 1982). There has been considerable controversy in the medical literature about the necessity of monitoring ICP and the associated risks of the monitoring systems. Several studies of human patients have demonstrated an improved outcome when ICP is measured, but critics have argued that the coincident attention to improved cerebral oxygenation and overall patient monitoring and management may be responsible for the results. Measurement of ICP is especially useful in patients in which neurologic signs cannot be used to detect deterioration or improvement, either because the patient is severely injured and has lost all monitored neurologic functions or because sedative and paralytic agents are being used in patient management. Complications that may be associated with ICP monitors include focal edema, hemorrhage, parenchymal injury, and infection.

Other Neurologic Monitoring Tools

Continuous oximetry of the jugular vein has proved a reliable method of monitoring cerebral circulation and oxygen extraction in humans. This is a sensitive and specific test for detecting global cerebral ischemia. Episodes of jugular oxygen desaturation are associated with an increased risk of poor neurologic outcome in humans (Robertson, 1993). Although oximetry of the jugular vein has not been evaluated in veterinary patients, it may provide a useful, minimally invasive parameter for monitoring cerebral oxygenation.

Other monitoring tools that have a place in the management of craniocerebral trauma include somatosensory evoked potentials (e.g., brain stem auditory evoked responses), electroencephalography, and transcranial Doppler sonography. These tools are not yet widely used in veterinary medicine, although electroencephalography and brain stem auditory evoked responses have been used to determine brain death.

TREATMENT

The goal of cerebral dehydration has been largely abandoned and replaced by the goal of maintaining brain tissue oxygen delivery. This approach requires attention to and maintenance of adequate circulating blood volume, systemic arterial blood pressure, and oxygen carrying capacity (see Table 2). One study of human patients reported that improved fluid resuscitation, increased use of intubation and mechanical ventilation, and increased vigilance reduced the prevalence of craniocerebral hypotension and hypoxia by 43%, with a similar improvement in outcome (Gentleman and Jennett, 1992).

It should always be assumed that the victim of traumatic brain injury has cerebral ischemia, and early resuscitation with volume replacement is necessary to promote blood flow to the brain. Although furosemide was once a mainstay of therapy because of its ability to promote diuresis and cause cerebral (and systemic) dehydration, it is no longer recommended unless sodium or water retention is

suspected and natriuresis or diuresis is necessary. In mild cases of head trauma, the administration of crystalloid fluids may be adequate. The volume should be selected on the basis of an assessment of the patient's hemodynamic status and an estimation of blood loss. When the patient is semicomatose or comatose, it is especially important to maximize oxygen delivery and also to minimize the risk of fluid overload. This is best accomplished by monitoring central venous pressure (CVP), systemic arterial blood pressure (indirect or direct), blood gases, pulse oximetry, body temperature, heart rate and rhythm (electrocardiogram), respiratory rate and rhythm, and urine output. Patients should be resuscitated to a state of normovolemia to slight hypervolemia, as the risks associated with hypovolemia and hypotension far outweigh those associated with slightly overzealous fluid administration.

Fluid Therapy

The administration of hypertonic and hyperosmotic solutions provides small-volume restoration of cardiac output and systemic arterial blood pressure, with a concomitant beneficial dehydrating effect on brain tissue. Extensive animal studies have shown that hypertonic saline administration (3 to 5 ml/kg of 7.5% NaCl over 5 minutes) reverses shock, decreases ICP, improves CBF and oxygen delivery, and increases survival following head injury (Prough et al, 1985; Shackford et al, 1992). The hypertonicity created by resuscitation with hypertonic saline draws fluid from the interstitial and intracellular spaces into the intravascular space and by doing so decreases the volume of red blood cells and endothelial cells in capillary walls, improving blood flow (rheology). Hypertonic saline should be avoided in systemic dehydration. The effects of hypertonic saline administration alone are short-lived (15 to 60 minutes), and it is recommended that colloids be administered to maintain the intravascular volume. Colloid solutions contain high molecular weight solutes (>60,000 D) that are larger than the pore size of most capillaries (see p. 66 and p. 131). This property allows colloids to remain in the vascular space and exert a prolonged effect. Synthetic colloid solutions currently available for veterinary use are hydroxyethyl starch (Hespan) and dextrans, and the standard dose is 20 ml/kg per 24 hours. Fresh-frozen plasma administration also provides colloidal effects and is indicated when coagulation factors are depleted.

The CVP should be maintained at 5 to 7 cm H_2O. If restoration of adequate CVP does not restore MAP to 80 to 100 mm Hg, administration of a vasopressor agent (i.e., dopamine at 2 to 10 μg/kg per minute) may be indicated.

Oxygen and Ventilation

Hypoxemia can contribute to cerebral vasodilation and increased cerebral blood volume, as well as neuronal injury. The PaO_2 should be maintained at a minimum of 80 mm Hg. Oxygen supplementation is never contraindicated in brain-injured patients and should always be administered if there is evidence of suboptimal oxygenation on blood gas analysis or pulse oximetry. A decrease in oxygen content because of anemia has a similar detrimental effect on cerebral vasculature. If the hemoglobin content of the blood is less than 7 gm/dl, a red blood cell transfusion should be considered.

When chemical autoregulation in the brain is intact, increases in $PaCO_2$ cause cerebral vasodilation and decreases in $PaCO_2$ cause cerebral vasoconstriction. Hyperventilation leads to decreases in $PaCO_2$, resulting in cerebral vasoconstriction, decreased cerebral blood volume, and a rapid decrease in ICP. Hyperventilation may decrease cerebral blood volume by up to 36%, whereas hypoventilation can cause an increase in cerebral blood volume of up to 170%. It is important, therefore, to maintain normoventilation, but hyperventilation is not always indicated. Hyperventilation-induced vasoconstriction may cause shunting of blood flow from areas of the brain with intact autoregulation to the more damaged areas of the brain tissue that have lost CO_2 reactivity. These effects, if excessive, may exacerbate global cerebral ischemia as well as focal areas of edema. Continuous hyperventilation is not recommended and should be used only when pulmonary injury or hypoventilation is causing hypercapnea ($PaCO_2$ >40 mm Hg) or hypoxia unresponsive to oxygen supplementation. Intermittent short periods of hyperventilation to achieve hypocapnea ($PaCO_2$ <30 mm Hg) may be useful as an emergency means of reducing ICP when neurologic deterioration is evident (i.e., in preparation for definitive therapy such as surgical decompression). When the decision is made to begin hyperventilation therapy, pretreatment with intravenous lidocaine (2 mg/kg for dogs, 0.25 mg/kg for cats) may be used to blunt the increase in ICP that may accompany the intubation process. The $PaCO_2$ should be maintained between 25 and 35 mm Hg. When mechanical ventilation is applied, positive end-expiratory pressure should be avoided, as it increases intrathoracic pressure, CVP, and, indirectly, ICP.

Head Elevation

Elevation of the head facilitates venous outflow from the cerebral vasculature and may promote CSF displacement into the spinal subarachnoid space. Because blood must be pumped uphill when the head is elevated, there may be a concomitant decrease in CPP and CBF, which must be prevented in order to minimize secondary brain injury. Elevation of the head to 30 degrees produces maximal gravitational decreases in ICP without significantly compromising CPP or CBF (Feldman et al, 1992). It is also important to prevent obstruction to venous outflow from pressure on the neck (i.e., from pillows, catheter wraps).

Mannitol

Mannitol, a six-carbon sugar, has multiple beneficial effects when used in the management of increased ICP and cerebral edema. Mannitol decreases the hematocrit and blood viscosity, which improves cerebral perfusion, promoting cerebral vasoconstriction, and lowering ICP. The hyperosmolality of mannitol draws fluid from the cerebral interstitium, causing some degree of cerebral dehydration, which also lowers ICP. The effect of mannitol on ICP can

be sustained by the concomitant administration of a colloidal fluid. Mannitol is also a free radical scavenger and may play a role in limiting the development of vasogenic cerebral edema following tissue ischemia. The hypertonicity of mannitol has an immediate plasma-expanding effect that increases total blood volume as well as cerebral blood volume. Mannitol may therefore have a role as a resuscitation fluid; however, the transient (5-minute) increase in ICP associated with the increased cerebral blood volume may be dangerous to patients with intracranial hypertension. In patients with severe injury, resuscitation should first be attempted with hypertonic saline and colloid or crystalloid fluid administration, and a short period of hyperventilation should be considered before mannitol is administered. Mannitol should be administered slowly (over 20 minutes) to minimize the initial increase in ICP. As mannitol begins to promote osmotic diuresis, the effect on blood volume resolves and the beneficial effects become more significant.

There has been speculation that mannitol administration may be detrimental in areas of the brain where the blood-brain barrier has been damaged. Mannitol may cross the barrier and accumulate in the brain interstitium, causing a reverse in the osmotic fluid shift and increased cerebral edema. This hypothetical consideration has never been proved and is unlikely to occur unless repeated doses or continuous infusions are administered. In addition, the global beneficial effects of mannitol probably override the risks associated with the development of focal areas of vasogenic edema. Mannitol is most effective and safest when administered as a bolus rather than as a continuous infusion. Repeated doses and continuous rate infusions of mannitol may lead to hyperosmolarity of the serum and promote fluid retention, especially if there is decreased renal function. There is also the potential for excessive diuresis and systemic hypovolemia if fluids are not administered to replace those lost. Single doses or several well-spaced intermittent boluses of mannitol can be administered safely in most cases and have beneficial effects that justify its use in most patients. The recommended dosage is 0.25 to 1.0 gm/kg over 15 minutes, no more than every 4 to 6 hours, until clinical improvement is noted. If significant cerebral hypertension is suspected or documented by CT or ICP measurement, higher doses (2 gm/kg) may be administered. Repeated administrations of this higher dosage (more than two or three in 24 hours) should be avoided unless serum osmolality can be measured. Osmolality should not exceed 320 mOsm/kg.

Corticosteroids

Glucocorticoids have long been used in the treatment of head trauma. Corticosteroid administration is theoretically beneficial for many reasons. These drugs stabilize lysosomal membranes and inhibit lipid peroxidation, thus potentially inhibiting the progression of secondary brain injury. Glucocorticoids also reduce cerebral edema formation and modulate the inflammatory response. Despite these advantages and encouraging results in laboratory studies, clinical trials have failed to show a significant effect of corticosteroid administration on neurologic outcome or mortality in head-injured human patients. In fact, corticosteroids have been shown to potentiate neuronal damage when ischemia is present and inhibit remyelinization of injured neurons (Sapolsky, 1985). Aggressive efforts to improve cerebral oxygen delivery and limit secondary brain injury appear to be of more importance and benefit than is the use of corticosteroids.

If corticosteroids are employed, the timing of administration appears to be important. The administration of glucocorticoids should be aimed at interrupting the development of brain swelling and increased ICP. High-dose methylprednisolone has been associated with improved outcome and survival when administered shortly after brain injury in laboratory animals (Hall, 1985). In a clinical trial, human patients administered high-dose methylprednisolone at the accident site had improved survival and neurologic outcome (Jane et al, 1982). However, several studies on human patients receiving corticosteroids after reaching the hospital have shown no clear beneficial effect but rather several possible detrimental effects, including gastrointestinal bleeding and hyperglycemia (Gudeman et al, 1979). The progressive brain ischemia, lipid peroxidation, and resultant edema formation, which develop quickly following brain injury, are mostly irreversible. This suggests that methylprednisolone should be administered within the first 6 hours only, if at all, following traumatic brain injury. The dosage regimen that has been recommended is an initial 30 mg/kg bolus, followed by a 15 mg/kg bolus 2 hours later, and every 6 hours for 24 to 48 hours. However, dosing beyond the initial 6-hour period is probably unnecessary. Alternatively, sodium prednisolone succinate (5 to 10 mg/kg IV) or dexamethasone (2 mg/kg IV) may be administered as a single dose.

Aminosteroids are synthetic nonglucocorticoid steroids that are potent inhibitors of lipid peroxidation and chelators of iron but lack the detrimental side effects of the glucocorticoids. In experimental animal studies, aminosteroid administration has been associated with an improved outcome following traumatic brain injury (Hall et al, 1988), but preliminary clinical trials in human patients have not confirmed this finding.

Barbiturates

Barbiturate administration can be used following traumatic brain injury to induce coma, which decreases cerebral metabolism and consequently decreases CBF and ICP. Pentobarbital administered to human patients with refractory intracranial hypertension significantly decreased mortality (Eisenberg et al, 1988). Barbiturate administration is not generally used as a first line of therapy for increased ICP but has been recommended for patients that do not respond to conventional medical therapy. Barbiturate administration can cause myocardial or respiratory depression and may induce hypotension. In addition, the complete loss of consciousness associated with barbiturate-induced coma removes any ability to assess neurologic deterioration from clinical signs. Pentobarbital (5 to 15 mg/kg to effect, then CRI of 0.2 to 1 mg/kg per hour) is a commonly used barbiturate protocol in small-animal patients. If a barbiturate coma is induced, the patient should be intubated and blood gas analysis performed frequently to prevent hypoventilation and hypoxemia. Systemic arterial blood pressure and CVP should also be monitored. The optimal length of time that a patient should be maintained in a barbiturate coma has not been determined, but a 24- to 48-hour period has been recommended.

Experimental Therapeutics

Hypothermia decreases the cerebral metabolic rate of oxygen consumption ($CMRO_2$) and consequently decreases ICP and CBF in severely head-injured patients. Controlled hypothermia (31° to 34°C) has been demonstrated in animal studies to improve neurologic outcome and survival (Pomeranz et al, 1993; Shiozaki et al, 1993). Detrimental effects of hypothermia include cardiac arrhythmias, coagulation abnormalities, and the possibility for rebound increases in CBF and ICP during rewarming (which may lead to brain herniation). Shivering in response to hypothermia may increase ICP and should be treated with muscle relaxants or paralysis (atracurium, 0.2 to 0.5 mg/kg IV followed by an IV CRI of 3 to 8 µg/kg per minute) if it occurs. Hyperbaric oxygen therapy is also being evaluated for use in head trauma patients, but few practices have the equipment for this treatment.

There are several drug therapies that have been investigated for use in the prevention and treatment of secondary brain injury. Glutamate, an excitatory neurotransmitter, is stored in postsynaptic vesicles and released during brain injury or ischemia. This release triggers an influx of calcium into cells and promotes membrane injury and free radical release. Glutamate receptor (NMDA) antagonists (such as dextromethorphan, nitroglycerin, and other experimental compounds) are being evaluated for use in cases of brain injury. Dimethyl sulfoxide (DMSO) is a free radical scavenger that stabilizes lysosomal membranes and has anti-inflammatory activity (see *CVT XII*, p. 68). The administration of DMSO (0.5 to 1.0 gm/kg IV over 30 minutes) has been shown to decrease ICP and improve outcome in laboratory animals following brain injury (Karaca et al, 1991). Acetylcysteine is an antioxidant, and its administration has been shown to improve neuronal survival and vascular reactivity during the reperfusion phase that follows periods of cerebral ischemia (Ellis et al, 1991). Tromethamine is a weak base and has been used as a buffer in the treatment of cerebral acidosis. It has shown some beneficial effects in preventing cerebral vasoconstriction during prolonged hyperventilation therapy (Muizelaar et al, 1991). Deferoxamine mesylate (25 to 50 mg/kg IM or slowly IV) is an iron chelator and an inhibitor of lipid peroxidation reactions and therefore may have a role in the early prevention of reperfusion injury (see *CVT XII*, p. 67). All these agents are intended to prevent the development of secondary brain injuries and should therefore be administered early in the treatment regimen.

Nutritional Support

Nutritional support has been shown to improve and hasten neurologic recovery in human patients (Young et al, 1987) and should be considered essential in the management of all patients with craniocerebral trauma. The preferred route of administration is enteral nutrition. If gastric emptying is adequate, peptide-rich compounds (e.g., Clinicare, Abbott Laboratories; 40 to 60 kcal/kg per day) should be administered via a nasogastric tube. If the gastrointestinal tract cannot be used, and the patient is not expected to be able to tolerate enteral feeding within 48 hours, parenteral feeding should be instituted. Hyperglycemia should be avoided in patients with moderate to severe brain injury or multiple-system trauma with unstable cerebral perfusion, or both. Hyperglycemia promotes anaerobic metabolism, which may result in lactic acid accumulation and cerebral acidosis. If hyperglycemia develops during parenteral nutrition administration, a decreased rate of administration of the nutritional solution or the administration of insulin should be considered.

Supportive Care Considerations

Nursing care strategies should be followed as for any recumbent animal. Physical therapy is essential to prevent limb contracture, although special care must be taken in cases of suspected spinal injury. The patient should be turned every 4 hours to prevent atelectasis of lung lobes. Ample padded bedding should be provided to prevent pressure sores. The eyes should be lubricated to prevent corneal ulceration. If a mechanical ventilator is used, strict precautions should be taken to prevent nosocomial pneumonia, and adequate sedation should be provided to prevent coughing and struggling against the ventilator, which would increase ICP.

Fever, pain, and seizures may all contribute to elevated ICP. If a fever develops, it is important to investigate for an underlying cause. Antibiotics should be administered if there is concern for infection (e.g., hemorrhage in ear canals or nose suggestive of open skull fractures, gastrointestinal bleeding, lacerations). Nonsteroidal anti-inflammatory agents can be used to treat fever. Hyperthermia is treated with cool fluids, wet blankets, and ice packs. Patients with multiple musculoskeletal injuries or skull fractures are likely to have pain and should be provided adequate analgesia. Seizures should be rapidly controlled with intravenous administration of diazepam (0.25 to 0.5 mg/kg IV) and then prevented with barbiturate administration.

Surgery

A specific description of surgical techniques for cranial decompression can be found elsewhere (Shores, 1993). Surgery is indicated in cases of depressed skull fractures, subdural hematomas, or severe intracranial hypertension (evidenced on CT) and in cases of neurologic deterioration despite aggressive medical management. If surgery is elected, anesthetic induction should be performed quickly, with the use of thiopental sodium or propofol, and endotracheal intubation achieved rapidly to prevent unnecessary increases in ICP. Hyperventilation with 100% oxygen will promote immediate decreases in ICP. Maintenance of anesthesia may be achieved with inhalant anesthetics. Isoflurane is the inhalant agent of choice, as halothane may cause increases in ICP.

References and Suggested Reading

Bagley RS: Intracranial pressure in dogs and cats. Compend Cont Educ Pract Vet 18:605, 1996.

Chestnut RM, Prough DS, eds: Critical care of severe head injury. New Horizons 3:365, 1995.
A series of articles devoted to head trauma in human patients that provides a comprehensive review of the various methods of monitoring and treatment modalities.

Dewey CW, Downs MO, Aron DN, et al: Acute traumatic intracranial haemorrhage in dogs and cats. Vet Clin Orthop Trauma 6:153, 1993a.

Dewey CW, Downs MO, Crowe DT: Management of a dog with an acute traumatic subdural hematoma. J Am Anim Hosp Assoc 29:551, 1993b.

Eisenberg HM, Frankowski RF, Contant CF, et al: High dose barbiturate control of elevated intracranial pressure in patients with severe head injury. J Neurosurg 69:15, 1988.

Ellis EF, Dodson LY, Police RJ: Restoration of cerebrovascular responsiveness to hyperventilation by the oxygen radical scavenger N-acetylcysteine following experimental traumatic brain injury. J Neurosurg 75:774, 1991.

Feldman Z, Kanter MJ, Robertson CS, et al: Effect of head elevation on intracranial pressure, cerebral perfusion pressure, and cerebral blood flow in head injured patients. J Neurosurg 76:206, 1992.

Fenner WR: Diseases of the brain. In: Ettinger SJ, Feldman EC, eds: Textbook of Veterinary Internal Medicine, Diseases of the Dog and Cat, 4th ed. Philadelphia: WB Saunders, 1995, p 578.
A review of the neurologic examination and localization of brain lesions.

Gentleman D, Jennett B: Causes and effects of systemic complications among severely head injured patients transferred to a neurosurgical unit. Int Surg 77:297, 1992.

Gudeman SK, Miller JD, Becker DP: Failure of high-dose steroid therapy to influence intracranial pressure in patients with severe head injury. J Neurosurg 51:301, 1979.

Hall ED: High-dose glucocorticoid treatment improves neurological recovery in head-injured mice. J Neurosurg 62:882, 1985.

Hall ED, Yonkers PA, McCall JM, et al: Effect of the 21-aminosteroid U74006F on experimental head injury in mice. J Neurosurg 68:456, 1988.

Hopkins AL, Wheeler SJ: Subdural hematoma in a dog. Vet Surg 20:413, 1991.

Jane JA, Rimel RW, Pobereskin LH, et al: Outcome and pathology of head injury. In: Grossman RG, Gildenberg PL, eds: Head Injury: Basic and Clinical Aspects. New York: Raven Press, 1982.

Karaca M, Bilgin UY, Akar M, et al: Dimethylsulfoxide lowers ICP after closed head trauma. Eur J Clin Pharmacol 40:113, 1991.

Mandellow AD, Teasdale GM, Russell T, et al: Effect of mannitol on cerebral blood flow and cerebral perfusion pressure in human head injury. J Neurosurg 65:43, 1985.
Describes a study that illustrated the multiple beneficial effects of mannitol in head-injured patients.

Muizelaar JP, Marmarou A, Ward J, et al: Adverse effects of prolonged hyperventilation in patients with severe head injury: A randomized clinical trial. J Neurosurg 75:731, 1991.

Pomeranz S, Safar P, Radovsky A, et al: The effect of resuscitative moderate hypothermia following epidural brain compression on cerebral damage in a canine outcome model. J Neurosurg 79:241, 1993.

Prough DS, Johnson JC, Poole GV, et al: Effects on intracranial pressure of resuscitation from hemorrhagic shock with hypertonic saline versus lactated Ringer's solution. Crit Care Med 13:407, 1985.

Robertson C: Desaturation episodes after severe head injury: Influence on outcome. Acta Neurochir 59:98, 1993.

Sapolsky RM: Glucocorticoids potentiate ischemic injury to neurons: Therapeutic implications. Science 229:1397, 1985.

Saul TG, Ducker TB: Effect of intracranial pressure monitoring and aggressive treatment on mortality in severe head injury. J Neurosurg 56:498, 1982.

Shackford SR: Fluid resuscitation in head injury. J Intensive Care Med 5:59, 1990.
A review of the effects of fluid resuscitation on brain injury, including the use of crystalloids, colloids, and osmotic agents.

Shackford SR, Zwang J, Schmoker J: Intravenous fluid tonicity: Effect on intracranial pressure, cerebral blood flow, and cerebral oxygen delivery in focal brain injury. J Neurosurg 76:91, 1992.

Shiozaki T, Sugimoto H, Taneda M, et al: Effect of mild hypothermia on uncontrollable intracranial hypertension after severe head injury. J Neurosurg 79:363, 1993.

Shores A: Intracranial surgery. In: Slatter D, ed: Textbook of Small Animal Surgery, 2nd ed. Philadelphia: WB Saunders, 1993.

A description of intracranial surgery, including indications, techniques, and monitoring recommendations.

Young B, Ott L, Twyman D, et al: The effect of nutritional support on outcome from severe head injury. J Neurosurg 67:668, 1987.

Medical Management of Acute Spinal Cord Disease

KARL H. KRAUS

North Grafton, Massachusetts

The spinal cord can be acutely injured by four basic mechanisms: anatomic disruption, compression, concussion, and ischemia. Anatomic disruption of the parenchyma of the spinal cord is physical laceration or other direct disruption of the spinal cord parenchyma and axons, the effects of which are currently considered clinically not treatable. Compression is a mass effect leading to increased pressure in the spinal cord, commonly caused by disc extrusion or tumors, with its effect focused primarily in the white matter of the spinal cord. Concussion is an acute impact to the spinal cord, such as a vertebral fracture or explosive disc extrusion, that causes the initiation of a cascade of autodestructive events precipitated by an ischemic episode in the central gray matter. Ischemia is a disruption of the arterial blood supply to the spinal cord, such as with fibrocartilaginous emboli, which can be permanent or transient. To date, the only clinically proven therapy for acute spinal cord disease is the administration of glucocorticosteroids, although many other interventions show theoretical and experimental promise. However, the formulation, dosage, and timing of glucocorticosteroid therapy are dependent on the specific type of spinal cord injury. Compression and concussive injuries have different effects on the spinal cord and should be understood as distinct entities. Ischemia, if transient, is very similar to concussion in its effects on the spinal cord and treatment approaches.

COMPRESSIVE SPINAL CORD INJURY

Slow compression of the spinal cord occurs when an epidural mass (tumor, protruding disc, spondylosis, fracture callus, epidural abscess) progressively impinges on the spinal cord over days, weeks, or months. The spinal cord is housed within nonexpandable vertebrae, and compression tends to distribute pressure throughout the spinal cord cross section. This effect is not limited to the area adjacent to the offending mass. The pressure within the spinal cord causes dysfunction. Interestingly, spinal cord blood flow and tissue oxygen levels are maintained until compression is severe. The order in which nerve fibers are affected relates to susceptibility to compressive effects, rather than location within the spinal cord segment. The tension on the surface membranes is related to pressure and the cross-sectional diameter of the fiber. Larger diameter fibers are preferentially affected by compression. Proprioceptive fibers are large, fast conducting fibers located within the dorsal and dorsolateral white columns. Experimentally, pathologic changes are first seen in these areas. Correspondingly, loss of proprioception is the first clinical sign seen in animals with spinal cord compression. Progressively smaller nerve fiber sizes are those associated with motor, superficial pain, and deep pain axons. It is in this order that function is lost with spinal cord compression.

Early histologic hallmarks of slow compression are vacuolization, loss of myelin, and axonal swelling of the white matter. The gray matter of the spinal cord is relatively preserved in this process. Although early in compression blood flow to the spinal cord is preserved, the ability of the spinal cord to regulate blood flow throughout ranges of systemic arterial blood pressures and carbon dioxide levels is diminished. The spinal cord appears to attempt to preserve itself by sacrificing myelin and axons to accommodate the offending mass. However, once white matter axons are lost, functional deficits tend to be permanent. Axonal loss is directly related to the degree and duration of spinal cord compression.

Late in the course of slow compression, the white matter becomes edematous. The edema comes from stenosis or obstruction of the epidural venous plexus and impairment of venous drainage. Venous stasis and subsequent vasogenic edema in the spinal cord play an important role in development of clinical signs (Ushio et al, 1977). Although a mass may be slowly impinging on the spinal cord over several weeks, clinical signs may progress acutely, within hours or days following the development of spinal cord edema. At this point, spinal cord blood flow decreases and damage can become permanent.

CONCUSSIVE SPINAL CORD INJURY

A concussive injury occurs when a rapid force is applied to the spinal cord without residual compression. If the applied force causes physical disruption of the spinal cord parenchyma, loss of function is immediate and permanent. Interestingly, forces far less severe than those that cause immediate damage can initiate a cascade of events that will lead to progressive destruction of spinal cord tissue and permanent damage.

Following impact injury, spinal cord blood flow decreases. The resultant hypoxia is a hallmark of impact injury, and the disruption to function is virtually identical to that produced by occlusion of spinal cord blood supply (Kraus et al, 1990). The effect is especially damaging to the gray matter of the spinal cord, which has a six-fold greater oxygen demand and consequently greater blood supply than that of white matter. The cause of ischemia following concussive injury is probably due to multiple factors, including catecholamine-induced vasospasm, direct microvascular damage and vasospasm, excessive activation of excitatory amino acid neurotransmitters, accumulation of intracellular calcium, and lipid peroxidation. The spinal cord loses its autoregulatory function that preserves blood flow and becomes susceptible to additional compromises in systemic arterial blood pressure, blood oxygen content, and blood carbon dioxide levels.

Ischemia results in a loss of microvascular endothelial integrity and the extravasation of fluid and cellular components of blood into the gray matter parenchyma. The result is hemorrhagic nonperfusion. The adjacent white matter is relatively resistant to the effects of ischemia and may even develop a hyperemic response. Thus, within a single cross section of spinal cord, early after spinal cord impact, there may be areas of nonperfusion and hypoperfusion concentrated in the gray matter, along with hyperperfused areas within the white matter. This situation establishes that there are sufficient prerequisites for oxygen free radical–induced lipid peroxidation, that is, reperfusion injury. This lipid peroxidation is generally accepted as the principal factor for propagation of traumatic hemorrhagic necrosis of the spinal cord following concussive injury (Hall, 1993).

Although quite complex, the sequence of events of reperfusion injury is well understood. In essence, ischemia results in the accumulation of metabolites and enzymes that, when reintroduced to oxygen, results in the accumulation of negatively charged oxygen-containing free radicals. These free radicals preferentially attack the lipids of cellular membranes, a process known as lipid peroxidation. Cellular injury begins in the gray matter and extends circumferentially (Fig. 1).

Once traumatic hemorrhagic necrosis extends into the white matter and disrupts ascending and descending axons, additional pathophysiologic events ensue. Disruption of the axon results in flow of axoplasm toward the lesion. The severed end of the axon tends to seal, but the axoplasmic flow continues. Dilation of the axon occurs more proximal (or distal) to the severed axon. The dilated axon is called a terminal club (Kao et al, 1977). The terminal club will rupture, releasing axoplasm rich in lysosomal enzymes, which then will involve adjacent axons, perpetuating the pathologic process. Thus, traumatic hemorrhagic necrosis starts within the gray matter and propagates circumferentially. Once white matter tracts are involved, necrosis is propagated axially along the spinal cord.

Investigations of concussive injury to the spinal cord have demonstrated that a "programmed cell suicide" (apoptosis) results in progressive loss of spinal cord parenchymal cells, primarily oligodendrocytes. Loss of these cells causes loss of axonal myelin and resulting dysfunc-

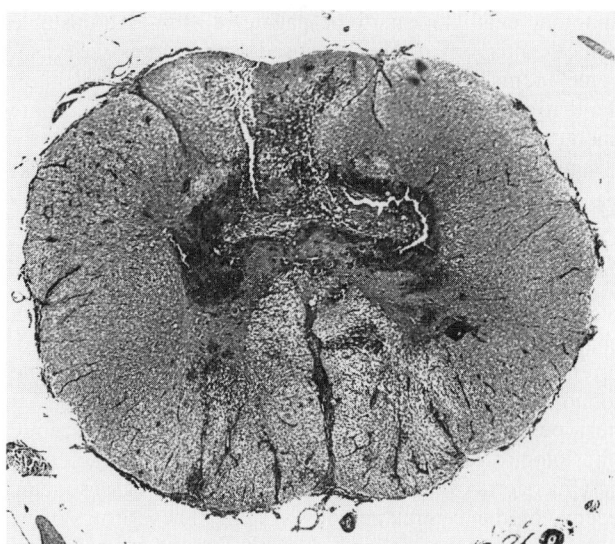

Figure 1. Photomicrograph of a cross section of the spinal cord of a dog in the area of a vertebral fracture 48 hours after a vehicular accident. Hemorrhagic necrosis is seen principally within the gray matter of the spinal cord and involves the adjacent white matter. Lateral white matter tracts are much less affected.

tion. The deprivation of trophic factors, including insulin-like growth factor and brain-derived growth factor, appears to be the cause of oligodendrocytes and motoneurons entering a process of apoptotic cell death. Interestingly, the propagation of apoptosis appears to predominate within the white matter of the spinal cord and may contribute to ascending and descending white matter degeneration (Li et al, 1996). Supplying spinal cord cells with neurotrophic factors after concussive injury has been shown to inhibit apoptotic cell death.

COMBINED COMPRESSIVE AND CONCUSSIVE SPINAL CORD INJURY

The categorization of spinal cord injury is helpful in describing pathophysiology, but pure forms of injury rarely occur clinically. With intervertebral disc extrusion, for example, the disc extrudes, concusses the spinal cord, causes transient ischemia, and remains as a compressive mass. With vertebral fractures, the initial injury causes parenchymal damage and concussive injury, while bone fragments or malalignment may result in continued spinal cord compression. Spinal cord injury in clinical patients is often a result of a combination of mechanisms. The combined effects of compression and concussion are difficult to study in experimental models; however, assumptions can be proposed regarding the pathophysiology of combined types of spinal cord injury.

The effects of compression contribute to the propagation of concussive injury. The vasogenic edema associated with compression increases intraparenchymal pressure, exacerbating the ischemic events of concussive injury. Also, the losses of autoregulation seen with compression and concussion probably act together to destabilize spinal cord metabolism.

Concussive injury affects primarily the gray matter of the spinal cord and extends to the white matter, where apoptotic death appears to propagate cell loss. An unstable white matter environment, caused by compressive vasogenic edema, is likely to further disrupt axonal and oligodendritic exposure to trophic agents and exacerbate apoptosis.

TREATMENT OF COMPRESSIVE SPINAL CORD INJURY

The capacity of a compressed spinal cord to regulate blood flow is compromised, along with its ability to tolerate changes in blood flow, blood gases, and manipulation. An offending mass should be surgically removed with little to no manipulation of the spinal cord and with special perioperative attention to maintaining proper systemic physiologic factors.

Glucocorticosteroids are effective in treating vasogenic edema of the central nervous system. These drugs have been shown to be effective in the treatment of spinal cord compression, resulting in a return of function without removal of the offending mass. The development of vasogenic edema of the white matter of the spinal cord is an important factor in slow spinal cord compression, especially when the progressive compression occludes the epidural venous plexus. Vasogenic edema causes further compression beyond that of the offending mass. This consideration explains the improvement in function often seen with the initiation of glucocorticosteroid therapy in long-standing spinal cord compression. There appears to be a direct dose-response relationship for the use of glucocorticosteroids in the treatment of spinal cord compression. Therefore, lower dosages can be used to treat mild compression, while high dosages should be used for treatment of animals demonstrating clinical signs of severe compression.

Dexamethasone is the most widely studied and used glucocorticosteroid for the treatment of spinal cord compression. It is also associated with a high incidence of side effects. If spinal cord injury is known, or strongly suspected to be caused strictly by compression (e.g., spondylopathy or epidural tumors), dexamethasone sodium phosphate is slowly administered at a dose of 2.2 mg/kg IV. Doses of glucocorticosteroids used for compression are typically an order of magnitude less than the doses used to treat concussive spinal cord injury. Although dosages ranging from 1.5 to 10 mg/kg have been reported, the use of dexamethasone in the treatment of spinal cord injury can cause adverse side effects, including gastric ulceration and colonic perforation. For this reason, it seems prudent to use the lowest effective doses. Since the duration of action of dexamethasone is 32 to 48 hours, more frequent dosing should be discouraged. Treatment of this form of spinal cord injury should focus on removal of the offending mass, if possible. There are situations when compressive spinal cord injury must be treated medically for long periods of time. An example is caudal cervical instability, where surgical decompression and stabilization is not reasonable. In these cases, oral prednisolone or prednisone can be administered. Since the potency of prednisolone is approximately one sixth that of dexamethasone, doses of prednisolone as high as 60 mg/kg have been recommended. To prevent potential adverse side effects of glucocorticosteroids, the lowest effective dosage should be used. Initially, prednisolone or prednisone should be administered orally at 2.5 mg/kg b.i.d. The dosage should be lowered over 3 or 4 days to the lowest effective dosage, for example, 2.5 mg/kg PO e.o.d.

A compressed spinal cord should be decompressed as soon as possible to enhance functional recovery. The loss of axons appears to be directly related to the degree and duration of compression. If axons are lost, the deficits tend to be permanent. The urgency of decompression in animals with compressive spinal cord injury from conditions such as intervertebral disc disease, vertebral fracture, and tumor impingement is still a matter of debate. For example, should a dog with disc extrusion and 2-day, nonprogressive neurologic signs of paresis with preserved deep pain perception be operated on within hours or days? Most clinical data suggest that surgical intervention sooner is better. However, surgical decompression should not be performed at the expense of adequate consideration for anesthetic and other perioperative care issues that might have an impact on outcome. In addition, the presence of long-standing spinal cord compression does not preclude the potential benefits of decompressive surgical intervention. Although the chance of functional recovery worsens with time (axonal loss), improvement in function can be seen with late decompression in long-standing spinal cord compressive diseases.

TREATMENT OF CONCUSSIVE SPINAL CORD INJURY

Concussive spinal cord injury *initiates* a cascade of events that leads to an autodestructive process. Thus, there is hope that by thwarting the autodestructive process, the resulting destruction of the spinal cord can be averted, with improved functional recovery. Although most investigations have concentrated on pharmacologic agents, many other factors are important, including the timing of medical and surgical interventions, the use of neuroprotective anesthetic protocols and hypothermia, surgical technique, the use of intraoperative monitoring, and postoperative physical therapy. There has been only one controlled clinical study (in human patients) involving the administration of a pharmacologic agent, methylprednisolone sodium succinate, that has demonstrated significant improvement in neurologic outcome (Bracken et al, 1992).

Lipid peroxidation is an important factor in post-traumatic spinal cord degeneration following acute impact trauma, and glucocorticosteroids are known to inhibit this event. Lipid peroxidation begins very early in the course of events following concussive injury and may be quite advanced in progression as soon as 8 hours following injury. Although rapid in onset, lipid peroxidation often continues to play a role in spinal cord injury for 24 to 48 hours or longer. Most studies indicate that progressive, and possibly permanent, destruction of spinal cord tissue is well established by 8 hours after impact. Therefore, any pharmacologic therapy used for the purpose of blocking the autodestructive events of impact must be initiated as early as possible. This requirement implies that the primary care clinician should be the individual who initiates medical therapy.

The action of methylprednisolone is not unique among the glucocorticosteroids. However, this well-studied drug is a water-soluble, fast-acting formulation that demonstrates a rapid, high concentration to the central nervous system. In experimental studies on cats with spinal cord injuries, methylprednisolone has demonstrated a very specific dosing requirement of 30 mg/kg IV; higher dosages of 60 mg/kg did not demonstrate increased efficacy, and lower dosages of 15 mg/kg were not effective. These results are contrasted with the use of glucocorticosteroids for the treatment of compressive spinal cord injury, in which these drugs have a direct dose-response relationship.

The Second National Acute Spinal Cord Injury Study involving a multicenter, randomized controlled trial was the first to demonstrate a significant effect of the use of any agent on clinical outcome in human patients (Bracken et al, 1992). Although the results of this study received substantial attention, the limitations of the study are telling (Young, 1993; Ducker and Zeidman, 1994). First, the positive effects of the administration of methylprednisolone were demonstrated only when the drug was administered within 8 hours following injury. In fact, administration of the drug more than 8 hours after injury resulted in worse neurologic recovery than that after placebo administration in some groups of patients.

Although the results of this study were significant and important, the observed improvements were, at best, quite modest. The most substantial improvement in patients treated with methylprednisolone was observed for recovery of motor function at 1 year after injury. A motor score scale of 0 (no function) to 70 (complete function) was used in this study. For patients receiving placebo, the mean admitting motor score was 23.8 and increased by 9.1 to a score of 32.9 by 1 year. For patients receiving methylprednisolone within 8 hours of injury, the admitting motor score was 21.1 and increased by 14.8 to 35.9 at 1 year. Certainly, scores of 32.9 versus 35.9 of 70 may be statistically valid, but they reveal the limitations of current pharmacologic intervention in patients with spinal cord injury.

Additional pharmacologic interventions that block at least one of the steps of the autodestructive cascade initiated after concussive spinal cord injury have shown promise in laboratory research but have yet to be proved to be clinically significant. These agents include 21-aminosteroids (Hall, 1993), calcium channel blockers, DMSO, and superoxide dismutase as well as neuroprotective anesthetics and hypothermia. The effectiveness of these approaches has not been substantiated with controlled clinical investigations. These interventions may have a finite time limit for efficacy and important dosing requirements. As with methylprednisolone, inappropriate dosing or timing of administration may be detrimental to clinical outcome, and the use of these promising approaches cannot be recommended for clinical patients at this time.

TREATMENT OF COMBINED COMPRESSIVE AND CONCUSSIVE SPINAL CORD INJURY

Acute spinal cord injury, occurring over hours to days, usually has some component of concussive injury. As such, methylprednisolone sodium succinate (30 mg/kg IV) should be administered as soon as possible. A compressive mass may accompany concussive injury, and methylprednisolone at this dosage is also an effective and appropriate intervention; for example, if acute spinal cord injury is concussive, yet actually due to an acute manifestation of compressive spinal cord injury, the administration of methylprednisolone is still appropriate. However, if a strictly compressive lesion is assumed when actually a concussive lesion is present, the administration of another glucocorticosteroid, such as dexamethasone at a low dosage, will not be effective against the concussive component of the spinal cord injury.

After the initial dose of methylprednisolone, there is controversy as to whether additional doses should be administered. There is substantial data that support the presence of lipid peroxidation continuing for at least 24 to 48 hours following a concussive injury. This finding would support continued administration of methylprednisolone for that duration, although there are no clinical data supporting prolonged use. In cases in which surgical decompression is not performed, or is unsuccessful in completely decompressing the spinal cord, prolonged administration of glucocorticosteroids should be considered. Usually, prednisolone or prednisone is administered orally, as described for compressive spinal cord injury.

References and Suggested Reading

Bracken MB, Shepard MJ, Collins WF, et al: Methylprednisolone or naloxone treatment after acute spinal cord injury: Results of the Second National Acute Spinal Cord Injury Study. J Neurosurg 76:23, 1992.
  This multi-institutional, blind, and randomized study demonstrated significant improvement in motor function in human patients 1 year following spinal cord injury with the administration of methylprednisolone given within 8 hours of injury.
Ducker TB, Zeidman SM: Spinal cord injury: Role of steroid therapy. [Review]. Spine 19:2281, 1994.
  A review of the use of glucocorticosteroids in spinal cord injury with an analysis of the First and Second National Acute Spinal Cord Injury Study.
Hall ED: Neuroprotective actions of glucocorticoid and nonglucocorticoid steroids in acute neuronal injury. [Review]. Cell Mol Neurobiol 13:415, 1993.
  A thorough description of the role of lipid peroxidation in concussive spinal cord injury and treatments.
Hall ED: Lipid antioxidants in acute central nervous system injury. Ann Emerg Med 22:1022, 1993.
  A description of experimental and clinical application of methylprednisolone as a lipid antioxidant in acute spinal cord injury, and the potential use of 21-aminosteroids for the same purpose.
Kao CC, Chang LW, Bloodworth JMB: Electron microscopic observations of the mechanisms of terminal club formation in transected spinal cord axons. J Neuropathol Exp Neurol 36:140, 1977.
  Description and mechanisms of terminal club formation that explain the mechanism of ascending and descending propagation of spinal cord injury.
Kraus KH, Pope ER, O'Brien DO, et al: The effect of aortic occlusion on transcranially induced evoked potentials in the dog. Vet Surg 19:341, 1990.
  Using electrophysiologic criteria, this study demonstrated that after ischemia, events occurred during reperfusion of the spinal cord that lead to dysfunction. These events primarily involved spinal cord gray matter.
Li GL, Brodin G, Farooque M, et al: Apoptosis and expression of Bcl-2 after compression trauma to rat spinal cord. J Neuropathol Exp Neurol 55:280, 1996.
  Apoptotic cell death occurred in longitudinal white matter tracts cranial and caudal to the area of acute compressive spinal cord injury. Neurons of the gray matter did not present signs of apoptosis.

Ushio Y, Posner R, Posner JB, et al: Experimental spinal cord compression by epidural neoplasms. Neurology 27:422, 1977.
  An experimental study in rats characterizing compressive spinal cord injury and treatment with dexamethasone.
Young W: Strategies for the development of new and better pharmacologi-cal treatments for acute spinal cord injury. [Review]. Adv Neurol 59:249, 1993.
  Description of the potential for developing treatment for concussive spinal cord injury and critique of the Second National Acute Spinal Cord Injury Study.

Recognition and Treatment of Disseminated Intravascular Coagulation

BERNARD F. FELDMAN
Blackburg, Virginia

REBECCA KIRBY
Milwaukee, Wisconsin

MARCO CALDIN
Padua, Italy

Intravascular coagulation was reported after transfusion with incompatible blood as early as 1876. A bleeding diathesis, most likely disseminated intravascular coagulation (DIC), was reported in a wounded soldier in Korea in 1951. Since this time, DIC has been widely recognized in humans and animals as a secondary, life-threatening complication (Ruiz de Gopegui et al, 1995).

The hemostatic response should be considered a defensive function: It prevents or avoids blood loss from damaged vasculature (hemorrhage) and ensures adequate blood flow, keeping the vascular tree free of obstruction (thrombosis). DIC represents loss of hemostatic equilibrium. Of all descriptors of this condition, the term *DIC* is given preference—it describes the dynamic process of disseminated coagulation taking place intravascularly. This is expressed as both hemorrhage and thrombosis, leading to impairment in blood flow, ischemia, and multiorgan failure. Because DIC is associated with diffuse thrombosis in the microvasculature, it is sometimes called diffuse intravascular thrombosis. It is also known as a consumption coagulopathy, an inappropriate descriptor because, although some coagulation proteins, factors, inhibitors, and platelets are consumed, most factors and other plasma constituents are biodegraded by plasmin (Jandl, 1991). Another descriptor, defibrination syndrome, could be more appropriately retitled "defibrinogenation syndrome" because fibrinogen is both consumed and biodegraded.

Any disease process characterized by capillary stasis, loss of vascular integrity, red cell hemolysis, inappropriate particulate matter in blood, or necrotic tissues with release of tissue thromboplastin into the vasculature can produce this life-threatening complication. It should be realized at the outset that initiating processes present differently along a continuum of events. DIC may occur at any point in the continuum and, depending on the position therein, patients may have radically different clinical and laboratory findings.

ETIOLOGY AND PATHOPHYSIOLOGY

Depending on the activation rate of the hemostatic system, DIC may occur as an acute and life-threatening clinical event or in a chronic form without severe thrombosis or hemorrhage. Procoagulant activity (inactive hemostatic proteins) is modulated or inhibited by several mechanisms. The equilibrium between activation and inhibition of hemostasis depends on interaction among endothelial cells, platelets, other circulating blood cells, and coagulation activators and inhibitors. DIC may be initiated by a single cause or by multiple causes occurring sequentially or simultaneously. The anticipated events inducing DIC in most conditions are related to (1) tissue factor or thromboplastin-like substances liberated into the circulation, (2) damaged endothelium or monocytes converting procoagulants (coagulation factors) into active forms (activated procoagulants-factors), (3) blood flow interruption preventing hemodilution of activators, and (4) impaired removal of activated procoagulants by the mononuclear phagocytic system, which resides mainly in the liver and spleen.

DIC may be considered an uncontrollable burst of thrombin generation and activation, followed by plasmin and kinin generation and complement activation. This massive activation overwhelms hemostatic inhibitors, depletes procoagulants and platelets, induces thrombosis and, as a final result, severely damages tissues. Thrombus formation and subsequent ischemia and necrosis may activate an enhanced fibrinolytic response that can impair platelet function and further deplete coagulation factors (Schrier, 1996).

The inflammatory response interacts with hemostasis, either activation or inhibition, through (1) neutrophil activation; (2) release of cytokines, tumor necrosis factor-alpha, and interleukin-1 (IL-1); and (3) complement activation through terminal components C5b-9. Neutrophil activation results in the release of substances that negatively affect antithrombin (AT) concentrations and

TABLE 1. Conditions Associated With Disseminated Intravascular Coagulation

Intravascular Hemolysis
  Hemolytic transfusion reaction
  Hemolytic anemia
Septicemia (see Table 2)
  Gram-negative bacteria (endotoxin)
  Gram-positive bacteria (bacterial coat mucopolysaccharide)
Viremia (see Table 2)
Parasitic infections
  Protozoal infection
  Metazoal infection
Obstetric Complications
Miscellaneous
  Gastric dilatation-volvulus
  Diabetes mellitus
Neoplasia
Massive Tissue Injury
  Burns
  Trauma
  Surgical procedures
  Heat stroke
Venoms and Toxins
  Snake bite
  Insect stings
  Aflatoxin
Hepatic Disease
Pancreatitis

may activate platelets. The release of cytokines affects endothelial integrity and accelerates platelet adhesion (and loss of circulating platelets). Activation of the terminal components of complement induces platelet procoagulant activity and platelet activation.

CLINICAL FINDINGS

DIC is expected in patients who have (1) a significant hypotensive crisis, (2) impaired blood flow to a major organ, or (3) release of vasoactive agents into the vasculature. Disease states in which DIC must be anticipated include those causing systemic inflammatory response syndrome (e.g., heat stroke, sepsis, pancreatitis, splenic tumors, chronic heartworm disease, immune hemolytic anemia, snake bite, diffuse neoplasia, crush trauma), severe and prolonged hypotension, polycythemia, and severe volume depletion. Specific clinical disease states and causative agents are listed in Tables 1 and 2. The ability to anticipate this deadly complication, prior to obtaining a definitive

TABLE 2. Bacteria and Viruses Incriminated in Disseminated Intravascular Coagulation

Bacteria	Viruses
Gram-Negative Bacteria	Infectious canine hepatitis
Escherichia coli	Canine distemper
Pasteurella haemolytica	Canine herpesvirus
Pasteurella multocida	Feline infectious peritonitis
Salmonella spp.	Feline panleukopenia
Gram-Positive Bacteria	
Staphylococcus spp.	
Streptococcus spp.	
Clostridium spp.	
Mycobacterium spp.	

diagnosis of the initiating disease state, is crucial to survival.

Although the classically described presentation of DIC includes fever, acidosis, hypoxemia, proteinuria, bleeding, shock, and evidence of multiple organ failure, it is essential to note there is considerable variability in clinical findings. Clinical signs can range from absent to thrombosis to bleeding.

DIC can be peracute, acute, or chronic depending on whether the underlying illness is acute (decompensated DIC) or chronic (compensated DIC). Patients with peracute disease may show laboratory changes but no overt clinical signs. In the acute phase, venipuncture oozing, mucous membrane hemorrhage, petechiae, ecchymosis, purpura, hematoma formation, and hemarthrosis are commonly encountered clinical signs. Physical findings in the peracute and acute phases of microthrombosis-associated DIC are associated with decreased organ perfusion.

Multiple organ dysfunction is a consequence of the acute phase of DIC. Hepatic failure is reported as common. Renal thrombosis or microthrombosis can lead to severe renal dysfunction. Gastrointestinal thrombosis causes submucosal necrosis and ulceration. This often results in spontaneous gastrointestinal hemorrhage clinically expressed as hematemesis, melena, hematochezia, or occult fecal blood. Pulmonary function may be compromised by microvascular thrombosis in DIC, resulting in tachypnea, hypoxemia, and acute respiratory distress syndrome. Cerebral microvascular thrombosis often leads to altered mentation or consciousness, convulsion, or coma. Organ ischemia, organ failure, and death are inevitable when DIC is fulminant. Compensated DIC develops in patients with illness that produces low-grade or intermittent procoagulant release stimulus, as in some dogs with dirofilariasis. This allows longer periods during which consumed or degraded coagulants, anticoagulant proteins, and platelets may be replenished. This compensated state may become unbalanced by stress, concurrent diseases, or worsening of the primary disease.

LABORATORY DIAGNOSIS

The diagnosis of DIC is made based on clinical suspicion, knowledge of associated diseases, and serial laboratory coagulation tests. It is vital to make an early diagnosis because therapy during the peracute phase provides the best results. Repetitive data accumulation is critical to recognizing and treating DIC appropriately. Clinicians must have the capability of examining the hemogram and hemostatic analytes virtually at will. Changes can occur rapidly. No single test will diagnose DIC, but the following tests are useful. The *platelet count* and *activated clotting time* (ACT) are the minimal laboratory analytes to be monitored in the practice setting. Other helpful laboratory tests include blood smears for red cell morphologic features and platelets, plasma fibrinogen concentration, prothrombin time (PT), and activated partial thromboplastin time (APTT) along with plasma concentrations of fibrin and fibrinogen degradation products (FDPs), D-dimers, and AT.

Schistocytosis

Schistocytes (fragmented red cells) result from mechanical damage to the red cell membrane from microvascular fibrin strands. Schistocytosis is more prominent in compensated DIC. In peracute DIC, the process is too fulminant to result in much red cell damage. Other conditions that potentially can produce schistocytosis include Heinz body anemia, iron deficiency, and artifacts resulting from operator handling.

Thrombocytopenia-Thrombocytopathia

Platelet counts are variable in DIC. This is because most systemic inflammatory states cause platelet counts to increase, a condition called reactive thrombocytosis. Nevertheless, simply examining *repeated* blood smears and estimating platelet counts is easy and essential. Appropriate platelet numbers are 10 to 13 per oil immersion field. Platelet counts that are within the low-normal reference interval in animals with severe systemic inflammation should be viewed with suspicion, especially in the presence of macroplatelets that suggest increased platelet turnover. In the future, increased concentrations of platelet factor 4 and beta-thrombomodulin could become pathognomonic features of platelet destruction associated with DIC.

Dysfunctional platelets, resulting in thrombocytopathia, are caused by FDPs coating platelet membranes, which causes the release of platelet procoagulant materials. Buccal mucosal bleeding time is relatively insensitive to thrombocytopathies induced by this mechanism and should not be performed in patients with thrombocytopenia, as the test results will be prolonged.

Fibrinogen

DIC causes consumption of fibrinogen when coagulation is activated, and fibrinogen is biotransformed into fibrin. Because fibrinogen is an acute-phase inflammatory protein, acute focal or systemic inflammation can increase fibrinogen concentration. Thus, *even low-normal concentrations with systemic inflammation should be suspected of indicating DIC*. Measuring fibrinogen kinetically—the biotransformation from fibrinogen to fibrin—allows more accurate fibrinogen determination and prevents interference from FDPs. In the dog, when plasma fibrinogen concentration is reduced to less than 75 mg/dl, the PT and APTT will be prolonged. A decrease in fibrinogen concentration often precedes thrombocytopenia.

Prothrombin Time

The PT examines factors VII, X, V, II, and I—the extrinsic and common coagulation pathways. Prolongation in the PT occurs when any factor within these pathways is decreased to less than 30% of its normal plasma activity (compared with a species-specific plasma pool considered to have 100% of each factor). Loss of factor I (fibrinogen) by biotransformation, plasmin degradation of factor V, or interference with fibrin polymerization by FDPs can result in prolongation of the PT. In the early stages of decompensated DIC, the PT can actually be shorter than control values.

Activated Partial Thromboplastin Time and Activated Coagulation Time

The APTT and ACT examine factors XII, XI, IX, VIII, X, V, II, and I—the intrinsic and common coagulation pathways. Prolongation in the APTT occurs when any factor within these pathways is decreased to less than 30% of its normal plasma activity. Shortening or prolongation of the APTT occurs for the same reasons as for the PT (see earlier). Prolongation of ACT is observed only with more profound decreases in factor concentrations. If the ACT is prolonged, it is meaningful; however, if the ACT is normal, testing of the APTT is required to detect more "subtle" coagulopathies. Repeated ACT testing is most useful in clinical practice (Ruiz de Gopegui et al, 1995).

Fibrin and Fibrinogen Degradation Products

Plasmin degradation of fibrin and fibrinogen produces FDPs. Hence, the appearance in blood of FDPs implies the presence of plasmin. FDPs are composed of fragments identified as X, Y, D, and E. Most commercial FDP tests examine blood for the presence of fragments D and E. The presence of FDPs is important diagnostically and physiologically. Physiologically, the presence of increased quantities of FDPs is associated with an increased tendency for hemorrhage. FDPs act as anticoagulants by interfering with the biotransformation of fibrinogen to fibrin.

The presence of FDPs is not pathognomonic for DIC. FDPs are present in hepatic failure, major focal vascular thrombosis, dysfibrinogenemia, and excessive fibrinolysis. FDPs also can be artifactually elevated during specimen handling. Conversely, an absence of FDPs does not preclude a diagnosis of DIC. Inactive fibrinolysis, excessive release of leukocyte proteases (elastase and collagenase) causing degradation of FDPs to unrecognizable fragments, and specimen handling may result in undetectable FDP concentrations. FDPs are easily and inexpensively ascertained "in-house" and should be so determined.

D-Dimers

D-Dimers are the product of fibrin degradation. D-Dimers directly imply fibrinolytic activity secondary to coagulation. To date, only one commercial test has been validated for use in the dog. This test exhibited good sensitivity and specificity (Caldin et al, 1997).

Antithrombin

AT—an alpha$_2$-globulin, acute-phase protein produced in the liver—is the natural inhibitor of serine proteases in the coagulation pathways (factors II, VII [inhibition of this factor is slight], IX, X, XI, XII, along with the kinin and kallikreins). When a patient is in a hypercoagulable state and prothrombin is being actively converted to thrombin, the AT concentration will be low (<80%). The affinity of AT for the serine proteases is enhanced 100-fold by the administration of heparin. Measurement of the AT concentration guides replacement and heparin therapy for DIC.

In a series of 157 critically injured human trauma patients, low AT concentrations were predictive of DIC (Owings et al, 1996). The patients with DIC had lower AT concentrations at each sample time period (hours 0, 8, 16, 24, and 48 and days 3, 4, 5, and 6) than did those without DIC. Other causes of low AT, such as protein-losing diseases, must be ruled out. However, reduced AT from any cause leaves the patient hypercoaguable and susceptible to thrombosis or DIC. AT levels may be elevated in inflammatory processes.

DIFFERENTIAL DIAGNOSIS OF DISSEMINATED INTRAVASCULAR COAGULATION

Alterations in the coagulation laboratory test results can be due to causes other than DIC. Hetastarch administration prolongs PT and APTT, whereas it leaves the platelet count and fibrinogen, AT, and FDP concentrations within normal ranges. Hetastarch does not cause clinical bleeding unless excessive quantities are administered. Dextran administration prolongs bleeding times and the PT and APTT. Animals that have had gastrointestinal or splenic vascular impairment (e.g., splenic torsion) may have platelet sequestration in affected vessels and frequently demonstrate a moderate thrombocytopenia and schistocytosis. The ACT may be mildly prolonged in these patients. Evaluation of AT concentrations will help identify hypercoagulability and early DIC. After successful therapy for the primary problem, it is often possible to restore platelet counts to reference intervals quickly and without administration of additional specific therapeutics in patients with normal AT concentrations.

THERAPY FOR DISSEMINATED INTRAVASCULAR COAGULATION

Successful therapy for DIC is dependent on early suspicion and detection of the condition. There are four treatment priorities: (1) promotion of capillary blood flow; (2) elimination of the initiating cause; (3) support of target organs at risk for hemorrhage, microthrombi, or ischemia; and (4) replacement plasma therapy and heparin administration, as needed.

Once DIC is suspected, the first treatment priority is to promote capillary blood flow and tissue oxygenation. Aggressive intravascular volume resuscitation may be required (see p. 140). During the peracute (hypercoaguable) phase of DIC, the administration of dextran (10 to 20 ml/kg IV in dogs; 5 to 15 ml/kg IV slowly in cats) is considered in conjunction with the administration of crystalloids (20 to 40 ml/kg IV). Dextrans decrease platelet adherence and increase blood flow through small vessels. However, if the patient has a systemic inflammatory response syndrome disease (see p. 131; also see *CVT XII*, p. 139), hetastarch would be the synthetic colloid of choice during any phase of DIC (10 to 20 ml/kg IV in dogs; 5 to 15 ml/kg IV slowly in cats) to improve and sustain systemic arterial blood pressure and cardiac output.

The administration of positive inotropic agents or vasodilators is indicated if crystalloid and colloid administration does not improve capillary blood flow adequately. Dobutamine (5 to 10 μg/kg per minute in dogs; 2.5 to 5 μg/kg

per minute in cats) or dopamine (2 to 5 μg/kg per minute) can be used for positive inotropic and slight chronotropic effect. Should there be adequate intravascular volume expansion (hypertension) accompanied by continued inadequate tissue blood flow, sodium nitroprusside (1 to 10 μg/kg per minute IV) could be titrated to effect. Careful systemic arterial blood pressure and central venous pressure monitoring is required with sodium nitroprusside administration (see p. 194).

Rapid elimination of the underlying disease state is the second priority. Unfortunately, many causes, such as pancreatitis, heat stroke, heartworm disease, and hematologic diseases, take time for correction, requiring careful patient support in the interim.

The lungs, kidneys, mononuclear phagocytic system, gut, and pancreas are targets for microthrombosis and ischemia or hemorrhage. This occurs because of the large capillary networks and the ability of these organs to produce and release vasoactive substances. These organs must be supported while definitive therapy is employed. Oxygen supplementation and ventilatory support can be required for pulmonary insufficiency. Afferent glomerular arteriolar dilatation may be caused by dopamine administration (1 to 3 μg/kg per minute) and may provide renal support. Enteral nutrition and sucralfate administration will help protect the gut, and appropriate systemic antibiotic therapy should be employed when breakdown of the gut mucosal barrier is suspected (see p. 136).

Blood component replacement and heparin therapy are the fourth priority. AT concentrations can be used to guide therapy (Table 3). Experimental studies of animals have shown that when AT was administered to subjects infused with a potent thromboplastin, the natural anticoagulant abilities of the blood were maintained and were protective against DIC and death (Taylor et al, 1988). Fresh-frozen plasma, fresh whole blood, cryoprecipitate, and stored whole blood are currently the only clinically available sources of AT. AT should be activated by heparin prior to adding more coagulation factors (plasma or blood transfusion) into a hypercoagulable environment.

Several methods have been proposed to activate AT using heparin, and at this time, the most appropriate method has not been identified. Heparin therapy has been reported as ineffective in the treatment of DIC and is often the cause of severe hemorrhagic complications. It is

TABLE 3. Using Antithrombin Values to Guide Therapy for Disseminated Intravascular Coagulation

Antithrombin Value	Interpretation	Therapy
>90%	Normal	Continue to monitor
<80%	Low—potential for hypercoagulation	Monitor closely; consider heparin
<60%	Very low—at risk for thrombosis and DIC	Requires AT replacement and heparin
<30%	Critical—immediate risk of thrombosis	Requires aggressive, immediate AT replacement and heparin

DIC, disseminated intravascular coagulation; AT, antithrombin.

anticipated that most of the poor responses to heparin are the result of heparin administration when there have been inadequate circulating concentrations of AT. In the absence of AT, heparin has only weak antithrombotic effects that are related to heparin-heparin cofactor II activity against thrombin. At the present time, we recommend the heparin dose (50 to 200 U/kg) be placed into the plasma or whole blood volume to be transfused. Incubating for 30 minutes prior to administration allows activation of AT prior to infusion of the coagulation proteins.

Two to five plasma infusions may be required to bring the AT concentration into an effective range. Once the AT concentrations are greater than 60%, heparin is continued alone at 50 to 100 U/kg administered subcutaneously every 8 hours. Should further plasma or blood transfusions be required, additional pretreatment (incubation) heparin should not be necessary because the animal should be heparinized. To prevent thrombosis, heparin therapy must be tapered over 48 hours before being discontinued.

When administered alone, heparin can actually diminish AT concentrations. Acidosis also inactivates AT, and tissue perfusion must be re-established, along with correction of blood pH, prior to heparinization. Without heparin activation of AT, providing coagulation factors via plasma transfusion could potentiate additional intravascular thrombosis.

References and Suggested Reading

Caldin M, Furlanello T, Berzo D, et al: Preliminary investigation of D-dimer concentrations in normal dogs and in dogs with disseminated intravascular coagulation. J Vet Intern Med 11:130, 1997.

Jandl JH: Blood: Pathophysiology. Boston: Blackwell Scientific, 1991, p 510.
Discussion of the pathophysiology of DIC.

Owings JT, Bagley M, Gosselin R, et al: Effect of critical injury on plasma antithrombin activity: Low antithrombin levels are associated with thromboembolic complications. J Trauma 41:396, 1996.
Critical examination of the effect of AT decrease.

Ruiz de Gopegui R, Suliman HB, Feldman BF: Disseminated intravascular coagulation: Present and future perspectives. Comp Haem Int 5:213, 1995.
Complete review of DIC.

Schrier SL: Disorders of hemostasis and coagulation. Sci Am V:1, 1996.
Excellent review of DIC with focus on pathophysiology and basis of therapy.

Taylor FB Jr, Emerson TE Jr, Jordan R, et al: Antithrombin-III prevents the lethal effects of *Escherichia coli* infusion in baboons. Circ Shock 26:227, 1988.
Treatment of DIC with AT.

Sodium Nitroprusside: Uses and Precautions

JEFFREY PROULX

NISHI DHUPA

North Grafton, Massachusetts

Sodium nitroprusside (disodium pentacyanonitrosylferrate(2-)dihydrate) has been used in human medicine for the treatment of hypertensive crises and catastrophic congestive heart failure and in surgical procedures in which controlled hypotension is beneficial. Because of the lack of knowledge and the difficulty in monitoring patients during sodium nitroprusside administration, its use in veterinary patients has been limited.

Sodium nitroprusside belongs to the nitrovasodilator class of medication, which also includes amyl nitrite, nitroglycerin, isosorbide, and nitric oxide. It is composed of a ferrous ion center in complex with five cyanide groups and a nitrosyl group. Common to all nitrovasodilators is the formation of nitric oxide (formerly known as endothelial-derived relaxation factor in vivo) (Fig. 1). Sodium nitroprusside undergoes a spontaneous one-electron reduction by reaction with any sulfhydryl group present on cell membranes to produce nitric oxide and free cyanide molecules. To a lesser degree, this same reaction can occur with oxyhemoglobin, with the subsequent production of methemoglobin.

Sodium nitroprusside–derived nitric oxide diffuses through the endothelial cell layer and, similar to endogenously produced nitric oxide, affects vascular smooth muscle tone. Through direct activation of cytosolic guanylate cyclase, guanosine triphosphate is converted to cyclic guanosine monophosphate, effecting a decrease in free cytosolic calcium. In addition, nitric oxide inactivates the myosin light-chain kinase. Both actions effect vascular smooth relaxation (see Fig. 1), resulting in decreases in systemic arterial vascular resistance (decreased afterload) and in-

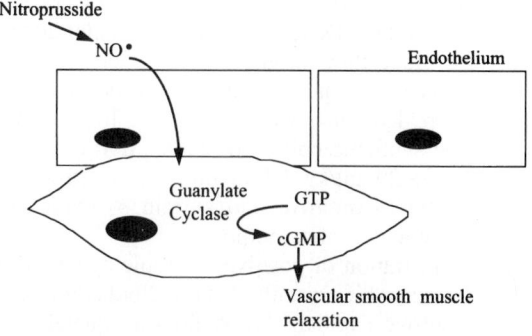

Figure 1. Sodium nitroprusside mechanism of action.

creases in systemic and pulmonary venous capacitance (decreased preload).

METABOLISM AND TOXICITY

Metabolism

The metabolism of sodium nitroprusside is outlined in Figure 2. On infusion, sodium nitroprusside reacts with sulfhydryl groups in erythrocytes and other cell membranes, and minimally with oxyhemoglobin to release five cyanide groups and the vasodilating compound nitric oxide. The methemoglobin produced has a high affinity for cyanide and combines to form cyanomethemoglobin, which exists as a nontoxic pool of cyanide for slow release and definitive cyanide metabolism. Free plasma cyanide is converted to thiocyanate either by thiocyanate oxidase in erythrocytes or via a transulfuration reaction with thiosulfate by the rhodanese enzyme within the liver. Thiocyanate from either source is freely filtered at the glomerulus and excreted in the urine.

Oxidative Injury

Feline erythrocytes have increased susceptibility to oxidative injury because of the greater amount of sulfhydryl groups on hemoglobin and a reduction in the ability to convert methemoglobin to oxyhemoglobin. The use of sodium nitroprusside in cats may increase Heinz body formation and methemoglobin levels at lower dosage rates when compared with other species. Although no studies have examined the results of sodium nitroprusside infusion in feline patients, methemoglobin levels and erythrocyte cytologic examination for Heinz bodies may be useful in monitoring these patients. Therefore, both total dose and rate of administration should be carefully monitored in feline patients.

Cyanide and Thiocyanate Toxicity

Cyanide toxicity results from binding to and inactivation of the cytochrome oxidase enzyme necessary for oxidative phosphorylation. The result is diffuse tissue energy depletion and secondary lactic acidosis. In human patients, clinical cyanide toxicity occurs at concentrations greater than

40 μM. Clinical signs range from mental depression to stupor and coma, seizures, cardiac arrhythmias, and severe metabolic acidosis. Venous oxygen and lactate levels rise secondary to nonuse of oxygen and consequent anaerobic metabolism. Patients that are predisposed to cyanide toxicity include those with limited thiosulfate stores (pediatric patients) or insufficient rhodanese enzyme levels or function (chronic malnutrition and liver insufficiency). Although the development of cyanide toxicity depends on many factors, clinical signs very rarely develop with the use of sodium nitroprusside over 2 or 3 days.

Treatment of cyanide toxicity includes discontinuance of sodium nitroprusside infusion and correction of metabolic acidosis. Supplemental oxygen is of little benefit, as the defect lies in oxygen utilization and not in oxygen delivery. In humans, hydroxycobalamin (vitamin B_{12a}) infusion allows binding of free cyanide to form cyanocobalamin, which is freely filtered by the kidney and limits plasma cyanide binding to cytochrome oxidase. The dosage in human patients is 1.5 mg/kg by IV infusion over 4 hours. Three percent sodium nitrate at 5 mg/kg by slow IV injection will convert hemoglobin to methemoglobin, allowing for free cyanide binding and a decrease in the toxic pool of cyanide. Measured methemoglobin levels should remain less than 10%. Caution is necessary when inducing methemoglobin formation in critically ill feline patients, as oxygen delivery may already be lowered because of higher baseline methemoglobin levels. In addition, sodium thiosulfate injection at 150 mg/kg IV over 15 minutes will provide substrate for production of thiocyanate from cyanide.

Thiocyanate is 100 times less toxic than cyanide, but its excretion represents a concern in the patient with renal insufficiency. Clinical signs of thiocyanate toxicity include nausea, vomiting, mental depression, lethargy, and seizures or coma. Blood levels of 60 μg/ml are consistent with signs of toxicity in human patients. Thiocyanate also has the potential to induce clinical hypothyroidism as a result of antagonism with iodine uptake by thyroid tissue. Treatment of thiocyanate toxicity includes the use of peritoneal dialysis.

INDICATIONS

Properties that make sodium nitroprusside ideal for the treatment of hypertensive crises and catastrophic heart failure include its rapid onset of action (2 to 3 minutes) and short duration of action (3 to 5 minutes). These two properties allow for an ease of dose titration to effect. Through nitric oxide production, vascular smooth muscle relaxation in arterial and venous circuits occurs in both the systemic and the pulmonary vasculature. The end result is a controlled reduction in afterload and preload.

Other than the potential for cyanide and thiocyanate toxicity with continued use, the main adverse effect of sodium nitroprusside use is hypotension. This fact underscores the importance of continuous blood pressure monitoring and a committed staff member for patient care. Ideally, an intra-arterial catheter is placed for continuous direct arterial blood pressure monitoring. Alternatively, oscillatory or Doppler blood pressure monitoring may be utilized on a frequent basis (every 2 to 5 minutes). This monitoring allows safe and accurate titration to a predeter-

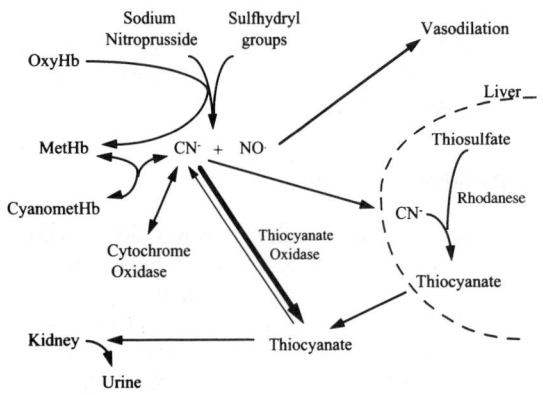

Figure 2. Metabolism of sodium nitroprusside.

mined effect. In addition, blood pressure monitoring should be complemented with monitoring by electrocardiography and pulse oximetry or blood gas analysis. The heart rate, respiratory rate and effort, and indicators of peripheral perfusion (capillary refill time, mucous membrane color, and extremity temperature) should also be monitored.

Sodium nitroprusside injection (Nitropress, Abbott; Nipride, Roche Laboratories) is available as a dry powder in a 50-mg quantity. Five percent dextrose in water is used for reconstitution; no other diluent solutions or additives should be used. The reconstituted color is red-brown and any other color should prompt the user to immediately discard the solution. Since sodium nitroprusside is extremely light-sensitive, intravenous lines and fluid containers should be wrapped with an opaque material such as aluminum foil. The infusion rate should be controlled by an IV fluid pump, and saline flushes should never be used, as even a small bolus of sodium nitroprusside can result in profound hypotension.

Hypertensive Crises

Sodium nitroprusside is indicated in the treatment of hypertensive crises with either evidence of or a significant risk of an end-organ pathologic condition. These changes include damage to the retina (edema, hemorrhage, and detachment), kidneys (hematuria and proteinuria), heart (ST segment changes and arrhythmias), and brain (generalized depression or focal signs possibly indicating intracranial hemorrhage). Because these organs are sensitive to systemic arterial blood pressures beyond the normal autoregulatory range, immediate controlled reduction of blood pressure is necessary. Sodium nitroprusside should be considered in dogs or cats with acute elevations in systolic arterial pressure above 200 mm Hg. If left untreated, hypertension can result in serious consequences to these organs because of microvascular damage.

Sodium nitroprusside infusion is initiated in dogs at 1 to 2 μg/kg per minute and cats at 0.5 μg/kg per minute with incremental increases every 3 to 5 minutes until a predetermined target blood pressure is attained. In a chronically hypertensive patient, the cerebral autoregulation of blood flow is shifted to higher systemic arterial blood pressure (Fig. 3). Autoregulation in a normotensive patient will be between 60 and 140 mm Hg mean systemic arterial blood pressure, whereas autoregulation in a chronically hypertensive patient will occur between higher values. It

can be envisaged that a rapid and aggressive reduction of systemic arterial blood pressure in a chronically hypertensive patient will result in hypoperfusion should the target systemic arterial blood pressure fall to less than this higher autoregulatory range. A reduction of 25% of the starting systemic mean arterial pressure over a 4-hour period, with slow reductions afterward, is recommended to allow re-adaptation of cerebral blood vessels so that autoregulation can occur within a normal range. A patient with acute hypertension (previously normotensive) will tolerate rapid reductions of systemic arterial blood pressure to normal values. After oral maintenance antihypertensive treatment is initiated and takes effect, sodium nitroprusside infusion may be slowly withdrawn to ensure continued systemic arterial blood pressure control. Coadministration of oral antihypertensive therapy with the initiation of sodium nitroprusside infusion limits the total dose and, therefore, limits the potential for cyanide and thiocyanate toxicity.

Catastrophic Heart Failure

In fulminant pulmonary edema caused by left-sided heart failure, sodium nitroprusside administration allows acute reductions in afterload and preload. This is especially useful in heart conditions with a component of mitral regurgitation. Systemic vascular resistance is often greatly elevated in congestive heart failure, and by decreasing afterload several effects occur. These effects include improved cardiac output, a reduction in the mitral regurgitant fraction, and a decrease in myocardial oxygen demand. Increased venous compliance decreases preload and abrogates pulmonary edema. Because of increased cardiac distensibility induced by the action of nitric oxide, end-diastolic pressure is reduced without changing end-diastolic volume, the result being conserved volume for cardiac output with a lowered risk for pulmonary edema.

Patients requiring sodium nitroprusside for catastrophic heart failure often require supplemental oxygenation, ventilatory support, and intensive monitoring. The administration of sodium nitroprusside must be titrated with fine tune control. The goal of treatment is to decrease or maintain the systemic mean arterial pressure at a level that supports vital organ function (approximately 70 mm Hg or a systolic arterial blood pressure that is between 85 and 95 mm Hg). Sodium nitroprusside infusion is initiated and titrated in a manner similar to treatment of hypertensive crises. Concurrent use of inotropic agents such as dobutamine (1 to 5 μg/kg per minute in cats and 5 to 10 μg/kg per minute in dogs) to increase cardiac output is often indicated and is crucial to therapy of severe left-sided heart failure caused by dilated cardiomyopathy.

CONTRAINDICATIONS

The administration of sodium nitroprusside should never be undertaken when high systemic arterial blood pressure exists as a compensatory mechanism to support cerebral perfusion (Cushing's reflex). Intracranial disease processes with associated systemic hypertension should be approached with the primary aim of controlling the increased intracranial pressure. In addition, sodium nitroprusside

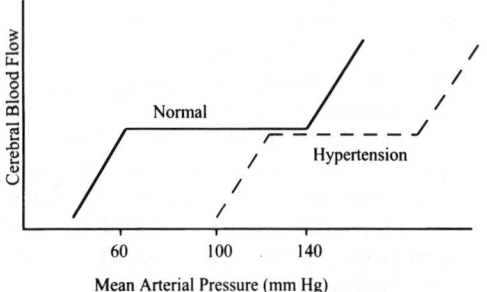

Figure 3. Cerebral blood flow autoregulation in normotensive and chronically hypertensive patients.

should be used with caution in the patient with renal or hepatic insufficiency due to a decreased ability for hepatic conversion of cyanide to thiocyanate or decreased renal clearance of thiocyanate. Severe left-sided congestive heart failure, when associated with pre-existent hypotension (e.g., systolic arterial blood pressure <90 mm Hg; mean arterial blood pressure <70 mm Hg), represents a relative contraindication to vasodilator therapy. This situation often indicates cardiogenic shock, and it is most often observed in dogs or cats with dilated cardiomyopathy. Should the arterial blood pressure remain low following initial treatment with cage rest, oxygen, and a diuretic, treatment with dobutamine or dopamine should be initiated to increase the arterial blood pressure before starting an infusion of sodium nitroprusside. Although sodium nitroprusside can increase cardiac output by reducing ventricular afterload, the arterial blood pressure often declines because of the prominent vasodilating effects of this drug.

References and Suggested Reading

Abdelwahab W, Frishman W, Landau A: Management of hypertensive urgencies and emergencies. J Clin Pharmacol 35:747, 1995.
   A review of parenteral agents currently being used in the treatment of acute hypertension.

Curry SC, Arnold-Capell P: Toxic effects of drugs used in the ICU. Nitroprusside, nitroglycerin, and angiotensin-converting enzyme inhibitors. Crit Care Clin 7:555, 1991.
   A review of the pathophysiology, toxic doses, diagnosis, and treatment of vasodilator toxicity in the intensive care patient.

Friederich JA, Butterworth JF IV: Sodium nitroprusside: Twenty years and counting. Anesth Analg 81:152, 1995.
   A review of the chemical properties, metabolism, toxicity, and clinical use of sodium nitroprusside in human patients.

Harrison DG, Bates JN: The nitrovasodilators: New ideas about old drugs. Circulation 87:1461, 1993.
   A review of the chemistry and mechanism of action of sodium nitroprusside and nitroglycerin.

Heesch CM, Hatfield BA, Marcoux L, et al: Predictors of pressure and stroke volume response to afterload reduction with nitroprusside in patients with congestive heart failure secondary to idiopathic dilated cardiomyopathy. Am J Cardiol 74:951, 1994.
   A prospective clinical study that examines baseline cardiovascular parameters in patients with dilated cardiomyopathy and their relationship to response with sodium nitroprusside treatment.

Ignarro LJ: Physiologic and pathophysiologic significance of nitric oxide. In: Ayres SM, ed: Textbook of Critical Care. Philadelphia: WB Saunders, 1995, p 208.
   A review of the chemistry, regulation of production, mechanism of action, and physiologic roles of nitric oxide in health and disease.

Zerbe NF, Wagner BK: Use of vitamin B_{12} in the treatment and prevention of nitroprusside-induced cyanide toxicity. Crit Care Med 21:465, 1993.
   A review of the safety and efficacy of hydroxycobalamin in the prevention and treatment of cyanide toxicity in patients with renal or hepatic disease.

Transvenous Pacing

LEE GARROD

Brentwood, New Hampshire

JOHN E. RUSH

North Grafton, Massachusetts

Transvenous cardiac pacing uses repetitive low-voltage impulses to maintain a hemodynamically stable cardiac rhythm. These pacing impulses are delivered by a catheter, usually placed in the right ventricle, which exits through the skin and is attached to an external pacing device. In most animals, transvenous (temporary) cardiac pacing is used to treat bradyarrhythmias until a normal cardiac rhythm is re-established or a permanent pacemaker can be implanted. Transvenous cardiac pacing is a minimally invasive technique that can be performed within a short time. This technique can be a lifesaving intervention in critical care environments. Advances in the level of veterinary care have led to additional situations in which temporary pacing techniques might be indicated. Veterinarians who practice in emergency or critical care environments may find it useful to understand the indications, technical logistics, and potential complications of transvenous cardiac pacing.

INDICATIONS

The indications for permanent cardiac pacing are reviewed on p. 719. Severe bradycardia and asystole are recognized complications of anesthetic induction for pacemaker implantation. Placement of a transvenous pacing catheter is often desirable immediately prior to implantation of a permanent cardiac pacemaker to avoid this complication. This article, however, concentrates on the indications and use of transvenous cardiac pacing in the emergency and critical care setting. These cases often fit into one of three categories: bradyarryhthmia without congestive heart failure, bradyarrhythmia with congestive heart failure, or bradycardia encountered during cardiopulmonary arrest.

Bradyarrhythmia Without Congestive Heart Failure

Although bradycardias are commonly encountered in clinical practice, not all bradyarrhythmias require immediate cardiac pacing. Animals with these arrhythmias often exhibit significant cardiomegaly on thoracic radiographs, yet they have no physical or radiographic evidence of congestive heart failure. In such cases, transvenous cardiac pacing may not be required. Some patients with sinus bradycardia are responsive to atropine or infusion of dopamine or dobutamine. Cardiac pacing is indicated in animals with atrioventricular block or sinus arrest and very slow ventricular escape rhythms (less than 35 to 40 per minute). Pacing is especially appropriate when these slow heart rates are poorly tolerated and result in patient weakness or syncope. Animals with long pauses (e.g., >6 seconds) in cardiac rhythm that result in weakness, collapse, or syncope should also be paced. Transvenous cardiac pacing can also be used as an ancillary, temporary treatment for drug-induced bradycardias (e.g., atrioventricular block following overdose with a calcium channel blocker) or for support during anesthesia, which typically suppresses escape activity.

The bradyarrhythmias that most commonly result in clinical signs of syncope, weakness, or collapse are sinus arrest and advanced forms of atrioventricular block. Sinus arrest is commonly seen in association with supraventricular tachyarrhythmias and is described as "sick sinus syndrome." In animals with sick sinus syndrome, clinical signs most commonly occur during the long pauses of sinus arrest. Fortunately, this syndrome rarely results in sudden death. Patients with frequent, severe, or prolonged episodes of syncope are candidates for transvenous cardiac pacing on an emergent basis. Pacing is especially indicated when pharmacologic management (anticholinergics or sympathomimetics) has proved unrewarding. In contrast, third-degree atrioventricular block is recognized to be associated with sudden death. Animals with frequent syncope (more than once a day) should have transvenous pacing until permanent pacemaker implantation can be scheduled. When definitive treatment with a permanent pacemaker is anticipated, attempts at pharmacologic management of the arrhythmia should be limited. The concerns associated with the potential proarrhythmic effects of catecholamines argue for the placement of a transvenous pacing catheter rather than the use of sympathomimetics in this setting. Once the transvenous pacing lead has been placed, the rate on the pulse generator is usually set between 70 and 90 pulses per minute for dogs. This rate is usually adequate to prevent syncope and meet the hemodynamic demands of the patient at rest.

Bradyarrhythmia With Congestive Heart Failure

In animals with bradycardia and evidence of congestive cardiac failure, transvenous pacing can be a successful adjunct to standard heart failure treatments and can prevent hypotension. Congestive heart failure may be evident from physical examination findings (ascites with jugular distention, dyspnea with pulmonary crackles, delayed capillary refill time, and so on) or from thoracic radiographs. Femoral pulse quality in these animals may be normal or brisk because of an increase in stroke volume and pulse pressure often found in animals with chronic bradycardia. Radiographic findings may include cardiomegaly, pleural effusion, pulmonary venous distention, and perihilar interstitial or alveolar infiltrates. In this setting, transvenous pacing is usually performed for 2 to 4 days until signs of congestive heart failure have resolved. Following resolution of congestive heart failure, the animal is a better candidate for

anesthesia and permanent pacemaker implantation. After placement of the pacing lead, the external pulse generator is usually set at a rate between 120 and 140 pulses per minute until signs of heart failure begin to resolve.

Several arrhythmias and clinical situations are recognized to result in the combination of bradycardia and congestive heart failure. The presence of chronic third-degree atrioventricular block or "high-grade" second-degree atrioventricular block can eventually lead to congestive heart failure. Dogs with sinus arrest and congestive heart failure often have concurrent chronic mitral valvular disease. Persistent atrial standstill (see *CVT XI*, p. 786), often seen in English springer spaniels, can lead to congestive heart failure and concurrent bradycardia. Many other forms of heart disease (e.g., neoplasia, myocarditis, dilated cardiomyopathy in cats) can lead to bradycardia and result in congestive heart failure. Echocardiography is used to identify severe underlying cardiac disease, which might indicate or preclude cardiac pacing.

Cardiopulmonary Arrest

In patients that develop bradyarrhythmias during cardiopulmonary arrest, early identification of bradycardia and rapid placement of a transvenous pacing lead can result in a greater likelihood of a successful outcome. Arrhythmias that may benefit from cardiac pacing include severe sinus bradycardia, advanced atrioventricular block, slow ventricular escape rhythms, and asystole. Cardiac pacing is not effective in animals with pulseless electrical activity or electromechanical dissociation. Transvenous pacing is usually attempted when atropine and repeated doses of epinephrine administration have failed to increase the ventricular firing to a rate that is capable of providing adequate perfusion for the patient.

For transvenous pacing to be successful, ventricular capture must occur. Myocardial stimulation with a pacing catheter becomes less efficacious because of underlying ischemia, hypoxia, acid-base disturbances, and electrolyte abnormalities once cardiopulmonary arrest has exceeded 15 minutes. When this happens, ventricular capture may still occur (pacing stimulus results in a QRS-T complex on the electrocardiogram [ECG]), but electromechanical dissociation is common. The stimulated QRS complex results in no effective blood flow. Eventually, ventricular stimulation with the pacing lead is no longer possible because of irreversible myocardial injury.

Placement of the transvenous catheter during cardiopulmonary arrest is usually performed without fluoroscopy, and with the motion artifact that occurs on the ECG during CPR, placement of the catheter can be exceedingly difficult. However, if open chest cardiopulmonary resuscitation has been performed, the heart can often be paced directly by placing the pacing lead on the epicardial surface of the heart. The heart can be paced via this technique until the patient's cardiac rhythm is stable or the jugular vein access has been secured for transvenous placement of the lead. Some newer defibrillators have transcutaneous pacing capabilities, and this technique is preferred to transvenous pacing in the setting of cardiopulmonary arrest.

TRANSVENOUS PACING TECHNIQUE

Patient Preparation and Sedation

A temporary pacemaker can usually be placed with the patient under light sedation and local anesthesia. Opiates, combined with a benzodiazepine, produce excellent mild sedation (i.e., oxymorphone, 0.05 to 0.1 mg/kg IV, or buprenorphine, 0.005 to 0.01 mg/kg IV in combination with diazepam, 0.1 to 0.2 mg/kg IV). After the procedure has been completed, naloxone (0.04 mg/kg IV or IM) can be administered to reverse the sedative effects of the narcotic if necessary.

The right or left jugular vein or the femoral vein can be used as vascular access for placement of the pacing lead. In large dogs, a 5F pacing wire may be successfully advanced up the lateral saphenous vein. The authors prefer the jugular vein, as vascular access is easier and the lead is less likely to migrate or dislodge and require repositioning from this location. Although the right jugular vein is the more direct route to the right atrium and ventricle, the left jugular vein or femoral vein should be used for temporary lead wire placement if a future permanent transvenous pacemaker implantation is anticipated. The skin over the target vein is clipped and infiltrated with 2% lidocaine, and the skin is cleaned with antiseptic solution. The vessel can be accessed via a cutdown technique or by vascular puncture using a catheter sheath introducer system (6 to 8.5F Percutaneous Sheath introducer sets, Arrow International, Reading, PA, and other suppliers) and a modified Seldinger approach. Once vascular access is secured, the pacing lead is passed into the vessel and toward the heart. Continuous electrocardiographic monitoring is performed during lead insertion to identify correct pacing lead placement and any episodes of asystole (failure to capture) or ventricular ectopy that might require repositioning of the catheter.

Placement Using Fluoroscopy

Under fluoroscopic guidance, the pacing catheter is advanced into the right atrium and directed ventrally across the tricuspid valve into the right ventricle. Passage of the pacing lead across the tricuspid valve is facilitated by placement of a 45-degree bend in the tip of the catheter. The pacing catheter is advanced until the tip of the catheter rests at the apex of the right ventricle (Fig. 1). The terminal of the external pacing device can then be connected to the lead to initiate pacing. The external pulse generator is set in the "demand" mode so that spontaneous ventricular activity can be sensed and impulses are not delivered during the electrically vulnerable period of ventricular repolarization. Ventricular capture should be confirmed and is identified on the ECG by a high-frequency pacing spike at the front of each ventricular-paced QRS-T complex. The pacing rate is set as previously described. The paced rhythm and heart rate, detectable via the ECG, should result in accompanying palpable arterial pulses at the same rate.

Placement Without Fluoroscopy

When fluoroscopic guidance is not available or not practical (e.g., during cardiopulmonary resuscitation),

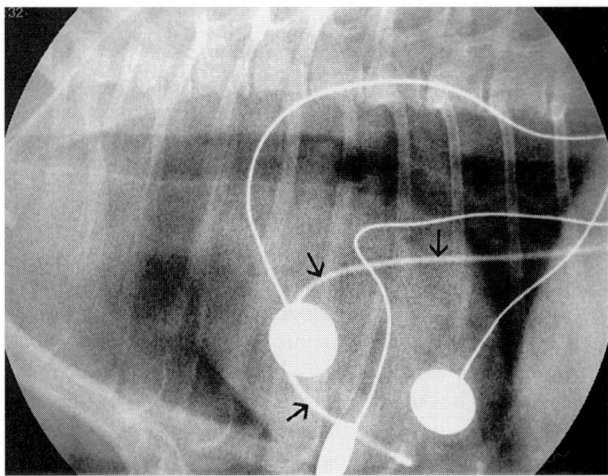

Figure 1. Lateral radiographic projection of the thorax of a dog. A pacing lead has been passed from the femoral vein into the right ventricle. Arrows mark the path of the pacing lead from the caudal vena cava into the apex of the right ventricle. Additional circular and linear metal densities are cutaneous electrodes and leadwires used for ECG monitoring.

transvenous pacing can still be performed successfully. This technique is challenging, and prior experience with transvenous pacemaker implantation using fluoroscopy is advantageous. Placement of the catheter from the femoral vein without fluoroscopy is difficult and not recommended. Vascular access is secured as described earlier. The approximate distance to the right atrium to the site of the incision or sheath introducer in the jugular vein is measured, and this distance is identified on the pacing catheter. When available, a flow-directed balloon-tipped, bipolar catheter (Xemex temporary pacing catheter, ZEON Medical Corp., White Plains, NY) may be helpful so that the balloon can be inflated to facilitate catheter passage across the tricuspid valve. The lead is connected to the external pulse generator, and the pulse generator is turned on to full output at a rate that is at least 10 to 20% faster than the patient's intrinsic ventricular rate. It can be helpful to set the pulse generator at a rate that is faster than the patient's intrinsic atrial rate because this will permit identification of the catheter location once it reaches the atrium (atrial capture should occur). As the lead is advanced into the vein and toward the heart, the ECG is observed. The ECG is used to detect capture, and once the electrode reaches the right ventricular endocardium a paced rhythm is observed on the ECG. Similarly, if the catheter has passed through the right atrium and is in the caudal vena cava at the level of the diaphragm, diaphragmatic pacing may occur. The lead may coil within the right atrium, and repeated withdrawal and insertion of the lead with a twisting motion may facilitate passage of the lead across the tricuspid valve and into the right ventricle.

Postoperative Monitoring

Once placement is determined to be successful, the rate of the pulse generator is adjusted to meet the patient's needs as previously described. The current is set between 2 and 5 mA (or approximately twice the current needed to maintain consistent ventricular capture). The lead is secured to the patient's neck (or rear leg) by placing water-proof tape on the catheter lead at the skin exit site and suturing the tape to the animal's skin. Finally, the insertion site is wrapped with a light bandage to protect it from external contamination. The excess pacing catheter is included in the wrap of the neck (or rear leg), and the pulse generator is placed in a backpack or wrapped in a bandage around the dog's thorax.

Postoperatively, sedation and patient immobilization should be maintained to minimize the chance of lead displacement resulting from patient motion. Many cardiologists recommend administration of broad-spectrum antibiotics routinely. The bandage should be changed and the insertion site checked for signs of inflammation or infection every 48 hours until the pacing lead is removed. The use of continuous electrocardiographic monitoring allows close observation of successful pacing and early identification of failure to capture, or pace, the ventricle.

COMPLICATIONS

The complications occurring during temporary transvenous pacing can result in abrupt deterioration or even death of the patient. The most common problem is failure to pace the ventricle. This can occur as a result of migration of the lead away from the ventricular wall or out of the ventricle, fracture of the pacing lead, and battery or pulse generator failure.

When failure to capture is encountered, the following approach can be used to identify the source of the problem.

1. It is necessary to be certain that the pacing rate is set at more than the patient's intrinsic heart rate.
2. The next step is to check the battery to make certain that it is functioning normally (always have a spare battery available).
3. The connections of the pacing lead to the terminals of the pulse generator should be checked to ensure good electrical contact, and the exposed portions of the lead should be evaluated for areas of fatigue or fractures. A cervical and thoracic radiograph may be necessary to detect breaks or to determine that the lead needs to be repositioned within the ventricle.
4. The current (output) from the pulse generator can be slowly increased while observing the ECG to determine whether successful capture results. This technique is most likely to be successful when the lead tip has migrated away from the ventricular wall, leading to loss of ventricular capture. Repositioning the patient within the cage may also solve this problem by placing the lead back into contact with the ventricular myocardium.
5. Many pulse generators have an asynchronous mode, which overrides the sensing and inhibition functions of the pulse generator. By using the asynchronous mode, the pulse generator will deliver a pacing spike regardless of intrinsic ventricular activity. Although this can lead to serious arrhythmia if a pulse is delivered in the vulnerable period of the T wave, this is rare, and this technique can be used to identify the location of the pacing lead and disorders in the sensing function of the pulse generator.

Additional complications that can occur in association with temporary transvenous pacing include cardiac dysrhythmias, anesthetic complications, vascular or ventricular perforation with the lead tip, intravascular thrombosis around the pacing catheter, and infection. Implantation of a permanent pacemaker is recommended by the third day of temporary pacing in order to reduce the risk of a catheter-related infection. In human patients, the prevalence of pacemaker-related complications can range as high as 20%, and they are more common in patients requiring pacing for more than 48 hours. With appropriate precautions and meticulous technique, the potential complications associated with temporary pacing can be minimized.

References and Suggested Reading

Bonagura JD, Helphrey ML, Muir WW: Complications associated with permanent pacemaker implantation in the dog. J Am Med Vet Assoc 182:149, 1983.
Brown KK: Bradyarrhythmias and pacemaker therapy. In: Kirk RW, ed: Current Veterinary Therapy VI. Philadelphia: WB Saunders, 1977, p 354.
Darke PGG, McAreavey D, Been M: Transvenous cardiac pacing in 19 dogs and one cat. J Small Anim Pract 30:491, 1989.
Helphrey ML, Schollmeyer M: Pacemaker therapy. In: Kirk RW, ed: Current Veterinary Therapy VIII. Philadelphia: WB Saunders, 1983, p 373.
Jafri SM, Kruse JA: Temporary transvenous cardiac pacing. Crit Care Clin 8:713, 1992.
Le K, Goldschlager N: Temporary cardiac pacing in the intensive care unit. J Intensive Care Med 11:57, 1996.
Lombard CW, Tilley LP, Yoshioka M: Pacemaker implantation in the dog: Survey and literature review. J Am Anim Hosp Assoc 17:751, 1981.
Rush JE, Ross JN: Cardiac pacing. In: Murtaugh RJ, Kaplan PM, eds 5: Veterinary Emergency and Critical Care Medicine. St. Louis: Mosby-Year Book, 1992, p 657.
Silver MD, Goldschlager N: Temporary transvenous cardiac pacing in the critical care setting. Chest 93:607, 1988.

Bacterial Translocation: Clinical Implications and Prevention

DOUGLASS K. MACINTIRE
Auburn University, Alabama

Sepsis is the most common cause of death in human trauma patients surviving more than 48 hours after the initial traumatic insult (Wilson, 1985). In many critically ill patients dying of sepsis, no source of infection can be found. Gram-negative bacteria are the most common organisms cultured from these patients. These observations have led many researchers to suspect that the gut is the reservoir of pathogenic bacteria and endotoxins that initiate the systemic host response leading to shock and organ failure (Beal and Cerra, 1994).

PATHOGENESIS

Bacterial translocation (BT) is defined as the passage of viable indigenous bacteria from the gastrointestinal (GI) tract to the mesenteric lymph nodes, liver, spleen, and blood stream (Deitch et al, 1996). Numerous animal and human studies have clearly documented that microorganisms and toxins normally present in the GI tract can translocate from inside the lumen to extraintestinal sites (Deitch et al, 1985, 1987, 1988). The clinical significance of BT was called into question, however, when researchers were unable to culture bacteria from the portal or systemic blood in a series of human trauma victims (Moore et al, 1991). In addition, the results of a multicenter trial in critically ill human patients evaluating selective gut decontamination were somewhat disappointing (Van Saene et al, 1992). When antimicrobial agents were used to aggressively depopulate the gut of pathogenic gram-negative bacteria and fungi, no improvement in survival was noted, although there was a 50% reduction in the number of infectious complications in these patients.

It is now believed that many bacteria that translocate to the intestinal lymphatic tissue are killed by the host, thereby initiating a massive proinflammatory response characterized by the release of cytokines, vasoactive substances, complement, and other immunomodulators (Deitch et al, 1996). Furthermore, gut-derived endotoxemia may be the signal that triggers, perpetuates, or exacerbates the hypermetabolic response seen in the systemic inflammatory response syndrome (SIRS). Endotoxins are known to stimulate cytokine release and can cause impairment of the immune system, the coagulation system, and the GI mucosal barrier. It is therefore not necessary to culture viable bacteria from the blood stream or distant organs to implicate the gut as the most probable cause of SIRS.

Splanchnic ischemia may play a central role in the development of multiple organ failure because there is a strong correlation between decreasing intramucosal pH and morbidity and mortality (Silverman and Tuma, 1992). It is believed that intestinal ischemia leads to the loss of barrier function, which results in exposure of the gut-associated lymphoid tissue (GALT) to bacteria and toxins and the ensuing release of massive amounts of cytokines and endotoxins. If the reticuloendothelial system is overwhelmed, systemic endotoxemia or bacteremia may result.

GI Mucosal Barrier

Under normal conditions, the gut provides an effective mechanical and functional barrier to systemic absorption of intraluminal bacteria and toxins. For BT to occur, bacteria must first adhere to the intestinal mucosa. Adherence is reduced by intestinal peristalsis and mucus production. Enhanced BT has been shown to occur in conditions associated with decreased peristalsis, such as intestinal ileus and obstruction. Administration of vasopressors, corticosteroids, and nonsteroidal anti-inflammatory drugs (NSAIDs) can result in decreased mucus production and the loss of the protective mechanical barrier. Conditions of poor perfusion, such as the splanchnic ischemia associated with shock, also result in decreased epithelial cell turnover, cell death, and enhanced potential for mucosal breakdown. Stress gastritis and ulceration are common in critical patients.

The gut is the largest immunologic and endocrine organ in the body. The GALT consists of Peyer's patches, lymphoid follicles, lamina propria lymphocytes, intraepithelial lymphocytes, and mesenteric lymph nodes. Secretory IgA is produced by antigen-primed lymphocytes that line the intestinal mucosa. These immune mechanisms are critical in defending the host against bacterial invasion. Immunosuppressed patients are therefore predisposed to BT. Poor nutrition of enterocytes can result in decreased IgA production and impaired GI immune defenses.

A final factor that helps maintain the normal GI mucosal barrier is the protective role of the normal indigenous microflora. Anaerobes are the most numerous bacteria in the GI tract. These bacteria compete with potential pathogens for nutrients and mucosal attachment sites, thereby inhibiting bacterial overgrowth with gram-negative bacteria. Antibiotic therapy often upsets the delicate balance of the GI microflora by selecting for gram-negative organisms and resistant organisms while suppressing the more sensitive indigenous anaerobes (Deitch et al, 1985). Other interventions that may disrupt the normal flora in critical patients include the use of H_2 blockers, which can result in bacterial overgrowth and colonization of the stomach, and the use of hyperosmolar enteral diets.

IMPORTANCE OF NUTRITION

For many years, the GI tract was ignored in the management of critically ill patients. The primary function of the

GI tract was seen as the absorption of nutrients, which was considered necessary for supporting adequate wound healing and host response to injury or infection. Concern over possible aspiration, vomiting, ileus, or lack of enteral access led many clinicians to pursue a course of "bowel rest." We now know that bowel rest can lead to mucosal atrophy, altered permeability, and loss of the trophic effects of GI hormones (see p. 136). It has been shown in experimental models that starvation and malnutrition alone do not induce BT, but they may predispose to mucosal damage and the development of a potentially lethal septic state of gut origin during periods of systemic inflammation. Currently, there is significant interest and ongoing research to identify the effects of individual nutrients and to use enteral nutrition as a modulator of metabolic and inflammatory processes.

CLINICAL SIGNIFICANCE

Based on experimental studies in animal models, three primary mechanisms leading to enhanced BT have been identified: (1) intestinal bacterial overgrowth, (2) deficiencies in host immune defenses, and (3) damage to the GI mucosal barrier. Aggressive prevention of BT must therefore address these three concerns as well as provide nutritional support of the gut.

Animal research models and human clinical reports have shown that BT can be promoted by thermal injury, immunosuppression, trauma, hemorrhagic shock, endotoxin, acute necrotizing pancreatitis, total parenteral nutrition (TPN), neutropenia, intestinal obstruction, and intestinal ischemia. These same conditions would be likely to promote BT in critically ill veterinary patients. In addition, dogs with severe parvoviral enteritis are uniquely predisposed to developing BT, sepsis, and endotoxemia because of the combination of neutropenia and breakdown of the GI mucosal barrier.

PREVENTION

Prevention of BT, sepsis, and multiple organ failure is an area of ongoing research. The most important factor for preventing BT is preservation of an intact GI mucosal barrier, as experimental studies have shown that BT can be prevented largely by limiting mucosal injury. For this reason, therapeutic measures are aimed at (1) decreasing the likelihood of mucosal disruption, (2) limiting the consequences of disruption if it occurs, and (3) supporting the gut so that mucosal defects can be rapidly repaired. The following recommendations can be made.

Improving Gut Oxygenation. It appears that most mucosal damage in critical patients is initiated by ischemia and potentiated by reperfusion injury. Oxygen delivery to the gut should be maximized with effective, aggressive hemodynamic resuscitation (see p. 140). Adequate fluid therapy with crystalloid and/or colloid fluids should be administered to maintain adequate blood pressure and GI perfusion. Positive inotropes such as dobutamine or dopamine may be necessary to maintain blood pressure in septic patients (Silverman and Tuma, 1992). Supplemental

oxygen should be administered if the pulse oximetry reading drops below 90 to 95%. If the hemoglobin concentration drops below 10 to 12 gm/100 ml, a blood transfusion or bovine hemoglobin solution can be administered to improve the oxygen-carrying capacity of the blood. If available, gastric tonometry is the best way of monitoring intramucosal pH and determining whether GI perfusion is adequate (Silverman and Tuma, 1992; see *CVT XII*, p. 133).

Broad-spectrum bactericidal antibiotics should be administered to any animal exhibiting clinical signs of sepsis. Early diagnosis and surgical correction of areas of devitalized gut or abscess drainage is paramount to successful case management (see p. 272).

Reperfusion injury may be experimentally prevented with allopurinol or superoxide dismutase. Vitamins C, E, and A, selenium, and beta-carotene as well as the amino acids cystine, glycine, and glutamine all are involved in the body's antioxidant defense network. Dietary supplementation with antioxidants may be beneficial. Although research is currently underway to identify agents that selectively improve GI perfusion, to date none have been found. Catecholamines such as norepinephrine and epinephrine, which induce splanchnic vasoconstriction, should be avoided.

Limiting the Consequences of Mucosal Injury. The use of antacids and H_2 receptor blockers to reduce stress ulcers and gastritis in critical patients may result in bacterial overgrowth and an increased prevalence of hospital-acquired pneumonia in ventilated patients (Van Saene et al, 1992). The use of sucralfate and nasogastric suctioning is currently recommended for decreasing gastric injury without increasing the gastric pH.

The use of selective gut decontamination appears to reduce the prevalence of hospital-acquired infections but has not been shown to increase survival in critically ill humans (Van Saene et al, 1992). Although not often used in veterinary patients, a combination of amikacin, amphotericin B, and polymyxin B is commonly used in human patients (Cockerill et al, 1992). In rats, orally administered neomycin alone prevented mortality and reduced BT after thermal injury (Oca et al, 1993). A combination of oral polymyxin B, charcoal, and Kaopectate has been used to bind lipopolysaccharide endotoxin (Fink and Fiddian-Green, 1989). In addition, anecdotal accounts of the use of dilute chlorhexidine or Betadine (povidone-iodine) enemas in puppies with parvoviral enteritis have been reported.

A polyvalent equine-origin antiserum against lipopolysaccharide endotoxin is available for use in small animals (SEPTI-serum, Immvac, Inc., Columbia, MO 75201). The dosage is 4.4 ml/kg diluted 1:1 with intravenous crystalloid fluids and administered slowly over 30 to 60 minutes. Although clinical trials are lacking with this product, it should be most effective if administered prior to antibiotic therapy, because circulating endotoxin concentrations will increase dramatically when bacteria are killed. Patients receiving equine-origin antiserum must be observed closely during administration for signs of anaphylaxis.

Supporting the Gut With Enteral Nutrition

The importance of providing nutrition to critically ill patients is well documented. However, in recent years, the importance of "feeding the gut" through early enteral nutrition has become more apparent.

Studies have shown that compared with enteral nutrition, TPN is associated with increased mortality and infection rates. Not only does TPN result in mucosal atrophy, but also the lipid emulsions have been shown to promote immunosuppression through depressed lymphocyte blastogenesis. In addition, omega-6 fatty acids are precursors of prostaglandins and leukotrienes that may promote inflammation. The current recommendation for TPN is that it should be used only when a true contraindication to enteral feedings exists.

Enteral nutrition exerts its beneficial effects on gut function by strengthening the immune system (lymphocytes and macrophages), increasing IgA and mucin secretion, and maintaining gut mass through its trophic effects.

The preferred metabolic fuel for cells lining the small intestine is glutamine. Glutamine has been considered a "conditionally essential" nutrient in critically ill patients. It is essential for lymphocyte mitogenesis and enhances gut barrier function. Many studies have shown the beneficial effects of adding glutamine to parenteral or enteral solutions (reduced BT, thicker GI mucosa, increased survivability), although some results are disappointing. Glutamine supplementation is safe, but unfortunately glutamine is very unstable and must be added to solutions immediately prior to feeding. In patients with extensive mucosal injury, glutamine supplementation may be beneficial (see p. 136). It is available as a powder (Cambridge Neutraceuticals, 1-800-265-2202) and can be given at a dosage of 10 mg/kg per day. Glutamine can be added to the drinking water of recovering animals or added to the enteral diet and administered through a nasoesophageal, gastrostomy, or jejunostomy tube. Other dietary additives that may reduce BT include omega-3 fatty acids (fish oil products), arginine, nucleic acids, and antioxidants.

The preferred fuel of colonocytes is short-chain fatty acids. These substances are produced through fermentation of nondigestible carbohydrates, commonly referred to as fermentable fibers (pectin, beta-glycan, and lactulose). Insoluble fibers, such as cellulose, have trophic effects on the GI mucosa by promoting mucus production and epithelial cell growth and preserving the growth of normal microflora. Insoluble fiber is thought to stimulate the release of trophic gut hormones that enhance gut barrier function. Current recommendations regarding optimal fiber type and dose are lacking, but research is ongoing. A number of preliminary animal studies indicate decreased BT, prevention of mucosal atrophy, and avoidance of cecal bacterial overgrowth with the addition of bulk fiber additives to enteral diets. Other research is focusing on hormones, such as bombesin, that exert protective trophic effects on the GI mucosa. Definitive dietary recommendations await the results of this exciting area of research.

References and Suggested Reading

Beal AL, Cerra F: Multiple organ failure syndrome in the 1990's: Systemic inflammatory response and organ dysfunction. JAMA 271:226, 1994.
An excellent overview of current theories and definitions of SIRS and MODS.

Cockerill FR, Muller SP, et al: Prevention of infection in critically ill patients by selective decontamination of the digestive tract. Ann Intern Med 117:545, 1992.
A randomized clinical trial showing decreased infection rates in ICU patients in the treatment group.

Deitch EA, Berg R, Specan R: Endotoxin promotes the translocation of bacteria from the gut. Arch Surg 122:185, 1987.
A study in mice implicating endotoxin in the pathogenesis of bacterial translocation.

Deitch EA, Bridge SW, Baker J: Hemorrhagic shock–induced bacterial translocation is reduced by xanthine oxidase inhibition or inactivation. Surgery 104:191, 1988.
A study showing enhanced BT in rats following hypotensive shock that can be prevented by allopurinol.

Deitch EA, Maejima K, Berg R: Effect of oral antibiotics and bacterial overgrowth on the translocation of the GI-tract microflora in burned rats. J Trauma 25:385, 1985.
A study in rats showing enhanced bacterial translocation when GI microflora is disrupted.

Deitch EA, Rutan R, Waymack JP: Trauma, shock and gut translocation. New Horizons 4:289, 1996.
An excellent review of the current thinking regarding the relationship between shock, trauma, bacterial translocation, and multiple organ failure.

Fink MP, Fiddian-Green RG: Care of the gut in the critically ill. In: Marston A, et al, eds: Splanchnic Perfusion and Multiple Organ Failure. London: Edward Arnold, 1989, pp 377–386.
A nice review of care and feeding of the gut in critical patients.

Mainous MR, Block EFJ, Deitch EA: Nutritional support of the gut: How and why. New Horizons 2:193, 1994.
An excellent review of current research supporting early enteral nutrition.

Moore FA, Moore FE, Paggetti R, et al: Gut bacterial translocation via the portal vein: A clinical perspective with major torso trauma. J Trauma 31:629, 1991.
No evidence of endotoxemia or portal vein bacteremia was found in 29 trauma patients.

Oca J, Millat E, et al: Selective bowel decontamination, nutritional therapy, and bacterial translocation after burn injury. Clin Nutr 12:355, 1993.
A study in rats showing the prevention of BT following burn injury with oral neomycin.

Silverman HJ, Tuma P: Gastric tonometry in patients with sepsis: Effects of dobutamine and packed red blood cell transfusions. Chest 102:184, 1992.
A study that uses gastric tonometry to show that dobutamine increases intramucosal pH in septic human patients.

Van Saene HKF, Stoutenbeek CC, Stoller JK: Selective decontamination of the digestive tract in the intensive care unit: Current status and future prospects. Crit Care Med 20:691, 1992.
A review of various clinical trials that documents a decrease in the number of nosocomial infections, but no improvement in survivability.

Wilson RF: Special problems in the diagnosis and treatment of surgical sepsis. Surg Clin North Am 65:965, 1985.
A review article documenting the relationship between sepsis and critically ill surgical patients.

Toxicologic Disorders

MICHAEL J. MURPHY

Consulting Editor

Summary of Small Animal Poison Exposures in a Major Metropolitan Area

Carl S. Hornfeldt
Minneapolis, Minnesota

Michael J. Murphy
St. Paul, Minnesota

The Hennepin Regional Poison Center (HRPC) is one of 51 poison centers nationally designated as a regional poison center by the American Association of Poison Control Centers (AAPCC, 1996). Since 1989, in addition to serving the lay public and medical professionals, the HRPC has actively promoted a Pet Poison Information Service to veterinary professionals in the State of Minnesota (Hornfeldt and Jacobs, 1991). These efforts appear to be well received, as nearly 7,000 animal-related exposures will be documented by this center in 1996. This article briefly describes the types and relative incidence of small animal poison exposures encountered by the HRPC. Please note that an exposure is an actual or a suspected contact with any substance that has been ingested, inhaled, or absorbed by, applied to, or injected into the body (Hornfeldt and Murphy, 1992). Thus, each exposure does not necessarily represent a toxicosis.

During 1995, the HRPC documented 6,091 poison exposures in small animals. There were 4,960 (81.4%) poison exposures in dogs, 1,000 (16.4%) exposures in cats, and 131 (2.2%) exposures in other species, such as rodents and lagomorphs, birds (parrots, cockatiels), reptiles (iguanas), nondomesticated (squirrels) and exotic (ferrets, pot-bellied pigs) animals.

Of 6,091 total exposures, 5,963 (97.9%) were of an accidental nature, 43 were a result of therapeutic error, 22 were environmental (exposure to contaminated air, soil, or water), 10 were adverse drug reactions, 7 were food poisoning, 4 were malicious in nature, and 42 were designated as other or unknown. Acute exposures constituted 6,068 (99.6%) cases, while 13 were considered chronic (exposure over a period of more than 8 hours), 8 were acute-on-chronic (i.e., an animal overdosed on its own medication), and 2 were unknown.

The site of exposure in 6,000 (98.5%) cases was a private residence, generally assumed to be the animal owner's home. In contrast, 4,103 (67.4%) of calls to the poison center originated from a private residence, while 1,856 (30.5%) came from a veterinary hospital or clinic. Other exposure and call sites included workplaces, health care facilities, schools, and other public areas.

The most prevalent route of exposure was oral ingestion (5,857, 93.9%) followed by dermal (250, 4.0%), inhalation (51, 0.8%), ocular (26, 0.4%), bites or stings (14, 0.2%), parenteral (5, 0.08%), and aspiration (2, 0.03%), and 32 (0.5%) were exposures by other or unknown routes (total exposures exceed the total number of cases due to multiple routes of exposure for some cases).

During 1995, the monthly call volume ranged from a low of 384 cases in March, increased to a peak of 618 in July, and gradually decreased through the fall and winter. Daily call volume peaked from 4:00 to 6:00 PM, when it is speculated that many animal owners return home to unkenneled animals.

The incidence of poison exposures in dogs, cats, and other species by poison category is described in Table 1, where it may be noted that exposures to pesticides, plants, and human medications constituted nearly two thirds of all exposures in small animals, and plants made up almost 30% of all exposure calls in cats.

TABLE 1. Incidence of Poison Exposures in Small Animals

Poison Category	Dog	Cat	Other	Total	Percent
Pesticides	1,036	165	25	1,226	20.1
Plants	535	293	46	874	14.3
Prescription drugs	734	87	6	827	13.6
OTC drugs	667	63	3	733	12.0
Household products	357	127	14	498	8.2
Miscellaneous	359	68	6	433	7.1
Food-related	285	9	3	297	4.9
Lawn and garden products	219	33	7	259	4.3
Personal care products	199	20	4	223	3.7
Veterinary products	107	48	4	159	2.6
Automotive products	114	18	6	138	2.3
Construction products	90	31	1	122	2.0
Art and craft products	101	6	2	109	1.8
Chemicals	84	22	2	108	1.8
Tobacco products	18	4	1	23	0.4
Bites or stings	20	2	0	22	0.4
Drugs of abuse	22	0	0	22	0.4
Fumes or gases	7	3	1	11	0.2
Industrial products	6	1	0	7	0.1
TOTAL	4,960	1,000	131	6,091	100.0

OTC, over-the-counter.

References and Suggested Reading

American Association of Poison Control Centers Membership Directory 1996, 3201 New Mexico Avenue NW, Suite 310, Washington DC, 20016.

Hornfeldt CS, Jacobs MR: A poison information service for small animals offered by a regional poison center. *Vet Hum Toxicol* 33:339, 1991.

Hornfeldt CS, Murphy MJ: 1990 Report of the American Association of Poison Control Centers: Poisoning in animals. *J Am Vet Med Assoc* 200:1077, 1992.

Treatments Used in Small Animal Toxicoses

AVA FIRTH

St. Paul, Minnesota

This article discusses issues of use of, need for, and availability of both specific and nonspecific therapeutics used in the management of small animal poisonings. How many different antidotes does a veterinarian actually need to keep in stock? How and where does one obtain the more unusual antidotes, how much do they cost, and are they really necessary? While each veterinarian's requirements for antidotes may vary slightly, some recommendations may be made for both general practice and emergency referral practices. Furthermore, both kinds of practices may benefit from a systematic approach to therapeutics used in the management of poisonings.

Three categories of agents are used in the management of poisonings. The first category is specific—antidotes—of which there are only a few. Current recommendations for use and inventory holdings of these antidotes are summarized in Table 1. Antidotes that are no longer considered to be commonly required are listed in Table 2.

The second, broader category includes drugs used in supportive management of clinical signs and that are part of our routine therapeutic stock. Drugs such as atropine, sedatives, and steroids fall into this category (Table 3).

The third category encompasses nonspecific decontaminants, such as activated charcoal, cathartics, and emetics.

TABLE 1. Recommended Antidote Inventory

Name	Used For	Trade Name, Manufacturer, Distributor	How Supplied	Dose	Recommended Practice Holdings (General, Emergency, or Both)
2-PAM	Organophosphate toxicity	Protopam, Wyeth-Ayerst	1-gm vials, box of 6 50 mg/ml	10–15 mg/kg IM or SC q8–12 hr, 36 hr minimum	Emergency
4-Methylpyrazole, fomepizole	Ethylene glycol toxicity	Antizol-Vet, Orphan Medical, Inc.	1.5-gm vial of dry powder to be reconstituted	*Dogs:* 20 mg/kg IV initial dose, 15 mg/kg IV q12hr × 2 doses, 5 mg/kg IV at 36 hr	Both
Acetylcysteine	Acetaminophen, other oxidant injuries	Mucomyst, Mead-Johnson	10-ml ampules of 200 mg/ml, box of 10	5% solution (50 mg/ml), 140 mg/kg initially, then 70 mg/kg IV q4hr × 12–24 hr	Both
Atropine	Organophosphate toxicity	Atropine, USP	Vials of 0.4, 0.5, or 1 mg/ml	0.2 to 0.5 mg/kg; ¼ of the dose IV (balance IM or SC)	Both
Calcitonin	Cholecalciferol toxicity	Rhone-Poulenc, Sandoz	200 IU/ml in 2-ml vials	4–6 IU/kg SC q2–3 hr until serum calcium levels are normalized	Emergency
Calcium EDTA	Lead, zinc toxicity	Calcium Disodium Versenate, 3M Pharmaceuticals	5-ml ampules of 200 mg/ml, box of 6	25 mg/kg SC q6hr × 2–5 days, diluted in 5% dextrose to decrease local irritation	Both
D-Penicillamine	Lead, heavy metal toxicities	D-Panamine	125- or 250-mg tablets	50–100 mg/kg/day PO × 1 wk minimum, can divide daily dose to reduce nausea	Neither
Deferoxamine	Iron toxicity	Desferal, Ciba-Geigy	500-mg vials of dry powder to be reconstituted	10 mg/kg IM or IV q8hr for 24 hr	Emergency
Ethanol	Ethylene glycol toxicity	Abbott, McGaw	5% alcohol in 5% dextrose and water, 1000 ml	*Dogs:* 5% ethanol, 22 ml/kg IV q4hr × 24 hr, then q6hr × further 24 hr. Alternatively, set up CRI to run 5.5 ml/kg/hr. *Cats:* 5% ethanol CRI of 5 ml/kg/hr	Both
Vitamin K₁	Anticoagulant rodenticides	Veta-K₁, others	5-mg tablets, 25-mg gel capsules, injectable solutions	2.5–5.0 mg/kg × 2–3 wk (depends on specific anticoagulant)	Both

CRI, constant-rate infusion.

207

TABLE 2. Antidotes No Longer Commonly Required

Rare Antidotes	Toxin
Physostigmine	Curare
Edrophonium	Curare
Sodium nitrite	Cyanide
Sodium thiosulfate	Cyanide
Calcium borogluconate	Fluoride
Diphenylthiocarbazone	Thallium
Prussian blue	Thallium

This article makes recommendations for antidote holdings by both general practice and emergency referral practices and briefly identifies the common therapeutics and nonspecific decontaminants that warrant a place in virtually every practitioner's cupboard.

SPECIFIC ANTIDOTES

Rational Management of Antidotes

Rational use of antidotes first requires an understanding that antidotes are no substitute for life-support measures. Administration of the antidote should be performed as soon as possible, but only after the patient has been stabilized, history and exposure have been confirmed, and steps have been taken to hasten excretion of the poison from the body. General information on the management of poisons can be found in *CVT XII* (Dorman, 1995), as well as in other textbooks (Firth, 1995). Identification of at least the class of poison is necessary before the use of an antidote can be justified. This identification may be based on product package identification or, more commonly, on classic, characteristic clinical signs.

TABLE 3. List of Common Therapeutics Useful in Symptomatic and Supportive Treatment of Poisonings

Drug	Use
Acepromazine	Sedation
Ammonium chloride	Urinary acidification
Atropine	Bradycardia
Beta-blockers	Tachycardias
Calcium gluconate	Hypocalcemia
Dexamethasone	Anti-inflammatory
Dextrose solution	Treatment of hypoglycemia
Diazepam	Sedation/anticonvulsant
Glyceryl guaiacolate	Mild sedation
Mannitol	Treatment of cerebral edema
Milk of magnesia	Gastrointestinal protectant
Sucralfate	Gastrointestinal protectant
Buprenorphine or butorphanol	Gastrointestinal discomfort
Dopamine	Renal perfusion support
Doxapram	Respiratory stimulant
Furosemide	Diuresis
Naloxone	Reversal of opioid agonists
Pentobarbital	Long-term anesthesia/heavy sedation/anticonvulsant
Potassium chloride	Treatment of hypokalemia
Prednisolone	Nonspecific anti-inflammatory, mild diuresis
Sodium bicarbonate	Correction of metabolic acidosis

The question then arises as to which antidotes a veterinary practitioner should stock. It would seem prudent and rational for any general practice to have antidotes on hand for the most common pesticides used in the geographic region. For example, warmer climates may have a high frequency of organophosphate use; colder climates may have a seasonal peak of rodenticide use. Ethylene glycol use is ubiquitous, and every practitioner should be ready to manage that particular toxicosis.

Most practices, when geographically at risk, should keep at least one dose of antidotal drugs, such as antivenins that are required for *immediate* management of patients. Tablet and oral forms of antidotes, such as vitamin K_1 and various chelating agents, are generally not required in an acute situation, because injectable forms can maintain the patient for 24 to 48 hours until an oral form can be obtained from suppliers or pharmacies.

Fortunately, the advent of express and overnight shipping has decreased the isolation once so characteristic of many veterinary practices and consequently has reduced the large range of inventory that a veterinary practice now needs to hold. Suppliers are now able to provide most inventory items in 24 hours or less. Unfortunately, practices that are more remote are still obliged to keep larger stocks of the less-available antidotes. Emergency practices that operate after hours and are "cut off" from suppliers during the weekend may also need to maintain a stock of antidotes. The availability of an emergency referral practice also can impact which antidotes a general practice keeps on hand, since an emergency referral practice, in support of a large number of general practices, will have significantly broader inventory requirements.

Criteria

Criteria helpful in deciding whether to stock a particular antidote are as follows:

- How many patients per year require this drug?
- How much did I use last year?
- What is the time frame of required therapy—less than 12 hours, 12 to 24 hours, or days?
- What is the availability of this drug from my suppliers—do they stock it routinely, how fast can they ship it?
- Is this drug routinely held by other local hospitals or pharmacies from which I may obtain an emergency supply?

Administration, Usage, and Holding

This section briefly outlines current recommendations for administration, usage, and holding of commonly used antidotes. References direct the reader to more detailed information on the various toxins and antidotes. See Table 1 for a summary as well as manufacturer and supply information.

Anticoagulant Rodenticides

Vitamin K₁

Usage. Vitamin K_1 is the antidote of choice for anticoagulant rodenticide toxicities. It provides an active form of vitamin K_1 to the liver beyond the point of inactivation caused by warfarin-coumarins. However, administered vitamin K_1 is then incorporated into the inactive pool, which means that the administration of active vitamin K_1 must be maintained *for as long as the anticoagulant substance is present* in the body. Assurance of effective therapy is best guided by assessment of the prothrombin time, measured 2 to 5 days after therapy has ceased.

Injectable vitamin K_1 should be administered only by subcutaneous injection to prevent anaphylaxis. Oral absorption of vitamin K_1 is enhanced when it is given with a small, fatty meal, such as a teaspoon of canned dog food. The dosage and duration of therapy vary, depending on the exact class of anticoagulant ingested. Vitamin K_3 is not recommended (Felice and Murphy, 1995; see the next article).

Recommended Holding. Each practice should have at least the injectable form on hand. Vitamin K_1 tablets or capsules are widely available and can be ordered from suppliers or prescribed to an outside pharmacy.

Ethylene Glycol

Ethanol

Usage. Ethanol is the only recommended antidote for ethylene glycol toxicity in cats and is still commonly used in dogs. The administration of ethanol is based on the principle of preventing toxic metabolite formation in the liver by providing the pivotal enzyme, alcohol dehydrogenase, with a competing substrate. Even though ethanol also induces signs of alcohol intoxication, including central nervous system depression and increased serum osmolality, it remains in common use owing to wide availability (Thrall et al, 1995; *CVT XII*, p. 232).

Recommended Holding. Inhibiting the formation of toxic metabolites is a *time-critical* process. Even a few hours can make a significant difference in patient outcome. For this reason, it is recommended that every practice maintain stocks of 20% ethanol to provide immediate treatment.

4-Methylpyrazole (4-MP)

Usage. 4-MP is the antidote of choice for ethylene glycol toxicity in dogs, but until recently its use has been hampered by the lack of a commercially available product. Like ethanol, 4-MP is a competitive inhibitor of alcohol dehydrogenase but does not cause central nervous system depression or hyperosmolality. 4-MP is not recommended for use in cats (Bahri, 1991; Dial et al, 1989).

Recommended Holding. As 4-MP becomes widely available, every practice should be able to maintain stocks, as for ethanol.

Lead, Zinc, Iron, and Copper

Calcium EDTA (Calcium Disodium Edetate)

Usage. Calcium EDTA exerts an antidotal action against lead and zinc by binding with them to form more water-soluble complexes, which are easily excreted in the urine (chelation). Although the incidence of lead toxicity is decreasing, the widespread use of zinc in nuts, bolts, and United States pennies has led to zinc intoxication ranking among the top 25 canine toxicities (Buck, 1995). Calcium EDTA is now recommended for use in zinc toxicity at dosages recommended for the treatment of lead toxicity (Meurs and Breitschwerdt, 1995). The major disadvantage of calcium EDTA is its availability in only an injectable form (see D-penicillamine, below).

Recommended Holding. Calcium EDTA has application to management of both acute and chronic lead and zinc toxicities. Although the incidence of these toxicities may be low, providing just symptomatic and supportive therapy may well fail. Zinc toxicity also appears to be more rapidly progressive than lead toxicity, and immediate treatment is warranted. Calcium EDTA should be available within 12 hours of diagnosis, which means that most practices should keep it in stock.

Deferoxamine

Usage. Deferoxamine is used in the treatment of iron toxicity. Compared with other chelating agents, it is the most effective chelator of iron. Iron toxicity is increasing in frequency owing to iron's wide use as a component of dietary and multivitamin supplements, which are often contained in palatable tablets, and may be ingested in large quantities (Greentree and Hall, 1995).

Recommended Holding. Deferoxamine should be administered as soon as possible, and certainly within 12 hours of ingestion. While iron toxicity is not as common as some other toxicities, it is another situation wherein antidotal therapy may be lifesaving and supportive therapy may not. Thus, it is recommended that general practices maintain a source capable of supplying deferoxamine within 12 hours of ingestion. Emergency practices may need to maintain their own supply.

D-Penicillamine

Usage. D-Penicillamine is another chelating agent with wide application to the treatment of metal toxicities. It is recommended for use in lead toxicity as well as copper, gold, and mercury toxicities. Primary use occurs as an oral chelating agent, for long-term outpatient therapy (Bratton and Kowalczyk, 1989).

Recommended Holding. There are few conceivable instances in which penicillamine treatment would commence without the veterinarian's knowing blood lead concentrations; therefore, it has little role as an emergency drug. Practices should be able to obtain it from pharmaceutical suppliers within 48 hours of diagnosis.

Cholinesterase Inhibitors

Pralidoxime Chloride (2-PAM)

Usage. 2-PAM is widely recommended for the treatment of the nicotinic signs associated with acute organophosphate toxicity, such as muscle fasciculations. 2-PAM does in fact relieve the muscarinic signs (salivation, bronchospasm) as well, but atropine (see Table 1) is generally adequate for this purpose. 2-PAM is also suggested for cats suffering from prolonged organophosphate exposure. Treatment reactivates the cholinesterase (CE) enzyme by destroying the otherwise stable CE-phosphate bond. 2-PAM is not appropriate therapy for carbamate toxicities, since it is unable to break the CE-carbaryl bond and will bind instead to the available sites on any unaffected CE enzyme, thus worsening the signs (Hansen, 1995).

Recommended Holding. 2-PAM is most effective if given within 24 hours of exposure, before the CE-phosphate bond has "aged" and become resistant to competitive binding. In actual practice, few organophosphate toxicities seem to require more than mild sedation and atropine on an emergency basis. Furthermore, 2-PAM will not make the difference between life and death. It would be reasonable for a practice to have access to 2-PAM within 12 hours of diagnosis, without actually stocking it.

Antivenins

The stocking of antivenins is an individual practice decision. The decision should be made based on the frequency of envenomation patients, seasonality of incidence, and availability of antivenin from other sources, such as human hospitals and neighboring veterinary practices. A common approach for practices in rural areas is to have one vial of antivenin on hand, with arrangements to obtain additional supplies within 12 hours if required.

Acetaminophen

N-Acetylcysteine

Usage. Acetaminophen toxicity still ranks in the top 25 most common toxicities of the cat (Oehme, 1986; Ilkiw and Ratcliffe, 1987).

Recommended Holding. There is only a short time available for effective intervention in acetaminophen toxicity. All practices should have acetylcysteine on hand or readily available from a 24-hour pharmacy.

TABLES OF ANTIDOTES

The list of true antidotes that are required, proven efficacy, and commercially or easily available is remarkably short. As various poisons become rarer, the antidotes for them also fall out of general availability; for example, thallium and cyanide.

Table 1 lists the antidotes discussed in the previous section, which are considered to be the ones with common application in veterinary medicine as a whole. The reader is encouraged to consult more specific pharmaceutical references for specific product availabilities and manufacturers. While manufacturers tend to be multinational, distributors and costs may vary considerably. The last column indicates whether the antidote is a recommended stock item

for general practice (G), emergency referral practice (E), or both (B).

SUPPORTIVE TREATMENT AGENTS

Many of the drugs required for supportive treatment will be routinely held in veterinary practices as normal therapeutics. Table 3 lists those drugs. Doses can be found in the Appendix of this edition or in specific articles describing usage. Familiarity with the general approach to management, as discussed in *CVT XII* (Dorman, 1995) or other textbooks (Firth, 1995), is essential.

NONSPECIFIC DECONTAMINANTS

Each practice should also maintain stocks of substances required for decontamination of the gastrointestinal tract. These fall into three broad categories: emetics, adsorbents, and cathartics. Emetics are a vexing problem, with apomorphine (0.02 to 0.04 mg/kg IV or IM) being withdrawn from the veterinary market.* Other emetic alternatives include xylazine, syrup of ipecac (2 to 6 ml PO or 1 to 2 ml/kg PO to a maximum of 15 ml/dog), and hydrogen peroxide (5 ml of 3% solution PO). Each practice should also have on hand a supply of activated charcoal. Powder or liquid forms are more efficacious than tablets. Activated charcoal (Acta-char, 1 to 4 gm/kg diluted in water, or Charcodote, 6 to 12 ml/kg) is also supplied by some companies as a prepack with sorbitol. Cathartics are replacing gastric lavage in human medicine, owing to the problems of aspiration pneumonia, incomplete emptying of the stomach, and concerns about intubating the patient. These concerns are no less real in veterinary medicine. However, it is rational to consider an increased use of cathartics, since so much of what we deal with has no specific antidote, the intoxicant has usually been ingested, and the agent may be of large particle size. Cathartics include mineral oil (2 to 10 ml for cats; 5 to 30 ml for dogs) and sodium sulfate (1 gm/kg).

References and Suggested Reading

Atkins CE: Hypertonic sodium phosphate enema intoxication. In: Kirk RW, ed: Current Veterinary Therapy IX. Philadelphia: WB Saunders, 1986, p 212.

Bahri LE: 4-Methylpyrazole: An antidote for ethylene glycol intoxication in dogs. Compend Cont Educ 13:1123, 1991.

Bailey EM, Szabunicwiez M: The use of glyceryl guaiacolate ether in the treatment of strychnine poisoning in the dog. Vet Med Small Anim Clin 70:170, 1995.

Bratton GR, Kowalczyk DF: Lead poisoning. In: Kirk RW, Bonagura JD, eds: Current Veterinary Therapy X. Philadelphia: WB Saunders, 1989, pp 152–159.

Buck WB: Top 25 generic agents involving dogs and cats managed by the National Animal Poisons Control Center in 1992. In: Bonagura JD, Kirk RW, eds: Current Veterinary Therapy XII. Philadelphia: WB Saunders, 1995, p 210.

Dial SM, Thrall MA, Hamar DW: 4-Methylpyrazole as treatment for naturally acquired ethylene glycol intoxication in dogs. J Am Vet Med Assoc 195:73, 1989.

Dorman DC: Emergency treatment of toxicoses. In: Bonagura JD, Kirk RW, eds: Current Veterinary Therapy XII. Philadelphia: WB Saunders, 1995, p 211.

Felice LJ, Murphy MJ: CVT update: Anticoagulant rodenticides. In:

---

*Conjunctival capsules may still be available (Island Pharmacies, Inc.).

Bonagura JD, Kirk RW, eds: Current Veterinary Therapy XII. Philadelphia, WB Saunders, 1995, p 228.

Firth AM: Poisonings. In: Bistner SI, Ford RB, eds: Handbook of Veterinary Procedures and Emergency Treatment. Philadelphia: WB Saunders, 1995, p 169.

Greentree WF, Hall JO: Iron toxicosis. In: Bonagura JD, Kirk RW, eds: Current Veterinary Therapy XII. Philadelphia: WB Saunders, 1995, p 240.

Hansen SR: Management of organophosphate and carbamate insecticide toxicosis. In: Bonagura JD, Kirk RW, eds: Current Veterinary Therapy XII. Philadelphia: WB Saunders, 1995, p 245.

Ilkiw JE, Ratcliffe RC: Paracetamol toxicity in a cat. Aust Vet J 64:245, 1987.

Meurs KM, Breitschwerdt EB: CVT update: Zinc toxicity. In: Bonagura JD, Kirk RW, eds: Current Veterinary Therapy XII. Philadelphia: WB Saunders, 1995, p 238.

Oehme FW: Aspirin and acetaminophen. In: Kirk RW, ed: Current Veterinary Therapy IX. Philadelphia: WB Saunders, 1986, p 188.

Thrall MA, Grauer GF, Dial SM: Antifreeze poisoning. In: Bonagura JD, Kirk RW, eds: Current Veterinary Therapy XII. Philadelphia: WB Saunders, 1995, p 232.

CVT Update: Rodenticide Toxicosis

MICHAEL J. MURPHY
St. Paul, Minnesota

The rodenticides most frequently encountered by pets are anticoagulant rodenticides, cholecalciferol, strychnine, zinc phosphide, and bromethalin. The anticoagulant rodenticides continue to cause a substantial percentage of calls to poison centers and veterinary clinics (see p. 206). Cholecalciferol is reviewed in the article on nephrotoxins in this section. Brief updates for anticoagulant rodenticides, strychnine, and bromethalin follow; more expansive discussions are available in *CVT XII* (p. 228), *CVT VIII* (p. 98) and *CVT X* (p. 147). Zinc phosphide, which has been substituted for strychnine in some gopher baits, also is discussed here.

ANTICOAGULANT RODENTICIDES

Anticoagulant rodenticides act by inhibiting the recycling of vitamin K_1, which leads to a reduction in circulating activity of factors II, VII, IX, and X. Activity of one or more of these factors is most commonly measured by activated coagulation time (ACT), one-stage prothrombin time (OSPT), or activated partial thromboplastin time (APTT). Prolongation of these times, beyond the expected value of the laboratory, indicates a coagulopathy. Each of these tests is abnormal in anticoagulant rodenticide toxicity.

Anticoagulant rodenticides should be considered in any dog or cat with dyspnea or exercise intolerance, when other possibilities in the differential diagnosis are not clearly present, because intrathoracic and intrapulmonary hemorrhages are common occurrences in animals with anticoagulant rodenticide toxicosis. Prolonged bleeding from venipuncture sites, hematomas, hematemesis, melena, hemoptysis, and hematuria are other signs easily attributable to a coagulopathy.

Anticoagulant rodenticide-induced coagulopathies may be distinguished from other coagulopathies by specific testing (see *CVT XII*, p. 457) or response to vitamin K_1 treatment. Each of the above coagulation parameters are dramatically shortened within 24 hours of starting vitamin K_1 treatment, if an anticoagulant rodenticide is responsible for the coagulopathy. Detection of the anticoagulant rodenticide in the serum of an affected animal is the most specific means of diagnosing an anticoagulant rodenticide toxicosis. Such testing is now available in many veterinary diagnostic laboratories throughout the United States.

Animals with a packed cell volume of less than 15 with severe bleeding, or demonstrating complications of anemia need fresh whole blood immediately. Animals with a moderate coagulopathy may respond well to vitamin K_1 therapy alone. Clotting factor increases may be measurable 12 hours after vitamin K_1 dosing and should have returned to normal within 36 hours of initiation of vitamin K_1 treatment. The bioavailability of vitamin K_1 is greatest when given orally, so this route is the one preferred for any nonvomiting animals. Vitamin K_1 may be given subcutaneously but should not be given intramuscularly or intravenously because of the increased risks of massive intramuscular hemorrhage and anaphylaxis, respectively. Doses of 2.5 to 5.0 mg of vitamin K_1/kg body weight per day have been shown to correct coagulopathies due to anticoagulant rodenticides on the market today. Treatment may needed for 2 to 4 weeks for the long-acting products, *brodifacoum, chlorophacinone,* and *diphacinone.*

Strychnine

Strychnine inhibits the postsynaptic "buffering" effect of glycine on sensory stimulation of motoneurons and interneurons. Consequently, strychnine-poisoned animals appear apprehensive, tense, and stiff within minutes to hours of exposure. Signs progress to tonic extensor ridigity, especially after stimulation with light, sound, or touch. Animals often die in opisthotonos owing to paralysis of respiratory muscles.

Urine in a live animal and stomach contents in a dead animal are the samples of choice for analytic confirmation of exposure to strychnine. Exposure to strychnine-containing baits and the excitatory clinical signs described above support a clinical diagnosis.

Sedating the animal to prevent seizures while strychnine is metabolized is the primary aim of treatment. Pentobarbital, to effect, is commonly used as a sedative. Methocarbamol may be used for muscle relaxation at a dosage of 55 to 220 mg/kg IV, one half administered rapidly, then the remaining half slowly to effect. Do not exceed 330 mg/kg per day. Although diazepam is normally the drug of choice for seizuring animals, its efficacy for strychnine-induced seizures is variable. Activated charcoal may be administered to reduce further absorption, provided that precipitation of seizures is avoided.

Zinc Phosphide

Within minutes to hours of ingestion of a toxic dose of zinc phosphide, animals progress through anorexia, lethargy, dyspnea, vomiting (occasionally with hematemesis), ataxia, weakness, recumbency, and death.

Elevated serum zinc concentrations or zinc phosphide detection in samples of vomitus supports a diagnosis in live animals, but such measurements are rarely obtainable in a time frame useful for determining treatment. The stomach contents of a dead animal *may* confirm the presence of zinc phosphide, although volatility may preclude such confirmation. Supportive histologic lesions may be detected in the liver, lungs, and gastrointestinal tract.

No specific antidote exists. Treatment is aimed at removing zinc phosphide from the stomach in known cases of ingestion via emetics, reducing phosgene liberation by gastric lavage with 5% sodium bicarbonate—taking care to prevent bloat—and IV fluid and hepatic supportive agents. Consult poison-control specialists.

Bromethalin

Bromethalin acts by uncoupling oxidative phosphorylation and gives rise to hyperexcitability in the acute phase and depression during the chronic phase. Hyperexcitability, muscle tremors, seizures, hindlimb hyperreflexia, depression, and death may be observed approximately 10 hours after a 5 mg/kg or higher exposure to bromethalin. Tremors, depression, ataxia, and recumbency may be observed 1 to 3 days after an exposure of 2.5 mg/kg or less, but signs may last up to 12 days.

Analysis of bait, stomach contents, or vomitus is possible to confirm exposure to bromethalin in a live animal. Analysis of tissues, including fat, may be used to confirm exposure in a dead animal.

No specific antidote exists. Aggressive charcoal therapy is aimed at reducing absorption and possible enterohepatic circulation of bromethalin. Mannitol and glucocorticoids have been used to reduce cerebrospinal fluid pressure, but they may not reliably reverse clinical signs.

Nephrotoxins

WILSON K. RUMBEIHA
East Lansing, Michigan

The kidney is a frequent target of toxic chemicals. Although the kidneys constitute less than 1% of body weight in the majority of mammalian species, they receive about 25% of the total cardiac output. This abundant blood supply explains the high renal exposure to xenobiotics. These chemicals may reach relatively high concentrations in the ultrafiltrate bathing the epithelial cells. The kidneys possess an elaborate apparatus for metabolism of drugs and other chemicals. Although metabolism of these compounds generally leads to detoxification, bioactivation of some chemicals causes nephrotoxicity.

Toxic-induced acute renal failure is a commonly encountered problem in small animals. Younger animals are the most frequently involved. In dogs, the most common causes of nephrotoxicosis are exposure to ethylene glycol, ingested or administered nonsteroidal anti-inflammatory drugs, eating bait containing cholecalciferol, and veterinarian-administered aminoglycoside antibiotics. Ethylene glycol and cholecalciferol are the most frequent causes of nephrotoxicosis in cats; however, there is an increasing incidence of Easter lily (*Lilium longiflorum*) plant-induced acute renal failure in cats. Only the most common causes of nephrotoxicosis are discussed in this article. The clinician should be advised, however, of the potential of other nephrotoxins in small animals (Table 1). It is also important to realize that certain factors predispose animals or increase the susceptibility of animals to the nephrotoxic effects of xenobiotics. In general, young and geriatric animals are more susceptible to the nephrotoxic effects of xenobiotics because young animals do not have a fully developed detoxifying system and old animals have a diminished capacity to detoxify xenobiotics compared with that of young adults. Malnutrition, dehydration, pre-existing renal conditions, and concurrent exposure to multiple nephrotoxins are some of the factors that increase the potential for nephrotoxicity.

ETHYLENE GLYCOL AND DIETHYLENE GLYCOL

Ethylene glycol (EG) is a sweet-tasting, colorless liquid widely used as a solvent in several commercial products, including antifreeze, paints, and polishes. Diethylene glycol (DEG) is also a widely used organic solvent in commercial products. Antifreeze is the most common source of EG exposure in pets. Commercial antifreeze contains 95% EG.

TABLE 1. Some Possibilities in the Differential Diagnosis of Acute and Chronic Renal Failure in Dogs and Cats

Household Products and Pesticides
Cholecalciferol (see text)
Sodium fluoride, superphosphate fertilizer
Rodenticides (e.g., phosphorus, thallium)
Herbicides (e.g., paraquat)
Industrial Compounds
Ethylene glycol (see text)
Chlorinated hydrocarbons (e.g., carbon tetrachloride, chloroform, hexachlorobutadiene)
Heavy Metals
Mercury, cadmium, lead, arsenic, chromium
Pharmaceuticals, Diagnostic Aids, and Anesthetics
Aminoglycoside antibiotics (see text)
Cephalosporins (e.g., cephaloridine, cefazolin, cephalothin)
Polymixins
Sulfonamides (e.g., sulfapyridine, sulfathiazole, sulfadiazine)
Amphotericin B
Nonsteroidal anti-inflammatory drugs (see text)
Lithium
Phosphorus-containing urinary acidifiers
Cyclosporine
Antineoplastics (e.g., methotrexate, cisplatin)
Methoxyflurane
Chelating agents (e.g., D-penicillamine, EDTA [ethylenediaminetetraacetic acid])
Radiologic contrast media
Gold salts
Diuretics (e.g., thiazides, furosemide)
Vitamin D₃ analogues (psoriasis medications)
Natural Toxins
Easter lily (*Lilium longiflorum;* see text)
Mycotoxins (e.g., ochratoxin A, citrinin)
Snake venom
Mushrooms (e.g., amatoxins)
Ischemic Renal Injury
Severe volume depletion
Hemolytic compounds (e.g., zinc toxicosis, acetaminophen toxicosis in cats)
Thromboembolism of renal arteries in cats
Infectious Conditions
Acute nephritis (e.g., leptospirosis) or pyelonephritis
Chronic tubulointerstitial nephritis
Primary Renal Diseases
Chronic renal disease (idiopathic)
Amyloidosis
Familial renal diseases
Obstructive Uropathy
Ruptured Urinary Conduit

Ethylene glycol toxicosis is reported all year round but is most frequently encountered from late fall to early spring. Ingestion is the most widely reported route of exposure. Ethylene glycol is rapidly absorbed from the gut, with peak plasma concentrations achieved 2 to 3 hours after ingestion. The plasma half-life of EG in small animals is about 3 hours. It is predominantly metabolized in the liver, with the reaction proceeding as follows: EG to glycoaldehyde to glycolate to glyoxalate. Glyoxalate is finally converted to several final metabolites, including oxalate, glycine, and formate. The conversion of EG to glycoaldehyde is catalyzed by alcohol dehydrogenase, while that of glycoaldehyde to glycolate is catalyzed by aldehyde dehydrogenase. The conversions of EG to glycoaldehyde and of glycoaldehyde to glycolate require NAD as a cofactor. Lactate dehydrogenase and glycolic acid oxidase catalyze the conversion of glycolate to glyoxylate. The conversions of EG to glycoaldehyde and of glycolate to glyoxalate are the rate-limiting steps in the metabolism of EG. Ethylene glycol itself is mildly toxic, but its metabolic products, especially glycoaldehyde, glycolate, and oxalate, are potentially lethal.

Toxicity and Signs

Cats are more sensitive to EG toxicity than are dogs. The minimum lethal dose of undiluted EG is 1.4 ml/kg in the cat and 4.4 ml/kg in the dog. The clinical presentation of EG toxicosis in dogs and cats can be divided into three phases. The first phase starts about 30 minutes after exposure and lasts up to about 8 hours. The predominant clinical signs during this phase are vomiting, depression, and ataxia. These signs are attributed to EG and glycoaldehyde. The latter reaches peak plasma concentration 6 to 12 hours after EG ingestion. The second phase starts at about 8 hours after exposure and lasts up to 24 hours. Depression, anorexia, tachycardia, and pulmonary congestion are the predominant clinical signs during this phase. If the animal survives these two initial phases, the third phase begins about 24 to 72 hours after EG ingestion. The predominant signs during the third phase reflect acute renal failure and include vomiting, anuria or oliguria, and uremia. Acidosis (increased anion gap), hyperosmolality, elevated blood urea nitrogen (BUN) and creatinine, hypocalcemia, polydipsia, and isosthenuria are hallmarks of EG toxicosis in small animals. Glycolic and lactic acids are the main causes of acidosis in EG toxicosis. Lactic acid formation is favored by the increase in the ratio of NADH to NAD, which drives the lactate dehydrogenase reaction. Acidosis can be detected as early as 3 to 4 hours after EG ingestion. Acute renal failure is the consequence of the direct toxic effects of EG metabolites on renal epithelial cells and of the tubular obstructive effects of calcium oxalate crystals.

Diagnosis

Diagnosis consists of a history consistent with EG exposure and the presence of clinical signs involving gastrointestinal upset, central nervous system depression, cardiopulmonary involvement, and acute renal failure. Blood samples can be taken for EG measurement and for determinations of anion gap (see *CVT XII,* pp. 121 and 956), BUN, creatinine, and total calcium concentrations. Urine is also valuable in the diagnosis of EG toxicosis. Microscopic examination of urine sediments reveals calcium oxalate crystals, although such crystals may be observed in the urine of healthy animals. In anuric animals, urine may be collected from the urinary bladder by passage of a catheter. The kidneys of dead animals should be analyzed for EG and total calcium and histologically for the presence of calcium oxalate crystals. Dogs and cats that die of EG poisoning generally have renal calcium concentrations greater than 1,000 ppm, although they may be as low as 600 ppm (normal <350 ppm). High renal calcium concentration is not pathognomonic of EG toxicosis because other conditions, such as cholecalciferol toxicosis and hypercalcemia of malignancy, may cause similar changes. Renal ultrasound may demonstrate striking echogenicity in the cortex, although this finding is not pathognomonic.

Treatment

Treatment of EG toxicosis should be prompt and is most successful if performed within 12 hours of ingestion. Gastric decontamination consists of inducing emesis followed by administration of activated charcoal and should be performed if the patient is presented within 4 to 6 hours of ingestion. Until recently when 4-methylpyrazole was approved by the FDA, ethanol was the drug of choice for treatment of EG toxicosis in dogs and cats. Ethanol is a preferred substrate of alcohol dehydrogenase and is used therapeutically to inhibit EG metabolism. The benefit of ethanol is probably minimal if the patient is presented more than 12 hours after EG ingestion. Twenty percent ethanol is given intravenously at 5.5 ml/kg IV every 4 hours for 24 hours or as a constant-rate infusion of 1.4 ml/kg per hour (dogs) or 1.25 ml/kg per hour (cats). To be of benefit, it is necessary to maintain therapeutic blood ethanol levels for up to 72 hours to ensure that EG has been excreted. The benefit of ethanol treatment is in question, especially in high-exposure situations and in comatose animals. 4-Methylpyrazole (4-MP) is another competitive inhibitor of alcohol dehydrogenase and is now approved for use in dogs (see *CVT XII,* p. 232). It is given as a 5% solution at 20 mg/kg IV initially. Twelve to twenty-four hours after the first dose, a second dose is given at 15 mg/kg. If necessary, a third dose is given 36 hours after the first one, and this is usually at 5 mg/kg. 4-Methylpyrazole given at doses that have been effective in dogs has not been beneficial in cats, and the drug is thus not recommended in felines. Although expensive and less accessible, hemodialysis is the recommended treatment of choice in situations of high EG exposure. Hemodialysis (alternative, peritoneal dialysis) appears beneficial even when started up to 24 hours after EG ingestion but is most effective if started 3 to 4 hours after ingestion. Further studies are needed to determine whether hemodialysis removes the more toxic metabolites of EG, the time frame over which it is beneficial, and whether 4-MP can be used in conjunction with hemodialysis. Because most patients are presented for treatment late in the course of disease, the mortality rate of EG toxicosis is higher than 70%. Other supportive treatment procedures for EG-induced nephrotoxicosis are summarized in Table 2 and on page 232.

Diethylene glycol (DEG) is also rapidly absorbed from the gut, with peak plasma concentrations reached in 1 to 2 hours. It is metabolized in the liver to 2-hydroxyethoxyacetic acid, its sole metabolite. Oxalate is not a metabolite of pure DEG. Diethylene glycol is excreted in urine either unchanged or as its metabolite. Toxicosis of DEG is characterized by renal failure, acidosis, and cardiac irregularities. The diagnosis of DEG nephrotoxicosis is difficult and can be supported only by its presence or that of its metabolite in blood or urine. Ethers of EG such as ethylene glycol butyl ether, a component of glass cleaners, may also cause oxalate-induced renal failure.

AMINOGLYCOSIDE ANTIBIOTICS

Among therapeutic compounds, aminoglycoside antibiotics are the most frequent causes of nephrotoxicosis in dogs and cats. Gentamicin, tobramycin, amikacin, kanamycin, and netilmicin are used for the treatment of gram-negative infections but have a narrow therapeutic index and should be used with caution in animals at high risk for nephrotoxic injury (as with dehydration). Aminoglycosides are not metabolized in vivo and, because of their low molecular weights and high water solubility, are excreted almost exclusively through the urine. In vivo, these antibiotics easily ionize to cationic complexes, which bind to anionic sites on the epithelial cells of the proximal tubules. Following binding, the drugs are internalized by pinocytosis. Renal cortical concentrations of aminoglycoside antibiotics may exceed the plasma concentration by 10-fold. In general, the toxicity of aminoglycoside antibiotics correlates positively with the number of ionizable groups of the drug molecule. For example, neomycin, which has six ionizable groups, is extremely nephrotoxic and is not used systemically. Gentamicin, tobramycin, amikacin, kanamycin, and netilmicin all have five ionizable groups and a high potential for renal toxicity when used systemically. Aminoglycoside antibiotics can cause acute tubular necrosis through a variety of mechanisms.

Aminoglycoside-induced renal failure is mostly iatrogenic (see *CVT XII,* p. 943). Under circumstances of therapy, animals are periodically monitored for the signs of renal disease with periodic urinalysis (protein, casts) and serum BUN and creatinine. For this reason, the mortality rate is low. Clinically affected animals have polyuria, proteinuria, azotemia, and high urinary N-acetyl-β-D-glucosaminidase activity. Animals receiving aminoglycoside therapy, especially those predisposed to nephrotoxic injury (dehydrated, receiving furosemide), should be monitored for the early signs of renal toxicosis and, if possible, for trough serum aminoglycoside concentrations. Nephrotoxicity can be prevented by increasing the dosage interval by a factor related to the serum creatinine concentration. For example, if the serum creatinine concentration is 3 mg/dl, the dose interval should be 3×8 hr = 24 hr, rather than the recommended 8-hour interval. The treatment of aminoglycoside-induced nephrotoxicosis consists of withdrawing the offending drug and other nonspecific measures, as summarized in Table 2 and discussed in the section on Urinary Disorders.

NONSTEROIDAL ANTI-INFLAMMATORY DRUGS

Although they share similar pharmacologic effects, nonsteroidal anti-inflammatory drugs (NSAIDs) have diverse chemical structures. Broadly, they can be classified into two groups: the carboxylic acids and the enolic acids. Aspirin, indomethacin, tolmetin, sulindae, naproxen, ibuprofen, and flunixin meglumine are examples of NSAIDs that belong to the carboxylic acid group. Phenylbutazone and piroxicam are examples of NSAIDs that belong to the enolic acid group. Nonsteroidal anti-inflammatory drugs are sold over the counter and are widely available in homes. Because of their wide availability, the accidental ingestion of these medications is commonly encountered in small-animal practice. Dogs are more frequently involved than are cats. Iatrogenic NSAID toxicosis is occa-

TABLE 2. Summary of General and Supportive Treatment of Toxic-Induced Acute Renal Failure

Keep the Patient Alive
If presented less than 6 hr after ingestion
  Emesis
    Apomorphine hydrochloride, 0.02–0.04 mg/kg IV or IM (if available);
    Syrup of ipecac, 2–6 ml PO; *or*
    3% hydrogen peroxide, 5 ml/dog or cat
  Activated charcoal
    Acta-Char, 1–4 gm/kg; *or*
    Charcodote, 6–12 ml/kg
  Cathartics
    Mineral oil, 10–50 ml/dog, 10–25 ml/cat q12hr PO; *or*
    Sodium sulfate, 1 gm/kg
Supportive treatment
  Hyperkalemia and acidosis
    Sodium bicarbonate, 10 mg/kg q8–12hr PO or BW (kg) $\times$ 0.3 $\times$ base deficit or $(20 - T_{CO_2})$ in mEq; half of this dose is given slowly
      IV in 15–30 min
  Fluid therapy
    Ideal fluid is 0.9% normal saline, or 2.5% dextrose in 0.45% saline; to enhance urinary excretion of toxin, correct electrolyte
      imbalances, manage moderate acidosis, dilute waste products normally excreted by the kidneys
  Diuretics to enhance toxin and metabolic waste products excretion
    Furosemide (avoid in gentamicin nephrotoxicity), 2–4 mg/kg as needed IV, IM, SC
    Mannitol, 1 gm/kg of 5–25% solution IV (avoid in pulmonary edema)
  Antiemetics or H$_2$ blockers to correct uremia-induced vomiting
    Metoclopramide, 0.2–0.5 mg/kg IV, IM, q6–8hr; *or*
    Cimetidine, 2.5–5.0 mg/kg IV q8–12hr
  Give proper nutrition: glucose supplementation, low-quantity but high-quality protein
  Peritoneal dialysis or hemodialysis if azotemia is progressive despite fluid therapy
Run Toxicology Tests to Identify and Remove Specific Underlying Causes
  Withdraw offending drug; eliminate sources (e.g., feed); give chelation therapy in cases such as exposure to heavy metals

Note: See also Treatments Used in Small Animal Toxicoses (p. 207).

sionally encountered and may be due to the higher sensitivity of some animals than others to these drugs.

The NSAIDs are a diverse group of compounds. In general, NSAIDs are well absorbed orally and are predominantly metabolized in the liver. Some NSAIDs, such as aspirin, require glucuronidation. Cats are especially sensitive to NSAID toxicosis because they have a reduced glucuronyl-conjugating capacity. Nephrotoxicity is just one of a diverse array of toxic effects caused by NSAIDs. Other effects include gastrointestinal irritation and ulceration, enhanced bleeding tendencies, and methemoglobinemia. Only the nephrotoxic effects are discussed here (see also Toxicity from Newer OTC Drugs, p. 227).

Mechanism

The nephrotoxic as well as the anti-inflammatory effects of NSAIDs pertain to the ability of these drugs to inhibit prostaglandin production. All NSAIDs inhibit cyclooxygenase, an enzyme responsible for the conversion of arachidonic acid to endoperoxides, which are intermediates in prostaglandin synthesis. Ibuprofen, mefenamic acid, and indomethacin reversibly inhibit cyclooxygenase. Aspirin, phenylbutazone, and some others cause irreversible inhibition of the same enzyme. It has been suggested that some NSAIDs may exert their pharmacologic and toxic effects through the blockade of prostaglandin receptors. Acute ingestion of large doses of NSAIDs induces acute renal failure characterized by oliguria and elevated BUN and creatinine concentrations. Chronic exposure to toxic doses of NSAIDs causes renal failure characterized by polyuria, which is a consequence of renal papillary necrosis. Dehydrated animals, animals in shock, and those with pre-

existing renal disease are most vulnerable to NSAID-induced nephropathy.

Diagnosis

The diagnosis of chronic NSAID-induced nephropathy is simple because it involves a history of exposure to these drugs usually for at least 14 days. The diagnosis of nephropathy caused by acute ingestion of toxic amounts of NSAIDs is more challenging. Usually, the presence of other signs attendant to acute NSAID toxicosis, such as gastrointestinal bleeding and ulceration, acidosis, mild elevations of hepatic enzymes in blood, and high levels of suspected drugs or their metabolites in blood and urine, helps support a diagnosis.

Treatment

The treatment of acute NSAID toxicosis should involve gastrointestinal decontamination with emetics and activated charcoal, intravenous fluid therapy to correct acidosis and maintain urine flow, and other life-support measures (see Table 2). In chronic toxicosis, the offending drug should be withdrawn. As far as recovery of renal lesions is concerned, the prognosis is generally good in acute renal injury but is guarded to poor in chronic exposure situations with renal papillary necrosis.

CHOLECALCIFEROL

Cholecalciferol (CCF, vitamin D$_3$) is a rodenticide compound that exerts its toxic effects by disrupting calcium homeostasis. Cholecalciferol toxicosis should always be considered whenever acute renal failure is observed in pets. Rat baits containing CCF are sold over the counter as Quintox, Rampage, and Muritan, among other proprietary names. Poisoning in pets occurs by bait ingestion through accidental contact or malicious acts. Although the median lethal dose (LD_{50}) of CCF in dogs is widely reported to be 43 to 88 mg/kg, the author's own studies have shown that as little as 10 mg/kg given once orally can be lethal. Dogs that ingest as low as 4 to 6 mg/kg of CCF once become sick. Clinically normal dogs that ingest single doses of 2 mg/kg of CCF develop hypercalcemia (>12.5 mg/dl). Starting from 1997, ingestion of human psoriasis medications containing vitamin D_3 analogues (calcipotriol, calcipotriene) and marketed as Davionex, Dovonex, or Psorcutan have emerged as common causes of vitamin D toxicosis in dogs.

Mechanism of Action

Following ingestion, CCF is rapidly absorbed and transported to the liver, where it is stored and metabolized slowly to 25-hydroxyvitamin D_3. In the kidney, the latter is metabolized to calcitriol (1,25-dihydroxyvitamin D_3), the active metabolite of CCF. Calcitriol stimulates calcium uptake from the gut. In conjunction with parathyroid hormone, calcitriol mobilizes calcium from bone tissue and conserves calcium by enhancing calcium reabsorption from distal tubules. It now is known that high serum concentrations of $25(OH)D_3$ will stimulate the $1,25(OH)D_3$ receptors and trigger similar events. The combined result of these effects is hypercalcemia and hyperphosphatemia. Calcification of soft tissues, especially the kidney, occurs when the calcium and phosphorus product (in mg/dl) is greater than 60. Renal calcification is the presumed cause of acute tubular necrosis and nonoliguric or oliguric renal failure. Hypercalcemia starts 12 to 18 hours after ingestion, but peak elevation is not observed until 48 to 72 hours after CCF exposure, coinciding with elevations in serum BUN and creatinine. Early signs of CCF toxicosis include anorexia, vomiting, melena, and depression.

Diagnosis

Diagnosis of CCF is based on a history of exposure, the presence of dark bloody feces, azotemia, elevated 25-hydroxyvitamin D_3, oliguria or polyuria, proteinuria, and glucosuria. Cholecalciferol-induced renal failure is easily differentiated from ethylene glycol– or soluble oxalate–induced toxicosis because the latter usually cause moderate hypocalcemia, whereas hypercalcemia and hyperphosphatemia are hallmarks of CCF renal toxicity.

Treatment

Treatment of CCF toxicosis can be challenging. The mortality rate is high because animals are often presented late in the course of disease, when substantial renal injury has already occurred. Nonspecific gastrointestinal tract decontamination procedures should be attempted if the animal is presented within 6 to 8 hours of known ingestion (see Treatments Used in Small Animal Toxicoses, p. 207, in this section). Specific therapy is aimed at lowering blood calcium to normal levels of 8 to 11 mg/dl with the use of salmon calcitonin. The recommended dose of calcitonin is 4 to 6 IU SC every 4 to 6 hours until the calcium level stabilizes (at least 3 weeks). Fluid therapy with normal saline is recommended to enhance urine flow and calcium excretion and to correct dehydration. Preliminary data from the author's studies in dogs treated with pamidronate disodium, 1.2 mg/kg (Aredia, Ciba-Geigy, Summit, NJ) by a slow saline infusion (2 hours), show promising results. Two intravenous infusions of pamidronate given 8 days apart were able to reverse a hypercalcemia of 16 mg/dl to normal levels for at least 28 days. Nonspecific treatment, which is frequently used in conjunction with calcitonin therapy, includes furosemide (2.5 to 4.5 mg/kg every 8 to 16 hours), prednisone (2 to 6 mg/kg IV, IM, PO every 24 hours) until blood calcium levels return to normal, and other measures, as summarized in Table 2.

TOXIC ORNAMENTAL PLANTS

Ingestion of leaves and/or flowers of the Easter lily (*Lilium longiflorum*) causes nephrotoxicity in cats. This was first reported in 1992 and has subsequently been reproduced experimentally. Shortly after eating leaves or flowers, cats develop signs of gastrointestinal upset (vomiting and diarrhea) and become depressed. Acute renal failure characterized by polyuria, dehydration, proteinuria, and glucosuria is usually observed 48 to 96 hours after exposure. The toxic mechanism or mechanisms and principle or principles have not been identified yet. The recommended nonspecific therapy includes gastrointestinal decontamination with the use of emetics, activated charcoal, and sodium sulfate, and fluid therapy to correct dehydration. This treatment approach is beneficial only if performed within 6 hours of plant ingestion.

References and Suggested Reading

Adams WH, Toal RL, Breider MA: Ultrasonographic findings in dogs and cats with oxalate nephrosis attributed to ethylene glycol intoxication: 15 cases (1984–1988). J Am Vet Med Assoc 199:492, 1991.

Austwick PK: Fungal nephrotoxins. Vet Res Commun 7:145, 1983.

Bach PH, Bonner FW, Bridges JW, et al, eds: Nephrotoxicity: Assessment and Pathogenesis. Somerset, NJ: John Wiley & Sons, 1982.
A review of the nephrotoxic effects of several xenobiotics in humans and several other species.

Brown SA, Engelhardt JA: Drug-related nephropathies: Part I. Mechanisms, diagnosis, and management. Compend Contin Educ Pract Vet 9:148, 1987.

Chew DJ, DiBartola S: Renal failure. In: Fenner WJ, ed: Quick Reference to Veterinary Medicine. Philadelphia: JB Lippincott, 1991, p 216.

Cronin RE, Bulger RE, Southern P, et al: Natural history of aminoglycoside nephrotoxicity in the dog. J Lab Clin Med 95:463, 1980.

Dial SM, Thrall MA, Hamar DW: Efficacy of 4-methylpyrazole for treatment of ethylene glycol intoxication in dogs. Am J Vet Res 55:1762, 1994.

Gunther R, Felice LJ, Nelson RK, et al: Toxicity of vitamin D_3 rodenticide to dogs. J Am Vet Med Assoc 193:211, 1988.

Hall JO: Nephrotoxicity of Easter lily (*Lilium longiflorum*) when ingested by the cat. J Vet Intern Med 6:121, 1992.

Kore AM: Toxicology of nonsteroidal anti-inflammatory drugs. Vet Clin North Am 20:419, 1990.

Werner M, Costa MJ: Nephrotoxicity of xenobiotics. Clin Chim Acta 237:107, 1995.

Hepatotoxins

STEPHEN B. HOOSER
West Lafayette, Indiana

The liver participates in many functions of the body, including the metabolism, detoxification, and excretion of foreign substances. Thus, it is frequently involved in poisonings, which may directly damage liver cells. For example, the liver plays a major role in toxicosis caused by antifreeze poisoning (ethylene glycol) and anticoagulant rodenticides (e.g., warfarin and brodifacoum); however, the primary tissue injury and clinical signs concern other organs. If one includes such metabolic transformation of therapeutic drugs, chemicals, poisonous plants, ethylene glycol, and anticoagulant rodenticides, approximately 25% of all poisonings affect the liver. However, since compounds such as ethylene glycol and anticoagulant rodenticides do not primarily cause liver damage, the actual number of clinical poisonings that result in liver damage is much lower. Although many toxins and chemicals have been reported to cause liver damage experimentally, this article discusses only the compounds that have been documented to cause poisoning in companion animals.

MECHANISMS OF HEPATOTOXICITY

The unique anatomy and physiologic functions of the liver make it particularly susceptible to damage by toxins. This susceptibility is highest when exposure is by ingestion (the majority of exposures). The liver normally receives 100% of the portal venous blood flowing from the stomach and intestines. Therefore, any poisons absorbed from the gastrointestinal tract go through the liver first. After absorption and transport to the liver, the arrangement of capillary sinusoids allows all hepatocytes contact with the contents of the blood. Some poisons, such as microcystin (from blue-green algae), and some toxins from *Amanita* sp. mushrooms cause highly specific liver damage because of selective uptake of these toxins by hepatocytes. Other poisons, such as phosphorus, are directly toxic to all cells but are associated with liver damage because hepatocytes are the first cells exposed following absorption from the intestines. Finally, some toxicants, such as acetaminophen, do not cause cellular damage until they are metabolized to more reactive forms inside the hepatocytes (or in other cells), resulting in liver damage. Species and male versus female differences in the metabolism of some chemicals also exist. For example, it is well known that cats have greater susceptibility to acetaminophen poisoning because of a relative deficiency in hepatic glucuronyl transferase, which results in reduced detoxification of the reactive metabolites formed in hepatocytes. As is true with all poisons, the dose of the toxin that an animal receives, route of administration (oral, dermal, inhalation, or intravenous), duration of exposure (whether single or multiple), and physiologic condition of the individual all contribute to the degree to which that individual is affected.

INDIVIDUAL HEPATOTOXINS

Although liver metabolism plays an important metabolic role in antifreeze and anticoagulant poisonings, severe hepatotoxicoses are uncommon in veterinary medicine. In a retrospective study of 1,800 cases of hepatobiliary disease in dogs in the Midwest over a 7-year period, approximately 2.5% were drug induced. Of these, about half were due to long-term anticonvulsant therapy. In addition to the anticonvulsants primidone, phenytoin, phenobarbital, and diazepam, other relatively common drugs that occasionally cause hepatotoxicity include thiacetarsamide (Caparsolate); diethylcarbamazine-oxibendazole; and trimethoprim-sulfadiazine. Although the use of corticosteroids in dogs results in variable degrees of hepatomegaly and increases in the serum activity of alkaline phosphatase and, to a lesser degree, alanine transaminase, these are not thought to contribute appreciably to clinical disease. Also, several case reports in the veterinary literature describe liver damage due to zinc (from ingestion of pennies or zinc oxide ointments) in dogs, and acetaminophen overdose in dogs and cats. While acetaminophen toxicosis is more common, the clinical syndrome is mainly due to the formation of methemoglobin and hemolysis, rather than the liver necrosis that occurs with high doses. Liver damage due to the ingestion of household cleaning products containing pine oil by cats and iron-containing mineral supplements by dogs also occurs sporadically. Dogs are also fairly sensitive to the hepatotoxic effects of aflatoxins; however, clinical cases of aflatoxicosis in dogs have only rarely been positively diagnosed in the United States. The remainder of the hepatotoxicants listed in Table 1 have been reported in the veterinary literature on only one or two occasions.

Anticonvulsants

Long-term treatment (from 6 months to 7 years) with primidone, phenytoin, and/or phenobarbital has been shown to occasionally result in liver damage in dogs. Of these, primidone alone or in combination with phenytoin or phenobarbital has been reported to result in greater liver damage, although all three drugs cause it to varying degrees. In relatively uncommon cases, these anticonvulsants have been associated with very severe liver damage and cirrhosis. In cats, administration of diazepam for 5 to 11 days (for treatment of inappropriate urination or aggression) was reported to cause idiosyncratic, severe hepatic necrosis in some (Center et al, 1996).

Thiacetarsamide (Caparsolate)

It has been estimated that 10 to 20% of dogs treated with thiacetarsamide for adult heartworms experience acute

217

TABLE 1. Reported Small Animal Hepatotoxicants

Toxicant	Species	Toxic Dose/Notes
Therapeutic Drugs		
More Common		
Primidone	Dog	165 mg/kg for 7.5 mo to 15 mg/kg for 7 yr
Phenytoin	Dog	200 mg/kg b.i.d. for 4 mo (with phenobarbital)
Phenobarbital	Dog	3 to 27 mg/kg for 5 to 82 mo
Diazepam	Cat	1 to 2.5 mg/kg for 5 to 11 days
Diethylcarbamazine-oxibendazole	Dog	Within 2 to 4 wk of starting daily dosing
Trimethoprim-sulfadiazine	Dog	30 mg/kg b.i.d. for 14 days (one report)
Thiacetarsamide	Dog and cat	2.2 mg/kg IV b.i.d. (toxicity usually after 1 or 2 doses)
Less Common		
Mebendazole	Dog	22 mg/kg for 5 days
Methoxyflurane	Dog	Repeated exposure
Halothane	Dog	Repeated exposure
Methotrexate	Dog	5 mg/m^2 PO 4 days/wk for 12 wk (with doxorubicin and cyclophosphamide)
Closantel	Dog	10 mg/kg for 3 days
Metals		
Zinc	Dog	Approx. 340 gm zinc oxide ointment (135 gm ZnO) or several post-1983 pennies
Iron	Dog	>20 mg/kg PO (possible to see tablets on radiographs)
Selenium	Dog	2.5 to 5 mg of selenium over 4 mo as vitamin E/selenium cattle preparation
Phosphorus	Dog	Secondary to eating opossums poisoned with 1% phosphorus bait in New Zealand
Biotoxins		
Aflatoxin	Dog	Moldy feed (can detect aflatoxins in feed)
Amanita sp.	Dog	About 2 mushrooms (40 gm)
Indospicine	Dog	Secondary to eating meat from horses poisoned by ingestion of *Indigofera linnaei* plants in Australia
Microcystin	Dog	Ingestion of water containing hepatotoxic blue-green algae
Pennyroyal oil	Dog	Approx. 60 ml applied dermally
Pine oil	Cat	Ingestion of household disinfectants containing pine oil
Lily of the valley (*Convallaria majalis*)	Dog	Ingestion of leaves

toxicity after the first or second dose. Unfortunately, it is difficult to predict which dogs will experience severe hepatotoxicity. Healthy cats treated with thiacetarsamide have also been reported to occasionally experience liver necrosis as well as severe pulmonary edema. This toxicosis should become less frequent with widespread use of melarsoprol.

Diethylcarbamazine-Oxibendazole

Idiosyncratic liver damage of varying degrees has been reported to occur in small numbers of susceptible dogs being given this combination heartworm-hookworm preventive. In these animals, one of two forms can be seen. In the first form, which can appear after 2 to 4 weeks of treatment, the dogs generally present with icterus, high serum alanine transaminase activity, and hepatic damage. The second form is more chronic and develops after 2 to 10 months of treatment. This chronic form is characterized by lethargy, with mild to moderate increases in serum liver enzyme activity. The liver damage generally resolves following discontinuation of the drug combination. There is speculation that the idiosyncratic hepatic damage may be due to the oxibendazole, since similar rare hepatotoxicoses have been reported with the related compound mebendazole, but not with diethylcarbamazine.

Trimethoprim-Sulfadiazine

This antibiotic combination has occasionally been reported to cause an idiosyncratic, moderate to massive hepatic necrosis in dogs. In the less severe cases, withdrawal of the drug has resulted in recovery.

Acetaminophen

Toxicoses in dogs and cats attributable to the use of acetaminophen are common. However, the major adverse clinical signs associated with this drug are related to the formation of methemoglobin and hemolysis. Although hepatic necrosis does occur, it generally represents a minor part of the clinical syndrome.

SIGNS

Although exposure to a wide variety of substances can result in hepatotoxicity, once this damage has occurred there are only a limited number of ways that the liver and the animal as a whole can respond to that damage. Therefore, the clinical signs and diagnosis of liver damage are similar for hepatotoxicity from all causes. Initially, these signs are nonspecific and may consist of anorexia, depression, weakness, vomiting, and diarrhea. In more severe

TABLE 2. Essentials of Hepatotoxicosis

Hepatotoxicoses in dogs and cats are relatively uncommon
The causes reported most often are
　Anticonvulsant drugs (primidone, phenytoin, phenobarbital,
　　diazepam)
　Diethylcarbamazine-oxibendazole
　Trimethoprim-sulfadiazine
Clinical signs are usually nonspecific
Diagnosis is based on history, signs, increased serum activities of
　hepatic enzymes, and histology
Treatment is primarily elimination of exposure, and symptomatic
　and supportive care
Many animals with drug-induced hepatotoxicities recover after
　cessation of the drug

cases or over longer periods of time, icterus, ascites, hemorrhage (through decreased production of clotting proteins), hyperammonemia, convulsions (hepatic encephalopathy), and death can occur.

DIAGNOSIS

The diagnosis of hepatotoxicity can be suspected on the basis of the following criteria:

- History of exposure and identification of the hepatotoxicant (if possible)
- Clinical signs consistent with liver injury
- Increased serum alanine transaminase and alkaline phosphatase activities during the period of exposure
- Decline in serum albumin (not attributed to other causes) and increases in serum bile acid (preprandial and postprandial)
- Discontinuation of treatment and/or exposure to the hepatotoxicant eliminates the adverse clinical signs, and hepatic serum enzyme activities return to normal

Additional criteria include the following:

- Histology from a liver biopsy or necropsy compatible with hepatotoxicosis
- Readministering the toxicant recreates the clinical syndrome (usually not justified clinically unless there is no substitute for the drug)

TREATMENT

For the causes of hepatotoxicity listed in this article (with the exceptions of acetaminophen and iron), no specific antidotes exist. Fortunately, the liver has remarkable regenerative capacity. Therefore, the treatment of hepatotoxicity should be aimed at the following (Table 2):

- Elimination of the source of exposure by ceasing treatment, or bathing (if dermal), or if the exposure was recent the use of emetics (if a gag reflex is present) or gastric lavage followed by activated charcoal (1 to 4 gm/kg in 50 to 200 ml of water PO) and a saline cathartic.

- Supportive care including intravenous fluids and, possibly, parenteral nutrition.
- Nutritional support to provide adequate calories and protein without exacerbating possible hyperammonemia and to ensure availability of energy substrates. A simple diet consisting of 1 cup of cooked rice, ½ cup of low-fat cottage cheese, vegetable oil, and a vitamin supplement would be suitable for an approximately 12-pound (5.4 kg) dog. For a more thorough and detailed review of nutritional support in hepatic disease, see Marks and colleagues (1994; also see CVT XII, pp. 749 and 752).
- In addition, specific antidotes for acetaminophen and iron are available. For acetaminophen use N-acetylcysteine (Mucomyst), 280 mg/kg PO or IV in 5% dextrose (for mild cases, start at 140 mg/kg). If the intravenous route is used, the dose is filtered and given slowly over 15 to 20 minutes. Follow with 70 mg/kg PO q.i.d. for a total of 6 doses after the loading dose. For iron toxicosis use deferoxamine mesylate (Desferal), which chelates iron, forming a water-soluble complex excreted by the kidneys. Initially, administer deferoxamine at 10 mg/kg IM or IV in two doses 2 hours apart. If a significant amount of iron was ingested, after the second dose the urine should appear reddish-orange. If a toxic amount was ingested, the deferoxamine should be continued at 10 mg/kg every 8 hours for 24 hours. The total dose should not exceed 80 mg/kg in 24 hours.

References and Suggested Reading

Beasley VR, Dorman DC: Management of toxicoses. Vet Clin North Am Small Anim Pract 20:307, 1990.
　Details of a wide variety of toxicoses and dosages for treatment.
Bunch SE: Hepatotoxicity associated with pharmacologic agents in dogs and cats. Vet Clin North Am Small Anim Pract 23:659, 1993.
　Review of drug-induced hepatotoxicity.
Bunch SE, Baldwin BH, Hornbuckle WE, et al: Compromised hepatic function in dogs treated with anticonvulsant drugs. J Am Vet Med Assoc 184:444, 1984.
　Experimental testing of primidone and phenytoin in dogs.
Center SA, Elstrom TH, Rowland PH, et al: Fulminant hepatic failure associated with oral administration of diazepam in 11 cats. J Am Vet Med Assoc 209:618, 1996.
　Case reports of severe hepatotoxicity in cats due to diazepam.
Dayrell-Hart B, Steinberg SA, Van Winkle TJ, et al: Hepatotoxicity of phenobarbital in dogs: 18 cases (1985–1989). J Am Vet Med Assoc 199:1060, 1991.
　Retrospective study of hepatotoxicity associated with long-term phenobarbital administration.
Hardy RM, O'Brien T, Adams LG, et al: Periportal hepatitis associated with the use of a heartworm preventive (diethylcarbamazine-oxibendazole) in 13 dogs. J Am Anim Hosp Assoc 25:419, 1989.
　Case reports of dogs with idiosyncratic liver damage related to administration of diethylcarbamazine-oxibendazole.
Marks SL, Rogers QR, Strombeck DR: Nutritional support in hepatic disease. Part II. Dietary management of common liver disorders in dogs and cats. Compend Cont Educ 16:1287, 1994.
　Thorough review of the diet to use for animals with liver disorders.
Papich MG: Toxicoses from over-the-counter human drugs. Vet Clin North Am Small Anim Pract 20:431, 1990.
　Includes iron toxicosis and treatment.
Thornburg LP: A study of canine hepatobiliary diseases. Part 5: Drug-induced hepatopathies. Comp Anim Pract 2:17, 1988.
　Review of drug-induced hepatopathies in dogs.

Grass, Poinsettias, and Nontoxic Plants

A. Catherine Barr

College Station, Texas

Pets left to their own devices sometimes chew on available plants. Most grasses are essentially nontoxic, and some small carnivores are known to eat grasses or other available plants. Such ingestion is occasionally followed by vomiting, although the relationship between the two acts is unclear. Frequent questions about poinsettias (*Euphorbia pulcherrima*) have highlighted the lack of dependable information regarding the safety to pets with respect to poten-

TABLE 1. Plants for Which No Reports of Small Animal Intoxications Were Found

Latin Name	Common Name(s)	Latin Name	Common Name(s)
Acanthus spinosus	Bear's-bush, bear's breech	*Fuchsia* hyb.	Fuchsia, lady's-eardrops
Achimenes hybrids (hyb.)	Hot-water plant, not orchid	*Gaillardia aristata*	Gaillardia, blanketflower
		Gardenia jasminoides	Gardenia, Cape jasmine
Aeschynanthus species (sp.)	Basket plant, lipstick plant	*Gazania* sp.	Gazania, treasure flower
		Gerbera jamesoni	Gerber daisy, Barberton, Transvaal daisy
Aphelandra hyb.	Zebra plant		
Araucaria heterophylla	Norfolk Island pine	*Hypoestes phyllostachya*	Freckle-face, polka-dot plant
Aster sp.	Alpine aster, Michaelmas daisy	*Impatiens* sp.	Garden balsam, impatiens, busy Lizzy, jewelweed
Beloperone guttata	Shrimp plant		
Bletia hyb.	Orchids	*Justicia carnea*	King's crown, Brazilian plume, flamingo plant
Bougainvillea glabra hyb.	Bougainvillea, paper flower		
		Laeliocattleya hyb.	Orchids
Bouvardia hyb.	Bouvardia	*Lagerstroemia indica*	Crape myrtle
Brassia hyb.	Orchids	*Leontopodium alpinum*	Edelweiss
Buddleia davidii	Buddleia, butterfly bush		
Cactaceae fam.	Rattail cactus, Peruvian torch, Christmas and Easter cacti	*Liatris spicata*	Gay-feather, blazing-star
		Lythrum salicaria	Purple loosestrife
Calathea sp.	Peacock plant	*Magnolia* sp.	Magnolias: laurel, Oyama, saucer, southern, star
Callisia elegans	Striped inch plant		
Callistephus chinensis	China aster	*Nandina domestica*	Nandina
Camellia sp.	Camellia	*Nephrolepis exaltata; N. cordifolia*	Boston fern, ladder fern, sword fern
Canna indica	Canna, Canna lily (*not* a true lily), Indian-shot		
		Odontoglossum hyb.	Orchids
Catalpa speciosa	Western Catalpa tree	*Oenothera* sp.	Primroses: Beach evening, Ozark, showy, white evening; fluttermills
Citrofortunella mitis hyb.	Calamondin		
		Oncidium hyb.	Orchids
Citrus limon 'Meyer'	Meyer's lemon	Palmae fam.	Palms: Areca, butterfly, coconut, date, fan, Weddell (*not* Cycads)
Clarkia (*Godetia*) *grandflora*	Godetia, satinflower		
Coreopsis grandiflora	Coreopsis, tickseed	*Pelargonium* sp. and hyb.	Geraniums: horseshoe, ivy-leaved, zonal
Cornus sp.	Cornelian cherry, dogwood, pink flowering dogwood	*Peperomia* sp.	Peperomia, emerald-ripple, pepper-face
		Phalenopsis hyb.	Moth orchids
Cosmos bipinnatus	Cosmos	*Philadelphus coronarius*	Mock orange, syringa
Crassula sp.	Silver jade plant, silver dollar, happiness tree, sickle plant		
		Phlox sp.	Phlox, moss pink, ground pink, moss phlox
Crossandra infundibuliformis	Firecracker flower		
		Photinia sp.	Photinia, red-tip photinia
Cymbidium hyb.	Orchids	*Phyllitis scolopendrium*	Hart's-tongue fern
Cyperus sp.	Egyptian paper plant, papyrus, umbrella plant		
		Portulaca sp.	Portulaca, purslane, rose moss
Cyrtomium falcatum	Japanese holly ferns	*Potentilla* sp.	Cinquefoils: bush, Himalayan, shrubby
Dahlia pinnata hyb.	Dahlia, dwarf dahlia	*Rosa* sp. and hyb.	Roses
Dendrobium hyb.	Orchid	*Saintpaulia ionantha* hyb.	African violets
Deutzia scabra	Deutzia		
Dianthus sp.	Alpine, pink, carnation, sweet William	*Sedum* sp.	Sedums, gold moss, stonecrop, wall pepper, October plant
Echeveria sp.	Baby echeveria, painted-lady, red echeveria		
		Sempervivum sp.	Hen-and-chickens, houseleek
Erica sp.	French heather, rose heath	*Setcreasea pallida* var. *purpurea*	Purple-heart, wandering Jew
Exacum affine	Persian violet		
Fittonia verschaffeltii	Mosaic plant	*Sinningia speciosa* hyb.	Gloxinia
Forsythia hyb.	Forsythia, golden bell, border forsythia		
Fortunella japonica	Marumi kumquat	*Tradescantia* sp.	Spiderwort, wandering Jew
Fraxinus ornus	Flowering ash, manna ash	*Zinnia elegans*	Zinnia, youth-and-old-age

tially toxic plants in the indoor and outdoor environments. Some ornamental plants, like poinsettias, were at one time toxic. Genetic selection for showy traits has decreased their potency to a level that is irritating, but usually not deadly. Many other attractive plants have a long history of safety in the home and garden, and veterinarians may consider recommending these species as alternatives to more dangerous plants.

To develop a guide to nontoxic plants, a list of generally available ornamental plants was compiled from Simon & Schuster's guides (Bianchini and Pantano, 1974; Chuisoli and Boriani, 1986). Toxic plants, trees, and shrubs were methodically eliminated from this article with the use of a series of texts (Cheek and Shull, 1985; Clarke and Clarke, 1967; Foster and Duke, 1990; Fowler, 1981; Kingsbury, 1964; Murphy, 1996; Norton, 1996). Information on the remaining plants was researched individually with the use of the Agricola database (Agricola, September 1996). Any plant mentioned as being toxic in any of these sources was excluded, and many plants were removed on the basis of their toxic relatives. Plants that present only a mechanical hazard were removed for the most part, although some families were retained because of widespread use (e.g., roses); commonsense must guide gardeners in these cases. With the caveat that idiopathic and allergic reactions vary considerably among individual animals, Table 1 lists relatively safe plants and trees for use as ornamentals where pets are kept.

References and Suggested Reading

Agricola on SilverPlatter. Beltsville: United States National Agricultural Library. Licensed to Evans Library, Texas A&M University, updated September 1996.

Bianchini F, Pantano AC: In: Perry F, ed: Simon & Schuster's Guide to Plants and Flowers. New York: Simon & Schuster, 1974, 354 pp.

Cheek PR, Shull LR: Natural Toxicants and Poisonous Plants. Westport: Avi Publishing Company, 1985.

Chuisoli A, Boriani ML: In: Schuler S, ed: Simon & Schuster's Guide to House Plants. New York: Simon & Schuster, 1986, 319 pp.

Clarke ECG, Clarke ML: Veterinary Toxicology. London: Ballière, Tindall, & Cassell Ltd, 1967.

Foster S, Duke JA: Peterson Field Guide to Eastern/Central Medicinal Plants. New York: Houghton Mifflin, 1990.

Fowler ME: Plant Poisoning in Small Companion Animals. St. Louis, MO: Ralston Purina Company, 1981.

Kingsbury JM: Poisonous Plants of the United States and Canada. Englewood Cliffs, NJ: Prentice-Hall, 1964.

Murphy MJ: A Field Guide to Common Animal Poisons. Ames: Iowa State University Press, 1996.

Norton S: Toxic effects of plants. In: Klaasen CD, ed: Cassarett & Doull's Toxicology: The Basic Science of Poisons. New York: McGraw-Hill, 1996, pp 841–854.

Lawn Care Products

ROGER A. YEARY
Delaware, Ohio

The most commonly used lawn care products consisting of fertilizers, herbicides, insecticides, and fungicides are shown in Table 1. In the residential environment, the rank order of use is fertilizer > herbicide > insecticide > fungicide. Highly toxic products are not registered by the Environmental Protection Agency (EPA) for use around homes. The greatest risk of intoxication for pets is exposure to *concentrated* formulations of products through inappropriate storage or use.

EXPOSURE TO TREATED LAWNS

Pesticide products applied to lawns are diluted prior to use. Ready-to-use formulations contain comparably low concentrations of active ingredients.

The residues of pesticides on turfgrass are low and generally range from 30 to 300 ppm or .003 to .03%. A cupful of fresh grass clippings weighs about 10 gm. Thus, a cupful of grass clippings containing a pesticide residue of 150 ppm would contain 1.5 mg of pesticide active ingredient.

EXPOSURE BY INGESTION

Table 1 presents the no observable effect level (NOEL), as determined from long-term dietary feeding studies in dogs. There is a large margin of safety when exposure by ingestion of grass is compared with the NOEL.

DERMAL EXPOSURE

Plants such as turfgrass are often more sensitive to direct contact with chemical substances than mammalian skin. Thus, phytotoxicity is readily seen when fertilizer or pesticides are applied at excessive rates (two to four times the recommended rate). It is highly unlikely that contact dermatitis or other forms of skin irritation will result in pets from their contact with treated lawns in the absence of phytotoxicity.

Percutaneous absorption of turf residues is negligible. Less than 10% of turfgrass residue is transferable or dislodgeable immediately following drying and less than 1% is dislodgeable after 24 hours (Hurto and Prinster, 1993).

COMMON MISCONCEPTIONS

Acute Renal Failure. None of the products used in lawn care have been shown to produce acute renal failure. Although the phenoxy herbicides (2,4-D, MCPA) may elevate blood urea nitrogen levels, there is no evidence that

TABLE 1. **Lawn Care Products and No Observable Effect Level (NOEL) in Dogs**

Common Name	Trade Name	NOEL ppm*	mg/kg
HERBICIDES			
Atrazine	Aatrex	150	
Benefin	Balan	5,000	
2,4-D	(Many)		1.0
DCPA	Dacthal	10,000	
Dicamba	Banvel		50.0
Glyphosate	Round-Up	2,000	
MCPA			0.2
Pendimethalin	Pre-M		12.5
Prodiamine	Barricade	200	
Triclopyr	Turflon		10.0
INSECTICIDES			
Carbaryl	Sevin	400	
Cyfluthrin	Tempo	160	
Diazinon	Diazinon Spectracide		4.3†
Imidacloprid		500	
Isofenphos	Oftanol	2.0	
Trichlorfon	Dylox	1,000†	
FUNGICIDES			
Flutolonil	Prostar		50.0
Iprodione	Chipco 26019	100	
Propiconazole	Banner	50	
Thiophanate-methyl	Cleary 3336F		50.0

*Dietary concentration.
†Subclinical cholinesterase depression occurred.

they produce clinically significant renal disease (Charles et al, 1996).

Seizures. Although organophosphate insecticides and phenoxy herbicides may produce neurologic signs, the products used in lawn care do not cause seizures.

Vomiting and Diarrhea. Concentrated formulations of most lawn care products are irritants and may produce vomiting and gastroenteritis. However, end-use aqueous dilutions (less than 1% active ingredient) are not irritants. Both untreated and treated grass may induce vomiting in dogs and cats.

Liver Disease. Several products (pendimethalin, dicamba, imidacloprid) may elevate liver enzymes at doses above the NOEL in long-term feeding studies, but they have not produced jaundice or other evidence of liver failure.

Carcinogenicity. A report linking 2,4-D to canine malignant lymphoma (Hayes et al, 1991) has been controversial. Hayes and colleagues reported a two-fold increased risk of canine malignant lymphoma with four or more yearly applications of 2,4-D. An industry task force rebutted Hayes' study (Carlo et al, 1992), and Hayes and associates rebutted the rebuttal (Hayes et al, 1995). The debate continues to be centered on issues related to the methods employed to determine exposure. Studies have not found 2,4-D to be carcinogenic in dogs (Charles et al, 1996).

WHERE CAN I GET MORE INFORMATION?

Most product Material Safety Data Sheets (MSDS) contain information on animal toxicity and should be available from pesticide applicators and major retailers. There are several useful resources on the Internet. EXTOXNET is a collaborative effort of the Cooperative Extension Offices of Oregon State University, Cornell University, Michigan State University, and the University of California, Davis. The EXTOXNET Universal Resource Locator (URL) address is http//ace.orst.edu/info/extoxnet. The EXTOXNET server maintains pesticide information profiles.

References and Suggested Reading

Carlo GL, Cole P, Miller AB, et al: Review of a study reporting an association between 2,4-dichlorophenoxyacetic acid and canine malignant lymphoma: Report of an expert panel. Regul Toxicol Pharmacol 16:245, 1992.

Charles JM, Dalgard DW, Cunny HC, et al: Comparative subchronic and chronic dietary toxicity studies on 2,4-dichlorophenoxyacetic acid, amine, and ester in the dog. Fundam Appl Toxicol 29:78, 1996.

Hayes HM, Tarone RE, Cantor KP, et al: Case control study of canine malignant lymphoma: Positive association with dog owner's use of 2,4-dichlorophenoxyacetic acid herbicides. J Natl Cancer Inst 83:1226, 1991.

Hayes HM, Tarone RE, Cantor KP: On the association between canine malignant lymphoma and opportunity for exposure to 2,4-dichlorophenoxyacetic acid. Environ Res 70:119, 1995.

Hurto KA, Prinster MG: Dissipation of turfgrass foliar dislodgeable residues of chlorpyrifos, DCPA, diazinon, isofenphos, and pendimethalin. In: Racke KD, Leslie AR, eds: Pesticides in Urban Environments: Fate and Significance. Washington, DC: American Chemical Society, 1993, p 86.

Common Household Chemical Hazards

David C. Dorman
Research Triangle Park, North Carolina

Jane Owens Clark
Groton, Connecticut

Since hazardous chemicals may be found throughout the home, there is a significant potential for companion animal exposure to these agents, resulting in poisoning. As with children, most veterinary cases are the result of an accidental exposure from the improper storage or handling of these household chemicals. This observation indicates the need for client education on the proper storage of hazardous chemicals in the home environment to prevent exposure of pets and children. Unlike drugs and other agents, many household products are formulated as complex chemical mixtures. The veterinarian must determine the most probable toxic ingredient or ingredients for each product. The correct identification of the most likely toxicant or toxicants and the establishment of the exposure history are critical steps in case management. In many cases, it is difficult to determine the precise exposure history, since only indirect evidence of exposure is noted by the owner (e.g., chewed product container, household chemical spill). On occasion, a retrospective diagnosis of poisoning is based on the historical finding of recent chemical use in a home and the development of appropriate clinical signs (e.g., liver failure resulting from phenol exposure).

Examination of the product container by the attending veterinarian is recommended. Signal words on product labels provide useful warnings regarding the toxicity of most household and commercial products. Although no warning label is required for products with an acute oral median lethal dose (LD_{50}) > 5 gm/kg, products with the signal words **Caution, Warning**, or **Danger: Poison** indicate an LD_{50} value of 0.5 to 5 gm/kg, 50 to 500 mg/kg, and 50 mg/kg, respectively. The Poison Prevention Packaging Act of 1970 further requires that corrosive agents with concentrations of active ingredients above 10% (or 2% by weight of free chemical) are required to be sold in child-resistant containers. The majority of these products are labeled as corrosive. In addition to product label information, toxicity data can be obtained through human and animal poison control centers. Both human and animal poison control centers can provide product formulation, trade name, and chemical name information.

SOAPS, SHAMPOOS, AND DETERGENTS

Soaps are salts of fatty acids and are typically sold as personal hygiene bars or liquids. Soap-flake dishwashing and handwashing products are also available. Soap-based hair shampoos have been largely replaced by nonionic and anionic surfactants. Most additives found in soaps (e.g., selenium, salicylic acid, resorcinol in antidandruff shampoo preparations, preservatives, fragrances, and coloring agents) are not present in concentrations high enough to contribute to systemic toxicity. One exception is zinc pyridinethione, which has been associated with retinal detachment, exudative chorioretinitis, and blindness following ingestion by dogs or cats. Industrial-strength rug shampoos and carpet-cleaning products are more toxic than shampoos intended for personal care. Many personal care products (e.g., hair shampoos) also contain methanol, isopropanol, or other alcohols.

Detergents have a wide variety of uses for general home cleaning and most contain phosphate, silicate, or carbonate surfactants that rarely contribute to systemic toxicity. Many abrasive cleaners also contain pumice, silica (e.g., sodium metasilicate), or borax. Detergents are commonly classified as nonionic, anionic, or cationic, depending on their chemical structure (Kore and Kiesche-Nesselrodt, 1990). Both the chemical form of the active ingredient or ingredients and their respective concentrations influence the detergent's toxicity. Most soaps and anionic or nonionic detergents have low oral toxicity, and systemic symptoms develop only after massive exposure. Toxicity after exposure to most anionic and nonionic detergents through intact skin is limited; however, these products may be absorbed following skin damage through the dermis and subcutaneous tissues. Highly alkaline detergents are more toxic and may cause corrosive gastrointestinal damage and corneal erosions following ingestion and ocular exposure, respectively. Cationic detergents (quaternary ammonium compounds) are considered to be highly to extremely toxic. Concentrated cationic solutions (10 to 15%) are caustic, and even dilute solutions (0.1 to 0.5%) can produce mucosal irritation and damage to the gastrointestinal tract. Quaternary ammonium compounds are readily absorbed from the gastrointestinal tract, and the presence of alcohol in these preparations may enhance absorption.

Signs

Significant ingestion of nonalkaline soaps and anionic or nonionic detergents may result in nausea, vomiting, diarrhea, and abdominal pain. Despite their generally low toxicity, intravascular hemolysis following oral exposure to anionic detergents has been reported (Coppock et al, 1989). In dogs, death has been reported after the ingestion of 0.5 to 2.5 gm/kg of metasilicate automatic dishwasher detergent (Coppock et al, 1989). The clinical signs associated with quaternary ammonium toxicosis include profuse salivation, emesis, muscle weakness or fasciculation, central nervous system depression, and seizures. The systemic signs of quaternary ammonium toxicosis following dermal exposure may occur if significant ingestion occurs (via grooming) or following absorption from damaged skin.

Thorough rinsing of hair and eyes is advised following significant dermal or ocular exposure. Treatment for oral exposure to soaps or detergents includes dilution with milk, water, or egg whites. Emesis should be induced only for nonalkaline (noncorrosive) soaps when the animal has ingested more than 20 gm of soap per kg body weight within 0.5 to 2 hours (Coppock et al, 1989). Emesis and gastric lavage may be required following significant ingestion of cationic detergents. Emesis and gastric lavage, however, are contraindicated if the concentration of cationic detergent in the consumed product is more than 7.5% or if the animal is depressed. Administration of activated charcoal and saline catharsis are also indicated for significant cationic detergent ingestion. Patients that ingest cationic detergents should be evaluated for esophageal corrosive damage if dyspnea, dysphagia, or prolonged salivation occur. General supportive care, including management of seizures, should be instituted, depending on observed clinical signs (Kore and Kiesche-Nesselrodt, 1990). Because all these agents commonly produce emesis, protracted vomiting may occur, thereby necessitating fluid and electrolyte therapy.

GENERAL PURPOSE CLEANERS (PINE OIL, TURPENTINE, AND PHENOLS)

Liquid household cleaners contain more toxic constituents (e.g., acids, glycol ethers, petroleum distillates, phenols, and pine oil) than most synthetic detergent products. Combination cleaners with pine oil and phenol are the most toxic formulations in this group. Pine oils are a mixture of terpene alcohols derived from the distillation of pine wood. Pine-scented formulations contain only small amounts of pine oil and therefore have minimal toxicity compared with Pine Sol (20 to 35% pine oil). Turpentine is a related hydrocarbon mixture of terpenes derived from pine oil rather than petroleum (crude oil) and may be used as a paint thinner. Dermal or mucous membrane contact with pine oil or turpentine produces direct local irritation, pain, and erythema. Oral exposure results in vomiting and hypersalivation. The oral LD_{50} of pine oil ranges from 1 to 2.5 ml/kg. Pine oil and turpentine are readily absorbed from the gastrointestinal tract and metabolized by the liver via glucuronidation. As with phenols, cats are highly sensitive to pine oil toxicosis. Intoxication often leads to signs of ataxia, weakness, central nervous system and respiratory depression, hypotension, myoglobinuria, renal failure, shock, and death. Pulmonary toxicity may result from aspiration pneumonia or chemical pneumonitis. Pine oil toxicosis in the cat is associated with renal cortical and hepatic necrosis. Exposed animals may have a turpentine or pine oil odor on their fur or breath.

Phenolics

Phenolic compounds are commonly used as disinfectants, household cleaners, antiseptics, germicides, and preservatives. In some formulations, the vehicle is more toxic than the germicide. For example, Lysol contains 79% ethanol, which is more toxic than the small concentration (0.1%) of o-phenylphenol. Toxicoses caused by phenolic compounds should be considered a medical emergency.

The oral LD_{50} of phenol in dogs is estimated to be 0.5 gm/kg. Cats are considerably more sensitive because of their limited glucuronide transferase activity. Dermal exposure to some phenolic compounds (e.g., phenol, cresol) may result in areas of coagulative necrosis and white plaques accompanied by intense pain, while ocular exposure may lead to significant corneal damage. Severe corrosion of the upper gastrointestinal tract may be observed following ingestion of phenolic compounds. These compounds are also hepatotoxic, nephrotoxic, and neurotoxic, depending on the specific class of compound involved. The clinical signs of toxicosis include ataxia, weakness, tremors, coma, seizures, methemoglobinemia, and respiratory alkalosis secondary to respiratory stimulation. Liver and kidney damage may be apparent within 12 to 24 hours following exposure. Excretion of phenolic metabolites may turn the urine green or black.

Treatment

Most ingestions of household cleaners require only dilution with milk, egg whites, or water followed by administration of activated charcoal and a saline or osmotic cathartic. Induction of emesis or gastric lavage is generally avoided in animals that ingest significant quantities of pine oil, turpentine, or phenol. Eyes and skin should be rapidly decontaminated owing to efficient absorption of phenolic compounds from these sites. Additional treatments suggested for the treatment of phenol toxicosis include N-acetylcysteine administration (140 mg/kg PO or IV initially; then 50 mg/kg every 4 hours for 17 doses) to prevent hepatic and renal toxicity (Coppock et al, 1989). Methemoglobinemia resulting from phenol exposure may be treated with a single slow intravenous infusion of methylene blue in dogs (4 mg/kg) or cats (1.5 mg/kg) or oral ascorbic acid (20 mg/kg) in both. Ascorbic acid may be ineffective in reversing severe methemoglobinemia (Rumbeiha and Oehme, 1992). In all cases, the acid-base status, cardiovascular function, renal function, and hepatic function should be monitored, and appropriate symptomatic and supportive therapy administered.

BLEACHES

Most household bleaches (e.g., Clorox) contain 3 to 6% sodium hypochlorite. Household liquid chlorine mildew remover contains up to 5% calcium hypochlorite, which is twice as toxic as common household bleach. Some industrial bleaches and swimming pool products may contain as much as 50% hypochlorite. Nonchlorine bleach preparations or colorfast bleaches may contain sodium peroxide, sodium perborate, or enzymatic detergents. When mixed with strong acid or ammonia solutions, chlorine bleaches give off chlorine or chloramine gases, respectively, which are severe respiratory and ocular irritants. Although chlorine and nonchlorine household bleaches usually have very low corrosive potential, concentrated forms may be highly corrosive. Ingestion of granular formulations is associated with increased mucosal contact time and subsequent damage. The clinical signs rarely include systemic disorders and are generally related to oropharyngeal and gastrointestinal irritation. Treatment should include rapid dilution with milk or water and additional symptomatic and supportive care (e.g., fluids, dietary support) given as needed.

CORROSIVES

Despite changes in product packaging, the incidence of caustic ingestion among human beings in the United States exceeds 25,000 cases per year. Corrosive products can most often be found in kitchens, bathrooms, and garages. Hydrochloric, phosphoric, fluoric, boric, and other acids may be found in rust removers, soldering fluxes, radiator cleaners, metal cleaners, and certain liquid drain and pipe cleaners. Potassium alum sulfate, found in styptic pencils, releases sulfuric acid during hydrolysis of the salt. Basic household chemicals ("lye") include caustic soda, caustic potash, sodium and potassium hydroxides, carbonates, oxides, and peroxides. Lyes are commonly used as cleaning agents and are present in many washing powders, some denture cleaners, and metal cleaners. Granular or liquid drain cleaners generally contain sodium hydroxide or, less commonly, sodium hypochlorite. Household ammonia contains 3 to 10% ammonium hydroxide, with weaker solutions (3%) having only irritant properties. However, exposure to higher ammonia concentrations may be significantly corrosive. Other sources of corrosive chemicals include Clinitest tablets (sodium hydroxide) used for the determination of glucose in urine, toilet bowl cleaners (sodium hydroxide), laundry and automatic dishwashing detergents (sodium tripolyphosphate, silicates, and carbonates), and button batteries (40 to 45% potassium hydroxide). Disk batteries range from 8 to 25 mm, and esophageal impaction and secondary esophageal perforation occur most commonly in children with disk batteries larger than 18 mm.

Signs

The ingestion of corrosive agents tends to produce severe injury, depending on the concentration, pH, viscosity, volume ingested, exothermic reactions, and duration of chemical contact with the exposed mucosa. Corrosive liquid formulations tend to cause wider and more severe injuries than do tablets. Alkalis are more penetrating than acids. Both dermal and oral exposure result in necrotizing chemical burns. Esophageal and occasionally gastric erythema, edema, and ulceration are observed within the first 24 to 48 hours after ingestion. Esophageal granulation tissue deposition occurs within 1 to 2 weeks, followed by esophageal stricture formation 3 to 4 weeks after ingestion. Direct evaluation of the esophagus by endoscopy is the most reliable method of ascertaining initial damage, since significant esophageal burns may occur in the absence of oral lesions. Severe esophageal injury manifested by ulcerations, white plaques, and circumferential sloughing of the mucosa is associated with the highest incidence of esophageal stricture formation. Esophagoscopy to the level of initial esophageal damage using a flexible endoscope may be performed safely within 24 to 48 hours of ingestion. Dysphagia, excessive salivation, gastroenteritis with hematemesis, refusal to drink, pain, and shock all are indicative of corrosive injury. Ingestion of corrosive agents

should be managed by rapidly diluting the corrosive with water or milk, along with demulcents and gastrointestinal protectants (e.g., sucralfate). Gastric tubes should be avoided. Steroids are controversial in these cases, and their use in controlled clinical trials in children with corrosive esophageal injury is associated with little or no demonstrable clinical benefit. Attempts to remove the ingested material by emesis or lavage, to absorb it with activated charcoal, or to neutralize it by the administration of a weak acid or alkali are contraindicated.

Most ingested disk batteries pass spontaneously without symptoms. These button batteries may be visualized radiographically. Any button battery lodged in the esophagus should be removed, preferably by endoscopy, as soon as possible. Asymptomatic animals may be followed as outpatients, with monitoring of the stool for the passage of the battery. Although a typical mercury button battery contains 15 to 50% mercuric oxide, ingestion is unlikely to result in mercury toxicosis.

PETROLEUM DISTILLATES

Petroleum distillates are complex chemical mixtures that may include aliphatic hydrocarbons (alkanes, alkenes, and acetylenes), cycloalkanes (e.g., cyclohexane), and aromatic hydrocarbons (e.g., benzene). Petroleum distillates are found in gasoline, motor fuels, solvents, paints and paint thinners, and cleaning agents and as vehicles for other agents (e.g., some pesticides). The most severe clinical effects of these products are related to aspiration pneumonia. As little as 0.5 ml/kg of petroleum distillates aspirated into the lungs is potentially lethal. Agents with low viscosity, such as petroleum ether, mineral spirits, and mineral seal oil, are most likely to produce severe pulmonary toxicity because of their low surface tension. More viscous products, such as tar and grease, do not penetrate into the small airways and have minimal potential to induce aspiration pneumonia. Petroleum products are also skin and eye irritants. Dermal exposure may lead to severe dermatitis and necrosis, presumably owing to the dissolution of lipids and cell membrane injury. Systemic signs of toxicosis may occur after dermal or oral exposure. Clinical signs of aspiration pneumonia may develop rapidly and include coughing, fever, dyspnea, cyanosis, central nervous system depression, and pulmonary edema. Animals that remain asymptomatic for 6 to 12 hours following ingestion of petroleum distillates are unlikely to develop toxicosis.

Treatment

The treatment for animals with aspiration pneumonia from ingestion of hydrocarbons remains controversial. The use of emetics and the administration of oils are generally contraindicated. Gastric lavage and the administration of activated charcoal should be reserved for large ingestion or when other toxicants (e.g., pesticides) are present. Oxygen therapy and cage rest are recommended for the treatment of aspiration pneumonia. The literature generally discourages prophylactic antibiotic therapy. Eyes and skin should be flushed with water. Detergents or hand degreasers may be needed to remove higher viscosity compounds from the skin. The use of other solvents or other hydrocarbons to remove petroleum distillates from the skin is not recommended.

ALCOHOLS

The most commonly encountered alcohols include ethanol, methanol, and isopropanol. Ethanol toxicosis may occur following the ingestion of ethanol-containing beverages and consumer products. Ethanol toxicosis may also occur in dogs and cats following ingestion of raw sourdough containing common baker's or brewer's yeast. Intoxication resulting from the dermal use of ethanol-containing shampoos has also been reported. Methanol (otherwise known as wood alcohol) ingestion may occur from the ingestion of methanol-based automotive windshield fluid antifreezes and other consumer products. Ethanol and methanol are metabolized by alcohol dehydrogenase to acetaldehyde or formaldehyde, respectively. These aldehydes are then metabolized by aldehyde dehydrogenases to acetate or formic acid. The oral lethal dose of ethanol or methanol in the dog is approximately 4 to 8 gm/kg.

Signs

Intoxication with either ethanol or methanol results in central nervous system depression, behavioral changes (e.g., vocalization, excitability), ataxia, hypothermia, and respiratory or cardiac arrest. Clinical signs of toxicosis are ascribed to the parent alcohols. Clinical signs observed in alcohol-poisoned animals generally begin within 1 hour of ingestion and resemble those seen in the earliest phases of ethylene glycol toxicosis. Ethanol-induced metabolic acidosis resulting in part from acetate accumulation has also been reported. In methanol-poisoned humans, formic acid is considered to be the toxic metabolite of methanol, since the accumulation of formate accounts for the development of metabolic acidosis and blindness. However, formate accumulation and subsequent blindness does not occur in dogs exposed to methanol. Determination of blood alcohol levels may assist in confirming a diagnosis of alcohol intoxication.

Treatment

No specific antidote exists for the management of alcohol-intoxicated animals. Management of the moderately poisoned animal is dependent largely on symptomatic and supportive care, including fluid therapy and assisted ventilation, when needed. Treatment of animals that have ingested potentially toxic amounts of alcohol includes the judicious use of an emetic following recent ingestion. Activated charcoal (2 gm/kg PO) is generally ineffective in absorbing low-molecular-weight chemicals such as ethanol and methanol. Sodium bicarbonate (1 to 3 mEq/kg) administered in lactated Ringer's solution or saline over 1 to 3 hours is effective in managing a large volume ingestion resulting in metabolic acidosis.

PROPYLENE GLYCOL

Propylene glycol has been incorporated into certain types of automotive radiator antifreezes. The acute oral LD$_{50}$ of propylene glycol in dogs is approximately 9 ml/kg (vs. ethylene glycol's LD$_{50}$ of 3.6 ml/kg in dogs). The toxic syndrome induced by propylene glycol is similar to that observed during the acute phase of ethylene glycol toxicosis (i.e., ataxia and central nervous system depression; see page 212). Treatment for propylene glycol ingestion is dependent largely on the application of symptomatic and supportive care. Treatment of animals that have ingested potentially toxic amounts of propylene glycol includes the use of an emetic and administration of activated charcoal (2 gm/kg PO) following recent ingestion. The use of ethanol or 4-methylpyrazole as an alcohol dehydrogenase inhibitor is not required. Propylene glycol cross-reacts with certain colorimetric tests used for the detection of ethylene glycol.

"NONTOXIC" HOUSEHOLD CHEMICALS

Ingestion of the following substances usually does not produce symptoms in children and, by extension, companion animals (see also Grass, Poinsettias, and Nontoxic Plants, p. 220). However, ingestion of packaging materials or large quantities of the agent may lead to mechanical obstruction of the gastrointestinal tract. Examples of items considered unlikely to result in toxicity following ingestion include cured cyanoacrylate glues (noncured glues may cause tissue adhesions), elemental mercury (e.g., thermometers), Elmer's glue, 3% hydrogen peroxide, pastes, petroleum jelly, Prussian blue, silica gel packets, and toilet water. Common nontoxic cosmetics and related products include bath oils, body conditioners, calamine lotion, lipstick, petroleum jelly, and deodorants. Children's toys and school supplies, including ballpoint pen inks, chalk, crayons, modeling clay, Play-Doh, Silly Putty, indelible markers, newspaper, indoor acrylic paint, water colors, and pencil lead (graphite), are also considered nontoxic (Mofenson and Greensher, 1970).

References and Suggested Reading

Coppock RW, Mostrom MS, Lillie LE: Toxicology of detergents, bleaches, antiseptics, and disinfectants. In: Kirk RW, ed: Current Veterinary Therapy X: Small Animal Practice. Philadelphia: WB Saunders, 1989, p 162.
  Review of the clinical toxicology of common household chemicals.
Dorman DC: Petroleum distillates and turpentine. Vet Clin North Am Small Anim Pract 20:505, 1990.
  Review article that examines the clinical toxicology, including management of hydrocarbon chemical toxicoses.
Kore AM, Kiesche-Nesselrodt A: Toxicology of household cleaning products and disinfectants. Vet Clin North Am Small Anim Pract 20:525, 1990.
  This article reviews the clinical toxicology of common household cleaning products, including caustic agents, soaps and detergents, disinfectants, and bleach.
Kuhns DW, Dire DJ: Button battery ingestions. Ann Emerg Med 18:293, 1989.
  Assessment of the toxicity of button batteries, including a useful discussion of clinical management.
Mofenson HC, Greensher J: The non-toxic ingestion. Pediatr Clin North Am 17:583, 1970.
  Discussion of household products that are generally considered to be nontoxic in pediatric patients.
Rumbeiha WK, Oehme FW: Methylene blue can be used to treat methe-

moglobinemia in cats without inducing Heinz body hemolytic anemia. Vet Hum Toxicol 34:120, 1992.
Research article that examines the use of methylene blue for the treatment of methemoglobinemia in cats, a species previously thought excessively sensitive to this drug.

Valentine WM: Short chain alcohols. Vet Clin North Am Small Anim Pract 20:515, 1990.
A useful review of the toxicity and clinical effects of ethanol, methanol, isopropanol, and other alcohols in dogs and cats.

Toxicities From Newer Over-the-Counter Drugs

JANE OWENS CLARK
Groton, Connecticut

DAVID C. DORMAN
Research Triangle Park, North Carolina

As of 1996, there were approximately 300,000 nonprescription over-the-counter (OTC) drugs on the market formulated from hundreds of active ingredients. Six of every ten medications bought in the United States are nonprescription (Physicians' Desk Reference for Nonprescription Drugs). The number and variety of OTC products are increasing because of the growing consumer self-care movement, product line extensions, a rise in the number of prescription drugs being switched to OTC status, the cost-effectiveness of OTC versus prescription drugs, and the practice of private labeling of products under store names at competitive prices. The highest selling product categories are analgesics, cold-sinus-cough drops, vitamins, antacids, and laxatives. Recent additions to the OTC market include ranitidine (Zantac 75, GlaxoWellcome), nizatidine (Axid AR, Whitehall-Robins HealthCare), cimetidine (Tagamet HB, SmithKline Beecham), famotidine (Pepcid AC, Johnson & Johnson Merck Consumer), clemastine fumarate (Tavist-D, Sandoz), clotrimazole (Gyne-Lotrimin, Schering-Plough), miconazole nitrate (Monistat 7, Ortho), ketoprofen (Orudis KT, Whitehall-Robins HealthCare; Actron, Bayer), and naproxen sodium (Aleve, Procter & Gamble).

According to a 1990 report from human poison centers, OTC drugs accounted for approximately one third of the fatal cases of animal poisonings (Hornfeldt and Murphy, 1992). Exposure to OTC drugs may occur from the administration of these drugs by a sympathetic and well-meaning owner, through a treatment prescribed by a veterinarian, or through accidental ingestions in the home. Many OTC drug exposures or overdoses are the result of oral ingestions and are manifested clinically as an exaggeration of the pharmacologic effects of the drug. The practitioner must determine whether the animal is experiencing a relatively harmless pharmacologic effect or a true toxicity and take the appropriate course of therapy. This article discusses several of the newer high-volume OTC drugs. Widespread use of these OTC products will probably be associated with an increased incidence of accidental and intentional companion animal exposure and toxicosis.

NONSTEROIDAL ANTI-INFLAMMATORY DRUGS (NSAIDs)

Products

A variety of aspirin-like NSAIDs, including ibuprofen, naproxen, and ketoprofen, are available over the counter. Other NSAIDs include diflunisal (Dolobid, Merck), indomethacin (Indocin, Merck), piroxicam (Feldene, Pfizer), and sulindac (Clinoril, Merck). The common NSAIDs can be divided into four chemical classes: acetic acids, fenamic acids, oxicams, and propionic acids. All the NSAIDs share a common mechanism of action, namely, inhibition of prostaglandin synthesis secondary to inhibition of cyclooxygenase (COX). Aspirin irreversibly inhibits COX, while the other commonly used NSAIDs (e.g., ibuprofen, naproxen) reversibly inhibit COX. Prostaglandins mediate a variety of normal physiologic functions, including renal blood flow regulation. Some prostaglandins are also vasodilatory and cytoprotective in the gastrointestinal tract.

Mechanism

The inhibitory activity of NSAIDs on COX activity explains not only their beneficial anti-inflammatory effects but also their platelet, gastrointestinal, and adverse renal effects. For example, piroxicam and indomethacin have high gastrointestinal toxicity and have their highest activity against the constituently expressed form of cyclooxygenase (COX-I). Drugs with higher potency against the inducible form of cyclooxygenase (COX-II) are effective anti-inflammatory agents that generally spare the gastrointestinal mucosa and kidney.

Pharmacokinetics

The pharmacokinetics of NSAIDs vary markedly between species. For example, the plasma elimination half-life of flurbiprofen has been reported to be 35 to 40 hours in dogs, 3 to 6 hours in rats, and $1\frac{1}{2}$ to 3 hours in monkeys.

Cats are thought to be more susceptible than dogs to some of the toxic effects of NSAIDs because of the prolonged half-lives of drugs that undergo glucuronidation in this species. Enterohepatic recycling of glucuronidated NSAIDs tends to be greater in the dog.

Signs

Ingestion of NSAIDs is a leading cause of poisoning in dogs and cats. Common clinical signs observed with NSAID toxicosis include vomiting, depression, anorexia, diarrhea, and ataxia. It is well recognized that dogs are particularly sensitive to the ulcerogenic effects of NSAIDs. Gastroduodenopathy from NSAID use can be associated with high-dose acute exposures as well as lower-dose chronic treatment. Cotherapy with glucocorticoids may be an additional risk factor for ulceration. Damage to the gastrointestinal tract following NSAID ingestion can occur rapidly. The onset of gastrointestinal upset is generally within the first 2 to 6 hours after ingestion, with the onset of gastrointestinal hemorrhage and ulceration occurring 12 hours to 4 days after ingestion. Severe gastric complications may occur, however, with only minimal symptomatology. Lesions associated with NSAID gastroenteropathy include perforations, erosions, ulcers, and hemorrhages in the upper (stomach and duodenum) and, on occasion, lower (colon) gastrointestinal tract. Gastric lesions may be detected by endoscopy. Oral sucrose administration in dogs, followed by the evaluation of urinary sucrose excretion, holds promise as a noninvasive method of assessing gastroduodenal integrity.

Massive NSAID ingestion is associated with renal failure characterized by oliguria and azotemia initially, followed by either an oliguric or anuric course. The onset of renal failure often occurs within the first 12 hours after massive exposure to an NSAID but may be delayed until 3 to 5 days after exposure. Seizures have also been reported following ingestion of a substantial amount of an NSAID.

Treatment

In massive exposures, airway control with assisted ventilation and supplemental oxygen may be required. Seizures should be treated with standard anticonvulsants, such as diazepam (2.5 to 5 mg/kg IV). Fluids (0.45% saline and 2.5% dextrose IV), whole blood, inotropic agents such as dopamine (1 to 2 μm/kg per minute), and electrolytes should be given to control hypotension and hemorrhage, manage acute bleeding ulcers, maintain renal function, and correct electrolyte abnormalities. Peritoneal dialysis may be necessary if unresponsive oliguric or anuric renal failure has developed. In general, the highly protein bound NSAIDs are not amenable to enhanced elimination by forced diuresis.

Induction of emesis is generally ineffective when performed more than 1 hour after ingestion. Activated charcoal combined with a saline or an osmotic cathartic is the preferred method of gastric decontamination following ingestion of a potentially toxic dose of an NSAID. Gastric lavage, followed by activated charcoal, is indicated after massive ingestion (e.g., ibuprofen ingestion >250 mg/kg).

Certain NSAIDs (e.g., indomethacin, sulindac, piroxicam) undergo extensive enterohepatic recirculation; therefore, repeated doses of activated charcoal are indicated. Occasionally, NSAID tablets or capsules may form concretions in the gastrointestinal tract; consequently, adsorbents, cathartics, and lavage procedures are sometimes of value even several hours after exposure.

Sucralfate and the H$_2$-receptor antagonists cimetidine, ranitidine, and omeprazole have pharmacologic properties that should, in theory, offer some protection against NSAID-induced gastric lesions. Sucralfate (0.5 to 1 gm every 8 to 12 hours PO in dogs; 0.25 gm every 8 to 12 hours PO in cats, cimetidine (10 mg/kg every 8 hours IM, IV, or PO), ranitidine (2 mg/kg every 8 hours IV or PO in dogs; 2.5 mg/kg every 12 hours IV, or 3.5 mg/kg every 12 hours PO in cats), and omeprazole (0.7 mg/kg every 24 hours PO in dogs) have been demonstrated to be of benefit in the management of gastric ulcers. Misoprostol (3 μg/kg PO every 8 hours), a synthetic prostaglandin E$_1$ analogue, has been demonstrated in dogs to be effective in the prevention of aspirin-induced gastric ulcers (Johnston et al, 1995) but is not recommended after ulcer formation. In addition, misoprostol may be associated with adverse side effects, such as abdominal pain, vomiting, and diarrhea. The effectiveness of misoprostol and these other drugs following an acute massive dose of an NSAID has not been evaluated. Metoclopramide (0.2 to 0.4 mg/kg every 6 to 8 hours PO or SC) may be helpful in controlling vomiting. Mild gastrointestinal irritation may be treated symptomatically with nonabsorbable antacids, such as magnesium or aluminum hydroxide. Bismuth subsalicylate antacid formulations are contraindicated.

Individual Examples

Ibuprofen. The most common form of ibuprofen is available over the counter as 200-mg tablets and pediatric liquid preparations under a number of proprietary names (Advil, Medipren, Midol, Motrin IB, Nuprin, Pamprin-IB). Prescription forms include capsules (200 to 800 mg), sustained-release capsules (100 and 200 mg), and 100-mg suppositories. Dogs that ingest single ibuprofen doses less than 100 mg/kg and cats that ingest less than 50 mg/kg generally remain asymptomatic. Repeated doses of ibuprofen in both dogs and cats increase the likelihood of development of clinical signs. Ibuprofen at 5 mg/kg every 12 hours PO has been used to reduce pain and inflammation in dogs, but this dose may also produce gastrointestinal irritation and hemorrhage. A single oral dose of ibuprofen greater than 125 mg/kg is associated with ulcers and erosions in the gastric antrum and pyloris. Common clinical signs of ibuprofen gastrointestinal toxicity include prolonged vomiting, anorexia, mild depression, hematemesis, and melena. Acute doses greater than 300 mg/kg in either dogs or cats have resulted in clinical signs of acute renal failure in addition to gastrointestinal toxicity.

Naproxen. Naproxen (Aleve, Procter & Gamble) is available over the counter as 200-mg tablets. Prescription forms (Anaprox and Naprosyn, Syntex; Naprelan, Wyeth-Ayerst) include oral suspensions; 250-, 375-, and 500-mg capsules; 375- and 500-mg delayed-release tablets; and

500-mg suppositories. Naproxen is approximately 10 times more potent than aspirin as a COX inhibitor. In dogs, the drug has a half-life of 74 hours, and naproxen probably undergoes extensive enterohepatic recirculation. Toxicosis in a dog given 5.6 mg/kg of naproxen for 7 days involved signs of anemia, melena, and renal and hepatic dysfunction.

Ketoprofen. Ketoprofen (Orudis KT, Whitehall-Robins HealthCare; Actron, Bayer) is available over the counter as 12.5-mg tablets. Prescription forms include capsules (25 to 100 mg), sustained-release capsules (100 and 200 mg), and 100-mg suppositories. Toxicology data are limited for ketoprofen in dogs and cats. The oral median lethal dose (LD_{50}) of ketoprofen in dogs is 2,000 mg/kg.

ANTIHISTAMINES

Products

Antihistamines (H_1 antagonists) such as diphenhydramine, chlorpheniramine, dimenhydrinate, and cyclizine are common ingredients in cough and cold medications. Diphenhydramine has also been used to control motion sickness and as a sleep aid. Clemastine fumarate (Tavist-D, Sandoz), also known as meclastine fumarate or mecloprodin fumarate, is an ethanolamine antihistamine that has been recently added to the OTC market for the relief of histamine-mediated allergic conditions. Each Tavist-D tablet contains 1.34 mg of clemastine fumarate for immediate release and 75 mg of phenylpropanolamine hydrochloride in a sustained-release form. H_1 antagonists compete with histamine at the receptor, thereby preventing the effects of histamine, but do not block its release.

Signs

Clinical signs of antihistamine intoxication are limited primarily to sedation, ataxia, vomiting, and diarrhea; however, central nervous system excitement or seizures may also be observed. The acute oral LD_{50} of clemastine is 175 mg/kg in the dog. In addition, the anticholinergic effects of H_1 antagonists may result in other clinical signs, including dry mucous membranes, tachycardia, urinary retention, and hyperthermia.

Treatment

Supportive treatment should include steps to limit absorption, such as an emetic and activated charcoal. Maintenance of hydration is important, as these agents are excreted primarily in urine (Papich, 1990). Serious anticholinergic effects may be treated with physostigmine (0.02 mg/kg IV) and diazepam administered for seizures every 12 hours (Plumb, 1995).

H₂ BLOCKERS

Products

The H_2 blockers famotidine, ranitidine, nizatidine, and cimetidine inhibit gastric acid secretion and are recent additions to the OTC market. The incidence of adverse reactions to these agents is low in humans owing, in part, to the limited function of H_2 receptors in organs other than the stomach and poor central nervous system penetration. In dogs anesthetized with nitrous oxide and halothane, intravenous doses of cimetidine greater than 3 mg/kg resulted in decreased heart rate, blood pressure, and left ventricular pressure, while cardiac output and coronary blood flow were affected only at doses of 30 mg/kg (Miyata et al, 1990). In laboratory animals, high doses of cimetidine have resulted in tachycardia and respiratory failure. Cimetidine is the only H_2 blocker that inhibits cytochrome P-450 activity, thereby slowing the metabolism of drugs that are substrates for cytochrome P-450. Cimetidine prolongs the half-life and thus increases the serum levels of phenytoin, theophylline, diazepam, lidocaine, procainamide, phenobarbital, propranolol, and warfarin. The dosage of these drugs should be adjusted, and the patient should have increased therapeutic monitoring (Plumb, 1995). Hepatic blood flow is also reduced, and this reduction may decrease the clearance of flow-limited drugs, such as propranolol and lidocaine. In addition, cimetidine-induced leukopenias and thrombocytopenia have been reported.

Ranitidine

Ranitidine, unlike cimetidine, has apparently minimal effects on hepatic metabolism. In laboratory species, doses greater than 200 mg/kg per day have been associated with muscular tremors, vomiting, and rapid respiration (Plumb, 1995).

Famotidine

Famotidine is reported to be safer than cimetidine in dogs, although it may produce a negative inotropic effect or exacerbate cardiac arrhythmias. In humans, 40 to 45% of the dose is absorbed. Massive oral exposure of famotidine (>2 gm/kg) may cause vomiting, restlessness, and hyperemia. Higher doses may cause cardiovascular changes and collapse.

Nizatidine

Nizatidine (Axid AR, Whitehall-Robins HealthCare) is well absorbed (>90%) in humans orally. Overdose in humans is characterized by cholinergic signs, including lacrimation, salivation, emesis, miosis, and diarrhea. The oral LD_{50} of nizatidine in the dog is 2,600 mg/kg. In acute toxicity studies, however, a single oral dose of 800 mg/kg was not lethal in dogs.

Treatment

Overdose with H_2 antagonists may be treated by limiting intestinal absorption and symptomatic therapy. If tachycardia and respiratory failure develop after cimetidine exposure, beta-adrenergic blockers and ventilatory support are suggested. Cholinergic signs seen with nizatidine may be treated with atropine and supportive therapy.

NICOTINE

Products

Several OTC nicotine-based 2- or 4-mg polacrilex chewing gums (Nicorette, SmithKline Beecham) and replacement transdermal patches (Nicotrol, McNeil; Nicoderm, Hoechst Marion Roussel; Habitrol, Basel Pharmaceuticals; and ProStep, Lederle) are available in the United States for the treatment of nicotine dependence. Nicotine polacrilex is a resin complex of nicotine and polacrilin that is a cation-exchange resin prepared from methacrylic acid and divinylbenzene. The gum also contains sorbitol as a sweetener and buffering agents to enhance buccal absorption of nicotine. The rate of release of nicotine from the resin complex in chewing gum is variable and depends on the vigor and duration of chewing. Nicotine transdermal patches contain 8.3 to 114 mg of the free alkaloid. All patches have significant residues of nicotine (2 to 83 mg) even after 24 hours of application. The Nicoderm patch consists of a drug reservoir containing nicotine in an ethylene–vinyl acetate copolymer matrix that delivers the drug via a rate-controlling polyethylene membrane. Other sources of nicotine include smokeless tobacco, cigarettes (contain approximately 15 to 25 mg of nicotine), cigars, and related products.

Toxicity and Signs

Nicotine is a cholinergic (nicotinic) receptor agonist that exhibits both stimulant (low-dose) and depressant (high-dose) effects in the peripheral and central nervous systems. Nicotine's cardiovascular effects are usually dose dependent. Nicotine may increase circulating levels of cortisol and catecholamines. Nicotine is one of the most toxic poisons (minimal oral lethal dose in dogs and cats is approximately 10 mg/kg), and the toxic effects develop rapidly after ingestion. Nicotine-induced clinical effects may include tremors, hypertension, tachycardia, tachypnea, vomiting, hypersalivation, central nervous system depression or excitation, mydriasis, ataxia, weakness, seizures, and death from respiratory paralysis. Interestingly, dogs that ingested one or two nicotine transdermal patches had only vomiting despite nearly complete nicotine absorption from the patch (Matsushima et al, 1995).

Treatment

Management of nicotine overdose generally involves gastric decontamination followed by symptomatic and supportive therapy. If vomiting has not occurred following an acute ingestion of nicotine, the stomach should be emptied immediately by inducing emesis or by gastric lavage. Activated charcoal and a saline cathartic should be given immediately following gastric emptying. Activated charcoal should be given every 6 to 8 hours following ingestion of transdermal patches, since delayed nicotine release may occur. Vigorous fluid support and additional appropriate therapy should be instituted if hypotension or cardiovascular collapse occur. Seizures should be treated with standard anticonvulsants such as diazepam. Atropine may be given for bradycardia, excessive bronchoconstriction, or diarrhea.

Assisted pulmonary ventilation may be necessary for the management of respiratory paralysis.

TOPICAL ANTIFUNGAL CREAMS

The imidazoles available over the counter, clotrimazole and miconazole, exert their antifungal mechanism through interference with ergosterol synthesis, resulting in disruption of cellular membranes. These agents inhibit fungal P-450–dependent lanosterol C_{14}-demethylase, thereby reducing the formation of ergosterol. The selective toxicity of the imidazole is due to the relative specificity for the fungal P-450. In mammals, side effects are due to inhibition of P-450, which is responsible for the conversion of lanosterol to cholesterol, and due to decreased synthesis of cortisol and reproductive steroids. Thus, in mammalian species some of these agents may decrease cholesterol, cortisol, androgen, and testosterone biosynthesis and induce hepatic P-450. Clotrimazole and miconazole are marketed as topical creams, as both of these drugs have poor oral absorption. Monistat cream (Ortho; miconazole) is one of the top-selling OTC drug preparations. The oral LD_{50} in the mouse is 872 mg/kg. The clotrimazole contained in Mycelex 7 (Bayer), Lotrimin (Schering-Plough), and Gyne-Lotrimin (Schering-Plough) has an oral LD_{50} in the dog of more than 2 gm/kg.

Another OTC imidazole, Femstat 3 (Procter-Syntex), is a newly approved 3-day yeast infection cream containing 2% butoconazole nitrate. In animals, increased liver enzymes and hepatocellular damage (cholangiohepatitis) have been reported with the prescription-only imidazole ketoconazole. Cats have been reported to be more prone to this hepatic toxicity than dogs. The imidazoles currently available over the counter are unlikely to produce systemic toxicity owing to their poor oral availability.

Should a massive overdose occur with an imidazole, supportive measures such as gastric lavage followed by activated charcoal would be appropriate.

MINOXIDIL

Rogaine topical solution (Pharmacia & Upjohn; minoxidil 2%) is available over the counter for the treatment of hair loss. Minoxidil stimulates vertex hair regrowth in several forms of alopecia when applied topically or orally. Tablet formulations containing 2.5 or 10 mg of minoxidil (Loniten, Pharmacia & Upjohn) are also available by prescription. The mechanism of hair regrowth has not been fully characterized, but the drug appears to act at the level of the hair follicle, perhaps by stimulating hair follicle epithelial growth. The vasodilatory effect on the scalp has not been consistently linked to hair regrowth. Minoxidil has also been used in the management of severe hypertension in humans, as it reduces peripheral vascular resistance and blood pressure.

In humans, minoxidil is absorbed rapidly from the gastrointestinal tract but is poorly absorbed from intact skin. Approximately 0.3 to 4.5% of a topically applied dose is systemically absorbed and is widely distributed to body tissues. The metabolism of minoxidil has not been fully described, but in humans a large portion of the oral dose is conjugated with glucuronic acid. Since cats do not adequately form glucuronides, the half-life of minoxidil may be prolonged in this species. Oral overdose in humans (>70 mg/kg) is characterized by pericardial effusion, tamponade, angina, generalized edema resulting from sodium retention, hypotension, reflex tachycardia, headache, and skin flushing. The alcohol base of the topical formulation may irritate mucous membranes. In dogs, short-term minoxidil administration has been reported to cause hemorrhagic and necrotic lesions in the heart. Long-term animal studies have demonstrated cardiac hypertrophy and other cardiac lesions. The acute oral LD_{50} of minoxidil in rats is 1,321 mg/kg.

Therapy for acute minoxidil ingestion should include gastric emptying and supportive treatment. Exposed mucous membranes should be flushed with copious cool water to reduce irritation. Tachycardia may be minimized by administration of a beta-adrenergic blocking agent, such as propranolol, while the sodium retention and edema may be treated with diuretics.

References and Suggested Reading

Hornfeldt CS, Murphy MJ: 1990 Report of the American Association of Poison Control Centers: Poisonings in animals. J Am Vet Med Assoc 200:1077, 1992.
   A review of animal poisoning cases reported to human poison control centers.

Johnston SA, Leib MS, Forrester SD, et al: The effect of misoprostol on aspirin-induced gastroduodenal lesions in dogs. J Vet Intern Med 9:32, 1995.
   An experimental study that demonstrated reduced gastrointestinal toxicity in dogs following subchronic (30-day) simultaneous misoprostol and aspirin administration.

Matsushima D, Prevo ME, Gorsline J: Absorption and adverse effects following topical and oral administration of three transdermal nicotine products to dogs. J Pharm Sci 84:365, 1995.
   An experimental study indicating that nicotine toxicity in dogs from the ingestion of transdermal patches is less severe than what would have been anticipated on the basis of nicotine content alone.

Miyata K, Kamato T, Fujihara A, et al: Cardiovascular and bronchial actions of famotidine in anesthetized dogs. Arzneimittel-forschung 40:1234, 1990.
   An experimental study comparing the cardiovascular and pulmonary effects of H_2 blockers.

Papich MG: Toxicoses from over-the-counter human drugs. Vet Clin North Am Small Anim Pract 20:431, 1990.
   A review article describing the toxicity of many commonly used OTC drugs in small animals.

Physicians' Desk Reference for Nonprescription Drugs, 17th ed. Montvale, NJ: Medical Economics Company, 1996.
   An annual publication containing human drug package insert information with some toxicity information is included. This reference also includes a product identification section that is very helpful in determining the active ingredient in many OTC and prescription products.

Plumb DC: Veterinary Drug Handbook, 2nd ed. Ames: Iowa State University Press, 1995.
   A comprehensive veterinary formulary including drug indications, adverse effects, and dosages for approved and nonapproved drugs.

Toxicity of Flea and Tick Products

PATRICIA TALCOTT
Moscow, Idaho

ORGANOPHOSPHATE AND CARBAMATE INSECTICIDES

The organophosphate and carbamate insecticides are still one of the most commonly abused parasiticidal compounds as a category (see *CVT XII*, p. 245). These compounds either are formulated singularly or are commonly used in conjunction with pyrethrins, pyrethroids, or insect growth regulators, for control of fleas, ticks, and mites on animals and premises. There are hundreds of formulations, with a resulting wide range of toxicities (Table 1).

Both organophosphate and carbamate compounds inhibit the enzyme acetylcholinesterase; therefore, clinical signs of overexposure are often a mixture of symptoms owing to overstimulation of the nicotinic receptors of the somatic nervous system (skeletal muscle), sympathetic and parasympathetic preganglionic junctions, all parasympathetic postganglionic junctions (few sympathetic postganglionic junctions), and some neurons within the central nervous system.

The onset of clinical signs can vary between a few minutes to several hours, depending on the dose and route of exposure (dermal versus oral versus inhalation). Commonly reported clinical signs include excessive salivation, anorexia, vomiting, diarrhea, excessive lacrimation, miosis or mydriasis, dyspnea, excessive urination, and bradycardia or tachycardia. Prominent nicotinic signs include ataxia, weakness, and muscle twitching. In massive acute oral exposures, seizures can occur within 10 to 20 minutes, with death resulting from respiratory paralysis and tissue hypoxia. Cats appear to be particularly sensitive to chlorpyrifos, and anorexia, muscle weakness, ataxia, and depression are the predominant features.

The diagnosis of organophosphate and carbamate toxicoses relies heavily on observing compatible clinical signs combined with known or suspected exposure. Inhibition of whole blood, plasma, serum, retinal, or brain cholinesterase activity (at least 25 to 50% of normal) supports an exposure to these compounds and toxicosis if the clinical signs are compatible. Cholinesterase testing can still be performed after the administration of atropine and may still be useful several days after exposure. Lack of inhibition cannot rule out exposure to carbamate compounds, owing to the reversibility of their binding to acetylcholinesterase. In addition,

TABLE 1. Common Active Ingredients of Flea and Tick Products

Chemical	Form of Product	Use
Cholinesterase Inhibitors		
Organophosphates		
Chlorpyrifos (Dursban)	Collar, dip, spray, shampoo, dust, fogger	Dog, cat, premises
Dichlorvos	Collar, fogger	Dog, cat, premises
Cythioate (Proban)	Tablets, oral liquid	Dog
Fenthion (Pro-Spot)	Topical liquid	Dog
Malathion	Dip	Dog, premises
Diazinon	Collar	Dog, cat
Tetrachlorvinphos	Collar, spray	Dog, cat, premises
Phosmet	Dip, dust	Dog
Carbamates		
Carbaryl (Sevin)	Dust, spray, powder, shampoo	Dog, cat, premises
Propoxur	Spray, collar, foam, fogger	Dog, cat
Methomyl	Collar	Dog, cat
Pyrethroids		
Permethrin, resmethrin, D-*trans*-allethrin, tetramethrin, S-bioallethrin, fenvalerate, sumethrin, cyfluthrin, cypermethrin, fluvalinate, tralomethrin	Dip, spray, cream rinse, shampoo, topical liquid, collar, dust, fogger	Dog, cat, premises
Botanicals		
Pyrethrins	Spray, shampoo, foam, gel, dip, mousse, dust, fogger	Dog, cat, premises, rabbit
Rotenone	Dust, dip, powder	Dog, cat
d-Limonene	Dip, spray, shampoo	Dog, cat, premises
Linalool	Shampoo, spray	Dog, cat, premises
Miscellaneous		
Methoprene	Collar, spray, dip, fogger, liquid concentrate	Dog, cat, premises
Lufenuron	Oral suspension and tablet	Dog, cat
Imidacloprid (Advantage)	Topical solution	Dog, cat
Fipronil (Frontline)	Spray	Dog, cat
Amitraz	Collar	Dog
Methoxychlor	Powder	Dog, cat
Orthoboric acid	Powder	Premises
Lindane	Dip, spray	Dog
N,N-Diethyl-m-toluamide (DEET)	Spray	Dog, cat

brain cholinesterase activity may be normal in the acutely poisoned patient owing to the acuteness in onset of signs and possible death and the inability of some compounds to readily traverse the blood-brain barrier. Tissue analysis of organophosphate or carbamate insecticides is reserved primarily for confirming an exposure during a postmortem examination. Stomach and intestinal contents, liver, kidney, and skin (in cases of suspected dermal exposures) should be collected, individually bagged and labeled, and kept frozen during shipment to a laboratory.

Treatment should be aimed at preventing further absorption through aggressive decontamination procedures and control of the muscarinic- and nicotinic-associated signs. In the asymptomatic orally exposed patient, emetics such as 3% hydrogen peroxide (1 ml/pound, not to exceed 10 ml in cats or 50 ml in dogs) or apomorphine can be used shortly after feeding a small amount of food. If vomiting is contraindicated, a gastric lavage can be performed after inducing anesthesia with a short-acting barbiturate, followed by the placement of a cuffed endotracheal tube. Induction of emesis or gastric lavage should always be followed by the use of activated charcoal and/or a cathartic (see p. 210). A mild detergent bath and thorough rinsing is recommended in cases of dermal exposure. In the topically exposed patient, particularly the cat, exposure may be both dermal and oral owing to excessive grooming. In such cases, benefit may be derived from both dermal and oral decontamination procedures.

Atropine sulfate, 0.20 to 0.50 mg/kg (one quarter IV, remainder SC or IM), is used to control the muscarinic signs (miosis, salivation, diarrhea, bradycardia, bronchoconstriction, respiratory depression). The dosage selected should be just enough to provide adequate atropinization, and atropine may be repeated at half the initial dose if signs return. Oxygen therapy with or without artificial respiration may be required until the patient is breathing normally on its own.

Seizures, muscle tremors, or agitation can be controlled with intravenous diazepam or phenobarbital. Pralidoxime chloride (2-PAM; 10 to 20 mg/kg IM or SC b.i.d. or t.i.d.) can help reduce muscle tremors resulting from nicotinic receptor stimulation by an organophosphate. A positive clinical effect should be observed within the first few days, and treatment should be continued as long as improvement is observed. Pralidoxime has it best effect if administered within 24 hours of an organophosphate exposure, but some benefits may occur, particularly in cases involving large exposures, if it is given within 36 to 48 hours. Rapid intravenous injection may cause tachycardia, muscle rigidity, transient neuromuscular blockade, and laryngospasm. Diphenhydramine use is somewhat controversial in the treatment of organophosphate and carbamate poisonings. The suggested effective dose of diphenhydramine in dogs is 2 to 4 mg/kg PO every 6 to 8 hours. However, there have been reports of excessive sedation or excitement and anorexia when used in poisoned dogs and cats.

Good supportive and nursing care, including intravenous fluids, adequate nutritional management, and maintenance of normal body temperature and electrolyte balance should also be considered in the acutely poisoned patient. Chlorpyrifos poisoning in cats requires special attention; poisoned cats often show signs of ataxia, anorexia, depression, and muscle tremors for several days or weeks after initial exposure (Fikes, 1992).

PYRETHRINS AND PYRETHROIDS

Pyrethrins are organic esters extracted with fat solvents from flower heads of the pyrethrum plant *Chrysanthemum cinerariifolium.* Pyrethroids, their synthetic cohorts, vary in both structure and potency (see *CVT XII*, p. 242). There are hundreds of pyrethin- and pyrethroid-containing formulations, often combined in mixtures along with organophosphates or carbamates, insect growth regulators, or insect repellents and synergists. Piperonyl butoxide is a common additive to pyrethrin products; it possesses limited insecticidal activity and also exerts a synergistic action in extending the pyrethrin's killing power. The mode of synergistic activity is not known. It is hypothesized that piperonyl butoxide may (1) prolong a pyrethrin's action by preventing rapid oxidation; (2) form complexes with the pyrethrin, leading to higher insecticidal activity; or (3) delay pyrethrin detoxification by the insect's tissue enzymes. *N*-Octyl bicycloheptene dicarboximide, di-*n*-propyl isocinchomeronate, and butoxypolypropylene glycol are insect repellents that are often present in pyrethrin- or pyrethroid-containing products at concentrations ranging from 0.34 to 15%. The toxicity of these mixtures may be attributed solely to the pyrethrins and pyrethroids or may be due to the combined effects of the insecticides plus the additives, synergists, and solvents.

Pyrethrins work by stimulating the insect's central nervous system. This action results in muscular excitation, convulsions, and paralysis. When dissolved in thin oils, pyrethrins readily penetrate through the hard, chitinous covering of the insect, and their insecticidal action is rapid. Both pyrethrins and pyrethroids affect nervous tissue in mammals by reversibly prolonging sodium conductance, producing increased depolarizing afterpotentials that result in repetitive nerve firing. In mammals, the toxicity of pyrethrins and pyrethroids is low, and when they are used according to label instructions no deleterious effects should occur. Toxicoses are commonly observed when these products are ingested or after overzealous heavy topical application, particularly in cats and small dogs.

Clinical signs are usually observed shortly after exposure and commonly include excessive salivation (oral sensory stimulation), muscle tremors, depression, ataxia, anorexia, and vomiting. Less commonly reported adverse effects include weakness, dyspnea, diarrhea, hyperthermia or hypothermia, hyperesthesia (ear flicking, paw shaking; repeated contractions of the superficial cutaneous muscles), and recumbency. Death is rarely reported in these poisonings.

The diagnosis of poisonings relies heavily on recent use and/or possible access to these products. The clinical signs closely mimic other poisonings (e.g., organophosphate and carbamate poisonings), and there are no specific clinico-pathologic abnormalities routinely observed in affected animals. Laboratory methods for analyzing pyrethrins or pyrethroid residues are not routinely available; the finding of residues in tissues (blood, urine, liver) merely confirms exposure—not necessarily toxicosis. Since clinical signs often mimic organophosphate or carbamate poisonings, blood or brain acetylcholinesterase measurement is recommended. Cholinesterase activity will not be inhibited in cases of pyrethrin or pyrethroid poisonings, whereas it may be in organophosphate or carbamate exposures and poisonings.

No specific antidote exists for pyrethrin and pyrethroid poisonings, and treatment should be aimed at decontaminating the animal to prevent further absorption, and supportive care. Bathing the animal in warm, soapy water, followed by a thorough rinsing, is recommended for topical exposures. Long-haired dogs and cats may require multiple bathings-dryings-brushings or clipping to remove residues from the hair. Oral ingestions can be treated with emetics, activated charcoal, and/or a cathartic. Muscle tremors can usually be controlled with diazepam (0.5 to 1.0 mg/kg IV, or to effect). Providing adequate hydration and maintaining normal body temperature and electrolyte status is important in achieving a positive outcome. Low doses of atropine sulfate (0.01 to 0.04 mg/kg IM or SC) can be used to help control the hypersalivation. The prognosis for the majority of pyrethrin and pyrethroid poisonings is excellent, with most animals recovering within 24 to 72 hours.

AMITRAZ

Amitraz, a formamidine pesticide, is present in some tick collars for dogs at a concentration of 9%, designed to kill ticks for 4 months. Ocular exposure to this compound can lead to mild irritation. Toxicosis usually occurs in dogs that ingest a substantial portion of, or the entire, collar. The clinical signs can be severe but are often transient and rarely fatal. A lethal dose of amitraz is estimated to be around 100 mg/kg PO, with toxic doses reported to be as low as 10 to 20 mg/kg. The entire collar weighs 27.5 gm, so each gram of collar contains approximately 90 mg of amitraz. However, the collar is a controlled-release device that releases amitraz in first-order kinetics over an effective period of more than 90 days. Release is therefore much higher when the collar is new than when its activity is nearly exhausted. The most common ingestion leading to toxicosis is when a young or small dog eats 2 gm or more of the collar during the first week of use. Amitraz is well absorbed by the gastrointestinal tract. Clinical signs of toxicosis usually begin within 1 hour of ingestion, sometimes as early as 30 minutes. The majority of clinical signs are associated with amitraz's alpha$_2$-adrenergic properties. Signs include depression (sedation), ataxia, bradycardia, mydriasis, hypothermia, vomiting, polyuria, and gastrointestinal stasis or diarrhea. Other signs that have been reported include hyperthermia, gastric dilatation, hypersalivation, dyspnea, anorexia, shock, tachycardia, urinary incontinence, disorientation, tremors, and coma (Duncan, 1993; Grossman, 1993; Hovda and McManus, 1993). Clinical laboratory data often reveal hyperglycemia. When aggressive treatment is instituted, most symptoms, whether in mild or excessive exposures, usually abate within 24 to 48 hours.

Treatment is aimed at decontamination to prevent further absorption, and reversal of the adrenergic agonist effects. In the asymptomatic patient, emesis should be induced with 3% hydrogen peroxide. Administering a nonoily laxative such as activated charcoal with cathartic is recommended as long as no diarrhea is present. An enema to evacuate the colon may be administered 12 to 18 hours after ingestion, if diarrhea has not occurred or the laxative does not produce the desired effect. If it is suspected that a coiled length of collar is lying in the gastrointestinal tract, or if depression or sedation is severe and prolonged, an abdominal radiograph is indicated. Retrieval of the collar or pieces of the collar can be performed with endoscopy, gastrotomy, or enterotomy. Xylazine and other alpha$_2$-agonists should be avoided owing to the possibility of exacerbating the hypotensive situation. All surgical procedures and anesthesia protocols should be carefully considered because of the potential to exacerbate pre-existing problems (e.g., gastric dilatation, bradycardia). The probability of having to perform these more invasive decontamination procedures is low.

Since amitraz is not a cholinesterase inhibitor, atropine and 2-PAM are contraindicated in the treatment of poisonings. In moderately or severely affected patients who cannot be aroused, yohimbine or atipamezole (both alpha$_2$-antagonists) may be administered at doses of 0.1 mg/kg IV or 50 µg/kg IM, respectively (Hsu and Hembrough, 1986; Hugnet et al, 1996). Both compounds should reverse amitraz-induced changes within 20 to 30 minutes. Since yohimbine's action is of short duration (half-life = 1.5 to 2.0 hours), it may need to be repeated until the dog's clinical condition improves significantly. Body temperature should be monitored following yohimbine use so as to prevent hyperthermia from occurring. Fluid therapy is also warranted in the bradycardic, dehydrated patient.

BOTANICAL OIL EXTRACTS

Various fragrant volatile oils have been isolated from a number of plant species currently marketed as having parasiticidal properties. The most popular of these oils include d-limonene and linalool and are sold as shampoos, sprays, and dips for flea and tick control for dogs and cats. These products are considered to be relatively nontoxic and are *generally regarded as safe* by the U.S. Food and Drug Administration (FDA). Both d-limonene and linalool are present in oils extracted from the skins of citrus fruits and have been associated with poisonings in dogs and cats only when used at excessive concentrations or rates.

With normal use, these compounds may cause temporary irritation of the eyes, skin, nose, throat, and respiratory tract. Adverse reactions to these compounds can occur following inhalation or excessive dermal and oral exposures. Clinical effects are often observed 15 to 30 minutes after exposure and include excessive salivation, muscle tremors, hypothermia, hypotension, ataxia, scrotal and perineal dermatitis, vomiting, and mydriasis. Death is rare and is presumed to be secondary to severe hypotension and hypothermia. There has been one report of erythema multiforme majus and disseminated intravascular coagulation in

a dog following dermal application of a d-limonene–containing dip (Rosenbaum and Kerlin, 1995).

Treatment is aimed at decontamination, with supportive care based on the clinical signs. Repeated bathings with warm, soapy water, followed by thorough rinsings, are recommended following topical applications; gastric lavage with activated charcoal and/or a cathartic is recommended following oral ingestions. Body temperature and blood pressure should be monitored to prevent hypotension and hypothermia. Diazepam has been used to control the muscle tremors, and fluid therapy is generally recommended to prevent dehydration. Most affected animals recover within 24 hours.

Pennyroyal oil has long been used as a flea repellent and is sold as a shampoo, a powder, or the pure oil itself. Pennyroyal is an herb consisting mainly of leaves from two different plants, *Mentha pulegium* and *Hedeoma pulegioides*. The oil is derived from the leaves and flowering tops of these plants. Pulegone constitutes approximately 85% of the pennyroyal oil and is metabolized to the toxic metabolite menthofuran by the liver. Toxicoses have been described in both animals and humans following dermal application and oral ingestion, with signs associated primarily with gastrointestinal upset and central nervous system effects. Clinical signs have included lethargy, vomiting, diarrhea, hemoptysis, epistaxis, dyspnea, miosis or mydriasis, seizures, and death (Anderson et al, 1996). Massive hepatic necrosis has been reported in dogs (Sudekum et al, 1992).

Pennyroyal oil ingestion is treated by decontaminating the stomach with gastric lavage and activated charcoal. Emesis is not suggested because of the rapid absorption of pennyroyal oil, the risk of developing aspiration pneumonia, and the potential for rapid onset of central nervous system depression. Repeated bathing with a mild detergent, followed by thorough rinsings, is recommended following topical applications. *N*-Acetylcysteine has been suggested in cases where there is a high risk of inducing a toxicosis—starting with a loading dose of 140 mg/kg and following with 70 mg/kg every 4 hours. *N*-Acetylcysteine therapy should be beneficial within the first few hours of poisoning and should be continued for at least 24 to 48 hours. Any additional therapy is supportive only and should be based on clinical signs. Complete blood count (CBC), serum chemistry and coagulation profile, and urinalysis should be performed to monitor organ function.

INSECT GROWTH REGULATORS AND OTHER MISCELLANEOUS PRODUCTS

Insect growth regulators constitute a relatively new category in the war against fleas and ticks. All act as analogues of juvenile growth hormones, thereby interrupting the normal growth patterns of the insect. *Methoprene* preferentially kills fleas and ticks in the larval stage by binding to and activating juvenile hormone receptors and thereby preventing larvae from developing into adult fleas. It is considered to be virtually nontoxic. *Lufenuron*, a benzoylphenyl urea, inhibits the synthesis, polymerization, and deposition of chitin in the eggs or exoskeleton of fleas. The recommended oral dosage is dependent on weight, at 30 mg/kg in the cat and 10 mg/kg in the dog, once a month.

Lufenuron is highly lipophilic and readily accumulates in adipose tissue. Lufenuron has shown no synergistic or additive effects when combined with other insecticides. It has proved to be safe at recommended dosage regimens in puppies and kittens as young as 6 weeks of age, as well as in lactating dogs and cats and their offspring. Various studies in dogs and cats using as much as 5 to 10 times the normal dose have shown no serious health effects over an exposure period of 1 to 9 months. A mild decrease in food consumption was reported in puppies (8 weeks to 10 months of age) exposed to 18 to 30 times the recommended dosage. However, the majority of studies have shown no significant adverse effects on food consumption, body weight, hematology, clinical chemistries, and urinalyses following excessive exposures. Few effects on fertility and reproduction have been reported. Administration of lufenuron to breeding male and female dogs at 90 times the recommended dosage of 10 mg/kg resulted in a reduced pregnancy rate compared with control subjects. Pups born to treated females exhibited nasal discharge, pulmonary congestion, diarrhea, dehydration, and sluggishness. It appears that lufenuron concentrates in the milk at a 60:1 milk-to-blood concentration ratio (Ciba-Geigy Corp.). Lufenuron, 90 mg/kg, was administered to breeding cats prior to mating, and through gestation and lactation. In kittens born to these cats, no adverse effects on health, growth, and survival were noted (Ciba-Geigy Corp., 1996; Shipstone and Mason, 1995). No cases of methoprene or lufenuron poisoning in pets have been reported in the literature to date, and treatment should be based on clinical signs and symptoms observed.

Fipronil is a pyrazole flea and tick adulticide currently marketed as a spray and topical liquid and has a wide margin of safety; thus, it can be used on dogs, cats, and puppies and kittens older than 8 weeks of age. Fipronil acts on the GABA-mediated chloride channels of invertebrates, thereby interrupting nervous transmission and leading to the rapid death of fleas and ticks. Mammals reportedly have receptors inside the chloride channel that are shaped differently from those of invertebrates, and fipronil is not thought to bind these for a long period of time. Following dermal application, fipronil is not considered systemically active and is thought to be sequestered in the pet's sebaceous glands. *Imidacloprid* is a topically used adulticide that reportedly binds specifically to postsynaptic nicotinic acetylcholine receptors of insects; it kills adult fleas and exhibits some larvicidal action. During toxicity testing, both fipronil and imidacloprid have shown no adverse effects when used at five times the maximal dose in dogs and cats. A few cases of alopecia and erythema have been observed following dermal application. No cases of systemic toxicosis from these two products have been reported in the literature to date. Theoretically, poisoning could occur by the oral route if the dosage or concentration was excessive. No specific antidote exists, and all treatment should be based on observed clinical signs and symptoms. Topically exposed pets should be bathed and rinsed, while orally exposed patients should be decontaminated with either emesis or lavage, followed by the use of activated charcoal and/or a cathartic.

References and Suggestive Reading

Anderson IB, Mullen WH, Meeker JE, et al: Pennyroyal toxicity: Measurement of toxic metabolite levels in two cases and review of the literature. Ann Intern Med 124:726, 1996.

Blagburn BL, Vaughan JL, Lindsay DS, et al: Efficacy dosage titration of lufenuron against developmental stages of fleas (*Ctenocephalides felis felis*) in cats. Am J Vet Res 55:98, 1994.

Blagburn BL, Hendrix CM, Vaughan JL, et al: Efficacy of lufenuron against developmental stages of fleas in dogs housed in simulated home environments. Am J Vet Res 56:464, 1995.

Campbell WR, Lynn RC: Tolerability of lufenuron (CGA-184699) in normal dogs and cats. J Vet Intern Med 3:2, 1992.

Ciba-Geigy Corporation: Program (lufenuron) for control of existing flea infestations. Adv Pract Vet, 1996, pp 1–8.

Ciba-Geigy Corporation: Summary of studies submitted as part of the new animal drug application, #141-035, for lufenuron tablets. Ciba-Geigy Corp., Greensboro, NC, 800-637-0281.

Duncan KL: Treatment of amitraz toxicosis. J Am Vet Med Assoc 208:1115, 1993.

Fikes JD: Organophosphorus and carbamate insecticides. Vet Clin North Am 20:353, 1990.

Fikes JD: Feline chlorpyrifos toxicosis. In: Kirk RW, Bonagura JD, eds: Current Veterinary Therapy XI: Small Animal Practice. Philadelphia: WB Saunders, 1992, pp 188–191.

Grossman MR: Amitraz toxicosis associated with ingestion of an acaricide collar in a dog. J Am Vet Med Assoc 203:55, 1993.

Hansen SR: Management of adverse reactions to pyrethrin and pyrethroid insecticides. In: Bonagura JD, Kirk RW, eds: Current Veterinary Therapy XII: Small Animal Practice. Philadelphia: WB Saunders, 1995, pp 242–245.

Hansen SR: Management of organophosphate and carbamate insecticide toxicoses. In: Bonagura JD, Kirk RW, eds: Current Veterinary Therapy XII: Small Animal Practice. Philadelphia: WB Saunders, 1995, pp 245–248.

Hansen SR, Buck WB: Treatment of adverse reactions in cats to flea control products containing pyrethrin/pyrethroid insecticides. Feline Pract 20:25, 1992.

Hink WF, Zakson M, Barnett S: Evaluation of a single oral dose of lufenuron to control flea infestations in dogs. Am J Vet Res 55:822, 1995.

Hooser SB: *d*-Limonene, linalool, and crude citrus oil extracts. Vet Clin North Am Small Anim Pract 20:383, 1990.

Hovda LR, McManus AC: Yohimbine for treatment of amitraz poisoning in dogs. Vet Hum Toxicol 35:329, 1993.

Hsu WH, Lu ZX, Hembrough FB: Effect of amitraz on heart rate and aortic blood pressure in conscious dogs: Influence of atropine, prazosin, tolazoline, and yohimbine. Toxicol Appl Pharmacol 84:418, 1986.

Hugnet C, Buronfosse F, Pineau X, et al: Toxicity and kinetics of amitraz in dogs. Am J Vet Res 57:1506, 1996.

Miller TA: Personal communication. Virbac, Inc, 3200 Meacham Blvd, Fort Worth, TX 76137.

Program (lufenuron): A Radical Breakthrough in Flea Control. Greensboro, NC: Ciba Animal Health, Ciba-Geigy Animal Health, 1995.

Rosenbaum MR, Kerlin RL: Erythema multiforme major and disseminated intravascular coagulation in a dog following application of a *d*-limonene–based insecticidal dip. J Am Vet Med Assoc 207:1315, 1995.

Shipstone MA, Mason KV: Review article: The use of insect development inhibitors as an oral medication for the control of the fleas *Ctenocephalides felis*, *Ct. canis* in the dog and cat. Vet Dermatol 6:131, 1995.

Sudekum M, Poppenga RH, Raju N, et al: Pennyroyal oil toxicosis in a dog. J Am Vet Med Assoc 200:817, 1992.

Valentine WM: Pyrethrin and pyrethroid insecticides. Vet Clin North Am 20:375, 1990.

Veterinary Pharmaceuticals and Biologicals, 9th ed. Lenexa, KS: Veterinary Medicine Publishing Co. K. Kanzler K, ed, 1995/1996, pp 841–843.

Whittem T: Pyrethrin and pyrethroid insecticide intoxication in cats. Compendium 17:489, 1995.

Pet Food Safety

E. Phillip Miller
Topeka, Kansas

Commercial foods, including pet foods, are not sterile and may contain microorganisms or other agents associated with foodborne illness. Contamination can occur at any stage of production, starting in the field and ending with storage in the home. The time intervals between the process of harvesting agricultural raw materials, pet food manufacturing, handling in the home, and consumption of the final product provide multiple opportunities for microbial populations to increase in number. These opportunities can result in spoilage or increased risk of foodborne illness. The addition of uncooked meat or table scraps to a commercial food also has the potential to introduce pathogens into the food. The earlier in the food production cycle the contamination occurs, the more widespread the outbreak potential.

When a pet exhibits signs of gastrointestinal disease, the owner often concludes that food must be the culprit. In the past, when pets relied on table scraps, carrion, garbage, and improperly cooked pet foods for sustenance, this conclusion was reasonable. Today, foodborne disease in household pets is rare. The 1990 annual report of the American Association of Poison Control Centers (AAPCC) indicated that of the 41,854 cases of dog and cat poisonings reported, foodborne illnesses accounted for only 1.7% of the total. This phenomenon can be attributed to the fact that most pets in developed countries depend on processed commercial pet foods for their daily diet, instead of fresh food or table scraps. Present-day commercial pet foods are much safer than those in the past because of modern manufacturing methods and a high degree of governmental regulation. Procedural breakdowns or oversights during the production or storage of a pet food product can have a catastrophic effect on company profits and reputation and even the future viability of a company.

INGREDIENTS

Modern pet foods are not composed of a single ingredient but are formulated from multiple ingredients, including grains, meats, meat by-products, vegetables, eggs, dairy products, fish, and other added nutrients. The use of many and varied ingredients tends to dilute any contamination in a particular commodity or ingredient. Commercial pet food manufacturers commonly use manufacturing techniques such as extrusion for dry foods and cooking in a commercial retort for canned foods to produce temperatures high enough to destroy most pathogens and heat-labile toxins. Improved packaging materials and a better knowledge of proper warehousing also help protect raw materials and finished products from moist conditions and possible contamination during storage. Furthermore, manufacturers use sensitive analytical techniques to verify that ingredients and final products are high quality and free from contami-

nants. The value of these efforts is supported by a study in which researchers analyzed 35 dog foods and 17 cat foods and found that most were remarkably free from toxic contaminants (Mumma et al, 1986).

Pet foods and individual pet food ingredients that are shipped across state or United States international boundaries are regulated by the U.S. Food and Drug Administration (FDA) under the authority of the Federal Food, Drug and Cosmetic Act (FFDCA). Section 402 of the Act states that foods, including pet foods, shall be considered adulterated when they contain an added substance (e.g., bacteria, mycotoxins, drugs, pesticides, metals) that may render the food injurious to health. The Act further empowers the Secretary of Health and Human Services to promulgate regulations and tolerances that limit the quantity of these unintentional added substances. The FDA monitors pet food and individual pet food ingredients for pesticides, mycotoxins, and heavy metals as part of its Feed Contaminants Program.

PESTICIDES

Pesticide tolerances for food ingredients and food products are unique in that they are not set by the FDA but instead fall under the jurisdiction of the U.S. Environmental Protection Agency (EPA) under the authority of the FFDCA and the Federal Insecticide, Fungicide and Rodenticide Act (FIFRA). They are developed by combining the results of crop and animal field trials with laboratory animal toxicity data. The EPA establishes and publishes pesticide tolerances for the various plant and animal commodities in 40 CFR 180. The U.S. Department of Agriculture (USDA) and the FDA jointly enforce the EPA pesticide tolerances.

ACTION AND ADVISORY CONCENTRATIONS

For contaminants not covered by a specific tolerance level, the FDA may choose to issue either an action or an advisory level. Both are considered maximal allowable levels; however, an action level is generally supported by more definitive safety data than is an advisory level. Action and advisory levels constitute nonbinding FDA guidance that the agency uses in exercising enforcement discretion when considering product adulteration. There may be circumstances that warrant enforcement below an action or advisory level or in which enforcement is not warranted even though an action or advisory level has been exceeded. For contaminants not covered by any of previously discussed limits (tolerance, action, or advisory level), the maximum remains theoretically at zero. However, the sensitivity of present-day analytical methods has progressed to the point that minuscule amounts can now be detected.

Fortunately, the FDA is able to exercise discretionary power when a contaminant is detected at a low level not considered to be a safety concern.

Finally, intrastate pet foods are less subject to federal scrutiny and fall under the authority of local and state officials. Many locally produced dry pet foods are pelleted instead of extruded. The manufacturing processes used for these products may not produce temperatures high enough to kill bacteria and inactivate heat-labile toxins. These products also frequently utilize locally procured raw materials that may hold more potential for undetected contamination.

BACTERIA

The bacteria of major concern for foodborne illnesses in people include the following: *Clostridium perfringens, C. botulinum, Staphylococcus aureus, Bacillus cereus, Salmonella* spp., *Listeria* spp., *Yersinia* spp., *Aeromonas* spp., *Campylobacter* spp., *Escherichia coli, Vibrio* spp., *Enterococcus faecalis, Enterobacter cloacae,* and *Klebsiella ozaenae.* These same organisms have the potential to cause disease in animals but usually at a lower incidence rate. The infective dose can vary greatly, depending on the animal species, food substrate, patient's immunologic status, and resistance of the normal intestinal flora. For example, dogs are apparently tolerant to a common cause of human food poisoning, staphylococcal enterotoxin. The author has observed that dogs remained asymptomatic following oral doses that were as high as 100 μg/kg body weight. Healthy adult dogs and cats are also fairly resistant to the pathogenic effects of the *Salmonella* spp.; however, the presence of these bacteria in food or water is indicative of poor hygiene and inadequate cooking. Racing greyhounds have been infected with salmonellae by diets supplemented with large amounts of raw meat from rendering plants. Although dogs are less susceptible to the effects of *Clostridium botulinum* toxin than are people, naturally occurring canine botulism has occurred (Barsanti et al, 1978). Toxins of *Escherichia coli,* strain 0157:H7, have been incriminated in an unusual clinical syndrome in racing greyhounds termed "Alabama rot" or "Greenetrack disease" (Fenwick et al, 1995).

MYCOTOXINS

Mycotoxins such as aflatoxin, deoxynivalenol, rubratoxin, and penitrem A can also be present in pet foods. These agents occur in raw ingredients and, in turn, in the final product. Aflatoxins are heat stable and are not destroyed by boiling, autoclaving, or other food-manufacturing methods. Therefore, the FDA has established an action level of 20 parts per billion (ppb) for total aflatoxins in pet food. Prevention strategies involve identification of raw materials with unacceptable levels (>20 ppb), maintenance of proper storage conditions, and assay of final feeds.

Vomitoxin, chemically known as deoxynivalenol (DON), is a mycotoxin produced by members of the genus *Fusarium.* Vomitoxin can be found in any grain but most commonly affects wheat and barley. Like most other mycotoxins, it is heat stable. Dogs are among the most suscepti-

ble species to the effects of vomitoxin and are affected at relatively low concentrations. The clinical signs include feed refusal, vomiting, and diarrhea. The 1993 FDA advisory level for DON in grains and grain by-products used in pet foods is 5 ppm with the added recommendation that these ingredients not exceed 40% of the diet (i.e., 2 parts per million [ppm] DON in the complete pet food). However, feed refusal in dogs has been reported at concentrations below 2 ppm. Therefore, a more practical maximal level is probably 1 ppm.

METALS

Pet foods may also be contaminated with metallic agents. Metals are unique in that they are never destroyed or created, just redistributed in the environment. They tend to accumulate in plant and animal matter, creating the possibility of toxic levels in food ingredients. Foods can also become contaminated during commercial manufacturing and in the home by the inadvertent addition of metal shavings, grease, oils, and other chemicals. Acidic foods can leach paint, soldered joints, or plating agents from the food container or food bowl. Most foodborne metal toxicities in dogs and cats involve lead, zinc, cadmium, and arsenic. These agents cause a variety of clinical syndromes, depending on age, dose ingested, and length of exposure.

Several studies have been conducted in an attempt to quantify such exposures from commercial pet foods. In one study, researchers analyzed 28 brands of commercial dog food and seven brands of cat foods and found that the average levels of lead, arsenic, and cadmium were 1.26, 0.37, and 0.22 ppm, respectively. A later study of 35 dog foods and 13 cat foods found that the average levels of lead, cadmium, and zinc were 0.88, 0.80, and 122.0 ppm, respectively. These studies confirm that low, nontoxic levels of metals may be present in pet foods; however, their presence at these levels would not support a diagnosis of metal toxicity. Instead, the diagnosis must be based on finding elevated concentrations in the food that correspond to elevated concentrations in blood, liver, or kidney.

DIAGNOSTIC PROTOCOL

If a diagnosis of foodborne illness seems feasible, extensive questioning about the animal's diet should be initiated. First, the veterinarian should discuss all possible food sources, including commercial foods and home preparation, feeding amounts, use of table scraps or raw meat, and the availability of unintentional food sources (e.g., garbage). This is also a good time to request that the client bring the food to the clinic for testing purposes. It is important that the entire food container be brought—not just a sample selected by the client. Sample collection, shipping, and so forth should follow the rules of physical evidence, even if the possibility of litigation seems remote, so that testing results are admissible in court if circumstances change.

Common questions about commercial foods should include the brand name, manufacturer, lot or date code, feeding method (e.g., meal fed, free choice), length of time that the pet has been consuming this brand of food, length of time the pet has been fed from the present container of food (e.g., bag or can), and storage method and whether water is mixed with the food. Any recent change in either the food source or food preparation should be queried further. The amount of food consumed should be compared with the manufacturer's recommended amount for an animal of similar size. If the amount consumed is markedly less than the calculated amount, it could mean that the animal does not like the food and may be foraging other food sources or garbage. Decreased intake may also indicate the feed refusal typical of vomitoxin contamination.

Contamination of a major brand of pet food usually produces an epizootic of sick pets with a wide geographic area. If other animals in the same household are consuming food from the same bag or container and are asymptomatic, implication of the food is diminished and other possible etiologies should be investigated. Commercial pet foods are often purchased from a veterinarian, so that individual would have first-hand knowledge of other animals consuming the same lot or batch of food. If the other patients are asymptomatic, the commercial food may again be discounted as the causative agent. However, even if it appears that the commercial food has been exonerated, one should not end the investigation there because the commercial food could still be involved if a supplier or client has compromised the product's integrity by improper storage or usage. The clinician should contact the manufacturer to determine whether similar cases have been reported. Company technical personnel can also aid in the differential diagnosis process by supplying key information about product testing, additional areas of investigation, and beneficial laboratory tests.

The relationship between microbial populations and the quality of pet foods can only be estimated and must be viewed with caution, especially when one considers that most sampling and microbial counting procedures possess inherent inaccuracies; however, measurement of microbial populations may yield information that is valuable in comparing one sample of a pet food to another sample of the same product. For example, it would be valuable to know whether bacterial numbers had increased dramatically while the food was in the pet's bowl. This knowledge could yield information about the hygiene and timeliness of the pet's feeding routine. In summary, the presence of an organism in a food alone does not establish the diagnosis but must be considered as one piece of the diagnosis puzzle.

If the client is feeding a commercial pet food, following label directions, and using proper storage procedures, the likelihood of pet food–borne illness is quite low. As stated previously, the failure to follow proper preparation, food hygiene, and storage procedures can increase the risk of foodborne disease for pets that consume commercial pet foods. A proper and complete laboratory evaluation of the patient, food, food containers, and food utensils helps establish or eliminate the possibility of pet food contamination. A thorough knowledge of the pet's environment also helps quantify the patient's exposure to other sources of toxicants and microbial agents. If the pet is allowed to roam freely outdoors, the risk of exposure to other foodborne pathologic agents increases greatly.

Owing to the sophistication of modern analytical methods, the isolation of a microorganism or detection of a toxic agent in a food sample is not a sufficient basis for diagnosis. A diagnosis with a high rate of confidence in one's accuracy must, instead, be based on a strong correlation between the factors: history, clinical signs, clinical laboratory values, food analytical results, pathology, microbial isolations, response to therapy, and the simultaneous elimination of other similar or complicating diagnoses.

References and Suggested Reading

Barsanti JA, Walser M, Hatheway CL, et al: Type C botulism in American foxhounds. J Am Vet Med Assoc 172:809, 1978.

Council for Agricultural Science and Technology: Mycotoxins, economic and health risks. Task Force Report No. 116, Ames, IA, 1989.

Edwards WC, McCoy CP, Coldiron VS: Lead, arsenic and cadmium levels in commercial pet foods. Vet Med/SAC 74:1609, 1979.

Fenwick B: Food safety for the canine athlete and their owners. In: The North American Veterinary Conference 1996 Proceedings. Orlando, FL, Gainesville, FL: Eastern States Veterinary Association, 1996.

Fenwick B, Hertzke D, Cowan L: Alabama rot: almost the complete story. In: Proceedings. Eleventh Annual International Canine Sports Medicine Symposium. Gainesville, FL: Center for Veterinary Sports Medicine, 1995, pp 15–21.

Hornfeldt CS, Murphy MJ: 1990 Report of the American Association of Poison Control Centers: Poisonings in animals. J Am Vet Med Assoc 200:1077, 1992.

Mumma RO, Rashid KA, Shane BS, et al: Toxic and protective constituents in pet foods. Am J Vet Res 47:1633, 1986.

Price WD, Lovell RA, McChesney DG: Naturally occurring toxins in feedstuffs: Center for Veterinary Medicine perspective. J Anim Sci 71:2556, 1993.

Van Houweling CD, Bixler WB, McDowell JR: Role of the Food and Drug Administration concerning chemical contaminants in animal feeds. J Am Vet Med Assoc 171:1153, 1977.

Adverse Drug Reactions

WILLIAM C. KELLER

NEAL BATALLER

Rockville, Maryland

Drugs are developed to provide therapeutic benefits when used appropriately. Historically, concurrently with the recognition within society that therapeutic drugs were of value came the recognition that any drug can conceivably have toxic or other undesired effects in an individual. Additionally, it was recognized that product defects or inappropriate use of therapeutic products may also result in adverse drug experiences. Consequently, in addition to a premarketing requirement to provide for safe and effective drugs is a requirement for the monitoring of marketed drug products. A regulatory framework for the monitoring of marketed drugs and a government agency to implement existing laws and regulations is found in most industrialized nations. A number of countries, including the United States, the European Community Union (ECU), and Australia, have adopted laws and regulations that provide for a similar government activity for animal drugs. The term most frequently applied to this monitoring activity is *pharmacovigilance*.

The purpose of this article is to briefly describe the pharmacovigilance program for animal drugs in the United States, provide comprehensive information on adverse experiences reported for animal drugs in companion animals, and answer some of the more commonly received questions about the reporting of adverse experiences.

PHARMACOVIGILANCE

Pharmacovigilance refers to the generation, collection, maintenance, and evaluation of information on spontaneous adverse drug experiences. Generally, pharmacovigilance is not associated with planned preapproval field trials or clinical studies. The information may be contributed from a variety of sources of varying reliability. In the United States, the reporting of adverse experiences by veterinarians is encouraged, but is strictly voluntary. The reporting to the U.S. Food and Drug Administration (FDA) of adverse experiences by industry is mandatory. The purposes of the FDA Center for Veterinary Medicine's (CVM) program are (1) to gather information to detect unreported adverse effects or clinical manifestations of drugs after they are marketed and introduced to large populations of animals, (2) to monitor for unsafe or defective products, and (3) to monitor for unsafe drug use practices.

SAFETY PROFILING

Despite the high standards for safety and effectiveness needed for FDA approval, not all is known about a drug when it is first marketed. Only the most common adverse drug events will be observed and included in product labeling at the time of FDA approval because of the limited size and controlled nature of premarketing clinical trials. Therefore, information on adverse effects that occur at a low rate, or that occur more frequently but primarily in a breed or population that was not included in investigational studies, would not be available from preapproval clinical trials or target animal safety testing. The number and variety of animals exposed during the investigational process is simply inadequate to detect anything beyond frequently occurring adverse events. A more accurate safety profile emerges after a product is marketed and the number and spectrum of animals receiving the drug increases. Tables 1 and 2 contain information on adverse reactions in dogs and cats compiled from pharmacovigilance reports received by CVM. Many are reports of adverse reactions or side effects not identified during preapproval investigations. Examples of adverse reactions that were of sufficient importance or severity to prompt label changes or notification of veterinary clinicians follow.

An example of adding safety information to product labeling through pharmacovigilance occurred with Otomax (Schering-Plough). This product was approved in 1993 for the treatment of canine otitis externa. It is a combination-drug product containing gentamicin sulfate, betamethasone valerate, and clotrimazole. During clinical trials there were no reports of hearing loss. The possibility of hearing dysfunction was included, as a standard statement in the precautions section of the package insert, although the location of the statement was not prominent. Following approval, adverse drug experience (ADE) reports suggested that use of the product may be associated with deafness in some dogs. The follow-up investigations suggested that the deafness is usually temporary if the ear is flushed when the problem is first noted and use of the product is discontinued. There was a clear pattern to the ADE reports, and in 1994 CVM requested that the sponsor submit a supplemental New Drug Application to add a label warning of deafness. The goal of this change was to heighten the awareness of prescribing veterinarians to the possibility of the problem and to ensure appropriate therapy if needed.

MANUFACTURING AND LABELING DEFECTS

Unsafe products include both manufacturing defects and product labeling defects. A manufacturing defect might result in a subpotent product lacking efficacy or an extrapotent product that is toxic. A defect might stem from the lack of sterility in an injectable product or particulate matter in a solution. An example of a product defect occurred with a prednisone aqueous suspension that was the subject of complaints regarding "syringeability" (difficulty in filling and discharging the syringe). The problem

TABLE 1. Adverse Drug Experiences Reported in Dogs

Autonomic and Central Nervous System Drugs

Acepromazine (oral)	Death, collapse, ineffectiveness
Acepromazine (parenteral)	Death, prolonged recovery
Butorphanol (oral)	Sedation, anorexia, increased liver enzymes, ataxia
Butorphanol (parenteral)	Death, apnea, cardiac arrest, cyanosis
Droperidol, fentanyl	Head bobbing, aggression, death, convulsions, nervousness, lethargy, panting
Isoflurane	Ineffectiveness, cardiac arrest, facial swelling, death, shock, dyspnea, apnea
Ketamine	Ineffectiveness, death, prolonged recovery, apnea, cardiac arrest, convulsions, ataxia
Meclofenamic acid	Vomiting, anorexia, diarrhea, death, bloody diarrhea
Pentobarbital, phenytoin	Ineffectiveness, hyperactivity
Tiletamine, zolazepam	Death, fever, turbulent or prolonged recovery, crying, convulsions, panting
Xylazine	Death, ineffectiveness
Yohimbine	Death, convulsions, nervousness, panting

Antiparasitic Drugs

Amitraz	Lethargy, death, vomiting, ataxia, convulsions, anorexia, diarrhea, fever, aggression, hypersalivation
Dichlorophene, toluene	Vomiting, ataxia, death, lethargy, hypersalivation, trembling, convulsions, diarrhea
Diethylcarbamazine	Vomiting, ineffectiveness, lethargy, diarrhea, anorexia
Diethylcarbamazine, oxibendazole	Increased liver enzymes, vomiting, lethargy, oxibendazole anorexia, liver lesions, ineffectiveness, death, diarrhea
Epsiprantel	Ineffectiveness, vomiting
Fenbendazole	Vomiting, lethargy, death, anorexia, diarrhea
Fenthion	Skin reactions, vomiting, lethargy, trembling, death, alopecia, ataxia, hypersalivation
Ivermectin	Lethargy, vomiting, ataxia, mydriasis, anorexia, diarrhea, death, convulsions
Ivermectin, pyrantel	Vomiting, lethargy, diarrhea, death, ineffectiveness
Lufenuron	Vomiting, lethargy, diarrhea, pruritus, anorexia, urticaria
Mebendazole	Vomiting, anorexia, increased liver enzymes, death, lethargy, diarrhea, liver lesions
Milbemycin	Lethargy, vomiting, death, anorexia, ataxia, convulsions, diarrhea
Praziquantel	Injection site reactions, lameness
Pyrantel	Death, vomiting, convulsions, diarrhea, ineffectiveness
Thiacetarsamide	Death, vomiting, lethargy, anorexia

Antimicrobial Drugs

Amoxicillin (oral)	Death, lethargy, vomiting, anemia, skin rash
Amoxicillin (parenteral)	Injection site pain
Amoxicillin, clavulanate	Vomiting, lethargy, anorexia, death, hematuria, icterus
Betamethasone, clotrimazole, gentamicin	Deafness, aural irritation, ineffectiveness
Clindamycin	Convulsions, vomiting, lethargy, bloody diarrhea, anorexia, ataxia, petechiae, confusion
Enrofloxacin (oral)	Convulsions, lethargy
Ormetoprim, sulfadimethoxine	Lethargy, fever, thrombocytopenia
Sulfadiazine, trimethoprim	Lethargy, anorexia, fever, anemia, vomiting

Hormones

Triamcinolone	Anaphylaxis, death, vomiting

was resolved by placing a statement on the product label indicating a minimum needle gauge compatible with the product. An example of a labeling defect is a misprint that incorrectly lists product strength or, even, mislabeling of a product. For example, a printing error occurred resulting in "gm" being substituted for "mg" on the label of a production lot of trimethoprim-sulfadiazine. The sponsor recalled the product and relabeled it with the proper label and notified veterinarians by mail.

UNSAFE USE

Unsafe use practices may involve some type of extra label product use. An example of an unsafe use practice would be the use of injectable cattle ivermectin (Ivomec, Merek AgVet) in dogs. This practice has resulted in numerous reports of death in dogs. In response to these reports, a Caution Statement was placed in the product insert indicating that the product was for use in cattle and reindeer only, and that adverse reactions, including fatalities in dogs, had been reported when it was used in other species. Another particularly noteworthy example occurred with

isoflurane. Human anesthesiology reports had indicated that carbon monoxide accumulation may arise owing to infrequent changing of the calcium carbonate in the adsorption chamber. A warning statement was placed on the human labeled product but, unexplainably, not on product labeled for animal use. In response to a letter from a veterinary practitioner, the Center investigated the difference in labeling and the manufacturer readily agreed to add the warning to the veterinary product.

COMMONLY ASKED QUESTIONS

The Center responds to a number of frequently asked questions regarding the pharmacovigilance program.

What Is an ADE? In common terms, an adverse drug experience (ADE) is either an undesired side effect or the lack of a desired effect. The CVM defines an ADE as "any side effect, injury, toxicity, or sensitivity reaction (or failure to perform as expected) associated with use of an animal drug, *whether or not determined to be attributable to the drug.*"

TABLE 2. Adverse Drug Experiences Reported in Cats

Autonomic and Central Nervous System Drugs

Butorphanol (parenteral)	Death
Diazepam	Lethargy, death, vomiting
Ketamine	Ineffectiveness, death, prolonged recovery, apnea, cardiac arrest, convulsions, ataxia
Tiletamine, zolazepam	Death, prolonged recovery, dyspnea, ataxia, pulmonary edema

Antiparasitic Drugs

Dichlorophene, toluene	Vomiting, ataxia, lethargy, hypersalivation, death
Epsiprantel	Ineffectiveness, ataxia
Lufenuron	Vomiting, lethargy, anorexia
n-Butyl chloride	Vomiting
Praziquantel	Death, injection site alopecia, ambulatory problems, anaphylaxis, dyspnea

Antimicrobial Drugs

Amoxicillin (oral)	Vomiting, alopecia, skin congestion, diarrhea
Amoxicillin (parenteral)	Pain at injection site
Amoxicillin, clavulanate	Vomiting, anorexia, diarrhea, hypersalivation
Bacitracin, neomycin, polymyxin B	Corneal ulcers, conjunctivitis
Cefadroxil	Vomiting
Clindamycin	Petechiae, blood on mouth or lips, vomiting
Griseofulvin	Leukopenia, diarrhea, lethargy, fever, anorexia, death, vomiting
Iodine (topical)	Anorexia, lethargy

Hormones

Methylprednisolone	Dyspnea, polydipsia, polyuria, hyperglycemia

What Are the FDA Center for Veterinary Medicine's Specific Areas of Interest? The primary purpose of our ADE monitoring system is to detect problems, or "side effects" associated with the use of FDA-approved animal drugs. Lack of effectiveness is also considered an adverse experience. The majority of reports of this nature involve anesthetics, tranquilizers, and anthelmintics. These reports can be difficult to evaluate, but a group of similar reports will prompt further investigation. The CVM gives careful consideration to any reports of adverse experiences occurring in humans as a direct result of the use or administration of an animal drug or in other situations involving accidental human exposure. Any unintended effect on the environment and/or wildlife would also be considered an adverse event.

Does CVM Review Reports That Involve Extralabel Use of Animal Drugs? The reporting of ADEs associated with extralabel use is important to the veterinary profession. Under the Animal Medicinal Drug Use Clarification Act of 1994, veterinarians can administer drugs more freely in an extralabel manner. About one third of the reports on file involve extralabel use. We are also interested in ADEs involving human drugs used in veterinary practice and in ADEs involving animal drugs marketed without FDA approval.

Who Monitors Reports of ADEs for Products Used to Treat Animals? The FDA Center for Veterinary Medicine monitors reports of ADEs for animal drug products, medicated feeds, and animal devices under the Federal Food, Drug and Cosmetic Act. Animal vaccines and most biologicals (e.g., rabies vaccines) are regulated by the United States Department of Agriculture (USDA). Most of the products used topically for the control of ectoparasites and insects on animals are regulated by the Environmental Protection Agency (EPA). The United States Pharmacopeia (USP) operates an independent, nongovernmental reporting program called the Veterinary Practitioner's Reporting Program. The USP will forward reports of ADEs to the appropriate regulatory agency and to the drug company, at the discretion of the person reporting. This program has the support and endorsement of the American Veterinary Medical Association. The USP program is not affiliated with the FDA.

Are There Any Laws That Require Reporting of ADEs? Reporting by veterinary medical professionals is entirely voluntary. However, federal regulations require that drug companies send to the FDA all information concerning adverse drug experiences reported to, or coming to the attention of, the company. The reporting requirements for products regulated by the USDA and EPA are not the same as those for animal drugs. Veterinarians at the CVM evaluate about 4,400 reports annually. This estimate includes reports of product defects. Approximately 95% of ADE reports are submitted by drug companies after they have learned of the adverse experience from a veterinarian or an animal owner. The other 5% of reports are submitted directly to the CVM by veterinarians and animal owners.

If I Decide to Report an ADE, Who Should I Contact? You should first call the drug company. Inform them that you wish to report an ADE, and ask to speak to a technical services veterinarian. The technical services veterinarian should ask a series of questions about the experience, complete a form called the FDA 1932, and forward the report to the CVM. We suggest the drug company as your first point of contact because many companies will also offer clinical advice or diagnostic assistance. The CVM does not provide these services. Drug company phone numbers can be obtained from the publications *Compendium of Veterinary Products* (North American Compendiums Inc., Port Huron, MI) and *Veterinary Pharmaceuticals and Biologicals* (Veterinary Medicine Publishing Company, Lenexa, KS).

If you wish to confirm that your report was forwarded, or if you prefer not to call the drug company, you may contact the CVM directly toll-free at (888) FDA-VETS. Please ask to speak to one of the veterinarians responsible for the ADE monitoring program. We can also provide a supply of prepaid mailers (Form FDA 1932a). These mailers are available by writing to or telephoning the CVM and are also distributed at veterinary medicine meetings and seminars. If the ADE involves a product other than a drug, the following numbers may be useful: to reach the USDA regarding biologicals dial (800) 752-6255; to reach the EPA regarding topical insecticides dial (800) 858-7378; to reach (the independent) United States Pharmacopeia regarding any veterinary product dial (800) 4-USPPRN.

What Happens After I Report an ADE? Each ADE report is evaluated by a veterinarian and entered into a database. The reviewer enters a brief clinical description of the ADE and makes an assessment of whether the event is judged to be drug related by using an algorithm scoring system. The CVM publishes an annual summary of this ADE database. The information is limited to reports assessed as at least "possibly drug related." The publication is available from the FDA Center for Veterinary Medicine. The CVM also provides a cumulative ADE annual summary on the CVM World Wide Web Internet server. Other information and reports from the database can be requested on an individual basis by filing a written Freedom of Information (FOI) request. For more information about filing a request, you can contact the CVM Communications staff at (301) 594-1755.

What Actions Result From Reports of ADEs? A group of similar reports submitted in a short period of time may alert the CVM and the drug company to a problem with a particular lot of drug. Investigation may result in a product recall of the affected lot. Another outcome might be a label change to include new information gleaned from reported ADEs. In very rare instances, a drug may be removed from the market owing to problems discovered by ADE reporting. At times, the CVM may require the involved drug company to issue a "Dear Doctor" letter to veterinarians informing them of the type of actions that resulted from ADE reports.

Why Should Veterinarians in Practice Care About Reporting an ADE? Veterinarians in practice depend on the information available in drug labeling to make informed choices about the risks and benefits associated with the use of a drug. The purpose of ADE monitoring is to ensure that animal drug labeling is adequate and accurate. An accurate safety profile emerges only after a product is marketed and the number and spectrum of animals receiving the drug increase. Practicing veterinarians are in a unique position to observe adverse clinical outcomes. The pharmacovigilance program for animal health products is composed of a partnership of three elements: industry, veterinarians and their clients, and regulatory agencies. Of all the elements in the pharmacovigilance process, the veterinary clinicians' participation is the most critical.

Acknowledgment
The authors wish to express their appreciation to all past and current members of the CVM who have contributed to the pharmacovigilance program and, ultimately, this article. In particular, we wish to thank Douglass Oeller, Walter Sessions, Mukund Parkhie, Robert Schmidt, Michael Talley, Steven Gustavson, Mohammad Sharar, Edward Spenser, Vitolis Vengris, and Randall Lovell for their contributions.

Infectious Diseases

EDWARD B. BREITSCHWERDT

Consulting Editor

***Still Current Information Found in* Current Veterinary Therapy XII:**

Why Are Infectious Diseases Emerging?

EDWARD B. BREITSCHWERDT
Raleigh, North Carolina

STEVEN W. DOW
Denver, Colorado

As an introduction to the section on infectious diseases, we are pleased to have the opportunity to address the question: Why are infectious diseases emerging? In the future, when historians examine the numerous events that have contributed to the acquisition of knowledge related to infectious diseases during the latter portion of the 20th Century, it is probable that contributions generated during this period will be considered of unique medical importance (Gao and Moore, 1996; Levins et al, 1994). Several decades ago, coinciding with the development of new, more potent broad-spectrum antimicrobials, research momentum related to infectious diseases diminished considerably. For the most part, physicians and veterinarians completing their education during the 1970s were left with the mistaken impression that medically relevant knowledge of most infectious diseases was complete. Hopefully, in contrast, it has been impressed on recent medical college graduates that knowledge related to the pathogenesis, diagnosis, treatment, and prevention of many infectious diseases remains considerably incomplete. In addition, based on the identification of numerous, previously unrecognized pathogens during recent years, it seems obvious that many insidious pathogens remain unidentified. It is possible that as yet unrecognized pathogens contribute to the etiopathogenesis of numerous immune-mediated, inflammatory, or degenerative diseases.

Although numerous factors have contributed to the recognition of emerging infectious diseases or to the re-examination of the relevance of known infectious organisms, five factors are of central importance.

1. The rapid emergence of a large population of immunodeficient individuals infected with the human immunodeficiency virus has led to the recognition of "new" infectious agents and to the identification of patterns of disease that had not been associated with known infectious organisms. Research momentum and new scientific techniques generated in retrovirology and related research laboratories were rapidly transmitted to laboratories studying opportunistic infectious agents that proved to be important cofactors in the progression of acquired immunodeficiency syndrome (AIDS).
2. The rapid evolution of highly sophisticated molecular-based techniques has greatly enhanced the accuracy of microbial detection and classification schemes as well as the approach to diagnostic, therapeutic, and preventive strategies for many infectious diseases.
3. Complex social, economic, and ecologic forces have enhanced the risk of human infection with infectious organisms, such as *Escherichia coli* O157 during food processing, cryptosporidiosis through transmission as a fecal or waterborne pathogen, and *Borrelia burgdorferi* and other vector-borne infections, as humankind increasingly encroaches on the habitats of other animals. With rare but notable exceptions, such as the human immunodeficiency virus, it should be emphasized that the emergence of most newly recognized infectious diseases is related to societal changes rather than spontaneous changes in the pathogens themselves.
4. The rapid evolution in our understanding of the host's immunologic response to infection has promoted the importance of infectious agents in the pathogenesis of chronic insidious diseases of undetermined cause. It is perhaps this area of research that holds the greatest promise for enhanced understanding of diseases of uncertain etiology—diseases such as inflammatory bowel disease, systemic lupus erythematosus, rheumatoid arthritis, pulmonary granulomatosis, and others.
5. Finally, the increased recognition of the importance of infectious diseases, particularly AIDS, to societal health has resulted in enhanced funding of infectious disease research. As a result of these and other factors, the comparative medical importance of organisms that infect both animals and human beings has been recognized with much greater clarity in recent years.

The utility of molecular-based detection of novel infectious agents has been demonstrated repeatedly in recent years (Gao and Moore, 1996; Levins et al, 1996). An excellent example of a single application of molecular technology for this purpose is the use of polymerase chain reaction amplification of highly conserved eubacterial genes, such as the 16S rRNA gene, for identifying previously unculturable bacteria. For nearly a decade, numerous, previously unculturable, argyrophilic bacteria were observed in an unusual vascular endothelial proliferative lesion (bacillary angiomatosis) in AIDS patients. In 1990, Relman and colleagues reported the use of this technology for amplification of eubacterial DNA from patients with bacillary angiomatosis. When the amplified product was sequenced, the argyrophilic bacteria were found to be most closely related to *Rochalimaea* (now *Bartonella*) *quintana*, the cause of trench fever. Following this observation, there has been a rapid and ongoing expansion of our understanding of diseases of comparative medical importance caused by members of the genus *Bartonella*. The role of *B. henselae*, *B. clarridgeiae*, and *B. vinsonii* as zoonotic or canine pathogens, respectively, will be considered in subsequent articles.

It is probable that current research efforts have only begun to define the importance of infectious organisms in the development of many "noninfectious" disease states.

244

For example, it is well recognized that systemic illness frequently precedes the onset of juvenile diabetes mellitus. Immunologic reactivity to a heat shock protein (hsp 65), which is expressed when bacterial or animal cells are heat stressed, has been shown experimentally to cause diabetes mellitus in mice (Cohen, 1992). Concurrent administration of hsp 65 and a monoclonal antibody directed against hsp 65 prevents the development of diabetes mellitus. Similarly, absorption of intestinal bacteria or bacterial antigens into the systemic circulation has been strongly implicated as a cause of "immune-mediated" polyarthritis in humans and presumably contributes to many of the idiopathic polyarthritides observed in cats and dogs. Based on a rapidly growing body of literature, immune activation by bacterial DNA has been proposed as a cause of systemic lupus erythematosus and the induction of anti-DNA antibodies (i.e., antinuclear antibodies) (Pisetsky, 1997). During the past decade, *Helicobacter pylori* has emerged as an important cause of chronic superficial gastritis, peptic ulcer disease, and antibiotic-responsive gastric mucosa-associated lymphoid tissue lymphoma in human patients. The role of various *Helicobacter* species as pathogens of veterinary importance, or as cofactors in the development of gastric or hepatic adenocarcinoma in humans, continues to be defined (see *CVT XII,* p. 720).

It is becoming increasingly obvious that disease expression is frequently influenced by a genetically predetermined immunologic response of an individual within a population to an infectious pathogen (Kotb, 1995; Lucey et al, 1996). Of potential comparative medical importance, the study of companion animal breed-specific tendencies for the development of infection with pathogens such as *Pneumocystis carinii* in long-haired red dachshunds or *Mycobacterium avium* in Siamese cats and basset hounds, might facilitate enhanced understanding of host-pathogen interactions. Unfortunately, unless studied as an animal model of a human infectious disease or as a source of zoonotic infection, funding for companion animal infectious disease research is limited. This factor partially explains why there has not been a rapid and simultaneous recognition of new infectious diseases in companion animals.

If one considers the limited financial resources that have been available historically to support veterinary versus human medical research, infectious disease research contributions from the veterinary community have been impressive, and current research efforts continue to facilitate enhanced understanding of diseases caused by comparable human pathogens. For example, retroviruses were identified in several animal species long before the description of a human retrovirus. Similarly, infection with *Ehrlichia* in-volving a variety of animal species has been recognized for several decades, whereas human infection with monocytic and granulocytic *Ehrlichia* species was first described in the United States in 1986 and 1994, respectively. The recent recognition of *Babesia microti* as a human pathogen was predated by a considerable body of clinical and research literature on babesiosis in several animal species. These examples are meant to emphasize the potential comparative medical importance of the study of infectious diseases in domestic and wild animals. Enhanced environmental exposure of animals to vector, soil, and waterborne pathogens are distinct advantages for the future identification and characterization of novel organisms that infect animals and potentially humans. In addition, the ability to study natural disease outbreaks in herds, kennels, or catteries, as well as the opportunity to reproduce infectious diseases using a controlled experimental approach are distinct advantages for the veterinary researcher. In conclusion, as in the past, the future for veterinary infectious disease research holds considerable promise for the improvement of both animal and human health.

References and Suggested Reading

Cohen IR: Autoimmunity to hsp 65 and the immunologic paradigm. Adv Intern Med 37:295, 1992.
  This article reviews the concept that autoimmunity is primarily a physiologic process, and only when it is aberrant does a pathologic process evolve.

Gao SJ, Moore PS: Molecular approaches to the identification of unculturable infectious agents. Emerg Infect Dis 2:159, 1996.
  This article discusses recent advances in the use of molecular biologic techniques to detect and identify unculturable infectious diseases.

Kotb M: Bacterial pyrogenic exotoxins as superantigens. Clin Microbiol Rev 8:411, 1995.
  This review considers the role of microbial proteins produced by bacteria and viruses, known as superantigens, as mediators of acute life-threatening inflammatory diseases as well as chronic debilitating autoimmune diseases.

Levins R, Awerbuch T, Brinkman U, et al: The emergence of new diseases. Am Sci 82:52, 1994.
  This article considers the diverse factors that have contributed to emergence or recognition of new infectious diseases.

Lucey DR, Clerici M, Shearer GM: Type 1 and type 2 cytokine dysregulation in human infectious, neoplastic and inflammatory diseases. Clin Microbiol Rev 9:532, 1996.
  This article provides an excellent review of cytokine dysregulation in the development of infectious, neoplastic, and inflammatory diseases.

Pisetsky DS: Immune activation by bacterial DNA: A new genetic code. Immunity 5:303, 1997.
  This article considers recent evidence for the role of bacterial DNA as a molecular immunogen.

Relman OA, Loutit JS, Schmidt TM, et al: The agent of bacillary angiomatosis: An approach to the identification of uncultured pathogens. N Engl J Med 323:1573, 1990.

Molecular Biology of Infectious Disease

Nicholas J.H. Sharp

Raleigh, North Carolina

Infectious organisms are usually invisible to the naked eye, but in the last 100 years we have learned how to "see" them in a number of different ways. We first saw bacteria by using the light microscope and later saw viruses under the electron microscope. We then learned how to "see" organisms by putting visible labels on antibodies raised against their proteins. More recently we have used bacterial plasmid DNA as a genetic fingerprint to trace the spread of antibiotic resistance among gram-negative bacilli. With the advent of the polymerase chain reaction (PCR), not only are we able to examine an organism's genetic fingerprint more thoroughly but also we can multiply its DNA so that it actually becomes visible to the naked eye as a band on a gel! The phenomenal power of the PCR to amplify tiny amounts of DNA has been eloquently described as "detecting a needle in a haystack and then making a haystack of those needles" (Klingeborn, 1992).

There are four general applications of molecular techniques to the diagnosis of infectious disease. They can be used to demonstrate how closely related two strains of an organism are, to provide insight into the virulence of a particular strain, to identify new agents for previously unknown diseases, and to facilitate a clinical diagnosis. The last application is obviously of most relevance to clinicians and will therefore form the basis of this article. I shall first give a brief overview of molecular techniques before giving specific examples in the diagnosis of canine and feline infectious diseases. Table 1 provides a brief definition of commonly used terms. I shall then outline the problems that must be considered in using these tests and end with a discussion of what these tests will mean to the future of infectious disease diagnosis in veterinary medicine.

SPECIFIC MOLECULAR METHODS

There is not space in this article to provide a complete introduction to molecular biology, and I refer the reader to the reviews provided in the reference section (Alleman, 1996; Rosenthal 1994a, 1994b, and 1994c; Rosenthal 1995). The most important molecular techniques are summarized in the following sections.

Southern Analysis of DNA

One way of examining an organism's DNA is to perform Southern analysis. In this procedure, named after its inventor E.M. Southern, DNA is extracted and then cut into small pieces using bacterial enzymes called restriction endonucleases. The resultant DNA fragments are then size-fractionated by gel electrophoresis and transferred (or blotted, hence the term Southern blot) to a nylon membrane for ease of handling and storage. This Southern blot is usually hybridized with a labeled probe to identify DNA from a specific organism.

Probes and Hybridization

A probe is a piece of DNA that fulfills two basic criteria. It is complimentary to the target DNA, and therefore binds to it very strongly, and it is also labeled so that it produces a detectable signal under suitable conditions. Probes can be labeled in a number of different ways such as by incorporating a radioactive phosphate (^{32}P) into the probe DNA. Nonradioactive probes may be less sensitive than radioactive ones, but they are safer to use. Nonradioactive methods for probe labeling include the use of biotin, which can be made to produce a color reaction using a streptavidin–alkaline phosphatase conjugate; digoxigenin, which can produce either color or a chemiluminescent reaction; or a fluorescent marker. Labeled probes can be applied to Southern blots made from genomic DNA, plasmid DNA, or PCR products. The labeling of probes forms a crucial step for in situ hybridization (Jackwood, 1994).

In Situ Hybridization

Although probe hybridization on a nylon membrane can identify a specific organism within a mixture of DNA molecules extracted from a clinical sample, it does not necessarily identify that organism as the cause of the disease. In situ hybridization, in contrast, uses histologic sections instead of a nylon membrane as the template for the hybridization reaction. The signal obtained using a labeled probe allows DNA or RNA from a specific pathogen to be detected within the histologic lesion, thereby confirming the diagnosis (Naber, 1994). This technique is superior to immunohistochemistry for the diagnosis of parvovirus enteritis.

Polymerase Chain Reaction

The PCR is a powerful tool to amplify a precisely defined segment of target DNA. The target DNA to be amplified is specified by the design of the two PCR primers (Rosenthal, 1994b). If the two primers are located 500 base pairs apart on the target DNA, the PCR product will be 500 base pairs long. The target DNA undergoes logarithmic amplification and is effectively doubled after each of the 30 to 40 PCR cycles. Even after just 22 cycles, the target DNA has been amplified 1 million times. These copies of target DNA are called *amplicons* or simply the *PCR product*. Each reaction must be run together with a positive and a negative control in order to interpret the significance of any PCR product that is generated (see problems, below).

TABLE 1. Glossary of Terms

16S RNA: Part of the ribosomal RNA gene.

Amplicon: See PCR product.

cDNA: A DNA copy of an RNA strand, which is termed the *complementary DNA* (cDNA).

Complementary: A single strand of DNA is made up of individual bases of adenine (A), guanine (G), cytosine (C), and thymine (T) on a sugar and phosphate backbone. Two complementary strands are held together by hydrogen bonding between either the As and Ts or the Cs and Gs.

Cycle: A cycle of PCR amplification consists of a denaturation step, in which the DNA strands are separated; an annealing step, in which the primer is allowed to hybridize to the target DNA; and the extension step, in which the DNA polymerase synthesizes more DNA using the target strand as a template.

DNA: Deoxyribonucleic acid.

Electrophoresis: The separation of nucleic acids in an agarose gel by applying an electrical current across the two ends of the gel. Because DNA is a negatively charged molecule, it migrates toward the anode.

Eubacterial primer: PCR primers that can amplify DNA from any species of bacteria because of the shared sequence within parts of the 16S ribosomal RNA gene.

Hybridize: Process of mixing a probe with the target DNA under suitable conditions so that the two are able to base-pair to each other.

Label: Technique used to render a probe detectable in some way.

mRNA: Messenger RNA or RNA transcript that contains the genetic code required to build a particular protein. The mRNA is actually an RNA copy of the coding region contained within a gene.

Nested PCR: A second round of PCR performed after the first round using primers that are still complementary to the target DNA but are slightly inside the first set of primers. This not only subjects the target DNA to more rounds of amplification but also increases the specificity of the PCR.

PCR: The polymerase chain reaction is used to amplify a specific segment of DNA called the target DNA. The exact segment to be amplified is specified by the two PCR primers.

PCR primer: A short length of single-stranded DNA, usually 18 to 25 bases in length, that is complementary to the beginning or the end of the target DNA sequence.

PCR product: The product of a PCR amplification, also known as an amplicon.

Probe: A variable length of DNA that is complementary to the target DNA or region of interest and that has also been labeled.

Restriction endonuclease: One of a wide range of bacterial enzymes, each of which cuts DNA at a specific sequence.

Reverse transcriptase: The enzyme that makes a DNA copy of an RNA template.

Genome: the entire genetic information for a particular organism.

RNA: Ribonucleic acid.

RT-PCR: Reverse transcriptase PCR, employs a reverse transcriptase step to convert an RNA template to its cDNA before the PCR is performed.

Southern blot: Technique in which DNA is separated by electrophoresis on a gel and then transferred to a nylon membrane.

Target DNA: The region of DNA to be amplified by PCR or to be detected using a labeled probe.

Universal primer: Primers that are able to amplify DNA from a wide range of species of bacteria or viruses.

Detection of Polymerase Chain Reaction Products

After electrophoresis on an agarose gel, the DNA is made to fluoresce under ultraviolet light in the presence of ethidium bromide. Confirming that a PCR product is of the expected size is an important part of the detection process but is not usually enough for a definitive diagnosis. The PCR product could have been derived from one of the many other millions of DNA molecules in the sample, some of which may be similar enough to the target se- quence for the primers to hybridize. Sometimes this chance event can produce a PCR product of the same size as the target segment. More specific tests are usually employed to confirm the origins of the PCR product. The product can be sequenced, but this is too cumbersome for routine diagnostic use. The identity of a product can be checked by Southern analysis using a labeled cDNA probe. The PCR product can also be digested with a restriction endonuclease to produce a specific pattern of DNA fragments for each PCR product. If the desired PCR product is not seen using one of these techniques, it usually means that the target segment of DNA was not present in the starting specimen. Several variations of the standard PCR reaction are now in use; these will be discussed along with the diseases to which they have been applied.

DIAGNOSIS OF SPECIFIC DISEASES

Many organisms have been amplified using PCR, those causing disease in dogs and cats are listed in Table 2. Most of these PCR techniques have only been used in a research rather than a clinical setting, but this will eventually change. For example, the Synbiotics Corporation is now offering several PCR tests through a small number of veterinary laboratories, but the number of laboratories participating in molecular diagnostic testing is likely to grow rapidly.

The application of PCR to the diagnosis of infectious diseases is considered in four categories. They include

TABLE 2. Common Canine and Feline Pathogens for Which a Polymerase Chain Reaction Technique Has Been Developed

Organism	Type of Polymerase Chain Reaction	Specimen
*Toxoplasma**	1	CSF, aqueous humor, serum, blood
Neospora	1	Direct from organism
Haemobartonella	?	Blood
*Ehrlichia**	1	Blood macrophages
Rickettsia	1 or 2	Blood, urine
*Bartonella**	1 or 4	Heart valve, blood
Borrelia	1 or 2	CSF, urine, blood
Mycobacterium	1	CSF, lymph node
Yersinia	?	Not specified
Wide range of bacteria*	4	Joint fluid
FeLV*	1	Blood, gingiva, fixed tissue
FIV	1 or 2	CSF, serum, bone marrow
Pseudorabies*	1 or 2	Direct from organism†
Feline herpes*	1	Conjunctiva, cornea, throat swab, ganglia, optic nerve
Canine herpes	1	Tonsil, lumbosacral ganglia, salivary gland, liver
Canine distemper	3	Blood, bone
Rabies	3 or 2 and 3	CSF, saliva
Feline coronavirus	2 and 3	Serum, various body fluids
Parvovirus*	1	Feces, fixed tissues

FeLV, feline leukemia virus; FIV, feline immunodeficiency virus; 1, single PCR; 2, nested PCR; 3, RT-PCR; 4, PCR with eubacterial primers; CSF, cerebrospinal fluid.

*Currently used for clinical diagnosis.
†Described in a Florida panther.

diseases that are best detected using (1) a single round of PCR, (2) nested PCR, (3) reverse transcriptase polymerase chain reaction (RT-PCR), or (4) universal primers.

Single-Round Polymerase Chain Reaction Amplification

The most common type of PCR is single-round PCR amplification; it is used for the majority of agents shown in Table 2. Organisms detected in this way include *Toxoplasma gondii*, *Neospora caninum*, *Ehrlichia canis*, *Rickettsia rickettsii*, *Bartonella* species, *Borrelia burgdorferi*, *Mycobacterium* species, feline leukemia virus (FeLV), feline immunodeficiency virus (FIV), and both the feline and canine herpes viruses and parvoviruses. The most widely used PCR in veterinary medicine is for feline herpesvirus as a cause of ulcerative keratitis. This test does appear to have a high rate of positive results, which makes it difficult to interpret. The same is true, but to a lesser extent, for *T. gondii* in aqueous humor, in which 19% of cats with uveitis have positive results by PCR but 9% of normal cats do also. Even when appropriate controls are used, it is important to realize that these organisms could be present *but may not be causing disease.*

A PCR for FIV has been used to identify viral DNA in the blood and bone marrow of seronegative cats that were housed with FIV-infected animals. A PCR for FeLV is as accurate as enzyme-linked immunosorbent assay for diagnosis. Retrospective PCR examination of archival tissue embedded in paraffin blocks has even detected FeLV DNA in post mortem tissue of FeLV-negative cats that died of lymphoma. A PCR for parvovirus has also been used on fixed tissue, but this test has the most impact for the rapid diagnosis of parvovirus enteritis using fecal samples.

The PCR for *E. canis* is slightly less sensitive than an indirect fluorescent antibody test or Western blot, but PCR is much faster. For this and other organisms that grow extremely slowly, such as *Bartonella* species, PCR has obvious advantages for diagnosis. A single round of PCR can also be used to detect *B. burgdorferi,* but for some samples such as cerebrospinal fluid (CSF) the sensitivity is much higher using a nested reaction rather than a single round of PCR.

Amplification of DNA by Nested Polymerase Chain Reaction

A standard PCR reaction employs 30 to 40 cycles of amplification. Sometimes this is not enough to detect target templates that are present at very low concentrations. In such cases, it may be necessary to perform a second round of amplification. This is carried out in a new reaction tube, as the original enzyme is usually ineffective by the end of the first PCR. In addition to adding new reagents, the second round of amplification can be made more efficient by choosing primer sequences that are slightly inside the sequences of the first-round primers. This technique is often termed a *nested PCR.* Its main disadvantage is that the two separate rounds of amplification take longer and give greater opportunity for PCR contamination (see the problems associated with molecular diagnosis section further on).

Nested PCR is often applied to *B. burgdorferi* DNA, but even this very sensitive approach may not detect the organism in CSF from humans with neuroborreliosis. Amplification from urine gives more reliable results, but some asymptomatic humans excrete *Borrelia* in their urine. A single-round PCR for Lyme disease has been reported in the veterinary literature, but its clinical efficacy has not been studied, and it is likely that the sensitivity problems encountered in diagnosing human borreliosis will also apply to dogs and cats.

Amplification of RNA by Reverse Transcriptase Polymerase Chain Reaction

RT-PCR is used to amplify an RNA template such as the RNA virus of canine distemper. This RNA must first be turned into a cDNA copy using an enzyme called *reverse transcriptase.* The technique is therefore called reverse transcriptase PCR (RT-PCR) and it is mainly used to amplify RNA viruses such as canine distemper-rabies and feline infectious peritonitis (FIP). The cause of FIP is a feline enteric coronavirus, which also causes a common subclinical infection in cats. At present, there is no way to distinguish between pathogenic and nonpathogenic strains of this virus. It was hoped that PCR would be able to provide a definitive test for FIP, but unfortunately this has not proved to be the case thus far. The first round of RT-PCR for feline enteric coronavirus is often followed by a nested reaction, which can then detect the organism readily. The problem, similar to serologic testing, is that PCR is unable to differentiate a virus causing FIP from the nonpathogenic feline enteric coronavirus. The extreme sensitivity of PCR also means that it detects the ubiquitous coronavirus easily; therefore, this is a very poor diagnostic and prognostic test. Consequently, a PCR result should not be used as the sole indication to euthanize a cat with possible FIP.

RT-PCR has also been used to determine if an organism is actively making mRNA as a template for new proteins. This test has been proposed as a way of differentiating between an organism that is latent in tissue from one causing disease.

Amplification of Unknown Organisms

Primers for a PCR reaction are usually designed to be as specific as possible for a given organism. The opposite approach has been used to identify organisms for which no DNA sequence is available. There are regions of a genome, such as parts of the ribosomal genes (the 16S ribosomal RNA gene), that are so crucial that their sequences are the same in all bacterial species. Between these highly conserved regions of the 16S gene are sequences that are not so important and have evolved to be very different between genera, and even between different species within a genus (Persing, 1993). By deliberately designing so-called eubacterial primers to be complimentary to two of the conserved regions, the PCR can be made to amplify across the variable regions of the 16S gene. The sequence of the PCR product in the variable region will then be specific for only one organism. By applying eubacterial primers to a previously unknown organism growing on an agar plate, or even to tissue samples from an unknown disease, the variable region for that organism can be amplified and the sequence for that novel organism characterized. This is now an accepted microbiologic technique, which in veterinary medicine has been used to identify a new *Bartonella* species as a cause of canine endocarditis.

A different use for eubacterial primers has been in the diagnosis of septic arthritis caused by a wide range of gram-positive or gram-negative bacteria. Within a few hours, this PCR can determine if bacteria or bacterial DNA are present in the fluid or not. As these primers work for most species of bacteria, the test has broad applicability and could be used as a rapid screening test for bacteremia.

PROBLEMS ASSOCIATED WITH MOLECULAR DIAGNOSIS

The biggest problem with PCR is also a direct result of its ability to generate huge numbers of PCR products or amplicons (Persing, 1993). As DNA is a stable molecule, amplicons can quickly build up until they contaminate every surface in the laboratory. These amplicons drift into any PCR reaction set up in that laboratory, which means that each reaction will be positive irrespective of whether the sample contained the target organism or not. This situation can be confirmed by deliberately setting up blank PCR reactions with everything except DNA in the reaction mixture. These blank tubes are left open on the bench for 30 minutes before the lids are closed and the reactions started. In severely contaminated laboratories, these blank reactions will be positive because the amplicons that contaminate them are a perfect target for further amplification. This type of contamination is a problem only if the original primer pair is still being used; amplicons from one primer pair do not generally cause false-positive results for a different primer pair unless they share a common sequence. Amplicon contamination is a particular problem with nested reactions, as the tube is often opened between the first and second rounds of PCR.

Several steps can be taken to reduce the risk of false-positive results from this type of contamination. These steps include physically separating the room where a reaction is set up from the room where the finished reaction is opened for analysis (thereby liberating amplicons in the process). Chemical methods also exist to "sterilize" amplicons and prevent them from acting as targets for future amplifications, and at least one of these methods should be incorporated into every diagnostic PCR protocol (Persing, 1993). Even when taking all these precautions, it is also important to include appropriate negative controls with each sample, such as the blank reaction described previously. A negative control that omits the reverse transcriptase step must also be incorporated for RT-PCR.

There is another potential problem when interpreting a positive PCR result—even if contamination has been ruled out as a potential factor. The organism may indeed be present in the clinical specimen, but it may be latent, as can occur with herpes viruses, *T. gondii,* and some retroviruses. False-positive results can also occur if PCR is used in place of culture to monitor response to antimicrobial therapy. The PCR result may still be positive after successful therapy

because it can amplify organisms that are no longer viable but contain nucleic acid.

False-negative PCR results are generally less of a problem than are false-positive results, but they can also occur. One example of a false-negative result is when an organism such as *B. burgdorferi* is still present in neural tissue, but the host's immune response has been able to clear the organism from the CSF sample used in the PCR. Another cause of false-negative results is when PCR inhibitors are present in the sample, the most common inhibitor being heme derived from hemoglobin.

FUTURE OF MOLECULAR DIAGNOSIS

As PCR technology is applied to the diagnosis of more and more infectious diseases, the problems that have plagued all previous diagnostic tests will also apply to PCR. These problems include what type of sample to collect, what volume and in what preservative if any to collect it in, how to transport the sample and how to avoid potential inhibitory substances. Several other important questions will also need to be answered. Since PCR technology can be associated with a number of technical problems, how does a clinician decide which laboratory is sufficiently competent to run each test? Have the appropriate positive and negative controls been run with each sample, and how does the laboratory report the results of these controls? Does the laboratory take adequate precautions against contamination? All of these precautions and controls will obviously add to the expense of each test. If a laboratory tries to reduce the cost of a PCR by economizing on controls for contamination, the result that it provides may well be meaningless. In addition to all these problems, guidelines will need to be developed on how to interpret the PCR results for each disease, especially for organisms with latency or for ubiquitous organisms like feline enteric coronavirus. Furthermore, how long after vaccination will a PCR result be positive as a result of the vaccinal strain of organisms like canine distemper virus? Although PCR will become extremely important to veterinary medicine during the next few years, clinicians will be faced with almost as many questions about PCR as PCR will provide answers about infectious disease diagnosis.

References and Suggested Reading

Alleman AR: Molecular tools for the diagnosis of animal diseases. Vet Clin North Am 26:1223, 1996.
  Excellent introduction to molecular biology and basic diagnostic techniques.
Jackwood MW: Biotechnology and the development of diagnostic tests in veterinary medicine. JAVMA 204:1603, 1994.
  Excellent overview of labeling techniques, sequencing, and PCR.
Naber SP: Molecular medicine. Molecular pathology—diagnosis of infectious disease. N Engl J Med 331:1212, 1994.
  Very good descriptions of in situ hybridization and PCR.
Persing DH: Diagnostic molecular microbiology. Current challenges and future directions. Diagn Microbiol Infect Dis 16:159, 1993.
  Great perspective of problems associated with PCR and the implementation of molecular diagnostics.
Rosenthal N: Molecular medicine. DNA and the genetic code. N Engl J Med 331:39, 1994a.
  An outstanding short description of the basics of molecular biology.
Rosenthal N: Molecular medicine. Tools of the trade—recombinant DNA. N Engl J Med 31:315, 1994b.

Amplification of DNA by bacterial cloning or by PCR, with excellent descriptions of both techniques.
Rosenthal N: Molecular medicine. Stalking the gene—DNA libraries. N Engl J Med 331:599, 1994c.

Excellent descriptions of cloning and making DNA libraries.
Rosenthal N: Molecular medicine. Fine structure of a gene—DNA sequencing. N Engl J Med 332:589, 1995.
Excellent description of sequencing.

Vaccines and Vaccinations: Issues for the 21st Century

RICHARD B. FORD
Raleigh, North Carolina

RONALD D. SCHULTZ
Madison, Wisconsin

The rapid proliferation of companion animal vaccines, recent technologic advances in vaccine development, and concerns over vaccine safety are clearly among the key issues practicing veterinarians will face as we enter the next century. Although many would argue that these are already issues, the future promises to be especially challenging as the vaccines we currently use and the protocols we currently recommend undergo unprecedented change.

ANNUAL VACCINATION

In 1989, the American Veterinary Medical Association's Council on Biologic and Therapeutic Agents published immunization guidelines for dogs and cats (American Veterinary Medical Association's Guidelines, 1989). In that report, booster vaccinations for all canine and feline vaccines were recommended annually (*vaccines for canine coronavirus, Lyme disease, and feline infectious peritonitis were not available at the time these recommendations were published*). As recently as 1996, a survey of vaccination practices conducted in veterinary schools throughout North America indicated that annual revaccination of adult dogs and cats was routinely performed (Mansfield, 1996). It is reasonable to assume, therefore, that most practitioners currently recommend annual booster vaccinations to the owners of their companion animal clientele.

However, recent publications (Smith, 1995; Bowlin, 1996; Larson and Bradley, 1996), as well as recommendations outlined by a panel convened by the American Association of Feline Practitioners and the Academy of Feline Medicine suggest that current guidelines fail to address realistic duration of immunity data. At issue is the fact that a protective immune response is, depending on the antigen, likely to persist for several years following vaccination. Despite the absence of duration of immunity studies, representative suggestions for booster vaccination include administering core vaccines (e.g., feline panleukopenia, herpesvirus 1, calicivirus, canine distemper, parvovirus, adenovirus 2, and rabies) at up to 3-year intervals in adult animals.

Yet, despite current recommendations, several vaccines routinely used in companion animal practice, such as parainfluenza virus, *Bordetella bronchiseptica*, *Leptospira*, and feline *Chlamydia psittaci* probably do not provide protective immunity for 12 months (Mansfield, 1996) and that realistic risk assessment may dictate revaccination at intervals more often than yearly in selected animals.

Companion animal vaccination guidelines are currently undergoing critical scrutiny by representatives from private practice, industry, and academia. Despite widespread recommendations for annual revaccination, information available today suggests that current vaccination practices in North America do not necessarily correspond with the body of knowledge pertaining to duration of immunity derived from licensed vaccines. As a direct result, companion animal practitioners should expect significant changes in the current standard of practice pertaining to the administration of vaccines to dogs and cats.

Among the most significant changes anticipated in the future will be the recommendation to discontinue routine administration of annual booster vaccinations to adult dogs (distemper virus and parvovirus) and cats (panleukopenia, feline herpesvirus 1, and feline calicivirus). The incidence of canine distemper, canine parvovirus, canine adenovirus, and feline panleukopenia among vaccinated adults (>1 year of age) is virtually zero. The correlation among vaccination, the development of a "positive" antibody response, and protection from exposure to virulent virus is excellent. Furthermore, protection derived from immunization is sustained for periods as long as 5 or 6 years or more. Future vaccination standards for adult dogs and cats are likely to center around vaccination intervals of every 3 years.

Vaccines intended to protect against diseases such as *B. bronchiseptica*, canine parainfluenza virus, leptospirosis, Lyme disease, and feline chlamydiosis are not known to provide measurable protection against challenge for sustained periods. Annual boosters are likely to be recommended for those animals considered by the clinician to be *at risk of exposure.*

SELECTION OF ANTIGENS

Not only is it perceived that dogs and cats are vaccinated too often, it also has been suggested that pets are inoculated with too many different antigens in combination (multivalent) vaccines. The issue at hand for the future is to determine which vaccines are, in fact, indicated. Surveys of companion animal practitioners and veterinary teaching hospitals on vaccination protocols indicate there is considerable diversity within the profession about which vaccines should and should not be administered.

In the future, vaccination protocols for dogs and cats will likely center around recommendations for administering so-called *core* and *noncore* vaccines. Core vaccines are those vaccines recommended for administration to every animal presented to the practice. Recommendations to designate a particular vaccine "core" centers around diseases that are particularly severe, are highly transmissible to other animals, or represent a significant zoonotic potential. Noncore vaccines, in contrast, would be recommended to clientele when a known or likely risk of exposure is anticipated or when the animal's lifestyle represents a reasonable risk of exposure to the infectious agent, for example, feline leukemia virus (FeLV), feline infectious peritonitis virus, and canine coronavirus. Although annual boosters are still recommended, the actual risk:benefit ratio derived from FeLV and feline infectious peritonitis virus vaccination does not appear to justify annual vaccination with these products.

Another issue pertaining to selection of antigens is the administration of modified-live versus killed vaccines. Although recommendations against the administration of multivalent, modified live vaccines have been in place for several years (Tizard, 1990), most veterinarians continue to administer modified live biologics whenever there is a choice. Neither scientific data nor specific recommendations addressing the value of killed vaccine products over live, attenuated vaccines have been published.

VACCINE SAFETY

Among the most important issues facing practitioners today is that of vaccine safety. For most vaccines on the market today, it must still be assumed that the benefits of vaccination, when performed in accordance with currently published standards, far outweigh the risk of vaccine-induced illness or disease. However, recent reports have raised serious concerns within the profession over the relationship between vaccination and delayed adverse events, specifically vaccine-associated fibrosarcoma in cats (Kass et al, 1993; Hendrick et al, 1994) and immune-mediated hemolytic anemia in dogs (Duval and Giger, 1996). Determining which vaccines represent a specific risk to which animals, and when, simply cannot be determined with the information available today, yet it is still the practitioner who assumes responsibility not only for recommending a particular vaccination protocol but also for any consequences that might arise as a result of administering a vaccine (see liability section later).

Concern over the safety risks of attenuated (modified live) vaccines, such as disease caused by residual virulence, or disease attributed to contamination during manufacture,

has sustained a market for inactivated (killed) products. However, there are significant advantages of attenuated vaccines—such as rapid-onset, sustained protection; the ability to stimulate cell-mediated immunity; and the ability to immunize by way of natural routes—that may not justify the decision to offer only killed vaccines to companion animal patients.

Adverse Events

Information on the behavior of individual vaccines used under everyday field conditions is maintained by the manufacturers and reported to the United States Department Agriculture Center for Veterinary Biologics.* Such postmarketing surveillance also serves as an alert system for the rapid detection of vaccine-related events that appear to be unusual in nature or frequency. However, the single most significant factor that serves to compromise the effectiveness of the postmarketing surveillance program is the lack of adverse event reporting by practitioners.

An adverse event is any undesirable occurrence following the use of an immunobiologic product, including illness or reaction, whether or not the event was caused by the product. Anecdotal surveys suggest that adverse event reports from veterinarians dramatically underrepresent the number of reactions observed and regarded to be vaccine-associated. Despite efforts to categorize adverse events, there are still no uniform standards used by practitioners, manufacturers, or the United States Department of Agriculture to classify frequency and type of event.

Although there are few reports that specifically address the various causes of adverse events, reactions have been attributed to preservatives, contaminants, adjuvant, route of administration, concurrent administration of other vaccines, and the ordinal number of the vaccine (most immediate reactions occur subsequent to administration of the first vaccine as opposed to the second or third vaccine dose in a series). Neither the cause nor the exact frequency of delayed reactions, such as tumor formation or immune-mediated hemolytic anemia, are known.

Reporting of adverse events is the responsibility of the practitioner who administers the vaccine or observes the reaction. Reports should be made directly to the vaccine manufacturer, usually to the technical services section. The information to include in an adverse event report is summarized in Table 1.

Multidose (TANK) Vials

Veterinarians are advised to administer vaccine from *single-dose vials* only. Administering vaccine from a multidose, or TANK, vial (typically 10 doses per vial) containing killed virus vaccine carries the risk of delivering a significantly larger concentrations of adjuvant on administration of the last vial dose compared with the first. Furthermore, repeat penetration of the capped vial increases the chance of contamination.

---

*Animal Immunobiologic Vigilance. Brochure published by the United States Department of Agriculture, Center for Veterinary Biologics, 223 S. Walnut Avenue, Ames, IA 50010 (November 1996).

TABLE 1. Adverse Event Reporting Criteria to Be Reported to the Vaccine Manufacturer

Patient Information
Patient signalment (age, breed, sex)
Pertinent history
Case identification number (if applicable)
Adverse Event
A description of the event (e.g., onset of signs following inoculation; clinical signs-lesions)
Supporting laboratory data—include normal and abnormal findings (if applicable)
Date of inoculation
Date signs were first noticed
Outcome
A list of *all* immunobiologic products administered* that might be associated with the adverse event, to include:
　Product brand name
　Serial or lot number
　Product code number
Administration information (each vaccine administered):
　Dose
　Route
　Site
　Needle size
　Administration of concurrent (nonbiologic) drugs
　Date vaccine was reconstituted
Personal Information
Name, address, and phone number of veterinarian
Name, address, and phone number of owner-agent

*For combination products, list the product code and serial number of each vial as well as the product code of the combination package.

LIABILITY

Discussions with vaccine manufacturers, practicing veterinarians, attorneys, and representatives from the American Veterinary Medical Association's Liability Trust suggest that there is considerable confusion among practicing veterinarians over (1) the use of vaccines in a manner not specifically recommended by the manufacturer (as published in the package insert) and (2) the liability assumed when a vaccine causes, or is presumed to cause, a serious or expensive injury to the patient.

It is reasonable to assume that vaccination protocols for companion animals vary considerably throughout North America. Furthermore, it is the veterinarian who, after assessing the various risk factors unique to the individual patient, makes recommendations as to which type of vaccine and which antigens are to be administered. Veterinarians are *not* obligated to follow the recommendations outlined in the package insert for a specific product. Despite the label recommendations, discretion in the selection of which vaccine antigens to administer and when to administer them is the responsibility of the veterinarian. Such discretion is appropriate as long as it meets provisions defined by "standard of practice."

RISK ASSESSMENT

Providing effective immunoprophylaxis to the companion animal population does not require that all animals presented for vaccination be inoculated with each of the antigens for which a vaccine is currently licensed. Factors related to the individual patient, both intrinsic and extrinsic, as well as factors unique to the infectious agent should be taken into consideration when establishing recommendations or when assigning a vaccination protocol to an individual dog or cat.

Some vaccines, designated *core vaccines,* are appropriately recommended for all young dogs or for all cats. Recommendations for determining which antigens are deemed *core* should be based on the following: (1) the consequences of infection are particularly severe (e.g., feline panleukopenia), (2) infection is zoonotic and potentially puts human health at risk (e.g., rabies), or (3) the disease is prevalent and easily transmitted so that it poses a risk to the population of animals at large (e.g., feline herpesvirus and calicivirus).

The decision to vaccinate an animal with a vaccine that is *not* core should be based on the clinician's assessment of the individual animal's *risk profile* and takes into consideration information about the (1) animal's health status, (2) the environment, and (3) the infectious agent or agents to which the animal is likely to have been exposed.

Host Factors

Suboptimal response to vaccination is possible among animals that are malnourished, have concurrent infection or illness, or are receiving regular doses of immune suppressive drugs. Additional intrinsic factors considered to influence the outcome of infection include heritable resistance (and possible susceptibility) factors and stress. Age at the time of exposure is an important, independent variable in assessing an individual's risk to an infectious agent. Although no age group can be considered entirely free of risk, kittens (less than 6 months of age) are generally more susceptible to infection following exposure than are adult cats and therefore represent the principal target population for feline vaccination protocols.

The presence of maternal antibody is an intrinsic host factor known to protect a kitten or puppy following exposure to an infectious agent. However, interference of vaccine antigen by maternal antibody is the most likely cause of vaccination failure. Failure to vaccinate a kitten or puppy at an age when maternal antibody has declined sufficiently (approximately 12 weeks of age) will increase an animal's risk.

Environmental Factors

Population density and opportunity for exposure to other animals (free-roaming or "indoor-outdoor" activity) are among the most critical issues affecting the risk of exposure to an infectious agent. Puppies and kittens living within cluster households are at substantially higher risk of infection than are pets living in a household with only one or two other pets. Furthermore, the frequent introduction of new animals into a household cluster poses a potential risk to the entire population, despite vaccination. Geographic distribution of various infectious agents may represent significantly different exposure risks to animals living in different parts of the United States and should be considered when determining which *noncore* vaccines would be appropriate.

In multiple-cat households, sustained high ambient temperatures and humidity, in addition to housing environments with fewer than 12 air exchanges per hour, increase the risk of exposure to respiratory pathogens. In kennels, a single puppy with parvovirus puts all other nonvaccinates at risk for several months.

Agent Factors

A multitude of independent, agent-associated variables, such as virulence, dose, and mutation, influence the outcome of infection but are difficult to objectively assess in the clinical setting. However, in the domain of risk assessment, it is the interaction between the agent and the host that dictates the outcome following exposure and infection. The severity of an infection, particularly a viral infection, is highly variable within a population of animals with similar exposure to the same agent. Clinical illness may range from inapparent or mild to severe, acute illness to chronic or latent infection. Considering the advances in molecular and genetic biology made in the past few years, it is feasible that in the future it will be possible actually to predict the relative risk a particular virus poses to various genetically typed individuals.

RECOMBINANT VACCINES

Recombinant vaccines are among the newest products in the rapidly emerging biotechnology market and involve isolating and splicing (or recombining) gene-sized DNA fragments from one organism and transferring them to another. It has already been demonstrated that the hybrid organism resulting from the in vitro exchange of genetic material has the ability to deliver safe, immunogenic DNA into the host animal and, as such, represents a truly new generation of vaccine development for the veterinary profession. The recombinant vaccines currently being introduced into companion animal practice appear to provide exceptional safety. Efficacy, however, still must be determined on a case-by-case basis. In the 21st century, the introduction of even more refined DNA vaccines, for example, naked DNA, can be anticipated.

The technology behind recombinant or DNA vaccines is sophisticated and has quickly moved routine vaccination of dogs and cats to the subcellular level and away from the practice of administering attenuated live or killed organisms (Veterinary Exchange, 1997). As we enter the 21st century, new recombinant vaccines can be expected to enter the companion animal marketplace. Veterinarians are encouraged to become familiar with recombinant vaccines and understand the basic technology behind their development and the advantages they offer the companion animal population.

References and Suggested Reading

American Veterinary Medical Association's Council on Biologic and Therapeutic Agents: Canine and feline immunization guidelines. J Am Vet Med Assoc 195:314, 1989.

Bowlin CL: Proceedings from Perspectives on Vaccines in Feline Practice, eighth annual Feline Practitioners Seminar. Columbus, OH, July, 1996.

Duval D, Giger U: Vaccine-associated immune-mediated hemolytic anemia in the dog. JVIM 10:290-295, 1996.

Hendrick MJ, Kass PH, McGill LD, et al: Postvaccinal sarcomas in cats. J Natl Cancer Inst 86:341, 1994.

Kass PH, Barnes WG, Spangler WL, et al: Epidemiologic evidence for a causal relation between vaccination and fibrosarcoma tumorigenesis in cats. J Am Vet Med Assoc 203:396, 1993.

Larson RL, Bradley JS: Immunologic principles and immunization strategy. Comp Cont Ed Pract Vet 18:963, 1996.

Mansfield PD: Vaccination of dogs and cats in veterinary teaching hospitals in North America. J Am Vet Med Assoc 208:1242, 1996.

Smith CA: Are we vaccinating too much? J Am Vet Med Assoc 207:421, 1995.

Tizard I: Risks associated with use of live vaccines. J Am Vet Med Assoc 196:1851, 1990.

Veterinary Exchange: Recombinant vaccine technology. Compend Cont Educ Pract Vet 19(suppl):5, 1997.

Vaccination of the Immunocompromised Animal

RANCE K. SELLON
Pullman, Washington

There are few things as routine in veterinary practice as the administration of vaccinations. Although the benefits of vaccination in healthy pets are obvious and uncontested, the benefits and risks of vaccination in immunocompromised pets are not as clear. Immunodeficiencies may be congenital or acquired and affect either the nonspecific or specific immune system (see *CVT XII*, p. 560 and p. 516). Acquired causes of immune compromise (Table 1) are most commonly encountered in veterinary practices. Although there is little scientific data to address the capacity of immunocompromised pets to respond to antigenic challenge, several general issues should be considered before vaccinating an animal with immune deficiency.

First is *the nature of the deficiency*. Animals with congenital defects of the nonspecific immune system are generally capable of responding to vaccination. Since the specific immunologic machinery (B cells and T cells) is intact, these animals should receive vaccinations. Administration of vaccines should occur between clinical episodes of infection. Patients with acquired nonspecific immune dys-

TABLE 1. Common Acquired Causes of Compromised Function of the Specific Immune System in Dogs and Cats

Drugs
  Antineoplastics
  Corticosteroids
  Other immunosuppressive agents (e.g., azathioprine, gold salts)
Malnutrition
  Intestinal parasitism
  Inflammatory bowel disease
  Protein-calorie deficiency
  Obesity
Infections
  Viral infection (FeLV, FIV, FIP, CDV, parvovirus)
  Ehrlichia canis
Endocrine disease
  Hyperadrenocorticism
  Diabetes mellitus
Neoplasia
Miscellaneous
  Neonatal animals
  Colostrum deprivation

FeLV, feline leukemia virus; FIV, feline immunodeficiency virus; FIP, feline infectious peritonitis; CDV, canine distemper virus.

function, however, require careful consideration because many of these diseases are associated with defects in specific immunity as well.

The question of whether to vaccinate animals with deficiencies of the specific immune system depends again on the nature of the immune deficiency. Dogs with severe combined immunodeficiency are unsuited for vaccination. Dogs with selective IgA deficiency should receive parenterally administered vaccinations; however, vaccines designed to stimulate mucosal immunity directly, such as intranasally administered products, are less likely to have a beneficial effect and could have adverse consequences (e.g., clinical signs). For the patient with an acquired defect of the specific immune system, correction of the underlying problem should be attempted whenever possible before administration of vaccines.

The second issue to be considered before vaccinating a patient with compromised immune function is the relative *risk versus benefit* of vaccination. To assess risk and benefit, a number of questions can be asked:

What is the prevalence of the disease for which I am vaccinating and what are the chances that my patient will be exposed to the organism? Or, what is the risk of not vaccinating my patient? A high disease prevalence would increase the likelihood that the patient will contract the disease if it is at risk of being exposed. Vaccination of this animal may be deemed more important than if disease prevalence or risk of exposure is low. In some instances, the risks associated with contracting a disease, even if the disease prevalence is low, may outweigh any inherent risks associated with vaccination of the immunocompromised pet; rabies is a good example.

How long has it been since my patient was last vaccinated? What type of vaccines has my patient received? Was my patient last vaccinated during a period of potential immune compromise? Few studies have investigated the duration of immunity following vaccination of dogs or cats. A long duration of immunity (years) is achieved in

most animals following vaccination with modified live virus (MLV) products (Fishman and Scarnell, 1976; Gorham, 1966). Immunity after vaccination with killed or inactivated products is not as long as that provided by MLV vaccines. The immunity conferred by intranasally administered vaccines is also considered to be of shorter duration than that of parenterally administered vaccines. The duration of immunity provided to patients vaccinated during periods of immune system compromise cannot be reliably predicted. For these patients, it is safer to presume that immunity from previously administered vaccines will not be as lasting as in normal dogs and cats.

Will the vaccine be harmful to my patient? There are several risks associated with vaccination (Table 2), both known and suspected. The risks of adverse side effects following vaccination are not necessarily diminished in the immunocompromised pet. Other risks, such as injection site abscesses, could have more serious consequences in immunocompromised patients.

Will the vaccine be beneficial to my patient, that is, will my patient be able to mount an immune response to the vaccine? Within a population of "normal" animals, there will be some that respond less than optimally to immunization. The likelihood of a less than optimal response is greater still in immunocompromised patients. Additionally, it is difficult to predict the response of any one patient to vaccination. The safest assumption is that vaccination of immunocompromised pets is not as protective as vaccinations given to immunocompetent patients.

What are the local laws and human health risks associated with failure to vaccinate? Rabies vaccination is required by most state or local laws. Because of the zoonotic potential that exists for rabies, the serious consequences of rabies infection or even rabies exposure for the pet and its human contacts, the increasing prevalence of rabies in many areas of the United States, and the safety and efficacy of current rabies vaccinations, it is this author's opinion that no animal should be exempt from rabies vaccination. Patients vaccinated during a period of immunocompromise may need a booster vaccination earlier than the 3-year interval permitted in many states after immunization with some rabies vaccines.

VACCINATION RECOMMENDATIONS FOR SOME SPECIFIC CONDITIONS ASSOCIATED WITH COMPROMISED IMMUNE FUNCTION

Administration of Immunosuppressive Drugs

A common cause of immune system compromise in veterinary practice is the administration of corticosteroids or other immunosuppressive drugs. Few clinical studies

TABLE 2. Known and Suspected Adverse Consequences of Vaccination

Vaccine-induced disease (e.g., distemper)
Injection site sarcomas
Hypersensitivity reactions
Immune-mediated anemia-thrombocytopenia
Infection with contaminating agent (e.g., blue tongue virus)
Injection site infection

have addressed immune responses in animals receiving immunosuppressive drugs. Those that exist suggest that short (3 weeks or less) courses of immunosuppressive doses of corticosteroids do not impair immune responses or increase the risk of disease induced by vaccines (Nara 1979). Humans receiving prolonged (>2 weeks) courses of immunosuppressive doses of corticosteroids are advised to postpone vaccinations until they are no longer receiving such doses, and it would be prudent to follow such advice when possible for veterinary patients. If vaccination is deemed important for the patient that has received prolonged courses of immunosuppressive drugs, killed products would be safest because of the theoretical risk that MLV products could cause clinical disease.

Few studies have been conducted on the effects of antineoplastic drugs on the canine and feline response to vaccination. Administration of methotrexate prior to vaccination has impaired immune responses in dogs (Slater, 1970). In humans, MLV products may be given to adults who have not had antineoplastic drugs for at least 3 months. The interval between the discontinuation of antineoplastic drugs and the return of ability to respond to vaccines is unknown but has been estimated at between 3 months and 1 year. Children receiving antineoplastic drugs are generally not vaccinated with MLV products but are instead given killed products or toxoids. Routine vaccinations for children or adults may be administered between courses of chemotherapy or after induction of chemotherapy. Thus it is likely to be safe to vaccinate a dog or cat being treated for neoplasia or immune-mediated disease during the maintenance phase of many protocols, but vaccination during the induction phase of chemotherapy would not be recommended.

Hyperadrenocorticism

Whether or not animals with long-standing, untreated hyperadrenocorticism mount adequate immune responses to vaccination is not currently known. The assurance of an adequate immune response would likely be greater after control of the disease through treatment. If, however, vaccination is deemed necessary for the animal with uncontrolled hyperadrenocorticism, vaccination with killed products would be safer. The duration of immunity in hyperadrenocorticoid animals is unknown but may be suspected to be shorter than normal, especially if killed products are used.

Cats With Feline Immunodeficiency Virus or Feline Leukemia Virus

Experimentally, cats infected with feline leukemia virus or feline immunodeficiency virus (FIV) can mount detectable antibody responses to administered antigens, although detection of immunoglobulin may be delayed, and the magnitude of the response smaller, than that seen in uninfected cats. Theoretically, cats that test positive for retrovirus should receive some protection from vaccinations. Because both these viruses are lymphotropic, and virus production is enhanced by cell replication, the antigenic stimulation of vaccination (which is accompanied by lym-

phocyte proliferation) has the potential to increase virus production and foster progression of the infection. Conversely, some studies suggest that there are beneficial effects of antigenic stimulation on FIV infection without progression of FIV-related disease (Reubel et al, 1994). There is some evidence that cats infected with feline leukemia virus or FIV may be at increased risk for the development of vaccine-related infections: cats in the acute phase of FIV infection that were vaccinated with an MLV panleukopenia vaccine acquired clinical signs of panleukopenia (Buonavoglia et al, 1993). For cats that test positive for retrovirus and can be isolated from other cats, the risk of acquiring infections for which vaccines are given would seem low, and vaccination of these cats may not be warranted. It would seem prudent to vaccinate only those cats at high risk of exposure to infectious disease and when possible to use killed products. The recommendation to use killed vaccines is in keeping with the advice given to humans with human immunodeficiency virus infection.

Pregnant Animals and Orphan Animals

Pregnancy is associated with some degree of immunocompromise. More importantly, two goals of preventive medicine for breeding programs are somewhat at odds with each other: assurance that colostral antibodies against the infectious agent are high and protection of the fetuses from adverse effects of vaccination of the dam or queen. Ideally, dams and queens are vaccinated immediately prior to breeding. Alternatively, vaccination is withheld until the third trimester of gestation, and then only killed products are administered. Parenterally administered MLV products should not be given to pregnant animals, although intranasally administered vaccines, with the possible exception of feline infectious peritonitis (FIP) vaccine in cats, are probably safe.

Although not necessarily immunocompromised, orphan animals are presumed to be colostrum-deprived or from a questionable maternal immunologic background and therefore unprotected against infectious disease. However, adequate colostrum ingestion may have occurred, with maternal antibodies potentially interfering with early vaccine responses. Vaccinations should start as soon as possible after 10 days of age, and boosters administered every 3 weeks until the animals are 15 to 16 weeks of age. Killed products should be used in puppies and kittens less than 6 weeks of age, after which vaccination with MLV products is preferred.

Aged Animals

It has been proposed, based on limited in vitro studies of canine lymphocyte responses to mitogenic stimulation, that dogs older than 7 years may have compromised immune function, and thus should be vaccinated on a yearly basis. At present, the author is unaware of any definitive evidence to suggest that antibody responses or antibody levels diminish solely as a result of aging in dogs or cats. Aged animals may of course have other diseases that secondarily affect immune function.

In the absence of clinical data that address the preceding

issues, veterinarians must rely on a basic understanding of immune responses, the conditions that have the potential to alter immune responses, and the unique circumstances of each patient to guide vaccination decisions. It should also be emphasized that vaccination of a patient known to be immunocompromised may constitute an extralabel use of the vaccine. Immunocompromised patients deserve a few moments of thought before they are subjected to any routine procedure. Vaccination schedules and the vaccines administered should address the specific needs of the individual animal.

References and Suggested Reading

Buonavoglia C, Marsilio F, Tempesta M, et al: Use of a feline panleukopenia modified live virus vaccine in cats in the primary stage of feline immunodeficiency virus infection. Zentralb Vet 40:343, 1993.
Cats in the primary phase of FIV infection were susceptible to vaccine-induced panleukopenia.
Centers for Disease Control: Update on adult immunization: Recommendations of the Immunization Practices Advisory Committee (ACIP). MMWR Morbid Mortal Wkly Rep 40:1, 1991.
Contains guidelines for the immunization of immunocompromised humans.
Duval D, Giger U: Vaccine-associated immune-mediated hemolytic anemia in the dog. J Vet Int Med 10:290, 1996.
A retrospective study that indentifies a temporal relationship between vaccination and the development of immune-mediated hemolytic anemia and thrombocytopenia.
Fishman B, Scarnell J: Persistence of protection after vaccination against infectious canine hepatitis virus. Vet Rec 99:509, 1976.
Dogs vaccinated once with an MLV CAV-1 vaccine and isolated from exposure to field strains maintained titers for up to 11.5 years without additional vaccination.
Gorham JR: Duration of vaccination immunity and the influence on subsequent prophylaxis. J Am Vet Med Assoc 149:699, 1966.
Summarizes studies indicating that most dogs maintain titers for upward of 3 to 4 years or longer following vaccination with MLV canine distemper vaccine.
Nara PL, Krakowka S, Powers TE: Effects of prednisolone on the development of immune responses to canine distemper virus in beagle pups. Am J Vet Res 40:1742, 1979.
Puppies treated for 3 weeks with tapering regimens of prednisolone and dosages of 10 mg/kg mounted protective immune responses following vaccination with MLV canine distemper vaccine.
Reubel GH, Dean GA, George JW, et al: Effects of incidental infections and immune activation on disease progression in experimentally feline immunodeficiency virus–infected cats. J Acquir Immune Defic Syndr 7:1003, 1994.
FIV-positive cats exposed to feline pathogens and given vaccinations had no evidence of enhanced disease progression during the 3-year study.
Slater EA: The response to measles and distemper virus in immunosuppressed and normal dogs. J Am Vet Med Assoc 156:1762, 1970.
Dogs treated with methotrexate at the time of vaccination failed to mount protective immunity to infectious canine distemper virus challenge.
Wernicke D, Trainin Z, Ungar-Waron H, et al: Humoral immune response of asymptomatic cats naturally infected with feline leukemia virus. J Virol 60:669, 1986.
FeLV-positive cats immunized with a synthetic antigen mounted humoral immune responses, but peak titers were delayed and reduced when compared with FeLV-negative cats.

Lyme Disease Vaccination

MAX J.G. APPEL
Ithaca, New York

Lyme disease or Lyme borreliosis, is a tick-borne disease caused by the spirochete, *Borrelia burgdorferi.* Although it has a worldwide distribution, the disease in humans and dogs is restricted to certain areas in the United States. More than 90% of human cases are reported from 10 states in the northeastern United States, with foci in other parts of the country. Vaccination of dogs against Lyme disease, therefore, should be considered only in endemic areas or in dogs that travel to endemic areas. Lyme disease is also known to affect horses, cows, and cats; however, since vaccines are not available for these species, this discussion is restricted to vaccination of dogs.

With an ever-increasing number of canine vaccines and some concern about adverse reactions from vaccination, the question arises whether any dog should be vaccinated against Lyme disease. Although up to 80% of dogs become infected and are seropositive in endemic areas, it is estimated that only about 5% of seropositive dogs show clinical signs of lameness, the most common form of Lyme disease symptoms in dogs. In addition, dogs respond well to antibiotic treatment, and the antibiotic-resistant form of Lyme arthritis seen in humans is rarely seen in dogs.

There are some strong arguments in favor of vaccination of dogs against Lyme disease. When dogs become infected by tick exposure, the infection persists for years, probably for a lifetime. With the vaccines currently available, the persistent infection is not cured if the vaccine is given after infection. Vaccines prevent infection only in naive dogs. As mentioned previously, only about 5% of seropositive dogs show signs of lameness. However, even in the absence of clinical lameness, a mild polyarthritis was found by histopathologic study in dogs experimentally exposed to infected ticks, which might lead to sluggishness and reluctance to move (Appel et al, 1993). In addition, a fatal nephritis caused by *B. burgdorferi* has been reported in some dogs, especially in Labrador retrievers, for which antibiotic treatment has little effect (Levy et al, 1993).

Although it is generally believed that antibiotic treatment cures Lyme disease in dogs, that may not be true. The most commonly used antibiotics for Lyme disease in dogs are doxycycline and amoxicillin. In a recent study in dogs experimentally infected with *B. burgdorferi,* treatment with doxycycline or amoxicillin for a 4-week period at the recommended dose reduced the joint lesions but *B.*

burgdorferi infection was not cleared. Recurrent disease and lameness, therefore, could result from persistent infection even after antibiotic treatment.

For these reasons, it appears advisable to vaccinate dogs that will be exposed to ticks in endemic areas before they become infected, as recommended by vaccine companies. The question is, which vaccine should be used?

There are currently two different types of Lyme vaccine for dogs available. One type, which has been available for several years, consists of completely killed *B. burgdorferi* in a proprietary adjuvant (Chu et al, 1992). Although there appear to be few immediate adverse reactions to this vaccine in dogs, it is undesirable to have multiple components in the vaccine that are not involved in protection from infection and that have a potential to induce delayed adverse responses. Hamsters immunized with this bacterin and challenged by infected ticks acquired arthritis several weeks or months later (Lim et al, 1994). This concern has precluded development of a whole cell bacterin from consideration as a human vaccine.

The other type of vaccine consists of a recombinant outer surface protein A (OspA) of *B. burgdorferi,* which is responsible for the induction of specific borreliacidal antibody in the host (Chang et al, 1995; Coughlin et al, 1995; Straubinger et al, 1995). This vaccine became available for dogs in 1996 and it is currently being tested by two companies in field trials for humans (Wormser, 1995; van Hoecke et al, 1996).

The mode of protection of the OspA vaccine appears to involve spirochetal killing in the tick. OspA induces borreliacidal antibody in dogs. When ticks attach and engorge, a 24- to 48-hour feeding period is needed before the *Borrelia* migrate from the midgut of the tick to the salivary gland to invade the new host. When ticks engorge blood containing borreliacidal antibody, this migration is blocked and the new host does not become infected.

Why don't borreliacidal antibodies clear infection from previously infected dogs? There appears to be a shift in expression of OspA by *B. burgdorferi* from the low-temperature tick to the high-temperature mammalian host. After entering the mammalian host, OspA expression is replaced by OspC expression, as can be seen in western blot patterns with mammalian sera, including that of the dog. It might be desirable to include OspC in a Lyme vaccine to have an effect in the host after natural infection. However, OspC antibody is not as borreliacidal as OspA antibody, and experiments in mice have shown that elimination of persistent infection cannot be achieved by OspC antibody. Furthermore, there is an early and strong antibody response to OspC in dogs and other mammalian hosts after tick exposure. Obviously, this antibody does not eliminate persistent infection.

A caveat in vaccination with OspA or OspC is the fact that there are antigenic variations among different serotypes of *B. burgdorferi sensu stricto* and between different species. In Europe, where *B. burgdorferi sensu lato* (*B. garinii* and *B. afzelii*) are predominant, both OspA and OspC are rather heterogenous proteins (Wilske et al, 1996). This is less of a problem in North America, where only *B. burgdorferi sensu stricto* appears to exist with probably more than 90% of isolates of one serotype for OspA

(Lovrich et al, 1994). OspC appears to show a greater diversity.

Another experimental approach to vaccination appears to be promising. Antibodies against a *B. burgdorferi*–binding protein protected mice from challenge. These antibodies restrict migration of spirochetes. However, this research is in its early stages.

There have been several attempts to link cellular immune responses to protection from infection. Results have been less convincing than have results with antibody induction. It may well be that cellular responses restrict persistent infection. It is well known that macrophages ingest and degrade spirochetes, and T-cell responses may be important. However, the infection, once established, does persist in dogs and humans. Clearance of the spirochetes, therefore, is only partial.

Duration of immunity after vaccination and recommendations for booster inoculations are important questions. Yearly revaccinations are currently recommended for existing vaccines. Besides protocols from industry, duration of immunity studies in dogs are limited. We have tested and found complete protection in dogs 6 months after OspA vaccination. It would be advisable to vaccinate dogs in early spring before the tick season.

One drawback of vaccination is that it complicates interpretation of serologic studies. In nonvaccinated dogs, a positive enzyme-linked immunosorbent assay or fluorescent antibody titer indicates infection. In vaccinated dogs, these tests are not sufficient to determine whether dogs that test positive for *B. burgdorferi* were only vaccinated or were also infected by tick exposure. A Western blot is needed to differentiate between vaccination and tick exposure. Although after tick exposure, dogs have a wide range of antibodies to different *Borrelia* proteins, vaccinated dogs have only an OspA response if vaccinated with OspA vaccine or a limited number of *Borrelia*-specific antibodies, including OspA, if vaccinated with a killed bacterin.

It remains unresolved whether vaccination of seropositive dogs has a beneficial or hazardous effect, or no effect at all. We only know that persistent infection is not cured if either the bacterin or the OspA vaccine is given after tick infection, and major health problems have not been reported. Dogs can be tested by serologic methods before vaccination. If seropositive, dogs could be treated with antibiotics before vaccination.

The question is frequently asked whether dogs with Lyme disease can be seronegative. Because the onset of antibody response in humans and dogs may take 3 or 4 weeks, early signs of Lyme disease (erythema migrans) in humans are frequently seen in seronegative patients. The first sign of Lyme disease in dogs is usually arthritis, which occurs after the onset of antibody response. Under experimental conditions, we have not seen a seronegative dog with Lyme arthritis. Another reason for seronegative Lyme disease in humans could be related to early antibiotic treatment, which might suppress antibody production but may not eliminate the spirochetes. In addition, other infections may mimic Lyme disease in dogs and humans, for example, granulocytic ehrlichiosis. The causative agent, *Ehrlichia equi* or a close relative, is transmitted by the same ticks that transmit Lyme disease.

References and Suggested Reading

Appel MJG, Allan S, Jacobson RH, Lauderdale T-L, et al: Experimental Lyme disease in dogs produces arthritis and persistent infection. J Infect Dis 167:651, 1993.
A general description of the biology of canine Lyme's disease under experimental conditions.

Chang Y-F, Appel MJG, Jacobson RH, et al: Recombinant OspA protects dogs against infection and disease caused by *Borrelia burgdorferi*. Infect Immun 63:3543, 1995.
A report of a study in dogs vaccinated with OspA and protected from infection.

Chu H-J, Chavez LG Jr, Blumer BM, Sebring RW, et al: Immunogenicity and efficacy study of a commercial *Borrelia burgdorferi* bacterin. J Am Vet Med Assoc 201:403, 1992.
A report of a study in dogs vaccinated with a whole cell bacterin and protected from disease.

Coughlin RT, Fish D, Mather TN, et al: Protection of dogs from Lyme disease with a vaccine containing outer surface protein (Osp)A, OspB, and the saponin adjuvant QS21. J Infect Dis 171:1049, 1995.
A report of a study in dogs vaccinated with OspA and protected from infection.

Levy SA, Barthold SW, Dombach DM, et al: Canine Lyme borreliosis. Comp Cont Ed 15:833, 1993.
A general description of the biology of canine Lyme's disease under natural conditions.

Lim LCL, England DM, DuChateau BK, et al: Development of destructive arthritis in vaccinated hamsters challenged with *B. burgdorferi*. Infect Immun 62:2825, 1994.
A study in hamsters that developed arthritis after vaccination with whole cell bacterin followed by challenge with live B. burgdorferi.

Lovrich SD, Callister SM, Lim LCL, et al: Seroprotective groups of Lyme borreliosis spirochetes from North America and Europe. J Infect Dis 170:115, 1994.
A report of five distinct seroprotective groups of B. burgdorferi from North America and Europe.

Straubinger RK, Chang Y-F, Jacobson RH, et al: Sera from OspA-vaccinated dogs, but not those from tick-infected dogs, inhibit in vitro growth of *Borrelia burgdorferi*. J Clin Microbiol 33:2745, 1995.
A description of an assay that detects high levels of borreliacidal antibody in OspA vaccinated dogs and low levels in tick exposed dogs.

Van Hoecke C, Comberbach M, De Grave D, et al: Evaluation of the safety, reactogenicity and immunogenicity of three recombinant outer surface protein (OspA) Lyme vaccines in healthy adults. Vaccine 14:1620, 1996.

Wilske B, Busch U, Fingerle V, Jauris-Heipke S, et al: Immunological and molecular variability of OspA and OspC. Implications for *Borrelia* vaccine development. Infection 24:208, 1996.
A description of the variability of OspA and OspC from different isolates of B. burgdorferi.

Wormser GP: Prospects for a vaccine to prevent Lyme disease in humans. Clin Infect Dis 21:1267, 1995.
A discussion of the potential of OspA as a human vaccine.

Disinfectant and Antiseptic Use in Small Animal Practice

BRENDA C. LOVE
Columbus, Ohio

DWIGHT C. HIRSH
Davis, California

Although scientists in the mid-1800s were debating whether diseases were caused by microorganisms, disinfectant* and antiseptic† use began in medieval times, probably for controlling foul odors and for wound antisepsis. By the mid-1800s, medical doctors realized that hand washing and disinfectant use could reduce the spread of disease through medical wards and protect surgical patients from infection. Although disinfectant use is widespread today, the threat of nosocomial infections persists. Knowing which disinfectant or antiseptic is appropriate to use, and the proper way to use it, may help reduce the risk of both nosocomial and postsurgical infections in a small animal practice.

EVALUATION PROCEDURES

There are two main categories of test design: the first tests the antimicrobial activity of the product in a suspension (in vitro tests) and the second tests the product in a simulated "real-life" situation (practical tests). Practical tests can be performed on carrier models (e.g., glass or skin) or on surfaces (steel, linoleum). Neither of these methods (in vitro or practical) may be truly indicative of how a disinfectant will perform in practice. There are many variables that may affect the test outcome, including the test organism used, the method of preparation of the organism, and the subculture method used. Test organisms may undergo spontaneous inactivation on certain carriers, making the disinfectant appear more effective than it is. Formulations of antiseptics and disinfectants contain one or more active compounds together with inactive ingredients such as perfumes and colorants. The method of formulation can affect the properties of the chemical; thus, it is not adequate to assume that because a specific amount of chemical has been included, a product will be effective in use. *Disinfectants are registered with the Environmental Protection Agency (EPA) as pesticides, and neither the EPA nor the Food and Drug Administration verifies disinfectant efficacy data that is submitted for registration.* Research has been conducted on many pathogens using nonstandard

---

*An agent that destroys infective agents or renders them inactive, used in the context of inanimate objects.

†A substance that inhibits the growth and development of microorganisms without necessarily destroying them, used in the context of living tissue.

laboratory methods in an effort to add realism to efficacy data. These tests evaluate the effect of pH, temperature, hard water, and organic matter on specific disinfectants.

SPECTRUM OF ACTIVITY

There is a general scale of "innate" resistance of microorganisms to disinfectants. From least resistant to most resistant, the scale is vegetative bacteria, vegetative fungi and fungal spores, enveloped viruses, nonenveloped viruses, protozoal spores, mycobacteria, and bacterial spores. An EPA-registered disinfectant with a claim of a particular activity (e.g., virucidal) can be expected to also be effective against less resistant categories (e.g., fungi and vegetative bacteria).

RESISTANCE MECHANISMS

As with antibiotic resistance, resistance of microorganisms to disinfectants can be innate or acquired. Bacterial spores and mycobacteria are naturally resistant because of their cell wall structure. Some bacteria (*Staphylococcus aureus*, some members of the family Enterobacteriaceae) carry genes that encode disinfectant resistance. These genes are often carried with other genes that encode antibiotic resistance, and they are potentially mobile DNA elements (i.e., they can be transferred among bacteria). There are reports of the apparent development of resistance of "resident" bacteria in a hospital to the most frequently used disinfectant, with a decrease in numbers of bacteria cultured from surfaces and hospital workers after a change in disinfectant. Despite these reports, it seems that the primary reason for inactivity of a disinfectant against a given microorganism is either innate resistance of the organism or inappropriate use of the disinfectant (e.g., presence of organic matter or other inactivating substance).

PRODUCTS-CHEMICALS: CHEMICAL-PHYSICAL ATTRIBUTES

Quaternary Ammonium Compounds

Quaternary ammonium compounds are cationic detergents. The activity of quaternary ammonium compounds decreases in the presence of hard water, and they are usually formulated with a chelating agent (e.g., ethylenediaminetetraacetic acid) to remove calcium and magnesium ions. Activity is also decreased by organic matter (e.g., blood or pus), and they are not compatible with anionic detergents and soaps. If anionic detergents or soaps are used for cleaning, care must be taken to rinse well before using a quaternary ammonium compound. Factors that enhance the activity of quaternary ammonium compounds include a slightly alkaline pH, higher temperatures, and ethanol. Quaternary ammonium compounds are irritating to conjunctiva and mucous membranes, and repeated use may result in hypersensitivity and contact dermatitis. Oral ingestion is poisonous. Strong concentrations can be corrosive to steel or iron. Consult Table 1 for the microbiologic activity of these compounds and of the other disinfectants and antiseptics discussed in the balance of this article.

Phenols

Phenol itself is rarely used as a disinfectant today because it is highly toxic and corrosive, but newer synthetic compounds are commonly used. Hexachlorophene is a phenol derivative that has been used for skin preparation before surgery. It has a prolonged residual activity but a slow onset of action. It has been shown to be neurotoxic and teratogenic with prolonged exposure through the skin. Cats are particularly sensitive to the toxic effects of phenols, and small doses absorbed through the skin or swallowed can be fatal.

Bisguanides

The most commonly used chemical in this class is a bisbiguanide, chlorhexidine gluconate. It is used at concentrations of 4% or less as a skin cleanser and antiseptic and for cold sterilization of surgical instruments. It has a rapid onset of action and a long residual effect. The residual effect may be decreased in the presence of alcohol. The chlorhexidine molecule has strongly cationic groups and is inactivated by anionic compounds (e.g., chloride and soaps). Activity is somewhat reduced in the presence of organic matter and is completely absent in the presence of

TABLE 1. Effectiveness of Disinfectants and Antiseptics Against Various Microorganisms

	Quaternary Ammonium	Phenol	Bisguanide	Chlorine	Iodine	Alcohol	Peroxygen	Aldehyde
Bacteria								
Gram-negative	±*	+	±	+	+	+	+	+
Gram-positive	+	+	+	+	+	+	+	+
Spores	−	−	−	+	±	−	+	+
Mycobacterium	−	+	−	+	+	+	+	+
Fungus	±	+	+	+	+	+	+	+
Virus								
Enveloped†	+	+	+§	+	+	+§	+	+
Unenveloped‡	−	±	±	+	±	±	+	±
Protozoa	±	?	?	+‖	+	?	+	?

*±, Some strains are affected, others are not; +, affected; −, not affected.
†Canine distemper virus, rabies virus, feline leukemia virus, feline immunodeficiency virus.
‡Canine infectious hepatitis virus; canine parvovirus; feline panleukopenia virus.
§Rabies virus not affected.
‖*Cryptosporidium* spp. not affected.

gross fecal contamination. Chlorhexidine has been shown to be cytotoxic to fibroblasts in vitro at concentrations lower than are effective for bactericidal activity. For this reason, solutions less than 0.05% are recommended for wound lavage. There is extremely low, if any, percutaneous absorption through normal skin, and chlorhexidine has an extremely low irritant potential for human skin. Oral toxicity is low because of poor absorption through the intestinal mucosa. Overall, chlorhexidine has been shown to be a safe, effective antiseptic and disinfectant.

Halogen-Releasing Products

Chlorine

Sodium hypochlorite (household bleach) is a commonly used and effective disinfectant. It acts through the release of hypochlorous acid in aqueous solutions. The bactericidal activity seems to be from oxidation of key enzymes within the cell membrane or cytoplasm. Active concentrations are expressed in terms of available free chlorine. Effective concentrations range from 0.05 to 5 ppm available chlorine, which will kill vegetative bacteria within 15 seconds to 5 minutes, to 200 ppm, which will kill a substantial number of bacterial spores within 5 minutes. Recommendations in human medicine are to use a 500-ppm solution to achieve levels capable of killing tuberculous or human immunodeficiency virus organisms (this corresponds to a 1:100 dilution of household bleach). These concentrations are nontoxic and have little environmental impact, although high concentrations are corrosive to skin, metals, and other materials. Sodium hypochlorite solutions are relatively unstable and decompose easily. Factors that decrease stability include an acidic pH, exposure to light, heavy metal ions, and high temperatures. Formulations are usually alkaline and are provided in light-proof containers to increase shelf life. Solutions of sodium hypochlorite do not wet surfaces well and as a result have been formulated with detergents, which do not affect their microbicidal activity. Sodium hypochlorite should *never be mixed with acids,* as this results in the release of toxic chlorine gas. The instability of sodium hypochlorite at acidic pH results in their being more effective microbicides in these conditions (pH 6 to 7). This is due to the potentiation of oxidation and to being able to penetrate the cell membrane more easily. However, the sporicidal activity is enhanced in the presence of 1.5 to 4% w/v NaOH. Factors that decrease the activity of hypochlorite solutions are the presence of organic matter, which it readily oxidizes, thus reducing the oxidizing power against microorganisms, and cationic detergents. The calcium and magnesium ions in hard water do not inactivate chlorine disinfectants, but ferrous or manganous cations, and nitrate and sulfide anions do. Sodium hypochlorite solutions are cytotoxic in vitro. Use of these solutions in wound lavage is recommended at concentrations of 0.125%, although no studies have evaluated the effect of this concentration on wound healing in animals.

Iodine

Aqueous iodine and tinctures of iodine (2% iodine in 50% ethyl alcohol) are no longer used frequently because of their corrosiveness and capacity for skin irritation. Rather, iodine that has reacted with neutral polymers (polyvinylpyrrolidone) or ethoxylated surfactants, called iodophors or povidone-iodine, are used. Iodophors have a wide spectrum of activity. In general, iodophors work best in a slightly acidic environment, and formulations are stabilized with acids or acidic buffers. Iodophors are inactivated by hard water and organic matter, including blood. The activity of iodophors is dependant on the level of free molecular iodine in the solution. The activity of iodine follows a bell-shaped curve, peaking at 24 ppm (achieved in a 0.07% solution) and decreasing with either higher or lower concentrations. Thus, dilutions of the commercially available stock solutions are more potent than are the stock solutions. Povidone-iodine is also available as a presurgical scrub. The detergent in this scrub should be used only on intact skin. This product exhibits rapid microbial killing and has a residual antimicrobial activity of 4 to 6 hours, which is reduced in the presence of alcohol or organic matter. The efficacy of povidone-iodine is comparable to that of chlorhexidine. Contact dermatitis occurs in a substantial percentage of dogs with iodophor use and may result in increased postsurgical infection rates. Systemic absorption of iodine is also a potential problem, especially when used to lavage open wounds or the peritoneal cavity. The presence of peritonitis decreases the lethal dose of 10% povidone-iodine from 8 ml/kg (without peritonitis) to 2 ml/kg. Iodine is excreted primarily by the kidney, and caution should be exercised when using povidone-iodine in animals with renal insufficiency. Recommendations are to use povidone-iodine at concentrations of 0.1 to 1.0% for wound lavage, and its use should be avoided in animals with burns or large wounds. Iodophors are effective for ''cold sterilization'' of medical equipment, although the corrosive effects on the equipment should be considered.

Alcohols

In Europe, alcohols have been the standard by which all hand and skin antiseptics are judged. In the United States, alcohols are not routinely used for this purpose, although they are used commonly for other disinfecting purposes. The most useful alcohols are ethanol and the propanols; *n*-propanol is the most active, isopropanol somewhat less, and ethanol is the least. A key point to remember when using alcohols to disinfect is that the presence of water is necessary for microbial killing. Generally, concentrations of 60 to 80% (v/v) are necessary for ethanol and somewhat less (30 to 40%) for the propanols. High concentrations (90% up to absolute alcohol) are less effective. Organic matter decreases the activity of alcohol, although prolonging the exposure time has been shown to compensate for this effect. Alcohol may potentiate the activity of other disinfectants, although hexachlorophene is inactivated by alcohols. Increased temperature intensifies the antimicrobial activity. Percutaneous absorption of alcohols through intact skin is negligible but may cause intoxication in very young animals. Alcohols are cytotoxic in open wounds and should never be used for wound lavage. Prolonged exposure to high concentrations may cause drying and irritation of the skin, although, in general, alcohols are relatively safe and effective when used properly.

Peroxygen-Based Products

Hydrogen peroxide is considered a high-level disinfectant. Concentrations of 10–25% are considered sporicidal within minutes, and lower concentrations (3%) are effective at killing vegetative bacteria. Increasing the temperature also increases the efficacy of hydrogen peroxide. Hydrogen peroxide solutions must be stabilized through adjusting pH to 5 and adding phosphonates, because they are extremely reactive. Hydrogen peroxide is often used to clean wounds. While a 3% solution was not shown to adversely affect wound healing, this concentration has been shown to be toxic to human fibroblasts in culture. Hydrogen peroxide is commonly used for sterilization of endoscopes. Care must be taken to thoroughly rinse the endoscope after sterilization, as enteritis may develop as a result of residual peroxide entering the gastrointestinal tract.

Aldehydes

The most common aldehyde-based disinfectant in use is glutaraldehyde. Activity is nonspecific, and is just as effective on mammalian cells as on microorganisms. However, glutaraldehyde solutions are used to treat dermatophytes in human patients, with no adverse effects noted. Prolonged exposure times (of several hours) may be required. The activity of glutaraldehyde is potentiated by cations, such as calcium and magnesium, and by ultrasonics. Alkaline conditions enhance the activity of glutaraldehyde, although they also contribute to the increased breakdown of the chemical. For this reason, acidic formulations are provided, which must be converted to an alkaline solution at the time of use. Organic soiling has little effect on the activity of glutaraldehyde. This is one of the agents of choice for cold sterilization of medical equipment such as endoscopes. A 2 to 3% solution is used, and contact times of up to 3 hours are recommended for complete destruction of bacterial spores. Thorough rinsing with sterile (not tap) water is necessary before use to remove all residual glutaraldehyde. Aldehydes have also been formulated with quaternary ammonium compounds and phenols to achieve a synergistic effect. Glutaraldehyde causes toxicity, the most severe of which is respiratory and ocular irritation from vapors and allergic contact dermatitis. The oral toxicity is less than the dermal toxicity. There does not seem to be any teratogenic, mutagenic, or carcinogenic effect.

APPLICATIONS

Hand Washing and Surgical Hand Scrub

Hand washing is considered one of the mainstays for the control of nosocomial infections. However, some studies have shown that hand washing itself may contribute to the spread of infections through a hospital because mechanical scrubbing of the skin results in the shedding of squames, which carry with them the resident bacteria. Also, frequent hand washing can result in irritation, which can change the ecology of the skin, resulting in an increase in gram-negative bacteria. In order to have a positive effect on the control of the spread of infection, an antimicrobial soap (as opposed to plain soap and water) must be used.

Some of the chemicals used in antimicrobial soaps can be irritating to the skin, however. For hand washing between patients, an agent that kills microorganisms very rapidly is needed. Alcohol and alcoholic chlorhexidine solutions seem to be best suited for this purpose.

Surgical hand scrubs are intended to decrease the numbers of both transient flora (those microorganisms picked up from the environment) and resident flora (those microorganisms that reside in the deeper layers of the skin). The most important source of microorganisms on a surgeon's hands is the subungual space, and care must be taken to specifically remove this source. Surgical hand scrubs should ideally have both an immediate effect and a residual effect that lasts several hours.

Surgical Preparation

Preparation of a surgical site is carried out to minimize the risk of postsurgical infection. Typically, preparation involves removal of the hair or fur, scrubbing, and application of an antiseptic. Again, the goal is to remove transient and resident flora, both immediately and residually. Reports indicate that even with this preparation, up to 20% of the resident flora remain. Because clipping the site can cause significant skin irritation, it may be helpful to do this 1 to 2 days before the surgery, if possible. Also, treatment of the area with an antiseptic solution and wrapping with an occlusive bandage the day before surgery may be of benefit. In humans, whole-body bathing with an antiseptic the day before surgery has been shown to decrease the incidence of postsurgical infections.

Povidone-iodine and chlorhexidine gluconate scrubs are used extensively in veterinary practice; they are virtually equal in reducing bacterial colony counts both immediately and several hours after application.

Care should be taken when using antiseptics for lavage of open wounds or body cavities, as several antiseptic chemicals are toxic to cells in vitro and may cause systemic toxicity.

Cleaning Surfaces

The most important factor in disinfecting surfaces (countertops, floors, feeding utensils) is the prior removal of all organic material and thorough rinsing to remove residual soaps, which may inactivate the disinfectant. The potential for damage to the surface by the disinfectant (e.g., chlorine- and iodine-releasing compounds) must also be considered. Currently, the recommendation in the human medical field is to use "low-level" disinfectants (such as quaternary ammonium compounds)—which are effective against vegetative bacteria, some viruses, and fungi—for cleaning of surfaces. The recommendation in dentistry is to use "intermediate-level" disinfectants, which are effective against nonenveloped viruses and mycobacteria. Examples of intermediate-level disinfectants are iodophors, chlorine-releasing agents, and phenolic compounds that contain more than one phenolic agent.

The effectiveness of cleaning and disinfection protocols can be ascertained by periodic assessment of bacterial numbers on surfaces. This is usually carried out by using "contact plates," which are specially designed Petri plates that have been slightly overfilled above the rim so that the agar can be placed in contact with a surface. Some commercially available plates (PML Microbiologicals, Tualatin, OR) have bacteriologic media with relatively wide microbial appeal (tryptic soy agar) containing substances that inactivate disinfectants and antiseptics (lecithin for quaternary ammonium compounds; polysorbate 80 for phenolics and biguanides; both lecithin and polysorbate inactivate ethanol). At our institution, contact plate assessment is made monthly, and surfaces with a bacterial count of greater than three colonies/cm² are recleaned and disinfected.

Cleaning Equipment

Equipment that is reused but not amenable to heat sterilization, and that comes in contact with mucous membranes or nonintact skin but does not enter vascular systems, can be disinfected with "high-level" disinfectants. Equipment of this nature includes thermometers, endoscopes, and endotracheal tubes. Appropriate disinfectants include 2% glutaraldehyde, iodine formulations, and stabilized 6% hydrogen peroxide. Each of these agents has the potential to cause irritation (glutaraldehyde and hydrogen peroxide) or to be corrosive to equipment (iodine). Thorough rinsing with sterile water—not tap water, which may contain microorganisms (such as *Cryptosporidium* spp.)—is recommended before use.

Suggested Reading

Ascenzi JM, ed: Handbook of Disinfectants and Antiseptics. New York, Marcel Dekker, 1996.

Bacterial Resistance

MARK G. PAPICH
Raleigh, North Carolina

Bacterial drug resistance in human medicine has been considered by some a crisis (Neu, 1992). New drug development had kept pace with emerging resistant populations steadily since the discovery of penicillin. However, in the last 10 years that trend has changed. Bacteria, such as *Staphylococcus aureus*, *Streptococcus pneumoniae*, *S. pyogenes*, and *Haemophilus influenzae*, that were once susceptible to many antibiotics now have a high rate of resistance. Bacteria such as enterococci and *Mycobacterium tuberculosis* are a significant problem because there are no new drugs to treat resistant infections. In veterinary medicine, bacterial resistance has not reached these proportions, but therapeutic problems caused by drug-resistant bacteria are increasing.

Veterinary medicine presents unique limitations to dealing with resistant bacteria because when resistance occurs, therapy usually requires administration of the newer, expensive antibiotics. Because many of the more active drugs require IV infusions several times a day, they are impractical to administer in some clinical settings. There are also public health concerns about administering extended-spectrum antibiotics developed for humans to animals. If veterinarians are to enjoy the effectiveness of most of our antibacterial drugs, careful surveillance, rational prescribing, and strict practices to prevent the spread of resistant bacteria are necessary.

WHAT DEFINES RESISTANCE?

Bacteria are considered resistant when an in vitro test shows that it is not susceptible to antibacterial drugs for which it would ordinarily be susceptible. Some bacteria exhibit *inherent resistance* (intrinsic resistance), which should not be confused with *acquired resistance*. Bacteria have intrinsic resistance if they are not susceptible to certain antibacterial drugs even though they have not acquired a resistant plasmid or chromosomal mutation. For example, if a patient has an infection caused by *Pseudomonas aeruginosa*, a veterinarian may suggest that the patient has a "resistant" infection when it is actually just the wild strain of *Pseudomonas* that has inherent resistance to most beta-lactam antibiotics, macrolides, tetracyclines, and trimethoprim-sulfonamide combinations. Another example of inherent resistance is that exhibited by streptococci and enterococci to fluoroquinolones.

Not all nosocomial infections are resistant infections and vice versa. Nosocomial infections are acquired in a hospital. However, because of antibiotic selection, many nosocomial infections are resistant to commonly used antibacterial drugs.

Acquired resistance is the emergence of resistance in a previously susceptible species. Bacteria identified as resistant have an minimal inhibitory concentration (MIC) greater than a defined breakpoint (see p. 33) or a small zone of inhibition on the agar disc diffusion test defined by accepted standards (National Committee for Clinical Laboratory Standards, 1995). Mechanisms by which bacteria become resistant are shown in Table 1. These mechanisms can be grouped into three broad categories: (1) decreased antibiotic entry into bacteria, (2) altered target site, or (3) synthesis of enzymes that modify the drug.

TABLE 1. **Important Resistance Mechanisms for Antibacterial Agents**

Drug	Mechanism	Example
Beta-lactams		
Penicillins*	Decreased entry	Gram-negative bacteria
	Altered target (PBP†)	Resistant enterococci and staphylococci
	Production of enzymes	Synthesis of beta-lactamase enzyme
Cephalosporins‡	Decreased entry	*Pseudomonas aeruginosa*
	Altered target (PBP)	Resistant enterococci
	Production of enzymes	*Escherichia coli*
Chloramphenicol	Production of enzymes	Synthesis of acetyltransferase by many bacteria
	Decreased entry	*P. aeruginosa*
Aminoglycosides§	Production of enzymes	*Escherichia coli,* enterococci
	Decreased entry	*P. aeruginosa*
	Altered target (ribosomes)	Gram-negative bacteria
Erythromycin	Decreased entry	Most gram-negative bacteria
	Altered target (ribosome)	Staphylococci
Lincomycin, clindamycin	Altered target (ribosome)	Gram-negative bacteria, staphylococci
Fluoroquinolones‖	Altered target (gyrA)	*E. coli, P. aeruginosa,* staphylococci
Trimethoprim-sulfonamides	Altered target	Many bacteria
Tetracycline	Altered target (ribosomes)	Many bacteria
	Increased (active) efflux	Many bacteria
Vancomycin	Altered cell wall target	Enterococci

*Includes penicillin G, ampicillin, amoxicillin, and derivatives.
†PBP, penicillin-binding proteins.
‡Includes cefazolin, cephalothin, cephalexin.
§Includes gentamicin, tobramycin, kanamycin, amikacin.
‖Includes ciprofloxacin, enrofloxacin, difloxacin, and orbifloxacin.

MANAGING RESISTANT INFECTIONS

When a bacterial infection is believed to be caused by resistant bacteria, switching among antibiotics without any justification will prolong the problem and most likely will be expensive. Veterinarians should use a consistent, rational approach to dealing with resistant infections. Initially, it should be established whether the lack of response is caused by a bona fide resistant bacteria or other factors. Recall that susceptibility tests assume that the drug plasma concentration is approximately equal to the tissue fluid concentration and do not take into consideration the local factors that may account for treatment failure. A summary of other reasons for drug failure is shown in Table 2.

Obtaining a Valid Culture of the Bacteria

Whenever possible, a culture should be obtained to assess an infection suspected to be caused by resistant bacteria. Second, the susceptibility of antibacterial drugs should be tested in a valid laboratory that uses recognized protocols. In-house methods, although convenient, may not adhere tightly enough to rigid procedural guidelines that are necessary to obtain a verifiable susceptibility result for resistant bacteria. Whenever possible, one should adhere to the guidelines of the National Committee on Clinical Laboratory Standards (National Committee for Clinical Laboratory Standards, 1995) for interpreting test results.

Should Resistant Bacteria Always Be Treated?

The difference between *colonization* and *infection* must be recognized. Resistant bacteria may be cultured from a catheter tip, endotracheal tube, or a swab of tissue or fluid.

In many instances, the bacteria cultured represent local colonization and not a serious infection. *(Just because a bacteria is cultured from an endotracheal tube does not mean that the patient has pneumonia.)* The decision to expose the patient to potent, and potentially toxic, antibiotics must be made carefully. Good clinical judgment and experience are the best guides to determine the significance of a culture result.

TABLE 2. **Reasons for Drug Failure Other Than Drug Resistance**

Mechanism of Drug Failure	Clinical Example
Anatomic barriers to diffusion	Treating an infection associated with a large abscess
Immune deficiency	Treating patient that has neutropenia or feline leukemia virus
Drug antagonism	Administration of penicillin combined with tetracycline may result in drug antagonism
Failure to recognize infection caused by anaerobic bacteria	Drugs such as fluoroquinolones have poor activity against anaerobes
Failure to recognize infection caused by fungus or virus	Unresponsive skin infections are often associated with dermatophytes
Failure to consider local factors that may decrease drug activity	Infection contaminated with pus or cellular debris will not respond well to drugs such as aminoglycosides or glycopeptides
Presence of foreign material	Bacteria associated with foreign body are protected from antibiotics and patient's defense mechanisms
Confusing bacterial sepsis with other diseases	Immune-mediated disease, vasculitis, or thromboembolism may appear as bacterial infection

PROBLEM BACTERIA

Pseudomonas aeruginosa

Pseudomonas aeruginosa is a problem bacteria by virtue of its ability to rapidly develop high-level resistance. It is a water-loving bacteria and thrives in moist environments such as dog's ears, urine, and locations in the hospital such as water baths, sinks, and animal runs. *P. aeruginosa* has even been known to survive in disinfectant solutions, irrigation solutions, ointments, and soap dishes.

P. aeruginosa has inherent resistance to many drugs because it lacks high-permeability porin proteins by which antibiotics gain access to bacteria. Without these porin channels, many antibiotics cannot gain access to the sites of action or will pass through so slowly as to be ineffective. *P. aeruginosa* also becomes resistant via beta-lactamase synthesis and an efflux system that can pump some antibiotics out of the cell. Beta-lactamase from *P. aeruginosa* inactivates penicillins and cephalosporins and is not affected by clavulanate.

A wild strain of *P. aeruginosa* will likely be resistant to most common drugs but susceptible to amikacin, gentamicin, or tobramycin; extended-spectrum penicillins (ticarcillin, piperacillin); some selected third-generation cephalosporins (ceftazidime or cefoperazone); carbapenems (imipenem-cilastatin, Primaxin, Merck & Co.); and perhaps a fluoroquinolone (enrofloxacin, difloxacin, or orbifloxacin). However, *P. aeruginosa* may develop resistance to any or all of these drugs. In one veterinary survey (Hariharan et al, 1995), the only drugs that had a high degree of activity against *P. aeruginosa* among those tested were tobramycin, amikacin, ceftazidime, and cefoperazone. Only 50% were sensitive to enrofloxacin, and 70% were sensitive to carbenicillin.

Treatment

A valid susceptibility test is necessary to consider possible antimicrobial drug choices. If a beta-lactam or aminoglycoside is used, animal studies have shown that a combination of ticarcillin (Ticar, Smithkline Beecham) plus either gentamicin (Gentocin, Schering-Plough), tobramycin (Nebcin, Lilly), or amikacin (Amiglyde-V, Fort Dodge) are more effective than single drugs. Moreover, data from studies in humans indicate that treatment with a beta-lactam alone (e.g., ticarcillin or ceftazidime) is associated with increased emergence of resistance. Including an aminoglycoside reduces this risk. For this reason, it is recommended, at least during the initial phase of treatment, that a combination of these two drug groups be administered. We recommend either ticarcillin or ceftazidime in combination with one of the aminoglycosides. This combination should not be mixed in the same syringe or vial because incompatibility will cause drug inactivation. In some cases, the only drug identified for which *Pseudomonas* is susceptible is the carbapenem imipenem-cilastatin sodium.* If imipenem is used, consult a reliable drug reference or the package insert because there is a strict procedure for preparing and administering this drug.

Administration of Aminoglycosides. Several studies in human medicine and laboratory animals indicate that once-daily dosing is at least as effective and perhaps not as toxic as doses administered twice or three times daily (Freeman et al, 1997). In addition, once-daily dosing may be more bactericidal and less likely to cause resistant bacterial strains (see p. 33). Unfortunately, there are no published clinical reports to support these dose rates in small animals, but evidence from other species is so persuasive that our dosing regimens in small animals usually employ a single daily dose. As an example of a single-dose regimen used in our hospital, we administer gentamicin (Gentocin, Schering-Plough) at a dose of 7 to 10 mg/kg and amikacin (Amiglyde-V, Fort Dodge) at a dose of 10 to 15 mg/kg. Either drug is administered once daily (preferably in the morning) IV, SC, or IM.

Administration of Fluoroquinolones. *Pseudomonas* may be susceptible to the fluoroquinolones, but it is important to note that the MIC may be higher than for other susceptible gram-negative bacteria (such as *Escherichia coli*), and this will necessitate doses at the highest end of the range (Walker et al, 1992).* Because we anticipate a high MIC for *P. aeruginosa* in our hospital, we routinely initiate treatment with enrofloxacin (Baytril, Bayer) at a minimum dose of 10 mg/kg every 24 hours. If the MIC is 1.0 µg/ml, 20 mg/kg every 24 hours, or 10 mg/kg every 12 hours is used. If orbifloxacin (Orbax, Schering-Plough) or difloxacin (Dicural, Fort Dodge) is used instead of enrofloxacin, the highest dose in the range is administered.*

Ear Infections. Ear infections present the most common situation in which resistant *P. aeruginosa* is identified in small animals. The moist environment and previous drug therapy aimed at yeasts and other competing organisms cause *Pseudomonas* to thrive in the external and middle ear. When this infection is chronic, the organism often has become resistant to many antimicrobials.

Some veterinarians have experienced success with topical administration of enrofloxacin for otitis externa caused by *Pseudomonas*. For these cases, a 22.7 mg/ml injectable solution of enrofloxacin has been mixed with saline, water, or other topical ear solution in a 1:1 to 4:1 ratio (e.g., 4 parts saline, 1 part enrofloxacin). Stability studies by this author have confirmed these solutions to be stable for 2 weeks at room temperature. The admixture is instilled into the ear canal two or three times daily for 2 weeks. When it is believed that there is an infection of the middle ear, and the tympanum is intact, topical treatment alone is not sufficient and systemic treatment for *Pseudomonas* as described earlier should be used.

Enterococci

Enterococci are gram-positive cocci that have emerged as important causes of infections, especially those that are nosocomial. The most common species identified are *Enterococcus faecalis* and *E. faecium*. Until 1984, these bacteria were in the genus *Streptococcus*, but they are

---

*The author has provided doses for all drugs discussed in this article in the Appendix of this book.

*The author has provided doses for all drugs discussed in this article in the Appendix of this book.

now recognized as a unique genus. Enterococci carry the Lancefield group D streptococcal antigen. The most common sites of infection are the urine, wound infections, and blood stream. *E. faecalis* is more common, but *E. faecium* is usually the more resistant. Wild-strain enterococci may still be sensitive to penicillin G and ampicillin or amoxicillin. The enterococci have an inherent resistance to cephalosporins and fluoroquinolones, although newer generations of fluoroquinolones are being developed that have better activity against enterococci.

Enterococci can develop high-level resistance to both aminoglycosides and the penicillins. Resistance to beta-lactam antibiotics is caused by production of a low-affinity penicillin-binding protein (PBP) (PBP-5), which assumes the role of cell wall synthesis when other PBPs have been inhibited. These strains also are usually resistant to trimethoprim-sulfonamide combinations, clindamycin, and erythromycin. Susceptibility test results for cephalosporins, beta-lactamase–resistant penicillins (e.g., oxacillin), trimethoprim-sulfonamide combinations, and clindamycin can give misleading results. Even if isolates are susceptible on the basis of an in vitro test to a fluoroquinolone, this class of drugs may not be a good alternative for treatment.

The emergence of enterococci resistance in people has been linked to overuse of cephalosporin and fluoroquinolone antibiotics, neither of which has activity against enterococci. Most recently in people, strains of enterococci have been identified that are resistant to vancomycin because of plasmids that carry the *vanA* gene. This leaves virtually *no* drugs available to treat these infections. In Europe, enterococcal resistance to glycopeptides has been associated with administration of these drugs to food animals. (Note: It is illegal to administer glycopeptides to food animals in the United States.)

Treatment

Treatment is frustrating because there are so few drug choices. If the *Enterococcus* isolated is sensitive to penicillins, amoxicillin or ampicillin should be administered at the high end of the dose range* because protocols for interpreting susceptibility test results allow enterococci to have a higher MIC than other susceptible organisms (National Committee for Clinical Laboratory Standards, 1995). Whenever possible, an aminoglycoside should be combined with a beta-lactam antibiotic when treating serious infections. Each drug is poorly bactericidal against enterococci when used alone, but synergistic when administered in combination.

Occasionally, one of the carbapenems (imipenem-cilastatin) or an extended-spectrum penicillin (e.g., piperacillin) can be considered for treatment of *E. faecalis* (but not *E. faecium*). Usually, however, when strains are resistant to beta-lactam antibiotics and aminoglycosides, the only active drugs will be the glycopeptides.

Of the glycopeptides, vancomycin is the only one used in veterinary medicine. Teicoplanin is used in Europe but is not available in the United States. Vancomycin (Vancocin, Lilly) should be given only as an IV infusion administered over 30 to 60 minutes. It is not absorbed orally and is too painful when injected intramuscularly. The dose to maintain concentrations within the therapeutic range, and avoid toxicity is 15 mg/kg, every 6 to 8 hours, IV. For successful therapy, especially when treating endocarditis, an aminoglycoside such as gentamicin or amikacin should be administered with vancomycin.

Is Treatment Always Necessary? Not all enterococcal infections must be treated (Nichols and Mizik, 1992). *Enterococcus* may not be pathogenic except when it occurs in the blood stream. When it occurs at other sites, especially wound infections or in the abdomen, studies have failed to demonstrate an important role. Usually these infections are polymicrobial. In experimental animals, when drugs are administered that are active against other organisms in the mixed infection, but not necessarily active against *Enterococcus*, the animal has a good chance for cure (Nichols and Mizik, 1992). However, if the infection is in the blood stream or central nervous system, or if there is a strong likelihood that the infection could seed a blood stream infection, it should be treated aggressively.

Staphylococcus

Staphylococcus aureus, and occasionally other staphylococcal species, have become among the most dangerous of the resistant bacteria causing nosocomial infections in humans. Most staphylococci produce a beta-lactamase enzyme that hydrolyzes the beta-lactam ring of penicillin and other penicillins. The development of beta-lactamase–resistant penicillins (oxacillin, dicloxacillin), cephalosporins (e.g., cephalexin), and beta-lactamase inhibitors (clavulanic acid) has allowed physicians and veterinarians to treat these infections effectively. However, another resistance mechanism has emerged. An altered target, the penicillin-binding protein 2a (PBP 2a), renders all of the beta-lactam antibiotics ineffective. Because these bacteria are resistant to even the beta-lactamase–resistant penicillins, they are referred to as methicillin-resistant staphylococci (MRSA when it involves *S. aureus*).

Although there is no direct mechanism to cause cross-resistance, MRSA also is usually resistant to clindamycin, erythromycin, fluoroquinolones, and tetracyclines. In most cases, these bacteria can be treated only with a glycopeptide antibiotic (e.g., vancomycin).

Fortunately, in small animal veterinary medicine, most staphylococcal infections are caused by *S. intermedius*. Isolation of pathogenic *S. aureus* is unusual. According to reports of canine *S. intermedius* susceptibility, resistance to first-generation cephalosporins (e.g., cephalexin, cefadroxil), amoxicillin-clavulanate (Clavamox, Pfizer Animal Health), and beta-lactamase–resistant penicillins (oxacillin, cloxacillin) is rare. It is also encouraging that despite widespread use of these antibiotics in small animals, the pattern of resistance to these drugs has not changed in the last 10 years (Lloyd et al, 1996). If patients have been previously treated with antimicrobial drugs (e.g., because of recurrent pyoderma), clinical reports indicate that there is a greater likelihood that *S. intermedius* will be resistant to clindamycin, lincomycin, tetracyclines, and chloramphenicol.

---

*The author has provided doses for all drugs discussed in this article in the Appendix of this book.

Treatment of Resistant Infections

If staphylococci are resistant to oxacillin or methicillin, they should be considered resistant to all other beta-lactams, regardless of the susceptibility test result. Staphylococcal infections in small animals resistant to the beta-lactam antibiotics listed earlier should be tested for susceptibility to clindamycin or a fluoroquinolone. Occasionally, these drugs may still be active. In some instances, the only drug that is active for treatment will be a glycopeptide such as vancomycin. Doses for vancomycin were discussed earlier for enterococci.

Coliform Bacteria

Coliform bacteria, which are enteric gram-negative bacilli, have often been associated with resistance problems. The prolific rate at which they develop resistance is because of their ability to transfer plasmids. The most common location for infections caused by these bacteria has been the urine, but infections also may occur in the respiratory tract and soft tissues. The bacteria most often implicated in resistance problems have been *E. coli*, *Klebsiella pneumoniae*, *Enterobacter* spp., and *Proteus* spp. Of the *Proteus* species, *P. mirabilis* is indole-negative and usually susceptible; *P. vulgaris* is indole-positive and usually more resistant.

Newer drugs in use in the last 10 years have improved our ability to treat resistant infections. Strains that were resistant to penicillins, aminoglycosides, and first-generation cephalosporins have been sensitive to fluoroquinolones, extended-spectrum cephalosporins, and carbapenems. However, some resistant strains have emerged. Some strains produce extended-spectrum beta-lactamase that inactivates even the third-generation cephalosporins.

Treatment

After obtaining a valid culture, it must be determined which drug is the most rational to use. In some instances, fluoroquinolones such as enrofloxacin, difloxacin, or orbifloxacin may be used, but high-level resistance is possible. A culture report should be examined for susceptibility against imipenem, a second-generation cephalosporin (e.g., cefoxitin) or a third-generation cephalosporin (e.g., cefotaxime) because in some instances these may be the only active drugs.* There are some extended-spectrum beta-lactamases produced by these bacteria that may inactivate first- and third-generation cephalosporins but not second-generation cephalosporins or imipenem. Therefore, one must use a susceptibility test that provides a complete spectrum of choices.

Since most second- and third-generation cephalosporins and the carbapenems are only administered parenterally, an oral drug is valuable when convenience is needed to treat resistant infections on an outpatient basis. Cefixime (Suprax) is one of the only two oral third-generation cephalosporins. It is available as a liquid suspension and tablets

and has been administered to dogs (10 mg/kg, every 12 hours) when oral therapy is desired.

Anaerobic Bacteria

Ordinarily, most anaerobes are highly susceptible to penicillins, (including ampicillin), clindamycin, chloramphenicol, and metronidazole, but *Bacteroides* is an exception. The inducible beta-lactamase from *B. fragilis* also is a cephalosporinase (not inhibited by clavulanate), but the beta-lactamase from other anaerobes usually can be inhibited by clavulanate. Some organisms from this group can be resistant to metronidazole but metronidazole resistance is rare. *Bacteroides* that were more likely to be sensitive, and were found primarily in infections of the head, neck, and mouth, are now in the genera *Prevotella* and *Porphyromonas* (the "pigmented *Bacteroides*"). Those that are now included in the *B. fragilis* group can cause resistant infections, especially in the abdomen.

In a veterinary survey of anaerobic bacteria isolated from dogs and cats, most of the anaerobic organisms identified belonged to the *B. fragilis* group, *Peptostreptococcus*, *Fusobacterium*, or *Porphyromonas*. All were sensitive to the combination of clavulanic acid and amoxicillin (Clavamox, Pfizer Animal Health) and chloramphenicol. Most were sensitive to metronidazole. However, the authors found that there was a trend toward a higher percentage of *Bacteroides* isolates that were resistant to ampicillin and clindamycin, compared with previous surveys (Jang et al, 1997).

Treatment

Treatment of anaerobic infections caused by the *B. fragilis* group is complicated by a lack of standardized susceptibility tests. Second-generation cephalosporins resistant to beta-lactamase (e.g., cefoxitin and cefotetan*) will be active and are a good choice, particularly when there is a mixed infection with gram-negative bacilli. Clindamycin (Antirobe, Pharmacia and Upjohn) also may be active against anaerobes that are resistant to beta-lactams.

PREVENTION AND CONTROL OF RESISTANCE

We cannot prevent resistance. It will always occur. To minimize the development of resistance, effective use of antimicrobial drugs is critical. Antibacterial drugs must be administered at appropriately high doses and irrational combinations must be avoided (see p. 33). Routine use of extended-spectrum cephalosporins and carbapenems (e.g., imipenem) should be avoided because these drugs can induce beta-lactamase–mediated resistance. When administering prophylactic antibiotics, they should be administered immediately before surgery and not sooner. It was shown in one study that when cefazolin was administered too long before a surgical procedure, postoperative infections had a higher likelihood of being resistant to cefazolin. Antibiotics

---

*The author has provided doses for all drugs discussed in this article in the Appendix of this book.

*The author has provided doses for all drugs discussed in this article in the Appendix of this book.

should not be administered for longer than 24 hours after an uncontaminated or uninfected surgical procedure. There is no rational basis for longer courses of therapy.

In animal hospitals, precautions should be taken to prevent the spread of resistant infections. Animals that have resistant infections should be isolated if they will be staying in the hospital. In a hospital, a color-coded tagging system can be used to identify the patient's record and cage when there is a resistant infection. This will alert hospital staff handling this animal that it has a resistant infection and identify the cage for thorough disinfection after the patient has been discharged. When performing routine treatments, animals with resistant infection should be treated as the last in a series. Hospital staff should be instructed to wear disposable gloves and practice careful hygiene when handling fluids or excreta from these patients. Finally, whenever possible, the hospital stays for these animals should be short.

References and Suggested Reading

Freeman CD, Nicolau DP, Belliveau PP, et al: Once-daily dosing of aminoglycosides: Review and recommendations for clinical practice. J Antimicrob Chemother 39:677, 1997.
This is one of the most current comprehensive references that cites evidence for once-daily dosing of aminoglycosides.

Hariharan H, McPhee L, Heaney S, et al: Antimicrobial drug susceptibility of clinical isolates of *Pseudomonas aeruginosa*. Can Vet J 36:166, 1995.
This is one of the few references that reports on the susceptibility pattern of Pseudomonas isolated from veterinary species.

Jang SS, Breher JE, Dabaco LA, et al: Organisms isolated from dogs and cats with anaerobic infections and susceptibility to selected antimicrobial agents. J Am Vet Med Assoc 210:1610, 1997.

Lloyd DH, Lamport AI, Feeney C: Sensitivity to antibiotics amongst cutaneous and mucosal isolates of canine pathogenic staphylococci in the UK, 1980–1996. Vet Derm 7:171, 1996.
This is one of the most recent and useful references that describes staphylococcal susceptibility patterns from isolates of dogs.

National Committee for Clinical Laboratory Standards (NCCLS): NCCLS Document M7-A3. Vol. 15, No. 14. National Committee for Clinical Laboratory Standards, 771 East Lancaster Ave., Villanova, PA. 19085, 1995.
This is a critical document for performing and interpreting culture and sensitivity results for resistant infections.

Neu HC: The crisis in antibiotic resistance. Science 257:1064, 1992.
This is a thorough and often-quoted reference that summarizes the current problem in antibacterial drug resistance that has caused serious problems in human medicine.

Nichols RL, Mizik AC: Enterococcal infections in surgical patients: The mystery continues. Clin Infect Dis 15:72, 1992.
This reference is helpful for veterinarians to understand the importance of enterococcal infections in animals.

Walker RD, Stein GE, Hauptman JG, et al: Pharmacokinetic evaluation of enrofloxacin administered orally to healthy dogs. Am J Vet Res 53:2315, 1992.

Antimicrobial Therapy for the Neutropenic Dog and Cat

ANTHONY C.G. ABRAMS-OGG
STEPHEN A. KRUTH
Guelph, Ontario, Canada

Neutropenia most commonly results from impaired granulopoiesis or overwhelming infection (for specific causes of neutropenia see *CVT XII,* p. 452 and p. 447 in this volume). No clinical signs are caused by neutropenia itself; signs are due to the underlying disease and infection. There is an increased risk of bacterial and fungal infections developing during neutropenia, and established infections are more difficult to treat. Most neutropenic animals acquire a fever when infections occur. Occasionally, only lethargy, inappetence, and tachycardia are present. Animals may present in septic shock with severe infections. The signs of local inflammation are subtle if granulopoiesis is impaired, and the site of infection may be difficult to identify.

Several factors affect the risk and outcome of infection, the most important of which are severity and duration of neutropenia. Animals should be considered at risk for opportunistic infections when neutrophil counts fall to less than $2.0 \times 10^9/L$ (2,000/μl). The risk increases exponentially with worsening neutropenia; so, animals are at moderate, high, and very high risk for infection with neutrophil counts less than or equal to $1.0 \times 10^9/L$ (1,000/μl), $0.5 \times 10^9/L$ (500/μl), and $0.2 \times 10^9/L$ (200/μl), respectively. Falling neutrophil counts are associated with a higher risk of infection than are stable neutrophil counts. Infections are less likely to develop in cats with low neutrophil counts than in dogs with similar counts.

Most infections can be controlled with appropriate antimicrobial therapy when neutropenia is of short duration (less than 7 days). Infections complicating neutropenia of moderate duration (7 to 14 days) are more difficult to treat. Infections in patients with prolonged neutropenia (longer than 14 days) are even more difficult to treat, especially if the neutrophil count is less than $0.2 \times 10^9/L$ (200/μl).

Disruption of natural barriers and immunosuppression increase the risk and severity of neutropenic infections. Natural barriers are disrupted with gastrointestinal damage during parvoviral infections and anticancer chemotherapy, facilitating invasion by enteric bacteria. Intravenous catheterization increases the risk of infection with cutaneous organisms. Immunosuppression may be present concurrent with myelosuppression because of the primary disease, malnutrition, or therapy. There is an increased risk of infection in neutropenic humans if there is concurrent lymphopenia or monocytopenia.

MICROBIOLOGY

Infections secondary to neutropenia may be due to environmental, nosocomial, or contagious organisms, but the greatest source of infection is the patient's own flora, especially that of the intestinal tract. Organisms most frequently isolated are gram-negative enteric bacilli (*Escherichia coli*, *Klebsiella* spp., *Enterobacter* spp.), followed by gram-positive cocci (*Staphylococcus* spp., *Streptococcus* spp.). *Pseudomonas* spp. are less frequently isolated but are of concern because of antimicrobial resistance. Although anaerobic bacteria occur in large numbers in the intestinal tract, they are not commonly the first invaders in opportunistic infection during neutropenia. There is evidence, however, that *Clostridium perfringens* contributes to sepsis during parvoviral infections (Turk et al, 1992). Clostridia are important nosocomial pathogens in some veterinary hospitals, but their role in causing sepsis during neutropenia is unknown.

The most common sites of infection are the blood stream (bacteremia) and the lung. Pneumonia may be due to upper respiratory flora or translocation of intestinal bacteria. Local cellulitis may occur, manifesting as edema of one or more limbs. Other possible sites of infection include the oral cavity, gastrointestinal tract, urinary tract, heart, and central nervous system.

Fungal infections with *Candida* spp. and *Aspergillus* spp. may occur, especially with prolonged antibacterial therapy. The prevalence of fungal infections in animals appears to be low in contrast to humans. This difference is partially due to the use of less aggressive anticancer chemotherapy protocols in veterinary medicine.

PATIENT MANAGEMENT

Neutropenia in dogs and cats is usually of short duration and mild to moderate severity. Prompt therapy with familiar antibiotics and good supportive care results in a successful outcome in most cases.

Isolation reduces the risk of acquiring infection. Neutropenic animals not requiring critical care should be maintained at home and confined to the house and yard. In the veterinary hospital, contact with the general patient population should be avoided. Hands should be washed thoroughly and laboratory coats changed prior to handling neutropenic animals; gloves and isolation gowns should be considered for severe cases. Thermometer use should be restricted to the particular patient. Only canned foods should be fed to dogs and cats with severe neutropenia; table scraps should be avoided.

Antimicrobial Therapy

Antimicrobial therapy remains the cornerstone of management of neutropenia. It can be divided into three catego-

ries: (1) prophylactic therapy, (2) empirical treatment during febrile episodes, and (3) treatment of documented infection.

Prophylactic Therapy

Antimicrobial prophylaxis in the asymptomatic patient should be considered whenever a neutrophil count less than $0.5 \times 10^9/L$ ($500/\mu l$) is present or anticipated. Antimicrobial therapy is directed at the intestinal flora, with the principal objective of reducing the gram-negative and gram-positive organisms most often responsible for infections. The anaerobic population should be left relatively undisturbed, as it contributes to resistance to fungal overgrowth and colonization by pathogens. A second objective of prophylactic therapy is to provide sufficient tissue drug levels to contain an incipient bacterial infection. Choices for prophylactic therapy are presented in Table 1.

Antimicrobial prophylaxis is controversial. Potential advantages include a reduced infection rate, an increased time to onset of infection, and a reduced speed in which an incipient infection develops into overwhelming sepsis. These benefits facilitate home management of neutropenic animals and improve quality of life. Prophylactic therapy is most likely to be beneficial during severe, prolonged neutropenia. Potential disadvantages include emergence of resistant organisms and drug-induced inappetence, vomiting, and diarrhea, especially in cats (Kunkle et al, 1995). Antimicrobial prophylaxis may also be an unnecessary expense, although treating sepsis is more expensive than preventing it.

We currently use cephalexin prophylaxis for dogs receiving sequential chemotherapy of lymphoma with L-asparaginase, vincristine, cyclophosphamide, and doxorubicin (Matus, 1989), although the benefit is not proven. We do not routinely use antimicrobial prophylaxis during other chemotherapy protocols—for example, cyclophosphamide, vincristine (Oncovin), and prednisone (COP); vincristine, doxorubicin (Adriamycin), and cyclophosphamide (VAC); or single-drug protocols. Prophylaxis is initiated in any asymptomatic animal when a neutrophil count less than $0.5 \times 10^9/L$ ($500/\mu l$) is noted during pretreatment evaluation and is continued until recovery of the count to greater than $2 \times 10^9/L$ ($2,000/\mu l$). Chemotherapeutic drugs are withheld until neutrophil recovery. Animals that have had an episode of chemotherapy-induced sepsis are also given antimicrobial prophylaxis during additional treatments. We also use prophylactic therapy when severe and prolonged neutropenia is anticipated, such as with pancytopenia caused by phenylbutazone in dogs and retroviral infections in cats. Antifungal prophylaxis with nystatin, itraconazole, or fluconazole is used in humans but does not appear to be necessary for animals.

Empirical Treatment of Febrile Neutropenic Patients

Asymptomatic neutropenic animals and animals at risk for neutropenia should have their body temperatures monitored. Depending on anticipated risk, this may vary from measuring temperature when animals show signs of leth-

TABLE 1. Prophylactic Oral Antimicrobial Therapy for the Neutropenic Dog and Cat

Antimicrobial Agent	Dosage	Comment
Trimethoprim-sulfamethoxazole (Apo-Sulfatrim, Apotex)	15 mg/kg (combined dose) q12h	Inexpensive No prophylaxis against *Pseudomonas* spp. Risk for keratoconjunctivitis sicca with prolonged use May retard marrow recovery following severe myelosuppression
Trimethoprim-sulfadiazine (Tribrissen, Schering-Plough)	15 mg/kg (combined dose) q12h	As with trimethoprim-sulfamethoxazole, but more expensive
Ormetoprim-sulfadimethoxine (Primor, Pfizer)	55 mg/kg on first day, then 27.5 mg/kg q24h	As with trimethoprim-sulfamethoxazole, but more expensive
Enrofloxacin (Baytril, Bayer)	5–10 mg/kg q12h	Expensive Prophylaxis against *Pseudomonas* spp. More inappetence and vomiting than at higher doses with other choices?
Ciprofloxacin (Cipro, Bayer)	7.5–15 mg/kg q12h	As with enrofloxacin Smaller tablets with higher strength than enrofloxacin
Orbifloxacin (Orbax, Schering-Plough)	2.5–5.0 mg/kg q12h	Less well evaluated than enrofloxacin and ciprofloxacin
Cephalexin (Novo-Lexin, Novopharm)	30 mg/kg q12h	Expensive No prophylaxis against *Pseudomonas* spp. Better bioavailability of capsule formulation compared with tablets?
Amoxicillin (Moxilean, MTC)	10–20 mg/kg q12h	Inexpensive No prophylaxis against *Pseudomonas* spp. Not first choice, acceptable for cats not tolerating other choices Ampicillin causes more intestinal disturbance than does amoxicillin
Amoxicillin-clavulanate (Clavamox, Pfizer)	12.5–25 mg/kg q12h	Expensive No prophylaxis against *Pseudomonas* spp. Not first choice, acceptable for cats not tolerating other choices Increased activity against *Staphylococcus* spp., *Klebsiella* spp., *Escherichia coli*, and *Bacteroides* spp. compared with amoxicillin

Modified from Abrams-Ogg ACG, Kruth SA: Infections associated with neutropenia in the dog and cat. In: Prescott JF, Baggot JD, eds: Antimicrobial Therapy in Veterinary Medicine, 2nd ed. Ames, IA: Iowa State University Press, p 383, 1993, with permission.

argy or inappetence to monitoring two to four times daily. Axillary temperature measurements facilitate home monitoring and are 0.5 to 1°C (1 to 2°F) lower than rectal temperature measurements. A rectal temperature greater than 39°C (102.2°F) in dogs and 39.2°C (102.6°F) in cats should be regarded with suspicion. A rectal temperature greater than 39.5°C (103.1°F) should be considered to be a true fever.

Fever or unexplained depression and inappetence in a neutropenic animal should be considered bacterial in origin until proved otherwise. The animal should be examined carefully for subtle signs of inflammation, and an appropriate specimen obtained for culture. Blood cultures should be considered if there is no obvious site of infection. Our protocol is to obtain two simultaneous blood samples for culture of 5 to 15 ml with blood obtained from different veins (Reller, 1994). However, blood cultures are expensive. Furthermore, results take 2 to 7 days and are often negative and frequently do not alter initial therapy. For these reasons, we do not always perform blood cultures during anticancer chemotherapy when the anticipated duration of neutropenia is short, nor do we routinely perform them in animals with parvoviral infections. Blood cultures should always be performed if the cause of neutropenia is not known or if the animal is severely ill.

Additional tests are required in an effort to localize infection and characterize the severity of illness. We obtain serum glucose, urea, and electrolyte levels and urine specific gravity in all patients. Thoracic radiographs should be obtained and culture of airway (transtracheal or bronchoalveolar) lavage samples performed when respiratory signs are present and when the cause of neutropenia is not known. We routinely obtain thoracic radiographs in cancer patients and perform an airway lavage culture if there are radiographic signs of pneumonia. However, normal thoracic radiographs do not rule out pneumonia, and an airway lavage should be considered if the animal is severely ill without localizing signs, if respiratory signs develop, or if the animal does not respond to antimicrobial therapy.

Urinalysis and urine culture should be performed if there are any historical or physical signs of urinary tract disease. Cystocentesis should not be performed if the platelet count is less than or equal to 50×10^9/L (50,000/μl), and catheterization should be avoided because of the risk of introducing infection. Free catch samples submitted for quantitative culture suffice in these cases. A serum chemistry profile should be obtained and abdominal radiographs or abdominal ultrasonographic examination performed if the animal is vomiting or exhibits abdominal pain. These tests are also performed if the cause of neutropenia is not known or if the animal is severely ill. Results of the tests may prompt invasive biopsy procedures.

Empirical antimicrobial therapy should be initiated while awaiting culture results. The drugs chosen should be bactericidal and have limited marrow toxicity and should be active against gram-negative enteric bacilli, *Pseudomonas* spp., and gram-positive cocci. Drug selection may be assisted by previous culture results, localizing signs, Gram staining of body fluid, and antibiotic susceptibility testing of nosocomial pathogens. If there is a history of fluoroquinolone prophylaxis, a febrile episode likely is caused by a gram-positive or anaerobic organism. Standard drug dosages are employed. A representative selection of antimicrobial drugs is presented in Table 2. Historically, combination therapy has been preferred over a single agent to increase the antibacterial spectrum, take advantage of additive and synergistic effects while minimizing toxicity, and reduce resistance. Most approaches have combined an aminoglycoside with a beta-lactam antibiotic. Other approaches have been advocated to avoid aminoglycoside nephrotoxicity

and improve efficacy. When enrofloxacin is used, it should be noted that it has limited activity against gram-positive and anaerobic organisms, especially in neutropenic patients (see p. 41). For infections complicating the episodes of neutropenia usually encountered by veterinarians, the various protocols are probably of equivalent efficacy. We currently use enrofloxacin plus cefazolin in cancer patients; ampicillin plus gentamicin, or cefoxitin, for parvoviral infections; and imipenem-cilastatin for initial therapy in animals with overwhelming sepsis associated with severe neutropenia of undetermined cause.

Intravenous administration is preferred initially. Intravenous catheterization is better tolerated than repetitive venipuncture for drug injection and is often necessary for fluid therapy. However, there must be strict adherence to asepsis during catheter placement. Povidone-iodine ointment should be placed over the skin entry site and the site bandaged. Injection ports should be cleaned with alcohol and allowed to dry prior to injection. The catheter should be removed promptly and cultured if signs of phlebitis

TABLE 2. Empirical Antimicrobial Therapy for the Febrile Neutropenic Dog or Cat

Antimicrobial Drug	Comment
Combination Therapy	
Aminoglycoside + cefazolin or cephalothin (first-generation cephalosporin)	Commonly used in veterinary medicine
	Relatively inexpensive
	Spectrum may not cover *Pseudomonas* spp.
	Cephalosporin increases risk of nephrotoxicity?
Aminoglycoside + ampicillin	Commonly used for treatment of parvoviral infections
	Relatively inexpensive
	Spectrum may not cover *Pseudomonas* or *Staphylococcus* spp.
	Increased activity against anaerobes over preceding combinations
	Disturbance of gastrointestinal flora common
Aminoglycoside + antipseudomonal penicillin or ceftazidime	More expensive than preceding combinations
	Synergy against *Pseudomonas* spp. and Enterobacteriaceae
	Less activity against gram-positive organisms
	Can prevent beta-lactamase activity by using ticarcillin-clavulanate
Enrofloxacin substituted for aminoglycoside in preceding combinations	Less well evaluated than are aminoglycoside combinations
	More expensive than aminoglycosides
	Avoids aminoglycoside nephrotoxicity
	Combinations more likely to be additive than synergistic
Combination of two beta-lactam antibiotics*	Avoids aminoglycoside nephrotoxicity
	Resistance more likely to develop?
	Prolongation of neutropenia?
	Potential antagonism
Single Agents	
Cefoxitin (second-generation cephalosporin [cefamycin])	Substitute for aminoglycoside + ampicillin
	Not effective against *Pseudomonas* spp.
	Effective against anaerobes
	Disturbance of gastrointestinal flora common
Ceftazidime (third-generation cephalosporin)	Expensive
	Less activity against gram-positive organisms than combination therapy
Imipenem-cilastatin (carbapenem)	Expensive
	Active against complete antimicrobial spectrum

*For example, first-generation cephalosporin + antipseudomonal penicillin; first-generation cephalosporin + ceftazidime; ceftazidime + antipseudomonal penicillin.

Doses: *All IV injections are given as a slow push over 15 to 20 min unless indicated otherwise.* Optimal doses in recommended dose ranges are not known. In order to reduce the risks of nephrotoxicity when using aminoglycoside antibiotics, we prefer to use the lower doses and once daily administration. We avoid their use in dehydrated animals and in animals receiving furosemide. *Aminoglycosides:* amikacin (Amiglyde-V, Ayerst) 5–10 mg/kg q8h or 15–20 mg/kg q24h IV, IM, or SC; gentamicin (Gentocin, Schering-Plough) 2–4 mg/kg q8h or 5–6 mg/kg q24h IV, IM, or SC; netilmycin (Netromycin, Schering) 2–4 mg/kg q8h IV; tobramycin (Nebcin, Lilly) 2 mg/kg IV, IM, or SC. *Cephalosporins:* cefazolin (Cefazolin, Novopharm) 20–30 mg/kg q6–8h IV, IM, or SC; cephalothin (Keflin, Lilly) 25–40 mg/kg q6–8h IV, IM, or SC; cefoxitin (Cefoxitin, Novopharm) 20–40 mg/kg q6–8h IV; ceftazidime (Fortaz, Glaxo) 25–30 mg/kg q8h IV or SC. We usually dose these cephalosporins at 30 mg/kg q8h IV. *Antipseudomonal penicillins:* piperacillin (Pipracin, Wyeth-Ayerst) 50–70 mg/kg q6–8h IV or IM; ticarcillin (Ticar, SmithKline Beecham) 40–75 mg/kg q6–8h IV or IM; ticarcillin-clavulanate (Timentin, SmithKline Beecham) 30–50 mg/kg q6–8h IV. *Miscellaneous:* Ampicillin (Ampicin, Bristol-Myers Squibb) 20–40 mg/kg q6–8h IV, IM, or SC; enrofloxacin (Baytril, Bayer) 5–10 mg/kg q12h IV or IM; imipenem-cilastatin (Primaxin, Merck Sharp & Dohme) 3–10 mg/kg IV q8h (1-hour infusion). We usually use 5 mg/kg.

Modified from Abrams-Ogg ACG, Kruth SA: Infections associated with neutropenia in the dog and cat. In: Prescott JF, Baggot JD, eds: Antimicrobial Therapy in Veterinary Medicine, 2nd ed. Ames, IA: Iowa State University Press, p 386, 1993, with permission.

develop. If the duration of catheterization is anticipated to be more than a few days, a jugular catheter may be preferred.

Animals receiving aminoglycosides should be monitored for evidence of renal tubular damage (casts, glucosuria, azotemia), especially when the duration of therapy is longer than 5 days. Netilmicin is the least nephrotoxic aminoglycoside, followed by amikacin, tobramycin, and gentamicin, but it is also the most expensive drug. Enrofloxacin should be avoided in animals less than 6 months of age because of the possibility of inducing cartilage defects, although the risk for such defects following short courses of therapy at standard doses is not known. Many antibiotics inhibit platelet function (Catalfamo and Dodds, 1988). This effect is most pronounced with penicillins, and animals so treated should be observed for hemorrhage if there is concurrent thrombocytopenia, especially if the platelet count is less than or equal to $20 \times 10^9/L$ (20,000/μl). Fluoroquinolones have minimal effects on platelet function. Cefazolin does not inhibit platelet function in normal dogs (Wilkens et al, 1995).

Reduction of fever is expected within 72 hours of initiation of antimicrobial therapy, and the animal should appear more alert. (Increased depression accompanying a falling temperature may be a sign of impending septic shock.) The duration of antibacterial therapy is controversial. Prolonged therapy increases the expense, duration of hospitalization, and risk of fungal infection. Therapy should be continued for a minimum of 1 day, to a maximum of 7 days, beyond recovery of the neutrophil count to greater than 1.0 $\times$ $10^9/L$ (1,000/μl) and resolution of fever. Changing from intravenous therapy to oral therapy (see Table 1) during this period reduces expense and promotes earlier discharge from the hospital. For cancer patients without a documented site of infection during a febrile episode, we discontinue intravenous antimicrobial drugs the day following recovery of the neutrophil count to greater than or equal to 1.0 $\times$ $10^9/L$ (1,000/μl) and resolution of fever. We continue oral antimicrobial prophylaxis in animals that were receiving it and initiate oral therapy for 7 days in animals that were not receiving prophylaxis. Animals recovering from parvoviral infections generally do not require oral antimicrobial agents. In animals with pancytopenia in which prolonged neutropenia is anticipated, antimicrobial therapy is continued a minimum of 10 days beyond the resolution of fever.

Pyrexia may not resolve promptly if (1) it is not bacterial in origin, (2) the organism is not sensitive to the antimicrobial agent or agents, and (3) host defenses are sufficiently compromised that the infection and associated fever will not resolve with any antimicrobial agent. This last situation occurs during prolonged, severe neutropenia and is infrequently encountered in veterinary medicine. Initial culture results, if obtained, may assist therapeutic decision-making with unresponsive fever. If a resistant organism is documented, antimicrobial therapy may be changed based on susceptibility testing. Occasionally, the organism involved may be sensitive to the current medication, or a bacterial cause of the fever may not be documented, in which case another empirical judgment will be necessary. If the animal is stable, the current medication may be continued until resolution of fever and recovery of

the neutrophil count as previously discussed. If the animal's clinical status is deteriorating, different antimicrobial drugs should be employed and are usually added to existing therapy. The choice of additional drugs depends on which drugs were used for initial therapy. Failure of response to cefoxitin or an aminoglycoside plus first-generation cephalosporin would prompt additional therapy against *Pseudomonas* spp. with ticarcillin, piperacillin, ceftazidime, or imipenem-cilastatin. A resistant gram-negative enteric organism should be suspected if there are signs of intestinal damage—choices for additional therapy include an aminoglycoside, enrofloxacin, cefoxitin, ceftazidime, and imipenem-cilastatin. A resistant gram-positive organism should be suspected if there are signs of phlebitis or injury to the skin or oral cavity. The additional drug of choice in animals is clindamycin (Dalacin C Phosphate, Pharmacia & Upjohn), 10 mg/kg IV, SC every 12 hours, although the drug is bacteriostatic. Vancomycin and teicoplanin are the drugs of choice for resistant gram-positive infections in humans, but there is limited veterinary experience with these drugs. A nonresponding fever may also be due to an anaerobic infection, especially in cats. Additional therapy could include metronidazole (Flagyl, Baxter), 10 to 15 mg/kg every 8 hours IV (1-hour infusion), clindamycin, cefoxitin or imipenem-cilastatin. Although imipenem-cilastatin is expensive, it is less expensive than combined administration of enrofloxacin, cefazolin, and metronidazole and may be substituted for the latter.

The preceding recommendations may not be feasible because of cost restrictions or the inability of the owner to return the animal to the hospital. In such cases, initial therapy with oral antimicrobial agents is chosen if the animal is stable. In addition, oral antimicrobial therapy may be chosen for treatment of neutropenic animals that have been febrile and stable for several days. For animals with moderate to severe neutropenia or pyrexia, enrofloxacin or ciprofloxacin plus cephalexin or amoxicillin-clavulanate is recommended. For animals with mild neutropenia and mild pyrexia, therapy as described in Table 1 is recommended. Therapy with tetracyclines for *Ehrlichia canis*–induced neutropenia may also control secondary infections. Doxycycline is recommended because it causes less disturbance of intestinal colonization resistance than tetracycline or oxytetracycline. In all cases, the animal should be observed closely for clinical deterioration, and arrangements should be made to initiate parenteral therapy. Oral antimicrobial therapy is not appropriate when the animal is hypovolemic, is vomiting, or there is disruption of the intestinal mucosa.

Empirical antifungal therapy is not commonly used in dogs or cats. If neutropenia and antibacterial therapy persist beyond 10 days, stools should be monitored by cytologic studies or culture for *Candida* spp. overgrowth, especially if antibacterial agents are being used that disturb intestinal colonization resistance (e.g., amoxicillin, cefoxitin, metronidazole).

Therapy for Documented Infections

Therapy for documented bacterial infections should consist of bactericidal antibiotics, with the choice based on susceptibility testing. The guidelines for choosing intravenous or oral routes of administration are the same as previously discussed for empirical therapy. The guidelines for duration of therapy for animals with documented bacteremia but no localization into other organs are also as previously discussed. Therapy for documented pneumonia and urinary tract and soft tissue infections should be continued a minimum of 7 days beyond recovery of the neutrophil count to at least 1.0×10^9/L (1,000/μl) and resolution of clinical and radiographic signs. An infection may appear to become worse as the neutrophil count recovers and increased inflammation develops. However, fever should be resolving if the antimicrobial agents selected are effective. The guidelines for intensifying therapy if fever is not resolving are similar to those previously discussed.

Amphotericin B is the therapy of choice for *Aspergillus* spp. infection. Amphotericin B can also be used for systemic candidiasis, but ketoconazole or itraconazole therapy may suffice. Intestinal candidiasis can be treated with nystatin, ketoconazole, or itraconazole. Fluconazole is the drug of choice for urinary candidiasis, but its use is often cost-prohibitive. (For specific treatment recommendations see *CVT XII*, p. 327.)

References and Suggested Reading

Abrams-Ogg ACG, Kruth SA: Infections associated with neutropenia in the dog and cat. In: Prescott JF, Baggot JD, eds: Antimicrobial Therapy in Veterinary Medicine, 2nd ed. Ames, IA: Iowa State University Press, 1993, p 378.
A review of the causes and treatment of neutropenia and associated infections in dogs and cats with references to human medical literature.
Catalfamo JL, Dodds WJ: Hereditary and acquired thrombopathias. Vet Clin North Am Small Anim Pract 18:185, 1988.
A review of platelet dysfunction including the effects of antimicrobial agents.
Couto CG: Management of complications of cancer chemotherapy. Vet Clin North Am Small Anim Pract 20:1037, 1990.
A discussion of diagnosis and therapy of infections complicating neutropenia in veterinary cancer patients.
Kunkle GA, Sundlof S, Keisling K: Adverse effects of oral antibacterial therapy in dogs and cats: An epidemiologic study of pet owners' observations. J Am Anim Hosp Assoc 31:46, 1995.
A study of the adverse effects of oral antimicrobial agents in dogs and cats with various disorders.
Legendre AM: Antimycotic drug therapy. In: Bonagura JD, ed: Current Veterinary Therapy XII Small Animal Practice. Philadelphia: WB Saunders, 1995, p 327.
A review of antimycotic drugs and treatment guidelines for specific fungal infections.
Matus RE: Chemotherapy of lymphoma and leukemia. In: Kirk RW, ed: Current Veterinary Therapy X Small Animal Practice. Philadelphia: WB Saunders, 1989, p 452.
A description of the chemotherapy protocol for lymphoma for which we are currently using oral antimicrobial prophylaxis.
Reller LB: What the practicing physician should know about blood cultures. In: Koontz F, ed: Blood Culture Controversies—Revisited. Iowa City, IA: American Society of Microbiology Audioconference, 1994, p 1.
A review of the diagnosis by blood culture of bacteremia and fungemia in humans.
Turk J, Fales W, Miller M, et al: Enteric *Clostridium perfringens* infection associated with parvoviral enteritis in dogs: 74 cases (1987–1990). J Am Vet Med Assoc 200:991, 1992.
A retrospective study of necropsy accessions documenting clostridial proliferation in the intestinal tracts of dogs with parvoviral enteritis.
Weiss DJ: Leukocyte disorders and their treatment. In: Bonagura JD, ed: Current Veterinary Therapy XII Small Animal Practice. Philadelphia: WB Saunders, 1995, p 452.
A comprehensive review of the causes and management of neutropenia in the dog and cat.
Wilkens B, Sullivan P, McDonald TP, et al: Effects of cephalothin, cefazolin, and cefmetazole on the hemostatic mechanism in normal dogs: Implications for the surgical patient. Vet Surg 24:25, 1995.
A study investigating the effects of three cephalosporin antibiotics on platelet function and coagulation in dogs.

Therapeutic Management of Sepsis

ELIZABETH M. HARDIE
Raleigh, North Carolina

The search for new treatments for life-threatening bacterial infection has been fraught with problems. Therapies designed to block endotoxin or inflammatory mediators worked well in endotoxin models but did not increase survival in the older, often compromised, septic human population. Drugs that blocked inflammatory mediators sometimes actually led to increases in mortality, probably because they resulted in a depressed immune response to infection. These drug failures have directed researchers toward more detailed study of the septic patient to more fully understand how to enhance the host's immunologic response to infection. Current therapeutic recommendations are surprisingly traditional: give appropriate antibiotics, provide cardiovascular support, increase tissue oxygenation, protect against oxygen radical damage, remove the focus of infection, and manage organ failure. Methods of enhancing endotoxin clearance without affecting the inflammatory cascade may also show promise.

The speed with which sepsis is recognized and treated is critical. Human septic patients treated early have a 92% survival rate. Patients who develop septic shock, in which hypotension persists despite adequate fluid resuscitation, have a survival rate of 54%. A recent study (Hauptman and Walshaw, 1996) demonstrated that for dogs, a 97% sensitivity and 64% specificity for the diagnosis of sepsis were obtained if at least two of four clinical criteria (Table 1) were present. A second study (Swann and Hughes, 1996) of dogs and cats demonstrated that the presence of a pH less than 7.2, a P_{CO_2} greater than 55 mm Hg, a glucose concentration of less than 50 mg/dl, or a lactate concentration of greater than 5.5 mmol/L in an abdominal fluid sample had a sensitivity of 71 to 86% and a specificity of 100% for the diagnosis of bacterial peritonitis versus nonbacterial effusion. The treatment regimens for both dogs and cats have been reviewed (see *CVT XII,* p. 139); the present discussion provides therapeutic updates (see also p. 140).

ANTIBIOTICS

Numerous studies in human medicine have demonstrated that early administration of appropriate antibiotics is a critical factor in the survival of the septic patient. Administration of a single broad-spectrum antibiotic has been shown to be as effective as using multiple drugs in peritonitis, provided that the single drug kills *Bacteroides* spp. and Enterobacteriaceae. In septic patients, increased drug doses are often needed because of altered drug pharmacokinetics. Optimal treatment regimens are still under investigation, but doses and dosing frequencies have changed considerably for some drugs that have traditionally been used to treat sepsis (Table 2). Antibiotics result in differing degrees of endotoxin release when killing gram-negative organisms and retrospective human clinical studies have shown that this effect may cause harm. When other factors were equalized, treatment of septic trauma patients with endotoxin-releasing antibiotics such as aztreonam, ceftazidime, and cefotaxime sodium resulted in higher mortality than did treatment with similar non–endotoxin-releasing antibiotics. These drugs should probably be avoided until prospective studies can define the true extent of this problem (Sibbald and Vincent, 1995).

Two organisms deserve special mention. First, there has been debate as to whether *Enterococcus* is a significant pathogen in intra-abdominal infection. It has been shown that the presence of *Enterococcus* in human intra-abdominal infection *is* a predictor of treatment failure, probably because it becomes an important pathogen of colon origin in elderly, highly compromised patients. Highly compromised peritonitis patients should thus be treated with drugs that have marked activity against resistant gram-positive organisms. Second, a toxic shock syndrome associated with a group G streptococci has been described in dogs, and inappropriate treatment with enrofloxacin appeared to play a role in the progression of the disease (Miller et al, 1996). Dogs with signs of this syndrome (necrotizing fasciitis, respiratory distress) should be treated with beta-lactam or macrolide antibiotics.

CARDIOVASCULAR SUPPORT

Colloids are routinely used in sepsis to maintain vascular volume without producing tissue edema (Table 3; see

TABLE 2. Intravenous Antibiotic Doses for Septic Dogs or Cats

Drug	Dose (IV)
Ampicillin	20–40 mg/kg q6–8hr
Ampicillin-sulbactam	20 mg/kg q6hr
Ticarcillin-clavulanic acid	40–50 mg/kg q6–8hr
Cefazolin	20–25 mg/kg q4–8hr
Cefoxitin	30 mg/kg q5hr
Cefotetan	30 mg/kg q5–8hr
Imipenem	0.7–1.1 mg/kg q8hr
Vancomycin	15 mg/kg q6hr
Gentamicin	6 mg/kg q24hr
Amikacin	20 mg/kg q24hr
Enrofloxacin	5–20 mg/kg q12hr
Metronidazole	15 mg/kg q12hr
Clindamycin	11 mg/kg q12hr

pp. 63 and 131). Hydroxyethyl starch (HES) appears to be superior to other colloids, including human albumin (Bolt et al, 1996). Hydroxyethyl starch prevents activation of endothelial cell coagulation and decreases plasma concentrations of soluble adhesion molecules in septic patients. Improved splanchnic perfusion is seen in patients treated with HES. Cats and dogs differ in their response to HES (Kirby, 1996). Rapid administration of HES causes vomiting and hypotension in the cat; thus, bolus volumes used for resuscitation must be given slowly. After initial resuscitation, cats with sepsis require 0.5 to 1.5 ml/kg per hour for 1 to 2 days, after which their capillaries abruptly seal and volume overloading can occur rapidly. Dogs tolerate rapid administration of HES but take longer to regain vascular integrity during sepsis and require 0.8 to 1 ml/kg per hour for as long as 3 to 4 days.

When volume therapy does not resolve hypotension, inotropes and vasopressors are used to increase blood pressure in septic patients (see *CVT XII*, p. 188). There is little agreement among the experts as to when inotrope or vasopressor treatment should be initiated (before hypotension develops or only in its presence) and which class of drugs should be used first. Dobutamine increases overall tissue oxygen delivery and norepinephrine improves splanchnic oxygen utilization, compared to dopamine (see Table 3). Although epinephrine reliably increases blood pressure, this drug has been associated with worsening of lactic acidosis in sepsis and should probably be avoided as a first-line drug.

TISSUE OXYGENATION

Optimizing tissue delivery of oxygen is a treatment goal for septic patients. This goal is accomplished by maximizing cardiovascular function, providing red blood cells or hemoglobin to transport oxygen, increasing the inspired oxygen concentration, and preventing the development of microthrombi (see Table 3). Controversies about this goal surround the need to push septic patients to supranormal values for tissue oxygen delivery. Aggressive fluid therapy may lead to pulmonary and tissue edema in some some patient populations. This topic continues to be hotly debated, and until a consensus is reached veterinarians should probably err on the side of achieving supranor-

TABLE 1. Criteria Indicating the Presence of Sepsis in Dogs

Measurement	Value
Body temperature	<38°C, >39°C
Heart rate	>120 beats/minute
Respiratory rate	>20 breaths/minute
WBC count or	<6, >16,000 d/μl
band neutrophils	>3%

TABLE 3. Sample Therapies for a Septic Dog or Cat

Goal	Drug or Treatment	Drug Dose	Comments
Remove infection	Antibiotics, surgery	See Table 2	Continue antibiotics until white blood cell count is normal
Restore vascular volume	Replacement crystalloid therapy	As needed for resuscitation, then up to 15 ml/kg/hr IV	Reduce 40–60% if colloids are used
	Hydroxyethyl starch	As needed for resuscitation, then 15–30 ml/kg/24 hr IV	Resuscitate with 5 ml/kg boluses, give slowly in cat (see text)
Normalize glucose, electrolytes	Dextrose, potassium, calcium, magnesium	According to need	
Increase cardiac output	Dobutamine	5–10 μg/kg/min (dog), 2.5–5 μg/kg/min (cat)	Use early in sepsis
Increase blood pressure	Norepinephrine	0.5–1 μg/kg/min	Protects gut after volume replacement
Maximize oxygen delivery	Packed red cells or hemoglobin substitutes nasal oxygen	To obtain PCV >25%, hemoglobin >10 gm/dl	
		4–8 hr 100% oxygen; 40% oxygen thereafter	Continue until resolution of sepsis
Prevent microthrombi	Heparin	100 IU/kg SC q8hr	
Restore plasma proteins	Fresh frozen plasma	To maintain albumin >2 gm/dl	
Scavenge oxygen radicals	Deferoxamine	5–15 mg/kg IV	Give slowly, monitor for hypotension
Protect intestinal mucosa	Early enteral feeding	Begin with 2–5 ml of liquid food q4–6hr	Place jejunostomy tube if vomiting-regurgitating
Treat ileus	Nasogastric suction	Suction q4–6hr	
	Metoclopramide	0.2–0.5 mg/kg q6–8hr, 0.01–0.02 mg/kg/hr IV	
Treat respiratory failure	Place on respirator		Perform early, not late
Treat oliguria	Mannitol	0.1 gm/kg IV	Volume and blood pressure normalized first
	Dopamine	1–3 μg/kg/min	Use with furosemide
	Furosemide	1 mg/kg/hr IV for 4 hr	

mal values. A recent roundtable (Sibbald and Vincent, 1995) concluded that hemoglobin concentrations should be maintained above 10 gm/dl in human patients whose intravascular volume has been normalized. This level would correspond to a packed cell volume (PCV) of at least 20%, and many clinicians would argue for maintaining it above 25%. A study of septic mice has helped clarify the effect of oxygen enrichment (Gennari and Alexander, 1996). Mice given short-term hyperoxia (4 to 8 hours of 100% oxygen) had improved short-term, but not long-term, survival. Mice given 100% oxygen for 8 hours plus 5 days of 40% oxygen had better gut barrier function, decreased bacterial translocation, and improved long-term survival.

The best regimens for early detection and prevention of microthrombi are being intensively investigated, because occult thrombosis appears to be a critical factor in the development of multiple organ failure. In septic rats, coadministration of heparin and antithrombin III prevents thrombocytopenia, ameliorates organ damage, and improves survival (Yang and Hauptman, 1994). Antithrombin III is too expensive for most veterinary patients, but administration of heparin (see Table 3) and possibly plasma (see p. 190) appears to be rational.

The best method of measuring oxygen delivery in septic patients has yet to be determined. Gastric mucosal P_{CO_2} and pH_i (see *CVT XII*, p. 133) appear to be sensitive indicators, but methodologic problems have prevented these measurements from being widely used. The recent development of a fiberoptic intramucosal carbon dioxide sensor (Paratrend 7, Biomedical Sensors, High Wycombe, UK) may allow continuous monitoring. Using current technology, the goal is a pH_i greater than 7.25 in dogs.

Blood lactate is often used as a global measurement of perfusion (goal = <2.5 mmol/L). A problem with lactate measurements is that septic patients consume oxygen, produce pyruvate, and oxidize pyruvate at a much faster rate than healthy subjects (Gore et al, 1996). A by-product of increased pyruvate is increased lactate production; thus, lactic acidosis can be due either to poor oxygen delivery or to altered metabolism. If steps have been taken to maximize oxygen delivery, metabolic acidosis or high lactate values may thus represent ongoing metabolic alterations, rather than inadequate therapy.

OXYGEN RADICAL SCAVENGERS

Increased production of oxygen-derived free radicals is thought to play a major role in the pathophysiology of sepsis. Septic patients that survive have a higher plasma antioxidant potential than nonsurvivors, indicating that the ability to scavenge free radicals is critical to survival. Early administration of oxygen radical scavengers has been shown to improve survival in experimental models. Deferoxamine (Desferal, Ciba Geigy Corp) given early in the course of sepsis may thus have beneficial effects (see Table 3). Other available scavengers include allopurinol, mannitol, dimethyl sulfoxide, quinacrine hydrochloride, corticosteroids, and adenosine.

REMOVING THE FOCUS OF INFECTION

Removal of the septic focus is accomplished with the use of surgical debridement, excision, or drainage. Severe abdominal contamination can be managed with either an open abdomen technique or a closed drainage technique with planned reoperation. In human patients, percutaneous drainage of abscesses under computed tomography (CT) or ultrasound guidance has become routine. This method probably has limited application in dogs, who do not tend to form abdominal abscesses, but may be of use in selected cases. Cats tend to form abscesses readily, but the body cavity most affected is the thorax, which may be more safely accessed with an open approach.

ORGAN FAILURE

Multiple organ failure occurs in septic patients when accumulating microcirculatory insults result in a cascade of compromised organ function. Learning to prevent these insults will be critical to the future treatment of septic patients. Currently, clinicians must recognize and treat organ failure as quickly as possible. Failure of the gut is now recognized to be a "trigger" for the development of other organ failures, since bacterial translocation (see p. 201) and release of endotoxin occur once the gut fails. Similarly, lung failure (which can be due to aspiration pneumonia, pulmonary thromboembolism, or respiratory distress syndrome) may serve to initiate a cascade of organ failure if oxygen delivery is compromised. Dogs with peritonitis commonly develop gut failure, pancreatitis, and respiratory failure. Renal failure may occur as a terminal event. Cats often develop respiratory failure early in the course of sepsis.

Early enteral feeding (see *CVT XI*, p. 117; see p. 136) of the septic patient is important in preventing gut failure. There is no need to give large volumes of feeding solutions to these patients because small amounts of food are equally protective. Since regurgitation and vomiting are often present, feeding tubes must enter the small intestine. Both jejunostomy and gastrojejunostomy tubes can be used, but the latter are more expensive. Feeding products should contain glutamine and fiber to preserve mucosal health. Impaired intestinal absorption is common in septic patients, and feeding solutions containing peptides may be needed. Enteral feeding should not be discontinued if pancreatitis develops, since feeding below the pancreas has been shown to be an acceptable method of treatment for pancreatitis.

Vomiting and regurgitation may contribute to respiratory failure, and placement of a nasogastric suction tube (*CVT XI*, p. 32) allows aspiration of stomach contents before accidental inhalation may occur. Metoclopromide is used to combat ileus (see Table 3). Septic dogs with evidence of pulmonary dysfunction ($PaO_2 < 60$ mm Hg on room air, $PaCO_2 > 60$ mm Hg) or respiratory exhaustion should be placed on a respirator early in the course of the disease—do not wait until respiratory failure becomes severe (*CVT XI*, p. 98).

BLOOD FILTRATION AND ENDOTOXIN BINDING

After the failure of clinical trials testing mediator blockers in the treatment of sepsis, some researchers returned to an old idea: since endotoxin and other bacterial products initiate much of the inflammatory cascade in sepsis, getting rid of these products will prevent many of their deleterious effects. While hemofiltration with increasingly sophisticated filters is being used in most experimental studies, one study (Read et al, 1995) indicated that substantially improved endotoxin clearance was obtained with intravenous infusion of lipids (Intralipid, Kabivitrum Inc., 1 gm triglyceride/kg). Lipid-bound endotoxin was cleared by the hepatocytes, while unbound endotoxin was cleared by macrophages. Improved survival in the lipid-treated rats was associated with reduced mediator release.

References and Suggested Reading

Bolt J, Muller M, Heesen M, et al: Influence of different volume therapies and pentoxifylline infusion on circulating soluble adhesion molecules in critically ill patients. Crit Care Med 24:385, 1996.
One study examining the role of hydroxyethyl starch in septic patients; also reviews the topic.

Gennari R, Alexander JW: Effects of hyperoxia on bacterial translocation and mortality during gut-derived sepsis. Arch Surg 131:57, 1996.
Defines the role of oxygen supplementation in the prevention of gut organ failure.

Gore DC, Jahoor F, Hibbert JM, et al: Lactic acidosis during sepsis is related to increased pyruvate production, not deficits in tissue oxygen availability. Ann Surg 224:97, 1996.
Defines the cause of lactic acidosis during sepsis.

Hauptman JG, Walshaw R: Evaluation of the sensitivity and specificity of diagnostic criteria for sepsis in the dog. Proceedings of the sixth annual ACVS Symposium, San Francisco, 1996, p 26.
Defines the utility of clinical criteria for the diagnosis of sepsis.

Kirby R: Synthetic colloids. Proceedings of the fifth IVECC Symposium, San Antonio, 1996, p 884.
Describes the various colloids and outlines the differing responses of septic dogs and cats to colloid therapy.

Miller CW, Prescott JF, Mathews KA, et al: Streptococcal toxic shock syndrome in dogs. J Am Vet Med Assoc 209:1421, 1996.
A description of streptococcal toxic shock in seven dogs.

Read TE, Grunfeld C, Kumwenda ZL, et al: Triglyceride-rich lipoproteins prevent septic death in rats. J Exp Med 182:267, 1995.
Examines the effect of infusing a lipid emulsion after cecal ligation and puncture in rats.

Sibbald WJ, Vincent JL: Roundtable conference on clinical trials for the treatment of sepsis. Crit Care Med 23:394, 1995.
Review of current therapies for human sepsis, ranking them according to the scientific evidence supporting their use.

Swann H, Hughes D: Use of abdominal fluid pH, pO₂, pCO₂, [glucose], [lactate] to differentiate bacterial peritonitis from non-bacterial causes of abdominal effusion in dogs and cats. Proceedings of the fifth IVECC Symposium, San Antonio, 1996, p 884.
Defines the criteria for the diagnosis of bacterial peritonitis.

Yang S, Hauptman JG: The efficacy of heparin and antithrombin III fluid-resuscitated cecal ligation and puncture. Shock 2:433, 1994.
Heparin and antithrombin III infusion was associated with reduced organ failure in septic rats.

Ocular Manifestations of Systemic Infectious Diseases

Brian C. Gilger

Raleigh, North Carolina

It has been stated many times that the eye is the "window to the soul." Indeed, the eye should also be considered the window to the body, for there is no other site in the body where a clinician can directly and noninvasively observe vasculature or extracellular space. The fine vasculature in the eye tends to filter out infectious organisms from the blood, and this, coupled with the fact that the eye is a sensitive organ, may explain why the eye is frequently the first organ system to be involved in a systemic infection.

The clinician should consider an ocular examination as an important diagnostic tool when evaluating an animal with a possible systemic illness, and it should be included in each physical examination. To fully use this diagnostic "test," the clinician must be able to interpret ocular signs correctly. For example, one must be able to differentiate between conjunctival hyperemia due to conjunctivitis and injected episcleral vessels due to glaucoma. Proper use of tonometers, ophthalmoscopes, and magnification during the ocular examination is critical to performing an accurate examination and to differentiating between similar ocular signs.

In general, treatment of ocular disease occurring secondary to systemic infectious diseases is primarily by specific treatment for the primary infectious disease and nonspecific control of ocular inflammation. Often it is the secondary inflammatory response, and not the infectious agent, that destroys vision in the eye. Steroidal and nonsteroidal medications are frequently used to control intraocular inflammation. Mydriatic medications (e.g., Atropine, tropicamide) are used to relieve intraocular pain (by paralyzing the spasming ciliary musculature) and prevent adhesions and other intraocular complications (Table 1).

CONJUNCTIVITIS (Table 2)

Canine Distemper Virus

Canine distemper virus, which occurs primarily in young dogs, may cause a transient conjunctivitis accompanied by mucopurulent ocular and nasal discharge. The conjunctivitis is generally followed by lethargy, anorexia, and neurologic signs consisting of focal seizures and progressive paresis. In the nontapetal ocular fundus, well-defined silver-tan focal retinitis lesions may be visible. Retinitis or retinochoroiditis lesions may also be seen, but less commonly, in the tapetal fundus. They appear as gray, hyporeflective lesions with a hyperpigmented ring. Chronic lesions may appear as hyperreflective discs, indicating retinal scarring. Optic neuritis may also occur, resulting in mydriasis and blindness. Diagnostic tests for canine distemper include conjunctival cytologic studies (identification of intracytoplasmic inclusion bodies and fluorescent antibody testing) and serologic studies (fluorescent antibody) on both serum and cerebrospinal fluid.

Feline Herpesvirus

Feline herpesvirus (feline rhinotracheitis virus) may cause up to 80% of the surface inflammatory conditions of the cat's eye. Most cats are exposed to this virus early in life. In adolescent cats, the virus usually causes conjunctivitis and rhinitis, which are self-limited, running a course of approximately 21 days. In adult cats, the virus can cause chronic conjunctivitis and a pathognomonic dendritic keratitis. Diagnosis of this condition involves a history, clinical signs, and diagnostic conjunctival cytologic studies. Diagnostic tests using the polymerase chain reaction are specific and sensitive and probably the most useful for confirming herpesvirus infection, although asymptomatic cats may also test positive. Treatment of the conjunctivitis is palliative and uses broad-spectrum antibiotics (e.g., oxytetracycline) to prevent secondary infection. Treatment of severe keratitis, in which herpesvirus has been confirmed, is with specific antiviral medication (trifluridine, Viroptic), as discussed further on page 1057.

Other less common infectious causes of conjunctivitis in cats include chlamydiosis (*Chlamydia psittaci*) and mycoplasmosis (*Mycoplasma felis*). These organisms cause a conjunctivitis that appears similar to that produced by herpesvirus. Diagnosis is by conjunctival cytologic studies or culture of the organism. Intracytoplasmic inclusion bodies in conjunctival epithelial cells may be seen with chlamydia. Topical oxytetracycline (Terramycin) is effective against both organisms.

TABLE 1. Nonspecific Therapy for Inflammatory Ocular Diseases

	Dose
Topical Steroidal Ophthalmic Medications	
Prednisone acetate 1.0%	b.i.d.–q.i.d.
Dexamethasone HCl 0.1%	b.i.d.–q.i.d.
Topical Nonsteroidal Ophthalmic Medications	
Flurbiprofen sodium 0.03%	b.i.d.–q.i.d.
Suprofen 1%	b.i.d.–q.i.d.
Diclofenac 0.1%	t.i.d.
Mydriatic Medications	
Atropine 1%	Every 24 hr, p.r.n.
Tropicamide 0.5%	q.i.d.

TABLE 2. **Systemic Infectious Diseases Associated With Ocular Clinical Signs**

Ocular Clinical Sign	Infectious Disease	Diagnostic Test
Dog		
Conjunctivitis	Canine distemper	IFA on conjunctive cytologic studies, serologic tests
Corneal edema	Infectious canine hepatitis	Serologic tests
Uveitis	Infectious canine hepatitis	Serologic tests
	Brucellosis	
	Leptospirosis	
	Blastomycosis	Serologic (AGI); cytologic studies
	Coccidioidomycosis	Serologic (complement fixation); cytologic studies
	Toxoplasmosis	Serologic (ELISA)
	Leishmaniasis	Serologic tests
	Rocky Mountain spotted fever	Serologic (microimmunofluorescence)
	Ehrlichiosis (*E. canis*)	Serologic (IFA)
	Cyclic thrombocytopenia (*E. platys*)	Serologic (IFA)
	Dirofilariasis	Knott's test, ELISA
Retinitis, chorioretinitis	Blastomycosis	AGI; cytologic studies
	Histoplasmosis	Serologic (CF)
	Cryptococcosis	Cytologic studies, serologic tests
	Coccidioidomycosis	Serologic (CF); cytologic studies
	Toxoplasmosis	Serologic tests
	Leishmaniasis	Serologic tests
	Rocky Mountain spotted fever	Serologic tests
	Ehrlichiosis (*E. canis*)	Serologic (IFA)
	Protothecosis	Cytologic studies, culture
	Aspergillosis	Cytologic studies
Cat		
Conjunctivitis	Feline herpesvirus	Cytologic (PCR)
	Chlamydiosis	Cytologic studies
	Mycoplasmosis	Cytologic studies
Keratitis, corneal edema	Feline herpesvirus	Cytologic (PCR)
Uveitis	Feline leukemia virus	
	Feline immunodeficiency virus	
	Feline infectious peritonitis	
	Blastomycosis	AGI; cytologic studies
	Coccidioidomycosis	Serologic (CF); cytologic studies
	Toxoplasmosis	Serologic (ELISA, IgM, IgG, antigen)
	Leishmaniasis	
Retinitis, chorioretinitis	Feline infectious peritonitis	
	Blastomycosis	Serologic (AGI); cytologic studies
	Histoplasmosis	Serologic (CF)
	Cryptococcosis	Cytologic studies, serologic tests
	Coccidioidomycosis	Serologic (CF); cytologic studies
	Toxoplasmosis	Serologic tests

AGI, agar gel immunodiffusion; CF, complement fixation; IFA, indirect fluorescein antibody; PCR, polymerase chain reaction.

CORNEA

Infectious Canine Hepatitis

Approximately 20% of dogs recovering from infectious canine hepatitis (canine adenovirus type 1) may acquire corneal edema, which occurs suddenly and is usually transient. Mild anterior uveitis may also accompany or immediately precede the corneal edema and may occur, although rarely, after vaccination with canine adenovirus type 1 (0.4%), or less commonly with canine adenovirus type 2 vaccines. Afghan hounds appear to be particularly sensitive. The corneal edema usually resolves without treatment; however, nonspecific use of topical anti-inflammatory medications (see Table 1) is helpful for treatment of the uveitis.

UVEITIS

Rocky Mountain Spotted Fever

Rocky Mountain spotted fever (RMSF), caused by *Rickettsia rickettsii* and transmitted by ticks, is primarily a disease involving infection of vascular endothelium and perithelial smooth muscle. Ocular clinical signs (subconjunctival hemorrhage, hyphema, anterior uveitis, retinal petechiae, retinal edema, and perivascular inflammatory cell infiltrate) are related to this vascular infection (Davidson, 1989). Generally, the ocular signs are mild and resolve with systemic tetracycline therapy. Diagnosis is confirmed by serologic tests (microimmunofluorescence).

Ehrlichiosis

The ocular signs of ehrlichiosis (*Ehrlichia canis*) are similar to RMSF but are more severe and widespread. Anterior uveitis, hyphema, serous and exudative retinal detachments, chorioretinitis, and retinal perivascular exudation are typical ocular signs of *E. canis* infection. Ocular lesions result from inflammatory vascular disease or thrombocytopenia. Diagnosis is made using serologic tests (indirect fluorescein antibody testing).

E. platys, the causative agent for canine infectious cyclic thrombocytopenia, may also cause anterior uveitis. Other characteristic findings with *E. platys* infections include thrombocytopenia, anemia, platelet inclusion bodies, and elevated serum titer (indirect fluorescein antibody). Treatment for either type of *Ehrlichia* infection involves nonspecific ocular anti-inflammatory medications and systemic tetracycline.

Feline Leukemia Virus

The role of feline leukemia virus (FeLV) in causing uveitis in cats is controversial. Whether the virus directly causes uveitis or whether the uveitis associated with FeLV-positive cats is associated with FeLV-associated lymphoma, or both, is not known. Pupillary light response abnormalities causing a "spastic pupil" syndrome are associated with FeLV infection. Other ocular signs (hyphema, retinal hemorrhage, anterior uveitis) in FeLV-positive cats may not be a direct result of FeLV infection but instead may be due to FeLV-associated anemia or secondary infections.

Feline Immunodeficiency Virus

Feline immunodeficiency virus may cause primary ocular signs consisting of anterior uveitis, glaucoma, or pars planitis (English, 1990). Anterior uveitis is most common, consisting of aqueous flare, peripheral iridal hyperemia, and hypotony. Pars planitis is a less common sign in feline immunodeficiency virus–positive cats. Pars planitis appears as white, punctate infiltrates in the anterior vitreous. Nonspecific treatment of the ocular inflammation using topical corticosteroids may help keep the cat comfortable.

Feline Infectious Peritonitis

Feline infectious peritonitis (FIP) is caused by a coronavirus. Several clinical forms of FIP are generally recognized (effusive, noneffusive, and mixed). Ocular signs are usually seen with the noneffusive form. Ocular disease may develop initially without other systemic clinical signs. A pyogranulomatous uveitis is typical, consisting primarily of retinal vasculitis, retinal detachment with exudative subretinal fluid, and retinal hemorrhage. Anterior segment lesions may include severe aqueous flare, "mutton-fat" keratic precipitates, hyphema, hypopyon, miosis, swollen iris, synechiae, and hypotony. Diagnosis of FIP is by clinical signs, recognizing elevated serum proteins, and by tissue biopsy (which is nonspecific). Many times, diagnosis is made by exclusion of other causes or at necropsy. Treatment of ocular FIP is nonspecific (see Table 1).

Blastomycosis

Blastomyces dermatitidis is a fungus and most commonly affects young adult dogs living in endemic areas of the Mississippi and Ohio River valleys. Approximately 30% of dogs with a systemic blastomycosis infection have ocular involvement (Brooks, 1991). Ocular signs of blastomycosis include anterior uveitis, blepharospasm, photophobia, epiphora, miosis, aqueous flare, chorioretinitis, subretinal granulomas, optic neuritis, endophthalmitis, and possibly secondary glaucoma. Diagnosis of blastomycosis is most reliably determined by identifying the organism in lymph node aspirates, cytologic studies of cutanous lesions, or from an aspirate of the subretinal space. Serologic tests, using agar gel immunodiffusion, can also be used to help confirm blastomycosis. Itraconazole has been used for successful treatment of blastomycosis. Nonspecific therapy (see Table 1) is used for ocular inflammation. If the eye has severe endophthalmitis (i.e., the entire eye is inflamed) or secondary glaucoma, enucleation is the treatment of choice.

Blastomycosis in cats is less common than in dogs. However, cats in endemic areas may become infected, and the most common clinical sign is dyspnea or chronic cough. Retinal granulomatous lesions are the most common ocular lesions in cats. Diagnosis and treatment is similar to that in dogs.

Cryptococcosis

Cryptococcosis is a systemic mycotic disease caused by *Cryptococcus neoformans*. Inhalation is the usual route of initial infection. Disseminated cryptococcosis may have ocular involvement. Common ocular clinical signs include chorioretinitis, granulomatous retinitis, retinal detachment, and optic neuritis. The chorioretinitis has a typical appearance: multifocal lesions in the tapetal fundus with a dark center, clear periphery, and a dark peripheral ring ("bull's-eye" or "target" appearance). Other clinical signs may include neurologic signs (e.g., depression, seizures) from meningoencephalitis. Diagnosis is by identifying the organism in fluid aspirates (e.g., cerebrospinal fluid, vitreous, subretinal fluid) or by serologic tests (latex agglutination for cryptococcal antigen). There have been several reports of successful treatment of cryptococcosis using ketoconazole in dogs and cats. Itraconazole or fluconazole have also been reported to be effective for treatment of cryptococcosis and may have fewer side effects than does ketoconazole (see p. 815). A rapid decrease in the serologic titer may indicate an improved prognosis. Generally, other than systemic antifungal therapy, no specific ocular treatment is required for the ocular disease.

Toxoplasmosis

Toxoplasma gondii is an intracellular coccidian organism. The cat is the primary host. A high percentage of cats may be exposed, but the disease, toxoplasmosis, is usually uncommon. *T. gondii* may also infect dogs, humans, and other species of animals. In cats, toxoplasmosis may cause anterior uveitis or chorioretinitis. Several reports have implicated toxoplasmosis as the most common infectious cause of uveitis in cats. Diagnosis of toxoplasmosis is complicated; however, enzyme-linked immunosorbent assay for *T. gondii*–specific IgM, IgG, and circulating antigens may be useful. An antibody titer of greater than or equal to 1:64 of IgM or IgG, or a positive enzyme-linked immunosorbent assay antigen in serum has been considered a positive result for toxoplasmosis.

The role of toxoplasmosis in eye disease is poorly understood and is controversial. Treatment for uveitis is usually nonspecific (see Table 1) unless there are signs of systemic illness. If chronic systemic signs are present, oral clindamycin (Antirobe) may be administered with the following precaution: experimental studies have indicated that clindamycin decreases macrophagic function and may worsen the disease in acute cases (Davidson et al, 1996). Furthermore, with the waxing and waning nature of clinical toxoplasmosis in cats, the effectiveness of clindamycin therapy is unknown.

Leishmaniasis

Leishmaniasis is caused by a protozoal organism (*Leishmania donovani*) that is endemic to the Mediterranean area and rare in the United States. Systemic leishmaniasis commonly invades the eye, resulting in severe nongranulomatous anterior uveitis, retinitis, retinal hemorrhage, and retinal detachment. Characteristic clinical signs and serologic tests are the basis for diagnosis.

RETINITIS-CHORIORETINITIS

Histoplasmosis

Histoplasma capsulatum is a mycotic organism that primarily causes pneumonia in dogs and cats. Disseminated histoplasmosis may cause ocular signs consisting of multifocal retinitis and chorioretinitis in the dog and cat. Ocular signs are nearly always associated with systemic illness (dyspnea, skin lesions, lethargy). Diagnosis is made using serologic tests (complement fixation) or identification of the organism by cytologic studies. Ketoconazole, itraconazole, or fluconazole may be effective treatments for disseminated histoplasmosis.

Coccidioidomycosis

Coccidioides immitis is a soil fungus found in the desert southwestern United States. Infection can occur in dogs; the primary site is the lungs, resulting in pneumonia. Ocular lesions can occur with disseminated infection and typically cause anterior uveitis, granulomatous chorioretinitis and retinal detachment, and granulomatous endophthalmitis. Diagnosis is made by serologic tests (complement fixation test), identification of the organism on cytologic samples, or by histologic features. Ocular inflammation is treated using nonspecific anti-inflammatory medication, and the systemic infection is treated with ketoconazole. The eye may need to be enucleated if the infection is severe and nonresponsive to treatment.

Protothecosis

Prototheca zopfii and *P. wickerhamii* are achlorophyllous algae that are the causative agents of protothecosis in dogs and are found in the coastal regions of the southeastern United States. Systemic infection with *Prototheca* causes bloody diarrhea, progressive weight loss, and lethargy. Ocular signs in disseminated infections primarily involve the posterior segment (vitreous, retina, and choroid) of the eye, including chorioretinitis, retinal detachment, retinal hemorrhage, and in some cases, panuveitis-endophthalmitis. Diagnosis is made by identifying the organism in cytologic specimens (ocular aspirates, feces), culture of the organism, and ultimately by histopathologic characteristics. Treatment of dogs with disseminated protothecosis with a variety of antibiotics or antifungal agents (amphotericin B and tetracycline, ketoconazole, itraconazole, clotrimazole) has usually been unsuccessful.

Aspergillosis

Disseminated aspergillosis infection may cause ocular involvement. The most common ocular signs are panuveitis and granulomatous retinal detachments. The upper respiratory tract is usually infected in these dogs. Diagnosis is made by identifying the septate hyphae by ocular aspiration, cytologic studies, serologic tests, or histopathologic features. Amphotericin B and ketoconazole have been used with limited success for the treatment of disseminated aspergillosis.

References and Suggested Reading

Brooks DE, Legendre AM, Gum GG, et al: The treatment of canine ocular blastomycosis with systemically administered itraconazole. Prog Vet Comp Ophthalmol 1:263, 1991.
A retrospective study describing a large number of cases of ocular blastomycosis and its treatment with itraconazole.
Davidson MG, Lappin MR, Rottman JR, et al: Paradoxical effect of clindamycin in experimental, acute toxoplasmosis in cats. Antimicrob Agents Chemother 40:1352, 1996.
A research paper of ocular toxoplasmosis describing treatment effects of clindamycin.
Davidson MG, Nasisse MP, Breitschwerdt EB, et al: Ocular effects of canine Rocky Mountain spotted fever. J Am Vet Med Assoc 194:777, 1989.
A retrospective study of ocular effects of RMSF with comparison to ehrlichiosis.
English RV, Davidson MG, Nasisse MP, et al: Intraocular disease associated with feline immunodeficiency virus infection in rats. J Am Vet Med Assoc 196:1116, 1990.
A retrospective study with excellent descriptions of FIV-induced uveitis with comparisons to other cases of feline uveitis.
Martin CL: Ocular infections. In: Greene CE, ed: Infectious Diseases of the Dog and Cat. Philadelphia: WB Saunders, 1990, pp 197–214.
An excellent review of infectious ocular diseases.

CVT Update: Feline Leukemia Virus

ALICE M. WOLF

College Station, Texas

GENERAL CONCEPTS

Feline leukemia virus (FeLV) is a type-C oncornavirus of the retrovirus group. Both horizontal and vertical transmission occur. Virus is excreted in many secretions; excretions with saliva are the most important for transmission. FeLV is very unstable in the environment and is viable for only a few hours under the most favorable conditions. Close, intimate contact between cats is required for transmission. The reported incidence of FeLV infection in cat populations varies, depending on the source of the information, but averages less than 3% in suburban cats to as much as 30% in endemic multiple-cat households and catteries. In the author's practice, we are seeing fewer FeLV-infected cats because almost all purebred catteries (previously the largest source of infected cats) are now FeLV free, most shelters and animal rescue groups are not adopting out FeLV-positive cats, most individual cat owners are having kittens or cats tested before allowing them into their households, and more owners tend to keep their cats confined. Although vaccination may have had some impact on the incidence of FeLV, epidemiologic studies suggest that with the efficacy rates of available FeLV vaccines and vaccination rates of cats, other factors are more important.

The outcome of exposure to FeLV is highly variable and depends on a number of important host factors, including age, immunocompetence, and the presence of concurrent diseases. Outcome is also affected by the virulence of the viral strain and the dose and duration of exposure. Influenced by these factors, FeLV-infected cats may develop a regressive infection, leading to clearing of the infection and immunity (transient infection), or a progressive infection that results in persistent viremia. During infection, transcribed viral DNA inserts into the host cell genome. Even transiently infected cats have latent (nonreplicating) virus-infected cells for some time. These latently infected cells are usually cleared after a number of months to years. During this time of latency, all routine FeLV diagnostic tests are negative. However, it is possible that the infection may reactivate if the cat is stressed. FeLV-negative lymphomas may also develop later in life in some transiently infected cats.

The clinical signs and laboratory findings associated with persistent FeLV infection have been well described. Illness in affected cats usually results from either the direct effects of the virus on the bone marrow (bone marrow suppression, myeloproliferative disease) or lymphoid tissue (lymphoma) or, more often, from the effects of viral immunosuppression resulting in life-threatening secondary infections. FeLV may also directly affect the nervous system, causing unusual signs, such as periodic anisocoria or urinary incontinence (see p. 288).

DIAGNOSTIC TESTING FOR FeLV

Which Feline Leukemia Virus Antigen Test Should Be Used?

All FeLV tests are based on detection of p27 viral antigen. The controversy over which FeLV test is the best is long-standing. A number of highly reliable FeLV antigen tests have been developed for both in-clinic testing and at commercial laboratories. Which test is selected for an individual patient depends on the tests and procedures available to the practitioner, knowledge about the pathogenesis and progression of FeLV infection and how it relates to the outcome of various tests (Table 1), the population of cats being tested (e.g., healthy kittens versus sick adult strays from a shelter facility), and the reliability and interpretation of various test results. Ideally, the FeLV status of every cat should be known. The American Association of Feline Practitioners and the Academy of Feline Practice have developed a set of guidelines that address various situations and give recommendations for how and when cats should be tested for FeLV (Table 2). However, clinicians should tailor their FeLV testing recommendations as best suits the needs of their own individual patients and practice philosophy.

Which Cats Should Be Tested and How?

The immunofluorescent antibody (IFA) test on peripheral blood is considered by many to be the the gold standard for FeLV testing. A positive IFA test confirms well-established FeLV infection in the bone marrow and correlates well with persistent infection for life. Drawbacks to this test are (1) slightly reduced sensitivity compared with peripheral blood enzyme-linked immunosorbent assay (ELISA) tests, (2) the fact that this test must be run by an outside commercial laboratory, resulting in a time delay in obtaining test results, and (3) higher cost compared with most other FeLV tests. For these reasons, the author recommends the use of the more sensitive peripheral blood ELISA test for routine screening (or prevaccination testing) of all sick or healthy cats and reserves the use of the IFA for confirmatory testing of cats with positive ELISA results or for evaluating FeLV status on the basis of bone marrow specimens.

Microwell peripheral-blood ELISA test kits are more cost-effective if a large number of tests are performed at the same time. However, these tests are also more frequently subject to technical error unless they are being performed by excellently trained personnel. Membrane ELISA tests are much less prone to error and are more useful if only one test is run at a time. Some data suggest that using whole blood for testing (rather than serum or

TABLE 1. Pathogenesis of FeLV

Following infection, FeLV has a specific pattern of replication that affects the results of FeLV testing and the clinical signs that may be seen in an individual cat.

STAGE I: Days 2–4
Replication: In local lymphoid tissue (retropharyngeal, tonsil, gastrointestinal mucosa)
Clinical signs: None to mild viral (fever)
FeLV status: All tests negative at this time
Prognosis: Majority recover

STAGE II: Days 1–14
Replication: Few circulating lymphocytes and mononuclear cells (primary viremia)
Clinical signs: None, or mild viral signs
FeLV status: Serum ELISA becomes positive, PCR may be positive, (IFA, saliva, tears negative)
Prognosis: Most recover, possible latency (6–30 mo)

STAGE III: Days 3–12
Replication: Systemic lymphoid centers (germinal centers)
Clinical signs: None, or mild to moderate viral signs
FeLV status: Serum ELISA positive, PCR positive (IFA, saliva, tears negative)
Prognosis: Recovery for many, possible future lymphosarcoma

STAGE IV: Days 7–21
Replication: Bone marrow stem cells, epithelial cells
Clinical signs: Peripheral blood alterations, viral signs
FeLV status: Serum ELISA, PCR, bone marrow IFA positive (peripheral-blood IFA positive or negative, saliva, tears negative)
Prognosis: Likely to progress to persistent infection

STAGE V: Days 14–28
Replication: Marrow origin, general viremia
Clinical signs: All associated hematologic and systemic FeLV signs possible
FeLV status: Serum ELISA, PCR, bone marrow, and peripheral-blood IFA positive (saliva, tears negative)
Prognosis: Persistent viremia, recovery from this stage of infection is rare

STAGE VI: Days 28–?
Replication: Marrow viremia, widespread epithelial and lymphoid replication
Clinical signs: Any associated with FeLV
FeLV status: Serum ELISA, PCR, BM and peripheral blood IFA, ELISA on saliva and tears may be positive
Prognosis: Long term prognosis is grave, 85% of cats die within 3 years in multicat households, longevity is increased for single cats with good veterinary care

plasma) may slightly increase the sensitivity of some ELISA tests. Cell debris may produce false-positive results in some test systems; thus, this substrate should be used only with a test kit that has been approved for the use of whole blood. Several of these test systems have built-in positive and negative controls so that any technical problem or cross-reactivity is immediately evident. One test system is also available as a combined FeLV–feline immunodeficiency virus (FIV) test so that an adult cat can be tested for both diseases simultaneously. A comparative study showed no significant differences in specificity and sensitivity among four FeLV antigen ELISA test systems, with most having sensitivities and specificities of approximately 98% (Hawks et al, 1991).

Even with the high quality of the test systems available, the *incidence of disease* in the population of cats being tested must be taken into account when one is interpreting FeLV test results. Given an incidence of FeLV in the test population of only 1%, as might be expected in a typical "healthy" suburban cat population, and a test with a sensitivity and specificity of 98%, the reliability of a positive test result is only approximately 33%. Therefore, two of the three positive results obtained from testing 100 healthy cats are false-positive results. An apparently healthy cat or kitten should never be condemned on the basis of a single positive ELISA test result. However, when one uses the same test on a sick cat population with an incidence of FeLV of 30%, the reliability of a positive test result is 99.7%.

If the peripheral-blood ELISA test is positive, an IFA test can be performed to confirm infection and help determine the stage of the infection. Alternatively, an ELISA test can be repeated in 3 or 4 months. If the cat is in an early stage of FeLV infection, regression of the infection and termination of viremia should occur within that period of time and the test will produce a negative result when repeated. Cats remaining persistently positive for FeLV antigen after 3 or 4 months will usually remain antigenemic for life. A small number of cats test consistently positive on peripheral-blood ELISA tests, but negative on peripheral-blood IFA. This group of "discordant" cats may have a sequestered infection in some organ or tissue. Viral antigen apparently leaks into the blood, but virus-infected cells are not being released from bone marrow. It is not known where the virus is sequestered (and it could be the salivary glands or oral tissue); thus, the author treats these discordant cats like any other FeLV-positive cat and considers them to be potentially infectious to other cats.

The saliva FeLV ELISA test is attractive because samples can usually be collected easily and the test can be run quickly while the physical examination is proceeding. This advantage may allow one to make a more rapid diagnosis of FeLV infection, discuss the problem with the owner immediately, and take appropriate precautions in handling the patient. The saliva test is somewhat less sensitive and specific than is blood or serum testing. Tears can also be used as the substrate for testing for FeLV antigen; however, epithelial tissue infection is the last stage of FeLV progression. The lower sensitivity of antigen detection in tears is a serious drawback, and this test cannot be recommended for routine use. All positive or negative saliva or tear tests must be confirmed with a peripheral-blood ELISA or IFA test.

The polymerase chain reaction (PCR) is a technique used to detect minute amounts of viral antigen. Several studies have compared PCR test results to serum ELISA test results in populations of both sick and healthy cats. In these studies, FeLV PCR results correlated nearly 100% with ELISA results. There seems to be no diagnostic advantage to the use of this test, it cannot be performed in clinic and is more than twice as expensive as ELISA testing. In addition, PCR could not be successfully performed on 20% of the samples submitted in one study. PCR testing may have an advantage in a symptomatic cat suspected of having FeLV infection whose routine FeLV test (ELISA, IFA) results are repeatedly negative. If PCR can detect latent virus, it may be possible to confirm infection in such a patient. Bone marrow would probably be a better target tissue than peripheral blood for attempting to identify latent infection in these cats.

TABLE 2. American Association of Feline Practitioners–Academy of Feline Medicine Recommendations for Feline Leukemia Virus Testing

1. The feline leukemia virus (FeLV) status of all cats should be known. FeLV infection is global in occurrence, with prevalence rates varying by location.[1] FeLV is transmitted contagiously among cats and is associated with the illness and death of more cats than any other pathologic condition.[2]
2. Testing and identifying positive cats is the mainstay of managing FeLV infection; this is not supplanted by vaccination. The best means of preventing disease is by preventing exposure to FeLV-infected cats.[1]
3. Testing should occur in the following:
   a. new kittens or cats before introduction into a household to prevent exposing existing cats
   b. newly adopted kittens or cats, even if they are the only cat in the household, for the following reasons:
      i. the strong emotional bond that forms between pet owners and pets justifies knowing the FeLV status because of the future ramifications
      ii. statistically, most cats do not remain the only cat in a household, so future exposure is very likely to occur
      iii. even cats that are meant to be kept indoors may escape and expose other cats
   c. cats in existing households where the FeLV status is not known because carriers can remain asymptomatic for years and expose all other cats in the household
   d. cats in which a recent exposure (known or potential) has occurred—regardless of previous negative test results—because the FeLV status can change
   e. ill cats because FeLV has been associated with a great variety of illnesses in cats
   f. cats presented for FeLV vaccination should have a known FeLV status prior to vaccination because:
      i. vaccination does not affect the carrier state or the development of disease in cats with existing infection
      ii. existing carriers remain an exposure risk
      iii. an existing carrier can subsequently become ill and appear to be a "vaccine failure"
4. The principle of FeLV testing is the detection of p27 core antigen or other antigens of the virion. The ELISA detects p27 in whole blood, serum, plasma, tears, or saliva, whereas the IFA detects antigen within leukocytes and platelets.[a]
5. Kittens can be tested at any age; maternal immunity in young kittens does not interfere with FeLV diagnostic tests.[1]
6. Vaccination with FeLV vaccines does not interfere with FeLV diagnostic testing. The diagnostic tests assay for viral antigens; so, immune response to the vaccine is not detected.[1]
7. The ELISA test is recognized as the preferred screening test for FeLV.[1] The IFA test is more appropriate as a confirmatory test for FeLV.[1] The ELISA kit tests are accurate and allow for rapid in-clinic testing.[2]
8. After screening by use of an ELISA test, a positive or equivocal result should be repeated.[1] The FeLV ELISA systems are most reliable when serum or plasma is tested.[1] If an ELISA test is positive using whole blood, saliva, or tears, the test should be repeated using a serum or plasma sample.
9. ELISA tests using saliva or tears have a disproportionate number of both false-positive and false-negative results.[1] Therefore, these tests cannot be recommended for routine screening of individual cats.
10. One should always run a validated IFA test to confirm results on a healthy positive cat before considering it persistently viremic.[1]
11. No test is 100% accurate at all times and under all conditions; therefore, a critical decision about the care of a patient—whether healthy or ill—should never be based solely on a single test result.[3]
12. All kittens or adult cats that test negative by the first ELISA screening test—but with a known or suspected exposure to FeLV—should be retested. This is done to rule out possible negative results obtained during incubation of the FeLV virus. Although the majority of cats will test positive within several weeks, final retest of negative cats should be no sooner than 90 days after exposure. Clients should be counseled on the potential risk of FeLV exposure when adding a cat with one negative test result to an FeLV-negative household.
13. Discordant results are defined as conflicting test results, usually being an ELISA-positive and IFA-negative result.[1] Discordancy can occur owing to testing in the early phase of infection; antigenemia without viremia (no intact virus); or a false-positive ELISA due to faulty technique or cross-reactive antigens. These cats should be monitored by both ELISA and IFA assays at 4- to 8-week intervals for at least 90 days.[2]
14. Periodic (e.g., annual) testing of cats "at risk" is justifiable. Cats at risk are defined as those with known or potential exposure to FeLV. These include outdoor cats; fighting cats; strays; cats with bite wounds; escapees; recently mated females if the FeLV status of the male is unknown; cats in open multiple-cat households; cats in closed multiple-cat households with any other cats of unknown FeLV status; cats in households having a known FeLV-positive cat.
15. All FeLV-negative exposed cats in a multiple-cat household (in which an FeLV carrier is found) should be retested at 3-month intervals until all cats within the household or facility test FeLV negative on at least 2 consecutive tests and the risk of exposure to FeLV infection is past. All FeLV-positive cats should be immediately isolated or removed at the time of diagnosis.[1, 4]
16. Other confirmatory tests, such as methodologies utilizing polymerase chain reaction (PCR), may be useful but are currently unvalidated. Although PCR offers a promising approach to FeLV testing, currently neither production of PCR reagents (primers) nor testing protocols are standardized or consistent.
17. Latent infections with FeLV are undetectable with ELISA or IFA testing. PCR testing can offer a new means of detecting these cases.[5] Shedding of FeLV or development of FeLV-related diseases can be a consequence in latently infected cats, but is felt to be a rare clinical occurrence.[2]
18. FeLV-positive healthy cats may live for months to years. The question of euthanizing a positive cat is one that must be addressed in each individual case, in consultation between veterinarian and client. Effective FeLV case management involves measures aimed at preserving the health of the infected cat; preventing the spread of FeLV infection; and early recognition and aggressive treatment of FeLV-associated disease. The quality of life and clinical status of FeLV-positive cats can be enhanced through the concerted efforts of the pet owner and the attending veterinarian.

[a]All recommendations regarding IFA testing are based on studies done by a VALIDATED IFA test run by National Veterinary Laboratories.
[1]Colloquium on FeLV/FIV: Tests and vaccination. J Am Vet Med Assoc 199(10):1275–1276, 1991.
[2]Loar AS: Feline leukemia virus tests: Evaluation and interpretation. In: August J, ed: Consultations in Feline Internal Medicine. Philadelphia: WB Saunders, 1991, pp 535–541.
[3]Barr MC: Feline immunodeficiency virus tests and their interpretation. Feline Health Top Vet 8(3):1–5, 8, 1993.
[4]Rojko JL, Hardy WD, Jr: Feline leukemia virus and other retroviruses. In: Sherding R, ed: The Cat: Diseases and Clinical Management, 2nd ed. New York: Churchill Livingstone, 1994, pp 361–375.
[5]Kremer KA, Thompson JP: Polymerase chain reaction detection of feline leukemia virus in naturally infected cats. In: ACVIM abstract, Proceedings of the 12th ACVIM Forum, San Francisco, CA, 1994, p 1007.

MANAGEMENT OF THE FeLV-POSITIVE CAT

Husbandry

It is not necessary to euthanatize a healthy FeLV-infected cat if the owner understands the long-term implications of this infection. Many of these animals remain healthy for a long time if kept in a protected environment and provided with good nutrition and excellent health care. FeLV-infected cats should not be allowed to roam freely outdoors because they have the potential to spread the infection and they themselves may be exposed to injury, environmental hazards, or diseases from other animals they encounter. FeLV-infected cats should be kept indoors in a single-cat household, or if there are multiple cats the infected cat or cats must be separated from the other cats in the house. Although FeLV vaccination may provide some protection for the uninfected housemates, no vaccine is 100% effective and the best way of avoiding any risk of transmission is to keep the infected cat isolated. Routine vaccinations against feline parvovirus (panleukopenia), feline herpesvirus, feline calicivirus, and rabies should be given on an appropriate schedule. Vaccination of FeLV-infected cats with an FeLV vaccine is not necessary or beneficial. Because FeLV-associated immunosuppression is the major cause of morbidity and mortality in FeLV-infected cats, any signs of illness should be recognized and treated promptly. Secondary bacterial infections are treated with antibiotics (see p. 269).

Specific Treatment Strategies

Immunomodulators

Immunosuppression is a major feature of FeLV infection; thus, there is great interest in immunomodulator therapy and a number of these therapies have been used to treat FeLV-infected cats (see p. 287). Most reports on immunomodulators have been uncontrolled clinical studies, so it is difficult to critically evaluate their efficacy. Reports such as these must be treated as anecdotal because we know that clinical improvement in FeLV-infected cats can occur with symptomatic therapy alone and spontaneous seroconversion to FeLV-negative status does occur.

Staphylococcal protein A (Protein A, Pharmacia Biotech) has been used at a dose of 10 μg/kg IP twice weekly to treat FeLV-infected cats. One report recorded clinical improvement in some cats and a few that reverted to FeLV-negative status. This study was not controlled, and it is not known how many cats would have improved or seroconverted without SPA treatment. In a controlled study with SPA, there was no seroconversion and no improvement in humoral immune responses with a similar protocol (20 μg/2.75 kg IP twice weekly for 8 weeks).

In an uncontrolled study, acemannan (Carrington Laboratories) was given at a dose of 2 mg/kg IP once weekly for 6 weeks. Some of the treated cats clinically improved; however, there were no untreated control subjects with which to compare these results. In blinded, controlled studies with acemannan conducted at Texas A & M University, no differences were seen in clinical signs or mortality in treated and untreated FeLV-infected cats. Similar controlled studies on FIV-infected cats showed no significant change

in their CD4/CD8 ratios (a quantitative measure of cell-mediated immunity) after 8 weeks of acemannan treatment.

In an uncontrolled clinical study of a killed *Propionibacterium acnes* preparation (Immunoregulin, ImmunoVet) given at 0.5 ml (per cat) IV once or twice weekly, clinical improvement was reported in some of the treated cats. However, other treatments were used in addition to *P. acnes,* and it is difficult to determine what actually produced the improvement.

In experimental trials, human recombinant interferon alpha (rHuIFN-α; Roferon, Roche), given at a dose of 1,000 to 10,000 U/kg IM every 24 hours, has been demonstrated to enhance lymphocyte responses in normal cats. Another study in FeLV-infected cats demonstrated a reduction in viral load with the use of similar rHuIFN-α doses. Even a temporary reduction in viral load might allow an affected cat's immune status to improve sufficiently to recover from a secondary infection or bone marrow insult. This study also demonstrated that antibodies developed against heterologous rHuIFN-α limit high-dose parenteral rHuIFN-α therapy to a 3- to 7-week course. A combined trial with high-dose rHuIFN-α, as previously described, and the antiviral drug 3′-azido-3′-deoxythymidine (zidovudine [formerly AZT]; Retrovir, Glaxo Wellcome) demonstrated that a combination of these agents was no more effective than rHuIFN-α alone in reducing the magnitude of FeLV viremia in asymptomatic cats. Low-dose (30 U every 24 hours) oral administration of rHuIFN-α is used by a number of clinicians to treat FeLV-infected cats, and anecdotally it appears to reduce clinical signs and improve well-being in some infected cats. Given at this dosage and by this route, interferon therapy appears to be safe, does not stimulate antibody production, is inexpensive, and is convenient for the owner to administer. Recent experimental studies suggest that interferon gamma (IFN-γ) may be even more immunostimulatory and produces fewer side effects at high doses than does rHuIFN-α. No clinical trials with IFN-γ have yet been completed.

Most studies evaluating immunomodulators have been performed on symptomatic FeLV-infected cats. Immunomodulators do not seem to have harmful effects when given for short periods, but proof of their superiority compared to symptomatic treatment alone is lacking because of the paucity of well-controlled studies. Whether long-term treatment of asymptomatic cats with immunomodulators is helpful or will prolong the asymptomatic period or longevity of FeLV-infected cats is unknown. Clearly, immunomodulators are not panaceas, and controlled clinical studies using these agents are badly needed.

Antiviral Drugs

Use of either the antiviral drug zidovudine, at 15 mg/kg PO every 12 hours, or 9-(2-phosphomethoxyethyl)adenine (PMEA), at 2.5 mg/kg SC every 12 hours, has reduced clinical symptoms in some ill FeLV-infected and FIV-infected cats. No change in their virus status was observed. These drugs are toxic to the bone marrow, and cats being treated with either zidovudine or PMEA should have hemograms evaluated frequently. Treatment with these drugs at these doses should be limited to a 3-week course to avoid marrow toxicity. Zidovudine was used at a dosage of 5 mg/kg PO every 8 hours in a controlled study of symptomatic cats with natural FIV infection. Six of nine treated cats had a complete remission of clinical signs after 4 to 6 weeks of treatment. Side effects of zidovudine included transient anemia and hyperglobulinemia in five cats, and hyperglycemia with persistent anemia in one cat. Interestingly, the control group in this study was treated with antibiotics and immunomodulators alone, and all five of these cats experienced remission of symptoms within 10 to 14 days. This obviously demonstrates the difficulty of doing comparative trials in clinical patients. Zidovudine, 15 mg/kg PO every 12 hours, or diethylcarbamazine citrate (DEC), 3 mg/kg PO every 24 hours, delayed the onset of tumor development and improved survival times in cats experimentally infected with a lymphoma-producing FeLV virus strain compared with untreated control subjects. Another antiviral agent related to PMEA, 9-[(2R,5R-2,5-dihydro-5-phosphonomethyoxy)-2-furanyl]adenine (D4API), demonstrates excellent in vitro retroviral inhibition. Unfortunately, this drug is an accumulative toxin causing widespread hepatic and lymphoid necrosis in vivo in cats.

All these antiviral drugs have significant toxic effects in cats, and a decision to use them must be considered carefully. Antiviral agents can reduce the FeLV viral load and may improve clinical signs of illness and reduce immuno-suppression associated with this infection. Their use should probably be limited to short-term administration to patients with severe clinical signs in which symptomatic therapy alone may not be lifesaving.

References and Suggested Reading

Jackson ML, Haines DM, Taylor SM: Feline leukemia virus detection by ELISA and PCR in peripheral blood from 68 cats with high, moderate, or low suspicion of having FeLV-related disease. J Vet Diagn Invest 8:25, 1996.
 Compares results between these two techniques.
Hawks DM, Legendre AM, Rohrbach BW: Comparison of four test kits for feline leukemia virus antigen. J Am Vet Med Assoc 199:1373, 1991.
Lubkin SR, Romatowski J, Zhu M, et al: Evaluation of feline leukemia virus control measures. J Theor Biol 178:53, 1996.
 Demonstrates a mathematical model for predicting efficacy of vaccination and test and removal procedures in various cat populations.
Sellon R, Novotney C, Devera C, et al: Therapeutic effects of diethylcarbamazine and 3'-azido-3'-deoxythymidine on feline leukemia virus lymphoma formation. Vet Immunol Immunopathol 46:181, 1995.
Zeidner NS, Myles MH, Mathiason-DuBard CK, et al: Alpha interferon (2b) in combination with zidovudine for the treatment of presymptomatic feline leukemia virus–induced immunodeficiency syndrome. Antimicrob Agents Chemother 34:1749, 1990.
 Demonstrates efficacy of and development of antibodies against rHu-INFα given at high doses parenterally to cats.

CVT Update: Feline Immunodeficiency Virus

JULIE K. LEVY
Gainesville, Florida

Feline immunodeficiency virus (FIV) is a lymphotrophic lentivirus that, like HIV in humans, causes an acquired immunodeficiency syndrome (AIDS) in domestic cats. FIV is related morphologically and biochemically to HIV but is antigenically distinct. Both viruses also share a similar pattern of pathogenesis, characterized by a long period of clinical latency during which immune function gradually deteriorates. During this time, the number of T helper (CD4+) cells decreases, resulting in an inverted ratio of CD4+ cells to cytotoxic-suppressor (CD8+) cells. It has been reported that concurrent with the loss of important T-cell subsets, the production of cytokines (interleukins-12 and -2) critical for the development of a strong cell-mediated immune response to pathogens are decreased, whereas a suppressive cytokine (interleukin-10) is increased. Eventually, AIDS develops and is accompanied by opportunistic infections, systemic disease, and malignancies. It is the close relationship between HIV and FIV that has kindled interest in the use of FIV as an animal model for the study of human HIV pathogenesis. Because of this, FIV has been intensively studied, and much has been learned since the first description of the virus a decade ago.

VIRAL TRANSMISSION

Although the existence of FIV was first reported in 1987, there are extensive data indicating that cats have carried this virus for a much longer time. FIV has a worldwide distribution in domestic cats, with infection rates approaching one third of the cats in some populations. Altered strains of the virus are also found to infect at least 17 species of wild felidae. The greater diversity of viral nucleic acid sequences and the decreased pathogenicity of wild cat strains compared with those of domestic cats suggest that nondomestic felids may have been living with the virus for a longer time and that domestic cat virus strains may have originated with wild cats (Carpenter and O'Brien, 1995). These observations are similar to the belief that HIV infection in humans may have arisen recently (less than 100 years ago) from a related virus of nonhuman primates. Over time, host resistance and viral attenuation usually develop so that the host-parasite relationship becomes less destructive, as is the case for FIV.

Epidemiologic studies of domestic cats have long suggested that most cases of FIV infection are acquired by horizontal transmission among adult cats. Worldwide, adult male cats living outdoors consistently compose the majority of FIV-infected cats, and the risk is highest for sexually intact males. The fighting and biting behavior of this group of cats is believed to be the main cause of transmission. Infectious virus is found in the saliva of FIV-positive cats, and the virus has been successfully transmitted via experimental bite wounds. Interestingly, sexual transmission, the most common mode of transmission of HIV, appears to be unusual in FIV, even though the semen of infected cats frequently contains infectious virus. In large surveys of stray and feral cats in the United States, overall prevalence rates of 2 to 4% are usually reported. Of 850 feral cats presented to a spay-neuter clinic in Raleigh, NC, over a 16-month period, 20 cats were FIV-positive (2.3%); of these, 75% were males. In another study, 80% of 826 naturally infected cats examined at North American veterinary teaching hospitals were males, and 78% were at least 2 years old at the time of presentation. In an interesting model of FIV transmission within colonies of free-roaming cats, it has been suggested that FIV has little impact on the total population. A low rate of transmission, the long asymptomatic stage of infection, and the high death rate from other causes combine to minimize the effect of the virus on these cats. Such colonies usually exist at the carrying capacity of the habitat, regardless of whether FIV infection exists in the group. The low impact of FIV is taken as further evidence that FIV infection of domestic cats arose long ago.

Vertical transmission, which is perhaps the most common route of infection of FeLV, appears to be infrequent in FIV in nature. Neonatal kittens are known to be susceptible to infection by oral inoculation of FIV or by nursing on acutely infected queens. Likewise, certain strains of FIV, but not others, are capable of crossing the placenta to infect fetuses if the queen is infected during pregnancy. More recently, queens chronically infected with certain FIV strains have been shown to produce infected offspring, particularly if the maternal CD4+ cell count is less than 200 cells/μl and if the queen has clinical signs of immunodeficiency. In contrast to the relative ease with which kittens can be experimentally infected via their mothers, in nature, FIV-positive queens rarely infect their offspring. This is believed to result from the biologic characteristics of the virus, in which a high viral burden is produced for only a few weeks after infection. After the acute stage of infection, the plasma antibody titer rises, circulating virus is often undetectable, and vertical transmission becomes unlikely.

The practical aspect of transmission research arises when clients present kittens for routine testing or when one of the cats in a household is found to be infected with FIV. Although kittens that nurse chronically infected queens are unlikely to become infected, they readily absorb colostral antibodies against FIV. Testing such a kitten will result in a false-positive result, because diagnostic enzyme-linked immunosorbent assay (ELISA) or Western blot tests detect antibodies, not antigen. Most such kittens are truly uninfected, and colostral antibody titers decline over a period of several months. Therefore, a diagnosis of FIV infection should not be made on the basis of an antibody test before the age of 6 months. Because transmission by casual contact, such as sharing litter boxes and food dishes is uncommon, it is relatively safe to keep an FIV-positive pet in a household with other cats if the cats do not fight.

DIAGNOSIS

The mainstay of clinical screening for FIV infection is ELISA detection of circulating antibodies against FIV.

Routine screening for viral antigens is not possible because after the acute infection stage, circulating viral burden is low and difficult to detect. Because FIV produces a persistent infection from which few cats recover, the detection of specific antibodies is adequate for the diagnosis of infection. The exception to this occurs in kittens that have acquired anti-FIV antibodies by passive transfer in colostrum. ELISAs have the potential for occasional false-positive results, so the Western blot is used to confirm infections in low-risk cats. Some cats fail to produce detectable antibodies to FIV following infection, and these cats will have false-negative results on ELISA or Western blots. More sensitive tests for the detection of viral nucleic acids, such as the polymerase chain reaction (PCR), or infectious virus (viral culture) are used routinely in research laboratories, but patent restrictions have prevented their use as diagnostic tests in the United States. An interesting form of infection that escapes detection by routine tests is seen in cats that appear to mount a strong cell-mediated immune response to the virus. Some cats experimentally challenged with FIV appear to resist infection in that no circulating FIV antibodies or antigens are detected and that PCR and viral culture results of peripheral blood mononuclear cells are negative. In some of these cats, however, removal of CD8+ cytotoxic-suppressor cells from blood samples prior to viral culture unmasks FIV infection. It appears that in these cats, CD8+ T cells are strong inhibitors of virus replication. This observation not only implies that some cats have acquired partial immunity against FIV but also suggests a mechanism by which vaccination strategies or immunomodulatory therapeutics may be developed against FIV.

EMERGING DISEASE SYNDROMES

The course of clinical disease following infection with FIV is dependent on a number of factors, including the age and health of the cat at the time of infection, the dose and route of virus inoculation, the strain of the virus, and the immunologic background of the cat. Experimental infections of cats with different backgrounds have helped to differentiate primary viral effects from those that develop only in the presence of disease cofactors. For instance, there are marked differences in the development of disease syndromes in laboratory-reared specific pathogen–free (SPF) cats compared with random-source cats previously exposed to common feline pathogens such as upper respiratory infections and parasites. In one report of cats followed for 4 years after experimental FIV infection, both SPF and random-source cats experienced immunodeficiency marked by progressive inversion of the CD4+:CD8+ cell ratio and decreased mitogen responses. The random-source cats went on to acquire an AIDS-like syndrome characterized by stomatitis, recurrent respiratory disease, diarrhea, and weight loss. In contrast, several SPF cats developed B-cell lymphomas or neurologic disease, which are believed to represent direct viral effects, but not AIDS. This suggests that various infectious cofactors have a profound influence on the clinical course of cats infected with FIV (English et al, 1994).

During natural FIV infection, most cats experience a prolonged asymptomatic period of several years following seroconversion. The age of 826 FIV-positive cats presented for evaluation at veterinary teaching hospitals since 1988 peaked at 10 to 15 years. In contrast, most of the other feline patients seen at these centers were less than 7 years old. The most common disease syndromes diagnosed in the FIV-positive patients were stomatitis, neoplasia (especially lymphoma and cutaneous squamous cell carcinoma), ocular inflammation (uveitis and chorioretinitis), anemia and leukopenia, opportunistic infections, renal insufficiency, lower urinary tract disease, and endocrinopathies such as hyperthyroidism and diabetes mellitus.

Feline Immunodeficiency Virus–Associated Nephropathy

FIV-infected cats are at increased risk for the development of chronic renal insufficiency when compared with uninfected cats. In a study of 155 cats with natural FIV infection examined at the North Carolina State University College of Veterinary Medicine, FIV-infected cats were much more likely to be azotemic and proteinuric than were age-matched FIV-negative cats. In a similar study of 97 SPF cats with experimental FIV infection, FIV-positive cats were more likely to have renal dysfunction than were FIV-negative SPF cats, although the severity of azotemia and proteinuria was less than that of the naturally infected cats. Renal biopsy specimens were examined in a subset of each group. Renal lesions were more common in FIV-positive cats, with thickened Bowman's membrane, glomerulosclerosis, microcystic tubular dilatation, and mononuclear interstitial infiltrates and fibrosis being the most common findings. Human patients with HIV infection are also at increased risk for the development of renal disease. HIV-associated nephropathy affects up to 40% of HIV-infected patients and is characterized by a prolonged course of proteinuria, followed terminally by rapidly progressive end-stage renal disease. The histopathologic lesion of HIV-associated nephropathy is a distinctive focal segmental glomerulosclerosis and microcystic tubular dilatation. The similar renal syndromes that develop in both cats and humans with these viral infections suggest a common pathogenesis, but extensive efforts to identify an infectious agent or specific molecular cause have been unsuccessful.

Neurologic Disease

Both central and peripheral neurologic disease complicates the course of HIV infection of humans, and the same is true of FIV (see p. 288). The dementia of human AIDS is often characterized by a slight decline in cognitive ability or behavior, changes that may be too subtle to recognize in cats. In some cats, however, obvious central and peripheral neurologic disease occurs and may take the form of seizures, striking behavior changes, anisocoria, or paresis. Sensitive electrodiagnostic tests such as nerve conduction velocities and brain stem auditory evoked potentials may detect abnormalities in clinically normal FIV-infected cats. Experimentally, neurologic expression of FIV infection is highly strain-dependent. Neurologic abnormalities tend to respond favorably to treatment with zidovudine (AZT) (15

mg/kg PO every 12 hours); in many cases, there is marked improvement within the first days of therapy. Neurologic disease represents one of the most AZT-responsive clinical syndromes associated with FIV infection.

Ulceroproliferative Stomatitis

Chronic ulceroproliferative stomatitis is one of the most common disease syndromes induced in cats with long-standing FIV infection. Interestingly, this syndrome occurs only in cats that are also exposed to other infectious agents in addition to FIV, and does not develop in SPF cats. Concurrent calicivirus infection is often identified in the oral cavity of cats with FIV-associated stomatitis and may be one of the infectious cofactors capable of inducing stomatitis in combination with FIV. The proliferative mucosal lesions associated with FIV characteristically originate in the fauces and gradually spread rostrally, especially along the maxillary teeth. The lesions are often painful and infected, and tooth loss is common. Histologically, the mucosa is invaded by plasma cells and lymphocytes, accompanied by variable degrees of neutrophilic and eosinophilic inflammation. The cause of the syndrome is uncertain, although the histologic findings suggest an immune response to chronic antigenic stimulation or immune dysregulation. In addition, the circulating lymphocytes of cats with stomatitis have higher than normal expression of inflammatory cytokines, further implicating immune activation in the pathogenesis of this condition. Repeated treatment with dental cleaning, antibiotics, or corticosteroids may offer palliative relief but is rarely sufficient to resolve the lesions or to halt additional tooth loss. The most effective treatment is extraction of the molars and premolars, paying careful attention to removal of all of the roots of the teeth. In almost all cases of stomatitis in FIV-positive cats, long-term resolution of inflammation is achieved, and cats return to eating a normal diet, including kibble. Persistent lesions may develop over remnants of incompletely removed tooth roots or may resolve only after extraction of the canines and incisors in addition to the cheek teeth.

PREVENTION OF FELINE IMMUNODEFICIENCY VIRUS INFECTION

Many approaches have been taken toward the development of an effective vaccine against FIV, but the same hurdles facing HIV prevention also apply to the feline virus. Both viruses have error-prone reverse transcriptases, which enhance the mutation rate of replicating virus and increase the opportunity for escape from immune surveillance. The viruses also take advantage of specific antibody formation, often using these antibodies to enhance viral pathogenicity or to enter cells via immune complexes. Although neutralizing antibodies are of some importance in resistance to HIV and FIV, most work has focused on vaccines that induce a strong antiviral cell-mediated immune response. Various approaches have been taken to the development of FIV immunity, including passive transfer of antibodies and immune cells, inactivated whole virus, fixed infected cells, viral subunits, viral and plasmid vectors, DNA transfer, mucosal vaccination, mutant strains, and various adjuvants. To date, no approach has been completely successful in preventing infection of a challenge inoculum, and in some cases immunization paradoxically enhances viral replication and disease expression. In cases in which a vaccine does prove effective, prevention is usually conferred only to the homologous strain from which the vaccine is derived. Vaccine failure is especially prominent when the challenge virus is from another FIV subtype or "clade." Complicating the evaluation of vaccine efficacy is the recent report of latent infectious virus isolated from necropsy tissues of cats that had tested negative by PCR for circulating virus for more than a year past vaccination and challenge.

Until an effective vaccine is developed, the only truly effective means of preventing disease transmission is to keep cats indoors where they will not encounter other infected cats. Spaying and neutering cats that do go outdoors also limits the spread of FIV by decreasing fighting and roaming behavior. Cats that are already infected should be kept indoors to reduce the risk to other cats as well as to reduce their exposure to secondary infectious diseases.

TREATMENT

Immune Modulator Therapy

Immunomodulators are proposed to benefit FIV-infected cats by restoring compromised immune function, thereby enabling cats to reduce the viral burden and its associated clinical syndromes. Two currently used immunomodulators, acemannan (Carrisyn, Carrington Laboratories) and *Propionibacterium acnes* (Immunoregulin, Immunovet), are proposed to stimulate the immune system via nonspecific activation of macrophages and the subsequent production of interleukin-1, tumor necrosis factor, and interferon gamma production. Low-dose interferon alpha (Intron-A, Schering Plough, 0.5 to 30 U/cat PO every 24 hours for 5 days on alternate weeks) has also gained interest as a potential, but unproven, immune stimulant. The mechanism by which interferon alpha may act is unknown, but the product is not believed to be present in the blood or oral cavity at sufficient concentrations to achieve an antiviral effect. It is possible that interferon alpha binds to mucosal receptors, triggering an immunologic cascade with advantageous systemic responses. However, in our laboratory, five cats with ulceroproliferative stomatitis caused by chronic FIV infection failed to respond to oral interferon alpha treatment with either improved clinical signs or CD4$^+$:CD8$^+$ cell ratio correction. One concern that has arisen over the use of nonspecific immune stimulation in FIV-positive or HIV-positive patients is the possibility of enhanced viral replication and disease progression that typically follows lymphocyte activation and division. This may be unwarranted, however, since neither viral burden nor disease progression was accelerated in FIV-positive cats sequentially stimulated by polyproline immunogens, rabies virus vaccination, *Toxoplasma gondii*, herpesvirus, *Haemobartonella felis*, calicivirus, and diptheria, tetanus, and pertussis vaccination (Reubel et al, 1994). Unfortunately, there is scant literature reporting controlled trials of immunomodulators for the benefit of FIV-infected cats. Overall, those that have been performed have been disappointing.

Antiviral Therapy

AZT (Retrovir, Burroughs Wellcome), remains the only drug currently available with proven efficacy and safety in the treatment of experimental and natural FIV infection. An inhibitor of the retroviral enzyme, reverse transcriptase, AZT (15 mg/kg PO every 12 hours) effectively aborts experimental infection when treatment is started at the time of virus inoculation. In a double-blind, placebo-controlled trial of AZT (5 mg/kg SC every 12 hours) in cats with natural FIV infection and stomatitis, AZT-treated cats had significant improvements in stomatitis, overall clinical condition, and CD4$^+$:CD8$^+$ cell ratios after 3 weeks of therapy, whereas the cats receiving placebo continued to deteriorate (Hartmann, et al, 1992). AZT (5 mg/kg PO or SC every 8 to 12 hours) has also been reported to be effective in naturally infected cats with clinical signs of FIV disease (respiratory infections, diarrhea, stomatitis) treated with AZT for up to 2 years. Although response was variable, most of the reported cats had sustained clinical improvement and increased CD4$^+$:CD8$^+$ cell ratios throughout the treatment. The most common complication of AZT treatment is anemia. If the packed cell volume drops to less than 20%, treatment should be stopped until it returns to normal, usually in 1 to 2 weeks. The AZT can then be restarted at half the previous dose and increased to the original dose after 1 to 2 more weeks. In most cases, such cats will eventually tolerate return to the initial dose. As in HIV, chronic AZT treatment can enhance the mutation rate of FIV, which might eventually lead to AZT-resistant strains and drug resistance. The recent advances in antiviral therapy yielded by a new class of drugs known as protease inhibitors have altered the standard of care for HIV-positive patients. Unfortunately, these protease inhibitors appear to be highly species-specific, and in vitro screening of several different protease inhibitors for anti-FIV activity has been disappointing.

References and Suggested Reading

Carpenter MA, O'Brien MA: Coadaptation and immunodeficiency virus: Lessons from the Felidae. Curr Opin Genet Dev 5:739, 1995.
  Review of the coadaptation of host and virus at the individual and population level, in disease outbreaks, and during spread to related host species.
English RV, Nelson P, Johnson CM, et al: Development of clinical disease in cats experimentally infected with feline immunodeficiency virus. J Infect Dis 170:543, 1994.
  A prospective study of the long-term disease expression of random source and SPF cats during FIV infection.
Hartmann K, Donath A, Beer B, et al: Use of two virustatica (AZT, PMEA) in the treatment of FIV and of FeLV seropositive cats with clinical symptoms. Vet Immunol Immunopathol 35:167, 1992.
  A double-blind, placebo-controlled clinical trial of AZT and 9-(2-phosphonylmethoxyethyl) adenine (PMEA) treatment of 33 clinically ill FIV-infected cats.
Proceedings of the Third International Feline Retrovirus Research Symposium, Fort Collins, Co, March 6–9, 1996.
  Abstracts of 99 current worldwide research projects on the epidemiology, virology, immunology, pathogenesis, treatment, and prevention of FIV infection.

Proceedings of the Fourth International Feline Retrovirus Research Symposium, Glasgow, Scotland, May 28–30, 1998.
Abstracts of 81 international research projects on FIV and FeLV.
Reubel GH, Dean GA, George JW, et al: Effects of incidental infections and immune activation on disease progression in experimentally feline immunodeficiency virus–infected cats. J Acquir Immune Defic Syndr 7:1003, 1994.
Virologic and immunologic response during immune stimulation of FIV-infected cats and the relationship to progression of clinical disease.

Retroviral Infection of the Nervous System

ELISABETH ZENGER
San Francisco, California

Among the clinically notable and biologically intriguing aspects of retroviruses are their effects on the central nervous system (CNS). In addition to opportunistic CNS infections and neoplasms predisposed to retrovirus-associated immunodeficiency, there is also a unique syndrome of neurologic impairment that appears to result from a more fundamental effect of the retrovirus itself. Although lentiviruses, including feline immunodeficiency virus (FIV), human immunodeficiency virus (HIV), simian immunodeficiency virus, and others, seem to be the more clinically relevant retroviral neuropathogens, the oncornavirus feline leukemia virus (FeLV) has been associated with neurologic syndromes as well. The high incidence of neurologic dysfunction from HIV infection has led to heightened interest in retrovirus-associated neuropathogenesis, including that associated with feline retrovirus infections. Although neuropathogenesis of FeLV is still not well characterized, FIV has been shown to cause a disease syndrome in cats remarkably similar to that associated with HIV infection in humans. An extensive introduction to neurologic disease associated with feline retroviral infection can be found elsewhere (see *CVT XI,* p. 1010). Following is an updated summary of retroviral infections of the CNS including information on their neuropathogenesis.

CLINICAL NEUROLOGIC DISEASE AND PATHOLOGY

In common with all retroviruses, FeLV and FIV are neuroinvasive and neurovirulent to various degrees. The incidence of FeLV-associated neurologic disease is uncommon and most often due to lymphosarcoma (LSA). Other, more unusual neurologic manifestations associated with FeLV infection include myelopathy, urinary incontinence, and intermittent anisocoria without visual deficits.

Close observation specifically looking for evidence of neurologic dysfunction has shown that FIV-associated neurologic disease may not be uncommon. Neurologic dysfunction was observed in nearly one third of FIV-infected cats studied over a 3-year period (Dow et al, 1992). The nature of the neurologic abnormalities tends to be behavioral rather than motor, although a wide range of deficits has been described. Reported clinical behavioral abnormalities encompass subtle to overt changes, including docility, agitation, confusion, loss of litterbox training, dementia or psychotic behavior (hiding, rage, excessive aggression), and compulsive (i.e., repetitive, purposeless) motor movement or roaming. Specific neurologic defects have included anisocoria, nystagmus, delayed pupillary reflex, ataxia, paresis, paralysis, delayed or absent righting, and other abnormal postural reflexes. Focal seizures seem to be a common finding and are characterized as twitching of a specific muscle group. These are frequently facial muscles, but flank muscle involvement has also been reported. Epileptiform convulsions and intention tremors have also been observed. Alterations in sleep patterns have been reported in cats experimentally infected with FIV, and decreased rapid eye movement sleep with associated fatigue and malaise may contribute to decreased quality of life in these cats as it does in HIV-infected patients.

Although the majority of FIV-infected cats do not manifest clinically observable neurologic dysfunction, a much higher proportion have microscopic CNS lesions. However, as occurs with HIV, there is often poor correlation between the histopathologic lesions and detected clinical neurologic abnormalities. Experimental infection with Petaluma strain FIV consistently causes gliosis and inflammatory cell infiltration in the CNS, but these lesions usually are not associated with clinical disease. In contrast, experimental infection with Maryland strain FIV causes rapid onset of neurologic signs but only mild CNS lesions (Podell et al, 1993). It has also been our experience with FeLV that there may be considerable neurologic dysfunction documented clinically with no detectable lesions on routine histopathologic examination. Therefore, the clinician should not be dismayed by a lack of histopathologic changes at postmortem examination.

NEUROPATHOGENESIS OF RETROVIRUS INFECTIONS

Although there has been a surge of information during the last several years, many questions regarding retrovirus-associated neuropathogenesis are unanswered. Lentiviruses seem to be the more important retroviral neuropathogens, although there are reports that FeLV is also associated with neurologic syndromes (see *CVT XI,* p. 1010). FeLV has been recovered from the cerebrospinal fluid (CSF) of cats with neurologic disease, and experimentally FeLV has been shown to infect the CNS and induce spinal cord dysfunction. Neuropathogenesis of FeLV apart from that caused by LSA is poorly understood and has been attributed to polyneuropathy. There is evidence that FeLV envelope proteins may be directly neurotoxic via altered calcium homeostasis, although the in vivo significance of this is yet to be substantiated.

Despite nearly a decade of research, the CNS target cells and alterations responsible for neurologic dysfunction from FIV are yet to be definitely identified. In vivo and in vitro studies suggest that neuroglia, the support cells of the CNS, rather than neurons are the principal cellular targets for lentiviruses. The observed neurologic dysfunction likely involves an intricate web of subcellular pathways and neurotoxic factors affecting neurons but produced by infected neuroglia, specifically microglia and astroglia. Microglia, macrophages, and derivative multinucleated cells have been identified as the major HIV-expressing cells in the brain. However, the number of these cells is small relative to the widespread neuropathologic condition. Nonproductive infection of astroglial cells may play a major role in the development and progression of lentivirus-associated neurologic dysfunction although in vivo productive infection of astroglia seems to be rare. Prominent nonexclusive hypotheses to explain possible indirect mechanisms of retrovirus-induced neuronal dysfunction include direct toxicity of viral proteins, excitotoxicity from accumulation or potentiation of excitatory neurotransmitters such as glutamate, and immunologically mediated damage from toxic products such as tumor necrosis factor, nitric oxide, or free radicals.

Investigations of FIV's effects on microglia have been few. In vitro FIV infection of microglia is relatively noncytopathic, and altered function or cytokine release has not been demonstrated. Results of experiments examining HIV-infected microglia suggest that despite widespread belief in the importance of microglia in lentivirus-associated neuropathogenesis, there are likely to be other players of at least as much significance. Astroglial functions in the maintenance of CNS homeostasis include regulation of ion concentrations, uptake and metabolism of certain neurotransmitters such as the excitotoxic amino acid glutamate, and development and maintenance of the blood-brain barrier. Disruption of any of these astroglial functions could lead to neuronal damage. In vitro studies suggest a critical role for altered astroglial function in the progression of FIV-associated neurologic disease. FIV infection of astroglia causes significant toxic effects at the subcellular level (Zenger et al, 1995), including decreased mitochondrial membrane potential and cell-cell communication via gap junctions, perturbed calcium homeostasis, plasma membrane fluidity, and intracellular glutathione concentration. Exposure to FIV enhances sensitivity to the excitotoxic effects of glutamate in primary feline mixed neuronal-glial cultures (Meeker et al, 1993). Whether this results from impaired glutamate uptake by astroglia or is caused by a synergistic effect of the virus and the excitatory amino acid is uncertain, and it may actually be a combination of both. We have demonstrated a significant decrease in the ability of astroglia to take up glutamate as early as 1 day following infection with FIV.

DIAGNOSIS OF RETROVIRUS-ASSOCIATED NEUROLOGIC DISEASE

The diagnostic tests that may be useful in differentiating opportunistic infections and neoplasia from primary effects of the retrovirus are outlined in Table 1. Despite some differences in the pattern of primary disease versus secondary effects, direct virus-induced neurologic dysfunction is diagnosed by exclusion of other causes. Clinicians must be careful not to ascribe all clinical diseases in retrovirus-seropositive cats to the virus. Although opportunistic infection seems to be a surprisingly rare cause of retrovirus-associated neurologic disease, it is worth considering in the diagnostic work-up because of the potential for treatment. The initial data base in cases of suspected retrovirus-associated neurologic disease should include complete physical, ophthalmic, and neurologic examinations; a complete blood cell count; serum chemistry panels; and serum enzyme-linked immunosorbent assays for FeLV and FIV. Results may help dictate what ancillary tests are appropriate. For both FeLV and FIV, immunodiagnostic testing of serum may produce negative results despite the presence of virus infection; negative FeLV and FIV test results do not exclude these as causes of retrovirus-associated neurologic disease.

Cryptococcosis, toxoplasmosis, and feline infectious peritonitis virus infections are the most common secondary infections resulting in neurologic disease in retrovirus-infected cats (Lappin, 1995). The incidence of cryptococcosis in FIV-infected cats compared with uninfected cats suggests that coinfection is coincidental rather than opportunistic. Infection with feline infectious peritonitis appears to be strongly associated with FeLV but not with FIV. Although FIV infection potentiates *Toxoplasma gondii* repli-

TABLE 1. Diagnostic Approach for Retrovirus-Associated Neurologic Disease

Cause (Rule Out)	Diagnostic Evaluation
Opportunistic infection, e.g., toxoplasmosis, FIP, bacterial meningitis or abscess	Physical-neurologic examination—fever, nonlocalizing deficits
	Serum or CSF titers for antibodies to specific organisms
	CSF analysis—mild increased protein and mononuclear cells, may show organisms or inflammatory cells
	EEG—irritative pattern
	CT and MRI—generally not useful
Primary CNS neoplasia, e.g., oligodendroglioma	Neurologic examination may indicate focal lesion
Secondary neoplasia, e.g., nasal adenocarcinoma with CNS invasion	CSF analysis—supportive but generally not diagnostic; increased protein and mononuclear cells
	CT and MRI—mass lesion
Primary retroviral effects	Neurologic examination—may show anisocoria, delayed pupillary reflex, gait abnormalities, abnormal postural reflexes
	CSF—increased lymphocytes with normal to mildly increased protein
	EEG—diffuse slow wave
	CT and MRI—generally not helpful, may show cortical atrophy

FIP, feline infectious peritonitis; CSF, cerebrospinal fluid; EEG, electroencephalogram; CT, computed tomography; MRI, magnetic resonance imaging.

cation (Lin et al, 1992), *T. gondii* infection of the CNS seems to be a rare cause of FIV-associated neurologic disease. The antemortem differentiation of cause is difficult in cases of CNS infection. CSF analysis, although not generally diagnostic by itself, may be useful when combined with other findings.

FeLV-associated extradural LSA is the most common tumor to induce spinal cord dysfunction in cats. Although retrovirus-associated oncogenesis occurs more commonly with oncornaviruses, it does occur with lentiviruses as well. However, lentivirus-associated neoplasias are often considered opportunistic and frequently include unusual types of cancer. CNS tumors described in FIV-infected cats include meningioma, oligodendroglioma, and spinal choroid plexus, or cortical LSA (Bendinelli et al, 1995; Hurtrel et al, 1992; Callanan et al, 1996). Meningioma is the most common CNS tumor in the cat and is likely a coincidental finding in an old FIV-infected cat, but the others are remarkable. Secondary neoplasia causing neurologic dysfunction must also be considered. For example, CNS extension of a highly invasive nasal adenocarcinoma was diagnosed in an FIV-infected cat presented for evaluation of neurologic dysfunction as the single detectable abnormality reported by the client (Zenger, 1990). Neuroradiologic imaging techniques are invaluable in the diagnosis of CNS neoplasia.

Electroencephalography has been shown to be a sensitive indicator of neurologic dysfunction in FIV-infected cats, with abnormalities detected as early as 3 months after infection. Abnormalities ranged from asymmetrical or diffuse high-amplitude activity to marked alterations in sleep patterns with predominant slow wave activity. The electroencephalogram may be useful in differentiating opportunistic infections or neoplasms from primary effects of the retrovirus because of its ability to distinguish irritative from degenerative processes. With CNS inflammation, there is generally low voltage activity and spikes, whereas high-voltage slow wave activity is associated with neuronal degeneration. Neuroradiologic evaluation has also been performed in FIV-infected cats. Although an insensitive indicator of FIV-associated neurologic abnormalities, magnetic resonance imaging may reveal subtle abnormalities, including ventricular enlargement and focal white matter lesions (Podell et al, 1993).

TREATMENT

If a secondary cause of retrovirus-associated neurologic disease can be identified, treatment should be directed at the specific cause. However, treatment for opportunistic infections or tumors may need to be modified to take into account an impaired immune system. For example, treatment for cryptococcosis in cats seropositive for FeLV or FIV has a high likelihood of failure compared with treatment in otherwise uncompromised cats (Jacobs et al, 1997). The optimal therapy for cryptococcal meningitis remains unresolved, although initial treatment with amphotericin B, followed by lifelong maintenance therapy with fluconazole, appears promising in HIV-infected patients.

Results of antiretroviral therapy trials in FeLV- or FIV-infected cats have been mixed, and unfortunately well-controlled studies have been few (see *CVT XI*, p. 211 and *CVT XII*, p. 280 for review). Zidovudine (AZT) and protease (PR) inhibitors, alone or in combination, reduce the signs of HIV-associated dementia. During treatment, AZT has been shown to reach effective concentrations in the CSF of cats and to affect FIV and FeLV viremia, suggesting that it may be of use for managing FIV-induced encephalopathy. Myelosuppression and hepatotoxicity may be dose-limiting adverse effects of AZT in cats. In vitro data suggest that PR inhibitors effective against HIV PR are generally less efficient inhibitors of FIV PR by a factor of 100 or more, although PR inhibitors effective against a broad range of PR variants are being investigated. Cytokine therapy with human recombinant interferon alpha may be an effective means of minimizing drug toxicity and exploiting an additive antiviral effect. Combination of AZT with interferon alpha has been shown to be superior to AZT alone in controlling FeLV viremia. Anecdotal reports and studies have demonstrated improvement of the appetite and activity level of cats infected with FeLV or FIV, or both, treated solely with low-dose interferon (Weiss et al, 1991). Other treatments under investigation for retroviral infections include other viral enzyme inhibitors and chemokine receptor antagonists. Whether any of these drugs are effective in retrovirus-infected cats that show signs of neurologic dysfunction is yet to be reported.

An effective treatment that will limit neurologic signs associated with retrovirus infections has not been identified. Symptomatic therapy of seizures or behavioral problems may offer relief to certain patients, but treatment of the underlying neuropathologic condition is most likely to be more effective for the majority of patients. There is a great deal of evidence implicating certain neurotoxic mechanisms. Among the candidates are altered calcium homeostasis, enhanced toxicity of excitatory neurotransmitters such as glutamate, and oxidative damage. In vivo studies with glutamate antagonists are ongoing in HIV-infected patients, and the utility of cytoprotective agents such as antioxidants and calcium channel blockers is under consideration. These types of therapies hold potential to prevent or correct the neurologic dysfunction, but it is likely to be several years before specific agents are available for routine clinical use.

References and Suggested Reading

Bendinelli M, Pistello M, Lombardi S, et al: Feline immunodeficiency virus: An interesting model for AIDS studies and an important cat pathogen. Clin Microbiol Rev 8:87, 1995.
Excellent review of the biology of FIV, including clinical manifestations.
Callanan JJ, Jones BA, Irvine J, et al: Histologic classifications and immunophenotype of lymphosarcomas in cats with naturally and experimentally acquired feline immunodeficiency virus. Vet Pathol 33:264, 1996.
Report of eight FIV-infected cats with LSA, most of which were considered unusual in their distribution.
Dow SW, Dreitz MJ, Hoover EA: Exploring the link between feline immunodeficiency virus and neurologic disease in cats. Vet Med Dec:1181, 1992.
Review of FIV-associated encephalopathy, including a diagnostic approach and therapeutic options.
Henriksen SJ, Prospero-Garcia O, Phillips TR, et al: Feline immunodeficiency virus as a model for study of lentiviral infection of the central nervous system. Curr Top Microbiol Immunol 202:167, 1995.
Extensive review of FIV model for study of lentivirus infection of the CNS.

Hurtrel M, Ganiere J-P, Guelfi J-F, et al: Comparison of early and late feline immunodeficiency virus encephalopathies. J AIDS 6:399, 1992.
Report of neuropathologic changes detected during the first year of FIV infection.

Jacobs GJ, Medleau L, Calvert C, Brown J: Cryptococcal infection in cats: Factors influencing treatment outcome and results of sequential serum antigen titers in 35 cats. J Vet Intern Med 11:1, 1997.
Treatment results of 35 cats with cryptococcosis.

Lappin MR: Opportunistic infections associated with retroviral infections in cats. Semin Vet Med Surg (Small Anim) 10:244, 1995.
Review of the diagnosis, treatment, and zoonotic potential of the common opportunistic agents associated with feline retroviral infections.

Lin D-S, Bowman DD, Jacobson RH: Immunological changes in cats with concurrent *Toxoplasma gondii* and feline immunodeficiency virus infections. J Clin Microbiol 30:17, 1992.
Study examining immunologic changes brought about by acute infections with FIV and T. gondii.

Meeker RB, Hayward JN, English R, et al: Enhanced excitotoxicity in primary feline neural cultures exposed to feline immunodeficiency virus. Proceedings of the International Symposium of Feline Retrovirus Research, North Carolina State University, 1993, p 26.
Abstract of an in vitro study examining excitotoxicity enhancement by FIV.

Podell M, Oglesbee M, Mathes L, et al: AIDS-associated encephalopathy with experimental feline immunodeficiency virus infection. J AIDS 6:758, 1993.
Neurodiagnostic evaluation of cats experimentally infected with FIV.

Weiss RC, Joseph MC, Richards AB: Low-dose orally administered alpha interferon treatment for feline leukemia virus infection. J Am Vet Med Assoc 199:1477, 1991.
Review of reported use of interferon for FeLV and other infections.

Zenger E: Clinical findings in cats with feline immunodeficiency virus. Feline Pract 18:25, 1990.
Report of clinical and hematologic abnormalities in 32 cats testing positive for FIV.

Zenger E, Collisson EW, Barhoumi R, et al: Laser cytometric analysis of FIV-induced injury in astroglia. Glia 13:92, 1995.
In vitro study of toxic effects of FIV in cultured feline astroglia.

Diagnosis and Prevention of Feline Infectious Peritonitis

ALFRED M. LEGENDRE
Knoxville, Tennessee

The definitive diagnosis of feline infectious peritonitis (FIP) requires the histopathologic study of diseased tissues. A tentative diagnosis constitutes an acceptable standard of practice if it is well supported by historical, physical, and laboratory findings. There is no specific test that establishes the clinical diagnosis; rather, the diagnosis relies on a combination of supportive findings of FIP and the exclusion of other diseases.

Approximately 75% of cats with FIP have ascites or pleural effusion. The effusive or "wet form" of FIP is easiest to diagnose. In cats with FIP, there is a viscous, clear to yellow exudate. The abdominal or pleural effusion contains few nucleated cells ($<20,000/\mu l$), which differentiates the effusion from a septic exudate (pyothorax). The fluid is rich in protein, approaching the protein concentrations of serum. Albumin:globulin ratios and protein electrophoresis of the effusions are helpful in supporting a diagnosis. In Sparkes' study (1994), all 16 cats with FIP had fluid protein concentrations greater than 3.5 gm/dl, with globulins constituting greater than 50% of the proteins. Shelly's study (1988) showed that 10 of 12 cats with FIP had fluid gamma globulin concentrations that were greater than 32% of the total fluid protein. Globulin-rich fluids are expected in FIP, so cats with a fluid albumin:globulin ratio greater than 0.81 are unlikely to have FIP. Other causes for pleural effusion and ascites, such as heart failure, should be excluded with chest radiographs and ultrasonography. Diffuse abdominal neoplasia and lymphocytic cholangitis may produce protein-rich effusions, but these cats are usually middle aged or older. Effusive forms of FIP occur most often in cats younger than 2 years of age. Fever is more common in FIP than in other diseases that produce protein-rich effusions. The combination of historical and clinical findings is necessary to support a diagnosis of FIP. In cats in which the diagnosis is still uncertain, exploratory laparotomy or ultrasonography-guided biopsy are required.

The noneffusive or "dry form" of FIP presents a greater diagnostic challenge. Anorexia, fever unresponsive to antibiotics, and weight loss are common signs. More than 45% of these cats have ocular involvement or neurologic disease, or both. Serum globulins are often increased, especially when the disease is chronic. Any chronic infectious or inflammatory condition (e.g., chronic bronchitis) can produce a hypergammaglobulinemia, but FIP is the most likely suspect. Enlarged kidneys should alert the clinician to the possibility of FIP. A pyogranulomatous cellular infiltrate found on needle aspiration of the kidney is supportive of FIP. Hematologic and serologic studies, urinalysis and urine culture, and serum chemistry findings are not diagnostic for FIP but can help identify other causes for an antibiotic resistant fever. Titers help support the diagnosis of FIP, but a definitive diagnosis requires biopsy of involved tissues.

SERUM ANTIBODY TITERS TO FELINE CORONAVIRUSES

Serum antibody titers are sometimes helpful, but they *should not* be used as the sole criterion for making a diagnosis. The enzyme linked immunosorbent assay

(ELISA) and indirect immunofluorescence assay (IFA) identify antibodies to coronaviruses and are not specific for FIP. Feline enteric coronavirus (FECV), canine coronavirus, transmissible gastroenteritis virus of swine, and feline infectious peritonitis virus (FIPV) all produce antibodies measured by the IFA and ELISA tests for coronavirus. Although cats with FIP usually have high antibody titers, there is an overlap in titers between cats with FIP and normal cats infected with FECV. The absence of antibodies to coronavirus makes FIP less likely but does not exclude FIP. One study (Sparkes et al, 1994) identified only 1 of 28 cats with FIP that had no measurable antibodies by IFA. Young cats with acute infections or cats in the terminal stages of FIP may not have antibodies. A negative ELISA SNAP test (Idexx Laboratories, Westbrook, ME) for FIP does not mean an absence of antibodies because the test is designed to show only high concentrations. An IFA or an ELISA that measures small amounts of antibodies is required to identify cats free from coronavirus antibodies.

There is no standardization of coronavirus antibody tests among laboratories. This makes interpretation of titers difficult, and the results of each laboratory must be interpreted using the reference values for that laboratory. In Sparkes' study, high IFA antibody concentrations ($>$1:1,280) were more common in cats with FIP (25%) than in cats with other diseases (5%), but there is still considerable overlap in antibody titers between normal and diseased cats.

POLYMERASE CHAIN REACTION

The latest diagnostic test proposed for the definitive diagnosis of FIP uses the molecular biology technique of polymerase chain reaction (PCR). This technique amplifies a portion of the genome of the coronavirus until a DNA band can be seen on a gel. This technique can identify small numbers of coronavirus found in effusions, plasma, or stool. This sensitive technique suffers from the same limitations as the antibody titers in that the currently used primers cannot differentiate FECV from FIPV. Many laboratories are trying to identify the genetic differences between avirulent FECV and the pathogenic FIPV, but as yet these differences have not been defined. Until these viruses can be differentiated, a positive PCR result means that the cat has *a* coronavirus, not necessarily FIPV.

Previously, it was believed that only pathogenic coronaviruses (FIPV) became systemic, whereas avirulent FECV remained in the intestine. Herrewegh and colleagues (1995) using a PCR technique detected coronavirus in the plasma of asymptomatic cats that remained well for more than 8 months. These cats were from a cattery where FECV was endemic. Li and Scott (1994) identified feline coronavirus by PCR in the tissues of 7 of 8 cats with suspected FIP, but they also found coronavirus in the tissues of 51 of 84 cats that died of diseases other than FIP.

PREVENTION OF FELINE INFECTIOUS PERITONITIS

To advise cat owners about decreasing the incidence of FIP in their catteries, the veterinarian must understand the transmission and behavior of coronaviruses. FIP is mainly

a disease of catteries and multiple cat households. In households with only 1 or 2 cats, the incidence of FIP is estimated to be 1 in 5,000. In coronavirus endemic environments with many cats, an FIP mortality rate of 5% is expected.

FIP does not occur without exposure to feline coronavirus. Eighty to 90% of cats in catteries have antibodies to feline coronaviruses, suggesting exposure or infection with this family of viruses. There is widespread avirulent FECV in most catteries. Studies by Foley and colleagues (1997) using a reverse transcriptase-polymerase chain reaction (RT-PCR) technique showed that 41% of cattery cats at anytime were shedding virus in the stool. Most cats shed virus intermittently, but some cats were persistent virus shedders. Young cats were more likely to continually shed virus. Most cats appear to have cycles of infection that result in fecal virus shedding, recovery, and subsequent reinfection. Antibody titers were not useful in identifying persistent virus shedders.

FECV infection produces no signs of disease in adult cats and simply a few days of diarrhea in kittens. FECV is a highly contagious virus, transmitted mainly through ingestion of feces, but the virus also is found in urine and saliva. Current thinking supports a scheme in which the FECV grows in the intestinal epithelium of the cat and occasionally mutates into FIPV. The FIPV readily enters macrophages, where it replicates and is distributed by the macrophages throughout the body. The various FIPV isolates differ in virulence. A competent immune system may prevent infection with less pathogenic strains of FIPV, but the cat's genetic susceptibility, the numbers of ingested organisms, or the immunosuppressive effects of concurrent feline leukemia virus infection or stress may allow infection with less virulent strains.

This scheme is supported by the findings of Addie and co-workers (1995) who showed that kittens born into households that had had FIP-infected cats were at no greater risk for the development of FIP than were kittens born into FECV-endemic households without FIP. This supports a theory that FIPV is not spread cat to cat and that a kitten with FIP poses no greater risk than one infected with FECV. There are obviously some strains of FIPV that can spread throughout catteries producing epidemics (Panzero, 1992). In the cattery of Cornish rex cats studied by Panzero, 17 of the 39 cats died within 6 months of introducing a kitten with FIP. This rapid movement of FIPV through the cattery is atypical behavior for FIPV.

To remove the threat of FIP, FECV must be eliminated from the cattery. This will be impossible in households where strict isolation of cats cannot be carried out. Serologic testing for feline coronaviruses of 10% of the cats in the household will identify infected environments. FECV is transmitted by direct contact between cats and by fomites. It has been transmitted on shoes and clothing, as well as by improperly washed food and litter pans. Feces, which contain the highest concentration of virus, present the greatest hazard. Young, recently infected cats shed the largest amount of virus, but some cats become chronic virus shedders. Some cats that have eliminated the infection can be reinfected and resume virus shedding. The recommendations from the FIP Workshop (Pedersen et al, 1995) give detailed procedures for FECV control.

Isolation of pregnant queens and weaning of kittens by 5 weeks of age was shown by Addie and Jarrett (1995) to produce FECV-free kittens from queens that were serologically positive for coronavirus. This technique allows the breeder to produce kittens from chronically infected queens, thereby preserving those genetic characteristics of the queens that make them champions. Queens must be isolated from other cats 2 weeks before giving birth. The queen and kittens must remain isolated until the kittens are weaned. Infected queens have antibodies against FECV that are passed in the colostrum and prevent infection of the kittens until they are 4 to 6 weeks of age. Early weaning around 5 weeks of age protects the kittens from a queen that might be shedding FECV. The kittens must be isolated as a litter, away from all other cats, to prevent FECV infection. The success of the isolation procedure is verified by serologic testing at 16 weeks when all maternally derived antibodies against FECV are gone. Antibody-free kittens can be confidently sold into single cat households or coronavirus-free catteries. The prevalence of FECV in most catteries, and the contagiousness of the FECV, makes it difficult to maintain an isolation area free of FECV.

Vaccination is the logical solution to protection of seronegative kittens, but there is controversy about the value of the only FIPV vaccine currently available—Primucell FIP (Pfizer Animal Health, Exton, PA). Primucell FIP is a modified live vaccine that is given intranasally. The virus is temperature-sensitive, and growth is restricted to the cooler areas of the upper respiratory tract. The intent is to produce mucosal and cell-mediated immunity without production of IgG antibodies that may increase the likelihood of the development of clinical FIP and accelerate the course of the disease. Field studies have shown the vaccine to be safe in seropositive and seronegative cats (Gerber, 1995). Challenge studies by Scott and colleagues (1995) have shown that accelerated disease occurred when kittens were challenged with high doses of virus, but low-dose challenge demonstrated protection. An excellent natural exposure study by Reeves (1995) showed a 50 to 75% protection rate when seronegative kittens were vaccinated and exposed in a multicat environment. Other studies by Hoskins and colleagues (1995) showed protection of seronegative kittens against challenge with a virus similar to the vaccine virus, but McArdle and colleagues (1995) in England showed no protection when kittens were challenged with a British isolate of FIPV. A Swiss vaccine study (Fehr et al, 1995) in cats from households chronically infected with feline coronoviruses showed no protection

against FIP. The conclusions from these studies suggest that the Primucell FIP vaccine is not effective in cats already exposed to FECV but that it does offer a reasonable degree of protection to seronegative cats. The protection may vary from one geographic area to another. In endemic situations, kittens are infected with FECV by 6 to 7 weeks of age, and the vaccine is not recommended until 16 weeks of age. Early vaccination has been recommended by Panzera (1992) in an FIP-endemic population, but the safety in young kittens is not known. With an incidence of FIP in single cat households of 1 in 5,000, the cost:benefit ratio of vaccination in this population must also be considered.

References and Suggested Reading

Addie DD, Jarrett O: Control of feline coronavirus infections in breeding catteries by serotesting, isolation and early weaning. Feline Pract 23:92, 1995.

Addie DD, Toth S, Murray GD, et al: Risk of feline infectious peritonitis in cats naturally infected with feline coronavirus. Am J Vet Res 56:429, 1995.

Fehr D, Holznagel SB, Hauser B, et al: Evaluation of the safety and efficacy of a modified live FIPV vaccine under field conditions. Feline Pract 23:83, 1995.

Foley JE, Poland A, Carlson J, et al: Patterns of feline coronavirus infection and fecal shedding from cats in multiple-cat environments. J Am Vet Med Assoc 210:1307, 1997.

Gerber JD: Overview of the development of a modified live temperature-sensitive FIP virus vaccine. Feline Pract 23:62, 1995.

Herrewegh AA, de Groot RJ, Cepica A, et al: Detection of feline coronavirus RNA in feces, tissues, and body fluids of naturally infected cats by reverse transcriptase PCR. J Clin Microbiol 33:684, 1995.

Hoskins JD, Taylor HW, Lomax TL: Independent evaluation of a modified live feline infectious peritonitis virus vaccine under experimental conditions. Feline Pract 23:72, 1995.

Li X, Scott FW: Detection of feline coronavirus in cell cultures and in fresh and fixed feline tissues using polymerase chain reaction. Vet Microbiol 42:65, 1994.

McArdle F, Tennant B, Bennett M, et al: Independent evaluation of a modified live FIPV vaccine under experimental conditions. Feline Pract 23:67, 1995.

Panzero RA: An outbreak of feline infectious peritonitis in a colony of Cornish rex cats. Feline Pract 20:7, 1992.

Pedersen NC, Addie D, Wolf A: Recommendations from working groups of the International Feline Enteric Coronavirus and Feline Infectious Peritonitis Workshop. Feline Pract 23:108, 1995.

Reeves NP: Vaccination against naturally occurring FIP in a single large cat shelter. Feline Pract 23:81, 1995.

Scott FW, Corapy WV, Olsen CW: Independent evaluation of a modified live FIPV vaccine under experimental conditions. Feline Pract 23:74, 1995.

Shelly SM, Scarlett-Krans J, Blue JT: Protein electrophoresis on effusions from cats as a diagnostic test for feline infectious peritonitis. J Am Anim Hosp Assoc 24:495, 1988.

Sparkes AH, Gruffydd-Jones TJ, Harbour DA: An appraisal of the value of laboratory test in the diagnosis of feline infectious peritonitis. J Am Anim Hosp Assoc 30:345, 1994.

The Rabies Pandemic

CHERIE L. DRENZEK
CHARLES E. RUPPRECHT
Atlanta, Georgia

From antiquity to the present, rabies has been regarded as one of the most terrifying zoonotic diseases, especially in the context of transmission from the human's historical companion animal—the dog. In the developing world, uncontrolled canine rabies remains a serious problem and results in an excess of 35,000 human deaths per year. In the United States, the number of rabies cases in domestic animals has decreased steadily since the 1940s, when effective vaccines became available and widespread canine vaccination control programs were implemented. In concert, human rabies cases declined from 10 to 12 cases annually in the 1940s to a mean of 3 cases per year in the 1990s. Since 1960, rabies has been reported more frequently in wild animals than in domestic animals in the United States; in 1995, wildlife rabies accounted for 92% of all reported animal rabies cases (Krebs et al, 1996). Currently, most human rabies cases in the United States are associated with either exposure to indigenous insectivorous bats or to dogs abroad in areas highly enzootic for rabies. The veterinarian serves an important role in rabies prevention not only by promulgation of domestic animal vaccination but also by possessing a knowledge of current issues in rabies control that provide a basis for public health decisions. These issues include the epidemiology of wildlife rabies and the appropriate management of wildlife and exotic pets involved in possible human exposures, indirect human exposures via domestic animals, and situations in which administration of rabies postexposure prophylaxis (PEP) should be considered.

WILDLIFE RABIES

Epidemiology

Although the rabies virus can potentially infect any mammal, four terrestrial mammals (raccoons, foxes, skunks, and coyotes) and bats are the dominant wildlife reservoirs of rabies in the United States. Eight genetically distinct rabies virus variants are recognized within broad geographic regions of the United States in these terrestrial hosts. These include variants in raccoons (*Procyon lotor*) in the eastern United States, in red (*Vulpes vulpes*) and Arctic (*Alopex lagopus)* foxes in Alaska and New England, in gray foxes (*Urocyon cinereoargenteus*) in Arizona and Texas, in coyotes (*Canis latrans*) in southern Texas, and in skunks (primarily *Mephitis mephitis*) in California, the north central states, and the south central states.

The most commonly reported wild animal with rabies in the United States is the raccoon; the variant of rabies virus associated with raccoons has been present in the southeastern United States since the 1950s and was introduced into the mid-Atlantic region in the mid-1970s, probably as the result of animal translocation. The epizootic

continued to spread throughout the region so that the southeastern and mid-Atlantic foci converged in the state of North Carolina in 1994, resulting in one large epizootic affecting the entire eastern seaboard. Although westward progression of the epizootic has been slowed by geographic barriers such as lakes, rivers, and mountains, the first indigenous case of raccoon rabies was detected in the state of Ohio in 1996 (Centers for Disease Control, 1997b). Once rabies becomes established in raccoon populations in the Ohio Valley, the potential for rapid spread across the Midwest exists. There have been no documented human rabies cases in the United States associated with the raccoon rabies virus variant. This may reflect both the accurate recognition of exposure to humans and appropriate administration of rabies PEP, as well as the barrier to human infection provided by widespread domestic animal vaccination programs.

Besides the terrestrial reservoirs, multiple independent rabies reservoirs exist in several species of insectivorous bats in the United States. Cases of bat rabies have been reported in more than 30 different species from all 48 contiguous states. Bats are increasingly implicated as significant wildlife reservoirs for variants of rabies virus transmitted to humans. During the period from 1980 to 1996, 17 (53.1%) of the 32 cases of human rabies diagnosed in the United States were associated with insectivorous bats. Twelve (70.6%) of these 17 cases were associated with the silver-haired bat, *Lasionycteris noctivagans*, a solitary, migratory species infrequently submitted to laboratories for rabies testing and with a preferred habitat of old growth forest.

Rabies Postexposure Prophylaxis Recommendations

Since clinical signs of rabies cannot be interpreted reliably in wildlife, PEP is recommended for humans with bite, scratch, or mucous membrane exposure to any wild mammal (especially bats, raccoons, skunks, foxes, and coyotes) unless the animal is available for testing, with negative results for rabies (Centers for Disease Control, 1991). Rodents and lagomorphs are rarely found to be infected with the rabies virus, and exposure to such animals constitutes a low risk of rabies virus transmission, with the exception of woodchucks (*Marmota monax*) in areas of the United States affected by the raccoon rabies epizootic (resulting from spillover from infected raccoons). Indirect human exposures, such as caring for wounds inflicted by a wild animal to a pet dog or cat, do not constitute a high risk of exposure to rabies by the caregiver and have never resulted in a documented human fatality. In unclear cases, the state or local health department should be consulted to assist in the decision to recommend PEP to an individual.

Investigations of recent human rabies cases associated with bats suggest that seemingly insignificant contact with rabid bats may result in virus transmission, even in the absence of a clear history of bite or scratch. Bat teeth are very small and sharp, and the bite wounds may not necessarily draw blood, thus going unnoticed. Furthermore, some bat rabies virus variants reportedly possess certain biologic characteristics that may enhance transmission (Morimoto et al, 1996). Therefore, PEP is also recommended when there is a reasonable probability that a bat bite or scratch occurred, even if a lesion is not physically demonstrable. For example, when a sleeping person awakes to find a bat in the room, if an adult witnesses a bat in a room with a previously unattended child, or a bat is found in the presence of a mentally challenged or intoxicated individual, PEP should be considered unless prompt testing of the bat results in a negative diagnosis of rabies.

EXOTIC PETS

Ferrets

The European ferret (*Mustela putorius*) has become increasingly popular as a companion animal in the United States. However, public health officials have been reluctant to endorse the ferret as a pet because of reports of serious injuries inflicted by ferrets on young children and a lack of data on the pathogenesis of rabies in ferrets. Rabies is rarely reported in ferrets; since 1958, only 22 cases of rabid ferrets have been documented in the United States. Rabies infection in pet ferrets appears to be a result of spillover from wildlife rabies reservoirs, such as raccoons or skunks. Nevertheless, since the viral shedding period and clinical signs of rabies are unknown in ferrets, those animals that bite humans are frequently euthanized and tested for rabies, even if the ferret has been vaccinated against rabies. Studies investigating rabies pathogenesis in ferrets inoculated with a skunk rabies virus variant were initiated (Niezgoda et al, 1995) to assist in the development of public health recommendations regarding the suitability of a quarantine and observation period in lieu of immediate euthanasia for ferrets that bite humans. Preliminary results indicate that (1) the incubation period ranged from 2 weeks to more than 3 months, (2) typical clinical signs included paresthesia, fever, weight loss, ataxia, and ascending paralysis, (3) the period between the onset of clinical signs and death was approximately 4 to 5 days, and (4) rabies virus could be isolated from the salivary gland of only one rabid ferret at necropsy. Although these data are preliminary and based on a single rabies virus variant, they suggest that quarantine and observation periods may be a management consideration for ferrets that bite humans; however, further

studies are warranted. Current recommendations for management of ferrets that bite humans depend on the circumstances of the bite, the epidemiology of rabies in the area, the ferret's history, current health status, and potential for exposure to rabies (Centers for Disease Control, 1997a).

Wolves and Wolf Hybrids

Reports of rabies in wolves and wolf hybrids are rare; only two cases in wolf hybrids have been documented in the United States, and reports of rabies cases in wolves averaged less than one per year during the period from 1980 to the present. No rabies vaccines are currently licensed for parenteral use in wolves, wolf hybrids, or any other captive wild animal. In addition, no laboratory-based studies of rabies virus pathogenesis, clinical presentation, and viral shedding periods in wolves and their hybrids have been performed. Without such data, public health officials often recommend euthanasia and testing as management for wolves and wolf hybrids that bite humans. Current, albeit controversial, mammalian taxonomic revisions (Wilson and Reeder, 1993) have removed the species designations separating the gray wolf (*Canis lupus*) and the domestic dog (*Canis familiaris*). These revisions have led to questions as to whether wolves and wolf hybrids should be vaccinated against rabies with currently licensed canine vaccines and managed in the same manner as domestic dogs after a human bite. Although no simple answer exists, taxonomic changes do not in themselves substitute for pathogenetic, clinical, and epidemiologic studies of rabies in wolves and wolf hybrids and, as such, caution is still warranted. Again, management of these animals when they bite humans depends on the circumstances of the bite, the epidemiology of rabies in the area, the biting animal's history, and its potential for exposure to rabies.

References and Suggested Reading

Centers for Disease Control: Rabies prevention—United States, 1991: Recommendations of the Immunization Practices Advisory Committee (ACIP). MMWR Morbid Mortal Wkly Rep 40(RR-3), 1991.

Centers for Disease Control: Compendium of animal rabies control. MMWR Morbid Mortal Wkly Rep 45(RR-4), 1997a.

Centers for Disease Control: Update: Raccoon rabies epizootic—United States, 1996. MMWR Morbid Mortal Wkly Rep 45:1117, 1997b.

Krebs JW, Strine TW, Smith JS, et al: Rabies surveillance in the United States during 1995. J Am Vet Med Assoc 204:2031, 1996.

Morimoto K, Patel M, Corisdeo S, et al: Characterization of a unique variant of bat rabies responsible for newly emerging human cases in North America. Proc Natl Acad Sci (USA) 93:5653, 1996.

Niezgoda M, Briggs D, Shaddock J, et al: Rabies pathogenesis in the domestic ferret. Presented at the 99th annual meeting of the United States Animal Health Association, Reno, NV, Oct 28 to Nov 3, 1995.

Wilson DE, Reeder DM: Mammal Species of the World. Washington DC: Smithsonian Institution Press, 1993.

Ticks as Vectors of Companion Animal Diseases

S.A. EWING
Stillwater, Oklahoma

Ticks are ancient ectoparasitic arthropods that, along with mites, compose the order Acarina. Many individuals mistakenly think of them as insects owing in part no doubt to their role as vectors of disease agents. Mosquitoes, which *are* insects, are the only arthropods that rival ticks in importance as agents of disease transmission. In the case of companion animals, ticks far exceed mosquitoes in their importance as vectors.

CLASSIFICATION

There are fewer than 850 species of ticks, and the vast majority are assigned to one of two families, the Ixodidae and Argasidae; a third family, Nuttalliellidae, has only a single species, and it does not parasitize companion animals. The largest of the families, the Ixodidae or "hard ticks," consists of approximately 650 species, fewer than 60 of which have been reported in the United States. The Argasidae or "soft ticks" is made up of about 170 species, about 20 of which have been reported in the United States. Only a fraction of these ticks affect companion animals, and the ixodids are more important than the argasids by far.

LIFE CYCLE

Ticks have four stages in their life cycle: egg, larva, nymph, and adult (male and female). Larvae are six-legged, whereas nymphs and adults have eight legs. Sexual dimor-phism (two forms) is marked in ixodids but not in argasids. Life cycle patterns involve variations on a theme among the various species of both argasids and ixodids, but all species ingest multiple blood meals in the course of their development.

Ixodids

The hard ticks are mostly three-host ticks (about 600 of the 650 species), that is, larvae feed on one host, nymphs on another, and adults on a third. A few species are two-host ticks (whereby larvae and nymphs feed on one host and adults on a second), and there are several one-host ixodids. Species of the latter group find their hosts as larvae and feed through the three successive stages without leaving the host to molt, dropping off finally as adult ticks. Although the same animal may be attacked successively during each of the three feeding stages of a three-host tick species (e.g., *Rhipicephalus sanguineus* [the brown dog tick] may attack a single dog), the more usual pattern is exploitation of a wider host range. Such behavior naturally contributes to the success of three-host ticks as vectors of disease agents. Among the few (about 50) ixodids with one-host and two-host cycles, none is important as a vector for companion animal diseases in the United States.

Larvae, nymphs, and adult females all feed to repletion and then drop from the host; larvae and nymphs then molt to the next stage, whereas females lay eggs. Male ixodids

TABLE 1. Infectious Diseases of Companion Animals Associated With Ixodid Ticks

Disease	Species of Tick	Common Name	Route of Transmission
Canine babesiosis	*Rhipicephalus sanguineus*	Brown dog tick	Transovarial
Canine haemobartonellosis	*R. sanguineus*	Brown dog tick	Transstadial
Canine hepatozoonosis	*R. sanguineus*	Brown dog tick	Transstadial
Classic canine ehrlichiosis (*Ehrlichia canis*)	*R. sanguineus*	Brown dog tick	Transstadial
Canine granulocytic ehrlichiosis (*E. ewingii*)	*Amblyomma americanum*	Lone star tick	Transstadial
Canine granulocytic ehrlichiosis (*E. equi*)	*Ixodes scapularis*	Black-legged tick	Transstadial
Canine Rocky Mountain spotted fever	*A. americanum*	Lone star tick	Transstadial
	Dermacentor andersoni	Rocky Mountain wood tick	Transstadial
	D. variabilis	American dog tick	Transovarial, transstadial
	I. pacificus	Western black-legged tick	Transstadial
Feline cytauxzoonosis	*Dermacentor andersoni*	Rocky Mountain wood tick	Transstadial
	D. variabilis	American dog tick	Transstadial
Lyme borreliosis	*I. ricinus* complex		
	I. dammini (or *I. scapularis*)	Black-legged tick	Transstadial
Tularemia	*D. andersoni*	Rocky Mountain wood tick	Transstadial
	D. occidentalis	Pacific Coast tick	Transstadial
	D. variabilis	American dog tick	Transstadial
	I. pacificus	Western black-legged tick	Transstadial
	I. scapularis	Black-legged tick	Transstadial

consume far less blood than do females and are more likely to switch from one host to another and to mate multiple times. Many female ixodids will engorge only partially until they are mated, after which they feed to repletion. Nymphs and females usually feed slowly at first and then engorge rapidly for about the last 12 to 24 hours before detachment. Once replete, females leave their host and seek sheltered locations where the blood meal is digested and eggs are deposited; subsequently the tick dies. Embryonization and hatching of eggs is temperature-dependent and may vary from a few days to weeks or months; the period is longer when oviposition occurs in late autumn in a temperate climate. Accordingly, some life cycles are annual and others are biennial. For a species like *R. sanguineus,* there can be more or less continuous cycling in the United States because in this country the tick feeds almost exclusively on dogs and is well adapted to living in climate-controlled homes and kennels where it can complete an entire cycle in about 2 months.

Argasids

The terms *one-, two-,* and *three-host ticks* are not appropriately used in connection with argasids. Rather, these ticks are more generally thought of as multihost ticks because they feed intermittently and for short periods. (An exception is the spinose ear tick, *Otobius megnini,* which remains on a single host continuously as larva and nymph; the replete nymph drops from the host to molt, and adults, which mate on the ground, do not feed at all.) Unlike ixodids, nymphal argasids may feed and molt repeatedly before finally metamorphosing to adults.

VECTOR POTENTIAL

Several features of the biology of ticks account for their great potential to serve as vectors of infectious agents. Foremost among these, of course, is their obligatory dependence on blood as a food source in all feeding stages. Requiring a blood meal in every feeding stage of the life cycle ensures that ticks will frequently acquire certain infectious agents that routinely circulate in the blood of their vertebrate hosts. Furthermore, the probability is great that the opportunity for transmission to another host will occur during a subsequent feeding. Not surprisingly, a number of routes of pathogen transmission have evolved

TABLE 2. Noninfectious Diseases of Companion Animals Associated With Ixodid Ticks

Diseases	Species of Tick	Comment
Tick paralysis	*Amblyomma americanum* *A. maculatum* *Dermacentor andersoni* *D. occidentalis* *D. variabilis* *Ixodes pacificus* *I. scapularis*	Although reported for many species of ticks, it is probably most often associated with *Dermacentor* spp.
Gotch ear	*A. maculatum*	More commonly seen in cattle than in dogs

TABLE 3. Diseases of Companion Animals Associated With Argasids

Disease	Species	Common Name	Comment
Relapsing fever spirochetosis	*Ornithodoros talaje* *O. turicata*	None Relapsing fever tick	Relapsing fever; more common in human beings, but has been reported in dogs
Otoacariasis and possibly tick paralysis	*Otobius megnini*	Spinose ear tick	Tick paralysis more commonly associated with ixodids, especially *Dermacentor* spp.

over time, including transstadial (stage-to-stage), transovarial (female-to-offspring) and, in at least one instance, a virus that is passed venereally. The most common route of entry into a new host is through the tick salivary gland while the tick feeds, but other mechanisms include ingestion of an infected tick while the host grooms, and contamination of a wound by tick feces or secretions from the coxal glands.

Ixodids

A feature of feeding behavior that enhances the spread of organisms via the salivary glands involves the alternate sucking of blood and tissue fluid and the discharge of salivary secretions into the host. As feeding progresses, these activities alternate periodically, often every 5 to 30 seconds. The feeding mechanism appears marvelously well suited for transfer of pathogens between and among hosts. Indeed, hard ticks transmit pathogens of many types, including both prokaryotes and eukaryotes. Viruses, bacteria (including rickettsiae, spirochetes, and less specialized bacteria), protozoa, and helminths can be transmitted. Furthermore, during the time that blood meals are digested and molting occurs, many pathogens undergo maturation or multiplication within the tick. Specific examples are given in Table 1. Noninfectious diseases that are associated with ixodids are listed in Table 2.

Argasids

Soft ticks are far less abundant than are hard ticks, and the variety of pathogens transmitted is not as great. Nevertheless, soft ticks are well adapted for transmitting infectious agents. Moreover, because some argasid species are very long-lived, they can also be regarded as reservoir hosts. Specific examples of diseases associated with soft ticks are found in Table 3.

References and Suggested Reading

Cupp EW: Biology of ticks. In: Hoskins JD, ed: Tick-transmitted diseases. Vet Clin North Am 21:1, 1991.
This 26-page introductory chapter to a 202-page book cites 73 references and offers an overview of ticks that includes anatomy, life cycles, and behavior, in addition to a brief discussion of the evolution of ixodids and argasids.

Hoskins JD, Cupp EW: Ticks of veterinary importance: Part I. The Ixodidae family: Identification, behavior, and associated diseases. Compend Contin Educ Pract Vet 10:564, 1988.
This paper provides an extensive treatment of hard ticks and includes eight tables that detail tick identification and summarize diseases transmitted to mammals and birds by ixodids.

Hoskins JD, Cupp EW: Ticks of veterinary importance: Part II. The Argasidae family: Identification, behavior, and associated diseases. Compend Contin Educ Pract Vet 10:699, 1988.
This paper details identification of ticks and a summary of diseases transmitted to mammals and birds by argasids (six tables).

Kaufman WR: Tick-host interaction: A synthesis of current concepts. Parasitol Today 5:47, 1989.
In this review, salivary gland function and ixodid tick feeding mechanisms are discussed in detail, together with the tick-host interactions that influence the likelihood of pathogen transmission.

Strickland RK, Gerrish RR, Hourrigan JL, et al: Ticks of Veterinary Importance. Handbook No. 485. Washington, DC, Animal and Plant Health Inspection Service, US Department of Agriculture, 1976, p 122.
This manual is designed as a training aid and has life history summaries, extensive drawings of ticks, and five schematic diagrams that depict life cycles and patterns of disease transmission. It provides a checklist of ticks found in the United States as well as information in tabular form regarding diseases transmitted by ticks.

Granulocytic Ehrlichioses

BARBARA GREIG
Eden Prairie, Minnesota

The ehrlichioses are veterinary and human tick-borne diseases caused by bacteria of the genus *Ehrlichia*, family Rickettsiaceae. The organisms are gram-negative, pleomorphic, obligate intracellular parasites. Within their mammalian hosts, the bacteria demonstrate tropisms for leukocytes and multiply within endosomes, producing cytoplasmic inclusions called *morulae* (Fig. 1). There are two main types of ehrlichiae: monocytic ehrlichiae, which primarily infect lymphocytes and monocytes, and granulocytic ehrlichiae, which infect neutrophils and eosinophils. Sequencing of the 16S ribosomal RNA (rRNA) gene has been used to phylogenetically classify ehrlichial organisms into groups of closely related species: *E. canis* genogroup (*E. canis, E. ewingii, E. chaffeensis, E. muris*), *E. phagocytophila* genogroup (*E. phagocytophila, E. equi, E. platys*) and *E. risticii* genogroup (*E. risticii, E. sennetsu*) (Dumler and Bakken, 1995).

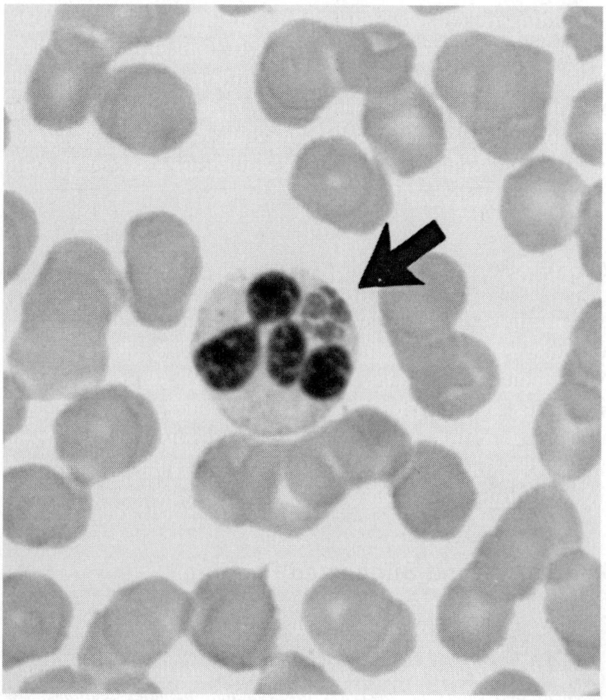

The diseases caused by *Ehrlichia* are characterized by acute febrile syndromes of varying clinical presentations but with similar laboratory features. The diseases tend to be regional and seasonal because the disease pattern is determined by the geographic range and feeding activity of the particular tick vector. Following a tick bite, the incubation period for all ehrlichioses is 1 to 3 weeks. Although there has been a dramatic increase in the recognition of veterinary and human ehrlichial infections over the last 5 years, the pathogenesis of disease is largely unknown. What is understood is that fatal and severe cases of human ehrlichiosis tend to occur in immunocompromised and elderly patients, and there is evidence for chronic infection following therapy or latent infection that may reactivate. Canine and human seroprevalence studies in the United States also indicate that the incidence of subclinical ehrlichial infections in both dogs and humans is far greater than the incidence of clinical disease.

DOGS

There are two canine granulocytic ehrlichial diseases. Canine granulocytic ehrlichiosis (GE) caused by *E. ewingii* and canine GE caused by an agent nearly identical to *E. equi* (equine granulocytic ehrlichiosis).

Ehrlichiae ewingii

Canine GE caused by *E. ewingii* was discovered in 1971 in the southern United States. *E. ewingii* is closely related to *E. canis* and is only known to be a canine pathogen.

Figure 1. Multiple *Ehrlichia* morulae *(arrow)* in a peripheral blood neutrophil (Wright's stain) (magnification, × 1,000).

Cases have been reported from the southern United States (Arkansas, Missouri, Mississippi, Oklahoma, Tennessee, and North Carolina). Ill dogs present with an acute polyarthritic syndrome characterized by a sudden onset of fever, lethargy, anorexia, lameness, or muscular stiffness. Dogs may be lame in one or more limbs, have generalized or pelvic stiffness, or may be reluctant or unable to stand. Joint fluid analyzed within the first 3 to 4 days of the onset of clinical signs reveals inflammatory joint disease. Ehrlichial morulae may be found within synovial fluid neutrophils. The tick vector for *E. ewingii* is *Amblyomma americanum,* which actively feeds year round and, hence, there is no seasonal disease incidence. Abnormal hematologic findings include mild nonregenerative anemia, mild to moderate thrombocytopenia, and monocytosis and eosinophilia. The white blood cell count, neutrophil count, and lymphocyte count may be normal, increased, or decreased. Ehrlichial morulae, when present, are found in less than 1 to 9% of circulating neutrophils. Mild elevation in serum alanine aminotransferase activity is frequent. To test for anti–*E. ewingii* antibodies, *E. canis* serologic tests are used, because *E. ewingii* and *E. canis* have cross-reactive antigens.

Ehrlichiae equi

E. equi was identified in California in the early 1960s as the causative agent of equine granulocytic ehrlichiosis. Experimentally, the organism has successfully infected dogs, cats, and nonhuman primates. Natural canine *E. equi* infection was reported in 1982 in two California dogs receiving immunosuppressive therapy; *E. equi* infection was confirmed by successfully transmitting the ehrlichial agent from one of the dogs to several horses, which became ill with signs typical of equine granulocytic ehrlichiosis. No other suspected canine *E. equi* infections were reported until GE was discovered in Sweden and the midwestern United States in 1989 and 1990, respectively. Genetic analysis has revealed that the granulocytic ehrlichial diseases of Swedish dogs and those of the midwestern United States are caused by the same ehrlichial agent, which is distinct from *E. ewingii* and nearly identical to *E. equi*. This ehrlichial agent has also been identified in horses of Sweden and the midwestern United States.

Dogs infected with the *E. equi*–like agent present with an acute febrile illness characterized by anorexia and lethargy. Clinical signs attributable to a specific body system are rare. The severity of disease varies, with some dogs so severely lethargic the owners are fearful their pets are dying. The black-legged tick, *Ixodes scapularis* (also called the deer tick, *I. dammini*), is the vector of *E. equi*–like GE in the upper midwestern United States, and the seasonal occurrence of disease in early spring through early summer and again in autumn corresponds with the peak feeding periods of the tick. The disease is rarely seen midsummer and has never been diagnosed midwinter. Ill dogs do not have pathognomonic clinical pathologic abnormalities, but there are supportive findings. Hematologically, 86% have mild to moderate thrombocytopenia and 67% are lymphopenic. The neutrophil count, similar to that in *E. ewingii* infections, is not diagnostically helpful. Eighty percent of ill dogs have normal neutrophil counts, whereas 7% are

neutropenic, 13% are neutrophilic, and 20% have a regenerative left shift. Morulae are found in less than 1 to 24% circulating neutrophils. Clinical chemistry findings can be helpful in making a diagnosis of *E. equi*–like infection in a dog. All ill (100%) dogs have elevated serum alkaline phosphatase activity, and 50% have elevated serum amylase activity. Forty-four percent are hypoalbuminemic and 38% are proteinuric. Serologically, infected dogs acquire antibodies to *E. equi* antigen and seroconversion to *E. canis* antigen does not take place.

Of importance, human granulocytic ehrlichiosis (HGE) caused by the *E. equi*–like agent was also discovered in the upper midwestern United States in 1990. HGE has subsequently been found in human patients in the northeastern United States, and human serologic studies suggest it exists in Europe. Considering the broader United States geographic distribution of HGE and of the *I. scapularis* tick, canine GE caused by the *E. equi*–like agent will likely soon be reported elsewhere outside the upper midwestern United States and Sweden.

CATS

There is a single published case of monocytic ehrlichiosis in a cat and no published reports of natural feline GE, although cats have been successfully infected with *E. equi* experimentally. There are unpublished reports of feline GE in ill cats, with preliminary evidence suggesting that the causative agent is identical to the upper midwestern *E. equi*–like organism (personal communication, Martha A. Mellencamp, St. Joseph, MO, and Allen R. Cahill, PRL-DyNAgenics, Neosho, MO).

DIAGNOSIS

A diagnosis of ehrlichiosis should begin with suspicion based on compatible clinical signs in an animal that has been living in a tick endemic region for 1 to 3 weeks prior to illness. The most rapid method for diagnosing ehrlichiosis is finding the cytoplasmic morulae within infected circulating leukocytes. Morulae are frequently observed in circulation during granulocytic ehrlichiosis and, in contrast, are rarely observed during monocytic ehrlichiosis.

Serologic tests, specifically indirect immunofluorescence, is the mainstay for diagnosing ehrlichial infections, but has several drawbacks. First, identification of a fourfold seroconversion (increase) to the appropriate antigen (i.e., a specific *Ehrlichia* species) is retrospective and, thus, a poor tool for therapeutic decision-making in acute illness. A single seropositive test is *not* diagnostic because seropositive healthy dogs and humans are often found in endemic areas. In addition, closely related ehrlichiae may induce cross-reactive antibodies.

After many years of research, in vitro cultivation of granulocytic ehrlichiae from blood was accomplished in 1995, but the method is not widely available for veterinary diagnostic use. As with serologic testing, culture is not very helpful in therapeutic decision-making, because it usually takes 5 to 12 days to isolate the organism. Ehrlichiae will not grow in specimens from tetracycline-treated animals and, hence, culture is also not a good retrospective test.

Polymerase chain reaction (PCR) amplification of the ehrlichial 16S rRNA gene from blood is the most sensitive diagnostic procedure. Experimentally infected animals are positive for *Ehrlichia* on PCR before they are bacteremic, and they remain positive several days after the bacteremic phase. This method of testing is not performed by many veterinary reference-diagnostic laboratories. One laboratory that offers PCR assays for *E. equi, E. equi*–like organism from the upper Midwest (HGE agent), and *E. ewingii* is DyNAgenics Veterinary Diagnostics in Neosha, MO (phone: 417-451-0201).

TREATMENT

All veterinary ehrlichioses are treated with tetracycline antibiotics (tetracycline and doxycycline). Dogs with GE caused by *E. ewingii* or the *E. equi*–like agent are treated identically. Ill dogs undergo defervescence, with an abatement of clinical signs, within 12 to 48 hours of initiating therapy. There are no reported cases of canine fatalities. Tetracycline is administered at 22 mg/kg every 8 hours PO for 14 to 21 days, and doxycycline is given at 5 to 10 mg/kg every 12 hours PO for 7 to 10 days.

References and Suggested Reading

Anderson BE, Greene CE, Jones D, et al: *Ehrlichia ewingii* sp.nov., the etiologic agent of canine granulocytic ehrlichiosis. Int J Sys Bacteriol 42:299, 1992.
  A brief clinical and genetic description of E. ewingii.
Bakken JS, Krueth J, Wilson-Nordskog C, et al: Clinical and laboratory findings of human granulocytic ehrlichiosis. JAMA 275:24, 1996.
  A good review of HGE in the Midwest.
Dumler JS, Bakken JS: Ehrlichiae diseases of humans: emerging tick-borne infections. Clin Infect Dis 20:1102, 1995.
Greig B, Asanovich KM, Armstrong PJ, et al: Geographic, clinical, serologic, and molecular evidence of granulocytic ehrlichiosis, a likely zoonotic disease. J Clin Microbiol 34:44, 1996.
  A summary of the preliminary findings of natural canine GE in the Midwest.
Stockham SL, Schmidt DA, Curtis KS, et al: Evaluation of granulocytic ehrlichiosis in dogs of Missouri, including serologic status to *E. canis, E. equi,* and *Borrelia burgdorferi.* Am J Vet Res 53:63, 1992.
  A summary of findings of natural cases of canine GE in Missouri.
Stockham SL, Tyler JW, Schmidt DA, et al: Experimental transmission of granulocytic ehrlichial organisms in dogs. Vet Clin Pathol 19:99, 1990.
  A summary of experimental E. ewingii infections (not speciated when written).
Walker DH, Barbour AG, Oliver JH, et al: Emerging bacterial zoonotic and vector-borne diseases. Ecological and epidemiological factors. JAMA 275:24, 1996.
  A good summary of tick-borne diseases infecting people.

Bartonella vinsonii Infection in Dogs

BRANDEE L. PAPPALARDO
EDWARD B. BREITSCHWERDT
Raleigh, North Carolina

Bartonella vinsonii subspecies *berkhoffii*, a bacteria first isolated in 1993, is the only member of the genus *Bartonella* that has been isolated from dogs. The organism causes endocarditis and granulomatous lymphadenitis.

EPIDEMIOLOGY

According to a seroepidemiologic survey conducted by our laboratory, risk factors associated with an increased likelihood of exposure to *B. vinsonii* in dogs include (1) dogs that spend their time outdoors with freedom to roam the neighborhood, (2) dogs from rural environments (especially farms), and (3) dogs from multidog households. These dogs are likely to have had heavy ectoparasite infestation (fleas and especially ticks) (Table 1). Furthermore, a high serologic correlation has been found between exposure to *B. vinsonii* and exposure to *Ehrlichia canis* or *Babesia canis* in dogs. These findings implicate a role for *Rhipicephalus sanguineus*, the only documented vector of *E.canis* or *B. canis*, in transmission of *B. vinsonii* to dogs (Table 2). As the previously mentioned epidemiologic factors are inconsistent with sole exposure to a domestic tick species (i.e., one associated primarily with kennels and households), it appears likely that other field tick species (*Dermacentor, Amblyomma, Ixodes*) or other ectoparasites may be vectors for transmission of the organism between wildlife hosts and from these hosts to dogs. *R. sanguineus* may then play a role in the transmission of *B. vinsonii* from dog to dog in multidog households.

PATHOGENESIS

In humans, various species of *Bartonella* (formerly *Rochalimaea*) cause disease manifestations ranging from mild lymphadenopathy (seen in cat scratch disease) to endocarditis. Lesions of nearly every organ system (heart, bone, bone marrow, muscle, soft tissue, liver, spleen and central nervous system) have been associated with *Bartonella* infections. Unique to this genus are lesions characterized by endothelial cell proliferation with neovascularization. Little is known about the disease manifestations associated with *B. vinsonii* infection in dogs, although disease manifestations recognized to date have paralleled those associated with human disease. Vegetative endocarditis involving the aortic and mitral valves was diagnosed in the first dog from which *B. vinsonii* was isolated. Although this has

TABLE 1. Association Between Canine Seropositivity to *Bartonella vinsonii* and Potential Environmental Risk Factors*

Risk Factors	Odds Ratio†	95% Confidence Interval for the Odds Ratio
Horse exposure (versus no exposure)	1.2	(1.03, 1.34)
Roaming (versus confinement)	4.8	(2.39, 9.79)
Multidog household:		
1–3 additional dogs	2.5	(1.19, 5.37)
>3 additional dogs	6.0	(2.01, 18.15)
Heavy flea exposure (versus no fleas)	5.6	(1.82, 18.01)
Rural (versus urban) environment	7.1	(2.13, 25.00)
Farm (versus no farm)	7.2	(2.76, 19.37)
Outdoors (versus indoors)	8.5	(3.39, 21.71)
Cattle exposure (versus no exposure)	9.3	(1.76, 65.83)
Heavy tick exposure (versus no ticks)	14.2	(4.63, 45.38)

*The odds ratio and the 95% confidence interval for the odds ratio are shown.

†An odds ratio (OR) is a measure of likelihood that indicates the direction and magnitude of the effect. An OR greater than 1 indicates an increased likelihood, an OR less than 1 indicates a decreased likelihood, and an OR equal to 1 indicates no association between the environmental factors and the serologic status of the dog (seronegative versus seropositive).

been the only reported case of *B. vinsonii* infection in a dog, the organism has subsequently been isolated from dogs in Georgia, North Carolina, Virginia, and Tennessee. Serologic evidence of exposure to *B. vinsonii* has been obtained for dogs from the Virgin Islands, Israel, and Italy. Our laboratory has identified eight additional dogs with culture-negative endocarditis and high reciprocal *B. vinsonii* antibody titers (≥4096) or detection of *B. vinsonii* DNA by polymerase chain reaction, or both. Additionally, the organism has been implicated as the cause of pyogranulomatous lymphadenitis in a dog that was seropositive (reciprocal titer 128) to *B. vinsonii* and in which DNA was detected by polymerase chain reaction from a peripheral blood sample and from a lymph node biopsy specimen.

DIAGNOSIS

Dogs with *B. vinsonii* endocarditis may have a protracted illness with the eventual development of a heart murmur. Weight loss is gradual and frequently severe. A

TABLE 2. Classification of Several Dog Populations Based on Prior Tick Exposure (to Either *Dermacentor variabilis* or *Rhipicephalus sanguineus*) and Percentage of Seropositivity to *Bartonella vinsonii*

Population	Tick Vector	% Seropositive (to *B. vinsonii*)
Dog sera		3.6% (69/1920)
Rickettsia rickettsii seropositive	D. variabilis	7.8% (11/141)
Ehrlichia canis seropositive	R. sanguineus	36.0% (54/151)*
Babesia canis seropositive	R. sanguineus	57.1% (4/7)

*Additionally, sera from 68 of the 69 dogs seropositive for *B. vinsonii* were assayed against *E. canis* antigen by indirect fluorescent antibody testing: 24 of 68 (35.2%) were seroreactive to both agents.

shifting leg lameness has been reported in several dogs, which may be due to polyarthritis or poorly localized bone pain. These disease manifestations are recognized in human patients infected with *Bartonella* spp.

Results of hematologic and biochemical evaluations are nonspecific, and values may often lie within the normal reference ranges. Therefore, obtaining historical information on the lifestyle of a dog suspected of having *Bartonella* infection combined with serologic testing may prove crucial to diagnosis. Dogs with *B. vinsonii* endocarditis may present with clinical, hematologic, and biochemical abnormalities consistent with gram-negative sepsis (see p. 272). Mild anemia, thrombocytopenia, neutrophilia with a mild left shift, mild to absent neutrophil toxicity, and hypoglycemia can be detected at initial presentation. Vegetative lesions have most frequently involved the aortic valve, and arrhythmias or conduction abnormalities are not uncommon.

Serologic Testing

Detection of antibodies to *Bartonella* spp. is the most convenient method of diagnosis. An indirect fluorescent antibody assay IgG antibody titer greater than 64 is considered indicative of past or present exposure to the organism. Seroprevalence to *B. vinsonii* antigens in 1,920 sick dogs from North Carolina and Virginia was 3.6%, indicating a relatively low degree of exposure to the organism and suggesting reasonable specificity of the assay. The extent to which exposure to *B. henselae*– or *B. clarridgiae*–infected cat fleas might induce a cross-reactive antibody response has not been established. Antibody titers derived from dogs with clinical abnormalities can overlap with those from seemingly healthy dogs. Our findings suggest that dogs may experience prolonged asymptomatic infection or that considerable pathogenic variability may exist among different strains of *B. vinsonii* subspecies *berkhoffii*. The reciprocal indirect fluorescent antibody assay titers derived from clinically ill dogs have ranged from 128 to 8192. One limitation of serologic testing concerns the inability to determine whether the antibody response represents active, subclinical, or past infection. Additionally, the degree of canine cross-reactivity to various *Bartonella* spp. or to other bacteria such as *Chlamydia psittaci*, which cross-reacts with *Bartonella* antigens in human serum samples, has not been established. In our laboratory, following experimental inoculation of dogs with a single intravenous injection of *B. vinsonii* subspecies *berkhoffii*, IgG antibody titers quickly became elevated between days 3 and 11 postinoculation and persisted for the remaining 8 months of the study.

Blood Culture

Bartonella spp. have been difficult to culture from canine or human blood. The lysis centrifugation blood culture system (Wampole Laboratories, Cranbury, NJ) has proved more sensitive and has increased the likelihood for isolation of the organism. Positive cultures have been obtained from human patients by direct plating of ethylenediaminetetraacetic acid–treated blood, lymph node tissue, or aspirates of involved organs. Optimal in vitro conditions for growth of *B. vinsonii* require incubation in an enriched carbon dioxide atmosphere, at 35 to 37°C, on medium supplemented with blood. When grown on solid medium, colonies are usually white to off-white, raised, and often pitted into the agar. In most clinical microbiology laboratories, blood cultures are carried out in broth medium and are routinely disposed of after 1 week. *Bartonella* spp. may require extended incubation of the primary culture plates, which can require up to 2 months to visualize growth. Therefore, culture-negative results following conventional processing of blood samples do not necessarily indicate lack of active infection. Prior freezing of aseptically collected ethylenediaminetetra-acetic acid–treated blood samples has enhanced recovery of *B. henselae* from cat blood and may facilitate isolation of *B. vinsonii* from dogs.

Special Stains

Bartonella can be visualized by light microscopy using a variety of stains. Gram staining the organism reveals gram-negative, slightly curved, pleomorphic rods. Wartharin-Starry silver stain facilitates detection of *Bartonella* spp. in tissue samples. With this staining technique, the rod-shaped organism appears black on an orange background. Acridine orange and Gimenez stains have been helpful in visualizing the organism in samples derived from blood culture bottles or when using tissue culture systems.

TREATMENT

Definitive antimicrobial efficacy has not been established for the treatment of *B. vinsonii* in dogs. Using in vitro antibiotic susceptibility testing, *Bartonella* species are susceptible to amoxicillin, third-generation cephalosporins, tetracyclines, macrolides, and rifampicin. In human patients and experimentally infected cats, however, relapses have been reported following a 2- to 4-week course of antibiotic therapy (doxycycline or enrofloxacin).

PREVENTION

It is probable that many aspects of *Bartonella*-induced disease in dogs remain uncharacterized. Future improvements in microbial isolation techniques or molecular detection of the organism in clinical specimens as well as an enhanced understanding of the role of serologic testing are needed to facilitate diagnostic conformation of *Bartonella* infection in dogs. With regard to prevention of *Bartonella* infection, vaccination may prove to be an appropriate strategy in the future. Currently, efforts to prevent exposure to fleas and ticks and rapid elimination or removal of feeding ticks may help to prevent transmission of the organism to dogs. To date, there is no evidence that *B. vinsonii* subspecies *berkhoffii* is a zoonotic infectious disease.

References and Suggested Reading

Adal KA, Cockerell CJ, Petri WA: Cat scratch disease, bacillary angiomatosis, and other infections due to *Rochalimaea*. N Engl J Med 330:1509, 1994.

Breitschwerdt EB, Kordick DL, Mararkey DE, et al: Endocarditis in a dog due to infection with a novel *Bartonella* subspecies. J Clin Microbiol 33:154, 1995.

Maurin M, Raoult D: Antimicrobial susceptibility of *Rochalimaea quintana, Rochalimaea vinsonii,* and the newly recognized *Rochalimaea henselae.* J Antimicrob Chemother 32:587, 1993.

Pappalardo BL, Correa MT, York CC, et al: Epidemiologic evaluation of the risk factors associated with exposure and seroreactivity to *Bartonella vinsonii* in dogs. Am J Vet Res 58:467, 1997.

Bartonella Infections in Domestic Cats

DORSEY L. KORDICK
EDWARD B. BREITSCHWERDT
Raleigh, North Carolina

EPIDEMIOLOGY AND PATHOGENESIS

Organism

The genus *Bartonella,* which includes the former *Rochalimaea* and *Grahamella* organisms, is currently composed of 11 species. *Bartonella* are facultative intracellular, gram-negative, argyrophilic (silver-staining) coccobacilli or slightly curved rods of approximately 1 to 2 μm in length. Polar flagella have been observed in two species (*B. bacilliformis, B. clarridgeiae*) by negative staining techniques. Pili are present on initial isolation but diminish during subsequent passaging of the bacteria. *Bartonella* spp. are hemotropic and have been observed attached to or within erythrocytes but are distinct from *Haemobartonella* spp., which are rickettsial pathogens that are similarly associated with erythrocytes. Only *B. henselae* and *B. clarridgeiae* have been isolated from domestic cats, and both are of zoonotic importance. Asymptomatic bacteremic cats constitute a major reservoir of these two species. Chronic subclinical infection suggests that the domestic cat can serve as a reservoir host for *B. henselae* and *B. clarridgeiae,* but little is known about the life cycle. Until recently, most efforts to culture these organisms from cats have been in the continental United States; however, feline *Bartonella* isolates have also been obtained in the Hawaiian islands, Japan, Israel, Australia, France, and the Netherlands.

Human disease has been associated with several *Bartonella* spp., most notably *B. bacilliformis* (Oroya fever, verruga peruana) and *B. quintana* (trench fever). Following years of controversy, it appears that *B. henselae* and *B. clarridgeiae* are responsible for the majority of cat scratch disease (CSD) cases. In a review of 1,200 CSD case reports, more than 90% contained a historical association with cats. *B. henselae* is now recognized as the primary cause of CSD in immunocompetent humans and of potentially fatal bacillary angiomatosis in immunocompromised humans. Endocarditis, visceral peliosis, septicemia, granulomatous hepatitis or splenitis, osteolysis, and retinitis have also been attributed to human infection with *B. henselae*. To date, *B. clarridgeiae*, which is the most recently recognized pathogenic species, has been associated only with CSD. A *Bartonella* etiology for these conditions has been corroborated by *Bartonella*-specific serologic assays, culture of the organism from blood or tissue homogenates, or documentation of *Bartonella* DNA in reactive lymph nodes, various other affected tissues, and the CSD skin test antigen.

Prevalence of Infection

It is now apparent that cats are not merely mechanical but also biologic vectors. The prevalence of feline *Bartonella* infection has been examined by several investigators using blood culture and serologic tests. In North Carolina, *Bartonella* were cultured from 7 of 25 (28%) healthy cats with no association of CSD and 17 of 19 (89%) cats associated with CSD. Blood culture studies from California revealed that 25 to 41% of cats were bacteremic with *Bartonella*. In northern California, 81 of 205 (40%) cats were positive to *Bartonella* by blood culture, whereas 166 of 205 (81%) had detectable *B. henselae*–specific immunoglobulins (reciprocal titer ≥64). Substantial numbers of seroreactive cats have also been identified in other seroepidemiologic studies. Jameson and colleagues (1995) reported seroreactivity against *B. henselae* in the United States ranging from 5 of 128 (4%) in the Rocky Mountain region and 4 of 60 (7%) in the Midwest to 32 of 80 (40%) along the Pacific Coast, 10 of 19 (53%) in Hawaii, and 46 of 77 (60%) in the Southeast. In Japan, 3 of 48 (6%) cats in the northeastern area of the country, compared with 13 of 59 (22%) in central Japan were seropositive. In separate studies, *Bartonella* exposure was reported in cats from Israel, France, the Netherlands, Egypt, and Portugal. A comparison of results suggests that *Bartonella* exposure is related to climate and vector distribution. Cat fleas (*Ctenocephalides felis*) have recently been identified as a vector of *B. henselae*. Fleas are more commonly found in warm, humid climates, which may partially explain the higher rates of seroreactivity in those regions of the world. Feral cats tend to have higher rates of seroreactivity.

Animals with impaired immune responses have increased susceptibility to opportunistic infections. Three groups have examined retrovirus-infected cats for evidence of coinfection with *Bartonella* spp. Contrary to expectations, no significant difference in the incidence of *Bartonella* bacteremia or seroreactivity was detected between retrovirus-infected and retrovirus-free cats. This is in contrast to an increased incidence of *H. felis* infection in cats infected with feline immunodeficiency virus or feline leukemia virus. Among bacteremic cats, however, IgG titers in retrovirus-infected cats were lower than in retrovirus-free cats, which could be due to an impaired ability of the immunodeficient cat to produce *Bartonella*-specific antibodies. The potential pathogenic importance of concurrent retroviral and *Bartonella* infection has not been adequately evaluated. Controlled experimental studies are needed to determine if retroviral infection enhances the pathogenicity of *Bartonella* infections in cats, as appears to be the case in human immunodeficiency virus–infected humans.

Historically, CSD is more often associated with exposure to young cats or kittens. Several studies have investigated the prevalence of *Bartonella* seroreactivity or bacteremia in cats 1 year of age or younger, and results are inconsistent. Most investigators report no significant difference in the age of the cat relative to the prevalence of *Bartonella* infection. Therefore, the relationship between human infection and young cats may result from the type of contact humans have with younger cats, which increases the likelihood of traumatic exposure through bites, scratches, or licks.

Transmission

Bartonella spp. can successfully colonize cats following intradermal or subcutaneous inoculation with plate-grown bacteria or intramuscular or intravenous administration of infected blood. Oral challenge with bacteria or infected blood has not been studied. Various arthropods have been identified as vectors in the transmission of other *Bartonella* spp. Recently, Chomel and co-workers (1996) demonstrated *C. felis* to be a competent vector in the horizontal transmission of *B. henselae* between cats. As few as five fleas infected with *B. henselae* were able to transmit infection to specific-pathogen-free (SPF) kittens, resulting in bacteremia within 2 weeks of exposure. It is unknown whether flea-borne transmission occurs via flea regurgitation, scratching of flea feces into the inoculation site, or ingestion of infected fleas. The dose of *B. henselae* required to transmit infection to humans has not been established. *C. felis* is the most common flea found on cats and dogs, accounting for approximately 97% of the fleas found on cats. Although *C. felis* readily bites humans, flea bites are rarely present in the medical history of *Bartonella*-infected individuals. Since *B. henselae* can be cultivated from 9-day-old flea feces, it is likely that contact with this material may be important in the transmission of organisms to humans. Claws containing infected flea feces may function to inoculate infectious material beneath the skin. The transmission of *Bartonella* to humans without a history of a traumatic wound from a cat could potentially occur following exposure to flea feces on cats, furniture, or carpeting. Tick involvement in the transmission of *B. henselae* or *B. clarridgeiae* has not been systematically examined; however, anecdotal reports of human *B. henselae* infection following tick exposure exist. Considering the large number of cats infected with *B. henselae* or *B. clarridgeiae*, or both, transmission to humans appears to be inefficient.

Bite wounds inflicted by cats have occasionally been associated with human *Bartonella* infection. Since stomatitis is frequently encountered in cats, it is conceivable that a blood-borne organism could be present in the saliva and transmitted to either cats or humans via biting or licking. In fact, *B. henselae* has been detected in the saliva of a bacteremic cat using species-specific polymerase chain reaction (PCR). Unlike the epidemiologic features of feline immunodeficiency virus infections, *B. henselae* seroreactivity or bacteremia does not appear to be strongly related to roaming or fighting behavior or the sex of the cat; therefore, although the possibility exists for transmission via saliva, it is probably not a predominant method for transmission between cats.

Vertical transmission of *Bartonella* spp. from queen to kittens was evaluated in three litters of kittens. Both bacteremic and abacteremic kittens were found; however, these animals were also heavily infested with fleas. Chomel and colleagues (1996) observed two kittens housed with five chronically bacteremic cats in a flea-free environment to determine the efficiency of transmission during casual contact between cats. Naive kittens did not undergo seroconversion or become bacteremic after 21 weeks of cohabitation.

Duration of Infection

The pathogenesis of *B. henselae* or *B. clarridgeiae* infection in the cat is not yet clarified. Cats have been experimentally challenged with laboratory-cultivated bacteria or blood from infected donor cats. When cultured *Bartonella* is administered, bacteremia is transient, whereas infection with blood results in a prolonged, relapsing bacteremia. Cats experimentally infected with blood and individually housed in an ectoparasite-free isolation facility for 454 days experienced periods of bacteremia interspersed with culture-negative periods. Culture-negative intervals occurred randomly and ranged in length from 1 to 4 months. No cyclic pattern was identified. In two instances, bacteremia was documented xenodiagnostically when *Bartonella* infection was transferred from culture-negative donors to recipient cats via blood transfusion. This indicates that very low levels of bacteremia are difficult to detect by current blood culture methods.

Natural infection in cats can also apparently be of long duration. Asymptomatic carriers have been identified as bacteremic for up to 21 months. These naturally exposed cats were housed outside a controlled environment, however, and may have been rechallenged repeatedly rather than chronically infected.

Coinfection with *B. henselae* and *B. clarridgeiae* has been documented in one naturally infected cat donated for long-term study. Blood transfusions from this cat transmitted *B. henselae* to recipients on one occasion and *B. clarridgeiae* on another. A recent report describing the isolation of *B. clarridgeiae* from a cat owned by a human with bacteremic infection from *B. henselae* could also reflect dual infection in the cat.

CLINICAL MANIFESTATIONS

Clinical Signs

The clinical syndrome known as CSD as it appears in humans has not been reproduced in cats following inoculation of purulent material from lymph nodes, cultivated bacteria, or infected blood. Greene and colleagues (1996) described a raised lesion at the site of intradermal inoculation of cultivated bacteria that persisted for 2 to 4 weeks; however, no fever or lymphadenopathy was observed. Regnery and co-workers (1996) observed slight swelling at the inoculation site of two cats that received bacterial inoculum intradermally and subcutaneously, but not in 25 cats that received subcutaneous challenge. Other investigators have noted fever and lymphadenopathy following the intravenous or intramuscular administration of infected blood or cultured bacteria. No readily discernible clinical signs of *Bartonella* bacteremia in cats have been described. Clinical abnormalities observed in experimentally infected cats include intermittent fever, lymphadenopathy, and transient, mild anemia. Brief febrile episodes lasting 2 to 6 days were observed within approximately 2 weeks after experimental challenge with infected blood or bacterial cultures.

Despite being a relatively uncommon clinical problem in cats, we have observed transient neurologic deficits in three cats with bacteremia from *B. henselae* (one natural infection, two experimentally infected). These cats appeared disoriented and demonstrated diminished tactile sense and conscious proprioception. A return to normal function occurred within 2 days without treatment. Analysis of the cerebrospinal fluid obtained during these episodes did not reveal bacteria and was within the normal range for protein and cell numbers. It is perhaps noteworthy that *Bartonella*-specific antibodies have been detected in the cerebrospinal fluid of human immunodeficiency virus patients presenting with progressive neurologic disease. Ophthalmoscopy of one cat immediately following resolution of central nervous system signs disclosed a focal equatorial cataract, but the lesion resolved within 5 weeks. Cataractous lens lesions were eventually observed in six of eight SPF cats experimentally challenged with *Bartonella*. Although the cats were not littermates, a hereditary component cannot be ruled out. No accompanying uveitis was observed; however, this could be due to the extended periods between ophthalmologic examinations.

Stress or intercurrent infection might influence the clinical presentation or potentiate the persistence of *Bartonella* infection. Four apparently healthy cats that were presented for neutering (three castration, one ovariohysterectomy) became febrile during the immediate postoperative period. *B. henselae* was subsequently recovered from all four cats by blood culture. Whether the temporal associations of fever, stress of the surgical procedure, and *B. henselae* bacteremia were related remains undetermined. An attempt to produce a recrudescence of detectable bacteremia in experimentally infected cats with latent infections using corticosteroids was unsuccessful. Four days after the administration of a single intramuscular dose of methylprednisolone acetate (20 mg/kg), blood cultures for *Bartonella* were negative. The leukogram reflected a typical response to corticosteroids, but these indices returned to normal within 1 month.

Clinical Pathologic Features

Although *Bartonella* infections in cats are associated with erythrocytes, they do not result in an acute, life-threatening hemolytic anemia that is the hallmark of clinical hemobartonellosis. Examination of seroreactive, naturally exposed cats has not revealed anemia as a common abnormality. In contrast to controls, experimentally infected cats experienced a decrease in packed cell volume (PCV) of 10 to 36% of baseline values within 14 to 21 days of receiving blood inoculum from infected cats. A regenerative response was marked by anisocytosis, polychromasia, and occasional nucleated erythrocytes. PCV returned to normal within 2 to 3 weeks. Fluctuations in PCV did not appear to correlate with severity of bacteremia, and plasma protein levels remained within normal range throughout the study period. Relapses of bacteremia were not accompanied by increased body temperature or decreased PCV.

Pathogenic Findings

Nonmalignant lymphadenopathy of undetermined cause, associated with lymphoid hyperplasia or the presence of argyrophilic intracellular bacteria, has been reported in cats. Several experimentally challenged cats have experienced transient lymph node enlargement. Although no bacteria have been detected histologically, regional lymphoid and splenic hyperplasia have been observed in cats acutely or chronically infected with *B. henselae* or *B. clarridgeiae*. Since *Bartonella* can be visualized using silver impregnation stains, these organisms should be considered in the differential diagnosis of nonmalignant lymphadenopathy in cats.

Tissue pathologic conditions have been reported in association with *Bartonella* infection in cats. Histologic patterns indicative of an infectious process were observed in tissues recovered from cats experimentally infected with *B. henselae* or *B. clarridgeiae*. Tissue specimens obtained from acutely infected cats disclosed multifocal splenic and hepatic neutrophilic infiltrates, multifocal myocarditis, focal pyogranulomatous nephritis, and hepatic abscesses. Post mortem studies performed on chronically infected cats revealed biliary and hepatic lesions consisting of multifocal lymphocytic cholangitis or pericholangitis. Focal accumulations of lymphocytes and plasma cells were also observed in the myocardium.

DIAGNOSIS

Blood Films

Diagnosis of *Bartonella* infection by light microscopy is difficult. Peripheral blood films prepared from bacteremic cats and stained with a Romanowsky-type stain such as Diff-Quick do not reveal *Bartonella*. *Bartonella* organisms can be visualized in blood smears with acridine orange staining and fluorescent microscopy; however, this method is not routinely available in most veterinary clinics, the technique nonspecifically labels DNA, and interpretation of fluorescence can be difficult.

The intradermal skin test, which has been employed for many years in the diagnosis of CSD in humans, does not appear to be useful in cats. Skin test antigen material is prepared from pooled fluid aspirated from CSD patients, homogenized, sterilized, and diluted. Cats are poor delayed-type hypersensitivity responders, and common macroscopic indications of exposure such as erythema and induration are often transient or not detectable. Evaluation of 16 experimentally infected cats revealed only two weakly positive responders.

Serologic Findings

Both indirect immunofluorescent antibody and enzyme-linked immunosorbent assays are currently available for serum analysis.* The sensitivity and specificity of both methods is similar. The various species share several immunoreactive surface antigens and as a result, cross-reactivity among *Bartonella* species has been described by many investigators. Although immunoglobulin kinetics have not been defined, serologic tests can be helpful in determining if a cat has been exposed to *Bartonella*. Chomel and colleagues (1995) evaluated the usefulness of indirect immunofluorescent antibody serologic tests in determining the status of bacteremia in cats. Their results indicated a positive predictive value of 46.4% and a negative predictive value of 89.7%. Rarely some bacteremic cats fail to produce detectable antibodies; however, a negative serologic test result against both *B. henselae* and *B. clarridgeiae* can generally be interpreted as not infected. Positive test results may be more difficult to interpret. Cats can remain seroreactive but blood culture–negative. This may be due to an inherent insensitivity of our blood culture systems to isolate these fastidious organisms or the periodic sequestration of *Bartonella* in other tissues. Given this situation, the potential infectivity of a cat cannot accurately be determined by serologic tests; however, the compilation of data from several studies indicates that higher titers are frequently accompanied by bacteremia.

Bacteriologic Culture

Bacteriologic culture of the blood remains the most reliable tool for the diagnosis of *Bartonella* infection. However, since culture-negative intervals during chronic infection can confound attempts to demonstrate the presence of the bacteria, specimens from cats may need to be cultured on repeated occasions. Ideally, 1.5 ml of blood aseptically obtained by jugular venipuncture is placed in an Isolator tube for processing within 24 hours.† Isolator tubes contain sodium polyanetholesulfonate (SPS), saponin, and polypropylene glycol to aid in recovering bacteria intimately associated with erythrocytes. If Isolator tubes are unavailable, blood can be placed in ethylenediaminetetra-acetic acid (EDTA)-treated tubes. Freezing of EDTA-treated blood has enhanced bacterial recovery in one study. The sample is streaked on chocolate or blood (rabbit, sheep, or horse) agar plates and incubated at 35°C with 5% carbon dioxide. Colonies are commonly visualized within 10 to 14 days; however, cultures should be maintained for 60 days before discarding them as negative because some strains require substantially longer incubation times. *Bartonella* spp. may be recovered using conventional blood culture bottles, but as the organisms produce little carbon dioxide, growth is

---

*Tick-borne Disease Laboratory, NCSU-CVM, Room C-321, 4700 Hillsborough St, Raleigh, NC 27606.
†Wampole Laboratories, Cranbury, NJ 08512.

not easily detected in these systems. Blind subcultures and acridine orange staining of bottle contents are recommended. Primary isolation of *Bartonella* has also been achieved using endothelial cell co-cultures or liquid media.

Members of the genus *Bartonella* are gram-negative, catalase-negative, oxidase-negative, and urease-negative organisms. Biochemical testing of *Bartonella* isolates for preformed enzymes and carbohydrate utilization is generally unremarkable. *Bartonella* can be difficult to identify to the species level unless PCR-based assays such as gene sequencing or PCR-restriction fragment length polymorphism (RFLP) analysis of various genes are used. These techniques are not readily available outside of research institutions.

Detection of Organisms or Antigen

Organisms can be visualized in tissue specimens using Warthin-Starry or Steiner silver stains. This technique is not specific for *Bartonella*, however, and will detect any argyrophilic bacteria. Polyclonal and monoclonal antibodies are also available for immunocytochemical identification of *Bartonella* spp. in various specimens. Recently developed molecular techniques can be used to detect *Bartonella* DNA in blood or tissue specimens without culturing. Molecular diagnostic tests with increased sensitivity and specificity are being refined and should aid in diagnosing the chronic carrier state; however, availability to the veterinary practitioner is limited. An antigen enzyme-linked immunosorbent assay has not yet been developed but would be clinically useful for identifying infected cats.

THERAPY

Antimicrobial Efficacy

Limited studies have been performed to assess the efficacy of antimicrobial agents against *Bartonella* infections in cats. In vitro, *Bartonella* species are susceptible to most antimicrobial agents; however, in vivo efficacy may be poor, even when antibiotics with good intracellular penetration are used. Bacterial clearance is difficult to assess because the bacteremia can be relapsing and the organism's growth characteristics fastidious, and blood cultures are not uniformly sensitive. In clinical or experimental studies, one negative blood culture result does not necessarily equate to antimicrobial blood sterilization. Drugs reported to have limited success eliminating feline *Bartonella* infections are enrofloxacin (Baytril, Miles Inc., Animal Health Products) at a dosage of 22.7 mg every 12 hours PO, doxycycline hyclate (Danbury Pharmacal, Inc.) at a dosage of 25 mg every 12 hours PO, and amoxicillin (AmoxiTabs, Pfizer Animal Health) at a dosage of 100 to 200 mg every 12 hours PO, when administered for 1 to 4 weeks. The benefits of a longer course of treatment remain uncertain. Regnery and co-workers (1996) reported no improvement over controls when cats were treated with amoxicillin or enrofloxacin; a persistent bacteremia was also seen, but a decrease in colony count was observed with erythromycin or tetracycline. Long-term clinical trials are indicated to determine the response to treatment more accurately. Efficacy may be dependent on the species, the bacterial load, the duration of treatment, or the chronicity of infection.

Antibiotic clearance of infection in cats would be beneficial to prevent the spread of *Bartonella* between cats and to humans. Conflicting reports exist, however, regarding the possibility of reinfection if cats are challenged. Long-term administration of antibiotics to cats infected with bacteria of apparently low pathogenicity for the feline host and with the potential for reinfection should be approached judiciously. These drugs are important for the eradication of more serious pathogens, and the risk of development of resistant strains of *Bartonella* or other bacteria is a possibility. If a cat is owned by, or in frequent contact with, someone who is immunosuppressed, treatment with enrofloxacin, doxycycline, or amoxicillin for 4 weeks seems prudent. Blood cultures should be performed 2 to 4 weeks following completion of treatment and periodically thereafter to monitor bacteremia status. The opportunity for reexposure to *Bartonella* should be decreased by keeping the cat indoors, away from other cats, and by rigorous flea and tick control measures.

Protective Immunity

Humoral protection appears to be lacking, but antibodies may have a role in the control of bacteremia. In one study, a progressive decrease in the antibody titer was observed prior to relapses of bacteremia, and a decrease in colony count was usually accompanied by an increase in antibody titer. The existence of protective immunity following recovery from infection is questionable. Greene and colleagues (1996) attempted to reinfect previously bacteremic cats with a secondary challenge of homologous inoculum containing laboratory-cultivated *B. henselae*. A 4-week observation period failed to detect bacteremia in the recipients. Regnery and colleagues (1996) were also unable to document reinfection of *B. henselae*–challenged cats previously exposed to laboratory-cultivated *B. henselae*, but they successfully transmitted *B. henselae* to cats previously exposed to *B. quintana*. In contrast, using *B. henselae* or *B. henselae*– and *B. clarridgeiae*–infected blood as inoculum, the authors observed bacteremia in one cat challenged with a homologous strain of *B. henselae* and one cat exposed to a heterologous strain of *B. clarridgeiae*.

PUBLIC HEALTH IMPLICATIONS

Zoonosis Prevention Program

In light of the increasing immunocompromised human population resulting from infectious diseases, cancer, organ transplantation, and senescence, veterinarians are relied on to advise owners of the zoonotic risks involved with pet ownership. It was recently estimated that up to 40% of immunocompromised individuals own pets. Whether owners are immune compromised or not, pets fulfill an important role as companions, and euthanasia is not recommended for *Bartonella*-infected cats. Relative to *Bartonella* infection, several recommendations can be made. These should include good hygienic practices such as washing hands with soap following cat contact and refraining from behaviors that might lead to biting or scratching by the cat.

Kissing cats or allowing them to lick open wounds on a human should also be discouraged. Onychectomy is not recommended. Several case reports of *Bartonella* infection in association with declawed cats exist. Contact with an infected cat may be sufficient to transmit *Bartonella* if breaks in the skin are present. Transmission of infection to cats following inoculation of urine sediment from bacteremic cats was unsuccessful; however, the medical literature contains reports that suggest this may be an occasional route of *Bartonella* transmission. If possible, cleaning of the litterbox should be attended to by someone other than the ill individual. Clinical signs or symptoms of human exposure to *Bartonella,* including febrile episodes, persistent lesion following a cat scratch or bite, lymphadenopathy, blood-filled papules, myalgia, or unexplained lethargy, should be brought to the attention of a physician. Although in most cases involving immunocompetent individuals, the course of the disease is self-limited, immunocompromised patients appear to benefit from the administration of antimicrobial therapy.

PREVENTION AND CONTROL

Iatrogenic Transmission

Given the prevalence of asymptomatic bacteremia and the success of experimental transmission studies using blood inoculum or infected fleas, the opportunity for iatrogenic transmission by blood transfusion is high. We recommend screening potential blood donors by culture techniques and serologic tests. Blood from cats that are culture-positive or culture-negative with a high antibody titer is not recommended for blood transfusion therapy.

Ectoparasite Control

Since flea-borne *B. henselae* and presumably *B. clarridgeiae* can be transmitted between cats and possibly to humans, regular flea control should be stressed. In consideration of the as yet undefined role of ticks in the transmission of *B. henselae* and *B. clarridgeiae*, the environment should also be kept tick-free.

Vaccination

A vaccine against *B. henselae* and *B. clarridgeiae* is not commercially available. The development of a vaccine that will prevent infection, and therefore curtail human disease, is being pursued by several investigators.

References and Suggested Reading

Childs JE, Rooney JA, Cooper JL, et al: Epidemiologic observations on infection with *Rochalimaea* species among cats living in Baltimore, MD. J Am Vet Med Assoc 204:1775, 1994.
A retrospective study of 592 feline sera previously analyzed for reactivity against FIV and Toxoplasma gondii.
Chomel BB, Abbott RC, Kasten RW, et al: *Bartonella henselae* prevalence in domestic cats in California: Risk factors and association between bacteremia and antibody titers. J Clin Microbiol 33:2445, 1995.
A prospective epidemiologic study of 205 cats illustrating the usefulness of serologic screening to identify abacteremic but not necessarily bacteremic cats.
Chomel B, Kasten RW, Floyd-Hawkins K, et al: Experimental transmission of *Bartonella henselae* by the cat flea. J Clin Microbiol 34:1952, 1996.
Results of this study provide convincing evidence that the cat flea plays an important role in the transmission of B. henselae *between cats.*
Greene CE, McDermott M, Jameson PH, et al: *Bartonella henselae* infection in cats: Evaluation during primary infection, treatment, and rechallenge infection. J Clin Microbiol 34:1682, 1996.
A transmission study using laboratory-cultivated B. henselae *as inoculum to infect and rechallenge random source cats.*
Jameson PH, Greene CE, Regnery RL, et al: Seroprevalence of *Rochalimaea henselae* in pet cats throughout regions of North America. J Infect Dis 172:1145, 1995.
A serosurvey of cats from various regions of the continental United States, Alaska, and Hawaii depicting high seroreactivity that coincides with warm, humid environments and probably flea prevalence.
Kordick DL, Breitschwerdt EB: Relapsing bacteremia after blood transmission of *Bartonella henselae* to cats. Am J Vet Res 58:492, 1997.
Results from this transmission study using blood from bacteremic donors illustrate the relapsing nature of Bartonella *bacteremia in asymptomatic cats.*
Kordick DL, Wilson KH, Sexton DJ, et al: Prolonged *Bartonella* bacteremia in cats associated with cat-scratch disease patients. J Clin Microbiol 33:3245, 1995.
The results of this study support the conclusion that Bartonella *spp. are responsible for human CSD and are transmitted by cats that can be chronically infected for periods exceeding 1 year.*
Regnery RL, Rooney JA, Johnson AM, et al: Experimentally induced *Bartonella henselae* infections followed by challenge exposure and antimicrobial therapy in cats. Am J Vet Res 57:1714, 1996.
A transmission study using laboratory-cultivated B. henselae *as inoculum to infect and rechallenge SPF cats.*
Schwartzman WA: Infections due to *Rochalimaea:* The expanding clinical spectrum. Clin Infect Dis 15:893, 1992.
An excellent review article describing the history of Bartonella *(previously* Rochalimaea*) associated human disease and recent advances in our understanding of these microorganisms.*
Zangwill KM, Hamilton DH, Perkins BA, et al: Cat scratch disease in Connecticut: Epidemiology, risk factors, and evaluation of a new diagnostic test. N Engl J Med 329:8, 1993.
Sera from CSD patients and appropriate controls were analyzed by IFA for B. henselae*–specific antibodies, and risk factors for CSD were identified.*

Leptospirosis

Linda A. Ross

Virginia Rentko

North Grafton, Massachusetts

Over the past 5 years, several reports have suggested an apparent change in the epizootiology of canine leptospirosis. *Leptospira interrogans* serovars *pomona* and *bratislava,* and *Leptospira kirschneri* serovar *grippotyphosa* have been identified as important causes of canine leptospirosis. The dog is an incidental host for these serovars, and therefore transmission between dogs is poor. The maintenance hosts for serovars *grippotyphosa* and *pomona* include skunks, raccoons, and opossums. Pigs are the maintenance hosts for serovar *bratislava.*

DIAGNOSIS

Leptospirosis should be considered in all dogs presenting because of acute renal failure, with or without concurrent evidence of hepatic disease. To facilitate the diagnosis, appropriate serum, urine, or tissue samples for diagnostic testing, or a combination of the three, should be obtained as early in the course of the disease as possible.

Serologic Findings

The microscopic agglutination test (MAT) remains the standard, most frequently used serologic test for leptospirosis; it evaluates the presence of serum antibodies to leptospiral antigens. It is important to determine the MAT for the serovars that are common in a given geographic region because there is some cross-reactivity of antibodies to different leptospiral serovars, and because dogs may be infected by any one of the many serovars of *Leptospira.* The MAT should generally include serovars *canicola, icterohaemorrhagiae, pomona, grippotyphosa, hardjo,* and possibly *bratislava.* In general, the infecting serovar is assumed to be the one to which the highest antibody titer is obtained. Cross-reactivity usually occurs within 6 weeks of the onset of the disease, after which time the titer of the infecting serovar predominates. Leptospiral serologic testing is performed at a number of veterinary diagnostic laboratories throughout the United States.

The MAT should be interpreted in light of the duration of disease, prior antibiotic therapy, and vaccination status of the animal. A single high titer (>1:800) in an animal with compatible clinical and laboratory abnormalities is considered diagnostic. However, because the titer may be negative early in the course of the disease, measurement of a convalescent titer 2 to 4 weeks after the acute titer may be necessary. A fourfold increase in the convalescent titer indicates recent infection with that serovar. However, antibiotic therapy early in the course of the disease may blunt the rise in antibody titer. Commercial canine bacterins are derived from serovars *canicola* and *icterohaemorrhagiae.* Postvaccinal titers are usually low (1:100 to 1:400),

although occasionally they may rise as high as 1:3,200. High titers will decrease with time, although they can persist for 6 months or longer after vaccination. The antibodies produced by vaccination may cross-react with other serovars but at a low titer (<1:100). There has been some question about cross-reactivity between antibodies to *Leptospira* and *Borrelia burgdorferi*; however, studies have failed to support any substantial degree of cross-reactivity.

Histopathologic Findings

Histopathologic study of renal tissue obtained by an ultrasonogram-guided, automated biopsy gun has been a useful early aid in diagnosis (see *CVT XII,* p. 933). In the authors' experience, dogs with acute renal failure and biopsy findings of acute lymphocytic, plasmacytic, and neutrophilic interstitial nephritis (without significant glomerular or tubular pathologic findings) have almost all been confirmed serologically as suffering from leptospirosis. The availability of ultrasonography for guided biopsies and the turnaround time for histopathologic results will determine the usefulness of this test in a practice situation.

Demonstration of Leptospires

In the past, direct visualization of leptospires in urine by darkfield microscopy was recommended as a method for early diagnosis of leptospirosis. However, this test is no longer recommended because of its technical difficulty and low specificity (other spirochetes, such as *B. burgdorferi,* may also appear in urine). Similarly, demonstration of leptospires by silver staining of renal biopsy tissue was recommended in the past. However, this technique has both low sensitivity and low specificity and therefore is no longer recommended.

Two newer techniques (fluorescent antibody testing and polymerase chain reaction [PCR]–based assays) may be useful in detecting the presence of leptospires, especially early in the course of the disease. Both of these tests can be performed on either urine or tissue samples. Fluorescent antibody test results must be interpreted in light of the fact that leptospires may not be shed into the urine until 4 to 10 days after the onset of clinical signs and that antibiotic therapy eliminates leptospiruria rapidly. In most laboratories, fluorescent antibody testing does not identify the serovar of *Leptospira* that has caused disease; additional serologic testing is still necessary for this determination. Fluorescent antibody testing for leptospirosis is currently being performed by several diagnostic laboratories in the United States.

Amplification of DNA by PCR techniques has recently been used to develop PCR-based assays for both the detection of leptospires and the identification of the infecting serovar. The technique is specific and sensitive. A disadvantage of PCR testing is that false-positive results may occur from contamination if it is not performed under strict quality control. PCR testing is not yet readily available for private practitioners but should become available as the technology improves.

EPIZOOTIOLOGY

The incidence of canine leptospirosis may be underreported. Retrospective studies based on serologic testing that considered a single antibody titer of 1:3,200 or a fourfold increase in a convalescent titer diagnostic may not have included dogs with acute renal failure in the early phase of disease with negative or low titers (Rentko et al, 1992; Scanziani et al, 1994). However, more recent studies have shown that dogs may have a negative titer during the acute phase of the disease and subsequently have diagnostic titers during the convalescent phase (Harkin and Gartrell, 1996; Levitan, manuscript in preparation).

The clinical manifestations of leptospirosis have been reported to be serovar-dependent. Reports of dogs infected with serovar *grippotyphosa* have described primarily renal involvement, or renal disease with only mild hepatic involvement. A recent epizootic associated with serovar *grippotyphosa* in more than 100 dogs on Long Island, New York, was characterized by acute renal failure with dramatic hepatic involvement (Levitan, 1996, personal communication). Hyperbilirubinemia ranged from 3 to 50 mg/dl, with associated increases in serum alkaline phosphatase and alanine aminotransferase activity. As in previous reports, cross-reactivity with other serovars at low titers was noted. Particularly interesting in this outbreak was the severe hepatic involvement, as well as the large number of dogs affected. The outcome of these cases was similar to previously reported studies in that successful outcome was dependent on early clinical recognition.

Serologic data for leptospirosis testing at the Tufts Veterinary Diagnostic Laboratory from June 1992 through October 1996 identified 345 serum samples from 303 dogs tested. Samples were submitted by clinicians at Tufts University Foster Hospital for Small Animals and by small animal practitioners from New England, which shows that clinicians have an increased awareness of leptospirosis. Serovars tested were *hardjo*, *icterohaemorrhagiae*, *grippotyphosa*, *canicola*, and *bratislava*. Thirty of the 303 dogs had a single titer of 1:3,200 or higher or a fourfold increase in convalescent titer. Serovars *grippotyphosa* and *pomona* most commonly induced the predominant titers. Serologic evidence of infection with serovar *grippotyphosa* was evident in 21 dogs, serovar *pomona* was evident in 7 dogs, and serovars *icterohaemorrhagiae* and *canicola* in 1 dog each. Serovar *bratislava* was tested in 95 of the 303 dogs. Four dogs that had a titer ($\geq$1:12,800) compatible with active infection by serovar *bratislava* also had a titer of greater than or equal to 1:12,800 to serovar *grippotyphosa*. Cross-reactivity between these two serovars could not be ruled out.

THERAPY

Animals with acute renal failure due to leptospirosis should be managed with appropriate fluid therapy and other supportive measures, as described on p. 173. Leptospirocidal antibiotic therapy should be instituted immediately in any animal in which the clinical presentation is consistent with leptospirosis, after appropriate diagnostic samples have been obtained. Early antibiotic therapy hastens resolution of renal failure or hepatic disease and shortens the duration of urine shedding of the organism. Two phases of antibiotic therapy are necessary—the first to eliminate leptospiremia and the second to eliminate the organism from renal tubular cells and the renal carrier state. Penicillin (25,000 to 40,000 U/kg every 12 to 24 hours IV or IM for 14 days) remains the antibiotic of choice to eliminate leptospiremia. The dose should be adjusted downward if the animal has renal failure. A rough clinical approximation of dosage adjustment can be obtained by dividing the dose by the serum creatinine concentration. The renal carrier state is best eliminated by dihydrostreptomycin; however, this drug is no longer available. Instead, doxycycline (5 to 10 mg/kg b.i.d. PO) is administered for an additional 14 days following penicillin therapy. Because doxycycline is not excreted by the kidneys, no dosage adjustment is necessary.

The prognosis for animals with renal failure caused by leptospirosis is guarded. Although some animals recover completely, others, even with prompt and appropriate therapy, die of their disease or recover only partial renal function and remain azotemic. The best prognostic indicator is the rate of decrease of the serum creatinine concentration in response to penicillin and fluid therapy.

ZOONOTIC POTENTIAL

Animals with leptospirosis may pose a threat of infection to other animals or to humans. Animals suspected of having the disease should be isolated, and the individuals handling them should wear gloves and practice careful hygiene when handling blood, urine, and tissue. Iodine-based solutions are effective for disinfection of contaminated areas and equipment. Infection of one domestic animal by another is apparently rare; however, both may have been exposed to the same source. Therefore, if leptospirosis is suspected in one animal, it may be prudent to immediately vaccinate others with which it has had contact. Owners or hospital personnel, especially those who are immunosuppressed for any reason, should seek advice from their physician if they have had contact with an infected animal.

Infection with or exposure to leptospires was recently reported in individuals living in inner city environments. Their exposure was suggested to be from rat urine because 90% of rats trapped in these areas were found to carry leptospirosis by PCR (Vinetz et al, 1996). There is concern that leptospirosis in humans is being underdiagnosed or that the disease is re-emerging in humans as well as in dogs.

IMMUNIZATION

Immunization for leptospirosis is relatively serovar-specific. Therefore, although commercial bacterins for dogs are available, they provide protection against serovars *canicola* and *icterohaemorrhagiae* only. Despite this, immunization is recommended, especially for dogs living in areas in which leptospirosis has been reported.

References and Suggested Reading

Bal AE, Gravekamp C, Hartskeerl RA, et al: Detection of leptospires in urine by PCR for early diagnosis of leptospirosis. J Clin Microbiol 32:1894, 1994.
A description of the diagnostic test for detection of leptospires and identification of the infecting serovar.

Bolin CS: Diagnosis of leptospirosis: A reemerging disease of companion animals. Semin Vet Med Surg (Small Anim) 11:166, 1996.
A review of the methods of laboratory diagnosis of leptospirosis and their interpretation.

Brown CA, Roberts AW, Miller MA, et al: *Leptospira interrogans* serovar *grippotyphosa* infection in dogs. J Am Vet Med Assoc 209:1265, 1996.
A review of 11 cases of canine leptospirosis attributed to serovar grippotyphosa, *including isolation of the organism from two dogs.*

Harkin KR, Gartrell CL: Canine leptospirosis in New Jersey and Michigan: 17 cases (1990–1995). J Am Anim Hosp Assoc 32:495, 1996.
A retrospective review of the serologic and clinical findings of canine leptospirosis.

Levitan D: An epizootic of canine leptospirosis on Long Island, New York (100 cases), 1996, personal communication.
A description of the serologic and clinical findings in an epizootic of leptospirosis in New York.

Nielsen JN, Cochran, GK, Cassells JA, et al: *Leptospira interrogans* serovar *bratislava* infection in two dogs. J Am Vet Med Assoc 199:351, 1991.
A report describing infection with Leptospira interrogans *serovar* bratislava *in two dogs.*

Rentko VT, Clark N, Ross LA, et al: Canine leptospirosis. A retrospective study of 17 cases. J Vet Intern Med 6:235, 1992.
A review of serologic, clinical and clinicopathological findings of canine leptospirosis.

Scanziani E, Calcaterra S, Tagliabue S, et al: Serological findings in cases of acute leptospirosis in the dog. J Small Anim Pract 35:257, 1994.
A review of the serologic findings of canine leptospirosis in Italy.

Van Den Broek AHM, Thrusfield MV, Dobbie GR, et al: A serological and bacteriological survey of leptospiral infection in dogs in Edinburgh and Glasgow. J Small Anim Pract 32:118, 1991.
A survey showing the importance of serovar bratislava *in the dog in Scotland.*

Vinetz JM, Glass GE, Flexner CE, et al: Sporadic urban leptospirosis. Ann Intern Med 125:794, 1996.
Report of recent cases of leptospirosis in humans, and infection rate in rats in an inner city environment.

Canine Hepatozoonosis

DOUGLASS K. MACINTIRE
Auburn, Alabama

NANCY VINCENT-JOHNSON
San Antonio, Texas

Hepatozoonosis has been reported in dogs from Africa, Asia, Europe, the Middle East, Japan, Malaysia, the Philippines, and the United States. In most parts of the world, the disease is diagnosed by detecting gametocytes on a blood smear. The gametocyte stage of the organism appears as an intracellular, oblong, encapsulated inclusion body in the cytoplasm of neutrophils or monocytes. The pathogenicity of the disease has been questioned by researchers in Africa, Japan, and Israel, where gametocytes are commonly found in asymptomatic dogs. A recent serologic survey in Israel revealed that 33% of apparently healthy dogs sampled had positive immunofluorescent antibody titers against *Hepatozoon canis*. These findings have led many researchers to conclude that hepatozoonosis is not pathogenic unless the infection is overwhelming or the dog is immunosuppressed or has concurrent disease.

Experience with the organism identified as *H. canis* has been radically different in the United States, where hepatozoonosis appears to cause a distinct clinical syndrome characterized by chronic myositis, debilitation, and death. The disease was first reported in Texas in 1978 and for many years appeared to be localized to the Texas Gulf Coast region. In 1996, however, we reported the disease in 22 dogs from Alabama and Georgia. Since that report we have continued to see infected dogs at our hospital, including dogs from Alabama, Georgia, Florida, and Tennessee.

Our experience leads us to believe that the disease is becoming more widespread geographically and that many practitioners are currently unfamiliar with the disease. The purpose of this discussion is to describe the clinical syndrome of hepatozoonosis as it appears in domestic dogs in the United States. The causative agent of American hepatozoonosis has recently been identified as a new species, *Hepatozoon americanum*, which is separate and distinct from *H. canis*.

LIFE CYCLE, TRANSMISSION, AND PATHOGENESIS

The hepatozoon organism requires two hosts to complete its life cycle. The definitive host of *H. canis* is *Rhipicephalus sanguineus*, the brown dog tick, but oocysts of *H. americanum* have been identified in *Amblyomma maculatum* (Gulf Coast tick). The tick ingests gametocytes while feeding on the intermediate host (the dog). The gametocytes fuse within the tick to form an ookinete, which eventually develops into an oocyst containing many sporocysts. Each sporocyst in turn contains 12 to 24 sporozoites. Thus, one infected tick contains hundreds of infective organisms. The dog must ingest the tick to become infected because the organisms cannot migrate to the mouth parts of the tick. Once ingested, the sporozoites are released and penetrate the intestinal tract of the dog and are carried by blood or lymph to various tissues throughout the body where they are ingested by mononuclear phagocytes. Once within the cells, the organisms form schizonts, which then undergo asexual division. Merozoites are formed within the schizonts and are released to form more schizonts or to infect leukocytes and become circulating gametocytes. The life cycle is completed if a tick ingests the gametocytes.

The cyst is the most common stage of the organism found in infected dogs. It most commonly appears as a round to ovoid structure, 250 to 500 μm in diameter, with pale blue laminar membranes, giving it an "onion skin" appearance. Often, a single nucleus is present in the cyst, but sometimes multiple developing meronts can be seen within the schizont. Cystic structures are found in cardiac and skeletal muscle, lymph nodes, spleen, and pancreas, and they usually are not associated with an inflammatory response. It is theorized that after the cysts mature, they rupture, releasing numerous merozoites. These merozoites are phagocytized by macrophages and initiate a marked pyogranulomatous response. Multifocal pyogranulomas composed of neutrophils and macrophages, many containing merozoites, can be found in great abundance in cardiac and skeletal muscle and occasionally in pancreas, lymph nodes, kidneys, liver, and lung. Grossly, the pyogranulomas may appear as multiple white to tan foci, 1 to 2 mm in diameter, diffusely scattered throughout these organs. Pyogranulomas can also be found in the fascia and periosteum surrounding bones, resulting in increased osteoblastic and osteoclastic activity, exostoses, and thickening of bone surfaces. Vascular lesions, including fibrinoid degeneration of vessel walls, mineralization and proliferation of vascular intima, and pyogranulomatous vasculitis, may result in thrombosis. Renal lesions consisting of pyogranulomas; lymphocytic, plasmacytic, interstitial nephritis; and mesangioproliferative glomerulonephritis may be seen in chronic cases. Chronic disease may also result in amyloid deposition in the spleen, lymph nodes, small intestine, liver, and kidney.

CLINICAL SIGNS

The most common clinical signs associated with *H. americanum* infection are fever, chronic weight loss, mucopurulent ocular discharge, pain, and gait abnormalities. The clinical signs may wax and wane with the degree of pyogranulomatous inflammation. Rectal temperature often fluctuates between normal and highs of up to 41.11°C (106°F), but fever is nonresponsive to antibiotics. Many dogs have been treated for fever of unknown origin with several courses of antibiotic therapy before it becomes evident that the waxing and waning course of the disease is not a positive response to treatment. Chronic weight loss most likely results from muscle atrophy and increased caloric demands associated with the chronic inflammatory state. The ocular discharge may be secondary to inflammation of extraocular muscles or destruction of the lacrimal gland from pyogranulomatous inflammation. Approximately one third of the dogs have decreased tear production on a Schirmer test in addition to the matted eyes. The pain that accompanies the myositis may manifest as cervical,

back, joint, or generalized pain. Hyperesthesia, stiffness, neck guarding, and fever can easily be mistaken for meningitis or discospondylitis, but analysis of the cerebrospinal fluid is usually unremarkable. Gait abnormalities can include stiffness, generalized weakness, rear limb paresis and ataxia, and an inability or unwillingness to rise. Many of the dogs with *H. americanum* referred to our hospital are referred to our neurology service for suspected neurologic disease.

LABORATORY FINDINGS

The most consistent hematologic finding is marked leukocytosis composed primarily of a mature neutrophilia. In 22 dogs with hepatozoonosis examined at Auburn University, the initial white blood cell count ranged from 27,800 to 196,000/μl, with a mean leukocyte count of 85,700/μl. Other common hematologic findings include mild nonregenerative anemia and normal to elevated platelet counts. Thrombocytopenia generally does not occur with *H. americanum* infection unless there is concurrent disease with ehrlichiosis, babesiosis, or Rocky Mountain spotted fever.

The most common abnormalities detected on serum chemistry panels include mildly increased serum alkaline phosphatase activity, hypoglycemia, and hypoalbuminemia. The increase in serum alkaline phosphatase activity may be secondary to periosteal activity associated with inflammatory myositis. Hypoglycemia, generally in the range of 40 to 60 mg/dl, is thought to be the result of in vitro metabolism of glucose by white blood cells. When sodium fluoride is used as the anticoagulant to block glucose metabolism by the cells, the blood glucose value is usually in the normal reference range. Hypoalbuminemia is a consistent finding and may be associated with decreased protein intake, chronic inflammation, or renal loss. With chronic disease, dogs may develop glomerulonephritis characterized by marked proteinuria and elevated urine protein:creatinine ratios. Blood urea nitrogen (BUN) values are often low in affected dogs. Decreased BUN values may represent reduced protein intake or disordered protein metabolism secondary to negative nitrogen balance and production of inflammatory proteins. Although hypoglycemia, hypoalbuminemia, and low BUN are often associated with liver disease, serum bile acids are usually normal or only mildly elevated in dogs with *H. americanum* infection.

DIAGNOSIS

A tentative diagnosis of hepatozoonosis can be made if clinical signs and laboratory findings are suggestive and other causes of fever, pain, and leukocytosis are ruled out. A definitive diagnosis requires identification of the organism. Gametocytes may be detected on a blood smear, but the number of infected cells rarely exceeds 0.1% of the leukocytes. The gametocytes can easily be missed because of poor stain uptake by the parasite nucleus. Gametocytes may exit the host cell after blood is drawn, leaving behind an empty capsule that is difficult to visualize. When they are seen, gametocytes appear as oblong intracellular inclusion bodies in the cytoplasm of white blood cells, measuring approximately 11 μm × 5 μm, with a clear to pale blue capsule.

Because examination of blood smears is often laborious and unrewarding, muscle biopsy has been used to detect cysts, merozoites, or pyogranulomas in skeletal muscle of infected dogs. The tissue state appears to be widespread in the dog, and muscle biopsy is more likely to yield a positive diagnosis than is examination of blood smears. We generally take two to three small (2 cm × 2 cm) wedge biopsies from the biceps femoris, semitendinosus, or epaxial muscles. An incision is made to reveal the muscle fascia. The muscle belly is then grasped with a towel clamp, and a small piece is removed and preserved in formalin. Several samples are submitted for histopathologic examination to increase the chances of detecting the organism.

At present, no serologic test is available to definitively diagnose the *H. americanum*. Israeli researchers developed an immunofluorescent antibody titer assay that detects antibodies against *H. canis* gametocytes, but preliminary serologic results in American dogs were inconsistent, with a high incidence of false-negative results. Inability to grow the hepatozoon organism in cell culture has hindered development of serologic tests or vaccination.

Radiographs can be used as a screening test to provide supportive data for a diagnosis of hepatozoonosis. Periosteal proliferation is often evident on various bones. Lesions may be subtle or marked and can range from irregular proliferative exostoses to smooth lamellar thickening of the periosteum (Fig. 1).

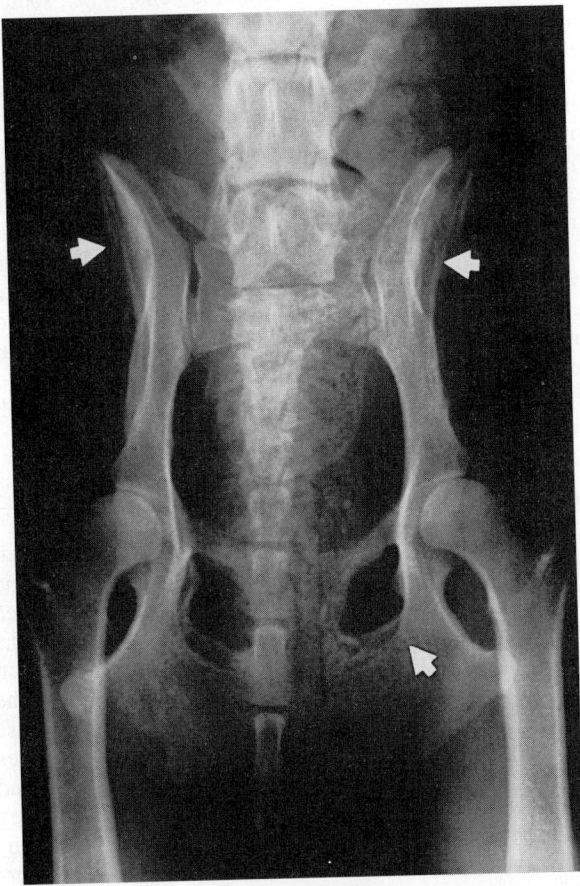

Figure 1. Pelvic radiographs may reveal characteristic periosteal proliferation (*arrow*) of various bones in dogs with hepatozoonosis.

TREATMENT

Occasionally dogs with extreme debilitation or high fevers require treatment with intravenous fluids and nutritional support. Many dogs with hepatozoonosis may have other tick-borne diseases, and a course of doxycycline (5 mg/kg every 24 hours for 14 days) may be warranted.

There is currently no treatment for hepatozoonosis that will reliably eliminate the organism from the host. Remission of clinical signs can usually be obtained by combination therapy with trimethoprim sulfa (15 mg/kg PO every 12 hours), pyrimethamine (0.25 mg/kg PO every 24 hours), and clindamycin (10 mg/kg PO every 8 hours) for 14 days. In addition, nonsteroidal anti-inflammatory drugs can be used as palliative therapy to relieve the symptoms of fever and pain. Although the response to treatment is often dramatic, most dogs experience relapse of clinical signs within 2 to 6 months following treatment. It is theorized that exacerbation of clinical signs occurs when merozoites are released from the cysts, thereby initiating pyogranulomatous inflammation in the tissues. Preliminary data from our hospital suggest that remission can be prolonged by daily administration of decoquinate (Decox, Rhone-Poulenc, Athens, GA) at a dose of 10 to 20 mg/kg twice daily. Decoquinate is a coccidiostat marketed for use in food animals. Studies have shown the drug to be safe in dogs when administered at various dosages daily for up to 2 years. Decoquinate is available as a powder and can be mixed in the food according to the dosage schedule in Table 1. Preliminary findings in 24 dogs seem to indicate that the drug is safe and effective in preventing relapses if administered daily. In several dogs, clinical signs of disease returned when owners discontinued the medication. It appears that the treatment has to be continued long term (more than 1 year) to prevent relapses in dogs infected with *H. americanum*. Decoquinate is available in 50-pound bags from most feed stores or can be obtained in smaller amounts from Duran Farm Supply (334–745–7964).

Other drugs that have been used to treat hepatozoonosis include imidocarb dipropionate, diminazene aceturate, primaquine phosphate, and toltrazuril. Imidocarb (Schering-Plough Animal Health, Union, NJ) has recently been approved for use in the United States. The recommended dosage is 5 mg/kg SC given twice, 14 days apart. Pretreat-

TABLE 1. Decoquinate Dosage

Weight of Dog*	Amount of Powder to Mix in Food Twice Daily
1–10 lb.	¼ tsp.
11–20 lb.	½ tsp.
21–30 lb.	¾ tsp.
31–40 lb.	1 tsp.
41–50 lb.	1¼ tsp.
51–60 lb.	1½ tsp.
61–70 lb.	1¾ tsp.
71–80 lb.	2 tsp.
81–90 lb.	2¼ tsp.
91–100 lb.	2½ tsp.

*If borderline, move to next 10-lb. increment.
Recommended dosage = 10–20 mg/kg every 12 hours.
10 mg/kg = 1/4 tsp/10 lb.

ment with atropine 30 minutes prior to the injection may prevent the occurrence of parasympathomimetic side effects (salivation, nausea, diarrhea, abdominal cramping). The other drugs are not readily available in North America, and none has been shown to eliminate the parasite completely. Spontaneous remission has been reported in approximately 20% of dogs, but the majority undergo a chronic waxing and waning course characterized by cachexia, intermittent fever and pain, and renal disease. The average survival time reported is 10 to 12 months. The use of decoquinate has extended the survival time, with all treated dogs still living.

PREVENTION

In endemic areas, tick prevention with effective acaricides is paramount to preventing the disease. The tendency for cases to cluster around certain geographic areas may also suggest a wildlife reservoir. It is not known whether *H. americanum* can be transmitted through ingestion of infected tissue, similar to toxoplasmosis. Until more is known about the possibility of such transmission, consumption of raw meat from wildlife in endemic areas should be avoided.

Approximately half of the dogs diagnosed with *H. americanum* at our hospital have concurrent disease. It is not known whether the stress of concurrent disease causes exacerbation of a subclinical *H. americanum* infection or whether the debilitating effects of *H. americanum* infection make dogs more susceptible to other diseases. Effective management involves recognition and treatment of concurrent disease. Current research is focused on differentiating the American form of hepatozoonosis from that seen in other parts of the world.

References and Suggested Reading

Baneth G, Shkap V, Presentey BZ, Pipano E: *Hepatozoon canis:* The prevalence of antibodies and gametocytes in Israel. Vet Res Commun 20:41, 1996.
  A paper describing the occurrence of subclinical H. canis *infections in Israeli dogs.*
Barton CL, Russo EA, Craig TM, et al: Canine hepatozoonosis: A retrospective study of 15 naturally occurring cases. J Am Anim Hosp Assoc 21:125, 1985.
  A description of the clinical syndrome seen in Texas dogs with hepatozoonosis.
Craig TM, Smallwood JE, Knauer KW, et al: *Hepatozoon canis* infection in dogs: Clinical, radiologic, and hematologic findings. J Am Vet Med Assoc 173:967, 1978.
  First report of hepatozoonosis in dogs in the United States.
Craig TM: Hepatozoonosis. In: Greene CE, ed: Infectious Diseases of the Dog and Cat. Philadelphia: WB Saunders, 1990, pp 778–785.
  An overview of the current knowledge of pathogenesis, diagnosis, and treatment.
Elias E, Homans PA: *Hepatozoon canis* infection in dogs: Clinical and hematological findings—treatment. J Small Anim Pract 29:55, 1988.
  A good description of H. canis *infection in Israeli dogs.*
Macintire DK, Vincent-Johnson N, Dillon AR, et al: Hepatozoonosis in dogs: 22 cases (1989–1994). J Am Med Assoc 210:916, 1997.
  A report of 22 infected dogs from Alabama and Georgia.
Murata T, Inoue M, Taura Y, et al: Detection of *Hepatozoon canis* oocyst from ticks collected from the infected dogs. J Vet Med Sci 57:111, 1995.
  A report of the detection of H. canis *oocysts in ticks other than* Rhipicephalus *spp. in Japan.*
Nordgren RM, Craig TM: Experimental transmission of the Texas strain of *Hepatozoon canis.* Vet Parasitol 16:207, 1984.
  Proof that H. canis *can be transmitted to dogs through ingestion of infected* R. sanguineus *ticks.*
Vincent-Johnson N, Baneth G, Macintire D: Canine hepatozoonosis: Pathophysiology, diagnosis and treatment. Compend Cont Educ 19:51, 1997.
  A review paper describing the differences between hepatozoonosis in the United States and that worldwide.
Vincent-Johnson N, Macintire D, Lindsay D, et al: A new hepatozoon species from dogs: description of the causative agent of canine hepatozoonosis in North America. J Parasitol 83:1165, 1997.
  A paper describing H. americanum *as a separate species distinct from* H. canis.

Canine Cutaneous Pythiosis

GARY J. SPODNICK
Cary, North Carolina

Pythium spp. are important plant pathogens, but *Pythium insidiosum*, in contrast to other species of *Pythium*, has developed the ability to cause disease in animals and humans. The terminology used in the literature regarding infections caused by *Pythium* spp. and other fungal organisms is confusing. Pythiosis is caused by *P. insidiosum;* the disease was formerly known as phycomycosis. The term *phycomycosis* should not be applied to infections caused by *P. insidiosum* because this organism belongs to the order Peronosporales, phylum Oomycota, and kingdom Protista. Organisms that cause phycomycosis (the term *zygomycosis* has replaced the term phycomycosis and is the preferred term for describing fungal infections caused by Mucor,

Absidia, Rhizopus, and Mortierella) are classified in the kingdom Fungi. Beyond semantics, this information is clinically relevant because the dissimilarity between Zygomycetes and *P. insidiosum* is believed to account for differences in the therapeutic response of these organisms to antifungal chemotherapeutic agents.

CLINICAL DISEASE

Pythiosis primarily affects young, large breed dogs and is most common in warm aquatic environments such as the subtropical regions of the United States, including the Gulf

Coast states and the southeastern United States. Cutaneous disease usually develops during the summer months. *P. insidiosum* is considered a true pathogen, rather than an opportunistic organism, since affected dogs are not immunosuppressed and are otherwise healthy. Although gastrointestinal pythiosis is the most commonly reported form of the infection in dogs (see *CVT XII*, p. 324), cutaneous pythiosis appears to be an emerging form of the disease that can be extremely difficult to treat successfully. Exposure to the organism is postulated to occur when animals stand in stagnant fresh water containing newly emerged zoospores of *P. insidiosum*. The zoospores are motile and possess the ability to chemotactically orient themselves toward aquatic plants or animal hair. It is unknown whether zoospores can penetrate intact skin or whether infection can occur from direct inoculation of mycelial elements into damaged tissues. It is assumed that infection occurs when zoospores enter a pre-existing wound in the skin or mucosa. Although development of cutaneous lesions may be associated with a history of exposure to standing or stagnant fresh water, not all dogs with cutaneous pythiosis have a compatible history or the opportunity for such exposure in their environment.

The cutaneous lesions of pythiosis are fairly typical in appearance and consist of rapidly enlarging, destructive ulceroproliferative lesions with a superficial serosanguineous exudate. Lesions are commonly found on the extremities, base of the tail, perineum, and ventral trunk. They may or may not be pruritic. Lesions are often present for weeks or months before diagnosis and have been unresponsive to antibiotic therapy. Frequently, regional lymph nodes draining the site are enlarged. The ulceroproliferative lesion is often accompanied by considerable peripheral swelling secondary to lymphaticovenous obstruction.

DIAGNOSIS

Confirmation of cutaneous infection with *P. insidiosum* requires concomitant isolation of the organism from tissue (not exudate) and demonstration of tissue invasion by a morphologically compatible organism. The organisms may be difficult to see or may be unrecognizable in tissue sections stained with hematoxylin and eosin. The histologic appearance of the lesion is characterized by pyogranulomatous to granulomatous inflammation containing large numbers of epithelioid macrophages and multinucleate giant cells. Intense tissue eosinophilic infiltration is also characteristic of pythiosis. The diagnosis of pythiosis should be considered in biopsies from dogs with granulomatous inflammation accompanied by eosinophils in the skin and subcutis. Gomori's methenamine silver stain should be used on tissue sections when pythiosis is suspected. Fungal hyphae of *P. insidiosum* are irregularly branching and have thick, almost parallel walls. The hyphae range in diameter from 4.8 to 7.2 μm and have few thick septa.

Aseptically collected tissue specimens should be used to inoculate fungal culture media. Sabouraud dextrose agar, blood agar, and cornmeal agar media will all support rapid fungal mycelial growth at 35 to 37°C (95 to 98.6°F). Failure to grow the organism may be due to improper sample handling. Cooling or freezing the tissues will rapidly kill the organism. When the sample needs to be shipped to a diagnostic laboratory or when a delay between sample collection and plate inoculation is necessary, the sample should be washed with sterile saline and transported in sterile saline-ampicillin (100 μg/ml) solution at room temperature by next-day delivery. Positive identification of *P. insidiosum* can also be achieved by an indirect immunoperoxidase staining technique on sections of paraffin-embedded fixed tissues. This test (available through the Louisiana Veterinary Medical Diagnostic Laboratory, School of Veterinary Medicine, LSU, Baton Rouge, LA, 70803) may be a helpful ancillary test for confirmation of the diagnosis of pythiosis when attempts to culture the organism fail.

TREATMENT

The prognosis for dogs with cutaneous pythiosis is poor. Wide surgical excision offers the best opportunity for successful treatment of cutaneous pythiosis. Unfortunately, involvement is often extensive by the time a definitive diagnosis is established, making successful treatment unlikely. Therefore, the key to successful treatment is early recognition; the index of suspicion for pythiosis should be high based on the appearance and clinical behavior of the lesion. For lesions involving an extremity, amputation should be considered. For truncal lesions, wide en bloc surgical excision using oncologic surgical principles should be performed. Factors that influence prognosis include the location and size of the lesion and the duration of the infection. Small lesions of short duration or lesions located in areas that permit wide, complete surgical excision usually have the best prognosis. Recurrence of the lesion is common if the infected tissues are incompletely excised.

Attempts to treat cutaneous pythiosis in the dog with amphotericin B and ketoconazole alone or in combination with surgery have been unsuccessful. Although successful management of gastrointestinal pythiosis in the dog has been reported using itraconazole, the cutaneous form of the disease has been poorly responsive to itraconazole, and no cures have been reported to date. The disappointingly poor response to antifungal chemotherapeutic agents may be attributable to the fact that Oomycetes have plasma membranes that lack ergosterol and cell walls composed of cellulose and other glucans rather than chitin. The antifungal effect of the imidazoles, such as ketoconazole, and the triazoles, such as itraconazole, results from the inhibition of ergosterol synthesis in formation of the plasma membrane by these drugs. The lack of efficacy of amphotericin B is less well understood because this drug directly damages the plasma membrane. Immunotherapy using a phenolized, ultrasonicated autogenous preparation of *P. insidiosum* has been reported in horses and at least one dog. A poor response was noted in the dog. A lysosomal formulation of nystatin (Nystatin, IV, Argus Pharmaceuticals, Inc., Woodlands, TX) has been used in clinical trials for the treatment of systemic fungal infections in humans and cutaneous pythiosis in dogs. The use of nystatin, a polyene antibiotic, incorporated in liposomes for treatment of fungal infections has two distinct advantages: (1) it decreases the toxicity of nystatin and (2) it targets a significant fraction of the drug administered to the monocyte-macrophage system, which plays a major role in the inflammatory response to fungal infections, thereby potentially improving drug delivery to the site of infection. Further investigation is required to determine the efficacy of this drug and other treatment modalities as we strive to develop a rational therapeutic approach for the management of cutaneous pythiosis in dogs.

CVT Update: Therapy for Nasal Aspergillosis

Autumn P. Davidson
Davis, California

Kyle G. Mathews
Raleigh, North Carolina

Canine nasal aspergillosis, characterized by colonization and invasion of the nasal passages and frontal sinuses by a ubiquitous, saprophytic fungus, is most commonly treated topically. Oral administration of azole antifungal agents is effective in only 43 to 70% of cases, requiring protracted treatment (months), which is costly. Topical administration of the synthetic imidazole derivative clotrimazole, as described in *CVT XII,* p. 899, has met with a high degree of success (Davidson and Pappagianis, 1995).

The infusion of clotrimazole into the nasal passages and frontal sinuses described previously required trephination for placement of infant feeding tubes used as catheters, a somewhat invasive procedure requiring surgical expertise (Davidson et al, 1992). Based on subsequent studies of the distribution of topical agents in the frontal sinuses and nasal passages (Richardson and Mathews, 1995), a new technique for topical administration of clotrimazole in canine nasal aspergillosis was evaluated and found to be equally effective and less invasive.

The response to topical administration of the antifungal medication clotrimazole was evaluated in 60 dogs with confirmed nasal aspergillosis (Mathews et al, 1998). All dogs were anesthetized during treatment, and a cuffed endotracheal tube was used to prevent aspiration. The final outcome was determined by telephone conversation with owners and referring veterinarians. Based on this study, a newer method of clotrimazole administration is preferable.

Twenty-seven dogs were treated with a single topical application of clotrimazole in polyethylene glycol 200 delivered via surgically placed frontal sinus and nasal catheters (group 1) using a previously described technique (Davidson et al, 1992).

Eighteen dogs were treated by a single intranasal infusion of clotrimazole (group 2). All catheters were placed with the group 2 dogs in lateral recumbency. A 24F Foley catheter was placed by mouth so that the tip of the catheter lay dorsal to the soft palate. This process was aided initially by grasping the catheter tip with a pair of right-angle forceps (Meeker) or long-handled needle holders so that the catheter tip was directed rostrally. A mouth gag was placed, and an assistant pulled the tongue rostrally to improve visualization during catheter placement. The catheter was advanced until the balloon was dorsal to the junction of the hard and soft palates. The balloon of the Foley catheter was then inflated to occlude the nasopharynx. The balloon was palpated through the soft palate to confirm its position just caudal to the hard palate. Moistened laparotomy sponges were counted and then placed in the pharynx so that the catheter could not migrate caudally and to absorb any infusion that might escape around the balloon. During sponge placement, the index finger of the opposite hand was used to maintain balloon position. The mouth gag was removed. One 10F polypropylene infusion catheter was then advanced through each nostril. Beginning dorsomedially, each catheter was advanced into the dorsal nasal meatus to the level of the medial canthus of the ipsilateral palpebral fissure. A Foley catheter (12F) was then inserted into each nostril and the balloons were inflated so that they lay just caudal to, and occluded, the nostrils (Figs. 1 and 2). Occasionally, a nylon suture was placed across each nostril to prevent cranial migration of the nasal balloons. The three Foley catheters (one nasopharyngeal, two nasal) were placed, and their balloons inflated to slow the leakage of clotrimazole from the nasal cavity and frontal sinuses. The dogs were then repositioned in dorsal recumbency, and an additional laparotomy sponge was placed just caudal to the upper incisors between the endotracheal tube and the incisive papilla to control leakage of clotrimazole through the incisive ducts.

One gram of clotrimazole in 100 ml of polyethylene glycol 200 (1% solution) was then evenly divided between two 60-ml syringes (50 ml per syringe). The clotrimazole was slowly infused over a 1-hour period (50 ml per infusion catheter). The polypropylene catheters were maintained in a horizontal position, parallel to the table, throughout infusion. When fluid was noted within the lumen of a Foley catheter, it was clamped shut. Each animal was positioned so that its nose protruded beyond the edge of the treatment table, which allowed clotrimazole escaping around the nasal catheters to drip into a receptacle.

While the dogs' bodies were maintained in dorsal recumbency, their heads were rotated and maintained in the following positions to ensure drug contact with all nasal surfaces: dorsal recumbency (15 minutes), left lateral re-

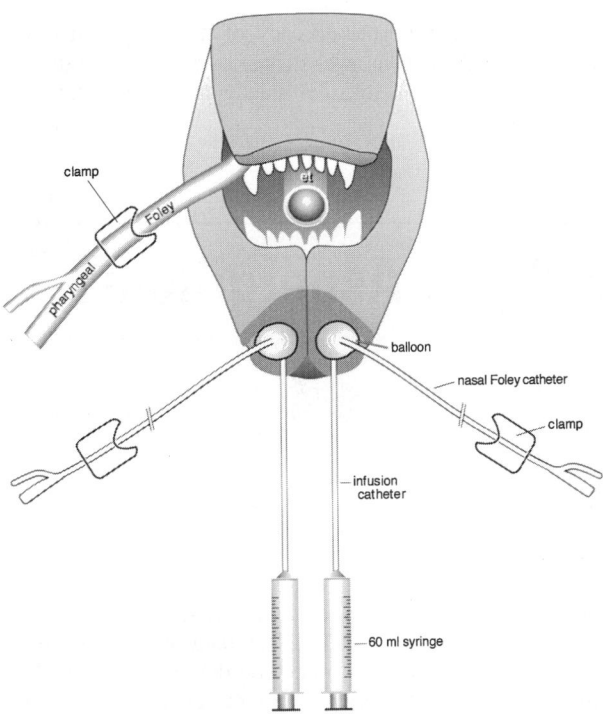

Figure 1. Catheter position with the dog in dorsal recumbency. A Foley catheter with the balloon inflated in the nasopharynx and pharyngeal gauze sponges (not shown) minimize leakage of infusion caudally. A cuffed endotracheal tube (et) further diminishes the risk of aspiration. Sixty-milliliter syringes are used to inject infusion into the dorsal nasal meatus via polypropylene infusion catheters. Inflated Foley catheter balloons obstruct the nares to diminish leakage of infusion rostrally. Tubing clamps on Foley catheters are closed when fluid is observed within the catheter lumen. (Adapted from Mathews KG, Koblik PD, Richardson EF, et al: Computed tomographic assessment of noninvasive intranasal infusions in dogs with fungal rhinitis. Vet Surg 25:309–319, 1996.)

cumbency (15 minutes), right lateral recumbency (15 minutes), and dorsal recumbency (15 minutes). The dogs were then placed in sternal recumbency, the catheters and sponges were removed and counted, the medication was allowed to drain rostrally, and the pharynx and proximal esophagus were suctioned. The dogs were then allowed to recover from general anesthesia.

Some dogs with advanced disease may require multiple 1-hour clotrimazole infusions. Most will experience resolution of nasal discharge after one treatment. Two cases in group 1 had serious complications that eventually resulted in euthanasia. Neither case had a pretreatment computed tomographic scan performed. The most common post-treatment complication in dogs treated by trephination of the

frontal sinuses was subcutaneous emphysema in seven cases (26%).

The results of this study indicated that the topical application of clotrimazole, using either technique, is an effective treatment for dogs with nasal aspergillosis. The success rate with one or more topical clotrimazole applications was 86%. Pretreatment computed tomographic scans are encouraged so that the extent of the disease can be determined and the integrity of the cribriform plate can be evaluated. The use of the noninvasive intranasal infusion technique for administration of topical clotrimazole eliminates the need for surgical trephination of the frontal sinuses in many cases of canine nasal aspergillosis and was associated with fewer complications and less expense.

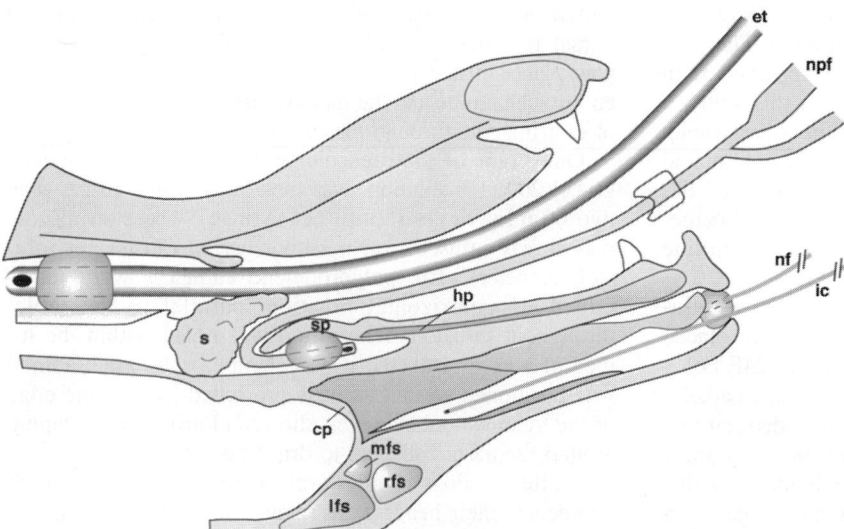

Figure 2. Sagittal section showing the position of the endotracheal tube (et), nasopharyngeal Foley catheter (npf), pharyngeal sponges (s), infusion catheter (ic), and rostral nasal Foley catheter (nf) in relation to the hard palate (hp), soft palate (sp), cribriform plate (cp), rostral frontal sinus (rfs), medial frontal sinus (mfs), and lateral frontal sinus (lfs). (From Mathews KG, Koblik PD, Richardson EF, et al: Computed tomographic assessment of noninvasive intranasal infusion in dogs with fungal rhinitis. Vet Surg 25:309–319, 1996.)

Based on a previous study in cadavers, the average volume of the frontal sinuses in breeds predisposed to fungal rhinitis was 25 ml per side (Richardson and Mathews, 1995). Flooding the nasal cavity and sinuses with a larger volume of infusion (50 to 60 ml per side) results in distribution of the infusion to all areas of the nasal cavity and frontal sinuses. In addition, a 1% formulation of clotrimazole (Lotrimin, Schering Corporation, Kenilworth, NJ) is readily available in a 30-ml vial, making treatment with two vials per side convenient. At present, our recommendation is to use 50 to 60 ml per side in middle to large breed dogs regardless of head size.

Topical administration of clotrimazole into the frontal sinuses and nasal passages is generally well tolerated. A favorable response to clotrimazole therapy is usually indicated by resolution of nasal discharge by 2 weeks after therapy. Unabated persistence of nasal discharge 2 weeks after therapy is an indication for repeat treatment. Patients selected for topical therapy should have aspergillosis limited to the frontal sinuses and nasal passages, without central nervous system involvement.

References and Suggested Reading

Davidson AP, Pappagianis D: Treatment of nasal aspergillosis with topical clotrimazole. In: Bonagura JD, ed: Kirk's Current Veterinary Therapy XII: Small Animal Practice. Philadelphia: WB Saunders, 1995, pp 899–901.

Davidson AP, Komtebedde J, Pappagianis D: Treatment of nasal aspergillosis with topical clotrimazole. In Proceedings of the Tenth Annual Veterinary Medicine Forum, San Diego: American College of Veterinary Internal Medicine, 1992, p 307.

Mathews KG, Davidson AP, Richardson EF, et al: Topical clotrimazole therapy in dogs with nasal aspergillosis—comparison of intranasal vs. surgical infusions: 60 cases (1990–1996), J Am Vet Med Assoc (in press).

Richardson EF, Mathews KG: Distribution of topical agents in the frontal sinuses and nasal cavity of dogs: Comparison between current protocols for treatment of nasal aspergillosis and a new noninvasive technique. Vet Surg 24:476, 1995.

Endocrine and Metabolic Disorders

MARK E. PETERSON

Consulting Editor

Still Current Information Found in Current Veterinary Therapy XII:

CVT Update: Interpretation of Endocrine Diagnostic Test Results for Adrenal and Thyroid Disease

ROBERT J. KEMPPAINEN

ELLEN N. BEHREND

Auburn, Alabama

The following questions represent frequent inquiries received by our endocrine diagnostic laboratory. In previous editions of this book (see *CVT X,* p. 961 and *CVT XII,* p. 335) protocols and interpretation of common endocrine tests were described. Reference ranges mentioned are used by the Auburn University Endocrine Diagnostic Service (World Wide Web home page: http://www.vetmed.auburn.edu/endo/). Refer to the Table "Systeme International (SI) Units in Clinical Chemistry" in the Appendices for conversions between SI (e.g., nmol/L) and mass units (e.g., (gm/100 ml).

ADRENOCORTICOTROPIC HORMONE STIMULATION TEST

- *I am having difficulty locating a source for adrenocorticotropic hormone (ACTH) gel. What should I do?* We recommend the use of Cortrosyn (synthetic ACTH or cosyntropin, Organon, Inc., West Orange, NJ). Cortrosyn costs approximately $140 for a package of 10 vials (250 μg ACTH per vial). The dose for dogs is 5 μg/kg IV (maximal dose, 250 μg; Peterson et al, 1996); for cats the dose is 125 μg IV. In dogs and cats, a pre-ACTH sample is collected, ACTH is injected, and one post-ACTH sample is collected 1 hour later. Once a Cortrosyn vial is reconstituted, it can be stored in the refrigerator for up to 4 months and reused. ACTH gel is still available from Rhone-Poulenc Rorer, Collegeville, PA, who sell H.P. Acthar Gel at 80 USP U/ml. We have encountered vials of ACTH gel from other sources that seem to lack biologic activity. Consequently, it is best to test ACTH gel for activity in healthy dogs prior to use.
- *I performed an ACTH stimulation test to evaluate a dog for Addison's disease and the post-ACTH cortisol value was greater than normal. Could this dog actually have hyperadrenocorticism?* Unlikely. It is not uncommon to find a mild to moderately elevated post-ACTH cortisol concentration in dogs tested for Addison's disease (in dogs that do *not* have the disease). Presumably, a normal physiologic response to recent (or chronic) stress is the cause of the elevation, so we consider this response to be indicative of a normal pituitary-adrenal axis. In true cases of Addison's disease, cortisol concentrations both pre- and post-ACTH are usually very low (both less than 10 nmol/L).
- *Can recent steroid therapy affect the ACTH stimulation test?* Yes, glucocorticoids can affect the results in two ways. First, some glucocorticoids cross-react in the cortisol assay and can be detected as immunoreactive cortisol.

In our assay, cross-reacting steroids include hydrocortisone, prednisone, and prednisolone. In general, we recommend waiting at least 24 hours after (oral) administration to allow these drugs to clear. Second, glucocorticoid therapy may suppress the pituitary-adrenal axis, causing reduced cortisol concentrations pre- and post-ACTH administration. The severity of the suppression is related to dose, potency, frequency of use, and chemical form (e.g., repositol versus oral) of the glucocorticoid therapy.

- *I treated a dog suspected of having Addison's disease with steroids yesterday, and now I want to perform an ACTH stimulation test. Will the results be meaningful?* Yes, they probably will be useful. A single injection (or infusion) of glucocorticoids may lower the cortisol values in the ACTH stimulation test. However, this type of short-term, nonrepositol treatment will only moderately (about 25%) lower the cortisol values relative to the normal range. Most dogs with Addison's disease have very low plasma cortisol concentrations and fail to show any increase in cortisol in response to ACTH.
- *How do I monitor the efficacy of mitotane therapy?* Periodic ACTH stimulation testing is recommended in all dogs with hyperadrenocorticism treated with mitotane. "Ideal" cortisol concentrations in a dog receiving treatment are between 30 and 110 nmol/L in both pre- and post-ACTH samples. If values are mildly to moderately greater than 110 nmol/L (e.g., in the 110- to 250-nmol/L range) one should consider increasing the dose (approximately 25%) if maintenance therapy is being given or continuing daily loading therapy for a few additional days. If values are higher, it is likely that 5 to 7 days of daily mitotane will be necessary to reduce the adrenal cortical mass to the target level. Clinical condition and recurrence of signs must be considered in the choice of therapy.
- *How long should I wait between performing a dexamethasone suppression test and an ACTH stimulation test?* We suggest waiting at least 48 hours after a low dose of dexamethasone (0.01 to 0.015 mg/kg) and 5 days after a high dose of dexamethasone (0.1 to 1.0 mg/kg). No wait is necessary when performing the combined dexamethasone suppression–ACTH stimulation test (Kemppainen and Zerbe, 1989). Dexamethasone suppression tests can be performed the day after ACTH stimulation testing.

DEXAMETHASONE SUPPRESSION TESTING

- *What form of dexamethasone should I use for a dexamethasone suppression test?* Dexamethasone in polyethylene glycol or dexamethasone sodium phosphate can be used, but the dose is based on the amount of active dexamethasone in solution. For example, a 4 mg/ml solution of dexamethasone sodium phosphate provides about 3 mg/ml of active dexamethasone. The dexamethasone can be given IV or IM, although we prefer the IV route.

- *I think I injected the dexamethasone outside the vein. What should I do?* It is best to wait 48 hours (low dose) or 72 hours (high dose) and repeat the test.
- *The calculated (low) dose of dexamethasone is only 0.03 ml for this poodle. How do I accurately administer such a small volume of dexamethasone?* It is important to administer the correct dose. Dilute the dexamethasone (e.g., make a 1:20 dilution by mixing 0.2 ml of dexamethasone with 3.8 ml of sterile saline or sterile water) so that a reasonable volume is given. (For Azium, a 1:20 dilution will make the solution 0.1 mg/ml.)
- *Can I use the results of the low-dose dexamethasone suppression test to both diagnose and differentiate hyperadrenocorticism in dogs?* Sometimes the results can strongly indicate a diagnosis of pituitary-dependent hyperadrenocorticism (but never adrenal-dependent hyperadrenocorticism). Normally, cortisol concentrations after dexamethasone administration (both 4 and 8 hours) are less than 30 nmol/L. If one or both postdexamethasone cortisol concentrations are greater than 30 nmol/L and one or both of these values is less than 50% of the predexamethasone cortisol concentration, pituitary-dependent hyperadrenocorticism is likely.

GENERAL QUESTIONS CONCERNING THE DIAGNOSIS OF HYPERADRENOCORTICISM

- *Do normal results on an ACTH stimulation test or a low-dose dexamethasone suppression test rule out hyperadrenocorticism? Conversely, do abnormal results definitely diagnose the disease?* Results of the ACTH stimulation test will be in the normal range in about 20% of dogs with hyperadrenocorticism, whereas the false-negative rate with the low-dose dexamethasone test is somewhat lower. If results of one test are normal, but clinical suspicion for the disease is high, one should consider performing the other screening test. It is important to recognize that each test also has false-positives, particularly when dogs with nonadrenal disease are tested. Interestingly, of the two screening procedures, the low-dose dexamethasone suppression test seems more prone to this potential error. About 50% of dogs with nonadrenal illness had abnormal results (inadequate suppression of plasma cortisol) when tested with a low dose of dexamethasone (Kaplan et al, 1995). None of the dogs in that study had a clinical presentation or signs consistent with hyperadrenocorticism. Assessment of test results in dogs with nonadrenal illness in which a clinical suspicion of hyperadrenocorticism is also present is challenging. The predictive value for hyperadrenocorticism of a positive screening test result increases in direct proportion to the number and severity of clinical signs and biochemical changes typically occurring in the disease.
- *What is the best test for hyperadrenocorticism in cats?* We recommend the high-dose dexamethasone suppres-

sion test, administering the steroid at a dose of 0.1 mg/kg IV and collecting a predexamethasone sample and two samples after dexamethasone administration (at 4 and 8 hours).

- *How and why should I try to differentiate pituitary- from adrenal-dependent hyperadrenocorticism in dogs?* Unless results of the low-dose dexamethasone suppression test support pituitary-dependent hyperadrenocorticism, a differentiating test is recommended. Results of ACTH stimulation cannot differentiate the types. The two endocrine tests for this purpose are the high-dose dexamethasone suppression test (0.1 or 1.0 mg/kg) and endogenous ACTH measurement. If cortisol concentrations suppress (>50% decline from prevalue, or decline to <30 nmol/L) in response to dexamethasone, a diagnosis of pituitary-dependent disease is made. However, in about 15 to 20% of dogs with pituitary-dependent hyperadrenocorticism, cortisol is not suppressed by dexamethasone. Because cortisol is not suppressed by dexamethasone in dogs with adrenal-dependent disease and because pituitary-dependent disease is the most common form, failure to suppress to dexamethasone means the odds of having one form or the other are about 50:50. In other words, failure of cortisol concentrations to suppress in response to high-dose dexamethasone is not diagnostic for either form of spontaneous hyperadrenocorticism. Endogenous ACTH measurement can positively differentiate the forms, since circulating ACTH concentrations are low to nondetectable in adrenal-dependent disease and normal to high in pituitary-dependent disease. Accurate measurement of ACTH in plasma requires special sample handling (Kemppainen and Clark, 1995). Other means to differentiate hyperadrenocorticism include ultrasonography and other imaging modalities and surgical exploration. It is best to differentiate the forms because of differences in therapy and prognosis. Surgical removal of an adrenal tumor can be curative. If mitotane is used for chemical treatment, the therapeutic approach is different depending on the type of disease. In general, adrenal-dependent disease requires higher dosages and a longer induction phase (Kintzer and Peterson, 1989). The prognosis in dogs with a large adrenocortical carcinoma or with diffuse metastatic disease is poor.
- *What is the value in measuring a urinary cortisol:creatinine ratio (UCCR)?* This test is best used to determine if a dog does *not* have hyperadrenocorticism. Nearly 100% of dogs with spontaneous hyperadrenocorticism have an elevated UCCR. Unfortunately, many dogs with an elevated UCCR do not have hyperadrenocorticism. Consequently, a high ratio means that hyperadrenocorticism is possible and a more definitive screening test (ACTH stimulation, low-dose dexamethasone suppression test) is indicated. Therefore, a normal UCCR is valuable in ruling out hyperadrenocorticism.

CANINE HYPOTHYROIDISM

- *What is the value of measuring total thyroxine (T₄)?* Total T_4 can best be used to rule out the diagnosis of hypothyroidism. If the total T_4 is normal (i.e. >20 nmol/L), it is unlikely the dog is hypothyroid. If the T_4 is less than normal, the dog may or may not be hypothyroid.

Numerous nonthyroidal factors such as medications and chronic illness (i.e., euthyroid sick syndrome) can suppress T_4 to less than the normal range.

• *What is the value of measuring free T_4?* Free T_4 (FT_4) is the portion of total T_4 not bound to protein and represents about 0.1% of total T_4. The pituitary-thyroid axis functions to maintain free, not total, T_4 within a certain range, so measurement of FT_4 is a better test of thyroid function. Two methods are used to measure FT_4: analogue radioimmunoassay and equilibrium dialysis. Analogue radioimmunoassay is less expensive but is not reliable in dogs with euthyroid sick syndrome, providing no additional diagnostic value over measurement of total T_4 (Nelson et al, 1991). Equilibrium dialysis gives more reliable estimates of true FT_4 concentrations. Measurement of FT_4 can be the initial test for the diagnosis of hypothyroidism, or it can be used in dogs that have been found to have borderline low total T_4 concentrations. How the euthyroid sick syndrome or drugs affect FT_4 concentration is not fully known; however, chronic glucocorticoid therapy or hyperadrenocorticism can depress FT_4 levels (Ferguson and Peterson, 1992). Overall, in our experience, measurement of FT_4 by dialysis is more effective than total T_4 in distinguishing euthyroidism from hypothyroidism.

• *How would I know if autoantibodies to thyroid hormones are present and what is their significance?* Autoantibodies are usually suspected when total T_3 or T_4 concentrations are high in a sample from a dog evaluated for hypothyroidism. With procedures used by most diagnostic laboratories, the presence of autoantibodies causes false elevations in the apparent concentration. Total T_3 is most often affected; however, autoantibodies to T_3 are present in less than 1% of samples submitted to our laboratory. The exact clinical and prognostic significance of autoantibodies to thyroid hormones is unknown (Kemppainen and Young, 1992). If autoantibodies are present, it is best to measure FT_4 by equilibrium dialysis to better evaluate thyroid function. If the FT_4 concentration is normal, the patient should be scheduled for periodic (every 4 to 6 months) FT_4 determination. If the FT_4 level is low, hypothyroidism is likely.

• *How valuable is measurement of endogenous canine (thyroid-stimulating hormone [TSH])?* A relatively new assay is available to measure canine TSH. In dogs with primary hypothyroidism, TSH concentrations are expected to be elevated because of the loss of negative feedback by thyroid hormones on the pituitary. Indeed, thyroidectomized dogs had TSH levels approximately 30 times greater than normal (Williams et al, 1995). Since about 95% of canine hypothyroidism is of the primary type, measurement of TSH should be a useful test. Although thorough evaluation of the test is not yet available, preliminary data are somewhat discouraging. In one study, 4 of 62 normal dogs showed elevated TSH concentrations, and although 7 of 16 spontaneously hypothyroid dogs had clearly elevated TSH levels, 3 had only marginal increases and 6 had TSH concentrations within the normal range (Scott-Moncrieff et al, 1996). Another concern was that 5 of 26 dogs with euthyroid sick syndrome had elevated TSH concentrations. Thus, data so far suggest that concentrations of TSH are elevated in most but not all dogs with primary hypothyroidism and

that some healthy dogs and dogs with euthyroid sick syndrome have TSH concentrations greater than currently established normal ranges. Consequently, a sole determination of endogenous TSH concentration should not be used to diagnose hypothyroidism. The test should be used to supplement historical data and clinical examination findings in conjunction with measurement of total or FT_4 concentrations, or both.

• *The total T_4 concentration in a dog suspected of having hypothyroidism is less than normal. How certain can I be that this dog is hypothyroid?* A low total T_4 means that the dog may be hypothyroid; alternatively, a nonthyroidal factor could be depressing T_4 or this dog could simply have a lower than "normal" circulating total T_4 concentration (and be euthyroid). Some options exist for these patients: (1) FT_4 can be measured by equilibrium dialysis with or without measurement of endogenous TSH. These tests are more definitive than total T_4. This is the best option. (2) Total T_4 can be retested in a few months. If the dog is hypothyroid, the T_4 should continue to decline and clinical signs should become more profound. (3) Trial thyroid hormone replacement therapy can be attempted. The dog should be re-evaluated at 5 and 10 weeks of thyroxine therapy using objective criteria (e.g., regrowth of hair) to assess recovery. A postpill T_4 level should be evaluated after 5 weeks to ensure therapeutic blood levels of the hormone. Trial therapy is complicated by partial responders and the fact that thyroxine may have a pharmacologic effect to induce hair growth in some euthyroid dogs. Incorrect diagnosis can consign the owner to providing lifelong therapy, so the first two options are strongly recommended in preference to the third.

• *How do I test for hypothyroidism when a dog is on thyroid supplementation?* Trying to confirm a diagnosis of hypothyroidism after thyroid replacement therapy has been initiated can be difficult. Therapy should be withdrawn and the pituitary-thyroid axis allowed to recover. A total T_4, or better FT_4 by equilibrium dialysis, should be measured after 1 month. If the result is borderline, therapy should be withheld for an additional 4 weeks and the measurement repeated to see if there is continuing recovery. The time needed to allow full recovery of thyroid gland function after chronic suppression by exogenous T_4 is unknown.

FELINE HYPERTHYROIDISM

• *Does the finding of a normal T4 level in a cat rule out hyperthyroidism?* No. Cats with early or mild hyperthyroidism may have a T_4 concentration within the upper half of the normal range (i.e., 25 to 50 nmol/L). The T_4 level can fluctuate in and out of the normal range in such cats. Alternatively, nonthyroidal factors (illness) can suppress the T_4 level in a hyperthyroid cat into the normal range.

• *If the T_4 level is normal, but I am still suspicious of hyperthyroidism, what can I do?* If the T_4 level is less than 25 nmol/L, it is unlikely that the cat is hyperthyroid. If the T_4 level is in the upper normal range (25 to 50 nmol/L), further evaluation is warranted. In sick, older cats with a normal thyroid, low total T_4 concentrations are typically measured (Peterson and Gamble, 1990). Options to consider in hyperthyroid-suspect cats with T_4 values in the upper normal range follow: (1) The total T_4 measurement should be repeated; sometimes T_4 will fluctuate into and out of the normal range in hyperthyroid cats. (2) FT_4 should be measured by equilibrium dialysis (Peterson et al, 1995). (3) A T_3 suppression test or a thyrotropin-releasing hormone stimulation test should be performed (Graves and Peterson, 1994).

• *What is the value of measuring FT_4 in cats suspected of being hyperthyroid?* The rationale of using the FT_4 to diagnose hyperthyroidism in cats is the same as that for using this measurement in dogs—that the concentration of FT_4 is less affected by nonthyroidal factors. In this instance, FT_4 should be high in hyperthyroidism. Its use seems most appropriate for cats with mild or early hyperthyroidism or in cats suspected of being hyperthyroid with nonthyroidal illness and have total T_4 concentrations in the upper normal range (see earlier). In one study, FT_4 was elevated in 25 of 26 mildly hyperthyroid cats (96%) as compared with finding an elevated total T_4 in only 16 of these cats (62%) (Peterson et al, 1995). However, FT_4 may also be elevated in up to 12% of sick, euthyroid cats (Peterson et al, 1995; Mooney et al, 1996). In order to help discriminate between hyperthyroidism and euthyroid sick syndrome in cats, a total T_4 should be measured along with the FT_4. Hyperthyroid cats tend to have total T_4 concentrations in the upper half of the normal range, whereas sick, euthyroid cats have total T_4 values in the lower half of the normal range, even if they show elevated FT_4 (Mooney et al, 1996).

• *The total T_4 concentration in a cat I was testing for hyperthyroidism came back less than normal. Is the cat hypothyroid?* Unlikely. It is most likely the cat has the euthyroid sick syndrome, since hypothyroidism is rare in cats. Measurement of FT_4 will help differentiate hypothyroidism from the euthyroid sick syndrome.

References and Suggested Reading

Ferguson DC, Peterson ME: Serum free and total iodothyronine concentrations in dogs with spontaneous hyperadrenocorticism. Am J Vet Res 53:1636, 1992.
  Thyroid hormone measurement in 42 dogs with hyperadrenocorticism indicated that dogs with the disease had significantly lower total T_4, total T_3, and free T_4 (by equilibrium dialysis) concentrations than did normal dogs.
Graves TK, Peterson ME: Diagnostic tests for feline hyperthyroidism. Vet Clin N Am (Small Anim Pract) 24:567, 1994.
  Review of tests for the diagnosis of hyperthyroidism in cats.
Kaplan AJ, Peterson ME, Kemppainen RJ: Effects of disease on the results of diagnostic tests for use in detecting hyperadrenocorticism in dogs. J Am Vet Med Assoc 207:445, 1995.
  Study showing a high false-positive rate when screening tests for hyperadrenocorticism were applied to 59 dogs with a variety of nonadrenal illnesses.
Kemppainen RJ, Clark TP: CVT update: Sample collection and testing protocols in endocrinology. In: Bonagura JD, Kirk RW, eds: Kirk's Current Veterinary Therapy XII: Small Animal Practice. Philadelphia: WB Saunders, 1995, p 335.
  Update on the thyrotropin stimulation, T_3 suppression, and thyrotropin-releasing hormone tests as well as measurement of endogenous ACTH, free T_4, and urine cortisol:creatinine ratio.
Kemppainen RJ, Young DW: Canine triiodothyronine autoantibodies. In: Kirk RW, Bonagura JD, eds: Current Veterinary Therapy XI: Small Animal Practice. Philadelphia: WB Saunders, 1992, p 327.
  Discussion of the prevalence, detection, and significance of autoantibodies to T_3 in dogs.
Kemppainen RJ, Zerbe CA: Common endocrine diagnostic tests: Normal values and interpretation. In Kirk RW, Bonagura JD, eds: Current Veterinary Therapy X: Small Animal Practice. Philadelphia: WB Saunders, 1989, p 961.
  Description of commonly used endocrine diagnostic testing procedures in dogs and cats, including normal values.
Kintzer PP, Peterson ME: Mitotane (o,p'-DDD) treatment of cortisol-secreting adrenocortical neoplasia. In: Kirk RW, Bonagura JD, eds: Current Veterinary Therapy X: Small Animal Practice. Philadelphia: WB Saunders, 1989, p 1034.
  Description of the diagnosis of functional adrenocortical tumors and therapy using mitotane.
Mooney CT, Little CJL, Macrae AW: Effect of illness not associated with the thyroid gland on serum total and free thyroxine concentrations in cats. J Am Vet Med Assoc 208:2004, 1996.
  Comparison of total and FT_4 concentrations in healthy cats and cats with nonthyroidal illness.
Nelson RW, Ihle SL, Feldman EC, et al: Serum free thyroxine concentration in healthy dogs, dogs with hypothyroidism, and euthyroid dogs with concurrent illness. J Am Vet Med Assoc 198:1401, 1991.
  Study demonstrating that the diagnostic value of measurement of total T_4 was similar to that of measuring FT_4 using the analogue method when evaluating thyroid function in healthy, hypothyroid, and euthyroid dogs with nonthyroid illness.
Peterson ME, Gamble DA: Effect of nonthyroidal illness on serum thyroxine concentrations in cats: 494 cases (1988). J Am Vet Med Assoc 197:1203, 1990.
  Study showing that serum T_4 concentrations are suppressed in cats with nonthyroidal illness (compared with normal cats), and the degree of suppression is related to the severity of the illness.
Peterson ME, Liminana CM, Nichols CE: Determination of free T_4 by dialysis as an aid in diagnosis of mild hyperthyroidism in cats. J Vet Intern Med 9:183, 1995.
  Abstract reporting FT_4 concentrations measured by dialysis in healthy cats, cats with nonthyroidal illness, and cats with hyperthyroidism.
Peterson ME, Wallace MS, Kerl ME, et al: Dose-response relation between plasma concentrations of ACTH and cortisol after administration of incremental doses of cosyntropin for ACTH stimulation testing in dogs. J Vet Int Med 10:186, 1996.
  Abstract concerning the plasma cortisol response in dogs to varying doses of synthetic ACTH (cosyntropin).
Scott-Moncrieff JC, Nelson RW, Bruner JM, et al: Serum canine thyrotropin concentration (cTSH) in euthyroid, hypothyroid and sick euthyroid dogs. J Vet Intern Med 10:186, 1996.
  Abstract reporting TSH concentrations in healthy dogs, dogs with nonthyroidal illness, and hypothyroid dogs.
Williams DA, Scott-Moncrieff JC, Bruner J: Canine serum thyroid-stimulating hormone following induction of hypothyroidism. J Vet Intern Med 9:184, 1995.
  Abstract showing that TSH concentrations increased in dogs made hypothyroid using [131]I.

Clinical Use of the Vasopressin Analogue DDAVP for the Diagnosis and Treatment of Diabetes Insipidus

RHETT NICHOLS

Farmingdale, New York

Desmopressin (l-desamino-8-D-arginine vasopressin, or DDAVP) is a synthetic analogue of the natural antidiuretic hormone arginine vasopressin (AVP), which has antidiuretic and hemostatic properties. DDAVP has become the drug of choice for the treatment of central diabetes insipidus (DI) in humans. DDAVP has increased antidiuretic activity, prolonged duration of action, decreased pressor actions, and fewer side effects than AVP, the natural hormone. The results of experimental studies in normal dogs and in dogs and cats with central DI indicate that DDAVP is safe for use in small animals.

FORMULATIONS OF DDAVP

DDAVP is available for clinical use intranasally, orally, intravenously, and subcutaneously. The intranasal preparation (DDAVP, Rhone-Poulenc Rorer Pharmaceuticals) is supplied in 2.5- and 5-ml bottles containing 100 μg/ml of DDAVP. The 2.5-ml bottle is equipped with a small, calibrated plastic catheter or nasal tube so that exact amounts can be measured and deposited intranasally. With this delivery system, 1 drop of nasal solution corresponds to 1.5 to 4.0 μg of DDAVP. A tuberculin or insulin syringe may be used for more accurate dosing. The 5-ml bottle is equipped with a compression pump nasal spray. Each spray delivers 10 μg of DDAVP. Although administration of medication to dogs and cats via the intranasal route is possible, it is not tolerated in many cases. Drops placed in the conjunctival sac are a more suitable alternative.

The oral preparation of DDAVP (DDAVP Tablets, Rhone-Poulenc Rorer Pharmaceuticals) is available as 0.1-mg and 0.2-mg tablets. Each 0.1-mg tablet is comparable to 5 μg (1 large drop) of intranasal DDAVP.

The parenteral preparation (DDAVP Injection, Rhone-Poulenc Rorer Pharmaceuticals) is available in 1- and 2-ml ampules containing 15 μg DDAVP/ml and 1- and 10-ml ampules containing 4 μg DDAVP/ml. Parenteral administration of DDAVP is most useful in patients that will not tolerate or absorb the drug by the intranasal or conjunctival routes. Because the cost of the parenteral preparation of DDAVP is 20 times higher per microgram than the intranasal preparation, the intranasal form of DDAVP, although not designed for parenteral use, has been given to dogs and cats by injection with no apparent adverse effects; however, the intranasal form is not sterile, so clinicians may want to pass this preparation through a bacteriostatic filter. Clinically, the intranasal and injectable preparations of DDAVP induce indistinguishable responses when administered intravenously or subcutaneously.

DIAGNOSTIC TESTING FOR DIABETES INSIPIDUS

In the assessment of disorders of polyuria and polydipsia, diagnostic tests for confirming and differentiating central DI, nephrogenic DI, and psychogenic DI include the water deprivation test and the response to DDAVP. The water deprivation test is designed to determine whether endogenous vasopressin is released in response to dehydration, and whether the kidneys can respond normally to circulating vasopressin. This test should be performed after all other causes of polyuria and polydipsia have been ruled out (e.g., pyometra, hypercalcemia, diabetes mellitus, hyperthyroidism, pyelonephritis, renal failure, hyperadrenocorticism; see p. 831 for a full discussion), limiting the differential diagnosis to central DI, nephrogenic DI, and psychogenic polydipsia. Following water deprivation, if the animal fails to concentrate urine adequately (urine specific gravity >1.025) after losing 5% or more of its body weight, 5 μg of DDAVP may be given SC or IV, or 20 μg of DDAVP (approximately 4 drops of the 100 μg/ml intranasal preparation) can be administered as intranasal or conjunctival drops. Measurement of urinary concentrating ability (i.e., urine specific gravity or osmolality) is then monitored every 2 hours for 6 to 10 hours. Alternatively, aqueous vasopressin (Pitressin, Parke-Davis) may be given intramuscularly (0.5 U/kg of body weight, up to a maximum dosage of 5 U); urine specific gravity or osmolality should be monitored 1 and 2 hours after injection. Further increases in urine osmolality or specific gravity greater than 10% is suggestive of central DI. An increase in urine osmolality or a specific gravity less than 10% is suggestive of a vasopressin-resistant disorder (i.e., nephrogenic DI or psychogenic polydipsia). Because the instrumentation necessary for determination of urine osmolality is not readily available to most veterinarians, urine osmolality (mOsm/L) can be generally approximated by multiplying the last two numbers of the urine specific gravity by 36 (except in cases of proteinuria or glycosuria). For example, a urine specific gravity of 1.012 would be equivalent to a urine osmolality of 432 mOsm/L (12 × 36 = 432), although this method will not always be accurate.

As an alternative to the water deprivation test, or in animals in which this test fails to establish a definitive diagnosis, a closely monitored therapeutic trial with DDAVP can be performed. Again, all other causes of polyuria and polydipsia should be ruled out, limiting the differential diagnosis to central DI, nephrogenic DI, and psychogenic polydipsia. The pet owner should measure the animal's 24-hour water intake 2 to 3 days before the therapeutic trial with DDAVP is initiated, allowing free-choice water intake. The oral tablets (0.1 mg) or the intranasal preparation of DDAVP (1 to 4 drops placed into the conjunctival sac) are administered every 12 hours for 5 to 7 days. A reduction in water intake greater than 50% would strongly suggest a vasopressin deficiency and a diagnosis of central DI. There should be minimal improvement in dogs and cats with nephrogenic DI and psychogenic polydipsia. Rarely, DDAVP abolishes polyuria but has a delayed or no effect on thirst or polydipsia. Consequently, excess water is retained, with resultant hyponatremia. Water overload may occur in animals with psychogenic polydipsia or in animals with central DI that continue to drink inappropriately because of an associated defect in the thirst mechanism.

Occasionally, results obtained from the water deprivation test or a therapeutic trial with DDAVP are incorrectly interpreted. One of the most common causes of misinterpretation is the unsuspected case of hyperadrenocorticism. These patients may show (1) complete ability to concentrate urine after dehydration (suggesting psychogenic polydipsia), (2) incomplete ability to concentrate urine after dehydration followed by a further increase of 10 to 50% in urine concentration after aqueous vasopressin or DDAVP injection (suggesting central DI), or (3) a decrease in water intake greater than 50% after a therapeutic trial with DDAVP (suggesting central DI). Misdiagnosis of hyperadrenocorticism is most easily avoided by screening for this disorder (e.g., using adrenocorticotropic hormone stimulation or low-dose dexamethasone suppression testing) prior to initiating water deprivation or response to DDAVP supplementation (see p. 321).

TREATMENT OF CENTRAL DIABETES INSIPIDUS

Since the repositol vasopressin preparation (Pitressin tannate in oil, Parke-Davis) is no longer available, DDAVP has become the drug of choice for the treatment of central DI in dogs and cats. In affected patients, regardless of the severity or cause of the vasopressin deficiency, administration of the drug completely eliminates polyuria and polydipsia both acutely and during long-term therapy. Because of individual differences in absorption and metabolism, the dose required to achieve complete, around-the-clock control varies from patient to patient. Usually, however, 1 to 4 drops of the intranasal preparation administered once or twice daily in the conjunctival sac is sufficient to control

signs of central DI. Alternatively, the oral tablets can be used, but the treatment cost is much higher. The maximal effect of the drug occurs 6 to 10 hours after administration, and the duration of effect of DDAVP varies from 8 to 24 hours. Some animals may require only evening administration of the medication to control nocturia. Injectable DDAVP is used in humans for chronic therapy of central DI and the management of temporary polyuria following head trauma or surgery in the pituitary region. However, because of its short duration of action (8 to 24 hours), which would require repeated injections, and its high cost, the injectable form of DDAVP is not suitable for long-term management of central DI in veterinary medicine. As previously mentioned, if injectable administration of DDAVP is necessary or desired, the intranasal formulation can be administered safely parenterally. The parenteral dose of DDAVP is 2 to 5 μg administered SC once or twice daily.

DDAVP is safe for dogs and cats with central DI. The only complication of any importance is the induction of water intoxication (hyponatremia). This complication is uncommon and results from a failure to reduce water intake adequately because of damage to the inhibitory component of the thirst mechanism. To avoid this potential problem, it is recommended that subsequent doses of DDAVP be administered when polyuria returns. Ideally, if the cause of the patient's polyuria and polydipsia is uncertain, serum sodium levels should be monitored for several days after initiation of antidiuretic therapy. If hyponatremia develops, the treatment should be stopped and the diagnosis reevaluated. One major problem associated with the long-term treatment of central DI is the expense. The cost of treating a central DI patient with the intranasal preparation of DDAVP averages $65 to $80 per month.

References and Suggested Reading

Feldman EC, Nelson RW: Water metabolism and diabetes insipidus. In: Feldman EC, Nelson RW, eds: Canine and Feline Endocrinology and Reproduction. Philadelphia: WB Saunders, 1996, p 2.
An in-depth review of physiology of water metabolism, differential diagnosis of polyuria, diagnostic approach to polyuria, and the treatment of diabetes insipidus.
Nichols R: Diabetes insipidus. In: Kirk RW, ed: Current Veterinary Therapy X. Philadelphia: WB Saunders, 1989, p 973.
A review of the diagnosis and treatment of diabetes insipidus.
Nichols R, Hohenhaus AE: Use of the vasopressin analogue desmopressin for polyuria and bleeding disorders. J Am Vet Med Assoc 205:168, 1994.
In-depth review of historical aspects, pathophysiology, formulations, and antidiuretic and hemostatic applications of DDAVP.

Complications and Concurrent Conditions Associated With Hypothyroidism in Dogs

DAVID L. PANCIERA
Denver, Colorado

Hypothyroidism can lead to many different clinical abnormalities because of the widespread influence that thyroid hormones have on cellular metabolism. Typical clinical signs of hypothyroidism include lethargy, weight gain, seborrhea, and alopecia; however, many other complications can develop. Recognition of the varied complications and conditions associated with hypothyroidism leads to appropriate diagnosis and treatment.

NEUROLOGIC COMPLICATIONS

A variety of neurologic abnormalities are associated with hypothyroidism. Peripheral neuropathies are recognized with increasing frequency in hypothyroid dogs. Generalized neuropathy may result from impaired axonal transport secondary to decreased activity of the sodium-potassium–adenosine triphosphatase pump. Dogs with generalized peripheral neuropathies may present with generalized weakness, exercise intolerance, inappetence, or unilateral forelimb lameness. Physical examination findings include depression, proprioceptive deficits and ataxia predominately in the hind limbs, hyporeflexia, and pain in the shoulder of dogs with forelimb lameness. Electromyographic abnormalities consistent with denervation are present in affected dogs. In fact, electromyographic changes have been reported to occur frequently even in hypothyroid dogs without clinical signs of neuropathy or myopathy. A mild increase in protein may be found in the cerebrospinal fluid of affected hypothyroid dogs. Dogs with hypothyroidism and generalized peripheral neuropathy generally respond rapidly and completely to thyroid hormone supplementation, with an increase in strength noted within the first week and complete resolution within 3 to 8 weeks of initiating treatment.

Localized peripheral neuropathies involving the vestibular and facial nerves, often occurring concurrently, are also frequently recognized in hypothyroidism. Since most affected dogs do not show signs of generalized neuropathy, hypothyroidism must be differentiated from otitis media or otitis interna, idiopathic peripheral vestibular disease, and other causes of neuropathy. Localized neuropathy may result from metabolic neuropathy or compression of the vestibular and facial nerves as they pass through the internal acoustic meatus. Dogs typically present with an acute (occasionally more gradual) onset of head tilt, nystagmus, ataxia, and circling. Proprioception and segmental spinal reflexes are normal. Otic examination and radiographs of the tympanic bulla should be normal. Vestibular abnormalities respond more slowly to thyroid hormone supplementation than do other neuropathies; noticeable improvement may require 8 weeks. A residual head tilt may be present in some dogs.

Megaesophagus can occur in hypothyroid dogs, but the pathogenesis of the disorder is unclear. Because the megaesophagus only occasionally resolves following treatment, the role of hypothyroidism is unknown. Hypothyroidism could cause megaesophagus by inducing either a neuropathy or a myopathy. Alternatively, megaesophagus has been described in hypothyroid dogs with myasthenia gravis. In this case, the myasthenia and hypothyroidism could have an immune-mediated pathogenesis similar to that reported in humans. Regardless of the relationship of hypothyroidism and megaesophagus, the prognosis for recovery of normal esophageal function is guarded to poor, since few reports document resolution of megaesophagus following treatment of hypothyroidism.

Another localized neuropathy attributed to hypothyroidism is laryngeal paralysis. Although some dogs with laryngeal paralysis are hypothyroid, the vast majority are not, and a clear causal relationship remains to be established.

Central nervous system disease can occur subsequent to cerebral hypoxia resulting from atherosclerosis or from metabolic neuropathy similar to that found in peripheral nerves. Vestibular, facial, and trigeminal nerve paresis and paralysis, as well as hemiparesis and hypermetria, may occur. These signs resolve more slowly than most other manifestations of hypothyroidism, and residual neurologic deficits may remain.

Among the behavioral abnormalities that have been attributed to hypothyroidism, aggressive behavior has been reported to partially resolve following thyroid hormone supplementation in the small number of dogs that were probably hypothyroid. Because of the paucity of documented cases, the relationship between behavioral problems and hypothyroidism remains speculative.

It is important to interpret thyroid function tests cautiously in dogs with neurologic abnormalities, since euthyroid dogs with neuropathies and those with megaesophagus have been shown to have significantly lower basal serum T_4 concentrations than those seen in normal dogs.

REPRODUCTIVE COMPLICATIONS

Reproductive complications of hypothyroidism can develop in bitches. A variety of abnormalities, including prolonged anestrus, irregular cycle length, decreased libido, and abortion, have been suggested to occur in hypothyroid bitches. These abnormalities, however, have not been well documented. Galactorrhea occasionally occurs in intact females with hypothyroidism. Hypothyroid bitches may have severe galactorrhea during pseudopregnancy or galactorrhea that continues beyond the time expected for a normal pseudopregnancy. It may occur secondary to increased prolactin secretion in response to pituitary stimulation by thyrotropin-releasing hormone. Effects of hypothyroidism in male dogs is discussed on p. 940.

OCULAR COMPLICATIONS

Ocular complications of hypothyroidism are rare. Corneal lipidosis, corneal ulceration, lipid aqueous flare, uveitis, retinal detachment and hemorrhage, optic disc swelling, and keratoconjunctivitis sicca have been suggested to occur in hypothyroid dogs. Most of these abnormalities have not been definitively linked with hypothyroidism. Hyperlipidemia secondary to hypothyroidism can in rare cases result in corneal lipidosis, lipid aqueous flare, and chronic uveitis. Keratoconjunctivitis sicca has been reported to occur in hypothyroid dogs, although a clear connection has not been established. Retrospective studies of hypothyroidism have not identified a significant number of dogs with concurrent keratoconjunctivitis sicca, and experimental hypothyroidism for 6 months' duration failed to alter tear production or other ocular parameters. A common immune-mediated pathogenesis has been proposed for intercurrent hypothyroidism and keratoconjunctivitis sicca, but this has not been proved. It is recommended that dogs with ocular changes secondary to hyperlipidemia be evaluated for hypothyroidism by a thorough search for other evidence of hypothyroidism and evaluation of thyroid function tests. Dogs with keratoconjunctivitis sicca should have thyroid function tests performed if other evidence of hypothyroidism is found in the history and physical examination.

HYPERLIPIDEMIA AND ATHEROSCLEROSIS

Hyperlipidemia is a common complication of hypothyroidism. Serum cholesterol concentration is elevated in about 75% of affected dogs, whereas hypertriglyceridemia occurs less frequently. Hypothyroidism results in a decrease in low-density lipoprotein receptors, so entry of cholesterol-laden low-density lipoprotein into the liver and other cells is impaired. In addition to the decrease in clearance of cholesterol from the circulation, utilization of cholesterol is reduced and production is increased. Hyperlipidemia can lead to the development of atherosclerosis and ocular abnormalities.

Severe hypercholesterolemia (typically >700 mg/dl) can lead to the development of atherosclerosis in susceptible hypothyroid dogs. Clinical signs of atherosclerosis are related to ischemia or thromboembolism of multiple organs, including the brain, heart, kidneys, intestines, spleen, and pancreas. Lethargy, anorexia, weakness, dyspnea, collapse, vomiting, and neurologic signs result from end-organ hypoxia. The neurologic signs are often referable to cerebellar or brain stem involvement and deficits in cranial nerves V, VII, and VIII. Head tilt, nystagmus, hemiparesis, decreased facial sensation, hypermetria, and facial nerve deficits can all occur in hypothyroid dogs. Cardiac arrhythmias and congestive heart failure can occur rarely subsequent to coronary atherosclerosis and myocardial infarction. Some dogs may present for the signs of pancreatitis that occur frequently in dogs with atherosclerosis and hypothyroidism. Mild to moderate elevation of liver enzymes and azotemia are common findings.

Diagnosis of hypothyroidism in these cases may be difficult because some dogs lack typical signs of thyroid hormone deficiency. Thyroid function should be evaluated in any dog with unexplained hypercholesterolemia. Evidence of myocardial infarction such as ST segment elevation, a notched QRS complex, or atrial fibrillation is suggestive of atherosclerosis in a dog with marked hyperlipidemia. Radiographic studies may reveal aortic mineralization, and angiography may reveal thrombosis or narrowing of various arteries. Antemortem diagnosis of atherosclerosis is difficult, but the presence of multiorgan disease in a dog with hypercholesterolemia is supportive. Thyroid gland biopsy may aid in the diagnosis, since most dogs reported to have atherosclerosis have involvement of the thyroid artery. In fact, it is possible that hypothyroidism may occur in some dogs secondary to severe thyroid artery atherosclerosis and subsequent thyroid atrophy.

Treatment with thyroid hormone supplementation and a low-fat diet may result in improvement or complete resolution of signs if the end-organ damage is not severe. The atherosclerosis is not completely reversible, but proper treatment can reduce the severity of the lesions. The main factor in response to treatment is the severity of organ damage. Although clinically significant atherosclerosis is rare, early intervention can prevent this serious complication.

IMMUNOLOGIC COMPLICATIONS

Immunosuppression may occur in hypothyroidism. It may be responsible for the recurrent or persistent superficial and deep pyoderma, otitis externa, and poor response to antibacterial treatment for the skin infections present in some hypothyroid dogs. Because infections in other organs do not appear to occur more often than expected in hypothyroid dogs, hypothyroidism may primarily affect local cutaneous immunity rather than systemic immunity. In support of this, we were unable to document alteration of immune response as assessed by lymphocyte blastogenesis in response to phytohemagglutinin, pokeweed mitogen, and concanavalin A 22 weeks after inducing hypothyroidism experimentally (Panciera and Kurzman, unpublished data).

HEMATOLOGIC COMPLICATIONS

A mild nonregenerative anemia is found in 25 to 30% of hypothyroid dogs. However, there is little evidence to support hypothyroidism as a cause of abnormal hemostasis or increased bleeding tendency. Hypothyroidism can increase the platelet count and decrease platelet size without affecting platelet function or buccal mucosal bleeding time. A deficiency in von Willebrand's factor does not occur secondary to hypothyroidism in dogs without concurrent congenital von Willebrand's disease. Thyroid hormone supplementation does not increase von Willebrand's factor in euthyroid dogs and may decrease it in hypothyroid dogs. Thus, there is no rational basis for treatment of bleeding disorders with thyroid hormone supplementation.

MYXEDEMA COMA

Myxedema stupor or coma is perhaps the most serious complication of hypothyroidism. Although this manifestation is rarely recognized, it may be more common than thought. Many cases may go unrecognized because of the unusual presentation and the high mortality rate of the disease. Myxedema coma occurs following decompensation of chronic hypothyroidism, often brought on by a concurrent disease or drug administration. The metabolic consequences of hypothyroidism lead to many different compensatory physiologic responses. Peripheral vasoconstriction occurs in order to maintain core body temperature, which tends to become lower in response to decreases in metabolic rate, cardiac output, and vascular volume. Reduced beta-adrenergic responsiveness without a similar alteration of the alpha-adrenergic response contributes to the decreased vascular volume and to diastolic hypertension because of vasoconstriction. The decrease in renal blood flow (secondary to the cardiovascular changes) and increased arginine vasopressin secretion impair free water clearance in hypothyroidism. Depression of the respiratory response to hypercapnia as well as respiratory muscle weakness lead to hypoventilation and hypercapnia. In addition, the metabolism of many drugs is reduced in hypothyroid humans, which can lead to an increase in side effects if drugs are administered to a hypothyroid individual.

It is these compensatory responses to the hypothyroid state that set the stage for the severe nature of myxedema coma. Decompensation of hypothyroidism and myxedema coma are associated with altered mental status, abnormal thermoregulation, and a precipitating event or illness. Precipitating events in humans include congestive heart failure or other acute medical illness, infection, surgery, trauma, hypothermia, or administration of diuretics or of central nervous or respiratory system depressants. Clinical signs in dogs include an obtunded or comatose mental condition, hypothermia without shivering, bradycardia, hypotension, and hypoventilation as well as the typical signs of hypothyroidism and cutaneous myxedema. Clinicopathologic abnormalities include mild nonregenerative anemia, hypercholesterolemia, and hyponatremia. Pleural effusion and a pulmonary alveolar pattern have been observed by radiography. Treatment must be instituted immediately, often before receipt of thyroid function test results, so clinical signs of hypothyroidism combined with the preceding abnormalities should prompt the clinician to consider strongly myxedema coma as the diagnosis.

Appropriate treatment of myxedema coma involves management of the failed compensatory responses and thyroid hormone supplementation. Passive warming by covering the dog with blankets rather than active warming with a heating device is necessary to resolve the hypothermia without inducing peripheral vasodilation and exacerbating hypotension. Because the compensatory mechanisms of long-standing hypothyroidism result in a decrease in blood volume, any degree of hypotension should be considered serious and must be treated promptly. Direct or indirect measurements of blood pressure (see *CVT XII*, pp. 110 and 113) are preferable to estimates such as pulse quality and capillary refill time. Fluid supplementation with crystalloids should be instituted, being cautious not to induce hyponatremia, since free water clearance is reduced. Administration of colloids such as hetastarch or dextrans may be useful in some cases. Dogs with concurrent congestive heart failure are at increased risk for worsening fluid retention and pulmonary edema during intravenous fluid

administration. If other treatment does not relieve hypotension, dopamine infusion is indicated. Dopamine is preferable to other agents as it preserves coronary and renal blood flow.

Infection is the most common precipitating event for myxedema coma in humans. Thorough investigation for infection or other underlying disease is indicated in all dogs with decompensated hypothyroidism. Broad-spectrum antibiotics should be part of the initial treatment until the presence or absence of infection can be confirmed. Glucocorticoid supplementation in the form of hydrocortisone, prednisone, or dexamethasone sodium phosphate is recommended because of the reduced secretion of cortisol in response to stress in severe hypothyroidism. Hypoventilation can be recognized by hypercapnia seen on arterial blood gas monitoring. It should be treated with mechanical ventilatory assistance if severe.

Thyroid hormone replacement should be given intravenously to avoid any delay in absorption from the gastrointestinal tract. Although the dose and specific type of thyroid hormone to be administered is controversial, I recommend administration of a loading dose of intravenous levothyroxine (Synthroid Injection, Knoll Pharmaceutical, Mount Olive, NJ) that is three to five times the standard daily dose (0.066 to 0.11 mg/kg). If injectable thyroxine is not available, thyroxine should be administered orally. Triiodothyronine could also be administered but is less readily available. Subsequent treatment with levothyroxine can be given orally at the usual replacement dose of 0.022 mg/kg every 12 hours. The prognosis is guarded to poor, but recognition and treatment of any concurrent condition in concert with proper treatment of myxedema can resolve this severe complication of hypothyroidism in some cases.

POLYGLANDULAR ENDOCRINOPATHY

Polyglandular endocrinopathy results from an immune-mediated destruction of multiple endocrine glands, including the thyroid, adrenal cortex, pancreatic islet cells, and parathyroid glands. Concurrent hypoadrenocorticism and hypothyroidism are the most common manifestations of this syndrome in dogs. Clinical signs of hypoadrenocorticism predominate, but the presence of hypercholesterolemia (seen in 80% of dogs with both diseases) should alert the clinician to the possibility of concurrent hypothyroidism. In order to reduce the potentially confounding effects of nonthyroidal illness, thyroid function testing is best undertaken after resolving the hypoadrenal crisis.

Diabetes mellitus has been reported occasionally in hypothyroid dogs. Although it is possible that some cases occur as a manifestation of a polyglandular endocrinopathy with common immune-mediated pathogenesis, hypothyroidism causes glucose intolerance that could lead to the development of diabetes mellitus. The glucose intolerance induced by hypothyroidism is significantly greater than that caused by obesity. The insulin resistance in hypothyroidism may result from decreased tissue delivery of insulin, the presence of a postreceptor defect such as generation of intracellular signals or altered intracellular glucose metabolism, or reduced expression of the membrane glucose transporter. It seems unlikely that insulin resistance subsequent to hypothyroidism is a major factor in the pathogenesis of most cases of diabetes mellitus because of the infrequent concurrent incidence of the diseases. However, thyroid hormone deficiency can result in insulin resistance and difficulty in glycemic control in diabetic dogs. Hypothyroidism should be included in the list of potential causes of increasing insulin requirements or overt insulin resistance. Thyroid hormone replacement should be instituted gradually in dogs with diabetes mellitus, since insulin requirements will decrease and severe hypoglycemia may occur. Levothyroxine should be administered at 25% of the normal replacement dose, with an increase of 25% of the normal dose every 2 weeks. Full replacement doses may result in hypoglycemia within 2 weeks of instituting treatment. Urine glucose monitoring by the owner can help identify dogs at risk for hypoglycemia. Blood glucose curves should be obtained weekly or when urine glucose measurements are negative.

References and Suggested Reading

Dewey CW, Shelton GD, Bailey CS, et al: Neuromuscular dysfunction in five dogs with acquired myasthenia gravis and presumptive hypothyroidism. Prog Vet Neurol 6:117, 1995.
   A description of myasthenia gravis and megaesophagus in five dogs with abnormal thyroid function tests.
Ford SL, Nelson RW, Feldman EC, et al: Insulin resistance in three dogs with hypothyroidism and diabetes mellitus. J Am Vet Med Assoc 202:1478, 1993.
   Three cases of poorly controlled diabetes mellitus in hypothyroid dogs that improved following treatment of the hypothyroidism.
Jaggy A, Oliver JE, Ferguson DC, et al: Neurological manifestations of hypothyroidism: A retrospective study of 29 dogs. J Vet Intern Med 8:328, 1994.
   A retrospective study of a variety of neuromuscular findings in hypothyroid dogs.
Johnson CA: Reproductive manifestations of thyroid disease. Vet Clin North Am 23:509, 1994.
   A review of the known and suspected effects of hypothyroidism on reproduction in dogs and humans.
Miller PE, Panciera DL: Effects of experimentally induced hypothyroidism on the eye and ocular adnexa of dogs. Am J Vet Res 55:692, 1994.
   An evaluation of the effects of hypothyroidism on ocular parameters using an experimental model in dogs.
Nicoloff JT, LoPresti JS: Myxedema coma, a form of decompensated hypothyroidism. Endocrinol Metab Clin North Am 22:279, 1993.
   A review of the pathophysiology, clinical presentation, and treatment of myxedema coma in humans.
Panciera DL, Johnson GS: Plasma von Willebrand factor antigen concentration and buccal mucosal bleeding time in dogs with experimental hypothyroidism. J Vet Intern Med 10:60, 1996.
   Evaluation of plasma von Willebrand factor and buccal mucosal bleeding times before and after induction and treatment of experimental hypothyroidism.
Zeiss CJ, Waddle G: Hypothyroidism and atherosclerosis in dogs. Compend Contin Educ Pract Vet 17:1117, 1995.
   A retrospective compilation of clinical and pathologic findings in dogs with atherosclerosis and thyroid gland histologic features compatible with hypothyroidism.

Use of Endogenous Thyrotropin and Free Thyroxine Determinations for Monitoring Thyroid Replacement Treatment in Dogs With Hypothyroidism

DEBORAH S. GRECO
Fort Collins, Colorado

GUIDELINES FOR TREATMENT OF HYPOTHYROIDISM

Hypothyroidism is a gratifying disease to treat because of the ease and completeness of response to thyroid hormone administration. Once a diagnosis of hypothyroidism has been established, appropriate therapy is carried out with synthetic hormone or sodium L-thyroxine given at a recommended dosage (22 to 44 μg/kg daily to a maximum of 0.8 mg b.i.d.). Use of a brand name medication is recommended because the bioavailability of generic L-thyroxine can be variable. Although many dogs respond adequately to once daily administration of thyroxine, some may require twice daily treatment to achieve and maintain a clinically euthyroid state.

Therapy is usually monitored by assessing total thyroxine (TT_4) or total triiodothyronine (TT_3) concentrations, or both, 4 to 6 hours after oral L-thyroxine administration (postpill testing) and resolution of the clinical signs of hypothyroidism. However, a few dogs with hypothyroidism have T_4 autoantibodies, which makes postpill monitoring with TT_4 difficult. Furthermore, there is considerable variation in the dose required to physiologically supplement dogs with thyroid hormone. This discussion addresses monitoring thyroid hormone replacement therapy with endogenous thyroid-stimulating hormone (TSH) and free serum thyroxine (FT$_4$) concentrations. For a discussion of postpill monitoring using serum total T$_4$ and T$_3$ see *CVT XII,* p. 364.

GOALS OF THYROID HORMONE REPLACEMENT THERAPY

Resolution of clinical signs is the first and most important goal of thyroid hormone replacement therapy. Unfortunately, it is not always easy to define the optimal dose of thyroid hormone in an individual patient. Furthermore, the clinician may be using a therapeutic trial of levothyroxine to confirm a diagnosis of hypothyroidism. In this case, assurance of adequate serum concentrations of levothyroxine is important to rule out therapeutic failure.

In humans, early evidence of therapeutic response includes diuresis, regression of puffiness, and weight loss. In dogs, the first signs of improvement usually consist of increases in appetite, mental alertness, physical activity, heart rate, and body temperature. In dogs, resolution of skin and hair coat changes generally require several months of appropriate therapy. Unfortunately, even when a patient appears to be metabolically normal, a small increase in dose may effect still more improvement without inducing thyrotoxicosis. Conversely, subclinical thyrotoxicosis has been documented in humans undergoing levothyroxine replacement therapy and is manifested as decreased bone density or osteoporosis, heart disease, and increased levels of liver enzymes. Thyroid hormone oversupplementation is meticulously avoided in humans by closely monitoring endogenous serum thyrotropin (TSH) concentrations; the dose is reduced if endogenous TSH falls to less than the normal range. Some authors have suggested that dogs are immune to the development of thyrotoxicosis because the canine thyroid metabolism is more rapid than that of humans (Refsal and Nachreiner, 1995). However, we cannot tell currently if dogs suffer from being oversupplemented because we do not look for subtle or mild signs of thyrotoxicosis such as osteoporosis or occult cardiac hypertrophy. Therefore, therapeutic monitoring of TT$_4$, TT$_3$, FT$_4$, and endogenous canine TSH (cTSH) concentrations are important tools in determining the optimal dosage of T$_4$ for a given animal.

Pharmacokinetics

Pharmacokinetics is the study of absorption, distribution, elimination, and metabolism of a given drug. The relationship between dose and therapeutic response is not as direct as the relationship between serum concentration and therapeutic response because individuals differ in certain pharmacokinetic parameters. For levothyroxine, the most variable pharmacokinetic parameters are absorption and metabolism. In hypothyroid animals, the dose of thyroid medication necessary to predict a response is variable because maintenance of euthyroidism is dependent on absorption of a bolus of thyroid hormone rather than constant secretion of minute amounts of thyroid hormone from the thyroid gland. In humans undergoing thyroid hormone replacement therapy, serum T$_3$ concentrations vary widely and in general the T$_3$:T$_4$ concentration ratios are less than those found in normal subjects (Ingbar, 1985). When thy-

roid hormone is absorbed orally rather than secreted into the blood, a significant portion of drug undergoes first-pass metabolism through the liver, resulting in lower serum iodothyronine values. As a result of individual variation in pharmacokinetics of levothyroxine, postpill TT$_3$ and TT$_4$ determinations may vary significantly in animals receiving the same dosage of thyroid medication.

Pharmacokinetic parameters, such as postpill TT$_4$ and TT$_3$ concentrations, indicate if the drug is being absorbed from the intestinal tract and surviving first-pass metabolism in sufficient quantity to ensure therapeutic serum concentrations. Conversely, prepill monitoring predicts adequate duration of thyroid hormone concentrations in blood and if prepill TT$_4$ concentrations are low, this would suggest that more frequent administration of levothyroxine is indicated. Serum TT$_4$ or TT$_3$ concentrations do not tell the clinician that the animal is supplemented adequately to *predict a therapeutic response.*

Pharmacodynamics

Although postpill and prepill TT$_4$, TT$_3$, or FT$_4$ concentrations assess the pharmacokinetic status of thyroid hormone replacement, measurement of physiologic parameters such as basal metabolic rate (BMR) or endogenous cTSH indicate the pharmacodynamic response of the animal. Pharmacodynamics is the study of drug response, physiologic effects of drugs, and the mechanism of action of drugs. A pharmacodynamic parameter assesses the drug response at the molecular or cellular level. The ultimate pharmacodynamic goal of thyroid hormone replacement is to increase the basal metabolic rate of the hypothyroid animal. Pharmacodynamic indicators of response to levothyroxine include indirect calorimetry, which is a measure of basal metabolic rate, and suppression of endogenous cTSH concentrations, which indicates adequate negative feedback to the pituitary gland by thyroid hormone.

METHODS OF MONITORING THYROID HORMONE REPLACEMENT

Pharmacokinetic Methods: Serum Total Thyroxine, Total Triiodothyronine, Free Thyroxine, Free Triiodothyronine

For postpill monitoring, the serum TT$_4$ should be in the upper normal or greater than normal range 6 hours after dosing) (Refsal and Nachreiner, 1995). Some authors have suggested that TT$_3$ is more predictive of clinical response than is TT$_4$. However, in humans, normalization of baseline endogenous TSH was achieved when serum T$_3$ was similar to, and serum T$_4$ was higher than, controls (Ingbar, 1985). However, in humans, serum concentrations of TT$_3$, TT$_4$, and TT$_3$:TT$_4$ ratios did not predict response to therapy (Ingbar, 1985).

The unbound fraction of thyroid hormone, which is the form available to the tissues, is proportional to the action of thyroid hormone (see *CVT XII,* p. 360). Therefore, measurement of FT$_4$ is the most important thyroid diagnostic tool in humans. An estimate of FT$_4$ theoretically is not subject to drug-induced or protein-binding effects that may occur in TT$_4$ measurements (Ferguson, 1994). A small

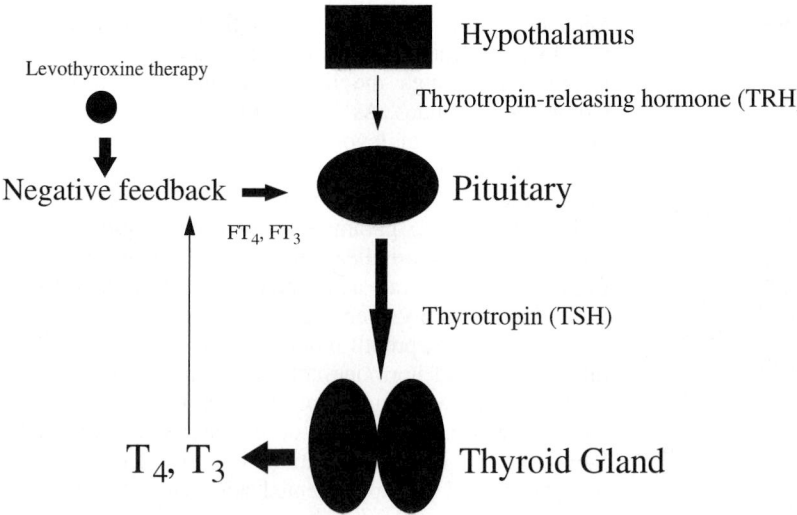

Figure 1. Diagram of the hypothalamic-pituitary-thyroid axis illustrating negative feedback during thyroid hormone supplementation.

percentage of hypothyroid dogs (<1%) exhibit TT_4 autoantibodies secondary to immune destruction of the thyroid gland. These dogs may have alterations in serum TT_4 (high or low levels) because of interference with the assay by the T_4 autoantibodies. In those animals, the diagnosis and monitoring of thyroid replacement therapy must be based on the serum FT_4 concentrations. The preference has classically been to measure FT_4 by dialysis because of inaccurate measurements of FT_4 by analogue methods. However, the inaccuracies in the FT_4 analogue assays occur at the low end of the FT_4 range because of optimization of the assay for human FT_4 concentrations. This author has found that the immunoassay FT_4 analogue assay is acceptable for monitoring FT_4 after thyroid hormone replacement therapy. As with serum TT_4, the FT_4 concentration should be in the middle to upper normal range 6 hours after dosing.

Pharmacodynamic Methods: Basal Metabolic Rate and Endogenous Canine Thyroid-Stimulating Hormone

BMR is a quantitative measure of total body energy production and is considered an index of the overall metabolic effect of thyroid hormone. Although BMR determinations have been replaced by biochemical thyroid testing, resting energy expenditure (REE) determinations by indirect calorimetry are used in studies of hypothyroidism to assess the pharmacodynamic *response to thyroid hormone replacement therapy.* A human patient is considered adequately supplemented with levothyroxine when the REE returns to the normal range.

The REE is defined as the energy expended by the animal when in a postabsorptive state under thermally

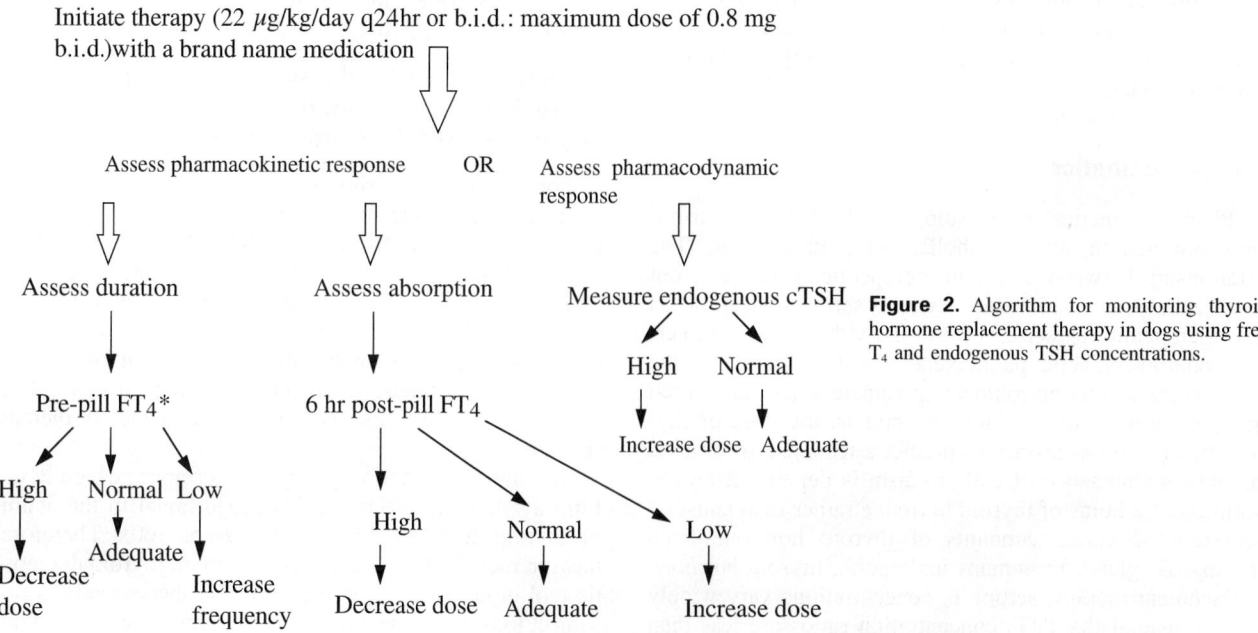

Figure 2. Algorithm for monitoring thyroid hormone replacement therapy in dogs using free T_4 and endogenous TSH concentrations.

neutral conditions. Noninvasive estimations of REE can be made by measuring oxygen consumption ($\dot{V}O_2$) and carbon dioxide production ($\dot{V}CO_2$) using indirect calorimetry. In a recent study of 40 hypothyroid dogs at our institution, the mean REE before L-thyroxine supplementation was 32.76 $\pm$ 9.53 kcal/kg/day or 82.6 $\pm$ 3.9 kcal/kg$^{0.75}$/day. The mean REE for the dogs after L-thyroxine supplementation was significantly higher than baseline (40.45 $\pm$ 13.0 kcal/kg/day or 99.1 $\pm$ 4.0 kcal/kg$^{0.75}$/day; $P <$ .05), indicating a metabolic response to thyroid hormone supplementation. These data support the contention that thyroid hormone supplementation increases the energy expenditure of apparently resting hypothyroid dogs.

Baseline serum concentrations of TSH are elevated in primary hypothyroidism, and normalization of TSH levels with thyroid supplementation provides an end point of appropriate negative feedback to the pituitary-thyroid axis (Fig. 1). In dogs, experience with the endogenous TSH assay is limited; however, in a recent study of 40 hypothyroid dogs at the author's institution, all dogs with initially elevated TSH (primary hypothyroidism) exhibited a significant decrease in mean cTSH concentrations (0.69 ng/ml versus 0.09 ng/ml; $P <$ .05) following thyroid hormone supplementation. Theoretically, the best method of determining if a dog with primary hypothyroidism is adequately supplemented is by assessing the suppression of the pituitary-thyroid axis by measuring endogenous cTSH. As in humans, endogenous cTSH should decrease into the normal range in dogs with primary hypothyroidism. One advantage of measuring serum endogenous TSH for monitoring thyroid hormone replacement therapy is that unlike postpill monitoring, the sample may be collected at any time during the day.

Recent studies in dogs with experimentally induced hypothyroidism also indicate that endogenous cTSH decreases in levothyroxine-supplemented dogs (Bruner et al, 1996). One caveat about cTSH monitoring is that the dog must have *primary* hypothyroidism with basal elevations in cTSH prior to monitoring in order to determine if the cTSH is suppressed. Another possible disadvantage of measuring cTSH is that this first-generation TSH assay may not be sensitive enough to determine if a dog is *oversupplemented* with levothyroxine. In human patients, overdosage is monitored via a highly sensitive third-generation TSH assay. A summary of levothyroxine monitoring using cTSH and FT$_4$ concentrations is shown in Figure 2.

References and Suggested Reading

Bruner JM, Scott-Moncrieff C, Williams DA: Diurnal fluctuations of serum canine thyroid stimulating hormone (cTSH) in euthyroid, hypothyroid and thyroxine-supplemented dogs. J Vet Intern Med 10:184, 1996.

Ferguson D: Update on the diagnosis of canine hypothyroidism. Vet Clin North Am Small Anim Pract 24:515, 1994.
Review of the latest developments in diagnostics for canine hypothyroidism.

Ingbar SH: The thyroid gland. In: Wilson JD, Foster DW, eds: Textbook of Endocrinology, 7th ed. Philadelphia: WB Saunders, 1985, pp 730–731.
Review of thyroid hormone supplementation in humans and monitoring methods.

Refsal KR, Nachreiner RF: Monitoring thyroid hormone replacement therapy. In: Bonagura JD, ed: Kirk's Current Veterinary Therapy XII. Philadelphia: WB Saunders, 1995, pp 364–368.
Review of post-pill TT$_4$ and TT$_3$ concentrations for monitoring thyroid hormone replacement therapy.

CVT Update: Medical Treatment of Hyperthyroidism in Cats

CARMEL T. MOONEY
Dublin, Ireland

KEITH L. THODAY
Edinburgh, Scotland

Hyperthyroidism (thyrotoxicosis) is recognized as the most common endocrine disorder of cats. Benign adenomatous hyperplasia (adenoma) of one or, more commonly, both thyroid lobes accounts for more than 98% of cases. Excessive production of the active thyroid hormones L-thyroxine (T$_4$) and L-triiodothyronine (T$_3$) results, having widespread systemic effects. Spontaneous remission of the condition has not been reported, and it is insidiously progressive, eventually resulting in emaciation, severe metabolic and cardiac dysfunction, and ultimately death. How-

ever, because of the benign nature of the thyroid lesion, the disease carries a favorable prognosis with effective therapy.

The fundamental cause of feline hyperthyroidism is not known, and methods for preventing or removing inciting causes are not yet available. Treatment is aimed at removing or destroying abnormally functioning thyroid tissue, pharmacologic inhibition of thyroid hormone synthesis and release, or amelioration of the impact of excessive T$_4$ and T$_3$ on peripheral tissues. To date, surgical thyroidectomy or thyroid ablation using radioactive iodine (see *CVT XII*, p.

372) are the only curative methods available. Pharmacologic or medical management prior to surgery decreases the metabolic and cardiac complications associated with hyperthyroidism. In addition, medical control of clinical signs is desirable if there is a delay prior to receiving radioactive iodine or a return to euthyroidism after treatment. Medical management alone is not curative but offers a practical, long-term treatment option for many patients. Medical therapy requires no advanced training, skills, or special licensing and is readily available and reasonably inexpensive. Treatment usually results in rapid clinical improvement, with an acceptable percentage of adverse reactions, and avoids occasional perioperative and postoperative complications such as cardiac arrhythmia, hemorrhage, hypoparathyroidism, and hypothyroidism. Potential drawbacks are the dependence on adequate owner and cat compliance for daily administration of the medication and regular biochemical monitoring to ensure the efficacy of treatment and minimize complications. Despite this, medical therapy may be the treatment of choice for some cats of advanced age and for those with concurrent diseases precluding surgery or radioactive iodine therapy. Medical treatment is indicated when radioactive iodine facilities are not available or when owners refuse other forms of therapy because of the potential for surgical complications, doubts about radiation therapy, or cost. In addition, because medical management has no long-term effects after withdrawal, it is the best option for trial therapy in cats when deterioration of renal function is a possibility once euthyroidism is restored (see p. 337).

Thyroid carcinomas may also be functional but account for less than 2% of feline cases. Medical management may assist in controlling the production or effects of excessive amounts of thyroid hormones, but the prognosis remains guarded if used alone. More aggressive treatment involving surgical thyroidectomy or radioactive iodine, either alone or in combination, is more appropriate.

AVAILABLE OPTIONS

Numerous pharmacologic agents may be employed in the medical management of feline hyperthyroidism. Indications, dosage regimens, and potential adverse reactions are summarized in Tables 1 and 2. A more detailed review of the mode and site of action of these drugs is available elsewhere (see CVT XI, p. 338).

Thioureylenes

The therapeutic mainstays in the medical management of hyperthyroidism include the thiouracils (propylthiouracil) and the imidazoles (methimazole [Tapazole, Eli Lilly] and carbimazole [NeoMercazole, Roche]). These drugs are actively concentrated by the thyroid gland and interfere with intrathyroidal thyroid hormone synthesis but not with iodide trapping or the release of preformed hormones. Propylthiouracil, the most widely available drug, has the added advantage of inhibiting T_4 to T_3 production both intrathyroidally and extrathyroidally; however, the drug is considered too toxic in cats and should not be used. Methimazole is available in the United States and Japan and carbimazole can be found in Europe.

Carbimazole exerts its antithyroid effect through immediate conversion to methimazole when administered orally (Peterson and Aucoin, 1993). Serum concentrations of methimazole achieved after carbimazole administration are less than after administration of an equal weight of methimazole, reflecting the molar ratio of the two drugs. Thus, a 5 mg dose of carbimazole is equivalent to approximately 3 mg of methimazole and may explain, at least in part, the differences in recommended dosages between the two agents and the apparent lower incidence of adverse reactions noted with carbimazole (Peterson et al, 1988; Mooney et al, 1992). Aside from this, there are no significant pharmacokinetic differences between the two drugs. Methimazole is well absorbed after oral administration with a high bioavailability and rapidly reaches peak concentrations with a half-life of approximately 4 to 6 hours (Trepanier et al, 1991). There is a trend in hyperthyroid cats toward faster elimination of the drug when compared with healthy cats, but this is not important clinically (Trepanier and Peterson, 1991). Despite the relatively short half-life of methimazole, the intrathyroidal residence time during which methimazole exerts its effect is likely to be approximately 20 hours in cats as it is in human patients. Thus, where a twice or three times daily dosing schedule is

TABLE 1. Indications and Dosages for the Drugs Most Commonly Used to Treat Hyperthyroidism in Cats

Drug	Indication	Daily Dosage Per Cat	Length of Therapy
Methimazole	Prior to surgery	10–15 mg divided twice or three times daily	2–3 wk
	Chronic management	7.5–10 mg divided twice daily	Long-term
Carbimazole	Prior to surgery	15 mg divided three times daily	2–3 wk
	Chronic management	10 mg divided twice daily	Long-term
Stable iodine	Prior to surgery	30–100 mg once or divided twice daily	10–14 days (combined with methimazole/carbimazole/propranolol)
Propranolol	Prior to surgery	7.5–15 mg divided three times daily	3–14 days (usually combined with methimazole/carbimazole/stable iodine)
	Prior to ¹³¹I therapy	7.5–15 mg divided three times daily	As required
Calcium ipodate	Prior to surgery	100 mg divided twice daily	2 weeks
	Chronic management	100 mg divided twice daily	Long-term (assess for relapse after 14 wk)

TABLE 2. Adverse Reactions Associated With Drugs Used Therapeutically in Feline Hyperthyroidism

Drug	Reaction	Approximate Percentage of Cats Affected	Time at Occurrence	Treatment Required
Methimazole	Vomiting, anorexia, depression	15	<4 wk	Usually transient
	Eosinophilia, leukopenia, lymphocytosis	15	<8 wk	Usually transient
	Self-induced excoriations	2	<4 wk	Withdrawal and glucocorticoid therapy
	Agranulocytosis, thrombocytopenia	<5	<3 mo	Withdrawal and symptomatic therapy
	Hepatopathy (anorexia, ↑ alanine aminotransferase, alkaline phosphatase)	<2	<2 mo	Withdrawal and symptomatic therapy
	Positive ANA	>50	>6 mo	Decrease daily dosage
	Acquired myasthenia gravis	Rare	<16 wk	Withdrawal or concomitant glucocorticoid therapy
Carbimazole	Vomiting, anorexia, depression	10	<3 wk	Usually transient
	Eosinophilia, leukopenia, lymphocytosis	5	<2 wk	Usually transient
	Self-induced excoriations	Rare	<4 wk	Withdrawal and glucocorticoid therapy
Stable iodine	Salivation and anorexia	Occasional	Immediate	Change formulation

difficult to implement chronically, once daily dosing may be effective. Further decreasing the frequency of dosing, however, may result in the recurrence of hyperthyroidism.

Indications and Method of Use

Administration of methimazole or carbimazole is the method of choice for the preoperative control of hyperthyroidism because of the consistent effect in controlling thyroid hormone production. The initial dose and frequency of administration of methimazole is titrated depending on the severity of the hyperthyroid state. By contrast, carbimazole appears to be most effective if administered at a dose of 5 mg per cat at strict 8-hour intervals. The time to achieve euthyroidism is relatively short, occurring, at least for carbimazole, within a mean ($\pm$SD) of 5.7 ($\pm$2.9) days and is correlated to the pretreatment serum total T_4 concentration (Mooney et al, 1992). For practical purposes, a 2- to 3-week course of therapy is initially prescribed, which allows time for more obvious clinical improvement and ensures the attainment of euthyroidism in most cats. At that time, a serum total T_4 concentration is measured, and if it is within or less than the reference range, surgery can be performed. As euthyroidism is achieved, there is an associated progressive decline in the serum concentrations of alanine aminotransferase and alkaline phosphatase. The measurement of these enzymes can serve as an alternative nonspecific indicator of therapeutic efficacy. In severely affected cats, a longer course of preoperative therapy may be required before these animals are considered good surgical candidates, and such patients should subsequently be managed chronically until surgery is performed. In a small number of cats, euthyroidism is not achieved during this initial treatment period. A gradual increase in the daily dosage (in 2.5- to 5-mg increments) up to 25 to 30 mg/cat/day has been recommended. However, in our experience, this problem is almost invariably due to poor owner or cat compliance, or both. Retraining of the owner or hospitalization of the cat with a longer pretreatment course is usually effective without increasing the daily drug dosage. To pre-

vent escape from the inhibitory effects of these drugs, the last tablet is administered on the morning of surgery.

Methimazole and carbimazole are currently the only drugs recommended for long-term medical control of thyrotoxicosis. Once euthyroidism has been achieved as outlined earlier, the daily dosage of methimazole is reduced in 2.5- to 5-mg decrements. Further dose adjustments are based on serum total T_4 concentrations assessed every 2 to 3 weeks. Most cats are successfully maintained on a total daily dose of between 7.5 and 10 mg of methimazole per cat, preferably divided twice daily. A few cats require as little as 2.5 to 5 mg/day, whereas some require 15 to 20 mg/day. A consistent dose of 5 mg per cat administered twice daily is required for carbimazole. Once stability is attained, serum total T_4 concentrations are measured every 3 to 6 months or as indicated clinically.

The use of methimazole and carbimazole prior to radioactive iodine therapy is controversial and has not been evaluated in cats exhibiting a delayed return to euthyroidism after treatment. In humans, these drugs are stopped at least 2 to 3 days prior to radioactive iodine administration and the calculated radiation dose is automatically increased by 25%. In early feline studies, prior antithyroid drug administration was considered to increase the radioresistance of thyroid tissue and was therefore not recommended. Although this has never been objectively addressed, Peterson and Becker (1995) perceived no difference in response to radioactive iodine treatment in cats that did not receive antithyroid medication and those in which the drugs had been stopped for the previous 1 to 2 weeks. Since waiting lists for radioactive iodine therapy are often lengthy, and control of thyrotoxicosis desirable in the interim, further work in this area is required.

Adverse Effects

Most clinical adverse reactions associated with antithyroid medication occur within the first 3 months of therapy and are summarized in Table 2. Vomiting, anorexia, and depression occur more frequently with methimazole and may be related to its bitter taste, whereas carbimazole is tasteless. Mild hematologic abnormalities, including eosinophilia, lymphocytosis, or leukopenia may also be noted. These reactions are transient and rarely require withdrawal of the drug. Self-induced excoriation of the head and neck occurs occasionally with methimazole and rarely with carbimazole. In humans, such effects may respond to antihistamine (H_1-receptor antagonist) therapy without withdrawal of the drug, but the latter is necessary in the cat together with symptomatic glucocorticoid therapy. More serious adverse reactions have not yet been reported with carbimazole. Agranulocytosis or thrombocytopenia are the most frequent major reactions associated with methimazole therapy, although other problems have been reported (see Table 2). Complete blood and platelet counts have been recommended every 2 weeks, at least for the first 3 months of therapy, in order to detect such reactions. However, because of the low frequency of these effects, together with their unpredictability, the cost-effectiveness of routine monitoring must be questioned. Monitoring hematologic parameters if and when clinical signs (overt bleeding, pyrexia) appear is probably more appropriate. A bleeding tendency has also been noted without the development of thrombocytopenia. Decreased platelet function is possible, but this mechanism has not yet been evaluated. Serum antinuclear antibodies (ANAs) develop in a high proportion of cats treated with methimazole for longer than 6 months. Clinical signs of a lupus-like syndrome have not been observed, but the daily drug dosage is decreased because most cats that develop antinuclear antibodies are receiving doses equal to, or in excess of, 15 mg/day. Once serious reactions are noted, an alternative form of therapy should be sought.

Serum total T_4 concentrations are frequently depressed to less than the reference range in cats treated with carbimazole or methimazole. Clinical signs of hypothyroidism do not develop, presumably because serum T_3 concentrations tend to remain within the reference range or possibly because drug dosage is adjusted, preventing the situation from continuing for a significant duration.

A deterioration in renal function has been described in hyperthyroid cats undergoing treatment. This is presumably related to a decrease in glomerular filtration rate, which unmasks latent renal disease (Graves et al, 1994). This potential effect is not specific to antithyroid medication but also occurs after radioactive iodine therapy or surgical thyroidectomy (DiBartola et al, 1996; see also next article). There are no obvious means available to predict the emergence of azotemia and uremia in individual cases. Renal function should be assessed if clinical signs of overt renal disease occur as euthyroidism is achieved. The decision to continue treatment for hyperthyroidism is based on which of the two diseases is more severe.

Trial Therapy

A positive clinical response to trial therapy with methimazole or carbimazole has been advocated as a means of diagnosing hyperthyroidism when serum total T_4 concentrations are equivocal. This is arguable unless recurrence of the clinical signs is demonstrated on subsequent withdrawal of the drug. A range of other, more definitive diagnostic tests are currently available for equivocal cases (see *CVT*

XII, p. 335 and p. 323 in this volume). Trial therapy, because of its reversibility, plays an important role in assessing the effect of treatment on renal function, particularly if there is pre-existing evidence of dysfunction. If there is no deterioration in renal function as euthyroidism is achieved, other more permanent treatment options (surgery, radioactive iodine) may be considered.

Stable Iodine

Large doses of stable iodine acutely decrease the rate of thyroid hormone synthesis (Wolff-Chaikoff effect) and release. These effects are at best inconsistent and short-lived, with rapid escape from inhibition and, at worst, result in exacerbation of the thyrotoxicosis because of potential enrichment of thyroid hormone stores within the gland. As such, stable iodine is usually used in combination with a beta-adrenoreceptor–blocking agent for 10 to 14 days prior to surgical thyroidectomy in cats intolerant to methimazole or carbimazole. The iodine is administered in aqueous solution either as a saturated solution of potassium iodide (SSKI, 100 gm potassium iodide/100-ml solution, yielding approximately 35 to 50 mg iodine/drop), or as Lugol's solution (5 gm iodine with 10 gm potassium iodide/100 ml solution, yielding approximately 6 mg iodine/drop). More long-term control has been achieved in human patients with mild thyrotoxicosis, but this has not been evaluated in cats. Stable iodine is contraindicated prior to radioactive iodine therapy but, at least in humans, is used as adjunctive therapy after treatment when escape from inhibition is less likely to occur. There is no synergistic action between stable iodine and methimazole or carbimazole. The addition of stable iodine to the antithyroid drug regimen is considered useful by some workers because of a consequent reduction in the vascularity and friability of the thyroid gland, making surgical excision less problematic. In humans, however, this is considered to be an effect seen only in patients treated with a beta-adrenoreceptor–blocking agent prior to stable iodine therapy.

The adverse reactions associated with potassium iodide purportedly result from its unpleasant brassy taste. These can be avoided through the use of gelatin capsules, dilution of SSKI to a 10 mg/ml solution, or by administering iodine-rich products such as kelp or, at least in the United Kingdom, potassium iodate tablets (85-mg tablets, yielding 50 mg free iodine, Cambridge Self Care Diagnostics).

Beta-Adrenoreceptor–Blocking Agents

Propranolol (Inderal, Zeneca) is the most frequently used beta-blocker in hyperthyroid cats. Propranolol has no direct effect on the thyroid gland but is useful in controlling the tachycardia, polypnea, hypertension, and hyperexcitability associated with hyperthyroidism. Propranolol is used when rapid control of clinical effects is required and is usually combined with methimazole or carbimazole or stable iodine. Since propranolol does not affect radioactive iodine treatment, it is a useful option for cats awaiting radiation therapy or when there is a delayed return to euthyroidism after treatment.

Propranolol is a nonselective beta-adrenoreceptor–

blocking agent and is therefore contraindicated in cats with pre-existing uncontrolled overt congestive cardiac failure or asthma. Atenolol (Tenormin, Stuart) offers some potential advantages over propranolol, including more selective beta$_1$-adrenoreceptor–blocking action, a longer duration of activity, and availability in syrup form. Atenolol is used at a dose of 6.25 to 12.5 mg/cat/day. The starting dose should be low and gradually increased to effect. These drugs should not be instituted immediately prior to anesthesia or surgery without a suitable period of dose titration.

Iodinated Radiographic Contrast Agents

Oral cholecystographic agents (e.g., calcium ipodate [Oragrafin, Squibb]) acutely inhibit peripheral T$_4$ to T$_3$ conversion and also decrease T$_4$ production, presumably mediated through iodine, which is released as ipodate is metabolized, or through direct inhibition of the effects of thyroid-stimulating hormone. The former effect has been clearly demonstrated in cats in which hyperthyroidism has been induced experimentally, and the drug appears to be well tolerated with few adverse reactions. Data on the use of calcium ipodate in naturally occurring cases are limited. Murray and Peterson (1997) treated 12 hyperthyroid cats with calcium ipodate, 8 of which exhibited a good response. Serum total T$_3$ concentrations decreased to within the reference range by 2 weeks of therapy and remained there for the entire study period of 14 weeks. This was associated with an improvement in clinical signs, weight gain, a decrease in heart rate, and reduced blood pressure in hypertensive cats. Four of these cats continued to do well in follow-up periods of between 5 and 6 months, whereas two had a relapse of hyperthyroidism by week 14 of therapy. Serum total T$_4$ concentrations were not affected by the therapy. Cats with severe hyperthyroidism were less likely to respond to the treatment despite doubling the daily dose, although the efficacy and safety of further dose adjustments were not assessed. As such, calcium ipodate serves as an alternative to stable iodine in the short-term preparation of hyperthyroid cats for surgical thyroidectomy. In addition, it is also a feasible medical alternative to carbimazole or methimazole, although further studies are required to assess the more long-term inhibitory effects of this drug.

References and Suggested Reading

Cooper DS: Treatment of thyrotoxicosis. In: Braverman LE, Utiger RD, eds: Werner and Ingbar's The Thyroid. A Fundamental and Clinical Text. Philadelphia: Lippincott-Raven, 1986, p 713.
   An overview of current concepts in the management of human thyrotoxicosis.
DiBartola SP, Broome MR, Stein BS, et al: Effect of treatment of hyperthyroidism on renal function in cats. J Am Vet Med Assoc 208:875, 1996.
   A prospective study of the effects of methimazole and radioactive iodine therapy on renal function in cats.
Graves TK, Olivier NB, Nachreiner RF, et al: Changes in renal function associated with treatment of hyperthyroidism in cats. Am J Vet Res 55:1745, 1994.
   The effect of surgical thyroidectomy on glomerular filtration rate in 13 hyperthyroid cats.
Mooney CT, Thoday KL, Doxey DL: Carbimazole therapy of feline hyperthyroidism. J Sm Anim Pract 33:228, 1992.
   A study on the efficacy of, and adverse reactions to, carbimazole therapy in hyperthyroid cats.
Murray LAS, Peterson ME: Ipodate as medical treatment in 12 cats with hyperthyroidism. J Am Vet Med Assoc, 211:63, 1997.
   A prospective study on the clinical and biochemical effects of calcium ipodate in 12 naturally occurring cases of feline hyperthyroidism.
Peterson ME, Aucoin DP: Comparison of the disposition of carbimazole and methimazole in clinically normal cats. Res Vet Sci 54:351, 1993.
   A study of the oral disposition of the antithyroid drugs methimazole and carbimazole.
Peterson ME, Becker DV: Radioiodine treatment of 524 cats with hyperthyroidism. J Am Vet Med Assoc 207:1422, 1995.
   A comprehensive study on the effect of radioactive iodine treatment in feline hyperthyroidism.
Peterson ME, Kintzer PP, Hurvitz AI: Methimazole treatment of 262 cats with hyperthyroidism. J Vet Intern Med 2:150, 1988.
   A study on the efficacy of, and adverse reactions to, methimazole therapy in hyperthyroid cats.
Trepanier LA, Peterson ME: Pharmacokinetics of methimazole in normal cats and cats with hyperthyroidism. Res Vet Sci 50:69, 1991.
   A study examining the effects of hyperthyroidism on methimazole pharmacokinetics in cats.
Trepanier LA, Peterson ME, Aucoin DP: Pharmacokinetics of intravenous and oral methimazole following single- and multiple-dose administration in normal cats. J Vet Pharmacol Ther 14:367, 1991.
   A study assessing the pharmacokinetics of methimazole in cats.

The Kidney and Hyperthyroidism

STEPHEN P. DiBARTOLA
Columbus, Ohio

SCOTT A. BROWN
Athens, Georgia

The clinical evaluation and management of geriatric cats with concurrent hyperthyroidism and chronic renal disease (CRD) is challenging. On one hand, the effect of nonthyroidal illness on serum thyroxine concentration makes the diagnosis of hyperthyroidism difficult in a cat with CRD. On the other hand, the presence of hyperthyroidism in a cat with CRD can increase glomerular filtration rate (GFR), decrease serum creatinine concentration, and mask underlying renal disease.

PATHOPHYSIOLOGY

Hyperthyroidism increases cardiac output and decreases peripheral vascular resistance, leading to increased renal plasma flow (RPF) and an increased GFR. Both GFR and RPF were increased in normal cats rendered hyperthyroid by administration of thyroxine for 30 days (Adams et al, 1995). Increased GFR reduces serum creatinine concentration, whereas increased body turnover of protein may increase blood urea nitrogen (BUN) concentration slightly. Mild proteinuria may occur as a consequence of increased GFR, especially if accompanied by intrarenal or systemic hypertension. Reduction in muscle mass decreases total body stores of potassium, and muscle weakness due to hypokalemia may occur in some hyperthyroid cats before or during therapy (Nemzek et al, 1994). This finding resembles thyrotoxic periodic paralysis in human patients with thyrotoxicosis, which is thought to result from episodic translocation of potassium from extracellular to intracellular fluid.

Progressive weight loss and reduction in muscle mass also contribute to lower serum creatinine concentrations in hyperthyroid cats, which, in turn, may mask underlying renal disease in some affected cats. Observed increases in serum creatinine concentration after treatment of hyperthyroidism may reflect unmasking of pre-existing renal dysfunction, a decrease in GFR with correction of the hyperthyroid state, weight gain with increased muscle mass, or some combination of these factors. Treatment of hyperthyroidism by bilateral thyroidectomy in cats resulted in the GFR decreasing from a mean of 2.5 ml/min/kg to 1.5 ml/min/kg 30 days after surgery (Graves et al, 1994). In this same study, mean serum creatinine and BUN concentrations increased from 1.3 to 2.0 mg/dl and 27 to 35 mg/dl, respectively. In another study, mean BUN and serum creatinine concentrations increased significantly from a combined baseline mean of 30 mg/dl for BUN and 1.6 mg/dl for serum creatinine to 36 mg/dl for BUN and 2.2 mg/dl for serum creatinine at day 30 and 37 mg/dl for BUN and 2.4 mg/dl for serum creatinine at day 90 after treatment of hyperthyroidism in cats by surgical thyroidectomy, radioiodine, or methimazole (Tapazole, Jones Medical Industries) (DiBartola et al, 1996). In yet another study, BUN and serum creatinine concentrations were increased 30 days after treatment of hyperthyroid cats with radioiodine (Adams et al, 1997). An interesting finding in the latter study was that many of the hyperthyroid cats had a decreased GFR before treatment with radioiodine. This observation is compatible with the clinical impression that hyperthyroidism and CRD occur concurrently in many geriatric cats. Whether this simultaneous occurrence in older cats is coincidental or the result of some pathophysiologic interaction between these two disorders is an intriguing but currently unanswered question.

Although the most emphasis has been placed on the potentially adverse effects of treatment of hyperthyroidism on renal function, it also is possible that hyperthyroidism in some way contributes to the development of CRD in older cats. In clinically normal cats, nearly 60% of renal perfusion pressure is transmitted to the glomerular capillary bed (Brown, 1993). Systemic hypertension accompanies hyperthyroidism in most hyperthyroid cats. If failure of autoregulation occurs, a substantial portion of systemic hypertension may be transmitted to glomeruli, resulting in intraglomerular hypertension and glomerular hyperfiltration. These factors are recognized as contributing to glomerular sclerosis and progression of renal disease in rats.

The possible pathophysiologic relationship between hyperthyroidism and CRD raises important questions about the treatment of hyperthyroidism. It could be argued that reducing serum thyroxine concentrations in older cats with mild hyperthyroidism and CRD should be avoided because treatment may reduce GFR and allow emergence of azotemia and uremia. Conversely, if an increased GFR results in glomerular hyperfiltration in hyperthyroid cats, it may contribute to progression of renal disease. If so, hyperthyroidism in older cats actually may predispose to CRD, and early effective treatment of hyperthyroidism may be important to prevent pathophysiologic changes in the kidney that could lead to progressive renal disease.

DIAGNOSIS

Ideally, the GFR should be measured in affected cats (see *CVT XII,* p. 931). The presence of a lower than normal GFR in a hyperthyroid cat indicates excess risk for adverse clinical outcome after treatment of hyperthyroidism (Adams, 1997). Unfortunately, methods for measurement of GFR are not widely available or practical. Consequently, careful evaluation of routine serum chemistry and urinalysis results must suffice in most instances. Cats with normal BUN, serum creatinine, and serum electrolyte concentrations and highly concentrated urine should be at minimal risk for adverse effects on renal function after treatment of hyperthyroidism. Serum creatinine concentration, however, should be evaluated in light of the cat's body condition and muscle mass. An emaciated cat is expected to have a somewhat lower serum creatinine concentration than is a well-muscled cat with similar renal function. Availability of previous serum creatinine determinations in the cat in question may be helpful in making this evaluation. Occasionally, cats with considerable renal disease retain surprising renal concentrating ability. Consequently, the clinician cannot assume that mild azotemia with concentrated urine in a geriatric cat necessarily is prerenal in origin. In most cats, abdominal palpation of the kidneys is easily performed and yields considerable information about the presence or absence of renal disease. Small, firm, irregular kidneys suggest end-stage renal disease. Renal ultrasonography should be considered if questions remain about the cat's renal function after physical examination and routine laboratory testing.

More difficult yet is establishing a diagnosis of hyperthyroidism in geriatric cats with CRD. This latter condition is one of several nonthyroidal illnesses that may decrease serum thyroxine concentrations to within the normal range, making the diagnosis of concurrent hyperthyroidism difficult. The extent to which the serum thyroxine concentration is decreased in cats with nonthyroidal illness is related more to the severity than to the nature of the illness. The clinician must therefore rely on the presence of a palpable thyroid nodule and use alternative diagnostic methods (e.g., T_3 suppression test, pertechnetate thyroid imaging) to establish a diagnosis of hyperthyroidism in some cats with

CRD. The ability to consistently palpate a thyroid nodule on physical examination is a practical and valuable clinical tool, and its importance in diagnosis should not be ignored.

TREATMENT

The effects of methimazole on thyroid function are rapidly reversible, and it is prudent initially to treat azotemic hyperthyroid cats with methimazole until it can be determined whether correction of the hyperthyroid state will worsen azotemia and result in uremia (see previous article). According to one protocol, affected cats are first treated with 2.5 mg methimazole PO b.i.d. for 2 weeks. If routine tests of renal function remain unchanged, the dosage is increased to 2.5 mg PO t.i.d. If renal function tests remain stable after an additional 2 weeks, the dosage is increased to 5.0 mg PO b.i.d. If renal function tests remain stable for 2 more weeks, the dosage of methimazole is increased to 5 mg PO t.i.d. if deemed necessary by serial monitoring of serum thyroxine concentration (Feldman and Nelson, 1996). If the cat's renal function remains stable or improves on this regimen, other treatments (e.g., surgery, radioiodine) may be considered. If renal function deteriorates at any point during this protocol, methimazole treatment is discontinued, and the cat's clinical condition reassessed. Some increase in serum creatinine and BUN concentrations after correction of the hyperthyroid state may be an unavoidable consequence of effective hyperthyroidism treatment in some cats. It is unknown what, if any, increase in serum creatinine concentration would be safe during treatment of feline hyperthyroidism. Many older cats with serum creatinine concentrations of 2.0 to 3.0 mg/dl do well clinically over a course of several years. Provided that their underlying renal disease is nonprogressive or only slowly progressive, cats with serum creatinine concentrations in this range after antithyroid therapy should be at minimal risk for an adverse clinical outcome.

Hypothyroidism is associated with a reduction in GFR, and treatment protocols that render hyperthyroid cats hypothyroid could pose a threat to renal function. During methimazole therapy, the clinician should carefully monitor serum thyroxine concentration to maintain the cat in a euthyroid state. Blood samples should be drawn at the same postpill interval (e.g., 4 to 6 hours) each time the cat is evaluated to ensure uniformity in serial comparison of serum thyroxine concentrations. Surgical thyroidectomy or radioiodine treatment also may render some treated cats hypothyroid. With all forms of therapy, the effect of nonthyroidal illness on serum thyroxine concentrations creates difficulty in assessing treated cats for later development of hypothyroidism. When clinical hypothyroidism and decreased GFR are suspected after treatment of hyperthyroidism, temporary thyroid hormone replacement using 0.1 mg thyroxine PO every 24 hours for several months may be helpful. In general, a cautious approach that combines the initial treatment of hyperthyroidism using a low but gradually increasing dosage of orally administered methimazole with careful serial monitoring of renal function and serum thyroxine concentration should minimize the adverse effects of treatment of hyperthyroidism on renal function in geriatric cats.

References and Suggested Reading

Adams WH, Daniel GB, Legendre AM: Investigation of the effects of hyperthyroidism on renal function in the cat. Proceedings of the Am Coll Vet Radiol. Honolulu, Hawaii, August 6–11, 1995, p 6/1.
Demonstration that excessive amounts of thyroxine can increase GFR and RPF in normal cats.

Adams WH, Daniel GB, Legendre AM, et al: Changes in renal function in cats following treatment of hyperthyroidism using [131]I. Vet Radiol and Ultrasound 38:231, 1997.
Demonstration that BUN and serum creatinine concentrations increase after treatment of hyperthyroidism by radioiodine.

Brown SA: Determinants of glomerular ultrafiltration in cats. Am J Vet Res 54:970, 1993.
Demonstration that a substantial portion of systemic arterial pressure is transmitted to the glomeruli in normal cats.

DiBartola SP, Broome MR, Stein BS, et al: Effect of treatment of hyperthyroidism on renal function in cats. J Am Vet Med Assoc 208:875, 1996.
Demonstration that BUN and serum creatinine concentrations increase after treatment of hyperthyroidism regardless of treatment modality.

Feldman EC, Nelson RW: Feline hyperthyroidism (thyrotoxicosis). In: Feldman EC, Nelson RW, eds: Canine and Feline Endocrinology. Philadelphia: WB Saunders, 1996, p 148.
Presentation of a protocol for the cautious administration of methimazole to hyperthyroid cats with abnormal renal function.

Graves TK, Olivier NB, Nachreiner RF, et al: Changes in renal function associated with treatment of naturally-occurring hyperthyroidism in cats. Am J Vet Res 55:1745, 1994.
Demonstration that GFR and RPF decrease markedly after treatment of hyperthyroid cats by surgical thyroidectomy.

Nemzek JA, Kruger JM, Walshaw R, et al: Acute onset of hypokalemia and muscular weakness in four hyperthyroid cats. J Am Vet Med Assoc 205:65, 1994.
Demonstration that the clinical course of hyperthyroidism in cats can be complicated by hypokalemia and muscle weakness.

Treatment of Hypoparathyroidism

Dennis J. Chew
Larry A. Nagode
Columbus, Ohio

PATHOPHYSIOLOGY AND DIFFERENTIAL DIAGNOSIS

Hypoparathyroidism is a state of absolute or relative deficit of parathyroid hormone (PTH) secretion that can be permanent or transient. Hypocalcemia and clinical signs referable to low ionized calcium are the hallmarks of advanced hypoparathyroidism. This latter condition is an uncommon cause of hypocalcemia in dogs and cats (Table 1), but it is the only condition requiring acute and chronic

TABLE 1. Conditions Associated With Hypocalcemia in Dogs and Cats*

Common
  Hypoalbuminemia (ionized calcium is normal)
  Chronic renal failure
  Puerperal tetany ("eclampsia")
  Acute renal failure
  Acute pancreatitis
  Undefined cause (mild hypocalcemia)
Occasional
  Hypoparathyroidism
    Primary
      Absence or destruction of parathyroid glands
        Idiopathic-spontaneous, immune
        Bilateral thyroidectomy
      Following sudden reversal of chronic hypercalcemia
        (atrophy of remaining parathyroid glands)
      Suppressed PTH secretion (without destruction of gland)
  Ethylene glycol intoxication
  Phosphate enema
  Following NaHCO₃ administration
  Soft tissue trauma, rhabdomyolysis
Uncommon
  Laboratory error
  Improper sample anticoagulant (EDTA)
  Rapid intravenous infusion of phosphates
  Acute calcium-free intravenous infusion (dilutional)
  Intestinal malabsorption, severe starvation
  Hypovitaminosis D
  Blood transfusion (citrated anticoagulant)
  Nutritional secondary hyperparathyroidism
  Infarction of parathyroid gland adenoma (dog)
  Hypomagnesemia
  Canine distemper virus affecting parathyroid gland
Human†
  Sepsis/critical illness
  Drug-induced hypoparathyroidism
    (aluminum, asparaginase, doxorubicin, cytosine
      arabinoside, cimetidine, ethanol)
  Antiresorptive agents
    (estrogen, plicamycin, calcitonin, bisphosphonates)
  Pseudohypoparathyroidism
  Parathyroid gland agenesis
  Osteoblastic bone neoplasia
  Hypercalcitonism
  ¹³¹I radiation damage

*Based on total serum calcium.
†Comparative causes in human patients; not yet documented in dogs or cats.
PTH, parathyroid hormone; EDTA, ethylenediaminetetra-acetic acid.

treatment to alleviate clinical signs associated with hypocalcemia. Hypoparathyroidism in dogs is most commonly an idiopathic or primary condition, whereas surgical removal or injury during thyroidectomy to correct hyperthyroidism is the most common condition in cats.

Inappropriately low levels of PTH cause hypocalcemia, hyperphosphatemia, and decreased levels of 1,25-dihydroxycholecalciferol (calcitriol). Hypocalcemia is explained by increased urinary loss (hypercalciuria), reduced bone mobilization, and decreased intestinal absorption (secondary effect) of calcium during periods of low PTH levels. Hyperphosphatemia results from the decreased urinary loss of phosphorus (hypophosphaturia), which overcomes decreased bone mobilization and intestinal absorption of phosphorus during periods of decreased PTH levels. PTH is a potent stimulator and phosphorus a potent inhibitor of the 25(OH)-cholecalciferol–1α-hydroxylase system in the renal tubules; consequently, the absence of PTH and the presence of hyperphosphatemia work together to decrease renal synthesis of calcitriol. Decreased levels of calcitriol contribute to hypocalcemia largely through decreased intestinal calcium absorption. A component of hypocalcemia that is unrelated to low PTH levels may arise from increased uptake of calcium into bone following rapid correction of long-standing hyperparathyroidism or hyperthyroidism, both of which are associated with loss of bone calcium prior to treatment (hungry bone syndrome).

Patients with hypoparathyroidism can be divided into three categories: (1) those with absence or destruction of parathyroid glands, (2) those with sudden correction of chronic hypercalcemia, or (3) those with suppressed secretion of PTH without parathyroid gland destruction. The most common category of hypoparathyroidism in dogs and cats is that associated with the absence or destruction of the parathyroid glands.

CLINICAL SIGNS

Clinical signs related to hypocalcemia are identical regardless of the underlying cause. Low plasma ionized calcium increases the excitability of neuromuscular tissue, which accounts for many of the clinical signs of hypoparathyroidism. Animals with mild decreases in ionized calcium generally display no obvious clinical signs. The duration and magnitude of the calcium depression, as well as the rate of calcium decline, interact to determine the severity of clinical signs. The most severe forms of hypocalcemia can cause death from harmful circulatory effects (hypotension and decreased myocardial contractility) and respiratory arrest from paralysis of respiratory muscles. Serum total calcium concentration of less than 4.0 mg/dl can cause death, especially if it has rapidly decreased to this level. Other electrolyte and acid-base abnormalities can either magnify or diminish the signs of hypocalcemia.

Patients with chronic hypocalcemia often display intermittent clinical signs despite a seemingly unchanging total serum calcium concentration. Although unpredictable, clinical signs often follow periods of exercise or excitement that may relate to respiratory alkalosis and reduction of the ionized fraction.

Clinical signs (Table 2) in dogs with chronic hypocalcemia caused by primary hypoparathyroidism are most commonly recognized in the form of seizures, muscle tremors or fasciculations, muscle cramping, stiff gait, and behavioral changes (restlessness and excitation, aggression, hypersensitivity to stimuli, disorientation). Neuromuscular signs in cats with chronic hypocalcemia associated with primary hypoparathyroidism are similar to those in dogs (muscle tremors, weakness, generalized seizures). Anorexia and lethargy seem more common in cats than in dogs with primary hypoparathyroidism. In cats, seizures have not been noted to be induced by excitement (as opposed to dogs), nor has prolapse of the third eyelid been a prominent finding (as has been noted in cats with acute hypocalcemia).

Clinical signs due to acute postoperative hypocalcemia are similar in dogs and cats and are related to excitation of neuromuscular tissues. Focal twitching of facial muscles and whiskers may be noticed prior to more generalized muscle tremors or seizures.

DIAGNOSIS

The diagnosis of hypoparathyroidism requires the evaluation of inclusionary and exclusionary criteria related to the causes of hypocalcemia (see Table 1). Although there are numerous causes of hypocalcemia, there is only one cause for the combination of low serum calcium, high serum phosphorus, and normal renal function (blood urea nitrogen [BUN] or creatinine) in the face of low PTH levels. Low serum calcium and high serum phosphorus levels can be encountered during nutritional secondary hyperparathyroidism, renal secondary hyperparathyroidism, following administration of a phosphate-containing enema, and with tumor lysis syndrome, but PTH is increased in all these conditions. A presumptive diagnosis of hypoparathyroidism can be made on the basis of low serum calcium, high serum phosphorus, normal renal function, and the absence of an obvious alternative diagnosis. The definitive diagnosis of hypoparathyroidism requires the finding of an inappropriately low PTH level during a time of hypocalcemia because hypocalcemia provides a strong stimulus to the normal parathyroid gland to secrete PTH at a high level. Since primary hypoparathyroidism requires lifelong treatment, confirmation of the diagnosis with PTH measurement is highly recommended.

TREATMENT

Treatment is individualized based on the severity of calcium-specific signs, the magnitude of the hypocalcemia, the rapidity of the decline in serum calcium levels, and trends toward a further decrease or stability in the serum calcium concentration. More aggressive treatment is prescribed for patients with severe signs of hypocalcemia, patients with severe ionized hypocalcemia with or without signs, and patients in which the serum calcium level appears to be steadily or rapidly declining. Acute, subacute, and chronic rescue treatment regimens are available using supplementation with calcium salts and vitamin D metabolites. The goal of therapy is to predictably and smoothly increase the serum calcium concentration to a level that alleviates the signs of hypocalcemia, lessens the likelihood of hypercalcemia developing later, and reduces the magnitude of hypercalciuria. For suspected temporary postsurgical hypoparathyroidism, it is desirable to keep serum calcium levels on the low side to maximize compensatory hypertrophy of remaining parathyroid glands.

No treatment regimen completely compensates for the full physiologic actions of absent PTH. Vitamin D metabolite treatment corrects the low intestinal absorption of calcium but does not completely protect the kidneys from hypercalciuria as would occur under the influence of PTH. Similarly, vitamin D metabolites do not exert as powerful an effect on bone in the absence of PTH. Replacement therapy with once-daily subcutaneous injections of human PTH-(1–34) to human patients was highly effective in providing good 24-hour calcemic control in a recent study. Better control of serum phosphorus and less hypercalciuria were additional benefits of PTH-(1–34) treatment compared with calcitriol treatments. Use of synthetic human PTH amino terminal compounds for treatment of veterinary patients is conceivable, since the amino-terminal portions of PTH appear to have been highly conserved in evolution and would be unlikely to elicit an immune response against the injected PTH.

Hypocalcemia that is severe enough to create clinical signs should be anticipated in dogs undergoing parathyroidectomy as treatment for hypercalcemia resulting from a parathyroid gland tumor. Those with very high levels of serum calcium, PTH, and serum alkaline phosphatase may

---

TABLE 2. Clinical Signs Associated With Hypocalcemia

Common
- Muscle tremors, fasciculations
- Seizures, status epilepticus
- Facial rubbing
- Muscle cramping
- Stiff gait
- Behavioral change
  - Restlessness, excitation
  - Aggression
  - Hypersensitivity to stimuli
  - Disorientation
  - Growling

Occasional
- Panting
- Pyrexia
- Lethargy, depression
- Anorexia
- Prolapse of third eyelid (cats)
- Posterior lenticular cataracts
- Electrocardiographic findings: Tachycardia/QRS alternans, QT interval lengthening

Uncommon
- None
- Polyuria, polydipsia
- Hypotension
- Respiratory arrest, death

be at greater risk for the development of postoperative hypocalcemia. In this instance, postoperative hypocalcemia is the consequence of acute hypoparathyroidism from chronic suppression of the remaining parathyroid glands as well as calcium uptake into "hungry bones." One should anticipate hypocalcemia in cats that undergo bilateral thyroidectomy, as up to 30% of patients can be expected to demonstrate a lower serum calcium level transiently.

We do not agree with any recommendation to wait for signs of tetany prior to instituting calcium-specific therapy to increase serum calcium. Pre-emptive therapy to increase serum calcium levels may be a good choice for patients with marked hypocalcemia despite an absence of clinical signs or for those in which calcium is steadily or rapidly declining. Prophylactic therapy to prevent hypocalcemia in dogs undergoing surgery for hyperparathyroidism should be considered, especially in those with more severe levels of hypercalcemia. Active vitamin D metabolites should be started before surgery in these instances because there is a lag until maximal effect; vitamin D metabolites given at the time of surgery or after surgery fail to prevent the development of hypocalcemia.

ACUTE MANAGEMENT OF HYPOCALCEMIA CAUSING TETANY OR SEIZURES

Tetany or seizures caused by hypocalcemia requires treatment with intravenous calcium salts. Calcium is given to effect at 5 to 15 mg /kg of elemental calcium (0.5 to 1.5 ml/kg of 10% calcium gluconate) over a 10- to 20-minute period. The percentage of calcium contained varies widely with the specific calcium salt (Table 3). There is no difference in the effectiveness of intravenous calcium salts to correct hypocalcemia when the dose is based on elemental calcium content. Calcium gluconate is often chosen as the calcium salt of choice because it is nonirritating if the solution is injected outside a vessel; calcium chloride is extremely irritating to tissues but provides more elemental calcium in each milliliter of solution (see Table 3).

The heart rate and electrocardiogram should be monitored during acute infusion of calcium salts. Bradycardia may signal the onset of cardiotoxicity from infusing calcium at too rapid a rate; sudden elevation of the ST segment, shortening of the QT interval, or premature ventricular complexes may also indicate cardiotoxicity from the calcium infusion. Not all clinical signs will immediately abate following acute correction of hypocalcemia, as reso-

lution of some signs may lag by as much as 30 to 60 minutes. Nervousness, panting, and behavioral changes may persist despite the return of normocalcemia during this period, perhaps reflecting a lag in cerebrospinal fluid equilibration with the calcium in extracellular water (as there is slow equilibration between calcium in extracellular water and that in cerebrospinal fluid). Hyperthermia that resulted from increased muscle tremor activity or seizures may also take some time to dissipate.

SUBACUTE MANAGEMENT OF HYPOCALCEMIA

The initial bolus injection of elemental calcium can be expected to decrease signs of hypocalcemia for a limited time, for as little as 1 hour to as long as 12 hours if the initial cause of the hypocalcemia persists. Vitamin D metabolites should be started as soon as possible because they require at least a few days before the effects to enhance intestinal calcium transport are maximized. Additional parenteral calcium salt administration will be necessary to maintain a required degree of calcemia until therapy with vitamin D metabolites is effective in maintaining serum calcium at acceptable levels.

Multiple intermittent intravenous injections of calcium salts can be given to control clinical signs, but this method is not recommended because wide fluctuations in serum calcium concentrations are likely to be encountered. The remaining two options are continuous infusion of calcium salts or the intermittent injection of subcutaneous calcium salts.

Continuous intravenous infusion of calcium is recommended at 60 to 90 mg/kg/day of elemental calcium (2.5 to 3.75 mg/kg/hr) until oral medications provide calcemic control. Initial doses in the higher range are administered to patients with more severe hypocalcemia, and the dose is decreased according to the level of calcemia achieved. The dose of intravenous calcium is tapered further as oral calcium salts and vitamin D metabolites become more effective.

Ten milliliters of 10% calcium gluconate provides 93 mg of elemental calcium. A convenient method to infuse calcium is available when intravenous fluids are given at a maintenance volume of 60 ml/kg/day (2.5 ml/kg/hour). Approximately 1 mg/kg/hr, 2 mg/kg/hr, or 3 mg/kg/hr of elemental calcium is provided by adding 10, 20, or 30 ml of 10% calcium gluconate respectively, to each 250-ml

TABLE 3. Treatment of Hypocalcemia With Parenteral Calcium*

Drug	Preparation	Available Calcium	Dose	Comment
Calcium gluconate	10% solution	9.3 mg of calcium/ml	Slow IV to effect (0.5–1.5 ml/kg)	Stop if bradycardia or shortened QT interval occurs
			OR	
			5–15 mg/kg/hr IV	Infusion to maintain normal calcium level
			OR	
			1–2 ml/kg diluted 1:1 with saline SC t.i.d.	May be given SC
Calcium chloride	10% solution	27.2 mg of calcium/ml	5–15 mg/kg/hr IV	Only given IV, as extremely caustic perivascularly

*Do not mix calcium solution with bicarbonate-containing fluids because precipitation may occur.

TABLE 4. **Treatment of Hypocalcemia With Oral Calcium Salts***

Drug	% Calcium Available	Preparation	Dose (mg/kg/day)	Comment
Calcium carbonate	40 (tablet)	Many sizes	25–50	Most common calcium supplement
Calcium lactate	13 (tablet)	325-, 650-mg tablets	25–50	
Calcium chloride	27	Powder	25–50	May cause gastric irritation
Calcium gluconate	10	Many sizes	25–50	

*When using oral calcium, calculate dose on elemental calcium content.

fluid bag. Obviously, the same rate of calcium infusion is provided by adding 20, 40, or 60 ml of 10% calcium gluconate to each 500 ml fluid bag to be infused at maintenance rates.

Calcium salts should not be added to fluid therapy preparations that contain lactate, acetate, bicarbonate, or phosphates because calcium salt precipitates can occur. Alkalinizing fluid therapy containing sodium bicarbonate decreases ionized calcium and may expose clinical signs of hypocalcemia in animals with borderline hypocalcemia and consequently should not be used.

Alternatively, fluids containing calcium can be administered subcutaneously. Calcium gluconate should be diluted at least 1:1 prior to subcutaneous injection; calcium chloride should not be used because it is highly irritating to tissues. The dose of calcium initially needed to control tetany can be given three to four times daily, or a dose of 60 to 90 mg/kg/day can be divided and given in subcutaneous fluids given several times a day. Doses of subcutaneous calcium should be tapered as described for continuous infusion of calcium.

SUBACUTE AND CHRONIC MAINTENANCE THERAPY

Supplemental elemental calcium is administered orally (Table 4) to guarantee adequate available calcium for intestinal absorption following activating effects from vitamin D metabolites. Oral calcium administered by pill or slurry is most important during initial treatment, especially if the animal is not eating. Active intestinal transport mechanisms of calcium uptake are under the control of calcitriol when calcium intake is low, but vitamin D–independent passive intestinal absorption of calcium occurs when calcium intake is high. One can take advantage of the passive mechanisms for intestinal calcium transport before vitamin D actions are effected in the intestine. Normal dietary intake

contains sufficient calcium to maintain adequate calcium levels in the presence of vitamin D metabolite treatment for most patients. Consequently, oral calcium salt supplementation can be tapered and discontinued in many instances as vitamin D compounds reach maximal effect.

Calcium carbonate is the most widely used oral preparation of the commonly prescribed calcium salts because it contains the greatest percentage of elemental calcium, and this translates into fewer pills administered. The degree of calcium ionization and bioavailability for absorption vary by the specific calcium salt and the conditions within the intestine; consequently, it is not simply a matter of determining the elemental calcium content of a specific oral calcium salt. Oral calcium is usually given at 25 to 50 mg/kg/day of elemental calcium divided over the day. Oral calcium carbonate serves as an intestinal phosphate binder in addition to providing additional calcium for intestinal absorption. It is advisable to continue oral calcium carbonate therapy for its intestinal phosphate-binding effects if serum phosphorus levels remain increased. Lower serum phosphorus concentrations may allow increased endogenous synthesis of calcitriol as the phosphate-mediated inhibition of the renal tubular 1α-hydroxylase system in the renal tubules is relieved.

Vitamin D preparations include ergocalciferol, cholecalciferol, dihydrotachysterol, 25(OH)-cholecalciferol (calcidiol), 1α-hydroxycholecalciferol, and 1,25-dihydroxycholecalciferol (Table 5). Ergocalciferol, dihydrotachysterol, and calcitriol are the preparations most commonly used in veterinary medicine. Lifelong treatment with some form of vitamin D metabolite is necessary for patients with primary hypoparathyroidism or those with postoperative hypocalcemia that fails to resolve.

Ergocalciferol is favored by some because of its low cost, but it has several features that make it the least attractive agent for calcemic actions. Ergocalciferol and its immediate metabolite 25-hydroxyergocalciferol have mini-

TABLE 5. **Treatment of Hypocalcemia With Vitamin D Compounds**

Preparation	Daily Dose	Time for Maximal Effect to Occur	Time for Toxicity Effect to Resolve
Vitamin D$_2$ (ergocalciferol)	*Initial:* 4000–6000 U/kg/day *Maintenance:* 1000–2000 U/kg once daily to once weekly	5–21 days	1–18 wk
Dihydrotachysterol	*Initial:* 0.02–0.03 mg/kg/day *Maintenance:* 0.01–0.02 mg/kg q24–48 hr	1–7 days	1–3 wk
1,25-dihydroxyvitamin D$_3$ (calcitriol)	*Initial:* 20–30 ng/kg/day × 3–4 days *Maintenance:* 5–15 ng/kg/day	1–4 days	2–7 days

mal vitamin D receptor avidity, and consequently high doses are employed to increase interactions with the vitamin D receptor. Calcitriol is about 1000 times as effective as the parent vitamin D and 500 times as effective as its precursor calcidiol (25-hydroxyvitamin D) in binding to the natural calcitriol receptor. Ergocalciferol is highly lipid-soluble, requiring weeks to saturate body stores in order to achieve maximal effect; it also has a long half-life. Consequently, prolonged periods of hypercalcemia occur after any overdose with ergocalciferol. Additionally, there is extreme individual variation in the dose of ergocalciferol required to achieve the target level of serum calcium. Loading doses reduce the time required to achieve maximal calcemic effect (see Table 3).

Dihydrotachysterol (DHT) is a synthetic vitamin D analogue with onset of maximal calcemic action between that of ergocalciferol and calcitriol, as is the half-life of its biologic action. DHT possesses both 1α and 25-hydroxy groups (after 25-hydroxylation in the liver) but lacks a 3β-hydroxyl, dramatically reducing the efficiency of 25-hydroxydihydrotachysterol in receptor binding. The polarity and lower dose requirements of DHT limit its storage in fat compared with ergocalciferol. Toxicity from hypercalcemia can still be prolonged (up to 30 days), however, and some patients still exhibit wide variation in the dose required to achieve target levels of serum calcium. Loading doses of DHT also reduce the time for maximal calcemic effects to occur.

Calcitriol is the vitamin D metabolite of choice to provide calcemic actions because it has the most rapid onset to maximal action and the shortest biologic half-life. The dose of calcitriol can be adjusted more frequently because of more "real-time" effects on serum calcium. Should hypercalcemia occur, it is likely to abate quickly following dose reduction. The half-life of calcitriol in blood is 4 to 6 hours, whereas its biologic half-life is 2 to 4 days, which facilitates the rapid correction of hypercalcemia should it occur. Loading protocols for the use of calcitriol in animals have not been reported, but it seems logical to employ one when more rapid calcium correction is desirable. A calcitriol dose of 30 to 60 ng/kg/day has been recommended; this dose may be satisfactory as a loading dose, but in our experience it is far too high for chronic maintenance therapy. Calcitriol doses for chronic maintenance therapy in humans range from 10 to 40 ng/kg/day, with mean doses of 10 to 20 ng/kg/day; doses are divided twice daily. We have employed loading doses of 20 to 30 ng/kg/day for the initial 3 to 4 days and maintenance doses of 5 to 15 ng/kg/day in most patients. The dose of calcitriol is divided twice daily to ensure sustained priming effects on intestinal epithelium for calcium transport. Calcitriol is commercially available in 0.25- and 0.50-μg capsules (250 and 500 ng per respective capsule; Rocaltrol, Hoffman-LaRoche). It is likely that reformulation of calcitriol in doses suitable for a variety of animal sizes will be necessary. It may be useful to prescribe calcitriol in liquid formulation so that small adjustments in dosage can be made accurately. A number of specialty pharmacies reformulate human drugs for veterinary use and can create any calcitriol doses needed.

Thiazide diuretics are sometimes used to treat humans with primary hypoparathyroidism as a maneuver to reduce hypercalciuria. This is especially useful in humans when hypercalciuria continues despite a serum calcium level that is within the low normal range. It would be likely that further reduction of the vitamin D metabolite dose would be necessary after starting thiazides because calcium levels would be higher because of more reclaimed calcium by the kidney. The effects of thiazide diuretics on urinary calcium excretion are debatable in dogs and unknown in cats.

FOLLOWING THE PATIENT AND MANAGING COMPLICATIONS

Periods of hypocalcemia and hypercalcemia occur sporadically in patients during initial efforts to manage serum calcium levels. Daily measurement of total serum calcium during the initial stabilization of serum calcium is necessary, and then weekly calcium measurements will suffice during maintenance therapy until the target level of calcium has been achieved and maintained. Quarterly measurement of total serum calcium is recommended thereafter in animals with permanent hypoparathyroidism. The target level for serum calcium ideally should be just below the reference range rather than the middle or upper range of normal calcium concentrations. This not only lessens the likelihood that hypercalcemia will develop but also reduces the level of hypercalciuria that occurs in patients missing the renal effects of PTH. Maintaining a mildly decreased level of serum calcium also ensures an ongoing stimulus for hypertrophy of any remaining parathyroid tissue in patients with postoperative hypoparathyroidism.

It is important to change the dose of vitamin D metabolite gradually following evaluation of serum calcium values and to make sure that enough time has been given to see its maximal effect before the dose is changed yet again. The time lag for this effect varies with the vitamin D metabolite employed (see Table 3). Dosage increases of 10 to 20% are recommended for most cases that are still below the desired calcium target level. Vitamin D metabolites and calcium salt supplementation should be temporarily discontinued in patients with hypercalcemia. Doses should be reduced until the serum calcium level falls to just less than the reference range.

Hypercalcemia is a serious side effect that can result in the death of the animal or chronic renal damage severe enough to cause both acute and chronic renal failure. Owners should be taught the early signs of hypercalcemia and instructed to seek veterinary attention so that serum calcium can be measured if signs suggest hypercalcemia. Signs of hypercalcemia that clients are likely to recognize include polydipsia and polyuria, anorexia, vomiting, and depression. Animals with severe hypercalcemia will require a combination of hospitalization, intravenous fluids, furosemide, steroids, and perhaps bisphosphonates or calcitonin initially (see next article). All patients with symptomatic vitamin D metabolite–induced hypercalcemia should be placed on a calcium-restricted diet because hypervitaminosis D is a form of hypercalcemia in which intestinal hyperabsorption of calcium contributes substantially to the development of hypercalcemia.

The long-term prognosis for quality and length of life have not been reported for dogs and cats during treatment of chronic hypoparathyroidism. Patients that have frequent episodes or long duration of hypercalcemia during treatment have poor prognoses. Patients that maintain calcium levels in the target zone are often managed successfully for years. It is our experience that patient management employing calcitriol is easier and more successful in inducing and maintaining target zone calcium levels than are older therapeutic approaches.

Hypercalciuria, nephrocalcinosis, urolithiasis, and reduced renal function have all been noted in human patients treated for chronic hypoparathyroidism. As many as 80% of human patients treated for 2 years or longer have decreased creatinine clearance. These abnormalities can be attributed to episodes of hypercalcemia and hyperphosphatemia as well as hypercalciuria that occurs in the absence of the full calcium-retaining actions of PTH at the level of the renal tubule. In the absence of PTH, hypercalciuria occurs more readily at all levels of serum calcium concentration and is especially severe as calcium concentrations approach the normal level, which increases the filtered load of calcium. Nephrocalcinosis, reduced renal function, and chronic renal failure have also been suspected in veterinary patients receiving long-term treatment for hypoparathyroidism, but the risk for these disorders has not been critically evaluated.

Great care is given to tailor the dosage of vitamin D metabolites in human patients to both the level of serum calcium and the degree of hypercalciuria achieved during treatment. Maintaining a mildly decreased serum calcium level does not guarantee that hypercalciuria will not occur. Hypercalciuria is monitored by measuring 24-hour millimolar urinary calcium excretion or by determination of the urinary calcium:urinary creatinine ratio. Guidelines to assess the magnitude of hypercalciuria in veterinary patients have not yet been developed.

Vitamin D metabolite treatment is gradually tapered and then discontinued in patients with postsurgical hypoparathyroidism because hypocalcemia is usually transient. Most cats are able to maintain normal levels of serum calcium 2 weeks after thyroidectomy, although some may take as long as 3 months. Dogs with hypocalcemia usually require 6 to 12 weeks of treatment following removal of a parathyroid gland tumor. We usually start tapering vitamin D metabolites 1 month into therapy. If serum calcium declines substantially, the previous dose is resumed and a taper attempted once again 1 or 2 months later. Permanent hypoparathyroidism is likely if failure to maintain reasonable levels of serum calcium occur following a taper of vitamin D metabolite at 3 months.

References and Suggested Reading

Berger B, Feldman EC: Primary hyperparathyroidism in dogs: 21 cases (1976–1986). J Am Vet Assoc 191:350, 1987.
  Provides further detail about the development of hypocalcemia following surgical removal of parathyroid gland adenoma as treatment for primary hyperparathyroidism in dogs.
Birchard SJ, Peterson ME, Jacobson A: Surgical treatment of feline hyperthyroidism: Results of 85 cases. J Am Anim Hosp Assoc 20:705, 1984.
  This is the original large series describing intracapsular techniques for surgical removal of thyroid glands and associated frequency of hypocalcemia and its duration.
Bruyette DS, Feldman EC: Primary hypoparathyroidism in the dog. J Vet Intern Med 2:7, 1988.
  Further detail is provided about the diagnosis and treatment of primary hypoparathyroidism in the dog.
Feldman EC, Nelson RW: Hypocalcemia and primary hypoparathyroidism. In: Feldman EC, Nelson RS, eds: Canine and Feline Endocrinology and Reproduction, 2nd ed. Philadelphia: WB Saunders, 1996, pp 497–516.
  Overview of hypocalcemia in general.
Kallet AJ, Richter KP, Feldman EC, et al: Primary hyperparathyroidism in cats: Seven cases (1984–1989). J Am Vet Med Assoc 199:1767, 1991.
  Original case series of cats with hyperparathyroidism.
Peterson ME: Hypoparathyroidism. In: Kirk RW, ed: Current Veterinary Therapy IX. Philadelphia: WB Saunders, 1986, pp 1039–1045.
  Good detail about the mechanisms of action of various vitamin D metabolites.
Welches CD, Scavelli TD, Matthiesen DT, et al: Occurrence of problems after three techniques of bilateral thyroidectomy in cats. Vet Surg 18:392, 1989.
  Review of possible advantages of one surgical technique over another during treatment of hyperthyroidism in cats.

Hypercalcemia and Primary Hyperparathyroidism in Dogs

EDWARD C. FELDMAN
RICHARD W. NELSON
Davis, California

Hypercalcemia is usually an abnormality serendipitously identified on serum biochemical analysis. Disorders associated with hypercalcemia in dogs include lymphosarcoma, acute and chronic renal failure, vitamin D toxicosis, hypoadrenocorticism, apocrine gland carcinomas of the anal sac, multiple myeloma, systemic mycoses, and primary hyperparathyroidism (PHP). Information from the history, physical examination, complete blood count (CBC), urinalysis, serum biochemistry analysis, thoracic and abdominal radiographs, abdominal ultrasonogram, and examination of cytologic and biopsy specimens usually provide adequate information to establish the diagnosis. A tentative diagnosis of PHP may be supported with measurement of the serum parathyroid hormone (PTH) concentration, and final diagnosis requires histologic confirmation of excised parathyroid tissue. PHP is a relatively uncommon cause of hypercalcemia and the diagnosis can be obvious or elusive. Many of the steps involved in the evaluation of a hypercalcemic dog fail to contribute to the final diagnosis because results from dogs with lymphosarcoma can mimic those from dogs with PHP. This discussion presents the diagnostic approach to hypercalcemic dogs with the final diagnosis being PHP.

DIFFERENTIAL DIAGNOSIS FOR HYPERCALCEMIA

Since hypercalcemia is almost always an unsuspected finding, it is never a mistake to obtain a second blood sample to be certain that laboratory error has been ruled out. In our experience, laboratory error is extremely uncommon. With confirmation of hypercalcemia, the veterinarian should review the signalment and history with the owner to identify clues not noted initially. Dogs with PHP are usually 6 years of age or older and of either sex; a breed predisposition in the Keeshound is suspected. Dogs with PHP, unlike dogs with most other diseases that cause hypercalcemia, are not usually ill. Their clinical signs are relatively mild and usually consist only of polyuria-polydipsia, muscle weakness, decreased activity, and decreased appetite.

From the history, one can attempt to identify an obvious explanation for the hypercalcemia, such as possible exposure to toxins containing vitamin D (some rodenticides), evidence of pain resulting from a lytic bone lesion (multiple myeloma or mammary tumor), difficulty eating because of oral lesions associated with renal failure, or a waxing and waning course of illness sometimes noted with hypoadrenocorticism. The physical examination should also be repeated in an attempt to identify the cause of hypercalcemia. The spine and long bones should be palpated to identify bone pain, and evaluation of the mammary chain for neoplasia, the oral cavity for rubber jaw or lesions consistent with renal failure, the rectal area for apocrine gland carcinoma, the heart rate and pulse for abnormalities consistent with hypoadrenocorticism, and the peripheral lymph nodes for enlargement suggestive of lymphoma should be carried out. Dogs with PHP have unremarkable physical examinations, and parathyroid masses are rarely palpable.

A thorough review of the CBC, serum biochemistry profile, and urinalysis should be completed. The urine specific gravity is commonly less than 1.020 in hypercalcemic dogs with renal disease, hypoadrenocorticism, and hyperparathyroidism. Urinary tract infection is common in these disorders. The CBC in PHP is usually unremarkable, as opposed to the normocytic normochromic nonregenerative anemia common in chronic renal failure, hypoadrenocorticism, and various neoplasias (such as lymphoma). The serum biochemistry profile is also available to assess the blood urea nitrogen and creatinine and serum phosphate levels for increases consistent with renal failure, hyperkalemia and hyponatremia consistent with hypoadrenocorticism, hyperglobulinemia consistent with myeloma, or ab-

normal liver enzyme activity in association with a variety of malignancies. Dogs with PHP usually have none of these abnormalities, aside from the small percentage that have mild increases in serum alkaline phosphatase or the small percentage with increases in blood urea nitrogen, creatinine, and phosphate. To this point, the only added expense has been the repeated serum calcium assay.

Assuming the review of the history, physical examination, and data base has not defined the cause for hypercalcemia, thoracic radiographs are the next diagnostic study. The primary purpose is to assess the cranial mediastinum and perihilar areas for a mass consistent with lymphoma. If lymphadenopathy is identified, biopsy specimens should be evaluated to confirm the diagnosis of lymphoma. Radiographs also provide an opportunity to evaluate the lungs for neoplasia or systemic mycoses, the spine and ribs for lytic lesions caused by neoplasia, and the heart for microcardia of hypoadrenocorticism. Thoracic radiographs in dogs with PHP are typically unremarkable. Abdominal radiographs can also be assessed, although ultrasonographic examination of the abdomen is preferred. The size and consistency of the liver, spleen, and mesenteric and sublumbar lymph nodes can be evaluated for abnormalities suggestive of malignancy (lymphoma). Diagnostic imaging to evaluate for malignancy (lymphoma) applies to a variety of tumors located in other organs, but tumors other than lymphoma are an uncommon cause of hypercalcemia. When possible, abnormal areas should be aspirated or biopsied to determine the presence or absence of neoplasia. The size and consistency of the kidneys can be assessed, although renal failure should have been ruled out by the initial blood test results. Dogs with PHP occasionally have renal mineralization and 30 to 40% have uroliths. Otherwise, the abdominal evaluation is typically unremarkable. If these studies fail to indicate a diagnosis other than PHP, the index of suspicion for this condition increases. However, until a specific cause for hypercalcemia is confirmed, lymphoma should never be ruled out.

CONFIRMATION OF PRIMARY HYPERPARATHYROIDISM

Additional testing is available to aid in confirming a diagnosis of PHP. Serum ionized calcium concentrations, when available, are persistently increased in dogs with PHP, whereas they are often normal to decreased in dogs with hypercalcemic renal failure. Serum PTH concentrations are commercially available, and normal to increased concentrations confirm the diagnosis of PHP in hypercalcemic dogs without renal failure. Dogs with renal failure may also have increased serum PTH concentrations, but within the context of the renal parameters, the serum phosphate concentration, serum ionized calcium concentration (usually normal to decreased in dogs with renal failure), and other pertinent information, it should be possible to distinguish PHP from renal failure. Serum PTH-related protein (PTHrP) concentrations that are increased in hypercalcemic dogs are most consistent with lymphoma or apocrine gland tumors of the anal sac. If a specific explanation for hypercalcemia remains elusive, we recommend response to treatment be a last-resort approach. Before any medication is given, aspiration or biopsy of lymph nodes, spleen, or liver, or a combination of these organs, should be considered in an attempt to rule out lymphoma. This condition is emphasized here because it can be a difficult diagnosis to confirm in some dogs. In addition, once a dog with lymphoma has been treated with glucocorticoids, for example, that diagnosis becomes even more difficult to confirm.

LOCALIZATION OF PARATHYROID TISSUE CAUSING HYPERPARATHYROIDISM

Once it is believed that the diagnosis of PHP is confirmed, the most cost-effective and expedient approach to patient management would be surgical exploration of the neck. Abnormal, autonomously secreting, parathyroid masses may not always be obvious at surgery, although experienced surgeons rarely have difficulty in identifying the parathyroid tissue causing hypercalcemia. The abnormal parathyroid adenoma, carcinoma, or adenomatous hyperplastic tissue is typically larger and darker than normal parathyroid glands. Surgeons may benefit from knowing which side of the neck or specific location within one side of the neck it is likely that a tumor or abnormal parathyroid tissue will be found.

Abnormal parathyroid tissue has been localized in humans using ^{99}Tc-sestamibi nuclear scintigraphy. Scintigraphy has been reported to be effective in two dogs with PHP. However, facilities for nuclear scintigraphy are not widely available, results in dogs with PHP have been inconsistent, and the cost of such a procedure may exceed that of cervical exploratory surgery.

Ultrasonographic examination of the cervical area has recently received attention because it is becoming widely available, is noninvasive, and is relatively cost-efficient. Ultrasonography, as much as any diagnostic tool used in veterinary medicine, is operator-dependent. The skill of the individual performing the examination is a major factor in assessing the value of any study. As facilities with equipment, various high-frequency transducers, and the experience of sonographers improve, this diagnostic tool will become even more useful. More than 90% of dogs with PHP that we have evaluated with ultrasonography have had a visible mass that has correlated with the size and location of the abnormal parathyroid tissue identified at surgery. Ultrasonographic examination of the cervical area has become a routine component of the diagnostic evaluation of dogs with hypercalcemia at our institution.

Recent attempts to localize the side of the neck in which abnormal parathyroid tissue was situated using selective venous sampling and measuring the serum concentration of PTH has not been satisfactory. Venous drainage from parathyroids is into the jugular veins. In theory, serum PTH concentrations from the contralateral jugular vein and the systemic circulation (cephalic vein) should be similar, but serum PTH concentration from the jugular vein on the side of the abnormal parathyroid tissue would be increased. The serum PTH concentrations from both jugular veins and one cephalic vein from a group of dogs with PHP were evaluated. An obvious gradient distinguishing the side of the abnormal parathyroid tissue was not obvious. Failure to find results consistent with the theory employed may be due to the fact that the venous drainage is not as expected, because the blood obtained was not below the site of

parathyroid drainage into the jugular veins, or some other factor. In any case, this procedure has not yet been demonstrated to be helpful.

INITIAL MANAGEMENT OF HYPERCALCEMIA

Hypercalcemia has the potential for impairing renal tubular concentrating ability, reducing renal flow and decreasing the glomerular filtration rate. Progressive renal injury leading to azotemia and renal tubular degeneration becomes more likely in animals with persistent elevations of ionized calcium, although dogs with PHP are typically (but not always) spared. Thus, a focused and expedient clinical and laboratory evaluation is important to minimize the lag between the initial identification of hypercalcemia and the start of specific therapy. In the interim, treatments that lower the serum calcium level may be indicated. Such therapy is particularly important in animals with azotemia or an "increased" calcium-phosphorus product (e.g., calcium $\times$ phosphorus >70). The severity of hypercalcemia alone is not an indication for intervention. Some of the dogs with PHP in our series have had total serum calcium concentrations in excess of 19 mg/dl and ionized calcium concentrations in excess of 2 mmol/L. These dogs have typically had serum phosphate concentrations less than 3 mg/dl and products much less than 60. These dogs have not had any clinical signs of hypercalcemia other than polyuria, polydipsia, and muscle weakness. They have been clinically stable, and their electrocardiograms have been unremarkable.

If treatment is needed, fluid therapy is the initial method to lower serum calcium and preserve renal perfusion. Once blood and urine have been obtained for analysis, an IV catheter should be placed and the patient rehydrated over the next 6 to 12 hours as required. Subsequent volume expansion with intravenous 0.9% saline can promote calcium excretion, and a saline diureses is initiated by infusing volumes of 120 to 180 ml/kg over 24 hours. This therapy is usually combined with administration of the loop diuretic furosemide (2 mg/kg IV every 8 hours), which potentiates calciuresis. To prevent iatrogenic hypokalemia, intravenous potassium chloride may be needed, and initial supplementation rates of 16 to 20 mEq of potassium chloride/L saline solution are usually adequate. These general measures reduce serum calcium to an acceptable range, although the effect on hypercalcemia may be modest in some patients and totally inadequate in others.

Should the preceding measures fail, other drugs may be needed to lower the serum calcium level. Glucocorticoids may effectively decrease serum calcium levels. Prednisolone (2 mg/kg PO or IM every 12 hours) increases calcium excretion in the urine, reduces intestinal absorption, and inhibits calcium resorption from bone. Glucocorticoids are particularly useful in the hypercalcemia associated with malignant lymphoma; however, this treatment can impede a definitive diagnosis by reducing neoplastic cell mass and should be withheld, if possible, until lymphoma has been ruled out. Refractory hypercalcemia can be treated with mitramycin or with calcitonin (5 U/kg, IM or SC every 8 hours). These are costly and more complex treatments. Veterinarians inexperienced in using these drugs should first consult an oncologist or internist about specific aspects of therapy and associated adverse effects.

TREATMENT OF PRIMARY HYPERPARATHYROIDISM

The treatment of dogs suspected of having PHP also serves to confirm the diagnosis. Complete exploratory surgery of the thyroid area is recommended, with an effort made to evaluate both sides of the neck and both the ventral and dorsal surfaces of the thyroid lobes. In most dogs with PHP, the abnormal parathyroid tissue is solitary, darker, and larger than normal parathyroid tissue and is easily recognized and extirpated. Only the abnormal parathyroid tissue is removed if possible, although the thyroid gland is usually removed along with abnormal internal parathyroid masses. If no parathyroid mass is observed and the diagnosis is thought to be correct, one thyroid-parathyroid complex should be removed and examined histologically. If two abnormal parathyroid glands are observed, both should be removed. Three or four abnormal parathyroid glands pose a dilemma and usually one gland is left in situ. The observation of two, three, or four abnormal parathyroid glands is atypical and suggests hyperplasia rather than adenoma.

If the presurgery serum calcium concentration is greater than 11.5 mg/dl but less than 14.0 mg/dl, we simply monitor serum calcium or ionized calcium concentrations twice daily for 5 to 7 days after surgery. Vitamin D therapy is instituted only if the serum calcium concentration decreases to less than 8.0 mg/dl, the ionized calcium decreases to less than 0.85 mmol/L, or clinical signs of tetany are observed (see preceding article). If the serum calcium concentration prior to surgery is ≥15 mg/dl, the incidence of postsurgical hypocalcemia is greater, and we initiate vitamin D therapy (dihydrotachysterol; 0.03 mg/kg/day; divided b.i.d., and then tapered to ever-decreasing dosages over a 2- to 6-month period) the morning before surgery or immediately after surgery. Monitoring of serum calcium is carried forth as described, and parenteral calcium is administered only if tetany occurs or is thought to be imminent.

References and Suggested Reading

De Vries SE, Feldman EC, Nelson RW, et al: Primary parathyroid gland hyperplasia in dogs: Six cases (1982–1991). J Am Vet Med Assoc 202:1132, 1993.
   Review of primary hyperparathyroidism caused by primary parathyroid gland hyperplasia.
Feldman EC, Nelson RW: Canine and Feline Endocrinology and Reproduction. Philadelphia: WB Saunders, 1996, pp 455–497.
   A review of the causes, consequences, and treatment of hypercalcemia in dogs, focusing on primary hyperparathyroidism.
Torrence AG, Nachreiner R: Intact parathyroid hormone assay and total calcium concentration in the diagnosis of disorders of calcium metabolism in dogs. J Vet Intern Med 3:86, 1989.
   Review of the causes for hypercalcemia and the use of PTH assay results for these conditions.
Wisner ER, Nyland TG, Feldman EC, et al: Ultrasonographic evaluation of parathyroid glands in hypercalcemic dogs. Vet Radiol Ultr 34:108, 1993.
   A review of ultrasound examination of the neck in hypercalcemic dogs.

CVT Update: Monitoring Treatment of Diabetes Mellitus in Dogs and Cats

KATHY L. CRENSHAW
New York, New York

Long-term monitoring of diabetic dogs and cats can be difficult for veterinarians and frustrating for pet owners. Diabetes is best evaluated by frequent measurement of the patient's blood glucose concentrations at home; however, this monitoring technique is not practical for diabetic pets. Therefore, other parameters need to be assessed by pet owners on a routine basis. Regular veterinary attention is also needed for proper regulation of most diabetic animals. There are clearly individual preferences among clinicians for long-term monitoring of diabetes. This article provides a review of available methods.

HOME MONITORING

The owner's observations of the pet's clinical signs of diabetes are extremely valuable and can provide an accurate assessment of the diabetic condition. In the diabetic animal, water consumption and urination appear to be closely linked to the degree of metabolic control. Most pet owners are able to distinguish these clinical signs accurately. Although some diabetic animals may not appear polydipsic (water intake >90 ml/kg/day for dogs; 45ml/kg/day for cats), their water consumption may be much higher than that considered normal for the particular animal.

Attitude, appetite, and activity level also are useful parameters that should be monitored closely by the pet owner. If possible, body weight should be measured at home on a weekly to biweekly basis.

Urine glucose testing has traditionally been recommended by most veterinarians as the best at-home method to evaluate insulin therapy in the diabetic animal. However, certain problems are associated with urine glucose testing (see *CVT XII,* p. 403): (1) the urine glucose concentration reflects the blood glucose level over the period of urine formation and is not indicative of the blood glucose level at the time the urine is voided and tested; (2) the renal threshold for glucose is variable in animals, ranging from 175 to 220 mg/dl in dogs and slightly higher in cats; (3) owner compliance is often poor with this test; (4) a Somogyi effect occurs; and (5) false-negative and false-positive results can occur. Despite these problems, urine testing can be helpful with diabetic regulation, especially if the urine is tested every day and more than once a day. Trends in urine glucose testing are much more meaningful as an aid in glucose regulation than are isolated urine samples.

RECHECK RECOMMENDATIONS

Diabetic pets should be examined on a regular basis by a veterinarian. A complete physical examination that includes measurement of body weight, and evaluation of home monitoring records should be performed every 3 to 6 months in stable patients. Often, animals need more frequent attention in the early stages of diabetic regulation. The owner's injection technique should be observed.

Blood testing should include evaluation of glucose homeostasis by the measurement of serum fructosamine or glycosylated hemoglobin as well as evaluation of the overall well-being of the animal (i.e., serum biochemical profile and complete blood count). A urine sample should be obtained for determination of glucose and ketone concentrations. It is usually not necessary to perform a glucose curve on a well-regulated diabetic patient.

Fructosamine

The term *fructosamine* refers to albumin and other plasma proteins that have been linked to a sugar (usually glucose) by a nonenzymatic chemical reaction, a process known as glycosylation. The serum fructosamine concentration is proportional to the blood glucose concentration over the life span of the glycated protein measured (e.g., in humans, 2 to 3 weeks in the case of albumin). Therefore, measuring the serum fructosamine concentration is a means of assessing the *average* blood glucose concentration in an individual over the preceding few weeks. Although the life span of albumin in cats is not known, it is assumed to be similar to that in dogs, approximately 1 to 2 weeks (Dixon et al, 1953).

Serum fructosamine can be measured quickly, easily, and economically, and the test has been shown to be useful in evaluating dogs and cats with diabetes. Recently completed studies suggest that the fructosamine concentration reflects metabolic control more objectively than do sporadic blood glucose measurements. Measurement of serum fructosamine should be included as part of the initial diagnostic work-up in the diabetic animal and should be monitored periodically during follow-up evaluations. This test is especially helpful in the cat because fructosamine is not affected by stress hyperglycemia, which commonly occurs during blood collection (Crenshaw et al, 1996). Healthy cats and nondiabetic sick cats typically have fructosamine concentrations of less than 400 μmol/L.

Glycosylated Hemoglobin

The nonenzymatic and irreversible binding of glucose with hemoglobin over the life span of erythrocytes is commonly thought of as the classic example of the glycation process and is a reflection of the average blood glucose concentration over the life span of the red blood cells (70 and 120 days in cats and dogs, respectively). The major problems with this test are (1) lack of universal reference standards for glycosylated hemoglobin assays for dogs and cats, (2) the falsely elevated levels that occasionally occur, (3) the limited availability of the test, and (4) the expense of the test. In addition, this test is not the best choice for assessment of long-term glycemic control in cats because feline hemoglobin and erythrocytes demonstrate certain peculiarities that may make the test invalid in this species. Normal glycosylated hemoglobin values in dogs are 4 to 8%, which may vary depending on the test method used and the laboratory. Poorly controlled diabetic dogs have values greater than 10%.

Glucose Curve

The difficult to control diabetic patient requires a more extensive evaluation, which usually includes serial glucose determinations throughout the day. A 12- to 24-hour in-hospital glucose curve may also be necessary when there are problems with blood glucose regulation. Glucose curves are commonly performed for the following reasons: (1) to document insulin overdosage (subclinical or overt hypoglycemia), (2) to document insulin resistance in patients receiving high doses of insulin (>2 U/kg per administration), and (3) to re-evaluate poorly controlled diabetes.

A glucose curve performed at home in the animal's natural environment will be a more accurate reflection of the actual glucose metabolism than an in-hospital curve. Many animals do not eat normally in the hospital and are frightened and stressed, especially cats. In some instances, an intravenous catheter may be placed at the hospital and the test performed in the animal's home. However, most animals will need to be in a hospital to have a glucose curve performed. The animal should be kept on as normal a routine as possible, that is, fed the usual food in the usual amount at the usual time of day. If possible, the owner should feed the animal, administer the insulin, and come to the veterinary hospital as soon as possible to begin the curve. Samples should be drawn every 1 to 2 hours for a period of 12 to 24 hours. Some animals may not need to have an indwelling intravenous catheter placed but rather samples can be obtained with a tuberculin syringe and small-gauge needle (a glucometer requires only a drop of whole blood for determination of glucose concentration). Results of the glucose curve should show the insulin effectiveness, the glucose nadir, and the duration of insulin action.

Insulin effectiveness is evaluated by the decrease in glucose concentration with respect to the dose and type of insulin administered (see *CVT XII,* p. 387). Ideally, the glucose concentration should range between 100 and 200 mg/dl throughout most of the day, although many diabetic animals will be considered well regulated by owners and veterinarians with a glucose determination ranging between

100 and 300 mg/dl. Resolution of clinical signs as perceived by the owner is also an important indicator of insulin effectiveness and must be evaluated in conjunction with the curve results.

If the glucose concentration does not decrease to within an acceptable range and the animal has clinical signs of diabetes, several problems should be considered: (1) the insulin dose may be too low, (2) the owner's administration technique may be incorrect, (3) the insulin may be biologically inactive (out of date, heat-inactivated), (4) the type of insulin may be inappropriate (a long-acting insulin such as Ultralente is less potent than an intermediate-acting insulin such as Lente or NPH), or (5) concurrent disease may be present, causing insulin resistance (see *CVT XII*, p. 390).

The glucose nadir, or lowest blood glucose concentration, should be approximately 75 to 100 mg/dl. If the glucose decreases to less than 65 mg/dl, the animal may be at risk for the Somogyi effect (hypoglycemia triggering the release of glucose-elevating hormones, leading to hyperglycemia), and the insulin dosage should be reduced. If the glucose nadir is greater than 120 mg/dl, the insulin dosage may need to be increased, depending on other findings such as body weight, resolution of clinical signs, and serum fructosamine concentration.

If results of the glucose curve indicate that blood glucose concentrations are out of the acceptable range for most of the day, the insulin type, dosage, or frequency of insulin administration needs to be changed. Insulin usually needs to be administered every 12 hours to both dogs and cats (intermediate-acting insulin, such as NPH or Lente, administered every 12 hours is a good initial insulin choice for both dogs and cats). Occasionally, in the cat, satisfactory control may be achieved using a long-acting insulin such as Ultralente given once daily.

Although the glucose curve theoretically is the test of choice when a diabetic is not well regulated, the procedure is labor intensive, and results are affected by a variety of factors that are difficult to control. Therefore, interpretation can be difficult and confusing. Extremely nervous or aggressive animals may not tolerate the procedure well, and results may be significantly altered by the pet's level of stress. Fructosamine or glycosylated hemoglobin levels may be a better alternative in these animals.

References and Suggested Reading

Crenshaw KL, Peterson ME, Heeb LA, et al: Serum fructosamine concentration as an index of glycemia in cats with diabetes mellitus and stress hyperglycemia. J Vet Intern Med 10:360, 1996.
Fructosamine is a meaningful test for diagnosis of diabetes, for differentiating diabetes from stress hyperglycemia, and for monitoring metabolic control in treated diabetic cats.

Dixon FJ, Maurer PH, Deichmiller MP: Half-lives of homologous serum albumins in several species. Proc Soc Exp Biol Med 83:287, 1953.
Describes half-life of albumin in animals.

Feldman EC, Nelson RW: Diabetes mellitus. In: Canine and Feline Endocrinology and Reproduction, 2nd ed. Philadelphia: WB Saunders, 1996, p 339.
In-depth review of disease, therapy, complications, and monitoring.

Hasegawa S, Sako T, Takemura N, et al: Glycated hemoglobin fractions in normal and diabetic dogs measured by high performance liquid chromatography. J Vet Med Sci 53:65, 1991.
Review of glycosylated hemoglobin in dogs.

Hasegawa S, Sako T, Takemura N, et al: Glycated hemoglobin fractions in normal and diabetic cats measured by high performance liquid chromatography. J Vet Med Sci 54:789, 1992.
Review of glycosylated hemoglobin in cats.

Jensen AL: Serum fructosamine as a screening test for diabetes mellitus in non-healthy middle-aged to older dogs. J Vet Med A 41:480, 1994.
Fructosamine used as screening test for diabetes in older, non-healthy dogs.

Kaneko JJ, Kawamoto M, Heusner AA, et al: Evaluation of serum fructosamine concentration as an index of blood glucose control in cats with diabetes mellitus. Am J Vet Res 53:1797, 1992.
Study of fructosamine to evaluate glycemic control in diabetic cats.

Miller E: Long-term monitoring of the diabetic dog and cat: clinical signs, serial blood glucose determinations, urine glucose, and glycated blood proteins. Vet Clin North Am (Sm Anim Pract) 25:571, 1995.
In-depth review of long-term monitoring.

Reusch CE, Liehs MR, Hoyer M, et al: Frustosamine: A new parameter for diagnosis and metabolic control in diabetic dogs and cats. J Vet Intern Med 7:177, 1993.
Fructosamine is a valuable parameter for diagnosis and metabolic control of diabetes in dogs and cats.

Treatment of Non–Insulin-Dependent Diabetes Mellitus in Cats Using Oral Hypoglycemic Agents

DEBORAH S. GRECO
Fort Collins, Colorado

Diabetes mellitus (DM) is one of the most common endocrine diseases of cats. Islet amyloid polypeptide is a recently discovered protein that may be involved in the pathogenesis of feline non–insulin-dependent diabetes mellitus (NIDDM) (O'Brien, 1993). The majority of cats with DM probably suffer from NIDDM; however, by the time clinical signs develop, the disease has often progressed to the point that there is little insulin reserve. The physiologic

TABLE 1. Oral Hypoglycemic Drugs Used in the Treatment of Non–Insulin-Dependent Diabetes Mellitus in Humans and Cats

Drug	Dose	Frequency	Side Effects	Mechanism of Action
Glipizide (Glucotrol)	2.5–5 mg/cat	b.i.d.–t.i.d., PO	Hepatotoxicity, hypoglycemia, vomiting	Increases insulin secretion and sensitivity
Glimeperide (Amaryl)	1–4 mg (H) Unknown (C)	q24 (H) Unknown (C)	Same as above but lower incidence	As above
Metformin (Glucophage)	500–750 mg (H) Unknown (C)	b.i.d. (H) Unknown (C)	Anorexia, vomiting	Inhibits hepatic glucose production
Precose (acarbose)	50 mg (H) 12.5–25 mg (C)	b.i.d.–t.i.d. with meals	Flatulence, soft stool	Alpha$_1$-glucosidase inhibitor, impairs glucose absorption from gut
Troglitazone	200–400 mg (H) Unknown (C)	q24 hr	Mild decreases in WBC, platelet, and Hb counts	Increases insulin receptor sensitivity
Chromium	1,000 µg (H) Unknown (C)	q24 hr	?	Increases insulin receptor sensitivity
Vanadium	0.2 mg/kg/day	q24 hr in food or water	Anorexia, vomiting	Increases insulin receptor sensitivity

H, human; C, cat; WBC, white blood count; Hb, hemoglobin.

abnormalities associated with NIDDM dictate the approach to therapy. The primary physiologic abnormalities of NIDDM are increased hepatic glucose production; insulin receptor and postreceptor resistance or defects; and impaired insulin secretion. The treatment of NIDDM is aimed at attenuating the physiologic abnormalities of NIDDM by decreasing hepatic glucose output and glucose absorption from the intestine, increasing peripheral insulin sensitivity, and increasing insulin secretion from the pancreas. This discussion considers the therapy for NIDDM in cats from a physiologic approach.

THERAPEUTIC GOALS OF ORAL HYPOGLYCEMIC THERAPY IN NON–INSULIN-DEPENDENT DIABETES

The therapeutic goals in the treatment of cats with NIDDM include amelioration of the metabolic abnormalities of diabetes and extension of life. These goals can be difficult to attain in cats with NIDDM because of the broader clinical spectrum of islet cell dysfunction. However, NIDDM does permit a greater choice of therapeutic options. For example, diet alone may be used or diet may be combined with oral hypoglycemic agents.

Human diabetic patients can be divided into three therapeutic categories according to beta-cell function: (1) type I—those who require exogenous insulin to control hyperglycemia (type I diabetes), (2) those who require only dietary therapy because of sufficient islet reserve and insulin sensitivity to maintain relatively normal glucose levels, or (3) those with sufficient islet reserve and insulin sensitivity to respond to oral hypoglycemic drugs. Human beings with NIDDM (type II diabetes) are often classified according to their beta-cell function based on provocative testing. In cats, the differentiation of these catagories is almost impossible prior to treatment; therefore, the clinician must rely on the *response* to oral hypoglycemic agents as a guide to whether the cat has sufficient beta-cell function to be managed with oral hypoglycemic agents.

ORAL HYPOGLYCEMIC AGENTS: INDICATIONS

Oral hypoglycemic agents include the sulfonylureas (glipizide, glyburide, glimeperide), biguanides (metformin),

thiazolidinediones (troglitazone), alpha-glucosidase inhibitors (acarbose), and transition metals (chromium, vanadium) as summarized in Table 1. Most of the oral hypoglycemic agents work either by increasing insulin secretion or decreasing insulin resistance, glucose absorption, or hepatic glucose production (Fig. 1). Indications for oral hypoglycemic therapy in cats include normal or increased body weight, lack of ketones, probable type II diabetes with no underlying disease (pancreatitis, pancreatic tumor) and the owner's willingness to administer oral medication rather than an injection.

Drugs That Enhance Insulin Secretion

The mechanism of action of the sulfonyureas is to increase insulin secretion and reduce insulin resistance; however, some of these agents also cause an increase in hepatic glucose output. This leads to delayed hyperinsulinemia, weight gain, and atherosclerosis in humans undergoing sulfonylurea therapy (Kahn and Shechter, 1990). By provoking insulin release, sulfonylureas may promote the progression of pancreatic amyloidosis and hence increase

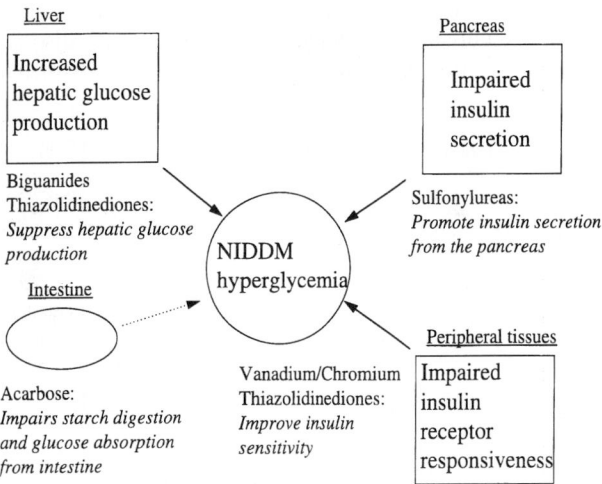

Figure 1. Diagram of the physiologic abnormalities that contribute to hyperglycemia in NIDDM in humans and cats, and the site of action of selected oral hypoglycemic agents.

the risk of long-term complications of diabetes. In cats, glipizide has been used to successfully treat DM at a dosage of 2.5 to 5 mg b.i.d. (see *CVT XII,* p. 401 for a full discussion). An outline for monitoring and managing cats undergoing glipizide therapy is shown in Figure 2. Side effects of oral hypoglycemic agents include severe hypoglycemia (rare in cats), cholestatic hepatitis, and vomiting. Gastrointestinal side effects, which occur in about 15% of cats treated with glipizide, resolve when the drug is administered with food (Ford, 1995). The author's personal experience with glipizide as an oral hypoglycemic agent in cats has been disappointing. However, this may be related to patient selection rather than to overt failure of the drug. Cats with early type II diabetes are most likely to respond to any oral hypoglycemic agent. Therefore, emphasis should be placed on identifying cats with NIDDM early in the development of the disease. A new sulfonylurea, glimepiride (Amaryl), has recently been introduced in the human market; this compound has fewer side effects and causes less fasting hyperinsulinemia than glipizide.

Drugs That Inhibit Hepatic Glucose Release

Metformin belongs to the biguanide group of oral hypoglycemic agents. These agents work by *inhibiting* hepatic glucose release and by improving peripheral insulin sensitivity (Kahn and Shechter, 1990). Biguanides may be used alone or in conjunction with other oral hypoglycemic agents to treat type II DM in humans (DeFronzo and Goodman, 1995). One advantage of the biguanides is that they do not promote insulin release; therefore, there is little potential for the development of hypoglycemia when metformin is used as a sole agent. Furthermore, metformin does not cause progression of pancreatic amyloid deposition (DeFronzo and Goodman, 1995). In a recent large randomized parallel group, double-blind control study, human patients with NIDDM underwent treatment with metformin or with placebo. Compared with patients in the placebo group, the metformin group had lower mean fasting plasma glucose concentrations and glycosylated hemoglobin values. Side effects of the biguanides include lactic acidosis and gastrointestinal signs such as nausea and diarrhea. Contraindications for metformin therapy in humans, and presumably in cats, include concurrent renal disease, liver dysfunction, or cardiac disease. Experience with this

drug as treatment for NIDDM in cats is limited. The author has treated two cats and observed no change in blood glucose concentrations at a dosage of 125 to 250 mg b.i.d. PO. Furthermore, the high dose (250 mg) was associated with severe gastrointestinal signs including vomiting and diarrhea.

Drugs That Impair Intestinal Glucose Absorption

The alpha-glucosidase inhibitors impair glucose absorption from the intestine by decreasing fiber digestion and hence glucose production from food sources (Kahn and Shechter, 1990). These drugs were initially developed as starch blockers to control obesity in humans and may have application to the treatment of obese diabetic cats. Acarbose is used as initial therapy in obese prediabetic patients suffering from insulin resistance or as adjunct therapy with sulfonylureas or biguanides to enhance the hypoglycemic effect in patients with DM. Side effects include flatulence, loose stool, and diarrhea at high dosages. One advantage of these medications is that they are not absorbed systemically and may be used in conjunction with other oral hypoglycemic agents. They are not indicated in patients of low or normal body weight because of their effects on nutrition. The author has had limited experience with acarbose at a dosage of one-quarter to one-half tablet per cat with meals; side effects are more common at the high end of the dose and include semiformed stool or in some cases overt diarrhea. The glucose-lowering effect of acarbose is mild, with blood glucose concentrations decreasing only into the 250 to 350 mg/dl range.

Drugs That Enhance Peripheral Insulin Sensitivity

A new class of oral hypoglycemic agents that are receiving attention in medicine are the thiazolidinedione compounds (Saltiel and Olefsky, 1996). These drugs facilitate the action of insulin in skeletal muscle and adipose tissue. Although the exact mechanisim of action is unknown, thiazolidinediones facilitate insulin-dependent glucose disposal and inhibit hepatic glucose output by attenuation of gluconeogenesis and glycogenolysis. In addition, the thiazolidinediones have been shown to have beneficial ef-

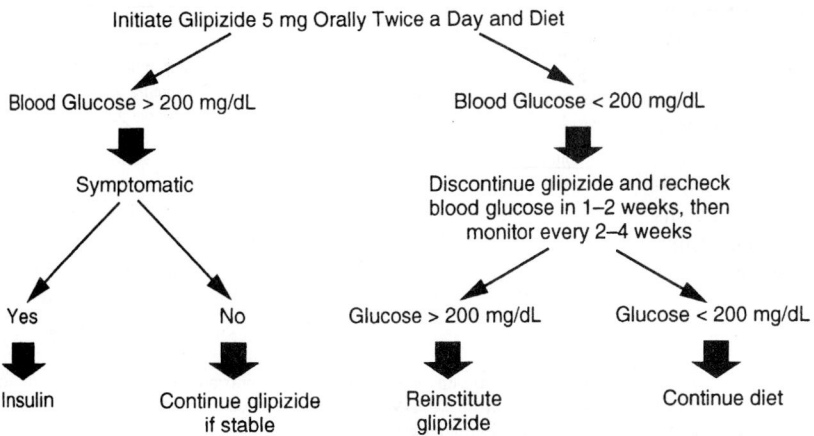

Figure 2. Possible clinical consequences of glipizide treatment. (From Ford SL: NIDDM in the cat: Treatment with the oral hypoglycemic medication glipizide. Vet Clin North Am Small Anim Pract 25[3]:611, 1995, with permission.)

fects on the lipid disturbances associated with NIDDM. Troglitazone is the thiazolidinedione compound that has progressed to clinical development for use in humans with NIDDM. In fact, some authors have suggested that the use of this drug early in the course of NIDDM may slow the progression of NIDDM (Saltiel and Olefsky, 1996). Side effects of troglitazone were minimal and included transient mild decreases in white blood cells, platelets, and hemoglobin (Berkowitz et al, 1996). No hypoglycemic reactions were described. The author as yet has no experience with these compounds in cats.

Compounds containing the metals vanadium and chromium have been shown to have extensive insulin-like properties when administered in the drinking water of mice suffering from experimentally induced DM (type I and type II). A recent United States Department of Agriculture study of 180 patients with NIDDM found that administration of 1,000 µg of chromium picolinate once daily resulted in amelioration of the classic signs of diabetes and normalization of blood levels of hemoglobin A1c. In Type I diabetes, vanadium decreases, but does not eliminate, the need for insulin (Cam et al, 1993). In type II diabetes, constant suppression of blood glucose is achieved with vanadium (Brichard et al, 1989). Studies have documented restoration of secretion of insulin in patients with type II diabetes treated with vanadium, suggesting reversal of "glucose toxicity" and disease progression. Oral vanadate causes a marked and sustained improvement in glucose homeostasis in NIDDM by exerting an insulin-like effect on peripheral tissues; furthermore, vanadium prevents the exhaustion of insulin stores in the pancreas. Vanadium compounds are currently being investigated as insulin-mimetic agents in humans, documenting their promise as a future therapy for type II diabetes.

Despite the efficacy of oral vanadium and chromium compounds in lowering blood glucose levels, the exact mechanism of action is unknown. Current research indicates that vanadium bypasses the insulin receptor and activates glucose metabolism within the cell (Shechter, 1990) By acting at a postreceptor site, vanadium is the ideal treatment for type II DM that results from a lack of insulin receptor responsiveness. Unlike insulin, vanadium and chromium do not lower blood glucose concentrations in normal animals.

Studies in our laboratory indicate that low doses (0.2 mg/kg/day) of oral vanadium will decrease blood glucose and serum fructosamine concentrations and alleviate the signs of diabetes (polydypsia, polyuria) in cats with *early* type II DM. Side effects include anorexia and vomiting initially; however, most cats showed no ill effects when vanadium therapy was reinstituted. Long-term toxicity of vanadium is related to the accumulation of the metal in organs such as bone, kidney, liver, adipose tissue, and pancreas. We have observed acute renal failure (blood urea nitrogen >100 mg/dl, creatinine >12 mg/dl) in one patient after 1 year of vanadium therapy; however, the cat recovered renal function (blood urea nitrogen <40 mg/dl, creatinine <3 mg/dl) after discontinuation of the metal. Humans ingest vanadium as a solution in juice and chromium as a tablet; however, cats will ingest vanadium more readily in food than in water.

INSULIN AND ORAL HYPOGLYCEMICS: DO THEY MIX?

A change from insulin to oral hypoglycemic agents or vice versa may be necessary in some diabetic cats. If a cat is particularly sensitive to insulin or exhibits transient diabetes because of reversal of "glucose toxicity," a change to an oral hypoglycemic agent should be considered. Conversely, if a cat is managed with oral hypoglycemic agents and ketosis develops, the cat should be switched to insulin therapy. Agents that impair glucose absorption from the intestine (acarbose) or increase insulin sensitivity (vanadium, metformin, troglitazone) may be combined with insulin to improve glucose control. Vanadium has been shown to be beneficial in conjunction with insulin in rat and mice models of IDDM (Shechter, 1990). In the case of brittle diabetes in which small incremental changes in insulin dose may precipitate hypoglycemia, addition of a drug that enhances the action of insulin may lead to a reduction in the insulin dosage required to attain euglycemia. In human patients, acarbose and metformin are commonly used in conjunction with insulin and other oral hypoglycemic agents (sulfonylureas) that cause insulin release (DeFronzo and Goodman, 1995). Caution should be used in combining any oral hypoglycemic agent with insulin, as hypoglycemic reactions may occur and greater experience is needed before firm recommendations can be advanced.

MONITORING HYPOGLYCEMIC AGENT THERAPY IN CATS

It appears that methods of assessing *long-term* glycemic control are better indicators of response to therapy with oral hypoglycemics than are spot glucose determinations or blood glucose curves. The author prefers to monitor the resolution of clinical signs of DM, such as polydipsia and polyuria and serum fructosamine concentrations in cats undergoing oral hypoglycemic therapy. Serum fructosamine concentrations less than 450 mg/dl are consistent with moderate to good long-term control of hyperglycemia. Body weight should increase or remain stable and polydipsia-polyuria should resolve with effective oral hypoglycemic therapy.

References and Suggested Reading

Berkowitz K, Peters R, Kjos SL, et al: Effect of troglitazone on insulin sensitivity and pancreatic beta-cell function in women at high risk for NIDDM. Diabetes 45:1572, 1996.
  Large clinical study of troglitazone treatment in women at high risk for NIDDM; few side effects observed in the treated group.
Brichard SM, Pottier AM, Henquin JC: Long term improvement of glucose homeostasis by vanadate in obese hyperinsulinemic fa/fa rats. Endocrinology 125:2510, 1989.
  Early work on the use of vanadium compounds in a model of type II diabetes in rats.
Cam MC, Pederson RA, Brownsey RW, et al: Long-term effectiveness of oral vanadyl sulphate in streptozotocin-diabetic rats. Diabetologia 36:218, 1993.
  Long-term study of glucose control by vanadium in rats with experimentally induced type I diabetes mellitus.
DeFronzo RA, Goodman AM: Efficacy of metformin in patients with non–insulin-dependent diabetes mellitus. N Engl J Med 333:541, 1995.
  Large controlled clinical trial in humans comparing placebo

and metformin or placebo and metformin combined with sulfonyl-ureas.

Ford S: NIDDM in the cat: Treatment with the oral hypglycemic medication, glipizide. Vet Clin North Am Sm Anim Pract 25:599, 1995.
Review of the use of glipizide in cats.

Kahn CR, Shechter Y: Insulin, oral hypoglycemic agents and the pharmacology of the endocrine pancreas. In: Goodman Gilman A, Rall TW, et al, eds: The Pharmacological Basis of Therapeutics, 8th ed. New York: Pergamon Press, 1990, pp 1463–1495.
Basic pharmacology, side effects, and clinical use of oral hypoglycemic agents in humans.

Saltiel AR, Olefsky JM: Thiazolidinediones in the treatment of insulin resistance and type II diabetes. Diabetes 45:1661, 1996.
Excellent recent review of thiazolildinedione drug family: possible uses in diabetes and other diseases.

Shechter Y: Insulin-mimetic effects of vanadate: Possible implications for future treatment of diabetes. Diabetes 39:1, 1990.
Review of the insulin-like effects of vanadium.

Unger RH, Foster DW: Diabetes mellitus. In: Wilson JD, Foster DW, eds: Textbook of Endocrinology, 7th ed. Philadelphia: WB Saunders, 1985, pp 1062–1064.
Textbook chapter on the treatment of NIDDM in humans.

Complications Associated With Insulin Treatment of Diabetes Mellitus

RICHARD W. NELSON
EDWARD C. FELDMAN
Davis, California

HYPOGLYCEMIA

Hypoglycemia is a common complication of insulin therapy. Signs of hypoglycemia are most apt to occur following sudden large increases in insulin dosage, with excessive overlap of insulin action in dogs and cats receiving insulin twice a day, during unusually strenuous exercise, following prolonged inappetence, and in insulin-treated cats that have reverted to a non–insulin-dependent state. In these situations, severe hypoglycemia may occur before the diabetogenic hormones (i.e., glucagon, cortisol, epinephrine, and growth hormone) are able to compensate for and reverse low blood glucose concentrations. Signs of hypoglycemia include lethargy, weakness, head tilting, ataxia, and seizures. The occurrence of clinical signs is dependent on the rate of blood glucose decline as well as on the severity of hypoglycemia. Treatment consists of glucose administered as food, sugar water, or dextrose intravenously. Insulin therapy should be reinitiated once glucosuria or hyperglycemia, or both, have been documented. Whenever signs of hypoglycemia occur, adjustments in insulin therapy must be made. The owner should be instructed to decrease the insulin dosage by 25 to 50%, continue that dose for 2 to 3 days, and then return to the veterinarian for the dog or cat to be evaluated with serial blood glucose determinations.

Persistent Euglycemia Following Hypoglycemia

Hyperglycemia and glucosuria may not recur until 2 to 5 days after hypoglycemia. In some diabetic dogs and cats, hyperinsulinemia caused by excessive insulin overdosage or too frequent insulin administration and subsequent accumulation of circulating insulin prevents recurrence of hyperglycemia. Impaired glucose counterregulation may also promote prolonged hypoglycemia. Secretion of the diabetogenic hormones, most notably epinephrine and glucagon, stimulates hepatic glucose secretion and helps counter severe hypoglycemia. A deficient counterregulatory response to hypoglycemia has been identified as early as 1 year after diagnosis of insulin-dependent diabetes mellitus in humans (White et al, 1983). As a consequence, when the blood glucose concentration approaches 60 mg/dl, there is no compensatory response by the body to increase the blood glucose, and prolonged hypoglycemia ensues. An impaired counterregulatory response to hypoglycemia has also been documented in dogs with insulin-dependent diabetes mellitus. Dogs with impaired counterregulation had more problems with hypoglycemia than did diabetic dogs without impaired counterregulation. This condition should be considered in a diabetic dog or cat that is exquisitely sensitive to small doses of insulin or with problems of prolonged hypoglycemia after administration of an acceptable dosage of insulin.

Transient Clinical Diabetes Mellitus

Failure of hyperglycemia to recur within a week of hypoglycemia suggests transient clinical diabetes mellitus. This condition occurs in approximately 20% of treated diabetic cats but is uncommon in diabetic dogs and is usually associated with the end of diestrus in bitches. Cats (and presumably dogs) with transient clinical diabetes have pancreatic islet pathologic features and impaired insulin secretory capabilities (Feldman and Nelson, 1996). Subclinical diabetes becomes clinical when beta-cell function is stressed by concurrent insulin antagonistic drugs or disease. Euglycemia and subclinical diabetes may be re-established after improving hyperglycemia with insulin therapy and treating concurrent insulin antagonistic disorders.

RECURRENCE OF CLINICAL SIGNS

Recurrence or persistence of clinical signs (i.e., lethargy, polyuria, polydipsia, polyphagia, weight loss) is perhaps the most common "complication" of insulin therapy in diabetic dogs and cats. Recurrence or persistence of clinical signs is usually caused by problems with the owner's technique of administering insulin; problems with insulin therapy as it relates to insulin type, dosage, species or frequency of administration; or problems with responsiveness to insulin caused by concurrent inflammatory, infectious, neoplastic, or hormonal disorders (i.e., insulin resistance).

Administration Technique and Insulin Activity Problems

Problems with insulin activity or the administration technique should be ruled out before insulin therapy is adjusted or a diagnostic evaluation for concurrent inflammatory, infectious, neoplastic, or hormonal disorders is undertaken. Failure to administer an appropriate dosage of biologically active insulin can mimic insulin resistance because of an unrecognized insulin underdosage. Such underdosage can result from administration of biologically inactive insulin (e.g., outdated, overheated, mixed by shaking), administration of diluted insulin, use of inappropriate insulin syringes for the concentration of insulin (e.g., U100 syringe with U40 insulin), or problems with the insulin administration technique (e.g., misunderstanding how to read the insulin syringe, inappropriate injection technique or site). The easiest ways to identify these types of problems are careful observation of owner administration technique and administration of new, undiluted insulin by the clinician and measurement of several blood glucose concentrations throughout the day. Changes in insulin therapy or a diagnostic evaluation, or both, to rule out causes of insulin resistance may be warranted, depending on the blood glucose results.

Insulin Overdosage and Glucose Counterregulation

An excess dosage of insulin may cause overt hypoglycemia, glucose counterregulation (Somogyi phenomenon), or insulin resistance. The Somogyi phenomenon results from a normal physiologic response to impending hypoglycemia induced by excessive insulin. When the blood glucose concentration declines to less than 65 mg/dl or when the blood glucose concentration drops rapidly regardless of the glucose nadir, direct hypoglycemia-induced stimulation of hepatic glycogenolysis and secretion of diabetogenic hormones, most notably epinephrine and glucagon, increase the blood glucose concentration, minimize signs of hypoglycemia, and cause marked hyperglycemia within 12 hours of glucose counterregulation (Feldman and Nelson, 1983). Diagnosis of insulin-induced hyperglycemia requires the demonstration of hypoglycemia (<65 mg/dl) followed by hyperglycemia (>300 mg/dl) within one 24-hour period following insulin administration. Therapy involves reducing the insulin dose. If the diabetic dog or cat is receiving an "acceptable" dose of insulin (i.e., ≤1.5 U/

kg in the dog; ≤5 U per cat), the insulin dosage should be decreased 10 to 25%. If the dog or cat is receiving a large amount of insulin (e.g., >2.2 U/kg), glycemic regulation should be reinitiated using the insulin dosage recommended for the initial regulation of the diabetic dog or cat. The glycemic effects of the new insulin dosage should be assessed 7 to 10 days later and adjustments made accordingly.

Secretion of diabetogenic hormones during the Somogyi phenomenon may induce insulin resistance, which can last 24 to 72 hours following the hypoglycemic episode. If serial blood glucose concentrations are evaluated on the day of hypoglycemia, the Somogyi phenomenon will be identified and the insulin dosage lowered accordingly. However, if blood glucose concentrations are monitored after secretion of the diabetogenic hormones, insulin resistance may be diagnosed and the insulin dosage increased, further exacerbating the Somogyi phenomenon. A cyclic history of 1 or 2 days of good glycemic control followed by several days of poor control should raise the suspicion of insulin resistance caused by glucose counterregulation. Establishing the diagnosis may require several days of hospitalization and serial blood glucose curves. An alternative approach that we prefer is to arbitrarily reduce the insulin dose and have the owner evaluate the patient's response (based on clinical signs) over the ensuing 2 to 5 days. If clinical signs of diabetes worsen following a reduction in the insulin dose, another cause for the insulin resistance should be pursued. However, if the owner reports no change or improvement in clinical signs, continued gradual reduction of the insulin dosage should be pursued.

Short Duration of Insulin Effect

In many diabetic dogs and cats, the duration of effect of intermediate and long-acting insulins is considerably less than 24 hours. As a result, hyperglycemia (>250 mg/dl) occurs for prolonged periods each day. This hyperglycemia may begin as early as 6 hours after insulin administration. Owners of these pets usually mention continuing problems with evening polyuria and polydipsia or weight loss. A diagnosis of short duration of insulin effect is made by demonstrating hyperglycemia (>250 mg/dl) within 18 hours or less of the insulin injection, whereas the lowest blood glucose concentration is maintained at greater than 80 mg/dl. The clinician must evaluate multiple blood glucose concentrations obtained throughout the day to establish the diagnosis. One or two afternoon blood glucose determinations consistently fail to identify the problem. Treatment involves changing the type of insulin or the frequency of administration, or both.

Inadequate Insulin Absorption

Subcutaneous administration of insulin does not guarantee that the insulin will be absorbed into the circulation for subsequent interaction with insulin receptors. Slow or inadequate absorption of subcutaneously deposited insulin is most commonly observed in diabetic cats receiving Ultralente insulin (Broussard and Peterson, 1994). Ultralente insulin is a long-acting insulin that has a slow onset and prolonged duration of effect. In approximately 20% of the cats seen in our practice, Ultralente insulin is absorbed from the subcutaneous site of deposition too slowly for it to be effective in maintaining acceptable glycemic control. In these cats, the blood glucose concentration may not decrease until 6 to 10 hours after the injection or, more commonly, the blood glucose concentration decreases minimally despite insulin dosages of 8 to 12 U given every 12 hours. As a consequence, the blood glucose concentration remains greater than 300 mg/dl for most of the day. We have had success by switching these cats from Ultralente to Lente or NPH insulin given twice a day.

When changing the type of insulin, a more potent insulin should be substituted for the previous insulin. We generally switch to the next most potent insulin and reduce the insulin dosage (usually to amounts initially used to regulate the diabetic dog or cat) to avoid hypoglycemia. For example, cats treated with Ultralente insulin are switched to Lente insulin at 1 to 2 U/injection, dogs treated with Lente insulin are switched to NPH insulin at 0.5 U/kg, and so forth. The duration of effect becomes shorter as the potency of the insulin increases, which may necessitate a change in the frequency of administration.

Circulating Insulin-Binding Antibodies

Insulin antibodies result from repeated injections of a foreign protein (i.e., insulin). The more divergent the insulin molecule being administered from the species being treated, the greater the likelihood that significant or worrisome amounts of insulin antibodies will form. The amino acid sequences of canine, porcine, and recombinant human insulin are similar, and the amino acid sequences of feline and bovine insulin are similar. All species of insulin available commercially are effective in most diabetic dogs and cats. However, insulin immunogenicity and production of insulin antibodies can alter the duration of insulin activity and, in some patients, the ability to decrease blood glucose concentrations (Bolli et al, 1984). Preliminary studies using enzyme-linked immunosorbent assay to detect insulin antibodies in insulin-treated diabetic dogs suggest that the prevalence of insulin antibodies is common in dogs treated with beef insulin and is associated with erratic glycemic control in some dogs. In these dogs, blood glucose concentrations typically fluctuate between 200 and 400 mg/dl and the status of glycemic control vacillates from day to day, but overt insulin resistance (i.e., blood glucose concentrations consistently >400 mg/dl) is not evident. Excessive insulin-binding antibodies causing insulin resistance characterized by blood glucose concentrations consistently greater than 400 mg/dl is uncommon. Insulin-binding antibodies can also cause erratic fluctuations in the blood glucose concentration, with no correlation between the timing of insulin administration and changes in blood glucose concentration. Fluctuations in blood glucose concentration presumably result from changes in the circulating free insulin concentration as antibody-binding affinity for insulin changes (Bolli et al, 1984). A sudden decrease in antibody-binding affinity results in increased concentrations of circulating free insulin and decreased blood glucose concentrations, and vice versa. In contrast, insulin antibody formation is infrequent in dogs treated with re-

combinant human insulin, and glycemic control often improves when the source of insulin is changed from beef to recombinant human insulin. In an attempt to avoid problems with insulin effectiveness, we prefer to use recombinant human insulin in diabetic dogs initially, recognizing that the probability of having to administer insulin twice each day is high.

Preliminary studies suggest that the prevalence of insulin antibodies is uncommon in cats treated with recombinant human insulin. Use of a longer-acting insulin takes priority over the species of insulin in cats. We prefer to use Ultralente insulin of recombinant human origin initially, in the hope of obtaining adequate glycemic control with administration of insulin once a day. Although beef and pork Lente and NPH insulin are effective in many cats, usually they must be administered twice a day. In some cats, the duration of effect of beef and pork Lente and NPH insulin is too short, and even twice daily administration is not effective in controlling clinical signs. For these reasons, we reserve the use of beef and pork Lente or NPH insulin for cats that do not respond to Ultralente insulin because of poor absorption from subcutaneous sites of deposition and for cats with suspected insulin resistance caused by excessive antibody production directed against human recombinant insulin.

Concurrent Disorders Causing Insulin Resistance

There are many disorders (see *CVT XII*, p. 390) that can interfere with the effectiveness of insulin and cause the persistence of clinical signs of diabetes (Table 1). Obtaining a complete history and performing a thorough physical examination are the two most important steps in identifying concurrent disorders. Abnormalities identified in the history or by a thorough physical examination may suggest a concurrent insulin-antagonistic disorder or infectious

TABLE 1. Recognized Causes for Poor Response to Insulin Treatment or Insulin Resistance in the Diabetic Dog and Cat

Caused by Insulin Therapy	Caused by Concurrent Disorder
Inactive insulin	Diabetogenic drugs
Diluted insulin	Hyperadrenocorticism
Improper administration technique	Diestrus (bitch)
Inadequate dose	Acromegaly (cat)
Somogyi phenomenon	Infection, especially oral cavity and urinary tract
Inadequate frequency of insulin administration	Hypothyroidism (dog)
Inadequate insulin absorption, especially with Ultralente insulin	Hyperthyroidism (cat)
Anti-insulin antibody excess	Renal insufficiency
	Liver insufficiency
	Cardiac insufficiency
	Glucagonoma (dog)
	Pheochromocytoma
	Chronic inflammation, especially pancreatitis
	Pancreatic exocrine insufficiency
	Severe obesity
	Hyperlipidemia
	Neoplasia

process and can give the clinician direction in the diagnostic evaluation of the patient. If the history and physical examination are unremarkable, a complete blood count, serum biochemical analysis, urinalysis with bacterial culture, serum thyroxine concentration (cat), and abdominal ultrasound (dog) should be obtained to screen further for concurrent illness. Additional diagnostic tests will depend on the results of these initial screening tests.

ALLERGIC REACTIONS TO INSULIN

Significant reactions to insulin occur in up to 5% of human diabetics treated with insulin and include erythema, pruritus, and induration at the injection site and, uncommonly, systemic manifestations characterized by urticaria, angioneurotic edema, or frank anaphylaxis (Kahn and Rosenthal, 1979). Atrophy or hypertrophy of subcutaneous tissue (i.e., lipoatrophy and lipodystrophy) may also occur at the insulin injection site. Many humans with insulin allergy have histories of sensitivity to other drugs as well. Allergic reactions are usually seen with injection of nonpurified animal insulins. The prevalence of allergic reactions has decreased with the increasing use of recombinant human insulins in humans.

Allergic reactions to insulin have been poorly documented in diabetic dogs and cats. Pain on injection of insulin is usually caused by inappropriate injection technique or the site of injection and not an adverse reaction to insulin per se. Chronic injection of insulin in the same area of the body may cause thickening of the skin and subcutaneous tissues, which may be caused by an immune reaction to insulin or some other protein (e.g., protamine) in the insulin bottle. Rotation of the injection site helps prevent this problem. Rarely, diabetic dogs and cats will experience focal subcutaneous edema and swelling at the site of insulin injection. Insulin allergy is suspected in these animals. Treatment includes switching to a less antigenic insulin (recombinant human insulin for dogs, beef or beef and pork insulin for cats) and to a more purified insulin preparation (e.g., regular crystalline insulin or regular and NPH insulin mixtures) in the hope of minimizing a potential immune reaction to the species of insulin or some contaminant in the insulin preparation. We have not yet identified systemic allergic reactions to insulin in dogs or cats.

References and Suggested Reading

Bolli GB, Dimitriadis GD, Pehling GB, et al: Abnormal glucose counterregulation after subcutaneous insulin in insulin-dependent diabetes mellitus. N Engl J Med 310:1706, 1984.
Retrospective study evaluating the effects of insulin-binding antibodies on plasma free insulin concentrations and the development of hypoglycemia in humans with insulin-dependent diabetes mellitus.

Broussard JD, Peterson ME: Comparison of two Ultralente insulin preparations with protamine zinc insulin in clinically normal cats. Am J Vet Res 5:127,1994.
Study that evaluated the pharmacokinetics of Ultralente and protamine zinc insulin in healthy cats.

Feldman EC, Nelson RW: Insulin-induced hyperglycemia in diabetic dogs. J Am Vet Med Assoc 180:1432, 1982.
Retrospective study describing the Somogyi phenomenon in a group of diabetic dogs.

Feldman EC, Nelson RW: Canine and Feline Endocrinology and Reproduction, 2nd ed. Philadelphia: WB Saunders, 1996.
Complete discussion of complications of insulin treatment in diabetic dogs and cats.

Kahn CR, Rosenthal AS: Immunologic reactions to insulin: Insulin allergy, insulin resistance, and the autoimmune insulin syndrome. Diabetes Care 2:283, 1979.
Discussion of the etiology, clinical manifestations, and treatment of immunologic reactions to insulin in human diabetics.

White NH, Skor DA, Cryer PE, et al: Identification of type I diabetic patients at increased risk for hypoglycemia during intensive therapy. N Engl J Med 308:485, 1983.
Retrospective study documenting impaired glucose counterregulation as a cause of recurring hypoglycemia in diabetic humans treated with insulin.

Treatment of Insulinoma in the Dog, Cat, and Ferret

KARELLE A. MELEO
Redmond, Washington

ELAINE R. CAPLAN
Ames, Iowa

Insulinoma, or functional beta-cell tumor, originates from the islet cells of the endocrine portion of the pancreas. Insulinoma has been described in dogs, cats, and ferrets. Although insulinoma cells produce a variety of polypeptides, most patients with insulinoma are examined because of clinical signs related to hyperinsulinism.

Insulinoma has been reported in dogs ranging from 3.5 to 15 years old but is most common in dogs 8 to 12 years old. A variety of breeds have been reported to be overrepresented, but any purebred or mixed-breed dog can be affected. Insulinoma is rare in cats, with four cats having been reported; these cats ranged in age from 12 to 17 years, and three of the four were Siamese. Insulinoma is common in domestic ferrets. The median age of ferrets with insulinoma in two recent studies was 5 years, and the range was 2 to 7 years. No sex predilection has been reported in dogs, but male ferrets may be more commonly affected than females.

CLINICAL SIGNS

The clinical signs in animals with insulinoma are caused by hyperinsulinism, which leads to hypoglycemia. In response to a low blood glucose concentration, epinephrine, glucagon, cortisol, and growth hormone are released. In clinically normal animals, these hormones, in conjunction with a decrease in the circulating insulin concentration, help prevent the development of a dangerously low blood glucose concentration. In animals with insulinoma, insulin continues to be secreted by the tumor, and the blood glucose level continues to fall.

Dogs with insulinoma may be examined because of clinical signs related to the following: (1) the neuroglycopenic manifestations produced by glucose deprivation of the central nervous system, (2) the adrenergic manifestations caused by epinephrine, or (3) a combination of these signs. The most common complaint for dogs with insulinoma is seizures. Other signs include collapse, lethargy, weakness, ataxia, mental dullness, muscle fasciculation, trembling, and nervousness. Similar signs have been reported in cats with insulinoma.

Ferrets with insulinoma also commonly show signs of weakness and lethargy. However, seizures are relatively uncommon in this species. Ptyalism is a clinical sign associated with insulinoma in ferrets that has not been described in dogs. The cause of this sign is not known, but ptyalism in ferrets may indicate nausea.

DIAGNOSIS

The first step in the diagnosis of insulinoma is the recognition of clinical signs associated with hypoglycemia. A plasma glucose concentration of 40 mg/dl or less supports the conclusion that the signs are caused by hypoglycemia. If the administration of glucose relieves the clinical signs, Whipple's triad (i.e., clinical signs of hypoglycemia, low plasma glucose, and resolution of signs with administration of glucose) is satisfied. Whipple's triad can be seen in animals with hypoglycemia for any reason and is not diagnostic of insulinoma. Other causes of hypoglycemia in mature animals include an extrapancreatic tumor, severe hepatic dysfunction, toxemia of pregnancy, sepsis, insulin overdose, hypoadrenocorticism, starvation, malabsorption, beta-cell hyperplasia, and hunting dog hypoglycemia. Many of these differential diagnoses can be quickly ruled out during the initial history and physical examination. After eliminating these diseases, insulinoma should be seriously considered in a mature patient with clinical signs of hypoglycemia.

Hyperinsulinism is best diagnosed by the interpretation of paired serum insulin and glucose concentrations. If the clinician suspects hyperinsulinism at the time of the initial examination of an animal with signs associated with hypoglycemia, serum samples can be obtained at that time. If attempting to document hyperinsulinism at a later date,

samples should be obtained after fasting when the glucose is less than 60 mg/dl (Steiner and Bruyette, 1996). It is essential that patients suspected of having hyperinsulinism fast under supervision to allow intervention should signs of hypoglycemia occur. Samples for blood glucose determination should be collected in sodium fluoride. It is also important that the insulin radioimmunoassay be validated for the species of interest. Reference ranges vary among laboratories and species.

A high insulin concentration in any animal with concurrent hypoglycemia is consistent with hyperinsulinism. If a hypoglycemic patient has an insulin concentration that is within the reference range, the animal should again fast and the test repeated when two consecutive blood glucose readings of 60 mg/dl or less are obtained.

A basic medical work-up (complete blood count, serum chemistry profile, and urinalysis) generally reveals no abnormalities, and thoracic radiography does not contribute to the diagnosis (thoracic metastases have not been reported in animals with insulinoma). Abdominal ultrasonography has occasionally been able to identify pancreatic masses in dogs, cats, and ferrets with insulinoma. This procedure may be helpful in patients in which the serum insulin concentration is not high at the time the animal is hypoglycemic. Abdominal ultrasonography may also be helpful in identifying abdominal metastases and in ruling out other neoplasms as a cause of hypoglycemia.

Although hyperinsulinism can be confirmed by clinical pathologic testing, histologic examination is required for a definitive diagnosis of insulinoma. Exploratory celiotomy is recommended in all patients with hyperinsulinism if the owner wishes to pursue treatment of the insulinoma.

THERAPY

Emergency Treatment

All patients with serious neurologic signs referable to hypoglycemia should be treated immediately by intravenous administration of dextrose at dosage of 1 to 2 ml/kg of a 50% solution. If the animal responds, continuous intravenous administration of fluids with a 5% dextrose solution should be considered.

Some clinicians prefer to dilute the initial dose in 5% dextrose or sterile water to create a 20% solution prior to injection and thereby reduce the osmolality of the infused solution.

Owners witnessing a hypoglycemic seizure may be instructed to rub a sugar solution (corn syrup) on their pet's gums. Most animals respond rapidly. Owners should be warned not to place their hands directly into the mouth of an animal having a seizure and not to pour a sugar solution into the mouth of an unconscious pet.

If the animal responds to intravenous or oral glucose administration, it should then be fed a small, high-protein meal and kept as quiet as possible. Owners who notice the pet becoming weak may prevent a hypoglycemic seizure by feeding.

Prolonged hypoglycemia can cause focal laminar and pseudolaminar necrosis of the cerebral cortex, which can result in an acquired seizure disorder. Anticonvulsants may be required long term for some animals recovering from hypoglycemic seizures (see p. 959).

In an emergency situation, if seizures persist despite the correction of hypoglycemia, cerebral hypoxia and edema may be responsible. Glucocorticoids, mannitol, or both, should be administered. Diazepam and phenobarbital may be required to control the seizures. The clinician should also consider the possibility that a condition other than hypoglycemia may be the cause of the seizures.

The uptake of glucose by cells is accompanied by the intracellular transport of potassium. The serum potassium concentration should be monitored in patients receiving dextrose infusions and supplemented in most cases (e.g., 16 mEq KCl/L of fluid). This is particularly important for animals who are unable to eat.

Surgery

Surgery is the treatment of choice for the initial management of animals with insulinoma. Exploratory celiotomy is useful in confirming the diagnosis, staging the patient, and removing the neoplastic tissue. All identifiable pancreatic nodules should be removed, and metastatic lesions should be resected. When possible, masses should be removed by partial pancreatectomy. The survival time for dogs undergoing partial pancreatectomy is longer than that for those undergoing nodulectomy. Whether or not metastatic lesions are visible, biopsy of the liver and mesenteric lymph nodes is recommended for staging. Details of the surgical technique are described elsewhere (Matthiesen and Mullen, 1990).

It can be difficult to localize a pancreatic nodule. Careful palpation of the entire pancreas and visualization of the liver and mesenteric lymph nodes should be performed. Intravenous infusion of methylene blue has been suggested as a means of enhancing the visibility of insulinomas, but this procedure has not been evaluated in a large study, and methylene blue can cause serious Heinz-body hemolytic anemia. Intraoperative ultrasonography is safe, but the accuracy of this technique depends on the experience of the ultrasonographer.

When a nodule cannot be identified intraoperatively, biopsy specimens should be taken from the pancreas, liver, and mesenteric lymph nodes. In dogs, insulinoma develops within the right and left pancreatic lobes with equal frequency, and occult nodules are most common in the body of the pancreas. Thus, there is no advantage to random removal of pancreatic tissue.

Nodules were identified during surgery in the four cats with insulinoma that have been described. One of these cats had a relapse of clinical signs 6 days after surgery, suggesting that occult nodules were present. A second cat, who had a very large tumor, died in the immediate postoperative period. The other two cats each had a single nodule identified and removed.

In ferrets, multiple pancreatic nodules are more common than solitary nodules. Occult insulinoma appears to be rare in ferrets. Full abdominal exploratory celiotomy is recommended in all species but is especially important in ferrets. Nonpancreatic neoplasia has been identified frequently in ferrets undergoing celiotomy for insulinoma. Adrenal tumors are the most common tumors seen.

The serum glucose concentration should be stabilized before induction of anesthesia and surgery. Frequent feedings or continuous intravenous infusion of dextrose solution (5% dextrose or higher), or both, are the best ways to accomplish this. If these methods are unsuccessful, more aggressive medical management (see section on medical management) should be considered.

It is important to monitor the serum glucose concentration throughout and after surgery. Surgical manipulation of insulinoma can enhance the release of insulin from the tumor or tumors. Anesthesia will mask the signs of neuroglycopenia, and thus the only way of preventing serious hypoglycemia is to monitor the patient carefully and administer dextrose as needed. While the surgeon is manipulating the pancreas and any metastatic lesions, the blood glucose concentration should be evaluated every 10 to 20 minutes. Since the patient may require several different concentrations of dextrose-containing solutions throughout the surgery and postoperative period, it is prudent to prepare such solutions in small quantities and to have supplies close at hand.

After surgery, the glucose concentration should be monitored every 30 to 60 minutes for the first 3 to 4 hours, and then every 2 to 4 hours until the glucose concentration has stabilized and the appropriate concentration of dextrose solution has been selected. The patient may have hyperglycemia after surgery, and intravenous fluids without dextrose may be appropriate.

In dogs, the most common postoperative complication is pancreatitis. During surgery, the pancreas should be handled gently, and the surgeon should pay special attention to preserving the blood supply to the pancreas when performing a partial pancreatectomy (Matthiesen and Mullen, 1990). Intravenous administration of fluids (e.g., lactated Ringer's with 5% dextrose) before, during, and after surgery will help ensure adequate pancreatic circulation. Dogs should be held off food and water for 36 to 48 hours after surgery or longer if clinical signs of pancreatitis are apparent. Small amounts of water and bland food may be started on the second or third day after surgery.

In some animals, the high concentration of circulating insulin secreted by the tumor suppresses the function of the normal beta cells, leading to hyperglycemia. As function of the beta cells returns, postsurgical hyperglycemia resolves. If treatment with insulin is required, the clinician and owner should be aware that endogenous insulin may eventually be produced either by the normal beta cells or by recurrent tumor cells. The owner should monitor the glucose in the urine several times per week, and serum glucose should be checked at least monthly to avoid an iatrogenic hypoglycemic crisis.

Postoperative pancreatitis and postoperative hyperglycemia appear to be uncommon complications in ferrets. Ferrets may be fed 24 hours after surgery. The prevalence of postoperative complications in cats undergoing surgery for insulinoma is not known. The conservative postoperative management described earlier is also recommended for cats.

When a patient who has previously undergone surgery for insulinoma begins to show signs of hypoglycemia, a second surgery may be attempted or medical management instituted. If all visible tumor can again be resected, animals may remain symptom-free for a number of additional months. It appears that ferrets whose first symptom-free interval was several months are the most likely to benefit from a second surgery.

Medical Management

Chemotherapy

Specific antineoplastic therapy can be considered in animals in which all the tumor cannot be resected and in animals that have undergone previous surgery and are again showing signs of hypoglycemia. Chemotherapy should be given only to patients with a confirmed histologic diagnosis of insulinoma.

Streptozotocin (Zanosar, Pharmacia & Upjohn, Kalamazoo, MI) is a chemotherapeutic drug that selectively destroys pancreatic beta cells. When given alone, this drug causes severe, acute renal failure in dogs. The drug can be safely administered if given with aggressive saline diuresis. Normal saline should be given at 18 to 20 ml/kg/hr for 7 to 8 hours. Streptozotocin is administered in the saline solution over the fourth and fifth hours at a dosage of 500 mg/m^2 intravenously. Antiemetic medications such as butorphanol (Torbugesic, Fort Dodge Laboratories, Fort Dodge, Iowa) should be administered at the end of the 7-hour period. Care should be taken to ensure that the dog does not become dehydrated in the days after therapy. Fluid support is strongly recommended if the dog is vomiting or is not drinking adequately.

At this time, streptozotocin should be considered investigational, and owners should sign an informed consent form before treatment is begun. It should be used in dogs with known metastatic disease or those with clinical signs of hypoglycemia. The estimated response rate in dogs treated with streptozotocin is 30%. The duration of response is variable and may be brief. There are no reports on the use of streptozotocin in cats or ferrets with insulinoma. Further study of this agent is needed in all species.

Alloxan (Research Organics, Cleveland, OH) is another drug that has a direct toxic effect on beta cells. It can cause renal tubular necrosis and should be administered only in combination with aggressive fluid therapy. A single treatment with 65 mg/kg intravenously was effective in controlling hypoglycemia for several months in four of eight dogs; however, hypoglycemia eventually recurred in all of these dogs (Feldman and Nelson, 1996). Toxicities associated with alloxan administration include renal tubular necrosis with subsequent renal failure, acute respiratory distress syndrome with pulmonary edema, and hepatic necrosis.

Doxorubicin (Adriamycin, Pharmacia & Upjohn, Kalamazoo, MI) alone has been reported to be effective in a few human patients with insulinoma. This drug is commonly used in veterinary oncology, but its efficacy against insulinoma is unknown. It is generally well tolerated by dogs, cats, and ferrets and thus could be considered as either a single agent or in combination with other drugs for the treatment of insulinoma. The accepted dosage for doxorubicin in dogs is 30 mg/m^2 intravenously every 2 to 3 weeks. For cats and ferrets, 1 mg/kg intravenously every 3 weeks is recommended. At this time, doxorubicin is the only drug discussed here that is known to be safe in cats and ferrets and thus would be reasonable to consider for further study in client-owned animals.

Combination protocols of streptozotocin with doxorubicin and streptozotocin with fluorouracil are also used in the treatment of human patients with insulinoma. Given the aggressive nature of the disease in veterinary patients, such protocols merit further investigation in animals.

Symptomatic Therapy

Symptomatic therapy is recommended for animals that are showing signs of hypoglycemia and have either previously undergone surgery or whose owners have declined surgery.

Animals with insulinoma should be fed a diet that is high in protein, fat, and complex carbohydrates. Simple sugars, often contained in semimoist pet foods, should be avoided. Dogs should be fed small meals three to four times daily. Cats may be fed free choice if they do not become obese. Ferrets may be fed free choice.

Glucocorticoids are recommended when frequent feedings are no longer successful in controlling clinical signs. These drugs inhibit glucose uptake in the peripheral tissues and stimulate glycogenolysis. Prednisone (or prednisolone) is started at 0.25 mg/kg PO twice daily. The dosage may be gradually increased as needed to control clinical signs or may be decreased if the disease is well controlled at the initial dosage. The clinician should be aware that dosages of 1.1 mg/kg twice daily or higher are considered immunosuppressive.

Diazoxide (Proglycem, Baker Norton Pharmaceuticals, Miami, FL) is a nondiuretic benzothiadiazide that decreases insulin secretion, promotes gluconeogenesis and glycogenolysis, and inhibits the cellular uptake of glucose. Diazoxide is currently available in tablet and liquid form. The recommended starting dosage is 5 mg/kg PO twice daily. As with prednisone, the dosage may be increased as needed to control clinical signs. The maximal recommended dosage is 30 mg/kg PO twice daily.

The most common side effects of diazoxide are anorexia, vomiting, and diarrhea. These signs may be avoided or lessened by giving the medication with food. Ferrets find the diazoxide suspension distasteful, but since only small volumes are required, owners are usually able to administer it. Other potential side effects of diazoxide are hyperglycemia, bone marrow suppression, and sodium retention. Because of the potential for sodium and fluid retention, this drug should be used with caution in patients with heart disease. Diazoxide is metabolized by the liver. Patients with hepatic dysfunction may exhibit side effects at lower dosages than do normal animals.

Thiazide diuretics enhance the effects of diazoxide. Hydrochlorothiazide at a dosage of 1.0 to 4.0 mg/kg once daily can be used in combination with diazoxide in patients that have not responded to diazoxide alone or have progression of their clinical signs despite other treatments.

Somatostatin is a polypeptide hormone that inhibits the secretion of insulin, glucagon, gastrin, secretin, and motilin. Octreotide acetate (Sandostatin, Sandoz Pharmaceuticals, East Hanover, NJ) is a long-acting somatostatin analogue that can be used in the management of patients with insulinoma.

Reports on the use of octreotide acetate in veterinary patients are limited. Of the eight reported dogs with insulinoma who were refractory to other forms of treatment, six dogs had improvement in their clinical signs. In three of these dogs, a decrease in the serum insulin concentration was documented. One dog acquired diabetes mellitus, but no other important side effects were observed. To our knowledge, no reports have been published on the use of octreotide acetate in ferrets or cats with insulinoma. We have used octreotide acetate to treat one ferret that was refractory to other forms of treatment, and clinical signs improved. The recommended dosage is 1 to 2 μg/kg subcutaneously two to three times daily. This drug is relatively expensive, but this may change. Only small amounts are needed in ferrets, so cost is not prohibitive in this species.

Currently, there is no way of predicting which patients will respond to octreotide acetate. This agent does appear to be safe and can be administered by owners at home, and thus it should be considered for the treatment of animals with insulinoma that are refractory to or unable to tolerate traditional medical or surgical therapy.

Other drugs that have met with variable success in the management of insulinoma in humans include L-asparaginase, phenytoin, propranolol, and calcium channel blockers. None of these agents has been studied in veterinary medicine and should be used only when other therapeutic options have failed.

PROGNOSIS

The short-term prognosis for dogs with insulinoma is good, although most will die of this disease. The median survival time for dogs with insulinoma who undergo surgery is approximately 1 year. In one study, dogs that had complete resection of all visible disease via partial pancreatectomy had a mean survival time of 17.9 months (range 3 to 51 months). The stage of disease is an important prognostic factor. Only 20% of dogs with metastatic disease live longer than 1 year. The prognosis for dogs who are treated medically is not known. In one study in which dogs with unresectable metastatic disease were treated with diazoxide, the mean survival time was approximately 8 months. Even in dogs in which all the disease cannot

be removed, cytoreduction may reduce the frequency and severity of hypoglycemic episodes.

The prognosis for cats with insulinoma cannot be accurately determined. Two of the four cats described who underwent surgery died in the perioperative period. One cat remained free of clinical signs for 7 months after surgery, and one had recurrence of clinical signs 10 months postoperatively. The last cat survived an additional 8 months while being treated with prednisone. Intermittent seizures persisted during this time.

As with dogs, it appears that surgery or a combination of surgical and medical treatment benefits most ferrets with insulinoma. The reported median postoperative survival time of ferrets with insulinoma is 15.8 to 17 months. The reported median symptom-free interval after surgery is 7.9 to 10.6 months Ferrets who do not undergo surgery or who have a relapse of their clinical signs after surgery may survive several months with medical treatment, but their clinical signs rarely resolve completely.

References and Suggested Reading

Caplan ER, Peterson ME, Mullen HS, et al: Diagnosis and treatment of insulin-secreting pancreatic islet cell tumors in ferrets: 57 cases (1986–1994). J Am Vet Assoc 209:1741, 1996.
Summary of clinical signs, diagnostic tests, and outcome after surgical and medical therapy for insulinoma in ferrets.
Ehrhart N, Withrow SJ, Ehrhart EJ, et al: Pancreatic beta cell tumor in ferrets: 20 cases (1986–1994). J Am Vet Assoc 209:1737, 1996.
Results of surgical management of insulinoma in ferrets.
Feldman EC, Nelson RW: Beta-cell neoplasia: Insulinoma. In: Feldman EC, Nelson RW, eds: Canine and Feline Endocrinology and Reproduction. Philadelphia: WB Saunders, 1996, p 422.
An in-depth overview of the diagnostic approach and treatment of insulinoma in animals.
Hawks D, Peterson ME, Hawkins KL, et al: Insulin-secreting pancreatic (islet cell) carcinoma in a cat. J Vet Intern Med 6:193, 1992.
A case report on a cat with insulinoma and a review of three other reported cases.
Matthiesen DT, Mullen HS: Problems and complications associated with endocrine surgery in the dogs and cat. Probl Vet Med 2:627, 1990.
Includes details of surgical techniques, as well as intraoperative and postoperative management of dogs with insulinoma.
Steiner JM, Bruyette DS: Canine insulinoma. Compend Contin Educ Pract Vet 8:13, 1996.
A review of the pathophysiology, clinical staging, diagnosis, treatment, and prognosis of dogs with insulinoma.

Effects of Nonadrenal Disease on Adrenal Function Tests in Dogs

Andrew J. Kaplan
Greenbrae, California

Mark E. Peterson
New York, New York

Hyperadrenocorticism, a disorder characterized by excessive production of cortisol by the adrenal cortex, is well recognized in dogs. Underlying causes include excess secretion of corticotropin (adrenocorticotropic hormone [ACTH]) by a pituitary neoplasm and, less commonly, autonomous production of cortisol by an adrenal cortical neoplasm (Peterson, 1984; Feldman, 1989). Diagnosis is best made by combining history, clinical signs, and results of routine laboratory testing (complete blood count, serum biochemical analysis, and urinalysis) with results of specific pituitary-adrenal function tests (Feldman and Peterson, 1987).

During the past few years, analysis of results of pituitary-adrenal function tests to diagnose hyperadrenocorticism in dogs has become routine because of the availability of appropriate hormone assays. We have observed that an increasing number of dogs without classic historical or clinical signs of hyperadrenocorticism undergo testing, despite the fact that many of these dogs are known to have other diseases. However, evidence from both human patients and dogs suggests that results of pituitary-adrenal function tests alone may be unreliable in diagnosing hyperadrenocorticism, especially in animals with concurrent nonadrenal disease.

In humans, a variety of conditions other than hyperadrenocorticism may affect the hypothalamic-pituitary-adrenal axis and cause abnormal results of pituitary-adrenal function tests. False-positive test results suggesting overactivity in the hypothalamic-pituitary-adrenal axis have been reported in human patients with chronic renal failure, diabetes mellitus, anorexia nervosa, protein-calorie malnutrition, and various critical illnesses. Administration of the anticonvulsants phenytoin and phenobarbital have also been associated with false-positive test results for hyperadrenocorticism. Test abnormalities observed in these studies varied and included high urinary cortisol excretion, high resting cortisol concentration, high ACTH-stimulated cortisol concentration, and inadequate cortisol suppression after dexamethasone administration.

The earliest study that evaluated pituitary-adrenal function tests in dogs with nonadrenal disease (e.g., diabetes mellitus, liver disease, or renal disease) found that false-positive test results were common (Chastain et al, 1986). In this study, the most common abnormality (17 of 33 dogs, 52%) was inadequate plasma cortisol suppression 8 hours after a "low dose" of dexamethasone was administered, and the second most common abnormality (12 of 33 dogs, 36%) was an exaggerated cortisol response (i.e., higher than reference range values) to ACTH stimulation.

In another study, in which the urinary cortisol:creatinine ratio was evaluated as a screening test for hyperadrenocorticism, a high proportion (22 of 28 dogs, 79%) of false-positive test results was reported in dogs with nonadrenal disease (Smiley and Peterson, 1993). Similarly, Basenji dogs with familial renal tubular dysfunction (Breitschwerdt et al, 1983) as well as many dogs with diabetes mellitus (Lester et al, 1981) were found to have exaggerated cortisol responses to ACTH stimulation.

In contrast to these studies, another report described 15 dogs with diabetes mellitus that were well regulated and had plasma cortisol concentrations within reference range limits before (baseline) and after ACTH stimulation (Zerbe et al, 1988). Therefore, false-positive test results are not universal findings in dogs with nonadrenal disease, at least not for the pituitary-adrenal function tests that have been evaluated.

In our recent study (Kaplan et al, 1995), we evaluated all three of the commonly used screening tests for hyperadrenocorticism (low-dose dexamethasone suppression test, ACTH stimulation test, and urinary cortisol:creatinine ratio) in 100 dogs, composed of three groups of dogs (59 dogs with nonadrenal disease, 20 dogs with proven hyperadrenocorticism, and 21 normal dogs). The purpose of our study was to investigate the supposition that diagnostic tests for hyperadrenocorticism in dogs with nonadrenal disease may yield false-positive results and to evaluate the effect of the severity of nonadrenal disease on test results.

False-positive results were observed for all three screening tests, but results of the low-dose dexamethasone suppression test and urinary cortisol:creatinine ratio were incorrect more frequently than were results of the ACTH stimulation test. Of the 59 dogs with nonadrenal disease, 20 (34%) had high baseline cortisol concentrations, and 22 (38%) and 33 (56%) had inadequate serum cortisol suppression at 4 and 8 hours, respectively, after administration of a low dose of dexamethasone. Compared with clinically normal dogs, dogs with nonadrenal disease had significantly higher mean serum cortisol concentrations at 4 and 8 hours after administration of a low dose of dexamethasone. However, significant differences were not detected between mean cortisol concentrations at 8 hours after administration for dogs with nonadrenal disease and for dogs with hyperadrenocorticism. Of the dogs with nonadrenal disease, 45 (76%) had a high urinary cortisol:creatinine ratio. When compared with normal dogs, dogs with nonadrenal disease had a significantly higher mean urinary cortisol:creatinine ratio, but significant differences did not exist between the mean urinary cortisol:creatinine ratio of dogs with nonadrenal disease and that of dogs with hyperadrenocorticism. After ACTH stimulation, only 8 of 59 (14%) dogs with nonadrenal disease had high serum cortisol concentrations, and significant differences did not exist between mean serum cortisol concentrations of clinically normal dogs and that of dogs with nonadrenal disease.

When dogs in our study were classified according to severity of disease, abnormal test results were more common in dogs with severe disease compared with those with mild and moderate disease. Such a relationship between severity of illness and diagnostic test results may help explain some of the discrepancies between studies. Of 15 dogs with well-controlled diabetes mellitus (Zerbe et al, 1988), all had plasma cortisol concentrations within reference range limits, including baseline concentrations and concentrations measured after ACTH stimulation. In contrast, in our study and the study conducted by Chastain and colleagues (1986), none of the diabetic dogs were well regulated and many had moderate or severe disease; accordingly, a much higher proportion of dogs had abnormal results for one or more pituitary-adrenal function tests.

Because false-positive results may occur with the three commonly used screening tests for hyperadrenocorticism (at least when dogs with nonadrenal disease are tested), positive test results must be viewed in light of the history and clinical signs in each dog. A definitive diagnosis of hyperadrenocorticism should never be made solely on the basis of results of these screening tests, especially in dogs without classic historical evidence of the disease (e.g., polyuria, polydipsia, and polyphagia), classic physical examination findings (e.g., abdominal enlargement, symmetrical alopecia, thin skin, hepatomegaly, and panting), and supporting biochemical abnormalities (e.g., high alkaline phosphatase and high cholesterol levels). Testing a sick dog for hyperadrenocorticism is inappropriate and should be avoided, if possible. It is best to wait until the dog has recovered from its nonadrenal disease before testing.

A complete history and thorough physical examination are essential components of good medical practice and are equally essential for effective use of laboratory testing. Experienced clinicians are justifiably suspicious of the results of many routinely performed laboratory screening procedures. Indiscriminate use of pituitary-adrenal function tests in dogs that do not have signs of hyperadrenocorticism or in dogs that have concurrent disease of nonadrenal origin is doomed to failure if prevalence of the disease in the general population is low, as it is for hyperadrenocorticism in dogs. By obtaining a complete history, performing a thorough physical examination, and carefully evaluating a routine minimal database (complete blood count, serum biochemical analysis, and urinalysis), clinicians can increase the prevalence of disease in the population tested, thereby increasing the predictive value of any test.

References and Suggested Reading

Breitschwerdt EB, Ochoa R, Waltman C: Multiple endocrine abnormalities in basenji dogs with renal tubular dysfunction. J Am Vet Med Assoc 182:1348, 1983.
Study demonstrating that many basenji dogs with renal tubular dysfunction have exaggerated serum cortisol responses to ACTH stimulation.

Chastain CB, Franklin RT, Ganjam VK, et al: Evaluation of the hypothalamic pituitary-adrenal axis in clinically stressed dogs. J Am Anim Hosp Assoc 22:435, 1986.
Study demonstrating that dogs with nonadrenal disease frequently have false-positive test results for the low-dose dexamethasone suppression test.

Feldman EC: Adrenal gland disease. In: Ettinger SJ, ed: Textbook of Veterinary Internal Medicine: Diseases of the Dog and Cat. Philadelphia: WB Saunders, 1989, p 1721.
Reviews causes of clinical features of, diagnostic approach to, and treatment of hyperadrenocorticism in dogs.

Kaplan AJ, Peterson ME, Kemppainen RJ: Effects of disease on the results of diagnostic tests for use in detecting hyperadrenocorticism in dogs. J Am Vet Med Assoc 207:445, 1995.
Study demonstrating that dogs with nonadrenal illness have false-positive results when tested for hyperadrenocorticism.

Lester SJ, Bellamy JEC, MacWilliams PS: A rapid radioimmunoassay method for the evaluation of plasma cortisol levels and adrenal function in the dog. J Am Anim Hosp 17:121, 1981.
Study demonstrating that many dogs with diabetes mellitus have exaggerated serum cortisol responses to ACTH stimulation.

Peterson ME: Hyperadrenocorticism. Vet Clin North Am Small Anim Pract 14:731, 1984.
Reviews causes of, clinical features, diagnostic approach to, and treatment of hyperadrenocorticism in dogs.

Peterson ME, Feldman EC: Diagnostic testing procedures for canine pituitary-adrenal disease: Proceedings of the Fifth Annual Veterinary Medicine Forum. Am Coll Vet Intern Med 5:635, 1987.
Reviews diagnostic workup for dogs with hyperadrenocorticism.

Smiley LE, Peterson ME: Evaluation of a urine cortisol:creatinine ratio as a screening test for hyperadrenocorticism in dogs. J Vet Intern Med 7:163, 1993.
Study demonstrating that dogs with moderate to severe nonadrenal disease frequently have false-positive test results for the urine cortisol:creatinine ratio.

Zerbe CA, Refsal KR, Schall WD, et al: Adrenal function in 15 dogs with insulin-dependent diabetes mellitus. J Am Vet Med Assoc 193:454, 1988.
Study demonstrating that dogs with well-regulated diabetes mellitus usually will show a normal cortisol response to ACTH stimulation.

CVT Update: L-Deprenyl in the Treatment of Canine Pituitary-Dependent Hyperadrenocorticism

DAVID S. BRUYETTE
Los Angeles, California

WILLIAM W. RUEHL
Overland Park, Kansas

MECHANISM OF ACTION AND RATIONALE

Canine hyperadrenocorticism is a common disorder in the dog and is likely the most common endocrinopathy encountered in geriatric patients. The majority of cases (90%) occur as the result of pituitary hypersecretion of adrenocorticotropic hormone (ACTH; corticotropin) (pituitary-dependent hyperadrenocorticism or Cushing's disease), which results in bilateral adrenal hyperplasia and overproduction of cortisol. Histologically, adenoma formation or areas of hyperplasia of ACTH-producing cells within the pars distalis or pars intermedia are the most frequently encountered findings.

In the pars distalis, ACTH secretion is regulated by a positive-feedback mechanism mediated via corticotropin-releasing hormone (CRH) and a negative-feedback mechanism mediated via glucocorticoids. Approximately 70% of cases of pituitary-dependent hyperadrenocorticism appear to arise from abnormalities within the pars distalis. ACTH release from the pars intermedia appears to be regulated primarily via tonic inhibition involving dopamine, although CRH-containing fibers have been observed in the canine pars intermedia. Approximately 30% of cases of canine pituitary-dependent hyperadrenocorticism are thought to arise from the pars intermedia.

Hypothalamic overstimulation of pituitary ACTH secretion could occur as a result of abnormalities in CRH production or secretion or problems related to CRH receptor function or signal transduction. In the dog, little evidence exists to implicate CRH as a factor in the development of pituitary-dependent hyperadrenocorticism. Alternatively, hypothalamic overstimulation of ACTH release may occur from loss of normal inhibition of the hypothalamic-pituitary-adrenal (HPA) axis. Finally, an increasing body of evidence points to hypothalamic dopamine deficiency as playing a role in the pathogenesis of pituitary-dependent hyperadrenocorticism in the dog.

Although dopamine appears to inhibit ACTH secretion primarily from the pars intermedia in normal dogs, it also appears to affect ACTH release from the pars distalis. Dogs treated with the dopamine antagonist, domperidone, had enhanced CRH-mediated ACTH release, and this response was only partially blocked when the dogs were pretreated with dexamethasone. Several reports have indicated that acute or chronic administration of dopamine antagonists (domperidone, haloperidol, metoclopramide) increases secretion of pro-opiomelanocortin peptides from the pars distalis of the dog, rat, and human. Pro-opiomelanocortin is the precursor from which a number of peptide hormones, including ACTH, are derived. Under the influence of dopaminergic blockade (or dopamine deficiency), an increase in ACTH secretion from the pars distalis may be related to the recruitment of previously nonsecreting corticotrophs or increased responsiveness to CRH. It is important to note that dopamine concentrations have been reported to be significantly decreased in the median eminence of dogs with pituitary-dependent hyperadrenocorticism when compared with control dogs and dogs treated with dexamethasone.

The neurotoxin L-methyl-4-phenyl-1,2,3,6-tetrahydropyridine (MPTP) results in parkinsonian signs and symptoms in several species including humans and dogs. MPTP is converted to the active metabolite methyl-phenyl-pyridine (MPP$^+$) via oxidation through monoamine oxidase B (MAO-B). MPP$^+$ then causes damage to nigrostriatal dopaminergic neurons, resulting in signs identical to those observed with spontaneous Parkinson's disease. Plasma ACTH and cortisol concentrations were found to increase 40% and 60%, respectively, in dogs treated with a single intravenous injection of MPTP, indicating that loss of dopaminergic neurons can result in activation of the HPA axis.

L-Deprenyl (selegiline hydrochloride; (R)-(-)-N,2-propinylphenylethylamine hydrochloride) is a selective and irreversible inhibitor of monoamine oxidase, type B (MAO-B), which is approved for treatment of dogs with pituitary-dependent hyperadrenocorticism in the US and Canada (Anipryl; Pfizer Animal Health, Inc). It is also approved for the treatment of humans suffering from Parkinson's disease, a neurodegenerative disorder characterized by dopamine depletion of the nigrostriatum and other brain regions. In the central nervous system, dopamine is rapidly metabolized by monoamine oxidases. MAO-B activity levels are known to increase not only with age but also particularly in certain neurodegenerative disorders such as Parkinson's disease and Alzheimer's disease. L-Deprenyl also increases dopamine concentrations by decreasing presynaptic dopamine reuptake, increasing the concentration of phenylethylamine, which potentiates the action of dopamine, and increasing the synthesis of the enzyme aromatic L-amino acid decarboxylase, which, in turn, increases dopamine synthesis.

A variety of additional effects of L-deprenyl may also play a therapeutic or prophylactic role in geriatric patients (see p. 53). L-Deprenyl decreases free radical production by increasing superoxide dismutase, catalase, and free radical scavenging activity. L-Deprenyl has been shown to have neuroprotective effects in addition to the mechanisms noted previously. Experiments in laboratory animals demonstrated that L-deprenyl enhanced the survival of neurons after nerve trauma or exposure to neurotoxin. The neuroprotective effects are clinically relevant because the drug has been shown to slow the actual progression of Parkinson's disease, rather than merely provide symptomatic relief. The majority of patients with Parkinson's disease do not show complete reversal or amelioration of their symptoms with L-deprenyl therapy. However, the majority of the dogs with pituitary-dependent hyperadrenocorticism treated with L-deprenyl demonstrated reversal or amelioration of their clinical signs, or both, indicating that L-deprenyl may be more efficacious in this disease in animals than in the management of human Parkinson's disease.

CLINICAL MANAGEMENT OF CANINE PITUITARY-DEPENDENT HYPERADRENOCORTICISM

Most dogs with pituitary-dependent hyperadrenocorticism are treated with the adrenolytic agent 1,1-dichloro-2-(*o*-chlorophenyl)-2-(*p*-chlorophenyl) ethane (*o,p'*-DDD, mitotane; Lysodren, Bristol-Myers), whereas some dogs are treated with the adrenal enzyme inhibitor ketoconazole (Nizoral, Janssen; see *CVT XII*, p. 416). Although efficacious (approximately 50% with ketoconazole and up to 80% with *o,p'*-DDD), side effects occur in up to a third of the dogs, which may necessitate withdrawal of the medications. Toxicities include gastrointestinal upset and transient (ketoconazole) or permanent (*o,p'*-DDD) hypoadrenocorticism. Approximately half of dogs experienced a relapse of hyperadrenocorticism during maintenance therapy with *o,p'*-DDD.

As a result of decreasing cortisol secretory capacity, these treatments palliate the clinical signs of pituitary-dependent hyperadrenocorticism but do not address the underlying pathophysiology of pituitary-dependent hyperadrenocorticism and may result in further dysregulation of the HPA axis. Based on the proposed pathogenesis of canine pituitary-dependent hyperadrenocorticism and the mechanisms of action of L-deprenyl, we have examined the safety and efficacy of L-deprenyl in the management of pituitary-dependent hyperadrenocorticism in more than 150 pet dogs. To the best of our knowledge, these were the first large scale prospective trials of the medical management of canine pituitary-dependent hyperadrenocorticism. Based on the results of these studies, the drug has been approved for treatment of dogs with pituitary-dependent hyperadrenocorticism in the US and Canada (Anipryl; Pfizer Animal Health, Inc) and is currently under review by the United States Food and Drug Administration Center for Veterinary Medicine. Much of this work has been recently summarized (Bruyette, 1997).

The owners of 88% of dogs treated with L-deprenyl felt that their pet's general health and quality of life had improved. In addition, 93% of the owners whose dogs completed the clinical trial elected to have their pets continue receiving the medication under a compassionate-use protocol. Final assessments provided by investigators indicated that 83% of the dogs had improved clinically, with 12% of the dogs showing stable disease and 4% showing progression of clinical signs during the 6-month trial. Adverse events thought to be related to the medication were uncommon.

SAFETY

In addition to the effects on the HPA axis, we also have examined the safety of chronic L-deprenyl treatment in 82 beagle dogs. During more than 2 years of treatment, no clinically significant differences between the L-deprenyl and placebo groups were seen with respect to routine laboratory parameters (complete blood counts, serum biochemistry profiles), liver function tests (bile acids), neurologic and behavioral examinations, ophthalmic examinations, and blood pressure measurements.

During the clinical trials in dogs with pituitary-dependent hyperadrenocorticism, adverse events were uncommon. During 13,057 treatment days, only one dog had an adverse event thought to be definitely related to L-deprenyl therapy. This consisted of three episodes of diarrhea. The diarrhea resolved following discontinuation of therapy, and the dose was lowered to 1.0 mg/kg/day; no further problems were reported. No other dogs experienced side effects that required dosage adjustment or discontinuation of therapy. This side effect rate is much lower than those reported in dogs treated with *o,p'*-DDD or ketoconazole.

INDICATIONS AND PRECAUTIONS

L-Deprenyl should be considered as the first-line treatment of dogs with uncomplicated, pituitary-dependent hyperadrenocorticism. Therapy with L-deprenyl is not indicated for treatment of dogs with iatrogenic disease or dogs with functional adrenal tumors. Endocrine function testing to confirm pituitary-dependent hyperadrenocorticism should be performed prior to initiation of therapy (see p. 321).

In our clinical trials, as well as in a recent retrospective study, failure to respond initially to either L-deprenyl or *o,p'*-DDD or deterioration following initial improvement may be due to concurrent disease. Therefore, if complications associated with pituitary-dependent hyperadrenocorticism or concurrent nonadrenal illness are evident at the time of diagnosis or develop during L-deprenyl therapy, the dog should be evaluated and managed appropriately. Although the drug has been used successfully in selected dogs with significant illness associated with pituitary-dependent hyperadrenocorticism (e.g., pancreatitis, diabetes mellitus) and in dogs with significant concurrent disease (e.g., renal disease or congestive heart failure), we have not studied such use in formal clinical trials. Concurrent use of L-deprenyl in conjunction with other forms of therapy for canine pituitary-dependent hyperadrenocorticism (*o,p'*-DDD, ketoconazole, or pituitary irradiation) has not been reported. The effect of L-deprenyl on reproduction in the bitch has not been determined. L-Deprenyl is contraindicated in patients with known hypersensitivity to this drug or other MAO inhibitors.

Concurrent use of L-deprenyl and other MAO inhibitors

(antidepressants) or medications in which MAO inhibition may play a role (Mitaban, Pharmacia & Upjohn) is not recommended. In humans, L-deprenyl is contraindicated for use with meperidine, and this contraindication is often extended to other opioids. Further experience in human patients has revealed adverse interactions between nonspecific MAO inhibitors and tricyclic antidepressants such as fluoxetine (Prozac, Merck). Although no such interaction has been reported for L-deprenyl in any nonhuman species, it seems prudent to avoid such combinations in dogs. During clinical trials, dogs treated with L-deprenyl for as long as 3 years were monitored for the occurrence of adverse drug interactions. No drug interactions were reported with a variety of antibiotics, anthelmintics, ectoparasiticides, heartworm medications, analgesics, and antihistamines.

DOSAGE AND ADMINISTRATION

Following confirmation of the diagnosis of pituitary-dependent hyperadrenocorticism, L-deprenyl is recommended orally once daily at an initial dose of 1 mg/kg (0.45 mg/lb) of body weight. During the first 2 months of therapy, the dog should be re-evaluated periodically for clinical response by history and physical examination. If no improvement in clinical signs or physical examination findings is evident by 2 months, the dose can be increased to 2 mg/kg once daily and the dog re-evaluated in similar fashion 1 month later. If there is still no improvement or if clinical signs progress, the dog should be evaluated for the presence of concurrent disorders, including performance of appropriate laboratory tests or other studies as warranted. As L-deprenyl is neither adrenolytic nor an inhibitor of adrenal steroidogenesis, ACTH stimulation testing and routine measurement of serum electrolytes are not helpful or necessary in evaluation. In dogs in which clinical signs of pituitary-dependent hyperadrenocorticism progress despite

L-deprenyl therapy (in the absence of concurrent disease), alternative therapy with o,p'-DDD should be considered.

References and Suggested Reading

Bruyette DS: Alternatives in the treatment of hyperadrenocorticism in dogs and cats. In: Kirk RW, ed: Kirk's Current Veterinary Therapy XII. Philadelphia: WB Saunders, 1995, p 421.
This chapter reviews a number of treatment options for managing hyperadrenocorticism in dogs and cats in addition to o,p'-DDD and ketoconazole.
Bruyette DS, Ruehl WW, Entriken TL: Spontaneous canine pituitary dependent hyperadrenocorticism: A potential model for neurodegenerative disorders. Prog Brain Res 106:207, 1995.
This article presents the results of a large, prospective clinical trial of L-deprenyl in dogs with pituitary-dependent hyperadrenocorticism.
Bruyette DS, Ruehl WW, Entriken TL, et al: Management of canine pituitary dependent hyperadrenocorticism with L-deprenyl (Anipryl). Vet Clin North Am Small Anim Pract, 27:273, 1997.
This chapter provides an overview on the rationale for L-deprenyl in the management of canine pituitary-dependent hyperadrenocorticism and summarizes the results of the various clinical trials.
Bruyette DS, Ruehl WW, Smidberg TL: Therapy of canine pituitary dependent hyperadrenocorticism with L-deprenyl. J Vet Intern Med 7:114, 1993 [abstract].
This abstract describes the initial pilot study of L-deprenyl in the treatment of canine pituitary-dependent hyperadrenocorticism.
Gerlach M, Riederer P, Youdim MH: The mode of action of MAO-B inhibitors. In: Szelenyi I, ed: Inhibitors of Monoamine Oxidase B: Pharmacology and Clinical Use in Neurodegenerative Disorders. Birkhauser, Basel, 1993, p 183.
This chapter provides an excellent overview of the mechanisms of action of L-deprenyl and its use in a number of neurodegenerative disorders.
Peterson ME, Palkovits M, Chiueh CC, et al: Biogenic amine and corticotropin-releasing factor concentrations in hypothalamic paraventricular nucleus and biogenic amine levels in the median eminence of normal dogs, chronic dexamethasone treated dogs, and dogs with naturally-occurring pituitary-dependent hyperadrenocorticism (canine Cushing's disease). J Neuroendocrinol 1:169, 1989.
This paper documents hypothalamic dopamine depletion in dogs with pituitary-dependent hyperadrenocorticism.

Diagnosis and Management of Large Pituitary Tumors in Dogs With Pituitary-Dependent Hyperadrenocorticism

MARIELLE GOOSSENS
EDWARD C. FELDMAN
ALAIN THÉON
Davis, California

The pituitary gland in dogs is suspended by a stalk-like projection (the pars tuberalis) from the ventral surface of the hypothalamus. A thin layer of dura mater, the diaphragma sella, covers the dorsal aspect of the pituitary gland, separating it from overlying structures. A large foramen in the center of this dura mater loosely encircles the

pars tuberalis. The remainder of the gland lies within a shallow depression in the basisphenoid bone, called the sella turcica. The sella turcica surrounds the ventral and lateral aspects of the pituitary. If a tumor causing hyperadrenocorticism arises within the pars distalis or pars intermedia of the pituitary, growth and expansion almost always follows the path of least resistance: dorsally through the incomplete diaphragma sella. Dorsal tumor expansion beyond the sella turcica (suprasellar extension) usually compresses or invades the hypothalamus, third ventricle, or thalamus. In contrast to what is observed in humans, large pituitary tumors in dogs tend to spare the optic chiasm.

LARGE PITUITARY TUMORS CAUSING CLINICAL SIGNS IN DOGS WITH PITUITARY-DEPENDENT HYPERADRENOCORTICISM

Large pituitary masses causing clinical signs occur in 10 to 20% of dogs with pituitary-dependent hyperadrenocorticism (PDH). Approximately 15% of dogs with neurologic signs caused by a large pituitary tumor have those signs when PDH is diagnosed; 35% exhibit signs 30 to 120 days after medical treatment for PDH has been initiated; and 50% exhibit signs more than 6 months after medical treatment for PDH has been initiated. It is not known whether clinical signs are the result of absolute mass size, mass size versus cranial vault volume, rate of tumor growth, specific tissue affected, presence of edema surrounding the abnormal tissue, or inflammation in this area. It is likely that all these factors have roles in development and severity of the signs observed. Veterinarians usually do not suspect or recognize signs caused by small pituitary tumors because the signs are extremely subtle. Almost every dog with obvious signs caused by a pituitary mass has had a tumor larger than 10 mm size at its greatest diameter. Further, tumors large enough to cause obvious clinical signs may be too large for surgical resection and have an unpredictable response to radiation therapy. Therefore, one goal in managing dogs with PDH might be to diagnose and treat pituitary tumors *before* the resulting clinical signs are severe.

Dogs that have had large pituitary tumors with dorsal growth resulting in compression or invasion of the hypothalamic area usually have problems that become progressively more obvious or worrisome to the owner. Those signs usually progress and worsen slowly. The signs we have observed in more than 50% of dogs with large pituitary tumors include mental obtundation, listlessness, inappetence or anorexia, apparent disorientation, aimless wandering, staring, and pacing. Less than 50% of dogs with large pituitary tumors exhibit ataxia, head pressing, circling, urinating or defecating in the home, or grand mal seizures. Rare problems attributed to large tumors include diabetes insipidus, aggressive behavior, thermoregulatory disturbances, or blindness. We emphasize that most dogs with clinical signs caused by a large pituitary tumor with suprasellar extension have subtle problems. It is also fair to state that these abnormalities are recognized by owners but not often confirmed by veterinarians. Therefore, these clinical signs may be obvious only to someone who is extremely familiar with the pet.

The most common clinical signs caused by a large pituitary tumor (listlessness, inappetence, dull behavior) are those most commonly attributed to hypocortisolism secondary to medical therapy. Thus, initial management should include discontinuing medical therapy while attempting to determine a cause for the clinical signs. A database (complete blood count, serum chemistry profile, urinalysis, thoracic radiography, and abdominal ultrasonography) may be warranted in an attempt to identify quickly any new or previously unsuspected problem. Dogs that have had or currently have hyperadrenocorticism may acquire diabetes mellitus with or without ketoacidosis, pancreatitis, infection, or a number of other conditions that could result in listlessness, dull behavior, or anorexia. If the database does not identify the cause for illness, an ACTH stimulation test should be completed, followed by several days of glucocorticoid administration. Dogs that have hypocortisolism typically have plasma cortisol concentrations (pre- and post-ACTH administration) that are less than or equal to 1.5 μg/dl (≤40 nmol/L) and they quickly improve with glucocorticoid therapy.

If the database, ACTH stimulation test result, and glucocorticoid therapy neither explain nor resolve the clinical signs, a large pituitary mass should be considered. Computed tomography (CT) or magnetic resonance imaging (MRI) can be employed to support or refute this diagnosis. It is appreciated that such sophisticated diagnostic equipment is not uniformly available to veterinary practitioners; however, there appear to be no other reliable methods for confirming the presence of a large pituitary tumor with suprasellar extension. If necessary, referral to colleagues with access to such facilities is recommended. MRI is superior to CT for visualizing small tumors (<5 mm), but either modality should be diagnostic for large tumors (≥8 mm at greatest diameter).

DIAGNOSIS OF PITUITARY TUMORS BEFORE THE DEVELOPMENT OF CLINICAL SIGNS

In an attempt to better understand the biologic characteristics of pituitary tumors in dogs with PDH, a randomly selected population was evaluated with pituitary MRI scans immediately following PDH confirmation and prior to any therapy. None of these dogs had *any* clinical signs consistent with the presence of a large, compressive, pituitary-hypothalamic mass. More than 50% of these dogs had easily visualized pituitary masses (≥4 mm in diameter). The endocrine evaluation of dogs with visible pituitary tumors was no different from results obtained from dogs without any visible intracranial lesion. More than one half of the dogs with PDH and no visible pituitary mass initially, had a visible mass 1 year later and most dogs with a visible tumor prior to treatment had obvious tumor growth 1 year later. Several dogs that had pituitary masses greater than or equal to 8 mm in diameter initially had clinical signs directly attributable to a growing pituitary tumor within a year of diagnosis and treatment for PDH.

TREATMENT

Following documentation of a "macro" pituitary mass that has grown dorsally, the only noninvasive method of treatment is irradiation with high-energy gamma (telecobalt) or x- (linear accelerator) rays of the pituitary area. Veterinary facilities for irradiation are not as available as we would like, but the use of these treatment methods is expanding. Current treatment protocols include 10 to 12 fractions given on alternate days over a 3- to 4-week time span, delivering a total of 44 to 48 Gy. Complications of radiation therapy are uncommon and, when they occur, are relatively mild and self-limiting. Mild problems we have encountered have included graying of the hair below the ears, scalp epilation, and otitis externa.

Successful radiation treatment with partial to complete resolution of clinical signs caused by a tumor less than or equal to 25 mm at greatest diameter, invading or compressing tissues, has been achieved in a majority of dogs. Results of radiation treatment in dogs with moderate clinical signs (dull, inappetent) caused by tumors larger than 25 mm have not been predictable, but good results are achieved in less than 25% of the cases. Finally, radiation is rarely helpful for dogs with severe clinical signs (head pressing, seizures) caused by a tumor larger than 25 mm in greatest diameter.

Radiation therapy has been most effective for dogs with no or minimal clinical signs (signs seen by the owner and not by the veterinarian) and a relatively small pituitary tumor (<15 mm in greatest diameter). In general, the more vague the clinical signs, the smaller the pituitary mass and the more likely it is that the dog will respond to pituitary irradiation. In a recent study, a population of dogs with recently diagnosed and untreated PDH was evaluated. All dogs had obvious clinical signs of hyperadrenocorticism, but none had clinical signs consistent with a large pituitary tumor. Each dog had been evaluated with a pituitary MRI scan prior to any therapy. Those dogs with a visible pituitary mass were treated with cobalt irradiation prior to any medical therapy. In contrast to the group of dogs treated medically, all these dogs had pituitary masses seen on MRI scan 1 year later; the masses were smaller than observed initially. None of these dogs had clinical signs suggestive of a growing or large pituitary tumor. However, although several of these dogs had transient resolution of the clinical signs attributable to PDH, almost all have required subsequent medical treatment of Cushing's syndrome. Therefore, pituitary irradiation successfully stopped tumor growth or caused the tumor to decrease in size, but excess secretion of ACTH was not permanently resolved.

In summary, when possible, veterinarians may consider CT or MRI of dogs diagnosed with PDH. Radiation of pituitary tumors greater than or equal to 8 mm in height is recommended. Since CT or MRI is not always feasible, veterinarians should be aware of the vague and subtle signs often associated with an expanding pituitary tumor. When owners observe such signs, a logical and practical evaluation of these dogs may lead to the suspicion of a pituitary macrotumor. Diagnosis confirmation requires pituitary CT or MRI, and radiation is the most reasonable treatment available.

References and Suggested Reading

Bertoy EH, Feldman EC, Nelson RW, et al: Magnetic resonance imaging of the brain in dogs with recently diagnosed but untreated pituitary-dependent hyperadrenocorticism. J Am Vet Med Assoc 206:651, 1995.
More than 50% of dogs with PDH have pituitary tumors that are greater than or equal to 3 mm at greatest diameter at the time of diagnosis.

Bertoy EH, Feldman EC, Nelson RW, et al: One-year follow-up evaluation of magnetic resonance imaging of the brain in dogs with pituitary-dependent hyperadrenocorticism. J Am Vet Med Assoc 208:1268, 1996.
A majority of dogs with PDH, treated medically, invariably have pituitary tumors that expand in size; in a minority, the tumor size appears to be static.

Dow SW, LeCouteur RA, Rosychuk RAW, et al: Response of dogs with functional pituitary macroadenomas and macroadenocarcinomas to radiation. J Sm Anim Pract 31:287, 1990.
One of the first studies of radiation therapy for large pituitary tumors in dogs.

Kipperman BS, Feldman EC, Dybdal NO, et al: Pituitary tumor size, neurologic signs, and relation to endocrine test results in dogs with pituitary-dependent hyperadrenocorticism: 43 cases (1980–1990). J Am Vet Med Assoc 201:762, 1992.
Article demonstrating that endocrine test results do not correlate well with pituitary tumor size.

Nelson RW, Ihle SL, Feldman EC, et al: Pituitary macroadenomas and macroadenocarcinomas in dogs treated with mitotane for pituitary-dependent hyperadrenocorticism: 13 cases (1981–1986). J Am Vet Med Assoc 194:1612, 1989.
Article reviews the signalment, endocrine test results, and necropsy findings in a small group of dogs with large pituitary tumors and PDH.

The Incidentally Discovered Adrenal Mass

CARLOS MELIÁN
Las Palmas de Gran Canaria, Spain

MARK E. PETERSON
New York, New York

A silent adrenal mass, or adrenal "incidentaloma," refers to an adrenal mass unexpectedly discovered during a radiologic examination or exploratory surgery for problems unrelated to adrenal function. In recent years, the comparatively wider availability of noninvasive diagnostic techniques in veterinary medicine, such as ultrasonography, computed tomography (CT), and magnetic resonance imaging (MRI) and the increasing success of veterinary ultrasonographers in detecting adrenal glands in dogs and cats, have resulted in the increasingly more frequent discovery of silent adrenal masses.

In humans, an adrenal mass is found in 1 to 10% of

patients who undergo imaging techniques for various reasons other than endocrine disease (Gross and Shapiro, 1993). Over the last 10 years, several studies of high numbers of patients have been done to evaluate the endocrine behavior of human adrenal incidentaloma. Although most of these patients have no clinical signs or endocrine screening test results consistent with adrenal disease, some patients have abnormalities of endocrine function indicating the existence of a preclinical state of adrenal disease (Reincke et al, 1992).

In veterinary medicine, few data are available regarding the incidence of these tumors or the functional endocrine status of affected dogs and cats. Therefore, the work-up and management of these patients are problematic.

DIFFERENTIAL DIAGNOSIS FOR THE INCIDENTALLY DETECTED ADRENAL MASS

Adrenal masses can originate from any zone of the adrenal cortex or from the adrenal medulla. These tumors may be functional, secreting normal or excessive amounts of one or more hormones, or nonsecretory. In addition, less common causes of adrenal masses include infiltrative disease (e.g., granulomatosis) and metastasis to the adrenal glands. Finally, one must also exclude lesions that produce the same signs and symptoms as those of adrenal lesions but, in reality, are adrenal pseudotumors arising from adjacent structures (e.g., kidney, pancreas, spleen, lymph nodes, or vascular structures; Table 1).

For functional tumors that arise from the adrenal gland, four diseases must be considered. These disorders include hyperadrenocorticism (Cushing's syndrome), pheochromocytoma, hyperaldosteronism, and hypersecretion of sex steroids.

TABLE 1. List of Possibilities in the Differential Diagnosis of an Incidentally Discovered Mass in the Adrenal Region

Adrenal Cortex
  Nodular hyperplasia
  Adenoma
  Carcinoma
Adrenal Medulla
  Pheochromocytoma
  Ganglioneuroma
Extra-adrenal Masses
  Extra-adrenal pheochromocytoma (paraganglioma)
Other Adrenal Masses
  Myelolipoma
  Granulomatous disease (fungal, feline infectious peritonitis)
  Teratoma
  Adrenal cyst
  Hematoma
Metastasis
  Mammary gland tumors
  Lymphoma
  Leukemia
  Pulmonary adenocarcinoma
  Other carcinomas (prostate, bladder, gastric)
Pseudoadrenal Masses
  Arising from kidney, pancreas, spleen, lymph nodes, and
    blood vessels
Technical Artifacts

Cushing's Syndrome

The most common cause of primary adrenal gland neoplasia in dogs and cats is a cortisol-secreting adrenal adenoma or carcinoma. These tumors are seen in approximately in 15 to 20% of dogs and cats with spontaneous Cushing's syndrome. Although a well-recognized syndrome exists in both dogs and cats, the number and intensity of clinical signs can vary greatly, and some of these animals may have only mild clinical signs of cortisol excess.

Pheochromocytoma

Tumors arising from the chromaffin cells of the adrenal medulla have the ability to hypersecrete catecholamines. Pheochromocytomas are uncommon in dogs and extremely rare in cats. The clinical signs are associated with hypertension and include episodic weakness, anorexia, weight loss, tachypnea, and syncope. Invasion of the caudal vena cava may cause signs of vascular obstruction. However, these signs occur in fewer than half of affected animals, and most pheochromocytomas are an unexpected finding at necropsy (Gilson et al, 1994).

Primary Aldosteronism

Primary aldosteronism, or Conn's syndrome, is a rare disorder in veterinary medicine (Ahn, 1994). However, it has been reported in both dogs and cats. The classic signs are often nonspecific and may include weakness, lethargy, ventral neck flexion, and nocturia. These signs are caused by an overproduction of aldosterone and are related to hypokalemia or systemic hypertension (resulting from sodium retention–induced hypervolemia), or both.

Sex Steroids Excess

Adrenocortical androgens, progesterones, and estrogens (e.g., estradiol, testosterone, progesterone, 17-hydroxyprogesterone, androstenedione, and dehydroepiandrosterone sulfate) can be autonomously secreted by an adrenocortical tumor (Rosenthal and Peterson, 1996). Such tumors have not been reported in either dogs or cats but are common in ferrets (see p. 372). The clinical signs detected in affected ferrets are bilaterally symmetrical alopecia, pruritus, vulvar enlargement, and muscle atrophy. The cause of the disease in ferrets is hypersecretion of one or more adrenal androgen or estrogen.

IMAGING CHARACTERISTICS OF THE INCIDENTALLY DETECTED ADRENAL MASS

Imaging characteristics may be helpful in determining whether an adrenal mass is malignant or benign, and whether the tumor should be removed. Four imaging procedures are available for imaging of the adrenal glands: radiography, ultrasonography, CT, and MRI.

Radiography

Large or calcified adrenal masses can be identified with the use of conventional abdominal radiography. Radiographically evident mineralization of the adrenal gland has been reported in approximately half of dogs with cortisol-secreting adrenal adenoma or carcinoma. Adrenal calcification is uncommon both in clinically normal dogs and cats and in animals with pituitary-dependent hyperadrenocorticism. Therefore, the radiographic finding of calcification in the area of one or both adrenal glands in a dog is highly suggestive of adrenocortical tumor (Pennick et al, 1988) or prior granulomatous infection.

Poor demarcation, irregular texture with mineralization, and large size of an adrenal mass all are characteristic of malignancy. However, an adrenocortical carcinoma can also be manifested as a small, well-demarcated, homogeneous mass. Therefore, radiographic differentiation between adrenocortical adenoma and carcinoma is usually impossible.

Ultrasonography

Imaging of the adrenal region has become part of a routine abdominal ultrasonographic examination in veterinary medicine. Abdominal ultrasonography is more sensitive than abdominal radiographs in identifying adrenal tumors in dogs. However, the accuracy of the procedure depends on the expertise of the sonographer.

Once an adrenal mass is identified, additional information should be obtained. The size of the contralateral adrenal gland is important, because it is usually large in dogs and cats with pituitary-dependent hyperadrenocorticism; small to undetectable in those with a unilateral, hyperfunctional cortisol-secreting tumor; and normal-sized in animals with a unilateral, nonfunctional or non–cortisol-producing adrenal mass.

The echogenicity of adrenal neoplasia varies compared with that of the renal cortex. Malignant tumors (e.g., adrenocortical carcinoma and pheochromocytoma) are more complex than benign tumors and range from hypoechoic to hyperechoic, whereas adenomas range from isoechoic to hypoechoic. Ultrasonography is also valuable in detecting local invasion of adjacent structures such as the kidneys or blood vessels, identifying regional or distant metastases, and evaluating organ changes related to chronic hormone excess (e.g., glucocorticoid-induced hepatopathy).

Computed Tomography

Computed tomography is a useful means of identifying adrenal masses in dogs and cats, but the disadvantages include its cost and the need for general anesthesia. Computed tomography can accurately differentiate between symmetrical bilateral adrenal enlargement and a unilateral adrenal mass. However, asymmetrical nodular hyperplasia associated with pituitary-dependent hyperadrenocorticism may give rise to a CT image that is indistinguishable from the CT image of an adrenocortical tumor (Voorhout et al, 1990). In addition, differentiation between a benign and a malignant adrenal mass by CT on the basis of size, shape, or contrast studies is not usually possible. However, more recent studies in human patients have shown that CT densitometry on delayed scans after contrast enhancement may be useful in distinguishing between a benign and a malignant adrenal gland tumor.

Magnetic Resonance Imaging

Magnetic resonance imaging has only recently been introduced for veterinary use, but in the future this technique may become the modality of choice for imaging adrenal glands. The use of MRI, as with CT, is limited by availability and cost. Magnetic resonance imaging makes a definitive contribution to adrenal imaging because of its improved soft-tissue contrast compared with CT. In human medicine, it has been reported that MRI techniques including T_2 measurements and chemical shift imaging aid in differentiating between benign and malignant adrenal masses (Gross and Shapiro, 1993).

DIAGNOSTIC WORK-UP OF THE INCIDENTALLY DETECTED ADRENAL MASS

Once an adrenal incidentaloma is observed, one should review the history and physical examination findings to identify any signs of hormone excess that may have been overlooked. A complete blood count, serum biochemical profile, and urinalysis are helpful for the detection of laboratory abnormalities consistent with adrenal disorders (see p. 321).

If any abnormality consistent with hyperadrenocorticism is found (e.g., high serum alkaline phosphatase activity or cholesterol concentration), the authors recommend first performing a *high-dose* dexamethasone suppression test to rule out adrenal-dependent hyperadrenocorticism. Even in the absence of classic clinical signs or laboratory abnormalities consistent with hyperadrenocorticism, the use of a high-dose dexamethasone suppression test can help exclude the disease, since a cortisol-secreting adrenal mass is the most common functional adrenal mass in dogs and cats. Commonly used tests for diagnosing hyperadrenocorticism (e.g., adrenocorticotropic hormone [ACTH] stimulation test, low-dose dexamethasone suppression test, and urinary cortisol:creatinine ratio) in dogs and cats are all *less specific* than the high-dose suppression test (i.e., all can show positive results even in the absence of a functional cortisol-secreting tumor). In addition, the ACTH stimulation test is not a very sensitive test for the diagnosis of hyperadrenocorticism in dogs and cats with unilateral adrenal tumors (i.e., 40 to 50% of animals with cortisol-secreting adrenal tumors have a normal test result).

If the results of a high-dose dexamethasone suppression test indicate that there is no suppression of serum cortisol concentration, the diagnosis of Cushing's syndrome is confirmed. Some dogs with pituitary-dependent Cushing's disease also fail to show adequate cortisol suppression after administration of a high dose of dexamethasone; therefore, documentation of atrophy of the contralateral adrenal gland with the use of imaging techniques is important. Alternatively, the finding of a low to undetectable plasma concentration of endogenous ACTH in an animal that fails to show suppression of serum cortisol concentration confirms adrenal-dependent hyperadrenocorticism.

If the results of the high-dose dexamethasone suppression test show adequate serum cortisol suppression, a functional cortisol-secreting adrenal tumor (i.e., adrenal-dependent Cushing's disease) is ruled out. The dog could still have pituitary-dependent hyperadrenocorticism with asymmetrical nodular adrenal hyperplasia, but the possibility of adrenal carcinoma is diminished. If mild Cushing's disease is still suspected clinically, the authors recommend the use of one or more of the screening tests for diagnosing hyperadrenocorticism (e.g., ACTH stimulation test, low-dose dexamethasone suppression test, and urinary cortisol:creatinine ratio).

Dogs that have an adrenal mass, but are not demonstrating clinical signs or laboratory abnormalities supporting hyperadrenocorticism, should have repeated measurements of blood pressure (see *CVT XII,* pp. 110 and 113). Normal blood pressure makes the diagnosis of pheochromocytoma or aldosteronoma less likely. However, in many dogs with pheochromocytoma, catecholamine secretion by the tumor, and thus systemic hypertension, have been shown to be episodic. Therefore, if signs suggestive of hypertension (e.g., episodic weakness, tachypnea, epistaxis, intraocular hemorrhage, or syncope) have been noted, multiple blood pressure measurements may be needed to document systemic hypertension. Determination of plasma and urinary concentrations of catecholamines and their metabolites should also be considered in animals in which pheochromocytoma is suspected. Unfortunately, most veterinary diagnostic laboratories do not perform catecholamine determinations; in addition, the technical difficulty in properly collecting the samples, the cost, and the lack of standard reference ranges for these tests severely limit their usefulness in animals.

Other causes of hypertension related to adrenal masses exist. Cushing's syndrome and Conn's syndrome (hyperaldosteronism) can increase blood pressure. In animals with hypertension, especially with concurrent hypokalemia, determination of basal and ACTH-stimulated aldosterone levels is recommended to confirm a diagnosis of primary aldosteronism.

Sex steroid–secreting masses of the adrenal gland are relatively common in ferrets (see p. 372) but have not been reported in dogs or cats. In ferrets, determination of adrenocortical androgens, progesterones, and estrogens is helpful diagnostically, and they should also be measured in dogs and cats that have an adrenal mass and signs compatible with an excess of a sex hormone.

In animals that have adequate cortisol suppression in response to a high-dose dexamethasone suppression test, normal blood pressure, and no clinical or laboratory evidence of either pheochromocytoma or aldosteronoma, a nonfunctional adrenal tumor is likely. If the results of imaging suggest malignancy (i.e., large size and vascular invasion), further endocrine testing should be performed. Otherwise, no further endocrine testing is indicated unless clinical signs suggesting hormone hypersecretion develop.

TREATMENT OF THE INCIDENTALLY DETECTED ADRENAL MASS

Surgical removal is the treatment of choice for all functional adrenal tumors in dogs, cats, and ferrets. Before surgery, it is important to document which hormone or hormones are secreted by the tumor so that adequate medical preparation can be made for the preoperative, operative, and postoperative periods. In patients with an autonomous cortisol-secreting tumor, glucocorticoids (e.g., dexametha-

sone) should be administered to avoid signs related to the sudden decrease of serum cortisol concentration after adrenalectomy. In animals with pheochromocytoma, one must control catecholamine-induced cardiac arrhythmias and hypertensive crisis before and during surgery with the use of beta- or alpha-adrenergic blockers.

Mitotane (*o,p'*-DDD) is the only available drug capable of causing selective, progressive necrosis of the adrenal cortex, and this drug is sometimes useful as an adjunct to treatment of adrenocortical tumors. Mitotane is especially useful in dogs in which the tumor is not resectable or dogs that are not suitable candidates for surgery. Although mitotane has been used primarily to treat dogs with cortisol-secreting tumors, the drug would be expected to have an adrenocorticolytic effect on any tumor that arises from the adrenal cortex. Under no circumstances, however, would mitotane be expected to be an effective treatment for animals with pheochromocytoma. In addition, mitotane appears to have only limited effectiveness in the cat with a cortisol-secreting adrenocortical tumor. The dosage of mitotane required to treat an adrenocortical tumor usually exceeds that commonly used to treat pituitary-dependent adrenal hyperplasia. Although not consistently correlated with tumor regression, serum cortisol concentration is one means of monitoring therapeutic response, with the goal of treatment a normal to low, preferably low, cortisol value. An imaging procedure (e.g., abdominal ultrasonography) should also be periodically repeated to monitor tumor regression.

When signs of adrenal disease are absent and blood pressure is normal, no treatment is initially recommended. However, the owner should be educated regarding the clinical signs of adrenal disease and should notify the veterinarian should problems become apparent. One should re-evaluate the mass with abdominal ultrasonography at 1- to 3-month intervals. If the tumor is growing rapidly, vascular invasion becomes apparent, or metastasis develops, surgical excision and biopsy should be considered.

References and Suggested Reading

Ahn A: Hyperaldosteronism in cats. Semin Vet Med Surg (Small Anim) 9:153, 1994.
Review article describing the pathophysiology, diagnosis, and treatment of hyperaldosteronism in humans and cats.

Gilson SD, Withrow SJ, Wheeler SL, et al: Pheochromocytoma in 50 dogs. J Vet Intern Med 8:228, 1994.
Description of the clinical, imaging, and pathologic features of 24 asymptomatic and 26 symptomatic dogs with pheochromocytoma.

Gross MD, Shapiro B: Clinical review 50: Clinically silent adrenal masses. J Clin Endocrinol Metabol 77:885, 1993.
A review article discussing how to approach an incidentally discovered adrenal mass in human patients.

Kintzer PP, Peterson ME: Mitotane treatment of 32 dogs with cortisol-secreting adrenocortical neoplasms. J Am Vet Med Assoc 205:54, 1994.
Mitotane, when administered at high dosages, is an effective and acceptable alternative to surgery in most dogs with cortisol-secreting adrenocortical tumors.

Pennick DG, Feldman EC, Nylan TG: Radiographic features of canine hyperadrenocorticism caused by autonomously functioning adrenocortical tumors: 23 cases (1978–1986). J Am Vet Med Assoc 192:1604, 1988.
Abdominal radiography can detect an adrenal mass in about half of the dogs with adrenal-dependent hyperadrenocorticism, but calcification does not distinguish between adenoma and adenocarcinoma.

Peterson ME, Birchard SJ, Mehlhaff CJ: Anesthetic and surgical management of endocrine disorders. Vet Clin North Am Small Anim Pract 14:911, 1984.
Review describing the preoperative and postoperative management of dogs and cats undergoing adrenalectomy.

Reincke M, Nieke J, Krestin GP, et al: Preclinical Cushing's syndrome in adrenal "incidentalomas": Comparison with adrenal Cushing's syndrome. J Clin Endocrinol Metabol 75:826, 1992.
A series of 68 human patients showing that the incidence of pathologic secretion of cortisol in asymptomatic patients with adrenal masses is more frequent than was previously assumed.

Rosenthal KL, Peterson ME: Evaluation of plasma androgen and estrogen concentrations in ferrets with hyperadrenocorticism. J Am Vet Med Assoc 209:1097, 1996.
Study that documents high concentrations of one or more of the following hormones (estradiol, 17-hydroxyprogesterone, and androstenedione) in 96% of affected ferrets with adrenal masses.

Voorhout G, Stolp R, Rijnberk A, et al: Assessment of survey radiography and comparison with x-ray computed tomography for detection of hyperfunctioning adrenocortical tumors in dogs. J Am Vet Med Assoc 196:1799, 1990.
Computed tomography is more sensitive than radiography in detecting adrenal masses but often cannot differentiate between benign and malignant tumors.

Widmer WR, Guptill L: Imaging techniques for facilitating diagnosis of hyperadrenocorticism in dogs and cats. J Am Vet Med Assoc 206:1857, 1995.
A good overview of the current status of techniques that can be used for adrenal gland imaging in dogs and cats.

Hyperadrenocorticism in the Ferret

KAREN L. ROSENTHAL
Farmingdale, New York

MARK E. PETERSON
New York, New York

Hyperadrenocorticism is a common problem in pet ferrets (3 years of age or older) in the United States (Rosenthal et al, 1993). The disease appears to be rare in other parts of the world where pet ferrets are also common. The most frequently observed clinical signs include alopecia in both sexes and a large vulva in females. Characteristic of the disease is unilaterally or, less commonly, bilaterally large adrenal glands producing abnormally high quantities of various androgens or estrogens, which are responsible for the observed clinical signs. It is important for clinicians to understand that this disease *is not Cushing's disease,* and that affected ferrets do not have consistently high concentrations of serum cortisol. Treatment is aimed at reducing the secretion of androgens or estrogens produced by the abnormal adrenal gland or glands.

CLINICAL SIGNS

Alopecia is seen in most ferrets with this hyperadrenocorticism. Hair loss typically begins on the rump, the tail, or the flanks and spreads to the sides, dorsum, and ventrum. Most spayed female ferrets develop an enlarged vulva, sometimes accompanied by a mucoid discharge. More than one third of affected ferrets are pruritic. Owners may also report that their ferret acts sexually aggressive toward other ferrets and has a musky odor. Infrequently, male ferrets develop dysuria because of urethral blockage, which develops when prostatic tissue surrounding the proximal urethra becomes hyperplastic or cystic and narrows the urinary conduit.

HEMATOLOGY AND BIOCHEMISTRY

Typically, results of a complete blood count are within normal limits. Rarely, adrenal disease in ferrets results in anemia and, even more rarely, pancytopenia. The results of serum biochemical analysis are also usually within reference range limits. Hypoglycemia caused by a pancreatic beta cell tumor may be found, since this disease is also common in old ferrets (see p. 357).

DIAGNOSIS

The diagnosis of hyperadrenocorticism in ferrets is made by a combination of history, clinical signs, detection of adrenal gland enlargement by means of abdominal ultrasonography, and demonstration of high plasma concentrations of adrenal androgens or estrogens. Very few other diseases in ferrets cause similar clinical signs. Radiographs are almost never diagnostic. Large adrenal glands can be detected only with ultrasonography performed by an experienced sonographer. Determination of baseline or adrenocorticotropic hormone (ACTH)–stimulated plasma cortisol concentration does not aid in the diagnosis of adrenocortical disease in ferrets because excessive cortisol secretion is not part of the disease in this species. Similarly, the dexamethasone suppression test is not helpful in the diagnosis of adrenal disease in ferrets.

If the diagnosis of adrenal gland disease is equivocal, the most useful assays are for concentrations of basal plasma androgens and estrogen. In ferrets with adrenal gland disease, some adrenal androgens and estrogen are produced in abnormally large quantities. The three hormones that are most commonly elevated include dehydroepiandrosterone sulfate (DHEAS), androstenedione, and 17-hydroxyprogesterone (Rosenthal and Peterson, 1996b).

In practice, the diagnosis of hyperadrenocorticism in ferrets is usually unambiguous. However, the diagnosis may be complicated in young female ferrets, because an

intact female ferret or one with a functional ovarian remnant may have a large vulva and minimal alopecia. If the ferret is intact or an ovarian remnant is present, inject 1,000 U of human chorionic gonadotropin (hCG) once and repeat this dose in 2 weeks to achieve a reduction in the size of the vulva, or use the adrenal androgen assay to differentiate between these two conditions.

TREATMENT

Surgery or medical treatment can be used, but surgery is preferred because medical treatment is usually ineffective. Thus, adrenalectomy should be recommended unless the ferret has concurrent disease (e.g., heart disease) that makes it a poor surgical candidate. Other factors to be considered include age, cost of treatment, and health status. In old ferrets with insulinoma, the pancreatic tumor or tumors can be removed at the same time that adrenalectomy is performed.

Most ferrets with hyperadrenocorticism are not seriously ill and do not need surgery immediately. Two serious, life-threatening conditions associated with adrenal gland disease in ferrets necessitate immediate attention: profound anemia (rarely observed) and urethral blockage.

Surgery

In most ferrets, surgery is curative because adrenal cortical tumors rarely metastasize and signs of the disease resolve after surgery. Signs recur if the contralateral adrenal gland becomes diseased or if the diseased gland is not entirely removed. Typically, removal of the left adrenal gland is a simple task, but right adrenalectomy is technically challenging.

Before surgery, the ferret should be kept NPO for at least 4 hours. A ferret with an insulinoma requires intravenous administration of fluids with dextrose during this time. If the ferret is severely anemic, a transfusion may be required.

During surgery, the abdomen should be fully explored. One should monitor the heart rate and rhythm, blood pressure, and fluid administration. At the time of surgery, both adrenal glands should be visualized, palpated for size and firmness, and compared with each other, since disease can be bilateral. The clinician should examine other organs, including the liver, lymph nodes, pancreas, kidneys, and spleen, and take appropriate biopsy specimens.

The technique of adrenalectomy in ferrets has been described (Mullen, 1992). The left adrenal gland is found cranial to the left kidney in fatty tissue. The clinician should dissect the left adrenal gland free from the fatty tissue while ligating one or more small vessels attached to the gland. Right adrenalectomy is more difficult, inasmuch as the right adrenal gland lies between the kidney and a liver lobe and is bound to the vena cava by fascial tissue. Removal of the entire right adrenal gland usually produces vena cava damage, resulting in severe hemorrhage. Alternatively, one can debulk as much tissue as possible from the right adrenal gland, leaving the vena cava intact, but this method leaves diseased tissue in the ferret.

If both glands are diseased, one option is to perform a complete adrenalectomy on one adrenal gland and a subtotal adrenalectomy on the other gland. One should completely remove the larger of the two glands or remove the entire left adrenal gland, since it is more accessible, and as much of the right as possible.

After surgery, the ferret should be given maintenance and replacement fluids, if needed, until it can be fed. Cortisol hypersecretion does not play a role in this syndrome; thus, postoperative glucocorticoid replacement is not usually necessary in a ferret that has had unilateral adrenalectomy. However, if the ferret appears lethargic after surgery for no apparent reason, or if parts of both adrenal glands have been removed, one can administer dexamethasone sodium phosphate (2 to 4 mg/kg IV).

The prognosis with surgical treatment is excellent. The complications include recurrence of the adrenal tumor because of metastasis (very rare), contralateral adrenal gland enlargement, or life-threatening vena cava bleeding.

Medical Treatment

Mitotane (Lysodren, Bristol-Myers) can be used to treat ferrets with hyperadrenocorticism that do not undergo surgery or do not have their adrenal tumor fully resected at surgery. However, mitotane is rarely successful in reversing signs—when it does, signs often recur. Owners should be forewarned that successful treatment with mitotane is uncommon, and if signs recur it is unlikely that reloading will be effective.

The mitotane regimen that the authors recommend is a loading dose of 50 mg/ferret daily for 1 week, followed by a maintenance schedule of 50 mg/ferret two to three times a week. The authors use a pharmacy that prepares 50-mg gelatin capsules of mitotane (Island Pharmacy, Wisconsin; (800) 328-7060). Ferrets are easily persuaded to swallow capsules coated with a substance such as Nutrical.

Mitotane treatment should be monitored by the progression or regression of clinical signs. If signs regress, the ferret can remain on mitotane or be weaned off the medication. If signs recur, daily administration of mitotane should be reinstated. The prognosis for adrenal gland disease with medical treatment is unknown but is poor if bone marrow suppression is present.

Urinary Blockage

Under the influence of high levels of circulating adrenal androgens, the prostatic tissue surrounding the proximal urethra may swell and narrow the urethra. This tissue is usually hyperplastic and cystic and often infected as well. Affected ferrets may have a history of chronic strangury but usually present with acute urinary obstruction. Abdominal radiography or ultrasonography rules out calculi as the cause of the urinary tract blockage. Occasionally, a soft tissue enlargement just caudal to the bladder is seen on radiographs.

Initially, the urinary blockage should be corrected by inserting a small catheter (e.g., 3.5 French red rubber) through the urethra into the bladder. To perform this procedure, one should anesthetize the ferret and exteriorize the penis. Entering the urethral opening may be hampered by the os penis. Care should be taken not to damage the delicate urethral tissue; magnifying loops aid in visualizing the urethral opening. If efforts to relieve the blockage are unsuccessful, cystocentesis with a 25-gauge needle attached to a syringe can be attempted. However, this procedure is risky and can cause rupture of the bladder.

Once the urethral catheter is secured in place, the bladder should be emptied and the metabolic status of the ferret ascertained. If the urinary blockage is long-standing, one can assume a serum electrolyte imbalance similar to that seen in blocked cats (see p. 849), and intravenous administration of fluids and electrolytes to stabilize the ferret is necessary.

Definitive treatment of prostatic enlargement is surgery to remove the affected adrenal gland or glands. Biopsy and bacterial culture of appropriate specimens should also be done. If the prostatic tissue is hyperplastic or cystic, removal of the adrenal gland usually causes the swollen tissue to return to normal size within a few days. The urinary catheter is left in place until the ferret can urinate on its own—usually 24 to 48 hours postoperatively. If infection is present, the hyperplastic prostatic tissue may

have to be marsupialized to the outside, because antibiotics and adrenalectomy alone may not resolve the problem. If the prostatic tissue is neoplastic, rather than hyperplastic and cystic (a rare comination), debulking of the prostatic tissue in addition to adrenalectomy may be necessary.

References and Suggested Reading

Mullen H: Surgical treatment of ferrets. In: Proceedings of the 27th Annual Meeting of the American College of Veterinary Surgeons. Miami, FL, 1992.
A review of surgical techniques in ferrets, including adrenalectomy.
Rosenthal KL, Peterson ME: Clinical case conference: Stranguria in a castrated male ferret. J Am Vet Med Assoc 209:462, 1996a.
Description of the prostatic disease associated with hyperadrenocorticism.
Rosenthal KL, Peterson ME: Plasma androgen concentrations in ferrets with adrenal gland disease. J Am Vet Med Assoc 209:1097, 1996b.
Study describing the association of ferret hyperadrenocorticism and high androgen concentrations.
Rosenthal KL, Peterson ME, Quesenberry KE, et al: Hyperadrenocorticism associated with adrenocortical tumor or nodular hyperplasia of the adrenal gland in ferrets: 50 cases (1987–1991). J Am Vet Med Assoc 203:271, 1993.
A retrospective study of the signs, diagnosis, and treatment of ferret hyperadrenocorticism.

Differential Diagnosis of Hyperkalemia and Hyponatremia in Dogs and Cats

PETER P. KINTZER
Springfield, Massachusetts

Hyperkalemia and hyponatremia are the classic electrolyte abnormalities found in dogs and cats with naturally occurring, primary hypoadrenocorticism (Addison's disease) and are seen in more than 95% of affected animals. In addition, a significant number of dogs with spontaneous secondary hypoadrenocorticism (isolated adrenocorticotropic hormone [ACTH] deficiency) are hyponatremic. Although a relatively uncommon disorder, hypoadrenocorticism is often the first disease that springs to mind when these serum electrolyte abnormalities are detected. The clinician cannot, however, rely on electrolyte disturbances alone for the diagnosis of hypoadrenocorticism. Definitive diagnosis of hypoadrenocorticism requires demonstration of inadequate adrenal reserve as evidenced by a low basal serum (or plasma) cortisol concentration coupled with a subnormal response or the absence of a response to exogenous ACTH administration.

The results of an ACTH stimulation test are considered the "gold standard" for the diagnosis of hypoadrenocorticism in both dogs and cats. Dogs *with* hypoadrenocorticism have a low to undetectable resting serum cortisol concentration, and the response to exogenous ACTH administration is diminished or absent (post-ACTH plasma cortisol concentration <50 nmol/L). In dogs *without* hypoadreno-

corticism (nonadrenal illness), the resting serum cortisol concentration may also be low if they have been treated with one or more doses of glucocorticoids (secondary to feedback inhibition of ACTH), but normal adrenocortical responsiveness will be maintained (post-ACTH plasma cortisol concentration >150 to 200 nmol/L).

The purpose of this article is to review the differential diagnosis of hyperkalemia and of hyponatremia in dogs that have normal cortisol responses after ACTH stimulation. In general, a wide variety of diseases more prevalent than hypoadrenocorticism may be associated with hyperkalemia and hyponatremia, such as renal disease, gastrointestinal disorders, heart failure, and acidosis.

DIFFERENTIAL DIAGNOSIS

Various disorders in dogs and cats are associated with hyperkalemia or hyponatremia (Table 1). While some of these disorders are not commonly recognized by the practicing veterinarian as causes of hyperkalemia or hyponatremia, they must be considered for the clinician to arrive at the correct diagnosis. The following compilation is not comprehensive, but does reflect clinically relevant situa-

TABLE 1. Common Causes of Hyperkalemia or Hyponatremia

Hyperkalemia
  Increased intake (oral or intravenous)
  Metabolic acidosis
  Severe tissue damage or cell breakdown
  Acute renal failure, especially oliguric renal failure
  Severe chronic renal failure
  Urethral obstruction
  Uroperitoneum
  Decreased effective circulating blood volume
    Gastrointestinal losses
    Peritoneal or pleural effusion
    Severe burns
    Severe congestive heart failure
  Hypoadrenocorticism
  Pseudohyperkalemia (e.g., thrombocytosis)
  Drug therapy (e.g., angiotensin-converting enzyme inhibitors)
Hyponatremia
  Diuretic therapy
  Congestive heart failure
  Renal disease (including nephrotic syndrome, ruptured urinary bladder, and urinary obstruction)
  Liver failure
  Gastrointestinal diseases
  Syndrome of inappropriate secretion of ADH (SIADH)
  Primary polydipsia
  Hypoadrenocorticism
  Postobstructive diuresis
  Diabetes mellitus
  Mannitol therapy
  Pseudohyponatremia
  Vasopressin therapy

tions. The reader is referred to Rose (1989) and Dibartola (1992) for complete reviews of disorders of sodium and potassium.

Renal and Urinary Tract

Hyperkalemia is commonly encountered in animals with acute renal failure, terminal chronic renal failure, urethral obstruction, and urinary tract rupture. Failure to excrete potassium is a fundamental mechanism in most of these cases. Renal failure can be difficult to differentiate from hypoadrenocorticism in some patients in the absence of an ACTH stimulation test, because more than 50% of dogs with hypoadrenocorticism have an impaired ability to concentrate their urine (specific gravity <1.030) in the presence of high blood urea nitrogen (BUN) and creatinine levels. In addition to increased serum potassium, hyponatremia can be associated with a ruptured urinary bladder, chronic renal failure, renal tubular disorders, diuretic-induced or osmotically induced diuresis, and nephrotic syndrome.

Digestive System

Digestive system disorders, particularly those characterized by vomiting and diarrhea, can result in hyperkalemia and hyponatremia and "pseudo-Addison's syndrome." Disorders reported to cause these electrolyte disturbances include trichuriasis, ancylostomiasis, salmonellosis, viral enteritis, hemorrhagic gastroenteritis, intestinal malabsorption, perforated ulcers, gastric torsion, hepatic cirrhosis,

and acute and chronic liver failure. Hyponatremia may be related to sodium loss combined with free water retention in response to low effective circulating blood volume. The mechanisms underlying hyperkalemia are not as well understood, but the condition is due, in part, to reductions in potassium excretion.

Acidosis

Any disorder resulting in moderate to severe acidosis can cause hyperkalemia because of the intracellular buffering of hydrogen ions. To maintain electroneutrality, potassium ions move into the extracellular space, resulting in hyperkalemia.

Cellular Trauma

Massive cellular damage can cause hyperkalemia as a result of the rapid release of intracellular potassium into extracellular fluid. The potential causes include crush injury, systemic arterial thromboembolism, widespread infection, heat stroke, tumor lysis syndrome, and extensive surgery.

Effusive Disorders

Low effective circulating volume can lead to hyperkalemia and hyponatremia, which are occasionally found in animals with effusive disorders. The author has identified these electrolyte abnormalities in animals with pleural and peritoneal effusions, as well as in cases of heart failure caused by pericardial effusion.

Other Disorders

Edematous states such as congestive heart failure or nephrotic syndrome may result in hyponatremia and, occasionally, in hyperkalemia (as a result of low effective circulating volume, continued drinking, and high vasopressin levels). Diuretic therapy—especially combination treatment with furosemide and a thiazide diuretic—potentiates the problem. Primary polydipsic disorders and the syndrome of inappropriate secretion of antidiuretic hormone (ADH), or SIADH, may be associated with hyponatremia. Iatrogenic causes of hyperkalemia or hyponatremia (altered intake or fluid or drug therapy) are usually apparent from careful review of the medical history. Examples include mild hyperkalemia from enalapril therapy, hyponatremia from treatment with exogenous vasopressin, and hyponatremia due to fluid therapy with sodium-depleted fluids (e.g., 5% dextrose solution).

Laboratory Artifact

Lipemia (hyperlipidemia) can lower the measured plasma and, less commonly, the serum sodium concentration. The erythrocytes of Akitas (and possibly related breeds) have a higher than normal intracellular potassium concentration. Delay in separation of serum from the clot can cause an artifactual hyperkalemia. Hypertonicity as well as extreme leukocytosis or thrombocytosis has been reported to falsely elevate the serum potassium concentration.

References and Suggested Reading

Dibartola SP, ed: Fluid Therapy in Small Animal Practice. Philadelphia: WB Saunders, 1992.
  A comprehensive review of renal disease and fluid and electrolyte disturbances in small animals.
Feldman EC, Nelson RW: Canine and Feline Endocrinology and Reproduction, 2nd ed. Philadelphia: WB Saunders, 1996.
  Includes an overview of the diagnosis and treatment of hypoadrenocorticism in dogs.
Kintzer PP, Peterson ME: Hypoadrenocorticism in dogs. In: Kirk RW, Bonagura JD, eds: Kirk's Current Veterinary Therapy XII. Philadelphia: WB Saunders, 1995, p 425.
  Overview of the diagnosis and treatment of hypoadrenocorticism in dogs.
Rose BD: Clinical Physiology of Acid-Base and Electrolyte Disorders, 3rd ed. New York: McGraw-Hill, 1989.
  A comprehensive review of fluid and electrolyte disturbances with detailed descriptions of mechanisms of hyperkalemia and hyponatremia.
Senior DF: Fluid therapy, electrolytes and acid-base control. In: Ettinger SJ, Feldman EC, eds: Textbook of Veterinary Internal Medicine, 4th ed. Philadelphia, WB Saunders, 1995, p 294.
  Review of potassium and sodium disorders in the dog and cat.

Growth Hormone Therapy in the Dog

JOHN F. RANDOLPH
Ithaca, New York

MARK E. PETERSON
New York, New York

NORMAL ACTIONS AND REGULATION OF GROWTH HORMONE

Growth hormone (GH, somatotropin) is normally synthesized and secreted by the somatotrophs of the adenohypophysis. The secretion of GH is episodic and controlled by two hypothalamic hormones: GH-releasing hormone (which stimulates production and secretion of GH) and somatostatin (which inhibits secretion of GH). Once in the circulation, GH exerts its effects directly, and indirectly through the elaboration of somatomedin C (also known as insulin-like growth factor I [IGF-I]). The indirect actions of GH, mediated by somatomedin C (IGF-I), are anabolic and include increased protein synthesis and growth of soft tissue (including skin) and bone. Experimentally, administration of GH to dogs with delayed union fractures enhances bone healing (Wilkens et al, 1996). In contrast, the direct effects of GH are predominantly catabolic (e.g., lipolysis and restricted cellular glucose transport).

DISORDERS TREATED WITH GROWTH HORMONE

In the dog, disorders treated with GH are rare and include hypopituitary dwarfism in puppies and GH-responsive dermatosis in adult dogs.

Hypopituitary dwarfism is most commonly associated with cystic distention of the craniopharyngeal duct (Rathke's pouch) in the pituitary gland, but it is unknown whether expansion of this pituitary cyst destroys adjacent adenohypophyseal tissue or whether a primary defect in the differentiation and secretory capability of the adenohypophyseal cells creates the cyst. Regardless, what ensues is a deficiency of GH, sometimes accompanied by concurrent deficiencies of adrenocorticotropin, thyroid-stimulating

hormone, and/or follicle-stimulating hormone and luteinizing hormone. This disorder is inherited as an autosomal recessive trait in German shepherds and Carelian bear dogs. Affected pups show growth retardation characterized by proportionately stunted short stature, and a soft, woolly haircoat with retention of secondary (lanugo) hairs and a lack of primary (guard) hairs that progresses to bilaterally symmetrical alopecia and skin hyperpigmentation with age. Growth hormone, and sometimes thyroid hormone, supplementation are necessary to improve the skin and haircoat of affected dogs. If dogs with hypopituitary dwarfism are treated with GH after epiphyseal closure, body size does not increase.

Growth hormone–responsive dermatosis in the adult dog is characterized by symmetrical truncal alopecia and hyperpigmentation, seen most commonly in normal-sized, young adult (1- to 5-year-old), male Pomeranians, Chow Chows, Poodles, Keeshonden, and Samoyeds. The pathogenesis of mature-onset GH-responsive dermatosis has been attributed to GH deficiency, but the actual cause of the disorder is unknown. Some investigators believe that affected dogs have mild hypopituitarism with resultant decreased production of GH, whereas others attribute the skin changes to mild hyperadrenocorticism with secondary suppression of GH secretion (Rijnberk et al, 1993). Work in Pomeranians suggests that the cause is adrenocortical hyperprogestinism or hyperandrogenism resulting in decreased GH production (Schmeitzel and Lothrop, 1990).

Most dogs with adult-onset GH-responsive dermatosis have hyposomatotropism documented by the finding of little to no increase in circulating GH concentrations following provocative stimulation with clonidine, xylazine, or GH-releasing hormone. However, other affected dogs have normal GH stimulation tests yet still respond to GH supplementation (Lothrop, 1988). In addition, some dogs with abnormal GH stimulation test results have normal somatomedin C levels, suggesting that these dogs are not really GH deficient (Lothrop, 1988; Rijnberk et al, 1993). These collective findings cast suspicion on the primary role of GH in this condition. Clinicians have successfully managed affected dogs with therapies other than GH supplementation, including *o,p'*-DDD (Lysodren, Bristol-Myers) or castration (Schmeitzel et al, 1995). Spontaneous regrowth of hair has occurred in some untreated dogs.

GROWTH HORMONE THERAPY

Preparations

Although ovine GH has been reported to be ineffective, human, bovine, and porcine GH preparations have been recommended for use in the dog. Historically, these preparations were made from pituitary extracts and were both difficult to obtain and expensive.

With the advent of recombinant DNA technology, the production of biosynthetic GHs escalated. Nevertheless, recombinant human GH still remains expensive and difficult to procure. An agreement between the manufacturers of recombinant human GH and the U.S. Food and Drug Administration (FDA) limits the supply to physician endocrinologists to avoid potential abuse of human GH as a body-building enhancer or growth promoter in children of normal short stature. Administration of human GH to dogs is discouraged because it appears to induce antibody formation that interferes with its effectiveness (van Herpen et al, 1994). Recombinant bovine GH (Posilac, Monsanto) is an inexpensive product, readily available in the veterinary field for increasing milk production in cows. Unfortunately, this product is marketed as a prolonged-release formulation designed for use in cattle and is not suitable for dilution to the smaller dose requirement for dogs. This product is also not approved for use in dogs. Furthermore, bovine GH may also cause immunogenicity problems when administered to dogs (Dr. F. C. Buonomo, Monsanto, personal communication). Subcutaneous implants containing recombinant canine GH have been used experimentally in dogs, but are not commercially available.

Porcine-origin GH can be purchased at a reasonable cost through Dr. A. F. Parlow, Pituitary Hormones and Antisera Center, Harbor-UCLA Medical Center, Torrance, CA. Porcine GH is immunologically similar to canine GH, so antibodies should not develop to thwart its efficacy in dogs.

Dose

The current guideline for treating canine hypopituitary dwarfism is 0.1 IU of GH/kg subcutaneously three times weekly for 4 to 6 weeks (Feldman and Nelson, 1996). Protocols for treating GH-responsive dermatosis in the adult dog include 2.5 IU of GH for dogs weighing less than 14 kg and 5 IU of GH for larger dogs subcutaneously every other day for a total of 10 treatments; 0.3 IU of GH/ kg weekly divided into two or three subcutaneous doses for 4 to 6 weeks (Feldman and Nelson, 1996; Schmeitzel

and Lothrop, 1990); or 4 IU of GH per Chow Chow dog subcutaneously every other day for three doses (Bell et al, 1993). With either disorder, GH retreatment (0.1 IU/kg subcutaneously three times weekly for 1 week) may be completed if dermatologic signs recur (Feldman and Nelson, 1996).

Side Effects

Because GH is a powerful diabetogenic hormone, dogs receiving GH should have blood glucose concentrations monitored weekly and urine glucose checked daily during treatment. Stop GH supplementation if glucosuria or hyperglycemia develops. The carbohydrate intolerance or diabetes mellitus resulting from GH therapy may be transient or permanent. Veterinarians who have used even small amounts of the prolonged-release bovine GH preparation in dogs have created diabetes mellitus that is difficult to control. Long-term overdosage of GH in dogs could induce acromegaly, with the resultant signs of inspiratory stridor (due to soft tissue overgrowth in the oropharyngeal region), prognathism, excessive skin folds around the head and neck, and increased size of the head and paws.

Hypersensitivity reactions to GH (e.g., angioedema) may also occur, although these reactions should be minimized with the use of the less immunogenic GH preparations.

References and Suggested Reading

Bell AG, Jones BR, Scott MF: Growth hormone–responsive dermatosis in three dogs. NZ Vet J 41:195, 1993.
   Report of three dogs with GH-responsive dermatosis successfully treated with recombinant human GH.
Feldman EC, Nelson RW: Canine and Feline Endocrinology and Reproduction, 2nd ed. Philadelphia: WB Saunders, 1996, p 38.
   Review of disorders of GH in the dog and cat.
Lothrop CD: Pathophysiology of canine growth hormone–responsive alopecia. Compend Cont Educ Pract Vet 10:1346, 1988.
   Review of the pathophysiology, diagnosis, and treatment of canine GH-responsive dermatosis.
Rijnberk A, van Herpen H, Mol JA, et al: Disturbed release of growth hormone in mature dogs: A comparison with congenital growth hormone deficiency. Vet Rec 133:542, 1993.
   A comparison of GH stimulation tests and IGF-I concentrations in two miniature Poodles with presumed mild hyperadrenocorticism resembling GH-responsive dermatosis and two German shepherds with congenital hypopituitary dwarfism.
Schmeitzel LP, Lothrop CD: Hormonal abnormalities in Pomeranians with normal coat and in Pomeranians with growth hormone–responsive dermatosis. J Am Vet Med Assoc 197:1333, 1990.
   A prospective study of hormonal abnormalities, including adrenal sex hormones in Pomeranians with normal coats and with GH-responsive dermatosis.
Schmeitzel LP, Lothrop CD, Rosenkrantz WS: Congenital adrenal hyperplasia–like syndrome. In: Kirk RW, Bonagura JD, eds: Kirk's Current Veterinary Therapy XII. Philadelphia: WB Saunders, 1995, p 600.
   Review of the pathogenesis, diagnosis, treatment, and prognosis of an adrenocortical sex hormone imbalance syndrome resembling mature-onset GH-responsive dermatosis.
van Herpen H, Rijnberk A, Mol JA: Production of antibodies to biosynthetic human growth hormone in the dog. Vet Rec 134:171, 1994.
   Report on the presumptive development of antibodies to recombinant human GH in four dogs.
Wilkens BE, Millis DL, Daniel GB, et al: Metabolic and histologic effects of recombinant canine somatotropin on bone healing in dogs, using an unstable ostectomy gap model. Am J Vet Res 57:1395, 1996.
   A study of the effect of recombinant canine GH on bone healing in dogs subjected to midradius ostectomy.

Hematology, Oncology, and Immunology

BRUCE R. MADEWELL

Consulting Editor

Interpretation of Cytograms and Histograms of Erythrocytes, Leukocytes, and Platelets

Harold Tvedten

East Lansing, Michigan

Michael Scott

G. Daniel Boon

Columbia, Missouri

HEMATOLOGIC INTERPRETATIONS

The same basic rules and approaches used for interpretation of numerical hematologic data and blood smear evaluation are used to interpret the computer-generated graphics (cytograms and histograms) of newer hematology analyzers. Veterinarians need not learn new concepts to diagnose conditions such as regenerative anemias, toxic left shifts, leukemia, and thrombocytopenia. The graphic reports of the newer hematologic instruments simply make diagnosis easier by allowing us to better visualize the abnormal populations of cells. The saying, "One picture is worth a thousand words," emphasizes the benefit of these graphics. A glance at some of the newer reports may allow instantaneous diagnoses of major hematologic abnormalities before even one number is read.

The initial shock when one first sees the magnitude of numerical and pictorial data of the newer hematologic reports (Fig. 1) can quickly be converted to enhanced understanding by learning to recognize the major hematologic alterations. The authors illustrate and describe the more important and common patterns to recognize, and minimize description of the technical aspects of the instruments. The two instruments discussed are the Bayer (Technicon) H-1 (Bayer Diagnostic Division, Tarrytown, NY) and the Abbott Cell-Dyn 3500 (Abbott Diagnostics, Abbott Park, IL 60064). The principles of interpretation can apply to graphic displays of other hematologic instruments.

Graphic illustrations of all cell populations permit more sensitive detection of diseases such as iron deficiency anemia and, importantly, allow laboratory personnel to identify laboratory errors that were undetected with simpler instruments. Simpler and earlier hematologic instruments often generated numbers without the graphic or numerical evidence to identify potential errors in the results. The scattergrams and histograms often permit laboratory personnel and experienced diagnosticians to recognize when small erythrocytes were counted as platelets; or when large platelets were not counted; or when cell debris and cytoplasmic fragments from intravascular hemolysis or lipemic droplets were counted as platelets.

Erythrocyte Scattergrams and Histograms

The three major morphologic patterns of erythrocyte alterations in canine anemia are macrocytic-hypochromic anemia, normocytic-normochromic anemia, and microcytic-hypochromic anemia (Fig. 2). The macrocytic-hypochromic erythrocytes are usually the immature erythrocytes, and their numbers reflect the magnitude of the bone marrow erythropoietic response. The number of macrocytic-hypochromic erythrocytes correlates well with the number of reticulocytes, especially at the peak of reticulocyte production, 4 or 5 days after the onset of severe anemia. The number of macrocytic-hypochromic erythrocytes is, moreover, a more consistent indicator of erythropoietic activity, especially after the peak reticulocyte response has passed and when reticulocytes are declining in numbers, or in species that do not have a strong or consistent reticulocyte response. This is an advantage of hematologic reports that can graphically display data and report the number of macrocytic-hypochromic erythrocytes (see Figs. 2 to 4).

In normocytic and normochromic anemia almost all (95 to 100%) erythrocytes are normal in size and hemoglobin concentration (Figs. 3 and 4). This lack of young macrocytic-hypochromic RBCs indicates a lack of significant bone marrow erythropoiesis and obviates the need for a

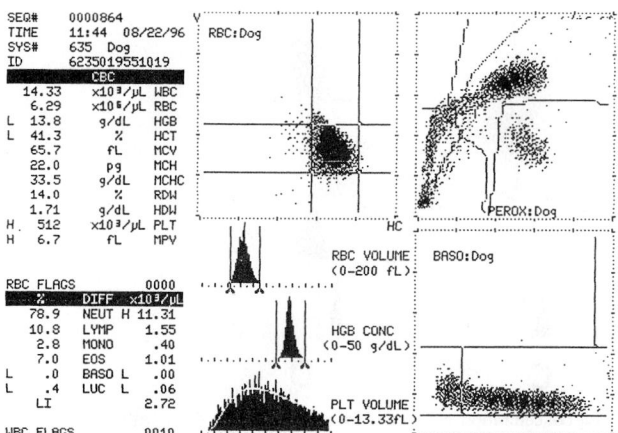

Figure 1. Bayer (Technicon) H-1 report from a relatively normal dog. The text and numerical results on the left are fairly standard except for a few new parameters (e.g., red-cell distribution width [RDW], hemoglobin distribution width [HDW], lobularity index [LI], and red blood cell [RBC] or white blood cell [WBC] flags; not discussed here). The automated leukocyte differential count on the lower left is based on the two leukocyte cytograms on the far right. The middle graphics are mainly the erythrocyte cytogram and histograms described in Figure 2. The platelet histogram is described in Figure 8. Note that the mean platelet volume (MPV) and platelet count are above the reference range and highlighted with an H (for high). The two WBC cytograms on the right are described in Figure 5.

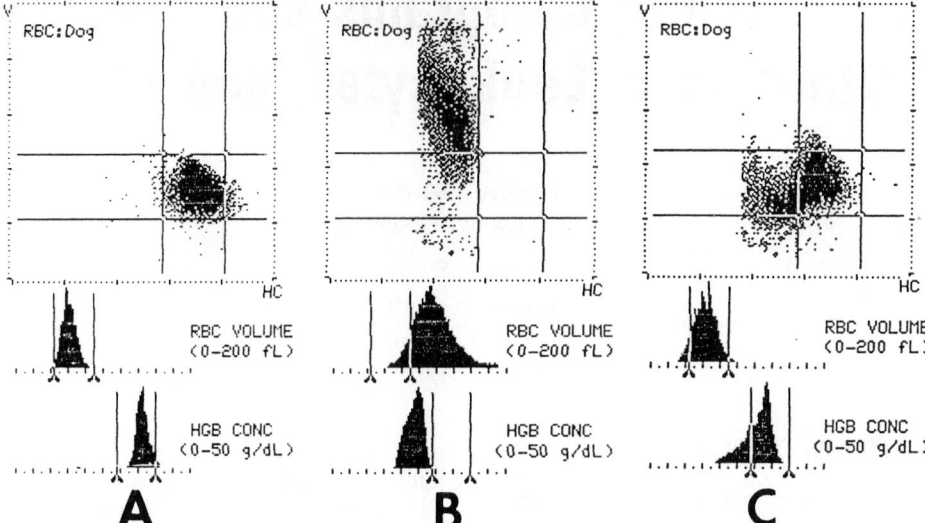

Figure 2. The red blood cell [RBC] cytogram, RBC volume histogram, and hemoglobin concentration histogram of three dogs. Dog *A* had a normocytic-normochromic anemia. Dog *B* had an unusually strong macrocytic-hypochromic anemia. Dog *C* had a microcytic-hypochromic anemia. The RBC cytogram has nine boxes based on the volume of the RBCs on the vertical axis and the hemoglobin concentration on the horizontal axis. RBCs of normal volume and hemoglobin concentration are displayed in the *center box*, as in the left cytogram. The volume and hemoglobin concentration of each RBC are determined, and each cell is displayed as a dot. Thousands of RBCs are displayed but overlie each other, creating a dark cluster. The relative number of RBCs of various volumes are displayed in the RBC volume histogram, with the peak approximating the mean corpuscular volume (MCV). The right and left lines depict the upper and lower limits of the reference range for volume. Similarly, the relative number of RBCs with various hemoglobin concentrations (HGB CONC) are displayed as a histogram. The RBC volume histogram of dog *B* indicates that almost all RBCs were larger (macrocytic) than normal, and the wide base of the histogram indicates that there was marked anisocytosis. Dog *B* had immune-mediated hemolytic anemia with predominantly young RBCs recently released from the bone marrow. Predominance of young RBCs is also reflected by the HGB CONC histogram showing that all RBCs were more hypochromic than normal. Dog *C* had two RBC clusters in the RBC cytogram. One consisted of normal RBCs in the center box. The other cluster was located to the lower left (microcytic-hypochromic). The dog had iron deficiency anemia, and the microcytic-hypochromic RBCs were best revealed by the RBC cytogram. The RBC volume histogram has a wider base (anisocytosis) but is not obviously microcytic. The HGB CONC histogram shows well that perhaps 20 to 25% of the RBCs were hypochromic. The specific percentage of RBCs in each of the nine boxes in the RBC cytogram can be obtained from the H-1.

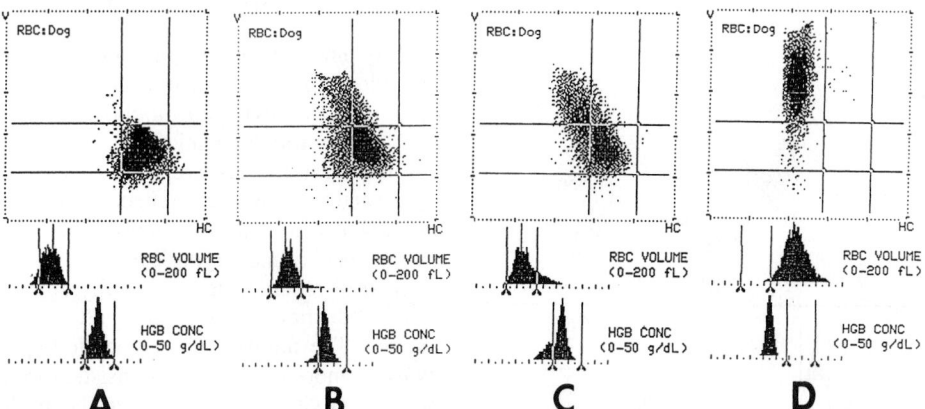

Figure 3. RBC cytogram, RBC volume histogram, and hemoglobin concentration histogram from four anemic dogs with variable degrees of erythropoiesis (regeneration). Dog *A* is similar to dog *A* in Figure 2 but does not have as uniform a population of normocytic-normochromic RBCs. Dog *A* was a Dalmatian with pancytopenia. Dog *D* is very similar to dog *B* in Figure 2 in that virtually all the RBCs were macrocytic and hypochromic (also an immune-mediated hemolytic anemia). These two cases had unusually strong regenerative responses. Dog *C* is more typical of a dog with a regenerative anemia in terms of the relative number of macrocytic hypochromic RBCs. The HGB CONC histogram shows that about 20% of the RBCs were young, hypochromic RBCs well defined to the left of the lower reference range. The RBC volume histogram has a similar number of macrocytic RBCs, with most extending to the right of the upper reference range for RBC volume. The RBC cytogram of dog *B* has macrocytic hypochromic RBCs that extend above and to the left of the normal RBC cluster, but one cannot judge the relative number of cells from the cytogram. The RBC volume histogram and HGB CONC histogram of dog *B* reveal few RBCs extended outside of the vertical lines representing the reference range. Histograms illustrate relative numbers well and show what was too weak a response to consider as indicative of a regenerative anemia. Regenerative anemias would fall in the range set by dogs *C* and *D*.

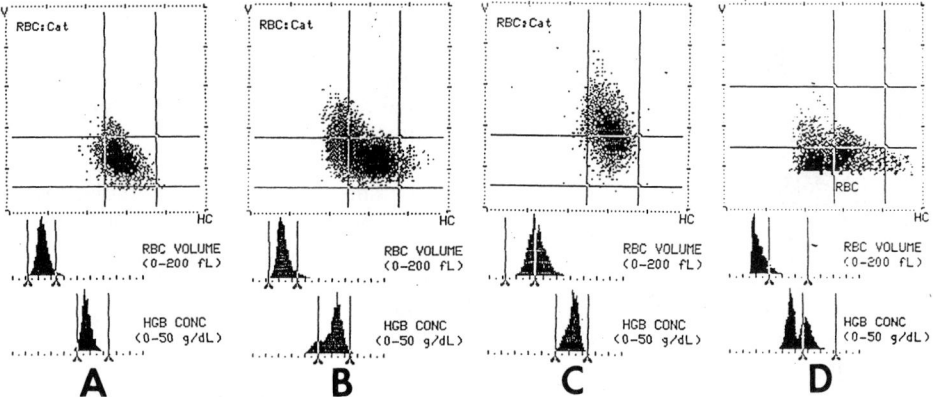

Figure 4. Feline erythrocyte patterns. Examples are similar to the canine examples in Figures 2 and 3. Dog 3A shows a nonregenerative, normocytic-normochromic anemia. Cat A had panleukopenia and a packed cell volume (PCV) of 10%. Cat B had a regenerative anemia (due to *Haemobartonella felis*) with macrocytic and hypochromic RBCs. Cat C had a macrocytic-normochromic anemia, but no increase in reticulocytes. This pattern is suggestive of feline leukemia virus infection. Cat C had acute lymphoblastic leukemia. Cat D was a 5-week-old kitten with nutritional iron deficiency anemia (milk diet). The cytogram and histograms appear different because human software was used, so the thresholds were set for the sizes of human RBCs, which are larger than feline RBCs. The HGB CONC histogram best shows the second population of hypochromic RBCs, but the two populations of RBCs are also seen on the RBC cytogram. The mean corpuscular volume (MCV) and mean corpuscular hemoglobin concentration (MCHC) were normal and thus would not have identified the iron deficiency without the cytogram and histograms. No examples with the feline software were available. The human software excluded (truncated) many of the smaller feline RBCs at the bottom to give the straight lower boundary.

reticulocyte count. It indicates that the anemia is nonregenerative or preregenerative.

Microcytic-hypochromic anemia usually indicates iron deficiency anemia in dogs and cats. Newer hematology analyzers are able to detect and measure the number of these microcytic cells and are more sensitive tests for iron deficiency than are the mean corpuscular volume (MCV) and mean corpuscular hemoglobin concentration (MCHC; see Fig. 4). The traditional MCV and/or MCHC often does not reveal the animal's production of microcytic-hypochromic erythrocytes because there may be too few abnormal RBCs to pull mean values out of a wide reference range, or large young RBCs may be present that offset the effect of the microcytes. About half of dogs with iron deficiency have reticulocytosis, so larger young RBCs are often present. About 70% of kittens at the age of weaning from an iron-deficient milk diet had iron deficiency anemia and microcytic-hypochromic erythrocytes in numbers too small to detect with just the MVC and MCHC (Weiser and Kociba, 1983). Somewhat of an exception is the microcytosis of portosystemic shunts in dogs in which microcytic erythrocytes are usually present—but these dogs also have serum iron abnormalities, perhaps reflecting something of a functional iron deficiency.

Many erythroid abnormalities, especially RBC shape changes, are not detected by the automated hematology analyzers. These abnormalities include canine spherocytes, blood parasites, acanthocytes, fragmentation, basophilic stippling, and Howell-Jolly bodies. Thus, the evaluation of blood smears in anemic animals remains important.

A few erythroid abnormalities may be suggested by graphic patterns. The changes described in this paragraph are illustrated elsewhere (Tvedten, 1993a, 1993b). Erythrocytes may appear hyperchromic and normocytic if they contain many Heinz bodies (Tvedten, 1996). Hyperchromasia usually indicates a sample or laboratory error, because mature erythrocytes are filled with hemoglobin.

Heinz bodies make the erythrocytes appear optically more dense in the H-1 laser counter, and so the cells seem to have an increased hemoglobin concentration. Nucleated erythrocytes may be detected on leukocyte scattergrams. On the H-1 peroxidase cytogram, nucleated RBCs fill the space between lymphocytes and the platelet-cell debris cluster. On the H-1 basophil cytogram, nucleated RBCs are usually hidden among the neutrophils but also appear to spray up from the "worm's back." RBC autoagglutination in the H-1 RBC cytogram is detected as either a very irregular array of cells or as a cluster of "seemingly macrocytic normochromic" RBCs above the normal RBCs.

Leukocyte Scattergrams and Histograms

The main information needed to evaluate a WBC response includes the absolute number of each type of WBC per unit of blood and the morphologic appearance of the cells. The H-1 and Cell-Dyn perform an automated differential leukocyte count to report relative and absolute numbers of WBCs. The H-1 automated differential count appears good for dogs but poor for cats (Tvedten and Haines, 1994; Tvedten and Korcal, 1996).

Detection of the presence and magnitude of a left shift is usually the most important and critical piece of information for evaluating inflammatory diseases in animals. The H-1 does not differentiate between mature and immature neutrophils, but the appearance of the basophil cytogram is an indicator of a left shift or toxic change (see Fig. 6). The basophil cytogram depicts the complexity of naked nuclei (cytoplasm is removed), and immature neutrophils or toxic neutrophils have a less dense chromatin pattern. See Figure 5 for the normal appearance of the H-1 basophil cytogram. It is most easily described as a worm. Normal dogs and cats have many mature neutrophils with dense chromatin, so the basophil cytogram extends greatly to the right, giving the "worm" a long, thin body. In toxic left

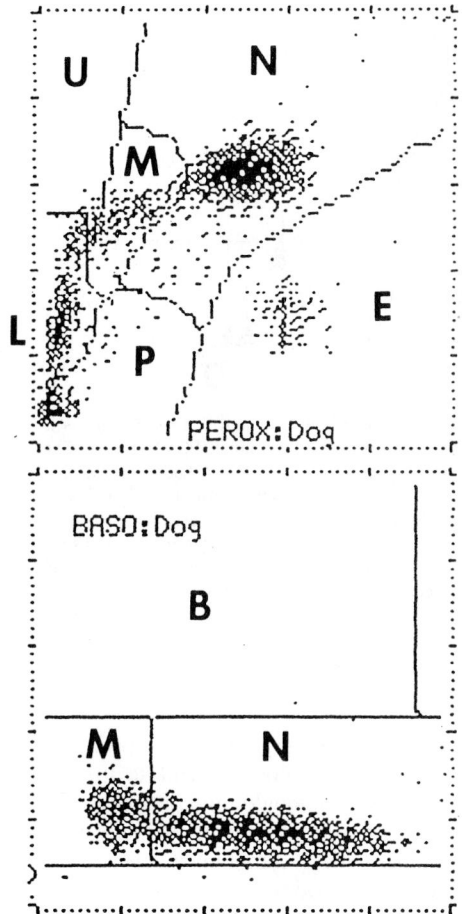

Figure 5. Normal canine leukocyte cytograms. The upper peroxidase cytogram displays WBCs based on peroxidase staining on the horizontal axis, and volume on the vertical axis. Neutrophils (N) and eosinophils (E) have strong peroxidase staining and form distinct clusters to the right. Monocytes (M) have weak-to-no peroxidase staining and may extend to the left into the large unstained cell area (labeled U in this figure) or lymphocyte (L) area. Large unstained cell (LUC is the abbreviation in the automated differential count) is a unique category that includes peroxidase-negative monocytes, large lymphocytes, and blast cells. Lymphocytes (L) are small, peroxidase-negative cells. Beneath the lymphocytes are platelets (P) and cell debris, and this area extends to the upper right to include platelet clumps that appear larger. The lower, basophil cytogram displays the nuclei of nucleated cells (usually WBCs). A reagent strips the cytoplasm off all WBCs (except human basophils and some animal basophils). The nuclei are displayed based on volume (vertical axis) and complexity or density (horizontal axis). The cells in the basophil cytogram resemble a worm. The head of the worm (M) is in the small box for mononuclear cells (lymphocytes and monocytes). The body of the worm in the long box to the lower right is usually mainly neutrophils (N) but may include eosinophils or nucleated RBCs. The automated differential is determined by the number of cells classified in both cytograms, and the results of each must match the other or an error is indicated. Cells in the large box (B) are counted as basophils but are not really basophils in the dog and cat. More often, blast cells or nucleated RBCs extend into the basophil area.

shifts, the neutrophils have lighter chromatin patterns and the worm contracts toward the head, giving it a teardrop to round shape (Fig. 6). This tendency to form a toxic ball of cells on the basophil cytogram is especially prominent and diagnostically useful in the horse. This tendency is not as prominent in dogs and cats and does not indicate the magnitude of either a left shift or a toxic change; in these species, the microscopic differential leukocyte count and the evaluation of a blood smear by an experienced observer is superior. The lobularity index of the H-1 was intended to indicate the presence of a left shift but has not been validated in animals.

Leukemia usually may be detected on the leukocyte cytograms (Fig. 7). It is easy to diagnose the fully leukemic forms, but one needs blood smear analysis and often special stains to specifically classify the type of leukemia. The basophil cytogram may show small numbers of blasts, including blast-transformed reactive lymphocytes, especially in young animals.

Platelet Histograms

Hematology analyzers now can provide total platelet counts, mean platelet volume (MPV), and a histogram of the relative number of platelets of various volumes, plus additional calculated information. Larger platelets represent an accentuated thrombocytopoietic stimulus. The presence of larger platelets may be detected by both an increase in the MPV and an extension of the platelet histogram to the right (Fig. 8). Increased platelet size is well known as an indicator of increased platelet shedding from megakaryocytes, but it is not very specific for a particular *cause* of thrombocytopenia. Increased MPV with large platelets may be seen in most forms of thrombocytopenia, including myelofibrosis of the bone marrow. With the newer instruments, an increased MPV with more large platelets seems to be noted more often in many nonthrombocytopenic situations (see Fig. 1). The cause is usually undetermined but is often stated to be due to "nonspecific bone marrow stimulation."

The presence of a *decreased* MPV and thrombocytopenia is also compatible with a clinical diagnosis of immune-mediated thrombocytopenia (IMT), as demonstrated in 16 of 17 dogs with decreased MPV (Northern and Tvedten, 1992).

An important use of platelet histograms and an H-1 RBC cytogram, illustrated elsewhere (Tvedten, 1993b), is the detection of errors in the platelet count. Sharp, narrow-based spikes on the platelet histogram indicate that cell fragments, rather than platelets, were included in the platelet count and laboratory error is expected. RBC cell fragments are most commonly seen in immune-mediated hemolytic anemias with intravascular hemolysis. The H-1 "Mie" cytogram displays all cells counted in the RBC channel, including RBCs, platelets, and WBCs. Laboratory personnel can check this research cytogram to determine whether there is overlap between small RBCs and platelet clusters or whether microcytic RBCs may have been counted as platelets. Large platelets are also revealed on this cytogram, and especially in the cat platelets may be larger than the size usually counted as platelets. This error is generally small, but in one cat with a myeloproliferative disorder the H-1 reported a normal platelet count, while the buffy coat was 4% of the blood volume and was composed mainly of large, bizarre platelets.

Bayer H-1 Examples

Diagnosticians use pattern recognition in the detection of many diseases. The visual displays of cytograms and

Text continued on page 389

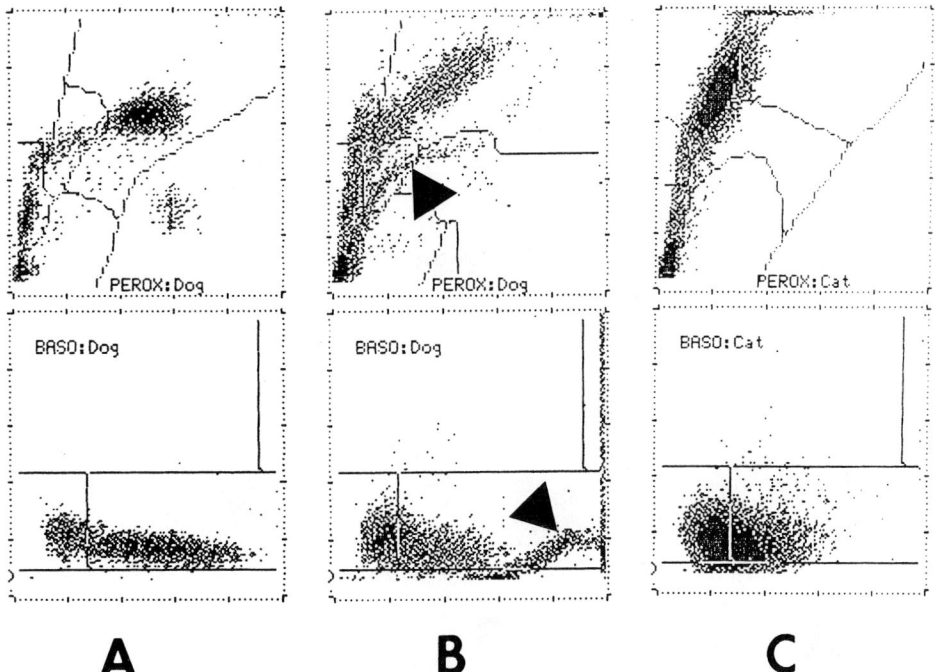

A   **B**   **C**

Figure 6. Leukocyte cytograms from two dogs and a cat. Dog *B* and cat *C* had toxic left shifts and severe inflammation. The lower, basophil cytograms are the most reflective of the presence of many immature and toxic neutrophils. Compare these with that for dog *A*, which had a normal basophil cytogram with the long, dark body to the "worm." This image reflects the mature, condensed, dense chromatin of normal neutrophils. Immature and toxic neutrophils have thicker nuclei with less condensed, more dispersed chromatin, and these neutrophils are displayed more to the left (nearer the head of the worm). The retraction of the normally elongated, basophil cytogram toward more of a ball shape is best seen in the cat on the right. Cat *C* had bacterial pyothorax with many more immature neutrophils than mature ones. All neutrophils were very toxic. The basophil cytogram of the dog in the middle was retracted into a teardrop shape because it had more immature neutrophils than mature ones and a strong toxic change in neutrophils. This teardrop shape is somewhat obscured by lipemic droplets that formed a thick, linear cluster coming up from under and behind the WBC cluster and extending to the upper right (see lower right part of *arrowhead*). The lipemic cluster looks like the tail of the worm. The lipemia in the peroxidase cytogram appears as a linear curve extending above and to the right of the platelet cluster at the lower left (see upper right part of *arrowhead*). The basophil cytograms depict severe left shifts or toxic change but are not as sensitive indicators of mild-to-moderate left shifts as blood smear analysis performed by an experienced observer.

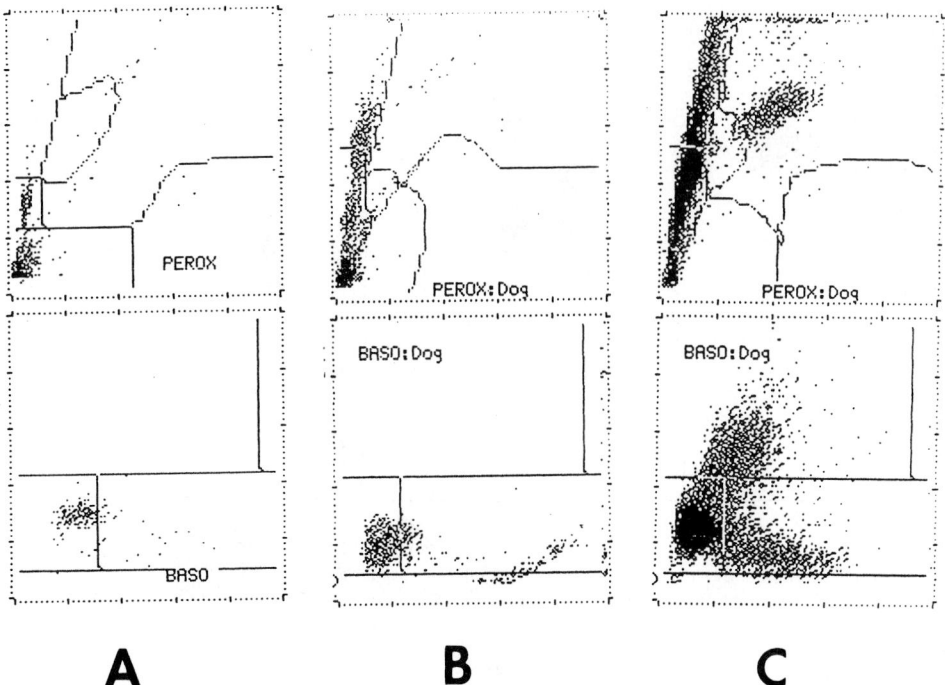

Figure 7. Leukocyte cytograms in three dogs. Dog *A* had ehrlichiosis and pancytopenia. The microscopic differential leukocyte count had 88% lymphocytes. This relatively pure lymphocyte population is illustrated clearly by the lymphocyte position on the cytograms. Almost all cells are in the lymphocyte box of the peroxidase cytogram or the head of the worm in the basophil cytogram. One can easily see the leukopenia and relative lymphocytosis. Dog *B* also had severe leukopenia (and pancytopenia), but the microscopic differential count indicated 68% lymphocytes and 21% monocytes. By comparison with dog *A*, the position of monocytes is illustrated. The mononuclear cells (lymphocytes plus monocytes) are still only the head on the basophil worm, as in the dog on the left, but the peroxidase cytogram displays the monocytes above the lymphocyte cluster. The basophil cytogram reveals lipemic droplets in a linear curve at the lower right, although not as strongly as in dog *B* in Figure 6. In both examples, the severe neutropenia and leukopenia are clearly evident before one reads the numerical data. In severe leukopenia cases, many more WBCs are shown on these two cytograms than one can find on a blood smear.

One can quickly diagnose leukemia in dog *C* by the pattern of the WBC cytograms. Blast cells come off the head of the worm at a 45-degree angle in numbers too large to be just reactive lymphocytes. The blast cells of this acute lymphoblastic leukemia extend in large numbers from the lymphocyte cluster high up into the LUC area. Large numbers of WBCs are indicated by the darkness of the cell cluster. The cytograms indicate a large number of blast cells and therefore acute blast cell leukemia. The myeloid leukemias with significant differentiation into peroxidase-staining cells may extend more to the right, reflecting peroxidase staining. Further diagnosis requires blood smear evaluation.

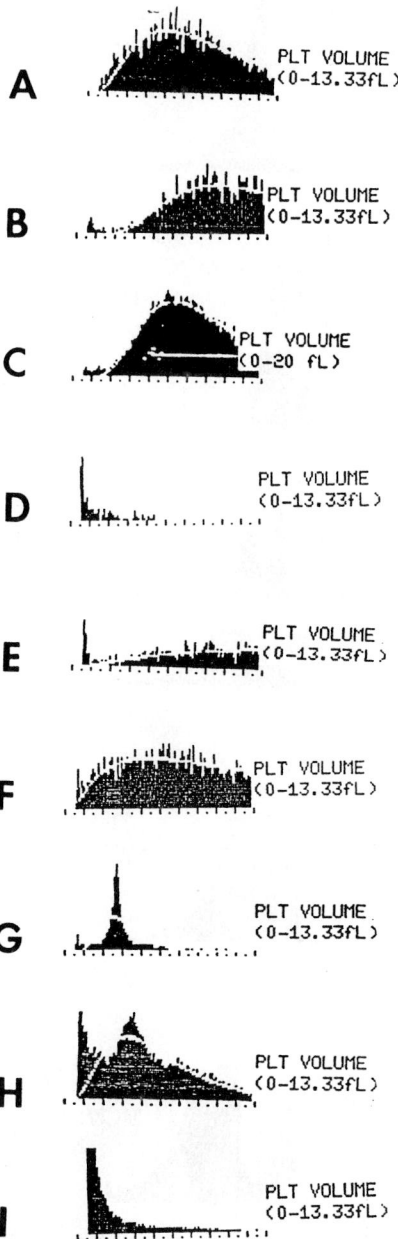

Figure 8. Platelet histograms illustrate the composition of the platelet population or suggest cell fragments or lipid droplets being erroneously included in the total platelet count. Histogram *A* displays a fairly normal canine platelet population. Histogram *B* illustrates that normal cats have platelets larger than those of dogs. Histogram *C* used human software and included platelets up to 20 fl, unlike the typical veterinary software displaying platelets up to 13.33 fl. Even this extended range up to 20 fl missed many platelets larger than 20 fl in this kitten with thrombocytosis due to iron deficiency anemia (as well as larger platelets in normal cats). Histogram *D* illustrates a great reduction in the number and size of platelets. The area under the curve reflects platelet numbers, as with other histograms, and the area was greatly reduced. The location of the remaining platelets way to the left indicates their relatively small size. This dog had immune-mediated thrombocytopenia and low mean platelet volume (MPV). Histogram *E* indicates a shift in the average platelet size to the right, with relatively more larger platelets and increased platelet shedding in this dog with thrombocytopenia. Histogram *F* is similar to *E* in illustrating increased numbers of larger platelets and increased platelet production, but this dog had a higher platelet count.

Platelet histogram *G* indicates the presence of a sharp, uniform spike of particles too narrow in width to be considered platelets. These were cytoplasmic fragments in a dog with intravascular hemolysis accompanying immune-mediated hemolytic anemia. These RBC fragments hid the severity of the thrombocytopenia because they were counted as platelets. Histogram *H* has a similar spike of particles more hidden among the platelets in a cat with autoagglutination and *Haemobartonella felis*. Another spike, probably representing cell debris, is at the far left (near 0 fl in size). This spike indicates probable error in the total platelet count. Histogram *I* was from a dog with lipemia and a "platelet" count of 2,439 × 10⁹/L (normal 164 to 510) and a MPV of 2.4 fl (normal 3.9 to 6.1). These were lipid droplets being counted, rather than platelets, which appeared normal in number on the blood smear.

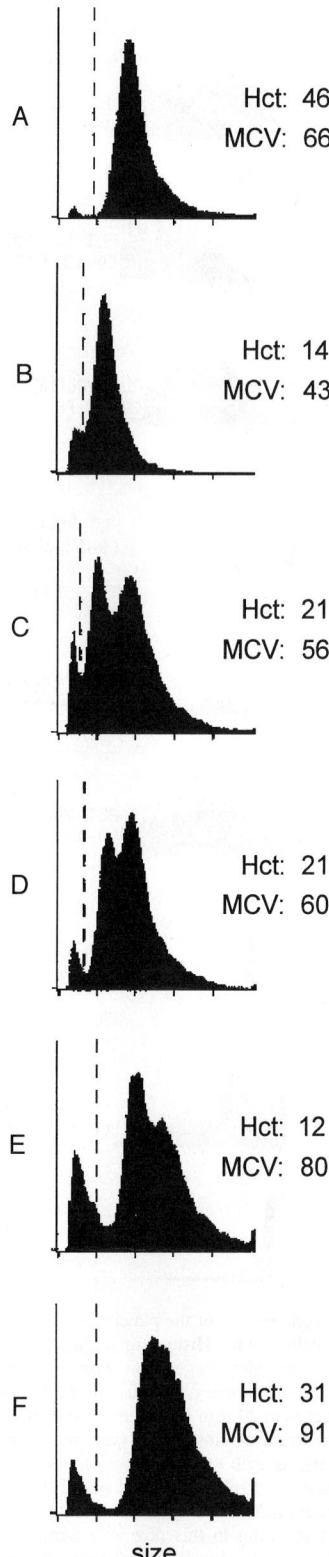

Figure 9. Cell-Dyn RBC histograms. These histograms depict the size distribution of RBC (to the right of the vertical dashed line) and platelet (leftmost peaks) populations. The vertical dashed lines represent the instrument's placement of the floating threshold between platelets and RBCs. A clear separation is present only in *A,* and the separation is worst with the marked microcytoses seen in *B* and *D.* Reference gates are not displayed, but the hatch marks along the horizontal axes (size) allow comparisons among histograms. Note that a normal RBC population is centered approximately over the second hatch mark from the left *(A),* while the microcytic population from a dog with iron deficiency anemia is shifted to the left *(B).* After treatment of this dog, microcytic and normocytic populations were apparent *(C).* A similar bimodal RBC distribution with a microcytic population of acanthocytes was repeatedly obtained from a dog with splenic hemangiosarcoma *(D).* Double populations may also occur owing to abnormal macrocytic populations, such as in a dog with nonregenerative anemia and ineffective erythropoiesis of undetermined cause *(E).* The entire RBC population may be macrocytic, as seen with this single broad peak from a dog with a transient macrocytosis that was temporally associated with transient, marked hypernatremia *(F).*

histograms depict patterns that permit rapid and often more sensitive detection of many hematologic diseases (see Figs. 1 through 8). These graphics do not depict all hematologic disorders, so evaluation of the blood smear is still required. The graphics do permit a very rapid diagnosis of many important disorders, however, and may offer better information than what was previously possible.

The Abbott Cell-Dyn 3500

The Abbott Cell-Dyn 3500, equipped with its Vet 2.0 software, generates information similar to that of the Bayer Technicon H-1, but uses different analytical methods, which result in different graphic displays. The Cell-Dyn uses aperture impedance to evaluate RBCs and platelets (Fig. 9), light scatter to differentiate unstained WBCs, and both impedance and light scatter measurements to count WBCs. The independent determination of total leukocyte concentrations by both impedance and optical methods is a form of quality control. The degree and nature of the differences between the two values are used to identify the presence of nucleated RBCs, osmotically resistant RBCs, and fragile WBCs. Because impedance methods do not measure individual RBC hemoglobin concentrations, the Cell-Dyn does not generate outputs analogous to the RBC cytogram and hemoglobin concentration histogram of the H-1 (see Figs. 1 through 4).

The Cell-Dyn's optical analyzer generates a five-part differential count by assessing the light scattered from each WBC at each of four different angles.* When the instrument cannot reliably discriminate between populations, default thresholds are used to determine the differential. The differential is then flagged, and the specific suspect populations are noted. The six possible cytograms that can be produced from the four scatter parameters are automatically generated, and as many as four of them may be displayed at one time on the instrument's monitor (Fig. 10). These pictorial displays allow the instrument operator to verify or refute proper delineation of the cell populations by the instrument's floating thresholds. This evaluation requires the instrument's color monitor or a color printer because the cell populations are color-coded and they cannot be completely differentiated with black-and-white printouts. As would be expected from the large number of cells counted, the precision of the automated differential count is excellent compared with manual methods. The accuracy of the differential count is a more difficult assessment, and a thorough evaluation of the accuracy of the differential count of animal blood with the use of the Cell-Dyn 3500 with Vet 2.0 software has not been published.

Cytograms and histograms from this instrument may offer clinically useful information. The leukocyte cytogram of size versus complexity appears to be useful for identifying toxic change (Fig. 11). Toxic change, but not left shifts alone, appears to be associated with an upward shift

*Size is assessed by 1- to 3-degree scatter, cellular complexity by 7- to 11-degree scatter, nuclear lobularity by 70- to 100-degree scatter, and cytoplasmic granularity by depolarized 70- to 110-degree scatter.

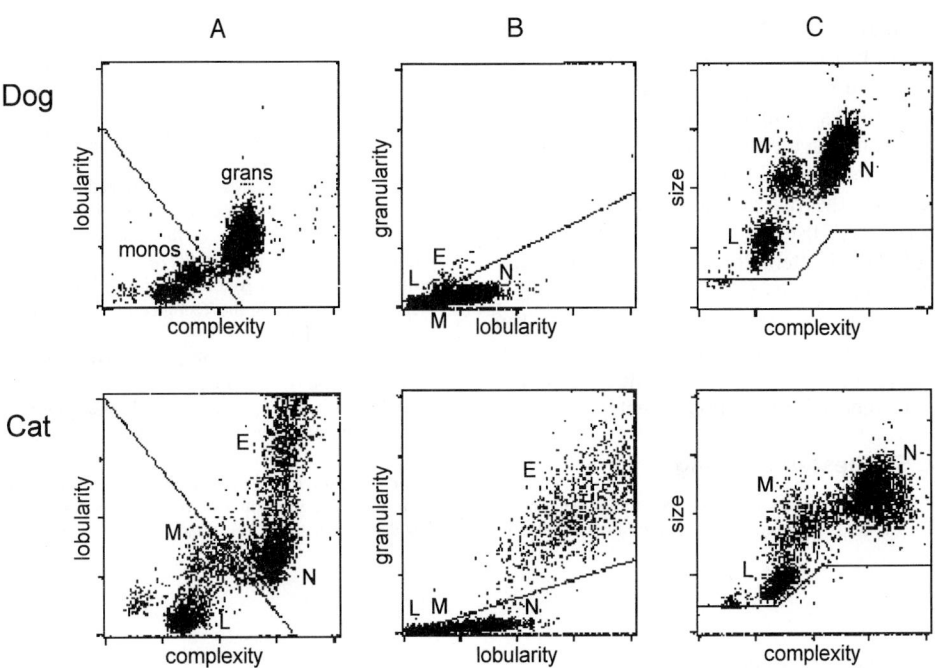

Figure 10. Cell-Dyn leukocyte cytograms from a normal dog *(top row)* and a cat with eosinophilia. The differential count is generated by first separating the unstained cells into granulocytes and "mononuclear cells" (including basophils) on the basis of nuclear lobularity and complexity *(A)*. Neutrophils are distinguished from eosinophils by plotting cytoplasmic granularity against nuclear lobularity; note that the cat *(B, bottom)* had many circulating eosinophils, while the dog had few. The mononuclear cells are separated into monocytes, lymphocytes, and degranulated basophils by plotting size against complexity to produce the cytogram *(C)* most comparable in appearance to the peroxidase cytogram of the H-1 (see Fig. 5). The eosinophils are interspersed with the neutrophils in *A* and *C*. The few basophils and the overlapping cell populations cannot be discerned without color imaging. Not shown are the other three cytograms that are available for each sample and generated by plotting the remaining combinations of the four scatter parameters (e.g., lobularity versus size). monos, mononuclear cells; grans, granulocytes; E, eosinophils; L, lymphocytes; M, monocytes; N, neutrophils.

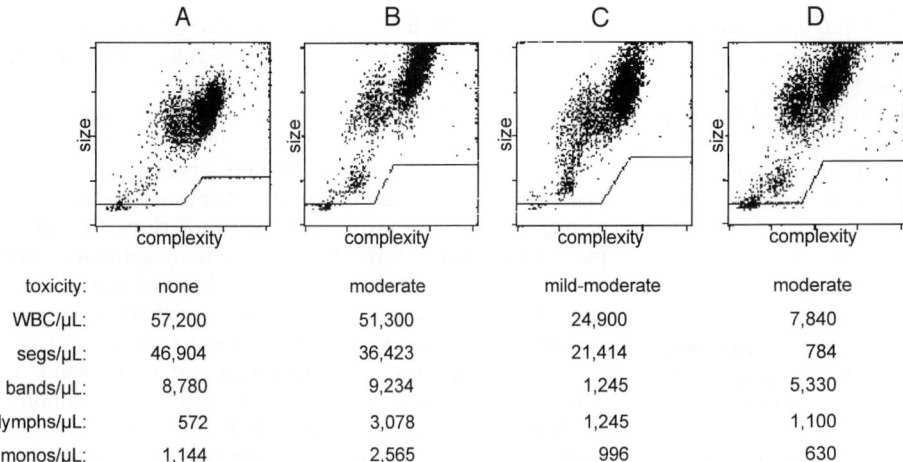

	A	B	C	D
toxicity:	none	moderate	mild-moderate	moderate
WBC/µL:	57,200	51,300	24,900	7,840
segs/µL:	46,904	36,423	21,414	784
bands/µL:	8,780	9,234	1,245	5,330
lymphs/µL:	572	3,078	1,245	1,100
monos/µL:	1,144	2,565	996	630

Figure 11. Leukocyte cytograms and manual differential leukocyte counts from four dogs with inflammatory conditions. Dogs *A* and *B* had leukocytoses and regenerative left shifts of similar magnitude. Note, however, that the neutrophil cluster is shifted upward (compare with Figure 10*C*) only for the dog with toxic change *(B)*. Upward shifts of the neutrophil cluster also occur when toxic change accompanies more mild left shifts *(C)* and with degenerative left shifts in the absence of leukocytosis *(D)*.

of the neutrophil cluster. This pattern is distinctly different from that of aged blood (mailed in samples), in which the neutrophil clusters are loosely arranged and unassociated with significant upward drift. As with the H-1 (see Figs. 2 and 4), the RBC size distribution histogram can be used to detect abnormal RBC populations that may or may not be sufficiently large to affect the RBC indices (see Fig. 9). Blood smears must then be evaluated to determine the specific abnormalities present. When evaluating the RBC histogram, it is important to recognize that the platelet peak is generated relative to the RBC peak, which has a constant height despite the packed cell volume (PCV). Therefore, peak heights do not correlate with the concentration of either platelets or RBCs. The RBC histogram does not appear to be particularly useful in identifying regenerative anemias, in part because of the right shoulder that is frequently present in samples from nonanemic animals (see Fig. 9*A*). Marked thrombocytopenias and thrombocytoses may be apparent on canine RBC histograms, but apparent inconsistencies between the platelet and RBC histograms have limited the authors' use of the platelet histogram. Clear separation of the platelets from the RBCs is often not possible with canine samples (see Fig. 9*B* to *F*), and it is rarely possible with feline samples. In such cases, the automated platelet concentrations should not be accepted, and platelet concentrations should be estimated by smear evaluations or determined with a hemocytometer.

References and Suggested Reading

Northern J Jr, Tvedten HW: Reports of retrospective studies. Diagnosis of microthrombocytosis and immune-mediated thrombocytopenia in dogs with thrombocytopenia: 68 cases (1987–1989). JAVMA 200:368 1992.
  Retrospective study that describes the unique finding of low mean platelet volume in dogs diagnosed as having immune-mediated thrombocytopenia and illustrates the platelet histogram changes in various diseases.
Tvedten HW: Advanced hematology analyzers: Interpretation of results. Vet Clin Path 22:72 1993a.
  A paper similar to this article—includes additional examples of diagnostic patterns.
Tvedten HW: Multispecies Hematology Atlas. Tarrytown, NY: Miles Inc., 1993b, p 44.
  Includes about 50 veterinary cases that illustrate hematologic changes well visualized with cytograms and histograms, describes more in-depth technical aspects of the H-1 analyzer, and has a section on interpretation of H-1 reports.
Tvedten HW: What is your diagnosis? Cat with Heinz body anemia after eating baby food. Vet Clin Path 25:148 1996.
  Case report that illustrates the unique RBC cytogram and hemoglobin histogram patterns of Heinz bodies in apparently hyperchromic RBCs; also shows how WBC cytograms demonstrate errors in the WBC count owing to Heinz bodies.
Tvedten H, Haines C: Canine automated differential leukocyte count: Study using a hematology analyzer system. Vet Clin Path 23:72 1994.
  Describes the accuracy of an automated differential WBC count in dogs and what errors are likely.
Tvedten H, Korcal H: Automated differential leukocyte count in horses, cattle and cats using the Technicon H-1E hematology system. Vet Clin Path 25:72 1996.
  Describes the accuracy of an automated differential WBC count in cats and what errors are likely.
Weiser MG, Kociba GJ: Sequential changes in erythrocyte volume distribution and microcytosis associated with iron deficiency in kittens. Vet Pathol 20:1, 1983.
  The first paper to document the frequent presence of microcytosis and iron deficiency in kittens. Newer, more sensitive hematology analyzer techniques were required to detect the disease.

Hematology Instrumentation for the In-House Laboratory

BARRY T. MITZNER
Miami, Florida

The complete blood count (CBC) is typically performed in the veterinary hospital or clinic using either manual methods or instrumentation. Manual methods have been extensively described elsewhere. The purpose of this article is to educate veterinarians about the types of hematology instruments available, the various features and limitations of each, and the responsibilities that come with performing in-house hematology. The informed veterinarian-consumer should choose hematology instruments that are truly appropriate to the needs of the particular practice.

The CBC is one of the most common tests performed by veterinarians and should be considered a part of every minimum database. The indications for CBC testing include diagnostic evaluation for numerous disease states as well as presurgical screening. The CBC should also be included in any geriatric or other well-animal screen. The author believes that CBC results are best obtained in-house and are often of greatest value when available on a STAT basis owing to the dynamic nature of whole blood.

METHODOLOGIES

The first blood-counting instruments used by veterinarians, perhaps as long as 30 years ago, were of the electronic-impedance type. Most were semiautomated Coulter Counters, which were manufactured for the human market but were found to perform reasonably well with animal specimens. These early impedance-type analyzers were limited in their diagnostic scope and could be troublesome to operate and maintain. With the increased use of microprocessor technology in the early 1980s, many of these problems were reduced or eliminated completely, greatly improving impedance counter operation and ease of use. Today, electronic impedance analyzers still constitute the majority of instruments used in both human and veterinary medical offices as well as hospitals and reference laboratories (Table 1).

The theory behind electronic impedance counting is based on the finding that cells are poor electrical conductors. When cells are diluted in a conductive solution (saline) and passed through an aperture having electrodes on each side, a measurable change in the current moving between the electrodes is produced by the resistance of the cell. The number of minute changes in the electrical current produced within a designated time interval corresponds to the number of cells in solution, while the magnitude of the resistance corresponds to the size of each individual cell. Further electronic refinements based primarily on cell size allow the impedance analyzer to pick and choose which cells are counted.

A second methodology, developed in the 1980s, uses quantitative buffy coat analysis. This methodology is based on the principle that different cell types have different densities. When whole blood is centrifuged at high speed in a narrow tube, cells tend to sediment based on their individual densities. In a spun microhematocrit tube, white blood cells are represented by a narrow line between the red blood cells and the plasma interface. This narrow line is referred to as the buffy coat. Quantitative buffy coat analysis relies on the *expansion* of this narrow line, or buffy coat, so that each individual cell layer can be visualized and measured. Of the current instruments available, one contains an expansion float that is inserted into the tube while supravital stains coating the inside of the tube aid the system in further delineating and recognizing each layer. A second method takes a direct reading from the nonexpanded buffy coat layer.

The final methodology, discussed here for the sake of completeness, is flow cytometry. Flow cytometry uses a laser beam through which cells are passed, resulting in a diffraction, or "scattering," of the light. The exact character of the scattering correlates with the size and granularity of the cell type. Although flow cytometry–based instruments offer perhaps the most accurate and precise methodology for counting animal specimens, the cost of these advanced systems is usually far beyond the means of all but perhaps the largest veterinary practices.

QUALITY-CONTROL PRODUCTS

Commercial quality-control (QC) products, that is, preassayed blood samples, are available for almost every analyzer. Although all of these products are manufactured for the human market with the exception of Multi-Trol (CDC Technologies), they are still capable of providing adequate precision checks on the instrument, reagent system, specimen preparation, and operator protocol. Since the variation inherent in animal samples would be beyond the scope of any single QC product, the blood smear must also be included as a necessary part of any QC program.

In 1988, the United States Congress initiated legislation known today as the Clinical Laboratory Improvement Act, or CLIA '88. This legislation effectively regulated all laboratory tests performed in physicians' offices and established strict guidelines for testing, including periodic inspection and certification of the office laboratory. Daily bilevel QC testing to ensure the accuracy of patient tests run that day was among the new requirements for physicians' offices. Although veterinary offices were exempted from this legislation, it is no less essential that veterinarians establish their own in-house QC program, as veterinarians are frequently called on to treat the most critically ill of patients,

TABLE 1. Feature Comparison of Selected Hematology Analyzers[1]

	Parameters	Specimen Required	Cycle Time (min)	Cost/Test[2] (Unburdened)	Methodology	Autodilution[3]	Multispecies Software	Space Required	Reagent[4] System	QC Product[5]	Service Provided	Suggested[6] Retail
ABBOTT Diagnostics												
Cell-Dyn 400[7]	Hct, RBC, WBC, Hgb, MCV	40 µl	<2	$0.40	Impedance	No	N/A	18" × 17"[8]	Open	Available	On site	$8,990
BIOCHEM Immunosystems												
Baker System 9010 + 9110	HCT, RBC, WBC, Hgb, MCV, MCH, MCHC, RDW, Plt, MPV	110 µl	<2	<$1.00	Impedance	Yes	29 species	24" × 17"	Closed	Available	On site	$36,000
CDC Technologies												
Hemavet 300	HCT, RBC, WBC, LY%&#, Plt	20 µl	5	$2.36	Impedance	Yes	Dog, cat, cow, horse	10.5" × 17"	Closed	Available	Ship out	$8,250
Hemavet 500	HCT, RBC, WBC, Hgb, MCV, MCH, MCHC, RDW, Plt, Ne/M/Ba%&#, Ly%&#, Eos%&#, Histograms	20 µl	5	$2.36	Impedance	Yes	Dog, cat, cow, horse	10.5" × 17"	Closed	Available	Ship out	$12,950
Hemavet 800	HCT, RBC, WBC, Hgb, MCV, MCH, MCHC, RDW, RSD, NRBC%,; NRBC#, Reticulocyte%&#, Plt, MPV, PCT, PDW, Ne%&#, Mo%&#, Ba%&# #, Ly%&#, EO%&#, Histograms	20 µl	5	$2.36	Impedance	Yes	13 species (Diff: dog and cat only)	10.5" × 17"	Closed	Available	Ship out	$15,950
COULTER Diagnostics												
Z2[9]	RBC, WBC, Plt	40 µl	1	N/A	Impedance	No	N/A	12" × 12"	Open	Available	On site	$18,000
DANAM Electronics												
5710 V	Hct, RBC, WBC, Hgb, MCV, MCH, MCHC, RDW	20 µl	<2	$0.50	Impedance	No	Dog, cat, horse	19" × 15"[8]	Open	Available	Ship out	$6,500
Excel 10 V	Hct, RBC, WBC, Hgb, MCV, MCH, MCHC, RDW, Plt, MPV	60–125 µl	1	$1.00	Impedance	Yes	Dog, cat, horse	18" × 17"	Closed	Available	Ship out	$14,875
IDEXX												
QBC-V Autoread	HCT, WBC, Hgb, MCHC, Plt, Gran%&#, Eos, Neut, Lym/Mono[10] Neu#,[11] Retic%,[10] Fibrinogen[12]	111 µl	<10	$3.36	QBC analysis	NR[13]	Dog, cat, cow, horse	15" × 17"	Closed	Cal tube[14,15]	Ship out	$10,800

	Parameters	Sample		Cost/test[2]	Method[3]		Species	Dimensions	Reagent system[4]	QC[5]	Installation	Price[6]
SYSMEX Corporation												
F520	Hct, RBC, WBC, Hgb, MCV	20 µl	2	$0.40	Impedance	No	N/A	18" × 13"[8]	Open	Available	On site	$12,700
F820	HCT, RBC, WBC, Hgb, MCV, MCH, MCHC, Plt, RDW, PDW, MPV, (Gran%&#, Ly%&#, Histograms[16])	20 µl	<1	$0.40	Impedance	No	N/A	23.5" × 16"[8]	Open	Available	On site	$22,700
Texas International Labs (TIL)												
H5	Hct, RBC, WBC, Hgb, MCV	20 µl	<2	$0.33	Impedance	No	N/A	18" × 18"	Open	Available	Ship out	$5,995
H18	Hct, RBC, WBC, Hgb, MCV, MCH, MCHC, Plt, MPV, RDW, Ly, Mono, Gran%and#, Histogram	32 µl	1	$0.14	Impedance	Yes	Dog, cat, horse, cow, human	18" × 15"	Closed	Available	Ship out	$16,500
ZYNOCYTE												
VS2000	Hct, WBC, Hgb, MCHC, Plt, TP, Ict, Lip, Hemolysis[17]	45 µl	12	$2.59	QBC analysis + photometric[18]	NR	Dog, cat, horse	9.5" × 12"	Closed	Cal tube[13]	Ship out	$5,950

Ba, Basophil; EO or Eos, eosinophil; Gran, granulocyte; Hct, hematocrit; Hgb, hemoglobin; Ict, icterus; Lip, lipemia; LY or Lym, lymphocyte; MCH, mean cell hemoglobin; MCHC, mean cell hemoglobin concentration; Mo or Mono, monocyte; MPV, mean platelet volume; MCV, mean cell volume; Ne or Neu or Neut, neutrophil; NRBC, nucleated red blood cell; PCT, plasma clotting time; PDW, platelet distribution width; Plt, platelet; RDW, red-cell distribution width; Retic, reticulocyte; RSD, red-cell standard deviation; TP, total protein.

[1] The analyzers listed have been selected for comparison on the basis of features, cost, and operational skills required. While this list is by no means all inclusive, it includes most well-known of the analyzers capable of meeting a variety of individual practice needs.

[2] The unburdened cost per test (cost/test) may not include consumables used for quality control, calibration, or preventive maintenance procedures.

[3] Systems that do not have this feature require that specimens be diluted prior to counting. This procedure is usually performed with an automatic dilutor; however, dilution can also be accomplished manually.

[4] Instruments with "open" reagent systems have more than one source for consumables and supplies. "Closed" systems require that consumables be purchased from a single manufacturer.

[5] QC products are commercial blood preparations with known assay values that are designed to mimic an actual patient specimen as it is processed through each step of the analytical procedure.

[6] Suggested retail pricing has been supplied by each manufacturer. Typical and promotional pricing tends to be lower to much lower, depending on the product.

[7] Cell-Dyn is manufactured for Abbott Diagnostics by Metertech. Metertech also manufactures a proprietary analyzer for nondomestic distribution under the Excell name.

[8] Includes space allotment for a separate dilutor.

[9] Sold primarily as a "particle counter" for use in analytical research, the Z2 has the ability to count animal cells and can store settings for as many as five custom-selected species.

[10] Canine only.

[11] Canine and feline only.

[12] Fibrinogen testing requires a software update and accessory precipitator (about $125.00).

[13] Testing is performed with a nondiluted specimen.

[14] The calibration (cal) tube checks only the computer and optical reader. Additional materials would be required for complete QC.

[15] Complete QC products are manufactured by both Becton Dickinson and Hematronix for use with the human version of the QBC AutoRead system.

[16] Human only, not yet available for veterinary species.

[17] Analysis is performed on plasma.

[18] Refers to a methodology utilized for quantitation of plasma constituents and hemoglobin.

and laboratory errors could have dire consequences. While daily QC testing may not be appropriate for all veterinary practices, it is important that a regular schedule be established and strictly adhered to; for without a QC program, laboratory results become just "numbers," instead of clinically useful answers.

IMPORTANCE OF THE BLOOD SMEAR

Although most practitioners would prefer to have differential counts performed automatically, the current state of veterinary hematology precludes the sole reliance on instrument-generated differential counts. While several reasonably priced instruments offer differential counts, partial differential counts, or differential-related information, without exception every operator's manual recommends a blood smear *to complete the hematologic picture.*

Among the more important reasons for this recommendation is the fact that "some disease states are characterized by the presence of abnormal white cell types or nucleated red blood cells and yet *may display total white cell counts in the normal range* as well as normal quantitative relationships of granulocytes to lymphocytes/monocytes."[*] In addition, "the [blood] film provides the necessary morphology to fully investigate the nature of the condition."[†] The issue of QC encompasses another important reason for performing the blood smear, as the blood smear can easily and graphically provide crosschecks on the instrument-derived measurements. "Since no single quality control technique can routinely provide sufficient data for effective quality assurance, the recommended QC program . . . includes manual review of patient samples."[‡] Although it would be profoundly beneficial to have an instrument that provides the practitioner with the equivalent of a complete blood smear evaluation, escaping the responsibility of performing a microscopic blood smear examination is neither compatible with high-quality practice nor an appropriate reason for investing in hematology instrumentation.

IMPEDANCE INSTRUMENTS

As mentioned earlier, impedance instruments make up the largest group in use today in both veterinary and physicians' offices. They are also the choice of most small to medium-sized reference laboratories, owing to the wide array of impedance instruments available. Among the manufacturers of impedance instruments (Table 2) applicable to office-based animal testing are (alphabetically) Abbott Diagnostics, BioChem Immunosystems (Baker), CDC Technologies, Coulter, Danam, Sysmex, and Texas International Laboratories (TIL).

When compared with human blood, the accurate enumeration and measurement of animal blood cells introduces a new set of technologic challenges. First and foremost, the system must have operator-adjustable settings to ac-

---

[*]QBC Autoread Operator's Manual. Sparks, MD: Becton Dickinson Primary Care Diagnostics, 1996, Sec. 7.2.1.

[†]QBC VetAutoread Owner's Manual. Westbrook, ME: Idexx Laboratories, 1995, Sec. A-3.

[‡]Mascot Product Reference Manual for Hemavet Series Multispecies Hematology Instruments. Oxford, CT: CDC Technologies, Inc., 1996, Secs. 1–2.

TABLE 2. Hematology Instrumentation Manufacturers

Abbott Diagnostics Division 850 Maude Avenue Mountain View, CA 94043 (800)933-5535	Danam Electronics 4230 Shilling Way Dallas, TX 75237 (800)433-0945
BioChem Immunosystems 100 Cascade Drive Allentown, PA 18103-9562 (800)345-3127	Idexx Laboratories One Idexx Drive Westbrook, ME 04092 (800)248-2483
CDC Technologies 1 Great Hill Road Oxford, CT 06478 (800)858-2324	Sysmex Corporation of America Gilmer Road, 6699 RFD Long Grove, IL 60047-9596 (800)379-7639
Coulter Corporation Particle Characterization 　Division M/C 19500/PO Box 169015 Miami, FL 33116-9015 (305)885-0131, X3911	Texas International Laboratories 5 Rain Hollow Houston, TX 77024 (713)464-6946
	Zynocyte, Ltd. 225 Water Street, Suite 212 Plymouth, MA 02360 (508)830-0054

*This list may not include some manufacturers and suppliers.

---

commodate the differences in cell size among the various animal species. Animal platelets, particularly in dogs and cats, are sensitive to clumping, which can interfere with counts. In addition, large immature platelets can interfere with RBC counts. Lysing reagents, which were originally formulated to lyse RBCs while sparing the relatively resistant human white blood cells (WBCs), must be sufficiently mild so as not to affect or completely destroy the more fragile animal WBCs.

Of the manufacturers listed previously, some offer human-based systems with available specialized veterinary software packages, while others simply offer instruments in nonveterinary packaging that provide the necessary requirements for testing of animal specimens. Since there is still no commercially available multispecies calibrator, the calibration parameters utilized by so-called multispecies hematology systems are based on statistical data derived from assaying multiple samples from each single species. One manufacturer, CDC Technologies, supplies only veterinary instruments and reagents, which the company claims have been specifically formulated to better handle animal specimens. The range of parameters available from impedance-type analyzers extends from entry level systems that perform just WBC, RBC, hematocrit (Hct), and hemoglobin (Hgb) all the way to systems that offer differential information, histograms, and other measurements such as platelet distribution width (PDW), red-cell distribution width (RDW), and mean platelet volume (MPV).

Entry-level impedance analyzers tend to be the simplest to operate and maintain. They are generally affordable and typically offer a low cost per test, often below 50 cents. The use of microprocessors has greatly improved performance and reduced reliance on extensive manual procedures to maintain the analyzer in peak operating condition.

Among the potential disadvantages of impedance analyzers is the concern that particle counters cannot easily distinguish between two different particles (cells) of the same size. This drawback can be a particular problem with feline specimens, which often include large platelets that are similar in size to the relatively small feline RBCs. Lower-cost instruments, in particular, tend to read these mixtures of platelets and RBCs as a single subpopulation, often making interpretation of results difficult. Some middle- and higher-priced instruments, however, are now offering histograms as well as other refinements that have aided in the interpretation of some of these difficult specimens. Other considerations include instrument size (some are physically quite large) and the fact that a variety of solutions and other consumables have to be inventoried and periodically checked for expiration dates. While the reliability of most impedance instruments has improved dramatically over the last decade or so, repairs, if necessary, can still be expensive.

BUFFY COAT ANALYZERS

Quantitative buffy coat (QBC) analyzers have been used as screening devices in veterinary practice since the middle to late 1980s. The first analyzer of this type to be marketed to the veterinary community was the QBC-V from Becton Dickinson. The first QBC-V was a manual system, requiring the operator to directly view the various sediment layers through an ocular viewer to establish each layer's thickness. The QBC-VetAutoread, manufactured by Becton Dickinson and distributed today by Idexx Laboratories, utilizes a computerized optical reader that automatically records measurements from a spinning capillary tube. Both the QBC-VetAutoread (veterinary version) and the QBC Autoread (human version) are manufactured by Becton Dickinson; however, Idexx Laboratories has developed an extensive veterinary software package to expand the utility of the system and to aid in the interpretation of results. Both the human and the veterinary versions can also measure fibrinogen levels, which requires a software update and an accessory precipitator. In addition, Idexx has developed a computer link that captures the results from the VetAutoread as well as the company's chemistry and electrolyte instruments, to provide a single, composite patient laboratory report.

A relative newcomer to the QBC analysis field is the newly released VS2000 from Zynocyte, Ltd. Utilizing a filled capillary tube similar to that used in the VetAutoread system, the VS2000 uses infrared laser analysis to generate values for HCT, WBC, and platelets. A built-in polychromatic reader simultaneously scans the plasma portion of the spinning tube for changes suggestive of lipemia, icterus, or hemolysis. Also included with the VS2000 is a built-in photometer that, at the option of the operator, can be used to determine Hgb, mean cell hemoglobin concentration (MCHC), and values for total solids.

Quantitative buffy coat analysis was developed in the early 1980s as a screening tool for use primarily in locales where skilled laboratory personnel might not be readily available. This use underscores the major advantage of the QBC methodology—simplicity. Other advantages of the QBC methodology include the analyzer's compact size, the low maintenance requirements, and the limited number of consumables laboratories must inventory. Repairs of these systems are relatively inexpensive because there are no pumps, tubing, or valves, as there are in impedance analyzers.

The potential disadvantages of buffy coat analyzers include the relatively high cost per test (relative to most impedance analyzers), slower turnaround time for results, and, for some systems, the absence of a true QC product that verifies the proper performance of all parts of the system. Quality control for both the VS2000 and the QBC-VetAutoread is currently limited to a permanent calibration tube that checks only the optical reader. Another consideration is the requirement that live specimens be used. This requirement precludes holding the specimen for several hours before analysis. For systems that use coated tubes (QBC-VetAutoread), attention must be paid to the open-vial stability of these products, which is independent of the expiration date. Lower-volume users may find themselves disposing of leftover tubes after 30 days or gambling on performance.

Buffy coat analysis was originally developed as an easy-to-use screening tool; thus, in the author's view, veterinarians should be cognizant of inherent limitations of this methodology. If these limitations are kept in mind, however, QBC analyzers may provide a viable alternative for some practices.

While the addition of in-house hematology studies can be a valuable asset for any practice, veterinarians should spend ample time considering the diagnostic needs and technical capabilities of their particular practice before making a purchasing decision. Sales representatives should be asked about the advantages, disadvantages, sample costs, and QC issues. Individual practice needs should also be considered. Will the instrumentation be used primarily to screen normal patients, or will abnormal and critically ill patients also be tested? How many tests will be performed each week or each month? Will blood smears be a part of every CBC? How will quality control be addressed and implemented? These are just a few of the questions that must be answered. There are undoubtedly many more. Most important, veterinarians must realize that they alone are responsible for the accuracy of the laboratory results they generate in their hospitals and must be willing to accept these responsibilities to the extent that any clinical action they take can be adequately validated.

References and Suggested Reading

Brown SA, Barsanti JA: Quantitative buffy coat analysis for hematologic measurements of canine, feline, and equine blood samples and for detection of microfilaremia in dogs. Am J Vet Res 49:321, 1988.
  A review of the QBC technology, correlation to reference methods, advantages, and limitations.
Carlson D: Hematology testing in the doctor's office laboratory. Clin Lab Med 6:273, 1986.
  A review of the methods commonly used to perform hematologic testing in the physician's office laboratory (POL).
Hart A: General Review of Different Blood Cells; Review of Mechanics of the Different Methods of Producing Blood Counts; Obtaining and Handling Specimens. Paper presented at 67th Annual Convention of the Florida Veterinary Medical Association, Orlando, September 20, 1996.
  The paper compares the QBC technology to other reference methods and discusses the importance of blood smear evaluation as an integral part of each CBC.

Knoll JS, Rowell SL: Clinical hematology: In clinic analysis, quality control, reference values, and system selection. Vet Clin North Am. Small Anim Pract 26:981, 1996.
    A review of the various methods for performing complete blood counts, including a description of some of the available automated hematology instruments used in both private practice and reference laboratories.
Rebar AH: Personal communication, February 7, 1997.

Tvedten H: Referral and in-office laboratories. In: Willard MD, Tvedten H, Turnwald GH, eds: Small Animal Clinical Diagnosis by Laboratory Methods. Philadelphia: WB Saunders, 1989, pp 1–13.
    A review of the components of the basic veterinary laboratory as well as discussions of quality control and cost comparison. The establishment of relationships with reference laboratories is also reviewed.

Blood Typing and Crossmatching to Ensure Compatible Transfusions

URS GIGER

Philadelphia, Pennsylvania

Transfusion therapy has assumed an increasingly important role in the life support of companion animals (Howard et al, 1992). Over the past decade, the use of blood products in treating critically ill animals has drastically increased (Callan et al, 1995; Griot-Wenk and Giger, 1995). Furthermore, the need for blood typing and crossmatching as well as testing of donors for transmittable diseases has now been recognized for ensuring safe and more efficacious transfusions (Cotter, 1991; Hohenhaus, 1992; Giger, 1997). Advances in blood compatibility testing in dogs and cats are reviewed, and practical recommendations are made.

CANINE BLOOD TYPES

Blood types are genetic markers on erythrocyte surfaces that are antigenic and species specific. A set of blood types of two or more alleles makes up a blood group system. More than a dozen blood group systems have been described in dogs (Bell, 1983). The various systems are referred to as dog erythrocyte antigens, with the abbreviation DEA followed by a number. For all blood group systems other than the DEA 1 system, red blood cells from a dog can be positive or negative for that blood type. For instance, for the DEA 7 system, a dog's cells can be DEA 7 positive or DEA 7 negative. These blood types appear to be codominantly inherited. The DEA 1 system, however, has at least two subtypes: DEA 1.1 (also known as A_1) and DEA 1.2 (A_2). Thus, a dog's red blood cells can be DEA 1.1 positive or negative, and DEA 1.1–negative cells can be DEA 1.2 positive or negative. An A_3 subtype has been described in Australia, but no reagents are available for comparative studies. Only limited surveys on the frequency of these blood types have been reported (Table 1). There may be geographic and breed-associated differences in the frequencies of these blood types (Giger et al, 1995).

Blood types that are strongly antigenic are of great clinical importance in dogs; the most antigenic blood type is DEA 1.1. Dogs can become sensitized after receiving a mismatched transfusion, that is, blood with a type different from that of the recipient. Transfusion of DEA 1.1–positive cells to a DEA 1.1–negative dog invariably elicits a strong alloantibody response. After a first transfusion, anti–DEA 1.1 antibodies develop after more than 4 days and may cause a delayed transfusion reaction. However, a previously sensitized DEA 1.1–negative dog will develop an acute hemolytic reaction after transfusion of DEA 1.1–positive blood (Giger et al, 1995). Transfusion reactions may also occur after a sensitized dog receives blood that is mismatched for a red blood cell antigen other than DEA 1.1. For instance, a Whippet developed an alloantibody against a common red blood cell antigen, resulting in a general incompatibility with any donor except a littermate (Callan et al, 1996).

A blood-typing card for classifying dogs as DEA 1.1 positive or negative has become available as a simple in-practice kit.* The assay requires a small amount of anticoagulated blood (0.1 ml) and is based on an agglutination reaction that occurs within 2 minutes when erythrocytes that are DEA 1.1 positive interact with a murine monoclonal antibody specific to DEA 1.1 (Andrews et al,

---

*DMS Laboratories, 2 Darts Mill Road, Flemington, NJ 08822, (800) 567-4DMS.

TABLE 1. Blood Type Frequencies in Dogs

Blood types	Percentage	
	Positive	*Negative*
DEA 1.1*		
1.1 (A1)	33–45	55–67
1.2 (A2)	7–20	35–60*
DEA 3 (B)	5–10	90–95
DEA 4 (C)	87–98	2–13
DEA 5 (D)	12–22	78–88
DEA 7 (Tr)	8–45	55–92

*DEA 1.1 *and* 1.2 negative dogs.
From limited surveys in Giger U, Gelens J, Callan MB, et al: An acute hemolytic transfusion reaction caused by dog erythrocyte antigen 1.1 incompatibility in a previously sensitized dog. J Am Vet Med Assoc 206:9, 1995.

1992; Kohn et al, 1998). Typing of donors for DEA 1.1 is strongly recommended because of the strong antigenicity of this antigen. Whenever it is possible, the recipient should also be typed, to allow the use of DEA 1.1–positive blood for DEA 1.1–positive recipients. Typing for DEA 1.1 can be done in practice or is available through most commercial and veterinary school laboratories as well as through the author's laboratory.

Caution should be exercised whenever the blood is autoagglutinating or has a very low hematocrit (<10%). It is recommended to check for autoagglutination of blood with saline on a slide. Autoagglutinating blood may first be washed with saline. However, true (persistent) auto-agglutination precludes typing because such a specimen will always look like DEA 1.1–positive blood. An animal with such blood should receive DEA 1.1–negative blood until the blood does not agglutinate anymore. Recently transfused dogs may show a mixed-field reaction, with only recipient or transfused cells agglutinating. Furthermore, DEA 1.1–positive blood from very anemic animals may not agglutinate when exposed to the DEA 1.1 reagent because of a prozone effect. In these cases, some of the patient's plasma may be discarded before a drop of blood is applied to the card. Finally, a very fine agglutination reaction may be observed with blood from DEA 1.1–negative, but DEA 1.2–positive, dogs (A. Hale, personal communication).

Typing service and polyclonal antisera are available for DEA 1.1, 1.2, 3, 4, 5, and 7 (blood types mentioned in Table 1).* Use of these blood-typing products, however, requires some expertise and experience. Some veterinarians recommend exclusive use of canine donors that are negative for all testable DEA except DEA 4 (98% of all dogs are positive) to prevent sensitization against these blood types (Hale, 1995). However, the author does not support the routine typing for other blood types, for the following reasons:

1. This protocol unnecessarily eliminates many active and potential donors. Based on the published frequencies, fewer than 1 in 10 dogs would be acceptable.
2. This extended blood-typing protocol would be cost prohibitive because many dogs would need to be typed for every negative dog.
3. Generally, humans are typed only for ABO and Rh, although many other blood types are known.
4. Typing for more than DEA 1.1 does not eliminate the need for crossmatching.
5. There are no supporting published clinical reports that transfusion reactions could be substantially reduced with routine typing for other blood types.

FELINE BLOOD TYPES

The AB blood group system is the only one recognized in cats and consists of three blood types: type A, type B, and type AB (Auer and Bell, 1981; Bell, 1983; Griot-Wenk et al, 1993). Their inheritance pattern is unique and of considerable importance to breeders with respect to neo-natal isoerythrolysis. The A allele is dominant over the B allele. Thus, only homozygous B/B cats express the type B antigen on their erythrocytes. Type A cats are either homozygous (A/A) or heterozygous (A/B) for the A allele (Giger et al, 1991a). Finally, the rare AB blood type is separately inherited as a third allele that is recessive to A and codominant to B (Griot-Wenk et al, 1996). The frequency of feline A and B blood types varies geographically and among breeds (Table 2). Although type A is the most common blood type, the frequency of type A and B in domestic shorthair cats varies worldwide and even among regions. Depending on the breed, the type B frequency may vary from none, as in the Siamese and related breeds, to 40%, as in the British shorthair and Devon Rex breeds. In contrast, type AB is extremely rare, with a frequency of less than 1% in domestic shorthair and some purebred cats.

In contrast to dogs, cats possess naturally occurring alloantibodies (also known as isoantibodies) against the blood type antigen they lack. In particular, all type B cats develop very strong anti-A antibodies with high hemolysin and agglutinin titers (>1:32) after a few weeks of age (Bücheler and Giger, 1993). These anti-A antibodies are responsible for the life-threatening incompatibility reactions, such as neonatal isoerythrolysis and acute hemolytic transfusion reactions.

A mismatched transfusion with type A blood given to a type B cat will result in a very serious acute hemolytic transfusion reaction (Giger and Bücheler, 1991). A first transfusion and as little as 1 ml of incompatible blood may cause a fatal reaction without prior sensitization. Affected cats may show anaphylactic signs of hypotension, brady-cardia, vomiting, and convulsions followed by hemolytic signs of pigmenturia and icterus without a transfusion-associated rise of the hematocrit. Thus, mismatched trans-fusions are dangerous as well as ineffective.

The A and AB kittens receiving anti-A alloantibodies through the colostrum from type B queens, including pri-miparous queens, during the first day of life are at risk for neonatal isoerythrolysis. Hemolysis of the newborn is characterized by dark pigmenturia, anemia, icterus, an-orexia, and sudden death within the first week of life.

In contrast to type B cats, type A cats have generally weak anti-B alloantibodies with low anti-B titers of 1:2. These antibodies cause shortened survival of transfused B cells in type A cats with relatively mild signs of acute hemolytic anemia. However, these anti-B antibodies have not been associated with neonatal isoerythrolysis in type B kittens born to type A queens.

A simple blood-typing card has become available for classifying cats as type A, B, or AB.* This test kit is similar to the canine blood-typing cards except that there are separate wells to detect type A and B cells. Serum from type B cats and a lectin (*Triticum vulgaris*) serve as anti-A and anti-B reagents and produce strong agglutina-tion reactions with type A and type B blood, respectively (Andrews et al, 1992a; Griot-Wenk et al, 1993; Kohn et al, 1997). As for canine typing, the same precautions regarding autoagglutinating and very anemic blood apply for cats. Feline blood typing is also available through most commer-

---

*From Dr. Robert Bull, B228 Life Sciences Building, Michigan State University, East Lansing, MI 48824; 517-355-4616.

*DMS Laboratories, 2 Darts Mill Road, Flemington, NJ 08822, 1-800-567-4DMS.

TABLE 2. **Blood Type A and B Frequencies in Cats**

Domestic Shorthair*	Percentage (%)		Purebred Cats	Percentage (%)	
	Type A	Type B		Type A	Type B
USA			Abyssinian	84	16
Northeast	99.7	0.3	American shorthair	100	0
North central	99.6	0.4	Birman*	82	18
Southeast	98.5	1.5	British shorthair*	64	36
Southwest	97.5	2.5	Burmese	100	0
West Coast	95.3	4.7	Cornish Rex	67	33
Other Countries			Devon Rex	59	41
Australia (Brisbane)	73.7	26.3	Exotic shorthair	73	27
Argentina	97.3	2.7	Himalayan	94	6
Europe			Japanese Bobtail	84	16
Austria	97.0	3.0	Maine Coon	97	3
England	97.1	2.9	Norwegian Forest	93	7
Finland	100	0	Oriental shorthair	100	0
France	85.1	14.9	Persian	86	14
Germany	94.0	6.0	Scottish Fold*	81	19
Italy	88.8	11.2	Siamese	100	0
Netherlands	96.1	3.9	Somali*	82	18
Scotland	97.1	2.9	Sphinx* (Canadian hairless)	83	17
Switzerland	99.6	0.4	Tonkinese	100	0

*Breeds with isolated type AB cats.

Adapted from Giger U, Bücheler J, Patterson DF: Frequency and inheritance of A and B blood types in feline breeds of the United States. J Hered 82:15, 1991, by permission of Oxford University Press; and Giger U, Griot-Wenk M, Bücheler J, et al: Geographical variation of the feline blood type frequencies in the United States. Feline Pract 19:5, 1991, with permission.

cial and veterinary school laboratories, including the author's laboratory, which has typed more than 12,000 cats. Blood that is typed as AB should be confirmed in a reference laboratory because unspecific agglutination may mimic the rare AB blood type. Typing is recommended (1) for feline donor and recipient cats to give matched transfusions and (2) for breeding cats to ensure blood-compatible mates.

BLOOD CROSSMATCHING TEST

Whereas blood-typing tests reveal the blood group antigens on the red blood cell surface, blood crossmatching tests indicate the serologic compatibility or incompatibility between donor and recipient (Giger, 1997). Thus, the crossmatching tests check for the presence or absence of naturally occurring and induced alloantibodies in serum (or plasma); these antibodies may be hemolyzing and/or hemagglutinating and can be directed against known blood groups or other red blood cell surface antigens. The major crossmatch tests for alloantibodies in the recipient's plasma against donor cells, whereas the minor crossmatch test looks for alloantibodies in the donor's plasma against the recipient's red blood cells. Autoagglutination or severe hemolysis may preclude crossmatch testing. A major crossmatch incompatibility is of greatest importance because it predicts that the transfused donor cells will be attacked by antibodies in the patient's plasma, thereby causing an acute hemolytic transfusion reaction that could be life-threatening. A minor crossmatch incompatibility is of lesser concern because the donor's plasma volume is small, particularly in packed red blood cell products, and is markedly diluted in the patient. It is important to recognize that the prediction and interpretation of crossmatch test results are different between dogs and cats (also see the next article for specific crossmatch techniques).

Dogs. The initial blood crossmatch between two dogs that have never before received a transfusion should be compatible, because dogs do not have naturally occurring alloantibodies. Therefore, one might omit a crossmatch before the first transfusion. Because the crossmatch does not determine the blood type of the patient and donor, a compatible crossmatch does not prevent sensitization of the patient against donor cells within 1 to 2 weeks. Therefore, previously transfused dogs should always be crossmatched, even when they receive blood from the same donor. The time span between the initial transfusion and incompatibility reactions may be as short as 4 days, and the risk of a reaction lasts for many years (i.e., years after the last transfusion, alloantibodies may be present). Obviously, any blood donor should never have received a blood transfusion.

Cats. The initial crossmatching test result before the first transfusion may already be incompatible because of the presence of naturally occurring alloantibodies in cats. Furthermore, based on the crossmatch results and knowledge of the donor's blood type, one might be able to predict the blood type of the patient. If the *major* crossmatch is strongly incompatible, the recipient is probably a type B cat, and the donor has type A (or AB) blood (because of the *recipient's* strong anti-A). If the *minor* crossmatch is strongly incompatible, the recipient is likely to be a type A (or AB) cat, and the donor has type B blood (because of the *donor's* strong anti-A). Finally, if both crossmatches are compatible, the donor and the recipient have the same blood type. Thus, if blood typing is not available in a timely fashion, at least a crossmatch test should be done. Owing to strong anti-A agglutinins, blood type incompatibilities in cats can be recognized by a simplified crossmatch procedure mixing 2 drops of plasma with 1 drop of blood from either the recipient or the donor on a slide at room temperature. The development of macroscopic agglutination within a minute documents an A-B incompatibility. In contrast, administration of a small amount of blood to test for incompatibility is no longer an acceptable procedure. Only 1 ml of AB-incompatible blood can result in life-threatening acute hemolytic transfusion reactions (Giger and Bücheler, 1991; Griot-Wenk and Giger, 1995).

ALTERNATIVES TO BLOOD TRANSFUSIONS

Alternatives to blood transfusions should be considered because of the risk of incompatibility reactions and the time and expense involved in blood typing and crossmatching. Administration of erythropoietin can stimulate erythrocyte production in animals with renal failure and cancer. Although the DNA sequence of canine and feline erythropoietin is known, only a human recombinant erythropoietin is available, and this substance, unfortunately, may induce antierythropoietin antibody production, thereby blocking any regenerative response. Species-specific recombinant erythropoietins are being tested for dogs and cats. For the acute management of an anemic animal, highly purified hemoglobin solutions offer immediate oxygen-carrying capacity and volume expansion. A multicenter clinical trial on the efficacy and safety of an ultrapurified bovine hemoglobin solution (Biopure Corporation, Boston) in the treatment of anemic dogs has been completed, and it received approval in 1998 by the U.S. Food and Drug Administration (Rentko, 1992; see p. 424).

References and Suggested Reading

Andrews GA, Chavey PS, Smith JS: Production, characterization and application of a murine monoclonal antibody to dog erythrocyte antigen 1.1. J Am Vet Med Assoc 201:1549, 1992.
An ideal typing reagent for DEA 1.1.

Andrews GA, Chavey PS, Smith JE, et al: N-Glycolylneuraminic acid and N-acetylneuraminic acid define feline blood group A and B antigens. Blood 79:2485, 1992a.
A biochemical description of the feline blood group system.

Auer L, Bell K: The AB blood group system in cats. Anim Blood Groups Biochem Genet 12:287, 1981.
An initial description of the feline AB blood group system in Australia.

Bell K: Blood groups of domestic animals. In: Agar NS, Board DG, eds: Red Blood Cells of Domestic Mammals. Amsterdam: Elsevier Press, 1983, p 137.
A comprehensive review of blood groups in dogs and cats.

Bücheler J, Giger U: Alloantibodies against A and B blood types in cats. Vet Immunol Immunopathol 38:283, 1993.
A characterization of feline anti-A and anti-B alloantibodies.

Callan MB, Jones LT, Giger U: Hemolytic transfusion reactions in a dog with an alloantibody to a common antigen. J Vet Intern Med 9:277, 1995.
A clinical report of a hemolytic transfusion reaction.

Callan MB, Oakley DA, Shofer FS, et al: Canine red blood cell transfusion practices. J Am Anim Hosp Assoc 32:303, 1996.
The use of canine red blood cell transfusions.

Casal ML, Jezyk PF, Giger U: Transfer of colostral antibodies from queens to their kittens. Am J Vet Res 57:1653, 1996.
A study on feline colostral and neonatal antibodies.

Cotter SM, ed: Comparative Transfusion Medicine. San Diego, CA: Academic Press, 1991.
A comprehensive book on veterinary transfusion medicine.

Giger U: Transfusion medicine. In: Morgan RV, ed: Handbook of Small Animal Practice. San Diego, CA: Harcourt Brace, 1997, p. 739.
A practical review of transfusion medicine.

Giger U, Bücheler J: Transfusion of type A and type B blood to cats. J Am Vet Med Assoc 198:41, 1991.
An experimental study on feline red blood cell transfusions.

Giger U, Bücheler J, Patterson DF: Frequency and inheritance of A and B blood types in feline breeds of the United States. J Hered 82:15, 1991a.
A study on the mode of inheritance of feline blood types.

Giger U, Gelens J, Callan MB, et al: An acute hemolytic transfusion reaction caused by dog erythrocyte antigen 1.1 incompatibility in a previously sensitized dog. J Am Vet Med Assoc 206:9, 1995.
A documented case of DEA 1.1 incompatibility.

Giger U, Griot-Wenk M, Bücheler J, et al: Geographical variation of the feline blood type frequencies in the United States. Feline Pract 19:5, 1991b.
A survey of blood type frequencies in domestic cats.

Griot-Wenk M, Pahlsson P, Chisholm-Chait A, et al: Biochemical characterization of the feline AB blood group system. Anim Genet 24:401, 1993.
Biochemical studies of the feline AB blood group system.

Griot-Wenk ME, Giger U: Feline transfusion medicine: Blood types and their clinical importance. Vet Clin North Am Small Anim Pract 25:1305, 1995.
A clinical review of feline transfusions.

Griot-Wenk ME, Callan MB, Casal ML, et al: Blood type AB in the feline AB blood group system. Am J Vet Res 57:1438, 1996.
A detailed description of the feline AB blood type.

Hale AS: Canine blood groups and their importance in veterinary transfusion medicine. Vet Clin North Am Small Anim Pract 25:1323, 1995.
A review of canine blood types.

Hohenhaus AE, ed: Problems in Veterinary Medicine, vol 4. Philadelphia: Lippincott-Raven, 1992.
An issue on transfusion medicine.

Howard A, Callan MB, Sweeney M, et al: Canine transfusion practice and costs. J Am Vet Med Assoc 201:1697, 1992.
A survey of canine transfusions in practice.

Kohn B, Reilemeyer S, Giger U: Bestimmung der Blutgruppe DEA 1.1 und deren Bedeutung beim Hund. Kleintierpraxis 43:77, 1998.

Kohn B, Niggemeier A, Reilemeyer S, Giger U: Blutgruppen bestimm ung bei der Katze mit Hilfe einer neuen Testkartenmethode. Kleintierpraxis 42:941, 1997.

Rentko VT: Red blood cell substitutes. In: Hohenhaus AE, ed: Problems in Veterinary Medicine, vol 4. Philadelphia: Lippincott-Raven, 1992, p 647.
A review on red blood cell substitutes.

Blood Transfusion Guidelines

BERNARD F. FELDMAN
Blacksburg, Virginia

RATIONALE FOR THERAPY

Whole blood is a mixture of cellular constituents suspended in a liquid transport medium. The cells have different functions. Erythrocytes carry oxygen and participate in host defense by surface adsorption and absorption of many materials, phagocytes control bacteria, platelets are required for hemostasis, and lymphocytes mediate immunity. The liquid medium also contains an array of dissolved substances: albumin, globulins, coagulation proteins, metabolic intermediates, electrolytes, organic anions, and trace elements. Practical techniques for the separation and concentration of some of the cellular constituents of whole blood are within the capabilities of all major veterinary blood donor centers. Modern transfusion therapy should be based on the use of specific components to treat specific deficiencies. There are a number of rationales for the preferential use of blood components (Barnes, 1993).

Consideration of the Limited Resource

The most cogent argument in support of component therapy is that blood is a precious resource, when one considers its therapeutic potential and the logistics and costs required in obtaining and delivering blood products. Separation into components permits a single donation to meet the individual needs of several patients. The eligibility criteria for screening blood donors should be sufficient to obtain a safe donation.

Kinetic Considerations

Following hemorrhage, homeostatic mechanisms restore the various blood constituents at differing rates, depending on the individual's capacity for synthesis, endogenous consumption, degradation, and distribution in various physiologic compartments. The half-life of canine and feline red blood cells is in terms of months, whereas the half-life of albumin is just 3 to 4 days. Surgical blood loss may require restoration of red blood cells. Albumin may not be required, as it will be restored within several days. Another consideration is tolerance. Loss of 50% of red blood cell mass is well tolerated in a healthy individual, whereas loss of 50% of blood volume can be fatal unless rapidly corrected.

Consideration of Adverse Effects

Other rationales in support of the use of blood components include the myriad of possible adverse effects that can result from transfusion of unnecessary blood constituents. *Any transfusion reaction means that the transfusion is not doing the intended job and, importantly, has impaired a patient already burdened by the physiologic state requiring transfusion.* Sensitization to blood cells can result in refractory results in subsequent transfusions. Transfusion of multiple units of whole blood sequentially to achieve a certain hematocrit may also produce pulmonary edema as a result of volume overload.

Blood Donor Screening

All blood donors should be given thorough physical examinations at each donation and should have annual hematologic, biochemical, and serologic screenings. Donors should be healthy, should be receiving adequate nutrition, and should be free from parasites. All donors should be blood-typed and current on appropriate vaccinations. Female donors should not have had puppies or kittens and preferably should have been neutered. In addition, all canine donors should be screened for brucellosis, heartworm microfilariae, ehrlichiosis, Rocky Mountain spotted fever, trypanosomiasis, and systemic mycoses. Feline donors should be house cats not allowed to roam. Cats should be screened for retroviruses, heartworm microfilariae, toxoplasmosis, and haemobartonellosis.

Blood Typing

The feline AB blood group system consists of three blood types: type A, type B, and type AB (see previous article). All type B cats have strong alloantibodies against type A red blood cells. Type A cats have weak but potent anti-B alloantibodies. These alloantibodies are responsible for transfusion reactions and neonatal isoerythrolysis in cats and can be detected by crossmatch procedures. Feline patients receiving blood products should receive donor products of the same blood type as the patient and should have had crossmatch testing that indicates compatibility. Cats with the rare AB blood type should receive AB blood (often quite difficult to obtain) or type A blood that is compatible or only slightly incompatible in the crossmatch. There are no feline "universal" donors.

The dog has eight different blood types, identified as dog erythrocyte antigens (DEA) 1.1, 1.2, 3, 4, 5, 6, 7, and 8 (see previous article). The use of DEA 1.1– and 1.2– positive blood products that are crossmatch-incompatible may cause hemolysis. Controversy exists as to whether DEA 7 is an important determinant in canine transfusion reactions. Ideally, canine blood negative for DEA 1.1, 1.2, and 7 should be used, as it conforms with the concept of universal donor blood; however, only a small percentage of the population fulfills this requirement. In random-source, first-time canine transfusion of noncrossmatched or nontyped blood, the transfusion reaction rate is approximately 15%. Again, transfusion reaction indicates that the materials transfused are not effective and are causing a physiologic burden on an already burdened patient—reasons to perform blood typing and crossmatching. There have been suggestions that the only significant canine antigen is DEA 1.1. Donor blood products negative for DEA 1.1 that are crossmatch-compatible have a much reduced chance of causing a transfusion reaction.

A simple "in-house" card test for feline red blood cell antigens A, B, and AB and canine DEA 1.1 has become available.* Other methods are discussed in the previous article.

The Crossmatch

Crossmatching reveals the presence of naturally occurring isoantibodies or antibodies generated in response to a previous incompatible transfusion. Crossmatching does not prevent sensitization of the patient to future transfusions. *Even with a specific blood donor that is crossmatch-compatible with the patient, if at least 5 days have elapsed since the first transfusion, another crossmatch must be performed when more blood products are to be administered and especially when the same donor blood products will be used.*

Crossmatching is a simple technique that can be performed with standard laboratory equipment. A major, minor, and autocontrol crossmatch should be performed, although the minor crossmatch is rarely used in dogs. The major crossmatch should always be compatible at room temperature and at 37°C. The following is a simple (nonpurist) *major crossmatch protocol (donor red blood cells and patient serum or plasma)*:

1. Centrifuge EDTA (ethylenediaminetetraacetic acid) or citrated *donor* blood at the *lowest* centrifugal rate possible on your centrifuge for about 10 minutes.
2. Remove 0.2 ml of packed erythrocytes and place in 4.8 ml of normal (0.9%) saline. Mix. (There are now 5.0 ml in the tube; this procedure essentially replaces the washing step.)
3. Place 0.1 ml of this mixture into *three small* test tubes.
4. Place 0.1 ml of *patient* serum or plasma into each of the three tubes described previously. Each tube now has 0.1 ml of the *donor* red blood cell–saline mixture and 0.1 ml of patient serum or plasma, a total of 0.2 ml each.
5. Incubate (for 15 minutes) one tube at 37°C, one at room temperature (25°C), and one at refrigerator temperature (4°C).
6. Centrifuge briskly (fastest centrifugal rate on clinical centrifuge) for 1 minute.
7. Examine the supernatant for any hemolysis. Any hemolysis indicates crossmatch incompatibility.
8. Examine the cell button. Flick or swish the test tube. The fluid in the tube should redden as red blood cells disperse. If the button is agglutinated or microagglutinated (examine a drop under low microscopic power), crossmatch incompatibility exists.
9. *To complete the minor crossmatch, use patient red blood cells and donor serum or plasma. To complete the*

autocontrol, use patient red blood cells and patient plasma. In dogs, the minor crossmatch is useful for a patient receiving multiple plasma product transfusions.

The Decision to Transfuse

Any transfusion therapy can produce only transient improvement in the patient's condition. More transfusions will be necessary unless the patient is able to produce the deficit component endogenously. Furthermore, transfusions dampen the physiologic response to deficiency of a blood constituent. For example, if a patient has a low red blood cell mass, tissue hypoxia results in increased erythropoietin production and the bone marrow responds with reticulocytosis. In this patient, red blood cell transfusion will result in a diminished and delayed reticulocyte response. Several questions should be considered when transfusion is an option.

- Is blood transfusion really necessary?
- What is the patient's particular clinical need?
- Does the prospective benefit justify the risks of transfusion?
- What blood component will effectively meet this special need at the lowest cost?
- (After transfusion) Did the transfusion result in the anticipated benefit for the patient?

Answers to these questions should be documented in the patient's record. As a minimum for red blood cell transfusion, a pretransfusion hematocrit and total protein should be followed by post-transfusion (24-hour) determinations.

Blood components may be conveniently classified according to their physiologic functions: oxygen transport, as an adjunct in intravascular volume maintenance, hemostasis, and phagocytosis. In veterinary medicine, support of phagocytosis with granulocyte transfusions has not been accomplished. Volume replacement requires maintenance of colloid oncotic pressure (COP) through the use of colloids (hetastarch, pentastarch, dextrans, gelatin products) in addition to plasma. Albumin administered in the form of plasma to hypo-oncotic (hypoalbuminemic) patients not receiving concurrent colloidal support will rapidly equilibrate with the extravascular space.

TRANSFUSION TO INCREASE OXYGEN TRANSPORT

There is no set hemoglobin or hematocrit concentration below which a patient needs red blood cells. The condition of patients, and patient care, dictate when red blood cells are required. A patient who has lost one third of its red cell mass acutely requires increased oxygen-carrying capacity. Patients with chronic processes may have dramatically low hematocrits and, if not stressed, may not require additional oxygen-carrying capacity. However, patients with underlying heart disease may not tolerate even a moderate anemia. In general, in both the dog and the cat, administering red blood cells to meet oxygen transport needs should be considered when the hemoglobin concentration is below 7 gm/dl (hematocrit of 21%). When considering transfusion

---

*Rapid Vet-H, Feline and Rapid Vet-H, Canine. DMS Laboratories, Inc., 2 Darts Mill Road, Flemington, NJ 08822.

in specific patients, the clinician should consider age, etiology and duration of anemia, hemodynamic stability, and presence of coexisting cardiac, pulmonary, or vascular conditions.

Products That Increase Oxygen Transport

Packed Red Cells (PRCs). PRCs are achieved when refrigerated whole blood is centrifuged in refrigeration and plasma is removed. Because the hematocrit will approximate 70 to 80%, PRCs are often mixed with sterile saline or with an additive solution to decrease viscosity. In the author's practice, we add a solution* that contains sodium chloride, adenine, dextrose, and mannitol to decrease PRC viscosity, prolong the storage life of red blood cells, and prevent red cell hemolysis.

Whole Blood. Acute massive blood loss exceeding 20% of blood volume (appropriate blood volume is 90 ml/kg for dogs; 70 ml/kg for cats), coagulopathy with massive blood loss, and some patients with disseminated intravascular coagulopathy (DIC; see p. 190) are the only valid indications for whole blood transfusion, which supplies both cells and volume at a rapid flow rate.

Effects of Red Blood Cell Transfusion. Hematocrit and hemoglobin will increase, but intravascular volume will return to baseline within 12 to 24 hours. Red blood cell transfusion blunts the erythropoietic response. Red blood cell viability depends on the maintenance of adenosine triphosphate (ATP) concentrations, but oxygen release to tissues depends on 2,3-diphosphoglycerate (2,3-DPG), which will be diminished in older stored red blood cell products. When oxygen transport is critical, older red cell products (more than 3 weeks of age) may be administered when sandwiched with fresher red cells (less than 2 weeks of age).

TRANSFUSION TO MAINTAIN HEMOSTASIS

Platelets. The logistics of significantly increasing and maintaining profoundly low platelet counts in an average-sized dog or cat with platelet-rich plasma should give one pause. Most often, it is an exercise in futility. Platelet transfusions are required every 6 to 8 hours for a minimum of several days, and immune activity against platelet-specific antigens is often swift.

Fresh-Frozen Plasma (FFP) and Stored-Frozen Plasma (SFP). FFP is plasma that is solidly frozen within 8 hours of donation. SFP is plasma frozen after more than 8 hours from the time of donation. The products are virtually identical. Cofactors V and VIII are diminished in SFP, and SFP and FFP can be used interchangeably unless the patient is deficient in factor VIII (hemophilia A) or has von Willebrand factor (vWF) deficiency. Both products have appropriate concentrations of vitamin K–dependent proteins and albumin.

---

*Adsol²-Fenwall Division, Baxter HealthCare Corp, Deerfield, IL.

Cryoprecipitate (Cryo). Cryo is produced by ultra-freezing plasma ($-70°C$) for 24 hours, thawing in a refrigerator ($4°C$) for 24 hours, and removing the cryoprecipitate-free plasma. Cyroprecipitate concentrates factor VIII, fibrinogen, von Willebrand factor (vWF), and fibronectin. Cryo is used to treat DIC, vWF deficiency, hemophilia A, and generalized sepsis. Fibronectin (plasma opsonic factor) is required to enhance mononuclear phagocytic function.

Cryoprecipitate-Free Plasma (CryoFree). This product is the result of removing Cryo and is virtually the same as FFP or SFP. In fact, the products can be used interchangeably. CryoFree is replete with albumin and has all the vitamin K–dependent proteins (with a modest, but not clinically significant, reduction in factor IX). Because CryoFree has diminished factor VIII, fibrinogen, vWf, and fibronectin, there are few situations in which FFP or SFP may be superior.

ADMINISTRATION OF BLOOD PRODUCTS

Blood products should always be administered warmed with an in-line blood filter (not an intravenous fluid set) because all blood products have microagglutinates. Blood products should not be warmed in excess of 37°C, as this will precipitate numerous proteins and will enhance lysis of red blood cells.

In a normovolemic patient, the recommended infusion rate for whole blood or plasma products is 22 ml/kg per 24 hours. In the hypovolemic animal, the rate should not exceed 22 ml/kg per hour. For patients with compromised cardiac function, the rate should not exceed 4 ml/kg per hour. In normovolemic patients receiving red blood cells, the hematocrit will increase over the baseline value immediately after transfusion and increase further within 24 hours with volume redistribution.

Cryo is Administered to Effect at 1 Unit/10 kg Every 12 Hours as Needed

To *determine anticipated hematocrit* in patients receiving red blood cells, calculate total blood volume (see section on whole blood above) and the total volume of red blood cells (calculated from the pretransfusion hematocrit). Determine the total blood volume after administering the transfusion (pretransfusion blood volume + volume of transfusion). Determine the new hematocrit by adding the volume of transfused red blood cells to the pretransfusion red cell volume. The anticipated post-transfusion hematocrit is the post-transfusion red cell volume divided by post-transfusion total blood volume.

TRANSFUSION REACTION

Transfusion reactions include immune-mediated and non–immune-mediated reactions. Transfusion reactions can be immediate or delayed (reactions can occur as late as a week or more after transfusion). Immediate reactions are the result of preformed antibody in the patient not detected by the crossmatch test. Delayed reactions are the result of an anamnestic response to an antigen to which the patient was previously sensitized.

Among immune transfusion reactions are hemolysis (including neonatal isoerythrolysis; post-transfusion purpura), fever (an increase of 1°C over pretransfusion temperature), allergic reactions, and graft-versus-host response.

Among non–immune-mediated transfusion reactions are hemolysis, circulatory overload, sepsis resulting from transfusion contamination, citrate toxicity (hypocalcemia, especially in cats), hyperammonemia, dilutional coagulopathy, and disease transmission (Kristensen and Feldman, 1995; Hohenhaus, 1992).

APPROACH TO THE PATIENT REQUIRING BLOOD PRODUCTS

The following 10 steps summarize the approach to the patient in need of blood products:

- Determine whether any clinical signs of blood component loss are present, or whether the patient is at risk from surgery, anesthesia, or other procedures.
- Determine the amount and type of current and expected losses.
- Determine which components are needed; calculate the dose.
- Blood-type and crossmatch.
- Obtain transfusion-relevant history.
- Inspect component.
- Warm component.
- Determine the appropriate access site, and calculate the administration rate.
- Slowly start the transfusion, and monitor the patient's response.
- Follow-up: Was the transfusion effective over the short term and the long term?

References and Suggested Reading

Barnes A: Blood component therapy. In: Bick RL, ed: Hematology: Clinical and Laboratory Practice. St. Louis: Mosby-Year Book, 1993, p 1649.
  A comprehensive review of human transfusion medicine.
Kristensen AT, Feldman BF, eds: Transfusion Medicine. Vet Clin North Am Small Anim Pract 25:6, 1995.
  A complete overview of canine and feline transfusion medicine.
Hohenhaus AE, ed: Transfusion Medicine. Problems in Vet Med 4:4, 1992.
  A multifaceted overview of canine and feline transfusion medicine.

Hematopoietic Cytokines: The Myelopoietic Factors

CHERYL LONDON
Boston, Massachusetts

Hematopoietic growth factors are glycoproteins that affect the growth and differentiation of bone marrow–derived cells, including erythrocytes, platelets, monocytes, granulocytes, and lymphocytes. Some of these growth factors are multikinetic, exerting their effects on multiple cell lineages, whereas others are cell lineage specific. Additionally, many of the growth factors possess overlapping and/or synergistic biologic activities (Fig. 1). Most of the known mouse-, rat-, and human-derived hematopoietic growth factors have been cloned and produced with the use of recombinant technology. These factors include granulocyte colony-stimulating factor (G-CSF), macrophage colony-stimulating factor (M-CSF), granulocyte-macrophage colony-stimulating factor (GM-CSF), stem cell factor (SCF), interleukin-3 (IL-3), erythropoietin (EPO, reviewed in *CVT XI*), and, most recently, thrombopoietin (TPO). The availability of recombinant growth factors has proved to be of great significance in human medicine, rapidly advancing the ability to treat serious diseases. While the most important application of these factors has been in the setting of bone marrow transplantation and chemotherapy-induced myelo-suppression, they are now being used in the treatment of a multitude of disorders. As of this writing, only EPO, G-CSF, and GM-CSF have been approved by the U.S. Food and Drug Administration, and most of the remaining factors are in advanced clinical trials.

Several of the canine hematopoietic growth factors have been cloned, but these are available only through clinical trials conducted at veterinary teaching institutions. The available recombinant human growth factors all should be used *with caution* in dogs and cats. Although often effective, they exhibit sufficient differences in protein structure from the corresponding protein in dogs or cats to induce the production of neutralizing antibodies. These antibodies are often cross-reactive, recognizing both the foreign (human) and the host (dog/cat) protein. This reaction can be deleterious to the affected animal, as it may eliminate any remaining host growth factor activity, thereby exacerbating the initial problem. As molecular technology improves and becomes less expensive, many of the canine—and potentially feline—growth factors may be commercially available, eliminating this problem.

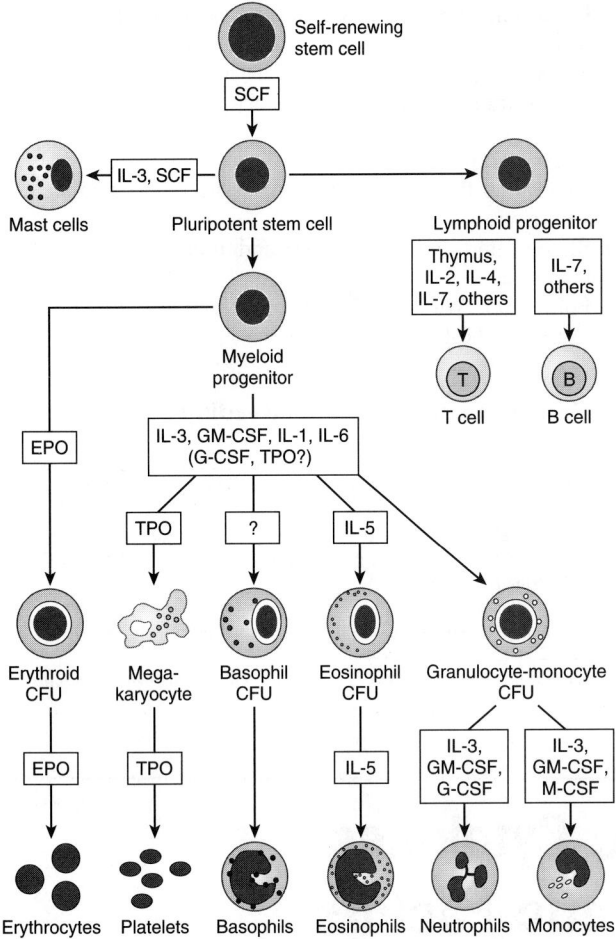

Figure 1. Maturation of hematopoietic cells. The maturation of different lineages of bone marrow–derived cells is regulated by several different cytokines, the functions of which sometimes overlap. CFU, colony-forming unit; IL, interleukin; GM-CSF, granulocyte-macrophage colony-stimulating factor; EPO, erythropoietin; SCF, stem cell factor; TPO, thrombopoietin.

GRANULOCYTE COLONY-STIMULATING FACTOR

Granulocyte colony-stimulating factor is a 20-kD glycoprotein produced by bone marrow stromal cells, monocytes/macrophages, and endothelial cells. The receptor for G-CSF is expressed primarily by granulocyte progenitor cells in the bone marrow and mature neutrophils. The primary activity of G-CSF is to stimulate the proliferation and maturation of neutrophil precursors, and, to a lesser degree, monocyte precursors, from the bone marrow. It also acts to prime neutrophils for cell killing by enhancing antibody-dependent cellular cytotoxicity, superoxide production, and Fc receptor expression. Furthermore, G-CSF promotes neutrophil migration across the vascular endothelium. While G-CSF initially appeared to be lineage specific, more recent work has demonstrated that at higher doses it may act in a multilineage fashion, stimulating the differentiation of several hematopoietic progenitors. This observation is supported by the fact that G-CSF receptor expression has been detected on CD34[+] hematopoietic progenitor cells. Canine G-CSF has been cloned (rcG-CSF) and produced, but is *not* commercially available.

Granulocyte colony-stimulating factor has been exten-

sively studied in research and clinical settings and is used routinely in human medicine. In both humans and dogs, G-CSF administration causes a dose-dependent rise in neutrophils, as well as a moderate increase in monocytes. In normal dogs, the response to subcutaneous injection of rcG-CSF is rapid, inducing a neutrophilia within 24 hours of administration (Mishu et al, 1992). After two doses of rcG-CSF at 1 μg/kg, the neutrophil count increased fourfold to $17,161 \pm 1,295/\mu l$ from $4,941 \pm 862/\mu l$; after 16 days of therapy, the neutrophil count increased sevenfold to $32,350 \pm 1,552/\mu l$. In this study, doses of 1, 2, or 5 μg/kg given subcutaneously every 12 hours were well tolerated, with only mild irritation at the injection site occasionally noted. Of interest, rcG-CSF was given to cats at a dose of 5 μg/kg/day SC and the same effect on neutrophil counts was noted (Obradovich et al, 1993). Furthermore, after 42 days of therapy, neutrophil counts remained high, indicating that neutralizing antibodies to the canine G-CSF had not been generated.

G-CSF is now routinely given to certain human cancer patients who are undergoing chemotherapy to help prevent episodes of severe neutropenia. Typically, G-CSF administration is begun 24 to 48 hours after treatment, permitting the neutrophil precursors not eliminated by chemotherapy to rapidly expand and mature. This approach leads to a decrease in both the magnitude and the duration of neutropenia. This effect of G-CSF has also been demonstrated in dogs. In a study conducted by Ogilvie and co-workers (1992), 10 normal dogs were given mitoxantrone at a dose of 5 mg/m² by intravenous injection. Five of the dogs were then given rcG-CSF at a dose of 5 μg/kg/day by subcutaneous injection beginning 24 hours after chemotherapy administration and continuing for 20 days. The median neutrophil counts dropped below normal (<3,000/μl) for 5 days in dogs that did not receive rcG-CSF, compared to 2 days in dogs that did receive rcG-CSF. Furthermore, four of the five dogs that did not receive rcG-CSF developed serious neutropenia (<1,500/μl); this condition did not occur in the rcG-CSF–treated group. Therefore, as in human medicine, G-CSF appears to reduce the duration and severity of chemotherapy-induced myelosuppression.

Although G-CSF administration appears to be useful in modulating chemotherapy-induced myelosuppression when used prophylactically, recent evidence suggests that it is not beneficial in the treatment of established afebrile or febrile neutropenia. In one study of 138 human patients with severe chemotherapy-induced afebrile neutropenia, treatment with G-CSF significantly reduced the median time to recovery of the absolute neutrophil count to 500/mm³, but there was no effect on the rate of hospitalization, number of days in the hospital, duration of treatment with parenteral antibiotics, or number of culture-positive infections. Similar results have been noted in the treatment of patients with established neutropenic fever, with most trials demonstrating no reductions in the duration of hospitalization, number of days of fever, or mortality (Walton, 1998). Consequently, recombinant human G-CSF (rhG-CSF) should probably not be used in dogs or cats for the treatment of established neutropenias.

Another application of rcG-CSF is in the treatment of cyclic neutropenia (cyclic hematopoiesis), an inherited disease of humans and grey collie dogs. This syndrome is characterized by recurrent episodes of neutropenia. In af-

fected people, neutropenic episodes occur every 20 to 24 days, while affected dogs have 12- to 14-day neutropenic cycles. Although the exact nature of the defect leading to this cycling is not known, it does not appear to be secondary to defects in G-CSF or the receptor for G-CSF. One study provided evidence of a defect in signal transduction after G-CSF binds its receptor in the neutrophils of affected dogs. When rhG-CSF is given to affected people, the mean neutrophil counts are increased, and the severity of neutropenia associated with the cycles is decreased. The same effect was noted in affected dogs given rhG-CSF, although neutralizing antibodies were generated after 25 days, leading to prolonged neutropenia (Lothrup et al, 1988). This problem was circumvented by giving rcG-CSF at a dose of 1 to 2.5 μg/kg every 12 hours (Mishu et al, 1992). In both humans and dogs, G-CSF does not completely eliminate the cycling of neutrophils or the clinical signs associated with disease, supporting the notion of a defect in receptor signaling, rather than in G-CSF itself.

In patients receiving bone marrow transplants, the time period before hematopoietic recovery is critical, as the absence of white blood cells, particularly neutrophils, leaves them susceptible to overwhelming bacterial infection. The administration of G-CSF after high-dose chemotherapy and autologous bone marrow transplantation improves the rate of peripheral blood neutrophil recovery, reducing the morbidity and mortality associated with febrile neutropenic episodes. In dogs given 350 cGy of total body radiation, the administration of G-CSF beginning immediately after treatment and continuing daily led to complete bone marrow reconstitution within 21 days (Schuening et al, 1989).

Another use for G-CSF in transplantation is in the mobilization of hematopoietic progenitors for collection prior to myeloablative therapy. After treatment with G-CSF for several days, high concentrations of progenitor cells are found in the peripheral blood (PBPCs). These PBPCs are collected by leukapheresis and administered to the patient after high-dose chemotherapy in place of marrow. Dogs given rcG-CSF or recombinant canine SCF (rcSCF), or both, developed significant increases in the levels of circulating hematopoietic progenitors (deRevel et al, 1994). Peripheral-blood mononuclear cells were collected from these dogs after 7 days of treatment with growth factors, and were given back to the dogs after 400 cGy of total body radiation. Bone marrow recovery was complete in four of five dogs that had received G-CSF or SCF alone, and in all dogs that had received both growth factors prior to leukapheresis. In human patients, clinical trials using G-CSF for progenitor cell mobilization and collection have demonstrated this therapy to be effective in reducing the period of absolute leukopenia following myeloablation and transplantation. Although controversial, G-CSF has also been used to expand hematopoietic cells in vitro prior to transplantation. This preparatory step may permit the generation of mature hematopoietic cells, as well as the expansion of progenitor cells, prior to bone marrow transplantation. This procedure could potentially allow multiple transplantations, helping to prevent failure of engraftment as well as providing mature cells to aid in the host's defense against infection.

Given the effect of G-CSF on neutrophil function, it may prove useful in the treatment of certain infectious diseases. This notion is supported by experiments in mice that have demonstrated that G-CSF given in combination with antibiotics significantly improved survival compared with antibiotics alone in the setting of overwhelming bacterial infection. Although it may seem intuitive to use G-CSF during parvoviral infection in dogs and in cats, such use may exacerbate disease because the virus replicates in actively dividing cells. Increasing the proportion of cycling neutrophil precursors may actually prolong the neutropenic period, owing to viral infection and destruction of these cells.

Given the propensity for the generation of neutralizing antibodies, the decision to use rhG-CSF in the dog must be made carefully. If no other options are available, rhG-CSF should be used on a short-term basis (less than 5 to 7 days). Repeated cycles of administration will be more likely to induce anti–G-CSF antibodies. A clinical trial is currently underway to determine whether short-term use of rhG-CSF in dogs to ameliorate chemotherapy-induced myelosuppression results in antibody formation.

GRANULOCYTE-MACROPHAGE COLONY-STIMULATING FACTOR

Granulocyte-macrophage colony-stimulating factor is a 10- to 30-kD glycoprotein (depending on the extent of glycosylation) that was named for its ability to stimulate the formation of granulocyte and macrophage colonies in semisolid cultures of bone marrow. It is produced by a wide variety of cells, including fibroblasts, endothelial cells, monocytes, and T lymphocytes, in response to several stimuli. The receptor for GM-CSF is expressed on several different hematopoietic progenitors, as well as on neutrophils, eosinophils, and monocytes/macrophages and antigen-presenting dendritic cells. GM-CSF has a number of significant biologic actions, which are summarized in Table 1. In general, it acts to prolong the survival of hematopoietic progenitors and mature neutrophils, eosinophils, and macrophages; it stimulates the proliferation of progenitor cells; and it enhances the functional capacity of the mature cells. Given its wide variety of actions, GM-CSF has a number of potential clinical applications.

Canine GM-CSF has been cloned, although the recombinant protein is not commercially available. Recombinant canine GM-CSF (rcGM-CSF) given to normal dogs at a dose of 25 μg/kg b.i.d. SC caused a significant increase in circulating neutrophils and monocytes, whereas the effect on circulating eosinophils was variable (Nash et al, 1994).

TABLE 1. Biologic Actions of GM-CSF

Enhances the survival of neutrophils, eosinophils, macrophages, and their progenitor cells

Stimulates the proliferation and differentiation of neutrophil, eosinophil, macrophage, megakaryocyte, and early erythroid progenitor cells

Stimulates the secretion of cytokines and inflammatory mediators from neutrophils and macrophages (IL-1, G-CSF, M-CSF, IL-6)

Increases phagocytosis and antibody-dependent cellular cytotoxicity of neutrophils, eosinophils, and macrophages

Enhances bactericidal activity in neutrophils and macrophages, and the killing of parasites in eosinophils and macrophages

Enhances the antigen-presenting activity of macrophages and Langerhans cells and stimulates immune responses to foreign antigens

Thrombocytopenia developed during treatment, but it resolved after rcGM-CSF was discontinued. Unlike G-CSF, GM-CSF was not effective in promoting hematopoietic recovery or improving survival in dogs given 400 cGy of total body radiation. However, experimental studies and clinical trials have demonstrated that administration of PBPCs and a combination of GM-CSF and G-CSF after high-dose chemotherapy significantly enhances neutrophil recovery.

In people, GM-CSF has been shown to decrease the duration and severity of chemotherapy-induced neutropenia. Although rhGM-CSF was shown to be active in dogs, inducing neutrophilia and eosinophilia, it produced variable results in dogs with chemotherapy-induced myelosuppression. As rcGM-CSF exhibits only 70% amino acid sequence homology with the human protein, higher doses than those used in human patients may be necessary to achieve an effect during treatment of myelosuppression. The most frequently occurring toxicity associated with systemic administration of GM-CSF is bone pain, probably secondary to the stimulation of hematopoiesis. Other side effects reported in human patients include fever and flu-like symptoms. However, at the doses currently used, the incidence of toxicity is quite low.

Perhaps one of the most important uses of GM-CSF is in the activation of monocytes and macrophages. After exposure to GM-CSF, these cells exhibit the ability to recognize and destroy malignant cells, both in vitro and in vivo. It is speculated that macrophage killing of tumor cells not only helps eliminate the tumor but also permits the presentation of tumor-derived antigens to helper T lymphocytes. Once activated, these tumor-specific helper cells can then stimulate tumor-specific cytotoxic T cells, thereby enhancing the antitumor immune response. Several studies in mice have demonstrated the ability of GM-CSF to generate an antitumor response, leading to the elimination of experimental tumors.

In an effort to deliver GM-CSF directly to the tumor, allowing local recruitment and activation of macrophages, researchers have designed DNA plasmid vectors that contain the coding sequence for GM-CSF. These vectors can be delivered to the tumor in a number of different ways, resulting in transfection of the tumor cells in vivo with the plasmid, and local production of GM-CSF. This approach has been used to treat oral malignant melanoma in dogs. The coding sequence for canine GM-CSF was cloned into a eukaryotic expression vector and injected directly into the oral melanomas of three dogs. Complete remission occurred in two of the three dogs, including regression of a submandibular lymph node metastasis in one dog.

Another method of inducing an antitumor immune response with the use of GM-CSF is to remove the primary tumor or a metastatic lesion, culture the tumor cells in vitro, and transfect them with a eukaryotic expression vector encoding GM-CSF. These tumor cells are then irradiated so that they cannot divide but can still produce GM-CSF, and are injected back into the affected individual in the form of an autologous tumor vaccine. Such approaches have been effective for certain tumors in mouse models. This approach was also undertaken in two dogs with oral malignant melanoma, and one of the two dogs achieved complete remission. The advantages of using eukaryotic

expression vectors encoding hematopoietic growth factors include the local production of cytokines leading to a more specific effect, the reduction or elimination of systemic side effects associated with administration of the growth factor, and the elimination of the need for large quantities of the recombinant growth factor. Clinical trials are now underway in human patients who have metastatic malignant melanoma using autologous melanoma cells transfected with the GM-CSF gene as a vaccine, similar to the approach used in mice and dogs. Clearly, GM-CSF has great potential in the treatment of malignancies in both veterinary and human medicine.

STEM CELL FACTOR

Stem cell factor (steel factor, mast cell growth factor, c-*kit* ligand) is a 30-kD glycoprotein produced primarily by stromal cells in the bone marrow, fibroblasts, and endothelial cells. It exists in both cell surface–associated and secreted forms. The receptor for SCF is encoded by the proto-oncogene c-*kit* and expressed on hematopoietic stem cells as well as on mast cells and melanocytes. With the exception of mast cells, as hematopoietic cells differentiate, they lose expression of c-*kit* and are no longer responsive to SCF. Stem cell factor acts in synergy with many other growth factors, including EPO, IL-3, IL-6, IL-7, G-CSF, and GM-CSF, to promote the production of early and intermediate precursors of erythroid, myeloid, and lymphoid lineages. The differentiation of specific lineages is not governed by SCF alone, but by the properties of the additional growth factors. For example, when SCF and EPO are added to human or murine bone marrow cultures, a population of erythroid progenitors is expanded. Conversely, addition of SCF alone or SCF and IL-3 to bone marrow cultures induces the differentiation and proliferation of mast cells.

Evidence of the action of SCF on hematopoietic progenitors is supported by work in mice, dogs, and nonhuman primates. When SCF is administered in vivo, a significant increase (2 to 100 fold) in hematopoietic progenitor cells in the bone marrow and blood is noted. This increase, in turn, leads to a rise in the number of peripheral red blood cells, granulocytes, monocytes, and lymphocytes. Therefore, SCF can act as a multilineage hematopoietic growth factor in vivo, reflecting its ability to work synergistically with other endogenous growth factors.

The administration of SCF is of potential benefit in several clinical settings. Conditions in which immature hematopoietic precursors are damaged or defective, such as aplastic anemia, myelofibrosis, or bone marrow toxicity secondary to drug- or radiation-induced damage (e.g., estrogen or melphalan toxicity), may be responsive to SCF therapy. Studies conducted in vitro suggest that SCF can significantly enhance the proliferation of bone marrow cells derived from patients with aplastic anemia when used in combination with other hematopoietic growth factors. Clinical trials in humans are underway to determine the efficacy of SCF administration in the treatment of such conditions. Another potential application is in patients receiving bone marrow transplantation. As discussed before, SCF can be used to aid in the mobilization of hematopoietic progenitor cells. Other uses include the expansion of autologous bone marrow with SCF in vitro, and the administration of SCF after bone marrow transplantation or chemotherapy to enhance hematopoietic recovery.

Although most work with SCF has been conducted in mice and humans, rcSCF has been used in dogs in both research and clinical settings. When given alone or in combination with rcG-CSF, rcSCF was shown to significantly increase the level of peripheral-blood hematopoietic progenitor and stem cells. Furthermore, when rcSCF was administered with rcG-CSF to dogs after total body radiation, the time to hematopoietic recovery was less than when either agent was given alone. Also, rcSCF has been used either alone or in combination with rcG-CSF to successfully treat grey collies with cyclic neutropenia (Dale et al, 1995). Long-term treatment of these dogs with rcSCF at doses of 10 to 30 μg/kg/day SC was generally well tolerated, supporting the notion that this therapy could be used safely to treat hematopoietic disorders of the dog.

One of the side effects of SCF therapy is an extensive proliferation of mast cells seen at the site of subcutaneous injection. Although this proliferation is reversible on discontinuation of therapy, SCF injections have been associated with hypersensitivity reactions. In humans receiving SCF, these reactions were successfully managed with appropriate therapy designed to prevent and treat mast cell degranulation (anaphylaxis). Of interest, feline SCF has been cloned.

THROMBOPOIETIN

Thrombopoietin is a 35-kD glycoprotein that is produced primarily by the liver. The ligand for TPO is encoded by the proto-oncogene c-mpl. The identification and cloning of TPO proved quite difficult because of the extremely low levels of the protein present even in rich physiologic sources, such as plasma from mice with experimentally induced thrombocytopenia. Thrombopoietin has several biologic functions, the most important of which is as a regulator of thrombopoiesis. In addition to its role as a late-acting megakaryocyte maturation factor, TPO is also a potent stimulator of hematopoietic progenitor cells, inducing them to undergo proliferation and differentiation into megakaryocytic colonies. Furthermore, it has the ability to promote the viability of and suppress apoptosis of primitive multipotential progenitor cells, in addition to those committed to the megakaryocytic lineage. Experiments in vitro have demonstrated that TPO can synergize with SCF and IL-3 to act on early multipotential progenitor cells.

Work in mice has demonstrated that TPO can stimulate enhanced platelet recovery and improve the recovery of other hematopoietic lineages after bone marrow transplantation. In addition, TPO has been shown to act synergistically with G-CSF in accelerating neutrophil recovery in mice after radiation or chemotherapy. Moreover, it appears as if TPO can be used alone or in combination with other growth factors for PBPC mobilization and leukapheresis prior to transplantation. Given the encouraging results in animal models, TPO has progressed rapidly from its cloning in 1994 to phase II clinical trials. It is probable that TPO will have a significant impact on the treatment of patients undergoing bone marrow transplantation, as well as those receiving chemotherapy. It is interesting to note that some investigators have demonstrated the development of myelofibrosis in mice receiving chronic high doses of TPO. In these mice, the levels of both transforming growth factor beta-1 and platelet-derived growth factor were increased two to five fold, supporting the belief that megakaryocyte-derived factors may be involved in the pathogenesis of this disorder. Further work with TPO may lead to a more complete understanding of myelofibrosis, generating the development of novel therapeutics.

OTHER HEMATOPOIETIC GROWTH FACTORS

Macrophage colony-stimulating factor is a 70- to 90-kD glycoprotein produced by monocytes and endothelial cells that stimulates the growth and differentiation of mononuclear phagocytic precursors from the bone marrow. It also promotes the survival and effector functions of monocytes and macrophages in a manner similar to that of GM-CSF. While M-CSF has been shown to help the cellular recovery of patients who have undergone bone marrow transplantation, it is not as effective as G-CSF or a combination of G-CSF and GM-CSF. M-CSF may prove useful in the treatment of fungal infections, as it stimulates the release of G-CSF, GM-CSF, IL-1, and interferon gamma from monocytes. To date, there are no reports of the use of M-CSF in dogs or cats.

Interleukin-3 is a 25-kD glycoprotein produced primarily by T cells that promotes the survival, proliferation, and development of multipotential hematopoietic stem cells, and of committed progenitors of the granulocyte-macrophage, erythroid, eosinophil, basophil, megakaryocyte, and mast cell lineages. Additionally, IL-3 enhances myeloid cell functions, including phagocytosis, antibody-dependent cellular cytotoxicity, and monocyte cytotoxicity. Interleukin-3 has been used in human patients and leads to multilineage expansion of myeloid cells, including platelets, neutrophils, and monocytes. Also, IL-3 has been used in combination with GM-CSF to treat chemotherapy-induced myelosuppression; however, the incidence of toxicity, including fever, fatigue, and headaches, was higher than when GM-CSF was given alone. When rhIL-3 was given to dogs with cyclic neutropenia, no effect was noted on the recurrent neutropenia, but a significant eosinophilia was induced. Recombinant IL-3 may prove useful in the treatment of hematopoietic disorders of progenitor cells, such as myelodysplasia or aplastic anemia.

References and Suggested Reading

Dale DC, Rodger E, Cebon J, et al: Long-term treatment of canine cyclic hematopoiesis with recombinant canine stem cell factor. Blood 85:74, 1995.
This study demonstrates that rc-SCF is synergistic with rcG-CSF in inducing neutrophilia and abrogating neutropenic episodes in dogs with cyclic neutropenia.
Lothrup CD, Jr, Warren DJ, Souza LM, et al: Correction of canine cyclic hematopoiesis with recombinant human granulocyte colony-stimulating factor. Blood 72:1324, 1988.
This study demonstrates that the administration of rhG-CSF to canine patients, although effective in ameliorating cyclic neutropenia in affected dogs, leads to the generation of neutralizing antibodies that cross-react with native canine G-CSF, leading to prolonged neutropenia.

Mishu L, Callahan G, Allebban Z, et al: Effects of recombinant canine granulocyte colony-stimulating factor on white blood cell production in clinically normal and neutropenic dogs. J Am Vet Med Assoc 200:1957, 1992.
  This study demonstrates that rcG-CSF administration to normal dogs, those with cyclic neutropenia, and those undergoing autologous bone marrow transplantation, is an effective way of stimulating granulopoiesis as well as myelopoiesis.

Nash RA, Schuening FG, Seidel K, et al: Effect of recombinant canine granulocyte-macrophage colony-stimulating factor on hematopoietic recovery after otherwise lethal total body irradiation. Blood 83:1963, 1994.
  This study demonstrates that although rcGM-CSF induces neutrophilia in the dog, it is not effective in promoting hematopoietic recovery when used as a single agent after lethal irradiation.

Obradovich JE, Ogilvie GK, Stadler-Morris S, et al: Effect of recombinant canine granulocyte colony-stimulating factor on peripheral blood neutrophil counts in normal cats. J Vet Intern Med 7:65, 1993.
  This study demonstrates that rcG-CSF is safe and effective for expanding the number of neutrophils in normal cats.

Ogilvie GK, Obradovich JE, Cooper MF, et al: Use of recombinant canine granulocyte colony-stimulating factor to decrease myelosuppression associated with the administration of mitoxantrone in the dog. J Vet Intern Med 6:44, 1992.
  This prospective study demonstrates that rcG-CSF reduces the duration and severity of mitoxantrone-induced myelosuppression in dogs.

deRevel T, Appelbaum FR, Storb R, et al: Effects of granulocyte colony-stimulating factor and stem cell factor, alone and in combination, on the mobilization of peripheral blood cells that engraft lethally irradiated dogs. Blood 83:3795, 1994.
  These studies demonstrate that both G-CSF and SCF dramatically increase the level of peripheral-blood hematopoietic progenitor and stem cells and support the view that these factors can act synergistically.

Schuening FG, Storb R, Goehle S, et al: Effect of recombinant human granulocyte colony-stimulating factor on hematopoiesis of normal dogs and on hematopoietic recovery after otherwise lethal total body irradiation. Blood 74:1308, 1989.
  This study documents the effectiveness of rG-CSF administration in inducing full hematopoietic recovery after radiation, demonstrating the activity of G-CSF on several hematopoietic lineages.

Walton SM: Therapeutic use of colony-stimulating factors for established neutropenic fever. W V Med J 94:26, 1998.

Hematopoietic Cytokines: The Interleukin Array

STUART C. HELFAND

Madison, Wisconsin

Of all the biologic sciences, perhaps none has advanced more in recent years than the field of immunology. The explosion of information has revealed new paradigms of how the immune system works, which in turn have presented novel opportunities for clinical medicine. Some of the most important advances focus on the proteins secreted by activated cells of the immune system, which form complex networks of intercellular signaling molecules in response to immunologic stimulation. Collectively, these proteins are called interleukins, and they are produced mainly by activated monocytes and lymphocytes. In a more general sense, the interleukins constitute only a subset of signaling molecules, referred to as cytokines, that include interleukins, interferons, and colony-stimulating factors, produced not only by leukocytes but also by cells of numerous tissue origins. In this article, the discussion is limited primarily to interleukins produced by lymphocytes and monocytes.

By convention, interleukins are named by assigning ascending numbers corresponding to the chronologic order of their discovery. As of this writing, 17 interleukins have been described, but this number most assuredly will increase as our understanding of the immune system continues to grow. The bewildering array of numbered proteins presents a challenge to students of the immune system who seek to understand the actions and interactions of these molecules. In addition, recently discovered interleukins that function upstream in the immune response of earlier described interleukins will have a higher numerical designation. Thus, a classification of the interleukins based on numbering, while descriptive, is not always informative in explaining their biologic interactions.

Interleukins—and cytokines in general—mediate functions that are pleiotropic, redundant, synergistic, and antagonistic. This action allows them to regulate immune responses in a coordinated, interrelated way. Grouping interleukins on the basis of the effects on target immune cells that they mediate in common and on interleukin profiles associated with specific types of immunologic responses provides a physiologic perspective of this system and is the approach used in this presentation. Where appropriate, the interleukins with the greatest potential for clinical use are discussed.

NATURAL SOURCES OF INTERLEUKINS

Interleukins are secreted predominantly by activated helper T (Th) lymphocytes and monocytes-macrophages. Together, these cells account for secretion of interleukin-1 (IL-1), IL-2, IL-3, IL-4, IL-5, IL-6, IL-8, IL-9, IL-10, IL-12, IL-13, and IL-15. Secretion by these cells is inducible in response to a variety of natural and artificial stimuli. With appropriate stimulation, secretion of interleukins follows a cascading network regulating activation, proliferation, differentiation, or secretion of antibody or other interleukins by a variety of cells. In general, the effects of interleukins are mediated by binding to specific receptors expressed on the cell membranes of responding target cells. Binding to receptors can be autocrine or paracrine. In health, only a small percentage (e.g., $\leq$ 15%) of circulating immune cells express interleukin receptors, thereby guarding against overzealous immune responses. However, interleukin receptors are also inducible following appropriate antigenic stimulation, enabling the immune response to become amplified when necessary. Thus, it can be seen that natural immune responses regulated by interleukins are antigen driven.

A number of established lymphoid cell lines secrete various interleukins such as mouse EL-4 thymoma cells, which constitutively secrete IL-2 and IL-4. Malignant lymphocytes from a dog were found to secrete IL-2 and express IL-2 receptors as well (Helfand et al, 1995).

PHARMACOLOGIC SOURCES OF INTERLEUKINS

The convergence of molecular biology techniques and a better understanding of how the immune system works has incited the quest to produce interleukins in the laboratory. This effort has led to the cloning of numerous genes that encode many cytokines, including the interleukins. There are many commercial sources of recombinant mouse and human interleukins, primarily for laboratory studies. Human recombinant IL-2 is licensed for human cancer patients. In veterinary medicine, a number of interleukins have been cloned, with gene sequences deposited in the National Institutes of Health genetic sequence database, the National Center for Biotechnology Information GenBank, available on the World Wide Web (http://www.ncbi.nlm.nih.gov/Web/Genbank/index.html). In the dog, these interleukins include IL-1β, IL-2, IL-6, IL-8, IL-10, and IL-12 as well as tumor necrosis factor alpha (TNF-α) and interferon gamma (IFN-γ); while in the cat, they are IL-1β, IL-2, IL-4, IL-6, IL-10, and IL-12. A number of biotechnology companies have cloned genes for canine cytokines as well. At this time, there are no commercial sources for recombinant canine or feline interleukins.

CYTOKINE PROFILE OF THE CELL-MEDIATED IMMUNE RESPONSE: IL-1, IL-2, IFN-γ, TNF-α, IL-6, IL-8, IL-12, AND IL-15

Immune Cell Activation

In large part, concepts of cytokine profiles have come from studies of infectious disease, but those observations have far-reaching implications for the understanding of autoimmunity, inflammation, and tumor immunology. These studies have demonstrated that two major Th cell subsets, Th1 and Th2, can emerge from (antigen-)naive Th cells following antigenic stimulation. The interaction between antigen-presenting cells (APCs) and T lymphocytes forms the basis for the triggering of cell-mediated immunity. Th cells recognize processed antigen with the use of a broad repertoire of T-cell receptors (TCR) when peptide antigen is bound and presented on a major histocompatibility complex (MHC) class II molecule by an APC

(macrophage, dendritic cell, or B cell). Cross-linking of T-cell co-stimulatory receptors (e.g., CD28) by APCs provides a necessary second signal for triggering T cells through the TCR. When additional requisite accessory signals are provided by macrophages (or other APCs), the Th cell is stimulated into an activated state (i.e., from G_0 to G_1 of the cell cycle). The nature of the T cell's primary response—that is, no response, or activation, anergy, or apoptosis—is determined by the intensity of the cross-linking of the TCR and co-stimulatory molecules as well as additional accessory signals.

Entry of the Th cell into G_1 is signaled by expression of a number of early-response genes, including those that encode IL-2 and the IL-2 receptor (composed of α, β, and γ subunits). IL-2 provides a proliferation signal that stimulates activated T cells to progress through the cell cycle, resulting in their proliferation and differentiation into effector T cells that regulate cell-mediated (Th1) or humoral (Th2) responses. The features of activated T cells include up-regulated expression of various types of adhesion molecules that assist with cell trafficking and production of a variety of interleukins. Activated T cells can traffic to sites of antigen concentration (e.g., infection or tumor cells) and elaborate large quantities of their specific interleukin repertoire, which was programmed during priming. Some of the progeny of activated T cells function as antigen-specific memory T cells. These cells have the capacity to mount a more robust secondary immune response on subsequent exposure to the priming antigen. In this way, the immune system presents a strategy so that the host does not need to generate a "fresh" immune response when the same antigen is encountered again at a later time.

Th Subsets

The two major Th cell subsets, Th1 and Th2, elaborate cytokines that drive the immune response to a cell-mediated or humoral pathway, respectively (Fig. 1). The signature cytokines of Th1 cells are IL-2 and IFN-γ. Tumor necrosis factor beta is also part of the Th1 cytokine profile. These cytokines are considered proinflammatory because they are found in relatively high concentrations at sites of inflammation. IL-2 and IFN-γ, in particular, are responsible for induction of cellular functions such as delayed-type hypersensitivity and activation of cytotoxic T lymphocytes (CTLs, T_c, CD8$^+$). Each of these cytokines contributes to the generation of cellular immunity through unique and overlapping activities. The functions of these cytokines have been described in detail. IL-2 induces clonal expansion of antigen-primed Th cells, amplifying the interleukin response, and augments cytotoxicity mediated by CTLs and natural killer (NK) lymphocytes. IFN-γ up-regulates MHC class I and II molecules (potentiating antigen presentation) and is a potent monocyte-macrophage activator. The positive-feedback loop created between IFN-γ–secreting Th1 cells and target macrophages increases the response by stimulating macrophage-enhanced secretion of IL-1, IL-6, IL-8, and IL-12. Strictly speaking, IL-6 and IL-8 are not usually considered Th1 cytokines; however, they are included in this discussion because of their obvious association with cell-mediated responses. Curiously, the pleiotropic activities of IL-6 also contribute to antibody production,

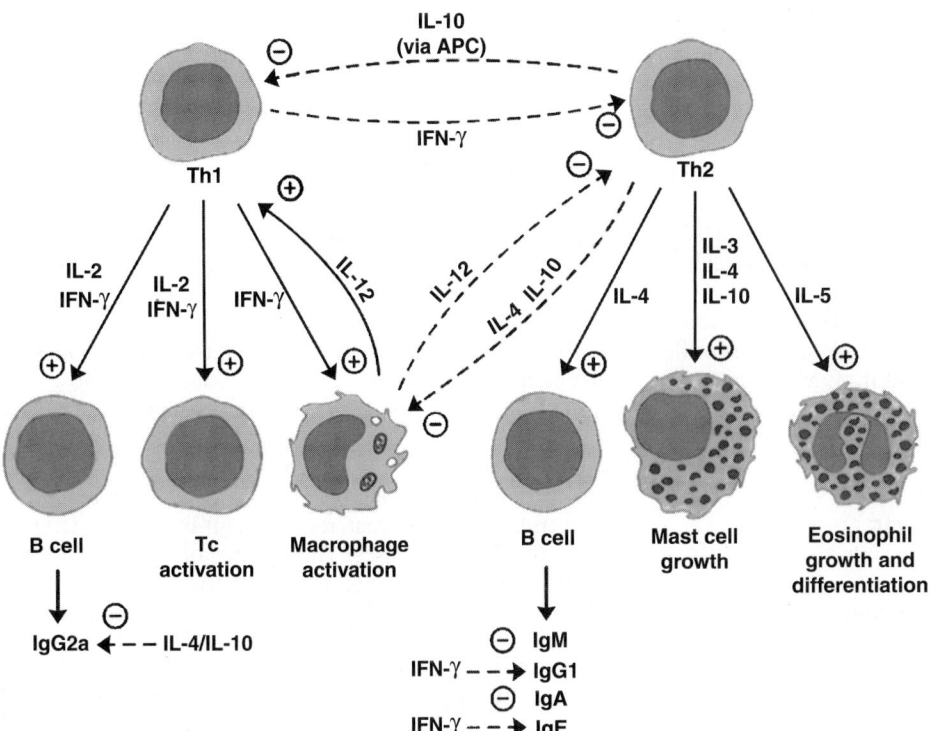

Figure 1. Cross-regulatory effects of interleukins secreted by Th1 lymphocytes, Th2 lymphocytes, and macrophages on the generation of cell-mediated and humoral immune responses. *Solid lines* represent stimulatory pathways; *dashed lines* indicate inhibitory effects. (Adapted from *Immunology*, 2nd edition, by Kuby. © 1994 by W.H. Freeman and Company. Used with permission.)

prompting some to consider IL-6 as a Th2-type cytokine. Functionally, activated macrophages acquire enhanced antitumor cytotoxic activity, and the secretion of IL-8 promotes neutrophil chemotaxis and activation (i.e., release of lysosomal enzymes and respiratory burst) that broadens the arsenal of cytotoxic immune cells in the response. In the presence of antitumor antibody of the IgG2a isotype, which is the only type of antibody induced by Th1 interleukins (see Fig. 1), neutrophil killing of tumor cells is markedly augmented (Helfand et al, 1994a). IL-15, a product of both activated monocytes and Th cells, has been described with biologic activity similar to that of IL-2. Seemingly, it appears that the function of IL-2 is so important in generating cell-mediated responses that nature has provided a "back-up" in the form of IL-15.

Interleukin-12 Is Critical

A dominant role for IL-12 in the induction of Th1 cells has been described. IL-12 is secreted primarily by activated monocytes-macrophages. Its presence early in an immune response forces commitment and expansion of undifferentiated Th cells into the Th1 phenotype. The activity of IL-12 is remarkable in that it is also the most potent inducer/activator of NK cell- and CTL-mediated killing of tumor cells. It increases proliferation of NK and T lymphocytes and induces production of IFN-γ by Th1 cells, which, in turn, propagates macrophage activation and further stimulates IL-12 secretion. Clearly, IL-12 is preeminent in the genesis of cell-mediated immunity.

Clinical Correlates (Table 1)

Understanding the basic biologic activities of interleukins has generated interest and enthusiasm for the use of both interleukins and their antagonists for therapeutic gain.

Interleukin-2

IL-2 has received more attention than any other interleukin for therapy. The potential use of IL-2 for cancer therapy is based on its ability to augment direct cell-mediated lysis of tumor cells by NK cells and CTLs. Killer lymphocytes that have been activated by IL-2 are said to acquire lymphokine-activated killer (LAK) activity. The interspecies activity of human recombinant IL-2 (hrIL-2) in the dog and cat has facilitated investigations of this molecule for veterinary patients.

In the dog, hrIL-2 binds to lymphocytes with high affinity and induces LAK activity in vitro and in vivo. It has been administered to dogs subcutaneously by injection or infusion pump, intravenously by continuous infusion through a peripheral vein, by hepatic and splenic artery infusion, and by inhalation of liposomes containing IL-2. As in human patients, it appears that hrIL-2 has activity in treating canine malignant melanoma. However, relatively few clinical and no controlled studies have been done with hrIL-2 in canine oral melanoma to establish an exact role for IL-2 in this disease. The author's laboratory reported that hrIL-2 activates the immune system in normal dogs (Helfand et al, 1992, 1994b, and 1994c), and this also appears to be the case in dogs with advanced, metastatic melanoma (Fig. 2). However, administering an immune modulator such as IL-2 to animals with bulky disseminated disease is probably not the ideal setting for testing this modality, as the immune system is greatly outnumbered in this scenario.

The place for IL-2 in clinical practice will probably be in combination with other forms of immunotherapy. Preliminary data in dogs supports this approach. IL-2, in combination with hrTNF-α, induced objective responses in 5 of 13 dogs with oral malignant melanoma (Moore et al,

TABLE 1. Interleukins of Clinical and Investigational Interest in Small Animal Medicine 1998*

Interleukin	Natural Source	Clinical Interest

IL-2	Activated helper T lymphocytes	Cancer immunotherapy in the dog
		Infectious disease
		Deficient in:
		  canine demodicosis
		  feline immunodeficiency virus (FIV)
		  feline leukemia virus (FeLV)
		  canine leishmaniasis
		  canine retrovirus–like infection associated with immunosuppression
		Treatment of FeLV infection

IL-6	Activated monocytes and macrophages	Cancer immunotherapy: increased in dogs and cats treated with the monocyte-macrophage activator L-MTP
		Infectious disease: increased in FIV-infected cats
		Hematopoiesis: stimulant of canine megakaryocytopoiesis, thrombocytopoiesis, and platelet activation
		Inflammatory conditions
		Increased in canine:
		  joints with osteoarthritis
		  postischemic reperfusion of myocardium
		  local inflammation
		  recurrent fever of unknown origin—Shar pei dog

IL-8	Activated monocytes and macrophages	Increased in canine pulmonary inflammation
IL-12	Activated monocytes and macrophages	Cancer immunotherapy in the dog

*These examples were selected from the literature.
L-MTP, liposome-encapsulated muramyl tripeptide.

1991). Responses were also seen in dogs with cutaneous mast cell tumor. The potential to combine hrIL-2 with antimelanoma monoclonal antibodies to target activated canine immune cells also appears to have promise in the dog based on in vitro observations (Helfand et al, 1994a).

Liposome encapsulation is an interesting approach to the delivery of IL-2 that potentially increases IL-2 half-life and bioavailability in vivo. Inhalation of IL-2 liposomes directly into the pulmonary tree in normal dogs activates the tumoricidal function of pulmonary alveolar cells (Khanna et al, 1996). This effect is potentially important in the treatment of primary and metastatic pulmonary disease, and preliminary studies in several dogs with metastatic osteosarcoma treated with inhaled IL-2 liposomes suggest that durable regression of metastatic foci is possible.

Several IL-2 fusion proteins have been constructed with the use of molecular biology techniques. One construct links hrIL-2 to diphtheria toxin for the treatment of lymphohematopoietic malignancies that express IL-2 receptors. Because these receptors can bind and internalize IL-2, the diphtheria toxin is delivered intracellularly, where it is lethal. The approach has shown promise in human lymphoma/leukemia, and it is a strategy worth considering in canine lymphoma because IL-2 receptors are also expressed on malignant canine lymphocytes.

A number of dosage regimens for hrIL-2 in the dog have been published. In interpreting these data, one problem is that units of IL-2 have not been standardized between studies. In the earlier work, IL-2 was measured in Biological Response Modification Program (BRMP) units (from the National Cancer Institute), especially in studies with Hoffmann-LaRoche hrIL-2. Other work using IL-2 from Cetus was measured on a different IL-2 unit scale, with one Cetus unit biologically equivalent to 2 Roche (BRMP) units. At this time, the only clinical grade hrIL-2 in the United States is Proleukin, from Chiron (Emeryville, CA), with activity expressed in International Units (IU). Three IU are approximately equal to 1 BRMP unit; so for example in a study from the author's laboratory using Hoffmann-LaRoche hrIL-2, dogs were dosed at 3×10^6 (BRMP) units/m^2/day (days 1 to 4 and 8 to 11) by continuous intravenous infusion (Helfand et al, 1994b). If one uses the newer Chiron IL-2 formulation in IU, the dose would be 9×10^6 IU/m^2/day (see Fig. 2). This is important to keep in mind, as hrIL-2 in very high doses induces clinically significant hypotension in the dog (Kilbourn et al, 1994); however, if hrIL-2 is given at doses such as 9×10^6 IU/m^2/day, toxicity is minimal and consists of mild gastrointestinal signs (Helfand et al, 1994b). It should also be said that it is inevitable that dogs will eventually develop antibodies against this foreign protein because these forms of IL-2 are based on the human gene sequence. This reaction has been seen in dogs after 30 days of inhaled liposome hrIL-2 (Khanna C, personal communication, 1996).

Because IL-2 is so fundamental to eliciting a cellular immune response, a role for it in treating several infectious diseases in dogs and cats has been considered. This approach is especially exciting for the treatment of infections where Th2 cytokine profiles have been associated with disease progression, while Th1 cytokine patterns are associated with more effective containment of an infection. For example, in dogs with natural and experimentally induced *Leishmania* infection, animals that are asymptomatic or resistant manifest cell-mediated immune responses exclusively, but no antibody production against *Leishmania* antigen (Th1 response) predominates (Pinelli et al, 1994). On the other hand, symptomatic dogs with leishmaniasis fail to mount cell-mediated responses but develop high (nonprotective) antibody titers to leishmanial antigens (Th2 response). Thus, a therapeutic window exists for treatment of affected dogs with IL-2 (and/or IL-12) to shift to a cell-mediated immune response and potentially contain the infection in these dogs.

Similarly, dogs with generalized demodectic mange show decreased cell-mediated responses (Th1) but heightened antibody production. Production of IL-2 by T cells from dogs with generalized demodicosis is decreased and fewer T lymphocytes express IL-2 receptors, suggesting a T cell defect (Lemarie and Horohov, 1996). Treatment of dogs with generalized demodicosis with the use of IL-2 awaits clarification; however, given these observations,

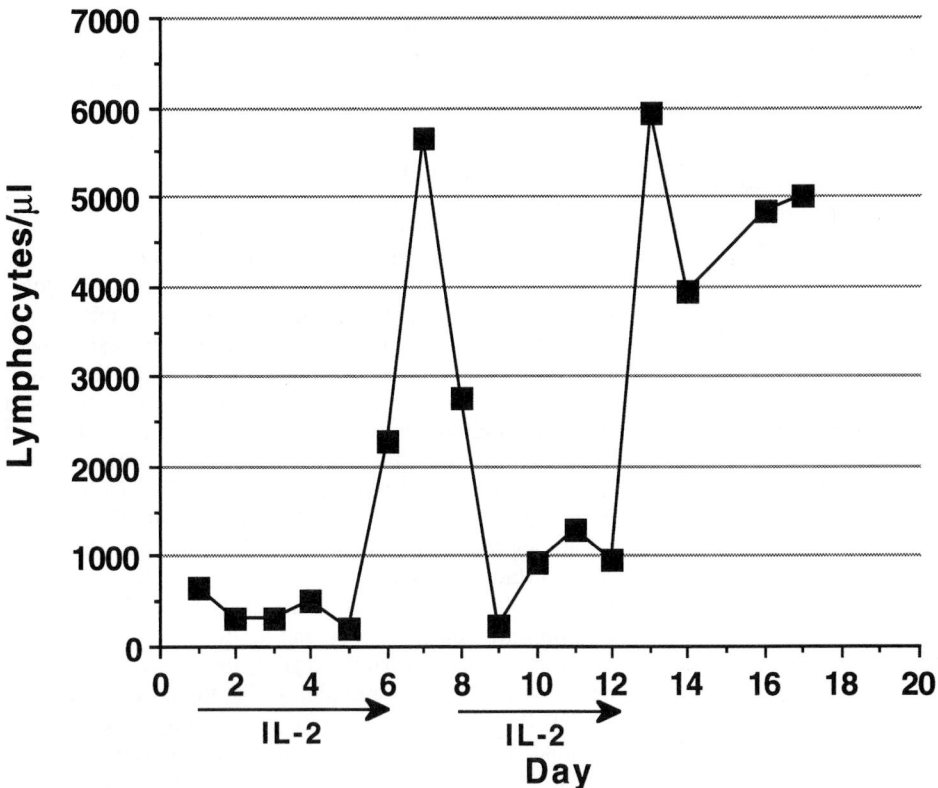

Figure 2. IL-2–induced lymphocyte proliferation in a dog with widely disseminated malignant melanoma when the cytokine was given by continuous multiday intravenous infusion (*arrows*; IL-2, 9 × 10⁶ IU/day). During days of IL-2 administration, the IL-2–responsive lymphocytes leave the circulation and multiply within lymph nodes and other reticuloendothelial tissues. After the IL-2 is discontinued, a rebound lymphocytosis occurs.

induction of cell-mediated responses by administration of hrIL-2 alone (or combined with IL-12) is an approach that may have merit. Without a doubt, more clinical manifestations of infectious disease in veterinary medicine will be explained on the basis of inappropriate Th cell cytokine profiles, and treatment opportunities will become apparent.

IL-2 has a central role in initiating cellular immune responses; thus, it may possibly be the lowest common denominator in mounting an immune response. For this reason, IL-2 has been used to treat human and veterinary patients for infectious diseases associated with immunodeficiency, such as retroviral infections. The objective of this approach is to reconstitute the immune system by providing an alternative source of Th1 interleukin help that is missing in these patients, owing to the demise of CD4 T cells by virus. In cats experimentally infected with feline leukemia virus (FeLV), combination treatment that included IL-2–activated T cells (so-called adoptive immunotherapy) resulted in clearance of FeLV infection in 4 of 9 cats (Zeidner et al, 1993). Similarly, lymphocytes from cats infected with feline immunodeficiency virus demonstrate depressed IL-2 production after stimulation, providing a rationale for treating these cats with IL-2. Although hrIL-2 activates feline lymphocytes, the cloning of feline IL-2 (Cozzi et al, 1993) offers hope that more specific feline IL-2–based therapy may become available in the future.

Interleukin-6

IL-6 is a multifunctional cytokine with effects on a variety of cellular targets. It activates B cells, T cells, and hematopoietic precursors. Its release from activated monocytes-macrophages is associated with the acute-phase response of inflammation. Serum elevation of IL-6 in dogs with cancer may mediate antitumor responses in dogs treated with the monocyte-macrophage activator liposome-encapsulated muramyl tripeptide (L-MTP) (Shi et al, 1995). Human rIL-6 has the capacity to stimulate megakaryocyte proliferation and differentiation within the bone marrow and exhibits cross-species activity in the dog; thus, it has been given to dogs (80 μg/kg/day) to activate and augment platelet counts (Peng et al, 1994). It has also been given to dogs (18 μg/kg/day) in the setting of total body radiation to promote reconstitution of bone marrow megakaryocytes, resulting in earlier increases in thrombocyte counts. As a "footprint" of an inflammatory process, elevation of IL-6 within synovial fluid has been associated with induction and progression of canine osteoarthritis (Hay et al, 1997). Elevations of serum IL-6 in the dog have also been associated with a febrile condition in the Chinese Shar pei dog (Rivas et al, 1992).

Interleukin-8

IL-8 is a product of activated monocytes-macrophages and is a potent neutrophil chemoattractant and activating factor. It enhances neutrophil adhesion to endothelial cells and connective tissue matrix proteins. These actions support a cell-mediated inflammation-promoting activity for IL-8. In the dog, a number of studies have documented a central role for IL-8 in the generation of inflammatory lung disease. Human rIL-8 also activates canine neutrophils. Thus, it is conceivable that antagonists of IL-8 could find a role in the treatment of inflammatory lung disease in the dog. On the other hand, hrIL-8 might also play a clinical role in treating dogs with neutrophil defects, such as Weimaraners.

Interleukin-12

IL-12 is a key cytokine in immune regulation. It promotes activation of NK cells, CTLs, and B cells. Great excitement surrounds the use of IL-12 for oncology because of its potent antitumor effects in rodent models. It also has direct antiangiogenic effects, a property important for inhibiting tumor growth. Human rIL-12 is in clinical trials in humans, and the author's laboratory has recently shown activity of hrIL-12 on canine immune cells (unpublished, 1998). Hopefully, the cloning of both subunits of canine IL-12 will lead to the availability of canine IL-12 for study. There is also growing interest in IL-12 as an inducer of autoimmune disease mediated by induction of Th1 cytokines. An immune-mediated etiology has now been clarified for a number of diseases in experimental models, such as insulin-dependent diabetes mellitus and rheumatoid arthritis (Trembleau et al, 1995). IL-12 promotes highly destructive cell-mediated inflammatory reactions at organ-specific sites, such as the pancreas or within joints. Therefore, ameliorating these intense cellular reactions with IL-12 antagonists (e.g., IL-10) may represent a specific therapeutic strategy directed at the cause of some autoimmune diseases.

CYTOKINE PROFILE OF THE HUMORAL IMMUNE RESPONSE: IL-4, IL-5, IL-6, IL-10, AND IL-13

The generation of the humoral immune response is mediated by a Th2-type cytokine profile. The hallmark cytokines are IL-4, IL-5, IL-6, IL-10, and IL-13. IL-13 shares many of the properties of IL-4. Several of these interleukins have effects that are antagonistic to Th1 cytokines (see Fig. 1). For example, IL-10 inhibits IL-12 secretion, thereby preventing Th1-cell induction. NK cells and CTLs do not mediate cytotoxic activities in the presence of IL-10 and IL-4. Instead, these interleukins synergize to activate and provide help to B lymphocytes for the purpose of antibody production of the IgE, IgG1, IgG3, and IgG4 isotypes. Curiously, in contrast with Th1 cytokines, secretion of the Th2 interleukins is stimulated by large extracellular pathogens, such as helminths. Apparently, host defenses have evolved to favor antibody-mediated responses for protection from these pathogens compared with the cell-mediated immune responses that viruses and bacteria evoke. On the other hand, inappropriate dominance of Th2 patterns can be harmful to the host, as illustrated by the examples of *Leishmania* and *Demodex* infections, discussed earlier. Viruses such as Epstein-Barr virus may encode IL-10 in their genome, apparently as a strategy for tipping the host's immune response away from cell-mediated surveillance to that of antibody-mediated surveillance, thereby favoring survival of the virus. Some autoimmune diseases mediated by production of autoantibodies, such as autoimmune thyroiditis, result in part from IL-4 and IL-5 stimulation of B cells specific for thyroid antigen. Thus, a

role for IL-4 as a regulator of the balance between humoral and cell-mediated responses has emerged.

Clinical Correlates

IL-4 and IL-10 are anti-inflammatory in vivo because they antagonize the effector functions of IFN-γ. The ratio of IL-4 to IFN-γ is apparently important in determining which pattern of cytokine production prevails. Thus, there is enthusiasm for the use of IL-4 in the treatment of diseases characterized by autoreactive or exaggerated delayed-type hypersensitivity responses, but trials in the clinical setting await evaluation. Curiously, IL-4 has been used to treat human cancer patients. As of this writing, feline—but not canine—IL-4 has been cloned.

THE INTERLEUKIN TEETER-TOTTER

Most immune responses do not stimulate an absolute Th1 or Th2 pattern, but rather functional dominance either by Th1 or Th2 interleukins. The polarized patterns of interleukins secreted by Th1 and Th2 cells probably represent extreme examples. In fact, a third type of Th cell, Th0, has been described with the capacity to secrete both Th1 and Th2 type cytokines. A number of factors probably determine which cytokine profile dominates. These variables include the nature of the stimulating antigen, dose of antigen, nature of the antigen-presenting cell (e.g., macrophages present to Th1 cells while B cells present antigen to Th2 cells), and anatomic site where antigen presentation occurs. Fortunately, it appears that in the majority of instances, the Th1-Th2 teeter-totter falls toward the side likely to generate an interleukin profile that benefits the host.

References and Suggested Reading

Cozzi PJ, Padrid PA, Takeka J, et al: Sequence and functional characterization of feline interleukin 2. Biochem Biophys Res Commun 194:1038, 1993.
Describes cloning of feline IL-2 cDNA and synthesis of bioactive recombinant feline IL-2.

Hay CW, Chu Q, Budsberg SC, et al: Synovial fluid interleukin-6, tumor necrosis factor, and nitric oxide values in dogs with osteoarthritis secondary to canine cranial cruciate ligament rupture. Am J Vet Res 58:1027, 1997.
Prospective study of inflammatory mediators IL-6, TNF, and nitric oxide in synovial fluid from stifle joints of dogs with cranial cruciate ligament disease that could contribute to cartilage injury.

Helfand SC, Modiano JF, Moore PF, et al: Functional interleukin-2 receptors are expressed on natural killer–like leukemic cells from a dog with cutaneous lymphoma. Blood 86:636, 1995.
Constitutive expression of IL-2 receptors and aberrant production of IL-2 by canine leukemic cells with dermatotropism suggest an autostimulatory mechanism for this malignancy.

Helfand SC, Modiano JF, Nowell PC: Immunophysiological studies of interleukin-2 and canine lymphocytes. Vet Immunol Immunopathol 33:1, 1992.
Characterizes bioactivity of hrIL-2 in the dog and investigates IL-2–dependent pathways in canine peripheral blood lymphocytes.

Helfand SC, Soergel SA, Donner RL, et al: Potential to involve multiple effector cells with human recombinant IL-2 and antiganglioside monoclonal antibodies in a canine malignant melanoma immunotherapy model. J Immunother 16:188, 1994a.
Investigates expression and targeting of gangliosides on canine melanoma by IL-2–activated canine leukocytes directed against melanoma antigens with antiganglioside antibodies.

Helfand SC, Soergel SA, MacWilliams PS, et al: Clinical and immunological effects of human recombinant interleukin-2 given by repetitive weekly infusion in normal dogs. Cancer Immunol Immunother 39:84, 1994b.
A relatively well-tolerated regimen of IL-2 in dogs induces dramatic increases in lymphocyte numbers and activation, associated with augmentation of their in vitro antitumor reactivity.

Helfand SC, Soergel SA, Modiano JF, et al: Induction of lymphokine-activated killer (LAK) activity in canine lymphocytes with low-dose human recombinant interleukin-2 in vitro. Cancer Biother 9:237, 1994c.
Examines the ability of a clinically relevant (low) dose of hrIL-2 to enhance the tumoricidal properties of canine peripheral blood lymphocytes in vitro.

Khanna C, Hasz DE, Klausner JS, et al: Aerosol delivery of interleukin 2 liposomes is nontoxic and biologically effective: Canine studies. Clin Cancer Res 2:721, 1996.
Novel delivery of hrIL-2 encapsulated in liposomes directly into pulmonary tree by inhalation enhanced tumoricidal activity of canine pulmonary leukocytes in vitro.

Kilbourn RG, Owen-Schaub LB, Cromeens DM, et al: NG-methyl-L-arginine, an inhibitor of nitric oxide formation, reverses IL-2–mediated hypotension in dogs. J Appl Physiol 76:1130, 1994.
Shows that hypotension, the major dose-limiting toxicity of IL-2 in humans, also occurs in dogs at very high IL-2 doses and is mediated by induction of nitric oxide.

Lemarie SL, Horohov DW: Evaluation of interleukin-2 production and interleukin-2 receptor expression in dogs with generalized demodicosis. Vet Derm 7:213, 1996.
Determines lymphocytes from dogs with generalized demodicosis produce less IL-2 and express fewer IL-2 receptors than normal dogs, suggesting a Th1-deficient response.

Moore AS, Theilen GH, Newell AD, et al: Preclinical study of sequential tumor necrosis factor and interleukin 2 in the treatment of spontaneous canine neoplasms. Cancer Res 51:233, 1991.
Shows objective tumor responses in dogs with oral melanoma and cutaneous mast cell tumors treated with TNF followed by IL-2.

Peng J, Friese P, George JN, et al: Alteration of platelet function in dogs mediated by interleukin-6. Blood 83:398, 1994.
Determines that IL-6 enhanced responsiveness of canine platelets to activating stimuli and increased platelet numbers in normal dogs.

Pinelli E, Killick-Kendrick R, Wagenaar J, et al: Cellular and humoral immune responses in dogs experimentally and naturally infected with *Leishmania infantum*. Infect Immun 62:229, 1994.
Describes a number of immunologic parameters in dogs with chronic Leishmania infantum *infection that exhibited either patterns of progressive disease or apparent resistance.*

Rivas AL, Tintle L, Kimball ES, et al: A canine febrile disorder associated with elevated interleukin-6. Clin Immunol Immunopathol 64:36, 1992.
Describes a multiple immunodeficiency, involving antibody- and cell-mediated responses in Chinese Shar pei dogs.

Shi F, Kurzman ID, MacEwen EG: In vitro and in vivo production of interleukin-6 induced by muramyl peptides and lipopolysaccharide in normal dogs. Cancer Biother 10:317, 1995.
Measures IL-6 activity induced by muramyl dipeptide and lipopolysaccharide in vitro and by liposome-encapsulated muramyl tripeptide-phosphatidylethanolamine in vivo in normal dogs; findings suggest that IL-6 may play an important role in the biologic response observed in canine cancer patients treated with L-MTP-PE.

Trembleau S, Germann T, Gately MK, et al: The role of IL-12 in the induction of organ-specific autoimmune diseases. Immunol Today 16:383, 1995.
Review examines the role of interleukin-12 in the induction of autoimmune diseases and discusses potential immunointervention strategies.

Zeidner NS, Mathiason-Dubard CK, Hoover EA: Reversal of feline leukemia virus infection by adoptive transfer of lectin/interleukin-2–activated lymphocytes, interferon alpha, and zidovudine. J Immunother 14:22, 1993.
Examines the hypothesis that combination chemoimmunotherapy might induce the clearance of FeLV infection; results suggest that combined treatment that uses IFN-α and adoptive lymphocyte transfer induced the reversal of retroviremia.

Hereditary Erythrocyte Disorders

URS GIGER

Philadelphia, Pennsylvania

Anemia is one of the most common clinical signs and abnormal laboratory test results in companion animals. Although acquired conditions, such as infections, immune disorders, intoxication, blood loss, and chronic organ failure, represent the main causes of anemia, hereditary blood diseases leading to anemia are also important in clinical practice. Several hereditary erythrocyte defects have been reported in companion animals, and much new information has emerged since the past review of this topic (Giger, 1989). In a few instances, the molecular bases of the erythrocyte defects have now been determined. Erythrocyte defects in companion animals are reviewed in this article.

CANINE AND FELINE ERYTHROCYTES

Although the major structural features and functions of erythrocytes are similar among mammals, some noticeable differences exist between canine and feline erythrocytes (for review see Agar and Board, 1983; Harvey, 1997).

Feline erythrocytes are smaller than canine erythrocytes; therefore, the biconcave disk shape, which allows for easy deformability through the microvasculature and provides a large surface area for oxygen delivery, is reflected only by a small central pallor in feline erythrocytes. Normal variations observed in many Akitas and Miniature Poodles are erythrocyte microcytosis and macrocytosis, respectively. In addition to the common aggregated reticulocytes that are observed for approximately 1 day in circulation, cats also have punctate reticulocytes that are recognized in blood circulation up to 3 weeks after release from the bone marrow, until complete maturation occurs. The normal life spans of erythrocytes in dogs and humans are similar (100 to 120 days), but erythrocyte life span is only 75 days in cats. The half-life can be assessed best by biotinylation or ^{14}C-cyanate labeling of erythrocytes; in contrast, the apparent half-life of ^{51}Cr-labeled cells is generally shorter.

Devoid of a nucleus and mitochondria, erythrocytes have a limited and specialized metabolism that enables them to survive in the circulation and to adequately transport oxygen. Genetic polymorphism of various erythrocytic enzymes has been observed in dogs and cats. Energy is generated almost exclusively through anaerobic glycolysis, also known as the Embden-Meyerhof pathway, a process that also plays an essential role in ancillary pathways. The hexose monophosphate shunt reduces pyridine nucleotides and glutathione, which are necessary for degradation of oxidants, thereby preventing membrane damage and hemoglobin denaturation. In addition, the methemoglobin or cytochrome-b_5 reductase system reduces heme iron from the ferric (Fe^{3+}) to the ferrous (Fe^{2+}) form. The Rapoport-Luebering pathway is responsible for the synthesis of 2,3-diphosphoglycerate (DPG), which influences the oxygen affinity of canine—but not feline—hemoglobin. The erythrocytic DPG concentration is similar in dogs and humans but very low in cats.

Dogs and cats apparently have embryonic, but no fetal, hemoglobin. With the exception of some Japanese breeds, which have two hemoglobins (HbA and HbB), only one adult hemoglobin has been found in dogs. However, further studies are needed to characterize canine hemoglobin. In cats, two major adult hemoglobins were described with a large variation of the HbA-to-HbB ratios. Recent studies, however, revealed that adult cats have one alpha-globin and six different beta-globins. With each cat having one to four different beta-globins, at least 17 hemoglobin patterns were recognized that could be explained by a two-gene beta-globin region with two to six alleles (Kohn et al, 1998a, b).

The erythrocyte membrane consists of a lipid bilayer, affixed to a membrane skeleton, which determines cell shape and deformability. Various transmembrane glycoproteins function as receptors or transporters. Canine and feline erythrocytes lose their Na^+,K^+-ATPase during late maturation in the bone marrow, owing to proteolysis, with the exception of erythrocytes from Akitas and some mongrel dogs in Japan (Inaba and Maede, 1986). Therefore, erythrocytes' high-sodium and low-potassium concentrations are similar to those of serum electrolytes. Consequently, hyperkalemia generally does not occur after intravascular hemolysis unless stress reticulocytes or erythrocytes from Japanese dogs are lysed. In fact, Akitas' erythrocytes are "leaky" in vitro, and pseudohyperkalemia has been observed in serum that has not been separated immediately from its clot (Degen, 1987). Finally, canine erythrocytes have been noted to be uniquely fragile under alkaline conditions, compared with erythrocytes from cats and other species, presumably because of a facilitated calcium entry under these conditions. This pH sensitivity may explain the tendency of canine erythrocytes to lyse in uncapped tubes in the laboratory.

CLASSIFICATION OF HEREDITARY DISORDERS

Inherited erythrocyte defects form a large heterogeneous group of diseases. Each erythrocyte disorder is observed only rarely, although a particular defect may occur frequently within a family or breed. If the same disorder is recognized in several breeds, it is probably caused by different mutations of the same gene. The mode of inheritance is autosomal recessive, with the exception of feline porphyria, which is inherited as a dominant trait. Although the degree of characterization is varied, many seem to be homologues of hereditary disorders in humans. These disorders have been classified into four groups: (1) heme defects and hemoglobinopathies, (2) cytosolic enzyme deficiencies, (3) membrane abnormalities, and (4) production and maturation defects (Table 1); a few specific disorders are discussed later, in more detail.

Hemoglobin

In contrast to the common occurrence of thalassemia and sickle cell anemia in people, *no hemoglobinopathies have been documented in dogs and cats*. A presumed β-thalassemia in a severely anemic domestic cat was later recognized to have one of the many normal feline beta-globin patterns (Giger et al, 1994). An electrophoretically abnormal hemoglobin was seen in a dog that exhibited exercise intolerance but no anemia. Isolated cases of methemoglobinemia associated with cytochrome-b_5 reductase deficiency were found among dogs of various breeds (Harvey et al, 1991, 1994) and a domestic shorthair cat (Harvey et al, 1997). Defects of heme synthesis known as porphyrias have been reported in anemic Siamese and nonanemic domestic shorthair cats with pigmented and pink-fluorescent teeth and bones (Haskins and Patterson, 1987).

Membrane

Elliptocytosis and microcytosis resulting from a deficiency of the protein band 4.1, which strengthens the interaction between spectrin and actin in the cytoskeleton, have been characterized at the molecular level in an inbred, nonanemic mongrel dog (Smith et al, 1983; Conboy et al, 1991). Other presumed membrane abnormalities include stomatocytosis in Alaskan malamutes (Fletch et al, 1975), in a Dutch breed with gastritis (Slappendel et al, 1994), and in Miniature Schnauzers (Giger et al, 1988; Brown et al, 1994); nonspherocytic anemia in Beagles (Maggio-Price et al, 1988; Hinds et al, 1989); and erythrocytes with increased osmotic fragility in an English Springer spaniel (Rand and O'Brien, 1987) and in Abyssinian and Somali cats (Kohn et al, 1996).

Enzymes

Deficiencies of the two key regulatory glycolytic enzymes result in distinctly different forms of hemolytic anemia. The classic pyruvate kinase (PK) deficiency initially reported in Basenjis (Whitney and Lothrop, 1995; Giger and Nobel, 1991) is now seen in several other breeds and cats (Giger et al, 1997). Phosphofructokinase (PFK) deficiency is frequently reported in English Springer spaniels (Giger and Harvey, 1987; Smith et al, 1996) and has also been observed in a Cocker spaniel and a mixed-breed dog (Giger et al, 1992). Although glucose-6-phosphate dehydrogenase deficiency is the most common erythroen1-6zymopathy in humans, screening of more than 3000 dogs revealed only one healthy Weimaraner to have a partial enzyme deficiency of this sort (Smith et al, 1976).

TABLE 1. Inherited Erythrocyte Defects

Defects	Breed	Inheritance	PCV % (Range)	Reticulocyte % (Corrected)	Erythrocyte T 1/2 (d)	Erythrocyte Morphology	Specific Tests	Clinical Features
Erythroenzymopathies								
Pyruvate kinase (PK) deficiency	Basenji, Beagle, West Highland White terrier, and Cairn terrier, Miniature Poodle	AR	11–25	10–45	4–9	Polychromasia, echinocytes	DNA test for Basenji and West Highland White terrier; Abnormal M-PK, PK-kinetic and stability and glycolytic intermediates	Hemolytic anemia, myelofibrosis, osteosclerosis
	Abyssinian, Somali, DSH cats	AR	10–33	1–33	U	Polychromasia	PK-activity <20%, DNA test	Intermittent hemolytic anemia
Phosphofructokinase (PFK) deficiency	English Springer spaniel, Cocker spaniel	AR	11–18	5–23	4	Polychromasia	DNA test; PFK activity 8–22%	Inducible hemolytic crises, mild myopathy, pigmenturia
Glucose-6-phosphate dehydrogenase (G6PD) deficiency	Weimaraner	U	N	N	U	Unremarkable	G6PD activity 40%	None
Hemoglobin Synthesis Defects								
Hemoglobinopathies	None							
Cytochrome-b_5 reductase (Cb_5R) deficiency	Many isolated cases	U	High	N	U	Unremarkable	Cb_5R activity 0–30%; Methemoglobin >10%	Cyanosis, mild polycythemia, exercise intolerance
Porphyria	Siamese	AD					Porphobilinogen deaminase deficiency	Anemia, discolored teeth
	DSH cats	AD						Discolored teeth, no anemia

Membrane and Other Abnormalities

Disorder	Breed	Inheritance				Blood smear	Diagnostic test	Clinical signs
Elliptocytosis (band 4.1 deficiency)	Mixed-breed dog	AR	34	2	16–23	Elliptocytes	Membrane protein electrophoresis	None
Stomatocytosis	Alaskan malamute, Miniature Schnauzer	AR	N	3–7	6–18	Stomatocytes, polychromasia	Stomatocytes, increased osmotic fragility	Chondrodysplasia in malamutes, none in Schnauzers
Increased osmotic fragility	English Springer spaniel, Mixed-breed dog	U	N	2–5	U	Polychromasia, poikilocytosis	Increased osmotic fragility, unknown	Exercise-induced hyperthermia
	Abyssinian, Somali	U	8–35	1–14	U	Macrocytosis	Increased osmotic fragility	Intermittent anemia, splenomegaly
High-potassium erythrocytes	Akita Japanese mongrels	U	N	N	U	Unremarkable	Increased erythrocyte and serum potassium	None, pseudohyperkalemia
Nonspherocytic hemolytic disorders	Beagle	AR	29–12	8–23	7–15	Polychromasia	Calcium ATPase pump (?)	None, mild anemia
Poikilocytosis	DSH cats	U	7–12	10–30	U	Severe poikilocytosis	Poikilocytosis	Severe anemia
Familial microcytosis	Akita	U	N	N	U	Microcytosis	Erythrocyte indices	None

Production and Maturation Defects

Disorder	Breed	Inheritance				Blood smear	Diagnostic test	Clinical signs
Cyclic hematopoiesis	Gray collie	AR	N	0–8	N	Intermittent	Serial complete blood cell counts	None related to erythrocytes, recurrent infection, bleeding
Selective cobalamin malabsorption	Giant Schnauzer Border collie	AR	20–31	0	U	Nonregenerative megaloblasts, hypersegmented neutrophils	Low serum cobalamin (B_{12}), urinary organic acids	Cachexia, dementia, responsive to parenteral vitamin B_{12}
Familial macrocytosis and dyshematopoiesis	Poodle (miniature and toy)	U	N	N	U	Macrocytes, hypersegmented neutrophils	Macrocytosis, normal osmotic fragility	None, gingivitis

Data collected from references and author's unpublished observations.

N, normal; U, unknown; AR, autosomal recessive; AD, autosomal dominant. M-PK, M-type pyruvate kinase; PK, pyruvate kinase; PCV, packed cell volume.

Erythropoiesis

Whereas the previous defects resulted in shortened erythrocyte survival and regenerative anemias, the production and maturation disorders are reflected not only in a nonregenerative anemia but also in changes in other bone marrow–derived cells. Cyclic hematopoiesis of Gray collies is the classic example (Jones, 1983). Selective cobalamin (vitamin B_{12}) malabsorption resulting from an ileal intrinsic cobalamin receptor defect has been reported in Giant Schnauzers (Fyfe et al, 1989, 1991) and Border collies (Outerbridge et al, 1996). Familial macrocytosis of Poodles is a presumed maturation defect and can be associated with leukopenia, neutrophil hypersegmentation, and thrombocytopenia, but not anemia (Schalm, 1976).

CLINICAL SIGNS

Because the shortening of the erythrocyte life span and erythropoietic response differ among erythrocyte defects, the clinical features of hemolytic anemia also vary, ranging from severe hemolytic crises to well-compensated hemolysis without clinical signs. Typical signs of anemia, including lethargy, exercise intolerance, pallor, icterus, pigmenturia, and tachycardia, may be noted at a few weeks to months of age. Because these disorders are chronic, affected animals usually have adapted well and show only minimal overt signs. However, certain environmental conditions and other diseases (e.g., infections) may exaggerate these features, as is best exemplified in canine PFK deficiency. Hepatosplenomegaly may result from severe extravascular hemolysis and extramedullary hematopoiesis. Furthermore, erythrocyte defects may be part of a multisystemic syndrome caused by the pleiotropic effects of a single mutant gene, for instance, chondrodysplastic Alaskan malamute dwarfs with stomatocytosis.

LABORATORY DIAGNOSIS

Although the signalment, type, and severity of the anemia and the pleiotropic effects observed may provide clues to an inherited erythrocyte defect, a full laboratory evaluation is essential in validating the diagnosis or discovering new inherited disorders. In fact, in a few breeds, more than one erythrocyte disorder has been recognized. Routine hematologic laboratory tests are used to detect hematologic abnormalities and to rule out acquired anemia. An inherited erythrocyte defect should be considered in animals with Coombs-negative hemolytic anemia, a lack of toxin exposure or infection, and adequate kidney as well as liver function. A careful examination of a peripheral blood smear is pivotal in recognizing any poikilocytosis, such as elliptocytosis and stomatocytosis, although most erythrocyte defects cause no change in cell shape and are historically known as nonspherocytic hemolytic anemias. The degree of reticulocytosis is often marked, even in the case of PK deficiency with osteosclerosis, and is proportional to the shortened survival of defective erythrocytes. Thus, a bone marrow examination rarely provides new information. The signs of hemolysis may be mild owing to the chronicity and low-grade hemolysis. Bilirubinuria and bilirubinemia are generally noted. Low serum haptoglobin concentrations, hemoglobinemia, or hemoglobinuria, which indicate intravascular hemolysis, have been reported in PFK deficiency. Some defective erythrocytes appear extremely fragile in vitro, resulting in artificial lysis in blood tubes.

Special laboratory tests for defining the nature of an intrinsic erythrocyte defect can be divided into general screening tests, used to characterize unknown erythrocyte disorders, and specific screening tests for known defects. Both are performed only in specialized laboratories (e.g., Josephine Deubler Genetic Disease Testing Laboratory at the School of Veterinary Medicine, University of Pennsylvania, Philadelphia).

The erythrocyte osmotic fragility test, membrane protein electrophoresis, and ion transport studies are used for membrane defects. Various hemoglobin separation methods and shape changes in the hemoglobin-oxygen dissociation curve may be useful in discovering new hemoglobinopathies. Finally, cytosolic enzyme deficiencies are identified by demonstrating a decrease in the activity of an enzyme, the absence of immunologic cross-reacting material, abnormal enzyme kinetics, accumulation of enzyme substrates, and a lack of products. For instance, erythrocyte DPG concentration is decreased in PFK deficiency but is increased in PK deficiency in dogs. Unfortunately, these tests are time-consuming as well as demanding and require specific shipping instructions and submission of a control sample from a healthy animal.

More recently, molecular genetic screening tests have become available for identifying erythrocyte defects caused by specific mutations. Such tests can be developed whenever a causative mutation in a defective gene has been identified. These tests are mutation-specific, and so they are generally also breed-specific; that is, the same enzyme deficiency in various breeds may be caused by different mutations. Currently, DNA tests are available for PK deficiency in Somali and Abyssinian cats and Basenjis and West Highland White terriers—but not for PK deficiency in other breeds—and for PFK deficiency in English Springer and American Cocker spaniels. These DNA-based tests are also most valuable in identifying carriers (heterozygotes) that are asymptomatic but pass on the mutant allele.

THERAPY AND PREVENTION

Hemolysis resulting from erythrocyte defects may be well compensated for by marked erythropoiesis, thereby causing no or only minimal clinical signs and allowing the animal to have a normal life expectancy. Furthermore, affected animals may have adapted well to the chronic anemia (e.g., PK-deficient dogs show mild clinical signs despite severe hemolytic anemia, but die before 5 years of age because of anemia, osteosclerosis, and hepatic failure). In contrast, some disorders are associated with severe hemolytic crises for which animals may need to receive supportive therapy, including blood-typed, compatible transfusions. Cats with increased erythrocytic osmotic fragility or PK deficiency have marked splenomegaly and may be helped with splenectomy by removing a major site of erythrocyte destruction; however, it appears that PK- and PFK-deficient dogs have not benefited from this procedure.

Experimentally, allotransplantation of bone marrow has been shown to correct the aforementioned enzymopathies in dogs. Furthermore, hemolytic crises in PFK-deficient dogs may be prevented by avoiding panting, strenuous exercise, and heat. Finally, affected and carrier animals should not be used for breeding, to prevent the further spread of these disorders.

SPECIFIC ERYTHROCYTE DISORDERS

Phosphofructokinase (PFK) Deficiency

This glycolytic enzyme deficiency is common in field-trial English Springer spaniels in the United States, Great Britain, and Denmark but has also been reported in bench dogs as well as a Cocker spaniel and a mixed-breed dog. It is caused by a missense mutation of the muscle-type PFK that results in a truncation and instability of the enzyme, thereby leading to a complete muscle-type PFK deficiency (Smith et al, 1996).

The disorder is characterized by hemolytic crises and exertional myopathy (Giger and Harvey, 1987). Sporadic dark pigmenturia resulting from severe hemoglobinuria and bilirubinuria is a key feature and commonly develops after episodes of excessive panting and barking, extensive exercise, and high temperature. Hyperventilation-induced alkalemia results in intravascular lysis of PFK-deficient erythrocytes. During these crises, affected dogs may become severely anemic and icteric, and show fever, lethargy, and anorexia, which usually resolve within days. Situations triggering hemolytic crises should be avoided. PFK-deficient dogs may have a normal life span, but have persistent bilirubinuria and reticulocytosis despite a normal hematocrit because of the high hemoglobin oxygen affinity of PFK-deficient erythrocytes. Furthermore, affected dogs totally lack PFK activity in muscle; therefore, they have a metabolic myopathy characterized by exercise intolerance, occasional muscle cramps, and mildly increased serum creatine kinase (CK) activity. They thus will perform poorly as field-trial dogs (Giger et al, 1989).

A simple polymerase chain reaction (PCR)–based DNA test accurately diagnoses PFK-deficient and carrier dogs. English Springer and Cocker spaniels with suspicious signs should be screened for PFK deficiency before field-trial training and breeding.

Pyruvate Kinase (PK) Deficiency

Although PK deficiency was first, and best, characterized in the Basenji breed (Giger and Noble, 1991), the clinical features and biochemical abnormalities appear very similar in other canine breeds. Despite the severity of the anemia, the clinical signs, except for pallor, are mild. The anemia is highly regenerative, with numerous circulating metarubricytes and reticulocyte counts as high as 90%. An unexplained progressive myelofibrosis and osteosclerosis of the bone marrow and generalized hemosiderosis with associated hepatic failure develop, causing death usually before 5 years of age. Erythrocytes completely lack the adult erythrocyte isozyme form of PK known as R-PK. Instead, they express a fetal M-PK form that is also present in the spleen and white blood cells. However, M-PK appears unstable and malfunctions in erythrocytes in vivo, as shown by the shortened erythrocyte survival and abnormal erythrocyte metabolite pattern. The molecular genetic basis of PK deficiency has been identified in Basenjis (Whitney et al, 1994; Whitney and Lothrop, 1995) and West Highland White terriers (Chapman and Giger, 1990; Giger, unpublished), and PCR-based tests are available for these breeds, but not for others. Thus, a cumbersome PK-enzyme test with isozyme characterization is required to define PK deficiency in other breeds. Carriers do not express the M-PK form and have half the normal PK activity; however, differentiation between carriers and homozygous normal dogs based on enzyme activity can be difficult. PK deficiency has also been reported in Beagles (Giger et al, 1991), Cairn terriers (Schaer et al, 1992), and recently in the author's laboratory in Miniature Poodles. It appears probable that the previously described nonspherocytic hemolytic anemia and osteosclerosis in Poodles was caused by a PK deficiency (Randolph et al, 1986).

In cats, PK deficiency causes intermittent anemia with a moderate regenerative response, but cats do not develop osteosclerosis (Ford et al, 1992; Giger et al, 1997). Cats have splenomegaly, and splenectomy appears to ameliorate the clinical signs of intermittent anemia, the oldest such cat reaching 8 years of age. Erythrocyte PK activity is severely reduced, and there is no M-type PK expression, thereby simplifying the diagnosis. Furthermore, a molecular screening test for PK deficiency in Abyssinian and Somali cats has recently been developed in the author's laboratory.

Increased Osmotic Fragility

Increased osmotic fragility of erythrocytes suggests a membrane or ion transport defect. Chondrodysplastic Alaskan malamute dwarfs with stomatocytosis were the first dogs described with fragile erythrocytes, but the exact mechanism is still unknown (Fletch et al, 1975). Miniature Schnauzers with stomatocytosis had no skeletal abnormalities, and both breeds had only mild anemia based on hemoglobin measures (Giger et al, 1988). Furthermore, stomatocytosis and gastritis have been described in the Dutch breed (Slappendel et al, 1994).

A marked osmotic fragility of erythrocytes associated with intermittent anemia, severe splenomegaly, and hyperglobulinemia has been observed in Abyssinian and Somali cats (Kohn et al, 1996). Although the cause has not been identified, affected cats with marked splenomegaly may benefit from prednisone treatment and splenectomy. However, the osmotic fragility of erythrocytes in vitro does not appear to improve.

References and Suggested Reading

Agar NS, Board PC: Red Blood Cells of Domestic Animals. Amsterdam: [North Holland] Elsevier, 1983.
   The most comprehensive review of comparative erythrocyte physiology.
Brown DE, Weiser MG, Thrall MA, et al: Erythrocyte indices and volume distribution in a dog with stomatocytosis. Vet Pathol 31:247, 1994.
   A description of stomatocytosis in a Miniature Schnauzer.

Chapman BL, Giger U: Inherited pyruvate kinase deficiency in the West Highland White Terrier. J Small Anim Pract 31:610, 1990.
The only case report of a PK-deficient West Highland White terrier.

Conboy JG, Shitamoto R, Parra M, et al: Hereditary elliptocytosis due to both qualitative and quantitative defects in membrane skeletal protein 4.1. Blood 78:2438, 1991.
A molecular characterization of elliptocytosis.

Degen M: Pseudohyperkalemia in Akitas. J Am Vet Med Assoc 290:541, 1987.
A description of leaky high-potassium erythrocytes.

Fletch SM, Pinkerton PH, Brueckner PJ: The Alaskan malamute chrondrodysplasia (dwarfism-anemia) syndrome: A review. J Am Anim Hosp Assoc 11:353, 1975.
A description of stomatocytosis in Alaskan malamutes.

Ford S, Giger U, Duesberg C, et al: Inherited erythrocyte pyruvate kinase (PK) deficiency causing hemolytic anemia in an Abyssinian cat. J Vet Intern Med 6:123, 1992.

Fyfe JC, Jezyk PF, Giger U, et al: Inherited selective malabsorption of vitamin B_{12} in giant schnauzers. J Am Anim Hosp Assoc 25:533, 1989.
A clinical report of the hematologic changes associated with cobalamin deficiency.

Fyfe JC, Giger U, Hall CA, et al: Inherited selective intestinal cobalamin malabsorption and cobalamin deficiency in dogs. Pediatr Res 29:24, 1991.
A metabolic study of hereditary cobalamin deficiency.

Giger U: Hereditary disorders of canine erythrocytes. In: Kirk RW, ed: Current Veterinary Therapy X: Small Animal Practice. Philadelphia: WB Saunders, 1989, p 429.
A review of canine erythrocyte defects.

Giger U, Harvey JW: Hemolysis caused by phosphofructokinase deficiency in English springer spaniels: Seven cases (1983–1986). J Am Vet Med Assoc 191:453, 1987.
Clinical description of PFK deficiency.

Giger U, Noble NA: Inherited erythrocyte pyruvate kinase deficiency in Basenji dogs. J Am Vet Med Assoc 198:1755, 1991.

Giger U, Amador A, Meyers-Wallen V, et al: Stomatocytosis in miniature schnauzers. ACVIM Proc 1988, p 754.
First report of stomatocytosis in Miniature Schnauzers.

Giger U, Argov Z, Schnall M, et al: Metabolic myopathy in canine muscle-type phosphofructokinase deficiency studied by ^{31}P-NMR. Muscle Nerve 11:1260, 1989.
A characterization of the metabolic myopathy in PFK-deficient dogs.

Giger U, Rajpurohit Y, Wang P, et al: Molecular basis of erythrocyte pyruvate kinase deficiency in cats. Blood 90:S5b, 1997.
A report of clinical, hematologic, and molecular features of PK-deficient cats.

Giger U, Reilly M, Chin M, et al: Beta-thalassemia in the cat. Blood 84:364a, 1994.
An anemic cat with severe poikilocytosis.

Giger U, Smith BF, Woods CB, et al: Inherited phosphofructokinase deficiency in the American Cocker spaniel. J Am Vet Med Assoc 201:1569, 1992.
A report on PFK deficiency in American Cocker spaniels.

Giger UG, Mason GD, Wang P: Inherited erythrocyte pyruvate kinase deficiency in a Beagle dog. Vet Clin Pathol 20:83, 1991.
A report on PK-deficient Beagles.

Harvey JW: Erythrocyte metabolism. In: Kaneko JJ, ed: Clinical Biochemistry of Domestic Animals, 4th ed. New York: Academic Press, 1989.

Harvey JW: The erythrocyte: Physiology, metabolism and biochemical disorders. In: Kaneko JJ, Harvey JW, Bruss KL: Clinical Biochemistry of Domestic Animals, 5th ed. San Diego, CA: Academic Press, 1997, p 157.

Harvey JW, Dahl M, High ME: Methemoglobin reductase deficiency in a cat. J Am Vet Med Assoc 205:1290, 1994.
A case report of methemoglobin reductase deficiency in a cat.

Harvey JW, King RR, Berry CR: Methemoglobin reductase deficiency in dogs. Compar Haematol Int 1, 1991.
A review of methemoglobin reductase deficiency.

Haskins ME, Patterson DF: Inherited metabolic diseases. In: Holzworth J ed: Diseases of the Cat. Philadelphia: WB Saunders, 1987, p 808.

Hinds TR, Hammond WP, Maggio-Price L, et al: The activity of the red blood cell Ca pump is decreased in hemolytic anemia of the beagle dog. Blood Cells 15:421, 1989.
Characterization of erythrocyte abnormalities in Beagles with hemolysis.

Inaba M, Maede Y: Na,K-ATPase in dog red cells. J Biol Chem 261:16099, 1986.
Characterization of canine erythrocyte membrane pumps.

Jones JB: Cyclic hematopoiesis: Animal models. Exp Hematol 11:571, 1983.
A review on cyclic hematopoiesis.

Kohn B, Hohenhaus A, Giger U: Hemolytic anemia caused by increased osmotic fragility of erythrocytes in cats. ACVIM Proc 1996, p 760.
A clinical report on a new hemolytic disorder in cats.

Kohn B, Henthorn PS, Rajpurohit Y, et al: Feline adult β-globin polymorphism reflected in restriction fragment length patterns. Submitted, 1998a.
A molecular characterization of the feline beta-globins.

Kohn B, Reilly MP, Asakura T, et al: Polymorphism of feline β-globins studied by high-performance liquid chromatography. Am J Vet Res, in press, 1998b.
A novel explanation of the feline hemoglobin polymorphism.

Maggio-Price L, Emerson CL, Hinds TR, et al: Inherited nonspherocytic hemolytic anemia in beagle dogs. Am J Vet Res 49:1020, 1988.
A clinical description of a hereditary hemolytic disorder in Beagles.

Outerbridge CA, Myers SL, Giger U: Hereditary cobalamin deficiency in Border Collie dogs. ACVIM Proc, 1996, p 751.
A clinical report of vitamin B_{12} malabsorption.

Rand JS, O'Brien PJ: Exercise-induced malignant hyperthermia in an English springer spaniel. J Am Vet Med Assoc 190:1013, 1987.
A clinical report of osmotically fragile erythrocytes.

Randolph JF, Center SA, Kalfelz FA, et al: Familial nonspherocytic hemolytic anemia in poodles. Am J Vet Res 47:687, 1986.
The initial report of a hemolytic anemia and osteosclerosis in Poodles.

Schaer M, Harvey JW, Calderwood-Mays M, et al: Pyruvate kinase deficiency causing hemolytic anemia with secondary hemochromatosis in a Cairn terrier. J Am Anim Hosp Assoc 28:233, 1992.
A report of PFK deficiency in a Cairn terrier.

Schalm OW: Erythrocyte macrocytosis in miniature and toy poodles. Canine Pract December, 1976, p 55.
A clinicopathologic description of an unexplained macrocytosis.

Slappendel RJ, Renooij W, deBruijne JJ: Normal cations and abnormal membrane lipids in the red blood cells of dogs with familial stomatocytosis–hypertrophic gastritis. Blood 84:904, 1994.
A description of stomatocytosis in dogs.

Smith BF, Stedman H, Rajpurohit Y, et al: The molecular basis of canine muscle type phosphofructokinase deficiency. J Biol Chem 271:20070, 1996.

Smith JE, Ryer K, Wallace L: Glucose-6-phosphate dehydrogenase deficiency in a dog. Enzyme 6:21, 1976.
A large screening study identified one deficient dog without clinical signs.

Smith JE, Moore K, Arens M, et al: Hereditary elliptocytosis with protein band 4.1 deficiency in the dog. Blood 61:373, 1983.
A case report of an elliptocytosis.

Whitney KM, Lothrop CD: Genetic test for pyruvate kinase deficiency of Basenjis. J Am Vet Med Assoc 207:918, 1995.
A molecular screening test for diagnosing PK deficiency.

Whitney KM, Goodman SA, Bailey EM, et al: Molecular basis of canine pyruvate kinase deficiency. Exp Hematol 22:866, 1994.
A description of the molecular defect in PK-deficient Basenjis.

Disorders of Feline Red Blood Cells

MARY M. CHRISTOPHER
Davis, California

Erythrocyte, or red blood cell (RBC), disorders are detected through alterations in the number, size, shape, and color of RBCs, and the presence of inclusions or organisms. In general, feline RBC disorders are similar to those of other species. There are, however, a few unique RBC abnormalities in cats that require special consideration in regards to diagnosis and treatment (see the previous article). These include Heinz body anemia (associated with drugs, diet and disease), poikilocytosis (associated with hepatic disease and doxorubicin administration) and macrocytic anemia (associated with feline leukemia virus infection).

HEINZ BODY ANEMIA

Pathophysiology of Heinz Body Formation in Cats

Heinz bodies are clumps of precipitated hemoglobin inside RBCs that result from oxidative damage. Oxidation (oxidative stress) is caused by increased production (or decreased detoxification) of highly reactive chemical moieties called free radicals, which interact with and damage surrounding cell components. Free radicals can be spontaneously generated from oxygen (which is in high concentration inside RBCs) or can result from drugs, chemicals, or plants with oxidant properties. Hemoglobin oxidation may result in methemoglobin or Heinz body formation. Heinz bodies damage RBCs and can contribute to anemia. In cats, Heinz bodies had previously been called "erythrocyte refractile (ER) bodies" or Schmauch bodies; they are a prominent RBC feature in all members of the family Felidae.

Feline hemoglobin is particularly sensitive to oxidation because it contains a high number of free thiol (SH) groups, which are prime targets for oxidative damage. Thiol oxidation causes reconfiguration of globin chains and their eventual denaturation into Heinz bodies. Feline hemoglobin dimers also dissociate more readily than those of other species, and glutathione, a thiol protector, is unstable and readily depleted in feline RBCs. The net result is the remarkable ease with which Heinz bodies form in feline RBCs in association with drugs, diet, and disease. Because globin structure is closely linked to heme oxidation, methemoglobinemia often accompanies or precedes the formation of Heinz bodies.

Heinz bodies are also much more likely to be observed in cats because of the nonsinusoidal structure of the feline spleen. Unlike dogs, cats have relatively generous splenic openings that permit free passage of RBCs even when rigid inclusions such as Heinz bodies are present. Therefore, feline spleens do not affect the rate of removal of Heinz body–containing RBCs from the circulation. Heinz bodies themselves shorten RBC survival, but the degree of anemia

that results, if any, is dependent on the rapidity of Heinz body formation, their size and number, and the severity of damage to the RBC membrane.

Causes of Heinz Bodies in Cats

Drug-Induced Heinz Bodies

Oxidant drugs that induce Heinz body formation include acetaminophen (Tylenol; paracetamol), phenacetin, phenazopyridine, methylene blue, and DL-methionine. All these drugs may cause concurrent methemoglobinemia. Benzocaine (Cetacaine, Cetylite) causes methemoglobinemia without Heinz body formation. Oxidant drugs are much more likely to cause Heinz body hemolytic anemia than are other causes of Heinz bodies because of the rapid rate at which Heinz bodies form and the likelihood of additional oxidative damage to the RBC membrane. Acetaminophen is most often implicated in Heinz body anemia in cats, owing to the inability of cats to detoxify the drug by glucuronidation. Acetaminophen toxicity is dose dependent, and a *single 325-mg tablet* is sufficient to result in toxicity. In general, oxidant drugs cause toxicity in cats at lower doses than those required for other species. Careful questioning of the client is often necessary to establish a diagnosis of drug toxicity.

Diet-Induced Heinz Bodies

Dietary elements that cause Heinz bodies in cats include onions, propylene glycol (a food additive), and some fish-based diets. Diet-induced Heinz bodies may be accompanied by a normal hematocrit or may result in mild to moderate anemia. The rate and degree of Heinz body formation is related to food intake and the amount of oxidant ingested. With small amounts of oxidant, the bone marrow has sufficient time to compensate for shortened RBC survival. Cats that ingest dietary oxidants may be more susceptible to oxidant drugs. For example, acetaminophen is more toxic in cats that consume diets containing propylene glycol.

Onions (fresh, cooked, dehydrated or powdered) cause Heinz bodies in a dose-dependent manner; large amounts can cause hemolytic anemia. Some commercial meat-based baby foods (e.g., Gerber) contain enough onion powder to result in more than 50% Heinz bodies and, in some cases, anemia, depending on food intake. Baby foods with onion powder should especially be avoided in cats with diabetes or other diseases in which Heinz bodies are already increased and may have an additive effect. Some commercial cat foods contain minuscule amounts of onion powder or salt, which are unlikely to cause any increase in Heinz body formation. One or more thiol compounds in onions are responsible for oxidizing hemoglobin.

Until recently, propylene glycol was added to semi-moist cat foods as a carbohydrate source and preservative. Cat foods no longer contain propylene glycol because it causes Heinz bodies; however, dog foods may still contain the additive. Some feline snacks contain propylene glycol, but the amount ingested with a treat is very small and is unlikely to have an effect on Heinz body formation. The mechanism by which propylene glycol causes oxidation is unknown; it is dose dependent, and high doses can cause mild to moderate anemia. Fish-based diets have also been associated with Heinz bodies and may cause anemia, especially in kittens. The specific components of fish responsible for Heinz body formation have not been investigated.

Disease-Associated Heinz Bodies

In cats, several diseases have been associated with increased numbers of Heinz bodies, most prominently, diabetic ketoacidosis. Ketoacidotic cats (including those with ketoacidosis independent of diabetes) may have as many as 70 to 80% large Heinz bodies, and most have more than 30% (Christopher et al, 1995). Nonketotic diabetic cats also develop increased numbers of Heinz bodies, but to a lesser extent (5 to 20%). The mechanism of diabetes-induced Heinz body formation is unknown. The number of Heinz bodies correlates with the blood ketone concentration, so some relation with ketosis is probable.

Hyperthyroidism and neoplasia, especially lymphoma, are also consistently associated with increased numbers of Heinz bodies, although the Heinz bodies are usually smaller and fewer than those in diabetic cats. Diabetes, hyperthyroidism, and neoplasia result in increased ketogenesis, gluconeogenesis, and protein catabolism, suggesting a common mechanism of increased oxidative stress. Hepatic disease, renal disease, urologic disease, upper respiratory disease, stomatitis, pharyngitis, and intestinal disorders may also cause increased numbers of Heinz bodies in some cats. Hypophosphatemia has been associated with Heinz bodies in cats, but it is not clear whether the condition is a primary cause of hemoglobin oxidation or whether it is simply a concurrent finding in certain disease conditions, such as ketoacidotic diabetes.

Disease-induced Heinz bodies frequently result in mild to moderate, sometimes severe, anemia because of their large size and number and because the primary disease often secondarily impairs erythropoiesis. Acute hemolysis is not generally observed, since disease-associated Heinz body formation is usually slower than drug-induced Heinz body formation. Cats with disease-induced Heinz bodies may also be more susceptible to other oxidants. For example, diabetic or hyperthyroid cats fed baby food with onion powder appear to have more Heinz bodies than would be expected on the basis of ingestion of onions or disease alone.

Diagnosis of Heinz Body Anemia

Quantitation of Heinz Bodies

Cats with anemia should always be evaluated for the presence of Heinz bodies. Similarly, cats with Heinz bodies noted on blood smears should always be evaluated for

anemia. In addition, all cats with ketosis (as detected by urine dipstick) should be evaluated for Heinz bodies. Heinz bodies should be quantitated as a percentage (%) of 1,000 RBCs with the use of a supravital new methylene blue stain (Christopher and Harvey, 1992). Rapid evaluation of Heinz bodies—and reticulocytes—can also be done by placing a drop of new methylene blue on a dried blood smear and covering it with a coverslip. Sometimes, Heinz bodies are seen as pale inclusions in Wright-Giemsa–stained smears, particularly if they are large enough to bulge from the RBC periphery. Some RBCs may appear to be extruding a Heinz body. Heinz bodies can also result in the formation of "ghost cells," which result from partial RBC lysis and leakage of hemoglobin. Ghost cells appear as hollow RBC rims with an attached Heinz body. Unlike those in dogs, Heinz bodies in cats are usually single and uniform in size and can become very large (occupying as much as one third of the cell volume). Oxidant drugs may cause multiple Heinz bodies. Many large Heinz bodies can artifactually increase the mean cell hemoglobin concentration (MCHC) and total leukocyte count as measured by some automated cell counters; double peaks or left shoulders may be seen on leukocyte histograms.

The dogma that Heinz bodies are "normal" in cats derives from a lack of understanding about the causes and implications of Heinz bodies in this species. Truly healthy cats have less than 5% Heinz bodies, and cats on strictly controlled diets have less than 1 to 2%. Although absent in newborn kittens, Heinz bodies have no other association with age, sex, or breed. Cats with more than 10% Heinz bodies should be evaluated for possible drug, dietary, or disease causes of Heinz bodies. Cats with more than 50% Heinz bodies and no evidence of drug exposure should be carefully evaluated for diabetes, ketoacidosis, or ingestion of onions.

Methemoglobinemia and Anemia

Oxidant drugs almost always result in Heinz body hemolytic anemia, which may range from mild to severe and is often accompanied by methemoglobinemia. Cats with acetaminophen toxicity generally present with depression, vocalization, salivation, facial edema, vomiting, hyperventilation, icterus, and cyanosis (owing to methemoglobinemia). Occasionally, hemoglobinuria may be observed. Methemoglobinemia is easily evaluated with the use of a "spot test" (when methemoglobin content is 15% or more, a drop of blood on white absorbent paper will appear brown in comparison to a drop of normal blood) or by laboratory quantitation of methemoglobin concentration (Christopher and Harvey, 1992). Diet- and disease-associated Heinz bodies do not usually cause methemoglobinemia.

Heinz bodies associated with diet and disease variably cause anemia, depending on the size and number of Heinz bodies and the rate at which they formed. Cats with disease-associated Heinz bodies are usually more anemic (especially cats with ketoacidotic diabetes) than cats with the same diseases but without Heinz bodies. The greater the number and size of Heinz bodies, the greater the likelihood of anemia. However, it is possible for cats to have 100% Heinz bodies and a normal hematocrit, particularly if Heinz bodies are small or the rate of Heinz body formation (and shortened RBC survival) was slow enough for the bone marrow to compensate for their production. Although Heinz bodies usually form more slowly with diet or disease than with drugs, they can subsequently reach a much larger size. Anemia is more probable when Heinz bodies are large and affect more than 30% of RBCs. It may be difficult to separate the effect of Heinz bodies on the hematocrit from that of the primary disease.

Reticulocyte counts should be done in all cats with Heinz bodies to evaluate the regenerative response. Drug-induced Heinz body hemolytic anemia is often accompanied by reticulocytosis, whereas increased numbers of punctate reticulocytes may provide evidence of subtle or chronic hemolysis. Other causes of anemia should not be ruled out, even when Heinz bodies are present. In diabetic cats, for example, serum phosphorus should be measured to differentiate hypophosphatemia-induced hemolysis from Heinz body anemia. In acetaminophen toxicity, hepatic enzymes should also be monitored, since a few cats may develop fulminant hepatic failure that can result in death.

Treatment of Heinz Body Anemia

Treatment of drug-induced Heinz body anemia is both antidotal and supportive. First, the source of the oxidant must be identified and removed. Second, supportive care should be directed toward adequate tissue perfusion. A transfusion may be required if the hematocrit is extremely low (<12%), but care should be taken to avoid stressing the cat. Oxygen therapy and a quiet, dark cage with a minimum of handling and stress are often sufficient. Third, antioxidant therapy is aimed at restoring depleted glutathione and is particularly useful in cases of acetaminophen toxicity. Treatment with N-acetylcysteine (Mucomyst, Apothecon; or Mucosil, Dey Labs) provides the best response, since it can speed the clearance of acetaminophen as well as replenish thiol groups. N-Acetylcysteine comes as a 10 or 20% solution. It should be administered at a dosage of 140 mg/kg PO or IV initially, followed by 70 mg/kg every 4 hours for three to five additional treatments. Sodium sulfate (a 1.6% solution) is also effective at 50 mg/kg IV every 4 hours. Some cats (especially females) may benefit from methylene blue therapy for reversal of methemoglobinemia (Rumbeiha et al, 1995). Contrary to popular opinion, methylene blue can be used safely in cats, provided that it is administered only once (1.0 to 1.5 mg/kg IV); additional doses may exacerbate Heinz body formation. Ascorbic acid has also been recommended for the treatment of methemoglobinemia, but its uptake by feline RBCs is so slow that it is probably of limited benefit.

It is possible that N-acetylcysteine, ascorbic acid, and even vitamin E could benefit cats with diet- or disease-induced Heinz body formation, but no prospective studies have been designed to test their efficacy. It is most important to identify and eliminate the offending dietary component, or to treat the underlying disease and provide supportive care as needed. Once the oxidizing principle is removed, Heinz bodies usually disappear gradually over a period of 1 to 4 weeks. Cats should be carefully monitored for the development of anemia, which may occur if RBC removal is rapid because of the large size and/or number

of Heinz bodies. All cats with Heinz body anemia due to any cause should be monitored with sequential hematocrit, reticulocyte, and Heinz body counts to document the disappearance of Heinz bodies and the regeneration of RBCs.

POIKILOCYTOSIS

Erythrocyte shape abnormalities (poikilocytes) are much less common in cats than in dogs, owing, in part, to the smaller size of feline RBCs. For this reason, poikilocytes are more specific indicators of disease or drug therapy in cats and can provide useful diagnostic and prognostic information.

Poikilocytosis in Hepatic Disease

More than 50% of cats with hepatic disease develop poikilocytosis characterized primarily by acanthocytes and ovalocytes (elliptocytes; Christopher and Lee, 1995). Lower numbers of keratocytes, schistocytes, and blister cells may also be observed. While these morphologic changes also occur in dogs with hepatic disease, the rarity of poikilocytosis in cats imparts a greater diagnostic and prognostic importance to these findings. Poikilocytosis tends to persist or increase in cats with worsening hepatic disease and decreases with disease regression and normalization of other laboratory data.

Cats with hepatic lipidosis are significantly more likely to have poikilocytosis than are cats with other types of hepatic disease. In addition, cats with moderate (2+) to marked (4+) poikilocytosis are more likely to be anemic, with hematocrits averaging 5% lower than those of cats with hepatic disease but no poikilocytosis. Poikilocytosis in hepatic disease is probably associated with altered RBC membrane lipids and is more prominent in cats with hypercholesterolemia. Other possible mechanisms include increased oxidative damage resulting from vitamin E deficiency (from malabsorption secondary to cholestasis) and microangiopathy. Numbers of Heinz bodies are sometimes increased in hepatic disease, but they are most often observed with lipidosis secondary to diabetes mellitus.

Poikilocytosis Caused by Doxorubicin Treatment

Doxorubicin administration causes RBC poikilocytosis similar to that observed in hepatic disease, with a mixture of ovalocytes, echinocytes, keratocytes, acanthocytes, schistocytes, and blister cells (O'Keefe and Schaeffer, 1992). The degree of poikilocytosis increases from slight (1+) to marked (4+) with sequential treatments of the drug. The severity of poikilocytosis caused by doxorubicin is considerably greater in cats than in dogs, and in cats poikilocytes are notably increased after only one treatment with the drug. This effect after one treatment may be due, in part, to the oxidant sensitivity of feline RBCs. Anemia does not generally develop in cats treated with doxorubicin.

MACROCYTIC ANEMIA

Macrocytic anemia is often observed in cats infected with feline leukemia virus (FeLV), with a mean cell volume of more than 50 fl (Shelton and Linenberger, 1995). Although macrocytic anemia can also be caused by reticulocytosis (owing to the larger size of immature RBCs), in this case it appears to result from a defect in RBC production, and polychromasia is not observed. A mean cell volume (MCV) greater than 55 fl in the absence of polychromasia is a good positive predictor of FeLV infection (see p. 280). Increased MCV, usually without anemia, is observed in some cats with hyperthyroidism.

References and Suggested Reading

Christopher MM, Broussard JD, Peterson ME: Heinz body formation associated with ketoacidosis in diabetic cats. J Vet Intern Med 9:24, 1995.
A prospective study of biochemical abnormalities and Heinz body formation in cats with spontaneous diabetes mellitus.
Christopher MM, Harvey JW: Specialized hematology tests. Semin Vet Med Surg (Small Anim) 7:301, 1992.
A useful description of hematologic techniques, including reticulocyte counts, Heinz body counts, and methemoglobin determination.
Christopher MM, Lee SE: Red cell morphologic alterations in cats with hepatic disease. Vet Clin Pathol 23:7, 1995.
An evaluation of the type and amount of poikilocytosis and other laboratory abnormalities in different types of hepatic disease in cats.
O'Keefe DA, Schaeffer DJ: Hematologic toxicosis associated with doxorubicin administration in cats. J Vet Intern Med 6:276, 1992.
A prospective study of red blood cell, neutrophil, and platelet changes associated with several cycles of doxorubicin treatment.
Rumbeiha WK, Lin Y-S, Oehme FW: Comparison of N-acetylcysteine and methylene blue, alone or in combination, for treatment of acetaminophen toxicosis in cats. Am J Vet Res 56:1529, 1995.
Recent experimental data on optimal treatment protocols for acetaminophen toxicity in cats.
Shelton GH, Linenberger ML: Hematologic abnormalities associated with retroviral infections in the cat. Semin Vet Med Surg (Small Anim) 10:220, 1995.
A comprehensive review of the hematologic abnormalities associated with feline leukemia virus and feline immunodeficiency virus infections.

Practical Use of a Blood Substitute

VIRGINIA RENTKO
North Grafton, Massachusetts

BASIS FOR USE

A variety of clinical states are associated with a decreased oxygen-carrying capacity of the blood. Among the most important are anemia, low blood volume, and poor blood flow. Physiologic compensation for these conditions often involves increasing cardiac output to maintain tissue oxygen delivery. The increase in cardiac output partially compensates for the decrease in the unit quantity of oxygen carried by the blood. Clinical signs of anemia, such as pallor, lethargy, and tachycardia, reflect both the stresses associated with impaired oxygen delivery and the cardiovascular responses to acute anemia. The prognosis of an animal with acute anemia depends on the animal's ability to compensate for the condition as well as the cause and the severity of the underlying disorder that is causing the anemia.

The oxygen-carrying capacity of transfused blood is lifesaving in cases of severe anemia. However, the problem of limited availability of disease-free, compatible blood for transfusion plagues practitioners. A hemoglobin solution that carries oxygen in the plasma has been approved by the U.S. Food and Drug Administration (FDA). Use of a hemoglobin-based oxygen-carrying (HBOC) solution in the treatment of anemia permits adequate quantities of oxygen to be delivered to tissues without an associated increase in cardiac workload.

CHARACTERISTICS OF AN OXYGEN-CARRYING SOLUTION

Oxyglobin (hemoglobin glutamer-200 [bovine]) is an ultrapurified, polymerized hemoglobin solution of bovine origin (13 gm/dl) in modified Ringer's lactated solution. It is a sterile solution for intravenous administration with a physiologic pH (7.8) and osmolality (300 mOsm/kg). The viscosity is low compared with that of blood: 1.3 versus 3.5 centipoise (cp), respectively. Oxyglobin contains a distribution of hemoglobin polymers with an average molecular weight of 200 kilodaltons (kD). Less than 5% is unstabilized tetramer ($\leq$65 kd); approximately 50% is 65 to 130 kD; and at most 10% is greater than 500 kD. The concentration of methemoglobin, the inactive form of hemoglobin, is at most 10%. It is stable for at least 2 years when stored under ambient temperatures (2° to 30°C). Oxyglobin requires no preparation for use. Its intravascular half-life is dose dependent, typically 30 to 40 hours at 30 ml/kg in healthy dogs. The hemoglobin will carry oxygen for as long as it is present in the plasma. More than 90% of the administered dose is expected to be eliminated from the body in 5 to 7 days following infusion. The oxygen half saturation pressure (P-50) of Oxyglobin is greater than that of canine blood: 38 versus 30 mm Hg, respectively. The increased P-50 corresponds to a greater efficiency of releasing oxygen to the tissue relative to hemoglobin in the red blood cells. Oxyglobin's oxygen dissociation curve is hyperbolic, compared with the sigmoidal shape of the curve for blood. The polymerization process of Oxyglobin restricts the conformational changes of hemoglobin that are responsible for the sigmoidal shape of the hemoglobin-oxygen dissociation curve of blood (Fig. 1).

INDICATION FOR USE

The increased oxygen content of the blood supplied by Oxyglobin via plasma hemoglobin is effective in relieving the clinical signs of anemia. Oxyglobin was tested in a

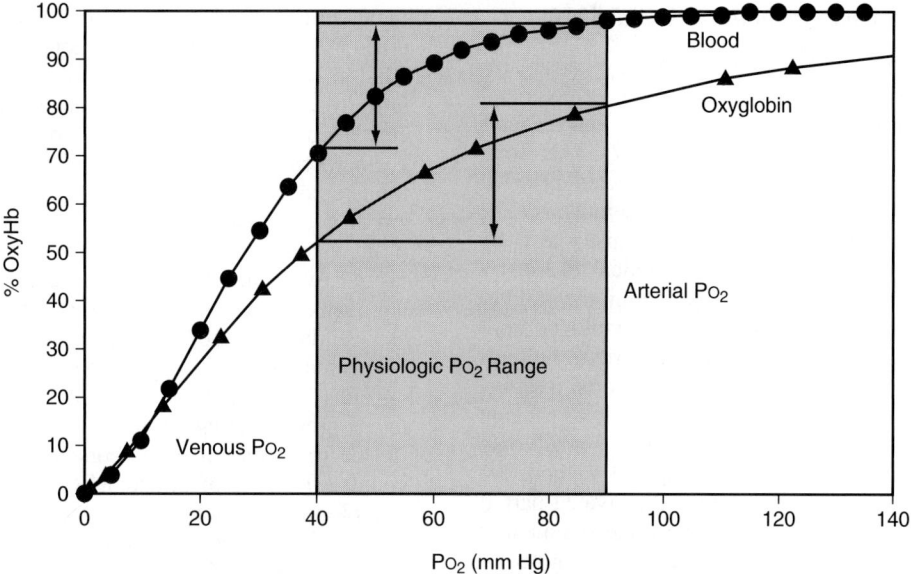

Figure 1. Oxygen equilibrium curves for red blood cells and Oxyglobin as measured by a Hemox Analyzer at 37°C, pH 7.4. The vertical arrows represent the oxygen delivery capacity at the physiologic Po_2 limits.

multicenter clinical trial in dogs with moderate to severe anemia (packed cell volume [PCV], 6 to 23%) due to blood loss (n = 25), hemolysis (n = 30), or ineffective erythropoiesis (n = 9) (Rentko et al, 1996). Thirty dogs were randomized to the Oxyglobin group, and 34 dogs to an untreated control group. Dogs in both groups were monitored for a decrease in total hemoglobin or a deterioration in physical condition, at which time they received additional oxygen-carrying support. If additional oxygen-carrying support was needed, Oxyglobin-treated dogs received packed red blood cells (PRBCs; n = 1), and untreated control dogs received Oxyglobin (n = 22). Treatment success was defined as lack of the need for additional oxygen-carrying support for 24 hours. The success rate in treated dogs (95%) was significantly greater than the success rate in control dogs (32%; α = 0.05). Overall, this marked difference in success rates between treated and control dogs was seen regardless of the cause of anemia (Fig. 2).

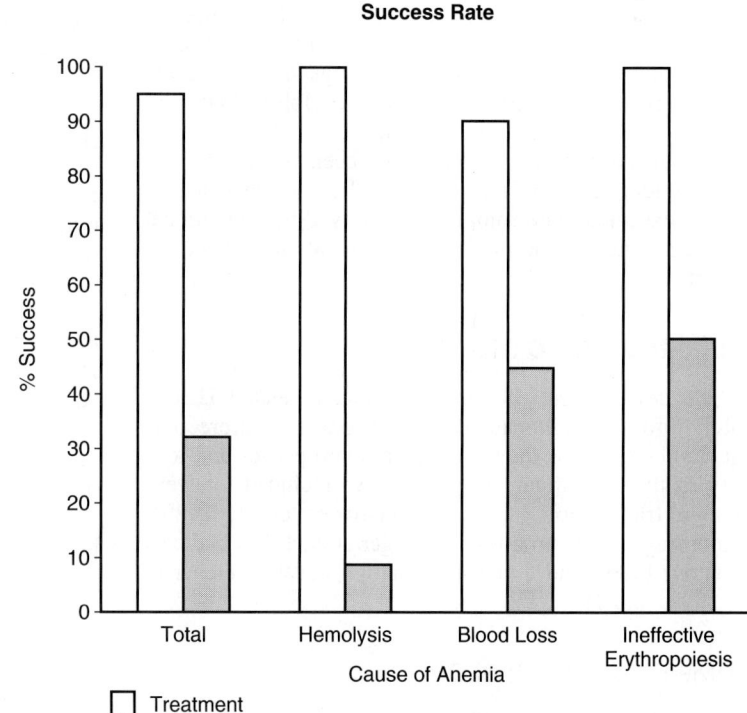

Figure 2. Success rates in Oxyglobin-treated and control groups stratified by cause of anemia in a clinical trial of 64 dogs.

EFFECTS OF HEMOGLOBIN IN THE PLASMA

The presence of Oxyglobin in serum may cause artifactual increases or decreases in the results of serum chemistry tests, depending on the type of analyzers and reagents used (Moreira et al, 1997; Callas et al, 1997). Therefore, blood samples for analysis should be collected prior to infusion. The interference is *not* typical of hemolysis. The product labeling includes a list of valid chemistry tests by analyzer. Before interpretation of any clinical chemistry test performed on serum containing Oxyglobin, the validity of the test in the presence of Oxyglobin should be confirmed. In general, all tests that use colorimetric techniques are *invalid*. Other methodologies also show some interferences. Some interferences last until Oxyglobin is cleared from the blood. No interference is seen with hematologic or coagulation parameters except when optical methods are used for measuring prothrombin time and activated partial thromboplastin time. Examination of the urine sediment is accurate; however, dipstick measurements (pH, glucose, ketones, protein) are inaccurate while gross discoloration of the urine is present.

SAFETY

Treatment with Oxyglobin is associated with transient discoloration (yellow to brown) of the mucous membranes, sclera, urine, and sometimes skin. At the recommended dose of 30 ml/kg, a potential exists for overexpansion of the vascular volume. In the clinical trial, rates of administration of 10 ml/kg per hour in normovolemic dogs increased central venous pressure, which was sometimes associated with pulmonary edema or other respiratory signs of circulatory overload. Vomiting occurred in approximately one third of the dogs that were treated with Oxyglobin. Diarrhea, fever, and death were also seen in approximately 15% of the dogs treated with Oxyglobin; however, the association with Oxyglobin or the underlying disease could not be determined. These findings occurred most frequently in dogs treated with Oxyglobin that had immune-mediated hemolyic anemia.

Repeated use of Oxyglobin has not been evaluated clinically. A long-term preclinical study of its repeated use in dogs is expected to be completed in early 1999. No clinical data regarding the use of Oxyglobin in cats have been reported.

PHARMACOLOGIC STUDIES

The development of Oxyglobin and a related HBOC solution for use in humans has included testing in preclinical studies to assess the pharmacologic properties and toxicity of these solutions. The tests have included total exchange transfusion in sheep (Vlahakes et al, 1989), hemorrhagic shock in dogs (Harringer et al, 1992) and cats (Walton, 1996), and tumor oxygenation in rats (Teicher et al, 1993a and 1993b).

COMPARISON WITH BLOOD

The effects of an HBOC solution compared with blood have also been evaluated. In a model that mimics the clinical situation of severe blood loss, Standl and colleagues (1996) compared the effects of autologous stored red blood cells (RBCs), fresh whole blood, and an HBOC solution on the hemodynamics and tissue oxygenation of skeletal muscle in dogs. After isovolemic hemodilution to hematocrits of 20, 15, and 10%, each solution was administered to increase total hemoglobin in increments of 1 gm/dl until tissue oxygenation was restored to baseline. Hindlimb muscle partial pressure of oxygen (Po_2) was measured with an Eppendorf microelectrode histographic technique. Cardiac index increased with hemodilution and subsequently decreased during retransfusion in all groups, as expected. Tissue oxygenation decreased similarly in all groups during hemodilution but increased differently between groups during retransfusion ($P < .05$). Restoration of tissue oxygenation to baseline measurements required 2.5 and 2.0 gm/dl of stored RBC hemoglobin and fresh whole blood hemoglobin, respectively. Tissue oxygenation increased above baseline measurements with administration of approximately 0.7 gm/dl of total hemoglobin in the group receiving an HBOC solution. The data show that the HBOC solution provided higher tissue oxygen tensions per unit of hemoglobin compared with stored or fresh RBCs after marked hemodilution. This advantage may be clinically important in acute tissue hypoxia due not only to anemia but also to other low-flow conditions.

Harringer and associates (1992) studied the efficacy of an HBOC solution in dogs during resuscitation from hemorrhagic shock (systolic arterial pressure ≤ 50 mm Hg for 60 minutes). Allogeneic PRBCs or 10% human serum albumin (HSA) were the controls. Resuscitation with an HBOC solution restored stable hemodynamics and corrected acidosis in a manner comparable to treatment with PRBCs. Oxygen transport was maintained at a higher level than that in dogs treated with HSA. The HBOC solution restored the blood volume without cardiopulmonary collapse, bronchospasm, pulmonary vascular spasm, or other significant cardiovascular effects.

Walton (1996) evaluated the effects of an HBOC solution, autologous whole blood, or 6% hydroxyethyl starch (HES) in cats during resuscitation from hemorrhagic shock (mean arterial pressure 40 mm Hg for 60 minutes). The HBOC solution and autologous blood were equally effective in restoring oxygen transport variables, including heart rate, arterial and venous oxygen contents, oxygen extraction, and blood gases. Cardiovascular parameters, that is, arterial blood pressure and pulmonary artery pressure, returned to normal in cats treated with whole blood or the HBOC solution. Peripheral perfusion also improved equally in these groups, as evidenced by an increase in arterial pH and a decrease in blood lactate levels. Resuscitation with HES resulted in restoration of blood pressure, but oxygen transport parameters remained decreased. This study showed that all three resuscitation fluids restored blood pressure, but only whole blood and an HBOC solution normalized oxygen transport successfully.

FUTURE USE

Expanded clinical uses of an HBOC solution are now being explored. Experimental studies offer a foundation for the rationale of clinical use. However, additional clinical data are needed to evaluate the utility of an HBOC solution in a variety of clinical situations. Its use in the dog is dictated by the immediate requirement for oxygen-carrying ability. A solution that is easily stored and delivers oxygen without the necessity for crossmatching or blood typing fills this important clinical need.

References and Suggested Reading

Callas DD, Clark TL, Moriera PL, et al: In vitro effects of a novel hemoglobin-based oxygen carrier on the routine chemistry, therapeutic drug, coagulation, hematology, and blood bank assays. Clin Chem 43:1744, 1997.
This study reports how the presence of an HBOC solution in serum interfered with a variety of clinical assays.
Harringer W, Hodakowski GT, Svizzero, et al: Acute effects of massive transfusion of bovine hemoglobin blood substitute in a canine model of hemorrhagic shock. Eur J Cardiothorac Surg 6:649, 1992.
This study describes the effectiveness of an HBOC solution in resuscitation after major blood loss in dogs.
Moreira PL, Lansden CC, Clark TL, et al: Effect of Hemopure® on the performance of Ektachem and Hitachi clinical analyzers. Clin Chem 43:1790, 1997.
This technical brief describes the effects of an HBOC solution on serum chemistry tests with two commonly used analyzers.
Rentko VT, Wohl J, Murtaugh R, et al: A clinical trial of a hemoglobin-based oxygen carrier (HBOC) fluid in the treatment of anemia in dogs. J Vet Intern Med 10:177, 1996.
This abstract reports the efficacy and safety of an HBOC solution in a clinical trial in anemic dogs.
Standl T, Horn P, Wilhelm S, et al: Bovine hemoglobin is more potent than autologous red blood cells in restoring muscular tissue oxygenation after profound isovolaemic hemodilution in dogs. Can J Anaesth 43:714, 1996.
This report compares the effects of stored RBCs, fresh blood, and an HBOC solution on hemodynamics and tissue oxygenation in dogs.
Teicher BA, Holden SA, Menon K, et al: Effect of hemoglobin solution on the response to intracranial and subcutaneous 9L tumors to antitumor alkylating agents. Cancer Chemother Pharmacol 33:7, 1993a.
This report examined the effects of increasing the oxygenation of a solid tumor on the response of the tumor to alkylating agents.
Teicher BA, Schwartz GN, Sotomayor EA, et al: Oxygenation of tumors by a hemoglobin solution. J Cancer Res Clin Oncol 120:85, 1993b.
This study evaluated the oxygen tensions of solid tumors in response to the administration of an HBOC solution while the subject was breathing various compositions of oxygen.
Vlahakes GJ, Lee R, Jacobs EE, et al: Hemodynamic effects and oxygen transport properties of a new blood substitute in a model of massive blood replacement. Eur J Cardiothorac Surg 100:379, 1989.
This report describes an exchange transfusion with an HBOC solution in awake sheep to a hematocrit of 3%.
Walton RS: Polymerized hemoglobin versus hydroxyethyl starch in an experimental model of feline hemorrhagic shock. Proceedings of the 5th IVECC Symposium, 1996.
This abstract reports the efficacy of an HBOC solution in resuscitation from hemorrhagic shock in cats.

CVT Update: Diagnosis and Treatment of Immune-Mediated Hemolytic Anemia

ELLEN MILLER
Fort Collins, Colorado

PATHOPHYSIOLOGY

Immune-mediated hemolytic anemia (IMHA) is a life-threatening hematologic disease of dogs and cats. Erythrocytes are destroyed by a type II hypersensitivity reaction that results in extravascular or intravascular hemolysis. Extravascular hemolysis occurs when immunoglobulin- or complement-coated erythrocytes are removed by phagocytic cells of the mononuclear phagocyte system. If the red blood cells are coated with enough immunoglobulin G (IgG) or M (IgM) molecules to fix complement, intravascular hemolysis may result. Ten to twenty percent of dogs with IMHA have the intravascular form.

Immune-mediated hemolytic anemia has been classified in several ways. One method for classifying subtypes of IMHA is based on etiology. Primary IMHA is a true autoimmune reaction against red blood cells. The majority of dogs with IMHA are thought to have this form of the disease, as no underlying etiology can be identified. In secondary IMHA, erythrocytes are destroyed as innocent bystanders in an immune reaction against some foreign protein that may be adherent to the erythrocyte surface. In this form, no true autoantibody exists. Usually, the trig-gering protein is a result of viral or bacterial infection, drug administration, or neoplastic processes. Secondary IMHA is the more common form of this disease in cats.

A second method of classification is based on the type of antibody causing the hemolysis. Class I disease results from antibodies, called in-saline acting agglutinins, capable of causing autoagglutination of erythrocytes. Clinically, this class is identified by positive slide agglutination. Class II IMHA results from antibodies capable of fixing complement and causing intravascular hemolysis. These antibodies are usually of the IgM class but may be of the IgG class. Classes I and II are the most severe forms of IMHA. Class III IMHA is the most common form of IMHA in dogs and results from antibodies that cause extravascular hemolysis. This antibody is detected only by the direct Coombs' test. Classes I to III all are caused by warm-reacting antibodies that have their effect at body temperature. These antibodies are more common than cold-reacting antibody forms of the disease. Class IV IMHA is caused by cold-reacting agglutinating antibodies, while class V disease is caused by cold-reacting intravascular hemolysins.

Research by Barker and colleagues (1991) has eluci-dated erythrocyte autoantigens that may possibly be re-

TABLE 1. Causes of Hemolytic Anemia in Dogs and Cats

Inherited Causes
Pyruvate kinase deficiency
Phosphofructokinase deficiency
Chondrodysplasia/anemia
Nonspherocytic hemolytic anemia
Immune-Mediated Causes (Primary)
Primary (idiopathic) IMHA
IMHA associated with systemic lupus erythematosus
Neonatal isoerythrocytolysis
Incompatible transfusions
Metabolic Causes
Hypophosphatemia
Neoplastic Causes
Microangiopathic anemia associated with hemangiosarcoma
   or lymphosarcoma
Infectious Causes
Babesia canis
Babesia gibsoni
Haemobartonella canis
Haemobartonella felis
Dirofilaria immitis
Bacterial endocarditis
Feline leukemia virus
Leptospirosis
Cytauxzoon felis
Ehrlichia canis
Toxin- or Drug-Related Causes
Onion toxicity
Zinc toxicity
Methylene blue
Copper toxicity
Propylthiouracil
Methimazole
Sulfa drugs
Penicillins and cephalosporins
Quinidine

sponsible for IMHA in dogs. Immunoprecipitation techniques utilizing antierythrocyte autoantibodies obtained from dogs with IMHA have identified seven distinct erythrocyte autoantigens. It is thought that these autoantigens may be glycophorins (glycoproteins that bear blood group antigens in people) or may be the canine equivalent of the Rhesus antigen, a glycoprotein complex necessary for the maintenance of erythrocyte viability. Identification of the autoantigens and autoantibodies is an important step toward our understanding of IMHA and, ultimately, our therapeutic control of the disease.

It is important to realize that hemolytic anemia is not only caused by immunologic mechanisms. Other diseases, drugs, or toxins associated with hemolytic anemia are listed in Table 1. The diagnostic approach to the patient with hemolytic anemia should address other potential etiologies (see *CVT XII*, pp. 437 and 447).

DIAGNOSIS OF IMMUNE-MEDIATED HEMOLYTIC ANEMIA IN DOGS

Clinical Presentation

Signalment

Immune-mediated hemolytic anemia is a disease of middle-aged dogs (mean age of affected dogs is approximately 6.5 years). Although any breed may be affected, Cocker

spaniels, English Springer spaniels, collies, Poodles, Old English sheepdogs, and Irish setters are overrepresented. Most reports of canine IMHA have shown a predominance of female dogs. Of the dogs affected at less than 1 year of age, males are more common.

Clinical Signs

Table 2 summarizes the historical and physical examination abnormalities in dogs with IMHA. The clinical signs associated with IMHA are a reflection of the inflammatory reaction and the resultant anemia. The onset of IMHA can be acute or insidious. Lethargy, depression, and anorexia are the most common signs. Vomiting and diarrhea are reported occasionally. Sudden collapse or syncope are less common signs. The owner may note discolored urine. Most often, discoloration is due to bilirubin content, but occasionally port wine–colored urine is seen, consistent with the intravascular form of the disease. A few dogs may have signs of respiratory distress prior to presentation. Klag and associates (1993) noted a seasonal incidence of disease. The most frequent diagnoses of IMHA occurred in the spring and summer months, with 40% of the patients being presented in the months of May and June. An additional study found that 26% of dogs had received vaccinations within the month prior to the diagnosis of IMHA, suggesting a possible relationship with vaccination and the development of IMHA (Duval and Giger, 1996).

The findings on physical examination include pallor, icterus, depression, and weakness. Tachycardia is present in approximately one third of the dogs. Occasionally, cardiac murmurs are noted secondary to severe anemia or underlying heart disease. Hepatosplenomegaly can often be noted on abdominal palpation. The hair in the perineal area or around the penis may be discolored by the bilirubin or hemoglobin in the urine. Petechial hemorrhages may be noted in mucous membranes and in the skin in those animals that have a concurrent thrombocytopenia or vasculitis. Fever and lymphadenopathy are sometimes present.

Laboratory Results

The typical results of laboratory evaluation are listed in Table 3. Complete blood counts consistently reveal anemia, which can be moderate to severe. Packed cell volumes (PCVs) can be as low as 6%. As many as 50% of the

TABLE 2. Common Clinical Signs in 42 Dogs With IMHA

Clinical Sign	Percentage Affected
Anorexia	90
Lethargy	86
Pallor	76
Weakness	67
Icterus	50
Tachycardia	33
Hepatosplenomegaly	25

Adapted from Klag AR, Giger U, Shofer FS: Idiopathic immune-mediated hemolytic anemia in dogs: 42 cases (1986–1990). J Am Vet Med Assoc 202:783, 1993, with permission.

TABLE 3. Laboratory Findings in 17 Dogs With IMHA

Laboratory Parameter	Mean (SD)	Range
Packed cell volume (%)	15.7 (6.3)	6–35
MCV (fl)	78.4 (11.9)	60–129
Reticulocyte count ($\times 10^3/\mu$l)	173.7 (188.6)	0–1,102.5
WBC ($\times 10^3/\mu$l)	31.0 (21.1)	5.4–109.5
Platelet count ($\times 10^3/\mu$l)	185 (170)	1–922
Bilirubin (mg/dl)	7.2 (13.2)	0.01–63.6
BUN (mg/dl)	31.5 (23.4)	8–85
Creatinine (mg/dl)	0.78 (0.36)	0.3–1.6
Glucose (mg/dl)	94.5 (26.2)	37–128
Calcium (mg/dl)	9.0 (0.6)	8.1–10.4
Phosphorus (mg/dl)	5.0 (1.6)	3.2–9
ALP (IU/L)	792.2 (1,344.2)	21–5,570
ALT (IU/L)	132.2 (251.8)	20–1,072
Albumin (gm/dl)	3.03 (0.48)	2.3–3.8
Globulin (gm/dl)	2.99 (0.86)	2.1–6
TcO$_2$ (mEq/L)	14.7 (4.1)	7.2–21.8

ALP, alkaline phosphatase; ALT, alanine transaminase; BUN, blood urea nitrogen; MCV, mean cell volume; TcO$_2$, total carbon dioxide; WBC, white blood cells.

dogs with IMHA have nonregenerative anemia based on reticulocyte index. Erythrocyte morphology is important in the diagnosis of IMHA. Spherocytosis is a common but nonspecific finding in dogs with IMHA. Spherocytes are small, dense erythrocytes with decreased deformability formed when macrophages remove a portion of the erythrocyte membrane that is coated with antibody and/or complement. Spherocytosis implies an underlying immune mechanism but does not indicate whether the etiology is primary or secondary. Spherocytosis may also be hereditary in certain breeds of dogs (see p. 414). Polychromasia, anisocytosis, and nucleated red blood cells are present on blood smears from dogs with an appropriate regenerative response. In addition, macrocytosis is common in dogs with strongly regenerative anemias. Microscopic autoagglutination is noted in blood smears from some dogs with IMHA. The erythrocytes clump, owing to antibody coating, and appear as clusters of grapes.

The total leukocyte count can range from low to extremely high. Leukopenia may result from antibody-mediated neutropenia, sepsis, or decreased bone marrow production. Very high counts (up to 100,000/μl) have been attributed to the inflammatory reaction, cytokines that act as colony-stimulating factors for various cell lines, and general activation of the bone marrow secondary to anemia.

Thrombocytopenia is a concurrent finding in approximately 70% of dogs with IMHA. Thrombocytopenia can be a result of immune-mediated destruction of platelets or consumptive processes, such as sepsis or disseminated intravascular coagulation (DIC; see the following articles).

Autoagglutination is considered the hallmark of class I IMHA and negates the need for direct Coombs' testing. In a retrospective study of 105 cases of canine IMHA by the author, 70 of the 73 dogs tested had blood samples that were positive for autoagglutination. Erythrocytes coated with high titers of warm antibody and complement can spontaneously agglutinate. To ensure that the agglutination is real autoagglutination, and not the result of rouleaux formation, one drop of EDTA (ethylenediaminetetraacetic acid)-anticoagulated blood is placed with one to two drops of saline on a glass microscope slide. The slide is gently rocked to mix the blood and saline, and if agglutination is still present a presumptive diagnosis of IMHA can be made. This test gives information similar to that produced by the Coombs' test and is not specific for IMHA (see later).

There are no consistent serum biochemical abnormalities that aid in the diagnosis of IMHA. Serum biochemical parameters often reflect hemolysis, dehydration, and hypoxic damage to organs. More than two thirds of dogs with IMHA exhibit hyperbilirubinemia. Variable concentrations of conjugated and unconjugated bilirubin are found. Prerenal azotemia can be noted in patients that are severely affected. Azotemia secondary to acute renal failure is rare but can result from renal ischemia, DIC, sepsis, and hemoglobin (pigment) nephropathy. Mild to moderate elevations in serum hepatic transaminases have been attributed to hepatocyte hypoxia. Serum alkaline phosphatase may be increased because of cholestasis from mononuclear phagocyte system hyperplasia or extramedullary hematopoiesis within the liver. Low total carbon dioxide (TcO$_2$) or serum bicarbonate concentration may reflect probable lactic acidosis associated with decreased tissue oxygen delivery. Hyperglobulinemia is occasionally noted and may be indicative of the inflammatory response.

Bilirubinuria is the most common finding on urinalysis. In dogs with intravascular hemolysis, hemoglobinuria is evident as a dark red color, which persists following centrifugation. Additional abnormalities may include proteinuria, hematuria, and cylinduria. Bacteriuria and pyuria are indicative of concurrent urinary tract infection. Any signs of urinary tract infection warrant further work-up, as bacterial endocarditis can result in urinary tract infection and a secondary IMHA. The urine is usually concentrated if the dog is dehydrated; however, the urine specific gravity can be isosthenuric if acute or chronic renal failure is present.

Direct Coombs' Test

The direct Coombs' test detects the presence of antibodies and/or complement on the erythrocyte surface. The test should be run at 37°C and 4°C to detect both warm- and cold-reacting antibodies. The Coombs' reagents are *species-specific* antisera against canine IgG and IgM and the C3 component of complement. Ideally, the test should use separate antisera; however, some laboratories utilize a combined antisera, which produces a positive test result if any one of the three immune factors (IgG, IgM, or C3) are present on the erythrocyte surface. Most dogs with IMHA have IgG or IgG and C3 on the surface of their red blood cells. Intravascular IMHA may be expected to be IgM mediated because of the efficiency with which IgM fixes complement. Dogs with positive direct Coombs' test results based on C3 alone are more likely to have diseases other than primary IMHA (Slappendale, 1979).

The Coombs' test result is positive in 35 to 60% of dogs with IMHA. False-negative results occur as a consequence of prior therapy, the use of weak antisera, the use of antisera that is too strong (prozone effect), remission of disease, and the presence of low amounts of erythrocyte autoantibody, below the threshold of detection. False-positive test results can be produced by concurrent disease states such as neoplasia, haemobartonellosis, babesiosis, bacterial infections; administration of certain drugs; previous transfusion; improper antisera preparation; and nonspecific adsorption of serum proteins on damaged red blood cells. It is important to interpret the test results in light of the individual patient and realize that a positive test result is consistent with, but not diagnostic for, IMHA.

Additional Diagnostic Tests

Arterial blood gas analysis is important in the dyspneic dog. Profound hypoxemia with normocapnia and normal acid-base balance is consistent with pulmonary thromboembolism (see *CVT XII*, p. 891). The calculated alveolar arterial oxygen gradient is markedly increased in these dogs.

Coagulation parameters can be abnormal in dogs with IMHA. Elevations in activated clotting time, one-stage prothrombin time, activated partial thromboplastin time, and fibrin degradation products may be indicative of DIC. Buccal mucosal bleeding times should be normal unless the dog is thrombocytopenic or has concurrent von Willebrand's disease. Antithrombin III levels can be decreased in cases with DIC.

Bone marrow examination may be useful, especially in cases in which the regenerative response is poor. Evaluation of bone marrow aspirates from the majority of dogs with IMHA shows erythroid or generalized marrow hyperplasia. Erythrophagocytosis is occasionally seen and may be indicative of immune-mediated red cell destruction within the bone marrow. Erythrocyte hypoplasia or erythroid maturation arrest can also be seen. In a study of nonregenerative IMHA by Jonas and colleagues (1987), the bone marrow was examined in six dogs. Maturation arrest occurred at the metarubricyte to prorubricyte stages of erythrocyte development in five of the six dogs. The authors postulated that the stage of arrest is probably determined by the target erythrocyte autoantigen. Common antigen expression on mature red blood cells and red blood cell precursors defines which cells are destroyed. In addition, the authors proposed that serum factors present in dogs with IMHA may have inhibitory effects on erythropoiesis.

Radiographs of the thorax and abdomen are warranted in some animals with IMHA. Thoracic radiographs aid in ruling out underlying diseases such as neoplasia and infection that may be associated with secondary IMHA. Routine radiography may also detect evidence of pulmonary thromboembolism in dyspneic or hypoxemic dogs. A pronounced interstitial pattern is most commonly noted; however, a patchy alveolar pattern and pleural effusion can also be seen (Klein et al, 1989). Hepatosplenomegaly can be detected by abdominal radiography. In addition, evidence of abdominal neoplasia, gastric foreign bodies, or other intraabdominal abnormalities may be detectable by radiography or ultrasonography.

Pulmonary perfusion can be assessed with nuclear scintigraphy in dogs with IMHA and suspected pulmonary thromboembolism. This modality is the most accurate, though generally unavailable, method of detecting thromboembolism. Irregular distribution of radiolabeled macro-aggregated albumin is consistent with vascular obstruction by thromboemboli.

DIAGNOSIS OF IMMUNE-MEDIATED HEMOLYTIC ANEMIA IN CATS

As mentioned previously, primary IMHA is extremely rare in cats. The high incidence of concurrent disease, especially feline leukemia virus infection and *Haemobartonella felis* infection, should prompt the clinician to search for an underlying cause. When true IMHA occurs in cats, the age at onset and clinical signs are expected to be similar to those in dogs. Most affected cats are castrated males. Hemogram abnormalities are variable in cats with IMHA, showing regenerative or, less commonly, nonregenerative anemia. Reticulocytosis, if present, is mild to moderate. Spherocytes are rarely detected because of the difficulty in distinguishing these cells from the normally small feline erythrocytes. The white blood cell count is usually within normal limits. Thrombocytopenia may be noted in some cats. Autoagglutination of erythrocytes can occur, but it is not diagnostic for IMHA in cats. In the author's experience, most cats with autoagglutination test positive for feline leukemia virus infection in the peripheral blood or bone marrow. A Coombs' test that uses feline reagents can aid in the diagnosis of IMHA in cats; however, as in dogs, results must be interpreted with caution. False-positive results can occur with feline leukemia virus infection, *H. felis* infection, feline infectious peritonitis virus infection, myeloproliferative diseases, other neoplastic diseases, and chronic bacterial infections. As many as 40% of normal cats in one study had weakly positive Coombs' test results (Dunn et al, 1984). Very little is known about primary IMHA in cats, its definitive diagnosis, treatment, and prognosis, because of the paucity of reports.

THERAPY FOR IMMUNE-MEDIATED HEMOLYTIC ANEMIA

The therapy for dogs with IMHA is both supportive and specific for the disease. Supportive care is necessary for patients with severe IMHA, such as the intravascular or autoagglutinating forms of the disease. There have been no controlled clinical studies supporting the use of specific therapeutic regimens. Therefore, the treatment approach varies with the clinician (see *CVT XII*, p. 152).

Supportive Care

Supportive care primarily involves maintenance of hydration, acid-base balance, and organ perfusion. In addition, diuresis is indicated in patients with intravascular hemolysis to prevent hemoglobin nephrosis. Although the role of free hemoglobin as a nephrotoxin is controversial, a significant portion of dogs with intravascular IMHA in the author's experience have clinical laboratory data suggestive of acute renal failure and have necropsy evidence of hemoglobin (pigment) nephrosis. Subcutaneous fluid administration may be adequate; however, this route is contraindicated in dogs that are severely thrombocytopenic, owing to the risk of subcutaneous hemorrhage. Intravenous catheter placement in a peripheral vein is recommended but has been identified as a risk factor for the development of pulmonary thromboembolism. Jugular vein catheterization may not be advisable because of potential coagulopathies, both hemorrhagic and hypercoagulable states.

Attention to aseptic technique and the use of latex gloves when one handles dogs with IMHA is extremely important. Immunosuppressive therapy increases the risk of sepsis in these patients. Although prophylactic antibiotic therapy is not necessary, routine monitoring for sepsis is mandatory. A dog that is being treated with immunosuppressive doses of glucocorticoids may not be able to generate a fever, so body temperature is not an accurate means of identifying sepsis.

Dogs should be walked outside to urinate several times daily, if possible, to minimize urine retention and the potential for urinary tract infections. Cages should be well padded to aid in the prevention of decubital ulcers.

Specific treatment may be indicated in patients with vomiting related to IMHA or to the immunosuppressive therapy. Gastrointestinal ulceration may be prevented by the early use of histamine H_2 blockers or prostaglandin analogues (see *CVT XII,* p. 706). Antiemetics, such as metoclopramide, may be necessary for controlling vomiting (see *CVT XII,* p. 679).

Blood Transfusion

Unique risks are associated with transfusions in dogs with IMHA. Although blood transfusion should never be contraindicated, sometimes the risks of transfusion outweigh the benefits. The presence of autoantibodies in the patient shortens the survival of the transfused erythrocytes, reducing the benefit of the transfusion. Rarely, transfusion may actually worsen hemolysis and result in clinical deterioration of the patient. Transfusion may suppress the erythropoietic response of the patient, prolonging the time to erythroid recovery. Transfusions have been suspected of increasing the risk of pulmonary thromboembolism in dogs with IMHA (Klein et al, 1989). This risk is significant in that many dogs with IMHA that develop pulmonary thromboembolism will die.

Pretransfusion testing, that is, crossmatching, is difficult to interpret because of the presence of autoagglutination. As a general rule, an autocontrol (patient's plasma with patient's washed red blood cells) should be run along with the major and minor crossmatch (see p. 396). If the crossmatches agglutinate more than the autocontrol, the patient and donor have incompatible blood types. When autoagglutination is present at the same degree in all three samples, the test is uninterpretable.

Individual patient selection is important; there is no exact PCV that indicates transfusion. The patient's need for transfusion is determined by clinical evaluation of laboratory parameters and the clinical signs associated with the anemia. Frequent assessment of the PCV is important in determining the trend (up or down) and the rate of the change. Patients undergoing severe, rapid hemolysis should be monitored more frequently. If the PCV is stable, transfusion may not be warranted. Clinical parameters including patient attitude, exercise tolerance, respiratory rate, and heart rate may indicate the need for a transfusion. In general, if the dog is stable and comfortable at rest, transfusion is not necessary. However, transfusion may be indicated in cases of severe weakness or obtundation, respiratory distress due to anemia, and cardiac arrhythmias.

If blood transfusion is indicated, the clinical status of the dog must be taken into consideration in choosing the best blood product for the animal. In general, if the patient has not been typed, blood from DEA 1.1– and 1.2–negative donors should be used (see p. 400). If red blood cells are the only component needed by the patient, fresh packed red blood cells may be given to reduce the risk of transfusion reactions to plasma proteins present in whole blood. The recipient will gain the most benefit from a fresh unit. Storing blood products results in aging of erythrocytes, which are removed from the circulation by the recipient's mononuclear phagocyte system and, therefore, are unavailable to the patient. If the dog has a coagulopathy such as DIC in conjunction with anemia, fresh whole blood or packed red blood cells and fresh-frozen plasma may be needed. Administration of blood products should be initiated cautiously (0.5 to 1.0 ml/kg per hour for the first 30 minutes), and the patient monitored closely for signs of transfusion reactions. If no reactions are noted, the rate can be increased so that the full unit is completely administered within the next 4 hours. Blood can be administered at a rate of 20 to 80 ml/kg per hour in life-threatening situations. If the patient has reduced cardiovascular function, transfusion rates should not exceed 4 ml/kg per hour. Recently approved hemoglobin solutions may also be considered in patients requiring increased oxygen delivery to tissues (see prior article).

Immunosuppressive Therapy

Glucocorticoids

Glucocorticoids are the mainstay of therapy in the majority of dogs with IMHA and may be the sole drug used in the treatment of this disease. The major therapeutic effect of glucocorticoids in IMHA is to decrease Fc receptor–mediated erythrocyte destruction within the mononuclear phagocyte system. Glucocorticoids also inhibit complement activation and reduce circulating levels of cytokines, thereby diminishing the amplification of the immune response. Although there is much debate over which glucocorticoid to use, no controlled clinical trials support the use of one over another. Some authors suggest the use of dexamethasone initially, especially in dogs with severe anemia; however, one retrospective study of 105 dogs treated at Colorado State University failed to document any obvious benefit. Prednisone or prednisolone acetate is recommended at immunosuppressive doses of 1 to 2 mg/kg twice daily orally or by injection, respectively. This dose is maintained until the patient shows clinical improvement (rising PCV) for at least 5 to 7 days. At this point, the dosage can be reduced by 25 to 50% every 4 weeks if the complete blood count supports the view that remission is maintained. If at any time there is any indication of relapse such as return of autoagglutination or a reduction in PCV, the dose of prednisone is increased to the next higher dose and future dose tapering is slowed. In severe relapses, initial immunosuppressive doses may need to be reinstituted. When the dose of prednisone is reduced to 0.5 mg/kg per day, alternate-day therapy may be initiated at the next monthly recheck evaluation if remission has been maintained. Although no clinical trials have been completed to assess the need for lifelong therapy, relapse of IMHA does occur. Recurrences of IMHA may be more difficult to control in some patients.

Cytotoxic Drugs

In severe cases of IMHA (intravascular or autoagglutinating) or in cases unresponsive to glucocorticoids alone, the addition of cytotoxic drugs may be necessary. Cyclophosphamide and azathioprine have been used individually or together in these situations. Although the mechanisms of action of the two drugs are different, the end result is suppression of T cell–dependent B-cell responses, reducing the number of lymphocytes available for immune reactions and decreasing the amount of autoantibody produced. Cyclophosphamide also suppresses neutrophil and macrophage function. Studies in laboratory animals and in vitro data suggest a lag between the onset of administration of these drugs and their effect. Furthermore, the time to onset of action is unknown in dogs. It has been shown that cyclophosphamide is more effective against the humoral immune response, particularly IgM-mediated disease, and azathioprine is more effective against cell-mediated disease. The role of autoantibody in the pathogenesis of IMHA and the role of IgM in the intravascular form of the disease support the use of cyclophosphamide in the treatment of IMHA. However, a recent retrospective study failed to show a benefit of combination cyclophosphamide-prednisone therapy when compared to simple prednisone therapy in the treatment of extravascular IMHA (Mason et al, 1997).

Cyclophosphamide (Cytoxan, Bristol-Myers Squibb) is dosed at 50 mg/m² for 4 consecutive days of each week of therapy. It should be given in the morning, and the dog should be given several opportunities to urinate before bedtime to help prevent hemorrhagic cystitis. The diuresis induced by prednisone is probably somewhat protective and also reduces the concentration of toxic metabolites in the urine. Cyclophosphamide is continued at a consistent dose until the dose of prednisone is reduced to alternate-day administration. At this time, if a complete blood count indicates that the disease is still in remission, cyclophosphamide can be discontinued. The side effects of cyclophosphamide include gastrointestinal upset, bone marrow suppression, poor hair growth, and hemorrhagic cystitis.

The dose of azathioprine (Imuran, Glaxo Wellcome) is 2 mg/kg given daily or on alternate days. If azathioprine is used in place of cyclophosphamide, it can be discontinued in a similar manner. When the prednisone dose is reduced to alternate-day administration, azathioprine can be given on the days when prednisone is not given. If after 4 weeks remission is maintained, the azathioprine can be discontinued. In dogs that are sensitive to the side effects of glucocorticoids, azathioprine can be used on alternate days to maintain remission. The side effects of azathioprine include gastrointestinal upset, bone marrow suppression, poor hair growth, and pancreatitis.

Danazol

Danazol (Danocrine, Sanofi Winthrop Pharmaceuticals), an attenuated androgen used in the treatment of IMHA and immune-mediated thrombocytopenia in human patients, has been recommended in the therapy for IMHA in dogs. Danazol reduces autoantibody and complement binding to platelets and erythrocytes in people (Ahn et al, 1985). Dosages range from 5 mg/kg PO twice daily to 4 mg/kg PO three times a day. A double-blind clinical study of the use of danazol in dogs with IMHA was recently completed by the author. Eighteen dogs with extravascular IMHA were divided into two groups, a treatment (prednisone, azathioprine, and danazol) group or a control (prednisone, azathioprine, and placebo) group. There was no difference in survival between the two groups. Danazol did not offer any advantages over the standard therapy in this study; however, it may still have a role in the management of long-term remissions of IMHA.

Cyclosporin A

Cyclosporin A is a potent immunosuppressive drug directed at cell-mediated immune responses (see *CVT XII*, p. 73). Cyclosporin A blocks the expression of the interleukin-2 and interferon gamma genes within T lymphocytes, thereby blocking the amplification of the immune response at a crucial step in T-cell activation. This action results in suppression of cell-mediated immunity and a reduction in antibody production by T cell–dependent B-cell mechanisms. Cyclosporin A has been used effectively alone or in combination with other immunosuppressive therapies in dogs with IMHA with some success; however, several issues preclude its widespread use. The cost is relatively high compared with other immunosuppressive agents. Treatment of a 10-kg dog costs approximately $11 per day. Because of variability in gastrointestinal absorption, predictable blood levels are difficult to attain, necessitating the determination of serum drug concentrations for accurate dosing. This testing adds further to the cost of administration of the drug. The side effects can be severe. In dogs, the most common side effects include vomiting, diarrhea, and anorexia. For these reasons, the use of cyclosporin A is reserved for patients with severe disease that is unresponsive to other medications. In the author's experience, cyclosporin A in combination with cyclophosphamide and prednisone may have a role in the treatment of dogs with intravascular IMHA. Therapy with cyclosporin A (Sandimmune, Sandoz Pharmaceuticals) is initiated at a dose of 10 mg/kg PO every 12 to 24 hours. Ideally, therapeutic drug monitoring is recommended at 2- to 4-week intervals. A trough concentration of 100 to 300 ng/ml as measured by high-performance liquid chromatography is recommended (Vaden et al, 1995). Cyclosporin A can be discontinued when remission has been maintained for at least 2 weeks.

Intravenous Gamma Globulin

Intravenous gamma globulin (IVGG) administration has been used to treat several immune-mediated diseases in people, specifically IMHA, immune-mediated thrombocytopenia, and immune-mediated neutropenia. Recently, administration of IVGG to dogs with IMHA has been reported (Scott-Moncrieff et al, 1997). The mechanism by which IVGG suppresses the immune destruction of erythrocytes is thought to be due to blockade of macrophage Fc receptors and possibly anti-idiotypic down-regulation of autoantibody production. When given at a dose of 1.0 gm/kg IV over 6 to 12 hours, a profound reticulocytosis occurs followed by a more slowly rising PCV. Side effects are minimal; however, preliminary work suggests a high incidence of pulmonary thromboembolism in dogs with IMHA treated with this product. More investigation of IVGG in IMHA is warranted.

COMPLICATIONS OF IMMUNE-MEDIATED HEMOLYTIC ANEMIA IN DOGS

The complications of IMHA are severe and life-threatening. They include refractory anemia, hemorrhage, bacterial or fungal infections, acute renal failure, and pulmonary thromboembolism. It is difficult to glean from the literature the proportions of dogs that die from specific causes. In a retrospective study by the author at a referral institution, 40% of the dogs with IMHA responded to treatment and survived. Sixty percent died or were euthanatized, because of refractory anemia, relapse of anemia, or other complications of the disease or its treatment. The cause of death as determined by necropsy was available in 25 dogs. Three dogs with intravascular hemolysis had evidence of acute renal failure secondary to hemoglobin nephrosis. One dog died of sepsis. Pulmonary thromboembolism was found in 22 dogs.

Refractory anemia is common in dogs with IMHA. Failure of the dog to respond to immunosuppressive agents often leads to spontaneous death or to the owner's decision to euthanatize the pet. This frustrating sequela of IMHA often follows a great expense incurred by the owner, as many of these dogs are hospitalized for extended periods, receive multiple blood transfusions, and have multiple drugs prescribed. Clearly, continued investigation into new and effective therapeutic protocols is needed.

The complications of IMHA also include hemorrhage, which may result from the disease itself or its treatment. Gastrointestinal hemorrhage is commonly seen and can result from the combined effects of ischemia, thrombocytopenia, DIC, and drug-associated alterations in epithelial cell turnover and gastric acid and mucus production. Thrombocytopenia alone is rarely severe enough to lead to significant hemorrhage in the absence of other factors.

Therapy for IMHA is still crude and nonspecific. Unfortunately, immunosuppressive drugs inhibit not only aberrant immune responses but also immune responses necessary to protect the host from infection. Disseminated bacterial, fungal, and protozoal infections have contributed to the deaths of dogs with IMHA.

Pulmonary thromboembolism is a common cause of death in dogs with IMHA. In a study by Klein and associates (1989), 32% of 31 dogs with IMHA died of pulmonary thromboembolism, based on findings at necropsy. The authors postulated that hypercoagulability is most probably responsible for thrombus formation. Documentation of hypercoagulability is lacking, however. Potential causes of hypercoagulability may include an imbalance in procoagu-

lant and naturally occurring anticoagulant factors, DIC, endothelial cell–mediated coagulation triggered by anti-erythrocyte antibodies, and procoagulant factors released from damaged erythrocytes. Hyperbilirubinemia, hypoalbuminemia, intravenous catheter placement, and severe thrombocytopenia ($<50,000/\mu l$) have been identified as risk factors for the development of thromboembolism (Klein et al, 1989; Carr and Panciera, 1996). The clinical signs of acute dyspnea, orthopnea, and profound anorexia should prompt further evaluation. Sudden death without prior clinical signs also occurs. Clinical evaluation of arterial blood gases and thoracic radiographs was discussed earlier. Nuclear scintigraphy is the definitive diagnostic procedure. Therapy with heparin and streptokinase often fails to alter the progression of thromboembolic disease. Prophylactic therapy has been recommended in dogs with IMHA; however, to date, no effective protocols have been published. In the author's experience, heparin at dosages of 50 to 75 U/kg SC three times daily has not consistently prevented the development of thromboembolism. The addition of aspirin at a dose of 1 to 5 mg/kg once daily may be of benefit. Until the underlying mechanisms promoting thrombus formation are identified, it is unlikely that an effective therapeutic protocol will be developed.

References and Suggested Reading

Ahn YS, Harrington WJ, Mylvaganam R, et al: Danazol therapy for autoimmune hemolytic anemia. Ann Intern Med 102:298, 1985.
   A retrospective study of the use of danazol in humans with IMHA.
Barker RN, Gruffydd-Jones TJ, Stokes CR, et al: Identification of autoantigens in canine autoimmune haemolytic anaemia. Clin Exp Immunol 85:33, 1991.
   Describes methods of determining canine erythrocyte autoantigens important in the pathophysiology of IMHA.
Carr AP, Panciera DL: Immune-mediated hemolytic anemia in dogs: A retrospective study with emphasis on hemostatic parameters. Proceedings of the Fourteenth American College of Veterinary Internal Medicine Forum. Denver: ACVIM, 1996, p 754.
   A retrospective study of risk factors associated with IMHA in dogs.
Dunn JK, Searcy GP, Hirsch VM: The diagnostic significance of a positive direct antiglobulin test in anemic cats. Can J Comp Med 48:349, 1984.
   A retrospective study of the results of Coombs' tests in normal and anemic cats.
Duval D, Giger U: Vaccine-associated immune-mediated hemolytic anemia in the dog. Proceedings of the Fourteenth American College of Veterinary Internal Medicine Forum. Denver: ACVIM, 1996, p 754.
   A retrospective study correlating the onset of IMHA with recent vaccination.
Jonas LD, Thrall MA, Weiser MG: Nonregenerative form of immune-mediated hemolytic anemia in dogs. J Am Anim Hosp Assoc 23:201, 1987.
   A retrospective study of bone marrow evaluation in dogs with nonregenerative IMHA.
Klag AR, Giger U, Shofer FS: Idiopathic immune-mediated hemolytic anemia in dogs: 42 cases (1986–1990). J Am Vet Med Assoc 202:783, 1993.
   A retrospective study of 42 cases of IMHA in dogs.
Klein MK, Dow SW, Rosychuk RAW: Pulmonary thromboembolism associated with immune-mediated hemolytic anemia in dogs: Ten cases (1982–1987). J Am Vet Med Assoc 195:246, 1989.
   A retrospective study of dogs with IMHA and pulmonary thromboembolism, with particular emphasis on risk factors.
Mason NJ, Duval D, Giger U: Evaluation of combined cyclophosphamide and prednisone versus prednisone alone in the treatment of canine immune-mediated hemolytic anemia. Proceedings of the Fifteenth American College of Veterinary Internal Medicine Forum. Denver: ACVIM, 1997, p 677.

Scott-Moncrieff JC, Reagan WJ, Snyder PW, et al: Treatment of canine immune-mediated hemolytic anemia with human intravenous immunoglobulin. J Am Vet Med Assoc 210:1623, 1997.
A study of the use of human gamma globulin for the treatment of IMHA in dogs.
Slappendale RJ: The diagnostic significance of the direct antiglobulin test (DAT) in anemic dogs. Vet Immunol Immunopathol 1:49, 1979.

A retrospective study of the results of Coombs' tests in dogs with anemia due to a variety of causes.
Vaden SL, Breitschwerdt EB, Armstrong PJ, et al: Effects of cyclosporine versus standard care in naturally occurring glomerulonephritis in dogs. J Vet Intern Med 9:259, 1995.
A study of the use of cyclosporin A in the treatment of glomerulonephritis in dogs.

Von Willebrand's Disease and Other Hereditary Coagulopathies

ANTHONY P. CARR
Blue Mounds, Wisconsin

DAVID L. PANCIERA
Denver, Colorado

A large number of inherited bleeding disorders have been identified in dogs. For some of the most common disorders, inheritance patterns are known, whereas for others heredity remains obscure. This information must be obtained before appropriate breeding recommendations can be made to reduce the frequency of disease.

VON WILLEBRAND'S DISEASE

Von Willebrand's disease (vWD) is the most common inherited bleeding disorder in dogs. It is caused by a lack of von Willebrand factor (vWF). Von Willebrand factor is an adhesive glycoprotein that is produced by endothelial cells and megakaryocytes. Unlike platelets in other species, canine platelets do not contain large amounts of vWF in their alpha granules. Extracellular vWF is found in the subendothelium and circulating in plasma in multimeric form. The multimers vary in size from 0.5 to 20 million D (daltons), with the larger multimers being more hemostatically active. The multimers are composed of identical 270,000 D subunits joined by disulfide bonds.

The predominant function of vWF is to promote the adhesion of platelets to exposed subendothelium, especially in areas of high shear stress. The vWF can come from the plasma, endothelial cells, or the subendothelium. Von Willebrand factor also plays a role in platelet-to-platelet aggregation in conjunction with platelet receptor and fibrinogen. When platelets become activated, they express a receptor that can bind several adhesion molecules, including vWF. This binding then allows other platelets to bind to the vWF molecule, forming an aggregate. The other major function of vWF is to form a tightly bound complex with factor VIII, thereby prolonging the half-life of factor VIII.

Three basic forms of vWD are found in dogs. In type I vWD, all multimers are present, but in considerably reduced quantity. This form of vWD is most common. It has been identified in more than 50 breeds of dogs. Breeds

associated with type I vWD and a hemorrhagic tendency include Doberman pinscher, Standard Poodle, Shetland sheepdog, and German shepherd dogs. The hemorrhagic tendency, while variable, often manifests as increased bleeding associated with surgical procedures or after trauma. Spontaneous mucosal bleeding (epistaxis, urogenital bleeding) can occasionally be seen. Other stressors that suppress hemostasis can precipitate bleeding, such as the transient thrombocytopenia noted to occur after vaccination with a modified live vaccine or the administration of nonsteroidal anti-inflammatory agents that inhibit platelet activity. In severely affected animals, spontaneous hemorrhage can be protracted. In some breeds, decreased vWF has been documented, but a bleeding tendency does not seem to exist. Type I vWD probably represents a heterogeneous group of diseases with marked breed variation. In type II vWD the larger, more effective multimers are absent and bleeding can be severe. This form of the disease has been identified in German shorthaired and German wirehaired pointers. The most severe form of vWD is type III in which all multimers are absent. This form of the disease is associated with life-threatening hemorrhagic episodes. It has been reported to occur in Scottish terriers, Chesapeake Bay retrievers, and Shetland sheepdogs.

The manner of inheritance of vWD is largely unknown. An autosomal mode of inheritance must be present, as males and females are equally affected. An autosomal dominant mode of inheritance with incomplete penetrance has been suggested (Brooks, 1992). It has been proposed that in Doberman pinschers the disease may be produced by a single gene defect (Moser et al, 1996b), with each allele being responsible for 50% of the vWF level the dog has. A defective allele would result in less than 15% of normal vWF production. Type II vWD in German wirehaired pointers probably is inherited as an autosomal recessive trait (Brooks et al, 1996). Variation and overlap in vWF levels exist; thus, it is sometimes difficult to definitively establish genotype on the basis of a single vWF measurement alone. Just as disease expression is heterogeneous, it is likely that the genetic basis of the disease varies.

Diagnostic Testing

At present, diagnosis of vWD is predominantly through determination of vWF levels. Progress is being made toward identifying the underlying genetic abnormalities associated with vWD. DNA analysis is now available for certain breeds of dogs (VetGen, Ann Arbor, MI). The validity of the assay has not yet been published. When vWF is analyzed, the patient's vWF is reported as a percentage of a control canine pool. The pool is considered to represent 100%, often expressed as 100 U (units). Blood for analysis should be anticoagulated with 3.2% citrate at a 9:1 ratio of blood to anticoagulant or with 15% EDTA (ethylenediaminetetraacetic acid) at a ratio of 1:100. Hemolyzed samples are not to be used, as hemolysis causes a significant decrease in vWF levels (Moser et al, 1996a). The blood is centrifuged immediately and is then frozen for storage prior to analysis. The sample should be shipped frozen on dry ice to prevent thawing. In the process of thawing, some proteolysis may occur. This breakdown of protein would tend to artificially elevate vWF when an antigenic assay is used because breaking up large multimers into smaller subunits exposes more antigenic sites (Stokol and Parry, 1995).

Testing of vWF is usually by means of either an electroimmunoassay or an ELISA with the concentration expressed as vWF:Ag (antigen). Using an enzyme-linked immunosorbent assay (ELISA), workers at the Comparative Hematology Laboratory of Cornell University established the following ranges: normal range, 70 to 180% vWF:Ag; borderline range, 50 to 69% vWF:Ag; abnormal range, 0 to 49% vWF:Ag (Brooks, 1992). These assays do not determine biologic activity or multimeric distribution. When this system is used, dogs in the normal range are considered free from vWD and are unlikely to transmit the disease. Dogs in the abnormal range are diagnosed as carriers of vWD and can transmit the trait to offspring. Dogs in the borderline range cannot be classified definitively. Daily variation in vWF:Ag concentration can be high, so multiple measurements may be necessary to establish the von Willebrand status of a dog.

Multimeric distribution can be determined with the use of electrophoresis, although it usually is only available as a research tool. This modality is of value in that the larger multimers are thought to be more hemostatically active. It is also possible to measure the ability of certain substances to form platelet aggregates, which, in some circumstances, is dependent on the presence of vWF. Botrocetin (a snake venom) cofactor analysis (BCf) assesses the ability of vWF to induce platelet agglutination, with the larger multimers having greater activity. Usually the value derived from BCf closely parallels vWF:Ag values. An exception is in type II vWD, in which BCf is lower than expected compared with vWF:Ag, possibly because the more active larger multimers are deficient in these dogs. A platelet-agglutination kit based on BCf has been marketed, but its clinical use is limited because of methodologic difficulties (Johnson et al, 1988).

Bleeding times can be measured in patients to determine whether a defect of primary hemostasis is present. Both the cuticle bleeding time (CBT; duration of hemorrhage from a toenail that is cut short enough to bleed) and the buccal mucosal bleeding time (BMBT; see p. 442) are prolonged in vWD. The BMBT is the preferred test, as the CBT is also prolonged in coagulopathies such as hemophilia A and B. The BMBT is measured by determining the duration of hemorrhage from small standardized cuts in the upper lip (Johnson et al, 1988). The clinician folds back the patient's upper lip using gauze tied around the maxilla. This maneuver exposes the inner surface of the upper lip and causes mild vascular engorgement. A disposable, spring-loaded device (Simplate II, American Diagnostics) is used to make two small standardized incisions in the mucosa. Visible blood vessels are avoided when one chooses the site to incise. As blood is shed, it is blotted with filter paper at 5-second intervals below the incisions to prevent formation of a fibrin coagulum over the wound. This blotting should not disturb the wounds, otherwise the forming platelet plug will be disrupted. The end point for the test is cessation of hemorrhage from the incisions. The values obtained from the two incisions can be averaged. Normal dogs have a BMBT of less than 4 minutes. When one evaluates BMBT results, it is important to remember that BMBT is a global test of primary hemostasis. Not only vWD, but also thrombocytopenia, platelet function defects, and vasculitis result in a prolonged BMBT.

Physiologic Factors Affecting vWF:Ag

A variety of factors are known to affect measured vWF:Ag levels. Within individuals, levels can vary substantially over time, making classification into affected, carrier, or disease-free categories very difficult if based on a single sample (Moser et al, 1996a). When blood is drawn from a cephalic vein, vWF:Ag levels are greater than when it is drawn from a jugular vein (Moser et al, 1996a). Strenuous exercise, epinephrine, and pregnancy raise vWF levels (Moser et al, 1996a). The effect of thyroid status has been debated; however, recent studies show no association between hypothyroidism and acquired vWD (Panciera and Johnson, 1996).

Therapy

The mode of therapy employed to treat vWD is dependent on the presenting situation. Many times, the clinician needs to plan for protracted hemorrhage during a surgical procedure in a patient with vWD. Less often, a patient is presented with spontaneous hemorrhage that is difficult to control. Blood products are the undisputed form of therapy in either scenario. If anemia is not severe, the use of fresh plasma, fresh-frozen plasma, or cryoprecipitate (CP) is recommended. Cryoprecipitate is especially valuable, since the clinician can give larger quantities of vWF without having to be concerned about volume overload, as can occur with plasma products. Administration of CP significantly increases vWF levels within 30 minutes of administration in Doberman pinschers with type I vWD, an effect that remained apparent for at least 4 hours (Ching et al,

1994). The BMBT was similarly rapidly improved, but by 4 hours it was at the same level as before treatment. In animals given fresh plasma, the vWF level increased in a manner similar to that of patients given CP, but no improvement in BMBT occurred. The significance of this observation is unclear, as fresh plasma is effective in the treatment of vWD, based on clinical experience.

DDAVP (desmopressin acetate) can also be useful in the treatment of vWD, especially in situations in which therapy is initiated to prevent or control hemorrhage in association with surgery. DDAVP is used extensively in humans with vWD and appears to have a variety of effects that promote hemostasis, including the release of stored vWF from endothelial cells. In humans, a significant increase in vWF occurs in most patients with vWD. In dogs, this rise is much less pronounced, especially in those with vWD. Despite the insignificant increase in vWF in dogs with type I vWD given DDAVP, the BMBT decreases (Kraus et al, 1989). This decrease appears to be the result of a preferential increase in the larger, more hemostatically active multimers that occur after DDAVP administration. The onset of activity occurs in 30 minutes, and the duration of effect is approximately 2 hours. DDAVP releases stored vWF; thus, repeating the DDAVP injection has significantly less effect than the initial treatment. If DDAVP is used prior to surgery, the authors recommend rechecking the BMBT 20 to 30 minutes prior to the procedure to ensure that the drug has been effective. In the case of a nonemergency surgery, the authors have routinely administered DDAVP 1 to 2 days before the procedure and performed a BMBT. If the animal fails to respond, other means of treatment should be available at the time of surgery. DDAVP can be given to donor dogs to maximize vWF levels prior to phlebotomy. Although an intravenous product is available, its cost has led to the successful use of an intranasal product given subcutaneously at 1 to 4 μg/kg.

HEMOPHILIA A

Hemophilia A is an X chromosome-linked recessive inherited disease caused by factor VIII deficiency. Generally, the female is the carrier, and only males express signs of the disease. However, a mating between a carrier female and an affected male would result in affected females. The disease has been diagnosed in most dog breeds and also in mixed-breed dogs. A higher prevalence is observed in German shepherd dogs. The clinical manifestations vary, depending on the degree of deficiency. As with most coagulopathies, body cavity hemorrhages (abdomen, thorax, and joints) and extensive bruising are the most common manifestations. In severely affected individuals, death at birth can result from umbilical cord hemorrhage. In others, the first clinical manifestation may be seen during teething. Since factor VIII is involved in the intrinsic coagulation pathway, prolongations of activated clotting time (ACT) and activated partial thromboplastin time (APTT) are seen. The diagnosis is verified by specific factor analysis. Factor VIII activity varies from 0 to 25% in affected animals. The results of a BMBT would be normal, whereas the CBT would be prolonged. A mild decrease in factor VIII activity can be seen in animals afflicted with vWD. This decrease occurs because factor VIII circulates bound to vWF, which

prolongs its half-life. Dogs with hemophilia A tend to have increased levels of vWF.

Therapy for hemophilia A consists of administration of blood products. If red blood cells are needed because of anemia, whole blood can be given. Fresh-frozen plasma or cryoprecipitate is preferred if anemia is not present. Therapy with anabolic steroids has been suggested to increase factor VIII activity in humans. Unfortunately, anabolic steroids also increase fibrinolysis, leading to more rapid clot lysis. As a result, human hemophiliacs treated with anabolic steroids tend to have increased factor VIII activity but need more transfusions, possibly because blood clot lysis is accelerated.

HEMOPHILIA B

Hemophilia B (Christmas disease) results from factor IX deficiency. The disease has an X chromosome–linked recessive mode of inheritance and has been identified in 15 breeds of dogs. Factor IX is a vitamin K–dependent protein produced in the liver. The clinical signs of hemophilia B mimic those encountered with hemophilia A. The clinical manifestations vary in severity from mild to fatal hemorrhages. Unlike dogs with hemophilia A, dogs with factor IX deficiency invariably have less than 1% of normal factor activity detected. Both ACT and APTT are prolonged in dogs with this disease because factor IX is a part of the intrinsic pathway of coagulation. The final diagnosis depends on specific factor analysis.

Therapy for factor IX deficiency consists of the administration of blood products. Fresh-frozen plasma or cryosupernatant are indicated when anemia is not marked. Factor IX is also found in serum, so it could also be given.

OTHER HEREDITARY COAGULOPATHIES

A variety of other coagulopathies have been identified in dogs (Fogh and Fogh, 1988). In some, the only clinical manifestation is an alteration of routine hemostatic tests without an associated bleeding tendency. Definitive diagnosis requires testing by reference laboratories involved in research on coagulation disorders in animals. Hypofibrinogenemia (factor I deficiency) has been identified in Saint Bernard dogs associated with a prolongation of one-step prothrombin time (OSPT; extrinsic pathway of coagulation) and marked bleeding diathesis in severely affected animals. An autosomal recessive factor II (prothrombin) deficiency has been identified in a family of Boxer dogs with prolongation of OSPT. Bleeding was severe in some pups, but was generally mild in adults. Factor VII deficiency has been identified as an autosomal dominant disease in Beagle dogs. Bleeding is rarely reported, although OSPT values are prolonged. In Cocker spaniels, factor X deficiency has been reported as an autosomal dominant trait with a variable expression of the hemorrhagic tendency. Both APTT and OSPT are prolonged in this disease. Severely affected animals generally do not survive. Factor XI deficiency has been seen in Kerry Blue terriers, Great Pyrenees, and English Springer spaniels as an autosomal recessive trait. The disease manifests as a prolongation of APTT and a variable bleeding tendency. Factor XII (Hageman factor)

deficiency has been identified in Miniature Poodles, but is much more commonly identified in cats. Deficiency of this factor causes a prolongation of APTT, but it is not associated with a bleeding tendency. Prekallikrein deficiency has been seen in a variety of breeds. It causes a prolongation of APTT, apparently without an associated tendency toward hemorrhage.

THERAPY WITH BLOOD PRODUCTS

Whole Blood

In cases in which anemia is a significant problem, fresh whole blood (less than 6 hours since collection) is the product of choice. Factor VIII, vWF, and factor V are inactive when blood has been stored, but the vitamin K–dependent factors (factor II, VII, IX, and X) retain their activity. Donors should be negative for canine red cell antigens DEA 1.1, 1.2, and 7 (see p. 396). The volume of transfusion depends on the severity of the anemia, but a general guide is 12 to 24 ml/kg, which would be expected to raise the packed cell volume (PCV) by 5 to 10%. The major drawback in treating a coagulopathy with blood is the volume overload that can occur, even though the quantity of coagulation factors given is small. Blood products containing red blood cells should be reserved for animals with significant anemia, as transfusion can lead to sensitization to red cell antigens. Such sensitization could preclude safe administration of red cells at a later date, when they may be vitally needed.

Fresh and Fresh-Frozen Plasma

Plasma harvested from whole blood within 6 hours of collection is termed fresh plasma. If this plasma is transfused within the 6-hour time frame, all vital coagulation protein activity is retained. Rapid separation from whole blood preserves the activity of factors V and VIII and vWF. Fresh plasma also contains albumin, complement proteins, antithrombin III, and immunoglobulins. Plasma frozen within 6 hours of the blood collection is termed *fresh-frozen plasma* and can be stored frozen (preferably at −70°C) and retain its coagulation activity for as long as 1 year. Usually, 6 to 10 ml/kg is transfused, and this amount can be administered every 8 hours as needed. Volume overload is a consideration with plasma administration, especially when an animal is severely affected with vWD and needs multiple transfusions.

Stored or Frozen Plasma

Stored plasma results when plasma is separated from red blood cells more than 6 hours after collection. When frozen, this plasma is termed *frozen plasma*. It is deficient in factors V and VIII and vWF activity but does have the other coagulation factors present (including factor IX). It is generally not used in the treatment of coagulopathies.

Cryoprecipitate

When fresh-frozen plasma is slowly thawed (at 4°C), a precipitate is formed, called cryoprecipitate (CP). Most of the factor VIII, fibrinogen, and vWF in the plasma is contained in the CP. It generally is only one tenth of the volume of the original plasma. The remainder of the plasma is called cryo-free plasma or cryosupernatant. Cryosupernatant still contains most of the other active coagulation factors and plasma proteins. Cryoprecipitate and cryo-free plasma can be frozen again and stored for as long as 1 year. The reported concentration of vWF in CP varies from approximately 4 times that in the original plasma (Stokol and Parry, 1995) to 20 times the original (Ching et al, 1994). The larger multimers appear to preferentially precipitate (Ching et al, 1994). Both a slow defrost (4°C) and a fast defrost (37°C) of frozen CP resulted in equal retention of factor VIII and vWF activity. Interestingly, a decrease in activity was not seen when the thawed CP was stored for 24 hours at room temperature (Stokol and Parry, 1995). This finding is in sharp contrast with human CP, for which as much as a 54% decrease has been reported. The therapeutic efficacy of CP stored at room temperature was not reported, and it is of some concern that CP might not be effective in vivo. The high level of vWF determined may have reflected proteolysis induced by the conditions to which the CP was subjected. Proteolysis fragments larger multimers into smaller fragments, causing increased detection when an antigen-based assay is used. Although they register on the in vitro assay, it is unknown how their in vivo effectiveness in controlling hemorrhage would compare. A dose of 1 U of cryoprecipitate (cryoprecipitate produced from 150 ml of plasma) per 10 kg body weight has been recommended. Cryoprecipitate can be obtained from commercial animal blood banks.

References and Suggested Reading

Brooks M: Management of canine von Willebrand's disease. Probl Vet Med 4:636, 1992.
  Good review of vWD, including basic science, genetics, and treatment options.
Brooks M, Raymond S, Catalfamo J: Severe, recessive von Willebrand's disease in German Wirehaired Pointers. J Am Vet Med Assoc 209:926, 1996.
  Case series characterizes autosomal recessive type II vWD in this breed.
Ching YN, Meyers KM, Brassard JA, et al: Effect of cryoprecipitate and plasma on plasma von Willebrand factor multimers and bleeding time in Doberman Pinschers with type-I von Willebrand's disease. Am J Vet Res 55:102, 1994.
  Study shows that plasma and cryoprecipitate increase vWF:Ag when given to dogs with vWD and that cryoprecipitate administration decreased BMBT.
Fogh JM, Fogh IT: Inherited coagulation disorders. Vet Clin North Am Small Anim Pract 18:231, 1988.
  Extensive listing of all coagulopathies identified in small animal species at the time the article appeared.
Johnson GS, Turrentine MA, Kraus KH: Canine von Willebrand's disease: A heterogeneous group of bleeding disorders. Vet Clin North Am Small Anim Pract 18:195, 1988.
  Good review with information on laboratory evaluation, basic science of vWF, and specific aspects of vWD in certain dog breeds.
Kraus KH, Turrentine MA, Jergens AE, et al: Effect of desmopressin acetate on bleeding times and plasma von Willebrand factor in Doberman Pinscher dogs with von Willebrand's disease. Vet Surg 18:103, 1989.
  Study of the effect of DDAVP on vWF:Ag, BCf, and BMBT in 12 Doberman pinschers.
Moser J, Meyers KM, Meinkoth JH, et al: Temporal variation and factors

affecting measurement of canine von Willebrand factor. Am J Vet Res 57:1288, 1996a.
Study looks at vWF:Ag as it varied over time in the same individual animal and how it was influenced by hemolysis, hyperlipidemia, blood collection site, anticoagulant, duration of vascular occlusion, centrifugation speed, storage time, and freeze-thawing.

Moser J, Meyers KM, Russon RH: Inheritance of von Willebrand factor deficiency in Doberman Pinschers. J Am Vet Med Assoc 209:1103, 1996b.
Prospective study of Doberman pinschers and mixed-breed dogs suggesting that a single gene defect is responsible for the inheritance of vWD in this breed.

Panciera DL, Johnson GS: Plasma von Willebrand factor antigen concentration and buccal mucosal bleeding time in dogs with experimental hypothyroidism. J Vet Intern Med 10:60, 1996.
Experimental study shows that induction of hypothyroidism does not lead to a defect in primary hemostasis or reductions in vWF:Ag.

Stokol T, Parry BW: Stability of von Willebrand factor and factor VIII in canine cryoprecipitate under various conditions of storage. Res Vet Sci 59:152, 1995.
Study looks at the concentration of vWF:Ag in cryoprecipitate and the effect of repeated freeze-thaw cycles, freezer temperature, and storage at room temperature on this concentration.

Infectious and Immune-Mediated Thrombocytopenia

CAROL B. GRINDEM
Raleigh, North Carolina

Thrombocytopenia is the most common platelet disorder observed in dogs and cats. The prevalence of thrombocytopenia (<200,000 platelets/μl) at North Carolina State University College of Veterinary Medicine is approximately 5% in dogs and 2% (unpublished update from 1990 to 1996) in cats (Grindem et al, 1991; Jordan et al, 1993). There, the etiologic classification of canine thrombocytopenia revealed 5% idiopathic immune mediated, 13% neoplasia, 23% infectious or inflammatory diseases, and 59% miscellaneous causes. Similarly, the etiologic classification of feline thrombocytopenia revealed 2% idiopathic immune mediated, 20% neoplasia, 29% infectious diseases, 7% cardiac diseases, 22% multiple etiologies, and 20% unknown causes.

The focus of this article is thrombocytopenia associated with inflammatory disorders, including infectious and idiopathic immune-mediated diseases. Primary immune-mediated thrombocytopenia, also called idiopathic thrombocytopenic purpura (ITP), is considered to be a secondary manifestation of unidentified causes. Therefore, infectious causes must be diligently searched for and ruled out before one makes the diagnosis of ITP.

MECHANISM OF THROMBOCYTOPENIA

Simply put, thrombocytopenia can be caused by decreased production and/or decreased availability of platelets due to increased utilization, destruction, or sequestration. Although the mechanisms of thrombocytopenia may be multifactorial and vary during the course of the disease, usually one mechanism predominates. Knowledge of this mechanism, especially in the setting of infectious diseases, facilitates patient management and selection of diagnostic tests. Decreased production occurs with suppression or destruction of megakaryocytes, myelophthisic diseases, and idiopathic or secondary immune-mediated disorders. De-

creased availability results from increased utilization (disseminated intravascular coagulation [DIC] or blood loss), increased destruction (immune-mediated mechanism, endotoxin, viruses), or increased sequestration (spleen, liver, and lungs). Platelet sequestration is usually transient.

Most of the immune-mediated thrombocytopenias in dogs and cats are secondary to infectious agents, neoplasia, transfusions, or drug therapy. Remember, ITP is uncommon and can be diagnosed only after other causes of thrombocytopenia have been eliminated (Lewis and Meyers, 1996).

CLINICAL EVALUATION OF THE THROMBOCYTOPENIC PATIENT

A thorough physical examination and complete medical history are necessary for immediate patient management, including appropriate selection of diagnostic tests and therapeutic regimens. Hemorrhage is inconsistently associated with thrombocytopenia. Most thrombocytopenic patients do not bleed overtly. Rather, they are presented for lethargy, weakness, fever, or clinical signs related to the underlying cause of the thrombocytopenia. The thrombocytopenia is often first identified on the routine complete blood cell count (CBC).

The most common physical examination finding specific for a thrombocytopenic coagulopathy is petechial or ecchymotic hemorrhages on the mucous membranes or skin. Other clinical signs may include epistaxes, hematuria, hematochezia, hematemesis, and melena. The probability of clinically evident bleeding increases as the platelet count decreases below 50,000/μl. Spontaneous hemorrhage rarely occurs until the platelet count is lower than 30,000/μl. The occurrence of bleeding also relates to the rapidity of the decrease in platelet number, vascular integrity, and the incidence of traumatic events.

Splenomegaly and hepatomegaly are features of platelet

sequestration (hypotension, shock, hypothermia, and endo-toxemia) or platelet phagocytosis (immune-mediated disorders). Classically, ITP occurs in middle-aged purebred female dogs. A high prevalence of ITP is reported in Cocker spaniels, German shepherds, Poodles, and Old English sheepdogs. However, ITP has been reported in dogs 8 months to 15 years of age, in male dogs and mixed-breeds (Lewis and Meyers, 1996).

Like anemia, thrombocytopenia is a laboratory abnormality—not a specific disease. The importance of a careful inquiry regarding drug ingestion, exposure to toxins, or previous illnesses cannot be overemphasized. Without this information, thrombocytopenia caused by drugs, toxins, or previous infections may be erroneously attributed to ITP.

DIAGNOSTIC APPROACH TO INFECTIOUS OR IMMUNE-MEDIATED THROMBOCYTOPENIA

Collect and save an EDTA (ethylenediaminetetraacetic acid) anticoagulated blood sample and a serum sample prior to treatment. Then, stabilize the patient and proceed with the diagnostic evaluation. Pretreatment samples are important for establishing baselines for therapeutic monitoring and for providing the best diagnostic specimens for detecting infectious agents (identifying hemic parasites, culturing bacteria, performing serologic or polymerase chain reaction [PCR] tests) and for detecting antiplatelet antibodies.

Confirm the thrombocytopenia by performing a CBC that includes an automated platelet count and a blood smear examination of the platelets. Electronic platelet counts are not valid when platelets clump (activated platelets, cat platelets, poor venipunctures), when platelet size overlaps with red cell size, and when platelet counts are outside instrument linearity (very low or very high counts). Therefore, a smear should always be evaluated to confirm an automated platelet count and to evaluate platelet morphology. To estimate a platelet count from a blood smear, multiply the mean platelet number of 5 to 10 fields (at $100\times$ oil in the unilayer area of the smear) by $15,000/\mu l$. If platelets are clumped at the feathered edge, the platelet estimate will be inaccurate, but clumping usually indicates that the number of platelets is adequate to prevent hemorrhage. If patients with petechial or ecchymotic hemorrhages have normal or increased platelet counts, the clinician needs to pursue platelet function defects or vascular disorders, rather than thrombocytopenia (see next article).

Next, evaluate platelet size. Large platelets are often associated with increased platelet turnover, and a responding bone marrow with increased numbers of megakaryocytes. Normal-sized or small platelets are often associated with acute disorders, before the bone marrow has had time to respond, or nonresponsive disorders such as aplastic anemia or some forms of ITP.

The leukogram and erythrogram are helpful in distinguishing production problems from utilization or destructive disorders. Infectious diseases that cause decreased production of platelets (e.g., feline leukemia virus [FeLV], feline immunodeficiency virus [FIV], feline panleukopenia virus [FPV], *Ehrlichia canis*) often cause decreased leuko-cyte and red cell production characterized by a peripheral leukopenia, without a left shift, and possibly a nonregenerative anemia. Anemia is expected only with diseases that cause a long-term decrease in red cell production (e.g., FeLV but not FPV) because the red cell life span is relatively long (110 days in dogs, 68 days in cats). An inflammatory leukogram characterized by neutrophilia or neutropenia with a left shift or toxic change indicates inflammation with increased utilization or destruction of platelets. Chronic inflammatory diseases (bacterial abscesses, systemic lupus erythematosus) cause a nonregenerative iron-sequestering anemia, whereas immune-mediated diseases, hemic parasites (*Haemobartonella felis*, *H. canis*, *Babesia canis*, *B. gibsoni*, *Cytauxzoon felis*), and other infectious agents can cause hemolytic anemias. Additionally, red cell morphology may give clues to the mechanism of thrombocytopenia (e.g., schistocytes indicate DIC or vasculitis).

A bone marrow aspiration (cytology) or core (histopathology) biopsy is necessary for identifying causes of thrombocytopenia that are not apparent from the routine clinical work-up. Thrombocytopenia is not a contraindication to bone marrow biopsy. In fact, it may be the only way of establishing a diagnosis or prognosis. Thrombocytopenic patients rarely have any hemostatic complications associated with bone marrow biopsy. However, it is wise to choose a biopsy site, such as the proximal humerus, where hemorrhage is easily controlled with a pressure wrap and muscle masses are avoided. If the patient is already bleeding, consider transfusion before the bone marrow biopsy. Increased numbers and immaturity of megakaryocytes indicate a regenerative response, whereas decreased numbers of megakaryocytes indicate an unresponsive marrow or one that has not had time to respond (a bone marrow response should be seen by 3 to 5 days after an acute thrombocytopenic episode).

Analysis of the history, physical examination findings, and baseline laboratory data is mandatory for selecting the next logical diagnostic step. Blood cultures should be done in animals that appear seriously ill or that are immunocompromised. Enlarged organs (lymph nodes, liver, spleen), and exudates or effusions should be examined cytologically or histopathologically. Paired serum samples should be submitted for serology when viral or rickettsial diseases are suspected.

A coagulation profile—prothrombin (PT), activated partial thromboplastin time (APTT), and fibrin degradation products (FDPs)—should be obtained in any patient with thrombocytopenia to determine whether the thrombocytopenia is accompanied by other hemostatic abnormalities, such as a consumptive coagulopathy, which often occur with overwhelming sepsis, vasculitis, or acute hemolysis. The marked increase in FDPs and prolonged PT and APTT help distinguish thrombocytopenia associated with DIC from thrombocytopenia (usually mild) associated with hemorrhage (factor deficiency or warfarin toxicity). The coagulation profile is also invaluable for monitoring heparin therapy for DIC. Additional tests that are affected by thrombocytopenia include mucosal bleeding time (prolonged), clot retraction (poor), and, possibly, activated clotting time (ACT; time prolonged).

Tests that have been used to confirm an immune-mediated component (idiopathic or secondary) include antiplatelet antibody tests, antimegakaryocytic antibody tests, platelet factor 3 assay, antinuclear antibody test, and Coombs' test (Feldman et al, 1988). The diagnosis of ITP is challenging because no test or clinical finding is specific. Helpful criteria besides signalment include severe thrombocytopenia (<50,000 platelets/μl), microthrombocytosis, increased numbers of bone marrow megakaryocytes, detection of antiplatelet antibodies, and response to immunosuppressive glucocorticoid therapy. Ultimately, however, the diagnosis is made by excluding all other etiologies for thrombocytopenia.

INFECTIOUS ETIOLOGIES ASSOCIATED WITH THROMBOCYTOPENIA

Infectious diseases that can cause thrombocytopenia are listed in Table 1 (Breitschwerdt, 1988; Greene, 1990). The mechanisms by which these viral, bacterial, fungal, and parasitic agents cause thrombocytopenia are often multifactorial and incompletely understood. Many infectious diseases can induce DIC; especially noteworthy are gram-negative sepsis, infectious canine hepatitis (ICH), leptospirosis, salmonellosis, and babesiosis. Vascular endothelial cell damage causes thrombocytopenia in endotoxemia, septicemia, heartworm disease, feline infectious peritonitis (FIP), ICH, canine herpesvirus infection, Rocky Mountain spotted fever (RMSF), relapsing fever borreliosis, and bartonellosis. Bone marrow suppression occurs in FeLV, FIV, and feline and canine parvoviral infections, and ehrlichiosis. Platelets sequester in the spleen, liver, and lungs with hemolytic crises (babesiosis, hemobartonellosis, cytauxzoonosis) and shock (septicemia, endotoxemia).

In addition to clinical signs and history, the distinguishing features of infectious diseases associated with thrombocytopenia include geographic location and severity of thrombocytopenia. Geographically, babesiosis, ehrlichiosis, RMSF, and cytauxzoonosis are more common in the southern states, whereas histoplasmosis occurs primarily in the major river valleys. Severe thrombocytopenias are seen most often with ITP and overwhelming sepsis. The thrombocytopenia of ehrlichiosis is generally more severe than that of RMSF, perhaps as low as 1,000 platelets/μl. *Ehrlichia platys*, the only platelet-specific infectious agent, causes a severe, cyclic thrombocytopenia in dogs, but it is generally not associated with illness in the United States. Thus, illness with *E. platys* suggests the presence of another agent, such as *Ehrlichia canis*, *E. equi*, or *Babesia canis*.

Serology or PCR amplification of bacterial DNA, when available, may be the only way of confirming a specific diagnosis because these agents may seldom be observed on blood smears (*E. canis*, *E. equi*, *E. platys*) and may be difficult to culture. Cytauxzoonosis, which can be confused with the ring form of *Haemobartonella*, is usually fatal in domestic cats but can be confirmed with histopathology. Babesiosis can also be confirmed with histopathology. Unfortunately, serology is not available for *H. felis* and *H. canis*, and no pathognomonic lesions are present on histopathology. Therefore, *Haemobartonella* spp. should be diligently sought on blood smears. The role of other chronic blood-borne pathogens, such as *Bartonella henselae* and

Rochalimaea felis, as a cause of infectious thrombocytopenia in cats awaits clarification.

Modified live virus vaccines (e.g., canine distemper vaccine) can produce mild to severe thrombocytopenia 1 to 21 days after vaccination. Elective surgeries, such as ear trims, ovariohysterectomies, and castrations, are not recommended during this postvaccination period.

Infectious diseases can have an immunologic component; thus, they can be confused with immune-mediated diseases. Antierythrocyte antibodies (Coombs' reaction) have been reported with haemobartonellosis, ehrlichiosis, babesiosis, and bacterial endocarditis. Therefore, a complete work-up is necessary before one rules out infection as the cause of thrombocytopenia.

THERAPY

The goals of therapy are to stop any bleeding, halt ongoing platelet destruction, and treat the underlying disorder. Therapy may include a combination of the following: fresh whole blood or platelet-rich transfusions to stop the immediate bleeding; vincristine (Oncovin, Lilly), 0.010 to 0.025 mg/kg IV, one dose, to increase platelet counts; anticoagulant therapy to manage DIC; gastrointestinal protectants to stop or prevent melena (see *CVT XII*, p. 706); glucocorticoid therapy to prevent platelet destruction; supportive therapy to treat shock; and *pathogen-specific drug therapy* to eliminate the underlying disease (see Table 1; Greene, 1990). Avoid bone marrow suppressive drugs and drugs that are associated with immune-mediated platelet destruction, if possible. Transfusions are often not rewarding (lasting only hours) because they fail to slow the accelerated platelet destruction, inadequate numbers of platelets are transfused, or alloantibodies develop. Vincristine is indicated only if other forms of therapy have failed and if adequate numbers of megakaryocytes are present in the bone marrow. Therapy for DIC is discussed on page 190.

A general approach to the ITP patient is to start immunosuppressive doses of glucocorticoid: prednisone (Prednisone, Barr) or prednisolone (Delta-Cortef, UpJohn), 1 to 3 mg/kg PO every 12 hours, or dexamethasone (Azium, Schering), 0.1 to 0.6 mg/kg PO or IV every 24 hours. If platelet counts normalize in less than a week, decrease the dose of glucocorticoid over 1 to 3 months to 0.5 to 1 mg/kg every 48 hours. If the platelet count remains low, add azathioprine (Imuran, Glaxo-Wellcome), 2 mg/kg PO every 24 hours), cyclophosphamide (Cytoxan, Bristol-Myers Squibb Oncology), 1.5 to 2.5 mg/kg PO or IV every 24 hours for 4 days each week, or vincristine, 0.02 mg/kg IV once each week, to the therapy regimen. If platelet counts normalize after 1 or 2 weeks, discontinue the vincristine or cyclophosphamide but continue to reduce the dose of glucocorticoid or azathioprine for an additional 1 to 2 months. Frequent monitoring of platelet counts is critical to the appropriate choice of drugs and drug dosages to control the thrombocytopenia yet avoid deleterious drug side effects. Long-term maintenance treatment with alternate-day azathioprine may be considered as an alternative to glucocorticoids to avoid the serious side effects of high-dose glucocorticoid therapy. Danazol (Danocrine, Sanofi Winthrop), 5 to 10 mg/kg PO every 12 hours, has also

TABLE 1. Infectious Causes of Thrombocytopenia in Dogs and Cats

Disease Categories*	Species	Mechanism	Diagnostic Tests†	Therapy†
Viral				
Canine distemper‡ (morbillivirus)	C	U	Serology, virus isolation	Supportive
Canine herpesvirus infection	C	V	Serology, virus isolation	Supportive
Canine parvovirus infection	C	P	Serology, virus isolation, fecal EM	Supportive
Infectious canine hepatitis	C	U, V	Serology, virus isolation	Supportive
Feline immunodeficiency virus infection	F	P	Serology	Supportive
Feline infectious peritonitis (coronavirus)	F	U, V	Serology, histopathology	Supportive
Feline leukemia virus infection	F	P	Serology, virus isolation	Supportive
Feline panleukopenia (parvovirus)	F	P	Serology, virus isolation	Supportive
Rickettsial				
Ehrlichiosis	C	D, P, S	Serology, blood smear examination	Tetracycline (22 mg/kg PO q8hr for 14 days), or doxycycline (5–10 mg/kg PO q12–24hr for 10 days)
Haemobartonellosis	C, F	D, S	Blood smear examination	Tetracycline (dog, 40 mg/kg PO q8hr for 2 wk; cat 22 mg/kg PO q8hr for 2–3 wk) ± blood transfusion, ± glucocorticoids
Rocky Mountain spotted fever	C	V	Serology	Tetracycline (22 mg/kg PO q8hr for 14 days), or doxycycline (10–20 mg/kg PO q12hr for 14 days)
Bacterial				
Bacteremia or septicemia	C, F	D, U, V	Blood, urine, or organ culture	Supportive therapy and appropriate antimicrobial drug
Leptospirosis	C, F	D, U, V	Urine darkfield microscopy, culture, serology	Penicillin G (25,000–40,000 U IM or IV q12hr for 2 wk) followed by streptomycin (15 mg/kg IM q12hr for 2 wk)
Salmonellosis	C, F	D, U, V	Fluid and tissue culture	Chloramphenicol (dog, 25–50 mg/kg IV, IM, SC, or PO q6–8hr; cat, 50 mg/kg IV, IM, or SC q12 hr), or trimethoprim-sulfonamides (15–30 mg/kg PO, SC, or IV q12hr), or amoxicillin (20–25 mg/kg IV, IM, SC, or PO q8hr)
Protozoal				
Babesiosis	C§	U, S	Serology, blood smear examination, histopathology	¶,‖Diminazene aceturate (3.5 mg/kg [10% solution] IM one injection), or phenamidine isethionate (15 mg/kg [5% solution] SC q12hr for 2 days), or imidocarb dipropionate (2–6 mg/kg IM or SC one injection)
Bartonellosis	C	D	Serology, blood culture	Not clearly established
Cytauxzoonosis	F	U, S	Blood smear, histopathology	Supportive, almost always fatal. Parvaquone (10–30 mg/kg IM or SC q24hr for 2–3 days) or thiacetarsamide (0.1 mg/kg IV q12hr for 2 days)
Leishmaniasis	C	U	Cytology, histopathology	‖Meglumine antimonate (100 mg/kg IV or SC q24hr for 3–4 wk), or sodium stibogluconate (30–50 mg/kg IV or SC q24hr for 3–4 wk)
Relapsing borreliosis	C	D	Blood smear, serology, culture	Doxycycline (5 mg/kg q12hr for 14 days)
Toxoplasmosis	C, F	U	Cytology, histopathology, serology	Clindamycin (dog, 10–20 mg/kg PO or IM q12hr for 2 wk; cat, 12.5–25 mg/kg PO or IM q12hr for 2 wk)
Nematodal				
Dirofilaria immitis infection	C	D, U, V	Knott's test, filter test, serology, radiology	Thiacetarsamide (2.2 mg/kg IV q12hr for 2 days) or melarsomine (2.5 mg/kg IM q24hr for 2 days) followed in 4 wk by ivermectin (0.05 mg/kg PO one dose)
Fungal				
Disseminated candidiasis	C, F	U	Fungal culture, histopathology	Ketoconazole (dog, 5–11 mg/kg PO q12hr for 4 wk; cat, 50–100 mg [total] PO q12–24hr for 4 wk)
Histoplasmosis	C, F	U	Cytology, histopathology	Ketoconazole (dog or cat, 10–15 mg/kg PO q12hr for 4–6 mo; cat, 50 mg [total] PO q24hr for 4–6 mo), or amphotericin B (0.25–0.5 mg/kg IV q48hr for cumulative dose of 5–10 mg/kg in dogs or 4–8 mg/kg in cats)

*Disseminated intravascular coagulation and drug therapy may cause thrombocytopenia in patients with other infectious diseases.
†Refer to Greene CE: *Infectious Diseases of the Dog and Cat*, and Breitschwerdt EB: Infectious thrombocytopenia in dogs. Compend Cont Educ 10:1177, 1988, for more details on diagnostic tests and therapy; see also Section 4 of this volume.
‡Infection or after vaccination with modified live virus vaccine.
§*Babesia felis* is not reported in the United States.
¶No drug is completely efficacious for *B. gibsoni*; *B. canis* may respond to supportive therapy.
‖Contact the Centers for Disease Control and Prevention (CDC), Atlanta, GA.
C, canine; F, feline; EM, electron microscopy; D, destruction; P, production decrease; S, sequestration; U, utilization increase; V, vascular damage.

shown promise in combination with immunosuppressive doses of prednisone. Splenectomy should be considered in refractory cases of thrombocytopenia (Feldman et al, 1988).

References and Suggested Reading

Breitschwerdt EB: Infectious thrombocytopenia in dogs. Compend Contin Educ Pract Vet 10:1177, 1988.
A review of the pathophysiology, etiology, and treatment of infectious causes of canine thrombocytopenia.

Breitschwerdt EB, Nicholson WL, Kiehl AB, et al: Natural infections with *Borrelia* spirochetes in two dogs from Florida. J Clin Microbiol 32:353, 1994.
A report of a Borrelia *species (not the Lyme disease agent) that causes thrombocytopenia and disease.*

Breitschwerdt EB, Kordick DL, Malarkey DE, et al: Endocarditis in a dog due to infection with a novel *Bartonella* subspecies. J Clin Microbiol 33:154, 1995.

A report of a newly recognized canine pathogen that caused endocarditis and thrombocytopenia.

Feldman BF, Thomason KJ, Jain NC: Quantitative platelet disorders. Vet Clin North Am Small Anim Pract 18:35, 1988.
An overview of the various causes of quantitative platelet disorders, including specific diagnostic tests and therapeutic recommendations.

Greene CE: Infectious Diseases of the Dog and Cat. Philadelphia: WB Saunders, 1990.
A textbook providing in-depth information on the diagnosis, treatment, and prevention of specific infectious agents.

Grindem CB, Breitschwerdt EB, Corbett WT, et al: Epidemiologic survey of thrombocytopenia in dogs: A report on 987 cases. Vet Clin Pathol 20:38, 1991.
A study on the prevalence and causes of thrombocytopenia in dogs.

Jordan HL, Grindem CB, Breitschwerdt EB: Thrombocytopenia in cats: A retrospective study of 41 cases. J Vet Intern Med 7:261, 1993.
A study on the prevalence and causes of thrombocytopenia in cats.

Lewis DC, Meyers KM: Canine idiopathic thrombocytopenic purpura. J Vet Intern Med 10:207, 1996.
A review of the pathophysiology, diagnosis, and treatment of immune-mediated thrombocytopenia.

Platelet Dysfunction

MARJORY BROOKS

JAMES L. CATALFAMO

Ithaca, New York

Platelets are small, anucleate cell fragments, yet their active participation is crucial for initiating and regulating hemostasis. This article describes the clinical management of bleeding diatheses caused by thrombopathia, or platelet dysfunction.

NORMAL PLATELET FUNCTION

Platelets circulate in the vascular compartment as discrete, nonadhesive, smooth disks. When a blood vessel is injured, platelets are rapidly transformed into adhesive spiny spheres that attach to the damaged subendothelial surface and to each other. The adherent platelets release numerous substances from platelet storage organelles. These substances accumulate locally and recruit additional platelets to the injury site. As platelet numbers increase, platelet aggregates accumulate and bridge the zone of vascular damage to form a hemostatic plug. The plug is stabilized by the generation of a thrombin-mediated platelet fibrin meshwork that traps platelets and red blood cells (RBCs). The growing clot is later consolidated by the action of platelet contractile proteins that retract the clot (Colman et al, 1994).

The ability of platelets to respond to injury-induced stimuli is central to their role in maintaining vascular integrity (Fig. 1). These stimuli initiate platelet activation by mediating a change in concentration of intracellular second messengers, such as ionized calcium, inositol triphosphate, diacylglycerol, and arachidonic acid metabolites. Prostacyclin (PGI_2), prostaglandin E_2 (PGE_2), and PGD_2 are endoperoxides synthesized by endothelial cells and released into the vascular space. Prostacyclin inhibits platelet reactivity by elevating intraplatelet cyclic adenosine monophosphate (cAMP) and decreasing free ionized calcium and inositol phosphate formation. Endothelium-derived nitric oxide can also reduce platelet responsiveness by raising the level of intracellular cyclic guanosine monophosphate (cGMP).

The rapid transition from nonadhesive disk to adhesive sphere requires that platelets recognize cell adhesion molecules in plasma and subendothelial matrix. Adhesion (platelet–subendothelial matrix interactions) and aggregation (platelet-platelet association) depend on integrin and other platelet glycoprotein receptors. Integrin receptors are composed of alpha and beta subunits. The GPIIb-IIIa ($\alpha_{IIb}\beta_3$) complex is the most abundant platelet integrin and functions as the activation-dependent receptor for fibrinogen, fibronectin, and von Willebrand factor (vWF). The binding of fibrinogen to this receptor is essential for normal platelet aggregation. Platelet adhesion and aggregation at high shear rates depend on vWF binding to GPIIb-IIIa ($\alpha_{IIb}\beta_3$). Platelet adhesion to collagen is supported by its binding to the integrin receptor GPIa-IIa ($\alpha_2\beta_1$). This receptor is also involved in signaling collagen-induced platelet activation.

CLINICAL SIGNS OF PLATELET DYSFUNCTION

The characteristic signs of platelet dysfunction include cutaneous ecchymoses, bleeding from mucosal surfaces

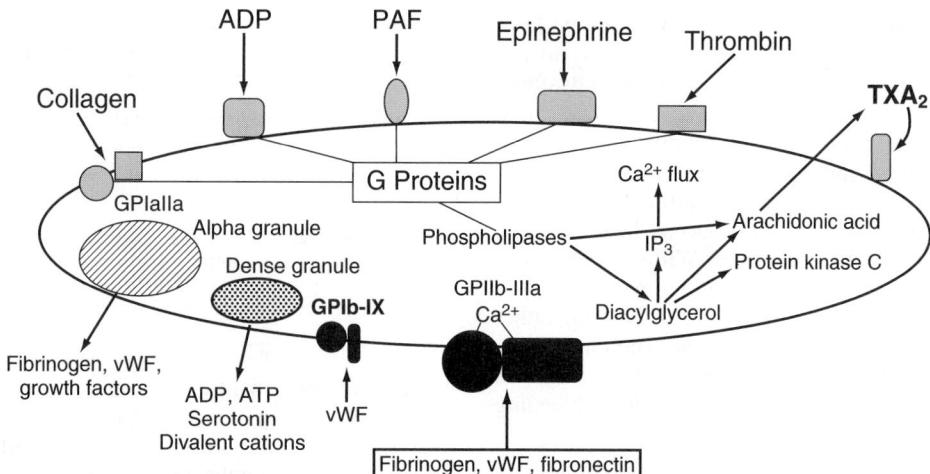

Figure 1. Receptors and second messengers involved in platelet activation. Platelet stimuli bind to specific cell surface receptors activating phospholipase C via coupled G proteins, including the integrin receptor for collagen, GPIaIIa. Activated phospholipase C hydrolyzes phosphoinositides to generate inositol 1,4,5-triphosphate (IP_3), and diacylglycerol (DAG) and to mobilize ionized calcium from platelet storage sites. Ca^{2+} also activates phospholipase A_2 to release arachidonic acid, which is converted to thromboxane A_2 (TXA_2). Thromboxane is released and activates other platelets via its surface receptor. DAG stimulates protein kinase C to phosphorylate intraplatelet proteins critical for platelet function, including dense and alpha granule release. Von Willebrand factor binds to either GPIb-IX or GPIIb-IIIa to support platelet adhesion to damaged subendothelium. Platelet aggregation is mediated by bound fibrinogen bridging GPIIb-IIIa receptors on adjacent platelets. The release of dense granule constituents amplifies platelet reactivity. Alpha granules secrete hemostatic proteins and other factors to support platelet adhesion and wound healing. The elevation of intraplatelet cAMP blocks ionized calcium mobilization and phosphoinositide hydrolysis. PAF, platelet-activating factor.

(gingival hemorrhage, epistaxis, melena, hematuria), and prolonged or excessive bleeding at the sites of surgery or trauma. Pinpoint hemorrhage or petechiae are more commonly seen in thrombocytopenic patients, but there are no pathognomonic signs to differentiate platelet dysfunction from other primary hemostatic disorders. The systemic diseases that cause acquired platelet dysfunction often cause concurrent deficiency or inhibition of the coagulation cascade. In these cases, the bleeding diathesis is more severe than that caused by platelet dysfunction alone and may include hematoma formation or spontaneous hemorrhage into the central nervous system (CNS) or pleural or peritoneal spaces. The most obvious findings on initial examination are frequently signs of acute or chronic blood loss anemia. Identification of an underlying defect of platelet function therefore requires an index of suspicion that a bleeding diathesis is present and a diagnostic plan for evaluating hemostatic pathways.

DIAGNOSTIC APPROACH

The initial evaluation of bleeding in dogs and cats should be directed at differentiating blood loss caused by injury to a local or focal group of vessels from a systemic bleeding diathesis. A thorough history and physical examination, in some cases including ancillary diagnostics (radiography, ultrasonography, endoscopy), is usually sufficient for locating the source and underlying cause of hemorrhage from large vessels. A history of repeated episodes of hemorrhage, bleeding at multiple sites, and concurrent disease known to affect hemostasis suggests the presence of a systemic bleeding diathesis. A systematic evaluation of preliminary screening tests should then be performed to rule out the more common bleeding disorders, before one pursues detailed studies of platelet function. Table 1 lists

screening tests of hemostasis and definitive tests for identifying platelet dysfunction.

Preliminary Evaluation

Thrombocytopenia and coagulation factor deficiencies are the most common bleeding diatheses in dogs and cats. A platelet estimate from a blood smear and/or platelet count, and coagulation screening tests, are therefore performed as the first step in evaluating any patient suspected of having a bleeding disorder. Determination of plasma vWF concentration provides a rapid screening test for von Willebrand disease (vWD). This defect of primary hemostasis is clinically indistinguishable from platelet dysfunction and should be ruled out in dogs and cats before one moves on to platelet function studies. A complete drug

TABLE 1. Diagnosis of Platelet Dysfunction

Initial Screening Tests	Specific Platelet Studies
1. Platelet count	1. Dilute whole blood clot retraction
2. Coagulation assays: APTT, PT, TCT, or fibrinogen	2. Platelet aggregation studies: ADP, collagen, arachidonate, and epinephrine
3. von Willebrand factor antigen	3. Platelet secretion studies: serotonin, ATP, ADP
4. Bleeding time tests: buccal mucosa, cuticle	4. Platelet membrane glycoprotein composition: GPIb, GPIIb, GPIIIa
5. Fibrin degradation product titer	5. Platelet ultrastructure (electron microscopy)
6. Antithrombin III	

APTT, activated partial thromboplastin time; PT, prothrombin time; TCT, thrombin clotting time; ADP, adenosine diphosphate; ATP, adenosine triphosphate; GP, glycoprotein.

history and metabolic profile are included in the preliminary evaluation to identify disease processes likely to impair platelet function and to direct therapy. Platelet dysfunction commonly accompanies the disseminated intravascular coagulation (DIC) process. Tests for defining or characterizing DIC complete the initial laboratory screening process (see p. 438). An in vivo assessment of primary hemostasis is performed by measuring buccal mucosa bleeding time (BMBT; see p. 434) (Forsythe and Willis, 1989). The finding of a long bleeding time, normal platelet count, and normal vWF concentration is compatible with either acquired or inherited platelet dysfunction. The clinical severity of bleeding caused by platelet dysfunction, however, does not always correlate with prolongation of bleeding time.

Specific Platelet Function Testing

Platelet response and specific platelet defects are characterized by performing a series of in vitro tests for evaluating platelet structure and function (see Table 1). Test procedures must be adapted and validated for use in dogs and cats to accommodate species-specific differences. Accurate measurement of platelet function in aggregation and release studies requires that samples be analyzed within 3 hours of collection to ensure the viability of patient platelets. This requirement necessitates patient referral to the clinic or center where testing is performed. Platelet aggregation in response to different agonist compounds is measured by detecting changes in light transmission of platelet-rich plasma samples or changes in electrical impedance of whole blood samples. Whole-blood aggregation studies utilize small sample volume and are simple to perform—features useful for detecting dysfunction in patients that have acquired disorders secondary to disease or drug administration. Aggregation studies that utilize platelet-rich plasma are more difficult to perform, but they provide more detailed information for characterizing and defining platelet response in patients having inherited platelet function defects. Special platelet function testing is available at the authors' laboratory and at other veterinary teaching hospitals (including Auburn University and the University of Pennsylvania).

SPECIFIC DISORDERS

Acquired Platelet Dysfunction

Platelet dysfunction occurs in association with many common diseases or as a result of drug administration. The clinical significance of impaired platelet function is highly variable under these conditions. The clinician should be prepared to closely monitor and, if needed, treat patients that have hemorrhagic complications. Conversely, if hemorrhage due to platelet dysfunction is suspected, a thorough search to identify underlying disorders or drug administration is indicated.

Platelet Dysfunction Secondary to Disease

The disorders most commonly associated with platelet dysfunction are listed in Table 2. Complex and variable

TABLE 2. Diseases Associated With Acquired Platelet Dysfunction

Anemia
  Chronic regenerative or nonregenerative
Disseminated intravascular coagulation
Liver disease
  Cholestasis and acquired or inherited shunts
Paraproteinemias
  Lymphocytic leukemia, multiple myeloma, benign macroglobulinemia, polyclonal gammopathies
Uremia

patterns of abnormalities are often seen in platelet function studies of these patients, and the mechanisms underlying platelet dysfunction are likely to be multifactorial. Factors extrinsic to the platelet may predominate, such as impairment of platelet adhesion due to changes in blood viscosity in anemic patients, or the presence of paraproteinemia. Uremia is believed to cause an intrinsic platelet function defect by altering prostaglandin metabolism, in addition to an extrinsic defect related to an increase in plasma levels of dialyzable metabolites.

Platelet Dysfunction Secondary to Drug Administration

Many drugs demonstrate platelet inhibitory effects in vitro; however, clinically significant impairment of hemostasis has been reported for relatively few of these products. Aspirin and other nonsteroidal anti-inflammatory drugs (NSAIDs) are most commonly implicated in cases of drug-induced platelet dysfunction in dogs and cats. These drugs block production of thromboxane, a potent platelet agonist, by inactivating platelet cyclooxygenase. The effects of aspirin on platelet function are irreversible, lasting as long as 7 days, whereas inhibition caused by NSAIDs is transient, lasting for only a few hours (Grauer et al, 1992). The drugs listed in Table 3 have proven or potential platelet inhibitory effects, and should be used cautiously, if at all, for patients undergoing surgery or demonstrating signs of abnormal hemostasis.

Inherited Platelet Dysfunction

Inherited disorders of platelet function can be classified broadly into disorders of platelet membrane glycoproteins, defects involving platelet storage granules, and defects of intracellular signaling; Boudreaux et al, 1996). Inherited platelet defects are rare and are often breed specific (Table 4). In some cases, affected dogs and cats can be maintained as pets, provided that they are managed carefully with intermittent transfusion therapy.

TREATMENT OF PLATELET DYSFUNCTION

Effective treatment of platelet dysfunction includes control of hemorrhage from the sites of active bleeding, stabilization of the patient to ameliorate signs of hypovolemia or blood loss, and correction of any underlying disease that may cause or exacerbate the hemostatic defect. Acquired platelet dysfunction is by far more common than inherited

TABLE 3. Drug-Induced Platelet Dysfunction

Category	Drug	Mode of Action
Antibiotics	Carbenicillin	Unknown
	Cephalothin	Membrane*
	Moxalactam	Membrane
	Sulfonamides	Membrane
Anti-inflammatory drugs	Aspirin	Prostaglandin inhibition†
	Ibuprofen	Prostaglandin inhibition‡
	Naproxen	Prostaglandin inhibition‡
	Phenylbutazone	Prostaglandin inhibition‡
Cardiac or respiratory drugs	Aminophylline	Phosphodiesterase§
	Isoproterenol	Membrane
	Propranolol	Membrane
	Theophylline	Phosphodiesterase
	Verapamil	Prostaglandin inhibition‡
Miscellaneous	Barbiturates	Signal transduction¶
	Dextran	Membrane
	Heparin	Unknown
	Hydroxyethyl starch	Membrane

*Interacts or interferes with platelet membrane receptors.
†Irreversible acetylation of platelet cyclooxygenase.
‡Reversible inhibition of prostaglandin metabolites.
§Inhibitor of phosphodiesterase causing increased intraplatelet cAMP.
¶Interferes with the rise of intraplatelet calcium levels.

platelet disorder, and the long-term management of dogs and cats with acquired disorders is dictated by the specific primary disease process (see Table 2). Initial treatment for both acquired and inherited disorders can be divided into transfusion and nontransfusion support.

Transfusion Therapy

In contrast to management of thrombocytopenic patients, limited transfusion support is often effective in controlling hemorrhage caused by platelet dysfunction. The physical presence and any residual function of thrombopathic platelets enable them to participate in the formation of hemostatic plugs initiated by the normal, transfused platelets.

Blood Collection and Processing for Platelet Transfusions

Blood products that supply active platelets include fresh whole blood (FWB), platelet-rich plasma (PRP), and platelet concentrates (PCs). Special collection and processing techniques are needed to maintain maximal platelet viability and prevent the formation of platelet aggregates (Mooney, 1992). The most important of these include (1) maintenance of blood products at room temperature throughout collection, processing, and storage; (2) use of plastic bags or syringes and citrate-based anticoagulants, rather than glass receptacles and heparin anticoagulant; and (3) transfusion within 24 hours of collection (FWB) or within 3 days (PRP, PC). Special care is given to aseptic collection technique because platelet transfusions are maintained at room temperature. It is ideal to administer these products as soon as possible after collection.

Platelet-rich plasma is prepared by centrifugation of FWB for less time and at a lower speed (soft spin) than routinely used for separation of fresh plasma. Platelets remain suspended in the supernatant plasma, with an expected yield of about 80% of the platelets in whole blood. Platelet concentrates are prepared by centrifugation of PRP using a high speed (hard spin) to form a platelet pellet, and then suspending the pellet in a small volume (50 to 75 ml) of plasma (Abrams-Ogg et al, 1993). The PRP and PC prepared in this manner have some contamination with donor red and white blood cells, albeit at a much lower concentration than that of the whole blood from which they are prepared. The equipment and supplies for production of PRP and PC are readily adapted for dogs, but the short storage life of these products limits their use primarily to the referral centers where they are prepared. Transfusion of platelet components in feline medicine has been reported only in research, rather than clinical trials.

Guidelines for Platelet Transfusion

Donor Selection. Donors should be blood-type compatible with recipients because all platelet replacement prod-

TABLE 4. Inherited Platelet Dysfunction

Type Defect	Breed	Features*
Glanzmann's thrombasthenia (membrane GP)	Otter hound, Great Pyrenees	Abnormal platelet adhesion; absent or trace aggregation to most stimuli; abnormal clot retraction; absent or reduced GPIIb-IIIa complex
Storage pool	Persian cat	Associated with Chédiak-Higashi syndrome; reduced number of dense granules; failure to secrete ADP and serotonin; abnormal platelet aggregation; normal clot retraction
	American Cocker spaniel	Normal number dense granules; abnormal storage and secretion of ADP; abnormal platelet aggregation to ADP and collagen; normal clot retraction
Signal transduction	Basset hound	Abnormal platelet adhesion; absent or trace platelet aggregation in response to most stimuli; normal clot retraction, normal levels of GPIIb-IIIa complex; abnormal cAMP metabolism
	Spitz	Abnormal platelet adhesion; absent or trace platelet aggregation in response to most stimlui; normal clot retraction, normal levels of GPIIb-IIIa complex; abnormal signaling pathway
Signal transduction and storage pool	Collie	Associated with cyclic neutropenia and primitive stem cell disorder; normal platelet aggregation to ADP, partially impaired for other stimuli; defective uptake and storage of serotonin; abnormal platelet protein phosphorylation

*Inherited platelet disorders are associated with variable clinical signs, ranging from mild to severe bleeding tendency.

ucts (FWB, PRP, PC) contain red cells. Feline donors and recipients should be matched for blood type A or B, whereas dogs negative for DEA 1.1 and DEA 1.2 (see p. 397) can be used as "universal donors" for platelets. Greyhounds are not recommended as donors for production of PRP, because it is difficult to obtain high yields of their platelets with the use of routine centrifugation protocols. Recipients likely to need repeated transfusions over long periods of time (months) are at risk for developing alloantibodies to foreign platelet antigens. Sequential donations from a single donor, rather than pooled platelet donations, are likely to delay the immunization process (Slichter et al, 1986).

Platelet Administration. Intravenous catheters should be placed in peripheral veins of thrombopathic patients because catheterization of the jugular vein might cause perivascular hemorrhage and interfere with respiration. If intravenous catheter placement is impossible, transfusion via the intraosseous route is an acceptable alternative for platelet replacement. Intraperitoneal transfusion and intraoperative salvage of blood are not effective means of supplying active platelets. In-line blood filters should be used for FWB and platelet component transfusions. An appropriate rate for transfusion is 6 ml/min for dogs, with the transfusion completed over the period of 1 to 2 hours for both dogs and cats. Routine pretreatment with corticosteroid or antihistamine is not required.

Clinical Indications. Platelet transfusion is always indicated to provide rapid control of hemorrhage in critical functional sites such as the CNS or respiratory tract. A single transfusion is often sufficient to control epistaxis or other mucosal bleeds, whereas transfusion support for patients undergoing surgery is more intensive. A first transfusion is given preoperatively, within 1 to 2 hours of the procedure. A second dose is given postoperatively for major surgery, or if any excess hemorrhage is noted. Close monitoring of the surgical site and serial determinations of hematocrit should be performed for the first 24 hours after surgery, and an additional platelet transfusion given if required. It is unusual for rebleeding to occur if hemostasis is adequate at 24 hours after surgery. The BMBT is not an accurate predictor of perioperative bleeding complications.

Fresh whole blood is the optimal product for treating thrombopathic dogs or cats having signs of acute blood loss anemia and active hemorrhage. Platelet components (PRP, PC) are ideal for preoperative prophylaxis and for thrombopathic patients requiring repeated transfusion within a 24-hour period. Platelet concentrates provide most of the active platelets, in less than one half the volume, of the PRP from which they are prepared. Nevertheless, transfusion of PRP is usually sufficient to supply effective numbers of platelets without volume overload, and the extra time and expense in preparing PC is rarely worthwhile when one treats acquired or inherited platelet dysfunction. Table 5 presents general dosage guidelines for platelet replacement. The most successful transfusion strategy is to treat with an initial high dose of blood products to supply enough active platelets for hemostatic plug formation.

Transfusion Reactions

Transfusion of platelet products may be complicated by any of the acute, chronic, immune or nonimmune reactions associated with transfusion of whole blood. Acute reactions are treated by stopping the transfusion and administering symptomatic or supportive care. Febrile reactions are the most common complication. These reactions tend to be self-limited and are probably mediated by white blood cells in the platelet products. Procedures for removing contaminant white blood cells (special centrifugation techniques, leukocyte filters) also reduce platelet yield. Urticaria and anaphylaxis are uncommon acute immune transfusion reactions. Urticaria may be a reaction to plasma proteins, and this condition is treated with administration of antihistamine and short-acting corticosteroid. Anaphylaxis may result from transfusion of incompatible red blood cells or transfusion of large aggregates of activated platelets. These complications are prevented with the use of only type- and crossmatch-compatible platelet donors, careful collection techniques, and transfusion through blood filters. Dogs having inherited platelet function defects that have received repeated transfusions throughout their lives are at greatest risk for alloimmunization causing shortened platelet survival.

Nontransfusion Therapy and Supportive Care

No drug or hormonal therapy can substitute for platelets' structural and metabolic roles in initiating primary hemostasis. In human medicine, desmopressin acetate [DDAVP; 1-deamino(8-D-arginine) vasopressin] is used as adjuvant therapy for patients with mild or nonspecific signs of defective primary hemostasis. This drug may be applicable for the treatment of dogs and cats (see p. 337), but there are no controlled studies demonstrating clinical efficacy.

For secondary or drug-induced platelet dysfunction, treatment of the underlying disorder or discontinuation of the suspected drug may be sufficient to prevent or control hemorrhage and obviate the need for transfusion. In these cases, invasive procedures should be avoided or delayed, pending the response to specific treatment.

Local treatment of surgical or traumatic wounds can eliminate or reduce the transfusion requirements of thrombopathic patients. Procedures for improving local hemostasis include electrocautery, ligation of small vessels, multilayer closure of incisions, and application of pressure wraps. Topical tissue adhesives are very effective in controlling hemorrhage from small wounds on cutaneous or mucosal surfaces, provided that bleeding is first controlled

TABLE 5. Guidelines for Platelet Transfusion

Product	Dose	Frequency
Fresh whole blood	12 to 20 ml/kg	q24h (volume overload limits interval)
Platelet-rich plasma (PRP)	5 to 10 ml/kg	q6–12hr
Platelet concentrate (PC)	1 U*/15 kg	q6–12hr

*One unit is defined as the platelet concentrate produced from 450 ml of fresh whole blood.

with direct pressure and the tissues are dry. Oral tissues are rich in fibrinolysins and are likely to bleed. To minimize hemorrhage from gingival injuries and tooth extraction sites, these wounds can be packed with absorbable sponges and sutured.

References and Suggested Reading

Abrams-Ogg ACG, Kruth SA, Carter RF, et al: Preparation and transfusion of canine platelet concentrates. Am J Vet Res 54:635, 1993.
A descriptive study detailing the preparation, efficacy, and safety of platelet concentrates used to treat severe thrombocytopenia induced by bone marrow irradiation in five dogs.

Boudreaux MK, Kvam K, Dillon AR, et al: Type I Glanzmann's thrombasthenia in a Great Pyrenees dog. Vet Pathol 33:503, 1996.
A description of a newly identified congenital canine thrombopathia, including a comprehensive battery of tests used to characterize platelet dysfunction and a complete reference list of inherited thrombopathias in animals.

Colman RW, Marder VJ, Salzman EW, et al: Overview of hemostasis. In: Colman RW, Hirsh J, Marder VJ, et al, eds: Hemostasis and Thrombosis. Philadelphia: Lippincott-Raven, 1994, p 3.
A concise presentation of the role of platelets and fluid-phase coagulation factors in the process of hemostasis.

Forsythe LT, Willis SE: Evaluating oral mucosa bleeding times in healthy dogs using a spring-loaded device. Can Vet J 30:344, 1989.
A standardized technique for measuring bleeding time of dogs or cats.

Grauer GF, Rose BJ, Toolan LA, et al: Effects of low-dose aspirin and specific thromboxane synthetase inhibition on whole blood platelet aggregation and adenosine triphosphate secretion in healthy dogs. Am J Vet Res 53:1631, 1992.
A description of the antiplatelet effects of aspirin and the use of whole-blood aggregometry in a controlled study utilizing 20 laboratory Beagles.

Mooney SA: Preparation of blood components. In: Hohenhaus AE, ed: Problems in Veterinary Medicine, Transfusion Medicine. Philadelphia: Lippincott-Raven, 1992, p 594.
A comprehensive description of the procedures, equipment, supplies, and sources for the production of canine blood components.

Slichter SJ, O'Donnell MR, Weiden PL, et al: Canine platelet alloimmunization: the role of donor selection. Br J Haematol 63:713, 1986.
A prospective study comparing platelet recovery and survival in recipient dogs transfused with one of five different transfusion programs in order to identify the most effective method of providing long-term platelet support.

Overview of Neutrophil Dysfunction in Dogs and Cats

KENNETH S. LATIMER
Athens, Georgia

Neutrophils are the primary phagocytic cells that defend the body against bacterial infection. Successful elimination of bacterial infection requires complex, carefully orchestrated interactions between plasma- and tissue-derived proteins, endothelial cells, and neutrophils. Collectively, these interactions of biologically active proteins, blood vessels, and leukocytes constitute the inflammatory response (Cotran et al, 1994).

OVERVIEW OF INFLAMMATION AND NEUTROPHIL FUNCTION

The inflammatory process has three essential components. First, bacterial invasion and tissue perturbation cause transient vasoconstriction of arterioles, which is followed quickly by vasodilation of the microvasculature or capillary beds. Blood flow to the infected tissue increases, causing both tissue heat and redness. Second, the permeability of the microvascular bed increases, usually as the result of endothelial cell contraction, cytokine-induced changes in endothelial cell junctions, endothelial cell necrosis and detachment, or leukocyte-mediated injury of the endothelial cells (Breider, 1993; Cotran et al, 1994). Ultimately, increased vascular permeability allows the escape of intravascular, protein-rich fluid into the tissues, with concomitant slowing of blood flow through the affected tissue. Clinically, fluid exudation, or edema, is reflected as tissue swelling. Third, slowing of blood flow allows leukocytes, especially neutrophils, to marginate within and emigrate from capillaries into the tissues in an attempt to eliminate bacterial infection.

As blood flow slows during inflammation, leukocytes fall, or marginate, from the main stream of circulation toward the endothelial surface. Following margination, neutrophils first roll along and then adhere, or stick, to the endothelial cell surface. These activities are mediated by expression of selectin and integrin molecules on the neutrophil and endothelial cell plasma membranes. Neutrophil rolling is promoted by expression of selectin molecules (L-selectin on neutrophils and P- and E-selectin on endothelial cells), while neutrophil adherence results from tighter binding between integrin molecules—CD11-CD18 complex and VLA-4 on neutrophils, and intracellular adhesion molecules (ICAM-1, ICAM-2) and vascular cell adhesion molecules (VCAM-1) on endothelial cells.

Neutrophils subsequently extend a pseudopod between endothelial cells, digest a small portion of the basement membrane, and emigrate from the microvasculature into the interstitium of the tissue. Although neutrophils may remain viable for 24 to 48 hours in healthy tissues, their life span can be shortened considerably in disease. Senescent neutrophils subsequently are phagocytosed, or engulfed, by monocyte-macrophages or lost from mucosal or wound surfaces following transmigration.

Within the tissues, neutrophils follow a chemotactic gradient to the site or sites of infection. Chemotactic factors to which neutrophils respond are diverse and include complement components, arachidonic acid metabolites, kinin system derivatives, and fibrin split products. These products may be generated following tissue injury, inflammation, or infection (Latimer, 1995).

As neutrophils encounter bacteria, these pathogens are readily recognized if they have undergone opsonization, or have been prepared for phagocytosis, by neutrophils. Opsonins include both immunoglobulin G (IgG) and fragments of the third component of complement (C3). The specific cell receptors responsible for neutrophil recognition of opsonized bacteria include the FcγR receptor, which detects the Fc portion of IgG, and complement receptors 1, 2, and 3 (CR1, 2, 3), which detect both C3b and C3bi (the stable form of C3b).

Following recognition, the opsonized bacteria are phagocytosed as the neutrophil concurrently experiences a respiratory burst (Bender and Chickering, 1983). Phagocytosis involves attachment of the bacterium to the neutrophil plasma membrane, extension of pseudopods around the organism, and fusion of neutrophil membrane. Following phagocytosis, the internalized bacterium is encased in an inverted plasma membrane sac called a phagosome. Subsequently, the phagosome fuses with neutrophil primary (azurophilic) and secondary (specific) granules to form a phagolysosome.

Bacterial killing is accomplished primarily by oxygen-dependent mechanisms involving the interaction of elemental oxygen, enzymes, and halide ions. The respiratory burst involves the generation of various toxic oxygen radicals used in bacterial killing. Oxygen and the reduced form of nicotinamide adenine dinucleotide phosphate (NADPH), in the presence of NADPH oxidase, produce superoxide anion. Superoxide anion is a highly reactive oxygen radical that spontaneously degrades to form hydrogen peroxide. Hydrogen peroxide is converted to hypochlorous acid in the presence of chloride ions by myeloperoxidase, an enzyme obtained from the primary neutrophil granules. Hypochlorous acid is essentially dilute bleach (e.g., Clorox), which is extremely toxic to bacteria. Bacterial killing by oxygen-dependent mechanisms is accomplished by covalent binding of chloride ions or other halides to intracellular protein or by membrane lipid peroxidation and oxidative cross-linking of membrane proteins by toxic oxygen radicals (Weiss, 1991).

Although the majority of bacterial killing is accomplished by the hydrogen peroxide–myeloperoxidase–halide system, neutrophils also may kill bacteria by oxygen-independent mechanisms. These mechanisms involve enzymes such as lysozyme or cationic proteins such as bactericidal permeability–increasing protein and defensins. Lysozyme, which is present in both primary and secondary granules, hydrolyzes muramic acid–N-acetylglucosamine bonds in the bacterial glycoprotein coat. Defensins, which are present in the primary granules, are highly cytotoxic, arginine-rich, cationic proteins. Defensins form voltage-gated ion channels in the bacterial cell membrane, resulting in increased permeability (Evans and Harmon, 1995).

Following bacterial killing, acid hydrolases from the primary neutrophil granules digest the bacteria. Hydrolase digestion is promoted by decreasing the pH (pH 4 to 5) within the phagolysosome.

NEUTROPHIL DYSFUNCTION

A major problem in documenting neutrophil dysfunction in dogs and cats is a lack of awareness of this condition and inadequate laboratory facilities for testing all aspects of neutrophil function. Complete laboratory testing of patients with suspected neutrophil dysfunction should include both serum and cellular parameters. Testing of all these parameters is available only in a few research laboratories; however, one can purchase commercial kits for quantitating immunoglobulins, some complement components, and nitroblue tetrazolium (NBT) dye reduction.

Neutrophil dysfunction may be hereditary or acquired. Such deficiencies may involve abnormalities in opsonic activity or chemotactic factor generation of serum or abnormalities in neutrophil adherence, chemotaxis, phagocytosis, or bactericidal activity. Congenital neutrophil dysfunction should be suspected in neonates or closely inbred families of dogs or cats that experience recurrent, occasionally severe to life-threatening bacterial infections in the presence of a normal to markedly increased neutrophil count. The clinical signs include periodontitis or gingivitis, poor wound healing, and lymphadenopathy. Cytologic preparations from presumed sites of infection may be deficient in neutrophils, especially if abnormalities of neutrophil adherence or chemotaxis are present. Acquired neutrophil dysfunction may occur in both juvenile and adult animals that experience recurrent bacterial infections in the presence of dermatologic or metabolic disease, viral infection, or toxicosis.

Numerous instances of congenital and acquired neutrophil dysfunction have been described and studied in humans. In contrast, reports of neutrophil dysfunction in dogs and cats are rare (Table 1). As interest in neutrophil function increases in veterinary medicine, more instances of neutrophil dysfunction will be recognized. The following brief discussion summarizes the published information concerning neutrophil dysfunction in dogs and cats.

Congenital or Familial Neutrophil Dysfunction

Canine CD11-CD18 Adhesion Protein Deficiency. Canine CD11-CD18 adhesion protein deficiency (canine leukocyte adhesion molecule deficiency, canine granulocytopathy syndrome) was first observed in 1974 in an Irish setter puppy with recurrent infections and defective neutrophil bactericidal activity. However, the molecular basis of the disease was not elucidated until 1986, when the absence of CD11-CD18 adhesion protein was demonstrated. CD11-CD18 is an integrin that allows neutrophils to adhere to endothelium and other matrix proteins. Therefore, a deficiency of this molecule affects neutrophil adherence, chemotaxis, and phagocytosis.

TABLE 1. Congenital and Acquired Neutrophil Dysfunction in Dogs and Cats

Dysfunction	Species
Chemotactic Factor Generation	
Congenital	
C3 deficiency (Brittany spaniel)	Dog
Adherence	
Congenital	
CD11-CD18 adhesion protein deficiency (Irish setter)	Dog
Acquired	
Diabetes mellitus (poorly regulated)	Dog
Chemotaxis	
Congenital	
C3 deficiency (Brittany spaniel)	Dog
CD11-CD18 adhesion protein deficiency (Irish setter)	Dog
Chédiak-Higashi syndrome (Persian)	Cat
Pelger-Huët anomaly? (Foxhound)	Dog*
Primary ciliary dyskinesia (Pointer)	Dog
Recurrent infections (Weimaraner)	Dog
Acquired	
Bacterial pyoderma	Dog
Demodicosis (serum inhibitor?)	Dog
Feline leukemia virus infection	Cat
Feline infectious peritonitis	Cat
Hyperalimentation-induced hypophosphatemia	Dog
Protothecosis (serum inhibitor?)	Dog
Phagocytosis	
Congenital	
C3 deficiency (Brittany spaniel)	Dog
CD11-CD18 adhesion protein deficiency (Irish setter)	Dog
Recurrent and persistent infections (Weimaraner)	Dog
Acquired	
Continuous-flow centrifugation and filtration-leukapheresis collected neutrophils	Dog
Hyperalimentation-induced hypophosphatemia	Dog
Bacterial Killing	
Congenital	
CD11-CD18 adhesion protein deficiency (Irish setter)	Dog
Cyclic neutropenia (Gray Collies)	Dog
Recurrent and persistent infections (Weimaraner)	Dog
Rhinitis-pneumonia syndrome (Doberman pinscher)	Dog
Acquired	
Feline leukemia virus infection	Cat
Hyperalimentation-induced hypophosphatemia	Dog
Lead toxicosis	Dog
Turpentine-induced inflammation	Dog

*Neutrophil chemotaxis was tested in only one of four English-American (Walker) Foxhounds with Pelger-Huët anomaly; defective chemotaxis has not been found in other dogs, including Foxhounds, with the anomaly.

CD11-CD18 adhesion protein deficiency has been infrequently reported in Irish setter and Irish setter–cross puppies in the United States and Sweden. This disorder is transmitted as an autosomal recessive trait. Evidence of recurrent bacterial infection is present before 12 weeks of age (Trowald-Wigh et al, 1992). The clinical signs include gingivitis, superficial pyoderma, deep skin wound infections, pododermatitis, omphalophlebitis, lymphadenopathy, pneumonia, and lameness. Marked neutrophilic leukocytosis ($\leq$208,000 white blood cells/μl) may occur. Paradoxically, cytologic preparations from sites of infection reveal a paucity of neutrophils. The lack of CD11-CD18 adhesion molecules within the neutrophil plasma membrane is associated with profoundly decreased neutrophil adherence, aggregation, and chemotaxis. Although oxidative function of neutrophils is normal, the cells have impaired phagocytosis of opsonized particles, including bacteria. In the living animal with CD11-CD18 adhesion protein deficiency, bacterial infection may not be eliminated because the neutrophils are unable to reach the site or sites of infection or cannot phagocytose the bacteria efficiently.

C3 Deficiency in Brittany Spaniels. The third component of complement (C3) is a hepatic-derived plasma protein that participates in both the classic and the alternative pathways of the complement cascade. C3 is of crucial importance in both pathways, being ultimately responsible for opsonization of bacteria (C3b, C3bi), generation of a potent chemoattractant for neutrophils (C5a), and production of the membrane attack complex (C5b6789) that can lyse some organisms. Therefore, severe congenital C3 deficiency predisposes to the development of severe infections.

C3 deficiency has been described in Brittany spaniels and is transmitted as an autosomal recessive trait (Winkelstein et al, 1982). Dogs that are homozygous for C3 deficiency may develop life-threatening bacterial infections, such as pneumonia, septicemia, and pyometra. Isolated bacteria often include *Clostridium* sp., *Escherichia coli*, and *Klebsiella* sp. Laboratory testing of clinically affected dogs reveals severely decreased to absent serum C3 concentration, inability to generate chemotactic factors (C5a) for neutrophils, and inability to opsonize bacteria. Therefore, neutrophil chemotaxis and phagocytosis may appear abnormal.

Recurrent Infections in Weimaraners. Recurrent and persistent bacterial infections have been described in Weimaraners from Australia, the United States, and Belgium (Hansen et al, 1995). The dogs from Australia were often related, suggesting a familial or an inherited disorder of neutrophil function. Although this disease has not been characterized completely, neutrophil defects include decreased neutrophil chemiluminescence, suggesting a reduced production of oxygen radicals for bacterial killing. In addition, defective neutrophil phagocytosis and an inability to kill *Staphylococcus aureus* have been found in two dogs.

Chronic Rhinitis and Pneumonia in Doberman Pinschers. Eight closely related Doberman pinschers have been described with chronic respiratory disease, including rhinitis and pneumonia (Breitschwerdt et al, 1987). Limited laboratory testing indicates that neutrophils phagocytose bacteria normally but have impaired bactericidal activity. Abnormal bacterial killing of *Staphylococcus epidermidis* is related to the inability of neutrophils to generate toxic oxygen radicals after appropriate cellular stimulation. Affected neutrophils also fail to reduce nitroblue tetrazolium dye or produce superoxide. Defective opsonization of pathogens is not responsible for defective phagocytosis because immunoglobulin and complement concentrations are within the reference interval or elevated. The disease state apparently shares some similarities with chronic granulomatous disease or complement receptor deficiency in humans; however, more in-depth study of affected dog neutrophils will be necessary to identify the molecular basis of this disease.

Chédiak-Higashi Syndrome in Cats. Chédiak-Higashi syndrome (Chédiak-Steinbrinck-Higashi anomaly, congenital giantism of peroxidase granules) has been reported in Persian cats with an indistinct smoke-blue haircoat and yellow-green irises. This disorder, transmitted in an autosomal recessive pattern, is characterized by enlarged cytoplasmic granules in circulating leukocytes and melanocytes. The enlarged granules in leukocytes result from the fusion of more normally sized pre-existing lysosomes and, on Romanowsky-stained blood smears, appear as pink to magenta cytoplasmic inclusions 2 μm in diameter. Although defective neutrophil chemotaxis has been reported, affected cats apparently are not predisposed to infection, as are human beings (Brickman et al, 1984). Mild neutropenia has been documented in experimental studies, but usually it is not discerned in a routine clinical setting (Latimer and Robertson, 1994).

Cyclic Hematopoiesis of Gray Collies. Cyclic hematopoiesis is a hereditary stem cell disease of Gray Collies that is transmitted in an autosomal recessive manner. In affected collies, the haircoat is a diluted color (silver-gray, beige, or charcoal). Although leukocyte, platelet, and reticulocyte counts cycle regularly, profound neutropenia is responsible for the most severe clinical consequences. Repetitive, severe neutropenia is associated with life-threatening bacterial infection. In addition, secondary systemic amyloidosis results from repeated infections. Affected collies usually die within the first year of life. Long-term survival is possible only with bone marrow transplantation. Although neutrophils from Gray Collies can phagocytose bacteria adequately, bacterial killing is compromised severely because of myeloperoxidase deficiency (Chusid et al, 1975).

Pelger-Huët Anomaly of Dogs and Cats. Pelger-Huët anomaly is a congenital disorder of leukocyte development characterized primarily by granulocyte nuclear hyposegmentation in the presence of a mature nuclear chromatin pattern. Nuclear hyposegmentation gives the appearance of a degenerative left shift in the stained blood smear. This anomaly has been reported in a variety of dog breeds and in domestic shorthair cats. The anomaly is presumed to be transmitted in an autosomal dominant manner in dogs and cats. However, the author's recent data in Australian shepherds suggest that transmission of the anomaly is incompletely dominant, being governed by two or more genes.

Defective neutrophil migration into skin abrasion sites has been reported in one English-American (Walker) Foxhound. However, more recent studies of the anomaly in five dogs indicate that affected neutrophils demonstrate normal neutrophil adherence, random movement, chemotaxis, phagocytosis, and bactericidal activity (Latimer et al, 1989). Clinical evidence of neutrophil dysfunction generally has not been reported in dogs or cats with the anomaly (Latimer and Robertson, 1994). A large recent study of human beings with Pelger-Huët anomaly also has failed to disclose abnormalities in neutrophil function.

Acquired Neutrophil Dysfunction

Numerous instances of acquired neutrophil dysfunction have been reported in humans with sepsis, viral infection, diabetes mellitus, malnutrition, drug therapy, systemic lupus erythematosus, and rheumatoid arthritis. In contrast, only a few reports of acquired neutrophil dysfunction in dogs and cats have been published (see Table 1).

Conditions with acquired neutrophil dysfunction in dogs include poorly controlled diabetes mellitus, bacterial pyoderma, demodicosis, lead intoxication, hypophosphatemia associated with hyperalimentation, inflammation, and protothecosis. Decreased neutrophil adherence may be partially responsible for the increased incidence of infections in poorly regulated diabetics. Putative inhibitors of neutrophil chemotaxis have been reported in both demodicosis and prototothecosis. Bacterial pyoderma, especially infection with *Staphylococcus* sp., has been associated with defective neutrophil chemotaxis. Lead toxicosis has been associated with decreased neutrophil bactericidal activity from acquired myeloperoxidase deficiency. Transient deficits in neutrophil bactericidal activity have also been observed in inflammation. Multiple defects in neutrophil function, as exemplified by hyperalimentation-induced hypophosphatemia, may be discerned if all major aspects of neutrophil function are evaluated simultaneously.

Thus far, neutrophil dysfunction has been reported only in cats with viral infections. Decreased neutrophil chemotaxis has been found in clinically ill, viremic cats with feline leukemia virus (FeLV) infection (Kiehl et al, 1987). In contrast, decreased neutrophil chemotaxis was not observed in cats with subclinical FeLV infection or in sick cats without FeLV infection. A previous study also suggested that bacterial killing might be decreased because of an inability to generate oxygen radicals adequately. Defective neutrophil chemotaxis has also been demonstrated in some cats with feline infectious peritonitis (Tsuji et al, 1989). The molecular basis of cell dysfunction in these viral infections has not been elucidated.

LABORATORY EVALUATION OF NEUTROPHIL FUNCTION

Documentation of neutrophil dysfunction by laboratory testing is expensive, complex, and labor intensive and requires appropriate control neutrophil preparations. Unfortunately, many bioassays of neutrophil function are subject to great variability or have inherent limitations. Therefore, subtle impairments of neutrophil function may not be detected. Furthermore, neutrophil function may be influenced by inflammation, infection, and drug administration. To minimize these latter effects, it is preferable to examine neutrophil function in the patient during periods of disease remission and in the absence of any medication. In instances of suspected neutrophil dysfunction, tests should be performed to evaluate opsonization activity and generation of chemotactic factors from serum as well as neutrophil adherence, chemotaxis, phagocytosis, and bacterial killing.

Opsonization is evaluated by quantitation of immunoglobulin (especially IgG) and complement (C3) concentrations in the patient's serum and by testing the ability of the serum to support phagocytosis of bacteria. If IgG concentrations are subnormal, antibody generation to T lymphocyte–dependent (tetanus toxoid) and T lymphocyte–independent (*Brucella abortus* antigen, sheep erythrocytes) antigens should be determined. In addition, the prudent clinician may obtain quantitation of circulating immune complexes to assess antibody catabolism.

Generation of chemotactic factors can be evaluated by quantitating the chemotaxis of control neutrophils to patient serum that has been "activated" by previous exposure to yeast (zymosan) or purified endotoxin.

Adherence is measured by determining the percentage of the patient's neutrophils that adhere to nylon-fiber columns. If defective adherence is documented, flow cytometry and fluorescein isothiocyanate (FITC)–conjugated monoclonal antibodies can be used to evaluate CD11-CD18 integrin expression on the neutrophil plasma membrane.

Chemotaxis may be measured in vitro by neutrophil migration under agarose or by transmigration of a polycarbonate membrane in a blindwell (modified Boyden chamber) in response to a chemotactic gradient. In vivo assessment of chemotaxis may be performed by quantitating neutrophil migration into skin windows or chambers at sites of minor cutaneous abrasion. The chemoattractant is usually endotoxin- or zymosan-activated pooled serum. In contrast to several animal species including the human, dog and cat neutrophils do not respond to N-formyl-methionyl-leucyl-phenylalanine (f-MLP), a synthetic chemotactic tripeptide.

Neutrophil phagocytosis may be quantitated by light microscopy or flow cytometry. Neutrophils are fed opsonized fluorescent latex spheres, nitroblue tetrazolium–impregnated latex spheres, or bacteria. Flow cytometry can quantitate the percentage of the neutrophil population that is phagocytic and accurately quantitate as many as five fluorescent latex spheres per cell. Light microscopy can quantitate these parameters as well, but it is more labor intensive. However, light microscopy may allow a distinction to be made between bacterial attachment to the cell membrane and actual engulfment or phagocytosis of the organisms. The importance of nitroblue tetrazolium dye reduction is explained below.

Bactericidal activity of neutrophils can be quantitated directly or indirectly. Indirect assessment of putative bactericidal ability may be accomplished by measuring protein iodination (^{125}I) by the hydrogen peroxide–myeloperoxidase–halide reaction, nitroblue tetrazolium dye (yellow) reduction to formazan (blue) by oxygen radicals, chemoluminescence with luminol as superoxide emits light when it makes the transition from an excited to a resting state, and cytochemical staining or chemical analysis for myeloperoxidase activity. Direct assessment of bactericidal activity is accomplished by feeding the neutrophils opsonized pathogenic bacteria in log phase growth. Bacterial killing is usually quantitated by examining neutrophil lysates for viable bacteria by agar plate culture.

MANAGEMENT OF NEUTROPHIL DYSFUNCTION

Specific therapy for congenital defects in neutrophil function is rarely possible. However, the diagnosis of neutrophil functional disorders allows the clinician to anticipate bacterial infections and plan the medical management of these complications in advance. Bone marrow transplantation is curative in some congenital disorders, such as Gray Collie syndrome, but has only been accomplished in

a research setting. Bone marrow transplantation is impractical in a clinical setting because major histocompatibility and blood type matching are required, patients must be prepared for transplantation by total body irradiation and chemotherapy, and bacterial infections may be difficult to manage during engraftment. These considerations make bone marrow transplants both involved and expensive.

The clinician can best manage acquired states of neutrophil dysfunction by eliminating or controlling the underlying disease. This approach may include appropriate antibiotic therapy in bacterial pyoderma, precise insulin regulation in diabetics, and phosphorus regulation in animals on hyperalimentation regimens.

References and Suggested Reading

Bender HS, Chickering WR: Superoxide, superoxide dismutase and the respiratory burst. Vet Clin Pathol 12:7, 1983.
A review of toxic oxygen products in bacterial killing.

Breider MA: Endothelium and inflammation. J Am Vet Med Assoc 203:300, 1993.
An overview of the importance of the endothelium in inflammation.

Breitschwerdt EB, Brown TT, DeBuysscher EV, et al: Rhinitis, pneumonia, and defective neutrophil function in the Doberman pinscher. Am J Vet Res 48:1054, 1987.
Neutrophil dysfunction in Doberman pinschers.

Brickman TJ, Kier AB, Collier LL: In vitro demonstration of defective neutrophil chemotaxis in Chediak-Higashi affected cats. Fed Proc 43:390, 1984.
Abnormal chemotaxis in cats with Chédiak-Higashi syndrome.

Chusid MJ, Bujak JS, Dale DC: Defective polymorphonuclear leukocyte metabolism and function in canine cyclic neutropenia. Blood 46:921, 1975.
Neutrophil dysfunction in grey collies.

Cotran RS, Kumar V, Robbins SL, eds: Robbins Pathologic Basis of Disease, 5th ed. Philadelphia: WB Saunders, 1994, p 51.
An overview of inflammation and repair.

Evans EW, Harmon BG: A review of antimicrobial peptides: Defensins and related cationic peptides. Vet Clin Pathol 24:109, 1995.
An overview of cytotoxic proteins and peptides.

Hansen P, Clercx C, Henroteaux M, et al: Neutrophil phagocyte dysfunction in a Weimaraner with recurrent infections. J Small Animal Pract 36:128, 1995.
Neutrophil dysfunction in a Weimaraner.

Kiehl AR, Fettman MJ, Quackenbush SL, et al: Effects of feline leukemia virus infection on neutrophil chemotaxis in vitro. Am J Vet Res 48:76, 1987.

Latimer KS: Leukocytes in health and disease. In: Ettinger SE, Feldman EC, eds: Textbook of Veterinary Internal Medicine: Diseases of the Dog and Cat, 4th ed. Philadelphia: WB Saunders, 1995, p 1892.
An overview of leukocyte responses in dogs and cats.

Latimer KS, Robertson SL: Inherited leukocyte disorders. In: August JR, ed: Consultations in Feline Internal Medicine 2. Philadelphia: WB Saunders, 1994, p 503.
Hereditary leukocyte disorders in cats.

Latimer KS, Kircher IM, Lindl PA, et al: Leukocyte function in Pelger-Huët anomaly of dogs. J Leukoc Biol 45:301, 1989.
Neutrophil function in canine Pelger-Huët anomaly.

Trowald-Wigh G, Håkansson L, Johannisson A, et al: Leucocyte adhesion protein deficiency in Irish setter dogs. Vet Immunol Immunopathol 32:261, 1992.
Canine CD11-CD18 adhesion protein deficiency.

Tsuji M, Goitsuka R, Hirota Y, et al: Chemotactic responses of neutrophils in cats with spontaneous feline infectious peritonitis. Jpn J Vet Sci 51:917, 1989.
Defective chemotaxis in cats with viral infections.

Weiss DJ: White cells. Adv Vet Sci 36:57, 1991.
An overview of granulocyte production and function.

Winkelstein JA, Johnson JP, Swift AJ, et al: Genetically determined deficiency of the third component of complement in the dog: In vitro studies on the complement system and complement-mediated serum activities. J Immunol 129:2598, 1982.
C3 deficiency in Brittany spaniels.

Modern Diagnostic Strategies for Cancer: Sampling Guidelines

BRUCE R. MADEWELL
STEPHEN M. GRIFFEY
Davis, California

The diagnosis of cancer is based on interpretation of the often subjective morphologic attributes of a tumor on hematoxylin and eosin–stained tissue sections. For some tumor types, such as mammary cancer, precise histologic diagnosis and clinical stage are the most reliable indicators of prognosis; however, hormonal receptor status, cytoskeletal structure, DNA ploidy, cellular proliferation index, oncogene expression (e.g., c-*erb* B2), expression of *p*-glycoprotein, and intratumoral microvessel density are now being tested for their usefulness in clinical practice.

These new tests are rapidly being introduced into the veterinary diagnostic laboratory to describe unique attributes of tumors useful for diagnosis and patient management. Immunohistochemistry has become an everyday tool in diagnostic pathology, and molecular pathology is now also having an impact in the diagnostic laboratory. Often based on small clinical specimens derived from minimally invasive procedures, these and other new laboratory tests are being developed and used as specific and sensitive markers of cancer. In time, these tests not only will optimize clinical diagnosis and staging but also will allow identification of affected patients and/or those at risk for disease, reflect tumor burden, have value as prognostic indicators, be predictive of tumor recurrence, and serve as aids for the selection of effective treatment strategies.

Although new technologies have expanded the diagnostic repertoire of the clinician and pathologist, they have also increased the responsibilities of the persons who collect and handle the specimens. The clinical veterinarian can no longer simply place all specimens destined for the pathology laboratory in neutral buffered formalin. Communication between the clinical veterinarian and the diagnostic pathologist ensures that specimens are collected and handled in the most appropriate manner, particularly for neoplasms that pose diagnostic challenges. The purpose of this article is to provide guidelines for the collection and preparation of clinical specimens for the diagnostic laboratory, so that the clinician can take full advantage of the diagnostic repertoire of the pathology laboratory. These recommendations for sample collection and handling affect not only specimens used in cancer diagnosis but also those that are analyzed with many of the molecular diagnostic methods used in genetics, hematopathology, virology, and microbiology and for coagulation and mitochondrial DNA disorders. Because sample preparation is so important for ultrastructural studies, a few comments regarding the collection and fixation of tissues for electron microscopy are also included.

GENERAL SAMPLING GUIDELINES FOR THE ROUTINE DIAGNOSTIC LABORATORY

Biopsy Guidelines for Routine Processing. The following procedures are recommended for tissues being collected for routine processing in the diagnostic laboratory. These procedures (Fig. 1) may vary somewhat from laboratory to laboratory, depending on the individual preferences of personnel, but general recommendations comprise the following:

- Include adjacent normal tissues in the specimen to allow examination of the relationship of the lesion to the adjacent tissues. An exception to this general rule is when sampling bone lesions suspected of representing primary bone tumors, where studies have demonstrated that specimens collected from the center of the lesion are more likely to be representative of the neoplasm and less likely to reflect reactive bone.
- Gently rinse any blood or debris from the tissue surface with saline to allow proper fixation.
- If the tissue specimen is more than 1.0 cm in diameter, and the transit time is going to be more than 24 hours, section partially through the tissue with a sharp scalpel or razor blade to allow proper fixation of the specimen. Written descriptions or diagrams can be useful for orientation, especially for tissues collected from areas of complex anatomy, such as the head and neck. Craniocaudal and mediolateral orientations are particularly important for large tissue specimens, such as those procured from mammary glands. If surgical excision of a tumor is found to be inadequate by histologic examination, it is imperative that the surgeon know where residual tumor remains to allow additional treatment planning.
- The fixation container should hold a 10:1 ratio of fixative to tissue volume. Avoid containers with narrow necks, and do not force the tissue through the container opening if the opening is too small. Small tissue specimens will intumesce and become harder during fixation, making removal of the tissue from narrow-necked containers difficult or impossible without breaking the container. In general, tissues should not remain in formalin for more than 24 to 48 hours before additional processing.
- For routine histology, refrigerate the tissue until fixation; never freeze the specimen before placing it in fixative. If the tissue is frozen, place it in fixative to thaw.
- When labeling, label both the container and the lid. If only the lid is labeled, samples may become inadvertently mixed during examination and processing by the pathologist.

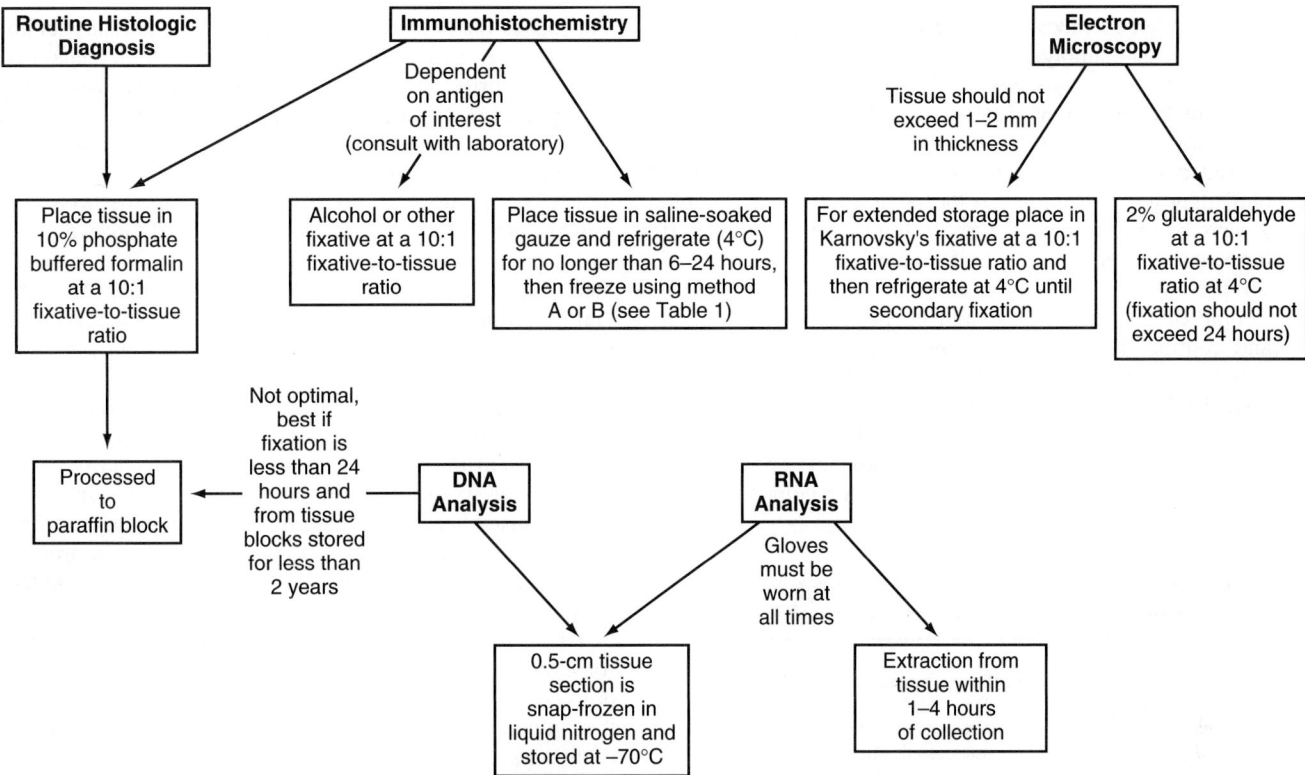

Figure 1. Proper handling of tissues for different diagnostic strategies.

- If you are submitting multiple tumors that are similar in characteristics (size, shape, and consistency), they should be placed in separate containers to help the pathologist distinguish each during the examination. Alternatively, additional specimens may be placed in separate, properly labeled tissue cassettes and included in the same formalin container, provided that the 10:1 ratio of fixative to tissue is maintained.
- Good communications with the diagnostic laboratory that you are using should be established to ensure proper handling of tissues and to maximize the benefit of laboratory examination.

IMMUNOHISTOCHEMISTRY

Immunohistochemistry is used for the evaluation of poorly differentiated neoplasms. It is an important tool for tumor typing, and its applications have improved the understanding of cellular differentiation. Immunohistochemistry often allows precise determination of the histogenesis of a neoplasm that would otherwise be characterized as undifferentiated on the basis of morphologic examination. The predominant sample in diagnostic pathology has been the formalin-fixed specimen processed to paraffin wax, sectioned and mounted on glass slides. Undoubtedly, this system will continue to be used most often for clinical specimens because of the need to rapidly establish a diagnosis based on histomorphologic criteria. For immunohistochemistry, however, an important problem is that the procedures necessary for making the paraffin block and processing tissue sections to slides often have detrimental effects on the tissue components of interest. Loss,

diffusion, reduction, chemical alteration, or masking of the antigen may result in negative immunohistochemical results.

Another factor that may influence the results of immunohistochemical staining procedures in the laboratory is storage of the unstained specimen on glass slides. In a study involving human breast cancer specimens collected in formalin, paraffin-embedded, and immunostained for the p53 antigen, the staining intensity was markedly reduced when the unstained glass slides were stored at room temperature (Jacobs et al, 1996). After 2 weeks, the staining intensity decreased to 31% of that recorded on day 0, by 4 weeks the staining intensity was 18% of that originally recorded, and by 12 weeks some cases originally considered positive were scored as negative. Storage of the unstained tissues on slides at 4°C did not prevent antigen loss, although the decline in immunoreactivity was not as rapid as that of the specimens stored at room temperature. Loss of staining intensity was also demonstrated for factor VIII antigen, estrogen receptor, and *bcl*-2 protein on slides stored at room temperature. Formalin-fixed specimens embedded in paraffin and stored at room temperature do not appear to lose antigenicity. Although antigen loss associated with storage of specimens is generally not a problem with clinical specimens when laboratory studies are done within a few days of collection, these results demonstrate, however, that slides destined for immunohistochemical studies should not be pre-cut and stored, but rather prepared anew from the original paraffin blocks for any procedures that are to be delayed for more than just a few days.

Tissue Processing. For immunohistochemical procedures, tissues need to be handled promptly by freezing or other fixation methods to preserve tissue antigens without allowing tissue autolysis to occur. Tissues can remain unfixed for 6 to 24 hours, with little deterioration, as long as they are handled properly following excision. For short-term storage, fresh tissues should be wrapped in saline-soaked gauze and refrigerated at 4°C (not frozen in ice) until they are transported to the laboratory. Saline should always be used to preserve the isotonicity of the tissue. If tap water is used, cellular artifact can result. For freezing, a representative area of the tissue should be cut, while a sample of the specimen should be preserved for fixation and routine morphologic examination. Table 1 outlines methods for snap-freezing of tissue specimens for immunohistochemical studies used in the authors' hospital.

Cryostat sections of frozen tissues offer the best opportunity for the demonstration of the broadest spectrum of antigens. Frozen sections are required for comprehensive

TABLE 1. Methods for Snap-Freezing of Tissue Specimens for Immunohistochemical Studies

Method A

1. Plastic cassettes (Tissue Tek, Baxter Diagnostics, Inc., McGaw Park, IL) are labeled with a marker pen.
2. Tissues to be placed in the cassettes should be no larger than two thirds of the capacity of the cassette used. The tissue is placed into the cassette, with the surface to be sectioned facing downward.
3. The tissue is then completely covered with optimal cutting temperature (OCT) embedding material (Tissue Tek, Baxter Diagnostics, Inc., McGaw Park, IL), filling the cassette well and minimizing bubble formation.
4. The cassette is placed in a beaker of isopentane (2-methylbutane) that has been cooled in liquid nitrogen. The isopentane has reached an adequately cool temperature when it begins to freeze on the inner surface of the beaker and it resembles Styrofoam. The tissue block should be left in the isopentane for 45 seconds.
5. Once frozen, the blocks are double-bagged in freezer bags to prevent desiccation and are stored in liquid nitrogen or in a freezer at −70°C.
6. When blocks are required for sectioning, they are taken from storage and placed in the cryostat. The temperature of tissues at the time of sectioning should not rise above −20°C. When the blocks have reached −20°C, the tissue specimen in the surrounding medium can be pushed out of the cassette onto a block holder with additional OCT medium for sectioning.
7. Once sections are taken, the tissue block and surrounding medium are double bagged and returned to cold storage.

Method B

1. Label 2.5-ml polyethylene sample vials with a marker pen and fill them one-half to one-third full with OCT medium, minimizing bubble formation.
2. Tissue specimens should be no larger than 10 × 10 × 5 mm and should be completely submerged in the OCT medium, oriented correctly to obviate the necessity of thawing the tissue for cutting.
3. The cap should be placed securely on the vial, which is then submerged directly into liquid nitrogen for at least 30 to 45 seconds.
4. Once frozen, the vials are double-bagged in freezer bags to prevent desiccation and are stored in liquid nitrogen or in a freezer at −70°C.
5. When vials containing tissue specimens are required for sectioning, they are taken from storage and placed in the cryostat. The temperature of tissues at the time of sectioning should not rise above −20°C. When temperature of the vial has reached −20°C, the tissue pellet in the surrounding medium can be pushed out of the vial and mounted on a block holder with additional OCT medium for sectioning.
6. Once sections are made, the tissue pellet and surrounding medium can be placed back into the vial, covered with OCT medium, and returned to cold storage.

analysis of the hematopoietic tumors because many leukocyte surface differentiation antigens are often denatured after even brief contact with formaldehyde. Further, many cell type markers, such as desmin, keratins, and vimentin, are also seen in higher numbers of tumor cells in frozen sections than in formaldehyde-fixed tissues. Many of the newly developed immunohistochemical methods for growth factors and/or their receptors, and oncogene-encoded proteins, often require frozen sections. On the other hand, more and more antibodies are becoming commercially available for formalin-fixed tissues. Furthermore, some markers require formaldehyde fixation and cannot be demonstrated on acetone- or alcohol-fixed frozen sections, because they are apparently soluble to those fixatives and are washed away. Among these are antigens such as S-100 protein, neuron-specific enolase, and alpha$_1$-antitrypsin. Duration of fixation in formaldehyde may also influence immunohistochemical results; for example, prolonged fixation of the specimen in formaldehyde will compromise immunohistochemical staining for proliferating cell nuclear antigen (PCNA). In some cases, alcohol fixation may be better than formaldehyde for preserving some antigens; for example, the antigenicity of intermediate filaments is preserved with ethanol and methanol fixation, including their modifications (Carnoy's fixative), and the advantages of this method over frozen section are convenience and better preservation of morphology.

Although the antigenicity of many epitopes are abolished or decreased after formalin fixation, some antigens are only hidden by the cross-linking nature of formaldehyde fixation and can be released by microwave or proteolytic enzyme predigestion; commonly used enzymes include trypsin, pronase, and pepsin. Because actual tissue fixation varies within different parts of the specimen, optimal immunostaining is often achieved in only a portion of the specimen, giving a patchy immunostaining pattern. Antigen retrieval methods pose an additional methodologic consideration, however, when one interprets the results of immunohistochemistry. Antigen retrieval procedures can result in an increase in reactivity of the target antigen by lowering the detection threshold for immunoreactivity. This may be an important consideration when one examines oncogene or tumor suppressor gene proteins, such as c-*erb*B2 or p53, when the stained slide is viewed in semiquantitative fashion as an index of gene expression.

Cytologic Immunostaining. Although not routinely done in veterinary medicine, immunostains of cytologic preparations may assist in the diagnostic process. If sufficient clinical material is procured, the specimen can be fixed in B5 fixative and prepared as a cell block. Cell blocks can be prepared from material washed out of the syringe with phosphate-buffered saline. For specimens too sparsely cellular for preparation of cell blocks, cytospin preparations can be prepared.

ELECTRON MICROSCOPY

Electron microscopic examination allows precise diagnosis when there are specific submicroscopic features of differentiation. For example, ultrastructural studies may assist in the diagnosis of malignant melanoma when melanin produced by the tumor cells is minute and is not readily discerned by routine electron microscopy. The melanocytic nature of malignant melanoma may be confirmed in these cases by detection of melanosomes or premelanosomes.

Fixation of the specimen is the most important single procedure in the processes involved in biologic electron microscopy. *Commercial formaldehyde, as used routinely in histologic preparations, is a poor fixative* for ultrastructure because its methanol content may act as a coagulative fixative and protein denaturant. The ideal fixation preserves every detail of cellular ultrastructure as it was in life the instant before the specimen was collected. Fixation must be rapid and certain, and optimally fixation should occur within seconds of collection. Tissues are carefully sliced into small cubes not exceeding 1 to 2 mm in thickness with the use of a sharp razor or scalpel blade and are placed immediately into the proper fixative. Two-stage fixation procedures that use glutaraldehyde buffered with phosphate of cacodylate followed by osmium tetroxide are almost universally used. Two percent glutaraldehyde (10 parts fixative per 1 part tissue) in a 0.05 to 0.1 M phosphate buffer at pH 7.2 is a superior fixative for ultrastructural detail, but it slowly penetrates into tissue, which may allow the center of thick specimens to autolyze. Glutaraldehyde fixation is optimized when the fixative is stored at 4°C or is prepared fresh, the pH adjusted and allowed to warm to room temperature immediately before the tissue is introduced. After 1 or 2 hours at room temperature, the specimen in the tissue fixative is again cooled to 4°C, the total primary fixation time being 1 to 3 hours to overnight.

Karnovsky's fixative, a combination of paraformaldehyde and glutaraldehyde, combines the fixation potency of glutaraldehyde and the rapid fixation advantage of formaldehyde. A modification of Karnovsky's fixative is used in the authors' hospital. The fixative is 2.5% glutaraldehyde and 2% paraformaldehyde, in a 0.05 to 0.1 M phosphate or cacodylate buffer. The specimen is otherwise handled as noted previously for glutaraldehyde with postfixation in osmium tetroxide.

DIAGNOSTIC MOLECULAR TECHNIQUES

Increasing data regarding genetic changes that are often specifically associated with particular types of tumors are being derived from molecular oncology. These tests are based on demonstration of molecular changes, at the nucleotide level, that occur in tumor cells. These procedures involve the isolation of DNA, RNA, or protein from tumor cells and the analysis of their components for abnormalities related to the presence, absence, or amplification of a specific gene or its products or other alterations such as chromosome translocation.

One important consideration in the use of molecular techniques to detect or characterize tumor cells is the lower limit of detection of the tumor cells within the host's constituent tissues or within the inflammatory or scirrhous response to that tumor. This issue may prove to be important for the clinical veterinarian, as new technologies are applied to specimens collected from regions previously treated for cancer or, perhaps, from sites of possible metastasis such as the regional lymph nodes, that is, for the detection of minimal residual disease and/or metastasis. In

comparative studies, reverse transcriptase-polymerase chain reaction (RT-PCR) was more sensitive than immunohistochemical techniques, although in other studies that used rigorous immunohistochemical or immunofluorescent procedures comparable results were obtained (Pelkey et al, 1996). For example, using anticytokeratin antibodies or melanoma-specific or epithelial-specific antibodies in immunohistochemical procedures, the lower limit of detection of the respective tumor cells in model systems ranged from $1/10^4$ to $1/10^6$ (tumor cells detected/nucleated hematopoietic cells). Using RT-PCR for the detection of prostate-specific antigen within prostate tumor cells, or tyrosine hydroxylase mRNA within melanoma cells, or tyrosine hydroxylase mRNA within neuroblastoma cells, the lower limit of detection was within the range of $1/10^6$ to $1/10^7$.

DNA-Based Techniques. The DNA-based techniques used most often in diagnostics include Southern (dot or slot) hybridization, PCR, ligase chain reaction, in situ hybridization, in situ PCR, and DNA sequencing. In Southern hybridization, nucleic acid probes are employed to analyze genetic material in clinical specimens with the use of electrophoretic blotting techniques. Probes are used to diagnose neoplastic, infectious, or genetic diseases. Difficulties with the use of Southern blot analysis in diagnostic pathology are its low sensitivity for the detection of altered DNA (1 to 5%), the need to obtain DNA from fresh tissues, and the length of time required for a result (several days). The PCR is an in vitro enzymatic method, allowing several million-fold amplification of a specific nucleic acid sequence. Polymerase chain reaction facilitates nucleic acid–based detection systems for genetic disorders, as well as for diseases caused by viruses, bacteria, and other pathogens, and is particularly suited to clinically procured specimen because unlike other biologic procedures it does not require high-molecular-weight DNA for successful amplification. Ligase chain reaction is a technique that is exceptionally well-suited for the detection of known mutations. In situ hybridization is used to demonstrate nucleic acid sequences within cells; it is used for localizing nucleic acid targets in the context of histomorphology. In situ hybridization detects and identifies DNA (or RNA) and is analogous to immunohistochemistry, giving a detectable reaction product that can be visualized and correlated with corresponding tissue or cell morphology. In situ PCR combines PCR with in situ hybridization and permits the localization of specific amplified DNA segments within isolated cells and sections of tissue.

RNA-Based Techniques. For RNA, the most popular techniques include RT-PCR, in situ hybridization, RNase protection assay, and Northern blot hybridization. Changes in cellular mRNA levels constitute an important feature of gene expression; examination of these changes facilitates understanding of the mechanisms by which regulated gene expression contributes to the control of biologic functions. A variety of methods are used to quantitate mRNA levels, including Northern dot or slot blots, in situ hybridization, and quantitative RT-PCR. Northern blot analysis is not sufficiently sensitive to detect low-abundance mRNA and has relatively limited clinical use because of the relative instability of RNA and the fact that it requires relatively large amounts of RNA and, therefore, a large number of cells (10^8 or 10^9). In situ RNA hybridization has the advantage of detecting specific mRNAs in individual cells, but it is time-consuming and it does not allow accurate quantitation of mRNA levels. Quantitative RT-PCR methods are now available as extremely sensitive techniques for the detection of low-abundance mRNA. RT-PCR allows detection of minute quantities of mRNA from submicrogram amounts of total mRNA, and it is the preferred method for the detection and quantitation of mRNA when the particular transcript is very rare or restricted in its cellular distribution. The RNase protection assay is a sensitive technique used to detect and measure low-abundance, specific mRNAs in a sample of total cellular RNA. The RNase protection assay is now considered the most reliable method for the detection and quantitation of mRNA levels (Ma et al, 1996).

HANDLING OF TUMOR MATERIAL

Solid Tumors. If it is anticipated that the specimen collected will be used for genetic analysis, for either additional clinical tests, or for research purposes, it may be useful to divide the freshly isolated tumor into two equal portions with a sterile disposable scalpel. Slices taken from the outer, visible, cellular region of one half of the specimen are snap-frozen in liquid nitrogen, whereas corresponding slices from the other half are prepared for histopathologic examinations.

In the laboratory, frozen tissue samples are thawed quickly. The DNA yield is enhanced if the tissue is first minced or chopped as finely as possible. This chopping should be done as quickly as possible on a cold surface to minimize DNA degradation by any nucleases present.

For tissues submitted for DNA-based tests, it is often important to know that the DNA test is being done on the appropriate piece of tissue. One way of making certain that the tissue is appropriate is to snap-freeze the tissue in liquid nitrogen. Before DNA analysis, obtain a thin section, 6 μm, of the tissue and stain it with hematoxylin and eosin. Have a pathologist examine the specimen by light microscopy to ascertain the tissue contains the cells of interest.

Retrospective analysis of DNA is often possible with the use of fixed tissues because of the fact that part of the cellular DNA is intact in paraffin-embedded, fixed tissues, as previously demonstrated by flow cytometry or in situ hybridization studies (Crisan and Mattson, 1993). The ability to perform genetic analysis on formalin-fixed tissues has allowed investigators access to the vast archival resource of well-characterized tissues. Indeed, the use of decades-old archival tissues for PCR has been shown to be feasible (Iwamoto et al, 1996). DNA derived from fixed tissues is generally less efficient for molecular analyses than either purified DNA or DNA in crude extracts from fresh tissues. The best fixative for retrospective DNA analysis is neutral buffered formalin, although 25 to 50% of specimens collected in formalin may not yield good, high-molecular-weight DNA. Tissues fixed in methanol or ethanol also contain extractable DNA, and indeed even air-dried Romanowsky-stained smears of blood or bone marrow may also be used as sources of DNA. Fixation-induced DNA

degradation, for formalin-fixed tissues, is due primarily to cross-linking of proteins to DNA. Other fixatives containing mercuric acid, such as B5 and Zenker's, result in more extensive degradation of DNA. The extraction of DNA from fixed tissues roughly parallels the methods used to extract high-molecular-weight DNA from fresh tissues. It must be remembered, however, that DNA extracted from tissues actually represents the DNA derived from a heterogeneous collection of different types of cells and phenotypes, and the extracted DNA represents an average phenotype. All spatial relationships and subtle differences in cellular phenotypes, which are often critical for histologic diagnosis, are lost.

Fixation times influence the resultant extractable DNA. Fixation time also influences the ability to amplify DNA. Fixation of the tissue specimen in neutral buffered formalin generally yields abundant amplification products from tissues fixed up to 24 hours, but reduction in amplification efficiency occurs for tissues fixed for longer periods, reducing the product yield (Greer et al, 1991). Also, the length of time the tissue block is stored may influence results. Although DNA was still derived from tissues stored in paraffin for 5 years or more, the size of the DNA fragments obtained from blocks stored 2 years or more was smaller than that of DNA fragments derived from blocks less than 2 years old (Goelz et al, 1985).

The use of microdissected archival material (tissue dissected from glass slides) is not without drawbacks, however, and difficulties arise from small sample size and poor quality of DNA. The degraded DNA derived from fixed tissues is usually a mixture of fragments ranging in size from 100 to 2,400 base pairs (bp), although in some cases the DNA is so degraded that it is not useful for some procedures, such as Southern hybridization or PCR. One way of overcoming the problem of degraded DNA for PCR is to amplify short regions of less than 200 bp. Another difficulty is that oligonucleotide primers are usually designed to analyze genomic DNA, rather that paraffin-embedded material. It is important to determine how well these oligonucleotides will perform with archival material. If DNA degradation and low quantity are issues, it may be necessary to use nested primers. This technique involves an initial amplification that produces a small amount of a specific product, usually undetectable on ethidium bromide–stained gels. A small portion of this first PCR product is then amplified in a second amplification step initiated with primers that hybridize to sites within the original set.

The general procedure for PCR extraction from paraffin-embedded tissues involves de-waxing and purification of DNA by proteinase K digestion, followed by phenol-chloroform extraction. The goal of these procedures is to make available DNA of good quality—double stranded, high molecular weight, and cleavable by restriction endonucleases.

Blood. Blood is a commonly used source of biologic material for diagnostic purposes. Porphyrin compounds derived from heme are inhibitors of PCR, and PCR samples that contain enough hemoglobin to produce a slightly red discoloration show inhibition (Panaccio et al, 1994). Heparin is also reported to inhibit PCR amplification. These problems can be overcome by purifying DNA from white blood cells prior to PCR. Blood for DNA-based testing should be collected in EDTA (ethylenediaminetetraacetic acid, lavender-top) or ACD (acid-citrate-dextrose, yellow-top) tubes. The red blood cells are then lysed with a detergent such as ammonium chloride, or by separation of the nucleated cells by buffy coat preparation. For DNA, 10^6 cells will yield 5 to 10 μg of DNA, which is sufficient for a single lane on a Southern blot and adequate for many PCR amplifications (at 100 ng per amplification). It is important to extensively rinse the nuclear pellet prior to PCR processing. If DNA is extracted from nucleated blood cells, a patient with a normal leukocyte count will provide good DNA yields, in the range of 10 to 40 μg/ml of whole blood (Farkas et al, 1996). DNA can also be procured from clotted blood (red-top tube), but the specimen needs to be homogenized to disrupt the clot. Similarly, high-quality DNA can be obtained from bone marrow aspirates; it is best to refrigerate the specimens until DNA extraction begins, and particles and fragments should first be disrupted by homogenization.

Of particular interest in hematology is extraction of DNA from blood smears. A suitable way of preserving blood and bone marrow aspirate samples for retrospective DNA analysis is to make air-dried smears on slides and to store them at ambient temperature. The smears may also be ethanol- or methanol-fixed on the slides. One important consideration in the use of blood smears for DNA extraction is the number of nucleated cells on the smear; several smears are needed because whole blood contains fewer nucleated cells than does bone marrow aspirates. It was estimated that with a total leukocyte count of 5,000/μl of blood, a 100-μl blood smear contained about 500,000 cells, or approximately 3 μg of nuclear DNA (Crisan and Mattson, 1993).

Handling and Storage of DNA. DNA is relatively stable. Long-term storage should occur at temperatures that range from −70° to −140°C; all chemical reactions essentially stop at −140°C. DNA remains stable in solid tissue kept at −70°C for at least 2 years (Farkas et al, 1996). DNA processed from the tumor is stable for up to 26 weeks at 23° to 25°C and up to 1 year if contaminating nucleases are absent. Prolonged storage of processed DNA after the initial testing has been completed should be at −70°C, where it will remain stable for as long as 7 years. EDTA buffer is the ideal solvent for long-term storage of DNA. EDTA in TE buffer chelates divalent cations, which are necessary cofactors for nuclease activity. DNA is protected from the activity of nucleases at temperatures below 0°C, but as solutions are thawed, nucleases may act, even in the presence of EDTA. The specimen should be divided into portions of proper unit size for storage to avoid repeated freeze-thaw cycles.

Procedures to properly label and track specimens must be clearly established so that the specimens are not lost in the laboratory. Temperatures, freeze-thaw cycles, desiccation, and contamination all may affect the quality of the stored specimens. The extent to which these factors will influence subsequent procedures probably varies with the type of specimen stored and the type of test subsequently conducted; nevertheless, good laboratory practices should be in place so that the specimens are not rendered useless as a consequence of improper storage.

Handling and Storage of RNA. For RNA, its lability and the ubiquity of RNases demand special precautions. The specimen should be handled with gloves. Solid tissues should be quickly snap-frozen; however, if snap-freezing cannot be accomplished, RNA extraction should commence in the laboratory within 1 to 4 hours. RNA will remain stable in solid tissues stored at 23° to 25°C for only 5 minutes or less, and for only 1 hour when stored at 2° to 8°C. Solid tissues for subsequent RNA analysis should not be stored long term at −20°C, but rather at −70°C, at which temperature it will remain stable for as long as 2 years. For long-term storage of processed RNA, it is best stored as a precipitate in ethanol at −70°C, at which temperature it will remain stable indefinitely. RNA should be stored in sterile, hydrophobic plastic tubes that have not been handled with ungloved hands and that optimally have been treated with diethylcarbonate water to rid the tubes of RNases, which are stable, ubiquitous proteins that function without cofactors. The most common source of RNases is the skin, and so gloves must be worn at all times in the laboratory when one works with RNA.

RT-PCR is a widely used technique for studying mRNA derived from tumor specimens. The mRNA is extracted from blood or bone marrow cells or tumor, usually with the use of guanidinium thiocyanate–phenol–chloroform techniques or variations of this method. The mRNA is then converted into cDNA through the use of specific primers and the enzyme reverse transcriptase. The cDNA is then amplified by PCR, and after gel electrophoresis of the PCR product the presence of the amplified product is identified either by ethidium bromide staining and examination under ultraviolet light or by Southern blot analysis with labeled hybridization probes.

TRENDS

In recent years, there has been a marked change in the role of the clinical pathologist and pathologist in clinical oncology. The modern pathologist has expanded his or her domain from tumor classification to a more interactive role with the surgeon, radiation oncologist, and medical oncologist. The diagnostic pathologist–clinical pathologist has been instrumental in bringing techniques derived from basic research into the diagnostic laboratory, and sophisticated technologies like flow cytometry, immunohistochemistry, and molecular oncology are now being used for patient management in diagnosis, treatment planning, and assessment of prognosis. Although specimens obtained by small needle biopsy, often procured in the outpatient clinic, have expedited clinical sampling, these small specimens have created additional problems for both clinicians and laboratory personnel. The small sample size has resulted in a considerable increase in the responsibilities of the workers handling these specimens. To ensure that analytic tests can be done effectively and accurately, methods such as those highlighted in this section of the book for sample collection, transport to the laboratory, and storage in the laboratory must be in place. It is anticipated that these newly understood attributes of neoplasms, based on biologic and molecular parameters, in concert with the histomorphologic diagnosis, will influence the management of veterinary cancer patients.

References and Suggested Reading

Crisan D, Mattson JC: Retrospective DNA analysis using fixed tissue specimens. DNA Cell Biol 12:455, 1993.
Critically evaluates the factors that influence the quality of DNA that can be derived from formalin-fixed, paraffin-embedded tissues.

Farkas DH, Kaul KL, Wiedbrauk DL, et al: Specimen collection and storage for diagnostic molecular pathology investigation. Arch Pathol Lab Med 120:591, 1996.
Describes methods for collection and storage of specimens used in diagnostic molecular techniques.

Goelz SE, Hamilton SR, Vogelstein B: Purification of DNA from formaldehyde fixed and paraffin embedded human tissue. Biochem Biophys Res Commun 130:118, 1985.
Describes methods for extraction of DNA from formalin-fixed, paraffin-embedded tissues.

Greer CE, Peterson SL, Kiviat NB, et al: PCR amplification from paraffin-embedded tissues: Effects of fixation and fixation time. Am J Clin Pathol 95:117, 1991.
Examination of effects of fixatives and fixation times on DNA derived from paraffin-embedded tissues for amplification procedures.

Iwamoto KS, Mizuno T, Ito T, et al: Feasibility of using decades-old archival tissues in molecular oncology-epidemiology. Am J Pathol 149:399, 1996.
Feasibility and limitations of using decades-old archival materials for molecular epidemiologic studies.

Jacobs TW, Prioleau JE, Stillman IE, et al: Loss of tumor marker–immunostaining intensity on stored paraffin slides of breast cancer. J Natl Cancer Inst 88:1054, 1996.
Critical study of the loss of p53 (and other antigen) immunostaining from tissues cut onto glass slides and stored for short periods at room temperature.

Ma YJ, Dissen GA, Rage F, et al: RNase protection assay. Methods 10:273, 1996.
Reviews the RNase protection assay for the detection and quantitation of mRNA.

Miettinen M: Immunohistochemistry of solid tumors: Brief review of selected problems. APMIS 98:191, 1990.
Reviews selected problems associated with immunohistochemistry involving solid tumors.

Panaccio M, Good RT, Reed MB: A road map for PCR from clinical material. J Clin Lab Anal 8:315, 1994.
Reviews methods for collecting clinical specimens for polymerase chain reaction to minimize inhibitory substances.

Pelkey TJ, Frierson HF, Bruns DE: Molecular and immunologic detection of circulating tumor cells and micrometastases from solid tumors. Clin Chem 42:1369, 1996.
Compares the lower limits of detection of tumor cells in biologic material with the use of immunologic and molecular methods.

Nutritional Support of the Cancer Patient

GLENNA E. MAULDIN
Baton Rouge, Louisiana

Cancer cachexia is the unique form of protein-calorie malnutrition that commonly occurs in both human and veterinary cancer patients. Evidence of cancer cachexia is present in as many as 80% of humans with cancer, although the reported incidence varies with the type of malignancy and the sensitivity of the means of nutritional assessment. The syndrome is typically characterized by one or more of three clinical findings: diminished host nutrient intake; progressive host weight loss; and the presence of numerous distinctive clinicopathologic abnormalities.

The detrimental effects of protein-calorie malnutrition in human patients are well documented and include anemia, hypoproteinemia, delayed wound healing, decreased immunocompetence, and compromise of gastrointestinal, pulmonary, and cardiovascular function. Severe debilitation and eventual death are the result in affected individuals. Therefore, it is not surprising that the presence of cancer cachexia also carries great clinical significance. In fact, along with tumor type, stage of disease, and performance status, weight loss has been shown repeatedly to be an independent determinant of prognosis in the human cancer patient. Thus, the importance of accurate nutritional assessment and early nutritional intervention in malnourished patients with neoplastic disease cannot be overemphasized. This article briefly reviews the current understanding of the pathophysiology of cancer cachexia, discusses some practical methods of nutritional assessment for veterinary patients, and makes specific recommendations for the nutritional support of the small animal cancer patient.

THEORETICAL CONSIDERATIONS

Weight loss occurs in the tumor-bearing host for two basic reasons: (1) nutrient intake is often reduced because of the physical effects of the tumor itself or the therapies used to treat it; and (2) alternatively or concurrently, metabolic changes secondary to the presence of the malignancy result in inefficient energy utilization. It is clear that many tumors have a negative impact on host nutritional status, simply owing to their location or size: for instance, large intraoral masses may prevent normal food intake, while diffuse neoplastic infiltration of the small bowel may significantly disrupt normal digestion or absorption of nutrients. It is also well established that decreased food intake may occur secondary to various anticancer therapies. Cancer treatment in human patients is often associated with important abnormalities in nutrient intake, digestion, and absorption because of the nausea, vomiting, mucositis, and diarrhea caused by radiation or chemotherapy.

While the potential role of physical factors such as those described previously is immediately apparent, the unique biochemical alterations associated with the tumor-bearing state have proved to be the most intriguing aspect of cancer cachexia. Certain specific metabolic abnormalities play an incompletely defined role in the pathogenesis of cancer cachexia: it is hypothesized that they are associated with inefficient energy utilization by the host, which results in accelerated weight loss. Many investigators have studied both human cancer patients and rodents bearing implanted tumors in great detail, in an attempt to further elucidate these mechanisms. A number of important principles have emerged from this work. First, tumor cells have an obligate requirement for glucose and are incapable of significant fat oxidation or aerobic glycolysis: they must derive energy from anaerobic glycolysis. Glucose consumed by tumor glycolysis is lost to the host, and furthermore host hepatocytes then resynthesize glucose from the lactate produced. This version of the Cori cycle operates entirely at the expense of the host's energy. Second, many tumor cells are characterized by high metabolic activity and rapid growth. Accelerated catabolism of host lean body mass is necessary to provide a constant supply of amino acids for these functions. Mobilized amino acids are utilized for energy, after being metabolized by the host to glucose through gluconeogenesis, as well as for various anabolic processes within the tumor cell. Finally, numerous host hormones and cytokines are released in response to the presence of neoplastic disease, and these compounds can have both local and distant effects on host metabolic processes. Inefficient energy utilization in wide-ranging host tissues may be the outcome.

Numerous specific and characteristic abnormalities in the intermediary metabolism of all three energy substrates—carbohydrate, protein, and lipid—have been demonstrated in human cancer patients as well as tumor-bearing rodents, and they are not described in detail here; the reader is referred to several excellent reviews on this subject (Brennan, 1977; Kern and Norton, 1988; Ogilvie, 1996). However, each of these changes is ultimately the result of the disruptions in host metabolism described previously and appears to be associated with processes resulting in host weight loss. Both lean body mass and adipose stores are affected. Interestingly, recent work by veterinary investigators suggests that very similar metabolic perturbations are present in dogs with naturally occurring neoplastic disease. Dogs with lymphoma have been studied in greatest detail (Vail et al, 1990; Ogilvie et al, 1994). Canine lymphoma is useful as a potential model of cancer cachexia, because it is a naturally occurring disease in an outbred patient population. Some caution must be exercised in translating the results of these studies to cachectic human patients, because many of the dogs studied to date do not show significant weight loss. Nonetheless, the close similarities in demonstrated biochemical abnormalities in these dogs compared with human cancer patients certainly makes them worthy of further study. Weight-stable dogs with lymphoma have been demonstrated to have increased resting serum lactate concentrations; increased lactate production in response to infusion of intravenous dextrose solutions; hyperinsulinism and insulin resistance, presumably the result of a post–insulin receptor defect; altered serum amino acid profiles; increased serum concentrations of triglycerides, nonesterified fatty acids, and very-low-density lipoprotein (VLDL); and

decreased serum concentrations of high-density lipoprotein (HDL). Less is known regarding other tumor types, but preliminary results suggest that disruption of normal energy metabolism is likely in dogs and cats with a wide variety of neoplastic diseases and may contribute to clinically significant weight loss.

Theoretically, host energy expenditure should be altered as a consequence of the changes in flux through the various metabolic pathways described earlier. Increased metabolic activity and futile cycling, such as that which may occur through the Cori cycle, should result in increased host energy expenditure. The ultimate result would be host weight loss. Accordingly, both human and veterinary investigators have measured host energy expenditure, primarily by indirect calorimetry, in an attempt to quantify the potential energy lost through these pathways. Unfortunately, the results of these studies are variable and difficult to interpret. Energy expenditure seems to vary with tumor type and stage of disease. It appears to be increased in some studies, is apparently unchanged in others, and may actually be decreased in still others. One valid conclusion must be that significant variation exists in energy expenditure and the manifestations of cancer cachexia, not only between tumor types but also between individuals with the same tumor, depending on the stage of their disease. However, one must also consider several additional explanations for these findings. First of all, the methodology involved in indirect calorimetry is complex, and results may be difficult to consistently reproduce. Second, selection of the best controls for such studies is problematic; some authors compare their cachectic cancer patients to young, healthy, weight-stable control subjects, while others insist that the only appropriate comparison is between weight-losing cancer patients and weight-losing patients with nonmalignant disease. Finally, the analysis of results is further complicated in veterinary patients, because the true energy requirements of even healthy dogs and cats are controversial and incompletely defined. It is hoped that ongoing work by both veterinary and human investigators in this area will clarify some of the current inconsistencies.

NUTRITIONAL ASSESSMENT

Understanding the pathophysiology of cancer cachexia serves no practical purpose for the veterinary clinician, unless there is some means by which to identify affected animals. A systematic method allowing determination of the etiology and severity of malnutrition, identification of patients requiring specialized nutritional intervention, and prediction of patients at greatest risk for the development of malnutrition and its related complications would allow initiation of the most appropriate, specific, and presumably successful nutritional therapy possible. In human clinical nutrition, the process of gathering data to answer these questions is called nutritional assessment. It involves obtaining a detailed dietary history, a complete physical examination, and morphometric, hematologic, and biochemical evaluations. This science is still in its infancy in small animal veterinary medicine, but enough is known that some general recommendations can be made.

A detailed diet history and physical examination are the initial components of a complete nutritional assessment.

The diet history must include specific information about the quantity and content of the patient's present diet, as well as the animal's diet prior to illness (these may differ significantly), and any medications or nutritional supplements currently being administered by the owner. Physical examination of the cat or dog suffering from cancer cachexia may reveal one or more nonspecific clinical signs of malnutrition, including muscle wasting, pallor, poor haircoat, hepatomegaly or splenomegaly, evidence of chronic infections, lymphadenopathy, or peripheral edema. Specific or pathognomonic clinical signs of malnutrition are unfortunately much rarer, but a good example is the central retinal degeneration and dilated cardiomyopathy characteristic of taurine deficiency in the cat.

In human patients, lean body mass and body fat stores are evaluated primarily through morphometric measurements such as triceps skinfold thickness and midarm circumference. Adapting these specific techniques for use in cats and dogs is difficult, because of the large variation in body size and conformation among different breeds. However, careful monitoring of body weight as well as consistent use of a standardized body condition scoring system provides the veterinarian with much of the same information. Body condition scoring systems generally utilize a five- or nine-point system, where each point corresponds to a particular body condition with defined criteria; that is, "cachectic" (no obvious body fat), through "optimal" (ribs easily palpable), to "obese" (large deposits of subcutaneous and abdominal fat). These classifications provide at least an initial assessment of a small animal patient's lean body mass and adipose stores (Kronfeld et al, 1991).

Finally, although relatively insensitive as nutritional markers, several hematologic and biochemical parameters easily available to the veterinarian can provide additional information. Cancer cachexia and the effects of protein-calorie malnutrition may result in anemia and decreased total lymphocyte counts in some patients. Animals suffering from significant protein deficiency may also have decreased serum albumin concentrations. However, the serum half-life of this protein is relatively long (approximately 8 days in the dog); thus, an extended period of protein deprivation is required before concentrations fall below the normal range. A more sensitive means of nutritional assessment, at least in the cat, may be determination of serum creatine kinase concentrations. Recent work has shown that serum creatine kinase concentrations increase rapidly in the cat during anorexia, and decrease dramatically after initiation of supportive alimentation (Fascetti et al, 1997). Further study is required to determine whether serum creatine kinase concentration is a useful marker of nutritional status in the dog.

DIETARY RECOMMENDATIONS

Specifically targeted nutritional support should help improve body condition in veterinary cancer patients identified through nutritional assessment as being malnourished, or at risk for becoming malnourished. Palatable, highly digestible, or energy-dense diets could reverse some of the deleterious nutritional effects of neoplastic disease and cancer treatment. Potential benefits to the cancer patient include improved ability to tolerate aggressive antineoplastic therapy, enhanced quality of life, and, even, increased survival times. Rations can also be designed to take advantage of the metabolic differences between tumor cells and normal host tissues. Diets with a relatively high fat content are preferred, because they should preferentially provide energy to the patient. Diets that are high in carbohydrate should be avoided. Readily available sugars may supply additional energy to the tumor; furthermore, host utilization of carbohydrate calories may be inefficient because of insulin resistance. Beneficial effects have been documented in human cancer patients fed such diets, including improved weight gain, improved energy and nitrogen balance, improved preservation of body adipose stores, and decreased glucose intolerance.

The optimal dietary protein intake in small animal patients with neoplastic disease is unknown, and somewhat controversial. Some authors recommend relative protein restriction, in an effort both to limit the nitrogen available to the tumor for anabolism and to decrease the host's rate of gluconeogenesis from amino acids. Obviously, each patient must be carefully evaluated on an individual basis, but the protein content of any ration fed to a cat or dog with cancer also needs to be adequate to meet the potentially increased requirements that may be encountered when neoplastic disease is complicated by systemic conditions such as sepsis. Investigators studying hospitalized canine patients with a variety of critical illnesses were recently able to document high rates of urinary nitrogen loss, a reflection of accelerated protein catabolism (Michel et al, 1997). Loss of lean tissue among many of the dogs in this study who had no food intake was over 200 gm per dog per day. It seems probable that critically ill canine and feline cancer patients have equally high protein requirements, and thus they may require as many as 30 to 50% of their total daily calories as protein. This requirement should be especially true in critically ill feline patients, who rapidly develop life-threatening protein-calorie malnutrition. Cats are unable to effectively conserve lean body mass, because the potentially increased protein requirements of illness are superimposed on an unusually high basal protein requirement in this species. This requirement is the result, in part, of obligatory gluconeogenesis from amino acids and continuous cycling of hepatic transaminases and urea cycle enzymes.

Based on these theoretical and practical considerations, a high-fat (i.e., greater than 40 to 50% of calories), restricted-carbohydrate, highly palatable and digestible ration that contains ample protein is recommended for use in small animal cancer patients. Definitive recommendations regarding the specific dietary intake of other nutrients such as glutamine, arginine, omega-3 fatty acids, and antioxidants must await the publication of controlled studies. Either canned or dry foods may be appropriate, although it is useful to remember that dry foods are often more energy dense than canned products. Rations should be complete and balanced: a commercial pet food produced by a reputable manufacturer is the safest and most convenient way of avoiding micronutrient deficiencies or excesses. In general, the types of rations most likely to fit the outlined profile include "premium" canned or dry products for cats or dogs, canned or dry products designed for use during performance or stress, and dry or canned kitten or puppy foods.

SUPPORTIVE ALIMENTATION

It is vital to recognize that many of the veterinary cancer patients who would benefit most from the types of dietary therapy outlined previously are unwilling or unable to eat for themselves, and have inadequate voluntary food intake. Every effort should be made to encourage animals to eat on their own, including hand-feeding of highly palatable foods. Provision of small, frequent meals may also improve food intake in animals with inconsistent appetites. However, despite these measures, caloric intake will still be marginal in many patients. Feeding tubes or catheters should be placed without hesitation in animals with persistent anorexia, to ensure maintenance of optimal nutrient intake.

The use of pharmacologic appetite stimulants for anorectic small animal cancer patients is advised by some authors (see p. 69). Various benzodiazepine derivatives, most commonly diazepam (Valium, Roche Laboratories), as well as the drug cyproheptadine (Periactin, Merck Sharp & Dohme), have been reported to increase food intake in dogs and cats. However, objective evidence supporting the clinical efficacy of these compounds is generally lacking. Careful monitoring of actual food intake frequently reveals that although consumption may be transiently increased immediately after drug administration, the overall food intake over longer periods is unchanged. Furthermore, appropriate and necessary placement of feeding tubes is frequently delayed while the clinician awaits a response to medication. For these reasons, it is difficult to recommend the routine use of these drugs in anorectic dogs and cats with cancer.

Enteral Nutrition

Reviews describing enteral nutrition in veterinary patients have been published (Davenport, 1995; Wheeler and McGuire, 1989). With few exceptions, enteral feeding is superior to parenteral or intravenous feeding. Enteral nutrition helps prevent intestinal mucosal atrophy and bacterial translocation from the gut (p. 139), is cheaper and technically less complex than parenteral feeding, and has fewer potential complications. The potential disadvantages of enteral nutrition include extended periods of transition, and contraindication in situations in which the gastrointestinal tract is nonfunctional.

Several different types of feeding tubes are available for delivery of enteral nutrition in small animal cancer patients. Nasoesophageal tubes are indicated for relatively short-term support in patients who are anorectic but have normal gastrointestinal function, in patients who have oropharyngeal disease that prevents normal food intake, and in patients who are too critically ill to tolerate the general anesthesia required for placement of most other types of feeding tubes. Gastrostomy tubes are a better choice for those patients who require long-term nutritional support, because they can often be left in place indefinitely. They are also useful in animals who are anorectic but have normal gastrointestinal tract function, and in patients with oropharyngeal disease. Jejunostomy tubes allow bypass of the entire upper gastrointestinal tract, including the stomach and pancreas, and so they can be used to support animals with persistent vomiting, gastric outflow obstructions, and pancreatitis.

The ideal tube feeding formula for canine and feline cancer patients has the same characteristics as the ideal commercial ration: high in fat, ample protein calories, relatively restricted simple carbohydrates, and complete and balanced with regard to micronutrients. A very-calorie-dense formula (i.e., high fat) also minimizes the volume that must be fed through the tube. Liquid commercial veterinary products specifically designed for tube feeding (CliniCare, Abbott Laboratories) are generally the best choices for nasoesophageal and jejunostomy tubes, while paste-type formulations (Eukanuba Nutritional Recovery Formula/Canine & Feline, The Iams Company; Hill's Prescription Diet Canine/Feline a/d, Hill's Pet Products, Inc.) or canned cat or dog food that has been put through a blender may be fed through gastrostomy tubes. It is important to remember that human enteral feeding products are not complete and balanced for use in dogs and cats. Initial bolus feeding should be administered every 2 hours, with the use of a small volume of dilute formula. If this ration is well tolerated, the concentration and volume can gradually be increased until the patient is finally receiving the full target volume in 4 to 6 daily feedings. This process usually takes at least 3 to 4 days, and in some patients it takes even longer. Constant-rate infusion, rather than bolus feeding techniques, is preferred with jejunostomy tubes.

Parenteral Nutrition

Parenteral nutrition is the only option for nutritional support in small animal cancer patients that cannot tolerate enteral feeding (see p. 80). The primary indication for parenteral nutrition is a nonfunctional intestinal tract, such as may occur with intractable vomiting, gastrointestinal obstruction, or severe ileus. Parenteral nutrition is also considered primary therapy for certain types of inflammatory gastrointestinal lesions, such as pancreatitis or severe inflammatory colitis. The major advantage of parenteral nutrition in these situations is that it permits complete bowel rest. Parenteral nutrition can also be utilized in patients that are too critically ill to tolerate the general anesthesia that may be required for the placement of some enteral feeding tubes. Finally, coma is another potential indication—the risk of aspiration is significantly decreased when intravenous feeding is used to support such patients. However, regardless of the underlying disease being treated, parenteral nutrition is usually not considered unless a veterinary patient is expected to require support for at least 3 to 5 days, because of its cost and complexity.

The major disadvantages of parenteral nutrition are the development of significant intestinal mucosal atrophy after long-term use; an increased incidence of bacterial translocation from the gut; the necessity for specialized equipment, products, and care; and increased expense. In addition, an increased potential for complications exists with parenteral nutrition compared with enteral feeding. The possible complications include an increased risk of sepsis, mechanical complications such as catheter disconnection and twisted intravenous lines, and biochemical complications such as hyperglycemia and hyperlipidemia.

The parenteral nutrition prescription for a dog or cat with cancer should be designed to follow the same principles as the enteral diets described previously. The dextrose content should be relatively restricted, providing a maximum of 30 to 40% of nonprotein calories. The fat content should be relatively increased, providing 60 to 70% of nonprotein calories. Sufficient protein must be supplied to meet requirements, and this level is currently estimated to be 4 to 6 gm/kg per day in canine cancer patients with normal hepatic and renal function, and 6 gm/kg per day in feline cancer patients with normal hepatic and renal function. If parenteral nutrition is continued for longer than 5 to 7 days, appropriate vitamin and mineral supplements must be administered to ensure a complete and balanced nutrient intake.

References and Suggested Reading

Brennan MF: Uncomplicated starvation versus cancer cachexia. Cancer Res 37:2359, 1977.
   A classic review of the differences between uncomplicated starvation and the syndrome of cancer cachexia.
Davenport DJ: Enteral and parenteral nutritional support. In: Ettinger SJ, Feldmon EC, eds: Textbook of Veterinary Internal Medicine. Philadelphia: WB Saunders, 1995, p 244.
   A practical review of supportive alimentation, including methods of enteral nutrition.
Fascetti AJ, Mauldin GE, Mauldin GN: Correlation between serum creatine kinase activities and anorexia in cats. J Vet Intern Med 11:9, 1997.
   A study examining the utility of serum creatine kinase concentration as a method of nutritional assessment in the cat.
Kern KA, Norton JA: Cancer cachexia. JPEN 12:286, 1988.
   A detailed review of the underlying pathophysiology of cancer cachexia in human patients and rodent models.
Kronfeld DS, Donoghue S, Glickman LT: Body condition and energy intakes of dogs in a referral teaching hospital. J Nutr 121:S157, 1991.
   A study describing the practical application of a body condition scoring system.
Michel KE, King LG, Ostro E: Measurement of urinary urea nitrogen content as an estimate of the amount of total urinary nitrogen loss in dogs in intensive care units. J Am Vet Med Assoc 210:356, 1997.
   A prospective study quantifying urinary nitrogen losses and protein catabolism in critically ill dogs.
Ogilvie GK, Ford RB, Vail DM, et al: Alterations in lipoprotein profiles in dogs with lymphoma. J Vet Intern Med 8:62, 1994.
   A study describing abnormalities in lipid metabolism in dogs with lymphoma.
Ogilvie GK: Metabolic alterations and nutritional therapy for the veterinary cancer patient. In: Withrow SJ, MacEwen EG, eds: Small Animal Clinical Oncology, 2nd ed. Philadelphia: WB Saunders, 1996, p 117.
   A detailed review of the pathophysiology of cancer cachexia in the small animal cancer patient.
Vail DM, Ogilvie GK, Wheeler SL, et al: Alterations in carbohydrate metabolism in canine lymphoma. J Vet Intern Med 4:8, 1990.
   The first study describing hyperlactatemia and hyperinsulinism in dogs with lymphoma.
Wheeler SL, McGuire BH: Enteral nutritional support. In: Kirk RW, ed: Current Veterinary Therapy X: Small Animal Practice. Philadelphia: WB Saunders, 1989, p 30.
   A concise review of enteral nutrition in dogs and cats.

Practical Mechanics of Drug Delivery

ERIC R. SIMONSON
SUSAN A. KRAEGEL
Davis, California

The goal of this article is to provide detailed instructions for practitioners who intend to administer antineoplastic drugs in their practice. The guidelines provided are those used by the Oncology Service at the University of California, Davis, Veterinary Medical Teaching Hospital. The authors recognize that alternative methods may be employed by other clinicians in the administration of these drugs. General safe handling guidelines used in the preparation and disposal of chemotherapeutic agents are described in *CVT XII,* page 475.

GENERAL ADMINISTRATION GUIDELINES

A few recommendations apply universally to the administration of all chemotherapy agents.

1. Prior to using each drug, the clinician should review the drug insert provided by the manufacturer.
2. All equipment should be ready before the infusion is started.
3. It is safest to use preservative-free 0.9% saline as a flush just prior to and immediately after the use of any agent because many drugs react with heparin or preservatives.
4. Preservation of veins for multiple therapies is critical:
   a. All blood for diagnostic purposes should be drawn from the jugular veins to preserve peripheral veins for chemotherapy administration.
   b. Chemotherapy drugs should be administered only through catheters that are freshly placed with one clean stick into the vein. Following unsuccessful catheter placement, additional attempts should be made on another limb or at a spot clearly proximal to the site of failed placement.
   c. Following catheter removal, a pressure bandage should be placed at the catheter site to prevent hematoma formation and maintain vein patency for future injections.

SPECIFIC DRUG ADMINISTRATION PROTOCOLS

Doxorubicin

The administration-related side effects of doxorubicin include perivascular necrosis if the drug is extravasated and anaphylaxis during drug administration. Extravasation can be prevented with careful catheter placement. Anaphylaxis is rare in properly premedicated animals and, in the authors' experience, is seen only in dogs.

1. Thirty minutes prior to drug administration, inject diphenhydramine (Benadryl, Parke-Davis) at 2 mg/kg SC in dogs and 1 mg/kg SC in cats.
2. Draw up doxorubicin into a syringe and dilute it with preservative-free 0.9% sodium chloride (NaCl) to a volume of 10 ml for small cats and dogs (20-ml syringe) and 20 ml for large dogs (35-ml syringe).
3. Immediately prior to administration, place an indwelling intravenous catheter (20 or 22 gauge) in a peripheral vein with an intermittent infusion plug. The catheter should be secured with tape, but the insertion site of the catheter and the limb area proximal to the catheter site should be visible at all times so that catheter patency can be monitored.
4. Start a rapid drip of normal saline (0.9% NaCl) into the catheter through an intravenous administration set.
5. Confirm catheter patency by aspiration and by unimpeded flow of the saline.
6. Inject dexamethasone sodium phosphate, 0.2 mg/kg, intravenously into the side port of the administration set.
7. Connect the doxorubicin syringe to the side port of the intravenous set with an 18-gauge needle and wrap the connection site with an alcohol-soaked gauze pad.
8. Slowly inject doxorubicin through the side port while continuing the intravenous saline drip over 5 to 10 minutes.
9. Observe the animal for signs of distress, including erythema of the pinna, pruritus, and urticaria. If these signs develop, stop the doxorubicin infusion. When the signs cease, resume the infusion at a slower rate. If the signs continue, administer diphenhydramine, 1 mg/kg slowly IV (dogs only), followed by dexamethasone sodium phosphate at 2 mg/kg IV. Resume infusion if rapid and complete resolution of the signs occurs. If signs do not resolve quickly or if disease progression is noted, do not resume doxorubicin infusion and treat for shock as needed (see *CVT XII*, p. 150). Anecdotally, some generic doxorubicin compounds have been related to an increased incidence of anaphylaxis episodes; this outcome can be prevented by switching brands.
10. When doxorubicin injection is complete, turn off the intravenous set, and carefully withdraw the doxorubicin syringe, keeping the gauze in place to catch small drops of the drug. After disconnecting the syringe, start the intravenous set again and continue saline administration until the intravenous line is absolutely clear.
11. Disconnect the intravenous administration set from the intermittent infusion plug, inject 6 ml of normal saline into the catheter, and then remove the catheter and apply a pressure wrap to the catheter site.

Cisplatin

Major considerations in the administration of cisplatin are vigorous diuresis to prevent irreversible renal tubular damage and antiemetics to prevent nausea and vomiting. In addition, aluminum needles should not be used because they react with cisplatin.

1. Place an intravenous catheter (20 gauge) into a peripheral vein and secure the catheter.
2. Give 0.9% NaCl intravenously at 18.3 ml/kg per hour for 4 hours using an intravenous pump and an administration set with a buretrol (Ogilvie et al, 1991).
3. Take the dog out to urinate as needed during the 4-hour infusion and immediately prior to cisplatin administration.
4. Give butorphanol, 0.4 mg/kg SC, immediately prior to cisplatin.
5. Inject the correct dose of cisplatin into an empty buretrol and dilute it with enough 0.9% NaCl to bring the total volume in the buretrol to 1 hour's maintenance fluid volume. Administer this cisplatin-saline mixture over 30 minutes.
6. Administer 0.9% NaCl intravenously at 18.3 mg/kg per hour for 2 additional hours, taking the dog outside to urinate every hour. All urine evacuated after cisplatin infusion should be considered biohazardous.
7. Remove the catheter and apply a pressure wrap to the catheter site.

Vincristine, Vinblastine, Cyclophosphamide, Methotrexate (Butterfly Catheter)

These drugs can generally be given through a butterfly catheter. Vincristine and vinblastine are vesicants and cause tissue damage when extravasated.

1. Assemble a 23-gauge, ¾-inch (0.65 × 19 mm), winged infusion set with 12-inch tubing (Surflo Winged Infusion Set, Terumo Medical Corporation, Elkton, MD), chemotherapy drug, two 6-ml syringes filled with preservative-free 0.9% NaCl, and dry cotton balls and tape for a pressure wrap after infusion. Loosen needles on all syringes so that they can be disconnected with one hand, and preflush the catheter with 0.9% NaCl.
2. Insert the catheter into a peripheral vein, making sure that the catheter is fully threaded and securely seated in the vein. Do not secure the catheter with tape, as any tension on the insertion site is likely to result in catheter dislodgement.
3. Throughout the procedure, hold the catheter by the syringe attachment connection only, and do not place any tension on the catheter tubing. Ideally, the syringe attachment connection and the patient's limb are held in one hand so that sudden patient movement will not dislodge the needle.
4. Connect the syringe holding the preservative-free 0.9% NaCl to the butterfly syringe attachment point, and aspirate blood at least half way into the infusion tube to ensure good patency. Slowly infuse 1 to 2 ml of the

saline into the catheter to also assess patency. If any question as to patency exists, a larger volume of saline (5 to 10 ml) will help in assessment. If placement of the catheter fails, remove it and place a catheter in another vein.

5. For all syringe changes, clamp or kink the butterfly tubing adjacent to the syringe attachment point to prevent the contents of the catheter from leaking.
6. Slowly infuse one third to one half of the chemotherapeutic drug.
7. Again assess patency by aspirating blood into the tube and making sure that it flows freely.
8. Slowly infuse the remainder of the drug, checking patency by aspiration as needed.
9. Flush the catheter with 1 to 2 ml of preservative-free normal saline directly after completing the drug infusion. Do not aspirate the catheter first, as this maneuver will cause any drug remaining in the butterfly infusion line to become diluted in the saline flush.
10. After all of the drug has been flushed into the patient with normal saline, assess catheter patency by aspirating blood into the infusion tubing and flushing with the remainder of saline.
11. Remove the catheter, and apply a pressure wrap to the site.

Actinomycin D, Carboplatin, 5-Fluorouracil, Mitoxantrone (IV Push)

Actinomycin D is given by IV push because it is a severe vesicant and will cause necrosis if extravasated. For the other drugs, this method is convenient because of the volume to be infused. For carboplatin, aluminum needles should not be used, as they react with the drug.

1. Immediately prior to administration, place an indwelling intravenous catheter (20 or 22 gauge) in a peripheral vein with an intermittent infusion plug. The catheter should be secured with tape, but the insertion site of the catheter and the limb area proximal to the catheter site should be visible at all times so that catheter patency can be monitored.
2. Place a 23-gauge, ¾-inch (0.65 × 19 mm), winged infusion set with 12-inch tubing (Surflo Winged Infusion Set, Terumo Medical Corporation, Elkton, MD) through the intermittent infusion plug into the catheter.
3. Aspirate through the butterfly tubing and infuse 5 to 10 ml of preservative-free 0.9% NaCl to check patency.
4. For all syringe changes, clamp or kink the butterfly tubing adjacent to the syringe attachment point to prevent the contents from leaking.
5. Slowly administer the chemotherapeutic drug through the butterfly infusion line into the indwelling catheter.
6. Infuse 5 to 10 ml of preservative-free normal saline to clear all remaining drug from the butterfly catheter and remove the butterfly catheter.
7. Infuse 1 to 2 ml of preservative-free normal saline directly into the indwelling catheter through an intermittent infusion plug to flush any residual drug, then remove the catheter and apply a pressure wrap to the catheter site.

L-Asparaginase

L-Asparaginase is a protein with the potential to cause anaphylaxis. The incidence of anaphylaxis with L-asparaginase administration is rare when appropriate premedication is given.

1. Thirty minutes prior to drug administration, inject diphenhydramine at 2 mg/kg SC in dogs and 1 mg/kg SC in cats.
2. Immediately prior to L-asparaginase administration give dexamethasone sodium phosphate, 0.2 mg/kg IV or IM.
3. Inject L-asparaginase SC.
4. Observe the animal for 30 to 60 minutes to monitor for anaphylaxis.
5. If anaphylaxis occurs, follow standard anaphylactic shock guidelines (see *CVT XII*, p. 150).

Mechlorethamine

Mechlorethamine has specific handling requirements that make administration beyond the capabilities of most general practices. It decomposes rapidly in solution. Administration requires special precautions and must be followed by immediate neutralization of all remaining solution and all administration equipment according to manufacturer directions. In addition, mechlorethamine causes severe skin necrosis if extravasated and, on rare occasions, dogs may vomit during the infusion. Routine use of antiemetics, however, is not necessary.

1. Mechlorethamine should be prepared immediately before use. After reconstitution, mechlorethamine is not stable.
2. Immediately prior to administration, place an indwelling intravenous catheter (20 or 22 gauge) in a peripheral vein with an intermittent infusion plug. The catheter should be secured with tape, but the insertion site of the catheter and the limb area proximal to the catheter site should be visible at all times to monitor catheter patency.
3. Start a rapid drip of normal saline (0.9% NaCl) into the catheter through an intravenous administration set.
4. Confirm catheter patency by aspiration and by unimpeded flow of the saline.
5. Connect the mechlorethamine syringe to a side port of the intravenous set with an 18-gauge needle and wrap the connection site with an alcohol-soaked gauze pad.
6. Slowly inject mechlorethamine through the side port while continuing the rapid intravenous saline drip over a few minutes.
7. When mechlorethamine injection is complete, turn off the intravenous set, wrap an alcohol-soaked gauze pad around the connection between the mechlorethamine needle and the intravenous line infusion port, and carefully withdraw the mechlorethamine syringe, keeping the gauze in place to catch small drops of the drug. After disconnecting the syringe, start the intravenous set again and continue saline administration until the intravenous line is flushed.

8. Disconnect the intravenous administration set from the intermittent infusion plug, inject 6 ml of normal saline into the catheter, then remove the catheter, and apply a pressure wrap to the site.

9. The catheter, syringe, intravenous lines, empty vials, any surface contaminated with mechlorethamine, and any remaining drug must be neutralized following administration. Mechlorethamine should not be used if this step is not completed. An aqueous solution with equal volumes of sodium thiosulfate (5%) and sodium bicarbonate (5%) is prepared. All contaminated items, including tubing and syringes, are soaked in this solution for 45 minutes in a zip-lock bag. Any leftover mechlorethamine solution is mixed with an equal volume of sodium thiosulfate and sodium bicarbonate solution and allowed to stand for 45 minutes.

EXTRAVASATION

Extravasation of vesicant antineoplastic agents (doxorubicin, mechlorethamine, actinomycin D, vincristine, vinblastine) can cause local reactions that range from minor irritation to severe necrosis. While every precaution should be taken to prevent drug extravasation, all personnel handling these drugs should also be familiar with the steps to be taken during a known or suspected extravasation event (Ringlein, 1991):

1. Stop the infusion.

2. Leave a catheter or butterfly catheter in place.
3. Attempt to withdraw extravasated fluid from the injection site through the catheter.
4. Remove the catheter.
5. Specific therapies by drug:
   a. Doxorubicin or actinomycin D: Apply ice to the site for 30 minutes q.i.d. for 72 hours.
   b. Vincristine or vinblastine: Administer 1 to 6 ml (150 U/ml) of hyaluronidase (Wydase, Wyeth-Ayerst) subcutaneously at the site. Follow with warm compresses.
   c. Mechlorethamine: Administer 5 to 6 ml of isotonic sodium thiosulfate 2.6% subcutaneously at the site.
6. Document the incident.
7. Use an appropriate means of preventing the patient from licking the site.
8. Follow the patient for 2 weeks and consult with a surgeon should necrosis develop.

References and Suggested Reading

Ogilvie GK, Straw RC, Powers BE, et al: Prevalence of nephrotoxicosis associated with a short-term saline solution diuresis protocol for the administration of cisplatin to dogs with malignant tumors: 61 cases (1987–1989). J Am Vet Med Assoc 199:613, 1991.
  Evaluates the effectiveness of the 6-hour diuresis protocol in preventing renal toxicity.
Ringlein JW: Management of nausea and vomiting and other acute side effects of cancer chemotherapy. In: Skeel RT, ed: Handbook of Cancer Chemotherapy. Boston: Little, Brown, 1991, p 502.
  Offers recommendations for the treatment of drug extravasation.

CVT Update: Anticancer Drugs and Protocols Using Traditional Drugs

Barbara E. Kitchell
Ravinder S. Dhaliwal
Urbana, Illinois

Medical treatment of cancer has been improved and refined over the last 40 years. Despite significant advances in therapy, cure rates for veterinary patients with disseminated cancers remain very low. Progress is hampered in veterinary oncology by the lack of randomized prospective trials. Economic factors and psychological and cultural biases against the treatment of cancer in animals prevent large clinical trials. Despite these impediments to clinical research, anticancer chemotherapy is now a commonly accepted form of treatment. Malignancy can be viewed as a chronic, manageable condition for many companion animals with a variety of different diseases that fall under the broad category of "cancer."

Widespread acceptance of chemotherapy in veterinary medicine is limited by the anticipation of unacceptable toxicities. Anticancer chemotherapeutic agents have selective toxicity against *rapidly dividing cell populations*—not necessarily selective toxicity against cancer cells. The drugs cause some level of toxicity to rapidly dividing normal cells, including those of bone marrow, gastrointestinal epithelium, and, in some breeds, hair follicles. Toxicities to these and other replicating cells are the basis of common side effects: immunosuppression, myelosuppression, anemia, vomition, delayed wound healing, reproductive failure, and alopecia. In addition to toxicity to rapidly dividing cells, toxicities such as cardiotoxicity, nephrotoxicity, and neurotoxicity are induced by individual drugs.

Combination Chemotherapy. Chemotherapy drugs are most commonly used in combination. The guidelines for combination drug protocol design are as follows: (1) give drugs with efficacy as single agents against the tumor type in question; (2) combine drugs with different mechanisms of action, to facilitate cell killing; and (3) combine drugs with different dose-limiting toxicities to minimize adverse effects, especially bone marrow and gastrointestinal reactions. Many of the anticancer drugs have yet to be validated as effective single agents against veterinary cancers. However, combination therapy is expected to produce similar responses in spontaneous human and animal cancers.

Dose Intensity. Cancer cells are killed when they are exposed to adequate concentrations of effective drugs for a sufficient time. Anticancer drugs kill by first-order kinetics (i.e., the dose of drug that reduces a tumor burden of 10^8 cells to 10^6 will reduce 10^6 cells to 10^4). This observation led to the most common hypothesis of protocol design: to kill cancer cells optimally, one must give the *maximum tolerated dose* of drug at the *closest possible interval* between doses. Oncologists who advocate treatment based on dose intensity would argue that it is inappropriate to reduce the doses of chemotherapy to ineffective levels, or to stop treatment before the disease has been totally eradicated. In the dose-intense therapy model, the most "toxic" effect of treatment is death from insufficient treatment. This argument is particularly compelling when the subject undergoing treatment is a young individual with the potential for substantial life prolongation if cured. However, the majority of veterinary cancer patients are geriatric. The potential for depriving patients of an acceptable quality of life in a situation limited by the basic chronobiology of the organism should be considered. If all parties understand that the goal of therapy is the maintenance of a good quality of life for as long as possible, chemotherapy with overtly palliative intent is an appropriate treatment goal. Newer information about molecular drug resistance mechanisms would suggest that cancer cells may be intrinsically resistant to classes of anticancer drugs, and that they may also be resistant to apoptosis, or programmed cell death. Molecular mechanisms of drug resistance help explain the low cure rates for disseminated solid tumors, regardless of the dose intensity of the drug protocol instituted (DeVita et al, 1997).

Issues in Drug Selection. Anticancer drugs have narrow therapeutic indices; thus, chemotherapy doses should be adjusted to the metabolic weight of the patient. This adjustment is important in veterinary oncology, because we treat a variety of animal shapes and sizes, from Chihuahuas to Irish wolfhounds. However, the small-animal square-meter (m^2) body surface area (BSA) tables currently available are flawed. In human medicine, m^2 BSA is based on kilograms of body weight and height, whereas in veterinary medicine the conversion formula involves weight alone. In clinical practice, the errors in the square-meter conversion formula are manifested as potential for increased toxicity in very small dogs, and shorter survival in large dogs treated for lymphoma with square-meter–based dosing (Ogilvie and Moore, 1995). Veterinary pharmacologists are currently re-evaluating the most appropriate dose regimens for anticancer drugs; for most drugs and in most individuals, the square-meter dosing guidelines are still appropriate. Veterinary oncologists must consider the consequences of inadequate drug dosing (lack of remission, short remission

durations) or prolonged interval between drug doses (repopulation of neoplastic cells, acquired drug resistance) versus the potential for toxicity inherent in dose-intense protocols. Additional considerations in protocol selection include pre-existing diseases in the patient that could impact drug pharmacology and cost and convenience to the client. Anticancer chemotherapeutics are not approved for use in veterinary medicine at this time and are not likely to become so soon, because of the high costs involved with drug licensing. Owners should be made aware of this and also that anticancer drugs have a low therapeutic index, with idiosyncratic reactions possible. However, published protocols available in the veterinary literature are generally associated with mild and predictable toxicities. Anticancer drugs must be handled and administered with care and attention to detail (see *CVT XII,* pp. 478 and 482; see also previous article).

CLASSES OF CHEMOTHERAPY DRUGS

General classes of chemotherapy drugs are based on mechanisms of action. The classes include alkylating agents, platinum analogues, antimetabolites, plant alkaloids, antitumor antibiotics, hormones, and miscellaneous agents.

Alkylating Agents. Alkylating agents have the common property of dissociating a positively charged, electrophilic alkyl group capable of reacting with negatively charged, electron-rich, nucleophilic centers on DNA, proteins, and small molecules such as glutathione. Alkylators form a variety of DNA adducts at the N-7 position of the guanine. Adduct formation results in DNA strand breaks that interfere with DNA replication and the production of mRNA and ATP. Alkylating agents are cell cycle dependent but are not cell cycle phase specific. Alkylators damage both proliferating and resting cells, but cycling cells are more sensitive than cells in G_0 phase of the cell cycle.

Cyclophosphamide. Cyclophosphamide (Cytoxan [CTX]) is often used to treat various veterinary neoplastic and non-neoplastic (autoimmune) diseases. CTX is activated in vivo by liver microsomal enzymes to 4-hydroxycyclophosphamide (4-HC). 4-HC spontaneously breaks down to phosphoramide mustard and acrolein, both of which cause DNA damage. As much as 90% of the parent drug and metabolites are excreted in the urine. Elevated blood levels of CTX have been observed in human patients with renal failure; dose modification for renal insufficiency should be considered. CTX is commonly used in combination chemotherapy for lymphoma. Efficacy is also seen in combination therapy for the treatment of mast cell tumor, mammary carcinoma, and hemangiosarcoma. CTX is used to treat autoimmune diseases such as systemic lupus erythematosus, rheumatoid arthritis, immune-mediated hemolytic anemia, immune-mediated thrombocytopenia, and pemphigus vulgaris.

CTX can be administered orally at the dose of 50 mg/m^2 every second or third day; on a 4 days on, 3 days off schedule; or as an intravenous injection of 200 to 250 mg/m^2 once weekly. The CTX tablet contains a core of active ingredient sealed within a compression coating. The distribution of the active ingredient may not be uniform if tablets are split or crushed for administration to cats and small dogs. Common adverse effects of CTX include myelosuppression and gastrointestinal toxicity. Sterile hemorrhagic cystitis and transitional cell carcinoma of the bladder secondary to CTX therapy have been reported in dogs and cats. Hemorrhagic cystitis with CTX therapy is due to acrolein, which causes mucosal ulceration, edema, and necrosis of the bladder. Administration of prednisone on the same day as the CTX may decrease the rate of hemorrhagic cystitis, since prednisone induces diuresis and also inhibits the activation of CTX by hepatic microsomal enzymes. More aggressive measures for the treatment of sterile hemorrhagic cystitis include intravesical instillation of acetylcysteine (which inactivates acrolein) and the use of sodium 2-mercaptoethanesulfonate (mesna) and prostaglandin $F_{2\alpha}$. Irrigation of the bladder with 1% formalin in anesthetized patients has proved effective. Intravesical administration of 50% dimethyl sulfoxide (DMSO) has been used in human beings and dogs to treat CTX-induced cystitis. The treatment of CTX-induced cystitis should initially include discontinuation of the drug and the substitution of alternative alkylating agents, such as chlorambucil.

Chlorambucil. Chlorambucil (Leukeran) is a widely used bifunctional alkylating agent. This drug forms biadducts that are mainly interstrand DNA cross-links. Other bifunctional alkylating agents include melphalan and busulfan. Chlorambucil is well absorbed after oral administration. Peak plasma levels are reached in 1 hour. The current recommended doses for oral chlorambucil range from 2 to 8 mg/m² on alternate days. Chlorambucil may also be administered at a dose of 20 mg/m² PO every 21 days. Higher doses are associated with a greater potential for myelosuppression and gastrointestinal toxicity. The uses of chlorambucil in veterinary medicine include the treatment of chronic lymphocytic leukemias and of mast cell tumors and as a maintenance agent in the management of lymphomas in dogs and cats.

Melphalan. Melphalan (Alkeran) is a bifunctional alkylating agent that causes interstrand, intrastrand, and DNA-protein cross-linking. Unlike cyclophosphamide, this drug does not require hepatic activation. Melphalan combined with prednisone is the treatment of choice for multiple myeloma. The adverse effects are primarily gastrointestinal and hematopoietic. Melphalan can be administered orally, intravenously, or intraperitoneally. The dosages are as follows: 2 mg/m² every 24 hours for 7 to 10 days, then 2 to 4 mg/m² PO every 48 hours; or 6 to 8 mg/m² PO for 4 or 5 days, repeated every 21 days.

Busulfan. Busulfan (Myeleran) is a bifunctional alkylating agent that interacts with cellular thiol groups. It is used for the treatment of chronic myelogenous leukemia and polycythemia. Leukopenia may be a side effect. Busulfan is given at a dose of 3 to 4 mg/m² PO daily. This dose is then used intermittently to maintain the white blood cells at 15,000 total cells/μl.

Plant Alkaloids. Vincristine and vinblastine are the most commonly used plant alkaloids in veterinary medi-

cine. These alkaloids were isolated from the common periwinkle plant (*Catharanthus roseus*). Several semisynthetic vinca alkaloids are currently entering clinical trials in both Europe and the United States. Vinca alkaloids are cell cycle phase–specific drugs that cause metaphase arrest of dividing cells by binding to dimeric tubulin. Tubulin crystallizes when bound by the vinca alkaloids, resulting in the dissolution of the mitotic spindle and cell cycle arrest at M phase. The abundance of tubulin in platelets makes these drugs useful in the treatment of immune-mediated thrombocytopenia. Both vincristine and vinblastine are metabolized primarily by the liver, with roughly 70% excreted in feces and 12% in the urine. Methotrexate accumulation is increased in tumor cells exposed in vitro to vincristine and vinblastine. This effect is mediated by vinca-induced blockade of methotrexate efflux from cells.

Vinca alkaloids are used for the treatment of lymphoreticular malignancies, mast cell tumors, and various sarcomas. A combination of vincristine with doxorubicin (Adriamycin) and cytoxan (VAC protocol) has been used for hemangiosarcoma and other malignancies. Vincristine is administered in combination with cyclophosphamide and prednisone, and many other drugs, as part of many lymphoma treatment combinations. Vincristine therapy can be curative for canine transmissible venereal tumor (TVT). Vinblastine is also used to treat lymphoma and mast cell disease.

The primary toxicities of vinca alkaloids include myelosuppression (especially vinblastine), gastrointestinal mucosal injury, and alopecia. Although reversible peripheral neuropathy (manifested as hyporeflexia and paresthesia) is commonly seen as a dose-limiting toxicity in human patients, it is an uncommon finding in veterinary patients. Cats given vinca alkaloids may develop reversible axon swelling (giant axon formation) and paranodal demyelination. Neurotoxicity can be associated with constipation and paralytic ileus, which may contribute to anorexia in cats undergoing vincristine therapy. Vincristine sulfate administered at the therapeutic dose (0.5 to 0.75 mg/m² BSA weekly) induces a transient mild decrease in platelet numbers, followed by a moderate increase in numbers, with peak platelet count 8 days after administration. Vinblastine is dosed at 2 mg/m² IV every 7 to 14 days and is much more myelosuppressive than vincristine. Both drugs are excreted in bile; 50% dose reduction in cases of bilirubinemia above 2 mg/dl is recommended (Ogilvie and Moore, 1995). Both vincristine and vinblastine are severe irritants if extravasated.

Antimetabolites. Antimetabolites are S phase–specific drugs that interfere with DNA synthesis or folic acid metabolism. They are structural analogues of purines, pyrimidines, or folic acid and interfere with pathways that utilize those molecules for DNA replication.

Methotrexate. Methotrexate acts as an inhibitor of the enzyme dihydrofolate reductase (DHFR). This enzyme is required for purine and thymidylate synthesis; methotrexate inhibits the synthesis of DNA by this mechanism. Leucovorin (D,L-N^5-formyl-5, 6, 7, 8-tetrahydrofolic acid) can be used to antagonize the effects of methotrexate (leucovorin rescue). Methotrexate is used in combination therapy for lymphoma and osteosarcoma. Dose reduction should be considered in cases of renal insufficiency, as this agent is renally cleared and induces renal tubular necrosis at high doses. The drug is protein bound; concurrent administration of other medications that can interfere with albumin binding (sulfa drugs, tetracyclines, aspirin, chloramphenicol, phenytoin) should be avoided. Methotrexate can be administered at a dose of 2.5 mg/m^2 PO every 48 hours, or 0.5 to 0.8 mg/kg IV every 7 to 14 days. Toxicities include myelosuppression, renal tubular necrosis, hepatotoxicity, and pneumonitis. Vomition is the most commonly induced side effect of methotrexate.

Cytosine Arabinoside. Cytosine arabinoside (Cytosar, Ara-C) is an arabinose nucleoside isolated from the sponge *Cryptothetya crypta*. Its antineoplastic activity is due largely to inhibition of DNA synthesis by incorporation into the growing DNA strand, with resultant chain termination. The active metabolite of cytosine arabinoside is a competitive inhibitor of DNA polymerase. Cerebrospinal fluid levels (approximately 20 to 40% of blood levels) are achieved after 2 hours of continuous infusion. The half-life of cytosine arabinoside in cerebrospinal fluid is much longer than that in blood because of the absence of deaminases; the drug may be administered by the intravenous or intrathecal route to treat central nervous system lymphoma. Subcutaneous administration results in lower peak concentrations than the same dose administered as an intravenous bolus, but a two-fold greater area under the curve is noted. In veterinary oncology, cytosine arabinoside is used to treat lymphoid malignancies and leukemias. Toxicities include myelosuppression and gastrointestinal effects. Dose regimens include 100 mg/m^2 as a continuous intravenous infusion for 48 to 96 hours, or 100 mg/m^2 divided t.i.d. to q.i.d. SC for 48 to 96 hours.

Fluoropyrimidines. Fluorouracil is the only drug in this family used in veterinary medicine. It is converted via multiple intracellular pathways to fluorouridine monophosphate (FUMP), then into either of the two active metabolites, fluorouridine triphosphate (FUTP) or 5-FdUMP. FdUMP inhibits the synthesis of the DNA precursor deoxythymidine triphosphate (dTTP). FUTP becomes incorporated into RNA and inhibits processing and function. Primary toxicities include dose-limiting myelosuppression, gastrointestinal toxicity, and neurotoxicity (leucovorin may enhance the gastrointestinal toxicity of 5-FU). Fluorouracil is used as a 1 or 5% topical cream or solution in humans and dogs for the treatment of superficial squamous cell and basal cell tumors. Severe, potentially fatal, neurotoxicity occurs in cats given 5-FU; its use is contraindicated even in the topical form. Indications include the treatment of canine mammary carcinoma (in combination with doxorubicin [Adriamycin] and cyclophosphamide [FAC protocol]), dermal squamous cell carcinoma, and treatment of tumors of the gastrointestinal tract. The dose is 150 mg/m^2 IV weekly, or 5 to 10 mg/kg IV weekly.

Hydroxyurea. Hydroxyurea inhibits DNA synthesis through interference with the ribonucleotide reductase system. It can be administered orally or intravenously. The most common use of hydroxyurea is as second-line therapy for dogs with chronic myelogenous leukemia no longer responsive to busulfan, and the in treatment of polycythemia. The dose is reported to be 50 to 80 mg/kg PO every 3 days. The toxicities include myelosuppression, especially thrombocytopenia, and pulmonary fibrosis.

Antitumor Antibiotics. Drugs in this class have in common their origin as fungal or bacterial products. The mechanisms of action and cell cycle phase specificity vary, depending on the drug. Most have complex mechanisms of action. Antitumor antibiotics used commonly in veterinary medicine include doxorubicin, mitoxantrone, actinomycin, and bleomycin.

Doxorubicin. Doxorubicin is one of the most commonly used chemotherapeutic drugs in veterinary oncology. Derived from *Streptomyces* sp., this drug is used as a single agent or in combination therapy to treat hemolymphatic malignancies, carcinomas, and sarcomas. The presence of antitumor antibiotics within the structure of DNA (intercalation) induces the failure of DNA replication and impaired protein production through interference with the transcription of mRNA. Through a series of complex reactions, the quinone and semiquinone side groups on this anthracycline produce hydroxyl free radicals that are highly damaging to molecular DNA and cell membrane lipids. Doxorubicin intercalation alters the helical structure of DNA and may trigger enhanced activity of topoisomerase II. The net result is a dramatic increase in chromosomal strand breaks.

Doxorubicin is a severe vesicant if extravasated. The drug is cleared through the bile almost exclusively in the dog and cat; dose reductions in the case of hyperbilirubinemia (<2 mg/dl) are indicated. Doxorubicin has been associated with renal insufficiency in cats when given at high doses. The dose in dogs is 30 mg/m^2 BSA IV every 21 days, and in cats 20 to 25 mg/m^2 IV every 21 days. Other dosing strategies used in veterinary medicine include dosing at 1 mg/kg IV every 21 days, and giving weekly doses of 10 mg/m^2 IV to minimize cardiotoxicity.

Doxorubicin has one of the widest adverse effect profiles of all the anticancer drugs. In addition to the standard concerns for alopecia and gastrointestinal and marrow toxicities, doxorubicin can induce anaphylactic reactions by causing mast cell degranulation. Some authors recommend premedication with antihistamines (diphenhydramine, 1 mg/kg SC) and a slow rate of infusion (over 20 to 60 minutes) to minimize allergic reaction (see previous article). Doxorubicin produces dose-limiting cardiac toxicity. Acute myocarditis-pericarditis syndrome can cause rhythm disturbances (supraventricular arrhythmias, heart block, and ventricular tachycardia) or failure (decreases in ejection fraction) and can lead to congestive heart failure. Some patients develop pericardial effusions. In addition, a cumulative dose-dependent cardiomyopathy can lead to congestive heart failure. A total dose of 550 mg/m^2 in humans and more than 240 mg/m^2 in dogs can result in noninflammatory cardiomyopathy. Cardiomyopathy at a cumulative dose of less than 90 mg/m^2 has been reported in dogs. Canine breeds that are predisposed to cardiomyopathy (Doberman pinschers, Boxers, Rottweilers, Great Danes) must be monitored closely during doxorubicin treatment. A chemoprotective iron-chelating agent, ICRF-187, has been found to minimize or block cumulative cardiotoxicity in humans and dogs. In cats, in addition to cardiac toxicity, renal dysfunction manifested by increasing azotemia and progressively dilute urine with confirmed histopathologic evidence of renal disease has been documented.

Mitoxantrone. Mitoxantrone is a completely synthetic anthracenedione DNA intercalator. Like doxorubicin, mitoxantrone is known to trigger topoisomerase II–mediated DNA strand breaks. The semiquinone free radical of the mitoxantrone molecule is unreactive, making this drug much less cardiotoxic than doxorubicin. Renal clearance accounts for less than 10% of the total dose administered. Mitoxantrone can be administered to cats with renal insufficiency, whereas doxorubicin may induce further renal damage. Mitoxantrone has been used alone or in combination with radiation therapy as a treatment for oral squamous cell carcinoma in both dogs and cats. Besides lymphoma and oral squamous cell carcinomas, mitoxantrone administration induces measurable regression in various other canine sarcomas and carcinomas. The dosage is 5.5 to 6.5 mg/m² IV every 21 days, in a 1- to 2-hour saline infusion.

Myelosuppression and gastrointestinal side effects are observed with single agent mitoxantrone protocols. However, perivascular sloughing is not observed if mitoxantrone is extravasated. The most common signs of mitoxantrone toxicosis observed in dogs and cats include vomiting, anorexia, diarrhea, lethargy, sepsis, and convulsions (reported in cats only). Toxicosis from the administration of the first dose is associated with signs of toxicosis during subsequent treatments.

Bleomycin. Bleomycin is a derivative of the fungus *Streptomyces verticullus*. This drug has a DNA binding site and an iron-binding protein at the other end of the molecule. The bound iron ion generates highly toxic superoxide and hydroxyl free radicals, which cleave DNA at the intercalation site of the DNA binding domain. This drug is renally cleared and requires dose reduction in renal insufficiency. Adverse effects to marrow and gastrointestinal tract are mild, but pulmonary fibrosis and allergic reactions may be noted. The drug is administered intramuscularly or subcutaneously at a dose of 0.3 to 0.5 mg/kg per week, or intravenously over 10 minutes. A total cumulative dosage of 125 to 200 mg/m² should not be exceeded because of the risk of increased pulmonary toxicity. Bleomycin has been used intralesionally in veterinary patients for the treatment of squamous cell carcinoma. Further indications for bleomycin therapy in veterinary oncology may be developed now that drug costs are lower than in the past.

Actinomycin D. Actinomycin D is another *Streptomyces* species derivative. This drug intercalates DNA, blocks DNA and RNA synthesis, and causes single-strand DNA breaks. The drug is excreted unchanged in bile. Myelosuppression and gastrointestinal toxicity with diarrhea are the most common adverse effects seen. This drug can cause perivascular reactions that are milder than those seen with doxorubicin. Actinomycin can be painful on injection and can cause acute vomiting if administered too rapidly. For this reason, intravenous infusion over 20 minutes is recommended. This drug has been used to treat lymphomas,

sarcomas, and carcinomas in dogs at a dose of 0.5 to 0.9 mg/m² IV every 2 or 3 weeks.

Platinum Compounds. The platinum coordination complexes are the most important group of agents currently in use in human oncology. Platinum agents have a unique mechanism of action and toxicity, and so they may be synergistic when used with other cancer drugs and radiation therapy. Cisplatin and carboplatin are the platinum-based anticancer drugs used in veterinary oncology. These drugs kill cancer cells by cross-linking DNA at the guanine bases, in a manner analogous to the bifunctional alkylating agents.

Cisplatin. Cisplatin (*cis*-diamminedichloroplatinum II) consists of a central platinum with two atoms each of ammonia and chloride arranged in a *cis* spatial configuration. The ammonia and chloride bond covalently to platinum at fixed bond angles. Cisplatin exerts its cytotoxic effect by an aquation reaction that displaces the chloride molecules. In extracellular fluid, the high chloride concentration maintains the unreactive dichloro form. The intracellular chloride concentration favors the aquation reaction, yielding the highly reactive form of cisplatin. Cisplatin binds to all DNA bases, but there is preferential bonding with the N-7 positions of guanine and adenine. The two chloride ligands react with the two different sites on DNA to produce intrastrand cross-links, which are thought to inhibit DNA replication and function. Cisplatin is cleared through the kidneys and is a nephrotoxin. Saline diuresis prevents damage by increasing the chloride concentration in the renal tubular epithelium, preventing aquation to the active form.

Cisplatin is used as an adjuvant therapy after amputation for appendicular osteosarcoma in dogs. Survival times are significantly longer in dogs treated with cisplatin following amputation or limb-sparing surgery compared with dogs treated with amputation alone. Cisplatin alternating with doxorubicin is also an effective adjuvant treatment for canine osteosarcoma. Cisplatin has been used in the treatment of transitional cell and squamous cell carcinomas in dogs. Cisplatin can be administered by intracavitary installation for malignant pleural or peritoneal effusions at a dosage of 50 mg/m² with saline diuresis. Toxicity with intracavitary cisplatin administration was slight. Intravenous cisplatin may also be helpful in the treatment of nasal carcinoma in dogs.

Several reports describe the intralesional use of cisplatin. Sustained-release cisplatin gel therapeutic implant is effective in treating canine sun-induced squamous cell carcinoma, oral melanoma, and other cutaneous malignancies in dogs. The combination of local hyperthermia and intratumoral cisplatin has proved safe and effective for the treatment of selected localized neoplasms. Cisplatin is used as a radiosensitizer in human malignancies such as head and neck carcinoma.

Several different protocols for cisplatin administration have been reported. The protocol that the authors prefer is cisplatin at a dose of 60 to 70 mg/m² IV over 20 minutes after 4-hour intravenous saline diuresis (0.9% NaCl at a rate of 18.3 ml/kg per hour). After cisplatin infusion, saline diuresis should be continued at the same rate for another 2 hours. Antiemetics must be administered prior to cisplatin infusion. Cisplatin (60 to 70 mg/m^2 IV every 21 days) can be given over 20 minutes after 0.9% saline diuresis for 3 hours at the rate of 25 ml/kg per hour. Saline diuresis should be continued at the same rate for an additional hour after cisplatin infusion. Hypertonic saline (7%) appears to be as effective as normal saline (0.9%) in the maintenance of renal function. The administration of a single dose of cisplatin in 3% saline solution to healthy dogs demonstrated no significant decrease in glomerular filtration rate.

Cisplatin is nephrotoxic. Methimazole at a dose of 40 mg/kg IV over 1 minute has been demonstrated to impart protection against cisplatin-induced renal disease in dogs. Cisplatin also induces vomition by direct stimulation of the chemoreceptor trigger zone. Several antiemetics can be used to control the nausea and vomiting induced by cisplatin. Commonly used pretreatment antiemetics include butorphanol (0.4 mg/kg IM), metoclopramide (0.1 mg/kg IV), and dexamethasone (0.25 mg/kg IV). Cisplatin induces an apparent species-specific dose-related pulmonary toxicity (fatal pulmonary edema) in cats, which is independent of saline fluid loading. The systemic use of cisplatin is contraindicated in cats.

Carboplatin. Carboplatin is a second-generation chemotherapeutic platinum compound. The mechanism of action is thought to be the same as that for cisplatin. However, with carboplatin there is an alteration in the chloride-bearing side chains of carboplatin that replaces the renal toxicity of cisplatin with myelosuppression as the dose-limiting toxicity. Carboplatin is renally excreted. Administration to patients with renal insufficiency prolongs the half-life and exacerbates marrow toxicity; dose reduction is indicated for carboplatin administration to renal patients. The indications for carboplatin administration are the same as for cisplatin. The systemic dose is 300 mg/m^2 IV every 21 days for dogs, and 180 to 260 mg/m^2 IV every 21 days for cats. Diuresis is not required. Intratumoral administration of carboplatin for the treatment of squamous cell carcinoma of the nasal planum in cats has been documented. Carboplatin for intratumoral administration was used at the dose rate of 100 mg/m^2 BSA.

MISCELLANEOUS AGENTS

Drugs with mechanisms of action that do not fit into the aforementioned categories are classed as miscellaneous agents, and the mechanisms of action vary accordingly.

Dacarbazine (Dimethyltriazenoimidazole Carboxamide [DTIC]). Dacarbazine is activated by hepatic microsomal enzymes to produce an alkylating-like effect through the formation of reactive carbonium ions. Dacarbazine also demonstrates antimetabolic activity by inhibition of purine nucleoside incorporation into DNA. Dacarbazine is activated when exposed to light. Since dacarbazine is activated by the liver and cleared through the kidneys, it should be used cautiously in patients with hepatic and renal dysfunction. Gastrointestinal toxicity (vomiting and diarrhea) is dose limiting. Other toxicities include myelosuppression (platelets), and phlebitis and venous spasm during intravenous administration. The use of a catheter to prevent perivascular tissue damage is recommended. A study in dogs

revealed that the administration of the entire dose (800 to 1,000 mg/m^2) over an 8-hour period or administering the total dose over a 5-day period (200 mg/m^2 IV daily) resulted in no significant difference in efficacy and toxicity. DTIC may be repeated every 21 days, provided that marrow recovery takes place. This drug is not recommended for use in cats because of lack of knowledge about the capacity of the feline liver to activate and break down the compound. Dacarbazine is effective in the treatment of relapsed canine lymphoma. It is useful in the treatment of melanoma and soft tissue sarcomas. This drug is thought to be synergistic in combination with doxorubicin.

L-Asparaginase. L-Asparaginase, an enzyme drug prepared from *Escherichia coli* and *Erwinia carotovora*, is specifically used for the treatment of lymphoid malignancies. L-Asparagine is an amino acid required for protein synthesis. Most normal cells and the majority of non-lymphoid cancer cells are able to synthesize L-asparagine via induction of the enzyme L-asparagine synthetase. Malignant lymphoid cells depend on preformed L-asparagine and are selectively vulnerable to its depletion. The drug L-asparaginase converts L-asparagine to aspartic acid and ammonia by hydrolysis, thus depleting the plasma, extracellular fluid, and cerebrospinal fluid of the amino acid. L-Asparaginase can cause an anaphylactic reaction because the enzyme is highly antigenic, especially when administered intravenously. Pretreatment of the patient with antihistamine prior to the administration of chemotherapy is recommended. Reversible elevation of liver enzymes, induction of hypercoagulability with thrombus formation, and cerebral dysfunction similar to hyperammonemia has been seen in human patients. An idiosyncratic and sometimes lethal acute hemorrhagic pancreatitis has been reported in humans and dogs. This drug is used as part of induction therapy for canine and feline lymphomas and mast cell disease at a dose of 10,000 IU/m^2 SC or IM in dogs and 400 IU/kg SC or IM in cats.

Nitrosoureas. Lomustine (chloroethylcyclohexlnitrosourea [CCNU]) and carmustine (bischloroethylnitrosourea [BCNU]) are nitrosoureas that have been used in veterinary oncology. These are highly lipid-soluble agents. The cytotoxic effect is through spontaneous chemical decomposition to two reactive intermediates, a chloroethyldiazohydroxide and an isocyanate group. The chloroethyldiazohydroxide further decomposes to yield carbonium ions, which form adducts with DNA bases (guanine) and cause DNA interstrand cross-links. CCNU exerts a preferential killing effect in early S and G$_1$ phases. BCNU must be administered intravenously, whereas CCNU is an oral preparation. These drugs are useful for central nervous system neoplasia owing to high lipid solubility. The elimination of nitrosoureas is primarily renal. These drugs are indicated for the treatment of brain tumors; partial remissions have been reported in the dog. The use of CCNU as a rescue agent for relapsed canine lymphomas (90 mg/m^2 PO every 21 days) for 4 to 5 cycles, then every 6 to 8 weeks thereafter has been reported. The most frequent toxicity seen is delayed myelosuppression. Pulmonary fibrosis has been reported in humans. Other adverse effects include gastrointestinal, hepatic, renal, and ocular (corneal de-epithe-lialization) toxicities.

Hormones. Glucocorticoids such as prednisone are the most commonly used (and abused) hormones in veterinary oncology. Glucocorticoids are indicated as a part of combination chemotherapy for lymphoid malignancies and mast cell disease. The exact mechanism by which corticosteroids cause lymphoblast lysis is not known. It is presumed that the activity involves interaction with a cytosolic receptor and translocation of this receptor to the nucleus. Glucocorticoids activate endonucleases that cleave DNA and cause cell death. The dose of prednisone varies with the protocol described; most protocols call for 20 to 40 mg/m² PO on alternate days. The adverse effects of long-term steroid administration are the well-known constellation of signs associated with cushingoid syndrome in the dog.

CANINE LYMPHOMA PROTOCOLS

The most commonly treated disseminated malignancy in veterinary oncology is lymphoma in the dog. One of the purposes of this article is to provide commonly used protocols to readers in an overview format. Thirty-eight published protocols were recently summarized in tabular form (Jeglum, 1996). Veterinary oncologists use many of the same drugs to treat canine lymphoma, but the dose and scheduling vary from one institution to another. In general, remission can be expected in about 75 to 80% of canine lymphoma patients, and the length of first remission ranges from 4 to 6 months. Maintenance and rescue protocols add to the duration of survival of these patients.

The authors have attempted to summarize published lymphoma protocols that differ in substantial ways from one another, whether in dose intensity, response or toxicity rates, or indications. Also included are survival statistics and toxicity data, when established. Comments regarding these protocols are based on the authors' practice experience and are included as a guide for the practitioner. Variations in dose regimens for a given protocol are indicated by the italicized word *"OR."* Multidrug regimens are used more often to treat lymphoma than are single-agent protocols, with the exception of doxorubicin as a single agent. The reader should select a lymphoma protocol based on his or her experience, the preference of referral oncologists who can support the practitioner with difficult cases or unexpected toxicities, and the therapeutic goals for the individual patient. Increased dose intensity increases the potential for long-term survival but also increases the potential for a significant adverse effect. A young dog in otherwise good health may be a better candidate for a dose-intense protocol, such as Madison-Wisconsin; a geriatric patient with other life-limiting conditions may be better treated with a milder, less dose-intense induction protocol, such as COPLA. Duration and quality of life are among the variables that should be discussed with clients when one selects one protocol over another. Concerns about cost may make substitution of dactinomycin for doxorubicin a logical choice, provided that the client understands the potential for poorer overall survival outcome. Mitoxantrone may be substituted for doxorubicin for patients with con-

current cardiac disease. The selection of doxorubicin as a single agent may improve convenience and the cost to the owner in other situations.

COP. COP (cyclophosphamide, Oncovin [vincristine], and prednisone) is one of the oldest and mildest protocols for the treatment of lymphoma. It may be used for low-grade lymphoma or in situations where the potential for pancreatitis from L-asparaginase and doxorubicin should be avoided. The median duration of remission with this protocol is reported to be 6 months.

- Cyclophosphamide: 50 mg/m² PO every other day for 8 weeks; *OR* 300 mg/m² PO every 3 weeks for 1 year, then every 4 weeks (treatment stopped after 78 weeks).
- Vincristine: 0.5 to 0.7 mg/m² IV once a week for 8 weeks; *OR* 0.75 mg/m² IV once a week for 4 weeks, then every 3 weeks for 1 year, then every 4 weeks.
- Prednisone: 20 mg/m² PO once a day for 1 week, then every other day until relapse or adverse corticosteroid effect, in which case taper and discontinue; *OR* 1 mg/kg PO daily for 4 weeks, then on alternate days for up to 78 weeks.

CHOP. CHOP (cyclophosphamide, doxorubicin [hydroxydaunomycin], Oncovin [vincristine], and prednisone) is recommended for high-grade lymphoma and lymphoma at extranodal locations. The median survival has been reported to be 216 days. The injectables in the protocol that follows can be repeated every 21 days for a maximum of six to eight cycles (MacEwen and Young, 1996).

- Cyclophosphamide: 50 mg/m² PO every other day for 8 weeks.
- Vincristine: 0.5 to 0.7 mg/m² IV on days 8 and 15.
- Prednisone: 20 mg/m² PO once a day for 1 week, then every other day until relapse.
- Doxorubicin: 30 mg/m² IV on day 1 of each cycle.

COAP. COAP is an older protocol that adds cytosine arabinoside to a standard COP protocol. This addition gives the combination the potential of utility in central nervous system lymphoma, or to facilitate eradication of lymphoblasts from the marrow. This protocol was originally published by Theilen (1987) and has been updated (Dobson and Gorman, 1994). The median duration of survival reported by Dobson is 25 weeks when the protocol is given for 8 weeks, then reduced to 1 week on therapy and 1 week off. At the end of 6 months of treatment, the vincristine was stopped. If sterile hemorrhagic cystitis was observed, melphalan was substituted for cyclophosphamide and the vincristine was continued for a further 3 to 6 months.

- Cyclophosphamide: 50 mg/m² PO every other day for 8 days.
- Vincristine: 0.5 mg/m² IV once a week for 8 weeks.
- Prednisone: 40 mg/m² PO once a day for 1 week, then 20 mg/m² PO every other day.
- Cytosine arabinoside: 100 mg/m² IV daily on days 1 to 4.

CDP. CDP (chlorambucil, dactinomycin, and prednisone) can be used for clients with financial concerns, as it substitutes the antitumor antibiotic dactinomycin for the more costly doxorubicin. It is not a dose-intense protocol, so severe toxicity and the necessity for costly hospitalization are not anticipated. Survival expectation is comparable to that seen with a COP protocol.

- Chlorambucil: 4 mg/m² PO every other day.
- Dactinomycin: 0.5 to 0.75 mg/m² IV every 2 to 3 weeks.
- Prednisone: 20 mg/m² PO every other day.

VCAA. This protocol has been used in conjunction with the canine monoclonal lymphoma antibody CL/MAb 231. It is associated with a 75% remission rate. When followed by the monoclonal antibody therapy, dogs have been reported to have a median survival duration of 591 days (Jeglum, 1996).

- L-Asparaginase: 400 IU/kg IP or SC, week 1.
- Vincristine: 0.75 mg/m² IV, week 2.
- Cyclophosphamide: 75 mg/m² PO daily for 4 days, week 3.
- Doxorubicin: 30 mg/m² IV, week 4.

Advanced Drug Combinations. The following protocols all vary with regard to dose and scheduling of the same five drugs: cyclophosphamide, vincristine, L-asparaginase, prednisone, and doxorubicin. All are associated with a remission rate of 75 to 80%, and median remission durations ranging from 175 to 369 days. Most of these protocols, when associated with rescue of relapse, are expected to provide close to 1 year median survival expectation (with the exception of T-cell lymphomas, or those associated with hypercalcemia or advanced stage). The Madison-Wisconsin protocol adds methotrexate to the other drugs and has the highest published proportion of patients with 2-year survival (30%; Keller et al, 1993).

COPLA. COPLA (cyclophosphamide, vincristine [Oncovin], prednisone, L-asparaginase, doxorubicin [Adriamycin]) is associated with a low rate of side effects and a reasonable duration of remission, owing to the addition of intensification with doxorubicin at the end of the induction protocol when the dogs are in complete clinical remission (Kitchell, unpublished data, 1997).

- Cyclophosphamide: 50 mg/m² PO every other day for 8 weeks, then substitute chlorambucil, 4 mg/m² PO every other day until relapse or 2 years of therapy.
- Vincristine: 0.5 to 0.7 mg/m² IV once a week for 8 weeks, then step down to every other week for two cycles, every third week for three cycles, then every 4 weeks thereafter until relapse or 2 years of therapy.
- Prednisone: 20 mg/m² PO once a day for 1 week, then every other day until relapse or adverse corticosteroid effect, in which case taper and discontinue.
- L-Asparaginase: 10,000 IU/m² IM or SC on days 1 and 8, and again at relapse.
- Doxorubicin: 30 mg/m² IV weeks 6, 9, and 12, and again at relapse.

ACOPA I and II. These protocols were developed by Cotter (Stone et al, 1991). They vary in the intensity of the induction phase, toxicity, and remission duration. In fact,

they are instructive as a comparison of dose intensity versus toxicity and remission duration. ACOPA I is a dose-intense protocol with a remission rate of 76%, a median duration of remission of 330 days, and 48% of patients in remission at 1 year. However, a 12% fatality rate due to toxicity on induction was observed. ACOPA II uses the same drugs in a different sequence. Toxicities were fewer, but so were remissions (65%) and median duration of remission (228 days; 34% of patients in remission at 1 year). Overall, ACOPA I is considered the more appropriate protocol for most patients, provided that vincristine is given the day before L-asparaginase.

ACOPA I. ACOPA I is maintained by repeating weeks 10 to 16 every 9 weeks until week 75. Melphalan is substituted for cyclophosphamide in the case of sterile hemorrhagic cystitis, as described earlier.

- Vincristine: 0.75 mg/m2 IV a week, weeks 1 to 4, then weeks 7, 10, 13, and 16.
- L-Asparaginase: 10,000 IU/m² IM a week, weeks 1 to 4, then weeks 7, 10, 13, and 16.
- Cyclophosphamide: 250 mg/m² PO, weeks 7, 13, and 16.
- Doxorubicin: 30 mg/m² IV, week 10.
- Prednisone: 40 mg/m² PO daily for 7 days, then every other day.

ACOPA II. This protocol maintained after week 29 by repeating weeks 10 to 16 every 9 weeks until week 75. Melphalan is substituted for cyclophosphamide in the case of sterile hemorrhagic cystitis, as described earlier.

- Vincristine: 0.75 mg/m2 IV, weeks 4, 10, 13, 16, 19, and 22.
- L-Asparaginase: 10,000 IU/m² IM, weeks 7, 8, 25, and 26.
- Cyclophosphamide: 250 mg/m² PO, weeks 4, 7, 13, 16, and 22.
- Doxorubicin: 30 mg/m² IV, weeks 1, 10, and 19.
- Prednisone: 40 mg/m² PO daily for 7 days, then every other day.

AMC 2. This protocol has a 6-week induction followed by repeats of weeks 4 to 6. Weeks 4 to 6 are repeated at 2-week intervals for two cycles, and then are repeated at 21-day intervals for two cycles (Greenlee et al, 1990).

- Vincristine: 0.7 mg/m² IV, weeks 1 and 4.
- L-Asparaginase: 400 IU/kg IP *OR* IM, week 1.
- Cyclophosphamide: 200 to 250 mg/m² IV, weeks 2 and 5.
- Doxorubicin: 30 mg/m² IV, weeks 3 and 6.
- Prednisone: 30 mg/m² PO daily, week 1; then 20 mg/m² PO daily, week 2; then 10 mg/m² PO daily, week 3.

VELCAP. After week 28, this protocol repeats weeks 12 to 18 every 9 weeks until 75 weeks. Doxorubicin administration is preceded by echocardiograms after the sixth treatment. Melphalan is substituted for cyclophosphamide in the case of hemorrhagic cystitis (Ogilvie and Moore, 1995).

- Vincristine: 0.75 mg/m² IV, weeks 1 to 3, 7, 12, 15, 18, 21, and 27.

- L-Asparaginase: 10,000 IU/m^2 IM (maximum dose 10,000 IU), weeks 7 to 9, 24, and 25.
- Cyclophosphamide: 250 mg/m^2 PO, weeks 7, 12, 15, 21, and 24.
- Doxorubicin: 30 mg/m^2 IV, weeks 2, 4, 18, and 27.
- Prednisone: 40 mg/m^2 PO daily, week 1, then every other day.

Madison-Wisconsin. After week 17, weeks 11 to 17 are repeated every 2 weeks until week 25, then every 3 weeks until week 49, and then every 5 weeks. Chlorambucil at 1.4 mg/kg PO replaces cyclophosphamide after week 11 for dogs in complete remission (Keller et al, 1993).

- Vincristine: 0.5 to 0.7 mg/m^2 IV, weeks 1, 3, 6, 8, 11, and 15.
- L-Asparaginase: 400 IU/kg IM, week 1.
- Cyclophosphamide: 200 mg/m^2 IV, weeks 2, 7, and 13.
- Doxorubicin: 30 mg/m^2 IV, weeks 4 and 9.
- Methotrexate: 0.5 to 0.8 mg/kg IV, week 17.
- Prednisone: 2 mg/kg PO daily, week 1; then 1.5 mg/kg PO daily, week 2; then 1.0 mg/kg PO daily, week 3; and then 0.5 mg/kg PO daily, week 4.

Rescue Protocols. Most dogs treated for lymphoma are expected to relapse at some point after induction of remission. Drug resistance may have been acquired by cells that have survived sublethal exposure to the previously encountered induction agents. The following protocols are used for reinduction of remission (Ogilivie and Moore, 1995).

ADIC. One of the oldest rescue protocols, ADIC combines doxorubicin with dacarbazine. These drugs are thought to be synergistic in combination. Care should be taken to screen for cardiac toxicity if high cumulative doses of doxorubicin have been administered in the initial induction protocol (more than 200 to 240 mg/m^2 total).

- Doxorubicin: 30 mg/m^2 IV every 21 days.
- Dacarbazine: 200 mg/m^2 IV daily for 5 days, *OR* 800 mg/m^2 administered as an 8-hour intravenous infusion.

MOPP. This is a very aggressive protocol with a high rate of myelosuppression and sepsis. Care should be taken to monitor these patients closely. The protocol given here includes dose modifications to decrease toxicity from the original protocol, which resulted in death in 35% of 17 dogs treated. This protocol is repeated at 28-day intervals.

- Mechlorethamine: 3 mg/m^2 IV, day 1.
- Vincristine: 0.7 mg/m^2 IV, day 1.
- Procarbazine: 50 mg/m^2 PO, days 1 to 14.
- Prednisone: 30 mg/m^2 PO, days 1 to 14.

References and Suggested Reading

DeVita VT, Hellman S, Rosenberg SA: Cancer: Principles and Practice of Oncology, 5th ed. Philadelphia: Lippincott-Raven, 1997, p 375.
  This is the *textbook in human oncologic medicine. A "must-read" for the true oncophile.*
Dobson JM, Gorman NT: Canine multicentric lymphoma 2: Comparison of response to two chemotherapeutic protocols. J Small Anim Pract 35:9, 1994.
  Compares COP with COAP in 90 dogs.
Greenlee P, Filippa D, Quimby F, et al: Lymphomas in dogs: A morphologic, immunologic and clinical study. Cancer 66:480, 1990.
  This article was very important in establishing the role of histology and immunophenotype in response of canine lymphoma to rotating sequential chemotherapy.
Jeglum KA: Chemoimmunotherapy of canine lymphoma with adjuvant canine monoclonal antibody 231. Vet Clin North Am Small Anim Pract 26:73, 1996.
  Provides a comprehensive overview of all the published canine lymphoma protocols in table form.
Keller ET, MacEwen EG, Rosenthal RC, et al: Evaluation of prognostic factors and sequential combination chemotherapy with doxorubicin for canine lymphoma. J Vet Intern Med 7:289, 1993.
  The Madison-Wisconsin protocol results in 30% long-term survivals of more than 2 years.
MacEwen EG, Young KM: Canine lymphoma and lymphoid leukemias. In: Withrow SJ, MacEwen EG, eds: Small Animal Clinical Oncology, 2nd ed. Philadelphia: WB Saunders, 1996, p 451.
  This textbook is currently the most comprehensive and up-to-date overview of veterinary oncologic medicine.
Ogilvie GK, Moore AS: Lymphoma. In: Ogilvie GK, Moore AS, eds: Managing the Veterinary Cancer Patient: A Practice Manual. Trenton, NJ: Veterinary Learning Systems, 1995, p 228.
  This chapter is highly readable and practical for the practitioner seeking to get a handle on the treatment of lymphoma in dogs.
Stone MS, Goldstein MA, Cotter SM: Comparison of two protocols for induction of remission in dogs with lymphoma. J Am Anim Hosp Assoc 27:315, 1991.
  Cotter and company compare ACOPA I and ACOPA II in the usual meticulous style.
Theilen GH, Madewell BR: Chemotherapy. In: Theilen GH, Madewell, BR, eds: Veterinary Cancer Medicine, 2nd ed. Philadelphia: Lea & Febiger, 1987, p 157.
  This chapter supplies good chemotherapy information for the veterinarian and provides a very comprehensive overview and historical perspective.

Anticancer Drugs: New Drugs or Applications for Veterinary Medicine

ANGELA E. FRIMBERGER

Worcester, Massachusetts

CHEMOTHERAPY DRUGS

Ifosfamide and Mesna

Ifosfamide (Ifex, Bristol-Myers Squibb) is a nitrogen mustard developed as a broad-spectrum analogue of cyclophosphamide. In human oncology, it is used in the treatment of lymphoma, osteosarcoma, and testicular carcinoma. Ifosfamide is less myelosuppressive than cyclophosphamide but consistently causes severe urothelial toxicity (hemorrhagic cystitis) when given alone. Concurrent administration of the thiol drug mesna (Mesnex, Bristol-Myers Squibb Oncology; see discussion on chemoprotective drugs, below) significantly prevents the urothelial toxicity. A dose escalation study in dogs with chemoresistant lymphoma and soft tissue sarcomas showed that ifosfamide, given in a saline diuresis protocol with mesna, was very well tolerated at doses of 350 to 375 mg/m². The dose-limiting toxicity was myelosuppression, with measurably decreased neutrophil counts and, occasionally, thrombocytopenia 1 week after administration, but without accompanying clinical signs in most cases. Small dogs appear to be more sensitive to the myelosuppression, so they should be treated at the low end of the dose range. The drug was found to be useful in salvage therapy for lymphoma; stable partial responses with significantly increased subjective well-being were seen, and this positive impact on quality of life and tolerability makes ifosfamide particularly appealing as a salvage drug. Its use in soft tissue sarcomas and osteosarcoma is being explored at this time. It is expected to be a useful addition to regimens for these diseases, as well as germ cell tumors, in dogs because of its activity in the analogous diseases in humans.

Nitrosoureas: Lomustine and Carmustine

The nitrosoureas are among the few chemotherapy agents that can be used to treat brain tumors, because by virtue of their lipophilic nature they have the unusual ability to cross the blood-brain barrier. They are also useful in the treatment of lymphoma because they are not substrates for the multidrug resistance protein P-glycoprotein, and they do not share cross-resistance with other alkylating agents.

Lomustine, or CCNU (CeeNU, Bristol-Myers Squibb), is a nitrosourea that has been used in human patients for the treatment of brain tumors and non-Hodgkin's lymphoma. In humans, the dosage interval is 6 weeks because of delayed myelosuppression occurring 3 to 4 weeks after administration. Vomiting 24 hours after administration is common in people. Clinical trials in dogs with brain tumors and lymphoma have demonstrated a different pattern of toxicity.

Vomiting has been seen only infrequently. Although myelosuppression is the dose-limiting toxicity, the neutrophil nadir appears to occur 1 week after administration, rather than the longer interval noted in human patients. Furthermore, dogs receiving prolonged treatment may develop thrombocytopenia cumulatively; therefore, the platelet count should always be monitored as part of the routine complete blood count (CBC) when this drug is being used. The recommended dose of lomustine in dogs is 90 mg/m² PO every 4 to 6 weeks, with a CBC performed 1 week after administration and immediately prior to the next dose. Discontinue use if platelet count is less than 200,000/μl and until thrombocytopenia is resolved. Objective responses have been seen in lymphoma resistant to other chemotherapy, in mast cell tumors, and in brain tumors of various histologic types.

Carmustine, or BCNU (BiCNU, Bristol-Myers Squibb), has also been evaluated for the treatment of brain tumors in dogs in one clinical trial. The dose used was 50 mg/m² IV every 6 weeks. Myelosuppression was the dose-limiting toxicity, with a neutrophil nadir 7 to 9 days after administration and lasting for 15 days. One dog developed subclinical pulmonary fibrosis, which is a recognized potential side effect of the drug in humans. Other toxicities in humans include myelosuppression and hepatotoxicity and nephrotoxicity. All dogs with glioma in this study had partial remissions, with survival times comparable to that expected following radiation therapy.

Carboplatin

Carboplatin (Paraplatin, Bristol-Myers Squibb Oncology) is an analogue of cisplatin. The spectrums of activity of these two drugs are similar. The main clinical difference between the drugs lies in their toxicity profiles: carboplatin is not nephrotoxic but is more myelosuppressive than cisplatin. The use of carboplatin in dogs can now be considered routine and is discussed elsewhere in this volume (see p. 470). However, this new drug has been somewhat of a breakthrough for cats that could not previously receive systemic platinum therapy at all. The appropriate dose is somewhat controversial: a trial in normal cats and one clinical trial have found the maximally tolerated dose to be 200 to 210 mg/m², while another clinical trial found the dose to be greater than 260 mg/m². Until this controversy is resolved, it would seem prudent to use the lower dose (210 mg/m²), every 3 to 4 weeks, as a slow intravenous bolus. The drug should be diluted to 10 mg/ml in 5% dextrose in water, rather than in 0.9% NaCl, because the presence of chloride ions in the diluent could favor the conversion of carboplatin to cisplatin in solution. Although

474

carboplatin is not nephrotoxic, it is renally eliminated, so the dose should be reduced in the presence of renal insufficiency, or toxicity will be increased. The dose-limiting toxicity is myelosuppression, which can occur as late as 21 days after administration; thus, a CBC should be evaluated before each dose is given, and the treatment should be delayed if the neutrophil count is below 3,000/ μl. Carboplatin has activity against a variety of carcinomas and soft tissue sarcomas in cats. Carboplatin has also been used for intralesional chemotherapy of facial squamous cell carcinoma in cats.

Lobaplatin

Lobaplatin is another non-nephrotoxic platinum analogue. The side effects in people include mild nausea, vomiting, and myelosuppression, and as with carboplatin dose reduction is needed in accordance with renal function. Lobaplatin is currently being used in a clinical trial of dogs with osteosarcoma, at a dosage of 35 mg/m² IV every 3 weeks initiated after surgery (either amputation or limb sparing). Preliminary data indicate that this dose is well tolerated overall, with the dose-limiting toxicity of myelosuppression occurring 7 to 10 days after administration, and transient depression and vomiting in the first 2 days and 7 to 10 days after administration. To date, the efficacy appears comparable to that of cisplatin and carboplatin.

Paclitaxel

Paclitaxel (Taxol, Bristol-Myers Squibb) has been studied extensively in people in recent years because of unprecedented efficacy in the treatment of some carcinomas, particularly breast and ovarian cancers. Although there was initial concern over the environmental impact of harvesting paclitaxel from yew trees, the drug can now be synthesized. This drug acts as a mitotic inhibitor by inhibiting microtubule disassembly, thereby "choking" the cell with microtubules (in contrast to the vinca alkaloids, which prevent microtubule assembly). Paclitaxel is hydrophobic; so the carrier Cremophor EL is used to solubilize it. Cremophor also has significant pharmacologic effects, particularly triggering severe mast cell degranulation in dogs and cats. Dogs must be extensively premedicated with prednisone (1 mg/kg PO for 5 days), and then given cimetidine (4 mg/kg IV), diphenhydramine (4 mg/kg IM), and dexamethasone sodium phosphate (1 mg/kg IV) 1 hour before paclitaxel infusion to ameliorate severe anaphylactoid reaction. Dogs must be observed closely during the infusion, since even with premedication, the rate of infusion must often be slowed to control reactions. The recommended dose is 165 mg/m², diluted to 0.6 mg/ml in 0.9% NaCl, given as a continuous intravenous infusion over at least 2 hours, and every 3 weeks. The toxicities include vomiting and diarrhea potentially severe within 1 week of administration, myelosuppression with a neutrophil nadir that appears to occur within 1 week of administration, and extremely profound alopecia. Objective responses have been seen in carcinomas and lymphoma; however, the response rate in sarcomas is extremely low.

Paclitaxel is also under investigation for use in cats.

Pretreatments and the expected toxicities are similar to those in dogs, but in addition cats also exhibit swelling of the ears and paws. The investigational dose in cats is 5 mg/kg (Ogilvie GK, personal communication, 1998).

Epirubicin

Epirubicin (Pharmorubicin, Pharmacia & Upjohn) is a stereoisomer of doxorubicin that has been used in clinical trials in humans and has been found to be less cardiotoxic than doxorubicin is (see *CVT XI*, pp. 392 to 395 for other details). A large, multi-institutional randomized clinical trial comparing epirubicin with doxorubicin as single agents in the treatment of canine lymphoma showed comparable efficacy between the two drugs. Epirubicin was found to be somewhat less cardiotoxic, based on myocardial histopathology, but echocardiographic and other changes associated with cardiotoxicity were seen with both drugs. The two drugs appear to be similar with respect to the acute dose-limiting toxicities, myelosuppression, and gastrointestinal toxicity. Epirubicin is not commercially available in the United States at this time; however, it is marketed in Canada.

Methoxymorpholino-doxorubicin

FCE-23762 (Pharmacia) is a new methoxymorpholino derivative of doxorubicin. This drug has been studied in large phase I and II clinical trials in tumor-bearing dogs (Sheafor et al, 1997), with quite favorable results. The drug has in vitro activity against tumor cells resistant to doxorubicin, and this finding was reflected in its efficacy as a rescue agent for chemoresistant lymphoma, with a 33% overall response rate. Dogs with untreated lymphoma had complete responses. Dogs with sarcomas had a 20% overall response rate, and those with carcinomas had an overall response rate of 33%. Toxicity consisted of mild to moderate myelosuppression and gastrointestinal toxicity. No cardiotoxicity was seen. The recommended dose is 80 μg/kg IV every 3 weeks (Sheafor SE, personal communication, 1998).

Topoisomerase I Inhibitors: 9-Aminocamptothecin

The camptothecins are the only chemotherapy drugs that work by inhibiting the DNA replication and transcription enzyme topoisomerase I. As such, they are unrelated to any other chemotherapy agent used to treat lymphoma in dogs. 9-Aminocamptothecin (Pharmacia & Upjohn) is under study for use in dogs with lymphoma. In human patients, the schedule of administration appears to be unusually important relative to toxicity and efficacy of the drug, and the same seems true in dogs. A total dose of 3.7 mg/ m² administered intravenously as a 72-hour continuous infusion resulted in a high rate of objective responses in dogs with lymphoma, and was well tolerated by most dogs. The dose-limiting toxicity is myelosuppression, which may be cumulative. Again, small dogs appear to be more susceptible to myelosuppression from this drug, so they should be treated with caution, possibly with the use of a lower dose. The dosage of this drug should perhaps be based on body weight rather than on body surface area; however, pharmacokinetic data have yet to be analyzed. Although the drug is known to be highly bioavailable when given orally, an appropriate oral dose has not yet been determined in dogs.

BIOLOGIC RESPONSE MODIFIERS

Piroxicam

Piroxicam (Feldene 10- and 20-mg tablets, Pfizer Laboratories; generics available) is a nonsteroidal anti-inflammatory drug (NSAID). This drug has been shown to have activity against a variety of tumors in humans and dogs. It has no direct antitumor effect in vitro and the primary activity is cyclooxygenase inhibition; thus, the mechanism of action is believed to be immunologic. In dogs, it has been used most extensively in the treatment of transitional cell carcinoma (TCC), where its efficacy as a single agent is comparable to that of cisplatin. Responses have also been observed in the treatment of squamous cell carcinoma (SCC), mammary adenocarcinoma, and transmissible venereal tumor (TVT). The dosage is 0.3 mg/kg PO every 24 hours, and the drug is well tolerated by most patients. As with most NSAIDs, the primary toxicity of piroxicam is gastrointestinal irritation; therefore, the drug should be given with food, and the addition of misoprostol (Cytotec 100- and 200-µg tablets, Searle) at a dose of 3 µg/kg PO every 8 hours should be considered in dogs that tolerate NSAIDs poorly. If signs of severe irritation or ulceration develop, the drug should be discontinued and treatment for gastric ulceration instituted (cimetidine and sucralfate were found to be effective). Once signs abate, it may be possible to administer piroxicam again, in combination with misoprostol. When piroxicam has been given alone, another known potential side effect of NSAIDs, renal papillary necrosis, has been noted on postmortem examination but has not been a clinical problem. However, when a combination of piroxicam and cisplatin was used for the treatment of canine bladder TCC, the piroxicam appeared to potentiate the nephrotoxicity of cisplatin. Therefore, until more data are available on the interaction of these two drugs, this drug combination should be used with extreme caution if at all. Piroxicam is a particularly attractive chemotherapeutic option for dogs because of its easy at-home administration and low toxicity. Furthermore, it is an analgesic as well; thus, it can play a palliative role even when it is not chemotherapeutically effective. Piroxicam has not been evaluated for use in cats.

L-MTP-PE

Liposome-encapsulated muramyl tripeptide phosphatidylethanolamine (L-MTP-PE) is a monocyte-macrophage activator derived from bacterial cell walls. Used in combination with chemotherapy, it has been shown to significantly improve outcomes compared with chemotherapy alone in canine splenic hemangiosarcoma and osteosarcoma (MacEwen and Kurzman, 1996). It is also currently in human clinical trials. Despite these encouraging results,

L-MTP-PE is not currently being marketed, although it may become commercially available in the future.

Retinoids: Etretinate and Isotretinoin
(see *CVT XII*, pp. 585 to 590)

Etretinate (Tegison 10- and 25-mg capsules, Hoffman-LaRoche) has been used for chemoprevention and as a differentiating agent in humans for a variety of tumors. Responses have been reported following the use of this drug to treat SCC and preneoplastic lesions (actinic keratoses), cutaneous lymphoma, and mycosis fungoides (epitheliotropic T-cell lymphoma), in dogs and cats, and various benign skin tumors including intracutaneous cornifying epitheliomas in dogs. Recommended doses are 1 mg/kg every 12 to 24 hours for 90 days to 6 months for dogs with benign and precancerous skin lesions, and 3 to 4 mg/kg every 24 hours or divided every 12 hours for cutaneous lymphoma and mycosis fungoides in dogs; and 10 mg/cat every 24 hours for cats.

Isotretinoin, or 13-*cis*-retinoic acid (Accutane 10-, 20-, and 40-mg caplets, LaRoche), has activity against cutaneous lymphoma and mycosis fungoides in dogs and cats, and various skin tumors in dogs. It is ineffective in the treatment of feline facial SCC. The recommended doses are 1 to 2 mg/kg every 24 hours for skin tumors and 3 to 4 mg/kg every 24 hours or divided every 12 hours for cutaneous lymphoma and mycosis fungoides in dogs, and 10 mg/cat every 24 hours for cutaneous lymphoma and mycosis fungoides in cats.

The toxicity profiles of these two drugs are similar. The most common adverse reaction to retinoids in dogs is keratoconjunctivitis sicca (KCS), although it has not been reported in cats receiving retinoids. Dogs receiving retinoids should have a baseline Schirmer tear test performed and then should be monitored monthly thereafter. If KCS develops, it may resolve when the drug is stopped, and cyclosporine ophthalmic drops have been reported to be helpful. Others toxicities and side effects are reversible when the drug is stopped, but dogs that have a history of pancreatitis, hepatitis, or diabetes mellitus should be treated with caution, if at all. Teratogenesis and decreased spermatogenesis are severe, and these effects can occur as long as 2 years after stopping the etretinate because of body fat storage of the drug; therefore, retinoids should not be used in breeding animals. Fortunately, most dogs exhibit no adverse effects, and when such sequelae do occur they are usually mild. Also, side effects occur more frequently with isotretinoin; therefore, when long-term therapy is used, etretinate is preferred. Cats are generally more tolerant of retinoids, rarely exhibiting any adverse effects except anorexia; however, a drug reaction consisting of reversible erythema and alopecia of the face, feet, abdomen, and perineum has been seen in cats receiving etretinate. If such a reaction is seen, the drug should be stopped or the dosage decreased.

CHEMOPROTECTIVE DRUGS

Mesna

Mesna (Mesnex, Bristol-Myers Squibb Oncology) is a thiol compound developed to prevent the urothelial toxicity (hemorrhagic cystitis) seen with ifosfamide and cyclophosphamide administration. None of the other toxicities of the drugs are prevented. Mesna forms dimers in the circulation that are broken down at the renal tubular epithelium to release free, active thiol groups into the urine, where they bind urotoxic metabolites. In humans, ifosfamide given without mesna causes such severe and consistent urothelial toxicity that the drug could not be used alone. In a clinical trial of ifosfamide in dogs, a dose of mesna equal to 20% of the ifosfamide dose was given three times with the infusion, and no incidences of hemorrhagic cystitis were seen. Mesna has been given with intravenous high-dose cyclophosphamide in dogs, at a dose of 40% of the cyclophosphamide dose, repeated six times every 3 hours, starting at the time of cyclophosphamide administration.

Dexrazoxane

Dexrazoxane (Zinecard, Pharmacia & Upjohn) is an iron chelator that significantly prevents the chronic cardiotoxicity caused by cumulative doxorubicin administration. Dexrazoxane does not change the pharmacokinetics of doxorubicin and does not prevent myelosuppression or gastrointestinal toxicity; therefore, it is thought unlikely to modify the antitumor effect. Its efficacy in preventing cardiotoxicity is proven in humans and dogs and is dramatic; however, cardiotoxicity can still occur at very high doses of doxorubicin. Dexrazoxane is given at a dose ratio to doxorubicin of 10 to 20:1; or in dogs, 25 mg/kg is administered intravenously 15 minutes before doxorubicin is given. Despite the obvious cardioprotective effect of dexrazoxane, it has still not been clearly shown that patients will derive long-term benefits such as improved overall survival from the use of this drug; therefore, the overall value of dexrazoxane therapy is still controversial.

PALLIATIVE DRUGS

Fentanyl Patch

A new transdermal delivery patch (Duragesic System, Janssen Pharmaceutical) has made administration of the narcotic analgesic fentanyl possible for outpatients for several days at a time. The patches are available in 25-, 50-, 75-, and 100-μg/hr sizes. In a clinical trial in humans, the patches were found to provide effective analgesia for the majority of outpatients. In a study (Kyles et al, 1996) of the pharmacokinetics of fentanyl after placement of the 50-μg/hr patch on normal Beagles, the plasma concentration rose to analgesic levels approximately 24 hours after placement and remained at a steady state until the patch was removed 72 hours after placement. After removal, plasma levels fell rapidly over the next 12 to 24 hours. None of the dogs in this study exhibited any opioid side effects, such as respiratory depression or sedation; however, they did exhibit marked individual variation in pharmacokinetics. Clinical experience with tumor-bearing dogs also indicates that the appropriate dose varies considerably, but that in general a 25-μg/hr patch for cats and small dogs, a 50-μg/hr patch for medium-sized dogs, and two 50-μg/hr patches for very large dogs, or 3 to 5 μg/kg per hour, will provide analgesia. The therapeutic margin for this drug is

wide, and if analgesia is not achieved at these doses and there is no sedation the dose can safely be increased; however, both occasional sedation and occasional agitation, which resolved when the patches were removed, have been seen in this dose range. To place the patch on animals, the inguinal area is clipped and wiped gently with alcohol, then the adhesive backing of the patch is exposed and pressed against the clipped skin. Others prefer placing the patch in the interscapular area, as ingestion of the patch can be dangerous (caution: inadvertent ingestion is also a hazard to children). Care should be taken to place the patch in such a way that it will not pull skin or hair. Because of the 24-hour lag time, the patch should be placed before pain occurs if it can be anticipated (i.e., the night before surgery). If immediate analgesia is needed, an intravenous bolus of fentanyl of 30 μg/kg can be given at the same time that the patch is placed. If analgesia will be needed for more than several days, a new patch is placed every 72 hours, and the old patch is not removed until the new one has been in place for 24 hours.

Piroxicam

Piroxicam (Feldene, Pfizer; generic available) is an NSAID that has antitumor effects (see earlier). It is also a well-tolerated analgesic and can used for palliation in dogs even when it is not indicated as a chemotherapeutic. See earlier discussion for dosage and side effects.

Butorphanol

Butorphanol (Stadol, Bristol) is a narcotic that has antiemetic effects in addition to its analgesic and antitussive effects. Despite the availability of other antiemetics, only butorphanol has been effective in preventing cisplatin-associated vomiting. In a randomized clinical trial, dogs given butorphanol (0.4 mg/kg IM) at the end of the cisplatin infusion had a 19% chance of vomiting, while dogs that received no antiemetic had a 89% chance of vomiting. In this setting, the butorphanol had no adverse effects, and it is recommended routinely with cisplatin therapy. Butorphanol at this dose may also help ameliorate the vomiting associated with other chemotherapy drugs.

Ondansetron

Ondansetron (Zofran, Glaxo) is a serotonin (5-HT$_3$) receptor antagonist that is a relatively new option for the treatment of chemotherapy (and anesthesia)-associated nausea and vomiting. This drug is remarkably effective in controlling nausea and vomiting in people and has greatly lessened the morbidity of chemotherapy for many patients. It has no effect on antitumor efficacy and, in humans, has fewer side effects than metoclopramide. There is no doubt that it is extremely effective in dogs as well, and the main deterrent to its use in veterinary oncology has been cost. This drug should be considered if vomiting cannot be controlled with more conventional antiemetics, and the cost should be reviewed on a case-by-case basis. The dosage is 0.1 to 1.0 mg/kg PO every 12 to 24 hours, or 30 minutes before and 90 minutes after starting cisplatin infusion.

Cyproheptadine

Cyproheptadine (Periactin, 4-mg tablets, Merck) has been recommended for appetite stimulation in cats and dogs. The doses reported for use in the cat are 1 to 4 mg/cat or 0.35 to 1 mg/kg, once or twice a day. The appetite stimulant action exceeds 18 hours in cats. In dogs, a dose of 0.1 to 0.2 mg/kg caused polyphagia in 25% of dogs in a double-blinded, placebo-controlled trial of cyproheptadine for allergic pruritus (it did not improve the pruritus). The agitation sometimes seen in cats will resolve when the dose is lowered or the drug is stopped.

NEW MODES OF ADMINISTRATION

Intracavitary Administration

Chemotherapy can be administered directly into the thoracic and peritoneal cavities for the treatment of tumors involving the serosal surfaces, such as mesothelioma and carcinomatosis. This method of administration is especially effective in cases in which effusion is a major clinical complaint, particularly in the thoracic cavity. Intracavitary chemotherapy administration has been best documented with cisplatin (Moore et al, 1991). The concentration of drug in the tumor cells is increased over what would be achieved with intravenous dosing for only the first 3 mm of tissue, so large bulky tumors are not treated appropriately with this method. The cisplatin is absorbed systemically, so the safe whole-body dose (see p. 470) should not be exceeded, and an intravenous saline diuresis protocol must be used as if the cisplatin had been given intravenously. Vomiting can also be seen, as it is with intravenous administration of cisplatin; thus, butorphanol or ondansetron should be used (see earlier). The calculated dose of cisplatin is diluted into 0.9% NaCl in a bag with an intravenous drip set attached (the line should be primed before adding the drug), in a volume of 250 ml/m^2 for thoracic administration and 1,000 ml/m^2 for peritoneal administration. If the thorax is to be treated, the preferred area for puncture is the intercostal spaces of the right side of the chest, in the area of the cardiac notch. If the abdomen is to be treated, the dog should be allowed to urinate before treatment (especially in light of the diuresis) and the puncture should be made along the midline, caudal to the umbilicus. Ultrasound guidance may be helpful in avoiding viscera when the catheter is placed. The area is clipped and scrubbed, and is blocked with lidocaine, and a rigid 14-gauge intravenous catheter is inserted. Before infusion, 10 to 20 ml of plain saline is infused to test the catheter; any coughing or discomfort indicates that the catheter is not correctly placed. The saline should flow easily. The area should be watched during administration for signs of subcutaneous leakage of fluid. After the delivery is complete, pressure should be applied to the area for a few minutes, then the patient should be walked to help distribute the fluid in the cavity.

Liposome-Encapsulated Drug Delivery

Liposomes are particles of synthetic lipid bilayer encapsulating an aqueous phase. In recent years, liposomes have been vigorously developed as drug-delivery vehicles because they can change the pharmacokinetics of drugs markedly. Liposomal encapsulation increases the circulation time of many drugs, increasing tumor cell exposure and, at the same time, decreasing toxicity by reducing peak plasma level. Simple liposomes are taken up rapidly by the reticuloendothelial system (RES), making them ideal for delivery of biologic response modifiers (e.g., L-MTP-PE), but not for chemotherapeutic drugs. However, liposome-encapsulated doxorubicin was evaluated in healthy dogs and found to be significantly less cardiotoxic than the native drug. Liposomes that incorporate polyethylene glycol (PEG) in the outer surface are not taken up by the RES, resulting in longer circulation times for more effective chemotherapy drug delivery. A PEG-ylated liposome-encapsulated doxorubicin formulation (Doxil, Sequus Pharmaceuticals) has been studied in clinical trials in cats and dogs. Preliminary results indicate decreased toxicity and significant antitumor efficacy at doses of doxorubicin similar to those used with native drug; however, a new cutaneous toxicity not seen with native doxorubicin has emerged and is dose-limiting. Liposome-encapsulated formulations of vincristine and cisplatin have also been developed and tested in a preclinical setting, and are in early veterinary trials. Liposomes can also be modified by the addition of antibodies to their surface to target them to a particular cell type, and specifically designed liposomes also show promise as vehicles for the delivery of cytokines and as transfection vectors for gene therapy.

References and Suggested Reading

Veterinary Cancer Society Proceeding of Annual Conferences.
The best overview of recent developments in veterinary oncology, containing abstracts relating to current clinical trials often a year or more before publication in journals. To receive VCS newsletters and proceedings contact Dr. Richard E. Weller, Treasurer, Veterinary Cancer Society, Developmental Toxicology Section, Batelle, Pacific Northwest Labs, P.O. Box 999, Mail Stop K810, Richland, WA 99352.
Ogilvie GK, Moore AS: Managing the Veterinary Cancer Patient. Trenton, NJ: Veterinary Learning Systems, 1995.
A user-friendly practice manual and thorough, up-to-date review of the literature relating to veterinary oncology.
Knapp DW, Richardson RC, Bottoms GD, et al: Phase I trial of piroxicam in 62 dogs bearing naturally occurring tumors. Cancer Chemother Pharmacol 29:214, 1992.
The largest published study to date of piroxicam therapy in veterinary patients.
Kyles AE, Papich M, Hardie EM: Disposition of transdermally administered fentanyl in dogs. Am J Vet Res 57:715, 1996.
A pharmacokinetic study of the fentanyl patch in normal dogs.
MacEwen EG, Kurzman ID: Canine osteosarcoma: Amputation and chemoimmunotherapy. Vet Clin North Am Small Anim Pract 26:123,1996.
Although specifically about osteosarcoma, this is the most recent veterinary publication by the group of researchers who have been studying L-MTP-PE in animals and have published their findings extensively in the veterinary and human medical literature.
Moore AS, Kirk C, Cardona A: Intracavitary cisplatin chemotherapy experience with six dogs. J Vet Intern Med 5:227, 1991.
The original description of the use of intracavitary chemotherapy in veterinary medicine.

Multidrug Resistance

PHILIP J. BERGMAN

Houston, Texas

For veterinarians involved in the treatment via chemotherapeutics of dogs with cancer, drug resistance is a common phenomenon and the most common cause of treatment failure. For example, many chemotherapeutic agents are capable of inducing rapid remissions in dogs with lymphoma; however, the ability to effectively treat these patients once they have relapsed is significantly impaired. This inability to effectively treat patients after relapse is probably due to a multitude of resistance factors, which have been elucidated over the last three decades. Multiple mechanisms of resistance are probably present in most normal cells, and their presence represents a level of redundancy for the protection of the cell and the organism. Unfortunately, many neoplasms have devised methods of employing these resistance mechanisms for their own protection.

Drug resistance is generally categorized into intrinsic and acquired forms, with probable overlap in mechanisms across these two categories. Additionally, resistance mechanisms can be looked at from organism and cellular levels. Although there are many recognized processes responsible for overall resistance, there are also many that we as clinicians can easily circumvent, including inappropriate underdosing of chemotherapeutics and improper scheduling of drugs. Other mechanisms, over which we may not have any control, include poor absorption and erratic bioavailability of oral drugs, decreased drug activation, increased repair of drug damage, increased drug extrusion, and poor penetration of the drug into the tumor. Over the past two decades, research has uncovered strategies for circumventing some of these previously untouchable resistance mechanisms; in fact, some have become clinically relevant resistance-reversal strategies. This overview focuses on some of the important cellular mechanisms of resistance.

P-GLYCOPROTEIN

The most researched form of cellular drug resistance is the overexpression of a plasma membrane protein given the name P (permeability)-glycoprotein, or P-170 (protein molecular weight of 160 to 180 kD). Resistance related to P-glycoprotein overexpression is one of the major factors leading to the multidrug resistance (MDR) phenotype. MDR is the phenomenon by which cancer cells acquire resistance to a variety of drugs commonly used in veterinary medicine, such as doxorubicin, vincristine, actinomycin D, and mitoxantrone (Table 1). Such drugs are typically developed from natural sources and are hydrophobic, but otherwise they have very few similarities in their mechanisms of action or their chemical structures. Not only will

cancer cells develop resistance to these chemotherapeutics, but also these same compounds will induce the formation of the MDR phenotype. P-glycoprotein genes have been found in bacteria, viruses, plants, insects, nematodes, and mammals; such extreme evolutionary conservation signifies the level of importance of this gene and its protein.

P-glycoprotein acts as a plasma-membrane drug-efflux pump that actively extrudes drugs from cancer cells, thereby limiting the cytotoxicity of the drug at its cellular site of action. The normal function of P-glycoprotein is not completely known, but it has been found to be expressed in normal adrenal gland, kidney, liver, colon, brain, lung, peripheral blood and bone marrow cells, and multiple fetal cell lines. It is therefore hypothesized that P-glycoprotein normally functions as a drug-efflux pump. Additionally, P-glycoprotein has been found to mediate resistance to complement-mediated cytotoxicity and electrochemical fluxes across the plasma membrane. Many tumors derived from the aforementioned anatomic locations express large amounts of P-glycoprotein, which may explain their commonly observed intrinsic resistance to chemotherapeutic agents. The clinical importance of MDR is demonstrated in human oncology by the observation that increasing levels of P-glycoprotein expression positively correlate with a lack of response or remission following appropriate forms of chemotherapy. Most research in P-glycoprotein has centered on its localization to the plasma membrane; however, recent work suggests that P-glycoprotein also functions as a cytoplasmic vacuole pump in the cancer cell to provide yet another way of decreasing the cytotoxicity of the chemotherapeutic inside the cell.

A potential explanation for why dogs with lymphoma treated with the chemotherapy protocol containing cyclophosphamide, vincristine (Oncovin), and prednisone (COP) have a shorter remission than those treated with doxorubicin alone may lie within the realm of MDR. Two of the drugs within the COP protocol are known to induce the MDR phenotype, whereas doxorubicin induces the MDR phenotype in single fashion. Similarly, the use of corticosteroids prior to the initiation of chemotherapy for canine lymphoma is a negative prognostic factor, probably related to the induction of P-glycoprotein expression via prednisone.

Two studies in veterinary medicine have demonstrated the importance of P-glycoprotein in dogs with lymphoma. In the first study (Bergman et al, 1996), the prevalence of positive staining of P-glycoprotein via immunohistochemistry was ascertained in 58 dogs with lymphoma. Dogs had samples evaluated prior to the initiation of chemotherapy, at the time of relapse, and at the time of necropsy, and in some dogs samples were evaluated at all three times. Consistent with previous findings in P-glycoprotein research in human oncology, P-glycoprotein expression levels significantly increased at relapse and necropsy com-

This work supported in part by the American Cancer Society (PRTA #40). Its contents are solely the responsibility of the author and do not necessarily represent the official views of the American Cancer Society.

TABLE 1. **Multidrug Resistance (MDR) Overview**

Drugs Exhibiting Cross-Resistance in MDR Due to P-Glycoprotein	Drugs Known to Modulate P-Glycoprotein Activity	Mechanisms of Multidrug Resistance
Vincristine	Verapamil	P-Glycoprotein
Vinblastine	Quinine	Multidrug resistance–related protein (MRP)
Doxorubicin	Cyclosporine	Lung resistance-related protein (LRP)
Daunorubicin	Reserpine	Glutathione and glutathione-S-transferase
Mitoxantrone	Chloroquine	Topoisomerases
Actinomycin D	Trifluoroperazine	Apoptosis resistance (e.g., Bcl-2)
Etoposide	Tamoxifen	Dihydrofolate reductase
Mitomycin C	Various surfactants	Thymidylate synthase
Taxol/Taxanes	Progesterone	O^6-alkylguanine-DNA-alkyltransferase
Corticosteroids	Corticosteroids	Aldehyde dehydrogenase
Others	Others	Others

pared with levels at the initiation of chemotherapy. This study also demonstrated that the level of P-glycoprotein staining prior to the initiation of chemotherapy was inversely correlated to both remission and survival times; whereas the level of P-glycoprotein staining at relapse was inversely correlated to the time from relapse to death. Therefore, patients with high pretreatment levels of P-glycoprotein had significantly shorter remission times and survival times, and patients with high P-glycoprotein levels at relapse had significantly decreased times from relapse to death. An additional striking observation was that P-glycoprotein staining at the initiation of chemotherapy was the most significant prognostic factor of any of those examined in the study (including, among others, stage, substage, presence of hypercalcemia, age, weight, and gender).

In the second study, Lee and colleagues (1996) identified expression of P-glycoprotein by immunohistochemistry, and pretreatment P-glycoprotein expression was found to be an independent negative predictor of overall survival. Additionally, P-glycoprotein expression after relapse was greater than that in pretreatment samples. When these studies are taken in concert, it appears that determination of P-glycoprotein expression in a prospective fashion for dogs with lymphoma represents a viable pretreatment and intra-treatment diagnostic tool. These works also suggest that canine lymphoma represents an excellent comparative model for human P-glycoprotein research. There is a need for future studies in canine drug resistance incorporating determination of P-glycoprotein expression as well as those resistance mechanisms listed below performed in a prospective fashion.

There are many ways of attempting to reverse P-glycoprotein–associated MDR; however, few treatments have yielded any significant clinical benefit. Many compounds can competitively bind to P-glycoprotein to inhibit its efflux actions (see Table 1). Unfortunately, many of these compounds have produced severe unexpected toxicities at the levels necessary for P-glycoprotein reversal. The dose-response curves of most cancer cells are very steep; thus, one way of circumventing resistance is to use higher doses of drugs. However, significant toxicity, especially myelosuppression, is usually the result. Since myelosuppression is often the dose-limiting toxicity for most chemotherapeutics, clinicians have taken the same gene that induces MDR in cancer cells and placed it inside bone marrow cells. Initial human studies indicate this procedure is a very

viable method of increasing the ability of the patient to tolerate remarkably dose-intensive chemotherapy protocols. Additionally, new drugs, liposome-encapsulated drugs, signal transduction agents, and drug conjugates are currently under study for their ability to intrinsically block P-glycoprotein–mediated MDR.

MULTIDRUG RESISTANCE–RELATED PROTEIN (MRP)

Multiple studies have shown that when P-glycoprotein is not present, an MDR phenotype is still possible, thereby suggesting that other resistance mechanisms are probably at work in MDR. The second most frequently examined form of drug resistance is that involving MRP. MRP is a 190-kD protein that localizes to the cytoplasm in most normal tissues, whereas plasma membrane localization is more common in neoplastic tissues, suggesting an excretory function in the cancer cell. The normal function of MRP has been identified as the carrier of glutathione-S conjugates and bilirubin glucuronides in the cell and then excretion of these conjugates out of the cell. Normal MRP appears to be most strongly expressed in various epithelia, macrophages, heart, and tissues with an excretory function such as liver, kidney, and others, which is very similar to the normal expression of P-glycoprotein. Therefore, MRP has been termed by many as the "toxic waste manager" of the cell for toxins conjugated by the glutathione system, which unfortunately is a common detoxification system for many of the frequently used chemotherapy agents in veterinary medicine (see glutathione section as well). As a measure of MRP's clinical importance, rats and humans with mutations in MRP have chronic conjugated hyperbilirubinemia (Dubin-Johnson syndrome).

To date, no studies have been published on MRP in veterinary oncology; however, the prognostic significance of MRP in human oncology is beginning to be realized. Many tumor cell lines co-express P-glycoprotein and MRP, whereas others with an MDR phenotype without P-glycoprotein expression can have strong MRP expression. It appears that acute leukemias, transitional cell carcinomas, and squamous cell carcinomas have the strongest MRP expression, suggesting that normal cells that undergo malignant transformation have retained their MRP expression. To date, no studies have been published concerning reversal strategies for MRP-associated MDR.

LUNG RESISTANCE-RELATED PROTEIN

Lung resistance-related protein (LRP) is a 110-kD protein originally isolated from a human lung cancer cell line that is a distant relative of P-glycoprotein and MRP. The normal function of this protein is a major "vault" protein that regulates transport of substances between the nucleus and the cytoplasm, suggesting that LRP may be involved in the transport of cytotoxic agents. LRP has been detected in numerous cancer cell lines and clinical specimens of many tumors, including acute myeloid leukemia, ovarian carcinoma, myeloma, fibrosarcoma, and others. Overexpression of LRP in ovarian carcinoma is associated with an unfavorable prognosis. To date, no studies have been published on the detection of LRP in veterinary patients, and no studies have been published on reversal strategies for LRP-associated drug resistance.

TOPOISOMERASES

DNA topoisomerase II (Topo II) is an essential enzyme that catalyzes various conformational changes in DNA which are necessary for normal steps in DNA metabolism. Topo II forms a transient double-strand DNA break followed by DNA strand passage and then re-ligation of the DNA. Inhibitors of Topo II prevent the re-ligation process by freezing the "cleavable complex" formed between the enzyme and the DNA, leading to cell death. Drugs that target Topo II include actinomycin D, epipodophyllotoxins (e.g., etoposide), anthracenediones (e.g., mitoxantrone), and anthracyclines (e.g., doxorubicin and daunorubicin). Drugs involved with Topo II–mediated MDR include all those in P-glycoprotein–associated MDR except the vinca alkaloids and taxanes. In contrast to P-glycoprotein–associated MDR, the decreased chemosensitivity associated with Topo II is due to *reduced* expression or activity of the enzyme. Attempts to circumvent Topo II–associated MDR have been typically met with difficulty; however, a newer generation of Topo II–targeting drugs are currently under evaluation.

GLUTATHIONE SYSTEM

The major role of glutathione-S-transferase (GST) and glutathione (GSH) is the detoxification of cytotoxic drugs. Many cancer cell lines and clinical cancer specimens have increased production of GST and GSH compared with normal tissues. It appears that doxorubicin, chlorambucil, cyclophosphamide, melphalan, nitrosoureas, and others are involved with GST/GSH-mediated MDR. To date, attempts at reversal of GST/GSH-mediated MDR with ethacrynic acid as a GST inhibitor and buthionine sulfoximine as a GSH synthesis inhibitor have been met with poor efficacy and significant toxicity. To date, no reports on GST/GSH-mediated MDR in veterinary oncology have been published.

APOPTOSIS RESISTANCE-RELATED MDR

Apoptosis,* or programmed cell death, is an internally programmed mechanism of cell death morphologically and biochemically distinct from necrosis that allows for noninflammatory single cell deletion. Most forms of chemotherapy and radiation kill cancer cells by inducing them to undergo apoptosis. Many normal endogenous activators and suppressors of apoptosis have been elucidated. Unfortunately, cancer cells have developed mechanisms of up-regulating or activating these suppressors of apoptosis. Although much is left to be learned about apoptosis and its relationship to cancer biology, it appears that apoptosis-resistant cancer cells are resistant to even the highest doses possible of chemotherapeutics and radiation. Therefore, based on the fact that such apoptosis regulators lie profoundly downstream from our therapeutic agents, a greater understanding of how apoptosis impacts resistance and cancer therapy in general is urgently needed. Such an understanding will open new and probably extremely clinically relevant therapeutic modalities for cancer as well as autoimmune, infectious, and degenerative diseases.

References and Suggested Reading

Beck WT, Grogan TM, Willman CL, et al: Methods to detect P-glycoprotein–associated multidrug resistance in patients' tumors: Consensus recommendations. Cancer Res 56:3010, 1996.
Workshop performed by the leaders in the field of human MDR research that reviews and contrasts the various methodologies of ascertaining P-glycoprotein levels and their respective importance in human tumor samples.
Bergman PJ, Ogilvie GK: Drug resistance and cancer therapy. Compend Contin Educ Pract Vet (Small Anim) 17:549, 1995.
Concise and general overview of the various mechanisms of neoplastic drug resistance and how such resistance impacts the treatment of cancer. Recommendations are made for the best way of treating veterinary cancer patients in light of these resistance mechanisms.
Bergman PJ, Ogilvie GK, Powers BE: Monoclonal antibody C219 immunohistochemistry against P-glycoprotein: Sequential analysis and predictive ability in dogs with lymphoma. J Vet Intern Med 10:354, 1996.
Immunohistochemical assessment of P-glycoprotein in 58 dogs with lymphoma. Levels of Pgp expression at the start of therapy, relapse, and necropsy were analyzed in relationship to various clinical end points, such as remission time, survival, and time from relapse to death.
Bergman PJ, Harris D: Radioresistance, chemoresistance, and apoptosis resistance: The past, present, and future. Vet Clin North Am Small Anim Pract 27:47, 1997.
Concise review of resistance mechanisms for radiation and chemotherapy, with a review of the relationship of programmed cell death (apoptosis) resistance as a significant mechanism of combined radiation-chemotherapy resistance.
Broxterman HJ, Giaccone G, Lankelma J: Multidrug resistance proteins and other transport-related resistance to natural product agents. Curr Opin Oncol 7:532, 1995.
Excellent review of current understanding of MDR in relation to the numerous natural-product chemotherapies in clinical use today.
Ford JM: Modulators of multidrug resistance. Hematol Oncol Clin North Am 9:337, 1995.
Examination of the various clinical and preclinical MDR modulators available.
Giaccone G, Pinedo HM: Drug resistance. The Oncologist 1:82, 1996.
Excellent clinically relevant review of the myriad of mechanisms of drug resistance in cancer cells.
Goldstein LJ: Clinical reversal of drug resistance. Curr Probl Cancer 19:65, 1995.
Review article covering the problems and difficulties encountered with MDR reversal strategies to date. Also concisely reviews the cancers for which effective MDR reversal has been realized.
Koc OM, Allay JA, Lee K, et al: Transfer of drug resistance genes into hematopoietic progenitors to improve chemotherapy tolerance. Semin Oncol 23:46, 1996.
Report on the use of infecting patients' bone marrow cells with MDR

*Pronounced with a silent second p.

genes to improve the bone marrow's ability to handle higher dose chemotherapy in hopes of increasing the cure rates for various human malignances.

Lee JJ, Hughes CS, Fine RL, et al: P-glycoprotein expression in canine lymphoma. Cancer 77:1892, 1996.
Immunohistochemical evaluation of P-glycoprotein in dogs with lymphoma with comparison to clinical end points.

Moore AS, Leveille CR, Reimann KA, et al: The expression of P-glycoprotein in canine lymphoma and its association with multidrug resistance. Cancer Invest 13:475, 1995.
Report on the use of Western blotting for the assessment of P-glycoprotein expression in dogs with lymphoma in comparison to response rates and times.

Pastan I, Gottesman M: Multiple-drug resistance in human cancer. N Engl J Med 316:1388, 1987.

Excellent older review of the MDR literature with special emphasis on the normal function, biochemistry, and potential clinical significance of P-glycoprotein in various human malignancies.

Roninson IB: The role of the MDR1 (P-glycoprotein) gene in multidrug resistance in vitro and in vivo. Biochem Pharmacol 43:95, 1992.
Review article particularly emphasizing the experimental research findings related to P-glycoprotein–associated multidrug resistance.

Thompson CB: Apoptosis in the pathogenesis and treatment of disease. Science 267:1456, 1995.
Concise review of the importance of apoptosis (programmed cell death) as a mechanism of cellular homeostasis to organisms ranging from nematodes to humans. Also reviews apoptosis in relationship to a variety of diseases, including cancer, neurodegenerative disorders, human immunodeficiency virus (HIV) infection, and other diseases related to apoptotic dysregulation.

Radiation Therapy: Systems of Application and Eligible Patients

MARGARET C. McENTEE

Davis, California

Radiation therapy is rapidly becoming more accessible and is increasingly utilized in the treatment of a wide range of neoplastic diseases. Radiation therapy sources in use include external beam radiotherapy, brachytherapy, and systemically administered radionuclides. The following is a review of available radiation sources and applications.

EXTERNAL BEAM RADIOTHERAPY

Most radiation therapy facilities utilize megavoltage teletherapy units, either cobalt 60 units or linear accelerators, for external beam radiotherapy. Other teletherapy units in use include orthovoltage, and cyclotrons for proton therapy or the generation of neutron beams.

Orthovoltage Units

Orthovoltage units deliver x-rays that are generated by bombarding a metallic target with high-energy electrons. An orthovoltage unit is a relatively low-energy radiotherapy source, typically 250 kVp (range 150 to 500 kVp). The other descriptor for orthovoltage x-rays is half-value layer (HVL), which is the thickness of material required to reduce the energy of the primary beam by one half. There is differential absorption of dose in tissue based on atomic number, so that there is a relatively higher deposition of dose in bone compared with soft tissue. As a result, there is an increased risk of damage to bone in an irradiated field and potential bone necrosis. Additionally, maximum dose deposition occurs at the skin surface, with dose decreasing exponentially with depth in tissue. No skin-sparing effect exists with orthovoltage x-rays, with resultant increased acute radiation skin reactions compared with megavoltage

radiotherapy units. Also, the source-to-skin distance with orthovoltage is shorter (50 cm) compared with megavoltage (e.g., 80 cm for cobalt 60), which limits the size of the radiation treatment field. The advantages of orthovoltage units include less expense incurred in obtaining and maintaining the equipment, and decreased shielding requirements because of the relatively low-energy radiation beam. The applications include irradiation of superficial skin tumors and mast cell tumors, and it has been used effectively in the treatment of nasal tumors. Cytoreductive surgery is required prior to irradiation of nasal tumors with the use of orthovoltage x-rays, owing to depth-dose characteristics, and the inability to penetrate the full depth of the nasal cavity. There are numerous reports in the veterinary literature of the use of orthovoltage units in the treatment of a wide range of tumors. Orthovoltage units should be used primarily for the treatment of relatively superficial tumors, particularly with the increasing availability of higher energy megavoltage radiotherapy units for large and more deeply seated tumors.

Cobalt 60 Units

Cobalt 60 megavoltage teletherapy units deliver gamma rays with an average energy of 1.25 MeV (approximately 10 times more energetic than orthovoltage x-rays). X-rays and gamma rays are equivalent forms of electromagnetic radiation but differ in how each is generated. Gamma rays are emitted as the result of decay of a radioactive nuclide. The cobalt 60 source has a diameter of approximately 2 cm and is housed in a shielded head in a drawer that moves the source to a position over the patient when the unit is on. The cobalt 60 units in use include column-mounted and isocentric units. For column-mounted units, one treatment field or parallel opposed treatment fields can be used. For parallel opposed fields, the patient is positioned for the first field, and then the patient has to be repositioned to set up the second field. The main advantage of isocentric units is the flexibility and increased accuracy of treatment field set-up. The patient is positioned on the bed, the initial treatment field is defined, and then the source can be rotated around the patient while the patient remains stationary. A multiplicity of treatment field set-ups is possible with 360-degree capability around the patient, with the caveat that more complex treatment fields require the use of a computed tomography (CT)–based computer-generated treatment plan. Cobalt 60 units require relatively minimal maintenance. The half-life of cobalt 60 is 5.25 years. As the radioactive source decays, the output from the source declines and treatment time increases, so the source is replaced approximately every 5 years. Cobalt 60 units are commonly obtained from human cancer treatment facilities that are replacing cobalt units with linear accelerators, but the cobalt 60 units can pose a problem because of the risk of equipment failure as older units become outdated. One advantage of cobalt 60 is the skin-sparing effect with a dose build-up region and maximum dose deposited starting at 0.5 cm below the skin surface. Additionally, with cobalt 60—as opposed to orthovoltage—there is not a differential absorption of dose in bone versus soft tissue, and it is possible to treat more deeply seated tumors. One disadvantage of cobalt 60 is the increased penumbra, or scatter, outside the radiation treatment field because cobalt 60 is a block of material, as opposed to a point source as is the case with linear accelerators as well as orthovoltage units.

Linear Accelerators

Linear accelerators are the most commonly used megavoltage radiotherapy units in human cancer treatment centers and are increasing in number at veterinary academic institutions and referral treatment facilities. Linear accelerators produce both high-energy electron beams and x-rays in the range of 4 to 25 MeV. The electron beam used in the treatment of superficial tumors is produced through the use of high-frequency electromagnetic waves that accelerate electrons to high energy through a microwave accelerator. Alternatively, if the high-energy electron beam strikes a target, an x-ray beam is produced for the treatment of deeply seated tumors. Linear accelerators in place in veterinary cancer treatment centers are either 4 or 6 MeV units. The advantages of linear accelerators include the ability to more uniformly treat large tumors, treatment of both superficial and deeply seated tumors, higher output allowing treatment of a higher case load per day, and less penumbra, or scatter, of radiation outside the treatment field. There is also a skin-sparing effect, which varies, depending on the energy of the linear accelerator (e.g., maximum dose is deposited at 1 cm for 4 MeV and 1.5 cm for 6 MeV linear accelerators). Linear accelerators are isocentric machines with the attendant capability to treat an area 360 degrees around the patient without the patient having to be repositioned after the first treatment field has been set up. The main disadvantage of linear accelerators is the higher cost and level of maintenance required, including frequent equipment calibration by a radiation physicist.

Megavoltage radiotherapy units are used in the treatment of a wide range of tumors and sites. A partial list of tumors commonly irradiated at veterinary cancer treatment facilities include *mast cell tumors, soft tissue sarcomas, nasal tumors, brain tumors, bone tumors, and a variety of oral tumors.* A multimodality approach to cancer management has become the accepted standard of therapy, and most patients treated with radiation therapy have also undergone or will undergo surgery or adjuvant chemotherapy, or both. In general, the responses to radiation therapy have been improved with the combination of surgery and irradiation. Patients are irradiated either preoperatively or postoperatively. The debate is ongoing as to the optimal approach with combination therapy. Mast cell tumors, soft tissue sarcomas, and the majority of other solid tumors are more effectively treated with a combination of radiation and surgery. Nasal tumors are treated effectively with megavoltage radiation therapy alone, and results are not improved by prior surgery. With megavoltage radiotherapy, there is a dose build-up region, and air cavities resulting from cytoreductive surgery prior to irradiation alter and impede dose delivery to nasal tumors. A fully fractionated course of definitive radiation therapy is used to treat patients, with the intent to cure. The application of palliative radiation therapy (coarsely fractionated radiation therapy) is increasing with the recognition of a subset of patients that are better served by this approach. Palliative radiation therapy is used to treat patients with painful bone metastases or large unresectable tumors with or without metastatic disease, and to relieve obstruction (e.g., airway) due to a tumor.

Other Units

Cyclotrons are in limited use in veterinary medicine. Cyclotrons are used to accelerate protons for proton beam therapy and are used in the generation of neutron beams. The advantage of proton beam therapy versus x-rays or gamma rays is that the dose decreases rapidly to zero at the end of the proton beam range. Cobalt 60 gamma rays or x-rays from a linear accelerator exhibit exponential energy loss with tissue penetration. The dose deposited in tissue with proton therapy increases slowly with depth in tissue and reaches a sharp maximum near the end of the particles' range, referred to as the Bragg peak, and then goes to zero at the end of the particles' range. Additionally, there is minimal side scatter of radiation with protons. One veterinary institution in Europe utilizes conformal proton beam therapy using protons of 177 MeV in the treatment of cancer in companion animals.

Boron neutron capture therapy (BNCT) has limited availability and is used primarily for the treatment of brain tumors. BNCT entails the intravenous administration of a stable nonradioactive isotope of boron (^{10}B), which preferentially concentrates in tumor cells. The tumor is then irradiated (single dose of radiation) with the use of a beam of low-energy neutrons that produce short-range radiation when absorbed or captured by the boron, with the generation of predominantly alpha particles. Alpha particles are characterized as high linear energy transfer (LET) radiation with a very short path length, minimal normal tissue damage, decreased dependence on the presence of oxygen for radiation damage to occur, and the ability to kill both dividing and nondividing tumor cells. The main disadvantage of BNCT—other than its limited availability—is that neutrons are attenuated rapidly by tissue; thus, it is difficult to treat tumors at any significant depth. It appears that BNCT is equivalent to conventional external beam irradiation in the management of canine brain tumors.

BRACHYTHERAPY

Brachytherapy refers to the use of radiation sources located at a short distance from the tissue to be irradiated. Brachytherapy utilizes radioisotopes typically in the form of seeds or needles that are placed on or in the patient. Two distinct forms of brachytherapy exist. Intracavitary brachytherapy refers to the placement of radiation sources in a body cavity in close proximity to the tumor. Interstitial brachytherapy utilizes radioactive seeds implanted directly into the tumor and is the main type of brachytherapy used for the treatment of veterinary cancer patients. Interstitial brachytherapy uses either temporary or permanent implants. The most commonly used radionuclide is iridium 192 as a temporary implant. The dose of radiation delivered depends on a number of factors, including the number and activity of the radioactive sources, their geometric distribution in the tumor, and the duration of time the implants are left in the patient. The two different techniques for interstitial brachytherapy include low dose-rate and high dose-rate brachytherapy. Low dose-rate brachytherapy utilizes radioactive sources of relatively low activity, which are placed in the tumor and typically deliver the radiation dose over a period of 6 to 8 days. In high dose-rate brachytherapy, high-activity radioactive sources are implanted in the tumor with the use of a remote-controlled afterloading device. With the patient under general anesthesia, catheters are implanted in the tumor. Orthogonal radiographs are made to visualize the placement of the radioactive sources with the use of dummy nonradioactive sources. The distribution and location of the sources are entered into a computer program to determine the dose distribution and treatment time. One application is given, with the duration of treatment dependent on radiation dose from the source or sources and time for delivering a tumoricidal radiation dose.

The advantages of interstitial brachytherapy include the ability to deliver a high local dose of radiation in a relatively short time period with minimal exposure to surrounding normal tissues. There is rapid fall-off of dose with the distance from the source, as described by the inverse square law (the dose from the point source varies inversely as the square of the distance). The disadvantages of interstitial brachytherapy include exposure of personnel to the radioactive sources in the process of placement and removal of the sources and in the care of patients during hospitalization. The risk associated with radiation exposure can be minimized through the use of remote-controlled afterloading devices, and isolation of patients during treatment. Catheters are placed in the tumor, dose calculations are performed, and then through a remote-controlled device the radioactive sources in the form of needles or seeds are placed in the catheters. Another disadvantage of interstitial brachytherapy is that placement of the radioactive sources involves a surgical procedure. The applications of brachytherapy in small animal veterinary oncology include tumors in the nasal cavity, skin, and subcutaneous tissues. Brachytherapy can be used to treat solid tumors, or the radioactive sources can be placed postoperatively to treat residual neoplastic disease after cytoreductive surgery.

Radioactive sources with a relatively short half-life can be left in the patient permanently. Iodine 125 is the most commonly used permanent interstitial implant. The advantages of the use of permanent implants include only one anesthetic episode for placing the sources and the patient can be discharged from the hospital with the sources in place.

Strontium 90

Another form of brachytherapy is plesiotherapy, or surface therapy, in which the radioactive source applicator is placed in contact with the surface of a tumor. Strontium 90 applicators are used to deliver beta particles to superficial tumors. Beta particles have limited penetration. The depth dose characteristics of strontium 90 irradiation limit its use to tumors of less than 2 to 3 mm in depth. Treatment is also limited to lesions of relatively small diameter, as the typical applicator has an active diameter of less than 1 cm. The half-life of strontium 90 is 28.9 years. Strontium 90 decays to yttrium 90 (^{90}Y), which emits beta particles with a maximum energy of 2.27 MeV. The 50% isodose line corresponds to a depth of 2 mm for most applicators, and all energy from beta particle irradiation is effectively absorbed within the first 4 mm of tissue. This form of radiation has been used primarily for the treatment of squamous cell carcinoma in cats with superficial cutaneous lesions. A relatively high dose of radiation is delivered, on the order of 100 to 200 Gy with one application, and treatment can be repeated as necessary. The acute reactions from irradiation are minimal and typically self-limiting, with minimal, if any, chronic radiation side effects.

RADIOISOTOPES

Radioactive Iodine (^{131}I)

The most frequently used radioisotope in veterinary medicine is radioactive iodine (^{131}I). This radioisotope is employed in the treatment of feline hyperthyroidism. Radioactive iodine is available at a number of treatment facilities, including private referral practices and academic institutions (see *CVT XII,* p. 372). Radioactive iodine is usually given as an intravenous bolus, but it is equally efficacious when administered subcutaneously. There is an oral form of ^{131}I, but treatment with this form requires a higher dose and administration can be problematic if the patient vomits. Several different methods are used to determine the dose of radioactive iodine that should be administered. The methods of dosing radioactive iodine range from a fixed dose (e.g., 4 mCi) to dose selection based on a combination of factors, including severity of clinical signs, thyroid size, and serum thyroxine (T_4) concentration, to more complex methods based on a tracer dose of radioiodine. The half-life of ^{131}I is 8 days. Radioactive iodine is taken up by and concentrated in hyperplastic thyroid tissue.

The primary cause of cell death is due to beta particles emitted by radioactive iodine, which can travel a maximum of 2 mm in tissue with an average distance of 400 μm. Normal thyroid tissue is protected because less radioactive iodine is taken up by suppressed thyroid tissue, and because beta particles travel only a short distance. Additionally, the parathyroid glands and other tissues from the cervical region are not damaged by [131]I. The ^{131}I not taken up by the thyroid is eliminated in the urine and, to a lesser extent, in the feces. The majority of cats become euthyroid within 2 weeks after a single dose of ^{131}I, with 90% euthyroid by 3 months after treatment. Radioiodine is the treatment of choice for feline hyperthyroidism.

The main disadvantage of treatment with radioiodine is the requirement for hospitalization for 1 to 3 weeks until the thyroid surface dose decreases to an acceptable level. Other potential disadvantages include transient dysphagia due to radiation thyroiditis, and hypothyroidism that can occur in a small subset of patients. Cats with malignant thyroid carcinomas that are hyperthyroid are still candidates for radioactive iodine treatment but require a higher dose of [131]I (10 to 30 mCi). It is recommended that hyperthyroid cats with malignant thyroid carcinomas be treated with a combination of cytoreductive surgery and high-dose radioiodine. In addition, ^{131}I has been used in the treatment of dogs with functional metastatic thyroid carcinomas, and in dogs with "nonfunctional" thyroid carcinoma with or without distant metastasis. Patients with extensive pulmonary metastasis are at risk for the development of radiation pneumonitis.

Phosphorus 32 (^{32}P)

Radioactive phosphorus (^{32}P) has a half-life of 14.3 days and is a pure beta particle emitter with a maximum energy of 1.71 MeV. Radioactive phosphorus delivered as sodium phosphate is preferentially taken up in bone and localizes at sites of increased cell proliferation in the bone marrow. The radioisotope has been used in a limited number of dogs with polycythemia rubra vera and essential thrombocythemia, with positive responses observed in a subset of patients. Radiophosphorus has been used in human cancer patients for palliation of the pain associated with bone metastasis, but it can be associated with bone marrow suppression. Radiophosphorus is not readily available for the treatment of veterinary cancer patients.

Colloidal suspensions of ^{32}P as chromic phosphate can be used for intracavitary instillation in the management of malignant effusions. Uptake by cells lining the serosal surface results in fibrosis and resultant decreased fluid production.

Samarium 153 ([153]Sm)

Samarium-153-EDTMP has been used primarily in the treatment of bone tumors in dogs. Samarium 153 is a radionuclide that emits both gamma rays and beta particles. When samarium 153 is bound to ethylenediaminetetramethylene phosphonate (EDTMP) and injected intravenously, it is taken up preferentially by metabolically active bone cells. The administered dose that has been used in dogs is 1.0 mCi/kg (37 MBq). The utility of this modality in managing bone tumors has yet to be defined, but there may be some efficacy in the management of both primary and metastatic bone tumors.

References and Suggested Reading

Burk RL, King GK (eds): Radiation Oncology. Vet Clin North Am Small Anim Pract 27:1, 1997.
A series of articles on veterinary radiation oncology. Topics covered include discussion of irradiation of specific tumor types and sites, radiation side effects, and basic principles of radiation biology and physics.

Gillette EL (guest editor): Radiation Oncology. Semin Vet Med Surg (Small Anim) 10:127, 1995.
A comprehensive series of articles on veterinary radiation oncology, including basic principles, applications, results of therapy, and treatment complications.

Lattimer JC, Corwin LA, Stapleton J, et al: Clinical and clinicopathologic response of canine bone tumor patients to treatment with samarium-153-EDTMP. J Nucl Med 31:1316, 1990.
Description of the treatment of 40 dogs with primary or metastatic bone tumors treated with one or two doses of the radionuclide samarium-153-EDTMP. Small lesions with minimal bone lysis, metastatic lesions, and axial skeleton lesions generally responded well. Large lesions with minimal bone formation responded poorly. The major side effects were thrombocytopenia and leukopenia, which persisted for as long as 4 weeks after treatment.

Peterson ME, Becker DV: Radioiodine treatment of 524 cats with hyperthyroidism. J Am Vet Med Assoc 207:1422, 1995.
Provides the results of subcutaneously administered radioiodine in a large series of hyperthyroid cats. Dose of radioiodine was based on severity of clinical signs, thyroid size, and serum thyroxine concentration. A good response to treatment was documented in 94.2% of the cats.

Smith M, Turrel JM: Radiophosphorus (^{32}P) treatment of bone marrow disorders in dogs: 11 cases (1970–1987). J Am Vet Med Assoc 194:98, 1989.
Report of the use of radiophosphorus for the treatment of bone marrow disorders, including eight dogs with polycythemia vera (five responded to a single treatment) and three dogs with essential thrombocythemia (two responded to a single treatment).

Thompson JP, Ackerman N, Bellah JR, et al: [192]Iridium brachytherapy, using an intracavitary afterload device, for treatment of intranasal neoplasms in dogs. Am J Vet Res 53:617, 1992.
A report of the use of brachytherapy in the treatment of eight dogs with nasal cavity tumors. The paper provides a discussion of the details of brachytherapy, including techniques and dosimetry.

Hyperthermia

Durham, North Carolina

INTRODUCTION

Reference to the use of hyperthermia as therapy for cancer can be found as early as the writings of Hippocrates. In modern times, hyperthermia has been extensively studied at both the biologic and the clinical levels. The scientific rationale for hyperthermia therapy, combined with radiation, chemotherapy, and cytokines, is multifactorial, and new justifications for its use are continuously being identified. Detailed discussion of the biologic rationale is beyond the scope of this article, and the reader is referred to outstanding recent publications on this topic (Seegenschmiedt et al, 1995 and 1996). Even though the biologic rationale is strong, and hyperthermia has been studied in phase I to III trials for the past 20 years, it has yet to become a widely accepted mode of therapy because (1) current hyperthermia technology cannot deliver adequate power to result in effective tumor heating of all sites; (2) the lack of noninvasive temperature measurement technology makes the technology too cumbersome, inaccurate, and expensive for routine use; (3) many potential clinical applications outside its use with radiation therapy have not been explored extensively; and (4) in the context of total body hyperthermia, there has been slow progress toward establishing a means of achieving therapeutic gain.

In practically all areas of clinical development, studies in pets with spontaneous malignancies have paved the way for or augmented human trials. In this article, emphasis is placed on the importance of those studies in the continued development of this method of therapy.

Four important developments have the potential to revolutionize the application of hyperthermia for the treatment of local and regional disease in human patients. First, recent positive results of three human European phase III trials (head and neck, chest wall recurrences from breast cancer, and melanoma), and one from the United States (previously untreated high-grade brain tumors), have shown the potential for this treatment method, when combined with radiation therapy, to improve local control of tumors. Collectively, these results justify the rationale for investing the time and resources to further improve the technology so that deeper-seated tumors can be approached. Interestingly, positive phase III trials in spontaneous pet animal tumors, comparing hyperthermia plus radiation to radiation alone, were reported as early as 10 years before the human studies.

Second, a method of documentation of the thermal adequacy of hyperthermia treatment has been identified from retrospective analysis of thermal data from phase II trials. Again, early concepts of this type were demonstrated previously in pet animal trials, and the similarity between the thermal dose-response relationships and the human trial results is notable.

Third, the clinical feasibility of noninvasive thermometry has been demonstrated, with the use of magnetic resonance imaging. Other noninvasive thermometry methods, such as ultrasound and impedance tomography, also show great promise and suggest that the clinical implementation of hyperthermia may eventually be less demanding in terms of personnel costs and involvement.

Fourth, significant developments in the modeling of power deposition and heat transfer in tumors may lead to powerful methods for pretreatment planning as well as treatment monitoring. Collectively, these developments raise the expectation that investment in new hyperthermia technology will probably lead to improved local-regional control of other tumors, extending even to deep-seated sites, and that the ease with which this technology can be utilized will represent a quantum leap over the current methods of application.

New areas of investigation in hyperthermia biology not only point to expanded rationale for its use with radiation, but also indicate its potential as a means of increasing sensitivity to a number of chemotherapeutic agents as well as augmenting new cancer treatment strategies, such as monoclonal antibodies, liposomal drug delivery systems, and gene therapy.

Thus, there is a strong rationale for the revived interest in hyperthermia and its continued development toward a legitimate method of cancer therapy.

PHASE III CLINICAL TRIAL RESULTS

During the period from 1970 to 1984, the results of several phase I and II human trials were published; these data indicated the potential for hyperthermia to increase the radiation response of superficially accessible tumors. Of particular interest was the series of studies that compared the responses of matched lesions. Although there was some variation from one study to the next, the overall improvement in response averaged a factor of 2, over what was achieved with radiation alone (Dewhirst et al, 1993). Based largely on these results, the Radiation Therapy Oncology Group initiated a phase III trial in 1981 (RTOG 81-04) that compared radiation alone with the combination of radiation therapy and hyperthermia. Unfortunately, the results of that trial were negative. The failure of RTOG 81-04 to show a therapeutic advantage for hyperthermia was probably related to problems with quality assurance. In 1984, the European Society of Hyperthermic Oncology recognized the limitations of the RTOG trial and adopted new quality assurance procedures that are quite similar to those now recommended by the RTOG (Seegenschmiedt et al, 1995 and 1996). These quality assurance guidelines were used in the conduct of published human phase III trials, which showed a therapeutic advantage to the use of hyperthermia in combination with radiation therapy,

486

compared with the use of radiation therapy alone (Vernon et al, 1996; Overgaard et al, 1995). In addition, a recent North American phase III trial for previously untreated high-grade gliomas showed a survival advantage for adjuvant hyperthermia when combined with brachytherapy compared with brachytherapy alone (Sneed et al, 1998).

IMPORTANCE OF THERMAL DOSIMETRY IN OPTIMIZING TREATMENT: ESTABLISHMENT OF MEANS FOR WRITING A THERMAL PRESCRIPTION

North American investigators have recognized the importance of recent positive clinical trials in superficial malignancies and are pushing for further development of the modality so that it can be tested as an adjuvant for more important, deep-seated tumors. The success of such an effort will depend on understanding how to optimize the therapy, since it is much more difficult to heat deep-seated lesions than superficial ones. Critical for continued progress in clinical hyperthermia is the development of a quantitative and reproducible thermal dosimetry system to make it possible to write and verify a thermal prescription (Dewhirst et al, 1993). Important advances have been made in this arena. The most cogent ones have formed the basis for the conduct of multi-institutional prospective thermal dose-escalation trials.

It is well recognized that temperature distributions that develop in tumors during hyperthermia treatment are nonuniform. The nonuniformity stems from two spatially varying sources: power deposition and tumor blood perfusion. Two commonly used descriptors of the measured temperature distribution, that have been related to treatment outcome, are the minimum tumor temperature and the 10th percentile (commonly referred to as the T_{90}), which is the temperature that is exceeded by 90% of measured points within the tumor. The cytotoxicity of hyperthermia is dependent on both temperature and time. Thus, the aforementioned descriptors have frequently been integrated with time and converted to an equivalent number of minutes at a reference temperature, such as 43°C (referred to as $EQ43T_{90}$). The time-integrated temperature descriptor has allowed for the development of thermal dosimetric concepts.

In 1984, it was demonstrated that the time-integrated descriptor, as it relates to the minimum monitored temperature, was related to both response rates and duration of local control in spontaneous pet animal tumors that were treated with thermoradiotherapy. Oleson and colleagues demonstrated that $EQ43T_{90}$ was related to response rates in three different types of disease in humans (superficially accessible tumors, soft tissue sarcomas, and deep-seated tumors). In a separate study, $EQ43T_{90}$ was found to be correlated with both response and duration of local control in nodular chest wall recurrences of breast cancer (Kapp et al, 1995). It was of particular interest to find that the dose-response relationships for human and canine trials were quite similar (Fig. 1). Similar results have now been published for chest wall recurrences and melanomas treated in phase III European trials. Collectively, these results suggest that currently available invasive thermometry, which typically involves implantation of one to three catheters for

thermometric access, can be used to form a basis for crude thermal dosimetry. However, the correlations with treatment outcome have been made retrospectively, so it is not known whether prospective control of delivered dose will lead to the identification of the same type of dose-response relationship.

One method that can be used to augment the thermal dose in tumors would be to use total body hyperthermia in combination with local hyperthermia. The logic behind the use of this approach is that heating of the blood entering the tumor will lead to less steep thermal gradients around the tumor and higher minimum temperatures. This approach was tested in a randomized trial in dogs with soft tissue sarcomas comparing radiation therapy with either local hyperthermia alone or local hyperthermia in combination with whole body hyperthermia (Thrall et al, 1996). While there were measurable differences in the minimum temperatures achieved in the tumors, there was no demonstrable difference in local tumor control between the two arms. In addition, there appeared to be a higher incidence of distant metastases in the group of dogs that received total body hyperthermia, compared with the group that received local hyperthermia alone. Thus, this approach to the augmentation of thermal dose has been abandoned. Importantly, this result obviated the need for a more expensive and risky trial of this combination therapy in humans.

Prospective thermal dose-escalation trials are currently being conducted, in both human and canine tumors, that address this question in a different way. In the current trials, both the number of hyperthermia fractions and the duration of heating per fraction are being varied. In addition, more attention is being paid to target temperatures, which may result in improvements in the minimum temperature achieved in the heated volume.

DEVELOPMENT OF NONINVASIVE THERMOMETRY AND MODELING TECHNIQUES

A key component needed for the continued development of hyperthermia is a method for noninvasively measuring temperature. Even though invasive methods have been shown to provide enough data to support thermal dosimetric concepts, these methods have a number of restrictions. First, the data that are acquired represent a small linear sample of the entire volume of tumor, and errors in sampling occur because the temperature distribution is quite nonuniform and three-dimensional. Second, catheter insertion into superficial tumors is usually simple, but for deep-seated tumors, it is much more problematic. Third, invasive procedures are intrinsically unattractive to patients and relatively costly because physician time is required.

Aside from the practical limitations of invasive thermometry described previously, there are also restrictions on hyperthermia applicator design and utilization that result from the limitations of invasive thermometry. Relatively sophisticated multisource devices are currently available that allow for greater control over power deposition. Examples include multielement ultrasound and radiofrequency (rf) arrays that have phase- and amplitude-shifting capabilities. Theoretically, these devices could be used to greatly enhance power deposition in tumors while they minimize

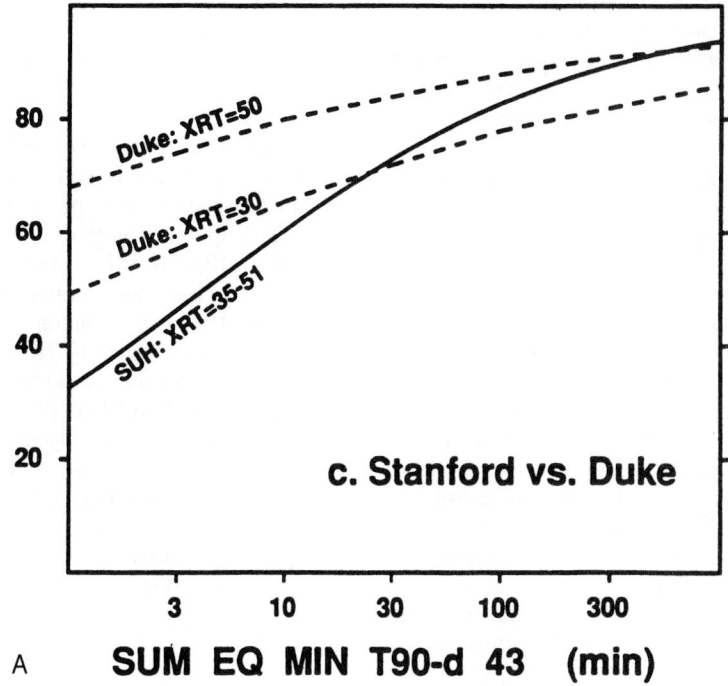

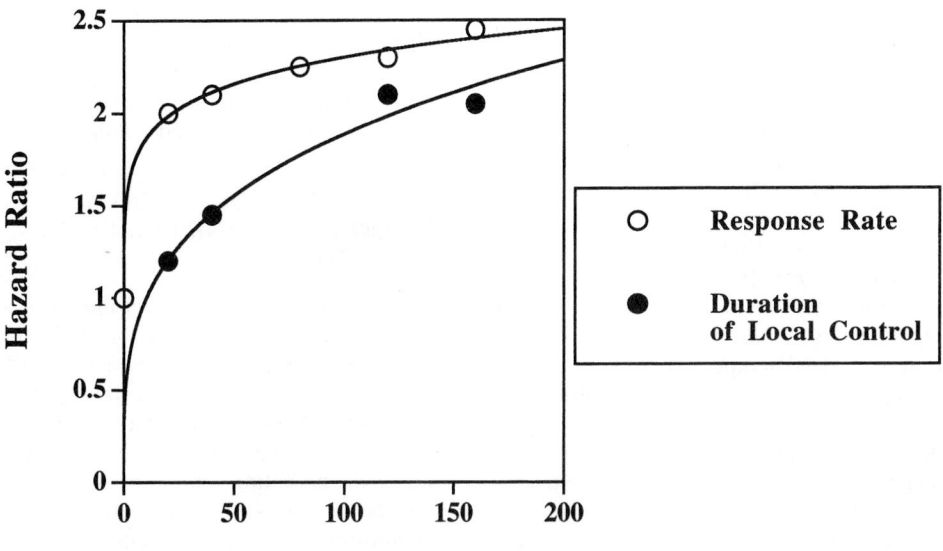

Figure 1. Clinical thermal dose-response relationships. *A,* Logistic regression model for initial complete response as influenced by the $EQ43T_{90}$ thermal dose parameter for superficial nodular recurrences of human breast cancer treated at Stanford (Stanford University Hospital) and miscellaneous superficial tumors (Duke University Medical Center). The dose-response curves from the two studies are quite similar. Two curves from Duke show the effect of radiation dose on response (30 versus 50 Gy). In the Stanford study, the same parameter also was predictive for duration of local control. *B,* Logistic regression models indicating a change in hazard rates for complete response rate and duration of local control for increasing EQ43CTmin in pet animal cancers treated with hyperthermia and radiation. The shapes of the hazard rate curves are quite similar to those shown for human studies *(A).* (Figure *A* from Kapp DS, Cox RS: Thermal treatment parameters are most predictive of outcome in patients with single tumor nodules per treatment field in recurrent adenocarcinoma of the breast [see comments]. Int J Radiat Oncol Biol Phys 33:887–899, 1995, with permission. Figure *B* redrawn from Dewhirst MW, Sim DA: The utility of thermal dose as a predictor of tumor and normal tissue responses to combined radiation and hyperthermia. Cancer Res Suppl 44:4772s–4780s, 1984, with permission.)

power deposition in normal tissues. However, none of these devices is being used to its full capacity because of limitations on thermometric data. The successful development of noninvasive thermometry will lead to the better use of these devices as well as the development of superior hyperthermia technology. Such improvements in technology can optimize power deposition in real time, so as to account for variations in factors such as tissue perfusion and patient movement.

The most developed method for noninvasive thermometry uses magnetic resonance imaging. Recent studies using the diffusion-weighted images have demonstrated the feasibility and accuracy of this method in phantom and in vivo studies. A more sensitive method is the magnetic resonance measurement of the chemical shift of water. It has been demonstrated that this method can yield 0.5°C resolution in 0.02 cm³ voxels in normal and malignant tissues. An example of this type of measurement in a canine patient with a soft tissue sarcoma of the foot is shown in Figure 2. This method has some limitations that need to be addressed as well, however. It is more sensitive to movement of the patient within the magnet bore, system stability, and possibly changes in perfusion. Techniques for correcting for these confounding effects are being investigated. Both magnetic resonance imaging methods have imaging times of 20 seconds for multislice data, so they are feasible for real-time monitoring of temperature. This capability means that they could be used for real-time phase and amplitude control of multielement hyperthermia devices.

Another limitation on the utilization of hyperthermia technology is the difficulty in deciding how to set the device to optimize power delivery to the tumor. Methods for real patient computer simulation of power deposition are under development, and clinical feasibility has been demonstrated. Once power deposition is known, the next step would be to use these data, in conjunction with measures of perfusion, so that the temperature distribution could be calculated (Fig. 3). This method may be an alternative to noninvasive thermometry, or it may be a powerful tool for pretreatment planning, particularly for the newer, more sophisticated multifactorial hyperthermia devices.

Collectively, the advances in noninvasive thermometry and modeling are likely to lead to better use of the currently available hyperthermia technology as well as the development of sophisticated, yet user-friendly methods that can vary power deposition in tumors both spatially and temporally.

TOTAL BODY HYPERTHERMIA

The logic behind the use of total body hyperthermia relates primarily to the fact that many cancers are systemic in nature. Thus, if one is to have an impact on the survival of the patient, it is necessary to consider augmentation of systemic chemotherapy. However, in the context of total body hyperthermia, it is difficult to readily recognize the potential for therapeutic gain, since most normal tissues will be at the same temperature as the tumor. Nevertheless, a number of studies were undertaken in dogs with spontaneous tumors to search for such effects.

One area of emphasis was in the use of platinum-containing drugs in combination with total body hyperthermia. Initial pharmacodynamic studies in normal animals suggested the potential for therapeutic gain because of differences in tissue disposition induced by the hyperthermia procedure (Page and Thrall, 1994). In particular, there seemed to be an augmentation of delivery of drug to the lungs, compared with other normal organs. These results suggested that this approach might be useful in diseases with a propensity to metastasize to the lungs. However, when corroborative studies were done in dogs that had pulmonary metastases, there was no evidence for enhanced uptake of platinum in the metastatic nodules, compared with normal lung. In addition, the use of whole body hyperthermia in combination with either cisplatin or carboplatin caused augmentation of normal tissue toxicities, which necessitated a reduction in dose from what could be achieved under normothermic conditions. The spectrum of toxicities seen with each drug was not different, just the dose at which the toxicities were observed. For 42°C hyperthermia, the dose reduction factor was 0.6 for cisplatin and 0.8 for carboplatin.

Additional trials of total body hyperthermia were conducted to test whether such therapy would augment the efficacy of doxorubicin and mitoxantrone as single agents for the treatment of non-Hodgkin's lymphoma in dogs. Phase I trials indicated no dose-modifying effect of total body hyperthermia on normal tissue tolerance to either of these drugs. A phase III study of doxorubicin total body hyperthermia showed decreased response in the arm with total body hyperthermia. These results are not in concert with the known effects of hyperthermia on doxorubicin toxicity, in vitro. Potential explanations for the lack of therapeutic gain include alterations in tissue distribution of drug, enhancement of drug resistance via induction of the heat shock response, or the induction of one or more cytokines or lymphokines that accelerated relapse. Of note are several recent studies that may provide a new rationale for therapeutic gain, when whole body hyperthermia is combined with chemotherapeutic agents and cytokines. For example, it has been shown in a murine tumor model that lower temperature, long-duration whole body hyperthermia, perhaps in combination with tumor necrosis factor-alpha (TNF-α), may provide a larger margin of safety. In addition, a number of cytokines are released during whole body hyperthermia that could be beneficial in terms of protecting critical normal tissues. Additional research in this arena is warranted.

RECENT DEVELOPMENTS IN HYPERTHERMIA BIOLOGY

This discussion focuses on new developments in hyperthermia biology that have implications toward the clinical application of hyperthermia. There are many exciting new developments related to the study of the stress response, and there is no question that the use of hyperthermia as a means of inducing cellular stress has been a useful tool for such study. Space limitations, however, do not allow for summary of this work here.

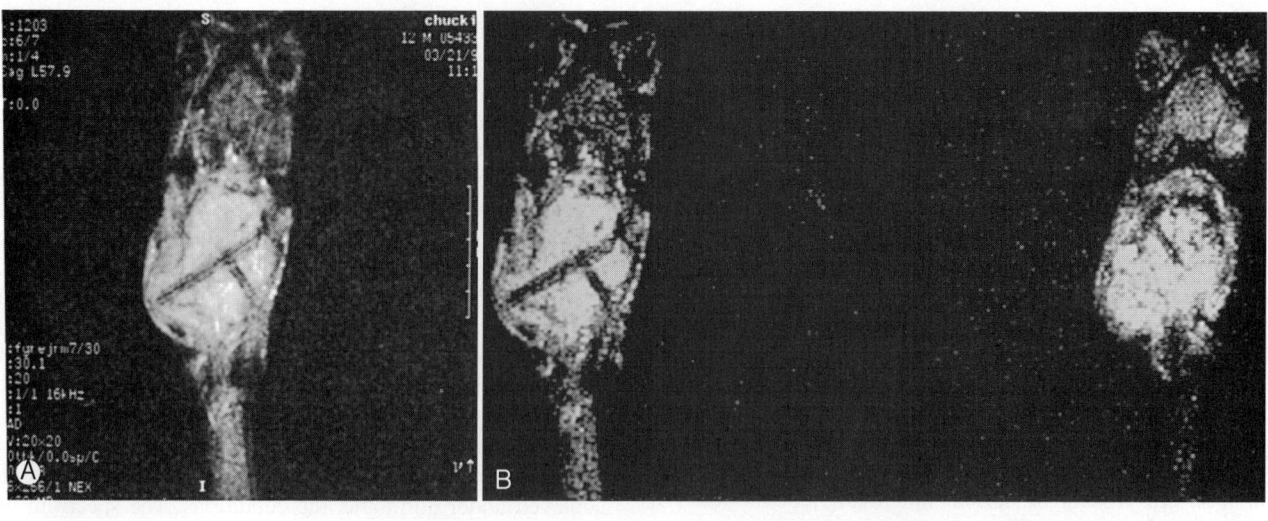

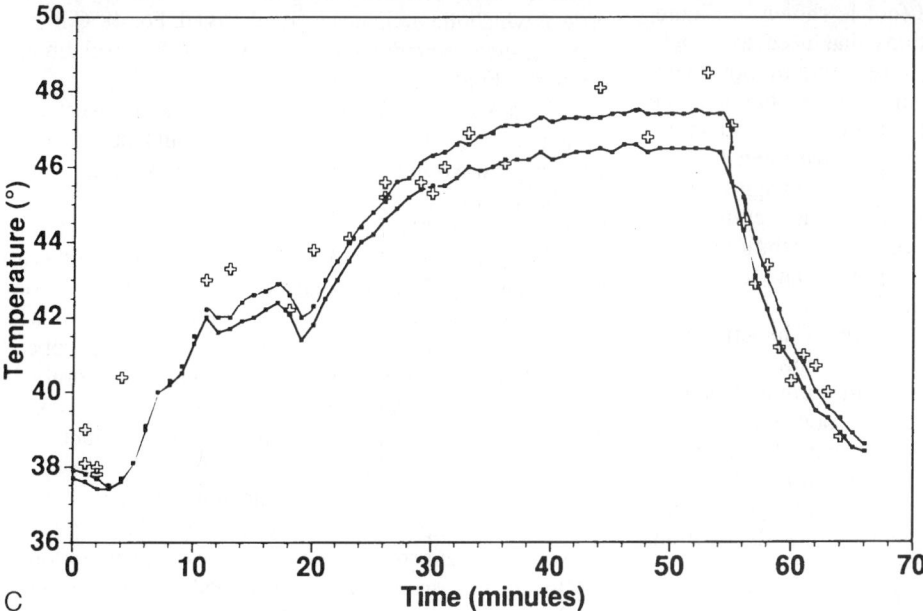

Figure 2. Magnetic resonance chemical shift images of a canine forepaw containing a soft tissue sarcoma. *A,* T2-weighted image of sarcoma, indicating the location of intratumoral catheters used for temperature monitoring. *B,* Two phase images in two planes of the tumor, taken during the steady-state portion of the hyperthermia treatment. The image to the left is in the same plane as that in *A*. The phase shift of water is temperature dependent, which forms the basis for this temperature measurement method. *C,* Comparison of temperatures measured with thermometers at the intersection of two catheters with the phase shift method. Good agreement was achieved, in terms of both the magnitude and temporal variation. (Data kindly provided by Drs. Samulski and Prescott.)

Effects of Hyperthermia on Tumor Oxygenation

Traditionally, it was believed that hyperthermia caused vascular damage to tumors and that this effect should be avoided when radiation is combined with hyperthermia. However, much of the early work was at thermal doses that are in excess of what can be achieved clinically. Furthermore, studies in human tumors suggested that human tumor vasculature is more resistant to thermal damage than its counterpart in rodents. It has been recognized that hyperthermia can actually cause tumor reoxygenation and that the degree of reoxygenation is related to the level of

cytotoxicity achieved. Further augmentation of reoxygenation can be achieved by adding carbogen breathing to the hyperthermia treatment.

In humans with soft tissue sarcoma treated with thermoradiotherapy, there has been no evidence of reoxygenation after 1 week of prehyperthermia radiation therapy, but one heat treatment leads to measurable reoxygenation 24 to 48 hours following a hyperthermia treatment. When reoxygenation occurs, it is positively correlated with percentage necrosis at the time of surgical resection (Brizel et al, 1996). This effect may not occur in all tumors, however, so further studies are needed to determine why it occurs and under what circumstances it might be expected. In

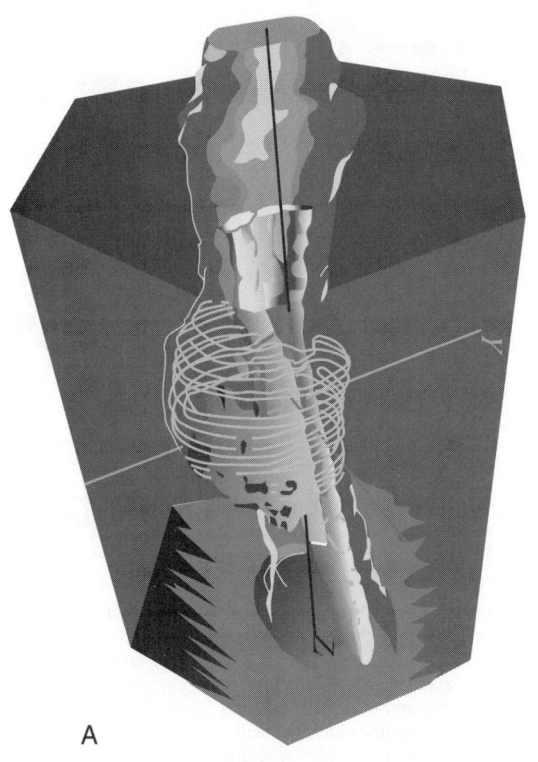

A

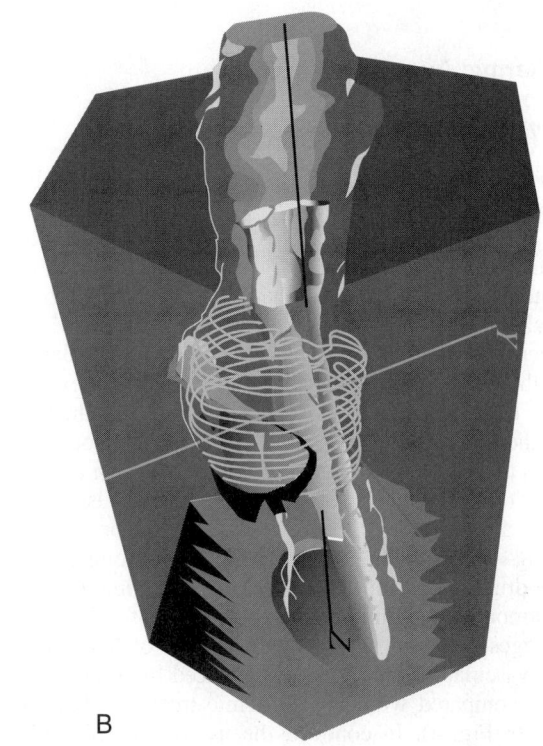

B

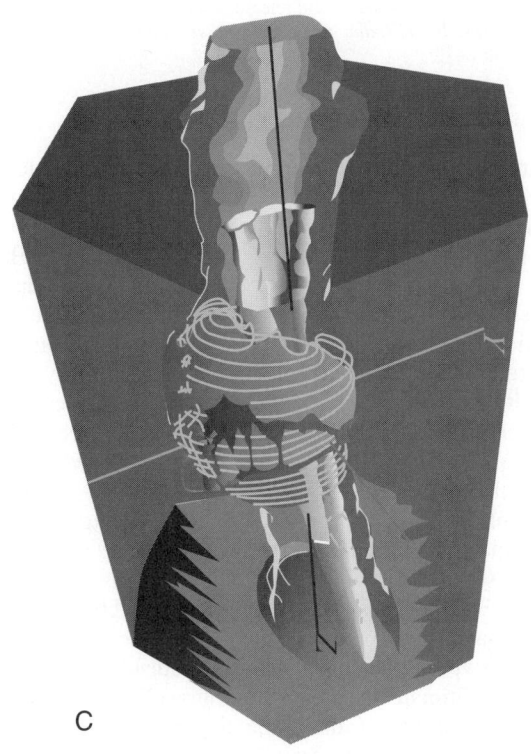

C

Figure 3. Computer simulation power deposition and temperature distributions from a radiofrequency (rf) phased array into the forelimb of a dog with an extremity sarcoma. *A,* Measurement of the relative perfusion index was performed using the magnetic resonance imaging contrast agent gadolinium. The light gray surface indicates the region of highest relative perfusion. The tumor region is indicated by the lined contours. These data were used in the simulation of temperature distributions shown in *(C),* below. *B,* Optimum power deposition into a tumor mass from an array of six microwave antennas in a hexagonal array surrounding the tumor. The light gray color represents the 25% maximum isopower contour. *C,* Resultant temperature distributions, as calculated from heat transfer models, for the optimized setting of phase and amplitude of the hexagonal array of antennas. The light gray color indicates the 42°C isotherm contour. The heat transfer models utilized actual measured temperature data, obtained during treatment, for simulation of the entire temperature distribution. (Figure kindly provided by Dr. Scott Clegg. The simulations were based on experiments conducted by Dr. Deborah Prescott.)

any case, reoxygenation may be another means by which hyperthermia augments the cytotoxicity of radiation therapy.

Hyperthermic Augmentation of Drug, Monoclonal Antibody, Liposome, and Viral Delivery

Years ago, it was recognized that hyperthermia could be used to augment the cytotoxicity of and reverse drug resistance to chemotherapeutic agents. Augmentation of cellular drug uptake was responsible, in part, for these effects. It has been recognized that hyperthermia may also provide additional advantages in regard to drug delivery, particularly when the drugs or their carriers are relatively large (greater than or equal to macromolecular size). For example, it has been demonstrated in several studies that the use of hyperthermia can enhance the delivery of monoclonal antibodies to tumors, with resultant improvement in antitumor effect (Hauck et al, 1995). Hyperthermia has also been shown to augment drug delivery and antitumor effects when drug-containing liposomes are used, in comparison with free drug or liposome-encapsulated drug administered under normothermic conditions. Work in the author's laboratory suggests that the rate of extravasation of liposomes from the vascular compartment is enhanced by a factor of 40 to 50, compared with normothermic treatment (Gaber et al, 1996; Fig. 4). In contrast, the use of hyperthermia does not seem to enhance drug uptake into tissue when it is administered in the free form. Thus, the use of hyperthermia shows considerable promise as an agent for increasing the delivery of novel cancer therapeutic agents. This approach could lead to substantial enhancement (1 to 2 orders of magnitude in drug delivery over what can be achieved with administration of free drug). In the future, these approaches could be used as a means of enhancing the selective delivery of gene therapy approaches as well.

Modification of Tumor Blood Flow and Microenvironment

There are also promising new approaches to enhancing the the cytotoxicity of hyperthermia that focus on temporary reduction in intracellular pH. It has been known for some time that acute intracellular acidification can lead to sensitization to hyperthermic cytotoxicity. However, it has been difficult to determine a safe way of achieving this effect in vivo. Early studies examined the feasibility of using hyperglycemia to achieve acidification. The logic behind this approach was that excess glucose availability would lead to an increase in anaerobic metabolism and a build-up in lactic acid. However, careful studies in rodents, in which glucose was administered intraperitoneally, indicated that tumor acidification was probably the result of decreased blood pressure and tumor perfusion. These effects were created by the hyperosmotic environment within the peritoneal cavity, which led to hypovolemia as well as changes in red blood cell rheology. More recent studies have indicated that it is possible to induce hyperglycemia, via the intraperitoneal route, that acidifies tumor without a drop in blood pressure. Studies using oral glucose adminis-

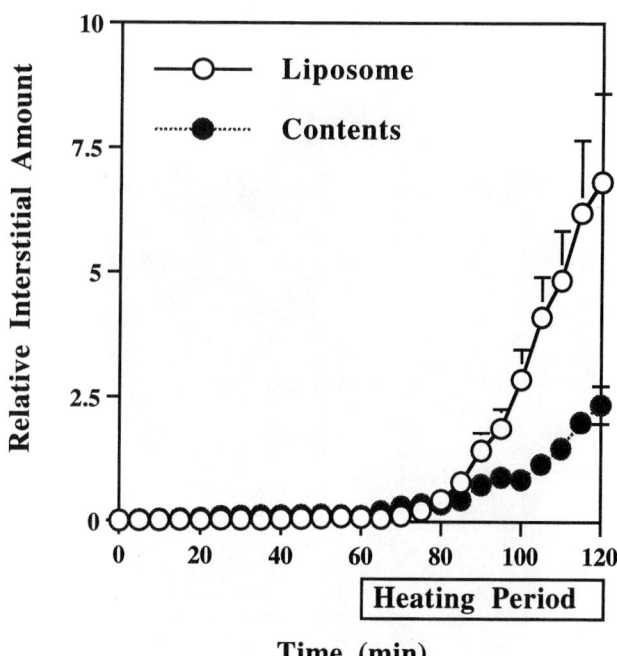

Figure 4. Quantitative fluorescence measurement of liposome extravasation out of tumor vasculature during normothermia (first 60 minutes) and hyperthermia (42°C for the last 60 minutes). The total amount extravasated after heating averages 40 times the amount extravasated after 60 minutes at normal temperature. The contents (doxorubicin) are self-quenched when inside the liposome, but will release on heating, which shows accumulation of fluorescence signal during the second 60-minute period. These particular liposomes were formulated to be thermally sensitive at 42°C. (Redrawn from Gaber MH, Wu NZ, Hong K, et al: Thermosensitive liposomes: Extravasation and release of contents in tumor microvascular networks. *Int J Radiat Oncol Biol Phys* 36:1177–1187, 1996, with permission.)

tration in humans have indicated adequate acidification in some patients, but the results have been inconsistent. Parenteral administration in dogs bearing soft tissue sarcomas did not result in a reduction of tumor intracellular pH.

More recently, Song and coworkers have shown that inhibitors of hydrogen ion pumps can lead to intracellular acidification, increased in vivo cytotoxicity, and enhancement of tumor growth delay, when combined with hyperthermia. It is also possible that intracellular acidification can be achieved via the use of vasoactive drugs, since such agents frequently cause a reduction in tumor blood flow. However, the successful use of such agents will require identification of one that does not require a significant reduction in blood pressure to achieve the desired effect. Additional studies with other vasoactive agents are currently underway, since identification of an effective agent could also have the benefit of causing increased temperatures during hyperthermia as a result of reduced heat transfer capacity. Ultimately, reduction in intracellular pH may require combinations of the three approaches described previously to achieve the desired result. The results of studies in this area of investigation may be important for other types of cancer therapy, including the use of some chemotherapeutic agents whose intracellular uptake is modified by changes in the pH gradient across the cell membrane.

References and Suggested Reading

Brizel DM, Scully SP, Harrelson JM, et al: Radiation therapy and hyperthermia improve the oxygenation of human soft tissue sarcomas. Cancer Res 56:5347, 1996.
Hyperthermia improves oxygenation of soft tissue sarcomas, which results in an improved antitumor effect.

Dewhirst MW, Griffin TW, Smith AR, et al: Intersociety Council on Radiation Oncology essay on the introduction of new medical treatments into practice. J Natl Cancer Inst 85:951, 1993.
This paper reviews the scientific and economic constraints on the development of new technology for cancer therapy.

Gaber MH, Wu NZ, Hong K, et al: Thermosensitive liposomes: Extravasation and release of contents in tumor microvascular networks. Int J Radiat Oncol Biol Phys 36:1177, 1996.
Hyperthermia greatly enhances the delivery of liposomes to target tissue as well as the release of contents.

Hauck ML, Zalutsky MR, Dewhirst MW: Enhancement of radiolabeled monoclonal antibody uptake in tumors with local hyperthermia. In: Torchilin VP, ed: Handbook of Targeted Delivery of Imaging Agents. Boca Raton, FL: CRC Press, 1995, p 335.
Reviews rationale and issues related to the enhancement of antibody delivery to tumors with hyperthermia.

Kapp DS, Cox RS: Thermal treatment parameters are most predictive of outcome in patients with single tumor nodules per treatment field in recurrent adenocarcinoma of the breast [see comments]. Int J Radiat Oncol Biol Phys 33:887, 1995.
This paper shows the relationships between thermal doses achieved and response rates and duration of local control of chest wall recurrences of breast cancer treated with hyperthermia and radiation.

Oleson JR, Samulski TV, Leopold KA, et al: Sensitivity of hyperthermia trial outcomes to temperature and time: Implications for thermal goals of treatment. Int J Radiat Oncol Biol Phys 25:289, 1993.

Overgaard J, Gonzalez Gonzalez D, Hulshof MCCM, et al: Randomised trial of hyperthermia as adjuvant to radiotherapy for recurrent or metastatic malignant melanoma. Lancet 345:540, 1995.
This paper reports the first positive phase III trial in humans, comparing radiation therapy alone to radiation therapy plus hyperthermia for the treatment of malignant melanoma.

Page RL, Thrall DE: Therapeutic hyperthermia: Contribution from clinical studies in dogs with spontaneous neoplasia. In Vivo 8:851, 1994.
This paper reviews the scientific contributions that studies in dogs have made to the overall progress in therapeutic hyperthermia.

Seegenschmiedt MH, Fessenden P, Vernon CC: Thermoradiotherapy and Thermochemotherapy, vol 1, Biology, Physiology, and Physics; vol 2, Clinical Applications. New York: Springer-Verlag, 1995 and 1996.
A recent two-volume set that reviews all aspects of hyperthermia, including basic biologic concepts, physical methods of application, and clinical trial results.

Sneed PK, Stauffer PR, McDermott MW, et al: Survival benefit of hyperthermia in a prospective randomized trial of brachytherapy boost ± hyperthermia for glioblastoma multiforme. Int J Radiat Oncol Biol Phys 40:287, 1998.

Song CW, Lyons JC, Makepeace CM, et al: Effects of HMA, an analog of amiloride, on the thermosensitivity of tumors in vivo. Int J Radiat Oncol Biol Phys 30:133, 1994.

Thrall DE, Prescott DM, Samulski TV, et al: Radiation plus local hyperthermia versus radiation plus the combination of local and whole-body hyperthermia in canine sarcomas. Int J Radiat Oncol Biol Phys 34:1087, 1996.
This paper demonstrates the lack of enhancement of the hyperthermia effect when whole body hyperthermia is added to local hyperthermia, in combination with radiation therapy, for the treatment of canine soft tissue sarcomas.

Vernon CC, Hand JW, Field SB, et al: Radiotherapy with or without hyperthermia in the treatment of superficial localized breast cancer: Results from five randomized controlled trials. International Collaborative Hyperthermia Group. Int J Radiat Oncol Biol Phys 35:731, 1996.
This paper reports positive phase III trial results for hyperthermia plus radiation therapy in the treatment of chest wall recurrences of breast cancer.

Gene Therapy for Cancer

ROBYN E. ELMSLIE
STEVEN W. DOW
Denver, Colorado

Gene therapy has been the subject of considerable debate recently, partly in response to excessive claims made by early proponents of gene therapy. In the midst of this ongoing debate, gene therapy has been rapidly moving into clinical trials. Nearly all human gene therapy trials underway are directed toward cancer treatment, primarily because the most impressive experimental gene therapy results thus far have come from cancer gene therapy studies. The purpose of this article is to review the current status of cancer gene therapy, including strategies that are being evaluated clinically, as well as the potential advantages and disadvantages of each. In addition, preliminary results from cancer gene therapy studies being conducted in dogs and cats are also discussed.

APPLICATION OF GENE THERAPY TO THE TREATMENT OF CANCER

At present, there are four general gene therapy approaches to cancer treatment (Table 1). These approaches include suicide gene therapy, genetic immunotherapy, tumor suppressor gene therapy, and administration of drug resistance genes.

Suicide Gene Therapy

Suicide gene therapy is accomplished by transfecting cancer cells with a gene whose protein product will convert an inactive prodrug into a compound that is toxic to the

TABLE 1. Approaches to Cancer Gene Therapy

Suicide Gene Therapy
Herpes simplex virus–thymidine kinase (HSV-tk)
Cytosine deaminase
Cytochrome P-450
Genetic Immunotherapy
Cytokines
Co-stimulatory molecules
Tumor Suppressor Gene Therapy
p53
Retinoblastoma gene
p21
BCL-x_s
Drug Resistance Gene Therapy
MDR1
Dihydrofolate reductase
Glutathione-S-transferase
O^6-Methylguanine-DNA-methyltransferase

transfected cancer cell. The best example of this method of gene therapy is the herpes simplex virus-thymidine kinase gene (HSV-tk) system. Tumor cells transfected with the HSV-tk gene are rendered sensitive to the cytotoxic effects of ganciclovir. Culver and colleagues (1992) determined that 11 of 14 glioma-bearing, ganciclovir-treated rats achieved complete remission when their tumors were directly injected with HSV-tk retroviral vector transfected fibroblasts. Toxicity to the adjacent brain tissue was not observed. Regression occurred in tumors containing as few as 10% of HSV-tk–transfected cancer cells. This "bystander" effect is believed to be mediated by host immune cells that secrete cytokines, such as interleukin-1 (IL-1) and tumor necrosis factor-alpha (TNF-α). The HSV-tk gene is currently being evaluated in clinical trials in humans for the treatment of ovarian cancer. Complete remission has been achieved in 2 of 14 patients with advanced-stage ovarian cancer. Also underway are human trials using this suicide gene for the treatment of brain tumors, with a 10% complete remission rate to date.

Cytosine deaminase is useful for suicide gene therapy, as it converts nontoxic 5-fluorocytosine (5-FC) to the toxic 5-fluorouracil (5-FU). 5-FU is converted to 5-fluorouracil monophosphate and 5-fluorouracil triphosphate, which block thymidylate synthetase and mRNA transcription, respectively. Significant tumor inhibition following treatment with 5-FC has been observed in mice bearing cytosine deaminase–transfected colon cancer and fibrosarcomas.

Other genes that hold promise for suicide gene therapy include the cytochrome P-450 enzyme and deoxycytidine kinase genes. Tumor cells transfected with these genes have significantly increased sensitivity to alkylating agents (cyclophosphamide and ifosfamide) and cytosine arabinoside, respectively.

Genetic Immunotherapy

Genetic immunotherapy for tumors seeks to achieve three goals: (1) attract T cells, macrophages, and dendritic cells to the tumor site; (2) enhance recognition of tumor-specific antigens and induce activation of immune effector cells; and (3) induce systemic antitumor immunity. In cases in which complete tumor eradication is not possible, continued immune surveillance by immune memory cells is necessary for detection and eradication of newly arising metastatic tumor cells and for continued control of the growth of the primary tumor.

Role of Co-stimulation in Tumor Rejection. The critical importance of the CD28-B7 interaction and the CD28 co-stimulatory signal in T-cell activation and tumor rejection has been confirmed by in vivo experiments. In the absence of the co-stimulatory signal delivered by B7 binding to CD28, T-cell receptor–mediated recognition of the peptide-MHC complex may induce T-cell anergy (unresponsiveness), involving a block in both IL-2 production and responsiveness to IL-4. Induction of T-cell anergy is thought to be one mechanism by which malignant cells evade recognition by the immune system. The anergic state can be prevented either by co-stimulation with B7 or by high doses of IL-2, resulting in gradual recovery of the activated, responsive state. Some studies in mice have shown that B7-transfected melanomas were rejected, whereas B7-negative tumors grew progressively. B7 expression by the transfected melanoma cells provided the co-stimulatory signal to its counter-receptor CD28, inducing IL-2 expression, T-lymphocyte proliferation, and clonal expansion, which resulted in CD8+-mediated killing of the tumor cells. B7 and other co-stimulatory molecules are also required for natural killer (NK) cell participation in tumor rejection.

The effect of B7 transfection on the tumorgenicity of several murine tumor cell lines has been investigated. B7 transfection of relatively immunogenic tumor cell lines such as RMA, E6B2, P815, EL4, and K1735 prevented tumor formation and protected against subsequent challenge with wild-type, nontransfected tumors. Clinical trials in human patients are currently underway to determine whether vaccination with B7-transfected autologous, irradiated human melanoma cells can stimulate systemic tumor immunity.

Transfection of tumor cell lines with a combination of B7 and IL-2 genes has also been studied. Expression of both B7 and IL-2 in the fibrosarcoma line CMS5 induces rejection of tumors in mice, whereas expression of either of these genes alone results in the rapid formation of tumors. Additionally, expression of either B7 or IL-2 alone has little effect on the tumorgenicity of the poorly immunogenic NC adenocarcinoma cell line, whereas the combined expression of B7 and IL-2 induces potent antitumor responses, including rejection of established tumors. The enhancement of antitumor responses observed with the combined expression of B7 and IL-2 may be due to the reversal of anergy. Studies have previously shown that high-level expression of IL-2 can prevent the onset of anergy and can reverse established anergy. IL-2 secretion by tumor cells also overcomes the abnormal signal transduction often seen in T lymphocytes from tumor-bearing mice. These findings emphasize the importance of studies evaluating the therapeutic relevance of combined expression of co-stimulatory genes with immunomodulatory cytokine genes.

Cytokines. Cytokine genes have been used in tumor cell vaccination experiments to enhance tumor immunity. In tumor cell vaccine experiments, tumor cells are transfected in vitro with a vector expressing the cytokine gene of interest. Transfected tumor cells are irradiated to prevent continued division, but the tumor cells can continue to produce cytokine proteins for several days before they die. These transfected, irradiated tumor cells are then injected into mice. Several weeks from the time of tumor vaccination, mice are challenged with wild-type (nontransfected, nonirradiated) tumor cells so that induction of tumor-specific immunity can be assessed. The most impressive results have been observed with tumor cells transfected with granulocyte-macrophage colony-stimulating factor (GM-CSF), IL-2, IL-4, IL-6, or IL-12.

Experiments involving the treatment of already established tumors constitute a more rigorous and clinically relevant evaluation of cancer gene therapy evaluation than do vaccination experiments. Mice are injected with wild-type (unmodified) tumor cells, which are then allowed to grow until a measurable tumor is established (7 to 14 days). The mice are then injected with the tumor cell vaccine to assess the vaccine's effect on regression of the tumor. Under these conditions, several cytokine genes have exhibited efficacy against small established tumors, including IL-2, IL-4, IL-6, IL-12, and GM-CSF. None of these cytokines demonstrated efficacy against large tumor burdens, raising some doubts about the ultimate benefit of this particular type of gene therapy for cancer treatment in humans with large tumor burdens. The failure to demonstrate efficacy against large tumor burdens may have resulted from insufficient potency of antitumor immunity, inability of effector cells to traffic into poorly vascularized, bulky tumors, or inability to overcome induction of high levels of peripheral immune tolerance by the large growing tumor. In some cases, the lack of efficacy against bulky disease may be related to tumor growth kinetics. In many experimental murine tumors, the rapid growth of the tumor simply outpaces the developing immune response. Cytoreduction of bulky tumors may therefore be beneficial when done prior to initiation of cytokine gene therapy.

A recent study reported by Mehtali and colleagues (1996) evaluated xenogeneic green-monkey kidney cells (Vero cells) transfected with the human IL-2 gene for the treatment of malignant melanoma in dogs and fibrosarcoma in cats. Animals were first treated with surgery and radiation therapy to reduce tumor burden to microscopic disease. The animals were then randomized to receive repeated injections of Vero cells transfected with human IL-2 DNA or no further therapy. At 16 months after therapy, 69% of control cats had recurrence of the fibrosarcoma, versus 31% in the Vero cell cohort. At 12 months after treatment, 6% of control dogs were still alive versus 37% of the Vero cell cohort.

By injecting xenogeneic human IL-2 transfected cells into the tumor site, an inflammatory reaction against the foreign cells was induced and local local expression of IL-2 enhanced the inflammatory response. The result was believed to be due to activation of NK cells. Phase I trials in humans are underway in Sweden and France to evaluate this gene therapy approach to cancer treatment.

Genes encoding cytokines may also be injected in vivo directly into the tumor mass, with the use of one of several delivery systems, including liposomes, synthetic conjugates, adenoviral vectors, and gene gun delivery. A poten-

tial advantage of this strategy is that the immunostimulatory gene of interest is expressed directly in the tumor environment, thereby bypassing the need for establishment of tumor cell lines and in vitro tumor cell transfection. Multiple cytokine gene administrations are generally required to induce an antitumor effect. Gene gun–mediated delivery of IL-12 DNA into established cutaneous mouse tumors was shown to induce complete tumor regression (RENCA carcinoma, L5178Y lymphoma), partial tumor regression (MethA sarcoma, SA-1 sarcoma), or attenuated tumor growth (P815 mastocytoma, B16 melanoma). These results are exciting inasmuch as it is the first time that direct DNA injection has been shown to induce consistent regression of established tumors in mice. In addition to tumor regression, treated mice developed systemic antitumor immunity, resulting in delayed onset of metastasis and increased survival times in most mice.

Recently, Elmslie and associates (1995) reported preliminary results of treating dogs with oral malignant melanoma with a series of direct intratumoral injections of plasmid DNA complexed to a cationic lipid formulation. Canine malignant melanoma is an extremely aggressive cancer in dogs. Aggressive surgery may induce prolonged survival in dogs with small tumors (diameter <2 cm), whereas the majority of dogs with larger tumors at the time of diagnosis succumb to lymph node and pulmonary metastases within 6 months of treatment. Radiation therapy may be palliative for dogs with advanced tumors. Chemotherapy has not demonstrated significant benefit in the treatment of melanoma in dogs.

In the canine melanoma genetic immunotherapy studies, two immunostimulatory genes were used in combination: a bacterial superantigen gene (*Staphylococcus* enterotoxin B; SEB) plus a cytokine gene (either GM-CSF or IL-2). SEB is a potent activator of both CD4+ and CD8+ T lymphocytes and triggers lymphocyte secretion of several cytokines, including interferon gamma (IFN-γ), TNF-α, IL-2, and IL-12. SEB-activated lymphocytes also develop strong tumor cytolytic activity and can induce tumor regression when adoptively transferred into tumor-bearing mice. In the dog studies, the cytokine gene was included to augment the antitumor effects induced by the superantigen gene. Animals were treated by twice-monthly intratumoral injections of plasmid DNA complexed to cationic lipids, for a total of 12 or more treatments.

Patients were evaluated for treatment-associated toxicity, tumor responses, and survival times. Bacterial superantigens are extremely potent molecules, and even very low concentrations (as little as 1 μg) are capable of inducing toxic shock syndrome in humans and other mammals, including dogs. However, adverse effects have not been observed in any of the more than 50 dogs treated with intratumoral injections of superantigen plus cytokine DNA. This lack of toxicity is most likely explained by the fact that local production of superantigens in tumor tissues was sufficient to induce local T-cell responses, but not sufficient to induce systemic toxicity.

Intratumoral SEB and cytokine treatment induced a high percentage of tumor responses in treated animals. The response rate (complete or partial remission) was 45% in dogs with stage III tumors (lymph node metastasis). Tumor biopsies obtained after DNA injection and evaluated by immunohistochemistry demonstrated a pronounced infiltrate of CD4 + and CD8 + T cells and macrophages. Thus, the local expression of superantigen and cytokine genes was sufficient to attract T cells and macrophages into the local tumor environment and activate them. Preliminary studies have also revealed evidence of T-cell activation in draining lymph nodes of treated dogs.

Treated dogs were also evaluated for evidence of a systemic antitumor response. Levels of antitumor cytotoxic T-lymphocyte activity in peripheral blood of treated stage III animals were high compared with those of untreated or nonresponding animals. Perhaps more important, survival times for treated dogs were significantly longer than those for historical control animals. Thus, direct intratumoral expression of potent immunostimulatory genes was capable of inducing not only local tumor control in dogs with a spontaneous and highly malignant tumor, but also systemic antitumor responses. Improvements in gene delivery and vector design can be expected to further improve the response to this type of genetic immunotherapy.

Tumor Suppressor Gene Therapy

The p53 tumor suppressor gene serves as an important negative regulator of cell division. Synthesis of the p53 protein is normally upregulated following DNA damage. The p53 protein, in turn, upregulates the production of p21, which prevents DNA replication by binding to proliferating cell nuclear antigen. The p21 protein also prevents phosphorylation of the retinoblastoma gene, which then, in turn, is able to sequester transcription factors that regulate cell proliferation, thereby maintaining the cell in a dormant state. The combined actions of these two tumor suppressor genes can prevent cellular proliferation and can maintain cell cycle control. Many tumors are associated with inactivating mutations in the *p53* gene, which lead to uncontrolled cell proliferation. Therefore, replacing the mutated *p53* gene with the functional gene has been one genetic approach to cancer treatment.

Lesoon-Wood and colleagues (1995) achieved marked regression of transplanted xenogeneic breast carcinomas in nude mice following systemic injection of a p53-liposome complex. Clinical trials in humans with hepatocellular carcinoma have yielded encouraging early results, with one of eight patients undergoing measurable tumor regression. One of nine patients with lung cancer recently achieved complete remission following in vivo *p53* gene therapy.

Drug Resistance Gene Therapy

To facilitate administration of higher doses of chemotherapy, drug resistance genes are inserted into patients' hematopoietic cells to decrease their sensitivity to the effects of chemotherapeutic agents. This form of therapy allows the use of increased doses of cytotoxic agents without the accompanying myelosuppressive effects. Hematopoietic cells transfected ex vivo with the multidrug resistance gene 1 *(MDR1)* gene have demonstrated increased resistance to a wide range of chemotherapeutic agents, including paclitaxel, vinca alkaloids, epipodophyllotoxins, and anthracyclines. Transfection with the dihydrofolate re-

ductase *(DHFR)* gene and the O^6-methylguanine-DNA-methyltransferase gene protects cells from antifolate drugs such as methotrexate and nitrosourea drugs such as carmustine, respectively. Most human clinical trials underway are investigating the effects of transfection with the *MDR1* gene, but preliminary results are not yet available.

METHODS OF GENE DELIVERY

The ideal gene delivery system should be capable of efficiently introducing the gene of interest into nearly 100% of target cells, resulting in efficient and long-term gene expression, and should do so by utilizing a gene delivery system that is both nontoxic and cost-effective. Although the optimal gene delivery system still has not been perfected, many methods for gene transfer and expression have been developed for both in vivo and in vitro applications (Table 2). Each system has advantages and disadvantages that must be considered when one designs a gene therapy strategy for cancer treatment.

Retroviral Vectors. Retroviral vectors are gene transfer constructs that utilize the replication and integration mechanisms of retroviruses to efficiently insert genes into the chromosomes of host cells. The ability of retroviral vectors to insert the gene of interest into the host cell chromosome represents a distinct advantage of retroviral vectors over other vectors, but it is also a potential risk. Once a cell has been transduced with a retroviral vector, all its progeny cells will also contain the transferred gene. However, the use of retroviral vectors for in vivo transfection is limited by their inability to integrate into nondividing cells.

There are three major safety concerns related to clinical use of retroviral vectors. First, the level of gene expression

TABLE 2. Methods for Delivering Genes into Mammalian Cells and Possible In Vitro and In Vivo Applications

Method	Application in Gene Therapy	
	In Vitro	In Vivo
Viral Vectors		
Retroviruses (MoMuLV, HIV, foamy virus)	+	+
Adenoviruses (Ad2, Ad5)	+	+
Adeno-associated virus (Dependovirus; AAV-2)	+	+
Herpes simplex virus (HSV)	+	+
Epstein-Barr virus (EBV)	+	+
Alphaviruses (Sindbis, Simliki forest virus)	+	+
Vaccinia virus	+	+
Parvoviruses	+	+
Nonviral or Viral-Assisted Techniques		
DEAE-dextran	+	−
Calcium phosphate co-precipitation	+	−
Electroporation	+	−
Cationic lipids	+	+
Microinjection	+	−
Naked plasmid DNA direct injection	−	+
DNA microprojectile bombardment	+	+
Receptor-mediated endocytosis	+	+

DEAE, diethylaminoethanol.

can vary greatly from cell to cell, depending on the particular site of proviral integration. Second, the insertion of retroviral vectors into host chromosomes is a random event; thus, there is the potential risk of insertional mutagenesis. For example, the presence of retroviral vector sequences could disrupt crucial upstream or downstream genetic regulatory sequences, leading to either cell death or cellular transformation and the generation of a malignant phenotype. Third, retroviral vectors propagated in vitro occasionally give rise to fully replication-competent retroviruses. These replication-competent viruses are capable of infecting and replicating extensively in the host, much as would a wild-type retrovirus. Therefore, viral stocks must be rigorously screened to ensure that they are free from replication-competent viruses.

A number of detailed reviews concerning the safety of retroviral vectors for gene therapy have been published over the years. All the data currently available indicate that the risks associated with their use are very low, particularly compared with the known risks of increased malignancy rates in humans following conventional therapies such as radiation therapy, chemotherapy, and immunosuppression.

Adenoviral Vectors. The ability of adenoviruses to efficiently infect nondividing cells increases the potential use of this vector system for in vivo gene delivery. For use in gene therapy, the adenovirus genome has been engineered to remove certain regions, including the E1A region, responsible for viral replication. The resulting modified adenovirus vectors infect cells very efficiently, and can be purified and concentrated to very high titers. Most important, unlike retroviruses, adenoviruses are able to introduce DNA into nonreplicating cells, where the introduced DNA remains in an episomal location, thereby eliminating the risk of insertional mutagenesis. One drawback with the use of adenovirus vectors is that the duration of expression in an adult immunocompetent host tends to be rather short (1 to 2 months). Moreover, it has thus far been difficult to successfully readminister adenovirus of the same serotype following an initial treatment because of the extreme immunogenicity of adenoviral vectors. Another major concern with the use of adenoviral vectors is that these vectors, although extensively modified, may still be able to replicate and cause disease in humans, who are the definitive hosts for adenoviruses.

Direct Introduction of Plasmid DNA. Recent attention has focused on techniques for introducing plasmid DNA into tissues in vivo. The impetus for this approach came from what were, at the time, startling observations suggesting that plasmid expression vectors utilizing strong mammalian promoters could be expressed in mammalian tissues in vitro. The technique of plasmid gene transfer offers significant advantages over virally mediated gene delivery in terms of biosafety and reduced vector immunogenicity. The major drawback is the relatively low efficiency of this technique relative to viral gene delivery. At present, there are three primary methods for introducing plasmid DNA into mammalian cells in vitro are as follows:

Gene Gun (Particle-Mediated Gene Transfer). DNA-coated submicron-sized silver or gold particles are accelerated to high speeds by a so-called gene gun to bombard a target cell or tissue. Gene transfer and expression are highly efficient in vitro, and feasibility has been demonstrated for a wide variety of cells and organs. This method of gene delivery is nontoxic and ideally designed for in vitro gene delivery to superficial tissues, such as skin. The major disadvantages are the inability to transfect cells deeper than a few microns, the cumbersome equipment required, and the expense associated with use of silver and gold particles.

Lipid-Mediated Gene Transfer. Plasmid DNA can be complexed to polycationic lipids based on charge interactions, and the lipid-DNA complexes can then be administered in vivo by several different routes. The lipid molecule fuses to the cell membrane, introducing the plasmid DNA into the cell, which then travels to the nucleus, where transcription takes place. Plasmid expression vectors are maintained extrachromosomally and do not integrate into the host cell chromosome. This feature of plasmid expression vectors eliminates a major safety concern associated with the use of retroviral vectors. By modifying the lipid composition, DNA can be delivered to respiratory epithelium by aerosolization, or to various internal organs (especially lung tissues) after intravenous injection. Specific organs (and tumors) can also be transfected by direct intraorgan (intratumor) injection of lipid-DNA complexes. Multiple administrations are typically required because of the transient expression of the DNA, and decreased efficiency of transfection compared with other delivery systems. This system lends itself well to in vivo administration because of the relative low costs and low toxicity. The authors have demonstrated the clinical usefulness of direct intratumoral DNA injection in dogs with malignant melanoma (see earlier).

Synthetic Conjugates. One factor that limits the efficiency of in vitro gene transfer of plasmid DNA is the bulk lysosomal degradation of DNA after entry into the cell. DNA degradation can be partially circumvented by complexing DNA to a cationic polypeptide, such as polylysine. These products increase the efficiency of DNA transfer and expression, but not the duration of expression. By coupling a cell-surface protein through a polylysine linkage to naked DNA, the uptake of plasmid DNA can be directed to target cells expressing the relevant receptor. Although this method of gene delivery holds great promise for tissue targeting, the in vitro effectiveness of such a targeting approach remains to be determined.

References and Suggested Reading

Culver KW, Ram Z, Wallbridge S, et al: In vivo gene transfer with retroviral vector-producer cells for treatment of experimental brain tumors. Science 256:1550, 1992.
Dow SW, Elmslie RE, Willson AP, et al: In vivo tumor transfection with superantigen plus cytokine genes induces tumor regression and prolongs survival in dogs with malignant melanoma. J Clin Invest 101:2406, 1998.
Elmslie RE, Dow SW: Genetic immunotherapy for cancer. Semin Vet Med Surg (Small Anim) 12:193, 1997.
Elmslie RE, Dow SW: Pilot study of intravenous gene delivery for

treatment of pulmonary metastatic disease. Proceedings of the Veterinary Cancer Society, 16th Annual Conference, October 20–23, 1996,
Pacific Grove, California, pp 83.
Lesoon-Wood LA, Kim WH, Kleinman HK, et al: Systemic gene therapy
with p53 reduces growth and metastases of a malignant human breast
cancer in nude mice. Hum Gene Ther 6:395, 1995.

Quintin-Colonna F, Devauchelle P, Fradelizi D, et al: Gene therapy of
spontaneous canine melanoma and feline fibrosarcoma by intratumoral
administration of histoincompatible cells expressing human interleu-
kin-2. Gene Ther 3:1104, 1996.
Roth JA, Cristiano RJ: Gene therapy for cancer: What have we done and
where are we going? J Natl Cancer Inst 89:21, 1997.

Feline Fibrosarcoma: Vaccine Associated

MATTIE J. HENDRICK
Philadelphia, Pennsylvania

Several reports support a strong association between the
administration of vaccines, particularly feline leukemia and
rabies, and the subsequent development of sarcomas in cats
at the site of vaccination. Although these sarcomas are
uncommon, with estimates of their occurrence ranging
from 1 in 1,000 to 1 in 10,000 cats receiving vaccinations,
they are aggressive, with significant morbidity and mortality. Such tumors have proved resistant to standard treatment
modalities, and many cats have multiple recurrences, with
euthanasia as the final outcome.

CLINICAL APPEARANCE AND BEHAVIOR

Most postvaccinal sarcomas arise in the interscapular
subcutis, but others occur along the dorsal and lateral
thorax and flank and in the musculature of the thigh,
reflecting less common vaccination sites. Typical tumors
are gray-white, firm, well demarcated, and partially encapsulated. Most tumors are larger than 4.0 cm in diameter
when found by the owner or veterinarian, and have a
necrotic center, giving them a cystic appearance. Despite
the circumscribed gross appearance of the tumor, there is
often histologic evidence of "tongues" of tumor extending
away from the mass along fascial planes. The majority of
postvaccinal sarcomas are fibrosarcomas, but malignant
fibrous histiocytomas (also called myofibrosarcomas or my-
ofibroblastic sarcomas), osteosarcomas, chondrosarcomas,
rhabdomyosarcomas, myxosarcomas, and liposarcomas
have been seen. Histologically, most vaccine-associated
fibrosarcomas have a high degree of nuclear pleomorphism,
cellular atypia, and multinucleated giant cells. Many, but
not all, have peripheral aggregates of lymphocytes and
macrophages. In some, the macrophages contain a globular
gray-brown material that has been shown to be aluminum,
a common adjuvant used in feline vaccines.

In one retrospective study (Hendrick et al, 1994), 62%
of the tumors recurred following excisional biopsy, most
within 6 months. A total of 22% of cats had fibrosarcomas
recur two, three, or four times. Based on published reports,
metastasis of postvaccinal sarcomas appears to be rare.
Some oncology centers have anecdotal evidence of higher
metastatic rates, but additional controlled studies must be
completed to determine the true metastatic rates of vaccine-
associated sarcomas.

PATHOGENESIS

Based on morphologic and immunohistochemical evidence, vaccine-associated sarcomas appear to arise from
primitive mesenchymal cells that have features of fibroblasts and myofibroblasts. The exact origin of myofibroblasts is controversial, but many believe they represent
a "transitional stage" through which fibroblasts or some
other primitive mesenchymal cells pass during the process
of wound healing. Injection of vaccines commonly results
in a localized granulomatous reaction that varies in severity
and duration, depending on the vaccine and adjuvant.

The increased incidence of fibrosarcomas in cats began
in the late 1980s, shortly following the introduction and
widespread use of killed aluminum-adjuvanted rabies and
leukemia virus vaccines not previously used in the cat.
Macy (1996) has documented that these vaccines consistently produce palpable inflammatory masses at the site of
injection in cats. Hypothetically, postvaccinal sarcomas
may arise from inappropriate or overzealous inflammatory
or immunologic reactions associated with the presence of
vaccine components in vaccination sites that lead to uncontrolled proliferation of fibroblasts and myofibroblasts. Despite the importance of feline leukemia virus (FeLV) and
feline sarcoma virus (FeSV) in many diseases and neoplasms in cats, these viruses do not appear to play a
role in the pathogenesis of postvaccinal sarcomas (Ellis et
al, 1996).

Research projects in the author's laboratory and others
are focusing on growth factors and oncogenes as likely
players in this neoplastic transformation. Many studies and
animal models support the hypothesis that growth factors
promote neoplastic transformation. A large percentage of
human tumors have been shown to have receptors for
growth factors that they themselves produce in an abnormal
or autonomous fashion. Termed *autocrine stimulation,* the
author and colleagues have documented this phenomenon
in feline postvaccinal sarcomas, using immunohistochemical methods. In addition, various oncogene products are
homologous to growth factors or their receptors, or to
other components involved in growth factor–induced signal
transduction in the cell. The overexpression of oncogenes
and their normal counterparts, proto-oncogenes, has been
shown to lead to neoplastic transformation of cells. The

proto-oncogene c-*jun*, which codes for a transcriptional protein implicated in cellular proliferation and oncogenesis in vitro, is overexpressed in feline postvaccinal sarcomas (unpublished data). Last, dysregulation of p53, a tumor suppressor protein, appears to be a feature of many feline fibrosarcomas, including those associated with vaccination (Helfand et al, 1995). Clearly, differences in host genome and alterations in oncogene and growth factor expression play a role in the pathogenesis of these tumors and should be the focus of future research.

TREATMENT AND PREVENTION

As mentioned previously, vaccine-associated sarcomas are aggressive tumors that frequently recur. Surgical excision, the most common treatment, has resulted in less than satisfactory results, with recurrence rates of 62%. In some instances, failure may be due to incomplete excision at the time of first surgery. It must be re-emphasized that although the tumor may appear on gross examination to be well circumscribed, small fingers of neoplastic cells that extend out from the tumor may be grossly indiscernible. Therefore, *wide margins in all directions* should be obtained, which in some cases may include partial scapulectomy or excision of epaxial muscles and dorsal cervical vertebral processes. Amputation of an involved limb should also be considered. One study comparing surgery alone versus surgery and radiation therapy (Davidson et al, 1997) showed that complete surgical excision of low-grade postvaccinal tumors resulted in a median tumor-free interval of 16 months, with survival times of more than 24 months. The animals that received radiation therapy had shorter median tumor-free intervals (4.5 months) and survival times (9 months), but in all cases radiation therapy was attempted much later in the course of the disease, after one or more prior surgeries. The results of another study (Cronin et al, 1998) suggest that low recurrence rates and long disease-free intervals can be achieved in cats that have received radiation therapy prior to surgical excision; however, further controlled prospective studies are needed. There are numerous anecdotal reports concerning the therapeutic effects of various chemotherapeutic agents and immunomodulatory drugs such as acemannan, but scant scientific evidence of efficacy.

A few centers across the United States are involved in studies evaluating carboplatin in tumor-bearing cats. Although in the preliminary stages, and with very low numbers of cases, one abstract reports complete or partial remission of vaccine-associated fibrosarcomas following carboplatin administration. Another study (Barber et al, 1996) focused on the effect of combined doxorubicin and cyclophosphamide therapy on nonresectable feline fibrosarcomas. Although not curative, this combination of agents did result in an objective decrease in the size of primary tumors and radiographic evidence of regression of metastatic lesions. Further evaluation of doxorubicin-based chemotherapy is warranted as a means of controlling postvaccinal tumors. Although acemannan is commercially available for use in animals with fibrosarcoma, its therapeutic effects have been inconsistent, often depending on the size of the tumor (best results in tumors <2 cm). However, given the probable role of inflammatory mediators such as cytokines and growth factors in the pathogenesis of vaccine-associated sarcomas, manipulation of the inflammatory and immunologic mechanisms at the injection site through the therapeutic use of galactomannans, cytokines (interleukin-2, tumor necrosis factor, interferons), and monoclonal antibodies against growth factor receptors may prove to be important in prevention as well as treatment.

As can be surmised, there is currently no successful treatment for vaccine-associated sarcomas in the cat. Research is ongoing to determine the best methods of prevention, control, and treatment. Until these methods can be determined, the following general guidelines offered by the Vaccine-Associated Feline Sarcoma Task Force* are presented, to further characterize the causal link and to facilitate the treatment of vaccine-associated sarcomas.

1. Veterinarians should standardize vaccination (and other injection) protocols within their practice and document the location of the injection, the type of vaccine or other injectable product administered, and the manufacturer and serial number of the vaccine in the patient's medical record.
2. It is recommended that
    a. Vaccines containing antigens limited to panleukopenia, feline herpesvirus type 1, and feline calicivirus (with or without *Chlamydia*) should be administered on the right shoulder, according to the manufacturer's recommendations
    b. Vaccines containing rabies antigen (plus any other antigen) should be administered on the right hindlimb as distally as possible, according to the manufacturer's recommendations
    c. Vaccines containing FeLV antigen (plus any other antigen except rabies) should be administered on the left hindlimb as distally as possible, according to the manufacturer's recommendations
    d. Injection sites of other medications should be recorded
3. The use of single-dose vaccine vials is encouraged
4. Vaccination is a medical procedure, and protocols should be individualized to the patient. Administration of any vaccine should proceed only after one has considered the medical significance and zoonotic potential of the infectious agent, the patient's risk of exposure, and germane legal requirements.
5. In addition to the veterinarian's reporting directly to the vaccine manufacturer, it is recommended that the United States Pharmacopeia (U.S.P.) Practitioners' Reporting Form from the American Veterinary Medical Association (AVMA) be used to report occurrences of vaccine-associated sarcomas or other adverse reactions. Information about the U.S.P. Practitioners' Reporting Program and a sample submission form are found in JAVMA, Vol. 208, No. 3, February 1, 1996, pages 361 to 363.

---

*The Vaccine-Associated Feline Sarcoma Task Force is a combined effort of the American Veterinary Medical Association, the American Animal Hospital Association, the American Association of Feline Practitioners, and the Veterinary Cancer Society. Its membership is composed of representatives from the aforementioned groups, veterinary researchers and clinicians, and representatives from the U.S. Department of Agriculture and the Animal Health Institute. The guidelines are based on discussions and materials provided by this group and the Academy of Feline Medicine and the California Veterinary Medical Association.

References and Suggested Reading

Barber LG, Sorenmo KU, Cronin KL, et al: Effect of combined doxorubicin and cyclophosphamide therapy on nonresectable feline fibrosarcoma. Proceedings of the 16th Annual Conference of the Veterinary Cancer Society, Pacific Grove, CA, 1996, p 53.
An abstract describing a retrospective study of the effects of combined doxorubicin and cyclophosphamide therapy on nonresectable fibrosarcomas in 10 cats.

Cronin KL, Page RL, Thrall DE: Radiation and surgery for fibrosarcoma in 33 cats. Vet Rad Ultrasound 39:51, 1998.
A retrospective study of 33 cats comparing the effectiveness of radiation therapy alone versus radiation and surgery.

Davidson EB, Gregory CR, Kass PH: Surgical excision of soft tissue fibrosarcomas in cats. Vet Surg 26:265, 1997.
A retrospective study evaluating differences in tumor-free intervals and survival times in cats that have had one surgery, more than one surgery, or surgery followed by radiation therapy.

Ellis JA, Jackson ML, Bartsch RC, et al: Use of immunohistochemistry and polymerase chain-reaction for detection of oncornaviruses in formalin-fixed, paraffin-embedded fibrosarcomas from cats. J Am Vet Med Assoc 209:767, 1996.
The authors attempt, unsuccessfully, to identify FeLV and FeSV antigens or expression in vaccine-associated tumors using immunohistochemistry and the polymerase chain reaction.

Helfand SC, Kisseberth WC, Wielgosh P, et al: Abnormal expression of p53 tumor suppressor protein in feline fibrosarcoma. Proceedings of the 15th Annual Conference of the Veterinary Cancer Society, Tucson, AZ, 1995, p 67.
An abstract discussing the role of p53 protein in neoplastic transformation in humans and cats.

Hendrick MJ, Shofer FS, Goldschmidt MH, et al: Comparison of fibrosarcomas that developed at vaccination sites and at nonvaccination sites in cats: 239 cases (1991–1992). J Am Vet Med Assoc 205:1425, 1994.
A retrospective epidemiologic study describing differences between vaccination-site fibrosarcomas and nonvaccination-site fibrosarcomas in regard to signalment of cat, size of the tumor, vaccines given, recurrence, metastasis, and final outcome.

Macy DW, Hendrick MJ: The potential role of inflammation in the development of postvaccinal sarcomas in cats. Vet Clin North Am Small Anim Pract 26:103, 1996.
An overview of the history and pathogenesis of postvaccinal sarcomas, with emphasis on the role of specific vaccines and the inflammatory responses they evoke.

Tumors of the Respiratory Tract

KEVIN A. HAHN

TAMMY E. ANDERSON
Knoxville, Tennessee

NASAL PLANE

Pathology and Natural Behavior

Malignant tumors of the nasal plane are common in the cat and rare in the dog (Table 1; Théon et al, 1995; Withrow and Straw, 1990). Squamous cell carcinoma is by far the most frequent malignant diagnosis and is the result of prolonged exposure of the nonpigmented planum to ultraviolet light. Solar-induced dermatitis followed by erythema, crusting, or ulceration of the planum is considered a preneoplastic process. While regional and distant metastases have not been reported, extensive local invasion of the nasal cavity with destruction of underlying soft-tissue structures and bone is common to all types of tumors of the nasal plane and explains their poor response to most conventional therapeutic approaches (e.g., superficial excision, localized irradiation).

Diagnostic Approach

With erosive or proliferative lesions, a deep wedge biopsy should be performed to determine the degree of invasion and the histologic type of disease. These superficial lesions tend to be inflammatory owing to tumor necrosis and bacterial contamination; thus, cytologic scrapings or superficial biopsies are of little value. Lymph nodes are rarely involved except in very advanced disease, and thoracic radiographs are invariably negative for metastasis.

TABLE 1. Malignant Tumors of the Canine and Feline Nasal Plane

Histologic Types	Natural Behavior	Signs and Symptoms	Diagnostic Findings	Treatment Options
Canine and Feline Squamous cell carcinoma *Infrequently Reported* Lymphoma Fibrosarcoma Melanoma Mast cell tumor Lymphomatoid granulomatosis	Slowly progressive, highly invasive lesions that may cause erythema or ulceration or swelling of the nasal plane Metastasis extremely rare No prognostic features have been identified	Sneezing Epistaxis Stertorous breathing pattern Nasal discharge Pain on examination Submandibular or prescapular lymphadenopathy	Neutrophilic leukocytosis Radiographic lysis of the nasal planar bone Neoplastic cells observed histologically from an incisional wedge biopsy of the affected region	*Surgery:* the median tumor-free survival time following aggressive local excision is 16 mo (1 to 27+ mo) for cats and 24 mo (range 14 to 48+ mo) for dogs *Radiation Therapy:* significant progression-free survival times can be achieved in cats

Treatment and Prognosis

Nasal plane tumors can be cured with aggressive surgical resection (Withrow and Straw, 1990). The entire non-haired nasal plane, deep cartilage, and turbinates should be removed, and any areas where deeper tumor invasion is suspected should be biopsied selectively or removed. Careful case selection is imperative, and advanced imaging procedures such as computed tomography, if available, may be helpful prior to definitive therapy to delineate more clearly the extent of tumor. Accurate assessment of the extent of the tumor is essential for determining whether clean surgical margins can be expected with resection of the nasal plane as well as for planning appropriate fields if radiation therapy is to be applied. In one series of cases in which nine cats and five dogs were treated with aggressive resection of the nasal plane, the median postoperative tumor-free survival period was 16 months (1 to 27 + months) for cats and 24 months (range 14 to 48 + months) for dogs (Withrow and Straw, 1990). Radiation protocols involving higher doses and modified dose-fractionation schemes have led to improvements in the survival times of cats with deeply invasive squamous cell carcinomas of the nasal plane (Théon et al, 1995). Following irradiation, 1- and 5-year progression-free survival rates were 60.1 and 10.3%, respectively.

NASAL CAVITY AND PARANASAL SINUSES

Pathology and Natural Behavior

In dogs, approximately two thirds of intranasal tumors are epithelial in origin, slightly fewer than one third are mesenchymal in origin, and only a few are of neuroendocrine origin (Table 2; Patnaik, 1989). Intranasal tumors are locally aggressive and while most animals present with signs referable to the upper respiratory system (e.g., epistaxis, nasal discharge, sneezing, reversed sneezing, dyspnea), some animals present with facial swelling (with or without exophthalmos) and neurologic signs (e.g., seizures, behavioral changes), suggesting extension beyond the nasal cavity and paranasal sinuses, that is, brain involvement (Hahn et al, 1992).

Intranasal tumor metastasis is infrequently reported at presentation; however, it appears that micrometastases do occur and may remain subclinical for 12 to 36 months following presumed definitive treatment (Hahn et al, 1997a). Metastatic sites may include the regional lymph nodes (e.g., medial retropharyngeal, submandibular, prescapular, hilar lymph nodes), lungs, liver, kidneys, or bone. The extremely rare canine patients with a neuroendocrine tumor usually present with metastatic lesions (>86%) and have a poor prognosis.

Although intranasal lymphomas and carcinomas occur more commonly in the cat than in the dog, the results of a retrospective study of 16 cats with intranasal neoplasia suggest that cats and dogs with intranasal tumors have similar biologic courses (O'Brien et al, 1996). In that study, metastasis was uncommon (i.e., lymph node metastasis occurred in only two cats; one with olfactory neuroblastoma, one with undifferentiated carcinoma), and local extension to the brain occurred in two cats (one with neuroblastoma, one with undifferentiated carcinoma).

Diagnostic Approach

When presented with a dog or cat with an intranasal neoplasm, a thorough head and neck palpation should be performed and radiographs of the thorax should be obtained to identify any metastatic lesions. Destruction of the nasal turbinates, evidence of septal deviation, and soft-tissue or fluid-density lesions are common abnormalities observed radiographically in dogs and cats with intranasal neoplasia.

TABLE 2. Malignant Tumors of the Canine and Feline Nasal and Paranasal Sinuses

Histologic Types	Natural Behavior	Signs and Symptoms	Diagnostic Findings	Treatment Options

Canine
Adenocarcinoma
  Differentiated
  Undifferentiated
Squamous cell
  carcinoma
Chondrosarcoma
Fibrosarcoma
Lymphosarcoma
Feline
Adenocarcinoma
Lymphoma
Infrequently Reported
Osteosarcoma
Hemangiosarcoma
Rhabdomyosarcoma
Leiomyosarcoma
Nerve sheath tumors
Neuroblastoma
	Slowly progressive and invasive destruction of the nasal and paranasal sinuses
	More common in older animals (8 to 10 yr of age); no breed or sex predilection
	Brain involvement is a poor prognostic sign
	Local extension to the brain and/or metastasis to regional lymph nodes, lung, or bone has been reported to occur 12 to 36 mo following definitive treatment; a probable result of slow-growing micrometastatic lesions present at the time of original presentation
		Early in the course of the disease the pet will present with unilateral signs, ultimately progressing to bilateral signs as the disease becomes more advanced
		Nasal discharge
		Postnasal drip
		Epiphora
		Sneezing
		Reversed sneezing
		Epistaxis
		Anorexia
		Halitosis
		Facial deformities
		Exophthalmos
		Pain on examination
		Seizures (secondary to cranial extension)
		Retropharyngeal or submandibular lymphadenopathy
			Neutrophilic leukocytosis
			Anemia of chronic disease
			Reactive, inflammatory, or neoplastic medial retropharyngeal, submandibular, prescapular, sternal, or hilar lymphadenopathy
			A soft-tissue mass, bony lysis, and/or septal deviation of the nasal turbinates observed radiographically or on CT or MRI examination
			Pulmonary nodular metastatic disease
			Neoplastic cells observed histologically on an incisional biopsy obtained during a rhinoscopic examination or exploratory rhinotomy
				Surgery: contraindicated unless combined with radiation therapy
				Radiation Therapy: radiotherapy with or without surgery is the treatment of choice; median survival rates vary from 8 to 36 mo in the dog and 1 to 36 mo in the cat with the use of teletherapy or brachytherapy protocols
				Chemotherapy: Platinol (cisplatin) has been reported to palliate clinical signs from 2 to 12 mo for nonhematopoietic tumors; combination chemotherapy is recommended for nasal lymphoma due to systemic disease

CT, computed tomography; MRI, magnetic resonance imaging.

However, advanced images such as those obtained with the use of computed tomography or magnetic resonance techniques, if available, are far better than conventional radiographic images to determine whether disease has extended beyond the nasal cavity and paranasal sinuses (Fig. 1).

A definitive diagnosis of intranasal neoplasia requires biopsy. Various biopsy methods such as core catheter biopsy or punch biopsy can effectively be combined with antegrade and retrograde rhinoscopy to attain an accurate diagnosis in about 80% of cases. Rhinoscopy-assisted biopsy is less invasive and less expensive and has less morbidity than an exploratory rhinotomy, which may be necessary if rhinoscopy-assisted biopsy fails to yield a diagnosis.

Treatment and Prognosis

Intranasal neoplasms generally have a quick clinical course following diagnosis (Hahn et al, 1992 and 1994). With or without turbinectomy, localized irradiation of the nasal cavity and paranasal sinuses is the accepted therapeutic approach and will substantially improve the medial survival time of dogs and cats with intranasal neoplasms. Median survival rates vary in the dog, from 8 to 36 months with the use of teletherapy (i.e., fractionated external beam) or brachytherapy (i.e., short-term implantation) protocols (Théon et al, 1993). The median survival time of dogs receiving no therapy is usually less than 6 months and does not improve after surgery alone. Systemic chemotherapy using cisplatin or cis-diamminedichloroplatinum II (Platinol; Bristol-Myers-Squibb, Syracuse, NY) at a dosage of

60 mg/m^2 IV once every 4 weeks (Hahn et al, 1992) has resulted in the palliation of clinical signs (e.g., epistaxis, pain secondary to facial deformity) in some dogs for as long as 12 months.

Few reports regarding the treatment of intranasal neoplasms in cats exist; however, in one study by Théon and colleagues (1994), survival times after 48 Gy of telecobalt or orthovoltage irradiation ranged from 1 to 36 months. The 1- and 2-year overall survival rates were 44.3 and 16.6%, respectively. Histologic type (10 carcinomas, 6 sarcomas) and clinical stage did not have prognostic value in this limited study.

LARYNX AND TRACHEA

Pathology and Natural Behavior

Tumors arising from the laryngeal, perilaryngeal, and tracheal tissues are rarely encountered in the dog and cat (Table 3; Hahn, 1996). In both dogs and cats, males are affected more commonly than females. No breed predilection has been identified in dogs or cats. Benign osteocartilaginous tracheal tumors are common in young dogs with active osteochondral ossification. Benign laryngeal oncocytomas also occur in young dogs. The most common type of canine tracheal tumor appears to be osteochondroma, which routinely arises in dogs younger than 1 year of age and may be amenable to complete resection. Most other canine tracheal tumors are malignant epithelial or mesenchymal tumors. Malignant epithelial and lymphoid tracheal tumors have been reported, rarely, in the cat. Epithelial tumors and rhabdomyomas (oncocytomas) are the most

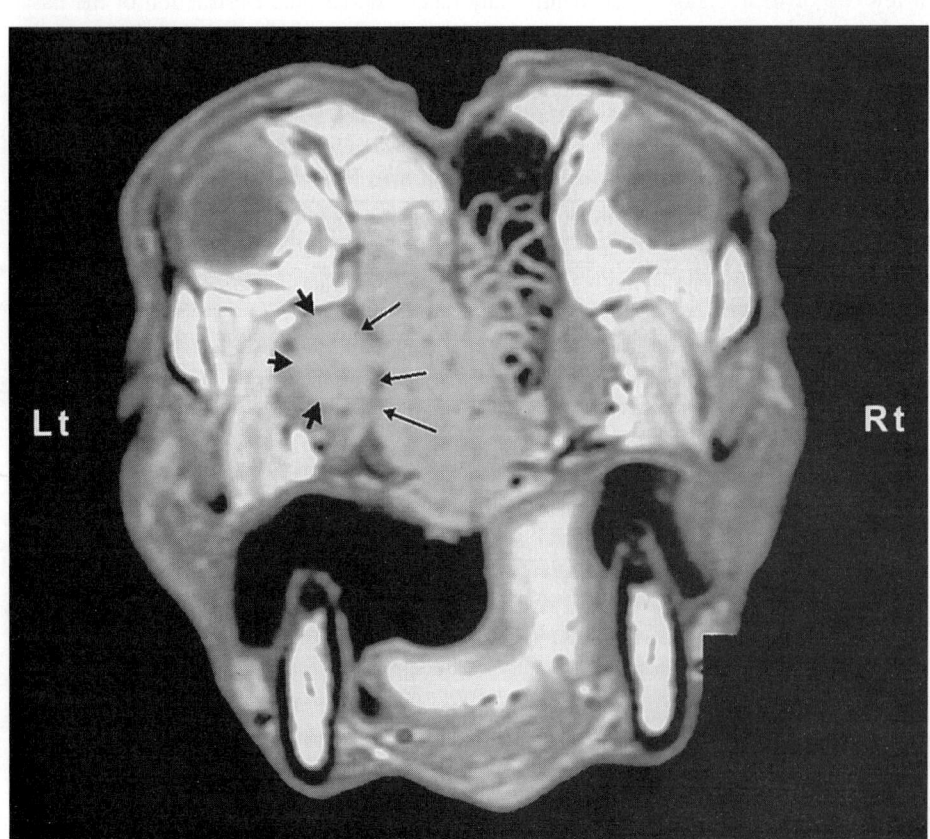

Figure 1. T1-weighted axial magnetic resonance image of the caudal nasal passage of a dog at the level of the orbit. A uniform medium signal intensity mass is present, filling the left nasal passage and extending through the cartilaginous nasal septum into the right nasal passage. The mass has eroded through the palatine bone *(small arrows)* into the orbit. A portion of the extranasal mass *(arrowheads)* effaces the medial pterygoid muscle. (Courtesy of Dr. William H. Adams, University of Tennessee.)

TABLE 3. **Malignant Tumors of the Canine and Feline Larynx and Trachea**

Histologic Types	Natural Behavior	Signs and Symptoms	Diagnostic Findings	Treatment Options

Tracheal Tumors
Lymphoma
Squamous cell
  carcinoma
Mast cell tumor
Chondrosarcoma
Adenocarcinoma
Osteosarcoma
Anaplastic carcinoma
Leiomyoma
Laryngeal Tumors
Lymphoma
Squamous cell
  carcinoma
Mast cell tumor
Osteosarcoma
Melanoma
Adenocarcinoma
Chondrosarcoma
Granular cell
  myoblastoma
Fibrosarcoma
Anaplastic carcinoma
Leiomyoma
	Extremely rare tumors
	Locally invasive
	No prognostic features
	  identified
	Metastasis is
	  uncommon, since
	  most animals are
	  euthanatized at
	  presentation
		Dyspnea
		Stridor
		Wheezing
		Coughing
		Dysphagia
		Change in or loss of
		  vocalization
		Palpable mass (rare)
		Prescapular
		  lymphadenopathy
			Abnormal lung sounds
			  secondary to aspiration
			  pneumonia
			Cough on tracheal palpation
			Neutrophilic leukocytosis
			Pale mucous membranes
			  secondary to anemia of
			  chronic disease
			Polycythemia secondary to
			  chronic hypoxia
			Soft-tissue radiographic lesion
			  narrowing the tracheal or
			  laryngeal lumen
			Reactive, inflammatory, or
			  neoplastic prescapular,
			  sternal, or hilar
			  lymphadenopathy
			Distortion of the arytenoid
			  cartilages
			Aspiration pneumonia
			Neoplastic cells may be
			  observed cytologically or
			  histologically from a fine-
			  needle aspirate or incisional
			  biopsy from the mass or
			  masses
				Surgery: localized,
				  relatively small tumors
				  are effectively treated
				  by removal of the
				  affected tracheal rings,
				  regional resection of the
				  trachea, or laryngectomy
				  followed by placement
				  of a permanent
				  tracheostomy
				Radiation Therapy: may
				  be indicated for
				  localized lymphoma of
				  the larynx or trachea
				Chemotherapy: indicated
				  for lymphoma of the
				  larynx or trachea due to
				  systemic disease

frequently reported types of malignant tumors of the canine larynx. In the cat, malignant epithelial tumors and lymphomas are more common.

Clinical signs for tracheal and laryngeal tumors are similar. Dyspnea, wheezing, coughing, and stridor are common complaints. Voice change may be noted in some animals affected by laryngeal tumors.

Diagnostic Approach

Radiographically, most animals have evidence of a distinct mass, although some show only a narrowing of the lumen at the tracheal laryngeal area. The veterinarian uses biopsy to make the definitive diagnosis after first performing laryngoscopy and tracheoscopy to assess the function and structure of the larynx and trachea.

Treatment and Prognosis

The prognosis for malignant tracheal tumors, although difficult to assess from historical information, is likely to be poor, especially if the tumor involves the adventitial surface of the trachea. Radiation therapy may be valuable as an addition to surgery or alone in the treatment of lymphoreticular tumors. Only tracheal osteochondromas appear to be amenable to complete resection.

LUNG

Pathology and Natural Behavior

Tumors originating within the lung parenchyma (primary lung neoplasia) are rare in dogs and cats (Table 4; Ogilvie et al, 1989a; Hahn et al, 1997b). The average age at presentation in dogs and cats with primary lung tumors

is 10 to 12 years. No breed or sex predisposition has been observed. The majority of primary lung tumors arise from the airways (e.g., bronchial adenocarcinomas). Fewer cases are classified as originating from the terminal airways or alveoli (bronchiolar-alveolar), and rarely are tumors identified as arising from the bronchial glands. Primary lung tumors of connective tissue origin are uncommon in the dog or cat (i.e., <2.5% of all primary lung tumors reported in the dog and cat). Primary nonepithelial tumors of the lung are uncommonly reported in other domestic species as well.

Weight loss, lethargy, dyspnea, and coughing are common owner complaints at the time of presentation to a veterinarian; however, such signs may not manifest until quite late in the course of the disease. Lameness has been reported to be a presenting sign in cats and may be associated with musculoskeletal metastases or with hypertrophic osteopathy.

Diagnostic Approach

Accumulation of thoracic fluid is an important factor contributing to dyspnea in many cases of primary lung neoplasia. If there is extensive accumulation of clear thoracic fluid, thoracocentesis may be necessary to allow radiographic pulmonary detail to be assessed accurately and to determine whether exfoliated neoplastic cells are present. Cytologic evaluation of effusive material can be helpful in differentiating primary lung neoplasia from other causes of clear fluids, such as cranial mediastinal lymphoma and cardiomyopathy (Hahn et al, 1997b).

Radiographic findings that justify a high index of suspicion for a primary lung tumor include the finding of a single circumscribed mass, marked lobar consolidation, or diffuse patterns containing severe peribronchial infiltration,

TABLE 4. Malignant Tumors of the Canine and Feline Lung

Histologic Types	Natural Behavior	Signs and Symptoms	Diagnostic Findings	Treatment Options
Canine Adenocarcinoma Squamous cell carcinoma *Feline* Adenocarcinoma *Infrequently Reported* Bronchoalveolar carcinoma Anaplastic carcinoma Malignant histiocytosis Lymphomatoid granulomatosis	Older animals (>10 yr of age) Metastases to regional lymph nodes and within the lung are common in the early course of the disease; musculoskeletal metastases are more frequent in the cat	May be asymptomatic (incidental finding) Chronic cough (productive or nonproductive) Anorexia Tachypnea Vomiting Diarrhea Dyspnea Weight loss Exercise intolerance Lethargy Lameness Wheeze Hemoptysis	Pale to ruddy-colored mucus membranes Abnormal breath sounds Neutrophilic leukocytosis Anemia of chronic disease Polycythemia secondary to chronic hypoxia Metabolic acidosis Reactive, inflammatory, or neoplastic sternal or hilar lymphadenopathy Solitary or multiple pulmonary nodules Pulmonary nodular metastatic lesions and/or pleural effusion Radiographic evidence of one or more bone metastases and/or hypertrophic osteopathy Neoplastic cells may be observed cytologically or histologically from a fine-needle aspirate or incisional biopsy from the mass or masses	*Surgery:* lung lobectomy is the treatment of choice in animals without enlarged regional lymph nodes or distant metastases; normal regional lymph nodes are associated with a longer survival than enlarged lymph nodes (345 vs. 60 days in the dog; 335 vs. 54 days in the cat)

a reticulonodular pattern, and alveolar filling. There is no correlation between the interpretation of thoracic radiographic images and the histologic type of tumor. The right caudal lung lobe and accessory lung lobe in dogs and the left caudal lung lobe in cats are the preferred sites of occurrence for primary lung tumors (Ogilvie et al, 1989a; Hahn et al, 1997b). The list of possibilities in the differential diagnosis of radiopaque lung lesions would include metastatic neoplasia, granuloma, cysts, infarcts, localized hemorrhage, localized pneumonia, torsion, and abscess.

If a mass is identified radiographically, cytologic evaluation of fine-needle aspiration material obtained from a pulmonary mass should be considered to resolve the diagnosis. Since the vast majority of primary lung tumors are epithelial in origin, carcinoma cells are likely to be observed. In one series of cats with primary lung tumors, a diagnosis was obtained in 80.0% of cases, prior to surgery or necropsy, when a fine-needle aspiration biopsy procedure was performed (Hahn et al, 1997b).

Treatment and Prognosis

Surgical resection (i.e., lung lobectomy) is the preferred treatment for lung tumors in dogs and cats (Ogilvie et al, 1989b; Hahn et al, 1998). Significant morbidity and mortality are associated with the surgical treatment of lung cancer; thus, it is important to identify and to exclude from primary surgical therapy the patients who will not benefit from attempts at resection. Dogs and cats *without* enlarged tracheobronchial lymph nodes observed radiographically or at the time of surgery have a significantly longer survival time compared with dogs and cats with enlarged lymph nodes (345 versus 60 days in the dog; 335 versus 54 days in the cat; Ogilvie et al, 1989b; Hahn et al, 1997c). The presence of pleural effusion or distant metastatic disease,

including dissemination to tracheobronchial lymph nodes, is a contraindication to pulmonary resection for cure in dogs and cats.

References and Suggested Reading

Hahn KA: Chondrosarcoma, larynx/trachea. In: Tilley LP, Smith FWK, eds: The 5 Minute Veterinary Consult. Baltimore: Williams & Wilkins, 1996.
  A diagnostic and therapeutic review of laryngeal and tracheal tumors in the dog and cat.
Hahn KA, Bravo L, Adams WH, et al: Naturally occurring tumors in dogs as comparative models for cancer therapy research. In Vivo 8:133, 1994.
  A review of common canine malignancies and current treatment methods.
Hahn KA, Knapp DW, Richardson RC, et al: The clinical response of nasal adenocarcinoma to cisplatin chemotherapy in 11 dogs. J Am Vet Med Assoc 200:355, 1992.
  A prospective study describing the palliative effects of cisplatin therapy.
Hahn KA, Adams WH, McGavin MD: Bilateral renal metastasis of nasal chondrosarcoma in a dog. Vet Pathol 34:352, 1997a.
  A case report and literature review regarding the late-onset metastatic behavior of nasal tumors in the dog.
Hahn KA, McEntee MF: Feline lung primary lung tumors: A retrospective review of 86 cases (1979–1994). J Am Vet Med Assoc 211:1257, 1997b.
  A clinical, radiographic, and pathologic review of cats with primary lung tumors.
Hahn KA, McEntee MF, Patterson MM, et al: Prognostic factors for tumor remission and survival in cats after surgery for primary lung tumor: 21 cases (1979–1994). Vet Surg 27:307, 1998.
  A review of the surgical approach and prognosis in cats with primary lung tumors.
O'Brien RT, Evans SM, Workman JA, et al: Radiographic findings in cats with intranasal neoplasia or chronic rhinitis: 29 cases (1982–1988). J Am Vet Med Assoc 208:385, 1996.
  A retrospective study in cats.
Ogilvie GK, Haschek WM, Withrow SJ, et al: Classification of primary lung tumors in dogs: 210 cases (1975–1985). J Am Vet Med Assoc 195:106, 1989a.

A clinical, radiographic, and pathologic review of dogs with primary lung tumors.

Ogilvie GK, Weigel RM, Haschek WM, et al: Prognostic factors for tumor remission and survival in dogs after surgery for primary lung tumor: 76 cases (1975–1985). J Am Vet Med Assoc 195:109, 1989b.
A review of the surgical approach and prognosis in dogs with primary lung tumors.

Patnaik AK: Canine sinonasal neoplasms: Clinicopathological study of 285 cases. J Am Anim Hosp Assoc 25:103, 1989.
A retrospective review regarding the natural behavior of nasal tumors in dogs.

Théon AP, Madewell BR, Harb MF, et al: Megavoltage irradiation of neoplasms of the nasal and paranasal cavities in 77 dogs. J Am Vet Med Assoc 202:1469, 1993.
The efficacy of radiotherapy alone or radiotherapy following partial tumor resection in dogs with carcinomas (58) or sarcomas (19) of the

nasal and paranasal cavity is reported along with a review of the current treatment literature.

Théon AP, Madewell BR, Shearn VI, et al: Prognostic factors associated with radiotherapy of squamous cell carcinoma of the nasal plane in cats. J Am Vet Med Assoc 206:991, 1995.
A prospective evaluation of prognostic factors affecting the radiation response of 99 cats with squamous cell carcinoma of the nasal plane.

Théon AP, Peaston AE, Madewell BR, et al: Irradiation of nonlympho-proliferative neoplasms of the nasal cavity and paranasal sinuses in 16 cats. J Am Vet Med Assoc 204:78, 1994.
The treatment, side effects, and prognosis of 16 cats with intranasal carcinomas and sarcomas is reported.

Withrow SJ, Straw RC: Resection of the nasal planum in nine cats and five dogs. J Am Anim Hosp Assoc 26:219, 1990.
A descriptive report regarding the surgical approach and prognosis of nasal planum tumors in dogs and cats.

Immunophenotyping in the Dog

PETER F. MOORE

VERENA K. AFFOLTER

WILLIAM VERNAU

Davis, California

INTRODUCTION

Immunophenotyping refers to the application of antibodies specific for differentiation antigens of lymphocytes and accessory immune cells in order to identify the lineages of these cells present in reactive (inflammatory) or neoplastic diseases involving the immune system. Immunophenotyping is an objective adjunct to conventional morphologic assessments. Immunophenotyping can be performed on snap-frozen tissue sections, formalin-fixed paraffin sections, unfixed cytologic smears, and unfixed blood smears, and also on fluids (e.g., blood) by flow cytometry. In a number of diseases, the application of immunophenotyping is a crucial element in either the attainment of an accurate diagnosis or the provision of an accurate prognosis; these diseases are discussed here. Immunophenotyping is not widely available outside of specialty laboratories within a few veterinary schools. However, we expect this to change as commercial pathology interests consolidate and explore the provision of enhanced services to clinicians on a nationwide basis. Therefore, this article provides sufficient background information to familiarize the reader with some basic concepts in this specialized area.

Cell Lineages in the Immune System

Lymphocytes fall within the confines of three distinct lineages: B (bursal), T (thymic), or NK (natural killer). T cells exist as two distinct families based on the T-cell receptor proteins expressed on their surfaces; these are $\alpha\beta$ T cells and $\gamma\delta$ T cells. The $\alpha\beta$ T cells contribute in a major way to the adaptive immune response to pathogens of all classes, cancer cells, and allografts. There are two

major subsets of $\alpha\beta$ T cells based on the expression of CD4 (helper-inducer subset) or CD8 (cytotoxic-suppressor subset) differentiation antigens. CD4 T cells respond to exogenously acquired peptide antigens presented by major histocompatibility complex class II antigens (MHC class II) on professional antigen-presenting cells, which are most often immune accessory cells of either dendritic antigen-presenting cell (APC) lineage, or macrophages. Activated B cells can also present peptide antigens to T cells via MHC class II molecules. CD8 T cells respond to endogenous peptide antigens presented by MHC class I antigens that are present on most cells of the body. Endogenous peptide antigens could, for instance, be derived from viral proteins present in virally infected cells or mutated host proteins in cancer cells. The $\gamma\delta$ T cells are a mysterious family of cells. They are infrequently encountered in blood and lymphoid organs. They occur in greater numbers at mucosal surfaces, where they have a tropism for epithelia. They are also found in relatively large numbers in the splenic red pulp in close association with the red pulp macrophages. The functions of $\gamma\delta$ T cells are still actively debated. They often lack expression of CD4 and CD8 accessory molecules and hence may not be MHC restricted in their interactions. Proposed functions include regulation of $\alpha\beta$ T-cell responses, regulation of repair processes in epithelia, and interaction with macrophages in innate immune responses to certain pathogens. B cells (and plasma cells) are the immunoglobulin (Ig)-producing cells of the immune system. The Ig classes produced by B cells in response to antigen are highly regulated, especially by functionally distinctive CD4 T-cell subsets termed T_H1 and T_H2 cells, which differ markedly in the cytokine profile produced following T-cell activation. Immunophenotyping can identify the presence of the different lymphocyte lineages, dendritic APCs and macrophages; it cannot be used to indicate the presence of neoplastic cells of any lineage, or to predict the functional program of a cell (e.g., T_H1 versus T_H2). Other assessments are needed in parallel with immunophenotyping to make these distinctions.

Most immunophenotyping is performed with monoclonal antibodies (Mab). Leukocyte antigen workshops have focused on clustering of Mab with similar patterns of reactivity in diverse cells and tissues. This systematic approach has led to the emergence of a common nomenclature for human antigens and their homologues in other species ("Cluster of Differentiation," or CD antigens). Workshops have been conducted in human, bovine, ovine, equine, porcine, and canine antigens, but not yet in feline. With few exceptions, Mab specific for leukocyte antigens label cells of diverse lineages. Hence, to identify specific cell types in lesions, it is often necessary to consider the results obtained with multiple Mabs.

Tissue Handling

Only a minority of Mabs specific for leukocyte antigens are reactive in formalin-fixed tissue, although important assessments can still be made with this material. More detailed work is possible in snap-frozen tissue. This procedure necessitates prospective planning. Fortunately, tissue handling requirements are very tolerant. The tissue must be harvested freshly, enveloped in a saline-soaked, surgical gauze pad, protected from desiccation in a sealed tube or zip-lock bag, and transported to the immunodiagnostic laboratory in an insulated foam box containing a frozen gel-ice pack. The transit time influences the results: less than 24 hours is best, although the authors have achieved diagnostic results in "tragic circumstances" after 4 days' transit time. Blood (at least 2 ml) for immunophenotyping of leukemia by flow cytometry should be provided in tubes containing acid citrate dextrose (ACD, yellow top—best) or EDTA (ethylenediaminetetraacetic acid; purple top—satisfactory).

Canine CD Antigens

The nomenclature and complexity of the biology of leukocyte antigens is intimidating. Currently, 166 CDs have been assigned in the human immune system, as well as many other defined molecules that have not yet been assigned to clusters of differentiation. Far fewer CDs have been assigned in the canine system (Cobbold and Metcalf, 1994), and of those CD molecules identified, not all are useful in immunodiagnostics. Table 1 consists of the CDs and related molecules of most importance in veterinary immunodiagnostics. Unless stated otherwise, the following molecules are detectable only in unfixed cells, which can include unfixed air-dried cytologic preparations, anticoagulated blood, and fresh tissue that has been carefully snap-frozen and sectioned.

CUTANEOUS ROUND CELL TUMORS

The most compelling need for immunophenotyping is the determination of the cell of origin in cutaneous "round" cell tumors of dogs. The overlapping morphologic appearances of histiocytoma, epitheliotropic cutaneous lymphoma (mycosis fungoides, or MF), nonepitheliotropic cutaneous lymphoma (NECL), histiocytic sarcoma, mast cell tumor, plasmacytoma, and transmissible venereal tumor (TVT) contribute to an alarmingly high frequency of mistaken diagnosis even by experienced veterinary pathologists. Immunophenotyping of routine formalin-fixed paraffin sections offers significant added value to the conventional assessment of these cases.

The skin is a complex, tertiary immunologic organ. The cellular components of skin-associated lymphoid tissue (SALT) include B and T lymphocytes, dendritic APCs, macrophages, mast cells, and NK cells. Skin-homing T cells are memory cells that predominantly express $\alpha\beta$ T-cell receptors in normal canine skin. Dendritic APCs or Langerhans' cells (LCs) of canine skin occur in two major locations: within the epidermis and within the dermis, especially adjacent to postcapillary venules. Langerhans' cells are best identified by their abundant expression of CD1 molecules, which together with MHC class I and MHC class II molecules are responsible for the presentation of peptides, lipids, and glycolipids to T cells. Epidermal and dermal LCs (dermal dendrocytes) are distinguishable by their Thy-1 (CD90) expression; epidermal LCs lack Thy-1 and dermal LCs express abundant Thy-1. Migration of LCs (as veiled cells) beyond the skin to the paracortex of lymph nodes occurs following contact with antigen. Langerhans' cells differentiate into potent APCs during this migration and change their surface phenotype accordingly. The interdigitating dendritic APCs of lymph node paracortex are derived in part from such migration.

Epitheliotropic Cutaneous Lymphoma

This disease is also known as mycosis fungoides (MF). Mycosis fungoides is a disease that affects old dogs (mean age 10 years). The topical cutaneous lesions of MF in dogs include erythema, scaling, pruritus, depigmentation, alopecia, infiltrative plaques, ulceration, crusting, and nodule or mass formation. Lesions occur throughout the skin, but a marked tendency to involve the mucocutaneous junctions (lips, eyelids, nasal planum, anorectal junction, or vulva) or oral cavity (gingiva, palate, or tongue) is apparent. In time, the mucocutaneous and cutaneous forms of MF merge with disease progression. Like human MF, canine MF can occur in three principal stages (patch, plaque, and tumor). Progression of canine MF to the tumor stage is more rapid in the dog. Spread beyond the skin to lymph nodes and other organs is also commonly observed in tumor-stage MF. Sézary syndrome, the leukemic variant of MF, has been observed in dogs, although it is extremely rare. The total clinical course of the authors' MF cases has ranged from 3 months to 4 years. The T-cell specific surface antigen CD3, which is part of the T-cell antigen receptor complex (TCR/CD3), is consistently expressed in MF. Neoplastic T cells express CD8 in about 80% of cases and in the remaining cases lack expression of CD4 or CD8 (Moore and Olivry, 1994). Also, canine MF is predominately a $\gamma\delta$ T-cell lymphoma (70% of cases). The pagetoid form of canine MF, which is initially totally confined to the epidermis, is exclusively a $\gamma\delta$ T-cell lymphoma. This

TABLE 1. Important CDs and Related Molecules in Veterinary Immunodiagnostics

CD1

Canine CD1a, CD1b, and CD1c molecules have been characterized. CD1 molecules are distantly related to MHC class I; they present peptide, lipid, and glycolipid antigens to T cells. CD1 molecules are expressed by cortical thymocytes, but not by mature T cells. CD1 molecules are the best markers of dendritic APCs, although subpopulations of B cells and monocytes express CD1c. The vast majority of histiocytic proliferative disorders in the dog involve dendritic APCs and are best defined by expression of CD1 molecules.

T-Cell Receptor/CD3

The TCR/CD3 complex is expressed only on the surface of mature T cells (and thymocytes). There are two types of TCR: $\alpha\beta$ and $\gamma\delta$. Each is associated with the CD3 complex (five polypeptides: CD3γ, CD3δ, CD3ϵ, CD3ζ, and CD3η), which is the signal transduction portion of the receptor complex in both TCR types. Mabs specific for the CD3ϵ component of the CD3 complex are available. CD3ϵ expression is limited largely to mature T cells, although activated human NK cells can express CD3ϵ in their cytoplasm. Evaluation of CD3 expression is possible in formalin-fixed tissue with the use of either an Mab (CD3-12, Serotec, Oxford, UK) or a rabbit polyclonal antibody (#A452, Dako, Carpinteria, CA) specific for a highly conserved peptide sequence from the cytoplasmic domain of CD3ϵ from diverse species (e.g., dog, cat, horse, human). Demonstration of CD3 expression is one of the most useful immunophenotypic analyses currently performed in veterinary immunodiagnostics and is used for the diagnosis of T-cell lymphoma. CD3 expression, with rare exceptions, confirms the presence of T cells in a lesion, although it does not distinguish $\alpha\beta$ and $\gamma\delta$ T cells. Mab specific for $\alpha\beta$ and $\gamma\delta$ T cells exist in the dog and can be used for this purpose.

B-Cell Antigen Receptor/CD79

The B-cell antigen receptor complex (BCR) consists of surface Ig (sIg) complexed with two invariant molecules that function as signal transduction molecules (CD79a, CD79b). CD79a (MB-1) is expressed throughout all stages of B-cell development and persists into the plasma cell stage (despite absent or diminished sIg on plasma cells). CD79a is a useful marker for establishing the diagnosis of B-cell lymphoma and leukemia, since it is present in the BCRs of all B cells regardless of the isotype of the sIg receptor. The background associated with Ig stains in tissues is also not an issue. CD79a is useful in the diagnosis of cutaneous plasmacytoma (about 80% have focal to diffuse expression). HM57 Mab (Dako) is specific for a cytoplasmic peptide sequence that is well conserved in diverse species (human and mouse) and is detectable in formalin-fixed tissue sections. HM57 also has good reactivity with B cells in dogs, cats, and horses, although CD79a sequence is unavailable in these species.

CD4

In the canine, CD4 is expressed by MHC class II restricted helper T cells. Canine neutrophils constitutively express CD4 and, in this respect, differ from neutrophils of all other species for which data are available. Macrophages and dendritic APCs can up-regulate CD4 in some instances.

CD8

CD8 is expressed by MHC class I restricted cytotoxic T cells. T cells usually express CD8$\alpha\beta$ heterodimers; although they can express CD8$\alpha\alpha$ homodimers. A subset of NK cells may also express CD8$\alpha\alpha$ homodimers.

CD11/CD18

The β_2 integrins (CD11/CD18) are the major leukocyte adhesion molecule family. The absence of β_2 integrins due to mutations in CD18 results in leukocyte adhesion deficiency syndrome (LAD-I) described in humans, Irish setter dogs, and Holstein cattle. Afflicted individuals are unable to mount effective inflammatory reactions and die of sepsis within a few months after birth. Most leukocytes express one or more members of this family. CD18 is the β_2 subunit, which pairs with one of four α subunits to form a heterodimer. Hence, staining for CD18 indicates the presence of the β_2 subunit but does not indicate which of the four integrin molecules is present. The four α subunits are CD11a (all leukocytes), CD11b (granulocytes, monocytes, some macrophages), CD11c (granulocytes, monocytes, dendritic antigen-presenting cells), and α_D (macrophages and T cells in splenic red pulp, and large granular lymphocytes). Macrophages and granulocytes express 10-fold more CD18 than do lymphocytes. Canine CD18 and α_D are detectable with Mab in formalin-fixed tissue sections. In the absence of CD3 or CD79a expression, abundant CD18 expression by large mononuclear cells is evidence of macrophage or dendritic APC differentiation. Frozen section or unfixed cytologic smears stained for CD1 would be necessary for confirmation.

CD21

CD21 is a C3dg receptor (CR2) that complexes with components of the B-cell antigen receptor complex (sIg, CD79a, CD79b), CD19 and CD35 (CR1). CD21 is expressed on mature B cells and follicular dendritic cells of the germinal center. Detection of CD21 is useful in the diagnosis of B-cell lymphoma and B-cell leukemia.

CD45

CD45 is the leukocyte common antigen family and all leukocytes express one or more CD45 isoforms. Alternative mRNA splicing generates eight possible isoforms from three alternatively spliced exons. CD45RA is one of these isoforms. Canine CD45RA is detectable with Mab in formalin-fixed tissue sections. CD45RA is expressed by all B cells and by 100% of B-cell lymphomas involving lymph nodes. Peripheral T-cell lymphomas usually occur in memory T cells in older individuals. Memory cells switch from expressing CD45RA to CD45RO. Memory cells preferentially traffic to cutaneous and mucosal sites, and T-cell lymphomas (CD3ϵ+) in these sites usually do not express CD45RA.

---

finding contrasts markedly with human MF, in which $\alpha\beta$ T cells predominate, and CD4 is expressed in about 90% of cases. The high prevalence of $\gamma\delta$ T cells in canine MF, coupled with the low frequency of $\gamma\delta$ T cells in normal blood and lymph nodes, makes flow cytometry for the detection of T-cell lineages in blood a valuable adjunct to morphologic assessment in predicting clinical progression of MF lesions in dogs.

Nonepitheliotropic Cutaneous Lymphoma

Canine NECL is usually a disease of old dogs (mean age 10 years). Often, NECLs are large cell lymphomas that occur as solitary or multiple nodules, and plaques. Involvement of the oral cavity also occurs. Many lesions are infiltrated by eosinophils, and this infiltration often leads to confusion of these lesions with undifferentiated mast cell tumor. Reactive dendritic APC and T cells are often prevalent within regions of NECL lesions; misdiagnosis of reactive (cutaneous histiocytosis) or neoplastic histiocytic proliferative disorders (histiocytic sarcoma) is common in these instances. Comprehensive immunophenotyping of frozen sections is necessary to resolve these complex cases, although in most instances paraffin section immunophenotyping is sufficient to indicate the presence of T-cell neoplasia. NECL is largely a T-cell lymphoma (85% of cases are CD3+; n = 24). B-cell lymphomas have been described infrequently. CD8 was expressed only in 44% of cases assessed (n = 16), and CD4 was expressed in only one case. The majority of cases were CD4− and CD8− (50%). Preliminary data indicate that TCR expression is less predictable in NECL than in MF. The existence of NK cell lymphomas (CD3−) in canine skin is likely. Proof of the existence of such lymphomas awaits the development of canine-specific NK cell markers. Progression of NECL is usually more rapid than that of MF; lymph node and systemic metastases are observed. Euthanasia is performed in many instances because of poor response to chemotherapy, or poor prognosis.

Histiocytic Diseases

Immunophenotypic analysis has shown that histiocytic proliferative diseases in dogs are derived largely from proliferation of dendritic APCs, rather than macrophages, based on the expression of CD1 molecules by the infiltrating cells. In paraffin sections, abundant CD18 expression coupled with the lack of expression of lymphoid markers (CD3 or CD79a) is good evidence of the presence of histiocytes (dendritic APCs or macrophages). Histiocytic diseases, which include cutaneous histiocytoma, cutaneous histiocytosis, systemic histiocytosis, malignant histiocytosis, and histiocytic sarcoma, are covered in more detail elsewhere in *CVT* (see p. 588). Cutaneous and systemic histiocytoses are reactive Langerhans' cell histiocytoses (LCHs) of dermal LCs (CD1+, CD11c/CD18+, MHC class II+, Thy-1+, CD4+) arising in the context of disordered immune regulation; they respond to immunosuppressive drugs administered episodically. In severe cases, continuous immunosuppression is necessary. Corticosteroids are effective in less than 30% of cases; the remainder require cyclosporin A or Leflunomide (Hoechst Marion Roussell, Wiesbaden, Germany). Cutaneous histiocytomas display an epidermal LC phenotype (CD1+, CD11c/CD18+, MHC class II+) and lack expression of Thy-1 and CD4. The pronounced epidermotropism often seen in histiocytomas can lead to confusion with more serious diseases, such as MF. Histiocytomas up-regulate expression of adhesion molecules that normally occur on activated normal LCs during migration from the skin to draining lymph nodes after contact with antigen. Migration of histiocytomas to lymph nodes with lymph node obliteration occurs rarely, and spontaneous regression without treatment also may occur in lymph nodes. Unfortunately, some dogs with migratory histiocytoma were euthanatized. Hence, the true incidence of spontaneous regression is unknown. Widespread metastasis of histiocytoma beyond lymph nodes has been documented in three recent cases. The syndrome of multiple histiocytomas is more common in Shar Pei dogs. The clinical progression of these lesions, which can be quite serious, is unpredictable. Delayed spontaneous regression (up to 9 months) has been observed. Malignant histiocytosis and histiocytic sarcoma are aggressive, malignant tumors of dendritic APC (CD1+, CD11c/CD18+, MHC class II+) that occur in spleen, lymph nodes, bone marrow, and lung. Involvement of skin and subcutis occurs rarely. Solitary lesions have been successfully surgically excised. Multicentric or disseminated histiocytic sarcoma (i.e., malignant histiocytosis) usually has a hopeless prognosis and responds poorly to chemotherapy.

Cutaneous Plasmacytoma

Plamacytoma is a common tumor in aged dogs and occurs preferentially on digits, lips, mouth, and ear canals. Marked cellular pleomorphism and the presence of multinucleated giant cells are disturbing cytologic features; however, the course is largely benign. The analysis of archival formalin-fixed specimens has revealed expression of antigens characteristic of B cells and plasma cells. CD79a, a component of the B-cell antigen receptor complex, and CD45RA are expressed in 80% and 90% of cases, respectively. These assessments are useful in distinguishing plasmacytoma from more serious diseases, such as malignant melanoma and histiocytic sarcoma.

LYMPHOMAS

Unlike the situation with cutaneous lymphoma, the diagnosis of lymphoma is usually not problematic in lymph node biopsy specimens. Even though the majority of canine lymphomas involve proliferation of B cells, about one third of cases are of T-cell origin. Hence, the incidence of T-cell lymphoma is higher in dogs than in people (20%). Immunophenotypic analysis does have value in the assessment of lymphoma involving lymph nodes. A study in which a multivariate analysis of prognostic factors in canine lymphoma was conducted, concluded that immunophenotype was correlated with prognosis. Specifically, T-cell lymphomas carried a far worse prognosis. The interval between attainment of complete remission with chemotherapy and disease relapse was significantly shorter, and overall survival was reduced (Teske et al, 1994).

LEUKEMIAS

Immunophenotypic analysis of leukemia is best performed by analysis of blood by flow cytometry. Staining is performed with Mab labeled with fluorescent dyes. Flow cytometry for leukemia diagnosis is currently available at two sites in the United States (University of California, Davis, and North Carolina State University). The most common form of leukemia in the authors' case series is chronic lymphocytic leukemia (CLL), which also has the best prognosis. Acute leukemias are less common and have an extremely poor prognosis. In this instance, there appears to be some benefit in distinguishing lymphoid and myeloid leukemias, although such differentiation is not always possible with the available tools (cytology, immunophenotyping, and enzyme cytochemistry). Acute myeloid leukemias are rapidly fatal despite chemotherapy. Some degree of remission is achievable in acute lymphocytic leukemia, although it is often of short duration.

Chronic Lymphocytic Leukemia

In humans, CLL is a common, often indolent leukemia affecting older adults, particularly males (male-to-female ratio is greater than 2:1). More than 95% of human CLL cases involve proliferation of B lymphocytes. Canine CLL occurs in older dogs (mean age 9.5 years; range 1.5 to 15 years; n = 50+ cases). Blood lymphocyte counts ranged from 15,000/μl to 1,200,000/μl. Surprisingly, 70% of CLL cases involved proliferation of T lymphocytes (CD3+), and 57% of CLL cases had large, granular lymphocyte (LGL) morphology; cases of LGL CLL were almost exclusively proliferations of T cells that expressed CD8 and $\alpha_D\beta_2$ (CD11d), and more frequently expressed TCR$\alpha\beta$ (65%) than TCR$\gamma\delta$ (35%). The non-LGL T-cell CLL cases (13% of CLL cases) involved proliferation of $\alpha\beta$ T cells in which no consistent pattern of CD4 or CD8 expression was found. B-cell CLL constituted 30% of canine CLL cases based on the expression of CD21 or CD79a.

Canine CLL is most often an indolent, slowly progressive disease. Several cases were discovered during routine complete blood count (CBC) analysis for other purposes. Other dogs presented with lethargy and reduced appetite. Splenomegaly and mild anemia were common findings. Thrombocytopenia was variably present, and absolute neutropenia was rare. Involvement of bone marrow in T-cell CLL with proliferation of LGL occurs relatively late in clinical disease. The neoplastic expansion in these instances appears to originate in the spleen, and the majority of cases exhibit expression of $\alpha_D\beta_2$, a leukocyte integrin (CD11d) that is expressed in splenic red pulp. The clinical course of CLL is highly variable, owing in part to the occult nature of the disease in its early stages and the potential for considerable delay in the initial diagnosis. The diagnosis of CLL can be difficult, particularly in early disease with mild lymphocytosis. Immunophenotyping can assist in the diagnosis, especially if aberrant phenotypes are present, although no clear influence of CLL phenotype on prognosis is apparent. Molecular genetic analysis, which documents clonal expansion in chronic lymphocytosis, is the most objective diagnostic test. This methodology is under development, but it is not yet available for use in dogs. Nevertheless, the prognosis in canine CLL is relatively favorable, even without therapy in some instances. Treatment should be reserved for individuals that are clinically ill, have significant anemia and/or thrombocytopenia, or have infiltrative disease leading to organomegaly. The mainstays of therapy are prednisone and chlorambucil (Leukeran). Many clinically ill dogs in the authors' series achieved complete remission with this therapy and prolonged survival is possible (longer than 3 years).

References and Suggested Reading

Cobbold SP, Metcalf S: Monoclonal antibodies that define canine homologues of human CD antigens: Summary of the First International Canine Leukocyte Antigen Workshop (CLAW). Tissue Antigens 43:137, 1994.
  Presents a good source of information on clustering analyses of canine leukocyte antigens.
Moore PF, Olivry T: Cutaneous lymphomas in companion animals. Clin Dermatol 12:499, 1994.
  Presents a detailed review of the clinical, pathologic, and immunophenotypic features of cutaneous lymphomas in dogs and cats.
Moore PF, Schrenzel MD, Affolter VK, et al: Canine cutaneous histiocytoma is an epidermotropic Langerhans cell histiocytosis which expresses CD1 and specific β_2 integrin molecules. Am J Pathol 148:1699, 1996.
  The first paper documenting the dendritic APC (Langerhans' cell) lineage of canine histiocytic diseases; it contains background information on the comparative biology and proliferative diseases of dendritic APCs.
Teske E, van Heerde P, Rutteman GR, et al: Prognostic factors for treatment of malignant lymphoma in dogs. J Am Vet Med Assoc 205:1722, 1994.
  A well-designed study that correlates clinical, morphologic, and immunophenotypic findings with prognosis in canine lymphoma.

Immunosuppressive Agents

CLARE R. GREGORY
Davis, California

Over the last half of the 20th century, immunosuppressive agents have evolved from nonspecific, myelotoxic drugs to agents that target specific enzymes that catalyze reactions required for normal immune function. Much of our current understanding of T-cell function was provided by research performed to understand the mechanism of action of cyclosporine. As each element of antigen recognition, T-cell activation, cytokine synthesis, and T cell–dependent cytolysis are unraveled, investigators are devising specific, less toxic, and more efficacious agents for interrupting the immune response. This process is termed *rational drug development,* and it replaces the selection of potential immunosuppressive agents based on their ability to lyse or inhibit the activation of T and B cells in vitro. Although specific immunosuppression with the use of naturally induced and genetically engineered antibodies, soluble receptor fragments, and other biologic methods are available for the treatment of human diseases, most are not applicable or available for use in the treatment of animal diseases. For the foreseeable future in clinical veterinary medicine, immunosuppression will continue to be accomplished with the use of chemotherapies. As the new immunosuppressive agents become more readily available and clinicians become familiar with their indications, effects, and side effects, immunosuppression should become more specific, effective, and safe.

MYELOTOXIC AGENTS

Cyclophosphamide

The major effect of cyclophosphamide results from alkylation of deoxyribonucleic acid (DNA) during the S phase of the cell cycle. The alterations in DNA structure can be lethal to the cell or may produce miscoding errors that inhibit cell replication or DNA transcription. Cyclophosphamide produces T- and B-cell lymphopenia and suppresses both T-cell activity and antibody production. Cyclophosphamide is administered to dogs for the treatment of corticosteroid-resistant autoimmune hemolytic anemia, corticosteroid-resistant thrombocytopenia, rheumatoid arthritis, and polymyositis (in conjunction with corticosteroids). Cyclophosphamide is administered to cats for the treatment of autoimmune hemolytic anemia and rheumatoid arthritis. Myelosuppression, gastroenteritis, alopecia, and hemorrhagic cystitis are the major complications associated with cyclophosphamide therapy.

Azathioprine

Azathioprine is a purine analogue that is metabolized to ribonucleotide monophosphates. Poor conversion to diphosphates and triphosphates leads to an intracellular accumulation of monophosphates that produces a feedback inhibition of the enzymes required for the biosynthesis of purine nucleotides. The triphosphate analogues that do form become incorporated into DNA and result in ribonucleic acid (RNA) miscoding and faulty transcription. Azathioprine has a greater effect on humoral than on cell-mediated immunity. For the treatment of immune-mediated diseases in dogs, azathioprine is generally administered in conjunction with a corticosteroid and/or cyclophosphamide. Azathioprine has been used for the treatment of autoimmune thrombocytopenia, autoimmune hemolytic anemia (see p. 509), autoimmune skin diseases (see p. 536), chronic hepatitis, myasthenia gravis, immune-mediated glomerulopathy, chronic atrophic gastritis, systemic lupus erythematosus (see next article), and inflammatory bowel disease (see CVT XII, p. 723). Although very myelotoxic in cats, azathioprine has been used for the treatment of feline autoimmune skin diseases. Azathioprine and prednisolone, when administered at maximally tolerated levels, do not effectively suppress the rejection response against canine major histocompatibility complex (MHC)–nonmatched renal allografts. However, when administered on an every-other-day schedule (1 to 5 mg/kg) with cyclosporine, azathioprine has been used to successfully maintain canine MHC-matched renal allografts. The primary complication encountered with the administration of azathioprine is bone marrow suppression that can result in leukopenia, anemia, and thrombocytopenia. Acute pancreatitis and hepatotoxicity may also occur.

Methotrexate

Methotrexate competitively inhibits folic acid reductase, which is necessary for the reduction of dihydrofolate to tetrahydrofolate and affects the production of both purines and pyrimidines. The effects of methotrexate occur during the S phase of the cell cycle. Methotrexate is used primarily as an antineoplastic agent in dogs and cats for lymphomas, carcinomas, and sarcomas. In human medicine, methotrexate is administered for the treatment of rheumatoid arthritis and psoriasis. Gastrointestinal toxicity is the most common complication encountered with the administration of methotrexate.

GLUCOCORTICOIDS

Prednisolone

Glucocorticoids, and in particular prednisolone, have both direct and indirect effects on the immune response. Glucocorticoids stabilize the cell membrane of endothelial cells and inhibit the production of local chemotactic factors, thus decreasing infiltration of neutrophils, monocytes, and lymphocytes. In allogeneic tissues, the secretion of destructive proteolytic enzymes such as collagenase, elastase, and plasminogen activator is inhibited. Glucocorticoids also inhibit the release of arachidonic acid from membrane phospholipids. This inhibition prevents the synthesis of prostaglandins, thromboxanes, and leukotrienes, which are major mediators of inflammation. Glucocorticoids redistribute monocytes and lymphocytes from the peripheral circulation to the lymphatics and bone marrow. This redistribution affects primarily T cells. T-cell activation and cytotoxicity are also reduced. Glucocorticoids suppress cytokine activity and alter macrophage function. Prednisolone and prednisone are considered to be the first-line immunosuppressive agents for the treatment of immune-mediated and chronic inflammatory diseases in dogs and cats because of their general efficacy and low cost. Autoimmune hemolytic anemia and thrombocytopenia, autoimmune and allergic skin diseases, myasthenia gravis, allergic pneumonitis and bronchitis, immune-mediated arthritis, and systemic lupus erythematosus are just some of the indications for corticosteroid therapy in animals. Prednisolone has been used in both dogs and cats to slow allograft rejection; when administered as a single agent, however, prednisolone is not capable of preventing allograft rejection.

Although inexpensive and often effective, the chronic use of corticosteroids in both human beings and animals can result in severe complications, usually manifested as signs of hyperadrenocorticism. This complication, in addition to the fact that corticosteroids suppress multiple elements of the immune response, has led to the search for *steroid-sparing* immunosuppressive protocols.

CALCINEURIN INHIBITORS

Cyclosporine

Cyclosporine is bound in the cytosol of lymphocytes by cyclophilins (cyclosporine-binding proteins). The cyclosporine-cyclophilin complexes associate with calcium-dependent calcineurin–calmodulin complexes to impede calcium-dependent signal transduction. Transcription factors that promote cytokine gene activation are either direct or indirect substrates of calcineurin's serine-threonine phosphatase activity. This enzymatic activity is reduced by association of the cyclosporine-cyclophilin bimolecular complex with calcineurin. Via this mechanism of action, cyclosporine inhibits early T-cell activation (G_0 phase of the cell cycle) and prevents synthesis of several cytokines, in particular, interleukin-2 (IL-2). Without stimulation by IL-2, further T-cell proliferation is inhibited, and T-cell cytotoxic activity is reduced (see *CVT XII,* p. 564). Cyclosporine may also exert an immunosuppressive effect as it stimulates mammalian cells to secrete transforming growth factor-beta (TGF-β) protein. TGF-β is a potent inhibitor of IL-2–stimulated T-cell proliferation and generation of antigen-specific cytotoxic lymphocytes. Cyclosporine is not cytotoxic or myelotoxic and is specific for lymphocytes. This specificity spares other rapidly dividing cells and allows nonspecific host defense mechanisms to continue to function.

Cyclosporine is gaining wide use in veterinary medicine. Combination cyclosporine and prednisolone immunosuppression has maintained normal function of MHC-nonmatched feline renal allografts for more than 6 years. Cyclosporine in combination with azathioprine, prednisolone, and antithymocyte serum has been used to maintain MHC-nonmatched canine renal allografts. Bone marrow transplantation has been successfully performed in cats with the use of cyclosporine immunosuppression. Cyclosporine has also been used to control corticosteroid-resistant autoimmune hemolytic anemia and thrombocytopenia in dogs. Cyclosporine is available in an ophthalmic preparation (Optimmune, Schering-Plough, Kenilworth, NJ) for the control of keratoconjunctivitis sicca in dogs (see *CVT XII,* pp. 1231 to 1239). Cyclosporine (10 to 20 mg/kg per day) was found to significantly reduce the size and depth of perianal fistulas in dogs (Mathews and Sukhiam, 1996). Most dogs did not require further therapy, either medical or surgical, after 6 to 8 weeks of therapy.

Cyclosporine is available in two oral formulations: Sandimmune and Neoral (Sandoz, East Hanover, NJ). Both contain cyclosporine in a concentration of 100 mg/ml, but the two solutions are not biologically equivalent. Sandimmune consists of an olive oil base, and adsorption of cyclosporine requires emulsification of the agent by bile salts and digestion by pancreatic enzymes. The absorption percentage can be as little as 4%, and there is a tremendous variation in dose-trough whole blood levels among individuals of the same species. Neoral is a microemulsion preconcentrate of cyclosporine that becomes a microemulsion when in contact with gastrointestinal fluids. The microemulsion is directly absorbed through the gut epithelium, resulting in more sustained and consistent blood levels of the drug. When Neoral replaces Sandimmune as treatment, most feline renal transplant recipients have had a reduction in the dose level necessary to maintain the same trough whole blood levels. In addition, feline renal transplant patients have been administered Sandimmune at a dose of 10 to 15 mg/kg over 24 hours to initiate immunosuppression at the time of surgery. To achieve the same trough whole blood levels of cyclosporine (approximately 500 ng/ml), Neoral is administered at a dose of 1 to 4 mg/kg over 24 hours. Neoral appears be a more effective immunosuppressant than Sandimmune owing to a more complete ab-

sorption, which results in a more sustained and predictable blood level. In addition, it is more economical to use.

To achieve immunosuppression with cyclosporine in dogs, the author recommends attaining a 12-hour whole blood trough level (measured just before the next oral dose) of at least 500 ng/ml. With Sandimmune, achieving this level requires an oral dose of 10 to 25 mg/kg over 24 hours divided into two doses. Neoral can be initiated at 5 to 10 mg/kg over 24 hours divided into two doses. With either formulation, gastrointestinal inflammation will increase the dose requirements, and blood levels of the agent must be measured starting 24 to 48 hours after initiation of therapy to ensure that adequate blood levels are achieved. Blood levels of cyclosporine should be measured at periodic intervals during the time of therapy. To reduce the cost of the cyclosporine necessary to treat medium-sized to large dogs, the author administers ketoconazole at a dose of 10 mg/kg over 24 hours in addition to the cyclosporine. Ketoconazole interferes with the hepatic metabolism of cyclosporine, and it will reduce the dose requirement of cyclosporine by as much as 60%. The author has not encountered any toxic effects with the coadministration of these agents, but it has been reported that the chronic administration of ketoconazole to dogs may result in cataract formation.

To achieve immunosuppression with cyclosporine in cats, the author recommends attaining a 12-hour whole blood trough level of 250 to 500 ng/ml. With Sandimmune, obtaining this level will require an oral dose of 4 to 15 mg/kg over 24 hours divided into two doses. Neoral can be initiated at 1 to 5 mg/kg over 24 hours divided into two doses. Again, it is imperative to measure blood levels 24 to 48 hours after initiation of therapy to ensure that adequate blood levels have been achieved. Blood levels must also be measured periodically during the course of therapy.

Whole blood or plasma levels of cyclosporine can be determined by high-pressure liquid chromatography, fluorescence polarization immunoassay, and specific monoclonal antibody radioimmunoassay. Most medical centers that serve human patients perform cyclosporine assays and will serve veterinary needs. The clinical pathology laboratory at the Veterinary Medical Teaching Hospital, University of California, Davis, is preparing to assay whole blood cyclosporine levels for veterinary patients using the monoclonal antibody radioimmunoassay method.

Unlike the situation in people, cyclosporine is not nephrotoxic or hepatotoxic in dogs and cats unless extremely high blood levels are maintained (>3,000 ng/ml). Levels higher than 1,000 ng/ml can cause inappetence in cats. If levels of 1,000 ng/ml are maintained for several weeks or months, opportunistic bacterial and fungal infections can occur. As in people, cyclosporine can promote the development of neoplasia, particularly lymphomas, in cats and dogs. The administration of high levels (1 to 2 mg/kg over 24 hours) of prednisolone with cyclosporine increases the likelihood of tumor formation. As in humans, cyclosporine has resulted in a marked increase in hair growth in several of the author's feline renal transplant recipients.

Cyclosporine has a distinctly unpleasant taste to both people and animals. It is necessary to administer the drug in gelatin capsules. Sandoz supplies capsules containing 25 mg or 100 mg of cyclosporine. For most cats, these capsules are too large. The author places the oral solution in No. 0 or No. 1 gelatin capsules. Some cats need only a very small dose of cyclosporine: 1 to 3 mg/dose. Measuring and administering this small amount (0.01 to 0.03 ml) of drug is very difficult and imprecise. Sandimmune can be diluted and stored in olive oil; the author usually makes a 1-to-10 dilution. Neoral can be diluted in any oral solution, but it must be administered immediately after it is diluted because it is a microemulsion concentrate. The author dilutes Neoral in tap water.

Cyclosporine is also available in an intravenous solution (Sandimmune IV) that must be diluted in 0.9% sodium chloride or 5% dextrose in water. The author administers a dose of 6 mg/kg over 4 hours in the calculated maintenance fluid requirement. Intravenous cyclosporine is administered to control organ rejection episodes or an acute hemolytic crisis, or during periods when a patient cannot tolerate oral medications.

Tacrolimus

Although tacrolimus, or FK-506 (Prograf, Fujisawa USA, Dearfield, IL), is structurally different from cyclosporine, it shares a similar mechanism of action. Tacrolimus binds in the cytosol of lymphocytes with an immunophilin, FK-binding protein (FKBP). As with the cyclosporine-cyclophilin complex, the tacrolimus-FKBP complex binds to calcineurin and inhibits its phosphatase activity. This inhibition directly and indirectly inhibits de novo expression of nuclear regulatory proteins and T-cell activation genes. The transcription of cytokines (IL-2, -3, -4, and -5, interferon-gamma [IFN-γ], TNF-α, and granulocyte-macrophage colony-stimulating factor [GM-CSF]) responsible for lymphocyte activation is suppressed, as is the expression of IL-2 and IL-7 receptors. Tacrolimus, in vitro, is 50 to 100 times more potent an inhibitor of lymphocyte activation than is cyclosporine. Tacrolimus also inhibits B-cell proliferation and production of antibody by unknown mechanisms. Tacrolimus decreases the hepatic injury associated with ischemia-reperfusion injury, perhaps by inhibiting production of TNF and IL-6 by hepatocytes, and stimulates hepatic regeneration following liver injury. Experimentally, allograft recipients from many species have been successfully treated with tacrolimus at doses several times less than those for cyclosporine. Tacrolimus has prolonged the survival of renal, liver, pancreas, heart, lung, and vascularized limb grafts in rodents, dogs, and nonhuman primates. In human organ recipients, tacrolimus is superior to cyclosporine for the reversal of ongoing rejection. Also, the steroid-sparing effect of tacrolimus seems to be greater than that of Sandimmune, but it may not be superior to that of Neoral. The toxicity of tacrolimus is similar to that of cyclosporine in people.

Little, if any, use of tacrolimus has been applied to veterinary patients, but based on its effectiveness in experimental animal trials it could be very effective in controlling a wide range of immune-mediated conditions. Tacrolimus may be particularly effective in controlling immune-mediated anemia, thrombocytopenia, and arthritis because of its inhibition of antibody synthesis, in addition to inhibition of T-cell proliferation. Despite the potential benefits of tacrolimus for treating diseases in dogs, a major concern is

the possible toxicity of the drug. A dose of 0.16 mg/kg per day IM or 1.0 mg/kg per day PO has been reported to be effective in prolonging renal allograft survival in Beagle dogs. The side effects included anorexia, vasculitis, and intestinal intussusception. In a study using mongrel dogs, the same doses were not effective in prolonging renal allograft survival, and most of the dogs developed severe vasculitis leading to fatal myocardial infarction, hepatic failure, and intussusception. Combination therapy with cyclosporine appears to have an additive effect, with less toxicity. Blood levels of tacrolimus are assayed at human medical centers with the use of monoclonal immunoassays. The effective serum trough level of tacrolimus in dogs is approximately 0.1 to 0.4 ng/ml—about 100 times lower than that of cyclosporine. Trough levels of 2.0 ng/ml or greater can result in death.

INHIBITORS OF CYTOKINE AND GROWTH FACTOR ACTION

Sirolimus

Sirolimus, or rapamycin (Rapamune, Wyeth-Ayerst, Philadelphia, PA), is a macrocyclic antibiotic with a structure similar to tacrolimus that also binds in the cell cytosol to FKBP. However, sirolimus and tacrolimus affect different and distinct sites in the signal transduction pathway. The immunosuppressive activity of sirolimus appears to be a consequence, in part, of the sirolimus-FKBP complex's blocking the activation of the 70-kD S6 protein kinases that are involved in cell proliferation. The kinase activity of additional cell cycle regulatory proteins, cyclin-dependent kinase-2 and -4, is also inhibited by sirolimus. Sirolimus blocks IL-2 and other growth factor–mediated signal transduction and the calcium-independent CD28-B7 co-stimulatory pathway. While cyclosporine and tacrolimus block T-cell cell cycle progression at the G_0 to G_1 stage, sirolimus prevents cells from progressing from G_1 to the S phase. Sirolimus blocks T-cell activation by IL-2, -4, and -6 and stimulation of B-cell proliferation by lipopolysaccharide (LPS). Sirolimus directly inhibits the B-cell immunoglobulin synthesis caused by interleukins. Sirolimus has been shown to prevent acute, accelerated, and chronic rejection of skin, heart, renal, islet, and small bowel allografts in rodent, rabbit, dog, pig, and nonhuman primate graft recipients. It has also been shown to be efficacious in models of autoimmunity: insulin-dependent diabetes and systemic lupus erythematosus. Sirolimus' antagonism of cytokine and growth factor action is not limited to cells of the immune system. Sirolimus inhibits the proliferation of fibroblasts, endothelial cells, hepatocytes, and smooth muscle cells induced by growth factors such as platelet-derived growth factor (PDGF) and fibroblast growth factor (FGF). Sirolimus has been very effective in preventing intimal smooth muscle proliferation (arteriosclerosis) following mechanical or immune-mediated arterial injury. Sirolimus is being evaluated in phase I and phase II clinical trials of human organ transplantation. Supplementation of a cyclosporine-based protocol was associated with a reduction in acute renal allograft rejection.

Mycophenolate Mofetil

Mycophenolate mofetil, also known as RS-61443 or mycophenolic acid (Cellcept, Roche Laboratories, Palo Alto, CA), is a prodrug hydrolyzed by liver esterases to mycophenolic acid. Mycophenolic acid is cytostatic for lymphocytes, owing to its inhibition of inosine monophosphate dehydrogenase (IMPDH), an enzyme necessary for de novo purine biosynthesis. Mycophenolic acid is a relatively selective inhibitor of T- and B-cell proliferation during the S phase of the cell cycle via its ability to prevent guanosine and deoxyguanosine biosynthesis. Mycophenolic acid has been shown to reduce allograft rejection in multiple animal models, being most effective when combined with cyclosporine, tacrolimus, and/or sirolimus. Mycophenolic acid was developed, in part, as a nonmyelotoxic replacement for azathioprine in human allograft patients. Early clinical trials in human renal allograft recipients showed a decrease in biopsy-proven acute rejection episodes in patients receiving mycophenolic acid in place of azathioprine. At therapeutic doses, mycophenolic acid can be toxic to animals. The primary dose-limiting effects are anemia and weight loss in rats; leukopenia, diarrhea, and anorexia in monkeys; and gastrointestinal hemorrhage, anorexia, and diarrhea in dogs. To reduce the toxic effects, the dose can be lowered or mycophenolic acid can be given in combination with other immunosuppressive agents. Mycophenolic acid can also inhibit growth factor–induced smooth muscle and fibroblast proliferation. Sirolimus and mycophenolic acid, in combination, are extremely effective in preventing arterial intimal smooth muscle proliferation following mechanical injury.

Leflunomide and Leflunomide Analogues

Leflunomide (Hoechst AG, Wiesbaden, Germany) is a synthetic organic isoxazole that the intestinal mucosa metabolizes to the active form, A77 1726. Leflunomide mediates at least part of its antiproliferative activity during the S phase of the cell cycle by inhibiting the de novo pathway of pyrimidine biosynthesis. The target of A77 1726 in this pathway is the enzyme dihydroorotate dehydrogenase. At higher concentrations, leflunomide is also an inhibitor of tyrosine kinases associated with growth factor receptors. In addition to T and B lymphocytes, leflunomide also has an antiproliferative effect on smooth muscle cells and fibroblasts, which also is due to inhibition of the pyrimidine biosynthetic pathway in these cells. Leflunomide is currently being evaluated in phase III trials for rheumatoid arthritis in Europe and the United States. It has been shown to be an effective disease-modifying antirheumatic drug free from the side effects commonly associated with currently approved immunosuppressants. In addition to its efficacy in people and animal models with autoimmune diseases, leflunomide has been found to control acute, ongoing, and chronic allograft rejection of the kidney, skin, heart, vessels, and lung in small and large animal models. The author has used leflunomide to successfully treat steroid-resistant autoimmune hemolytic anemia and systemic histiocytosis in dogs. In combination with cyclosporine,

leflunomide has completely prevented the rejection of canine MHC-nonmatched renal allografts in both experimental and clinical studies. At doses used in people, leflunomide causes gastrointestinal toxicity in dogs as a result of the accumulation of a metabolite, trimethylfluoroanaline (TMFA). Fortunately, the canine lymphocyte is far more sensitive than the human lymphocyte to the effects of the active agent, A77 1726, and much lower oral doses are equally effective in achieving immunosuppression. The author currently uses a dose of 4 mg/kg PO over 24 hours and adjusts the dose as needed to obtain a 24-hour serum trough level of 20 μg/ml. Early studies in the cat suggest that TMFA does not present the toxicity problem encountered in dogs; however, cats metabolize the drug much more slowly and require approximately half the oral dose to achieve effective blood levels. Leflunomide should soon be commercially available in Europe for the treatment of rheumatoid arthritis in people. Leflunomide analogues are being developed for transplantation applications.

COMBINATION THERAPY

Most of the currently used and the soon to be available immunosuppressant agents have differing mechanisms of action and are effective at different stages of the cell cycle. Experimentally and clinically, combining agents often results in more effective immunosuppression with fewer drug-induced side effects. In human transplant patients, cyclosporine and tacrolimus are considered to be the first-line immunosuppressive agents. To increase their effectiveness and decrease toxicity, azathioprine, prednisolone, or mycophenolic acid, or all three, are added to antirejection protocols. Sirolimus will soon be commercially available, and it shows excellent effectiveness in animal models when combined with either cyclosporine or tacrolimus. Few of the new nonmyelotoxic agents have been used in veterinary patients, but many published experimental animal trials investigating autoimmune disease and organ transplantation provide indications and insight into their use. Based on the author's experimental and clinical experience in canine MHC-nonmatched organ transplantation, cyclosporine and leflunomide are an extremely powerful and safe immunosuppressive combination.

References and Suggested Reading

Mathews KA, Sukhiam HR: OL27-400 (cyclosporine) treatment of canine perianal fistulas: A prospective, randomized, double-blind, controlled study. Vet Surg 25:433, 1996.

Morris RE: Mechanisms of action of new immunosuppressive drugs. Kidney Int 49:S-26, 1996.
   Describes the new immunosuppressive agents, the background of their development, experimental studies, and current use.

Plumb DC: Veterinary Drug Handbook, 2nd ed. Ames: Iowa State University Press, 1995.
   Gives the indications for use and dose levels for cyclophosphamide, azathioprine, methotrexate, and prednisolone.

Suthanthiran M, Morris RE, Strom TB: Immunosuppressants: Cellular and molecular mechanisms of action. Am J Kidney Dis 28:159, 1996.
   Describes how new immunosuppressive agents work at the molecular level to promote immunosuppression.

CVT Update: Diagnosis and Treatment of Systemic Lupus Erythematosus

STEVEN L. MARKS
Baton Rouge, Louisiana

CAROLYN J. HENRY
Columbia, Missouri

Systemic lupus erythematosus (SLE) is a multisystemic, immune-mediated disease reported infrequently in the dog and rarely in the cat. It is estimated that 0.03% of the canine population may be affected, while 0.06% of feline hospital visits were for SLE (Scott et al, 1995). First identified in the dog (Lewis et al, 1965), this disease has been studied extensively as an animal model for SLE in people. Multiple organ systems can be involved during the course of this disease; thus, SLE can mimic a variety of diseases, and clinical recognition may be difficult. SLE exhibits no consistent breed predisposition, although some breeds, including the Shetland sheepdog, Old English sheepdog, Afghan hound, collie, Beagle, German shepherd, Irish setter, and Poodle, are overrepresented (Halliwell and Gorman, 1989). In the cat, the Persian, Siamese, and Himalayan may be predisposed (Pedersen and Barlough, 1991). SLE exhibits no sex predilection in companion animals, whereas human SLE occurs more often in women. There is much debate on the pathogenesis and diagnostic criteria for SLE in the dog and cat.

ETIOLOGY AND PATHOGENESIS

Genetic, environmental, and transmissible factors have been implicated in the etiology of SLE, but a definitive cause remains unknown (Grindem and Johnson, 1982). The underlying pathology of SLE is related to the presence of high levels of circulating antigen-antibody complexes (type III hypersensitivity) or antibodies directed toward self-antigen on cells such as erythrocytes, thrombocytes, and leukocytes (type II hypersensitivity; Halliwell and Gorman, 1989). To a lesser degree, type IV hypersensitivity may be involved when cell-mediated activity is initiated against self-antigen. The inflammatory lesions caused by circulating antigen-antibody complexes are not specific for organ systems but can lead to disorders such as vasculitis, glomerulonephritis, polyarthritis, and dermatitis. Soluble immune complexes diffuse into vascular endothelium and initiate complement-mediated perivascular inflammation. Inflammatory mediators cause chemotaxis and increase vascular permeability, which may promote acute necrotizing vasculitis, fibrinoid deposition, and sclerosis. Immune complex deposition to the kidneys causes a membranous glomerulonephritis. Polyarthritis results when immune complexes diffuse into the synovium. In companion animals, as in people, abnormal immune activation and loss of self-tolerance appear to be the underlying events involved in development of SLE. Immune activation may be triggered by endogenous factors (genetic, hormonal, and metabolic) or exogenous factors (drugs, ultraviolet light, foods, and infectious agents such as viruses, bacteria, and parasites). The loss of self-tolerance and the expansion of an autoreactive B-cell population result in autoantibody-producing cells as well as memory B cells, which may be responsible for periodic disease flares.

CLINICAL SIGNS

Clinical signs with SLE can be quite variable, based on the number of different organ systems that can be involved. Classically, clinical signs are intermittent, and often animals are presented with a chronic history. However, some animals may present with apparent acute clinical signs.

The most common presenting complaint in the dog is gait abnormality, seen most often as a shifting lameness. This finding may be reflective of polyarthritis or polymyositis. Joints may be distended or painful on palpation, and myalgia with or without muscle wasting may also be present. Other abnormalities that may be found on physical examination include skin lesions with no specific distribution. The areas affected can include the limbs, body, head, ears, mucocutaneous junctions, and face. These lesions can be erythematous, ulcerative, crusting, oozing, or alopecic. Mucocutaneous junctions and oral cavity mucosa may develop ulceration. Erosive lesions may be evident in thin-skinned areas, such as the axillae, ventral abdomen, and periocular skin. In the dog, the clinical signs can be divided into major and minor signs (Table 1). Nonspecific complaints include lethargy, anorexia, and weakness. In the

TABLE 1. Diagnosis of Systemic Lupus Erythematosus*

Major Signs	Minor Signs	Serology
Skin lesions	Fever of unknown origin	Antinuclear
Polyarthritis	Central nervous system	antibody (ANA)
Hemolytic anemia	signs, seizures	Lupus
Glomerulonephritis	Oral ulceration	erythematosus
Polymyositis	Lymphadenopathy	(LE) cell
Leukopenia	Pericarditis	preparation
Thrombocytopenia	Pleuritis	

*Definite SLE: Two major signs with positive serology; one major sign; two minor signs with positive serology. *Probable SLE*: One major sign with positive serology; two major signs with negative serology.

From Gorman NT, Werner LL: Immune-mediated diseases of the dog and cat: I. Basic concepts on the systemic immune-mediated diseases. Br Vet J 142:395, 1986, with permission.

514

cat, the clinical signs include hematologic abnormalities, lymphadenopathy, polyarthritis, myopathy, oral ulceration, renal disease, fever, and neurologic signs (Scott et al, 1995; Pedersen and Barlough, 1991).

DIAGNOSIS

No single diagnostic test can reliably be used to diagnose SLE. The diagnosis of SLE is best based on clinical assessment and laboratory data. Serologic testing may be valuable in diagnosing SLE. The antinuclear antibody (ANA) test, which identifies serum antibodies to nuclear material, is considered by some to be the most sensitive test for SLE in the dog. This test has been less reliable in the cat, and false-negative and false-positive results can occur in either species. Diseases with similar clinical presentations, including pemphigus erythematosus, discoid lupus, generalized demodicosis, rheumatoid arthritis, feline leukemia virus, feline infectious peritonitis, immune-mediated hemolytic anemia, bacterial endocarditis, and immune-mediated thrombocytopenia, may also cause increases in ANA titers. The lupus erythematosus (LE) cell preparation is highly specific for SLE, but it is time-consuming and less sensitive than the ANA test for SLE. The LE cell test identifies opsonized nuclear material within neutrophils and macrophages.

No specific findings on the complete blood count (CBC) are pathognomonic for SLE. If a regenerative anemia is present and blood loss is excluded, a direct Coombs' test should be considered and evaluation of slides for spherocytosis should be performed. A positive Coombs' test identifies complement or antibody on red blood cells, consistent with the immunopathology of SLE, but such finding is not specific for the disease. Positive Coombs' test results may also be obtained with conditions such as ehrlichiosis, immune-mediated hemolytic anemia unrelated to SLE, and generalized demodicosis, all of which may have clinical presentations suggestive of SLE. If a nonregenerative anemia, leukopenia, or thrombocytopenia is present, bone marrow evaluation and rickettsial titers may be beneficial in excluding primary bone marrow disease or diseases such as ehrlichiosis. Other nonspecific abnormalities may include leukocytosis with neutrophilia and monocytosis. The serum chemistry profile may aid in identifying glomerulonephritis or myositis. Azotemia and hypoalbuminemia may indicate renal disease and should be further investigated with urinalysis. Proteinuria, if present, should be evaluated with a urine protein-to-creatinine ratio, as significant protein loss supports a diagnosis of glomerulonephritis. Immune complex deposition is demonstrable by direct immunofluorescence and histopathologic examination of renal biopsy specimens. Myositis is suggested by increases in aspartate aminotransferase and creatinine phosphokinase activity. Further evidence of myositis may be obtained by histologic examination of muscle biopsy in cases with supporting clinical signs and laboratory values. Hyperglobulinemia may be further characterized by serum electrophoresis. A polyclonal gammopathy is compatible with a diagnosis of SLE. Arthrocentesis should be performed if a joint effusion is detected, or suspected, or if a nonerosive arthritis is documented radiographically. Synovial fluid analysis results consistent with SLE include a sterile neutrophilic fluid

with decreased viscosity. Culture and sensitivity of synovial fluid should be performed if degenerate neutrophils or bacteria are found. Biopsy of the synovium may also help confirm a diagnosis of SLE. Skin biopsies should be performed if lesions are present and immune complex deposition can be demonstrated with immunofluorescence.

The diagnosis of SLE is based on the finding of multisystemic signs not explainable by other disease processes and on supporting laboratory data. This area is where most debate occurs among clinicians. Some authors suggest extrapolation from the criteria of the American Rheumatism Association. Others suggest that these criteria do not fit SLE in the dog and cat. Proposed diagnostic criteria for SLE in the dog are found in Table 1.

TREATMENT

Therapy for SLE is nonspecific and is directed toward reducing tissue inflammation. Concurrently, it is also important to manage any organ failure that is present. Generally, the initial drug of choice is prednisone or prednisolone (1 to 3 mg/kg PO b.i.d.) until clinical improvement is seen. If no improvement is seen after 7 to 10 days, additional immunosuppressive therapy can be instituted. In dogs azathioprine (1 mg/kg PO every 24 hours) can be used, and in cats chlorambucil (0.25 to 0.5 mg/kg PO every 24 to 48 hours) can be employed. Cyclophosphamide has also been used as an immunosuppressive agent in the dog. Once clinical remission occurs, drug dosages can be tapered to the lowest dosage where no clinical signs recur. Aspirin has been used to control pain and inflammation in both dogs and cats. Other nonsteroidal anti-inflammatory agents can also be considered for analgesia, as can opioids (see p. 57). Levamisole (3 to 7 mg/kg PO every other day for 4 months) has been used in some dogs with SLE, as has chrysotherapy. A report suggests remissions of as long as 9 years when levamisole was used in combination with corticosteroids and as a single agent (Fournel et al, 1992). Other drugs such as dapsone, colchicine, omega 3/6 fatty acids, and cyclosporine that have been used in people have not been evaluated in dogs and cats (Scott et al, 1995). Plasmapheresis has also been utilized to treat dogs with SLE. Pentoxifylline (Trental, Hoechst Marion Roussel) has been used to alter microvascular blood flow (Hargis and Mundell, 1992) and has anecdotally found some success in the treatment of vasculitis in the dog. It can be used at a dosage of 10 mg/kg PO t.i.d.

PROGNOSIS

Generally, the prognosis for this disease is guarded, but such prognosis must be based on clinical signs and the condition of the animal. Approximately 40% of dogs diagnosed with SLE are dead within 1 year, according to one source (Scott et al, 1995). However, a clinical study has been more optimistic, with more than 50% of dogs having long-term survival (Fournel et al, 1992). The most common causes of death are bronchopneumonia, septicemia, and euthanasia. The finding of organ failure and infection carries a poor prognosis. Dogs that respond to glucocorticoid therapy alone, seem to have the best prognosis. The prognosis for the cat is unclear because of the infrequent diagnosis, but 9 of 11 cats in one report responded to therapy (Pedersen and Barlough, 1991).

References and Suggested Reading

Fournel C, Chabannel L, Caux C: Canine systemic lupus erythematosus I: A study of 75 cases. Lupus 1:133, 1992.
Report of 75 cases of canine SLE suggesting that ANA titers correlated with severity of disease and that levamisole has produced long-term remissions.

Grindem CB, Johnson KH: Systemic lupus erythematosus: Literature review and report of 42 new canine cases. J Am Anim Hosp Assoc 19:489, 1983.
Excellent literature review and discussion of pathophysiology, clinical signs, and diagnosis of canine SLE.

Halliwell EW, Gorman NT: Veterinary Clinical Immunology. Philadelphia: WB Saunders, 1989, p 324.
Useful immunology textbook with excellent review of immune-mediated disease.

Hargis AM, Mundell AC: Familial canine dermatomyositis. Compend Contin Educ Pract Vet 14:855, 1992.
Review article of the pathogenesis, diagnosis, and treatment of canine dermatomyositis.

Jones DRE: Canine systemic lupus erythematosus: New insights and their implication. J Comp Pathol 108:215, 1993.
Review of the comparative immunopathology of SLE in dogs and people.

Lewis RM, Picut CA: Veterinary Clinical Immunology: From Classroom To Clinics. Philadelphia: Lea & Febiger, 1989, p 167.
Very helpful immunology textbook covering both the clinical and the immunologic aspects of canine SLE.

Lewis RM, Schwartz RS, Henry WB Jr: Canine SLE. Blood 25:143, 1965.
Original description of canine SLE.

Pedersen NC, Barlough JE: Systemic lupus erythematosus in the cat. Feline Pract 19:5, 1991.
Helpful review of feline SLE.

Scott DW, Miller WH, Griffin CE: Small Animal Dermatology. Philadelphia: WB Saunders, 1995, p 578.
Excellent dermatology textbook with concise review of immunologic skin diseases.

Hereditary and Acquired Immunodeficiency Diseases

PETER J. FELSBURG

Philadelphia, Pennsylvania

Immunodeficiency diseases are a diverse group of disorders caused by abnormalities in one or more components of the immune system that result in increased susceptibility to infections. Primary, or hereditary, immunodeficiencies are diseases in which the animal is born with a genetic defect involving the immune system, and any clinical disease observed in these animals is a direct consequence of the hereditary defect. Animals with secondary, or acquired, immunodeficiencies are born with intact immune systems, but their immune systems become transiently or permanently impaired as the result of some underlying disease process.

Animals with immunodeficiencies generally experience chronic or recurrent infections. The following conditions are suggestive of an underlying immunologic defect: (1) increased frequency or severity of infection, (2) chronic or prolonged course of infection, (3) incomplete clearing between episodes of infection, (4) incomplete or no response to treatment, and (5) infections with usually nonpathogenic organisms. The type of infection involved and the clinical signs are influenced by the severity of the defect and the particular component of the immune system affected. Defects in the B-cell (humoral immune) system usually predispose an animal to increased susceptibility to bacterial infections. Animals with T-cell (cell-mediated immune) deficiencies usually have an increased susceptibility to intracellular microorganisms such as fungi, protozoa, and viruses. It should be stressed that since a humoral (antibody) immune response is highly dependent on the T-cell system, certain T-cell deficiencies may also present as humoral immunodeficiencies even though the B-cell system itself may be normal. Disorders of the phagocytic and complement components of the immune system are usually associated with superficial or systemic infections with pyogenic organisms.

PRIMARY (HEREDITARY) IMMUNODEFICIENCIES

Although more than 40 primary immunodeficiency diseases have been documented in people, the study of these diseases in dogs and cats is still in its infancy. The primary immunodeficiencies discussed here are the hereditary disorders of the specific (lymphocytic) and nonspecific (phagocytic and complement) components of the immune system, which have been well documented in dogs and cats, and are associated with increased susceptibility to infections. The primary immunodeficiencies are hereditary; thus, the majority of affected patients are puppies and kittens or young adults. Although many of the following diseases have been described primarily in certain breeds, they most probably occur in all breeds. For example, IgA deficiency was originally described in Beagles and Shar peis, but it has since been observed in many breeds as well as in mixed-breed dogs.

X-Linked Severe Combined Immunodeficiency

Severe combined immunodeficiency (SCID) is the most severe of all the primary immunodeficiencies. The term

SCID describes a heterogeneous group of disorders that have the common feature of severely deficient humoral and cell-mediated immune responses resulting in an increased susceptibility to a wide spectrum of microbial agents, with untreated patients rarely surviving past infancy.

An X-linked form of SCID (XSCID) has been documented in the dog. Problems with infections in the neonatal period are rare because of the presence of maternal antibody. Recurrent or chronic infections begin to appear between 4 to 8 weeks of age, with clinical signs that include pyoderma, otitis, diarrhea, and respiratory infections. These infections, usually of bacterial origin, are nonresponsive to antibiotic therapy. A universal finding in affected dogs is a failure to thrive (stunted growth). On physical examination, there is an absence of any palpable lymph nodes, and tonsils are not noticeable. Affected puppies usually die before 3 to 4 months of age, either from overwhelming bacterial infections or viral infections. Several affected puppies vaccinated with a modified-live distemper vaccine died 2 to 3 weeks later of distemper induced by the vaccine.

XSCID is caused by mutations in the common gamma chain (γc) gene that encodes for an essential component of the receptors for interleukin-2 (IL-2), IL-4, IL-7, IL-9, and IL-15. The shared usage of the γc by receptors of cytokines essential for normal B- and T-cell development and function explains the profound immunologic abnormalities and clinical severity of this disease.

In XSCID, only males are affected, whereas females may be carriers of the disease. In the dog, approximately half of the males in a litter from a carrier female will be affected, and half of the females will be potential carriers. It is important to emphasize that carrier females show no clinical or immunologic abnormalities. When a male is diagnosed and the mutation determined, a polymerase chain reaction–based DNA test can be developed to detect female carriers of the disease within that family or line of dogs.

Lymphocyte counts are usually low, averaging 1,000/mm³, but they can be within the normal range. Affected dogs have normal or elevated proportions of peripheral B cells, and low to nearly normal proportions of nonfunctional peripheral T cells. Laboratory findings include normal serum concentrations of IgM, but low to absent serum IgG and IgA. IgG may be normal during the first few weeks as the result of maternal antibody. The patient's T cells fail to proliferate following mitogenic or antigenic stimulation in the lymphocyte transformation (blastogenesis) test. The typical postmortem findings are a very small thymus characterized by thymic dysplasia and a lack of lymph nodes, tonsils, and Peyer's patches.

The only successful means of treating XSCID is bone marrow transplantation. Although normal immune function can be successfully reconstituted in XSCID dogs following bone marrow transplantation. This treatment is currently not practical in veterinary medicine.

Selective IgA Deficiency

Selective IgA deficiency (IgAD) represents a heterogeneous group of diseases consisting of three major types: severe IgAD, as defined by undetectable IgA measured by radial immunodiffusion; partial IgAD, as defined by detectable IgA but less than two standard deviations of the mean value for age-matched normal dogs; and transient IgAD, as defined by undetectable or low IgA, with subsequent development of normal IgA concentrations. All three forms of IgAD have been documented in the dog. There does not appear to be a difference in the clinical manifestations between dogs with severe IgAD and dogs with partial IgAD. It has been suggested that IgAD alone in human patients with severe IgAD is sufficient to cause clinical disease, whereas in partial IgAD patients, a concomitant IgG subclass deficiency predisposes to disease. IgG subclasses have not been examined in canine IgAD.

The most common clinical problems in dogs with IgAD include recurrent infections, usually upper respiratory infections due to *Bordetella bronchiseptica* and canine parainfluenza virus, otitis, staphylococcal dermatitis, diarrhea, and atopic dermatitis. The infections associated with IgAD are usually not severe or life-threatening. Several dogs have experienced convulsive episodes. Older dogs may develop autoantibodies and, possibly, autoimmune disease. There appears to be a high incidence of IgAD in Shar peis, which may be a reflection of their predisposition to upper respiratory infections and atopic disease.

The only abnormal laboratory finding is an absence or a markedly low concentration of serum IgA compared with values in age-matched normal dogs. It is possible that some young dogs diagnosed as having IgAD may have a transient IgAD and will outgrow their tendency for recurrent infections as they become adults.

Treatment of IgAD is mainly symptomatic. Immune globulin, if available, is contraindicated, since IgAD patients have been reported to make anti-IgA antibodies, which may lead to an anaphylactic reaction when they are treated with immune globulin.

Immunodeficiency Syndrome in Shar Pei Dogs

This disorder is a recently described late-onset immunodeficiency that appears to be similar to common variable immunodeficiency in humans. The mean age at clinical onset in affected dogs is 3 years. The disease is characterized by intermittent fever and recurrent infection of the skin, respiratory system, and gastrointestinal system, including ulcerative colitis. In several of the reported cases, death occurred as the result of intestinal adenocarcinoma and lymphoma. Although the immunologic defect is unknown, both B- and T-cell abnormalities have been observed in affected dogs.

The laboratory findings include low serum concentrations of one or more of the serum immunoglobulins (IgG, IgM, and IgA). In about half the patients, the in vitro proliferative response of the lymphocytes to mitogenic stimulation is depressed.

Transient Hypogammaglobulinemia of Infancy

Transient hypogammaglobulinemia of infancy is a self-limited immunoglobulin deficiency resulting from an abnormally delayed onset of IgG and IgA production by the neonate or young puppy. Affected puppies are clinically normal during the time they possess maternal antibody. However, when the maternal antibody disappears, they have an increased susceptibility to infection, primarily chronic or recurrent bacterial infections of the respiratory tract. Spontaneous recovery occurs between 5 and 7 months of age when the animal's own humoral immune system begins to produce sufficient immunoglobulin. It may be necessary to treat the animal symptomatically during the period of hypogammaglobulinemia.

The only significant laboratory finding is markedly reduced concentrations of serum immunoglobulins after the disappearance of maternal antibody, around 2 months of age, that persists until their own humoral immune system becomes operational, usually between 5 and 7 months of age. It is essential to monitor the immunoglobulin concentrations of puppies diagnosed as immunoglobulin deficient to determine whether the defect is permanent or transient.

Hypotrichosis With Thymic Aplasia (Nude Kittens)

An autosomal recessive disease has been described in Birman cats that appears to be the homologue of the nude mouse. The disease is characterized by the lack of hair growth and thymic development, and a severe immunodeficiency. Kittens are born with no hair and fail to thrive, which results in death within a few days. Necropsy findings include the lack of a thymus and severely aplastic lymph nodes, if they are detected at all.

Canine Cyclic Hematopoiesis

Neutropenia is the most common disorder of the polymorphonuclear phagocytic system in people and results in increased susceptibility to severe bacterial infections and a poor response to antibiotic treatment. Cyclic hematopoiesis is characterized by a periodic production and maturation defect of hematopoietic cells in the bone marrow and can either be acquired or hereditary.

A hereditary form of cyclic hematopoiesis has been documented in collies that has an autosomal recessive mode of inheritance. Affected collies have hypopigmentation, and their coat appears silvery gray or light tan, thus the term *gray collie syndrome*. Unlike cyclic neutropenia in people, the disease in the dog is characterized by cyclic fluctuations of not only peripheral blood neutrophils but also all cellular blood elements, including platelets. The blood cell elements cycle at 10- to 14-day intervals, lasting for 2 to 4 days. The clinical signs are cyclic and are present only during the periods of severe neutropenia ($<1,000/\mu l$). Affected dogs experience severe, recurrent bacterial infections primarily involving the respiratory and gastrointestinal tracts. Epistaxis or profuse hemorrhage may be present, owing to the associated thrombocytopenia. Affected dogs rarely survive past 3 years of age.

The reason for the recurrent infections was originally thought to be the lack of sufficient numbers of functional neutrophils during the periods of neutropenia. It is now evident that metabolic abnormalities, including a myeloperoxidase deficiency and a defect in iodination, result in the impaired ability of neutrophils from affected animals to kill bacteria. No other immunologic abnormalities have been documented in this disorder.

The laboratory diagnosis is based on the demonstration of a cyclic neutropenia as well as an abnormal bactericidal assay. Treatment of this condition is primarily supportive antibiotic therapy to control infections. Although lithium carbonate has been shown to be effective in controlling the cycling of the neutrophils and platelets, it is only effective at high and toxic doses. Once treatment is stopped, the cycling of cells and clinical signs reappear.

Leukocyte Adherence Deficiency

For phagocytes to perform their major function of ingesting and killing microorganisms, they must be able to adhere to and migrate across the vascular endothelium, and bind to, phagocytose, and kill the microorganism. In addition, the effector function of cytotoxic T cells and natural killer (NK) cells requires adherence to the target cell. Many of these functions are regulated by glycoproteins of the integrin family that are found on the surface of leukocytes, including CD11a, CD11b, and CD11c and their common beta chain component, CD18. Leukocyte adherence deficiency (LAD) is caused by a deficiency of the common beta subunit, which results in the dysfunction of all three integrins and is characterized by defective phagocytic function and suppressed cell-mediated immunity. In people, LAD can have an X-linked as well as an autosomal recessive mode of inheritance.

An autosomal recessive form of LAD has been reported in Irish setters in the United States and Europe. Clinical signs begin at a few weeks of age and consist primarily of recurrent pyogenic infections, including pyoderma, pododermatitis, gingivitis, pneumonia, thrombophlebitis, and osteomyelitis. Poor wound healing is a common feature. Infection sites usually exhibit a localized cellulitis with minimal pus formation.

The laboratory findings include a persistent marked leukocytosis, with most of the cells being mature, hypersegmented neutrophils. Fluorescence-activated cell sorter (FACS) analysis of leukocytes with monoclonal antibodies shows a lack of CD11a to CD11b and/or CD18. Neutrophil function test results are uniformly abnormal. Lymphocytes from affected dogs also have a markedly suppressed blastogenic response following mitogenic stimulation.

Chédiak-Higashi Syndrome

Chédiak-Higashi syndrome is an autosomal recessive genetic disease of humans and other species, including blue-smoke Persian cats. It is characterized by the presence of abnormally large, eosinophilic granules in neutrophils, basophils, and eosinophils. Enlarged melanin granules are observed in the skin and hair shafts of affected animals.

Affected cats show an increased susceptibility to infection, particularly to neonatal septicemia and viral respiratory infections. Sudden death due to an increased bleeding tendency may occur. The tendency for increased bleeding is thought to result from abnormal platelet function and can result in major bleeding problems following even minor surgery and hematoma formation following venipuncture. The abnormal melanin granules cause abnormally light coat colors in affected blue-smoke Persian cats. Affected cats may also have light-colored irises, reduced fundic pigmentation, photophobia, and an increased incidence of congenital cataracts.

Neutrophils from affected cats exhibit impaired chemotaxis and a defect in intracellular killing of bacteria. Treatment is symptomatic.

C3 Deficiency

C3 is a component of the complement system important in the opsonization of bacteria. A C3 deficiency, with an autosomal recessive mode of inheritance, has been reported in the dog. Dogs that are homozygous for the trait have no detectable C3, whereas dogs that are heterozygous have C3 concentrations that are approximately 50% of normal. Clinical signs are observed only in dogs that are homozygous for the C3 deficiency and are related to an increased susceptibility to bacterial infections, including septicemia primarily involving gram-negative organisms and clostridia. Signs of renal failure and possibly amyloidosis may be present. The major immunologic abnormality is the absence of serum C3.

Miscellaneous Neutrophil Deficiencies

A neutrophil oxidative metabolic defect has been independently described by two groups of researchers in a total of 64 related Weimaraner dogs. The clinical signs included recurrent episodes of fever, vomiting, diarrhea, pneumonia, pyoderma, lymphadenopathy, and osteomyelitis. Neurologic signs consisting of disorientation, ataxia, head pressing, and seizures were observed in some of the dogs. The only abnormal immunologic finding appears to be the inability of the neutrophils to kill bacteria because of their metabolic defect.

A defect in the bacterial killing capacity of neutrophils has also been reported in eight related Doberman pinschers that had a history of recurrent respiratory infections since birth. These dogs had normal neutrophil counts, and laboratory tests of the B- and T-cell systems were normal.

SECONDARY (ACQUIRED) IMMUNODEFICIENCIES

Acquired immunodeficiencies can be classified into two major etiologic types: (1) those in which the immunosuppression is a biologic complication of another disease process, such as failure to receive colostrum, infections, metabolic diseases, and neoplastic diseases; and (2) those in which the immunodeficiency is due to complications of therapy for other diseases, such as chemotherapy or immunosuppressive therapy. Secondary immunodeficiencies can be seen in any age group because they are acquired. For example, failure to receive colostrum is a problem in the neonate, viral infections are problems in postweaning and young adult animals, and neoplasia is a disease of middle-aged to old animals.

Failure to Receive Colostrum

The immune system of the neonate is competent at birth. However, neonates have never been exposed to environmental antigens, and so any immune response they mount following their first exposure to antigens has to be a primary immune response. Thus, they are vulnerable to infections during the first few weeks of life. Maternal antibody helps protect the neonate while they develop their own immune response to the antigens in their environment. Puppies and kittens that fail to ingest colostrum may have problems with infections during the first 2 months of life, until their own immune system has produced sufficient antibody to protect them. These animals may have to be maintained on supportive antibiotic therapy.

Infections

Many viral infections are capable of producing an acquired immunodeficiency in dogs and cats, especially those that affect the lymphoid tissue. The viruses include canine distemper virus, canine parvovirus, feline leukemia virus, feline immunodeficiency virus, and feline panleukopenia virus. These viral infections cause primarily a T-cell deficiency as the result of a direct lytic effect on the lymphocytes or a disruption in the normal immunoregulatory cytokine network.

An acquired T-cell deficiency has been observed in some dogs with generalized demodicosis with secondary pyoderma. The immunosuppression in these dogs is a result of the secondary bacterial infection, rather than the parasitic infection itself. Severe endotoxemia or sepsis can cause immunosuppression, due to abnormal cytokine production.

Metabolic Disorders

A growth hormone deficiency has been reported in an inbred family of Weimaraner dogs that also had an associated T-cell deficiency. Affected puppies appear normal at birth, but at 6 to 7 weeks of age they develop a wasting syndrome that is characterized by emaciation, lethargy, growth failure, and recurrent infections, resulting in their death. The peripheral T cells from affected dogs fail to respond to mitogenic stimulation. The thymus is small and lacks cellularity. Replacement therapy with growth hormone results in a marked increase in size and cellularity of the thymus and a dramatic clinical improvement.

An acquired T-cell deficiency has been described in Bull terriers secondary to an abnormality in the absorption and metabolism of zinc. The clinical signs include skin lesions (acrodermatitis, chronic pyoderma, and paronychia), diarrhea, and recurrent respiratory infections. Affected dogs also have a lighter pigmentation at birth. The median survival time for affected dogs is 7 months, with bronchopneumonia as the major cause of death. Unlike other zinc deficiencies, affected dogs show little clinical improvement following zinc supplementation. Secondary T-cell deficiencies have also been reported in vitamin A, vitamin E, and selenium deficiencies.

Neoplastic Disease

Animals with advanced cancer are often susceptible to infections because of acquired immunodeficiencies. The immunodeficiencies associated with lymphoreticular tumors are usually due to replacement of normal lymphocytes with neoplastic lymphocytes or due to the interference with the growth and development of normal lymphocytes. Nonlymphoid cancers can be immunosuppressive by producing substances that interfere with lymphocyte development or function.

MANAGEMENT OF IMMUNODEFICIENCY DISEASES

Successful management of patients with immunodeficiency diseases depends on whether the deficiency is hereditary or acquired and which part of the immune system is involved. Acquired immunodeficiencies are usually the easiest to manage. If the primary disease process can be cured, the immunodeficiency will resolve itself. On the other hand, there is no practical cure for the hereditary immunodeficiency diseases in dogs and cats. Antibiotics are lifesaving for treating infectious episodes in patients with immunodeficiency disease, especially for patients with

antibody and neutrophil deficiencies (see p. 267). There is no practical way of treating T-cell deficiencies, other than symptomatic therapy. Early and aggressive broad-spectrum antibiotic therapy should be used even for what would usually be considered mild infections. The use of bactericidal antibiotics is often preferable. Depending on the severity of the deficiency, continuous antibiotic therapy may be required to control infections.

References and Suggested Reading

Blum JR, Cork LC, Morris JM, et al: The clinical manifestations of a genetically-determined deficiency in the third component of complement in the dog. Clin Immunol Immunopathol 24:304, 1985.

Felsburg PJ, Glickman LT, Jezyk PF: Selective IgA deficiency in the dog. Clin Immunol Immunopathol 36:297, 1985.

Felsburg PJ, Somberg RL, Perryman LE: Domestic animal models of severe combined immunodeficiency: Canine X-linked severe combined immunodeficiency and severe combined immunodeficiency in horses. Immunodeficiency Rev 3:277, 1992.

Felsburg PJ: Overview of the immune system and immunodeficiency disease. Vet Clin North Am Small Anim Pract 24:629, 1994.

Giger U, Boxer LA, Simpson PJ, et al: Deficiency of leukocyte surface glycoproteins Mo1, LFA-1, and Leu M5 in a dog with recurrent bacterial infections: An animal model. Blood 69:1622, 1987.

Rivas AL, Tintle L, Argentieri D, et al: A primary immunodeficiency syndrome in Shar-Pei dogs. Clin Immunol Immunopathol 74:243, 1995.

Diseases of the Spleen

DOMINIC J. MARINO
Plainview, New York

The spleen is a complex organ located in the left cranial quadrant of the abdomen. Its functions are varied and although they have been studied in detail, most of them remain only partially understood. The four basic areas of splenic function include storage, hematopoiesis, filtration, and immunity. It has long been recognized that the spleen is not essential for life. Its contributions to the maintenance of homeostasis are beginning to be appreciated as the pathophysiology of various disease processes becomes better understood. Splenectomy should not be regarded as a procedure without consequence and is indicated only in certain types of neoplasia, vascular pedicle compromise, and rupture from trauma or masses, and in some forms of immune-mediated disease. The hematologic changes seen in normal dogs after splenectomy include regenerative anemia, leukocytosis, and an increase in Howell-Jolly bodies, nucleated red blood cells, target cells, and platelets. Splenectomy can result in exacerbation of latent disease in dogs or cats infected with organisms such as *Haemobartonella* and *Babesia*. Experimental studies have shown that the spleen is able to maintain left ventricular performance during hemorrhage by mechanisms other than autotransfusion, thus indicating that splenectomized dogs may be at greater risk during periods of hemorrhage and shock than

are normal dogs (Horton et al, 1984). Most disorders of the spleen involve either generalized or localized splenomegaly, or trauma. The causes of generalized splenomegaly can be divided into infiltrative or congestive diseases (Table 1). The causes of localized splenomegaly can be divided into neoplastic and non-neoplastic diseases (Table 2).

FUNCTIONS

The reservoir capacity of the spleen differs between species, but reportedly it can store as much as 10 to 20% of the total blood volume in dogs and cats (Couto, 1989). Red blood cells circulating through the spleen can be divided into three "pools," based on their circulatory pattern. Ninety percent of the blood entering the spleen enters the "rapid" pool, traversing the spleen in 30 seconds. Nine percent of the circulation enters an "intermediate" pool, traversing the spleen in 8 minutes, and 1 percent enters a "slow" pool, traversing the spleen in 1 hour. During splenic contraction, 98% of the blood is shifted to the rapid pool, resulting in a significant increase in blood volume during times of stress, heavy exercise, or severe hemorrhage. Platelets are stored in the spleen in a slow pool, and as much as 30% of the entire platelet mass may be found

TABLE 1. Causes of Generalized Splenomegaly

Infiltration
   Inflammation
      Infectious
      Granulomatous
   Neoplasia
      Primary
         Lymphoma
         Mastocytosis
         Histiocytosis
      Metastatic
   Hyperplasia
      Extramedullary hematopoiesis
   Amyloidosis

Congestion
   Pharmacologic
      Phenothiazine tranquilizer
      Barbiturates
   Torsion of splenic pedicle
      Isolated
      With gastric dilatation–volvulus
   Portal vein/caudal vena cava hypertension
      Vascular anomaly
      Cardiac failure
      Hepatic cirrhosis
      Neoplasia

there at any given time. Iron is stored in the spleen as part of the recycling of sequestered and destroyed red blood cells awaiting transport to the bone marrow for use in the production of new red blood cells.

The spleen functions as an organ of hematopoiesis during fetal development. This activity normally ceases at birth in both dogs and cats. A limited capacity for hematopoiesis is preserved in the adult and is referred to as *splenic extramedullary hematopoiesis*. Splenic extramedullary hematopoiesis is rare in cats. In dogs, splenic extramedullary hematopoiesis occurs with infiltrative disease of the bone marrow or spleen or with excessive demands on bone marrow due to peripheral erythrocyte destruction. Splenic extramedullary hematopoiesis can result in generalized splenomegaly.

The spleen functions as an organ of filtration in both dogs and cats. Filtration is more efficient in the dog because of anatomic differences in vasculature (the dog's spleen is sinusal, and the cat's spleen is nonsinusal). The presence of rigid cytoplasmic inclusions on the normally pliant erythrocyte permits the removal and phagocytosis of the cytoplasmic inclusions as the cells traverse the sinusal architecture of the canine spleen. If the entire cell becomes nonpliant, as seen with spherocytes, acanthocytes, or senescent red blood cells, the entire cell is removed from circulation and phagocytosed. The liver also functions in filtering blood-borne bacteria; however, the spleen is particularly effective against poorly opsonized bacteria.

TABLE 2. Causes of Localized Splenomegaly

Neoplasia	Non-neoplasia
Hemangiosarcoma	Hematoma
Hemangioma	Nodular hyperplasia
Lymphosarcoma	Abscess
Leiomyosarcoma	
Fibrosarcoma	

The spleen is the principal site of IgM production in the dog and cat. IgM is one of the major immunoglobulins involved in the early immune response following exposure to infectious agents. In addition to phagocytosis and IgM production, other mediators of immunity are synthesized, enhancing both neutrophil phagocytosis and the activation of the complement pathway. The spleen functions effectively in controlling infections with intracellular organisms by the same method used to cull damaged or aged red blood cells, a process called "pitting."

GENERALIZED SPLENOMEGALY

Infiltration

Infiltrative splenomegaly refers to the accumulation of abnormal cells or substance in the spleen or the presence of cells in amounts in excess of normal. Inflammatory infiltration (splenitis) is usually infectious or granulomatous in nature and can be categorized according to predominant cell type. The clinical signs of disease manifested depend on the causative agent and are more readily recognized than are those resulting from generalized splenomegaly. Lymph nodes and bone marrow are more accessible sites of phagocytosis for biopsy than is the spleen and are typically affected in inflammatory diseases of the spleen. Hyperplasia of the spleen commonly occurs in response to blood-borne antigens or massive erythrocyte destruction and is the result of increases in the lymphoreticular population. Clinical signs attributable to splenic hyperplasia are rare and are more often related to the underlying disease process. Extramedullary hematopoiesis commonly results in generalized splenomegaly in dogs and can be caused by a variety of stimuli. Primary or metastatic neoplastic infiltration can cause generalized splenomegaly, although the former is more common. Myeloproliferative neoplasms, lymphosarcoma, and mastocytosis typically produce generalized splenomegaly, in contrast to the localized splenomegaly occurring with neoplasms of the connective tissue elements of the spleen. Mastocytoma and lymphosarcoma are the most common splenic neoplasms in cats.

Congestion

Congestive splenomegaly is most often seen after sedation with tranquilizers or barbiturates. Smooth muscle relaxation of the splenic capsule results in pooling of as much as 30% of the total blood volume in the spleen and significant decreases in packed cell volume. These factors should be considered when one interprets red blood cell parameters in blood obtained from anesthetized or tranquilized patients. Splenic torsion is a common cause of congestive splenomegaly and can occur with or without gastric dilatation-volvulus syndrome. Dogs with isolated splenic torsion most often present with acute abdominal pain, vomiting, anorexia, and depression, but they can present for chronic abdominal pain, weight loss, or hemolysis and hemoglobinuria. The treatment of choice for dogs with splenic torsion is splenectomy. Other causes of splenic congestion include portal vein or caudal vena cava obstruction, passive cardiac congestion, and chronic hepatic cirrhosis, all of which occur infrequently in dogs and cats.

LOCALIZED SPLENOMEGALY

Neoplastic

Localized splenomegaly or splenic masses are more common than generalized splenomegaly in dogs, while the opposite occurs in cats. Several recent studies have shown that non-neoplastic splenic masses are more common than neoplastic masses, and that they are indistinguishable at the time of surgery (Spangler and Culbertson, 1992; Marino et al, 1994). Hemangiosarcoma is the most common cause of splenic neoplasia in dogs and carries a poor long-term prognosis. Metastasis at the time of surgery is present in as many as 50% of dogs, but it does not influence survival after splenectomy and should not be used as a criterion for euthanasia (Johnson et al, 1989). Although surgery may not prolong survival, it does eliminate clinical signs attributable to the abdominal mass and often provides control of abdominal hemorrhage if the mass has ruptured. Other causes of localized splenic neoplasia include hemangioma, fibrosarcoma, leiomyosarcoma, lymphosarcoma (in dogs), and secondary metastasis.

Non-neoplastic

Hematoma and nodular hyperplasia are the most common causes of localized splenomegaly in the dog. Histologic evaluation of hyperplastic nodules and hematomas suggests that they may represent a continuum. The failure of marginal zone circulation secondary to nodular hyperplasia results in an accumulation of blood within the hyperplastic nodule, eventually leading to hematoma formation, hypoxia, and necrosis (Spangler and Culbertson, 1992). For nodular hyperplasia and hematoma, splenectomy is recommended at the time of diagnosis because both are indistinguishable from neoplasia at the time of surgery, and because of the possibility of rupture and life-threatening hemorrhage. The long-term prognosis is excellent for both nodular hyperplasia and hematoma after surgery. Splenic abscesses may result in localized splenomegaly. They occur infrequently in both dogs and cats and may be a sequela to severe splenitis.

TRAUMA

Splenic trauma may be relatively common, based on the prevalence of splenic pathology found during abdominal exploration and at necropsy, but rarely necessitates surgical intervention. Most splenic injuries are not life-threatening because the spleen is partially protected by the rib cage and a durable fibromuscular capsule and is relatively mobile within the abdominal cavity. The contractile ability of the fibromuscular capsule and the close proximity of the greater omentum seem to provide a rapid and efficient mechanism for stabilization of minor injuries. Severe crushing or avulsion injuries typically do not respond to conservative therapy, and require immediate surgical intervention. More sophisticated diagnostics, such as the diagnostic peritoneal lavage (see p. 162), have increased the ability of clinicians to detect internal injuries and decide on an appropriate course of therapy.

DIAGNOSIS

Physical Examination and Hematologic Findings

Most clinical signs in dogs and cats with disorders of the spleen are related to the underlying disease process—and not the splenomegaly. The clinical signs of splenomegaly include anorexia, weight loss, abdominal pain and enlargement, vomiting, weakness or collapse, and polyuria-polydipsia. The mechanism of polyuria-polydipsia is not understood; however, clinical signs usually resolve after splenectomy. Palpation of the spleen is easily accomplished in most patients and frequently results in the detection of localized splenomegaly. Palpation should be gentle because many localized masses are friable and can rupture, resulting in life-threatening hemorrhage. Lymphadenopathy frequently occurs in diseases resulting in infiltrative splenomegaly and can be readily palpated and biopsied. Other physical findings may include pallor, petechiae, tachycardia, and pulse deficits. Significant increases in white blood cell counts with left shifts are common in dogs with splenic torsion and hemangiosarcoma (Marino et al, 1994). Coagulation profiles and platelet counts are recommended because of the prevalence of disseminated intravascular coagulation with many underlying disease processes associated with splenomegaly (Hammer et al, 1991). Electrocardiograms are useful in cases of localized splenomegaly because of the high prevalence of ventricular arrhythmias in dogs with splenic masses (Knapp, 1993; Marino et al, 1994). Detection of ventricular arrhythmias at times necessitates antiarrhythmic therapy or modifications in the anesthetic protocol (see pp. 733 and 122). Other diagnostics, including bone marrow aspiration, may be helpful, depending on the underlying disease process, and should be selected on an individual case-by-case basis.

Diagnostic Procedures

The spleen is easily visualized radiographically, but its location can vary, owing to its mobility within the abdominal cavity. The size of the spleen is difficult to assess because of the passive splenic congestion produced when tranquilizers or anesthetics are used during radiography. Large localized splenic mass lesions usually appear in the middle abdomen, displacing the small intestines caudally. Abdominal ultrasound is extremely useful in detecting splenomegaly and for noninvasive characterization of the lesion and potential causes of splenic enlargement. Ultrasound can be used to further define the underlying disease process and to evaluate the abdomen for metastatic disease. Abdominal ultrasound can be used to detect vascular compromise with torsion of the splenic pedicle or portal vein congestion, as well as congestion secondary to cardiac or liver disease. Both computed tomography and magnetic resonance imaging are useful in evaluating splenomegaly and concurrent underlying disease processes. Neither modality is commonly used in the diagnosis of splenic disorders because of the time and financial commitments involved in utilizing either one. Splenic aspiration with cytologic evaluation is a minimally invasive procedure that can be done without sedation (O'Keefe and Couto, 1987). The area of localized splenomegaly can usually be manually isolated, and a 22-gauge, 1.5-inch needle attached to a 12-ml syringe can be used to aspirate the lesion. Abdominal ultrasound can be used to guide the aspiration if the localized splenomegaly is not easily palpated. Cytologic evaluation can be used to determine the need for surgery, further diagnostics, or therapy.

SURGERY

Partial Splenectomy

Partial splenectomy is indicated only when a portion of the spleen has been injured. A partial splenectomy is more difficult to perform than a total splenectomy, but it has the advantage of retaining splenic function. Hematologic abnormalities are less extreme in dogs that have had a partial splenectomy than those found in dogs that have undergone a total splenectomy. A total splenectomy should always be performed if neoplasia is suspected. Several partial splenectomy techniques utilizing different methods of separating splenic parenchyma have been described. Regardless of the technique, all begin with ligation of the hilar vessels that supply the area of spleen to be resected, and identification of the demarcation of ischemia. Splenic parenchyma can be divided digitally, clamped with forceps, transected, and sutured in a continuous pattern, or divided with a mattress pattern placed through the parietal and visceral surfaces of the spleen, and then transected. With either technique, digital pressure and individual sutures are occasionally needed to control hemorrhage after separation of the parenchyma. Automatic stapling devices (Thoracoabdominal Stapler [TA], United States Surgical Co., Norwalk, CT) are very effective in both separating the splenic parenchyma and placing a double row of staples in a single application. These devices decrease operating time and are strongly recommended when one handles critical cases. The carbon dioxide laser and ultrasonic cutting devices have been used to perform partial splenectomies in dogs in research applications and may become clinically useful as these modalities become more readily available.

Total Splenectomy

Total splenectomy is indicated in cases of splenic masses, torsion, severe trauma, and immune-mediated disease refractory to medical management. Several techniques have been described regarding ligation of the splenic vascular supply. Some suggest that splenectomy by individual ligation of the short splenic branches of the splenic artery and vein is advantageous because of preservation of the left gastroepiploic artery and short gastric arteries. Others recommend splenectomy by ligation of the splenic artery, left gastroepiploic artery, and short gastric arteries because of the decreased time and handling associated with this technique. The latter technique does not compromise gastric blood flow and, in the author's opinion, is technically easier to perform. Double ligatures are recommended to avoid the risk of hemorrhage after surgery. Automatic stapling devices (Ligate and Divide Stapler [LDS], United States Surgical Co., Norwalk, CT) place a double row of staples and divide the vessel between them. These devices

are helpful in facilitating a sometimes tedious process and are preferred by the author. Pedicle ligation can be difficult in cases of splenic torsion because of the tautness of the splenic pedicle, and manual ligation is usually required. Derotation of the spleen prior to vascular ligation must be avoided to prevent toxins from entering the blood stream. Intrasplenic injection of epinephrine to reduce the size of the spleen is not recommended because of the prevalence of ventricular arrhythmias in cases of splenic masses and splenic torsion.

Complications

In a recent study of 50 dogs having total splenectomy, 22 (44%) had ventricular tachycardia (Marino et al, 1994). Ventricular arrhythmias are the most common complication in dogs who have undergone splenectomy and usually begin approximately 5 hours after surgery. Some dogs have ventricular arrhythmias before or during surgery. Dogs with anemia, hypotension, leukocytosis, and splenic mass rupture concurrently have an increased prevalence of ventricular arrhythmias and should be monitored closely. The method of cardiac monitoring significantly influences the detection of ventricular arrhythmias. When continuous electrocardiographic monitoring was simultaneously compared with 1-minute electrocardiographic monitoring every 6 hours (ECG q6hr), half of the dogs experiencing more than 1,000 ventricular extrasystoles per hour went undetected by ECG q6hr (Marino et al, 1994). Most arrhythmias resolve within 10 days, and dogs rarely need antiarrhythmic therapy. Strict cage rest and supportive care decrease cardiac demand and decrease the risk of an acute crisis. Antiarrhythmic therapy should be reserved for dogs that exhibit the following: hemodynamic instability, multiform electrocardiographic complexes, very rapid ventricular tachycardia, or R-on-T complex.

Hemorrhage after splenectomy can be life-threatening and may require a second surgery. After total or partial splenectomy, ligatures should be examined for security, and additional ligatures should be applied if needed. Coagulation abnormalities can result in significant oozing from cut surfaces but rarely become life-threatening. Ischemic pancreatitis, sepsis, and gastric necrosis secondary to excessive tissue handling have been described; however, all are extremely rare, in the author's experience.

References and Suggested Reading

Couto CG: Diseases of the lymph nodes and spleen. In: Ettinger SJ, ed: Textbook of Veterinary Internal Medicine. Philadelphia: WB Saunders, 1989, p 2225.
Comprehensive review of the pathophysiology and treatment of lymph node and splenic disorders.
Hammer AS, Couto CG, Swardson C, et al: Hemostatic abnormality in dogs with hemangiosarcoma. J Vet Intern Med 5:11, 1991.
Clinical review of hematologic abnormalities in 24 dogs with hemangiosarcoma.
Horton JW, Longhurst JC, Coln D, et al: Cardiovascular effects of haemorrhagic shock in spleen intact and in splenectomized dogs. Clin Physiol 4:533, 1984.
Laboratory model evaluation of the splenic contribution toward hemodynamic stabilization in dogs with severe hemorrhage.
Johnson KA, Powers BE, Withrow SJ, et al: Splenomegaly in dogs. J Vet Intern Med 3:160, 1989.

Clinical review of splenomegaly in 100 dogs, with comparisons between hematologic findings and clinical outcome.

Knapp DW: Cardiac arrhythmias associated with mass lesions of the canine spleen. J Am Anim Hosp Assoc 29:122, 1993.
Review of medical records of 106 dogs with splenic masses and cardiac arrhythmias.

Marino DJ, Matthiesen DT, Fox PR, et al: Ventricular arrhythmias in dogs undergoing splenectomy: A prospective study. Vet Surg 23:101, 1994.
Prospective evaluation for cardiac arrhythmias in 50 dogs having splenectomy and a comparison of ECG monitoring techniques.

O'Keefe DA, Couto CG: Fine-needle aspiration of the spleen as an aid in the diagnosis of splenomegaly. J Vet Intern Med 1:102, 1987.
Description of a diagnostic procedure for splenomegaly and clinical results in dogs and cats.

Spangler WL, Culbertson MR: Prevalence, type, and importance of splenic diseases in dogs: 1480 cases (1985–1989). J Am Vet Med Assoc 200:829, 1992.
Review of records of splenic biopsies from a diagnostic laboratory with discussions of histologic evaluations and the pathophysiology of clinical findings.

Dermatologic Diseases

CRAIG GRIFFIN
WAYNE S. ROSENKRANTZ

Consulting Editors

Practical Laboratory Methods for the Diagnosis of Dermatologic Diseases

Milan, Italy

Laboratory procedures in veterinary dermatology are very useful for confirming a clinical diagnosis or excluding other disorders. Several of these procedures are quite easy to perform, even in the consulting room, are inexpensive (Table 1), and offer rapid or immediate results. Included among this group are skin scrapings, microscopic examination of hair (trichography), the collection and microscopic examination of scales and debris, cytologic examination of skin and cutaneous infiltrates, Wood's lamp examination of hair and skin, and fungal cultures. These practical tests can offer a great amount of information if performed correctly; thus, the practitioner needs to learn about and skillfully perform these techniques to obtain reliable results.

SKIN SCRAPING

Skin scraping should be performed in all cases of alopecia or scaling disease, in both dogs and cats. Scrapings can be performed with a scalpel blade (No. 20 with or without a handle) or a curet (e.g., Volkmann's curet with a double spoon, diameter of 5 to 7 mm). The skin of the chosen area should be clipped with scissors and moistened with a drop of mineral oil. Holding a skin fold between the thumb and the index finger, one should press the fold to squeeze as much material as possible out of the hair follicles, then repeatedly scrape in the direction of the hair growth on the

TABLE 1. List of Materials Needed for Most Common Diagnostic Procedures in Veterinary Dermatology

Scalpel blades N. 20
Curet, or double spoon of Vokmann
Mineral oil and/or chlorlactophenol and/or 10% or 20% KOH
Glass microscope slides and coverslips (20 × 60 mm and 20 × 20 mm)
Glue for glass mounting (Eukitt's)
Microscope with 4×, 10×, 40×, and 100× objectives and immersion oil
Sterile hemostats
New individually packed toothbrushes
Small, sterile paper envelopes
Dermatophyte Test Medium and Sabouraud's culture medium
Clear cellophane tape
Lactophenol cotton blue
Rubber-covered hemostats
Flea comb 12 teeth per centimeter
Syringes, 10 ml
Cotton swabs
Needles, 25 gauge
Needles, 21 gauge
Cytologic stains (Diff-Quik or New Methylene Blue)
Matches or lighter
Hair scissors

same site with the blade or the curet, holding the instrument at an angle of 45 to 90 degrees. The collected material should stick to the oil on the blade. The scraping should then be smeared on a microscope slide and diluted, if necessary, with one more drop of mineral oil. The sample is then emulsified with the oil on the slide until the sample is homogeneous, a coverslip is applied (best is 2 × 2 cm), and the sample is carefully examined under the microscope at 4× and at 10× magnification. The owners often request that the scraped area be disinfected; thus, although it is not necessary, it is good practice to perform a slight disinfection routinely. Different techniques of skin scraping are applied, depending on the ectoparasite suspected. If one is searching for *Demodex* mites or *Pelodera* larvae, both of which live in the hair follicles, one to three scrapings should be carried out, and scrapings should be performed until capillary oozing occurs (deep skin scrapings). Scraping can be difficult to perform in an animal that has pododemodicosis, because the procedure can be very painful, and bleeding is a consequence of even a very superficial scraping because of the inflammation and edema. In this case it is advisable to perform hair-plucking (see later) to look for the mites. Skin scrapings for *Demodex* mites should always be diagnostic, if performed correctly and provided that the animal has the condition and has not yet been treated. Reaching an adequate depth can be very difficult or even impossible in Shar pei dogs, because of the very thick dermis typical of this breed. In this case, if demodicosis is suspected and skin scraping has produced negative results, one should obtain a skin biopsy for histopathologic examination.

Skin scrapings for *Sarcoptes* mites in dogs should be performed over a larger area (ideally 20 cm²). After gently clipping all the hair with an electrical clipper, the skin is scraped in a superficial way, to collect as many scales as possible for microscopic examination. Scraping until capillary bleeding occurs is not necessary in this case. The best areas to scrape are the outer skin of the pinnae, the lateral elbows, and any other area that presents with thick scales or with papules and yellow crusts. *Sarcoptes* mites, eggs, or feces are not always found in skin scrapings of affected animals, even if the scrapings have been correctly performed. Therefore, a negative skin scraping does not exclude sarcoptic mange.

In feline scabies, *Notoedres* mites are easy to find and abundant in skin scrapings. These scrapings should be performed in a manner similar to that described for *Sarcoptes* mites in dogs. Superficial skin scrapings can also be performed to collect scales when infestation with *Cheyletiella* is suspected, although this technique is less sensitive than acetate tape impression or scale collection with a flea comb.

TABLE 2. Formulas of Solutions Used in Dermatology

Chlorphenolac
  Chloral hydrate, 50 gm
  Liquid phenol, 25 ml
  Liquid lactic acid, 25 ml
Chlorphenolac is not commercially available; ingredients are available from chemical suppliers. After mixing the ingredients, let the mixture stand for 24 to 48 hours, to allow all the crystals to dissolve.

Lactophenol Cotton Blue
  Phenol crystals, 20 gm
  Glycerine, 40 ml
  Lactic acid, 20 ml
  Distilled water, 20 ml
Gently heat the mixture over a water bath to dissolve all the ingredients. Then add 0.05 gm of cotton blue dye and mix well. This mixture is also commercially available.

Finally, the skin surface, especially in cases of greasy seborrhea, can be gently scraped to collect material to smear on a slide, stain, and examine for *Malassezia* (see discussion of microscopic examination of scales). As alternatives to mineral oil, chlorphenolac (Table 2) or 10 to 20% potassium hydroxide (KOH) can be used as clarifying agents. These substances are used primarily when one tries to find fungal hyphae or spores. Both clarifying agents are toxic to the skin; therefore, the scrapings should be performed with a dry blade and the material should then be mixed with a drop of chlorphenolac or KOH on the microscope slide. The preparation with KOH should be gently heated under a flame for 30 seconds or let stand for 30 minutes at room temperature before being examined under the microscope. Preparations with chlorphenolac can be examined immediately and need not be heated.

TRICHOGRAPHY

Microscopic examination of the hair is a valuable technique used with increasing frequency and complementary to other studies (Table 3). Hairs are collected with small rubber-covered hemostats and are pulled from the follicles in the direction of the hair growth. Rubber is used on the tips of the hemostats to grasp hair in all developmental stages—not just telogen hair, which is more easily epilated.

TABLE 3. Indications for In-Office Diagnostic Procedures in Veterinary Dermatology

Procedure	Indication
Wood's lamp	Infection with *Microsporum canis*
Skin scraping	Ectoparasitoses, dermatophytosis, infection with *Malassezia* (*Pityrosporon*)
Flea combing	Ectoparasites
Coat brushing	Collection of material for fungal culture
Acetate tape impression	Ectoparasitoses, infection with *Malassezia*
Hair-plucking and trichography	Demodicosis, dermatophytosis, lice, infection with *Cheyletiella*, alopecia
Cytology	Skin tumors, bacterial and fungal infections, *Malassezia*, pemphigus complex, eosinophilic granuloma complex

Hair is then put on a drop of mineral oil, chlorphenolac, or KOH on a microscope slide, covered with a coverslip, and examined under the microscope. Alternatively, the collected material can be fixed with clear acetate tape firmly pressed to the slide.

Trichography can be useful in the diagnosis of demodicosis, because very often mites are pulled out of the follicles with the hairs, and they can then be readily examined under the microscope at $4\times$ or $10\times$ magnification. The technique is also diagnostic for dermatophytosis, if spores or hyphae are observed in or on the hair shafts. This test is positive in 60 to 70% of cases of dermatophytosis. However, if test results are negative, the disease cannot be excluded, and a fungal culture must be performed (see later). In the search for dermatophytes, ideally one should collect the hairs that fluoresce under the Wood's lamp, broken stubby hair, or hair at the periphery of the lesions. Normal hair is clean and has an even surface, the cortex and medulla are readily recognized, and the tips are nicely tapered. Affected hair that has been invaded by hyphae has an irregular surface, the cortex and medulla are not distinguishable, and the tips are often broken into a "brush-like" surface. Spores appear as round, refractile bodies, arranged in chains or groups on the surface of the hair shaft, and have a diameter of 3 to 8 μm.

Trichography can also be a useful aid in canine and feline noninflammatory alopecia. Examination of the tips and roots can reveal whether the hair loss is self-induced (resulting from licking or scratching because of pruritus) or due to other reasons (endocrinopathies, hair dystrophies). If hairs have large, round, pigmented roots, which look soft, stretched, and bent owing to the hair-plucking (anagen stage, seen in normally growing hair), together with broken tips, the hair has most probably been licked or scratched off by the animal. If most or all of the roots are thin, club shaped, straight, and nonpigmented (telogen stage, typical of resting, nongrowing hair), and the hair tips are normally tapered, the alopecia is most probably due to a metabolic (e.g., hormonal) disorder. Abnormal distorted hair bulbs (compared with bulbs plucked from a healthy dog of the same breed and in the same molting season) can be observed in some cases of follicular dysplasia or in alopecia areata. Observation of the hair shaft can be diagnostic of color dilution alopecia. In normal hair, pigmented melanin granules are evenly distributed all along the shaft, giving a homogeneous color to the hair. In color dilution alopecia, the pigmented melanin granules are clumped together in macromelanosomes, which can distort and break the hair cuticle. These pigment abnormalities are observed in hairs plucked from all areas of the body, even in the yellow or red hairs, which do not show alopecia.

Focal abnormalities of the hair shafts, such as an irregular or a broken cuticle, can be observed in cases of malnutrition or repeated trauma to the hair (excessive grooming) or in the rare disease called trichorrhexis nodosa. In diseases that present with comedones or infundibular enlargement and with hyperkeratosis (including endocrinopathies, sebaceous adenitis, demodicosis, and vitamin A–responsive dermatosis), keratin follicular casts can be observed adherent to the hair shafts, and these disorders have to be differentiated from dermatophyte hyphae and spores. This material is amorphous, formed by several layers of keratin, and often contains thin wound-up secondary hairs, which, due to the keratin plug, are not able to reach the skin surface.

Lice nits and *Cheyletiella* eggs can be observed attached to the hair shaft, the latter being much smaller and less firmly glued to the shaft than the former.

MICROSCOPIC EXAMINATION OF SCALES

The microscopic examination of scales and debris can identify some ectoparasites, such as fleas, *Cheyletiella*, and lice. Scales can be collected by placing the animal on black or brown paper, briskly rubbing its coat, and collecting all material falling onto the paper. Alternatively, a metal flea comb with about 12 teeth per centimeter can be used. The material collected can be directly mixed with mineral oil, chlorphenolac, or KOH (see earlier) and observed under the microscope with a coverslip. *Cheyletiella* mites, lice, flea eggs, and flea feces can be easily recognized at 4× magnification. A concentrated preparation of large amounts of scales can be made by flotation. The collected material is heated briefly in a small amount of 10% KOH, then submerged in a saturated sugar solution or into a fecal examination flotation medium, and then centrifuged. The supernatant is collected with a pipette and put on a microscopic slide, covered with a coverslip, and observed at 4× magnification. This technique is particularly useful if one looks for *Cheyletiella*, because these mites are usually not abundant.

Scales can also be collected by pressing a strip of acetate tape repeatedly on the animal between the hairs. The tape is then pressed—the glued face down—on a microscope slide and observed under the microscope. This technique is also suitable for the collection of seborrheic material and, after cytologic staining (see later), for the search for *Malassezia* (*Pityrosporon*) on the keratin scales.

CYTOLOGY

Techniques

Glass slides should be cleaned with alcohol 70% beforehand to enhance specimen adhesion. Cytologic collection techniques differ, depending on the type of the lesion. The fine-needle aspirate technique is often used for solid lesions. After hair clipping and gentle surface disinfection, a 21-gauge needle connected to a 10-ml syringe is inserted into the center of the lesion, and a negative pressure of about 2 ml is applied. Without releasing the negative pressure, the needle is then moved back and forth into the lesion three or four times. Before the needle is withdrawn from the lesion, the negative pressure is released, to prevent the collected material from entering into the syringe cone. The syringe and the needle (containing the sample) are then separated, 10 ml of air is sucked into the syringe, before needle and syringe are connected again. Finally, the material is blown on a glass slide by rapidly pressing on the syringe plunger. If the material is abundant or very liquid, it can then be streaked with another glass slide. Aspiration with a syringe can also be performed to collect material from cysts, abscesses, large vesicles, or pustules.

Impression smears are useful in open, exudative lesions and greasy seborrheic surfaces and from freshly cut surfaces of skin biopsies or extirpated nodules. With this technique, the glass slide is simply pressed repeatedly (not streaked) on the lesion. In a similar way, one can collect pus from pustules and under crusts, after gently opening the pustules or the crusts with a small, 25-gauge needle.

Material for cytology can be collected with a swab from fistulas, deep pyoderma, ear canals, or, with a moistened swab, from a greasy skin surface. The swab is then gently rolled across the slide. All cytologic samples have to dry on the slide. Slides with greasy or waxy material or specimens collected with a moistened swab have to be lightly heated over a match or lighter flame before staining. Common rapid stains used in cytology include modified Wright's stains (Diff-Quik, Hemacolor) and new methylene blue. Other stains, which are convenient or require special laboratory equipment, such as Gram's, PAS (periodic acid–Schiff), and May-Grünwald-Giemsa stains, are rarely necessary.

After staining, slides are shortly rinsed under tap water, air-dried, and observed under the microscope at 10×, 40×, and 100× magnification (with oil immersion). To keep the preparations for a longer period, a coverslip can be glued on the glass slide with special glues (e.g., Eukitt or Accu-Mount 60, Baxter Healthcare Corp.). Acetate tape preparations can also be stained, rinsed, and pressed to a microscope slide with the sticky face on the slide.

Interpretation

The examination of samples from nodules can reveal the presence of inflammation (inflammatory cells such as neutrophils, macrophages, lymphocytes, and plasma cells) or neoplasia. In an inflammatory exudate, one can often observe the presence of bacteria and evaluate their number, shape, and position (intracellular versus extracellular). Bacteria seen in cytology usually are cocci (mostly *Staphylococcus*). Rarely, rods or mixed infections (cocci and rods) can be observed. Rods cannot be identified by cytology alone; thus, finding intracellular rods or mixed infections warrants a bacterial culture and sensitivity test. Only intracellular bacteria (usually in degenerated swollen neutrophils) are diagnostic of pyoderma. In most cases of deep pyoderma, few intracellular bacteria are observed, but many neutrophils and macrophages, and some lymphocytes and plasma cells, are found. Numerous extracellular bacteria are indicative of contamination or of a very superficial pyoderma (e.g., a "hot spot"). *Malassezia* yeasts are rarely seen in samples from normal skin, but they can be present in healthy ears and are often abundant in specimens from greasy seborrhea or ceruminal otitis. These yeasts are larger than most bacteria, have a bottle or peanut shape (budding yeast), and stain variably from light blue to dark violet when seen in modified Wright-stained samples. *Malassezia* is always extracellular and often sticks to corneocytes. Other microorganisms, such as agents of deep fungal infections or *Leishmania*, may be occasionally observed in samples from skin or lymph nodes. In cases of suspected cryptococcosis, it is very useful to mix a small drop of black China (or India) ink with the exudate to identify the mucinous capsule, which clearly stands out against the dark background.

Sterile pustules, with well-preserved neutrophils, variable numbers of eosinophils, and acantholytic cells are very suggestive of pemphigus complex diseases. Acantholytic cells are small, dark, round keratinocytes of the basal or spinous layer, which detach from the surrounding cells owing to the rupture of intercellular bridges. Large, clear cells with straight edges and corners cannot be considered acantholytic cells, but are normal desquamating corneocytes. True acantholytic cells are particularly abundant in feline pemphigus and are often grouped in rafts. A few acantholytic cells are sometimes observed in pustules due to bacterial infections. In this case, they are less numerous and do not group easily in rafts, and bacteria are clearly visible inside the neutrophils. Bacteria together with acantholytic cells are also observed in samples from pemphigus diseases collected from under a crust, which has most probably been secondarily infected. In these difficult cases, it is advised to obtain multiple skin biopsies and send them to a dermatopathologist for definitive diagnosis.

Eosinophils, as the main cellular type, are observed in lesions of the feline eosinophilic granuloma complex, in ectoparasitoses (scabies, fleas, nasal pyoderma due to arthropod bites), in some cases of canine food or contact allergy, and in the rare sterile eosinophilic pustulosis of the dog. Mature surface corneocytes can be observed in samples collected from the skin surface or from aspiration biopsies from follicular cysts. They are large, flat, light-blue, anucleated cells with sharp edges, which can look dark blue when rolled up in a cigar shape.

WOOD'S LAMP EXAMINATION

Examining the skin and hair with the Wood's lamp can be useful in the diagnosis of dermatophytosis caused by *Microsporum canis*. The Wood's lamp produces ultraviolet (UV) light with a wavelength of 253.7 nm, filtered through a cobalt or nickel filter. Lamps with a magnifying glass are preferred. The examination should take place in a completely dark room. In order for the lamp to reach the ideal wavelength, it has to be warmed up for 5 to 10 minutes. It is useful to spend this time in the dark room, allowing one's eyes to adapt to the conditions. Some 50% of the strains of *M. canis* fluoresce under UV light, as a result of the production of tryptophan metabolites. The positive fluorescence is typically apple-green in color and can be observed at the hair base, like a cuff surrounding the intrafollicular and extrafollicular portions of the hair shaft. Often, positive hairs are stubby or broken at the periphery of the lesions. Sometimes, positive scales may be observed. False-positive fluorescence is of a different color (white, light blue) and may be given by scales, debris, topical therapies, bacteria *(Pseudomonas)*, or keratin plugs around the hair shafts. To confirm a positive finding, it is advised to collect the fluorescing hairs, observe them under the microscope for fungal elements (see earlier), and use some of the sample for fungal culture.

Some fungal strains have to be irradiated several minutes before they develop the typical fluorescence. Thus, one should keep the lamp above the lesion for at least 5 minutes, before deciding that the test is negative. Half of the *M. canis* strains and all of the *Trichophyton* species that infect small animals do not exhibit fluorescence, so a negative Wood's lamp examination does not exclude dermatophytosis. In suspected cases, a fungal culture should be performed.

FUNGAL CULTURE

Fungal culture is imperative when one suspects a dermatophytosis, but trichography and Wood's lamp examination are negative. To avoid excessive contamination, the hair is clipped 1 cm from the skin, and the lesion is lightly disinfected with 70% alcohol, then allowed to dry. Broken, stubby hair, fluorescing hair, and scales and hair at the periphery of the lesion are collected with sterile hemostats and either placed in a small paper envelope for later inoculation or directly put on the culture medium. Care has to be taken to place as much of the collected material as possible in contact with the culture medium, because only spores that are in contact with the medium will develop a mycelium. In animals that do not have lesions (particularly suspected asymptomatic carrier cats, or animals on whom one is performing follow-up culture after a therapy cycle), the MacKenzie toothbrush technique is advised. New, single-packaged toothbrushes can be used, because in their original packaging they usually are mycologically sterile. The whole body of the animal has to be brushed, and particularly dermatophyte predilection sites, such as the face, the pinnae, and the anterior paws. Care has to be taken to also collect a small amount of hair with the toothbrush. The toothbrush is then gently pressed repeatedly onto the culture medium, and the hair is then distributed and pressed on the whole surface of the plate. Claws (nails) crushed into small pieces, and debris collected with a curet from the nail bed or under the concave face of the claw, can also be cultured for fungi. Inoculation of exudates, and material recently treated with topical antifungal therapy, are to be avoided. Inoculated plates or bottles have to be loosely closed and stored at room temperature (20 to 25°C) in a dark place, with a relative humidity not lower than 30%. A shoebox with a cup of water in it is a good homemade incubator. Cultures have to be inspected every day for at least 14 days. If no growth is visible after 2 weeks, the culture is probably negative.

The culture medium most often used is the dermatophyte test medium (DTM; see p. 526). This medium contains gentamycin and chlortetracycline against bacteria, and cycloheximide against saprophytic fungi, so that dermatophyte growth is favored. Some pathogenic fungi, such as *Cryptococcus*, some *Aspergillus* species, Zygomycota, and agents of phaeohyphomycosis, are sensitive to cycloheximide and do not grow on this culture medium. DTM also has phenol red as a pH indicator, which turns from yellow to red in an alkaline environment. Dermatophytic fungi first use proteins as nourishment, thus producing alkaline metabolites, which cause the indicator to turn red as soon as the mycelium growth is noticed. Saprophytic fungi use carbohydrates, first producing acid metabolites, which keep the indicators yellow. Eventually, if the culture is held long enough (10 days or more), and the medium is depleted of all carbohydrates, the saprophytic fungi will also use proteins as nourishment and turn the indicator red. It is important to notice that for saprophytic fungi, the change in color of the medium occurs *after* the mycelium has developed and has been clearly visible for some days. Therefore, one must observe the culture for fungal growth and color changes daily. Because other fungi, such as *Blastomyces*, *Sporothrix*, *Histoplasma*, *Coccidioides*, and some *Aspergillus* species, may also rapidly turn the DTM medium red, a macroscopic and microscopic evaluation of the culture must be performed to identify the fungal species. Macroscopic evaluation of the upper surface and underside of the culture is best performed when the sample is inoculated or subcultured on a Sabouraud plate in parallel with the DTM plate. *Microsporum canis* shows a whitish, cottony colony, with a yellow-orange center on the underside. *Microsporum gypseum* has a flat, pale-brown colony with a granular surface and a pale yellow underside. *Trichophyton mentagrophytes* shows a flat, white to gray, powdery colony with centrifugal radiation, and a brown underside. Saprophytic fungi often have black, gray, green, or dark-brown colonies, and some are completely white, without a yellow underside.

Microscopic evaluation of the macroconidia is best performed not sooner than 5 to 7 days from the first observation of mycelial growth, preferably on Sabouraud medium. Rapid sporulating media are also commercially available, but their advantage is doubtful. A piece of clear acetate tape is gently pressed on the colony surface, so that part of it can stick to the tape. The tape is placed on a drop of cotton blue lactophenol, with the glued face under, on a microscope slide and directly observed under the microscope at 10× and 40× magnification. Macroconidia of *Microsporum canis* are spindle shaped, have thick walls with six or more cells, and have knob-like ends. *Microsporum gypseum* has spindle-shaped macroconidia with thin walls, no knob-like ends, and six or less cells. Macroconidia of *T. mentagrophytes* can be difficult to find, are cigar shaped, and have thin walls. *Trichophyton mentagrophytes* is best recognized by its spiral hyphae and its grape-like microconidia, which are abundant and easy to observe.

References and Suggested Reading

Miller WH: What's "new" in clinical dermatology II: Trichography. Proceedings of the 12th ESVD Annual Congress, Barcelona, 1995, p 167.
   A short description of this diagnostic technique, its application, and the most frequent findings.
Scott DW, Miller WH, Griffin CE: Muller and Kirk's Small Animal Dermatology, 5th ed. Philadelphia: WB Saunders, 1995, pp 55–173.
   An in-depth review of all current diagnostic techniques used in veterinary dermatology.

Hypoallergenic Diets for Dogs and Cats

PHILIP ROUDEBUSH
Topeka, Kansas

Dermatologic manifestations of adverse food reactions in dogs typically occur as nonseasonal pruritic dermatitis that occasionally is accompanied by gastrointestinal signs. The pruritus is of varying severity, and the distribution of lesions is often indistinguishable from that seen with atopy: feet, face, axillae, perineal region, inguinal region, rump, and ears. A large number of dogs with adverse food reactions show lesions only in the region of the ears. This finding suggests that adverse food reactions should always be suspected in dogs with pruritic, bilateral otitis externa, even if accompanied by secondary bacterial or *Malassezia (Pityrosporum)* infections. In cats, dermatologic signs of adverse food reactions include several different patterns of clinical reactions, such as severe, generalized pruritus without lesions; miliary dermatitis; pruritus with self-inflicted trauma centered around the head, neck, and ears; traumatic alopecia; moist dermatitis; and scaling dermatoses. Angioedema, urticaria, or conjunctivitis often occurs in cats with adverse food reactions. Adverse reactions to food may also cause self-inflicted alopecia (psychogenic alopecia; neurodermatitis), eosinophilic plaques, and indolent ulcers of the lip in some cats.

DIETARY HISTORY

The dietary history of the patient should be carefully reviewed for ingredients that are thought to be commonly associated with adverse food reactions. The dietary history should include a list of specific commercial foods, commercial snacks or treats, supplements, chewable medications, chew toys, human foods routinely used as part of the regular diet or as treats, and access to other sources of food. As an example, a dog might be given a dry, commercial food as its main source of nutrition but the dog may also be given rawhide chews, commercial dog biscuits, and various foods left over from human meals and may have access to commercial food or the litter box provided for cats in the household. It is often helpful to have the owner of the pet keep a diary for several weeks that documents on a daily basis what types of food and other items are ingested by the animal. A good dietary history is also essential in determining what ingredients the elimination diet for an individual patient should or should not contain.

FOOD ALLERGENS

The specific food allergens that cause problems in animals have been poorly documented. In general, the major food allergens that have been identified in human beings are water-soluble glycoproteins that have molecular weights ranging from 10,000 to 60,000 daltons (D) and are stable to treatment with heat, acid, and proteases. Other physiochemical properties that account for their unique allergenicity are poorly understood.

A survey of veterinarians in North America incriminated food preservatives and dyes, wheat, beef, chicken egg, corn, poultry, soy, and dairy products as common causes of dermatologic signs of food allergy in dogs. It is interesting to compare these clinical perceptions with what has been documented in case studies in the literature. Ten different studies, representing a total of 253 dogs, have described cutaneous lesions associated with adverse reactions to specific foods or ingredients. In these studies, adverse reactions to beef, dairy products, and wheat have accounted for 68% of all the reported cases in dogs. Adverse reactions to chicken, chicken egg, lamb, or soy have accounted for approximately 25% of the reported canine cases.

Food allergens incriminated in North American cats with dermatologic disease include fish, beef, chicken or other kinds of poultry, dairy products, preservatives, and dyes. Seven different reports, representing a total of 45 cats, have described cutaneous lesions associated with adverse reactions to specific foods or ingredients. In these studies, adverse reactions to beef, dairy products, and fish have accounted for more than 80% of all the reported cases in cats.

Human allergy reference books often contain phylogenetic tables of animal and vegetable foods, and food-allergic persons are often advised to avoid other closely related foods. In clinical practice, human patients often report cross-reactivity among various fishes and among various crustaceans, but less cross-reactivity is reported within vegetable food groups. The results of oral food challenges in children demonstrate that clinically important cross-reactivity to legumes (peanuts, soybeans, green beans, lima beans, peas, lentils) is very rare. Wheat, rye, and barley show cross-reactivity in allergic human beings, but oat allergens appear to cross-react only weakly with these other three grains. Cross-reactivity between milk proteins from cows, goats, and sheep has been noted, and chicken egg–allergic children have also exhibited cross-reactivity with egg proteins of other birds. Certain allergens are apparently common to both foods and pollens. Common allergens have been reported in melon, banana, and ragweed pollen; celery and mugwort pollen; and apple and birch pollen. Cross-reactivity among food allergens has not been well investigated in pet animals.

NONIMMUNOLOGIC REACTIONS TO FOOD

Nonimmunologic reactions to food include food intolerance and dietary indiscretion. Food intolerance may mimic food allergy except that it can occur on the first exposure to a dietary substance, since nonimmunologic mechanisms are involved. The incidence of food intolerance versus food hypersensitivity or allergy is unknown.

Idiosyncratic adverse reactions to food additives are often described in human beings. Food additives that are frequently incriminated in human adverse reactions include sulfites, monosodium glutamate, tartrazine and other azo or nonazo dyes, benzoates, parabens, and spices. Few of the adverse reactions to food additives appear to have an immunologic mechanism, although IgE-mediated reactions may occur. Confirmed reactions to food additives are best described as food intolerance or food idiosyncrasy, because clinical signs resulting from their ingestion are thought to be nonimmunologically mediated. Examples are reactions to azo dyes, nonazo dyes, and antioxidants that can directly cause histamine release from leukocytes of some individuals.

While food additives are frequently incriminated as causing problems in dogs and cats, there are few data confirming this perception. Propylene glycol has been documented as causing hematologic abnormalities in cats and subsequently has been eliminated from cat foods sold in the United States and many other countries.

Some veterinary dermatologists have incriminated food colorants and other food additives as causes of erythema multiforme or other "drug-like" skin eruptions. Erythema multiforme is a pattern of cutaneous reactions of multifactorial etiology seen uncommonly in dogs and rarely in cats. Lesions include erythematous macules and papules that spread to produce annular target and arciform lesions. Involvement of the oral and nasal mucosa, pinnae, axillae, and groin areas is common. Most documented cases of erythema multiforme in dogs and cats are associated with drug hypersensitivity, while neoplasia and infection are less common initiators. Food additives have been suspected in some cases but the cases are poorly documented. Further studies are needed to document adverse reactions to pet food additives and the responsible mechanisms.

Another cause of food intolerance is pharmacologic reactions to substances found in food. Vasoactive amines such as histamine have been shown to cause clinical signs in human beings, when present in excessive levels in food. Scombroid fishes such as tuna, mackerel, skipjack, and bonito, which undergo bacterial spoilage before consumption, are a frequent cause of histamine toxicosis in human beings. The usual clinical signs include diarrhea, flushing, sweating, nausea, vomiting, urticaria, facial swelling, and erythroderma. Recent surveys of histamine in pet foods found the highest levels of histamine in canned fish-based cat foods or cat foods containing fish solubles. Other vasoactive amines such as tyramine, spermine, spermidine, phenethylamine, putrescine, and cadaverine have also been found in pet foods. What role histamine and other vasoactive amines play in food intolerance in animals is unknown. Vasoactive amines may not be present in levels high enough to cause clinical signs but could lower the threshold levels for allergens in individual dogs and cats. In allergic animals, commercial foods that contain fish ingredients should probably be avoided unless they are known to be free from vasoactive amines.

THE IDEAL ELIMINATION FOOD

Dietary elimination trials are the main diagnostic method used in dogs and cats with suspected adverse food reactions. Intradermal skin testing, radioallergosorbent (RAST) tests, and enzyme-linked immunosorbent assay (ELISA) testing for food hypersensitivity are considered unreliable in animals with dermatologic disease (see pp. 526 and 560).

The ideal elimination food should include a reduced number of novel, highly digestible protein sources, avoid protein excesses, avoid additives and vasoactive amines, and be nutritionally adequate for the animal's life stage and condition. Ingredients in an ideal elimination food should provide a limited number of novel protein sources. Preferably, the food should contain one to two different types of protein to which the animal has not been previously exposed, often including a commercial or homemade food with one animal protein source and one vegetable protein source. In the dermatologic patient, excess dietary protein levels should be avoided to reduce the amount of potential allergens to which the animal is exposed. Dietary protein level of 16 to 20% (dry matter basis) for adult dogs and 30 to 40% (dry matter basis) for adult cats are recommended. In patients with hypoproteinemia, hypoalbuminemia, and/or weight loss associated with severe gastrointestinal disease, a higher dietary protein level may be necessary for counteracting gastrointestinal losses.

Digestibility of the dietary protein is also an important consideration when one assesses an elimination diet. Complete digestion of food protein results in free amino acids and small peptides, which are poor antigens. Thus, an incompletely digested food protein has the potential to incite an allergic response because of residual antigenic proteins and large polypeptides. Protein digestibility has been documented for some commercial pet foods marketed as hypoallergenic or elimination diets. A protein digestibility of greater than 90% is recommended for such foods.

Although specific pet food additives have not been documented as causing adverse food reactions, generally food additives should be avoided in elimination diets. The ideal elimination diet should avoid ingredients, such as fish, that are known to contain higher levels of vasoactive amines, such as histamine.

Finally, although elimination trials are usually performed for only 4 to 12 weeks, the food used in the trial should be nutritionally complete and balanced for the intended species, age, and lifestyle of the animal. Many specialists recommend at least 6-week trials for cats and 8-week trials for dogs. Elimination food trials are often performed in young animals, in whom the use of nutritionally inadequate foods is more likely to result in nutritional disease.

HOMEMADE ELIMINATION FOODS

In a survey of veterinarians in the American Academy of Veterinary Dermatology, homemade foods were recommended most often as the initial test diets for dogs and cats with suspected food allergy. Homemade test diets usually include a single protein source or a combination of a single protein source and a single carbohydrate source. The ingredients recommended most often for homemade feline foods include lamb baby food, lamb, rice, and rabbit. The ingredients recommended most often for homemade canine foods include lamb, rice, potato, fish, rabbit, venison, and tofu.

In the previously mentioned survey, most of the homemade foods recommended for the initial management of dogs and cats with suspected food allergy were nutritionally inadequate for growth or adult maintenance. This failure to meet nutritional requirements occurs in most homemade foods because rations are devised to include a minimum of ingredients. In general, homemade foods lack a source of calcium, essential fatty acids, certain vitamins, and other micronutrients.

The use of nutritionally inadequate homemade foods in young dogs and cats for more than 3 weeks may result in nutritional disease. In experimental studies, clinical signs of anorexia and poor growth occur in puppies within 10 to 20 days of starting a thiamine-deficient diet. Anecdotally, many practitioners report similar signs in young dogs on 3 to 4 weeks of homemade diets. Anorexia and emesis also appear within 1 to 2 weeks of feeding a thiamine-deficient diet in cats. Many previously recommended homemade elimination diets have a severe inverse calcium-phosphorus ratio of 1:10. Diets with this severe mineral imbalance can cause skeletal disease in young dogs within 4 weeks and should not be fed for longer than 3 weeks. In young growing animals, a source of calcium, such as additive-free oyster shell calcium (calcium carbonate), should always be used in homemade recipes. Most homemade foods require a specific calcium supplement. When the protein fraction equals or is greater than the carbohydrate fraction, usually only calcium carbonate is needed, at a dose of 0.5 g/5 kg of body weight (BW) per day in cats and at least 2.0 g for a 15-kg dog. Additive free calcium carbonate, containing 40% calcium, is available in most grocery stores and pharmacies in tablets of various sizes. When the protein fraction is less than the carbohydrate fraction, an additive-free calcium phosphorus supplement is sufficient. Dicalcium phosphate contains approximately 18 to 24% calcium and 18% phosphorus and should be fed at the same dose as calcium carbonate.

Complete and balanced homemade food recipes are available in other references. Nonflavored, additive-free vitamin and mineral supplements that do not contain animal or vegetable protein are unlikely to be a source of ingested allergens and should be used in all homemade diets. Intolerance to calcium supplements in atopic children has been reported but is rare. Calcium supplementation should be routinely used in homemade recipes for dogs and cats younger than 10 months of age. A source of essential fatty acids, such as vegetable oil, should also be included in homemade rations. Studies show that human beings allergic to peanuts and soybeans can safely ingest peanut oil or soybean oil. This fact supports the concept that vegetable oils are not a routine source of ingested allergens and can be used in homemade rations. Fatty acid supplements that contain fish oils are more likely to be contaminated with trace amounts of protein. Recipes recommended for homemade foods should also provide the optimal amount of protein, and foods for cats should be supplemented with taurine, 250 mg daily for the average-sized cat.

COMMERCIAL ELIMINATION FOODS

A variety of limited and different protein foods are now being manufactured by several companies (Table 1). These commercial products are attractive because they are convenient, often contain novel protein sources, and are nutritionally complete and balanced for either dogs or cats. Protein digestibility has been compared for some of these commercial products and varies considerably. It is important to understand that few of these commercial foods have been adequately tested in dogs and cats with known adverse food reactions. To the author's knowledge, only a few commercial foods have undergone the scrutiny of a clinical trial in patients with dermatologic or gastrointestinal disease. In the published clinical trials using commercial foods, two thirds to three fourths of the patients with suspected adverse food reactions showed significant improvement in clinical signs.

TABLE 1. Commercial Pet Foods Marketed or Recommended as Hypoallergenic or Elimination Diets

	Manufacturer	Protein Sources*
Canine Canned Products		
Prescription Diet Canine d/d Lamb & Rice	Hill's	Rice, lamb, lamb liver
Prescription Diet Canine d/d Whitefish & Rice	Hill's	Whitefish, rice
Prescription Diet Canine u/d	Hill's	Chicken, egg, rice, pork liver
Prescription Diet Canine s/d	Hill's	Egg, pork liver
Limited Ingredient Lamb & Potato	IVD	Potato, lamb, lamb by-products, lamb liver
Limited Ingredient Venison & Potato	IVD	Potato, venison, venison by-products
Limited Ingredient Rabbit & Potato	IVD	Potato, rabbit, rabbit by-products
Limited Ingredient Duck & Potato	IVD	Potato, duck, duck by-products
Limited Ingredient Lamb & Potato	IVD	Potato, lamb, lamb by-products, lamb liver
Eukanuba Veterinary Diets Response Formula	Iams	Catfish, herring meal, potato, beet pulp
Lamb & Rice Diet	Lick Your Chops	Lamb, lamb liver, rice, quinoa, flax, kelp
Selected Protein Diet with Lamb & Rice	Waltham/Pedigree	Lamb by-products, lamb, rice, natural flavors
Selected Protein Diet with Chicken	Waltham/Pedigree	Poultry by-products, chicken, rice, natural flavors
Selected Protein Diet with Venison	Waltham/Pedigree	Venison, venison by-products, rice, natural flavors
Canine Anergen	Wysong	Lamb, lamb liver, brown rice, flax, yeast
Specific Dermil	Leo	Mutton, rice
Canine Dry Products		
Prescription Diet Canine d/d Rice & Egg	Hill's	Rice, egg
Prescription Diet Canine u/d	Hill's	Rice, egg, whey
Prescription Diet Canine d/d Rice & Salmon	Hill's	Rice, salmon
Prescription Diet Canine d/d Rice & Duck	Hill's	Rice, duck by-products
Limited Ingredient Lamb & Potato	IVD	Potato, lamb, lamb meal, lamb digest
Limited Ingredient Venison & Potato	IVD	Potato, venison, venison meal, venison liver
Limited Ingredient Duck & Potato	IVD	Potato, duck meal, duck, duck digest
Limited Ingredient Lamb & Potato	IVD	Potato, lamb, lamb meal, lamb digest
Non-Meat Kibble	Nature's Recipe	Rice, soy, barley, carrots
CNM HA-Formula	Purina	Modified soy protein, corn starch
CNM LA-Formula	Purina	Rice, salmon meat, trout, canola meal, yeast
Eukanuba Veterinary Diets Response Formula	Iams	Potato, herring meal, catfish, beet pulp, fish digest
Canine Anergen	Wysong	Lamb meal, chicken, brown rice, flax, quinoa, yeast, kelp
Specific Dermil	Leo	Egg, rice
Selected Protein Diet with Rice & Catfish	Waltham/Pedigree	Rice, catfish meal, rice gluten, catfish, natural flavor
Canine Hypoallergenic Formula	MediCal	Oat flour, duck meal, oat bran, yeast, potato protein, duck digest
Feline Canned Diets		
Prescription Diet Feline d/d	Hill's	Lamb lungs, lamb liver, rice
Prescription Diet Feline c/d	Hill's	Beef lungs, pork liver, corn, glandular meal
Limited Ingredient Lamb & Potato	IVD	Lamb, lamb by-products, lamb liver, potato
Limited Ingredient Venison & Potato	IVD	Venison, venison by-products, venison liver, potato
Limited Ingredient Rabbit & Potato	IVD	Rabbit, rabbit by-products, potato
Eukanuba Veterinary Diets Response Formula LB	Iams	Lamb liver, lamb tripe, barley, lamb meal, beet pulp
Feline Anergen	Wysong	Lamb, lamb liver, brown rice, kelp, quinoa
Lamb & Rice Diet	Lick Your Chops	Lamb, lamb liver, brown rice, kelp
Selected Protein Diet with Venison & Rice	Waltham/Whiskas	Venison, venison by-products, rice, natural flavors
Feline Dry Diets		
Prescription Diet Feline c/d	Hill's	Rice, poultry meal, corn, glandular meal
Limited Ingredient Lamb & Potato	IVD	Potato, lamb, lamb meal
Limited Ingredient Venison & Potato	IVD	Potato, venison, venison meal, venison liver, venison digest
Limited Ingredient Duck & Potato	IVD	Potato, duck, duck meal, duck digest
Feline Anergen	Wysong	Poultry, poultry meal, rice, oats, lamb meal, liver digest, flax, kelp, yeast
Feline Hypoallergenic/Gastro Formula	MediCal	Oat flour, duck meal, potato protein, duck digest, yeast, oat bran

*Sources obtained from ingredient list on information panel of package or manufacturer's technical information. (Modified from Roudebush P, Guilford WG, Shanley KJ: Adverse reactions to food. In: Hand MS, Thatcher CD, Remillard RL, eds: Small Animal Clinial Nutrition IV. Topeka, KS: Mark Morris Institute [in press], with permission.)

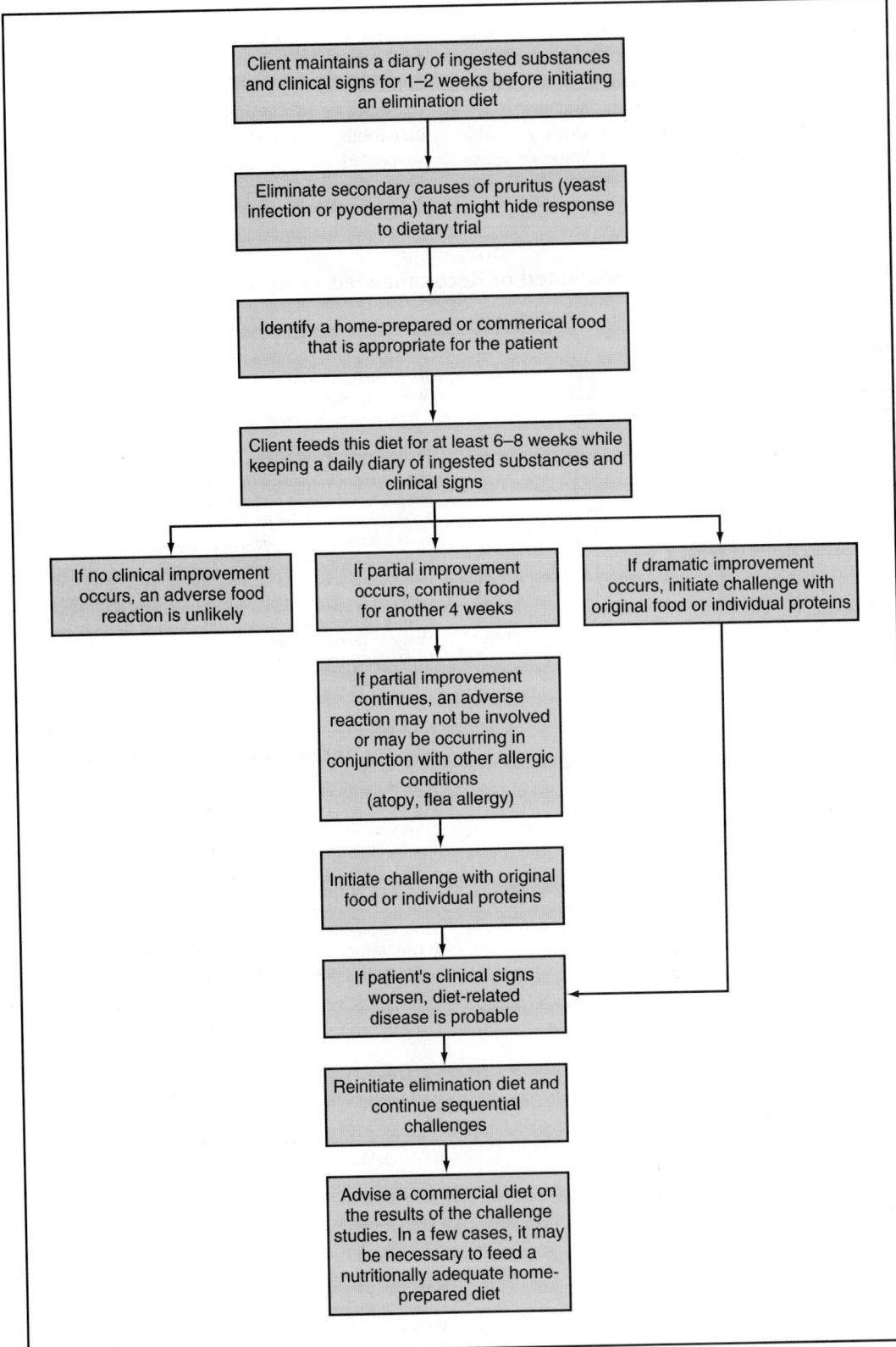

Figure 1. Preparation for and performance of an elimination trial in the patient with dermatologic disease. (Modified and redrawn from Roudebush P, Guilford WG, Shanley KJ: Adverse reactions to food. In: Hand MS, Thatcher CD, Remillard RL, eds: Small Animal Clinical Nutrition IV. Topeka, KS: Mark Morris Institute [in press], with permission.)

PERFORMING AN ELIMINATION TRIAL IN PATIENTS WITH DERMATOLOGIC DISEASE

Before an elimination diet is initiated, it is useful for the client to keep the dog or cat on its usual food for 7 to 14 days (Fig. 1). During this time, the client should record the type and amount of food ingested, any other ingested food items such as table scraps, treats, or snacks, and the occurrence and character of adverse reactions. Causes of pruritus such as *Malassezia* infection, flea infestation, or pyoderma should be eliminated before initiating the dietary trial. The patient is then placed on a controlled elimination food for 6 to 12 weeks. In addition to the dietary change, no other ingested substances, including treats, flavored vitamin supplements, chewable heartworm prevention tablets, fatty acid supplements, and chew toys, should be offered. Dogs or cats that roam or hunt outdoors should be confined during the trial. During the dietary elimination trial, the client should continue daily documentation of the type and amount of food ingested, and the occurrence and character of adverse reactions. This daily diary is important for documenting both the progression of clinical signs during the elimination trial and whether a strict elimination trial has been performed in the home environment. The diary often documents different findings from those offered to the clinician by the client during the recheck examination.

In dermatologic patients, a tentative diagnosis of an adverse food reaction is made if the level of pruritus markedly decreases. This improvement may be gradual and may take 6 to 12 weeks to become evident.

A diagnosis of adverse food reaction is confirmed if the animal's former diet and other ingested substances are subsequently offered as a challenge, with a return of clinical signs within 10 to 14 days. Reinstituting the elimination diet should resolve the clinical signs induced by the food challenge. Food challenge can be performed in an "open," "single-blind," or "double-blind" manner. In an open food challenge, both the client and the veterinarian are aware that a specific food or previous diet is being fed. In a single-blind food challenge, only the client is unaware of what food is being given. In a double-blind food challenge, both the client and the veterinarian are unaware of whether a specific food is being given. Double-blind, placebo-controlled food challenges are considered to be the "gold standard" for the diagnosis of adverse food reactions in human beings. Only half the human patients believed to be allergic to a food react to the food when they are challenged in controlled, blinded conditions. Unfortunately, all reports and most recommendations of food challenge in the veterinary literature have been open challenges. Open challenges will continue as the most practical method of establishing a tentative diagnosis of adverse food reaction in dogs and cats, but they are subject to false interpretation by both the client and the veterinarian.

Provocation involves introducing single dietary ingredients until as many positive reactions as possible can be documented. Clients and veterinarians are often reluctant to pursue challenge and provocation once clinical signs have improved or have been eliminated. Provocation may also be difficult in many dogs and cats because commercial pet foods contain such a large number of ingredients and because these ingredients often cannot be duplicated in challenge studies. As an example, use of chicken meat in a provocative food challenge may not duplicate the types of antigens found in poultry by-product meal.

Elimination trials are often difficult to interpret in some dogs and cats because of concurrent allergic skin disease. In several studies of food-allergic dogs and cats, 20 to 30% or more had concurrent hypersensitivities. The response to an elimination trial may be only partial in these patients. Flea-allergic dermatitis and atopy are the most common canine and feline allergies and should be eliminated through other diagnostic testing.

MONITORING THE PATIENT

For most adverse food reactions, avoiding the offending foods or food additives is the most effective treatment. How selective or meticulous an avoidance diet must be depends on the individual animal's sensitivity. Some dogs and cats may suffer adverse reactions to even trace quantities of an offending food or food additive, whereas others may have a higher tolerance level. Concurrent allergies influence the threshold level of clinical signs in some animals. Symptomatic therapy in pruritic animals can also include corticosteroids and antihistamines. Corticosteroids, along with dietary change, are often used in cats with inflammatory bowel disease.

One third of human beings on a strict avoidance diet for 1 to 2 years have tolerated the reintroduction of food allergens into their diet. This fact suggests that strict avoidance in animals with food allergy may allow some of these dogs and cats to tolerate exposure to certain food allergens later in life.

Both homemade and commercial foods can be used for long-term maintenance of patients with suspected food allergy. It is very important that any homemade recipe for long-term maintenance ensure a nutritionally adequate ration. An attempt should always be made to find an acceptable commercial food that will raise owner compliance with the dietary change and ensure a nutritionally adequate ration.

References and Suggested Reading

Brown CM, Armstrong PJ, Globus H: Nutritional management of food allergy in dogs and cats. Compend Contin Educ Pract Vet 17:637, 1995.
  Nutritionally complete and balanced homemade diet recipes are summarized.
Codner EC, Thatcher CD: The role of nutrition in the management of dermatoses. Semin Vet Med Surg 5:167, 1990.
  Nutritionally complete and balanced homemade diet recipes are summarized.
Remillard RL, Thatcher CD: Dietary and nutritional management of gastrointestinal diseases. Vet Clin North Am Small Anim Pract 19:809, 1989.
  Nutritionally complete and balanced homemade diet recipes are summarized.
Roudebush P: Pet food additives. J Am Vet Med Assoc 203:1667, 1993.
  A review of common pet food additives and their possible role in causing adverse food reactions in pets.
Roudebush P: Diagnosis and management of adverse food reactions. In: Bonagura JD, ed: Current Veterinary Therapy XII. Philadelphia: WB Saunders, 1995, p 59.
  A review of the terminology, pathophysiology, diagnosis, and treatment of adverse food reactions in dogs and cats.

Roudebush P, Cowell CS: Results of a hypoallergenic diet survey of veterinarians in North America with a nutritional evaluation of home-made diet prescriptions. Vet Dermatol 3:23, 1992.

Results of a diet survey that outlines the use of both commercial and homemade elimination diets for dogs and cats. Evaluations of homemade diet recipes recommended by veterinarians are also given.

Nonsteroidal Immunosuppressive Therapy

STEPHEN D. WHITE
Fort Collins, Colorado

The medications discussed in this article are used in veterinary dermatology to treat cases of *pemphigus, lupus erythematosus, bullous pemphigoid, erythema multiforme,* and other immune-mediated diseases. Although described as "immunosuppressive" drugs for the convenience of this article, they are perhaps better thought of as "immune-modulating" drugs, as their exact mechanism of action in the treatment of the preceding diseases has not been well documented in small animals. General aspects, uses, and adverse effects of the drugs are also discussed on page 509.

AZATHIOPRINE

Azathioprine (Imuran, Burroughs-Wellcome) is a purine analogue that was originally developed as an antineoplastic agent and is often used in the treatment of autoimmune disease in humans and dogs. Azathioprine is not always effective in inducing a remission of clinical signs of immune-mediated skin diseases and must be used in conjunction with corticosteroids. Because azathioprine is thus used as a means of maintaining a remission, it is often thought of as a "steroid-sparing" agent, allowing the clinician to decrease the initially high immunosuppressive dosages of corticosteroids used to induce remission or to eliminate the drug altogether. One may dramatically decrease the dosage of corticosteroids in many dogs once azathioprine is added to the treatment regimen; however, the point must be made that to the author's knowledge, there are no controlled studies in either human patients or dogs to support the concept of a steroid-sparing drug.

The most commonly used dosage in the dog is 2 mg/kg per day for 4 to 6 weeks; the frequency may then be reduced to every 48 hours. Azathioprine is available as a 50-mg tablet, which is easily broken in half. Azathioprine does not seem to reach full effectiveness until given for at least 3 to 6 weeks, during which time the clinician should try to slowly decrease the corticosteroid dosage as the disease is brought under control.

Side effects are relatively uncommon but include vomiting, bone marrow dyscrasias (especially thrombocytopenia), and rarely hepatotoxicity. These latter two side effects are somewhat surprising, as azathioprine has been used successfully in the dog as a treatment for immune-mediated thrombocytopenia (p. 438) as well as to induce immune suppression for experimental liver transplantation

in dogs. In humans, increases in myelosuppression are associated with low activity of an enzyme in the liver (thiopurine methyltransferase) that the body uses to detoxify the drug. The relevancy of this to dogs is uncertain. In humans, the drug allopurinol may interfere with another important azathioprine-metabolizing enzyme, xanthine oxidase, thus increasing myelosuppression; these two drugs should be used together with great caution. Because of the potential side effects, a complete blood count, platelet count, and liver enzyme panel should be performed once monthly during the first few months of azathioprine therapy, and ideally every 3 to 6 months thereafter. Some recommend more frequent monitoring of the complete blood count (e.g., every 2 to 3 weeks). The interpretation of the liver enzyme panel may be difficult, as the alkaline phosphatase will increase because of the concurrent use of corticosteroids. In general, the rapid elevation of alanine aminotransferase and gamma glutamyltransferase may be more reliable indicators of possible liver damage due to azathioprine.

It should be emphasized that, in the author's opinion, this drug is contraindicated in cats. It can induce a profound myelosuppression in this species, even at recommended dosages, and can be fatal. Chlorambucil or gold salts are the preferred drugs to use in the cat.

CHLORAMBUCIL

Chlorambucil (Leukeran, Burroughs Wellcome) is an alkylating agent similar to cyclophosphamide (p. 465). These drugs alter DNA synthesis and inhibit rapidly proliferating cells. Chlorambucil is administered orally at a dosage of 0.1 to 0.2 mg/kg every 24 hours (or 48 hours) in conjunction with prednisone or another oral corticosteroid. The small pill dose size of chlorambucil (2.0 mg) allows relatively easy dosing of small animals. Most cats require one-half tablet (1.0 mg) per day. Toxicities are uncommon but may include mild, gradual, and rapidly reversible bone marrow suppression. Anorexia, vomiting, and diarrhea have been reported but may resolve when the drug is changed from a daily to an alternate-day schedule.

Chlorambucil has been recommended as a routine treatment for feline pemphigus foliaceus and for severe recalcitrant cases of feline eosinophilic granuloma complex. Daily treatment in cats (0.1 to 0.2 mg/kg per day) is maintained until marked resolution of clinical signs has been achieved, or approximately 75% improvement is seen. This degree of improvement may require 4 to 8 weeks of treatment. Alternate-day chlorambucil is then initiated and maintained for several weeks provided that there is no exacerbation of clinical signs. After this, the concurrently used corticosteroid and chlorambucil are decreased alternately and gradually until the lowest possible maintenance dose is determined. Most cats do not require continued chlorambucil and may be maintained on low alternate-day doses of corticosteroids. However, each cat is unique and successful protocols vary. Animals should be monitored by complete blood and platelet counts every 2 weeks while receiving chlorambucil therapy. Dogs with pemphigus may be treated with the same protocol. Monitoring complete blood count and platelets in dogs may need to be carried out only once monthly.

NIACINAMIDE AND TETRACYCLINE

Niacinamide (the amide of niacin; nicotinamide in Europe) and tetracycline together have been effective in controlling approximately two thirds of the cases of discoid lupus erythematosus in dogs so treated by the author. These drugs in tandem have been shown to suppress neutrophil migration and histamine release by mast cells in vitro. How this relates to their efficacy in vivo is unclear. Dosage is 500 mg of each drug every 8 hours (in dogs weighing less than 10 kg, 250 mg of each drug every 8 hours; in dogs weighing less than 5 kg, 100 mg of each drug every 8 hours). Improvement is usually noted within 6 weeks. The ability to maintain improvement by decreasing the dosage or frequency is variable. Side effects are uncommon, but anorexia, lethargy, and vomiting (primarily due to the niacinamide) have been noted. This drug combination may occasionally be helpful in sterile pyogranulomas and idiopathic onychodystrophy.

GOLD

Gold salts have been used in humans, dogs, cats, and horses, primarily in the treatment of the pemphigus complex, and also in plasmacytic stomatitis and pharyngitis and plasmacytic pododermatitis of cats. Gold salts are contraindicated in cases of systemic lupus erythematosus, as their potential to cause blood dyscrasias and glomerulonephropathies may potentiate, trigger, or exacerbate these signs of systemic lupus erythematosus, or at any rate may confuse the clinician if they do occur. As with azathioprine and chlorambucil, corticosteroids must usually be used concurrently when treating pemphigus (see *CVT XII,* p. 636).

Gold salts have a wide range of effects, such as reduction of lysosomal enzymes, histamine, and prostaglandins. Gold salts are available in either injectable or oral forms. Aurothioglucose is available in 10-ml vials in a concentration of 50 mg/ml. Auranofin is available in a nonbreakable capsule of 3-mg strength. Of the injectable preparations, aurothioglucose (Solganal, Schering) is used most often in veterinary dermatology. The oral form, auranofin (Ridaura, Smith-Kline Beecham) does not seem to be as effective

and is more likely to cause gastrointestinal side effects; however, it is less likely to cause the severe side effects noted earlier, at least in humans. Aurothioglucose is used as a weekly intramuscular injection (the paraspinal muscles work best) at 1 mg/kg until 6 to 12 weeks of treatment, at which time the frequency may be decreased to biweekly and eventually once monthly if possible. Rarely, if the animal has been free of clinical signs for 6 months using once-monthly injections, the clinician may discontinue gold treatment. The author has used auranofin in dogs at a daily dose of 0.12 to 0.2 mg/kg b.i.d. Complete blood and platelet counts, serum enzyme profiles, and urinalysis (for evidence of glomerulonephropathy) should be performed once monthly for 2 to 3 months, then ideally every other month.

PENTOXIFYLLINE

Pentoxifylline (Trental, Hoechst-Roussel) is a methylxanthine derivative and has been found useful in the treatment of dermatomyositis, idiopathic ear margin dermatoses, rabies vaccination–induced alopecia, erythema multiforme, and atopy. Pentoxifylline has a number of actions, such as making the wall of the red blood cell more pliable and decreasing the ability of lymphocytes to adhere to keratinocytes. Pentoxifylline is available in 400-mg tablets and is best given with food. The dosage is 10 mg/kg b.i.d. The major side effect is vomiting. It may take 1 to 4 months to see an effect.

CYCLOSPORINE

Cyclosporine is a potent inhibitor of T-cell activation (discussed more fully on p.509; *CVT XII,* p. 73). In veterinary dermatology, cyclosporine has been used systemically in animals to treat pemphigus foliaceus (with limited success) and with sebaceous adenitis at a dose of 5 mg/kg b.i.d. The author has used cyclosporine topically in cases of discoid lupus erythematosus and idiopathic sterile granuloma of the muzzle or planum nasale. The drug is provided as a 1 or 2% ointment or solution. This is applied sparingly to the lesions two to three times daily until a positive response is seen (generally within 1 to 2 months); the frequency is then reduced to the lowest possible to maintain improvement. Side effects are uncommon, although with the immunosuppressive nature of this drug, one might expect focal infection of *Demodex canis, Malassezia pachydermatis,* dermatophytosis, or pyoderma if the solution is applied to the haired areas of the skin. Side effects noted with the systemic use of this drug (such as nephrotoxicity) have not been associated with topical use.

INTERFERON ALFA-2a

The drug interferon alfa-2a (Roferon-A, Hoffman-LaRoche) has been used in cats for treatment of indolent lip ulcers. Dosage in cats is 60 to 120 units/day orally or subcutaneously. Dosage is 1.5 to 2 million units/m^2 three times weekly, subcutaneously, when used to treat cutaneous T-cell lymphoma and for severe cases of oral and cutaneous papillomas. Malaise seems to be the primary but rare side effect. Mechanisms of action involve suppression of cell proliferation and enhancing antitumor activity in macrophages.

VITAMIN E

Vitamin E is an oil-soluble vitamin. It is composed of four fractions: alpha, beta, gamma, and delta. The alpha fraction is the most effective therapeutically and is available in *d* (natural), *dl* (synthetic), and mixed forms. Most of the work done with vitamin E has been with *d*-alpha-tocopherol acetate or succinate. In veterinary dermatology, vitamin E has been used to treat discoid lupus erythematosus, pemphigus erythematosus, dermatomyositis, epidermolysis bullosa, idiopathic acanthosis nigricans, and demodicosis.

The author generally uses vitamin E as adjunctive treatment in canine demodicosis, discoid lupus erythematosus, or acanthosis nigricans, at a dosage of 200 to 400 IU three times a day. Some advocate giving the vitamin on an empty stomach. Effectiveness is variable, but the vitamin appears relatively innocuous at these dosages.

References and Suggested Reading

Helton-Rhodes K: Feline immunomodulators. In: Bonagura JD, ed: Kirk's Current Veterinary Therapy XII. Philadelphia: WB Saunders, 1995, p 581.
A good review of various immune-modulating medications in the cat.
Kummel BA: Medical treatment of canine pemphigus-pemphigoid. In: Bonagura JD, ed: Kirk's Current Veterinary Therapy XII. Philadelphia: WB Saunders, 1995, p 636.
Good in-depth discussion of immunosuppressive agents useful in treating pemphigus and pemphigoid.
Rosenkrantz W: Immunomodulating drugs in dermatology. In: Kirk RW, Bonagura JD, eds: Current Veterinary Therapy X. Philadelphia: WB Saunders, 1989, p 570.
Previous review in this series with much still usable information, in particular mechanisms and pharmacokinetics.
Snow JL, Gibson LE: A pharmacogenetic basis for the safe and effective use of azathioprine and other thiopurine drugs in dermatologic patients. J Am Acad Dermatol 32:114, 1995.
An excellent introduction into the pharmacokinetics of adverse reactions of azathioprine in human beings.
White SD, Rosychuk RAW, Reinke SI, Paradis M: Tetracycline and niacinamide for treatment of autoimmune skin disease in 31 dogs. J Am Vet Med Assoc 220:1497, 1992.
Initial article on the use of these drugs in veterinary dermatology.

Essential Fatty Acids

RICHARD G. HARVEY
Coventry, United Kingdom

Essential fatty acid (EFA) supplementation is used increasingly in the management of dermatologic disease. In 1989, Muller and associates were advocating the empirical use of equal quantities of animal fat (lard) and vegetable fat as a supplement in cases characterized by a dull coat, scale, and chronic pruritus. This supplementation was sometimes accompanied by success. More recently, investigators have studied the use of supplements rich in linoleic acid (18:2n6 [LA]), gamma-linolenic acid (18:3n6 [GLA]), alpha-linolenic acid (18:3n3 [aLA]) and eicosapentaenoic acid (20:5n3 [EPA]), since these are the EFAs with the most promise as anti-inflammatory agents. This review considers the choices of EFA supplements available and the clinical use of these supplements in the management of dermatologic conditions in the dog and the cat.

SOURCES OF SUPPLEMENTAL ESSENTIAL FATTY ACIDS

Commercially prepared balanced diets, provided that they are properly stored and used within the product life, are adequately supplemented with EFAs for maintenance in almost all situations. Supplementation is usually part of a therapeutic strategy and the clinician has a number of disparate sources of EFA from which to choose, including those from specific animal, vegetable, fungal, and microbial sources. However, the principal sources of interest are those with high concentrations of the EFAs mentioned previously in a biologically available source. Suitable EFAs are found in oils from marine animals, particularly cold-water fish oils, and the seed oils of sunflower, evening primrose, borage, black currant, corn, flax, and other plants. A number of fungal sources such as oil of javanicus produced from *Mucor javanicus* are also rich in EFAs. Although these various oils are rich in EFAs, there is variation in the oil content, the proportion of the various EFAs, and the biologic availability of the EFAs among these products (Table 1).

Sunflower and Other Oils Rich in Linoleic Acid

Sunflower oil is high in LA and contains no GLA (see Table 1), but its anti-inflammatory effects have recently received attention. In addition to acting as substrate for subsequent biotransformation into other n:6 EFAs and eicosanoids, LA is important in its own right as a component of biologic membranes and for maintaining the integrity of the epidermal permeability barrier. One double-blinded clinical study (Harvey, 1993) demonstrated that sunflower oil was as efficacious as evening primrose oil in the management of feline inflammatory dermatoses, particularly papulocrustous (miliary) dermatitis. Furthermore, Campbell and associates (1992) demonstrated that the addition of

TABLE 1. A Comparison of the Levels of 18:2n6, 18:3n6, 18:3n3, and 20:5n3 in the Various Oils Available for Supplementation*

Oil Source	% Linoleic Acid 18:2n6	% Gamma-Linolenic Acid 18:3n6	% Alpha-Linolenic Acid 18:3n3	% Eicosapentaenoic Acid 20:5n3
Canola	21.1	0	9.1	0
Cold fish	3.58	3.8	0	57.90
Corn	59.0	0	0	0
Black currant	47.0	16.7	13.3	0
Borage	37.7	18.7	4.3	0
Flax	18.0	0	55.6	0
Evening primrose	72.0	10.0	0.2	0
Fungal (typical)	10.4	18.9	0	0
Safflower	76.05	0.47	0.5	0
Soybean	52.0	0	7.4	0
Sunflower	52.0	0	0.3	0

*Note: These are typical values; relative concentrations will vary from batch to batch.

sunflower oil to the diet of dogs with seborrhea was beneficial and resulted in normalization of the previously abnormal concentrations of fatty acids within the skin. It may be that sunflower oil acts to decrease the inflammatory milieu via hydroxy acid synthesis and membrane effects rather than through the more specific anti-inflammatory actions that have been suggested to explain the effects of fish oils and GLA. If LA does possess an anti-inflammatory action, its low cost makes it an attractive choice as a dietary supplement. However, more studies on the value of this oil in managing canine atopy, in particular, are necessary before it can be recommended without reservation. Other seed oils with a relatively high LA content include those derived from black currant, borage, corn, evening primrose, safflower, and soybean. The low cost of some these oils makes them attractive propositions, if proved efficacious.

Evening Primrose Oil, Rich in Gamma-Linolenic Acid

Evening primrose oil contains not only LA but also high concentrations of GLA (at 8 to 10% of the triglyceride fraction; see Table 1). Although evening primrose oil has an absolute level of GLA that is lower than that found in borage seed oil, there are stereochemical factors that appear to render it a better biologic source of GLA (Gunstone, 1992; Lawson and Hughes, 1988). The anti-inflammatory role of evening primrose oil is believed to result from the presence of GLA and its ability to act as a substrate for anti-inflammatory eicosanoid production. There are several clinical studies in both dogs and cats that have demonstrated usefulness in the management of inflammatory dermatoses, in particular atopy in the dog. There is little doubt that evening primrose oil has a useful anti-inflammatory effect, but the principal drawback against high-dose use of evening primrose oil is expense. One factor that has received little attention to date is the potential for interaction between LA and GLA. It may be that the concentration of these oils in the animal's normal diet has significant effects on the clinical efficacy of supplemental oils. This has been

suggested as an explanation for the poor clinical efficacy of evening primrose oil in some human studies.

Borage Seed Oil, Rich in Gamma-Linolenic Acid

Borage seed oil contains a high concentration of GLA in addition to LA (see Table 1). Although there is some evidence to suggest that stereochemical factors may reduce the biologic availability of this GLA, with such a high concentration, even a less efficient molecular structure may yield useful amounts of GLA for absorption. Borage seed oil certainly has been shown in experimental models to have measurable anti-inflammatory effects. At least one commercial presentation of borage oil, Viacutan (Boehringer-Ingelheim), is available for dogs and cats in the United Kingdom, and a double-blinded, placebo-controlled study has demonstrated its value in the management of atopy in dogs (Harvey, 1999).

Other Vegetable and Fungal Oils as Sources of n:6 Essential Fatty Acids

Other seed oils that have received attention in the human health supplement field include black currant seed oil and the various fungal oils. Their use is advocated on low cost, compared with the oil of evening primrose, and to a high GLA content (see Table 1). However, the efficiency of enzymatic cleavage of the various triglycerides, and hence their net potential for anti-inflammatory action, is not known. Although most of these oils are available as human supplements, there are limited data describing experimental anti-inflammatory potential or clinical efficacy in animals. Other vegetable oils rich in GLA that have the potential for use as supplements include gooseberry seed oil (10 to 12% GLA), red currant seed oil (4 to 5% GLA), and comfrey seed (26% GLA).

Some seed oils (e.g., soy, canola, and flax) contain both LA and aLA. Flax seed oil in particular is potentially useful because it contains large concentrations of aLA, which is unusual for a plant source. Controlled studies are necessary to screen these less expensive oils for clinical efficacy. Many microbes produce clinically useful concentrations of EFAs, and although these oils contain high concentrations of GLA it is often in association with lower concentrations of LA than is found in vegetable oils. Some of these oils are produced on a commercial basis, but there are no data on their use in animals.

Cold-Water Fish Oils as Sources of n:3 Essential Fatty Acids

Cold fish oils contain relatively high concentrations of n:3 EFA and their usefulness derives from the interaction of n:3-derived EFA as competitive substrate (competing with n:6 EFA) and as n:3-derived anti-inflammatory eicosanoids. Fish oils have been shown to be useful in experimental anti-inflammatory models and in a few controlled clinical studies. Logas and Kunkle (1994) showed that high doses (180 mg EPA and 120 mg docosahexaenoic acid per 4.55 kg weight PO every 24 hours) of marine fish oils were far superior to corn oil in controlling pruritus, self-trauma, and coat gloss in pruritic dogs—principally those with atopy or atopy and fleabite hypersensitivity. However, most work from experimental models and human studies appears to suggest that although n:3 EFAs are beneficial, they are much more efficacious if mixed with n:6 supplements (see further on). The big advantage of cold-water fish oils is that they are inexpensive. However, they are also rich in saturated fat, in addition to EFAs. Supplementing these oils in high doses may add to the total dietary fat and caloric intake of the animal considerably.

Vegetable Seed Oils as Sources of n:3 Essential Fatty Acids

Some seed oils contain n:3 EFA in addition to n:6 EFA. Examples include corn, canola, soybean, and particularly flax seed oils. Black currant seed oil contains the attractive mix of LA, GLA, and aLA, which suggests that it deserves further investigation in the clinical setting. Given the possibility that a combination of n:6 and n:3 oils may be more useful, from a clinical point of view, than either n:6 or n:3 oils used alone, the yet to be proven potential of these oils is apparent.

n:3 or n:6 Essential Fatty Acids?

The relative superiority of n:3 over n:6 as the sole EFA supplement is unresolved, principally because of the lack of a single, blinded study comparing n:3 and n:6 efficacy. The only blinded study comparing n:3 and n:6 efficacy (Logas and Kunkle, 1994) used corn oil as the n:6 EFA, arguably more of a placebo than a positive control and certainly not a source of n:6 EFA that would be chosen today if one was looking to demonstrate efficacy. This general paucity of published data on the clinical use of n:3 EFA supplements is in contrast to the situation with n:6 EFA, for which there have been several blinded studies investigating both n:6 and mixtures of n:6–n:3 supplementation in both dogs and cats.

In certain experimental inflammatory models, it has been clearly demonstrated that a mixture of n:6 and n:3 EFA is more effective than either n:6 or n:3 alone (Miller et al, 1991). Most of these studies recommend a ratio as high as 3 or 4 parts n:6 to 1 part n:3 as optimal for anti-inflammatory action. One of the problems experienced in determining ratios of n:6 to n:3 dietary supplements in practice is the composition of the diet of the animal, since it is the composition of the EFA in the diet as a whole that is important, rather than that of the supplement alone. In this regard, the controlled study by Vaughn and colleagues (1994) was most interesting. They concluded that a diet formulated to contain between 5 and 10 parts n:6 to one part n:3 demonstrated the most anti-inflammatory action in their canine model. Clearly these contradictions require resolution before firm recommendations can be made, but providing a diet with optimized EFA composition is obviously preferable to adding supplementary EFAs to a diet whose composition can only be guessed at.

INDICATIONS FOR SUPPLEMENTATION

Dogs With Atopy

Many atopic dogs respond well to immunotherapy. However, a significant proportion require adjunctive antipruritic therapy, and those dogs that do not respond to immunotherapy will require other treatment. There have been a number of clinical reports on the efficacy of supplemental EFAs in the management of canine atopy (Miller et al, 1989; Scarff and Lloyd, 1992; Harvey, 1999). Atopy is important in clinical practice, and there are both medical and client-driven pressures to avoid, or at least minimize, the chronic use of systemic glucocorticoids. Almost all studies into EFA supplementation in dogs have been performed using evening primrose oil as the source of n:6 EFA. The comments made earlier on other sources of EFA should be borne in mind, as it may be that other, less expensive, sources of n:6 EFA are equally effective in practice.

Consideration of the knowledge gleaned from clinical trials of EFA therapy in dogs with atopy suggests five basic rules to EFA supplementation in atopic dogs:

- EFAs will not be effective in the face of significant inflammation, be it due to bacteria, yeast, or xerosis.
- EFA response is dose-related.
- The effect of EFA is associated with a lag period of at least 3 weeks. Maximal benefit may not be appreciated until after 3 months of treatment, although this has recently been challenged (Scott et al, 1997).
- Additive effects (and possibly synergism) are apparent with certain antihistamines.
- Even if not able to alleviate systemic glucocorticoid therapy, EFAs can, in some cases, significantly reduce glucocorticoid requirement.

The most important guide to the management of atopic dogs is the recognition of the degree of pruritus that can result from microbial infection of the skin. Staphylococcal infection and colonization of the skin by *Malassezia pachydermatis* can result in severe inflammation, pruritus, and self-trauma (see p. 574). Thus adjunctive topical antimicrobial shampoos (e.g., those containing chlorhexidine and miconazole) and strategic use of systemic bactericidal and antibacterial agents are indicated in most atopic dogs. Extensive areas of alopecic and erythematous skin can become xerotic and pruritic. Topical humectant therapy can be beneficial in these cases (see *CVT XII,* p. 590). Control of these factors will result in much less inflamed skin and provide the best chance of a nonsteroidal anti-inflammatory agent (EFA or antihistamine) being effective.

The dose responsiveness of EFA therapy is somewhat unfamiliar to clinicians used to prescribing fixed dose rates according to data sheets. Clinicians should be wary, however, of recommending that supplemental oils be administered on a "higher the better" basis without making some effort to assess the animal's intake of total dietary fat and attendant calories. The author currently uses a commercial blend of evening primrose oil and fish oils (Efavet Regular Capsules, Efamol Vet) at an initial dose of four capsules per 10 kg weight every 24 hours PO, which provides 2.7 gm LA, 136 mg GLA, and 68 mg EPA per 10 kg body weight. Other veterinary products available include Dermcaps and 3V Caps (DVM Pharmaceuticals); EFA-CAPS (Allerderm/Virbac); Pet-Derm O.M. CAPS (SmithKline-Beecham); and Omega-3 Fatty Acid Capsules (Vet Solutions). It is important to remember the possibility of a lag period because very pruritic dogs cannot be expected to respond quickly. The author cautions owners not to expect any significant response for 3 to 4 weeks and explains that maximal response may take up to 3 months. Clients are often all too familiar with the rapid effect of systemic glucocorticoids and communication must be good. In some cases, a short (7- to 10-day) course of systemic glucocorticoid may be necessary to suppress severe pruritus (see *CVT XII,* p. 573).

If treatment with EFAs alone is not sufficient to control pruritus in atopic dogs, clinicians should consider adding an antihistamine to the treatment regimen (also see page 48). Studies in both North America and Europe have shown that additive effects (and possibly synergistic effects) appear to develop with these treatments (Paradis et al, 1991; Paterson, 1995). Chlorpheniramine (0.22 to 0.4 mg/kg PO every 8 hours), clemastine (0.1 mg PO every 12 hours), and hydroxyzine (2.2 mg/kg PO every 8 hours) are the antihistamines most likely to demonstrate additive activity. It is generally considered that a period of 2 to 3 weeks should be allowed before assessment of efficacy is made. Since each of the antihistamines listed is from a different class of drug, one may conclude that failure to respond to one does not preclude one or more drugs of the other two classes being effective. It seems reasonable to suggest that since EFAs take time to effect a response, the clinician should be aware of this before concluding that additive effects do not exist. Certainly a period of at least 4 weeks from the onset of EFA supplementation would appear prudent.

If EFAs alone or EFAs and antihistamines prove ineffective, and the dog has failed to respond to immunotherapy, the clinician may have to consider systemic therapy with prednisolone, prednisone, or methylprednisolone. Again, the preceding comments on control of infection and xerosis are pertinent. Bond and Lloyd (1994) demonstrated that concurrent use of EFAs allows a significant reduction in the dose of prednisolone necessary to control signs of atopy in dogs refractory to other treatments. These workers achieved a mean reduction in prednisolone dose on the order of 56%.

Dogs With Idiopathic Defects in Keratinization (Seborrhea)

Campbell and colleagues (1992) reported that supplementing the diet of dogs with idiopathic defects in keratinization with sunflower oil (1.5 ml/kg every 24 hours PO) was beneficial. They found that administration of oral sunflower oil resulted in the amelioration of clinical signs and changes in EFA both within the skin and in serum. Specifically, there was an elevation of 18:2n6 and 18:3n6 in the serum and skin samples and a fall in 20:4n6 in both the serum and skin. This is particularly interesting, as it suggests that sunflower oil (which is low in 18:3n6 but high in 18:2n6) can produce changes similar to those attributed to oils much richer in 18:3n6.

Pruritic Cats

Fleabite hypersensitivity, atopy, concurrent fleabite hypersensitivity and atopy, or idiopathic pruritus and bilateral alopecia are the most common feline conditions that have been treated with EFAs. Fleabite hypersensitivity is best treated with topical/systemic flea control combined with effective environmental treatments. Some cats will remain partially or totally refractory to flea control and may be suffering from concurrent atopy or their lifestyle may result in regular reinfection. These cats may well respond to therapy with EFAs. Patently, those cats with atopy that is not complicated by fleabite hypersensitivity are also suitable candidates for EFA therapy. These cats may present with a variety of clinical signs, such as crusted papules, bilateral alopecia, and pruritus. These dermatoses are generally not extremely pruritic, in contrast to eosinophilic plaque. Rasmussen and Svendsen (1991) reported some success in managing symmetrical alopecia and eosinophilic plaque with evening primrose oil, which is interesting because the author has found these conditions difficult to manage with EFAs alone. Most published studies of EFA therapy in cats have used a combination of evening primrose oil and fish oil at the dose of one capsule (delivering 675 mg LA, 34 mg GLA, and 17 mg EPA) per cat every 24 hours PO. Capsules may be placed directly into the cat's oropharynx or cut and mixed into the food. If the latter course of action is taken, the food should be eaten within a short time because the oils may oxidize if allowed to stand.

Both sunflower oil and evening primrose oil have been shown to be useful in the management of feline dermatoses characterized by crusting papules (Harvey, 1993). This is somewhat surprising because cats have little ability to metabolize 18:2n6 into 18:3n6, the putative anti-inflammatory component of evening primrose oil.

References and Suggested Reading

Bond R, Lloyd DH: Combined treatment with concentrated essential fatty acids and prednisolone in the management of canine atopy. Vet Rec 134:30, 1994.

Demonstrates that EFA supplementation can reduce steroid requirement.

Campbell KA, Uhland CF, Dorn GP: Effects of oral sunflower oil on serum and cutaneous fatty acid concentration profiles in seborrheic dogs. Vet Dermatol 3:29, 1992.
Demonstrates that sunflower oil can have effects on EFA metabolism.

Gunstone FD: Gamma linolenic acid—occurrence and physical and chemical properties. Prog Lipid Res 31:145, 1992.
Reviews natural sources of gamma-linolenic acid.

Harvey RG: A comparison of evening primrose oil and sunflower oil for the management of papulocrustous dermatitis in cats. Vet Rec 133:571, 1993.
Demonstrates that sunflower oil is as efficacious as evening primrose oil in the management of papulocrustous dermatitis in cats.

Harvey RG: A double-blinded, prospective, placebo-controlled paralled study into the efficacy of borage and fish oil in the management of canine atopy. Vet Rec 1999, in press.

Lawson LD, Hughes BG: Triacyl structure of plant and fungal oils containing linolenic acid. Lipids 23:313, 1988.
Explains why a high concentration of GLA does not necessarily mean that a given oil will have a high biologic yield.

Logas D, Kunkle GA: Double-blinded crossover study with marine oil supplementation containing high-dose eicosapentaenoic acid for the treatment of canine pruritic skin disease. Vet Dermatol 5:99, 1994.
The only clinical paper, to date, that compares fish oils with an n:6 EFA source.

Miller CC, Tang W, Ziboh VA, et al: Dietary supplementation with ethyl ester concentrates of fish oil (n-3) and borage oil (n-6) polyunsaturated fatty acids induces epidermal generation of local putative anti-inflammatory metabolites. J Invest Dermatol 96:98, 1991.
Demonstrates that mixtures of n:6 and n:3 EFAs may be more efficient, in an anti-inflammatory role, than either used alone.

Miller WH, Griffin CE, Scott DW, et al: Clinical trial of DVM Derm Caps in the treatment of allergic disease in dogs: A nonblinded study. J Am Anim Hosp Assoc 25:163, 1989.

One of the first publications to report that EFAs were useful in practice.

Muller GH, Kirk RW, Scott DW: Small Animal Dermatology, 4th ed. Philadephia: WB Saunders, 1989, p 725.
Standard text on dermatology.

Paradis M, Lemay S, Scott DW: Efficacy of clemastine (Tavist), a fatty acid-containing product (Derm Caps), and the combination of both products in the management of canine pruritus. Vet Dermatol 2:17, 1991.
Demonstrates that concurrent use of EFA and an antihistamine might have additive effects in dogs.

Paterson S: Additive benefits of EFAs in dogs with atopic dermatitis after partial response to antihistamine therapy. J Small Anim Pract 36:389, 1995.
Demonstrates that concurrent use of EFAs and antihistamines might have additive effects in dogs.

Rasmussen M, Svendsen AM: Katte med alopecia. Dansk Veterinærtidsskrift 74:15, 1991.
Demonstrates that EFAs are useful in the management of feline dermatoses, principally pruritic ones.

Scarff DH, Lloyd DH: Double blind, placebo controlled, crossover study of evening primrose oil in the treatment of canine atopy. Vet Rec 131:97, 1992.
The first publication to demonstrate that EFAs were superior to placebo in the management of atopy.

Scott DW, Miller WH, Reinhart GA, et al: Effect of an omega-3/omega-6 fatty acid containing commercial lamb and rice diet on pruritus in atopic dogs: Results of a single blinded study. Can J Vet Res 61:145, 1997.

Vaughn DM, Reinhart GA, Swaim SF, et al: Evaluation of effects of dietary n-6 to n-3 fatty acid ratios on leukotriene B synthesis in dog skin and neutrophins. Vet Dermatol 5:163, 1994.
Demonstrates that certain ratios of n:3 to n:6 EFAs appear to be superior to others in decreasing some components of the inflammatory response.

Pruritus Therapy in the Cat

LINDA M. MESSINGER
Denver, Colorado

Pruritus stems from *prurire,* which is Latin for "to itch." Pruritus has been defined as an "unpleasant sensation that provokes the desire to scratch." It is a sensation that is limited to the skin. The pathophysiology of pruritus is not well understood. The somatosensory receptor units involved in pruritus (and pain) are known as nociceptors and are supplied by the myelinated Aδ and nonmyelinated C fibers. Many mediators and modulators of pruritus exist, including histamine, eicosanoids, serotonin, platelet-activating factor, various proteases and peptides, and others. The pruritic stimulus travels from peripheral to central pathways, where processing occurs. In the sensory cortex, modification of the original stimulus may occur because of emotional factors (e.g., stress, boredom, anxiety) and other competing cutaneous sensations.

Physiologic pruritus is thought to be a well-adapted sensation that induces scratching to remove potentially noxious or damaging stimuli. Mild pruritus is encountered routinely in everyday life and is a trivial phenomenon. However, severe or intense pruritus can be extremely distressing and can interfere with one's quality of life. In veterinary medicine, quality of life issues are not limited to the pruritic animal. The quality of life of many owners is also affected by their pruritic pet. For example, many owners are kept awake at night by the constant scratching, rubbing, or licking noises made by the pet or are affected by the emotional distress of seeing their pet uncomfortable or alopecic.

Pruritus is a common chief complaint on presentation to a veterinarian and is a sign of many different diseases. Ideally, the underlying cause of pruritus in the cat should be identified and subsequently removed, treated, or avoided. Therapy with glucocorticosteroids has been the mainstay of treatment in alleviating pruritus in the cat (see *CVT XII,* p. 573). In addition to glucocorticosteroids, antipruritic therapies or devices used in the cat include antihistamines, fatty acids, psychotropic drugs, progestogens, immunotherapy, topical therapies, and mechanical barriers. The first choice of therapy for pruritus varies with the underlying disorder (see other articles in this section) and the experience of the clinician as well as other factors (e.g., concurrent diseases). The feline patient may be difficult to medicate, especially topically or orally. Owners should be instructed on how to properly medicate their cats, which enhances therapeutic success (see p. 21). Although the author has endeavored to provide accurate and comprehensive dosing guidelines, before prescribing, the clinician should read all label inserts for possible drug interactions, disease contraindications, and potential adverse effects.

GLUCOCORTICOSTEROIDS

Glucocorticosteroids are potent, broad-spectrum anti-inflammatory agents that are commonly used in the management of the pruritic feline patient. Anti-inflammatory dosages are higher than those used in the dog. Injectable methylprednisolone acetate (Depo-Medrol, Upjohn) is most commonly used; the typical dose is 20 mg per average 10-pound cat or 4 to 5 mg/kg subcutaneously or intramuscularly. Other glucocorticosteroids used to manage the pruritic cat include oral prednisone and prednisolone starting at 1.1 to 2.2 mg/kg every 24 hours and tapering to the lowest effective dose. A better response may be seen with prednisolone than with prednisone (Power, 1993/1994). Oral methylprednisolone (0.8 to 2.0 mg/kg every 24 hours and then tapered), oral dexamethasone (0.25 mg every 12 to 24 hours, then tapered to one to three times per week or less) and oral triamcinolone (0.5 to 0.75 mg/kg per day for 3 to 10 days and then tapered to every 3 to 4 days) are also used to treat the pruritic cat. If one steroid is not effective in a particular patient, other steroid types may be.

Fortunately, cats tend to tolerate glucocorticosteroids better than do dogs and humans. This difference may in part be due to the lower number and affinity of dexamethasone-binding receptors in the liver and epidermis of cats compared with dogs (van den Broek and Stafford, 1992). However, adverse effects from glucocorticosteroids may still be observed. The more common adverse effects include polyuria, polydipsia, polyphagia, weight gain, diabetes mellitus, and iatrogenic Cushing's disease. In addition, steroid tachyphylaxis may occur. Thus, when glucocorticosteroids are used on a chronic or frequent basis or when they are contraindicated by the presence of certain diseases or medications, nonsteroidal therapeutic options should be sought.

ANTIHISTAMINES

Antihistamines reversibly block H_1 receptors in the skin and other organs, thereby decreasing pruritus, erythema, and edema. Antihistamines may also have some local anesthetic actions and many cross the blood-brain barrier, causing sedative effects (see also p. 48). Greater benefit often is derived when the antihistamine is administered before histamine release. Thus, in the chronically pruritic patient, prophylactic use may be warranted instead of use on an as-needed basis. Antihistamine therapy tends to be more efficacious in the allergic cat than in the allergic dog. Generally, a 7- to 21-day trial period per antihistamine is advised.

The most commonly used antihistamine for the pruritic cat is chlorpheniramine maleate. In one study (Miller and Scott, 1990), 73% of the cats studied had an excellent response to chlorpheniramine dosed at 2 mg per cat PO every 12 hours. Reported response rates of pruritic cats given chlorpheniramine from noncontrolled studies or clinical impressions varied from 0 to 73%. The most common dose is 2 to 4 mg per cat PO every 12 hours. On rare occasions, maintenance therapy of 2 to 4 mg per cat PO every 24 hours may be maintained; alternate-day therapy was ineffective.

Adverse effects most commonly noted with chlorpheniramine maleate in cats include transient drowsiness and unpalatability. Occasionally, vomiting, diarrhea, and hyperexcitability have been observed. In the United States, chlorpheniramine can be purchased over the counter in 4- and 8-mg tablets (often scored) or in similar capsule strengths. To overcome the cat's aversion to the bitter taste of chlorpheniramine, the broken end of the split tablet can be dipped in tuna fish "juice," butter, or petroleum jelly to "seal" the end. Empty gelatin capsules may be purchased, and the split tablet may be placed in the gelatin capsules, or a pharmacist's assistance may be sought in reformulating the medicine in a more acceptable form. Some cats may readily accept the 8-mg time-released chlorpheniramine maleate capsules when the capsule is opened and one fourth to one half of its contents is sprinkled on or mixed with the cat's food.

Other antihistamines that have been used in the cat include hydroxyzine HCl, clemastine fumarate, cyproheptadine, diphenhydramine, cetirizine, and oxatomide (Table 1). Some of these agents have additional properties including antiserotonin, antidepressant, or anxiolytic activities, or a combination (see p. 48). In general, antihistamines are a safe alternative to chronic glucocorticosteroid or progestational therapy. The most commonly reported adverse effects include drowsiness and hyperexcitability. A fixed drug eruption of periocular erythema was noted in a cat given clemastine fumarate (Moriello KA, personal communication, 1994). Because of the teratogenic potential of antihistamines, precautions are warranted in pregnant queens.

PSYCHOTROPIC DRUGS

Psychotropic agents are commonly used in feline dermatology in the cat with psychogenic alopecia, although they can also be used in the pruritic cat. Tricyclic antidepressants (TCAs), serotonin reuptake inhibitors, and barbiturates are examples of the psychotropic (behavioral) medications. Diazepam or phenobarbital may also fall into this general category, and these drugs may be used in pruritic cats, although other safer antipruritic agents should be tried first.

TCAs block serotonin reuptake and many are potent H_1 and H_2 blockers. Amitriptyline is probably the most commonly used TCA for the pruritic cat; it is dosed at 5 to 10 mg per cat every 24 hours or 2.5 to 7.5 mg per cat every 12 to 24 hours. The success of amitriptyline varies widely. When discontinuing TCAs, they should be tapered over 1 to 3 weeks, as bizarre behavioral changes have been noted in humans and dogs when these drugs were stopped abruptly. Potential adverse effects include sedation, disorientation, hypersalivation, anorexia, vomiting, anticholiner-

TABLE 1. Antihistamines Used in Cats

Antihistamine	Common Oral Dose*	Adverse Effects
Cetirizine	5 mg per cat q12–24hr 10 mg per cat q24hr	None known
Chlorpheniramine maleate	2–4 mg per cat q12–24hr	Transient drowsiness Unpalatibility
Clemastine fumarate	0.34–0.68 mg per cat q12hr	Lethargy Diarrhea Fixed drug eruption
Cyproheptadine	2 mg per cat q12hr	Polyphagia Behavioral changes Increased blood urea nitrogen
Diphenhydramine	0.5 mg/kg q12hr	Hyperexcitability Liquid formulation is distasteful
Hydroxyzine HCl	1–2 mg/kg q8–12hr 5–10 mg/cat q8–12hr	Hyperexcitability Depression Behavioral changes Polydipsia
Oxatomide	30–60 mg q24hr	Polyphagia

*"Per cat" is based on the average 10-pound cat.

gic effects, ataxia, and cardiac conduction disturbances. TCAs should not be used concurrently with monoamine oxidase inhibitors. Amitriptyline *should be avoided* in patients with cardiac disease, a history of urinary retention, or seizures. A cardiac evaluation and baseline laboratory work (complete blood count and serum chemistry panel) are recommended as a standard pretreatment evaluation (Overall, 1997).

Fluoxetine (Prozac) is a selective reuptake inhibitor used occasionally to control pruritus in cats when most other therapies have failed. The dose ranges from 1 to 5 mg per cat every 24 hours. Potential adverse effects include irritability, nervousness, anxiousness, changes in elimination patterns, anorexia, and sleep disturbances. Pretreatment baseline laboratory work is advised.

Generally, the treatment trial period with psychotropic drugs should be 1 to 4 weeks to assess efficacy. Tapering may be done over 1 to 3 weeks for short-acting behavioral drugs and 6 to 8 weeks for the longer-acting ones (e.g., fluoxetine).

FATTY ACIDS

Supplementation with fatty acids theoretically shifts eicosanoids toward the less inflammatory mediators. Many formulations exist with varying ratios of omega-6 and omega-3 fatty acids (see previous article). Recently, a lamb and barley diet (LB Response, Iams) has become available that offers "built-in" omega-6 and omega-3 fatty acids in a ratio (5:1 to 10:1 of omega-6:omega-3) the manufacturer recommends based on proprietary research.

Variable success rates have been reported in pruritic cats given the various fatty acids supplements available. In one clinical trial, approximately 40% of the 22 cats with nonseasonal pruritus or pruritic miliary dermatitis had a good to excellent clinical response to supplementation with a product containing omega-3 and omega-6 fatty acids; no side effects were noted (Miller et al, 1993). Fatty acids are a safe alternative to glucocorticosteroid therapy. Some cats will show benefit within 1 to 2 weeks; however, it may take a therapeutic trial of 6 to 12 weeks before a favorable response is seen. Synergistic effects are reported when fatty acids are combined with antihistamines. When used in combination with glucocorticosteroids, less steroid therapy may be needed. Some cats may find fatty acids unpalatable. A chewable tablet form (VetriDerm, Bayer) may improve acceptance of fatty acid supplementation by the cat. Adverse effects are uncommon in cats and include vomiting, diarrhea, weight gain, and a "fish breath" halitosis. Cats allergic to fish may become more pruritic with marine oil fatty acid supplements.

PROGESTOGENS

Because of the potential serious adverse effects, progestogen therapy in the pruritic cat should be reserved as a last resort before euthanasia. As such, and because safer effective alternatives are available, progestogens are rarely used by veterinary dermatologists. Megestrol acetate (Ovaban, Megace) is an oral progestogen with antiestrogenic, glucocorticoid-like and behavior-altering effects. Adverse effects are common and include depression; pyometra; stump pyometra; diabetes mellitus; adrenocortical suppression; gynecomastia; mammary gland hypertrophy or adenocarcinoma, or both; polyuria; polydipsia; weight gain secondary to polyphagia; and temperament changes (aggression, increased affection). Mammary gland changes can occur in both male and female cats. Cutaneous changes such as alopecia, atrophic skin, and cutaneous xanthomatosis may occur with megestrol acetate use. Adverse effects occur with low or high doses for short or long treatment periods; some adverse effects resolve with discontinuation of the drug, whereas others do not.

Medroxyprogesterone acetate (Depo-Provera) is an injectable repository progestogen. Adverse effects are similar to those seen with megestrol acetate. However, because of its repository properties, it cannot be withdrawn quickly if side effects are evident.

IMMUNOTHERAPY

Immunotherapy (hyposensitization) is a biologic therapy that involves administering increasing doses of appropriate allergens to the atopic cat (see p. 564). The typical route of administration is subcutaneously. The mechanism of action is not well understood. A good to excellent response to immunotherapy has been reported in approximately 66 to 73% of atopic cats in studies conducted in the United States and France. The number of cats used in these studies ranged from 6 to 28. In the United Kingdom, however, in a study involving 12 cats over a 2-year period, the success rate was only 45% (O'Dair and Foster, 1995). "Good to excellent" meant fewer or no other concurrent therapies were needed to control the signs of atopy. Response can be seen after 1 to 4 months of beginning therapy; however it may take 8 to 12 months to see a positive response in some cats. During immunotherapy, a cat may require concurrent antipruritic therapy, albeit at decreased frequency or dosage from the cat's preimmunotherapy needs.

TOPICAL THERAPY

Many cats do not lend themselves as readily to topical therapy, especially baths, as dogs do. Also, because cats normally groom themselves, they may lick the medicines off; this may enhance systemic absorption of the topical therapy. An Elizabethan collar placed temporarily around the cat's neck may decrease licking the medicine off until it is properly absorbed, dried, or rinsed off.

For focal or local pruritic areas, topical corticosteroids may be beneficial. These topical steroids come in many formulations, including sprays, drops, creams, and ointments. Also, topical oatmeal sprays or lotions often offer temporary relief of pruritus (e.g., Relief Spray, OVM Pharmaceuticals; Dermacool-HC Spray, Allerderm/Virbac; Dermacool with Lidocaine Spray, Allerderm/Virbac; Heska Pramoxine Spray, Heska; or Dermal-Soothe Anti-Itch Spray, EVSCO Pharmaceuticals). Also available are sprays that contain lidocaine and oatmeal, lidocaine with hydrocortisone and oatmeal, or diphenhydramine and oatmeal. The cat should be distracted for 10 to 15 minutes after each application to allow the product to dry or work, or both.

Medicated shampoos with oatmeal may offer a temporary decrease in pruritus. Again, the cat must be amenable to baths. Most oatmeal shampoos should be shaken before they are applied to the cat, and then a 10- to 15-minute contact time should be allowed before rinsing well. Other antipruritic shampoo therapies include formulations that contain oatmeal with pramoxine, diphenhydramine, or hydrocortisone. Details of many of these products can be found in *CVT XII,* p. 590.)

Oatmeal conditioners or cream rinses are also available. These may be used after an oatmeal shampoo or other medicated bath. Some oatmeal cream rinses also contain pramoxine. Recently, leave-on conditioners (by Allerderm/Virbac) became available. These are of added benefit in that they offer a longer residual action. Formulation of such antipruritic leave-on conditioners include those with oatmeal, diphenhydramine, pramoxine, or hydrocortisone, or a combination.

MECHANICAL BARRIERS AND DEVICES

Elizabethan collars are often-used barrier devices. There are many types, including opaque plastic collars, clear plastic collars, soft foam-like collars, and the homemade varieties made from plastic plates, poster-board, and so on. Variations of the Elizabethan collar include bandannas placed around the cat's neck and neck wraps made of bandage material to prevent the cat from scratching a pruritic cervical area. Infant-sized or baby T-shirts have been used as mechanical barriers for the cat with truncal pruritus. Disadvantages of such devices include poor owner compliance and poor tolerance of the device by the cat.

Occasionally, nail trimming may be enough to decrease self-trauma to the skin by the pruritic cat. Booties and socks may be worn over the paws; these are generally poorly tolerated by the cat. Soft plastic nail caps called SoftPaws (SoftPaws, Inc.) are a good alternative. These nail caps are glued onto the cat's existing nails using the manufacturer's instructions and tend to be well tolerated by most cats. This product blunts the trauma induced by the nails from scratching.

References and Suggested Reading

Greaves MW: Pathophysiology and clinical aspects of pruritus. In: Fitzpatrick TB, Eisen AZ, Wolff K, et al, eds: Dermatology in General Medicine, 4th ed. New York: McGraw-Hill 1993, pp 413–421.
An overview of the pathophysiology and clinical aspects of pruritus in humans.
Halliwell REW: Pathogenesis and treatment of pruritus. J Am Vet Med Assoc 164:793, 1974.
An overview of the pathogenesis and treatment of pruritus.
Messinger LM: Therapy for feline dermatoses. Vet Clin North Am Small Anim Pract 25:981, 1995.
An overview of the therapies available for use in the cat with skin problems.
Miller WH, Scott DW: Efficacy of chlorpheniramine maleate for management of pruritus in cats. J Am Vet Med Assoc 197:67, 1990.
A prospective study on allergic cats treated with chlorpheniramine maleate.
Miller WH, Scott DW: Medical management of chronic pruritus. Compend Contin Educ 16:449, 1994.
An overview of treatment options in medically managing chronic pruritus in the dog and cat.
Miller WH, Scott DW, Wellington JR: Efficacy of DVM Derm Caps Liquid in the management of allergic and inflammatory dermatoses of the cat. J Am Anim Hosp Assoc 29:37, 1993.
A study investigating the efficacy of a fatty acid supplement in the cat with various dermatoses.
O'Dair HA, Foster AP: Focal and generalized alopecia. Vet Clin North Am Small Anim Pract 25:851, 1995.
An overview of causes of alopecia in the cat, including therapies.
Overall KA: Introduction to psychotropic drugs. Veterinary Proceedings, vol 10. The North American Veterinary Conference, Orlando, FL, 1997, pp 40–41.
An overview of the use of psychotropic drugs in veterinary medicine.
Paradis M, Scott DW: Non-steroidal therapy for canine and feline pruritus. In: Kirk RW, Bonagura JD, eds: Current Veterinary Therapy XI Small Animal Practice. Philadelphia: WB Saunders, 1992, pp 563–566.
An overview of alternatives to steroid therapy in the pruritic dog and cat.
Power HT: Tips/Questions. Practice tips. In: Roudebush P, ed: Derm Dialogue. Winter:7 1993/1994.
A clinical observation and tips.
Romatowski J: Use of megestrol acetate in cats. J Am Vet Med Assoc 194:700, 1989.
An overview of the use of megestrol acetate in cats.
Scott DW, Miller WH, Griffin CE: Muller and Kirk's Small Animal Dermatology, 5th ed. Philadelphia: WB Saunders, 1995.
A comprehensive review of small animal dermatology.
van den Broek AHM, Stafford WL: Epidermal and hepatic glucocorticoid receptors in cats and dogs. Res Vet Sci 52:312, 1992.
A study investigating glucocorticoid receptors in the skin and liver of dogs and cats.

Melatonin Therapy for Canine Alopecia

MANON PARADIS
Quebec, Canada

Melatonin is a hormone synthesized in the pineal gland, mainly at night, and is a product of the multistep conversion of L-tryptophan to serotonin and subsequently melatonin. It has been implicated in the regulation of a wide range of physiologic and behavioral processes in a wide array of vertebrate species. These processes include modulation of reproduction, especially in species that are seasonally reproductive; photoreception; thermoregulation; skin and pelage coloration; and fur growth cycles. In humans, clinical and basic research on the effects of melatonin involves antiaging, antioxidant (its free radical scavenger properties appear more powerful than those of vitamin E), oncostatic properties, sleeping disorders, jet lag syndrome, depression, and contraception.

Most knowledge regarding melatonin has been attained in the last two decades. Because of the wide array of its potential effects, a vast literature has developed on the topic; a Medline search on the textword "melatonin" yielded more than 3,000 references for articles published from the late 1980s to the late 1990s. However, melatonin is barely mentioned in human dermatology literature. This is interesting considering that the hormone was first isolated from bovine pineal glands in 1958 by Dr. Aaron Lerner, a dermatologist studying its effect on skin pigmentation. Although melatonin causes lightening of the skin of amphibian frogs (because of rapid melanosomal aggregation around the nucleus of the dermal melanocytes), and is responsible for growth of white winter pelage in weasels and Siberian hamsters (probably because of its anti–melanocyte-stimulating hormone effect), it does not seem to play a major role in human skin pigmentation. Concurrently, the oncostatic properties of melatonin are being actively evaluated in human patients with cancer, especially melanoma. Longer survival time has been reported in patients with melanomas treated with interleukin-2 (IL-2) and melatonin compared with patients treated with IL-2 alone. In addition, advanced solid neoplasms resistant to IL-2 may become responsive to IL-2 therapy by a concomitant administration of melatonin, which could act by enhancing IL-2 antitumor immune effect or by increasing the susceptibility of cancer cells to the cytolysis mediated by IL-2–induced cytotoxic lymphocytes, or both.

It has even been postulated that increased daily retinal exposure to artificial light in the 20th century, in contrast with earlier times, has resulted in decreased melatonin secretion, which, in turn, has contributed to an increased incidence of melanomas and other cancers.

In veterinary dermatology, little attention has been paid to melatonin. This substance is involved in the neuroendocrine control of photoperiod-dependent molting or pelage color in many mammals. However, the mechanism by which melatonin induces molting and fur growth is not entirely understood. The hormone may act directly on hair follicles, or within the central nervous system to alter secretion of melanocyte-stimulating hormone or prolactin secretion, or both.

Effects of melatonin on fur growth have been studied in mink and foxes. There are indications of a synergistic effect of prolactin and melatonin, two photodependent hormones, at the level of the hair follicle. The melatonin secretion pattern is an inverse function of day length, and circulating melatonin levels correlate inversely with prolactin levels. Melatonin secretion occurs during the hours of darkness, so the amount of melatonin biosynthesis is directly related to the length of the daily dark period. The quantity continues to increase in autumn until winter solstice.

Mink exhibit a seasonal fur growth cycle regulated by photoperiod. As the length of the photoperiod decreases, an increase in melatonin concentration (and a decrease in prolactin) results, initiating growth of the winter pelage, which begins in September in northern latitudes. In spring, the opposite occurs: the length of the photoperiod increases, resulting in an increase in prolactin concentration (and a decrease in melatonin), initiating the spring molt. Mink treated with implants of melatonin in June, when natural melatonin production is low; or exposed to an artificial 6L:18D photoperiod; or treated with bromocriptine, a dopamine agonist, have suppressed prolactin production and exhibit an early onset of autumn molt and produce prime winter pelage by mid-October, 6 to 8 weeks earlier than normal. For this reason, melatonin implants have been commercially available for several years to the fur industry for use in mink and foxes. This is to the best of this author's knowledge, the only commercial application of melatonin in veterinary dermatology. However, melatonin was implicated in the 1960s in the treatment of canine acanthosis nigricans. Recently, it has been used experimentally in dogs with recurrent flank alopecia, pattern baldness, and alopecia-X of Nordic breeds.

CANINE RECURRENT FLANK ALOPECIA

Clinical Features

Canine recurrent flank alopecia (CRFA) is a recently recognized skin disorder of unknown cause that is characterized by episodes of truncal hair loss that often occurs on a recurrent basis. It has previously been described under several synonyms: *seasonal flank alopecia, seasonal growth hormone deficiency, canine idiopathic cyclic flank alopecia, cyclic follicular dysplasia,* and *follicular dysplasia.* CRFA is most commonly seen in Boxers, bulldogs, and Airedale terriers but also occurs in several other breeds. Dogs of either sex and any reproductive status can be affected. CRFA is characterized by a nonscarring alopecia that is most often confined to the thoracolumbar region. Lesions are usually bilaterally symmetrical, but in occasional dogs (or episodes), only one side of the body is affected, or one side is more affected than the other. The alopecic lesions are annular, or "geographic" in shape with well-demarcated borders. The alopecic skin is often markedly hyperpigmented. Mean age at the onset of the first episode is 3.8 years, but can be variable (range: 8 months to 11 years). The onset of alopecia is not confined to the fall and winter months in males or to the spring months in females as was first reported. Instead, when all cases are combined, the majority of dogs have an onset of alopecia between November and March in the Northern hemisphere. The month of onset does not seem to be affected by breed, age, sex, or sexual status.

Spontaneous regrowth of hair occurs in 3 to 8 months in most cases and usually consists of normal pelage density, even though some dogs may grow darker hair in the previously affected areas (particularly boxers) or may grow a golden color (aurotrichia) as seen in some miniature Schnauzers. However, after several consecutive episodes of alopecia, some of the affected dogs will not experience complete hair regrowth before the onset of the next episode. Approximately 20% of these dogs will only have one isolated episode of flank alopecia in their life span in the experience of this author. However, the majority will develop recurrent alopecic episodes for years. Other dogs have an occasional year when the alopecia does not recur. The degree of alopecia is variable, with some dogs having a virtually identical hair loss (size and duration) year after year, and other dogs developing larger areas or longer episodes of hair loss, or both, as years go by.

Cause and Pathogenesis

The cause of CRFA remains obscure. To date, underlying causes, such as endocrinopathies, have not been identified. The seasonal nature and recurrence of CRFA suggests that photoperiod may be involved in the process. It is the author's belief that there is a higher incidence of CRFA at higher latitude (i.e., north of the 45th parallel), suggesting that CRFA might indeed be caused by a genetically influenced melatonin deficiency that is responsible directly or indirectly (by its effect on prolactin, androgen, estrogen, or growth hormone, or a combination) for the recurrent alopecia.

Treatment

Although several therapeutic agents have erroneously been proclaimed effective in treating CRFA, no treatment has yet been confirmed effective. Nevertheless, melatonin holds promise in the treatment of CRFA because initial therapeutic trials have produced encouraging results. However, the unpredictable course of CRFA and the spontaneous regrowth of hair render the evaluation of any therapeutic agent, used either to prevent or shorten an episode of alopecia, in CRFA extremely difficult. The only subjective reference we have used is the knowledge that a dog who has suffered at least three consecutive episodes of CRFA has a high likelihood (>80%) of having the alopecia recur the following year.

In the initial trial conducted to evaluate the efficacy of melatonin treatment in preventing CRFA, nine dogs who had previously suffered three or more consecutive episodes of CRFA were used (Paradis, 1995). Around the autumnal equinox (approximately 2 months before the next "expected" episode of CRFA) each received melatonin: three dogs received two SC injections of 12.5 mg of melatonin in soybean oil (2.5 mg/ml; this formulation is not available commercially) at 2-week intervals, and six dogs received three constant-release implants impregnated with 12 mg of melatonin (36 mg total, based on the 12 mg/fox dose) SC. None of the nine dogs treated with melatonin in the fall experienced large areas of alopecia in the winter after the melatonin treatment as they had done the previous years. Instead, two (two large male Airedale terriers) had a very discrete, unilateral, 1.5- to 2-cm-diameter area of hypotrichosis of less than a month's duration, which was different from their previous much larger areas of alopecia that usually lasted several months. One older female boxer who had had six consecutive episodes, with incomplete regrowth after the most recent, had no hair regrowth of that relatively small area of alopecia that had remained after melatonin administration, but did not develop new area of alopecia. Also of interest, several owners reported an overall noticeably denser hair coat than usual following melatonin administration.

Since the initial study, several veterinary dermatologists have used melatonin in CRFA either to prevent recurrence or to shorten the duration of an alopecic episode. Apparent success was obtained in several cases with melatonin administered either orally (tablets or capsules) or subcutaneously (aqueous injections or implants). To document the real benefit of melatonin therapy in this disorder, one should selectively treat dogs before or shortly after the onset of alopecia (although the use of melatonin as a preventive treatment is limited, considering that the chance of recurrence is 60 to 70% in any given year). A placebo-controlled, double-blinded study using oral melatonin is warranted, since this seems to be the treatment of choice for most owners and veterinarians.

CANINE PATTERN BALDNESS

Clinical Features

Canine pattern baldness (CPB) is a relatively common but poorly defined disorder. Three different syndromes have been recognized in dogs. The most common syndrome typically consists of an acquired alopecia developing at the postauricular regions; along the ventral neck, thorax, and abdomen; and on the caudomedial thighs. It is seen primarily in dachshunds but is also recognized in several short-coated breeds: Chihuahuas, miniature pinschers, whippets, greyhounds, Boston terriers, boxers, and so on. The hair loss usually starts around 6 months of age and gradually progresses over the following year but remains restricted to the described areas.

Treatment

Because CPB is a purely aesthetic problem, not much energy has been spent in finding a possible treatment for it. To date, no effective treatment has been reported aside from the possible beneficial effect of melatonin. Indeed, in this author's study evaluating the efficacy of melatonin in CRFA, two boxers with concurrent CPB experienced impressive hair growth in those areas in which the hair coat was previously sparse to absent (more specifically the chest and ventral neck). Based on these unexpected findings, a pilot study was conducted to evaluate the efficacy of melatonin in the treatment of canine CPB (Paradis, 1996). Eleven purebred dogs affected with CPB as described were treated either with one to three constant-release implants impregnated with 12 mg of melatonin (7 dogs) SC, or with one capsule containing 5 mg of melatonin in a lactose base given PO, every 24 hours for 30 days (4 dogs). All 11 dogs experienced hair growth (varying from mild to significant) in affected areas that was noticed as early as 1.5 months after the initiation of the treatment. Maximal growth was achieved 3 to 4 months later. Most owners were pleased with the results, and several reported an overall denser and more attractive hair coat. Results were less impressive in the two dachshunds and the two miniature pinschers of the trial, and for all dogs hair growth on the sternum was negligible, perhaps because of premature wearing or irreversible follicular atrophy.

Since the initial study, other CPB cases have been treated with melatonin by several veterinary dermatologists. Good results have been observed in several dogs (but not all), including Dachshunds and Boston terriers.

ALOPECIA-X OF THE NORDIC BREEDS

This is the name several veterinary dermatologists are now using to refer to the following diseases: pseudo-Cushing, adult-onset growth hormone deficiency, hyposomatotropism of the adult dog, growth hormone–responsive alopecia, castration-responsive dermatosis, gonadal sex hormone dermatoses, sex-hormone alopecia, sex hormone/growth hormone dermatosis, biopsy-responsive alopecia, adrenal sex hormone imbalance, congenital adrenal hyperplasia–like syndrome, Lysodren-responsive dermatosis, follicular dysplasia of Nordic breeds, Siberian husky follicular dysplasia, follicular growth dysfunction of the plush-coated breeds, and others.

A number of patients with "that disease" have been treated with melatonin by several veterinary dermatologists with apparent success in more than 50% of the cases. Criteria have not yet been established regarding the responsiveness for any given breed, sex, age, and so on.

SOURCE OF MELATONIN

Melatonin is easily synthesized and is therefore a relatively cheap hormone that can be administered orally (tablets or capsules) or systemically using aqueous SC injections or constant-release SC implants. Interestingly, melatonin is also present naturally in some plants. However, to absorb 3 mg of melatonin, one would have to eat 120 bananas or 30 large bowls of rice!

Melatonin tablets are sold over the counter in health stores and drugstores in the United States and several other countries, where it is considered a dietary supplement rather than a drug (so it is not regulated as such). It is found as 2- or 3-mg tablets under several brand names. However, only licensed products have guaranteed purity. Although less practical, capsules can be made from melatonin crystalline powder purchased at Sigma Chemical Company (P.O. Box 14508, St. Louis MO, USA, 63178-9916; approximately 40 US dollars per gram). The major concern with oral administration of melatonin is its short half-life and dose-dependent bioavailability. In a study, its apparent half-life in dogs was 18.6 minutes following administration of 3 mg/kg IV. An injectable aqueous melatonin (made from melatonin crystalline powder dissolved in ethanol and mixed with water and DMSO) has been available for several years, through Rickards Research Foundation (18001 Euclid Avenue, Cleveland, OH 44112) and has been used in the past for the treatment of acanthosis nigricans (Scott et al, 1995). This could be a valuable option, although no pharmacokinetic data are available. Constant-release implants impregnated with 2.5 mg and 12 mg of melatonin have been approved in several countries for use in mink and foxes, respectively, and are commercially available from Wildlife Pharmaceuticals (Fort Collins, Colorado 80524-2778). Unfortunately, some dogs who received the subcutaneous implants experienced sterile abscesses or granulomas at the site of implantation. This seems particular to dogs; in the fur industry, more than 10 million minks and foxes have received subcutaneous melatonin implants with no reports of adverse local reactions.

CLINICAL USE OF MELATONIN

The use of melatonin in dogs must be considered experimental at this time. There is no information on possible harmful long-term side effects in dogs or any other species. When human volunteers were fed 6 g (6,000 mg) of melatonin every night for 30 days, stomach discomfort and some residual sleepiness were the only reported side effects. Since melatonin has been shown to regulate light-mediated reproductive events in mammals, it is best to avoid its use in breeding dogs. However, since CRFA, CPB, and alopecia-X of Nordic breeds are most likely genetically programmed, it is better to avoid proliferating dogs affected with those conditions. For melatonin to be a valuable therapeutic option in some types of canine alopecia, its long-term effects will have to be evaluated. Myriad questions remain, such as: What is the optimal dose and route of administration, length of treatment, and the best time of year (or time of day for oral administration) for treatment to be initiated? It is not known whether its efficacy depends on a sustained high level or only a peak of melatonin produced in the initial stage, nor do we know the minimal number of days that the presence of melatonin is required to initiate the growth of hair. Finally, it is also not known if the animal will become insensitive or refractory to the formerly inductive melatonin signal after an extended period of exposure to high melatonin concentrations.

Studies are needed to corroborate the results of these preliminary trials investigating the effectiveness of melatonin therapy for varous types of canine alopecias. Meanwhile, if one wishes to try melatonin in dogs with alopecia, this author's recommendations for the time being are as follows: use 12-mg implants SC at the rate of one to four per dog. This is purely empirical and is based on the 12 mg/fox dose, which successfully produces precocious winter fur growth in that species. It has the advantage of being sustained-release, and it is possible that this may be important for therapeutic efficacy. Melatonin is released over a few months in foxes, so it may be administered once (CRFA) or twice (CPA?) a year, depending on the disease being treated. If implants are not an option, one can use oral melatonin, given daily for 4 to 6 weeks at as high a dose and frequency that one dares (e.g., 3 to 6 mg every 8 to 12 hours). It may later be revealed that this treatment regimen is excessive in dosage and duration. However, these current recommendations are based on the short half-life of orally administered melatonin in dogs, and on the knowledge that in mink, activation of hair follicles by melatonin occurs during a 4- to 6-week period. This photoperiodic signal does not seem necessary for later pelage growth and maturation. Melatonin appears to be safe, but owners should be made aware of the experimental nature of the treatment and sign a release form accordingly.

References and Suggested Reading

Curtis CF, Evans H, Lloyd DH: Investigation of the reproductive and growth hormone status of dogs affected by idiopathic recurrent flank alopecia. J Small Anim Pract 37:417, 1996.
  Results from 12 neutered dogs with idiopathic recurrent flank alopecia suggests that they have normal reproductive function and growth hormone levels.

Fontaine J, Beco L, Paradis M: Alopécie récidivante des flancs: Étude de douze cas chez le griffon Korthals. Point Vét 29:445, 1998.
  Clinical features of 12 griffon Korthals dogs affected with CRFA.

Miller MA, Dunstan RW: Seasonal flank alopecia in Boxers and Airedale terriers: 24 cases (1985–1992). J Am Vet Med Assoc 203:1567, 1993.
  Clinical features and dermatohistopathologic description of 24 dogs with this disease.

Paradis M: Canine recurrent flank alopecia: Treatment with melatonin. Proceedings of the annual meeting of the American College of Veterinary Dermatology and the American Academy of Veterinary Dermatology, Santa Fe, NM, 1995, p 49.
  A prospective study evaluating the efficacy of melatonin in canine recurrent flank alopecia.

Rose J, Stromshak F, Oldfield J, et al: Induction of winter fur growth in mink (Mustela vision) with melatonin. J Anim Sci 58:57, 1984.
  Mink treated with melatonin or a 6L:18D photoperiod molted the summer pelage and grew the winter pelage 6 weeks earlier than did controls.

Scott DW, Miller WH, Griffin CE: Acquired alopecia. In: Scott DW, Miller WH, Griffin CE, eds: Muller & Kirk's Small Animal Dermatology, 5th ed. Philadelphia, WB Saunders, 1995, pp 727–729.
  Description of various types of acquired canine alopecias, including CPB and "cyclic follicular dysplasia."

Paradis M: Melatonin therapy in canine pattern baldness. Proceedings of the Third World Congress of Veterinary Dermatology. Edinbourgh, Scotland, 1996, p 53.
  A prospective study evaluating the efficacy of melatonin in canine pattern baldness.

Valtonen M, Vakkuri P, Blomsted L: Autumnal timing of photoperiodic manipulation critical via melatonin to winter pelage development in mink. Anim Sci 61:589, 1995.
  Melatonin appears to be the photoperiodic signal to autumn molt but seems not to be necessary for later pelage growth and maturation.

Pyotraumatic Dermatitis ("Hot Spots")

WAYNE S. ROSENKRANTZ
Garden Grove, California

"Hot spots," more appropriately described as pyotraumatic dermatitis, are defined as a circumscribed moist exudative area brought on by self-trauma. The self-trauma results from attempts to alleviate pain or pruritus associated with an underlying disease that is creating this sensation.

The most common causes of hot spots are allergic conditions such as flea allergy, atopic dermatitis, food hypersensitivity, scabies, and anal gland problems (Table 1). Clipping or grooming complications can also create localized inflammation that results in pruritus and hot spot formation.

TABLE 1. Causes of Hot Spots

Common Causes	Uncommon Causes
Allergies—flea, atopy, food	Dermatophytosis
Parasitic—scabies, *Demodex*	Injection site reactions
Anal gland disease	Drug reactions
Clipping or grooming	Autoimmune disease
Result of deep pyoderma	Panniculitis
	Vasculitis

Occasionally, other infectious conditions (*Staphylococcus*, demodicosis, or dermatophytosis) can result in localized, multifocal areas of pain and pruritus leading to hot spot–like lesions. Other less common causes of hot spots are listed in Table 1.

Although any breed of dog can experience hot spots, some consider certain breeds to be predisposed. These include the golden retriever, Labrador retriever, St. Bernard, collie, and German shepherd. However, many of these breeds are actually predisposed to the common underlying causes of hot spots, such as allergies. Long hair coat length has also been thought to be involved with a predisposition to hot spots. However, in a report on 40 dogs, 50% had short hair and 50% had long hair (Schroeder et al, 1996).

The role of *Staphylococcus* in the development of hot spots remains controversial. *Staphylococcus* can be isolated from the skin of normal dogs. Higher numbers of these organisms are found in allergic dogs, even in those without active skin disease. Therefore, allergies may contribute to hot spots not only by the presence of pruritus but also by creating a favorable environment for larger numbers of staphylococci to flourish on the skin. One investigator proposes that hot spots are of two types based on histopathologic patterns (Reinke et al, 1987). One is a superficial lesion in which bacteria are considered surface colonizers. The other can be a deep lesion in which coagulase-positive *Staphylococcus* species, particularly *Staphylococcus intermedius,* acts more in a primary role. This same study showed a strong tendency for young dogs, golden retrievers, and St. Bernards to be predisposed to the deeper form of hot spots. In a more recent study, staphylococcus was isolated from all lesions before topical treatment. The condition in placebo vehicle control groups cleared completely within 7 days without topical antimicrobial treatment (Schroeder et al, 1996). The role of *Staphylococcus* as a primary cause in hot spots is certainly unclear.

CLINICAL FEATURES

The historical hallmark of hot spots is intense pruritus, and it represents one of the situations in which clients are generally correct when reporting that the lesion "just happened." The intense self-trauma can produce large lesions in minutes.

Regardless of the cause, most hot spots look similar clinically. They are generally well circumscribed, moist, erosive to ulcerated, erythematous, and usually painful lesions. The overlying hair is matted and coated with a serous to suppurative exudative discharge. Variable amounts of crusted debris may be present. Acute lesions tend to be edematous, whereas chronic lesions may be thickened with lichenified to scarred peripheral areas resembling an acral lick dermatitis.

The most common body locations for pyotraumatic dermatitis include the rump, the perineal-rectal area, and the lateral aspect of the face below the ear. The rump is the most common location and the condition here is usually associated with flea allergy. The perineal-rectal area lesions are generally due to anal gland disease (see p. 591). The lateral cervical facial lesions can be due to ear problems, atopy, or food allergy.

DIAGNOSIS

Diagnosis is generally made from the history and physical examination. The intensity of pruritus, body location, and physical appearance are often all that is necessary to make a diagnosis. Initially, skin scrapings and cytologic studies (see p. 526) should be considered to rule out *Demodex* infection and help select the initial therapeutic options. In more chronic or relapsing conditions, fungal and bacterial cultures, biopsies, and allergy work-ups (allergy testing and elimination diets) should be performed. If these tests do not lead to a diagnosis, laboratory testing for underlying immune-mediated or metabolic problems should be performed.

THERAPY

Topical Agents

Regardless of the cause and independent of what is used either topically or systemically, shaving the hair and cleansing the hot spot is the initial form of therapy. In order to shave or clean the wound, a topical desensitizing agent or sedation maybe necessary because of the pain and discomfort associated with the lesion. After the area is clipped, the full extent and nature of the lesion can be observed. An antimicrobial shampoo containing benzoyl peroxide (Oxydex, Sulf/Oxydex, DVM Pharmaceuticals; Pyoben, Allerderm/Virbac) or chlorhexidine (Chlorhexi Derm, DVM Pharmaceuticals; Hexadene, Allerderm/Virbac; Nolvasan, Fort Dodge) are the author's favorites. Over-the-counter antimicrobial shampoos such as those containing benzalkonium chloride can also be effective.

After the site is clipped and washed appropriately, additional topical and, in some situations, systemic treatment is needed. Occlusive vehicles should be avoided (ointments and creams). Nonocclusive vehicles (sprays, rinses, gels, and lotions) are preferable to allow exudation to occur and prevent occlusion of follicles and progression into a deeper folliculitis.

Many practitioners like to use an astringent for the first 24 to 48 hours on hot spots. Astringents precipitate proteins and usually do not penetrate deeply. These products do tend to dry out and decrease the exudation. Examples of astringents include 5% tannic acid, aluminum acetate solution (Burow's solution); Domeboro (Miles Pharmaceuticals) diluted 1:40 in cool water, 25% silver nitrate solution, and potassium permanganate 1:1000 to 1:30,000 solution. The author prefers Domeboro as it is tolerated best and does not stain compared with the other astringents.

The most common topical products used on hot spots are antipruritic sprays, gels, and lotions. Some of these products substitute another sensation for the pruritus such as heat or cold. Cooling tends to decrease pruritus. Examples include methol 0.12 to 1%, camphor 0.12 to 1%, thymol 0.5 to 1%, or cold ice packs. Other products use local anesthetic or desensitizing agents such as benzocaine, tetracaine, lidocaine, 1% pramoxine (Relief, DVM Pharmaceuticals; Dermacool, Allerderm/Virbac), benzoyl peroxide (Oxydex Gel, DVM Pharmaceuticals; Pyoben Gel, Allerderm/Virbac), and tars. These agents are short-acting. Topical antihistamines are considered effective in humans but, in the author's experience, have limited value in the dog. Anecdotal reports suggest that topical 2% diphenhydramine (Histacalm, Allerderm/Virbac) is effective in reducing pruritus in dogs with hot spots. Colloidal oatmeal rinses and shampoos can also give topical relief from pruritus. Commonly used products include Epi-Soothe (Allerderm/Virbac) and Aveeno (Rydelle). The most effective topical products in controlling the pruritus associated with hot spots are glucocorticoids. Hydrocortisone is the safest and very effective. Hydrocortisone, 1%, is considered particularly safe and can be used long term with no adverse topical or systemic side effects. The most commonly used veterinary products include CortiSpray (DVM Pharmaceuticals), Dermacool-HC (Allerderm/Virbac), PTD-HC (Veterinary Prescription), Cortisoothe (Allerderm/Virbac), and CortiCalm (DVM Pharmaceuticals).

Topical antimicrobial agents can be used alone or in combination with other ingredients. Alcohol-based products can be bactericidal and astringent but can also be irritating to ulcerated surfaces. The most commonly used alcohol product is 2% benzyl alcohol (PTD lotion, Veterinary Prescription). Some of the active agents mentioned in the shampoo section are also available in gel and solution forms and can be used on focal lesions. Chlorhexidine diacetate or gluconate and 2.5 to 5% benzoyl peroxide gels (Oxydex, DVM Pharmaceuticals; Pyoben, Allerderm/ Virbac) are examples. One of the oldest antimicrobials is iodine. The "tamed" iodines povidone-iodine (Betadine) and polyhydroxydine (Xenodine) are less irritating and less staining than their precursors but are generally not as effective as some of the other antimicrobials mentioned.

Surface-acting agents like the quaternary ammonium compounds (i.e., benzalkonium chloride) are good broad-spectrum antibacterial agents. Some products combine this agent with alcohol and 1% hydrocortisone (PTD-HC, Veterinary Prescription).

Many potent topical antibacterial agents are available. The author's favorite veterinary topical antibiotic is mupirocin (Bactoderm, Pfizer Animal Health) because of its high efficacy for coagulase-positive staphylococci and its ability to penetrate deeper pyodermas. Other products that can be helpful include neomycin, gentamicin, bacitracin, and polymyxin B.

Combination antibiotic and glucocorticoid products often produce the best results and quickest healing. A recent study supported this when neomycin, prednisolone, and neomycin-prednisolone products were compared. The combination product produced the quickest recovery (Schroeder et al, 1996). The most commonly used veterinary products include Tresaderm (Merial), Gentocin Topical Spray (Schering-Plough), Panolog (Solvay Animal Health), and Otomax (Schering-Plough). Because these products contain potent glucocorticoids, their use should be limited and are not for the long term.

Systemic Therapy

The need for systemic therapy for hot spots is variable on a case-by-case basis. Most dogs benefit from a course of systemic antibiotics, particularly if the hot spot represents a deeper folliculitis. Antibiotic selection should be based on proven efficacy for *Staphylococcus intermedius* and should

be used for a minimum of 14 days and generally continued 7 to 10 days beyond clinical cure. The author's personal favorites include cephalexin 20 to 30 mg/kg every 12 hours; ormetoprim-sulfadimethoxine (Primor, Roche), 55 mg/kg for the first 24 hours and then 27.5 mg/kg every 24 hours after that; amoxicillin-clavulanate (Clavamox, Pfizer Animal Health), 15 to 20 mg/kg every 12 hours; and enrofloxacin (Baytril, Bayer) 5 mg/kg every 24 hours.

The use of systemic glucocorticoid therapy is more controversial. Some dermatologists avoid glucocorticoids, especially for deeper pyotraumatic folliculitis, arguing the concern for immune depression. Certainly if the practitioner elects to use glucocorticoids, long-acting injectables should be avoided and only short courses of oral prednisone or prednisolone should be used to break the pruritic cycle (see *CVT XII*, p. 573). Suggested dosages would include anti-inflammatory doses (1 mg/kg every 24 hours for 3 to 5 days).

Ultimately, identifying, eliminating, or controlling the predisposing factors is the long-term goal for prevention of hot spots. The client should be educated about the various differentials, and work-ups should be performed accordingly. Lastly, the client should be warned about future lesions because this is commonly a recurring problem. Attention to increased episodes of pruritus after grooming and bathing should be stressed. Maintaining parasite control and routine examination of the ears and anal glands is also recommended.

References and Suggested Reading

Reinke SI, Stannard AA, Ihrke PJ, et al: Histopathologic features of pyotraumatic dermatitis. J Am Anim Hosp Assoc 190:57, 1987.
A series of cases describing two different histologic patterns of pyotraumatic dermatitis—a superficial form and a deeper pyotraumatic folliculitis.
Schroeder H, Swan GE, Berry WL, et al: Efficacy of a topical antimicrobial–anti-inflammatory combination in the treatment of pyotraumatic dermatitis in dogs. Vet Derm 7:163, 1996.
A prospective study evaluating topical antimicrobial–anti-inflammatory treatment for pyotraumatic dermatitis with clinical lesions, bacterial cultures, histopathological data, and recovery times compared.
Scott DW, Miller WH, Griffin CE: Muller and Kirk's Small Animal Dermatology, 5th ed. Philadelphia: WB Saunders, 1995, p 883.
A comprehensive review of pyotraumatic dermatitis.

Acral Lick Dermatitis

JOHN M. MACDONALD
DINO BRADLEY
Auburn, Alabama

Acral lick dermatitis (ALD) is a multifactorial condition characterized by excessive, compulsive licking at an area of the extremities resulting in a firm, proliferative, ulcerative, alopecic plaque or plaques. This condition, also referred to as *lick granuloma* and *acral pruritic nodule,* remains one

of the more challenging and frustrating problems seen by both the specialist and the private practicing veterinarian. One of the more difficult aspects of the treatment is related to the multifactorial etiology. Although environmental stress, such as boredom, confinement, loneliness, or separation anxiety, may contribute to the onset of the condition, this cause appears to be less important than other factors.

The lesion, by definition, is located on an extremity, and cases appear to be equally distributed between the front and the rear legs, most noticeably on the dorsal aspect of the carpus, metacarpus, tarsus, or metatarsus. Lesions usually begin with a small area of dermatitis and alopecia and progress to more extensive lesions through persistent licking. The expansion of the lesions may interfere with locomotion and has resulted in changes of the bony tissue underneath. This condition is more commonly seen in older (5 to 12 years old), large-breed dogs (Doberman pinscher, Great Dane, Golden retriever, Labrador retriever, German shepherd, and boxer), although the condition has been observed in other breeds, including the Dalmatian, English Setter, Shar Pei, and Weimaraner.

The development of ALD may be related to numerous causes. Constant licking of the affected area results in hair loss and erosion of the skin. Exposure of the sensory nerve endings causes the site to be pruritic, and the dog licks the affected area to alleviate the itching. This perpetuates a vicious cycle, resulting in the development of an ulcerated skin lesion, which does not heal because of the dog's constant licking. This condition should be approached as are other dermatologic problems in which a *primary disease* becomes complicated by *perpetuating factors* and results in persistence of the problem. Since there may be a number of simultaneous diseases and factors causing ALD, it is apparent that no single treatment will be effective in treating all cases. Symptomatic therapy may decrease the compulsive tendency of licking but is unlikely to resolve the lesion, particularly in one with a chronic history. Although conventional treatments such as intralesional injection with glucocorticoids (triamcinolone or methylprednisolone acetate) may produce an anti-inflammatory effect, they may actually intensify the infection that is almost always present. History taking becomes an important part of the diagnostic approach to these cases, and identifying an underlying disorder is truly the key to successful management.

PRIMARY FACTORS

Although boredom and stress factors have been considered predominant causes of ALD, they seem to be less important than other *primary* factors (Table 1). There is some variability with regard to certain breeds. The Great

Dane and Doberman pinscher often do not have an obvious coexisting problem or underlying disease associated with the ALD. In contrast, in many other breeds, allergy is the primary cause of the initial compulsive licking. Secondary bacterial folliculitis further potentiates and perpetuates the development of the lesion, especially in the Labrador retriever, Golden retriever, German shepherd, Shar Pei, and Dalmatian. Allergic diseases to be considered include canine atopy (see p. 560), food allergy, and flea allergy. Historical information about early-onset pruritic disease may be helpful in defining the relationship of allergy to the evolution of these lesions. Food allergy has notably been related to the development of ALD and may result from an abrupt onset of aggressive pruritus and occur spontaneously in the older dog (>6 years).

PERPETUATING FACTORS

Perpetuating factors may be as important as the primary cause and, if left untreated, will ultimately result in failure to control the problem (see Table 1). One of the most important of these factors is infection. The infectious agent most commonly isolated from lesions of ALD is *Staphylococcus intermedius*. Infection starts as an area of folliculitis and progresses further to furunculosis. Histologic and microbial assessments of ALD lesions almost always demonstrate infected tissue. Treatment for bacterial infection should routinely be included in the therapeutic regimen. Although lesions are not exudative, cultures of aseptically acquired tissue will almost always reveal a staphylococcal species and in chronic cases may include a gram-negative organism (*Pseudomonas*, *Proteus*, *Escherichia coli* spp).

It is well recognized that licking or scratching incites a cycle of irritation and intensifies pruritus. A theory of potentiation of this behavior suggests that endorphin release, as a consequence of chronic licking, induces repetition of the activity. Regardless of the mechanisms involved, the learned behavior of chronic licking may present an obstacle as a perpetuating factor that will impede resolution of the problem even if the primary and other perpetuating factors are no longer present. Thus, most ALD cases involve both primary factors and consequential perpetuating factors. If the problem were as simple as a psychogenic or obsessive-compulsive behavioral disorder, treatment with psychoactive drugs should demonstrate greater efficacy than is currently observed.

DIAGNOSTIC APPROACH

One of the common causes of failure in the treatment of ALD is the inability to identify either primary or perpetuating factors. The appearance of the lesion nearly always elicits a "knee-jerk" response with regard to the name of the problem and an oversimplistic approach. Associated and underlying factors are often overlooked. Routine topical or systemic therapy is instituted before understanding the relationships involved with the disease evolution and progression. Although ALD may be considered a purely psychogenic phenomenon, the diagnostic plan must include tests to rule out underlying causes of chronic licking and self-mutilation. Initial appraisal of focal or multifocal le-

TABLE 1. Primary Causes of and Perpetuating Factors in Acral Lick Dermatitis

Primary Factors	Perpetuating Factors
Allergic dermatitis	Bacterial infection
Arthropathies	Osteomyelitis
Foreign bodies	Keratin foreign bodies
Neuropathies	Periostitis
Trauma	Secondary arthritis
Neoplasia	Learned behavior
Mycotic infection	
Parasitoses (e.g., scabies)	
Psychogenic factors	

sions should include documentation of location and size. Calipers may be used to quantify the size and shape of the lesion. The use of acetate film or plastic kitchen wrap and an indelible felt-tip pen provides a convenient method for tracing the lesion. A permanent record may be kept for comparison during the treatment process. Routine blood work (complete blood count and survey profile), urinalysis, and a minimal database of skin scrapings and a dermatophyte test medium culture should be obtained. Suspicion of possible underlying disease should influence the direction of diagnostics for that individual animal. History of allergic episodes should direct the clinician toward pursuing allergic disease.

Skin Biopsy

Biopsy of lesions associated with ALD remains controversial among some dermatologists, although it is included as part of our diagnostic work-up. This provides a relatively expedient way to rule out neoplasia or mycotic infection with a similar cutaneous presentation. Mast cell tumor, histiocytoma, and squamous cell carcinoma are examples of tumors that may be associated with compulsive licking of the area. Likewise, infectious diseases, including superficial keratinophilic fungi (dermatophytosis), deep mycoses (blastomycosis), or sporotrichosis, may all be ruled out by this procedure. Tissue may also be sent for microbiologic evaluation (bacterial culture and susceptibility testing or fungal culture) during this procedure. Impression smears made from biopsy specimens should be obtained routinely, with the expectation of ruling out neoplasia or infective diseases.

Radiography

Depending on the chronicity and progression of the lesions, radiography may or may not be included in the initial diagnostic approach. This is certainly indicated with chronic and larger lesions or if there is concern about an underlying arthropathy associated with the problem. Radiography is most helpful when evaluating the prognosis. Those with more extensive radiographic evidence of bony involvement are least likely to be satisfactorily resolved.

Fine Needle Aspiration and Cytologic Studies

Fine needle aspiration should be included in the initial phase of the diagnostic work-up if biopsy specimens are not going to be acquired. This is to provide early recognition of cutaneous neoplasia, although lack of evidence does not rule it out. Cytologic examination of material acquired from the typical ALD lesion shows little cellularity aside from representative inflammatory cells. Impression smears of the surface exudate contain many different bacteria and white blood cells, demonstrating opportunistic colonization of an ulcerative lesion.

Bacterial Culture and Susceptibility Testing

Bacterial cultures are often included in the diagnostic work-up but must be obtained from an aseptically acquired biopsy punch specimen to offer credible results. Six-millimeter punch biopsy samples are submitted to a microbiology laboratory for maceration and inoculation on culture medium for identification of microorganisms. Transport media must be used if specimens cannot be taken to the laboratory promptly. There are several commercial products available that contain Stuart's transport media and are appropriate for this purpose. Culture may be helpful in chronic lesions, particularly when gram-negative organisms may be present. Culturing the *surface* of the lesion offers little diagnostic help in either antibiotic selection or understanding the relationship of perpetuating factors. Some clinicians use a culturette to sample the defect left by a punch biopsy, but in our experience this method is not reliable in identifying important microorganisms.

Electrodiagnostic Testing

Electrodiagnostic testing consisting of electromyography and motor-sensory nerve conduction velocities may be conducted to rule out the presence of an underlying neuropathy or nerve root lesion. Results of these studies are not generally useful, except in situations in which automobile accidents or other types of trauma may result in peripheral neuropathy.

Allergy Testing

Allergy testing should be considered a part of the diagnostic evaluation if canine atopy is suspected based on history and clinical symptoms. Intradermal allergy testing or in vitro allergy testing is desirable for identification of allergens with the anticipation of implementing antigen therapy (see p. 560). Although this will not provide an immediate effect on the active lesion, it may be helpful in the prevention of further lesions. Intradermal allergy testing may need to be deferred if repeated intralesional injection of glucocorticoids has been performed. Of course, treating the primary problem may not provide a measurable contribution if the perpetuating factors represent a large component. Food trials should be considered routinely in animals in which food allergy is suspected, particularly the Golden retriever, Labrador retriever, Shar Pei, Dalmatian, and German shepherd.

TREATMENT

There is no *one* specific treatment for ALD. Identifying and specifically treating the primary condition and the perpetuating factors is critical to its satisfactory resolution. Chronic unresponsive lesions have an extremely poor prognosis for resolution. Prevention of licking by introduction of mechanical barriers should be included in the initial phase of all therapy. Bandaging may have limited value because of rapid removal by the dog, but it may be helpful in certain cases. Wire muzzles and bandaging have proved a good combination for deterring continued licking. Elizabethan collars, although poorly accepted by most pet owners and their pets, can be effective. An alternative to the Elizabethan collar is the use of a plastic bucket with a hole cut in the bottom. This can be slipped over the head and secured to a collar. Some innovative pet owners and veterinarians have used modified polyvinyl chloride piping to cover lesions and provide sufficient air flow through perforations so as not to cause a dermatitis. Intermittent examinations are critical to determine response to therapy. We strongly recommend the use of a measuring mechanism to record changes in the size of focal lesions so that their progression can be followed.

Antibiotics

Antibiotics are one of the most important treatments of ALD. These agents should be used systemically and therapy may require a protracted period (4 to 6 months). The selection of antibiotics should be based on culture and susceptibility testing when available. Cephalosporins have been used commonly with more success than other antibiotics, for example, cephalexin (Keflex, Lilly), 30 mg/kg PO every 12 hours, or sulfadimethoxine/ormetoprim (Primor, Pfizer), 26 mg/kg for the first day and then 25 mg/kg once daily thereafter. Enrofloxacin (Baytril, Bayer), 5 mg/kg once daily, has been useful, particularly if there is a gram-negative organism present. Treatment of the animal should be carried out 3 to 4 weeks beyond regression of the lesion. Maintenance antibiotic therapy may be required in the event of incomplete resolution of the lesion or when the lesion recurs after the termination of antibiotic administration. Pulse therapy has been successfully used in some cases in which administration of antibiotics is alternated with periods of no antibiotics.

Treatment of Allergic Diseases

Antigen therapy should always be considered when canine atopy has been determined to be one of the primary factors. The decreased use of systemic glucocorticoids is an objective of treatment in chronically infected lesions, and antigen therapy may help accomplish this goal. It is important with any allergic condition to consider avoidance as an optimal treatment, but practically, this is limited to food or flea allergy. ALD predominantly affecting the rear legs with coexisting lesions over the pelvic area should be evaluated for flea allergy and treated with parasiticidal therapy regardless of gross observation of fleas. The products most helpful for this trial include "on-the-animal" adulticides such as imidacloprid and fipronil. Dietary trials and challenge should be used to identify the optimal food for routine feeding of the food-allergic or -intolerant animal. Owners should be cautioned about deviating from the restricted food.

Surgery or Cryotherapy

Surgical intervention is often met with postoperative complications and incomplete resolution of the problem. This is a salvage procedure and indicated if underlying arthropathy is identified in a location where arthrodesis may be used for joint stability and pain reduction. Foreign bodies are also treated surgically. Surgical excision of the lesion does not prevent recurrence. The primary disease must be treated.

Radiation Therapy

Radiation therapy has been used for treatment of ALD, with varying degrees of success. The earlier, less pronounced lesions with minimal fibrosis and inflammation demonstrate the best response, whereas larger, chronic lesions with underlying bony involvement do not respond as well. The cost factors and unavailability of treatment centers make radiation therapy impractical in the vast majority of cases unless the underlying lesion is a radiosensitive tumor with a difficult surgical approach.

Topical Antipruritic and Anti-inflammatory Treatment

The sole use of topical anti-inflammatory drugs has a limited effect in the majority of cases in our experience. They may be prescribed after initial resolution has been observed with antibiotic therapy. A variety of choices are available, including Tresaderm (Merck Ag Vet), Otomax (Schering Plough Animal Health), or the Synotic-Banamine combination. The latter is preferred, and preparation is made by placing 3 ml of Banamine (flunixin meglumine, Schering Plough) in a vial of Synotic (Syntex) with application made twice daily for 30 days. The use of capsaicin (Zostrix, GenDerm) has been helpful in some cases. This compound is a substance P inhibitor that is available as an antiarthralgic-myalgic preparation in ointment form for human application. The topical application on and around lesions may help decrease the reinforcing sensations but must be used consistently at a rate of three to four times per day. This drug is now available as a nonprescription item. It is formulated as a 0.025% and 0.075% ointment. A more concentrated formulation (Dolorac, GenDerm) contains 0.25% capsaicin. We have used this in combination with mupirocin antibiotic (Bactoderm, Pfizer) in a 1:1 mixture applied three times daily. The use of bitter apple and Heet Linament (Whitehall) in a ratio of two parts bitter apple to 1 part Heet has also been popular as a topical antipruritic therapy. Heet contains capsaicin (0.025%), methylsalicylate (15%), and camphor (3.6%) and has activity similar to that of the generic capsaicin or Zostrix (GenDerm). A substantial trial period is necessary (4 to 6 weeks) to evaluate these topical products. It must be stressed that this type of treatment by itself will have little impact on chronic lesions. Specific treatments of the primary and perpetuating factors are critical for any hope of resolving the lesions.

Intralesional Injection

Intralesional injections of glucocorticoids are *not* recommended, particularly in the early stage of disease management, because the vast majority of lesions are infected with *Staphylococcus* spp. and possibly by gram-negative microorganisms. Many acute lesions become chronic in nature with progression of the infection. Acute lesions should be treated with a regimen of antibiotic therapy before consideration of intralesional steroid therapy. Topical anti-inflammatory drugs are far more conservative and would be better employed in lieu of intralesional steroid therapy. We have seen cases that require protracted treatment with antibiotics (>13 months) when the lesion had been treated with glucocorticoid therapy. Intralesional steroid injections should be withheld at least until a complete appraisal of the case has been made and a course of antibiotic therapy evaluated.

CANINE ACRAL LICK DERMATITIS AND OBSESSIVE-COMPULSIVE DISORDER

There may be similarities between the uncontrollable licking experienced by dogs suffering from ALD and the uncontrollable actions of humans suffering from obsessive-compulsive disorder (OCD). This condition in humans is characterized by recurrent, persistent thoughts or impulses (obsessions) or by repetitive, unnecessary behavior (compulsions). OCD, expressed by acts such as chronic hair pulling (trichotillomania), hand washing, or nail biting, has been considered an exaggeration of normal grooming habits. Some feel that ALD is a manifestation of exaggerated grooming habits in animals.

Investigations into the etiology of OCD indicate that these patients have an abnormality in the pathway that links the frontal lobes of the cerebral cortex with the basal ganglia. The frontal lobes promote deliberation and judgment, with the basal ganglia serving as a relay station for planning and execution of movements. It is suspected that the caudate nucleus, a portion of the basal ganglia, is deficient in filtering messages from the frontal lobes to the rest of the brain.

Biochemically, it appears that serotonin is linked directly with the presence of obsessive-compulsive disorder. Simply stated, serotonin is a neuromodulator that plays a role in sensory perception, emotion, arousal, and higher cognitive functions. Serotonin-releasing fibers are distributed throughout the central nervous system, influencing the sleep cycle, sex drive, body temperature, appetite, respiration, cardiovascular activity, mood, and aggression.

After a meal, serotonin (5-hydroxytryptamine [5-HT]) is made from the amino acid L-tryptophan after it reaches serotonin-releasing neurons in the brain. Once synthesized, serotonin is enclosed within vesicles at the presynaptic terminal. An action potential at the presynaptic terminal releases the serotonin into the synaptic gap, allowing binding to specialized receptors on the postsynaptic neuron. The serotonin is removed from its binding site and transported back to the presynaptic terminal, where it is reused or degraded to its primary metabolite, 5-hydroxyindoleacetic acid.

Experimentally, it has been shown that the primary function of the brain serotonin system is to facilitate tonic motor actions and inhibit sensory information processing. In patients with OCD, serotonin neuronal activity is low, resulting in impairment of these functions. It is thought that the repetitive motor activities of an OCD patient serve to increase serotonin neuronal activity. These repetitive acts are a means of self-medication. As the pattern of exaggerated grooming behavior applies to canines, it would appear that the chronic licking of ALD may serve to increase serotonin neuronal activity as well.

Therapy Using Drugs That Modify Neurologic Activity

Recent clinical investigations indicate that certain medications effective in the treatment of OCD in humans have a similarly positive effect on dogs with ALD. The drugs that show the most promise are tricyclic antidepressants (TCAs) and selective serotonin reuptake inhibitors (SSRIs), which affect central serotonin neurotransmission. The specific mechanism of action is based on the prevention of removal of serotonin from the synaptic cleft, increasing the functional activity of the serotonin. TCAs block the reuptake of both norepinephrine and 5-HT by their presynaptic terminals. Adverse reactions in humans include cardiotoxicity, resulting in arrhythmias or heart block, or central nervous system toxicity. SSRIs are more specific in their mode of action, acting to block reuptake of 5-HT by presynaptic terminals. This eliminates many of the adverse effects noted with the use of TCAs.

Clomipramine (Anafranil, Ciba-Geigy), a TCA, administered orally at a dose of 1 to 3 mg/kg once daily, has shown some efficacy in the treatment of ALD in some dogs (also see p. 90). Because of the transient side effects of vomiting or diarrhea, we recommend treating the dog with 1 mg/kg PO for the first 3 days of therapy, with a gradual increase in dosage based on clinical response. The SSRI fluoxetine HCl (Prozac, Dista Products), administered at a dose of 1 mg/kg PO once daily, has been an effective treatment for ALD. Other SSRIs currently available for treatment of OCD in humans are paroxetine HCl (Paxil, SmithKline Beecham Pharmaceuticals) and fluvoxamine maleate (Luvox, Solvay Pharmaceuticals). Hydrocodone has been used in the treatment of ALD. The dosage is variable pending response and tolerance of the drug. The standard dosage is 5 mg/20 kg body weight twice daily and has also been used at 10 mg/20 kg body weight three times daily.

These drugs should also be efficacious in the management of ALD in dogs, but there are no publications evaluating the clinical application of these drugs for this particular condition. In any event, one should anticipate a lag phase of at least 4 to 5 weeks before any change in excessive grooming behavior is seen.

References and Suggested Reading

Brignac MM: Hydrocodone treatment of acral lick dermatitis. Proceedings of the 2nd World Congress of Veterinary Dermatology, Montreal, Canada, May 13–16, 1992. Columbus: Ohio State University. 2:50, 1992.
Reference relating to the treatment of acral lick dermatitis with hydrocodone in the dog.
Goldberger E, Rapoport JL: Canine acral lick dermatitis: Response to the antiobsessional drug clomipramine. J Am Anim Hosp Assoc 27:179, 1991.
Response of acral lick dermatitis to treatment with clomipramine.
Jacobs BL: Serotonin, motor activity and depression-related disorders. Am Scientist 82:456, 1994.
Review of relationship between serotonin and depression-related disorders, including OCD.
Luescher UA, McKeown DB, Halip J: Stereotypic or obsessive-compulsive disorders in dogs and cats. Vet Clin North Am 21:401, 1991.
Review of OCD in small animal medicine.
Marder AR: Psychotropic drugs and behavioral therapy. Vet Clin North Am 21:329, 1991.

Review of psychogenic therapy in small animal medicine.

Rapoport JL, Rylord DH, Kriete M: Drug treatment of canine acral lick dermatitis: An animal model of obsessive compulsive disorder. Arch Gen Psychiatry 49:517, 1992.
Description of canine acral lick dermatitis as an animal model for OCD in humans.

Rivers B, Walter PA, McKeever PJ: Treatment of canine acral lick dermatitis with radiation therapy: 17 cases (1979–1991). J Am Anim Hosp Assoc 29:542, 1993.
Report of a study using radiation therapy for the treatment of acral lick dermatitis in 17 dogs.

Scott DW, Walton DK: Clinical evaluation of a topical treatment for canine acral lick dermatitis. J Am Anim Hosp. Assoc 20:565, 1984.
Report of the use of Synotic and Banamine therapy in canine acral lick dermatitis.

Shanley K, Overall K: Psychogenic dermatoses. In: Kirk RW, Bonagura JD (eds): Current Veterinary Therapy XI. Philadelphia: WB Saunders, 1992, pp 552–558.
Review of psychogenic dermatoses including acral lick dermatitis and mechanisms relating to perpetuation of the problem through learned behavior.

Shoulberg N: The efficacy of fluoxetine (Prozac) in the treatment of acral lick and allergic inhalant dermatitis in canines. Proceedings of the annual members meeting of the American Academy of Veterinary Dermology and the American College of Veterinary Dermatology, Scottsdale, AZ, April 28–May 1. 6:31, 1991.
Report of the efficacy of fluoxetine in the treatment of acral lick dermatitis

White SD: Naltrexone for treatment of acral lick dermatitis in dogs. J Am Vet Med Assoc 196:1073, 1990.
Report of the effect of naltrexone in the treatment of ALD in the dog.

Therapy for Drug Eruptions

KENNETH V. MASON
Queensland, Australia

Cutaneous drug eruptions are uncommon and unpredictable but are a known risk in clinical practice. The clinician must be ever vigilant to the untoward effect of drugs prescribed. A cutaneous drug reaction can mimic any dermatosis. The mechanism of a drug-induced dermatosis may be either nonimmunologic or immunologic, although our current knowledge in many areas is deficient. Nonimmunologic reactions are predictable, dose-dependent toxicologic manifestations and are usually listed in standard reference sources. Immunologic mechanisms are unpredictable and depend on factors such as the capacity of the drug to elicit an allergic response, the host's possibly genetic susceptibility to respond in such a manner, the drug's capacity to interact with other drugs or host proteins, and a number of other poorly defined factors.

A variety of descriptive classifications are used for drug eruptions, depending on the clinical and histopathologic features. The classification based on the clinical features is most useful to the clinician. The criteria for making a diagnosis of a drug eruption are as follows:

- A history of exposure to the drug.
- Finding clinical signs that are consistent with a drug eruption and are not explained by another cause.
- Biopsy specimen with histopathologic features of a drug eruption.
- Resolution of clinical signs after drug withdrawal.
- A negative challenge with other concurrently used drugs.
- The value of and need to challenge with the suspect drug (which is the ultimate test of causative association) must be weighed against the risk of worsening clinical signs, even the possibility of a fatal outcome. The situation of life being dependent on the suspect drug and the unavailability of other drugs would warrant a special consideration.

The clinician must be diligent in searching for a possible drug cause. It must be remembered that reactions can also result from preservatives, medicaments, food fillers, dyes, and stabilizers used in preparation of drugs, food, or cosmetics. The clinician must also be aware that many different drugs share structural characteristics or metabolic products; these are potentially similar antigens.

All modes of application, including systemic (injectable and oral) and topical (ointment, shampoo, and rinses), should be considered in cases of suspected drug eruption. Any given drug may induce a variety of clinical presentations; conversely, a particular presentation can be a consequence of many different drugs. Rarely does a drug produce a stereotypic reaction, although there are some notable examples such as flucytosine, which produces pruritus.

PRURITUS, URTICARIA-ANGIOEDEMA, AND ANAPHYLAXIS

Pruritus, urticaria and angioedema, and anaphylaxis are grouped together because the immunopathogenesis is principally a type I, and occasionally a type II, hypersensitivity (Table 1). Also, there is a possibility of progression from pruritus alone to urticaria, and then anaphylaxis. However, each sign may occur alone or together with the other signs.

In general, pruritus and most urticarial eruptions carry a favorable prognosis. Angioedematous reactions affecting the respiratory passages or associated with systemic signs are more serious. Drug withdrawal and antihistamines may be all that is necessary for animals with pruritus alone; urticaria and angioedema necessitate glucocorticoids until symptoms abate. Anaphylaxis is serious and may be a fatal systemic manifestation of an allergic reaction to drugs. Most commonly, heterologous blood products are involved, and there may be no prior exposure before the reaction is elicited. Clinical manifestations occur soon after exposure and are sudden in onset. Vomiting, urination, and bowel

TABLE 1. Clinical Presentations of Drug Eruptions and Associated Drugs

Clinical Presentation	Associated Drug
Pruritus	Allergy immunotherapy vaccines, numerous drugs (systemic and topical), shampoos (benzyl peroxide, tar- and herbal-based) flucytosine, pyrethroid dips and sprays
Urticaria-angioedema	Biologic (vaccines, blood products, bacterins, and so on) Antibiotics (penicillins, sulfonamides, tetracyclines, and so on) Parasiticides (amitraz, levamisole, ivermectin) Barbiturates, contrast medium, flucytosine, amphotericin B, shampoo, benzyl peroxide
Maculopapular eruptions	Antibiotics, shampoos (citrus-based, herbal-based, coal tar–based, benzyl peroxide), levamisole
Erythroderma (exfoliative)	Shampoos (herbal-, citrus-, tar-, and benzoyl peroxide–based), dips (herbal and antiparasitic-based), antibiotics
Vesiculobullous lesions	Triamcinolone, antibiotics (penicillins, sulfonamides, tetracycline), parasiticides (levamisole, diethylcarbamazine), cimetidine, aurothioglucose, thyroxine, anticonvulsants
Epidermal necrosis	Antibiotics (cephalexin, trimethoprim-sulfadiazine, penicillins, griseofulvin), 5-flucytosine, aurothioglucose, antisera, D-limonene, levamisole, herbal flea shampoos
Injection-site reactions	Repositol glucocorticoids and progestogens, vaccines (rabies, distemper, hepatitis, and dermatophyte), antibiotics, and anthelmintic (praziquantel)
Purpura	Azathioprine, chlorambucil, cyclophosphamide Antibiotics (penicillin, sulfonamides, tetracycline), levamisole, aurothioglucose, estrogens, vitamin K analogues (overdose or poisoning)

movements commonly precede collapse and severe shock. Multiple organ failure or death may ensue quickly if rapid treatment is not instituted. First, all suspect medications must be stopped, oxygen must be provided, and intravenous fluid, antihistamines, soluble glucocorticoids, and epinephrine started (see CVT XII, p. 150). Mucous membrane color, blood pressure indices, and heart rate must be monitored and intravenous epinephrine titrated. If intravenous placement is not possible and an endotracheal tube was passed to administer oxygen, diluted epinephrine may be flushed down the endotracheal tube or delivered via cardiac puncture. Careful continuous monitoring will be necessary for many hours, although most improvement is noted in 1 to 3 hours. Administration of continuous high-volume fluids, while monitoring urinary output, is a good management practice unless there are signs suggesting pulmonary edema. Serum biochemical and blood gas values should be monitored and appropriate treatment adjustments made. Disseminated intravascular coagulation can be a sequela and should be suspected, especially in animals showing bloody diarrhea soon after emerging from the acute crisis.

MACULOPAPULAR LESIONS

Maculopapular lesions are common to many dermatoses. These lesions are easily missed because of the coat covering. They are usually revealed in the hairless ventral abdominal area or after clipping. Lesions are usually generalized to truncal and symmetrical. Pruritus is variable.

The reaction is usually self-limited and only rarely leads to serious consequences. If associated with mucocutaneous depigmentation, vesicles, or ulceration, a more serious variant of drug-induced erythema multiforme should be considered (see the section on vesicular bullous eruption further on).

The principal decision or dilemma facing the clinician about drug-induced maculopapular eruption is to differentiate lesions from purpura. The latter has a more serious prognosis and different treatment considerations. Differentiation is more a clinical skill than any specific test; however, diascopy can be used by pressing a glass slide on the lesion. If the skin becomes blanched, the erythema is due to vessel dilatation. If not, the lesion may be a hemorrhage. The finding of epistaxis or blood oozing from the gum line would also indicate a clotting disorder and thus imply purpura.

Once the clinician is satisfied that no serious sequelae are possible, all suspected drugs are withdrawn and, if pruritus is present, antihistamine and moderate-dose prednisolone (0.5 to 1.0 mg/kg) are administered, if required. The author prefers not to use prednisolone unless the animal is showing severe discomfort, as glucocorticoids mask the possibility that causes other than a drug eruption are present. Lesions dry up and crust in 5 to 7 days and completely resolve in 14 days after the offending drug has been discontinued. A hypopigmented or hyperpigmented macule may remain for some weeks thereafter and does not necessarily indicate a continuing active pathologic condition.

ERYTHRODERMA

Erythroderma is a generalized diffuse reddening of the skin that may be accompanied by variable amounts of scale (exfoliation), which often develops a week after the initial onset of erythroderma. The skin is often painful. Diascopy as described previously is useful to confirm that the erythema is due to vascular dilatation. Affected animals often show mild to moderate systemic signs of hyper- or hypothermia, depression, and general irritability, presumably due to cutaneous pain. A drug-induced erythroderma is suspected when the lesions appear suddenly while the animal is receiving drug therapy for some other disease for which erythroderma is not characteristic. Other causes of erythroderma include environmental and food allergies, generalized superficial Malassezia and Staphylococcus infection, and cutaneous epitheliotropic lymphoma. Erythroderma can represent a cutaneous sign of internal malignancy. Biopsy is of value only in diagnosing alternative causes of diffuse erythema.

Shampoo and dips are most commonly associated with erythroderma; the condition can be caused by systemic medications. Provided that a drug cause is recognized and the drug withdrawn within a reasonable time, most cases of erythroderma will resolve without major problems. For suspect typical reactions, thorough rinsing with water is indicated. Erythema usually resolves within 7 days, but diffuse scaling may continue for another 2 to 3 weeks and is often accompanied by extensive hair loss. Hair will regrow.

VESICULOBULLOUS PRESENTATIONS

Many autoimmune and immune-mediated diseases present with vesiculobullous lesions. Most of these serious diseases are rare. When confronted with vesiculobullous lesions, a drug cause should always be considered, no matter how characteristic the lesion and distribution might be for an autoimmune skin disease. Pemphigus foliaceus–like drug eruption is associated with penicillin-type antibiotics, diethylcarbamazine, and cimetidine. Bullous pemphigoid has been recorded from triamcinolone injections.

When confronted with vesiculobullous lesions in animals on drug therapy, appropriate samples for diagnostic tests (e.g., biopsy), are obtained first, after which all drugs are withdrawn, and supportive care is provided pending test results. Avoid immunosuppressive therapy if at all possible, as it may mask improvement due to resolution from drug withdrawal. This approach may prevent unnecessary lifelong immunosuppressive therapy if drugs are the cause. The author has encountered vesiculobullous lesions (classic for ulcerative dermatosis in a collie) that responded to a home-prepared meat-and-rice elimination diet. The disease had been in evidence for 3 months, was poorly responsive to prednisolone and azathioprine, and resolved completely with dietary change.

The prognosis and treatment of vesiculobullous drug eruptions are variable. A single confined area of affected skin, as with fixed drug eruption in which only a patch of skin—typically the scrotum—is affected, carries a good prognosis. Lesions often resolve after 2 weeks of drug withdrawal. At the other end of the spectrum is total body involvement or large areas of affected skin. This may occur in toxic epidermal necrosis or erythema multiforme major, which may result in a high mortality.

With drug-induced erythema multiforme minor, variable numbers of ulcerative and circular lesions on the trunk or mucocutaneous surfaces may be all that is present; however, anemia, thrombocytopenia, and hepatic necrosis occasionally occur. Thus, appropriate hematologic and biochemical tests should be performed. Therapy consists of immediate drug withdrawal and appropriate management of anemia and thrombocytopenia by transfusion accompanied by high-dose glucocorticoids. If large areas of skin are affected, supportive care as detailed further on for serious epidermal necrosis should be instituted.

EPIDERMAL NECROSIS

Drug-induced epidermal necrosis has many similarities and overlaps with the vesicular bullous drug eruptions. It requires an experienced clinician and dermatopathologist to distinguish these conditions, and even then consensus among experts is unlikely.

Superficial suppurative necrolytic dermatitis of Schnauzers is associated with natural flea shampoos and tar shampoos. Lesions appear within 5 days of application. Because of the method of application, lesions are extensive and generalized. Dogs are febrile and in pain and become secondarily infected. Most cases respond to fluid therapy, antibiotics, and corticosteroids. Consideration should be given to repeated tepid water rinsing, at least initially, to remove any residual shampoo products.

Drug-induced erythema multiforme major is a severe variant of the condition described earlier (in the sections on maculopapular and vesiculobullous lesions) but with extensive epidermal necrosis particularly involving the mucocutaneous surfaces. Large numbers of variably sized lesions may coalesce, leaving extensively de-epithelialized, dermis exposed. Animals are in pain and systemically ill, with some suffering from anemia, hypoproteinemia, thrombocytopenia, and occasionally liver and kidney damage. Eyelid, anal, and vulvar scarring causing distortion or obstruction may be sequelae.

Most cases that are not extensive will resolve with supportive care involving antibiotics and parental fluid and blood product replacement therapy. The essential feature of erythema multiforme is that affected animals may survive for long periods despite the extent of cutaneous lesions, which then allows time for diagnosis, drug discontinuation, and supportive care until lesions and symptoms resolve.

Toxic epidermal necrolysis is a rare, fulminating disease that can be caused by drugs, among other things. Initially, erythema may occur, but this sign is often masked by the coat. Eventually, extensive, full-thickness epidermal sloughing occurs after the slightest skin trauma. Affected animals are invariably ill and in pain, with signs of shock, pale to gray mucous membranes, depression, or coma. Death commonly occurs within 2 days, but inexplicably, some animals in whom the drug is not accidentally repeated may live long enough to allow treatment. Mucocutaneous ulceration predominates, with resultant distortion due to scarring in the occasional dog lucky enough to recover.

Provided that death does not occur during the acute shock stage, hypoproteinemia from extensive loss of epidermis, secondary infection, sepsis, and electrolyte imbalance are the principal therapeutic concerns. Treatment is similar to that of extensive third-degree burn patients and includes initial crystalloid or colloid treatment for shock, glucocorticoids, and careful monitoring (urinary output, blood pressure). Once the acute stage has passed, plasma replacement (with frequent protein, albumin, and globulin assessments), blood transfusions, intravenous antibiotics, and careful protection of denuded epidermal surfaces are required. Surface infection with *Pseudomonas*, which easily becomes blood-borne, is a major problem. Animals with extensive oral and mucosal sloughing will not eat or defecate and therefore need hyperalimentation and fecal softeners.

PURPURA

Purpura results from hemorrhage into dermal tissues. Hematoma results from substantial hemorrhage into subdermal tissues. Hemorrhage without substantial trauma occurs from either damage to blood vessels or clotting disorders (see p. 434). Although many diseases may cause both vasculitis and defects of clotting, drugs may also precipitate purpura. This may be a direct toxic effect of the drug, as with anticoagulant rodenticides, or may occur via bone marrow damage resulting from overdose of various immunosuppressive drugs. Thrombocytopenia may also develop by indirect immunopathologic reaction, from drugs binding to platelets, inducing a hypersensitivity reaction and consequent thrombocytopenia. Finally, drugs may induce a type III hypersensitivity with vasculitis. This can occur in dogs (especially Doberman pinschers) after administration of sulfonamides.

The skins will not blanch when diascopy is performed, confirming that hemorrhage into the tissues, and not simple vascular dilatation, is responsible for the lesion.

Therapy for bleeding disorders is discussed in Section 6. If an immunopathologic pathogenesis is suspected, high-dose immunosuppressive glucocorticoid therapy is necessary until all the inciting drug is cleared from the body and normal hematologic and vascular function has returned.

INJECTION-SITE REACTIONS

A number of reactions subsequent to various injections have been recorded. Commonly seen injection-site lesions are alopecia, crusting, ulceration, and necrosis. An uncommon but recent addition is fibrosarcoma (see p. 498).

Glucocorticoids and progesterones produce focal, well-circumscribed, rounded areas of alopecia 2 to 3 cm in diameter. The patch may be depressed, indicating atrophy, and either hypopigmented or hyperpigmented. Vascular effects of the long-acting adjuvants and granulomatous reaction to their presence may be part of the pathogenesis; however, persistent hormonal effects are also most likely involved.

Vaccines may also produce a similar lesion, but the reactions are more often associated with damage to the vascular supply underneath the lesion. Poodles are reported to be more susceptible to rabies vaccine reactions. Killed feline respiratory and enteritis virus vaccine can cause severe sterile abscess formation and subsequent alopecia and scarring.

Granulomas and fibrosarcomas have been reported to be associated with a wide variation of feline viral vaccines. Granulomas may occur from any injection but more commonly active substances (antibiotics, hormones, and so on) in long-acting or adjuvant vehicles.

Many cases are self-limited, although some leave scars or take many months to resolve. If a better cosmetic effect is required, surgical excision is indicated. Surgical intervention is required for more serious reactions and can be curative.

GENERAL TREATMENTS

When a drug eruption is suspected, the first principle of treatment is to withdraw the drug. In uncomplicated non–life-threatening cases, this may be all that is required.

If there is extensive denuding of cutaneous surfaces, topical medication may be required. Topical therapy should be aimed at controlling infection, removing scale and crusts, and aiding re-epithelialization. Moist bandages that inhibit bacteria aid re-epithelialization. Clipping, debriding, and removal of crusts may be required to aid visualization and topical treatment.

In animals with systemic signs, intensive fluid, plasma, and occasionally hematologic constituent replacement therapy may be necessary. Careful attention to protein loss and possible *Pseudomonas* septicemia are required with extensive denuded skin surfaces.

When considering which supportive drugs to prescribe, the clinician must be mindful of the drug's antigenic profile and metabolic pathways to ensure that it will not exacerbate the existing drug reaction. This issue is particularly relevant in antibiotic-induced drug reaction, as many antibiotics may cross-react antigenically.

References and Suggested Reading

Hendrick MJ, Shofer FS, Goldschmidt MH, et al: Comparison of fibrosarcomas that developed at vaccination sites and nonvaccination sites in cats: 239 cases (1991–1992). J Am Vet Med Assoc 205:1425, 1994.
The histologic and epidemiologic features of vaccination sarcomas.
Lester S, Clemett T, Burt A: Vaccine site associated sarcomas in cats: Clinical experience and laboratory review (1982–1993). J Am Anim Hosp Assoc 32:91, 1996.
A good review of the clinical features of vaccine-site sarcomas.
Malik R, Medeiros C, Wigney DI, Love DN: Suspected drug eruption in seven dogs during administration of flucytosine. Aust Vet J 74:285, 1996.
A recent report of dose-dependent drug eruption.
Mason KV: Cutaneous drug eruptions. Advances in clinical dermatology. Vet Clin North Am Small Anim Pract 20:1633, 1990.
A general review of the clinical, histologic, and pathophysiologic features of drug eruptions.
Rosenkrantz WS: Cutaneous drug reactions, In: Griffin CE, Kwochka KW, MacDonald JM, eds. Current Veterinary Dermatology, the Science and Art of Therapy. St. Louis: Mosby–Year Book, 1993, p 154.
A review of drug eruptions, including the clinical features and drugs commonly involved.
Scott DW, Miller WH Jr, Griffin CE: In: Muller and Kirk's Small Animal Dermatology, 5th ed. Philadelphia: WB Saunders, 1995, p 590.
A textbook summary of drug eruptions.

In Vitro Assays in the Diagnosis and Treatment of Atopic Disease

MONA J. BOORD
San Diego, California

IN VITRO ASSAYS

Atopic disease has been defined as the predisposition to developing IgE antibodies to environmental allergens, which results in allergic disease on re-exposure. IgE is a primary mediator of allergic disease. Current in vitro testing is based on this fact. In 1984, however, a non-IgE anaphylactic antibody, IgGd, was described in the dog. This has raised questions concerning the pathologic requirement for IgE and whether it is crucial to atopic disease. If there is a population of atopic animals whose disease is not mediated by IgE, this population could be missed with the current in vitro assays detecting allergen-specific IgE. Further discussion regarding IgGd follows further on. Specific issues related to atopy in cats are also considered in the next article.

DIAGNOSIS OF ATOPIC DISEASE

Multiple criteria must be met in the diagnosis of atopy, and many of these criteria overlap with those in other pruritic diseases. *The diagnosis of atopy is based on historical and physical criteria, as well as elimination of other appropriate differentials.* Willemse and colleagues (1985) proposed a listing of major and minor criteria that should be considered in the diagnosis of atopy. Pruritus (particularly of the face and paws) is one of the major features of atopy, but it also develops in several other diseases. One should keep in mind that a positive in vitro allergy test is considered only a minor criterion in the diagnosis of atopy. Thus, in vitro allergy testing should be performed only after the clinician has a high level of confidence in the diagnosis of atopy. The test results should then be supportive of the history and diagnosis. The major differential considerations include flea allergy, food allergies, scabies, pyoderma, and *Malassezia* dermatitis, among other disorders. Included here is a brief review of the criteria that define atopy and that should be considered before in vitro testing. It is emphasized that many of the features are also seen in other disorders.

Diagnostic Criteria

The signalment should include a breed predisposed to atopy. Breeds reported to be overrepresented often vary in different parts of the world. A minimal history should include the age at onset of the first clinical signs, whether the problem is seasonal or continual, the distribution of pruritus, whether other pets or humans are affected, and the pet's response to previous therapy. The average age at onset of atopic disease is between 6 months and 4 years.

When the onset of pruritus does not fall within this range, other differential diagnoses for pruritic disease should be strongly considered before in vitro allergy testing. The author finds that the most reliable clue to the diagnosis of atopy is a history of seasonal pruritus. Unfortunately, 70 to 80% of dogs with atopy present with continual disease. However, these patients may have seasonal exacerbation of clinical signs suggestive of atopy or flea allergy. If other pets are exhibiting pruritus, flea control or treatment of contagious diseases (particularly scabies) should be considered before undertaking in vitro testing. It is important to evaluate the patient's response to previous therapy. Glucocorticoids are so effective in the treatment of atopy that failure to respond to steroids makes atopy less likely to be the sole cause of pruritus.

Clinical evaluation of the patient initially reveals no primary skin lesions or only mild, diffuse erythema. Broken hairs or salivary staining may be seen. A papular, pustular rash with partial alopecia may develop with secondary pyoderma. Lichenification and hyperpigmentation develop following chronic self-trauma. The distribution of lesions is important. Rarely is the dorsal lumbosacral region involved unless there is concurrent flea allergy. Facial or pedal pruritus is common. Pruritus often variably involves the ears, axillae, flexor elbows, or groin. Recurrent otitis is commonly present (up to 75% of cases) and should be used as an indication that more than a flea hypersensitivity is occurring. Conjunctivitis and hyperhidrosis may also be noted.

After major differential considerations are ruled out, and the diagnostic criteria of atopy are satisfied, allergy testing and immunotherapy should be considered. Generally, atopy therapy variably involves glucocorticoids (see *CVT XII*, p. 573), antihistamines (see pp. 48 and 542), essential fatty acid supplementation (see p. 538), or immunotherapy. The latter especially is recommended for patients when the pruritic season extends beyond 3 months or if high levels of glucocorticoids are required to control signs (even for shorter periods). An elimination diet, prior to allergy testing, may be considered in patients with a year-round history of pruritus (p. 530). In vitro screening for food allergy is available and is discussed later in this article. The author often elects to perform allergy testing before an elimination diet for the following reasons. In non–flea-allergic animals with hypersensitivity, the prevalence of atopy is 70 to 90%, in contrast to that in food allergy (10 to 30% of cases). Up to 80% of patients with food allergy have concurrent atopy, and up to 10% of atopic dogs may have food allergy. The author does recommend an elimination diet first in cats with facial pruritus, in animals whose initial onset of pruritus was before 6 months or after 4 years of age, predisposed

TABLE 1. **In Vitro Allergy Laboratories**

Laboratory	Testing Technique	Reagent Used	Species	Antigen House	Allergens Tested	Number of Regions	Insect Testing	Current Cost
BioMedical	ELISA	Polyclonal anti-IgE	Canine Feline	Nelco Allergen	30 group	16	Yes Additional	$68.00
BioProducts	ELISA	Polyclonal anti-IgE	Canine	Iatric Allergen	14 group 36 singles	Canada only	No	$75.00 $82.50
Greer	ELISA	Polyclonal anti-IgE	Canine	Greer Allergen	45 singles	4	Yes Additional	$75.00
Heska	ELISA	Fc receptor	Canine	Heska Allergen	48 singles	5	No	$75.00
Spectrum	RAST	Polyclonal anti-IgE	Canine Feline	Nelco Allergen	24 groups	12	Yes Additional	$60.00
University of Pennsylvania	ELISA	Polyclonal anti-IgE	Canine	Greer	24 mixed groups and singles	1	No	$55.00
			Feline	Allergen	48 singles			$85.00
Veterinary Allergy Reference Laboratory	Liquid phase	Mixture of three monoclonal anti-IgE	Canine Feline	Greer Allergen	40 singles	25	Yes Included	$75.00

ELISA, enzyme-linked immunosorbent assay; RAST, radioallergosorbent test.

breeds, or animals with additional gastrointestinal signs. Clients are always informed that food allergy is a differential diagnosis and are given the option of performing an elimination diet before allergy testing. If a poor response to an elimination diet is found initially and a partial response to hyposensitization is obtained, the elimination diet may need to be repeated.

Allergy testing and immunotherapy are now more available to the private practitioner than ever before through the commercial availability of in vitro tests detecting allergen-specific IgE. Although in vitro allergy testing is less useful for confirming the diagnosis of atopy, and studies in the dog indicate that false-positive results are common, good clinical responses have been seen with immunotherapy based on in vitro results. Therefore, the value of the in vitro test is *not in diagnosing atopy but in selecting appropriate allergens* so that immunotherapy can be initiated. Because the test is being used to select appropriate allergens for hyposensitization, it is important that specific, sensitive, and reproducible results detecting allergen-specific IgE are obtained.

Available Tests

In vitro assays are now available to detect allergen-specific IgE produced by different laboratories and companies (Table 1). Because no two laboratories use the same testing technique or protocol, results vary. This makes comparisons among tests difficult. The radioallergosorbent test (RAST) was one of the first commercial tests available.* Most companies offer enzyme-linked immunosorbent assays (ELISAs). The techniques for both the RAST and ELISA involve incubating the patient's serum with the allergen, which is bound to a solid substrate. Laboratories may use various types of solid substrates. This has been shown to affect the level of non-specific IgE binding. The patient's allergen-specific IgE binds to the allergen. It is during this incubation period that nonspecific binding may occur. Ideally, rinsing removes immunoglobulins not specific for the allergen. Anticanine IgE, which is labeled with a radioisotope for the RAST or an enzyme substrate for

the ELISA, is then incubated with the allergen-antibody complex. After a final rinse, the remaining labeled anti-IgE antibody–allergen complex is measured. Samples are run concurrently with negative and positive control sera. The negative control is either water or pooled sera from clinically normal dogs. The positive controls are not standardized across tests and may vary markedly. The positive controls are usually obtained from clinically atopic, intradermal test–positive dogs. Some companies have a positive control for every allergen tested, whereas others may have only a single allergen positive control. Based on the reactivity of the controls, a standard curve is established and the reactivity of the patient's serum is assigned a score. The definition of a positive test result is somewhat arbitrary. Negative control sera will have some level of nonspecific binding, and the cutoff point for a positive result is often defined in terms of a multiple of the level of nonspecific binding. For these reasons, concordance of results among companies varies.

Previous studies have shown no difference in the degree or quantity of positive reactions in normal versus atopic dogs (Codner and Lessard, 1993). This has raised concerns about the specificity of these tests. Many of the newer companies have attempted to address this concern by offering tests with increased specificity. The Veterinary Allergy Reference Laboratory (VARL) uses newer liquid-phase technology. The patient's serum and the test antigens are incubated in a liquid phase. Because allergens are three-dimensional molecules with multiple antigenic sites, a single allergen can potentially interact with many different antibodies. It is proposed that while in the liquid phase more sites are exposed (versus being bound to the solid phase), thereby improving reactivity and sensitivity. The liquid-phase technology is also proposed to limit less nonspecific binding caused by electrostatic and hydrostatic forces associated with a solid substrate, thus yielding an increase in specificity. This test varies from the ELISA and RAST in that it has two negative controls to compensate for nonspecific binding. The first is pooled serum from clinically normal dogs similar to that used by other laboratories. The second evaluates the level of nonspecific binding for each allergen tested. It does so in the following manner. After the incubation period, the liquid contents are

---

*Spectrum Laboratory, Laguna Hills, CA.

transferred to two new wells. This prevents any nonspecific binding that may have occurred during the incubation period from being detected. In one well, the antigen-antibody complex is bound to the side of the test well via a chemical reaction. In the second well, only a buffer is added, which should not bind the allergen-antibody complex to the well. The samples are then rinsed. The rest of the test is similar to the ELISA except that the level of reactivity of the buffered sample is deducted from the reactivity of the sample chemically bound. This allows each reaction to have its own negative control of nonspecific binding.

Although intradermal testing may have problems, it is still considered the standard against which in vitro tests are compared. One of the difficulties with intradermal testing may be poor sensitivity. There is a population of small animals that fulfill the clinical criteria of atopy, yet have negative results on intradermal testing. The strength of the intradermal test appears to be specificity, and for this reason most dermatologists continue to perform intradermal testing in selecting allergens for immunotherapy. However, when drugs cannot be withdrawn or a poor intradermal test result is obtained, in vitro testing may be a more sensitive option for selecting allergens for immunotherapy. In vitro tests also offer the general practitioner an opportunity to perform allergy testing and prescribe immunotherapy without incurring the overhead costs or training required to perform the intradermal test properly. Additional studies are needed to evaluate the sensitivity and specificity of tests now available.

Available Reagents

Once the patient's specific IgE has been bound to the allergens of the in vitro assay, there are various reagents that can be employed to detect bound IgE. Polyclonal anti-IgE antibodies have been used since in vitro testing originated. Currently, there is neither standardization nor studies comparing reagents. As a consequence, one should not always expect the results from different companies to correlate. Reagents should be evaluated for cross-reactivity to other immunoglobulin classes. Previous studies have indicated that some of the polyclonal ELISA assays have 100% sensitivity. The problem had been poor specificity (increased false-positive results). This may be due to nonspecific binding and cross-reactivity with other antibody classes (IgG) or to measurement of IgE nonspecifically bound to the solid substrate. In an attempt to make the in vitro assay more specific, monoclonal anti–canine IgE antibodies are now used for in vitro assays. Each monoclonal anti-IgE antibody is produced from a single B-cell precursor and has identical variable regions and a limited number of epitopes with which it binds. Monoclonal-based assays do appear to have an increased specificity but also appear less sensitive (increased false-negative results; Peng et al, 1993). It is known that IgE immune complexes in the circulation can markedly alter IgE measurement, especially for the monoclonal anti-IgE antibodies. One study evaluating monoclonal versus polyclonal anti–human IgE determined that 20% of the IgE was detected by the monoclonal anti-IgE and 90% was detected by polyclonal anti-IgE (Ritter et al, 1991). In humans, certain races may have a mild variation of the IgE molecule, which does not

allow the monoclonal antibody to bind (Alaba, personal communication, 1997). This should be considered in veterinary medicine with the multiple breeds evaluated. A mixture of monoclonal antibodies may be a better solution to improve specificity without a loss of sensitivity, but additional studies are needed. The Veterinary Allergy Reference Laboratory offers a mixed monoclonal anti-IgE reagent with liquid-phase technology. At the time of this writing, other companies use polyclonal anti-IgE reagents, except Heska. Heska utilizes a high-affinity Fc epsilon receptor alpha chain (FcϵR1α) and ELISA technology. The alpha chain is one of three protein subunits forming the IgE receptor on mast cells and basophils. Other antibodies, IgA, IgM, IgG, do not bind to this receptor. This test detects only IgE able to bind to mast cells and basophils, which is the theory of atopy's etiology. Also if a subclass of IgG, such as IgGd, can bind to this receptor, it would be detected by this test, unlike anti-IgE reagents. In a study of 300 atopic dogs and 66 normal dogs comparing intradermal testing to the FcϵR1α system, the average accuracy was 90%. This study reported a sensitivity of 86% and specificity of 92% using the intradermal test as the gold standard (Bevier et al, 1997).

IgGd

As mentioned earlier, IgGd may play a role in the etiology of atopy. The University of Utrecht uses an antibody directed against IgGd reaginic antibody. A study evaluated 82 dogs diagnosed with atopy; 89% of 62 dogs that tested positive on intradermal tests had elevated IgGd levels and 55% of 20 dogs that tested negative on intradermal tests had elevated IgGd levels (Willemse et al, 1985). This group of dogs was not tested for allergen-specific IgE. Thus, if there is a population of dogs whose atopic disease is mediated by IgGd, the diagnosis would be missed by tests using anti-IgE reagents. Anti-IgGd reagent is not yet commercially available for testing and requires additional studies.

Feline Testing

Feline in vitro assays have been available for several years, and results have been controversial among dermatologists. The initial studies comparing in vivo versus in vitro allergy testing in the cat concluded that the ELISA had a poor predictive value and was not a useful test. The first report of a polyclonal antisera specific for feline IgE was not reported until 1995 (Gilbert and Halliwell, 1995). This group also reported their antisera and ELISA system to be a sensitive, specific, and reliable testing method in cats (Gilbert and Halliwell, 1996). Another group developed a polyclonal anti–feline IgE that they could separate into reagents recognizing 30 different epitopes and documented the polyclonal agent's ability to induce a reverse cutaneous anaphylactic reaction. However, the investigators found the majority of the reagents also reacted to IgA or IgM. They concluded that assays detecting feline IgE should be evaluated for the potential of cross-reactivity with other immunoglobulins (DeBoer et al, 1994). There are five laboratories offering feline in vitro assays; no comparative studies have been published at this time.

Allergens

There are four different manufacturers of antigens. There is no standardization of allergens and they may differ greatly among manufacturers. When producing allergens, the allergenic source should be specifically identified material that does not contain foreign substances. Pollen extracts may vary up to 10-fold in potency from year to year. Therefore, standardization based on biologic activity or mixtures of different harvest years are recommended. Mite extracts may be either pure mite bodies or whole mite cultures. The whole mite culture extract contains material from the mite bodies, eggs, larvae, and feces, which is the material a mite-allergic patient is exposed to naturally. The preparation of any allergenic extract should not denature or alter the proteins. The extraction process and source of allergen varies among companies and should never be assumed to be the same. The allergen source of each laboratory is listed in Table 1.

Allergens may be tested as individual extracts or group mixtures. When an animal is tested with group antigens and has a positive reaction, allergy may or may not exist to all the extracts included in that mix, making the selection of allergens for hyposensitization less specific. If group antigen testing is to be used, the allergens combined should be grouped by family and genus with allergens known to cross-react. Because the goal of testing is to specifically select allergens for immunotherapy, the author prefers individual allergen testing.

Food Allergens

The term *food hypersensitivity* is used to classify dogs with an adverse reaction to food. This term implies an immunologic reaction. The term *food intolerance* is also used and implies a nonimmunologic cause. To date, an immunologic mechanism in the dog has not been proved nor has the involvement of IgE. Controversy also prevails regarding the way antigens are selected for food allergy testing. Certainly cooking and processing foods, combined with digestion and absorption, alters the protein composition of the food and potentially the allergen. The positive and negative predictive values reported for in vitro food allergy tests have been poor in several studies and no studies have supported their use. In the author's hands, false-negative and false-positive results are common with both the intradermal testing and in vitro testing for foods; therefore, testing for foods is not recommended. Screening for food allergy is offered by several companies manufacturing in vitro tests. A food elimination diet, followed by a challenge with the original diet, is still the test of choice in the diagnosis of food allergy (see p. 530).

Insect Allergens

Multiple genera of insects may also induce an atopic dermatitis–like syndrome. Examples include housedust mites, ants, flies, cockroaches, mosquitoes, and moths. As previously mentioned, there is a population of pruritic dogs meeting the criteria of atopic disease yet having negative intradermal test results. In southern California, 202 suspected atopic animals were intradermally tested. Of those

tested, 4.5% tested positive only to the insect-arachnid group. They tested negative to all other 62 allergens used, including fleas and house dust mites. In Las Vegas, the percentage of insect-only reactors was 8.3% (Griffin, 1993). Another study evaluating the testing of insect allergens compared intradermal testing to the liquid-phase VARL assay using Western blot analysis as the standard. The sensitivity for the VARL assay was 77.4% and that for the intradermal test was 29%. The specificity of the VARL test was 62.5% and that for the intradermal test was 75% (Griffin et al, 1993). The preceding studies indicate the importance of evaluating the atopic patient for insect hypersensitivity and also that the VARL assay is of value when compared with Western blot analysis in detecting insect hypersensitivity. One should also realize that in animals that have negative test results and are suspected of having atopy, the failure to test for the causative allergens may be the reason for the negative results. One company includes insect allergens in its standard screen and several others have insect screens available for an additional fee (see Table 1). It is also important to keep in mind that clinically flea-allergic dogs with positive intradermal test results to flea often have negative flea allergy tests results on an in vitro assay. This is believed to be due to hypersensitivity triggered by mechanisms other than IgE.

IMMUNOTHERAPY

Immunotherapy (hyposensitization) is second only to steroids in the treatment of atopy. Furthermore, systemic glucocorticoids can be avoided 75% of the time when immunotherapy is used alone or in combination with other nonsteroidal therapy such as antihistamines (see p. 542) or fatty acid supplementation (see p. 538). The efficacy of immunotherapy has been reported to range from 50 to 100%. Realistically, 60 to 70% of canine patients have a good to excellent response when allergens are specifically selected. In the feline population, the response is 70 to 80%. Performing an allergy test for the selection of allergens is important, as animals treated nonspecifically for the most common reactors have a response rate comparable to placebo (15 to 20%). Multiple studies comparing in vivo versus in vitro hyposensitization success rates have found no statistically significant difference. It is important to realize that the efficacies quoted are reported by dermatology clinics. In these studies, the specialist has a high level of confidence in the diagnosis of atopy before selecting an in vitro test. The allergens are then carefully selected based not only on the test results but also on careful review of the history and knowledge of the region in which the patient lives. The animals are monitored closely for secondary factors and finally, immunotherapy is adjusted depending on the patient's response.

In vitro assays are certainly an invaluable tool when used correctly for the *selection of allergens*. The greatest concern is that these tests are being used improperly in the attempt to diagnose atopy. The greatest asset of the in vitro test is that a blood sample is all that is required, but there are inherent weaknesses to various tests, as discussed in this article. The clinician should not expect to achieve the success mentioned unless one is willing to select cases appropriately, perform follow-up, control secondary factors, and help the client and patient through the initial induction phase.

References and Suggested Reading

Bevier DE, Mondesire RL, et al: Fc∈R1α-based ELISA technology for in vitro determination of allergen-specific IgE in a population of intradermal skin-tested normal and atopic dogs. Supplement Compend Contin Educ Pract Vet 19(11), 1997.

Codner EC, Lessard P: Comparison of intradermal allergy test and enzyme-linked immunosorbent assay in dogs with allergic skin disease. J Am Vet Med Assoc 202:739, 1993.
A study evaluating the sensitivity and specificity of an ELISA allergy test using intradermal testing as the standard.

DeBoer DJ, Yue X, Donner R: Monoclonal antibodies against feline immunoglobulin E. Proceedings of the American Academy of Veterinary Dermatology/American College of Veterinary Dermatology, Charleston, SC, 1994.
Discusses the cross-reactivity of feline monoclonal IgE.

Gilbert S, Halliwell REW: The characterisation of feline IgE. Proceedings of the American Academy of Veterinary Dermatology/American College of Veterinary Dermatology, Santa Fe, NM, 1995.
Defines the characteristics of feline IgE.

Gilbert S, Halliwell REW: Assessement of an ELISA for the detection of allergen specific IgE in cats experimentally sensitized against house dust mites. Proceedings of the Third World Congress of Dermatology, Edinburgh, Scotland 1996.
Evaluates the sensitivity of ELISA testing in the cat.

Griffin CE: Insect and arachnid hypersensitivity. In: Griffin CE, ed: Current Veterinary Dermatology: The Science and Art of Therapy. St. Louis: Mosby–Year Book, 1993, p 133.
Discusses insect hypersensitivity as an atopic-like dermatitis.

Griffin CE, Rosenkrantz WS, Alaba S: Detection of insect/arachnid specific IgE in dogs: Comparison of two techniques utilizing western blots as the standard. In: Ihrke PJ, ed: Advances in Veterinary Dermatology, vol 2. Oxford: Pergamon Press, 1993, p 263.
Evaluates the sensitivity and specificity of the liquid phase assay in detecting insect allergens.

Peng Z, Simons FER, Becker AB: Measurement of ragweed-specific IgE in canine serum by use of enzyme-linked immunosorbent assays, containing polyclonal and monoclonal antibodies. Am J Vet Res 54:239, 1993.
Discusses the differences in using polyclonal versus monoclonal antibodies in an ELISA assay.

Ritter C, Battig M, Kraemer R, et al: IgE hidden in immune complexes with anti-IgE autoantibodies in children with asthma. J Allergy Clin Immunol 88:793, 1991.
Evaluates the sensitivity of monoclonal anti-IgE in detecting serum IgE levels.

Willemse A, Noordzij A, Van den Brom WE, et al: Allergen specific IgGd antibodies in dogs with atopic dermatitis as determined by the enzyme linked immunosorbent assay (ELISA). Clin Exp Immunol 59:359, 1985.
Discusses the value of using an ELISA with anti-IgGd reagent for identifying clinically atopic patients.

Feline Atopy

SONYA V. BETTENAY
Mount Waverley, Australia

Feline dermatitis that responded to hyposensitization, and was therefore considered suggestive of atopy, was first reported in 1982 (Reedy). Since then, it has been noted that a number of clinical syndromes are associated with atopy in cats and that these syndromes respond clinically to hyposensitization.

CLINICAL MANIFESTATIONS OF ATOPY

The predominant clinical sign in atopic cats is pruritus. In most cats, the presenting signs are the result of self-trauma, and the commonly recognized clinical syndromes include noninflammatory alopecia, miliary dermatitis, eosinophilic granuloma complex (indolent ulcer of the lip, eosinophilic granuloma, and eosinophilic plaque), facial and neck excoriation and ulceration, and (uncommonly) otitis externa. It cannot be emphasized enough that these clinical signs are *suggestive for* but *not pathognomonic of* atopy. There are many other possible causes of these signs (Table 1). It is of interest that the clinically affected sites frequently have less hair. There is evidence in humans that airborne allergens can exacerbate atopic dermatitis when placed in direct contact with the skin. This has not been studied in the cat.

Allergic asthma is seen as an uncommon clinical mani-

festation of atopy in cats, and a recent report (Halliwell, 1997) described six cats, presumptively diagnosed as asthmatic, that responded to hyposensitization. Rarely, affected cats will display several syndromes at the same time.

DIAGNOSIS OF FELINE ATOPY

The diagnosis of atopy in the cat is made predominantly on the basis of a careful clinical history and physical examination and ruling out other possibilities such as infectious and allergic causes (see Table 1). Once these other diseases have been eliminated, specific allergy testing can be performed (see previous article). Intradermal skin testing is used to confirm a diagnosis of atopy, but more importantly it identifies the offending allergens so treatment options may be expanded. The use of serum IgE tests to *confirm* a diagnosis is questionable because there are false-positive results reported with this test method.

The aforementioned review by Halliwell with regard to the feline radioallergosorbent test indicates that the serum IgE tests have value, as hyposensitization based on the test yielded significant response rates. These data were based on a mailed questionnaire that had a less than 50% return rate. The author uses intradermal allergy testing exclusively in cats at present, as the serum allergy test companies have

TABLE 1. Differential Diagnosis of the Etiology and Investigation of the Common Clinical Syndromes

Etiology	Mode of Diagnosis	M.D.	V.Alop	Eos.Com.	Head/Neck	O.Ext.
Allergies						
Flea bite hypersensitivity	Flea control / Intradermal skin test	√	√	√	√	
Food hypersensitivity	Elimination diet	√	?	√	√	√
Atopy	History and examination / Intradermal skin test	√	√	√	√	√
Ectoparasites						
Notoedres cati	Skin scraping / Ivermectin trial	√	√	?	√	√
Cheyletiella spp.	Skin scraping / Ivermectin trial	√	√	?	√	?
Trombiculids	Inspection	—	—	?	√	√
Pediculus	Inspection	√	—	—	√	—
Otodectes cynotis	Skin scraping / Ear swabs / Ivermectin trial	√	—	√	√	√
Nutritional						
Biotin deficiency	Biopsy / Supplementation	√	—	—	—	—
Essential fatty acid Deficiency	Biopsy / Supplementation	√	—	—	—	—
Infection						
Bacterial	Cytologic studies / Biopsy	√	—	√	√	√
Dermatophyte	Wood's light examination / Fungal culture / Biopsy	√	√	?	√	—
Malassezia	Cytologic studies / Biopsy	√	—	?	√	√
Demodex	Skin scraping	√	√	—	?	?

M.D., miliary dermatitis; V.Alop, ventral alopecia; Eos.Com., eosinophilic complex; O.Ext., otitis externa.

not yet published data to validate their tests. If skin testing is not available, serum allergy tests should be considered solely to select allergens for hyposensitization.

Intradermal Allergy Testing

Technique

The intradermal allergy test is regarded as the most accurate test method available, but it requires significant expertise in interpreting the results. The allergens lose potency with time, and so new test kits need to be made on a regular basis and the old kits discarded; thus, the caseload will affect financial practicality, and often these studies are obtained by referral. A stock test kit is made every 4 to 6 weeks and stored in sterile glass allergen vials. Fresh syringes are drawn weekly from these vials and any unused allergens are discarded. An additional consideration in cats is the possibility of feline immunodeficiency virus transmission; thus, needles must be changed between patients.

Intradermal injections are technically more difficult in the cat than in the dog or horse because of the thin skin of this species. To minimize elevated cortisol levels subsequent to the stress of handling, the cat must be sedated. The sedative of choice is a combination of ketamine, 5 mg/kg, and diazepam 0.25 mg/kg, intravenously or, alternatively, tiletamine-zolazepam (Telazol, A.H. Robbins, Richmond, VA), 4 mg/kg, intravenously. The lateral thorax is shaved with a No. 40 clipper blade, and injection sites are marked with a waterproof pen. Next, 0.05 to 0.1 ml of each allergen, a positive control (histamine), and a negative control (the allergen diluent, which contains 0.4% phenol) are then injected intradermally.

The degree of erythema, swelling, induration or firmness, diameter of the wheal, and appearance of pseudopod-like projections at the site are used to evaluate the response to the individual allergens. Wheals are evaluated by digital palpation and visualization. Erythema can usually be observed only in nonpigmented skin. A *subjective* comparison is used between the negative and positive controls. *All* positive controls are graded as 4+, negatives as 0, and the other results read subjectively in comparison to these scores.

The author initially reads feline skin tests in a dark room, as the wheal margins and heights are easier to observe when lit sideways by a point source of light. Feline skin test reactions are evaluated between 10 and 15 minutes after the injections. The technique requires experience and supervised training to master. False-positive or "irritant" reactions will occur unless the intradermal allergen extracts are appropriately diluted. The level at which the allergen fails to produce an irritant reaction has been investigated in the cat (Bevier, 1990) and is similar to that used in dogs. Prick testing, the method used in humans, has not been evaluated in cats. Some authors have proposed a fixed diameter for the positive and negative controls and allergen companies produce "reaction guides" that have circles

TABLE 2. Antihistamines and Oral Dosages

Antihistamine	Dosage	Further Information
Chlorpheniramine* (Piriton, Boots Co.)	2–4 mg/cat q12h	Antihistamine of choice in cats
Cyproheptadine (Periactin, Merck & Co.)	2–4 mg/cat q8h	Can cause PU/PD, increased appetite and vocalization
Promethazine (Phenergan, Rhone-Poulenc)	1–2 mg/kg q12h	
Diphenhydramine* (Benadryl, Parke Davis)	2 mg/kg q12h	
Diphenylpyraline (Histalert, 3M Corp.)	0.1–0.2 mg/kg q8h	
Terfenadine (Teldane, MarionMerrellDow)	2 mg/kg q12h	Nonsedating
Hydroxyzine (Atarax, Pfizer)	2 mg/kg q8h	Teratogenic, narrow margin of safety
Amitriptyline (Elavil, Zeneca)	10 mg q24h	

*Many other companies supply these drugs, including generics.
PU/PD, polydipsia/polyuria.

drawn on clear plastic "rulers" so that diameters can be easily assessed. On this basis, it is possible to grade histamine-positive controls as only 1+ or 2+.

Interpreting Positive Test Results

An accurate knowledge of important allergens and (in the case of pollen allergens) their pollination times in the cat's geographic area is essential to the interpretation of the test results. To obtain this information, the allergen laboratories, specialist dermatologists (preferably veterinary dermatologists), local government departments, and plant nurseries can be contacted. Books with the regional weeds, common grasses, and trees are available but are usually written for botanists, so they may not be limited to plants relevant to allergic disease.

When interpreting results, the author reviews the positive reactions in respect to the known environmental allergens and any seasonal reactions in the history. If skin test reactions do not correlate perfectly with the clinical and environmental history, one should consider the "allergic threshold" (that intangible level above which signs of allergy exist and below which the animal is clinically normal; i.e., the indoor cat that is allergic to dust mites and pollen but is asymptomatic in winter). Perhaps the cat has had *exposure to some allergens in the past,* causing positive reactions that are inconsistent with the current history. Interpretation of positive test results requires careful history taking and a knowledge of potential allergens.

TREATMENT OPTIONS

Once a presumptive diagnosis of atopy is reached, the owners have three therapeutic paths from which to choose. All three must be continued in the long term, as cures are not achieved with therapy. They can choose nonspecific symptomatic treatments such as corticosteroids, antihistamines, and supplementation with essential fatty acids, in which case the individual offending allergens do not need to be known. Alternatively, they can choose to try to identify the specific allergens with allergy tests and, based on the test results, to either avoid the offending allergen or if this is not possible (or practical) to administer "immunotherapy" or "hyposensitization" injections. Avoidance is possible with some environmental allergens, such as feathers and kapok (furniture stuffing), but is not practical for pets with dust mite allergy unless the felines are to be excluded from buildings. If the owners elect to proceed with hyposensitization, most cats need to receive concurrent symptomatic treatments in the initial stages (months) of the vaccine therapy. It is likely that hyposensitization therapy will be required for life, although a small percentage of patients have had their hyposensitization shots discontinued after years of therapy and remain in clinical remission.

Symptomatic Treatments

The treatment of pruritus in the cat can be rewarding using essential fatty acid supplementation, antihistamine therapy, and (in suitable cases) shampoos. Improvement may even occur in those patients that are clinically refractory to high-dose glucocorticosteroid therapy.

Essential Fatty Acids

The author uses an oral oil supplement that contains omega-3 fatty acids—OMEGA 3 (Biochemical Veterinary Research, Mittagong NSW),* 1 ml/7 kg PO every 24 hours. Other supplements containing omega-6 or both omega-3 and omega-6 fatty acids are EFAVET 2, 1 capsule per cat PO every 24 hours (Efamol, Kentville, Nova Scotia) and Dermcaps Liquid, 1 ml/9 kg PO (DVM) have also been reported as effective in the treatment of miliary dermatitis in cats (see p. 538 for further details of fatty acid supplementation).

Antihistamines

In the author's practice, a trial of antihistamine therapy is always offered in conjunction with essential fatty acid supplementation. The cats are prescribed two to three 10-day courses of different antihistamines (Table 2). The specific medication and frequency chosen varies with the cat's body weight and compliance. These antihistamines are taken consecutively with a 4-day washout to help determine whether any clinical improvement is directly related to the medication. Improvement may be coincidental—in which case there is no relapse on withdrawal of the antihista-

---

*Omega 3 constituents per 1 gm: eicosapentaenoic acid, 112.5 mg; docosahexaenoic acid, 75 mg, *cis*-linoleic acid, 70 mg; *dl*-alpha-tocopheryl acetate, 1 mg.

mines. Other details of antihistamine therapy are found on pp. 48 and 542.

Glucocorticoids

In the case of corticosteroid therapy, it is important to remember that cats need higher doses of glucocorticoids to achieve anti-inflammatory responses than do dogs. Although cats are relatively resistant to the development of hyperadrenocorticism, iatrogenic hyperadrenocorticism, pancreatitis, and liver disease do occur. Glucocorticoids may be administered concurrently with hyposensitization at anti-inflammatory dose rates. Prednisolone is used at the rate of 1 mg/kg PO every 12 hours tapered to every 48 hours or even to two separate days a week. Methylprednisolone acetate (20 mg/cat SC) is used by the author as a last resort in cats that do not respond to prednisolone in combination with essential fatty acids and antihistamines or that refuse oral medications. It is not recommended that more than two injections be given in a 4-month period. Cases of diabetes mellitus have occurred after only one such injection.

Avoidance

Allergens that can be specifically avoided include the following:

- House dust mites—by confining the animal to outdoors and providing it with a well-ventilated sleep and shelter area (not a dusty shed or outdoor room)
- Wool—by removing woolen items from the living areas of the pet (which is difficult in houses in which carpets are 100% wool)
- Kapok—by restricting access to rooms with kapok-stuffed furniture and cushions or identifying and removing them
- Tobacco—by having owners stop smoking
- Feathers—by replacing feather-filled pillows or doonas with synthetic fiber filling, or restricting access to these rooms

Pollens and mold spores are airborne allergens and are difficult to avoid. Some cats may be confined indoors throughout the pollen season to avoid direct contact with the plants and this may help minimize symptoms. However, even cats that are permanently indoors cannot completely avoid the windborne pollens. In cats that are allergic to pollen, mold spores, or house dust mites, the indoor confinement may decrease pollen but increase mold and dust mite exposure. In these cases, indoor confinement may produce no clinical improvement.

Allergen Hyposensitization

Hyposensitization offers an effective treatment alternative for cats. Reported success rates range from 60 to 78%. Before formulating an allergy vaccine, the offending allergens must be identified. A double-blind trial compared hyposensitization in canine atopic dermatitis using a standard mixture of allergens or allergens selected on the basis of positive skin test results (Willemse, 1993). Assessment was based on pruritus and the extent and severity of dermatitis. The group treated with the "standard" allergen mixture (containing dust mites, danders, and regional grasses) showed a median improvement of 18%, whereas 70% of the group hyposensitized with allergens based on the skin test results showed a greater than 50% reduction in symptoms. A previous study by the same author obtained a 20% response to placebo-treated atopic dogs (Willemse et al, 1984). These studies indicate the importance of careful evaluation and selection of allergens to be formulated in an allergen vaccine. Additional studies in dogs and humans have shown that sensitivity to allergens can be induced by their administration to previously nonsensitive individuals. This finding has the most relevance when formulating allergy vaccines based on a "grouped allergen serum" test. In a grouped allergen test, a number of separate allergens are placed together in the test well (see previous article). One, some, or all of the allergens tested in that well may be reactive, but there is no way to differentiate this. The author would prefer to leave an allergen out of the vaccine rather than include an allergen to which the cat is not currently allergic and risk actually sensitizing it! Thus, testing of individual allergens is of importance. If faced with the choice of a group test result or nothing, the allergens should be carefully chosen, as always, based on seasonal and environmental relevance.

In addition to the preceding criteria, the actual grade of reactivity or test score is also relevant. A study compared the success rates of hyposensitization in dogs with strong reactions to weak reactions. Those dogs with 1+ reactions to pollens showed a response rate of only 32%, whereas those with 3+ to 4+ reactions to pollens showed a 60% response rate. The author chooses 2+, 3+, and 4+ reactions on the basis of successful hyposensitization in patients that had 2+ only reactions, but there are others who restrict their selections to 3+ or 4+ grades.

There are numerous hyposensitization protocols described, with little evidence to suggest a best approach. Although there are no good controls, there is some evidence to suggest that increasing the protein nitrogen units and total numbers of allergens in the vaccines may alter the success rates of the therapies used. The protocol used by the author is outlined in Table 3. The injections are administered subcutaneously, and the owners are encouraged to perform the injections themselves at home. The commonly observed side effects of increased pruritus and exacerbation of the dermatitis are explained as dose-related, and the need for consultation with the veterinarian if they do occur is emphasized. Anaphylaxis is a rare adverse effect. The risk of anaphylaxis is explained before the initiation of the treatment, and written instructions are given so that the owner will administer the injection when veterinary service is immediately available and will be able to observe the cat for 30 minutes after each shot. Insulin syringes with swaged 27-gauge needles are used to avoid difficulty in handling, and "0.1 ml" is referred to as "10 units" in the client's schedule. It is recommended that asthmatic cats be admitted for hospital observation on the day of the injection (the author has never had a problem with an asthmatic cat nor heard reports of this from other dermatologists, but asthma can be life-threatening).

Time from onset to observed clinical response varies

TABLE 3. **Hyposensitization Schedule**

Week	Dose (ml) Subcutaneous Injection
Vial 1 (200 PNU/ml)	
1	0.1
2	0.2
3	0.4
4	0.8
5	1.0
Vial 2 (2000 PNU/ml)	
6	0.1
7	0.2
8	0.4
9	0.8
10	1.0
Vial 3 (20,000 PNU/ml)	
11	0.1
12	0.2
13	0.4
14	0.8
15	1.0
continue at 1.0 ml every 3 wk	

from between 1 and 8 months of therapy. An improvement of greater than 50% in reduction of pruritus and dermatitis is regarded as a satisfactory response. It must be stressed that regardless of the protocol selected, the individual response to that protocol must be carefully monitored. Modifications to the injection dose rate and frequency may need to be made during the course of hyposensitization. At the author's clinic, the following common scenarios are seen and subsequent actions taken:

A. For a few days after the shot, the cat becomes itchy. The itching subsides after a few days but flares again after the next shot.

Treat on the morning of the injection and for 1 to 2 subsequent days with antihistamines (see Table 2) or prednisolone, 1 mg/kg PO every 12 hours, if the cat is not already taking it.

B. The itching becomes worse throughout the course with no apparent change in signs in relation to the injections.

Stop the injections for 2 weeks to determine if the itching is related to the allergy shots, a coincidental flare, or a secondary infection. If it is coincidental, or concurrent infection is present, the cat will remain pruritic and will need more intensive adjunctive therapy; if the pruritus settles, restart the allergy shots but at a lower rate. If the cat relapses, repeat the process—stop, settle, and restart again at an even lower rate.

C. The cat continues to recrudesce even though the allergy shots in point B are increased.

Some cats never get to the "top of the schedule" dose. The clinical signs may be managed with doses of 0.1 ml of vial once per week. This will be determined by trial and error and discussions with the owners.

D. The cat was doing well until the treatment was extended to an injection every 3 weeks and then it developed

signs—these subside after the shot, but start to recur 1 to 2 weeks before the next shot.

This is a good sign—switch the frequency back to weekly or twice weekly. Use 0.3 to 0.5 ml per week and 0.7 ml every 2 weeks as initial alternative doses.

E. The cat shows no clinical response to the shots by week 32.

This cat needs a complete reassessment. It is possible for some animals to take 8 to 12 months to respond to hyposensitization regimens; others will be nonresponders or will have secondary infections or flea bite hypersensitivity complicating their pruritus and clinical appearance. All these factors need to be carefully assessed at this stage, and a physical examination is mandatory. Additionally, any of the preceding clues should be acted on.

There may be many reasons for discontinuation of the allergy shots, but once an owner has decided to discontinue hyposensitization it is often difficult to get him or her to initiate the shots again. That cat will then require lifelong symptomatic drug administration. This may be avoided by closer monitoring. The reasons many owners discontinue hyposensitization include:

- Impatience—why is it not working yet? This may develop into "It will not work, my cat is one of the failures, so I'll stop wasting my time now."
- Busy personal schedules—the owners forget and think they have mismanaged the schedule and will need to start (and possibly also pay) all over again.
- Concern for their pet—some owners are confused and believe that they should not administer other drugs concurrently. The cat is left without any treatment (as the allergy shots will not help for months initially in the majority of cats) and the condition progressively worsens. The owners cannot let their pet suffer and they seek alternative drug therapy, giving up on the vaccine.
- Failure to remember how bad the allergy was—an owner may perceive the vaccine as a failure when the veterinarian assesses it as successful. The author carefully records the current "itch" level and the medications the cat is taking when the vaccine is initiated. Furthermore, owner expectations may change. There may have been a partial improvement, but at that point the owner wants a complete "cure."

These reasons for discontinuing therapy are best avoided by providing detailed written instructions, knowledgeable telephone support, and a recall system that does not allow the cat to be forgotten. Recall appointments are really an essential component of the hyposensitization protocol. The author recommends a recheck at approximately week 32 of the 42-week course, at which stage they have reached 1 ml of vial 3–strength allergens and have given 3 injections at 3 weekly intervals. Other dermatologists prefer to see the pet for its initial "hyposensitization recheck" at week 16.

References and Suggested Reading

Bevier DE: The reaction of feline skin to the intradermal injection of allergenic extracts and passive cutaneous anaphylaxis using serum from skin test positive cats. In: von Tscharner C, ed: Advances In Veterinary Dermatology, vol 1. London: Bailliere Tindall, 1990, p 126.

Contains the recommended dilutions (which are essentially those the author uses for dogs).

Codner EC, Griffin CE: Serologic allergy testing for dogs. Comp Cont Ed Pract Vet 3:237, 1996.
An excellent review of serum allergy testing in dogs; many of the principles can be directly applied to the interpretation of feline serologic allergy test results.

Cohn LA: The influence of corticosteroids on host defense mechanisms. J Vet Intern Med 5:95, 1991.
For those interested in reviewing the effects of corticosteroids when used with standard vaccination practices, although the relevance of this to hyposensitization is not known.

DeBoer DJ, Saban R, Schultz KT, Bjorling DE: Feline IgE: Preliminary evidence of its existence and cross reactivity with canine IgE. In: Ihrke P, ed: Advances In Veterinary Dermatology, vol 2. Oxford: Pergamon Press, 1993, p 51.
An elegant scientific study.

Halliwell REW: Efficacy of hyposensitization in feline allergic diseases based upon results of in-vitro testing for allergen-specific IgE. J Am Anim Hosp Assoc 33:282, 1997.
Results of a questionnaire answered by general practitioners who diagnosed 81 cats on the basis of RAST and clinical signs. In 75.3% of cases, an improvement of at least 50% was seen.

Middleton E, ed: Allergy Principles And Practice, 3rd ed. St Louis: CV Mosby, 1988.
An outstanding reference text for those truly interested in allergic skin disease (there is a 4th edition).

Mueller RS, Bettenay SV: Long term immunotherapy of 146 dogs with atopic dermatitis—a retrospective study. Aust Vet Pract 26:128, 1996.

Reedy LM: Results of allergy testing and hyposensitisation in selected feline skin diseases. J Am Anim Hosp Assoc 18:618, 1982.
This was a landmark article. Reedy treated cases of miliary dermatitis and eosinophilic granuloma complex with hyposensitisation based on intradermal skin test results.

Willemse A: In vivo versus in vitro testing for canine atopy. In: Ihrke P, ed: Advances in Veterinary Dermatology, vol 2. Oxford: Pergamon Press, 1993, p 426.
A double blind trial comparing hyposensitization.

Willemse A, Van den Brom WE, Rijnberk A: Effect of hyposensitization on atopic dermatitis in dogs. J Am Vet Med Assoc 184:1277, 1984.
Includes a placebo controlled study.

Canine Papillomaviruses

MASAHIKO NAGATA

Tokyo, Japan

The papillomavirus was first described in 1933, when Shope recognized the causative agent responsible for cutaneous papilloma in the cottontail rabbit. Watrach first recognized the structural characterization of the canine papillomavirus in 1969. Yet this group of viruses has remained refractory to standard virologic study because to date all efforts aimed at tissue culture propagation of any of the papillomaviruses have remained unsuccessful. Since the mid-1980s, there has been a virtual explosion in research and interest in the papillomaviruses.

VIRAL PROPERTIES

The papillomaviruses are grouped together with the polyomaviruses to form the papovaviruses. The papillomavirus is a small, naked virus with double-stranded, circular DNA. The size of the canine papillomavirus has been estimated at 33 to 49 nm; the particles form closely packed crystalline structures within the nuclei. The lack of a lipid envelope may account for the relative resistance of the virus to physical or chemical destruction. Papillomavirus infections appear to be limited to the epidermis and epithelium. Epidermal DNA is present in the basal layer of the epidermis, and viral replication is dependent on epidermal cellular differentiation. The site of viral latency is in the basal layers, although complete viral particles are found at the granular level.

CLINICAL FEATURES

The clinical manifestation of papillomavirus is dependent on the host, the papillomavirus type, and the anatomic site infected. Transmission studies, immunohistochemistry, and in situ hybridization methods have suggested that dogs may be infected by four or more distinct papillomaviruses, although the most common outcome of papillomavirus infection may be asymptomatic infection.

Canine Oral Papilloma

Canine oral papillomatosis is a self-limited infectious disease that is normally confined to mucosal tissue of the oral cavity or lips in young dogs, but it can also produce papillomas on the conjunctiva and external nares (Sundberg, 1992). The disease is caused by the canine oral papillomavirus, which has been cloned and characterized. Canine oral papillomavirus–induced generalized papillomas may occasionally be the presenting sign in immunosuppressed dogs (Sundberg et al, 1994). The lesions begin as white, flat, smooth, shiny papules and plaques and progress to whitish gray, pedunculated or cauliflower-like hyperkeratotic masses. The lesions regress spontaneously in most cases, although malignant transformation to carcinomas has been reported.

Cutaneous Exophytic Papilloma

Cutaneous exophytic papillomas occur in older dogs and are more common in males (Scott et al, 1995). Transmission studies have shown the warts to be distinct from canine oral papilloma. Cutaneous exophytic papillomas may be single or multiple and occur mainly on the head, eyelids, and feet. They present as white, pink, or pigmented (brown to black); pedunculated or cauliflower-like; smooth to keratinous lesions. Microscopically, cutaneous papillomas consist of marked epithelial proliferation on numerous thin fibrovascular stalks. When undergoing regression, the papillomas become dark red and soft.

Cutaneous Inverted Papilloma

Another uncommon lesion associated with canine papillomavirus is the cutaneous inverted papilloma (Campbell et al, 1988). Tumors occur commonly on the ventral abdomen and the groin. Lesions present as single or multiple, small raised, firm masses covered by skin with a central pore opening to the surface. Light microscopy shows an inverted flask-like structure below the level of the normal epidermis. Canine inverted papillomas regress spontaneously (Shimada et al, 1993).

Canine Genital Papilloma

Venereal lesions are probably caused by a different canine papillomavirus, since neither the oral nor the cutaneous canine papillomaviruses induce tumors of the lower genital tract (Sundberg, 1992). This form of canine papillomavirus infection is less frequently reported and has yet to be given a properly detailed description.

Papillomavirus-Associated Canine Pigmented Plaques

Papillomavirus-associated canine pigmented plaques (PCPP) have been reported to occur in some pugs and miniature schnauzers during young adulthood (Nagata et al, 1995). PCPP develop progressively over time and never regress, even when affected dogs have not previously been prone to bacteria, fungal, or other viral infections. Lesions are multiple, scaly, deeply pigmented macules and plaques commonly seen on the ventral neck, trunk, and medial thighs. The potential for transformation to squamous cell carcinoma has also been reported. The presence of numerous papillomavirus particles within lesions and the presumed familial nature of PCPP strongly suggest that it is equivalent to epidermodysplasia verruciformis (EV) in humans. EV is considered to be genetically determined and caused by unusual susceptibility to infection by EV-specific human papillomaviruses related to the suppression of immunosurveillance exclusively against these viruses.

TREATMENTS

The search for an effective treatment against warts has been frustrated by our lack of adequate knowledge about canine papillomavirus infections. The mechanisms by which viral expression results in epidermal proliferation rather than cell death, the way in which canine papillomavirus maintains latency in the basal layer, and the nature of canine papillomavirus immunity are inadequately understood at this time to allow rational drug development. Fortunately, routine treatment of these lesions is not crucial. The majority of papillomavirus infections regress spontaneously without leaving a trace after the development of a cell-mediated immune response. Thus, the true effectiveness of a given therapy is difficult to assess because of

spontaneous regression on the one hand and recurrence on the other. Various reported therapies are described in the following sections.

Surgery

Surgical treatment has been used frequently for single warts. Procedures employed include excision, blunt dissection, curettage, and electrodesiccation. Great care must be taken to limit surgical manipulation in order to reduce the possibility of seeding the surgical site with virus particles. The patient should be rechecked for possible postoperative complications. A period of 90 days must be allowed to pass before assessing surgical results.

Cryotherapy

Cryotherapy effectively reduces temperature and the metabolic rate of injured tissue. This is the most widely used treatment for warts in humans. Freezing by liquid nitrogen or solid CO_2 (dry ice) is frequently used for heavily keratinized skin warts. Satisfactory results have been obtained by application of a cotton bud dipped in the fluid. The cotton bud may be made by twirling loose wisps of cotton wool by hand around one end of a small applicator stick. Treatment is repeated at least every 3 weeks when possible, as longer intervals are less effective. This may stimulate the development of an immune response. The main disadvantage of freezing is pain. Cryotherapy may be an effective treatment for skin warts in dogs, especially tumors on the eyelids and the bulbar conjunctiva and as additional therapy after surgical excision of squamous cell carcinomas.

Antimetabolites

5-Fluorouracil (5-FU) inhibits the enzyme thymidylate synthetase and results in thymidine deficiency, leading to inhibition of DNA synthesis. Application of a solution containing 0.5% 5-FU has been successful in human patients with widely dispersed warts. Topical application of 5-FU may be useful as part of the overall management for dogs with hyperkeratotic skin lesions. 5-FU is applied topically, using latex gloves, to focal lesions once daily for 5 days, and then once weekly for 4 to 6 weeks. An Elizabethan collar is used to prevent the dog from licking the medication. Topical application of 5-FU results in skin inflammation and irritant dermatitis in some cases, and the therapy may even cause systemic toxicity, including vomiting, diarrhea, pulmonary edema, respiratory failure, cardiac failure, central nervous system effects, and death (see p. 465).

Another therapeutic innovation has been the use of retinoids, referring to all chemicals, natural or synthetic, with vitamin A activity (see CVT XII, p. 585). Retinoids promote desquamation of hyperkeratotic skin and a normalization of deregulated proliferative activity. Etretinate is a synthetic retinoid that has been helpful in treating dogs with skin warts. Extensive hyperkeratotic PCPP lesions have been treated with daily oral doses of etretinate, 1 mg/kg every 24 hours (Nagata et al, 1995). Severe hyperkeratosis has been ameliorated after approximately 1 month of this treatment. This has been useful in temporarily relieving pruritus or disability due to exceptionally hyperkeratotic warts. Retinoid toxicity, including teratogenicity, conjunctivitis, hyperactivity, pruritus, pedal and mucocutaneous junction erythema, stiffness, vomiting, and diarrhea, has been observed.

Intralesional bleomycin has been shown to be another effective treatment. Bleomycin appears to inhibit DNA synthesis. Doses of this cytotoxic agent are given in units or in milligrams; 1 mg contains 1.5 to 2 U. Protocols vary in humans, although concentrations as low as 0.5 U/ml seem effective, with the volume per injected lesion ranging between 0.2 and 1.0 ml. Injections are painful and local anesthesia should be considered for sensitive sites. Although clinical experience with this therapy has been extremely limited, it may yet prove useful. Bleomycin has been applied intralesionally for management of recurrent gingival mucosal cauliflower-like epithelioma (Iwasaki, 1978). In this case, 5 mg of bleomycin was diluted with 3 ml of lidocaine and administered to the lesion once weekly. The tumor regressed after 8 weeks of the treatment. There was no evidence of local or systemic toxicity, and no papillomas reappeared after treatment.

Immunotherapy

Autogenous vaccines have been used especially for treatment of mucous membrane warts in humans and dogs. It has been demonstrated that systemic administration of a formalin-inactivated canine oral papilloma vaccine can protect against mucosal infection with canine oral papillomavirus (Bell et al, 1994). In this study, 26 dogs received two doses of phosphate-buffered saline intradermally, and 99 dogs received two doses of the inactivated vaccine. One month after the second dose, all dogs were challenged with infectious canine oral papillomavirus by scarification of the oral mucosa. All control dogs acquired papillomas 6 to 8 weeks after infection, whereas none of the vaccinated dogs did. The vaccine may be protective against canine oral papillomavirus epidermal infections that develop as a consequence of the spread of oral lesions to the haired skin in immunosuppressed dogs (Sundberg et al, 1994). In addition, the vaccination might have a role in protecting against the development of squamous cell carcinomas in dogs infected with canine oral papillomavirus.

Sensitization to dinitrochlorobenzene followed by an application of dinitrochlorobenzene to lesions and contact sensitization with diphenylcyclopropenone has been a useful treatment of cutaneous malignancies and refractory warts in humans. Such treatment, however, has been tried in only a limited number of human studies, and no studies have been conducted with dogs.

Antiviral Therapy

Interferons have antiviral, antiproliferative, and immunomodulating effects. In in vitro studies, interferon has been shown to reduce the number of papillomavirus genomes in mouse cells transformed by BPV-1. Intralesional and parenteral interferon therapy has been successful in treating human patients. These studies, however, are seldom directly comparable, and the use of interferons in treating warts is still experimental.

Laser Therapy

The CO_2 laser produces an infrared light (10,600 nm) that is invisible to the human eye and is strongly absorbed by water. These properties allow the CO_2 laser to make incisions by vaporizing cells in its path, but render it useless in pools of fluid or blood. These properties also make the CO_2 laser an excellent surgical scalpel, especially for superficial procedures. The CO_2 laser is effective in eradicating some difficult human warts, but causes significant postoperative pain, scarring, and temporary loss of function. There have been no studies in dogs with skin warts.

Photodynamic therapy (PDT) is a relatively new treatment advocated for a variety of skin cancers in animals. The technique involves the parenteral administration of a photosensitizing compound followed by activation of that compound by laser-generated light. A series of physical and chemical events is set in motion and oxygen radicals are generated. Two laser systems are used for PDT—gold vapor and argon-pumped dye lasers. Excellent responses to PDT have been seen in several tumors, and squamous cell carcinomas have been treated in dogs with PDT using profimer sodium. Clinical experience with wart treatments is limited at this time.

References and Suggested Reading

Bell JA, Sundberg JP, Ghim S, et al: A formalin-inactivated vaccine protects against mucosal papillomavirus infection. A canine model. Pathobiology 62:194, 1994.
The effects of systemically administered, formalin-inactivated vaccine against mucosal infection by canine oral papillomavirus and approaches for the development of human papillomaviruses vaccines.

Campbell KL, Sundberg JP, Goldschmidt MH, et al: Cutaneous inverted papillomas in dogs. Vet Pathol 25:67, 1988.
The original case report of cutaneous inverted papillomas in the dog.

Iwasaki T: A canine case of oral florid papillomatosis [Japanese]. J Jpn Vet Med Assoc 31:580, 1978.
The clinical experience of using intralesional bleomycin for gingival mucosal epithelioma in a dog.

Nagata M, Nanko H, Moriyama A, et al: Pigmented plaques associated with papillomavirus infection in dogs. Is this epidermodysplasia verruciformis? Vet Dermatol 6:179, 1995.
The original description of epidermodysplasia verruciformis–like dermatosis in the dog.

Scott DW, Miller WH Jr, Griffin CE: Muller and Kirk's Small Animal Dermatology, 5th ed. Philadelphia: WB Saunders, 1995, p 994.
A review of the cause, clinical findings, diagnosis, and clinical management of cutaneous papilloma.

Shah KV, Howley PH: Papillomaviruses. In: Fields BN, Knipe DM, eds: Fields Virology, 2nd ed. New York: Raven Press, 1990, p 1651.
A review of the history, infectious agent, biology, pathogenesis, clinical features, diagnosis, and management of papillomaviruses.

Shimada A, Shinya K, Awakura T, et al: Cutaneous papillomatosis associated with papillomavirus infection in a dog. J Comp Pathol 108:103, 1993.
First report of multiple canine inverted papillomas in an old dog.

Sundberg JP: Papillomaviruses. In: Castro AE, Heuschele WP, eds: Veterinary Diagnostic Virology: A Practitioner's Guide. St Louis: Mosby–Year Book, 1992, p 148.
A review of the viral properties, disease, diagnosis, and clinical management of canine papillomaviruses.

Sundberg JP, Smith EK, Herron AJ, et al: Involvement of canine oral papillomavirus in generalized oral and cutaneous verrucosis in a Chinese Shar Pei dog. Vet Pathol 31:183, 1994.
First report of corticosteroid-induced generalized canine oral papillomavirus infection in a dog.

Therapy for Sebaceous Adenitis

EDMUND J. ROSSER, JR.
East Lansing, Michigan

Sebaceous adenitis is an inflammatory disease process directed against the sebaceous glands of the skin and has an unknown etiology and pathogenesis (Rosser et al, 1987; Scott, 1986). In Standard Poodles, the results of pedigree analyses and prospective breeding studies of affected animals suggests that sebaceous adenitis is a heritable, autosomal recessive skin disease of variable expression (Dunstan and Hargis, 1995).

CLINICAL FEATURES

Sebaceous adenitis occurs primarily in young adult to middle-aged dogs, with no apparent sex predisposition. The disease can be divided into two major forms based on their differences in clinical presentation and histopathologic changes (Rosser, 1992).

The first form occurs in long-coated breeds and has been recognized most frequently in the Standard Poodle (*see CVT XII,* p. 619), Akita, and Samoyed. This form of the disease is characterized by a dull, brittle haircoat, alopecia, moderate to severe scaling, and the formation of follicular casts. Pruritus and malodor are variable and tend to be mild or absent early in the course of the disease and may become moderate to severe in advanced cases or when a secondary bacterial folliculitis develops. In Standard Poodles, the lesions most commonly affect the dorsal regions of the body, including the dorsal planum of the nose, top of the head, pinnae, dorsal trunk, and tail. When the disease is progressive, the affected areas develop tightly adherent scales (varying from silver-white to brown, depending on haircoat color) with small tufts of hair matted within the scales. The disease in Standard Poodles may present in several clinical forms: (1) a subclinical form (detectable only on histopathologic examination of skin biopsy specimens of apparently normal skin); (2) a localized, mild, and self-limiting form; (3) a progressive moderate to severe form; and (4) a cyclic form with periods of spontaneous improvement or worsening independent of any treatment. In Samoyeds, the alopecia, scaling, and follicular casts most commonly affect the entire trunk and pinnae. The disease in the Akita may represent its own variant of sebaceous adenitis in long-coated breeds of dogs, as it differs by the additional presence of greasiness of the skin and haircoat and the frequent presence of papules and pustules. Akitas may also show signs of systemic illness, such as fever, malaise, and weight loss (Power and Ihrke, 1990).

The second form occurs in short-coated breeds of dogs and has been most frequently recognized in the Vizsla. This form of the disease is characterized by "moth-eaten," annular, or diffuse areas of alopecia and mild scaling, affecting the trunk, head, and ears. Dogs usually do not have pruritus, and the development of secondary bacterial folliculitis is rare.

DIAGNOSIS

The breed affected, the historical development of the problem, and the physical findings are what first lead the clinician to suspect sebaceous adenitis. The diagnosis is confirmed by the histopathologic examination of several skin biopsy specimens that are representative of the different degrees of lesion severity noted during the physical examination. Sites selected for biopsy should include any apparently normal skin, mildly affected areas, and severely affected areas. The most common histologic finding is a nodular granulomatous to pyogranulomatous inflammatory reaction at the level of the sebaceous glands (Dunstan and Hargis, 1995; Gross et al, 1992).

TREATMENT AND MANAGEMENT

Long-term management of sebaceous adenitis can be a frustrating experience for owners and veterinarians because the response to therapy varies depending on the severity of the disease at the time of diagnosis; in addition there is a lack of a consistent response to any single treatment regimen. This problem has led to several treatment recommendations and much confusion about which treatments should be tried. For this reason, the author recommends a systematic approach to the treatment of sebaceous adenitis in dogs.

The goal of therapy should be to remove the excess scales, improve the luster of the haircoat, and regrow hair whenever possible (in Standard Poodles, the hair regrowth is usually straight rather than curled). When response to treatment is evident, some level of maintenance therapy is usually required to control the disease. In severe or chronic cases in which the sebaceous glands have been completely lost, the prognosis for accomplishing these goals is guarded. However, a successful response to treatment (White et al, 1995), as well as the reappearance of sebaceous glands (Dunstan, personal communication, 1997), can occur even when the initial histopathologic examination of skin biopsy specimens revealed follicular fibrosis and apparent loss of the sebaceous glands.

In mildly affected dogs, the regular use of antiseborrheic shampoos, conditioners, emollients, and essential fatty acid dietary supplements (see p. 538) may be effective. If the response is inadequate, the author's first recommendation is the consistent use of a combination of essential fatty acid dietary supplements (Derm Caps ES, Dermatologics for Veterinary Medicine, Inc.), one capsule PO every 12 hours, and evening primrose oil, 500 mg PO every 12 hours, per dog (Rosser, 1992). This treatment should be continued for 2 months before being considered ineffective. Occasionally observed side effects include vomiting, diarrhea, and flatulence. This treatment has been most effective in the Standard Poodle and Samoyed breeds and usually requires lifelong administration to control the disease. When this is ineffective, or in dogs with large areas of tightly adherent scales (as in Standard Poodles), a bath oil treatment can be recommended. This is carried out by mixing any light mineral oil–containing bath oil (e.g., Alpha Keri Bath Oil, Westwood Pharmaceuticals or generic bath oil) 50:50 with water and spraying over the entire coat (Blair, 1993). The bath oil is then rubbed well into the haircoat and allowed to soak into the coat for 1 hour. The dog should be put in a crate or kennel during the 1-hour soak. The bath oil is then removed by several bathings (usually three shampooings) using a liquid dishwashing detergent (e.g., Palmolive dish soap, Ivory dish soap) while scrubbing the haircoat with a soft hair brush. A conditioner or creme rinse (HyLyt, Dermatologics for Veterinary Medicine; Humilac, Allerderm/Virbac) should be applied after the final bath. This process results in the removal of a significant amount of the excess scaling, and this treatment alone may control the scaling and allow the regrowth of hair. This procedure is then repeated every 7 days for the first month and then every 14 to 30 days as needed. It must be mentioned that this procedure is relatively labor-intensive but can be effective. An alternative to this form of treatment is the use of a 50:50 or 75:25 mixture of propylene glycol and water applied once daily as a spray to the affected areas (Griffin, 1988).

When these treatments have been ineffective, the use of a synthetic retinoid may be considered (see *CVT XII*, p. 586). In the management of sebaceous adenitis in Vizslas, isotretinoin (Accutane, Roche) has been shown to be a most effective retinoid (Stewart et al, 1991; White et al, 1995). The recommended dosage of isotretinoin is 1 mg/kg PO every 12 to 24 hours, with improvement usually noticed within 6 weeks. If improvement is evident, an attempt can be made to decrease the dosage to 1 mg/kg PO every 24 to 48 hours for another 6 weeks. If improvement continues, the long-term goal is to control the disease with either 1 mg/kg PO every 48 hours or 0.5 mg/kg every 24 hours.

For management of refractory cases of sebaceous adenitis in long-coated breeds of dogs (primarily Standard Poodles and Akitas), either isotretinoin or etretinate (Tegison, Roche) can be recommended. A recent study indicated that it could not be predicted as to which of these two retinoids would be more effective in the treatment of sebaceous adenitis in any long-coated dog breeds (White et al, 1995). Therefore, these dogs can be treated initially with either isotretinoin (1 mg/kg PO every 12 to 24 hours) or etretinate (1 mg/kg PO every 12 to 24 hours) for an observation period of 6 weeks. If there is a poor response to therapy on the first chosen retinoid, the dog should be switched to the second retinoid for an observation period of 6 weeks. If improvement is noted using either of these retinoids, an attempt can be made to decrease the dosage to 1 mg/kg PO every 24 to 48 hours for another 6 weeks. If improvement continues, the long-term goal is to control the disease using either retinoid at a dosage of 1 mg/kg every 48 hours or 0.5 mg/kg PO every 24 hours.

A treatment option in the management of sebaceous adenitis that has been nonresponsive to retinoid therapy is the use of cyclosporine (Sandimmune, Sandoz Labs) at a dosage of 5 mg/kg PO every 12 hours (Carothers et al, 1991) (see p. 509 and *CVT XII*, p. 73 for a discussion of the side effects and toxicities in the use of cyclosporine in dogs).

Sebaceous adenitis appears to be relatively refractory to either anti-inflammatory or immunosuppressive dosages of corticosteroids. When a secondary bacterial folliculitis is present, the treatment should include the use of an appropriate systemic antibiotic along with a keratolytic, antibacterial, and follicular flushing shampoo (Sulf Oxydex, Dermatologics for Veterinary Medicine, Inc.).

References and Suggested Reading

Blair GL: Home therapy of sebaceous adenitis. Prog SA Research, Winter/Spring, 1993, p 4.
  Genodermatosis Research Foundation publication describing a bath oil treatment for sebaceous adenitis in Standard Poodles.
Carothers MA, Kwochka KW, Rojko JL: Cyclosporine-responsive granulomatous sebaceous adenitis in a dog. J Am Vet Med Assoc 198:1645, 1991.
  A case report of granulomatous sebaceous adenitis in a miniature pinscher successfully treat with cyclosporine.
Dunstan DW, Hargis AM: The diagnosis of sebaceous adenitis in standard poodle dogs. In: Bonagura JD, ed: Kirk's Current Veterinary Therapy XII. Philadelphia: WB Saunders, 1995, p 619.
  A review article of the clinical features, histologic characteristics, heritability, pathogenesis, and registry of sebaceous adenitis in Standard Poodles.
Griffin CE: Common dermatoses of the Akita, Shar Pei, and chow chow. Annual meeting of the American Academy of Veterinary Dermatology, Washington DC, 1988, p 31.
  The clinical description and treatment of sebaceous adenitis in Akitas.
Gross TL, Ihrke PJ, Walder EJ: Veterinary Dermatopathology. St. Louis: Mosby–Year Book, 1992, p 247.
  The histologic features of sebaceous adenitis in dogs.
Power HT, Ihrke PJ: Synthetic retinoids in veterinary dermatology. Vet Clin North Am Small Anim Pract 20:1525, 1990.
  A review of the pharmacology, clinical uses, and toxicities of synthetic retinoids used in veterinary dermatology.
Rosser EJ: Sebaceous adenitis. In: Kirk RW, Bonagura JD, eds: Current Veterinary Therapy XI. Philadelphia: WB Saunders, 1992, p 534.
  A review of the clinical features, diagnosis, and treatment of sebaceous adenitis in dogs.
Rosser EJ, Dunstan RW, Breen PT, Johnson GR: Sebaceous adenitis with hyperkeratosis in the standard poodle: A discussion of 10 cases. J Am Anim Hosp Assoc 23:341, 1987.
  A prospective study describing the clinical features, laboratory findings, and histologic features of sebaceous adenitis in 10 Standard Poodles.
Scott DW: Granulomatous sebaceous adenitis in dogs. J Am Anim Hosp Assoc 22:631, 1986.
  Clinical and pathologic features of sebaceous adenitis in dogs.
Stewart LJ, White SD, Carpenter JL: Isotretinoin in the treatment of sebaceous adenitis in two vizslas. J Am Anim Hosp Assoc 27:65, 1991.
  Two case reports of sebaceous adenitis in Vizslas successfully treated with isotretinoin.
White SD, Rosychuk RAW, Scott KV, et al: Sebaceous adenitis in dogs and results of treatment with isotretinoin and etretinate: 30 cases (1990–1994). J Am Vet Med Assoc 207:197, 1995.
  A review article on the signalment, clinical signs, histologic features, and the use of isotretinoin and etretinate in the treatment of sebaceous adenitis in 30 dogs of various breeds.

Malassezia Dermatitis

RUSSELL MUSE

Garden Grove, California

The role of *Malassezia* spp. as a causative agent in skin disease has been fraught with controversy since it was first implicated as a disease-causing organism. The organism as a pathogen was first described by Dufait, a Belgian veterinarian (Mason, 1996). This was followed years later by Mason, who implicated the organism as a cause of localized or generalized pruritus associated with inflammatory skin disease (Mason, 1996). Since that time, numerous studies have attempted to further define the role that *Malassezia* plays as both a normal resident and a disease-causing organism.

It is now known that several species of *Malassezia* have been isolated from diseased skin in animals (Guillot et al, 1996). At least two of these species have been isolated from small animals. *Malassezia pachydermatis* is a lipophilic, nonmycelial, saprophytic yeast that possesses a characteristic thick-walled oval or peanut shape. The typical peanut shape is caused by the unipolar budding of daughter cells from one site on the cell wall. The organism also contains a distinctive spiraling ridge on the inside layer of the cell wall. It is a normal resident of the skin and is commonly found in the ear canal, anal sacs, interdigital areas, lip, rectum, and vagina of dogs (Scott et al, 1995). *Malassezia* organisms may be found on truncal skin, but are present in low numbers. Cats may also carry *M. pachydermatis* as a resident organism in ear canals and anal sacs.

Another organism, *M. sympodialis*, has been recognized as a separate species (Bond et al, 1995). This organism is more rounded or bulbous and is slightly smaller than *M. pachydermatis*. *M. sympodialis* has been isolated in normal cats with wax accumulations and in cats with inflammatory ear disease. *Malassezia* spp. and commensal staphylococci have been shown to have an interesting symbiotic relationship (Mason, 1996). There is production of mutually beneficial growth factors that alter the microenvironment to benefit both organisms. Both have lipases that may alter the sebum balance to support growth of both organisms and discourage growth of other competitors. However, despite the fact that *Malassezia* growth has been shown to be enhanced in vitro by the presence of staphylococci, there is no dependency between the organisms. The inhibition of one organism does not inhibit the growth of the other.

PATHOGENESIS

Since the presence of *Malassezia* spp. on the skin of normal, nondiseased animals has been well documented, other factors must play a role before these organisms cause clinical disease. These factors may include both alteration in skin microclimate and host defenses, as well as numerous host "predisposing factors."

Excessive sebum or cerumen production, moisture accumulation, and disruption of the epidermal barrier may allow yeast proliferation. *Malassezia* has been shown to have an adherence mechanism to corneocytes, ensuring a hold on the host. This adherence factor may be a protein or glycoprotein moiety (Bond and Lloyd, 1996). This allows lipases and lipoxygenases produced by the organism to cause further changes in the sebum film, resulting in a more favorable microclimate to support yeast growth. Recent studies have also shown protease, urease, and phosphatase activity in some strains of *M. pachydermatis* (Mathieson et al, 1996). Zymogen is a cell wall component that may be released, causing severe inflammation by activating the complement cascade. In addition, *Malassezia* organisms produce a substance that inhibits other fungal organisms to further limit competition.

There has been speculation for some time that a hypersensitivity reaction to the organism may exist, since some animals show extreme pruritus and other clinical signs when relatively few organisms are detectable. Recent work has indeed shown that atopic dogs with skin disease had an IgE-mediated type 1 hypersensitivity reaction to intracellular protein extracts of *M. pachydermatis,* whereas normal, nonatopic dogs did not show significant levels of IgE-specific antibodies (Morris, 1995).

Predisposing factors present in the host that may facilitate yeast overgrowth include allergic disease, cornification disorders (seborrhea), bacterial skin disease, as well as long-term corticosteroid or antibiotic administration used to treat these disorders (White et al, 1996). A genetic basis for breed predisposition may be due to deficient T-lymphocyte responses to the yeast. It has been suggested that the following breeds are predisposed: the West Highland White terrier, Basset hound, Springer spaniel, German shepherd, Cocker spaniel, Silky terrier, Australian terrier, Maltese, Chihuahua, Poodle, Shetland sheepdog, Lhasa apso, and Dachshund (Scott et al, 1995).

The precise pathogenesis and the number of organisms required to cause disease is not clearly defined. Likely, some changes in the cutaneous microclimate or alterations of the host immunity because of endogenous or exogenous factors can result in *Malassezia* overgrowth on the skin surface and hair follicles, resulting in a cascade of events and subsequent disease.

CLINICAL SIGNS

Clinical signs associated with *Malassezia* dermatitis are variable but generally consist of erythema, mild to severe pruritus, yellow to gray scale or greasy wax associated with a "yeasty," rancid, offensive odor. Chronic infections may result in lichenification, hyperpigmentation, and traumatic alopecia. However, these clinical signs are present in other dermatologic disorders, so their presence is suggestive, but not diagnostic, of *Malassezia* dermatitis. The most common sites of involvement are the ears; lip; muzzle; interdigital areas; ventral cervical flexural surfaces of the forelegs; anal; and perianal areas. The diseased areas may be focal, multifocal, or generalized, with numerous areas of the body affected. There are also other specific clinical syndromes in dogs that have been attributed to excessive colonization of *Malassezia* organisms. The most commonly encountered and most widely known syndrome associated with *M. pachydermatis* is otitis externa. This condition in association with the finding of large numbers of *Malassezia* organisms has been shown to occur as a secondary finding to a large number of diseases. Folliculitis and furunculosis in the form of chin acne and interdigital cysts have been shown occasionally to be associated with increased *Malassezia* numbers (Scott et al, 1995). Recently, *Malassezia* organisms were shown to be associated with paronychia and brown staining of the claw in atopic dogs, sometimes resulting in residual pedal pruritus (Griffin, 1996). This syndrome may lead the clinician to falsely assume that the treatment of the atopic disease is ineffective or only partially effective. In reality, treatment of the *Malassezia* allows resolution of the clinical signs. *Malassezia* dermatitis, although uncommonly reported in the cat, has been associated with black waxy otitis externa, recalcitrant feline acne, generalized keratinization defects, and a generalized scaly dermatitis (exfoliative erythroderma) (Scott et al, 1995). Feline immunodeficiency virus and diabetes mellitus have reportedly been seen in association with cats that acquire recurrent generalized *Malassezia* dermatitis (Scott et al, 1995).

DIAGNOSIS

Controversy exists as to the best diagnostic techniques available. Skin cytologic studies are the diagnostic method of choice in clinical practice because they are quick and easily performed with materials that are readily available in a clinical setting. Several methods of obtaining cytologic preparations have been advocated. These include direct impression smear, tape impressions, skin scrapings, and cotton swab smears. The author generally prefers direct impression smears, especially when the desired area to be sampled has a greasy, waxy, and flat surface. The slide is repeatedly pressed against the skin and rubbed vigorously to obtain surface debris and exudate.

Cotton swabs or broken swab handles can be used to scrape the skin in areas not having a large flat surface area. The resultant matter is then transferred by rolling or smearing the debris onto a glass slide. Cotton swabs are generally preferred for the ears and sometimes for interdigital areas. However, some recent studies have shown "swabbing" to be less reliable in obtaining yeast organisms (White et al, 1996). Skin scrapings and tape impression smears may be more diagnostic when the sampled surface consists of dry scale. Clear tape is pressed firmly onto the diseased skin; multiple areas should be sampled. The tape is then placed "sticky side down" onto several drops of stain placed on a glass slide. In addition, "sticky" slides are now commercially available. These slides are pressed directly onto the skin surface.

Once material is collected onto the slide, heat fixation is required to "adhere" the organisms onto the slide and prevent them from falling into the stain. Heat fixation can be performed with matches or disposable lighters waved on the undersurface of the slide for 2 to 3 seconds. The slide is then stained routinely. Diff-Quik, New methylene blue stain (which does not require heat fixation), or Gram's stain may be used to stain yeasts. The slides are then examined under oil immersion. Most dermatologists will consider more than 1 to 2 organisms per oil immersion field as significant. However, care should be exercised in interpreting the results from cytologic studies. As previously discussed, some areas of the body may have increased numbers of yeast present normally. Increased numbers should be correlated with typical clinical signs to determine the significance of the yeast's presence. Culture is generally not recommended as a diagnostic tool in clinical practice. Although some culture techniques are used in a quantitative manner in research, they are not practical and are often unrewarding in the clinical setting. Skin biopsy, like cultures, is not extremely helpful as a routine diagnostic procedure. Even in areas in which impression smears show large numbers of *Malassezia*, routine processing of the biopsy sample may result in a loss of organisms. However, organisms may occasionally be detected on the surface or in follicular hyperkeratotic material. When organisms are found on histopathologic examination, their presence should be viewed as significant. Follicular openings or "ostia" may also be areas where yeasts may be seen. The cutaneous pattern may be variable but is generally manifested as a hyperplastic, spongiotic, superficial, and perivascular to interstitial dermatitis with lymphohistiocytic cells predominating. Lymphocytic exocytosis is often noted, as is a mixed infiltrate with eosinophils present.

Occasionally, the preceding diagnostic protocols will detect only rare *Malassezia* organisms or none. However, clinical experience, along with suggestive clinical signs, may still cause the clinician to be concerned about the possibility of yeast organisms causing disease. In these cases, a trial therapy of antifungal medications or topical treatments may be the only way of resolving whether these organisms are causing or adding to the clinical disease.

TREATMENT

Therapy in *Malassezia* cases must be directed at both the yeast and elimination of any detectable predisposing problems facilitating the yeast's growth. Since the organism is a normal resident, its complete elimination is probably not possible. Therefore, without correction of underlying disorders, recurrence of the yeast infection usually results. This leads to frustration for both the veterinarian and the owner. When no underlying cause can be discerned or controlled, chronic management is usually needed.

Topical and systemic therapy are both helpful in reducing the populations of *Malassezia* spp. from the skin. Topical therapy has been used widely; however, the author recommends it only occasionally as the sole form of therapy, and only then in localized cases. Even in localized cases, topical therapy may not always be effective. The author finds that generalized *Malassezia* dermatitis often is only partially responsive to topical therapy. However, topical management as an adjunctive therapy is helpful in resolving the dermatitis more quickly. Ideally, topical preparations should have degreasing activities, antifungal activity, and some residual activity to decrease the rate of recurrence. No single product has all these properties; thus, many dermatologists rely on combination therapy.

Benzoyl peroxide (Oxydex, DVM Pharmaceuticals; Pyoben, Allerderm/Virbac), benzoyl peroxide and sulfur (Sulf/Oxydex, DVM Pharmaceuticals), selenium disulfide (Selsun Blue, Ross Laboratories), and tar are shampoo ingredients with good degreasing abilities and may be used to eliminate excessive sebum, which provides a favorable environment for the organism's growth. Specific antifungal shampoos are also advocated. Chlorhexidene (Chlorhexiderm, DVM Pharmaceuticals; Hexedine, Allerderm/Virbac), at a concentration of at least 1%, is the most commonly used antifungal product in clinical practice and has been shown to be effective against Malassezia, although a concentration of 2 to 4% may be more effective. Other shampoo ingredients available for topical treatment include miconazole (Dermazole, Allerderm/Virbac) and ketoconazole (Nizoral, Janssen Pharmaceutica). These products have shown variable success in numerous trials. A newer product, Sebolyse (Dermcare-Vet), which contains 2% miconazole nitrate and 2% chlorhexidine gluconate, has shown good efficacy but is not currently available in the United States. Several important factors in the use of all shampoos are especially applicable when treating Malassezia dermatitis. Shampoo therapy must be used at least twice weekly, and some cases may require more frequent treatment. Contact time of 10 to 15 minutes with the skin surface is also an important factor in getting the best possible response to shampoo therapy. Since shampoos have poor residual activity, rinses that are left on to dry give additional antifungal activity. Enilconazole (Imaverol, Janssen Pharmaceutica), although also not licensed in the United States, has been reported to be effective. However, an offensive odor and difficult application may limit its appeal to many clients. Enilconazole cannot be used on cats. This product is available in Europe, Australia, and Canada. Selenium sulfide shampoo followed by enilconazole rinses have been reported to be effective (Scott et al, 1995). Since most antifungal shampoos and rinses are costly, some clinicians use an equal mixture of white vinegar (acetic acid) and water used as a rinse followed by creams, ointments, or lotions containing miconazole, clotrimazole, nystatin, enilconazole, chlorhexidine, or ketoconazole. "Spot" treatment is usually reserved for cases in which only a few areas are affected and those areas are conducive to application of topical medicaments (lip folds, ears, interdigital areas, and so on).

Systemic treatment is the most effective method for Malassezia dermatitis. The author uses systemic treatment for all but the most localized of cases to resolve the infection initially. Concurrent and subsequent topical therapy, as discussed, may then be helpful in keeping the disease controlled so that relapses are minimal. Ketoconazole, itraconazole, and fluconazole have all shown efficacy against Malassezia. Ketoconazole (Nizoral, Janssen Pharmaceutica) is the most widely used and least expensive of the three drugs. The dosage and treatment regimens for ketoconazole in Malassezia dermatitis are as varied as the number of clinicians and dermatologists who use them.

The general recommendation is 5 to 10 mg/kg every 12 hours for 2 to 4 weeks. However, many dermatologists find that a dose as low as 5 mg/kg every 24 hours for a similar period is effective in the vast majority of cases. The author often begins therapy with 5 to 10 mg/kg daily for 10 days followed by the same dosage on an alternate-day basis for an additional 10 days. This treatment protocol resolves the majority of Malassezia infections with minimal relapses. In addition, it may allow better client compliance because of the expense involved with using ketoconazole at higher dosages. However, if the condition is unresponsive or only partially responsive or if relapse occurs, higher dosages may be required. Pruritus generally resolves rapidly within the first week, whereas other clinical signs resolve in the following weeks of therapy. Ketoconazole should be administered with food because gastrointestinal absorption is enhanced in an acidic environment. Gastrointestinal upset and rarely a hepatotoxic reaction may occur as side effects to ketoconazole but are uncommon at the lower dosages. Some dermatologists monitor liver enzymes in dogs undergoing therapy. The author usually reserves blood monitoring for dogs receiving chronic drug therapy or higher dosages of ketoconazole. Itraconazole (Sporonox, Janssen Pharmaceutica) has been used at 5 to 10 mg/kg every 24 hours and fluconazole (Diflucan, Roerig) is dosed at 5 mg/kg every 24 hours. Both these drugs have also shown good results (Scott et al, 1995). However, they are substantially more expensive than ketoconazole, which limits their usefulness in clinical practice. Griseofulvin, which is used to treat dermatophyte infections in small animals, is ineffective at controlling bacterial pyodermas, which may facilitate the Malassezia infections.

References and Suggested Reading

Bond R, Lloyd DH: Factors affecting the adherence of Malassezia pachydermatis canine corneocytes in vitro. Vet Derm 7:49, 1996.
   This article examines various protein and carbohydrate moieties and their effects on adherence of organisms to canine corneocytes.

Bond R, Anthony KM, Dodd M, Lloyd DH: Isolation of Malassezia sympodialis from feline skin and mucosae. Proceedings of the 12th European Society of Veterinary Dermatology. Barcelona, Spain, 1995, p 220.
   The initial report detailing isolation of this organism on feline skin.

Griffin CE: Malassezia paronychia in atopic dogs. Proceedings of the 12th annual American College of Veterinary Dermatology/American Academy of Veterinary Dermatology meeting. Las Vegas, Nevada, 1996, p 51.
   This article evaluates clinical findings of Malassezia paronychia in atopic dogs and results of therapy with ketoconazole.

Guillot J, Chermette R, Gueho E: Unsuspected diversity of Malassezia yeasts recovered from animal skin. In: Kwochka KW, Willemse T, von Tscharner C, eds: Advances in Veterinary Dermatology, vol 3. Boston: Butterworth-Heinemann, 1996, p 533.
   This abstract reports on various species of Malassezia organisms that were isolated from numerous domestic and wild animals.

Mason KV: Malassezia dermatitis and otitis. In: Kirk RW, ed: Current Veterinary Therapy XI. Philadelphia: WB Saunders, 1992, p 544.
   Review of clinical, diagnostic, and treatment options for Malassezia dermatitis.

Mason KV: Malassezia: Biology, associated diseases and treatment. Proceedings of the 12th annual American College of Veterinary Dermatology/American Academy of Veterinary Dermatology meeting—concurrent Session Notes. Las Vegas, Nevada, 1996.
   A good review of the history and state of current knowledge about Malassezia.

Mathieson I, Fixter LM, Little CJL: Enzymatic activity of Malassezia pachydermatis. In Kwochka KW, Willemse T, von Tscharner C, eds:

Advances in Veterinary Dermatology, vol 3. Boston: Butterworth-Heinemann, 1996, p 532.
Demonstration of various enzymatic activities in strains of Malassezia pachydermatis *in vitro.*

Morris DO, Rosser EJ: Immunologic aspects of *Malassezia* dermatitis in patients with canine atopic dermatitis. Proceedings of the 11th annual American College of Veterinary Dermatology/American Academy of Veterinary Dermatology meeting. Santa Fe, New Mexico, 1995, p 16.
This article discusses the effects of various enzymatic extracts of Malassezia *used intradermally on normal and atopic dogs.*

Scott DW, Miller WH, Griffin CE: Small Animal Dermatology, 5th ed. Philadelphia: WB Saunders, 1995, p 357.
Review of clinical and therapeutic options for Malassezia *dermatitis.*

White SD, Bourdeau P, Blumstein P, et al: Comparison via cytology and culture of carriage of *Malassezia pachydermatis* in atopic and healthy dogs. Third World Congress of Veterinary Dermatology. Edinburgh, Scotland, 1996, p 37.
This study evaluated cytologic features by swab and scraping and compared them to cultures for the Malassezia *organism on normal and atopic dogs.*

Dermatophytosis

LINDA A. FRANK
Knoxville, Tennessee

Dermatophytosis is a cutaneous fungal infection that invades keratinized structures. The dermatophytes of veterinary importance are the zoophilic fungi (*Microsporum canis, Trichophyton equinum, T. mentagrophytes, T. verrucosum,* and *M. nanum*) and the geophilic fungus (*M. gypseum*). In general, dermatophytosis is a self-limited disease; however, it may take several months or longer to resolve, depending on the host involved and on the immune status of the individual.

CANINE DERMATOPHYTOSIS

Dermatophytosis in dogs is not nearly as common as might be suspected. Infection occurs more frequently in warm, humid, tropical areas and when animals are housed in conditions of poor sanitation and overcrowding. Younger animals and immunosuppressed animals have a higher incidence of disease. Transmission is most often from direct contact with an infected host, fomite, or contaminated environment. The incubation period may vary from 4 to 30 days. Some organisms can remain viable in a dry state for years.

Clinical Signs

Clinical signs associated with dermatophytosis are reflections of the host's response to the fungus. Well-adapted species (e.g., *M. canis*) produce minimal inflammation, whereas less-adapted species (e.g., *M. gypseum* or *T. mentagrophytes*) produce a more marked inflammation. The "classic" lesion is a circular patch of alopecia characterized by broken stubby hair, scaling, and mild erythema. Lesions appear to spread outward, often with central healing. Pruritus is variable. Dogs with dermatophytosis may also present with regional to generalized areas of alopecia, erythema, crust, and scale. The major differential diagnoses for dermatophytosis include superficial pyoderma and demodicosis. *Remember, dermatophytosis in dogs is usually overdiagnosed.*

Other clinical presentations include kerions and onychomycosis. A kerion is a nodular dermal reaction with ulceration and draining tracts. It is the result of an extreme inflammatory reaction or hypersensitivity to the dermal location of a less-adapted dermatophyte species (e.g., *M. gypseum*). Kerions are often seen on the face but may occur anywhere and are a result of the dog rooting in the soil. Differential diagnoses for this presentation include histiocytoma, deep pyoderma, neoplasia, and demodicosis. Onychomycosis is a rare infection of the keratin at the nail bed, usually caused by *T. mentagrophytes*. This presents as misshapen, brittle nails. Onychomycosis affects one to multiple nails; however, symmetrical nail disease would be unlikely. Seldom are the nails affected without cutaneous involvement.

FELINE DERMATOPHYTOSIS

M. canis is the most common feline dermatophyte and can become endemic in some catteries, especially Persian catteries. A good rule of thumb is that long-haired cats from catteries or of unknown origin are presumed to have dermatophytosis until proved otherwise.

Clinical Signs

Clinical signs include patches of alopecia, crusting, and scaling, especially of the face and ears. Generalized dermatophytosis can present with miliary dermatitis and is a differential diagnosis for feline miliary dermatitis due to allergy. Although dermatophytosis is seldom pruritic, some cats have intense pruritus associated with lesions. Clinical signs may be limited to kittens in a cattery, with adults being asymptomatic carriers.

Other less common presentations include recurrent chin folliculitis, chronic blepharitis, and kerions. Rarely, cats may present with pseudomycetomas—subcutaneous nodules with ulceration and draining tracts that result from deep dermal to subcutaneous invasion of the dermatophyte. This condition has only been described in Persian cats. Pseudomycetomas may occur in asymptomatic cats or in cats with known superficial dermatophytosis.

DIAGNOSIS

Wood's light examination is a common first approach to diagnosing dermatophytosis. Remember that the only species of veterinary importance to fluoresce is *M. canis,* and less than 50% of this species fluoresces. Some topical medications (e.g., iodine) may destroy fluorescence. To maximize positive results, the Wood's light should be allowed to warm up for approximately 5 minutes, and the examination should last 3 to 5 minutes in order for the reaction on the hairs to become visible (Moriello and DeBoer, 1995a). Wood's light examination is positive if it results in apple-green fluorescence of the *hair shaft.* False-positive results may be caused by medications on the hairs or, in some instances, bacterial infection. In addition, epidermal scales, especially those produced from *Staphylococcus intermedius* collarettes, may fluoresce apple-green; therefore, it is important to differentiate scale from hair when interpreting a positive fluorescence. *A definitive diagnosis of dermatophytosis should not be based on Wood's light examination alone.*

Direct examination of the hair under a microscope may reveal ectothrix spores on the hair shaft (see p. 526). Visualization may be aided by the use of a clearing agent (potassium hydroxide, chlorphenolac formula [50 gm chloral hydrate added to 25 ml liquid phenol and 25 ml liquid lactic acid]) before examination of the hair. Examining Wood's lamp–positive hairs also increases the success of this technique. In general, this technique is not rewarding and requires practice at identifying infected hairs.

The only reliable method to diagnose dermatophytosis is fungal culture using dermatophyte test medium. Broken hairs from the periphery of the lesion, Wood's light–positive hairs, or biopsied tissue from culturing pseudomycetomas or kerions, may be used for culture. Obtaining hairs from the periphery of a kerion or pseudomycetoma may result in false-negative results. Scales from the undersurface of a nail with suspected onychomycosis, or the entire avulsed nail, can be cultured to diagnose onychomycosis, which can be difficult. Specimens for culture in asymptomatic cats should be obtained using the sterile toothbrush technique. This involves combing the entire cat with a new or sterile toothbrush and then culturing the hairs collected in the brush.

A positive culture is suspected when the medium turns red at the *first* evidence of colony growth (see p. 526). Culture plates should, therefore, be examined daily for up to 3 weeks. Pigmented colonies, regardless of the medium color, are always something other than pathogens. In addition to observing colony growth and color change, it is important to identify the specific dermatophyte using acetate tape and lactophenol cotton blue. This allows confirmation that the colony is a dermatophyte and, by identifying the specific organism, the source of the infection can be determined.

In addition to culture, histopathologic examination may be useful for diagnosing dermatophytosis in some cases. This procedure is especially helpful for pseudomycetomas and kerions but may also offer a means for rapid diagnosis of superficial dermatophytosis.

Any animal with the generalized form of the disease or recurrent infection should have a complete work-up in order to identify any underlying disease process. Diagnostic tools should include a complete blood count, chemistry panel, and urinalysis as a minimal database. Feline leukemia virus and feline immunodeficiency virus (FIV) testing should also be performed on all cats. Thyroid evaluation and tests for hyperadrenocorticism should be performed if indicated.

TREATMENT

Because of the zoonotic potential, dermatophytosis in dogs and cats should never be left to resolve spontaneously without treatment. The aims of treatment are to decrease environmental contamination and human exposure and to hasten the animal's recovery.

Topical Therapy

Single lesions in dogs may be spot-treated with topical antifungal creams or lotions applied twice daily. Lesions should first be clipped and the hair disposed of to minimize environmental contamination, although clipping may spread the infection unless concurrent systemic therapy is given. Antifungal preparations can also be applied topically to kerions; however, these lesions often resolve without intervention. Products frequently used for local treatment include miconazole cream or lotion (Conofite, Mallinckrodt), clotrimazole cream (Veltrim, Bayer Corp.), ketoconazole cream (Nizoral, Janssen), and chlorhexidine ointment (Nolvasan, Fort Dodge). There appears to be no clear advantage of one product over the other. Drugs that are ineffective include tolnaftate, which is a product frequently used in human medicine, because it is not effective on the haired skin of dogs and cats, as well as nystatin, which is only effective against yeast. Combination products with corticosteroids should be avoided unless the lesions are highly inflamed. The reasons for this include (1) the anti-inflammatory properties of steroids could potentially hinder resolution of the infection and (2) adverse effects from topical steroids, including follicular atrophy, alopecia, and thinning of the skin, could result. In addition to local therapy, whole body treatment at least once with a topical shampoo and dip is beneficial (see further on) because dermatophyte-infected hairs can be found up to 6 cm from an active lesion. Cats should never be spot-treated because they frequently have infected hairs in areas otherwise unaffected by lesions.

Multiple lesions require whole body treatment. Lesions should be clipped as previously discussed. Long-haired cats should be shaved entirely. Care should be taken not to traumatize the skin, as worsening of the dermatitis may occur. Whole body shampoos and dips should be performed one to two times per week. Antifungal agents in shampoos include chlorhexidine (ChlorhexiDerm, 2 to 4%, DVM Pharmaceuticals; Hexedine, 2%, Allerderm/Virbac), miconazole (Dermazole, Allerderm/Virbac), and ketoconazole (Nizoral, Janssen) with the latter two treatments being more costly. Antifungal dips include lime sulfur (LymDyp, DVM Pharmaceuticals), enilconazole (Imaveral, Janssen [not available in the United States]), chlorhexidine solution (Nolvasan, Fort Dodge), povidone-iodine, and sodium hypochlorite (bleach). A study comparing the mycologic cure of dermatophyte-infected dog and cat hairs using various topical products twice weekly found lime sulfur (30 ml/L) and enilconazole (20 ml/L) rinses to be the most effective, resulting in negative cultures after 1 week (White-Weithers and Medleau, 1995). Chlorhexidine (25 ml/L of 2% solution) and povidone-iodine (42 ml/L) solutions required 2 weeks, whereas ketoconazole shampoo and sodium hypochlorite (50 ml/L) needed 4 weeks to kill the fungus. The use of captan (Orthocide, Chevron Chemicals) never resulted in negative fungal cultures. Another similar study found lime sulfur, enilconazole, and miconazole shampoo to be superior (Moriello and DeBoer, 1995a). This author prefers lime sulfur because it is effective, safe, and economical. Enilconazole is available in Europe but is not approved for use on cats. The safety of this product on cats is controversial (Moriello and DeBoer, 1995a). *Recent studies in cats have shown that topical therapy alone does not result in mycologic cure* (DeBoer and Moriello, 1995). Most dogs with multiple lesions also require systemic therapy.

Systemic Therapy

Griseofulvin is the drug of choice for treating dermatophytosis systemically. Griseofulvin is a fungistatic drug that becomes incorporated into newly formed layers of the epidermis and dermal appendages. Absorption is maximized by using a micronized form of the drug (Fulvicin-U/F, Schering-Plough) and administering it with a fatty meal. The dose of micronized griseofulvin is 50 mg/kg every 24 hours PO. This dose may be doubled in resistant cases. Griseofulvin must be administered daily to be effective. This product is available in a pediatric suspension for dosing small cats and dogs. There are no label age restrictions for the use of griseofulvin. It has been used safely in puppies and kittens 12 weeks of age or older. There are anecdotal reports of its use in puppies and kittens as young as 6 weeks of age. Whole body clipping is advised, and topical therapy should be used in conjunction with this treatment, as previously discussed. The most common adverse reactions include anorexia, nausea, and vomiting. The gastrointestinal symptoms may be minimized by dividing the dose every 12 hours and administering the drug with food. Cats may be more sensitive to this drug. In addition to gastrointestinal signs, bone marrow suppression may occur in cats. The neutropenia or panleukopenia may be associated with FIV-positive cats or may be idiosyncratic (Shelton et al, 1990). Therefore, all cats should be tested for FIV before this drug is used, and a complete blood count should be obtained before treatment and every 1 to 2 weeks while the drug is being administered. Griseofulvin is teratogenic and should not be given to pregnant animals.

Ketoconazole (Nizoral, Janssen) and itraconazole (Sporonox, Janssen) are also effective for treating dermatophytosis. These imidazoles are usually reserved for griseofulvin failures or animals that cannot tolerate the drug. Ketoconazole is dosed at 10 mg/kg every 24 hours PO and should be given with an acidic meal. The most common side effect is anorexia. Hepatotoxicity has also been reported and may be more common in cats than in dogs.

Therefore, liver enzymes should be monitored before treatment and monthly while this drug is being administered.

Itraconazole has been effective for treating dermatophytosis when dosed at 5 mg/kg every 24 hours PO for dogs and 10 mg/kg every 24 hours PO for cats. Although more expensive than ketoconazole, fewer side effects are reported. A recent study comparing itraconazole with griseofulvin found both drugs to be effective in achieving mycologic cure; however, itraconazole appeared to reach this end point slightly faster (56 versus 70 days) (Moriello and DeBoer, 1995b). Even though side effects are less common, liver enzymes should also be monitored before treatment and monthly while this drug is being given. Both onychomycosis and pseudomycetomas may be better managed with itraconazole. A prolonged course of therapy is required, with cures taking up to 10 months to be achieved (Medleau and Rakich, 1994).

Length of Therapy

Regardless of the choice of systemic treatment, the length of therapy is crucial to resolving the infection. Treatment usually continues for a *minimum* of 6 weeks—2 weeks beyond clinical cure *and* when two to three negative fungal cultures are obtained at weekly intervals. It is best to start obtaining cultures after 4 weeks of therapy. If lesions are not evident, the toothbrush technique for obtaining a culture should be used.

Environmental Cleaning

Remember, the environment is a source of infection. Thorough vacuuming and steam cleaning will help; however, steam cleaning will not kill fungal spores. Vents, filters, and drapes need to be addressed. Nonporous surfaces should be cleaned regularly with a 1:10 dilution of sodium hypochlorite.

Catteries represent a special situation that is beyond the scope of this article. The readers are referred to Moriello and DeBoer (1995a) for a discussion of this topic.

Fungal Vaccines

A fungal vaccine (Fel-O-Vax MC-K, Fort Dodge) has been newly introduced to help in the management of dermatophytosis. This vaccine has not been effective at preventing infection. It appears to have some efficacy in therapeutics and may be beneficial as adjuvant therapy with systemic or topical treatments, or both. Field trials by the company demonstrated that dermatophyte lesions decreased dramatically several weeks after vaccination. Unfortunately, it is not known if these cats truly become culture-negative or simply become asymptomatic carrier animals. Further work is needed in evaluating these vaccines. The major side effect that has been encountered is sterile abscess formation at the site of inoculation.

References and Suggested Reading

DeBoer DG, Moriello KA: Inability of two topical treatments to influence the course of experimentally induced dermatophytosis in cats. J Am Vet Med Assoc 207:52, 1995.

A prospective study comparing the efficacy of a topical glyceryl monolaurate treatment to a commonly used chlorhexidine treatment regimen in juvenile cats with experimentally induced dermatophytosis.

Medleau L, Rakich PM: *Microsporum canis* pseudomycetomas in a cat. J Am Anim Hosp Assoc 30:573, 1994.

A case report of a Persian cat in whom the superficial dermatophytosis and pseudomycetoma was treated successfully with surgical excision and itraconazole.

Moriello KA, DeBoer DJ: Feline dermatophytosis—recent advances and recommendations for therapy. Vet Clin North Am 25:901, 1995a.

A review of feline dermatophytosis: epidemiology, pathogenesis, immunology, diagnosis, and treatment including new and controversial therapies.

Moriello KA, DeBoer DJ: Efficacy of griseofulvin and itraconazole in the treatment of experimentally induced dermatophytosis in cats. J Am Vet Med Assoc 207:439, 1995b.

A prospective study comparing the efficacy of griseofulvin and itraconazole to a placebo control in juvenile cats with experimentally induced dermatophytosis.

Shelton GH, Grant CK, Linenberger ML, Abkowitz JL: Severe neutropenia associated with griseofulvin therapy in cats with feline immunodeficiency virus infection. J Vet Intern Med 4:317, 1990.

A case report of neutropenia from griseofulvin treatment in six cats with FIV infection.

White-Weithers N, Medleau L: Evaluation of topical therapies for the treatment of dermatophyte-infected hairs from dogs and cats. J Am Anim Hosp Assoc 31:250, 1995.

A prospective study comparing the ability of various topical antifungal preparations to sterilize hair from cats and dogs infected with Microsporum canis.

Feline Demodicosis

DANIEL O. MORRIS

KARIN M. BEALE

Houston, Texas

INTRODUCTION

Feline demodicosis is a heterogenous disease caused by two different species of demodicid mites. Each species inhabits a separate ecologic niche within the skin, a factor that is responsible for a widely variable presentation of clinical signs.

Demodex Cati

The original species of demodicid mite, first reported by Leydig in 1859 and later named *Demodex folliculorum* var. *cati* by Megnin in 1877, was renamed *D. cati* by Hirst in 1919. *D. cati* is a long, slender follicular mite that is morphologically comparable to *D. canis*, the causative agent of canine demodicosis. *D. cati* mites may be found in clinically healthy cats as part of the normal cutaneous fauna. Many comparisons have been extrapolated from the canine disease to its feline counterpart, including the life cycles, pathophysiology of infestation, and host immune response to the mites. However, with only 18 *detailed* case reports of feline disease caused by *D. cati* in the veterinary literature, comprehensive reviews have drawn from limited experience when compared with canine demodicosis, and comparable studies of host immune function are completely lacking.

Regardless, it is clinically apparent that *D. cati* infestation may be exacerbated by systemic or immunocompromising diseases. Cases that have occurred in conjunction with diabetes mellitus, feline immunodeficiency virus viremia, systemic lupus erythematosus, feline leukemia virus viremia, hyperadrenocorticism, and lymphopenia associated with chronic upper respiratory infection have been described (cases reviewed by Chesney, 1989). Causation is only assumed, although resolution of the parasitism in several of these cases was not possible without concurrent control of the underlying disease.

Skin lesions associated with parasitism in these cases were variable, but included alopecia, erythema, crusting, and ceruminous otic discharge most commonly. This mite showed a preference for the skin of the head (especially periocular and pinnal) and the distal limbs; however, truncal and generalized lesions occurred in some cases. Attendant pruritus was highly variable. Evidence of contagion between adult cats was not reported.

Demodex Species

A second species of demodicid mite infesting the domestic feline was first reported in 1982 (Conroy et al, 1982) but remains unnamed. This species dwells superficially within the stratum corneum and is short and broad morphologically, inviting comparison to *D. criceti,* which inhabits the epidermal folds of the hamster.

Eleven cases involving this superficial species, including three reported previously by one of the authors, have been described in the veterinary literature. Five of these cases occurred among two sets of housemates, suggesting that contagion between adult cats is possible. In one pair, a cat eventually died from systemic toxoplasmosis after suffering a relapse of the demodicosis, whereas the housemate's dermatitis resolved completely with treatment for the mites (Medleau et al, 1988). In a separate three-cat household, two Siamese siblings with food allergy (who had received numerous parenteral doses of methylprednisolone acetate), developed concurrent demodicosis. Their lesions resolved only after control of both problems. Their unrelated Siamese housemate, which developed pruritic demodicosis before any corticosteroid use, recovered completely with treatment for the mite infestation alone (Morris, 1996).

TABLE 1. Feline Demodicosis—15 Cases

Case/Breed	Age at Onset	Glucocorticoids	Concurrent Disease	Distribution of Mites and Alopecic Lesions
Demodex Cati				
1. Domestic shorthair	6 mo	MPA injection weekly*	*Demodex* species and food allergy	Trunk, face, neck (with crusts)
2. Domestic shorthair	2 yr	MPA injection twice	None identified	Trunk
3. Domestic shorthair	4 yr	MPA injection multiple	None identified	Face, pinnae, feet (with crusts)
4. Domestic shorthair	10 yr	MPA injection multiple	None identified	Face, pinnae
5. Domestic shorthair	16 yr	Oral dexamethasone	Feline immunodeficiency virus	Trunk, face, neck (with milia)
Demodex **Species**				
6. Siamese	12.5 yr	MPA injection once	Diabetes mellitus	Trunk, face, neck
7. Domestic shorthair	6 mo	MPA injection once	Feline acne	Forelimbs, flanks
8. Himalayan	1.5 yr	Oral triamcinolone†	None identified	Abdomen, feet, neck
9. Domestic shorthair	3.5 yr	MPA injection multiple	None identified	Abdomen, legs (4)
10. Domestic shorthair	8 mo	None	None identified	Trunk and external ear canals
11. Siamese	7.5 yr	MPA injection multiple	Food allergy	Trunk, flanks, neck
12. Cornish Rex	4 mo	MPA injection multiple	Actinic dermatitis	Trunk (multifocal plaques)
13. Domestic longhair	6 mo	None	Pending	Trunk
14. Domestic shorthair	13 yr	MPA injection twice	Food allergy	Abdomen (papular rash)
15. Cornish Rex	8 yr	Oral triamcinolone	Food allergy	Trunk (papular rash)

*Also received oral megestrol acetate twice weekly.
†Also received injectable medroxyprogesterone acetate twice.
MPA, methylprednisolone acetate.

Symmetrically self-induced alopecia, erythema, and self-excoriations of the thorax and abdomen were the lesions most commonly associated with infestation by the superficial *Demodex* species. Facial, acral, and ear canal involvement occurred less frequently. Intense pruritus was the most consistent unifying feature.

RECENT OBSERVATIONS OF FELINE DEMODICOSIS

The authors have documented a series of 15 cases of feline demodicosis between January 1, 1994 and December 31, 1996 (excluding the three previously reported cases of superficial demodicosis that were recorded in Michigan; Table 1). Eleven (73%) of the cats were infested by the superficial species, and five (33%) of the cases involved the follicular species. One cat was infested by both species concurrently. In addition, we have consulted with numerous veterinarians in our practice area regarding cases that have involved the superficial species, but none that have involved the follicular mite to our knowledge. It thus appears, at least in our practice area (Southeast coastal and Central Texas), that the superficial *Demodex* mite is a more common cause of dermatitis in cats.

Demodex Species

Of the cats affected by the superficial species of *Demodex*, there were two Siamese, two Cornish Rex, six domestic shorthairs, and one domestic longhair. The cats ranged in age of onset from 6 months to 13 years, with an average of 4 years. Concurrent (predisposing?) diseases included diabetes mellitus (one cat), food allergy (four cats, all of which had received parenteral methylprednisolone acetate plus or minus oral medroxyprogesterone acetate), and actinic keratosis (one cat). Five cats had no apparent concurrent disease.

The presenting complaint for all 11 cats was pruritic

behavior, resulting in barbering of hair and self-excoriations. Evidence of primary inflammation was subtle and limited to mild erythema in most cases, although two cats were affected with papular rashes. The distribution pattern was primarily truncal in all, with the ventral abdomen and lateral thorax being the most common targets. The limbs, feet, and periocular area were less commonly involved. In one cat, lesions were multifocal erythemic plaques with actinic damage.

Two cats lived with other feline housemates, none of which was pruritic. One cat lived with a feline housemate that was pruritic but was not examined by us before treatment with lime sulfur dips. After four dips each, both these cats received skin scrapings, which were negative for *Demodex* mites. However, *Dermanyssus gallinae* mites were found on the housemate, so it was not known which mite was the original cause of the pruritus.

Most of these cats were housed strictly indoors, although one became pruritic after escaping outdoors for several hours. Treatment of its mite infestation permanently resolved the dermatitis. Two of the 11 cats were obtained from shelters and became pruritic after adoption.

Demodex Cati

All five of the cats with the follicular species of *Demodex* were domestic shorthairs. They ranged in age from 6 months to 16 years with an average of 6.5 years. One cat was diagnosed with a concurrent disease (food allergy) and also had the superficial species present. This cat was extremely pruritic and had received numerous weekly injections of methylprednisolone acetate and twice-weekly oral treatment with medroxyprogesterone acetate. A second cat was feline immunodeficiency virus–positive and had received daily oral doses of dexamethasone to help alleviate pruritus. The other three cats, of which two were pruritic, recovered completely with treatment for the demodicosis, and concurrent diseases were not identified. None of these three cats has experienced a relapse.

The presenting complaint for two cats with *D. cati* was crusting and follicular plugging of the skin of the pinnae and periocular areas, and in one of these cats, all four feet were also involved. The other three cats presented with follicular plugging and thinning alopecia across the dorsum and ventrum of the trunk, and one was also affected with miliary and self-excoriative lesions.

DIAGNOSIS AND TREATMENT

In general, the treatment of feline demodicosis is not as difficult as making the initial diagnosis. It may present in a highly variable manner and may or may not be pruritic, which will depend largely on the species involved. Both broad, superficial scrapings and concentrated, deep scrapings should be performed in all cases of feline dermatitis. Samples should be placed on microscopic glass slides, cover-slipped, and observed under 10× power, as the superficial species is especially easy to overlook. In an ongoing dermatologic case with concurrent systemic disease, or when corticosteroids, progestational drugs, or other immunosuppressant agents are used, periodic scrapings should be repeated to monitor for exacerbation of mite infestation.

All 15 cats in the authors' series were treated with 2% lime sulfur dips (LymDyp, DVM Pharmaceuticals). Most required six dips at 5- to 7-day intervals for complete resolution of the condition and associated clinical signs. In two cats with superficial *Demodex*, the dips were improperly diluted to 1% and ½% respectively, and there was no decrease in mite populations after four dips. Resolution was obtained after correction of the dip formulation. With the exception of xerosis in one cat, there were no side effects reported by owners or observed by the authors for cats dipped at home or at our hospital, respectively.

A prior report has documented a case in which lime sulfur failed to resolve a case of *D. cati* infestation after four dips at weekly intervals. The cat recovered after the dipping regimen was changed to 0.0125% amitraz weekly, although initial side effects included sedation, ptyalism, and hiding behavior (Cowan and Campbell, 1988). There has also been some debate about the need to treat cases of *D. cati* because of anecdotal reports of spontaneous remis-

sion for both localized and generalized disease. In dogs, generalized cases of demodicosis are thought to represent a different pathophysiologic mechanism and host immune response than localized cases, and treatment recommendations for the two forms are vastly different (Scott et al, 1995). Evidence sufficient to support a homologous situation in cats is lacking.

It is the opinion of the authors that all cats presenting with dermatitis associated with *Demodex* infestation (especially when involving the superficial species) should receive the benefit of a safe treatment modality. We routinely recommend that 2% lime sulfur dips be the initial treatment of choice because of an apparent wide margin of safety. Adverse effects have been noted with lime sulfur when ingested by cats (Moriello and DeBoer, 1995), and an Elizabethan collar may be placed until the dip has dried on the body to prevent grooming. A series of four to six dips at 5- to 7-day intervals is usually sufficient. Dips are stopped only when repeated skin scrapings are completely free of eggs, mites, and mite fragments.

References and Suggested Reading

Chesney CJ: Demodicosis in the cat. J Small Anim Pract 30:689, 1989.
A comprehensive review with excellent charts detailing previously reported cases.
Conroy JD, Healey MC, Bane AG: New *Demodex* sp. infesting a cat: A case report. J Am Anim Hosp Assoc 18:405, 1982.
The first recognized report of the unnamed Demodex *species affecting a cat.*
Cowan LA, Campbell K: Generalized demodicosis in a cat responsive to amitraz. J Am Vet Med Assoc 192:1442, 1988.
A clinical description of treatment failure utilizing lime sulfur dip for the unnamed Demodex *species.*
Medleau L, Brown CA, Brown SA, et al: Demodicosis in cats. J Am Anim Hosp Assoc 24:85, 1988.
Four new, detailed case reports with a chart reviewing cases previously reported in the literature.
Moriello KA, DeBoer DJ: Feline dermatophytosis: Recent advances and recommendations for therapy. Vet Clin North Am Small Anim Pract 25:901, 1995.
A comprehensive review of feline dermatophytosis, with comments on the therapeutic use of lime sulfur.
Morris DO: Contagious demodicosis in three cats residing in a common household. J Am Anim Hosp Assoc 32:350, 1996.
Three detailed case reports in which apparent contagion is described.
Scott DW, Miller WH, Griffin CE: Parasitic skin diseases. In: Scott DW, Miller WH, Griffin CE, eds: Muller & Kirk's Small Animal Dermatology, 5th ed. Philadelphia: WB Saunders, 1995, p 392.
Comprehensive review of canine demodicosis that is helpful for comparison with the feline disease.

Ear Flushing Techniques and Therapeutic Importance

Dawn Logas
Winter Park, Florida

The most important first step in the management of any case of otitis is proper cleaning of the external ear canal and the flushing of the middle ear cavity if the tympanum is absent. The procedure should be performed at the initial visit after obtaining cytologic specimens and possibly a specimen for culture from the diseased ear. In mild cases of otitis, ear flushing may be performed with gentle restraint, but in most cases the ears are painful enough to warrant heavy sedation with propofol (Diprivan 1%, Zeneca, Inc., Wilmington, DE) or ketamine and diazepam. In more severe cases of otitis externa, and in most cases of otitis media, general anesthesia is necessary. In some of the most severe cases, in which the canals are extremely inflamed and swollen, systemic and topical therapy is initiated first and a 3- to 14-day delay is necessary before cleaning. This allows the canal to open and the tympanic membrane to be more easily visualized.

The flushing solution used depends on the degree of inflammation, the characteristics of the discharge, and the status of the tympanic membrane. Commonly used solutions are DSS (dioctyl sodium sulfosuccinate), CLEAR$_x$ Ear Cleansing Solution (DVM Pharmaceuticals), or Cerumene ([squalane], Evsco Pharmaceuticals) for waxy discharges. Epi-Otic (Allerderm/Virbac), Tris-EDTA (6.05 gm of edetate disodium, 12 gm of tromethamine qs to 1 L, adjust pH to 8.0; compounded by a local pharmacist), 0.05% to 0.2% chlorhexidine solutions (Chlorhexiderm Flush, DVM Pharmaceuticals; 2% chlorhexidine solution), and 2.5% acetic acid (50:50 vinegar:water) or saline for purulent discharges. All these solutions except saline have the potential to damage exposed middle ear structures, although the caseous or purulent material being removed from the middle ear probably poses a greater threat. When the tympanum is known to be absent, a gentle solution such as 2.5% acetic acid or saline should be employed if possible. Unfotunately, many times these solutions alone will not remove the debris, and a more caustic cleaning solution must be employed. At the end of the procedure, it is important to flush the caustic solution out of the canal and middle ear completely with water or saline to minimize any damage the solution may cause.

IN-OFFICE EAR FLUSHING

A bulb syringe (Davol, Inc., Cranston, RI) or a No. 3 to 12 French red rubber feeding tube attached to a 6- to 12-ml syringe is an excellent and relatively safe flushing apparatus for in-office use. The open end of the tube must be trimmed to accommodate the syringe hub. The tip is then cut off so the final length of the tube is 4 to 6 inches or one-half to two times the length of the ear canal. Both straight and curved dull buck ear curettes (Edward Week & Co., Research Triangle Park, NC) can be used to remove large pieces of wax and debris. Once the horizontal canal has been cleared, it is usually easier to assess the status of the tympanic membrane. In many cases of chronic otitis, the tympanum is still difficult to visualize because the canal is stenotic secondary to lichenification and fibrosis. If the tympanum cannot be visualized, its status can be assessed indirectly by observing the curette catching on any bony prominence, the tube tip disappearing from view, the use of excessive tubing and fluid in the canal, or the act of the patient swallowing after infusion of fluid. Any of these observations would indicate a false middle ear or imperforate tympanum. If the tympanum is visually intact, but this is a case of chronic otitis (>3 months' duration), a myringotomy using a 25- or 27-gauge needle may be necessary and a culture taken from the middle ear if there is any evidence of fluid behind the membrane or membrane opacity and fibrosis.

The hazards of deep ear cleaning include inadvertent rupture of the tympanum, vestibular dysfunction, auditory dysfunction, contact irritant and allergy, and introduction of other pathogens. The most common hazard is the potential rupture of the tympanic membrane. A normal tympanum is difficult to rupture; therefore, if the membrane ruptures with gentle manipulation it was probably weakened and diseased. The occurrence of vestibular auditory dysfunction is unpredictable. In the dog, it is uncommon and usually mild and most of the time lasts only a few hours to a couple of days. In the cat, it occurs more frequently than in the dog, and the signs are usually more pronounced and may be permanent. To avoid contact irritation, a gentle solution should be used whenever possible, or more caustic solutions must be rinsed out extremely well with water or saline. New pathogens can be introduced into an already inflamed ear via unsterilized ear cleaning equipment. Bulb syringes and feeding tubes should not be used for multiple patients. It is difficult to completely sterilize the rubber; therefore, resistant strains of *Pseudomonas*, *Escherichia coli*, and *Proteus* can propagate.

AT-HOME EAR FLUSHING

Once the ear has been cleaned in the office, a home treatment plan for the owners must be designed according to the organism or organisms found on cytologic studies or culture, the chronicity of the ear disease, and the presence of a tympanum. In many cases, a prepared solution in a squeeze bottle is all that is necessary. If there is a great deal of purulent material, a bulb syringe should be employed and the owners instructed in its appropriate use.

After each use, the bulb syringe should be rinsed out several times with 50:50 vinegar:alcohol to minimize bacterial overgrowth in the bulb. The bulb syringe should be changed every 2 to 5 weeks, depending on the severity of the infection.

In the case of severe otitis or in a fractious patient, a flushing device may temporarily be affixed to the animal. Heavy sedation or general anesthesia should be employed. The open end of a red rubber feeding tube is secured via sutures or glue to the dorsal skin of the neck and head. The tube is then placed into the ear canal rostrally through the area of pretragic incision and secured in place with glue or suture. The tip of the tube should be trimmed so that the end of the tube is one-half to three-quarters of the way down the horizontal canal, but not touching the tympanum or the middle ear cavity. The tube should be approximately one-half to three-fourths the diameter of the horizontal canal. This will help minimize tube movement and subsequently patient discomfort. There should be enough space around the tube for fluid to backwash out of the ear during flushing. This will prevent a build-up of water pressure and possible middle ear and vestibular damage. The tube can remain in place for 5 to 10 days. There should be an Elizabethan collar on the dog at all times. Owners should be instructed to flush the cleaning solution, chlorhexidine solution (0.05% to 2%), saline, or 50:50 vinegar:water, through the tube gently with a 6- to 12-ml syringe. Each time the canal is flushed, a total volume of 18 to 36 ml should be instilled. As much of the fluid as possible should be evacuated from the ear canal after each infusion. The ear should be flushed at least three times daily. Antibiotic solutions can also be instilled into the horizontal canal through this apparatus by infusing 0.5 to 2 ml of medication into the tube and then flushing the medication through the tube into the canal using air.

The type of solution and frequency of flushing prescribed for home care depend on the severity of infection, consistency of the discharge, chronicity of the otitis, presence of yeast or bacteria, and the presence or absence of a tympanum. For bacterial infections, chlorhexidine solution (0.05 to 0.2%) and saline are good, gentle flushes. For *Pseudomonas aeruginosa* infections, a 2- to 5-minute contact time with Tris-EDTA, 50:50 vinegar:water (2.5% acetic acid) or otic Domeboro solution (Bayer Pharmaceutical, West Haven, CT) is a better choice because these agents have bactericidal activity against *Pseudomonas*. It is important to remember that purulent discharge will inactivate many topical antibiotics; accordingly, the ear should be flushed before each application of antibiotic until the ear is producing little to no purulent material. Initially, the frequency of flushing for severe cases, especially resistant *Pseudomonas* infections, can be four to six times daily. In most less severe cases, one to three times daily will suffice. As therapy continues, the frequency should decrease to several times per week and then once weekly to every other week as a prophylactic.

As with bacterial otitis, flushing ears can be important in the treatment of yeast otitis. Flushing helps remove the waxy organism-filled debris, acidify, and then dry the horizontal canal, making the microenvironment of the canal unsuitable for yeast growth. The frequency of application again depends on the severity of otitis and chronicity of the disease. In severe cases, flushing may be one to two times daily but should quickly drop to two to three times weekly. Over time, it will drop further to a maintenance level of once weekly to once every other week. The agents most commonly used are Epi-Otic, DSS, and 50:50 vinegar with alcohol or water.

It is particularly important that dogs with chronic histopathologic ear canal changes, such as fibrosis, stenosis, and lichenification be placed on a maintenance flushing program. Ears with chronic changes usually have increased cerumen production, hyperplasia of the stratum corneum, and decreased epidermal migration (self-cleaning). This leads to an increased build-up of debris in the canal. Flushing the ears helps remove the debris and acidify the canal, which helps prevent recurrence of active infections. The frequency of flushing ranges from two to three times weekly to once every other week. The solutions commonly used are Epi-Otic, chlorhexidine flush, Otic Domeboro, and vinegar with alcohol or water (50:50).

Although flushing is extremely important in the management of both chronic and acute otitis, it is imperative that the clinician remember that flushing too vigorously and too frequently can also be detrimental to the otitic epidermis. The animal with severe otitis who is undergoing flushing numerous times per day should be checked frequently, and flushing should be varied, depending on the cytologic and otic examination. This will prevent the ear flushes from doing more harm than good.

References and Suggested Reading

Griffin CE: Otitis externa and otitis media. In: Griffin CE, Kwochka KW, MacDonald JM, eds: Current Veterinary Dermatology. St Louis, Mosby–Year Book, 1993, p 245.
  This is a good review of causes and therapies for otitis.
Rosychuk RAW: Management of otitis externa. Vet Clin North Am Sm Anim Pract 24:921, 1994.
  This reviews the therapeutic options for otitis.

Appropriate Use of Glucocorticoids in Otitis Externa

Dawn Logas
Winter Park, Florida

The basic clinical signs of acute otitis externa are similar to those of other inflammatory processes and may include erythema, edema, discharge, and pain. Almost any inflamed ear may benefit from corticosteroid therapy, regardless of the underlying cause of the inflammation. Glucocorticoids inhibit vasodilation and capillary leakage by sensitizing vascular walls to adrenergic agonists, diminishing erythema and edema. Pain is consequently decreased, since edematous tissue is no longer entrapping nerve fibers against the auricular cartilage. Glucocorticoids also inhibit the accumulation of white blood cells at the site of inflammation, thereby reducing discharge. This inhibition of white blood cells, particularly neutrophils and eosinophils, is the result of decreased margination, reduced adhesion to blood vessels, and inhibition of chemotaxis. Glucocorticoids also prevent leukocytes from producing or releasing histamine, eicosanoids, and lysosomes, mediators that can damage the otitic epithelium.

As the otitis becomes chronic, cerumen production increases, the epidermis thickens, and eventually fibrosis and stenosis of the ear canal occur. Glucocorticoids relieve these changes by inhibiting epidermal proliferation, decreasing fibroblast proliferation and metabolism, and reducing sebum production.

In the treatment of otitis, the question is not whether a steroid should be used—but which steroid preparation is appropriate in combination with ear cleaning (see the previous article) and other treatments (see *CVT XII*, p. 647, and the next article). Before the physician decides which steroid to use, the underlying cause, the presence of infectious agents, and the chronicity of the ear disorder should be considered. In general, the least potent topical steroids that will control the symptoms should be used. The most common topical steroids and their potencies are listed in Table 1. Table 2 summarizes which topical steroids are recommended for use with specific problems and when to use systemic prednisone.

Steroids benefit ears with secondary infections by diminishing edema and pain and decreasing discharge. By reducing the swelling, the antimicrobial agent is able to reach the deeper recesses of the canal. The reduction in pain translates into a more compliant patient that allows the ears to be treated. By decreasing the discharge, there is less of a chance of the topical antibiotic or antifungal becoming inactivated by the inflammatory and cellular debris. The steroid should always be combined with an appropriate antibacterial agent when one treats a bacterial infection. In acutely inflamed ears with a mild infection, hydrocortisone is sufficient, whereas in chronically inflamed ears with a mild infection more potent glucocorticoids may be necessary. Ears severely infected with bacteria, particularly *Pseudomonas* sp., should be treated topically with nothing more potent than hydrocortisone whenever possible (see the next article). This will decrease the inflammation without greatly reducing the antibacterial action of leukocytes. In severe cases in which the canal is swollen closed, high-dose systemic prednisone (1.1 to 2.2 mg/kg PO divided q12hr) is necessary for 3 to 10 days to open the canal and allow the ear to be properly cleaned and medicated.

TABLE 1. Topical Steroids and Their Potency

Product	Equivalent Therapeutic Concentrations (%)	Relative Duration of Effect (hr)
Hydrocortisone	1	8–12
Triamcinolone	0.1	36–48
Dexamethasone	0.1	36–54
Betamethasone	0.05	36–54
Fluocinolone	0.025	36–54

TABLE 2. Recommended Steroid Preparations for Otitis

	Topical Steroid	Oral Prednisone*
Bacterial Otitis		
Mild infections	Hydrocortisone (1–2.5%)	Usually not necessary
Acute	Dexamethasone (0.1%)	
Chronic	Dexamethasone (0.1%)	May be needed
	Triamcinolone (0.1%)	
	Betamethasone (0.1%)	
Severe infections (*Pseudomonas*)	Hydrocortisone (1–2.5%)	May be needed, but use as low a dose and short a time as possible

	Topical Steroid	Oral Prednisone†
Uncomplicated Allergic or Seborrheic Otitis		
Acute		
Allergic	Hydrocortisone (1–2.5%)	
	Dexamethasone (0.1%)	
	Triamcinolone (0.1%)	
Seborrheic	Dexamethasone (0.1%)	May be needed
	Triamcinolone (0.1%)	
	Betamethasone (0.1%)	
Chronic		
Allergic	Dexamethasone (0.1%)	Usually needed
	Triamcinolone (0.1%)	
	Betamethasone (0.1%)	
	Fluocinolone (0.01%)	
Seborrheic	Betamethasone (0.1%)	Usually needed
	Fluocinolone (0.01%)	

*Prednisone, 1.1 to 2.2 mg/kg divided q12hr for 3 to 10 days. Stop as soon as possible.
†Prednisone, 1.1 to 2.2 mg/kg divided q12hr for 7 to 14 days, then 0.55 to 1.1 mg/kg q24–72hr, as needed to control signs.

In the case of *Malassezia*, a mild infection may clear with glucocorticoids and flushing alone. In eliminating the inflammation, the steroids normalize the ear's microenvironment, making it less hospitable for yeast overgrowth. More severe infections need an antifungal agent (such as otic solutions with clotrimazole or miconazole) in combination with a topical steroid and even high-dose systemic prednisone (1.1 to 2.2 mg/kg PO divided q12hr).

Uncomplicated allergic and seborrheic otitis benefits from the use of glucocorticoids alone. Mild acute cases of either disease can be treated with hydrocortisone. Chronically and severely affected cases may need more potent topical preparations, such as fluocinolone or betamethasone. Severe cases of seborrheic otitis and allergic otitis may also require high doses of systemic prednisone (1.1 to 2.2 mg/kg PO divided q12hr) for 3 to 14 days to completely control the inflammation and reduce cerumen production. Once the inflammation has subsided, low-dose systemic prednisone (0.55 to 1.1 mg/kg PO q24–72hr) may be necessary to maintain the ear.

Although relatively safe, topical steroids are not without side effects. This is particularly true of the more potent preparations, which after prolonged periods of use can exhibit adverse effects both locally and systemically. These side effects include suppression of the adrenocortical axis, potential suppression of serum T_4 levels, suppression of antimicrobial defenses, and elevation of serum alkaline phosphatase activity. These changes may lead to the erroneous diagnosis of hypothyroidism, to iatrogenic Cushing's disease, and to the possibility of superinfection by extremely resistant strains of *Pseudomonas* and *Proteus*. Long-term use can also cause severe epidermal atrophy, along with the loss of normal epidermal migration. These changes impair the ear's ability to "self-clean." Debris begins to collect in the canal, promoting secondary infections. Thus, while steroids are very beneficial in the treatment of otitis externa, they must be used judiciously (also see *CVT XII*, p. 573).

References and Suggested Reading

Scott DW: Dermatologic use of glucocorticoids. Vet Clin North Am Small Anim Pract 12:19, 1982.
  Reviews the use of steroids in various dermatologic conditions.
Wilcke JR: Otopharmacology. Vet Clin North Am Small Anim Pract 18:783, 1988.
  Reviews the reactions and adverse reactions of many ingredients found in ear products.
Scott DW, Miller WH, Griffin CE: Small Animal Dermatology. Philadelphia: WB Saunders, 1995, p 244.
  Review of steroid use and potency.

Pseudomonas Otitis Therapy

CRAIG E. GRIFFIN
San Diego, California

CLINICAL FINDINGS

Gram-negative bacteria, especially *Pseudomonas* species, are particularly frustrating to treat when they are associated with otitis externa and otitis media. Occasionally, these bacteria may represent primary pathogens, although in most cases they are secondary invaders. Therefore, finding the primary disease, as well as other secondary or perpetuating factors that may be present, becomes critical to the long-term control of otitis (Griffin, 1993). Clinical findings in *Pseudomonas* otitis usually include erythema, edema, areas of erosion or ulceration, and abundant production of exudate. The exudate usually is of light mucous consistency and pale yellow or off-white.

Cytologic examination of the exudate typically reveals predominantly neutrophils, some mononuclear cells, and occasionally macrophages. The cells often have swollen nuclei and appear degenerated and toxic. Proteinaceous debris surrounds the cells, and numerous small rods are present. *Pseudomonas* species may be the only pathogens, although often multiple organisms may be seen. In the author's experience, organisms can usually be visualized. However, the preliminary results of a study by Cole and associates were reported in a workshop and suggested that 20% of otitis externa cases with gram-negative organisms identified by culture were negative for rods cytologically (Griffin and Song, 1996). They reported that 80% of *Pseudomonas*-related otitis media cultured positive but produced negative results on cytologic examination. The author also recommends repeating cytologic studies when the color or texture of the exudate changes as one goes deeper into the ear canal. Sometimes different organisms will be found. The experience of Cole and associates suggests that the middle ear should always be tested separately because 30% of the cases that tested positive for *Pseudomonas* from specimens from the middle ear failed to grow *Pseudomonas* on cultures from the external ear.

Culture and sensitivity testing of the ear is not routinely recommended in otitis, but when it is performed it should always be accompanied by cytologic examination. If the cytologic examination reveals suppurative inflammation with rods, or if no organisms are evident but the animal has not responded to appropriate topical and systemic antibiotic therapy for gram-negative organisms, culture and sensitivity testing may be indicated. The laboratory should also be sent a cytologic slide as well as information regarding organisms seen at the time of collection so that personnel will know if multiple organisms should be identified.

TABLE 1. *Pseudomonas* Treatment Options

Cleaning	In-office flushing, home flushing, or cleaning
Disinfectants	Acetic acid 2–2.5%
	Chlorhexidine 0.25%
Topical antibiotics	Neomycin, polymyxin
	Gentamicin
	Enrofloxacin
	Amikacin
	Silver sulfadiazine
	Tobramycin
	Ticarcillin
Glucocorticoids	*Topical*
	Hydrocortisone
	Dexamethasone
	Betamethasone
	Flucinolone
	Systemic
	Prednisone
	Dexamethasone
	Triamcinolone
Systemic antibiotics	Enrofloxicin
	Enrofloxicin, cephalexin
	Carbenicillin
	Gentamicin
	Amikacin
	Ticarcillin
	Tobramycin

THERAPEUTIC APPROACH

Therapy of *Pseudomonas* otitis usually requires an approach that involves two or more components from the list of treatment options (Table 1). Cleaning, topical disinfectants, and topical antibacterial treatments are routinely used. Cleaning the ears is required because *Pseudomonas* infections produce abundant exudate that interferes with the penetration and complete dispersion of topical therapies. Some antibiotics, such as polymyxin, are inactivated by purulent exudates. In some cases, home cleaning by the client each day or every other day may be required (see p. 583). Topical disinfectants are helpful because some strains of *Pseudomonas* are resistant to many antibiotics. Occasionally, topical disinfectants are used as the main topical therapy and should be used routinely during or after cleaning of the ear canal. Chlorhexidine and acetic acid are preferred. Acetic acid, 2 to 2.5%, is the preferred disinfectant when the tympanic membrane is ruptured. If acetic acid is the only topical agent used, cleaning the ears daily and flushing the ear with acetic acid four to six times a day is necessary. In some cases, this may be irritating, although the concurrent use of steroids (see previous article) may limit this irritation.

Topical Antibacterial Therapy

First-line antibiotics most commonly used for *Pseudomonas* should contain polymyxin, neomycin, and polymyxin (Forte-Topical, Upjohn; Cortisporin Otic, Burroughs Wellcome) or gentamicin (Gentocin Otic or Otomax, Schering-Plough). Ototoxicity has been reported with all these topical agents. However, similar to chlorhexidine, this concern may be overstated. A study by Strain and associates (1995) showed no vestibulotoxic or ototoxic effects from 21 days of otic gentamicin applied twice daily to ears with ruptured tympanic membranes. Second-line products used in more resistant cases are often compounded products containing enrofloxacin (Baytril injectable, Bayer). The current favorite of the author involves a 25% mixture of injectable enrofloxacin (22.7 mg/ml). Others report using injectable enrofloxacin undiluted or diluted 50%, mixed with water, injectable dexamethasone, propylene glycol, or other topical products such as Epi-Otic (Allerderm/Virbac), CLEAR$_x$ Ear Drying Solution (DVM Pharmaceuticals), Oticalm (DVM Pharmaceuticals), or Synotic (Syntex). Third-line therapy is most commonly chosen after the results of culture and sensitivity testing. Injectable amikacin (Amiglyde-V, Fort Dodge) may be applied directly or mixed with injectable dexamethasone. Tobramycin (Tobrex ophthalmic solution, Alcon Labs) drops used undiluted every 8 hours and ticarcillin equine intrauterine infusion (Ticillin, Pfizer Animal Health) applied undiluted every 8 hours have proved effective in some cases that were resistant to enrofloxacin and amikacin, but these agents are not routinely used on some sensitivity tests. Silver sulfadiazine, 1%, was reported to be an effective antimicrobial in experimentally induced cases of *Pseudomonas* otitis externa (Thomas, 1990). This solution is made by mixing 1 gm silver sulfadiazine with 100 ml sterile water and is applied at a dose of 0.5 ml per ear twice daily. A recent study showed silver sulfadiazine as low as 0.1% to still be efficacious (Noxon, 1997).

Glucocorticoids

Often antibiotics will be prescribed in conjunction with glucocorticoids. The glucocorticoids are beneficial in most cases because they decrease the formation of exudate as well as glandular secretions and inflammation and swelling. Any time there is moderate inflammation, or if the exudate cannot be controlled with cleaning and a topical antibacterial agent, topical glucocorticoids should be used (see preceeding article). If topical agents are not effective or if there is severe inflammation, ulceration, or proliferative change, a systemic glucocorticoid is indicated. Short-term therapy is initiated with a short-acting injectable glucocorticoid such as dexamethasone sodium phosphate (0.1 to 0.2 mg/kg IM) or prednisone sodium phosphate (1 to 2.2 mg/kg SC). Oral prednisone or triamcinolone (Vetalog, Fort Dodge) may also be used if more than 2 days of therapy is needed.

Systemic Antibiotics

Systemic antibiotics are used in the presence of otitis media or moderate or marked proliferative changes to the canal or when appropriate topical therapy and cleansing are ineffective. If antibiotic selection is empirical, enrofloxacin (Baytril, Bayer) at 5 mg/kg PO every 24 hours is prescribed. In some cases 10 mg/kg every 24 hours appears to be more efficacious. If this is not effective, sensitivity testing is recommended. If resistance is seen to all oral antibiotics, if sensitivity testing is declined, or if there are proliferative changes evident in the canal, enrofloxacin is continued with the addition of cephalexin at 22 mg/kg PO every 12 hours.

References and Suggested Reading

Griffin CE: Otitis externa and media. In: Griffin CE, Kwochka KW, MacDonald SM, eds: Current Veterinary Dermatology, the Science and Art of Therapeutics. St. Louis, Mosby–Year Book, 1993.
A review of the causes and factors one should consider in cases of otitis externa and media.

Griffin CE, Song M: Otitis workshop. In: Kwochka K, Willemse T, von Tscharner C, eds: Advances in Veterinary Dermatology, vol 3. Boston: Butterworth-Heinemann, 1996, p 369.
Published proceedings of an open discussion of problems related to otitis diagnosis and therapy that contains some preliminary information of a study conducted by Cole and associates.

Noxon JO, Kinyon JM, Murphy OP: Minimal inhibitory concentration of silver sulfadiazine on *Pseudomonas aeruginosa* and *Staphylococcus intermedius* isolates from the ears of dogs with otitis externa. 13th Proceedings of the American Academy of Veterinary Dermatology/ American College of Veterinary Dermatology, Nashville, 1997, p 72.

Strain GM, Merchant SR, Neer M, et al: Ototoxicity assessment of a gentamicin sulfate otic preparation in dogs. Am J Vet Res 56:532, 1995.
A controlled study that evaluated auditory and vestibular function after 3 weeks of therapy with gentamicin sulfate in normal dogs after myringotomy.

Thomas ML: Development of a bacterial model for canine otitis externa. Proceedings of the annual members meeting of the American Academy of Veterinary Dermatologists. San Francisco: American Academy of Veterinary Dermatology and American College of Veterinary Dermatology 6:28, 1990.
A study that evaluated the efficacy of silver sulfadiazine and sodium hypochlorite for the treatment of experimentally induced Pseudomonas *otitis externa.*

Canine Cutaneous Histiocytic Diseases

VERENA K. AFFOLTER
PETER F. MOORE
Davis, California

A variety of histiocytic proliferative diseases (HPD) have been recognized in the dog. This is a frustrating group of diseases because the distinction between histiocytic inflammation and lymphoma can be difficult based on clinical features and conventional histopathologic characteristics. Cutaneous histiocytoma, cutaneous histiocytosis (CH), systemic histiocytosis (SH), histiocytic sarcoma (HS), and malignant histiocytosis (MH) are syndromes categorized as HPD. The clinical presentation, behavior, and responsiveness to therapy vary, and the exact pathogenesis of each of these diseases is unknown. The histiocytoma is a largely benign neoplasm of the skin. CH and SH are reactive forms of canine histiocytosis and affect both the skin and the subcutis. However, SH behaves more aggressively, and additional lesions develop in other organ systems. MH and HS are malignant neoplastic processes. HS develops as a solitary mass and is often localized in the skin and subcutis. MH (disseminated histiocytic sarcoma) is characterized by a multicentric distribution and primarily affects lymphoid organs.

The proliferation of histiocytes is the common feature of these diseases. Histiocytes are either macrophages or dendritic cells. Both originate from a common precursor cell in the bone marrow. On differentiation, these cells develop along two phenotypically separate cell lineages with different tissue distribution and function. It is not clear at this point whether differentiated cells stay committed to one lineage or whether bidirectional changes are possible in a suitable microenvironment. Macrophages are primarily involved with phagocytosis and intracellular digestion of foreign antigens and as such they are important cells of the innate immune system. Dendritic cells are poorly phagocytic; they specialize in processing and presenting antigens to T lymphocytes to evoke an antigen-specific immune response, sharing this function with other cells that are categorized as antigen-presenting cells (APCs).

PHENOTYPES OF HISTIOCYTIC PROLIFERATIVE DISEASE

Immunohistologic examination enables phenotypic evaluation of the cell populations involved. The results are discussed more extensively elsewhere in this volume (see p. 505). The histiocytes coexpress CD1a, CD1b, CD1c, CD11c, and MHC II, which characterize the cells as dendritic APCs. In the human literature, proliferations of dendritic APCs are classified as Langerhans cell histiocytosis (LCH) or class I histiocytosis. Hence, *canine HPD represent canine LCH.*

Phenotypical differences distinguish the syndromes of canine LCH. Histiocytomas lack expression of CD4 and Thy-1 (CD90) and they have a tropism for the epidermis that is consistent with the phenotype of epidermal dendritic cells, called epidermal Langerhans cells (LCs). This suggests that histiocytomas originate from epidermal LCs. Dendritic cells in CH and SH consistently express Thy-1 and CD4. Thy-1 is expressed by normal dermal perivascular dendritic cells, and CD4 expression is observed in activated LCs and human LCH cells. Therefore CH and SH are consistent with an expansion of activated dermal LCs. The origin of the proliferating dendritic cells in MH and HS is unclear. Intralesional dendritic cells lack CD4 expression, and the majority do not express Thy-1. However, dendritic cells in these disorders do not display epidermotropism and are unlikely to originate from epidermal LCs, which otherwise are phenotypically identical.

PATHOGENESIS OF LANGERHANS CELL HISTIOCYTOSIS

Human LCH includes a variety of clinical syndromes. The pathogenesis of proliferations of dendritic APCs is not understood. The majority of cases are considered reactive proliferative disorders. However, a limited number of cases have been evaluated for clonality, a feature characteristic of neoplasia; all the cases tested thus far represent clonal expansions of dendritic cells. Dendritic APCs are rare in the peripheral blood but are widely distributed in lymphoid and nonlymphoid tissues. Factors such as granulocyte-macrophage colony-stimulating factor (GM-CSF), tumor necrosis factor-alpha and interleukin-4 induce and support the differentiation of dendritic cell lineage from a precursor cell in the bone marrow. Differentiated dendritic cells function as APCs; their interaction with helper T lymphocytes elicits a successful immune response.

The cause of canine LCH also is unknown. Genetic factors, immune dysregulations, and clonal expansion may all be involved in the complex pathogenesis of different forms of canine LCH. The histiocytoma is a largely benign cutaneous tumor that occurs with high frequency in the general dog population. CH, which is also not restricted to special breeds, is less common. SH and MH as well as HS develop in more confined subpopulations; this indicates the influence of genetic factors. Clinical behavior, lack of response to immunomodulatory drugs, and histologic features of MH and HS are consistent with a *malignant neoplastic* process; however, clonality has not been demonstrated as yet. Histologic features of canine CH and SH are more consistent with an *inflammatory* process, as these conditions respond to the administration of immunoregulatory drugs. Thus, CH and SH are considered reactive expansions of dendritic cells. Reactive histiocytosis is likely the result of a persistent antigen stimulus. However, special histologic stains to demonstrate infectious agents produce negative results and bacterial and fungal cultures are also negative. Reactive histiocytosis could be the result of an immune dysregulatory process. A disturbed local cytokine milieu, a defective interaction between dendritic APCs and T lymphocytes, or a combination of both may result in the accumulation of dendritic cells together with lymphocytes and neutrophils.

CLINICAL PRESENTATION AND MANAGEMENT OF CANINE LANGERHANS CELL HISTIOCYTOSIS

Canine Cutaneous Histiocytoma

Clinical Presentation. Canine cutaneous histiocytoma is a common benign neoplasm in young dogs. The incidence of histiocytomas drops markedly after the age of 3 years, but histiocytomas develop in older dogs as well. Most cases present with a solitary, nonpruritic and nonpainful intracutaneous plaque or dome-shaped nodule. It often becomes alopecic and ulcerates. The majority of the nodules are smaller than 2.5 cm in diameter. The areas most often affected are the head, ears, neck, and extremities. Based on our observations, there is no breed or sex predilection for solitary lesions. Histiocytomas are characterized by nonencapsulated, poorly demarcated, intracutaneous nodules with diffuse proliferations of fairly monomorphic round cells with big round to oval, indented or twisted vesicular nuclei. There is intraepithelial growth of the proliferating cells, and mitotic figures are frequent. Reactive cellular infiltrates are scant, except for the marked infiltration of CD8+ cytotoxic T cells at a later stage, which correlates with the spontaneous regression seen in the majority of histiocytomas. Once initiated, regression may be completed within days. Cases of multiple histiocytomas at different sites or recurrent histiocytomas are less common. Multiple histiocytomas are predominantly seen in Shar-pei or Shar-pei–mixed breed dogs and may persist longer. Although some nodules start to regress, new ones can develop, and the condition may persist over a period of several months; however, eventually all masses undergo spontaneous regression.

Regional lymph nodes are rarely enlarged because of migrating histiocytoma cells in either solitary or multiple histiocytomas. The lymph nodes are not painful and, in our experience, localized lymphadenopathy will disappear simultaneous with the regression of the skin nodule or nodules. In other cases, premature euthanasia has precluded follow-up of lymphadenopathy. Ulceration of the surface predisposes the animal to secondary bacterial infection. Subsequent development of bacterial septicemia has been observed in isolated cases.

Differential Diagnosis. Solitary histiocytomas in young dogs are seldom difficult to diagnose. In older dogs or when multiple lesions are present, the differential diagnosis includes other cutaneous round cell tumors, such as the mast cell tumor; cutaneous epitheliotropic lymphoma (mycosis fungoides); cutaneous nonepitheliotropic lymphoma; plasmacytoma; and melanoma. Epitheliotropic behavior is a characteristic of mycosis fungoides, histiocytomas, and some melanomas. Immunohistologic examination (see p. 505) enables differentiation among these three tumors.

Therapy. Most lesions spontaneously regress within weeks. Regression is initiated by the infiltration of numerous CD8+ T cells. The administration of immunomodulatory drugs, which would interfere with the infiltration of the T cells, is therefore contraindicated. In cases of delayed regression, surgical excision is recommended. This is especially true for ulcerated nodules, which should be surgically removed to avoid secondary bacterial infections and possible septicemia. Antibiotics are recommended in cases of ulcerated histiocytoma.

Prognosis. Histiocytoma is a benign cutaneous neoplasm that usually undergoes spontaneous regression. Surgical excision is curative in the remaining cases, and a good prognosis can be given for solitary lesions. Multiple histiocytomas usually persist over a longer period (up to 9 months); however, they regress eventually, and with successful prevention of secondary infections, a good prognosis can be given.

Cutaneous and Systemic Histiocytosis

Clinical Presentation. Canine reactive LCH includes CH and SH. Both present with identical lesions in the skin and subcutis. In CH, there is no breed or sex predilection, and the age of the patients ranges from 3 to 9 years. SH was first described as a disease of Bernese mountain dogs, primarily affecting males. However, SH has now been recognized in a variety of other breeds, such as the Rottweiler, Golden and Labrador retrievers, Belgian shepherd, Standard poodle, Border collie, Irish water spaniel, and mixed-breed dogs. There is no sex predilection in these breeds. The age of the dogs with SH ranges from 4 to 7 years. They show solitary or, more often, multiple haired or alopecic cutaneous plaques and nodules, predominantly located on the head, neck, perineum, scrotum, and extremities. Lesions on the trunk are less frequent. The nodules are neither pruritic nor painful. Lesions of CH and SH tend to wax and wane. Partial remission of nodules can be observed, whereas new ones may develop in other locations. The cutaneous nodules often extend deep into the subcutaneous tissue. These are characterized by a multifocal to diffuse infiltration of a mixed cell population. There are numerous large, pale, round to oval histiocytes, with large vesicular nuclei, which are often indented and twisted. Phenotypically, these cells are consistent with dendritic APCs. Numerous lymphocytes and neutrophils are admixed. Eosinophils and plasma cells are seen less commonly. The lesions tend to focus around vessels, and vasoinvasion with subsequent thrombosis and tissue necrosis is common. The histologic features of CH and SH are consistent with a reactive process.

Clinical and histologic features of cutaneous lesions in CH and SH are identical. Migrating lesional dendritic APCs may result in an enlargement of regional lymph nodes, especially in SH. A generalized lymphadenopathy can be observed in some cases of SH. SH also affects the nasal cavity, eyelids, and sclera. Additional lesions often develop in the lung, spleen, liver, and bone marrow. Occasionally, lesions may occur in other locations, for example, in the retro-orbital tissues or in the testicular tissue. Clinical symptoms vary, depending on the organ systems involved; stertorous respiration, for example, is noted with involvement of the nasal cavity.

Differential Diagnosis. The differential diagnosis of CH and SH in skin includes multifocal granulomatous infectious diseases and nonepitheliotropic cutaneous lymphoma. However, the waxing and waning course of the disease is uncharacteristic of a neoplastic process, and histopathologic features are consistent with a reactive, inflammatory process. Multifocal bacterial or fungal infections can be ruled out with special stains. Attempts to culture infectious organisms are not successful. Immunohistologic examination enables the diagnosis of reactive canine LCH, which is characterized by an expansion of activated dendritic APCs with admixed T lymphocytes and neutrophils. Vascular obstruction and thrombosis are more consistently observed in lesions of SH. The diagnosis of SH is based on the involvement of other organ systems in addition to the skin.

Therapy. Some lesions spontaneously regress in early stages of the disease. Surgical excision has been successful in a minority of cases. Approximately 50% of animals with CH respond to immunosuppressive doses of corticosteroids. The majority of cases of SH do not regress with administration of corticosteroids. Other immunoregulatory drugs, such as cyclosporin A (Sandoz) and leflunomide (Arava, Hoechst-Marion-Roussel) have been used successfully for treatment of SH and cases of CH that responded poorly to corticosteroids. Detailed information regarding immunosuppressive therapy with these drugs is discussed elsewhere in this volume (see pp. 509 and 536).

After cessation of therapy, some dogs remain free of clinical symptoms for an indefinite period. Development of new lesions requires readministration of cyclosporin or leflunomide until regression is observed. Other patients develop new lesions as soon as the therapy is stopped. They need continuous administration of immunosuppressive drugs.

Prognosis. A minority of dogs show spontaneous regression of the lesions. Some respond well to treatment and may stay free of symptoms. However, a guarded prognosis must be given because most cases of reactive canine LCH behave as slow episodically or continuously progressive processes and hence, require long-term administration of immunosuppressive drugs.

Canine Histiocytic Sarcoma

Clinical Presentation. HS presents as a rapidly growing, solitary, locally aggressive soft tissue mass. Flat-coated retrievers seem to be predisposed, but HS occurs in other breeds as well, for example, the Golden retriever, Labrador retriever, and Rottweiler. The age of most affected dogs ranges from 6 to 11 years old; however, HS has been found in dogs as young as 2 years of age. There is no sex predilection. In the majority of cases, the mass is located on an extremity, in close proximity to a joint. HS can arise from the skin and subcutaneous tissue and infiltrate underlying tissues, such as skeletal muscles, fascia, and joint capsules. Some HS seems to originate from deeper tissues, for example, joint capsule, and subsequently expand into subcutis and skin. In this instance, HS frequently grows circumferentially around the extremity. HS can develop in other locations, such as the spleen, lung, lymph node, gastric wall, and tongue. The smooth, homogeneously white, multinodular masses show locally aggressive behavior with destruction of adjacent tissues. They are characterized by a nonencapsulated, poorly demarcated proliferation of pleomorphic, large, individualized round cells or more densely packed spindle cells. The cells have a large amount of pale eosinophilic cytoplasm and big round to oval, indented or twisted, vesicular nuclei. Multinucleated giant cells and bizarre mitosis are common. Reactive cellular infiltrates are usually sparse and often consist of neutrophils. Metastasis into regional lymph nodes or distant sites can occur. Metastasis from HS on extremities tends to occur at a later stage only.

Differential Diagnosis. The differential diagnosis for the masses developing in skin and underlying tissues includes a variety of soft tissue tumors that have a tendency to infiltrate into or arise from deeper tissues, such as hemangiopericytoma, synovial cell sarcoma, and schwannoma. The identification of the tumor cell origin often is not possible based on conventional histologic appearance. Immunohistologic examination is a reliable tool to rule out other neoplastic processes by identifying the tumor cells as proliferating dendritic APCs. It is important to evaluate the patient for additional masses in other locations so that a multicentric process consistent with MH (disseminated HS) can be ruled out.

Therapy. Complete surgical excision is the therapy of choice. Complete excision of HS located on the legs often require amputation of the entire extremity. If a surgical approach is impossible, an oncologist should be consulted. HS observed in the tongue of a young dog was successfully treated with radiotherapy. Chemotherapy is often unrewarding.

Prognosis. A guarded prognosis must be given. Regional lymph nodes should always be evaluated histologically to rule out early metastasis. If the tumor can be removed in its entirety before lymph node involvement has occurred, a more favorable prognosis may be warranted.

Canine Malignant Histiocytosis

Clinical Presentation. MH (disseminated HS) is a multicentric neoplastic disorder with aggressive biologic behavior. It has been recognized in Bernese mountain dogs, Rottweilers, Golden retrievers, Labrador retrievers, and Flat-coated retrievers. The age at onset ranges from 3 to 11 years old, and there is no sex predilection. Spleen, lymph nodes, lung, and bone marrow are primarily affected. Patients with widespread disease present with additional lesions in other organ systems, such as liver, lungs, central nervous system, kidneys, skeletal muscle, stomach, and adrenal glands. The skin and subcutis are rarely affected. Clinical symptoms vary depending on the organ systems involved. Histopathologic features are identical to the changes described in HS. MH is a rapidly progressing, aggressive disease.

Differential Diagnosis. A primary differential diagnosis includes multicentric large cell lymphoma, which may present with a similar distribution. Lesions limited to the lung and bronchial lymph nodes have to be differentiated from primary anaplastic large cell carcinoma of the lung or granulomatous pulmonary disease. Immunohistologic examination identifies the cells as proliferating pleomorphic dendritic APCs.

Therapy and Prognosis. MH is characterized by a poor response to chemotherapy. Surgical excision is usually less of an option because of the multicentric distribution of MH. By the time a diagnosis is reached, the lesions are usually advanced. Because of the aggressive behavior and poor response to therapy, a poor prognosis must be advanced.

References and Suggested Reading

Calderwood Mays MB, Bergeron JA: Cutaneous histiocytosis in dogs. J Am Vet Med Assoc 188:377, 1986.
  Presents a good description of clinical and pathologic features of CH.
Gadner H: The histiocytic syndromes. In: Fitzpatrick TB, Eisen AZ, Wolff K, et al: Dermatology in General Medicine, 4th ed. New York, McGraw-Hill, 1993, p 2003.
  This chapter offers an excellent overview of human LCH—its clinical presentation, diagnosis, and therapy.
Moore PF: Systemic histiocytosis of Bernese mountain dogs. Vet Pathol 21:554, 1984.
  Original paper describing the syndrome of SH.
Moore PF, Schrenzel MD, Affolter VK, et al: Canine cutaneous histiocytoma is a epidermotropic Langerhans cell histiocytosis which expresses CD1 and specific β2 integrin molecules. Am J Pathol 148:1699, 1996.
  This was the first paper documenting the dendritic APC (Langerhans cell) lineage of canine histiocytic disease; it contains a review of clinical and histologic features of canine cutaneous histiocytoma and background information on the comparative biology and proliferative diseases of dendritic APCs.
Rosin A, Moore PF: Malignant histiocytosis in Bernese mountain dogs. J Am Vet Med Assoc 188:1041, 1986.
  Original paper describing the syndrome of MH with an emphasis on the clinical features.

Diseases of the Anal Sacs

MARK S. THOMPSON
Columbia, Missouri

The treatment of problems associated with the anal sacs has long been a part of small animal veterinary practice. Despite the frequency with which practitioners are confronted with these problems, the diagnosis and therapy of anal sac disease continues to be confusing and ill-defined. This confusion stems from the lack of knowledge about the normal appearance, contents, and function of anal sacs.

Anal sacs are paired cutaneous evaginations situated between the internal and external anal sphincter muscles. They are often referred to as *anal glands,* but that term is more appropriately used to refer to the anal apocrine glands, which are tubuloalveolar glands that are found in the submucosa at the anocutaneous junction. Each anal sac and its associated duct are lined with squamous epithelial cells. The duct opens to the skin surface just lateral to the anus. Abundant apocrine glands found in the fundus of each sac empty into the lumen. Sebaceous glands are less numerous and are confined to the ductal epithelium.

Anal sac secretions consist of apocrine gland secretions, desquamated epithelial cells, bacteria, and sebaceous secretions. The secretions are usually expressed from the sacs when the dog defecates. The normal color of these secretions varies from yellow to gray to brown, and the consistency varies from liquid to viscid. The fluid may be granular or flecked with solid material. This variation in visual appearance in normal dogs sometimes leads to misdiagnosis of impaction or sacculitis. The fluid usually has a fetid odor that is probably due to bacterial putrefaction of the contents within the sacs. This odor also may vary greatly among dogs. A popular belief is that anal sac secretions play a role in the marking of territory or in sexual attraction, but there are no studies to substantiate that opinion. One study of bitches in estrous showed that males were attracted to vaginal secretions and urine of the bitches but not the anal sac fluid (Doty and Dunbar, 1974a). Another study by the same authors showed no relationship between hormonal status of the dog and the color, odor, or volume of the anal sac secretions (Doty and Dunbar, 1974b).

PATHOPHYSIOLOGY

The pathophysiology of anal sac disease is poorly understood. It is divided into impaction, sacculitis, abscessation, and neoplasia. It has been contended that abscessation and sacculitis are an extension of impaction (Halnan, 1976). Predisposing factors for impaction may include decreased muscle tone in small and obese dogs, chronic diarrhea, and increased glandular secretion associated with generalized seborrhea. It is logical to assume that loose stools or stools that are decreased in volume may be less effective at naturally expressing the contents of the anal sacs. Additionally, since the duct of the anal sac is relatively small, any problem that leads to swelling or edema in the perianal region may predispose the animal to impaction by occluding or partially occluding the duct. The pathogenesis of anal sacculitis is even less clear. The retention of secretions with impaction may predispose the animal to sacculitis; however, impacted anal sacs do not always progress to sacculitis. Abscessation likely is a sequela to sacculitis.

CLINICAL FEATURES

The historical signs of anal sac disease are similar for impaction, sacculitis, or abscessation. The most common signs are licking or biting at the perianal area, "scooting," discomfort when sitting, and pain on manipulation of the tail. It is important to realize that many other diseases can have these same clinical signs. Flea allergy commonly causes pruritus of the tail head area, and atopy and food allergy can cause perianal pruritus. Other diseases noted to cause these signs include vaginitis, proctitis, perianal fistulas, and parasitic diseases. Dogs with sacculitis may have an increased frequency and volume of a fetid discharge from the anal sac ducts. This discharge is often purulent or even bloody in nature. Erythema over the affected anal sac and moist dermatitis of the perineum may be seen. The anal sacs are distended with impaction and may or may not be distended with sacculitis. Abscessed anal sacs are red, swollen, and painful and may present with a draining fistulous tract if the abscess has ruptured. Some are pyrectic.

Definitive diagnosis of anal sac disease is problematic because of the overlap between clinical features of anal sac disease and normal variation. Anal sac impaction is characterized by distention of one or both sacs with retention of secretion and no evidence of inflammation. Palpable anal sacs, however, are not necessarily impacted. Normal dogs have varying degrees of filling of the sacs, and the size of the sacs vary with the size of the dog. It is difficult, therefore, to diagnose impaction by palpation alone. The character of the secretion is generally much thicker and pastier with impaction and is usually gray to brown. Expression takes greater pressure than normal, and the secretion may extrude in a thin ribbon.

As previously discussed, however, the character of normal anal sac secretions varies greatly, and dogs without clinical signs may have a similar thickened discharge. The diagnosis, therefore, is best assumed if the dog's clinical signs respond to the expression of the sacs.

Anal sacculitis is an inflammation of the anal sac and is assumed to be a bacterial infectious process; accordingly, one would expect to find evidence of inflammation and infection on cytologic examination of expressed fluid. Microscopic examination of the sac contents in these cases does tend to show numerous neutrophils and many bacteria; however, studies of the normal cytologic character of anal sac contents are lacking. Culture of these secretions is likely to reveal mixed bacterial growth, but these same bacteria may be cultured from normal sacs. Thus, cytologic studies and culture may be difficult to interpret and may represent an unnecessary expense. The clinician should rely on clinical signs and response to therapy to reinforce the diagnosis, while always taking care to consider other causes of perianal pruritus. Abscessation is the easiest disorder to diagnose because of its typical clinical presentation. The skin over the affected sac may appear red, hot, swollen, or painful. If the abscess has ruptured, a draining tract with a serosanguineous to mucopurulent discharge will be present.

THERAPY

Therapy of anal sac impaction involves gentle, manual expression of the sacs. This may be accomplished externally by lifting the tail, placing the thumb and one finger of the other hand lateral to the anal sacs, and gently applying pressure. I prefer internal expression in which the index finger is inserted into the rectum and the anal sac is palpated and expressed through the rectum. With true impaction, this should resolve the problem, at least temporarily. In dogs that exhibit frequent recurrence of signs, a search for an underlying cause should be carried out. Obese dogs may benefit from weight loss, and high-fiber diets that encourage more voluminous stools may aid natural expression during defecation. Disease processes, such as allergy, that predispose to perianal swelling and edema occlude the ducts and should be identified and addressed. Frequent expression of anal sacs should be limited to dogs with recurrent impaction and should not be used as a preventive procedure in asymptomatic dogs. Routine expression by veterinarians, veterinary technicians, or groomers of palpable sacs may cause irritation and subsequent inflammation and should be discouraged.

Therapy for anal sacculitis involves expression of the sacs and flushing with sterile saline. Since these inflamed sacs are often painful, sedation and analgesia are usually required. After flushing, an antibiotic-based lotion may be infused into the sac through the duct. Intramammary and otic preparations are often used because they are easy to administer. It is important to remember that most commercially available otic drugs contain some form of a corticosteroid. Since anal sacculitis is assumed to be a bacterial process, the advisability of using a corticosteroid is questionable, although short-term reduction of inflammation may be beneficial. Anal sac abscesses, if open and draining, are treated by copious irrigation with saline or with saline and a mild disinfectant. If not open, hot packs are used until they point and they are then lanced ventrally and irrigated as described previously. An antibiotic ointment can be infused into the sac through the duct, but therapy with a broad-spectrum antibiotic such as cephalexin or amoxicillin-clavulanic acid is necessary.

Recurrent or refractory impaction, sacculitis, or abscessation may necessitate anal sacculectomy. The reader is referred to standard veterinary surgery textbooks for surgical techniques. Complications after these procedures are not common but may include fecal incontinence resulting from trauma to the anal branch of the pudendal nerve and fistula formation from incomplete removal of the sac. Because fecal incontinence is a severe problem that often leads to euthanasia in dogs, medical means of management should be tried before surgical treatment is considered. Neoplasia of the anal sacs is another indication for surgical excision.

Anal sacculectomy has traditionally been a component of the treatment of perianal fistulas in dogs. However, a recently published study indicates that surgical treatment of this disease—and the associated neurologic complications—may be avoided in many dogs through the use of immunotherapy with *cyclosporine* (Mathews and Sukhiani, 1997). This prospective, placebo-controlled investigation evaluated the response of 20 affected German shepherds to cyclosporine and 10 affected German shepherds to placebo. Cyclosporine-treated dogs experienced marked improvement, with significant reduction of involved skin surface area (by 78%) and decreases in the depth of the fistulas. The control group showed progression of disease during the same period. Complete healing of the perianal fistulas occurred in 85% of cyclosporine-treated dogs. Nonresponders, or dogs in which fistulas recurred after initial therapy (7 dogs), required treatment with either additional cyclosporine or with surgery (although less radical surgery was needed if preceded by cyclosporine therapy). These exciting initial results indicate a strong consideration of cyclosporine therapy for treatment of perianal fistulas before any surgical management of the condition (for additional information about cyclosporine, see p. 509).

NEOPLASIA

The only reported neoplasm of anal sac origin is the apocrine gland adenocarcinoma. This tumor occurs predominantly in older female dogs and typically presents as a firm mass in the area of one of the anal sacs. These tumors often secrete parathyroid hormone–related protein, which leads to hypercalcemia, hypophosphatemia, polydipsia, and polyuria. Surgical excision is the treatment of choice if the tumor has not metastasized to the iliac and sublumbar lymph nodes. Surgical excision of regional metastases may be attempted if metastasis has already occurred. Apocrine gland adenocarcinomas are highly malignant, and recurrence after removal is common. Chemotherapy has been tried in a small number of cases, but more cases are needed to establish efficacy.

Anal Sac Disease in Cats

Anal sac disease is much less common in cats, but impaction, sacculitis, and abscessation are all recognized. Feline anal sacs contain sebaceous and apocrine glands in the fundic portion of the sac. It has been theorized that the sebaceous gland secretions may prevent the anal sac fluid from becoming as viscid, thus preventing impaction. Treatment of anal sac problems in the cat are similar to that of the dog.

References and Suggested Reading

Doty RL, Dunbar I: Attraction of beagles to conspecific urine, vaginal, and anal sac secretion odors. Physiol Behav 12:825, 1974a.
   A study comparing the attraction of male dogs to female urine, vaginal, and anal sac secretions.
Doty RL, Dunbar I: Color, odor, consistency, and secretion rate of anal sac secretions from male, female, and early-androgenized female beagles. Am J Vet Res 35:729, 1974b.
   A study showing the normal variation of color and consistency of anal sac secretions in dogs.
Halnan CRE: The experimental reproduction of anal sacculitis. J Small Anim Pract 17:693, 1976.
   A study that attempted to produce anal sacculitis by instillation of bacteria into anal sacs with ligated and unligated ducts.
Mathews KA, Sukhiani HR: Randomized controlled trial of cyclosporine for treatment of perianal fistulas in dogs. J Am Vet Med Assoc 211:1249, 1997.
   Prospective controlled study regarding the use of cyclosporine for treatment of perianal fistulas.
Ross JT, Scavelli TD, Matthiesen DT, et al: Adenocarcinoma of the apocrine glands of the anal sac in dogs: A review of 32 cases. J Am Anim Hosp Assoc 27:349, 1992.
   A retrospective study examining the recurrence rate and survival time of dogs with apocrine gland adenocarcinoma.
van Duijkeren E: Disease conditions of canine anal sacs. J Small Anim Pract 36:12, 1995.
   A complete review of the literature on anal sac disease.

Gastrointestinal Disorders

D<small>AVID</small> C. T<small>WEDT</small>

Consulting Editor

Gastrointestinal Disorders

DAVID C. TWEDT

Consulting Editor

Esophageal Feeding Tubes

CHAD M. DEVITT
HOWARD B. SEIM III
Fort Collins, Colorado

INTRODUCTION

Nutritional support of small animal patients has received considerable attention over the past decade. Tube esophagostomy is a technique that allows enteral feeding through a large-diameter feeding tube that enters the gastrointestinal tract in a relatively innocuous location. The long-term effects of tube esophagostomy in horses are disturbing; reported complications include dissecting mediastinitis, permanent fistula formation, and traction diverticula formation. Until recently, reports have failed to provide information regarding long-term follow-up of small animal patients with tube esophagostomy. For this and other reasons, gastrotomy tubes have been advocated in dogs and cats (p. 84); however, there are indications for tube esophagostomy. The purposes of this article are to develop criteria for the use of tube esophagostomy, describe a technique for tube esophagostomy placement, and discuss its advantages and disadvantages over those of other techniques of enteral nutrition.

INDICATIONS

Nutritional support is indicated in patients unable to meet nutritional demands because of an inability or reluctance to consume a prescribed diet (pp. 80 and 136). Specific examples include procedures such as mandibulectomy, maxillectomy, or cleft palate repair. Reluctance to consume a prescribed diet may be due to poor palatability of a particular diet or to the primary disorder, or may result from a treatment or procedure (e.g., radiation therapy).

CONTRAINDICATIONS

Tube esophagostomy is contraindicated in patients with esophageal dysfunction, including megaesophagus, esophagitis, esophageal stricture, pancreatitis, gastric outflow obstruction, and persistent vomiting. Vomiting is not an absolute contraindication to the use of an esophagostomy tube. In a recent series of 22 clinical cases of tube esophagostomy, five patients vomited during the time the esophagostomy tube was in place (Devitt and Seim, 1997). One patient was a dog; the other four patients were cats. The dog vomited once and displaced the tube through the oral cavity. Four cats vomited multiple times, but the tube remained in the proper position. In one of the cats, the vomiting was due to placement of the tube through the lower esophageal sphincter, leading to reflux esophagitis. Repositioning of the tube resolved the vomiting. In the other three cats, vomiting was probably due to the primary disorder (hepatic lipidosis). Antiemetic therapy (metoclopramide, 0.2 to 0.5 mg/kg every 12 to 6 hr) via the esophagostomy tube 15 to 20 minutes prior to feeding was effective in controlling the vomiting episodes, and all cats resumed oral consumption of food. Because of the risk of tube displacement, caution should be exercised when one considers tube esophagostomy in patients likely to vomit.

TECHNIQUE

Patients are routinely anesthetized, preferably with inhalant anesthetics via an endotracheal intubation in order to maintain an airway and prevent inadvertent introduction of the esophagostomy tube into the trachea. An 18 to 20 F red rubber feeding tube (All-Purpose Catheter; Davol, C. R. Bard, Inc., Cranston, RI) is placed in all patients regardless of body size. The distal orifices of the tube are enlarged, as depicted in Figure 1. The tube is premeasured and marked from the point of insertion in the midcervical esophagus to the sixth or seventh intercostal space. Patients are placed in right lateral recumbency, and the left cervical region is prepared aseptically from the caudal angle of the mandible to the point of the shoulder. An ELD percutaneous feeding tube applicator (ELD Gastrostomy Tube Applicator; Jorgensen Laboratories, Inc., Loveland, CO) is used to place the tube (Fig. 2). The applicator has a trocar that retracts into the hollow shaft of the applicator. The applicator tip is lubricated, introduced into the oral cavity, and passed into the esophagus to the level of the midcervical esophagus (a point midway between the caudal angle of the mandible and the point of the shoulder; Fig. 3). An incision is made through the skin and subcutaneous tissue over the tip to the applicator (see Fig. 3A). The trocar is advanced through the esophageal wall and through the skin and subcutaneous incision (see Fig. 3B). If necessary, the esophageal stoma is enlarged to allow passage of the shaft of the applicator through the esophageal wall and out the skin and subcutaneous incision. A loop of 2-0 nylon (Dermalon; D&G Monofil Inc., Manati, Puerto Rico) is passed through the eyelet of the trocar and the enlarged orifice of the feeding tube (see Fig. 3C). The trocar is

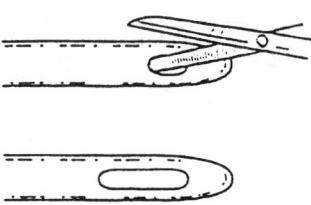

Figure 1. Modification of the distal orifice of the feeding tube with a scissors. The orifice is elongated 3 to 4 mm without compromising the strength of the tube. (From Devitt CM, Seim HB III: Clinical evaluation of tube esophagostomy in small animals. Am Anim Hosp Assoc 33:55–60, 1997, with permission.)

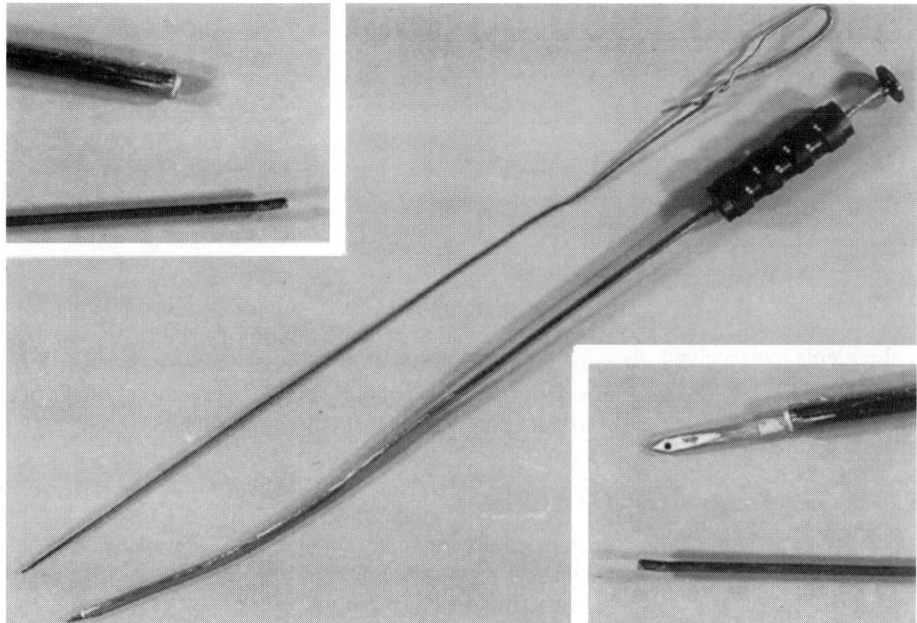

Figure 2. ELD percutaneous feeding tube applicator and stylet. *Upper Inset,* A close-up view to the distal tip of the applicator with the blade retracted. *Lower Inset,* A close-up view of the distal end of the applicator with the blade extended. Note the eyelet for securing suture material to the blade. (From Devitt CM, Seim HB III: Clinical evaluation of tube esophagostomy in small animals. Am Anim Hosp Assoc 33:55–60, 1997, with permission.)

retracted to approximate the tip of the applicator shaft and the tip of the feeding tube. The applicator and attached feeding tube are retracted through the skin, subcutaneous tissue, and esophageal wall into the esophagus and exteriorized through the oral cavity (Fig. 4A). The suture between the trocar and the feeding tube is transected. A heavy wire stylet is placed into the side orifice to rest against the tip of the feeding tube and is used to redirect the feeding tube aborally into the thoracic esophagus (see Fig. 4B). A stylet should not be used to introduce the

catheter in cats. The tube is pushed into the esophagus digitally. The feeding tube is retracted to the previously marked level (see Fig. 4C). The proximal aspect of the feeding tube is secured to the skin with No. 1 polybutester (Novafil; D&G Monofil Inc., Manati, Puerto Rico) in a Chinese finger-trap pattern. The tube entrance site is loosely bandaged with conforming gauze wrap.

Feeding can commence immediately through the feeding tube unless otherwise contraindicated. Diets available for use include Hill's A/D diet, blenderized canned diets, mo-

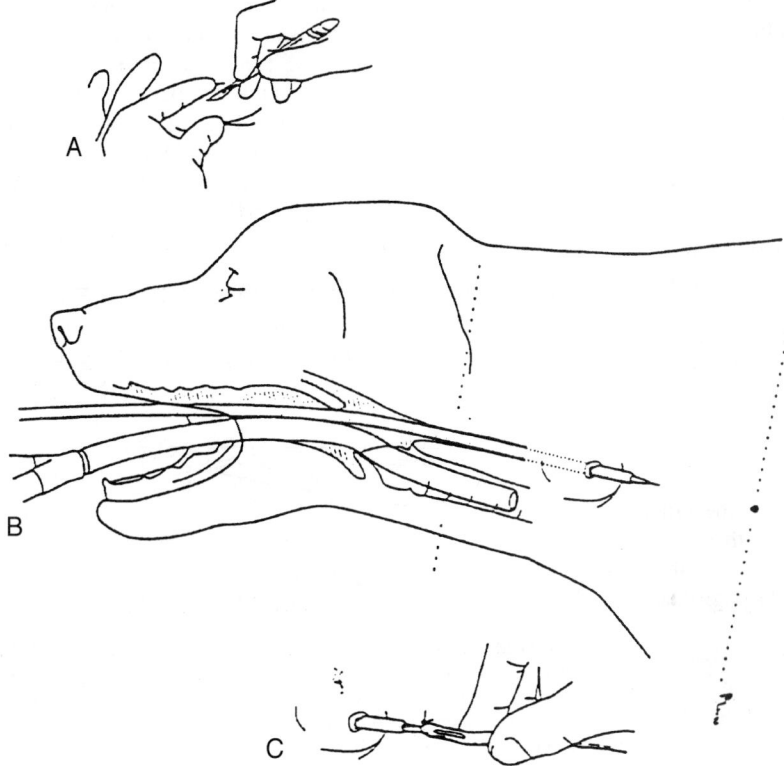

Figure 3. Insertion of ELD percutaneous feeding tube applicator to the midcervical esophagus. *A,* The distal tip is palpated, and an incision is made through the skin and subcutaneous tissue over the tip of the ELD. The trocar is advanced through the esophageal wall and directed through the incision. *B,* The remainder of the shaft is advanced through the esophageal wall. *C,* The distal end of the feeding tube is secured to the eyelet of the trocar with suture material. (From Devitt CM, Seim HB III: Clinical evaluation of tube esophagostomy in small animals. Am Anim Hosp Assoc 33:55–60, 1997, with permission.)

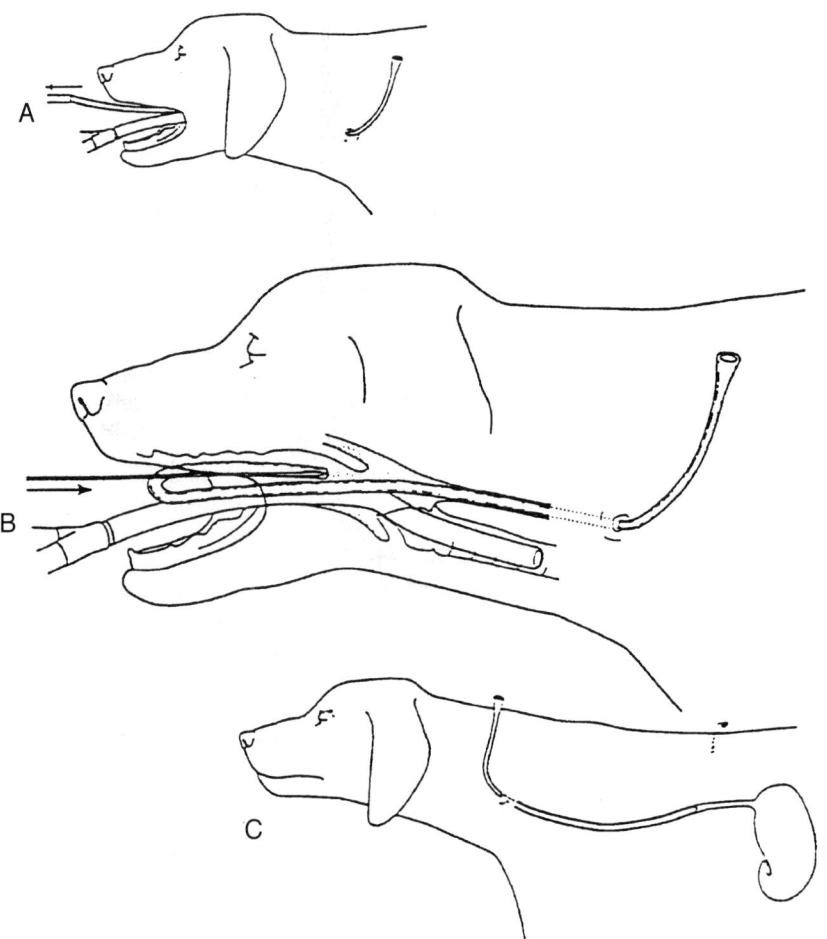

Figure 4. *A,* The ELD and attached feeding tube are retracted into the esophagus and exteriorized out the oral cavity. *B,* The feeding tube is redirected into the esophagus by inserting a wire stylet into the enlarged orifice and resting against the distal tip of the feeding tube. *C,* The tube is directed into the midthoracic esophagus and retracted to the previously marked level if necessary. (From Devitt CM, Seim HB III: Clinical evaluation of tube esophagostomy in small animals. Am Anim Hosp Assoc 33:55–60, 1997, with permission.)

nomeric diets, and polymeric diets. The tube entrance site should be maintained with daily inspection and cleaning with antiseptic solution (0.9% NaCl and 0.5% Betadine [povidone-iodine] solution). When nutritional support is no longer necessary, the tube is removed by cutting the retaining suture and pulling the tube. The esophagocutaneous fistula is allowed to heal by second intention and generally does so within 2 weeks.

ADVANTAGES

The technique of midcervical tube esophagostomy is economical and simple to perform and provides a large-diameter feeding tube. Tube esophagostomy is suitable in nutritionally compromised small animals with a functional esophagus and gastrointestinal tract. Tube esophagostomy should be placed from the midcervical esophagus to the midthoracic esophagus and should not cross the lower esophageal sphincter. Feeding via tube esophagostomy can commence immediately following tube placement. Long-term use of tube esophagostomy, in our experience, has not been associated with significant complications in dogs and cats. Following tube removal, the esophagocutaneous fistula heals readily by second intention.

Various methods are available for providing nutritional support in small animals, including nasogastric, nasoesophageal, pharyngostomy, gastrostomy, and jejunostomy tubes (pp. 84 and 136). Each method has advantages and

disadvantages. Although general anesthesia is required for placement, tube esophagostomy has the advantage over nasoesophageal or nasogastric tube in providing a large-diameter feeding tube, which eliminates the need for specialized diets. Tube esophagostomy has the advantage over nasogastric, nasoesophageal, and pharyngostomy tubes by being placed further caudad, eliminating the risk of aspiration or upper airway obstruction. Tube esophagostomy has the advantage over gastrostomy and jejunostomy tubes by eliminating the risk of peritonitis if the gastrostomy or jejunostomy tube is prematurely dislodged. The tube esophagostomy has advantages over a jejunostomy tube in that tube esophagostomy does not require laparotomy for placement, specialized diets, or expensive equipment for optimal usage.

References and Suggested Reading

Crowe DT Jr: Nutritional support for the hospitalized patient: An introduction to tube feeding. Compend Contin Educ 12:1711, 1990.
   A review of nutritional support methods in small animals.
Devitt CM, Seim HB III: Clinical evaluation of tube esophagostomy in small animals. J Am Anim Hosp Assoc 33:55, 1997.
   Prospective study of tube esophagostomy in 22 dogs and cats and guidelines for tube esophagostomy use.
Rawlings CA: Percutaneous placement of a mid-cervical tube esophagostomy: New technique and representative cases. J Am Anim Hosp Assoc 29:526, 1993.
   Another method of cervical esophagostomy tube placement in small animals.

Feline Stomatitis and Faucitis

LINDA J. DEBOWES
Manhattan, Kansas

The most common cause of oral inflammation is periodontal disease (gingivitis, periodontitis). Inflammation of the buccal mucosa (stomatitis) may be associated with severe periodontal disease. Eosinophilic complex–related disorders, neoplasia, trauma, irritation due to ingestion of noxious materials, immune-mediated diseases, and metabolic abnormalities are also potential causes of oral inflammation. Cats infected with feline leukemia virus or feline immunodeficiency virus that have altered immune function may have more severe periodontal disease or oral inflammation. Chronic calicivirus infection has been implicated as a factor in severe oral inflammation, especially in cats with faucitis. The gingiva adjacent to an odontoclastic resorptive lesion frequently is hyperplastic and inflamed.

Oral inflammatory disease of unknown cause is a common problem in cats. The degree of inflammation is variable and may be severe. These cats present a diagnostic and therapeutic challenge, and management is frequently frustrating for both the veterinarian and owner. Inflammation may involve the gingiva (gingivitis), buccal mucosa (stomatitis), glossopalatine arch (faucitis) or pharyngeal area (pharyngitis). Current knowledge about the cause of severe stomatitis and faucitis unrelated to periodontal disease in cats is limited. The condition has been referred to as lymphocytic-plasmacytic stomatitis based on the major cellular infiltrate present on histologic examination. The histologic description is compatible with a chronic inflammatory or immunologic response but does not provide a definitive diagnosis as to the primary cause. Cats with severe stomatitis and faucitis are often grouped together as all having the same unknown problem, yet based on clinical presentation and variable response to treatment, it is more likely that multiple factors are involved.

HISTORICAL AND CLINICAL SIGNS

Cats with severe oral inflammatory disease frequently present with a history of dysphagia, inappetence or anorexia, and pain when eating is attempted. The cat may appear interested in food but is unwilling to eat; it may attempt to eat but drops the food from its mouth or paws at its muzzle. The affected cat is usually reluctant to eat hard food but may eat soft fare. As the severity of the inflammation increases, the cat becomes more picky about what it will eat. The presence of blood-tinged saliva may be noted after eating. In severe cases, the cat may be in a great deal of pain, causing a reluctance to swallow and drooling (pseudoptyalism). Weight loss may be a significant problem, depending on the duration of anorexia. Affected cats may exhibit altered behavior, such as being less active, demonstrating aggressive behavior toward other pets or persons, or expressing an aversion to having their face or head touched. These cats may have an unkempt appearance resulting from a reluctance to groom because of oral pain.

ORAL EXAMINATION

Before examining the oral cavity, the regional lymph nodes should be palpated, and the mandible and maxilla should be examined for swellings or pain. It may not be possible to complete the initial oral examination if the cat has severe oral pain. In severe cases, the inflamed tissues may be ulcerated and bleed readily. Proliferation of oral tissues may make it difficult to visualize the teeth. Cats with severe stomatitis and faucitis may have extreme pain on opening the mouth; thus, the initial examination should be performed with the mouth closed while gently retracting the lips. This examination is performed slowly to minimize pain. The mouth is then opened gently if possible. Lesions of the oral cavity may include inflammation of the gingiva (gingivitis), oral buccal mucosa (stomatitis), and glossopalatine arch (faucitis). Often, a complete oral examination is not possible without benefit of sedation or general anesthesia.

DIAGNOSTIC EVALUATION

A complete blood count, biochemical profile, and urinalysis are performed to identify concurrent or contributory diseases. The complete blood count is usually unremarkable. Hyperglobulinemia has been identified in some cats with chronic stomatitis and faucitis. Serologic evaluation for feline leukemia virus antigen and feline immunodeficiency virus antibody should be performed. It is ideal to include virus isolation studies on specimens obtained from oral swabs of inflamed tissues in cats with stomatitis and faucitis. Although bacterial cultures are not part of a basic evaluation in most cases, bacterial culture and sensitivity testing may be helpful in chronic cases that do not respond to the antibiotics commonly used for oral infections. A specimen for biopsy of any lesion that appears neoplastic or of unknown cause should be obtained and submitted for histopathologic examination.

A complete oral and dental examination is performed with the cat under general anesthesia. The animal is evaluated for periodontal disease, odontoclastic resorptive lesions, and other problems that may cause oral inflammation. Dental radiographs are obtained to evaluate for alveolar bone loss (indicating periodontitis), locate odontoclastic resorptive lesions, and identify retained root tips.

MANAGEMENT

The goals of management are generally aimed at controlling plaque bacteria and decreasing the inflammatory and immunologic response. Controlling the plaque bacteria can be attempted by several methods, including scaling, topical antimicrobial application, systemic antimicrobial therapy, and tooth removal.

The author manages these cats initially with (1) complete scaling and polishing and extraction of teeth that show evidence of periodontitis or odontoclastic resorptive lesions extending beyond the enamel; (2) oral antibiotic administration for 4 to 6 weeks; and (3) methylprednisolone as described further on. Once the inflammation has decreased and the cat is eating, tooth brushing is instituted if the owners can brush the teeth adequately and the cat is cooperative. Many owners are not able to brush the teeth sufficiently to decrease plaque accumulation and prevent inflammation. To manage the inflammation and maintain appetite initially, most cats require methylprednisolone administration every 4 to 6 weeks and over time as frequently as every 3 weeks. The author informs the owners on the initial visit that we will try to manage the oral inflammation with frequent professional dental care and medical therapy, but that extractions may be the best long-term option.

Scaling and Polishing

The teeth should be scaled to remove plaque, bacteria, and calculus. Plaque bacteria may be a factor in the excessive inflammatory response present in these cats. The teeth should be polished after any scaling to smooth the tooth surface. Plaque will attach and become established on the tooth surfaces within several hours after the scaling and polishing procedures; therefore, continued measures should be taken to control plaque. Cats with severe oral inflammation are usually in too much pain for toothbrushing to be practical so that plaque control must be maintained initially with topical or systemic antimicrobial therapy. Once the oral inflammation is well controlled, the owner may attempt plaque control with toothbrushing. A finger toothbrush or small toothbrush designed for cats is used with an acceptably flavored veterinary dentifrice.

Antimicrobial Therapy

Antimicrobial therapy is best accomplished with systemic antibiotic administration. A variable response is observed with antibiotic therapy, although therapy of 4 to 6 weeks may result in improvement of clinical signs in some cats. Antibiotics as a single treatment are rarely effective in the initial management of inflammation, and combined treatment with antibiotics and glucocorticoids is usually required. Amoxicillin, amoxicillin–clavulanate acid (Clavamox, SmithKline Beecham), clindamycin (Antirobe, Upjohn), and metronidazole are useful antibiotics in managing these cats. Repeated treatment with antibiotics may be necessary. Complete resolution of clinical signs is unlikely, and relapses are common. Topical chlorhexidine may be used for adjunctive antimicrobial therapy in the initial management, especially at extraction sites. Long-term topical application is generally not well accepted or tolerated by the cat. Chlorhexidine gluconate appears to be accepted better than chlorhexidine acetate. Chlorhexidine gel works well for topical application.

Anti-inflammatory and Immunosuppressive Therapy

Immunosuppressive doses of glucocorticoids are required in most cats to decrease the inflammation and reduce pain sufficiently so that the cat will eat. Methylprednisolone acetate (Depo-Medrol, Upjohn) at 15 to 20 mg total dose IM is generally adequate, and cats usually demonstrate a decrease in the oral inflammation and a willingness to eat within 1 to 2 days. Satisfactory results are not often obtained with oral prednisone administration in cats with severe inflammation. For cats demonstrating moderate improvement after extractions and requiring further control of residual inflammation, oral prednisone (1 to 2 mg/kg every other day) may be sufficient. Yet, higher doses may be required, the ultimate dose being determined by the response. Gold salts are an alternative immunosuppressive therapy, although the author has limited experience with these in cats.

Extractions

Extractions may be indicated in cats with severe periodontitis. Teeth with odontoclastic resorptive lesions extending beyond the enamel should be extracted. In addition to extractions for treatment of related periodontal disease and odontoclastic resorptive lesions, removing healthy teeth may be an option for cats with severe oral inflammation (stomatitis, faucitis) of unknown cause. Plaque bacteria attaches to the tooth surfaces (crowns and roots). Extraction of the teeth removes the surfaces that are available for plaque retention and consequently decreases plaque and the associated inflammation. Extractions are successful in decreasing inflammation when the plaque is initiating the excessive inflammatory response. Retained roots may be a source of residual bacteria and, if found in association with oral inflammation, should be extracted as well. Dental radiographs are needed to confirm removal of all roots in cats with oral inflammation. Extractions are also a potential option when long-term medical management is not adequate or when side effects of drug therapy are unacceptable. Inflammation is frequently located adjacent to the premolars and molars, and extraction of all teeth distal to the canines may be beneficial. When inflammation is also present adjacent to the incisors and canines, a full mouth extraction may be necessary for maximal benefit. The response to extractions is variable, and not all cats respond satisfactorily; therefore, owners should be warned about this. Responses vary from complete resolution of the inflammation to no improvement. Cats tolerate extractions, even full mouth extractions, very well and can eat dry and moist cat food without teeth. After extractions, some cats may show significant improvement, and medical management may not be required to keep the cat free of clinical signs. Other cats may exhibit a partial response, requiring less aggressive medical management than that required before extractions. Another group of cats appears to have minimal response to extractions, and medical management is continued as before the extractions. In the author's practice, cats that responded poorly to full mouth extractions were those in which calicivirus was isolated from the oral cavity. In a report of 30 cats with gingivitis, stomatitis, and faucitis, the response to periodontal treatment and extraction of selected teeth, including retained root tips, was generally favorable (Hennet, 1994). Oral inflammation resolved completely in 60% (18 of 30) of the cats, with an additional 20% (6 of 30) responding with minimal residual inflammation and no oral pain. None of these 24 cats required medical treatment to manage oral inflammation after the treatment. Initial improvement requiring continued medical therapy to control clinical signs was found in 13% (4 of 30) and no improvement occurred in 7% (2 of 30) of the cats.

Reference

Hennet P: Results of periodontal and extraction treatment in cats with gingivo-stomatitis. Proceedings of the World Veterinary Dental Congress, Philadelphia, 1994, p 49.
A retrospective study of cats with gingivitis, stomatitis, and faucitis, reporting the response to periodontal treatment and extractions.

Canine Megaesophagus

ERICK A. MEARS
Tampa, Florida

ROBERT C. DeNOVO
Knoxville, Tennessee

Symptoms of esophageal disease occur when esophageal motility is disturbed or when there is obstruction to the movement of ingesta. Swallowing becomes difficult, even painful, and food will not go down. Regurgitation, dysphagia, and ptyalism are common signs, and aspiration pneumonia is a frequent complication. Typically, both liquid and solid foods pass poorly with motility disturbances of the esophagus, whereas liquids often pass easily with obstruction of the esophagus. A thorough physical examination and often an extensive diagnostic work-up are necessary for determining the cause of esophageal disease and for designing a treatment plan. Table 1 lists the primary causes of esophageal dysfunction in the dog.

FUNCTIONAL ANATOMY

The esophagus is not simply a tube through which food passes. It is an organ with complex innervation and patterns of motility designed to transport fluid and food efficiently from the pharynx to the stomach. The esophagus begins at the pharyngoesophageal junction, commonly referred to as the upper esophageal sphincter (UES), which prevents reflux and aspiration of ingesta from the esophagus. The body of the canine esophagus consists of two layers of skeletal muscle that propel ingesta to the stomach. The gastroesophageal junction, referred to as the lower esophageal sphincter (LES), is the distal limit of the esophagus and prevents reflux of gastric content into the esophagus.

The UES separates the pharynx from the cervical portion of the esophagus and is formed by the cricopharyngeus and thyropharyngeus muscles dorsolaterally and the cricoid cartilage ventrally. These striated muscles are innervated by the glossopharyngeal, pharyngeal, and recurrent laryngeal branches of the vagus nerve that originate in the brain stem nucleus ambiguus. The muscles of the sphincter remain contracted at all times, except during a swallow, when they relax momentarily to allow passage of a bolus. The muscles contract promptly to maintain closure of the sphincter and protect against esophagopharyngeal reflux and aspiration.

The entire length of the canine esophageal body consists of two oblique layers of skeletal muscle and is innervated by the somatic branches of the vagus nerve. The LES is a physiologic sphincter, rather than a true anatomic sphincter, because it does not consist of a distinct muscle mass. It consists of an outer layer of longitudinal striated muscle and an inner layer of circular smooth muscle that merge with the smooth muscle of the stomach. The LES remains closed except to allow passage of a bolus. Competence of the LES is maintained by the gastric rugal folds, the muscular sling of the right crus of the diaphragm, the oblique angle of the gastroesophageal junction, and gastric compression on the esophagus. This sphincter separates the esophagus from the cardia of the stomach and allows ingesta to pass into the stomach while preventing reflux of stomach content into the esophagus.

Esophageal peristalsis is initiated by the oropharyngeal phase of swallowing and the movement of food through the UES. Afferent vagal receptors in the pharynx and proximal esophagus are stimulated by the presence of food; solids are more effective than liquid in stimulating a swal-

TABLE 1. Disorders of the Esophagus

Motility Disorders	Obstructive Lesions
Megaesophagus	Foreign body
Congenital	Stricture
Acquired	Vascular ring anomaly
Primary (idiopathic)	Neoplasia
Secondary (see Table 2)	**Miscellaneous**
Dysautonomia	Diverticula
Hiatal hernia?	Bronchoesophageal fistula
Inflammatory Disease	
Esophagitis	
Gastroesophageal reflux	
Hiatal hernia	

lowing reflex. The origin of the vagus nerve, the nucleus ambiguus for striated muscle, initiates an efferent response via the somatic nerve fibers of the vagus. This neuronal pathway ends at the myoneural junction with a coordinated contraction of the UES and propagation of a peristaltic wave aborally along the body of the esophagus, through the LES, and into the stomach. The initial wave that begins at the pharynx is called *primary peristalsis*. Remaining intraluminal ingesta within the esophagus stimulate esophageal afferent receptors to initiate a secondary peristaltic wave to clear the lumen. Any disease or lesion affecting any part of this neuromuscular pathway can alter normal esophageal motility and cause megaesophagus (Table 2).

MEGAESOPHAGUS

Megaesophagus is a condition characterized by decreased or absent esophageal motility that usually results in diffuse dilatation of the esophagus. Megaesophagus occurs as a congenital disorder that becomes clinically apparent at or shortly after weaning, or it can occur as an acquired disorder in a previously normal adult. Acquired megaesophagus can be secondary to a variety of diseases that cause neuromuscular dysfunction, or it can occur as a primary disorder for which the cause is unknown (idiopathic megaesophagus).

Congenital Megaesophagus

Congenital megaesophagus occurs in both pure and mixed breed dogs. It is known to be inherited in the wirehaired fox terrier as an autosomal recessive trait and in the miniature schnauzer as either an autosomal dominant or autosomal recessive trait with partial penetrance. Congenital megaesophagus occurs with increased incidence in Great Danes, German shepherds, Labrador retrievers, Newfoundlands, Chinese Shar peis, and Irish setters. Al-

TABLE 2. Diseases Associated With and Causes of Megaesophagus in the Dog

Central Nervous System	Esophageal Musculature
Distemper	Esophagitis
Cervical vertebral instability with leukomalacia	Systemic lupus erythematosus
Brain stem lesions	Glycogen storage disease
Neoplasia	Polymyositis
Trauma	Dermatomyositis
Peripheral Neuropathies	Cachexia
Polyneuritis	Trypanosomiasis
Polyradiculoneuritis	Hypoadrenocorticism
Ganglioradiculitis	Hypothyroidism?
Dysautonomia	**Miscellaneous**
Giant cell axonal neuropathy	Pyloric stenosis
Spinal muscular atrophy	Gastric dilatation volvulus
Toxicity	Pituitary dwarfism
Lead	Thymoma
Thallium	Mediastinitis
Acrylamide	
Bilateral vagal damage	
Neuromuscular Junction	
Myasthenia gravis	
Botulism	
Tetanus	
Anticholinesterase toxicity	

though not proved, the predilection for megaesophagus in these breeds, in addition to reports of entire litters of German shepherds, Great Danes, Newfoundlands, and Shar peis being affected, suggests that a hereditary basis for megaesophagus does exist. For this reason, owners are best advised not to use affected dogs or those closely related to affected dogs for breeding. Clinical signs usually occur by 3 months of age; however, dogs with mild symptoms might not be presented until 1 year of age.

Although the pathogenesis of congenital megaesophagus is unclear, esophageal function studies of affected dogs indicate that defects exist in the vagal afferent innervation of the esophagus. Other studies have confirmed that vagal efferent innervation in affected dogs is normal but that esophageal motor function is decreased, possibly secondary to abnormal biomechanical properties of the esophageal muscle.

Acquired Megaesophagus

Secondary megaesophagus can be caused by any disorder that inhibits esophageal peristalsis either by disrupting esophageal neural pathways or by causing esophageal muscular dysfunction. Numerous central and peripheral neuropathies, diseases of the neuromuscular junction, and myopathies have been reported to cause megaesophagus (see Table 2). Most of these diseases are uncommon, and an exhaustive search to rule out all is unrealistic. Several diseases, however, should routinely be considered.

Myasthenia gravis (MG) is the most common cause of acquired megaesophagus in the dog. It occurs rarely as a congenital disease and more frequently as an acquired disease; both can cause megaesophagus. Acquired MG is an autoimmune disorder that interferes with normal neuromuscular transmission. Production of autoantibodies against nicotinic acetylcholine (Ach) receptors decreases the number of receptors available for normal neuromuscular transmission, resulting in skeletal muscle weakness. Diagnosis is made by measuring increased antibody titers to acetylcholine receptors.

Two forms of acquired MG, generalized and focal, have been identified. Generalized MG causes exercise-related generalized muscle weakness that worsens after exercise and improves with rest. Most dogs with generalized MG also have megaesophagus. Focal MG causes weakness that predominantly affects esophageal, pharyngeal, or facial muscles. Affected animals are usually presented to the clinician with symptoms of megaesophagus. It is important to note that many animals diagnosed as having "idiopathic" megaesophagus are likely to have focal MG. In a study by Shelton and associates (1990), serum samples from 152 dogs with idiopathic megaesophagus were tested for Ach receptor antibodies. Results confirmed that 40 of 152 (26%) had antibody titers diagnostic for MG. Of those affected, 48% had clinical improvement or remission of clinical signs with treatment.

Megaesophagus is occasionally observed in dogs with either primary or secondary hypoadrenocorticism. Impaired muscle carbohydrate metabolism and depletion of muscle glycogen stores resulting from glucocorticoid deficiency and decreased catecholamine activity have been suggested as possible causes. Megaesophagus has been reported to resolve with prednisone treatment in dogs with glucocorticoid-deficient hypoadrenocorticism.

Hypothyroidism has also been associated with several neuromuscular disorders in the dog, including megaesophagus. However, a definitive association between hypothyroidism and megaesophagus has not been proved. Few dogs with hypothyroidism acquire megaesophagus, and few reports of thyroid hormone–responsive megaesophagus exist. In one retrospective study of 29 hypothyroid dogs, 4 had megaesophagus; 1 dog showed clinical improvement in esophageal symptoms when treated with thyroid supplement. Radiographic evidence of a dilatated esophagus persisted in all four dogs (Jaggy et al, 1994). Difficulty in determining whether hypothyroidism causes megaesophagus has been compounded by the lack of a definitive test for hypothyroidism (see p. 327). Simultaneous measurement of endogenous thyroid-stimulating hormone and thyroxine concentrations, currently recommended as the test of choice for hypothyroidism, will hopefully improve diagnostic accuracy of hypothyroidism and help to clarify this issue.

Idiopathic Megaesophagus

Idiopathic megaesophagus is a severe and often fatal disease characterized by a large dilatated esophagus with no motility. It occurs spontaneously, usually in large-breed adult dogs between 5 and 12 years of age. There appears to be no sex or breed predisposition. Unfortunately, the majority of adult dogs with megaesophagus are diagnosed as having idiopathic megaesophagus. The etiopathogenesis of this disorder is unknown; however, recent studies have clarified that the abnormality appears to be neurogenic, rather than myogenic. Manometric studies have shown that the function of the UES and LES is normal in response to a swallow, indicating that the efferent innervation is intact. However, when the esophagus is distended with an intraluminal balloon to initiate secondary peristalsis, compliance of the esophagus is increased compared to normal dogs, the UES and LES fail to relax as in normal dogs, and inhibition of diaphragmatic electromyographic activity does not occur as in normal dogs. These observations indicate a defect of either afferent sensory innervation of the esophagus or of esophageal muscle function (Washabau, 1996).

Clinical Signs

Regurgitation is the most common clinical sign observed with megaesophagus. Most owners fail to recognize the difference between regurgitation and vomiting and report vomiting as the primary complaint. The clinician must differentiate between these clinical signs to ensure proper localization and diagnosis of the problem. Regurgitation is characterized as a passive evacuation of fluid, mucus, and undigested food from the esophagus. No consistent temporal relationship occurs between eating and regurgitation caused by esophageal disease. Other signs observed with megaesophagus include ptyalism, halitosis, and vomiting. Cough, nasal discharge, and dyspnea caused by aspiration pneumonia are frequent presenting complaints, especially in young or debilitated dogs. Some dogs appear normal on physical examination, whereas others are underweight to cachectic from poor nutritional intake, depending on the duration and severity of disease. Puppies with congenital megaesophagus are usually smaller than their littermates. Swelling of the ventral neck near the thoracic inlet from esophageal distention with ingesta is occasionally present. Other clinical signs may reflect diseases causing secondary megaesophagus. Careful examination should be performed for neuromuscular disease such as muscle weakness, pain, or neurologic deficits.

Diagnosis

Diagnosis of megaesophagus is based on radiographic identification of a dilatated or hypomotile esophagus. Survey thoracic radiographs confirm the presence of generalized megaesophagus in most cases and usually reveal an esophagus dilatated with air, fluid, or ingesta. In equivocal cases with mild or segmental dilatation, or if hypomotility without dilatation is suspected, a contrast esophagogram is indicated. Barium liquid and barium meal contrast studies must be performed to detect subtle hypomotility and to rule out a stricture, foreign body, or other obstructive lesion. Although the availability of fluoroscopy in practice is limited, good assessment of esophageal motility can be made with static contrast radiographs during and immediately after a swallow of contrast material. Esophageal retention of any contrast material in a dog that is symptomatic for esophageal disease is abnormal. Radiographic signs of aspiration pneumonia, even in the absence of clinical or radiographic signs of esophageal disease, should alert the clinician to the potential for esophageal disease and the need for a contrast esophagogram. Animals that have significant retention of contrast material in the esophagus are at risk for severe aspiration. They should be held in a vertical position for 5 to 10 minutes after the procedure and closely observed for at least an additional 30 minutes.

Esophageal motility is best evaluated using fluoroscopic, manometric, or scintigraphic procedures, which are usually limited to referral practices and teaching hospitals. Fluoroscopy provides visualization of swallow dynamics and helps to identify anatomic abnormalities of the esophagus. Manometry and scintigraphy provide quantative measures of esophageal motility. Manometry is most useful to evaluate subtle motility abnormalities that are not evident on fluoroscopy. Manometry uses a catheter passed into the esophageal lumen for dynamic measurement of esophageal pressures, transit rate, and lower esophageal pressures during a swallow. Scintigraphy is a newer quantitative technique used to measure the transit time of a radiolabeled food bolus as it moves through the esophagus. Scintigraphy has the advantage of evaluating the response of the esophagus to a normal bolus in an awake patient without the influence of foreign material such as barium or an esophageal catheter.

Once the presence of megaesophagus has been confirmed, the clinician must determine whether the disorder is primary (idiopathic) or secondary. Generally, most dogs with idiopathic megaesophagus have a very large, dilatated, aperistaltic esophagus. Contrast material is slow to move into the stomach and may not do so for hours. Dogs with secondary megaesophagus are often not as severely affected and will have less dilatation and some motility.

Formulating a logical and economic diagnostic plan can be challenging. The initial diagnostic plan should be broad and include a complete blood count, serum chemistry profile that includes a creatine kinase determination, electrolyte determination, urinalysis, and a fecal examination. Results of these tests will help determine which additional diagnostic tests should be considered. A complete blood count might provide a clue to the presence of hypoadrenocorticism, hypothyroidism, immune-mediated disease, lead toxicosis, or pneumonia. Serum chemistry profiles are useful to detect hypoadrenocorticism or myositis. Proteinuria is supportive of the diagnosis of systemic lupus erythematosus and a fecal examination might identify *Spirocerca lupi* in dogs from endemic areas. Patients with congenital or idiopathic megaesophagus generally have few, if any, laboratory abnormalities.

If results of the initial diagnostic tests are inconclusive, an Ach receptor antibody test should be performed to rule out focal or generalized MG. The immunoprecipitation radioimmunoassay (Comparative Neuromuscular Laboratory, University of California at San Diego, La Jolla, CA) is a specific and sensitive test. Although hypothyroidism is a questionable risk factor and hypoadrenocorticism is infrequently associated with megaesophagus, these diseases are potentially treatable causes of megaesophagus. Dogs with unexplained acquired megaesophagus should have thyroid function (thyroid-stimulating hormone–thyroxine) and adrenal function (adrenocorticotropic hormone stimulation test) evaluated.

Esophagoscopy usually is not helpful in determining the cause of megaesophagus. It is indicated if an obstructive lesion or foreign body is suspected but not confirmed by radiographs and to confirm the presence of esophagitis.

Other tests should be considered for individual cases if specific clinical signs or results of preliminary laboratory tests, or both, indicate the presence of a toxic, neurologic, or muscular disease. Lead, thallium, and anticholinesterase toxicities can be diagnosed by history, clinical signs, and toxicologic assay. Serum creatine kinase determinations, electromyography, and muscle biopsy are used to confirm the presence of myopathy or myositis. Systemic lupus erythematosus is diagnosed by the presence of systemic signs and positive antinuclear antibody or lupus erythematosus tests, or both. Symptoms of central nervous system disease can be evaluated with distemper titers, cerebrospinal fluid analysis, computed tomographic brain scans, or a combination of these methods. Such diseases are infrequent causes of megaesophagus.

Treatment

The goals in the management of megaesophagus are to identify and treat the primary cause, decrease the frequency of regurgitation, prevent overdistention of the esophagus, provide adequate nutrition, and treat complications such as aspiration pneumonia and esophagitis. Animals with secondary megaesophagus that can be treated specifically for underlying disease may show improvement of esophageal motility with time; however, responses are variable.

Treatment of animals in which an underlying cause cannot be found is entirely symptomatic.

Cases of focal and generalized MG are treated with long-acting anticholinesterase drugs. Either pyridostigmine bromide, 0.5 to 1.0 mg/kg PO every 8 to 12 hours, or neostigmine, 0.04 mg/kg IM every 6 hours (if oral medication is not tolerated), are effective. Improvement of clinical signs accompanied by a decrease in Ach receptor antibody concentration indicates a good response to treatment. Antibody concentrations should be checked every 4 to 6 weeks to determine the course of the disease and adjust therapy. Treatment should be continued until serum antibody titers are within the normal range. If clinical remission does occur, esophageal dilatation may completely resolve and medication can be discontinued; however, relapses do occur. The time course until remission can vary from 1 month to longer than 1 year. Some dogs with focal MG progress to generalized MG, usually within several weeks of the initial onset of clinical signs. Although myasthenia is an immune-mediated disease, the benefit of corticosteroid therapy has not been clearly determined. If response to anticholinesterase therapy is poor, addition of corticosteroids should be considered. Aspiration pneumonia should be ruled out before the use of corticosteroids, and the patient monitored closely for signs of developing infection.

Megaesophagus associated with hypoadrenocorticism resolves with corticosteroid and mineralocorticoid replacement. No well-documented reports of thyroxine-responsive megaesophagus in hypothyroid dogs exist; however, anecdotal information suggests that megaesophagus occasionally does improve if hypothyroidism is resolved. Immune-mediated polymyositis and polyneuritis and systemic lupus erythematosus may respond to immune suppression. Toxic causes of megaesophagus are treated by removal of the offending agent or by the use of specific antidotes, or by both.

The management of idiopathic megaesophagus as well as most cases of megaesophagus due to neurologic disease is entirely symptomatic and centers on special feeding techniques. A diet should be formulated using a high-calorie food to provide adequate nutritional intake. Meals should be fed in small portions several times daily and given to the dog in an upright position. This can be accomplished by placing the food on an elevated feeding platform or by simply holding the dog in a vertical position for several minutes after eating. Upright feeding provides surprisingly effective symptomatic control of regurgitation in many dogs.

Because dogs with megaesophagus vary in their ability to swallow foods of various consistencies, the type of diet fed should be tailored for each patient. Liquified foods tend to flow more easily with gravity than do solids, but liquids stimulate little peristaltic activity. Solids stimulate more peristalsis and perhaps pose less risk of aspiration. Barium contrast radiography using liquid, canned, and dry food might help determine the best consistency food for a particular patient. Ultimately, food trials are the best way of determining the consistency of food to be fed. In the authors' experience, feeding small meatballs made of canned food provides the best symptomatic control.

Some animals cannot tolerate oral feeding, especially if the esophagus is extremely distended, secondary esophagitis is present, or the patient is severely debilitated. Providing nutritional intake in these instances requires gastrostomy tubes for long-term feeding. Surgical, endoscopic, or nonendoscopic techniques for gastrostomy tube placement can be used (see p. 84). The authors have successfully managed the nutritional needs of large dogs with idiopathic megaesophagus for longer than 1 year using gastrostomy tube feeding. Esophagostomy tubes can exacerbate regurgitation and should not be used.

Aspiration pneumonia should be treated with broad-spectrum antibiotic therapy while culture and sensitivity results of a transtracheal wash are pending. Many dogs with megaesophagus appear to acquire esophagitis, which can worsen the clinical signs. Systemic antacid treatment with drugs such as ranitidine or omeprazole and protectant drugs such as sucralfate helps control symptoms in some patients.

Many types of drugs have been used, unsuccessfully, in an attempt to improve motility and esophageal emptying in dogs with megaesophagus. Anticholinergic drugs and calcium channel blocking drugs such as nifedipine have been used to decrease LES pressure. Little, if any, response has been observed. Anecdotal observations indicate that some dogs with megaesophagus improve clinically when treated with prokinetic drugs such as metoclopramide or cisapride (see p. 614). These observations have been questioned because the canine esophagus consists of striated muscle, and prokinetic drugs augment smooth muscle activity. In normal dogs, cisapride has actually been shown to decrease or slow the rate of transit of a food bolus through the esophagus (Mears, 1996). Therefore, cisapride and other prokinetic drugs cannot be recommended to improve esophageal motility in dogs with megaesophagus.

If reflux esophagitis is suspected as a cause of esophageal hypomotility or a complication of megaesophagus, a trial with prokinetic drugs should be considered. These drugs do increase LES pressure, potentially decreasing episodes of reflux and subsequent esophagitis.

Surgical treatment of congenital and idiopathic megaesophagus has not proved beneficial. Myotomy of the LES and techniques to plicate or resect the redundant esophagus may actually worsen the clinical signs. If radiographic evaluation of a patient shows failure of the LES to open and manometric studies confirm elevated sphincter pressures that did not relax in response to a swallow, a modified Heller's esophageal myotomy might be indicated.

Prognosis

The prognosis for megaesophagus is variable and difficult to predict. Successful outcome is dependent on early diagnosis and aggressive dietary management. Even with diligent care, owners should be warned that aspiration pneumonia is a frequent and often fatal complication.

Congenital megaesophagus has, at best, a guarded prognosis for the animal to become a healthy and functional pet. Reported recovery rates vary from 20 to 46%. Some animals improve with maturity, especially if the condition is recognized early and dietary management is begun before severe and irreversible dilatation occurs. Miniature Schnauzers appear to be an exception because most will acquire improved or normal esophageal function by 6 to 12 months of age.

Adult-onset idiopathic megaesophagus has a poor prognosis. Some affected animals respond to aggressive symptomatic management, but most die of aspiration pneumonia or are euthanized because of persistent regurgitation and debilitation within 5 months of the time of diagnosis. Spontaneous recovery rarely occurs.

The prognosis for dogs with secondary megaesophagus is good if the underlying disease can be treated successfully. This is especially true for MG in which clinical recovery can be expected to occur in at least 50% of the cases. Megaesophagus appears to respond well to corticosteroid therapy in dogs with hypoadrenocorticism. Some hypothyroid dogs respond to levothyroxine therapy; based on personal experiences, this response is unpredictable. Dogs with megaesophagus from polyradiculoneuritis, polymyositis, systemic lupus erythematosus, and botulism can recover esophageal function after successful treatment of the primary disease.

References and Suggested Reading

Bartges JW, Nielson DL: Reversible megaesophagus associated with atypical primary hypoadrenocorticism in a dog. J Am Vet Med Assoc 201:889, 1992.
Report and discussion of the pathophysiology of megaesophagus associated with glucocorticoid-deficient hypoadrenocorticism.
Boudrieau RJ, Rogers WA: Megaesophagus in the dog: A review of 50 cases. J Am Anim Hosp Assoc 21:33, 1985.
Good review of canine megaesophagus with classification of causes.
Bright RM, Burrows CF: Percutaneous endoscopic tube gastrostomy in dogs. Am J Vet Res 49:629, 1988.
Describes technique for endoscopic placement of gastrostomy feeding tubes in dogs.
Cox VS, Wallace LJ, Anderson VE, et al: Hereditary esophageal dysfunction in the miniature schnauzer dog. Am J Vet Res 41:326, 1980.
Discusses heritability and clinical course of esophageal hypomotility in Miniature Schnauzer dogs.
Dewey CW, Shelton GD, Bailey CS, et al: Neuromuscular dysfunction in five dogs with acquired myasthenia gravis and presumptive hypothyroidism. Prog Vet Neurol 6:117, 1995.
Report describes MG, hypothyroidism, and megaesophagus in five dogs; clinical signs resolved in two dogs after thyroid hormone therapy.
Diamant N, Szczepanski M: Idiopathic megaesophagus in the dog: Reasons for spontaneous improvement and a possible method of medical therapy. Can Vet J 15:66, 1974.
Discussion of idiopathic megaesophagus and observations on the clinical course of this disorder.
Guilford WG: Megaesophagus in the dog and cat. Semin Vet Med Surg Small Anim 5:37, 1990.
Good overview of the causes, clinical course, and treatment of canine and feline megaesophagus.
Holland CT, Satchell PM, Farrow BRH: Vagal afferent dysfunction in naturally occurring canine esophageal motility disorder. Dig Dis Sci 39:2090, 1994.
Study confirming normal efferent nerve function but abnormal afferent nerve function as the cause of congenital megaesophagus in the dog.
Holland CT, Stachell PM, Farrow BRH: Vagal esophagomotor nerve function and esophageal motor performance in dogs with congenital idiopathic megaesophagus. Am J Vet Res 57:906, 1996.
Study of congenital megaesophagus in dogs found normal vagal efferent innervation and decreased esophageal motor function.
Jaggy A, Oliver JE, Ferguson DC, et al: Neurological manifestations of hypothyroidism: A retrospective study of 29 dogs. J Vet Intern Med 8:328, 1994.
Good review of the neurologic manifestations of hypothyroidism in the dog, with a report of four cases of hypothyroid-related megaesophagus.

Mears EA, Jenkins C, Daniel G, et al: The effect of cisapride and metoclopramide on esophageal motility in normal beagles. Proceedings of the 14th American College of Veterinary Internal Medicine, San Antonio, TX, Forum 738(Abstract), 1996.
Describes the results of manometric and scintigraphic measurements of esophageal function in normal dogs treated with cisapride and metoclopramide.

Shelton GD: Canine myasthenia gravis. In: Kirk RW, Bonagura JD, eds: Current Veterinary Therapy XI. Philadelphia: WB Saunders, 1992, p 1039.
Good overview of the clinical manifestations and treatment of MG in the dog.

Shelton GD, Willard MD, Cardinet GH, et al: Acquired myasthenia gravis: Selective involvement of esophageal, pharyngeal, and facial muscles. J Vet Intern Med 4:281, 1990.

Report of the clinical features and outcome of acquired focal MG in dogs, with emphasis on esophageal hypomotility.

Tan BJ, Diamant NE: Assessment of the neural defect in a dog with idiopathic megaesophagus. Dig Dis Sci 32:76, 1987.
Esophageal function study in dogs with congenital megaesophagus indicates that a defect probably exists in the afferent pathway of the swallowing reflex, whereas the efferent pathway is normal.

Washabau RJ: Canine megaesophagus: Pathogenesis and therapy. Proceedings of the Tenth American College of Veterinary Internal Medicine Forum, San Diego, CA, 1992, p 671.
Describes the results of manometric measurements of the upper and lower esophageal sphincters and of the esophageal body during swallowing and during intraluminal distention in adult dogs with idiopathic megaesophagus. Results indicate that a defect probably exists in the afferent nerve pathway of the swallowing reflex.

Esophagitis

MICHAEL D. WILLARD

ELIZABETH A. WEYRAUCH

College Station, Texas

PATHOPHYSIOLOGY

Esophagitis (inflammation of the esophageal mucosa) is most often caused by gastric acid, caustic substances, or trauma from foreign objects. Iatrogenic esophagitis due to drugs (e.g., tetracycline) occurs in humans but is poorly documented in veterinary medicine. Cats occasionally lick disinfectants such as benzalkonium chloride off their fur and can sustain oral and esophageal lesions. Foreign objects usually produce focal lesions, whereas gastric acid and caustic agents typically cause more widespread inflammation.

Gastric acid is probably the most common cause of clinically serious esophagitis. The esophageal mucosa can be exposed to excessive acid because of gastroesophageal reflux (GER), frequent vomiting of normal amounts of acid (e.g., in parvoviral enteritis), or vomiting excessive amounts of acid (e.g., in gastrinoma). In GER, gastric contents move into the esophagus unrelated to vomiting. Normal animals may experience occasional GER, but no harm occurs because esophageal peristalsis quickly returns the acid to the stomach. If, however, sufficient acid persists in the esophagus, significant mucosal damage may occur. Anesthetized animals in particular can have GER that persists for relatively long periods (i.e., >15 to 20 minutes), and this may be one of the more common reasons for severe esophagitis in dogs and cats. Recent work has shown that the choice of preanesthetic agents, length of preoperative fasting, age, and intra-abdominal versus extra-abdominal procedures may influence the incidence of intraoperative GER (Galatos and Raptopoulos, 1995a, 1995b). Nonetheless, esophagitis due to anesthesia-associated GER occurs erratically and unpredictably. Interestingly, there was no association between patient positioning and GER in these studies. Finally, the esophagus may be infected by primary pathogens (e.g., pythiosis) or secondarily in immunodeficient patients (e.g., dogs being treated with immunosuppressive therapy for immune-mediated thrombocytopenia, immune-mediated hemolytic anemia, and so on). Fungal infections in particular may occur secondary to such immunosuppressive therapy. Occasionally, an esophageal tumor causes mucosal inflammation.

When the esophageal mucosa sustains a severe chemical "burn," motility can be impaired, allowing food to be retained and ultimately regurgitated. More importantly, poor esophageal motility allows the next aliquot of acid refluxed into the esophagus to remain, worsening the esophagitis. Thus, a positive feedback cycle may occur, perpetuating the problem. Lower esophageal sphincter dysfunction may occur secondary to the esophagitis, allowing more GER. If the mucosal damage is severe, healing may be accompanied by cicatrix and esophageal stricture. Most strictures resulting from GER occur between the thoracic inlet and the diaphragm, where GER will typically cause the most severe damage. Strictures cranial to the thoracic inlet are often caused by inflammation secondary to foreign objects.

CLINICAL SIGNS

The magnitude of clinical signs depends on the severity and depth of the esophageal inflammation and the presence and degree of stricture. Animals with esophagitis may regurgitate or be anorexic (ostensibly because of esophageal pain). The more severe the inflammation, the more severe the anorexia. Some pets appear hungry (i.e., expectantly go to the food bowl) but then refuse to eat. Blood is seldom present in the regurgitated material. If a caustic agent was ingested, there may be lingual and oral burns contributing to the anorexia.

Signs of esophagitis secondary to anesthesia-associated

GER often begin 2 days to 2 weeks after the anesthetic event. Esophagitis caused by trauma from a foreign object may result in immediate (due to inflammation) or delayed (due to stricture) signs. Animals with true profuse vomiting (e.g., an animal that shows prodromal signs, abdominal press, dry heaves, or bile or digested blood in vomitus) may begin to regurgitate concurrently. Regurgitation in animals that were previously vomiting suggests that esophagitis has developed secondary to the vomiting and persistent exposure of the esophageal mucosa to excessive gastric acid. Animals with previously asymptomatic esophageal disease (e.g., mild esophageal dilatation) that vomit (e.g., acute gastritis, foreign object) can retain substantial amounts of gastric acid in the dysfunctional esophagus. They may start regurgitating shortly after vomiting because of the resultant esophagitis.

Clinical signs of stricture depend on the tightness of the obstruction. In general, the more narrow the stricture, the more pronounced the signs. Mild to moderate strictures often allow the animal to ingest and retain liquids (if not drunk too fast), even though solid foods are expelled. Obstructions closer to the mouth usually cause more immediate regurgitation because of the smaller esophageal luminal reservoir proximal to the obstruction; therefore, retained material readily moves back to the cranial esophagus where it is regurgitated. Pain may be obvious as a food bolus is propelled toward the stomach and is abruptly stopped by a stricture. Modest obstructions cause no signs until the patient attempts to swallow a large food bolus or foreign object. Sometimes there is an obvious progression in severity as the stricture matures and causes greater obstruction.

DIAGNOSIS

Esophagitis or esophageal stricture may be suspected from the history (as described previously) or from clinical circumstance. Survey thoracic radiographs are seldom diagnostic, and esophagitis or stricture may not cause demonstrable esophageal dilatation. Contrast radiographs are often diagnostic; however, if mediastinum or focal pleural effusion is noted on plain thoracic films, perforation is likely and contrast films are seldom, if ever, needed. If a contrast study is performed, barium provides a more definitive study than does iodinated contrast media. Esophagitis is suggested by an irregular esophageal mucosa with some retention of barium. It is easy to miss mild to moderate strictures when using liquid barium (i.e., the barium may pass through the stricture without appreciable delay). Nonetheless, liquid barium should be administered first so that damage will be minimized if the patient regurgitates and aspirates. If no lesions are detected using liquid barium, barium mixed with canned food (this should be a "chunky" consistency) should be used next. Fluoroscopy is always preferred over static images because it may reveal partial obstructions not seen with the latter (i.e., a bolus may "squeeze" through a partial stricture in the period between the bolus being eaten and the radiograph being obtained). Barium paste offers no substantive advantage, misses lesions that are revealed by barium plus food, and, if aspirated causes more morbidity and mortality.

Hiatal hernia (a potential cause of GER and esophagitis) can be easy or extremely difficult to diagnose. Some animals have obvious abnormalities on plain thoracic radiographs, whereas others have normal barium-contrast studies, even when fluoroscopy is used. Diagnosis may require the administration of liquid barium and viewing the lower esophageal sphincter area fluoroscopically while applying pressure to the abdomen. This maneuver forces the gastric fundus through the hernia and into the caudal mediastinum, confirming the diagnosis. This technique may also reveal GER; however, it can be difficult to distinguish "innocent" from significant reflux.

Endoscopy is the most *sensitive and specific* way of detecting clinically significant esophagitis. Erythema, friability, and exudative pseudomembranes are usually obvious. Sometimes a distinctly roughened mucosal surface is evident, although the esophageal mucosa just aborad to the cricopharyngeal sphincter is normally a little rougher than the rest of the esophagus. Humans can have esophagitis that is only diagnosed histopathologically. We do not know if this occurs in dogs and cats, and if it does occur, whether it is important. Non-neoplastic canine esophageal mucosa (which has a stratified epithelium) is difficult to biopsy adequately with flexible endoscopic biopsy forceps. Rigid forceps or devices such as the Crosby capsule or Rubin tube are often necessary to obtain a biopsy specimen of canine esophageal mucosa that is not obviously diseased. Feline esophageal mucosa is a little more amenable to sampling with flexible forceps. Esophageal strictures are typically obvious at endoscopy; however, large dogs may have an esophageal stricture that decreases the luminal diameter by 50% or more and yet is missed by the endoscopist. The scope diameter can be so small when compared with the esophageal lumen of a larger breed dog that the tip of the scope will readily pass through a partial stricture without the operator noticing that the luminal diameter was diminished. This error is especially likely if the stricture is near the lower esophageal sphincter, where one may observe that the normal esophageal lumen narrows noticeably but think that the narrowing is simply the lower esophageal sphincter. This is particularly significant because many strictures occur near this sphincter.

THERAPY

Inflamed esophageal mucosa will usually heal if given the opportunity (i.e., protected from further damage). It is therefore important to eliminate predisposing factors (e.g., hiatal hernia), foreign objects, or predisposing drug therapy. For most patients, preventing further exposure to gastric acid is crucial. Esophageal mucosa is more easily damaged by acid than is gastric mucosa, as the esophagus does not have a mucus-bicarbonate pre-epithelial barrier and does not heal by epithelial restitution. Furthermore, endogenous prostaglandins are not as effective in protecting the epithelial surface of the esophagus, and the esophagus does not produce a "mucus cap" after epithelial injury (Orlando, 1996). Thus, minute amounts of acid have the potential to damage the esophagus significantly, and healing requires that the clinician prevent additional vomiting or GER. In humans, esophagitis usually results from GER, and the basis of effective therapy is to keep the stomach empty by administering prokinetic drugs (see p. 614) or to eliminate acid by prescribing inhibitors of gastric acid secretion (see pp. 48 and 616).

Studies in humans have demonstrated that although metoclopramide (Reglan, A.H. Robins) (a prokinetic agent effective in the stomach) is minimally effective in preventing esophagitis due to GER, cisapride (Propulsid, Janssen) is clearly beneficial (Klinkenberg-Knol et al, 1995). Cisapride is at least as effective as H_2 receptor antagonists (discussed further on), and cisapride plus an H_2 receptor antagonist is more effective than the latter by itself. The main disadvantage of cisapride therapy is that it is administered orally (and hence may never reach the stomach if the patient is regurgitating everything it ingests), whereas metoclopramide may be given parenterally. In humans, cisapride is particularly effective in preventing recurrence after esophagitis has been brought under control. The authors prefer cisapride at 0.25 mg/kg every 8 to 12 hours and use metoclopramide only if cisapride cannot be administered successfully.

H_2 antagonists inhibit gastric acid secretion, thus diminishing the volume that can be refluxed into the esophagus. These drugs are competitive inhibitors of gastric acid secretion and have been effective in treating the milder forms of human esophagitis but are not as useful in severe esophagitis. This is probably because H_2 antagonists may increase the gastric pH only to between 4 and 5, a level that is effective in treating gastric ulcers but may be inadequate when treating esophageal disease. Using larger and more frequent doses of the more potent H_2 antagonists (e.g., twice the recommended dose, every 6 to 8 hours, which is sometimes called a "reflux dose") is more effective because it causes greater suppression of acid secretion. The same is probably true in dogs and cats, but objective data are lacking.

Proton pump inhibitors are noncompetitive inhibitors and diminish gastric acid secretion to a much greater degree and for a much longer time than do the H_2 receptor antagonists. The two proton pump inhibitors currently available in the United States are omeprazole (Prilosec, Astra Merck) and lansoprazole (Prevacid, TAP). Therapy with omeprazole can produce near anacidity in the stomach and refluxed material. Consequently, these drugs are often effective in patients resistant to H_2 receptor antagonists (Klinkenberg-Knol et al, 1995). The authors prefer omeprazole 0.7 to 2.0 mg/kg every 12 to 24 hours. Twice-daily therapy lends itself to greater client compliance than does the schedule of every 6 to 8 hours required with some H_2 antagonists. Omeprazole is recommended anytime severe esophagitis is seen or anticipated. The medical therapy used by the authors in severely affected patients has been a combination of cisapride and omeprazole. The only disadvantage is that omeprazole is given orally and may be regurgitated before it reaches the stomach. The authors use H_2 receptor antagonists only if the oral omeprazole cannot be administered successfully. In humans, studies have shown that even though omeprazole is more expensive than H_2 receptor antagonists, it is ultimately more cost-effective because it is more effective. Lansoprazole has been tested in humans and found to be at least as effective as omeprazole.

If the esophagus is severely inflamed, a gastrostomy tube is recommended to ensure adequate nutrition while preventing as much irritation to the esophagus as possible. These tubes also allow administration of cisapride and omeprazole with confidence, instead of wondering whether the medications ever reached the stomach. Although of uncertain significance, esophagostomy and pharyngostomy tubes may perpetuate esophageal inflammation (via continued contact between the tube and the ulcerated mucosa) and are therefore not recommended in affected animals. Aggressive medical management (i.e., cisapride, omeprazole, and gastrostomy feeding tube; see p. 84) is strongly recommended for patients with severe disease or inflamed strictures; H_2 receptor antagonists and metoclopramide, although less expensive, also seem less effective.

Orally administered sucralfate (Carafate, Marion Merrell) has been used in patients with esophagitis and, although this therapy intuitively makes sense, studies in humans have demonstrated minimal or no benefit (Klinkenberg-Knol et al, 1995). One probably must time the administration of the sucralfate to coincide with high acid levels in the otherwise neutral esophagus if sucralfate is to function as desired. There is, therefore, some rationale for administering sucralfate and hoping that if GER does occur, the sucralfate will be carried back into the esophagus where it will be effective because of the now acid esophageal environment.

Corticosteroids are often administered to try to prevent stricture formation; however, they are of questionable efficacy. Humans who ingest caustic agents (resulting in a far more damaging lesion than is found in most dogs and cats) are not clearly benefited by such therapy and it might actually put them at increased risk of infection. Antibiotics are used to protect denuded esophageal mucosa from infection by bacteria normally found in oral secretions. These oral bacteria pass through the esophagus each time the patient swallows saliva. However, although antibiotics intuitively seem indicated in these patients, they have not clearly aided the healing of esophagitis lesions. If antibiotics are used, one should choose drugs that are effective against the anaerobic bacteria that are commonly found in the oral cavity, such as *Prevotella* spp, *Porphyromonas* spp, *Fusobacterium* spp, *Bacteroides* spp, and others.

Ballooning and bougienage are used to eliminate strictures. Surgical resection of esophageal strictures should be considered only as a last-ditch, salvage option because strictures commonly recur at the surgery site. Bougienage allows more force to be applied to the stricture than is possible with a balloon. This is important for patients with large amounts of thick, fibrous cicatrix that balloons cannot break down or strictures so small that balloons cannot be inserted through them. Studies in humans suggest that bougienage is essentially as effective as balloon dilation and about as safe (Cox et al, 1994; Yamamoto et al, 1992). Bougienage has the potential to be more traumatic (e.g., it can cause perforation); however, there is some thought that the incidence of side effects and complications is largely operator-dependent. Ballooning might be less likely to cause esophageal perforation, especially when performed by inexperienced operators. However, neither technique is completely safe. If ballooning is chosen over bougienage, the procedure is best performed by using over-the-wire or through-the-scope esophageal balloons. It is best not to pass a balloon catheter alongside the scope unless there is a flexible-tipped guidewire, which reduces the risk of iatrogenic esophageal trauma from the tip of the catheter cutting into the esophagus during inflation. Ballooning also allows the operator to visualize the dilation process while it is being performed. The esophagus should be evaluated after the procedure to detect any unexpected iatrogenic trauma. The animal's thorax should be radiographed after difficult procedures or if there is any hint of respiratory difficulty, to detect pneumothorax secondary to esophageal rupture. If the esophagus is traumatized by the dilation procedure or if pneumothorax develops, conservative medical care (which may include chest tubes) will often allow healing (Willard et al, 1994).

Optimally, the esophagitis patient without a stricture should be re-examined endoscopically after 5 to 8 days of medical therapy. If the esophagus has healed, one may start oral feedings. After the patient is able to eat normally without regurgitating, medical therapy can be discontinued. However, if the esophagitis was clearly due to a nonrecurring cause (e.g., foreign body that has been removed), repeat endoscopy is not crucial (unless signs suggesting stricture formation occur), and one may elect simply to start feeding the animal after 3 to 5 days of medical therapy. Animals with strictures but without esophagitis should be re-examined endoscopically 5 to 7 days after the dilation procedure. If the stricture has not recurred and the patient is eating without difficulty, a repeat examination is probably unnecessary. Alternatively, one may simply start feeding the animal after the stricture is broken down and observe if regurgitation recurs.

In contrast, repeat endoscopy 3 to 5 days after initiating therapy is necessary for patients with inflamed strictures as well as for those with severe esophagitis. Some of these patients will need only one dilation procedure, whereas others may need 5 to 10 dilations or more performed at regular intervals (e.g., two to three times per week) to prevent stricture reformation. Severely affected patients should undergo endoscopy at least twice weekly for examination of progress and redilation as necessary. The goal is not necessarily to eliminate the stricture altogether, but rather to achieve an esophageal lumen that is large enough to allow the animal to eat without fear of regurgitation. Concurrent esophagitis suggests that more procedures will be needed than if there was no inflammation. Occasional patients have additional strictures arise (usually close to the lower esophageal sphincter) while the first one is being treated.

PROGNOSIS

For patients with esophagitis without stricture formation, the prognosis depends on the underlying cause. Animals with congenital hiatal hernias that allow GER may require surgical correction of the hernia to resolve the esophagitis, but their prognosis is usually reasonably good.

There is currently no evidence that animals experiencing anesthesia-induced GER and subsequent stricture are at increased risk for recurrence if reanesthetized. If the animal is treated before the inflammation is severe enough to cause a stricture, the prognosis is usually good. Strictures accompanied by substantial inflammation are more difficult to resolve, and the owners should be prepared for multiple dilative procedures. Even animals with severe inflammation are typically salvageable if the owner can afford the multiple procedures that may be necessary. Animals with esophagitis caused directly or indirectly by neoplasms or fungal infections generally have a terrible prognosis. If the esophageal stricture cannot be resolved or if the stricture is due to a terminal malignancy, a permanent, low-profile gastrostomy device may be inserted to palliate the patient for as long as possible.

References and Suggested Reading

Cox JGC, Winter RK, Maslin SC, et al: Balloon or bougie for dilatation of benign esophageal stricture? Dig Dis Sci 39:776, 1994.
A discussion of the advantages and disadvantages of these two means of dilating esophageal strictures.

Galatos AD, Raptopoulos D: Gastro-oesophageal reflux during anaesthesia in the dog: The effect of age, positioning and type of surgical procedure. Vet Rec 137:513, 1995a.
A prospective study showing that age and type of surgical procedure affect the incidence of GER during anesthesia.

Galatos AD, Raptopoulos D: Gastro-oesophageal reflux during anaesthesia in the dog: The effect of preoperative fasting and premedication. Vet Rec 137:479, 1995b.
A prospective study documenting that age and anesthetic premedicants may affect the incidence of GER.

Harai BH, Johnson SE, Sherding RG: Endoscopically guided balloon dilation of benign esophageal strictures in 6 cats and 7 dogs. J Vet Intern Med 9:332, 1995.
A report of the treatment of 13 animals with esophageal strictures.

Klinkenberg-Knol EC, Festen HPM, Meuwissen SGM: Pharmacological management of gastro-oesophageal reflux disease. Drugs 49:695, 1995.
A comprehensive review of the treatment of GER in humans, with good discussions and comparisons of the different types of medical therapies.

Orlando RC: Why is the high grade inhibition of gastric acid secretion afforded by proton pump inhibitors often required for healing of reflux esophagitis? An epithelial perspective. Am J Gastroenterol 91:1692, 1996.
A good explanation of how the stomach and esophagus are affected by acid damage and why the proton pump inhibitors are so much more effective for treating esophagitis than are the H_2-antagonists.

Willard MD, Delles EK, Fossum TW: Iatrogenic tears associated with ballooning of esophageal strictures. J Am Anim Hosp Assoc 30:431, 1994.
Two case reports showing types of iatrogenic injury caused by esophageal dilation procedures and how to treat them conservatively.

Yamamoto H, Hughes RW, Schroeder KW, et al: Treatment of benign esophageal stricture by Eder-Puestow or balloon dilators: A comparison between randomized and prospective nonrandomized trials. Mayo Clin Proc 67:228, 1992.
A good study showing that bouginage is as effective and about as safe as ballooning but is probably more cost-effective in the long-term analysis.

Assessment of Gastrointestinal Motility

F. J. ALLAN
W. G. GUILFORD
Palmerston North, New Zealand

Gastrointestinal motility is rarely assessed by veterinarians despite the common occurrence of primary and secondary disorders of gastric and intestinal motility (Tables 1 and 2). Accurate diagnosis of these disorders allows clinicians to choose rational treatment modalities. The majority of the clinical signs of motility disorders are nonspecific (Table 3) and can be easily attributed to other causes. Potentially, this results in an underestimation of the prevalence of motility disorders.

Gastrointestinal myoelectrical activity is assessed directly by electrogastrography, manometry, and the use of electrodes and strain gauge transducers. These techniques are rarely used, however, for clinical diagnostic purposes because of their invasive nature. Rather, clinicians assess the functional correlate of coordinated gastrointestinal myoelectrical activity, which is the rate of movement of ingesta from one region of the alimentary tract to another. Veterinarians now have at their disposal a wide variety of methods to assess gastrointestinal motility (Table 4). The more practical of these methods are described in the following sections.

GASTRIC EMPTYING STUDIES

In recent years, a large number of diagnostic techniques have been employed to assess the rate of gastric emptying. None of these techniques meet all the criteria of the "ideal" method, but several offer useful clinical information. In medicine, radiographic studies of human patients have been superseded by more informative techniques such as scintigraphy. In veterinary practice, radiographic methods are still widely used because they are inexpensive and use equipment that is standard in most practices.

Radiographic Techniques

Survey Radiography

The dimensions of the stomach can be determined from right lateral recumbent radiographs, and this has been used

TABLE 1. Conditions That Cause Functional Abnormalities of Gastric Emptying*

Disorder	Functional Abnormalities
Mucosa	Gastric ulceration ↑ ↓
	Duodenal ulceration ↑ ↓
	Chronic gastritis ↓
	Inflammatory bowel disease ↓
	Adenocarcinoma ↓
Muscle	Polymyositis ↓
	Dermatomyositis ↓
	Muscular dystrophies ↓
	Carnitine deficiency ↓
	Gastric dysrhythmias ↓
	Gastric dilatation-volvulus ↓
Endocrine	Hypoadrenocorticism ↓
	Diabetes mellitus ↓
	Hypothyroidism ↓
	Hyperparathyroidism ↓
Metabolic	Acid-base imbalance ↓
	Electrolyte imbalance ↓
	Uremia ↓
	Hepatic failure ↓
	Malnutrition ↓
Iatrogenic	Abdominal surgery ↓
	Drugs ↑ ↓
Miscellaneous	Adynamic ileus ↓
	Idiopathic gastroparesis ↓
	Chronic intestinal pseudo-obstruction ↓
	Myenteric ganglionitis ↑
	Dysautonomia ↓
	Morbid obesity ↑
	Pain ↓

* ↓ indicates that the condition may cause delayed gastric emptying;
↑ indicates that the condition may result in an increased rate of gastric emptying; and
↑ ↓ indicates that the condition may cause both delayed and rapid gastric emptying.

TABLE 2. Primary or Secondary Motility Disorders of the Intestinal Tract

Adynamic ileus
　Major surgery, pain
　Electrolyte imbalance (hypokalemia, hypocalcemia)
　Pancreatitis, peritonitis, severe acute gastroenteritis
　Unrelieved mechanical obstruction
　Uremia
Dysautonomia
Iatrogenic
　Drugs (anticholinergic agents, prokinetic agents)
Idiopathic megacolon
Irritable bowel syndrome
Myenteric ganglionitis
Pseudo-obstruction syndrome

TABLE 3. Clinical Signs of Motility Disorders of the Stomach and Intestines

Abdominal discomfort
Abdominal distention
Anorexia
Borborygmus
Constipation
Diarrhea (small bowel or large bowel type)
Flatulence
Intestinal distention
Nausea
Tenesmus
Vomiting (often delayed for several hours after eating)

TABLE 4. Methods for Assessing Gastrointestinal Motility

Gastric Emptying and Motility
Standard clinical techniques
   Survey radiographs
   Barium suspensions
   Radiopaque markers
   Scintigraphy
Research or investigational techniques
   Applied potential tomography
   Drug absorption rates
   Electrode and strain gauge implantation
   Electrogastrography
   Fluoroscopy
   Gastric intubation
   Magnetic resonance imaging
   Manometry
   Metal detector
   Octanoic acid breath test
   Radiotelemetry
   Ultrasonography
Intestinal Transit and Motility
Standard clinical techniques
   Barium suspensions
   Breath hydrogen test
   Radiopaque markers
   Scintigraphy
Research or investigational techniques
   Electrode and strain gauge implantation
   Enteroclysis
   Fluoroscopy
   Manometry
   Metal detector

to assess the initiation and termination of gastric emptying of food in dogs and cats (Arnbjerg, 1992). Although this technique is likely to detect gross abnormalities in function, such as adynamic ileus, it is unlikely to detect subtle disturbances in gastric motility.

Positive Contrast Radiography

Positive contrast radiography involves obtaining abdominal radiographs at predetermined intervals after the oral administration of a positive contrast agent. The contrast agent is usually barium sulfate suspension, either given alone or mixed with food. Food is withheld for 12 to 24 hours before a positive contrast radiographic study to ensure that the stomach is empty; this should be confirmed by plain survey radiographs. The suspension can be administered by syringing it into the mouth or via a stomach tube. Radiographs are obtained immediately after administration, at 15 to 30 minutes, 60 minutes, and at 2, 3, and 6 hours.

Emptying of barium sulfate suspension from the stomach should begin within 15 minutes of administration. In nervous animals, however, the onset of emptying may be delayed for up to 45 minutes. Gastric emptying is considered abnormal if it has not started within 45 minutes. The stomach should be completely empty within 4 hours, but in most dogs, gastric emptying is complete within 1 to 2 hours (Hertage and Dennis, 1989).

The gastric emptying rate of a dry kibbled diet coated with a barium sulfate suspension has been determined in dogs (Miyabayashi and Morgan, 1984). The barium sulfate

separated from the food, however, which compromised the value of this technique as a method of assessing the gastric emptying of solids.

The initiation and termination of gastric emptying in cats fed a test diet of canned food mixed with a barium sulfate suspension has been determined in eight healthy cats (Steyn and Twedt, 1994). The mean plus or minus SD for the initiation and termination of gastric emptying was 42.5 ± 15.6 minutes and $11/6 \pm 0.9$ hours, respectively.

Positive contrast radiography studies provide little quantitative information about gastric emptying. The initiation and termination of gastric emptying can be established, but more reliable values, such as the time taken to empty 50% of the stomach's contents, cannot be determined. When barium sulfate suspension is used, only the gastric emptying of liquids can be assessed using these techniques. This is usually of less clinical relevance than is the gastric emptying of solids, which is controlled by mechanisms dependent on more complex (and more easily disrupted) physiology involving intimate coordination between the antrum, pylorus, and small intestine.

Fluoroscopy

Fluoroscopic examination of the barium-filled stomach allows direct assessment of the frequency of gastric contractions and the coordination of antropyloric movement. Species-specific objective criteria for evaluating gastric motility are lacking, however.

Radiopaque Markers

Radiopaque markers have been used for many years to quantify the gastric emptying rate of indigestible solids in humans and are now commercially available for use in dogs and cats (BIPS, MED-ID Systems Inc; Grand Rapids). The BIPS leave the stomach proportionately with a standard test meal and thereby provide an assessment of the gastric emptying rate of solid food (Guilford et al, 1997). Radiographs are obtained at convenient intervals (usually one set between 1 and 2 hours and one or two sets between 6 and 12 hours after ingestion) and the ratio of the number of markers that have left the stomach to the total number of markers administered is used to calculate the percent gastric emptying at each time point. This information is then compared with the manufacturer's published gastric emptying curves for healthy dogs and cats. The technique has been described in dogs (Allan et al, 1996) and cats (Chandler and Guilford, 1995).

For the radiopaque marker method to be accurate, a standard amount of a particular food must be fed and the markers thoroughly mixed through the food. The test meal must be standardized because the gastric emptying rate of the markers is influenced by the viscosity and flow rate of the ingesta in which they are suspended (Sirois et al, 1990). In addition, it is necessary to standardize the type of markers used because their physical characterisitics (especially size and density) determine their gastric emptying rate.

The principal advantage of the radiopaque marker technique is that it offers veterinarians in private practice a reliable and practical way of quantifying the gastric emptying rate of solid food. The main disadvantage of the technique is that it is an indirect assessment of the gastric emptying of ingesta. Unlike scintigraphy (see following section), the markers are not specifically attached to particular food components.

Scintigraphy

Scintigraphy provides a detailed, physiologic assessment of gastric emptying and is currently considered the "gold standard" technique for quantifying gastric emptying in human and veterinary medicine. The strength of scintigraphy lies in its ability to assess directly the gastric emptying of food labeled with a radioisotope. Conversely, radiographic techniques require the use of "nonfood" contrast media to indirectly assess the gastric emptying of ingesta. Radiolabels can be attached to solids, liquids, or both solids and liquids simultaneously. Unfortunately, the expense of the equipment and the technical difficulties associated with handling radioisotopes limits the availability of scintigraphy to referral institutions.

ASSESSMENT OF OROCOLIC AND SMALL INTESTINAL TRANSIT TIME

Orocolic and small intestinal transit times of dogs and cats are most commonly assessed by radiographic techniques and breath hydrogen testing.

Radiographic Techniques

Positive Contrast Radiography

In the absence of obstructive lesions, the rate of passage of barium sulfate suspension through the intestinal tract is determined by the frequency of peristaltic and segmental contractions of the intestine and the amount and viscosity of the contrast agent. As a result of these variables, intestinal transit time of barium suspensions is a poor measure of intestinal motility. The normal time for barium solutions to reach the colon varies from 90 to 240 minutes in dogs and 30 to 120 minutes in cats (Owens, 1995). In general, a transit time of greater than 4 hours is considered abnormal. When barium sulfate is mixed with canned food, the mean orocolic transit time in healthy cats is 4.1 ± 3.0 hours (Steyn and Twedt, 1994).

Fluoroscopy

Fluoroscopic inspection of the barium-filled intestinal tract allows direct assessment of the frequency of intestinal contractions, the coordination of peristaltic movement, and the manner in which contrast material is propelled through the intestinal tract. Unfortunately, this method is technically difficult and hampered by lack of species-specific objective criteria for evaluating bowel contractions.

Enteroclysis

Enteroclysis involves inflating the small intestine with a dilute solution of barium sulfate that has been administered through a tube placed directly into the duodenum under fluoroscopic guidance. Enteroclysis provides detailed information about small bowel morphologic features and limited information about motility. A uniform progression of barium through the intestinal tract is a better indicator of normal motility than of the exact transit time. Enteroclysis is technically difficult to perform in small animals.

Radiopaque Markers

Radiopaque markers (BIPS, MED-ID Systems Inc; Grand Rapids) can be used to determine the orocolic and small intestinal transit time of humans, dogs, and cats. The technique is similar to that described for evaluating gastric emptying except that the ratio of the number of markers that have entered the colon to the total number of markers administered is used to calculate the orocolic transit percent. This information is then compared with the manufacturer's orocolic transit curves for healthy dogs and cats. The small intestinal transit time is estimated by the difference in time between corresponding points on the gastric emptying and colonic filling curves.

Breath Hydrogen Testing

When carbohydrate is fermented in the gastrointestinal tract, it produces hydrogen gas. A small percentage of the hydrogen is absorbed into the blood stream and re-excreted in the breath where it can be measured. The time at which the breath hydrogen concentration first begins to rise over baseline values provides an estimate of orocolic transit time because under normal circumstances, hydrogen gas is generated predominantly in the large intestine. This test can be used in private practice because breath samples are easy to collect and they can be transported in capped syringes to laboratories that perform breath hydrogen analysis. The reliability of this test is affected by many variables such as the collection technique, the type of carbohydrate used, small intestinal bacterial overgrowth, flatulence, antibiotic use, and the criteria used to define a significant rise in breath hydrogen above baseline (Sparkes et al, 1996).

ASSESSMENT OF THE LARGE INTESTINAL TRANSIT

Evaluation of colorectal transit is of value in conditions such as idiopathic megacolon, constipation, and intractable diarrhea. Separate evaluation of transit through the different regions of the large intestine is advantageous to identify segmental lesions that may be amenable to surgical resection. Colonorectal transit can be evaluated by radiopaque marker studies or scintigraphy. Radiopaque marker studies of large bowel transit are performed in an analogous way to gastric emptying studies using radiopaque markers. The markers are fed in a standard diet (high-fiber diet), and radiographs are obtained at convenient intervals over the next 12 to 48 hours. The percentage of markers in each region of the large intestine is then compared with published reference values. The technique has been validated for use in cats (Fucci et al, 1995).

References and Suggested Reading

Allan FJ, Guilford WG, Robertson ID, et al: Gastric emptying of solid radiopaque markers in healthy dogs. Vet Radiol Ultrasound 37:336, 1996.
Describes use of barium-impregnated polyethylene spheres in dogs.

Arnbjerg J: Gastric emptying time in the dog and cat. J Am Anim Hosp Assoc 28:77, 1992.
Describes the use of plain survey radiographs in dogs and cats for the assessment of gastric transit times.

Chandler ML, Guilford WG: Assessment of gastric emptying and small intestinal transit in cats using radiopaque markers. J Vet Intern Med 9:192, 1995 (abstract).

Fucci V, Pechman RD, Hedlund CS, et al: Large bowel transit using radiopaque markers in normal cats. J Am Anim Hosp Assoc 31:473, 1995.
Describes a radiopaque marker technique to assess colonic transit in cats.

Guilford WG, Lawoko CR, Allan FJ: Accuracy of localizing radiopaque markers by abdominal radiography and correlation between their gastric emptying rate and that of a canned food in dogs. Am J Vet Res 58:1359, 1997.
Shows that the gastric emptying of the radiopaque markers is closely correlated with the gastric emptying of food in dogs.

Hertage ME, Dennis R: Contrast media. In: Lee R, ed: Manual of Radiography and Radiology in Small Animal Practice. Cheltenham: British Small Animal Veterinary Association, 1989, p 218.
Reviews the use of contrast media in radiology.

Miyabayashi T, Morgan JP: Gastric emptying in the normal dog. Vet Radiol 25:187, 1984.
Describes a technique for determining the rate of gastric emptying of a kibbled diet coated with barium sulfate.

Owens JM: Gastrointestinal diagnostic imaging. In: Bonagura JD, ed: Kirk's Current Veterinary Therapy XII, 1995, pp 659–664.

Sirois PJ, Amidon GL, Meyer JH, et al: Gastric emptying of nondigestible solids in dogs: A hydrodynamic model. Am J Physiol 258:G65, 1990.
Describes the variables influencing the rate of gastric emptying of indigestible solids.

Sparkes AH, Papasouliotis K, Viner J, et al: Assessment of orocaecal transit time in cats by the breath hydrogen method: The effects of sedation and a comparison of definitions. Res Vet Sci 60:243, 1996.
Discusses the use of breath hydrogen to assess orocolic transit time.

Steyn PF, Twedt DC: Gastric emptying in the normal cat: A radiographic study. J Am Anim Hosp Assoc 30:78, 1994.
Describes a technique for the radiographic evaluation of the gastric transit, gastric emptying, and small intestinal transit times in healthy cats.

Gastric Prokinetic Agents

JEAN A. HALL
Corvallis, Oregon

ROBERT J. WASHABAU
Philadelphia, Pennsylvania

GASTRIC PROKINETIC AGENTS

Delayed gastric emptying is a significant cause of upper gastrointestinal tract symptoms in dogs and cats (see preceding article). Dietary management and gastric prokinetic agents are used to treat delayed gastric emptying disorders, as surgical procedures are often unsuccessful. Dietary management is attempted initially. Dietary choices are made based on the knowledge that liquids are expelled from the stomach faster than solids, carbohydrates are expelled faster than protein, and protein is expelled faster than fats. Small amounts of a semiliquid, low-protein, and low-fat diet should be fed at frequent intervals. Cooked pasta or boiled rice can be added to the diet. Drug therapy with gastric prokinetic agents should be considered in animals that fail to respond to dietary management alone.

Some gastrointestinal prokinetic agents have effects throughout the gastrointestinal tract, whereas others exert action on the proximal or distal gastrointestinal tract. Gastrointestinal prokinetic agents work by many different mechanisms of action. Sites of activity and indications for use are summarized in Table 1. The discussion that follows is a more in-depth look at specific prokinetic agents used to treat gastric motility disorders.

Metoclopramide

Metoclopramide is prescribed as a gastric prokinetic and antiemetic agent (see *CVT XII*, p. 679). It is believed to exert its effects through antagonism of dopaminergic D_2 receptors and agonism of serotonergic 5-hydroxytryptamine 4 (5-HT$_4$) receptors. Metoclopramide hydrochloride is available in 5- and 10-mg tablets (Reglan, A.H. Robins), as an orange syrup containing 1 mg/ml, and for injection at 5 mg/ml (2- and 10-ml single dose vials or ampules, and 30-ml single-dose vials). The prokinetic dose of metoclopramide for use in the dog and cat is 0.2 to 0.5 mg/kg every 8 hours administered either orally or parenterally. Continuous intravenous infusions may also be administered at doses of 0.01 to 0.02 mg/kg every hour or 1 to 2 mg/kg every 24 hours.

Metoclopramide may be useful in the treatment of gastroesophageal reflux and reflux esophagitis in dogs and cats because it increases pressure in the lower esophageal sphincter and accelerates gastric emptying. Delayed gastric emptying promotes gastroesophageal reflux by increasing the gastric volume and pressure gradient.

Metoclopramide also increases the amplitude and frequency of antral contractions, inhibits fundic receptive relaxation, and coordinates gastric, pyloric, and duodenal motility, all of which should result in accelerated gastric emptying. However, the prokinetic effect of metoclopramide may be limited to gastric emptying of liquids.

Centrally, metoclopramide inhibits vomiting associated with activation of dopaminergic D_2 receptors in the chemo-

TABLE 1. Mechanisms, Sites of Activity, and Indications for Gastrointestinal Prokinetic Agents

Drug	Mechanisms of Action	Sites of Activity
Metoclopramide (Reglan, A.H. Robins)	D_2 dopaminergic antagonist	LES, stomach, intestine, CRTZ
	α_2-Adrenergic antagonist	Stomach
	β_2-Adrenergic antagonist	Stomach
	5-HT$_4$ serotonergic agonist	LES, stomach, intestine
	5-HT$_3$ serotonergic antagonist	Stomach, intestine
Domperidone (Motilium, Janssen)	D_2 dopaminergic antagonist	Stomach, CRTZ
	α_2-Adrenergic antagonist	Stomach
	β_2-Adrenergic antagonist	Stomach
Cisapride (Propulsid, Janssen)	5-HT$_4$ agonist	LES, stomach, intestine
	5-HT$_1$ antagonist	Stomach, intestine, emetic center
	5-HT$_3$ antagonist	Stomach, intestine, CRTZ
	5-HT$_2$ agonist	Colon
	Nonserotonergic mechanism	Canine antrum
Erythromycin (Erythromycin, Mylan)	Motilin agonist (cat)	Stomach, intestine
	5-HT$_3$ agonist (dog)	Stomach, intestine
Ranitidine (Zantac, Glaxo)	Acetylcholinesterase inhibitor	Stomach, intestine, colon
	M_3 muscarinic cholinergic agonist (?)	Stomach
Nizatidine (Axid, Eli Lilly)	Acetylcholinesterase inhibitor	Stomach, intestine, colon
	M_3 muscarinic cholinergic agonist (?)	Stomach

Drug	Indications
Metoclopramide (Reglan, A.H. Robins)	Vomiting disorders, gastroesophageal reflux, delayed gastric emptying, postoperative ileus, intestinal pseudo-obstruction
Domperidone (Motilium, Janssen)	Vomiting disorders, delayed gastric emptying (?)
Cisapride (Propulsid, Janssen)	Gastroesophageal reflux, delayed gastric emptying, postoperative ileus, intestinal pseudo-obstruction, constipation, chemotherapy-induced emesis
Erythromycin (Erythromycin, Mylan)	Delayed gastric emptying (liquids > solids)
Ranitidine (Zantac, Glaxo)	Delayed gastric emptying, intestinal pseudo-obstruction, constipation
Nizatidine (Axid, Eli Lilly)	Delayed gastric emptying, intestinal pseudo-obstruction, constipation

5-HT, 5-hydroxytryptamine; M, muscarinic; CRTZ, chemoreceptor trigger zone; LES, lower esophageal sphincter.

Modified from Washabau RJ, Hall JA: Diagnosis and management of gastrointestinal motility disorders in dogs and cats. Compend Contin Educ Pract Vet 19:721, 1997. Reprinted with permission.

receptor trigger zone. Peripherally, metoclopramide may diminish the severity of vomiting through its effects on motility by preventing gastric stasis and the retrograde peristalsis that precedes vomiting. Thus, metoclopramide is also indicated in the treatment of nausea and vomiting associated with delayed gastric emptying, gastroesophageal reflux, and reflux gastritis.

Metoclopramide should not be used when stimulation of gastrointestinal motility could be harmful, for example, in the presence of gastrointestinal hemorrhage, mechanical obstruction, or perforation. Metoclopramide should also be avoided in epileptics or in patients receiving other drugs that are likely to cause extrapyramidal reactions, since the frequency and severity of seizures or extrapyramidal reactions may be increased.

Atropine and the opioid analgesics may antagonize the action of metoclopramide. Additive sedative effects can occur when metoclopramide is given with narcotics or tranquilizers. Because chronic therapy with phenothiazines can produce side effects similar to those seen with metoclopramide, concomitant use of metoclopramide and phenothiazine drugs should be avoided. In diabetic patients, metoclopramide influences the delivery of food to the small intestine and thus the rate of absorption. Dosage and timing of insulin may need to be modified.

Domperidone

Domperidone is a peripheral dopamine antagonist that acts on dopaminergic D_2 receptors in the gastrointestinal tract and the chemoreceptor trigger zone. Domperidone has prokinetic and antiemetic properties similar to those of metoclopramide. Domperidone has not yet been approved for use in the United States, and there is little clinical experience with the drug in companion animal species. As a prokinetic agent, domperidone appears to be most effective in improving clinical signs—for example, anorexia and vomiting—associated with delayed gastric emptying. Domperidone may not be that useful as a gastric prokinetic agent in the dog, however. Domperidone is more potent than metoclopramide as an antiemetic agent for chemoreceptor trigger zone–mediated vomiting.

Cisapride

Cisapride is representative of a group of serotonergic or 5-HT drugs that bind 5-HT$_4$ receptors on enteric postganglionic cholinergic neurons and stimulate contraction of gastrointestinal smooth muscle. Cisapride also has 5-HT$_1$/ 5-HT$_3$ antagonistic effects on enteric cholinergic neurons and non–5-HT effects on canine antral cholinergic neurons.

Cisapride is the drug of choice for treating delayed gastric emptying, followed by erythromycin and ranitidine or nizatidine. The recommended dosage of cisapride for dogs and cats has been 0.1 to 0.5 mg/kg every 8 to 12 hours PO. It is available for oral use in 10- and 20-mg tablets (Propulsid, Janssen Pharmaceutical, Inc.). This dosage range was derived from studies of the effect of cisapride on normal gastric emptying in dogs. Higher dosages of cisapride (0.5 to 1.0 mg/kg) may be necessary to enhance gastric emptying in dogs with delayed gastric emptying.

Cisapride is indicated for the treatment of gastroesophageal (GE) reflux because it stimulates gastric emptying and increases GE sphincter pressure. It would appear to be a rational drug in the treatment of GE reflux disease in the dog and cat. Comparative studies have shown that cisapride is more potent than metoclopramide in stimulating gastric emptying and increasing GE sphincter pressure. Cisapride also stimulates distal esophageal peristalsis in those animal species (e.g., cat, humans, guinea pig) in which the distal esophageal muscularis is composed of smooth muscle. The obvious exception is the dog, a species in which the entire esophageal body is composed of striated muscle. A smooth muscle prokinetic agent would not be expected to have much effect on striated muscle function.

Cisapride accelerates gastric emptying in dogs by stimulating pyloric and duodenal motor activity, by enhancing antropyloroduodenal coordination, and by increasing the mean propagation distance of duodenal contractions. In this regard, cisapride appears to be superior to metoclopramide and domperidone in stimulating gastric emptying. Cisapride enhances cholinergic neurotransmission and motility in the canine antrum without activating 5-HT receptors; the neuronal receptor mediating this response has not been characterized.

Cisapride lacks the antidopaminergic properties typical of metoclopramide and domperidone. Thus, cisapride does not induce the hyperprolactinemia that is typical of metoclopramide and domperidone, and cisapride has only weak antiemetic effects against apomorphine-induced vomiting in dogs. Concurrent administration of anticholinergic compounds (e.g., atropine, aminopentamide, isopropamide) would be expected to compromise some of the beneficial effects of cisapride. Concurrent administration of cimetidine, in contrast, could lead to increased plasma cisapride concentrations because cimetidine inhibits cytochrome P_{450} enzyme systems. The facilitation of gastric emptying by cisapride could affect the rate of absorption of other drugs. Animals receiving drugs with narrow therapeutic ratios (e.g., digoxin, anticonvulsants) should be monitored closely.

Erythromycin

The antibiotic properties of erythromycin were discovered in the early 1950s. It was noted early on that erythromycin therapy was accompanied by frequent gastrointestinal side effects, for example, nausea and vomiting. The occurrence of these side effects suggested to researchers that erythromycin might have effects on gastrointestinal motility. In more recent times, it has been shown that much lower, microbially ineffective doses of erythromycin stimulate migrating motility complexes and antegrade peristalsis in a way similar to that induced by endogenous motilin.

Erythromycin accelerates gastric emptying by inducing antral contractions that are similar, but not identical, to those associated with phase III of the migrating motor complex. Phase III contractions, which usually occur only during the fasting state, empty the stomach of indigestible solids. Erythromycin accelerates gastric emptying of solids during the fed state so that food is inadequately triturated (i.e., food particles >0.5 mm) and emptied into the small intestine. Previous studies have shown that the stomach empties only 6% of solids as particles greater than 0.5 mm. Because of the small surface area:mass ratio associated with large chunks of food, the small intestine may inadequately digest and absorb these nutrients. Thus, erythromycin should be used as a gastric prokinetic agent with the understanding that it is inducing an interdigestive motor pattern and not restoring a normal fed pattern of gastric motility, and that food will not be expelled as normally digestible particles of small size. If large particles of food in the small bowel cause intestinal distress, use of this prokinetic drug may not lead to an improvement and could actually increase symptoms, despite more rapid gastric emptying.

Erythromycin is available in parenteral (erythromycin lactobionate; 100 mg/ml) and enteral forms (erythromycin stearate; erythromycin ethylsuccinate). The latter are available as enteric-coated tablets (250, 333, and 500 mg), film-coated tablets (250 and 500 mg), capsules (125 and 250 mg), oral drops (100 mg/ml), and oral suspension (25 and 50 mg/ml). The recommended antimicrobial dosage of erythromycin for dogs and cats is 10 to 20 mg/kg PO every 8 hours. However, the prokinetic dosage of erythromycin for dogs and cats is likely much lower, i.e., 0.5 to 1.0 mg/kg PO every 8 hours. No serious drug interactions have been reported in veterinary species.

Ranitidine

Ranitidine is a competitive, reversible, histaminergic H_2 receptor antagonist that was developed to inhibit gastric acid secretion. Ranitidine also stimulates gastrointestinal motility by inhibiting acetylcholinesterase activity and thus increasing the amount of acetylcholine available to bind smooth muscle muscarinic cholinergic receptors. Ranitidine may be useful in the treatment of gastric emptying disorders as well as gastric ulcers. Indeed, delayed gastric emptying is a consequence of gastric ulcer disease in the dog. Treatment with ranitidine would be beneficial not only in inhibiting gastric acid secretion but also in promoting gastric emptying. Ranitidine in the dosage range of 1 to 2 mg/kg every 12 hours inhibits anticholinesterase activity and stimulates gastric contractions. Thus, prokinetic effects would be expected at the clinically recommended dosages of ranitidine used for antisecretory activity. Ranitidine (Zantac, Glaxo Laboratories) is marketed for oral use as 75-, 150-, and 300-mg tablets and as a syrup at 15 mg/ml. Ranitidine is highly water-soluble and is available as an injection at 25 mg/ml or a premixed solution at 50 mg/50 ml.

Ranitidine was developed to improve on the perceived deficiencies observed with cimetidine. Ranitidine is reported to produce fewer adverse drug interactions and less systemic toxicity and to have greater potency. Differences in the chemical structure of ranitidine have reduced the androgenic effects, hepatic microsomal-enzyme inhibition, altered lymphocyte responsiveness, and cerebrospinal fluid penetration reported with cimetidine. Ranitidine has less affinity for the hepatic cytochrome P_{450} mixed-function oxidase enzymes, but still interferes with the metabolism of drugs normally removed by this system. The bioavailability of drugs with pH-dependent dissolution characteristics may be altered by ranitidine therapy. Otherwise, ranitidine would not be expected to alter the absorption of other drugs significantly, with the exception perhaps of ketoconazole.

Nizatidine

Nizatidine acts in a manner similar to cimetidine, ranitidine, and famotidine as a reversible, competitive H_2 receptor antagonist with gastric antisecretory properties. Nizatidine also stimulates gastric contractions and accelerates gastric emptying at gastric antisecretory doses. Thus, nizatidine, like ranitidine, may have clinical applications (i.e., gastrointestinal prokinetic therapy) not found with cimetidine or famotidine. Nizatidine (Axid, Eli Lilly) is marketed for oral use in 75-, 150-, and 300-mg capsules. The current recommended dosage of nizatidine is 2.5 to 5 mg/kg every 24 hours PO.

Nizatidine stimulates gastric motor activity and accelerates gastric emptying in a way comparable to cisapride. Nizatidine appears to have a wide margin of safety. Since nizatidine does not induce hepatic microsomal enzyme activity, there should be no interference with the disposition of other substances metabolized by the hepatic microsomal cytochrome P_{450} system. Concurrent administration of anticholinergic compounds such as atropine would be expected to block the beneficial prokinetic effects of nizatidine.

References and Suggested Reading

Hall JA, Washabau RJ: Gastrointestinal prokinetic therapy: Dopaminergic antagonist drugs. Compend Cont Educ Pract Vet 19:214, 1997.

Hall JA, Washabau RJ. Gastrointestinal prokinetic therapy: Motilin-like drugs. Compend Contin Educ Pract Vet 19:281, 1997.

Washabau RJ, Hall JA: Gastrointestinal prokinetic therapy: Serotonergic drugs. Compend Contin Educ Pract Vet 19:473, 1997.

Hall JA, Washabau RJ: Gastrointestinal prokinetic therapy: Acetylcholinesterase inhibitors. Compend Contin Educ Pract Vet 19:615, 1997.

Hall JA, Twedt DC, Burrows CF: Gastric motility in dogs. Part II. Disorders of gastric motility. Compend Cont Educ Pract Vet 12:1373, 1990.
A review of the various causes, diagnosis, and treatment of gastric motility disorders in dogs.

Mizumoto A, Fujimura M, Iwanaga Y, et al: Anticholinesterase activity of histamine H_2-receptor antagonists in the dog: Their possible role in gastric motor activity. J Gastrointest Motil 2:273, 1990.
An in vivo and in vitro research study in dogs on the anticholinesterase activity of cimetidine, ranitidine, and famotidine in relation to the enhancement of gastric motor activity.

Peeters TL: Erythromycin and other macrolides as prokinetic agents. Gastroenterology 105:1886, 1993.
In-depth review article.

Ueki S, Seiki M, Yoneta T, et al: Gastroprokinetic activity of nizatidine, a new H_2-receptor antagonist, and its possible mechanism of action in dogs and rats. J Pharmacol Exp Ther 264:152, 1993.
An in vivo and in vitro research study in dogs and rats on the antiacetylcholinesterase activity of nizatidine in comparison with cimetidine and famotidine.

Washabau RJ, Hall JA: Topics in drug therapy. Cisapride. J Am Vet Med Assoc 207:1285, 1995.
Clinical applications, pharmacokinetics, pharmacologic effects, and drug interactions for cisapride are reviewed.

Washabau RJ, Hall JA: Diagnosis and management of gastrointestinal motility disorders in dogs and cats. Compend Contin Educ Pract Vet 19:721, 1997.
Gastroenterology continuing education series of five articles on gastrointestinal prokinetic therapy.

Gastrinoma in Dogs

Kenneth W. Simpson
Ithaca, New York

A syndrome of gastric acid hypersecretion, fulminant peptic ulcer disease, and non–beta-islet cell tumors was first described in humans by Zollinger and Ellison (Zollinger-Ellison syndrome), who proposed that an ulcerogenic factor produced by the tumor caused these findings. This ulcerogenic factor was subsequently identified as the hormone gastrin, and the tumors became known as gastrinomas. The consequences of excessive gastrin secretion are hypersecretion of gastric acid, which causes gastrointestinal ulceration, esophagitis, and maldigestion (secondary to enzyme inactivation). Gastrin also has trophic effects on the gastric mucosa, and hypergastrinemia can cause hypertrophic gastropathy. Gastrinomas in dogs are rarely diagnosed, and only a few dogs have survived to undergo treatment. This article reviews the clinical findings, diagnosis, and treatment of gastrinoma in dogs. Data from the literature and six additional cases are presented.

DIAGNOSIS

Clinical Features

Gastrinoma has been reported in a wide variety of breeds of dog from 3.5 to 12 years of age (mean age of 16 dogs = 9 years). A sex bias has been suggested, but the review of 16 canine cases (7 females and 9 males) does not support this. Vomiting, weight loss, anorexia, depression, lethargy, and intermittent diarrhea are the most common clinical signs, with polydipsia, abdominal pain, melena, and hematemesis occurring less frequently (Table 1). Physical examination is often unremarkable, although poor body condition, abdominal pain, pallor, and melena may be detected. Some patients have signs of shock and acute abdomen secondary to gastrointestinal (GI) perforation. The diagnostic work-up is usually centered around the problems of vomiting, weight loss, and anorexia, and the pursuit

TABLE 1. Incidence of Clinical Findings of Gastrinoma in 23 Dogs and 2 Cats

Sign	Number of Animals	(%)
Vomiting	23/25	92
Weight loss	22/25	88
Anorexia	18/25	72
Lethargy, depression	16/25	64
Diarrhea	15/25	60
Polydipsia	6/24	25
Melena	6/25	24
Abdominal pain	6/25	24
Hematemesis	3/25	12
Hematochezia	3/25	12
Fever	2/25	8
Ravenous appetite	2/25	8
Abdominal mass	1/25	4
Tachycardia	1/25	4
Obstipation (alternating with diarrhea)	1/25	4

Adapted from Zerbe CA: Islet cell tumors secreting insulin, pancreatic polypeptide, gastrin or glucagon. In: Kirk RW, Bonagura JD, eds: Current Veterinary Therapy XI. Philadelphia: WB Saunders, 1992, pp 368–375, with permission.

of localizing findings such as melena, hematemesis, and abdominal pain.

Laboratory Findings

Laboratory findings are variable and nonspecific (Table 2). Decreased albumin concentrations and anemia are particularly frequent in older case reports and may reflect blood loss from GI ulceration, although some cases were complicated by the concurrent presence of *Ancylostoma, Dirofilaria, Capillaria,* or myelofibrosis. Findings such as hypokalemia, hypochloremia, and metabolic alkalosis, with or without aciduria, that are suggestive of an upper GI obstruction are present in some cases. When outflow obstruction is ruled out, these findings should prompt the consideration of gastrinoma. Elevations of alkaline phosphatase and alanine aminotransferase may reflect metastatic spread of gastrinoma to the liver. Occasional abnormalities include leukocytosis, hypoglycemia, hypocalcemia, and hyperbilirubinemia.

TABLE 2. Clinicopathologic Findings in 14 Dogs With Gastrinoma*

Clinicopathologic Finding	Number of Animals	(%)
Hypoproteinemia, hypoalbuminemia	8/14	57
Hypokalemia	6/14	43
Anemia	6/14	43
Increased alkaline phosphatase levels	6/14	43
Hypochloremia	5/14	36
Leukocytosis	5/14	36
Increased alanine aminotransferase levels	3/14	21
Hypoglycemia	1/14	7
Hyponatremia	1/14	7
Hyperbilirubinemia	1/14	7
Increased blood urea nitrogen levels	1/14	7
Hypocalcaemia	1/14	7

*Data compiled from the literature and six additional dogs with gastrinoma.

Radiography

Survey abdominal radiographs are usually unremarkable but may reveal prominent gastric rugae and loss of serosal detail if GI perforation has occurred. Contrast radiography may show gastroduodenal ulceration, gastric rugal hypertrophy, or outlet obstruction.

Endoscopy

Endoscopic findings include esophagitis, gastric or duodenal ulceration, hypertrophy of the gastric mucosa, and increased gastric juice. Gastric mucosal changes can appear similar to benign hypertrophic pylorogastropathy or mural thickening secondary to inflammation or neoplasia. When GI ulceration is present, and mastocytosis and metabolic, endocrine, and iatrogenic causes of GI ulceration such as nonsteroidal anti-inflammatory drugs have been ruled out (usually before endoscopy), these endoscopic findings should prompt the measurement of circulating gastrin.

Histologic examination of endoscopic biopsy specimens of prominent rugae in dogs with gastrinoma are often relatively normal, suggesting submucosal or muscular hypertrophy as the cause of rugal enlargement. Since neoplastic infiltration of rugae and benign hypertrophic pylorogastropathy can often elude endoscopic biopsy, these should also be considered. Ultrasonographic, contrast radiographic, or surgical evaluation of the stomach is necessary to define these mural lesions further.

Gastric pH or acid secretion has been infrequently measured in dogs with gastrinoma but has been indicative of acid hypersecretion when measured. Measurement of endoscopically collected unstimulated gastric juice demonstrated a low pH in the four cases in which it was evaluated (pH = 1.0, 1.0, 1.5, 0.99) and correlated with increased basal and stimulated acid secretion (two of two dogs). Thus, it seems prudent to recommend that when gastric juice is detected or seems increased, it should be collected for pH measurement. The demonstration of a low gastric pH and increased gastrin is useful for ruling out achlorhydria as a cause of hypergastrinemia.

Ultrasonography

Primary gastrinomas in the pancreas are almost invariably undetected because they are small, but metastases in regional lymph nodes or the liver may be evident. Objective information about gastric wall thickness and large ulcers can also be provided by ultrasonography.

Measurement of Circulating Gastrin

The most useful screening test for gastrinoma is probably measurement of circulating gastrin; it can be performed using commercial radioimmunoassay kits. Fasting blood samples are collected into ethylenediaminetetra-acetic acid, and plasma is separated, frozen, and stored. Gastrin concentrations in dogs with gastrinoma are reported to range from 3 to 10 times the upper limit of the reference range. The fasting gastrin concentration ($\pm$SD) in 18 healthy dogs evaluated at the Ohio State University was 43.4 ± 15.5 pg/

ml.* Gastrin concentrations in five dogs with gastrinoma evaluated at that laboratory ranged from 101 to 2550 pg/ml. The finding of a gastrin concentration greater than 1000 pg/ml is considered diagnostic for gastrinoma in humans. When gastrin concentrations are less markedly elevated, other causes of hypergastrinemia must be ruled out and provocative testing considered to confirm gastrinoma. Other causes of hypergastrinemia include a nonfasting sample, renal failure, achlorhydria (primary or secondary to omeprazole), Basenji enteropathy and, potentially, gastric outlet obstruction, G-cell hyperplasia, retained antrum, liver disease, and *Helicobacter* infection.

Provocative Testing

The evaluation of circulating gastrin at 0, 2, 5, 10, and 20 minutes after secretin (2 to 4 U/kg IV) may help confirm gastrinoma when fasting gastrin is normal or mildly elevated. An increase in gastrin of greater than 200 pg/ml or a twofold increase over basal levels within the first few minutes is considered a positive test result in humans. This test has been performed in only three dogs with gastrinoma, two of which showed greater than twofold increases and one of which exhibited a 1.4-fold increase. A syndrome similar to gastrinoma has been observed in a dog with a pancreatic polypeptide and insulin-secreting tumor. This dog had transient fasting hypergastrinemia (687 pg/ml) but normal secretin-stimulated gastrin concentrations. The release of gastrin in response to calcium infusion has also been recommended as a screening test for gastrinoma; however, calcium infusion is potentially more risky than

*Dr. T. O'Dorisio, Department of Endocrinology, The Ohio State University, Doan Hall, 410 W. 10th Ave., Columbus OH 43210.

secretin stimulation, which is the favored provocative test in humans with suspected gastrinoma.

Tumor Localization

A search for a gastrin-producing tumor is usually initiated on the basis of a high serum gastrin concentration and endoscopic features suspicious of gastrinoma.

Noninvasive Localization

Presurgical localization of metastasis may preclude a laparotomy in favor of medical management. Nonsurgical localization of gastrinomas in humans has until recently relied on ultrasonography (conventional and endoscopic), computed tomography, and magnetic resonance imaging, all of which fail to detect gastrinomas smaller than 1 to 2 cm and readily miss metastases. The development of a noninvasive technique using radiolabeled somatostatin analogues (indium lll–octreotide or –pentetreotide) that bind to receptors expressed on the tumor has greatly facilitated the localization of gastrinomas and their metastases in humans and has also enabled the identification of metastatic gastrinoma in a dog (Fig. 1). Positive scintigraphic images are consistent with somatostatin binding by receptors on tumor and suggest the possibility of a therapeutic response to somatostatin.

Intraoperative Localization

In contrast to humans, in whom the duodenum has been recognized as the most common site for gastrinomas (up to 77% of cases), gastrinomas in dogs have been exclusively of pancreatic origin, with most tumors located in the

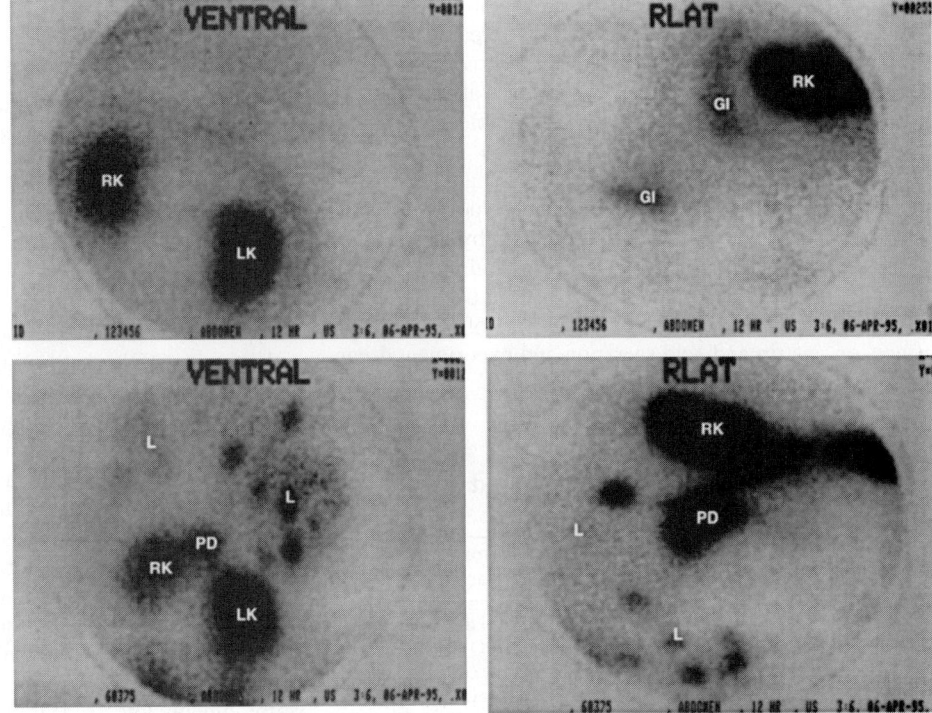

Figure 1. Pentetreotide scintigraphy in a healthy dog and a dog with gastrinoma. Multiple areas of uptake in the mid-ventral abdomen of a dog with gastrinoma (2nd row), which were consistently absent in the healthy control dog (1st row), were considered consistent with liver (L), pancreas/duodenum (PD) and possibly spleen (2nd row). Positive scintigraphic images were consistent with somatostatin binding by receptors on tumor tissue, which was subsequently confirmed by autoradiography *in vitro*. (From Altschul M, Simpson KW, Dykes NL et al. Evaluation of somatostatin analogues for the detection and treatment of gastrinoma in a dog. Journal of Small Animal Practice 38:286, 1997, with permission.)

right limb or the body. A tumor was detected in the liver but not the pancreas in one recent case, suggesting a nonpancreatic origin of gastrinomas in dogs. When a tumor is not visualized at surgery localization using ultrasonography, systematic palpation and exploration of the peripancreatic area may improve the detection rate.

Histopathologic Confirmation

Immunocytochemical confirmation of suspected gastrinomas can be performed using commercially available gastrin antisera by many referral pathology services. Assay of gastrin after extraction from the tumor and electron microscopic evaluation of secretory granules may also be used to confirm a diagnosis but are more specialized procedures.

TREATMENT

Management of patients with gastrinoma is aimed at tumor resection, if possible, and treatment of the excessive hormone secretion that creates the clinical syndrome of GI ulceration and abdominal pain.

Surgical Resection

Surgery has until recently been the only reliable method for detecting or confirming gastrinoma in dogs, and it is the treatment of choice for removing localized gastrinomas, tumor debulking, and removing metastases. The latter are common at the time of presentation and are most frequently reported in local lymph nodes and the liver. Resection of the right pancreatic lobe has been suggested for dogs in which a gastrinoma is suspected but cannot be localized. Intraoperative pancreatic ultrasonography and thorough evaluation of the duodenum and peripancreatic area should, however, be considered before blind pancreatic resection. Dogs undergoing surgery to confirm or remove a suspected gastrinoma should receive pre- and postoperative antisecretory therapy with omeprazole when possible (see further on) as well as adequate fluid therapy to minimize the risk of GI ulceration and perforation. Dogs undergoing pancreatic resection should be managed postoperatively like those with acute pancreatitis—nothing by mouth, fluid support, and careful monitoring. The pre- and postoperative administration of the somatostatin analogue octreotide may also be indicated in these patients because of its beneficial effects on gastrin and acid secretion and experimental pancreatitis in dogs.

TABLE 3. Therapeutic Agents Used to Treat Gastrinoma in Dogs

Drug Name (Trade Name)	Suggested Dosage for Dogs with Gastrinoma
Omeprazole (Prilosec)	0.7 mg/kg PO s.i.d.
Famotidine (Pepcid)	0.5–1.0 mg/kg PO b.i.d.
Sucralfate (Carafate)	0.5–1.0 gm PO t.i.d.
Octreotide (Sandostatin)	2–16 µg/kg SC t.i.d.

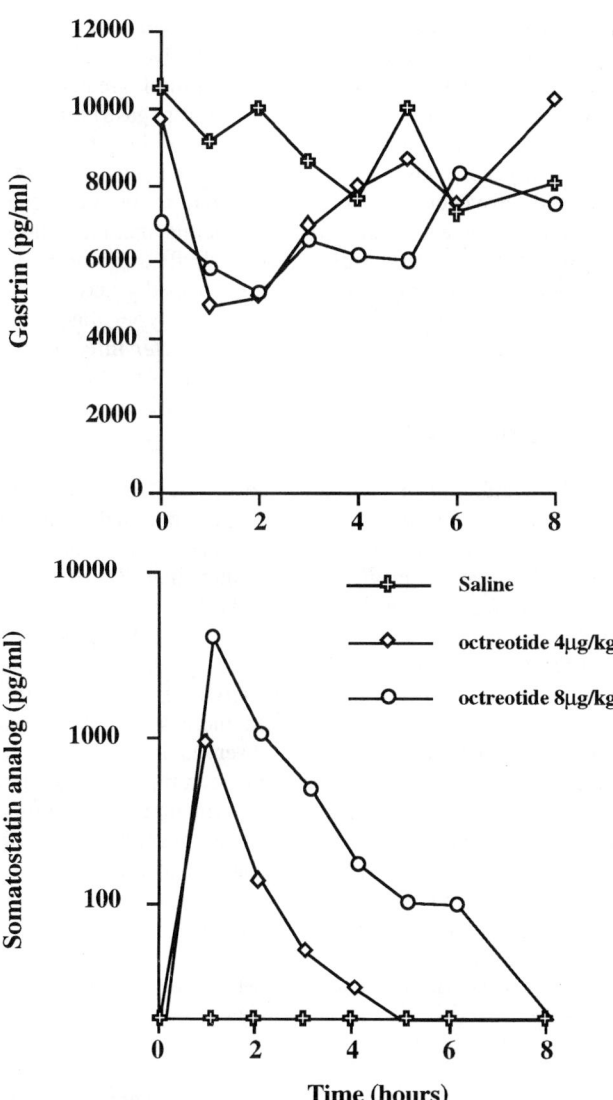

Figure 2. Plasma gastrin and somatostatin concentrations after the subcutaneous administration of octreotide (4 and 8 µg/kg) or saline. (Adapted from Altschul M, Simpson KW, Dykes NL et al. Evaluation of somatostatin analogues for the detection and treatment of gastrinoma in a dog. Journal of Small Animal Practice 38:286, 1997, with permission.)

Medical Management

Initial management consists of fluid and electrolyte therapy to correct abnormalities associated with vomiting. The hypersecretion of gastric acid and its loss in vomitus, rather than upper GI obstruction, may be responsible for the metabolic alkalosis observed in some patients and is treated with NaCl (0.9%) supplemented with KCl, given at a rate and amount to correct hypovolemia or dehydration, ongoing losses, and maintenance requirements. Symptomatic treatment of patients with suspected GI ulceration using gastric antisecretory drugs (usually an H_2 antagonist) and a mucosal protectant (e.g., sucralfate) is usually initiated before a definitive diagnosis of gastrinoma (Table 3). Blockade of acid secretion with antisecretory agents (see p. 609) may also help limit metabolic alkalosis associated with vomiting. The H^+/K^+ adenosine triphosphatase inhibitor omeprazole (see Table 3), or double doses of an H_2

antagonist (e.g., famotidine), should be given to dogs with endoscopic findings suggestive of gastrinoma (blood samples are obtained for gastrin analysis before antisecretory therapy) and to animals with confirmed or suspected gastrinoma managed medically or undergoing surgery. Early treatment is imperative because many dogs with gastrinoma have died as a result of complications related to hyperacidity, such as duodenal or esophageal perforation. Omeprazole has been used in combination with famotidine, octreotide, and sucralfate to enable a 14-month survival period in a dog with metastatic gastrinoma. The expense of omeprazole may preclude its use in some animals. In these patients, double doses (or higher) of H_2 antagonists may effect some control of acid secretion.

The long-acting somatostatin analogue octreotide has been beneficial in humans with gastrinoma. Octreotide binds to somatostatin receptors on the tumor and decreases gastrin release. Octreotide also directly decreases gastric acid secretion in response to gastrin and other secretagogues. Octreotide has been evaluated in combination with an H_2 antagonist or omeprazole, or both, and sucralfate in two dogs with metastatic gastrinoma. In one dog, a dose of 10 to 20 μg SC t.i.d. was associated with a good clinical response and patient survival for 10 months. Relapse was observed when octreotide was discontinued. In the other dog, increasing doses of octreotide (2, 4, 8, 16 μg/kg SC b.i.d. to t.i.d.; Fig. 2) caused a transient decrease in plasma gastrin, and combination therapy resulted in resolution of gastric ulceration and rugal hypertrophy at 5.5 months after the start of treatment and patient survival for 14 months. The relative longevity of these two dogs treated with a combination of antacids and somatostatin seems to be a significant advance on previous cases in which death occurred within 5 months of diagnosis.

Some dogs with gastrinoma have diarrhea that is a consequence of the destruction of pancreatic enzymes by excessive acid secretion. Diagnosis of secondary exocrine pancreatic insufficiency in these dogs requires the assay of fecal proteolytic activity rather than measurement of circulating trypsin-like immunoreactivity as secondary exocrine pancreatic insufficiency is caused by enzyme destruction and not pancreatic atrophy. Control of hyperacidity with omeprazole or H_2 antagonist may be effective in limiting enzyme inactivation in these cases.

PROGNOSIS

The long-term prognosis for gastrinoma is poor because metastases are common at the time of diagnosis. Many dogs with gastrinoma die before treatment is instituted or a diagnosis is made. Heightened awareness of gastrinoma and early diagnosis by endoscopy, assay of gastrin, and tumor localization and resection should improve survival. Early and aggressive treatment with acid-reducing agents, particularly omeprazole, and acid- and gastrin-reducing drugs such as octreotide also promise longer survival times.

References and Suggested Reading

Altschul M, Simpson KW, Dykes NL, et al: Evaluation of somatostatin analogues for the detection and treatment of gastrinoma in a dog. J Small Anim Pract 38:286, 1997.
A report describing the presence of somatostatin receptors on gastrinomas in dogs and the use of somatostatin analogues to detect and treat a dog with gastrinoma.

Gibril F, Reynolds JC, Doppman JL, et al: Somatostatin receptor scintigraphy: Its sensitivity compared with that of other imaging methods in detecting primary and metastatic gastrinomas. Ann Intern Med 125:26, 1996.
A report detailing the superiority of somatostatin receptor scintigraphy over ultrasound, magnetic resonance imaging, and computed tomography for the detection of gastrinoma in humans.

Lamberts SWJ, van der Lely AJ, de Herder WW, et al: Octreotide. N Engl J Med 334:246, 1996.
A detailed overview of the actions and applications of octreotide.

Lothrop CD: Medical treatment of neuroendocrine tumors of the gastroentero-pancreatic system with somatostatin. In: Kirk RW, ed: Current Veterinary Therapy X. Philadelphia, WB Saunders, 1989, p 1020.
An overview of the utility of somatostatin in the treatment of insulinoma and gastrinoma in dogs.

Metz DC, Pisegna JR, Fishbeyn VA, et al: Control of gastric acid hypersecretion in the management of patients with Zollinger-Ellison syndrome. World J Surg 17:468, 1993.
A report outlining strategies to control acid secretion in humans with gastrinoma.

Orloff SL, Debas HT: Advances in the management of patients with Zollinger-Ellison syndrome. Surg Clin North Am 75:511, 1995.
A recent review of the management of humans with Zollinger-Ellison syndrome.

Zerbe CA: Islet cell tumors secreting insulin, pancreatic polypeptide, gastrin or glucagon. In: Kirk RW, Bonagura JD, eds: Current Veterinary Therapy XI. Philadelphia, WB Saunders, 1992, p 368.
A detailed review with information on the prevalence of clinical findings in dogs and cats with gastrinoma.

Zerbe CA, Washabau RJ: Gastrointestinal endocrine disease. In: Ettinger SJ, Feldman EC, eds: Textbook of Veterinary Internal Medicine, 4th ed. Philadelphia, WB Saunders, 1995, p 1593.
A thoroughly referenced review of gastrinomas in dogs and cats.

Gastrointestinal Neoplasia

MICHAEL L. MAGNE
Rohnert Park, California

INTRODUCTION

Gastric and intestinal malignancies are relatively uncommon in companion animals, accounting for approximately 2% of all neoplasms. However, gastrointestinal (GI) tumors are often devastating in their impact on patients, owing to the advanced stage that is typical at the time of diagnosis and a very high metastatic rate. In cats, only 5% of GI neoplasms are benign, whereas approximately 35% are nonmalignant in dogs. Adenocarcinomas are by far the most commonly diagnosed GI malignancies in both dogs (71% of all GI malignancies) and cats (58%); lymphosarcoma is the second most common malignancy in both species, accounting for 10% of GI malignancies in dogs and 21% in cats. Although neoplasia may occur at any anatomic location within the GI tract, intestinal tumors are more common than gastric ones. Most patients with GI neoplasia are middle-aged (7 to 10 years). A sex predisposition has been reported in dogs for both adenocarcinoma and lymphosarcoma. In a large series of cases, 60% of adenocarcinomas and 70% of lymphosarcomas occurred in males; in the same study, however, no sex predisposition was apparent in the feline cases.

Patients with GI neoplasia typically present with a history of profound and chronic GI dysfunction. Clinical signs can include vomiting, hematemesis, hematochezia, melena, tenesmus or dyschezia, weight loss, lethargy, and, in some, edema due to protein-losing enteropathy. Clinical findings are related in part to the location and extent of organ involvement. In other patients, however, clinical signs are acute in onset and mimic GI obstruction caused by a foreign body, intussusception, or another GI disorder. Abdominal pain, either spontaneous or induced by palpation, may be found in some individuals. Perforation of GI neoplasms can occur, leading to septic peritonitis and a rapid deterioration in clinical status; perforation has also been seen during endoscopic examination of patients with gastric malignancies. Abnormalities found on physical examination variably include cachexia, a palpable abdominal mass or masses, diffuse bowel thickening, hepatomegaly, splenomegaly, regional or generalized lymphadenopathy, subcutaneous edema, abdominal pain, and pale mucous membranes. Examination should always include a gentle but thorough abdominal, as well as rectal, palpation to identify mucosal irregularities or masses.

Diagnostic evaluation in the patient with suspected GI neoplasia includes routine hematologic and biochemical testing, plain and barium radiographic studies, abdominal ultrasound, endoscopy, and surgical laparotomy. Hematologic abnormalities may be indicative of chronic GI blood loss and characterized by microcytic, hypochromic anemia; peripheral leukemia may occasionally be seen in the patient with GI lymphosarcoma. Although elevated leukocyte counts can be found in any patient with GI neoplasia, leukocytosis with a significant left shift increases the index of suspicion for perforation and peritonitis. The most common biochemical abnormalities are panhypoproteinemia due to protein-losing enteropathy and elevated liver enzymes owing to hepatic metastatic disease. Abdominal radiographs may be normal or may reveal signs of GI ileus or obstruction, abdominal effusion, organomegaly, lymphadenopathy, or an obvious mass lesion. Thoracic radiographs to screen for metastasis should be routine, although radiographic evidence of pulmonary metastases is relatively uncommon at the time of initial evaluation. Abdominal ultrasound is routinely required in suspect patients and is a valuable adjunct in eliminating other differential diagnoses. Ultrasound examination facilitates assessment of gastric or intestinal wall thickening or masses and guides fine-needle aspirate samples for cytologic analysis. Gastrointestinal endoscopy is an important aid in the diagnosis of neoplasms that are endoscopically accessible, for example, gastric, duodenal, colorectal, and perhaps ileal. In occasional patients, abdominal computed tomography (CT) scanning has been helpful as a diagnostic or preoperative evaluation technique. Laparotomy as a diagnostic maneuver is usually restricted to patients in which less invasive procedures are inadequate for diagnosis or staging. When surgery is contemplated, it should be planned with both a diagnostic and a therapeutic intent, that is, obtaining biopsy samples and anticipating bowel or mass resection.

GASTRIC NEOPLASIA

Adenocarcinoma accounts for approximately three fourths of the gastric malignancies diagnosed in dogs, but is very rare in the stomach of cats. Plain and positive-contrast radiographic abnormalities that are consistent with gastric adenocarcinoma include gastric wall thickening, abnormal rugal fold patterns, intraluminal mass, filling defects, and delayed gastric emptying. Ultrasound usually reveals similar findings and, for pragmatic reasons, is often done in preference to contrast radiography in clinical practice. Ultrasound is useful for identifying intra-abdominal metastatic disease (though the sensitivity and specificity are highly operator dependent) and guiding fine-needle or aspiration gun biopsy of identified lesions. This diagnostic procedure is minimally invasive compared to laparotomy. Gastroscopy often reveals a large ulcerated, indurated mass of the antral-pyloric region or lesser curvature, gastric retention of food or fluid, and abnormal rugal fold appearance. Although endoscopy allows for the collection of tissue biopsy samples, confirmatory histologic diagnosis can be difficult in some patients, and pathology may reveal only necrosis, inflammation, or fibroplasia. In such patients, laparotomy may be required for confirmation as well as therapeutic intervention and staging. Attempted surgical correction of gastric adenocarcinoma usually requires partial, subtotal, or total gastrectomy along with gastroduodenostomy or gastrojejunostomy and can be associated with appreciable patient morbidity. Unfortunately, established metastatic disease is common in adenocarcinoma patients; in one study of 26 gastric adenocarcinomas (personal observation), metastatic disease was found in regional lymph nodes in 95% and in the liver in 85% of patients at the time of surgery; additionally, most patients either died or were euthanatized within 6 months of diagnosis. These findings notwithstanding, surgical resection may be palliative in selected patients with localized disease and may cure animals with other forms of neoplasia (see below). Improved 5-year survival rates have been reported in human patients receiving adjuvant chemotherapy for gastric adenocarcinoma; however, effective chemotherapy for adenocarcinoma has not been reported for veterinary patients. In the unpublished study mentioned earlier (Magne), leiomyosarcoma was the second most common gastric malignancy presented for attempted surgical intervention, representing 42% of the surgical cases. Although the clinical symptomatology and tumor behavior was indistinguishable from that of adenocarcinoma, profuse gastric bleeding occurred in 55% of these patients necessitating single or multiple blood transfusions at the time of surgery.

Leiomyoma, of smooth muscle origin, is the most common benign neoplasm of the canine stomach and is usually seen in dogs of advanced age. These tumors grow slowly, are often pedunculated, and typically cause symptoms of gastric obstruction owing to a mass effect. These masses are usually pedunculated; therefore, surgical excision is relatively easy and often curative. Adenomatous polyps are also a relatively common, benign gastric lesion. Polyps may be associated with clinical signs owing to outflow obstruction, to altered gastric emptying, or occasionally to mucosal ulceration. Surgical excision, either endoscopically or via laparotomy, is the treatment of choice and is curative. In some patients, gastric adenomatous polyps may be multiple and can present a significant surgical challenge. Malignant transformation of gastric adenomatous polyps in dogs has not been reported.

INTESTINAL NEOPLASIA

Other than lymphosarcoma, intestinal adenocarcinoma is the most common GI malignancy, representing approximately 50% of GI neoplasia in cats and 25% in dogs. Although adenocarcinoma may occur at any location throughout the intestinal tract, the rectum in dogs and jejunum or ileum in cats appear to be the sites of predisposition. Several studies have suggested not only a sex predisposition for males but also perhaps a breed predisposition in Boxers, German shepherds, Collies, and Siamese cats. Adenocarcinoma typically occurs as an annular lesion of the bowel wall leading to stenosis and eventual obstruction, although polypoid, sessile forms may also be seen, perhaps more commonly in the canine colon or rectum. Occasionally, a diffuse, infiltrative variant may be diagnosed. Positive-contrast radiographic studies or ultrasound imaging are the most helpful diagnostic aids in patients with small intestine masses, whereas colonoscopy for visualization and biopsy is most valuable for patients with large bowel

tumors. Surgical intervention by laparotomy is the treatment of choice. In neoplasms of the small intestine, it may be indicated for diagnostic as well as therapeutic reasons. Occasionally, rectal tumors may be accessible with the use of a pull-through or prolapse technique.

Intestinal adenocarcinomas, of either small or large bowel origin, are also highly metastatic neoplasms; several studies have indicated metastatic rates of 60 to 70%, typically to regional lymph nodes, liver, lungs, and peritoneum. Notwithstanding the high metastatic rate, certain patients may have a significant symptom-free period of time following surgical resection. In one report of 23 cats with small intestinal adenocarcinoma treated with surgical resection and anastomosis, an interesting bimodal survival distribution was seen. Approximately 50% of the cats either died or were euthanatized within 2 weeks of surgery, whereas a mean survival time of 15 months was observed in the remaining cats. Five cats with demonstrated regional lymph node metastasis had a mean survival of 12 months. Adjuvant postoperative chemotherapy has demonstrated little benefit for veterinary patients with intestinal adenocarcinoma; however, intraoperative and external beam radiation therapy have been used with some encouraging results in canine patients with rectal neoplasms.

Adenomatous polyps are seen in the canine rectum and are often associated with tenesmus, hematochezia, or rectal or tumor prolapse. Surgical excision, by a pull-through approach or endoscopically, is again the treatment of choice and is potentially curative; however, recurrence can be problematic if adequate normal tissue margins are not attained at the time of surgery. Although malignant transformation of colorectal polyps occurs commonly in people, it appears to be a rare occurrence in dogs, having been reported only once in the veterinary literature.

GASTROINTESTINAL LYMPHOSARCOMA

The gastrointestinal tract represents the most common site of extranodal lymphosarcoma (LSA) in both dogs and cats. Cases of GI LSA may occur as focal, multifocal, or diffuse disease; however, in dogs LSA occurs most commonly as either multifocal or diffuse and accounts for approximately 10% of all GI malignancies in that species. Although the median age at time of diagnosis is approximately 7 years, there is a wide range, from the very young to the geriatric dog. As with other GI neoplasms, there appears to be a male predisposition; however, no breed predispositions are known. Hypoproteinemia due to protein-losing enteropathy is common in GI LSA, occurring in more than one half of affected patients. The diagnostic studies that are helpful in the evaluation for GI LSA are essentially the same as those discussed for other GI neoplasms. Radiographic or ultrasound studies may reveal bowel wall thickening due to neoplastic infiltration, focal masses, filling defects, or bowel obstruction. Significant hepatomegaly, splenomegaly, or visceral lymphadenopathy found during these examinations is very suggestive of LSA as opposed to other GI malignancies. The sonographic appearance of hepatic or splenic LSA lesions is typically described as hypoechoic or lucent-centered. Ultrasound-guided aspiration or biopsy of intra-abdominal organs, including the GI tract per se, is often adequate for establishing a diagnosis of GI LSA. Further studies, such as endoscopy or laparotomy, may allow for a more thorough biopsy and staging of disease extent in some cases. Because of the limited size of tissue samples obtained via endoscopy, there can be significant diagnostic error with this procedure. Additionally, histopathology reveals that most GI LSA lesions are associated with non-neoplastic lymphoid cell infiltrates, and the histologic differentiation between severe, non-neoplastic lymphoid infiltrate, that is, "inflammatory bowel disease," and LSA may be difficult in some cases. With further development of sophisticated cell-marker technology, accurate diagnosis of GI LSA may be simplified. As with other GI malignancies, exploratory laparotomy may be required for diagnostic purposes in some patients, and in those with focal disease surgery may also serve a therapeutic or palliative intent. Because of the typically multifocal or diffuse nature of GI LSA in dogs, combination chemotherapy is usually recommended as definitive treatment (p. 465). Although there is little published literature as to the efficacy of combination chemotherapy, prolonged remission times have been reported in some cases.

In cats, GI LSA lesions represent 20% of all GI malignancies and approximately 15% of all cases of LSA in that species. Although a majority of cats with other forms (multicentric, thymic) of LSA are positive for feline leukemia virus, only about one fourth or less of cats with GI LSA are positive for the leukemia retrovirus. Affected feline patients typically have either solitary or diffuse disease, and it has been suggested that renal involvement may be frequent in cats with GI LSA. Solitary lesions can occur anywhere throughout the GI tract and may or may not be associated with mesenteric lymph node involvement. The diffuse or multifocal form, on the other hand, typically is accompanied by lymph node involvement and perhaps also by neoplastic infiltrates of the liver or spleen. The diagnostic applications and limitations in feline LSA patients are similar to those discussed earlier for canine patients. Staging of feline GI LSA with the use of the World Health Organization system may be misleading, since all forms of extranodal LSA, including GI, would be classified as stage V and thus warrant a poor prognosis, yet solitary GI LSA in feline patients may carry a significantly better prognosis than diffuse forms. Reports of therapeutic response to combination chemotherapy are limited in the veterinary literature, and results are difficult to interpret because, often, different anatomic forms and treatment protocols are combined in statistical analysis. Even with aggressive chemotherapy, it would appear that median remission times with diffuse GI LSA are on the order of approximately 6 months or less; whereas patients with solitary gastric LSA following surgical resection may remain free from symptoms or

disease for appreciably longer periods. Although little is known regarding the results of nonsurgical, chemotherapeutic treatment of solitary GI LSA in cats, there is anecdotal evidence to suggest that favorable responses and prolonged remission times may be accomplished. Many individuals hold the opinion that LSA in all patients should be considered a systemic disease, and thus chemotherapy is routinely advocated as an adjunctive treatment, even in patients without objective evidence of disease beyond the focal site. An interesting observation that merits consideration is the finding in human patients of solitary gastric LSA ("maltoma") that regresses following treatment of the associated *Helicobacter pylori* infection.

References and Suggested Reading

Brodey RS: Alimentary tract neoplasms in the cat: A clinicopathologic survey of 46 cases. Am J Vet Res 27:74, 1966.
A review of various GI neoplasms in cats.
Grooters AM, Johnson SE: Canine gastric leiomyoma. Compend Contin Educ Small Anim Pract 17:1485, 1995.
Details the clinical presentation and treatment results in dogs with gastric leiomyomas.
Kaser-Hotz B, Hauser B, Arnold P: Ultrasonographic findings in canine gastric neoplasia in 13 patients. Vet Radiol Ultrasound 37:51, 1996.
Use of ultrasound as a diagnostic imaging technique with gastric tumors.
Kosovsky JE, Matthiesen DT, Patnaik AK: Small intestinal adenocarcinoma in cats: 32 cases (1978–1985). JAVMA 192:233,1988.
Review of clinical signs and treatment outcome in feline intestinal adenocarcinoma.
Mahony OM, Moore AS, Cotter SM, et al: Alimentary lymphoma in cats: 28 cases (1988–1993). JAVMA 207:1593, 1995.
Review of clinical presentation and treatment results of feline GI LSA.
Patnaik AK, Hurvitz AI, Johnson GF: Canine gastric adenocarcinoma. Vet Pathol 15:600, 1978.
The pathology of gastric carcinomas in dogs.
Patnaik AK, Hurvitz AI, Johnson GF: Canine gastrointestinal neoplasms. Vet Pathol 14:547, 1977.
Pathology of various GI malignancies in dogs.
Patnaik AK, Liu S-H, Johnson GF: Feline intestinal adenocarcinoma: A clinicopathologic study of 22 cases. Vet Pathol 13:1, 1976.
Clinical and pathological characteristics of feline intestinal adenocarcinoma.
Penninck DG, Nyland TG, Kerr LY, et al: Ultrasonographic evaluation of gastrointestinal diseases in small animals. Vet Radiol 31:134, 1990.
Original article describing the use of ultrasound in the diagnosis of GI diseases, including neoplasia.
Priester WA: The occurrence of tumors in domestic animals. Natl Cancer Inst Monogr 54:1, 1980.
A cataloging of all tumors occurring in domestic animals.
Theilen GH, Madewell BR: Tumors of the digestive tract. In: Theilen GH, Madewell BR, eds: Veterinary Cancer Medicine. Philadelphia: Lea & Febiger, 1979, pp 307–331.
Textbook review chapter on GI neoplasia.
Twedt DC, Magne ML: Diseases of the stomach. In: Ettinger SJ, ed: Textbook of Veterinary Internal Medicine, 3rd ed. Philadelphia: WB Saunders, 1989, pp 1289–1322.
Textbook review chapter on gastric diseases, including neoplasia.

Neonatal Diarrhea in Puppies and Kittens

JOHNNY D. HOSKINS
Baton Rouge, Louisiana

Neonatal diarrhea commonly occurs from birth to young adulthood in all breeds of dogs and cats in response to insults to the small intestine or large intestine, or a combination of insults to both the small and the large intestine. At this age, diarrhea may also occur secondary to many extraintestinal diseases. Diarrhea typically is of abrupt onset and has a short course that ranges from transient and self-limited to fulminating and explosive. Consideration of the animal's history, physical examination, and stool characteristics—frequency, volume, consistency, color, odor, and composition—can help localize the diarrhea to the small intestine or large intestine, or both, and a search for the cause and treatment can be undertaken (see Table 1). Although neonatal diarrhea may be associated with many different causes, the most common primary diseases are from dietary problems, infectious agents, and endoparasites.

CAUSES

Congenital-Related Diarrhea. Congenital disorders of the intestinal tract that could possibly contribute to neonatal diarrhea are rarely encountered in neonates, probably because most of these animals die at birth or become "fading" puppies or kittens. The congenital disorders that have been reported include atresia of an intestinal segment and duplication of an intestinal segment. These disorders in the newborn puppy or kitten are usually incompatible with life unless surgical correction is undertaken.

Dietary-Related Diarrhea. Successful rearing of nursing and motherless puppies and kittens requires providing them with a suitable environment; the correct quantities and quality of nutrients for different stages of growth; a regular schedule of feeding, sleeping, grooming, and exercise; and the stimuli that provoke micturition and defecation for the first 3 weeks of life. Feeding motherless puppies and kittens that still require milk can be quite rewarding. Mother's milk is always the ideal nourishment for nursing-aged offspring, but various modifications of homemade and commercially prepared formulas simulating mother's milk have been used with good success.

Commercially prepared milk replacement formulas sold specifically for use in nursing puppies or kittens are generally preferred, because they closely compare to mother's milk. The amount of milk replacement formula fed each day is determined by the individual puppy's or kitten's needs (usually 22 to 26 ml of formula per 100 gm of body weight given daily for the first 3 months of life) and is fed in equal portions three or four times daily. The amount of milk replacement formula fed is increased accordingly as the puppy or kitten gains weight and a favorable response to feeding occurs. Puppies should gain 1 to 2 gm/day/lb (2 to 4 gm/day/kg) of anticipated adult weight for the first 5 months of life. At birth, the kitten should weigh 80 to 140 gm (most weighing around 100 to 120 gm) and gain 50 to 100 gm weekly. After each feeding, the abdomen should be enlarged, but not overdistended. When a milk replacement formula is first fed, less than the prescribed amount per feeding should be given for the first feedings. The amount is then gradually increased to the recommended feeding amount by the second or third day.

The most common dietary reason nursing puppies or kittens develop neonatal diarrhea is overfeeding, that is, nursing too frequently or ingesting too much of mother's milk at each feeding. The most common dietary reasons that motherless puppies or kittens develop neonatal diarrhea include feeding a poorly formulated puppy or kitten milk replacement formula, feeding an improperly prepared milk replacement formula, providing inadequate amounts of water in the milk replacement formula (which alters the liquid-to-solid ratio in the formula), and overfeeding the milk replacement formula. When preparing the commercial milk replacement formula, always follow the manufacturer's directions on the label for its proper preparation, and keep all feeding equipment scrupulously clean. Once formula is prepared, it is best stored in the refrigerator at 4°C. The easiest and safest way of feeding a commercial milk replacement formula to puppies and kittens is by nipple bottle feeding or by tube feeding. The nursing and motherless puppy or kitten should be encouraged to begin eating growth food at 3 and 4 weeks of age, respectively. Once they are eating satisfactorily from a bowl, gradually reduce the amount of milk formula fed until only the puppy or kitten food designed for growth is being fed at least three times a day. Weaning should not be complete until they are 6 weeks of age or older.

Another contributing cause to neonatal diarrhea is malnutrition. Undernourishment with an accompanying diarrhea is commonly seen during the time when puppies and kittens depend entirely on their mother for their survival. The nursing puppy and kitten have similar nutritional requirements, and survival for each depends on the mother's ability to care for them, their ability to digest, absorb, and utilize nutrients, and the gradually increasing plane of nutrition provided. The puppy or kitten may ingest insufficient or inadequate milk because the mother dies or fails to care for her young or cannot adequately care for too large a litter, or there may be partial or complete lactation failure by the mother because of illness, mastitis, metritis, or underdeveloped mammae. In addition, the puppy or kitten may be born prematurely or underdeveloped; it may be so weak and sick that it cannot suckle normally, or it may have a congenital defect that precludes adequate milk intake. Failure to provide an adequate growth diet at 3 to 4 weeks of age can also result in inadequate nutrient intake

625

and fiber content to meet the demands of growth and a healthy developing intestinal tract.

The management of neonatal diarrhea resulting from inadequate nutrition for the nursing or motherless puppy and kitten generally requires that the proper amount and type of nourishment as well as fluids and electrolytes be provided. If diarrhea occurs despite receiving adequate amounts of mother's milk or properly prepared milk replacement formula, immediately reduce the amount of milk intake by one half. This can be done by reducing the time allowed for nursing on mother or diluting the milk replacement formula 1:1 with water or, preferably, with a mixture of equal parts of multiple electrolyte solution and 5% dextrose in water solution. As the condition of the feces improves, gradually increase the amount of milk ingested to the level required for adequate growth and the passage of formed stools. No type of milk replacement formula should be given to a weak and severely chilled puppy or kitten that displays a diminished sucking reflex or a rectal temperature below 35°C (95°F).

After weaning puppies and kittens completely to a growth diet, the dietary causes of neonatal diarrhea typically include an abrupt change in diet; intestinal overload from overeating; ingestion of rancid or spoiled foodstuffs; ingestion of indigestible and abrasive foreign material, e.g., bones, rocks, plants, wood, cloth, thread and sewing needles, and plastic objects; intolerance of lactose ingested as milk; and miscellaneous food intolerance, such as to fatty or spicy food. The incidence of ingesting foreign objects is much higher in young dogs and cats, probably because of their developmental chewing habits and curious natures. Trichobezoars (hairballs) are frequently encountered in the diarrheal stools of young long-haired cats and dogs. Many drugs (e.g., anti-inflammatory drugs, antimicrobial agents, and anthelmintics) and chemicals (e.g., heavy metals, cleaning agents, fertilizers, and herbicides) may cause diarrhea. Many ingested plants and plant toxins may also cause diarrhea.

Infectious Diarrhea. Many infectious agents are associated with varying degrees of neonatal diarrhea; the more likely causes of diarrhea are presented in Table 1. Bacteria (e.g., *Salmonella* spp., *Escherichia coli*, *Campylobacter* spp., *Yersinia enterocolitica*, *Bacillus piliformis*, and *Clostridium* spp.) and rickettsial agents (e.g., *Neorickettsia* spp.) reside in and often contribute to severe mucosal damage in the small or large intestine. Viruses—for example, canine distemper, canine parvovirus type 2 (CPV-2), canine parvovirus-type 1 (CPV-1), coronavirus, and rotavirus—are important causes of infectious diarrhea in young dogs. Other viruses that have been identified in unformed stools of dogs are astrovirus, herpesvirus, enterovirus, calicivirus, and parainfluenza viruses. Feline parvovirus (feline panleukopenia virus) and coronaviruses are the most prominent viruses in young cats; other viruses have been identified, including rotavirus, astrovirus, calicivirus, and reovirus. In refractory diarrheal problems or poorly growing kittens, feline leukemia virus (FeLV), feline immunodeficiency virus (FIV), and feline infectious peritonitis (FIP) virus should be considered. The primary fungi infecting the intestinal tract are *Histoplasma capsulatum*, *Aspergillus*

spp., and *Pythium* spp.; however, they are uncommon in dogs and cats younger than 6 months of age.

The newest cause of canine viral enteritis of young puppies is *canine parvovirus type 1* (CPV-1; also referred to as minute virus of canines or MVC), which was first isolated from the feces of military dogs. CPV-1 is distinctly differentiated from CPV-2 by its host cell range, spectrum of hemagglutination, genomic properties, and antigenicity. The physical and chemical properties of CPV-1 are, however, typical of parvoviruses. CPV-1 can be propagated on the Walter Reed canine cell line. The dog is the only known host, although it is likely that other members of Canidae are susceptible. Before 1985, CPV-1 was considered a nonpathogenic parvovirus of dogs; however, since 1985, clinical infections of CPV-1 in neonatal puppies have been encountered by practicing veterinarians and diagnostic laboratory personnel. It appears to be widespread in the dog population but is restricted to causing clinical disease in puppies younger than 6 weeks of age. It seems reasonable to assume that spread is similar to that of CPV-2.

The pathogenicity of CPV-1 for dogs is unclear at present. CPV-1 has been identified by immunoelectron microscopy in the feces of puppies and dogs with mild diarrhea. Four to six days after oral exposure, CPV-1 can be recovered from the small intestine, spleen, mesenteric lymph nodes, and thymus. The histologic changes in lymphoid tissue are similar to those observed in puppies infected with CPV-2 but are less severe. In addition, CPV-1 is capable of crossing the placenta and producing early fetal deaths and birth defects. CPV-1 has been observed infrequently in field dogs with mild diarrhea as well as in the feces of clinically healthy animals. Primarily, CPV-1 infection is a clinical disease in puppies between 5 and 21 days old. Affected puppies are usually presented with diarrhea, vomiting, dyspnea, and constant crying. Sudden death has also been observed.

CPV-1 infection should be considered in young dogs with mild diarrhea that are CPV-2 negative on routine "parvovirus tests" and also in unexplained fetal abnormalities, abortions, or fading puppies. CPV-1 has been observed by electron microscopy in fecal and rectal swab samples from field dogs. Immunoelectron microscopy is necessary for distinguishing CPV-1 from CPV-2. Inhibition of hemagglutinating activity in stool suspensions by specific antiserum is also diagnostic for CPV-1. Sera can be tested for specific antibody by use of virus neutralization or hemagglutination inhibition tests. Since only Walter Reed canine cell line supports growth of CPV-1, the availability of virus isolation and serum virus neutralization tests is limited. Once a diagnosis has been made, treatment of puppies with CPV-1 infection is unrewarding because of the rapid progression of the disease. However, mortality may be reduced by ensuring that the environmental temperature of newborn puppies is kept warm and adequate nutrition and hydration are provided. No vaccine is available at the present time.

Endoparasitic Diarrhea. Endoparasites generally do not produce intestinal lesions but contribute importantly to generalized unthriftiness, diarrhea, and weight loss or failure to gain adequate body weight. The younger the animal, the more frequently are endoparasites present and the more

TABLE 1. Causes of Neonatal Diarrhea in Puppies and Kittens

Causes	Basis for Diagnosis	Mode of Treatment
Dietary Abrupt change in diet Overfeeding Indiscretion: garbage ingestion, ingestion of abrasive or indigestible material Food intolerance Intolerance of lactose ingested as milk	History, response to diet modification	Control of diet fed
Drug- and Toxin-Induced Anti-inflammatory drugs Antimicrobials Anthelmintics Heavy metals: lead, arsenic, thallium Insecticides: organophosphates Plants	History of exposure	Eliminate exposure to the offending agent

Endoparasitic
Helminths
  Ascarids
  Hookworms
  Whipworms
  Strongyloides
Others: cestodes, trematodes, *Trichinella*
Protozoa
  Coccidia: *Cystoisospora, Cryptosporidium, Giardia*
  Others: *Pentatrichomonas, Entamoeba, Balantidium*
	Fecal examinations	Specific anthelmintics and antiprotozoal drugs

Viral Parvoviruses Coronaviruses Rotavirus Others: Canine distemper, FeLV, FIV, FIP	Clinical signs, demonstration of virus in feces, serology	Fluid therapy and other supportive care
Bacterial *Salmonella* spp. *Campylobacter* spp. *Yersinia enterocolitica* *Bacillus piliformis* Others: *E. coli, Clostridium* spp.	Specialized fecal cultures	Specific antimicrobial agents
Rickettsial Salmon poisoning disease	Clinical signs, endemic habitat, fecal examination for a fluke, eggs	Tetracycline-class drugs and other supportive care
Obstructive Intestinal foreign body Intussusception Intestinal volvulus	Clinical signs, abdominal palpation, contrast GI radiography	Surgery and supportive care
Idiopathic Chronic Diarrhea in Young Cats	Clinical signs, rule out other causes of diarrhea	Dietary management and time
Extraintestinal Renal failure Hepatic disease Hypoadrenocorticism Acute pancreatitis Diabetes mellitus	Serum or plasma biochemical profile, organ function tests	Various treatments to manage the underlying extraintestinal disease

severe the consequences of endoparasitism. Endoparasitism often complicates other existing intestinal disorders, such as virus- or bacteria-induced enterocolitis. The more common endoparasites that are identified in the intestinal tract of young dogs and cats are listed in Table 1.

Idiopathic Chronic Diarrhea in Young Cats. Young cats occasionally develop intractable idiopathic chronic diarrhea. Most affected cats recover spontaneously by approximately 6 to 12 months of age. The cats are usually bright and alert and still eat well. The diarrhea is most often watery and voluminous. Clinical signs of large intestine inflammation are occasionally present but are usually low grade. Little is known about the cause and pathogenesis of idiopathic diarrhea, but it is likely multifactorial. Early in life, the digestive and absorptive functions of the small intestine are not fully developed. In addition, the colon of the kitten cannot compensate for failure of the small intestine to absorb water and electrolytes. The intestinal dysfunction can then be exacerbated by poor feeding practices by owners or insults from various infectious or endoparasitic agents, resulting in chronic diarrhea. As with adults, young cats can develop diarrhea from a multitude of primary gastrointestinal diseases or diseases of other organs, and the diagnostic approach to the chronic diarrhea is similar in both young and adult cats. If no diagnosis is apparent after initial laboratory tests have been performed and antiparasitic therapy has been prescribed, and if no other warning signs of serious disease are apparent, it would be appropriate to feed a controlled diet (e.g., Iams dry kitten food) for 3 to 4 weeks to determine whether the diarrhea is food responsive. The diet probably should contain a single protein source that the cat has not been fed in the last several months. The addition of a small quantity of a fermentable fiber is also of value in the management of some cats. Frequent small feedings are advantageous.

Extraintestinal Diarrhea. Other disorders, including renal failure, hepatic disease, acute pancreatitis, neurologic disease, shock, sepsis, hypoadrenocorticism, diabetes mellitus, stress, and even altered behavior, may play a prominent role in the cause of neonatal diarrhea.

DIAGNOSIS

The diagnosis of neonatal diarrhea is usually made on the basis of history, signs, and physical findings, often without detailed diagnostic procedures. A review of dietary management, current medications, and possible exposure to chemicals or infectious diseases is warranted. Endoparasites, ingestion of milk replacement formula, questionable food or foreign material, and infectious diseases should always be considered the primary possible causes of diarrhea in the young dog or cat until proved otherwise. Animals that experience severe illness or fail to respond to symptomatic therapy usually require a more detailed medical and laboratory evaluation. Diagnostic efforts should then be aimed at the detection of an underlying extraintestinal disease as the contributing cause of the diarrhea. Diagnostic evaluations considered for short-term diarrhea are fecal identification of endoparasites, virologic tests, fecal cultures for bacteria, and abdominal radiographs for the detection of intestinal foreign material or an obstruction. Occasionally, a complete blood count (CBC) and serum biochemistries are obtained.

TREATMENT

Neonatal diarrhea is treated on the basis of the animal's history, signs, and physical findings. Symptomatic treatment is given initially for most cases of diarrhea. As with adults, most neonatal animals with diarrhea show improvement within 24 to 48 hours with little or no therapy and are usually treated on an outpatient basis. The basic principles in the treatment of neonatal diarrhea include removing the inciting cause; providing proper conditions for promoting mucosal repair; correcting fluid, electrolyte, and acid-base abnormalities; and alleviating secondary complications, for example, vomiting, abdominal pain, and sepsis.

Parenteral fluids are initiated when electrolyte or acid-base imbalances or dehydration occurs. The quantity of fluids given should be enough to supply daily maintenance needs (approximately 40 to 60 ml/kg per day), to correct existing dehydration, and to replace fluid losses that may occur with continued diarrhea (see *CVT XII*, p. 34). Neonatal diarrhea generally results in volume depletion and losses of sodium, chloride, bicarbonate, and potassium with metabolic acidosis. An isotonic, balanced electrolyte solution, such as lactated Ringer's solution, is usually recommended. Potassium levels are often depleted, particularly if inappetence has accompanied profuse diarrhea, and additional potassium chloride should be added to the fluids. The amount of potassium chloride added is based on the existing serum or plasma potassium levels.

Protectants are used frequently in the general treatment of diarrhea. Of the salicylates, bismuth subsalicylate appears to be effective as an oral antidiarrheal compound; however, it probably should be administered with caution in neonates and in young cats and should not be administered to animals younger than 3 months of age. The use of narcotic analgesics as antimotility drugs is warranted in the treatment of some diarrheas. These drugs effectively relieve abdominal pain and tenesmus and reduce the frequency of stools. The narcotic analgesics, such as diphenoxylate hydrochloride and loperamide hydrochloride, are the preferred motility modifiers to be used in the symptomatic treatment of diarrhea.

Because of the frequent occurrence of endoparasites as the primary or secondary cause of diarrhea in the young dog or cat, routine administration of an appropriate antiparasitic drug is recommended (see Appendix). The use of antimicrobial agents in the treatment of diarrhea is controversial. If antimicrobial agents only succeed in inhibiting the normal intestinal flora, they are detrimental. In diarrhea, antimicrobial therapy is warranted only when there is evidence of inflammation in the gastrointestinal tract (numerous inflammatory cells in the feces), damaged intestinal mucosa (blood in the stool), a systemic inflammatory reaction (fever and leukocytosis), or abnormal fecal culture results.

References and Suggested Reading

Hoskins JD: The digestive system. In: Hoskins JD, ed: Veterinary Pediatrics: Dogs and Cats From Birth to Six Months. Philadelphia: WB Saunders, 1995, pp 133–187.

Hoskins JD: Canine viral enteritis. In: Greene CE, ed: Infectious Diseases of the Dog and Cat. Philadelphia: WB Saunders, 1998, pp 40–49.

CVT Update: Diagnosis and Treatment of Parvovirus

Jennifer M. Rewerts
Leah A. Cohn
Columbia, Missouri

Canine parvovirus is probably the most common cause of infectious enteritis in dogs. Parvoviruses are single-stranded, nonenveloped DNA viruses that are ubiquitous in the environment and highly resistant to inactivation. A type 1 canine parvovirus (CPV-1) can be isolated from healthy dogs and is considered to be nonpathogenic except in neonates (see previous article). This article focuses on canine parvovirus type 2 (CPV-2), which emerged in 1978 as an important veterinary pathogen, most often resulting in severe enteritis.

TRANSMISSION AND PATHOGENESIS

Virus is shed in the feces of infected dogs, and transmission occurs via the fecal-oral route. Young puppies lacking sufficient antibody protection are most commonly affected.

As an essential part of its own replication, CPV-2 infects rapidly dividing cells. The cells most commonly affected include those of the lymphoid system, intestinal tract, and bone marrow. Disruption of intestinal epithelium, with necrosis of the intestinal villi and crypts, results in severe hemorrhagic diarrhea. Infection of marrow myeloprogenitor cells and direct infection of lymphoid cells contribute to leukopenia. When infection occurs in utero or shortly after birth, cardiac myocytes are destroyed, resulting in myocarditis and death in neonatal puppies. Although this presentation was common in the late 1970s and early 1980s, today neonatal death due to cardiac disease has become extremely rare because most adult bitches have some degree of immunity to parvovirus.

Following oronasal inoculation, viral replication occurs in the tonsils, retropharyngeal lymph nodes, and mesenteric lymph nodes (Meunier et al, 1985a). Viremia occurs 3 to 4 days after inoculation, at which time the virus begins intestinal shedding and can be detected in the feces. Animals may become febrile at the onset of viremia, but gastrointestinal signs lag behind viremia by 2 to 3 days as virus continues its rapid intracellular replication.

RISK FACTORS

Several risk factors for parvoviral enteritis have been identified. Parvovirus is primarily a disease of young dogs lacking protective antibody titers. Nonvaccinated puppies are at highest risk, although puppies that have not completed their series of vaccinations are also frequently affected. Although maternal antibody is protective during the first several weeks of life, it interferes with vaccine-induced development of a strong humoral immune response. Even

in vaccinated pups, there is a short period of time during which maternal antibody levels decline below protective levels but vaccine-induced immunity has not yet developed. This "window of susceptibility" often occurs shortly after weaning, when an increase in the mitotic rate of enterocytes makes them an especially prime target for CPV-2 infection.

A number of other risk factors have been identified as well. Rottweilers, Doberman pinschers, and Staffordshire terrier breeds are reported to have an increased risk of infection (Houston et al, 1996). Persistence of maternal antibody past the age at which vaccine series are usually completed or hereditary factors such as an altered humoral responsiveness have been speculated to contribute to breed-associated susceptibility. Intact male dogs are infected disproportionately to their population. Climate may be a risk factor as well, with an increase in cases reported between the months of July and September in temperate climates, while warmer climates see cases more evenly distributed throughout the year. Lastly, concurrent viral, bacterial, or parasitic infections may leave animals more susceptible to infection and worsen the prognosis for recovery after CPV-2 illness.

CLINICAL PRESENTATION

The clinical signs vary with the stage of illness and disease severity (Table 1). Severity is determined by the dose of viral inoculum, the virulence of the strain, and the host's immune response. Animals may become transiently febrile and lethargic at the time of initial viremia, with no associated gastrointestinal signs. Anorexia, depression, vomiting, and diarrhea generally follow 2 to 3 days later, when fever may or may not be present. Vomiting is often copious and protracted, and diarrhea is frequently characterized by large volumes of watery stools with mucous and

TABLE 1. Common Clinical Signs and Laboratory Abnormalities Associated With Canine Parvovirus

Clinical Signs	Laboratory Abnormalities
Fever	Leukopenia
Lethargy	Lymphopenia
Anorexia	Neutropenia
Vomiting	Anemia
Bloody diarrhea	Hypoproteinemia
Dehydration	Hypoglycemia
	Hypokalemia
	Hyponatremia
	Hypochloremia
	Metabolic acidosis

either frank or digested blood. Patients are often severely dehydrated on presentation.

Leukopenia is commonly associated with parvoviral infection. The initial leukopenia is the result of direct viral lymphocytolysis at the time of viremia. Although lymphocyte counts may rapidly rebound, profound neutropenia typically develops near the same time as the onset of gastrointestinal signs. Both peripheral neutrophil consumption (especially in the gastrointestinal tract) and destruction of progenitor cells within the bone marrow contribute to neutropenia.

Less consistent hematologic consequences of parvoviral enteritis include anemia, thrombocytopenia, and hypoproteinemia. Blood loss through the gastrointestinal tract can be severe and may lead to anemia and hypoproteinemia. Because young puppies have lower red blood cell counts to begin with, they are especially susceptible to anemia in association with hemorrhagic diarrhea. Thrombocytopenia occasionally results from increased platelet utilization in the gastrointestinal tract combined with destruction of megakaryocytic bone marrow precursors.

Several abnormalities are commonly identified on serum chemistry profiles. Hypoglycemia and hypokalemia may result from a lack of nutritional intake in young puppies. Vomiting, diarrhea, and dehydration may result in metabolic acidosis, hyponatremia, and hypochloremia. Less often, prerenal azotemia, elevated liver enzymes, and hyperbilirubinemia are observed to develop.

The complications of parvovirus that alter clinical signs and laboratory parameters either may be apparent at initial presentation or may develop during the course of therapy. Important complications include septicemia or endotoxemia, disseminated intravascular coagulation (DIC), and intestinal intussusception. Sepsis and DIC occur as the result of compromised intestinal barrier function and neutropenia. Intestinal hypermotility predisposes to intussusception, the clinical signs of which (vomiting and depression) could be easily mistaken for worsening viral illness. Careful and gentle daily physical examinations are a crucial part of care for the patient with parvovirus.

DIAGNOSIS

Confirmation of a diagnosis of CPV-2 consists of virus detection or determination of antibody titers (see *CVT XII,* p. 697). Virus detection via virus isolation, electron microscopy, fecal hemagglutination, or enzyme-linked immunosorbent assay (ELISA) for parvovirus antigen is often performed on fecal material, rectal swabs, or biopsies from the intestinal tract of affected animals. The most practical method for most veterinarians is the parvoviral ELISA antigen test (CITE, Idexx). The test is easily performed on fecal material from a rectal swab. Although the test is reasonably accurate, animals with suggestive clinical and laboratory signs but negative ELISA results should be handled as if they have parvovirus until proved otherwise. Because this test is often performed on recently vaccinated puppies, it is important to note that the manufacturers acknowledge that modified live parvoviral vaccines may result in a weak positive test result from 5 to 15 days after vaccination.

TREATMENT

The prognosis for survival in puppies infected with parvovirus is fair to good with supportive care. Average survival rates for dogs in the authors' hospital range between 80 and 90%. Previously noted breeds with an increased risk of contracting parvovirus may experience a higher mortality.

Fluid Therapy and Nutrition

Volume support with appropriate fluid therapy is a fundamental component of treatment for parvoviral enteritis. Dehydration is often rapid in onset and severe, especially in younger pups. Crystalloid fluids are the usual choice for correcting dehydration, providing maintenance fluid volumes, and replacing ongoing fluid losses. In the authors' hospital lactated Ringer's solution (LRS) is used most often. Because vomiting and anorexia often result in hypokalemia, fluids are supplemented with potassium chloride (e.g., 8 mEq of KCl/500 ml of fluid). Since hypoglycemia is common in young puppies, crystalloid fluids are supplemented with concentrated dextrose solution to make a 5% dextrose solution (e.g., 100 ml of 50% dextrose/L of fluids). An excellent review of fluid therapy in the puppy is found in *CVT XII,* p. 34. Anemia and hypoproteinemia may be sufficiently severe to warrant transfusion of packed red cells, whole blood, or plasma in addition to crystalloid or colloid fluid therapy.

Because feeding can exacerbate vomiting, most dogs with parvoviral enteritis should be withheld from food and water (NPO). Although adult dogs generally do well without food for several days, younger puppies may require nutritional support if they must to be kept NPO for more than a few days. Total parenteral nutrition (TPN) provides optimum support, but because of the needs for a central line, maintenance of complete asepsis, and frequent evaluation of electrolyte status, it may not be practical in all veterinary hospitals. A less cumbersome option is partial parenteral nutrition (PPN), which can be administered through a peripheral venous line (see p. 80). Enteral feeding is usually reinstituted after at least 24 hours have elapsed without vomiting. Initially, water is offered in small amounts, and if vomiting does not recur, small-volume, frequent feedings of a bland diet may be instituted. Several commercial diets are appropriate for this, including Hill's I/D (Science Diet; Topeka, KS), Iams Low Residue Diet (Eukanaba; Dayton, OH), and Purina EN (Purina, St. Louis, MO).

Antibiotics

Parenteral administration of broad-spectrum antibiotics is warranted in parvoviral enteritis because of the combination of severe disruption of the intestinal epithelial barrier (potentially allowing entry of bacteria into the blood stream) and peripheral neutropenia. A combination of either ampicillin (Omnipen-N, Wyeth) or a first- or second-generation cephalosporin and an aminoglycoside provide excellent broad-spectrum coverage (Table 2). Aminoglycosides are potentially nephrotoxic and should not be administered until hydration has been restored. Although they

TABLE 2. Drugs Used Commonly in the Treatment of Parvoviral Enteritis

Drug Name	Brand Name	Dosage
Antibiotics		
Ampicillin sodium	Omnipen Principen	10–40 mg/kg IV, IM, SC q6–8hr
Cephazolin sodium	Ancef Kefzol Cefazolin	22 mg/kg IV, IM, SC q6–8hr
Amikacin	Amiglyde-V	5–10 mg/kg IV, IM, SC q8hr
Gentamicin sulfate	Gentocin	2–4 mg/kg IV, IM, SC q6–8hr
Antiemetics		
Metoclopramide hydrochloride	Reglan	0.2–0.5 mg/kg IV,* IM, SC q6–8hr *or* 1–2 mg/kg/day constant-rate infusion
Prochlorperazine	Compazine	0.1–0.5 mg/kg IM, SC q6–8hr

*Slow IV injection.

possess a broad antimicrobial spectrum, fluoroquinolones should be used with caution (if at all) in growing animals. In the authors' experience, cefazolin (Cefazolin, Bristol-Myers Squibb) and amikacin (Amiglyde-V, Fort Dodge) is the antibiotic combination of choice.

Antiemetics

Medical control of vomiting is essential in many parvoviral-infected patients. Severe vomiting contributes to fluid loss and patient distress and makes enteral nutritional support impossible. Metoclopramide (Reglan, Robins) can be an effective centrally acting antiemetic that also increases gastrointestinal motility. In the authors' experience, constant-rate infusion of metoclopramide controls vomiting better than intermittent parenteral administration (see Table 2). Prochloperazine (Compazine, Schein) is the authors' preferred antiemetic. Its actions are entirely central. Although it causes a greater degree of sedation than metoclopramide, the authors have had very good results with minimal sedation at a dose of 0.1 to 0.5 mg/kg IM or SC every 6 to 8 hours.

Colony-Stimulating Factors

Colony-stimulating factors are cytokine growth factors that stimulate differentiation and maturation of specific hematopoietic cell lines in the bone marrow as well as prompt release of mature cells from the marrow (see pp. 403 and 408). Several hematopoietic factors have become commercially available in the recombinant human (rh) form. One of these, granulocyte colony-stimulating factor (rhG-CSF/filgrastim) (Nupogen, Amgen) has been used to good effect in the treatment of chemotherapy-induced neutropenia and has been advocated in the treatment of parvovirus-associated neutropenia as well. Granulocytic precursors are stimulated to mature, and the resulting neutrophils are released from the bone marrow storage pool into the peripheral circulation in response to G-CSF.

These effects have prompted the empirical use of rhG-CSF in dogs with parvoviral enteritis, although the merit of this therapy has not been established. Indeed, a controlled study in the authors' hospital (Rewerts et al, 1998) compared time to neutrophil count recovery, duration of

hospitalization, and survival rates in two equivalent groups of parvoviral enteritis puppies treated identically except for the administration of rhG-CSF (5 μg/kg every 24 hours SC) to one group. No advantage was found in any parameter including survival in the group treated with rhG-CSF. This may be because, unlike chemotherapy-induced neutropenia, by the time rhG-CSF treatment is begun parvoviral patients are already neutropenic. It is reasonable to expect that they will have already released stored neutrophils, and severe inflammatory disease coupled with neutropenia might elicit enough production of endogenous G-CSF that exogenous rhG-CSF provides little additional benefit.

Other Treatments

A number of less commonly used therapies have gained acceptance in some regions, based largely on anecdotal reports. Flunixin meglumine (Banamine, Schering-Plough) is a nonsteroidal anti-inflammatory drug commonly believed to provide beneficial effects in the treatment of endotoxemia. The adverse effects of flunixin meglumine may include gastrointestinal ulceration and nephrotoxicity, especially in dehydrated patients. Equine endotoxin antiserum (Endoserum, Immvac, Inc.) has been proposed as an effective and safe treatment in CPV-2 infections (Dimmitt, 1991). This equine-origin antiserum raised in response to a mutant *Salmonella typhimurium* bacterin-toxoid is proposed to provide cross-protective antiendotoxin antibodies and perhaps other unknown protections against gram-negative bacterial toxins. The authors are unable to recommend the routine use of either of these compounds at this time because of the potential for adverse effects and the lack of scientific studies that document effectiveness in the treatment of endotoxemia associated with parvoviral enteritis. Administration of GI protectants, H_2 blockers, or ion pump blockers is empirical and based on practitioner preference.

PREVENTION

Routine immunization is essential to the prevention of parvovirus infections. Vaccinations should begin at 6 to 8 weeks of age with boosters every 3 or 4 weeks until the animal reaches at least 16 weeks of age. Clients should be educated about the critical period during which maternal antibody has waned and vaccinal immunity is incomplete, and advised to limit exposure of pups to other dogs during this time. Vaccination at 20 to 22 weeks is recommended in "at-risk" breeds, including Rottweilers and Doberman pinschers. Previously unvaccinated adult dogs should receive two initial doses of modified live parvovirus vaccine 3 to 4 weeks apart. A newer generation of vaccines including those produced by Intervet (Progard-7, Intervet) may provide a stronger antibody response and therefore offer better protection against infection (McCaw et al, 1997). Until there is evidence to the contrary, the authors recommend following the directions of vaccine manufacturers to administer booster shots of vaccines yearly. A viable alternative to yearly revaccination is the assessment of protective antibody titer on a yearly basis. For more information on vaccinations refer to *CVT XI,* p. 202.

References and Suggested Reading

Dimmitt R: Clinical experience with cross-protective anti-endotoxin antiserum dogs with parvoviral enteritis. Can Pract 16:23, 1991.
A report on the use of equine antiserum in the treatment of dogs with parvoviral enteritis.
Houston DM, Ribble CS, Head LL: Risk factors associated with parvovirus enteritis in dogs: 283 cases (1982–1991). J Am Vet Med Assoc 208:542, 1996.
A retrospective study examining associated risk factors in dogs affected with parvovirus enteritis.
McCaw DL, Tate D, Dubovi EJ, et al: Early protection of puppies against canine parvovirus: A comparison of two vaccines. J Am Anim Hosp Assoc 33:244, 1997.
A comparison of two vaccines types based on individual immunologic response.
Meunier PC, Cooper BJ, Appel MJG, et al: Pathogenesis of canine parvovirus enteritis: Sequential virus distribution and passive immunization studies. Vet Pathol 22:617, 1985a.
A controlled study describing the pathogenesis of parvovirus from the onset of viremia through recovery.
Meunier PC, Cooper BJ, Appel MJG, et al: Pathogenesis of canine parvovirus enteritis: The importance of viremia. Vet Pathol 22:60, 1985b.
A description of the pathogenesis of parvovirus enteritis and the most commonly associated hematologic changes.
Rewerts JM, McCaw DL, Cohn LA, et al: Recombinant human granulocyte colony-stimulating factor for treatment of puppies with neutropenia secondary to canine parvovirus infection. J Am Vet Med Assoc 213:991, 1998.
Controlled clinical trial of G-CSF in dogs with parvovirus infection.

Dietary Sensitivity

EDWARD J. HALL
Bristol, United Kingdom

The management of dietary sensitivity is very simple: by feeding a diet that excludes the offending foodstuff the patient will be free from clinical signs. The key to treatment is the diagnosis and identification of the foodstuff that must be excluded, and it is here that difficulties arise. Yet, food allergy as a cause of both dermatologic and gastrointestinal (GI) disease is in vogue with pet owners, and the current growth industry in special veterinary exclusion diets would suggest that the condition is both common and readily diagnosed (see p. 530). Neither is true. Other causes of pruritus and diarrhea are more common, and as some of them respond to dietary manipulation (Table 1), they must be ruled out before an exclusion diet trial is performed.

MECHANISMS

Any repeatable adverse reaction to food that can be successfully managed solely by exclusion of a specific dietary component is defined as a true dietary sensitivity (Fig. 1). It may be a manifestation of either an immunologically mediated event, that is, a true food allergy, or a nonimmunologic event, that is, a food intolerance. Predisposition to both intolerances (through individual variations in the intestinal flora, enzyme activities, and permeability, and hepatic metabolism) and allergy may be influenced by genetic factors.

Current hypotheses of food allergy propose that there is an inadequate mucosal barrier and/or abnormal presentation of dietary antigens to the mucosal immune system, or that there is actual dysregulation of the immune system, or both. Either hypothesis could explain both genetic susceptibility to the development of allergy, and development of allergies after a primary GI insult. This would correlate with current clinical suspicions of apparent breed susceptibility, and development of allergies after diseases such as viral enteritis. Mechanisms of food allergy and tolerance

TABLE 1. Conditions That May Improve Clinically in Response to Dietary Modification

Food allergy
Food intolerance
Small intestinal bacterial overgrowth
Inflammatory bowel disease
Lymphangiectasia
Pancreatitis
Exocrine pancreatic insufficiency
Chronic gastritis
Gastroesophageal reflux
Gastric emptying disorders
Portosystemic shunt
Atopy
Flea-bite hypersensitivity?

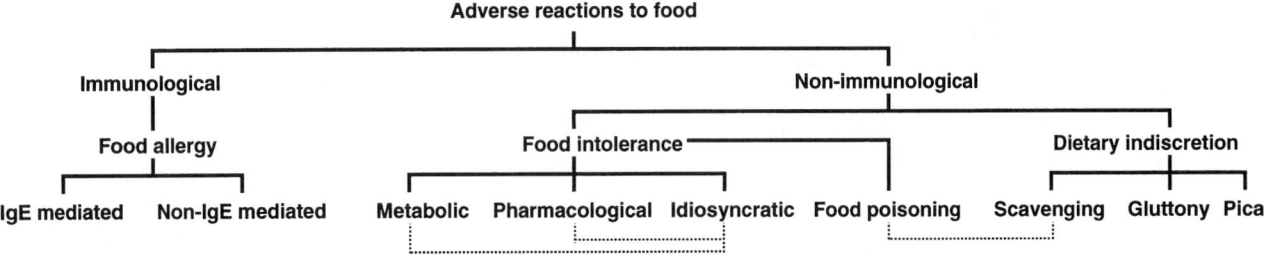

Figure 1. Classification of adverse reactions to food. Overlaps between categories are indicated by dotted lines. Food poisoning and dietary indiscretion are not necessarily repeatable and are therefore not true dietary sensitivities. (From Hall EJ: Gastrointestinal aspects of food allergy: A review. J Small Anim Pract 35:146, 1994, with permission.)

have been discussed previously in detail (see *CVT XII,* pp. 59 to 64).

In reality, whether a dietary sensitivity is an allergy or intolerance is largely irrelevant clinically; the signs may be similar and the diagnosis and treatment by dietary exclusion should be the same. Lactose "intolerance" is diagnosed in dogs and cats, but whether this represents a true intolerance (either a congenital lack of intestinal lactase activity or a relative lactase deficiency secondary to mucosal disease) or a true allergic reaction to milk protein is rarely defined; simple exclusion of dairy products resolves the clinical signs. Distinction between allergy and intolerance is only relevant if immunosuppressive drugs are indicated, or if there are allergic cross-reactivities that require related foodstuffs to be excluded.

MANIFESTATIONS

Clinical Picture

Although a positive response to dietary manipulation is crucial to the diagnosis, dietary sensitivity may be suspected clinically. A temporal association between ingestion of a particular food and signs is very suggestive, but acquired sensitivities to foods that have been in the normal diet for years also occur. Food allergy may be an recognizable immediate (type 1), IgE-mediated hypersensitivity. However, mixed or delayed reactions are probably more common, and the inevitable delay between food ingestion and the onset of signs obscures any causative link, particularly if repeated ingestion causes chronic disease.

Conflicting reports in the literature about possible breed predispositions to food allergic skin disease probably reflect the small numbers of documented cases, as well as geographic differences in the genetic pool and popularities of particular breeds. There are even fewer documented cases of diet-responsive GI disease; gluten-sensitivity has been documented in Irish setters and Soft-Coated Wheaten terriers but undoubtedly occurs in other breeds. Although there is an apparent predisposition for food allergic skin and GI disease in retrievers in the United Kingdom, this information cannot necessarily be extrapolated to other countries.

Food allergic skin disease can affect either sex but tends to occur in two different age groups; young animals (<1 year) and middle-aged to older dogs and cats. Allergy in young animals may develop because of an inadequate mucosal barrier, an immature immune system, and early wean-ing. Acquired sensitivity in older animals may follow a primary GI insult.

Clinical Signs

Food intolerances might be expected to produce primarily GI signs, although cutaneous signs could occur through nonimmunologic histamine release, pharmacologic effects, or photosensitization. In contrast, the majority of reports of food allergy in the veterinary literature have focused on cutaneous signs (see *CVT XII,* p. 59). However, it has been suggested recently that the co-existence of GI and cutaneous signs has been overlooked (Paterson, 1995). A survey of dogs with diet-responsive disease seen at the University of Bristol in 1996 revealed that 6 of 11 dogs with predominantly pruritic signs also had minor GI signs (H.A. Jackson, personal communication); 6 of 19 dogs with predominantly GI signs did have minor skin signs, but, apart from one dog with pruritus, all these signs could have been secondary to malnutrition. Gastrointestinal signs are seen in only 5% of human patients with gluten-sensitive skin lesions (dermatitis herpetiformis), although histologic examination shows a subclinical enteropathy in 95% of them. While the clinical signs are predominantly associated with the skin and GI tract, systemic signs may be seen and other organ systems are potential targets (Table 2). Anorexia and lethargy are nonspecific signs, while urticaria-angioedema and, very rarely, anaphylaxis are more specific and dramatic signs that may be caused by dietary sensitivity. Reports of food-responsive orthopedic, respiratory, behavioral, and central nervous system disease are anecdotal in veterinary medicine, but an exclusion diet could be tried if all else fails.

Skin Disease. Nonseasonal pruritus lacking any characteristic distribution is suggestive of food allergy. Localized pruritus of the face, ears, and feet are sometimes noted, but the itching can be generalized. A primary papular eruption may occur, but most visible skin lesions are the result of self-trauma, although secondary pyoderma and bilateral pruritic otitis externa are sometimes recognized. In cats, facial or generalized pruritus is characteristic, but miliary dermatitis, eosinophilic granuloma complex, and feline symmetrical alopecia may all, occasionally, be related to food allergy. No pathognomonic histologic changes are recognized on skin biopsy, although a perivascular eosinophil infiltrate may suggest an allergic etiology.

TABLE 2. Possible Clinical Signs of Food Allergies

Systemic Signs	Eosinophilic granuloma complex
Anorexia	(cats)
Lethargy	**Gastrointestinal Signs**
Peripheral lymphadenopathy	Vomiting
(cats)	Hematemesis
Urticaria-angioedema	Diarrhea
Anaphylaxis	"Small intestinal–like"
Cutaneous Signs	Profuse, watery
Primary papules	Borborygmi
Erythroderma	Melena
Pruritus	"Colitis-like"
Localized	Mucoid
Face	Bloody
Ears	Increased frequency and
Feet	tenesmus
Generalized	Abdominal pain/"colic"
Self-trauma	Weight loss and/or stunting
Erythema	Altered appetite
Alopecia	**Other Organ Systems**
Hyperpigmentation	Orthopedic?
Crusts and lichenification	Arthropathies
Excoriations	Respiratory?
Focal lick lesions	Rhinitis and conjunctivitis (cats)
Secondary pyoderma	Bronchoconstriction (asthma)
Scaling	CNS?
Pruritic otitis externa	Behavioral
Miliary dermatitis (cats)	Seizures

Gastrointestinal Disease. The signs of food allergic GI disease have not been well characterized and, unfortunately, are not specific. Vomiting, diarrhea, and abdominal pain are the signs most commonly associated with food allergy, but weight loss and failure to thrive may occasionally be seen even in the absence of the former localizing signs.

As with skin disease, no pathognomonic histologic changes are recognized on gut biopsy. Indeed, lack of any histologic changes is still consistent with dietary sensitivity; an intolerance is most likely to cause only a functional disturbance, and a type 1 hypersensitivity may resolve while food is being withheld before biopsy. Even if there are histologic abnormalities, there is an apparent overlap with changes seen in idiopathic inflammatory bowel disease (IBD).

DIAGNOSIS

The Problems

The cornerstone of the diagnosis of a dietary sensitivity is the response to dietary manipulation; remission with exclusion of a specific dietary component and relapse when challenged with the offending component are essential criteria for a definitive diagnosis. The problems are the paucity of objective criteria by which to judge response, and the fact that other diseases may respond to dietary manipulation (see Table 1). Furthermore, many cases are never satisfactorily followed through the challenge phase for positive proof, and often antibiotics are given for secondary pyoderma or small intestinal bacterial overgrowth (SIBO; see p. 637). Resolution of cutaneous signs with an exclusion diet may also be a reflection of a phenomenon called the allergic threshold. Atopic and flea-allergic dogs, when fed an exclusion diet, may be taken below this threshold

by a reduction in the overall antigenic load and therefore scratch less.

Preliminary Investigations

Although there may be an index of suspicion for a dietary sensitivity, there are no pathognomonic signs. Other major differential diagnoses should be ruled out before one begins an exclusion diet trial, as these conditions may be, at least partially, responsive to dietary change (see Table 1). Following a minimum database of hematology, serum biochemistry (including bile acids), and urinalysis to rule out systemic disease, specific investigations of the skin and GI tract should be performed.

Ectoparasites and skin infections as causes of pruritus should be diagnosed and treated before one considers a food trial. Ideally, flea-allergic dermatitis and atopy should also be excluded first, as an exclusion diet may take the pruritic patient below the allergic threshold, leading to a potentially incomplete diagnosis.

Preferably three fecal examinations should be performed to detect parasitism; alternatively empirical treatment with fenbendazole is given for possible occult *Giardia* or *Trichuris* infection. In young dogs, idiopathic SIBO is common but definitive diagnosis is difficult; therefore, empirical antibiotic therapy may be tried. Recurrent, antibiotic-responsive, chronic diarrhea beginning in adult dogs may also suggest a diagnosis of SIBO, but a search for an underlying cause, such as a partial obstruction, mucosal disease, or food allergy, should be made. Mucosal diseases, such as IBD or lymphangiectasia, are diagnosed by intestinal biopsy. However, many of the histologic changes seen in IBD can also be seen with food allergies.

Indirect Laboratory Tests

The difficulties and prolonged duration of diet trials have led to attempts to devise tests for food allergies. Unfortunately, none of the tests available to practitioners are particularly reliable. A low serum folate level appears to be a poor marker of food allergy; a study of 15 dogs with diet-responsive diarrhea found a low serum folate level in only one dog (Rutgers et al, 1995). In vitro measurement of antigen-specific serum antibodies is of questionable relevance in food allergy, as such antibodies are also found in normal individuals. Furthermore, cats and dogs frequently have circulating antibodies to beef antigens, as routine vaccinations usually contain bovine serum albumin. Food-specific IgE can be measured by radioallergosorbent test (RAST) and enzyme-linked immunosorbent assay (ELISA), but results are disappointing. It is claimed that a RAST is a good negative predictor (i.e., a negative tests indicates that a patient is not sensitive to that antigen), but further studies are needed to substantiate this claim. At present, available commercial tests do not represent good value for the money. Skin testing has proved unreliable in the diagnosis of food allergic skin disease. Finally, application of food antigens directly onto the gastric or rectal mucosa under endoscopic guidance and observation of immediate hypersensitivity reactions is technically demanding.

Principle of Food Trials

Exclusion. The principle of an exclusion (elimination) diet trial is simple: feed a diet consisting of a single protein and single carbohydrate source not found in the patient's diet (see p. 530). These must be the only things fed until it is certain that remission either has or has not been achieved. One key to the success of a diet trial is complete owner compliance; no scraps or treats can be fed, and it may be best to avoid veterinary vitamin supplements because they often contain meat and vegetable extracts. The prevention of scavenging by muzzling or even hospitalization may be required. Replacing tap water with bottled water is probably unnecessary, but ceramic food and water bowls are recommended.

Challenge. Once remission is achieved, challenge with the original diet should be performed to confirm the diagnosis. This is important if an animal is not to be committed unnecessarily to a lifelong special diet. Some animals may not relapse either because of misdiagnosis or because restoration of the mucosal barrier prevents further antigen access and/or there is waning of hypersensitivity. However, many clients are unwilling to risk recurrence of signs, particularly if diarrhea has been a chronic problem, and may even feed the exclusion diet indefinitely. While clinically acceptable, as long as a nutritionally balanced diet is being fed, it is preferable, through a systematic series of provocative tests, to identify the offending food or foods.

Rescue and Systematic Provocation. After reinduction of remission (i.e., rescue) with the exclusion diet, single foodstuffs are introduced sequentially for a provocation test. If there is no relapse, the food is identified as safe, and challenge with a new food can be started. If there is a relapse during provocation, assessed as recurrence of signs on at least 2 consecutive days, the food is noted. Rescue with the exclusion diet is repeated and further provocations are performed until either all the offending foods have been identified or enough safe foods are found to enable selection of a maintenance diet. Ideally, provocation should be repeated before any food is excluded forever.

Maintenance. A suitable commercial diet that excludes the food or foods responsible is selected for maintenance.

Choice of Diet for Food Trials

Exclusion Diet

Food Source. An exclusion diet is composed of single protein and carbohydrate sources. Lamb or chicken with rice have been standard choices for many years. However, the recent increase in the sophistication of petfood contents has led to the need to try more and more esoteric food sources. Commercial diets containing fish, venison, and duck with rice, corn (maize), tapioca, or potato are all marketed. Home-cooking permits the use of other ingredients, such as horse meat, cottage cheese, soya, tofu, and even ostrich or alligator as the protein source.

Food allergies to a number of different food antigens have been reported and occasionally multiple allergies exist, but information on what an individual patient has been eating is more important than the statistical likelihood of any particular antigen being responsible. Allergies to wheat, beef, pork, egg, and chicken in dogs and fish, beef, chicken, and dairy products in cats have been most commonly reported from around the world, but any protein is potentially allergenic. Geographic variations in the prevalence of particular sensitivities perhaps reflect differences in the popularity of certain foodstuffs. In North America, lamb is a often a successful exclusion diet because lamb was, until recently, rarely fed. In the United Kingdom, lamb is almost a staple food for some dogs and cats, and chicken- or fish-based exclusion diets are more likely to be successful. Often, a number of diets have been tried by the owners, usually under random, uncontrolled conditions, and it can be hard to obtain a complete dietary history and choose an appropriate exclusion diet. The suggestion that it has to be something the animal has never experienced in its life is probably unrealistic, but anything fed while the animal has been showing clinical signs should be avoided.

Palatability. Any exclusion diet will be successful only if the patient eats it. Most dogs will accept chicken-, lamb-, and fish-based diets, but if inappetence is a presenting sign, temporary administration of glucocorticoids may be necessary initially. However, the exclusion trial has to be extended beyond the time steroids finish. Palatability can be a significant problem in cats. Lamb and rice baby foods, rabbit, powdered rice baby food, and commercial diets containing venison and rice or lamb and barley are considered most palatable.

Home-Cooked Versus Commercial Diet. It has been argued that home-cooked diets should not be used, as they may be nutritionally inadequate (see *CVT XII,* p. 63). However, this possible inadequacy is of little significance in mature dogs and cats during the relatively short period of the exclusion trial. Attempts to supplement home-cooked diets with bone flour and vitamin-mineral preparations are likely to introduce an unwanted antigen accidentally. Conversely, it has been argued that home-cooked diets are better because the contents are simpler and can be controlled. There are reports of animals responding to home-cooked diets that relapsed when they were switched to similar commercial diets.

In practice, the choice is best made on which formulation is likely to produce owner compliance. Commercial diets are convenient but can be expensive, and must only be used if the clinician is certain of their ingredients. A commercial fish and potato diet has been introduced recently that has three claimed advantages as an exclusion diet: catfish which is low in histamine is the major protein source, pure potato starch is a protein-free carbohydrate source, and anti-inflammatory omega-3 fatty acids are supplemented. However, a small amount of pork fat is present and potentially contains sufficient pork protein to affect a sensitized animal.

There is no single diet that is universally acceptable in all patients, and no brand names are recommended. It is sensible for the clinician to have an arsenal of two or three familiar diets to use in all but those cases with a very bizarre dietary history. Chicken, lamb, or venison with rice, and fish with potato or maize (corn) offer sufficient alternatives for most cases.

Hypoallergenic Diets. A successful exclusion diet only needs to have a restricted antigen source, that is, the antigenic diversity—not the antigen concentration—is reduced. However, a number of veterinary diets are marketed as "hypoallergenic"; they are highly digestible so that the antigenic load is rapidly lowered during digestion, and some also have a restricted fat content. They are suitable diets for animals with malabsorption, but only some are true exclusion diets (i.e., single protein source) that can be used for an exclusion trial.

Gluten-Free Diets. There is uncertainty as to what constitutes a gluten-free diet. Strictly, gluten is the water-insoluble protein fraction of wheat germ, comprising alcohol-insoluble glutenins (responsible for making dough rise) and alcohol-soluble gliadins. Gliadins are a group of related proteins (α, β, γ, ω), all of which have the potential to elicit mucosal damage in gluten sensitivity in humans. Other cereals contain proteins that are often collectively termed gluten, but only the proteins in rye (secalins), barley (hordeins), and oats (avenins) are immunologically similar to gliadins. Thus, gluten sensitivity in humans usually encompasses sensitivity to wheat, rye, barley, and sometimes oats. The "gluten" in rice and corn (maize) is unrelated, and from an antigenic viewpoint they are gluten-free.

Challenge and Provocation Diets. Challenge is performed with the patient's original diet. For provocation trials, there is a choice between feeding new diets, such as changing from chicken and rice to lamb and rice, or simply adding one new ingredient to the exclusion diet. Provocative doses of 100 gm per animal or 0.6 gm/kg body weight have been suggested. The dose may be important in a food intolerance, but in food allergy the form of the ingredient (e.g., cooked versus uncooked) may be more important.

Protocol for Diet Trials

Exclusion Trial. The optimal duration for an exclusion diet trial has yet to be established, and 2 to 4 weeks has been arbitrarily chosen. However, there have been cases of food allergic skin disease requiring up to 10 weeks before resolution of signs were reported, although it is not known whether this amount of time is necessary for food allergic GI disease. If the manifestation of a food allergy is diarrhea, most clients are unwilling to persist with a diet trial even for 3 weeks, but if there are signs of partial resolution the trial should be continued.

Challenge and Provocation Trials. Challenge trials are usually conducted for up to 14 days, but they can be halted sooner if signs recur. In most cases, signs recur within a few hours to days, and 14 days is likely to be adequate. However, it must be remembered that children with gluten-sensitive enteropathy can take up to 2 years to relapse on gluten challenge.

Assessment of Response

The criteria for assessment of response are usually subjective, although objective criteria would be preferred, especially as most diet trials are open—not double-blinded.

Subjective Criteria. Often, the clinician has to rely on the remission of clinical signs to assess the response to an exclusion diet. Unfortunately, feeding an exclusion diet does not just provide a novel antigen source and thus solely test a patient's allergic potential. The fat and carbohydrate content of the diet are inevitably altered when different foodstuffs are fed, digestibility may be improved, and inclusion of substances such as fructo-oligosaccharides may affect the bacterial flora. All these factors have effects on the intestine's ability to digest and absorb nutrients, and consequently modify clinical signs such as diarrhea. Even cutaneous signs may be improved; for example, if the exclusion diet rectifies an undiagnosed micronutrient deficiency, provides essential fatty acids, or contains anti-inflammatory omega-3 fatty acids.

Objective Criteria

Intestinal Biopsy. Ideally, an abnormal intestinal biopsy is found while the animal is still fed its original diet, resolution of histologic changes should correlate with clinical remission, and repeat biopsy during challenge should document relapse. However, most owners are unwilling for three biopsies to be taken, and so far only gluten sensitivity in Irish setters has undergone such rigorous proof in companion animal medicine. Extrapolation from human gastroenterology and clinical experience suggests that certain histologic changes may represent dietary sensitivity (Table 3).

Histologic similarities between food allergy and idiopathic IBD probably mean that an exclusion diet trial should be tried before immunosuppression in most cases. In cases with mild to moderate signs, this is a reasonable option, and most clients are eager to try a diet before steroids. However, for expediency in severe cases, dietary modification and prednisolone administration are often performed simultaneously. Feeding a hypoallergenic exclusion diet treats any potential sensitivity, improves digestive function, and, by offering a novel "sacrificial" protein, may prevent the patient from developing an acquired sensitivity to its usual diet.

Intestinal Permeability. Indirect measurement of intestinal permeability, by quantifying urinary excretion of simple nondigestible sugars, assesses the integrity of the mucosal

---

TABLE 3. Histologic Changes in GI Biopsies That Are Sometimes Manifestations of Food Allergy But Are Also Seen in Other GI Diseases

Lymphoplasmacytic gastritis
Lymphoplasmacytic enteritis
Intraepithelial lymphocyte infiltration
Villus atrophy—partial or subtotal
Eosinophilic gastroenteritis

barrier and can monitor the response to dietary manipulation. Interestingly, in 15 dogs with diet-responsive diarrhea, five (all retrievers) showed normalization of permeability with clinical remission, but permeability remained high in the other 10. It was speculated that these divergent findings represented a difference between food allergy and intolerance.

TREATMENT

There are a number of gluten-free proprietary diets based on lamb, chicken, or fish that are often suitable for maintenance feeding once the offending food or foods have been identified. They are preferred over home-cooked diets, as they should be balanced. Assuming that the diagnosis is correct, management by diet alone should be completely successful. Treatment failure should lead to re-evaluation of the diagnosis. Desensitization has not been effective in food allergy. Medical therapy is reserved for cases in which a convenient diet cannot be found, owner compliance is poor, or the patient will not eat the prescribed food or scavenges. Prednisolone is recommended, but antihistamines and mast cell stabilizers (e.g., cromoglycate) can be tried.

References and Suggested Reading

Crowe SE, Perdue MH: Gastrointestinal food hypersensitivity: Basic mechanisms of pathophysiology. Gastroenterology 103:1075, 1992.
Review of the mechanisms of food allergy.
Guagère E: Food intolerance in cats with cutaneous manifestations: A review of 17 cases. Eur J Comp Anim Pract 5:27, 1995.
Clinical investigations in cats with food allergic skin disease.
Hall EJ, Batt RM: Dietary modulation of gluten sensitivity in a naturally occurring enteropathy of Irish setter dogs. Gut 33:198, 1992.
Proof of dietary sensitivity in dogs and influence of weaning.
Hall EJ: Gastrointestinal aspects of food allergy: A review. J Small Anim Pract 35:145, 1994.
Review of mucosal barrier, immune tolerance, and causation of allergy.
Harvey RG: Food allergy and dietary intolerance in dogs: A report of 25 cases. J Small Anim Pract 34:175, 1993.
A United Kingdom perspective of food allergic skin disease in dogs.
Paterson S: Food hypersensitivity in 20 dogs with skin and gastrointestinal signs. J Small Anim Pract 36:529, 1995.
Report of concurrent GI and cutaneous disease.
Rosser EJ: Diagnosis of food allergy in dogs. J Am Vet Med Assoc 203:259, 1993.
A United States perspective on food allergic skin disease in dogs.
Rutgers HC, Batt RM, Hall EJ, et al: Intestinal permeability testing in dogs with diet-responsive intestinal disease. J Small Anim Pract 36:295, 1995.
Monitoring permeability as an objective assessment of response to dietary exclusion.
White SD, Sequoia D: Food hypersensitivity in cats: 14 cases (1982–1987). J Am Vet Med Assoc 194:692, 1986.
A United States perspective on food allergic skin disease in cats.

Small Intestinal Bacterial Overgrowth

CHRIS L. LUDLOW
Overland Park, Kansas

DEBORAH J. DAVENPORT
Topeka, Kansas

The normal intestinal tract contains large numbers of bacteria. Bacterial numbers in the normal proximal small intestine of the dog range from 10^2 to 10^5 colony-forming units (CFU)/ml of intestinal fluid during the interdigestive phase. These numbers increase to 10^5 to 10^9 CFU/ml in the distal small intestine. By comparison, bacterial counts as high as 10^5 to 10^8 CFU/ml have been reported in normal feline proximal small intestine. Both aerobic and anaerobic flora are normally present, with aerobic organisms typically outnumbering anaerobes. By the current definition, small intestinal bacterial numbers exceed 10^5 CFU/ml or 10^4 anaerobic CFU/ml in dogs, small intestinal bacterial overgrowth (SIBO) exists. Affected dogs may be without clinical signs, or show weight loss, nutrient malassimilation, vomiting, diarrhea, borborygmus, and flatulence.

Much remains to be resolved in the diagnosis of SIBO. Feline bacterial numbers have been established with the use of different, more current bacteriologic methods, giving reason to question the validity of the defining point of 10^5 CFU/ml in dogs. Higher bacterial counts have been identified in clinically normal dogs. In addition, the importance of increased bacterial numbers and their relationship with the clinical syndrome of SIBO is currently unclear.

ETIOLOGY

The normal flora of the small intestine consists of a variety of aerobic bacteria (including *Escherichia coli*, *Staphylococcus* sp., *Streptococcus* sp., *Pasteurella* sp., *Proteus* sp., and *Corynebacterium* sp.) and anaerobic bacteria (including *Peptostreptococcus* sp., *Propionibacterium* sp., *Bacteroides* sp., and *Actinomyces* sp.). Small intestinal bacterial overgrowth may be associated with increased numbers of these species, or increases of more pathogenic bacteria. The latter may be directly damaging to the gut mucosa or produce enterotoxic or secretory compounds.

Overgrowth from normal flora or pathogens is prevented by the interaction of host and microbial factors that serve as the primary protective mechanisms of the gut. Host factors include intestinal motility, gastric acid secretion, pancreatic and biliary secretion, and intestinal immuno-globulin production. Anything that interferes with these defense mechanisms may predispose to SIBO. The clinical syndrome of primary SIBO, where host defense mechanisms are intact, is rarely recognized.

Normal intestinal motility serves to propel bacteria and intestinal contents aborad, preventing excessive bacterial colonization. Intestinal hypomotility has been associated with gastrointestinal parasitism, obstructive diseases (foreign bodies, intussusception), inflammatory and infectious intestinal diseases, neoplasia, and intestinal scarring. Surgical excision of the ileocolic sphincter alters normal GI motility, removes an important barrier to colonic bacteria, and will eventually result in SIBO. Bacterial overgrowth has been seen when motility has been disrupted owing to infectious or inflammatory diseases, such as viral gastroenteritis, and chronic enteropathies, such as lymphoplasmacytic and eosinophilic enteritis. In addition, these diseases may alter other mucosal factors, such as mucin production, mucosal immunity, and the normal bacterial flora, contributing to SIBO.

Few ingested bacteria survive the acid environment of the stomach. Gastric acid secretion inhibits bacterial growth in the proximal small intestine as well. After gastric surgery in human patients, small intestinal bacterial numbers tend to increase proportionally to gastric pH. Long-term antisecretory drug therapy has also been associated with increased bacterial numbers in the small intestine in humans. With more prevalent use of potent antisecretory drugs (newer H_2 antagonists, proton pump inhibitors) for treating gastric disease in animals (see *CVT XII*, p. 706), it is possible that associated SIBO will be recognized as well.

Pancreatic and biliary secretions (digestive enzymes, immunoglobulins) also have antimicrobial effects in the proximal small intestine. Using the conventional definition, approximately 70% of dogs with exocrine pancreatic insufficiency (EPI) develop SIBO. This condition causes a poor response to pancreatic enzyme replacement therapy, with improvement occurring when broad-spectrum antibiotics are included in the therapeutic regimen for these patients.

Immunoglobulin production, both at the mucosal level and in biliary secretions, is critical for control of microbial growth in the small intestine. Diseases that alter intestinal immune function may predispose to SIBO. Bacterial overgrowth has been well described in German shepherds and Beagles with IgA deficiencies. The relationships between SIBO, decreased IgA production, and other enteropathies (lymphoplasmacytic and eosinophilic enteritis) common in this breed are difficult to sort out. Clinical signs attributed to SIBO are commonly seen in human pediatric patients with immunosuppression secondary to human immunodeficiency virus (HIV) infection. While the feline immunodeficiency virus (FIV) does have a specific trophism for the GI tract and GI signs are common in FIV-positive cats, the prevalence of SIBO in FIV-infected cats is unknown.

In addition to host factors, microbial interactions within the intestinal lumen are responsible for limiting bacterial populations in the small intestine. Consumption of available nutrients, changes in pH from the production of short-chain fatty acids, production of growth inhibitors (bacteriocins), changes in redox potentials, and interference with bacterial mucosal adhesion may all limit colonization with anaerobes or pathogens. In addition, the indiscriminate use of antimicrobial drugs for the treatment of gastrointestinal disease may further upset this microenvironment, contributing to the development of SIBO.

PATHOPHYSIOLOGY

The process or processes by which SIBO causes clinical signs is not well understood and probably varies with the number and type of bacteria associated with overgrowth. Morphologic changes to the mucosal surface are rarely present with SIBO and, when present, are usually mild. Small intestinal bacterial overgrowth due to anaerobes is often associated with more severe histologic changes in the bowel. Villus atrophy and infiltration with lymphocytes and plasma cells have been described. With the use of biochemical techniques, alterations in brush border enzymes have also been identified in dogs with SIBO. These alterations lead to functional abnormalities of the enterocytes and malassimilation of nutrients and, if severe enough, may be responsible for clinical signs.

The effects of bacteria on intraluminal contents is probably of more importance. Bacteria compete for nutrients and may result in depletion and malabsorption of nutrients such as vitamin B_{12}, which are critical for protein metabolism. Dehydroxylation and deconjugation of bile salts by luminal bacteria results in decreased micelle formation and lipid maldigestion. Bacterial metabolism of lipids results in the production of hydroxylated fatty acids. These degradation products act as detergents, damaging the mucosal surface and mucus layer, leading to increased bacterial access to the mucosal surface. They also act as secretory agents in the colon. Bacterial degradation of carbohydrates leads to production of short-chain fatty acids and alcohols, which serve as osmotic agents, drawing fluid into the intestinal lumen. They may also be directly damaging to the mucosal surface. Any of the aforementioned mechanisms may disrupt intestinal electrical activity, leading to motility disorders. Whether primary or secondary, alterations of motility predispose to SIBO and exacerbate clinical signs.

Increased intestinal permeability has been identified in dogs with SIBO. With the use of differential sugar absorption tests and ^{51}Cr-labeled EDTA, increased permeability has been demonstrated in both research Beagles and naturally occurring SIBO in pet animals. Increases in intestinal permeability may lead to increased exposure of submucosal gut-associated lymphoid tissue to larger, more antigenic peptides capable of stimulating an immune response. Increased intestinal permeability is currently one of the most credible pathophysiologic mechanisms for the development of the immune reaction seen with inflammatory bowel disease. This is also consistent with the mononuclear inflammatory infiltrate seen in patients with SIBO.

Extraintestinal disease has been linked to SIBO. Increased numbers of intestinal bacteria have been associated with increased risk of sepsis due to translocation across the small intestinal mucosal barrier. Increased numbers of bacteria in mesenteric lymph nodes have been found in blind-loop models of SIBO in laboratory animals. Hepatic inflammation has also been described in rats with experimentally induced SIBO. Elevations in liver enzymes and histologic changes in these rats are thought to result from increased intestinal permeability and exposure to bacteria, bacterial cell wall components, and/or bacterial toxins that are present in higher amounts.

DIAGNOSIS

Suspicion of SIBO should be based on clinical signs of weight loss, vomiting, diarrhea, nutrient malassimilation, borborygmus, and flatulence. Since SIBO is rarely a primary condition, a complete diagnostic work-up should be performed to rule out underlying diseases. A complete blood count and serum chemistry profile help identify metabolic causes of hypomotility (e.g., diabetes mellitus) and also help assess the severity of derangements associated with nutrient malassimilation (e.g., anemia associated with vitamin B_{12} deficiency). Abdominal radiography and ultrasonography are helpful in ruling out obstructive diseases and intestinal neoplasia. They are also useful in crude assessment of gastrointestinal motility. Exocrine pancreatic insufficiency should be excluded by measurement of serum trypsin–like immunoreactivity assay. Often, intestinal biopsies are required for identifying underlying inflammatory or neoplastic intestinal disorders (e.g., lymphoplasmacytic gastroenteritis, lymphoma), although histologic changes are not diagnostic for SIBO. Measure of serum immunoglobulins may aid in the diagnosis of specific immunodeficiencies.

Many tests have been used to aid in the diagnosis of SIBO. Quantitative aerobic and anaerobic small intestinal bacterial cultures have long been considered the "gold standard" diagnostic test. These are seldom done in a practice setting because of the cost and difficulty in collecting, transporting, and performing quantitative aerobic and anaerobic intestinal juice cultures. Cultures may be obtained surgically by aspiration of proximal small intestinal fluid with a 22-gauge needle. Caution should be taken to remove air from the syringe as quickly as possible to preserve anaerobes. Intestinal fluid may also be collected endoscopically. It is necessary to properly sterilize the endoscope with gas or chemical sterilization (2% glutaraldehyde, 1.5% Zephiran [benzalkonium chloride]) prior to collection of the sample. Collecting a negative control sample (1 ml of sterile saline flushed through the endoscope) prior to specimen collection will help identify contamination of the endoscope. Some contamination of the endoscope probably occurs with introduction through the upper GI tract, but initial studies comparing endoscopically collected samples with those surgically collected show that differences between the two methods are not significant. As much fluid as possible should be collected, although often less than 1 ml is present. Samples should be cultured as soon as possible (within 30 minutes) and stored at 4°C if not cultured immediately to minimize bacterial loss. If this is not possible, your laboratory should be contacted to provide appropriate transport media. An alternative to collection of intestinal fluid is to culture intestinal biopsies. Specimen collection is technically easier, but difficulties still remain with transport and culturing techniques. Results are expressed as CFU/gm of tissue. At this time, normal levels of mucosal bacterial counts have not been established, so results are difficult to interpret.

Total bacterial counts of more than 10^5 CFU/ml and/or anaerobic counts of more than 10^4 CFU/ml have historically been considered diagnostic for SIBO in dogs. Unfortunately, often there is a poor correlation between increased bacterial numbers in the proximal small intestine and clinical signs of SIBO. Several explanations for this exist. Duodenal total bacterial counts of more than 10^5 CFU/ml and anaerobic bacterial counts of more than 10^4 CFU/ml have been frequently found in clinically normal research and pet dogs with no histologic evidence of small intestinal disease. This raises questions about the specificity of using conventional numerical values as diagnostic criteria for SIBO in those with clinical signs. Normal bacterial counts may need to be determined for each laboratory. It has also been demonstrated that there is a poor correlation between the numbers and types of organisms in small intestinal fluid and those associated with the intestinal surface as determined by culture of intestinal biopsies. There may also be wide variability between bacterial numbers at different locations in the proximal small intestine. Potential differences exist in the severity of histologic changes and the severity of clinical signs, depending on the types of bacteria involved in SIBO. We have much to learn if quantitative cultures are to continue to be the diagnostic gold standard. There exists a need to further clarify the significance of increased bacterial numbers in the proximal small intestine of normal dogs and dogs with clinical intestinal disease. In the authors' opinion, because of improvements in bacteriologic methods, the numerical breaking point needs to be re-evaluated. Bacterial populations need to be better characterized in both normal dogs and those with intestinal disease. The relationship between luminal and mucosal bacteria as well as their relative importance to small intestinal pathology must also be determined.

Other tests have been used as screening tools for SIBO. Measurements of fasting serum folate and vitamin B_{12} levels have been used in dogs and are readily available to practitioners. These tests are based on the principle that increased numbers of bacteria in the proximal small intestine produce increased amounts of folate and either utilize or interfere with the absorption of vitamin B_{12}. These effects will be reflected in serum vitamin determinations, resulting in increased serum folate and decreased serum vitamin B_{12} levels as the classic findings in patients with SIBO. Of the two, decreased serum vitamin B_{12} is the more consistent finding. Unfortunately, the specificity and sensitivity of serum folate and vitamin B_{12} levels, based on correlation with quantitative cultures, are not high. Parenteral vitamin supplementation will alter the serum level of both vitamins. It has been shown that dietary folate and vitamin B_{12} levels found in many commercially available pet foods when fed to normal dogs are high enough to cause elevations in fasting serum levels. Conversely, if proximal small intestinal pathology is severe enough, folate absorption may be reduced even in the setting of increased bacterial folate production, and serum folate levels may be normal to low even when SIBO is present. Not all bacteria associated with SIBO synthesize folate. Serum vitamin B_{12} levels may be reduced by diseases other than SIBO, including EPI and severe mucosal disease or atrophy at the site of absorption in the ileum.

The hydrogen breath test (HBT) has been used in human patients for many years as a noninvasive screening test for

SIBO. The HBT is based on the premise that unabsorbed carbohydrates are fermented by bacteria in the gut, resulting in the production of short-chain fatty acids and the gases hydrogen and carbon dioxide. Small but constant percentages of these gases are absorbed into the systemic circulation and excreted into expired air on first pass through the lungs. Therefore, changes in expired breath H_2 reflect changes in H_2 production in the gut. In the normal individual, bacterial numbers in the small intestine are not sufficient to produce a measurable rise in breath hydrogen, and the majority of breath hydrogen is attributed to fermentation in the colon. Increases in fasting breath hydrogen and an "early" rise of breath hydrogen after ingestion of test substrate have been reported in patients with SIBO. Fasting breath hydrogen levels are attributed to increased production and fermentation of intestinal glycoproteins. The early breath hydrogen rise is attributed to production from increased bacterial numbers in the proximal small intestine. This early rise must be clearly identified before the carbohydrate substrate could have been produced by colonic bacterial fermentation. While the HBT is simple and noninvasive, in people the sensitivity and specificity have varied markedly in different studies. Variability is due to differences in fermentation by bacterial populations; variability in small intestinal transit rates, which makes determination of an early rise difficult; and differences in carbohydrate substrates used in the test. In animals, the HBT is limited by the same variables, and availability of breath hydrogen measurement is very limited. It has yet to be proved valuable for the diagnosis of SIBO in animals.

Increased intestinal permeability has been demonstrated in dogs with SIBO. While measurement of intestinal permeability previously required handling and patient exposure to radioactive compounds (^{51}Cr-labeled EDTA), studies have shown that measurements from differential sugar absorption tests are reliable. These tests are based on differential absorption of normally nondigestible, nonabsorbable sugars to identify increased intestinal permeability (lactulose, rhamnose) and small intestinal absorptive function (xylose, 3-O-methylglucose). These sugars are administered per os, and urinary excretion is measured over a 5-hour period. Increased amounts of lactulose recovered relative to rhamnose indicate increased intestinal permeability, while decreased amounts of xylose relative to 3-O-methylglucose indicate decreased absorptive function. Studies in naturally occurring canine SIBO have shown increases in permeability and decreased absorptive function in the absence of histopathologic changes. Treatment with oral oxytetracycline resulted in decreased duodenal bacterial numbers, decreases in permeability, and increased absorptive function. Increased intestinal permeability is not specific for SIBO and may be present with other intestinal diseases associated with the development of SIBO. This makes measurement of permeability an unreliable screening test for SIBO, but it is useful in the assessment of the intestinal damage seen with SIBO and associated diseases. At this time, measurement of urinary sugar levels is not readily available to practitioners.

Measurement of serum unconjugated bile acids may prove to be a useful screening tool for SIBO. The test is based on the premise that increased bacterial numbers in the proximal small intestine result in increased deconjugation of bile salts, which are then readily absorbed. Increased serum levels of unconjugated bile acids have been demonstrated in human cases of SIBO. Current studies are underway to determine the sensitivity, specificity, and practicality of this test in animals.

Ultimately, owing to the lack of a sensitive and specific screening test, the response to antibiotic therapy remains a useful diagnostic aid. Once attempts to rule out underlying disease have been made and no response has been seen with appropriate dietary therapy and treatment of routine parasites, a 7- to 10-day antibiotic trial is a very reasonable step. Caution should be exercised because of the intermittent recurrent nature of many underlying diseases (e.g., lymphoplasmacytic gastroenteritis) and the possibility of a seeming, though unrelated, improvement with antibiotics leading to a false-positive response.

Definitive diagnosis of SIBO continues to be difficult. The identification of underlying diseases commonly associated with SIBO (e.g., EPI) should increase the index of suspicion. Elevated serum folate and decreased serum vitamin B_{12} levels are highly suggestive of SIBO and, in the presence of compatible clinical signs of SIBO, are sufficient reason to treat. In the presence of other GI diseases in which the response to initial therapy is poor, the addition of antimicrobial therapy may prove helpful.

TREATMENT

Once the diagnosis of SIBO has been made in a patient with compatible clinical signs, the first step in therapy is the identification and treatment of any underlying diseases. In patients with severe signs, or no readily identifiable underlying disease, antimicrobial therapy is the treatment of choice. The current recommendations include the use of a broad-spectrum antimicrobial effective against aerobes, coliforms, and anaerobes. Tetracycline, 5 to 10 mg/kg every 8 hours for 28 days, has proved effective in uncomplicated cases of SIBO. Metronidazole and tylosin (Tylan, Elanco) have been effective alternatives. Metronidazole, 10 to 20 mg/kg every 12 hours, has a primarily anaerobic spectrum and is not effective against aerobes. Tylosin, 10 to 20 mg/kg every 12 hours, has been used and is recommended in chronic cases, since it appears less susceptible to the development of antimicrobial resistance. Since tylosin is available only as a powder, it may be added to a gelatin capsule, or an empirical dose of 3 tsp/10 kg every 12 hours may be mixed with meals. The goal of therapy is to use the least possible amount to control clinical signs. Other broad-spectrum antimicrobials may be equally effective. Relapses may occur, necessitating therapy for as long as 6 weeks. This may be an indication that the primary cause of SIBO has yet to be identified.

Dietary therapy may be very helpful in controlling the clinical signs associated with SIBO. The idea is to reduce nutrients that predispose to the production of diarrheogenic compounds by intestinal bacteria and reduce the workload of the damaged intestinal mucosa. General recommendations are for a low-fat, highly digestible diet. Many commercially prepared and homemade recipes that fit this description are available. Parenteral supplementation with vitamin B_{12} may be necessary to return serum levels to normal. In addition to the use of diet to control clinical signs, dietary supplements such as oligosaccharides may prove an effective way of manipulating the intestinal microenvironment. These compounds are not digested or absorbed in the GI tract but are metabolized to varying degrees by the bacteria present there. Bacteria differ in their ability to utilize these compounds and grow in their presence, permitting manipulation of bacterial populations by preferentially feeding "good" bacteria. The use of a naturally occurring oligosaccharide added to a standard dog food fed for 2 weeks was shown to yield reduced bacterial counts both in intestinal fluid and at the mucosal surface in IgA-deficient German shepherds with increased duodenal bacterial. This reduction was primarily in aerobic bacteria. In this study, dogs were clinically normal, so care must be taken when one applies these results to dogs with clinical signs. Further studies will be necessary for establishing the importance of this therapy in SIBO.

References and Suggested Reading

Batt RM, Rutgers HC, Sancak AA: Enteric bacteria: Friend or foe? J Small Anim Pract 37:261, 1996.
A good review of normal enteric bacterial populations and the causes and pathophysiology of increased bacterial overgrowth; also reviews recent information about pathogenic enteric bacteria.

Davenport DJ: Small intestinal bacterial overgrowth: Need for a new definition? Proceedings of the 13th Forum of the American College of Veterinary Internal Medicine, 1996, pp 346–347.
Review summarizes the information, emphasizing the need for re-evaluation of bacterial numbers that define small intestinal bacterial overgrowth.

Delles EK, Willard MD, Simpson RB, et al: Comparison of species and numbers of bacteria in concurrently cultured samples of proximal small intestinal fluid and endoscopically obtained duodenal mucosa in dogs with intestinal bacterial overgrowth. Am J Vet Res 55:957, 1994.
Article compares bacterial populations and numbers and describes small intestinal histologic changes in IgA-deficient German shepherds.

Johnston K, Lamport A, Batt RM: An unexpected bacterial flora in the proximal small intestine of normal cats. Vet Rec 132:362, 1993.
Article describes the proximal bacterial flora in normal cats.

Rutgers HC, Batt RM, Elwood CM, et al: Small intestinal bacterial overgrowth in dogs with chronic intestinal disease. J Am Vet Med Assoc 206:187, 1995.
Study describes the results of quantitative cultures done on dogs with a variety of naturally occurring small intestinal diseases.

Rutgers HC, Batt RM, Proud FJ, et al: Intestinal permeability and function in dogs with small intestinal bacterial overgrowth. J Small Anim Pract 37:428, 1996.
Paper reports the results of measurements of intestinal permeability with the use of differential sugar absorption in dogs with increased small intestinal bacterial counts.

Willard MD, Simpson RB, Delles EK, et al: Effects of dietary supplementation of fructo-oligosaccharides on small intestinal bacterial overgrowth in dogs. Am J Vet Res 55:654, 1994.
Article describes the changes seen in small intestinal bacterial populations after the diet was supplemented with an oligosaccharide.

Willard MD, Simpson RB, Fossum TW, et al: Characterization of naturally developing small intestinal bacterial overgrowth in 16 German Shepherd dogs. J Am Vet Med Assoc 204:1201, 1994.
Good description of the bacteriologic and histologic findings in IgA-deficient German shepherds.

Protein-Losing Enteropathies

LISA ERIN MOORE
New York, New York

Protein-losing enteropathy (PLE) can be associated with a multitude of intestinal and systemic disorders. This group of disorders is characterized by a nonselective loss of proteins into the intestinal tract. The loss of proteins can be due to a loss of mucosal barrier function that results in increased intestinal permeability, such as in inflammatory or erosive disorders, or to malfunction or abnormalities of intestinal lymphatic drainage (Jeffries, 1983). Many diseases have been reported to cause PLE in dogs, including intestinal lymphangiectasia (primary or secondary), inflammatory disorders (lymphoplasmacytic, eosinophilic, granulomatous enteritides, and gluten-sensitive enteropathy), gastrointestinal ulceration, neoplasia (lymphosarcoma, intestinal carcinoma), intestinal fungal or parasitic infection (histoplasmosis, trichuriasis, ancylostomiasis), foreign bodies, chronic intussusceptions, acute viral enteritis (parvovirus), acute or chronic bacterial enteritis, immune-mediated and allergic diseases (systemic lupus erythematosus), constrictive pericarditis, and right-sided heart failure.

CAUSES OF PROTEIN-LOSING ENTEROPATHIES

Intestinal Lymphangiectasia

Intestinal lymphangiectasia (IL) is considered to be the most common disorder associated with PLE (Tams and Twedt, 1981). The disease is characterized by dilatated intestinal lymphatics, resulting in dilatated and ruptured lacteals in the villi and submucosa. This leads to a loss of proteins, lymphocytes, and chylomicrons into the intestinal lumen. IL can be primary or secondary. Primary IL is a congenital disease in which insufficient or malformed lymphatic vessels result in poor intestinal lymphatic flow and drainage. The disease can also be associated with systemic abnormalities of the lymphatic system (Fossum, 1989). Secondary IL usually results from obstruction to lymphatic flow, either in the lymphatic system (inflammatory lesions of the intestinal wall, neoplastic disorders) or subsequent to venous hypertension (congestive heart failure, portal vein thrombosis). Lipogranulomas are often observed around the lymphatics in inflammatory disorders (Van Kruiningen et al, 1984).

Inflammatory and Immune Disorders

Inflammatory and immune diseases of the intestines include lymphoplasmacytic, eosinophilic, and granulomatous enteritides. Lymphoplasmacytic enteritis is the most common cause of PLE in this category (Tams and Twedt, 1981). This disease is characterized by a diffuse infiltration of lymphocytes and plasma cells in the lamina propria of the intestinal mucosa. This is a chronic disorder for which no cause can be determined, but current theories are concentrating on defining immunologic abnormalities, including defective immunoregulation, dietary allergens, or other chronic antigenic stimuli (Guilford, 1996). Regardless of the cause or causes, the final pathway is inflammation that results in damage to the gastrointestinal tissue, which can, in some cases, result in protein loss.

Miscellaneous Disorders

As mentioned earlier, various other diseases can cause gastrointestinal protein loss (Tams and Twedt, 1981; Jeffries, 1983). Conditions resulting in erosion or bleeding of the intestinal mucosa, submucosa, or muscularis can result in loss of plasma or blood if the lesion is more severe. Examples would include erosion or ulceration due to foreign objects, drugs (most commonly nonsteroidal anti-inflammatory drugs), and intussusceptions. Infiltrative disorders such as histoplasmosis and lymphosarcoma are also reported causes of PLE. Acute and chronic infectious diseases should be included. Parvoviral enteritis can result in severe hypoproteinemia because of destruction of the villus and subsequent plasma leakage into the intestines. Various bacterial agents, including small intestinal bacterial overgrowth, and parasitic infections can cause PLE.

CLINICAL SIGNS

Clinical signs can be variable but almost always include weight loss. Other signs can be those associated with the gastrointestinal tract such as vomiting or diarrhea of a semisolid to watery consistency. It should be noted that not all animals with PLE have diarrhea; weight loss and hypoproteinemia can be the only signs. Other signs can be related to the hypoproteinemia. Ascites, peripheral edema, and dyspnea resulting from hydrothorax can all be seen. Abdominal palpation may reveal thickened intestinal loops, lymphadenopathy, or a mass. Thoracic auscultation may reveal cardiac abnormalities.

DIAGNOSIS

The hypoproteinemia seen with PLE is nonselective; therefore, albumin and globulin levels are decreased. Two notable exceptions include the PLE of basenji dogs and intestinal histoplasmosis. The basenji enteropathy is associated with hypoalbuminemia and hyperglobulinemia (Breitschwerdt, 1992). Intestinal histoplasmosis has also

been associated with a normal or elevated globulin fraction, presumably due to the inflammatory response (Williams, 1996). Other causes of hypoalbuminemia should be ruled out. Urinalysis and the urine protein:creatinine ratio are abnormal with renal protein loss. Decreased albumin production can be due to severe hepatic disease, and hepatic function testing such as bilirubin and bile acid analysis should be performed to eliminate this possibility. Protein loss can also occur with chronic blood loss, in which case anemia should be present. Radiography is useful to rule out obstructive lesions (foreign objects), cardiac disease, and metastatic or fungal lesions.

If all initial results are normal, the intestinal tract should be evaluated. Multiple fecal examinations (flotations and direct smears) should be performed. If all results are negative, empirical use of a broad-spectrum anthelmintic, such as fenbendazole, can be used before more expensive and invasive testing is carried out.

Intestinal function testing can be performed to detect malabsorption or maldigestion. Sudan staining of fecal material can be used to detect steatorrhea, which can indicate fat malassimilation. Oral D-xylose testing can indicate poor carbohydrate absorption. Barium series are helpful to delineate the location and severity of certain mucosal abnormalities, such as ulcerations. Cytologic examination of fecal smears or colonic scrapings may reveal fungal or protozoal organisms or leukocytes. Protein electrophoresis can determine which protein fraction is abnormal. Both albumin and globulin fractions are low with PLE. Determination of serum folate and cobalamin levels, along with breath hydrogen and intestinal permeability testing (if available), can further document gastrointestinal disease.

The gold standard for documenting intestinal protein loss is to quantitate radiolabeled (chromium-51) albumin in the feces after intravenous administration (Williams, 1996). For many reasons, the application of this test is limited in veterinary medicine. Another useful tool in human medicine, which has been studied in veterinary medicine more recently, is the measurement of alpha$_1$-antitrypsin (alpha$_1$-protease) in the feces (Williams, 1991). Alpha$_1$-antitrypsin has a molecular weight similar to that of albumin. This protein is present in the vascular and interstitial spaces and in lymph. Therefore, alpha$_1$-antitrypsin can be lost into the intestinal tract with PLE and is excreted in the feces intact. This protein can then be measured using an immunoassay and can give an indirect quantitation of protein loss. This can be of value in both diagnosis and monitoring of treatment.

Ultimately, intestinal biopsies are usually required to define the disease process causing PLE. Endoscopic biopsy or full-thickness biopsy via exploratory laparotomy can be performed. Laparotomy provides the advantage of being able to evaluate the entire intestinal tract, since some diseases may be focal, in addition to extraintestinal structures. Dilated lymphatics may be visualized as a milky web-like pattern on the serosal surface of the intestines and throughout the mesentery. Animals with PLE generally are malnourished and hypoproteinemic; therefore, they have delayed wound healing, which may lead to dehiscence. The chances can be minimized by using nonabsorbable suture material. In many cases, endoscopic biopsies are adequate to diagnose diffuse mucosal diseases. As hypoproteinemic animals tend to be hypovolemic because of reduced oncotic pressure, colloid support with plasma or synthetic colloids (e.g., hetastarch, Hespan; American Critical Care, McGaw Park, IL) should be considered before administration of anesthesia to avoid hypotension.

TREATMENT

Treatment should be aimed at any identifiable underlying disease. PLE from acute viral infections usually resolves with supportive care, and that due to bacterial or parasitic infections gets better with appropriate specific therapy. Other diseases should be treated accordingly (antifungal agents for histoplasmosis, chemotherapy for lymphosarcoma, and so on).

The mainstay of treatment for the two most common diseases causing PLE (IL, lymphoplasmacytic enteritis) is dietary control (Jeffries, 1983) and anti-inflammatory medication (Williams, 1996; Fossum, 1989). The diet should be low in triglycerides containing long-chain fatty acids, which must be transported into the circulation via the intestinal lymphatics. Short- and medium-chain triglycerides can be absorbed directly into the portal system. Commercially available diets can be used, such as Prescription diet r/d (Hill's Pet Products, Topeka, KS), or a homemade diet can be prepared (Fossum, 1989). The caloric density of the diet can be increased by adding medium-chain triglyceride (MCT) oil (Mead Johnson, Evansville, IN) at a dose of 1 to 2 ml/kg per day. MCT oil may be expensive, is unpalatable to some animals, and does not provide essential fatty acids. An alternative is the elemental supplement Portagen (Mead Johnson, Evansville, IN)—1.5 cups added to water makes a 1 quart mixture that contains 1 cal/ml (Fossum, 1989). This mixture is hypertonic and can cause vomiting and diarrhea.

Corticosteroids can prove effective in secondary IL and the inflammatory enteropathies. Prednisone at a dose of 2 to 3 mg/kg per day can be used with a slow taper once a response has been seen. A maintenance dosing schedule is usually required indefinitely, preferably on an alternate-day basis. If no response is seen with corticosteroids, immunosuppressive agents, such as azathioprine, can be used. Prognosis can be difficult to determine because few long-term studies have been performed in dogs and cats. In general, the prognosis should be guarded until a response is seen. Indefinite therapy is usually required and relapses occur.

References and Suggested Reading

Breitschwerdt EB: Immunoproliferative enteropathy of basenjis. Semin Vet Med Surg 7:153, 1992.
A review of this breed-specific disease.
Fossum TW: Protein-losing enteropathy. Semin Vet Med Surg 4:219, 1989.
A review of the diagnosis and treatment of PLE (primarily IL).
Guilford WG: Idiopathic inflammatory bowel diseases. In: Guilford WG, Strombeck DR: Strombeck's Small Animal Gastroenterology. Philadelphia: WB Saunders, 1996, p 451.
A review of the pathophysiology, diagnosis, and management of inflammatory bowel disease.
Jeffries GH: Protein-losing gastroenteropathy. In: Sleisenger MH, Fordtran JS, eds: Gastrointestinal Disease. Philadelphia: WB Saunders, 1983, p 280.
A review of intestinal causes of PLE in humans.
Jergens AE, Moore FM, Haynes JS, Miles KG: Idiopathic inflammatory bowel disease in dogs and cats: 84 cases (1987–1990). J Am Vet Med Assoc 201:1603, 1992.
A retrospective study of the clinical and pathologic findings in dogs and cats with inflammatory bowel disease.
Sherding RG: Intestinal Lymphangiectasia. In: Kirk RW, ed: Current Veterinary Therapy IX. Philadelphia: WB Saunders, 1986, p 885.
A review of the pathophysiology, diagnosis, and treatment of IL.
Tams TR, Twedt DC: Canine protein-losing gastroenteropathy syndrome. Comp Cont Ed Pract Vet 3:105, 1981.
A review of the pathophysiology, diagnosis, and treatment of various causes of PLE.
Van Kruiningen HJ, Lees GE, Hayden DW, et al: Lipogranulomatous lymphangitis in canine intestinal lymphangiectasia. Vet Pathol 21:377, 1984.
Description of four dogs with IL and lymphangitis.
Williams DA: Evaluation of fecal alpha-1-protease inhibitor concentration as a test for canine protein-losing enteropathy (PLE). J Vet Intern Med 5:133, 1991.
Abstract describing the use of an immunoassay in control dogs and three dogs with PLE.
Williams DA: Malabsorption, small intestinal bacterial overgrowth, and protein-losing enteropathy. In: Guilford WG, Strombeck DR: Strombeck's Small Animal Gastroenterology. Philadelphia: WB Saunders, 1996, p 367.
A review of the pathophysiology, diagnosis, and treatment of PLE.

Chronic Colitis in Dogs

MICHAEL S. LEIB
Blacksburg, Virginia

Chronic colitis is defined as inflammation of the colon that is present for at least 2 weeks. Although many different histologic forms of chronic colitis are recognized in dogs, the clinical signs, diagnostic plan, and therapy are similar for most forms. This chapter reviews the various histologic types of colitis, with emphasis on plasmacytic lymphocytic colitis. Following this is an overview of colitis, a discussion of the diagnostic plan that the author uses when evaluating chronic large bowel diarrhea, a brief review of the most important diseases (Table 1), and a discussion of therapy.

HISTOLOGIC FORMS OF COLITIS

Plasmacytic Lymphocytic Colitis

Plasmacytic lymphocytic colitis is the most common form of colitis seen in the author's practice (see Table 1).

TABLE 1. Diagnosis in 74 Cases of Chronic Large Bowel Diarrhea

Diagnosis	Number of Cases
Idiopathic	19
Plasmacytic lymphocytic colitis	15
Clostridium perfringens enterotoxicosis	10
Malignant neoplasia	10
Pyogranulomatous colitis	6
Histiocytic ulcerative colitis	3
Eosinophilic granulomatous colitis	2
Trichuris vulpis	1
Histoplasmosis	1
Miscellaneous	7

It may occur more commonly in males. The characteristic histologic lesion consists of increased numbers of plasma cells and lymphocytes in the mucosa. Concurrent involvement of the stomach or small intestine can cause vomiting or signs of small bowel diarrhea. Of the 15 dogs described in Table 1 with plasmacytic lymphocytic colitis, 7 had concurrent small bowel disease and 2 had gastric infiltration.

Pathophysiology

The pathophysiology of inflammatory bowel disease (IBD) is complex and not completely understood. It is unknown if IBD is caused by an inflammatory response to a foreign agent or if it is caused by an abnormal immunologic response to normal intraluminal antigens (such as food or bacteria). Most likely, the cause of IBD is multifactorial.

Increased mucosal permeability appears to be a central component of IBD in humans. A breakdown in the mucosal barrier allows increased access of antigens to mucosal immunologic defenses, causing a self-perpetuating inflammatory process. Inflammation leads to recruitment of additional inflammatory cells with release of potent inflammatory mediators (prostaglandins, leukotrienes, platelet-activating factor, interleukins, reactive oxygen metabolites, and several gastrointestinal peptides) that cause further damage to the mucosal barrier. This permits entry of additional intraluminal antigens across the mucosal surface, stimulating further inflammation and damage.

Increased permeability may be due to a primary mucosal defect or may result from damage secondary to infectious, metabolic, allergic, or toxic insults. Alternatively, faulty immunoregulation (decreased suppressor T-lymphocyte function) may occur, allowing normal intraluminal antigens to induce an exaggerated immune response that is not dampened and controlled by normal suppressor mechanisms.

Regardless of the cause of increased permeability, luminal antigens that normally are tolerated (do not induce an inflammatory response) by the intestinal immune system are capable of inciting a severe immune response. The therapeutic response to a hypoallergenic diet or antibiotics that occurs in some dogs may be due to limitation or reduction of luminal antigens that are secondarily involved in the inflammatory process.

Mucosal inflammation results in the clinical signs associated with IBD. Intestinal inflammation disrupts tight junctions between epithelial cells and reduces absorption and promotes the loss of nutrients, electrolytes, and water. Some inflammatory mediators stimulate intestinal secretion. Inflammation adversely affects motility by inhibiting segmental contractions and causing decreased fecal storage and frequent elimination of colonic contents. Goblet cells respond to inflammation by increasing secretion of mucus. Inflammation, erosion, or ulceration can lead to hemorrhage. The inflamed rectum becomes sensitized to stretch, initiating the urge to defecate and causing tenesmus. Inflammation in the duodenum and stomach stimulates receptors that trigger the vomiting reflex. Severe vomiting or profuse diarrhea can lead to dehydration from loss of fluid and electrolytes.

Endoscopy

In some cases, only subtle endoscopic abnormalities can be detected, which include a mild increase in mucosal granularity and friability (bleeding associated with routine endoscopic trauma). In other cases, visualization of submucosal blood vessels may be obscured or erosion of the mucosa observed. Ulceration, a deeper defect of the mucosa, occurs less commonly. In some dogs, the mucosa may appear normal, which emphasizes the importance of always collecting biopsy samples. The severity of endoscopic lesions can vary at different locations within the colon. In most cases, the severity of endoscopic lesions does not correlate with the severity of clinical signs.

Histopathologic Characteristics

The histologic criteria for establishing a diagnosis of plasmacytic lymphocytic colitis in dogs are controversial. Classification schemes have recently been proposed to provide some objective criteria that can be applied to the diagnosis of IBD.

All diagnostic classification schemes include as a central criterion the presence of increased numbers of plasma cells and lymphocytes within the mucosa. Lesser numbers of eosinophils and scattered neutrophils and macrophages are often found. In some cases, there are nearly equal numbers of eosinophils; these cases are classified as plasmacytic lymphocytic and eosinophilic colitis. Other histologic changes that occur in IBD include edematous separation of crypts, increased numbers of intraepithelial lymphocytes, cryptal abscessation, basophilia with flattening of surface epithelium, and erosion.

The major difficulty in interpreting the histopathologic changes in IBD lies at both ends of the spectrum. Mild lesions need to be differentiated from normal mucosa, and severe lesions must be distinguished from lymphosarcoma. Inflammatory infiltrates are commonly found in close proximity to neoplastic cells in lymphosarcoma. Thus, a small flexible endoscopic forceps biopsy may miss a neoplastic lesion.

Prognosis

The prognosis for most cases of plasmacytic lymphocytic colitis is good. In some dogs, medication or dietary therapy, or both, can be discontinued, whereas other dogs require long-term or lifelong treatment. Some dogs in which medication has been discontinued subsequently have recurrent clinical signs that require retreatment.

Eosinophilic Colitis

Eosinophilic colitis is much less common than plasmacytic lymphocytic colitis (no cases are included in Table 1). Dogs affected with eosinophilic colitis may be younger than those affected with plasmacytic lymphocytic colitis. Circulating eosinophilia may be present in some cases. Rectal cytologic specimens can contain eosinophils. Ulceration of the mucosa is more common. Infiltration of eosinophils can occur in any layer of the colonic wall. Lesser numbers of plasma cells and lymphocytes are often present.

Because of the eosinophilic infiltrate, gastrointestinal parasites should be considered a potential cause. Fecal examinations and therapeutic deworming are extremely important. Because of the possibility that migrating larvae of *Toxocara canis* might be a cause, a larvacidal dose of ivermectin, 200 μg/kg SC is indicated. Ivermectin should not be used in collies or related breeds because of its potential toxicity in these dogs. The prognosis is similar to that in cases of plasmacytic lymphocytic colitis.

A rare form of eosinophilic colitis, eosinophilic granulomatous colitis, was diagnosed in 2 of 74 cases (see Table 1). Large transmural granulomas develop in such cases. Masses may be palpated abdominally. The best treatment is surgical resection of the lesions, followed by medical management of the colitis. Unfortunately, lesions are usually advanced at the time of diagnosis, and surgery may not be possible. Prognosis is poor for this form of the disease.

Histiocytic Ulcerative Colitis

An uncommon form of colitis, histiocytic ulcerative colitis, occurs mainly in young boxer dogs; most are less than 2 years of age when clinical signs develop. The disease is characterized by progressive colonic ulceration that is histologically associated with a mucosal infiltrate of plasma cells, lymphocytes, and distended periodic acid–Schiff–positive macrophages.

Decreased appetite and lethargy may develop. Weight loss and debilitation occur as a result of chronic intestinal blood and protein loss (resulting in anemia and hypoproteinemia). A corrugated, thickened mucosa, hemorrhage, or pain may be evident on digital rectal examination.

If histiocytic colitis is advanced at the time of diagnosis, treatment often does not improve clinical signs, and a poor prognosis is warranted. However, if management is instituted early in the course of the disease, the prognosis is more favorable, although the disease is usually progressive, and lifelong therapy is required.

Pyogranulomatous Colitis

Pyogranulomatous colitis is an uncommon and poorly understood form of colitis. Clinical signs are uniformly severe. Endoscopically, proliferative masses of varying sizes ranging from 2 to 3 mm to 2 to 3 cm are found in the rectum. These masses can often be palpated rectally. Histologically, a mixture of inflammatory cells is found, including neutrophils, macrophages, and plasma cells, with varying amounts of fibrosis and vascular proliferation. Special stains have failed to identify fungal organisms. Sometimes there is also involvement of the anal area. Although it is not often possible, surgical resection of the abnormal mucosa is the best treatment. Most dogs do not respond to medical management.

HISTORY AND CLINICAL SIGNS

Chronic colitis usually develops in dogs less than 7 years of age. The mean age when clinical signs started in 221 dogs with colitis reported in the literature or studied by the author was 3.1 years. However, older dogs (up to 14 years of age) can be affected. Colitis occurs commonly in both males and females. Most breeds of dogs as well as mixed breeds can have colitis, although boxers are predisposed to a specific form—histiocytic ulcerative colitis.

The most common clinical sign is large bowel diarrhea. The frequency of defecation is increased, sometimes as often as 10 to 20 bowel movements per day. The amount of feces/movement is usually decreased. Fresh blood, or hematochezia, and excess mucus are often present. Straining to defecate, or tenesmus, occurs commonly. Owners may report straining when only a scant volume of feces or no feces at all is produced. Intermittent vomiting may occur but is usually less frequent and severe than the diarrhea. Weight loss is uncommon except in animals with IBD that also affects the small intestines or stomach. Lethargy and decreased appetite are uncommon.

The frequency and severity of diarrhea often progress. Initially, clinical signs may be sporadic and normal stools predominate. More frequent periods of diarrhea often develop. Some cases progress to constant diarrhea.

Physical examination is usually normal in cases of chronic colitis. Weight loss, if present, may be detectable. Rarely, a thickened colon may be palpated abdominally. Digital rectal examination may elicit pain. Blood can be present on the examination glove. An irregular mucosal surface can be detected in some cases.

DIFFERENTIAL DIAGNOSIS

The clinical signs of chronic colitis are indistinguishable from many of the other causes of large bowel diarrhea in dogs. Table 1 shows the clinical diagnosis in 74 cases of chronic large bowel diarrhea evaluated at the author's hospital. These cases came from a group of 116 consecutive dogs that underwent colonoscopy. Only 35% of the dogs with signs of chronic large bowel diarrhea had colitis (see Table 1). Because these cases were diagnosed at a referral hospital, the frequency of the diseases is different from that seen in private practice.

The two most common causes of chronic large bowel diarrhea in dogs, *Trichuris vulpis* and diet-responsive diarrhea, were not common in the dogs represented in Table 1. These referral animals did not have colonoscopy unless multiple fecal examinations and therapeutic deworming were performed and a diet trial with a highly digestible diet failed to eliminate clinical signs. Whipworms attach to the mucosa in the cecum and ascending colon and cause inflammation. Relatively few ova are shed, and only intermittently, making diagnosis difficult. The pathophysiology associated with diet-responsive diarrhea has not been studied because diarrhea resolves after minimal diagnostic testing and simple therapy. The characteristics of effective diets include high digestibility and low fiber (limiting the amount of nutrients that reach the colon) and a relatively low fat content. Unabsorbed fats can be metabolized by intestinal bacteria to hydroxy fatty acids that can promote diarrhea (see p. 632 for further information).

Although *Clostridium perfringens* enterotoxicosis has been reported to cause a catarrhal or suppurative colitis, less than 10% of the cases reported in Table 1 had histologic evidence of colitis. Thus, *C. perfringens* enterotoxicosis cases were not classified as a cause of colitis. *C. perfringens* type A spores contain an enterotoxin that causes diarrhea. The reasons for sporulation and enterotoxin formation are not known. Diagnosis is based on finding greater than three to four spores per oil immersion field in a rectal cytologic sample or identification of the toxin in feces with a reverse passive latex agglutination test (Pet RPLA *Clostridium perfringens*, Oxoid Limited, Hampshire, England).

Idiopathic large bowel diarrhea was diagnosed if all test results were within normal limits. Some of these cases could be classified as irritable bowel syndrome (see *CVT XI*, p. 604), whereas others were considered to have fiber-responsive large bowel diarrhea. The diagnosis of fiber-responsive large bowel diarrhea was based on a good or excellent clinical response to supplementation of the diet with the soluble fiber psyllium.

Adenocarcinoma and lymphosarcoma were the most common tumors found. Adenocarcinoma often occurs in older dogs and appears as an annular mass. Diagnosis requires biopsy of abnormal tissue. Lymphosarcoma occurs in middle-aged to older dogs. Often a diffuse infiltrative form occurs where the mucosa is thickened and roughened. Single or multiple masses can also be present. Concurrent involvement of the small intestines, stomach, and liver can occur. Diagnosis requires aspiration or biopsy of affected tissue. This series of cases did not contain any adenomatous polyps because dogs with polyps often do not have large bowel diarrhea but have hematochezia, excess mucus, and tenesmus.

DIAGNOSTIC PLAN

Only after following a thorough diagnostic plan, one that includes colonic biopsy, can a diagnosis of colitis be made. After chronic diarrhea has been localized to the large intestine (based on the historical description of the feces), some of the most common causes should be considered initially. Multiple fecal examinations should be performed to rule out the presence of whipworms. Because they are intermittent shedders of relatively low numbers of eggs, therapeutic deworming should be carried out even if results of fecal examinations are negative. The only time the author does not consider whipworms to be a likely cause of diarrhea is when the dog has received monthly

milbemycin for heartworm prophylaxis. Many products are effective in removing whipworms (see Appendix, p. 1239). The author often uses fenbendazole, 50 mg/kg SID PO for 3 days. If clinical signs resolve, the treatment should be repeated in 3 weeks and again in 3 months.

A rectal specimen should be obtained for cytologic study to evaluate for the presence of clostridial spores. A gloved finger should be used to abrade the rectal wall gently. The finger should be rolled gently across a microscope slide and the slide stained with a modified Wright's stain. Greater than three to four spores per oil immersion field is suggestive of *C. perfringens* enterotoxicosis. Treatment with amoxicillin, 10 to 20 mg/kg BID to TID for 7 to 14 days should resolve the diarrhea.

If whipworms or clostridial spores are not detected, and therapeutic deworming and amoxicillin therapy do not resolve clinical signs, a 3- to 4-week diet trial with a highly digestible diet is indicated (see p. 653). During this time, only the prescribed diet should be fed, and all forms of dietary indiscretion must be avoided. Although homemade diet recipes are available, most clients prefer prepared diets for convenience. Many acceptable diets are available and include i/d (Hill's Pet Products), EN (Ralston Purina), Low Residue Formula (Iams), and Low Fat (Waltham).

If diarrhea continues despite the dietary trial, further diagnostic testing is indicated. A minimum database consisting of a complete blood count, biochemical profile, and urinalysis, should be collected to rule out the presence of concurrent metabolic diseases and to assess the animal's risk if general anesthesia is used. Most dogs with colitis have a relatively normal database. Anemia and hypoproteinemia can develop if colonic ulceration is present. A fecal sample should be evaluated for clostridial enterotoxin with a reverse passive latex agglutination test. The author has seen cases that were negative for spores on cytologic examination and positive for toxin that responded to amoxicillin therapy. Finally, colonoscopic examination and histologic assessment of biopsy samples should be performed. The colon must be carefully prepared by withholding food for 24 hours and using a colonic lavage solution, such as GoLYTELY (Braintree Laboratories). Multiple tissue samples should be collected, even if the mucosal surface appears normal. The author routinely collects samples from the cecum, ascending and transverse colon, and the proximal, middle, and distal descending colon. The reader is referred to the reference list for a complete discussion of colonoscopic techniques.

TREATMENT

The optimal therapy for dogs with colitis often requires a combination of dietary and pharmacologic management that should be modified for each case. If initial therapeutic management does not improve clinical signs, other drugs and drug combinations should be instituted. When compared with the administration of a single drug, combination therapy often allows decreased drug dosages to be used, which reduces adverse drug effects. The initial treatment of choice varies greatly among clinicians, with some preferring dietary manipulations, whereas others use sulfasalazine, prednisone, or metronidazole. Regardless of the therapy selected, it should be continued 2 to 4 weeks past resolution of the clinical signs before dosage reduction is attempted. If the stool remains normal, further dosage reductions can be made at 2- to 4-week intervals. If diarrhea returns, the higher dosage that controlled clinical signs must be reinstituted. Reduction of drug dosage too soon may result in diarrhea that does not respond to the previously used dosage. Some animals require long-term or lifelong therapy.

Dietary Management

Hypoallergenic diets have been shown to alleviate diarrhea in several studies, and they are also successful in the author's experience. The diet must be highly digestible and contain a single protein that the dog has not previously eaten. The hypoallergenic diet must be the only source of nutrition that the dog receives during the 3- to 4-week trial period. Some dogs can be successfully managed with only a hypoallergenic diet. In other cases, the diarrhea improves, but medical therapy must be added to control clinical signs completely. In dogs that do not improve at all with hypoallergenic diet therapy, a highly digestible, low-fat, low-fiber diet should be fed. The reader is referred to the articles on Dietary Sensitivity (see p. 632) and Dietary Management of Diarrhea (see p. 653).

Sulfasalazine

If a hypoallergenic diet fails to control clinical signs, the author's drug of choice is sulfasalazine. This agent consists of mesalamine (previously called 5-aminosalicylic acid) linked by an azo bond to sulfapyridine. This linkage prevents absorption by the small intestine and allows delivery of approximately 70% of the drug to the colon. Bacteria in the distal small intestine and the colon break the azo bond, liberating both components. Sulfapyridine is absorbed, metabolized in the liver, and excreted by the kidney. It is not thought to have therapeutic effects in colitis and is responsible for some of the adverse reactions associated with sulfasalazine. Mesalamine acts topically in the colon to reduce mucosal inflammation due to antiprostaglandin and antileukotriene activity.

The recommended dosage range for sulfasalazine in dogs is 20 to 50 mg/kg up to a maximum of 1 gm t.i.d. High dosages are often needed in chronic cases. When treating a dog initially, a dosage of 20 to 30 mg/kg t.i.d. usually is effective. As previously discussed, the dosage can be slowly reduced at 2- to 4-week intervals if the stool remains normal. Initially, the author gives the same dose b.i.d., then 50% of the dose b.i.d then 50% of the initial dose s.i.d., and finally therapy is discontinued. In some dogs, sulfasalazine can be discontinued, whereas other cases require long-term therapy. Concurrent dietary management with a hypoallergenic or highly digestible diet may help control clinical signs with a lower dosage of sulfasalazine.

Vomiting and keratoconjunctivitis sicca are common side effects of therapy. Vomiting can usually be controlled by administering medication with food or using an enteric-coated preparation. If decreased tear production is detected early, reducing the dosage or discontinuing the drug may result in increased tear production and prevent progression to keratoconjunctivitis sicca. However, if decreased tear production is not detected early, it can become irreversible. The mechanism of action for this toxicity is unknown, but sulfapyridine may directly damage the lacrimal and nictitans tear glands, reducing production of the aqueous component of tears. When initiating sulfasalazine treatment, especially with high dosages, tear production should be monitored at 2- to 4-week intervals.

In order to reduce the toxicity associated with sulfasalazine, new drugs have been developed that deliver mesalamine to the colon without linkage to sulfapyridine. These drugs have been shown to be safe and effective in humans with IBD. Two have been approved for use in humans in the United States. Olsalazine (Dipentum, Kabi Pharmacia Laboratories) consists of two molecules of mesalamine linked with an azo bond. Asacol (Procter & Gamble Pharmaceuticals) consists of mesalamine coated with an acrylic resin that dissolves at a pH of 7 or greater, usually in the terminal ileum and colon. Although there are no firmly established guidelines for using these drugs in dogs with colitis, 10 to 20 mg/kg TID and 10 mg/kg TID, respectively, have been suggested.

These newer agents are less toxic than sulfasalazine in humans; approximately 80 to 90% of patients with sulfasalazine intolerance can be treated with these drugs without adverse effects. Although these drugs have not been used extensively in dogs, keratoconjunctivitis sicca has unfortunately been associated with Asacol use in a limited number of cases. The mechanism of toxicity is unknown. Because of their cost, and the fact that many dogs with colitis can be safely and effectively treated with sulfasalazine, Dipentum and Asacol should not be the initial drug used in dogs with colitis but should be reserved for those that have side effects associated with sulfasalazine.

Corticosteroids

Most dogs with colitis can be treated effectively by following the guidelines already described. Occasionally, other medications need to be used along with dietary management or in combination with sulfasalazine. The most common of these drugs are glucocorticoids or metronidazole. The efficacy of corticosteroids is thought to be due to their anti-inflammatory, antiprostaglandin, antileukotriene, and immunosuppressive effects. They inhibit cell membrane phospholipase A, suppressing the production of arachidonic acid and subsequently prostaglandin and leukotriene synthesis. Corticosteroids also increase sodium and water absorption and help regulate colonic electrolyte transport.

An initial dose of prednisone or prednisolone of 2 mg/kg per day often improves clinical signs. After normal feces have been produced for approximately 2 to 4 weeks, the dosage should be decreased by 50%. As long as diarrhea does not return, the dosage can gradually be reduced (at 2- to 4-week intervals) until the least amount that controls clinical signs is reached (alternate-day therapy). Some dogs require long-term treatment, whereas it is possible in others to discontinue prednisone within 3 to 4 months. When using prednisone with sulfasalazine, it may be possible to reduce the dosage of sulfasalazine when the prednisone dosage declines to 1 mg/kg every 48 hours. Side effects are common in dogs and often are dose-related. They include polyuria-polydipsia, polyphagia, iatrogenic hyperadrenocorticism, hypothalamic-pituitary suppression, gastrointestinal bleeding, acute pancreatitis, steroid hepatopathy, and predisposition to bacterial or fungal infections.

Metronidazole

Metronidazole possesses several properties thought to be beneficial in dogs with colitis. Besides antiprotozoal effects, it is a broad-spectrum antibiotic with excellent activity against anaerobic bacteria; it inhibits cell-mediated immunity, alters neutrophil chemotaxis, and may have other immunosuppressive effects. Ten to 20 mg/kg BID to TID has been recommended. Adverse effects at this dosage are uncommon, but severe neurologic toxicity has been reported with higher dosages. Peripheral neuropathy has developed in humans receiving long-term therapy. The author has found that the addition of metronidazole, for 2 to 4 weeks, to maintenance therapy may be beneficial in dogs that experience an unexplained bout of diarrhea.

References and Suggested Reading

Ewing GO, Gomez JA: Canine ulcerative colitis. J Am Anim Hosp Assoc 9:395, 1973.
The largest report of colitis cases.
Hall EJ, Rutgers HC, Scholes SFE, et al: Histiocytic ulcerative colitis in boxer dogs in the UK. J Small Anim Pract 35:509, 1994.
The most recent report of histiocytic colitis.
Leib MS, Matz M: Diseases of the intestines. In: Leib MS, Monroe WE, ed: Practical Small Animal Internal Medicine. Philadelphia: WB Saunders, 1997, p 685.
A complete discussion of all diseases of the intestines.
Leib MS: Colonoscopy. In: Tams TR, ed: Small Animal Endoscopy. St. Louis, CV Mosby, 1990a, p 211.
A complete description of colonoscopic techniques.
Leib MS: Fiber-responsive large bowel diarrhea. Proceedings of the American College of Veterinary Internal Medicine, Washington, DC, 1990b, p 817.
A presentation of cases and discussion of fiber-responsive diarrhea.
Leib MS, Hiler LA, Roth L, et al: Plasmacytic lymphocytic colitis in the dog. Semin Vet Med Surg 4:241, 1989.
A report of nine cases of colitis.
Nelson RW, Stookey LJ, Kazacos E: Nutritional management of idiopathic chronic colitis in the dog. J Vet Intern Med 2:133, 1988.
A clinical study showing the benefit of a restricted antigen diet.
Roth L, Walton AM, Leib MS, et al: A grading system for lymphocytic plasmacytic colitis in dogs. J Vet Diagn Invest 2:257, 1990.
A detailed histologic grading system for colitis.
Simpson JW, Maskell IE, Markwell PJ: Use of a restricted antigen diet in the management of idiopathic canine colitis. J Small Anim Pract 35:233, 1994.
A recent clinical study showing the benefit of a restricted antigen diet.
Twedt DC: *Clostridium perfringens*–associated enterotoxicosis in dogs. In: Kirk RW, Bonagura JD, eds: Current Veterinary Therapy XI. Philadelphia: WB Saunders, 1992, p 602.
A discussion of C. perfringens enterotoxicosis.

Feline Constipation and Idiopathic Megacolon

ROBERT J. WASHABAU

DAVID HOLT
Philadelphia, Pennsylvania

CLINICAL PRESENTATION

Constipation, obstipation, and megacolon may be observed in cats of any age, sex, or breed; however, most cases are observed in middle-aged (mean = 5.8 years) male cats (70% male, 30% female) of domestic shorthair (46%), domestic longhair (15%), or Siamese (12%) breeding (Washabau and Hasler, 1996). Affected cats are usually presented to the clinician because of reduced, absent, or painful defecation for a period ranging from days to weeks or months. Some cats are observed making multiple, unproductive attempts to defecate in the litter box, whereas other cats may sit in the litter box for prolonged periods without assuming a defecation posture. Dry, hardened feces are observed inside and outside of the litter box. Occasionally, chronically constipated cats have intermittent episodes of hematochezia or diarrhea due to the mucosal irritant effect of fecal concretions. This may give the pet owner the erroneous impression that diarrhea is the primary problem. The prolonged inability to defecate may result in other systemic signs, including anorexia, lethargy, weight loss, and vomiting.

Colonic impaction is the consistent finding on physical examination in affected cats. Other findings depend on the severity and pathogenesis of constipation. Dehydration, weight loss, debilitation, abdominal pain, and mild to moderate mesenteric lymphadenopathy can be observed in cats with severe idiopathic megacolon. Colonic impaction can be so severe in such cases as to render it difficult to differentiate impaction from colonic, mesenteric, or other abdominal neoplasia. Cats with constipation resulting from dysautonomia can have other signs of autonomic nervous system failure, such as urinary and fecal incontinence, regurgitation resulting from megaesophagus, mydriasis, decreased lacrimation, prolapse of the nictitating membrane, and bradycardia. Digital rectal examination should be performed carefully in all cats using sedation or anesthesia. Pelvic fracture malunion may be detected on rectal examination in cats with pelvic trauma. Rectal examination might also identify other unusual causes of constipation, such as foreign bodies, rectal diverticula, stricture, inflammation, or neoplasia. Chronic tenesmus may be associated with perineal herniation in some cases. A complete neurologic examination with special emphasis on caudal spinal cord function should be performed to identify neurologic causes of constipation, for example, spinal cord injury, pelvic nerve trauma, and Manx sacral spinal cord deformity.

ETIOLOGY AND PATHOGENESIS

Several authors have emphasized the importance of considering an extensive list of differential diagnoses (e.g., neuromuscular, mechanical, inflammatory, metabolic and endocrine, pharmacologic, environmental, and behavioral causes) for the obstipated cat. A review by Washabau and Hasler (1996), however, suggests that 96% of cases of obstipation are caused by idiopathic megacolon (62%), pelvic canal stenosis (23%), nerve injury (6%), or Manx sacral spinal cord deformity (5%). A smaller number of cases are caused by complications of colopexy (1%) and colonic neoplasia (1%); colonic hypo- or aganglionosis was suspected, but not proved, in another 2% of cases. Inflammatory, pharmacologic, and environmental and behavioral causes were not cited as predisposing factors in any of the original case reports. Endocrine factors (obesity, n = 5; hypothyroidism, n = 1) were cited in several cases but were not necessarily implicated in the pathogenesis of megacolon. Thus, although it is important to consider an extensive list of differential diagnoses in an individual animal, it should be kept in mind that most cases are idiopathic, orthopedic, or neurologic in origin (Washabau and Hasler, 1996).

The pathogenesis of idiopathic megacolon has been variably attributed to a primary neurogenic or degenerative neuromuscular disorder. Although it seems clear that a small number of cases (11%) result from neurologic disease, the vast majority (>60%) of cases have no evidence of such disease (Washabau and Hasler, 1996). These idiopathic cases may instead involve disturbances of colonic smooth muscle. Studies suggest that colonic smooth muscle function is impaired in cats affected with idiopathic megacolon (Washabau and Stalis, 1996; Hasler and Washabau, 1997). In vitro isometric stress measurements were performed on colonic smooth muscle segments obtained from cats with idiopathic dilatated megacolon. Megacolonic smooth muscle developed less isometric stress in response to neurotransmitters (acetylcholine, substance P, cholecystokinin), membrane depolarization (potassium chloride), and electrical field stimulation, when compared with healthy controls. These differences were observed in longitudinal and circular smooth muscle from both ascending and descending colon. No significant abnormalities of smooth muscle cells or of myenteric neurons were observed on histologic evaluation. These studies suggested that the disorder of feline idiopathic megacolon is a generalized dysfunction of colonic smooth muscle and that treatments aimed at stimulating colonic smooth muscle contraction

might improve colonic motility (Washabau and Stalis, 1996; Hasler and Washabau, 1997).

DIAGNOSTIC WORK-UP

Although most cases of obstipation and megacolon are unlikely to have significant changes in routine laboratory data (e.g., complete blood count, serum chemistry panels, urinalysis), these tests should nonetheless be performed in all cats presented for constipation. Metabolic causes of constipation, such as dehydration, hypokalemia, and hypercalcemia, may be detected in some cases. Basal serum thyroxine concentration and other thyroid function tests should also be considered in cats with recurrent constipation and other signs consistent with hypothyroidism.

Abdominal radiography should be performed in all constipated cats to characterize the severity of colonic impaction and to identify predisposing factors such as intraluminal radiopaque foreign material (e.g., bone chips), intraluminal or extraluminal mass lesions, pelvic fractures, and spinal cord abnormalities. The radiographic findings of colonic impaction cannot be used to distinguish among constipation, obstipation, and megacolon in idiopathic cases. First or second episodes of constipation in some cats may be severe and generalized but may still resolve with appropriate treatment.

Ancillary studies may be indicated in some cases. Extraluminal mass lesions can be further evaluated by abdominal ultrasonography and guided biopsy, whereas intraluminal mass lesions are best evaluated by endoscopy. Colonoscopy may also be used to evaluate the colon and anorectum for suspected inflammatory lesions, strictures, sacculations, and diverticula. Barium enema contrast radiography may be used if colonoscopy is not possible. Both colonoscopy and barium enema contrast radiography require colonic evacuation by enema before general anesthesia and must be done with care. Cerebrospinal fluid analysis and myelographic and electrophysiologic studies should be considered in animals with evidence of neurologic impairment. Finally, colonic biopsy or anorectal manometry is necessary to diagnose suspected cases of aganglionic megacolon.

THERAPY

The specific therapeutic plan will depend on the severity of constipation and the underlying cause (Washabau and Hasler, 1996). Medical therapy may not be necessary with first episodes of constipation. These episodes are often transient and resolve without therapy. Conversely, mild to moderate or recurrent episodes of constipation usually require some medical intervention. These cases may be managed, often on an outpatient basis, with dietary modification, water enemas, oral or suppository laxatives, colonic prokinetic agents, or a combination of these methods. Severe cases of constipation usually require brief periods of hospitalization to correct metabolic abnormalities and to evacuate impacted feces using water enemas or manual extraction of retained feces, or both. Follow-up therapy in such cases is directed at correcting predisposing factors and preventing recurrence. Subtotal colectomy will become necessary in cats suffering from obstipation or idiopathic dilatated megacolon. These cats, by definition, are unresponsive to medical therapy. Pelvic osteotomy without colectomy may be sufficient for some cats suffering from pelvic canal stenosis and hypertrophic megacolon of less than 6 months' duration (Schrader, 1992). An algorithm for the therapeutic approach to the constipated, obstipated, and megacolonic cat is outlined in Figure 1.

Removal of Impacted Feces

Rectal Suppositories

A number of pediatric rectal suppositories are available for the management of mild constipation (Table 1). They include dioctyl sodium sulfosuccinate (Colace, Mead Johnson; an emollient laxative), glycerin (a lubricant laxative), and bisacodyl (Dulcolax, Boehringer Ingelheim; a stimulant laxative). The use of rectal suppositories requires a compliant pet and a willing pet owner. Suppositories can be used alone or in conjunction with oral laxative therapy (see the section on laxative therapy further on).

Enemas

Mild to moderate or recurrent episodes of constipation may require the administration of enemas or manual extraction of impacted feces, or both. Several types of enema solutions may be administered, such as warm tap water (5 to 10 ml/kg), warm isotonic saline (5 to 10 ml/kg), dioctyl sodium sulfosuccinate (5 to 10 ml/cat), mineral oil (5 to 10 ml/cat), or lactulose (5 to 10 ml/cat). Enema solutions should be administered slowly with a well-lubricated 10F to 12F rubber catheter or feeding tube.

Manual Extraction

Cats that are unresponsive to enemas may require manual extraction of impacted feces. The cat should be ade-quately rehydrated and then anesthetized with an endotracheal tube in place to prevent aspiration should colonic manipulation induce vomiting. Water or saline is infused into the colon while the fecal mass is manually reduced by abdominal palpation. Sponge forceps may also be introduced rectally (with caution) to break down the fecal mass. It may be advisable to evacuate the fecal mass over a period of several days to reduce the risks of prolonged anesthesia and perforation of a devitalized colon. If this approach fails, colotomy may be necessary to remove the fecal mass. Laxative or prokinetic therapy, or both, may be instituted once the fecal mass has been removed.

Laxative Therapy

Bulk-Forming Laxatives

Most of the available bulk-forming laxatives are dietary fiber supplements of poorly digestible polysaccharides and celluloses derived principally from cereal grains, wheat bran, and psyllium. Many constipated cats will respond to supplementation of the diet with one of these products. Dietary fiber is preferable because it is well tolerated, more effective, and more physiologic than other laxatives. Fiber-supplemented diets (e.g., Prescription Diet w/d and r/d, Science Diet Lite, Hill's Pet Products) are available commercially, or the pet owner may wish to add psyllium (1 to 4 tsp per meal), wheat bran (1 to 2 tbsp per meal), or pumpkin (1 to 4 tbsp per meal) to canned cat food. Cats should be well hydrated before commencing fiber supplementation to maximize the therapeutic effect and to minimize the impaction of fiber in the constipated colon.

Emollient Laxatives

Emollient laxatives are anionic detergents that increase the miscibility of water and lipid in digesta, thereby enhancing lipid absorption and impairing water absorption.

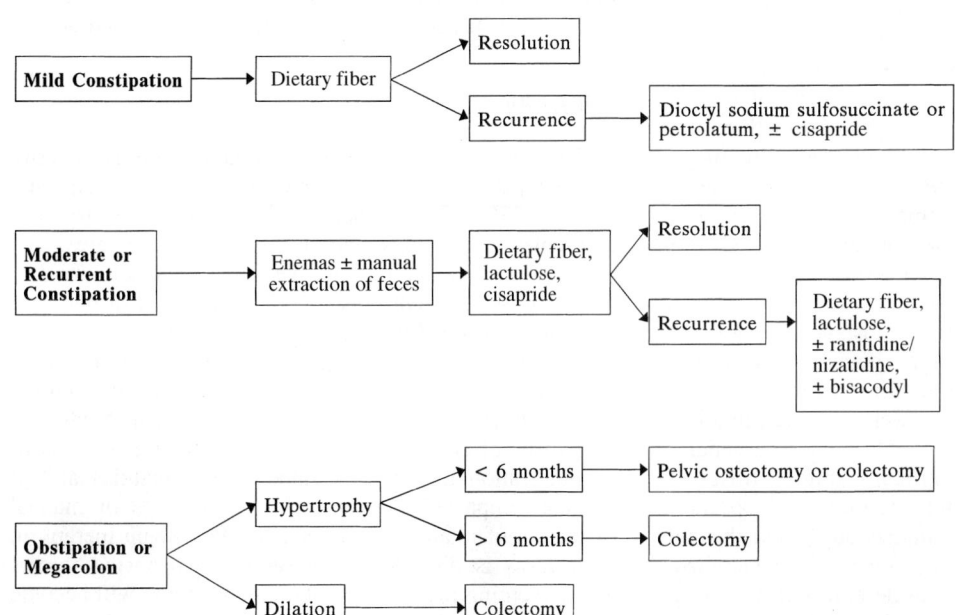

Figure 1. Management of mild, moderate, and recurrent constipation. (Modified from Washabau RJ, Hasler AH: Constipation, obstipation, and megacolon. In: August JR, ed: Consultations in Feline Internal Medicine, 3rd ed. Philadelphia: WB Saunders, 1997, p 108, with permission.)

TABLE 1. **Medical Therapy for Feline Constipation and Obstipation**

Drug Classification, Example, and Dosage	Dose
Rectal suppositories	
Dioctyl sodium sulfosuccinate (Colace, Mead Johnson)	1–2 pediatric suppositories
Glycerin (many manufacturers)	1–2 pediatric suppositories
Bisacodyl (Dulcolax, Boehringer Ingelheim)	1–2 pediatric suppositories
Enemas	
Warm tap water	5–10 ml/kg
Warm isotonic saline	5–10 ml/kg
Dioctyl sodium sulfosuccinate (Colace, Mead Johnson)	5–10 ml/cat
Dioctyl sodium sulfosuccinate	250 mg (12 ml) given per rectum as needed
Mineral oil (many manufacturers)	5–10 ml/cat
Lactulose (Cephulac, Merrell Dow; Duphalac, Reid Rowell)	5–10 ml/cat
Oral laxatives	
Bulk laxatives	
Psyllium (Metamucil, Searle)	1–4 tsp mixed with food q24hr or q12hr
Canned pumpkin	1–4 tbsp mixed with food q24hr
Coarse wheat bran	1–2 tbsp mixed with food q24hr
Emollient laxatives	
Dioctyl sodium sulfosuccinate (Colace, Mead Johnson)	50 mg q24hr PO
Dioctyl calcium sulfosuccinate	50 mg q24hr or q12h PO as needed
Lubricant laxatives	
Mineral oil (many manufacturers)	10–25 ml q24hr PO
Petrolatum (Laxatone, Evsco)	1–5 ml q24h PO
Hyperosmotic laxatives	
Lactulose (Cephulac, Merrell Dow; Duphalac, Reid Rowell)	0.5 ml/kg q8hr to q12hr PO as needed
Stimulant laxatives	
Bisacodyl (Dulcolax, Boehringer Ingelheim)	5 mg q24hr PO
Prokinetic agents	
Cisapride (Propulsid, Janssen)	0.1–1.0 mg/kg q8hr to q12hr PO
Ranitidine (Zantac, Glaxo)	1.0–2.0 mg/kg PO q8hr to q12hr
Nizatidine (Axid, Eli Lilly)	2.5–5.0 mg/kg PO q24hr

Dioctyl sodium sulfosuccinate and dioctyl calcium sulfosuccinate are examples of emollient laxatives available in oral and enema form. As with bulk-forming laxatives, animals should be well hydrated before emollient laxatives are administered. It should be noted that clinical efficacy has not been definitively established for the emollient laxatives. Dioctyl sodium sulfosuccinate, for example, inhibits water absorption in isolated colonic segments in vitro, but it may be impossible to achieve tissue concentrations great enough to inhibit colonic water absorption in vivo.

Lubricant Laxatives

Mineral oil and white petrolatum are the two major lubricant laxatives available for the treatment of constipation. The lubricating properties of these agents impede colonic water absorption and permit greater ease of fecal passage. These effects are usually moderate, however, and in general lubricants are beneficial only in mild cases of constipation. Mineral oil use should probably be limited to rectal administration because of the risk of aspiration pneumonia with oral administration, especially in depressed or debilitated cats.

Hyperosmotic Laxatives

Hyperosmotic laxatives consist of the poorly absorbed polysaccharides (e.g., lactose, lactulose), the magnesium salts (e.g., magnesium citrate, magnesium hydroxide, magnesium sulfate), and the polyethylene glycols. Lactulose (Cephulac, Hoechst-Marion-Roussel; Duphalac, Solvay) is the most effective agent in this group. The organic acids produced from lactulose fermentation stimulate colonic fluid secretion and propulsive motility. Lactulose administered at a dosage of 0.5 ml/kg body weight every 8 to 12 hours fairly consistently produces soft feces in the cat. Many cats with recurrent or chronic constipation have been managed well with this regimen of lactulose. The dosage may have to be tapered in individual cases if flatulence and diarrhea become excessive. Magnesium salts and polyethylene glycols are *not* currently recommended in the treatment of feline constipation and idiopathic megacolon (Washabau and Hasler, 1996).

Stimulant Laxatives

The stimulant laxatives are a diverse group of agents that have been classified according to their ability to stimulate propulsive motility. Bisacodyl, at a dosage of 5 mg every 24 hours PO, is the most effective stimulant laxative in the cat. It may be given individually or in combination with fiber supplementation for long-term management of constipation. Daily administration of bisacodyl should probably be avoided, however, because of injury to myenteric neurons with chronic use.

Colonic Prokinetic Agents

Cisapride (Propulsid, Janssen) enhances colonic propulsive motility through activation of colonic smooth muscle 5-hydroxytryptamine$_{2a}$ receptors in a number of animal species (Washabau and Hall, 1995; also see p. 614). In vitro studies have shown that cisapride stimulates feline colonic smooth muscle contraction (Washabau and Sammarco, 1996; Hasler and Washabau, 1997), although it has not yet been conclusively shown that cisapride stimulates feline colonic propulsive motility in vivo. Anecdotal experience at this time suggests that cisapride is effective in stimulating colonic propulsive motility in cats affected with mild to moderate idiopathic constipation; cats with longstanding obstipation and megacolon are not likely to show much improvement with cisapride therapy. The recommended dosage of cisapride for cats affected with mild to moderate idiopathic constipation has been 0.1 to 0.5 mg/kg every 8 to 12 hours PO. Higher dosages of cisapride (0.5 to 1.0 mg/kg) may be necessary in cats with moderate to severe constipation. At present, no significant side effects have been observed or reported in cats medicated with cisapride at dosages of 0.1 to 1.0 mg/kg every 8 to 12 hours PO.

Ranitidine and nizatidine, two members of the H_2 receptor antagonist drug class, are reported to stimulate colonic motility through inhibition of synaptic acetylcholinesterase (reviewed in Hall and Washabau, 1997). Ranitidine and nizatidine are selectively concentrated in gastrointestinal tract tissues, and they stimulate motility by increasing the amount of acetylcholine available to bind smooth muscle muscarinic cholinergic receptors. Other members of this same drug class (e.g., cimetidine, famotidine) do not have this effect. Thus, ranitidine and nizatidine may be useful colonic prokinetic agents in the treatment of constipated cats that have failed to respond to cisapride (Hall and Washabau, 1997).

Surgery

Idiopathic Dilated Megacolon

Colectomy should be considered in cats that are refractory to medical therapy (see *CVT XI,* p. 623). After a midline abdominal incision, the colon is exteriorized, fecal contents are moved from the operative site by gentle digital pressure, and the colonic lumen is occluded with a noncrushing clamp. Colectomy with colocolonic, ileocolonic, or jejunocolonic anastomosis may be performed, depending on the extent of disease. With routine colectomy, the ascending colon is transected 2 to 4 cm distal to the cecum, and the descending colon is transected 2 to 4 cm proximal to the pubis. The caudal mesenteric artery and vein should be left intact to maximize blood supply to the colon distal to the anastomosis. The colonic segments are anastomosed using a single layer of simple interrupted, appositional 4–0 polydioxanone sutures. The ileocolic junction should be preserved whenever possible (Sweet et al, 1994). Cats have a generally favorable prognosis for recovery after colectomy (Gregory et al, 1990; Rosin et al, 1988). Mild to moderate diarrhea may occasionally persist for weeks to months postoperatively, and some cats may suffer recurrences of constipation (Sweet et al, 1994).

Hypertrophic Megacolon

Pelvic osteotomy without colectomy has been recommended for cats with pelvic fracture malunion and hypertrophic megacolon of less than 6 months' duration (Schrader, 1992; see Fig. 1). Pathologic hypertrophy may be reversible with early pelvic osteotomy in such cases. Some surgeons still prefer colectomy in this instance because of the technical difficulty of some pelvic osteotomies (Matthiesen et al, 1991).

Subtotal colectomy is recommended in cats with pelvic fractures if hypertrophy and clinical signs have persisted for longer than 6 months (Schrader, 1992; Matthiesen et al, 1991). Hypertrophy is thought to be superseded by neuromuscular degeneration and pathologic dilatation in these cases. Pelvic osteotomy alone will not provide relief from obstipation in such cases; interestingly, many of these cats improve with colectomy alone.

References and Suggested Reading

Gregory CR, Guilford WG, Berry CR, et al: Enteric function in cats after subtotal colectomy for treatment of megacolon. Vet Surg 19:216, 1990.
Enteric function is preserved after subtotal colectomy in cats with idiopathic megacolon.

Hall JA, Washabau RJ: Gastrointestinal prokinetic therapy: Acetylcholinesterase inhibitors. Compend Contin Educ Pract Vet 19:615, 1997.
A review of ranitidine and nizatidine, inhibitors of synaptic acetylcholinesterase activity.

Hasler AH, Washabau RJ: Cisapride stimulates contraction of idiopathic megacolonic smooth muscle in cats. J Vet Intern Med 11:313, 1997.
Megacolonic smooth muscle is responsive to cisapride prokinetic therapy.

Matthiesen DT, Scavelli TD, Whitney WO: Subtotal colectomy for treatment of obstipation secondary to pelvic fracture malunion in cats. Vet Surg 20:113, 1991.
Colectomy without pelvic osteotomy is useful in some cats with pelvic fracture malunion.

Rosin E, Walshaw R, Mehlhaff C, et al: Subtotal colectomy for treatment of chronic constipation associated with idiopathic megacolon in cats. J Am Vet Med Assoc 193:850, 1988.
Colectomy is safe and effective in the management of feline idiopathic megacolon.

Schrader SC: Pelvic osteotomy as a treatment for obstipation in cats with acquired stenosis of the pelvic canal. J Am Vet Med Assoc 200:208, 1992.
Pelvic osteotomy without colectomy may be sufficient in cats with pelvic fracture malunion of less than 6 months' duration.

Sweet DC, Hardie EM, Stone EA: Preservation versus excision of the ileocolic junction during colectomy for megacolon: A study of 22 cats. J Small Anim Pract 35:358, 1994.
Cats have fewer postoperative complications if the ileocolic junction is preserved during colectomy.

Washabau RJ, Hall JA: Clinical pharmacology of cisapride. J Am Vet Med Assoc 207:1285, 1995.
A review of the clinical use of cisapride in the treatment of gastrointestinal motility disorders.

Washabau RJ, Hasler AH: Constipation, obstipation, and megacolon. In: August JR, ed: Consultations in Feline Internal Medicine, 3rd ed. Philadelphia: WB Saunders, 1997, p 104.
A review of the epidemiology, pathogenesis, and therapy of feline idiopathic megacolon.

Washabau RJ, Sammarco J: Effect of cisapride on feline colonic smooth muscle function. Am J Vet Res 57:541, 1996.
Cisapride stimulates contraction of feline colonic smooth muscle.

Washabau RJ, Stalis IH: Alterations in colonic smooth muscle function in cats affected with idiopathic megacolon. Am J Vet Res 57:580, 1996.
Feline idiopathic megacolon is a generalized disorder of colonic smooth muscle.

Nutritional Management of Diarrheal Diseases

Stanley L. Marks

Andrea J. Fascetti

Davis, California

The disciplines of nutrition and gastroenterology are intimately related by virtue of the primary role played by the gastrointestinal tract in the assimilation of food. The therapeutic approach to most gastrointestinal diseases involves a combination of pharmacologic and nutritional therapy. Unfortunately, the beneficial impact of nutritional therapy is often ignored in many patients, resulting in incomplete or delayed resolution of signs. Restriction or manipulation of individual dietary components is perhaps the single most important factor in the treatment of either acute or chronic gastrointestinal disturbances. Despite these recommendations, there is a paucity of information pertaining to the nutritional requirements of dogs and cats with gastrointestinal disorders.

ACUTE GASTROINTESTINAL DISEASE

The traditional dietary recommendations for managing dogs and cats with acute gastroenteritis include fasting the patient for 24 to 48 hours, followed by feeding a "bland," highly digestible, low-fat diet. The provision of bowel "rest" has been advocated to reduce the quantity of unabsorbed nutrients that could result in osmotic diarrhea, to decrease bacterial flora, and to attenuate antigenic stimulation of the mucosa. A low-fat diet is preferred in the refeeding period because malabsorbed fatty acids and bile acids may potentiate a secretory diarrhea in the large bowel. Boiled hamburger (with the fat poured off) and rice, cottage cheese and rice, or chicken and rice in an approximately 1:4 ratio are commonly used for managing acute gastroenteritis in dogs. Cats can be managed by offering small portions of cooked chicken or turkey alone for several days without adverse effect. Carbohydrates are usually deleted from the "bland" diet for cats, although baby rice cereal can be used if desired. The meals are typically offered in three to four small feedings per day to avoid overloading impaired digestive and absorptive functions. The animal's original diet may then be slowly reintroduced over a 2- to 3-day period provided that no adverse gastrointestinal effects have occurred. Recent studies have suggested that acquired food allergies to proteins ingested during acute gastroenteritis can delay recovery (Iyngkaran et al, 1978). The feeding of a "bland" diet containing a protein source different from that present in the patient's standard diet should theoretically reduce the likelihood of this problem occurring.

The novel concept of food-based oral rehydration and feeding-through-diarrhea has been well defined in humans and challenges the traditional dogma of bowel "rest" for managing acute diarrhea (Romatowski, 1985). Most oral rehydration solutions are isotonic and contain a carbohydrate source (glucose), an amino acid (glycine), an alkalinizing agent (sodium bicarbonate or sodium citrate), and electrolytes (sodium, potassium, chloride) (Zenger and Willard, 1989). Oral rehydration solutions act via a mechanism referred to as cotransport, or glucose-enhanced sodium resorption, in which active glucose and amino acid transport enhances the absorption of sodium and water. Patient selection for this mode of therapy is dependent on the presence of functional gastrointestinal epithelium and the absence of severe or intractable vomiting. The improper use of oral rehydration solutions can cause serious electrolyte imbalances, particularly hypernatremia. This condition is most likely to occur if insensible water losses are high, the kidneys' ability to excrete sodium is low, or the amount of oral rehydration solution offered exceeds the patient's deficits by a significant amount (Zenger and Willard, 1989). The induction of hypernatremia can be minimized by diluting two feedings of oral rehydration solution with one feeding of water (Zenger and Willard, 1989). Recommendations for dosage and administration technique vary; however, a minimal daily intake of 150 ml/kg every 24 hours has been advocated for small animals (Romatowski, 1985). The implementation of oral rehydration therapy in practice has been facilitated with the introduction of commercially manufactured veterinary oral electrolyte solutions such as Enterolyte (Pfizer, Inc., Exton, PA). Human oral electrolyte formulations should be avoided because of their high carbohydrate content and associated hyperosmolarity.

Feeding-through-diarrhea provides solid or semisolid food sufficient to meet the animal's caloric requirements. In humans, feeding-through-diarrhea has been shown to maintain greater mucosal barrier integrity and minimize malnutrition without prolonging the duration of the diarrhea (Brown, 1994). However, most of the studies in humans have involved secretory diarrhea, whereas dogs and cats with acute gastroenteritis usually have osmotic diarrhea. Furthermore, human studies indicate an increase in the frequency of stool production using this method, an adverse effect that may be unacceptable to owners of indoor pets. As a result, feeding-through-diarrhea may not be as successful in veterinary practice as the current recommendation of fasting the animal.

CHRONIC "SMALL BOWEL" DIARRHEA

Dietary modification is essential in the management of chronic diarrhea. For most chronic small bowel diarrhea, the diet selected should be (1) highly digestible, (2) low in fat and lactose, (3) gluten-free, (4) "hypoallergenic," and

653

(5) isotonic. The theoretic concerns with dietary fiber's "abrasive" effects on the inflamed intestinal tract and fiber's indigestibility are currently being reconsidered because the gelling and binding properties of fatty acids and deconjugated bile acids in soluble fibers may be beneficial in certain small bowel diseases.

Dietary Fat Content

A low-fat diet is important in the management of a variety of gastrointestinal diseases in dogs, even though fat is a valuable caloric source and enhances the palatability of the diet. Fat delays gastric emptying, and low-fat diets appear to be better tolerated in a variety of gastrointestinal diseases. In addition, fatty acids stimulate mucosal receptors to release cholecystokinin, a potent pancreatic secretagogue. For this reason, high-fat diets are relatively contraindicated in patients with pancreatitis. The assimilation of dietary fat is a relatively complex process and malabsorbed fatty acids are hydroxylated by intestinal and colonic bacteria. These hydroxy fatty acids stimulate colonic water secretion and exacerbate diarrhea and fluid loss. Fat malassimilation can also be associated with malabsorption of bile acids, resulting in deconjugation of unabsorbed bile acids and increased mucosal permeability and secretion. In contrast to dogs, cats with chronic gastrointestinal disease appear to be more tolerant of high-fat diets.

Dietary Lactose and Gluten Content

Intestinal disease frequently destroys or reduces mucosal brush border enzyme activity, particularly lactase, which is the most superficial enzyme. Milk or other lactose-containing substances should therefore be avoided in patients with enteric disease. Failure to digest lactose results in bacterial degradation of the sugar to volatile fatty acids, which can cause osmotic diarrhea. The use of yogurt for therapy of chronic diarrhea is not recommended because of its lactose content. In addition, orally administered bacteria in yogurt do not colonize the bowel and displace the "unfavorable" microorganisms in both normal and diseased intestines. Gluten is a component of wheat, oats, barley, and rye, all of which should be avoided in patients with inflammatory bowel disease (IBD) in the event that the diarrhea is due to a gluten enteropathy.

Dietary Protein Sources and Content

An attempt should be made to feed a highly digestible dietary protein source that the animal has not been previously exposed to. Excess dietary protein should be avoided to minimize dietary antigenicity and to limit the amount of malabsorbed protein, which can result in the generation of ammonia and contribute to colonic injury.

INFLAMMATORY BOWEL DISEASE

IBD in dogs and cats encompasses a spectrum of diseases that result in the accumulation of inflammatory cells within the mucosa and submucosa of the stomach, small intestine, or large intestine (see previous article). Although the pathogenesis of the syndrome is poorly understood, IBD is an inflammatory process thought to be initiated by dietary or microbial antigens in the gastrointestinal lumen. Because the presumed pathogenesis of IBD involves antigenic stimulation and an inflammatory response mediated by the mucosal immune system, therapy is aimed at removing any antigenic source of inflammation, followed by suppression of the cell-mediated inflammatory response in the gastrointestinal tract.

The goal of dietary management is to reduce antigenic stimulation of the intestinal immune system. Proteins, food colorings, and preservatives may all cause adverse gastrointestinal signs, but many of these reactions are direct and do not involve the immune system. Because antigenic determinants on proteins are incriminated as the causative factor in many cases of IBD, it is recommended that dogs and cats with IBD receive a "hypoallergenic" diet. The term *hypoallergenic* refers to a diet that is generally free of additives and preservatives and contains a single, novel protein source that is highly digestible. High-protein diets should be avoided because the excess dietary protein can lead to increased formation of antigen-antibody complexes in the intestinal wall. The protein should be highly digestible because intact proteins are far more antigenic than are polypeptides and amino acids.

There are no protein sources that are inherently hypoallergenic. Dogs and cats acquire immunologic sensitivities to dietary proteins that are eaten with some frequency. Wheat, corn, beef, milk, eggs, lamb, chicken, and fish can all be allergens promoting IBD in dogs and cats. The dietary strategy is to select a protein source that the animal has not eaten before. In dogs, a practical approach is to feed a homemade diet based on rice or potato. A single novel protein source such as cottage cheese, tofu, chicken, venison, rabbit, or lamb is added. In cats, homemade diets can include venison, rabbit, chicken, fish, or lamb. Cats do not readily accept cottage cheese and prefer baby rice cereal to cooked white rice. These diets must be balanced with essential fatty acids, calcium, minerals, vitamins, and taurine (cats) if they are to be fed for longer than several weeks. If the animal's clinical signs resolve on the homemade diet, one can then switch to a commercial diet with the same novel protein source (Table 1). It is important that the ingredients list of a potentially hypoallergenic diet be thoroughly evaluated because diets with several protein sources (lamb, beef, rice, and wheat) are commonly marketed with a claim to hypoallergenicity.

Diet Selection

The ideal diet for patients with chronic small bowel diarrhea is based on a highly digestible single protein and carbohydrate source that is gluten-free and low in fat and lactose. There are a limited number of commercial "hypoallergenic" diets currently available that fulfill these requirements (see Table 1), necessitating the use of computer-generated homemade diets in patients failing to respond to commercial diets (Table 2). Unfortunately, the increased use of commercial lamb-based formulas has diminished its application in many "hypoallergenic" diets, necessitating the selection of more "exotic" protein sources.

The concept of feeding a "sacrificial protein source" to

TABLE 1. Commercial Diets Containing Novel Protein Sources

Diet	Species	Protein Sources	Form
Hill's Prescription Diet d/d	Dogs	Whitefish	Canned
Hill's Prescription Diet d/d	Dogs	Lamb	Canned
Hill's Prescription Diet d/d	Dogs	Duck	Dry
Hill's Prescription Diet d/d	Dogs	Salmon	Dry
Hill's Prescription Diet d/d	Dogs	Egg	Dry
Hill's Prescription Diet d/d	Cats	Lamb	Canned
Waltham Selected Protein Diet	Dogs	Catfish	Dry
Waltham Selected Protein Diet	Dogs	Lamb	Canned
Waltham Selected Protein Diet	Cats	Duck	Dry
Waltham Selected Protein Diet	Cats	Venison	Canned
Innovative Veterinary Diets	Dogs	Duck	Canned/dry
Innovative Veterinary Diets	Dogs	Lamb	Canned/dry
Innovative Veterinary Diets	Dogs	Venison	Canned/dry
Innovative Veterinary Diets	Dogs	Rabbit	Canned
Innovative Veterinary Diets	Dogs	Whitefish	Canned
Innovative Veterinary Diets	Cats	Duck	Dry
Innovative Veterinary Diets	Cats	Lamb	Canned/dry
Innovative Veterinary Diets	Cats	Venison	Canned/dry
Innovative Veterinary Diets	Cats	Rabbit	Canned
Iams Eukanuba Response Formula	Dogs	Fish	Canned/dry
Iams Eukanuba Response Formula	Cats	Lamb	Canned
Nature's Recipe	Dogs	Lamb meal	Dry
Nature's Recipe	Dogs	Rabbit	Canned
Nature's Recipe	Dogs	Venison	Canned
Nature's Recipe	Dogs	Soybean	Canned/dry
Nature's Recipe	Cats	Rabbit	Canned
Natura California Natural	Dogs	Lamb	Dry
Ralston Purina CNM HA Formula	Dogs	Hydrolyzed soybean	Dry
DVM Pharmaceuticals EXclude	Dogs	Hydrolyzed casein and liver	Powder (water should be added)

small animal patients during the early phase of therapy is currently under investigation to minimize the likelihood of the patient becoming sensitive to the novel protein source while the intestine is still inflamed and more permeable to indigestible dietary proteins (Guilford, 1996). The first novel protein offered to the animal is referred to as a *sacrificial protein* because it is introduced while the gut mucosal barrier is abnormally permeable, increasing the likelihood of the patient acquiring an allergy to this protein. The sacrificial protein is fed for approximately 6 weeks, after which time a second novel protein source is offered. This diet change would coincide with the lowering of the prednisone dose from the immunosuppressive to the anti-inflammatory range.

A small number of animals with severe IBD will fail to respond to either commercial hypoallergenic diets or homemade formulations, despite aggressive pharmacologic therapy. These patients may benefit from human purified formulations in which the protein has been hydrolyzed to peptides or amino acids, carbohydrates are present as oligosaccharides, and lipid is present as essential fatty acids. Human liquid enteral formulations such as Vivonex T.E.N. (Novartis Nutrition, Minneapolis, MN), Ensure (Ross Laboratories, Columbus, OH), and Criticare H.N. (Mead Johnson, Evansville, IN) contain approximately 14 to 16% protein calories, and the relatively low protein content precludes their use for the long-term (longer than 3 weeks) feeding of cats. The lower protein formulas should be supplemented with protein (15 to 30 gm casein powder per 8 fluid ounce can) and taurine (250 mg per can) in cats. Commercial human formulations such as Impact (Novartis Nutrition, Minneapolis, MN) and Immun-Aid

(B. Braun/McGaw, Inc., Bethlehem, PA) are fortified with arginine and contain 22% and 32% protein and calories, respectively. Both formulations should be supplemented with taurine (250 mg per can), and Impact should be supplemented with additional protein (15 to 30 gm casein powder per 8 fluid ounce can) for the long-term management of cats with chronic diarrhea.

PROTEIN-LOSING ENTEROPATHY

The nutritional support of patients with protein-losing enteropathy should include additional high-quality protein to compensate for increased fecal losses. Fat is usually restricted because of the likelihood of increasing lymph flow (lymphangiectasia) or abnormal assimilation (IBD). Medium chain triglycerides can be used to increase the caloric density of the diet without stimulating lymph flow because they are primarily absorbed directly via the portal system. Portagen (Mead Johnson, Evansville, IN) or coconut oil fed at a rate of about 1 tsp per 400 gm of canned food provides an additional source of calories (8 kcal/ml) in dogs suffering from lymphangiectasia. Medium-chain triglycerides should be used with caution in cats because of the potential for inducing anorexia, hepatic lipidosis, and ketogenesis. Animals with concurrent IBD should receive a fat-restricted diet containing a novel protein source. There are currently no commercially available diets that fulfill these criteria, and computer-generated homemade formulations may be indicated in select patients. In addition, the use of commercial weight-reducing diets (high in fiber) for treatment of lymphangiectasia is contraindicated because these diets are too calorie-restricted and poorly digestible

TABLE 2. Controlled Homemade Diets for Dogs and Cats with Chronic Diarrhea

Diet 1: (Cottage Cheese–Based)

Ingredient	Amount for Dogs	Amount for Cats
Cooked white rice	1 cup	1¼ cups
Creamed cottage cheese	⅓ lb	4 ounces
Safflower oil	1 tsp	¼ tsp
Calcium phosphate dibasic	½ tsp	½ tsp
Calcium carbonate	⅛ tsp	—
Potassium chloride	¼ tsp	¼ tsp
Multivitamin and mineral tablets	1	½
Taurine	—	25 mg

Prepare the rice or cream of rice with water according to the package directions but do not add butter or salt. Combine all the ingredients, except for the multivitamin, and simmer for 10 minutes. Administer the multivitamin and taurine separately, or mix into the food just before serving.

This diet provides 430 kcal and 279 kcal of metabolizable energy for dogs and cats, respectively. The composition of the diet for dogs on a metabolizable energy basis is 18% protein, 19% fat, and 63% carbohydrates. For cats, the diet contains 26% protein, 22% fat, and 53% carbohydrate on a metabolizable energy basis.

Diet 2: (Whitefish-Based)

Ingredient	Amount for Dogs	Amount for Cats
Boiled potato with the skin	¾ lb	0.4 lb
Whitefish	0.2 lb	3 oz
Safflower oil	1 tsp	½ tsp
Potassium chloride	⅛ tsp	¼ tsp
Lite salt	1/16 tsp	—
Calcium phosphate dibasic	½ tsp	½ tsp
Calcium carbonate	¼ tsp	⅛ tsp
Multivitamin and mineral tablets	1	½
Taurine	—	25 mg

Boil the potatoes. Puree or blenderize the potatoes for cats. Poach or cook fish without added fat; retain juices. Combine fish, potatoes, and other ingredients except multivitamin, and simmer for 10 minutes. Administer the multivitamin and taurine separately, or mix into the food just before serving.

This diet provides 400 kcal and 269 kcal of metabolizable energy for dogs and cats, respectively. The composition of the diet for dogs on a metabolizable energy basis is 20% protein, 23% fat, and 57% carbohydrates. For cats, the diet contains 26% protein, 25% fat, and 49% carbohydrate on a metabolizable energy basis.

Diet 3: (Turkey-Based)

Ingredient	Amount for Dogs	Amount for Cats
Cooked white rice	1 cup	1.2 cups
Turkey flesh (precooked weight)	3 ounces	2.5 ounces
Safflower oil	2 tsp	¾ tsp
Potassium chloride	⅛ tsp	¼ tsp
Lite salt	⅛ tsp	—
Calcium phosphate dibasic	½ tsp	½ tsp
Calcium carbonate	¼ tsp	—
Multivitamin and mineral tablets	1	½
Taurine	—	25 mg

Prepare the rice or cream of rice with water according to the package directions but do not add butter or salt. Cook turkey without added fat; retain juices. Combine all ingredients except the multivitamin, and simmer 10 minutes. Administer the multivitamin and taurine separately, or mix into the food just before serving.

This diet provides 417 kcal and 256 kcal of metabolizable energy for dogs and cats, respectively. The composition of the diet for dogs is 18% protein, 21% fat, and 61% carbohydrate on a metabolizable energy basis. For cats, the diet contains 30% protein, 23% fat, and 48% carbohydrate on a metabolizable energy basis.

Diet Information

1. Diets for dogs were formulated with cooked white rice, whereas diets for cats were formulated with cream of rice cereal.
2. All diets may be stored in the refrigerator or freezer; simply warm before serving.
3. Potassium chloride may be provided through a salt substitute found in grocery stores. Ensure that it contains no sodium.
4. Select a human multivitamin and mineral supplement, preferably without additives or preservatives.
5. Calcium phosphate dibasic may be purchased from many feed stores or may be special-ordered through a pharmacy or chemical supply house.
6. Calcium carbonate may be obtained from pharmacies and grocery stores in the form of crushed oyster shells.
7. Maintenance energy requirements (MER) are calculated using the following formulas in cats and dogs: cats: 1.3 [Body weight (kg) × 30] + 70; dogs: 1.8 [Body weight (kg) × 30] + 70.

to support the increased protein and energy requirements of these patients.

ACUTE PANCREATITIS

Acute pancreatitis is managed by withholding food and water to minimize the synthesis and secretion of pancreatic enzymes. Fluid and electrolyte balance is maintained with crystalloids (usually lactated Ringer's solution), and colloid solutions such as dextran 70 or hetastarch are used to maintain oncotic pressure and help ensure adequate perfusion to the inflamed pancreas. Dietary amino acids and fatty acids are the most potent stimulators of pancreatic enzyme secretion and are thus avoided during the initial recovery period. Small amounts of water or ice cubes should be offered after the patient has stopped vomiting. If there is no recurrence of clinical signs, a diet rich in carbohydrate (rice, pasta, potatoes) and restricted in fat and protein should be gradually reintroduced. With continued clinical improvement, gradual introduction of a low-fat maintenance diet should be attempted. Animals with relapsing pancreatitis or severe necrotizing pancreatitis require prolonged hospitalization and attention to their nutritional status. Animals with prolonged anorexia may require enteral feeding via jejunostomy tube or total parenteral nutrition to maintain their metabolizable energy requirements. Dogs that have recovered from pancreatitis may need to be maintained on fat-restricted, highly digestible diets because of the association between high-fat meals, hyperlipidemia, and pancreatitis. The lack of commercially available fat-restricted, highly digestible diets may necessitate the use of computer-generated homemade diets in selected patients.

EXOCRINE PANCREATIC INSUFFICIENCY

Nutrient malabsorption in exocrine pancreatic insufficiency (EPI) arises as a consequence of a failure of intraluminal digestion and impaired function of intestinal mucosal enzymes. Most dogs and cats with EPI can be managed with dietary modification and pancreatic enzyme supplementation. A suboptimal response to enzyme supplementation usually reflects associated small bowel disease or bacterial overgrowth. Fat absorption does not return to normal despite appropriate enzyme replacement therapy in dogs and humans with EPI. This is usually compensated for by increasing caloric intake, necessitating an increase of approximately 20% above the calculated maintenance requirements. Experimental studies reveal that dietary fiber impairs pancreatic enzyme activity; therefore, high-fiber diets should be avoided. In addition, there is no evidence that reduced-fat diets are of value in patients with EPI. Patients who exhibit poor weight gain and do not tolerate diets with normal or high fat contents may benefit from supplementation with medium chain triglycerides. Pancreatic enzyme preparations containing low activities of fungal lipases and other proteases of nonpancreatic origin do not effectively treat patients with EPI. Furthermore, tablet preparations and enteric-coated formulations marketed for human patients are often ineffective in dogs and cats. Dogs should receive approximately 1 tsp of pancreatic extract per 20 pounds body weight per meal, whereas cats should

receive 1 tsp per meal. Studies have shown that no additional benefit is derived by preincubation of enzymes and food or by addition of bile salts or antacids to the food and enzyme mixture. Animals showing a suboptimal response to enzyme replacement therapy do not benefit from increasing the dose of enzyme given or by administering gastric acid secretion inhibitors to reduce intragastric destruction of enzyme. Raw pancreas obtained from healthy, inspected pigs, cattle, or sheep can be substituted for commercial dry pancreatic extract. Dogs require supplementation with 3 to 4 ounces of chopped pancreas per meal and cats require 1 to 3 ounces of pancreas per meal.

Serum concentrations of cobalamin (vitamin B_{12}) and of fat-soluble vitamins are often severely subnormal in cats with EPI (Williams, 1994). Cats with decreased serum cobalamin concentrations should receive supplementation with subcutaneously administered cobalamin at 100 to 250 μg, whereas dogs should receive subcutaneously administered cobalamin at 300 to 400 μg. The injections are administered on a weekly basis for 4 to 6 weeks, and the dosing schedule is then decreased to once every 6 to 12 months. Vitamin K malabsorption resulting in vitamin K–responsive coagulopathy has been documented in feline EPI and appears to be more common in affected cats than in affected dogs. Parenteral vitamin K_1 (2.5 mg/kg in divided doses every 12 hours) should be given when there is clinical or laboratory evidence of a coagulopathy. Serum concentrations of tocopherol (vitamin E) are also often severely subnormal in dogs and cats with EPI and can be resolved by supplementing tocopherol at 30 to 400 IU orally with food once daily.

CHRONIC LARGE BOWEL DIARRHEA

Dietary recommendations for the management of large bowel diarrhea are controversial. The response to dietary therapy can vary dramatically from one patient to another, with some animals showing improvement on low-residue, "hypoallergenic" diets, and others improving on less digestible diets containing soluble or insoluble fiber sources. Dietary fiber is composed mainly of the nonstarch polysaccharide and lignin portion of the plant cell wall. It may also contain oligosaccharides, polyphenolics, cutin, suberin, waxes, and inorganic constituents. Soluble fiber has a large water-holding capacity and is easily digested by gastrointestinal microflora. Pectin, mucilages, gums, and some hemicelluloses are considered soluble fiber. Insoluble fiber has a minimal ability to hold water and is not completely degraded by the microflora of the gastrointestinal tract. Cellulose and some hemicelluloses are classified as insoluble fiber. As a result of their different characteristics, soluble and insoluble fiber sources can have vastly different effects on the gastrointestinal tract, many of which improve fecal consistency (Leib et al, 1991). Soluble fiber delays the intestinal passage of ingesta, thereby permitting more water absorption. The bacterial flora and their by-products are increased secondary to microfloral fermentation of soluble fiber, resulting in increased fecal bulk. Insoluble fiber also increases fecal bulk because it is poorly digested. This ultimately results in colonic distention, which may help normalize colonic myoelectrical activity and segmentation. The result is a slower passage of stool through the colon, allowing for enhanced water absorption. Both types of fiber bind bile acids and aid in preventing deconjugated bile acids from causing large bowel diarrhea. In general, insoluble fibers have a low fermentability and soluble fibers tend to have high fermentability, although solubility does not always correlate with fermentability. Additional beneficial effects from fermentable fiber sources probably stem from their degradative products, such as butyrate, the principle energy source for the colonocyte, and other short-chain fatty acids (Simpson et al, 1994). In addition, short-chain fatty acids lower the colonic luminal pH, impeding the growth of pathogens.

The use of dietary fiber can have deleterious consequences. As dietary fiber increases, digestibility of essential nutrients decreases, which may result in nutritional imbalances, particularly if a marginal quality diet is being fed. If the animal becomes dehydrated, fecal bulk increases and constipation may result, especially if soluble fiber is fed. Dietary fiber should not be used when the provision of highly digestible nutrients is indicated (Bartges and Anderson, 1996). Examples of this include normal physiologic conditions such as pregnancy and lactation or disease states such as protein-losing enteropathies or lymphangiectasia. Table 3 lists sources and recommended amounts of dietary fiber for the treatment of large bowel diarrhea. The fiber source should be administered for several weeks before a final decision is made concerning its efficacy.

There is evidence to suggest that some forms of colitis may be associated with a dietary sensitivity similar to that observed with small bowel disease. Proteins, lipoproteins, glycoproteins, lipopolysaccharides, and carbohydrates can induce an immunologic or inflammatory response similar to that observed in the small intestine. The theoretic benefit for using highly digestible hypoallergenic diets for patients with colitis includes reducing the digestive challenge to the large intestine and minimizing the likelihood of dietary antigens actually reaching the colon, thus lessening the likelihood of an immunologic reaction (Simpson et al, 1994). In one study, clinical signs of colitis resolved in all dogs after the feeding of a low-residue, easily assimilated, relatively hypoallergenic diet (Nelson et al, 1988). Only two of the 13 dogs in the study tolerated refeeding of the same diet fed just prior to the onset of clinical signs.

The authors recommend feeding a complete and balanced commercial diet containing moderate amounts of a highly digestible protein source to which the animal has not been previously exposed (see Table 1). The supplementation of fermentable fiber sources such as psyllium or oat bran (see Table 3) may be necessary in animals showing partial resolution of their clinical signs. Failure to respond to these recommendations may necessitate selecting a hypoallergenic diet with a different novel protein source, adding insoluble fiber to the diet, or selecting a diet that is moderately fat restricted. A complete and balanced computer-generated homemade diet that is prepared by a veterinary nutritionist is a viable alternative for dogs and cats

TABLE 3. Dietary Fiber Sources

Fiber Source	Fiber Type	Amount
Coarse bran	Insoluble	1–3 Tbsp/day
Canned pumpkin	Insoluble	1–4 Tbsp/day
Bran cereals*	Insoluble	2–4 Tbsp/day
Oat bran	Soluble	1–2 Tbsp/day
Psyllium hydrocolloid†	Soluble and insoluble	1–3 Tbsp/day

*Includes human preparations such as Kellogg's All-Bran cereal.
†Includes human and veterinary medical fiber supplements such as Metamucil, Searle Consumer Products, Chicago, IL; Vetasyl, VRX Products, Harbor City, CA.
Modified from Dimski DS: Dietary fiber in the management of gastrointestinal disease. In: Kirk RW, Bonagura JD, eds: Current Veterinary Therapy XI. Philadelphia: WB Saunders, 1992, p 594, with permission.

that have not improved with conventional dietary recommendations.

References and Suggested Reading

Bartges J, Anderson WH: Dietary Fiber. Purina Nutrition Forum. Scientific Program Notes, 1996, p 1.
A review of the physiologic effects of fiber and its uses in small animals.
Brown KH: Dietary management of acute diarrheal disease: Contemporary scientific issues. J Nutr 124:455S, 1994.
A review of contemporary issues in the dietary management of children with acute diarrhea.
Guilford WG: Idiopathic inflammatory bowel diseases. In: Guilford WG, Center SA, Strombeck DR, et al, eds: Strombeck's Small Animal Gastroenterology, 3rd ed. Philadelphia: WB Saunders, 1996, p 451.
A textbook review of the classification, etiopathogenesis, diagnosis, and therapy of inflammatory bowel diseases in dogs and cats.
Iyngkaran N, Robinson MJ, Sumithran E, et al: Cow's milk protein sensitive enteropathy: An important factor prolonging diarrhea of acute infectious enteritis in early infancy. Arch Dis Child 53:150, 1978.
A study evaluating the role of cow's milk protein in prolonging diarrhea in 14 young infants with acute infective enteritis.
Leib MS, Monroe WE, Codner EC: Management of chronic large bowel diarrhea in dogs. Vet Med 922, 1991.
A review of the clinical signs, differential diagnoses, and therapeutic approaches to managing chronic large bowel diarrhea in dogs.
Nelson RW, Stookey L, Kazacos E: Nutritional management of idiopathic chronic colitis in the dog. J Vet Intern Med 2:133, 1988.
A study of the effects of diet in the pathogenesis of chronic colitis in the dog.
Romatowski J: Use of oral fluids in acute gastroenteritis in small animals. Mod Vet Pract 66:26, 1985.
A review of the use of oral fluids in the management of acute gastroenteritis.
Simpson JW, Maskell IE, Markwell PJ: Use of a restricted antigen diet in the management of idiopathic canine colitis. J Small Anim Pract 35:233, 1994.
A study evaluating the effectiveness of using a restricted antigen diet in the management of canine colitis.
Williams DA: Feline exocrine pancreatic insufficiency. In: Kirk RW, Bonagura JD, eds: Current Veterinary Therapy XII. Philadelphia: WB Saunders, 1995, p 732.
A textbook review of the etiology, pathophysiology, diagnosis, and treatment of feline exocrine pancreatic insufficiency.
Zenger E, Willard MD: Oral rehydration therapy in companion animals. Comp Anim Pract 19:6, 1989.
A review of the use of oral rehydration therapy in small animal practice.

Diagnostic Approach to Hepatobiliary Disease

PAUL R. HESS
Durham, North Carolina

SUSAN E. BUNCH
Raleigh, North Carolina

Assessing the small animal patient with suspected primary hepatobiliary disease is rarely a simple process because no single diagnostic test currently available has perfect sensitivity and specificity. The task is complicated by the liver's wide-ranging roles in digestion, intermediary metabolism, biosynthesis, and elimination, which make the signs of hepatic disease nonspecific and leave the liver vulnerable to injury from systemic disorders. To confound the process further, the causes of primary hepatobiliary diseases are diverse, and many are either poorly understood or unknown. Accordingly, most clinicians follow an implicit, algorithmic approach to hepatobiliary disease, tailored to the particular patient and tempered by clinical intuition. The purpose of this article is to provide a diagnostic approach and explain the thought processes behind it. We believe that the investigating clinician should consider three basic questions: (1) Can I make a strong case for hepatobiliary disease from the preliminary findings? (2) If so, does this represent primary or secondary hepatobiliary disease? and (3) What is the cause of the disease? Moving sequentially through this framework of inquiry, and understanding the pathophysiology of common liver disorders and the characteristic clinical and laboratory abnormalities they may cause, can provide a rational basis for test selection and interpretation, and the most efficient means of arriving at a correct diagnosis.

CAN I MAKE A STRONG CASE FOR HEPATOBILIARY DISEASE?

Hints of a hepatobiliary disorder in the dog or cat usually arise from historical and physical examination findings. Occasionally, laboratory evaluation performed as part of a routine geriatric evaluation or preanesthesia "screening" may identify the asymptomatic patient with hepatobiliary disease.

With the exception of acholic feces, the signs of hepatobiliary disease are nonspecific. Clinical presentations may range from apparent health to the icteric, septic, encephalopathic animal with ascites and melena. Because of the liver's great functional reserve, cases of long-standing, progressive hepatic injury may manifest acutely once that reserve is depleted. Clinical signs generally result from hepatobiliary inflammation, anatomic abnormalities (e.g., a palpable mass), cholestasis, chronic portal (venous) hypertension, or hepatocellular failure. Specific findings that are commonly observed in dogs and cats with hepatobiliary disease, and their pathogeneses, are listed in Table 1.

The suspicion for primary hepatobiliary disease may be heightened by additional historical findings. Prior treatment with a potentially hepatotoxic drug (e.g., phenobarbital, itraconazole) or, less commonly, consumption of a hepatotoxin (e.g., certain mushrooms) should be considered. Recognition of known or suspected breed predispositions (e.g., chronic hepatitis in American and English Cocker spaniels) should initiate scrutiny for these conditions when clinical findings are compatible. Occasionally, such recognition may diminish suspicion as well: the acutely ill, icteric, female Miniature Schnauzer with vomiting and cranial abdominal pain is most likely to have pancreatitis, not primary liver disease.

TABLE 1. Clinical Findings in Hepatobiliary Disease and Their Explanations

Finding	Explanation
Abnormal hepatic palpation	Mass; diffuse enlargement; irregular contour or consistency
Abdominal effusion	Portal hypertension (ascites); neoplasia (hemorrhagic or nonseptic exudate); ruptured bile duct or gallbladder (peritonitis); vasculitis secondary to feline infectious peritonitis (nonseptic exudate)
Anorexia, vomiting, and diarrhea	Mucosal edema and ulceration; hepatobiliary inflammation; malabsorption; accumulation of circulating emetogenic substances
Bleeding	Decreased coagulation factor synthesis; excessive fibrinolytic and anticoagulant activity; abnormal platelet function
Gastroduodenal ulceration	Hypergastrinemia (controversial); impaired mucosal perfusion
Jaundice	Failure of bilirubin elimination
Metabolic encephalopathy	Accumulation of "encephalotoxins": ammonia, mercaptans, short-chain fatty acids, γ-aminobutyric acid–like compounds
Polyuria and polydipsia	Impaired adrenal steroid metabolism, loss of renal medullary concentration gradient, altered portal vein osmoreceptor function (polyuria); encephalopathy (primary polydipsia)
Sedative or anesthesia intolerance	Impaired drug metabolism
Ulcerative, crusting dermatosis	Not known (suspected "nutritional abnormality")
Weight loss	Inadequate nutrient intake or assimilation; enhanced tissue catabolism (neoplastic or chronic inflammatory process)

A number of laboratory abnormalities may support clinical suspicions, so a minimal laboratory database (complete blood count, serum chemistry profile, urinalysis, fecal flotation) is a cost-effective, important next step in all cases in which a hepatobiliary disorder is suspected. Microcytosis (decreased mean corpuscular volume), without anemia, is seen commonly with congenital portosystemic shunt (PSS) in dogs and cats (and less commonly with primary hepatopathies), probably as a result of impaired iron transport. Blood smears from cats with PSS and other hepatopathies frequently exhibit poikilocytosis (altered erythrocyte morphologic characteristics); acanthocytes are most common, reflecting abnormal lipoprotein metabolism. Other morphologic variants observed in dogs include target cells. There are no particular leukocyte or platelet changes suggestive of hepatobiliary disease.

High serum liver enzyme activity (LEA) is frequently identified in hepatobiliary disorders; of these enzymes, alanine transaminase (ALT), alkaline phosphatase (ALP), and γ-glutamyl transferase (GGT) are the most commonly measured. Increases in ALT activity indicate hepatocyte membrane damage and leakage of this soluble, cytosolic enzyme (rarely, massive skeletal muscle necrosis can elevate ALT levels). The magnitude of ALT elevation roughly corresponds to the number of affected hepatocytes. Other routinely reported "leakage enzymes" (lactate dehydrogenase and aspartate transaminase) lack tissue specificity, and high values should be interpreted cautiously. Increases in the activity of ALP and GGT, which are membrane-bound enzymes found in hepatocytes and biliary epithelium, result from enhanced synthesis induced by certain drugs, or intra- or extrahepatic cholestasis. Discordance of these cholestatic enzyme activities sometimes is seen in cats (i.e., markedly increased ALP with normal to minimally increased GGT) and is consistent with hepatic lipidosis or, less commonly, extrahepatic bile duct obstruction. Comparing the relative magnitude of increases in ALT, ALP, and GGT levels allows characterization of the underlying disease process as primarily hepatocellular, primarily cholestatic, or mixed. Establishing this pattern can be important diagnostically, for example, the icteric dog with a 20-fold increase in ALT levels and normal ALP levels does not have obstructive cholelithiasis. An important caveat in making these comparisons, however, is that "pure" patterns rarely exist; for example, retained bile acids in primarily cholestatic diseases cause hepatocellular injury and ALT leakage, whereas cell swelling in primarily hepatocellular diseases causes obstruction of small bile ductules and ALP induction. Further, relatively minor elevations of ALP in the cat signify marked cholestasis, as the half-life and hepatic density of feline ALP are small fractions of canine values. It should be noted that there is no correlation between hepatic function and LEA, and normal LEA in the face of otherwise compelling signs of hepatobiliary disease should not deter further work-up. Patients with cirrhosis, congenital PSS, and metastatic neoplasia of the liver, for example, frequently have normal LEA. Such activity at less than reference range has no known clinical significance.

Several components of the routine chemistry profile serve as insensitive indicators of various hepatic functions. Hypoalbuminemia attributable to liver disease suggests chronic, marked (≤20% functional mass) liver dysfunction;

inhibition of albumin release due to hyperammonemia, and dilution in ascitic fluid, may further lower serum concentration. Similarly, hypoglycemia may result from diffusely impaired glycogen storage, gluconeogenesis, and insulin degradation, or rarely, as a hepatic paraneoplastic disorder. Deficient urea cycle function from reduced hepatic mass or portosystemic shunting may produce low blood urea nitrogen concentration. Serum cholesterol concentration is dependent in part on hepatic synthesis and conversion to bile acids; consequently, hypocholesterolemia may occur with decreased functional mass, whereas severe cholestasis may lead to hypercholesterolemia. Hyperbilirubinemia, in the face of normal heme degradation, signifies inadequate uptake or conjugation (hepatocellular disease) or inadequate excretion (biliary disease), or both. Neither the ratio of conjugated (direct):unconjugated (indirect) bilirubin fractions nor the measurement of urobilinogen has proved useful in differentiating between intra- and extrahepatic causes of hyperbilirubinemia. Urinalysis findings consistent with hepatobiliary disease include urate crystalluria or urolithiasis, persistently dilute urine, and in the cat, bilirubinuria. Bilirubinuria and bilirubin crystalluria may occur normally in the dog; however, excess bilirubin (>2+) in dilute urine is abnormal and suggests a hepatobiliary disorder in the nonanemic dog.

Although the clinical and laboratory signs of hepatobiliary disease are nonspecific, the presence of multiple signs occurring concomitantly, particularly in the absence of findings incriminating other organ systems, should strengthen early suspicions and provide justification for further diagnostic pursuit. Consideration also should be given to potential nonhepatic causes of the abnormalities identified to this point, such as the expected finding of microcytosis in Japanese Akita dogs.

IF THERE IS HEPATOBILIARY DISEASE, IS IT PRIMARY OR SECONDARY?

A number of diseases originating outside the hepatobiliary system affect the liver secondarily, producing disturbances in function and changes in LEA (see p. 668). Although the distinction between primary and secondary hepatobiliary disease in some cases can be made only after extensive investigation or liver biopsy, a concerted effort is made to rule out these conditions before performing more specific evaluation of the hepatobiliary system.

WHAT IS THE CAUSE OF THE DISEASE?

Further evaluation of the patient with presumptive primary hepatobiliary disease generally is necessary to characterize the cause and extent of the condition, to formulate a rational treatment plan, and to determine the prognosis for progression or resolution. In some cases, when it is recognized that the disease process likely represents an acute, reversible hepatic injury (e.g., adverse drug reaction), serial laboratory evaluation may be all that is needed if progressive improvement can be documented. In these instances, clinical recovery often is observed to precede resolution of laboratory abnormalities. Leakage enzymes, for example, do not decline strictly according to half-life, as increased

production and release occur during hepatocyte regeneration. Similarly, hyperbilirubinemia and icterus may persist after resolution of cholestasis because of the presence of bilirubin covalently bound to albumin (biliprotein); bilirubinuria will resolve, however, as biliprotein is not normally excreted into the urine.

Measurement of serum bile acid (SBA) concentration provides a sensitive indicator of hepatocellular, biliary, and portal circulatory function. Measurement of SBA is especially useful in confirming the hepatobiliary origin of suspicious laboratory abnormalities and in uncovering "occult" hepatobiliary disease when clinical signs are suggestive but other biochemical evidence is lacking. Evaluation of both fasting and postprandial SBA is particularly important in identifying conditions of abnormal hepatic blood flow. Substantial variation in SBA among individuals precludes correlating the magnitude of change between fasting and postprandial values with a specific disease. Further, SBA does not distinguish between primary and secondary hepatobiliary diseases; for example, low to moderate elevations in SBA (usually less than 60 μmol/L) may occur in canine steroid hepatopathy. The magnitude of a single SBA value only weakly corresponds with the severity of hepatic lesions; in general, however, there is a reasonable likelihood of finding histologic changes on a liver biopsy specimen if the fasting or postprandial SBA value exceeds 25 μmol/L. False-negative values (which occur rarely) may result from severe intestinal malabsorption or inadequate dietary provocation of bile release from the gallbladder. Although measurement of SBA is not needed to document hepatobiliary disease in the icteric, nonanemic patient, the liver's great functional capacity for bilirubin excretion (up to 30-fold over the normal heme load) makes hyperbilirubinemia an extremely insensitive scale for measuring changes in hepatic function. In some icteric animals, SBA can provide a useful, noninvasive means with which to monitor disease progression or response to therapy.

Beyond the laboratory database, SBA, and testing for causes of secondary liver disorders (e.g., hyperadrenocorticism, serum thyroxine levels in older cats), few other blood tests currently play a major role in the diagnosis of hepatobiliary disease. Although the fasting plasma ammonia level is a sensitive test of hepatic and portal circulatory function, it is our experience that false-positive results are not infrequently obtained because of the need for stringent handling requirements. Plasma ammonia is best reserved for rapid assessment of the critical patient with encephalopathic signs of unknown origin. Markedly elevated serum α-fetoprotein concentrations have been demonstrated in dogs with hepatic carcinoma and lymphoma (using an enzymetric kit for α-fetoprotein detection in human patients). In contrast, circulating antinuclear and antimitochondrial autoantibodies, which are important discriminatory markers in chronic inflammatory hepatopathies in human patients, have not shown similar diagnostic utility in the dog.

Diagnostic imaging of the liver and associated structures is an integral part of the evaluation of the animal with presumptive hepatobiliary disease. Because of its usefulness in imaging soft tissues, ultrasonography largely has supplanted plain film radiography in such studies. Abnormalities commonly identified by ultrasonography include diffuse or focal parenchymal disease, changes in hepatic size and margination, cystic lesions, vascular disorders, distention or abnormal contents of the gallbladder and biliary tree, perihepatic disease, and abdominal effusion. An important limitation of the technique is the requirement for a thorough, systematic examination by an experienced operator. Normal examination results do not exclude hepatobiliary disease; in one study, the sensitivity of ultrasonography in detecting canine hepatic lymphoma was 20%. Although in some instances a strong correlation can be made between changes in echogenicity and histologic findings (notably hepatocellular carcinoma in the dog and hepatic lipidosis in the cat), a definitive diagnosis cannot be made by ultrasonography. The principal utility of ultrasonographic imaging is to assist with biopsy planning, to identify surgically correctable vascular anomalies, and to differentiate intra- and extrahepatic causes of cholestasis. The ability of ultrasonography to diagnose extrahepatic bile duct obstruction is hampered by gallbladder distention and bile "sludging," which is often found in anorectic dogs and cats, and the persistent dilatation of bile ducts that may be observed after resolution of chronic obstruction. Scintigraphic studies may be helpful in certain cases but must be performed at referral centers or human hospitals. Clinically useful scintigraphic techniques have been established for determining patency of the biliary tract and the presence of macroscopic portosystemic shunting in dogs and cats.

In patients with abdominal effusion, fluid is collected for measurement of total protein content (or specific gravity), nucleated cell count, and cytologic examination. The appearance and composition of effusion resulting from portal hypertension varies somewhat, ranging from an amber to serosanguineous, modified transudate (<7000 cells/μl; ≥2.5 g/dl; 1.010 to 1.031) to a clear, colorless, pure transudate (<2500 cells/μl; ≤2.5 g/dl; <1.016) when complicated by marked hypoalbuminemia. In contrast to dogs, cats with severe liver disease rarely form ascites; the presence of abdominal effusion in a cat with apparent hepatobiliary disease should prompt further evaluation for pancreatitis, feline infectious peritonitis, or neoplasia. Patients with congenital PSS have normal portal pressures and consequently do not form ascites. Turbid, green-brown fluid with a high bilirubin content and neutrophilic inflammatory changes collected from an icteric animal suggest extrahepatic biliary tract rupture.

Once the initial suspicion for primary hepatobiliary disease has been validated by laboratory evaluation and imaging studies, pathologic examination of liver tissue usually is needed to reach a definitive diagnosis. Because of the technical ease of the procedure, minimal patient risk, low cost, and infrequent need for sedation, collection of a specimen for cytologic examination by fine needle aspiration (FNA) is a reasonable first step. Ultrasonographic guidance increases the probability of sampling discretely distributed lesions, avoiding inadvertent puncture of major biliary or vascular structures, and obtaining representative specimens in diffuse hepatobiliary disease. Cytologic findings of inflammation, cholestasis, necrosis, or hepatocyte hyperplasia or degeneration do not constitute a diagnosis but can provide objective evidence of liver disease and support for clinicopathologic data previously garnered.

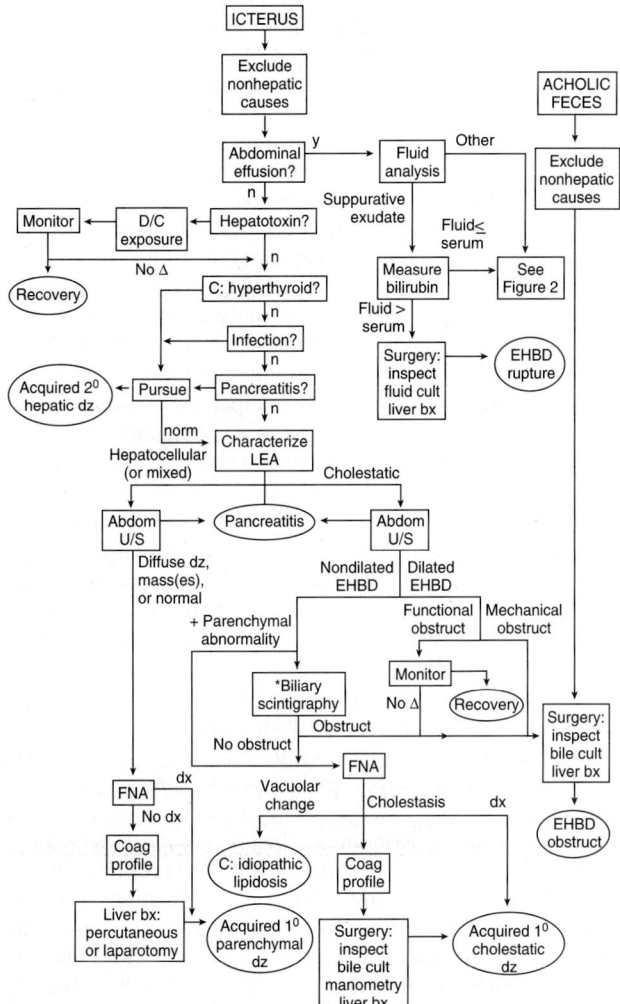

Figure 1. Diagnostic algorithm (logic circuit) for hepatobiliary disease in the dog and cat, beginning with chief complaints of icterus or acholic feces (other chief complaints are addressed in Figure 2). Initial problem divisions are not mutually exclusive; when occurring together, higher yield problems are pursued first (suggested order for all complaints: acholic feces → mass → icterus → effusion → increased LEA → nonspecific signs). Diagnostic procedures are enclosed in boxes; those marked with an asterisk are considered optional. Conditions enclosed in boxes and followed by a question mark indicate clinical suspicion. Ovals represent diagnostic end points. C, cat; D, dog; y, yes; n, no; s, suspect; norm, normal; abnorm, abnormal; d/c, discontinue; no Δ, no change; dx, diagnosis; bx, biopsy; dz, disease; 1°, primary; 2°, secondary; LEA, liver enzyme activity; FNA, fine needle aspirate cytologic examination; abdom U/S, abdominal ultrasonography; coag, coagulation; cult, culture; EHBD, extrahepatic bile duct; obstruct, obstruction.

Even in the case of a morphologic diagnosis, for example, vacuolar hepatopathy (e.g., lipidosis) in a cat, it should be remembered that a *clinical* diagnosis of idiopathic hepatic lipidosis is made only in the larger context of historical, physical examination, laboratory, and ultrasonographic findings. The value of FNA is that occasionally a definitive diagnosis of neoplasia (particularly round cell tumors or carcinomas) or infection can be established, obviating the need for more invasive and costly biopsy techniques. Despite the safety of FNA, there are some situations in which the procedure is contraindicated. Because of the possibility of tumor seeding into the abdominal cavity or along needle tracks, FNA of a solitary hepatic mass is not advocated if

surgical excision is planned. Similarly, we do not recommend routine FNA of gallbladder contents; in most instances when bile culture is indicated, a concurrent liver biopsy is also needed, and thus the risk of postprocedural bile leakage with this technique, although small, appears unjustified. Lastly, although not a strict contraindication to FNA, a bleeding diathesis represents additional patient risk and should be corrected, if possible, before the procedure.

Obtaining a liver biopsy is often the final step in evaluating an animal with presumptive primary hepatobiliary disease. Deciding whether a biopsy is needed, and if so, how the tissue sample should be collected, is an important part of the diagnostic process. Clinical judgment, biochemical characterization of the disease, and the results of imaging studies constitute the basis for these decisions. The indications for liver biopsy are the same as those for FNA: persistently high LEA, abnormal hepatic function, or ultrasonographically identified hepatic changes. Common means of liver biopsy include needle biopsy (blind or ultrasonographically guided percutaneous, keyhole, laparoscopic) and surgical biopsy (laparotomy). In general, needle biopsies are useful for primarily parenchymal diseases. Techniques for needle biopsy have been recently reviewed (Kerwin, 1995). A particular advantage of the percutaneous method, which can be rapidly and easily performed without general anesthesia, is the ability to collect serial biopsy specimens. Access to sequential tissue samples allows the clinician to gauge the success of therapy, which can be important in many chronic hepatobiliary diseases for which no specific cause is found. The principal limitation of needle biopsy is the relatively small sample size—it is not unusual for a specimen obtained with a 16-gauge needle, for example, to contain only four or five portal triads, without complete hepatic lobules or acini, making histopathologic interpretation difficult. Complications of needle biopsy include bleeding and bile peritonitis, although this occurs rarely with ultrasonographic guidance. Contraindications to needle biopsy include microhepatia, severe and uncorrectable coagulation abnormalities, large-volume ascites (which interferes with hemostasis), hepatic cyst or abscess, vascular tumor, or a lesion adjacent to the major bile ducts or porta hepatis. A surgical biopsy is warranted in such cases. Other indications for an operative procedure include a single, resectable hepatic mass, mechanical extrahepatic bile duct obstruction, presumptive congenital vascular anomaly or septic cholangiohepatitis, and diagnostic failure of a previous needle biopsy. Laparotomy, although invasive, offers a number of advantages over percutaneous biopsy techniques, including the ability to inspect the entire abdomen, prevent and control hemorrhage, collect bile for culture, perform manometry and portovenography, and correct certain conditions (e.g., tumor excision or congenital PSS ligation). There are disadvantages as well: many animals with chronic, severe hepatic dysfunction are in a relatively precarious state of compensation that is easily overwhelmed by seemingly straightforward procedures. As for any surgical candidate, suitability for anesthesia, potential for wound complications, and coagulation status are assessed preoperatively. We believe that adopting a standard approach to animals undergoing laparotomy for suspected hepatobiliary disease is useful. Complete exploration of the abdomen is routine. When portal hypertension is

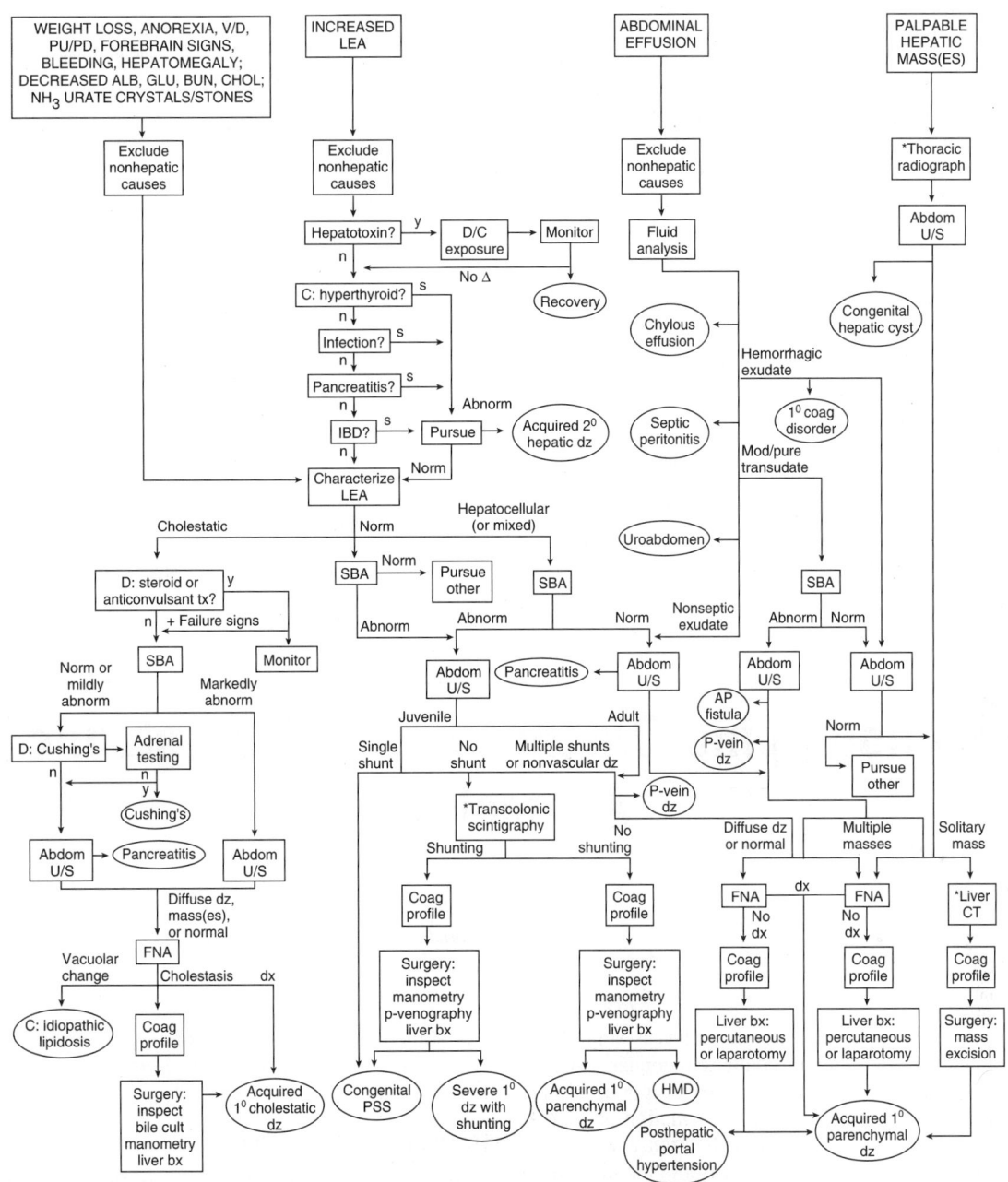

Figure 2. Diagnostic algorithm (logic circuit) for hepatobiliary disease in the dog and cat, beginning with four, distinct categories composed of typical chief complaints (other chief complaints are addressed in Figure 1). Initial problem divisions are not mutually exclusive; when occurring together, higher yield problems are pursued first (suggested order for all complaints: acholic feces → mass → icterus → effusion → increased LEA → nonspecific signs). Diagnostic procedures are enclosed in boxes; those marked with an asterisk are considered optional. Conditions enclosed in boxes and followed by a question mark indicate clinical suspicion. Ovals represent diagnostic end points. Abbreviations: C, cat; D, dog; y, yes; n, no; s, suspect; norm, normal; abnorm, abnormal; d/c, discontinue; no Δ, no change; dx, diagnosis; tx, treatment; bx, biopsy; dz, disease; 1°, primary; 2°, secondary; LEA, liver enzyme activity; SBA, pre- and postprandial serum bile acids; mod, modified; FNA, fine needle aspiration cytologic examination; CT, computed tomography; abdom U/S, abdominal ultrasonography; coag, coagulation; cult, culture; PSS, portosystemic shunt; HMD, hepatic microvascular dysplasia; p, portal; AP, arterioportal; obstruct, obstruction; v/d, vomiting/diarrhea; pu/pd, polyuria/polydipsia; alb, albumin; glu, glucose; BUN, blood urea nitrogen; chol, cholesterol.

suspected, manometry is performed immediately, as portal pressure declines substantially with anesthesia. The liver always is biopsied, even if the gross appearance is normal or if the disease appears to be primarily biliary or vascular. Surgical methods of biopsy include ligature, wedge resection, and punch biopsy techniques. Major bile ducts are evaluated for patency, and the gallbladder is expressed and

palpated for choleliths or masses. Bile for aerobic *and* anaerobic cultures is collected in all cats and in dogs with hematologic, biochemical, or ultrasonographic findings compatible with a primarily biliary disease pattern.

Histopathologic examination of a liver biopsy specimen may demonstrate a definitive cause, such as infection or neoplasia; more often, however, nonspecific changes, such as inflammation, cellular degeneration, cholestasis, bile ductule hyperplasia, regeneration, atrophy, or fibrosis are described. Additional characterization of the specimen should address the severity and chronicity of lesions, the pattern of changes in individual functional units, and the presumptive origin of the injury (i.e., primary or secondary disease). Special stains, such as rhodanine (for copper), trichrome (for fibrous connective tissue), and Congo red (for amyloid), may assist in formulating a morphologic diagnosis.

A summary of our diagnostic approach to dogs and cats with suspected primary hepatobiliary disease is presented in algorithmic form in Figures 1 and 2.

References and Suggested Reading

Biller DS, Kantrowitz B, Miyabayashi T: Ultrasonography of diffuse liver disease. J Vet Intern Med 6:71, 1992.
  A review of ultrasonographic findings in diffuse, parenchymal liver disease.
Center SA, Erb HN, Joseph SA: Measurement of serum bile acids concentrations for diagnosis of hepatobiliary disease in cats. J Am Vet Med Assoc 207:1048, 1995.
  An examination of pre- and postprandial bile acids, in conjunction with routine biochemical profiling, in the diagnosis of hepatobiliary disease in 108 cats.
Center SA, ManWarren T, Slater MR, et al: Evaluation of 12-hour preprandial and 2-hour postprandial serum bile acids concentrations for diagnosis of hepatobiliary disease in dogs. J Am Vet Med Assoc 199:217, 1991.
  An evaluation of the utility of pre- and postprandial bile acids, in conjunction with routine biochemical profiling, in the diagnosis of hepatobiliary disease in 170 dogs.
Kerwin SC: Hepatic aspiration and biopsy techniques. Vet Clin North Am 25:275, 1995.
  A thorough review of hepatic FNA and biopsy methods.
Kristensen AT, Weiss DJ, Klausner JS, et al: Liver cytology in cases of canine and feline hepatic disease. Compend Contin Ed Pract Vet 12:797, 1990.
  A well-illustrated but biased review and retrospective study of the diagnostic utility of hepatic cytologic studies.
Meyer DJ, Williams DA: Diagnosis of hepatic and exocrine pancreatic disorders. Semin Vet Med Surg 7:275, 1992.
  An excellent, interpretive discussion of liver enzyme activity and functional parameters in the diagnosis of hepatobiliary disease.
Roth L, Meyer DJ: Interpretation of liver biopsies. Vet Clin North Am 25:293, 1995.
  A discussion of histopathologic categories of liver disease and their significance.

Radiographic Diagnosis of Portosystemic Anomalies

PHILLIP F. STEYN
Fort Collins, Colorado

The diagnosis of portosystemic anomalies is suggested by radiographic or sonographic changes secondary to the shunt and is confirmed by visualization of portal blood shunting past the liver. Noninvasive confirmation of portosystemic shunts includes portovenography, transcolonic nuclear portography (scintigraphy), or ultrasonographic evaluation of the portal vein (Moon, 1990).

The portal vein is responsible for 75% of the hepatic blood flow in the mature animal and can be seen to shunt the blood into the caudal vena cava or the azygos vein at various levels both intra- and extrahepatically. Most of the dogs and cats with intrahepatic shunts have a persistent ductus venosus (Birchard and Sherding, 1992; Blaxter et al, 1988). In the fetus, the ductus venosus is responsible for shunting blood past the liver into the caudal vena cava. If the ductus venosus does not close after birth, the shunting persists during the postnatal phase. Extrahepatic shunting can occur when anomalous veins allow blood from the portal vein to drain directly into the caudal vena cava or the azygos vein without perfusing the liver parenchyma.

Acquired portosystemic shunts develop extrahepatically from vestigial portosystemic communications. The liver is typically small and the patient is generally (although not always) older. A history of chronic liver disease is present and some degree of ascites is often present because of the chronic portal hypertension resulting from the underlying liver disorder.

RADIOGRAPHIC SIGNS

Routine abdominal radiographs of these patients usually show small livers with significant cranial displacement of predominantly the pyloric part of the gastric axis. On the ventral-dorsal radiograph, the entire stomach may be displaced cranially due to hepatic atrophy. The oral administration of a small volume of barium sulfate suspension (5 to 10 ml) can often help in the radiographic evaluation of the liver by marking the location of the stomach. In some cases, the liver can be of normal size. Abdominal serosal detail is often poor because of emaciation of the patient. There is seldom a peritoneal effusion in congenital portosystemic shunts because of the absence of portal hypertension. The kidneys can be small, normal, or large. If ammonium biurate uroliths are present, they tend to be radiolucent.

PORTOGRAPHY

Several different radiographic techniques have been described to evaluate the flow of blood through the portal

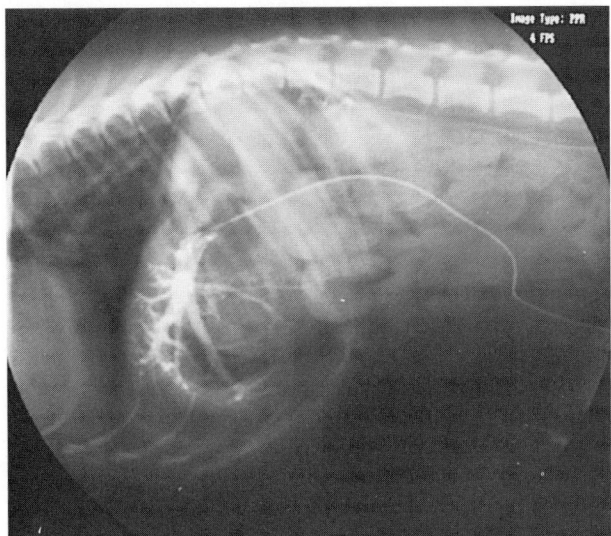

Figure 1. An intraoperative mesenteric portogram showing *normal hepatic perfusion* by portal blood. The catheter has been placed in a mesenteric vein and positive contrast can be seen in the liver.

vein (Birchard et al, 1989). All require general anesthesia and some degree of surgical intervention in terms of vessel catheterization. The end goals of these radiographic techniques is to produce a radiograph with positive contrast in the portal vein, showing either its normal hepatic arborization or its abnormal termination into the caudal vena cava, the azygos vein, or other systemic vein. The iodinated positive contrast medium is introduced (1) into the arterial blood supplying the bowel and radiographed during the portal phase (cranial mesenteric angioportography), (2) into a mesenteric vein draining the jejunum and radiographed during the portal phase (intraoperative mesenteric portography), or (3) into the pulp of the spleen and radiographed during the portal phase (splenoportography). Figure 1 is a radiographic image of an intraoperative mesenteric portogram showing normal hepatic perfusion by portal blood.

The catheter has been placed in a mesenteric vein, and positive contrast can be seen in the liver.

Cranial mesenteric angioportography (CMAP) is performed by selectively catheterizing the cranial mesenteric artery via a femoral artery using fluoroscopic guidance. The catheter tip is placed in the origin of the cranial mesenteric artery from the aorta, and a bolus (contrast medium, e.g., diatrizoate [Renografin] at 1.5 to 3 ml/kg) is injected using a pressure injector. The bolus of positive contrast (organic iodide) passes through the splanchnic vasculature and then accumulates in the portal vein as it proceeds to the liver. Radiographs are made at the rate of one or two per second as the contrast passes through the portal vein. Six radiographs are made during the arterial phase, which lasts about 4 to 10 seconds, and 10 radiographs are made during the portovenous phase, which lasts about 6 to 14 seconds. Clear visualization of the hepatoportal vasculature, followed by the caudal vena cava, is compatible with a normal study. Portocaval shunting is most commonly seen as a direct communication of the portal vein with the caudal vena cava (with little to no hepatoportal circulation seen). Various anatomic variations exist in the exact location of the shunting vessel; intrahepatic and extrahepatic portocaval shunts are most common, but portoazygous shunts also occur. Shunt vessels caudal to the 13th thoracic vertebra are most likely extrahepatic, and those cranial to the 13th thoracic vertebra are most likely intrahepatic portocaval shunts. The largest disadvantage of CMAP is the dilution of the contrast bolus by the time it reaches the portal vein. Radiographic subtraction techniques and digitalized fluoroscopy have made this technique more sensitive.

Intraoperative mesenteric portography is performed by catheterizing a splanchnic vessel (e.g., a jejunal vein) at surgery. Once the catheter is placed, the abdomen is closed. The patient is then transported to the radiology department where a hand injection of positive contrast (contrast medium, e.g., diatrizoate at 1 to 2 ml/kg) and a series of radiographs are made, approximately one per second for about 6 to 10 seconds. An advantage of this technique is that a concentrated bolus gives clear radiographic visualization of the portal vein. The interpretation of the study is basically the same as that for a CMAP. Figure 2 is a

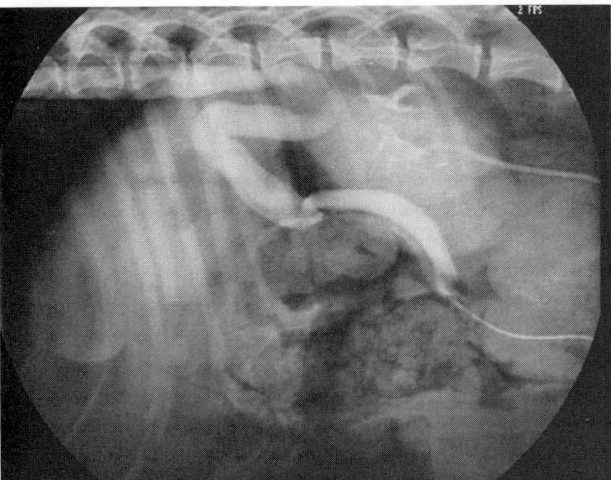

Figure 2. An intraoperative mesenteric portogram showing a *large portoazygous shunt.* A mesenteric vein has been catheterized. Positive contrast can be seen shunting dorsally to the azygos vein. Renal excretion of positive contrast is seen due to an earlier injection.

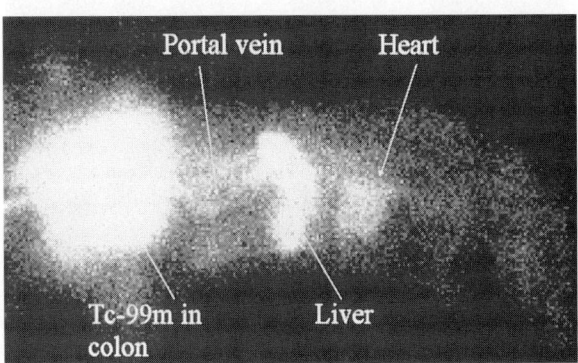

Figure 3. Transcolonic portal angiogram of a *normal dog.* A composite of 90 frames (each 2 seconds) allows clear visualization of the portal vein, liver, and heart. The large area of radioactivity in the colon represents unabsorbed technetium-99m.

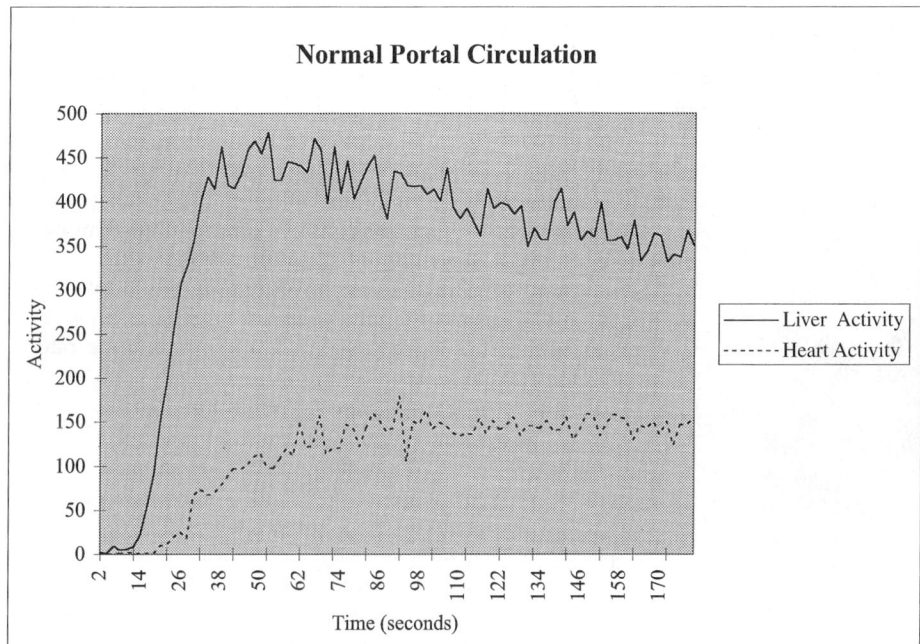

Normal Portal Circulation

Figure 4. A *normal* time activity curve for the regions of interest generated around the liver and heart. The radioactivity first enters the liver and then arrives at the heart about 8 seconds later.

radiographic image of an intraoperative mesenteric portogram showing a large portoazygous shunt.

Splenoportography is performed by injecting the positive contrast into the splenic pulp. The contrast is then taken up rapidly by the venous sinusoids into the portal system. The spleen can be injected either percutaneously with an over-the-needle type catheter (±26 gauge) or the spleen can be exposed by laparotomy and then injected directly. Either way, 1 ml/kg positive contrast is hand-injected into the splenic parenchyma, and a series of radiographs are made about 5 to 10 seconds later. Interpretation is the same as that for the CMAP. Advantages of splenoportography are that fluoroscopy, rapid injectors, and a rapid film changer are not required and hence it can be performed in most small animal hospitals. The disadvantage is that extrahepatic shunts caudal to the splenic vein will not be identified, resulting in possible false-normal diagnoses.

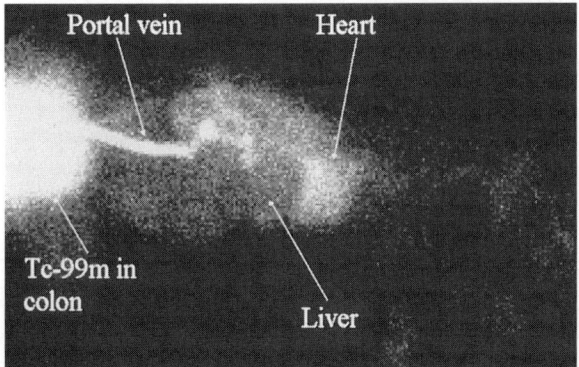

Figure 5. Transcolonic portal angiogram of a dog with a *moderate to severe portosystemic shunt.* A composite of 90 frames (each 2 seconds) allows clear visualization of the portal vein and the heart. The liver is not well visualized because of poor hepatoportal perfusion. The large area of radioactivity in the colon represents unabsorbed technetium-99m.

ULTRASONOGRAPHY

Longitudinal and transverse sonograms of the liver are made as the entire liver is evaluated. The liver often appears to be smaller than normal, with portal and hepatic veins reduced in size. Intrahepatic portosystemic shunts can sometimes be observed as vessels connecting the portal vein and the caudal vena cava. These abnormal vessels are best demonstrated while the dog is under general anesthesia (Wrigley et al, 1987) but can often be seen in awake patients. Color flow Doppler also enhances the diagnosis of portosystemic shunts, showing turbulence in the caudal vena cava where the shunting blood enters it. Extrahepatic shunts are more challenging but can sometimes be seen as abnormal tortuous vessels in the region between the kidneys and the liver.

TRANSCOLONIC NUCLEAR PORTOGRAPHY

Nuclear medicine imaging (scintigraphy) is available at most academic institutions and a few private clinics in the United States and is based on imaging the distribution of a radioactive tracer in the body of a patient. Various pharmaceutical agents, cells, or even antibodies can be attached to the radionuclide tracer, thereby determining its destination in the body. Images are made with a gamma camera, and patients are hospitalized until their radiation exposure levels are low enough to meet local release protocols. Physiologic imaging of the liver and portal system is best carried out with nuclear medicine techniques. This is especially true in the diagnosis and quantitation of portal systemic shunts and obstructive disorders of the biliary system (Daniel et al, 1991).

Five to 15 mCi of technetium-99m–pertechnetate is administered intracolonically and rapid frame image acquisition (90 × 2 second frames) is performed for 3 minutes with the patient in right lateral recumbency. Appropriate

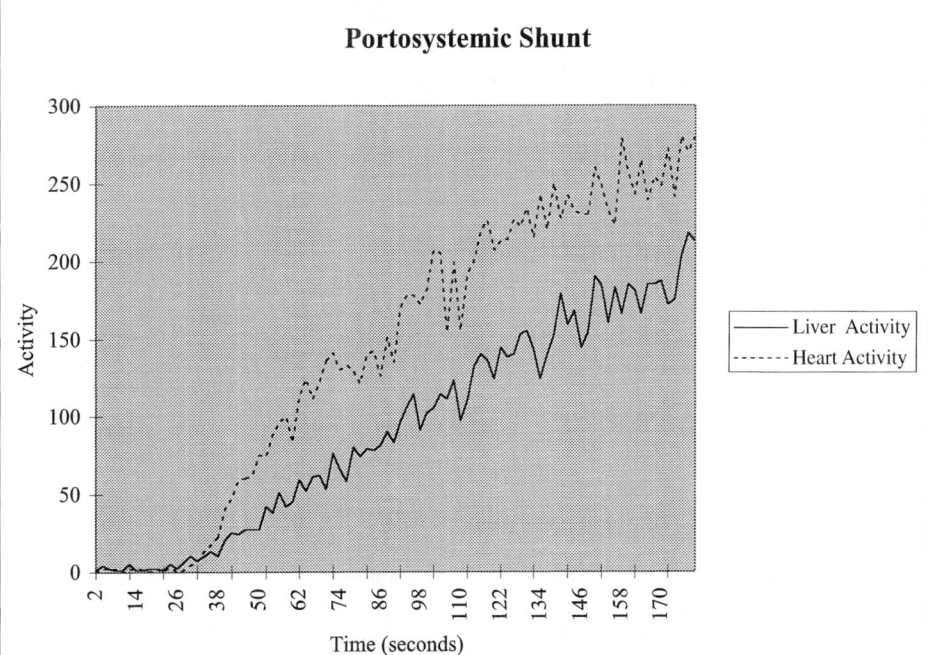

Figure 6. A time activity curve for the regions of interest generated around the liver and heart in a dog with a *moderate to severe portosystemic shunt.* The radioactivity arrives at the heart and the liver simultaneously, indicating that a certain fraction of the portal blood has bypassed the liver.

sedation should be considered if the patient cannot lie still for the duration of the study. The study is dynamic, so a repeat study can only be attempted 2 days later. A composite of these 90 frames is made (Fig. 3), regions of interest are drawn around the liver and heart and time activity curves are generated for these two regions of interest. Activity should be seen in the liver region of interest before the heart region of interest in the patient with a normal portal circulation. Figure 4 is a time activity curve showing the normal scenario in which portal blood first perfuses the liver and then goes to the heart. Patients with a portosystemic shunt (acquired or congenital) demonstrate tracer activity in the heart before the liver (Figs. 5 and 6). The percent shunt fraction can be calculated using the area under the curve of the liver and heart regions of interest and is categorized as mild, moderate, or severe, allowing the clinician to monitor the severity of the shunt or the response to treatment. Shunt fractions of up to 20% have been documented in normal dogs. Mild shunts range from 20 to 40%, moderate shunts from 40 to 60%, and severe shunts greater than 60%.

The extra- or intrahepatic position of a shunt may not be determined from this study. Multiple or large extrahepatic shunts are sometimes seen cranial to the kidneys, but in our practice this is not consistent enough to be reliably diagnostic. Complications are not expected from the pertechnetate study but could occur with the sedation that is sometimes necessary. Poor or nonuptake of the pertechne-

tate by the colon will result in a suboptimal study and can necessitate a repeat study. This would generally be scheduled for the following day. False-positive results have not been seen. False-negative results have been associated with microvascular shunting disorders.

References and Suggested Reading

Birchard SJ, Sherding RG: Feline portosystemic shunts. Compendium 14:1295, 1992.
Review article on portosystemic shunts in cats includes surgical approaches to therapy.

Birchard SJ, Biller DS, Johnson SE: Differentiation of intrahepatic versus extrahepatic portosystemic shunts in dogs using positive contrast portography. J Am Anim Hosp Assoc 25:13, 1989.
Discusses the value of portography in the diagnostic work-up of canine patients with portosystemic shunts.

Blaxter AC, Holt PE, Gibbs C, et al: Congenital portosystemic shunts in the cat: A report of nine cases. J Small Anim Pract 29:631, 1988.
Good retrospective review of clinical features, diagnosis, management and outcome of nine cats with portosystemic shunts.

Daniel GB, Bright R, Ollis P, Shull R: Per rectal portal scintigraphy using ^{99m}Tc pertechnetate to diagnose portosystemic shunts in dogs and cats. J Vet Intern Med 5:23, 1991.
Description of scintigraphic transcolonic portal angiography.

Moon ML: Diagnostic imaging of portosystemic shunts. Semin Vet Med Surg 5:120, 1990.
Review of various techniques, including radiographic, portographic, and sonographic methods.

Wrigley RH, Park RD, Konde LJ, et al: Subtraction portal venography. Vet Radiol 28:208, 1987.
Description of photographic subtraction technique.

Effect of Extrahepatic Disease on the Liver

DENNY J. MEYER
Boulder, Colorado

DAVID C. TWEDT
Fort Collins, Colorado

For the study of medical diseases of the liver, it is essential that the pathologist be apprised of the clinical findings and the results of laboratory tests and radiographic studies. The correct diagnosis is most likely to be reached by the pathologist and clinician working as a team.

KAMAL ISHAK, MD, PATHOLOGIST

Hepatic "reaction" and response to extrahepatic disease is appreciated with increasing frequency. Changes can occur in serum hepatic test results, as can histopathologic changes. The secondary hepatic involvement poses two diagnostic problems: (1) it mimics primary hepatic disease and (2) it diverts attention from the underlying extrahepatic disease. This article covers three areas relative to abnormal serum hepatic test results and associated histopathologic findings: (1) nonspecific hepatic reaction associated with extrahepatic inflammation and neoplasia, (2) hepatic response to selected extrahepatic diseases, and (3) histopathologic changes that develop during the biopsy procedure. Although somewhat arbitrary, and with obvious crossover of constituents, this approach is used to provide a simple framework for this discussion.

PHYSIOANATOMY

There are a variety of reasons why extrahepatic diseases secondarily involve the liver. The causes can be anatomic or functional. The liver has two blood supplies: the hepatic artery and the portal vein. The former provides oxygen and nutrition. The latter, which comprises approximately 80% of the total hepatic blood flow, delivers substances absorbed from the gastrointestinal tract and pancreatic hormones. The hepatic vein collects the blood that has percolated through the sinusoids before joining the inferior vena cava en route to the right atrium. Consequently, the liver can be affected secondarily by cardiovascular dysfunction, anemia, portosystemic shunts, enteritis, pancreatitis, and exposure to products in the systemic circulation from extrahepatic inflammation, neoplasia, and infection.

Hepatocytes reside in acini located in three diverse metabolic zones. Blood entering the liver, composed of a mixture of arterial and portal venous blood, flows from the portal triad, passing through zones 1, 2, and 3 before draining via the hepatic vein. Consequently, hepatocytes in zone 3 (centrilobular region) are most susceptible to hypoxic conditions such as anemia, right-sided heart failure, and shock. The metabolic diversity of the hepatic zones is necessary to accommodate the numerous homeostatic activities. Many of these functions are related to the intermediary role of hepatocyte metabolism between dietary sources of nutrients and extrahepatic tissue demands for energy. Therefore, metabolic diseases often involve the liver. Examples include hyperadrenocorticism, diabetes mellitus, and lipidoses.

The hepatocyte plays a pivotal role in the multistep, energy-dependent process of bile formation. Hyperthyroidism and extrahepatic infections can alter one or more of the complex steps, resulting in jaundice.

Another cell type that plays a role in the manifestations of extrahepatic disease is the Kupffer cell, a member of the monocyte-macrophage system. This cell is involved in the hepatic immune response and "filters" toxins and bacteria that enter the systemic and portal circulations. When this role is amplified in response to extrahepatic disease, focal suppurative and nonsuppurative hepatitis can result.

REACTIVE CHANGES

The liver often exhibits a variety of nonspecific secondary changes in response to disease elsewhere in the body. A variety of systemic infectious and inflammatory diseases secondarily affect the liver. In a review of 150 consecutive hepatic biopsies at Colorado State University, approximately 25% were classified as a "reactive secondary" or "degenerative" hepatopathy. In 95% of the cases, an underlying extrahepatic disease was identified (Table 1). In general, the serum alanine aminotransferase (ALT) activity was approximately twice the upper limit of the reference range and the serum alkaline phosphatase (ALP) activity was raised three to fourfold. The serum bile acid concentration remained in the reference range in patients in which it was measured (20% of the population studied).

The term *nonspecific reactive hepatitis* is often used to categorize the histopathologic findings, but replacing the term *hepatitis* with the word *changes* is recommended by some authors. The histopathologic features encompass a variable combination of portal and parenchymal changes that are usually of minor but occasionally of moderate degree and are distributed in a patchy, uneven manner. The findings include portal infiltration by mononuclear cells—primarily lymphocytes, fatty change, focal hepato-

TABLE 1. Extrahepatic Causes of Abnormal Hepatic Tests and Histologic Changes in the Liver

Enteritis, severe or chronic	Hypothyroidism(?)
Extrahepatic infections (bacterial, including rickettsial; septicemia)	Prolonged protein-restricted diet Congenital portosystemic shunts
Acute pancreatitis	Shock
Diabetes mellitus	Right-sided heart failure
Hyperthyroidism	Hyperadrenocorticism
	Hypoadrenocorticism

cellular necrosis, and lobular inflammation. The latter may consist of enlarged or hyperplastic Kupffer cells (sometimes forming small granulomatoid or lipogranulomatoid clusters) and small foci of other macrophages, neutrophils, or lymphocytes. Terms such as *periportal hepatitis, multifocal hepatitis,* or *hepatitis—chronic, active, mild* may be used to summarize the microscopic findings. The distinction between resolving acute hepatitis or a mild form of chronic hepatitis and reactive changes may be difficult and arbitrary without supportive clinical information.

Some of the hepatic histopathologic and biochemical changes that are caused by extrahepatic inflammatory diseases, that is, infections and neoplasia, are mediated by cytokines. These hormone-like molecules consisting of interferons, interleukins, and hematopoietic growth factors form a complex network of interactive signals. Tumor necrosis factor (also called *cachectin),* interleukin-1, and interleukin-6 have been shown to cause either hepatic histopathologic changes or biochemical changes. Interleukin-6 plays a prominent role in the regulation of hepatic-specific genes, resulting in the accelerated production of proteins referred to as *acute-phase reactants.* Fibrinogen is just one example of an acute-phase reactant protein of hepatic origin that is used as a marker of systemic inflammation. One consequence of the up-regulation of the acute-phase reactant proteins is a down-regulation of albumin synthesis through poorly understood mechanisms. The finding of a reduced serum albumin concentration as a functional consequence of chronic extrahepatic inflammation could be misinterpreted as a reflection of reduced hepatocellular mass.

Excessive concentrations of nitric oxide can also decrease albumin synthesis and alter other components of hepatic function. Endotoxin can stimulate the nitric oxide synthetase of blood vessels to increase the production of endothelium-derived nitric oxide as well as enhance nitrous oxide formation in both Kupffer cells and hepatocytes. The stimulation appears to be a direct effect on the Kupffer cell, whereas the hepatocyte requires the concurrent presence of excess interleukin-1 and tumor necrosis factor. Prolonged, excessive release of nitric oxide may mediate tissue damage directly or bind to heme-containing proteins, including cytochrome P_{450} enzymes, altering their activity and predisposing to drug-induced hepatotoxicity.

CHOLESTASIS OF SEPSIS

An impairment of bile flow (cholestasis) can also develop in association with extrahepatic bacterial infections (e.g., pneumonia, prostatitis, peritonitis, bite wounds). Clinically, the patients are icteric if the serum bilirubin concentration is greater than approximately 3 mg/dl, and often there is only a mild rise in serum hepatic enzyme test results despite a mild to marked rise in the serum bilirubin concentration. Serum bilirubin values in the 20- to 30-mg/dl range can develop and, in concert with serum hepatic enzyme values (200 to 500 IU/L), suggest extrahepatic obstructive disease. There are minimal histopathologic changes in the liver, with the exception of moderate to marked bile accumulation that includes canalicular plugs. The histopathologic features include a periportal lymphocytic infiltrate and scattered parenchymal foci of macrophages or neutrophils, sometimes surrounding individual necrotic hepatocytes. Successful management of the extrahepatic infection is associated with spontaneous resolution of the functional cholestasis. The pathophysiologic mechanisms responsible for this disorder are incompletely understood. Bacterial toxins and antibodies to bacterial cell wall components that cross-react with the canalicular membrane can "paralyze" the energy-dependent transport systems for bile acids. Since the excretion of bile acids is the primary driving force for bile flow, stagnation results in cholestasis. It has also been shown that selected acute-phase reactant proteins can interfere with hepatocellular uptake of bile acids, further impairing their pivotal role in facilitating bile flow.

INFLAMMATORY BOWEL DISEASE

Approximately 25% of dogs and cats with lymphocytic-plasmacytic enteritis are reported to have mildly raised serum ALT and ALP activities. Hepatic function test results are usually within the reference range. However, bacterial overgrowth can develop in chronic enteropathies and amplify the deconjugation of bile acids. The kinetics of unconjugated bile acids differ from conjugated bile acids in that unconjugated salts can be passively absorbed along the length of the intestinal tract and hepatic extraction from the sinusoidal blood is less efficient. This inefficient clearance can, on occasion, increase serum bile acid concentrations mildly, although we have documented values between 70 and 100 μmol/L. Microscopically, a periportal inflammatory infiltrate is found, suggesting a causal relationship between translocation of bacteria from the diseased intestinal tract into the portal circulation and the abnormal liver tests. A second possibility is that endotoxin lipopolysaccharide, a component of the cell wall of gram-negative bacteria, crosses the diseased intestinal wall and directly damages hepatocytes or stimulates the release of cytotoxic substances from activated Kupffer cells. Superoxides, toxic oxygen radicals, tumor necrosis factor, and platelet-activating factor can injure hepatocytes and endothelial cells in close proximity to the activated Kupffer cells. The more common microscopic findings include multifocal inflammatory foci and periportal inflammatory cell infiltrates consisting predominantly of lymphocytes and plasma cells with lesser numbers of macrophages and neutrophils. These findings again may prompt a diagnosis such as *hepatitis, chronic, active, mild.* The term *cholangiohepatitis* might even be used, considering the portal distribution of the cellular infiltrate. Bile ductular proliferation is usually mild but can be prominent secondary to chronic severe enteritis.

ACUTE PANCREATITIS

Acute pancreatitis can secondarily involve the liver in two ways: (1) by impairing bile flow in the common bile duct and (2) by directly injuring hepatocytes. There is a variable amount of peripancreatic inflammation associated with acute pancreatitis. When severe, it encompasses the common bile duct and causes clinical, biochemical, and histopathologic findings indicative of extrahepatic cholestasis. After resolution of the inflammatory process, the serum bilirubin level will decrease, often within 7 to 10 days. However, the formation of abundant fibrous tissue may cause a permanent obstruction to bile flow and can even necessitate surgical intervention. Biochemical and microscopic findings consistent with mild to moderate hepatocellular injury and intrahepatic cholestasis also develop in association with acute pancreatitis. In one study, approximately 60% of cats with acute pancreatitis had raised serum hepatic enzyme levels and hyperbilirubinemia. The incidence of abnormal serum hepatic test results may be misleadingly high because of the population that made up the study but serves as a reminder of the pancreas-liver relationship in disease. In an experimental dog study, the severity of the histopathologic changes were shown to be directly proportional to the intensity of the pancreatic inflammation (Andrzejewska, 1985). Microscopically, there is focal necrosis, Kupffer cell hyperplasia, periportal inflammatory cell infiltrates, and hepatocellular accumulation of bile pigment; subcellularly, there is mitochondrial degeneration. The pathophysiologic mechanisms responsible for these changes are speculative. One scenario is that the potent pancreatic proteases are released directly into the portal circulation, causing hepatocellular cytotoxicity. Alternatively, the products of the inflammatory process may be released into the portal circulation, "filtered" by the Kupffer cell, resulting in stimulation of the release of cytotoxic substances, as discussed earlier.

METABOLIC DISEASE

A variety of metabolic and endocrine diseases can cause abnormal liver test results and histopathologic changes. One of the more widely recognized hormonally associated diseases is hyperadrenocorticism. The canine liver is uniquely "responsive" to excessive glucocorticoids. There is often a moderate to marked rise in the serum ALP activity, without hyperbilirubinemia, and a foamy change in the hepatocyte cytoplasm caused by glycogen accumulation. The glycogen accumulation can be dramatic, resulting in hepatomegaly. In severe cases, focal accumulations of neutrophils can be found surrounding individual degenerating hepatocytes. Patients with diabetes mellitus can develop hepatic lipidosis with associated abnormal liver test results. Up to 80% of cats with hyperthyroidism have abnormal serum hepatic enzyme test results including hyperbilirubinemia. There are minimal to no microscopic hepatic lesions observed, and the biochemical changes spontaneously resolve with treatment, suggesting a functional hepatopathy. In dogs with hypothyroidism, the authors have occasionally observed an associated mild to moderately raised serum ALP activity with no to minimal histopathologic changes evident in the liver.

CONGENITAL PORTOVASCULAR ANOMALIES

Congenital portosystemic shunts (see p. 664) are often associated with a mild to moderate increase in the serum hepatic enzyme tests, a decrease in the biochemical markers of hepatic function (albumin, blood urea nitrogen, glucose), and a moderate to marked rise in the total serum bile acid concentration. The liver can appear normal histologically, or there can be mild to moderate vacuolar change, an absence of a portal vein in the portal tracts, and an increase in arteriolar-like structures in the portal area. Foci of pigment-filled macrophages (sometimes called *lipogranulomas*) occur with increased frequency in young dogs with congenital portosystemic shunts. The accumulation of hepatic iron (notably in Kupffer cells) is a common event and can be associated with a slight reduction in the hematocrit and the erythrocyte mean cell volume. The finding of increased iron in the biopsy specimen of a relatively young dog should stimulate the consideration of a congenital portosystemic shunt especially if foci of pigment-laden macrophages are present. Increases in plasma cortisol concentration, free cortisol concentration, and free cortisol fraction are present in dogs with portosystemic shunts, secondary to an altered hypothalamic-pituitary-adrenal axis, and may be responsible for the vacuolar change and raised serum ALP activity.

NODULAR HYPERPLASIA

Although nodular hyperplasia is an intrahepatic event, it is included because this relatively benign process is associated with abnormal serum hepatic enzyme test results and histopathologic changes that can be suggestive of chronic hepatitis or an extrahepatic metabolic disease such as hyperadrenocorticism. It is a common finding in older dogs and appears to be age-related. Nodules are found in some dogs by 6 years of age and, in one study, they were present in all dogs older than 14 years (Bergman, 1985). The expansile process compresses existing parenchyma, resulting in hepatocellular atrophy and approximation of the reticular fibers. Nonsuppurative inflammatory infiltrates and granulocytic extramedullary hematopoiesis occasionally located in the compressed portal tracts can mimic chronic active hepatitis. Grossly, their appearance mimics macronodular cirrhosis and neoplasia. The hepatocytes composing these nodules often develop a variety of cyto-

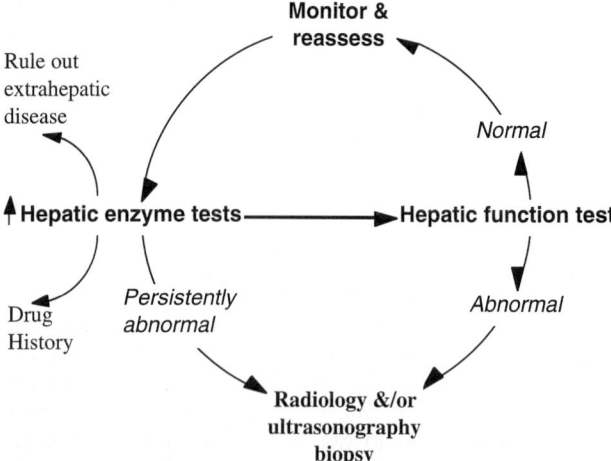

Figure 1. A flow chart illustrating a differential diagnostic approach to a patient with raised serum hepatic enzyme test results. (Modified from Meyer DJ, Harvey JW: Veterinary Laboratory Medicine: Interpretation and Diagnosis, 2nd ed. Philadelphia: WB Saunders, 1998, p 180, with permission.)

plasmic changes that morphologically include lipidosis, hydropic degeneration, and glycogen accumulation. Finding these changes in a needle biopsy specimen can be problematic because the actual identification of a nodule is difficult owing to size limitations, and the morphologic appearance can be suggestive of an extrahepatic metabolic disorder. The rise of the serum ALP activity and, less frequently, the serum ALT activity is usually mild to moderate.

CHANGES ASSOCIATED WITH THE BIOPSY PROCEDURE OR SITE

A biopsy specimen of the liver is often obtained to help define the reason for abnormal hepatic test results. Consequently, it is submitted with the expectation that an abnormality will be observed and, hopefully, offer an explanation for the abnormal hepatic test results. Certain histologic findings associated with the site of the biopsy or the age of the animal may be interpreted as abnormal. In other cases, histopathologic findings that could explain the cause of abnormal hepatic test results are missed because of the type of biopsy.

Needle Biopsy

Focal disease may be missed with a needle biopsy, which provides a core of tissue that represents approximately 1/50,000 of the whole organ. Multiple samples increase the probability of detecting the lesion, as does increasing the length of the specimen. An intact length of 1.5 cm is considered sufficient for recognition of chronic hepatitis in human patients. An intact needle biopsy that is at least 2 cm in length is suggested as minimally adequate for the recognition of bridging hepatic fibrosis, an important finding prognostically. It is also desirable for the identification of findings supportive of nodular regeneration.

A biopsy needle may "glance off" the fibrous septa of a cirrhotic liver and obtain relatively normal-appearing tissue of a regenerative nodule. The spring-driven cutting needles reduce this possibility.

Wedge Biopsy

The wedge biopsy provides ample tissue and permits examination of multiple portal tracts. Because of its superficial location relative to blood supply, the margin of the liver is predisposed to fibrosis that can mimic findings indicative of cirrhosis. In this location, fibrous septa join portal tracts to the subcapsular connective tissue or to each other. A superficial specimen of this tissue, for example, obtained by laparoscopy with a clam shell–type biopsy forceps, would give inaccurate findings suggestive of hepatic fibrosis. The subcapsular zone of the liver may show more extensive necrosis than would deeper parenchyma in chronic hepatitis, resulting in an overly pessimistic interpretation. Varying degrees of crush artifact at the periphery of the biopsy specimen further reduces the area available for evaluation.

In human patients, studies have shown that microscopic changes occur in biopsy specimens taken a period of time after the beginning of a surgical procedure secondary to tissue anoxia. Whether similar changes, referred to as *surgical hepatitis,* occur in veterinary medicine has not been studied adequately. Neutrophils can accumulate under the capsule, focally in liver cell plates, and in tight clusters around central veins. Along with isolated liver cell necrosis, these procedure-related changes would be indicative of suppurative hepatitis, resulting in a misdiagnosis. Less commonly, a mild increase in inflammatory cells may also be observed in portal tracts, giving the impression of cholangitis.

In summary, abnormal hepatic tests values and histopathologic changes can be associated with primary hepatic disease and extrahepatic disease. When a consequence of the latter, its management results in the resolution of the hepatopathy. Figure 1 illustrates one diagnostic strategy for a patient with raised serum hepatic enzyme test results.

References and Suggested Reading

Andrzejewska A, Dlugosz J, Kurasz S: The ultrastructure of the liver in acute experimental pancreatitis. Exp Pathol 28:167, 1985.
The histopathologic changes in the liver of dogs are described after the induction of pancreatitis.

Bergman JR: Nodular hyperplasia in the liver of the dog: An association with changes in the Ito cell population. Vet Pathol 22:427, 1985.
The clinical and histopathologic features of nodular hyperplasia in the dog are characterized.

Hill R, vanWinkle T: Acute necrotizing pancreatitis and suppurative pancreatitis in the cat. J Vet Intern Med 7:25, 1993.
Pancreatic histopathologic findings and clinical biochemistry changes in cats with acute pancreatitis are described.

Ishak K: Hepatic histopathology. In: Schiff L, Schiff ER, eds: Diseases of the Liver, 7th ed. Philadelphia: JB Lippincott, 1993, p 145.
The chapter presents a general approach to the examination of the liver biopsy and illustrates the findings for hepatic diseases.

Lichtman SN, Sartor RB, Keku J, et a:. Hepatic inflammation in rats with experimental small bowel bacterial overgrowth. Gastroenterology 98:414, 1990.
The histopathologic changes in the liver associated with bacterial overgrowth are described.

Meyer DJ, Harvey JW: Hematologic changes associated with serum and hepatic iron alterations in dogs with congenital portosystemic vascular anomalies. J Vet Intern Med 8:55, 1994.
The association between hematologic changes and hepatic iron accumulation in dogs with congenital portosystemic shunts is characterized.

Mochida S, Ohta Y, Ogata I, et al: Gut-derived substances in activation of hepatic macrophages after partial hepatectomy in rats. J Hepatol 16:266, 1992.
This article demonstrates that bacterial products of gut origin activate hepatic macrophages and contribute to hepatic injury.

Rothuizen J, Biewenga WJ, Mol JA: Chronic glucocorticoid excess and impaired osmoregulation of vasopressin release in dogs with hepatic encephalopathy. Domestic Anim Endocrinol 12:13, 1995.
This article documents an abnormal pituitary-adrenocortical axis resulting in hypercortisolemia in dogs with congenital and acquired portosystemic shunts.

Stark ME, Szurszewski JH: Role of nitric oxide in gastrointestinal and hepatic function and disease. Gastroenterology 103:1928, 1992.
This review article discusses the potentially deleterious hepatic effects of excessive nitric oxide production.

Taboada J, Meyer DJ: Cholestasis associated with extrahepatic bacterial infection in five dogs. J Vet Intern Med 3:216, 1989.
This article characterizes the clinicopathologic and histopathologic findings in dogs with a variety of extrahepatic infections.

Feline Cholangiohepatitis

Douglas J. Weiss
P. J. Armstrong
Josanne M. Gagne
St. Paul, Minnesota

Inflammatory liver disease (26%) is the second most common cause of feline liver disease (Gagne et al, 1996). Other common causes of liver disease are hepatic lipidosis (49%) and lymphosarcoma (7%). The terminology used to describe the histopathologic features of feline inflammatory liver disease is confusing. These terms include *suppurative cholangiohepatitis, chronic cholangiohepatitis, chronic nonsuppurative cholangiohepatitis, pericholangiohepatitis, chronic lymphocytic cholangitis, progressive lymphocytic cholangitis, sclerosing cholangitis, lymphocytic-plasmacytic cholangitis-cholangiohepatitis, lymphocytic cholangitis-cholangiohepatitis, lymphocytic portal hepatitis,* and *biliary cirrhosis.* Recent retrospective studies have clarified the classification of inflammatory liver disease (Jones, 1989; Center and Rowland, 1994; Gagne et al, 1996). The authors reviewed 175 feline liver biopsy specimens obtained from the University of Minnesota Veterinary Teaching Hospital (Gagne et al, 1996). Results of this study indicate that inflammatory liver disease can be divided into two general types: cholangiohepatitis and lymphocytic portal hepatitis. Cholangiohepatitis can be subdivided into acute (suppurative) and chronic forms.

ACUTE (SUPPURATIVE) CHOLANGIOHEPATITIS

Histopathologic features of acute cholangiohepatitis include infiltration of large numbers of neutrophils into portal areas of the liver and cholangitis (i.e., inflammation of bile ducts). Disruption of the periportal limiting plate results in an irregular border in portal areas, periportal necrosis, and infiltration of neutrophils into hepatic lobules. Bile duct hypertrophy and fibrosis are usually minimal or absent.

Acute cholangiohepatitis may begin as an ascending bacterial infection within the biliary tract. Organisms, including *Escherichia coli, Clostridia, Bacteroides, Actinomyces,* and alpha-hemolytic *Streptococcus,* can be isolated from some affected cats. Abnormalities of the biliary system, including choleliths and anatomic anomalies of the gallbladder, may predispose cats to cholangiohepatitis. In one retrospective study, 83% of cats with cholangiohepatitis had concurrent inflammatory infiltrates in the duodenum or jejunum, or both, and 50% had pancreatic lesions. Therefore, inflammatory bowel disease, pancreatitis, altered gallbladder structure or function, and cholelithiasis may predispose the animal to transient cholestasis and permit reflux of pancreatic secretions or retrograde bacterial invasion, or both.

Clinical signs associated with acute cholangiohepatitis are nonspecific. They include anorexia, weight loss, lethargy, vomiting, and fever (Table 1). Hepatomegaly can be detected in approximately half the cases. Ninety percent of cats with acute cholangiohepatitis had neutrophilia or a left shift consistent with an inflammatory response. Serum biochemical abnormalities include normal to slightly elevated alkaline phosphatase (ALP) activity, moderate to marked elevation of alanine aminotransferase (ALT) activity, and a moderate to marked increase in total bilirubin concentration. Fasting or postprandial bile acids, or both, are also abnormal in affected cats.

CHRONIC CHOLANGIOHEPATITIS

Chronic cholangiohepatitis is characterized histopathologically by a mixed inflammatory infiltrate in portal areas and bile ducts consisting of neutrophils, lymphocytes, and plasma cells. Periportal necrosis and moderate to severe bile duct hypertrophy and portal fibrosis are also present. In terminal stages, chronic cholangiohepatitis may progress to biliary cirrhosis.

Chronic cholangiohepatitis may have multiple causes. Some investigators postulate that chronic cholangiohepatitis is the chronic form of acute cholangiohepatitis, whereas others propose that it is a separate immune-mediated disease that is similar to primary biliary cirrhosis in humans. Other authors speculate that initial bacterial infection initiates immune-mediated hepatocellular injury or bile duct destruction, or both, which perpetuates the initial injury. The role of viruses, drugs, or chemicals as causes of chronic cholangiohepatitis have not been extensively evaluated. Agents that have been incriminated include feline infectious peritonitis virus, feline leukemia virus, toxoplasmosis, and liver flukes (i.e., *Amphimerus pseudofelineus*).

Clinical signs are similar to those for acute cholangiohepatitis; however, only 11% of affected cats (Gagne et al, 1996; Jones, 1989) were febrile (see Table 1). Frequent hematologic abnormalities include neutrophilia and a left shift. Serum biochemical abnormalities include moderate to marked increases in serum ALP and ALT activities and a moderate to marked increase in total bilirubin concentration. Fasting or postprandial bile acids, or both, are also abnormal in affected cats.

LYMPHOCYTIC PORTAL HEPATITIS

Lymphocytic portal hepatitis appears to be distinct from acute and chronic cholangiohepatitis based on infiltration of lymphocytes and plasma cells, but not neutrophils, into portal areas, lack of cholangitis, and the presence of an intact periportal limiting plate. Numbers of lymphocytes and plasma cells in portal areas vary from few (10 to 20)

TABLE 1. **Summary of Clinical Data for Cats With Acute and Chronic Cholangiohepatitis, Lymphocytic Portal Hepatitis, and Hepatic Lipidosis**

	Acute Cholangiohepatitis	Chronic Cholangiohepatitis	Lymphocytic Portal Hepatitis	Hepatic Lipidosis
Age (yr)	5.7	9.7	8.2	6.2
Fever (%)	71	11	28	6
Anorexia (%)	86	78	64	100
Weight loss (%)	86	33	56	88
Diarrhea (%)	0	11	28	19
Ascites (%)	14	0	4	6

to many (>100). In some cases, large lymphoid aggregates are present. Bile duct hypertrophy and portal fibrosis are present in most cases but do not progress to pseudolobule formation or biliary cirrhosis. Because the inflammatory infiltrate consists almost exclusively of lymphocyte and plasma cells, several authors have speculated that lymphocytic portal hepatitis is an immune-mediated disease (Jones, 1989; Center and Rowland, 1994; Gagne et al, 1996).

Anorexia and weight loss are frequent clinical signs associated with lymphocytic portal hepatitis (see Table 1). Vomiting, lethargy, fever, and diarrhea are less frequently observed. Liver size is large in approximately half of affected cats. Results of complete blood counts are unremarkable for most cats with lymphocytic portal hepatitis, with the exception of poikilocytosis, which is present in two thirds of affected cats. Typical serum biochemical abnormalities include mildly increased serum ALP activity, moderately increased ALT activity, and normal to mildly increased total bilirubin concentration (Tables 2 and 3). Fasting or postprandial bile acids, or both, are frequently abnormal.

MANAGEMENT OF ACUTE CHOLANGIOHEPATITIS

The treatment plan for cats with acute cholangiohepatitis includes antimicrobial therapy and restoring and maintaining normal fluid and electrolyte balance. When extrahepatic bile duct obstruction is identified, surgical decompression and biliary to intestinal diversion (i.e., cholecystojejunostomy) have been recommended (Center and Rowland, 1994).

Antimicrobial therapy is the major specific treatment for acute cholangiohepatitis. Whenever possible, bacterial culture and sensitivity testing on bile, liver aspirate or biopsy specimens, choleliths, or gallbladder should be used to select appropriate antimicrobial agents. The antibiotics used should be excreted in the bile in active form, be active against aerobic and anaerobic intestinal coliform bacteria, and should not be hepatotoxic. Penicillins, trimethoprimsulfa, aminoglycosides, and first-generation cephalosporins may not be effective because they are not excreted in bile in active form. Tetracycline, erythromycin, ampicillin, chloramphenicol, and metronidazole are excreted in the bile in active form and, therefore, may be more effective (Zawie and Garvey, 1984). However, tetracycline is hepatotoxic, erythromycin is not effective against gram-negative bacteria, and chloramphenicol may cause anorexia. Anorexia associated with chloramphenicol therapy can usually be avoided by administering a relatively low dose (50 mg PO every 12 hours). Ampicillin is a broad-spectrum antibiotic that is well tolerated by cats. Metronidazole is effective against anaerobes and coliform bacteria. Combination antibiotic therapy using ampicillin (20 to 40 mg/kg PO every 8 hours), chloramphenicol (50 mg PO every 12 hours) and metronidazole (10 to 25 mg/kg, maximum dose 50 mg, PO every 24 hours) has been recommended (Zawie and Garvey, 1984). Treatment with antibiotics for 3 months or longer is recommended.

Urodeoxycholic acid is a dihydroxy bile acid used for gallstone dissolution and for treatment of chronic cholestatic liver disease in human patients. In humans, urodeoxycholic acid treatment has resulted in remarkable clinical and biochemical improvement, probably because of a reduction in cell membrane injury associated with retention of bile acids. Urodeoxycholic acid has also been shown to reduce expression of class 2 histocompatibility antigens on hepatocytes and bile duct epithelium, which may be im-

TABLE 2. **Summary of Clinical Laboratory Test Results for Cats With Acute (n = 7) and Chronic (n = 9) Cholangiohepatitis, Lymphocytic Portal Hepatitis (n = 25), Hepatic Lipidosis (n = 25), and Hepatic Lymphosarcoma (n = 11)**

Test	Reference Range	Acute Cholangiohepatitis	Chronic Cholangiohepatitis	Lymphocytic Portal Hepatitis	Hepatic Lipidosis	Hepatic Lymphosarcoma
Packed cell volume (%)	25.8–41.8	33.1 ± 7.7	29.8 ± 9.9	32.7 ± 7.6	30.2 ± 5.9	29.3 ± 12.2
White blood cell count (×10³/μl)	3.80–19.00	14.51 ± 7.85	13.46 ± 7.61	11.02 ± 7.6	10.53 ± 3.55	20.33 ± 9.7
Segmenters (×10³/μl)	1.29–16.00	11.93 ± 7.0	11.37 ± 6.72	8.42 ± 7.19	8.62 ± 3.51	12.21 ± 8.39
Bands (×10³/μl)	0–0.19	0.47 ± 0.71	0.07 ± 0.12	0.08 ± 0.18	0.05 ± 0.14	0.06 ± 0.16
Serum alkaline phosphatase (U/L)	12–105	48 ± 41	200 ± 196	84 ± 82	426 ± 247	201 ± 176
Alanine amino transferase (U/L)	17–95	408 ± 540	359 ± 348	325 ± 592	349 ± 207	541 ± 311
Total bilirubin (mg/dl)	0.1–0.8	3.9 ± 4.5	5.4 ± 5.9	2.0 ± 4.4	6.8 ± 4.0	2.4 ± 3.0
Total protein (gm/dl)	4.8–8.7	8.6 ± 1.3	7.0 ± 1.3	7.5 ± 1.1	6.7 ± 0.6	7.59 ± 1.2

Values represent mean ± SD.

TABLE 3. Trends in Clinical Laboratory Test Results Potentially Useful in Differentiating Acute (n = 7) and Chronic (n = 9) Cholangiohepatitis, Lymphocytic Portal Hepatitis (n = 25), Hepatic Lipidosis (n = 25), and Hepatic Lymphosarcoma (n = 11)

Test	Acute Cholangiohepatitis	Chronic Cholangiohepatitis	Lymphocytic Portal Hepatitis	Hepatic Lipidosis	Hepatic Lymphosarcoma
White blood cell count >19,000/μl (%)	28	11	12	9	70
Segmenters >16,000/μl (%)	28	22	12	15	45
Bands >200/μl (%)	43	22	20	2	8
Serum alkaline phosphatase >200 U/L (%)	0	31	12	78	50
Alanine aminotransferase >200 U/L (%)	60	46	20	71	90
Total bilirubin >3.0 mg/dl (%)	50	58	16	71	20

portant in reducing immune injury to hepatocytes. Urodeoxycholic acid has been administered to cats at 10 to 15 mg/kg PO every 24 hours.

Some cats may require additional treatment if specific complications develop. Cats with acute cholangiohepatitis are often acutely ill and may have fluid and electrolyte derangements that should be corrected. Treatment with injectable vitamin K_1 (5 mg/cat IM every 1 to 2 days) can be given if bleeding diatheses develop. Hepatic encephalopathy can be managed by giving lactulose orally (2.5 to 5 ml/cat PO every 8 hours) with or without the addition of enteric antibiotics (neomycin 20 mg/kg PO every 8 to 12 hours).

Complete blood counts and chemistry profiles should be repeated frequently to monitor the progress of therapy. Persistent elevation of ALT activity and serum total bilirubin concentration or increasing serum ALP activity, or both, indicate that treatment has been inadequate.

MANAGEMENT OF CHRONIC CHOLANGIOHEPATITIS

The treatment of chronic cholangiohepatitis is similar to that of acute cholangiohepatitis. However, glucocorticoid therapy may be warranted in addition to antibiotics and urodeoxycholic acid. An immunosuppressive dose of prednisolone (2.2 to 6.6 mg/kg every 24 hours) should be administered initially. The dosage is then tapered to an alternate-day dose (2 to 4 mg/kg every 48 hours) for long-term maintenance.

MANAGEMENT OF LYMPHOCYTIC PORTAL HEPATITIS

Treatment of lymphocytic portal hepatitis is based on the hypothesis that the liver injury is immune-mediated. Lymphocytic portal hepatitis has been treated with immunosuppressive doses of corticosteroids as described earlier for chronic cholangiohepatitis. Anecdotal reports (Jones, 1989) indicate prolonged remission with prednisolone treatment; however, others report poor control of disease progression with such treatment (Center and Rowland, 1994). Azathioprine (0.3 mg/kg PO every 24 hours) has been tried, but side effects, including inappetence and leukopenia, limit its use. Low-dose weekly methotrexate therapy has been used in a few affected cats.

Response to treatment for lymphocytic portal hepatitis is difficult to assess because the disease is slowly progressive. Persistent increases in ALT activity or increasing total serum bilirubin concentration during corticosteroid treatment, or both, indicate that the disease is inadequately controlled. Switching to a nonsteroidal immunosuppressive drug may be beneficial.

PROGNOSIS FOR CHOLANGIOHEPATITIS

Of 16 cases of acute and chronic cholangiohepatitis included in the authors' retrospective study, 14 cases were treated with antibiotics and 10 cases were treated with immunosuppressive doses of corticosteroids. Of these cats, 47% survived 1 year or less, 40% survived between 1 and 5 years, and 13% survived longer than 5 years. Results of this study indicate that long-term survival can be expected if cats survive the first 3 months after diagnosis.

PROGNOSIS FOR LYMPHOCYTIC PORTAL HEPATITIS

Of 25 cases of lymphocytic portal hepatitis included in the authors' retrospective study, 13 were treated with antibiotics, 4 were treated with anti-inflammatory doses of corticosteroids, and 3 were treated with immunosuppressive doses of corticosteroids. Half the cats did not receive treatment with antimicrobials or corticosteroids. Of 23 cats that were available for follow-up, 30% survived less than 1 year, 44% survived between 1 and 5 years, and 26% survived longer than 5 years. Mean survival time for cats surviving more than 1 year was 51.8 months, with 22% of cases still alive at the time of follow-up.

References and Suggested Reading

Center SA, Rowland PH: The cholangitis/cholangiohepatitis complex in the cat. Proceedings of the 12th annual Veterinary Medical Forum. Orlando, FL, American College of Veterinary Internal Medicine, 1994, pp 776–771.
A review of diagnosis and treatment of feline cholangiohepatitis.
Gagne J, Weiss DJ, Armstrong PJ: Histopathologic evaluation of feline inflammatory liver diseases. Vet Pathol 33:521, 1996.
A retrospective study of the histopathologic features of cholangiohepatitis and lymphocytic portal hepatitis.
Jones BR: Feline liver disease. Aust Vet Pract 19:28, 1989.
A review of diagnosis and treatment of feline cholangiohepatitis.
Zawie DA, Garvey MS: Feline hepatic disease. Vet Clin North Am 2:1201, 1984.
A review of diagnosis and treatment of feline cholangiohepatitis.

Hepatic Nodular Hyperplasia

Lauren C. Prause

David C. Twedt

Fort Collins, Colorado

Hepatic nodular hyperplasia (HNH) is a common benign lesion observed in the livers of older dogs. It is characterized by a discrete accumulation of hyperplastic hepatocytes arising as either macroscopic or microscopic hepatic nodules. HNH does not appear to cause clinical signs of illness. The diagnosis of HNH is usually made as an incidental finding at necropsy or during a diagnostic work-up for other concurrent medical problems. These lesions may result in laboratory, ultrasonographic, and gross and microscopic hepatic changes that may lead to diagnostic errors in evaluating patients with diseases not related to the liver (Table 1). The purpose of this article is to describe the clinical aspects of this condition based on the current literature and a retrospective review of 57 dogs having HNH identified at Colorado State University.

ETIOPATHOGENESIS

Hepatic nodular hyperplasia has been reported in several species, including humans, mice, rats, dogs, and cats. HNH in the dog appears to be different from lesions observed in other species, and making comparisons may not be valid. In some species, HNH is suggested to be preneoplastic, but this has not been observed in dogs. Development of HNH in mice has occurred experimentally after feeding of a high-fat, low-protein diet (Fabry et al, 1982). The authors believe that nutritional aspects could possibly play a role in HNH in dogs; this belief is supported by one animal that developed extensive HNH with lipidosis after approximately a year of being fed a severely protein-restricted diet.

CLINICAL FEATURES

HNH is a common postmortem finding in older dogs and is reported to occur with increased incidence with advancing age of the animal. In one study, 70% of the dogs had HNH by 14 years of age (Fabry et al, 1982), whereas a second study described 50 consecutive necropsies, with 100% of the dogs 14 years or older affected (Bergman, 1985). In the authors' review of 57 cases, the mean age at diagnosis was 11 years. There was also no

TABLE 1. Key Facts of Hepatic Nodular Hyperplasia in the Dog

Common lesion in aged dogs

Affected dogs are asymptomatic

Most have abnormal serum ALP activity

Macroscopically can mimic cirrhosis or neoplasia

A needle biopsy often can not define hepatic nodular hyperplasia

Needle biopsy findings may suggest an underlying metabolic disease

ALP, alkaline phosphatase.

obvious gender or breed predisposition recognized in this series.

The authors identified a subgroup of 27 dogs with HNH and no history of drug therapy or concurrent disease that would affect liver-related laboratory data. These affected dogs with HNH had an increase in serum alkaline phosphatase (ALP) levels to greater than the normal reference range with no changes in mean total bilirubin, alanine aminotransferase, cholesterol, total protein, or albumin concentrations. The serum ALP activity in these dogs was 2.5 times higher than the upper limits of the reference range. Several dogs with HNH had ALP concentrations as high as 10 to 14 times normal. Bile acid concentrations were determined in a few cases and were normal. The most likely explanations for the raised serum ALP activity is increased production secondary to focal intrahepatic cholestasis within the hyperplastic nodules or from the direct mechanical compression by the nodules on surrounding hepatic parenchyma. Occasionally, a rise in the serum ALT activity was noted and may be the consequence of hepatocellular dropout due to altered microcirculation. It has also recently been shown that hepatocellular proliferation can result in a rise in the plasma aminotransferase activity; it is possible that the nodular proliferation is directly responsible for the rise.

Routine abdominal radiographs are generally unremarkable, and ultrasonographic findings are inconsistent because of the varied hepatocellular morphologic characteristics and the size of the nodules. The echogenicity is reported to be hypoechoic, hyperechoic, or mixed in appearance (Johnson, 1995). The nodules may also have echogenicity identical to normal parenchyma and thus be overlooked. Because some cases of HNH can present as multifocal, larger, macroscopic lesions, they may be mistaken for primary or secondary hepatic neoplasia (Voros et al, 1991). A less common ultrasonographic differential diagnosis might include cirrhosis with regenerative nodules.

The gross appearance of HNH viewed during laparoscopy or surgical exploration or at necropsy is varied. Some animals with microscopic hyperplasia may have normal-appearing livers. Macroscopic lesions may be distinct singular or multiple nodules. We found that the majority of HNH cases had macroscopic (84%) lesions ranging from one to several centimeters in diameter compared with microscopic (16%) lesions millimeters or less in size. Multiple nodules were found in most cases (86%), compared with singular lesions (14%), and were distributed randomly among the liver lobes, being superficial or deep within the parenchyma. There is one report describing an increase in frequency of nodules on the left lateral, right lateral, and right medial lobes (Bergman, 1985). The texture of the macroscopic nodules is often softer than the surrounding parenchyma and varies from yellow to pink to tan, which most likely reflects the cytoplasmic content of the nodules. Rarely, some HNH nodules can be as large as 5 cm in diameter or even larger.

CLINICAL DIAGNOSIS

HNH is a histologic diagnosis that requires representative hepatic tissue to demonstrate characteristic microscopic or macroscopic nodules. The nodules are composed of nonencapsulated hepatocytes that can have several morphologic appearances, including relatively normal hepatocytes or with variable vacuolar changes (fatty or hydropic degeneration). The vacuolar changes are thought to be due to fatty infiltration, glycogen, or water accumulation (Meyer, 1996). The latter is suggestive of glycogen accumulation similar to the metabolic effects of glucocorticoids on the hepatocytes in dogs. The nodules are characterized by more hepatocytes per unit area than seen in normal liver parenchyma, with a higher proportion of mitotic cells and a lower number of binucleate cells (Fabry et al, 1982). In severe cases, compression of the stromal structure can give the macroscopic and microscopic appearance of cirrhosis unless that liver is examined with special stains. Fibrosis and inflammation are not components of nodular hyperplasia but are in cirrhosis. The surrounding parenchyma is frequently compressed by the nodules, which alter sinusoidal portal tract position and cause atrophy. Degenerative changes such as focal congestion, vacuolization, hemosiderin deposits, and lipofuscinosis may also be present in adjacent tissues (Johnson, 1995). A common associated finding is the presence of lipogranulomas (pigment-laden macrophages) that stain brightly for iron.

A pathologist usually requires a surgical wedge biopsy specimen to make the diagnosis of HNH. Frequently, needle biopsies do not provide enough hepatic tissue to demonstrate the nodular hyperplasia and adjacent tissue distortion. A needle biopsy report may describe only hepatocyte vacuolar changes, suggesting to the clinician a reactive or metabolic condition such as hyperadrenocorticism or lipidosis. A needle biopsy sample also may not differentiate HNH from hepatic neoplasia, in particular hepatocellular carcinoma and adenoma.

CLINICAL SIGNIFICANCE

Our current understanding of HNH is that it has little significance in the morbidity of the canine patient but has considerable significance in the diagnostic evaluation of animals with HNH and other concurrent disease. Macroscopic nodules may also be wrongly mistaken for neoplastic lesions, and the authors are aware of several cases in which euthanasia was recommended based on gross inspection on the suspicion of metastatic neoplasia.

Dogs with HNH usually have increases in ALP concentrations, which often leads to extensive laboratory testing and other diagnostic methods to determine the cause of the persistent rise in serum ALP levels. HNH may consequently divert the clinician away from a correct diagnosis in the symptomatic dog with HNH and another disease. Hyperadrenocorticism appears to be the most often investigated disease in dogs with HNH and unexplained increases in ALP levels. Confusion is further compounded by the increased frequency of ultrasonographically guided needle biopsy failing to demonstrate the characteristic nodular nature of the lesions, thus sending the clinician on a search for causes of hepatic vacuolar changes. Thus, the primary purpose of this article is to raise the reader's awareness of HNH in older dogs.

References and Suggested Reading

Bergman JR: Nodular hyperplasia of the liver in the dog: An association with changes in the Ito cell population. Vet Pathol 22:427, 1985.
This article describes specific histologic changes associated with hepatic nodular hyperplasia.
Fabry A, Benjamin SA, Angleton GM: Nodular hyperplasia of the liver in the beagle dog. Vet Pathol 19:109, 1982.
Reports on macroscopic and microscopic findings on more than 400 dogs with hepatic nodular hyperplasia.
Johnson SE: Diseases of the liver. In: Ettinger SJ, Feldman EC, eds: Textbook of Veterinary Internal Medicine. Philadelphia: WB Saunders, 1995, p 1313.
A general review of liver disease, including hepatic nodular hyperplasia.
Meyer DJ: Hepatic pathology. In: Guilford WG, Center SA, Strombeck DR, et al, eds: Strombeck's Small Animal Gastroenterology. Philadelphia: WB Saunders, 1996, p 649.
Histologic characteristics are discussed, including comparisons to other hepatic changes.
Voros K, Vrabely L, Papp L, et al: Correlation of ultrasonographic and pathomorphologic findings in canine hepatic diseases. J Small Anim Pract 32:627, 1991.
A review of ultrasonographic changes occurring in liver disease.

Hepatic Fibrosis in the Dog

H. CAROLIEN RUTGERS
London, United Kingdom

Hepatic fibrosis is a common component of several chronic liver diseases in both humans and animals. It usually occurs as a sequel to hepatic parenchymal damage and inflammation and is often associated with cirrhosis. Treatment of such patients is therefore directed primarily toward the inflammatory liver disease rather than the fibrosis. Noninflammatory hepatic fibrosis has been described in humans with congenital hepatic fibrosis, cystic liver disease, and hepatoportal sclerosis, but similar syndromes had not been reported in the dog until recently. However, idiopathic hepatic fibrosis, not accompanied by obvious inflammation, is now increasingly recognized as a cause of chronic liver disease and portal hypertension in predominantly young dogs.

PATHOGENESIS

Hepatic fibrosis is characterized by an increased accumulation of collagen and other components (proteoglycans, elastin, and glycoproteins) of the hepatic extracellular matrix (ECM). It results from an imbalance between the synthesis, degradation, and deposition of matrix molecules; increased fibrogenesis appears to be the main factor. Collagen is the major constituent of the ECM, and treatment for hepatic fibrosis is therefore aimed at modifying collagen metabolism (Leveille and Arias, 1993). Collagens are triple helical proteins composed of polypeptide chains rich in proline, hydroxyproline, and lysine. Biosynthesis starts with intracellular formation of procollagen, which is then hydroxylated and glycosylated. Hydroxylation is necessary for formation of a stable triple helix, and interruption of this step will reduce procollagen formation. The procollagen molecule is then secreted extracellularly, where lysyl oxidase catalyzes collagen cross-linking and the formation of stable fibrils. Inhibition of this enzyme results in unstable collagen, which is then susceptible to increased degradation by extracellular proteases. Cross-linked collagen normally can be degraded only by specific collagenases.

Mechanisms of fibrogenesis in early and advanced liver disease probably are similar and involve activation and transformation of perisinusoidal lipocytes into myofibroblasts that produce large quantities of ECM. When tissue injury results in an inflammatory response, the stimulus to fibrogenesis is indirect and mediated by cytokines released from Kupffer cells, platelets, and neutrophils. In primary fibrogenesis, the agent itself or its primary metabolites cause intracellular generation of highly reactive compounds (such as acetaldehyde and products of lipid peroxidation), which may directly stimulate collagen production.

The ECM provides the structural framework for the liver and also affects the phenotypic expression of cells. Relatively subtle alterations of the matrix may have significant consequences. Increased deposition of ECM in the liver disturbs anatomic relationships and affects hepatocellular function. Portal hypertension occurs from sclerosis of central veins, deposition of matrix in the space of Disse (so-called capillarization of sinusoids), and compression of veins by fibrous bands. The ensuing perihepatic shunting of portal blood may lead to defective clearance of toxic compounds and hepatic encephalopathy (HE) and malnutrition of hepatocytes. Hepatocellular dysfunction is worsened further by perisinusoidal fibrosis, which becomes a barrier to diffusion and reduces transport of hepatocellular products. Portal hypertension may also result in renal retention of sodium and water and ascites.

The time course of hepatic fibrosis varies widely, depending on the underlying cause. Early fibrotic changes may be reversible, but advanced collagen changes, characterized by cross-linking and cirrhosis, are not. Early detection and modulation of hepatic fibrosis is therefore important so that progression to end-stage liver disease may be prevented.

HEPATIC FIBROSIS IN HEPATOBILIARY DISEASE

Hepatic fibrosis plays an important role in the development of end-stage liver failure in many hepatobiliary disorders (Table 1). In most of these conditions, it is associated with obvious inflammation. Fibrosis commonly occurs as a consequence of hepatic damage and inflammation in chronic hepatitis, regardless of the cause. Hepatic fibrosis due to toxins and chemicals is also usually associated with necrosis or inflammation, or both. There are probably few

---

TABLE 1. **Causes of Hepatic Fibrosis in the Dog**

Chronic hepatitis
  Hepatic copper accumulation
    Primary (Bedlington terriers, West Highland White terriers)
    Secondary (Doberman pinschers, Skye terriers)
  Infectious
  Drug-induced
    Primidone
  Metabolic
    Alpha$_1$-antitrypsin deficiency
  Others
    Lobular dissecting hepatitis
    Idiopathic chronic hepatitis
Toxins, chemicals
  Pyrrolidizine alkaloids, CCl$_4$
Postnecrotic fibrosis
Chronic congestive heart failure
Chronic cholangiohepatitis
Chronic biliary obstruction
Idiopathic hepatic fibrosis
  Perivenous
  Diffuse pericellular
  Periportal

---

compounds that have a direct fibrogenic effect on the liver in the dog. Postnecrotic fibrosis can follow severe parenchymal damage when all hepatocytes in acini are destroyed and the supporting framework collapses. Certain toxins primarily cause necrosis around central veins, which may result in pericentral fibrosis when this is not followed by regeneration. Pericentral fibrosis may also occur after prolonged passive congestion, as in chronic congestive heart failure.

Chronic cholangiohepatitis and bile duct obstruction may result in fibrosis with continuing inflammation in and around the bile ducts and portal areas and can culminate in biliary cirrhosis. Bacterial products absorbed from the intestine may cause mild portal fibrosis in the absence of inflammation. Inflammatory bowel disease has been associated with a number of hepatobiliary diseases in humans, including hepatoportal fibrosis, and with cholangiohepatitis in cats, but it is unknown whether this is the case in dogs.

IDIOPATHIC HEPATIC FIBROSIS

Types and Incidence

Idiopathic hepatic fibrosis encompasses a range of non-inflammatory fibrosing liver diseases, the cause of which is generally unknown. They have been categorized, based on the predominant location of the fibrosis, into central perivenous, diffuse pericellular, and periportal fibrosis (Rutgers et al, 1993).

Central perivenous fibrosis is characterized by an increase in perivenular fibrous connective tissue, which may compress the lumen and cause veno-occlusion. In some dogs, mural fibrosis is mild and no more than a thin collar of collagen around centrilobular veins. Liver architecture is generally maintained and portal areas are anatomically normal. *Diffuse pericellular fibrosis,* in contrast, is characterized by intense intralobular reticulin fibrosis that surrounds individual parenchymal cells and obliterates normal hepatic anatomy. Parenchymal cells may show atrophy, degeneration, and attempted nodular regeneration. In *periportal fibrosis,* there is marked fibrosis in portal areas, which is often associated with arteriolar and bile ductular proliferation. In some dogs, portal veins are small or absent, and in these animals it has been attributed to primary portal vein hypoplasia (Van den Ingh et al, 1995).

Idiopathic hepatic fibrosis is not a common disease, but it is probably underdiagnosed because of a lack of familiarity with its manifestations. It is most common in young dogs, with most less than 2 years of age when first presented, but has been diagnosed in dogs as young as 4 months and as old as 7 years (Table 2). Central perivenous fibrosis shows a marked breed predisposition for German shepherd dogs, and this breed is also overrepresented in cases of diffuse pericellular fibrosis. Periportal fibrosis has no breed predisposition. There is no apparent sex predisposition.

Etiology

The cause of central perivenous and diffuse pericellular fibrosis is as yet unknown. Central perivenous fibrosis resembles veno-occlusive disease, which is due to partial or total occlusive fibrosis of central or sublobular veins and is thought to develop from toxic damage to sinusoidal endothelium. The lesion in the dogs with central perivenous fibrosis differs from classic veno-occlusive disease in that it is associated with an expansion of mural connective tissue with no evidence of intimal damage. The young age

TABLE 2. Details and Outcome for 19 Dogs With Idiopathic Hepatic Fibrosis

Breed	Age	Sex	Treatment		Survival
			Supportive	*Antifibrotic*	
Central Perivenous Fibrosis					
GSD	2 yr	F	Symptomatic	Prednisolone	>4 yr
GSD	10 mo	M	Symptomatic	Colchicine	2 mo
GSD	15 mo	M	Symptomatic	Colchicine	2 mo
GSD	14 mo	M	Symptomatic	ND	>4 yr
GSD	2 yr	M	Symptomatic	ND	6 mo
Rottweiler	18 mo	F	Symptomatic	ND	Unknown
Rottweiler	4 mo	F	ND	ND	Euthanasia
Diffuse Pericellular Fibrosis					
GSD	7 mo	M	Symptomatic	Steroids	1 mo
Collie cross	18 mo	M, N	Symptomatic	ND	1 wk
Lhasa apso	4 yr	M	Symptomatic	ND	3 mo
GSD	5 mo	M	ND	ND	Euthanasia
GSD cross	11 mo	M	ND	ND	4 wk
Border collie	2 yr	F, N	ND	ND	1 day
Periportal Fibrosis					
GSD	6 yr	F	Symptomatic	Steroids	>3 mo
Golden retriever	7 yr	F	Symptomatic	Steroids	>4 yr
English setter	2 yr	F	Symptomatic	Colchicine	2 1/2 yr
GSD	9 mo	M	ND	ND	Euthanasia
GSDx Rottweiler	9 mo	M	Symptomatic	ND	1 wk
Toy Poodle	7 mo	M	Symptomatic	ND	1 wk

GSD, German shepherd dog; F, female; M, male; N, neutered; ND, not done.

of the affected animals and the predisposition for German shepherd dogs suggest congenital or genetic factors. There is no good human counterpart for diffuse pericellular fibrosis, which is found in a greater variety of breeds and affects a wider age range. In some dogs, it histologically resembles lobular dissecting hepatitis, which has been described as a cause of portal hypertension and jaundice in young dogs (Van den Ingh and Rothuizen, 1994). Lobular dissecting hepatitis is characterized by lobular infiltration of inflammatory cells as well as fibrosis, whereas pericellular fibrosis is not associated with inflammation. However, it is possible that both may represent a specific pattern of hepatic reaction to damage in the immature animal. Periportal fibrosis has been compared with human congenital hepatic fibrosis, but the latter disease is also associated with dilatation and irregularity of bile ducts, which is not a feature of the canine syndrome. Portal vein hypoplasia also has recently been suggested as a cause for hepatoportal fibrosis in dogs (Van den Ingh et al, 1995). In this study, gross or microscopic hypoplasia of the portal vein was suggested as the cause of portal hypertension in 42 dogs, 17 of which also had portal fibrosis. However, this may not explain all cases of periportal fibrosis, since in some dogs vascular structures appear well maintained.

Signs

Clinical signs in all dogs tend to be similar, independent of the histologic subclassification. Signs are predominantly due to the presence of portal hypertension and acquired portosystemic shunting, resulting in ascites or HE. Most dogs are presented for abdominal distention due to ascites and with vague gastrointestinal signs (vomiting, diarrhea, and anorexia) and weight loss. The duration of signs is variable, ranging from 1 or 2 weeks to several months. Some dogs are presented only when neurologic signs due to HE occur. Jaundice, a more obvious indicator for hepatocellular disease, is uncommon and is found mostly in dogs with diffuse pericellular fibrosis.

Diagnosis

Clinicopathologic findings are consistent with hepatic insufficiency and portosystemic shunting. Despite the absence of inflammation, liver enzyme activity is often elevated. Serum alkaline phosphatase activity is raised in the majority of dogs. Serum alanine aminotransferase levels are increased less frequently and to a lesser degree than is alkaline phosphatase, consistent with the histologic finding that this is not a primary hepatocellular abnormality. Hepatocellular changes in these dogs are relatively minor and appear to result from impaired blood flow interfering with hepatocyte nutrition and function, after which degenerative swelling of hepatocytes may lead to further impairment of sinusoidal circulation. Moderate hyperbilirubinemia may occur in dogs with diffuse pericellular fibrosis. Hypoproteinemia may be seen in up to a third of dogs and probably reflects the dilutional effects of renal water retention associated with ascites and renal hypoperfusion. Globulin concentrations tend to be reduced rather than elevated as in chronic hepatitis, in which acquired shunting of blood and

increased antigenic stimulation often lead to hyperglobulinemia. Erythrocyte microcytosis is common, similar to that found in dogs with congenital portosystemic shunts.

Liver function test results are abnormal in most dogs tested, but it should be noted that both resting ammonia and bile acid concentrations may be within the normal range in some animals. However, postprandial bile acid concentrations and ammonia tolerance test results are markedly abnormal, consistent with portosystemic shunting.

Abdominal radiography generally demonstrates small liver size. Hepatic ultrasonography usually does not show specific abnormalities in the hepatic parenchyma, but it may demonstrate multiple portosystemic shunts as enlarged tortuous vessels caudal to the liver. Color flow Doppler may demonstrate reduced portal flow, indicative of portal hypertension. Multiple shunts can be confirmed by contrast portography or at exploratory laparotomy. Portal pressure measurement at surgery further documents portal hypertension.

Liver biopsy is essential for definitive diagnosis. The small liver size makes blind percutaneous biopsy difficult, necessitating ultrasonographically guided biopsy, laparoscopy, or laparotomy. A good-sized sample is required for adequate evaluation of central veins and portal areas. Reticulin-stained preparations are useful in identifying the extent of fibrosis and hence the prognosis in biopsy specimens in which the amount of fibrosis is questionable. The degree of fibrosis does not always correlate with the severity of portal hypertension. Dogs with pericellular fibrosis tend to have more severe and progressive disease culminating in death or euthanasia.

Differential Diagnosis

Portal hypertension and multiple acquired portosystemic shunts are usually associated with chronic end-stage liver disease, which is more common in middle-aged to older dogs. Clinical and clinicopathologic findings can be similar to those of idiopathic hepatic fibrosis. Liver biopsy remains necessary for final diagnosis.

Hepatic arteriovenous fistulas are a rare but important cause of severe portal hypertension and acquired portosystemic shunts in young dogs. Ultrasonography demonstrates the fistulas as tortuous, anechoic tubular structures in the liver, and they can further be diagnosed by celiac arteriography or exploratory laparotomy.

Other rare causes of portal hypertension and multiple portosystemic shunts include partial occlusion of the portal vein (resulting from thrombosis, neoplasia, or extraluminal compression) or hepatic vein occlusion (a Budd-Chiari–like syndrome). A veno-occlusive type of disease associated with vascular spasm of hepatic vein sphincters has been described in a family of young American cocker spaniels, but it also has been considered a variant of vascular anomalies reported in this breed (Van den Ingh et al, 1995).

Sometimes acquired portosystemic shunts are found in young dogs with signs of hepatic dysfunction but with few abnormalities on liver biopsy. The mechanism for portal hypertension in these cases is uncertain. Hepatic fibrosis may be subtle and yet have major hemodynamic consequences; reticulin staining of biopsy specimens may help in its identification. Hypoplasia of the intrahepatic portal system has recently been suggested as a cause of portal hypertension in young dogs, with only minor abnormalities (such as reduced size of the portal vein and arteriolar proliferation in portal areas) evident on liver biopsy in some cases.

TREATMENT

Antifibrotic Therapy

The objective of antifibrotic therapy is to reduce the amount of collagen deposited in the liver. This may be achieved by modulating collagen synthesis or degradation (Table 3). When hepatic fibrosis is associated with inflammation, treatment with anti-inflammatory agents that alter cytokine production or the subsequent response of target cells is indicated, since inflammation is of paramount importance in the pathogenesis of fibrosis in these patients. Corticosteroids are then the drug of choice because they have anti-inflammatory, immune-modulating, and antifibrotic effects. One of their major actions is suppression of phospholipase A_2 activity, thereby decreasing conversion of membrane arachidonic acid to prostaglandins and leukotrienes. These arachidonic acid metabolites are potent inflammatory mediators and by suppressing them, a major stimulus for ongoing fibrogenesis is controlled. Corticosteroids also have a direct but milder antifibrotic effect through inhibition of the transcription of mRNA, thus decreasing procollagen mRNA synthesis, and by inhibition of prolyl hydroxylase activity, resulting in suppression of collagen formation. Corticosteroids may improve survival time in dogs with chronic hepatitis, but no data are available about their therapeutic benefit in reducing the progression of hepatic fibrosis. However, early antifibrotic therapy should be considered in animals with chronic hepatitis, since the prognosis worsens once bridging fibrosis is found in liver biopsy specimens. Corticosteroid therapy is probably not indicated in dogs with idiopathic hepatic fibrosis, since there is no obvious inflammation. Corticosteroids have been used in the management of some dogs with idiopathic fibrosis, including one dog with central perivenous fibrosis that survived more than 4 years, but these drugs probably are not instrumental in modifying the clinical course (Rutgers et al, 1993). Corticosteroid therapy may have undesirable side effects, such as steroid hepatopathy, greater susceptibility to infection, gastrointestinal ulceration, fluid retention, increased protein catabolism predisposing to HE, and iatrogenic hyperadrenocorticism. Azathioprine is an antimetabolite with immune-modulating effects that may be used as an adjunct to corticosteroid therapy when the latter is associated with too many side effects (see p. 509). It allows steroid doses to be reduced but has no direct antifibrotic actions.

Colchicine is an antifibrotic drug that inhibits the polymerization of microtubules, interferes with the synthesis and secretion of procollagen by fibroblasts, and induces the production of collagenase. It also inhibits leukocyte migration and thus has anti-inflammatory properties, whereas it may have a direct hepatoprotective effect by stabilizing hepatocyte plasma membranes. Its efficacy in the treatment of primary or secondary hepatic fibrosis in humans has been variable. It appears to be of limited, if any, benefit in human patients with primary biliary cirrhosis, but may be helpful in decreasing fibrogenesis associated with other forms of cirrhosis. In dogs, it usually has few side effects at the recommended dose (0.03 mg/kg per day), which has been extrapolated from human medicine, but anorexia, vomiting, and diarrhea have been reported. Controlled studies about its use in canine hepatic fibrosis are lacking. Colchicine has been used in the management of a dog with hepatic fibrosis and chronic hepatitis, in which it resulted in transient improvement of clinical signs and some reduction of hepatic fibrosis, although the dog eventually died of progressive liver failure. Colchicine therapy as an adjunct to supportive medical management seemed to have contained progression of hepatic fibrosis in a dog with hepatoportal fibrosis, but it did not appear to make a difference in two other dogs with central perivenous fibrosis (see Table 2). This drug deserves further evaluation in both primary and secondary fibrotic hepatopathies, but it should be used as an adjunct to aggressive symptomatic management.

D-Penicillamine is a drug better known for its cupruretic effects in patients with copper hepatotoxicosis, but it has

TABLE 3. Antifibrotic Drugs in Canine Hepatic Fibrosis

Drug	Dosage	Main Antifibrotic Mechanisms of Action	Major Side Effects
Prednisone	1–2 mg/kg/day PO, tapering to 0.5 mg/kg/day or every other day	Anti-inflammatory Inhibits mRNA transcription Inhibits prolyl hydroxylase	Polyuria, polydipsia Gastrointestinal ulceration Increased susceptibility to infection Iatrogenic Cushing's syndrome
Colchicine	0.03 mg/kg/day PO	Inhibits microtubular assembly necessary for extracellular secretion of procollagen Increases collagenase activity	Vomiting, diarrhea
Zinc acetate, gluconate	200 mg elemental zinc q24hr PO for 10- to 25-kg dog	Inhibits prolyl hydroxylase by competing with Fe^{2+} cofactor Cofactor for collagenase activity	Hemolysis if plasma zinc >1,000 μg/dl Vomiting (gluconate)
D-Penicillamine	10–15 mg/kg BID PO	Inhibits lysyl oxidase by chelating copper Disrupts cross-linking by interfering with products of lysyl oxidase reaction	Vomiting, diarrhea Anorexia

Modified from Leveille CR, Arias IM: Pathophysiology and pharmacologic modulation of hepatic fibrosis. J Vet Intern Med 7:73, 1993, with permission.

also been used as an inhibitor of collagen formation in patients with hepatic fibrosis. Its efficacy in humans is doubtful and its use in dogs is complicated by the frequent occurrence of gastrointestinal side effects.

Zinc is currently receiving much attention in the treatment of a variety of chronic liver disorders in humans, in whom serum and hepatic zinc concentrations are often low. In dogs, zinc is best known for its use in copper hepatotoxicosis because it inhibits intestinal absorption of copper. However, it also has antifibrotic properties resulting from inhibition of prolyl hydroxylase activity, and it may have direct hepatoprotective properties related to stabilization of lysosomal membranes and inhibition of lipid peroxidation. Zinc therapy has few side effects, although excessive administration may inhibit iron absorption, and toxic levels may cause hemolysis (see *CVT XII*, p. 238). Plasma zinc levels during treatment should be kept between 200 and 300 μg/dl. Zinc appears useful in the adjunct treatment of fibrotic hepatopathies, especially when associated with inflammation, but its antifibrotic efficacy remains to be demonstrated through clinical trials.

Oxidant liver injury is thought to play a role in the progression of chronic inflammatory or cholestatic liver disease. Free radical–initiated lipid peroxidation may also play a role in hepatic fibrogenesis (Britton and Bacon, 1994). Dietary supplementation with vitamin E, a naturally occurring antioxidant, has been shown to reduce carbon tetrachloride–induced hepatic fibrosis. Vitamin E doses of 100 to 400 IU PO every 12 hours have been suggested for the dog. Antioxidant therapy may be of value in secondary fibrotic hepatopathies, but its role in modulating fibrogenesis needs further research.

Symptomatic Therapy

Nonspecific medical management is aimed at supporting hepatic function, minimizing signs of HE, and controlling ascites and other complications of hepatic dysfunction (such as gastrointestinal bleeding). Therapeutic considerations for chronic hepatitis have been addressed in *CVT XII*, pp. 749 to 756 and elsewhere in this section. Symptomatic management appears particularly important in dogs with idiopathic hepatic fibrosis because these dogs may have relatively nonprogressive disease, with clinical signs predominantly due to portal hypertension. A moderately to severely protein-restricted diet is the keystone of therapy in all dogs, supplemented with lactulose and antibiotics as needed to control HE. Ascites tends to be a less consistent problem and usually can be managed with dietary sodium

restriction and diuretics. Coagulopathies are rare, but gastrointestinal ulceration and bleeding associated with portal hypertension occur and are managed with gastroprotectants and H_2 receptor antagonists (see *CVT XII*, p. 706). Surgical treatment of multiple extrahepatic portosystemic shunts has been proposed by attenuating the abdominal portion of the vena cava in order to create a pressure gradient with the portal vein and to increase hepatic perfusion. However, in dogs with naturally occurring portal hypertension due to severe intrahepatic disease, it has been unsuccessful in controlling clinical signs or improving survival and is not to be recommended (Boothe et al, 1996).

The prognosis for dogs with idiopathic fibrosis is guarded. However, some of these dogs may present with decompensated severe portal hypertension and fulminant HE, yet they may survive for long periods on symptomatic management. It is important for the clinician to be aware of this and to provide intensive supportive treatment. The role of antifibrotic management needs to be clarified with controlled studies.

References and Suggested Reading

Boothe HW, Howe LM, Edwards JF, et al: Multiple extrahepatic portosystemic shunts in dogs: 30 cases (1981–1993). J Am Vet Med Assoc 208:1849, 1996.
  Vena cava banding in dogs with multiple portosystemic shunts is not superior to medical and nutritional treatment.
Britton RS, Bacon BR: Role of free radicals in liver diseases and hepatic fibrosis. Hepatogastroenterology 41:343, 1994.
  Free radicals may play a role in initiating or perpetuating cellular damage and fibrosis in liver disease.
Leveille CR, Arias IM: Pathophysiology and pharmacologic modulation of hepatic fibrosis. J Vet Intern Med 7:73, 1993.
  A thorough review of the mechanisms of hepatic fibrosis and antifibrotic drugs.
Leveille-Webster CR, Center SA: Chronic hepatitis: Therapeutic considerations. In: Kirk RW, Bonagura J, eds: Current Veterinary Therapy XII. Philadelphia, WB Saunders, 1994, p 749.
  Review of specific and symptomatic treatment modalities for chronic hepatitis in the dog.
Rutgers HC, Haywood S, Kelly DF: Idiopathic hepatic fibrosis in 15 dogs. Vet Rec 133:115, 1993.
  Retrospective study describing clinical signs and follow-up in 15 young dogs with idiopathic hepatic fibrosis.
Van den Ingh TSGAM, Rothuizen J: Lobular dissecting hepatitis in juvenile and young adult dogs. J Vet Intern Med 8:217, 1994.
  Lobular dissecting hepatitis can cause portal hypertension in young dogs of many breeds.
Van den Ingh TSGAM, Rothuizen J, Meyer HP: Portal hypertension associated with primary hypoplasia of the hepatic portal vein in dogs. Vet Rec 137:424, 1995.
  Gross or microscopic portal vein hypoplasia as a cause of portal hypertension in young dogs with or without hepatoportal fibrosis.

Hepatoportal Microvascular Dysplasia

Sharon A. Center
Thomas Schermerhorn
Ithaca, New York

Ronald Lyman
Lesley Phillips
Ft. Pierce, Florida

The historical, clinical, clinicopathologic, and histologic features of congenital macroscopic portosystemic vascular anomalies (PSVA) in companion animals have been well described by many different authors since 1974 (Table 1; Ewing et al, 1974; Center, 1995). This diagnosis is usually straightforward once a clinician suspects the condition, pursues liver function testing, or discovers ammonium urate crystalluria. However, a group of dogs with abnormal total serum bile acid values, consistent with a diagnosis of PSVA, has been identified that, when referred for surgical correction, lack a demonstrable macroscopic vascular shunt despite hepatic histopathology consistent with PSVA. This disorder is referred to as *hepatoportal microvascular dysplasia* (MVD).

Hepatoportal microvascular dysplasia is a congenital and probably inherited hepatobiliary disorder that is well characterized in Cairn terriers but appears to be most prevalent among Yorkshire terriers (Schermerhorn et al, 1996; Phillips et al, 1996). We have also recognized MVD in other small-breed dogs (e.g., Miniature Schnauzer, Lhasa apso, Shih tzu, Dachshund, Maltese, Bichon frise, Pekinese, and Toy and Miniature Poodles). The histologic features of this disorder were first reported in 1985 (Zawie and Gilbertson, 1985; Baer et al, 1991). Clinical descriptions of

TABLE 1. Clinical, Clinicopathologic, and Diagnostic Imaging Features of Dogs With Macroscopic Portosystemic Vascular Anomalies and Dogs With Symptomatic and Asymptomatic Hepatoportal Microvascular Dysplasia

PSVA	Asymptomatic MVD	Symptomatic MVD
Clinical Signs	*Clinical Signs*	*Clinical Signs*
Signs <6 mo age	Few signs	Variable age, mostly adult
Stunted growth	Normal growth	Normal growth
Males often cryptorchidism	Rare drug intolerance	Variable signs:
Prominent kidneys		Polyuria/polydipsia
Polyuria-polydipsia		Vomiting/diarrhea
Vague GI signs		Food intolerance
Vomiting or diarrhea		Rare ammonium urate urolithiasis
Ammonium urate urolithiasis		Episodic seizures
Hepatic encephalopathy		Rare overt hepatic encephalopathy
Variable signs: e.g., lethargy, ataxia, weakness, abnormal behavior, seizures, coma		
Clinicopathologic Features	*Clinicopathologic Features*	*Clinicopathologic Features*
RBC microcytosis	Variable liver enzymes	Rare RBC microcytosis
↓ BUN, ↓ creatinine	↑ Serum bile acids	Rare ↓ cholesterol
↓ Cholesterol	↓ ICG plasma clearance	↑ Serum bile acids
↑ Serum bile acids		↓ ICG plasma clearance
↓ ICG plasma clearance		Rare hyperammonemia
Ammonia intolerance		
Survey Abdominal Radiograph	*Survey Abdominal Radiograph*	
Microhepatica	Normal liver size	
Prominent kidneys		
Abdominal Ultrasound	*Abdominal Ultrasound*	
Small liver	Normal to slightly small liver	
Hypovascular liver	Hypovascular liver	
Large kidneys	No anomalous vessels observed	
Anomalous vessel observed		
Colorectal Scintigraphy	*Colorectal Scintigraphy*	
Shunt fraction ≥80%	Shunt fraction ≤15%	
Radiographic Portography	*Radiographic Portography*	
Extrahepatic or intrahepatic PSVA	Uneven contrast distribution within liver lobes	
Poor to absent hepatic portal venous filling	Abnormally blunted tertiary portal vein branches	
	Abnormally prolonged tissue contrast "blush"	
	Absence of anomalous macroscopic shunting	

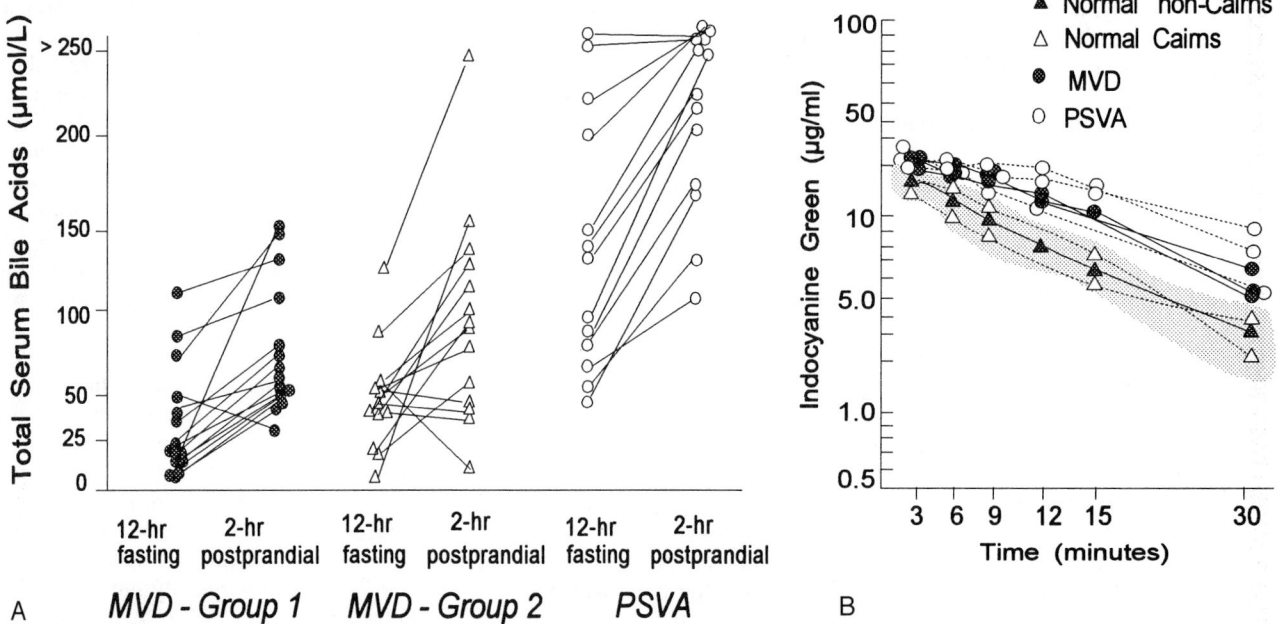

Figure 1. *A,* Total serum bile acid values after a 12-hour fast and 2 hours after feeding in dogs with hepatoportal microvascular dysplasia (MVD; group 1 = asymptomatic dogs; group 2 = symptomatic dogs) and dogs with portosystemic vascular anomalies (PSVA). Values for a single dog are connected. (Normal reference range: <25 μmol/L). *B,* Indocyanine green dye (ICG) plasma clearance curves in normal Cairn terriers, normal dogs of other breeds, Cairn terriers with microvascular dysplasia (MVD), and Cairn terriers with portosystemic vascular anomalies (PSVA). Values for an individual dog are connected. The shaded area represents the normal range of ICG clearance in healthy dogs.

typical features, diagnostic criteria, and histologic characteristics followed the identification of large numbers of dogs with abnormal liver function as bile acid assays became routinely used. Detailed studies in Cairn terriers were undertaken after breeders and consulting veterinarians suspected an increased incidence of PSVA in several kindreds. Estimation of liver function and perfusion with the use of fasting and postprandial serum bile acid measurements disclosed that as many as 70% of dogs in large kindreds had abnormally increased values. The subsequent evaluation of liver function with the use of indocyanine green (ICG) plasma clearance confirmed the presence of abnormal liver function and/or perfusion (Fig. 1). Contrast-enhanced radiographic, ultrasonographic, and scintigraphic imaging excluded the presence of macroscopic PSVA. The evaluation of hepatic histology disclosed features nearly identical to those found in dogs with PSVA.

Study of kindreds of Cairn terriers from across North America have disclosed that the disorder is common in this breed. Nearly every bloodline the authors have examined (n > 25) has had affected individuals. However, based on extensive clinical experience, the disorder is seemingly more common among Yorkshire terriers.

Clinical Features. The clinical hallmark of MVD is increased total serum bile acid concentrations. Dogs with MVD can be divided into two groups defined by the presence or absence of clinical symptoms (see Table 1; Center, 1995; Schermerhorn et al, 1996; Phillips et al, 1996).

Dogs in *group 1* have few clinical signs. Rarely, drug intolerance for substances metabolized or excreted by the liver is recognized. There are no consistent abnormalities

found on routinely evaluated clinicopathologic parameters. Unlike dogs with PSVA, these patients are not microcytic or hypocholesterolemic, do not have low serum urea nitrogen and creatinine concentrations, and rarely demonstrate increased liver enzyme activity or ammonium biurate crystalluria. However, these dogs have increased serum total bile acid values and reduced ICG plasma clearance (see Fig. 1). Serum bile acid values may show a pattern consistent with portosystemic shunting in which the fasting value may be within the normal reference range and the postprandial value moderately to markedly increased. Although the bile acid response test pattern is similar, absolute bile acid concentrations are usually lower than values typically associated with PSVA. Some dogs with MVD have been shown to have reduced ammonia tolerance; however, ammonia tolerance testing has not been rigorously pursued in this population.

The clinical signs in symptomatic dogs *(group 2)* include manifestations of hepatic encephalopathy, gastrointestinal abnormalities, and dysuria owing to ammonium urate urolithiasis. Hepatoencephalopathic signs may include any of the usual manifestations, including diffuse symmetric cerebral abnormalities and episodic seizures. Symptomatic hyperammonemia and ammonium biurate crystalluria may be concurrently recognized. Similar to dogs in *group 1*, these dogs also have increased serum total bile acid values (see Table 1). Some *group 2* dogs have a progressive decline in hepatic function accompanied by worsening signs. These dogs may develop portal hypertension, acquired portosystemic shunting, and ascites over several years. A few dogs have developed portal thromboembolism seemingly associated with coexistent inflammatory bowel disease. In the authors' experience, Yorkshire terriers, Maltese, and Bichon frise are at increased risk for these sequelae. Yorkshire terriers appear to outnumber other breeds within the *group 2* category.

Clinical and Definitive Diagnosis. Although hepatic biopsy is the only way of definitively confirming MVD, the histologic features are subtle and nearly identical to those associated with PSVA. Thus, the presence of a macroscopic PSVA must be ruled out to definitively confirm the underlying defect. A presumptive clinical diagnosis of MVD in *group 1–asymptomatic dogs* is based on the presence of increased fasting or postprandial serum bile acid values, signalment, and the absence of other clinical signs or clinicopathologic abnormalities. If a clinical diagnosis of MVD seems to fit, the authors do not recommend additional testing in asymptomatic dogs.

Symptomatic dogs (*group 2*) showing neurobehavioral abnormalities or other signs derived from urolithiasis (dysuria, stranguria) or vague gastrointestinal abnormalities (inappetence, vomiting) require full diagnostic evaluation to definitively rule out PSVA. In the authors' practice, these dogs often are referred with a suspicion of PSVA for surgical exploration or mesenteric portography.

Several noninvasive diagnostic evaluations can aid in the differentiation of MVD from PSVA. Abdominal ultrasonography performed by an experienced operator can recognize a "hypovascular intrahepatic portal vascular bed" in dogs with MVD as occurs in dogs with PSVA. Ultrasonography can also be used to subjectively estimate hepatic size. Liver size is very small in dogs with PSVA and is normal or only mildly reduced in size in dogs with MVD. The use of Doppler ultrasound permits visualization of abnormal blood flow turbulence at the site of communication between an anomalous shunting vessel and normal vasculature. However, a normal ultrasound examination does not definitively exclude the diagnosis of PSVA, as vascular malformations can be difficult to visualize owing to lack of patient cooperation or image interference caused by enteric gas. Although useful in the estimation of portal blood flow in the circumstance of hepatic cirrhosis, duplex-Doppler ultrasonography has not yet been proved as a clinical tool for differentiating PSVA from MVD (Nyland and Fisher, 1990).

Colorectal scintigraphy, in which technetium pertechnetate is administered in small volume per rectum and monitored with a computer-linked gamma camera, can be used to demonstrate macroscopic portosystemic shunting in dogs with PSVA (Daniel et al, 1991). Dogs with MVD have normal or only slightly increased "shunting fractions," while dogs with PSVA usually have shunting fractions greater than 60%.

Radiographic methods that include mesenteric or splenic contrast portography are the only methods that ensure that PSVA has not been overlooked. Mesenteric portograms completed in Cairn terriers with MVD have shown blunted or ill-defined terminal portal venules and an abnormally prolonged tissue blush, suggesting deranged portal venous or sinusoidal perfusion. Portions of liver lobes or entire lobes may fail to opacify with contrast. No macroscopic shunting vessels are observed, since the "shunting phenomenon" in dogs with MVD occurs at a microscopic intrahepatic level.

Hepatic Histology. Histologic changes in all species in which PSVA has been recognized (dogs, cats, foals, calves, piglets, rats, and humans) are similar. Lesions are subtle and may be overlooked if needle biopsies, rather than wedge biopsies, are collected. Abnormalities include the presence of juvenile-appearing portal structures, a notable paucity of blood in large branches of the portal veins with some vessels appearing collapsed, and prominent tortuous hepatic arterioles. The tortuosity of arterioles causes an increased number of cross-sectionally cut vessels. Increased numbers of ill-defined "vascular" channels between arterioles, portal veins, and adjacent sinusoids are commonly observed. Vacuolation of hepatocytes is variable and may have a multifocal or zonal distribution throughout hepatic lobules. Hepatic venules may demonstrate a prominence of vascular smooth muscle and appear constricted. Individual hepatocytes are atrophied, giving the appearance that portal triads are closer together than in normal tissue. In some dogs, increased quantities of connective tissue develop around hepatic veins and portal triads compared with what develops in dogs with surgically created portosystemic shunts (Schaeffer et al, 1986). A progressive accumulation of hemosiderin develops in Kupffer cells in randomly located lipogranulomatous lesions.

Histologic lesions observed in liver tissue from dogs with MVD include many of the features present in dogs with PSVA. Common features include increased numbers of juvenile-appearing, poorly formed portal triad structures, and increased cross sections of variably sized hepatic arterioles. There are increased numbers of small-caliber vessels devoid of blood components in the periphery of some portal triads. Microscopic examination of serial sections of hepatic tissue have disclosed unusual venous structures located adjacent to portal venules. These structures are seemingly derived from hepatic venules and may be communicating with portal triads. However, no distinct communications between these normally separated vascular beds have been demonstrable. Prominent vascular smooth muscle in hepatic venules is apparent in most dogs (Fig. 2). This may appear as a "sphincter-like" segmental constriction in transversely cut venous sections. Dilated vascular

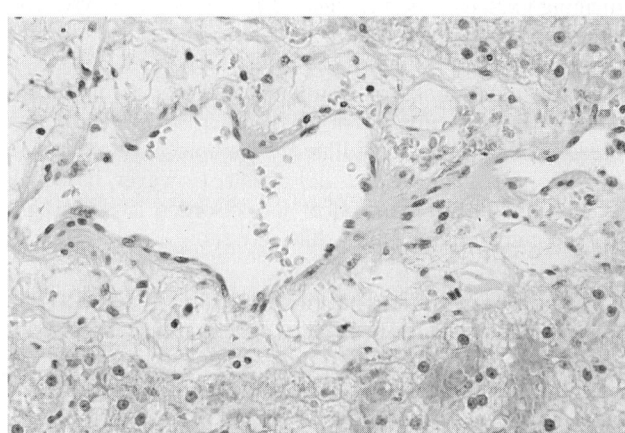

Figure 2. Photomicrograph of liver tissue from a dog with microvascular hepatoportal dysplasia showing the characteristic appearance of a hepatic venule. Notice the thickened smooth muscle and perivascular lymphatics (magnification 600×).

spaces lacking blood constituents, presumably lymphatics, often abut hepatic venules. Some dogs develop multifocal hepatic lipogranulomas containing hemosiderin identical to lesions observed in some dogs with PSVA. A variability in liver lobe involvement, as observed on portovenography, has been recognized for histologic lesions. Consequently, biopsy of a single liver lobe may overlook distinguishing lesions. Histologic lesions may also be missed if only very small biopsy specimens are examined (e.g., single needle biopsies). Some dogs with MVD are virtually indistinguishable from dogs with PSVA on the basis of hepatic histology. However, in dogs with MVD, portal vessels tend to be more obvious, contain more blood constituents, and hepatocytes do not appear to be atrophied.

Inheritance. Our breeding studies in Cairn terriers support a complex form of inheritance of MVD. The authors suspect this is a polygenic trait well ingrained in the breed genome. Breeders attempting to eliminate the trait from their kindreds have bred dogs with normal bile acid values verified by duplicate or triplicate testing, and still have produced affected dogs. A similar situation most certainly exists in the Yorkshire terrier also.

Treatment. There is no treatment that will rectify hepatic dysfunction in dogs with MVD. Dogs in group 1 require no treatment other than pharmacologic caution if adverse drug responses have been recognized. Dogs in group 2 are managed like any dog with PSVA demonstrating signs of hepatic encephalopathy. Dietary modification to less noxious protein sources (dairy and vegetable protein; see p. 693), inclusion of complex dietary carbohydrates, and treatment with lactulose to achieve several soft bowel movements each day (see *CVT XII*, p. 749), are the initial interventions. In dogs showing persistent neurobehavioral signs, inclusion of neomycin (22 mg/kg PO b.i.d.) or metronidazole (reduced dose, 7.5 mg/kg PO b.i.d.) is recommended. Caution is warranted in group 2 dogs to avoid drugs contraindicated in the circumstance of reduced hepatic function. These dogs must be monitored for worsening hepatic insufficiency and development of acquired portosystemic communications, ascites, and portal thromboembolism.

Relevance of MVD to Contemporary Veterinary Practice. Once understood, the inclusion of MVD as a differential diagnosis for dogs with abnormal serum bile acid values should temper the tendency to pursue expensive and invasive tests when the only recognized abnormality is the abnormal liver function test. This behavior would safeguard dogs in group 1 from iatrogenic complications. The authors believe that it is responsible to recognize affected dogs of at-risk breeds while they are young in order to avoid diagnostic errors in later life should these animals present for illnesses unrelated to the liver. Discovery of abnormal liver function in later life during illness can cause unnecessary diagnostic uncertainty and unwarranted invasive tests, such as liver biopsy and portovenography. How young dogs should be at the time of initial testing has not been established, as the authors have seen some dogs develop progressive increases in their bile acid values during the first 9 months of life. In most instances, the

authors have been able to discern affected dogs by 4 months of age. A reasonable approach would be to test suspect dogs at the time of their last pediatric vaccinations and at the time they are neutered. For the inquisitive breeder or owner, wedge liver biopsies from several different liver lobes could be collected at the time of ovariohysterectomy in females, although the authors do not currently recommend that this be done. Dogs in both groups may be monitored by serial evaluation of biochemical profiles that search for evidence of active hepatobiliary injury (increased liver enzyme activity) or loss of synthetic function. Serial determinations of serum bile acid values, once abnormal liver function is established in an MVD patient, do not serve a useful clinical purpose. Bile acid values do not quantitatively correlate with predictable degrees of liver injury owing to the fact that cholestasis, liver mass reduction, and diminished hepatoportal blood flow each impair bile acid clearance.

The existence of the MVD lesion explains why many dogs with PSVA, having undergone complete surgical ligation of their shunting vessel, never realize normalization of their serum bile acid tests, although they make a favorable clinical recovery (Lawrence et al, 1992). Biopsy of such animals, years after shunt occlusion, has demonstrated the persistence of the MVD lesion.

In conclusion, the authors have described a disorder of the hepatoportal microvasculature, characterized clinically by increased serum bile acid values, affecting a variety of small-breed dogs. Conservative management is indicated for asymptomatic dogs. A diagnostic work-up is required to rule out the likelihood of other acquired hepatic disorders and PSVA in symptomatic dogs. The relation between MVD and PSVA is not completely clarified. The authors believe that MVD and PSVA are genetically linked because of the associated high frequency of these defects in certain breeds (Meyer and Rothuizen, 1991; Schermerhorn et al, 1996), the similarity in their hepatic histologic features, and evidence suggesting that the histologic lesion of MVD curtails normalization of hepatic function in dogs with PSVA after complete surgical attenuation of their anomalous vessel.

The prognosis for *group 1 dogs* is excellent, based on the authors' prospective clinical evaluations of affected kindreds of Cairn terriers and clinical experience with geriatric affected dogs of other breeds. The prognosis for *group 2 dogs* is variable and depends on their response to treatments aimed at ameliorating signs of hepatic encephalopathy. Some group 2 dogs develop a progressive hepatic disorder associated with a poor prognosis.

References and Suggested Reading

Baer KE, Patnaik AK, MacDonald JM: Hepatic vascular dysplasia in dogs and cats (105 cases). In: Proceedings of the 42nd Annual Meeting of the American College of Veterinary Pathologists, Orlando, 1991, p 71.
Abstract of pathologic features of hepatoportal microvascular dysplasia in a large number of animals.

Center SA: Hepatic vascular diseases. In: Guilford WG, Center SA, Strombeck DR, et al, eds: Strombeck's Small Animal Gastroenterology, 3rd ed. Philadelphia: WB Saunders, 1995, pp 802–836.
Provides comprehensive clinical, diagnostic, and therapeutic information regarding portosystemic vascular anomalies and hepatoportal microvascular dysplasia.

Daniel GB, Bright R, Ollis P, et al: Per rectal portal scintigraphy using [99m]technetium pertechnetate to diagnose portosystemic shunts in dogs and cats. J Vet Intern Med 5:23, 1991.
Describes procedure and utility of colorectal scintigraphy for the diagnosis of portosystemic vascular shunting.

Ewing GO, Suter PF, Bailey CS: Hepatic insufficiency associated with congenital anomalies of the portal vein in dogs. J Am Anim Hosp Assoc 10:463, 1974.
Original description and characterization of portosystemic vascular anomalies in dogs.

Kantrowitz BM, Nyland TG, Fisher P: Estimation of portal blood flow with the use of duplex real-time and pulsed Doppler ultrasound imaging in the dog. Vet Radiol 30:222, 1989.
Description of a noninvasive method for estimating portal blood flow in dogs.

Lawrence D, Bellah JR, Diaz R: Results of surgical management of portosystemic shunts in dogs: 20 cases (1985–1990). J Am Vet Med Assoc 201:1750, 1992.
Description of the clinical and clinicopathologic features of dogs following surgical attenuation of congenital vascular anomalies.

Meyer HP, Rothuizen J: Congenital portosystemic shunts (PSS) in dogs are a genetic disorder. Tijdschr Diergeneeskd 116:809, 1991.
Report of suspected inherited portosystemic vascular anomalies in Irish wolfhounds.

Nyland TG, Fisher PE: Evaluation of experimentally induced canine hepatic cirrhosis using duplex Doppler ultrasound. Vet Radiol 31:189, 1990.
Specific application of portal blood flow estimation with the use of duplex Doppler ultrasound in distinguishing altered perfusion after development of hepatic cirrhosis.

Phillips L, Tappe J, Lyman R, et al: Hepatic microvascular dysplasia in dogs. Prog Vet Neurol 7:88, 1996.
Clinical characterization of microvascular hepatoportal dysplasia in symptomatic dogs.

Schaeffer MC, Rogers RR, Buffington CA, et al: Long-term biochemical and physiologic effects of surgically placed portacaval shunts in dogs. Am J Vet Res 47:346, 1986.
Clinicopathologic and histologic features of surgically induced portosystemic vascular shunting in dogs surviving for 50 weeks.

Schermerhorn T, Center SA, Rowland PH, et al: Characterization of microvascular dysplasia in a kindred of Cairn Terriers. J Vet Intern Med 10:219, 1996.
Clinical and pathologic characterization of hepatoportal microvascular dysplasia and portosystemic venous anomalies in a kindred of Cairn terriers.

Zawie DA, Gilbertson SR: Interpretation of canine liver biopsy: A clinician's perspective. Vet Clin North Am Small Anim Pract 15:67, 1985.
Defines the utility of liver biopsy for clinical diagnoses including the initial description of microvascular dysplasia.

CVT Update: Therapy for Hepatic Lipidosis

LARRY M. CORNELIUS
JOSEPH W. BARTGES
CHERYL C. MILLER
Athens, Georgia

Excessive accumulation of fat in the liver is termed *hepatic lipidosis* (HL). HL in cats may be secondary to diabetes mellitus, drugs (e.g., tetracycline therapy), chronic anorexia, and malnutrition, or it may be due to primary, idiopathic hepatic lipid (triglyceride) accumulation (idiopathic hepatic lipidosis [IHL]). Diagnosis of IHL in cats in the United States has increased markedly since the first reported cases and is now the most common hepatopathy reported in cats in this country. Whether this increase reflects a higher prevalence or better recognition of the clinical syndrome is unclear. Hepatic lipid accumulation in cats may cause severe hepatic dysfunction and death resulting from complications of liver failure. The primary objective of this article is to detail the management of IHL in cats. The principles of supportive care are usually applicable to secondary HL as well.

GENERAL CHARACTERIZATION OF IDIOPATHIC HEPATIC LIPIDOSIS IN CATS

IHL is a disorder of adult cats of either sex and any breed. One of the main keys to successful management of IHL is *early diagnosis*. Fortunately, certain risk factors for IHL are well recognized and should alert owners and clinicians. *Obesity* is nearly always present before the onset of IHL. Although more subjective, *stress* seems to play a

role in "triggering" the syndrome. Specific examples of stress are a diet change to a less preferred food, causing a decrease in food intake; a change in environment; or an infection such as bite wound cellulitis. Clinical findings include decreased or "picky" appetite, which may progress to complete anorexia over several days to several weeks. Significant weight loss (often >25% of usual body weight) and muscle wasting are common but may be obscured by continued obesity. Mild to moderate depression usually is present. Sporadic vomiting is common. The onset of icterus is gradual and may be missed until jaundice is fairly pronounced. Hepatomegaly is common but is generally mild. Signs of severe liver failure such as hepatic encephalopathy (ptyalism, depression, stupor) and overt clotting disorders may develop as the disorder progresses; these developments represent serious complications. Hepatic failure carries a guarded to poor prognosis.

Common laboratory abnormalities reflect cholestatic liver disease, and as the disorder progressively worsens, biochemical changes consistent with hepatic failure become evident. Serum alkaline phosphatase (ALP) activity is often markedly increased, but surprisingly gamma glutamyl transferase activity may be normal or only slightly increased (Center et al, 1993). Serum alanine aminotransferase (ALT) and aspartate aminotransferase activities are slightly to moderately increased in most cases but usually not of the magnitude of ALP elevation. Other indications of cholestasis and hepatic dysfunction are hyperbilirubinemia, bilirubinuria, and increased serum bile acid levels. Hypoglycemia, hypoalbuminemia, hyperammonemia, and abnormalities of coagulation may be associated with severe hepatic dysfunction.

Abdominal radiography of cats with uncomplicated IHL generally shows only mild hepatomegaly. The lipidotic liver has a generalized hyperechoic appearance on ultrasonography. Additionally, abdominal ultrasonography can help rule out extrahepatic biliary obstruction because normal-sized extrahepatic bile ducts are typical of IHL and pancreatitis (no evidence of peritoneal effusion and lack of typical mixed echogenic mass in the area of the pancreas; see p. 659).

Definitive diagnosis of IHL is best accomplished with a liver biopsy (percutaneous needle or wedge obtained during celiotomy). Cytologic evaluation of a percutaneous fine needle liver aspirate may allow a presumptive diagnosis of HL, and this procedure is usually safer for the patient than is open biopsy with general anesthesia and surgery.

PATHOPHYSIOLOGY OF IDIOPATHIC HEPATIC LIPIDOSIS

Unfortunately, little is known about the pathophysiologic mechanisms causing IHL in cats. Speculation has been concerned mainly with metabolic alterations associated with hepatic fat accumulation that results in liver failure (Dimski and Taboada, 1995). Although these events probably are important, mechanisms involved with persistent anorexia are not understood. It is remarkable, indeed, that obese cats, who previously ate excessively, become so persistently unwilling to eat. This issue may not be simple because multiple factors are involved in mediating food intake and energy balance, including central nervous system neurotransmitters such as neuropeptide Y, serotonin, and corticotropin-releasing hormone; peripheral hormones such as insulin, cholecystokinin, and stress hormones (catecholamines and glucocorticoids); and levels of cytokines such as tumor necrosis factor-alpha (TNF-alpha) and interleukin-1 (IL-1) (Ballinger, 1994).

Recent developments in understanding the complexities of appetite regulation in other species have been reported (Halmi, 1996). It now appears that adipocytes are integrally involved (Flier, 1995). Of particular interest is the recent discovery that TNF-alpha is overexpressed in adipose tissue of obese laboratory animals and human beings (Hotamisligil et al, 1995). It is now well documented that several members of the cytokine family, including TNF-alpha and IL-1 in high levels, cause anorexia and disturbances of lipid metabolism leading to increased lipolysis in adipose tissue (Grunfeld and Feingold, 1991). In laboratory animals, TNF-alpha has been shown to increase expression of the hormone leptin, the protein product of the obesity (ob) gene found in adipose tissue (Grunfeld et al, 1996). Leptin (the so-called thinness hormone) affects central nervous system centers and causes decreased food intake, possibly by decreasing levels of the neurotransmitter neuropeptide Y (Schwartz et al, 1996). Neuropeptide Y in the central nervous system is a potent appetite stimulant.

Preliminary work in the authors' laboratory has confirmed that obese cats have markedly increased levels of subcutaneous adipose tissue TNF-alpha when compared with cats of normal weight and that some cats with spontaneous IHL have significantly increased TNF-alpha levels in their subcutaneous fat. The clinical significance of these findings awaits further study.

TREATMENT

The management of cats with IHL is supportive and based on clinical experience and empirical observations. *Early diagnosis* and prompt attention to *nutritional support* probably account for a decline in the overall mortality rate from nearly 100% of cases when IHL was first recognized in cats to less than 30 to 40% observed today. Further gains may not occur until a more complete understanding of the cause or causes and metabolic derangements associated with IHL become available.

Standard medical management for cats with mild to moderate IHL not complicated by signs of severe liver failure such as hepatoencephalopathy and clotting disorders is summarized in Table 1. The major objective in managing these cats is to provide enteral nutrition efficiently and consistently using a high-protein, calorie-dense diet and feeding by the least stressful means possible until the cat is once again willing to eat adequate amounts on its own. This may take several days to a few months (average is 2 to 4 weeks in the authors' experience) and generally requires placement of a feeding tube. Appetite stimulants such as diazepam (Valium, Hoffman-La Roche) are seldom useful. In addition, chronic administration (>7 days) of diazepam PO to cats has been associated with fulminant hepatic necrosis (Center et al, 1996). Before placement of the feeding tube, the cat should be rehydrated with a balanced parenteral polyionic electrolyte solution such as lactated Ringer's or Ringer's solution preferably administered by the IV route. Since some anorectic cats are prone to the development of hypokalemia, serum potassium (K$^+$) should be measured. If hypokalemia (serum K$^+$ <3.5 mEq/L) is present, additional potassium in the form of potassium chloride should be added to the polyionic fluid. The authors generally add 16 mEq of K$^+$/L of lactated Ringer's solution to provide a final K$^+$ concentration of 20 mEq/L. The rate of IV administration of potassium should not exceed 0.5 mEq/kg per hour unless life-threatening hypokalemia (serum K$^+$ <2.5 mEq/L) is present. Low serum phosphorus concentrations (<2.5 mg/dl) resulting in hemolytic anemia occasionally occur in cats with IHL either before or after enteral tube feeding is begun. If needed, potassium phosphate should be added to either 0.9% saline or 5% dextrose solution and infused IV to correct hypophosphatemia. Reported effective doses of phosphate for hypophosphatemic cats ranged from 0.011 to 0.017 mmol of phosphate/kg per hour infused over a period of 6 to 12 hours (Adams et al, 1993). Initiation of enteral feeding of commercial cat food generally supplies adequate potassium and phosphorus to prevent further problems with hypokalemia and hypophosphatemia.

Several options are available for feeding tube placement including nasoesophageal, esophagostomy, and gastrostomy (see pp. 84 and 597). The particular tube chosen depends on several factors, including severity of illness and

TABLE 1. **Standard Medical Management for Cats With Signs of Mild to Moderate Idiopathic Hepatic Lipidosis**

Correct dehydration with lactated Ringer's or Ringer's solution IV.

Correct mild to moderate hypokalemia (serum K^+ 3.0–4.0 mEq/L) by adding 16 mEq of K^+ as potassium chloride to the lactated Ringer's or Ringer's solution (final K^+ concentration = 20 mEq/L). More K^+ may be added (up to 40 mEq/L) if the serum potassium is markedly decreased (serum K^+ <3.0 mEq/L). The rate of IV K^+ administration should not exceed 0.5 mEq/kg per hour without careful monitoring of serum K^+.

A gastrostomy tube is placed for long-term feeding. Prescription Diet a/d, c/d, and p/d (Hill's Pet Nutrition Inc.), CNM Feline CV Formula (Ralston Purina Co.), and Feline Nutritional Recovery Formula (Iams Co.) are acceptable.

For the first 12 hr, flush only small amounts of water (10–15 ml q6hr) through the gastrostomy tube, then begin food administration.

Estimated caloric needs = 1.5 × [30 × body wt (kg) + 70].

Determine quantity of diet needed to supply caloric requirements.

Mix 1 ounce of water with 1 ounce of food in a blender; warm to body temperature in a microwave oven and administer slowly over 10–15 min through the feeding tube. This mixture will meet daily maintenance fluid requirements.

Flush feeding tube with 10–15 ml of warm water after each feeding.

Administer estimated caloric requirements in six equally sized meals (q4h) for the first day or two. Thereafter, gradually increase the quantity per meal and decrease the frequency of feeding with the goal of feeding q8h by the owner at home. Always aspirate the feeding tube before each feeding. If the residual volume is >20% of the volume of the previous meal, skip the next feeding and start therapy with a prokinetic drug such as metoclopramide (Reglan, A.H. Robins Co.) or cisapride (Propulsid, Janssen Pharmaceutica, Inc.).

Use metoclopramide, 0.4 mg/kg q8h PO or SC or cisapride, 2.5–5 mg q8h PO 15–30 minutes before tube-feeding if needed to control vomiting or stimulate gastric motility and emptying, or both.

Re-evaluate the patient weekly for the first week or two, including history, physical examination, complete blood count, and serum biochemical profile. Thereafter, repeat measurement of serum ALT, ALP, and bilirubin every 2 or 3 weeks.

Have the owner periodically "challenge" the cat to eat by withholding one or two tube feedings and offering favorite foods.

Remove the gastrostomy tube when the cat is eating its estimated caloric needs voluntarily and has normal or nearly normal serum ALT, ALP, and bilirubin values.

ALT, alanine transaminase; ALP, alkaline phosphatase.

the preferences of the clinician and owner. Nasoesophageal tubes are more appropriate for short-term feeding (<5 to 7 days). General anesthesia is not required for their placement. Because of their relatively small diameter (5 to 8F), they may require the use of liquid diets such as Feline Clinicare (Pet-Ag, Inc.). However, an 8F red rubber catheter often can be placed, and grueled Prescription Diet a/d (Hill's Pet Nutrition, Inc.) or Feline Nutritional Recovery Formula (Iams Co.) administered through it. The authors use nasoesophageal tube feeding mainly in patients in which debility and serious liver failure are present, making anesthesia for placement of a gastrostomy feeding tube a serious risk. A few days of fluid and nutritional support may render such an animal an acceptable anesthetic risk, at which time a larger gastrostomy tube can be placed.

The authors prefer gastrostomy tubes (see p. 84) over esophagostomy tubes (p. 597) in cats mainly because feline patients often are uncomfortable with esophagostomy tubes and the associated neck wrap. This is evidenced by gagging, drooling, and facial expressions consistent with discomfort and stress. Since avoidance of stress is one of the major concerns, the authors seldom use esophagostomy tubes for enteral nutrition in cats. Major advantages of a gastrostomy tube for enteral nutrition in feline IHL are the large-diameter tube (up to 18F), the ability to administer through the tube easily commercial cat foods that have been put through a blender, and the apparent patient comfort with the tube because a light bandage wrap or no wrap at all can be used. In the authors' experience, cats typically become so adapted to gastrostomy tube feeding that the clinician needs to withhold tube feeding periodically to evaluate the cat for a return of appetite.

Several methods of gastrostomy tube placement have been described, including surgical (celiotomy), percutaneous endoscopic gastrostomy, and nonendoscopic percutaneous placement. The authors prefer a special rod-like instrument (Eld percutaneous gastrostomy feeding tube applicator—Jorgensen Laboratories) to place gastrostomy tubes percutaneously in cats. All the preceding methods of feeding tube placement require general anesthesia, but with experience such placement can be accomplished rapidly (5 to 20 minutes). Isoflurane (Aerrane, Ohmeda PPD, Inc.) anesthesia is preferred because hepatic metabolism is not required and the anesthetic agent is quickly eliminated once delivery is discontinued. Some clinicians prefer to confirm appropriate placement of the gastrostomy tube by radiographing the abdomen after tube placement. Tube visualization can be enhanced by instilling a small amount of iodinated contrast medium into the tube before radiography. The tube exit site is covered with a sterile 4 × 4 gauze to which a small amount of antibiotic ointment, such as bacitracin zinc–polymyxin B sulfate (E. Fougera Co.), has been applied. An elastic wrap is then applied, which can be partially removed at the time of each feeding.

For the first 12 hours, only small amounts of water should be flushed through the gastrostomy tube (10 to 15 ml every 6 hours). During this time, energy requirements should be estimated and a feeding plan developed. An accepted formula for estimating energy requirements is:

$$1.5 \times [30 \times \text{body weight (kg)} + 70].$$

Therefore, a cat weighing 5 kg needs approximately 1.5 × [30 × 5 + 70] = 330 kilocalories (kcal) per day. The feeding plan should include which food will be fed, how much will be fed, and how often it will be administered. The authors have used several diets, including canned Prescription Diets c/d, p/d, and a/d (Hill's Pet Nutrition, Inc.), canned CNM Feline CV Formula (Ralston Purina Co.), and Feline Nutritional Recovery Formula (Iams Co.). We believe that all of these diets are acceptable unless the patient shows clinical evidence of hepatic encephalopathy, in which case a protein-restricted diet, such as Prescription

Diet k/d (Hill's Pet Nutrition, Inc.) is indicated (see p. 693. The authors have not found any obvious clinical benefit from adding supplements such as carnitine, arginine, citrulline, fish oils, and zinc to the diet. After determining the caloric content of the diet, the quantity of food needed is determined. One half of a 15.5 ounce can of Prescription Diet c/d contains about 300 kcal. Therefore, in the previous example, approximately one-half can is needed to supply 330 kcal. Most canned cat foods require mixing with water in a blender (1 ounce of water for each ounce of food) into a slurry, although Hill's Prescription Diet a/d and Iams Feline Nutritional Recovery Formula Diet usually can be administered directly through the tube. Feedings should be divided preferably into six equal portions for the first day or two in order to allow for gradual patient acclimation. Before each feeding, the tube should be aspirated and the amount of residual food and water measured. If the quantity aspirated is significant ($>20\%$ of the volume of the previous meal), a feeding should be skipped to lessen the chances of vomiting from excessive gastric distention. Feeding smaller amounts at more frequent intervals and using a prokinetic drug to improve gastric emptying (see further on) also may be indicated. After food administration, the tube should be flushed with 10 to 15 ml of warm water and capped. This regimen supplies approximately 1 ml of water per milliliter of food slurry administered. Therefore, it is generally unnecessary to administer additional fluids for maintenance.

After 1 or 2 days, the amount per feeding is gradually increased, and the frequency of feeding is decreased with the goal of three daily feedings by the time the cat is sent home. This may take an additional 3 to 5 days. The most common complication is vomiting after feeding. Frequency of vomiting can be reduced by slowing the rate of food administration (10 to 15 minutes per feeding), warming the food to body temperature in a microwave oven, and pretreating with a prokinetic drug (see p. 614) such as metoclopramide [Reglan, A.H. Robins Co.]) or cisapride (Propulsid, Janssen Pharmaceutica, Inc.). While the patient is hospitalized, the authors generally use metoclopramide administered SC at 0.4 mg/kg every 8 hours about 15 minutes before three of the daily tube feedings. If sporadic vomiting continues at home, either metoclopramide (0.4 mg/kg every 8 hours) or cisapride (2.5 to 5 mg per cat every 8 hours) can be administered through the gastrostomy tube about 30 minutes before tube feeding. The clinician should be vigilant and, if indicated, pursue other potential causes of vomiting such as worsening liver failure, pancreatitis, or complications associated with the feeding tube (cellulitis, abscess, peritonitis). Table 2 shows drugs that are used for problems sometimes associated with IHL in cats.

Owner education and periodic rechecks while the gastrostomy tube is in place are especially important. Owners need to thoroughly understand all aspects of food preparation and administration, including flushing of the tube with water after each feeding. They should visually inspect the tube exit site daily and gently clean off accumulated debris with a warm water compress. They should report the development of excessive, foul-smelling material to the veterinarian to circumvent complications from the development of purulent cellulitis. If serious wound infection develops, it is prudent to perform culture and sensitivity testing and begin systemic antibiotic therapy for several days.

Rechecks should be performed weekly to assess the patient's progress, to ascertain if the owner is having any difficulty feeding the cat, and to evaluate the feeding tube site. A complete blood count and serum biochemical panel should be performed during the first or second recheck. Thereafter, if the patient is doing well, it may only be necessary to recheck liver tests such as serum ALP, ALT, and bilirubin. The authors generally expect to see a significant decline in these values within 1 to 2 weeks of the initiation of tube feeding. However, complete normalization of liver tests can take several weeks. Increasing serum ALP, ALT, and bilirubin values along with vomiting and continuing patient lethargy are causes for concern. Radiography and ultrasonography of the abdomen are indicated to re-evaluate the liver, biliary tree, and pancreas and tube placement. Referral to an internist for a second opinion should also be offered.

TABLE 2. **Treatment of Problems Associated With Idiopathic Hepatic Lipidosis in Cats**

Drug	Trade Name, Source	Dosage, Frequency, Rate	Comments
Vitamin K_1	AquaMEPHYTON, Merck & Co.	1–2 mg/kg q12hr SC	Improve coagulation abnormality caused by poor absorption of vitamin K
Cimetidine	Tagamet, Pfizer, Inc.	5–10 mg/kg q8hr PO, SC	Treat gastroduodenal ulceration; may suppress hepatic P_{450} enzymes*
Ranitidine	Zantac, Glaxo Co.	2–4 mg/kg q12hr PO	Treat gastroduodenal ulceration; may suppress hepatic P_{450} enzymes*
Famotidine	Pepcid, Merck & Co.	0.5 mg/kg q24hr PO	Treat gastroduodenal ulceration; no effect on hepatic P_{450} enzymes
Sucralfate	Carafate, Marion Merrell Dow Co.	0.25 g per cat q12hr PO	Treat gastroduodenal ulceration
Metoclopramide	Reglan, A.H. Robins Co.	0.4 mg/kg q8hr PO, SC	Decrease vomiting; increase upper gastrointestinal tract motility and improve gastric emptying
Cisapride	Propulsid, Janssen Pharmaceutica Co.	2.5–5 mg/cat q8hr PO	Increase gastrointestinal tract motility and improve gastric emptying
Lactulose	Cephulac, Marion Merrell Dow Co.	0.3–0.5 ml/kg q8hr PO	Treat hepatoencephalopathy
Neomycin	Biosol, Upjohn Co.	22 mg/kg q8hr PO	Treat hepatoencephalopathy
Metronidazole	Flagyl, Searle Co.	7.5 mg/kg q8–12hr PO	Treat hepatoencephalopathy

*The authors have not observed adverse clinical effects when using either cimetidine or ranitidine in cats with idiopathic hepatic lipidosis.

If the patient's progress is good, the owner should periodically withhold one or more feedings in order to "challenge" the cat to eat on its own. Offering the cat's favorite foods or special treats is one way of evaluating whether the animal may be regaining its appetite. Some owners are understandably reluctant to withhold tube feeding, but it is the authors' experience that some cats become content to allow the owner to feed them through the tube unless tube feeding is temporarily discontinued. This transition may be facilitated by repeating measurements of serum liver enzyme activities. Once the serum ALP and ALT values and serum bilirubin concentration normalize, the cat usually begins to eat voluntarily within 1 to 2 weeks if sufficiently motivated. If the cat does begin to eat, the owner should carefully estimate how much food is being consumed so that adequacy of caloric intake can be determined. When the cat is consuming all or almost all its daily caloric needs, the gastrostomy tube should be removed. This usually can be carried out simply by restraining the patient and pulling on the tube using steady traction. *A note of caution:* removing the tube too soon after placement (<7 days) before formation of adequate adhesions between the stomach and peritoneum, could result in leakage of gastric contents into the peritoneal cavity and peritonitis. After the tube is pulled, the wound should be inspected and cleaned, but left open. The tube exit site will generally seal over and heal within 4 to 7 days without complication.

PROGNOSIS

The prognosis for feline IHL remains guarded, but with early diagnosis and aggressive enteral nutritional support, most cats survive and have no residual liver damage. The authors have not personally seen recurrence of IHL in a patient. Nonetheless, we advise owners not to allow the cat to become obese again. This may be best accomplished by careful attention to how many calories are being fed daily and periodic monitoring of body weight. Prevention and management of obesity in cats should not be forced by changing to an unpalatable diet. If the obese cat refuses to eat adequate amounts, induction of IHL may occur. Rather, it may be more prudent to allow the cat to eat its favorite foods in smaller quantities.

References and Suggested Readings

Adams LG, Hardy RM, Weiss DJ, et al: Hypophosphatemia and hemolytic anemia associated with diabetes mellitus and hepatic lipidosis in cats. J Vet Intern Med 7:266, 1993.
A retrospective clinical study of five cats with diabetes mellitus and one with IHL showing hypophosphatemia-associated hemolytic anemia.

Ballinger A: Appetite control in health and disease. Br J Hosp Med 51:327, 1994.
An editorial summarizing biochemical mechanisms of appetite regulation in health and disease.

Center SA, Crawford MA, Guida L, et al: A retrospective study of 77 cats with severe hepatic lipidosis: 1975–1990. J Vet Intern Med 7:349, 1993.
A retrospective study summarizing the physical findings, pathophysiological characteristics, and survival rates of 77 cats with either idiopathic or secondary hepatic lipidosis.

Center SA, Elston TA, Rowland PH, et al: Fulminant hepatic failure associated with oral administration of diazepam in 11 cats. J Am Vet Med Assoc 209:618, 1996.
A retrospective study in 11 cats documenting an association between chronic (>7 days) administration of diazepam PO and diffuse hepatic necrosis and fulminant hepatic failure.

Dimski DS, Taboada J: Feline idiopathic hepatic lipidosis. Vet Clin North Am 25:357, 1995.
A review of the clinical features, diagnostic criteria, pathophysiological mechanisms, and management of feline IHL.

Flier JS: The adipocyte: Storage depot or node on the energy information superhighway? Cell 80:15, 1995.
A review of major components of the body weight regulatory system, including appetite regulation.

Grunfeld C, Feingold KR: The metabolic effects of tumor necrosis factor and other cytokines. Biotherapy 3:143, 1991.
A review of the metabolic effects of TNF-alpha, IL-1, and other cytokines, with emphasis on their effects on lipid metabolism.

Grunfeld C, Zhao C, Fuller, J, et al: Endotoxin and cytokines induce expression of leptin, the ob gene product in hamsters. J Clin Invest 97:2152, 1996.
A study of the role of TNF-alpha, IL-1, and the hormone leptin in anorexia associated with infection.

Halmi KA: Eating disorder research in the past decade. Ann NY Acad Sci 789:67, 1996.
A review of significant results of research studying various eating disorders.

Hotamisligil GS, Arner P, Caro JF, et al: Increased adipose tissue expression of tumor necrosis factor-α in human obesity and insulin resistance. J Clin Invest 95:2409, 1995.
A study documenting overexpression of TNF-alpha in adipose tissue, associated with insulin-resistance, in obese humans.

Schwartz MW, Baskin DG, Bukowski TR, et al: Specificity of leptin action on elevated blood glucose and hypothalamic neuropeptide Y gene expression in ob/ob mice. Diabetes 45:531, 1996.
A study of the effects of systemic administration of the hormone leptin on food intake, body weight, blood glucose, and expression of hypothalamic neuropeptide Y in a mouse model of obesity (ob/ob mice).

Ursodeoxycholic Acid Therapy

CYNTHIA R. LEVEILLE-WEBSTER
North Grafton, Massachusetts

For many years, practitioners of Eastern medicine have known of the healing powers of Chinese black bear bile. The major bile acid in this bear's bile, ursodeoxycholic acid (UDCA), has been commercially synthesized and marketed as a hepatoprotective agent in Japan since the 1930s. It was not until the 1970s that Western medicine began to appreciate the medicinal value of UDCA when this bile acid received approval from the Food and Drug Administration (Actigall, Ciba-Geigy) to be marketed for the dissolution of cholesterol gallstones in humans. In the 1980s, physicians noticed that UDCA therapy in patients with concurrent gallstones and chronic hepatic disease resulted in improvement in liver function test results. Since then, interest in the use of UDCA as a hepatoprotective agent has increased markedly, and several human clinical trials have addressed the value of UDCA in the therapy of various chronic hepatopathies.

HEPATOTOXICITY OF BILE ACIDS

One of the most compelling reasons to consider the use of UDCA in treating chronic hepatic disease is the growing awareness of the role of hydrophobic bile acids as hepatotoxins. Numerous studies have documented that bile acids are cytotoxic to hepatocytes. Since serum and hepatic retention of bile acids accompanies most hepatobiliary disorders, it stands to reason that retained hydrophobic bile acids contribute to ongoing hepatic damage.

The mechanisms whereby hydrophobic bile acids damage hepatocytes are not fully understood. Bile acids are biologic detergents whose physiologic function is to solubilize biliary lipids and facilitate absorption of fats in the intestine. Exposure of hepatocytes to bile acid concentrations that are normally present in the biliary ducts or intestine (1 to 2 mM) results in rapid cell lysis because of solubilization of cell membranes. At lower concentrations in the micromolar range, such as those readily obtainable in serum and hepatic tissue during cholestatic disorders, hydrophobic bile acids are still capable of disrupting biologic membranes. Accumulating evidence suggests that the major target of hydrophobic bile acids is the mitochondrial membrane. In isolated hepatocytes, exposure to hydrophobic bile acids disrupts mitochondrial electron transport and leads to increased generation of cytotoxic oxygen free radicals. Bile acid–induced mitochondrial damage also results in depletion of cellular adenosine triphosphate stores. Several nondetergent mechanisms of bile acid hepatocellular toxicity have been proposed. Bile acids are proinflammatory. They increase the generation of free radicals in neutrophils, degranulate mast cells, and stimulate leukotriene production in intestinal cell lines. Bile acids also increase hepatocyte intracellular calcium concentrations, which, in turn, have been linked with a loss of cell viability.

HEPATOPROTECTIVE ACTIONS OF URSODEOXYCHOLIC ACID

Mammalian bile acids are actually a family of amphipathic molecules that share a steroid nucleus with hydroxylation at the 3 position. The primary bile acids synthesized in the liver, chenodeoxycholic acid and cholic acid, are characterized by additional hydroxylations at the 7 and the 7 and 12 positions, respectively. These primary bile acids are conjugated in the liver with either glycine or taurine. These chemical modifications are important determinants of bile acid toxicity because both conjugation and hydroxylation decrease the molecule's hydrophobicity and, in general, the more hydrophobic the bile acid, the greater the tendency for hepatotoxicity.

UDCA is a relatively hydrophilic bile acid by virtue of its degree of hydroxylation and the orientation of these hydroxyl groups around the steroid nucleus. Several clinical trials in human patients with chronic hepatopathies have suggested that long-term UDCA therapy is hepatoprotective. Although the mechanism or mechanisms responsible for this hepatoprotective effect are the subject of much controversy in the human literature, the following beneficial actions have been proposed: (1) replacement of the more hydrophobic hepatotoxic bile acids in the circulating pool, (2) induction of choleresis, and (3) immunomodulation.

The major bile acids in humans are the relatively hydrophobic bile acid glycochenodeoxycholate and the more hydrophilic bile acid glycocholate. In cats and dogs, the major circulating bile acid is taurocholate, which is more hydrophilic and less hepatotoxic than is glycochenodeoxycholate. Administration of UDCA to human patients with chronic liver disease results in bile enriched in UDCA. By replacing glycochenodeoxycholate, UDCA may help to ameliorate the toxic effects of the latter. In small animals, the benefit of replacing taurocholate with UDCA may not be as great because both bile acids are relatively nontoxic. There is also evidence to suggest that UDCA's hepatoprotective effect may be mediated at the level of the intestinal lumen, where it may inhibit ileal uptake of toxic secondary bile acids formed in the lumen by bacterial modification of primary bile acids.

Unconjugated UDCA increases bile flow. The mechanism by which UDCA promotes choleresis is known as cholehepatic shunting. Unconjugated UDCA is secreted into bile, where it becomes protonated, leading to the generation of bicarbonate ion. Protonated UDCA is then passively absorbed by the biliary epithelial cells leaving the net secretion of one bicarbonate ion. The bicarbonate then serves as an osmotic draw for biliary water secretion. By inducing this choleresis, UDCA may protect hepatocytes from the accumulation of potentially toxic compounds normally secreted into the bile, such as copper, leukotrienes, cholesterol, and bilirubin.

Several immunomodulating effects of UDCA have been reported. UDCA decreases the production of immunoglobulin by B lymphocytes and interleukin-1 and -2 by T lymphocytes in response to nonspecific stimuli. UDCA treatment also decreases expression of hepatocyte cell surface membrane HLA class I molecules. Preliminary studies suggest that UDCA may bind to and stimulate the hepatocyte glucocorticoid receptor and that this action may account for its immunomodulatory activity.

CLINICAL USE OF URSODEOXYCHOLIC ACID IN HUMAN HEPATIC DISEASE

The therapeutic efficacy of UDCA has been investigated in several chronic hepatopathies in humans with varying results. The most extensively studied disease to date, and the one in which UDCA therapy appears to have the greatest benefit, is primary biliary cirrhosis (PBC). PBC is a chronic disorder of middle-aged women characterized by immune-mediated destruction of bile ducts. The disease has a variable age of onset and usually a long course (years), ultimately resulting in hepatic failure and the need for liver transplantation. A recent meta-analysis of several clinical trials exploring the use of UDCA to treat PBC revealed beyond any doubt that the bile acid has favorable effects on biochemical indicators of hepatobiliary disease, but it failed to show any conclusive effect on primary end points such as histologic progression, survival, or the need for liver transplantation.

Since the aim of these clinical trials was to demonstrate that UDCA could reverse the disease process or, at the very least, slow progression of disease, the failure of these trials to demonstrate convincingly an effect on primary end points is somewhat concerning. This failure may be the result of the slow and somewhat unpredictable nature of the disease. It may be that patients need to be followed over a longer period. In addition, many patients with late-stage disease were recruited into these studies, and some evidence exists to suggest that UDCA is ineffective in advanced disease and may actually worsen symptoms and biochemical test results.

Since UDCA alone fails to induce complete remission or to prevent progression in some patients with PBC, recent trials have addressed the possibility of combination therapy with UDCA. Several studies comparing the use of UDCA and colchicine to UDCA alone in PBC have failed to demonstrate that the addition of colchicine provides any benefit over the use of UDCA alone. The results of these trials need to be interpreted with the knowledge that UDCA could alter the pharmacokinetics of drugs such as colchicine, which undergoes biliary excretion. A preliminary study evaluating the use of UDCA along with low-dose immunosuppressive therapy versus the use of UDCA alone found that combination therapy resulted in a further improvement in serum enzyme activity and in the overall score of clinical disease activity.

UDCA has been of some therapeutic benefit in other chronic hepatic disorders in humans. Most notable are patients with biliary disease secondary to cystic fibrosis in which the choleretic action of UDCA may prevent the bile inspissation that characterizes this disorder. Another study suggests that UDCA may be beneficial in the treatment of nonalcoholic steatohepatitis. A 12-month course of therapy in individuals with this disorder resulted in both a decrease in serum enzymes and a reduction in the degree of hepatic lipidosis on histologic examination. The drug has received mixed reviews in therapeutic trials for the treatment of other hepatobiliary diseases such as idiopathic chronic hepatitis, autoimmune hepatitis, primary sclerosing cholangitis, and alcoholic hepatitis.

CLINICAL OBSERVATIONS ON THE USE OF URSODEOXYCHOLIC ACID IN VETERINARY PATIENTS

There have been limited reports on the use of UDCA in veterinary patients. No controlled clinical trials have been conducted. In a single case report, the use of UDCA at 15 mg/kg per day in a dog with chronic hepatitis resulted in enrichment of this bile acid in the serum and was associated with biochemical and clinical improvement. There have been anecdotal reports of similar success in treating other dogs with chronic hepatitis and in treating cats with chronic lymphocytic plasmacytic cholangiohepatitis.

The safety profile of UDCA has been fairly well established in healthy dogs and cats. Extensive toxicologic studies for Food and Drug Administration approval of UDCA performed in healthy dogs by the drug's manufacturer did not reveal any serious side effects of therapy. A study in 15 normal cats revealed that daily administration of 15 mg/kg PO of UDCA for 14 days did not result in any adverse clinical side effects. In a separate study, no adverse reactions were noted when UDCA was administered to five healthy cats at 10 mg/kg per day PO for 3 months. Anecdotal clinical impressions from several veterinary hepatologists who have been using this drug in feline and canine patients with hepatic disease corroborate these experimental findings. The only side effects reported with any frequency are rare instances of vomiting and diarrhea.

Limited experimental evidence is available on the effect of daily oral administration of UDCA on circulating bile acid pools in the dog and cat. In a single case report, administration of UDCA at 15 mg/kg PO resulted in enrichment of this bile acid in serum. In cats, daily administration of 10 mg/kg PO for 3 months resulted in an increase in total serum bile acid concentrations, and both UDCA and its taurine conjugate were detected in the serum at 1 and 2 months after treatment. At 3 months, however, increases in UDCA or its taurine conjugate were detected in only two of five cats treated. The reason for this is unknown but may have been associated with enhanced metabolism of UDCA or technical difficulties in measuring serum bile acid levels. In humans, dogs, and cats, administration of UDCA suppresses hepatic synthesis of cholesterol, thereby leading to a decrease in serum cholesterol levels.

There is some concern in human patients that chronic administration of unconjugated UDCA might potentiate taurine depletion in some patients with hepatic disease. This may be an important consideration in UDCA therapy in cats because they are obligate taurine conjugators. In addition, some cats with hepatic disease have increased urinary excretion of taurine-conjugated bile acids, which

would further predispose them to depletion of total body stores of taurine. Although dogs also conjugate the majority of their bile acids with taurine, they are capable of shifting to glycine conjugation and would be less likely to become depleted.

CURRENT RECOMMENDATIONS

It is currently unknown whether UDCA has any therapeutic benefit in treating canine or feline hepatobiliary disorders. The answer to this question awaits the results of prospective clinical trials. Extrapolation of information generated in the human literature suggests that this bile acid might be beneficial in some instances. The choleretic action of UDCA should be of benefit in acute and chronic hepatobiliary disorders marked by intrahepatic cholestasis. The possibility of extrahepatic biliary obstruction should always be ruled out before starting therapy because the use of choleretics is contraindicated in this instance. The long-term hepatoprotective and immunomodulating actions of the drug should be of benefit in the treatment of chronic inflammatory hepatopathies in both the dog and cat. It is the author's belief that UDCA is not a panacea for all chronic inflammatory hepatic disorders but may be of some benefit in slowing the progression of disease, especially when used at an early stage. Until controlled prospective clinical trials on the use of UDCA in chronic hepatopathies are performed, the author's current recommendation is to use UDCA monotherapy along with appropriate therapeutic measures to manage the complications of hepatobiliary disease (see *CVT XII*, p. 749) in animals with chronic

inflammatory disorders for 3 to 4 months to see if improvements in biochemical markers of hepatocellular injury occur. If improvement is seen, UDCA therapy is continued. If biochemical progression occurs, UDCA therapy is terminated or additional medications to slow progression, such as colchicine or glucocorticoids, are added.

UDCA is available as a 300-mg capsule for oral administration. The cost of therapy can be high. At the author's institution, the cost of treating a 30-kg (66-lb) dog or a 5-kg cat at a dose of 10 mg/kg per day is $90 and $15 per month, respectively. The recommended dose, 10 to 15 mg/kg per day PO, is extrapolated from human medicine.

References and Suggested Reading

Anwer MS, Meyer DJ: Bile acids in the diagnosis, pathology and therapy of hepatobiliary disease. Vet Clin North Am 25:503, 1995.
   A review of the structure and function of bile acids with an emphasis on the hepatotoxicity of bile acids and the hepatoprotective actions of UDCA.
Center SA: Serum bile acids in companion animal medicine. Vet Clin North Am 23:625, 1993.
   A comprehensive review of bile acid structure and metabolism with a discussion of the pathologic, diagnostic, and therapeutic potential of bile acids.
Green RM, Crawford JM: Hepatocellular cholestasis: Pathobiology and histological outcome. Semin Liver Dis 15:372, 1995.
   An excellent review of the pathophysiology of cholestatic liver disorders.
Jones DE, James OF, Bassendine MF: Ursodeoxycholic acid therapy in primary biliary cirrhosis. Hepatology 21:1469, 1995.
   A commentary on the results of three clinical trials of UDCA therapy in primary biliary cirrhosis with a critical evaluation of several other trials as well.

Nutritional Management of Liver Disease

DOROTHY P. LAFLAMME
Millstadt, Illinois

The role of dietary management in patients with hepatic disease is to maintain an adequate plane of nutrition to support hepatic regeneration and provide symptomatic relief for clinical signs. Correction of malnutrition can improve liver function and enhance the liver's functional reserve (Levinson, 1995). Thus, the patient evaluation should specifically seek to identify evidence of malnutrition and to identify clinical signs that may benefit from dietary management (Table 1).

NUTRITIONAL EVALUATION

Before instituting a dietary change in any animal, a thorough nutritional evaluation should be completed. Understanding how the nutritional needs of animals may be affected by existing disease conditions, along with a thorough evaluation of the patient and its current diet and feeding management, allows an appropriate dietary recom-

mendation. Such recommendations should take into account the needs of the patient and client preferences, as well as economics. Changes in feeding management should be considered a part of total patient management. As with any aspect of medical management, the animal should be re-evaluated at appropriate intervals to assure achievement of desired results.

Patient Evaluation

A complete medical history should be available and a thorough physical examination conducted, including body weight and body condition score. The skin and haircoat are considered. Thin, brittle hair and dry, flaky skin may be signs of nutritional deficiencies, such as protein or vitamin A deficiency. Abnormalities in the serum biochemistry profile may provide evidence of clinical or subclinical problems that may benefit from dietary modification as part

TABLE 1. **Dietary Implications of Hepatic Dysfunction**

Manifestation	Metabolic Disorder	Nutrient	Dietary Implication
Loss of lean muscle mass, hyperammonemia, hypoalbuminemia, ascites	Increased protein catabolism, decreased hepatic protein synthesis	Protein	Avoid protein restriction (i.e., at least 20% protein for dogs, 30% for cats on dry basis); feed several times daily to avoid prolonged fasting
Hepatic encephalopathy	Urea cycle dysfunction, hyperammonemia	Protein	Control GI bleeding; avoid meat, use dairy or soy protein; restrict dietary protein (i.e., 12 to 16% for dogs, 26 to 32% for cats on dry basis)
Increased serum triglycerides, cachexia	Decreased lipoprotein lipase activity	Fat	Provide calories from protein and carbohydrates; avoid excess fat (i.e., less than 15%); feed several times daily
Diarrhea ± steatorrhea	Cholestasis with fat malabsorption	Fat	Restrict fat (i.e., less than 10% from LCTs); consider MCTs for energy; supplement fat-soluble vitamins
Glucose intolerance, increased serum free fatty acids	Low insulin activity; increased lipolysis	Carbohydrate	Avoid simple sugars; use complex carbohydrates
Protein catabolism and muscle wasting, hypoglycemia	Glycogen depletion	Carbohydrate	Provide frequent meals; assure adequate energy intake
Ascites	Portal hypertension, excess sodium retention	Sodium	Restrict sodium (i.e., less than 0.25% of diet dry matter)
Hepatic encephalopathy, glucose intolerance, hypokalemia	Deficiency from low intake, diuresis, vomiting or diarrhea	Potassium	Avoid excessive diuretic therapy; assure adequate intake (i.e., at least 0.6% of diet dry matter); supplement with 2 mEq/day PO as potassium gluconate
Fibrosis	Toxicity from heritable metabolic defect	Copper	Use copper chelators (D-penicillamine 10–15 mg/kg PO q12hr) or zinc acetate (50–100 mg PO q12hr)
Anorexia, encephalopathy, hepatic fibrosis	Deficiency	Zinc	Consider oral supplementation with zinc gluconate (3 mg/kg/day) or zinc sulfate (2 mg/kg/day) divided into three doses
Coagulopathies	Deficiency from fat malabsorption	Vitamin K	Provide parenterally if severe fat malabsorption is present, 0.5 mg/kg SC or IM every 7–20 days as K_1

LCTs, long-chain triglycerides; MCTs, medium-chain triglycerides.

of medical management; for example, hypoalbuminemia (protein supplementation), hypoglycemia (small, frequent meals), or hypokalemia (potassium supplementation).

Increases or decreases in body condition should trigger further evaluation. If weight loss is evident, determine if it is associated with increased or decreased intake. A detailed dietary history and evaluation are warranted. Hepatic dysfunction or hepatic encephalopathy (HE) may affect appetite, as may a number of pharmaceutical agents used in these patients.

Clients should be queried about stool volume and character, as this may provide indications of fat malabsorption. Animals with fat malabsorption have different dietary needs than do those able to digest and absorb dietary fat.

Dietary Evaluation

Before concluding that a dietary change is needed, it is important to evaluate the food that is currently fed. This includes the normal diet, as well as other foods to which the patient might have access. The nutritional characteristics of the diet and the pet's acceptance of the diet are assessed. The transition to a new diet can be difficult for a sick animal, and this should be carried out only if needed. If the food is not one that the clinician is familiar with, the client should be asked to bring in the package. The manufacturer can be contacted and asked for information about the product, such as typical calorie and nutrient content, digestibility, and animal testing for nutritional adequacy.

Feeding Management Evaluation

Knowing what diet is fed does not indicate whether or not it is fed appropriately and eaten acceptably. This is especially true when animals have health problems. One must determine how much and how often each of the identified foods are fed, whether the patient is fed measured amounts of food or "free choice"; how well the animal accepts the food, and any changes in appetite. This information is important in determining the adequacy of the current dietary situation, and it is important in planning a dietary recommendation that will receive good client acceptance and compliance.

NUTRITIONAL IMPACT OF HEPATIC DYSFUNCTION

Protein Metabolism

Many serum proteins, including albumin and numerous transport proteins, normally produced by the liver are decreased in hepatic failure. They may be further decreased by inadequate protein intake, as may occur if protein is restricted to control HE. Certainly, reduction of excess dietary protein reduces the potential for hyperammonemia and HE. However, excess protein restriction leads to catabolism of endogenous proteins and increased ammonia production, loss of skeletal mass with decreased capacity for detoxification of ammonia, and increased potential for HE. Protein should be restricted only as needed to control HE.

If protein restriction is necessary, a minimal intake of at least 2.1 gm protein/kg body weight per day is recommended for dogs and 4 gm/kg per day for cats. However, it is important that protein adequacy (e.g., serum albumin) be monitored to assure that protein depletion does not occur.

Dietary proteins from soybeans and milk proteins are well tolerated by animals with liver failure. Meat and blood, including endogenous sources as in gastrointestinal hemorrhage, are poorly tolerated, perhaps because of high ammoniagenic potential. Because of amino acid imbalances often reported in liver failure (see *CVT XII*, p. 1153), sources of branched chain amino acids (BCAAs) have been used in the management of HE, but with inconsistent clinical results. Enteral and parenteral solutions enriched with BCAAs are considerably more expensive than standard solutions and do not generally provide better results than providing adequate nutrition using standard solutions. Use of BCAA-enriched solutions is recommended only if HE cannot be controlled in other ways (Levinson, 1995).

Carbohydrate Metabolism

Glycogen storage and glucose synthesis often decrease in advanced hepatic disease, contributing to fasting hypoglycemia. Depleted glycogen stores result in premature protein catabolism to supply amino acids for gluconeogenesis. The longer an animal with hepatic failure spends in the fasting state, the greater the loss of muscle tissue and protein depletion. Nitrogen balance and nutritional status can be improved by the consumption of several small meals, including a bedtime snack (Swart et al, 1989).

Fat Metabolism

Lipid metabolism can be compromised in hepatobiliary disease, resulting in hepatic lipidosis, hyperlipidemia, and either hyper- or hypocholesterolemia. In addition, hepatic dysfunction can interfere with the digestion and absorption of dietary fats and fat-soluble compounds.

Bile acids from the liver are important for the normal digestion and absorption of long-chain triglycerides (LCTs)—the normal lipids found in most diets. In the complete absence of bile acids, LCT absorption can drop to 30 to 50% of normal. Even when fat malabsorption is not clinically apparent, fat digestion may be somewhat reduced. Hydroxylation of unabsorbed fatty acids by colonic microflora can contribute to diarrhea in these patients, perhaps enhancing problems with deficiencies of fat-soluble vitamins and essential fatty acids.

In animals with suspected fat malabsorption, restriction of LCTs is recommended, although adequate essential fatty acids must be provided (i.e., dietary LCTs to equal between 5 and 10% of diet dry matter). Medium-chain triglycerides (MCTs) have been used successfully as an alternative energy source because these shorter fatty acids are more readily absorbed despite a lack of bile acids. Diets containing MCTs at levels not to exceed 50% of the dietary fat may be beneficial for these animals. Examples of commercially available diets are CNM EN-Formula and CNM HA-Formula (Ralston Purina Co.).

Vitamins and Minerals

Few vitamin deficiencies are recognized in veterinary patients with hepatic disease, with the exception of vitamin K (Michel, 1995). Coagulopathies secondary to vitamin K deficiency should be treated with two to three doses of vitamin K$_1$ (AquaMEPHYTON, Merck) at 0.5 mg/kg SC every 12 hours. The same dose may be given once every 7 to 21 days, as needed, based on coagulation test results. Vitamin C, which is not usually recognized as an essential nutrient for dogs or cats because of endogenous synthesis, may be deficient in some animals. Oral supplementation with 25 mg vitamin C/kg body weight per day has been recommended. In animals maintained on commercially produced pet foods, additional vitamin supplementation should be necessary only in the case of severe fat malabsorption. Patients maintained on home-prepared diets should receive complete vitamin and mineral supplements and should be monitored carefully for evidence of nutrient deficiencies.

Copper storage diseases are a well-known cause of hepatic failure in genetically predisposed dogs (see *CVT XII*, p. 757). Copper may also accumulate in the liver secondary to other hepatobiliary diseases, especially cholestatic disorders. Secondary copper accumulation rarely exceeds 2,000 ppm in liver tissue, compared with normal levels of less than 400 ppm and primary copper storage disease with accumulation of 2,000 to 10,000 ppm (Rolfe and Twedt, 1995). Treatment should address reducing the accumulation of hepatic copper, regardless of the cause, because excess copper can cause further hepatocellular damage. Hepatic copper excretion can be enhanced by copper-chelating agents (e.g., D-penicillamine [Cuprimine, Merck], 10 to 15 mg/kg PO every 12 hours; see *CVT XII*, p. 757).

Zinc deficiency is common in patients with hepatic disease, and can contribute to HE via altered nitrogen metabolism. Zinc supplementation also may reduce lipid peroxidation and have antifibrotic properties. Zinc gluconate (3 mg/kg per day) or zinc sulfate (2 mg/kg per day) divided into three doses can be given as a dietary supplement although zinc sulfate is associated with gastric irritation.

Hypokalemia is a common precipitating cause of HE in animals with hepatic disease. It is also linked to glucose intolerance, which is common in hepatobiliary disease. Hypokalemia can result from profuse vomiting or diarrhea, poor intake, or excessive use of diuretics for the management of ascites. Patients should be monitored for evidence of hypokalemia or acid-base imbalances. Cats with idiopathic hepatic lipidosis (IHL) may be particularly susceptible to potassium depletion. Potassium supplementation (2 to 6 mEq/cat per day PO as potassium gluconate) should be considered for cats with IHL, especially those that are glucose-intolerant or show evidence of hypokalemia. Potassium citrate should be avoided because of its alkalinizing properties and alkalosis can aggravate HE.

CLINICAL INDICATIONS FOR DIETARY THERAPY

Commercial pet foods are available to meet the needs of most patients with hepatic disease and should be used whenever possible. Selection of an appropriate product

TABLE 2. Recipes for Homemade Diets for Dogs and Cats with Liver Disease

Ingredient	Amount for Dogs	Amount for Cats
Rice, cooked without salt	2 cups	1/2 cup
Low-fat cottage cheese	2 cups	1/2 cup
Large egg, boiled		1
Soybean oil	1 tbsp	1/2 tsp
Bone meal	1 1/2 tsp	1/2 tsp
Lite salt (KCl)	1/2 tsp	1/8 tsp

The canine recipe provides approximately 1000 kcal, 27% calories from protein, 24% from fat, and 49% from carbohydrates. The feline recipe provides approximately 300 kcal, 29% calories from protein, 32% from fat, and 39% from carbohydrates. Protein can be reduced as needed by increasing the proportion of rice to cottage cheese, or increased by substituting one boiled egg for 1/4 cup cooked rice. Refrigerate unused food and warm before feeding. Give a multivitamin and mineral supplement daily. Use of commercially prepared pet foods is strongly encouraged for long-term use.

depends on the specific clinical signs observed. Home-prepared diets (Table 2) may be used if necessary. However, these diets are less likely to provide complete nutrition, and long-term use of such diets is discouraged.

A number of pharmaceutical agents used in the management of hepatobiliary diseases are associated with side effects that may have an impact on dietary needs. Glucocorticoids used in the management of chronic progressive hepatitis may cause or aggravate ascites, HE, glucose intolerance, and gastrointestinal ulceration. Colchicine, used to inhibit fibrosis, has been associated with nausea, vomiting, and hemorrhagic diarrhea. Anorexia and vomiting may also accompany therapy with D-penicillamine or other copper chelators. Diarrhea may result from excessive lactulose administration. These effects should be taken into consideration when planning total patient management. Introduction of a new diet while an animal is nauseated may lead to a learned aversion to that food. Ideally, the animal should be stabilized before introducing a food intended for long-term feeding.

Hepatic Encephalopathy

It is important to correct acid-base and electrolyte disorders and to maintain body weight in patients with liver failure in order to reduce the risk of HE. In the absence of a functional liver, the skeletal muscle serves a primary role in detoxifying ammonia. To help maintain muscle mass, protein should be restricted only as needed to prevent

HE. Use of lactulose and supplementation with highly digestible, nonmeat proteins may allow an increase in protein intake in encephalopathic patients (see p. 693). Vegetable proteins, such as those from soybeans, and milk proteins, such as casein, cottage cheese, and whey, are superior sources of protein for patients susceptible to HE. Serum proteins should be monitored regularly and supplemental protein provided if necessary.

Frequent, small meals should be fed to limit the time between meals. This can improve nutritional status and decrease catabolism in cirrhotic patients. It may also enhance intake in partially anorectic patients.

Diet digestibility appears to be important. Of the several dietary studies that seemed to "prevent" HE in dogs with portosystemic shunts, high digestibility was common among diets. Conversely, dietary fiber (soluble) may help acidify the colonic contents and minimize ammonia absorption. Commercial high-fiber diets contain primarily insoluble fiber, which is poorly fermented and unlikely to be beneficial. Lactulose is a nonabsorbable carbohydrate that serves as a soluble fiber and is fermented in the colon. Lactulose is dosed to effect to stimulate the passage of two soft stools daily (see *CVT XII*, pp. 753 and 1156).

Feline Idiopathic Hepatic Lipidosis

Successful treatment of IHL depends on providing the animal with adequate nutritional support (see p. 693). Although a trial with a chemical appetite stimulant may be attempted, tube feeding is usually indicated. Forced feeding is contraindicated in this and most disease conditions because adequate nutrition is rarely provided by this method. Tube feeding provides an effective, less stressful means of providing nutritional support. Endoscopic and nonendoscopic methods of placing gastrostomy tubes have been described (see *CVT XII*, p. 669 and also p. 84). If the cat cannot be safely anesthetized for placement of a gastrostomy tube, a nasoesophageal tube should be placed and a liquid, enteral nutrition product (e.g., CliniCare, Abbott Laboratories) used until the cat is stabilized.

A good quality, complete, balanced cat food of adequate nutrient density can be made into a gruel and administered via the gastrostomy tube (Table 3). If HE is present, any acid-base imbalance or potassium deficiency should be determined and corrected. A protein-restricted diet, such as intended for management of patients with chronic renal

TABLE 3. Guidelines for Tube Feeding Patients With Feline Idiopathic Hepatic Lipidosis

1. A kitchen blender, strainer, water, and a good quality complete and balanced cat food are needed to prepare an appropriate gruel for gastrostomy tube feeding. Combine one can cat food (e.g., one 5.5-ounce can CNM CV-Formula Feline Diet [Ralston Purina]) with one can water and blend together at high speed for 30 sec. Strain once through a kitchen strainer before administering through a 16F or larger feeding tube. Store under refrigeration. This example would supply the nutritional needs of a typical inactive cat for 1 day, including 20 gm protein, 12 gm fat and 0.6 gm potassium.
2. Always check placement and patency of gastrostomy feeding tube by passing 3 to 6 ml of sterile water first. If water leaks around the tube-skin site, do not proceed with feeding.
3. Introduce enteral feeding gradually, beginning with 50% of the daily energy needs, divided into four to six feedings. Gradually increase to 100% of calorie needs, divided into two to four feedings per day.
4. Enteral gruel diets should be fed between room and body temperature and should be administered slowly. The animal should be watched closely during feeding and for 10 to 15 minutes afterward for signs of nausea or vomiting.
5. Feed gruel diet exclusively for 1 to 2 weeks. Thereafter, offer fresh, palatable food before each feeding. Once the cat has voluntarily consumed at least 50% of its caloric needs for at least 3 consecutive days, tube feeding can be discontinued and the tube removed.

failure, may be needed until the encephalopathy can be resolved.

References and Suggested Reading

Laflamme DP, Allen SW, Huber TL: Apparent dietary protein requirements of dogs with portosystemic shunt. Am J Vet Res 54:719, 1993.
Research in dogs with surgically created portosystemic shunts.
Levinson MJ: A practical approach to nutritional support in liver disease. Gastroenterologist 3:234, 1995.
A review of the human medical approach to nutrition in cirrhotic patients.
Marks SL, Rogers QR, Strombeck D:. Nutritional support in hepatic disease. Part I. Metabolic alterations and nutritional considerations in dogs and cats. Compendium 16:971,1994.
A review of metabolic alterations in canine and feline liver patients.
Michel KE: Nutritional management of liver disease. Vet Clin North Am 25:485, 1995.
A review of the nutritional management of canine and feline liver patients.
Rolfe DS, Twedt DC: Copper-associated hepatopathies in dogs. Vet Clin North Am 25:399, 1995.
Review of the pathogenesis and treatment for this condition.
Swart GR, Zillikens MC, van Vuune JK, et al: Effect of late evening meal on nitrogen balance in patients with cirrhosis of the liver. Br Med J 299:1202, 1989.
A clinical trial showing benefit of frequent meals and bedtime snacks.

Canine Pancreatitis

DAVID A. WILLIAMS

JÖRG M. STEINER
College Station, Texas

Pancreatitis is a common disorder in dogs but, as in human patients, treatment of canine patients with pancreatitis is a challenge. This is in part related to the variation in severity and unpredictable course of pancreatitis as well as to the fact that the cause of pancreatitis remains elusive in many cases. The tremendous variation in pancreatic necrosis, and the degree of systemic involvement in particular, makes controlled studies to evaluate new therapeutic measures extremely difficult. Despite these limitations, many patients can be managed successfully based on existing knowledge of the pathophysiology of pancreatitis and clinical experience. For reviews of the etiology, pathogenesis, clinical features, and diagnosis, the reader is referred to reviews of this subject (Simpson, 1993; Williams, 1996).

The classification system for pancreatitis in humans has recently been updated (Bradley, 1993). Since there is no commonly accepted classification system currently in place in veterinary medicine, we employ the human system when possible. According to this classification system, acute pancreatitis is an acute inflammatory condition of the pancreas that, after removal of the inciting cause, is completely reversible. Pancreatic biopsy specimens do not show any signs of fibrosis. Chronic pancreatitis, conversely, is a longstanding inflammation of pancreatic tissue associated with irreversible histopathologic changes—most importantly, fibrosis and reduction in acinar cell mass. Both acute and chronic pancreatitis can be either mild or severe. The updated classification also defines pancreatic complications of pancreatitis such as infected necrosis and pseudocyst. Based on this classification system, this article discusses the treatment of severe pancreatitis, followed by the treatment of mild pancreatitis, and finally the treatment of pancreatic complications.

TREATMENT OF SEVERE PANCREATITIS

Severe pancreatitis is characterized by extensive pancreatic necrosis and multiple organ involvement (perhaps even organ failure) and is often associated with a poor prognosis. Severe pancreatitis can occur in patients with acute disease or as an exacerbation of chronic pancreatitis.

Removal of Inciting Cause

Unfortunately, the cause remains unknown in many cases of canine pancreatitis. However, every possible effort should be made to identify a cause and either remove or counteract it. Several causes and risk factors have been identified for pancreatitis in dogs.

Nutrition

There is much anecdotal but little scientific evidence that a fatty meal may cause pancreatitis. This may arise as a consequence of hyperlipoproteinemia and hypertriglyceridemia, factors that have been implicated in the genesis of pancreatitis in both humans and dogs. Therefore, a low-fat formula should be used for nutritional support independent of the route of administration, and certainly high-fat formulas should be avoided.

Toxins and Drugs

Drugs that either hyperstimulate pancreatic secretion or, conversely, block normal secretory mechanisms cause pancreatitis in experimental animals. Cholinesterase inhibitors and cholinergic agonists such as bethanechol have been associated with spontaneous pancreatitis. Potential exposure to organophosphates should be established in patients with suspected pancreatitis and further exposure avoided. Few cause-and-effect relationships between other drugs and pancreatitis have been conclusively demonstrated in humans or dogs because rechallenge with the drug in question cannot be justified for ethical reasons. Drugs used in veterinary medicine that have been implicated in causing pancreatitis in humans include thiazide diuretics, furosemide, estrogens, azathioprine, L-asparaginase, sulfonamides, tetracycline, metronidazole, cimetidine, ranitidine, acetaminophen, procainamide, and nitrofurantoin (Steinberg and Tenner, 1994). Corticosteroids do not appear to cause pancreatitis, although they do increase serum lipase activity (but decrease serum amylase activity) in dogs without causing pancreatitis. Corticosteroid therapy is of no proven benefit in pancreatitis and may be harmful in patients with severe pancreatitis. Therefore, the authors believe that corticosteroids should not be used, except in the treatment of severe shock.

Trauma and Hypoperfusion

Several cases of pancreatitis after traffic accidents and similar traumatic injuries have been reported. Surgical trauma has also been implicated as a cause of pancreatitis. However, evidence from the human literature as well as experimental data would suggest that hypoperfusion of the gland secondary to hypotensive states, such as may occur during anesthesia, rather than trauma to the pancreas per se is responsible for pancreatitis.

Other Causes

Hypercalcemia has been shown to cause pancreatitis in several species and should be rectified by appropriate management when identified. Pancreatitis can also occur in association with neoplastic infiltration by pancreatic adenocarcinoma.

Supportive Care

Aggressive fluid therapy is the mainstay of treatment for pancreatitis and must be individualized depending on the needs of the animal. The fluid rate chosen is dependent on the estimated degree of dehydration, estimated ongoing fluid losses in vomitus and diarrheic fluid, and the calculated daily maintenance rate. Careful attention to maintenance of a normal serum potassium concentration is particularly important because anorectic, vomiting patients with pancreatitis are particularly prone to hypokalemia. Although hypocalcemia is often noted, it is usually mild, and calcium supplementation should be reserved for those rare animals that manifest clinical signs in association with serum calcium concentrations less that 6.5 mg/dl. Acid-base imbalances are common in dogs with pancreatitis. Since either acidemia (most common) or alkalemia may develop, blind correction of suspected acid-base imbalance should not be attempted. Arterial blood pH, P_{CO2}, and bicarbonate should be measured.

Metabolic Support

It is still common practice to give nothing by mouth to human as well as veterinary patients with pancreatitis. This recommendation is sensible in patients that are vomiting. However, the importance of this therapeutic strategy remains scientifically unproved. The authors currently recommend withholding food and water from newly diagnosed patients for about 2 to 4 days. When vomiting ceases, small amounts of water can be offered several times per day. If vomiting does not recur, small amounts of a diet with a low-fat and moderate-protein content (rice, pasta, potatoes, or a commercial diet) can subsequently be given. If vomiting does not subside and oral feeding is withheld for more than 2 to 4 days, the nutritional needs of the patient has to be evaluated in order to decide whether alternative metabolic support is needed. If such support is thought to be desirable, jejunostomy tube placement has been recommended traditionally because of the minimal stimulation of exocrine pancreatic secretion that is likely when nutrients are given by this route. However, it is not known if mild to moderate stimulation of exocrine pancreatic secretion is truly harmful in patients with pancreatitis, and indeed there is some experimental evidence that mild stimulation may be beneficial. Total parenteral nutrition (see p. 80) is an alternative route for delivering nutrients but may be associated with other complications and should probably be reserved for animals with severe intractable vomiting. The authors have also found feeding via a gastrostomy tube to be a useful option in animals that do not vomit but refuse to eat.

Symptomatic Therapy

Analgesic Therapy

Some dogs with pancreatitis exhibit signs of extremely severe abdominal pain. Such patients need to be treated with analgesic agents such as meperidine hydrochloride (Demerol, Winthrop-Breon) at a dose of 5 to 10 mg/kg every 2 to 4 hours IM or SC or butorphanol tartrate (Torbutrol, Fort-Dodge) at a dose of 0.2 to 0.4 mg/kg every 6 hours SC.

Antiemetics

Antiemetics are not needed in most cases. Since cessation of vomiting is one sign of recovery from pancreatitis and an indicator that feeding may be reintroduced, antiemetic therapy should be considered only if vomiting is intractable or frequent. However, caution should be exercised when using antiemetics such as phenothiazine tranquilizers, which may induce hypotension that may be particularly harmful in patients with pancreatitis. Metoclopramide hydrochloride (Reglan, Robins) at a dose of 0.2 to 0.4 mg/kg every 6 to 8 hours IM or SC is a reasonable antiemetic of first choice.

Other Symptomatic Measures

Release of trypsin and other inappropriately activated digestive proteases and phospholipases into the blood may lead to a multitude of systemic complications, such as pulmonary edema, respiratory failure, cardiac arrhythmias, hypotension, acute renal failure, central neurologic deficits, disseminated intravascular coagulation, and multiorgan failure (see CVT XII, p. 12). All these potentially life-threatening conditions are poor prognostic signs that must be treated aggressively once they occur.

Plasma Therapy

Alpha₂-macroglobulin, one of the scavenger proteins for activated proteases in plasma, is depleted rapidly in severe pancreatitis, with resultant uninhibited protease activity leading to acute disseminated intravascular coagulation, hypotensive shock, and death. Fresh frozen plasma not only replenishes alpha₂-macroglobulin but also supplies albumin, which has several beneficial effects, including maintenance of plasma oncotic pressure. The authors therefore recommend daily treatment with fresh frozen plasma (50 to 250 ml), unless there are specific contraindications, until the patient is improving.

Antibiotic Therapy

There is no evidence to support routine antibiotic therapy in canine patients with pancreatitis, and given the lack of reports of septic complications of pancreatitis in dogs, it would seem unlikely that such therapy would be of value. Although such complications are a major cause of death in human patients several weeks after the onset of pancreatitis, this pattern of disease does not appear to occur in dogs. Inappropriate antibiotic therapy may actually increase the risk of antibiotic-resistant infections, so the authors do not recommend routine antibiotic treatment. If an infectious complication is suspected, efforts should be made to identify the causative organism before initiating treatment with an appropriate broad-spectrum antibiotic agent. Enrofloxacin (Baytril, Bayer) at a dose of 2.5 mg/kg every 12 hours IM is a suitable antibiotic that has been shown to penetrate well into canine pancreas.

Other Treatment Strategies

Anti-inflammatory Drugs

There is no evidence to support the usefulness of corticosteroids or nonsteroidal anti-inflammatory drugs in the treatment of canine pancreatitis, and corticosteroids have not been conclusively excluded as a cause of pancreatitis. Treatment with corticosteroids should therefore be reserved for use in cases of severe shock and should be used only for a short time in concert with other aggressive supportive measures. Recent studies in human patients have indicated that antagonists of inflammatory mediators, such as the platelet activating factor antagonist lexipafant, hold some promise for the future.

Protease Inhibitors

The value of protease inhibitors such as aprotinin (Trasylol, Bayer) in pancreatitis is supported by experimental data in dogs. Clinical trials in human patients led to disappointing results, however, perhaps because of the far greater potency of aprotinin in dogs than in humans. The authors currently do not use aprotinin because of its prohibitive cost, but experimental data would support the use of a dose of 250 mg (1.5 × 10⁶ kallikrein inhibitory units [KIU]) per dog by intraperitoneal injection every 6 to 8 hours. Some veterinary textbooks report the use of 5000 KIU/kg IV every 6 hours, but intraperitoneal administration

is preferable. Other protease inhibitors, such as the synthetic products gabexate mesylate and nafamostat mesylate, have also shown promise in experimentally produced pancreatitis in dogs but are not readily available for clinical use.

Selenium

In a recent report, there were only three deaths (18%) of 17 canine patients with pancreatitis treated with standard supportive care and supplemented with selenium (0.1 mg/kg selenium every 24 hours by IV infusion, equivalent to 0.3 mg/kg selenious acid or sodium selenite) compared with seven deaths (54%) in a group of 13 historical control patients that did not receive selenium (Kraft et al, 1995). These are small numbers, and retrospective controls cannot be used to assess therapy, but this method of treatment merits further investigation, including prospective clinical trials. To the authors' knowledge, the only injectable selenium preparation available in the United States is selenious acid at a concentration of 40 μg/ml (supplied by many manufacturers, including American Regent and McGuff.

Miscellaneous Treatment Strategies

Many other treatment strategies have been evaluated in human or veterinary patients with pancreatitis. Antisecretory agents, such as anticholinergics, calcitonin, and glucagon have all failed to show any beneficial effect. Nasogastric suctioning and inhibition of gastric acid secretion also have not proved effective. Somatostatin has shown promise in reducing complications in human patients with pancreatitis, but its use has not been reported in veterinary patients. Peritoneal lavage may also be beneficial in those few patients with marked accumulations of peritoneal fluid because it removes significant amounts of active pancreatic enzymes, reducing the burden on the plasma protease inhibitor system.

TREATMENT OF MILD PANCREATITIS

Mild pancreatitis is associated with minimal pancreatic necrosis and few systemic effects and is usually followed by complete recovery. It is likely that many animals recover spontaneously without medical intervention after a few days of mild depression and inappetence. However, some animals present with repeated signs of vomiting, abdominal discomfort, and depression, with evidence of either recurrent acute or chronic pancreatitis. Such animals may ultimately acquire diabetes mellitus or exocrine pancreatic insufficiency if sufficient pancreatic tissue is destroyed. Unfortunately, although management of these last two conditions is well documented, little is known about treatment of mild chronic pancreatitis and prevention of progression toward end-stage disease. As with acute pancreatitis, an effort should be made to identify the cause and rectify it if possible. It should be remembered that miniature schnauzers commonly exhibit hypertriglyceridemia or chronic pancreatitis, or both. If serum triglyceride concentrations are increased, feeding a low-fat diet may help reduce triglyceride levels and improve clinical signs. Chronic abdominal pain is one of the most important problems in human patients with chronic pancreatitis and may affect some canine patients as well (Steer et al, 1995). If pain is suspected, the animal can be given 0.5 to 2 tsp of dried pancreatic extract (Viokase, Fort-Dodge or Pancreozyme, Daniels) with each meal on a trial basis for 1 to 2 months. Although these patients do not have exocrine pancreatic insufficiency and do not require enzyme replacement for digestive purposes, the feedback effect of digestive proteases within the gut lumen appears to reduce the drive on pancreatic secretion and perhaps reduce the pancreatitis-associated discomfort.

TREATMENT OF PANCREATIC COMPLICATIONS

Pancreatic complications of pancreatitis are acute fluid accumulations around the inflamed pancreas (previously known also as pancreatic phlegmon), infected necrosis, pancreatic pseudocyst, and pancreatic abscess.

Acute Fluid Accumulation

Acute accumulation of small amounts of fluid in the region of the pancreas is common in canine pancreatitis. There is still controversy as to whether there is any benefit in draining larger amounts of fluid that are localized to the peripancreatic region, as long as it is sterile. Ultrasonographically guided aspiration of this fluid for culture should be attempted if an infectious complication is suspected.

Infected Necrosis

Some authors consider cases of infected necrosis in human patients a clear indication for surgical intervention, consisting of removal of necrotic tissue, copious lavage of the pancreatic region, and drainage of the area concurrent with aggressive antibiotic management. However, the authors are not aware of any reports of infected necrosis in dogs, suggesting that this complication, if it occurs at all in dogs, is rare. Increased use of ultrasonographically guided needle aspiration may change this clinical impression in the future.

Pancreatic Pseudocyst

A pancreatic pseudocyst is a collection of sterile pancreatic juice, enclosed by fibrous or granulation tissue. Pancreatic pseudocysts in humans are treated by surgical correc-

tion when the pseudocysts enlarge or do not regress. Successful surgical intervention has also been reported for a dog with a pancreatic pseudocyst and may be considered in canine patients in which pseudocysts fail to regress.

Pancreatic Abscess

A pancreatic abscess is a collection of pus with little or no pancreatic necrosis, occurring most commonly in close proximity to the pancreas; it can be either sterile or infected. Pancreatic abscess has been described as a complication of pancreatitis in humans and dogs, although reports of infected canine pancreatic abscess are rare. Surgical intervention with removal of the abscess, copious lavage, drainage, and aggressive antibiotic therapy are the treatments of choice in humans as well as dogs with pancreatic abscess (Salisbury et al, 1988).

References and Suggested Reading

Banks PA: Medical management of acute pancreatitis and complications. In: Go VLW, DiMagno EP, Gardner JD, et al, eds: The Pancreas: Biology, Pathobiology and Disease, 2nd ed. New York: Raven Press, 1993, p 593.
Comprehensive review of the treatment of acute pancreatitis in humans.
Bradley EL: A clinically based classification system for acute pancreatitis. Arch Surg 128:586, 1993.
Summary of the classification system for pancreatitis in humans agreed on at an international symposium.
Kraft W, Kaimaz A, Kirsch M, et al: Behandlung akuter Pankreatiden des Hundes mit Selen. Kleintierpraxis 40:35, 1995.
Study (written in German) reporting beneficial effects of selenium in the treatment of dogs with severe pancreatitis.
Salisbury SK, Lantz GC, Nelson RW, et al: Pancreatic abscess in dogs: Six cases (1978–1986). J Am Vet Med Assoc 193:1104, 1988.
Case reports of six dogs with pancreatic abscess.
Simpson KW: Current concepts of the pathogenesis and pathophysiology of acute pancreatitis in the dog and cat. Comp Cont Ed Pract Vet 15:247, 1993.
Brief review of the etiology and pathophysiology of pancreatitis in dogs and cats.
Steer ML, Waxman I, Freedman S: Medical progress: Chronic pancreatitis. N Engl J Med 332:1482, 1995.
Review of classification, etiology, diagnosis, and treatment of chronic pancreatitis in humans.
Steinberg W, Tenner S: Medical progress: Acute pancreatitis. N Engl J Med 330:1198, 1994.
Review of the epidemiology, etiology, diagnosis, and treatment of acute pancreatitis in human patients, summarizing many studies of novel therapeutic measures.
Williams DA: The pancreas. In: Strombeck DR, Guilford WG, Center SA, et al, eds: Small Animal Gastroenterology, 3rd ed. Philadelphia: WB Saunders, 1996, p 381.
Comprehensive discussion of exocrine pancreatic disease in the dog and cat.

Feline F ... eatic Disease

The incidence of exocrin
tionally been considered l
large retrospective study (
of 6,504 feline pancreat:
lesions. In contrast, of 1
nary Medical Data Ba
year period, only 1,07
crine pancreatic disc
cats suffer from d'
quently, these disor

PANCREATITIS

Classification

There hav(
velop a simp'
ley, 1993). ?
nary medic
system wl
tory cond
after rer
pancrea
change
and a(
of p:
necr
oft(
as'
o'

... pancreatitis. Traumatic pancreatitis (resulting ... affic accidents or falls from heights) has been re- ... . Infectious agents have been shown to cause feline ... creatitis, with the strongest evidence for a causal rela- ...ship for *Toxoplasma gondii* and rare cases of *Amphi- ...rus pseudofelineus* infestation. Weaker evidence has ...een presented for feline parvovirus infections in kittens ...nd infections with feline herpesvirus I and feline infec- ...ious peritonitis virus. Two cases of feline pancreatitis after topical use of fenthion, an organophosphate cholinesterase inhibitor, have been reported. Many other pharmaceutical compounds have been implicated in causing pancreatitis in humans and dogs (see preceding article), including azathio- prine, chlorothiazide, hydrochlorothiazide, estrogens, furo- semide, tetracycline, sulfonamides, L-asparaginase, 6-mer- captopurine, methyldopa, pentamidine, nitrofurantoin, dideoxyinosine, valproic acid, and procainamide; however, no cases have been reported in the cat. Cholangitis and cholangiohepatitis may coexist in feline patients with pan- creatitis, but there is no evidence that they play a causative role. Finally, more than 90% of all cases of feline pancreati- tis are idiopathic.

:-
d-
:ri-
.ion
.ıma-
rsible
.hronic
.ıthologic
.ıly fibrosis
Mild forms
pancreatic
.f the patient
.ıcreatitis are
.osıs and multiple
.ıor prognosis.

Clinical Picture and Diagnosis

Clinical signs in cats with pancreatitis are nonspecific. In a recent report of 40 cats with severe pancreatitis, lethargy was reported in 100% of cases, anorexia in 97%, dehydration in 92%, hypothermia in 68%, vomiting in 35%, abdominal pain in 25%, a palpable abdominal mass in 23%, dyspnea in 20%, ataxia in 15%, and diarrhea in 15% (Hill and Van Winkle, 1993). Especially remarkable is the *low incidence* of vomiting and abdominal pain, both of which are common clinical signs in human and canine pancreatitis patients. Other clinical signs, such as polypha- gia, constipation, fever, icterus, polyuria, polydipsia, and adipsia have also been reported. Concurrent conditions, including hepatic lipidosis, inflammatory bowel disease, interstitial nephritis, diabetes mellitus, and cholangiohepa- titis, occur frequently (Akol et al, 1993).

A complete blood count and serum chemistry profile often show mild and nonspecific changes. Serum activities of lipase and amylase are within the reference ranges in most cases. Radiographic changes seen in some cases in- clude a decreased contrast in the cranial abdomen and displacement of the duodenum laterally and dorsally, the stomach to the left, and the transverse colon caudally. Abdominal ultrasonography is useful in the diagnosis of feline pancreatitis. Changes identified include pancreatic swelling, increased echogenicity of the pancreas, fluid ac- cumulation around the pancreas and, less frequently, a mass effect in the area of the pancreas. Abdominal computed

...ıtal pancreatitis in cats ...ıe generally accepted hy- ...cells ultimately respond in ... of harmful stimuli. Briefly, ...tion of pancreatic enzymes is followec ... abnormal cytoplasmic vacuoles in which the co... of lysosomes and zymogen granules co-localize. This leads to an inappropriate intracellular acti- vation of trypsin and subsequently of other digestive zymo- gens. These activated digestive enzymes lead to local ef- fects, such as inflammation, hemorrhage, acinar cell necrosis, and peripancreatic fat necrosis. Digestive en- zymes released into the blood stream may cause systemic effects, including systemic inflammatory changes, systemic vasodilatation leading to hypotension, pulmonary edema, disseminated intravascular coagulation, central neurologic deficits, respiratory failure, renal failure, and even multi- organ failure.

Several diseases and risk factors have been associated

tomography is a routine procedure in humans suspected of having pancreatitis, and although it would likely be of great benefit in the diagnosis of feline pancreatitis, it is currently only rarely used.

A radioimmunoassay for the measurement of serum trypsin-like immunoreactivity in feline serum (fTLI), currently only available through the authors' laboratory, has been evaluated as a diagnostic tool for feline pancreatitis. Initial data suggest an increase in serum fTLI in many cats with pancreatitis (Steiner and Williams, 1996). Assays for trypsinogen-activation peptide and for trypsin-alpha$_1$-protease inhibitor complexes may aid in the diagnosis of feline pancreatitis in the future.

A definitive diagnosis of feline pancreatitis can be made by pancreatic biopsy at exploratory laparotomy or laparoscopy. Although pancreatic biopsy per se is safe, this intervention is expensive and may be contraindicated in some patients because of high anesthetic risk.

Therapy

Supportive Therapy

Whenever possible, the inciting cause should be removed. Exposure to unnecessary drugs, especially those implicated in causing pancreatitis, should be avoided. Aggressive fluid therapy is the mainstay of supportive therapy. Fluid, electrolyte, and acid-base imbalances need to be assessed and corrected as early as possible.

Alimentation

The traditional recommendation for any animal with pancreatitis is to give nothing by mouth for 3 to 4 days. This recommendation is justified in animals that vomit, but there is little evidence to justify this strategy in those that do not. This issue is complicated further by the fact that cats with pancreatitis often have concurrent hepatic lipidosis (Akol et al, 1993). The authors think that the proven benefit of nutritional support for cats with hepatic lipidosis overrides the notion to withhold food from patients with pancreatitis. The preferred route of alimentation is a jejunostomy tube. However, a jejunostomy tube is impractical in many cases, and a gastrostomy tube or even a nasogastric tube is an acceptable alternative (see p. 84) if the patient does not vomit. However, if the cat vomits and if there is no evidence to support concurrent hepatic lipidosis, the cat should be given nothing by mouth for 3 to 4 days. After this time, water is reintroduced slowly, followed by small amounts of a carbohydrate-rich, low-fat diet (e.g., Purina CNM OM-formula or Hill's feline w/d). A low-fat diet suitable for tube feeding is outlined in Table 1.

Analgesia

Even though abdominal pain is uncommon in cats with pancreatitis, the patient should be carefully evaluated for abdominal discomfort. If abdominal pain is thought to be present, analgesic drugs are indicated. Meperidine (Demerol, Winthrop-Breon) at a dose of 1 to 2 mg/kg every 2 to 4 hours can be given IM or SC. Butorphanol tartrate (Torbutrol, or Torbugesic, both Fort-Dodge) at a dose of

TABLE 1. Low-Fat Diet Suitable for Tube Feeding Cats With Pancreatitis

Vital (Ross)	One package
Promod (Ross)	2 tbsp
Arginine*	500 mg
Taurine*	500 mg
Choline*†	350 mg
Liquid vitamin B supplement	1–2 ml

Reconstitute the Vital low-fat elemental diet with 355 ml (12 ounces) of water (to prevent excessive hyperosmolality) and add the remaining ingredients. The final solution contains 0.87 kcal/ml. The diet as prepared is still hyperosmolar, and patients are prone to the development of diarrhea.

*Available from health food stores.
†Optional ingredient in cats with concurrent hepatic lipidosis.
Information courtesy of Dr. Kathy Michel, Veterinary Hospital of the University of Pennsylvania.

0.2 to 0.4 mg/kg every 6 hours given subcutaneously can be used alternatively.

Plasma

Studies in dogs suggest that when alpha$_2$-macroglobulin, one of the scavenger proteins for activated proteases in serum, is depleted, death ensues rapidly. Fresh frozen plasma (FFP) or fresh whole blood not only contains alpha$_2$-macroglobulin but also albumin, which has many beneficial effects in patients with pancreatitis. Unfortunately, a clinical trial in human pancreatitis patients failed to show a benefit of plasma. However, because of the authors' own experience and anecdotal reports of beneficial effects of FFP in canine patients with pancreatitis, we recommend the use of FFP or fresh whole blood in cats with severe pancreatitis.

Antibiotic Therapy

There is no evidence to recommend the routine use of antibiotic agents in cats with pancreatitis. Even though several recent articles suggest an increased survival of human pancreatitis patients with early antibiotic intervention, careful examination of these studies reveal that only a small subset of patients benefit from antibiotic intervention, namely, patients with infectious complications. However, judged by necropsy results, infectious complications are rare in cats with pancreatitis. The authors do not recommend the routine use of antibiotics. However, in the rare instance when infectious complications are identified, efforts should be made to identify the agent and the patient should be treated with a broad-spectrum antibiotic therapeutic agent.

Anti-inflammatory Agents

There are no data on the use of anti-inflammatory agents in cats with severe pancreatitis. No benefit was found in human patients. In cats with severe pancreatitis, corticosteroids should be used only in cases of secondary cardiovascular shock. However, corticosteroids may be needed to treat cats with inflammatory bowel disease and concurrent mild chronic pancreatitis, and they do not appear to be harmful in these patients.

Dopamine

Dopamine has been shown to have beneficial effects in experimental cases of feline pancreatitis when given in the first 12 hours after induction. There was no beneficial effect when given after 12 hours. In addition, dopamine must be used carefully in patients with cardiac arrhythmias and may also cause nausea, vomiting, and seizures. Therefore, it cannot be recommended for routine use in feline patients with pancreatitis.

Other Therapeutic Strategies

Many other therapeutic strategies, such as the administration of trypsin-inhibitors (e.g., Trasylol), antacids, antisecretory agents (i.e., anticholinergics, calcitonin, glucagon, somatostatin), or selenium and peritoneal lavage all have been evaluated in human patients with pancreatitis (see preceding article). With the exception of selenium, none of these strategies has shown any beneficial effect at this point and should therefore be avoided until evidence for their usefulness is provided. The efficacy of selenium should be evaluated in cats with pancreatitis.

It should also be remembered that many cats have mild forms of chronic pancreatitis. Often, these cats have concurrent conditions, most notably inflammatory bowel disease. Little is known about appropriate therapy for these animals, and management is often limited to evaluation and treatment of the concurrent condition as well as close monitoring of the pancreatitis.

Prognosis

The prognosis for cats with severe pancreatitis is directly related to the severity of the disease, the extent of pancreatic necrosis, the occurrence of systemic and pancreatic complications, the duration of the condition, and the presence of concurrent disease.

EXOCRINE PANCREATIC INSUFFICIENCY

Exocrine pancreatic insufficiency (EPI) is a syndrome caused by insufficient synthesis and secretion of digestive enzymes by the exocrine portion of the pancreas, leading to insufficient activity of digestive enzymes in the lumen of the small intestine (Williams, 1994).

Etiology and Pathogenesis

As in human patients, chronic pancreatitis is the most common cause of EPI in the cat. Other, less commonly observed causes are *Eurytrema procyonis* infestation and idiopathic acinar atrophy. Most of the functional capacity of the exocrine portion of the pancreas has to be lost for clinical signs to develop. The lack of digestive enzymes in the duodenum leads to maldigestion. In addition, however, there are secondary disturbances of intestinal mucosal transport mechanisms. Altogether these changes lead to

voluminous soft stools, steatorrhea, and weight loss. Decreased assimilation of fat may also lead to hypovitaminoses of fat-soluble vitamins.

Clinical Picture and Diagnosis

Cats with EPI often present with a chronic history of polyphagia, diarrhea, and weight loss. The high fat content in the feces can lead to a greasy appearance of the hair coat, especially in the perineal and tail region. The complete blood count, serum chemistry profile, and urinalysis are almost always within the reference range. Abdominal radiographs and abdominal ultrasonography also do not reveal any abnormalities in most cases. The most reliable test for the diagnosis of EPI in the cat is the newly developed radioimmunoassay for fTLI (Steiner et al, 1996). The control range for this assay is 17 to 49 μg/L, and values of less than or equal to 8 μg/L are consistent with EPI (Steiner and Williams, 1996). Cats with EPI commonly have depleted body stores of cobalamin and less frequently of folate. Serum cobalamin and folate concentrations should therefore be determined in all cats with suspected EPI.

Management

Pancreatic Enzyme Supplementation

As in dogs, pancreatic enzyme supplementation is the mainstay of therapy for cats with EPI. Dried powdered extracts of bovine or porcine pancreas can be used. Initially 1 tsp, mixed into the meal should be given twice daily (Viokase, Fort-Dodge or Pancrezyme, Daniels). If the cat refuses to eat food with pancreatic extract, the enzymes can be packed into gelatin capsules, or raw beef or pork pancreas can be given. One to 3 ounces (30 to 90 gm) of chopped raw pancreas (can be kept frozen for a long time without losing enzymatic activity) is given with each meal initially. If the cat also refuses to eat raw pancreas, a fish-based liquid formulation of the enzyme supplement can be prepared; this is readily taken by most cats. Tablets, capsules, and enteric-coated products should be avoided. Pre-incubation of the food with pancreatic enzymes, supplementation with bile salts, or concurrent antacid therapy is unnecessary. After clinical signs have resolved, the dose of pancreas extract can be decreased gradually until a minimal effective dose has been reached. This dose differs among cats and may also change with different batches of the pancreatic supplement.

Dietary Considerations

Unfortunately, fat digestion does not normalize with enzyme supplementation because some of the lipase in the supplement is irreversibly denatured by the low pH in the feline stomach. A diet particularly low in fat can further deprive the animal of essential fatty acids and fat-soluble vitamins and should be avoided. Because some types of dietary fiber interfere with pancreatic enzyme activity, diets high in fiber should also be avoided. Any high quality maintenance diet is a good choice for cats with EPI.

Vitamin Supplementation

Most cats with EPI are severely cobalamin-deficient. Some of these cats do not respond well to enzyme supplementation until cobalamin is also supplemented. Initially 100 to 250 μg of cobalamin (cyanocobalamin injection, Elkins-Sinn, Goldline, and others) is given subcutaneously once a week. After a couple of months of treatment, the serum concentration of cobalamin should be rechecked and, if it has normalized, the dosing schedule can be changed to monthly, then bimonthly, and finally to every 6 months, with annual serum cobalamin and folate determinations.

Treatment of Concurrent Conditions

Hypovitaminoses of fat-soluble vitamins are uncommon but have been reported and should be anticipated as potential complications. Hypovitaminosis K can be especially life-threatening. Some cats with EPI do not respond appropriately to enzyme and cobalamin supplementation. Many of these cats have concurrent inflammatory bowel disease, as evidenced by decreased serum folate concentrations, and must be evaluated and treated appropriately for this condition. Finally, some cats with EPI have concurrent diabetes mellitus and need to be managed accordingly.

Prognosis

EPI is associated with an irreversible loss of pancreatic acinar tissue in most cases, and complete recovery is therefore improbable. However, with appropriate management and monitoring, these patients usually gain weight quickly, pass normal stools, and can go on to live a normal life for a normal life span.

EXOCRINE PANCREATIC NEOPLASIA

Pancreatic adenomas are benign tumors of the exocrine pancreas. Pancreatic adenocarcinoma is the most common malignant neoplastic condition of the exocrine pancreas in the cat (Andrews, 1987). A few cases of spindle cell sarcoma and lymphosarcoma have also been reported in feline patients.

Pathogenesis

Pancreatic adenomas are usually subclinical but may lead to clinical signs because of the transposition of other abdominal organs. In addition to transposition of abdominal organs, pancreatic adenocarcinomas can also lead to obstruction of the pancreatic duct and acinar atrophy, tumor necrosis followed by clinical signs of pancreatitis, and also clinical signs related to dysfunction of other organs due to metastatic disease.

Clinical Signs and Diagnosis

The presentation of feline patients with exocrine pancreatic neoplasia is nonspecific. In a case series of 58 cases, clinical signs most commonly reported were anorexia in 46%, weight loss in 37%, lethargy in 28%, vomiting in 23%, icterus in 14%, constipation in 9%, and diarrhea in 3% (Andrews, 1987). Clinical signs reported in other cases include polyuria, steatorrhea, fever, dehydration, and a distended cranial abdomen. Finally, clinical signs related to metastatic lesions, such as dyspnea, lameness, bone pain, or alopecia, may also be observed.

Routine blood test results are usually unremarkable. Serum lipase and amylase activities have been reported in only a few cases and have only rarely been elevated. Radiographic findings are also nonspecific in most cases. Ultrasonographic examination of the abdomen is helpful in these cats. A soft tissue mass can be identified in most cases in the region of the pancreas, but continuation with pancreatic tissue can rarely be demonstrated conclusively. Even though most pancreatic adenocarcinomas exfoliate poorly into the peritoneal fluid, peritoneal effusion, if present, should be aspirated and evaluated cytologically. Fine-needle aspiration or transcutaneous biopsy under ultrasonographic guidance can be attempted when suspicious masses are identified; however, the lack of exfoliation decreases the level of success of fine-needle aspiration. Overall, the final diagnosis in most cases is made at exploratory laparotomy or even at necropsy examination.

Therapy and Prognosis

Pancreatic adenomas are benign and theoretically do not need to be treated unless they cause clinical signs. However, the final distinction between pancreatic adenoma and adenocarcinoma is often made at exploratory laparotomy, and a partial pancreatectomy should be performed at that time, even in cases of pancreatic adenoma. The prognosis in these cases is excellent.

Pancreatic adenocarcinomas often present at a late stage of the disease. Metastatic disease has been reported to occur in 81% of cats with pancreatic adenocarcinoma at the time of diagnosis. In the few cases in which metastatic lesions are not identified at the time of diagnosis, surgical resection of the adenocarcinoma can be attempted. However, owners should be forewarned that clean surgical margins are only rarely achieved. Total pancreatectomy and pancreaticoduodenectomy, although theoretically possible, have not been described in cats. Extrapolation from experimental animals and from human patients suggests high morbidity and mortality for these procedures. Also, the complicated postsurgical lifelong management of EPI and diabetes mellitus make this procedure less than desirable. Chemotherapy or radiation therapy have shown little success in humans or veterinary patients with pancreatic adenocarcinomas. Overall, the prognosis for cats with pancreatic adenocarcinoma is grave.

PANCREATIC BLADDER

A pancreatic bladder is an abnormal extension of the pancreatic duct that forms a sac. Only a few feline cases have been described in the literature. These cats presented with clinical signs compatible with biliary duct obstruction. Appropriate management has not been studied, but surgical reconstruction may be most suitable in cats presenting with clinical signs.

PANCREATIC PARASITES

Eurytrema procyonis

The pancreatic fluke of the cat, *Eurytrema procyonis*, has been found in pancreatic ducts of cats, foxes, and raccoons. The parasites can lead to ductular thickening and fibrosis of acinar tissue. A significant decrease of pancreatic secretions has been shown in some cases. However, clinical signs of EPI in cats infested with *Eurytrema procyonis* are rare. Diagnosis is made by identification of eggs in fresh feces. Fenbendazole (Panacur, Hoechst) at a dose of 30 mg/kg PO once a day has been recommended for 6 consecutive days.

Amphimerus pseudofelineus

The hepatic fluke of the cat, *Amphimerus pseudofelineus,* can also infest the pancreas and can cause pancreatitis. Diagnosis is possible by identification of eggs on fecal examination by formalin–ethyl acetate sedimentation. In one clinical report, treatment with praziquantel (Droncit, Bayer), 40 mg/kg PO once daily for 3 consecutive days was successful. However, it should be noted that this dose is extremely high.

PANCREATIC PSEUDOCYST

Pancreatic pseudocyst, a collection of sterile pancreatic juice enclosed by fibrous or granulation tissue, is a recognized complication of pancreatitis in human patients and has recently been documented in a cat (Hines et al, 1996). Clinical signs observed in the cat were similar to those in cats with pancreatitis. Abdominal ultrasonography revealed a cystic structure in close proximity to the left lobe of the pancreas. Pancreatic pseudocysts in humans are treated by surgical correction when the pseudocyst enlarges or does not regress. Surgical intervention was also successful in the management of the cat reported.

PANCREATIC ABSCESS

A pancreatic abscess is a collection of pus with little or no pancreatic necrosis, most commonly in close proximity to the pancreas. Pancreatic abscess has been described as a complication of pancreatitis in humans and dogs but not in cats. However, the authors are aware of one feline patient with pancreatic abscess confirmed by histopathologic examination. Surgical intervention and aggressive antibiotic therapy are the treatments of choice in humans and dogs with pancreatic abscess, and such therapy was successful in treating the cat mentioned.

References and Suggested Reading

Akol KG, Washabau RJ, Saunders HM, et al: Acute pancreatitis in cats with hepatic lipidosis. J Vet Intern Med 7:205, 1993.
Case series of cats with hepatic lipidosis suffering from concurrent pancreatitis.
Andrews LK: Tumors of the exocrine pancreas. In: Holzworth J, ed: Diseases of the Cat. Philadelphia: WB Saunders, 1987, p 505.
Largest case series of cats with exocrine pancreatic neoplasia.
Bradley EL: A clinically based classification system for acute pancreatitis. Arch Surg 128:586, 1993.
Summary of the classification system for pancreatitis in humans agreed on at the International Symposium on Acute Pancreatitis in Atlanta, GA in 1992.
Hill RC, Van Winkle TJ: Acute necrotizing pancreatitis and acute suppurative pancreatitis in the cat. A retrospective study of 40 cases (1976–1989). J Vet Intern Med 7:25, 1993.
Largest case series of well-documented cases of feline pancreatitis.
Hines BL, Salisbury SK, Jakovljevic S, et al: Pancreatic pseudocyst associated with chronic-active necrotizing pancreatitis in a cat. J Am Anim Hosp Assoc 32:147, 1996.
The only report of a case of pancreatic pseudocyst in a cat.
Steiner JM, Williams DA: Feline trypsin-like immunoreactivity in feline exocrine pancreatic disease. Comp Cont Educ Pract Vet 18:543, 1996.
Summary of the current knowledge about the usefulness of fTLI in the diagnosis of exocrine pancreatic disorders in cats.
Steiner JM, Medinger TL, Williams DA: Development and validation of a radioimmunoassay for feline trypsin-like immunoreactivity (fTLI). Am J Vet Res 57:1417, 1996.
Report about the only immunoassay available to determine trypsin-like immunoreactivity in the cat.
Williams DA: Feline exocrine pancreatic insufficiency. In: Kirk RW, Bonagura JD, ed: Current Veterinary Therapy XII. Philadelphia: WB Saunders, 1994.
Comprehensive and still current discussion of EPI in cats.
Williams DA: Exocrine pancreatic disease. In: Strombeck DR, Guilford WG, Center SA, et al, ed: Small Animal Gastroenterology, 3rd ed. Philadelphia: WB Saunders, 1996, p 381.
Comprehensive and in-depth discussion of disorders of the exocrine pancreas in dogs and cats.

Cardiopulmonary Diseases

BRUCE W. KEENE
LINDA B. LEHMKUHL

Consulting Editors

Uses of Computed Tomography in Cardiopulmonary Disease

Amy S. Tidwell

North Grafton, Massachusetts

BACKGROUND

Computed tomography (CT) is an effective, noninvasive method of imaging the thorax. In humans, the use of CT to evaluate the mediastinum, pleural cavity, and chest wall is widely accepted. The role of CT in cardiopulmonary disease, however, is less clear and appears to be rapidly evolving as CT technology continues to improve. Historically, conventional CT scanners were ill-suited for imaging of the heart because scan times were too slow to prevent blurring from cardiac motion. Furthermore, the inability to resolve this motion made the assessment of cardiac function impossible. Likewise, CT images of the lung suffered from inadequate detail and from motion blurring due to patient respiration. Even with breath-holding techniques, inconsistent filling of the lungs from one CT slice to the next caused small lesions to be missed. Gradual improvements in scanning parameters and innovations such as dynamic scanning, electrocardiographic (ECG) gating, and high-resolution techniques (known as high-resolution CT or HRCT) eventually made CT of the heart and lungs feasible. However, it was only after the introduction and continued clinical application of state-of-the-art spiral (helical) and electron-beam (ultrafast or cine) technology that CT began to assume an essential role in the diagnosis of cardiopulmonary disease.

Few veterinarians currently have access to spiral or electron-beam CT scanners. The use of CT in cardiopulmonary disease in animals will not surpass that of radiography or ultrasonography. Nevertheless, animals may benefit from conventional CT of the heart and lungs in some circumstances, especially if dynamic scanning modes and HRCT are available. This article examines the clinical indications of conventional CT in the evaluation of cardiopulmonary disease in animals. Clinical and research applications of spiral (Costello, 1995) and electron-beam CT (Skorton et al, 1996) are briefly discussed in an attempt to illustrate the profound potential of CT for imaging the heart and lungs.

COMPUTED TOMOGRAPHY OF THE HEART

Imaging patients with cardiac disorders begins with plain thoracic radiographs followed by an echocardiogram. Unlike cardiac CT, echocardiography does not require anesthesia or the use of iodinated contrast medium and is not restricted to one imaging plane or window. The heart's orientation does not conform to the transverse plane of the body; thus, true short- and long-axis images of the heart are not readily obtained during CT, making assessment of chamber size and wall thickness difficult. Furthermore, CT does not depict the heart and its motion in real-time and therefore cannot confer the types of functional data derived from echocardiography.

Despite advances in echocardiographic techniques, such as Doppler imaging and the use of microbubble contrast agents, occasionally echocardiography does not provide a definitive diagnosis. Computed tomography may prove useful when the echocardiographic window to some or all of the heart is suboptimal because of a congenital deformity or trauma to the thoracic wall, pneumothorax, or severe lung hyperinflation. Even with an appropriate acoustic window, the full extent of some paracardiac abnormalities such as heart base masses or pericardial thickening may not be depicted with echocardiography. Likewise, diagnosis of some complex congenital heart diseases or vascular anomalies may require the use of routine CT or CT angiocardiography.

The performance of CT cardiac applications is highly dependent on the capabilities of the scanner. The walls of the heart and the blood within the chambers cannot be discerned without the use of iodinated contrast medium. In order to minimize motion blurring and optimize contrast medium concentration, scanning should be performed at as rapid a rate as possible. Many conventional scanners can acquire up to 8 to 12 scans/min using a dynamic scanning mode. The cardiac chambers and walls, the interventricular septum, and the great vessels should be consistently visualized; individual heart valves, however, will be less appreciable. Paracardiac masses do not opacify on early postcontrast images, distinguishing them from focal cardiac or vascular bulges. In the author's experience, visualization of the normal pericardium is inconsistent and relies on the presence of an adequate amount of underlying epicardial fat. The thickness of the normal pericardium should be no more than 1 to 2 mm. The identification of gross pericardial thickening or rare calcification may be used to support a clinical diagnosis of constrictive pericarditis when echocardiographic findings are equivocal.

Electron-beam CT scanners produce simultaneous, ECG-triggered images of multiple anatomic levels of the heart at subsecond (e.g., 50 msec) speeds. By manipulating the position of the patient relative to the scanning plane, true short- and long-axis images of the heart can be "frozen" at multiple points in the cardiac cycle with minimal loss of detail, thus allowing for both qualitative and quantitative assessment of cardiac anatomy and function. Current clinical and investigational applications in humans include assessment of ventricular mass and thickness, cardiac chamber volume, ventricular function, myocardial perfusion, valvular regurgitation, coronary artery stenosis, aorta and pulmonary artery disease, cardiac masses, pericardial disease, and congenital heart disease (Skorton et al, 1996).

COMPUTED TOMOGRAPHY OF THE LUNGS

Computed tomography may be used to evaluate the lungs when thoracic radiographs are normal but clinical suspicion of pulmonary disease is high, or when radiographic abnormalities need further clarification. Pulmonary CT also assists in cancer staging and therapy planning.

The CT image is free from superimposition and has superior density discrimination; thus, pathologic changes that are not apparent on thoracic radiographs may be depicted on CT. In humans, HRCT (a technique that employs edge-enhancement filters and thinly collimated, 1- to 2-mm slices targeted to a subsection of lung) has been used to detect or further characterize diffuse diseases, such as interstitial inflammation or fibrosis and emphysema, when radiographic changes are absent or minimal. The HRCT appearance of interstitial disease includes irregular margins of the vessels, bronchi, and pleura; thickened septa; well-defined nodules; a spider web–like network of lines; honeycomb cysts; and hazy or "ground-glass" patches of increased density (Webb, 1991). Emphysema appears as multifocal areas of very low density lacking visible walls, or as discrete bullae. The aforementioned processes are frequently patchy in nature; therefore, CT localization of affected areas may be useful prior to open lung biopsy or resection. Although the CT appearance of diffuse lung diseases in animals, such as interstitial pneumonitis or fibrosis, has not been established, findings are probably comparable to those in humans.

Computed tomography may also be used to differentiate pleural, extrapleural, or mediastinal tissues from the lung or to provide an unobstructed view of the lung when pleural effusion is present. Although fluid is readily depicted with ultrasonography, the underlying lung cannot be imaged unless consolidation or a mass near the periphery of the lung displaces its air. On a CT image, the lung is readily visualized and can be differentiated from the effusion either by the air within it or by its opacification following intravenous administration of contrast medium. In this regard, one clinical application of CT is determining the cause of atelectasis when effusion obscures the lung on thoracic radiographs. Although pleural effusion alone will cause a lung lobe to passively collapse, the presence of trapped fluid around the lung or shifting of the mediastinum toward the fluid suggests that the lobe itself (or bronchus to the lobe) may be diseased, preventing full inflation. In this instance, CT may help to diagnose bronchial obstruction by identifying a bronchial mass or a twisted lung lobe.

Even in the absence of pleural effusion, neoplasia of the lung may be radiographically silent. In humans, non-calcified interstitial nodules smaller than 6 mm in diameter generally will not be seen on plain radiographs. Nodules due to metastatic neoplasia tend to be subpleural and peripheral, which may make them harder to see. Routine CT

can detect nodules as small as 2 to 3 mm; with HRCT, nodules 1 to 2 mm in diameter may be seen (Webb, 1991). Therefore, if the presence of metastasis would influence therapy, pulmonary CT should be considered as a screening test for tumors that have a high propensity for lung metastasis. HRCT is time-consuming and impractical for scanning of the entire thorax; thus, routine CT studies should be performed, followed by regional HRCT if needed.

In addition, CT may assist cancer staging and therapy planning by identifying hilar lymph node enlargement in animals with primary lung tumors. Computed tomography can be used to guide aspiration biopsy of both the primary tumor and hilar lymph nodes (Tidwell and Johnson, 1994). Intravenous administration of iodinated contrast medium during the biopsy procedure helps to distinguish enlarged nodes from vascular or cardiac structures. If needle access to the lymph nodes is safe, biopsy of the nodes should have priority over the primary tumor because it enables simultaneous diagnosis and staging.

Spiral CT permits scanning of an entire thorax during one suspended (e.g., 32-second) respiration, eliminating motion and misregistration artifacts caused by inconsistent lung inflation from one slice to the next. Within a spiral CT scanner, the patient is advanced through a continuously rotating gantry; movement of the x-ray tube around the patient can therefore be likened to the threads of a screw. This process results in acquisition of a true volume of data, so sections can be reconstructed and overlapped at any level, producing high-quality two- and three-dimensional images. Rapid image acquisition also allows for scanning during optimal contrast medium opacification. Thus, with spiral CT, pulmonary disease can be diagnosed with improved accuracy. An example of an important application of spiral CT in humans is the noninvasive diagnosis of acute and chronic pulmonary embolism (Costello, 1995). During spiral CT angiography, emboli can be directly depicted as intraluminal filling defects within the pulmonary arteries without the use of selective catheterization.

References and Suggested Reading

Costello P: Thorax. In: Zeman RK, Brink JA, Costello P, et al, eds: Helical/Spiral CT: A Practical Approach. New York: McGraw-Hill, 1995, p 105.
A review of techniques and current applications of thoracic spiral CT in humans.
Skorton DJ, Schelbert HR, Wolf GL, et al, eds: Marcus Cardiac Imaging: A Companion to Braunwald's Heart Disease. Philadelphia: WB Saunders, 1996, p 793.
A comprehensive textbook of state-of-the-art cardiac imaging in humans.
Tidwell AS, Johnson KL: Computed tomography–guided percutaneous biopsy in the dog and cat: Description of technique and preliminary evaluation in 14 patients. Vet Radiol Ultrasound 35:445, 1994.
A description of the technique of CT-guided biopsy and examples of its use for thoracic and other lesions in dogs and cats.
Webb WR: High-resolution lung computed tomography: Normal anatomic and pathologic findings. Radiology Clin North Am 29:1051, 1991.
A review of the indications of pulmonary HRCT in humans and the HRCT appearance of normal and pathologic lung.

Nutritional Management of Heart Disease

PHILIP ROUDEBUSH
Topeka, Kansas

LISA M. FREEMAN
North Grafton, Massachusetts

For many years, the role of nutrition in the management of heart disease consisted primarily of treating nutrient deficiencies, such as thiamine, selenium, and, more recently, taurine. We now know that deficiencies are not the only concerns in patients with cardiac disease, but also that excessive levels of certain nutrients can be a problem. Nutrients also are now known to have potential interactions with cardiac medications that must be considered. Finally, pharmacologic dosages of some nutrients may have benefits above and beyond their nutritional effects.

GENERAL NUTRITIONAL CONCERNS IN CARDIAC PATIENTS

Changes in Body Condition

Cachexia

Cardiac cachexia, the muscle wasting associated with congestive heart failure (CHF), is a common disorder in patients with cardiac disease. It is present in more than 50% of dogs with dilated cardiomyopathy (DCM). The weight loss that occurs in these patients is unlike that seen in simple starvation. Primarily, adipose tissue is lost in simple starvation, while cachexia is distinguished by a loss of lean body mass. Loss of lean body mass can have direct and deleterious effects on strength, immune function, and survival.

The loss of lean body mass in cachexia is the result of a number of factors, including anorexia, increased metabolic requirements, and alterations in metabolism. The anorexia may be directly related to the CHF itself (i.e., fatigue, dyspnea) or may be due to iatrogenic factors (i.e., digoxin toxicity, abrupt dietary change). Increased energy requirements of up to 30% above normal have been documented in people with CHF. While these factors play a role in the loss of lean body mass, another major factor is the metabolic alterations that occur. Patients with CHF have elevations in the cytokines, tumor necrosis factor, and interleukin-1. These inflammatory mediators are known to directly cause anorexia, to increase energy requirements, and to increase breakdown of lean body mass. In addition, both cytokines have negative inotropic effects.

Cardiac cachexia is most commonly seen in dogs with DCM, especially those with right-sided CHF. Loss of lean body mass is usually noted first in the epaxial, gluteal, scapular, or temporal muscles, and may be very subtle initially. Nutritional therapy of cardiac cachexia consists primarily of nutritional support for anorexia and nutritional modulation of cytokine production. In animals that are anorectic, digoxin toxicity or other medication intolerances should be considered. Medication adjustment also may help animals that are tachycardiac or dyspneic by decreasing energy expenditure. Switching to a more palatable food can be important in anorectic patients. A common mistake is to insist that an owner feed only a severely sodium-restricted food, even if dietary intake of this food is inadequate. While sodium and chloride restriction is important in CHF patients, it should not be imposed to the detriment of overall nutrient intake. Changing to a different therapeutic food or a homemade food may be a more beneficial solution for some patients. Other methods of increasing food palatability include switching from dry to canned food (or canned to dry in some pets), warming the food, or adding flavor enhancers (low-sodium soup or tomato sauce, tuna juice, honey, or corn syrup). Especially in dogs with DCM, appetite may be cyclical, with respect both to overall appetite and to food preferences. A dedicated owner is required for these patients, and a trial-and-error approach must be used with different foods that are mildly to moderately sodium-restricted. A well-balanced homemade food may be a good solution for some of these patients.

Modulation of cytokine production is another potential means of managing anorectic or cachectic patients. Reduction of cytokines is known to be correlated with survival in dogs with CHF. One method of decreasing the production and effects of cytokines is with omega-3 fatty acid supplementation (see later). Supplementation of fish oil, which is high in omega-3 fatty acids has been shown to decrease cytokine production in dogs with CHF and to improve muscle mass. In some, but not all dogs with CHF-induced anorexia, fish oil supplementation can cause marked improvements in food intake.

Obesity

An estimated 30 to 50% of dogs and cats in the United States are overweight, so many small animal patients with cardiac disease have concurrent obesity. Obesity can have profound cardiovascular consequences. From a cardiovascular perspective, obesity is a disease of blood volume expansion with elevated cardiac output, increased plasma and extracellular fluid volume, increased neurohumoral activation, reductions in urinary sodium and water excretion, increased heart rate, abnormal systolic and diastolic ventricular function, exercise intolerance, and elevated blood pressure.

The tendency toward blood volume expansion and neurohumoral activation in animals with obesity parallels the compensatory changes that often occur in individuals with cardiac disease. This finding suggests that obesity may

711

have adverse effects in individuals with concomitant cardiovascular disease.

Obese patients with evidence of cardiovascular disease should undergo dietary management with a calorie-restricted food and client education should focus on the importance of achieving an ideal body weight. The potentially damaging effects of obesity in patients with heart disease should be emphasized to clients to enlist their active participation in a successful weight management program. These changes should be initiated as early as possible in the course of the disease (i.e., when a murmur is first detected in a dog with chronic valvular disease) when dietary modification is more easily accomplished.

Nutrient-Drug Interactions

Drug-drug interactions have received considerable attention in the past, but few clinicians think about how food or nutrient levels can affect drugs and their actions. Since many cardiac patients are treated with a combination of therapeutic foods and drugs, awareness of potential nutrient-drug interactions is important.

Nutrient-Diuretic Interactions

Blood volume contraction and circulatory impairment are potential complications of aggressive diuretic therapy. These complications can exacerbate pre-existing renal disease, alter excretion of drugs dependent on renal elimination, and reduce cardiac output by reducing cardiac filling pressures. Reduced levels of dietary sodium may contribute to volume depletion from excessive diuresis, although this theory has not been proved. Fractional excretion of sodium in the urine actually decreases in normal dogs fed a sodium-restricted food. The influence of diuretics on sodium and chloride balance in dogs with CHF fed sodium- and chloride-restricted foods has not been evaluated.

Furosemide has been implicated in the production of hypokalemia and hypomagnesemia due to increased urinary loss of potassium and magnesium. Hypokalemia and hypomagnesemia can contribute to arrhythmias both directly and by potentiation of the arrhythmogenic effects of digitalis toxicosis. Hypokalemia is not as common a finding in dogs and cats treated with furosemide compared to people taking the same drug. One veterinary study found that furosemide-treated dogs with CHF had significantly lower serum levels of magnesium and potassium than those of age-matched healthy control subjects; however, this has not been found in other studies of dogs with CHF. Therefore, while hypokalemia and hypomagnesemia are possible, they are not common electrolyte abnormalities in most dogs and cats with cardiac disease. In patients with arrhythmias, however, serum electrolyte analysis and treatment of any abnormalities is important.

Increased urinary loss of water-soluble vitamins is another potential nutritional problem with long-term furosemide therapy. One study, for example, found thiamine deficiency in more than 90% of human patients with CHF who were treated with furosemide compared to patients not receiving furosemide. The deficiency appeared to be the result of excessive urinary losses. Therefore, animals re-

ceiving chronic diuretic therapy should be supplemented with thiamine and other water-soluble vitamins or should be fed a commercial food with increased concentrations of these vitamins. Veterinary medical foods designed for patients with cardiac and renal disease are usually formulated with increased levels of water-soluble vitamins to offset excessive urinary losses.

Several studies have shown that in human patients with moderate CHF, the renin-angiotensin-aldosterone (RAA) system is not activated in the absence of diuretic therapy. The major increase in plasma renin activity and plasma aldosterone concentration occurs with the introduction of diuretic drugs, rather than as a result of the disease process itself. Furosemide apparently stimulates renin release by inhibiting chloride transport in the ascending limb of the loop of Henle, even if blood volume contraction is prevented. Treatment of normal geriatric dogs with moderate doses of furosemide profoundly stimulates the RAA system, irrespective of the dietary sodium level. Use of furosemide in conjunction with either hydralazine or enalapril also stimulates the RAA system in dogs with heart failure due to acquired mitral valve regurgitation.

Although diuretics will remain important first-line drugs for the management of pulmonary edema and chronic fluid retention, the profound stimulation of the RAA system by diuretics suggests that diuretics also have an important role in the progressive self-perpetuating cycle of CHF. Because of these effects on the RAA system, diuretic monotherapy for the management of CHF is no longer considered ideal. Diuretics should be reserved for the management of more advanced stages of CHF and should be used chronically only in conjunction with dietary sodium restriction, angiotensin-converting enzyme inhibitors (ACEI), or digoxin, or a combination of these therapies. Use of foods that avoid excess dietary sodium and chloride may allow lower dosages of diuretics to be used for control of the clinical signs of CHF.

Nutrient-ACEI Interaction

Captopril, enalapril, lisinopril, and other ACEIs have emerged as the drugs of choice for treating many dogs and cats with CHF. Inhibition of angiotensin II results in vasodilation and decreased circulating plasma aldosterone concentrations. Both angiotensin II and aldosterone play important roles in the maintenance of vascular volume and potassium balance by increasing the reabsorption of sodium and chloride and, in the case of aldosterone, by promoting the excretion of potassium.

The use of ACEI in human patients with severe renal insufficiency or in those given potassium supplements may increase the risk of the development of hyperkalemia. In one study, more than half of the dogs with CHF developed mild elevations in serum potassium concentration when treated with a commercial sodium-restricted veterinary medical food, furosemide, and captopril. Therefore, potassium supplementation is contraindicated in patients receiving ACEI. Although clinically significant hyperkalemia (serum potassium >6.5 mEq/L) is uncommon, feeding foods with a high potassium content to dogs receiving ACEIs may increase the risk of hyperkalemia. Routine monitoring of serum potassium levels in patients receiving ACEIs is important.

Functional renal insufficiency has been documented in as many as one third of salt-restricted human patients with severe CHF treated with ACEIs and diuretics. This decline in renal function has been attributed to the loss of angiotensin II–mediated systemic and intrarenal vasoconstrictor effects that maintain renal perfusion pressure and glomerular filtration rate in low-output CHF. Functional renal insufficiency appears to be alleviated in human patients by replenishing body stores of sodium through reduction of diuretic dosage and liberalizing dietary sodium intake. Renal insufficiency is a potential complication of ACEI therapy in dogs with CHF, but the role of sodium chloride restriction is unknown. However, treatment of canine CHF with furosemide and enalapril results in more frequent azotemia than does the use of furosemide alone. In patients with CHF, drug-induced azotemia is treated by reducing the diuretic dose (usually in half), by reducing the ACEI dose (usually in half), by increasing the dietary intake of sodium chloride to the next level (Table 1), or by using a combination of these tactics.

Nutrient–Cardiac Glycoside Interactions

Absorption of the cardiac glycosides is influenced by the formulation of the drug and when it is administered in relationship to meals. Because administration of digoxin or digitoxin with food may result in up to a 50% reduction in serum concentrations, these drugs are best given between meals. The body condition of the animal can also influence the pharmacokinetics of these drugs. Digoxin is minimally distributed in adipose tissue, so in obese individuals the dosage of the drug should be based on the lean body weight. Therefore, obese patients should receive a lower dose than that based strictly on weight. Digitoxin is more lipid soluble than digoxin, and its dosage need not be adjusted for obesity.

Metabolic derangements associated with an increased risk of digoxin toxicosis include hypokalemia, hypomagnesemia, hypercalcemia, renal insufficiency, and hypothyroidism. Serum electrolyte concentrations should be measured and corrections made before one initiates cardiac glycoside therapy. In addition, routine monitoring and dosage adjustment are important during therapy, especially when body condition changes.

SPECIFIC NUTRIENT CONSIDERATIONS
Minerals and Electrolytes

Congestive heart failure is associated with retention of sodium, chloride, and water; thus, these nutrients are of primary importance in patients with cardiovascular disease. Excess dietary sodium is easily eliminated by normal dogs and cats. Within a few hours of ingesting high levels of dietary sodium, the excess is excreted in the urine. Early in the course of cardiac disease, however, this response may be blunted because of compensatory responses to decreased cardiac output. As heart disease worsens and CHF ensues, the ability to excrete excess dietary sodium becomes more severely depressed.

Early in the course of heart disease, before CHF is present, rigid dietary sodium restriction is probably unnecessary. As heart disease progresses and CHF appears, however, sodium restriction is a key component of treatment even with the concurrent use of diuretics. Well-controlled studies in people have demonstrated that with a high sodium intake, loop diuretics such as furosemide fail to achieve a negative sodium balance. Despite an impressive natriuresis for several hours after furosemide administration, there is a compensatory increase in sodium reabsorption in the remaining 24-hour period that exactly matches the earlier losses. Thus, it may be essential to limit sodium intake to ensure negative sodium balances. Balance studies in normal human beings have demonstrated that significant negative sodium balance can predictably be obtained with loop diuretics if sodium intake is limited to 20 mEq/day (equivalent to 460 mg of sodium or 1.2 gm of sodium chloride per day). This level of sodium restriction in people is equivalent to that achieved with the use of veterinary medical foods formulated for veterinary patients with cardiovascular disease ("cardiac foods").

In the past, retention of sodium was primarily implicated in the pathogenesis of CHF. It is now known that the interaction of sodium with other ions, including chloride, in the diet also is important. In human hypertension, the full expression of disease depends on the concomitant administration of both sodium and chloride. This finding

TABLE 1. Classification of Commercial Dog Foods by Sodium Content

Category		Average Sodium Content in % Dry Matter (Range)
High	Popular (grocery store), canned	1.13 (0.60–2.22)
Moderate	Popular (grocery store), dry	0.40 (0.15–0.59)
	Premium/superpremium, canned	0.40 (0.25–0.64)
	Premium/superpremium, dry	0.40 (0.27–0.65)
Low	Geriatric/senior, canned and dry	0.22 (0.17–0.26)
	Canine renal foods, canned and dry	0.22 (0.22–0.23)
	Feline renal foods, canned and dry	0.26 (0.25–0.28)
Very low	Canine cardiac foods, canned and dry	0.10 (0.08–0.15)
Minimum sodium allowance (adult canine maintenance)		0.06
Minimum sodium allowance (adult feline maintenance)		0.20

suggests that both sodium and chloride are nutrients of concern in patients with CHF. There are a number of ways of restricting sodium and chloride intake in cardiac patients. It is not always necessary to prescribe a severely restricted food initially, especially when CHF is not yet present. Sometimes just switching to a food that is lower in sodium and chloride than the current food may have benefit, and more severe restriction can be achieved as the disease progresses (see Table 1). Owners, however, should be cautioned against feeding pet foods or table food that is high in sodium and chloride. Many owners need very specific instructions regarding the foods that are low in salt, and most will appreciate recommendations for acceptable, low-salt treats.

Potassium and magnesium are nutrients of concern in cardiac patients because depletions of these electrolytes can cause cardiac arrhythmias, decreased myocardial contractility, and profound muscle weakness, and can potentiate the adverse effects of cardiac medications. In addition, electrolyte homeostasis can be affected by medications used for the treatment of CHF. Potassium should be routinely monitored in CHF patients, and therapy should be adjusted accordingly. Serum magnesium concentrations can be measured but are a very poor indicator of total body stores, since only 1% of total body stores are found extracellularly in the circulation. Nonetheless, serial evaluations in an individual patient may be useful, especially in patients with arrhythmias, or in those taking high dosages of diuretics.

Taurine

The role of taurine deficiency in feline DCM has been well described. Despite this knowledge and the dramatic decline in the incidence of the disease over recent years, it is still unclear why some cases of DCM appear to be independent of taurine status and why there is variability in resistance to the development of DCM in taurine deficiency. Still, taurine deficiency should be suspected whenever the diagnosis of feline DCM is made. Whole blood taurine (which is a more reliable index of long-term status than plasma taurine) should be analyzed, and treatment with taurine (125 to 250 mg PO every 12 hours) should begin concurrent with medical therapy. The owner also should be counseled to switch to a food higher in taurine. Potassium depletion may contribute to taurine deficiency, and so hypokalemia also should be corrected if present.

Based on the association between taurine and feline DCM, it was a logical next step to examine the role of taurine in canine DCM. Low taurine concentrations have been documented in some American Cocker spaniels with DCM, which improved with taurine and carnitine supplementation. Sporadic cases of taurine deficiency based on plasma and whole blood taurine concentrations have been found in dogs with DCM, but the significance of this finding is unknown. In the authors' experience, taurine supplementation in these patients has been unrewarding. Nonetheless, taurine supplementation in dogs with *documented* taurine deficiency probably is worthwhile. Whether taurine deficiency plays a role in canine DCM, however, remains to be determined.

L-Carnitine

L-Carnitine, a compound synthesized from the amino acids lysine and methionine, is concentrated in the skeletal and cardiac muscle and is critical for fatty acid metabolism and ATP production. Carnitine deficiency may be due to decreased synthesis, decreased intake, decreased intestinal absorption, increased renal loss, or transport defects. Limited renal reabsorption of carnitine and probable transport defects in dogs may make this species particularly vulnerable to carnitine deficiency. Dogs are therefore thought to require dietary carnitine to maintain normal body stores.

Carnitine deficiency is associated with primary myocardial disease in a number of species, and was first shown to be associated with canine DCM in a family of Boxer dogs. Although anecdotal reports exist regarding the efficacy of carnitine in canine DCM, no blinded prospective studies have been done. It appears that a subset of dogs with DCM may have myocardial or systemic carnitine deficiency and may respond to carnitine supplementation, but it is difficult at this point to identify these patients. Most dogs with carnitine deficiency require an endomyocardial biopsy and expert sample analysis for diagnosis, which is obviously not feasible in all patients. Carnitine supplementation has few side effects; the major problem is the high cost, which can be prohibitive in some patients. The authors currently offer owners of dogs with DCM the option of carnitine supplementation (50 to 100 mg/kg PO every 8 hours), but do not consider it obligatory (although it is highly recommended in Boxer dogs and Cocker spaniels).

Nutriceuticals

Veterinary nutriceuticals currently have no legal definition, but they generally are considered to be substances that are "produced in a purified or extracted form and administered orally to patients to provide agents required for normal body structure and function and administered with the intent of improving the health and well-being of animals." Nutriceuticals, unlike the individual nutrients listed previously, are not provided to correct an absolute deficiency and often are administered at pharmacologic, rather than physiologic, levels.

Omega-3 Fatty Acids

The omega-3 fatty acids, eicosapentaenoic acid (EPA) and docosahexaenoic acids (DHA), are long-chain, polyunsaturated fatty acids in which the first double-bond is at the position of the third carbon from the methyl end (versus the omega-6 fatty acids, linoleic, linolenic, and arachidonic, in which the first double bond is at the sixth carbon). This difference conveys a different structure and different characteristics to the fatty acid. Omega-3 fatty acids normally are found in very low concentrations in the plasma membrane compared to the omega-6 fatty acids, but can be increased by a food or supplement enriched in omega-3 fatty acids. The benefit of having a higher concentration of omega-3 fatty acids in the membranes is that breakdown products of the omega-3 fatty acids (eicosanoids) are, in general, less potent inflammatory mediators than eicosanoids derived from omega-6 fatty acids. This decreases the production of cytokines and other inflammatory mediators in both people and dogs. Fish oil also has been shown to directly suppress gene expression of cytokines. In addition, dogs with CHF have been shown to have plasma fatty acid abnormalities (decreased EPA and DHA compared to normal dogs). In one study of dogs with DCM and CHF, fish oil supplementation normalized plasma fatty acid concentrations, decreased cytokine production, and improved muscle mass. In some dogs, fish oil supplementation also improved appetite. Another potential benefit of fish oil is that experimental evidence suggests that fish oil has antiarrhythmic effects. Fish oil will not benefit all dogs and cats with heart disease, but may be useful in those with muscle loss, anorexia, or arrhythmia. The authors currently recommend a dosage of EPA of 40 mg/kg and of DHA of 25 mg/kg. Fish oil capsules that contain 180 mg of EPA and 120 mg of DHA can be purchased at most pharmacies. Higher dosages, usually 300 mg of EPA and 180 mg of DHA, can be obtained from medical supply catalogs and often are more feasible for large dogs. Fish oil capsules that contain other supplements are not recommended. Prospective studies are needed to demonstrate efficacy and impact on major end points, such as survival and quality of life.

Coenzyme Q10

Coenzyme Q10 is a cofactor in a number of reactions required for energy production. It also is a very potent antioxidant and exhibits some protection against experimental myocardial ischemic injury. Some human studies have shown encouraging results with regard to beneficial effects of coenzyme Q10 supplementation on clinical signs and echocardiographic parameters in DCM; however, the results have not been uniform. Some veterinary clinicians use coenzyme Q10 in canine DCM at a dosage of 30 mg PO every 12 hours up to 90 mg PO every 12 hours in large dogs. Nonetheless, controlled, prospective studies are necessary for an accurate judgment of the efficacy of this product.

Antioxidants

Antioxidants vitamins have received a great deal of attention recently with reference to the prevention of human cardiac disease. While their potential to prevent free radical damage appears promising, most of the research in human cardiology has been done on coronary artery disease. Some evidence, however, points to increased free radical activity without a compensatory antioxidant capacity in CHF. Therefore, while much research remains to be done in this area, antioxidant supplementation may hold promise for the future in the treatment of CHF.

FEEDING STRATEGIES

Commercial Foods

There are a number of commercial veterinary medical foods designed for dogs and cats with cardiac disease (cardiac foods). The specific characteristics of these foods vary, but they generally are lower in dietary sodium and chloride and contain increased levels of B vitamins. The levels of protein, magnesium, phosphorus, and potassium vary, depending on the individual food. Selection of the optimal food for each patient depends on the stage of disease, clinical signs, laboratory parameters, and appetite. There also are a number of other foods on the market not designed specifically for animals with heart disease but that are reduced in sodium (foods designed for animals with renal disease and "senior" foods). It is important, however, to evaluate these foods to determine whether they are appropriate for the patient. Some of these foods may have characteristics that make them inappropriate for a given individual (i.e., too low in protein for cachectic patients or too high in potassium for patients receiving an ACEI).

Homemade Foods

In the majority of patients, a commercial food is the optimal choice. Some patients, however, have particular characteristics that make a homemade food more appropriate. These include unwillingness to eat a commercial food, persistent anorexia, or laboratory abnormalities that make the use of cardiac foods inappropriate (i.e., hyperlipidemia). The successful use of homemade diets requires a dedicated owner who is willing to undertake this time-consuming task and be counseled about ingredients that are low in salt. The client must be willing to follow the prescribed recipe. Finally, a well-balanced recipe must be specifically prescribed because there are a number of nutritionally unbalanced recipes available in the popular press.

Changing Foods

All dietary changes should be done gradually over a period of 4 or 5 days. It may be difficult to make major dietary changes while the patient is sick or hospitalized. It often is better to wait several days until the patient's condition has improved, and then initiate the change. Food aversions are known to develop in ill people, and such aversion may prevent adequate intake of the food over the long term. It also is important to specifically instruct the owner to notify you if the patient does not eat adequate amounts of the new food. It is preferable to have the animal eat a somewhat less than optimal food than to eat inadequate amounts.

Initiating and Monitoring Dietary Therapy

A serum biochemistry profile and urine specific gravity should be obtained in all dogs and cats with cardiac disease before any dietary and drug therapy is initiated. Patients with CHF and evidence of pre-existing renal disease, including isosthenuria, may be at increased risk for developing azotemia during combined dietary-drug therapy. No universal recommendations exist for controlled levels of dietary sodium, chloride, magnesium, or potassium for animals with cardiovascular disease. Rather, each patient should be monitored frequently (weekly for the first 2 weeks or after a change in medication, then bimonthly). Monitoring should include measurements of body weight and body condition, serum electrolyte and magnesium concentrations, and renal function. Adjustment of nutrient levels in the food and changes in drugs or drug dosages should be made according to changes in patients' clinical signs and laboratory parameters. Finally, alterations in body condition, either obesity or cachexia, should be treated early to avoid the complications associated with these condition.

References and Suggested Reading

Alexander JK: The heart and obesity. In: Hurst JW, ed: The Heart, 6th ed. New York: McGraw-Hill, 1986, p 1452.
Reviews the cardiovascular effects of obesity.
Boegehold MA, Kotchen TA: Relative contributions of dietary Na⁺ and Cl⁻ to salt-sensitive hypertension. Hypertension 14:579, 1989.
Reviews studies of human and animal blood pressure responses to dietary sodium loading without chloride.
Cobb M, Michell AR: Plasma electrolyte concentrations in dogs receiving diuretic therapy for cardiac failure. J Small Anim Pract 33:526, 1991.
Study of electrolyte concentrations in dogs with congestive heart failure.
Freeman LM, Roubenoff R: The nutrition implications of cardiac cachexia. Nutr Rev 52:340, 1994.
A review of the pathogenesis and treatment of cardiac cachexia.
Freeman LM, Rush JE, Kehayias JJ, et al: Nutritional alterations and the effect of fish oil supplementation in dogs with heart failure. J Vet Intern Med 12:65, 1998.
Study of the effects of fish oil on body composition, cytokine production, and survival in dogs with dilated cardiomyopathy and heart failure.
Keene BW: L-Carnitine deficiency in canine dilated cardiomyopathy. In: Kirk RW, Bonagura JD, eds: Current Veterinary Therapy XI. Philadelphia: WB Saunders, 1992, p 780.
A review of the pathogenesis, diagnosis, and treatment of carnitine deficiency.
Pion PD, Kittleson MD, Rogers QR: Myocardial failure in cats associated with low plasma taurine: A reversible cardiomyopathy. Science 237:764, 1987.
The first report of the role of taurine deficiency in feline dilated cardiomyopathy.
Roudebush P, Allen TA, Kuehn NF, et al: The effect of combined therapy with captopril, furosemide and a sodium-restricted diet on serum electrolyte concentrations and renal function in normal dogs and dogs with congestive heart failure. J Vet Intern Med 8:337, 1994.
A study examining nutrient-drug interactions in dogs with congestive heart failure.

Cardiovascular Complications of Thyroid Disease

DAVID L. PANCIERA
Blacksburg, Virginia

Thyroid hormones play an integral role in the function of the cardiovascular system. It is important to consider their effects on the heart and peripheral circulation when one evaluates and treats dogs and cats with disorders of the thyroid glands. Treatment of the underlying thyroid hormone excess or deficiency is generally all that is required for resolution of the cardiovascular abnormalities associated with these disorders. In some cases, however, more extensive clinical evaluation and specific treatment of the cardiovascular complications are necessary. In some cases, these changes are so profound that early descriptions of hyperthyroidism in humans attributed the disease to a primary cardiac disorder.

PATHOPHYSIOLOGY

Left ventricular hypertrophy and increased cardiac contractility and heart rate occur in hyperthyroidism as a result of direct and indirect effects on the heart (Klein, 1990; Polikar et al, 1993). Thyroid hormones induce production of a myosin isoform that increases the speed of myosin-actin interaction and thus increases contractility. Increased activity of the sarcoplasmic reticulum Ca⁺-ATPase and an augmented number of sarcolemmal calcium channels also increase contractility. The number of cardiac beta-adrenergic receptors is increased in hyperthyroidism, which may

contribute to increased contractility, and cardiac hypertrophy.

Perhaps more important than the direct effects of thyroid hormones on the heart are effects on the peripheral circulation. Hyperthyroidism increases metabolic rate by increasing oxygen and substrate consumption in thyroid-responsive tissues. Peripheral vascular resistance decreases in order to meet the peripheral tissue needs for blood flow, possibly through release of vasodilatory substances in tissues where oxygen consumption is increased. The decrease in diastolic blood pressure subsequent to reduced peripheral vascular resistance results in an increase in cardiac output mediated by increasing contractility and heart rate. In addition, the blood volume is increased in hyperthyroidism.

Hypertension occurs commonly in hyperthyroidism, probably as a result of increased cardiac output and blood volume. The exact pathogenesis of hypertension in hyperthyroidism remains to be determined.

The electrical activity of the heart is also altered by thyroid hormones. Increased heart rate and arrhythmias may result from increased cardiac beta-adrenergic receptors, myocardial hypertrophy, Na⁺,K⁺-ATPase activity, or direct effects of thyroid hormones.

The effects of hypothyroidism on the heart are generally the opposite of hyperthyroidism, but the changes are less profound. Decreased cardiac output, increased systemic vascular resistance, decreased blood volume, and bradycardia develop to varying degrees. Hypothyroidism can also contribute to the development of atherosclerosis, with resultant impaired cardiac function related to myocardial ischemia or infarction and cerebrovascular infarction.

CARDIOVASCULAR COMPLICATIONS OF HYPERTHYROIDISM

Clinical Findings

Thyroid hormone excess results in a number of cardiovascular abnormalities that are detectable on clinical evaluation. A systolic heart murmur or gallop rhythm is detected in about 50% of hyperthyroid cats. Sinus tachycardia is a common finding, whereas other arrhythmias are infrequent. Polyuria, reported in about one third of cases, may result primarily from increased renal blood flow. Tachypnea, dyspnea, orthopnea, lethargy, weakness, and anorexia can occur in congestive heart failure. Today, heart failure is found in only 2% of affected cats, compared with 12% in 1983 (Broussard et al, 1995). The large decrease in the frequency of heart failure associated with hyperthyroidism is probably the result of diagnosis of the disorder at a much earlier stage than in the 1980s. Weak femoral pulses, hepatomegaly, jugular venous distention, muffled heart and lung sounds, pulmonary crackles, a pleural fluid line, and cyanosis can be found variably in cats with congestive heart failure secondary to hyperthyroidism.

Electrocardiographic abnormalities include elevated R-wave amplitude consistent with left ventricular enlargement in about 34% of cases and sinus tachycardia in 7% (Broussard et al, 1995). Other arrhythmias that are occasionally found include supraventricular and ventricular premature contractions or tachycardia. QRS duration is occasionally prolonged. Conduction abnormalities can occur, particularly left anterior fascicle block, right bundle branch block, atrioventricular block, and ventricular pre-excitation. Some of these conduction disturbances may be unrelated to the thyroid condition, as conduction disease is relatively common in older cats.

Cardiomegaly is often evident on thoracic radiographs, primarily owing to left ventricular and atrial enlargement. Generalized cardiomegaly with pleural effusion or pulmonary edema are typical of cats with congestive heart failure. The most common echocardiographic changes are hypertrophy of the left ventricular free wall and interventricular septum, left atrial enlargement, and left ventricular dilatation (Bond et al, 1988). Ventricular hypertrophy is sometimes asymmetrical, with hypertrophy isolated to the interventricular septum (which can also occur in older cats without hyperthyroidism). Left ventricular outflow obstruction can be found in a small number of hyperthyroid cats with asymmetrical hypertrophy. It is unclear whether asymmetrical septal hypertrophy is the result of concurrent hypertrophic cardiomyopathy. Contractility measured echocardiographically is often increased in hyperthyroid cats. Generalized cardiac dilation may be observed in cats with heart failure, and overt dilated cardiomyopathy has been reported in a small number of hyperthyroid cats with congestive heart failure (Jacobs et al, 1986). It is not clear whether this occurs as a consequence of the hyperthyroid state or whether the hypocontractility is a manifestation of a primary dilated cardiomyopathy. Congestive heart failure and reversible dilated cardiomyopathy have been documented in some humans with long-standing hyperthyroidism (Umpierrez et al, 1995). An echocardiogram is essential in determining the most appropriate course of treatment of the hyperthyroid cat with congestive heart failure.

Aortic Thromboembolism

Despite the common occurrence of cardiac hypertrophy in hyperthyroid cats, aortic thromboembolism is a rare complication of this disease, when one considers the overall prevalence of hyperthyroidism in cats. The reasons are unclear but may be related to the less severe atrial enlargement and myocardial hypertrophy and higher cardiac outputs that occur in hyperthyroidism compared with idiopathic hypertrophic cardiomyopathy.

Systemic Hypertension

Hypertension has been reported in 20 to 87% of hyperthyroid cats (Kobayashi et al, 1990; Stiles et al, 1994). Hyperthyroid cats are relatively resistant to the retinal changes that occur in hypertension associated with renal failure and other causes. Hypertension is most commonly manifested as a retinopathy. Ophthalmic examination may reveal retinal edema, subretinal effusion, retinal hemorrhages, retinal arterial tortuosity, hyphema, and retinal detachment. Blindness can occur if the changes are severe. Other consequences of uncontrolled systemic arterial hypertension include progressive renal disease and central nervous system hemorrhage. Measurement of systolic, and if possible diastolic, blood pressure as well as an ophthalmic examination should be performed on all hyperthyroid cats. Prompt treatment may resolve even severe ocular complications of hypertension in some cases. Definitive treatment of the hyperthyroidism does not necessarily resolve the hypertension. Some cats will require continued antihypertensive treatment after euthyroidism has been established (see p. 838).

TREATMENT OF THE CARDIOVASCULAR COMPLICATIONS OF HYPERTHYROIDISM

Reversal of the hyperthyroid state results in resolution of most of the cardiovascular complications of hyperthyroidism. However, several weeks may be required before euthyroidism can be established, and management of the complications of hyperthyroidism is sometimes necessary.

Congestive Heart Failure

Treatment of the hyperthyroid cat with congestive heart failure is similar to treatment of a euthyroid cat (Keene and Rush, 1995). Although most affected cats have left ventricular hypertrophy and hyperkinetic function, there is often concurrent right atrial enlargement. Furthermore, it is essential to determine whether the patient has the rare dilated cardiomyopathy, which carries a poor prognosis. Furosemide, 2 to 4 mg/kg IV every 6 to 12 hours (Lasix,

Hoechst Marion Roussel; Disal, Fermenta Animal Health), oxygen, avoidance of stress, and sometimes nitroglycerin, ¼ inch every 6 hours (Nitro-Bid, Hoechst Marion Roussel), form the mainstay of treatment of cats that present on an emergency basis. Cats with biventricular heart failure and pleural effusion should undergo thoracentesis. Maintenance treatment for heart failure includes furosemide, 1 mg/kg every 12 to 48 hours, with the clinician using caution not to cause the dehydration common with excessive diuretic administration. Enalapril, 0.5 mg/kg every 24 hours (Enacard, Merck AgVet), is administered to cats with refractory heart failure. Enalapril may be contraindicated in cats with asymmetrical ventricular hypertrophy and left ventricular outflow tract obstruction, although this is unresolved. Antithyroid treatment such as methimazole (see p. 333) should be instituted at the time of diagnosis. Medications administered for heart failure can be gradually withdrawn as the heart failure is controlled and euthyroidism is established. Some hyperthyroid cats have concurrent idiopathic hypertrophic cardiomyopathy and have persistent cardiac disease requiring long-term treatment.

Hyperthyroid cats with the rare dilated cardiomyopathy should be administered treatment similar to that outlined earlier, including enalapril or benazepril. In addition, digoxin (Lanoxin, Glaxo Wellcome) should be administered to cats without renal dysfunction. The initial dose should be one fourth of a 0.125-mg tablet every other day. Dosage adjustments should be made on the basis of serum digoxin concentration obtained after 7 to 14 days of treatment. The treatment of these cats is commonly protracted, and the prognosis is guarded.

Arrhythmias

Sinus tachycardia, the most common arrhythmia in hyperthyroid cats, rarely requires treatment. Mild atrial arrhythmias such as supraventricular premature contractions or paroxysmal supraventricular tachycardia with a heart rate less than 240 beats/min may not require treatment. If severe atrial or ventricular arrhythmias are present, beta-adrenergic blocking drugs such as propranolol, 2.5 mg/cat PO every 8 to 12 hours (Inderal, Wyeth-Ayerst), or atenolol, 6.25 mg/cat PO every 12 to 24 hours (Tenormin, Zeneca Pharmaceuticals), should be administered. Dosage can be increased on a weekly basis if the response is inadequate. Beta-blockers should be used only after signs of heart failure have been controlled for 5 to 10 days unless the arrhythmia is life-threatening. Calcium channel blocking drugs such as diltiazem, 7.5 mg/cat every 8 hours (Cardizem, Hoechst Marion Roussel), or Cardizem SR, 20 mg/cat every 24 hours, can be used for the treatment of atrial arrhythmias if beta-blockers are contraindicated because of concurrent conditions, such as bronchitis, asthma, or aortic thromboembolism. Most arrhythmias resolve after the congestive heart failure and hyperthyroidism have been controlled, and so antiarrhythmic treatment should be used conservatively.

Aortic Thromboembolism

Fortunately, aortic thromboembolism is uncommon in hyperthyroid cats. Efficacious and safe treatment of aortic thromboembolism remains to be established. If thromboembolism is discovered within 6 hours of occurrence, treatment with tissue plasminogen activator or streptokinase may be effective. Unfortunately, mortality due to reperfusion injury or hemorrhage is very high, and clinical experience with these agents is limited. Further clot formation may be reduced by administration of heparin, 220 IU/kg IV, followed by 66 mg/kg SC every 6 hours, to maintain the activated partial thromboplastin time 1.5 to 2 times the pretreatment level. Aspirin, 25 mg/kg every 72 hours, or warfarin (Coumadin, DuPont Pharma) can also be administered to prevent clot formation. Acepromazine, 0.1 to 0.4 mg/kg SC every 8 hours (PromAce, Fort Dodge), or hydralazine, 0.5 mg/kg PO every 8 hours), can be administered in an attempt to cause vasodilation and increase collateral circulation. The efficacy of these treatments remains to be determined. Recovery is protracted, and the prognosis is guarded to poor.

Systemic Hypertension

Antihypertensive therapy should be reserved for cats that have moderate to severe hypertension (systolic blood pressure greater than 200 mg Hg) or those with signs consistent with hypertension. The calcium channel blocking drug amlodipine (Norvasc, Pfizer) appears to be the most effective antihypertensive agent available. Amlodipine, 0.625 mg/cat PO every 24 hours, is administered initially. If hypertension persists after 7 days of treatment, enalapril should be added to the amlodipine treatment. Hypertensive retinopathy should be managed by lowering blood pressure and by administration of topical and systemic glucocorticoids.

CARDIOVASCULAR COMPLICATIONS OF HYPOTHYROIDISM

Clinical Findings

The effects of hypothyroidism on the heart are generally less dramatic than those present in hyperthyroidism. Bradycardia, weak femoral pulses, a weak apex beat, and muffled heart sounds are found in some hypothyroid dogs. Electrocardiographic abnormalities include decreased amplitude of the R wave (<1 mV) in 50% of cases, sinus bradycardia, first-degree atrioventricular block, T-wave inversion, and a shift in the mean electrical axis (Panciera, 1994). These ECG changes partially resolve following 8 weeks of thyroid hormone replacement therapy. Ventricular arrhythmias occur rarely and may result from myocardial ischemia in dogs with atherosclerosis. Recently, atrial fibrillation has been documented to occur with increased frequency in hypothyroid dogs. This and other anecdotal reports support the presence of significant electrophysiologic effects in hypothyroidism.

Hypothyroidism is associated with impaired myocardial contractility. Decreased left ventricular shortening fraction combined with variable increases in left ventricular end-diastolic diameter or decreases in left ventricular end-systolic diameter is found in hypothyroid dogs. The decrease in contractility is generally mild but may be of considerable importance in dogs with pre-existing cardiac disease.

Atherosclerosis is a rare complication of canine hypothyroidism. It results from severe hypercholesterolemia and lipoprotein abnormalities that occur in some dogs with hypothyroidism. Arterial accumulation of lipid and macrophages combined with smooth muscle proliferation results in formation of atherosclerotic plaque. As plaques accumulate, they impair blood flow and may cause local ischemia. In addition to the typical signs of hypothyroidism and hypercholesterolemia, hypothyroid dogs with atherosclerosis may have signs of multiple organ involvement, including collapse, vomiting, lethargy, and neurologic abnormalities (Zeiss and Waddle, 1995). Pancreatitis, iliac thrombosis, and central nervous system infarction are common. The prognosis is poor, since most dogs have advanced disease at the time of diagnosis.

TREATMENT OF THE CARDIOVASCULAR COMPLICATIONS OF HYPOTHYROIDISM

Specific treatment of the cardiovascular abnormalities due to hypothyroidism is rarely necessary. The changes generally are sufficiently mild not to require more than thyroid hormone replacement. Dogs with congestive heart failure and hypothyroidism should be treated as appropriate for the cardiac disease and clinical signs. Levothyroxine replacement should be initiated at 25% of the typical dose: that is, 0.0055 mg/kg PO every 12 hours, with an increase of 0.0055 mg/kg every 2 weeks until serum thyroxine (T_4) and thyroid-stimulating hormone (TSH) concentrations are in the appropriate range. Although hypothyroid humans are at increased risk for digoxin toxicity, the pharmacokinetics of digoxin in hypothyroid dogs is not different from that in euthyroid dogs, so no dose adjustment appears necessary. Other antiarrhythmic treatment is rarely indicated in hypothyroid dogs with arrhythmias unless concurrent cardiac disease is present. Atherosclerosis should be managed with appropriate hormone supplementation and a low-fat diet in addition to management of the clinical manifestations of the disease.

References and Suggested Reading

Bond BR, Fox PR, Peterson ME, et al: Echocardiographic findings in 103 cats with hyperthyroidism. J Am Vet Med Med Assoc 192:1546, 1988.
Broussard JD, Peterson ME, Fox PR: Changes in clinical and laboratory findings in cats with hyperthyroidism from 1983 to 1993. J Am Vet Med Assoc 206:302, 1995.
Jacobs G, Hutson C, Dougherty J, et al: Congestive heart failure associated with hyperthyroidism in cats. J Am Vet Med Assoc 189:52, 1986.
Keene BW, Rush HE: Therapy of heart failure. In: Ettinger SJ, Feldman EC, eds: Textbook of Veterinary Internal Medicine, 4th ed. Philadelphia: WB Saunders, 1995, p 867.
Klein I: Thyroid hormone and the cardiovascular system. Am J Med 88:631, 1990.
Kobayashi DL, Peterson ME, Graves TK, et al: Hypertension in cats with chronic renal failure or hyperthyroidism. J Vet Intern Med 4:58, 1990.
Panciera DL: An echocardiographic and electrocardiographic study of cardiovascular function in hypothyroid dogs. J Am Vet Med Assoc 205:996, 1994.
Polikar R, Burger AG, Scherrer U, et al: The thyroid and the heart. Circulation 87:1435, 1993.
Stiles J, Polzin DJ, Bistner SI: The prevalence of retinopathy in cats with systemic hypertension and chronic renal failure or hyperthyroidism. J Am Anim Hosp Assoc 30:564, 1994.
Umpierrez GE, Challapalli S, Patterson C: Congestive heart failure due to reversible cardiomyopathy in patients with hyperthyroidism. Am J Med Sci 310:99, 1995.
Zeiss CJ, Waddle G: Hypothyroidism and atherosclerosis in dogs. Compend Contin Educ Pract Vet 17:1117, 1995.

Bradyarrhythmias

MARK RISHNIW
Ithaca, New York

WILLIAM P. THOMAS
Davis, California

Bradycardia is the general term used to describe a heart (ventricular) rate that is slower than normal for a given species. The term *bradyarrhythmia* is used to describe any of several arrhythmias accompanied by bradycardia. Normal heart rate varies by species and is influenced by body size, age, and physiologic state; thus, a precise definition of the minimum normal rate is difficult in any individual animal. A sinus rhythm rate less than 60 beats per minute (bpm) is usually considered bradycardic in awake adult dogs. In cats, the minimum normal awake heart rate has been reported to be between 90 and 120 bpm. It is important to recognize that these limits are arbitrary, and that a heart rate below these limits may not always be pathologic or cause clinical signs.

Bradyarrhythmias may result from primary cardiac disease affecting mainly the conducting system or by more generalized cardiac disease (e.g., valvular or myocardial disease), or may be secondary to extracardiac factors, or both, that lead to a decreased rate of discharge of the sinoatrial (SA) node or interrupted propagation of atrial impulses to the ventricles. Some rhythms are caused or influenced by an autonomic imbalance between the sympathetic nervous system (SNS) and the parasympathetic nervous system (PNS), and are often called *vagally mediated.*

Bradyarrhythmias may also result from certain extracardiac disorders that affect cardiac electrophysiology, such as hyperkalemia, hypothermia, or hypothyroidism.

CLINICAL SIGNS

Bradyarrhythmias may be subclinical or may result in clinical signs that are generally related to the severity of the associated hemodynamic disturbance. Most vagally mediated bradyarrhythmias are found coincidentally during routine physical examination and are not severe enough to produce clinical signs. The lack of reported signs does not uniquely distinguish these patients, however, since many animals with pathologic bradyarrhythmias also show no obvious clinical signs. This is especially true for cats, who are very good at limiting their activity to compensate for hemodynamic limitations and whose subsidiary (escape) pacemaker rates are often fast enough to prevent clinical signs at rest.

Many bradyarrhythmic animals are *apparently* subclinical; that is, observers fail to recognize subtle clinical signs associated with the bradyarrhythmia. Most of the clinical bradyarrhythmias occur in older animals, and so owners often attribute subtle clinical signs to the normal effects of aging. However, most owners report significant and often surprising clinical improvement (increased alertness and activity level) in these older animals after the bradyarrhythmia is treated. Therefore, dramatic clinical signs are not a prerequisite for recommending treatment of these patients.

There are no unique or pathognomonic clinical signs of bradyarrhythmias, and signs may initially suggest a neurologic or neuromuscular disorder. Clinical signs (in order of increasing severity) include lethargy or reduced activity, fatigue or exercise intolerance, episodic weakness or disorientation, collapse or syncope (loss of consciousness, fainting), and, occasionally, generalized seizures (occurring after a period of syncope). Most animals appear outwardly normal at rest but may be unable to tolerate moderate or even mild physical activities. The more severe clinical signs result from cerebral hypoxia caused by decreases in cardiac output, arterial pressure, and cerebral perfusion. Normally, when heart rate decreases, stroke volume increases to compensate and maintain total cardiac output. However, if a maximum stroke volume is reached and heart rate decreases further, cardiac output decreases. The resulting decrease in mean arterial pressure may be mild and tolerable when the animal is resting or during mild activity. However, with increased activity, peripheral (muscular) vasodilation and increased oxygen demand outstrip circulatory delivery, causing muscular fatigue and exercise intolerance. If cerebral perfusion and oxygen delivery also decrease, the more severe clinical signs of altered mentation or consciousness may occur.

Owners may present an animal for evaluation of intermittent and transient ataxia or behavioral abnormalities (brief periods of confusion, staring or "spacing out"). These signs are similar to the symptoms of *presyncope* in humans. Presyncope refers to the feelings of momentary weakness, light-headedness, dizziness, and tunnel vision, similar to the sensations of orthostatic (postural) hypotension. In presyncope, cerebral perfusion is restored before the patient loses consciousness and collapses. Since animals cannot report symptoms, we usually describe any similar observable signs in dogs and cats as episodic or intermittent weakness or disorientation.

Cessation of cardiac output and loss of cerebral perfusion for more than 6 to 8 seconds usually causes loss of consciousness and syncope. Syncopal attacks are usually brief, lasting from 1 to 10 seconds. There is an abrupt loss of consciousness with collapse that may be preceded by a brief period of incoordination, excitement, anxiety, or confusion. Vocalization, loss of autonomic control of visceral functions (voiding, defecating, salivating), and tonic-clonic activity are much less common than in animals with generalized seizures but can occur. Recovery is usually rapid, with no postictal period, and animals often resume normal activity quickly, seemingly oblivious to the episode. Prolonged cerebral hypoxia may occasionally result in a seizure during the syncopal episode. It may be difficult to determine whether the seizure is caused by a central nervous system disorder or a bradyarrhythmia, especially if the arrhythmia is intermittent and infrequent. It is important to try to differentiate between cardiac and central nervous system signs, as the subsequent diagnostic and therapeutic approaches are quite different.

Physical findings in bradycardic animals include exaggerated arterial pulses (unless the bradycardia is related to hypoadrenocorticism) and audible periods of bradycardia. These periods may take the form of intermittent pauses in an otherwise normal rhythm or a persistently slow, regular or irregular rhythm. Tachyarrhythmias (premature beats, paroxysmal tachycardia) may also be present in some patients (see later). In animals with atrioventricular (AV) block, fourth heart sounds associated with isolated atrial contractions and nonconducted P waves, are sometimes audible. Other findings reflect the presence or absence of underlying structural heart disease. In the absence of coexisting valvular or myocardial disease, signs of congestive heart failure are uncommon, although ascites and other signs of right heart failure have been observed in a few active, persistently bradycardic dogs without apparent underlying structural cardiac disease.

CHARACTERIZATION OF BRADYARRHYTHMIAS

Although an experienced clinician may suspect a specific bradyarrhythmia by physical examination, confirmation requires electrocardiographic (ECG) examination. Lead II is the most popular lead used for rhythm analysis in dogs and cats, but it is advisable to record all standard limb and chest leads and to examine every lead, especially when the rhythm is difficult to identify in lead II. In particular, recognition and timing of P waves is critical in identifying the specific arrhythmia, which is important for determining prognosis and treatment options. After identifying the arrhythmia, an attempt should be made to evaluate its etiology and clinical importance to the individual patient.

VAGALLY MEDIATED BRADYARRHYTHMIAS

Vagally mediated bradyarrhythmias arise from an imbalance of the autonomic nervous input to the heart. Affected animals usually have no major structural or conduction tissue pathology but, instead, have increased parasympathetic (vagal) and/or decreased sympathetic tone. Specific arrhythmias that may occur with high vagal tone include (1) *sinus bradycardia,* (2) *respiratory and nonrespiratory sinus arrhythmia,* (3) *SA block or arrest,* (4) *second-degree AV block,* and (5) *third-degree AV block* (rare). Escape beats may occur if the ventricular rate decreases enough to allow subsidiary (junctional or ventricular) pacemakers to spontaneously discharge. First-degree AV block (prolonged PR interval) may also be present. The most commonly encountered vagally mediated bradyarrhythmia is respiratory sinus arrhythmia (RSA), characterized by a rhythmic increase and decrease in heart rate during inhalation and exhalation, respectively. In most cats and many dogs, the rate variation is very mild. Some dogs, especially middle-aged to older small breeds or those with respiratory disease, can show very marked changes in respiratory rate (Fig. 1*A*). A wandering pacemaker, characterized by phasic changes in amplitude of P waves (in lead II P-wave amplitude increases during inhalation and decreases during exhalation), is also commonly present. Comparison of respiratory phase with heart rate by auscultation or ECG will identify most cases of RSA.

NONVAGAL BRADYARRHYTHMIAS

Clinically important nonvagal bradyarrhythmias are usually associated with pathology in the cardiac conducting system but may also result from certain metabolic disorders. These arrhythmias result from a failure to propagate an impulse in the SA node, or a failure to conduct the impulse to the atrial or ventricular myocardium.

Sinoatrial Nodal Disorders

The failure to generate an SA impulse can result in *sinus bradycardia,* intermittent *sinoatrial arrest,* or persistent *atrial standstill.* These conditions may result from primary disorders of the SA node or extrinsic disorders that affect SA nodal electrical properties. Primary disorders of the SA node include *sick sinus syndrome* (SSS) and *persistent atrial standstill.* Occasionally, infiltration or destruction of myocardium by neoplasia or a cardiomyopathy may affect the myocardium and SA node. Extrinsic disorders causing abnormally slow SA activity include metabolic disorders such as hyperkalemia or hypothermia, endocrine disorders such as hypothyroidism and hypoadrenocorticism, and autonomic system disorders such as feline and canine dysautonomia. Noncardiac clinical signs usually predominate with the extrinsic disorders, and therapy should be directed primarily at the underlying disorder.

Sick Sinus Syndrome

Sick sinus syndrome (SSS) is the term used to describe primary conduction abnormalities that produce erratic, inconsistent SA depolarizations, inadequate subsidiary escape rhythms, and clinical signs of bradycardia. The resulting bradyarrhythmias may include inappropriate sinus bradycardia, SA block, or intermittent SA arrest. Electrocardiographically, it is characterized by an unpredictable sinus rhythm that is interrupted by periods of SA slowing, pauses, or arrest, with inconsistent junctional or ventricular escape complexes. Variable degrees of first- and second-degree AV block may also be present. Some animals have premature atrial or ventricular depolarizations or periods of supraventricular (sinus or atrial) tachycardia (see Fig. 1*B*), suggesting more generalized conduction system involvement. This condition occurs predominantly in small breeds of dogs, including Miniature Schnauzers, American Cocker spaniels, and West Highland White terriers. The bradyarrhythmias of SSS typically show widely varying degrees of responsiveness to vagolytic drug administration.

Recently, bradyarrhythmias have been reported in some Doberman pinschers with dilated cardiomyopathy and syncope (Calvert et al, 1996). These dogs develop a profound sinus bradycardia or SA arrest associated with excitement or exercise, similar to vagally-mediated neurocardiogenic syncope in humans. However, drug therapy effective at controlling neurocardiogenic syncope in humans (beta-adrenergic blockade) has been unsuccessful in controlling clinical signs in these dogs, suggesting a different etiology (see *CVT XII,* p. 799).

Persistent Atrial Standstill (Atrioventricular Muscular Dystrophy)

Persistent atrial standstill is an uncommon condition that has been recognized predominantly in Springer spaniels and Old English sheepdogs. It has also been reported in a few Siamese cats with advanced dilated cardiomyopathy. In dogs, it has been compared to certain human muscular dystrophies (Emery-Dreifuss muscular dystrophy, fascioscapulohumeral muscular dystrophy) and has been called *atrioventricular muscular dystrophy* (see *CVT XI,* p. 786). Electrocardiographically, the rhythm is characterized by a primary junctional or idioventricular escape rhythm without detectable P waves (see Fig. 1*C*). Incomplete forms with

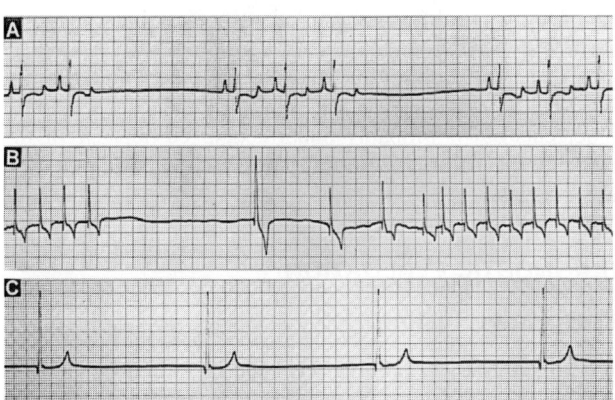

Figure 1. *A,* Lead III ECG from a Beagle dog with chronic lower airway disease, demonstrating pronounced respiratory sinus arrhythmia. Paper speed = 50 mm/sec. *B,* Lead II ECG from a Miniature Schnauzer with sick sinus syndrome. A period of sinoatrial arrest is followed by a single ventricular escape complex, two junctional beats, and then a burst of supraventricular tachycardia. Paper speed = 25 mm/sec. *C,* Lead II ECG from a Labrador retriever with atrial standstill, characterized by complete absence of P waves and a junctional escape rhythm at a rate 45 beats/min. Paper speed = 50 mm/sec.

small, barely detectable P waves and complete AV block may also occur. Intra-atrial electrograms typically show no, or only focal, atrial electrical activity. This disorder is unique in that there is progressive atrial and ventricular muscular degeneration and fibrosis, often resulting in congestive heart failure. The condition is usually fatal within 12 to 18 months of initial diagnosis.

Hyperkalemia

Increasing serum potassium concentration causes brady-arrhythmias that range from simple sinus bradycardia (serum K^+ 6 to 7 mEq/L) to a *sinoventricular rhythm* (serum K^+ ≥7 to 8 mEq/L). On the ECG, sinoventricular rhythm looks identical to, and is often initially called, atrial standstill. However, in hyperkalemia the rhythm originates in the SA node, but the impulse propagates through specialized atrial conduction fibers to the AV node and ventricles without depolarizing the atrial myocardium, resulting in loss of visible P waves on the ECG. Sinoventricular rhythm is usually distinguishable from primary atrial standstill by other clinical findings associated with severe hyperkalemia and its underlying cause.

DISORDERS OF CARDIAC CONDUCTION

Failure of an SA node impulse to conduct to the atrial or ventricular myocardium is the most commonly diagnosed type of *conduction block*. These disorders are usually separated into SA and AV blocks.

Sinoatrial Block and Arrest

Sinoatrial exit block occurs when normally generated SA impulses fail to exit the SA node. The resulting ECG shows one or more missing P waves, and the duration of the resulting pauses are multiples of the prevailing interval between normally conducted P waves. *Sinoatrial arrest* is diagnosed when the SA pauses are longer than 2 normal P-P intervals. Because of the high incidence and marked variability of RSA in many normal dogs, it is especially difficult to distinguish between normal and pathologic sinus arrhythmias (RSA, SA exit block, and SA arrest) in dogs. Fortunately, the causes, evaluations, and treatments are similar. Differentiation between vagally-mediated and non-vagal SA arrest is usually accomplished with provocative testing (see later).

Atrioventricular Block

Atrioventricular block is present when SA impulses are inhibited from conducting normally to the ventricular myocardium. Three degrees of severity of AV block are distinguished: first-degree AV block (prolonged AV conduction, prolonged P-R interval); second-degree, incomplete AV block (intermittent AV conduction, one or more nonconducted P waves); and third-degree, complete AV block (no AV conduction, asynchronous and independent P waves and QRS complexes; Fig. 2A and B). Only second- and third-degree AV blocks produce bradyarrhythmia. First- and second-degree AV blocks may be vagally-mediated (see earlier), drug-induced (digoxin, beta-blockade), or pathologic. In third-degree AV block, the pulse rate is

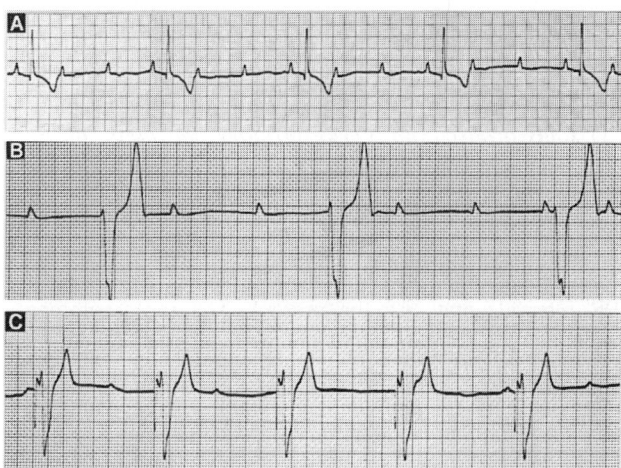

Figure 2. *A*, Lead II ECG from a mixed-breed dog with high-grade second-degree AV block. Only every third P wave is conducted to the ventricles (3:1 block). *B*, Lead II ECG from a German Shepherd dog with third-degree (complete) AV block. There is complete atrioventricular dissociation, with an atrial rate of 120 beats/min and a ventricular escape rhythm at a rate of 40 beats/min. *C*, Lead V$_4$ ECG obtained from the same dog as in *B* after transvenous pacemaker implantation. The atrioventricular dissociation persists, but the paced ventricular rate is 75 beats/min. Pacing spikes can be seen at the beginning of each ventricular complex. Paper speed for all tracings = 50 mm/sec.

determined by the rate of the subsidiary junctional or ventricular escape rhythm. Pathologic (nonvagal, nonpharmacologic) AV block is due to disease affecting the AV node or His-Purkinje system and is diagnosed much more often in dogs than in cats. Although the block may be acute and transient (e.g., trauma, sepsis, thrombosis, or iatrogenic causes), most cases of high-grade second- and third-degree AV block are pathologic, idiopathic, and permanent. Histologically, there may be fibrosis of the cardiac conduction tissue without an identifiable etiology. Reports have demonstrated possible associations between third-degree AV block and acquired myasthenia gravis (Hackett et al, 1995) or seropositivity for *Borrelia burgdorferi* (Levy and Duray, 1988) in dogs. Other potential associations include hyperthyroidism in cats, cardiomyopathies in dogs and cats, and congenital disease (Johnson and Sisson, 1993). Idiopathic AV block is occasionally observed in older cats but is probably underrecognized because of the intermittent nature or more rapid escape rate noted in this species.

DIAGNOSTIC EVALUATION

Provocative Testing

Once a bradyarrhythmia has been identified by ECG, it is advisable to determine whether it is wholly or partially autonomic in origin. This is done by provocative testing to alter vagal and/or sympathetic tone either physiologically (exercise, excitement) or pharmacologically (usually by atropine response testing).

Physiologic testing of bradyarrhythmias uses exercise to decrease vagal tone and increase sympathetic tone in response to an increased demand for cardiac output. Because physiologic testing is difficult to standardize and because animals with severe bradycardia may be reluctant to exercise, the authors do not advocate exercise testing of these patients. It is generally easier and more consistent to manipulate autonomic balance pharmacologically.

Chemically increasing sympathetic tone and heart rate is possible with the use of intravenous infusion of isoproterenol or dopamine. However, this method requires a constant-rate infusion and strict attention to infusion rate to prevent the development of tachyarrhythmias. This treatment is most useful therapeutically as a short-term, interim measure for increasing the junctional-ventricular escape rate in severely bradycardic animals that are being prepared for pacemaker implantation or other procedures. For routine testing of SA rate and AV conduction in bradycardic animals, it is usually much simpler and safer to pharmacologically decrease vagal tone with a vagolytic drug.

The atropine response test involves recording the ECG before and after the administration of parenteral atropine to reduce or abolish vagal tone. There is no single, standardized protocol recognized for atropine testing in animals, so clinicians should understand the range and sequence of anticipated responses to this drug, especially in dogs. In normal dogs, complete vagolysis results in a very regular sinus rhythm (no sinus arrhythmia) with a normal PR interval and no P-wave variability (wandering pacemaker). Incomplete responses are commonly recorded, especially following subcutaneous administration or use of low doses, or if the ECG is recorded too soon after administration (Rishniw et al, 1996). In dogs, the authors currently recommend administering atropine, 0.04 mg/kg IV, and recording the ECG after 10 to 15 minutes. A normal response is indicated by a heart rate increase of at least 100% or an increase to a rate more than 140 bpm. If a partial response is recorded after 15 minutes, the test is repeated with a second 0.04 mg/kg IV dose. Although the authors have much less experience testing cats (because of the relative rarity of serious bradyarrhythmias in cats), they use a similar protocol.

It is important to recognize when the response to atropine is abnormal and when it is normal but incomplete. In dogs, atropine appears to block vagal input to the SA node before the AV node. If the ECG is monitored continuously after administration, it is common to first observe an increased P-wave rate with first- and second-degree AV block. After several more minutes or following a second dose, AV conduction improves and normal, regular sinus rhythm or sinus tachycardia is observed without AV block. If this sequence is not understood, a partial response can be erroneously interpreted as pathologic. Whenever there appears to be a partial response, especially when a bradyarrhythmia is strongly thought to be vagally mediated, an additional dose of atropine should be administered and monitoring continued.

The expected atropine response of the common bradyarrhythmias should also be understood. In most animals with pathologic second- and third-degree AV block, vagolysis increases the atrial (P) rate, but AV conduction does not improve and the ventricular (QRS) rate does not increase significantly (there may be a slight increase in the number of conducted impulses in second-degree AV block or in the ventricular escape rate in third-degree AV block). Dogs with atrial standstill usually show little or no ECG response to atropine administration. The most variable response to

vagolysis occurs in dogs with SSS. A few dogs with SSS show no response, while most show at least a partial response to atropine administration. Some of these dogs show a normal initial response with resumption of regular sinus rhythm for several minutes, but then begin to develop SA pauses with or without AV block. Some dogs develop regular, but ectopic atrial or junctional rhythms. Some dogs with SSS may even appear to be completely responsive to atropine, making differentiation of a purely autonomic arrhythmia from a pathologic arrhythmia very difficult.

When an atropine-responsive bradyarrhythmia is identified, causes of increased vagal tone should be considered. Vagally mediated bradyarrhythmias usually occur in normal healthy individuals, and may be pronounced in highly athletic and brachycephalic breeds. The pathologic causes of increased vagal tone include chronic respiratory disease (chronic bronchitis, collapsing trachea, brachycephalic syndrome), central neurologic disease (brain tumors, encephalitides), gastrointestinal disease, hypothyroidism, drugs (e.g., xylazine, digoxin, beta-blockers), systemic hypertension, and ocular or retrobulbar disease. The authors have also seen a case of hypoadrenocorticism associated with a vagally-mediated third-degree AV block that resolved with treatment of the primary disorder. Vagal bradyarrhythmias usually do not cause clinical signs, and treatment to increase heart rate is rarely indicated.

Cardiac Evaluation

If a bradyarrhythmia fails to correct following administration of atropine, potential endocrine or metabolic diseases (hyperkalemia, hyperthyroidism, hypothyroidism, myasthenia gravis) or other major medical disorders (borreliosis) should be ruled out with appropriate laboratory tests. An echocardiogram and chest radiographs should be obtained to identify any valvular, myocardial, or other structural cardiac or thoracic disease that may underlie the conduction disorder and affect prognosis and response to treatment. Most dogs with pathologic AV block have no major underlying structural disease and respond well to treatment to raise heart rate. In rare cases, neoplasia, endocarditis, or other discrete pathology may be identified by echocardiography. Dogs diagnosed with persistent atrial standstill, on the other hand, always have atrial dilatation and may have ventricular dilatation and subnormal systolic function (decreased left ventricular shortening fraction) as indicators of an underlying degenerative myocardial disease. Many of the smaller breed dogs with SSS are middle-aged or older and have mild or moderate degenerative valvular disease with mitral and tricuspid regurgitation. Although comparatively rare, many cats with bradyarrhythmias have serious underlying myocardial disease that may limit their survival and response to raising heart rate. In each case, the evaluation is aimed at uncovering any underlying or additional medical problems that may affect the appropriateness and type of treatment offered.

Additional Electrophysiologic Testing

In some cases, the history and clinical signs, resting ECG, and response to atropine provocation give results that are equivocal or inconclusive. Additional evaluations may be indicated when (1) a suspected arrhythmia in a symptomatic animal cannot be documented on resting ECGs, (2) an arrhythmia appears to be mild and cannot be convincingly associated with reported clinical signs, or (3) an arrhythmia that appears to be clinically significant is abolished by atropine administration. To improve the chances of recording an intermittent or variable arrhythmia, continuous, 24-hour ambulatory ECG tape recording (Holter monitoring; see *CVT XII*, p. 792) is recommended.

In rare cases, intracardiac electrophysiologic (EP) study may provide additional proof of SA nodal dysfunction or abnormal AV conduction. In humans with suspected SSS, SA conduction time (SACT) and SA node recovery time (SNRT) are often measured prior to pacemaker implantation. Electrode catheters are inserted into the right atrium, and the atrium is paced at various rates. The SNRT is measured after sudden cessation of rapid atrial pacing, and the SACT is measured as the time taken for an impulse to conduct from the SA node to the low atrial myocardium. Similar studies have not been reported in animals with spontaneous bradyarrhythmias.

MANAGEMENT OF BRADYARRHYTHMIAS

The primary goal of treatment of symptomatic bradyarrhythmias is to increase the ventricular rate to a level that abolishes or markedly reduces clinical signs and improves the quality of life. This objective is accomplished either with drug treatment or by implantation of an artificial pacemaker. After a specific rhythm abnormality has been diagnosed, the first decision to be made is whether treatment is indicated, based on the type and severity of the arrhythmia and its expected natural history, the nature and severity of clinical signs, the presence of other cardiac or medical problems, the desires of the owner, and the availability of facilities and expertise for pacing. If an underlying cause is identified (e.g., hyperthyroidism, hypoadrenocorticism, brain tumor, urinary obstruction), therapy should be directed at first resolving or controlling this condition before a commitment to long-term treatment of the arrhythmia is made. Many cats and some dogs with bradyarrhythmias show no obvious clinical signs, even to a very observant owner. However, such signs may be subtle, making it difficult to determine the relative merits of treatment versus nontreatment. In such situations, knowledge of the natural history of each type of arrhythmia and experience with similar patients are often the keys to an informed decision.

The natural histories and risks of the common bradyarrhythmias are quite variable. Although there are occasional exceptions, vagally mediated bradyarrhythmias usually do not cause overt clinical signs, are not progressive, and do not require medical therapy. Some dogs with suspected SSS may show few clinical signs, and some appear to have a normal response to atropine administration. In these dogs, SSS can be strongly suspected if the signalment is typical (e.g., middle-aged or older Miniature Schnauzers, American Cocker spaniels). Routine monitoring of heart rate and rhythm, as well as educated observation by the owner, should be initiated. Fortunately, the risk of sudden death in SSS appears to be low, so there is little urgency to advise extensive diagnostic tests or to intervene immediately in dogs with equivocal or very mild and infrequent signs. However, dogs with SSS can develop serious, drug-resis

tant bradyarrhythmias when put under general anesthesia. In these dogs, anesthesia should be performed only after preoperative placement of a transvenous temporary pacing lead and control of the heart rate by external pacing.

Most animals with high-grade second- and third-degree AV blocks *are* symptomatic, although syncope may not be observed and other signs may be subtle and unrecognized by owners. In the authors' experience, dogs with idiopathic AV block and uniform, regular, and consistent escape rhythms have had a low risk of sudden death. Dogs with irregular, multiform, and unpredictable escape rhythms have had a greater incidence of both sudden death and life-threatening complications during anesthesia (cardiac arrest or ventricular fibrillation). Dogs with atrial standstill usually have regular, consistent escape rhythms and have a low risk of sudden death. However, they are at very high risk for developing progressive myocardial failure and congestive heart failure within 6 to 24 months after their bradyarrhythmia has been diagnosed.

Drug Treatment

Pharmacologic agents used to increase heart rate are either anticholinergic-vagolytic drugs or sympathomimetic-adrenergic drugs (Sisson, 1989; Tilley, 1992). These drugs are variably effective in dogs with SSS and are generally ineffective in animals with third-degree AV block or atrial standstill. The most commonly prescribed anticholinergic agents include propantheline bromide (Pro-Banthine, Searle; in dogs, 7.5 to 30 mg PO every 8 hours; in cats, 7.5 mg PO every 8 to 12 hours) or isopropamide (in dogs, 0.2 to 0.4 mg/kg PO every 8 to 12 hours). Prescribed sympathomimetic agents include theophylline (in dogs, 9 mg/kg PO every 6 to 8 hours; in cats, 4 mg/kg PO every 8 to 12 hours), aminophylline (in dogs, 11 mg/kg PO every 8 hours; in cats, 5 mg/kg PO every 8 to 12 hours), or terbutaline (Brethine, Geigy; in dogs, 0.2 mg/kg PO every 8 to 12 hours; in cats, 0.625 mg PO every 12 hours). In some dogs with SSS, the frequency or duration of sinus pauses and resulting clinical signs may be reduced during treatment with either type of drug. These drugs are usually well tolerated, but improvement is usually partial and often temporary, lasting from several weeks to several months. Rarely, these drugs may exacerbate an arrhythmia and clinical signs.

Some human patients with third-degree AV block have demonstrated improvement when treated with theophylline or aminophylline (Kragie and Sekovski, 1992), but these drugs are usually prescribed only in patients who are poor candidates for permanent pacing. These drugs may be given to animals with high-grade second- or third-degree AV block or atrial standstill, but they usually cause no or only a slight increase in the ventricular rate. There is also some unpublished evidence that high-grade AV block may occasionally improve or recover in response to glucocorticoid therapy, suggesting that an inflammatory disorder may underlie the AV nodal dysfunction in some cases (e.g., Lyme disease). The authors have rarely observed a significant response in symptomatic AV blocks and atrial standstill to oral anticholinergic or sympathomimetic drug administration, and have little experience with the use of corticosteroids for these arrhythmias. Nevertheless, medical therapy is a very poor substitute for pacing, and clients

interested in pacing should not be delayed in obtaining more effective therapy for their pets.

Pacemaker Implantation

Permanent implantation of an artificial pacemaker to provide electrical pacing of the ventricles is the most consistently effective treatment for symptomatic bradyarrhythmias, whether originating in the SA node, atrium, or AV node (see Fig. 2C). The pacing system consists of a pulse generator and a flexible, Silastic-coated lead wire that attaches to the heart. Early clinical reports of pacemaker implantation in dogs described the use of lead wires attached to the left ventricular epicardium via lateral thoracotomy (pulse generator positioned subcutaneously) or transdiaphragmatically via laparotomy (pulse generator positioned in the abdomen). In the past 10 years, however, transvenous endocardial pacing has become the approach of choice in dogs. With this method, the electrode wire is inserted into a jugular vein and maneuvered via fluoroscopy into the right ventricle, where the tip is secured against the endocardium. The pulse generator is positioned subcutaneously over the neck or back. The procedure is not technically difficult, although fluoroscopy is required. Greater expertise is required to be able to evaluate pacemaker function postoperatively and to troubleshoot malfunctioning systems. The authors usually set the resting pacemaker rate to about 80/min for a large dog, up to about 100/min for a small dog. Newer-generation pacemakers allow a range of rates to be programmed, permitting the heart rate to vary with the physiologic demands of the patient (so-called rate-responsive pacemakers). Transvenous pacemaker implantation in dogs carries a relatively low risk of major complications, and the clinical response is almost always favorable (for more procedural and technical details, see *CVT X*, 1989, p. 286). There are only a few reports of pacemaker implantation in cats with symptomatic bradyarrhythmias. The small size of the jugular veins in cats and their tendency to spasm when manipulated make transvenous implantation more difficult; thus, transthoracic (epicardial) implantation may be required. Modern pacemakers have projected life spans of 6 to 8 years or more, so an animal must survive for several years before encountering battery depletion and requiring pulse generator replacement.

When one considers pacemaker implantation, the same relative risks versus benefits noted earlier must be considered, plus the significant costs of the procedure and associated equipment. The authors recommend against pacemaker implantation for animals with equivocal clinical signs and ECG findings. Candidates for pacing should show convincing clinical signs or have a disorder that is known to cause significant physical limitations (e.g., high-grade AV block) or to worsen over time (e.g., atrial standstill). Fortunately, most bradyarrhythmias in animals do not carry a high risk of sudden death without prior clinical signs. The justification for pacing, therefore, is more about improving quality of life than preventing death, although improving longevity is also a factor, especially in complete AV block. The prognosis should be discussed prior to implantation. For example, owners of Springer spaniels with atrial standstill should understand that the dog probably has a cardiomyopathy that will progress and cause clinical deterioration over time, despite the improved heart rate afforded by pacemaker therapy (pacing may markedly improve the quality of life for these dogs for many months). On the other hand, pacemaker implantation for SSS or third-degree AV block often results in a markedly improved quality of life for the animal for several years.

The authors believe that all dogs with high-grade second- or third-degree AV block, even those whose owners are not aware of any clinical signs, benefit from pacemaker implantation. Owners consistently report significant and often surprising improvement in their pets' general attitude and activity level after pacing is instituted. The authors also recommend pacing as the most effective treatment for dogs with symptomatic SSS, as this disorder is permanent and sometimes progressive. Follow-up surveys of owners of dogs with uncomplicated transvenous pacemaker implants have indicated a high level of satisfaction with the procedure and the outcome, especially the consistently improved quality of life for their pet.

References and Suggested Reading

Calvert CA, Jacobs GJ, Pickus CW: Bradycardia-associated episodic weakness, syncope, and aborted sudden death in cardiomyopathic Doberman Pinschers. J Vet Intern Med 10:88, 1996.
Contains examples of bradycardic sinus node dysfunction in Doberman pinschers with cardiomyopathy.

Hackett TB, Van Pelt DR, Willard MD, et al: Third-degree atrioventricular block and acquired myasthenia gravis in four dogs. J Am Vet Med Assoc 206:1173, 1995.
Describes findings in four dogs that had both third-degree AV block and acquired myasthenia gravis.

Johnson LR, Sisson DD: Atrioventricular block in cats. Compend Contin Educ 15:1356, 1993.
An excellent description of the causes, clinical and electrocardiographic presentation, and treatment of AV blocks in cats.

Kragie L, Sekovski B: Theophylline: An alternative therapy for bradyarrhythmia in the elderly. Pharmacotherapy 12:324, 1992.
A prospective study on the use of theophylline in humans with various symptomatic bradyarrhythmias.

Levy SA, Duray PH: Complete heart block in a dog seropositive for *Borrelia burgdorferi*: Similarity to human Lyme carditis. J Vet Intern Med 2:138, 1988.
Describes an association and the pathological findings in a dog with third-degree AV block that was seropositive for Lyme disease.

Miller MS, Tilley LP, Atkins CE: Persistent atrial standstill (atrioventricular muscular dystrophy). In: Kirk RW, Bonagura JD, eds: Kirk's Current Veterinary Therapy XI. Philadelphia: WB Saunders, 1992, p 786.
A detailed discussion of AV muscular dystrophy in Springer spaniels.

Moise NS, Defrancesco T: Twenty-four-hour ambulatory electrocardiography (Holter monitoring). In: Bonagura JD, ed: Kirk's Current Veterinary Therapy XII. Philadelphia: WB Saunders, 1995, p 792.
An excellent description of Holter monitor use in dogs, including protocols for data acquisition, data analysis, and indications.

Rishniw M, Tobias AH, Slinker BK: Characterization of chronotropic and dysrhythmogenic effects of atropine in bradycardic dogs. Am J Vet Res 57:337, 1996.
Describes some of the responses that can occur with atropine administration in small doses or by different routes.

Sisson DD: Bradyarrhythmias and cardiac pacing. In: Kirk RW, ed: Kirk's Current Veterinary Therapy X. Philadelphia: WB Saunders, 1989, p 286.
Provides information about pacing techniques in small animals.

Sisson DD, Thomas WP, Woodfield JA, et al: Permanent transvenous pacemaker implantation in 40 dogs. J Vet Intern Med 5:322, 1991.
Describes the technique, complications, and outcomes of transvenous pacing in dogs with various bradyarrhythmias.

Tilley LP: Essentials of Canine and Feline Electrocardiography, 3rd ed. Philadelphia: Lea & Febiger, 1992.
Defines the limits for normal heart rates in dogs and cats.

Assessment and Treatment of Supraventricular Tachyarrhythmias

KATHY N. WRIGHT
Cincinnati, Ohio

Once considered relatively benign rhythm disturbances, supraventricular tachyarrhythmias (SVTs) are now known to be a potential cause as well as a result of structural heart disease. SVTs can cause a variety of clinical signs, including weakness, syncope, and even congestive heart failure. Sustained or frequently recurrent SVTs may lead to tachycardia-induced cardiomyopathy, indistinguishable from idiopathic dilated cardiomyopathy (DCM), but potentially reversible with effective long-term control of the SVT. SVTs may rarely even precipitate sudden death if resultant myocardial ischemia leads to ventricular tachycardia or fibrillation, or antiarrhythmic drugs used to treat SVTs have a proarrhythmic effect. Insights into SVT mechanisms provided by electrophysiologic studies during the past decade and the ability to cure certain SVTs have improved the diagnosis, treatment, and recognition of complications of these common arrhythmias.

DEFINITIONS

Supraventricular tachyarrhythmias are rapid rhythms either originating in the atria or using the atria or atrioventricular (AV) junction above the bundle of His as a crucial component of the tachycardia circuit. The term *paroxysmal atrial tachycardia* was used generically by some cardiologists to mean SVT. This general term has become outdated as we learn the multiple mechanisms that are responsible for SVTs. One useful classification scheme with diagnostic and therapeutic applications broadly divides SVTs into atrial or junctional tachyarrhythmias (Wathen et al, 1993). Atrial tachyarrhythmias are SVTs using atrial tissue alone for initiation and maintenance of the arrhythmia. Junctional tachyarrhythmias are SVTs that require the AV junction as an essential component of the tachycardia's initiation or maintenance, while the atrium may or may not be needed. Physiologic sinus tachycardia is in a unique class by itself, not included as a form of SVT.

ASSESSMENT OF SUPRAVENTRICULAR TACHYARRHYTHMIAS

Clues From the History and Physical Examination

History and signalment can provide useful initial information in determining the mechanism of SVT. The physical examination should include careful evaluation for underlying structural heart disease and heart failure. A clinician should strongly suspect the presence of an accessory AV pathway and AV reciprocating tachycardia in young to middle-aged animals that present with rapid, narrow QRS

complex tachycardia (see *CVT XII*, p. 807) without apparent structural heart disease. Based on what is known about humans with similar clinical histories, AV nodal reentrant tachycardia and AV reciprocating tachycardia are the most common SVTs in this group. Animals with DCM and SVT may have SVT resulting from DCM, or, more commonly than previously recognized, DCM resulting from sustained SVT. Often, reassessment of the structural heart disease after weeks to months of strict arrhythmia control is the only reasonable means of determining which disease process came first. If the structural heart disease involves primarily atrial dilation, intra-atrial reentrant tachycardia, automatic atrial tachycardia, atrial flutter, and atrial fibrillation should be carefully considered.

Surface Electrocardiographic Features

A logical, mechanistic-based approach to the surface electrocardiogram (ECG) is necessary when one evaluates SVTs. Supraventricular tachyarrhythmias characteristically exhibit narrow QRS complexes. In rare cases, however, a bundle branch block (preexistent or tachycardia-dependent) or conduction from atria to ventricles over an accessory AV pathway produces a wide QRS complex tachyarrhythmia that is supraventricular in origin. It is emphasized, however, that the vast majority of tachyarrhythmias with wide QRS complexes are ventricular tachyarrhythmias, not aberrantly conducted SVTs. Once narrow QRS complexes occurring at a rapid rate have been identified, one must decide whether the QRS complexes occur in a regular, regularly irregular, or irregularly irregular pattern. Atrial fibrillation is classically irregularly irregular. Other commonly encountered SVTs have regular patterns. Variable degrees of AV block of an atrial tachyarrhythmia produce irregularity in the occurrence of QRS complexes, but the ventricular response may still have a pattern (i.e., it is regularly irregular).

Identification of P′ waves* is the next important step in assessing the tachyarrhythmia; however, P′ waves may be very hard to identify during a rapid SVT. This task is made more difficult when one examines only one or two limb leads. Instead, all possible leads should be run at both normal and maximal sensitivities. P′ waves are often more easily identified in precordial (chest) leads than in standard limb leads. If an ECG machine is not equipped for precordial leads or if P waves remain obscure, the right and left arm electrodes of the standard ECG can be placed in various positions along the sternal borders of the chest wall

---

*P′ waves indicate atrial depolarization that does not originate in the sinoatrial node.

(Lewis leads) while monitoring the "lead I" channel to better demonstrate atrial activity. Esophageal leads are also valuable, but lack of patient cooperation limits their use.

The presence or absence of visible P′ waves, P′ wave morphology, and the relationship of a P′ wave to the preceding QRS complex all are helpful in SVT diagnosis (Fig. 1). The absence of visible P′ waves during a regular SVT, despite employment of all of the tactics previously discussed, is suggestive of typical AV nodal reentrant tachycardia, during which atrial and ventricular activation occur simultaneously. If the P′ wave is closer to the preceding QRS complex than to the subsequent QRS complex, so that the RP′ interval is less than or equal to 50% of the RR interval, the SVT is classified as a short RP′ SVT. If,

on the other hand, the P′ wave is closer to the subsequent QRS complex, with the RP′ interval more than 50% of the RR interval, the SVT is known as a long RP′ SVT. Figure 1 and Table 1 review the ECG characteristics and mechanisms of the more common SVTs.

Initiation and termination of the tachyarrhythmia are also important diagnostic features. Sudden onset and offset of SVT, without gradual rate acceleration and deceleration, respectively, are most characteristic of reentrant SVTs. Automatic SVTs (i.e., from discrete ectopic foci) exhibit a "warm-up" (rate acceleration on initiation) and "cool-down" (rate deceleration prior to termination) period. If a ventricular premature complex successfully terminates an SVT, it is almost certainly a junctional tachyarrhythmia.

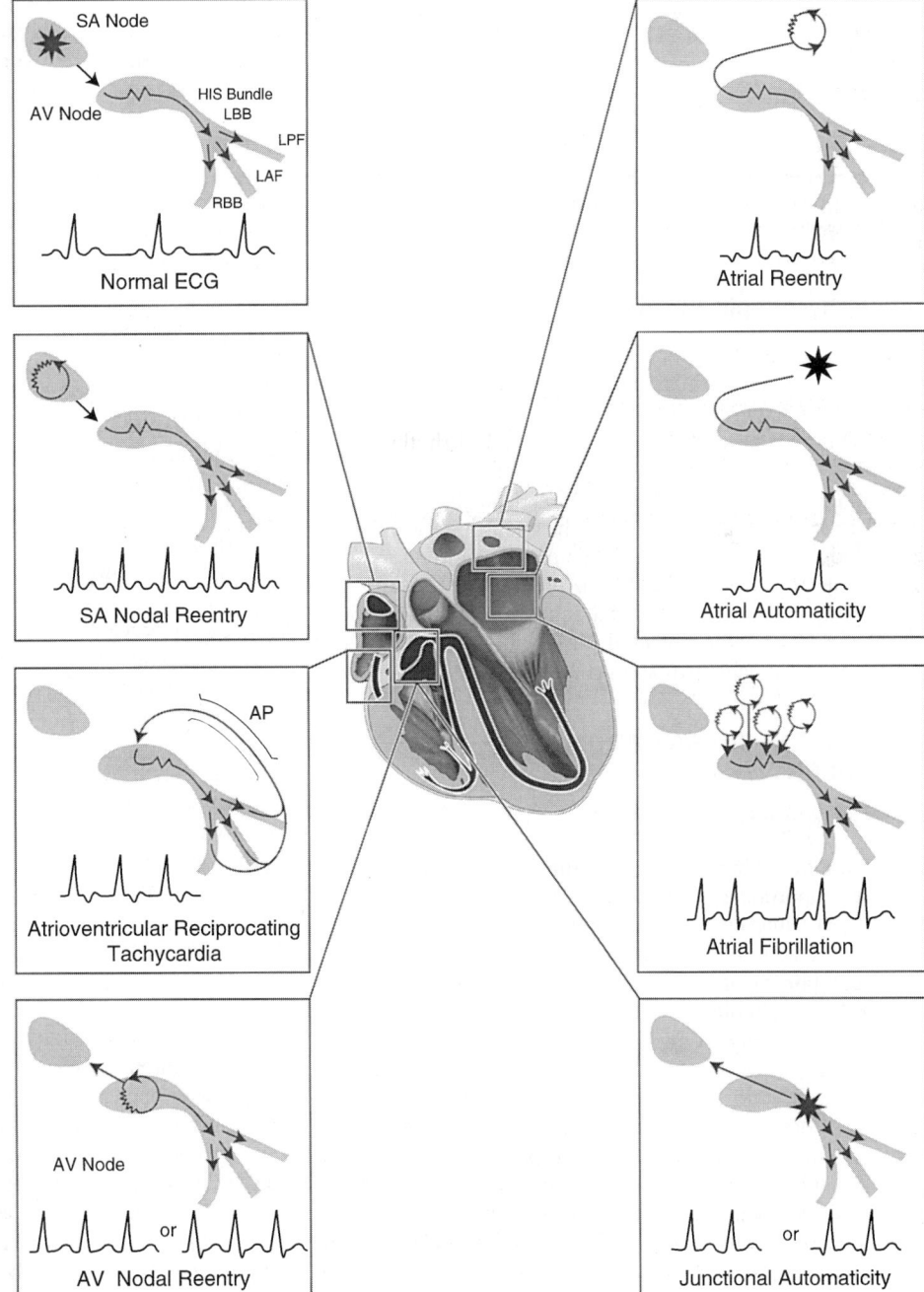

Figure 1. Illustration of the mechanisms and characteristic electrocardiographic features of the most common supraventricular tachyarrhythmias. ECG, electrocardiogram; SA, sinoatrial; AV, atrioventricular; LBB, left bundle branch; LPF, left posterior fascicle; LAF, left anterior fascicle; RBB, right bundle branch; AP, accessory pathway.

TABLE 1. **Typical Electrocardiographic Characteristics of Supraventricular Tachyarrhythmias**

SVT Mechanism	Visible P′ Waves	P′ Wave Morphology	RP′ Interval (vs. RR Interval)	Initiation/ Termination	Response to AVB
Atrial					
SNRT	Yes	Same as sinus P	Long	Abrupt onset/offset at SVT rate	SVT continues
AAT	Yes	Variable, differs from sinus P	Often long, but varies with SVT rate	Gradual rate acceleration/ deceleration	SVT continues
IART	Yes	Variable, differs from sinus P	Often long, but varies with SVT rate	Abrupt onset/offset at SVT rate	SVT continues
Atrial flutter	Flutter (F) waves	Identical saw-toothed F waves	Not applicable	Abrupt onset/offset at SVT rate	SVT continues
Atrial fibrillation	No. Fibrillation (f) waves may be seen	Not seen	Not applicable	Abrupt onset/offset at SVT rate (often incessant)	SVT continues
Junctional					
Common AV nodal reentrant tachycardia	Generally no. May be seen as pseudo-S wave in II, III, aVF	Retrograde (if seen): (−) in II, III, aVF	Short	Abrupt onset/offset at SVT rate, critical PR prolongation to initiate	SVT terminates
OAVRT	Yes. Within the ST-T segment	Retrograde: (−) in II, III, aVF	Typically short	Abrupt onset/offset	SVT terminates
AJT	Generally yes. AV dissociation common	Variable	Variable	Gradual rate acceleration/ deceleration	SVT continues with AV dissociation

SVT, supraventricular tachyarrhythmia; AVB, atrioventricular block; SNRT, sinus nodal reentrant tachycardia; AAT, automatic atrial tachycardia; IART, intra-atrial reentrant tachycardia; AV, atrioventricular; OAVRT, orthodromic atrioventricular reciprocating tachycardia; AJT, automatic junctional tachycardia.

Electrophysiologic Testing

Within the past 15 years in human cardiology, electrophysiologic testing with the use of percutaneously placed multipolar catheters has become commonplace. This valuable tool is available at certain veterinary referral centers and has been an important addition in both the diagnosis and the treatment of particular SVTs. Catheters are advanced to strategic locations in the heart through accessed veins (and occasionally arteries) for pacing and recording. The response of a patient's SVT to programmed electrical stimulation, the sequence of atrial activation, and the location of the His bundle potential during the SVT are used to diagnose its mechanism and "map" its location.

THERAPY FOR SUPRAVENTRICULAR TACHYARRHYTHMIAS

Acute Management

Division of SVTs into atrial and junctional tachyarrhythmias has important implications for management (Wathen et al, 1993). Junctional tachyarrhythmias may be successfully treated with single-agent therapy directed at any essential component of the circuit. Successful elimination of atrial tachyarrhythmias, on the other hand, requires "dual therapy." One drug is used initially to slow AV nodal conduction, then a second drug is used to terminate the atrial tachyarrhythmia itself. The site or sites of antiarrhythmic drug actions are shown in Figure 2. Vagal maneuvers lasting no more than 5 seconds (ocular pressure, gag reflex, single carotid sinus massage) may be helpful both diagnostically and therapeutically. These maneuvers may increase vagal tone, primarily slowing sinus nodal discharge and prolonging AV nodal conduction time and refractoriness.

If an SVT abruptly terminates in response to a vagal maneuver, AV nodal reentrant tachycardia, orthodromic AV reciprocating tachycardia, or sinus nodal reentrant tachycardia are most probable. Unfortunately, even SVTs using the sinus or AV nodes as essential circuit components typically fail to terminate with any vagal maneuver. Rare complications, such as ventricular fibrillation, may result, particularly from aggressive vagal maneuvers, so careful ECG monitoring during the procedure is essential.

Intravenous antiarrhythmic drug therapy may be used to treat a rapid SVT causing hemodynamic compromise. Hemodynamic (blood pressure) and ECG monitoring are important whenever one treats SVTs with intravenous agents. Diltiazem (Cardizem, Hoechst Marion Roussel; 0.125 to 0.35 mg/kg IV) now comes in a parenteral formulation and is being used widely in human and small animal patients. Its abilities to rapidly slow AV nodal conduction and prolong AV nodal refractoriness make diltiazem ideal for slowing the ventricular response to rapid atrial tachyarrhythmias and for terminating junctional tachyarrhythmias (except automatic junctional tachycardia). Diltiazem causes negative inotropic effects, necessitating the cautious use in the setting of left ventricular dysfunction; however, human clinical studies support its effective and safe use in patients with class III and IV heart failure and rapid SVTs (Heywood et al, 1991; Goldenberg et al, 1994). The author has used intravenous diltiazem in dogs with dilated cardiomyopathy who present with rapid, hemodynamically compromising SVT (often atrial fibrillation), after initial treatment with parenteral furosemide if congestive heart failure is present. Diltiazem is as effective and appears to have far fewer adverse effects than parenteral verapamil.

Adenosine (Adenocard, Fujisawa USA, Inc.) is another parenteral antiarrhythmic drug that slows AV nodal conduc-

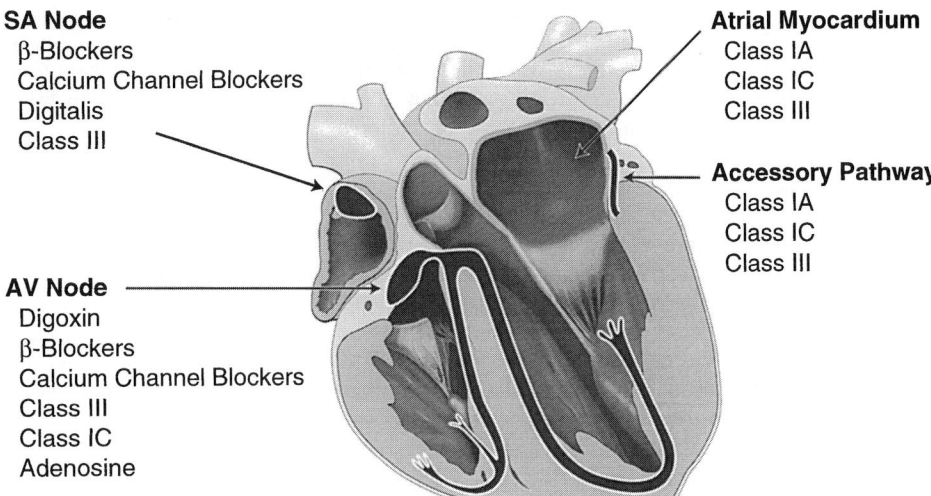

SA Node
β-Blockers
Calcium Channel Blockers
Digitalis
Class III

Atrial Myocardium
Class IA
Class IC
Class III

Accessory Pathway
Class IA
Class IC
Class III

AV Node
Digoxin
β-Blockers
Calcium Channel Blockers
Class III
Class IC
Adenosine

Figure 2. Sites of action of antiarrhythmic drugs, highlighting their utility for specific supraventricular tachyarrhythmias. SA, sinoatrial; AV, atrioventricular.

tion in humans. It must be administered as a rapid intravenous bolus, ideally through a central vein. Although the drug of choice for terminating SVTs (or distinguishing SVT from ventricular tachycardia) in human medicine, this agent has not been effective in dogs. Adenosine dosages up to 2 mg/kg did not slow AV nodal conduction in dogs in a recent study (unpublished data). In a limited number of cases, dosages of 0.5 mg/kg IV rapidly have failed to terminate junctional SVTs, which would consistently terminate in a person at one third of that dosage. An ultrashort-acting, selective beta₁-blocker, esmolol (Brevibloc, Ohmeda) at 0.5 mg/kg IV over 1 minute, has been used to slow AV nodal conduction and interrupt certain SVTs. Because its half-life is so brief compared to the longer-acting intravenous propranolol, esmolol is the preferred parenteral beta-blocker, as adverse effects are also short-lived. Nonetheless, it should be used cautiously in animals with ventricular dysfunction. Esmolol appears less effective than parenteral diltiazem in terminating canine junctional SVTs and has become the author's second choice of intravenous AV nodal–blocking drugs.

Procainamide is a class IA antiarrhythmic available in a parenteral formulation (Pronestyl, Elkins-Sinn, Inc.), which prolongs the refractory periods of atrial and ventricular myocardium, retrograde AV nodal pathways, and accessory AV pathways. Dosages of 6 to 8 mg/kg IV over 3 minutes or 6 to 20 mg/kg IM have been successful in terminating atrial tachyarrhythmias (after drugs to slow AV nodal conduction have been administered) and AV reciprocating tachycardia in dogs. There is far less experience with parenteral procainamide in cats. The adverse effects include hypotension with rapid intravenous administration and gastrointestinal upset. Myocardial contractility is not impaired except at higher doses (although the drug can cause vasodilation); therefore, procainamide can be used in animals with left ventricular dysfunction.

Chronic Antiarrhythmic Drug Therapy

Chronic antiarrhythmic drug therapy for atrial tachyarrhythmias may involve "dual" therapy, as discussed earlier,

or, with persistent atrial fibrillation, combination therapy to slow the ventricular response rate. The animal in congestive heart failure is placed on digoxin (Lanoxin, Glaxo Wellcome, or Cardoxin, Evsco Pharmaceuticals) at 0.005 to 0.01 mg/kg PO every 12 hours (dogs) or 0.0312 mg PO every 24 to 48 hours (cats) as an initial AV nodal–blocking drug. One exception is the cat with hypertrophic cardiomyopathy and atrial tachyarrhythmias, in which diltiazem is considered the drug of choice. The ventricular response rate is not sufficiently slowed in most animals with digoxin alone. The addition of a second AV nodal–blocking agent generally produces the targeted ventricular response. The choice is between a calcium-channel blocking and a beta-blocking drug. There are theoretical reasons for supporting either choice. Currently, the author chooses diltiazem, 0.5 to 1.5 mg/kg PO every 8 hours (dogs) and 7.5 mg PO every 8 hours (cats) because animals in congestive heart failure subjectively appear to tolerate this drug better than the dose of beta-blocker required to achieve equivalent ventricular rate control. Other clinicians prefer beta-blockers. The vasodilator properties of calcium-channel blockers may partially offset their negative inotropic effects in the failing heart (Falk, 1996). Also, in a small percentage of cases, diltiazem has converted an atrial tachyarrhythmia (presumed to be caused by triggered activity) to sinus rhythm.

Oral procainamide—Pronestyl, 10 to 20 mg/kg PO every 4 to 6 hours (dogs) and 3 to 8 mg/kg PO every 6 to 8 hours (cats)—has been used as one agent in dual-therapy regimens for atrial tachyarrhythmias and as single-agent therapy for junctional tachyarrhythmias. Higher dosages (up to 40 mg/kg PO every 6 hours) have been required for controlling junctional SVTs in some dogs. Gastrointestinal side effects and proarrhythmic concerns (particularly in animals with structural heart disease) are the major factors limiting chronic procainamide use in small animals. Antiarrhythmic drugs currently being investigated for utility in the management of atrial and junctional SVTs include amiodarone (Cordarone, Wyeth-Ayerst), with the widest spectrum of antiarrhythmic actions, and sotalol (Betapace, Berlex Laboratories), with beta-blocking and class III antiarrhythmic properties.

Nonpharmacologic Therapy

A few veterinary referral centers offer the possibility of curing, rather than simply controlling, certain SVTs. Transvenous catheter ablation with the use of radiofrequency energy has revolutionized the treatment of SVTs in human patients. This procedure follows the "mapping" of an SVT circuit using multiple electrode catheters. A specialized catheter with a 4- to 5-mm distal-tip electrode is positioned at a critical site within the circuit, and radiofrequency energy is delivered through the distal electrode causing thermal destruction of a small volume of tissue, sufficient to cause interruption of the tachyarrhythmia. This technique has been used with great success in human patients, and has been used by this author and others in a few canine cases.

References and Suggested Reading

Chakko S, Kessler KM: Recognition and management of cardiac arrhythmias. Curr Probl Cardiol 6:59, 1995.
General review of SVT mechanisms, diagnosis, and management.
Falk RH: Pharmacologic control of heart rate in atrial fibrillation. Cardiol Clin 14:521, 1996.
A discussion of the benefits and risks of various antiarrhythmic drugs that slow AV nodal conduction.
Goldenberg IF, Lewis WR, Dias VC, et al: Intravenous diltiazem for the treatment of patients with atrial fibrillation or flutter and moderate to severe congestive heart failure. Am J Cardiol 74:884, 1994.
A randomized, double-blind, placebo-controlled study of 37 human patients with atrial fibrillation and congestive heart failure. The beneficial and adverse effects of diltiazem are discussed.
Heywood JT, Graham B, Marais GE, et al: Effects of intravenous diltiazem on rapid atrial fibrillation accompanied by congestive heart failure. Am J Cardiol 67:1150, 1991.
Original study of nine men with congestive heart failure and a rapid ventricular response to atrial fibrillation who were treated with intravenous diltiazem.
Wathen MS, Klein GJ, Yee R, et al: Classification and terminology of supraventricular tachycardia. Cardiol Clin 11:109, 1993.
A review of the confusion in SVT terminology and presentation of a new classification scheme with diagnostic and therapeutic utility.
Wright KN: Novel techniques in the treatment of arrhythmias. Emerg Sci Technol 1:16, 1995.
A description of electrophysiologic testing and catheter ablation techniques in companion animals.
Zipes DP: Management of cardiac arrhythmias: Pharmacological, electrical, and surgical techniques. In: Braunwald E, ed: Heart Disease: A Textbook of Cardiovascular Medicine. Philadelphia: WB Saunders, 1996, p 593.
A review of various treatment modalities for SVTs.
Zipes DP: Specific arrhythmias: Diagnosis and treatment. In Braunwald E, ed: Heart Disease: A Textbook of Cardiovascular Medicine. Philadelphia: WB Saunders, 1996, p 640.
Specific mechanisms of SVT are discussed in more detail.

Reason Must Supersede Dogma in the Management of Ventricular Arrhythmias

DAVID H. KNIGHT
Philadelphia, Pennsylvania

Detection of ventricular ectopic beats often raises concern out of proportion to existing clinical circumstances. Consequently, antiarrhythmic drugs are frequently dispensed unnecessarily, based on unrealistic expectations for both the benefits of therapy and the actual risks directly related to the rhythm disturbance. To understand this orientation and encourage reconsideration of this practice, it may be helpful to consider the apparent origins of these attitudes and review what the experience has actually been with these common clinical events.

CONDITIONED ATTITUDES AND SOURCES OF CONFUSION

From the earliest, most impressionable stages of clinical training, veterinary students are taught to recognize the distinctive QRS morphology of ventricular ectopic beats. To justify this exercise, these electrocardiographic (ECG) patterns tend to be inseparably linked to the presence of cardiac disease or the potentially adverse clinical consequences that ventricular arrhythmias may provoke or exacerbate. This connection between occurrence and complications is reinforced in virtually all veterinary textbooks by seamless transitions between passages dealing with recognition of ventricular ectopic beats and those detailing the properties of antiarrhythmic drugs. Guidance for dispensing these drugs focuses on their pharmacologic characteristics and dosing protocols. Comment, if any, on the merits of therapy tends to project worst-case scenarios for untreated arrhythmias and neglect to address the difficulty in suppressing ectopic beats and the lack of tangible benefit from attempting to do so. Common notions regarding therapy are neither supported by veterinary clinical trials nor challenged with insights from actual experience. With few exceptions, the implication is usually unambiguous and simple: it is prudent to suppress ventricular arrhythmias. Consequently, it is not surprising that this response has become reflexive and widely adopted as conventional wisdom.

Myocardial infarction due to coronary artery disease (CAD) is the most frequently cited example in which death is often preceded by ventricular ectopy. The period immediately following infarction is a particularly vulnerable time during which human patients are at great risk for cardiogenic shock, ventricular arrhythmias, and sudden death. Although CAD is a major cause of morbidity and mortality in humans, it is not a significant entity in companion animals. Furthermore, the substrate of myocardial damage from CAD is unique and causes greater vulnerability to electrical instability than generally exists in other conditions. Veterinary clinicians have been inordinately influenced by the natural history of ventricular arrhythmias in human patients with CAD and electrophysiologic studies of iatrogenic myocardial ischemia in dogs. Despite the lack of correspondence in terms of acute onset, severity of cardiac complications, and potential risk of life, there is a common tendency to extrapolate from this high-profile disease to any other in which ventricular arrhythmias occur. These erroneous assumptions are widely accepted and have become entrenched as dogma.

Traditionally, the potential risk of ventricular ectopic beats triggering sudden death has been classified on the basis of their prematurity, frequency of occurrence, and morphologic diversity. This descriptive approach to the QRS complex facilitates easy recognition and stratification by type. However, ventricular arrhythmias in many disorders represent *dependent risk factors* and lack specificity as predictors of clinical outcome (Packer, 1992). Failure to consider the extent of underlying structural heart disease and cardiac dysfunction contributes to the erroneous assumption that all multiform, closely coupled, and repetitive ventricular ectopic beats are equally dangerous. This nondiscriminatory approach encourages frequent and often irrational administration of antiarrhythmic drugs.

EXAMINING THE EVIDENCE

Ventricular ectopic beats occurring singularly or in short runs are common and ubiquitous. In certain clinical circumstances, they can be a destabilizing force, but generally they are transient, benign events causing no appreciable clinical signs. Although supraventricular tachycardias (SVTs), such as atrial fibrillation and paroxysmal atrial tachycardia, tend to be viewed more tolerantly, they are usually associated with substantial structural heart disease that compromises cardiac function and frequently requires medical therapy. The difference in attitude toward ventricular arrhythmias as opposed to supraventricular arrhythmias stems from the perception that sudden death may be a consequence of the former, but not the latter, even though dogs with SVT are often significantly more compromised and may also die suddenly.

The traditional objectives for suppressing ventricular arrhythmias are (1) to relieve clinical signs of distress directly attributable to the cardiac rhythm and (2) to prevent sudden death triggered by fatal electrical instability. In the absence of clinical signs, suppressing frequent and even complex ventricular ectopic beats provides no benefit to apparently healthy people (Kennedy et al, 1985). However, signs as mild as the sensation of palpitations may cause sufficient discomfort or anxiety to justify treatment. In animals, the clinical signs must be more overt to be recognizable. Signs such as syncope, transient weakness, hypotension, blanched membranes, or acute exacerbation of heart failure, if directly linked to changes in rhythm, justify treatment. Therapy can be judged successful and worthy of continuation only if some control of related signs is achieved. Reduction in the number of ectopic events can be used as a measure of pharmacologic efficacy—but not therapeutic benefit.

There is no evidence that traditional drug treatment of ventricular arrhythmias prevents sudden death in dogs or cats. Speculation with regard to the utility of certain class I antiarrhythmic drugs for this purpose in human patients was ended by the Cardiac Arrhythmia Suppression Trial (CAST, 1992) conducted to test the hypothesis that suppression of asymptomatic and mildly symptomatic ventricular rhythms in patients surviving myocardial infarction would decrease the incidence of sudden death and improve overall survival. The conclusion drawn from the results of this trial is that antiarrhythmic drugs do not prevent malignant ventricular arrhythmias or sudden cardiac death. This axiom appears to be universal, since the same conclusion has been drawn from earlier studies of human patients with other cardiac diseases (Chakko and Gheorghiade, 1985). No comparable clinical trials have been conducted in veterinary patients, but there is no fundamental reason why they should respond differently.

Frequent ventricular ectopic beats and runs of nonsustained ventricular tachycardia in dogs are encountered most frequently in injured or ill patients with no independent evidence of heart disease. Trauma patients often display ventricular arrhythmias, even when the injury does not directly involve the heart (Macintire and Snider, 1984). The widely held supposition that these arrhythmias are a manifestation of "traumatic myocarditis" is an unfortunate misconception that continues to misguide the medical management of these patients by conveying legitimacy to the notion that consequential myocardial damage is present or will develop. Although myocardial damage appears not to be the cause, the mechanism of these arrhythmias remains an enigma. Ventricular arrhythmias also occur commonly with gastric dilatation-volvulus (GDV) (Brockman et al, 1995) and splenic masses (Marino et al, 1994). Ventricular arrhythmias seldom are a direct cause of hemodynamic instability in these instances, and although these rhythms may be responsive to drugs (Knapp et al, 1993) the value of such treatment is unproven. Furthermore, spontaneous reversion to normal sinus rhythm generally occurs within a few days without antiarrhythmic drugs, if the inciting disease process is dealt with successfully.

Accelerated idioventricular rhythm is one of the most common examples of a benign arrhythmia erroneously accorded pathologic status sufficient to justify antiarrhythmic therapy (Fig. 1). Typically, the ventricular ectopic pacemaker rate is slightly faster than the slowest phase of the accompanying sinus arrhythmia. Whenever the sinus rate slows, the ectopic pacemaker emerges and captures the heart beat. At times, the rhythm may be dominated by nonsustained runs of ectopic beats. The rate of this nonparoxysmal ventricular tachycardia is nearly the same as the sinus rhythm and seldom exceeds 170 beats/min. Passive ventricular filling is ordinarily not compromised significantly at this heart rate, unless, independently, ventricular function is severely depressed. Even when ventricular ectopy takes the form of frequent, single-complex premature beats, cardiac output is usually not adversely affected despite some pulse deficits, unless the ectopic beats are very

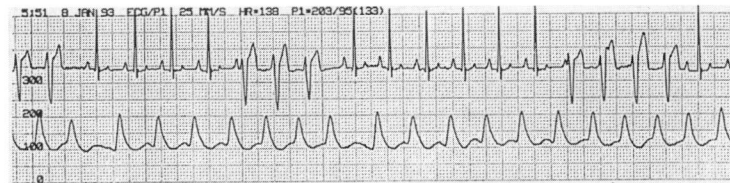

Figure 1. Long-axis electrocardiogram and metatarsal arterial blood pressure of a dog with a fractured femur, a ruptured kidney, and uroperitoneum. A slight sinus arrhythmia (HR, ~134) alternates with runs of accelerated ventricular rhythm (HR, ~150). The transition between rhythms is not a perfect example of the description in the text, but the recording does illustrate preservation of blood pressure and, indirectly, the stroke volume, during the ventricular beats. Pressure scale (mm Hg); chart speed (25 mm/sec).

premature and are especially numerous. It is not the frequency of the ectopic beats per se, but their clinical effect that is important.

Whether the myocardium is transiently injured as a consequence of neurohumoral factors, metabolic imbalances, or transient myocardial ischemia, survival depends on skillful and timely medical and surgical attention to the primary clinical problem—not antiarrhythmic drug therapy. Ventricular arrhythmias may trigger the moment of death but seldom are responsible for the preceding clinical deterioration. In a large retrospective study of GDV dogs (Brockman et al, 1995), antiarrhythmic drug therapy did not improve survival. More compelling causes of death are usually evident from an objective evaluation of all the clinical evidence. The fact that the most severely injured or ill patients with the worst prognoses for survival may also have ventricular ectopy does not justify blaming the rhythm disturbance for deaths that in all probability are not preventable. As self-evident as these assertions are to those who take this approach, skeptics will hold out for double-blind, placebo-controlled prospective studies in animals to confirm the mounting evidence in defense of these principles that has been accumulating in the human literature.

In other clinical settings, ventricular ectopic beats are a distinct risk factor for sudden death, independent of their immediate hemodynamic effect or frequency of occurrence. This association has been made in many cases of dilated cardiomyopathy, especially in the Doberman pinscher breed (see p. 756) and in dogs with subaortic stenosis (see *CVT XII*, p. 822). Both ventricular arrhythmias and sudden death are relatively common in the late stages of these conditions but are not always linked. Concern for these patients is both real and justified. However, the prospects for positively influencing their clinical course with antiarrhythmic drugs is problematic, at best, and may create additional clinical problems (Calvert et al, 1996). Even more ominous is the occurrence of ventricular ectopy in certain German shepherd dogs without structural heart disease but having a hereditary predisposition to developing fatal ventricular arrhythmias (Moise et al, 1994). These examples of dogs at real risk for arrhythmia-induced sudden death are recognizable by their special circumstances and clinical signs, and are not representative of the more commonplace cases in which ventricular ectopy is ordinarily not hazardous.

A MORE RATIONAL APPROACH

When ventricular arrhythmias are identified, a methodical approach should be followed to determine an appropriate medical response.

Determine the Nature of the Problem. Ventricular ectopy is usually a secondary manifestation of disease, not a primary etiologic factor. The clinical context in which the arrhythmia occurs usually distinguishes between the asymptomatic or benign rhythms and those exerting a destabilizing effect. The often transient appearance of ventricular arrhythmias may require ambulatory ECG monitoring (see *CVT XII*, p. 792) to establish a cause-and-effect relationship between changes in rhythm and episodic clinical signs.

Focus on the Primary Clinical Problems. When ventricular ectopy accompanies a noncardiac disease, it is usually self-limited, if the primary problem is addressed successfully. If cardiovascular function is compromised, it should be supported appropriately with fluid and electrolyte replacement, blood transfusion, or heart failure therapy as circumstances may warrant. Unless the arrhythmia directly impairs ventricular function, any attempt to suppress it is likely to be an unproductive digression. In most instances, when antiarrhythmic drug therapy is administered, it is in the context of acute medical support delivered in the hospital as part of a critical care protocol. In a well-equipped and adequately staffed intensive care unit (ICU), direct arterial blood pressure monitoring is frequently already in place and available for providing an objective beat-to-beat assessment of cardiac function. Although less precise, Doppler methods of blood pressure measurement may also be informative. Specific treatment protocols are addressed in the next article.

Justify Your Choices. The prospects for improving the patient's condition by modifying cardiac rhythm should be realistic. The additional drugs and professional time such a strategy requires should be considered in the cost-benefit analysis.

Be Fully Committed If Antiarrhythmic Therapy Is Elected. There is no assurance that the first drug and dosage chosen will produce a pharmacologic or therapeutic benefit, without methodical titration. The frequency and pattern of ventricular arrhythmias are unpredictable; thus, a reduction in ectopy can be assessed objectively only with diligent in-hospital and ambulatory outpatient monitoring. Protracted treatment of ventricular arrhythmias is usually not necessary, and its need should be challenged by periodic discontinuation. Casual treatment of ventricular arrhythmias is likely to produce misleading results that only perpetuate the misconceptions that have confused and misdirected management of this category of cardiac rhythm disturbance.

References and Suggested Reading

Brockman DJ, Washabau RJ, Drobatz KJ: Canine gastric dilatation/volvulus syndrome in a veterinary critical care unit: 295 cases (1986–1992). J Am Vet Med Assoc 207:460, 1995.
A comprehensive retrospective review of risk factors, including cardiac arrhythmias.

Calvert CA, Pickus CW, Jacobs GJ: Efficacy and toxicity of tocainide for the treatment of ventricular tachycardias in Doberman pinschers with occult cardiomyopathy. J Vet Intern Med 10:235, 1996.
Documents serious adverse side effects and limited pharmacologic efficacy without resolving the issue of long-term therapeutic efficacy.

Chakko CS, Gheorghiade M: Ventricular arrhythmias in severe heart failure: Incidence, significance, and effectiveness of antiarrhythmic therapy. Am Heart J 109:497, 1985.
Documents failure to prevent sudden death by treating asymptomatic complex ventricular arrhythmias in congestive heart failure patients who had ischemic or idiopathic dilated cardiomyopathy.

Echt DS, Liebson PR, Mitchell LB, et al: Mortality and morbidity in patients receiving encainide, flecainide, or placebo (The Cardiac Arrhythmia Suppression Trial). N Engl J Med 324:781, 1991.
Watershed study documenting the inherent risks of class 1C antiarrhythmic drug therapy and its failure to prevent sudden death in human survivors of myocardial infarctions.

Kennedy HL, Whitlock JA, Sprague MK, et al: Long-term follow-up of asymptomatic healthy subjects with frequent and complex ventricular ectopy. N Engl J Med 312:193, 1985.
Documents the benign nature of complex ventricular arrhythmias in people with otherwise normal hearts.

Knapp DW, Aronsohn MG, Harpster NK: Cardiac arrhythmias associated with mass lesions of the canine spleen. J Am Animal Hosp Assoc 29:122, 1993.
Noncontrolled study failing to distinguish between the clinical course of ventricular arrhythmias treated with antiarrhythmic drugs and the natural course of similar arrhythmias in untreated dogs.

Macintire DK, Snider TG III: Cardiac arrhythmias associated with multiple trauma in dogs. J Am Vet Med Assoc 184:541, 1984.
Case summaries of 10 dogs treated for ventricular arrhythmias in anticipation of complications, 8 of which survived and returned to normal sinus rhythm.

Marino DJ, Matthiesen DT, Fox PR, et al: Ventricular arrhythmias in dogs undergoing splenectomy: A prospective study. Vet Surg 23:101, 1994.
Detection of rapid (rate unspecified) ventricular tachycardia increased with splenic rupture and intensity of monitoring.

Moise NS, Meyers-Wallen V, Flahive WJ, et al: Inherited ventricular arrhythmias and sudden death in German shepherd dogs. J Am Coll Cardiol 24:233, 1994.
Detailed evaluation of fatal ventricular tachycardias (illustrated) suspected of being induced by imbalance of the sympathetic nervous system.

Packer M: Lack of relation between ventricular arrhythmias and sudden death in patients with chronic heart failure. Circulation 85:(suppl I):50–56, 1992.
Advances the thesis that antiarrhythmic drugs should not be added to the treatment of human heart failure patients with asymptomatic ventricular arrhythmias, no matter how frequent and complex the rhythm disturbance.

CVT Update: Ventricular Arrhythmias

N. Sydney Moïse
Ithaca, New York

VENTRICULAR ARRHYTHMIAS TO TREAT

When antiarrhythmic drugs are used, the assumption is that the frequency of the arrhythmias will be reduced, the risk of death lessened, and clinical signs abolished. However, these beneficial results do not always occur—instead, adverse consequences may develop. Proarrhythmia, heart failure, and noncardiovascular side effects can follow the use of antiarrhythmics. Therefore, only dogs exhibiting clinical signs or those at the highest risk for sudden death should be targeted for specific antiarrhythmic treatment.

The clinical problem is deciding which arrhythmias are dangerous and may result in sudden death. As indicated in the previous article, recommendations in veterinary medicine are based primarily on testimonial experiences without adequate scientific proof or extrapolating evidence from studies in human patients (Link et al, 1996). The general recommendation for treating ventricular arrhythmias is that single premature ventricular complexes (PVCs) usually are not treated, while ventricular tachycardia (VT), especially if very rapid or causing hypotension, usually is treated. However, standard electrocardiographic (ECG) recordings may not reveal the presence of VT because of the brevity of the monitoring. Ventricular tachycardia may only be revealed by 24-hour ECG monitoring. Not all VTs are considered dangerous. Ventricular rhythms that are considered lower risk are VTs (1) that are approximately the rate of the underlying sinus rhythm, (2) that are nonsustained (less than 30 seconds in duration), (3) that have a long coupling interval to the preceding normal beat, and (4) that are monomorphic. Conversely, the categorization of dangerous VT is based on the constellation of characteristics that include (1) rapid heart rate, (2) sustained rhythm, (3) short coupling interval, and (4) polymorphism.

Although limited information is available, certain clinical scenarios are more likely to demand that ventricular arrhythmias be treated, while others are usually self-limited. In human patients, myocardial dysfunction is the major determinant of risk, and this extrapolation is most likely true for dogs. Moreover, even before the development of myocardial failure, Boxers with VT (Boxer cardiomyopathy) and a history of syncope have a substantial risk of sudden death. These Boxers may not have VT documented, but may have other ventricular arrhythmias (frequent PVCs and shortly coupled pairs and triplets) that signature the potential for VT and ventricular fibrillation. German shepherd dogs with very rapid nonsustained VT are at risk for death until 18 months of age, whereas those with only PVCs or those older than 18 months are at low risk (Moise et al, 1997). Alternatively, a young dog hit by a car that has slow (and hemodynamically tolerated) sustained VT or an elderly dog that has occasional polymorphic PVCs are both at low risk. Therefore, understanding the circumstances in which ventricular arrhythmias occur can be just as important as the assessment of the rhythm itself.

ROLE OF THE AUTONOMIC NERVOUS SYSTEM

The neurogenic and humoral sympathetic influence not only affects the generation of the ventricular arrhythmias but also can modify the effectiveness of antiarrhythmic drugs (Podrid et al, 1990). Regardless of the mechanism underlying the arrhythmia, elevations in sympathetic tone can be arrhythmogenic. Not only can arrhythmias be triggered by adrenergic stimulation, but the antiarrhythmic effects of drugs can be nullified by catecholamines, as has been demonstrated with class I antiarrhythmic drugs.* Class I drugs such as mexiletine may actually have improved antiarrhythmic effects when combined with a beta-adrenergic blocker. Moreover, the prolongation of the action potential caused by class III antiarrhythmics may be optimal only when sympathetic tone is not elevated. Therefore, the combination of a beta-adrenergic blocker and class III action (e.g., amiodarone and sotalol) may be required. The major problem when one uses beta-adrenergic blockers with antiarrhythmic agents occurs in patients with myocardial failure.

TREATMENT PLAN

The treatment of arrhythmias demands a systematic approach. First, the most likely cause should be determined. The frequency of the ventricular arrhythmia must be documented to establish a baseline ectopic complex number. Ideally, this requires a minimum of a 24-hour ECG monitor. This monitoring is important for later interpretation of drug efficacy or proarrhythmic effect. Serum electrolyte concentrations (Na$^+$, K$^+$, Cl$^-$, Mg^{++}) should be measured. Hypokalemia can potentiate or cause VT and, in cats, may be a correctable cause of VT. If a drug can be tested for efficacy in an acute situation, the resulting findings may provide some information as to the effectiveness of the drug and potential side effects. During the short-term follow-up, which for most drugs is based on reaching steady state at 2 to 10 days, an evaluation of drug efficacy can be made. Finally, the long-term evaluation should be planned, because the disease state can change and arrhythmias may spontaneously lessen or increase.

DRUG SELECTION

Some general considerations of drug selection are clinically relevant. In the selection of an antiarrhythmic, a specific drug may not effective, but this does not mean that another drug within the same Vaughn Williams class (classes I through IV) will not be beneficial. Moreover, the treatment response is not concordant when a compound is administered by different routes. That is, just because a

drug is effective intravenously does not ensure that the compound given orally will give the same salutary effect. During chronic oral treatment, the accumulation of active metabolites and different myocardial concentrations may account for some of the differences that can occur between the routes of administration.

Drugs Most Often Used for Acute Treatment

Lidocaine. The most consistently effective drug to use intravenously for the rapid conversion of life-threatening, hemodynamically unstable, incessant VT is lidocaine (Stanton, 1995). Lidocaine can be given as a bolus or as an intravenous infusion. An initial bolus of 1 to 2 mg/kg can be given to judge response. Higher doses may be required, but rarely as high as 4 mg/kg. The bolus can be given rapidly within seconds; however, it is probably wiser to administer the bolus over 30 seconds. The effectiveness of lidocaine is short-lived and abates in approximately 10 to 15 minutes, if not sooner. Once the effectiveness of the lidocaine has been established, a constant-rate infusion can be started. It takes 3 to 6 hours for lidocaine to reach a steady-state concentration; thus, boluses of lidocaine will need to be repeated to maintain the antiarrhythmic effect. These boluses can be repeated at approximately 10-minute intervals. To prevent toxic side effects, the total dose given over approximately 1 hour should not exceed 8 mg/kg. As an alternative to repeated bolus treatment, the lidocaine infusion detailed below can be delivered at twice the maintenance dose for the first hour of treatment.

The dosage range for an infusion of lidocaine is wide, 25 to 80 µg/kg per minute, and one should adjust the dosage to effectiveness without causing toxicity. The infusion rate should be decreased in animals with liver disease or congestive heart failure. To prepare a constant-rate infusion with a midrange dose of 50 µg/kg per minute, 25 ml of fluid is removed from a 500-ml bag of fluids (e.g., lactated Ringer's solution). This fluid is replaced with 25 ml of 2% (20 mg/ml) lidocaine, which will provide a concentration of 1,000 µg/ml. The drip rate is calculated at the same rate that is used for administering a standard maintenance amount of fluids (approximately 70 ml/kg per 24 hours) for the dog. The infusion rate may be increased by delivering an increased amount of fluid or by making the infusion solution more concentrated. When it is believed that the infusion is no longer necessary, the infusion may be stopped without tapering. Lidocaine is stored in adipose tissues and continues to be released for several hours. Because the fluid and drug rate must frequently be more individualized, the dosing formula (next page) can be used to more precisely adjust the constant-rate infusion.

Lidocaine may be given intramuscularly to dogs at a dose of 4 mg/kg. In humans, therapeutic plasma levels occur within 10 to 15 minutes, with effects lasting about 90 minutes. Lidocaine should not be used intramuscularly in the presence of shock, because absorption from the site of injection may be erratic.

Lidocaine can cause central nervous system signs characterized by twitching, tremors, anxiousness, and seizures. Cats are especially sensitive to neurotoxic effects. These problems are usually avoided with careful selection of dosage, and treated by stopping the lidocaine and adminis-

---

*This class includes lidocaine, mexiletine, procainamide, and quinidine.

$$
\left.\begin{array}{l}\text{Volume (ml) of fluid to be removed from}\\ \\ \textit{and}\\ \\ \text{Volume (ml) of drug to be added back}\\ \\ \textit{to the fluid bottle or bag}\end{array}\right\} = \dfrac{\left[\dfrac{\text{CRI dose }(\mu g/kg/min)}{1{,}000\ \mu g/mg}\right] \times \text{Body weight (kg)} \times \begin{array}{c}\text{Volume of}\\ \text{fluids (ml)}\\ \text{to be given}\end{array} \times 60\ \text{min/hr}}{\begin{array}{c}\text{Drip rate of}\\ \text{fluids (ml/hr)}\\ \text{to be given*}\end{array} \times \begin{array}{c}\text{Concentration of}\\ \text{drug (mg/ml)}\end{array}}
$$

*For routine maintenance, the volume of fluid to be administered approximates 2.5 ml/kg/hr (adjust according to patient hydration, urine output, etc.).

tering diazepam if signs do not quickly abate. Lidocaine does not alter hemodynamics except transiently after intravenous bolus when there is pre-existing myocardial dysfunction. However, more profound effects at high doses can result in depression of blood pressure and cardiac output. This type of effect may then result in sinus tachycardia, although severe sinus bradycardia has been occasionally reported in humans and observed in cats.

Procainamide. Commonly in veterinary medicine and historically in human medicine, when lidocaine is ineffective in controlling VT, procainamide is administered intravenously as the second-choice drug. Recently, however, procainamide given intravenously was more effective in terminating sustained monomorphic VT than was lidocaine in humans. Whether lidocaine or procainamide is more beneficial in the treatment of a particular VT probably depends on the underlying mechanism of the arrhythmia, which usually cannot be determined in the canine patient. Procainamide is used more commonly for the treatment of ventricular arrhythmias than is quinidine because it has less physical side effects, less prolongation of the QT interval, and no interaction with digoxin, and causes less hypotension.

Procainamide can be given as an intravenous bolus at 10 to 15 mg/kg over 1 to 2 minutes. The bolus is administered slowly because it can cause hypotension, although in animals with normal myocardial function serious hypotension is uncommon. When continued parenteral administration is needed, a constant-rate infusion at 25 to 50 µl/kg per minute can be used. To prepare such an infusion, 5 ml of fluid is removed from a 500-ml bag of lactated Ringer's solution and then 5 ml of 10% (100 mg/ml) procainamide is added. This results in a concentration of 1,000 µg/ml. When given at a maintenance rate of 70 ml/kg per 24 hours (3 ml/kg per hour), a dose of 50 µg/kg per minute will be delivered. The constant-rate infusion formula can also be used. Using procainamide intramuscularly does not offer any benefit over oral medication unless the animal is unable to take oral medication, because the time to reach peak plasma levels approximates that of oral therapy.

Drugs Most Commonly Used for Chronic Treatment

Procainamide (and Quinidine). Procainamide, 10 to 20 mg/kg PO every 6 hours) is usually preferentially selected over quinidine in the treatment of VT in dogs. Oral quinidine frequently has more side effects than does procainamide, although depression and anorexia still plague both drugs. Both are relatively inexpensive, and although the sustained-release preparations cost more the added convenience offsets the modest drug expense. However, obtaining adequate blood levels is variable in dogs treated with the sustained-release procainamide (Procan SR, 10 to 20 mg/kg PO every 8 hours). If adequate arrhythmia control is not obtained, drug concentrations should be obtained to see whether subtherapeutic blood levels are present. In humans, procainamide, and especially quinidine, are less frequently used today because of the proarrhythmic effects. However, the real proarrhythmic threat in dogs with spontaneous arrhythmias from these drugs is not known.

Mexiletine. Mexiletine (Mexitil, Boehringer Ingelheim) may be used as a first-line antiarrhythmic drug for the oral treatment of VT in dogs. Currently in the United States, mexiletine is procurable only for oral use, but an intravenous form is available in Europe. Additionally, a sustained-release capsule (*Perlongets*) is available only in Europe. Mexiletine's electrophysiologic properties (i.e., onset-offset kinetics, sodium channel blockade, preferential effects in certain tissues) are similar to those of lidocaine; thus, the antiarrhythmic effectiveness and side effects of both drugs are comparable. Usually, VT that has been treated successfully with lidocaine may be most effectively treated with mexiletine. However, the effect of lidocaine does not always predict the response to mexiletine.

Adequate information is not available to conclusively state that mexiletine is superior to other drugs such as procainamide in the treatment of VT in dogs. However, some studies in humans substantiate the improved antiarrhythmic effect of mexiletine over procainamide and quinidine. Also, mexiletine may have less myocardial depressant effects on left ventricular function, and this may be beneficial in dogs with myocardial failure. Currently, at the author's hospital, mexiletine, 4 to 8 mg/kg PO every 8 hours, combined with atenolol, 0.5 mg/kg PO every 12 to 24 hours, is the first choice for the oral treatment of dangerous ventricular arrhythmias. Mexiletine costs substantially more than either procainamide or quinidine, but fewer side effects may reduce the overall cost of treatment. The side effects (trembling, seizures, anxiousness, depression) of mexiletine are similar to those of lidocaine at toxic doses. Gastrointestinal side effects can usually be limited by giving mexiletine with food. Mexiletine has less proarrhythmic effects than the commonly used class Ia drugs.

Beta-Adrenergic Blockers. The advantages of beta-adrenergic blockade in humans as an adjuvant treatment of

VT has been acclaimed because of the decrease in mortality. Beta-adrenergic blockers can decrease PVCs and VT, particularly those related to excessive catecholamines such as occur during certain anesthetic regimens (halothane) and exercise and in patients with hypertrophic cardiomyopathy. However, it has been argued that the use of the frequency of PVCs as a surrogate indicator of long-term beneficial versus adverse results (death) is not reliable. More specifically, it has been shown in humans that beta-adrenergic blockade alone only modestly affects the incidence of PVCs, but it does decrease mortality. The latter is most likely because of the antifibrillatory effects of beta-adrenergic blocking activity. Again, these studies are from humans or from dogs with experimentally induced infarctions, and the applicability to the canine patient with spontaneous arrhythmia is not known.

Different beta-adrenergic blockers are comparable in their antiarrhythmic effect, and, therefore, the selection of a particular agent is determined by other characteristics. For example, in humans metoprolol is the beta-adrenergic blocker that has shown benefit in congestive heart failure. This effect combined with the decrease in arrhythmias during metoprolol treatment may make this the beta-adrenergic blocker of choice in congestive heart failure. Commonly used beta-adrenergic blockers in veterinary medicine include atenolol and propranolol. However, the use of beta-adrenergic blockers during congestive heart failure must be weighed against the potential side effects, especially depression of myocardial function.

Newer Drugs for Chronic Treatment

Amiodarone and Sotalol. Only anecdotal information, with mixed results, is available regarding the use of these class III agents in the treatment of dogs with spontaneous VT. The varied experiences most likely reflect the variation in the dog population treated and the different doses used.

In humans, sotalol (Betapace, Berlex) and especially amiodarone (Cordarone, Wyeth-Ayerst) were previously reserved as last-chance treatments; however, these agents are more frequently used as first-line drugs today. The more frequent use of these two drugs is the result of favorable clinical trials. Although the empirical use of amiodarone or sotalol in dogs has been proposed because of these clinical trials, their use may be more effective for patients with coronary artery disease than for patients with cardiac failure or hypertrophic cardiomyopathy. Since coronary artery disease is rare in the dog, the value of these drugs is as yet unproven. Moreover, whether these drugs are more effective in dogs than the combination of mexiletine and a beta-adrenergic blocker or procainamide is unknown. Conversely, recent experience with sotalol in Boxers with dangerous UT has been positive. A recent study in humans showed that d,l-sotalol was more effective in suppressing arrhythmias than the combination of a class I drug with a beta-adrenergic blocker; however, no differences were found in survival between the two groups (O'Callaghan and McGovern, 1996). It should be emphasized that amiodarone and d,l-sotalol are not pure class III agents. Both have beta-adrenergic action that appears pivotal in the effectiveness of these drugs, and amiodarone also possesses class I and class IV activity.

Determining the dosing regimen of amiodarone is difficult because of its complex pharmacokinetics. Amiodarone is highly lipophilic and highly protein bound and has a high volume of distribution. Amiodarone given orally has a delayed and highly variable onset of action, making determination of clinical response difficult. Monitoring plasma concentrations of amiodarone may not be of benefit in determining the proper dose. Amiodarone potentially has severe and lasting side effects; thus, the goal should always be to use the smallest effective dose possible. In humans, many of the adverse effects initially reported were the result of excessively high doses. In dogs only very limited experience guides us. The following are recommended only as guidelines derived from the testimonial experiences of a few patients, from experimental studies of ischemic dog models, and from the mg/kg dosing recommended in the human pediatric population. A dose of 10 mg/kg PO every 24 hours was given to dogs in experimental studies (Patterson et al, 1983). This dose is given as a loading dose for 7 to 10 days followed by a maintenance dose of 5 mg/kg every 24 hours or three times per week.*

Studies in humans treated with amiodarone revealed no relationship between dose and efficacy of PVC suppression. Furthermore, controversy is evident with regard to the value of monitoring plasma levels. Despite these conflicts, plasma drug concentrations may be of some benefit in determining whether effective levels have been reached. Reverse triiodothyronine (T_3) levels have been used to monitor amiodarone therapy in humans because it blocks the conversion of thyroxine (T_4) to T_3. Elevated levels of reverse T_3 have been associated with adverse effects. It is recommended that liver and thyroid function, as well as routine serum biochemistries, should be monitored every 6 months. For amiodarone (and sotalol) the heart rate, QT interval, and PR interval should be examined. These changes develop proportionately with the dosage of sotalol.

The commercially available preparation of sotalol is the racemic mixture of d- and l-sotalol. The beta-adrenergic blocking activity of d,l-sotalol is about 30% that of propranolol. The beta-adrenergic blocking action occurs at lower doses than those for the class III action. Sotalol differs from amiodarone in that it does not bind to plasma proteins, is eliminated through the kidneys, is hydrophilic, lacks active metabolites, and has no effect on digoxin concentrations, and long-term administration does not alter its kinetics with plasma concentrations proportional to the dose. Pharmacokinetic studies have been done in the dog (Gomoll et al, 1990). Extensive studies of the dose responses of sotalol in the dog have been investigated (Bristol-Myers Squibb, unpublished observations) and thoroughly reviewed (O'Callaghan and McGovern, 1996). A general guideline dosage would be 0.5 to 2 mg/kg PO every 12 to 24 hours.

In addition to high expense, amiodarone and sotalol have potential side effects that hinder more extensive use. The numerous side effects (gastrointestinal, pulmonary fibrosis, hyperthyroidism, hypothyroidism, ocular opacities, and hepatic failure) of amiodarone and proarrhythmic and negative inotropic effects of sotalol are probably related to excessive doses. The use of low-dose amiodarone has been

---

*See page 756 for other canine dosages.

touted as a means of still achieving adequate antiarrhythmic effects. The risk of torsades de pointes, a severe form of VT, in humans has been related to the dosage of sotalol. Amiodarone and sotalol have potential problems in the setting of congestive heart failure.

Combination Therapy

Although combining antiarrhythmics can be dangerous, a potential exists for combinations to have synergistic effects. Studies in humans and experiments in the dog have shown that when monotherapy is ineffective, antiarrhythmic combinations can be effective in reducing VT and the induction of ventricular fibrillation. Moreover, combination therapy at moderate doses may be better tolerated than maximal dosages of monotherapy. A common combination is a class Ia drug (procainamide or quinidine) with class Ib drugs (lidocaine and mexiletine). Class Ia or class Ib drugs are potentially more antiarrhythmic when either is combined with a beta-blocker. For example, the effectiveness of mexiletine can be enhanced when given with a beta-blocker (atenolol, propranolol, nadolol, metoprolol). Procainamide or quinidine combined with sotalol has experimentally been effective in the treatment of ventricular arrhythmias. As mentioned earlier, some drugs that are classified as class III drugs (d,l-sotalol, amiodarone) actually exhibit some antiarrhythmic actions characteristic of beta-blocking drugs, thereby actually providing combination therapy.

Problems do exist with the use of antiarrhythmic drug combinations. Determining the effective dose of each drug may be more difficult than dosage calculation with monotherapy. The only statement that can be wisely made with regard to the dosage is to start lower than the dose used for each drug alone. Adverse effects may require the withdrawal of both drugs, although only one drug is really detrimental. Although the reason for drug combinations is synergism, adverse reactions can occur directly from the drugs or because of drug elimination.

RESPONSE TO TREATMENT

To judge a true reduction in the frequency of ventricular arrhythmias ideally requires a minimum of 24 hours of ECG monitoring, rather than just the standard rhythm-strip ECG that only lasts a few minutes (Moise and De Francesco, 1995). The latter cannot provide adequate information with regard to the baseline and post-treatment frequency of ventricular arrhythmias. The inadequacies of an ECG that is less than 24 hours are underscored by the studies that demonstrate the hourly spontaneous variability in the frequency of arrhythmias. This variability is greater when the frequency of PVCs is low (<200 beats/hr) than when the PVC counts are high (>1,000 beats/hr). Moreover, when the interval between recordings is increased, the spontaneous variability in arrhythmias varies even more. Therefore, to clearly demonstrate a positive drug effect, re-examination should be made within a short period of time, the percent reduction of arrhythmias should be stringent, long-term follow-up may include examination with the patient off drug treatment, and the limitations of monitoring

must be considered in diagnostic and therapeutic decision-making. Given the limitations, Holter monitoring can be a critical assessment in the treatment of ventricular arrhythmias.

In addition to reducing the frequency of ventricular arrhythmias, other means of assessing successful treatment are important. Under some circumstances, the VT may not be eliminated but the rate of the tachyarrhythmia may be reduced enough that it is more hemodynamically tolerated. The reduction of the frequency of an arrhythmia does not ensure that sudden death will be prevented. Drugs can be antiarrhythmic, with only minimal antifibrillatory effects. Conversely, the fibrillation threshold can be increased and the frequency of the arrhythmia stable. Drug concentrations may be of value, but the usefulness varies with the specific drug (Woosley, 1988).

References and Suggested Reading

Campbell RWF: Class IB antiarrhythmic agents. In: Podrid PJ, Kowey PR, eds: Cardiac Arrhythmias: Mechanisms, Diagnosis, and Management. Baltimore: Williams & Wilkins, 1995, p 391.
Review of class Ib antiarrhythmic drugs and their use in humans.
Gomoll AW, Lekich RF, Bartek MJ, et al: Comparability of the electrophysiologic responses and plasma and myocardial tissue concentrations of sotalol and its d-stereoisomer in the dog. J Cardiovasc Pharmacol 16:204, 1990.
Reference for drug dosing in an experimental dog model.
Link MS, Homoud M, Fote CB, et al: Antiarrhythmic drug therapy for ventricular arrhythmias: Current perspectives. J Cardiovasc Electrophysiol 7:653, 1996.
Review article that provides up-to-date information concerning the drug treatment of ventricular arrhythmias.
Moise NS, De Francesco T: Twenty-four-hour ambulatory electrocardiography (Holter monitoring). In: Bonagura JD, Kirk RW, eds: Kirk's Current Veterinary Therapy XII. Philadelphia: WB Saunders, 1995, p 792.
Instructions on the use, application, and interpretation of Holter monitoring in the dog.
Moise NS, Gilmour RF Jr, Riccio ML, et al: Diagnosis of inherited ventricular tachycardia in German shepherd dogs. J Am Vet Med Assoc 210:403, 1997.
Review (complete references of syndrome given) of the inherited sudden death that occurs in young German shepherds.
O'Callaghan PA, McGovern BA: Evolving role of sotalol in the management of ventricular tachyarrhythmias. Am J Cardiol 78:54, 1996.
Information in humans on how sotalol rose from a last-chance antiarrhythmic to one of the most favored in the treatment of ventricular arrhythmias.
Patterson E, Eller BT, Abrams GD, et al: Ventricular fibrillation in a conscious canine preparation of sudden coronary death: Prevention by short- and long-term amiodarone administration. Circulation 68:857, 1983.
Reference for the determination of dosing of amiodarone.
Podrid PJ, Fuchs T, Candinas R: Role of sympathetic nervous system in the genesis of ventricular arrhythmias. Circulation 82(Suppl I):I-03, 1990.
Reviews the important role that sympathetic tone plays in the triggering of arrhythmias and how this influences treatment.
Stanton MS: Class I antiarrhythmic drugs: Quinidine, procainamide, disopyramide, lidocaine, mexiletine, tocainide, phenytoin, moricizine, flecainide, propafenone. In: Zipes DP, Jalife J, eds: Cardiac Electrophysiology: From Cell to Bedside. Philadelphia: WB Saunders, 1995, p 1296.
Complete review of class I antiarrhythmic drugs.
Woosley RL: Role of plasma concentration monitoring in the evaluation of response to antiarrhythmic drugs. Am J Cardiol 62:9H, 1988.
Although an older paper, it contains valuable information regarding measuring drug concentrations and relating the results to treatment.

Feline Congenital Heart Disease

Rebecca L. Stepien
Madison, Wisconsin

Helio Autran de Morais
Londrina, Paraná, Brazil

PREVALENCE

Malformations of the heart and great vessels—congenital heart disease (CHD)—appear to be less common in cats than in dogs. Studies in the late 1970s and 1980s have shown an overall prevalence of CHD of about 0.2% in cats presented to clinics and 1.9 to 2.8% in necropsy studies (Liu, 1977; Harpster and Zook, 1987). Diagnosis of feline CHD may be more frequent today because of increased awareness of CHD in general and improvements in noninvasive diagnostic testing. The ability of many cats to live a relatively normal life despite the presence of congenital cardiac malformations makes accurate diagnosis of these abnormalities an important part of clinical practice.

Prevalence of CHD varies with breed popularity and region, but mitral dysplasia (MD) and ventricular septal defects (VSD) are the most common overall. Other common defects in cats are tricuspid valve dysplasia (TD), patent ductus arteriosus (PDA), vascular abnormalities, aortic (AS) or subaortic stenosis (SAS), tetralogy of Fallot (TF), atrial septal defects (ASD), common atrioventricular canal (endocardial cushion defects, ECD), and pulmonic stenosis (PS). Although endocardial fibroelastosis was the third most common CHD in one review (Harpster and Zook, 1987), in the authors' practices this abnormality is rare. In dogs, many cases of CHD have a genetic basis, but no systematic genetic studies have been published regarding cats with CHD. Cats show less breed predilection for specific CHD than dogs.

INITIAL ASSESSMENT

The clinical diagnosis of CHD in cats may be hampered by the difficulties inherent in auscultation of small patients, the ability of cats to maintain a relatively "normal" lifestyle in the presence of significant heart disease, and the variety of malformations and severity of abnormalities that may be encountered in the feline population. Although cardiac murmurs are the most common presenting sign of CHD, some forms of CHD do not have audible murmurs (e.g., mitral stenosis, some TF); occasionally, acquired diseases, especially hypertrophic cardiomyopathy, may cause murmurs at a very young age. Nevertheless, detection of a cardiac murmur is an important first step in the diagnosis of most cases of feline CHD.

Cardiac Murmurs

Cardiac murmurs are most frequently discovered during initial vaccination-related physical examination. Because many cats are diagnosed with CHD in the absence of overt clinical signs, the differentiation of "innocent murmurs" from murmurs likely to represent CHD is important. A systematic approach should be followed when one examines a young cat with a murmur. The timing of the murmur should be determined, as well as the point of maximal intensity, and the radiation of the murmur (Table 1). Murmurs can occur during systole or diastole or throughout the cardiac cycle (continuous murmurs). Most CHD in cats results in systolic murmurs. Murmurs that occur only during diastole are uncommon in cats with CHD, whereas a continuous murmur strongly suggests the presence of PDA. Murmurs are graded on an intensity scale of I to VI, with grade I applicable to the softest detectable murmur and grade VI applied to murmurs audible without a stethoscope. In some defects, the intensity of the murmur may be related to the severity of the defect (i.e., louder or higher grade murmurs may be associated with more severe abnormalities), but this is not true in every case. Owners should not be given a poor prognosis based on the presence of a loud murmur alone.

"Innocent" Murmurs

Kitten murmurs, innocent murmurs, and *flow murmurs* all refer to systolic murmurs of young (<16 weeks of age) kittens. The etiology of these murmurs remains obscure, but innocent murmurs appear to be less prevalent in cats than dogs (perhaps because of the difficulties of accurate auscultation of very small kittens). These murmurs present a clinical dilemma; the practitioner must decide whether to recommend further cardiac diagnostic testing immediately or wait for possible resolution of the murmur. The characteristics of the murmur and the clinical situation help guide this decision (Table 2). When a murmur with the characteristics of an innocent murmur is heard prior to the age of 16 weeks, re-examination at the age of 16 weeks or older is recommended. If the murmur persists, further diagnostic testing can be pursued at that time. If the murmur has characteristics not typical of an innocent murmur or if the kitten shows clinical signs of heart disease or heart failure, diagnostic testing should be pursued at an earlier age. Reliable clinical indicators of moderate to severe congenital malformations include lethargy (may be interpreted as a "quiet" animal), poor growth (as compared to littermates), cyanosis, or signs of congestive heart failure (CHF) accompanying a consistent murmur.

DIAGNOSTIC TESTING

Many cases of CHD can be tentatively diagnosed on the basis of clinical, radiographic, and electrocardiographic

TABLE 1. Clinical Findings in Feline Congenital Heart Disease

CHD*	Murmur Timing/PMI	Murmur Radiation	Radiographic Abnormalities	ECG Abnormalities	Echo Abnormalities
ASD	Systolic L base (murmur of relative PS)	Dorsal	RAE RVE Enlarged pulmonary aa/vv	RVE R axis shift	Dilated RA/RV/PA Echo drop-out at level of septal defect Low-velocity flow across defect
AS or SAS	Systolic L base	R base	LAE LVE	LVE LAFB	Thickened LV wall, septum Visible aortic/subaortic obstruction High-velocity flow across obstruction ± MR
ECD	Systolic ± diastolic or continuous Right sternal border ± left apex	Variable	Severe cardiomegaly (4 chamber) Enlarged pulmonary aa/vv	LVE RVE IVCD	Four-chamber dilation Echo drop-out: low atrial and high ventricular septa ± common atrioventricular valve MR/TR
MD	Systolic L apex	Dorsocranial	LAE LVE	LVE	Dilated LA/LV Valve/chordal abnormalities Papillary muscle abnormalities MR
PDA	Continuous L base† ± 2° MR murmur	R base	LAE LVE Aortic "ductus bump" Enlarged pulmonary aa/vv	LVE	Dilated LA/LV/PA Continuous turbulent flow in PA ± image ductus
PS	Systolic L base ± 2° TR murmur	Dorsal	RAE RVE	RVE R axis shift	Thickened RV wall, septum Dilated RA Visible pulmonary outflow obstruction High-velocity flow across pulmonic valve ± TR
TD	Systolic R apex	Cranial	RAE RVE	RVE R axis shift	Dilated RA/RV Valve/chordal abnormalities Papillary muscle abnormalities TR
TF	Systolic L base	Variable	RVE Small pulmonary vessels	RVE R axis shift	Thickened RV wall, septum Large VSD Overriding aorta Pulmonary outflow obstruction
VSD	Systolic R sternal border ± 2° relative PS murmur	L sternal border	LAE LVE Enlarged pulmonary aa/vv	LVE	Dilated LA/LV/PA Echo drop-out at level of septal defect High-velocity flow across defect if small

*Individual variation and combinations of malformations may lead to variable findings in any CHD.

†In some cats, diastolic murmur is barely audible.

Abbreviations of various types of CHD listed are found in the text. PMI, point of maximal intensity; ECG, electrocardiogram; Echo, echocardiogram; L, left; R, right; LAE, left atrial enlargement; LVE, left ventricular enlargement; RAE, right atrial enlargement; RVE, right ventricular enlargement; PA, pulmonary artery; aa, arteries; vv, veins; CHF, congestive heart failure; MR, mitral regurgitation; TR, tricuspid regurgitation; 2°, secondary.

findings; but definitive diagnosis may require the use of two-dimensional and Doppler echocardiography or cardiac catheterization. Accurate early diagnosis is especially important for animals with malformations that are amenable to surgical palliation (e.g., PDA) or are severe and limit survival. From the owner's point of view, discriminating among life-threatening, lifestyle-affecting, and clinically silent cardiac malformations in a kitten with a heart murmur is often the most important result of the diagnostic work-up.

Initial Work-Up

The most common feline congenital heart malformations and their pertinent clinical findings are listed in Table 1. After recognition and characterization of the murmur, a differential diagnosis list may be generated. In general practice, recommendations are based on clinical examination and radiographic and electrocardiographic examination. Two-dimensional and Doppler echocardiography, if available, usually provide the definitive diagnosis. Thoracic radiographs are used to support the most likely diagnosis and, in conjunction with physical examination findings, estimate the severity of disease and diagnose heart failure, if present. The severity of cardiac enlargement noted on

TABLE 2. Characteristics and Clinical Signs Associated With "Innocent" Murmurs Versus Murmurs Associated With CHD

Innocent Murmur	Congenital Heart Disease
Grade usually < III/VI	Grade ≥ III/VI
Systolic	Any timing possible
PMI: usually left base	PMI: any possible
Murmur characteristics change with animal position	Similar murmur characteristics in all positions
Decreased intensity with age	Same or increasing intensity up to and beyond 16 wk of age
Inaudible after ~16 wk of age	Persists after ~16 wk of age
Animal clinically normal	Stunting, unthriftiness, cyanosis, or signs of heart failure present

PMI, point of maximal murmur intensity.

thoracic radiographs usually correlates to the severity of CHD, and signs of CHF are easily detected. Animals with suspected CHD and clinical signs of CHF should be stabilized medically until they can be evaluated further. Electrocardiography provides additional information regarding the presence or absence of ventricular enlargement patterns and dysrhythmias. In some cases, the initial work-up suggests a mild abnormality, and the owner can be informed of the relatively minor risk of development of serious complications. Most severe malformations are detected on the initial work-up, but certain types of severe diseases (e.g., some cyanotic diseases, AS, or SAS) may be missed or their severity underestimated without echocardiographic diagnosis.

Cardiology Referral

Referral to a veterinary cardiologist should be considered when a clinician experienced in CHD is not available in the primary practice, or when echocardiographic examination by an individual experienced in CHD is not available. Identification and definitive diagnosis of mild congenital abnormalities is especially important in young animals under consideration for breeding programs. In animals with more severe CHD, a complete diagnostic work-up allows better prediction of survival and complications based on clinical experience with animals with similar disease severity. Early referral is recommended when clinical findings are confusing, dysrhythmias are present, or clinical signs are rapidly progressive.

TABLE 3. Indications, Recommended Therapy, and Cautions for Feline CHD

CHD	Indications and Recommended Therapy	Palliative or Definitive Therapy Available	Cautions

ASD	Pleural effusion, ascites
	  Thoracentesis
	  Furosemide
	  Enalapril
	Poor systolic function
	  Dobutamine (acutely)
	  Digoxin (chronically)
		Palliative surgery (pulmonary artery banding)	Furosemide predisposes to hypokalemia and hypomagnesemia, especially if animal is inappetent
			Use caution with enalapril (low doses; close monitoring of clinical condition, renal function, potassium concentration, and blood pressure)
			Dobutamine is used with caution in cats to avoid toxicity (seizures)

AS or SAS	Dyspnea, pulmonary edema
	  Nitroglycerin ointment (2%)
	  Furosemide
	  ± Enalapril
	Decreased diastolic function
	  CCB
	  BB
		Palliative balloon dilation (may be limited by small size of patient)	Extreme caution with enalapril (very low doses) to avoid hypotension in the presence of outflow obstruction
			Concurrent use of BB *and* CCB is contraindicated
			Monitor heart rate when using BB or CCB to avoid excessive decreases (below 130 bpm in hospital)

MD	Dyspnea, pulmonary edema (as for AS above) Poor systolic function late in disease (as for ASD above)	None	Enalapril used with caution in dehydrated animals or animals receiving high doses of diuretics

PDA	Dyspnea, pulmonary edema
	  Nitroglycerin ointment
	  Furosemide
	  Enalapril
		Surgical ligation recommended even in absence of clinical signs in cat <2 yr of age
		Asymptomatic cats >2 yr of age should be referred for evaluation
			CHF signs may need to be medically managed prior to surgical correction

PS	Pleural effusion, ascites
	  Thoracocentesis
	  Furosemide
	Poor systolic function (as for ASD above)
	Decreased diastolic function (as for AS above)
		Palliative balloon valvuloplasty (may be limited by small size of patient)
		Surgical dilation or expansion of outflow tract
			Avoid excessive decreases in heart rate
			Avoid use of BB, CCB when CHF is present

TD	As for ASD	None	As for ASD

TF	Cyanosis
	  BB to decrease dynamic component of outflow obstruction
	Polycythemia
	  Therapeutic phlebotomy when PCV exceeds 65–70%
		Palliative surgical procedures
		Create left-to-right shunt to increase pulmonary blood flow and decrease hypoxemia	

VSD	Dyspnea, pulmonary edema (as for AS above), may see pleural effusion if biventricular CHF Thoracentesis Poor systolic function (as for ASD above)	Palliative surgery (pulmonary artery banding)	

Disease abbreviations as for Table 1.
BB, beta-blockers; CCB, calcium channel blockers; CHF, congestive heart failure.

TABLE 4. Dosages for Medications Commonly Used in the Treatment of Feline Congenital Heart Disease

Medication	Approximate Dosages
Atenolol	6.25–12.5 mg PO q12–24 hr
Digoxin	0.0035–0.0055 mg/kg PO q12–24 hr
Diltiazem	0.5–2.0 mg/kg PO q8–12 hr
Dobutamine	2.5–10 µg/kg/min constant-rate infusion
Enalapril	0.25–0.5 mg/kg PO q12–48 hr
Furosemide	1–4 mg/kg IV, IM, SC, PO q8–12 hr
Nitroglycerin ointment (2%)	2–4 mg applied to skin q12–24 hr
Propranolol	2.5–5.0 mg PO q8 hr

THERAPY

No Clinical Signs Present

Surgical ligation of PDA is recommended in kittens even in the absence of clinical signs because of the risk of developing CHF or myocardial dysfunction. Therapy for asymptomatic animals with other defects is more controversial. Animals with known hypertrophic diseases (e.g., SAS, AS, PS) may be treated with beta-blockers or calcium channel blockers to slow heart rate and increase diastolic filling. To date, little published information is available regarding the risks and benefits of long-term therapy with these drugs in asymptomatic cats with normal sinus rhythm. In many cases of CHD, no therapy is used unless the animal has clinical signs of inadequate cardiac function or dysrhythmias are present.

Congestive Heart Failure and Dysrhythmias

Animals with CHD that have signs of CHF require palliative or curative procedures or aggressive medical therapy to maintain a reasonable quality of life. The types of feline CHD amenable to surgical correction or interventional catheterization as palliative therapy are listed in Table 3. If the CHD remains undetected until CHF or other clinical signs are present, the patient is stabilized with medical therapy until invasive procedures can be safely performed. In many cases of CHD, however, no definitive or palliative therapies are routinely available, so medical management of clinical signs is necessary for the life of the patient. The choice of medical therapy is based on the type of abnormality and dynamic dysfunction present (Table 4). Malformations that lead to a volume-loaded state—typically atrioventricular dysplasias and left-to-right shunts

(e.g., PDA, VSD, ECD)—usually require therapy with diuretics and vasodilators. Vasodilators should be used with caution in cats with TD or ASD; some reduction of afterload may be tolerated, but even "normal" doses of arterial dilators may result in arterial hypotension in animals with right-sided CHF. In most cases, angiotensin-converting enzyme inhibitors (ACEIs) provide relief of fluid retention with a level of vasodilation that can be tolerated by most animals. Caution is recommended if ACEIs are used with moderate to high doses of diuretics; concurrent use of higher doses of these drugs may result in dehydration and prerenal azotemia. If systolic dysfunction is present (poor pulse strength, hypotension, fractional shortening decreased on echocardiogram), positive inotropic drugs may be used acutely (e.g., dobutamine) or chronically (e.g., digoxin). Outflow tract obstructions (e.g., SAS, AS, PS) may show clinical improvement in exercise tolerance when treated with beta-blockers (e.g., atenolol [Tenormin, Zeneca]) or calcium channel blockers (e.g., diltiazem, [Cardizem, Hoechst Marion Roussel]). No published studies regarding the use of these drugs for treating congenital outflow tract obstruction in cats have been published, but careful titration of doses to control sinus tachycardias has resulted in clinical improvement in cats with these defects in the authors' practice. Both atenolol and diltiazem may decrease systolic function; the use of these drugs should be reserved for animals no longer in CHF. Complex CHD (e.g., multiple defects) or right-to-left shunts are treated for their predominant abnormalities. Dysrhythmias complicating CHD are treated in a fashion similar to that for dysrhythmias complicating acquired heart disease.

References and Suggested Reading

Bonagura JD: Cardiovascular diseases. In: Sherding RG, ed: The Cat: Diseases and Clinical Management, 2nd ed. New York: Churchill Livingstone, 1994, p 819.
An extensive and well-illustrated article summarizing clinical diagnosis and treatment of congenital and acquired feline cardiovascular disease.

Darke PGG, Bonagura JB, Kelly DF: Color Atlas of Veterinary Cardiology. London: Mosby-Wolfe, 1996.
Well-illustrated atlas of cardiovascular disease, including photographs of and clinical data on examples of feline congenital lesions.

Harpster NK, Zook BC: The cardiovascular system. In: Holzworth J, ed: Diseases of the Cat: Medicine & Surgery. Philadelphia: WB Saunders, 1987, p 871.
A review of congenital heart disease in cats, including the prevalence of congenital heart disease based on clinical and necropsy diagnoses over a 23-year period.

Liu SK: Pathology of feline heart disease. Vet Clin North Am 7:323, 1977.
A review of cardiac lesions and the prevalence of congenital and acquired heart disease in cats based on necropsy findings over a 14-year period.

Interventional Cardiology: Catheter Occlusion of Patent Ductus Arteriosus in Dogs

MATTHEW W. MILLER
College Station, Texas

INTRODUCTION

In its broadest sense, interventional cardiology or interventional catheterization refers to any catheterization during which some type of therapeutic procedure is undertaken. In medicine, the most common application of interventional cardiology is dilation or stenting of coronary artery stenosis. Interventional catheterization was first applied to congenital heart disease in children in 1966, when Dr. William Rashkind reported the use of balloon catheters to create atrial septal defects in children with transposition of the great vessels. Since that time, guidelines have been established for pediatric therapeutic catheterization covering indications and contraindications for balloon and blade atrial septostomies, balloon dilation of all four cardiac valves, balloon dilation of peripheral vessels including the aorta and pulmonary arteries, implantation of occlusion devices, foreign body retrieval, and ablation of abnormal conduction pathways (Allen et al, 1991). In veterinary medicine, interventional catheterization procedures include those in which obstructive lesions are dilated (ballooned), abnormal vascular communications are occluded, abnormal conduction pathways are interrupted (catheter ablation), or foreign bodies are retrieved. This article addresses only balloon dilation and catheter occlusion.

BALLOON DILATION

The application of balloon dilation to treat canine congenital pulmonic, subaortic, and tricuspid stenosis has been reported. In 1987, Bright and colleagues reported the successful use of balloon dilation to treat pulmonic stenosis in a dog. Since that time, several reports (Sisson and MacCoy, 1988; Brown and Thomas, 1995) have confirmed the safety and efficacy of this procedure. The long-term efficacy of balloon dilation of subaortic stenosis (SAS) is less universally accepted. Delellis and colleagues reported the results of balloon dilation in nine dogs with SAS and suggested that balloon dilation was beneficial (Delellis et al, 1993); however, long-term results have been less encouraging. Preliminary results from others suggest that despite favorable early results, a gradient reduction of at least 50% is maintained in less than half the dogs 6 months after they have undergone balloon dilation (Lehmkuhl and Bonagura, 1995). Important questions that remain unanswered regarding balloon dilation of SAS include whether balloon dilation improves the quality or quantity of life and whether the incidence of sudden death is significantly altered by the procedure. Readers are referred to excellent reviews of

these procedures for more information (see *CVT XII*, pp. 817–821 and 822–827). Broader application of balloon dilation procedures is expected. The author has used balloon dilation to successfully relieve the obstruction associated with cor triatriatum dexter and is aware of at least one other successful application in the treatment of that lesion.

CATHETER OCCLUSION

Occlusion of abnormal vascular communications (typically congenital) represents an important application for interventional catheterization. The two most common congenital vascular malformations in veterinary medicine are portosystemic shunts (PSS) and patent ductus arteriosus (PDA). There is a single case report of successful transvenous occlusion of an intrahepatic portosystemic shunt in a dog (Partington et al, 1993). In this case report, multiple procedures were utilized to sequentially deploy Gianturco vascular occlusion coils to gradually occlude an intrahepatic shunt. One of the potential complications associated with occlusion of PSS is the development of portal hypertension. This potentially catastrophic complication must be overcome before this procedure will enjoy widespread application. The author has recently developed a transvenous approach for identifying and catheterizing PSSs. Improved visualization and assessment of the hemodynamics associated with PSS should increase our ability to occlude them percutaneously.

There have been several recent reports describing the application of vascular occlusion devices in the therapy for left-to-right shunting PDA (Miller et al, 1995; Snaps et al, 1995; Grifka et al, 1996). These reports have suggested that percutaneous ductal occlusion is a viable alternative to surgical ligation. Although there are several devices available for percutaneous ductal occlusion, many of these devices are costly or must be delivered with large-sized catheters, precluding their use in young dogs. In veterinary medicine, the most viable occlusion device currently available is the Gianturco vascular occlusion coil (Cook, Inc., Bloomington, IN). This device is a stainless steel coil interwoven with Dacron fibers. The coil is delivered transarterially via catheter into the lumen of the vessel to be occluded. The thrombogenic characteristics of the Dacron fibers promote clot formation and maturation with subsequent vascular occlusion. The author and colleagues have successfully occluded left-to-right shunting PDAs in 35 dogs ranging in size from 2.1 to 25 kg using Gianturco vascular occlusion coils. The continued development of

742

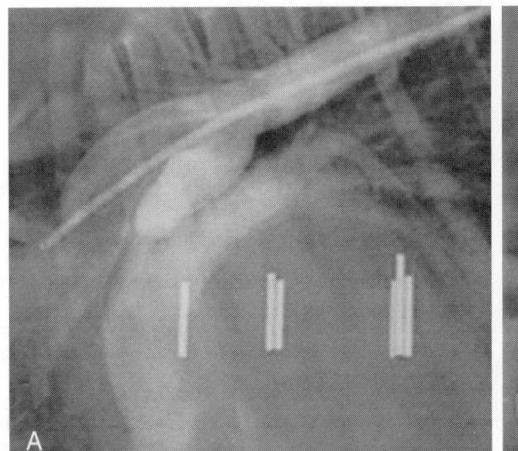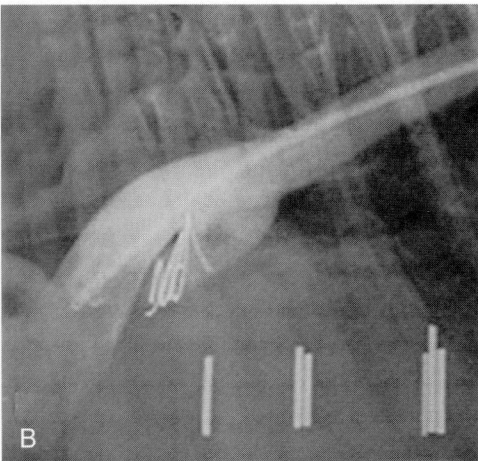

Figure 1. *A,* Right lateral aortic angiogram demonstrating a left-to-right shunting PDA. Notice that the aorta and pulmonary artery are equally and simultaneously opacified. *B,* Right lateral aortic angiogram made 15 minutes after deployment of two Gianturco vascular occlusion coils. Notice that there is no residual shunting. Radiographic markers at the bottom of the illustrations are 1, 2, and 3 mm in width.

improved occlusion devices will probably make percutaneous ductal occlusion more commonplace.

The success of the procedure is predicated on the deployment of an appropriately sized coil in the correct position within the ductus. Knowledge of ductal anatomy is paramount, as morphologic variations of the ductus may preclude appropriate coil engagement. It is also imperative to accurately determine minimal ductal diameter to decide whether the patient is a candidate for percutaneous ductal occlusion. Currently, the only way of reliably evaluating ductal morphology is angiography. Despite easy identification of the ductus with transthoracic echocardiography, critical description of the three-dimensional anatomy of the ductus with this imaging modality is limited. Transesophageal echocardiography may provide anatomic information, obviating the need for angiography.

Angiography is performed from the femoral artery with a multiple–side hole catheter advanced to the level of the descending aorta. Rapid, high-pressure injection of contrast material is essential in adequately outlining the ductus (Fig. 1*A*). If ductal anatomy is such that a coil can be safely deployed, a catheter is advanced into the ductus and the coil deployed. Coils are chosen that have an outside diameter at least twice the minimal diameter of the PDA. In most patients, occlusion occurs rapidly (less than 15 minutes) with the use of one or two coils (see Fig. 1*B*). Once the

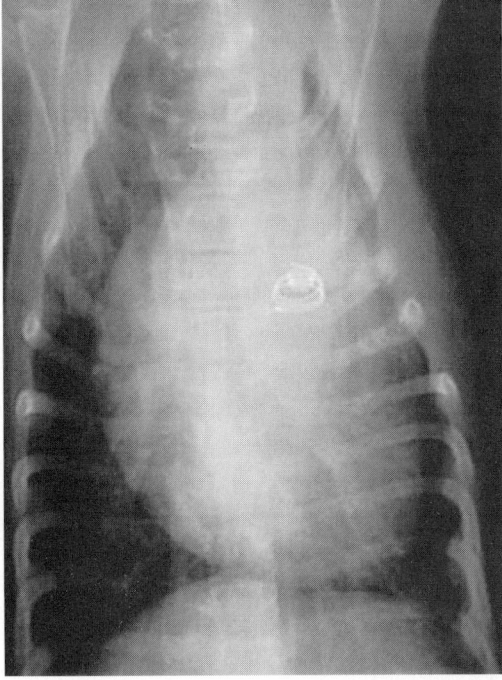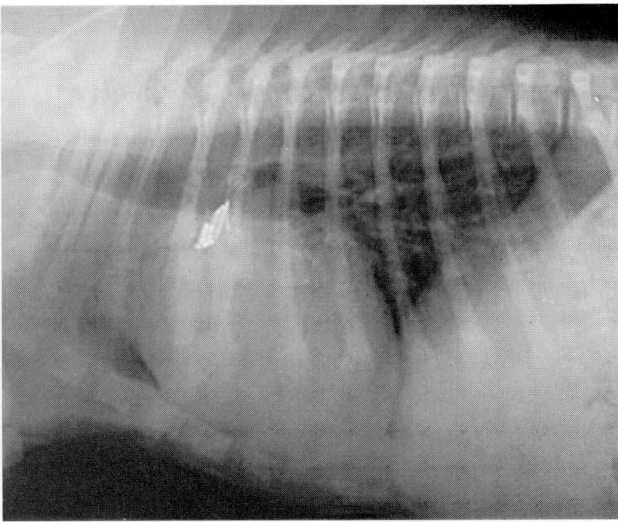

Figure 2. Ventrodorsal and lateral radiographs obtained from the patient in Figure 1, 24 hours after percutaneous ductal occlusion. The individual coils can readily be seen within the ductal ampulla.

coils have been deployed, dislodgment is very uncommon. Since the coils are stainless steel, their position can be readily evaluated with thoracic radiography (Fig. 2). In some patients, trivial residual flow is present even after coil deployment. This flow is not associated with an auscultable murmur but is rather detected with color-flow Doppler techniques. The importance of this hemodynamically trivial residual flow is the subject of much debate (Thilen et al, 1997). It has been the author's experience in dogs and that of other investigators in children that the vast majority of patients with persistent left-to-right shunting have complete resolution of residual flow within 12 months of coil deployment (Shim et al, 1996).

Complications associated with the procedure include local hemorrhage at the arterial access site, trace residual shunting as described earlier, and suboptimal deployment of the coil resulting in either pulmonary or systemic embolization. Although most coils embolized to the pulmonary circulation have not been retrieved, they have not been associated with any demonstrable clinical signs. Assessment of pulmonary vascularity with nuclear perfusion scanning suggests minimal long-term alterations in pulmonary perfusion. The author and co-workers have experienced three arterial embolizations. These coils have lodged in the distal aorta and were easily retrieved percutaneously through the femoral arterial sheath without apparent clinical consequences.

FUTURE DIRECTIONS

Although the application of interventional catheterization techniques is appealing, it is imperative not to embrace these techniques simply because they are less invasive and potentially less costly. We must critically evaluate the safety and efficacy of these techniques. This is especially true when interventional catheterization techniques are applied to disease processes for which established successful therapies are available (Birchard et al, 1990).

References and Suggested Reading

Allen HD, Driscoll DJ, Fricker FJ, et al: Guidelines for pediatric therapeutic catheterization. Circulation 84:2249, 1991.
Detailed recommendations as put forth by a subcommittee of the American Heart Association regarding indications and contraindications for pediatric interventional catheterization.
Birchard SJ, Bonagura JD, Fingland RB: Results of ligation of patent ductus arteriosus in dogs: 201 cases (1969–1988). J Am Vet Med Assoc 196:2011, 1990.
Retrospective evaluation of the clinical outcome of 201 cases of patent ductus arteriosus treated with surgical ligation.
Bright JM, Jennings J, Toal R, et al: Percutaneous balloon valvuloplasty for the treatment of pulmonic stenosis in a dog. J Am Vet Med Assoc 191:995, 1987.
Single case report detailing the diagnosis and percutaneous dilation of pulmonic stenosis in a dog.
Brown WA, Thomas WP: Balloon valvuloplasty of tricuspid stenosis in a Labrador retriever. J Vet Intern Med 9:419, 1995.
Single case report detailing the diagnosis and percutaneous dilation of tricuspid stenosis in a dog.
Delellis LA, Thomas WP, Pion PD: Balloon dilation of congenital subaortic stenosis in the dog. J Vet Intern Med 7:153, 1993.
Reports the technique and short-term hemodynamic and clinical results of balloon dilation in nine dogs with subaortic stenosis.
Grifka RG, Miller MW, Frischmeyer KJ, et al: Transcatheter occlusion of a patent ductus arteriosus in a Newfoundland puppy using the Gianturco-Grifka vascular occlusion device. J Vet Intern Med 10:42, 1996.
Single case report detailing percutaneous occlusion of PDA in a dog with a Gianturco-Grifka vascular occlusion device.
Lehmkuhl LB, Bonagura JD: CVT update: Canine subaortic stenosis. In: Bonagura JD, Kirk RW, eds: Kirk's Current Veterinary Therapy XII: Small Animal Practice. Philadelphia: WB Saunders, 1995, p 822.
Reports the technique and both long- and short-term hemodynamic and clinical results of balloon dilation in 20 consecutive dogs with subaortic stenosis.
Miller MW, Bonagura JD, Meurs KM, et al: Percutaneous catheter occlusion of patent ductus arteriosus. Proceedings of the 13th Annual Forum, American College of Veterinary Internal Medicine, 1995, p 308.
Describes the technique and initial clinical results of percutaneous ductal occlusion in dogs with Gianturco vascular occlusion coils.
Partington BP, Partington CR, Biller DS, et al: Transvenous coil embolization for treatment of patent ductus venosus in a dog. J Am Vet Med Assoc 202:281, 1993.
Single case report detailing the technique and clinical outcome of percutaneous occlusion of a PSS in a dog with Gianturco vascular occlusion coils.
Shim D, Fedderly RT, Beekman RH, et al: Follow-up of coil occlusion of patent ductus arteriosus. J Am Coll Cardiol 28:207, 1996.
Reports the prevalence and fate of residual ductal shunting following coil occlusion of patent ductus arteriosus in 75 people.
Sisson DD, MacCoy DM: Treatment of congenital pulmonic stenosis in two dogs by balloon valvuloplasty. J Vet Intern Med 2:92, 1988.
Reports the technique and clinical outcome of balloon dilation in two dogs with pulmonic stenosis.
Snaps FR, Mc Entee K, Saunders JH, et al: Treatment of patent ductus arteriosus by placement of intravascular coils in a pup. J Am Vet Med Assoc 207:724, 1995.
Single case report detailing percutaneous occlusion of a PDA in a dog with multiple Gianturco vascular occlusion coils.
Thilen U, Astrom-Olsson K: Does the risk of infective endarteritis justify routine patent ductus arteriosus closure? Eur Heart J 18:364, 1997.
Retrospective study of endocarditis associated with PDA challenging the current belief that the risk of endocarditis is a valid reason for occlusion of hemodynamically insignificant PDA.

Current Indications for Cardiac Surgery

E. CHRISTOPHER ORTON

Fort Collins, Colorado

Cardiac surgery is increasingly becoming an option for the management of congenital and acquired cardiac conditions in small animals. Some cardiac surgeries are widely available, whereas other surgeries, particularly those requiring cardiopulmonary bypass, are currently performed only at regional referral centers. Advances in cardiac surgery, veterinary anesthesia, and critical care have dramatically increased the operative success rate of cardiac surgery in animals. Cardiopulmonary bypass and open cardiac repairs can be performed successfully in dogs as small as 5 kg in weight. Unfortunately, cardiopulmonary bypass currently is not an option for domestic cats, although other methods for open cardiac repair, such as venous inflow occlusion or whole body hypothermia, have been performed successfully in cats. The success and availability of cardiac surgery in small animals will undoubtedly increase as experience is gained in this emerging area of veterinary medicine. This article reviews the current state of cardiac surgery in small animals, emphasizing current indications and expected outcomes.

PATENT DUCTUS ARTERIOSUS

Patent ductus arteriosus (PDA) is a persistent patency of the fetal communication between the pulmonary and the systemic circulation. Most animals with PDA experience premature death from progressive left-sided heart failure. Over time, secondary mitral insufficiency and volume overload–induced cardiomyopathy may contribute to the progression of heart failure. With few exceptions, surgical ligation is indicated in all dogs and cats with PDA. Surgical ligation can be undertaken any time after 8 weeks of age (>0.5 kg body weight). The surgery is curative when it is performed in animals 6 months of age. Mitral insufficiency and secondary cardiomyopathy, if present, are generally reversible when the surgery is performed early. These changes may not be reversible in animals older than 9 months of age, particularly in large-breed dogs. ACE inhibitor therapy may be indicated after surgery in animals with mitral insufficiency or myocardial failure to reduce neurohormonal activation and the progressive decline of myocardial function. Animals that present in congestive heart failure should be treated aggressively with furosemide (Lasix, Hoechst Marion Roussel), 1 to 4 mg/kg IV, IM, SC, or PO every 8 hours, and then should undergo surgical ligation once they are stable, usually within 24 to 48 hours. Digitalization is not necessary prior to surgery unless the animal has atrial fibrillation. Animals with pulmonary hypertension can undergo PDA ligation if pulmonary artery pressures have not reached systemic pressure levels. Surgical ligation of a right-to-left shunting PDA is contraindicated.

Operative mortality associated with PDA ligation is directly related to the surgeon's experience. The greatest risk associated with surgery is rupture of the ductus during dissection and severe hemorrhage. The operative success rate for experienced veterinary surgeons can exceed 98%.

PULMONIC STENOSIS

Pulmonic stenosis in dogs is usually valvular, but supravalvular and subvalvular defects also occur. Valvular stenosis may be *simple,* consisting of fusion of the valve leaflets, or *dysplastic,* characterized by a hypoplastic valve annulus and thickened immobile valve leaflets. More than 80% of dogs with valvular pulmonic stenosis have some degree of valve dysplasia. The prognosis for dogs with valvular pulmonic stenosis depends on the magnitude of the obstruction and the degree of compensatory right ventricular hypertrophy present. The severity of the stenosis can be assessed by recording the systolic pressure gradient between the right ventricle and pulmonary artery either directly by right-heart catheterization or indirectly by Doppler echocardiography. Doppler echocardiography is noninvasive and can be performed without sedation or anesthesia. A systolic pressure gradient across the obstruction of more than 80 mm Hg in an awake animal indicates severe pulmonic stenosis. Intervention is indicated in these patients to decrease the risk of premature sudden death or progressive right-sided heart failure.

The surgical options for severe pulmonic stenosis include dilation valvuloplasty and patch-graft valvuloplasty. Balloon-dilation valvuloplasty is accomplished with specially designed balloon catheters that are positioned across the stenosis and inflated during cardiac catheterization. The procedure is performed at many cardiology referral centers in North America. Alternatively, dilation valvuloplasty can be performed surgically by closed transventricular passage of a dilating instrument. Balloon-dilation valvuloplasty is less invasive and is generally regarded as more effective, and therefore is preferred when it is available. Dilation valvuloplasty should be regarded as a palliative, rather than curative, procedure for pulmonic stenosis. The degree of palliation is reflected in the degree of pressure gradient reduction achieved. Pressure gradients are rarely returned to normal by dilation valvuloplasty procedures, and initial gradient reductions may not be sustained. Dilation procedures are most effective for simple valvular pulmonic stenosis that is not associated with extensive hypertrophy of the right ventricular outflow tract. Dilation valvuloplasty can be performed with relatively low operative risk.

Patch-graft valvuloplasty is indicated for dogs with severe pulmonic stenosis characterized by valvular dysplasia or simple valvular stenosis with dynamic outflow obstruction secondary to outflow tract hypertrophy. Most often patch-graft valvuloplasty is considered for dogs that have failed to be adequately palliated by balloon-dilation valvuloplasty. Several surgical techniques for applying a patch-graft to the right ventricular outflow tract without the aid of cardiopulmonary bypass have been described. Open pulmonary patch-graft valvuloplasty placement during mild hypothermia and venous inflow occlusion generally results in substantial and sustained pressure-gradient reduction. However, this procedure is associated with an operative mortality rate of approximately 25%. A patch-graft valvuloplasty can be accomplished with the aid of a cardiopulmonary bypass. Cardiopulmonary bypass reduces operative risk and allows for a more deliberate placement of the graft, thereby enhancing the effectiveness of the procedure. Cost, limited availability, and slightly increased postoperative morbidity are the disadvantages of using cardiopulmonary bypass.

English bulldogs and boxers with pulmonic stenosis present a dilemma because of the possibility of an anomalous left coronary artery. In dogs with this defect, the left coronary artery originates from the right coronary ostia, courses across the right ventricular outflow tract, and is at risk for injury during valve dilation or patch-graft valvuloplasty. All English bulldogs and Boxers with pulmonic stenosis should undergo cardiac catheterization to assess coronary artery anatomy prior to therapeutic intervention. A conduit placed between the right ventricle and pulmonary artery is the only surgical option for this condition.

SUBVALVULAR AORTIC STENOSIS

Subvalvular aortic stenosis (SAS) is a common congenital defect in certain large and giant breed dogs. The defect occurs with widely disparate morphologic variation and degrees of severity. The typical defect consists of a discrete subvalvular fibrous membrane located 1 to 3 mm below the aortic valve leaflets that courses across the ventricular septum and reflects on to the septal mitral valve leaflet. The defect is often complicated by varying degrees of muscular septal hypertrophy and narrowing of the outflow tract. As with pulmonic stenosis, the severity and prognosis are determined by the magnitude of the Doppler echocardiography-estimated systolic pressure gradient across the defect. Dogs with a peak systolic pressure gradient greater than 100 mm Hg have a substantial risk of premature sudden death, often occurring before 3 years of age.

The surgical options for severe SAS include dilation valvuloplasty and open resection of the membrane. Dilation procedures, both percutaneous by balloon catheter and surgical via a closed transventricular approach, have been used for the treatment of SAS. Unfortunately, pressure gradient reduction after these procedures has been inconsistent, modest, and sometimes not sustained. Based on these results, there is little reason to believe that dilation of SAS offers any significant palliation of the disease unless objective, case-controlled, data are advanced to support the procedure. Currently, open resection of the stenosis (i.e., membranectomy with or without septal myectomy) during cardiopulmonary bypass is the most promising treatment for severe SAS in dogs. The surgery results in sustained pressure gradient reductions of 60 to 90% in dogs with severe SAS. Surgeries on dogs with systolic pressure gradients greater than 200 mm Hg have been successful. The

overall operative mortality associated with the surgery is currently less than 20% at Colorado State University and continues to decline as experience with the operation is gained. In human patients, this surgery reduces, but does not eliminate, the risk for sudden death and therefore is considered palliative, rather than curative. Dogs that have undergone successful surgery and gradient reduction have experienced sudden death as late as 40 months after surgery. Thus, the surgery should be considered palliative in dogs as well.

VENTRICULAR SEPTAL DEFECT

Ventricular septal defect (VSD) is an important congenital defect in dogs and cats. *Perimembranous defects* are located adjacent to the membranous septum, medial to the septal tricuspid leaflet, and ventral to the crista supraventricularis. *Infundibular (supracristal) defects* occur in the outlet muscular septum dorsal to the crista supraventricularis. *Muscular defects* occur in the inlet or trabecular muscle septum.

The pathophysiologic consequences of VSD depend on the size and location of the defect. A large VSD overloads the left and possibly right ventricle, and leads to progressive heart failure. Rarely, high shunt flows may cause a progressive left-sided congestive pulmonary arteriopathy, leading to increased pulmonary vascular resistance and right-to-left shunt flow *(Eisenmenger's syndrome)*. Last, a juxta-aortic location of the defect can result in aortic leaflet prolapse and progressive aortic insufficiency. Thus, surgical correction of a VSD is indicated for large defects to prevent progressive heart failure and pulmonary hypertension or when progressive aortic insufficiency is present even if the VSD is otherwise small.

The diagnostic findings suggestive of a hemodynamically significant VSD include radiographic evidence of pulmonary vascular enlargement, radiographic or echocardiographic evidence of left ventricular dilation, or a Doppler-measured shunt flow velocity less than 3.5 m/sec. Animals with these changes should undergo cardiac catheterization to determine the pulmonary-to-systemic flow $(Q_p:Q_s)$ ratio and pulmonary vascular resistance. Animals with a $Q_p:Q_s$ ratio greater than 2:1 or pulmonary vascular resistance greater than 4 U/m^2 should be considered for surgery.

Surgical options for VSD are pulmonary artery banding or definitive closure of the defect. Pulmonary artery banding is a palliative correction that involves surgical placement of a constricting band around the pulmonary artery. The intended result is an increase in right ventricular systolic pressure and a decrease in left-to-right shunt flow across the defect. The procedure thereby provides some protection against both progressive heart failure and pulmonary hypertension. Pulmonary artery banding has been largely abandoned in humans in favor of definitive repair. The procedure is a viable option in cats or dogs when definitive repair of the defect is not feasible. Limited information on the degree of long-term palliation achieved with the procedure is available in small animals, although anecdotal statements in the literature suggest that 10 years of life after the procedure is possible. Possible complications associated with pulmonary artery banding include over-tightening of the band, leading to reversal of shunt flow and tricuspid insufficiency.

Definitive closure of VSD can be accomplished under cardiopulmonary bypass in dogs weighing more than 5 kg body weight. Correction is considered curative. Complete atrioventricular block secondary to injury to conduction tissues is a possible complication associated with surgery.

ATRIAL SEPTAL DEFECT

Atrial septal defects (ASDs) result in a volume overload of the right heart. Echocardiography generally allows diagnosis of ASD without cardiac catheterization. The decision to perform surgery to correct an ASD is based on clinical signs and the hemodynamic significance of the defect. As with VSD, cardiac catheterization to determine the $Q_p:Q_s$ ratio has been the gold standard for evaluation of ASD. Atrial septal defects with a $Q_p:Q_s$ ratio greater than 2:1 are considered hemodynamically significant and require surgical closure of the defect to prevent premature death from heart failure. A transatrial septal blood flow velocity of more than 0.45 m/sec suggests a $Q_p:Q_s$ ratio greater than 2:1.

Open surgical correction of ASD can be undertaken with the aid of cardiopulmonary bypass. The septal defect is closed with autogenous pericardium.

TETRALOGY OF FALLOT

Tetralogy of Fallot is composed of a large ventricular septal defect, pulmonic stenosis, right ventricular hypertrophy, and an overriding aorta. The pathophysiologic consequences of tetralogy depends on the relative magnitude of the two physiologically significant defects: pulmonic stenosis and VSD. At one end of the spectrum are animals with a large VSD and insignificant pulmonic stenosis. The functional result is similar to an isolated large VSD. At the other end of the spectrum are animals with severe pulmonic stenosis, suprasystemic right ventricular systolic pressure, and right-to-left shunt flow. The result is moderate to severe cyanosis, exercise intolerance, and progressive polycythemia. Premature death from complications related to chronic hypoxemia, polycythemia, and thromboembolism are frequent in these animals. In the middle of the spectrum are animals in which the pulmonic stenosis and VSD are balanced, analogous to a VSD after pulmonary artery banding. A predominantly left-to-right shunt is termed *acyanotic tetralogy*, and animals with this condition may function reasonably well as long as the shunt flow is insufficient to result in left heart failure. Progression of right ventricular outflow tract obstruction due to infundibular hypertrophy can cause some animals to develop cyanosis later in life.

Acyanotic animals that have reasonably balanced defects should be followed for progression, but generally they do not require surgical intervention. Surgery should be considered for cyanotic animals that have a resting arterial oxygen saturation less than 70%. Palliative surgeries for tetralogy include isolated correction of the pulmonic stenosis or creation of a systemic-to-pulmonary shunt. Isolated correction of the pulmonic stenosis risks overcorrection of the stenosis, resulting in an overwhelming left-to-right shunt. From this standpoint, a dilation valvuloplasty would be preferred over a patch-graft procedure. Several systemic-to-pulmonic shunts have been devised for palliation of tetralogy, including the Blalock-Taussig (subclavian-to-pulmonary artery), Potts (aorticopulmonary anastomosis), Waterston (aorta-to-right pulmonary artery), and Glenn (venopulmonary arterial) shunts. Different modifications of the Blalock-Taussig shunt have been used to successfully palliate dogs with tetralogy. Harvesting the left subclavian artery as a free autogenous graft and placing it between the ascending aorta and the main pulmonary artery is preferred by the author. Definitive repair of tetralogy can be undertaken in dogs with the aid of cardiopulmonary bypass.

CARDIAC VALVE REPLACEMENT

Cardiac valve replacement is an emerging option for dogs with hemodynamically significant cardiac valve insufficiency. The possible indications for heart valve replacement in dogs include aortic valve endocarditis, degenerative mitral valve disease, and congenital tricuspid valve dysplasia. The options for cardiac valve replacement include fresh or cryopreserved allografts, glutaraldehyde-fixed bioprostheses, and mechanical valves. In addition, techniques for repair of the native valve have recently been perfected for humans, and these techniques could have application in dogs.

Dogs with aortic insufficiency secondary to bacterial endocarditis are potential candidates for valve replacement. If the animal is hemodynamically stable, it should undergo intense antimicrobial therapy before surgery is undertaken. Surgery is indicated when dogs become symptomatic for heart failure or when left ventricular end-systolic diameter measurements suggest that secondary cardiomyopathy is developing. A viable allograft is the method of choice for humans in this setting because of its durability, resistance to infection, and lack of need for anticoagulation to prevent thromboembolic complications. Valve allografts are well tolerated in humans; however, limited experimental studies suggest that allografts may undergo some degree of rejection in dogs, potentially reducing their durability.

Acquired mitral valve disease is an extremely important problem in small- and toy-breed dogs. Recent development of small, hemodynamically-efficient, bileaflet mechanical valves (Carbomedics, Inc.), and refinement of a cardiopulmonary bypass for small dogs, have increased the prospects for surgical treatment of this condition. Mitral valve replacement is indicated in dogs with medically refractory congestive heart failure, but the procedure must be undertaken before secondary cardiomyopathy has become irreversible. Early experience suggests that small dogs are capable of remarkable reversal of ventricular dilation and myocardial dysfunction after mitral valve replacement. Mitral valve replacement is contraindicated in dogs with refractory chronic respiratory disease. Replacement of the mitral valve with a mechanical prosthesis necessitates lifetime anticoagulation therapy with warfarin. An international normalization ratio (INR) of 2.0 to 2.5 is recommended in humans with bileaflet mechanical valves. Repair of the mitral valve is an attractive option in dogs because it eliminates the need for postoperative anticoagulation therapy and an expensive prosthesis. However, the advanced nature of the disease by the time surgery is likely to be undertaken, as well as the extensive surgical experience required to accomplish consistent repairs, will probably limit its application in dogs.

References and Suggested Reading

Gravlee GP, Davis RE, Utley JR, eds: Cardiopulmonary Bypass: Principles and Practice. Baltimore: Williams & Wilkins, 1993.
A comprehensive review of theory, pathophysiology, and techniques for cardiopulmonary bypass.
Kirlin JW, Barratt-Boyes BG, eds: Cardiac Surgery, 2nd ed. New York: Churchhill Livingstone, 1993.
Definitive review of indications, techniques, and outcomes for cardiac surgery in humans.
Monnet E, Orton C, Gaynor J, et al: Open resection of subvalvular aortic stenosis in dogs. J Am Vet Med Assoc 209:1255, 1996.
Surgical technique and outcome in 17 dogs undergoing surgery for subvalvular aortic stenosis.
Orton EC: Small Animal Thoracic Surgery. Baltimore: Williams & Wilkins, 1995.
A review and illustrations of cardiac surgery techniques in small animals.
Orton EC, Bruecker KA, McCracken TO: An open patch-graft technique for correction of pulmonic stenosis in the dog. Vet Surg 19:148, 1990.
Surgical technique and outcome in dogs undergoing patch-graft valvuloplasty for pulmonic stenosis.
Stark J, de Level M, eds: Surgery for Congenital Heart Defects, 2nd ed. New York: Grune & Stratton, 1994.
Comprehensive review of the indications for, technique of, and expected outcomes of surgery for congenital heart defects in children.

Outpatient Management of Chronic Heart Failure

WENDY A. WARE
Ames, Iowa

BRUCE W. KEENE
Raleigh, North Carolina

The clinical syndrome of heart failure can be the end result of a variety of heart diseases that affect companion animals; most commonly, chronic valvular heart disease and dilated cardiomyopathy in dogs, and hypertrophic cardiomyopathy in cats. Although the cause and pathophysiology of each of these diseases are different, the body's neurohormonal responses as well as the heart's reaction to those neurohormonal responses is similar. Neurohormonal responses (primarily activation of the sympathetic nervous and renin-angiotensin-aldosterone systems) are effective short- and intermediate-term "compensatory mechanisms" that maintain cardiac output and blood pressure during acute volume depletion or hemorrhage. However, the long-term activation of these mechanisms from chronically reduced cardiac function is generally detrimental to the patient. Although the benefits to patients from the inhibition of these responses theoretically should be relatively independent of the cause or pathophysiology of the underlying heart failure, clinical benefits in both humans and dogs have been best established in the setting of dilated cardiomyopathy (see *CVT XII*, p. 780).

As a result of the realization that the "compensatory mechanisms" activated by a variety of heart diseases are actually detrimental to long-term survival, therapeutic strategies for chronic heart failure now commonly incorporate angiotensin-converting enzyme inhibitors (ACEIs) and/or drugs that reduce or block sympathetic nervous system activity, regardless of the underlying etiology. Exceptions to this generality include an underlying cause of heart failure that can be directly addressed and corrected (e.g.,

pericardial disease and some congenital heart diseases), individual patient contraindications to any of these drugs, or socioeconomic factors.

RESPONSES TO CARDIAC DYSFUNCTION

When stimulated by reduced pump function, the sympathetic nervous, renin-angiotensin-aldosterone, and antidiuretic hormone (vasopressin) systems act together to increase vascular volume (by retaining sodium and water and increasing thirst) and vascular tone. The enhanced cardiac output and arterial blood pressure that result can be beneficial in acute heart failure; however, in the setting of significant, chronic heart disease, this volume retention often causes pulmonary edema or body cavity effusions. Systemic arteriolar vasoconstriction increases the workload on the heart, can reduce forward cardiac output, and can exacerbate valvular regurgitation. Chronic neurohormonal activation also appears to cause further deterioration in cardiac function directly by damaging both the myocardial interstitium and muscle cells.

Chronic exposure to increased sympathetic stimulation decreases the number and sensitivity of the heart's beta-receptors that are coupled to stimulatory G proteins but appears not to affect those that are coupled to inhibitory G proteins (the recently described beta$_3$-receptors). Although this probably represents a protective mechanism against the potentially cardiotoxic and arrhythmogenic effects of catecholamines, reduced ventricular performance and exercise intolerance result. Beta-blocking agents (or agents that otherwise reduce sympathetic nerve traffic) can help restore beta-receptor numbers and sensitivity but may worsen heart failure in some cases.

Decreased exercise capacity with heart failure probably results from several mechanisms, including reduced ventricular diastolic function, inadequate forward output, pulmonary edema or pleural effusion, and skeletal muscle weakness and loss. Abnormalities involving the peripheral vasculature are also important. Local endothelial factors as well as generalized neurohormonal activation can contribute to the impaired skeletal muscle vasodilatory capacity occurring with chronic heart failure. The improvement in exercise capacity shown in humans and dogs after chronic ACE inhibition suggests that the renin-angiotensin system may play an important role.

STRATEGIES FOR CHRONIC HEART FAILURE MANAGEMENT

The goal of chronic therapy is to improve the patient's quality of life as well as the duration of life. Treatment of chronic heart failure centers on blocking the chronic neurohormonal activation that characterizes advanced heart failure and controlling venous pressures, while ensuring that cardiac output remains adequate for routine activity and modest exercise. Edema and/or body cavity effusions are controlled to maintain patient comfort, and arrhythmias are managed as needed to maintain hemodynamic stability and, if possible, reduce the risk of sudden death. Therapy is individually tailored as the disease progresses by adjusting dosages, adding or substituting drugs, and further modifying lifestyle or diet; intensification of therapy is to be expected with advanced disease (Table 1). Episodes of acute, decompensated congestive heart failure requiring hospitalization and diuresis often develop in patients with chronic, progressive heart failure.

TABLE 1. Treatment Strategies for Common Complications of Advanced Heart Failure

Refractory Pulmonary Edema and Ascites
  Gradually maximize dose of ACEI
  Gradually maximize dose of furosemide
  Further restrict sodium intake; ensure adequate protein (increase if low albumin)
  Add low-dose hydralazine (especially if primary mitral regurgitation)
  Add spironolactone or hydrochlorothiazide-spironolactone
Collapse or Syncope
  Screen for (routine or ambulatory ECGs) and treat arrhythmias
  Reduce activity or excitement as much as possible
  If cough-syncope, consider cough suppressant if pulmonary edema is well controlled
Persistent Cough
  Screen for underlying airway or pulmonary causes if pulmonary edema appears well controlled
  For cough induced by mechanical irritation from enlarged left atrium: control pulmonary edema, use ACEI ± hydralazine to reduce regurgitant fraction as much as possible, cough suppressant (e.g., hydrocodone) as needed
Pleural Effusion or Chylothorax
  Drain fluid as completely as possible; intensify medication to slow reaccumulation

See text for dosage recommendations.
ACEI, angiotensin converting enzyme inhibitor; ECGs, electrocardiograms.

General Therapeutic Strategies

Angiotensin-Converting Enzyme Inhibitors (ACEIs)

ACEIs allow vasodilation and reduce sodium and water retention by blocking the formation of angiotensin II and decreasing circulating aldosterone (see *CVT XII*, p. 786). Their effects may be enhanced by vasodilator kinins normally degraded by ACE and inhibition of ACE within vascular walls. The ACEIs have advantages over direct arteriolar dilators (e.g., hydralazine) because they moderate excess neurohormonal responses. In conjunction with a diuretic and digoxin, ACEIs promote sustained clinical improvement in heart failure due to myocardial disease or volume overload, while prolonging survival. Although these drugs are generally safe and effective, the potential adverse effects of ACEIs include hypotension, gastrointestinal upset, deterioration of renal function, and hyperkalemia (especially when used with a potassium-sparing diuretic or a potassium supplement).

Currently, enalapril is the only ACEI approved for use in the United States for the treatment of heart failure in veterinary patients (Enacard, Merck Agvet), although other ACEIs are approved for this purpose in humans, and benazepril (Lotensin, Novartis) has been approved for this use in dogs in Canada and parts of Europe. The recommended starting dose of enalapril is 0.5 mg/kg every 24 hours for dogs, although some dogs respond better when dosed twice daily. A dose of 0.5 mg/kg every 24 hours can be used in cats. Benazepril (0.25 to 0.5 mg/kg every 24 hours), captopril (0.5 to 2.0 mg/kg every 8 to 12 hours; Capoten, Bristol-Myers Squibb), and lisinopril (0.5 mg/kg every 12 to 24 hours; Prinivil, Merck) are other ACEIs that have been used in veterinary patients.

Dietary and Exercise Considerations

Sodium Intake. Restriction of sodium intake reduces cardiac workload regardless of the underlying cause of heart failure. Since heart failure impairs sodium and water excreting ability, dietary salt restriction is recommended to help control fluid accumulation. Once fluid accumulation has occurred, moderate restriction is usually recommended initially (e.g., Hill's k/d, Purina CNM NF-formula, Science Diet Canine Senior, Purina CNM GL-formula). As heart failure progresses, more stringent sodium restriction may be helpful (e.g. Hill's h/d, Purina CNM CV-formula, or homemade low-sodium recipes), although the risk of azotemia rises when stringent salt restriction is combined with ACE inhibition and relatively high doses of diuretics. Non-softened or distilled water may be helpful in areas where much sodium is present in the drinking water. Very severe sodium restriction may exacerbate neurohormonal activation and contribute to hyponatremia, however.

Other Dietary Considerations. Obesity increases cardiac metabolic and hemodynamic demands; furthermore, excess thoracic fat can mechanically interfere with respiration and contribute to cor pulmonale. A reducing diet should be recommended for grossly overweight pets with heart disease, preferably before signs of heart failure develop.

Inappetance is common with advanced heart failure; increased respiratory effort, malaise, and adverse medication effects can contribute. In addition, poor splanchnic perfusion, bowel and pancreatic edema, and secondary intestinal lymphangiectasia may reduce nutrient absorption and promote protein loss. Strategies to increase food intake include warming the food; adding small amounts of palatable "people" foods (e.g., nonsalted meats or gravy, reduced sodium soups), salt substitutes, garlic powder or other spices; hand-feeding; and providing several small meals daily. Any diet changes should be instituted gradually. Cardiac cachexia is a poor prognostic indicator. Loss of lean body mass is associated with weakness, fatigue, and reduced immune function. While multiple factors appear to be involved (see p. 711), certain cytokines, especially tumor necrosis factor-alpha and interleukin-1β, are known to suppress appetite and cause hypercatabolism. Dietary omega-3 fatty acids theoretically reduce the production of these cytokines; the effects of omega-3 fatty acid supplementation in animals with heart failure are currently being evaluated.

Amino Acid Supplements. Supplementation of specific amino acids may be important in some cases of dilated cardiomyopathy. Low blood taurine concentrations and myocardial L-carnitine deficiency have been identified in some dogs with dilated cardiomyopathy. Measurement of plasma concentrations of taurine is recommended in any "unusual" (usually small-breed) dog with dilated cardiomyopathy. Myocardial carnitine deficiency was observed in approximately 40% of animals with dilated cardiomyopathy in a pilot study, although only a small percentage of those with myocardial carnitine deficiency mount a dramatic clinical response to supplementation. Dogs shown to be deficient in carnitine or taurine should be supplemented. Endomyocardial biopsy is invasive and not widely available (and plasma carnitine levels are an insensitive indicator of myocardial carnitine concentrations); thus, a 3-month therapeutic trial of L-carnitine supplementation may be offered to individual dog owners. The average dose of L-carnitine for a large- or giant-breed dog (2 gm t.i.d.) costs approximately $100.00 a month, and the owner must understand that therapy with L-carnitine is not likely to be beneficial in dogs that are not deficient. Dilated cardiomyopathy in American Cocker spaniels has been associated with both carnitine and taurine deficiency (see p. 761); supplementation with L-carnitine (1 gm PO every 8 to 12 hours) and taurine (500 mg PO every 12 hours) is recommended in addition to traditional pharmacotherapy for American Cocker spaniels with this disease.

Cats with dilated cardiomyopathy should be supplemented with taurine (250 to 500 mg PO every 12 hours) at least until it is known whether they suffer from plasma taurine deficiency. Most commercial and prescription cat foods now contain adequate amounts of taurine to prevent taurine-responsive dilated cardiomyopathy; thus, most cats with dilated cardiomyopathy are no longer taurine-deficient or -responsive.

Activity. Although strenuous exercise can provoke respiratory symptoms, fatigue, and/or collapse, *regular* mild to moderate exercise is thought to be beneficial. An activity level that does not cause excessive panting, shortness of breath, or weakness is encouraged. The animal should never be forced to continue exercise.

Diuretic Therapy

Diuretic therapy is indicated for the initial treatment and chronic prevention of fluid retention and can be lifesaving in the treatment of cardiogenic pulmonary edema. When present, a large-volume pleural effusion or tense ascites should be drained enough to normalize respiration before chronic diuretic therapy is begun. The lowest dose of furosemide that prevents development of edema or effusion is used for chronic therapy. This dose is individualized (usually 0.5 to 2 mg/kg per day) and may change over time as the disease progresses. In earlier stages of heart failure, following initial diuresis, daily furosemide may not be needed, especially with concurrent ACEI administration. Test doses of furosemide (e.g., 1 to 3 mg/kg PO every 12 to 24 hours) can be useful for differentiating signs of left heart failure (pulmonary edema) from primary respiratory disease in certain cases; prompt improvement of signs accompanies resolution of pulmonary edema, although the response is not always clear-cut. Furosemide is no longer recommended as the sole agent for treatment of chronic heart failure, primarily because it is associated with activation of the renin-angiotensin-aldosterone system, and with decreased survival compared to ACEI in human studies. Nevertheless, as congestive heart failure progresses, the clinician generally will need to prescribe higher doses of diuretics. Respiratory rate and pattern, hydration, body weight, exercise tolerance, renal function, serum electrolyte concentrations, and arterial blood pressure are used to monitor response to diuretic treatment. Adverse effects are usually related to excessive fluid and/or electrolyte losses.

When maximal doses of furosemide and vasodilators do not control fluid accumulation in refractory heart failure, another diuretic such as spironolactone (1 to 2 mg/kg PO every 12 hours) or spironolactone hydrochlorothiazide (1 to 2 mg/kg of the combination 25 mg/25 mg product) can be added (see p. 752). Spironolactone is a potassium-sparing aldosterone antagonist and must be used cautiously in patients receiving an ACEI or a potassium supplement. Peak diuresis occurs within 2 to 3 days; serum electrolytes as well as renal function are carefully monitored, usually at 3 to 4 days, 1 week, and periodic intervals thereafter. Spironolactone may decrease the clearance of digoxin.

Digoxin

Digoxin is indicated in heart failure from dilated cardiomyopathy as well as advanced atrioventricular valve insufficiency. The benefits of digoxin include a modest positive inotropic effect, supraventricular arrhythmia suppression, and a direct sensitizing effect on arterial baroreceptors and reduction in sympathetic nerve traffic. Oral maintenance doses of digoxin (dogs: 0.005 to 0.01 mg/kg every 12 hours, up to a maximum of 0.375 or, rarely, 0.5 mg/day; cats: 0.007 mg/kg every 48 hours) are used to initiate therapy. Doses are based on calculated lean body weight, especially in obese animals, since digoxin has poor lipid solubility. Therapeutic serum concentrations are reached in 2 to 5 days in dogs and about 10 days in cats.

Serum digoxin concentration is measured 5 to 10 days after drug initiation or dosage change; serum is drawn 8 to 10 hours after the dose. The therapeutic serum concentration range is 1 to 2 ng/ml, although some prefer values nearer to 1.3 ng/ml. If the serum concentration is less than 0.8 ng/ml, the digoxin dose is increased by up to 30%, and the serum concentration measured again. If serum concentration cannot be measured and toxicity is suspected, the drug should be discontinued for at least 1 to 2 days, then reinstituted at half of the original dose.

Digoxin intoxication may be signaled by loss of appetite, vomiting, diarrhea, or cardiac rhythm disturbances. Conservative doses and serum digoxin concentration measurement help prevent toxicity. Serum drug concentration increases with reduced renal function. Digoxin exhibits significant binding to skeletal muscle; thus, animals with reduced muscle mass as well as those with compromised renal function can easily become toxic at the usual calculated doses. It is important to remember that quinidine (and certain other drugs) can increase serum digoxin concentration and that hypokalemia potentiates its toxic effects.

Non-ACEI Vasodilators

The direct arteriolar vasodilator hydralazine can improve cardiac output and reduce mitral regurgitant fraction and is often used in hospital treatment of severe pulmonary edema. Direct vasodilators can also be chronically used to control pulmonary edema in cases of valvular insufficiency or myocardial failure. However, these drugs can contribute to the enhanced neurohormonal response in heart failure, which makes it less desirable for chronic use. The combination of hydralazine (0.5 to 2 mg/kg PO every 12 hours) and a nitrate (e.g., nitroglycerin ointment, ½ to 1½ inches every 8 to 12 hours cutaneously, or isosorbide dinitrate, 0.5 to 2 mg/kg PO every 8 hours) may provide a balanced vasodilating effect when an ACEI is not well tolerated or affordable. Nitrates may increase venous capacitance and reduce cardiac filling pressures, but high dosages, frequent application, or long-acting formulations are likely to be associated with drug tolerance.

Hydralazine can be cautiously used to intensify the treatment of dogs with refractory pulmonary edema from mitral insufficiency that is no longer responsive to ACEI, diuretic, and digoxin therapy. Hypotension and reflex tachycardia are potential adverse effects.

Re-evaluation of the Heart Failure Patient

Periodic re-evaluation of the heart failure patient often allows early detection of complications. The clinician should discuss various issues with the owner, including medications and dosage schedules, potential adverse drug effects, problems with drug administration, the pet's appetite, diet, activity level, and any other concerns. The client is instructed to monitor the pet's respiratory (and heart) rate when it is quietly resting at home. Resting respiratory rates are usually no more than 30 breaths per minute; pulmonary edema causes faster, more shallow respirations by increasing lung stiffness. A persistent increase of at least 20% in resting respiratory rate or the inability to sleep comfortably can be an early sign of worsening heart failure.

Likewise, a persistent increase in resting heart rate can signal the heightened sympathetic tone of decompensating failure.

Besides a careful physical examination, tests that may be indicated on re-evaluation include arterial blood pressure measurement, an electrocardiogram (especially if an arrhythmia is auscultated or suspected), thoracic radiographs, serum biochemistries (especially for evaluating renal function and electrolytes), an echocardiogram (although serial echocardiograms are not highly cost-effective in dogs), and serum digoxin concentration. Aside from the history, physical examination, blood pressure measurement, and routine chemistries, clinicians should use their judgment when selecting diagnostic studies.

FELINE HYPERTROPHIC CARDIOMYOPATHY

Increased ventricular stiffness and impaired filling characterize hypertrophic and also restrictive cardiomyopathies. Tachycardia further interferes with ventricular filling, predisposes to myocardial ischemia, and promotes venous congestion by shortening the diastolic filling period. Secondary mitral regurgitation can exacerbate heart failure. When present, dynamic left ventricular outflow obstruction (hypertrophic obstructive cardiomyopathy) increases wall stress and myocardial oxygen demand. Therapy is aimed at facilitating ventricular filling, reducing congestion, controlling arrhythmias, minimizing ischemia, and preventing arterial thromboembolism.

Guidelines for Therapy

Stress, activity level, and if possible sodium intake should be minimized. Ventricular filling is improved by slowing the heart rate and enhancing relaxation. Diltiazem or a beta-adrenergic blocker represents the foundation of chronic oral therapy; which agent is chosen may depend on characteristics of the individual's disease, medication response, or clinician preference. Cats without overt pulmonary edema may respond well to one of these drugs alone. Diltiazem (1.75 to 2.5 mg/kg PO every 8 hours) is well tolerated and seems effective in many cases, but t.i.d. dosing is difficult for many clients. Alternatively, pharmacodynamic studies indicate that some sustained-release preparations of diltiazem (Dilacor, Rhone-Poulenc Rorer) are suitable for cats at a dose of 30 mg (total dose) every 12 hours. Potential benefits include coronary vasodilation, enhanced ventricular relaxation, and mild reductions in heart rate and contractility. It may decrease a systolic outflow gradient if peripheral vasodilation does not enhance ventricular shortening.

The beta-adrenergic blockers often decrease heart rate more than diltiazem, are useful in controlling tachyarrhythmias, and reduce systolic outflow obstruction and myocardial oxygen demand (through their negative inotropic effect). Reduction in heart rate and myocardial ischemia resulting from beta-blocker therapy may indirectly improve left ventricular diastolic function. The nonselective beta-blocker propranolol (2.5 to 5 mg/cat every 8 hours) has been widely used, but can be associated with bronchospasm, lethargy, or depressed appetite in some cats. The $beta_1$ selective blocker atenolol (6.25 to 12.5 mg/cat every

12 to 24 hours) may be better tolerated and has a longer duration of effect. The authors favor atenolol over diltiazem for cats with severe outflow obstruction or paroxysmal arrhythmias. Sometimes, a beta-blocker is added to diltiazem therapy (or vice versa) in advanced cases; for example, when progressive hypertrophy is complicated by severe outflow obstruction or tachyarrhythmias. This combination must be used cautiously to avoid bradycardia or hypotension.

Pulmonary edema is treated with furosemide at the lowest dose that controls signs, as discussed previously. Significant pleural effusion should be removed by thoracentesis. Digoxin is generally contraindicated for hypertrophic cardiomyopathy, since increased myocardial oxygen demand and dynamic outflow obstruction could result. Drugs that increase heart rate or cause hypotension are to be avoided.

Enalapril has been used primarily in cats with refractory pulmonary edema or recurrent pleural effusion. Intitially low doses are gradually increased to the usual maintenance dose of 0.5 mg/kg every 24 hours (or every 12 hours if necessary); blood pressure and renal function should be monitored when one initiates or adjusts ACEI therapy. Other strategies useful for refractory heart failure include increasing doses of furosemide (up to 4 mg/kg every 8 hours), maximizing the dose of diltiazem or beta-blocker, or adding another diuretic such as hydrochlorothiazide/ spironolactone (2 to 3 mg/kg of the combination per day). Renal function and serum electrolytes should be monitored frequently. In advanced cases of congestive heart failure, mild to moderate azotemia may represent the price paid to prevent life-threatening edema or effusion. Digoxin could also be considered for refractory right heart failure in the absence of outflow obstruction.

More detailed information on the treatment of feline myocardial diseases as well as strategies for thromboembolism prevention and management can be found in previous volumes of *CVT*.

References and Suggested Reading

COVE Study Group: Controlled clinical evaluation of enalapril in dogs with heart failure: Results of the cooperative veterinary study group. J Vet Intern Med 9:243, 1995.
Multicenter randomized clinical trial documenting the benefits of enalapril.

Ferguson DW: Digitalis and neurohormonal abnormalities in heart failure and implications for therapy. Am J Cardiol 69:24G, 1992.
Review of the role of digoxin in reducing sympathetic nervous activation and restoring baroreceptor sensitivity in heart failure.

Hamlin RL, Benitz AM, Ericsson GF, et al: Effects of enalapril on exercise tolerance and longevity in dogs with heart failure produced by iatrogenic mitral regurgitation. J Vet Intern Med 10:85, 1996.
Experimental study documenting the positive effect of enalapril on exercise tolerance in heart failure.

IMPROVE Study Group: Acute and short-term hemodynamic, echocardiographic, and clinical effects of enalapril maleate in dogs with naturally acquired heart failure: Results of the invasive multicenter prospective veterinary evaluation of enalapril study. J Vet Intern Med 9:234, 1995.
Multicenter randomized clinical trial documenting the hemodynamic benefits of enalapril in acute heart failure.

Johnston CI, Fabris B, Yoshida K: The cardiac renin-angiotensin system in heart failure. Am Heart J 126:756, 1993.
Review of the implications of activation of the renin-angiotensin-aldosterone system in heart failure.

Kittleson MD, Keene B, Pion PD, et al: Results of the Multicenter Spaniel Trial (MUST): Taurine- and carnitine-responsive dilated cardiomyopathy in American Cocker Spaniels with decreased plasma taurine concentration. J Vet Intern Med 11:204, 1997.
Results of a multicenter radomized clinical trial comparing the efficacy of the combination of taurine and L-carnitine supplementation to placebo in the treatment of dilated cardiomyopathy in American Cocker spaniels.

Roudebush P, Allen TA, Kuehn NF, et al: The effect of combined therapy with captopril, furosemide, and a sodium-restricted diet on serum electrolyte levels and renal function in normal dogs and dogs with congestive heart failure. J Vet Intern Med 8:337, 1994.
Experimental study documenting the potential decrease in renal function when severe sodium restriction is combined with ACEI and high doses of diuretics.

Ware WA, Lund DD, Subieta AR, et al: Sympathetic activation in dogs with congestive heart failure caused by chronic mitral valve disease and dilated cardiomyopathy. J Am Vet Med Assoc 197:1475, 1990.
Results of a study that present evidence of activation of the sympathetic nervous system in dogs with heart failure.

Medical Management of Refractory Congestive Heart Failure in Dogs

DAVID SISSON
Urbana, Illinois

ASSESSING DOGS WITH REFRACTORY HEART FAILURE

When confronted with a refractory heart failure patient, the practicing veterinarian should first determine that all medications are prescribed at appropriate dosages and that they are routinely administered as prescribed. It is also important to establish that the diet is appropriately sodium-restricted. Substantive changes in the animal's attitude or activities should be noted and recorded for future reference. A meticulous physical examination should be performed in all patients with refractory heart failure. Many dogs with recurring signs of congestive heart failure have an identifiable systemic disorder that precipitates decompensated heart failure. Some relevant examples include systemic hypertension, systemic inflammation, neoplasia, hypothyroidism, hyperthyroidism or excessive thyroid supplementation, anemia, pneumonia, hyperadrenocorticism, pulmonary thromboembolism, and renal failure. Signs of congestive heart failure are often alleviated when these complicating disorders are identified and remedied or effectively palliated. With this in mind, it is always advisable to (1) measure blood pressure, (2) obtain red and white blood cell counts, serum electrolytes, and routine serum chemistries, (3) test for any suspected endocrine diseases, and (4) carefully inspect the thoracic radiographs for indications of coexisting respiratory disease. A simple urinalysis often helps determine owner compliance with dietary restrictions and prescribed diuretics. In some cases, it is important to measure the plasma concentration of certain administered drugs, for example, digoxin and certain antiarrhythmic drugs, either to ensure dosing compliance or to exclude toxicity.

The cause of sudden cardiac decompensation in an individual patient may become obvious when the examiner discovers a new arrhythmia, a new or changing murmur, pericardial effusion, or evidence of systemic or pulmonary thromboembolism. The condition of dogs with previously compensated heart disease often rapidly deteriorates when atrial fibrillation develops; atrial pressures rise rapidly, resulting in pulmonary congestion, and cardiac output declines, resulting in reduced exercise capacity. Atrial or ventricular tachycardia, heart block, and other serious rhythm disturbances can also exacerbate signs of heart failure. Appropriate treatment of the arrhythmia often suffices to alleviate signs of heart failure (see pp. 726 and 733).

The precise cause of worsening heart failure is difficult or impossible to identify in many dogs. Consultation with or referral to a cardiologist should be considered whenever this resource is available and the owner is willing. By this mechanism, a more complete cardiac evaluation may be performed and a greater variety of treatment options can be explored. Echocardiography is usually a desirable, if not mandatory, procedure in dogs with refractory heart failure. Other specialized diagnostic procedures, including ambulatory electrocardiographic recordings and invasive measurement of intracardiac or vascular pressures, are sometimes required to guide therapy. A variety of drug combinations unfamiliar to the skilled generalist may be required to achieve a successful result, and such therapy engenders the unavoidable possibility of adverse drug reactions and often unexpected drug interactions. In dogs with refractory heart failure, the inherent risks and complications of treatment are virtually always greater than those encountered in less severely affected patients treated with conventional drugs. In these circumstances, diagnostic and therapeutic strategies are best designed and implemented by or with the advice of a specialist.

PROGRESSION OF HEART FAILURE

Heart disease often progresses over time from an asymptomatic state to a severe and eventually refractory condition. In dogs with degenerative valvular disease or dilated cardiomyopathy, therapy for moderate to severe chronic congestive heart failure generally includes diuretics (typically furosemide), an angiotensin-converting enzyme

(ACE) inhibitor such as enalapril (Enacard, Vasotec, Merck) or lisinopril (Zestril, Zeneca; Prinivil, Merck), and digoxin. Standard therapy should be optimized in dogs with progressively worsening heart failure before additional drugs are prescribed. With progression of the underlying disease and the continued operation of certain deleterious physiologic responses, the signs of heart failure eventually recur. Congestive signs usually predominate, but progressive fatigue or organ-system dysfunction, most often renal failure, also develops as a consequence of declining cardiac output. In most cases, refractory pulmonary edema is best remedied by altering the diuretic or vasodilator arms of therapy (combination therapy) with the goal of reducing venous pressure. Many different strategies have been devised for managing such patients, and there is no consensus on the best approach. Refractory low-output heart failure is more difficult to treat except when it is precipitated by excessive dosing of diuretics. In this circumstance, the first priority of treatment is to optimize preload by moderating diuretic usage. In hypertensive or normotensive dogs, cardiac output can sometimes be improved by afterload reduction. Arterial vasodilators, such as hydralazine or amlodipine, are often selected for this purpose, but they should be avoided in dogs with low-output heart failure and hypotension. Hypotensive dogs with low-output heart failure are more likely to improve with the infusion of a potent positive inotrope.

ACE INHIBITORS AND VASODILATORS

Angiotensin-converting enzyme inhibitors are the most effective drugs yet identified for the successful management of chronic heart failure. An optimal dose has not been identified for any ACE inhibitor drug, and the "optimal dose" undoubtedly varies from patient to patient. Enalapril and lisinopril are effective when administered to dogs at a dosage of 0.5 mg/kg b.i.d. (The IMPROVE Study Investigators, 1995; Hamlin and Nakayama, 1998). If the clinical response to this dosage regimen is inadequate, the dose of either drug may be increased to 0.75 mg/kg b.i.d., assuming the patient is appropriately monitored and that renal dysfunction and other adverse effects (hypotension) are not evident.

When ACE inhibitors are not tolerated, the combination of hydralazine (Apresoline HCl, Novartis) and a nitrate can be substituted. While this drug combination is not as efficacious as ACE inhibitors, it has been shown to reduce symptoms and to prolong life in humans with heart failure. In dogs, hydralazine is usually initiated at 0.5 mg/kg b.i.d. The dose is gradually titrated upward to a maximum dose of 1.5 mg/kg or until clinical signs are alleviated. Hydralazine causes hemodynamic improvement in dogs with mitral insufficiency, but it has the unfortunate disadvantage of inducing tachycardia. This adverse effect can be minimized by concurrent administration of digoxin or, in select cases, by low doses of a beta-receptor blocking drug. Hydralazine and a nitrate can also be added to conventional (ACE inhibitor) therapy in dogs with refractory congestive heart failure. The safety and efficacy of this approach has not been critically evaluated. The safest approach is to first add a nitrate; hydralazine can be added subsequently, if necessary. When combining vasodilating drugs, it is extremely important to use a low dose initially and to titrate the dose slowly upward. Blood pressure should always be monitored to guide therapy. General targets are systolic pressures of 90 to 110 mm Hg, although many patients appear to tolerate slightly lower pressures.

Nitroglycerin and the organic nitrates act primarily as venous and coronary artery vasodilators with a less pronounced effect on the systemic arterioles. Nitroglycerin, applied as a 2% ointment to the inner surface of the pinna, is commonly used to treat dogs and cats with acute and chronic congestive heart failure. The efficacy of this treatment is unknown, and the administered dose is largely guesswork (1/4 to 3/4 inch every 6 to 8 hours). In humans, the absorption of cutaneously applied nitroglycerin varies with the site of administration, the amount of ointment used, and the size of the area to which the drug is applied. None of these variables have been critically studied in dogs or cats. Human patients quickly learn to adjust the dose and method of application of nitroglycerin ointment, as this drug formulation is used mainly to alleviate chest pain. Such adjustments are not possible in dogs and cats with congestive heart failure. For these reasons, the author prefers the use of orally administered organic nitrates, acknowledging that the doses of these compounds are not well established (McDonald et al, 1993; Jugdutt et al, 1995).

Isosorbide dinitrate is available in a sublingual formulation, in a standard oral formulation, and as a controlled-release capsule and tablet. Based on studies performed in dogs with experimentally-created myocardial infarcts, the estimated dose of isosorbide dinitrate varies from 0.5 to 2.0 mg/kg every 6 to 8 hours when the standard oral tablet is used (Isordil, Wyeth-Ayerst). A dosage-free interval, typically 10 to 12 hours long, is advised in human patients with angina to avoid the phenomenon of tolerance. The utility of this maneuver in dogs or cats with heart failure is unknown. Isosorbide mononitrate (ISMO, Wyeth-Ayerst), the major metabolite of isosorbide dinitrate, is also available for oral therapy. The estimated dose of isosorbide mononitrate is 0.25 to 2.0 mg/kg every 6 to 8 hours.

Amlodipine (Norvasc, Pfizer), a member of the 1,4-dihydropyridine family of calcium channel blocking drugs, is a vasodilating drug that reduces symptoms and improves exercise tolerance in humans with congestive heart failure (Packer et al, 1996). In contrast to many other calcium channel blocking drugs, amlodipine does not increase cardiovascular morbidity or mortality, and it seems to prolong survival in human patients with dilated cardiomyopathy. The efficacy of this compound in dogs with dilated cardiomyopathy or degenerative valve disease has not been determined. Preliminary observations suggest that amlodipine is efficacious in dogs with heart failure complicated by systemic hypertension and in normotensive dogs with refractory heart failure.

A safe and effective dose of amlodipine for treating dogs with heart failure has not been established. In a renal hypertensive dog (RHD) model, a single 1.0 mg/kg oral dose of amlodipine substantially reduces blood pressure with a peak effect (31 mm Hg reduction in blood pressure) at 8 hours after administration (Burges et al, 1989). This large dosage is accompanied by tachycardia unless a beta-receptor blocking drug is given simultaneously. Once-daily

treatment with amlodipine at 0.05 mg/kg caused a more modest and more gradual reduction in mean blood pressure (approximately 20 mm Hg decline) in the RHD model. The peak effect is observed in 4 to 7 days, reflecting the 30-hour half-life of this drug in dogs. In another experiment involving RHD, the acute dose required to lower systolic and diastolic blood pressure by 30 mm Hg was 0.3 and 0.4 mg/kg, respectively (Yamanaka et al, 1991). Chronic once-daily administration of amlodipine at 0.2 mg/kg effectively lowered blood pressure in RHD without causing tachycardia. Based on these observations, the experience in humans, and our own preliminary results in a small number of dogs, it is reasonable to attempt to palliate refractory heart failure in dogs with the addition of amlodipine to standard therapy using an initial dose of 0.05 and titrating upward to 0.20 mg/kg once daily, as needed.

DIURETICS

Some patients with chronic congestive heart failure become resistant to orally administered furosemide. The causes of diuretic resistance include dietary indiscretion, poor compliance, impaired bioavailability, impaired delivery or secretion (transport) of furosemide into the renal tubules, drug interference, worsening heart failure, and target-organ resistance (Ellison, 1991; Cody et al, 1994). The clinical efficacy of diuretics depends on adherence to a restricted-sodium diet. In most dogs with heart failure, moderate restriction of sodium intake (16 to 20 mg/kg BW per day) is adequate. In dogs with severe, refractory congestive heart failure, more severe sodium restriction may be helpful (6 to 8 mg/kg BW per day).

Compared to normal dogs, the rate of sodium excretion in response to furosemide administration is reduced in patients with heart failure. Renal blood flow and glomerular filtration rate decline with progressive reductions of cardiac output, and delivery of furosemide to its site of action decreases as heart failure worsens. This fundamental limitation of diuretic therapy is further complicated during chronic therapy by hypertrophy of the distal renal tubule. This adaptive change increases the rate of distal sodium reabsorption, diminishing the natriuretic effect of furosemide. Contraction of the extracellular fluid volume following bolus administration of furosemide further stimulates the renal tubules to retain sodium chloride until the next dose is administered. These limitations can often be alleviated by increasing the dose or frequency of administration of furosemide.

In patients with severe congestive heart failure, the rate of absorption of furosemide is reduced, resulting in reduced peak blood and urine concentrations and inadequate diuresis. This problem can be overcome by parenteral drug administration with the use of escalating doses until signs of congestive heart failure are eliminated. Most dogs with refractory congestion can be successfully treated in this fashion during a 1- or 2-day hospital stay. When the response to large, intermittent doses of parenteral furosemide (>4.4 mg/kg) proves inadequate, continuous intravenous infusion of the same daily dose of furosemide should be considered. The amount of sodium and water loss is substantially increased by this method. In this circumstance, the clinician must take particular care that diuretic-induced plasma volume contraction is not accompanied by progressive renal compromise, particularly in the patients concurrently treated with an ACE inhibitor. Renal function and serum electrolytes must be closely monitored, and the dose of diuretics modified accordingly. It may be necessary to monitor pulmonary capillary wedge pressure and systemic arterial pressure in order to optimize preload and cardiac output. Intermittent oral therapy can often be resumed after 1 or 2 days of infused furosemide.

To exert its diuretic effect, furosemide must be transported to the tubular lumen via the organic acid pathway. Uremic toxins and nonsteroidal anti-inflammatory drugs (NSAIDs) compete for these pathways and may reduce drug transport. Furosemide binds to albumin; thus, the efficacy of furosemide may be further reduced in animals with substantial proteinuria. Treating renal failure, eliminating NSAIDs, and increasing the dose of furosemide often improve the rate of sodium excretion in these circumstances. Very high doses of furosemide (250 to 4,000 mg/day) have been successfully used to treat human patients with reduced renal function and severe refractory heart failure (Gerlag and van Meijel, 1988). High-dose furosemide treatment has certain liabilities, including rapid dehydration and renal failure, hypokalemia, and, potentially, ototoxicity. Patients treated in this fashion should be initially hospitalized and carefully monitored. Body weight, sodium and water consumption, serum electrolytes, renal function, and urine production should be carefully measured when high-dose furosemide is used, particularly when ACE inhibitors are used concurrently.

For chronic outpatient treatment, diuretic combinations are an attractive alternative to high-dose or continuously infused furosemide. The addition of a different class of diuretics can block the adaptive, distal tubular responses that limit single-agent therapy, resulting in a synergistic effect. In humans with refractory congestive heart failure, metolazone, a thiazide-like drug, is commonly used in combination with furosemide or bumetanide. In dogs and cats, the author usually combines either chlorothiazide (Diuril, Merck), 20 to 40 mg/kg every 12 to 24 hours, or hydrochlorothiazide (HydroDIURIL, Merck), 2.0 to 4.0 mg/kg, with furosemide. Daily combined treatment with furosemide and a thiazide diuretic shares the same liabilities as high-dose furosemide therapy, namely, dehydration, renal failure, and electrolyte depletion. The addition of a thiazide diuretic to the standard therapeutic regimen every 2 or 3 days usually resolves refractory pulmonary congestion without causing dehydration. Hypokalemia can be prevented with this aggressive diuretic regimen by oral potassium supplementation or by adding spironolactone (Aldactone, Searle), 2.0 mg/kg every 12 hours. Spironolactone is a mineralocorticoid antagonist that in combination with an ACE inhibitor causes marked diuresis and symptomatic improvement in humans with heart failure (Pitt, 1995). Spironolactone is a reported cause of serious hyperkalemia in human patients receiving ACE inhibitors, but this complication appears uncommon in dogs. Nonetheless, serum potassium concentrations should be monitored shortly after initiating therapy. Spironolactone is thought to reduce myocardial fibrosis, and it has recently been shown to prevent the inhibitory effects of aldosterone on carotid sinus baroreceptors (Wang et al, 1992). The potential bene-

fits of these actions include improved diastolic function and a decreased heart rate. The clinical importance of these actions is uncertain at the present time, but a large clinical trial evaluating the efficacy of spironolactone in humans is currently in progress.

Substantial volumes of fluid often accumulate in the chest or abdomen or within the pericardial sac of dogs or cats with biventricular or right-sided heart failure. This fluid may need to be manually drained, and drug therapy should be adjusted to prevent the re-accumulation of fluid. Some patients with refractory right-heart failure require periodic centesis to remain comfortable. This procedure is easy to accomplish and is well tolerated by most dogs, many of which will survive months or years in this condition.

TREATMENT WITH POSITIVE INOTROPIC DRUGS

Intermittent infusions of milrinone or dobutamine have been used to treat human patients with acute, decompensated, or chronic heart failure (Baker et al, 1994; ACC/AHA Task Force, 1995). In patients with chronic, intractable heart failure, positive inotropic infusions are often administered as part of a comprehensive outpatient program, emphasizing patient education and close follow-up. Dobutamine (Dobutrex, Lilly) infusion is sometimes helpful for treating dogs with dilated cardiomyopathy and intractable heart failure. Using a low-dose protocol, dobutamine is infused at a dose of 2.0 to 5.0 μg/kg per minute for 12 to 24 hours. The infusion is repeated at 2- to 6-week intervals, as determined by the needs of the individual patient. Substantial clinical improvement occurs in some patients treated in this fashion, but there is no evidence that life is prolonged by this therapy. There is an unknown and probably substantial risk of sudden death from ventricular arrhythmia. This risk is acceptable because other remedies available to humans, such as heart transplantation and cardiomyoplasty, are not feasible alternatives for dogs. Milrinone infusions have been used in this same fashion in humans with refractory heart failure.

References and Suggested Reading

Baker DW, Konstam MA, Bottorff M, et al: Management of heart failure: I. Pharmacologic treatment. JAMA 272:1361, 1994.
  Review article of the drug therapy for heart failure due to left ventricular systolic dysfunction.
Burges R, Dodd MG, Gardiner DG: Pharmacologic profile of amlodipine. Am J Cardiol 64:10I, 1989.
  Reviews pharmacodynamics of the calcium channel blocker amlodipine.
Cody RJ, Kubo SH, Pickworth KK: Diuretic treatment for the sodium retention of congestive heart failure. Arch Intern Med 154:1905, 1994.
  Review article summarizing the rationale and current use of diuretics for the treatment of sodium retention and edema.
Ellison DH: The physiologic basis of diuretic synergism: Its role in treating diuretic resistance. Ann Intern Med 114:886, 1991.
  Reviews the sites and mechanisms of action of commonly used diuretics and combinations.
Gerlag PGG, van Meijel JJM: High-dose furosemide in the treatment of refractory heart failure. Arch Intern Med 148:286, 1988.
  Clinical study illustrating the successful use of high-dose furosemide to treat refractory heart failure in 35 human patients.
Hamlin RL, Nakayama T: Comparison of some pharmacokinetic parame-

ters of 5 angiotensin-converting enzyme inhibitors in normal beagles. J Vet Intern Med 12:93, 1998.

The IMPROVE Study Investigators: Clinical effects of enalapril maleate in dogs with naturally acquired heart failure: Results of the invasive multicenter prospective veterinary evaluation of enalapril. J Vet Intern Med 9:234, 1995.
Results of a blinded, placebo-controlled trial detailing the hemodynamic efficacy of enalapril.

Jugdutt BI, Khan MI, Jugdutt SJ, et al: Impact of left ventricular unloading after late reperfusion of canine anterior myocardial infarction on remodeling and function using isosorbide-5-mononitrate. Circulation 92:926, 1995.
Research study demonstrating improved ventricular function and decreased remodeling in dogs with late reperfusion of acute anterior myocardial infarction treated with isosorbide-5-mononitrate.

McDonald KM, Francis GS, Matthews J, et al: Long-term oral nitrate therapy prevents chronic ventricular remodeling in the dog. J Am Coll Cardiol 21:514, 1993.

Research study documenting attenuation of ventricular remodeling by long-term oral nitrate therapy in a dog model of discrete myocardial damage.

Packer M, O'Connor CM, Ghali JK: Effect of amlodipine on morbidity and mortality in severe chronic heart failure. N Engl J Med 335:1107, 1996.
Results of a randomized, placebo-controlled trial of amlodipine in human heart failure.

Pitt D: ACE inhibitor co-therapy in patients with heart failure: Rationale for the Randomized Aldactone Evaluation Study (RALES). Eur Heart J 16(Suppl N):107, 1995.

Wang W, McClain JM, Zucker IH: Aldosterone reduces baroreceptor discharge in the dog. Hypertension 19:270, 1992.

Williams JF Jr, Bristow MR, Fowler MB, et al: Report of the American College of Cardiology/American Heart Association Task Force on Practice Guidelines (Committee on Evaluation and Management of Heart Failure). J Am Coll Cardiol 26:1376, 1995.

Yamanaka K, Suzuki M, Ishiko J: Antihypertensive effects of amlodipine, a new calcium antagonist. Nippon Yakurigaku Zasshi 97:115, 1991.

CVT Update: Doberman Pinscher Occult Cardiomyopathy

CLAY A. CALVERT
Athens, Georgia

KATHRYN M. MEURS
Columbus, Ohio

Doberman pinscher (DP) cardiomyopathy (CM) is a common, insidious, slowly progressive primary myocardial disease that affects both genders and exhibits strong familial tendencies. A male preponderance has been observed in some, but not all, studies (Calvert et al, 1998; Calvert et al, 1997; O'Grady and Horne, 1995). In this breed, CM is characterized by a protracted (2 to 3 years and occasionally longer) occult or pre–congestive heart failure (CHF) phase in which ventricular and, occasionally, atrial premature contractions appear, followed by progressive left ventricular dysfunction and a tendency for progressively more severe ventricular tachyarrhythmias (VTA; Fig. 1). Sudden death, due to ventricular tachycardia-fibrillation, intervenes during the pre-CHF phase in approximately 25 to 30% of affected dogs, usually approximately 1 year prior to the time when CHF would otherwise occur (Calvert et al, 1997). Once overt CHF (usually left sided) develops, survival times are usually short (2 to 4 months) with at least a 90% 1-year mortality. When present at the time of diagnosis of CHF, atrial fibrillation or bilateral CHF is associated with increased mortality during the first month (Calvert et al, 1998). Also, the emergence of these two sequelae in dogs previously stabilized from CHF heralds accelerated deterioration. After CHF onset, death is usually the result of intractable CHF but is sudden in 25 to 30% of the dogs (O'Grady and Calvert, 1998).

PREVALENCE

The DP is affected with CM more than any other breed, accounting for at least 50% of all cases (Ettinger et al,

1992). Several studies have found that approximately 20 to 30% of overtly healthy adult DPs have probable markers (including echocardiographic abnormalities or heart rhythm disturbances) for CM on their first examination (Calvert, 1991; O'Grady and Horne, 1992, 1995; Smucker et al, 1990). Serial follow-up examinations of dogs with no initial abnormalities reveal an increasing prevalence of markers up to 8 to 10 years of age, and the cumulative incidence exceeds 50% in some families (O'Grady and Calvert, 1998). However, clinical CM may not appear until advanced age, and some old affected dogs die of concomitant diseases without manifesting overt signs of CM.

ETIOLOGY

The etiology of DPCM is poorly understood, but a genetic component is suspected. Although nutritional deficiencies, including taurine and carnitine, have occasionally been demonstrated to cause CM in some breeds, known deficiencies do not appear to be the sole inciting cause in the DP (Keene, 1992; Kramer et al, 1995). In some species, viral infection can cause systolic dysfunction and left ventricular dilation; however, histopathologic analysis of myocardial samples taken from affected DPs does not support a viral etiology (Keene, 1993; Calvert et al, 1997).

Myocardial biochemical studies indicate that impairment of intracellular energy homeostasis is central to the pathogenesis of DPCM. Progressive loss of cardiac performance parallels the loss of cellular-ATP production. Deficits of

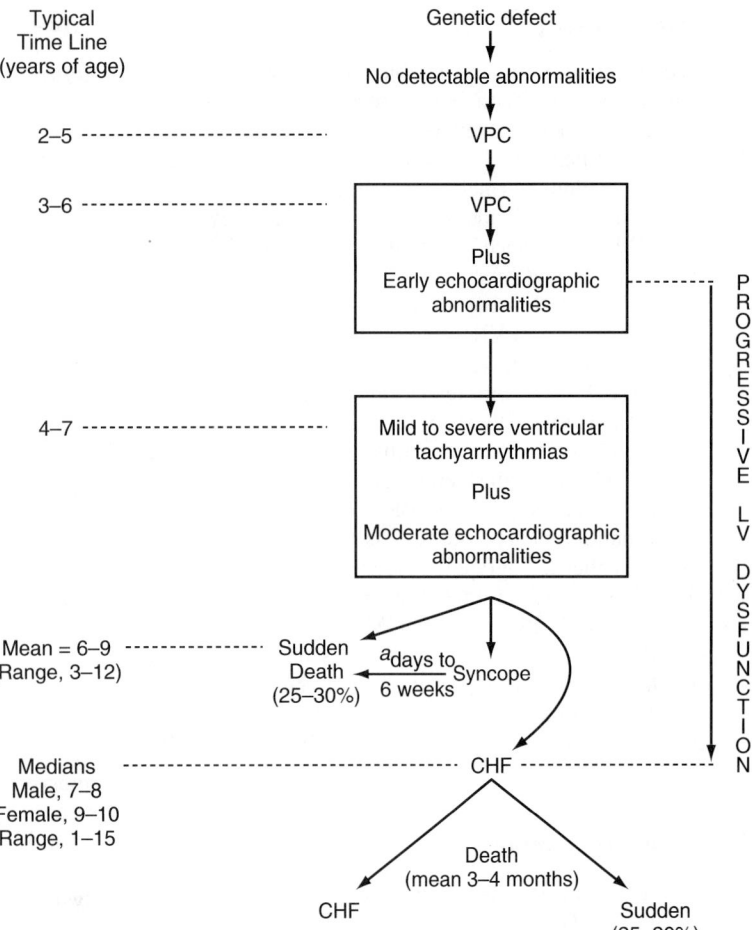

Figure 1. Proposed clinical evolution of Doberman pinscher cardiomyopathy in untreated dogs. Heart rhythm disturbances and echocardiographic changes can begin at less than 1 year or at more than 10 years of age. Untreated dogs experiencing pre-CHF syncope due to ventricular tachycardia are unlikely to survive to CHF. Once the $LVID_d$ reaches approximately 53 to 55 mm and the FS is 19 to 20%, CHF occurs in approximately 1 year unless sudden death intervenes. Congestive heart failure can occur from 1 to 15 years of age. [a], If syncope due to ventricular tachycardia.

specific enzyme gene expression may lead to abnormalities in that enzyme system and resultant cellular energy deficiency (O'Brien, 1997).

A hereditary component to the etiology of DPCM seems likely when one considers the high prevalence and frequent familial clustering of cases. Identification of an inheritance pattern is complicated by the lack of information on many family members, the adult onset of the disease, and the potential for occult disease in older dogs. The authors have seen a number of affected cross-bred Dobermans, both male and female. The Doberman parent was sometimes the sire and sometimes the dam. The high prevalence, sporadic occurrence in some families, wide age range at the time of onset of overt signs, common occurrence in both genders, and occurrence in mixed-bred DPs have made it difficult to determine the mode of inheritance of this disease.

IDENTIFICATION OF OCCULT (PRE-CHF) CARDIOMYOPATHY

Overt CHF represents the end stage of disease and is difficult to treat; survival times are generally short. Early detection is important in maximizing treatment options. Analyses of combined long-term (24-hour) ambulatory electrocardiographic (Holter) and echocardiographic recordings provide a means of identifying affected dogs long before clinical signs develop. Annual screening of overtly healthy adult dogs has been recommended because of the high prevalence of disease in this breed.

Holter Recording

Holter recording is a valuable diagnostic test for the detection of occult CM, particularly when coupled with echocardiography. The presence and frequency of VTA can be quantitated (with more than 80 to 90% accuracy), provided that a quality recording is obtained and analyzed by state-of-the-art computer technology.

The number of ventricular premature contractions (VPCs) considered to be abnormal in DPs has not been defined. Although a few VPCs can be normal, they can also be consistent with very early CM. The proportion of overtly healthy DPs with normal echocardiograms whose random 24-hour Holter recordings contain some VPCs (fewer than 50) is as low as 20% in dogs younger than 4 years of age and as high 50 to 70% in dogs older than 4 years of age. More than 100 VPCs in a 24-hour period should be considered abnormal, particularly when pairs, triplets, runs, or ventricular tachycardia (VT) are present (Calvert, 1991). Unless CM is detected in the very early stages, most affected DPs have at least several hundred and often several thousand or more VPCs in a 24 hour period.

Echocardiography

The echocardiogram is a valuable diagnostic test, particularly when coupled with Holter recording. Moderate to severe abnormalities are relatively easy to identify, but a definitive identification of early abnormalities is more difficult. The absolute normal measurements for this breed have been difficult to define because of the high prevalence of occult CM and reliance on linear estimates of global left ventricular function (Smucker et al, 1990; O'Grady and Horne, 1992). For this breed, the normal left ventricular internal dimensions (LVIDs) from the right parasternal sagittal plane have been reported as LVID less than 46 mm in diastole (LVID$_d$) and less than 39 mm in systole (O'Grady and Horne, 1995). A left ventricular shortening fraction (FS) greater than or equal to 30% is normal, whereas 26 to 29% is considered equivocal by the authors. The E-point septal separation (EPSS) is not sensitive to early dysfunction and should be less than 9 mm. Normal or equivocal echocardiographic results coupled with a high-quality Holter recording containing more than 100 VPCs per 24 hours is indicative of early CM, unless an alternative cause of the VPCs is evident. Any VPCs observed during ultrasound examination are strongly associated with CM, although their absence does not rule out CM. Progression of myocardial failure is best monitored by serial LVID, EPSS, and left atrial measurements, rather than FS.

Static Electrocardiography

The electrocardiogram is not sensitive as an early marker of CM. However, any VPCs recorded on an extended (6-minute) electrocardiographic rhythm strip are strongly suggestive of CM (O'Grady and Calvert, 1998). The absence of VPCs does not rule out CM. The frequency of or absence of VPCs on short electrocardiographic strips cannot be used to determine the risk of sudden death. Prolonged P-wave duration (>0.04 second) and QRS duration (>0.06 second) develops only with advanced CM and indicates that CHF is present or, without treatment, will probably occur within 6 to 9 months.

Radiography

Radiography is not sensitive for the detection of mild to moderate left heart enlargement. Left atrial enlargement is associated with advanced CM, and CHF generally will occur in less than 1 year in untreated dogs.

SUDDEN DEATH

Sudden death is often the first overt manifestation of DPCM. Many dogs do not survive the first episode of VTA-induced collapse, most do not survive a second episode, and surviving a third is unlikely. When the condition goes untreated, the interval between the first collapse and sudden death seldom exceeds 6 weeks, is often less than 2 weeks, and is statistically associated with a history of sustained VT and moderate-to-severe left ventricular dysfunction (Calvert et al, 1997). Affected dogs with normal or equivocal echocardiographic measurements rarely, if ever, experience severe VTA or sudden death.

TREATMENT

Occult Cardiomyopathy

The question is often asked as to when to intervene medically if occult CM is detected. Unless screened on an annual basis, most affected dogs will have significant myocardial failure when first identified clinically. A consensus regarding specific treatments for DPs with occult disease is lacking.

Myocardial Failure

There has been considerable interest in early therapy in asymptomatic patients with reduced left ventricular performance in order to retard disease progression. The authors recommend angiotensin-converting enzyme inhibition in DPs with echocardiographic evidence of moderate left ventricular dysfunction because such treatment may support contractility, retard left ventricular dilation, and prevent myocardial fibrosis; however, such therapy does not exert an obvious influence on VTA. Digoxin may exert a modest positive influence on contractility but may aggravate VTA, and the authors reserve it for use in dogs with atrial fibrillation, gallop rhythm (S$_3$), and severe left ventricular dysfunction. In the absence of echocardiography, early drug intervention is recommended if there is radiographic or electrocardiographic evidence of left atrial or left ventricular enlargement. Regular furosemide therapy is recommended when there is evidence of severe left ventricular dysfunction, pulmonary lobar vein distention, or pulmonary edema, or if a gallop rhythm is detected.

Carvedilol (Coreg, SmithKline Beecham) is a mildly beta$_1$-selective blocking drug that also has arteriolar dilating activity (alpha-adrenergic blockade) and antioxidant activity. In human patients, carvedilol exerts a favorable influence on the survival of patients with CM. Improved survival times are the result of not only a favorable influence on progressive myocardial failure but also decreased numbers of cases of sudden death. The beta-blocking and antioxidant properties retard myocardial degeneration, while the vasodilation offsets the negative inotropic action of the beta-blocker by reducing afterload. The beta-blocking action appears to confer some protection against arrhythmic sudden death. Carvedilol can be prescribed early in the disease evolution, but caution is advised when myocardial failure is advanced because of the drug's beta-blocking activity. There are no published studies of efficacy in DPs. Preliminary experience indicates that a dosage of approximately 0.3 mg/kg b.i.d. (12.5 or 18.75 mg b.i.d. for DPs between 36 and 43 kg) is well tolerated in those with an LVID$_d$ less than 55 mm, an FS greater than or equal to 20%, and an EPSS less than 15 mm. A dosage of 25 mg b.i.d. usually causes lethargy and weakness. The authors usually initiate therapy at 6.25 mg and titrate the dosage upward after 1 week. Carvedilol can be used in conjunction with digoxin and angiotensin-converting enzyme inhibitors, as well as antiarrhythmic drugs, including amiodarone. The influence of carvedilol on the survival of DPs with occult CM awaits controlled studies.

Controlled studies are needed to determine whether nutritional supplementation (particularly L-carnitine and taurine) influences disease progression (see p. 711). It has been the authors' experience that coenzyme Q10, vitamin E, or selenium supplementation does not exert an obvious positive influence on survival.

Ventricular Tachyarrhythmias

The treatment of VTAs is controversial for a number of reasons, including the absence of proven sustained efficacy and the failure to prevent sudden death, negative inotropism, and the proarrhythmic actions of most antiarrhythmic drugs (see p. 730). The goals of therapy are to prevent sudden death, eliminate VT, reduce the number of VPCs by 70% or more, and eliminate or prevent symptoms such as syncope, exercise intolerance, and behavioral changes associated with VTA.

Approximately 25 to 35% of DPs with moderate to severe left ventricular dysfunction are at high risk for sudden death. If rapid sustained VT, syncope associated with many VPCs, or an abnormal signal-averaged electrocardiogram (Fig. 2) is identified, antiarrhythmic therapy is recommended. When overt symptoms of VTA and sudden death have occurred, most dogs have had more than 8,000 to 10,000 VPCs per 24 hours, LVID$_d$ is greater than 50 mm, and FS is less than 23%. Unfortunately, sudden death can occur in the absence of any prior clinical signs, in dogs with as few as 500 to 1,000 VPCs per 24 hours (recorded by Holter monitoring within days to a few weeks prior to death) and in dogs with a recently recorded and normal signal-averaged electrocardiogram.

Although some dogs at high risk for sudden death can be identified, others cannot. Furthermore, frequent re-eval-uation is required in order to detect either progressive or more severe VTA, whether the dog is receiving antiarrhythmic drugs or not. While initially satisfactory responses to procainamide, quinidine, mexiletine, and tocainide are usual, loss of efficacy of these drugs after 3 to 6 months is common and sudden death has occurred in many DPs receiving these medications. Furthermore, many of these drugs exert a negative inotropic action, particularly procainamide and quinidine, and this must be taken into account in dogs with moderate to severe myocardial failure.

Beta-adrenoreceptor blocking drugs may improve the quantitative control of VTA when combined with commonly prescribed single agents, but they are not singularly effective. When prescribed at recommended dosages for dogs with moderate to severe myocardial failure, beta-blockers may embarrass left ventricular function. Sotalol (Betapace, Berlex) is a newer complex antiarrhythmic drug with beta-blocker activity. Sotalol may exert less negative inotropism than older beta-blockers and may confer protection against sudden death. Nonetheless, the authors have observed a negative influence on contractility in dogs with moderate to severe myocardial failure that were administered dosages of 40 or 80 mg b.i.d. Prospective studies of this drug are needed.

Amiodarone (Cordarone, Wyeth-Ayerst) is a unique antiarrhythmic drug that could be more effective at preventing sudden death than traditional antiarrhythmic drugs. The authors' experience is that the initial goals of antiarrhythmic treatment are usually achieved, although long-term efficacy remains unproved. Using a dosage of 10 mg/kg b.i.d. for 1 week and then 8 mg/kg once daily, recommended serum concentrations (1 to 2.5 μg/ml) are achieved

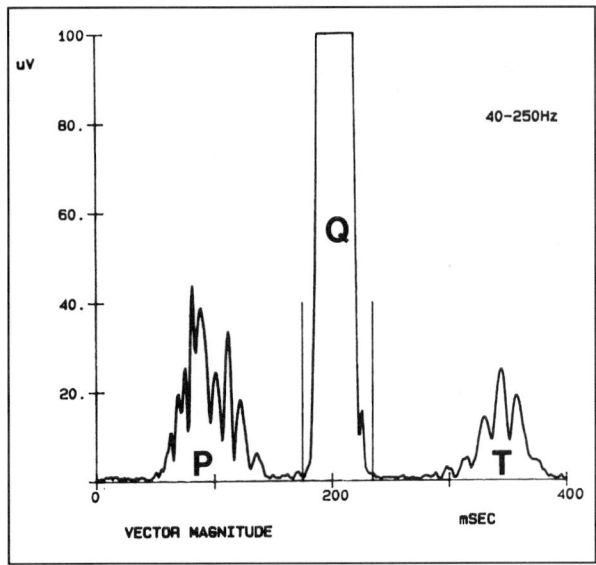

A

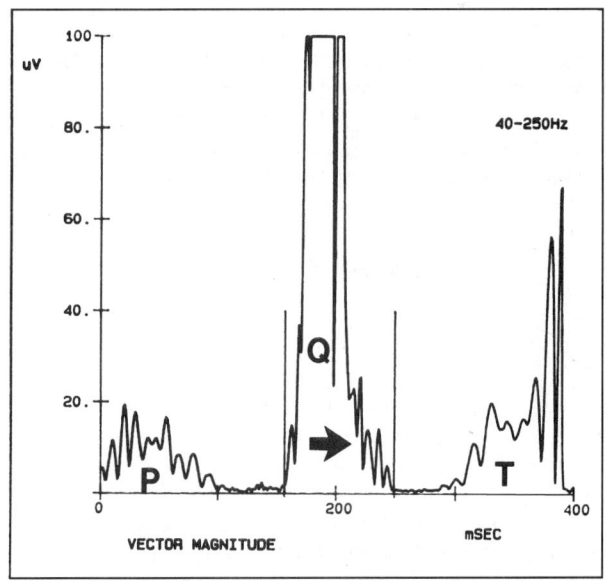

B

Figure 2. Normal *(A)* and abnormal *(B)* signal-averaged electrocardiogram from two Doberman pinschers. High-frequency, low-voltage signals appear in the terminal QRS complex and early ST segment *(arrow)* that may be ventricular late potentials. Ventricular late potentials may identify patients at high risk for sustained ventricular tachyarrhythmia. Their absence, however, does not rule out the risk of sudden death, even within the ensuing 1 to 2 months. P, P wave; T, T wave; Q, QRS complex. (From Calvert CA: Diagnosis and management of ventricular tachyarrhythmias in Doberman pinschers with cardiomyopathy. In: Bonagura JD, Kirk RW, eds: Kirk's Current Veterinary Therapy XII. Philadelphia: WB Saunders, 1995, p 804.)

within 1 week and maintained during chronic therapy. Measuring serum concentrations is not routinely done because tissue concentrations are most important. Higher dosages can produce hepatotoxicity and neutropenia, which resolve after drug withdrawal. The authors recommend monthly monitoring of the complete blood count and liver enzyme activities. Thoracic radiographs should be examined every 3 months for pulmonary fibrosis, a potential adverse effect that the authors have yet to encounter. Because of long-lasting tissue concentrations, after 6 months of good antiarrhythmia control, efficacy may be maintained at a reduced dosage of 5 mg/kg once daily. For severe VTA, following stabilization with lidocaine if necessary, the authors initiate mexiletine (Mexitil, Boehringer-Ingelheim) at 5 to 8 mg/kg t.i.d. for 1 week in combination with amiodarone, confirm efficacy, and then wean the patient off the mexiletine.

FUTURE GOAL

Assuming a genetic basis and considering the high prevalence and late onset of overt disease, it is difficult, if not impossible, to "breed out" the defect. A practical genetic test that can be performed on puppies is needed. It is possible, however, that few nonaffected dogs will be found.

References and Suggested Reading

Calvert CA: Long-term ambulatory electrocardiographic (Holter) monitoring as an aid in the diagnosis of occult cardiomyopathy in Doberman pinschers. Proceedings of the 9th Annual Veterinary Medicine Forum, New Orleans, LA. ACVIM, Madison, WI: Omnipress, 1991, pp 691–692.
A quantitation of VPCs in normal and cardiomyopathic DPs.
Calvert CA, Hall G, Jacobs G, et al: Clinical and pathologic findings in Doberman pinschers with occult cardiomyopathy that died suddenly or developed congestive heart failure: 54 cases (1984–1991). J Am Vet Med Assoc 210:505, 1997.
Echocardiographic and Holter data, histopathologic descriptions, and incidence of sudden death in DPs with ocult cardiomyopathy.
Calvert CA, Jacobs GJ, Pickus CW, et al: Signalment, survival, and prognostic factors in Doberman pinschers with end-stage cardiomyopathy. J Vet Intern Med 11:323, 1998.
Signalment, survival curves, and the influence of atrial fibrillation and bilateral CHF in DPs with overt heart failure.
Ettinger S, Lusk R, Brayler K, et al for the Cooperative Veterinary Enalapril (COVE) Study Group: Evaluation of enalapril therapy in dogs with heart failure in a large multicenter study. Proceedings of the 10th Annual Veterinary Medicine Forum, San Diego, CA. ACVIM, Madison, WI: Omnipress, 1992, pp 584–585.
A prospective study on the safety and efficacy of enalapril in treating dogs with moderate to severe heart failure.
Keene BW: Carnitine deficiency in canine dilated cardiomyopathy. In: Kirk RW, Bonagura JD, eds: Kirk's Current Veterinary Therapy XI. Philadelphia: WB Saunders, 1992, p 780.
A review of the role of L-carnitine in myocardial function, diagnosis of carnitine deficiency, and summary of therapeutic results.
Keene BW: Evidence for the role of myocarditis in the pathophysiology of dilated cardiomyopathy. Proceedings of the 11th Annual Veterinary Medicine Forum, Washington, DC. ACVIM, Madison, WI: Omnipress, 1993, p 565.
A review of the role of virus infection in myocarditis and cardiomyopathy.
Kramer GA, Kittleson MD, Fox PR, et al: Plasma taurine concentrations in normal dogs and in dogs with heart disease. J Vet Intern Med 9:253, 1995.
A comparison of plasma taurine concentrations in dogs with cardiomyopathy, acquired valvular disease, and control dogs.
O'Brien PJ: Deficiencies of myocardial troponin-T and creatine kinase MB isoenzyme in dogs with idiopathic dilated cardiomyopathy. Am J Vet Res 58:11, 1997.
A comparison of the myocardial concentrations of isoenzymes of creatine kinase in cardiomyopathic DPs and control dogs.
O'Grady MR, Horne R: Occult dilated cardiomyopathy: An echocardiographic and electrocardiographic study of 193 asymptomatic Doberman pinschers. J Vet Intern Med 6:112, 1992. (Abstract.)
A description of echocardiographic data among a large number of overtly healthy DPs.
O'Grady M, Horne R: Outcome of 103 asymptomatic Doberman pinschers: Incidence of dilated cardiomyopathy in a longitudinal study. J Vet Intern Med 9:199, 1995. (Abstract.)
A longitudinal study of the incidence of cardiomyopathy, pertinent echocardiographic data, and sudden death incidence among a population of DPs.
O'Grady M, Calvert CA: Canine myocardial diseases. In: Fox PR, Sisson D, Moise NS, eds: Textbook of Canine and Feline Cardiology, 2nd ed. Philadelphia: WB Saunders, 1998.
An overview of canine myocardial diseases with emphasis on dilated cardiomyopathy.
Smucker ML, Kaul S, Woodfield JA, et al: Naturally occurring cardiomyopathy in the Doberman pinscher: A possible large-animal model of human cardiomyopathy. J Am Coll Cardiol 16:200, 1990.
A comparison of echocardiographic and cardiac catheterization data between overtly healthy DPs and mongrel dogs.

Taurine- and Carnitine-Responsive Dilated Cardiomyopathy in American Cocker Spaniels

MARK D. KITTLESON
Davis, California

Following Pion, Kittleson, and colleagues' discovery that taurine deficiency causes dilated cardiomyopathy (DCM) in domestic cats in 1987, we and others started to look for taurine deficiency in dogs with DCM. With the group at the Animal Medical Center in New York, we examined the prevalence of taurine deficiency in dogs with DCM (Kramer et al, 1995). In that study of 76 dogs examined with DCM, 13 (17%) had a plasma taurine concentration less than 25 ng/ml and so were severely systemically deficient. Only one dog without DCM had a plasma taurine concentration less than 25 ng/ml. Only 1 of 33 Doberman pinschers was taurine-deficient. No other purebred dog belonging to a breed commonly associated with DCM was deficient. Conversely, all three American Cocker spaniels with DCM were deficient, and four of six Golden retrievers were deficient. The other five deficient dogs were mixed-breed dogs or dogs of breeds that do not commonly develop DCM.

Once the American Cocker spaniels were identified as taurine-deficient, we started to administer supplements to these dogs, hoping that their myocardial function would normalize in a manner similar to that observed in cats after supplementation. The first two dogs were supplemented with 500 mg of taurine every 12 hours and observed clinically and echocardiographically over the following 4 to 6 months. Neither dog had a demonstrable response. An endomyocardial biopsy from one of these dogs was analyzed for carnitine content and was low. The dog's plasma carnitine concentration was normal, a condition diagnostic of myopathic or myocardial carnitine deficiency. The author and others had previously identified myocardial carnitine deficiency in other breeds, including Boxers and Doberman pinschers with DCM. Carnitine supplementation was occasionally effective in partially reversing the disease in these dogs. In what turned out to be a pilot study, supplementation with the combination of taurine and L-carnitine, in addition to conventional pharmacotherapy for heart failure, resulted in sustained clinical and echocardiographic improvement in three American Cocker spaniels at two different centers (improvement sustained after withdrawal of conventional pharmacotherapy). As a result of these findings, a multicenter placebo-controlled trial was initiated (Kittleson et al, 1997).

Over the course of 2 years, we enrolled 14 dogs into a randomized trial of placebo versus supplementation with taurine and L-carnitine. Despite some methodologic problems associated with the trial, the data generated were statistically conclusive that the American Cocker spaniels with DCM in the trial were taurine-deficient (plasma taurine concentration <50 ng/ml) and responsive to taurine and L-carnitine supplementation. Based on the results of this trial and the author's experience in treating other American Cocker spaniels with DCM, it appears that while myocardial function does not return to normal in most American Cocker spaniels treated with taurine and L-carnitine, it does improve sufficiently to allow discontinuation of cardiovascular drug therapy. Furthermore, treated dogs maintain a normal quality of life for months to years, depending on the age of the dog at the time it was entered into the study. Most dogs are older and die of other disease.

TREATMENT RECOMMENDATIONS

American Cocker spaniels with DCM should be supplemented with 500 mg of taurine every 12 hours and 1 gm of carnitine every 12 hours. Both substances can be purchased in a health food store. Although these substances were administered every 8 hours in the study, the author has found that twice-daily administration is adequate. Plasma concentrations of taurine and carnitine can be measured. The plasma concentration of taurine is uniformly low, and the plasma carnitine concentration is uniformly normal. Consequently, measurement of either substance is not an absolute requirement. Following the onset of supplementation, echocardiograms should be repeated every 1 or 2 months. Once the shortening fraction exceeds 20% (usually within 3 to 4 months), the patient can be weaned off all cardiovascular drugs (e.g., angiotensin-converting enzyme inhibitors, digoxin, furosemide). The author has had regression of myocardial function in one patient whose owners became negligent with supplementation. Owners must be informed that supplementation is a lifelong process and that the supplements must be administered twice a day. Taurine is an inexpensive substance. Carnitine, however, can be expensive. Consequently, some owners hesitate to administer carnitine for long periods. Carnitine supplementation costs an average of $50.00 to $100.00 per month, depending on the source. The author has received anecdotal reports of American Cocker spaniels that have responded to taurine or carnitine supplementation alone. The author has also observed this response to taurine alone in at least three dogs in the clinic at the School of Veterinary Medicine, University of California, Davis (Gavaghan et al, 1997). Consequently, if an owner cannot afford carnitine supplementation, the author recommends that taurine supplementation be tried first. If no response is identified, carnitine supplementation can be added later.

Having not tried lower doses of carnitine in patients, the author does not know whether they might be efficacious.

References and Suggested Reading

Gavaghan BJ, Kittleson MD: Dilated cardiomyopathy in an American Cocker spaniel with taurine deficiency. Aust Vet J 75:862, 1997.

Kittleson MD, Keene B, Pion PD, et al: Results of the Multicenter Spaniel Trial (MUST): Taurine and carnitine responsive dilated cardiomyopathy in American cocker spaniels with decreased plasma taurine concentration. J Vet Intern Med 11:204, 1997.

A prospective blinded and placebo-controlled clinical trial of supplementing taurine and carnitine in taurine-deficient American Cocker spaniels with DCM.

Kramer GA, Kittleson MD, Fox PR, et al: Plasma taurine concentrations in normal dogs and in dogs with heart disease. J Vet Intern Med 9:253, 1995.

A prospective study designed to identify taurine deficiency in dogs with DCM.

Pion PD, Kittleson MD, Rogers QR, et al: Myocardial failure in cats associated with low plasma taurine: A reversible cardiomyopathy. Science 237:764, 1987.

The first report of taurine deficiency causing DCM in cats.

CVT Update: Therapy for Feline Myocardial Diseases

PHILIP R. FOX

New York, New York

DEFINITIONS

Cardiomyopathy defines a variety of structural or functional myocardial disorders. *Idiopathic (primary) cardiomyopathy* describes the myocardium as the sole source of heart disease when etiology cannot be identified, whereas *secondary cardiomyopathy* relates the heart muscle disorder to an identifiable systemic or metabolic abnormality. Classification is facilitated by clinical, pathologic, or physiologic information related to (1) morphologic phenotype (e.g., hypertrophic or dilated cardiomyopathy), (2) etiology (e.g., taurine deficiency myocardial failure, thyrotoxic heart disease), (3) myocardial function (e.g., systolic or diastolic dysfunction), (4) pathology (e.g., infiltrative cardiomyopathy), and (5) pathophysiology (e.g., restrictive cardiomyopathy). Unfortunately, any scheme is self-limited, and many cases have overlapping features or do not readily fit into one category. Despite these and other difficulties in diagnosis and classification, there remains the practical problem of treating heart failure and clinical abnormalities associated with myocardial disease. As long as one recognizes that categories have no sharply defined boundaries, categorization into hypertrophic, restrictive, and myocardial failure (or dilated) cardiomyopathies continues to have clinical utility.

CLINICAL FEATURES AND DIAGNOSIS

The manifestations of feline myocardial diseases are highly variable but often include arrhythmia, heart failure, arterial thromboembolism, and sudden death. A high-quality two-dimensional and M-mode echocardiogram is usually required for definitive diagnosis, although a full database is important for patient evaluation. This database includes an insightful history, complete physical examination, thoracic radiographs, electrocardiogram, arterial blood pressure determination, and certain clinical laboratory tests (e.g., serum triiodothyronine (T_3), thyroxine (T_4), blood urea nitrogen (BUN), creatinine, electrolytes, and hematocrit). *Hypertrophic cardiomyopathy (HCM)* is typified by a hypertrophied, nondilated left ventricle in which the ventricular septum and/or left ventricular free wall measured at end-diastole is more than 6 mm thick. Left atrial enlargement (usually greater than 16 mm) is usually present. *Restrictive cardiomyopathy (RCM)* is currently poorly characterized, but there are several relevant two-dimensional and M-mode echo characteristics: left atrial dilation (>16 mm, frequently >20 mm) in the absence of severe volume overload, such as mitral regurgitation; left ventricular internal dimension normal at end-systole (<12 mm), and normal (<21 mm) or slightly dilated at end-diastole; left ventricular shortening fraction normal (>30%) or slightly decreased (26 to 29%); occasionally, focal left ventricular wall thinning associated with myocardial infarction or scar. From Doppler echocardiography, a pattern of restrictive mitral inflow velocity represents a classic finding. This is typified by increased early diastolic filling velocity (i.e., E wave >1 m/sec), and decreased atrial filling velocity (i.e., A wave <0.4 m/sec) when E and A waves are not summated. *Cardiomyopathy characterized by myocardial failure, including dilated cardiomyopathy (DCM),* is manifested by mild to moderate left atrial enlargement (>16 mm); dilated left ventricular internal dimensions (end-systolic >12 mm, end-diastolic >21 mm); and reduced left ventricular fractional shortening (<30%, typically <25%). Myocardial infarction is common, especially involving the left ventricular free wall. *Endomyocardial fibrosis* is characterized by severe left atrial enlargement (frequently >22 mm); left ventricular myocardial speckling or bright, focal lesions; and a midventricular, bright, hyperechoic, endocardial, "band-like" plaque. In these disorders, variable right-heart enlargement and other structural and functional features are present.

TREATMENT OF ASYMPTOMATIC CATS AND PREVENTION OF DISEASE PROGRESSION

In asymptomatic cats that have never had congestive heart failure, diuretics are not indicated. Diuretics activate the renin-angiotensin-aldosterone system (RAAS), which can be potentially detrimental. Currently, there are no long-term clinical trials to indicate which is the most optimal therapy, whether combined therapy is more advantageous than monotherapy, or, for that matter, whether therapy is significantly better than no therapy at all. Similarly, it has not been determined whether drugs protect against sudden death or delay disease progression and improve prognosis in asymptomatic cases. Many cats with asymptomatic cardiomyopathies remain asymptomatic for years and appear to have normal longevity. Consequently, drugs are administered on an empirical basis, with the clinician relying on clinical experience, preferences, and theoretical benefits. There are several situations where treatment of asymptomatic cats would seem justified, as follows.

Myocardial Infarction. Suspicion is enhanced by echocardiographic evidence of regional left ventricular hypokinesis or dyskinesis, wall thinning (<2 mm), and ST-segment elevation (electrocardiogram). In human patients with chronic infarction, beta-blockers reduced long-term mortality by their antiarrhythmic effects and by prevention of reinfarction, particularly when decreased contractility and ventricular arrhythmias were present. Propranolol (Inderal, Wyeth-Ayerst), 2.5 to 5 mg PO every 8 to 12 hours, and atenolol (Tenormin, Zeneca), 6.25 to 12.5 mg/cat PO every 24 hours, have been used in cats suspected of having ischemic myocardial injury. Because of their potential negative inotropic and chronotropic effects, the echocardiogram and electrocardiogram should be monitored. Angiotensin-converting-enzyme (ACE) inhibitors have also been advocated on the basis of human trials showing reduced cardiovascular remodeling and improving hemodynamics. Enalapril (Enacard, Merial Ltd.), 0.5 mg/kg PO every 24 hours, is probably the most commonly used agent, although other ACE inhibitors are also available including benazepril (Lotensin, Novartis), 0.25 to 0.5 mg/kg PO every 24 hours, lisinopril (Prinivil, Merck), 0.25 mg/kg PO every 24 hours, and captopril (Capoten, Bristol-Myers Squibb), 3.12 to 6.25 mg/cat PO every 8 to 12 hours. Relative drug contraindications include bradyarrhythmias or severe myocardial failure (beta-blockers) or systemic hypotension (beta-blockers or ACE inhibitors).

Tachyarrhythmias. Ventricular tachyarrhythmias in the setting of myocardial diseases are usually associated with some degree of myocardial necrosis and fibrosis. Atrial tachyarrhythmias generally accompany marked left atrial enlargement. Some cases of tachycardia precipitate weakness or syncope. Beta-blockers (propranolol, 5 to 10 mg PO every 8 to 12 hours; atenolol, 6.25 to 12.5 mg PO every 12 to 24 hours) may be useful for treating paroxysmal ventricular tachycardia or frequent multiform ventricular arrhythmias. While digoxin (Lanoxin tablets [Glaxo Wellcome], generally 0.031 mg [one quarter of a 0.125-mg tablet] per 4.5-kg cat PO every 48 hours) or diltiazem may be tried for atrial tachyarrhythmias, control of ventricular heart rate usually requires the addition of a beta-blocker (beginning with half of the above dose).

Massive Left Ventricular Hypertrophy (Severe HCM). Morbidity and mortality are generally related to greatly increased left ventricular mass (i.e., maximal end-diastolic ventricular septal or left ventricular free wall thickness >7.5 mm). A number of drugs have been advocated, but their comparative effectiveness has not been compared in a large-scale clinical trial. Beta-blockers have historically been chosen for several attributes: negative chronotropism; indirect improvement of diastolic filling; reduction of dynamic outflow tract obstruction; decreased myocardial oxygen utilization; antiarrhythmic effects; and blunting of sympathetic myocardial stimulation. For an average-sized cat (4.5 kg), atenolol (6.25 to 12.5 mg PO every 24 hours) or propranolol (5 to 10 mg PO every 12 hours) usually reduces resting heart rate to 140 to 160 beats/min. Occasionally, dosage frequency must be increased (atenolol, every 12 hours; propranolol, every 8 hours) to achieve this effect. The calcium channel blocker diltiazem (Cardizem tablets, Hoechst Marion Roussel), 7.5 mg every 8 to 12 hours, is often selected for its effect of directly improving ventricular diastolic relaxation and filling, a desirable attribute for conditions characterized by diastolic dysfunction such as HCM. Diltiazem may slow the heart rate in some cases but this effect is generally much weaker than that observed with beta-blockers. Other diltiazem formulations have also been used. One is a long-acting form, Cardizem CD capsules (Hoechst Marion Roussel), 10 mg/kg every 24 hours. More recently, an extended-release formulation, Dilacor XR (Rhone-Poulenc Rorer) has become popular. Dilacor XR 240-mg capsules contain four controlled-released 60-mg tablets; the starting dosage is 15 to 30 mg every 12 to 24 hours. Some cats may tolerate 60 mg daily, although emesis is a common side effect.

ACE inhibitors blunt neuroendocrine (RAAS) activation and may prevent deleterious cardiovascular remodeling. The merits of ACE inhibitors for treating feline HCM have a theoretical scientific basis, but efficacy remains to be demonstrated.

Myocardial Failure. Taurine supplementation (250 mg PO every 12 hours) is initiated whenever myocardial failure is detected, even if blood taurine cannot be immediately assayed. Ideally, analysis of blood taurine concentration should ultimately be determined from a blood sample drawn and frozen prior to taurine administration (plasma taurine: normal >60 nmol/ml, at risk <30 nmol/ml; whole-blood taurine: normal >200 nmol/ml, at risk <100 nmol/ml). ACE inhibitor monotherapy is administered in cases of mild myocardial failure (percent fractional shortening [%FS] 23 to 29%; left ventricular internal dimensions at end-systole [LVIDs] 12 to 14 mm) with normal blood taurine concentration and sinus rhythm. The rationale is based on the actions of ACE inhibitors to counteract RAAS activation and prevent deleterious left ventricular remodeling. The latter often accompanies sustained or progressive myocardial failure, particularly when associated with myocardial infarction. Digoxin may be added if contractility deteriorates or if supraventricular tachyarrhythmias develop, particularly atrial tachycardia or atrial fibrillation. Digoxin is excreted by the kidney; thus, renal function and serum digoxin concentration should be monitored. Beta-blocker therapy may be beneficial if myocardial infarction is suspected, or if a tachyarrhythmia warrants control of ventricular heart rate despite other therapies. These drugs may also restore or "up-regulate" beta-adrenergic receptor numbers and sensitivity, and protect myocytes from the deleterious effects of excess catecholamines. One must be very mindful, however, of the potential negative chronotropic and inotropic effects of these agents. Therefore, a low starting dose of propranolol (2.5 mg PO every 12 hours) or atenolol (3.15 mg every 24 hours) may be initiated, followed by patient monitoring for fluid retention (chest radiograph), heart rate (by electrocardiogram), and myocardial contractility (i.e., left ventricular %FS) by echocardiography.

Restrictive Cardiomyopathy and Endomyocardial Fibrosis. There are no proven efficacious medical therapies. Consideration may be given to ACE inhibitors on the basis of preventing ventricular remodeling; to beta-blockers, particularly when myocardial infarction is suspected or tachyarrhythmias are present; or to aspirin when left atrial enlargement is severe.

TREATMENT OF SYMPTOMATIC CATS AND CONGESTIVE HEART FAILURE

The emergency treatment goals are to (1) eliminate congestion (edema, effusions) and associated clinical signs; (2) reduce or abolish serious tachyarrhythmias; (3) improve cardiac contractility (systolic function) or ventricular relaxation and filling (diastolic function); (4) prevent or manage arterial thromboembolism; and, occasionally, (5) eliminate the syncope or exercise intolerance associated with dynamic left ventricular outflow tract obstruction or tachyarrhythmia. The long-term goals are (1) prolongation of life by optimizing drug therapies that maintain cardiac compensation; (2) treatment of the underlying etiology, if known; (3) prevention of arterial thromboembolism; and, (4) theoretically, halting, slowing, or reversal of the myocardial dysfunction.

Hypertrophic and Restrictive Cardiomyopathies (Diastolic Dysfunction)

Cardiovascular emergencies usually result from left-sided heart failure (pulmonary edema), biventricular failure (pulmonary edema and effusions), or arterial thromboembolism; less common emergencies involve tachyarrhythmias, syncope, pericardial tamponade, or systemic venous congestion. In the severely dyspneic cat, care must always be taken to avoid stress.

Emergency Treatment. Acute pulmonary edema is rapidly progressive and life-threatening. Furosemide is administered to rapidly reduce left ventricular filling pressures. Peak diuresis occurs within 30 minutes when furosemide is administered intravenously (1.0 to 2.0 mg/kg every 4 to 8 hours). Resolution of severe pulmonary edema may be enhanced by adding 2% nitroglycerin cream (Nitro-Bid Ointment, Hoechst Marion Roussel), 1/4 to 1/2 inch every 6 to 8 hours cutaneously to the inside of the pinna for the first 24 to 36 hours. This measure provides additional preload reduction. A nitrate-"free" interval of 12 hours may help prevent development of tolerance. Supplemental oxygen (40 to 60% oxygen-enriched inspired gas) may be beneficial in improving pulmonary gas exchange. Clinical improvement is indicated by a reduction in the rate and work of breathing, reduced or resolved auscultatory lung crackles, and radiographic clearing of alveolar infiltrates by 24 to 36 hours after therapy. Respiratory distress from a large pleural effusion requires thoracentesis. This procedure may be safely accomplished with the use of a 23-gauge butterfly needle. Pulmonary edema and pleural effusion often coexist, although pleural fluid hampers radiographic detection of edema.

Maintenance Therapy. Dehydration and hypokalemia can result from overzealous diuresis, especially in the anorectic cat. Once congestion has been eliminated, furosemide is changed from intravenous or intramuscular to oral administration (typically, 6.25 mg PO every 12 to 24 hours). It is then gradually reduced to the lowest effective dosage over approximately 2 weeks. Some cats remain stable on 1.1 to 2.2 mg/kg PO given every other day. Occasionally, diuretics may be discontinued safely.

Beta-adrenergic blockers such as propranolol (5 to 10 mg PO every 8 to 12 hours) or atenolol (6.25 to 12.5 mg PO every 12 to 24 hours) are frequently added. These drugs reduce cardiac sympathetic stimulation, decrease heart rate, left ventricular contractility, and systolic myocardial wall stress, and thereby reduce myocardial oxygen requirements. Dynamic left ventricular outflow tract obstruction is often reduced or abolished. Left ventricular diastolic compliance may be improved indirectly by reducing heart rate and myocardial ischemia. In addition, control of certain tachyarrhythmias may be enhanced.

Calcium-entry blockers may be beneficial in managing some cases of HCM. They may reduce heart rate (verapamil much more so than diltiazem) and blood pressure; exert a mild negative inotropic effect (reducing myocardial oxygen consumption); and improve rapid diastolic ventricular filling. Diltiazem (7.5 mg PO every 8 to 12 hours) has been used most commonly. Two additional preparations include the extended-release formulation, Dilacor XR (each 240-mg capsule contains four controlled-released 60-mg tablets; starting dosage is 15 to 30 mg every 12 to 24 hours), or Cardizem CD capsules (10 mg/kg PO every 24 hours).

Since neurohumoral activation plays an important role in cardiac decompensation, ACE inhibitors, which blunt the RAAS may be beneficial. The optimal timing for their introduction, and dosage and frequency of administration are undetermined. While some clinicians use an ACE inhibitor as the primary therapy for HCM with or without furosemide, ACE inhibitors are more commonly added to beta-blocker or calcium channel blocker therapy, especially if right-sided heart failure is present or if pulmonary edema recurs. To date, the fewest untoward effects have been achieved with enalapril (0.25 to 0.5 mg/kg PO every 24 hours), benazepril (0.25 to 0.5 mg/kg PO every 24 hours), and captopril (3.12 to 6.25 mg/cat PO every 12 hours).

Recurrent and Refractory Congestive Heart Failure. When pulmonary edema or biventricular failure with predominantly pulmonary edema recurs, emergency treatment may require parenteral administration of furosemide (1 to 2 mg/kg IV or IM every 4 to 8 hours) and application of 2% nitroglycerin cream. Cardiac drug therapy is then modified to either (1) increase the dosage of the "primary" drug (i.e., beta-blocker, calcium channel blocker, or ACE inhibitor), (2) change to a different class of primary drugs, or (3) add a second primary agent. When congestion is refractory to these pharmacologic manipulations, particularly with severe, chronic effusions, upward dose titration of furosemide (2.2 to 4.4 mg/kg PO every 8 to 12 hours) may be required. Refractory right-sided heart failure may respond to the synergistic effects of a second diuretic agent that is active at a distal site in the nephron; for example, hydrochlorothiazide (HydroDIURIL, Merck), 1 to 2 mg/kg PO every 12 to 24 hours, or hydrochlorothiazide-spironolactone (Aldactazide, Searle), 2.2 mg/kg per day PO. Cats must be closely monitored for dehydration, azotemia, hyponatremia, and hypokalemia when combination diuretics are used. Digoxin may be prescribed when right-sided heart failure is unresponsive to diuretics, ACE inhibitors, or other therapy. If renal function is relatively normal, 0.031 mg (one quarter of a 0.125-mg digoxin tablet PO) is administered every 48 hours to the average-sized cat (i.e., 4.5 kg) and titrated by assessing serum digoxin concentration in 10 to 14 days; 1 to 2 ng/ml represents a therapeutic range when the sample is drawn 8 to 12 hours after the last dose after steady-state levels have been achieved. Hypokalemia and azotemia predispose to intoxication. For refractory congestive heart failure, several additional steps should be taken: (1) re-evaluate the database (electrocardiograms, radiographs, echocardiography, clinical pathology), (2) assess serum T_3 and T_4 (cats >6 years), (3) ascertain that prescribed drugs are being administered according to directions, and (4) refer the patient to a cardiologist.

CARDIOMYOPATHY CHARACTERIZED BY MYOCARDIAL (SYSTOLIC) FAILURE

Emergency Treatment. Initial therapy is directed toward reducing or eliminating pulmonary and systemic venous congestion, improving myocardial contractility, and promoting increased forward cardiac output. If breathing is compromised by severe pleural effusion, immediate thoracentesis is required. Furosemide is administered (1.0 to 2.0 mg/kg IV or IM every 8 to 12 hours) to reduce congestion, but the clinician must be mindful that overzealous diuresis can severely reduce ventricular filling (preload), and decrease cardiac output, causing azotemia and electrolyte abnormalities and prolonging renal clearance of digoxin.

Taurine supplementation is safe and effective in cases of taurine deficiency myocardial failure and is empirically administered (250 mg PO every 12 hours). The use of positive inotropes is based on the presumption that adequate myocardial or contractile reserve exists. Digoxin may be initiated if renal function is normal; dosage is guided by body weight. For a cat weighing 2 to 3 kg, 0.031 mg

(i.e., one quarter of a 0.125-mg tablet) is given PO every 48 hours; those 4 to 5 kg in weight receive 0.031 mg PO every 24 to 48 hours; cats weighing more than 6 kg are given 0.031 mg PO every 24 hours. The reported biologic half-life of digoxin in healthy cats given a single intravenous injection was 33.3 ± 9.5 hours; whereas mean half-life after chronic oral elixir administration (0.05 mg/kg every 12 hours) was 79 hours. In DCM cats given oral digoxin in tablet form (0.007 to 0.014 mg/kg every 48 hours), mean half-life was about 64 hours and steady state was reached after about 10 days. Renal insufficiency reduces digoxin clearance and increase serum concentration because digoxin is eliminated by renal excretion.

Synthetic sympathomimetic amines are stronger and more rapid-acting than digoxin. These inotropes provide finer control for acute management of cardiogenic shock. Dobutamine (Dobutrex, Lilly), 1 to 10 μg/kg per minute constant-rate infusion, is a direct-acting inotrope whose primary action is derived from stimulating myocardial beta-adrenergic receptors. It has comparatively mild chronotropic, hypertensive, arrhythmogenic, and vasodilative effects, especially compared with dopamine, and is usually the preferred of these two agents. Seizures are a potential side effect during administration, requiring dosage reduction or substitution with dopamine. The starting dose (1 to 2 μg/kg per minute) is titrated upward every 2 to 4 hours to achieve clinical improvement (e.g., stronger femoral arterial pulses, normalization of arterial blood pressure if initially depressed, stronger precordial apex beat, louder heart sounds, reduced lethargy, and normalization of core body temperature). Dopamine (Dopamine Hydrochloride Injection, Elkins-Sinn), 1 to 5 μg/kg per minute constant-rate infusion, directly stimulates cardiac beta$_1$-adrenergic receptors as well as causing release of myocardial norepinephrine stores. At low doses (1 to 2 μg/kg per minute), it stimulates renal dopaminergic receptors, promoting renal cortical blood flow and diuresis. Higher doses (>5 μg/kg per minute) stimulate beta$_1$-adrenergic receptors with undesirable increases in systemic arterial and venous pressures.

Vasodilators or ACE inhibitors may be useful in reducing congestion and improving cardiac performance. Nitroglycerin ointment (2%), which has significant venodilating effects and some activity on arteriolar beds, is best reserved for severe pulmonary edema. Perhaps more useful for decompensated myocardial failure are ACE inhibitors (e.g., enalapril, 0.25 to 0.5 mg/kg PO every 24 hours), which reduce preload and afterload by blunting the effects of the RAAS. While the effects of vasodiators and ACE inhibitors on morbidity and mortality have not been evaluated in feline clinical trials, proven efficacy in human and canine studies warrants their use. Anorexia, hypotension, and azotemia are potential side effects, especially in cats depleted by diuretics.

General supportive measures may be helpful. Hypothermia is common, and controlled external environmental heating may be beneficial. Judicious fluid therapy helps some cats with cardiogenic shock or circulatory failure. Potassium chloride must often be supplemented (e.g., 5 to 7 mEq for each 250 ml of fluids) when anorexia is prolonged. Blood pressure, serum electrolytes, and renal function should be monitored.

Maintenance Therapy. When pulmonary congestion is controlled, furosemide is tapered to the lowest effective dose and may be interrupted or discontinued if azotemia, anorexia, or dehydration develops. Chronic, refractory effusions may ultimately require gradually increasing doses of furosemide (2.2 to 4.4 mg/kg PO every 8 to 12 hours). A combination of hydrochlorothiazide and spironolactone may be added (2.2 mg/kg PO every 24 hours) in chronic, refractory cases. ACE inhibitors are continued, and in cases of severe, refractory pleural or abdominal effusions administration may be increased from once to twice daily. Serum digoxin concentration should be evaluated 10 to 14 days after initiating therapy. When blood is drawn 10 to 12 hours after administration, a serum concentration of 1 to 2 ng/ml is presumed to be therapeutic. Anorexia and depression are early signs of toxicity; electrocardiographic evidence of digoxin toxicosis may include ST-segment changes, first-degree atrioventricular block and/or PR-interval prolongation; more severe toxicity may cause advanced atrioventricular block, bradycardia, and ventricular arrhythmias. Clinical signs of toxicity may last up to 96 hours in normal cats given toxic doses, or up to 7 days in azotemic cats.

Taurine deficiency is uncommon but when encountered, myocardial failure is generally reversible with taurine supplementation and standard management of heart failure. For decompensated idiopathic myocardial failure, the prognosis is poor. The prognosis with concomitant thromboembolism is grave.

ARTERIAL THROMBOEMBOLISM

Clinical Signs

Thromboembolism is a common sequela to cardiomyopathy. The pathogenesis involves circulatory stasis and altered blood coagulability. The risk factors include severe left atrial enlargement (>20 mm), blood stasis (particularly evident by spontaneous echocardiographic contrast—especially when myocardial failure or atrial fibrillation are present), and endocardial fibrosis. However, less severely affected cats may also develop thromboemboli. The clinical signs are attributable to congestive heart failure and injury to the tissues or organs that are embolized (e.g., azotemia from renal infarction); more than 90% of affected cats present with a lateralizing posterior paresis due to saddle embolus at the distal aortic trifurcation. Anterior tibial and gastrocnemius muscles are often firm or become so by 10 to 12 hours after embolization from ischemic myopathy. Occasionally, a single brachial artery is embolized, causing monoparesis (usually of the right front leg). Coronary renal, mesenteric, or pulmonary embolization may be rapidly fatal. Intermittent claudication is rarely reported preceding clinical thromboembolism. Most affected cats are clinically dehydrated on presentation to the hospital. Serum concentrations of alanine aminotransferase (SGPT) and aspartate aminotransferase (SGOT) are elevated by about 12 hours and peak by 36 hours after embolization. Lactate dehydrogenase (LDH) and creatine phosphokinase (CPK) enzymes are greatly increased shortly after embolization. Echocardiography provides rapid assessment of cardiac structure and function, may detect intracardiac thrombi, facilitates diagnosis, and assists with therapy and prognosis.

Therapy

The optimal therapy for preventing arterial thromboembolism is unknown. Treatment is directed toward (1) managing the concomitant congestive heart failure that is often present; (2) general patient support, including nutritional supplementation; and (3) adjunctive therapies to either limit thrombus growth or formation or induce thrombolysis and analgesics. Beta-blockers should probably be avoided during acute therapy. Affected cats are a high surgical risk because of congestive heart failure, hypothermia, disseminated intravascular coagulation, and arrhythmias. Thus, embolectomy is generally contraindicated, and reported results have generally been poor.

Various medical treatments have been used for acute and chronic management, although most are empirical and efficacy is unsubstantiated. Arteriolar dilation with acepromazine maleate and hydralazine (Apresoline, Novartis) has been proposed. However, arterial dilation may not be uniform, these agents are potentially hypotensive, and they have not been shown to alter the platelet-induced reduction of collateral flow caused by vasoactive chemicals, such as serotonin.

Thrombolytic agents have caused high morbidity and mortality in limited unpublished trials. Streptokinase (Streptase, Astra) and urokinase (Abbokinase, Abbott) act by generating the nonspecific proteolytic enzyme plasmin through conversion of the proenzyme plasminogen. This enzyme causes a generalized lytic state with the attendant risk of bleeding. Tissue plasminogen activator (Activase, Genentech) has a higher specificity. It binds to fibrin in a thrombus and converts the entrapped plasminogen to plasmin, which initiates a local fibrinolysis with limited systemic proteolysis. Used in a small number of cats, it produced variable results.

Anticoagulants (heparin, warfarin [Coumadin]) have no effects on established thrombi. Their use has been based on the premise that by retarding clotting factor synthesis or accelerating their inactivation, thrombosis from activated blood clotting pathways can be prevented. Heparin (heparin sodium [Liquaemin, Organon]) binds to antithrombin III, enhancing its ability to neutralize activated factors XII, XI, X, and IX and thrombin; this action prevents activation of the coagulation process. Reported dosages vary widely. It may be administered as an initial intravenous dose (1,000 USP units), followed 3 hours later by subcutaneous injection (50 USP units/kg), repeated every 6 to 8 hours. The dose is then adjusted to prolong clotting time 2 to 2.5 times pretreatment baseline index values. Bleeding is a major complication, and clotting profiles (partial thromboplastin time [PTT]) should be monitored.

Warfarin (Coumadin Tablets, DuPont) impairs hepatic vitamin K metabolism, a vitamin necessary for the synthesis of procoagulants (factors II or prothrombin, VII, IX, and X). The initial oral dosage (0.25 to 0.5 mg/day) is adjusted to prolong the prothrombin time to twice the normal value; alternatively, it is adjusted by the International Normalization Ratio (INR = [Cat PT/Control PT][ISI]) to maintain a value of 2.0 to 3.0 (the laboratory should provide an index of thromboplastin reagent sensitivity, called international sensitivity index [ISI]). It should ideally be overlapped with heparin therapy for 3 days. Some cardiologists have proposed warfarin for chronic oral maintenance in cases of advanced myocardial disease. Others advise more caution, or reserve the drug for cases of actual arterial embolism. In cats who have suffered previous thromboembolism, or in patients with a predisposition for thrombosis, anticoagulant therapy may decrease the risk of thromboembolism in exchange for increased risk of major hemorrhage. Warfarin therapy should not be attempted without vigilant monitoring and appropriate patient selection (see *CVT XII*, p. 872).

Anti–platelet-aggregating drugs are theoretically beneficial during and after a thromboembolic episode in that they prevent further embolic events. Aspirin induces a functional defect in platelets by inactivation, through acetylation, of cyclooxygenase, an enzyme critical in thromboxane A_2 synthesis. The latter is an arachidonic acid derivative that induces platelet activation. This activation occurs mainly through platelet adenosine diphosphate release, the common pathway in platelet aggregation. Vasoconstriction results from released platelet thromboxane A_2 and serotonin.

Aspirin (25 mg/kg, or one quarter of a 5-grain tablet, PO every 48 to 72 hours) effectively inhibits platelet function for 3 to 5 days. Prostacyclin, the major cyclooxygenase product in vascular endothelium, causes arterial vasodilation and inhibits platelet aggregation. The optimal aspirin dose that inhibits thromboxane A_2 production but spares vascular endothelial prostacyclin synthesis has not yet been established in cats.

Adjunctive therapy includes maintenance of hydration, electrolyte balance, and nutritional support. Serum potassium should be monitored, as reperfusion can lead to rapid increases in serum potassium (which leaks from damaged muscle cells). Aspirin is also useful for the myalgia associated with ischemic myopathy, although it will not control the severe pain often associated with thromboembolism. This pain should be managed with suitable opiate analgesia, such as butorphanol or buprenorphine (see p. 57), for at least 24 to 36 hours. Epidural analgesia is often effective. Most affected cats are anorectic, dehydrated, and hypokalemic. Vitamin B and folate supplementation and correction of hypercysteinemia, when present, are emergent therapies. When congestive heart failure has been stabilized, placement of a nasoesophageal feeding tube for nutritional support may be helpful, particularly during the first week of therapy.

Prognosis. Motor ability may begin to return within 10 to 14 days. By 3 weeks, significant motor function (i.e., hock extension and flexion) has often returned, typically better in one leg than in the other. Motor function may be completely normal by 4 to 6 weeks, although a conscious proprioceptive deficit or conformational abnormality (e.g., extreme hock flexion) may persist in one leg. The short-term prognosis depends on the nature and responsiveness of the cardiomyopathic disorder, heart failure, and the severity of rhabdocytolysis. Acute hyperkalemia may result from reperfusion injury and confers a grave prognosis. Unfortunately, most cats experience additional thromboembolic episodes within 1 to 12 months.

References and Suggested Reading

Atkins CE, Gallo AM, Kurzman ID, et al: Risk factors, clinical signs, and survival in cats with a clinical diagnosis of idiopathic hypertrophic cardiomyopathy: 74 cases (1985–1989). J Am Vet Med Assoc 201:613, 1992.
Retrospective study describing clinical signs and prognosis in 74 cats with hypertrophic cardiomyopathy.

Bonagura JB, Fox PR: Restrictive cardiomyopathy. In: Bonagura JB, ed: Kirk's Current Veterinary Therapy XII: Small Animal Practice. Philadelphia: WB Saunders, 1995, p 863.
A clinical presentation proposing pathophysiology and suggested therapy for feline restrictive cardiomyopathy.

Bright JM, Golden AL, Gompf RE, et al: Evaluation of the calcium channel-blocking agents diltiazem and verapamil for treatment of feline hypertrophic cardiomyopathy. J Vet Intern Med 5:272, 1991.
Prospective study evaluating the clinical effects of diltiazem, verapamil, and propranolol on clinical outcome in cats with idiopathic hypertrophic cardiomyopathy.

Fox PR: Feline myocardial disease. In: Fox PR, ed: Canine and Feline Cardiology. New York: Churchill Livingstone, 1988, p 435.
A description of feline myocardial diseases, including etiology, pathophysiology, clinical diagnosis, and therapy.

Fox PR, Liu SK, Maron B: Echocardiographic assessment of spontaneously occurring feline hypertrophic cardiomyopathy: An animal model of human disease. Circulation 92:2645, 1995.
A prospective study recording the phenotypic characterization, gross pathology and microscopic findings, and clinical outcome of 47 cats with idiopathic hypertrophic cardiomyopathy.

Keene BW, Rush JE: Therapy of heart failure. In: Ettinger SJ, Feldman EC, eds: Textbook of Veterinary Internal Medicine: Diseases of the Dog and Cat, 4th ed. Philadelphia: WB Saunders, 1995, p 867.
A summary and update of drug indications for, use of, and overall strategies for managing congestive heart failure in the dog and cat.

Quinones M, Dyer DC, Ware WA, et al: Pharmacokinetics of atenolol in clinically normal cats. Am J Vet Res 57:1050, 1996.
Study to determine the pharmacokinetics of atenolol given intravenously and orally in nine clinically normal cats.

Sharpe N: Beta-blockers in heart failure. Heart Failure Rev 1:5, 1996.
Rationale for the use of beta blockade in heart failure, including neurohumoral alterations and clinical trials are reviewed.

Sisson DD, Thomas WP: Myocardial diseases. In: Ettinger SJ, Feldman EC, eds: Textbook of Veterinary Internal Medicine: Diseases of the Dog and Cat, 4th ed. Philadelphia: WB Saunders, 1995, p 995.
A review of the causes of, pathophysiology of, and therapies for canine and feline cardiomyopathies.

Spirito P, Seidman CE, McKenna WJ, et al: The management of hypertrophic cardiomyopathy. N Engl J Med 336:775, 1997.
A review of clinical presentations of hypertrophic cardiomyopathy in humans and corresponding treatment strategies.

CVT Update: Infectious Endocarditis

Teresa C. DeFrancesco

Raleigh, North Carolina

Infectious endocarditis is an uncommon but often devastating disease caused by microbial infection of the endothelial lining of the heart, which usually develops into a vegetation on the heart valves. These vegetative lesions consist of a fibrin and platelet matrix overlaying colonies of microorganisms, rendering them inaccessible to the host defense systems and resistant to penetration by antimicrobial agents. Not only is infectious endocarditis difficult to treat, but also the diagnosis is often complex and uncertain because of the inaccessibility of the intracardiac lesion and the variable and nonspecific nature of clinical manifestations. Recent advances in echocardiography (Durack et al, 1994) and the identification of new causative microorganisms from apparent "culture-negative" endocarditis have enhanced our diagnostic ability. The advent of newer and more potent antimicrobial agents and improved therapy for congestive heart failure may lead to improved survival and prognosis. The following discussion is focused on recent, clinically applicable advances in the diagnosis, treatment, and prevention of infectious endocarditis. For a more complete review of the pathogenesis and clinical features of infectious endocarditis, please refer to *Current Veterinary Therapy XI* (pp. 752 to 755).

HOST SUSCEPTIBILITY

Most retrospective reviews report the prevalence of infectious endocarditis in hospital- or necropsy-based populations of dogs with cardiovascular disease to be low, ranging between 0.1 and 6.6%, depending on the population studied (Showse and Meier, 1956; Calvert, 1982). Little information is available about the prevalence of infectious endocarditis in cats, but it appears to be an extremely rare feline disease. Endocarditis most often affects male large-breed dogs older than 4 years of age. Boxers, German shepherds, Golden retrievers, Rottweilers, and Doberman pinschers appear to be predisposed.

Congenital heart disease predisposes both humans and dogs to infectious endocarditis, and the similarities in the breeds predisposed to both endocarditis and subaortic stenosis reflect an important factor in causation, rather than coincidence (Kienle et al, 1994). Subaortic stenosis results in high-velocity blood flow in the left ventricular outflow tract, which roughens the surfaces of the aortic valve leaflets and facilitates colonization of bacteria. In a review examining the natural history of subaortic stenosis, Kienle reported that 6.3% of dogs, usually with mild to moderate stenosis, developed infectious endocarditis (Kienle et al, 1994). Ventricular septal defects and patent ductus arteriosus are rarely associated with endocarditis. Although mitral valve disease (endocardiosis) could theoretically predispose to infectious endocarditis, no such correlation has ever been established in dogs. In humans, mitral valve prolapse increases the risk of infectious endocarditis five to eight fold. Previous infectious endocarditis, intracardiac surgery, and transvenous pacemaker implantation are other substantial risk factors.

Recurrent bacteremia also increases host susceptibility to endocarditis. Severe gingivitis or periodontal disease, urinary or prostatic infection, dermatitis, gastrointestinal mucosal compromise, or a chronic traumatic wound may also predispose to endocarditis. Although the purported link between dental and valvular disease in dogs has never been demonstrated in a clinical study, abnormalities that impair the host defense systems, including chronic corticosteroid administration, Cushing's disease, or diabetes mellitus, may also enhance the risk of endocarditis, especially in the presence of additional risk factors (e.g., subaortic stenosis [SAS]).

CAUSATIVE ORGANISMS

Although a wide variety of organisms can cause infectious endocarditis, only a few species account for the majority of infections. *Streptococcus* spp., *Staphylococcus* spp., and *Escherichia coli* cause more than half of the infections in the dog (Calvert, 1982). Other bacteria such as *Corynebacterium* spp., *Pseudomonas aeruginosa*, (Sisson, 1994), *Proteus* spp., *Pasteurella* spp., and *Erysipelothrix rhusiopathiae* also cause endocarditis (Sisson, 1994).

Culture-Negative Endocarditis

Conventional bacterial cultures may fail to grow bacteria in a patient that has clinical and echocardiographic criteria for infectious endocarditis. *Diagnoses other than endocarditis should be meticulously excluded before a diagnosis of culture-negative endocarditis is accepted.* A working diagnosis is based on clinical manifestations, progression, and response of the disease to empirical treatment. Prior antimicrobial therapy, inappropriate culture techniques, chronic endocarditis with encapsulated vegetative lesions, fastidious, slow-growing bacteria, and fungal infections are potential causes of the failure to isolate an organism by conventional culture techniques. *Bartonella* spp. have been reported to cause apparent culture-negative endocarditis in humans (Spach et al, 1995). *Bartonella* spp. are fastidious, gram-negative bacilli that were previously known as Rickettsia and *Rochalimaea* and are increasingly recognized as causes of human disease (e.g., cat-scratch disease). Bartonella reside within or on the surface of erythrocytes, making them difficult to isolate from blood and requiring special culture techniques. *Bartonella* endocarditis was recently reported in a 3-year-old Labrador retriever in which all routine aerobic and anaerobic bacterial culture results were negative (Breitschwerdt et al, 1995). Blood cultured simultaneously by the lysis centrifugation technique, which lyses red blood cells prior to culture, grew *Bartonella vinsonii*. Presumably, *Bartonella* spp. are an uncommon cause of endocarditis in humans and dogs, although the failure to grow *Bartonella* by conventional culture techniques may account for some culture-negative endocarditis. Most cases of *Bartonella* infection have extremely high serum immunofluorescent antibody titers, which may be diagnostically useful. Gene amplification by the polymerase chain reaction (PCR) and other molecular techniques holds promise for the isolation of the organisms that cause endocarditis and other infectious diseases (see p. 246).

CLINICAL PRESENTATION

Endocarditis is often termed the great imitator because of the many organs it affects and the diversity of clinical signs it produces. Owner complaints are often vague, such as lethargy, shivering, anorexia, weakness, weight loss, and shortness of breath. The physical examination findings can be as variable as the historical observations. Common findings include fever, cardiac murmur, arrhythmias, and lameness. Fever (>103°F) is reported in approximately 50 to 70% of patients.

Cardiac Manifestations

A cardiac murmur is present in approximately 50 to 75% of dogs with endocarditis. The murmur may be caused by either preexisting cardiac disease or by structural damage to the valve from the infectious process. Infection may cause perforations, tears, deformities, and rupture of the valve leaflets and/or chordae tendineae, which would lead to the changes associated with valvular insufficiency. The mitral and aortic valves are most often affected in the dog; therefore, the murmurs most often heard are those associated with mitral and aortic insufficiency. The combination of fever in a dog with a blowing diastolic murmur and hyperdynamic arterial pulse is strongly suggestive of endocarditis. The diastolic murmur of aortic insufficiency may be difficult to hear because of its low intensity; however, it can be enhanced by auscultating over the aortic valve area while the dog is positioned in left lateral recumbency. A systolic murmur in a febrile dog is not as predictive of endocarditis because functional murmurs and degenerative mitral valve disease are so common. The development of a new or changing murmur in a febrile dog or cat should raise the suspicion of infectious endocarditis. Arrhythmias and conduction disturbances are common findings in endocarditis, and may include premature ventricular depolarizations, paroxysm or sustained ventricular and supraventricular tachycardia, and atrioventricular block (first-, second-, and third-degree). Congestive heart failure is the single most important complication of infectious endocarditis because it exerts a critical influence on long-term prognosis.

Embolic Manifestations

Septic emboli shed from valvular vegetations may lodge in the vascular beds of the kidneys, spleen, brain, heart (coronary arteries), intestines, and skin. These emboli may cause infarction and spread of infection and can result in myriad physical abnormalities. Neurologic complications are seen in about 30% of humans affected with endocarditis. In veterinary medicine, neurologic signs are not recognized as commonly. Seizures, sudden-onset paresis, or cranial nerve or postural reaction deficits may be noted. Emboli may cause peripheral arterial obstruction, leading to pain, absence of pulse, pallor, and decreased temperature in the limb affected. Abdominal pain may be related to infarction of the spleen, kidneys, or intestines. Other abnormalities potentially associated with embolic phenomena include septic arthritis, hematuria, retinal hemorrhages, hyphema, petechia (skin and mucous membranes), and epistaxis.

Immunologic Manifestations

The persistent bacteremia of endocarditis stimulates both humoral and cell-mediated immune responses. Splenomegaly is common in endocarditis and may be associated with the presence of activated immune responses. Antibodies of the IgG, IgM, and IgA classes are increased in endocarditis and can form immune complexes. Positive antinuclear antibody tests have been observed. Circulating immune complexes can lead to polyarthritis, causing joint pain and effusion as well as glomerulonephritis.

DIAGNOSIS

If the signalment, history, and physical examination are suggestive of endocarditis, blood cultures and an echocardiogram are the most essential elements in the diagnosis. Other diagnostic tests are helpful, but not specific.

Mild to moderate, nonregenerative, normocytic, normochromic anemia occurs in about 50% of dogs with endocarditis. Leukocytosis may also be seen, generally characterized by neutrophilia or monocytosis, or both. Azotemia is the most common serum biochemical abnormality and may reflect renal compromise resulting from embolization or congestive heart failure. Urinalysis often shows proteinuria or microscopic hematuria. Joint taps may yield a septic or sterile, suppurative, arthritis. An electrocardiogram should be performed to rule out conduction disturbance (atrioventricular block) or arrhythmia. The most significant information provided by thoracic radiographs in the assessment of endocarditis is to determine whether the patient has volume overload or congestive heart failure, as these findings negatively impact prognosis and affect management.

Blood Cultures

Isolation of an organism from the blood is an important step in the diagnosis and treatment of infectious endocarditis. Blood cultures should be considered in all dogs with significant fever of unknown origin. Three separate blood samples are drawn aseptically at least 1 hour apart, from different sites. For each culture, 10 ml of blood should be drawn and divided equally between an aerobic and anaerobic medium. Cultures should be incubated for at least 3 weeks, and Gram's stains made at intervals even if no growth is apparent at inspection. In addition to routine culture techniques, lysis centrifugation cultures enhance the yield of fastidious microorganisms. Empirical antimicrobial therapy should be initiated as soon as cultures are obtained.

Echocardiography

Echocardiography is important in the diagnosis of infectious endocarditis, but it should never replace blood cultures in the diagnostic evaluation. Echocardiography allows visualization of most established vegetative lesions, in addition to cardiac complications such as chordal rupture, ventricular dilation, and valvular insufficiency. The sensitivity and specificity of echocardiography vary with the quality and detail of the study and expertise of the sonographer. The quality of the image is an important factor in the sensitivity of echocardiography in the diagnosis of infectious endocarditis. For this reason, transesophageal echocardiography is prefered to transthoracic echocardiography in human medicine. The sensitivity of transesophageal echocardiography in the diagnosis of infectious endocarditis is 90% compared to approximately 60 to 70% for transthoracic studies (Durack, 1994). Transesophageal echocardiography is rarely available in veterinary medicine. New diagnostic criteria were developed for human infectious endocarditis utilizing specific echocardiographic findings in combination with blood culture and physical findings (Durack et al, 1994). The new Duke diagnostic criteria has been shown to decrease both over- and underdiagnosis of endocarditis in humans. Valve thickening or valve nodules were not considered to be major evidence of endocarditis. The application of these criteria to veterinary echocardiography seems reasonable in evaluating patients with suspected endocarditis. The *major criteria* are defined as follows:

1. Positive results of blood cultures for infective endocarditis
   a. *Typical* microorganisms from two separate blood cultures, *or*
   b. Persistently positive blood culture results (three separate cultures) with a microorganism consistent with infective endocarditis
2. Evidence of endocardial involvement
   a. Positive echocardiogram for endocarditis
      (i) *oscillating intracardiac mass* on valve or supporting structure, *or*
      (ii) periannular abscess (echolucent region adjacent to the valve annulus)
   b. New valvular regurgitation (worsening or change of preexisting murmur not sufficient)

The *minor criteria* are defined as follows:

1. Predisposition (predisposing heart condition)
2. Fever
3. Vascular phenomena (arterial embolism or infarction, intracranial hemorrhage)
4. Immunologic phenomena (glomerulonephritis, polyarthritis)
5. Echocardiogram (findings consistent with endocarditis but not meeting major criteria noted earlier)

6. Microbiologic evidence (positive blood culture results but not meeting major criteria noted earlier, or positive serologic evidence of active infection with a microorganism consistent with endocarditis)

Clinically, definitive endocarditis is diagnosed by the presence of either two major criteria, *or* one major and three minor, *or* five minor criteria. Possible endocarditis is defined as findings consistent with infective endocarditis that fall short of "definite" but are not rejected. A diagnosis of endocarditis should be rejected if a firm alternative diagnosis is made or there is resolution of the manifestations of endocarditis with antibiotic therapy for 4 days or less, or no pathologic evidence of infective endocarditis at surgery or necropsy after antibiotic therapy for 4 days or less.

Echocardiography may also be helpful in the prognosis and treatment of endocarditis. Human studies have shown that patients with vegetations larger than 10 mm are at higher risk for developing embolic phenomenon (Durack, 1994). In addition, an increase in vegetation size during antibiotic therapy predicts a prolonged healing phase and an increased risk of complications (e.g., congestive heart failure), independent of blood culture results.

TREATMENT

General Principles

The primary goals of treatment are to kill the infecting organism and to prevent or manage the consequences of infection. Appropriate, long-term bactericidal therapy is crucial to ensuring the eradication of the microorganism and to preventing relapse. The valvular infection is difficult to cure because of poor penetration of antimicrobials into the infected vegetation, altered metabolic state of the bacteria within the lesion, and absence of an adequate host-defense cellular response that could enhance antimicrobial action.

Antimicrobial Treatment

Route of Administration: Oral Versus Parenteral

Although the American Heart Association specifically recommends against oral therapy, treatment with parenteral antimicrobials for 4 to 6 weeks is next to impossible for most veterinary patients. The potential disadvantages of oral therapy include decreased compliance, gastrointestinal upset, and variable bioavailability, any of which could sabotage treatment. Despite these potential problems, carefully selected oral antibiotics offer the potential for equally effective therapy with shorter and less expensive hospitalization, without the risk of catheter-related phlebitis or infections. Several small human clinical trials have shown oral treatment of endocarditis either alone or as a follow-up to a short course of intravenous therapy to be efficacious. If the veterinary patient requires hospitalization because of its debilitated state or the rapid progression of clinical signs, the author recommends short-term (5 to 10 days) intravenous therapy followed by protracted oral antimicrobial treatment. However, if the patient does not otherwise require hospitalization, oral treatment may be considered.

Choice and Dose of Drug and Duration of Treatment

The chosen antimicrobial agent should be bactericidal, if possible, and the dose must maintain serum concentrations above the minimum inhibitory concentration (MIC) of the pathogen for most of the dosing interval. If blood cultures isolate an organism, the MIC or minimum bactericidal concentration (MBC) obtained from the sensitivity test should be used to ensure that the infecting organism is killed by—and is not resistant to—the agent or agents used. If blood cultures are negative, empirical therapy with a combination of broad-spectrum antimicrobials is recommended for expanding the spectrum of antibiotic coverage. For example, in animal models of endocarditis (usually rabbits), combinations of pencillins with aminoglycosides eradicate organisms from the vegetation more rapidly than do penicillins alone. The optimal antimicrobial therapy for *Bartonella* endocarditis is controversial. Ciprofloxacin, gentamicin, ceftriaxone, doxycycline, erythromycin, and azithromycin all have been shown to be clinically effective in humans (Spach et al, 1995). The third-generation cephalosporins show promising results for monotherapy for endocarditis. They retain the gram-positive activity of the first- and second-generation agents with expanded gram-negative activity and minimal adverse effects. Ceftriaxone sodium and cefixime are potentially useful third-generation cephalosporins.

Initial or Empirical Parenteral Antimicrobial Recommendations (Canine)

Enrofloxacin (Baytril, Bayer), 2.5 to 5 mg/kg IV or IM every 12 hours, *or*

Amikacin sulfate (Amiglyde-V, Fort Dodge), 11 mg/kg IV, SC, or IM every 12 hours for 5 days,

and

Ampicillin sodium (various trade names and manufacturers), 22 mg/kg IV every 6 to 8 hours, *or*

Cefazolin sodium (various trade names and manufacturers), 22 mg/kg IV or SC every 6 to 8 hours

Oral Antimicrobial Recommendations (Canine)

Amoxicillin–clavulanic acid (Clavamox, Pfizer Animal Health), 22 mg/kg PO every 8 to 12 hours, *or*

Cephalexin (Keflex, Dista), 22 mg/kg PO every 8 hours,

and

Enrofloxacin (Baytril, Bayer), 2.5 to 5 mg/kg PO every 12 hours

For Documented Resistance Against or Other Contraindications for Fluoroquinolones and Aminoglycosides (Canine)

Imipenem-cilastatin sodium (Primaxin, Merck), 0.7 to 1.1 mg/kg IV every 8 hours, *or*

Ceftriaxone sodium (Rocephin, Roche), 20 mg/kg IV every 12 hours, *or*

Cefixime (Suprax, Lederle), 10 mg/kg PO every 12 hours

To assess the efficacy of antimicrobial therapy, frequent physical examinations and follow-up blood cultures and echocardiography are recommended. Physical examinations should focus on changes in heart and lung sounds and cardiac rhythm, or signs of new cardiac, embolic, or immunologic complications. Ideally, follow-up blood cultures should be performed shortly after initiation of antimicrobial therapy (3 to 5 days) to ensure eradication of the infecting organism in vivo. Blood cultures are also recommended 2 to 4 weeks after the completion of therapy to detect a relapse. Echocardiography is also helpful in assessing the efficacy of therapy, as an increase in size of the vegetation or the appearance of a new lesion after prolonged antimicrobial therapy should prompt reassessment of therapy. Repeat echocardiography is recommended just prior to the completion of the antimicrobial therapy, or whenever clinical signs recrudesce.

Role of Aspirin?

Experimental animal evidence suggests that an antiplatelet dose of aspirin (5 mg/kg PO every 24 hours) reduces the weight of the infectious vegetations and improves the rate of bacterial sterilization when used in combination with antimicrobial therapy (Nicolau et al, 1995). At this point, it is premature to make concrete recommendations regarding the use of aspirin in the treatment or prevention of endocarditis, and further clinical studies are needed to define the risks and benefits of aspirin in clinical endocarditis.

PREVENTION

Antimicrobial agents may be effective in preventing infectious endocarditis by decreasing the magnitude of bacteremia associated with traumatic procedures, such as dental prophylaxis or intestinal surgery. Antibiotic prophylaxis is recommended in dogs with cardiovascular defects that predispose to endocarditis such as subaortic stenosis or previous endocarditis. Parenteral antibiotics should be administered approximately 1 hour prior to the surgical procedure. The following protocols are recommended:

Ampicillin sodium (generic), 30 mg/kg IV 1 hour prior and 6 hours after the procedure

Clindamycin phosphate (Cleocin, Pharmacia & Upjohn), 10 mg/kg IV 1 hour prior and 6 hours after the procedure

References and Suggested Reading

Anderson CA, Dubielzig RR: Vegetative endocarditis in dogs. J Am Anim Hosp Assoc 20:149, 1982.
A retrospective study of infective endocarditis in 40 dogs.
Bayer AS, Ward JI, Ginzton LE, et al: Evaluation of new clinical criteria for the diagnosis of infectious endocarditis. Am J Med 96:211, 1994.
Describes improved diagnostic accuracy with the new clinical criteria in infectious endocarditis.
Breitschwerdt EB, Kordick DL, Malarkey DE, et al: Endocarditis in a dog due to infection with a novel *Bartonella* subspecies. J Clin Microbiol 33:154, 1995.
The first case report of Bartonella *endocarditis in a dog from the North Carolina area.*

Calvert CA: Valvular bacterial endocarditis in the dog. J Am Vet Med Assoc 180:1080, 1982.
   A retrospective study of the clinical and pathologic features of infectious endocarditis in 61 dogs.

Durack DT: Infectious and noninfectious endocarditis. In: Schlant RC, Alexander RW, eds: Hurst's The Heart. New York: McGraw-Hill, 1994, p 1681.
   A thorough and up-to-date book chapter about the pathophysiology and clinical manifestations of infectious endocarditis in humans.

Durack DT, Lukes AS, Bright DK, and the Duke Endocarditis Service: New criteria for diagnosis of infectious endocarditis: Utilization of specific echocardiographic findings. Am J Med 96:200, 1994.
   Describes the new clinical and echocardiographic criteria for the diagnosis of human endocarditis.

Kienle RD, Thomas WP, Pion PD: The natural clinical history of canine congenital subaortic stenosis. J Vet Intern Med 8:423, 1994.
   Describes the long-term follow-up of 96 dogs with subaortic stenosis and its association with endocarditis.

Nicolau DP, Marangos MN, Nightingale CH, et al: Influence of aspirin on development and treatment of experimental *Staphylococcus aureus* endocarditis. Antimicrob Agents Chemother 39:1748, 1995.
   Experimental evidence supporting the use of aspirin in the treatment and prevention of infectious endocarditis.

Showse CL, Meier H: Acute vegetative endocarditis in the dog and cat. J Am Vet Med Assoc 129:278, 1956.
   One of the original clinical and pathologic descriptions of endocarditis in dogs and cats.

Sisson D: Bacterial Endocarditis. In: Proceedings for the Waltham/OSU Cardiology Symposium. Vernon, CA: Waltham USA, 1994, p 79.
   An excellent overview of the current knowledge regarding bacterial endocarditis in veterinary medicine.

Spach DH, Kanter AS, Daniels NA, et al: *Bartonella (Rochalimaea)* species as a cause of apparent "culture-negative" endocarditis. Clin Infect Dis 20:1044, 1995.
   A discussion and review of case reports of Bartonella *endocarditis in humans.*

Diagnosis and Treatment of Pericardial Effusion

FRANCIS W.K. SMITH, JR.
Lexington, Massachusetts

JOHN E. RUSH
North Grafton, Massachusetts

Pericardial disease in dogs and cats includes congenital (e.g., peritoneopericardial diaphragmatic hernia) and acquired diseases (e.g., pericardial effusion, constrictive pericarditis, and pericardial tumors). Pericardial effusion is the most common pericardial disorder and the one that most frequently affects cardiac function. Pericardial effusion is an increase in the volume of fluid within the pericardial sac. The term *cardiac tamponade* describes the clinical situation in which pericardial effusion has caused a rise in intrapericardial pressure sufficient to cause hemodynamic compromise. At the Foster Small Animal Hospital of the Tufts University School of Veterinary Medicine, pericardial effusion was recognized in 7% of the cardiology caseload (8% of canine cases and 6% of feline cases). While the overall incidence of pericardial effusion may be similar in these two species, symptomatic pericardial effusion is common in dogs and rare in cats.

PATHOPHYSIOLOGY

As fluid accumulates within the pericardial sac, the elastic or stretching capabilities of the pericardial sac are eventually exceeded. Further accumulation of pericardial fluid leads to high intrapericardial pressure, which can collapse the right atrium and/or ventricle, and restricts cardiac filling (tamponade). Cardiac preload is reduced as a result of cardiac tamponade. Low cardiac preload results in low forward blood flow and low cardiac output. As intrapericardial pressures rise further, left atrial and left ventricular filling is also affected by direct compression or from shifting of the ventricular septum into the left ventricle.

Chronic Pericardial Effusion

As the result of the compensatory mechanisms activated in any low cardiac output state, neurohumoral activation leads to fluid retention and, eventually, signs of congestive heart failure. High systemic venous pressure also contributes to heart failure. Signs of congestive heart failure are typically manifested as right-sided congestive heart failure with ascites, hepatomegaly, jugular distention or pulsation, and, in some cases, pleural effusion.

Acute Pericardial Effusion

When there is a sudden bleed into the pericardial sac (e.g., right atrial hemangiosarcoma with an acute bleed, left atrial tear secondary to chronic valvular disease), there is an abrupt rise in intrapericardial pressure. In these situations, the acute nature of the hemodynamic responses predominates, and since time is required for the body to retain sodium and water, fluid retention is usually not evident. Compression of cardiac chambers leads to an abrupt drop in preload and a commensurate drop in cardiac output. The clinical presentation reflects acute cardiovascular collapse owing to an abrupt decrease in cardiac output with collapse, weakness, hypotension, pallor, and delayed capillary refill time. Syncope may occur.

CAUSES OF PERICARDIAL EFFUSION

Neoplasia and idiopathic pericardial effusion cause 90% of the cases of pericardial effusion in dogs, with neoplasia being the most common cause, especially in older dogs. The most common neoplasm associated with pericardial effusion is hemangiosarcoma of the right atrium. Other tumors include mesothelioma, aortic body tumor (chemodectoma), ectopic thyroid carcinoma, and metastatic neoplasia. Other causes of pericardial effusion include coagulopathies (vitamin K antagonist), infection (coccidioidomycosis, trypanosomiasis, bacterial pericarditis), congestive heart failure, hypoalbuminemia, uremia, pericardial cysts, left atrial tear, and pericardial foreign body.

Feline infectious peritonitis (FIP) is the most common cause of pericardial effusion in cats in some reports. Congestive heart failure is another common cause, especially in cats with pleural effusion and severe cardiac enlargement. Other causes of pericardial effusion in cats include bacterial pericarditis, uremia, coagulopathies, lymphoma and metastatic neoplasia, left atrial tear, and idiopathic pericarditis.

CLINICAL PRESENTATION

Signalment

Pericardial effusion is most commonly diagnosed in large-breed dogs older than 5 years of age. The younger the dog, the more likely the cause is idiopathic pericardial effusion. The cause in dogs older than 7 years is commonly related to a neoplasm. Golden retrievers, German shepherds, and Labrador retrievers are predisposed to right atrial hemangiosarcoma. Golden retrievers, German shepherds, and male dogs appear predisposed to idiopathic pericardial effusion. Boxers, English bulldogs, and Boston terriers are predisposed to chemodectomas, but represent only a small percentage of dogs with pericardial effusion.

Clinical Signs

Chronic Pericardial Effusion

Chronic pericardial effusion causes right-sided congestive heart failure. Lethargy, anorexia, weakness, collapse, abdominal distention, tachypnea, restlessness at night, and muscle wasting may be described by owners. Common but variable findings on physical examination include ascites, muffled heart sounds, weak arterial pulses, pulsus paradoxus, tachypnea, pleural fluid line, tachycardia, and jugular venous distention. The physical finding of pulsus paradoxus, caused by an exaggerated fall in blood pressure during inspiration, is identified by palpation of a strong pulse during expiration and a very weak pulse on inspiration. Mucous membrane pallor and prolonged capillary refill time may also be noted. Fever is uncommon but may be evident in cases of septic pericarditis.

Acute Pericardial Effusion

In cases of acute pericardial effusion, the clinical presentation is usually one of sudden collapse. Syncope may be described. The owner may report a short period of lethargy, anorexia, or weakness prior to collapse. With rapidly developing effusions, most animals are extremely weak and may be reluctant or unable to stand. Arterial pulses are weak, and pulsus paradoxus may be present. Mucous membrane pallor is usually evident, and capillary refill time may be slowed. Tachycardia, tachypnea, and jugular vein distention are usually present.

DIAGNOSTIC TESTS FOR PERICARDIAL EFFUSION

Laboratory Tests

Dogs with hemangiosarcoma may have anemia, nucleated red blood cells, schistocytes or acanthocytes, and thrombocytopenia. Cats with FIP may have neutrophilia and lymphocytopenia. The serum biochemistry profile is usually normal; however, mild to moderate elevation of liver enzymes due to chronic passive congestion may be present. Mild azotemia, which is typically prerenal, may also be noted. Dogs with chronic pericardial effusion and ascites may have mild hypoproteinemia, hyponatremia, hypochloremia, or hyperkalemia. Hyperglobulinemia is often noted in cats with FIP. The urinalysis is usually normal. Coccidioidomycosis serology should be done on dogs from endemic areas. Some assessment of clotting time (e.g., activated clotting time, activated partial thromboplastin time, one-stage prothrombin time) should be performed prior to pericardiocentesis if coagulopathy is suspected clinically.

Radiography

Mild to severe enlargement of the cardiac silhouette is observed on thoracic radiographs. In cases of acute bleeding into the pericardial sac, the degree of enlargement is usually mild. In cases of chronic pericardial effusion, there may be severe enlargement. The cardiac silhouette is often globoid, or rounded, in appearance. It is usually difficult to identify specific cardiac chamber enlargement, with the exception of a left atrial tear in dogs with chronic valvular disease. On the dorsoventral view, the edges of the cardiac silhouette are often very "sharp" owing to a lack of cardiac motion artifact. Mild to moderate pleural effusion may be noted, and pulmonary metastatic disease is present in some cases. Pulmonary edema is typically absent. Other findings include tracheal elevation (especially with chemodectomas), dilation of the caudal vena cava, and pulmonary undercirculation. Abdominal radiographs may reveal hepatosplenomegaly or ascites. Dogs with right atrial hemangiosarcoma may have evidence of a splenic mass.

Electrocardiography

Sinus tachycardia is often present, and ventricular or supraventricular arrhythmias are possible. In dogs, low-voltage QRS complexes (QRS <1 mV in all limb leads

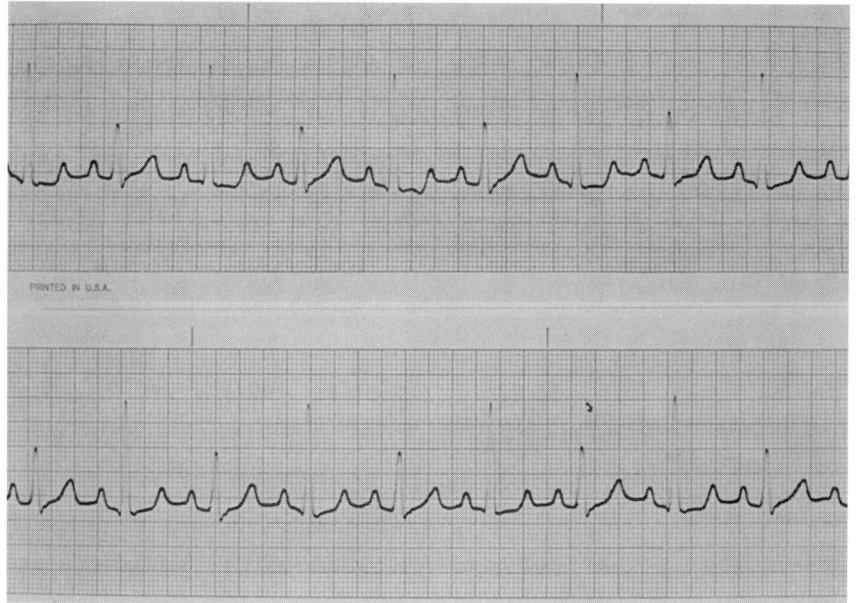

Figure 1. A lead II electrocardiogram recorded at 50 mm/sec from a dog with pericardial effusion. The heart rate is 160 bpm, and the rhythm is sinus with electrical alternans present.

and thoracic leads) may be identified. Less commonly, electrical alternans or ST-segment elevation is observed. Electrical alternans, which results from the heart swinging to and fro within the pericardial sac, typically results in a regular, or repeating, variation in QRS or T-wave height or morphology (Fig. 1) but is only found in large effusions. While electrical alternans has been reported in cats, the electrocardiogram is rarely helpful in diagnosing pericardial effusion in cats. An elevated ST segment is suggestive of pericarditis. A normal electrocardiogram does not rule out a diagnosis of pericardial effusion.

Echocardiography

Echocardiography is the best diagnostic test for confirming the presence of pericardial effusion. An echo-free space can be clearly identified between the pericardium and the epicardial surface of the heart, even with a very small volume of pericardial effusion (Fig. 2). Diastolic

collapse of the right atrium and/or right ventricle confirms a clinical diagnosis of cardiac tamponade. The heart may be seen to swing to and fro within the pericardial sac if the effusion is large in volume. Cardiac mass lesions may be identified. Echocardiography should be performed from the right and left hemithoraces to increase the likelihood of identifying cardiac masses. Cardiac mass lesions are more easily identified when large effusions are present; in cases of mild tamponade in which patient deterioration does not seem imminent, it is preferable to perform echocardiography and search for a cardiac mass prior to pericardiocentesis.

Pericardial Fluid Analysis

Most effusions in dogs are hemorrhagic, and cytologic evaluation of these effusions is usually unrewarding. Reactive mesothelial cells can mimic neoplastic cells, making differentiation between the two cell types very difficult.

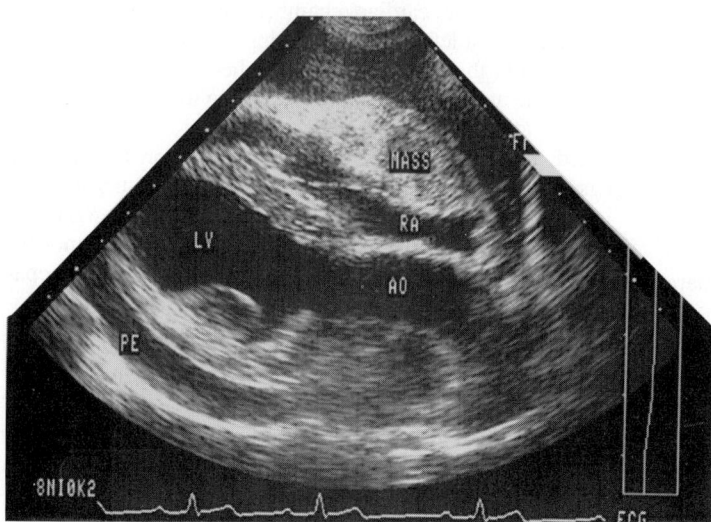

Figure 2. Two-dimensional long-axis echocardiographic view showing the right atrium (RA), left ventricle (LV), and aorta (Ao) from a dog with pericardial effusion and right atrial mass (MASS). Pericardial effusion (PE) is identified as the echo-free space between the pericardium and the cardiac walls. (Courtesy of Dr. Donald P. Schrope.)

In cases of fungal (e.g., coccidioidomycosis) or bacterial pericarditis, the organism may be identified. In cats, pericardial fluid analysis may be more useful because of the higher incidence of lymphoma, metastatic neoplasia, bacterial infections, or FIP. In cases of congestive heart failure leading to pericardial effusion, analysis of pericardial fluid usually reveals a nonspecific modified transudate. A pure transudate may also be observed in dogs with heart base masses that obstruct lymphatic drainage. In dogs, evaluation of the pH of the pericardial fluid may help discriminate between neoplastic and inflammatory causes of effusion. When pericardial fluid pH is measured by an acid-base analyzer, a pH less than 7.2 is most likely the result of an inflammatory condition, whereas a pH above 7.3 is more likely due to neoplasia (Edwards, 1996).

TREATMENT OVERVIEW

Pericardiocentesis

With the exception of active bleeding into the pericardial sac, pericardiocentesis is the best and most expedient treatment for returning the patient to a nearly normal hemodynamic status. In patients with idiopathic pericardial effusion, pericardiocentesis may be the only treatment required in up to 50% of affected dogs. In certain situations (see surgical management), pericardiocentesis may be followed by surgery or by administration of systemic or intrapericardial medications.

Pericardiocentesis can be performed with the patient in either sternal or right or left lateral recumbency. The authors' preference is for sternal recumbency, as this position seems to be best tolerated by hemodynamically unstable patients. Pericardiocentesis is usually performed from the right side of the thorax to reduce the risk of lacerating the left coronary artery. It is strongly advised that simultaneous electrocardiographic monitoring be used to identify arrhythmias that may result from contact between the needle or catheter and the myocardium. Echocardiography can be useful in identifying the best intercostal space and needle angulation for pericardiocentesis; however, echocardiography is not required. In the absence of echocardiography, pericardiocentesis is performed at the fifth intercostal space just below the costochondral junction at a point where the cardiac impulse is most prominent.

The haircoat is clipped and aseptically prepared between the third and eighth intercostal spaces from above the costochondral junction and extending ventrally to the sternum. Local anesthetic block improves patient comfort, and some patients benefit from a low dose of systemically administered opiates. A long (2 cm or longer) large-gauge (18 gauge or larger) catheter is advanced perpendicular to the body wall, through the skin and intercostal muscles into the pericardial sac.

As the needle is advanced, clear or sanguineous pleural fluid may be obtained before the catheter enters the pericardial sac, especially in animals with long-standing pericardial effusion. In most dogs, the pericardial fluid obtained during the pericardiocentesis is hemorrhagic and has a very dark red appearance. Some dogs have a serous or serosanguineous effusion. The appearance of pericardial effusion in cats depends on the underlying disease. If the source of the fluid is in question (intrapericardial versus intracardiac), check to see whether the fluid clots and check the hematocrit of the fluid. In animals with hemorrhagic pericardial effusion, the fluid does not clot unless the hemorrhage is active or very recent. A spun hematocrit of pericardial fluid is usually different from the animal's peripheral hematocrit, and the supernatant of this spun hematocrit may be xanthochromic.

In the absence of active bleeding (e.g., vitamin K antagonism or left atrial tear), remove as much pericardial fluid as possible. In patients with left atrial tear, remove only as much fluid as is required to resolve tamponade. Monitor the electrocardiogram while draining the pericardium. If frequent arrhythmias are identified, the needle or catheter should be repositioned.

Close observation of the patient and electrocardiographic monitoring are advised following pericardiocentesis. In animals with active hemorrhage into the pericardial sac, continued hemorrhage may leak through the window created during pericardiocentesis and lead to hemothorax and clinical deterioration of the patient. In the authors' practice, ventricular arrhythmias are commonly identified after pericardiocentesis and sometimes are severe enough to warrant antiarrhythmic therapy. For these reasons, pericardial effusion is usually followed by overnight hospitalization and monitoring.

Surgical Management

In selected dogs with pericardial effusion, surgery may be useful in providing relief of clinical signs and definitive treatment. Subtotal pericardiectomy below the phrenic nerve is useful in dogs with recurrent idiopathic pericardial effusion and selected tumors. This procedure allows the fluid that is accumulating in the pericardial sac to drain into the thoracic cavity, which has a better ability to absorb fluid than does the pericardial sac. In a small percentage of cases with idiopathic pericardial effusion, recurrent pleural effusion may occur following surgery. The pericardium should always be biopsied to exclude the possibility of mesothelioma, even in cases of presumed idiopathic pericardial effusion. Partial pericardiectomy (i.e., pericardial window) is not recommended when a thoracotomy is performed; however, successful use of partial pericardiectomy performed with the use of thoracoscopy has been reported (Richter et al, 1996). Balloon catheter dilation of pericardial effusion has been performed, but it has not been employed widely.

Heart Failure Management

Pericardiocentesis is the definitive treatment for correcting the hemodynamic consequences of pericardial effusion. Diuretic therapy should not be used in place of pericardiocentesis in an attempt to mobilize ascitic fluid. While diuretics may be helpful in reducing fluid accumulation, especially following pericardiocentesis or pericardial surgery, they reduce preload and cardiac output. Diuretics can lead to progressive azotemia, weakness, and collapse or syncope. Animals with moderate to severe ascites can be treated with diuretics following pericardiocentesis. If diuretics are used, furosemide or spironolactone should be used in low doses and with caution. Digitalis, vasodilators, and angiotensin-converting enzyme (ACE) inhibitors are relatively or absolutely contraindicated in dogs with pericardial effusion. Digitalis is usually not required, as inotropic function is usually normal, and vasodilators including ACE inhibitors can cause hypotension and limit the animal's ability to respond to stressful situations.

DISEASE-SPECIFIC TREATMENT AND PROGNOSIS

The therapy and prognosis for pericardial disease depends on the underlying cause. Unfortunately, most dogs with pericardial effusion have neoplasia and most cats have severe systemic disease or cardiomyopathy; thus, a poor long-term prognosis is usually appropriate. However, the prognosis for some diseases, such as idiopathic pericardial effusion, is good.

Cardiac Neoplasia

Hemangiosarcoma is highly malignant and has usually metastasized by the time it is identified as the cause of pericardial effusion. Periodic pericardiocentesis, pericardial window, or percutaneous balloon pericardiotomy (Cobb et al, 1996) may provide short-term relief to the patient, but the prognosis is poor. Some clinicians do not advise pericardiectomy in patients with right atrial hemangiosarcoma, as exsanguination is possible. Surgical removal of the tumor is usually unrewarding, and complications are commonly encountered during the postoperative period. The authors have used intrapericardial injections of cisplatin in a few cases; however, the long-term follow-up regarding significant case numbers is not available. Combination chemotherapy reduced the size of a right atrial hemangiosarcoma in a single case report (de Madron et al, 1987).

In dogs with chemodectomas, pericardiectomy may be useful in relieving the signs of cardiac tamponade. These tumors are often slow-growing and slow to metastasize; therefore, alleviation of clinical signs resulting from pericardial effusion may improve patient comfort and survival. These tumors usually cannot be surgically removed, as they are closely adherent to the great vessels. When these tumors are of sufficient size that they are compressing cardiac structures, surgery is less likely to provide long-term symptomatic improvement. Survival times of up to 3 years have been reported following pericardiectomy.

Mesothelioma is difficult to diagnose prior to surgery, and the surgical procedure performed in most instances is subphrenic pericardiectomy. Following surgery, mesothelioma often spreads to the pleural surface. At this stage, periodic thoracentesis may be necessary, and intrathoracic administration of cisplatin can be attempted to slow the rate of fluid accumulation.

Cats with pericardial effusion secondary to lymphosarcoma often respond favorably to combination chemotherapy (see p. 465).

Idiopathic Pericardial Effusion in Dogs

Approximately 50% of cases of idiopathic pericardial effusion resolve after one or two pericardiocenteses. In the remaining cases, pericardial effusion may recur any time from 10 days to 5 years after pericardiocentesis. Systemic or intrapericardial corticosteroids have been advocated for use in idiopathic pericardial effusion, but their efficacy has not been documented, and so they cannot be recommended. Additionally, one preliminary report suggested that azathioprine (Imuran, Glaxo Wellcome) limited the recurrence of idiopathic pericardial effusion (Bussadori, 1995). If pericardial effusion recurs following pericardiocentesis, corticosteroids (prednisone, 1 mg/kg every 24 hours for 2 to 3 weeks and then tapered) or possibly azathioprine (1 mg/kg every 24 hours for 3 months) can be considered, although neither treatment has been evaluated by prospective clinical trial. Follow-up echocardiography every 10 to 14 days for 2 months is recommended when idiopathic pericardial effusion is the suspected diagnosis. Pericardiectomy is recommended after the third recurrence of pericardial effusion. Following surgery, most dogs are asymptomatic, but a very small number of dogs have recurrent pleural effusion.

Infectious Pericarditis

For patients with fungal or bacterial pericarditis, aggressive therapy is warranted. Appropriate antimicrobials, based on microbial identification and/or culture and sensitivity testing, are administered for the susceptible organisms. Placement of an indwelling pericardial catheter for drainage and lavage may be helpful, but surgical therapy and pericardiectomy are the best treatments. The prognosis for infectious pericarditis is generally guarded to poor, and constrictive pericarditis is a major complication.

Left Atrial Tear

Pericardiocentesis is performed only in patients with unstable tamponade, and small volumes of fluid are serially removed until clinical signs improve. Prognosis is poor in these patients. While the tear may heal, animals are prone to recurrent tears and generally have advanced heart disease at the time they develop pericardial effusion. In cases of traumatic atrial rupture and recurrent effusions, surgical intervention may be warranted.

Miscellaneous Causes

Vitamin K_1 and fresh plasma transfusion is indicated for the treatment of animals with pericardial hemorrhage secondary to poisoning with vitamin K antagonists. Pericardial effusion secondary to congestive heart failure is usually treated with cardiac drugs appropriate for the underlying cardiac disease. There is no good therapy for cats with FIP, and the prognosis is poor.

References and Suggested Reading

Buchanan JW: Causes and prevalence of cardiovascular disease. In: Kirk RW, Bonagura JD, eds: Current Veterinary Therapy XI. Philadelphia: WB Saunders, 1992, p 647.
Review of causes and prevalence of congenital and acquired cardio-

vascular disease in dogs and cats, including tables on disease prevalence by breed.

Bussadori C: Idiopathic haemorrhagic pericarditis: Update on clinical evaluation. Proceedings of the 13th ACVIM Forum, Lake Buena Vista, FL, 1995, p 225.
Brief review of the pathophysiology, diagnosis, and treatment of idiopathic hemorrhagic pericarditis.

Cobb MA, Boswood A, Griffin GM, et al: Percutaneous balloon pericardiotomy for the management of malignant pericardial effusion in two dogs. J Small Anim Pract 37:549, 1996.
Case report describing the technique and outcome of balloon pericardiotomy in two dogs with malignant pericardial effusion.

de Madron E, Helfand SC, Stebbins KE: Use of chemotherapy for treatment of cardiac hemangiosarcoma in a dog. J Am Vet Med Assoc 190:887, 1987.
Case report of a dog with right atrial hemangiosarcoma that was treated with combination chemotherapy and had a reduction in tumor size.

Edwards J: The diagnostic value of pericardial fluid pH determination. J Am Anim Hosp Assoc 32:63, 1996.
A study looking at the diagnostic value of pericardial fluid pH for differentiating neoplastic from non-neoplastic causes of pericardial effusion in dogs.

Reed JR: Pericardial diseases. In: Fox PR, ed: Canine and Feline Cardiology. New York: Churchill Livingstone, 1988, p 495.
Review of pericardial diseases in dogs and cats, including numerous radiographs.

Richter KP, Jackson J, Hart JR: Thoracoscopic pericardiectomy in 12 dogs. Proceedings of the 14th ACVIM Forum, San Antonio, TX, 1996, p 746.
Abstract describing the technique and outcome of thoracoscopic pericardiectomy in 12 dogs.

Rush JE, Keene BW, Fox PR: Pericardial disease in the cat: A retrospective evaluation of 66 cases. J Am Anim Hosp Assoc 26:39, 1990.
Retrospective study of 66 cats with pericardial disease looking at the causes and incidence of pericardial disease in this species.

Sisson D, Thomas WP, Ruehl WW, et al: Diagnostic value of pericardial fluid analysis in the dog. J Am Vet Med Assoc 184:51, 1984.
A study looking at the value of pericardial fluid analysis in determining the etiology of pericardial effusion in dogs.

Thomas WP, Sisson D, Bauer TG, et al: Detection of cardiac masses in dogs by two-dimensional echocardiography. Vet Radiol 25:65 1984.
A review of the technique and utility of two-dimensional echocardiography in the diagnosis of pericardial effusion and the etiology of the effusion.

CVT Update: Heartworm Testing and Prevention in Dogs

DAVID H. KNIGHT

Philadelphia, Pennsylvania

Few, if any, diseases are better known to dog owners than heartworms (*Dirofilaria immitis*). Heartworm awareness has been promoted to the veterinary profession and the public for many years by the American Heartworm Society, the American Veterinary Medical Association and its state affiliates, and highly competitive commercial interests. The remarkable spread of heartworm infection in the past 40 years and its well-known potential health consequences provide justifiable reasons for being familiar with this disease. The momentum that originally grew out of health concerns is now sustained by powerful economic interests as well, since an affluent dog-fancying public represents a major market for the diagnostic tests and antifilarial drugs that have become major sources of income for veterinarians and the companies that supply them. Heartworm disease is a dynamic area of interest, and each new development has expanded our options and necessitated reconsideration of how we deal with different aspects of this condition. In recent years, clinicians in most geographic regions have been primarily engaged in prospectively screening asymptomatic dogs for early detection of heartworm infection and in dispensing chemoprophylaxis. The discussions that follow are consistent with the most recent recommendations of the American Heartworm Society (Seward and Knight, 1999) but express the author's personal viewpoint and emphasis.

PROSPECTIVE SCREENING

Heartworm infection is a potential, if not already established, entity in most communities in the continental United States. Although heartworms can spread through vector transmission directly from the borders of endemic zones, those living in seemingly isolated regions must be alert to the importation of already infected dogs. The resolve with which screening is conducted varies, depending on the perceived threat of heartworm infection. Even if infection has not been detected in the local population, some monitoring of dogs with the greatest opportunity for exposure to infective mosquitoes is important for ensuring timely awareness should the disease become endemic. In particular, dogs brought from elsewhere into communities with a low prevalence of infection should be tested as they are identified, since each reservoir in that environment may have important consequences.

Heartworm Antigen Testing

Since 1992, the American Heartworm Society has recommended that antigen testing be the primary mode of screening for heartworm infection. Very few dogs have circulating microfilariae without also having detectable antigenemia. When this situation does occur, it is generally a transient phase in lightly infected cases at about 6.5 months after infection when microfilariae begin to appear. Most of these dogs will become antigenemic by the time they are scheduled for retesting. Microfilariae are frequently absent in antigenemic dogs, however, and the diagnosis of heartworm disease will be missed in perhaps 20 to 25% of cases if it is based entirely on parasitologic findings. Heartworm infection in dogs without microfilaremia is referred to as being "occult."

Occult Infections

Etiology. Serologic testing was originally developed to identify microfilaria-negative dogs that had immune-mediated hypersensitivity to microfilariae. These dogs are frequently the same ones that display clinical signs of heartworm allergic pneumonitis or chronic pulmonary heart disease. Although still one of the most important types of occult infection, it may no longer be the most common now that monthly chemoprophylaxis has become widely practiced. The majority of dogs receiving chemoprophylaxis are given one of the macrolide endectocides, ivermectin or milbemycin oxime. Both drugs are microfilaricidal at prophylactic doses and also suppress microfilariae production (Lok and Knight, 1995). Infected dogs treated with these drugs either fail to become microfilaremic, or eventually become permanently microfilaria-negative. Additionally, infections composed of only one sex, or light infections in which the sexes are physically separated, will not produce microfilariae. Finally, prepatent infections are an important category of occult heartworm infection, since they are usually also antigen-negative in addition to being amicrofilaremic.

Occult Infections Detected by Antigen Tests. None of the commercial antigen test kits are able to detect infections composed only of male heartworms. However, each possesses a high degree of sensitivity for infections containing female worms. Prepatent infections generally produce insufficient antigen until about 5.5 to 6 months after infection, but some false-negative test results should be anticipated until the female worms reach maturity at about 7 months after infection. The amount of antigen in circulation bears a direct, though nonlinear, relationship to the number of mature females. Infections consisting of three or more mature females are generally detected (McTier, 1994; McTier et al, 1995). Given these caveats, immune-mediated, drug-induced, and female unisex occult infections should be reliably detected by antigen testing.

Role of Antigen Testing in Heartworm Prevention

Testing is an integral component of a concerted program of chemoprophylaxis. Ordinarily, it is the first step in such a program unless the dog has yet to be exposed, or exposure is too recent for antigenemia (or microfilaremia) to have developed. It is imperative that the infection status be known at the start of chemoprophylaxis if infection due to subsequent lapses in protection is to be distinguished from pre-existing infections. In highly endemic regions, it is prudent to obtain a second negative test result a year after starting chemoprophylaxis before one assumes that the program has begun effectively. Thereafter, surveillance should be continued by retesting periodically (every 2 to 3 years), or after an appropriate interval following a lapse in protection.

Test Timing for Best Results. At certain times, testing is pointless. The testing window does not open until the

heartworms are sufficiently mature to produce detectable levels of circulating antigen (or microfilariae). In dogs that are destined to become antigen-positive, antigen will not be found consistently until 7 months after infection. Therefore, 7 months is the absolute minimum age any puppy born during the transmission season should attain before being tested. Before infection is ruled out on the basis of a negative antigen test result, this latent period should be added to the last date on which infection is considered possible. An awareness of the local heartworm transmission season is a prerequisite for making such calculations (see Heartworm Transmission Season later in this article).

In practices doing a high volume of testing, it is difficult to schedule all dogs to come back for retesting in the same 2- to 3-month period of time before transmission resumes. Many clinicians, who insist on retesting annually, stagger the dates throughout the year, not realizing that (depending on the timing) they may partially defeat their goal of early detection. Consider the implications in an area where the transmission season ranges from the middle of June to late September, which is typical for most of the United States. In the event that infection occurred at the earliest possible date and the dog is on a December annual testing schedule, that infection would be near the end of its latent period in December and therefore probably would not be detected before the next December, 18 months after infection. A similar interval would pass for a dog infected in late September and tested in early April. Testing yearly on the same schedule does not shrink this overlap. The fact of the matter is that if a dog is thought to be getting macrolide endectocide chemoprophylaxis when it really counts, annual retesting is unnecessary. Adequately protected dogs should be retested periodically, but a 2- to 3-year interval is sufficient.

Interpretation of Antigen Test Results

Widespread testing and chemoprophylaxis have had a noticeable effect on the morbidity of heartworm disease. Both the prevalence and the severity of infection have decreased, and more cases are being diagnosed before either physical or radiographic signs become evident. Consequently, the only indication of infection may be a weakly positive antigen test result. Contrary to what many would think, the reliability of these tests is not based on their ability to identify most infected dogs (sensitivity) but on their ability to hardly ever misdiagnose uninfected dogs (specificity). This low false-positive rate is critically important because the prevalence of heartworm infection in many communities is less than 5%, and may be much less than 1% in clinic populations in which prophylaxis is promoted and widely practiced. In the latter circumstance, even a false-positive rate of only 1% (99% specificity) reduces the predictive value of a positive test result to less than 50% (more false- than true-positive results), less informative than flipping a coin. If therapy is initiated on the basis of a false-positive result, considerable financial, if not medical consequences, will be incurred. On the other hand, the failure to identify a lightly infected dog with low antigenemia is unlikely to jeopardize its health and only temporarily delays recognition, assuming that the dog is retested and becomes positive in the interim. Fortunately, the specificity of the enzyme-linked immunosorbent assay (ELISA) and immunochromatographic antigen assays is sufficiently high to make them useful for testing dogs not expected to be infected.

Positive antigen test results should always be verified, especially if the test is only weakly positive. If *D. immitis* microfilariae are found in the blood, the diagnosis is confirmed. However, microfilariae may be absent, at least at that time, and there may be no convincing physical or radiographic signs of disease. In these instances, the antigen test should be repeated, with close attention paid to technical procedure, if the assay is performed at the hospital. It may also be useful to confirm the result by retesting with a different test format. Visualization of worms in the main pulmonary artery and proximal ends of its interlobar branches can be attempted by two-dimensional echocardiography, but this is very unlikely to be helpful in lightly infected dogs. Whenever the antigen test result is in conflict with the preponderance of the clinical evidence, the diagnosis should be considered suspect. Chemoprophylaxis can be prescribed if it was under consideration, and the patient should be treated as a normal dog pending further antigen testing in several months time.

Antigen Test Selection

Antigen tests have become progressively more accurate and easier to use for on-site testing. Several commercial kits utilizing different methods and test formats are available (Table 1).

Although reference laboratories provide this service, the semiquantitative estimate of antigenemia that can be assessed from visual inspection of the ELISA and ICT assays is not usually reported. This additional information complements the physical examination and radiographic evaluations of disease by providing an indication of the current severity of infection. The degree of parasitism is an important consideration in developing a management strategy for infected dogs and, in those that are treated, in evaluating adulticide efficacy 4 months after administration.

Other references should be consulted for a more detailed description and comparison of the different antigen tests (McTier, 1994; McTier et al, 1995). Each has special attributes that may make it preferable to another in certain circumstances. Following are some of the factors that the clinician should consider when selecting one or two tests that best match the needs of a particular practice.

Accuracy. The accuracy of all the commercial kits is good to excellent. Small differences in sensitivity alone should not define suitability. Both the sensitivity and the specificity of the ELISA and ICT assays are better than those of the hemagglutination test, which lacks the endpoint resolution of the other two methods. The lower specificity of the hemagglutination test, in part because of difficulty in distinguishing agglutination from red blood cell rouleaux formation in some samples, makes this test less reliable for screening dogs with a low probability of infection. Statistics comparing accuracy should be evaluated critically, since many evaluations are not side by side comparisons on the same samples and the data may not reflect the latest test refinements.

Batch Versus Stat. Testing. When batch testing of large numbers of samples is desirable, the microwell systems are most efficient and cost-effective. However, they also require the most technical expertise. These tests are considered the benchmark because they are the only tests that include both true-positive and true-negative controls.

Performance Time. Except for the microwell systems, all the other tests are designed for individual stat. testing, although limited batching is possible with the ELISA and ICT stat. kits. The VetRED test provides the most prompt results but is critically time dependent and cannot be performed simultaneously with other tasks.

Convenience. The technical features of the antigen tests have been greatly simplified. The sample pretreatment step has been eliminated for the microwell systems and the test devices that accept plasma, serum or whole blood. In particular, the SNAP and ICT Gold devices have automated certain steps, thereby further reducing the possibility for operator error. The membrane on which the reaction develops in these tests can also be removed and preserved as a permanent record for comparison with subsequent positive results when infected dogs are tested serially.

To achieve the results these tests are capable of delivering, they must be performed as directed on high-quality fresh or frozen samples. These tests utilize immunochemical and enzymatic reactions; thus, it is critical that all reagents be brought to room temperature before the tests are performed.

Microfilaria Testing

The only time that microfilaria testing supersedes antigen testing is when chemoprophylaxis with diethylcarbamazine (DEC) is started or resumed, since this drug can be hazardous for microfilaremic dogs. A concentration (Knott or filter) test for microfilariae should be run to confirm each positive antigen test result, especially in asymptomatic dogs without other confirming evidence of infection, and to determine whether this life cycle stage need also be targeted as part of the filaricide therapy.

TABLE 1. Some Antigen Tests

Enzyme-Linked Immunosorbent Assays (ELISA)		
Microwell:	DiroCHEK	Synbiotics Corp., San Diego, CA
	PetCHEK HTWM PF	IDEXX, Westbrook, ME
Membrane:	SNAP Heartworm PF Antigen Test Kit	IDEXX
	UNI-TEC CHW	Synbiotics
Wand:	ASSURE/CH	Synbiotics
Colloidal Gold Technology		
Membrane:	ICT GOLD HW	Synbiotics
	WITNESS HW	Synbiotics
Hemagglutination		
Plate well:	VetRED Canine Heartworm Antigen Test Kit	Synbiotics

Species identification is usually apparent from the tapered shape of the head of *D. immitis* microfilariae.

CHEMOPROPHYLAXIS

Heartworm infection is easily prevented but can be difficult as well as costly to cure. Chemoprophylaxis should be encouraged whenever a reasonable chance of infection exists. Two classes of drugs are available. The monthly administered macrolide endectocides ivermectin (Heartgard-30 and Heartgard-30 Plus, Merial Ltd.) and milbemycin oxime (Interceptor, Novartis Animal Health US, Inc.) are currently the most popular choices. These products provide the advantages of greater convenience of administration, safety, and assurance of protection. Although once the mainstay of heartworm chemoprophylaxis, the daily administered piperazine derivative DEC (Filaribits and Filaribits Plus, Pfizer Animal Health and other brands) has been largely displaced by the macrolide endectocides.

Macrolide Endectocides. The prophylactic doses of both ivermectin (6 to 12 µg/kg) and milbemycin oxime (0.5 to 1.0 mg/kg) are nontoxic, even in Collie dogs that are sensitive to high doses. Despite the short half-lives, macrolide administration at monthly intervals has a prompt and complete filaricidal effect on precardiac (fourth stage) heartworm larvae before they mature to the pathologic adult stage. Where transmission pressure is heavy, continually aborted trickle infections may stimulate a degree of protective immunity that complements the efficacy of chemoprophylaxis. Once dogs are weaned, administration should be scheduled to begin within 1 month following the anticipated start of transmission and continue to within 1 month following the end of transmission. The retroactive efficacy of the macrolide endectocide, invermectin, has been documented to be as long as 4 months after infection, when monthly administration is continued for an additional 12 months (McCall et al, 1995). This extended period of protection increases the margin of safety and should not be encroached on by lengthening the normal interval of administration. However, in instances when a dog is already well into the transmission season before chemoprophylaxis has begun, the chance of infection may still be substantially reduced if chemoprophylaxis is promptly started. Furthermore, if adulticide therapy is declined or will be indefinitely delayed for a dog with a patent infection, monthly chemoprophylaxis can still be instituted, provided that the same precautions and monitoring normally follow when eliminating microfilariae are observed.

Diethylcarbamazine Citrate. Chemoprophylaxis with DEC is critically dependent on faithful adherence to daily administration (6.6 mg/kg) beginning in anticipation of exposure to infective mosquitoes and continuing for 2 months beyond the end of the transmission season. The omission of only a few doses can void protection. None of the creative flexibility accorded to the macrolides can be duplicated safely with DEC.

Heartworm Transmission Season

Transmission Model. Heartworm transmission requires the fortuitous convergence of microfilaremic canids acting as reservoirs of infection, mosquitoes that feed on dogs and are capable of serving as competent intermediate hosts and vectors, and a climate conducive to rearing mosquitoes and incubating microfilariae to the infective larval stage. While each is essential, climate is the controlling factor. The average daily temperature threshold for incubating infective larvae is 18°C (57°F). A prerequisite heat exposure must accumulate before larvae will mature to the infective stage. This maturation can take as few as 8 days at 30°C (86°F) or as many as 29 days at 18°C (65°F). At the lower ambient temperatures, mosquitoes seek hosts less actively and may not survive long enough for infective larvae to mature. Therefore, wherever transmission is possible in the Northern Hemisphere, it usually will be heaviest in July and August (Knight and Lok, 1995; Slocombe et al, 1995). The actual duration of transmission may be continuous in the subtropical climate of southern Florida or as brief as 3 months in the higher latitudes of northern Minnesota. Except for the Southeastern and Gulf States, transmission in the continental United States is estimated to be 6 months or less (Fig. 1). These projections are based on analysis of temperature data collected over a 30-year weather cycle and represent the extreme earliest and latest transmission dates (Knight and Lok, 1995). Based on limited field observations (McTier et al, 1992; Knight and Lok, 1995), the guidelines have provided a margin for error of several weeks. The maps in Figure 1 indicate the months in which first-day administration of macrolide chemoprophylaxis will follow the beginning or end of transmission within 30 days.

Policy Decisions. The key to heartworm prevention is motivating clients to administer chemoprophylaxis to their dogs. It is true that people sometimes forget the monthly schedule, but catastrophe is not necessarily the consequence of inconsistency. As a result of being overly wary that heartworm transmission might occur at any time, such as during a brief period of unseasonably warm weather in the off-season, and convinced that they must compensate for any possibility that their clients might forget to regularly treat their dogs, some clinicians have begun recommending chemoprophylaxis be continued all year. The first assumption behind this practice is incorrect, and the second is arguable at best. The time may be nearing when immunoprophylaxis or sustained-release drugs will put more control in our hands. In the meantime, a well-intentioned, perhaps, but misguided and self-serving policy that incurs considerable additional and unnecessary expense to clients is not good medicine, no matter how it is rationalized. Our duty is to provide medically sound advice in ways that our clients can comprehend. They must be convinced by real risks and make an informed, voluntary commitment to this effort. After clients have been provided with the means and our support, it becomes their responsibility to carry out the program. There is no evidence that a strategy of overkill, which obscures awareness of when caution is justified, will prevent critical lapses in protection. Unless heartworm transmission is clearly a threat at least 9 or 10 months a year, energy should be focused on providing protection during the time heartworm infection is actually possible.

Macrolide Heartworm Chemoprophylaxis
Estimated Timing of First Monthly Dose

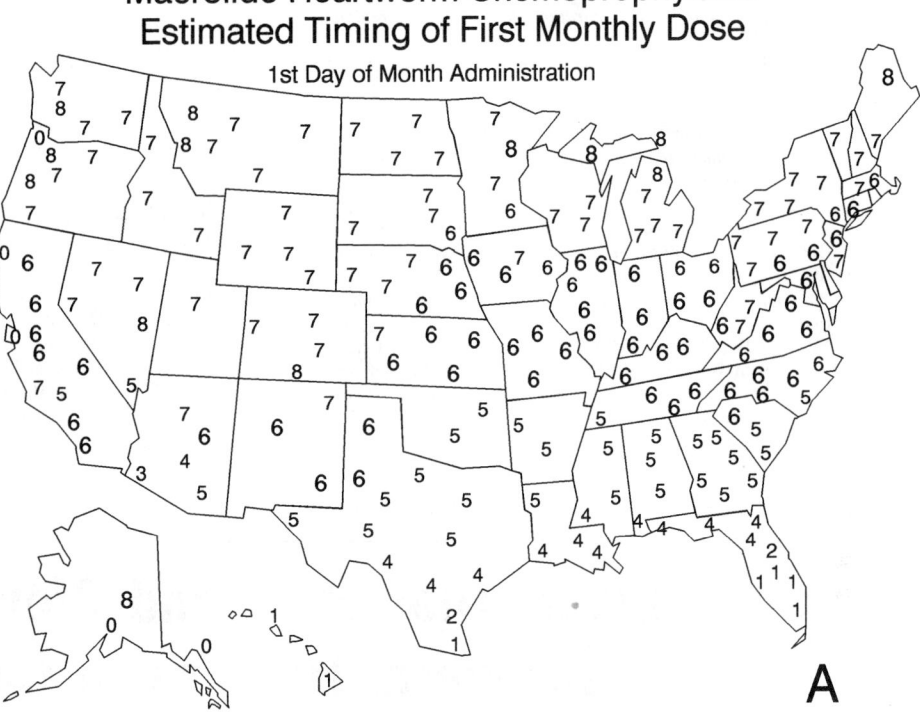

Figure 1. Numbers indicate the months in which the first (*A*) and last (*B*) doses of monthly administered heartworm chemoprophylaxis should be given to prevent infection under conditions most conducive to transmission. Numerals appear at the sites of nearly 200 weather stations. A one (1) for the first and last months indicates continuous all-year administration and zero (0) indicates no transmission. (From Knight DH, Lok JB: Seasonal timing of heartworm chemoprophylaxis in US. In: Soll MD, Knight DH, eds: Proceedings of the Heartworm Symposium 1995. Batavia, IL: American Heartworm Society, 1995, p 37. Reproduced with the permission of the American Heartworm Society.)

Macrolide Heartworm Chemoprophylaxis
Estimated Timing of Last Monthly Dose

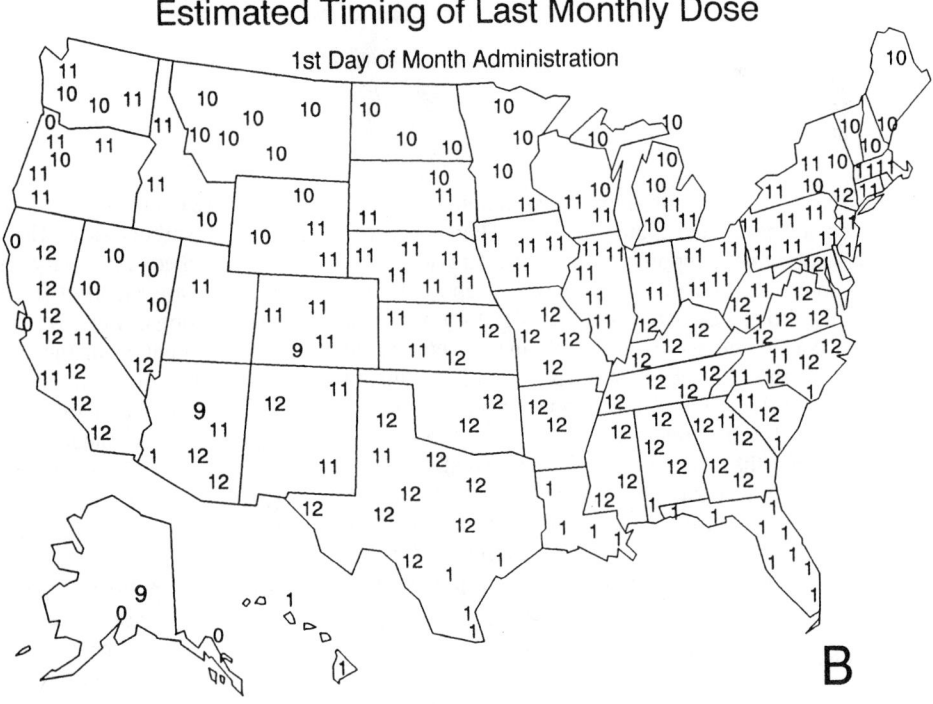

References and Suggested Reading

Knight DH, Lok JB: Seasonal timing of heartworm chemoprophylaxis in the United States. In: Soll MD, Knight DH, eds: Proceedings of the Heartworm Symposium '95. Batavia, IL: American Heartworm Society, 1995, p 37.
A preliminary survey based on temperature analysis defines regional transmission cycles.

Lok JB, Knight DH: Macrolide effects on reproductive function in male and female heartworms: Implications for diagnosis and treatment. In: Soll MD, Knight DH, eds: Proceedings of the Heartworm Symposium '95. Batavia, IL: American Heartworm Society, 1995, p 165.
Describes the mechanism of drug-induced occult infections and the utility of antigen testing in these circumstances.

McCall JW, McTier TL, Supakorndej N, et al: Clinical prophylactic activity of macrolides on young adult heartworms. In: Soll MD, Knight DH, eds: Proceedings of the Heartworm Symposium '95. Batavia, IL: American Heartworm Society, 1995, p 187.
Defines the limits of retroactive efficacy for ivermectin and milbemycin oxime.

McTier TL, McCall JW, Dzimianski MT, et al: Epidemiology of heartworm infections in beagles naturally exposed to infection in three southeastern states. In: Soll MD, ed: Proceedings of the Heartworm Symposium '92. Batavia, IL: American Heartworm Society, 1992, p 47.

Most important field study of seasonal heartworm transmission ever published.

McTier TL: A guide to selecting adult heartworm antigen test kits. Vet Med 89:528, 1994.
Excellent discussion of test attributes and selecting a test that fits individual needs.

McTier TL, McCall JW, Supakorndej N: Features of adult heartworm antigen test kits. In: Soll MD, Knight DH, eds: Proceedings of the Heartworm Symposium '95. Batavia, IL: American Heartworm Society, 1995, p 115.
Most recent and comprehensive comparison of all the commercial antigen test kits currently in production.

Slocombe JOD, Srivastava B, Surgeoner GA: The transmission period for heartworm in Canada. In: Soll MD, Knight DH, eds: Proceedings of the Heartworm Symposium '95. Batavia, IL: American Heartworm Society, 1995, p 43.
Detailed analysis of the effects of latitude and vector species on seasonal transmission.

Seward RL, Knight DH, eds: Recommended procedures for the diagnosis, prevention, and management of heartworm (*Dirofilaria immitis*) infection in dogs. In: Proceedings of the Heartworm Symposium '98. Batavia, IL: American Heartworm Society, 1999.
Concise and explicit guidelines based on a synthesis of the most recent clinical and experimental information.

CVT Update: Diagnosis and Prevention of Heartworm Disease in Cats

CLARKE E. ATKINS
Raleigh, North Carolina

WILLIAM G. RYAN
Iselin, New Jersey

Infection of a cat with *Dirofilaria immitis* was first recognized in the United States in 1922. There have been numerous subsequent reports, with a recent review (Ryan and Newcomb, 1996a) of 156 previously reported cases. Despite this, feline heartworm disease (FHWD) has generally been considered a novelty, with many veterinarians still believing that the cat is not at risk. This is an unfortunate misconception, as not only is the cat susceptible, but also its clinical signs are more severe than those of the dog, even when the worm burden is quite small. In recent years, increasing awareness has brought the development of better diagnostic tests, efforts at establishing a satisfactory adulticidal therapy, increasing public awareness, and, recently, the registration of a feline heartworm preventive.

PREVALENCE IN THE UNITED STATES

Heartworm infection is less common in cats than in dogs, approximating 5 to 20% of the canine prevalence in a given geographic area (Ryan et al, 1996b). This has led to a low index of suspicion for FHWD, with resultant underdiagnosis. In addition, the diagnosis of FHWD is often obscured because (1) cats are frequently amicrofilar-

emic; (2) serologic tests (respectively, the enzyme-linked immunosorbent assay [ELISA] antigen and antibody tests) have lacked sensitivity or specificity in cats; (3) worm burdens are small; (4) aberrant sites are more common than in dogs; and (5) clinical signs are often nonspecific and different from those seen in dogs. For these reasons, despite recent efforts at defining the scope of this problem in cats, the exact prevalence of FHWD is unknown and likely underestimated.

A review of studies reporting feline heartworm infection (FHWI) and a survey of veterinary practitioners revealed that the diagnosis has been made in 38 of the 50 United States (Fig. 1; Ryan et al, 1996b; American Heartworm Society, unpublished data). Not surprisingly, the greatest numbers of cases have been reported from the southeastern United States, the Eastern Seaboard, and the Gulf Coast and within the Mississippi River valley. Prevalence studies have focused mainly on cats from shelters. While this population choice has allowed the use of the relatively sensitive and very specific postmortem diagnosis, these studies are not necessarily applicable to pet cats, even in the same geographic region. These 12 studies, from 10 southeastern states, have revealed a prevalence of FHWI

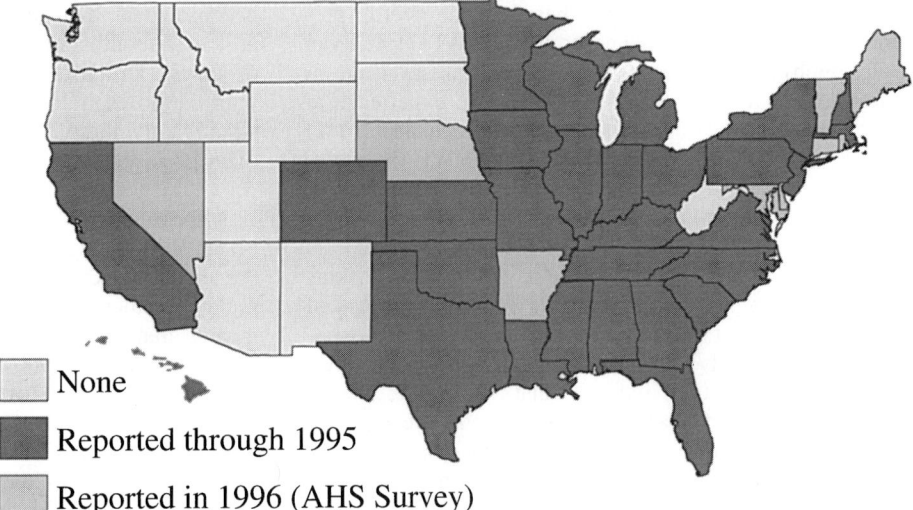

Figure 1. Map of the United States depicting the states that have reported feline heartworm infections through 1995 and those disclosed in a 1996 survey of members of the American Heartworm Society (AHS).

None

Reported through 1995

Reported in 1996 (AHS Survey)

ranging from 0 to 16% (Fig. 2). There are limited data in pet cats, but a joint study, performed on such cats presented to the teaching hospitals of North Carolina State University (NCSU) and Texas A&M University for evaluation of cardiorespiratory signs, demonstrated an infection prevalence of 9% and an exposure rate of 26%, the latter figure based on antibody titers (Atkins et al, 1996). A number of serologic surveys, largely in asymptomatic cats, have demonstrated exposure rates (antibody seropositivity) of 5 to 36%, even in areas not considered heavily heartworm endemic and as high as 43% in asymptomatic cats (Atkins, 1998a).

DIAGNOSIS

The diagnosis of FHWI or FHWD poses a unique and problematic set of issues. First, the clinical signs in cats are often quite different from those in dogs. Then, the diagnostic effort is often inadequate because the suspected

incidence in cats is low. Furthermore, the diagnosis is often elusive because eosinophilia is transient or absent; electrocardiographic findings are minimal; and most cats are amicrofilaremic. Radiography, while helpful, is neither adequately sensitive nor specific and requires expertise in interpretation. Echocardiography shows promise in terms of specificity but is costly and only moderately sensitive, and requires special equipment and expertise. Currently, the most useful tests include ELISA serologic tests. These too are imperfect. The antigen test is very specific but is inadequately sensitive, missing over 50% of natural infections (McCall, 1995). On the other hand, a recently developed feline antibody test is very sensitive, but its specificity is low, meaning that a positive test indicates exposure, but not necessarily adult infection (McCall et al, 1995).

Signalment, History, and Clinical Signs

While no breeds of cat have been shown to be at increased risk for FHWI, most authors do suspect a male

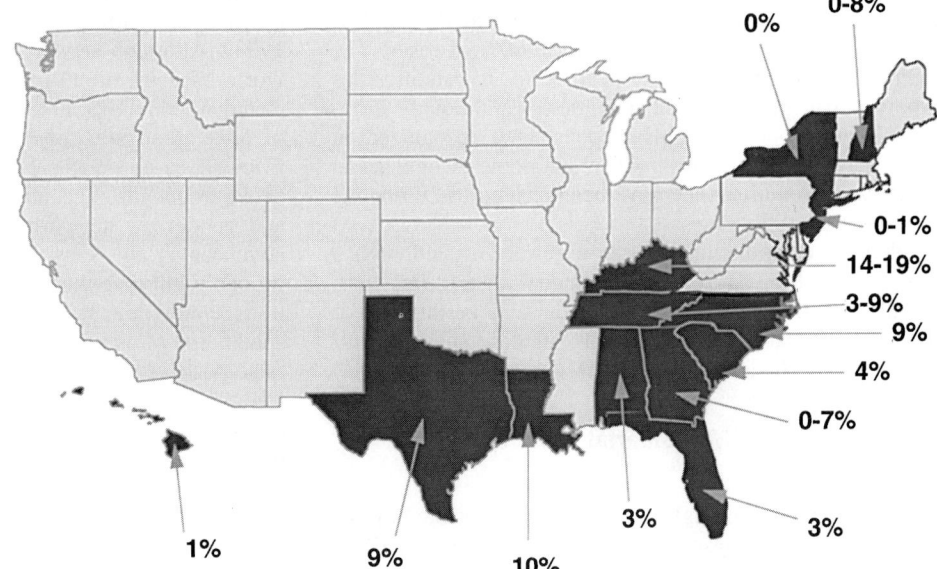

Figure 2. Map of United States depicting prevalence of *D. immitis* heartworm infection in cats, determined by postmortem or clinical surveys.

0%

0-8%

0-1%

14-19%

3-9%

9%

4%

0-7%

1%

9%

10%

3%

3%

predisposition. This suspicion is based on the overall preponderance of male cats diagnosed with FHWI (71%; Ryan et al, 1996b) and the greater experimental infection rate in males than in females (McTier, 1993). The experience at NCSU suggests, however, that while more males (61%) than females are indeed diagnosed with FHWI, the male-to-female ratio is not significantly different from that of the general population of cats seen at a teaching hospital (53% male; Atkins et al, 1998b) or the population of cats presented with cardiorespiratory signs (60% male; Atkins et al, 1996). The typical cat with FHWI is 4 to 6 years of age (range <1 to 19 years). The history of outdoor exposure would logically predict a heightened risk of FHWI; the experience at NCSU indicates that this is true. Nevertheless, one third of heartworm-infected cats are reported by their owners to be housed totally indoors. This may mean that owners misinterpret the question as to whether their pet goes outdoors or that indoor cats can be infected, or both. Although a seasonal incidence (August to December) has been suggested for FHWD (Guerrero et al, 1992), other studies do not support this contention (Atkins et al, 1998b).

Heartworm-infected cats may be asymptomatic, and clinical manifestations, when present, may take either an acute (often cataclysmic) or a chronic (often waxing and waning) course. Acute or peracute presentation is usually due to dead worm embolization or migration of worms to the central nervous system, and signs variably include salivation, tachycardia, shock, dyspnea, cough or hemoptysis, vomiting and diarrhea, syncope, dementia, ataxia, circling, head tilt, blindness, seizures, and death. Sudden death, with little or no premonitory signs, has been observed in approximately 23% of cases (Ryan et al, 1996b). Postmortem examination typically reveals pulmonary infarction with congestion and edema. Vena caval syndrome has also been recognized in cats.

Findings in chronic FHWD may include cough, dyspnea, anorexia, weight loss, lethargy, exercise intolerance, vomiting, and signs of right-heart failure. Cough is a relatively consistent finding (>50% of cases, compared with 15% in cats with cardiorespiratory signs, but not FHWI) and, when noted in cats in endemic areas, should increase the suspicion of FHWD. Likewise, dyspnea, though less specific than cough, is present in 40 to 60% of cases. The pulmonary response to in situ heartworms in cats includes type II cell hyperplasia and activation of pulmonary intravascular macrophages. This response, not recognized in dogs, may explain the asthma-like syndrome recognized in some cats, even after they have been cleared of *D. immitis* (Dillon et al, 1996).

Physical examination is often unrewarding, although a murmur, gallop, and/or diminished or adventitial lung sounds may be noted. In addition, cats may be thin and/or dyspneic. If heart failure is present, jugular venous distention, pleural effusion, and rarely ascites are detected.

Hematology and Microfilarial Tests and Serology

Hematology. Although the presence of eosinophilia or basophilia may increase the index of suspicion for FHWI, tests for these conditions are of limited value. This is true because these hematologic changes are transient (present at 4 to 7 months after infection) and present in only 33% of cases (Dillon, 1984). In a prospective study of cats with cardiorespiratory signs, those with FHWD were not significantly more apt to have eosinophilia or basophilia than those not shown to be infected (Atkins et al, 1996).

Microfilarial Tests. A definitive diagnosis of FHWI can be made by the detection of circulating microfilariae, using the modified Knott test, millipore filter, direct smear, or microhematocrit techniques. A recent literature review indicated that 36% of 45 cats with FHWD were microfilaremic (Ryan et al, 1996b), while other reports have indicated no more than 20% of infected cats are microfilaremic (Dillon, 1984; Atkins et al, 1996). This discrepancy probably reflects the fact that at the time of early reports diagnostic methods were limited to microfilarial tests and postmortem examination. While increasing the volume of blood samples, multiple testing, and drawing evening samples may increase the diagnostic efficiency of the microfilaria-dependent tests, the low percentage of cats that become microfilaremic, the transient nature of microfilaremia, and the low microfilarial numbers seriously limit their utility.

Antigen Tests. Although virtually 100% specific, ELISA antigen tests have been of somewhat limited use in cats because of the inability of these tests to detect low worm burdens (≤2 worms); in general, infected cats have 1 to 12 (most often 1, almost always <5) worms. Additionally, current tests detect antigens presumably produced in the reproductive tracts of mature female worms; thus, they do not detect immature (<7 months) or all-male infections. These factors may result in false-negative results, and their importance is underscored by a recent review of 108 naturally occurring cases of FHWD that revealed that 53% harbored single-worm infections and 18% had all-male infections (Ryan et al, 1996b). Furthermore, it is now clear that clinical signs may exist prior to worm maturation, at a time when cats are antigen negative. These limitations are demonstrated in two studies. First, in a study of six commercial ELISA antigen tests, positive test results were obtained, 36 to 93% of the time, from the sera of 31 known positive cats harboring 1 to 7 female worms (McTier et al, 1993). Although sensitivity increased with greater female worm burdens, no all-male heartworm infections were detected. Second, a commercial antigen test allowed detection of fewer than 40% of necropsy-proven natural infections (McCall et al, 1995). False-negative antigen test results occur frequently, depending on the test used, the maturity and gender of the worms, and the worm burden. Recent advances in the sensitivity of ELISA antigen tests will probably improve their efficiency in the diagnosis of infections containing at least 1 female worm. Although the specificity of antigen tests is well accepted, the risk of false-positive results increases with low prevalence. Therefore, positive test results should be confirmed by a second test or supported by the presence of appropriate clinical findings (e.g., cough, radiographic lesions, echocardiography).

Antibody Tests. There are now three commercially available, "send-off" ELISA antibody tests, designed specifically for the diagnosis of FHWI (Animal Diagnostics, Inc., St. Louis, MO, HESKA Corporation, Fort Collins, CO, and Antech Diagnostics, Farmingdale, NY) and two ELISA antibody tests (ASSURE/FH, Synbiotics Corp, San Diego, CA, and Solo Step PH, HESKA Corp, Fort Collins, CO) designed for "in-house" use. There is now published documentation only on the "send-off" tests, suggesting higher specificity than has been found with previous antibody tests (McCall, 1998). Although less specific than the antigen tests, the commercial ELISA antibody test is capable of detecting male-only and immature infections and has been shown to be useful in the detection of FHWI, even when antigen test results are negative (McCall et al, 1995). The antibody tests were shown to be 100% specific in determining cats to be heartworm negative prior to infection and detected 80% of experimental infections by 2 months, 97 to 100% by 3 months, and 100% by 4 months after infection (McCall et al, 1998). The antibody test was used to screen 215 random-source cats and detected 7 of 8 necropsy-proven cases (sensitivity = 88%) but at the same time gave "false-positive" results for 21 cats (90% specificity). The strength of this test is in *ruling out infection* (>99% negative predictive value), but a positive test clearly does not always indicate mature or current infection

(positive predictive value = 25%). A negative antibody test indicates either no infection or an early (<50- to 60-day) infection. A positive test result is thought to mean that (1) adults are present in the heart and/or pulmonary arteries, (2) past resolved infection with antibodies is still present, (3) precardiac late larva 4 (L4) or immature L5 infection exists, or (4) ectopic infection is present. Ideally, a positive test result should be confirmed with an antigen test, echocardiography, or angiography and supported by the presence of appropriate clinical findings (e.g., cough, radiographic lesions). In addition to aiding in making a diagnosis of FHWI, the antibody test may be useful as a marker for exposure to heartworms, even in cats that never develop mature infection. Finally, the antibody test is currently the most logical screening test for asymptomatic cats.

Imaging: Radiography and Echocardiography

Radiography. Radiographic findings of FHWD (Fig. 3) include enlarged caudal pulmonary arteries, often with ill-defined margins; pulmonary parenchymal changes, including focal or diffuse infiltrates (interstitial, bronchointer-

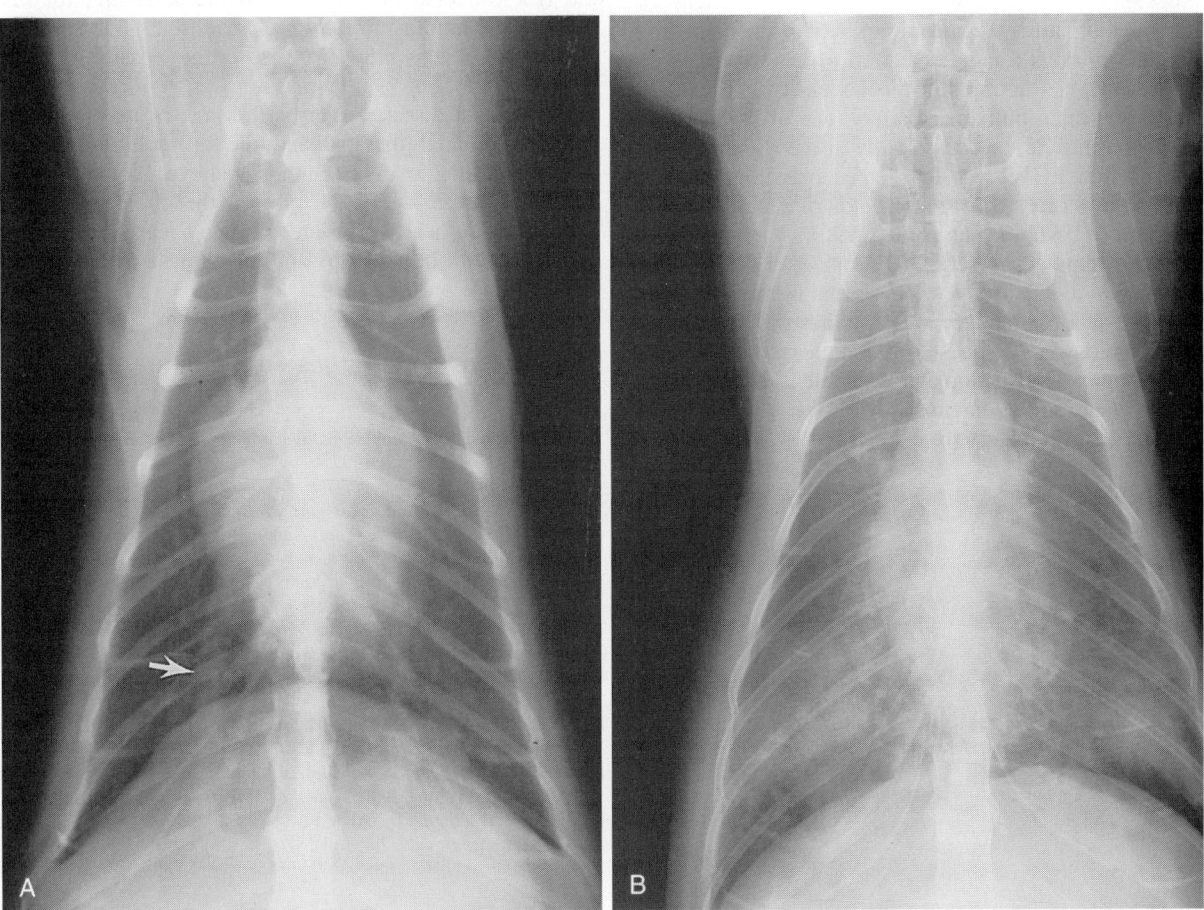

Figure 3. *A,* Thoracic radiograph from a cat with mild radiographic signs of heartworm disease. Note the right caudal pulmonary artery (*arrow*). The arrow is located in the ninth intercostal space, the site for comparison of the ninth rib with the pulmonary artery (*right or left side*). If the pulmonary artery is greater than 1.6 times the size of the rib, it is suggestive of heartworm disease (Schafer and Berry, 1995). *B,* Thoracic radiograph obtained from a more severely affected cat. Note the alveolar infiltrate in the caudal lung lobes. (From Schafer M, Berry CR: Cardiac and pulmonary artery mensuration in feline heartworm disease. Vet Radiol Ultrasound 36:499, 1995, with permission.)

stitial, or even alveolar); perivascular density; and, occasionally, atelectasis or pleural effusion. Pulmonary hyperinflation and right-heart enlargement may also be evident. Thoracic radiography has been suggested as an excellent screening test for FHWD. However, while often helpful, thoracic radiography is neither sensitive nor specific in making the diagnosis of FHWD. The single most sensitive radiographic criterion (left caudal pulmonary artery diameter greater than 1.6 times that of the ninth rib at the ninth intercostal space) can be identified in only 53% of cases (Schafer and Berry, 1995) and may also be noted in cats with heart failure, but not FHWI. Likewise, pulmonary parenchymal changes are only detectable radiographically in approximately 50% of natural cases (Schafer and Berry, 1995). Even though most cats with clinical signs have some radiographic abnormality, the findings are not specific for FHWD, are variable, and are often transient (Selcer et al, 1996). Lastly, radiographic abnormalities have been detected in experimentally exposed cats that ultimately resisted heartworm maturation and were negative on postmortem examination (i.e., false-positive; Selcer et al, 1996). On the other hand, pulmonary angiography can be used to make a definitive diagnosis by the demonstration of radiolucent intravascular "foreign bodies," as well as enlarged, tortuous, and blunted pulmonary arteries.

Echocardiography. Echocardiography is more sensitive in cats than in dogs for the detection of heartworm infection. Typically, a "double-lined echodensity" (Fig. 4) is evident in the main pulmonary artery, one of its branches, or the right ventricle, or occasionally at the right atrioventricular junction. FHWI was detected echocardiographically in 7 of 9 natural cases and 12 of 16 experimental infections (Atkins et al, 1996; Selcer et al, 1996). A retrospective review of a larger case series (DeFrancesco et al, 1998) revealed a lower sensitivity when worms were not specifically sought and, particularly, when studies were performed by noncardiologists. This observation underscores the need for a high index of suspicion and expertise if this technique is to be of value in the diagnosis of FHWI.

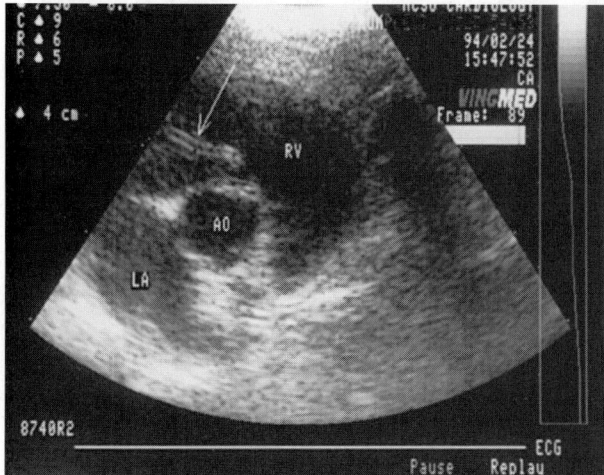

Figure 4. A two-dimensional echocardiogram obtained from a cat with heartworm disease. A double-lined density (adult heartworm, indicated by arrow) is evident and is diagnostic for heartworm infection. Ao, aorta; RV, right ventricle; LA, left atrium.

PREVENTION

Ivermectin, administered as a single dose of 24 μg/kg (Longhoffer et al, 1996), and milbemycin oxime, administered at 500 μg/kg in two doses 1 month apart (Stewart et al, 1992), effectively prevent FHWI when exposure has occurred during the previous month. In late 1996, the FDA approved ivermectin as a feline heartworm preventive for administration in a chewable formulation (Heartgard for Cats, Merial, Iselin, NJ). Ivermectin has been demonstrated to have an excellent safety profile, with no adverse effects in kittens at doses exceeding 110 μg/kg and doses of at least 750 μg/kg in adults (Longhoffer et al, 1996; Clark et al, 1992). Although not marketed for cats, milbemycin has recently received FDA approval as a feline heartworm preventive at a dosage of 2000 μg/kg.

Even though there is no reason to expect adverse reactions to prophylaxis in cats with existing FHWI, it could be useful to know the heartworm status of cats prior to the administratioan of a preventive. The current ELISA antigen tests have not yet been shown to be adequately sensitive for this purpose, unless the client is properly educated as to the limitations of the test. The ELISA antibody test (alone or with an antigen test) is currently more appropriate because of its higher sensitivity and ability to identify cats at risk (infected or exposed). While screening for FHWI before the administration of a preventive is not absolutely necessary, client education as to the possibility of pre-existing infection is imperative.

Based on disease severity, the lack of an effective and safe adulticidal therapy, and the difficulty in making a definitive diagnosis, the authors believe that cat owners in endemic areas should be offered the choice of their pet receiving a heartworm preventive. Clearly, cats already infected with heartworms and their house mates should be placed on a preventive.

References and Suggested Reading

Atkins CE, DeFrancesco TD, Miller M, et al: Prevalence of heartworm infection in cats with signs of cardiorespiratory abnormalities. J Vet Med Assoc 212:517, 1997.
   A prospective survey of the prevalence of heartworm infection in North Carolina and Texas cats with cardiorespiratory abnormalities. Prevalence, risk factors, and comparisons of diagnostic tests are provided.
Atkins CE: Veterinary CE Advisor: Heartworm disease: An update. Vet Med (Suppl) 93:12:2, 1998a.
   A comprehensive and very current review of the diagnosis and prevention of heartworm infection in dogs and cats.
Atkins CE, DeFrancesco TD, Coats J, et al: Feline Heartworm Disease: The North Carolina Experience. In: Soll MD, Knight DH, eds: Proceedings of the American Heartworm Symposium '98. Batavia, IL: American Heartworm Society, 1998b.
   Retrospective analysis of the risk factors, clinical presentation, diagnostic test results, and survival of 50 cats with heartworm infection.
Clark JN, Pulliam JD, Alva R, et al: Safety of orally administered ivermectin in cats. In: Soll MD, ed: Proceedings of the Heartworm Symposium '92. Batavia, IL: American Heartworm Society, 1992, p 103.
   Documents the safety of high-dose ivermectin in adult cats.
DeFrancesco TD, Atkins CE, Miller MW, et al: Diagnostic utility of echocardiography in feline heartworm disease. In: Soll MD, Knight DH, eds: Proceedings of the American Heartworm Symposium '98. Batavia, IL: American Heartworm Society, 1998.
   A review of a number of reports of the efficacy of echocardiography in the diagnosis of feline heartworm infection.

Dillon AR: Feline dirofilariasis. Vet Clin North Am 114:1184, 1984.
An overall review of the pathogenesis, risk factors, clinical signs, diagnosis, and treatment of feline heartworm disease.

Dillon AR, Warner AE, Molina RM: Pulmonary parenchymal changes in dogs and cats after experimental transplantation of dead *Dirofilaria immitis*. In: Soll MD, Knight DH, eds: Proceedings of the Heartworm Symposium '95. Batavia, IL: American Heartworm Society, 1996, p 97.
Describes electron micrographic and perfusion scan findings in dogs and cats with transplanted heartworms. Cats demonstrated type II cell hyperplasia and activation of pulmonary intravascular macrophages, unlike dogs, possibly explaining intraspecies differences in clinical presentation.

Guerrero J, McCall JW, Dzimianski MT, et al: Prevalence of *Dirofilaria immitis* infection in cats from the southeastern United States. In: Soll MD, ed: Proceedings of the Heartworm Symposium '92. Batavia, IL: American Heartworm Society, 1992, p 91.
A review of cases of feline heartworm disease seen through the Veterinary Medical Data Base, at Louisiana State University, and in three shelters in the Southeast. Comparisons of feline and canine prevalence, clinical signs, diagnostic efficiency, and feline worm burdens are provided.

Longhoffer SL, Daurio CP, Plue RE, et al: Ivermectin for the prevention of feline heartworm disease: Efficacy and safety. In: Soll MD, Knight DH, eds: Proceedings of the Heartworm Symposium '95. Batavia, IL: American Heartworm Society, 1996, p 177.
Describes the use of ivermectin as a heartworm and hookworm preventive in 2,500 cats, worldwide. Demonstrates the safety and efficacy of this drug in cats.

McCall JW, Nonglak S, Ryan W, et al: Utility of ELISA-based antibody test for detection of heartworm infection in cats. In: Soll MD, Knight DH, eds: Proceedings of the American Heartworm Symposium '95. Batavia, IL: American Heartworm Society, 1995, pp 127–133.
A prospective study of the usefulness of antibody and antigen tests in naturally occurring feline heartworm infection.

McCall JW, Guerrero J, Supakorndej P, et al: Evaluation of antigen and antibody tests for detection of heartworm infection in cats. In: Soll MD, Knight DH, eds: Proceedings of the American Heartworm Symposium '98. Batavia, IL: American Heartworm Society, 1998.

A prospective study of the usefulness for detecting experimental feline heartworm infection, comparing three antibody tests to each other and to two antigen tests.

McTier TL, Supakorndej N, McCall JW, et al: Evaluation of ELISA-based adult heartworm antigen test kits using well-defined sera from experimentally and naturally infected cats. In: Proceedings of the 38th Annual Meeting of the American Association of Veterinary Parasitologists, Minneapolis, 1993, p 37. (Abstract.)
Demonstrates the utility of ELISA antigen tests for the diagnosis of feline heartworm infection with a female worm or worms, but not all-male infections.

Ryan WG, Newcomb KM: Prevalence of feline heartworm disease: A global review. In: Soll MD, Knight DH, eds: Proceedings of the Heartworm Symposium '95. Batavia, IL: American Heartworm Society, 1996a, p 79.
Exhaustive review of all reported cases of heartworm infection in cats worldwide.

Ryan WG, Gross SJ, Soll MD: Diagnosis of feline heartworm infection. In: Soll MD, Knight DH, eds: Proceedings of the Heartworm Symposium '95. Batavia, IL: American Heartworm Society, 1996b, p 121.
Review of diagnostic tests, their utility and weaknesses, as well as risk factors and clinical signs.

Schafer M, Berry CR: Cardiac and pulmonary artery mensuration in feline heartworm disease. Vet Radiol Ultrasound 36:499, 1995.
Comparison of intrathoracic measurements and subjective comparisons between normal and heartworm-infected cats, demonstrating the utility of some measurements for making a diagnosis of heartworm disease.

Selcer BA, Newell SM, Mansour MS, et al: Radiographic and 2-D echocardiographic findings in eighteen cats experimentally exposed to *D. immitis* via mosquito bites. Vet Radiol Ultrasound 37:37, 1996.
Study of echocardiographic findings and serial radiographic changes in experimentally infected cats, showing development and progression or regression of abnormalities of feline heartworm disease.

Stewart VA, Hepler DI, Grieve RB:. Efficacy of milbemycin oxime in chemoprophylaxis of dirofilariasis in cats. Am J Vet Res 53:2274, 1992.
Study of the efficacy and safety of milbemycin oxime in 45 cats experimentally exposed to heartworms.

Current Uses and Hazards of Melarsomine

CLARENCE A. RAWLINGS
JOHN W. MCCALL
Athens, Georgia

Melarsomine dihydrochloride was released in September 1995 and has replaced thiacetarsamide as the agent for killing adult heartworms. This transition occurred quickly in the United States and was based on experiences gained from extensive clinical trials in the United States and several years of use in practice in Australia and Europe. The advantages of melarsomine are minimal hepatic and renal toxicity, greater efficacy at killing immature and adult heartworms, and the option of an alternative dosage, which distributes drug-induced thromboembolism over two periods instead of being concentrated after a single series of treatments. Acceptance of melarsomine has been smooth because its role in heartworm disease management is essentially the same as for thiacetarsamide.

USE OF MELARSOMINE DIHYDROCHLORIDE

Efficacy

The brand name for melarsomine dihydrochloride is Immiticide, a product that was developed by Rhone-Merieux. Melarsomine, a trivalent thioarsenite like thiacetarsamide, kills adult heartworms in a fashion similar to that of thiacetarsamide. The toxicity and efficacy of these arsenals are different, probably because of different pharmacokinetics. Intramuscular injection can be used because one half of the melarsomine injected into lumbar muscles is absorbed within 5 minutes. Maximal blood concentrations of arsenic are reached within 10.7 minutes. The recommended dosage of 2.5 mg/kg injected intramuscularly twice, 24 hours apart, yields a total dosage of 5 mg/kg, with a 0.75 mg/kg dose of elemental arsenic. In comparison, four thiacetarsamide injections deliver approximately twice as much arsenic, with 8.8 mg/kg of drug containing 1.56 mg/kg arsenic (Raynaud, 1992). Despite a treatment of less than half the arsenic dosage of thiacetarsamide, melarsomine kills more worms. Melarsomine produces a mean arsenic retention five times longer and a body clearance three times lower than that of thiacetarsamide. These differences between the thioarsenites may be related to the arsenic distribution in blood. Thiacetarsamide binds extensively to red blood cells; in contrast, no arsenic is detected in red blood cells during the first 6 hours after melarsomine injection. Arsenic bound to red blood cells is not thought to be ingested by or to effect heartworms (Raynaud, 1992).

The ability of melarsomine to kill heartworms has been evaluated in dogs that have had worms of known ages and gender transplanted into them, in dogs with naturally acquired infections that are obtained for research from random sources, and in those dogs that belong to clients. In the transplant model, melarsomine at 2.5 mg/kg given twice at a 24-hour interval killed more than 90% of both adult and 4-month-old worms. A single melarsomine injection kills nearly 90% of the male and 20% of the female worms, resulting in death of approximately one half of the worms. When the single injection was followed by the full two-injection treatment in 1 to 2 months (alternate regimen), 100% of male and 98% of female worms were killed (Immiticide, 1995; Keister et al, 1992). In contrast, thiacetarsamide produces kill rates as low as one third of young female heartworms and only slightly more than 90% for male worms of all ages (Rawlings et al, 1983).

Efficacy in client-owned dogs can be established by decreased antigen concentration and clinical improvement. Clinical improvement has been confirmed in all melarsomine studies. Client-owned dogs studied in the United States by Rhone-Merieux had an 80% or higher seroconversion rate from the previously positive antigen test results (Immiticide, 1995; Miller et al, 1995). Antigen presence was determined at 4 months after melarsomine using more modern and sensitive test kits. The average antigen concentration was reduced to approximately 1% of pretreatment concentrations, indicating nearly complete elimination of worms. In contrast, thiacetarsamide produced seroconversion in approximately two thirds of the dogs, and the antigen concentration was reduced to approximately 10% of pretreatment concentrations (Miller et al, 1995). When a less sensitive test system was used, seroconversion from positive test results after melarsomine treatment exceeded 98% (Vezzoni et al, 1992).

Patient Evaluation Before Administration

Since melarsomine is more effective than thiacetarsamide in killing heartworms, and heartworm death produces thromboembolism, it is critical that patients be more thoroughly evaluated before melarsomine treatment. When a greater number of heartworms are killed, thromboembolism increases pulmonary disease (Rawlings et al, 1993). We compared the thromboembolism in a controlled study of two groups of dogs: one group was treated with melarsomine and the other group was treated with thiacetarsamide.

In this controlled study, there was no difference in the severity of thromboembolism (Rawlings et al, 1993), but there are clinical reports of dogs with severe embolism after melarsomine treatment. These client-owned dogs with severe thromboembolism after melarsomine therapy frequently have been recently acquired or have had no preventive treatment. Most dogs had not had radiography. Thorough evaluation might have predicted that such dogs carried a heavy infection.

Before any heartworm treatment, the clinician should obtain a thorough history, complete a physical examination, and evaluate a microfilarial concentration test, a heartworm antigen test, thoracic radiographs, a urinalysis, and a complete blood count. In theory, an antigen concentration test could predict the severity of thromboembolism, as antigen concentration correlates with the number of female worms. Such an antigen test is not commercially available. However, although a rapid change to a positive test result in available kits may be suggestive of a high antigen concentration. Although there is a positive correlation between the number of female heartworms and antigen concentration, dogs infected with young heartworms may have no or low antigen concentrations. Since melarsomine can kill young heartworms, even some dogs with low antigen concentrations may experience severe thromboembolism after treatment. The intensity of pretreatment evaluation should depend on the dog's age, the local heartworm incidence, and clinical signs. Older patients and patients with either clinical signs (respiratory, cardiovascular) or coexistent conditions may need more diagnostic studies, particularly a serum chemistry profile, platelet count, and coagulation studies. The goal for this evaluation is to characterize the severity of heartworm disease and to detect other diseases.

A classification system was developed to customize melarsomine treatment. Class 1 dogs are asymptomatic or have mild clinical signs. Class 2 dogs have moderate signs that usually include coughing, radiographic evidence of pulmonary disease, mild anemia, or mild proteinuria. Class 3 dogs have severe pulmonary or cardiac dysfunction, that is, dyspnea or ascites. Class 4 dogs have caval syndrome and should undergo surgery to remove heartworms (Immiticide, 1995).

Administration

Class 1 and 2 dogs are treated with the 2.5 mg/kg intramuscular injections on consecutive days, whereas class 3 dogs are given only one initial injection. One to 2 months after the initial single injection of melarsomine, class 3 dogs receive the standard two injections, an approach called the *alternate regimen*. It is the judgment of the clinician as to whether some class 1 or 2 or even all patients should be treated by the alternate regimen. Melarsomine is packaged as 50 mg of dry powder that is reconstituted with 2 ml of water and given at 1 ml/10 kg of body weight. Care should be taken to inject all the melarsomine deeply into the epaxial muscle and avoid leaving a subcutaneous tract. This is performed with 22-gauge 1.5-inch needles in dogs greater than 10 kg and 23-gauge 1-inch needles in smaller dogs. An injection needle should replace the needle used to aspirate melarsomine from the vial. The injection should be completed before needle withdrawal from the lumbar muscle. These details are well illustrated in the product information. Some practitioners have been concerned about injecting more than 5 ml into a single intramuscular injection site. These practitioners are advised to inject into two sites, with one being approximately two lumbar vertebrae cranial to the initial site. Supportive care should be provided as previously practiced with thiacetarsamide. Exercise and stress must be limited during the 4 weeks after each melarsomine treatment.

The assignment of classification with the decision to use the alternate-dose regimen and the use of supportive care is based on the veterinarian's interpretation of clinical disease. Sick dogs may be symptomatically treated either before or after melarsomine administration. Ancillary treatments for complications of canine heartworm disease are reviewed in the previous edition (see *CVT XII*, p. 879). Short (e.g., 1 week) to moderate courses of prednisone at anti-inflammatory doses (0.5 mg/kg once or twice daily) are useful for controlling pulmonary complications of heartworm disease (e.g., pneumonitis) before or during melarsomine treatment. Pulmonary medications including bronchodilators and cough supressants may be considered in the occasional case that fails to respond to corticosteroid therapy and killing of adult heartworms. Severe pulmonary or cardiac dysfunction is also likely to benefit from supplemental oxygen and cage rest. Administration of aspirin (5 mg/kg per day) or low-dose heparin in dogs with severe pulmonary vascular disease to prevent further vascular injury or thrombosis is still considered investigational, although the approach is used by some experienced clinicians. Congestive heart failure is not nearly as common as pulmonary parenchymal injury but, when present, is managed by weeks of strict exercise restriction or cage rest, furosemide (2 to 4 mg/kg SC, IM every 8 to 12 hours initially, then PO), and modest sodium restriction. Oxygen also reduces pulmonary vascular resistance in some dogs, but this therapy is limited to the hospital. Digoxin (0.005 mg/kg PO every 12 hours) and angiotensin-converting enzyme inhibitors (see p. 780) are generally limited to dogs that are unresponsive to diet, rest, and furosemide.

A few thousand dogs have been treated by practitioners, and many ancillary treatments have been used without reported adverse drug interactions with melarsomine. The biggest improvement in patient management procedures was found to be the use of the alternate regimen in a large series of Italian dogs treated for heartworm disease. This approach probably has a greater impact on treatment success than any other treatment (Vezzoni et al, 1992). The advantages of the alternate regimen are the spread of thromboembolism over two treatments and a higher heartworm kill rate than occurs with the standard regimen. The only disadvantages to treating all dogs as class 3 (alternate dosage) are cost and a concern about whether the client will return for the complete series. Melarsomine's greater safety and efficacy may modify our approach for killing adult heartworms in individual dogs because treatment of older and diseased dogs should be safer with the alternate dosage of melarsomine than with thiacetarsamide.

Management After Administration

Recommendations to identify and treat circulating microfilaria, when present, remain unchanged. Ivermectin (50 μg/kg PO) and milbemycin (0.5 mg/kg PO) remain effective microfilaricides given approximately one month after melarsomine. Neither is approved as a microfilaricide by the U.S. Food and Drug Administration. When microfilaricides are given, a microfilarial concentration test should be performed 3 weeks after microfilarial treatment. A preventive program should be initiated within 1 month of the microfilaricide administration. At 3 to 4 months after the melarsomine treatment, an antigen test can be performed to document the efficacy of adult heartworm death. When using an immunodiagnostic test with high sensitivity, positive test results may be produced by a small number of remaining female worms. The currently recommended antigen test systems can detect infection by a single female worm. Since melarsomine is much more effective in killing worms, dogs with persistent positive antigen test results should be retreated *only* if they are performance dogs or have persisting clinical signs.

HAZARDS OF MELARSOMINE ADMINISTRATION

Complications with thiacetarsamide include injection reactions, hepatic and renal toxicity, and pulmonary thromboembolism after heartworm death. The complication rate of injection reactions is low with phlebitis after intravenous thiacetarsamide administration and myositis after intramuscular melarsomine administration. The frequency of injection reactions is similar between the two arsenical drugs (Immiticide, 1995). Melarsomine has produced essentially no direct drug toxicity, but a few dogs have been reported as receiving an inappropriate dosage. Apparently the thiacetarsamide dosage (1 ml/10 pounds) was administered instead of the melarsomine dosage (1 ml/10 kg). The typical sign in overdosed dogs is panting. The toxic dosage of melarsomine is 2.5 to 3 times the recommended dosage, with the toxic signs related to noncardiogenic pulmonary edema. Intramuscular dimercaprol (3 mg/kg) reverses toxicity if administered early (Atwell et al, 1989), but dogs receiving the appropriate melarsomine dosage should not require dimercaprol.

The higher efficacy of melarsomine in killing young worms makes it likely that the thromboembolism after melarsomine administration would be greater in dogs with young worms than if these dogs were given thiacetarsmide. One study found that there was no difference in thromboembolism between the two adult heartworm–killing agents in dogs with similar types of infections, even though more worms were killed by melarsomine (Rawlings et al, 1993). Some protection may be provided by the different effects of these two agents on pulmonary vascular reactivity. The best method to reduce thromboembolism after treatment for adult heartworms should be the alternate-treatment regimen. Thromboembolism after melarsomine is managed with rest and anti-inflammatory doses of prednisone by the same procedures used for thiacetarsamide (see *CVT XII*, p. 879). An advantage of melarsomine is that the thromboembolism can be spread over two separate episodes by the alternate regimen. When a clinician has concerns that the treatment regimen will be complicated, the alternate regimen should be strongly considered.

References and Suggested Reading

Atwell RB, Sheridan AD, Buoro IBJ, et al: Effective reversal of induced arsenic toxicity using BAL therapy. Proc Am Heartworm Soc 155, 1989.
  Clinical signs and treatment of toxic dosages of melarsomine are described.
Immiticide Sterile Powder Package Insert (melarsomine dihydrocholoride): Rhone-Merieux, 1995.
  This insert presents full disclosure information about melarsomine.
Keister DM, Dzimianski MT, McTier TL, et al: Dose selection and confirmation of RM340, a new filaricide for the treatment of dogs with immature and mature *Dirofilaria immitis*. Proc Am Heartworm Soc 225, 1992.
  This is a summary of data of efficacy studies.
Miller MW, Keister DM, Tanner PA, et al: Clinical efficacy and safety trial of melarsomine dihydrochloride (RM340) and thiacetarsamide in dogs with moderate (class 2) heartworm disease. Proc Am Heartworm Soc 233, 1995.
  A clinical study of 104 class 2 dogs treated with melarsomine is discussed.
Rawlings CA, Keith JC Jr, McCall JW: Thiacetarsamide efficacy: One more study, using a different research model. Proc Am Heartworm Soc 141, 1983.
  The efficacy study of thiacetarsamide is discussed.
Rawlings CA, Raynaud JP, Lewis RE, et al: Pulmonary thromboembolism and hypertension after thiacetarsamide versus melarsomine dihydrochloride treatment of *Dirofilaria immitis* infection in dogs. Am J Vet Res 54:920, 1993.
  This article presents research comparing thromboembolism after thiacetarsamide versus melarsomine in dogs with heartworm infection.
Rawlings CA, Tonelli Q, Lewis RE, et al: Semiquantitative test for *Dirofilaria immitis* as a predictor of thromboembolic complications associated with heartworm treatment of dogs. Am J Vet Res 54:914, 1993.
  This article presents research comparing thromboembolism in dogs with high versus low heartworm antigen concentration.
Raynaud JP: Thiacetarsamide (adulticide) versus melarsomine (RM340) developed as macrofilaricide (adulticide and larvicide) to cure canine heartworm disease in dogs. Ann Rech Vet 23: 1, 1992.
  This presents a review of the development of melarsomine, particularly the pharmacokinetics, efficacy, and safety.
Vezzoni A, Genchi C, Raynaud JP: Adulticide efficacy of RM340 in dogs with mild and severe natural infections. Proc Am Heartworm Soc 231, 1992.
  This article presents a clinical study of 382 heartworm infected dogs treated with melarsomine.

Airway Management

JOAN C. HENDRICKS
LESLEY G. KING
Philadelphia, Pennsylvania

GENERAL CONSIDERATIONS

The respiratory tract has evolved a variety of sophisticated defense mechanisms to ensure that it is protected from the daily onslaughts of inhalation of dry, cold, contaminated air. In the normal animal, air traveling through the nasal turbinates is warmed and saturated with water vapor before it reaches the pharynx. The turbulent air flow in the turbinates causes particles larger than 10 μm to collide with the mucous surfaces, and they can then be removed. Clinical techniques that bypass the nasal turbinates, such as tracheostomy, nasopharyngeal or tracheal administration of oxygen, and positive-pressure ventilation all result in considerable damage to the respiratory mucosa. In the normal animal, once past the turbinates, smaller particles can penetrate deep into the trachea and bronchioles, but collide with the mucus layer of the ciliated epithelium, and are carried up to the pharynx by the delicate cilia of the mucociliary escalator.

The airway responds to inflammation in a stereotypical way, with proliferation of goblet and Clara cells, and the production of increased amounts of airway mucus. The mucociliary escalator may be unable to effectively transport abnormally viscous mucus toward the pharynx. Inflammation can also result in destruction and loss of epithelial cells, with subsequent loss of effective ciliary activity. Edema and infiltration of inflammatory cells leads to airway narrowing and an increase in airflow turbulence. This combination causes hypoxia due to ventilation-perfusion mismatch, and the inability to clear infections because the natural defense mechanisms have been crippled. In addition, increased mucus production poses some serious management problems when the airway is instrumented with endotracheal or tracheostomy tubes.

Efforts to preserve airway function are directed at support of two of the most important defense mechanisms of the respiratory tract. First, the function of the mucociliary escalator must be optimized by ensuring that respiratory mucus is fluid and easily moved in an orad direction by the fragile cilia of the respiratory epithelium. Second, the cough mechanism must be encouraged, as it is one of the most important means by which material can be eliminated from the airway.

Hydration

Systemic Hydration

Since 90% of airway mucus consists of water, the most important way of optimally maintaining airway clearance and normal airway hygiene is to maintain normal hydration. Systemic dehydration results in drying of the mucus and mucociliary layer, and should be carefully avoided. The clinician must walk a fine line between overhydration and resulting pulmonary edema, and the extent of hydration required for optimizing airway clearance. In the presence of inflammatory conditions such as bronchopneumonia, maintenance of adequate hydration is vital. Intravenous fluid therapy is usually beneficial, and diuretics should be avoided unless the patient is in severe distress. In contrast, noninflammatory conditions such as pulmonary edema or hemorrhage may be associated with relatively little additional mucus production, and in this case the lungs and airway should be maintained in a much dryer state.

Humidification

The second option for increasing the moisture content of airway mucus is humidification of inspired air. The term *humidification* refers to the saturation of air with water vapor. The amount of water vapor is determined by the temperature of the inspired gas—the warmer the air, the more water vapor it contains. Normally, air passing through the turbinates is humidified and warmed to body temperature as it contacts the mucosal surface. If the turbinates are bypassed, the airway mucosa is damaged by cold, dry air. Even in an airway that was otherwise normal, such irritation leads to increased mucus production, damage to the respiratory epithelial cells, influx of inflammatory cells, and edema. This injury may be even more profound in the previously injured airway. Humidification of inspired air may be achieved in several ways.

Most commonly, supplemental oxygen is humidified by bubbling through water prior to administration to the patient. Oxygen is bubbled through a flowmeter (Pressure-Compensated Flowmeter, Ohmeda International, 9065 Guilford Road, Columbia, MD 21046), to which a Jet Humidifier (Ohio Medical Products, Airco Inc, Madison, WI 53707) is attached. By bubbling through the water at room temperature, the oxygen is passively humidified and can therefore assist in preserving the integrity of the respiratory mucosa. This type of humidification should be used whenever supplemental oxygen is being administered to the awake patient.

A number of different options are available for the anesthetized and intubated patient. Specially designed heated humidifiers can be inserted into the breathing circuit (Cascade 1a humidifier, Puritan Bennett International Inc, PO Box 25905, Overland Park, KS 66226). By heating the inspired air to body temperature, the content of water vapor is increased, closely approximating the action of the turbinates. An alternative, less expensive option for short-term anesthesia is the use of an "artificial nose" in the breathing circuit. These are small, disposable plastic, heat and moisture exchangers that are attached to the end of the endotracheal tube (Humid-Vent 1, Glbeck Respiration, PO Box 711, 5-194; 27 Upplands Vasby, Sweden).

Nebulization

While humidification saturates the air with water vapor, nebulization loads the inhaled air with small spherical droplets of water or saline. The droplets are then deposited at various levels of the respiratory tract, depending on their size. The smaller the droplet, the deeper it penetrates, impacting the airway mucosa as a result of brownian motion, gravity, and changes in direction of air flow. Droplets larger than 10 μm impact the mucosa of the upper airway

and trachea. In contrast, droplets smaller than 0.5 μm are small enough to reach the alveoli and are exhaled rather than showering out on the mucosal surface. Most nebulizers in clinical use create droplets in the range of 2 to 5 μm, with some variability in the size of the droplets that are produced. In this size range, the droplets penetrate and impact the mucosa at the level of the small airways. The most commonly used nebulizers create droplets by use of ultrasound (UltraNeb99, Devilbiss Healthcare Worldwide, Somerset, PA 15501). Alternatively, disposable nebulizers are available that are driven by gas pressure from an oxygen source (Adjustable Entrainment Nebulizer Adaptor and Sterile 0.45% NaCl source, Automatic Liquid Packaging Inc, Woodstock, IL 60098). Disposable nebulizers offer the potential advantages of a minimal risk of transmission of infection between patients, and the option to provide oxygen supplementation simultaneously with nebulization.

Various solutions can be administered by nebulization. Bland solutions such as sterile water or saline are most commonly used, with 0.9% saline solutions thought to be most effective for moistening secretions. The animal should inhale the nebulized solution for 15 to 20 minutes, four to six times daily, and coupage (clapping the thorax with cupped hands) should be performed at the same time to stimulate coughing. Acetylcysteine is a mucolytic agent that decreases the viscosity of airway mucus by breaking down disulfide bonds in mucus glycoproteins. This drug can be added to the nebulization solution at a dose of 2 to 5 ml of the 10% solution. Some patients treated with nebulization, especially if acetylcysteine is added to the solution, may suffer from short-term bronchospasm and transient hypoxia. This adverse side effect can be prevented by administration of bronchodilators prior to nebulization.

Although the benefits of nebulization have not been documented in veterinary patients, clinical experience suggests that it is very beneficial for patients with viscous respiratory tract secretions, particularly those with bronchopneumonia. With the exception of gentamicin therapy for acute tracheobronchitis caused by *Bordetella bronchiseptica*, drugs such as antibiotics and bronchodilators are not commonly added to nebulization solutions. Questions exist regarding the effective distribution of aerosolized drugs, with much of the drug being swallowed after deposition in the pharynx, or being distributed to normal, rather than abnormal, bronchi. Since systemic drug therapy is usually effective and should never be replaced by aerosolized drugs, additional nebulization of drugs is generally unnecessary.

Coupage and Physical Therapy

It is impossible to overemphasize the importance of the cough mechanism for clearance of respiratory tract secretions, particularly in the presence of bronchopneumonia. Coughing promotes movement of material into the pharynx, where it can be swallowed or expectorated. Once the secretions have been moistened, the simplest way of stimulating coughing is by inducing an increased tidal volume during respiration by having patients engage in mild exercise, such as walking, if they are stable.

Coupage is performed by repeatedly and firmly striking the chest wall with a cupped hand, which stimulates the cough reflex and helps to "break up" secretions in the airways; this procedure is usually well tolerated. Patients with bronchopneumonia should be coupaged for 5 to 10 minutes several times daily, especially if they are unable to stand and move around. As an alternative that may save time in the busy veterinary clinic, vibrating massagers designed for human use are readily available and inexpensive, and when wrapped around the chest, seem to be effective in the mobilization of secretions. The use of postural drainage may also be helpful in some patients. To maximize gravitational drainage from the bronchi, coupage can be performed with the patient in lateral recumbency with the worst lung uppermost. Since this manipulation may worsen hypoxia, it may not be well tolerated by the most unstable patients.

POSTOPERATIVE CARE OF PATIENTS WITH TRACHEOSTOMIES

Introduction

The successful care of small animal patients who have received tracheostomies is largely a matter of common-sense and vigilance. However, experience has also provided some lessons for the postoperative management of these patients to ensure a happy outcome.

General considerations apply to any patient with a tracheostomy. However, there are differences between the management of a patient with a tracheostomy site that is expected to be a temporary measure and the care of a patient whose stoma is intended to be permanent.

General Considerations

Every measure should be taken to replace normal airway functions, with an awareness that all such efforts will be imperfect. Some damage to the tracheal epithelium is inevitable from the flow of dry, cool air; and the risk of infection is always present.

Humidification and Warming of Inspired Air

Artificial Nose. Unfortunately, some problems have limited the usefulness of this device in tracheostomized patients. First, for some weak or impaired patients the added dead space adds unacceptably to the work of breathing. Second, because of extended length of the tube, some patients catch or occlude the end of it more frequently than a standard tracheostomy tube that is flush to the skin. Finally, if the patient is producing large amounts of mucus or pus, the "nose" quickly becomes occluded.

Instilling Saline. A simple, inexpensive method of humidification is the instillation of a few drops of warm sterile saline into the tube using a 1-ml syringe (needle removed!) every 2 to 4 hours. This is an acceptable method, although the fluid may trigger an undesirably vigorous cough reflex.

Nebulization. If a nebulizer is available, this method is nearly ideal because it does not add to the dead space and

the fine mist does not trigger a cough reflex. A patient with copious secretions may benefit from coupage and/or suction after nebulization.

Humidifying the Room. In a hospital without a nebulizer, or at the owner's home, the patient can be placed in a small room such as a bathroom and hot water run to steam up the room for approximately 20 minutes every 4 hours.

Minimizing Infection

Contamination will inevitably be introduced into any tracheostomy site. Caretakers can prevent the aspiration of gross secretions or foreign material, and monitor the patient carefully for evidence of aspiration and/or infection. They can also optimize the patient's own reflexes by keeping secretions moist, by providing both airway humidification and appropriate systemic hydration.

In tracheostomized patients, it is easy to collect airway secretions through the stoma and perform cytology daily. Inflammation will virtually always be present; thus, if infection is suspected, it is prudent to submit the sample for culture.

Problems Related to the Stoma

Preventing Occlusion

Occlusion of the intratracheal portion of the tube can occur when pus or mucus accumulates, if a patient flexes its neck so that the tracheal wall seals off the internal opening, or if a strong, large dog bends and kinks the tube. The external opening can also be occluded. If the patient is very weak or is not fully alert, the appropriate protective reflexes can be deficient. It also seems that some of the patients who have been accustomed to chronic airway obstruction have minimal awareness of occlusion and do little to defend themselves. A practical approach to preventing such problems is to ensure that the patient is centrally located and that personnel monitor it constantly. Most patients learn, with time, to adjust their position when an occlusion occurs. Monitoring devices such as a pulse oximeter, or a carbon dioxide monitor attached to the end of the tracheostomy tube, are very helpful because their alarms will signal an occlusion in most cases.

Reducing Harmful Defense Mechanisms

Paradoxically, vigorous defense mechanisms can be a problem. The normal airway defensive response to a foreign object and local trauma to the airway are mucus production, cough, anxiety, and increasing respiratory efforts. All of these responses are detrimental when a tracheostomy tube is in place, causing more inflammation and increasing the risk of obstruction. In addition to the measures discussed above—warming and humidifying the air and guarding against infection—the best approach to avoid triggering these responses is to minimize manipulation of the tube, minimize suctioning or instilling foreign materials into the tube, and keep the animal calm. In the Intensive

Care Unit of the Veterinary Hospital of the University of Pennsylvania, we suction airways relatively rarely, preferring to use other means of removing secretions (removing and cleaning the tube; coupage). Although a suctioning apparatus (either a cannula attached to wall suction or a simple red feeding tube) should be available, vigorous suctioning increases tracheal trauma and patient discomfort. Additionally, profuse secretions cannot be removed by suctioning alone, but rather may require removal and replacement of the entire tracheostomy apparatus. To keep the patient from becoming anxious and hyperventilating and coughing, soothing the patient and holding its head and neck at an angle that reduces the tendency to internal occlusion and trauma is a far better approach than the use of sedatives, simply because sedation increases the risk of occlusion. However, when an animal is frantic or when the requisite personnel are unavailable, sedation with acepromazine (PromAce, Fort Dodge), 0.03 to 0.05 mg/kg IM, SC, or IV, or diazepam (Valium, Roche), 0.5 mg/kg IV, may be helpful. If long-term sedation is required because the necessary personnel are not available, it is wise to consider referring the patient to a facility with 24-hour trained nursing care.

Wound Care

Tracheostomy wounds are usually simple, open wounds. Although they are contaminated, they usually heal well. However, twice-daily inspection of the wound margins is very important. Internal tracheitis or tracheal necrosis may be signaled by an increase in purulent or bloody secretions or coughing. A wash and aspiration for cytology and culture, and/or direct inspection via bronchoscopy, may be necessary for diagnosis.

Different Considerations for Temporary and Permanent Tracheostomies

Temporary Tracheostomies

The reasons for a temporary tracheostomy are extremely variable and dictate different approaches to postoperative management. In the simplest instances, the tracheostomy tube is left in place simply as a precaution after airway surgery, but after recovery from anesthesia it may well be possible to remove it. Where airway trauma has been extensive or chronic, a longer period of observation and time for wound healing may be necessary. A tracheostomy for ventilation performed to deal with a life-threatening problem will have to be maintained until the underlying problem resolves. The patient's history, including occurrences of problems during surgery and anesthesia, may modify the level of vigilance for complications, such as aspiration pneumonia, and will also determine the timing and means of weaning the patient from its artificial airway.

Weaning and removal of the tube is simplest when the patient is fully alert and calm, has a competent and untraumatized respiratory system, and has a narrow tube in place. In these instances, the clinician should choose a time when the patient can be observed without distraction for at least an hour. Manually occlude the tube while holding a

hand or the tubing from a carbon dioxide end-tidal monitor near the nose and mouth to confirm air flow through the upper airways. If airflow is apparent and the patient does not seem distressed by a 30-second occlusion, tape the opening closed and allow the patient to breathe around the tube for several minutes. If the patient seems completely comfortable after 20 to 30 minutes, you may try additional stresses by introducing exercise or food; or simply remove the tube and continue to observe for several more hours.

When a tube that fills the airway is in place, for example a cuffed tube used for ventilation, occlusion is not an option. The clinician will have to remove the tube in order to assess the patient's response. In such cases, the patient should be fully alert but calm, if possible. Personnel should be available to assist the patient for several hours, and blood gases should confirm that it is possible to maintain normal blood gases without the tube in place. For the first several hours after tube removal, the patient is monitored for any signs of discomfort, increased effort, stridor, or hypoxia. A pulse oximeter can provide early warning of hypoxia. The patient should be observed while it adopts various postures; eats and drinks; and sleeps. All of these behaviors present risks of occlusion.

At discharge, owners should be shown how to clean the site to remove secretions gently with a gauze pad moistened with clean water or sterile saline. They should also be instructed to observe for any increased cough, discharge, noises, local discomfort, swelling, and smell and, most especially, any difficulty in breathing. Bathing or swimming are prohibited until the wound has healed. Suture removal or a final inspection of the wound at 7 to 10 days after the surgery is routine.

For the long term, the owner should be aware that all tracheostomies narrow the airway slightly during the healing process. This is not ordinarily a problem because the normal cross-sectional area of the trachea is far greater than what is needed for quiet respiration. In the more unusual case in which there have been multiple airway surgeries, congenital airway narrowing, or extensive resection, the narrowing that occurs during healing may result in clinical signs such as stridor and exercise intolerance.

Permanent Tracheostomies

A variety of situations require a permanent tracheostomy. Some examples are an upper airway tumor that required wide resection; chronic airway obstruction leading to laryngeal collapse; or severe tracheal collapse.

In most cases, the local care of the tracheostomy is a very simple matter. All caretakers must be aware of the fragility of the wound site and take care not to interfere with the desired healing between the trachea and skin; thus, manipulation of the wound site should be as rare as possible and very gentle. However, in contrast to the temporary tracheostomy, the long-term goal is to promote squamous epithelialization of the trachea so that the problematic airway defenses—mucus production and coughing—are reduced. Epithelialization will occur over a period of several days' time as a response to exposure to cool, dry air. Thus, warming and humidifying the inspired air is done to the minimum extent necessary for preventing violent coughing and discomfort.

The risk of external occlusion with a chronic tracheostomy site is generally less than that with temporary sites. However, the airway may be occluded by the patient. Thus, all patients must be observed as they recover from anesthesia to note their responses to the new opening. Most patients learn to adjust their postures within a few hours.

On discharge, owners must be made aware that their pet now has an exposed airway. As well as general instructions to observe the pet closely for signs of infection (secretions, increased coughing) and occlusion (distress, stridor, increased respiratory effort), specific instructions (for example, no swimming and extremely careful bathing!) should be issued in writing as well as in person. Ideally, the owner should be able to observe the pet and its care in the hospital for a period of time to learn what to expect, and to provide

time for questions to nurses or doctors before the patient is sent home. The discharge should include a reasonable discussion about the measures the owner should take in case of emergency. Routine gentle cleansing of the wound, and attention to grooming to prevent occlusion with hair, are mandatory. In some patients, the level of secretions declines with time, so little is necessary in this regard after several months.

The owner should also be aware that stenosis and aspiration pneumonia can be expected in patients with a chronic tracheostomy. Some patients require repeated surgeries to enlarge the opening. These later surgeries need not be major, but the owners should be aware that the chronic tracheostomy is a procedure that may require additional surgeries for maintenance.

Feline Respiratory Tract Polyps

ERIC R. POPE

GHEORGE M. CONSTANTINESCU

Columbia, Missouri

Feline respiratory tract polyps are non-neoplastic masses that most commonly develop within the tympanic cavity or in the auditory tube close to its junction with the tympanic cavity. Clinical signs are usually related to extension of the masses into the nasopharynx or external ear canal or both. Synonyms for respiratory tract polyps include *feline inflammatory polyps, nasopharyngeal polyps, pharyngeal polyps,* and *middle ear polyps.* Feline inflammatory polyps are most common in young cats but also occur in middle-aged and old cats. Inflammatory polyps are now reported to be the most common mass in the external ear canal of cats.

HISTORY AND CLINICAL SIGNS

The historical findings vary, depending on the location of the polyp or polyps. Cats with nasopharyngeal masses typically present because of respiratory signs, while cats with external ear canal polyps have a history consistent with otitis externa. Cats with lesions in either or both of these locations may also have historical information indicative of middle ear involvement. Occasionally, inflammatory polyps are subclinical and are found either on routine examination or when endotracheal intubation is performed during anesthetic induction.

The clinical signs of nasopharyngeal masses include stertorous respiration, nasal discharge, sneezing, voice change, dyspnea, and dysphagia. Nasal discharge and infection associated with rhinitis and sinusitis may occur secondary to the obstruction of normal airflow. The clinical signs of masses in the external ear canal include otorrhea (dark brown ceruminous or purulent exudate), head shaking, and a mass in the ear canal. The signs of otitis media or interna, such as head tilt, nystagmus, and dysequilibrium, may be present.

DIAGNOSTIC WORK-UP AND TREATMENT

Ventral displacement of the soft palate or a pharyngeal mass may be evident on oral examination. Thorough examination of the nasal cavity and/or nasopharynx and radiography usually requires general anesthesia. Inflammatory polyps typically appear as oval-shaped pedunculated masses extending from the auditory tube into the nasopharynx or from the middle ear into the external ear canal, or both. Therefore, both areas should be inspected in all cases. If no mass is present in the ear canal, the tympanic membrane should be evaluated for evidence of middle ear involvement. The tympanic membrane may appear reddened or may bulge out into the ear canal if polyps are present in the middle ear or if secondary otitis media is present. If access is adequate, myringotomy may allow limited visualization of the middle ear or collection of material for culture and sensitivity testing. This approach may be impractical in small cats. Radiographically, nasopharyngeal polyps are best visualized on the lateral view as a soft-tissue density in the pharynx. Radiographic evaluation of the tympanic bullae should always be performed. Common radiographic changes include enlargement of the bulla or bullae, bony changes, and increased soft-tissue density within the bulla or bullae.

If radiographic changes in the bulla are documented, bulla osteotomy in conjunction with removal of the polyp should be recommended to reduce the likelihood of recurrence. The bulla osteotomy should be performed first, so that the attachment site can be clearly identified and completely excised. Masses in the nasopharynx or ear canal are then removed by simple traction. If signs of middle ear involvement are not present or if economic constraints preclude bulla osteotomy, removal of the nasopharyngeal or ear canal mass by traction alone can be performed and the cat followed for evidence of recurrence. Recurrence rates range up to 37% in patients treated with traction avulsion alone, compared to 2% in cases treated with bulla osteotomy.

Any cat with respiratory distress should be considered at risk for complications during anesthetic induction. The author (ERP) recommends a smooth and rapid induction that allows immediate access for airway intubation. Preoxygenation for 5 to 10 minutes prior to induction may increase the margin of safety in case there is difficulty in gaining control of the airway or if respiratory arrest occurs. Inflammatory polyps in the nasopharynx should be completely removed during the initial anesthetic period because of the risk of respiratory obstruction. The frequency of other lesions mimicking the appearance of inflammatory polyps is low, so it is difficult to justify incisional biopsy for histologic confirmation prior to complete excision.

Traction Avulsion. The nasopharynx is evaluated by retracting the soft palate rostroventrally with a spay hook or stay sutures. Once the palate is retracted, the masses can be displaced from the nasopharynx into the oropharynx. The author (ERP) has not had to incise the soft palate to gain exposure even with bilateral masses. His preference is to grasp the stalk of the polyp or polyps as close to the base as possible with Meeker right-angle forceps (or a similar instrument) and then apply traction to avulse the entire polyp from its attachment in the auditory tube or middle ear. Alternatively, a portion of the mass can be excised, with the clinician making sure to leave enough of the stalk so that it can be securely grasped while avulsing the remaining attachments. Hemorrhage is generally minimal and can be controlled with digital pressure. Bilateral masses are removed similarly.

Polyps in the ear canal are removed by grasping the mass with forceps and applying traction until the mass avulses from its attachment. A lateral ear canal resection can be performed if exposure is inadequate or if the mass cannot be grasped in the intact ear canal.

Ventral Bulla Osteotomy. Ventral bulla osteotomy is indicated when radiographic evidence of middle ear involvement is present, and is probably justified in all cases because of the likelihood that the polyps originate in the middle ear. Excellent descriptions of the surgical anatomy (Little and Lane, 1986) and operative technique (Ader and Boothe, 1979) have been published previously.

Ventral bulla osteotomy is performed with the cat in dorsal recumbency and the head and neck extended. The cat's tympanic bulla is a large and easily palpable landmark. A paramedian skin incision is made just medial to the digastricus muscle (i.e., approximately midway between the midline and the ventral border of the mandible). The incision should be centered midway between the angular process of the mandible and the wing of the atlas. The incision is continued through the subcutaneous tissue and platysma muscle. Blunt dissection is continued between the digastricus muscle laterally and the styloglossus and hyoglossus muscles medially. The hypoglossal nerve and lingual artery should be identified on the lateral border of the hyoglossus muscle and retracted medially. Exposure of the bulla is maintained with hand-held (e.g., Senn) or self-retaining (e.g., Gelpi) retractors. Soft tissue overlying the bulla is separated with a periosteal elevator. An opening is made into the bulla with a bur and pneumatic handpiece or a Steinmann pin in a hand chuck. If a Steinman pin is used, the opening can be enlarged with rongeurs. If exudate is present, samples should be collected for culture and sensitivity testing.

The tympanic bulla contains a transverse septum that divides the cavity into dorsolateral and ventromedial compartments (Fig. 1). The initial opening into the bulla exposes the ventromedial compartment. The sympathetic nerves lie on the surface of the promontory (dorsomedial wall) in this compartment and are easily damaged by curettage. The ventral portion of the transverse septum must be removed to evaluate the dorsolateral compartment, which is where most polyps originate. The septum can be removed in a manner similar to that used for the outer wall. This bone is thin and fragile, so care must be exercised to avoid iatrogenic damage to surrounding structures. The attachment of the polyp is gently teased from the wall of the bulla. The tympanic cavity is gently but thoroughly lavaged with sterile saline. A closed suction drain can be placed if infection is suspected. If thorough lavage is performed, the necessity for drains is questionable. The drain is exited through a separate incision adjacent to the primary incision line. The primary incision line is routinely closed in layers. Drain removal is based on the quantity and character of the exudate.

Postoperative Care

The cat should be closely monitored during the immediate postoperative period for respiratory distress resulting from edema of the pharyngeal tissues. Excessive manipulation or trauma to the pharyngeal mucosa can result in edema. If pharyngeal edema is noted, corticosteroids are administered. Intravenous fluids should be continued until the cat has recovered from anesthesia and is able to drink voluntarily. Food and water are offered the first day after surgery. Antimicrobials are administered, based on the results of culture and susceptibility testing. When one considers the organisms most commonly recovered, amoxicillin-clavulanic acid is a good choice for empirical treatment.

Horner's syndrome is a frequently observed complication after excision of feline inflammatory polyps. Horner's syndrome can occur following simple traction avulsion of nasopharyngeal or ear canal masses and is extremely common when bulla osteotomy is performed. In most instances, Horner's syndrome resolves in weeks to months. Even when Horner's syndrome is permanent, functional impairment is uncommon. Overzealous curettage of the bulla causing damage to the round (cochlear) window, oval (vestibular) window, or vestibulocochlear apparatus will result in signs of otitis interna. Damage to the cochlear apparatus would probably not be clinically detectable unless it oc-

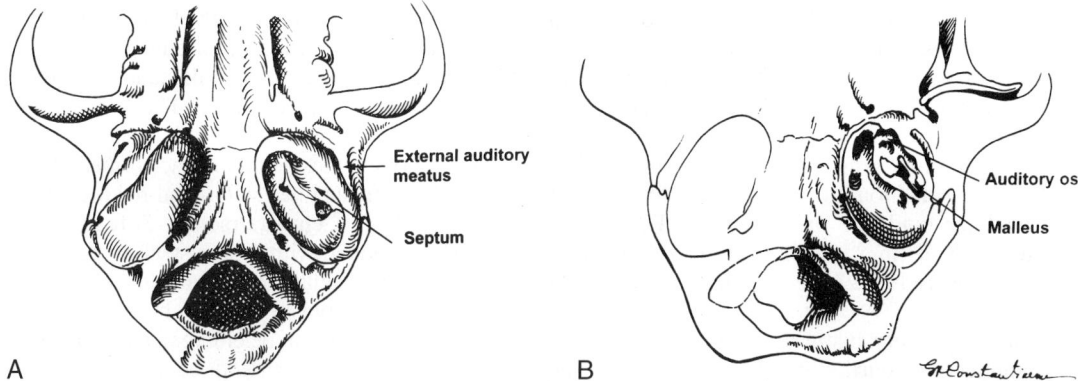

Figure 1. *A,* The ventral wall of the bulla has been removed, exposing the large ventromedial compartment. The intact septum obscures the contents of the dorsolateral compartment. *B,* The transverse septum has been removed to show the contents of the dorsolateral compartment. The tympanic membrane attaches to the manubrium of the malleus centrally. Many polyps arise at or near the opening of the auditory (eustachian) tube into the tympanic cavity.

curred bilaterally. Damage to the vestibular apparatus can result in head tilt, nystagmus, and/or ataxia. The prognosis for patients with inflammatory polyps is excellent following complete removal.

References and Suggested Reading

Ader PL, Boothe HW: Ventral bulla osteotomy in the cat. J Am Anim Hosp Assoc 6:757, 1979.
   A description of the surgical technique, including good pictures.
Kapatkin AS, Matthiesen DT, Noone KE, et al: Results of surgery and long-term follow-up in 31 cats with nasopharyngeal polyps. J Am Anim Hosp Assoc 26:387, 1990.
   A retrospective study that includes the results in cats treated by both traction avulsion and ventral bulla osteotomy.
Little CJL, Lane JG: The surgical anatomy of the feline bulla tympanica. J Small Anim Pract 27:371, 1986.
   An excellent description of the surgical anatomy (including pictures) that stresses the anatomic landmarks and structures that should be avoided to minimize complications.
Pope ER: Feline inflammatory polyps. Semin Vet Med Surg Small Anim 10:87, 1995.
   A complete review of pathophysiology, diagnosis, treatment, and prognosis for feline inflammatory polyps.

Management of Tracheal Collapse

MICHAEL E. HERRTAGE
RICHARD A. S. WHITE
Cambridge, England

Tracheal collapse is a syndrome characterized by dorsoventral flattening of the tracheal rings with laxity of the dorsal tracheal membrane. The syndrome is associated with clinical signs of cough and varying degrees of dyspnea and is most frequently encountered in middle-aged to old toy or miniature dogs. Considerable controversy surrounds the precise cause of the syndrome and, consequently, there is still little agreement as to the most effective approach to its management. Much attention has been focused on refining methods for surgical reconstruction of the collapsed trachea, but it is by no means clear that all cases require or benefit from surgery. A clearer understanding of the cause of the syndrome and the role played by the secondary factors that initiate the symptomatic state are probably the most urgent goals for future research.

ETIOLOGY

The cause of tracheal collapse is complex and it is best regarded as a syndrome with multifactorial causes, many of which are incompletely understood. The development of the clinical condition appears to require the presence of both a primary cartilage abnormality, resulting in weakness of the tracheal rings, together with secondary factors capable of initiating progression to the symptomatic state.

The primary defect responsible for the intrinsic weakness of the tracheal rings is considered to be a reduction in the glycoprotein and glycosaminoglycan content of the hyaline cartilage of the tracheal rings. This, together with other pathologic changes in the matrix, is responsible for reducing the capacity of the cartilage to retain water, consequently diminishing its functional rigidity (Dallman et al, 1985). The evidence to suggest that these underlying abnormalities of the matrix have a congenital origin is compelling. Both the onset of clinical signs during puppyhood in some dogs and the presence of clinical signs in most symptomatic dogs long before middle age, when the disease is classically recognized, support this concept. It seems likely, therefore, that affected dogs begin life with an abnormal trachea, and, conversely, dogs with normal tracheas are rarely susceptible to the disease.

Many toy and miniature dogs with the anatomic tendency to tracheal collapse can remain asymptomatic throughout life unless secondary or exciting factors initiate the clinical syndrome. These potential factors may include obesity, recent endotracheal intubation, respiratory infection, cardiomegaly, cervical trauma, and inhalation of irritants or allergens (Fig. 1). The precise role of upper airway obstruction in the etiology of the syndrome remains unclear. The presence of laryngeal paralysis or collapse in some affected dogs has led to the view that these conditions can precipitate the tracheal changes. Conversely, chronic obstructive disease of the lower airway is capable of promoting upper airway collapse, and hence the interrelation of both conditions remains controversial.

The dynamic changes of tracheal collapse may be confined to either the cervical or thoracic region of the trachea or may involve its entire length. Frequently, the changes are most pronounced at the cervicothoracic junction. Collapse of the cervical tracheal segment occurs on inspiration because of the decreased pressure within the trachea, whereas the thoracic portion tends to collapse during the expiratory phase of respiration or during coughing as a consequence of increased intrathoracic pressure. In severely affected dogs, these changes may also be detected more distally in the bronchi. As a consequence of the flattened configuration of the tracheal rings, the dorsal membrane becomes widened, pendulous, and flaccid. The dorsal membrane contributes to the dynamic obstruction of the airway as it is drawn into the tracheal lumen during the respiratory cycle.

Once clinical signs are apparent, the syndrome is perpetuated by the cycle of chronic inflammation of the tracheal mucosa, which exacerbates and, in turn, is exacerbated by the cough. Persistent inflammation of the tracheal mucosa leads to loss of epithelium, fibrinous membrane formation, and squamous metaplasia with polypoid proliferation in advanced cases. The population of ciliated cells is significantly reduced by the metaplastic changes in the mucosa, and the hyperplastic subepithelial glands secrete increasingly viscid mucus. As a consequence, normal ciliary function is progressively replaced by cough as the major tracheobronchial clearing mechanism. Once the condition becomes symptomatic, the changes in the dorsal membrane and cartilage are believed to progress beyond those of the original anatomic abnormality; however, it has proved difficult to document these worsening changes in individual cases.

INCIDENCE

Tracheal collapse is almost exclusively confined to toy and miniature breeds and is only sporadically encountered in medium- to large-breed dogs. The Yorkshire terrier is the most commonly affected breed, but other commonly affected breeds include the miniature poodle, Chihuahua, and Pomeranian. Typically, the patient is presented for evaluation at 6 to 7 years of age, although careful investigation will usually reveal that signs referable to the condition

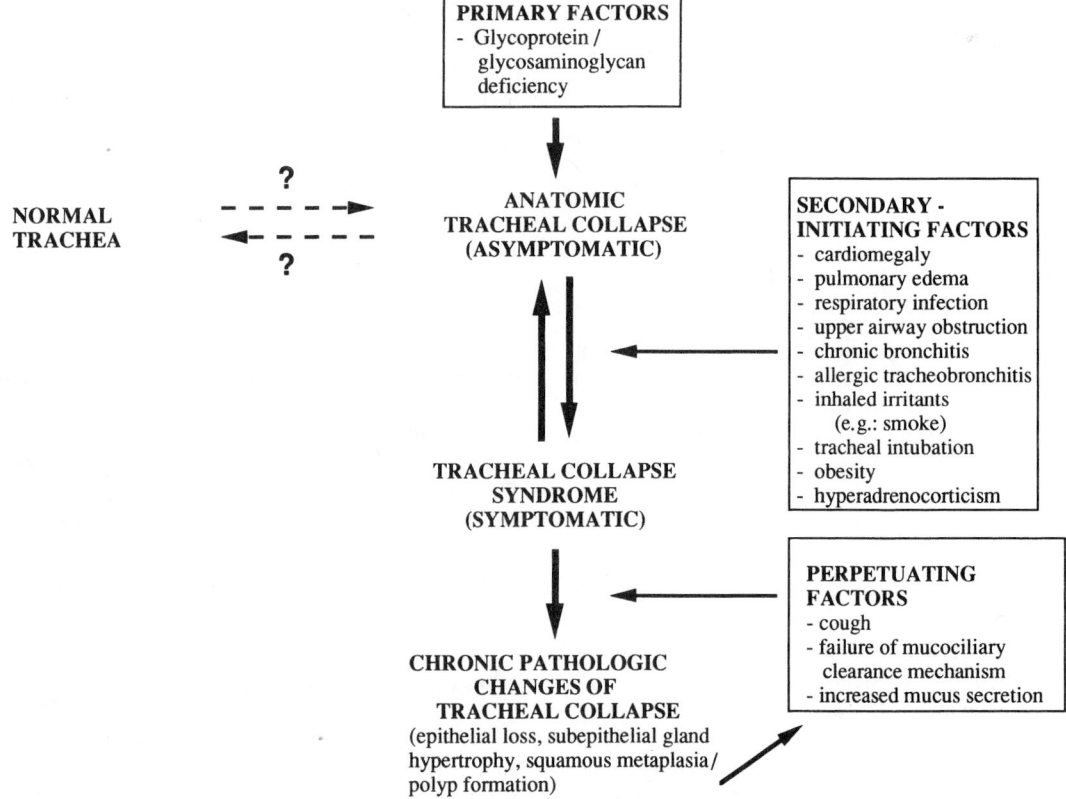

Figure 1. Interrelation of probable factors involved in the etiology of tracheal collapse.

have been present for some years before presentation. Approximately 25% of affected dogs are symptomatic by the age of 6 months. The syndrome is equally distributed between the sexes.

CLINICAL SIGNS

Tracheal collapse syndrome is characterized by a chronic, paroxysmal cough precipitated by excitement, anxiety, or pulling on the leash. The cough is typically harsh, dry, and nonproductive and is easily elicited on tracheal palpation. A "goose honk" cough is a frequent, but not consistent, finding. Affected dogs may be otherwise asymptomatic and are often able to sustain prolonged periods of exercise without any clinical signs. More severely affected dogs, however, may show varying degrees of tachypnea or even respiratory distress due to the severity of airway obstruction. Cyanosis or syncope due to hypoxemia may be noted in advanced cases. The severity of clinical signs does not relate directly to the severity of the anatomic changes, and classification systems describing the degree of tracheal collapse are of limited help in this respect.

On physical examination, turbulent air flow may be detected on auscultation directly over the cervical trachea, whereas referred musical or wheezing sounds may be heard on thoracic auscultation. The lung sounds in tracheal collapse may be normal or increased; however, in many cases the bronchovesicular sounds may be obliterated by referred sounds from the trachea. In dogs with tracheal collapse, the heart rate is usually normal or slow at rest with pronounced sinus arrhythmia, whereas dogs with left ventricular heart failure often lose sinus arrhythmia because of increased sympathetic tone, and the heart rate is often increased. The cough in left ventricular heart failure is typically soft, moist, and productive compared with the harsh, dry cough of tracheal collapse; however, left atrial enlargement can also cause left bronchial compression, which can mimic signs of tracheal collapse. Some dogs with tracheal collapse acquire pulmonary hypertension, which may result in a prominent or split second heart sound.

DIAGNOSIS

Confirmation of the diagnosis of tracheal collapse syndrome requires the combination of a persistent cough, a response to tracheal palpation, and demonstration of intratracheal changes, preferably by endoscopy. The dynamic dysfunction of the trachea can be demonstrated by a variety of diagnostic methods, including palpation, radiography, ultrasonography, or tracheoscopy.

Physical Examination

Collapse of the cervical portion of the trachea is usually readily appreciated on physical examination by careful palpation. The tendency of the dorsal membrane to invert into the tracheal lumen can be appreciated by gentle digital pressure once the trachea has been rolled laterally. More significantly, in affected dogs, this maneuver will usually initiate a cough.

Radiographic Examination

Radiography can be useful in demonstrating dynamic tracheal collapse during the different phases of the respiratory cycle. The most useful radiographic examinations include lateral projections of the thoracic inlet exposed during the inspiratory and expiratory phases, a tangential rostrocaudal (skyline) projection of the thoracic inlet, and fluoroscopic investigation to demonstrate movement of the dorsal membrane during the respiratory cycle. Luminal narrowing of the cervical trachea is seen on the lateral projection during inspiration, whereas ballooning of the same segment may be seen on expiration. These changes may be visible during expiration for the thoracic segment. These dynamic changes, including "fluttering" of the dorsal membrane during the respiratory cycle are best viewed in real time using image-intensified fluoroscopy. In the skyline projection, the flattened trachea is seen as an oval, "C" or crescent shape. The cross-section of the trachea at the thoracic inlet may, in severe cases, be narrowed to a slit-like opening. It should be emphasized that radiography may not highlight the dynamic changes of collapse in all cases.

Ultrasonography

Like fluoroscopy, ultrasonography provides real-time imaging that can be used to demonstrate dynamic changes in the tracheal profile. The technique has the distinct advantages of being noninvasive and safe and can be performed on minimally sedated or unsedated animals (Rudorf et al, 1997). A high-frequency transducer with a stand-off is required for imaging of the larynx and trachea. The transducer is positioned ventrally over the trachea just caudal to the cricoid cartilage and, with the neck in a neutral position, a transverse scan is made of the air shadow between the cricoid and first tracheal ring. Beginning from this point, the transducer is moved caudally, imaging the profile of the tracheal air shadow during the phases of the respiratory cycle and during hyperextension of the neck. Interpretation requires some experience.

Endoscopy

Tracheoscopic examination of the tracheal lumen should be regarded as the "gold standard" for the purposes of completing a diagnosis. Tracheoscopy is useful to confirm not only the presence of the anatomic abnormality but also changes in the dorsal membrane along its entire length. The ventrodorsal movement of the dorsal membrane during the respiratory cycle can be appreciated in lightly anesthetized dogs. In some dogs with severely obstruction, there may be an increased anesthesia risk, but this rarely proves to be a problem.

Microbiologic and Cytologic Studies

Tracheoscopy also permits the recovery of bacteriologic and cytologic samples from the lower respiratory system. Samples should be cultured for bacterial isolation and sensitivity, and cytologic studies should be performed to identify any cellular changes suggestive of an inhaled allergic or inflammatory airway response.

Other Tests

The identification of specific allergens or irritants often is not practical, although removal of the dog from cigarette smoke in the environment (or vice versa) for a test period is often useful in investigating this as a common initiating cause.

THERAPY

The clinician must be prepared to pursue several therapeutic avenues in the management of the individual dog in order to deal with the complex and multifactorial etiology of the syndrome (White and Williams, 1994). Since anatomic collapse alone does not guarantee a symptomatic state, every effort should be made to identify and correct any secondary causes. Successful long-term medical management is possible for the majority of patients provided the initiating factor or factors can be identified. This route should always be thoroughly investigated before a surgical solution is considered.

The Acute Case

The dog presenting in acute respiratory distress should be regarded as a medical emergency, and all diagnostic tests should be postponed until the dog has been stabilized. The dog should be sedated with acepromazine (ProMACE, Fort Dodge) at a dose of 0.02 to 0.2 mg/kg IV, IM, or SC as required and subjected to as little stress as possible. Oxygen therapy administered via a face mask may be the most practical means of improving the patient's oxygen status initially, but nasal intubation often causes the patient less anxiety for long-term management. The authors have used tracheostomy intubation as a temporary means of establishing an airway in hyperexcited dogs with severe obstruction with seemingly few long-term complications. In some dogs, the tachypnea may promote hyperthermia, exacerbating the dyspnea. The dog should be kept in a cool environment or ice-packs applied in severe cases to counter this problem. Short-acting glucocorticoids, for example, dexamethasone (Azium, Schering-Plough) given once at a dose of 1 mg/kg IV, may be helpful for dogs with laryngeal edema or tracheal inflammation. Opioid agonist-antagonists such as butorphanol (Torbutrol, Fort Dodge) at a dosage of 0.05 to 0.11 mg/kg every 6 to 12 hours IV, IM, or SC or buprenorphine hydrochloride (Buprenex, Reckitt and Colman) at a dosage of 0.01 to 0.02 mg/kg every 12 hours IM are useful mild cough suppressants that cause little respiratory depression.

Management of Secondary Initiating Causes

Weight Reduction. Many dogs with tracheal collapse are obese, and their intrathoracic adipose deposits may interfere with respiratory excursion, causing a reduction in thoracic wall compliance. Weight reduction should be pursued aggressively in all overweight patients; the clinical response can be dramatic in some cases. The daily caloric intake should be based on a high-fiber, low-calorie diet and restricted to 60% of the total daily requirement based on a lean body mass. Exercise restriction may limit the rate of weight loss. The veterinarian should monitor progress and encourage owner compliance with the regimen.

Congestive Heart Failure. Heart failure with pulmonary edema may initiate or exacerbate the clinical signs of tracheal collapse by increasing the volume of tracheobronchial secretions. Additionally, the cough may be promoted by pressure of the enlarged left atrium on the left mainstem bronchus. Reduction of preload by diuresis and the use of angiotensin-converting enzyme inhibitors reduces pulmonary edema. Digitalization may also be effective in suppressing the cough associated with congestive heart failure (see. p. 748).

Inhaled Irritants. There is good evidence to suggest that in some dogs the clinical syndrome of collapse is initiated by the inhalation of irritants or allergens. The removal of cigarette smoke from the dog's environment is an essential, although often difficult, part of the management regimen. The recognition and removal of other inhaled allergens is less straightforward but may prove beneficial in some dogs.

Respiratory Infections. Infections of the lower respiratory tract should be treated by appropriate antibacterial therapy based on the results of bacterial culture from bronchoalveolar lavage. Treatment should be continued for a minimum of 14 days and in selected cases may need to be continued for prolonged periods for the control of deep-seated chronic infection.

Collars. The use of collars, particularly of a sliding chain design, should be discouraged because repeated external pressure on the trachea may initiate mucosal irritation and promote coughing. Body harnesses are an alternative, although these may still pose some risk.

Management of the Coughing Animal

Antitussive Agents. Cough suppressants are recommended to reduce chronic irritation or damage to the tracheal epithelium caused by collapse of the dorsal membrane and to reduce shearing forces within the lung associated with chronic coughing. A variety of drugs are available, but the authors have had greatest success using co-phenotrope (Lomotil, Searle), which contains diphenoxylate hydrochloride and atropine.* The diphenoxylate acts as a narcotic antitussive agent and the atropine reduces the volume of mucus secreted into the lower respiratory tract and also acts as an antimuscarinic bronchodilator. The recommended dosage of co-phenotrope is 0.2 to 0.5 mg of diphenoxylate/kg PO every 12 hours; this dosage can be

---

*Co-phenotrope is not in widespread use as an antitussive agent in the United States, and no clinical trials demonstrating its efficacy and safety for this indication have been published. The potential adverse effects of atropine on the viscosity of airway secretions warrant further investigation before its widespread application.

maintained for extended periods until clinical signs subside. Constipation is an occasional problem but can usually be controlled by adding a stool softener to the diet. Other narcotic antitussive agents such as hydrocodone (Russigan, Daniels Pharmaceuticals) (0.22 mg/kg PO every 6 to 12 hours), codeine phosphate (Bronlex, Procter and Gamble Pharmaceuticals) (0.5 to 2.0 mg/kg PO every 12 hours) or butorphanol (Torbutrol, Fort Dodge) (0.5 to 1.0 mg/kg PO every 6 to 12 hours) may be used but are rarely as effective as co-phenotrope.

Glucocorticoids. Glucocorticoids should be used judiciously in the management of tracheal collapse. They may be beneficial in reducing laryngeal, tracheal, or bronchial inflammation, but should be used for short periods only because their extended use may exacerbate bacterial infections, promote tachypnea, or cause iatrogenic hyperadrenocorticism. Glucocorticoids also promote weight gain and may make weight reduction difficult to achieve. Prednisolone (Prednistab, Vedco) may be used initially at a dosage of 0.5 mg/kg PO every 12 hours. Since the benefits of glucocorticoids are normally apparent within 7 to 10 days, the dosage should be tapered and withdrawn within this period.

Bronchodilators. The use of bronchodilators in the management of tracheal collapse is regarded as controversial by some authors. The rationale for their use is based on the dilation of pulmonary airways which decreases intrathoracic pressure during expiration, thereby decreasing the tendency to tracheal narrowing during expiration. This is particularly important for patients with coexisting small airway disease, having increased intrathoracic pressure on expiration and hence a greater tendency to tracheal collapse. Methylxanthine bronchodilators (theophylline) may be beneficial in achieving bronchodilation, improving mucociliary clearance, and reducing diaphragmatic fatigue in dogs with tracheal collapse. The preparations most commonly used include sustained-release theophylline (Theodur, Key Pharmaceuticals) at a dosage of 20 mg/kg PO every 12 hours and theophylline ethylenediamine (aminophylline, Roxane and Alpharma) at a dosage of 8 to 10 mg/kg PO every 8 hours.

Beta$_2$-adrenergic agonists can also be used for bronchodilation. Terbutaline (Brethine, Ciba Geneva) (1.25 to 5 mg/dog every PO 8 to 12 hours) and albuterol (Proventil, Schering; Ventolin, Glaxo-Wellcome) (50 μg/kg PO every 8 hours) have been recommended for use in dogs. Signs of beta-agonist toxicity include hypotension and tachycardia; therefore, care should be taken when using these drugs in animals with congestive heart failure.

Surgical Management

Surgical management of tracheal collapse is appropriate for dogs who remain persistently symptomatic despite vigorous medical management and attempts to eradicate all potential initiating factors. Candidates for reconstruction of the trachea should be selected carefully and should be free of other medical complications, including congestive heart failure and collapse of the lower airway because these dogs rarely improve with surgical intervention.

A variety of surgical techniques has been described for the management of tracheal collapse. The majority of these techniques, including tracheal ring chondrotomy, plication of the dorsal membrane, prosthetic mesh support, and intraluminal prosthetic supports, have little foundation in success and are no longer considered of practical application. Placement of external prosthetic supports is currently the preferred technique for surgical management of tracheal collapse, and both ring (Hobson, 1976) and spiral (Fingland et al, 1986) prostheses manufactured from polypropylene are used. Most authors suggest reconstruction of the cervical and, when affected, the thoracic segment. However, the results of surgical management of the thoracic portion of the trachea is frequently unrewarding because of the high morbidity associated with this procedure. A number of complications have been associated with implantation of prosthetic tracheal supports, including loosening or failure of the implant, infection, laryngeal paralysis, and tracheal necrosis. Isolation of the tracheal blood supply to accommodate the application of prostheses has been demonstrated to result in significant impairment of the tracheal blood flow, risking necrosis (Kirby et al, 1991). However, a modified dissection of the lateral pedicles permits preservation of the vascular supply to one side of the trachea and avoids serious ischemic complications (Coyne et al, 1993). Arytenoid lateralization at the time of surgical reconstruction of the trachea may improve the results of surgery (White, 1995). The prognosis for older dogs (>6 years of age at the time of surgery) is significantly worse than that for younger dogs, even though the degree of tracheal collapse, as assessed by tracheoscopy, may be less severe (Buback et al, 1996). As emphasized previously, the severity of the grade of collapse does not appear to have any prognostic significance.

References and Suggested Reading

Buback JL, Boothe HW, Hobson P: Surgical treatment of tracheal collapse in dogs: 90 cases (1983–1993). J Am Vet Med Assoc 208:380, 1996.
Retrospective survey of cases designed to determine factors associated with long-term outcome in dogs with tracheal collapse and extraluminal polypropylene C-shaped stents.

Coyne BE, Fingland RB, Kennedy GA, et al: Clinical and pathologic effects of a modified technique for application of spiral prostheses to the cervical trachea of dogs. Vet Surg 22:269, 1993.
This article discusses an experimental study demonstrating how the tracheal blood supply can be preserved during spiral prosthesis reconstruction.

Dallman MJ, McClure RC, Brown EM: Normal and collapsed trachea in the dog: Scanning electron microscopy study. Am J Vet Res 46:2110, 1985.
The changes in tracheal cartilage between normal and affected dogs are discussed.

Fingland RB, DeHoff WD, Birchard SJ: Surgical management of cervical and thoracic tracheal collapse in dogs using extraluminal spiral prostheses: Results in seven cases. J Am Anim Hosp Assoc 23:173, 1986.
The technique for tracheal reconstruction using spiral prostheses is described.

Hobson HP: Total ring prosthesis for the surgical correction of collapsed trachea. J Am Anim Hosp Assoc 12:822, 1976.
The original technique for ring prosthetic reconstruction of the trachea is described.

Kirby BM, Bjorling DE, Rankin JHG, et al: The effects of surgical

isolation and application of polypropylene spiral prostheses on tracheal blood flow. Vet Surg 20:49, 1991.
This article describes an experimental study showing that complete isolation of the tracheal blood supply during prosthetic reconstruction risks ischemic necrosis.

Rudorf H, Herrtage ME, White RAS: The use of ultrasonography in the diagnosis of tracheal collapse. J Small Anim Pract 38:513, 1997.
The technique for ultrasonographic examination of the trachea, comparing normal and affected dogs, is described.

White RAS, Williams JM: Tracheal collapse in the dog—is there really a role for surgery? A retrospective study of 100 cases. J Small Anim Pract 35:191, 1994.
This retrospective study of 100 dogs with tracheal collapse showed that medical management resulted in long-term resolution of signs in 71% of cases.

White RN: Unilateral arytenoid lateralisation and extraluminal polypropylene ring prostheses for correction of tracheal collapse in the dog. J Small Anim Pract 36:151, 1995.
This retrospective study of 25 cases suggests that laryngeal dysfunction may influence prognosis after ring prosthetic reconstruction.

CVT Update: Canine Chronic Bronchitis

LYNELLE JOHNSON
Columbia, Missouri

Chronic bronchitis is characterized by inflammation of the conducting airway and results in a chronic cough for which no specific cause can be identified. In humans, chronic bronchitis is most often related to cigarette smoking, which causes a dramatic reduction in the ability of the host to clear organisms from the tracheobronchial tree by increasing the volume and viscosity of respiratory secretions, decreasing ciliary function, and altering the immune response. Acute exacerbations of disease are often associated with infection by *Haemophilus influenzae,* pneumococcal species, or *Mycoplasma* (Ball, 1995; Murphy and Sethi, 1992) Large-scale epidemiologic studies have not been carried out to investigate possible risk factors for the development of chronic bronchitis in dogs, despite substantial morbidity in the canine population. Environmental pollutants or inhaled irritants could be partly responsible for the induction of inflammatory airway disease in dogs; however, the role of bacterial infection in the generation or exacerbation of chronic bronchitis in dogs has not been established. Until further studies are performed, treatment of the disease must be based on all clinical information that can be gathered from the individual animal.

Chronic airway inflammation induces neutrophilic infiltration of the bronchial mucosa, with release of proteases, elastases, and oxidizing products. Mucosal injury is repaired by proliferation of the epithelium and hyperplasia of the surrounding tissue. Ongoing injury leads to a vicious cycle of airway injury and repair. These changes result in accumulation of mucus within the airway, which obstructs air flow and leads to clinical signs of cough and exercise intolerance. On histologic examination, chronic bronchitis is characterized by hypertrophy and hyperplasia of mucus glands and goblet cells, smooth muscle hypertrophy, fibrosis of the lamina propria, and epithelial erosion with squamous metaplasia. The character of these lesions confirms the chronicity of disease. When a diagnosis of chronic bronchitis is made, it must be recognized that therapy is directed only at controlling clinical signs; once initiated, this disease cannot be cured.

CLINICAL FINDINGS

Chronic bronchitis is defined by the presence of a daily cough for at least 2 months of the year and lacks a specific cause. Generally, the cough is described as a dry hacking cough, but it can be moist or productive when copious amounts of respiratory secretions are produced. The cough may be overshadowed by a "goose honk" cough in small-breed dogs that have concurrent tracheal collapse. Often, the dog has coughed for several years before it is brought to the veterinarian—an acute onset of worsening signs may cause the owner to seek veterinary attention. Acute on chronic bronchitis may be due to progression of inflammatory lung disease or pulmonary infection.

Classically, chronic bronchitis is considered a disease of small-breed dogs, and it is frequently diagnosed in poodles, terriers, and dachshunds. However, the diagnosis should not be overlooked in large-breed dogs. Usually, animals are middle-aged to older when the diagnosis is made, but the onset of cough may be at a relatively young age (3 to 4 years).

On physical examination, dogs with chronic bronchitis appear in generally good health and are often overweight. Coarse, diffuse crackles are reported most commonly, and these are typically harsher and louder than those associated with pulmonary edema or pneumonia. Pulmonary sounds in the dog may be normal at rest; however, auscultation generally reveals post-tussive crackles and wheezes. Tracheal sensitivity is usually present because of nonspecific airway inflammation. Concurrent tracheal collapse may be detected by the characteristic goose honk cough or by a snapping sound heard over the thoracic cage as the intrathoracic airway collapses on expiration. Dogs severely affected by bronchitis can have prolonged expiration with an expiratory push, and these animals may have a history of intermittent cyanosis or collapse.

DIAGNOSIS

The diagnosis of chronic bronchitis is one of exclusion. The history of a long-term cough in a small-breed dog is suggestive of chronic bronchitis; however, pneumonia, congestive heart failure, tracheal collapse, and pulmonary neoplasia can cause similar clinical signs. Therefore, the diagnosis is based on the history, clinical findings, chest radiographs, and airway sampling. Clinicopathologic abnormalities are typically absent.

Thoracic radiography is an important part of the diagnostic work-up, both to confirm the likelihood of chronic bronchitis and to rule out other conditions. Classically, a generalized increase in interstitial or peribronchial infiltrates is found in dogs with chronic bronchitis. End-on bronchi (doughnuts) and airways seen in longitudinal section (tram lines) represent airway walls thickened by inflammation. Increased linear markings should not be assumed to reflect "aging changes" because radiographic abnormalities are most likely indicators of a pulmonary pathologic condition. In the author's opinion, normal chest radiographs are found relatively often in dogs with chronic bronchitis and do not rule out the diagnosis. The presence of alveolar infiltrates suggests concurrent pneumonia or pulmonary edema.

Collecting airway samples by transtracheal wash or bronchoscopy is recommended to characterize the cellular infiltrate in the airway and to rule out infectious causes of cough. Bronchoscopy is particularly useful when typical radiographic findings of bronchitis are lacking. Dogs with chronic bronchitis have erythema, the airway appears rough, and the majority have increased mucus lining the airway. In animals with long-standing bronchitis, fibrous nodules can be seen protruding into the bronchial lumen.

Cytologically, chronic bronchitis is characterized by a preponderance of nondegenerate neutrophils. The presence of neutrophils does not confirm a septic process, and infection is likely only when toxic neutrophils or intracellular bacteria are present. A smaller percentage of animals have a predominance of eosinophils in airway washings. This may indicate systemic hypersensitivity (e.g., related to gastrointestinal parasites or ectoparasite infestation) or may suggest an allergic basis for disease. Alternatively, increased eosinophils in airway fluid may reflect the stage of disease. In humans, increased eosinophils are seen in airway samples of patients with acute exacerbation of disease, suggesting that noninfectious irritants, viruses, and *Mycoplasma* should be ruled out as causes of acute inflammation (Saetta et al, 1994). The importance of an eosinophilic infiltrate has not been investigated in dogs with chronic bronchitis. Increased mucus is present in many airway samples, and Curschmann's spirals (bronchial casts of airway mucus) are sometimes noted. Epithelial cells and squamous metaplasia may also be seen on cytologic examination.

The presence of suppurative inflammation on cytologic examination makes it tempting to ascribe clinical disease to an infectious condition, although in the author's opinion, bacterial infection is not a significant problem in most dogs with chronic bronchitis. The trachea and large airway of dogs are not sterile; therefore, various species of commensal bacteria and oral flora can be found in tracheal wash or bronchoalveolar lavage samples despite careful attention to technique. It then becomes difficult to determine whether the airway is colonized and infected, or contaminated, as is the dilemma in human cases of bronchitis (Ball, 1995;

Murphy and Sethi, 1992). Previously stable animals with bronchitis that have an acute exacerbation of disease may be experiencing true bacterial infection. Dogs with chronic bronchitis can aspirate oral bacteria during episodes of coughing or panting. Aspirated bacteria become trapped in the mucus of the lower airway and may overwhelm host defenses because of the abnormal environment in the lower airway and cause infection. A *septic* suppurative inflammation would be seen on cytologic examination. Heavy growth of a single bacterial species or an atypical resistance pattern would also support the diagnosis of bronchial infection.

Ancillary tests may be performed at a referral hospital to assess the severity of gas exchange or gas flow abnormalities and to follow therapy. Arterial blood gas analysis generally shows only mild to moderate hypoxemia. Hypercarbia is not detected until late in the disease when respiratory failure ensues. Nuclear ventilation scans can be performed and may reveal patchy areas of deficient ventilation (Padrid et al, 1990). Flow volume loops are commonly performed in human patients to assess maximal air flow. Tidal breathing flow volume loops have been performed in anesthetized dogs with chronic bronchitis and have shown reductions in expiratory flow and loop shapes similar to those seen in humans with chronic bronchitis (Padrid and Amis, 1992); however, these tests are not widely available. (For further discussion of canine bronchitis, see "Diagnosis and Therapy of Canine Chronic Bronchitis," *CVT XII*, p. 908.)

THERAPY

Anti-inflammatory Agents

Clinical signs of chronic bronchitis are due to airway inflammation, and therapy with glucocorticoids is successful in resolving clinical signs in the majority of patients. It is essential that infectious diseases be ruled out before the initiation of anti-inflammatory treatment. Also, it would seem wise to control coexisting diseases, such as severe dental disease or congestive heart failure, before using glucocorticoids.

Dosing of glucocorticoids should be tailored to the individual, with the severity of clinical signs, chronicity of disease, and general systemic health considered in decisions regarding treatment. Short-acting steroids such as prednisone or prednisolone are generally safe and effective in dogs with uncomplicated bronchitis. In the early stages of disease, dogs often require dosages of glucocorticoids ranging from 0.5 to 1.0 mg/kg every 12 hours for 5 to 7 days to induce remission of clinical signs. The dosage should be decreased by half every 5 to 7 days and, when possible, drugs should be administered on an alternate-day basis to allow normalization of the pituitary-adrenal axis. Long-term therapy (2 to 3 months) can be anticipated for chronic cases, although discontinuation of medication earlier may be possible. When disease worsens in the early stages of treatment, a return to the higher dose of glucocorticoid that controlled clinical signs is generally required. Alternatively, treatment with bronchodilators or antitussive agents can be added (see further on). Long-acting glucocorticoids such as dexamethasone, triamcinolone, and methylprednisolone acetate do not have a therapeutic advantage over prednisone and are associated with more severe derangements of the pituitary-adrenal axis. The author has not used cytotoxic drugs in the treatment of chronic bronchitis.

Antihistamines are occasionally efficacious in controlling signs in some patients with chronic bronchitis; however, they can dehydrate the mucus layer causing inspissation and blockage of the airways. In the author's experience, response to antihistamines is extremely variable, and multiple drug trials may be performed before any drug is deemed beneficial to the patient. Inhaled anti-inflammatory agents and mast cell stabilizers are used commonly in the treatment of human bronchitis patients with air flow obstruction. Medicated aerosol therapy has not met with widespread success in dogs because the thickness of the airway mucus may preclude penetration by drugs. Current research indicates that leukotrienes, substance P, and adhesion molecules are important in the induction and perpetuation of inflammatory pulmonary disease in human patients. Future therapy in humans may be directed against these mediators and may eventually prove beneficial in animals.

Bronchodilators

It is unclear whether bronchoconstriction plays a role in canine chronic bronchitis. Baseline pulmonary resistance increased in an experimental model of lung inflammation induced by *Bordetella bronchiseptica;* however, airway responsiveness as assessed by histamine challenge was unchanged (Cormier et al, 1993). The baseline increase in resistance was probably related to the presence of inflammatory products and mucosal edema rather than airway hyperreactivity. A subset of human bronchitis patients suffer from significant air flow limitation, and it is possible that certain dogs also have expiratory flow limitation. Bronchodilators are often clinically helpful in reducing signs in dogs with bronchitis or in allowing a reduction in the dosage of glucocorticoid required to control signs. Both methylxanthine derivatives and beta-agonists seem to act synergistically with glucocorticoids in the control of inflammatory lung disease. Bronchodilators may provide other beneficial effects by improving pulmonary perfusion, enhancing cardiac performance, reducing dyspnea, and stimulating mucociliary clearance. In dogs that fail to respond adequately to glucocorticoids, a 2-week trial on a bronchodilator is a reasonable therapeutic option.

The two main classes of bronchodilators used in veterinary medicine are methylxanthine derivatives and beta$_2$-agonists (for further discussion, see "Current Uses and Hazards of Bronchodilator Drugs," *CVT XI,* p. 660) Methylxanthine drugs were originally thought to act through phosphodiesterase inhibition, which causes smooth muscle relaxation through accumulation of cyclic adenosine monophosphate. Current research suggests that the clinical effects of methylxanthines result from adenosine antagonism. Long-acting theophylline products (Theo-Dur Tablets [Key Pharmaceuticals], 20 mg/kg PO every 12 hours; Slo-Bid Gyrocaps [Rhone-Poulenc Rorer], 20 to 25 mg/kg PO every 12 hours) have been shown to achieve plasma levels in dogs that approximate the human therapeutic range of 10 to 20 μg/ml. Although generic theophylline products have shown equal bioavailability in humans, this has not been researched in veterinary species. Therefore, when bronchodilators are prescribed, no generic substitution should be allowed initially. If a dog responds favorably to Theo-Dur or Slo-Bid but cost is prohibitive, owners may elect to try a generic sustained-release theophylline product.

Adverse effects of methylxanthines are probably also related to adenosine antagonism and include gastrointestinal upset, tachycardia, and hyperexcitability. It is essential to individualize drug therapy because there is a wide variation in the dose that causes side effects. Theophylline metabolism is influenced by many elements, including fiber in the diet, smoke in the environment, congestive heart failure, and the use of other drugs. The author recommends starting therapy with half the recommended dose (10 mg/kg every 12 hours) for the first week to reduce adverse side effects. If clinical signs improve and the dog tolerates the drug, the dosage may be increased as needed.

Beta$_2$-agonists such as terbutaline and albuterol have been used successfully in dogs with chronic bronchitis. Terbutaline is available through a wide number of pharmaceutical companies. Small dogs receive 0.625 to 1.25 mg PO every 12 hours, medium-sized dogs are given 1.25 to 2.5 mg PO every 12 hours, and larger dogs receive 2.5 to 5 mg PO every 12 hours. Albuterol at 50 μg/kg PO every 8 hours was efficacious in reducing cough in almost half the dogs evaluated in a review of canine chronic bronchitis (Padrid et al, 1990). Interestingly, the bronchodilator also resulted in a reduction in the severity of the pulmonary infiltrate. As with methylxanthines, beta-agonists may result in excitability or tremors during initial therapy, but animals usually become accustomed to the drug.

Anticholinergic agents are among the most commonly prescribed bronchodilators in human medicine. They are potent bronchodilators and are relatively free of side effects because they are administered only by inhalation. This feature limits their usefulness in veterinary patients.

Antitussive Agents

The cough reflex is of major importance to the dog with bronchitis because it serves the essential function of clearing viscid secretions from the airway. Although instantaneous mucociliary clearance is reduced in human patients with chronic bronchitis, the long-term removal of secretions is actually higher than in healthy humans because of potent clearance by the cough reflex. Suppression of this reflex before resolution of inflammation can be deleterious because of mucus trapping. Prolonged contact between inflammatory mediators in the mucus and epithelial cells perpetuates airway inflammation. When clinical signs suggest that inflammation is resolving, cough suppression is desirable because chronic coughing can lead to repeated airway injury and syncopal events. Over-the-counter dextromethorphan-containing compounds are efficacious in some animals. When more potent suppression of a dry cough is required, narcotic agents should be prescribed. The author prefers hydrocodone (Tussigon [Daniels Pharmaceuticals], 0.22 mg/kg PO every 6 to 12 hours) or butorphanol (Torbutrol [Fort Dodge], 0.05 to 1.0

mg/kg PO every 6 to 12 hours). These agents must be given at an interval that suppresses coughing without inducing excessive sedation. Long-term therapy may be required in some patients, particularly when tracheal collapse is also present.

Antibiotics

When infection has been documented through appropriate culturing techniques, and cytologic findings confirm the likelihood of infection, antibiotic treatment is warranted. In humans, antibiotics shorten the duration of acute disease and are routinely prescribed for patients who suffer recurrent exacerbations (more than four episodes per year) of disease (Ball, 1995). Biologic response modifiers (oral or aerosolized extracts of bacteria) are employed in chronic cases with frequent exacerbations to enhance natural immunity to bacteria and reduce inflammation within the lung. (Lusuardi et al, 1993).

Antibiotic choice should be based on culture and sensitivity results whenever possible. Drugs should have a broad spectrum of activity against bacteria commonly found in the lung, such as *Bordetella, Pasteurella, Staphylococcus, Streptococcus*, and various gram-negative species. The antibiotic chosen should be lipophilic to facilitate penetration of the airway and should be relatively free of side effects. When possible, the author prefers chloramphenicol (50 mg/kg PO every 8 hours), doxycycline (2.5 to 5 mg/kg PO every 12 hours), or enrofloxacin (Baytril [Bayer], 2.5 to 5 mg/kg PO every 12 hours). Enrofloxacin inhibits metabolism of theophylline, and the concurrent use of the two drugs results in toxic plasma levels of theophylline (Intorre et al, 1995). At least a 30% reduction in theophylline dose is recommended when enrofloxacin is required to treat coincident infection. Length of treatment depends on whether pneumonia is present or bronchial colonization and infection is suspected. True pneumonia generally requires 3 to 6 weeks of antibiotic therapy, whereas 5 to 10 days of treatment will usually resolve signs related to bronchial colonization.

In patients with concurrent bronchiectasis, infection plays a predominant role, and in these patients, long-term antibiotic therapy is indicated. Bronchiectasis is defined as a dilatation of the lower airways with suppuration. It may occur as a sequela to uncontrolled airway inflammation or infection. Mucus trapping and obstruction of the airway is severe, and recurrent pneumonia is commonly encountered. Chronic antibiotic therapy is often required in these patients, and broad-spectrum antibiotics or combinations of antibiotics should be chosen because infection may involve various gram-negative bacteria (especially *Pseudomonas*) and anaerobes. Chloramphenicol, trimethoprim-sulfa (15 mg/kg PO every 12 hours), or clindamycin (Antirobe [Pharmacia & Upjohn], 11 mg/kg PO every 12 hours) combined with enrofloxacin can be helpful in resolving long-standing pulmonary infection.

ADDITIONAL THERAPY

Obesity worsens clinical signs in dogs with chronic bronchitis by decreasing thoracic wall compliance, increas-

ing the work of breathing, and increasing abdominal pressure on the diaphragm. Improvements in exercise tolerance and arterial oxygenation can be seen with weight loss alone. Owners should be given reasonable goals for the dog's optimal weight and the time in which weight loss can be achieved. A 2 to 3% weight loss per week is desirable. This can be achieved through the use of a high-fiber, low-fat diet and by providing gradually increasing amounts of exercises.

Animals with concurrent tracheal collapse or marked tracheal sensitivity may benefit from a harness instead of a collar. When stresses in the environment are encountered, such as cigarette smoke, pollutants, heat, or humidity, the animal should be removed to a cool, clean area.

Some patients may benefit from clearing airway secretions with intermittent airway humidification via steam inhalation or nebulization. An ultrasonic nebulizer is preferred for respiratory therapy because it produces sufficiently small particles of water to penetrate deep into the airways. Humidified, oxygenated air can be provided to the patient by attaching the nebulizer to an oxygen cage or a standard cage covered with acrylic, or a hand-held nebulizer can be attached to the oxygen line of an anesthesia machine and air is then delivered via a face mask. Coupage of the chest or gentle exercise after nebulization facilitates clearance of secretions.

PROGNOSIS

Owners should be aware that bronchitis is a chronic disease that may be controlled but never cured. The majority of animals have residual cough and exhibit clinical signs periodically throughout life. The presence of fibrosis and chronic inflammation on biopsy specimens confirms the irreversibility of airway disease. The goals of therapy are to control inflammation, thus limiting clinical signs; diagnose and treat infection when it occurs; and prevent worsening airway disease that might lead to debilitating sequelae such as bronchiectasis and cor pulmonale.

References and Suggested Reading

Ball P: Epidemiology and treatment of chronic bronchitis and its exacerbations. Chest 108:43S, 1995.
　The role of bacterial infection in human bronchitis and the use of antibiotics is reviewed.
Cormier Y, Whitton R, Boulet LP, et al: Effect of inflammation on peripheral airway reactivity in dogs. Clin Sci 84:73, 1993.
　Airway inflammation caused by Bordetella bronchiseptica *resulted in changes in baseline pulmonary function tests.*
Intorre L, Mengozzi G, Maccheroni M, et al: Enrofloxacin-theophylline interaction: Influence of enrofloxacin on theophylline steady-state pharmacokinetics in the Beagle dog. J Vet Pharmacol Ther 19:352, 1995.
　Concurrent administration of enrofloxacin and theophylline was shown to result in toxic plasma levels of theophylline.
Lusuardi M, Capelli A, Carli S, et al: Local airways immune modifications induced by oral bacterial extracts in chronic bronchitis. Chest 103:1783, 1993.
　This study demonstrated the ability of an orally administered bacterial extract to enhance macrophage activity within the airway in human patients with bronchitis.
Murphy TF, Sethi S: Bacterial infection in chronic obstructive pulmonary disease. Am Rev Respir Dis 146:1067, 1992.
　This is a comprehensive review of the properties of bacteria that play a role in the induction of chronic bronchitis in humans.

Padrid PA, Amis TC: Chronic tracheobronchial disease in the dog. Vet Clin North Am 22:1203, 1992.
This is a concise review of diagnostics and therapeutics for dogs with disease of the conducting airway.

Padrid PA, Hornof W, Kurpershoek C, et al: Canine chronic bronchitis: A pathophysiologic evaluation of 18 cases. J Vet Intern Med 4:172, 1990.
The complete clinical assessment of 18 dogs suffering from chronic bronchitis is detailed.

Saetta M, DiStefano A, Maesterelli P, et al: Airway eosinophilia in chronic bronchitis during exacerbations. Am J Respir Crit Care Med 153:1646, 1994.
Airway eosinophilia was detected in association with acute exacerbations of disease in a group of human patients with chronic bronchitis.

CVT Update: Feline Asthma

PHILIP PADRID
Chicago, Illinois

Asthma is a disorder characterized in humans by cough and wheeze. These clinical signs are caused by spontaneous bronchoconstriction, which may resolve either spontaneously or in response to therapy. Additional defining features of asthma include airway inflammation and "airway hyperreactivity," a condition that results in decreased air flow after exposure to stimuli that cause no significant change in air flow in normal individuals. A remarkably similar condition in cats, "feline asthma" has been recognized in the veterinary literature since at least 1911. This early description by Hill included increased airway mucus associated with airway inflammation and the clinical signs of labored breathing and wheezing (Padrid et al, 1996).

The diagnosis of asthma in cats is based on clinical criteria. The most important findings used to make the diagnosis typically include the following:

1. A history of acute onset of labored breathing. This is usually quickly relieved with some combination of oxygen, bronchodilators, and steroids. In some cases, however, the only clinical problem is chronic cough.
2. Radiographic evidence of bronchial wall thickening, which is usually described as "doughnuts" and "tramlines," and air trapping.
3. Clinicopathologic evidence of airway inflammation, including the finding of large numbers of eosinophils recovered from tracheobronchial secretions.

These clinical findings, including reversible bronchoconstriction and airway inflammation, are strikingly similar to the clinical findings in human asthma. Additional similarities include hyperplasia and hypertrophy of the mucus-secreting apparatus and airway smooth muscle hyperplasia. Epithelial erosion also is frequently found in association with an eosinophilic infiltrate. Airway hyperreactivity, a defining feature of human asthma, has also been shown in cats with clinical signs of asthma. These striking clinical and histologic parallels between both species demonstrate that some cats with signs of lower airway disease meet the criteria for the diagnosis of asthma in humans. Nevertheless, 86 years after Hill's description of feline asthma, we are just beginning to increase our recognition of the clinical disease, and our understanding of the mechanism or mechanisms that may participate in the pathogenesis of asthma in cats.

The purpose of this article is to (1) review our current understanding of the pathophysiology of asthma in cats, (2) review common clinical signs and diagnostic tests, and (3) suggest rational and novel approaches for treating cats with this debilitating and frequently confusing airway disorder.

PATHOPHYSIOLOGY

Although the potential causes of asthma are numerous, the airways are capable of responding to noxious stimuli in only a limited number of ways. Airway epithelium may hypertrophy, undergo metaplastic change, erode, or ulcerate. Airway goblet cells and submucosal glands may hypertrophy and produce excessive amounts of viscid mucus. Bronchial mucosa and submucosa are usually infiltrated with variable numbers and types of inflammatory cells and may become edematous. Bronchial smooth muscle may remain unaffected, become hypertrophied, or spasm. In almost all cases, the unifying and underlying problem is chronic inflammation, whereas the exact cause remains unproved.

The resulting clinical signs of cough, wheeze, and lethargy are due to limitation of air flow from excessive mucus secretions, airway edema, airway narrowing from cellular infiltrates, and airway smooth muscle constriction. A 50% reduction in the luminal size of an airway results in a 16-fold reduction in the amount of air that flows through that airway. Clearly then, small changes in airway luminal diameter result in dramatic changes in air flow. The clinical implication of this finding is twofold. First, relatively small amounts of mucus, edema, or bronchoconstriction can partially occlude airways and cause a dramatic fall in air flow. Conversely, therapy that results in relatively small increases in airway size may cause a dramatic improvement in clinical signs.

Cough may also result from stimulation of mechanoreceptors located in inflamed and contracted airway smooth muscle. Inappropriate airway smooth muscle contraction, in turn, seems fundamentally linked to inflammation. Importantly, asthmatic human airways show evidence of chronic ongoing inflammation whether or not the patient is symptomatic. Although many inflammatory cell types are found within asthmatic airways of humans and cats, eosinophils appear to be primary effector cells in the development of asthmatic airway pathophysiology in both species. Highly charged cationic proteins within eosinophil granules are released into airways and cause epithelial disruption and sloughing. Additionally, these granular proteins can make airway smooth muscle more "twitchy" and prone to contraction after exposure to low levels of stimulation (airway hyperreactivity).

Eosinophil–T Lymphocyte Interactions

The pathogenesis of asthmatic airway hyperreactivity is clearly multifactorial and complex. Investigations suggest that the interaction between T lymphocytes and eosinophils within airways may play a particularly important role in the generation of eosinophilic airway inflammation and airway hyperreactivity in human asthma (Beasley et al, 1989; Bradley et al, 1991). Increased numbers of eosinophils and activated T lymphocytes are found in bronchoalveolar lavage specimens and bronchial mucosa of patients with asthma, and the presence of these cells is correlated with disease severity. Data suggest that activated T cells are recruited into the airways of asthmatic individuals when they are exposed to aeroallergens. CD4+ interleukin-5 (IL-5) secreted from T cells promotes eosinophilopoiesis, survival, activation, and recruitment into airways.

WHAT DO WE KNOW NOW?

Although coughing and wheezing cats have been identified by owners and veterinarians for more than 80 years, it is only since 1993 that we have begun to study the disorder in earnest. Dye and associates at the University of Illinois School of Veterinary Medicine have identified pulmonary function abnormalities in cats with signs of chronic lower airway inflammation (Dye et al, 1996). Some of these cats have increased pulmonary resistance that resolves after treatment with terbutaline, a beta$_2$-agonist, indicating the presence of reversible bronchoconstriction in these patients. Additionally, some of these cats experience dramatic bronchoconstriction after exposure to low levels of methacholine, a drug with minimal effects on pulmonary function when used in equivalent doses in nonasthmatic cats. This is important as the first demonstration of spontaneous, naturally occurring airway hyperreactivity in a nonhuman species. We also know that in cats, like humans, bronchoconstriction is reversible with beta-adrenergic agonists. Additionally, histologic changes in airways from asthmatic cats include epithelial erosion, goblet cell and submucosal gland hyperplasia and hypertrophy, and an increased mass of smooth muscle, which are all features of human asthmatic airways.

EXPERIMENTALLY INDUCED FELINE ASTHMA

Studies of cats with naturally occurring asthma are critical to our understanding of the disease in the feline population and can lead to the formulation of rational treatment strategies. However, these tests are available only in university settings and require that cats are first anesthetized. This has caused reluctance by owners to allow their pets to be used in these studies, and our understanding of the pathogenesis and natural course of asthma in cats has been hampered as a result. In an attempt to begin to understand the immunologic mechanisms that may be operative in the pathogenesis and perturbation of asthma in cats, and as a means to determine objective data regarding response to therapy, the author has developed an antigen (*Ascaris suum*)–sensitized and challenged model of feline asthma. These cats develop persistent airway eosinophilia and hyperresponsiveness to nebulized acetylcholine. There is a constellation of changes in airway wall structure, including an eosinophil infiltrate within epithelium, occasional foci of ulceration, hypertrophy and hyperplasia of epithelial goblet cells, hyperplasia of submucosal glands, and an increase in airway smooth muscle thickness. We have previously reported that these antigen-sensitized cats have elevated serum levels of soluble receptor for IL-2 found within 24 hours of antigen challenge. These animals also have a decrease in the CD4+:CD8+ peripheral blood T cell ratio compared with values obtained before antigen challenge. These findings suggest T-cell activation in asthmatic cats similar to the findings in humans with asthma.

Recognition of the potential role of activated T cells in the pathogenesis of the asthmatic airway and animal studies showing the effect of cyclosporin A (CsA) to inhibit late-phase responses have led to the clinical use of CsA to treat patients with severe asthma. However, the full potential therapeutic effect of CsA to inhibit T-cell activation and cytokine synthesis has been limited in part by the relatively low dose that can be used safely in humans (Alexander et al, 1995). Interestingly, the feline species is resistant to the harmful side effects of CsA even when administered in high doses for long periods.

To determine the role of products of activated T cells in the development of experimentally induced asthma in cats, the author treated *Ascaris suum*–sensitized and challenged cats with high doses of CsA 2 weeks before antigen challenge and then daily for the entire 6-week antigen challenge period. Because CsA blocks T-cell production of multiple cytokines, we reasoned that this drug might inhibit recruitment of activated eosinophils into airways and the development of airway hyperreactivity. We found that treatment with CsA dramatically inhibited the pathologic changes in airway structure and function seen in cats not treated with CsA (Padrid et al, 1996). These results are consistent with the use of CsA in humans with asthma and suggest a potential role for CsA in the treatment of chronic severe asthma in cats (see "Therapy" further on).

The author has shown that serotonin is a primary mediator in feline mast cells that contributes to airway smooth muscle contraction in vitro (Padrid et al, 1995). This mediator is absent in human, equine, and canine airways. During an acute asthmatic attack, inhaled antigens within airways cause acute mast cell degranulation and release of preformed serotonin, and this causes sudden contraction of airway smooth muscle. Interestingly, it has long been assumed that histamine released from feline mast cells caused acute bronchoconstriction. This assumption has recently been challenged by the finding that histamine nebulized into cat airways has an unpredictable effect from one cat to another. Specifically, histamine may have no effect, it may cause bronchoconstriction, and it may actually dilate feline airways. These findings have potential therapeutic applications (see the section on therapy).

CLINICAL FINDINGS

Incidence and Prevalence

There are currently no reliable data regarding the incidence and prevalence of asthma in cats. The prevalence of lower airway disease in the general adult cat population is estimated to be approximately 1%; prevalence in the Siamese breed may be 5% or greater. Anecdotal information and one published study suggest that the Siamese breed may actually be genetically susceptible to the development of asthma.

Clinical Signs

Clinical signs include cough, wheeze, and decreased play and hunting activity. In mild cases, symptoms may be limited to occasional and brief coughing. Some cats with asthma may be asymptomatic between occasional episodes of acute airway obstruction. Severely affected cats may have a persistent daily cough and experience many episodes of life-threatening acute bronchoconstriction. A common problem for the practitioner is to distinguish between chronic bronchitis and asthma as the cause of a chronic cough in cats. Although these two disorders are frequently lumped together under the title of *chronic bronchial disease* or *lower airway disease*, the two disorders require different therapeutic approaches and have different prognoses. *Chronic bronchitis* is a condition that causes a chronic cough for which other causes of cough, such as pneumonia, heartworm infestation, bronchopulmonary neoplasia, or heart failure, have been ruled out. *Asthma* is a disorder characterized by spontaneous bronchoconstriction that may resolve spontaneously or in response to therapy. All cats with chronic bronchitis, by definition, have symptoms of cough on most days throughout the year. Some cats with asthma may be asymptomatic between occasional episodes of acute airway obstruction. Other asthmatic cats may cough occasionally and demonstrate frequent tachypnea. Importantly, asthmatic cats, but not bronchitic cats, may benefit from bronchodilator treatment (see the section on therapy).

DIAGNOSTIC TEST FINDINGS

Physical Examination

There are no physical examination findings that can be relied on to make the diagnosis of asthma. In fact, cats with asthma may have a normal physical examination at rest. Conversely, respiratory distress primarily during the expiratory phase of breathing is the hallmark of asthma in cats. Adventitious sounds, including crackles and, more commonly, wheezes, are found in many cats with bronchial asthma.

Thoracic Radiographs

Routine survey chest radiographs may be normal and should not cause the practitioner to abandon the diagnosis of asthma. Frequently, however, radiographs may demonstrate diffuse prominent bronchial markings consistent with inflammatory airways. Radiographic signs of increased lung lucency and flattening and caudal displacement of the diaphragm represent hyperinflation and suggest air trapping. In the author's experience, approximately 10% of asthmatic cat radiographs have increased density within the right middle lung lobe associated with a mediastinal shift to the right. This is evidence of atelectasis.

Tracheobronchial Culture

The presence of a mixed population of aerobic bacteria in airways has previously been reported in cats with asthma. However, neither the lower airway nor lung parenchyma of healthy cats are sterile. Organisms usually considered to be pathogens such as *Klebsiella* and *Pseudomonas* can be recovered from healthy feline airways. Studies designed to correlate the clinical status of asthmatic cats with the presence or absence of bacteria within the airway have not, to the author's knowledge, been attempted or published. It is the author's opinion that bacteria isolated from the asthmatic feline airway most commonly reflect colonization rather than true infection. The role of *Mycoplasma* may be an exception to this. *Mycoplasma* (and certain viruses) can degrade neutral endopeptidase, which is an enzyme that is responsible for biodegradation of substance P, a protein capable of causing bronchoconstriction and edema in the feline airway. *Mycoplasma* might then indirectly prolong the effects of substance P on airway smooth muscle. It is tempting to speculate that *Mycoplasma* or viruses such as herpes, which can remain dormant in feline airways, might be responsible for increasing the levels of substance P in cat airways and contribute to spontaneous bronchoconstriction.

Tracheobronchial Washings

Until the 1980s, it was generally assumed that eosinophils played only a beneficial role in the immune system by protecting against parasite infestation. Within the last 20 years, however, it has become clear that the presence of these cells in the wrong place at the wrong time can result in significant cellular and tissue damage. It is therefore of great interest that eosinophils can be recovered in large numbers from the tracheobronchial washings of many healthy cats. These cells seemingly cause no damage to the host or the local tissue environment and should not by themselves be viewed as markers of allergy or parasitism.

NEW TREATMENT STRATEGIES

The primary signs of asthma include cough and wheeze, and these signs are frequently the result of some degree of airway smooth muscle contraction. It is tempting to treat these signs of asthma by using bronchodilators to relax the airway smooth muscle contraction. Although this is a central method of treatment when acute signs develop, it is critically important to understand that human (and perhaps feline) asthmatic airways show evidence of chronic ongoing inflammation whether or not the patient is symptomatic. Therefore, treatment strategies are most successful if they are directed toward decreasing the underlying inflammatory component of the disease in addition to the acute clinical signs of cough, wheeze, and increased respiratory effort.

There is currently no consistently reported or accepted strategy to treat cats with asthma. Additionally, there are no data to determine which treatments are most effective, in which setting, and for how long. The following approaches represent the author's suggested practical and theoretical strategies to treat cats with asthma.

High-Dose, Long-Term Corticosteroids

The most effective long-term treatment of human asthma is oral corticosteroids. This class of drugs is most likely to reproducibly suppress asthmatic inflammation, a process orchestrated by a network of proteins (cytokines) that act on circulating and structural airway cells. An important effect of steroids is to inhibit the synthesis of genes for cytokines that are important in generating asthmatic airway inflammation. However, the side effects of these medications in humans are often extreme and preclude the routine use of these systemic drugs. Fortunately, inhaled steroids have become available that do not cause systemic side effects, and this treatment has greatly enhanced the physician's ability to successfully treat patients with asthma. This same approach to the treatment of cats with asthma is not routinely available or practical. Luckily, compared with humans, the incidence of health-threatening side effects in cats from oral steroids is remarkably reduced. This is important because *the most consistent, most reliable, and most effective treatment for feline asthma is high-dose, long-term oral corticosteroids.* The author begins treatment of asthmatic cats with prednisone, 1 to 2 mg/kg PO every 12 hours for 10 to 14 days. At this point, the majority of newly diagnosed cats have greatly diminished signs. The dose of steroids is then tapered slowly, over at least 2 to 3 months. This approach is much more effective than low doses of prednisone given for short periods and in response to acute flare-ups.

Injectable Steroids

If clinical signs are not greatly improved within 7 days, the author re-evaluates the diagnosis. If I am still reasonably certain of the diagnosis of asthma, I administer a long-acting repository steroid (methylprednisolone acetate [Depo-Medrol], 10 to 20 mg IM every 2 to 4 weeks). The rationale for this approach is based on my assumption that the lack of clinical response is most likely because the owner is (1) unable to give the medication or (2) unaware that the patient is not ingesting the pills. A good response within 2 days of injection confirms my suspicions. At this point, I review with the owner the technique involved in "pilling" cats, and together we decide if this is a feasible approach. If not, the less desirable method of periodic injection of repository steroids is used.

Parenteral Terbutaline at Home

Terbutaline is a bronchodilator that stimulates beta$_2$-receptors in airway smooth muscle. This causes phosphorylation of certain proteins within the nucleus of smooth muscle and results in smooth muscle relaxation (bronchodilation). Beta$_2$-agonists are the most effective bronchodilators available and their use results in rapid relief of asthma symptoms in some cats. Many veterinarians use terbutaline only in an emergency to treat asthmatic cats that present in respiratory distress. Humans with asthma also routinely use inhaled terbutaline when acute symptoms develop, and this common practice precludes the need to visit an emergency room. The author proposes that we teach clients to give terbutaline subcutaneously to their asthmatic pets just as we teach them to give insulin to their diabetic pets. The indication for use of this drug in this clinical setting is acute respiratory difficulty at home. The dose I use is 0.01 mg/kg SC or IM. An obvious beneficial response occurs within 15 to 30 minutes. This may be repeated if a significant benefit is not observed after one dose. To determine if the drug has been absorbed and if a beneficial effect has occurred, heart rate and respiratory rate and effort are monitored before drug administration. A heart rate that approaches 240 beats per minute suggests that the drug has been absorbed. A respiratory rate or effort, or both, that drops by 50% or more suggests a beneficial effect.

The author believes this strategy will routinely prevent the need for inconvenient and costly (for the owner and practitioner alike) late-night emergency clinic visits.

Antibiotics

There is no objective evidence that bacterial infection plays a significant role in the cause or continuation of feline asthma. Similarly, there is no objective evidence that antibiotic therapy has any effect on the duration or intensity of signs displayed by the cat with asthma. It is important to remember that the clinical signs of asthma in cats frequently wax and wane in severity as well as in frequency of occurrence. There are many anecdotal reports describing the therapeutic effect of antibiotics in controlling asthmatic symptoms, but these reports are consistent with the "waxing and waning" nature of the symptom in nontreated cases.

A positive culture result obtained from a tracheobronchial wash does not necessarily imply the presence of a clinically significant airway infection and should not automatically prompt the clinician to initiate antibiotic therapy. In the author's opinion, antibiotics are rarely indicated for cats with asthma and are appropriate only when there is good evidence of superimposed airway infection. This may be inferred from the growth of a pure bacterial culture on a primary culture plate from material obtained from tracheobronchial secretions. This is because the concentration of aerobic bacteria recovered from the airways of healthy cats rarely exceeds 5×10^3 organisms/ml. In contrast, growth of a single organism recovered without the use of enrichment broth implies greater than 10^5 organisms/ml, and this is consistent with an "infected" airway in humans. Antibiotic therapy is then based on sensitivity data. Prophylactic or long-term therapy should be avoided unless there is documentation of a chronic airway infection, which is extraordinarily uncommon in feline asthma.

One possible exception to these statements involves *Mycoplasma* spp. *Mycoplasma* has been isolated from the airway of as many as 25% of cats with signs of lower airway disease, but *Mycoplasma* has not been cultured from the airway of healthy cats. For this reason, and because *Mycoplasma* has the potential to cause significant structural damage to airway epithelium, it may be prudent to treat any cat with a *Mycoplasma*-positive airway culture with an appropriate antibiotic.

Cyproheptadine

Cyproheptadine (Periactin) is marketed as an antihistamine; however, it has been used for years as an appetite stimulant for depressed or anorectic cats. This latter effect is actually due to its antiserotonin properties. As mentioned earlier, serotonin is a primary mediator released from activated mast cells into feline airways and causes acute smooth muscle contraction (bronchoconstriction) in cats but not in humans. The author has shown that the ability of cyproheptadine to block serotonin receptors in muscle cells is effective in preventing antigen-induced airway smooth muscle constriction in vitro. Limited clinical studies of asthmatic cats have supported these in vitro findings. The primary indication for this drug is the chronic symptomatic asthmatic cat on maximal doses of terbutaline and corticosteroids. Cyproheptadine comes in both pill and liquid form and is dosed at 2 mg PO every 12 hours. A beneficial therapeutic response may not be seen for 4 to 7 days, but depression, the primary side effect of this drug, may be seen 24 hours after administration. Depression is not life-threatening but may cause the owner to discontinue cyproheptadine therapy.

Cyclosporine

Evidence that activated T lymphocytes may play an important role in the generation of eosinophilic airway inflammation has revived interest in the use of CsA to treat human patients with asthma. In limited clinical trials in patients with moderate to severe asthma, CsA has improved lung function and acted as a steroid-sparing agent. For the small subpopulation of patients with chronic severe asthma who require large doses of corticosteroids or are steroid-resistant, CsA may be a useful adjunct to therapy. More widespread use of this drug to treat asthmatic patients is limited by the wide profile of side effects that results from administration of this agent. Because cats are relatively immune to the side effects of CsA reported in humans, veterinarians are not as limited in the doses they can prescribe for their asthmatic patients. In an experimental model of feline asthma, CsA was administered in high doses and was effective in preventing both histologic and clinical asthmatic changes. The indication for use of this drug is limited to the severe uncontrolled asthmatic cat, the kind of case in which euthanasia is being considered. The author uses an initial dose of 10 mg/kg PO every 12 hours. Oral absorption of CsA is unpredictable; therefore, blood levels must be checked at least weekly until a stable dose is achieved to maintain trough blood levels between 500 and 1,000 ng/ml. This blood test (radioimmunoassay) is available at most local and all referral human hospitals.

Anti–Interleukin-5 Antibody

As mentioned previously, eosinophils are primary effector cells in the pathogenesis of asthmatic airways. A number of elegant experimental studies have strongly implicated IL-5 in the pathogenesis of eosinophilic airway inflammation. The author has recently isolated the gene that codes for feline-specific IL-5. This cytokine product is secreted from feline-activated T lymphocytes and may have a principal role in causing activated eosinophils to migrate into feline airways and participate in the pathogenesis of asthmatic airway inflammation.

The author's laboratory is currently studying the effects of treating asthmatic cats with an antibody to IL-5. Nebulization of anti–IL-5 antibody results in resolution of 90% of the airway eosinophilia in experimentally induced asthma, and this effect persists for at least 45 days. The author's hypothesis is that blockage of this eosinophil chemotactic and activating factor will decrease the clinical signs and histologic derangements that characterize the asthmatic cat's airway. Antibodies to IL-5 are also currently being used in phase I clinical trials to treat human asthmatic patients. Clearly, this experimental approach requires increased study before it can be recommended for use in clinical veterinary patients.

References and Suggested Reading

Alexander AG, Barnes NC, Kay AB, et al: Clinical response to cyclosporine in chronic severe asthma is associated with reduction in serum soluble interleukin-2 receptor concentrations. Eur Respir J 8:574, 1995.
The therapeutic effects of cyclosporine in patients with severe asthma are documented.
Beasley R, Roche WR, Roberts JA, et al: Cellular events in the bronchi in mild asthma and after bronchial provocation. Am Rev Respir Dis 139:806, 1989.
This was one of the first reports to demonstrate inflammation in airways of mild asthmatics, even when the symptoms of asthma are not present.
Bradley BL, Azzawi M, Jacobson B, et al: Eosinophils, T lymphocytes, mast cells, neutrophils, and macrophages in bronchial biopsies from atopic asthma: Comparison with atopic non-asthma and normal controls and relationship to bronchial hyperresponsiveness. J Allergy Clin Immunol 88:661, 1991.
This was one of the first reports to demonstrate that airway inflammation is related to airway hyperresponsiveness.
Dye JA, McKiernan BC, Rozanski EA, et al: Bronchopulmonary disease in the cat: Historical, physical, radiographic, clinicopathologic and pulmonary functional evaluation of 24 affected and 15 healthy cats. J Vet Intern Med 10:385, 1996.
This is the only thorough review of naturally occurring bronchial disease in cats, and documents airway hyperresponsiveness in feline asthma.
Padrid PA: Animal models of asthma. In: Liggett SB, Meyers DA, eds: The Genetics of Asthma: Lung Biology in Health and Disease. New York: Marcel Dekker, 1996, pp 211–233.
This is a comprehensive review of the advantages and disadvantages of multiple animal species used in asthma research.
Padrid PA, Cozzi P, Leff AR: Cyclosporine A attenuates the development of chronic airway hyperresponsiveness and histologic alterations in immune-sensitized cats. Am J Respir Crit Care Med 154:1812, 1996.
Experimentally induced asthma is completely inhibited in cats treated with maximal doses of cyclosporin A for 6 weeks.

Padrid PA, Mitchell RW, Ndukwu IM, et al: Cyproheptadine-induced attenuation of type-I immediate hypersensitivity reactions of airway smooth muscle from immune-sensitized cats. Am J Vet Res 56:109, 1995.

This article describes the first report that serotonin within feline mast cells contracts feline airway smooth muscle in vitro and that cyproheptadine blockade of serotonin receptors prevents airway smooth muscle contraction in vitro.

Noncardiogenic Pulmonary Edema

KENNETH J. DROBATZ
H. MARK SAUNDERS
Philadelphia, Pennsylvania

Pulmonary edema is defined as an abnormal accumulation of transudate in the extravascular spaces of the lung. It is a dynamic clinical syndrome attributable to a variety of disease processes. Noncardiogenic pulmonary edema is due to an increase in vascular endothelial permeability, rather than a result of increased vascular hydrostatic pressure as seen in cardiogenic pulmonary edema.

Increased permeability in noncardiogenic pulmonary edema (NPE) originates from an injury to the pulmonary microvascular endothelium that separates the intravascular compartment from the pulmonary interstitium and alveoli. The increase in permeability results in an extravascular fluid that is relatively high in protein compared to hydrostatic or cardiogenic pulmonary edema. Also, the increased permeability leads to an increase in extravascular lung water content at lower hydrostatic pressures than in cardiogenic pulmonary edema.

NPE can reflect the pulmonary response to a primary pulmonary injury only, or to disease processes elsewhere in the patient. The common causes of primary pulmonary epithelial injury include aspiration of gastric contents, near-drowning, inhalation of smoke or toxic gases, blunt trauma, or high inspired oxygen concentrations for prolonged periods. Extrapulmonary-mediated insults include systemic sepsis, neurogenic pulmonary edema, pancreatitis, uremia, systemic inflammatory response syndrome, and pulmonary embolism.

DIAGNOSIS

NPE is a reasonable differential diagnosis in any critical animal that is showing signs of respiratory distress. The clinical difficulty is to distinguish this form of pulmonary edema from that of cardiac origin, as treatment will vary, depending on the etiology. The form of pulmonary edema is not always clear, and on rare occasions both cardiogenic and noncardiogenic pulmonary edema may be present simultaneously. In the absence of direct measurement of pulmonary artery wedge pressures, clinical acumen and experience are essential to reaching a diagnosis, beginning with a thorough history and physical examination.

The history may provide information for a diagnosis, such as exposure to electrical cords, head or chest trauma, airway obstruction, exposure to toxins, or inhalation of smoke. A thorough physical examination should include all organ systems to detect the presence of systemic disease. Evaluation of the pulmonary and cardiovascular systems is essential for determining the presence and severity of pulmonary edema. There are no pathognomonic physical signs for NPE. Particular attention should be given to the presence of cardiac abnormalities, such as a cardiac murmur, gallop, or arrhythmia, poor pulse quality, jugular pulse, and prolonged capillary refill time. Secondary cardiac signs may occur from NPE or mediators from systemic inflammation, confusing the physical determination of cardiogenic versus noncardiogenic pulmonary edema. Unfortunately, when animals present with severe respiratory distress, restraint can be stressful and detrimental to the patient. Therefore, a thorough physical examination may not be possible until the animal has been stabilized.

When the animal is stabilized, thoracic radiographs should be obtained to aid in differentiating cardiogenic from noncardiogenic pulmonary edema. The initial radiographs will also determine the extent and severity of pulmonary edema, reveal additional abnormalities and complications, and serve as a reference point after the institution of treatment. Cardiogenic pulmonary edema is often located in the perihilar region, although it can be diffuse, and is seen concurrently with left-sided cardiomegaly and pulmonary venous distention. Early NPE will typically appear radiographically as an interstitial pulmonary edema, although by the time animals with acute edema are radiographed, the disease may have already resulted in a mixed interstitial-alveolar or alveolar pattern. Although the distribution of NPE in the lateral view is typically in the caudodorsal lung quadrant, diffuse involvement can also occur. Symmetrical or asymmetrical distribution may depend on the inciting cause of the edema. For example, extrapulmonary-mediated insults are more likely to cause symmetrical involvement; inhalation of toxic fluids or near-drowning (primary pulmonary) may cause asymmetrical pulmonary edema.

Arterial blood gases are not characteristic of NPE but often reflect pulmonary dysfunction, revealing hypoxemia due to ventilation-perfusion mismatch. The $Paco_2$ initially is low, owing to hyperventilation in response to the pulmonary parenchymal disease and, if severe, hypoxemia. In the later stages, compromised pulmonary compliance can interfere with the animal's ability to ventilate, causing hypercapnia. A complete blood count, serum chemistry profile, and urinalysis round out the initial diagnostic tests searching for an underlying cause of NPE.

In summary, the diagnosis is not achieved by measuring one parameter. It involves assessing a combination of the history, physical abnormalities, thoracic radiographs, arterial blood gas measurements, and clinical laboratory test results. The measurement of pulmonary capillary wedge pressure is sometimes necessary for ruling out an increased hydrostatic cause of the pulmonary edema. However, such measurements are not yet routine in veterinary critical care.

INITIAL APPROACH AND MANAGEMENT

Ideally, the identification and elimination of the inciting cause of NPE might result in dissipation of the pulmonary edema. Corticosteroids and blockers of the cyclooxygenase and leukotriene pathways have not been proved to definitely resolve the pulmonary inflammatory process occurring in most patients with NPE. In lieu of specific therapies for the underlying disease process or resolution of the pulmonary endothelial inflammation, a nonspecific approach involving supporting the respiratory and cardiovascular systems is the current mainstay of treatment.

An animal that is presented in severe respiratory distress is a challenge; the restraint required for diagnosis and treatment could result in death. When possible, an intravenous catheter should be placed to allow rapid vascular access. Immediate oxygen therapy by oxygen cage, nasal oxygen, or intubation and ventilation can be lifesaving during the initial assessment and stabilization. The veterinarian may immediately be faced with the decision whether to sedate and/or anesthetize the patient for intubation and ventilation support. The acute, critical nature of some cases of NPE is such that ventilation may be required for obtaining initial stabilization.

Positive pressure ventilation (PPV) opens collapsed alveoli and small airways to increase the number of ventilated alveoli, thereby decreasing intrapulmonary shunting. NPE decreases lung compliance so that greater than normal inspiratory pressures (20 cm H_2O) are usually necessary for generating adequate tidal volumes of 10 to 20 ml/kg.

Inspired oxygen concentrations of more than 50% for 12 hours or longer might cause oxygen toxicity. Maintaining the animal on the lowest oxygen concentration possible to correct hypoxemia minimizes the chances of toxicity. Positive end-expiratory pressure (PEEP) is often used as an adjunct to mechanical ventilation with the goal of providing an adequate PaO_2 at a low mean airway pressure and low inspired oxygen concentration. It can also be used in spontaneously breathing patients. PEEP increases functional residual capacity, prevents alveolar and small airway collapse between breaths, and allows more alveoli to participate in gas exchange. The adverse effects of PEEP and PPV are similar. Both of these treatments can cause a decrease in venous return and cardiac output. Additionally, barotrauma and pneumothorax are not unusual sequelae in patients with NPE receiving high PEEP and end-inspiratory pressures from PPV.

Oxygen delivery to the tissues can be maintained despite hypoxemia if cardiac output is increased. Cardiac function

in animals with NPE can be adversely affected by hypovolemia, depressed myocardial contractility, and vasoconstriction. Low blood volume results in poor venous return to the heart, poor cardiac output, and systemic hypotension. Fluid administration to increase blood volume, cardiac preload, and subsequent cardiac output helps improve tissue perfusion. The major concern with fluid infusion is the very real potential that fluid therapy may increase pulmonary edema in patients with NPE. The choice of crystalloids versus colloids is a continuing controversy. The decrease in intravascular oncotic pressure and the increase in hydrostatic pressure associated with crystalloid infusion promote pulmonary edema in patients with increased pulmonary capillary permeability. On the other hand, colloid solutions do not necessarily decrease the incidence of pulmonary edema, and may be hazardous in the setting of altered pulmonary capillary permeability. The loss of colloid particles into the pulmonary interstitium would result in increased interstitial oncotic pressure and a subsequent increase in extravascular lung water. The relative permeability of the pulmonary microvasculature during disease states cannot be predicted clinically. A test infusion of a colloidal solution and monitoring the intravascular colloid osmotic pressure (see p. 116) might provide insight into the vasculature's ability to retain the infused colloids. No improvement, or a rapid decrease in colloid osmotic pressure, suggests that the colloid is rapidly lost from the vasculature and its use in the patient should be restricted. Existing data are thus contradictory on the comparative benefits of crystalloids and colloids with regard to pulmonary function in patients with NPE. Until more information is available, the choice of fluid therapy must be made on a patient-by-patient basis and according to the clinician's preference and experience.

Blood transfusions can optimize oxygen delivery. The authors recommend transfusion of whole blood or packed red blood cells to animals with NPE up to a packed cell volume of 30%. As the packed cell volume rises above 30%, the associated increase in blood viscosity and its deleterious effects on blood flow tend to negate any increases in oxygen delivery caused by the higher hemoglobin concentration.

High pulmonary microvascular hydrostatic pressure enhances fluid transudation across the vessel wall and worsens pulmonary edema. The goal is to achieve a normal pulmonary hydrostatic pressure (measured by pulmonary capillary wedge pressure, PCWP) and to maintain tissue oxygen delivery. In the absence of PCWP measurement, measurement of central venous pressure (CVP) might be useful, keeping in mind that the CVP might not reflect PCWP in patients with pulmonary or cardiac disease. CVP and PCWP measure hydrostatic pressure and therefore may be poor criteria for predicting the development or monitoring the progression of pulmonary edema in animals with a permeability defect.

Diuretics and vasodilators may be used to decrease pulmonary microvascular hydrostatic pressure. Our first choice for a diuretic is furosemide. In dogs, the initial dose is a 2 mg/kg bolus intravenously or intramuscularly if intravenous access is not available. This dose is repeated every 6 to 8 hours. Continuous intravenous infusion of furosemide has been demonstrated to have an improved diuretic response in critically ill patients. The authors use a dose of 0.1 mg/kg per hour of furosemide as a continuous infusion. If PCWP is very high, a systemic vasodilator such as nitroprusside (1 to 10 µg/kg per minute constant-rate infusion) can rapidly lower PCWP (see p. 194). Systemic hypotension and decreased tissue oxygen delivery must be avoided if diuretics or vasodilators are being used as part of therapy. Monitoring blood pressure is warranted, particularly when one uses vasodilators. Systemic hypotension (mean arterial pressure <80 mm Hg) in an animal with adequate blood volume indicates the need for a positive inotrope. Both dopamine (5 to 10 µg/kg per minute) and dobutamine (5 to 20 µg/kg per minute) can be used to increase myocardial contractility and improve cardiac output, and may prevent the volume overloading associated with excessive fluid therapy.

MONITORING THE EFFECTIVENESS OF THERAPY

Frequent assessment of mucous membrane color, capillary refill time, heart rate, pulse quality, thoracic auscultation, and respiratory rate and effort provides vital subjective information on the response to therapy. Serial pulse oximetry and arterial blood gas measurement provide more objective information about pulmonary function. Total thoracic compliance can be measured in intubated patients. A decrease in this measure often precedes the clinical signs of pulmonary edema from fluid overload in human patients. The resolution of NPE on thoracic radiographs is characterized by a shift from an alveolar to a mixed alveolar-interstitial and finally an interstitial pattern. Improvement of the radiographic pulmonary pattern lags behind the animal's clinical improvement.

Patients with NPE often have multiple organ problems and therefore warrant intensive monitoring of extrapulmonary organs, such as the cardiovascular, central nervous, and renal systems. Measurement of blood pressure, cardiac rhythm, and more extensive cardiovascular parameters such as CVP, PCWP, cardiac output, systemic vascular resistance, oxygen delivery, and oxygen consumption provides more detailed information regarding the patient's cardiovascular status. Urine output, serial urinalyses, and serum creatinine and blood urea nitrogen (BUN) provide assessment of renal function. In patients with systemic inflammation or sepsis, coagulation parameters should be serially evaluated for disseminated intravascular coagulation. The degree of monitoring should reflect the severity of the disease process, with the more severely affected patients requiring the most intensive monitoring.

References and Suggested Reading

Demling RH, LaLonde C, Ikegami K: Pulmonary edema: Pathophysiology, methods of measurement, and clinical importance in acute respiratory failure. New Horizons 1:371, 1993.
  A thorough review of the pathophysiology of pulmonary edema, the methods of measurement, and the clinical significance in humans.
Drobatz KJ, Concannon K: Noncardiogenic pulmonary edema. Compendium 16:333, 1994.
  A review of the pathophysiology, diagnosis, and treatment of noncardiogenic pulmonary edema.
Drobatz KJ, Saunders HM, Pugh CR, et al: Non-cardiogenic pulmonary edema: 26 cases (1987–1993). JAVMA 206:1732, 1995.
  A retrospective study of dogs and cats with neurogenic pulmonary edema.
Marinelli WA, Ingbar DH: Diagnosis and management of acute lung injury. Clin Chest Med 15:517, 1994.
  A thorough review of the diagnosis and management of human patients with acute lung injury.
Sibbald WJ, Cunningham MD, Chin DN: Non-cardiac or cardiac pulmonary edema? A practical approach to clinical differentiation in critically ill patients. Chest 84:453, 1983.
  An in-depth review of the differentiation of cardiogenic and noncardiogenic pulmonary edema.

Bacterial Pneumonia

RICHARD B. FORD
Raleigh, North Carolina

Pneumonia associated with the colonization of bacteria in the airway or the pulmonary interstitium is a complex infection characterized by inconsistent clinical signs that can range from subtle or chronic to acute and fulminating. Despite the potentially diverse nature of the clinical signs, the health of any animal with bacterial pneumonia is significantly compromised. Failure to diagnose and effectively intervene may have fatal consequences.

Bacterial pneumonia is more common in dogs than in cats, and its treatment is complicated by the fact that airway or pulmonary infections may involve a single type of organism or multiple organisms. Pathogenic bacteria may localize in a small portion of a single lung lobe or they can be disseminated throughout the entire lung. In many cases, respiratory complications associated with bacterial pneumonia are potentially life-threatening, and treatment must be initiated without a knowledge of the organism involved.

MANAGEMENT CONSIDERATIONS

Bacterial pneumonia is as much a *sign* as it is a *disease*. This fact has both diagnostic and therapeutic implications in the clinical management of affected patients. Although the identification of bacterial pneumonia is based on owner observations, physical examination, and laboratory and radiographic changes, bacterial pneumonia is unlikely to be a *primary* infection. The clinical evaluation, therefore, must include efforts to identify an underlying disorder that might predispose the animal to *secondary* or opportunistic bacterial infection of the lower respiratory tract. In addition, establishing the presence of an underlying disorder has important prognostic value. Several chronic diseases, for example, bronchitis, bronchiectasis, or megaesophagus commonly predispose animals to recurrent bacterial pneumonia. Recurrent infections in the same animal are expected to be more difficult to manage than the initial infection.

Under ideal conditions, the decision to administer antimicrobial therapy to a patient with bacterial pneumonia is based on the knowledge of the infecting organism or organisms. However, obtaining diagnostic samples from the lower respiratory tract can be difficult and, depending on the animal's condition, delaying therapy while waiting for bacterial culture and sensitivity test results may not be in the best interest of the animal. It is common, therefore, for clinicians to initiate antimicrobial therapy in dogs and cats suspected of having bacterial pneumonia despite the fact that laboratory confirmation of the agent involved is not available. Under emergency circumstances, empirical antimicrobial therapy is clearly indicated and can be lifesaving. However, the clinician who prescribes empirical therapy is obligated to assess the patient's response to treatment regularly and thoroughly, establish the presence or absence of a predisposing disease or diseases, and be willing to modify therapy in the event the animal's condition does not improve.

PATIENT ASSESSMENT

The presenting signs of noninfectious bronchopulmonary disease in dogs and cats can be difficult to distinguish from those of bacterial pneumonia. Although the signs of bacterial pneumonia are characterized by cough (more common in dogs than in cats), nasal discharge, sneezing, exercise intolerance, and tachypnea or dyspnea (Hawkins, 1998; Dye et al, 1996; Henik and Yeager, 1994), patients with noninfectious bronchopulmonary disease can present with similar signs. The presence of a mucopurulent nasal discharge, fever, abnormal pulmonary sounds, and characteristic patterns apparent on thoracic radiographs supports a clinical diagnosis of lower respiratory tract infection or bacterial pneumonia. However, it is important to note that dogs and cats with bacterial infections localized within a single lung lobe may not manifest overt signs of respiratory disease.

Diagnostic confirmation of bacterial pneumonia is based on the evaluation of lower respiratory secretions collected by invasive procedures such as tracheal wash (dog or cat), transtracheal aspiration (dog), bronchoalveolar lavage, or bronchoscopy. Diagnostic samples cannot be consistently recovered from the specimens taken from the nose or oral cavity. Secretions collected for diagnostic testing should be submitted for bacterial culture and sensitivity testing, Gram staining, or cytologic studies. The technique for these pro-cedures is described elsewhere in the veterinary literature (Hawkins, 1992; Padrid, 1992).

Efforts to identify a causative organism and establish a sensitivity profile are justified despite the fact that test results from specimens submitted for bacterial culture can take 3 to 5 days or longer. In the event a patient's condition does not improve subsequent to the administration of empirical antimicrobial therapy, knowledge of the specific bacterial isolate, and its sensitivity, could be critical to a successful outcome in the event it becomes necessary to modify the treatment regimen.

BACTERIAL ISOLATES

Several studies have confirmed the fact that bacterial isolates from dogs with clinical evidence of lower respiratory infection include a predominance of aerobic gram-negative bacteria (especially species belonging to the family Enterobacteriaceae) and obligate anaerobes (Angus et al, 1997). *Escherichia coli* is among the most common isolates, followed by *Pasteurella* spp., *Klebsiella pneumoniae, Bordetella bronchiseptica, Pseudomonas aeruginosa, Staphylococcus* spp., and *Streptococcus* (hemolytic and nonhemolytic) (Hawkins, 1998).

In cats with signs of lower respiratory disease, isolates from the lower respiratory tract are frequently consistent with bacteria isolated from the oral cavity and include a wide spectrum of organisms. *Moraxella* spp., *Mycoplasma* spp., and *Pasteurella multocida* are commonly reported; gram-negative, nonfermentative bacilli are commonly isolated from both healthy and affected cats, clouding the interpretation of these isolates (Moise et al, 1989; Dye et al, 1996) (Table 1).

TREATMENT

One of the fundamental principles of medicine dictates that therapy is best guided by an accurate diagnosis. In the clinical setting, however, there are times when the need for therapeutic intervention supersedes diagnostic precision. Intuition and experience guide the clinician when the animal's condition would be jeopardized by a delay in treatment. Empirical therapy, or prescribing treatment in the absence of a definitive diagnosis, is not often optimal, but it is occasionally necessary and, in many cases, lifesaving. The guidelines presented in Tables 2 and 3 address initial

TABLE 1. Common Bacterial Isolates Recovered From the Lower Respiratory Tract of Dogs and Cats With Bronchopulmonary Disease

Canine Respiratory Pathogens	Feline Respiratory Pathogens
Escherichia coli	*Moraxella* spp.
Streptococcus spp.	*Pasteurella multocida*
Pasteurella spp.	*Streptococcus*
Klebsiella pneumoniae	*Escherichia coli*
Pseudomonas aeruginosa	*Klebsiella pneumoniae*
Bordetella bronchiseptica	*Bordetella bronchiseptica*
Staphylococcus spp.	*Proteus* spp.
Obligate anaerobes	*Mycoplasma*

TABLE 2. Guidelines for Administration of Empirical Antimicrobial Therapy in Dogs Suspected of Having Bacterial Pneumonia*

Presenting Complaint and Site	Likely Organisms	First Treatment Choice	Alternative Choice
Stable Animal Cough, lethargy, decreased exercise tolerance, possibly fever but still eating	A mixed bacterial population is likely; gram-negative organisms may predominate	Trimethoprim-sulfonamide, 15–30 mg/kg PO or SC q12hr	Cephalexin, 20–40 mg/kg PO q8hr, *or* amoxicillin-clavulanate, 22 mg/kg PO q8–12hr, *or* chloramphenicol, 50 mg/kg PO or IV or SC q6–8hr
Unstable Animal Respiratory distress, fever, leukocytosis and a left shift	Aerobic gram-negative (enterics), especially *Escherichia coli*	Cefazolin, 15–25 mg/kg IV q6–8hr	Ampicillin,† 20–40 mg/kg IV or SC q6–8hr, *with* enrofloxacin,‡ 2.5 mg/kg slowly IV§ (or IM) q12hr

*Unless the patient's condition continues to deteriorate, empirical treatment should be administered at least 48 to 72 hours before the decision is made to select an alternative antimicrobial.

†Clindamycin, 10 to 20 mg/kg IV or SC q12hr; is an excellent alternative to ampicillin, particularly if an anaerobic organism is suspected.

‡Enrofloxacin should not be administered to dogs younger than 6 months of age unless the infection is considered to be life-threatening and a suitable alternative drug is not available.

§*Note:* Enrofloxacin is *not* labeled for IV administration but has been recommended in animals with life-threatening infections. The calculated dose is administered as an IV bolus over 1 to 2 minutes.

IV, intravenous; SC, subcutaneous; IM, intramuscular; PO, per os (to be administered orally).

empirical therapy of companion animals suspected of having bacterial pneumonia. However, as is the case with any set of prescribed guidelines, the recommendations outlined are not a template for success in all animals. The clinician who is willing to institute empirical therapy must be willing to modify the therapy at any time to best meet the needs of the animal. Empirical therapy is a starting point—it is planned with the animal's immediate needs in mind and must never be prescribed in lieu of a sound diagnostic strategy.

The Stable Patient

Not all patients with bacterial pneumonia have life-threatening infections and, therefore, do not necessarily require hospitalization and parenteral therapy. Depending on the underlying cause, a broad-spectrum antibacterial agent can be prescribed for oral administration at home. However, it is recommended that follow-up physical examination and thoracic radiographs be completed 48 to 72 hours after the onset of treatment. If the animal is eating

well, fever is absent, and thoracic radiographs are not worse than at the time of the initial examination, treatment is continued for at least 1 week beyond the time the patient appears to have recovered. Other than adequate rest, reasonable exercise, and a high-quality food, no other treatment is required.

Conversely, if the animal's physical condition deteriorates within 48 to 72 hours after the initial evaluation, it is appropriate to classify the patient as unstable (see further on) and recommend hospitalization, administration of parenteral fluid and antimicrobial therapy, and reassessment of the antibacterial agent of choice. If not already obtained, samples of secretions from the lower airway should be obtained and submitted for bacterial culture.

The Unstable Patient

Dogs and cats suspected of having bacterial pneumonia are designated unstable if tachypnea or dyspnea at rest is observed. Other signs that justify categorizing the animal as unstable include audible, abnormal pulmonary sounds

TABLE 3. Guidelines for Administration of Empirical Antimicrobial Therapy in Cats Suspected of Having Bacterial Pneumonia*

Presenting Complaint and Site	Likely Organisms	First Treatment Choice	Alternative Choice
Stable Animal Cough, decreased activity, increased respiratory effort, associated with radiographic changes	Gram-negative: *Pasteurella multocida, Moraxella* spp., *Escherichia coli, Klebsiella*	Amoxicillin-clavulanate, 10–20 mg/kg PO q8hr	Trimethoprim-sulfonamide, 15–30 mg/kg PO or SC q12hr, *or* cephalexin, 22–44 mg/kg PO q8hr
Unstable Animal Respiratory distress (tachypnea, dyspnea) associated with radiographic changes	Same as above	Cefazolin, 33 mg/kg IV q8–12hr	Ampicillin, 20–40 mg/kg IV or SC q8hr. *Note:* may be used in combination with enrofloxacin, 2.5 mg/kg slowly IV† q12hr

*Unless the patient's condition continues to deteriorate, empirical treatment should be administered at least 48 to 72 hours before the decision is made to select an alternative antimicrobial.

†*Note:* Enrofloxacin is *not* labeled for IV administration but has been recommended in animals with life-threatening infections. The calculated dose is administered as an IV bolus over 1 to 2 minutes.

IV, intravenous; SC, subcutaneous; PO, per os (to be administered orally).

on auscultation, fever greater than 40°C (104°F), and leukocytosis with an increased number of immature (band) neutrophils.

It is recommended that affected animals be hospitalized, with intravenous fluid and antibacterial therapy initiated immediately. In dehydrated animals, fluid therapy enhances mucociliary clearance, which subsequently improves ventilation and facilitates delivery of the antimicrobial agent to the lung by augmenting perfusion. Recommendations for administering parenteral antibacterial therapy are outlined in Tables 2 and 3.

Additional supportive therapy can be considered, depending on the cause of the bacterial pneumonia and the animal's health status. Airway humidification using a room nebulizer or vaporizer facilitates clearance of viscous secretions from the lower airway, particularly in dogs that are able to cough (see p. 790). Treatments lasting at least 15 to 20 minutes should be administered three to four times daily. Bronchodilator therapy may be of some value in both dogs and cats, particularly in the presence of generalized lung involvement; however, the clinical benefits derived from oral administration of albuterol and terbutaline are variable. Frequent, gentle chest percussion, also referred to as *coupage*, administered every hour throughout the day, is recommended to facilitate expectoration of mucous secretions from the lower airway. Supplemental oxygen, administered continuously by nasal tube, is reserved for animals that have low a Po_2 or elevated Pco_2 and are in respiratory distress. Animals receiving nasal oxygen are deemed at high risk and should be monitored for the duration of oxygen administration.

References and Suggested Reading

Angus JC, Jang SS, Hirsh DC: Microbiological study of transtracheal aspirates from dogs with suspected lower respiratory tract disease: 264 cases (1989–1995). J Am Vet Med Assoc 210:55, 1997.
This is a comprehensive clinical study on bacterial infections of the lower respiratory tract of dogs.

Dye JA, McKiernan BC, Rozanski EA, et al: Bronchopulmonary disease in the cat: Historical, physical, radiographic clinicopathologic, and pulmonary functional evaluation of 24 affected and 15 healthy cats. J Vet Intern Med 10:385, 1996.
This article discusses an investigation of diagnostic procedures and treatment of cats with lower respiratory tract disease compared with healthy, untreated cats.

Hawkins EC: Disorders of the pulmonary parenchyma. In: Nelson RW, Couto CG, eds: Small Animal Internal Medicine, 2nd ed. St. Louis: Mosby–Year Book, 1998, p 285.
The management of bacterial pneumonia in dogs and cats is reviewed.

Hawkins EC: Diagnostic tests for the lower respiratory tract. In: Nelson RW, Couto CG, eds: Essentials of Small Animal Medicine. St. Louis: Mosby–Year Book, 1992, p 185.
The procedures for diagnostic assessment of dogs and cats with lower respiratory disease are reviewed.

Henik RA, Yeager AE: Bronchopulmonary diseases. In: Sherding RG, ed: The Cat: Diseases and Clinical Management, 2nd ed. New York, Churchill Livingstone, 1994, p 979.
This chapter presents a general review of lower respiratory disease in the cat.

Moise NS, Wiedenkeller D, Yeager AE, et al: Clinical, radiographic, and bronchial cytologic feature of cats with bronchial disease: 65 cases (1980–1986). J Am Vet Med Assoc 194:1467, 1989.
This article describes a comprehensive study of cats with defined lower respiratory disease, including bacterial pneumonia.

Padrid P: Chronic lower airway disease in the dog and cat. Probl Vet Med 4:320, 1992.
This is a clinical perspective on the management of disorders predisposing dogs and cats to bacterial pneumonia.

Diagnosis and Treatment of Fungal Diseases of the Respiratory System

ALFRED M. LEGENDRE
ROBERT L. TOAL
Knoxville, Tennessee

Most systemic fungal infections enter through the respiratory tract and establish an initial focus of infection in the lungs before disseminating. This is true for blastomycosis, histoplasmosis, and coccidioidomycosis. Cryptococcal organisms and *Aspergillus* species initially colonize the nasal passages.

DIAGNOSIS

The clinician should suspect fungal pneumonia when antibiotic treatment has been ineffective; when eye, bone, skin, lymph nodes, intestinal tract, or brain are concurrently affected; or when characteristic radiographic lung patterns are seen.

Thoracic radiographic abnormalities of fungal pneumonia vary with the organism and with the severity of disease. Typically, there are unstructured linear to nodular interstitial and occasionally alveolar pulmonary infiltrates (Fig. 1). At times, single or multiple well-marginated soft tissue to cavitary nodules (>4 mm) are present (Fig. 2). These resemble the interstitial lesions seen with pulmonary metastasis. Hilar or mediastinal lymphadenopathy is inconstant and may be present with or without parenchymal lesions. Sternal lymphadenopathy is infrequent. Pleural thickening is a nonspecific change that is often present in fungal pneumonias as well as in other diseases.

Radiographically, blastomycosis and coccidioidomycosis have similar diffuse nodular interstitial to mixed bron-

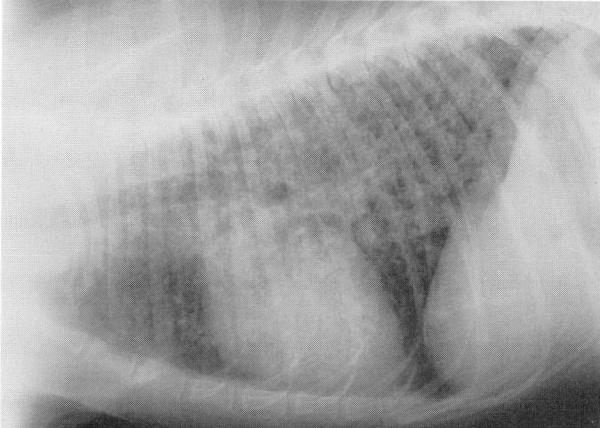

Figure 1. Typical diffuse unstructured to nodular interstitial pattern of fungal disease.

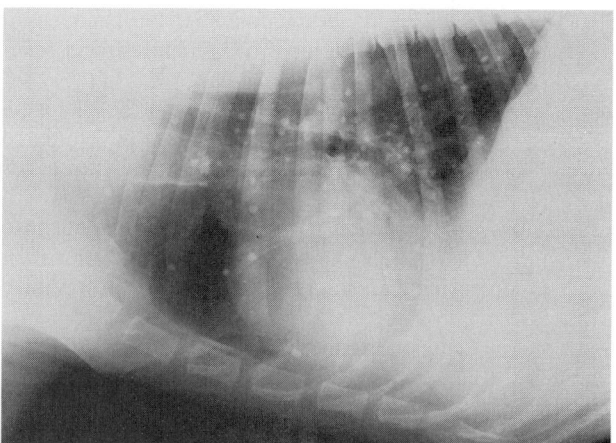

Figure 3. Calcification of histoplasmosis.

chointerstitial-alveolar infiltrates as well as variable degrees of pleural thickening. Tracheobronchial lymphadenopathy is more often seen with coccidioidomycosis (85%) than with blastomycosis (20%). Histoplasmosis generally has a more finely nodular interstitial infiltrate than does blastomycosis or coccidioidomycosis and less often exhibits alveolar disease (10%). Tracheobronchial lymphadenopathy occurs often in dogs with histoplasmosis (50%) but is uncommon in cats. Calcified pulmonary nodules and hilar nodes, 60% and 40%, respectively, are strongly suggestive of chronic, inactive histoplasmosis (Fig. 3). In some dogs with severe hilar lymphadenopathy and associated fibrosis, there is focal narrowing of the tracheal lumen or mainstem bronchus, resulting in airway obstruction and air trapping during expiration (Fig. 4). This is more common in histoplasmosis but also occurs in coccidioidomycosis. Air trapping causes an overinflated lung that appears radiographically as a hyperlucent thorax.

Cryptococcosis in the cat frequently affects the nasal passages with sneezing and nasal discharge. The skin of the head is often infected, with lung, eye, and brain disease seen less frequently. Radiographically, the nasal cavity lesions of cryptococcosis are usually nondestructive and have an increased fluid opacity in the nasal passages and frontal sinuses. The overlying incisive bones and maxillae may have variable lysis and soft tissue swelling (Fig. 5). Pulmonary lesions, when present, range from large solitary or multiple nodules to finely granular micronodular granulomas.

Aspergillosis in dogs occurs most commonly in German shepherds as a chronic rhinitis that is refractory to antibiotic treatment. Radiography is helpful in differentiating aspergillosis from nasal tumors. There is focal destruction of nasal concha, producing the radiographic changes of punctate holes to larger areas of conchal lysis. This may falsely mimic neoplasia. Unlike tumors, however, erosion of the vomer bone and nasal septum is unusual in all but advanced cases of aspergillosis. Occasionally, a mixed pattern characterized by bone destruction and soft tissue proliferation is present (Fig. 6).

Although pulmonary infection is common in blastomycosis, coccidioidomycosis, and histoplasmosis, retrieval of

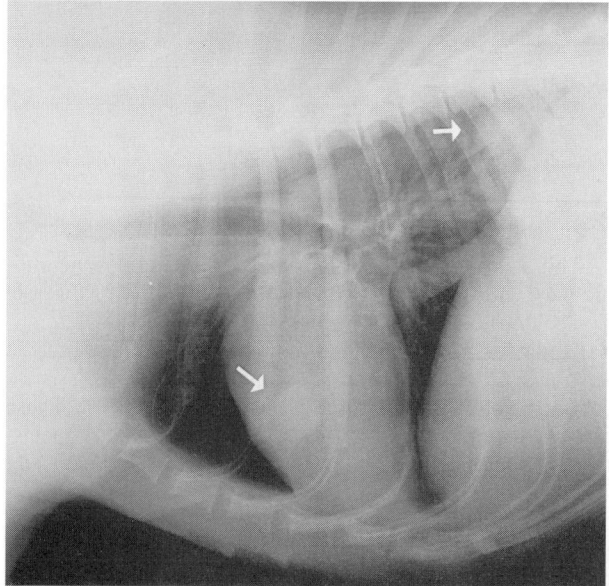

Figure 2. These soft tissue pulmonary nodules (*arrows*) are granulomas secondary to blastomycosis.

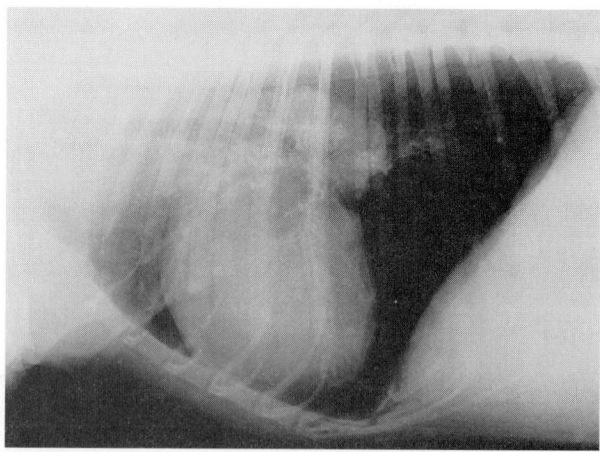

Figure 4. Tracheobronchial lymphadenopathy and hyperlucent lung with histoplasmosis.

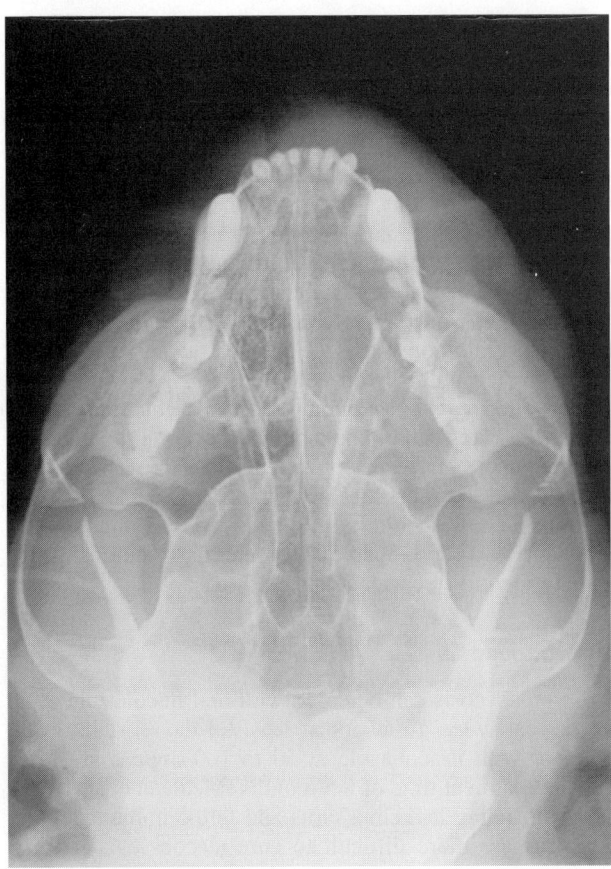

Figure 5. Cryptococcosis nasal lesions.

organisms from the respiratory tract is not consistent. Tracheal washes and bronchoalveolar lavage may recover the organism, but many dogs with prominent pulmonary lesions do not shed organisms into their bronchial secretions. Pulmonary aspirates may be required in some dogs, but in dogs with pre-existing dyspnea this is a slightly hazardous procedure. The organisms are usually easier to find in aspirates from enlarged lymph nodes, impression smears of skin lesions, bone biopsies, or enucleated blind eyes. Because of the long and costly treatment necessary for cure, a *definitive* diagnosis by cytologic or histopathologic studies or culture is preferred to a presumptive diagnosis from a positive serologic test result.

In cats with cryptococcosis, the organisms are usually plentiful in the thick, mucinous nasal material that can be obtained by examining the nasal passages with an otoscope speculum. Aspirates or biopsy specimens from swellings on the dorsum of the nose or from intranasal granulomas can also identify organisms.

Aspergillus mycelium can be found in some dogs in biopsy specimens taken from the nasal tissue through an otoscope speculum. A cavernous, open space in the nose is suggestive of the turbinate destruction seen in aspergillosis. A positive culture from infected turbinates support a diagnosis of aspergillosis, but recovery of a single colony may be a contaminant unless organisms are seen histologically in tissues. An open biopsy of the nasal passages may be necessary to remove necrotic material and obtain adequate biopsy specimens for diagnosis.

When organisms cannot be found directly, serologic studies are helpful in diagnosing systemic fungal infections. A positive agar gel immunodiffusion test is strongly supportive of a diagnosis of histoplasmosis or blastomycosis. This test lacks sensitivity, with up to 25% or more of dogs with early blastomycosis having negative test results. There may be cross-reactivity between blastomycosis and histoplasmosis, but a positive test result is supportive of a fungal infection. In coccidioidomycosis, the complement fixation test is an excellent aid to making a diagnosis because the organisms are difficult to recover. It is important to remove serum from the red cells quickly after the tube has clotted. Serum that remains on the red blood cells is more likely to be anticomplementary, thereby making it impossible to perform the assay. In cryptococcosis, the latex agglutination test for capsular antigens identifies most of the infected cats and strongly supports the diagnosis. Serologic tests for aspergillosis are supportive of a diagnosis but may produce negative results even with extensive disease.

TREATMENT

Blastomycosis

Blastomycosis in dogs and cats is best treated with itraconazole at a dose of 5 mg/kg per day for dogs and 10 mg/kg per day for cats. Treatment should be continued for at least 60 to 90 days or for at least 30 days after all

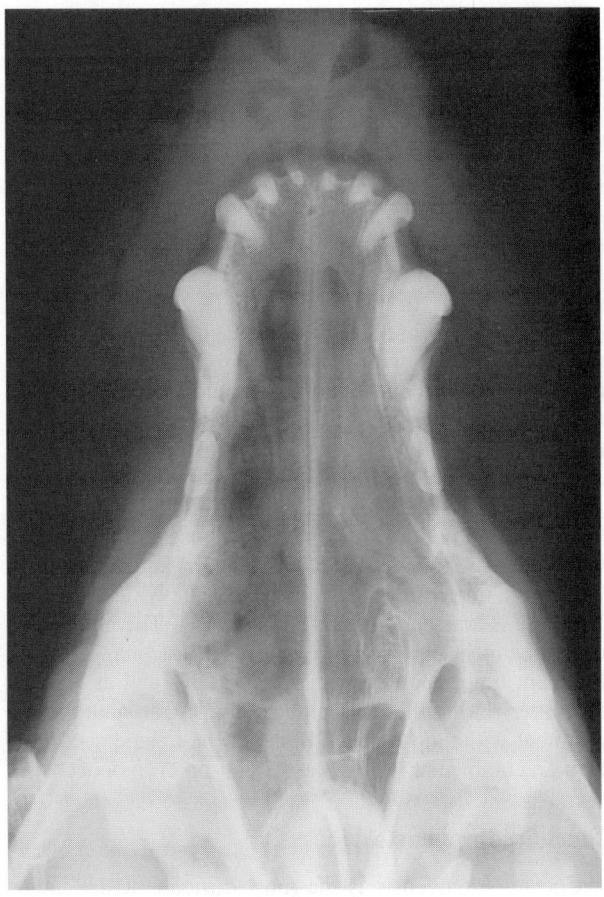

Figure 6. Aspergillosis destructive rhinitis.

signs of disease have resolved. Titers are not useful in determining duration of treatment. Itraconazole should be given with food to maximize absorption of the drug. Absorption varies greatly from animal to animal, and serum concentrations may need to be measured if a good response to treatment does not occur. The most common adverse effect of itraconazole treatment is anorexia from drug-induced hepatic toxicity. Serum alanine aminotransferase activity (ALT) should be measured monthly or if the animal loses its appetite. Itraconazole treatment should be stopped when the animal becomes anorectic and restarted at half the dose when the appetite returns to normal. Vasculitis occurs in some dogs receiving itraconazole therapy (Legendre et al, 1996). This results in circular necrotic skin changes and sometimes edema of the limbs. The changes resolve when therapy is discontinued.

Treatment of dogs with respiratory signs of blastomycosis may result in the worsening of respiratory signs 2 to 3 days after beginning the antifungal treatment. This complication occurs with itraconazole and amphotericin B and is probably attributable to inflammation secondary to the release of fungal components from dying organisms. These inflammatory changes can produce life-threatening dyspnea. Prednisone at a dose of 1 mg/kg twice a day for 3 or 4 days can be considered in dogs with worsening dyspnea after starting treatment. The benefits of steroid therapy are difficult to measure because many dogs with severe respiratory compromise die regardless of treatment. Dogs treated with steroids should be continued on itraconazole therapy for 2 to 4 weeks beyond the usual treatment times. Early diagnosis is important for improving the survival rate.

Histoplasmosis

Histoplasmosis occurs as a respiratory disease and as an intestinal tract and liver infection. Dogs and cats with mainly respiratory tract involvement are best treated with itraconazole, 10 mg/kg per day, given with food. One must be aware of the adverse effects discussed in the section on the treatment of blastomycosis. Dogs with intestinal histoplasmosis do not absorb itraconazole well and should be treated initially with amphotericin B at a dose of 0.5 mg/kg every 48 hours. The drug should be given intravenously over 3 to 4 hours in a 5% dextrose solution that does not contain electrolytes. Blood urea nitrogen concentrations should be measured before each dose is given. The severity of renal toxicity varies greatly among individual animals and cannot be predicted from the response to the first two or three doses. Usually, after six doses of amphotericin B, the dog is improved and gaining weight, which suggests that there is adequate intestinal absorption. The amphotericin B treatment can then be changed to itraconazole. Total treatment times should be at least 90 days and at least 30 days after resolution of all clinical signs. Cats that require treatment with amphotericin B should be treated according to the recommendations in the section on cryptococcosis.

Coccidioidomycosis

Coccidioidomycosis is the most difficult of the fungal diseases to cure, and lifelong therapy may be required,

especially when there is bone or central nervous system involvement. In dogs with severe, life-threatening coccidioidomycosis, initial treatment with fluconazole at 10 mg/kg twice a day may be more effective than ketoconazole therapy. After the crisis is resolved, therapy can be continued with ketoconazole at a dosage of 10 mg/kg given with food twice a day. Ketoconazole is considerably less expensive than fluconazole and appears equally effective in the long-term treatment of coccidioidomycosis. The dose should be reduced if anorexia and liver toxicosis occur, but it may be possible to return slowly to full therapeutic doses. Coccidioidomycosis of the central nervous system is best treated with fluconazole at 10 mg/kg twice a day. Response to treatment is monitored using complement fixation titers. Titers should be monitored every 2 to 3 months, and treatment can be discontinued when the lesions have resolved and the titers are low (1:2 to 1:4) or negative for 3 months. Titers should be measured every 3 months after treatment is discontinued for 1 year or if clinical signs recur to identify recurrence of the disease.

Cryptococcosis

Cryptococcosis can be cured with oral fluconazole at 50 mg per cat twice a day for at least 90 days (Malik et al, 1992) or with itraconazole at 50 to 100 mg/cat/day for a median treatment time of 8.5 months (Medleau et al, 1995). Cats with feline leukemia virus and feline immunodeficiency virus are more difficult to cure (Jacobs et al, 1997). The presence of ocular or central nervous system disease also makes cure less likely, but the disease can usually be controlled with continuing treatment. The cryptococcal organisms are likely to develop resistance to antifungal drugs. If the disease progresses, the treatment must be changed. Flucytosine at a dose of 100 to 125 mg/kg per day divided into three doses can be added to the fluconazole or itraconazole if the response is inadequate. The triazole drugs (itraconazole and fluconazole) can be switched because resistance to one triazole does not predict resistance to the other drug. Cats resistant to these drugs can be treated with amphotericin B. This agent is considered a dangerous drug in cats because of their sensitivity to amphotericin B–induced renal failure. Intravenously administered amphotericin B should be given at a dose of 0.25 mg/kg over a period of at least 3 to 4 hours every other day. The blood urea nitrogen should be monitored before each dose. Malik has proposed a new and somewhat unorthodox approach to amphotericin B treatment in the cat in which he gives the drug at 0.5 mg/kg every other day subcutaneously in 400 ml of 2.5% dextrose and 0.45% saline solution (Malik et al, 1996). In his hands, this has produced excellent responses without significant renal toxicity.

The latex agglutination test for cryptococcal capsular antigen is not only an excellent diagnostic test but also an excellent tool to monitor the response to treatment in the cat. Jacobs and colleagues (1997) showed that titers decrease to 10% or less of the initial titer within 2 months of starting effective treatment. Cats that maintain high titers despite therapy should be treated with a different drug. Titers are also helpful in determining when therapy can be discontinued. Long-term treatment of months to years is expected in cats with cryptococcosis, especially when there is central nervous system disease. Often, titers decrease to low levels (1:2 or 1:4) and remain at that level long after all clinical signs have resolved. If titers are low for several months, the drug can be discontinued and titers monitored monthly. Drug therapy can be reinstituted when titers start to increase or when clinical signs recur.

Nasal Aspergillosis

Treatment of nasal aspergillosis can be carried out with itraconazole given at 5 mg/kg per dose twice a day for at least 90 days. This produces a cure rate of 60 to 70% in previously untreated dogs. At this itraconazole dose, about 15% of animals have anorexia, requiring adjustment of the dose. Eight percent of dogs have ulcerative dermatitis due to vasculitis (Legendre et al, 1996). Although itraconazole treatment is the easiest route, the cost of long-term therapy of large dogs requires the consideration of a more cost-effective treatment. A technique of infusion of 1% clotrimazole into the nasal passages and sinuses is described in another article in this text (see p. 315). After treatment,

persistent nasal discharge is common because the damaged nasal mucosa is predisposed to secondary bacterial infection. Periodic treatment with antibiotics may be necessary.

Acknowledgment
Special thanks to Drs. Nita Gulbas and Donald Levesque for their help with the section on coccidioidomycosis.

References and Suggested Reading

Davidson AP, Pappagianis D: Treatment of nasal aspergillosis with topical clotrimazole. In: Bonagura JD, Kirk RW, eds: Kirk's Current Veterinary Therapy XII. Philadelphia: WB Saunders, 1995, pp 899–901.
Jacobs GJ, Medleau L, Calvert C, et al: Cryptococcal infection in cats: Factors influencing treatment outcome, and results of sequential serum antigen titers in 35 cats. J Vet Intern Med 11:1, 1997.
Legendre AM, Rohrbach BW, Toal RL, et al: Treatment of blastomycosis with itraconazole in 112 dogs. J Vet Intern Med 10:365, 1996.
Malik R, Wigney DI, Muir DB, et al: Cryptococcosis in cats: Clinical and mycological assessment of 29 cases and evaluation of treatment using orally administered fluconazole. J Vet Med Mycol 30:133, 1992.
Malik R, Craig DI, Martin P, et al: Combination chemotherapy of canine and feline cryptococcosis using subcutaneously administered amphotericin B. Aust Vet J 73:124, 1996.
Medleau L, Jackobs GJ, Marks MA: Itraconazole for the treatment of cryptococcosis in cats. J Vet Intern Med 9:39, 1995.

Medical and Surgical Management of Pleural Effusion

ELEANOR C. HAWKINS
Raleigh, North Carolina

THERESA W. FOSSUM
College Station, Texas

INITIAL MANAGEMENT OF PLEURAL EFFUSION

Respiratory distress from pleural effusion is caused by the inability of the lungs to expand; therefore, immediate thoracocentesis is indicated to stabilize these animals. Thoracocentesis is also indicated for diagnostic purposes in animals with pleural effusion, and fluid for analysis should be collected *before* initiating antimicrobial therapy. The primary risk of thoracocentesis is laceration of underlying lung tissue, resulting in pneumothorax, hemothorax, or pulmonary hemorrhage in an already compromised animal. This risk is minimized by a well-restrained animal, careful technique, and appropriate catheter selection. Local anesthesia or manual restraint alone is often adequate when performing thoracocentesis, but mild sedation facilitates restraint in animals that are anxious or fractious.

Thoracocentesis is usually performed between the seventh and ninth intercostal spaces, above the costochondral junctions. Location of focal accumulation of fluid is identified radiographically or ultrasonographically. If available,

ultrasonographic guidance facilitates insertion of the needle into localized pockets of fluid.

Butterfly catheters are commonly used because they are inexpensive, readily available, and convenient. Attached extension tubing prevents movement at the syringe from resulting in movement of the needle in the chest. A three-way stopcock facilitates retrieval of fluid and prevents the entrance of outside air into the thorax. The hand of the operator that holds the wings of the catheter should always rest gently on the body wall to minimize movement of the needle with respect to the body wall and be prepared for immediate withdrawal if the surface of the lungs is felt through the needle or restraint of the animal is lost. Specialized catheters for thoracocentesis are also available (Argyle Turkel Safety Thoracocentesis System, Sherwood Medical, St. Louis). Although they are more expensive, these catheter systems have safeguards to prevent damage to thoracic viscera. Alternatively, over-the-needle catheters can be used (e.g., 3.25-inch or 5.25-inch 16- or 18-gauge Angiocath, Becton Dickinson Vascular Access, Sandy, Utah) and have several advantages over butterfly catheters. Once over-the-needle catheters are in place, there is no needle in the thorax to lacerate the lung; it is even safe to reposition the animal to maximize retrieval of fluid. These catheters are also available in long lengths, which may be necessary to reach the pleural space in large-breed or obese dogs. Extension tubing and a three-way stopcock should be attached to the catheter to facilitate fluid removal. Side openings can be added to the catheter so that obstruction of a single opening is avoided. Gloves are worn and a surgical blade is used to shave one or two side holes in the catheter while maintaining sterility. To prevent the catheter from breaking off in the pleural space on removal, holes should be no greater than one third the circumference of the catheter, spaced apart from each other, and have no rough edges. After thoracocentesis, the modified catheter should be removed with care.

As much fluid is removed from the pleural space as is possible, except in animals with acute hemothorax. Respiratory distress in animals with hemothorax is often multifactorial (e.g., inadequate oxygen delivery, hypoventilation), and the blood within the pleural space can be reabsorbed. These animals benefit from restoration of oxygen-carrying capacity and blood volume, with thoracocentesis performed only as essential to allow lung expansion. Hemothorax may be diagnosed based on a history of acute trauma. Otherwise, obtaining frank blood during thoracocentesis can also indicate a traumatic tap. Free blood in the pleural space is distinguished from a traumatic tap by the following: failure of the blood to clot, low packed cell volume relative to peripheral blood, and erythrophagocytosis identified cytologically.

Fluid retrieved from the pleural space should always be analyzed cytologically. Total cell count, protein quantitation, and examination of a concentrated slide preparation allow fluid to be classified as a transudate, modified transudate, septic or nonseptic exudate, or hemorrhagic effusion. Slides should be scrutinized for infectious agents or abnormal cell populations. Fluid is saved for further characterization as indicated by history, gross examination, or cytologic findings. If pyothorax is suspected, Gram staining is performed and aerobic and anaerobic cultures are obtained. If chylothorax is among the differential diagnoses, fluid triglyceride concentrations are measured and compared with triglyceride concentrations in a serum specimen obtained at the time of thoracocentesis.

In addition to managing respiratory compromise, the cardiovascular and systemic needs of the animal are met, including fluid therapy for dehydration or shock or antibiotics for sepsis syndrome. A complete diagnostic evaluation is undertaken after stabilization. Test selection is based on the history, physical examination, and cytologic characteristic of the effusion. When a primary cause is identified that can be directly managed (Table 1), thoracocentesis is performed as needed to maintain the comfort of the animal until the underlying problem has resolved. The remainder of this article addresses the management of pyothorax, chylothorax, and malignant effusions.

PYOTHORAX

The diagnosis of pyothorax is confirmed by the identification of a septic exudate through thoracocentesis. The

TABLE 1. Causes of Pleural Effusion That Are Managed Directly

Heart failure (modified transudate or chyle)
  Heartworm disease
  Cardiomyopathy
  Pericardial disease
  Tricuspid insufficiency
  Congenital heart disease
Obstruction or thrombosis at cranial vena cava
Hypoproteinemia (pure transudate)
  Protein-losing enteropathy
  Protein-losing nephropathy
  Liver failure
Feline infectious peritonitis (nonseptic exudate)
Coagulopathy (hemorrhagic effusion)
  Rodenticide toxicity
  Factor deficiency
Trauma (hemorrhagic effusion or chyle)
Lung lobe torsion (nonseptic exudate or hemorrhagic effusion)
Diaphragmatic hernia (modified transudate, nonseptic exudate, or hemorrhagic effusion)
Pulmonary thromboembolism (modified transudate, nonseptic exudate, or hemorrhagic effusion)

diagnosis is generally straightforward when pleural fluid has been obtained before the initiation of antibiotic therapy, with organisms often visible cytologically. If antibiotics have already been given, the effusion may have the characteristics of a nonseptic exudate. Gram staining is helpful for characterizing organisms before culture results are available. A mixed infection, with anaerobes and aerobes, is generally present.

Often, no source of infection is identified, especially in cats. In some of these cases, pulmonary infection or a puncture wound may be the initiating event. A foreign body is another cause of pyothorax and can interfere with the successful medical management of the disease. Although pyothorax is often idiopathic in dogs, the presence of foreign material is of greater concern in dogs than in cats.

It is necessary first to stabilize patients that are presented with severe dehydration, electrolyte imbalances, or sepsis. Thoracocentesis is performed for diagnostic and therapeutic purposes. Intravenous fluids and antibiotics are administered. Antibiotic recommendations are discussed later.

The two key components of successful treatment for pyothorax are drainage and antibiotics. Routine supportive care is also indicated. Aggressive treatment is begun immediately after the diagnosis of pyothorax to minimize the formation of adhesions, which interfere with drainage and decrease the likelihood of successful medical management. Drainage is achieved through indwelling chest tubes. Intermittent thoracocentesis is not nearly as effective as draining through chest tubes but can be considered in animals in which euthanasia is the only other option.

One chest tube is placed initially. The tube should be as large as can fit between the intercostal spaces to avoid obstruction of the tube with fibrin. Thoracic radiographs are evaluated after removal of as much fluid as possible through the tube. If remaining effusion is minimal, the one tube is sufficient for treatment. However, if effusion persists on the opposite side, a second tube should be placed immediately. Inadequate positioning of a chest tube can result in persistent fluid on the ipsilateral side. Repositioning or replacement of the tube is warranted. The continued presence of fluid despite multiple attempts to improve tube placement is suggestive of adhesions. Medical management can be attempted for 2 to 3 days, but the continued presence of localized fluid is an indication for thoracotomy and surgical debridement.

Continuous or intermittent suction of the chest tubes can remove the exudate from the pleural space. Continuous suction offers the advantage of maximal drainage, whereas intermittent suction is more simple logistically. Continuous suction is provided with a suction pump attached to a collection system that collects retrieved fluid, controls suction pressure, and maintains a one-way closed system. Convenient disposable collection systems are commercially available (e.g., Thora-Seal III, Sherwood Medical, St. Louis). Alternatively, a three-bottle reusable system can be made. The reusable system consists of three airtight bottles attached to each other in series. The first bottle is connected to the chest tube and collects fluid. The second bottle controls the suction pressure. This bottle is partially filled with water. A straw enters the top of the jar, open to room air. The end of the straw within the bottle is placed beneath the surface of the water at a depth equal to the amount of suction pressure desired, for example, 10 to 15 cm to begin. The third bottle creates a water seal, preventing the entrance of air from beyond that point into the thorax. The water seal is created by passing the tube from the second jar into the third jar and submerging the end in water. The exit tube leaves from the top of the bottle and is attached to the suction unit.

Continuous suction does not greatly decrease the time required to manage pyothorax. Frequent monitoring is necessary to detect any problems with the system. Any leaks between the pleural cavity and the water seal can be rapidly and silently fatal. The system must also be evaluated periodically for obstructions due to kinking of tube or clogging with fibrin and debris.

Intermittent suction by syringe can be used successfully as long as the period between drainage attempts is short. Initially, suction should be performed every 2 to 4 hours. As the volume of fluid produced decreases, often within the first few days, the interval can be lengthened. Ideally, arrangements should be made for drainage to occur through the evening hours during the first 24 to 48 hours. If such arrangements are not feasible, the chest should be drained last thing in the evening and again first thing in the morning to minimize the time that fluid is allowed to accumulate.

Twice-daily lavage of the pleural space with sterile 0.9% saline helps maximize drainage. There is no obvious benefit from the addition of antibiotics, antiseptics, or enzymes. The chest is drained as thoroughly as possible. A maximal volume of 10 ml/kg body weight saline that has been warmed to body temperature is slowly infused into the chest. Less volume is used if discomfort is noted. The animal is slowly rolled from side to side for several minutes and the fluid is then removed. The expected recovery is approximately 75% of the infused volume. Recovery of a greater volume of cloudy fluid may indicate that a pocket of exudate was reached. Recovery of much less volume suggests pocketing of fluid in a region that is not getting

adequate drainage through the existing tubes. Such findings are confirmed with radiographic evaluation.

It is important to maintain sterile technique whenever the system is opened to prevent the entrance of hospital-origin pathogens. Adapter ports are covered with sterile caps when not in use and are wiped with hydrogen peroxide before use.

Initial antibiotic selection is based on coverage for both gram-negative organisms and anaerobes. Culture and sensitivity data are used once they become available to make modifications in the treatment plan if a resistant organism is detected. Negative culture results can occur despite the presence of organisms and should not be used to exclude a diagnosis of pyothorax. Antibiotics are administered intravenously until the patient is alert and eating well and are then given orally. Treatment with antibiotics is continued for 4 to 6 weeks after removal of the chest tube.

Ampicillin can be used initially, but is ineffective against *Bacillus fragilis* because of production of beta-lactamase. This resistance can be overcome using amoxicillin with clavulanate (Clavamox, Pfizer Animal Health, 22 mg/kg every 8 hours). Since amoxicillin with clavulanate is not available for intravenous administration, ampicillin with sulbactam can be used initially (Unasyn, Pfizer Animal Health). The drug is dosed based on the ampicillin component (22 mg/kg every 8 hours). Clindamycin (Antirobe [Pharmacia & Upjohn], 11 mg/kg every 12 hours) has good activity against anaerobes, including *B. fragilis*, but a second drug must be added to treat gram-negative organisms. Enrofloxacin (Baytril [Bayer], 2.5 to 5 mg/kg every 12 hours) or aminoglycosides can be used. Enrofloxacin is preferred because it can be administered safely for prolonged periods.

Special antibiotic considerations must be made if "sulfur granules" are visible grossly in removed pleural fluid or branching filamentous organisms are seen cytologically, indicative of *Actinomyces* or *Nocardia* spp. Acid-fast staining can help characterize the organisms. Acid-fast organisms are assumed to be *Nocardia*, although some *Nocardia* do not stain positively. Otherwise, the more common *Actinomyces* is assumed, pending results of culture. The final diagnosis is made through culture, and special techniques are required if these organisms are suspected. *Actinomyces* are generally susceptible to penicillin derivatives. *Nocardia* are less predictable, but prolonged therapy with trimethoprim-sulfa drugs, tetracyclines, or aminoglycosides can be tried.

It is extremely important to monitor patients regularly to ensure that days are not being wasted while the system is not providing adequate drainage, to determine the time to remove the chest tubes, and to determine whether surgical exploration is needed. Attempts to save money by forgoing regular monitoring often result in added expense in lengthened hospital stays or complications. Lateral and ventrodorsal or dorsoventral thoracic radiographs are evaluated at least every other day. Pockets of fluid that persist or increase in size indicate the need for replacement of chest tubes or surgical intervention if tube placement has been optimized. The volume of fluid recovered is measured, and a slide of the effusion is examined microscopically every day. The chest tube can be removed when the fluid has resolved radiographically, the volume of fluid recovered decreases to approximately 2 ml/kg body weight per day, and signs of infection have resolved cytologically. Cytologic resolution is indicated by the absence of organisms. In addition, neutrophils decrease in numbers and lose their degenerative appearance, and macrophages appear. If these criteria for tube removal have not been met within 1 week of aggressive therapy, surgical exploration is considered.

Complete blood count and serum biochemical analysis are performed as indicated by the general condition of the animal. Electrolyte abnormalities are common until the animal is eating well.

Animals are discharged with oral antibiotics after removal of chest tubes. Re-evaluation is indicated approximately 1 week after removal of the tubes and again approximately 1 week after discontinuation of antibiotics. Ideally, an additional re-evaluation occurs 1 month later. Thoracic radiographs are evaluated at these times. The purpose of these radiographs is to identify early recurrence of effusion. Early identification of recurrence greatly facilitates the ability of the surgeons to find a localized nidus of infection or foreign body. Thorough exploration of the chest cavity is extremely difficult, particularly in animals with a history of exudative disease. Localizing the disease provides a distinct advantage to the surgeon and increases the likelihood that a foreign body or nidus of disease can be found and removed.

Exploratory surgery is indicated for removal of a suspected foreign body or nidus of infection, for breakdown of adhesions when adequate drainage cannot be achieved, and for patients who do not show great improvement after 1 week of aggressive medical management. A sternotomy is performed so that both sides of the thorax can be accessed, unless an obvious lesion is visible radiographically. Fibrin tags are broken down, grossly abnormal lung lobes are removed, and a search for foreign material is performed. As previously mentioned, most foreign material is extremely difficult to identify at surgery. A chest tube is placed for continued drainage after thoracotomy. The tube is pulled based on the criteria described with medical management, usually after 1 to 3 days.

The prognosis for pyothorax is fair to good. Animals that receive aggressive treatment early in the course of disease can recover with no further complications. The majority of animals that do not survive either die or are euthanized during the first few days when they are systemically ill or the owner declines treatment. When a foreign body is present, recurrence is likely, unless surgical removal of the affected lung lobe or tissue is accomplished. Initial conservative treatment of pyothorax with oral antibiotics alone or with occasional thoracocentesis most often leads to adhesions, necessitating surgical debridement.

CHYLOTHORAX

Chyle is the term used to denote lymphatic fluid arising from the intestine and therefore containing a high quantity of fat; *chylothorax* is a collection of chyle in the pleural space. In most animals, abnormal flows or pressures within the thoracic duct (TD) are thought to lead to exudation of chyle from intact, but dilated, thoracic lymphatic vessels (known as *thoracic lymphangiectasia*). These dilated lymphatic vessels may form in response to increased lymphatic

flow resulting from increased hepatic lymph formation or decreased lymphatic drainage into the venous system because of high venous pressures, or both factors acting simultaneously to increase lymph flow and decrease drainage. Any disease or process that increases systemic venous pressure may cause chylothorax. Trauma is an uncommonly recognized cause of chylothorax in dogs and cats because the TD heals rapidly after injury and the effusion resolves without treatment within 1 to 2 weeks.

Possible causes of chylothorax include anterior mediastinal masses (i.e., mediastinal lymphosarcoma, thymoma), heart disease (e.g., cardiomyopathy, pericardial effusion, heartworm infection, right-sided congenital heart disease), fungal granulomas, venous thrombi, and congenital abnormalities of the TD. It may occur in association with diffuse lymphatic abnormalities, including intestinal lymphangiectasia and generalized lymphangiectasia with subcutaneous chyle leakage. In a majority of animals, the underlying cause is undetermined (idiopathic chylothorax) despite extensive diagnostic work-ups. Because the treatment of this disease varies considerably depending on the underlying cause, it is imperative that clinicians attempt to identify concurrent disease processes before instituting definitive therapy.

Chylothorax typically causes respiratory distress due to the pleural effusion or cough, or both. Coughing is often the first (and occasionally the only) abnormality noted by owners until the animal becomes dyspneic. Many owners report that they first noticed coughing months before presenting the animal for veterinary care; therefore, animals that cough and do not respond to standard treatment of nonspecific respiratory problems should be evaluated for chylothorax. Coughing may be a result of irritation caused by the effusion, or may be related to the underlying disease process (i.e., cardiomyopathy, thoracic neoplasia).

Any breed of dog or cat may be affected; however, a breed predisposition has been suspected in the Afghan hound for a number of years. More recently, it has been suggested that the Shiba Inu breed may also be predisposed to this disease. Among cats, Oriental breeds (i.e., Siamese and Himalayan) appear to have an increased prevalence. Chylothorax may affect animals of any age; however, in one study older cats were more likely to have chylothorax than were young cats. This finding was believed to be indicative of an association between chylothorax and neoplasia. Although this disease appears to develop in Afghan hounds in middle age, most affected Shiba Inu dogs have been less than 1 year of age. A sex predisposition has not been identified.

Most animals with chylothorax present with a normal body temperature unless extremely excited or severely depressed. Additional findings in patients with chylothorax may include muffled heart sounds, depression, anorexia, weight loss, pale mucous membranes, arrhythmias, and murmurs. Although the finding of a murmur suggests the presence of underlying cardiac disease, all animals with chylothorax should undergo a complete cardiac work-up because cardiac causes represent potentially treatable causes for chylothorax. Finding a noncompressible cranial thorax, particularly in cats, may indicate the presence of a mediastinal mass (e.g., lymphosarcoma). As with cardiac disease, such a finding means that the treatment of the underlying disease should be pursued rather than treatment of the chylothorax (other than to palliate the animal with intermittent thoracocenteses).

Diagnostic Approach to Animals With Chylothorax

If the animal is not overtly dyspneic, thoracic radiographs should be obtained to confirm the diagnosis of pleural fluid. Ultrasonography should be performed before fluid removal because the fluid acts as an "acoustic window," enhancing visualization of thoracic structures. Ultrasonography is used to evaluate cardiac function, valvular lesions and function, congenital cardiac abnormalities, the presence of pericardial effusion, cardiac entrance of the cranial vena cava, and mediastinal masses. Occasionally, heartworm infestation can be identified on echocardiography. The presence of pleural fluid often prevents satisfactory radiographic evaluation of the structures of the thoracic cavity. Since adequate visualization of the entire thorax is necessary to rule out anterior mediastinal masses such as lymphosarcoma or thymoma, radiographs should be repeated after removal of most of the pleural fluid.

Animals with collapsed lung lobes that do not appear to re-expand after removal of pleural fluid should be suspected of having underlying pulmonary parenchymal or pleural disease, particularly fibrosing pleuritis. Although the cause of the fibrosis is unknown, it apparently can occur subsequent to any prolonged exudative or blood-stained effusion. Fibrosing pleuritis is difficult to diagnose. The atelectatic lung lobes may be confused with metastatic or primary pulmonary neoplasia, lung lobe torsion, or hilar lymphadenopathy. In addition to animals with radiographic evidence of pulmonary parenchyma that fails to re-expand after removal of pleural fluid, fibrosing pleuritis should be considered in animals with persistent dyspnea in the face of minimal pleural fluid.

Chylous effusions are routinely classified as exudates. The color varies depending on fat content of the diet and the presence of concurrent hemorrhage. The protein content is variable and often inaccurate because of interference of the refractive index by the high lipid content of the fluid. The total nucleated cell count is usually less than 10,000/µl and consists primarily of small lymphocytes or neutrophils, with lesser numbers of lipid-laden macrophages. Chronic chylous effusions may contain low numbers of small lymphocytes because of the inability of the body to compensate for continued lymphocyte loss. Nondegenerative neutrophils may predominate with prolonged loss of lymphocytes or if multiple therapeutic thoracocenteses have induced inflammation. Degenerative neutrophils and sepsis is an uncommon finding resulting from the bacteriostatic effect of fatty acids but can occur iatrogenically because of repeated aspirations. Finding lymphoblasts in the pleural fluid suggests mediastinal lymphosarcoma; however, care should be taken to differentiate neoplastic cells from reactive mesothelial cells or normal lymphocytes.

To help determine if a pleural effusion is truly chylous, several tests can be performed, including comparison of fluid and serum triglyceride levels, Sudan III staining for lipid droplets, and ether clearance test. The most diagnostic test is comparison of fluid and serum triglyceride levels. *If the effusion is truly chylous, it will contain a higher concentration of triglycerides than simultaneously collected serum.*

Pseudochylous effusion is a term that has been misused in the veterinary literature to describe effusions that look like chyle but in which a ruptured TD is not found. Given the known causes of chylothorax in dogs and cats, this term should be reserved for effusions in which the pleural fluid cholesterol is greater than the serum cholesterol concentration and the pleural fluid triglyceride is less than or equal to the serum triglyceride. Pseudochylous effusions are extremely rare in veterinary patients but may be associated with tuberculosis.

Medical Management

If an underlying disease is diagnosed, it should be treated and the chylous effusion managed by intermittent thoracocentesis. If the underlying disease is effectively treated, the effusion often resolves; however, complete resolution may take several months. Surgical intervention should be considered only in animals with idiopathic chylothorax or in those that do not respond to medical management. Chest tubes should be placed only in animals with suspected chylothorax secondary to trauma (very rare!), with rapid fluid accumulation, or after surgery. Electrolytes should be monitored, as hyponatremia and hyperkalemia have been documented in dogs with chylothorax undergoing multiple thoracocentesis. A low-fat diet may decrease the amount of fat in the effusion, which may improve the animal's ability to resorb fluid from the thoracic cavity.

Commercial low-fat diets are preferable to homemade diets; however, if commercial diets are refused, homemade diets are a reasonable alternative. Medium-chain triglycerides (once thought to be absorbed directly into the portal system, bypassing the TD) are transported via the TD of dogs. Thus, they may be less useful than previously believed. It is unlikely that dietary therapy will "cure" this disease, but it may help in the management of animals with chronic chylothorax. Owners should be informed that with the idiopathic form of this disease, there is no effective treatment that will stop the effusion in all animals. However, the condition may spontaneously resolve in some animals after several weeks or months. Benzopyrone drugs have been used for the treatment of lymphedema in humans for years. Whether these drugs are effective in decreasing pleural effusion in animals with chylothorax is not known; however, preliminary findings suggest that greater than 25% of animals treated with benzopyrones (e.g., rutin, 50 mg/kg PO every 8 hours, available at health food stores) had complete resolution of their effusion at 2 months after initiation of therapy. Determination of whether the effusion resolved spontaneously in these animals or was associated with the drug therapy requires further study. Because the efficacy and potential side effects of this drug have not been determined in a large clinical study, it should be used with caution.

Surgical Treatment

Surgical intervention may be warranted in animals that do not have underlying disease and in whom medical management becomes impractical or is ineffective. Surgical options in animals that do not have severe fibrosing pleuritis include mesenteric lymphangiography and TD ligation, passive pleuroperitoneal shunting, active pleuroperitoneal or pleurovenous shunting, and pleurodesis. Only TD ligation and active pleuroperitoneal shunting are recommended by the authors. The mechanism by which TD ligation is purported to work is that after TD ligation, abdominal lymphaticovenous anastomoses form for the transport of chyle to the venous system. Therefore, chyle bypasses the TD and the effusion resolves. Unfortunately, TD ligation results in complete resolution of pleural effusion in only about 50% of animals undergoing operation. The advantage of TD ligation is that if it is successful, it results in complete resolution of pleural fluid (as compared with palliative procedures such as passive or active pleuroperitoneal shunting). Disadvantages are that operative time is long (which is problematic in debilitated animals), there is a high incidence of continued or recurrent chylous or nonchylous (from pulmonary lymphatics) effusion, and mesenteric lymphangiography may be difficult to perform (particularly in cats). Without mesenteric lymphangiography, complete ligation of the TD cannot be assured; however, this technique may not be uniformly successful in verifying complete ligation of the TD. Some small branches of the TD system may be present and yet not fill with dye during lymphangiography.

NEOPLASTIC EFFUSION

Any intrathoracic neoplasia can potentially result in pleural effusion through obstruction to lymphatic or venous drainage, inflammation, secondary infection, or hemorrhage. Effusion is most often associated with mediastinal lymphoma, pleural mesothelioma, and metastatic carcinoma.

Mediastinal lymphoma is a common tumor of cats and is treated with combination chemotherapeutic protocols as recommended for multicentric lymphoma. Response is often dramatic, with significant resolution of respiratory difficulties in 48 to 72 hours. Pending response, thoracocentesis is used to remove as much fluid from the thorax as possible. Stress is minimized, and an oxygen-enriched environment or nasal oxygen is provided as needed. Local radiation therapy can be administered when available and provides a similarly rapid response. Rates of remission as high as 92%, with durations as long as 29 months (median 6 months), have been reported for cats receiving combination chemotherapy (Cotter, 1983).

Remission is less likely in animals with mesothelioma and carcinoma involving the pleural surfaces. However, clinical signs in dogs can sometimes be relieved for prolonged periods through control of effusion with palliative therapy using intracavitary cisplatin (Platinol, Bristol Laboratories) or carboplatin (Paraplatin, Bristol Laboratories) therapy, with or without additional systemic treatment. Moore and associates (1991) reported resolution of pleural effusion in four dogs treated with intracavitary cisplatin. Effusion resolved in three dogs after one intracavitary treatment and in the fourth dog after two treatments. Recurrence of effusion ranged from 129 to greater than 306 days in a dog still alive and free of effusion at the time of the report. Two other dogs subsequently treated by the same author had decreased volumes, but not resolution, of effusion (Moore, 1992).

Cisplatin is able to reach high concentrations in tissues within a few millimeters of the contact surface. It is most likely to be effective before actual nodules have formed. Systemic chemotherapy can be administered in addition to intracavitary treatment to reach the interior of larger, vascularized nodules. The combination of intracavity cisplatin and systemic doxorubicin has been proposed for treatment of mesotheliomas (Moore, 1992).

The protocol for intracavitary delivery of cisplatin is not difficult. Dogs are administered 0.9% sodium chloride intravenously for 4 hours before treatment and for 2 to 4 hours after treatment at a rate of 10 ml/kg per hour. Cisplatin is given at a dose of 50 mg/m^2 diluted in 0.9% sodium chloride to a total volume of 250 ml/m^2. The solution is warmed to body temperature before administration. A 16-gauge over-the-needle catheter is placed into the pleural space using sterile technique, and as much fluid as possible is removed. Cisplatin is slowly infused into the pleural space through the same catheter and the catheter is removed. Carboplatin (200 mg/m^2) may be substituted for cisplatin, obviating the need for concurrent saline diuresis. The efficacy of either agent appears equivalent, but controlled studies are lacking.

Treatments were scheduled every 4 weeks in the study by Moore and associates (1991), and additional systemic treatment was sometimes given. The current protocol being used at our institution is to administer intracavitary carboplatin every 3 to 4 weeks as needed to control effusion. If the effusion resolves completely, intracavitary therapy is discontinued after the fourth treatment. Therapy is reinstituted if effusion recurs.

Nonlymphomatous malignant effusions are rare in cats, and standard treatment has not been established. Cisplatin is not recommended for administration in cats because of acute pulmonary toxicity. Carboplatin has not been associated with pulmonary toxicity and has the potential to be effective as an intracavitary infusion. Systemic doxorubicin can also be considered.

Pleurodesis has been proposed to control malignant effusions in dogs and cats. Unfortunately, a consistently effective technique has not been established.

The therapeutic response to any of these palliative measures is based primarily on clinical response, with the goal of therapy being a good quality of life with normal respiratory efforts. Thoracic radiographs can be taken for objective determination of progress. Animals with slowly forming effusion can be further managed with intermittent thoracocentesis. Placement of pleuroperitoneal shunts may provide symptomatic relief to patients requiring frequent thoracocentesis. By creating a path for pleural fluid to cross into the abdominal cavity, more space is available within the thoracic cavity for expansion of the lungs. Pleuroperitoneal shunts are discussed in detail by Lee and associates (1994).

References and Suggested Reading

Cotter SM: Treatment of lymphoma and leukemia with cyclophosphamide, vincristine, and prednisone. II: Treatment of cats. J Am Anim Hosp Assoc 19:166, 1983.

The rate and duration of remission for 53 cats with lymphoproliferative disease treated with combination chemotherapy is discussed. Twelve cats had mediastinal lymphoma.

Fossum TW, Birchard SJ, Jacobs RM: Chylothorax in 34 dogs. J Am Vet Med Assoc 188:1315, 1986.
This article discusses the signalment, history, etiology, and clinical findings in dogs with chylothorax.

Fossum TW, Evering WN, Miller MW, et al: Severe bilateral fibrosing pleuritis associated with chronic chylothorax in 5 cats and 2 dogs. J Am Vet Med Assoc 201:317, 1992.
The pathophysiology of fibrosing pleuritis associated with chylothorax in dogs and cats is reviewed.

Fossum TW, Forrester SD, Swenson CL, et al: Chylothorax in cats: 37 cases (1969–1989). J Am Vet Med Assoc 198:672, 1991.
This article describes a retrospective study of cats with chylothorax, including cause, clinical findings, and outcome.

Fossum TW, Miller MW, Rogers KS, et al: Chylothorax associated with right-sided heart failure in 5 cats. J Am Vet Med Assoc 204:84, 1994.
The history and clinical findings in five cats with heart failure and chylothorax is reviewed along with a discussion of the possible pathophysiologic mechanisms causing the effusion in these animals.

Kerpsack SJ, McLoughlin MA, Birchard SJ, et al: Evaluation of mesenteric lymphangiography and thoracic duct ligation in cats with chylothorax: 19 cases (1987–1992). J Am Vet Med Assoc 205:711, 1994.
This article discusses the technique and reviews the success of thoracic duct ligation in cats.

Lee KA, Harvey JC, Reich H, et al: Management of malignant pleural effusions with pleuroperitoneal shunting. J Am Coll Surg 178:586, 1994.
This article discusses the indications and use of pleuroperitoneal shunts in humans with terminal malignant pleural effusions.

Moore AS: Chemotherapy for intrathoracic cancer in dogs and cats. Probl Vet Med 4:351, 1992.
This is a complete review of chemotherapy for all intrathoracic cancers, with specific discussion of intrathoracic chemotherapy.

Moore AS, Kirk C, Cardona A: Intracavitary cisplatin chemotherapy experience with six dogs. J Vet Intern Med 5:227, 1991.
This article discusses the results of intracavitary treatment with cisplatin in six dogs with thoracic or abdominal effusion associated with neoplasia.

Turner WD, Breznock EM: Continuous suction drainage for management of canine pyothorax: A retrospective study. J Am Anim Hosp Assoc 24:485, 1988.
Presentation, laboratory findings, and response to treatment in 15 dogs with pyothorax are discussed.

Pneumothorax in the Dog

AMY K. VALENTINE
Springfield, Oregon

DANIEL SMEAK
Columbus, Ohio

Pneumothorax is the accumulation of air within the pleural space. The air source is usually from disruption of the thoracic wall, bronchial tree, pulmonary parenchyma, or esophagus, resulting from injury or disease. Clinical signs of pneumothorax may include tachypnea, dyspnea, abdominal breathing, or cyanosis. Auscultation reveals diminished lung sounds and increased resonance with percussion. Radiographic features of pneumothorax include air density within the pleural space, retraction of lung edges from the thoracic wall and diaphragm, and displacement of the cardiac silhouette away from the sternum on the lateral view. Pathophysiologic effects of pneumothorax include decreased lung expansion with subsequent ventilation-perfusion mismatch, hypoxia, and loss of intrapleural pressure gradients that impair the thoracic pump and venous return. These changes ultimately result in reduction of ventilatory capacity and cardiac output. Pneumothorax may be classified based on cause (traumatic or spontaneous) and pathophysiology (open or closed, simple or tension).

TRAUMATIC PNEUMOTHORAX

Traumatic pneumothorax, the most common type of pneumothorax in the dog, occurs in nearly half of all traumatic chest injuries (Kramek and Caywood, 1987). Traumatic pneumothorax is classified as open when it involves a penetrating injury to the chest wall, from, for example, a bite or stab wound, gunshot, or shearing injury. A closed traumatic pneumothorax is usually associated with blunt trauma resulting in laceration of the airway or pulmonary parenchyma. Simple, closed pneumothorax is characterized by *nonprogressive* loss of intrapleural negative pressure. In contrast, tension pneumothorax develops when a disrupted airway, lung parenchyma, or chest wall functions as a one-way valve. This leads to *progressive* air leakage and elevation in intrapleural pressure, and rapid deterioration of the patient.

Management

Management of traumatic pneumothorax is predicated on multiple factors, including the volume, source, and flow of air within the intrapleural space (Orton, 1993); the clinical condition of the patient; the severity of concurrent injury; and the availability of critical care resources. The most important means of stabilizing a patient in distress with pneumothorax, regardless of the cause, is evacuation of free pleural air and re-establishing normal thoracic pressure gradients. This may be accomplished by various techniques, including thoracentesis, tube thoracostomy with intermittent or continuous suction, or a Heimlich flutter valve (Butler, 1975). Additional therapies include supplemental oxygen, intravenous fluids, and intravenous antibiotics, depending on the overall condition of the patient.

Open Pneumothorax

The thoracic wound should be covered immediately with a clean cloth, bandage, or glove during initial patient evaluation and transportation to the treatment area. The wound is inspected briefly, clipped free of hair and debris, and a sterile, occlusive bandage with antiseptic ointment is applied to seal the wound. Immediate thoracentesis should be performed to evacuate air from the intrapleural space if the dog is dyspneic. Thorough wound debridement and reconstruction can be performed after the patient has been stabilized. Tube thoracostomy with intermittent or continuous suction should be considered if the pneumothorax progresses after initial thoracentesis.

Simple Pneumothorax

Simple pneumothorax, if not too severe, usually responds well to conservative management. Bilateral thoracentesis should be performed if there is clinical indication of tachypnea (respiratory rate >80 breaths per minute), dyspnea, or hypoventilation (cyanosis, abnormal arterial blood gas measurements, or decreased oxygen saturation). Most pleural injuries seal within hours after thoracentesis and cage rest are instituted. Patients should be monitored closely for several days for recurrence or progression of pneumothorax.

Tension Pneumothorax

Tension pneumothorax causes severe pathophysiologic consequences and may be rapidly fatal. Dogs with tension pneumothorax have severe and progressive dyspnea and distress, weakness, shallow respirations, abdominal breathing, and a barrel-shaped chest wall. Thoracic radiographs reveal a large amount of free air with flattening and displacement of the diaphragm caudally. Treatment should be rendered quickly and should include immediate thoracentesis followed by tube thoracostomy with intermittent or continuous suction. A flutter valve may be used as an alternative to continuous suction; however, efficacy of the valve may be decreased by blood or effusion or in dogs weighing less than 15 kg (Orton, 1985). An exploratory thoracotomy for definitive treatment should be considered only after aggressive medical management has failed to stabilize the animal. It is often difficult to identify the site of injury causing the pneumothorax at surgery, and general anesthesia puts the dog at additional risk. A median sternotomy is the preferred surgical approach to visualize both sides of the thorax (Bjorling, 1994).

Esophageal Perforation

Pneumothorax associated with esophageal perforation is usually caused by trauma from a sharp, intraluminal foreign body; a gunshot injury, a bite wound, or is iatrogenically induced via endoscopic procedures. Pneumothorax from esophageal injury is often accompanied by pneumomediastinum and an inflammatory pleural effusion. Diagnosis of the perforation is confirmed using endoscopy or positive contrast radiography with an organic (iodinated) contrast agent. Medical treatment for esophageal perforation is dis-

cussed elsewhere (Johnson and Sherding, 1994). Pneumothorax and pleural effusion are treated initially with chest tube drainage. Thoracotomy is reserved for significant esophageal injury or when esophageal healing is not progressing despite appropriate medical management.

SPONTANEOUS PNEUMOTHORAX

Spontaneous pneumothorax is defined as accumulation of air within the pleural space that is not associated with traumatic injury to the respiratory tract or chest wall. In contrast to traumatically induced pneumothorax, spontaneous pneumothorax rarely occurs in dogs. Numerous causes for spontaneous pneumothorax in dogs have been reported, including parasitism, bacterial pneumonia, neoplasia, and pulmonary abscess rupture. Ruptured subpleural blebs in conjunction with bullous emphysema have been reported as the most common cause of spontaneous pneumothorax in dogs; however, 50% of the cases in a recent study had underlying (nonemphysematous) lung disease. Management and prognosis for spontaneous pneumothorax are, in part, determined by the underlying cause (Valentine et al, 1996).

Management

Initial management of spontaneous pneumothorax should include thoracentesis, followed by tube thoracostomy pending evaluation of the dog's clinical response. A general diagnostic screen to identify underlying disease is recommended and should include a complete blood count, serum chemistry profile, examination for *Dirofilaria*, fecal flotation and sediment examination, and thoracic radiography. Serial evaluation of thoracic radiographs may be necessary after chest evacuation to help identify pulmonary disease.

Underlying Parenchymal Disease

Diagnosis of underlying pulmonary disease is important for appropriate treatment of dogs with spontaneous pneumothorax. Parasitic disease, such as dirofilariasis or paragonimiasis, should be treated medically; the pneumothorax usually responds well to conservative (chest drainage) therapy. Underlying metabolic disease such as renal failure or immune-mediated vasculitis may be refractory to treatment and therefore associated with a poorer prognosis for recovery and long-term survival. Pulmonary masses documented with thoracic radiographs may be further defined with ultrasonography (difficult with the presence of free pleural air), bronchoscopy, fine needle aspiration and cytologic studies, or exploratory thoracotomy. The mortality rate for dogs with spontaneous pneumothorax from confirmed neoplasia, bacterial or fungal pneumonia, and pulmonary abscess is high (Valentine et al, 1996).

Bullous Emphysema

A presumptive diagnosis of bullous emphysema should be considered if no other pulmonary disease can be identified after the general diagnostic screen (listed earlier) is performed. Radiographic confirmation of pulmonary bullae in dogs is not reliable (Yoshioka, 1982), since most bullae that have ruptured and are actively leaking are not visible on plain radiographs. Initial treatment may include thoracentesis followed by tube thoracostomy for 24 to 48 hours. The long-term resolution rate of spontaneous pneumothorax with pleural evacuation alone is low (less than 30%) compared with surgical exploration and excision of the affected lung (Valentine et al, 1996). Therefore, early exploratory thoracotomy is recommended for dogs with no evidence of pulmonary disease on radiographs and suspected bullous emphysema lesions.

A median sternotomy is recommended to evaluate the entire lung field (Yoshioka, 1982). After the thoracic cavity is filled with saline, the ruptured bulla is usually identified, as air bubbles leak from the affected lung during positive pressure ventilation. Partial or complete lung lobectomy should be performed. Histopathologic examination and bacterial or fungal culture, or both, should be considered if clinically indicated. Mechanical (gauze sponge) or chemical (tetracycline, sterile talc) pleurodesis may be performed if diffuse bullous emphysema is observed; however, the efficacy of this form of treatment for spontaneous pneumothorax in dogs is unknown (Orton, 1993). The overall long-term recurrence rate in dogs with spontaneous pneumothorax due to bullous emphysema after surgery is 12.5% (Valentine et al, 1996).

References and Suggested Reading

Bjorling DE: Management of thoracic trauma. In: Birchard SJ, Sherding RG, eds: Saunders Manual of Small Animal Practice. Philadelphia: WB Saunders, 1994, p 593.
This is a quick clinical guide to the diagnosis and treatment of thoracic trauma in small animals.
Butler WB: Use of a flutter valve in treatment of pneumothorax in dogs and cats. J Am Vet Med Assoc 166:473, 1975.
This article describes a clinical retrospective study describing application of flutter (Heimlich) valves for treatment of pneumothorax in dogs and cats.
Holtsinger RH, Beale BS, Bellah JR, et al: Spontaneous pneumothorax in the dog: A retrospective analysis of 21 cases. J Am Anim Hosp Assoc 29:195, 1993.
This article describes a retrospective analysis of the etiology, treatment, and prognosis for spontaneous pneumothorax in 21 dogs.
Johnson SE, Sherding RG: Disease of the esophagus and disorders of swallowing. In: Birchard SJ, Sherding RG, eds: Saunders Manual of Small Animal Practice. Philadelphia: WB Saunders, 1994, p 637.
This is a clinical guide to the diagnosis and treatment of esophageal perforation in small animals.
Kramek BA, Caywood DD: Pneumothorax. Vet Clin North Am 12:2, 1987.
This article presents a review of causes, pathophysiology, and treatment of pneumothorax in the dog and cat.
Orton EC: Pleura and pleural space. In: Slatter D, ed: Textbook of Small Animal Surgery. Philadelphia: WB Saunders, 1985, p 556.
This chapter presents a description of the clinical application of continuous suction and Heimlich valve techniques.
Orton EC: Pleura and pleural space. In: Slatter D, ed: Textbook of Small Animal Surgery, 2nd ed. Philadelphia: WB Saunders, 1993, p 381.
This chapter presents an anatomic and clinical review of surgical management of pleural diseases in small animals.
Valentine AK, Smeak DD, Allen D, et al: Spontaneous pneumothorax in dogs. Compend Contin Educ 18:1, 1996.
This article presents a clinical retrospective study of the etiology, diagnosis, treatment, and prognosis for spontaneous pneumothorax in the dog.
Yoshioka MM: Management of spontaneous pneumothorax in twelve dogs. J Am Anim Hosp Assoc 18:57, 1982.
This is a retrospective study of the etiology, clinical features, surgical management, pathologic findings, and therapeutic results in 12 dogs with spontaneous pneumothorax.

Urinary Disorders

JEANNE A. BARSANTI

Consulting Editor

Diagnostic Approach to Polyuria and Polydipsia

Jeanne A. Barsanti
Athens, Georgia

Stephen P. DiBartola
Columbus, Ohio

Delmar R. Finco
Athens, Georgia

NORMAL WATER BALANCE

Every animal must remain in water balance. If water intake exceeds output, positive water balance, which may be manifested by edema, develops. If water output exceeds input, dehydration occurs. Voluntary water and moist food intake are the major sources of input. Water intake varies with environmental temperature and humidity, with exercise, and with individual preference. In dogs and cats, normal water intake varies from 20 to 70 ml/kg per day. In calculating total water intake, one must consider water in food, especially when the animal's diet is commercial canned foods, which are at least 70% water. Cats are slower to correct dehydration by voluntary water intake than are dogs (Anderson, 1982). Urine formation is the major method of water output, with feces as a minor component. In dogs, water may also be lost by panting, especially with exercise and increased environmental temperature. Normal urine output is slightly less than intake because of nonurinary sites of water loss. Normal urine output in dogs and cats varies between 20 and 45 ml/kg per day.

Water balance is regulated primarily by antidiuretic hormone (ADH) acting on the collecting ducts of the kidneys. The hypothalamus produces ADH and releases it via the posterior pituitary gland. The major physiologic stimuli for ADH release are hypertonicity and volume depletion. ADH release is more sensitive to changes in osmolality than to changes in circulatory volume: an increase of only 1 to 2% in serum osmolality induces maximal release of ADH, whereas circulating volume must decrease by 5 to 10%. After release, ADH binds to receptors on the basolateral membrane of the collecting ducts of the kidneys. This binding initiates a series of intracellular events, leading to water reabsorption. The half-life of ADH is short (minutes), so the body can adjust rapidly to changes in water balance. Although ADH is required for water to enter collecting duct cells, water movement is also dependent on a high osmotic gradient within the renal medulla. High urea and sodium chloride concentrations maintained by the loops of Henle and vasa recta are responsible for this osmotic gradient.

DEFINING THE PROBLEM

Greater than normal urine output is referred to as polyuria. Owners are likely to detect polyuria in indoor pets that require litterbox or paper changing or that require being released or walked outside to urinate. Owners may particularly notice polyuria when the pet wakes them up to be let out or has "accidents" when confined for long hours. A thorough history must be obtained to separate the problem of polyuria from dysuria, behavioral problems with urination, and urinary incontinence. An owner may report the problem as "incontinence" whenever a pet urinates inappropriately in the house. The owner should be asked to describe exactly what the animal is doing. Whether urination is observed and whether it appears normal are important. The normal daily routine of the pet in regard to urination should be ascertained. An incontinent animal will dribble urine while sleeping (leaving wetness where it slept) or while walking about without being in a urination posture. Polyuric dogs, in contrast, consciously urinate inappropriately in the house if not allowed out frequently enough because their bladders have become uncomfortably full.

An animal with polyuria should also have polydipsia, or it will be dehydrated. Owners are likely to detect polydipsia if the animal drinks from a water source, such as a bowl, that requires more frequent refilling. Owners are usually accurate when they present an animal for increased water intake, although they may not know whether the amount drunk is excessive. The history should include the source of water and the owner's perception of the quantity of water intake. The type of food being fed and any recent changes in feeding regimen are also important because wet food can be an important water source in small animals and because low-protein foods may result in decreased medullary tonicity via decreased urea generation.

Any changes in the activity of the pet or in its environment are also important in assessing water intake and urine output. Since polyuria-polydipsia can result from many systemic causes, a complete general history is necessary as is a problem-specific one. The occurrence of vomiting, diarrhea, coughing, oculonasal discharge, and estrous cycles in intact bitches should be determined. A general history as to the presence of other medical problems will be important in determining the cause of polyuria-polydipsia.

To confirm that the problem is polyuria-polydipsia, water intake and urine specific gravity should be measured. Measurement of urine output is useful but is usually difficult to accomplish in a practice setting. The simplest step while the pet is in the office is to measure urine specific gravity. If the specific gravity is less than 1.030, the problem should be pursued. If water intake is reported to be excessive, but urine is concentrated to at least 1.030, there must be an extrarenal site of water loss or the owner's observation of polydipsia is incorrect. If the specific gravity is greater than 1.030, but the owner believes the animal is polyuric, the history should be re-evaluated to be sure the problem is not dysuria, a behavioral problem causing inappropriate urination, or incontinence.

DIFFERENTIAL DIAGNOSIS

Once the problem has been defined to be polyuria-polydipsia, the question arises as to which came first. There are diseases that result in polyuria, necessitating polydipsia for maintenance of water balance, diseases that cause polydipsia and thus polyuria, and diseases that do both (Table 1). The most common causes of polyuria-polydipsia in dogs are renal failure, hyperadrenocorticism, and diabetes mellitus, whereas the most common causes in cats are renal failure, diabetes mellitus, and hyperthyroidism.

Primary Polyuria

Diseases that cause primary polyuria are more common than those that cause primary polydipsia. Diseases that cause primary polyuria involve an abnormality in the ADH–renal tubule concentrating mechanism. A complete lack of ADH (pituitary origin diabetes insipidus) results in severe polyuria with hyposthenuria (specific gravity

TABLE 1. Causes of Polyuria-Polydipsia

Primary Polyuria	Primary Polydipsia
Lack of ADH	Hyperthyroidism
Pituitary-origin diabetes insipidus	Hypercalcemia
ADH inhibition (nephrogenic diabetes insipidus)	Hypokalemia
Pyometra	
Bacterial pyelonephritis	Hepatic failure
Escherichia coli septicemia	"Psychogenic"
	Hypothalamic lesion (thirst center)
Hypoadrenocorticism	
Hypokalemia	
Hypercalcemia	
Hyperadrenocorticism-glucocorticoid therapy	
Congenital lack of ADH receptors	
Renal inability to respond to ADH	
Generalized renal failure	
Increased solute load	
Generalized renal failure	
Diabetes mellitus–renal glycosuria	
Increased salt intake	
Posturethral obstruction	
Hypoadrenocorticism	
Diuretics	
Decreased medullary tonicity	
Hepatic failure	
Very low-protein diet	
Hypokalemia-hyponatremia	

ADH, adrenocorticotropic hormone.

<1.008). Partial deficiencies of ADH production result in less severe polyuria and require assessment of ADH concentrations in response to water deprivation to diagnose definitively. Diabetes insipidus can be congenital or acquired. Acquired causes include trauma, inflammation, and neoplasia of the hypothalamus or posterior pituitary gland.

In other diseases that cause polyuria, ADH is present in normal amounts, but its action at the surface of or within the collecting duct cell is inhibited. Bacterial endotoxins, especially those associated with *Escherichia coli*, can compete with ADH for its binding sites on the tubular membrane. Infections that have been associated with polyuria through this mechanism include pyometra, prostatic abscessation, pyelonephritis, and septicemia. Hypercalcemia also inhibits binding of ADH to its receptor site. Glucocorticoids and increased calcium concentrations inhibit the intracellular production of cyclic adenosine monophosphate (cAMP), which is normally stimulated by ADH. Aldosterone inhibits phosphodiesterase, the enzyme that degrades cAMP. Thus, in the absence of aldosterone (as in hypoadrenocorticism), ADH action is inhibited. Hyponatremia has also been associated with impaired renal concentrating ability in dogs (Tyler et al, 1987). This, and medullary washout, are other mechanisms whereby hypoadrenocorticism may result in inadequate urine concentration. A lack of ADH receptors at the collecting duct has been described in dogs as a congenital defect. The term *primary nephrogenic diabetes insipidus* is used to describe the absence of receptors, whereas the conditions listed previously in which ADH activity at the renal tubular receptor site is inhibited are referred to as acquired or secondary nephrogenic diabetes insipidus.

Renal failure in which there is a greater than 66% decrease in functional nephron number is also characterized by decreased renal concentrating ability. In renal failure, a reduced number of nephrons must excrete the same quantity of solutes as when the kidney was normal. To accomplish this, each nephron must excrete more water (obligatory polyuria). Specific gravity decreases gradually to the isosthenuric range as further nephron destruction occurs. This increased obligatory water loss prevents the kidney from conserving water when extrarenal water losses (vomiting, diarrhea, and so on) occur or when voluntary water intake is limited. Dehydration develops much more rapidly in an animal with renal failure than in a normal animal.

In a manner similar to that seen in renal failure, the kidney must excrete more water whenever it must excrete an increased solute load. An example is diabetes mellitus in which an increased glucose load must be excreted. Another example is increased salt intake. A similar situation exists after relief of urethral obstruction. The solutes retained during obstruction must be excreted, necessitating increased water loss. Natriuresis may also partially explain the polyuria in hypoadrenocorticism.

Hepatic failure can result in polyuria through at least two postulated renal mechanisms. One is decreased hepatic production of urea, a major contributor to medullary hypertonicity. Without urea, the osmolality of the renal medulla decreases, reducing the ability of the kidney to reabsorb water. Another postulated mechanism is that increased serum concentrations of ammonia, resulting from decreased hepatic conversion of ammonia to urea, is a direct renal tubular toxin. Low-protein diets may also result in decreased urea production and decreased medullary tonicity.

Hypokalemia is also associated with an inability to concentrate urine well. This is thought to be due to an inability to establish the normal osmolar gradients in the medullary interstitium, to suppression of cAMP generation, and to blunting of release of ADH from the neurohypophysis in response to hypertonicity (Rutecki et al, 1982).

Primary Polydipsia

Causes of primary polydipsia include hyperthyroidism, hypercalcemia, hypokalemia, hepatic failure, and lesions within the thirst center of the hypothalamus. One mechanism for polydipsia in liver failure is postulated to be a lack of catabolism of substances such as renin and angiotensin II, which directly stimulate the thirst center.

Some dogs and cats drink excessive water compulsively or intermittently for unknown reasons (psychogenic polydipsia). These animals have normal ability to concentrate urine when water is deprived unless medullary washout of solute has developed.

DIAGNOSTIC PLAN FOR POLYURIA AND POLYDIPSIA

Once the problem is documented to be polyuria-polydipsia, the history should be reviewed. Has the animal been receiving any drugs, such as diuretics, glucocorticoids, anticonvulsants, or thyroid hormone supplementation, which could induce polyuria? In intact bitches, when was the last estrus? Has the diet been changed recently?

On physical examination, the liver and kidneys should be palpated and size and contour noted. Endocrine alopecia or a pendulous abdomen, or both, may suggest hyperadrenocorticism. Lymphadenopathy may indicate lymphosarcoma, which may result in pseudohyperparathyroidism and hypercalcemia in some dogs. The neck in cats should be carefully palpated for thyroid enlargement. The sudden onset of cataracts suggests diabetes mellitus. If any abnormalities are found on physical examination, they should be pursued by appropriate diagnostic tests.

If there are no definitive abnormalities on physical examination, a complete urinalysis, complete blood count, blood chemistry profile, urine culture, and abdominal radiography or ultrasonography should be performed. The blood chemistry profile should include determinations of blood urea nitrogen, creatinine, liver enzymes, calcium, phosphorus, glucose, total protein, albumin, sodium, and potassium levels for all dogs and cats, and serum thyroxine concentrations in cats. These tests will determine whether systemic or urinary infections, azotemic renal failure, hepatic disease, hypercalcemia, diabetes mellitus, hyponatremia, hypokalemia, or hyperthyroidism is present. A blood urea nitrogen value that is less than normal suggests that medullary washout due to decreased urea production may be the cause of polyuria. Hyperadrenocorticism may be suggested by a stress leukogram, elevated liver enzyme levels, mildly elevated blood glucose levels, and urinary tract infection without pyuria. Hypoadrenocorticism may

be suggested by hyperkalemia, hyponatremia, and lack of a stress leukogram in spite of signs of a stressful illness. If either hyperadrenocorticism or hypoadrenocorticism is suspected, further adrenal function tests should be conducted. Abdominal radiography or ultrasonography, or both, are useful to assess liver, kidneys, uterus, prostate gland, and adrenal glands.

Urine specific gravity may suggest likely differential diagnoses. Markedly hyposthenuric urine (specific gravity <1.006) excludes generalized renal dysfunction, as renal function up to the distal tubule must be normal for urine to be dilute. Hyposthenuric urine suggests that lack of ADH, inhibition of ADH action, or psychogenic polydipsia is most likely. A urine specific gravity greater than 1.020 tends to exclude pituitary-origin diabetes insipidus and congenital lack of ADH receptors. If the urine specific gravity is 1.008 to 1.029 and proteinuria is present, renal insufficiency and hyperadrenocorticism should be the primary differential diagnoses considered.

If the cause of polyuria and polydipsia is still unknown (all laboratory test results are normal, except urine specific gravity), it may be useful to have the owner quantitate water intake at home for 5 to 7 days to confirm the consistency of the problem and as a baseline for comparison during further diagnostic and therapeutic efforts. Determination of water intake at home prevents potential reduction in water intake precipitated by the stress of hospitalization.

The next diagnostic step in the animal that is normal except for increased water intake and a low urine specific gravity is to perform either an abrupt or gradual water deprivation test. Water deprivation testing is *contraindicated* if the animal is dehydrated, azotemic, or hypercalcemic, or has any major systemic disease. Laboratory work should *always* be performed before water deprivation. The test should be carefully conducted as follows: the bladder should be emptied voluntarily or by catheterization at the beginning of the test, urine specific gravity measured, and a serum and urine sample submitted for osmolality if possible. The accuracy of the refractometer should be checked by ensuring that a reading of 1.000 is obtained with distilled water. The animal should be weighed (the same scale should be used throughout the test) and the time recorded. With the abrupt test, all water and food are removed and the animal should be monitored for dehydration every 2 to 4 hours by reweighing and examining skin turgor and mucous membrane moisture. Urine specific gravity should be recorded and the animal allowed to empty its bladder at each time point. The test is continued until there is a 5% decrease in body weight or until the specific gravity is greater than 1.035. Serum and urine osmolalities are measured at the end of the test. The major difficulty with water deprivation testing is that the duration of the test is unpredictable, and one is often faced with night approaching and an animal that has not yet reached 5% dehydration. In this situation, one can transfer the animal to a facility with overnight care so that sampling can continue or one can provide the animal with a maintenance water amount (calculated at 2.75 ml/kg per hour that the animal is to be unobserved). The following morning the animal is weighed, specific gravity is measured, water is again withdrawn, and the test is continued until the original target weight (indicating 5% dehydration) or a specific gravity greater than 1.035 is reached.

With a gradual water deprivation test, water intake is decreased from the original measured intake to 60 ml/kg over 3 days (Feldman and Nelson, 1996), followed by complete deprivation as described previously. The animal's body weight and urine specific gravity should be measured before beginning the test and at an increasing frequency as the restriction of water intake becomes more severe and the degree of weight loss approaches 5%. The authors generally perform abrupt, rather than gradual, water deprivation testing. However, a gradual test is performed if the results of the abrupt test are ambiguous (urine specific gravity 1.020 to 1.029) in order to rule out the possibility that medullary washout of solute from prolonged polyuria has prevented maximal urine concentration.

To evaluate the water deprivation test, one considers how rapidly dehydration occurred, what final specific gravity was reached, and how the pre- and post-test serum and urine osmolalities compare. Ninety-five percent of normal dogs and cats reach a urine specific gravity of 1.048 before they lose 5% of their body weight (Hardy and Osborne, 1979; Ross and Finco, 1981). Normal animals may require 2 to 4 days to become dehydrated, even with abrupt deprivation, whereas animals with diabetes insipidus may become dehydrated within a few hours. In normal animals, urine osmolality rises rapidly with minimal change in serum osmolality. If the animal does not concentrate urine (specific gravity <1.035) and becomes 5% dehydrated, an abnormality in the ADH–renal concentrating mechanism is confirmed. If the animal concentrates urine to greater than 1.035 but polydipsia has been previously documented, the most likely possibility is psychogenic polydipsia. If the animal concentrates urine to 1.030 to 1.035, a partial ADH deficiency, partial renal tubular defect, or psychogenic polydipsia with a degree of medullary washout may be present. If the animal concentrates urine to 1.030 with water deprivation, water restriction to maintenance amounts is usually adequate therapy, and no further diagnostic tests are usually performed.

If the patient does not concentrate urine to greater than 1.020 with water deprivation, an ADH response test should be performed. ADH in oil (vasopressin tannate) is no longer available. The authors currently use desmopressin acetate (DDAVP, Rhone-Poulenc-Rorer), 10 to 20 µg. At the University of Georgia, the sterile intranasal preparation is transferred via sterile procedures to a sterile vial and the dose is administered IV (Greene et al, 1979). The intranasal preparation is used because it is less expensive; however, an injectable preparation is available from the same company. The urine specific gravity should be checked every 1 to 2 hours for 8 hours and then at 12 and 24 hours. Response to intravenous desmopressin usually begins within 30 minutes, with maximal response at 4 to 8 hours after administration; in some animals, some effect may be evident up to 24 hours. Urine osmolality should be checked just before administration and at the time the specific gravity is highest. Water consumption can also be measured. The authors do not generally withhold water during ADH response testing unless the test is conducted immediately after water deprivation. There is potential danger of

overhydration if an animal with pituitary diabetes insipidus consumes large amounts of water just as ADH is administered.

A positive response to ADH is a rise in urine specific gravity to greater than 1.020 or a fivefold rise in urine osmolality (Hardy and Osborne, 1982). In an animal with an inability to respond to water deprivation, a positive response to ADH confirms pituitary diabetes insipidus. If urine specific gravity or osmolality does not rise significantly, an abnormality in renal tubular response to ADH is confirmed. Exogenous ADH administration consistently stimulates less urine concentration than does the endogenous response to water deprivation. The reasons for this are not known, but this difference is the reason that water deprivation is the preferred initial test. The results of water deprivation and ADH response testing are not always straightforward. Measurement of plasma ADH concentrations improves diagnostic accuracy but is not yet widely available in veterinary medicine. The most common diseases that result in a urine specific gravity of 1.015 to 1.029 after abrupt and gradual water deprivation and minimal further response after ADH administration are preazotemic, chronic, generalized renal failure and atypical hyperadrenocorticism (canine Cushing's disease with minimal dermatologic or serum chemistry changes). In these cases, measurement of serum cortisol concentrations in conjunction with adrenocorticotropic hormone stimulation or dexamethasone suppression or measurement of serum adrenocorticotropic hormone concentrations, or both, should determine whether Cushing's disease exists. A urine cortisol:urine creatinine ratio determination could also be performed; if the results are normal, hyperadrenocorticism would be unlikely. An exogenous creatinine clearance test (see *CVT XII,* p. 931) should be performed to determine whether renal dysfunction is the cause of the polyuria (Finco et al, 1982).

References and Suggested Reading

Anderson RR: Water balance in the dog and cat. J Small Anim Pract 23:588, 1982.
  A study of water intake and output in normal dogs and cats.
DiBartola SP: Fluid Therapy in Small Animal Practice. Philadelphia: WB Saunders, 1992, pp 17–29.
  A complete review of the many influences on water intake and urine output in dogs and cats.
Feldman EC, Nelson RW: Canine and Feline Endocrinology and Reproduction. Philadelphia: WB Saunders, 1996, pp 2–37.
  A complete review of the physiology of ADH and the pathophysiology of diabetes insipidus.
Finco DR, Coulter DB, Barsanti JA: Procedure for a simple method of measuring glomerular filtration rate in the dog. J Am Anim Hosp Assoc 18:804, 1982.
  Description of the method of measuring the glomerular filtration rate with exogenously administered creatinine, which is more accurate than endogenous creatinine clearance.
Greene CE, Wong PL, Finco DR: Diagnosis and treatment of diabetes insipidus in 2 dogs using 2 synthetic analogs of antidiuretic hormone. J Am Anim Hosp Assoc 15:371, 1979.
  The first report of the use of desmopressin acetate in assessment of clinical cases of polyuria-polydipsia.
Hardy RM, Osborne CA: Water deprivation test in the dog: Maximal normal values. J Am Vet Med Assoc 174:479, 1979.
  This study determined the response of normal dogs to water deprivation.

Hardy RM, Osborne CA: Aqueous vasopressin response test in clinically normal dogs undergoing water diuresis: Technique and results. Am J Vet Res 43:1987, 1982.
This study developed the use of aqueous vasopressin in assessment of polyuria.

Lage AL: Apparent psychogenic polydipsia. In: Kirk RW, ed: Current Veterinary Therapy VI. Philadelphia: WB Saunders, 1977, pp 1098–1102.
This review presents nine cases of psychogenic polydipsia in dogs, including results of all diagnostic tests performed, and remains the basis of our clinical understanding of this condition.

Ross LA, Finco DR: Relationship of selected clinical renal function tests to glomerular filtration rate and renal blood flow in cats. Am J Vet Res 42:1704, 1981.
This study assessed the urine concentrating ability of cats in relation to renal function.

Rutecki GW, Cox JW, Robertson GW, et al: Urinary concentrating capacity and antidiuretic hormone responsiveness in the potassium-depleted dog. J Lab Clin Med 100:53, 1982.
This study assessed the effect of potassium on renal concentrating ability.

Tyler RD, Qualls CW, Heald RD, et al: Renal concentrating ability in dehydrated, hyponatremic dogs. J Am Vet Med Assoc 191:1095, 1987.
Hyponatremia was found to impair urine concentrating ability in dogs.

Diagnosis of Systemic Hypertension in Dogs and Cats

SCOTT A. BROWN
Athens, Georgia

ROSEMARY A. HENIK
Madison, Wisconsin

DELMAR R. FINCO
Athens, Georgia

The care of a growing population of geriatric pets involves the recognition and treatment of multiple, simultaneously occurring medical problems. One of these problems is often high blood pressure, usually secondary to another disease process. Establishing a diagnosis of systemic hypertension is becoming increasingly important in veterinary practice.

DEFINITIONS

During each cardiac cycle, the pressure within systemic arteries rises during systole and falls during diastole. The systolic and diastolic pressures are the upper and lower limits, respectively, of these periodic oscillations. The mean arterial pressure is the time-averaged value for blood pressure in systemic arteries. Because systole is short, the mean pressure is not midway between systolic and diastolic pressures but is closer to diastolic pressure. In a normal dog or cat at rest, mean pressure can be approximated by the formula: mean pressure = diastolic pressure + one-third pulse pressure. However, this method for estimating mean arterial pressure is not reliable in animals with tachycardia, bradycardia, or certain cardiovascular disorders.

NORMAL AND ABNORMAL BLOOD PRESSURE

The average values for systemic arterial blood pressure (systolic/mean/diastolic) in calm, unsedated dogs and cats are approximately 125/100/80 mm Hg. These values are modified by sympathetic nervous system stimulation that is often associated with stress or fright. Systemic hypertension is persistent, abnormal elevation of blood pressure. In an animal with systemic hypertension, the systolic pressure or the diastolic pressure, or both, may be elevated. In the absence of other clinical signs of hypertension (e.g., retinal hemorrhage or detachment), it is advised that several blood pressure readings be taken on an individual animal, over several days if possible, rather than relying on a single measurement as the basis of treatment. Only animals with a marked elevation of systemic arterial blood pressure, particularly those with a disease commonly associated with systemic hypertension, should be considered candidates for therapy (see the next article, "Therapy for Systemic Hypertension in Dogs and Cats").

METHODS OF BLOOD PRESSURE MEASUREMENT

Blood pressure may be measured by either direct or indirect methods. Direct blood pressure measurement is the "gold standard" and usually involves placement of a needle or indwelling catheter into a peripheral artery. The needle or catheter is attached to a calibrated pressure transducer, and pressure is displayed on a screen or recording chart. This technique is technically difficult in unsedated small animals and may be painful. In addition, complications such as hematoma formation may develop. The indirect techniques are more applicable to a clinical setting because they require less restraint and are technically easier to perform. Indirect methods of blood pressure measurement include the auscultatory, ultrasonic Doppler, oscillometric, and photoplethysmographic methods.

All these indirect techniques employ an inflatable cuff wrapped around an extremity. The pressure in the cuff is measured with the aid of a manometer or a pressure transducer. A squeeze bulb is used to inflate the cuff to a pressure in excess of systolic blood pressure, thereby occluding the underlying artery. As the cuff is gradually deflated, changes in arterial flow are detected by one of several means. The value for cuff pressure at various levels of deflation is then correlated with systolic, diastolic, or mean blood pressure. This detection method varies among different indirect methods (see *CVT XII*, pp. 110 and 113).

For the auscultatory method, a stethoscope is placed over the artery distal to the cuff, and the listener hears a tapping sound when the inflation pressure falls below systolic pressure. As inflation pressure continues to fall, more blood escapes under the cuff with each beat, and eventually the sounds disappear, representing diastolic pressure. The low amplitude and frequency of the arterial (Korotkoff) sounds make the auscultatory technique difficult in dogs and cats.

Doppler flowmeters detect blood flow as a change in the frequency of reflected sound (Doppler shift) due to the motion of underlying red blood cells. Blood pressure is read by the operator from an aneroid manometer connected to the occluding cuff placed proximal to the Doppler transducer.

Devices using the oscillometric technique detect pressure fluctuations produced in the occluding cuff resulting from the pressure pulse. Machines using the oscillometric technique generally determine systolic, diastolic, and mean arterial pressures as well as pulse rate.

The most recently developed device for measuring blood pressure indirectly is the photoplethysmograph, which measures arterial volume by attenuation of infrared radiation and is designed for use on the human finger. It can be employed in cats and small dogs weighing less than 10 kg.

The Association for Advancement of Medical Instrumentation has established minimal criteria for accuracy and precision for instruments that measure blood pressure. Machines that do not meet these criteria are not generally accepted for clinical use in humans. Unfortunately, none of the currently available machines for detection of blood pressure in dogs and cats has been shown to meet these criteria for accuracy or precision. Consequently, caution must be employed in interpreting the results of measurement of blood pressure using these devices.

The ultrasonic Doppler and the oscillometric methods have been evaluated in conscious dogs and cats. Both these methods are equally reliable in dogs. In cats, the ultrasonic Doppler method is preferred because the oscillometric device is less accurate. In both species, the oscillometric devices tend to underestimate blood pressure by increasing amounts as the blood pressure increases. Another problem with the oscillometric devices is the excessive time required to obtain readings in cats. The major limitation of the Doppler technique is the imprecise discrimination of the sounds designating the diastolic, and therefore mean, pressure. Because of this, the Doppler method of blood pressure measurement may be unreliable for the routine

diagnosis and surveillance of animals with diastolic hypertension.

When the photoplethysmograph was evaluated in anesthetized cats, it had less of a tendency to underestimate blood pressure at high pressures and overestimate blood pressure at low pressures than did the Doppler and oscillometric devices. Disadvantages of the photoplethysmograph device include its cost, the need to reposition the cuff frequently for optimal traces, and the fact that its use is limited to cats and dogs weighing less than 10 kg.

On the basis of studies in conscious animals, devices using the Doppler principle are recommended at present for use in cats; either the oscillometric or Doppler devices are recommended in dogs.

CHOICE OF CUFF

An oversized cuff may give erroneously low recordings, and an undersized cuff, a falsely high reading. In dogs, indirect blood pressure measurement studies should employ a cuff width that measures 40% of the circumference of the limb (30 to 40% in cats). If the ideal cuff width is midway between two available sizes, the larger cuff should be used because it will theoretically produce the least error.

SITE OF CUFF PLACEMENT

The cuff may be placed around the brachial, median, cranial tibial, or medial coccygeal arteries. For the Doppler technique, the cuff is generally placed over the median artery and the transducer is placed between the carpal and metacarpal pad. Clipping of hair and application of acoustic gel at the site of transducer placement may enhance the signal. For the oscillometric technique, the median artery in cats and the coccygeal artery in dogs provide more reliable values than do other sites.

The cuff should be placed at the level of the aortic valve. If not, a compensation can be made for gravitational effect with a 1.0-mm Hg rise in blood pressure expected for each 1.3 cm of vertical distance between the level of the cuff and the level of the aortic valve.

ANXIETY-INDUCED ARTIFACT: THE "WHITE COAT EFFECT"

The visit to the veterinary clinic, hospitalization, presence in a strange environment, restraint in the examination room, clipper noise and vibration, cuff placement, cuff inflation, and other unusual stimuli in the setting of a veterinary hospital may induce anxiety in an animal during blood pressure measurement. As a consequence, a falsely elevated value for blood pressure may be obtained secondary to catecholamine release associated with this anxiety. Unfortunately, the magnitude of this effect varies widely among animals and among visits in the same animal.

RECOMMENDED PROCEDURE

Despite the relative ease of use, obtaining reliable values from an indirect device is not easy. Measurement of blood pressure should be viewed as a session, not a simple, singular procedure. Many measurements using a variety of cuff placements are required. It is preferable, although not always financially feasible, to use two different indirect devices during each session.

There are several limitations to the use of indirect devices that must be recognized by the practicing veterinarian as a standard protocol for blood pressure measurement is devised. First, these units require operator practice to master. Simply applying the cuff and cycling the machine through a standard procedure will result in poor reliability of values obtained. In many practices, because of available time or patience, or both, a technician may be preferred over the veterinarian as the individual responsible for blood pressure measurements. Consistency in personnel is critical. Failure to use the same technician can lead to artifactual changes in blood pressure. Second, because of the variability of anxiety-induced hypertension and the difficulty of obtaining reliable values in moving animals, blood pressure should be measured in a calm, motionless animal maintained in a quiet room, away from other animals, humans, and background noise. The owner should be present if possible to calm the pet. If a forelimb is used for cuff placement, the animal can be allowed to rest calmly in its own carrying crate, although the cuff must be carefully observed throughout the measurement sequence. Blood pressure should be measured before the physical examination but after the animal has had sufficient time (at least 10 minutes) to acclimate to its surroundings. Several readings must be taken on an individual animal, over several days if possible, rather than relying on a single measurement for the basis of treatment. Because errors in cuff placement can alter the values obtained, the cuff should be removed and replaced at least once during a blood pressure measurement session. If markedly different values are obtained with the new cuff placement, a third or fourth cuff positioning is required.

Conscious Animal Blood Pressure Measurement Procedure

1. Environment: Quiet, away from other animals, owner present.
2. Equilibration time: 10 minutes.
3. Device: Doppler principle in cats; oscillometric or Doppler principle in dogs; both devices if available. For comparative purposes, the same device should be used each time in an individual animal.
4. Cuff width: 40% of limb circumference in dogs; 30 to 40% of limb circumference in cats. The cuff width should be noted in the medical record for future reference.
5. Site of cuff placement: median artery for Doppler device; coccygeal artery (dog) for oscillometric device. For comparative purposes, the same site for cuff placement should be used each time in an individual animal and recorded in the medical record.
6. Personnel: Same individual (preferably a technician) performs all blood pressure measurements following a standard protocol.
7. Patient: should be calm, motionless.
8. Measurements: Five to seven consistent measurements from cuff placement; five to seven consistent measure-

ments from second cuff placement site; repeat as necessary if measurements from cuff sites do not agree; average all values to obtain blood pressure estimate; note site of cuff placement for future reference.
9. If in doubt, repeat measurement session on another day and at another site (e.g., forelimb and rear limb).

WHICH PATIENTS TO ASSESS: SIGNALMENT AND HISTORY

It is reasonable to measure blood pressure in all clinical patients, although currently few veterinarians follow this path. Thus, patient selection becomes an issue. Most dogs and cats with severe systemic hypertension are older (cats usually >12 years of age), presenting with signs such as blindness or hyphema, seizure, ataxia, or sudden collapse (signs compatible with cerebrovascular hemorrhage or stroke), and (rarely) labored breathing (signs related to heart failure). Cats suffering from acute, severe systemic hypertension may have a syndrome of progressive stupor, head pressing, seizures, and death. If a diagnosis is established early, these clinical signs resolve rapidly (<24 hours) with effective antihypertensive therapy.

If the veterinarian measures blood pressure only in animals suspected of having complications secondary to hypertensive injury, the opportunity for early identification of hypertension and intervention is lost. Although it is critical to measure blood pressure in animals with clinical signs that might be referable to systemic hypertension, animals at risk also should be assessed. Systemic hypertension in dogs and cats is nearly always secondary to another disease. In cats, chronic renal disease and hyperthyroidism are most commonly implicated, and the majority of cats with these diseases are hypertensive. Similarly, population surveys suggest that most dogs with chronic renal disease exhibit systemic hypertension. Other diseases in which blood pressure measurements are indicated include hypercortisolism (endogenous or exogenous), mineralocorticoid-secreting tumor, and pheochromocytoma. Primary or essential hypertension may occur in animals, although it is thought to be rare.

References and Suggested Reading

Binns SH, Sisson DD, Buoscio DA, et al: Doppler ultrasonographic, oscillometric sphygmomanometric, and photoplethysmographic techniques for noninvasive blood pressure measurement in anesthetized cats. J Vet Intern Med 9:405, 1995.
A critical appraisal of the utility of indirect techniques in cats, emphasizing the utility of photoplethysmography in anesthetized cats.
Coulter D, Keith J: Blood pressures obtained by indirect measurement in conscious dogs. J Am Vet Med Assoc 184:1375, 1984.
The results of the application of the oscillometric technique to normal dogs and to dogs with various abnormalities, including chronic renal failure, demonstrating the ability of this technique to detect expected changes.
Cowgill LD, Kallet AJ: Recognition and management of hypertension in the dog. In: Kirk RW, ed: Current Veterinary Therapy VIII. Philadelphia, WB Saunders, 1983, p 1025.
A review of the diagnosis and management of systemic hypertension in dogs with various clinical conditions.
Grandy JL, Dunlop CI, Hodgson DS, et al: Evaluation of the Doppler ultrasonic method of measuring systolic arterial blood pressure in cats. Am J Vet Res 53:1166, 1992.
An evaluation of the Doppler indirect technique for the diagnosis of systemic hypertension in cats.
Labato MA, Ross LA: Diagnosis and management of hypertension. In:

August JR, ed: Consultations in Feline Internal Medicine. Philadelphia, WB Saunders, 1991, p 301.
A review of the diagnosis and management of systemic hypertension in cats.

Remillard RL, Ross JN, Eddy JB: Variance of indirect blood pressure measurements and prevalence of hypertension in clinically normal dogs. Am J Vet Res 52:561, 1991.
An evaluation of the effects of the measurement of blood pressure in the clinical setting versus at home.

Snyder PS, Henik RA: Feline systemic hypertension. Proceedings of the twelfth annual Veterinary Medicine Forum. San Francisco, 1994, p 126.
An overview of the pathophysiology and management of systemic hypertension.

Tabaru H, Watanabe H, Tanaka M, et al: Non-invasive measurement of systemic arterial pressure by Finapres in anesthetized dogs. Jpn J Vet Sci 52:427, 1990.
Measurement of blood pressure with photoplethysmography in dogs.

Valtonen MH, Eriksson LM: The effect of cuff width and accuracy of indirect measurement of blood pressure in dogs. Res Vet Sci 11:258, 1970.
An evaluation of the effects of cuff width on the reliability of indirect blood pressure measurements in dogs.

Wessale JL, Smith LA, Reid M, et al: Indirect auscultatory systolic and diastolic pressures in the anesthetized dog. Am J Vet Res 46:2129, 1985.
Use of the auscultatory technique to indirectly assess blood pressure in dogs. This method was of utility in anesthetized dogs.

Therapy for Systemic Hypertension in Dogs and Cats

SCOTT A. BROWN
Athens, Georgia

ROSEMARY A. HENIK
Madison, Wisconsin

Antihypertensive agents may induce a variety of side effects, such as excess sodium and water loss, leading to dehydration and volume depletion; systemic hypotension, leading to weakness, syncope, and renal dysfunction; and kaliuresis, leading to hypokalemia and associated clinical signs. Consequently, the clinician should be confident of the diagnosis before embarking on treatment of hypertension. Diagnosis of systemic hypertension requires reliable measurement of blood pressure (see previous article on diagnosis of systemic hypertension in dogs and cats). Similarly, the effectiveness of therapy should be judged on the basis of repeated blood pressure measurements.

RATIONALE FOR TREATMENT

Systemic hypertension can damage a variety of tissues. A clear association exists between ocular injury and marked systemic hypertension in dogs and cats. However, most other adverse effects of systemic hypertension in dogs and cats are theorized on the basis of extrapolation from clinical studies in humans or experimental studies in laboratory rodents or dogs.

The eyes are the organs most commonly reported to be affected by hypertension in dogs and cats. The findings associated with hypertensive injury include hemorrhage of the retina, vitreous, or anterior chamber; retinal detachment and atrophy; retinal edema; perivasculitis; retinal vessel tortuosity; and glaucoma.

The kidney is susceptible to hypertensive injury. However, preglomerular arterioles usually constrict whenever blood pressure is elevated, serving to protect the renal glomerulus from hypertensive injury. In dogs and cats

with renal insufficiency, these preglomerular arterioles are dilated and poorly responsive to changes in blood pressure. Thus, the elevated blood pressure is transmitted directly to the glomerular capillary bed. This increase in glomerular capillary pressure is referred to as glomerular hypertension, which may produce glomerular damage and a progressive fall in renal function unless hypertension is effectively treated.

The heart is working against an increased arterial pressure (i.e., afterload), and so left ventricular hypertrophy and secondary valvular insufficiency may be observed. Tachycardia is not a common finding with hypertension, although some primary diseases that lead to secondary hypertension, such as hyperthyroidism, may lead to an elevated heart rate. Left ventricular hypertrophy may regress with antihypertensive treatment.

The signs consistent with cerebrovascular hemorrhage (head tilt, depression, seizures) have been seen clinically in cats and dogs with uncontrolled hypertension, and are associated with a poor prognosis.

SELECTION OF ANIMALS TO BE TREATED

In light of the uncertainty and the difficulties associated with blood pressure measurement in dogs and cats (see prior article), only the animals with marked elevations of indirectly measured blood pressure and/or with clinical abnormalities directly attributable to hypertensive injury should be considered candidates for treatment. Considering the association of marked systemic hypertension with ocular injury, the authors believe that antihypertensive treatment is indicated in any dog or cat with a sustained systolic blood pressure greater than 200 mm Hg or diastolic blood pressure greater than 120 mm Hg, regardless of other clinical findings. In both species, an animal with a systolic/diastolic blood pressure that consistently exceeds 170/100 mm Hg should be considered for treatment if clinical evaluation has identified abnormalities (e.g., retinal lesions, chronic renal disease, left ventricular hypertrophy) that could be caused or exacerbated by systemic hypertension. In animals in which the blood pressure is moderately elevated (systolic/diastolic blood pressure that consistently exceeds 170/100 mm Hg) and no clinical abnormalities related to systemic hypertension are identified, the rationale for therapy is less clear. Currently, some clinicians recommend treatment for animals in this range, while others do not.

RECOMMENDATIONS

1. Animals with markedly elevated blood pressure (systolic blood pressure greater than 200 mm Hg, and/or diastolic blood pressure greater than 120 mm Hg) are candidates for antihypertensive therapy.
2. Animals with moderately elevated blood pressure (systolic blood pressure 170 to 200 mm Hg, and/or diastolic blood pressure 100 to 120 mm Hg) and clinical signs referable to systemic hypertension are candidates for antihypertensive therapy.
3. Animals with no clinical signs and moderately elevated blood pressure (systolic blood pressure 170 to 200 mm Hg, and/or diastolic blood pressure 100 to 120 mm Hg) can be considered for treatment.
4. Animals with no clinical signs and mildly elevated blood pressure (systolic blood pressure 120 to 170 mm Hg, and diastolic blood pressure 80 to 100 mm Hg) should not be treated.
5. Animals with normal blood pressure *or in which blood pressure has not been measured* should not be treated with antihypertensive agents.

DURATION OF TREATMENT

The diagnosis of hypertension associated with chronic renal disease necessitates life-long antihypertensive treatment with periodic dosage adjustments based on blood pressure measurements.

Hypertension associated with hyperthyroidism and hyperadrenocorticism can be expected to resolve within 1 to 3 months following effective treatment of the underlying condition, unless chronic renal failure is also present. Occasionally, dogs with well-controlled hyperadrenocorticism remain hypertensive.

In other patients, the duration of treatment cannot be predicted, although it may be required for life. Periodic dosage adjustments based on blood pressure measurements are indicated.

THERAPEUTIC GOAL

It is usually not possible to restore blood pressure to normal values when one treats a hypertensive animal. It should be the veterinarian's goal to lower the blood pressure to within 30 to 50 mm Hg of the normal ranges for blood pressure. If an oscillometric unit is employed, the systolic, mean, or diastolic blood pressure can be used to judge the effectiveness of therapy. If a Doppler ultrasonic device is used, the systolic blood pressure should be used for monitoring the effectiveness of treatment. In general, the Doppler ultrasonic device is most reliable in cats and either unit provides equivalently reliable results in dogs (see previous article).

ANTIHYPERTENSIVE THERAPY

General

Systemic arterial blood pressure (blood pressure) is the product of cardiac output and total peripheral resistance, so antihypertensive therapy is generally aimed at reducing cardiac output or total peripheral resistance, or both. Therapy may be loosely classified as nutritional and pharmacologic.

Treatment is generally guided by sequential trials. Dosage adjustments or changes in treatment should be instituted no more frequently than every 3 weeks, unless extreme hypertension or severe clinical signs necessitate emergency treatment. When one uses pharmacologic agents, a wide range of dosages should be considered, with initial dosages at the low end of the range. If an agent or a combination of agents is incompletely effective, the dosage or dosages may be increased or additional agents added. Often, especially in dogs, multiple agents are used concurrently.

Dietary

The first recommendation is to institute a low-sodium diet that provides no more than 0.25% sodium on a dry-weight basis. A diet with a low chloride and a moderately elevated potassium content may provide further blood pressure-lowering benefit. It should be emphasized that these nutritional maneuvers alone are *very unlikely* to return blood pressure to reasonable and safe levels in a markedly hypertensive animal. Frequently, dietary sodium restriction is employed as a first step in order to enhance the efficacy of pharmacologic agents. In animals with chronic renal disease and hypertension, it may be more important to maintain adequate caloric intake, rather than to insist that a low-sodium diet be fed.

Obesity can elevate systemic arterial pressure in humans and dogs and, perhaps, in cats. Consequently, weight loss is desirable in obese, hypertensive animals. However, the effect of obesity on blood pressure is relatively modest and, by itself, would be difficult to appreciate with devices that indirectly estimate blood pressure. Weight loss will probably be of some benefit, and it should be a long-term goal of medium priority in obese, hypertensive cats and dogs.

Pharmacologic Agents

Medical treatment of hypertension in dogs and cats has, until recently, been extrapolated from human protocols. The recommendations for medical therapy have included diuretics, vasodilators, and beta-blockers; these agents are generally given in concert with dietary sodium restriction.

Vasodilators

Some drugs classified as calcium channel blockers reduce total peripheral resistance, leading to a decrease in blood pressure. Amlodipine besylate (Norvasc), a long-acting dihydropyridine calcium antagonist, has been used successfully as a single agent in hypertensive cats at a dosage of 0.625 mg/cat PO every 24 hours (Henik et al, 1994). Some larger cats (>4 kg) or those with severe hypertension may require dosages as high as 1.25 mg twice daily, although it is essential to titrate the dose carefully, guided by repeated blood pressure determinations. Blood pressure decreases significantly during amlodipine treatment, and significant adverse effects (i.e., azotemia, hypokalemia, weight loss) are infrequently identified. Amlodipine has a slow onset of action, and so adverse effects such as hypotension and loss of appetite are usually avoided. In dogs with chronic renal disease, a dosage of 0.05 to 0.10 mg/kg given orally once daily lowered blood pressure in initial pharmacokinetic trials. In many hypertensive dogs, however, amlodipine appears to be less effective, even at dosages as high as 0.25 mg/kg twice daily.

An inhibitor of angiotensin-converting enzyme (e.g., 0.5 mg/kg of enalapril or benazepril PO every 12 hours) lowers blood pressure; in cats, a higher dosage may be required and the results do not seem as predictable as with amlodipine. The co-administration of an angiotensin-converting enzyme inhibitor (ACEI) and a calcium channel antagonist may prove efficacious when monotherapy is not sufficient in lowering blood pressure.

Alpha-blockers, such as prazosin (1 to 4 mg PO every 12 to 24 hours) or phenoxybenzamine, may lower systemic arterial blood pressure by lowering peripheral vascular resistance. These drugs are infrequently used.

Concern has been raised about the potential for deleterious effects with the use of calcium channel antagonists. These concerns arise from studies in humans and diabetic dogs in which renal injury and/or proteinuria is exacerbated during therapy with calcium channel antagonists. In addition, there is a theoretic rationale for preferring the use of an ACEI over other antihypertensive agents in animals with pre-existing renal disease. However, the co-administration of a calcium channel antagonist and an ACEI apparently blocks any adverse effects of calcium channel antagonism alone, at least in diabetic dogs (Brown et al, 1993). In addition, because calcium channel antagonists are usually very effective in cats with systemic hypertension, they can be considered appropriate agents for use in affected cats until further information regarding their long-term effects on renal function in cats becomes available.

Beta-Blockers

Beta-blockers exert an antihypertensive effect by reducing cardiac output and decreasing renin release. A cardio-specific (beta$_1$) antagonist, such as atenolol, is preferred, with a starting dose of 0.5 mg atenolol/kg PO every 12 to 24 hours. These agents can be combined with vasodilators and/or diuretics. Beta-blockers may also be useful in hypertension associated with hyperthyroidism in cats.

Diuretics

Diuretics, such as the thiazides (e.g., 1 mg hydrochlorothiazide/kg PO every 12 to 24 hours), can be used in hypertensive dogs and cats. These agents lower extracellular fluid volume and cardiac output. Hypokalemia may occur with loop diuretics as well as thiazides, so potassium concentrations should be carefully monitored in all animals with chronic renal disease that are receiving a diuretic. The addition of spironolactone (1 to 2 mg/kg PO every 12 hours), a potassium-sparing diuretic, may be helpful in limiting potassium loss.

Emergency Management of Hypertension

Animals with neurologic signs or severe ocular manifestations of hypertension, such as retinal detachment or intraocular hemorrhage, warrant aggressive treatment. Sodium nitroprusside, an arterial and venous vasodilator acting as a donor of nitric oxide inside vascular smooth muscle cells, can be used for the initial treatment of a hypertensive crisis (see p. 194). This drug must be given by constant-rate infusion, can be titrated very precisely according to the blood pressure response, and usually does not cause reflex tachycardia.

If a constant rate of infusion and intensive monitoring are not available in a veterinary hospital, hydralazine plus furosemide can be used in combination or single-agent treatment with diltiazem (0.5 mg/kg PO every 6 hours) can be used. If blood pressure is not lowered within 12 hours by either of these approaches, a beta-blocker (e.g., atenolol) should be added.

Regardless of the initial therapy chosen for the management of an acute hypertensive crisis, a drug of choice for long-term management of systemic hypertension (e.g., amlodipine in cats; ACEI in dogs) should be instituted soon after presentation in order to facilitate the eventual transition to short-term or long-term maintenance therapy.

Follow-Up Care and Additional Medications

In all animals treated for systemic hypertension, routine examination should include a fundic examination, evaluation of any underlying diseases, and measurement of body weight, blood pressure, and serum concentrations of creatinine and electrolytes. The owner should be questioned for evidence of drug toxicity, which may include lethargy, increased time spent sleeping, ataxia, or anorexia. Animals on multiple-drug regimens are more likely to exhibit adverse effects than are those on a single antihypertensive agent. Once blood pressure is controlled, the animal should be evaluated at 3-month intervals. A complete blood count, serum biochemical panel, and urinalysis should be evaluated at least once every 6 months.

Many hypertensive animals have renal disease. Other treatments for chronic renal disease should accompany antihypertensive therapy, as appropriate. Potassium supplementation is often needed in cats with chronic renal disease. Animals with renal dysfunction generally have an impaired ability to adapt to sudden changes in sodium input; thus, the administration of electrolyte solutions can lead to volume overload, worsened systemic hypertension, and pleural effusion (or peripheral edema) in animals with renal failure. These problems are complicated by moderate to severe anemia, which can tax cardiac reserves. These clinical findings may be difficult to differentiate from right-sided congestive heart failure. Similarly, a sudden reduction in dietary sodium intake in an animal with renal failure can lead to extracellular fluid volume depletion. Some treatments, such as recombinant erythropoietin administered to elevate hematocrit (see *CVT XII,* p. 961), may exacerbate systemic hypertension and should not be used until systemic hypertension is controlled.

References and Suggested Reading

Brown SA, Walton CL, Crawford P, et al: Long-term effects of antihypertensive regimens on renal hemodynamics and proteinuria. Kidney Int 43:1210, 1993.
  Experimental study comparing the efficacy of a calcium channel blocker and an inhibitor of angiotensin-converting enzyme as renoprotective agents in a model of diabetic nephropathy in dogs. The profile of responses suggested that the converting enzyme inhibitor was preferred in this model of renal disease.
Henik RA, Snyder PS, Volk LM: Amlodipine besylate therapy in cats with systemic arterial hypertension secondary to chronic renal disease (abstract). Proceedings of the 12th ACVIM Forum, San Francisco, CA, 1994, p 976.
  Results of the use of amlodipine (a calcium channel blocker) in cats with systemic hypertension and chronic renal failure, demonstrating the potent antihypertensive effects of this agent.
Kibosh DL, Peterson ME, Graves TK, et al: Hypertension in cats with chronic renal failure or hyperthyroidism. J Vet Intern Med 4:58, 1990.
  Survey of cats with spontaneous hyperthyroidism demonstrating the
prevalence of systemic hypertension and some of the potential sequelae in these animals.*
Labato MA, Ross LA: Diagnosis and management of hypertension. In: August JR, ed: Consultations in Feline Internal Medicine. Philadelphia: WB Saunders, 1991, p 301.
  Overview of the diagnosis and treatment of spontaneous systemic hypertension in cats.
Littman MP: Chronic spontaneous systemic hypertension in dogs and cats. Proceedings of the 8th ACVIM Forum, Washington DC, 1990, p 209.
  Results of studies of spontaneous systemic hypertension in dogs and cats.
Littman MP: Spontaneous systemic hypertension in 24 cats. J Vet Intern Med 8:79, 1994.
  Detailed clinical study of systemic hypertension in cats afflicted with marked systemic hypertension. Considerable prospective information is provided.
Morgan RV: Systemic hypertension in four cats: Ocular and medical findings. J Am Anim Hosp Assoc 22:615, 1986.
  Ocular effects of severe systemic hypertension in a group of affected cats.
Ortega TM, Feldman EC, Nelson RW, et al: Systemic arterial blood pressure and urine protein/creatinine ratio in dogs with hyperadrenocorticism. J Am Vet Med Assoc 209:1724, 1996.
  Results of a study of the prevalence and possible adverse effects of systemic hypertension in dogs with hyperadrenocorticism.
Snyder PS, Henik RA: Feline systemic hypertension. Proceedings of the 12th Annual Veterinary Medical Forum, San Francisco, 1994, p 126.
  Overview of the pathophysiology and management of systemic hypertension in cats.
Stiles J, Polzin DJ, Bistner SI: The prevalence of retinopathy in cats with systemic hypertension and chronic renal failure or hyperthyroidism. J Am Anim Hosp Assoc 30:564, 1994.
  Discussion of the ocular abnormalities associated with systemic hypertension in cats with chronic renal failure or hyperthyroidism.
Turner JL, Brogdon JD, Lees GE, et al: Idiopathic hypertension in a cat with secondary hypertensive retinopathy associated with a high-salt diet. J Am Anim Hosp Assoc 26:647, 1990.
  Discussion of the ocular manifestations of systemic hypertension in cats and the possible effects of a high-salt diet on blood pressure.

Summary of Dietary Recommendations in Urinary Diseases

JOSEPH W. BARTGES
Knoxville, Tennessee

SCOTT A. BROWN
Athens, Georgia

A wide variety of urinary tract disorders are important in the clinical practice of veterinary medicine. Unfortunately, our understanding of dietary considerations for dogs and cats with urinary tract diseases is limited primarily to animals with chronic renal failure and those with urolithiasis, although dietary modification has been proposed in the treatment of protein-losing nephropathy and hypertension. The role of diet in the management of cats with idiopathic lower urinary tract disease unassociated with crystalluria is unknown.

The purpose of this article is to provide information on selected currently available commercial diets that may be useful in the management of various urinary tract disorders in dogs and cats. The information is provided in tabular format: Tables 1 and 2 present potential, but not necessarily proved, indications of selected diets, and Tables 3 and 4 present data on the composition of these selected diets. The information presented in Tables 1 and 2 is based on published articles that have evaluated some of these diets, information provided by manufacturers of these diets, and theoretic, but unproven, benefits of dietary modification for certain diseases. Information regarding additional medical

Text continued on page 846

TABLE 1. Potential Indications for Selected Diets Formulated for Treatment of Urinary Tract Diseases in Dogs

Chronic renal failure
Early Stage§
Advanced Stage§
   k/d* #
   Low Protein† ‡‡
   Medium Protein† ‡‡
   Modified Formula**
   NF‖ ††
   u/d* #

Protein-losing nephropathy
k/d* #
   Low Protein† ‡‡
   Medium Protein† ‡‡
   Modified Formula‡ **
   NF‖ ††
   u/d* #

Hypertension
   CV‖ ††
   h/d* #

Urolithiasis—calcium oxalate
Dissolution
   none available
Prevention
   DCO††
   k/d* #
   Low Protein† ‡‡
   Medium Protein§ ‡‡
   Modified Formula‡ **
   NF‖ ††
   u/d* #
   w/d* #

Urolithiasis—cystine
Dissolution
   u/d* #
Prevention
   u/d* #

Urolithiasis—struvite
Dissolution
   s/d* #
Prevention, sterile struvite
   c/d* #
   Control Formula**

Urolithiasis—urate
Dissolution
   k/d* #
   u/d* #
Prevention
   k/d* #
   u/d* #

§Eukanuba Diets, Iams Company, Dayton, OH; diet information as of October, 1998.
*#Prescription Diets, Hill's Pet Nutrition, Inc., Topeka, KS; diet information as of January, 1998.
**Select Care Diets, Innovative Veterinary Diets, Division of Nature's Recipe, diet information as of October, 1998.
††‖CNM Diets, Ralston Purina, Co., St. Louis, MO; diet information as of February, 1998.
‡‡†Veterinary Diets, Waltham, Leicestershire, England; diet information as of May, 1998.

TABLE 2. Potential Indications for Selected Diets Formulated for Treatment of Urinary Tract Diseases in Cats

Chronic renal failure
k/d*#
Low Protein† ‡‡
Mature Formula‡ **
Modified Formula‡ **

Hypertension
CV§ ††
h/d*#

Idiopathic lower urinary tract disease
If associated with struvite crystalluria—see information for struvite urolithiasis

Urolithiasis—calcium oxalate
Dissolution
  none available
Prevention
  c/d oxl#
  Control Formula‡ **
  k/d*#
  Low Protein† ‡‡
  Mature Formula‡ **
  Moderate pH/o§
  Modified Formula‡ **
  NF§ ††
  w/d*#
  Weight Formula‡

Urolithiasis—cystine
Dissolution
  none available
Prevention
  k/d*#

Urolithiasis—struvite
Dissolution
  s/d*#
Prevention
  c/ds#
  Control Formula‡ **
  Control pHormula† ‡‡
  Low pH/s§
  UR† ††

Urolithiasis—urate
Dissolution
  k/d*#
Prevention
  k/d*#

Information provided by pet food manufacturers.
§Eukanuba Diets, Iams Company, Dayton, OH; diet information as of October, 1998.
*#Prescription Diets, Hill's Pet Nutrition, Inc., Topeka, KS; diet information as of January, 1998.
**Select Care Diets, Innovative Veterinary Diets, Division of Nature's Recipe Pet Foods, diet information as of October, 1998.
†† §CNM Diets, Ralston Purina, Co., St. Louis, MO; diet information as of February, 1998.
‡‡ †Veterinary Diets, Waltham, Leicestershire, England; diet information as of May, 1998.

TABLE 3. Approximate Nutrient Profiles From Selected Diets Formulated for Treatment of Urinary Tract Diseases in Dogs*

Diet	Kcal/Serving†	As Fed						Dry Matter					Amount/100 kcal				
		Water (%)	Crude Protein (%)	Crude Fat (%)	Crude Fiber (%)	NFE (%)	Sodium (%)	Crude Protein (%)	Crude Fat (%)	Crude Fiber (%)	NFE (%)	Sodium (%)	Crude Protein (gm)	Crude Fat (gm)	Crude Fiber (gm)	NFE (gm)	Sodium (mg)
c/d‡	413/cup	7.34	20.20	19.50	2.30	46.6	0.25	21.80	21.04	2.48	50.3	0.27	4.86	4.69	0.55	11.2	0.06
	473/15.25 oz can	72.81	6.20	6.50	0.20	13.2	0.08	22.80	23.91	0.74	48.6	0.29	5.68	5.95	0.18	12.1	0.07
CV§	638/12.5 oz can	67.22	5.84	10.44	0.45	16.3	0.04	17.82	31.85	1.37	49.8	0.12	3.25	5.81	0.25	9.1	0.02
Control Formula#	2369/cup	8.00	19.50	16.40	2.50	48.9	0.28	21.20	17.83	2.72	53.1	0.30	4.88	4.10	0.63	12.2	0.07
	436/14 oz can	75.00	5.70	4.90	0.630	13.1	0.06	22.80	19.60	1.20	52.4	0.24	5.20	4.47	0.27	12.0	0.05
h/d‡	429/cup	7.56	15.90	19.30	0.80	51.9	0.06	17.20	20.88	0.87	56.1	0.06	3.68	4.47	0.19	12.0	0.01
	583/15.25 oz can	72.25	4.80	8.00	0.20	13.5	0.03	17.30	28.83	0.72	48.7	0.11	3.57	5.94	0.15	10.0	0.02
HiFiber Formula#	278/cup	6.00	22.30	9.30	14.50	41.5	0.20	23.72	9.89	15.43	44.2	0.21	6.61	2.76	4.30	12.3	0.06
	352/14 oz can	77.00	5.80	1.80	3.50	11.0	0.07	25.22	7.83	15.22	47.8	0.30	6.55	2.03	3.95	12.4	0.08
k/d‡	414/cup	7.53	13.50	18.00	0.70	56.9	0.19	14.60	19.47	0.76	61.5	0.21	3.24	4.32	0.17	13.7	0.05
	571/15.25 oz can	72.97	4.00	7.40	0.20	14.8	0.06	14.80	27.38	0.74	54.8	0.22	3.03	5.61	0.15	11.2	0.05
Low Protein**	310/cup	9.00	12.70	9.80	0.50	62.0	0.20	13.96	10.77	0.55	68.1	0.22	3.49	2.69	0.14	17.0	0.05
	650/13.6 oz can	65.00	6.60	9.20	0.30	20.0	0.22	18.86	26.29	0.86	57.1	0.63	3.92	5.47	0.18	11.9	0.13
Mature Formula#	319/cup	8.00	18.30	7.80	5.40	55.3	0.23	19.89	8.48	5.87	60.1	0.25	5.38	2.29	1.59	16.3	0.07
	370/14 oz can	75.00	5.40	2.70	1.30	14.6	0.05	21.60	10.80	5.20	58.4	0.20	5.80	2.90	1.40	15.7	0.05
Medium Protein**	320/cup	9.80	17.00	14.40	1.10	57.5	0.20	18.85	15.96	1.22	63.8	0.22	4.68	3.96	0.30	15.8	0.06
	540/13.6 oz can	57.50	7.30	9.80	0.40	10.0	0.20	17.18	23.06	0.94	23.5	0.47	5.22	7.01	0.29	7.2	0.14
Modified Formula#	362/cup	7.64	13.30	18.10	1.90	54.6	0.26	14.40	19.60	2.06	59.1	0.28	3.39	4.62	0.48	13.9	0.07
	525/14 oz can	71.43	4.80	6.30	0.40	16.3	0.06	16.80	22.05	1.40	57.0	0.21	3.64	4.77	0.30	12.3	0.05
NF§	415/cup	8.50	13.66	15.02	0.96	57.2	0.21	14.93	16.42	1.05	62.5	0.23	3.46	3.80	0.24	14.5	0.05
	516/12.5 oz can	69.31	5.08	7.76	0.47	16.6	0.07	16.55	25.29	1.53	54.1	0.23	3.49	5.34	0.32	11.4	0.05
s/d‡	621/15.25 oz can	71.05	2.20	7.60	0.80	17.0	0.37	7.60	26.25	2.76	58.7	1.28	1.53	5.30	0.56	11.9	0.26
u/d‡	346/cup	7.53	8.60	19.10	2.20	59.9	0.22	9.30	20.66	2.38	64.8	0.24	1.91	4.23	0.49	13.3	0.05
	644/15.25 oz can	72.17	3.20	7.60	0.40	16.0	0.07	11.50	27.31	1.44	57.5	0.25	2.15	5.11	0.27	10.8	0.05
w/d‡	226/cup	8.98	15.20	6.30	15.30	50.5	0.19	16.70	6.92	16.81	55.5	0.21	5.16	2.14	5.19	17.1	0.06
	390/15.25 oz can	73.46	4.30	3.20	3.60	14.4	0.07	16.20	12.06	13.56	54.3	0.26	4.78	3.55	4.00	16.0	0.08

*Based on information provided by pet food manufacturers.

†Cup = one 8-ounce measuring cup.

‡Prescription Diets, Hill's Pet Nutrition, Inc., Topeka, KS; diet information as of January, 1998.

§CNM Diets, Ralston Purina, Co., St. Louis, MO; diet information as of February, 1998.

#Select Care Diets, Vet's Choice, Santa Monica, CA; diet information as of October, 1998.

**Veterinary Diets, Waltham, Leicestershire, England; diet information as of May, 1998.

Eukanuba Diets, Iams Company, Dayton, OH; diet information as of October, 1998.

TABLE 4. Approximate Nutrient Profiles From Selected Diets Formulated for Treatment of Urinary Tract Diseases in Cats*

Diet	Kcal/Serving†	As Fed						Dry Matter					Amount/100 kcal				
		Water (%)	Crude Protein (%)	Crude Fat (%)	Crude Fiber (%)	NFE (%)	Sodium (%)	Crude Protein (%)	Crude Fat (%)	Crude Fiber (%)	NFE (%)	Sodium (%)	Crude Protein (gm)	Crude Fat (gm)	Crude Fiber (gm)	NFE (gm)	Sodium (mg)
c/d‡	519/cup	7.50	32.00	23.20	0.70	32.0	0.34	34.6	25.08	0.76	34.59	0.37	7.35	5.33	0.16	7.35	0.08
	603/15 oz can	71.00	12.70	8.50	0.50	5.7	0.11	43.8	29.31	1.72	19.66	0.38	8.97	6.00	0.35	4.03	0.08
CV	223/5.5 oz can	70.66	12.48	7.86	0.29	6.77	0.06	42.5	26.79	0.99	23.07	0.20	8.74	5.51	0.20	4.74	0.04
Control Formula#	410/cup	6.00	31.40	21.50	1.20	34.9	5.00	33.4	22.87	1.28	37.13	5.32	7.61	5.21	0.29	8.46	1.21
	432/14 oz can	77.00	10.60	7.10	0.20	3.9	1.20	46.1	30.87	0.87	16.96	5.22	9.76	6.53	0.18	3.59	1.10
Control pHormula**	378/cup	7.45	34.7	16.9	1.8	32.4	0.79	37.49	18.26	1.94	34.95	0.85	9.38	4.57	0.49	217.1	0.21
	207/6 oz can	81.00	7.4	8.7	0.1	1.1	0.23	38.95	45.79	0.53	5.79	1.21	7.18	8.45	0.10	10.6	0.22
h/d‡	542/15 oz can	71.00	12.60	7.80	0.10	6.9	0.07	43.6	26.99	0.35	23.88	0.24	9.90	6.13	0.08	5.42	0.06
k/d‡	519/cup	7.47	26.00	25.30	1.20	35.4	0.26	28.1	27.34	1.30	38.26	0.28	6.12	5.95	0.28	8.33	0.06
	624/15 oz can	72.01	8.20	11.50	0.70	6.3	0.07	29.3	41.09	2.50	22.51	0.25	5.60	7.85	0.48	4.30	0.05
Low Protein**	385/cup	6.20	25.00	23.60	3.00	45.0	0.10	26.6	25.16	3.20	47.97	0.11	5.90	5.57	0.71	10.62	0.02
	250/6 oz can	74.00	9.00	13.30	0.20	2.0	0.15	34.6	51.15	0.77	7.69	0.58	6.13	9.07	0.14	1.36	0.10
Mature Formula#	335/cup	7.00	27.20	15.60	2.00	43.2	0.35	29.3	16.77	2.15	46.45	0.38	7.61	4.36	0.56	12.09	0.10
	478/14 oz can	78.00	9.10	9.30	0.40	1.9	0.07	41.4	42.27	1.82	8.64	0.32	7.57	7.74	0.33	1.58	0.06
Modified Formula#	440/cup	6.36	26.50	20.70	1.40	41.0	0.26	28.3	22.11	1.50	43.78	0.28	6.50	5.08	0.34	10.06	0.06
	618/14 oz can	73.42	9.30	14.10	0.40	2.0	0.06	35.0	53.05	1.50	7.52	0.23	5.98	9.07	0.26	1.29	0.04
NF§	398/cup	7.40	28.50	11.90	1.14	46.9	0.18	30.8	12.85	1.23	50.63	0.19	6.51	2.72	0.26	10.70	0.04
s/d‡	521/cup	7.51	32.00	24.00	0.60	30.3	0.66	34.6	25.95	0.65	32.76	0.71	7.50	5.63	0.14	7.10	0.15
	591/15 oz can	71.01	12.00	9.90	0.50	4.6	0.25	41.4	34.15	1.72	15.87	0.86	8.65	7.14	0.36	3.32	0.18
UR§	366/cup	8.66	32.36	10.60	1.36	41.4	0.22	35.4	11.60	1.49	45.28	0.24	8.04	2.63	0.34	10.27	0.05
	493/12.5 oz can	70.71	12.12	10.70	0.03	4.8	0.13	41.4	36.53	0.10	16.49	0.44	8.73	7.70	0.02	3.48	0.09
w/d‡	246/cup	8.93	35.70	8.60	8.10	33.3	0.25	39.2	9.44	8.89	36.57	0.27	11.13	2.68	2.52	10.38	0.08
	390/15 oz can	75.49	10.00	4.20	3.10	5.7	0.12	40.8	17.14	12.65	23.26	0.49	10.92	4.59	3.39	6.23	0.13
Weight Formula#	357/cup	7.00	31.90	11.40	4.40	40.9	0.39	34.3	12.26	4.73	43.98	0.42	8.37	2.99	1.16	10.74	0.10
	337/14 oz can	79.00	8.60	3.80	1.00	6.4	0.07	41.0	18.10	4.76	30.48	0.33	10.15	4.48	1.18	7.55	0.08

*Information provided by pet food manufacturers.
†Cup = one 8-ounce measuring cup.
‡Prescription Diets, Hill's Pet Nutrition, Inc., Topeka, KS; diet information as of January, 1997.
§CNM Diets, Ralston Purina Co., St. Louis, MO; diet information as of October, 1996.
#Select Care Diets, Vet's Choice, Santa Monica, CA; diet information as of January, 1997.
**Veterinary Diets, Waltham, Leicestershire, England; diet information as of May, 1997.

or surgical therapy for these diseases is found elsewhere in this section. In Tables 3 and 4, diet composition is presented on an "as-fed" basis, a "dry-matter" basis, and nutrient amount per 100 Kcal of food as fed. For conversion of Kcal to KJ, 1 Kcal = 4.2 KJ. This information was provided by the manufacturers of these diets.

In general, dietary modification for selected urinary tract diseases include the following:

- Chronic renal failure: reduced protein, reduced phosphorus, alkalinizing, and, for cats, adequate potassium
- Protein-losing nephropathy: reduced protein, reduced sodium
- Hypertension: reduced sodium
- Urolithiasis—calcium oxalate: reduced protein, reduced sodium, alkalinizing; increased fiber; induction of diuresis
- Urolithiasis—cystine: reduced protein, reduced sodium, alkalinizing
- Urolithiasis—struvite: reduced protein, reduced phosphorus, reduced magnesium, acidifying, induction of diuresis
- Urolithiasis—urate: reduced protein, alkalinizing, induction of diuresis
- Idiopathic lower urinary tract disease in cats: if associated with struvite urolithiasis, reduced protein, reduced phosphorous, reduced magnesium, acidifying, induction of diuresis

---

Adverse Effects of Drugs on Formation of Canine and Feline Crystalluria and Uroliths

CARL A. OSBORNE
JODY P. LULICH
LISA K. ULRICH
St. Paul, Minnesota

GLENN W. AUSTIN
Orlando, Florida

IMPACT OF DRUGS ON FORMATION OF UROLITHS

Diagnostic and therapeutic drugs may potentiate urolithiasis in one or a combination of ways, including (1) alteration of urine pH in such fashion as to create an environment that is less soluble for some lithogenic substances; (2) alteration of glomerular filtration, tubular reabsorption, or tubular secretion of drugs or other substances that promote or inhibit urolithiasis; or (3) precipitation (e.g., drugs or their metabolites) to form a portion or all of a urolith (Tables 1 and 2). The prevalance of uroliths that contain drugs or their metabolites in dogs, cats, and other animals is unknown. It is probable that uroliths containing drugs are often unrecognized because they are not suspected and because of limitations associated with commonly used methods of quantitative urolith analysis. For this reason, the authors recommend that the relevant drug history of patients be included when uroliths are submitted for analysis.

SULFONAMIDE ANTIMICROBIALS

Risk Factors

Various types of commonly used sulfonamides are excreted primarily by glomerular filtration. Although sulfonamide crystalluria was a frequent problem associated with the use of older generations of sulfonamides, newer forms of this class of drug are far less frequently associated with the clinical signs attributed to sulfonamide crystalluria.

Factors that predispose to the precipitation of sulfonamides, and especially their acetylated derivatives, in the urinary tract include the administration of high doses of

TABLE 1. Some Drugs That May Contribute to Urolithiasis

Drugs that promote hypercalciuria
  Acidifiers
  Calcitriol
  Corticosteroids
  Furosemide
  Sodium chloride
Drugs that may decrease solubility of lithogenic substances
  Urine acidifiers
  Urine alkalinizers
Drugs that may promote hyperoxaluria
  Ascorbic acid
Drugs that may promote hyperxanthinuria
  Allopurinol
Drugs and their metabolites that may form portions or all of a urolith
  Urographic contrast agents
  Magnesium trisilicate
  Phenazopyridine
  Primidone
  Sulfamonamides and their metabolites
  Tetracyclines

TABLE 2. Factors Predisposing to Precipitation of Drugs in Urine

Reduced volume of highly concentrated urine
Stasis of urine
High rate of urinary excretion of drugs that are poorly soluble in urine
Prolonged treatment with high doses of potentially lithogenic drugs

these drugs for prolonged periods. In addition, acid urine and highly concentrated urine are risk factors.

Epidemiology

Using polarizing light microscopy and infrared spectroscopy, the authors detected sulfadiazine or its metabolites in uroliths formed by 20 dogs and 4 cats, and a urethral plug formed by a cat. In our series, all uroliths were located in the lower urinary tract, except for one canine ureterolith. Most animals had a history of long-term empirical treatment with a combination of sulfadiazine and trimethoprim for suspected bacterial urinary tract infection. Some dogs and cats were concomitantly given drugs or diets designed to acidify urine.

In eight dogs and two cats, sulfadiazine or its metabolites, or both, were the only crystalline component detected in the uroliths. In four dogs, sulfadiazine or its metabolites, or both, were mixed throughout the urolith with either calcium oxalate (two dogs), ammonium urate (1 dog), or magnesium ammonium phosphate (one dog). In one cat, sulfadiazine metabolites were observed to be mixed with ammonium urate. In eight dogs, sulfadiazine or its metabolites, or both, were observed as a surface layer over calcium oxalate (five dogs), ammonium urate (two dogs), and silica (one dog). In one cat, metabolites of sulfadiazine were observed in a shell covering sterile struvite.

Three of the four affected cats were of the domestic shorthaired breed. Of the four cats with uroliths, three were neutered females, and one was a neutered male. The mean age of the affected cats was 7 years (range = 6 to 8 years). A metabolite of sulfadiazine was found as the primary crystalline component in a urethral plug removed from a 2-year-old neutered male domestic shorthaired cat.

In our series, 15 of 20 canine uroliths were formed by 15 different breeds of dogs. Their mean age at the time of diagnosis was 7 years (range = 1 to 11 years). Canine sulfadiazine uroliths affected neutered (seven) and intact (six) males more frequently than they affected neutered (four) and intact (three) females.

Clinical Relevance

Epidemiologic studies of case records at the Minnesota Urolith Center indicate that older age, male gender, and formation of acidic urine are risk factors for calcium oxalate urolithiasis in dogs and cats. The authors hypothesize that the higher prevalence of sulfa-containing uroliths in older animals, especially male dogs, is confounded by unsuccessful attempts to use sulfa-containing antimicrobials to eradicate signs of lower urinary disease suspected to be caused by bacteria in dogs and cats with noninfectious metabolic uroliths (calcium oxalate, ammonium urate, and silica).

It is also likely that sulfadiazine is more likely to precipitate in patients with pre-existing uroliths. This phenomenon is known as heterogeneous nucleation and is somewhat analogous to the precipitation of water vapor around dust particles in the atmosphere.

On the basis of available data, the authors suggest avoiding the use of sulfadiazine to treat lower urinary tract signs empirically, especially in dogs (1) known to have uroliths, (2) known to be at increased risk for metabolic uroliths, and (3) known to be forming acidic or highly concentrated urine, or both.

Tetracycline Antimicrobials

Tetracycline made up 90% of multiple small, yellowish, friable urocystoliths removed from a 3-year-old male English Bulldog admitted to the University of Minnesota Veterinary Teaching Hospital. The dog had been receiving large quantities of orally administered tetracycline hydrochloride for at least 6 months before to surgery in an attempt to eradicate a recalcitrant *Proteus* spp. urinary tract infection. Approximately 1.5 years later, uroliths recurred in the urinary bladder, left kidney, and left ureter. The owners had apparently continued to give the dog a variety of antibiotics, including tetracycline, obtained from several veterinary hospitals. These uroliths also contained tetracycline. Subsequently, studies of human patients revealed that orally administered oxytetracycline could be found in calcium-containing uroliths.

Primidone

The authors observed primidone as the only crystalline component in a urethrolith removed from an 8-year-old neutered male domestic longhaired cat. According to the referring veterinarian, the cat had been treated for seizures during the past 7 years with orally administered primidone (Mysoline) tablets (25 mg/kg given every 12 hours). Primidone crystalluria has been observed in humans.

Drug-Associated Crystalluria

Crystalluria may occur as a result of urinary excretion of several drugs. Sulfonamides may form different types of crystals, including those described as (1) centrally or eccentrically waisted sheaves composed of needle-like crystals (Fig. 1), (2) shocks of wheat composed of slender sheaves that grow in such a way as to form two half-circles with central binding, (3) rosettes formed when the two half-circles just described finally close, (4) globules with a conspicuous radial striation, (5) wedge-shaped crystals with one sharp point and pronounced serrated or "saw-toothed" edges on one or both sides, and (6) transparent ovoid crystals with serrations on one or both edges.

The authors observed wheat sheaf–like crystals, presumed to be ampicillin, in the urine of a dog that was given large doses of ampicillin. The authors also observed wheat sheaf–like crystals in canine urine containing sodium diatrizoate (Hypaque 50, Winthrop Laboratories). Although

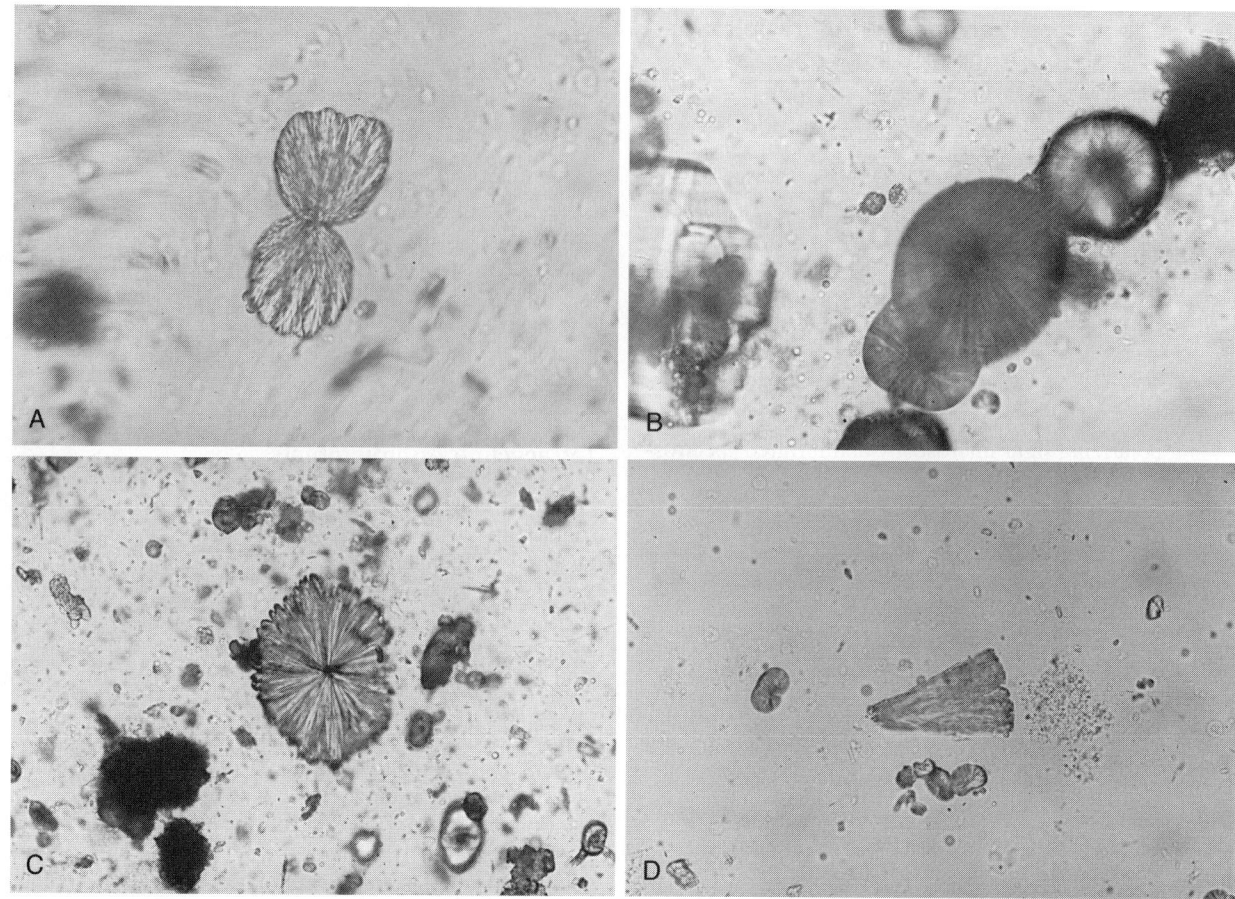

Figure 1. Photomicrographs of urine sediment from a 4-year-old male mixed-breed dog given subcutaneous injections of trimethoprim-sulfadiazine. *A*, Centrally waisted sheaves composed of needle-like crystals of sulfadiazine (original magnification, ×100). *B*, Rosettes of sulfadiazine with radial striations (original magnification, ×100). *C*, Rosette composed of needle-like sulfadiazine crystals (original magnification, ×100). *D*, Needle-like crystals of sulfadiazine that have formed a fan-shaped structure and rosettes of sulfadiazine (*arrows*) (original magnification, ×100).

wheat sheaf–like ampicillin and sodium diatrizoate crystals resemble sulfa crystals, urine containing these crystals produces negative results by lignin testing; when sulfas are present in urine, these results are positive.

Other drug-associated forms of crystalluria reported in humans include fluoroquinolones, 5-fluorocytosine, 6-mercaptopurine, methenamine mandelate, nalidixic acid, and theophylline. Methods of identifying crystals suspected of being composed of drugs include infrared spectroscopy, gas or liquid chromatography, and mass spectrometry.

References and Suggested Reading

Bailey DN, Jatlow PL: Chemical analysis of massive crystalluria following primidone overdose. Am J Clin Pathol 58:583, 1972.
This article contains photomicrographs of primidone crystals.
Jones HM, Schrader WA: Ampicillin crystalluria. Am J Clin Pathol 58:220, 1972.
This article contains photomicrographs of ampicillin crystals.
Koneman EW, Schessler J: Unusual urinary crystals. Am J Clin Pathol 44:358, 1965.
This article contains photomicrographs of sodium diatrizoate crystals.
Mulvaney WP, Beck CW, Qureshi MA: Occurrence of tetracycline in urinary calculi. J Urol 94:187, 1965.
This article describes factors involved in the incorporation of tetracycline into uroliths.
Osborne CA, Oldroyd NO, Clinton CW: Etiopopathogenesis of uncommon canine uroliths: Xanthine, drugs, and drug metabolites. Vet Clin North Am Small Anim Pract 16:217, 1986.
This article provides additional information about drugs and drug metabolites in uroliths.

Urologic Emergencies

San Marcos, California

THERAPY FOR A UREMIC CRISIS IN POLYURIC RENAL FAILURE

The first goal in treating a uremic crisis is to correct fluid volume deficit. A balanced electrolyte solution should be used to correct dehydration within in 4 to 6 hours (see *CVT XII*, p. 951). Always collect blood and urine *before* administering fluids. Once rehydration has been achieved, fluids should be administered at a rate of one and one-half to three times the maintenance rate in an attempt to expand volume, which will increase renal blood flow and facilitate the loss of uremic toxins (Chew, 1992; Rubin, 1995). Potassium chloride should be added to fluids so that hypokalemia is not induced. As long as the animal is not hyperkalemic, 10 to 20 mEq of potassium chloride can safely be added per liter of fluids. Care should be taken not to administer potassium chloride faster than 0.5 mEq/kg per hour.

Diuresis with an osmotic or loop diuretic may increase the excretion of uremic toxins by increasing urine flow. Some authors believe that this is theoretically feasible, whereas others believe that there is no theoretical basis to support the use of diuretics in polyuric chronic renal failure (Chew, 1992; Rubin, 1995). If a diuretic is used for this purpose, care should be taken to avoid inducing dehydration. Before a diuretic is administered, a fluid load is provided equal to 3 to 5% of the animal's body weight over 1 hour to expand volume. The diuretic is administered after the fluid load has been administered. Central venous pressure should be monitored and fluid administration should be decreased if the central venous pressure exceeds 13 cm H_2O or if it increases by more than 2 cm H_2O in any 10-minute period.

TREATMENT OF OLIGURIC RENAL FAILURE

Acute renal failure can be precipitated by renal ischemia, nephrotoxins (e.g., ethylene glycol), infection, or rupture or obstruction of the urinary conduit. Therapy for nonobstructive oliguric renal failure is aimed at keeping the patient alive while promoting renal blood flow and urine production with fluid therapy until kidney function is restored. Initial therapy involves the rapid replacement of fluid deficits and expansion of the blood vascular system. An indwelling urinary catheter is placed and fluid input and urine output are monitored. The animal is weighed after fluid replacement. Rehydration and volume expansion are achieved with a balanced electrolyte solution within 4 to 6 hours. If there were severe fluid losses previously or fluid losses are continuing because of vomiting and diarrhea, and the animal is in shock, fluid may need to be administered at a rate of 70 to 100 ml/kg body weight per hour for 2 to 4 hours to attain rehydration and volume expansion. Central venous pressure should be monitored.

After this initial fluid therapy, further therapy is dependent on insensible losses (22 ml/kg body weight per day), continuing losses via vomiting and diarrhea, and urine losses. One must continually monitor the patient's hydration.

After rehydration, animals should be producing approximately 3 ml of urine/kg body weight per hour. Failure to produce this amount of urine could be due to poor initial assessment of hydration status or primary oliguric renal failure. If the animal is appropriately rehydrated and is in oliguric renal failure, a diuretic may be administered at this time in an attempt to induce diuresis. Further volume expansion in oliguric animals is likely to induce pulmonary edema.

Diuretics have been reported to induce vasodilatation, decrease tubular reabsorption (therefore reducing the possibility of plugging tubules with cells, debris, crystals, and so on), and decrease renin release. Osmotic diuretics will also prevent and reduce kidney cell swelling and increase extracellular fluid volume, thus increasing renal perfusion. A single dose of mannitol (1 g/kg of a 5 to 25% solution IV) or furosemide (2 to 6 mg/kg, IV), or both, is recommended in an oliguric animal that fails to respond to fluid repletion. A single dose of either or both is unlikely to do harm and occasionally induces diuresis.

Reports indicate that dopamine and furosemide work synergistically to induce diuresis. If furosemide does not induce diuresis by itself, dopamine may be administered at a dose of 1 to 4 μg/kg per minute. Furosemide should also be given at the normal dose and dosage interval (1 to 2 mg/kg IV every 6 to 8 hours) during the dopamine infusion (Forrester, 1997; Grauer and Lane, 1995). If diuresis has not occurred by this time, dialysis is probably needed to maintain physiologic balance and prevent volume overload until the re-establishment of renal function (see p. 859).

A common cause of early death in oliguric renal failure is hyperkalemia. Rehydrating the animal with a potassium-free fluid will reduce serum potassium concentrations. Sodium bicarbonate at a dose of 2 to 3 mEq/kg body weight given IV over 30 minutes or a 20 to 30% dextrose solution given IV to effect, or both, can be used to reduce serum potassium concentrations in the event of more severe hyperkalemia. Both bicarbonate and glucose drive potassium intracellularly within minutes and the effects last hours. A 10% calcium gluconate solution administered IV can be given over 10 to 15 minutes if the patient is in danger of eminent death. The dose should not exceed 0.5 to 1 ml/kg. Calcium protects the heart from the adverse effects of hyperkalemia.

TREATMENT OF OBSTRUCTIVE UROPATHY

Obstructive uropathy (see also pp. 866, 868, and 870) may be due to a structural or functional impairment of

849

urine flow. Structural obstructions are most often caused by either urolithiasis or strictures but can also be caused by urethral mucus and crystals, neoplasia, blood clots, extrinsic mass lesions, trauma, or hernia. Functional obstructions are most often caused by neurologic disorders or chronic inflammation (Finco, 1995).

Complete outflow obstruction results in uremia in 1 to 3 days and death within 5 to 6 days. Urinary tract infection in the face of obstructive uropathy can result in pyelonephritis, acute renal failure, septicemia, and a rapid fulminating course leading to death. Finding a large distended bladder on abdominal palpation in an animal unable to void is diagnostic of obstructive uropathy.

Rapidly decompressing the bladder via cystocentesis in animals with structural obstructions or catheterization in animals with functional obstructions may be lifesaving. Urine should be submitted for urinalysis and culture. Polyionic, isotonic fluids are provided IV for dehydration and the solute diuresis that will occur after relief of the obstruction. Both hyperkalemia and acidosis rapidly correct themselves after the obstruction is eased. If anesthesia is needed for relieving the obstruction, it should be given only *to effect*.

Indications for leaving the catheter in place are severe depression and uremia, poor urine flow through the urethra, and a hypotonic bladder. Life-threatening hyperkalemia is managed as described in the previous section, beginning with sodium bicarbonate infusion. Once the obstruction is relieved and the animal is stable, the underlying cause of the obstruction is treated. If bacterial infection is present, an appropriate antibiotic is administered for 3 to 4 weeks. If there is no detectable bacterial infection, an antibiotic is administered for 5 to 7 days after the catheter is removed.

TRAUMA TO THE URINARY TRACT

Causes of trauma to the urinary tract include being hit by a car, urinary catheterization, penetrating wounds, and physical abuse. Hematuria is commonly seen in urinary tract trauma.

Renal trauma should be suspected in any animal with abdominal trauma. Fluid in the peritoneal cavity or in the retroperitoneal space may be an indication of renal hemorrhage. Radiographic signs of renal trauma include intra-abdominal effusion, retroperitoneal density changes, intestinal ileus, displacement or asymmetry of the kidneys, and loss of renal shadow. Excretory urograms may be needed in some cases. Abdominocentesis confirms the presence of blood in the abdominal cavity. Indications for exploratory abdominal surgery in cases of suspected renal trauma include deterioration of physical status, inability to control shock from continued blood loss, detection of free urine in the abdominal cavity, radiographic evidence of extravasation of dyes into the perirenal space, disruption

of the renal pelvis, shock, and an expanding sublumbar soft tissue swelling.

Urinary bladder trauma is the most common urinary tract injury. Rapid abdominal distention after fluid therapy is a common finding in animals with bladder rupture. Clinical signs of bladder rupture include abdominal pain resulting from chemical peritonitis and vomiting resulting from uremia. Uremia usually develops within 1 to 3 days. Abdominal fluid has a high urea nitrogen and creatinine concentration when compared with serum concentrations. Radiographic findings include ascites, ileus, and peritonitis. Retrograde positive cystography is the recommended contrast radiographic study to perform if a bladder rupture is suspected.

The patient with a ruptured bladder is stabilized by providing adequate IV polyionic fluids. Abdominal drains are useful to remove urine from the abdominal cavity. Peritoneal dialysis may help reduce the azotemia and make the animal a better surgical candidate. Placing a urinary catheter may also help remove urine. Surgical repair of the ruptured bladder is required. Urine should be collected during surgery for culture and sensitivity testing.

Rupture of the ureter and urethra may also occur. Ruptured ureters are usually treated with unilateral nephrectomy. Small urethral tears may heal with the placement of an indwelling urethral catheter for 7 to 21 days. Larger tears require surgical correction. Urethral stricture is the most common complication of urethral trauma.

References and Suggested Reading

Chew DJ: Fluid therapy during intrinsic renal failure. In: Dibartola SP, ed: Fluid Therapy in Small Animal Practice. Philadelphia: WB Saunders, 1992, p 554.
An in-depth discussion of the theory and practice of fluid therapy for animals in renal failure.

Finco DR: Obstructive uropathy and hydronephrosis. In: Osborne CA, Finco DR, eds: Canine and Feline Nephrology and Urology. Baltimore, Williams & Wilkins, 1995, p 889.
An outline of the current information on the pathophysiology and treatment of animals with urethral obstruction.

Forrester SD: Diseases of the kidney and ureter. In: Lieb MS, Monroe WE, eds: Practical Small Animal Medicine. Philadelphia, WB Saunders, 1997, p 282.
A general discussion of the treatment of both acute and chronic renal failure.

Grauer GF, Lane IF: Acute renal failure: Ischemic and chemical nephrosis. In: Osborne CA, Finco DR, eds: Canine and Feline Nephrology and Urology. Baltimore, Williams & Wilkins, 1995, p 441.
A general discussion of the current information on the treatment of acute renal failure.

Rubin SI: Managment of fluid and electrolyte disorders in uremia. In: Bonagura JD, Kirk RW, eds: Kirk's Current Veterinary Therapy XII: Small Animal Practice. Philadelphia, WB Saunders, 1995, p 951.
In-depth discussion of the treatment of animals with uremic crisis.

Wingfield WE, Van Pelf DR, Barker S: Physical injuries to the urinary tract. In: Osborne CA, Finco DR, eds: Canine and Feline Nephrology and Urology. Baltimore, Williams & Wilkins, 1995, p 895.
In-depth discussion of the causes and treatment of trauma to the kidney, ureters, urinary bladder, and urethra.

CVT Update: Canine Glomerulonephritis

GREGORY F. GRAUER
Fort Collins, Colorado

INTRODUCTION

Glomerulonephritis is the term used to describe glomerular cell proliferation and thickening of glomerular capillary walls. Glomerulonephritis is usually caused by the presence of immune complexes within the glomerulus. The hallmark clinicopathologic sign of glomerulonephritis is proteinuria (see *CVT XII*, p. 937). Use of the urine protein-to-creatinine ratio to quantitatively estimate proteinuria has greatly facilitated the diagnosis and treatment of canine glomerulonephritis; however, a definitive diagnosis of glomerulonephritis requires histologic examination of renal biopsy specimens. The treatment objectives for dogs with glomerulonephritis include (1) identification and elimination of underlying causative antigens and/or inflammation responsible for the immune complex formation, (2) immunosuppression, and (3) reduction of the glomerular response to the presence of immune complexes. Without treatment, glomerulonephritis can cause irreversible damage to the glomerulus by way of fibrin deposition and glomerulosclerosis. Irreversible glomerular damage renders the entire nephron nonfunctional and can eventually lead to renal insufficiency and failure.

ETIOLOGY AND PATHOPHYSIOLOGY

Soluble circulating antigen-antibody complexes may be deposited or trapped in the glomerulus when a mild antigen excess exists or when antigen and antibody molecules are present in the plasma in approximately equal numbers. Immune complexes may also form in situ when circulating antibodies react with antigens that have been incorporated in the glomerular capillary wall. These antigens may localize in the glomerular capillary wall as a result of electrical charge interaction or biochemical affinity. For example, glomerulonephritis in dogs with dirofilariasis probably occurs in part as the result of immune complex formation (Grauer et al, 1989).

After formation or deposition of immune complexes in the glomerulus, several factors, including activation of the complement system, platelet adhesion and aggregation, infiltration of polymorphonuclear leukocytes, and activation of the coagulation system with fibrin deposition, contribute to glomerular damage. Platelet adhesion and aggregation occur secondary to vascular endothelial damage or antigen-antibody interaction. Platelets, in turn, exacerbate glomerular damage by release of thromboxane and by facilitation of the coagulation cascade. There is increasing evidence to suggest that thromboxane is an important mediator of the inflammation and proteinuria associated with immune complex glomerulonephritis (Grauer et al, 1988 and 1992; Longhofer et al, 1991). The glomerulus responds to this injury by cellular and mesangial matrix proliferation and thickening of the glomerular basement membrane (Center et al, 1987; Jaenke and Allen, 1986).

CLINICAL SIGNS

There are often no clinical signs associated with glomerulonephritis that causes only mild to moderate proteinuria. If clinical signs are present, they are usually nonspecific, such as weight loss and lethargy. If proteinuria is severe and persistent with serum albumin concentrations less than 1.5 to 1 gm/dl, edema and/or ascites may occur. The combination of significant proteinuria, hypoalbuminemia, ascites or edema, and hypercholesterolemia is defined as the nephrotic syndrome. Hypertension and hypercoagulability are frequent complications in dogs with nephrotic syndrome. If glomerular damage is extensive, rendering three fourths of the nephrons nonfunctional, renal failure and resultant azotemia, polydipsia-polyuria, anorexia, nausea, and vomiting may be observed. Occasionally, signs associated with an underlying infectious, inflammatory, or neoplastic disease may be the reason that owners seek veterinary care for their pet. Rarely, dogs may be presented with acute dyspnea or severe panting caused by pulmonary thromboembolism.

DIAGNOSIS

Persistent, significant proteinuria with an inactive urine sediment or one that contains hyaline casts is the hallmark clinicopathologic abnormality associated with glomerulonephritis. The urine protein-to-creatinine ratio is used to quantitate the magnitude of the urine protein loss. In a review of 106 dogs with glomerulonephritis, the average urine protein-to-creatinine ratio was 11.1 (Cook and Cowgill, 1996). Glomerular amyloidosis also causes significant proteinuria, and differentiation of glomerulonephritis from glomerular amyloidosis requires evaluation of renal cortical histology. Thus, definitive diagnosis requires a renal biopsy (see *CVT XII,* p. 940).

MANAGEMENT

The generation of immune complexes depends on the presence of antigen; therefore, the most important treatment for glomerular disease is identification and correction of any underlying disease processes (Table 1). Dental tartar with gingivitis, bacterial pyoderma, dirofilariasis, ehrlichiosis, borreliosis, and systemic lupus erythematosus are examples of treatable diseases that may be associated with glomerulonephritis. In many cases however, an antigen source or underlying disease process is not identified or is

TABLE 1. Diseases Associated With Glomerulonephritis in Dogs

Infectious
  Canine adenovirus type 1
  Bacterial endocarditis
  Brucellosis
  Dirofilariasis
  Ehrlichiosis
  Leishmaniasis
  Pyometra
  Borreliosis
  Chronic bacterial infections
Neoplasia
Inflammatory, noninfectious
  Pancreatitis
  Systemic lupus erythematosus
  Other immune-mediated diseases
Other
  Hyperadrenocorticism and long-term high-dose
    corticosteroids
  Idiopathic
  Familial
  Nonimmunologic—hyperfiltration?
  Diabetes mellitus?

identified but is impossible to eliminate. Therefore the second arm of treatment, immunosuppressive drugs, is often used in dogs with glomerulonephritis (Table 2). Corticosteroids, azathioprine, cyclophosphamide, and cyclosporine have been used clinically or experimentally to prevent immunoglobulin production by B cells or to alter the function of helper T cells or suppressor T cells. Unfortunately, almost all the immunosuppressive drug recommendations come from the human literature; there are no controlled clinical trials that demonstrate the efficacy of immunosuppressive drugs in the treatment of canine glomerulonephritis. The association between hyperadrenocorticism (and long-term exogenous corticosteroid therapy) and glomerulonephritis and thromboembolism in the dog, as well as the lack of consistent therapeutic response to treatment of glomerular disease with corticosteroids, indicates that corticosteroids should be used with caution in dogs with glomerulonephritis. The exception would be a

TABLE 2. Treatment Guidelines for Canine Glomerulonephritis

1. Identify and correct any underlying disease processes
2. Immunosuppressive treatment? (use with caution, see text)
   a. Cyclophosphamide, 50 mg/m² s.i.d. for 3 or 4 days, and then discontinue for 4 or 3 days, respectively (or every other day), or
   b. Azathioprine, 50 mg/m² s.i.d. or every other day (dogs only), or
   c. Cyclosporine, 15 mg/kg s.i.d. (dogs only)
3. Anti-inflammatory-hypercoagulability treatment
   a. Aspirin, 0.5–5.0 mg/kg s.i.d. to b.i.d. (dogs); 0.5–5.0 mg/kg q48hr (cats)
4. Supportive care
   a. Dietary: sodium reduction, low quantity of high-quality protein
   b. Systemic hypertension: dietary sodium restriction; enalapril, 0.25–0.5 mg/kg s.i.d. to b.i.d.—often has antiproteinuric effects also
   c. Edema/ascites: dietary sodium restriction; furosemide, 2.2 mg/kg t.i.d. to s.i.d. if necessary for severe ascites

corticosteroid-responsive underlying disease process, such as systemic lupus erythematosus. If immunosuppressive drugs are used, the urine protein-to-creatinine ratio should be measured at least monthly to assess the effects of treatment. If the magnitude of proteinuria increases with treatment, immunosuppressive treatment should be changed or discontinued.

The third arm of treatment of glomerulonephritis is to decrease the glomerular response to immune complexes. There is increasing evidence that platelets and thromboxanes are integrally involved in the pathogenesis of glomerulonephritis. Beneficial responses to antiplatelet therapy with aspirin have been demonstrated in several experimental studies. Low-dose aspirin (0.5 to 5 mg/kg orally once to twice daily for dogs and every 48 hours for cats) can theoretically selectively inhibit platelet cyclooxygenase-mediated production of thromboxane, whereas it has a lesser effect on the formation of prostacyclin by endothelial cells. Specific thromboxane synthetase inhibitors have attenuated naturally occurring and experimental canine glomerulonephritis, as evidenced by decreased proteinuria, decreased glomerular cell proliferation and infiltration, decreased fibrin deposition, and preservation of glomerular filtration rate (Grauer et al, 1988; Longhofer et al, 1991; Grauer et al, 1992). It is anticipated that thromboxane synthetase inhibitors will soon be marketed in the United States for the treatment of coronary arterial disease in humans and that they will have an important role in the treatment of canine glomerulonephritis. In addition to antiplatelet therapy, treatment of glomerular disease with prostaglandin analogues or dietary supplementation with omega-3 polyunsaturated fatty acids to enhance prostacyclin activity and decrease production of thromboxanes and leukotrienes has also generally attenuated glomerular disease in experimental studies. However, additional work in this area is necessary before specific treatment recommendations can be made.

It was demonstrated that treatment with enalapril decreases proteinuria, improves renal function, and prolongs survival in male Samoyed dogs with hereditary nephritis (Grodecki et al, 1995). This primary glomerular disease results in chronic renal failure and death in affected dogs prior to 1 year of age. In addition, in dogs with unilateral nephrectomies and experimentally induced diabetes mellitus, another angiotensin-converting enzyme inhibitor (ACEI), lisinopril, reduced glomerular transcapillary hydraulic pressure and glomerular cell hypertrophy as well as proteinuria (Brown et al, 1993). Treatment with ACEI probably decreases proteinuria and preserves renal function associated with glomerular disease by several mechanisms in addition to decreasing intraglomerular hypertension and cellular proliferation. In rats, administration of enalapril prevents the loss of glomerular heparan sulfate that can occur with glomerular disease. Heparan sulfate is a glycosaminoglycan-proteoglycan that contributes to the negative charge of the glomerular capillary wall, which in turn hinders the filtration of negatively charged proteins such as albumin. In humans, administration of ACEI is also thought to attenuate proteinuria by decreasing the size of glomerular capillary endothelial cell pores. Attenuation of proteinuria alone may be renoprotective inasmuch as a correlation between proteinuria and renal functional decline has been observed in humans. In addition, the antiprotein-uric and renal protective effects of ACEI may be associated with improved lipoprotein metabolism. Lipid deposition in the glomerular mesangium can contribute to proteinuria and glomerulosclerosis. In humans with nephrotic-range proteinuria, administration of ACEI not only decreases proteinuria but also reduces plasma concentrations of low-density lipoprotein (LDL)-cholesterol and triglycerides. Based on these promising results, prospective, controlled clinical trials evaluating the effects of enalapril on naturally occurring glomerulonephritis in dogs are underway at this time.

Supportive therapy is important in the management of dogs with glomerulonephritis and should be aimed at de-creasing systemic hypertension, edema, and the tendency for thromboembolism to occur. Sodium-reduced diets should be strongly recommended, and vasodilators may be used as necessary. Enalapril is recommended as the first line of defense against sodium retention and systemic hy-pertension (see pp. 835 and 838). Protein-reduced diets improve the efficacy of ACEI treatment and should be recommended in an attempt to decrease glomerular hyper-filtration and the nonimmunologic progression of glomeru-lar disease. Replacing urine protein loss with supplemental dietary protein is not recommended, as it tends to exacer-bate proteinuria.

Measurement of plasma antithrombin III and fibrinogen concentrations may be helpful in determining which pa-tients should be treated with anticoagulant therapy. Dogs with antithrombin III concentrations less than 70% of nor-mal and fibrinogen concentrations greater than 300 mg/dl are candidates for therapy. Antiplatelet drugs, heparin, and coumadins have been used for anticoagulant therapy. Inas-much as antithrombin III deficiency is marked in some patients with protein-losing nephropathies, coumadin should be more effective than heparin in reducing hyper-coagulability. Warfarin is highly protein-bound, and its dosage must be individualized. An initial dosage of 0.1 mg/lb PO once daily has been recommended. Prothrombin time should be monitored and the dosage of warfarin ad-justed so that prothrombin time is maintained at 1.5 times baseline or the INR is 2.0 to 3.0 (see *CVT XII,* p. 868). Low-dose aspirin is easily administered on an outpatient basis and does not require extensive monitoring, as does coumadin treatment, and therefore is the author's treatment of choice for hypercoagulability. Since fibrin accumulation within the glomerulus can be a consequence of glomerulo-nephritis, anticoagulant treatment may serve a dual pur-pose.

Monitoring the urine protein-to-creatinine ratio is im-portant after any treatment has been initiated. For example, immunosuppressive treatment could alter the antigen-to-antibody ratio and exacerbate the glomerular lesions and proteinuria. In this case, treatment should be changed or discontinued. In addition, the serum creatinine and urea nitrogen concentrations should be monitored in patients with glomerulonephritis. In some volume-dependent dogs, treatment with ACEI can be associated with decreased renal excretory function, which tends to be reversible when treatment is discontinued. Although classically proteinuria occurs before the onset of azotemia, glomerulonephritis can lead to chronic renal insufficiency and failure. As renal failure develops, glomerular filtration decreases and therefore proteinuria usually also decreases.

References and Suggested Reading

Brown SA, Walton C, Crawford P, et al: Long-term effects of antihyper-tensive regimens on renal hemodynamics and proteinuria. Kidney Int 43:1210, 1993.
  A discussion of the benefits of controlling systemic hypertension in patients with glomerular disease.
Center SA, Smith CA, Wilkinson E, et al: Clinicopathologic, renal immu-nofluorescent, and light microscopic features of glomerulonephritis in the dog: 41 cases (1975–1985). J Am Vet Med Assoc 190:81, 1987.
  A retrospective case series of canine glomerulonephritis.
Cook AK, Cowgill LD: Clinical and pathological features of protein-losing glomerular disease in the dog: A review of 137 cases (1985–1992). J Am Anim Hosp Assoc 32:313, 1996.
  A retrospective case series of canine protein-losing nephropathies.
Grauer GF, Culham CA, Dubielzig RR, et al: Effects of a specific thromboxane synthetase inhibitor on development of experimental *Dirofilaria immitis* immune complex glomerulonephritis. J Vet Intern Med 2:192, 1988.
  Description of the effects of a thromboxane synthetase inhibitor on the development of heartworm-induced glomerulonephritis in dogs.
Grauer GF, Culham CA, Dubielzig RR, et al: Experimental *Dirofilaria immitis*–associated glomerulonephritis induced in part by in situ for-mation of immune complexes in the glomerular capillary wall. J Parasitol 75:585, 1989.
  Description of an in situ model of canine glomerulonephritis induced with heartworm antigens.
Grauer GF, Frisbie DD, Snyder PS, et al: Treatment of membranoprolifer-ative glomerulonephritis and nephrotic syndrome in a dog with a thromboxane synthetase inhibitor. J Vet Intern Med 6:77, 1992.
  A case report of canine glomerulonephritis treated with a thromboxane synthetase inhibitor.
Grodecki K, Gaines M, Jacobs R, et al: Ace inhibitor treatment of chronic renal failure in a canine model of hereditary nephritis. Vet Pathol 32:555, 1995.
  Description of the effects of angiotensin-converting enzyme inhibition treatment in dogs with hereditary glomerular disease.
Jaenke RS, Allen TA: Membranous nephropathy in the dog. Vet Pathol 23:718, 1986.
  A retrospective case series of canine membranous glomerulonephritis that focuses on histology.
Longhofer SL, Frisbie DD, Johnson HC, et al: Effects of thromboxane synthetase inhibition on immune complex glomerulonephritis. Am J Vet Res 52:480, 1991.
  Description of the effects of a thromboxane synthetase inhibitor on the development of concanavalin A–induced glomerulonephritis in dogs.

Cutaneous and Renal Glomerulopathy of Greyhound Dogs

Laine A. Cowan
Everett, Washington

Donna M. Hertzke
Marshfield, Wisconsin

Cutaneous and renal glomerular vasculopathy (CRGV) is a syndrome of skin ulceration, edema, and renal dysfunction that was first reported in Greyhounds in 1988 (Carpenter et al, 1988). Because the syndrome was first noted in racing dogs on the Greenetrack in Alabama, the syndrome has been referred to as *Greenetrack disease* or *Alabama rot*. This problem has been observed subsequently in almost every state where Greyhounds race or train. The clinical syndrome is characterized by deep, well-demarcated cutaneous ulcers primarily of the limbs. A small proportion of Greyhounds with cutaneous lesions experience acute renal failure. The true prevalence of CRGV and the frequency of renal failure is unknown.

CLINICAL FINDINGS

Signalment and History

Cutaneous and renal glomerular vasculopathy has been recognized almost exclusively in young adult (0.9 to 5 years of age) racing or training Greyhounds, although a few pet Greyhounds, recently adopted from racing Greyhound kennels, have been affected. Often, multiple dogs from a kennel are affected. Male and female dogs appear to be affected with equal frequency. The majority of Greyhounds appear healthy except for the skin lesions; in the remaining dogs, inappetence, vomiting, or lethargy is observed. Before examination by a veterinarian, Greyhound caretakers often administer various topical and systemic therapies (primarily antimicrobial medications) with no apparent beneficial effect toward the resolution of the cutaneous lesions.

Physical Examination

In the majority of dogs, cutaneous ulcers and pitting edema are the only abnormalities detected on physical examination. Cutaneous, well-demarcated ulcers occur primarily on the limbs, with some involvement of the tail and inguinal regions; the head and mucocutaneous junctions are spared. The number of cutaneous ulcers is variable, ranging from a single lesion to more than 15 on an individual Greyhound, with ulcer diameters ranging from 0.5 to 3.0 cm in most dogs, with a few dogs having extensive ulcerations (up to 25 cm in diameter). Before sloughing of the skin occurs, focal reddened cutaneous areas are apparent. In the minority of dogs, limbs with ulcers also have pitting edema involving the distal two thirds of the limb,

usually in one or two limbs. No other abnormalities are detected on physical examination in most dogs. Occasionally, dogs appear to be systemically ill (lethargy, inappetence), and all these dogs are uremic.

Clinicopathologic Evaluation

In a series of 18 dogs with CRGV (Cowan et al, 1997), all dogs were thrombocytopenic for a variable period (range, 1 day to more than 1 week) while the skin lesions were present. The magnitude of the thrombocytopenia ranged from 6,000 to 165,000 platelets/μl. Assessments of coagulation (prothrombin and activated partial thromboplastin times and fibrinogen and fibrin degradation products) were within reference ranges. Mild to severe anemia (hematocrit 11 to 48%) with evidence of microangiopathic hemolysis was detected in most Greyhounds, and hypoalbuminemia (1.3 to 1.9 g/dl) and proteinuria (urine protein:creatinine ratios of approximately 1.2 to 7.0) were present in many. Mildly increased serum alanine aminotransferase levels (up to three times the upper limit of the reference range) were detected in most dogs.

The prevalence of renal azotemia in Greyhounds with CRGV is unknown, but it likely occurs in a minority of dogs. When renal failure occurs it is acute, the dogs are uremic and, usually, oliguric or anuric. In the few dogs in which it was assessed (Cowan et al, 1997; Hertzke et al, 1995), subclinical renal involvement (decreased glomerular filtration rate or ultrastructural alterations) was present in affected Greyhounds without azotemia. Greyhounds with CRGV and renal failure had lower hematocrits, platelet counts, and serum albumin concentrations; higher serum creatine kinase concentrations and numbers of neutrophils per microliter; and were more likely to have proteinuria than were Greyhounds with CRGV without renal failure.

Progression

In most Greyhounds, no new ulcers form after the initial skin lesions heal. When the skin over joint surfaces is involved, the re-epithelialization over the ulcer bed may be prolonged (weeks). In some dogs, healed lesions remain alopecic. Based on an evaluation of 18 dogs with CRGV (Cowan et al, 1997), there were no clinical or clinicopathologic variables that could be used to predict which dogs would become azotemic. Renal azotemia was not detected, however, without concurrent decreasing platelet numbers or thrombocytopenia.

PATHOLOGIC FINDINGS

Although there are histologic abnormalities in several tissues (Hertzke et al, 1995), the renal lesions are most consistent and helpful in diagnosis. With light microscopy, the cutaneous lesions are characterized by epidermal necrosis, with subcutaneous edema and hemorrhage, and fibrinoid necrosis of arterioles. In the kidney, glomerular lesions predominate, with global necrosis, congestion, and hyalin thrombi in afferent arterioles and glomerular capillaries. Variable, multifocal tubular alterations are present with degeneration and necrosis of the epithelium and medullary congestion. Glomerular ultrastructural changes include endothelial degeneration, necrosis, and loss, followed by platelet adhesion. Gastrointestinal lesions characterized by rare thrombi and hyalinization of submucosal arterioles occur, but rarely.

HYPOTHESIZED PATHOGENESIS

Lesions similar to the microangiopathic lesions in CRGV have been recognized in disseminated intravascular coagulation, hemolytic-uremic syndrome, and thrombotic thrombocytopenic purpura. With normal coagulation profiles, normal fibrinogen and fibrin degradation products, and lesions primarily restricted to the skin and kidney, disseminated intravascular coagulation is considered unlikely. The ultrastructural progression of the lesions, with evidence of denuding of the endothelium and platelet adherence, and microangiopathic hemolytic anemia in CRGV is remarkably similar to that occurring in children with classic hemolytic-uremic syndrome (HUS) (Kaplan and Proesmans, 1987). In affected children, renal vascular endothelial necrosis is a result of bacterial Shiga-like toxin binding to and damaging the cells. In children, outbreaks of HUS have been associated with ingestion of food, primarily undercooked beef products, contaminated with *Escherichia coli* O157-H7 or other Shiga toxin–producing bacteria (Bell et al, 1994).

The pathogenesis of CRGV in Greyhounds is unknown. Although genetic susceptibility may be a factor, environmental factors in racing and training Greyhounds are unique and may be of greater importance. These dogs are fed raw ground beef that has been designated unfit for human consumption. This diet may be a source of exposure to Shiga toxin–producing *E. coli*. Additionally, preliminary studies have identified Shiga toxin receptors in Greyhound kidneys. The combination of potential Shiga toxin exposure, the presence of renal binding sites, the ultrastructural lesions, and the microangiopathic hemolytic anemia suggest the etiology and pathogenesis of CRGV may be similar to that of classic HUS in children.

OTHER EXCLUSIONS FOR CUTANEOUS ULCERS

Trauma, burns, bite wounds, deep pyoderma, drug eruption, immune-mediated vasculitis, erythema multiforme, pemphigus vulgaris, and toxic epidermal necrolysis may cause skin lesions that appear similar to those of CRGV. History, distribution of lesions, and the absence of systemic signs in Greyhounds without renal azotemia should help prioritize these other diagnoses. Biopsy and light micro-scopic evaluation of the lesions may be necessary for a definitive diagnosis.

TREATMENT AND PROGNOSIS

Edema and Cutaneous Ulcers

There is no specific treatment for the skin lesions. Daily cleansing of the affected areas in a whirlpool bath containing dilute povidone-iodine to remove crusts and exudate appears to hasten the healing of the ulcers. Minimization of additional trauma to pressure points by providing padded bedding and bandaging ulcers on the tip of the tail may be beneficial. Because no histologic or culture evidence of bacteria has been detected, antimicrobial therapy is not indicated. The majority of Greyhounds with CRGV and no renal azotemia survive. They may have alopecia over the healed skin lesions. Although the dogs may return to training, their subsequent racing performance is unknown.

Renal Failure

The management of acute renal failure in Greyhounds with CRGV is not unique to this syndrome. Maintenance of sufficient intravascular volume to assure adequate renal perfusion, normalization of plasma electrolytes and acid-base status, and controlling vomiting, if excessive, with an H_2 antagonist or a centrally active antiemetic should be considered. Based on the treatment of a limited number of cases, once renal failure is detected the prognosis is poor with standard supportive therapy. It is unknown if dogs with CRGV and renal failure, supported by hemodialysis or peritoneal dialysis, can recover adequate renal function. Based on the results of treatment in children with hemolytic-uremic syndrome, a disorder with suspected similar pathogenesis of renal damage, hemodialysis or peritoneal dialysis may be beneficial in stabilizing the uremic dogs during acute renal failure.

References and Suggested Reading

Bell BP, Goldoft M, Griffin PM, et al: A multistate outbreak of *Escherichia coli* O157:H7–associated bloody diarrhea and hemolytic uremic syndrome from hamburgers. JAMA 272:1349, 1994.
  A description of a large outbreak of E. coli–associated disease resulting in hemolytic-uremic syndrome in humans.
Carpenter JL, Andelman NC, Moore FM, et al: Idiopathic cutaneous and renal glomerular vasculopathy of greyhounds. Vet Pathol 25:401, 1988.
  A descriptive report of historical and physical examination findings in 160 Greyhounds with CRGV with additional clinicopathologic and pathologic results from a few dogs.
Cowan LA, Hertzke DM, Fenwick BF, et al: Clinical and clinicopathologic abnormalities in Greyhounds with cutaneous and renal glomerular vasculopathy: 18 cases (1992–1994). J Am Vet Med Assoc 210:789, 1997.
  A description of clinical and clinicopathologic abnormalities in Greyhounds with CRGV with comparisons between dogs with renal failure and dogs without the condition.
Hertzke DM, Cowan LA, Schoning P, et al: Glomerular ultrastructural lesions of idiopathic cutaneous and renal glomerular vasculopathy of greyhounds. Vet Pathol 32:451, 1995.
  A description of light microscopic and ultrastructural lesions in 12 Greyhounds with CRGV.
Kaplan BS, Proesmans W: The hemolytic uremic syndrome of childhood and its variants. Semin Hematol 24:148, 1987.
  A review article describing the incidence, epidemiology, clinical manifestations, pathogenesis, and treatment of hemolytic-uremic syndrome in children.

Differentiation of Acute From Chronic Renal Failure

SHELLY L. VADEN

Raleigh, North Carolina

The differentiation of acute renal failure (ARF) from chronic renal failure (CRF) is important for both prognostic and therapeutic reasons. It is more likely that an animal with ARF will recover than will an animal with CRF. Animals with ARF have not had time for the compensatory and adaptive mechanisms of remaining nephrons to become fully operational, whereas in animals with CRF, these mechanisms have most likely have had ample time to develop. Because the condition is potentially reversible, accurate and early identification of ARF is crucial to allow the institution of aggressive treatment, thereby affording the best chance for the animal's survival.

Despite the importance of this differentiation, there is not a "gold standard" that distinguishes ARF from CRF. Certain clinical findings may be useful (Table 1); however, it is often difficult to make the differentiation based on these factors alone. This difficulty is further compounded by the fact that some animals have acute exacerbations of CRF, a condition referred to as acute-on-chronic renal failure. The purpose of this article is to review the clinical findings that can be used to aide in the differentiation of ARF from CRF.

SIGNALMENT

In one study, dogs with ARF were more likely to be intact males and in the non–sporting breed group (American Kennel Club grouping: Boston terriers, bulldogs, Lhasa apsos, Poodles) than were dogs in a normal, reference population; no single age group was overrepresented (Vaden et al, 1997). Intact male dogs may have been at greater risk because they are more likely to wander, a behavior that offers greater exposure to infectious or toxic environmental hazards. There may have been a greater likelihood of dogs in the non–sporting breed group to be managed at a secondary or tertiary care facility, allowing these breeds to be artifactually overrepresented in the study. There are no published clinical studies describing the signalment and clinical findings of ARF in cats.

In a retrospective study of cats with CRF, cats older than 7 years of age were overrepresented and cats younger than 3 years of age were underrepresented in the CRF population when compared with a reference population (DiBartola et al, 1987). A gender difference was not detected and the authors were unable to assess breed representation. Similar data for CRF in dogs are not available.

TABLE 1. Diagnostic Aids for the Differentiation of Acute Renal Failure and Chronic Renal Failure*

	Acute Renal Failure	Chronic Renal Failure	Caveats
History	Ischemic episode Toxicant exposure Nephrotoxic drug use Trauma Acute illness	Long-standing signs of weight loss, polyuria-polydipsia, nocturia, vomiting, diarrhea Prior episodes of illness Prior renal disease-insufficiency	Animals with ARF developing secondary to another disease may have long-standing signs Urine output does not differentiate ARF from CRF
Body condition	Good	Poor	Some animals with ARF have a poor body condition from another disease process Some animals with CRF look fine
Kidneys	Normal to large Smooth contour May be painful	Small Irregular contour	Some chronic renal diseases cause renal enlargement
Osteodystrophy	Absent	Sometimes present	
Packed cell volume	Normal to increased	Decreased (nonregenerative)	Animals with ARF may have nonregenerative anemia
Urine sediment	May be active	Often inactive	Many animals with ARF have inactive urine sediments
Serum creatinine	Recently within reference range	Previously increased	Previous prerenal and postrenal factors could also have caused increase
Serum potassium	Normal to increased	Normal to decreased	Urine output is a major determinant of serum potassium concentrations
Metabolic acidosis	More severe	Less severe	
Histopathologic features	Acute tubular necrosis Acute inflammation	Interstitial fibrosis Glomerulosclerosis Chronic inflammation	Chronic renal lesions can be an incidental finding
Carbamoylated hemoglobin	Normal to mild increase	Increased	

*The clinician should be aware that there are many caveats to using these aids.
ARF, acute renal failure; CRF, chronic renal failure.

When a young animal presents in renal failure, it is more likely to have ARF than CRF. The exceptions are animals known to be predisposed to familial nephropathies.

HISTORY

Certain historical information may be helpful in the diagnosis of ARF versus CRF. Prolonged duration of decreased appetite, vomiting, diarrhea, weight loss, or a combination of these states, is more consistent with a diagnosis of CRF. However, because ARF often develops secondary to another disease process, some animals with ARF may appear to have a more protracted clinical course. An example is a dog with lymphosarcoma that acquires ARF secondary to hypercalcemia.

Urine output cannot be used to differentiate ARF from CRF. Oliguria and anuria are more commonly associated with ARF but can occur terminally in CRF or during acute exacerbations of CRF. Furthermore, nonoliguric ARF, in which an oliguric phase is never recognized, may be more common in dogs and cats than it was once thought to be. Polyuria-polydipsia and nocturia are cardinal signs of CRF but may occur during the recovery phase of ARF. A long-standing history of polyuria-polydipsia or nocturia, or both, is, however, supportive of CRF.

There are risk factors or pre-existing conditions, or both, that may predispose an animal to ARF (Table 2). If present, these factors corroborate a diagnosis of ARF. In a retrospective study of 99 dogs with ARF, ischemic events were the most commonly identified disorders associated with the development of ARF, followed by nephrotoxicant-toxin exposure (Vaden et al, 1997). The most commonly identified disorders that may have caused ARF or predisposed these dogs to ARF were pancreatitis, ethylene glycol inges-

tion, disseminated intravascular coagulation, sepsis, hypovolemic-hypotensive shock, liver failure, and decreased cardiac output. Nephrotoxicant exposure and advanced age were the most common inciting causes identified in a retrospective study of hospital-acquired ARF in 29 dogs (Behrend et al, 1996).

PHYSICAL EXAMINATION FINDINGS

Clinical signs (e.g., depression, gastrointestinal ulceration) may be more severe in animals with ARF than in those with CRF for any given magnitude of azotemia. Thinness, poor coat quality, and pallor are more common in animals with CRF. In general, animals with CRF may have small, firm, and irregularly shaped kidneys bilaterally, whereas animals with ARF may have normal to enlarged, smooth, and possibly painful kidneys bilaterally. However, several diseases associated with CRF may lead to enlarged kidneys (e.g., hydronephrosis, renal cysts, renal neoplasia, glomerulonephritis, amyloidosis). Overt signs of renal osteodystrophy ("rubber jaw," pathologic fractures) occur uncommonly in animals with CRF but not at all in animals with ARF.

CLINICOPATHOLOGIC FINDINGS

Perhaps the strongest supportive evidence for a diagnosis of ARF is knowing that serum creatinine concentrations were within the normal reference range in the weeks preceding the onset of renal failure. Likewise, serum creatinine concentrations returning to the reference range after treatment of renal failure is supportive of a diagnosis of ARF. The time needed to recover from ARF and return to a nonazotemic state can vary, taking up to 60 days in one study.

The presence of nonregenerative anemia has long been accepted as an indicator of CRF; however, nonregenerative anemia also can occur in patients with ARF. In one study, 32% of dogs with ARF were anemic (Vaden et al, 1997). Mild to moderate anemia was present at diagnosis or developed during hospitalization in 95% of humans with ARF (Hales et al, 1994). Suggested mechanisms for the development of the anemia included shortened red blood cell survival, mild hemolysis, external blood loss, and decreased red blood cell production.

Classically, hyperkalemia or normokalemia is said to occur in patients with ARF, whereas hypokalemia or normokalemia is said to occur in patients with CRF. Because the urine flow rate is a major determinant of serum potassium concentration, an animal presenting with polyuric ARF may be hypokalemic, whereas an animal with anuric CRF may be hyperkalemic.

Animals with ARF may have a more active urine sediment when compared with animals with CRF. However, lack of an active urine sediment does not preclude a diagnosis of ARF. Detection of a large number of urinary casts is indicative of an active disease process, but casts are shed into the urine intermittently. Urinary casts were detected in only 31% of dogs with ARF, and of those dogs, 80% had fewer than 5 casts per low-power field (Vaden et al, 1997). Animals with CRF also shed casts into the urine, although

---

TABLE 2. Partial List of Common Risk Factors or Conditions That May Predispose an Animal to Acute Renal Failure

Pre-existing renal disease
Advanced age
Ischemic event
    Pancreatitis
    Hypovolemic-hypotensive shock
    Sepsis
    Decreased cardiac output
    Liver failure
    Deep anesthesia
    Disseminated intravascular coagulopathy, renal
      vascular thrombosis
    Trauma
Nephrotoxicant exposure
    Ethylene glycol
    Aminoglycoside
    Hypercalcemia
    Cisplatin
    Thiacetarsamide
    Amphotericin-B
    Nonsteroidal anti-inflammatory drugs
    Tetracycline (use of outdated or deteriorated product)
Miscellaneous
    Hypokalemia
    Acidosis
    Leptospirosis
    Pyelonephritis

presumably in fewer numbers. Glucosuria with euglycemia is an expected finding in animals with proximal tubular defects. It was found in 23% of dogs with ARF (Vaden et al, 1997) but also would be expected with some forms of chronic renal disease–CRF (e.g., familial Fanconi syndrome). Likewise, proteinuria may occur in dogs with ARF or CRF. Proteinuria was detected in 66% of dogs with ARF, although in most cases the magnitude of proteinuria was mild (Vaden et al, 1997). Because acute glomerular diseases are uncommon in veterinary medicine, finding heavy proteinuria is supportive of CRF.

RADIOGRAPHIC AND ULTRASONOGRAPHIC FINDINGS

Survey radiographs may assist in the differentiation of ARF and CRF by providing information about kidney size and shape. Radiographic evidence of renal osteodystrophy, supportive of CRF, includes skeletal decalcification and soft tissue calcification (kidneys, stomach). Renal ultrasonography can be used to characterize renal size and shape further and also provides information about the renal parenchyma. Increased overall renal echogenicity and decreased corticomedullary distinction can be seen with, but are not diagnostic for, CRF. Dogs with ethylene glycol–induced ARF have bright renal cortices.

RENAL HISTOPATHOLOGIC FINDINGS

Renal biopsy may be required to differentiate ARF from CRF. Acute tubular necrosis, sometimes with regeneration, or acute inflammation, or both, is supportive of the diagnosis of ARF. Extensive tubular atrophy, calcification of basement membranes, interstitial fibrosis, and chronic inflammation or glomerulosclerosis, or both, are supportive of the diagnosis of CRF. Pre-existing renal disease is a risk factor for the development of ARF, and animals can have evidence of chronic renal pathology yet have an acute onset of renal failure.

CARBAMOYLATED HEMOGLOBIN

Urea exists in equilibrium with cyanate when in solution. Isocyanate, the reactive form of cyanate, irreversibly combines with the terminal valine group of both alpha- and beta-hemoglobin (Hb) chains to form carbamoylated hemoglobin (CarHb). The degree of carbamoylation is determined by measuring the amount of valine hydantoin that is formed by acid hydrolysis of Hb. The CarHb content appears to accumulate throughout the life span of the erythrocyte. Carbamoylated hemoglobin has been shown to aid in the differentiation of ARF from CRF in humans. In humans with stable CRF, CarHb concentrations correlate with the time-averaged urea concentration during the previous 2- to 3-month period. Carbamoylated Hb concentrations were significantly higher in dogs with CRF than in dogs with ARF. Using a cutoff value of 100 μg valine hydantoin/gm Hb, the sensitivity and specificity of CarHb for differentiating ARF from CRF was 96.1% and 84.2%, respectively. The time required to reach steady-state CarHb concentrations in dogs has not been determined.

TOENAIL CREATININE CONCENTRATIONS

Measurable amounts of creatinine are present in human toenails and canine claws. Fingernail creatinine is significantly higher in humans with CRF than in those with ARF; the latter group does not differ from normal. Increased toenail creatinine may reflect serum creatinine values several months previously and result from elevated serum creatinine concentrations during nail formation. In fact, there is a time delay between alterations in serum creatinine concentrations and subsequent changes in nail creatinine (Bergamo et al, 1993). Therefore, fingernail creatinine might be used to identify a recent onset of azotemia; however, similar studies have not been reported in dogs and cats.

References and Suggested Reading

Behrend EN, Grauer GF, Mani I, et al: Hospital-acquired acute renal failure in dogs: 29 cases (1983–1992). J Am Vet Med Assoc 208:537, 1996.
This article describes clinical findings in 29 dogs that developed ARF while hospitalized.

Bergamo RR, Laidlaw SA, Kopple JD: Fingernail creatinine as a predictor of prior renal function. Am J Kidney Dis 22:814, 1993.
This reference discusses the method used to extract creatinine from toenails.

DiBartola SP, Rutgers HC, Zack PM, et al: Clinicopathologic findings associated with chronic renal disease in cats: 74 cases (1973–1984). J Am Vet Med Assoc 190:1196, 1987.
This article describes clinical findings in 74 cats with CRF.

Hales M, Solez K, Kjellstrand C: The anemia of acute renal failure: Association with oliguria and elevated blood urea. Renal Failure 16:125, 1994.
This article describes a clinical study of anemia in humans with ARF.

Vaden SL, Levine J, Breitschwerdt EB: A retrospective case-control study of acute renal failure in 99 dogs. J Vet Intern Med 11:58, 1997.
This article describes clinical findings in 99 dogs with ARF.

CVT Update: Peritoneal Dialysis

LISA ANN DZYBAN
San Carlos, California

MARY ANNA LABATO
LINDA A. ROSS
North Grafton, Massachusetts

Peritoneal dialysis is a process that therapeutically removes toxic solutes from body fluids and normalizes endogenous solutes whose aberrant concentrations disrupt normal physiology. In this process, an electrolyte solution is infused into the abdominal cavity, where it equilibrates with plasma by osmosis across the peritoneal membrane. The solution is then drained from the abdomen, removing excess solutes and water. This process is repeated as needed, depending on factors such as resolution of uremic symptoms, normalization of hydration, electrolyte and acid-base status, or removal of a toxin from the body.

Peritoneal dialysis has been used to treat acute renal failure in humans since 1923. Today, peritoneal dialysis is used in humans to manage both acute and chronic renal failure, as well as to remove dialyzable toxins (e.g., ethylene glycol, ethanol, barbiturates), to reduce severe metabolic disturbances (e.g., hypercalcemia, hyperkalemia, hepatic encephalopathy), and to treat peritonitis, pancreatitis, uroabdomen, hypothermia, hyperthermia, and fluid overload secondary to heart failure.

In veterinary medicine, acute renal failure is the prevailing indication for dialysis. The specific application of peritoneal dialysis has been previously described (see *CVT XI*, p 865). There is, however, a tendency for veterinarians to consider peritoneal dialysis a "heroic" technique and to use it only in animals with a grave prognosis. This perception of peritoneal dialysis has been partly due to the complications that can occur with this technique. Recent advances in the technique and equipment for peritoneal dialysis may make two common complications, catheter failure and hypoalbuminemia, less problematic in the future.

NEW CATHETER DESIGN

One of the most common causes of catheter failure in small animal medicine is catheter obstruction by omentum, resulting in failure of dialysate to drain from the abdomen. This was a consistent problem with coiled, Tenckhoff, and straight silicone catheters used for short-term dialysis. Longer dialysis (greater than 3 days) was best conducted with a surgically implanted column disc catheter (Lifecath and Vetcath, Quinton Instruments) combined with a full or partial omentectomy. However, this catheter has recently been discontinued, and currently there are no manufacturers of the column disc–style catheter.

An alternative catheter style called the fluted-T (Ash Advantage Peritoneal Catheter, Medigroup, Aurora, IL) (Fig. 1) has shown good results in dogs. In one study, 17 dogs had fluted-T catheters placed by peritoneoscope and were dialyzed with 2 L of fluid/day. Only four catheters had outflow failure; these failures occurred 7 to 18 days after catheter placement. The remaining catheters functioned for the entire study period of 60 days, at which time they were removed by peritoneoscopy. In the same study, Tenckhoff catheters in the dogs were obstructed by omentum 2 to 4 days after placement.

The fluted-T catheter is currently available for veterinary use (see Fig. 1). The flutes are designed to offer minimal resistance to influx and outflux of fluid while preventing omental adhesions. This catheter is made of silicone and

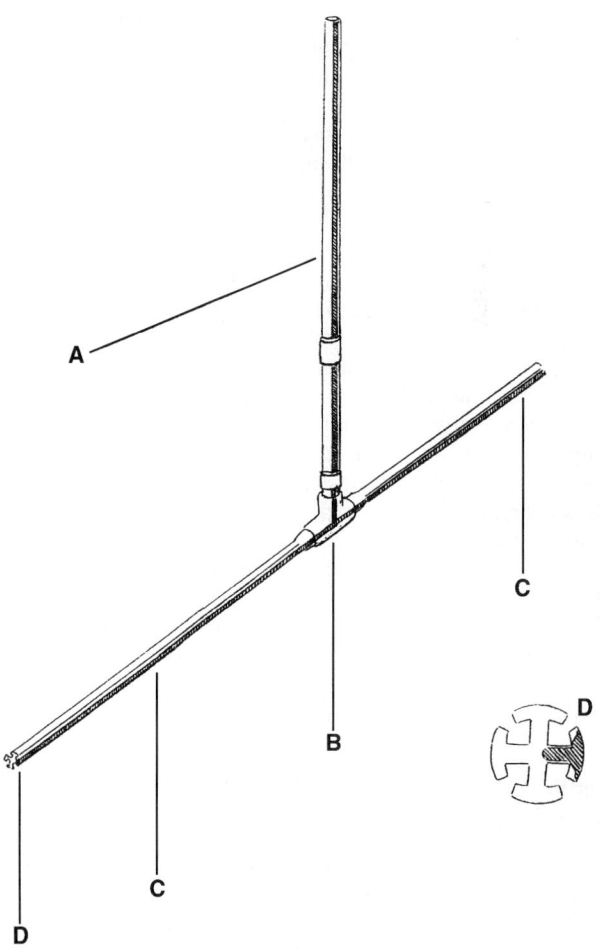

Figure 1. Fluted-T peritoneal dialysis catheter. A, transabdominal tube; B, transition tube; C, intraperitoneal fluted sections; D, cross-section view of flutes/slots. (Ash Advantage Peritoneal Catheter, Copyright © Medigroup Inc., Aurora, IL [800 323-5389].)

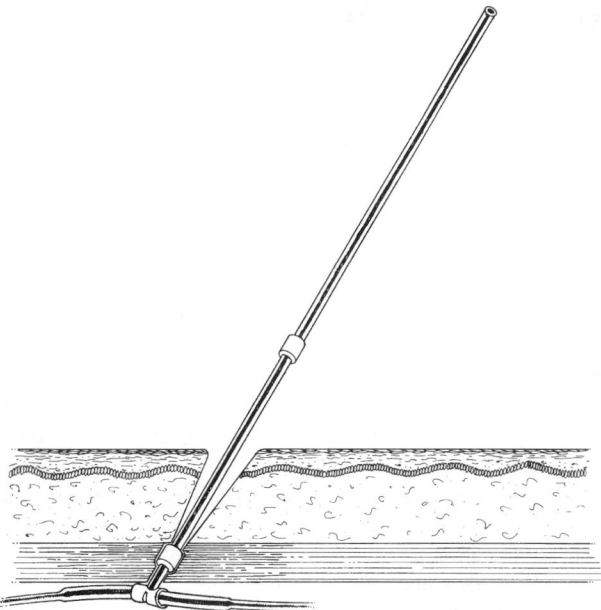

Figure 2. Insertion of the fluted-T catheter through the abdominal wall. The short arm of the "T" folds to allow catheter placement by laproscope. (Copyright © Medigroup Inc., Aurora, IL [800 323-5389].)

has two Dacron cuffs. When the cuffs are implanted in the rectus muscle and subcutaneous layers, the ingrowth of fibroblasts anchors the catheter into position. The T junction of the catheter is to be placed against the parietal peritoneum and oriented in a cranial-to-caudal plane. The catheter is flexible and designed to fold at the crosspiece temporarily to facilitate placement by peritoneoscope or laparoscope (Fig. 2). The fluted aspect of the adult catheter is 30 cm in length, but it can be cut to a shorter length for small patients. In humans, it is placed in a paramedian location, with the long aspect directed toward the inguinal ring. A subcutaneous tunnel is directed either laterally or inferiorly for the placement of the superficial cuff and the exit site of the catheter.

An alternative to the fluted-T catheter is the fluted Blake surgical drain (Johnson & Johnson, Arlington, TX). Although not specifically designed for peritoneal dialysis, the Blake drain would be expected to function in a manner similar to the fluted-T catheter and has been used for peritoneal dialysis in human infants (Ash and Janle, 1993). Neither the fluted-T peritoneal dialysis catheter nor the Blake surgical drain has yet to undergo published clinical trials in veterinary patients. However, the use of the fluted-T catheter in a canine model showed promising results and warrants further investigation.

NEW TECHNIQUE IN NUTRITIONAL SUPPORT

Hypoalbuminemia is a common complication of peritoneal dialysis because of low dietary protein intake, gastrointestinal or renal protein loss, loss in dialysate fluid, uremic catabolism, and concurrent diseases. Usually, the animal can maintain normal serum protein levels if nutritional intake is adequate (2.0 gm/kg per day of protein in the dog). However, anorexia and vomiting are common

with uremia, and adequate enteral nutrition may be difficult to maintain. Therefore, supportive measures to maintain positive nitrogen balance often must be used. Nutritional support includes feeding tubes, partial parenteral or total parenteral nutrition (see sections 1 and 2 of this volume), and a new technique of peritoneal dialysis using 1.1% amino acid solutions.

Amino acid dialysate solutions have been described in the research literature for more than 25 years. However, the results of clinical studies varied with regard to efficacy. Recently, controlled clinical studies in peritoneal dialysis in humans have provided convincing evidence to support the therapeutic role of amino acid dialysate in some patients. These solutions are currently approved for use in human patients in Europe, and approval by the Food and Drug Administration is currently pending in the United States (Baxter, McGraw Park, IL). Amino acid dialysate solutions use amino acids as the osmotic agent instead of the dextrose of standard dialysate solutions. A 1.1% amino acid solution has an osmolarity of 365 mOsm, similar to a 1.5% dextrose solution. Seventy to 90% of the amino acids are absorbed, depending on the dwelling time in the abdomen and the characteristics of the patient's peritoneal membrane. Therefore, a 2-L bag of a 1.1% amino acid solution would provide about 14 gm of amino acids to the body for protein metabolism (Jones, 1995).

The patient expected to benefit from this technique would be in negative nitrogen balance and not receiving adequate protein by enteral routes. One study of humans undergoing one to two dialysis exchanges per day with the amino acid solution (in addition to standard dialysis) showed that their nitrogen balance became strongly positive within 5 days and remained positive for the duration of time that they received the amino acid exchanges. Plasma amino acid levels increased within 10 days, and average total protein levels rose from 5.97 to 6.27 within 20 days. Overall, the treatment was well tolerated. Nausea and vomiting were reported in one patient; this patient proceeded to do well when the number of amino acid exchanges was reduced from two to one per day (Kopple et al, 1995). There is little beneficial effect of amino acid solution dialysis if the patient is not receiving adequate caloric intake, presumably because the amino acids are metabolized as an energy source. Therefore, it is recommended that the amino acid exchange be performed postprandially when carbohydrates and lipids are concurrently available to the body.

The major limitation of amino acids as osmotic agents is that they generate nitrogenous waste, and therefore the amount that can be administered to a patient in renal failure is limited. The ideal amount of amino acid dialysate would be that which would, in combination with enteral and parenteral nutrition, provide adequate daily protein intake without causing a significant rise in blood urea nitrogen or metabolic acidosis.

The use of amino acid dialysis is still under investigation. The unique protein requirements of each species mandate further studies. Current formulations for amino acid dialysate do not include taurine, an essential amino acid for cats; it would probably have to be supplemented in feline patients. Amino acid dialysis as a supportive nutritional technique is currently promising for both dialysis and nondialysis patients. It would be less costly than intravenous nutritional support and would result in less water load than elemental diets used for enteral tube feeding.

References and Suggested Reading

Ash SR, Janle EM: T-fluted peritoneal dialysis catheter. Adv Perit Dial 9:223, 1993.
   Description of the T-fluted catheter and a brief discussion of a pilot study using the catheter in 20 dogs for 7 to 60 days.
Cowgill LD: Application of peritoneal dialysis and hemodialysis in the management of renal failure. In: Osborne CA, ed: Canine and Feline Nephrology and Urology. Philadelphia: Lea & Febiger, 1995, p 573.
   A good overview of the application of peritoneal and hemodialysis in small animals.
Jones MR: Intraperitoneal amino acids: A therapy whose time has come? Perit Dial Int 15(Suppl):S67, 1995.
   A review article on the history, physiology, and clinical experience of amino acid intraperitoneal nutrition in human patients undergoing chronic ambulatory peritoneal dialysis.
Kopple JD, Bernard D, Messana J, et al: Treatment of malnourished CAPD patients with an amino acid based dialysate. Kidney Int 47:1148, 1995.
   A clinical study comparing a 15-day baseline metabolic balance of 19 human patients undergoing chronic ambulatory peritoneal dialysis to their metabolic balance while receiving an amino acid dialysate solution for 20 days.

Recent Developments in the Management of Progressive Renal Failure

Delmar R. Finco
Scott A. Brown
Jeanne A. Barsanti
Joseph W. Bartges

Athens, Georgia

Chronic renal failure is an irreversible condition characterized by the progressive loss of renal function and the eventual development of terminal uremia. In humans, dialysis and renal transplantation are used routinely to prevent death from uremia. However, great emphasis is placed on conservative management of renal failure before intervention because of the limited number of human kidneys available for transplantation and because of the cost of dialysis and transplantation procedures.

Dialysis and renal transplantation are emerging as modes of therapy for dogs and cats with renal failure, but economics dictate that treatment of most patients will be limited to conservative medical management. The objective of conservative management is to prolong life for the pet and maintain relative comfort without undue economic or husbandry obligations for the owner.

More recent developments in managing progressive renal failure suggest that the efficacy of some treatments previously employed were not substantiated during controlled laboratory studies. Other traditional aspects of therapy appear to warrant more emphasis, and several new approaches to therapy are under development.

DIETARY CONSIDERATIONS

Protein

Restriction of dietary protein has been advocated for patients in renal failure for two distinctly different reasons. Once azotemia occurs, signs of uremia may be ameliorated by dietary restriction of protein, presumably because some products of protein catabolism have extrarenal toxicity. There is general agreement among veterinary nephrologists that this is a valid reason for restricting dietary protein, but the level of azotemia at which restriction should be implemented is debatable. Most veterinary nephrologists believe that protein restriction for this purpose should be implemented when the blood urea nitrogen level exceeds 75 mg/dl.

The other justification for protein restriction is based on the theory that dietary protein restriction has benefits specifically on the kidneys. In male rats of certain susceptible strains, renal lesions develop spontaneously as the rats mature. The rate of development of renal lesions is accelerated by reduction of renal mass (remnant kidney model). Restriction of dietary protein intake in remnant kidney rats slows the progression of renal lesions. These observations led to the conclusion that reduction of renal mass leads to self-perpetuating renal lesions and that protein restriction slows the progression.

Reduction of renal mass in dogs also leads to the progressive development of renal lesions and deterioration of renal function, but restriction of protein intake does not alter the development of renal lesions nor does it preserve renal function. Lack of beneficial effects of protein restriction has been documented both in young dogs with marked reduction in renal mass (Finco et al, 1992; Polzin et al, 1993) and in old dogs with uninephrectomy (Finco et al, 1994).

Considering these findings, the authors do not recommend reduction of dietary protein in dogs with renal disease or reduced renal function in order to achieve renoprotective effects. Once moderate azotemia develops (blood urea nitrogen level >75 mg/dl), protein restriction should be employed for extrarenal benefits.

Phosphorus

Studies in azotemic dogs with reduced renal mass have indicated that dietary restriction of phosphorus has several beneficial effects (extrarenal in nature) that result in an increased duration of survival (Finco et al, 1992). These studies clearly indicate that phosphorus restriction is required once chronic renal failure has progressed to the point of azotemia. Potential benefits from phosphorus restriction have not been assessed in either cats or dogs before the onset of azotemia.

Considering that foods low in protein content are usually also low in phosphorus content, both protein restriction and a degree of phosphorus restriction can be achieved using commercial foods prepared for dogs and cats with renal failure. Unfortunately, the degree of phosphorus restriction in these diets is not adequate to maintain normal phosphorus homeostasis. For this reason, phosphate binders should be used as an adjuvant to dietary phosphorus restriction (see subsequent discussion).

Lipids

Some changes in plasma lipid profiles are observed in dogs with chronic renal failure, but the relevance of these changes to the progression of renal disease remains unclear. A recent study in dogs with induced chronic renal failure compared the addition of three sources of lipids to a standard, fat-free diet (Brown et al, 1998). The addition of omega-6 unsaturated fatty acids (safflower oil) was associated with more severe renal lesions than with the addition of saturated fatty acids (white fat), whereas the addition of omega-3 fatty acids (menhaden fish oil) was associated with milder renal lesions when compared with saturated fatty acids. The extremes in fatty acid composition by these additions are unlikely to be experienced with commercially available diets. However, the results suggest that dietary lipid intake may be important in the progression of renal damage in dogs and suggest that further research in this area may be fruitful. Products currently available with modified omega-3/omega-6 ratios have not been tested under controlled conditions to determine whether they are effective.

Calories

Several studies in rats and one study in cats suggest that caloric restriction may be beneficial in slowing the progression of renal failure. Conversely, a sustained lack of food intake could cause protein malnutrition and endogenous protein catabolism and acidosis in addition to caloric deficit. From data available at present, it is doubtful that purposeful restriction of caloric intake is advisable in dogs and cats with chronic renal failure. Since many of the diets formulated for dogs and cats with chronic renal failure are somewhat unpalatable, the question arises as to whether the patient is better served by reduced intake of "renal" diets or by adequate intake of "nonrenal" diets. Data are not currently available to resolve this issue, but the authors believe that adequate food intake, even if not protein- or phosphorus-restricted, is preferable to the potential for negative protein balance and suboptimal caloric intake that may be associated with unpalatable diets.

CALCITRIOL THERAPY

Calcitriol (1,25-dihydroxycholecalciferol) concentrations in blood may be decreased during chronic renal failure because of the role of the normal kidneys in hydroxylation of 25-hydroxycholecalciferol. Calcitriol plays an important role in normal animals in several biologic processes, including bone metabolism. Calcitriol also is known to cause a calcium-independent suppression of parathyroid hormone (PTH) secretion. Some evidence has accumulated that PTH has adverse effects on several body systems, including the kidneys. Administration of calcitriol to dogs and cats with chronic renal failure has been advocated to prevent the multiple-system toxicity attributed to PTH (Nogade et al, 1996).

In research on dogs with induced chronic renal disease, the authors eliminated PTH by performing parathyroidectomy. A group of these dogs was then compared with dogs that had intact parathyroid glands but had the same decrement of renal dysfunction. As expected, the dogs that underwent parathyroidectomy had undetectable plasma concentrations of PTH, whereas the other group had marked elevations of plasma PTH levels. After a study period of 2 years, the authors found no benefit to any body system attributable to parathyroidectomy except for higher bone mineral density in the dogs that underwent parathyroidectomy (Finco et al, 1997).

In other studies on dogs with induced chronic renal failure, the authors found that calcitriol was not consistently effective in suppressing plasma PTH concentration and that the margin between a suppressive dose and a dose that caused hypercalcemia was narrow. Results of these studies indicate that the risk of calcitriol use in chronic renal failure in dogs outweighs any potential benefits, and the authors do not recommend its use in either dogs or cats for this purpose.

PHOSPHATE BINDERS

Based on the authors' studies of dietary phosphorus restriction and the effects of PTH, we propose that dietary phosphorus has direct deleterious effects on dogs with renal failure rather than these effects being mediated via PTH. Lack of normalization of phosphorus homeostasis with "renal" diets necessitates further therapy with intestinal phosphorus binders. Comprehensive controlled studies are lacking on the efficacy and adverse effects of phosphate binders in dogs and cats. Aluminum salts have been used in humans but have been largely discontinued because of the deposition of aluminum in bone, worsening renal osteodystrophy. The authors administered an aluminum carbonate gel (240 mg/kg per day Al(OH)$_3$ equivalent) to dogs with mild induced renal failure for 2 months and subsequently analyzed tissues for aluminum. The authors were unable to demonstrate aluminum deposition in tissues, suggesting that short-term use of aluminum products may be acceptable.

Calcium salts have been advocated as phosphate binders to circumvent the toxicity of aluminum. However, lesser efficacy and potential toxicity from hypercalcemia have been cited as disadvantages of their use. The authors tentatively recommend initial use of aluminum salts for intestinal binding of phosphate for dogs and cats, with the goal of reducing the plasma phosphate concentration to the upper limit of the reference range. The dose of binder required to achieve this control must be determined in each animal individually. Consideration should be given to the use of calcium salts for phosphate binding if therapy is carried beyond 2 months. The authors have used up to 1.0 gm of calcium carbonate ($CaCO_3$) per kg body weight per day, but animals should be monitored for development of hypercalcemia, which occasionally develops.

ANGIOTENSIN-CONVERTING ENZYME INHIBITORS

Angiotensin is a potent systemic vasoconstrictor that has intrarenal effects apart from its vasoactive properties. An intrarenal system for generation of angiotensin exists, and intrarenal effects of angiotensin on the generation of growth factors and on salt balance have been shown. In some studies of human patients with renal failure from a variety of causes, administration of angiotensin-converting enzyme (ACE) inhibitors has been associated with a reduction in the degree of proteinuria and a slowing in the progression of renal failure. In rats with reduced renal mass, the same effects have been documented for ACE inhibitors but not for other antihypertensive agents, seemingly pointing to a renal effect apart from the effects of ACE inhibitors on systemic hypertension.

ACE inhibitors were found superior to calcium channel blockers for renoprotective effects in dogs with induced diabetes mellitus and seemed to reduce proteinuria and slow the development of lesions in dogs with reduced renal mass (Brown et al, 1993). Controlled clinical trials to determine if ACE inhibitors are of benefit in chronic renal disease in dogs and cats have not been reported, although some trials are ongoing. Although available information on the use of ACE inhibitors is encouraging, pharmaceutical companies that market ACE inhibitors have not yet sought approval from the Food and Drug Administration for labeling to allow their use to slow the progression of renal failure.

ENDOTHELIN INHIBITORS

Endothelin is a vasoconstrictor that is more potent than angiotensin, and the vasculature of the kidney is particularly vulnerable to its actions. Endothelin is generated by vascular endothelium throughout the body and also by renal tubular cells. In addition to a potential role in the control of systemic blood pressure, endothelin has some effects on the renal excretion of water and electrolytes.

Studies in rats with reduced renal mass, in mice with lupus nephritis, and in rats with induced diabetes or amino-glycoside nephrosis indicate beneficial effects from an oral endothelin inhibitor. Studies have not been reported on the effects of endothelin inhibitors on induced or naturally occurring renal diseases of dogs or cats.

SYSTEMIC HYPERTENSION

Systemic hypertension has been reported as a relatively frequent occurrence in dogs and cats with chronic renal failure, although limitations of common indirect measurement procedures should lead to caution in making this diagnosis (see article on diagnosis of hypertension of dogs and cats, in this section).

The relationship between hypertension as a cause versus an effect of chronic renal disease remains poorly defined, but marked hypertension warrants correction because of extrarenal adverse effects. Since chronic renal failure is not invariably associated with hypertension, each patient must be evaluated as an individual at intervals during management. Routine use of antihypertensive agents without reliable measurements of blood pressure are unwarranted and potentially dangerous. If measurement of blood pressure by indirect means indicates the presence of hypertension, appropriate therapy should be initiated (see article on treatment of systemic hypertension in dogs and cats, in this section).

ACID-BASE STATUS

Anecdotal evidence, as well as controlled case studies, provides a strong basis for a major role for metabolic acidosis as a factor in management of patients with renal failure. Studies on the effects of acidosis on the progression of renal lesions have not indicated an adverse effect in cats (Polzin et al, 1998); studies have not been reported in dogs. However, acidosis in several species is associated with extrarenal effects, including protein catabolism, anorexia, and precipitation of a uremic crisis.

Canine and feline patients with chronic renal failure should be monitored at regular intervals for acid-base status (plasma bicarbonate or TCO_2 determination) and acidosis should be suspected if anorexia occurs. Oral treatment with sodium bicarbonate or potassium citrate is indicated to keep plasma bicarbonate within reference range.

References and Suggested Reading

Brown SA, Brown CA, Crowell WA, et al: Effects of dietary fatty acid composition on the course of chronic renal disease in dogs. J Lab Clin Med 131:447, 1998.
Data demonstrating adverse and protective renal effects from diets with extreme variation in fatty acid composition.
Brown SA, Walton CL, Crawford P, et al: Long-term effects of antihypertensive regimens on renal hemodynamics and proteinuria. Kidney Int 43:1210, 1993.
Experimental data from dogs with induced diabetes mellitus, demonstrating the advantage of ACE inhibitors in ameliorating the progression of renal lesions.
Finco DR, Brown SA, Crowell WA, et al: Effects of dietary phosphorus and protein in dogs with chronic renal failure. Am J Vet Res 53:2264, 1992.
Experimental data indicating that phosphorus, but not protein, affected survival and renal function.
Finco DR, Brown SA, Crowell WA, et al: Effects of aging and dietary

protein intake on uninephrectomized geriatric dogs. Am J Vet Res 55:1282, 1994.
Data demonstrating that geriatric dogs fed a high-protein diet for 4 years did not have adverse renal effects.
Finco DR, Brown SA, Crowell WA, et al: Effects of parathyroidectomy on induced renal failure in dogs. Am J Vet Res 58:188, 1997.
Experimental data indicating that PTH is not a toxin in uremia but that mineral imbalances are the primary problem.
Nogade LA, Chew DJ, Podell M: Benefits of calcitriol therapy and serum phosphorus control in dogs and cats with chronic renal failure. Vet Clin North Am 26:1293, 1996.
Data supporting the use of calcitriol in the treatment of dogs with chronic renal failure.
Polzin DJ, Osborne CA, O'Brien TD, et al: Effects of protein intake on progression of canine chronic renal failure (CRF). Proceedings of the 11th annual Veterinary Medicine Forum, 1993, p 938.
Experimental data indicating that protein intake did not affect the generation of renal lesions in dogs with induced renal failure.
Polzin DJ, et al: Personal communication, 1998.
Changes in glomerular filtration rate in cats with induced renal failure fed acidifying diets.

Gastrointestinal Complications of Uremia

RHONDA L. SCHULMAN
DONALD R. KRAWIEC
Urbana, Illinois

The gastrointestinal tract is commonly affected in renal failure, leading to signs of anorexia, nausea, vomiting, weight loss, diarrhea, constipation, stomatitis, and uriniferous breath. These signs reflect both direct effects on the gastrointestinal tract and interactions among other organ systems. Gastrointestinal disturbances are often the signs that most concern the owner and may be the reason the pet is presented to a veterinarian. The dramatic nature of gastrointestinal tract disturbances strongly affects an owner's perception of the pet's quality of life.

ANOREXIA

Anorexia occurs for a variety of reasons (Table 1). Veterinarians or owners may want to blame unpalatable restricted protein and salt diets. However, given the number of animals who first present to veterinarians with a complaint of anorexia, dietary restrictions are only one of the potential reasons for a pet's refusal to eat (Polzin et al, 1995). Human patients with chronic renal failure (CRF) report nausea that waxes and wanes throughout the day but is often worse in the morning (Valenzuela, 1983). Many veterinary patients will eat small meals at various times of day, indicating a similar problem.

WEIGHT LOSS

Weight loss may be caused by physiologic abnormalities as well as an anorexia-induced inadequate caloric intake. CRF can result in a metabolic acidosis resulting from either inadequate excretion of acid or impaired reabsorption of bicarbonate. Metabolic acidosis promotes a state of protein malnutrition by increasing the rate of protein catabolism (Bergstrom, 1995). This proteolysis is in addition to the impaired insulin-stimulated protein synthesis found in uremic patients (Polzin et al, 1995). Weight loss may also reflect a low-grade malabsorptive syndrome resulting from gastroenteritis. Other potential causes of weight loss include the still vaguely defined "uremic toxins," especially the guanidine compounds (Chew and DiBartola, 1989).

VOMITING

Vomiting is a frequent complaint in renal failure. Many factors lead to vomiting, including hypokalemia and acidosis. Uremic gastroenteritis (discussed further on) can cause vomiting and possibly hematemesis. Mucosal irritability resulting from hyperacidity is one component of the gastroenteritis. Vomiting also results from the effects of uremic toxins on the chemoreceptor trigger zone.

STOMATITIS

One of the hallmark clinical signs of renal failure is stomatitis. Azotemia results in the increased excretion of urea into the oral cavity. Bacterial ureases degrade urea into ammonia, which causes the stomatitis (Krawiec, 1996). Oral ulcerations, when present, are typically seen on the buccal mucosa and the tongue. The tongue may have a brownish discoloration, or the anterior portion may be necrotic and slough as the result of fibrinoid arteritis with focal ischemia. Erosions may be present throughout the length of the gastrointestinal tract because of ammonia being liberated from urea. Uriniferous breath is a common finding. Xerostomia (dry mucous membranes) may also be noted. These problems may be exacerbated by the poor oral hygiene typical of veterinary patients.

TABLE 1. Causes of Anorexia in Chronic Renal Failure

Polyuria-polydipsia	Hypergastrinemia
Hypokalemia	Secondary hyperparathyroidism
Metabolic acidosis	Uremic toxins
Nonregenerative anemia	Gastric hyperacidity

UREMIC GASTROENTERITIS

As mentioned earlier, gastroenteritis is one of the causes for vomiting in the animal with renal failure. Uremic gastroenteritis can also be manifested as diarrhea or anorexia. There are many components to the pathophysiology underlying uremic gastroenteritis. Gastrin is cleared by the kidneys and therefore accumulates in renal failure. The hypergastrinemia stimulates the parietal cells to release more hydrochloric acid. Back diffusion of acid and pepsin through the stomach wall creates a viscious cycle by creating inflammation and hemorrhage, which stimulates mast cells to release histamine. This histamine then stimulates the parietal cells to release more hydrochloric acid. Thinning of the protective mucous layer in the stomach further increases the back diffusion of hydrochloric acid. Ischemia due to vascular lesions may also complicate gastroenteritis.

Hypergastrinemia can lead to pyloric sphincter incompetency and biliary reflux (Lazarus, 1991). Other motility disorders, including delayed gastric emptying and gastroesophageal reflux, have been noted in humans with CRF. The abnormal motility may result from electrolyte alterations, disturbances in gastrointestinal hormones, or autonomic nervous system dysfunction (Doherty, 1992).

Histopathologic changes in the gastrointestinal tract include glandular atrophy and mast cell infiltration. Edema of the lamina propria is also seen, as is fibroplasia and mineralization. Submucosal arteritis is another histologic finding.

CONSTIPATION

Constipation, mainly attributable to dehydration, is far more frequent in cats with CRF than in dogs with CRF. Phosphate binding agents used in the management of CRF may also cause constipation.

ANEMIA

Anemia is largely attributable to decreased erythropoietin production by the kidneys (Cowgill, 1995). Gastrointestinal hemorrhage, either from gastroenteritis or platelet dysfunction, can worsen the degree of anemia. Anemia in CRF patients contributes to weight loss because of a general feeling of unwellness. Anemic animals often have depressed appetites and their decreased caloric intake aggravates the state of malnutrition caused by the uremia. Malnutrition can then exacerbate the anemia even further.

DIAGNOSIS

That renal failure is the cause of gastrointestinal disturbances is elucidated with a laboratory database (complete blood count, chemistry profile, urinalysis). Clinical signs of uremia are not manifested until greater than 75% of renal function is lost.

TREATMENT

Successful management of gastrointestinal disturbances in animals with renal failure hinges on satisfactory treatment of renal failure in general. Correcting dehydration and hypokalemia improves the patient's overall well-being. Animals should be enticed to eat multiple small meals throughout the day. The palatability of the diet may be increased by warming the food. Dietary management is a cornerstone in the successful management of CRF; however, dietary restrictions may further discourage patients from eating. Gradually changing the diet to a more restricted food as opposed to abruptly switching foods may improve the situation. Sometimes flavoring agents such as garlic, dehydrated cottage cheese, low-salt butter, or clam juice may improve palatability. If an animal continues to lose weight, despite aggressive management of CRF, the diet should be re-examined to see if protein has been too severely restricted.

Specific medications can be used to treat vomiting and uremic gastroenteritis. As mentioned previously, hypergastrinemia leads to hyperacidity. Medications such as the H_2 receptor antagonists cimetidine and ranitidine can interrupt this pathway. Because of an increase in the elimination half-life of H_2 receptor antagonists, standard dosages should be halved (Table 2). It is also recommended to taper the dosage of these medications after the patient has been on one for a minimum of 2 weeks (Polzin et al, 1995).

Because of the effects of uremic toxins on the chemoreceptor trigger zone, some animals may require centrally acting antiemetics. Metoclopramide (Reglan, Robins) can be given orally at a dosage of 0.2 to 0.4 mg/kg three to four times daily (see Table 2). The lower end of the dosing scale is advisable because metoclopramide is excreted renally. Metoclopramide also has prokinetic effects on the gastrointestinal tract, which may be beneficial if the animal is suffering from altered motility (Krawiec, 1996). Another choice for patients with motility disorders is cisapride at 0.1 to 0.5 mg/kg PO t.i.d. (Propulsid, Janssen) (see p. 614).

The decrease in the mucous protective layer enables more back diffusion of acid through the stomach wall and allows erosions and ulcers to form. This can be combated using sucralfate (Carafate, Marion), which becomes charged in an acid environment and binds to the gastric proteins (see Table 2). Because this medication works by physically binding to the gastric mucosa, dissolving the medicine in a few milliliters of water may improve its efficacy.

References and Suggested Reading

Bergstrom J: Nutrition and mortality in hemodialysis. J Am Soc Nephrol 6:1329, 1995.

TABLE 2. Renal–Gastrointestinal Tract Drugs Used to Manage Gastrointestinal Effects of Uremia

Drug	Dosage	Route
Cimetidine	c-5 mg/kg q8–12 hr f-2.5–5 mg/kg q8–12 hr	PO, SC, IM, IV
Ranitidine	1–2 mg/kg q12hr	PO, IV
Metoclopramide	0.2–0.4 mg/kg q6–8hr 1–2 mg/kg/24hr	PO IV (as CRI)
Cisapride	0.1–0.5 mg/kg q8–12hr	PO
Sucralfate	0.25–1 gm q8–12hr	PO

c, canine; CRI, constant-rate infusion; f, feline.

Causes and predictive factors for protein malnutrition in human hemodialysis patients.

Chew DJ, DiBartola SP: Diagnosis and pathophysiology of renal disease. In: Ettinger SJ, ed: Textbook of Veterinary Internal Medicine. Philadelphia: WB Saunders, 1989, p 1893.
Comprehensive overview of renal disease.

Cowgill LD: CVT Update: Use of recombinant human erythropoietin. In: Bonagura JD, ed: Current Veterinary Therapy XII. Philadelphia: WB Saunders, 1995, p 961.
Discusses the clinical applications of r-HuEPO in dogs and cats with renal failure.

Doherty CC: Gastrointestinal effects of chronic renal failure. In: Cameron S, Davison AM, Grunfeld JP, et al, eds: Oxford Textbook of Clinical Nephrology. New York, Oxford University Press, 1992, p 1278.
This text reviews the effects of CRF on the human gastrointestinal tract; it is organized according to the section of the gastrointestinal tract being discussed.

Krawiec DR: Managing gastrointestinal complications of uremia. In: Polzin DJ, ed: The Veterinary Clinics of North America: Renal Dysfunction. Philadelphia: WB Saunders, 1996, p 1287.
The effects and management of CRF are reviewed as they relate to the gastrointestinal tract; it is organized according to the section of the gastrointestinal tract being discussed.

Lazarus H: Medical aspects of hemodialysis. In: Brenner BM, Rector FC, eds: The Kidney. Philadelphia: WB Saunders, 1991, p 2254.
This text discusses gastrointestinal complications in human CRF patients treated with dialysis.

Osborne CA, Polzin DJ: Pathophysiology of renal failure and uremia. In: Osborne CA, Finco DR, eds: Canine and Feline Nephrology and Urology. Baltimore: Williams & Wilkins, 1996, p 335.
Comprehensive discussion of the pathophysiology of renal disease, focusing on areas currently being studied.

Polzin DJ, James KM, Osborne CA: Metabolic acidosis in renal failure: Consequences, diagnosis, and treatment. In: Bonagura JD, ed: Current Veterinary Therapy XII. Philadelphia: WB Saunders, 1995, p 956.
A review of the underlying pathophysiology of, problems resulting from, and treatment of acidosis in renal failure.

Polzin DJ, Osborne CA, Bartges JW, et al: Chronic renal failure. In: Ettinger SJ, Feldman EC, eds: Textbook of Veterinary Internal Medicine. Philadelphia: WB Saunders, 1995, p 1734.
Overview of the pathophysiology and treatment of chronic renal failure.

Valenzuela J: Gastrointestinal abnormalities. In: Massry SG, Glassock RJ, eds: Textbook of Nephrology. Baltimore: Williams & Wilkins, 1983, p 759.
This text reviews the effects of CRF on the human gastrointestinal tract; it is organized according to the section of the gastrointestinal tract being discussed.

Indications for Nephrectomy and Nephrotomy

ELIZABETH ARNOLD STONE

JODY GOOKIN

Raleigh, North Carolina

NEPHRECTOMY

Nephrectomy is an irreversible treatment for unilateral renal disease that eliminates any contribution to total renal function by that kidney. Nephrectomy may be performed because of renal or ureteral neoplasia, end-stage hydronephrosis, renal calculi in a nonfunctional kidney, uncontrollable renal hematuria, and severe renal trauma. The entire ureter is removed with the kidney. When a clinician decides to perform a nephrectomy, the following presumptions are made: (1) the diseased kidney is more of a liability than a benefit to the animal's health and (2) the function of the contralateral kidney is sufficient to sustain life.

Determining the relative contribution to total renal function by the diseased and contralateral kidney can be difficult. If the diseased kidney is making any contribution to total renal function, the presence of azotemia is a contraindication for nephrectomy. In an azotemic animal, further loss of functional renal mass by nephrectomy would be life-threatening because total renal function is already reduced by at least 75%. Persistent isosthenuria may also be a contraindication to nephrectomy because it correlates with a two-thirds loss of total renal function. An exception might be the animal with acute disease in one kidney before the other kidney has had time to achieve compensatory hypertrophy. However, even in this instance, it may be difficult to maintain the animal's health after nephrectomy until the remaining kidney reaches maximal function. In addition, during acute disease, the presence of even a nonfunctional kidney may provide a greater stimulus for compensatory hypertrophy in the opposite kidney than if the nonfunctional kidney was removed.

In a nonazotemic animal, the degree of reduction in total glomerular filtration rate (GFR), which would be an absolute contraindication to nephrectomy, has not been defined. In animals with unilateral renal disease of short duration (e.g., 2 to 4 weeks), the potential for compensation by the remaining kidney should be considered. Within 4 to 6 weeks after nephrectomy in clinically normal dogs, GFR in the remaining kidney stabilized at 75% of total preoperative GFR.

Preoperative evaluation of dogs undergoing nephrectomy would ideally include an assessment of relative renal GFR. Renal nuclear scintigraphy provides information about preoperative renal function, but few facilities have this capability. Excretory urography provides a gross assessment of renal function, but it does not provide a quantitative estimate of the number of functioning nephrons.

In humans, studies have consistently demonstrated that renal function is well preserved for prolonged periods after nephrectomy provided that the remaining kidney is intrinsically normal. No progressive deterioration in renal function was seen for up to 20 years after surgery, and survival rate was not significantly different in kidney donors from that of the general population. In an experimental study in clinically normal geriatric dogs, GFR remained stable during the 2-year follow-up period. In cats that were kidney donors, renal and erythropoietic function was clinically preserved 2 to 5 years after nephrectomy.

NEPHROTOMY

Nephrotomy is used to examine and correct diseases of the renal pelvis. In the authors' experience with clinically normal dogs, nephrotomy did not significantly reduce single-kidney GFR as measured by nuclear scintigraphy and inulin clearance. The nephrotomy technique the authors use is different than that described in the 1970s, which was associated with a 20 to 40% decrease in renal function. In the former procedure, the kidney parenchyma was incised as far as the renal pelvis. The kidney was reapposed with 2–0 chromic gut mattress sutures. In contrast, in the currently used technique (Stone and Barsanti, 1992), an incision is made with the scalpel blade through the midline renal capsule only. The renal parenchyma is atraumatically separated with the blunt end of the scalpel handle as far as the renal pelvis. Any interlobar vessels encountered during the bisection are ligated and severed. The length of incision does not extend further than the length of the renal pelvis. No mattress sutures are used in the closure; instead, simple continuous synthetic suture material is placed in the capsule while the kidney halves are apposed with thumb and forefinger.

INDICATIONS WITH SPECIFIC DISEASES

Pyelonephritis

Preoperative criteria for performing nephrectomy as a treatment for chronic pyelonephritis have not been established. The authors have found that a diagnosis of pyelonephritis based on abdominal ultrasonography or excretory urography is *not* always confirmed by histologic diagnosis of the nephrectomized kidney. Results of bacterial culture or Gram staining of urine collected during surgery from the affected kidney have been confirmed by histologic findings. In the future, ultrasonographically guided aspiration of urine from the renal pelvis may provide a more accurate preoperative diagnosis.

In the authors' experience, nephrectomy does not consistently resolve urinary tract infection attributed to chronic unilateral pyelonephritis. Continued infection may be the result of undiagnosed pyelonephritis in the remaining kidney, failure of antimicrobial treatment, or iatrogenic or spontaneous reinfection. Nephrotomy may be useful in the pyelonephritic kidney that also has renoliths not amenable to medical dissolution.

Hydronephrosis

Determining the cause of hydronephrosis is important in the decision of whether or not to remove the kidney. When there is functional parenchyma remaining and the obstructive lesion can be reversed, the kidney should be preserved. The potential for return of some renal function exists as long as the kidney is spared. Nephrotomy may be useful to examine the renal pelvis and possibly remove the cause of the obstruction (e.g., renolith).

Renal Neoplasia

Primary renal tumors have a high metastatic rate. The decision to perform nephrectomy is based on no evidence of metastasis, the ability to achieve tumor-free excision margins (even removing body wall musculature, if necessary), and prevention of tumor seeding of the wound. Dogs with embryonal nephroma have a better prognosis than do dogs with other types of primary renal tumors, and nephrectomy is indicated. Using a nephrotomy incision to debulk a renal tumor has little benefit. In rare instances, nephrotomy may be useful for removing benign tumors or polyps.

Renoliths

Reasons for surgical removal of renoliths include renal pelvic obstruction, uncontrollable infection, progressive calculus enlargement, and deterioration in renal function. In some animals, particularly elderly animals, a nephrolith will not cause sufficient damage to the kidney during the animal's life span to warrant surgical removal.

In one study, renal scintigraphy supported the decision to perform nephrectomy rather than nephrotomy for the treatment of nephroliths when the affected kidney contributed less than 33% to the total GFR (Gookin et al, 1996) after noninvasive methods have been exhausted. One risk in removing a kidney as a treatment for nephroliths is that nephroliths may occur in the remaining kidney, even with preventive treatment. This may be more of a risk with calcium oxalate uroliths; greater than 50% of dogs with calcium oxalate uroliths had recurrence within 3 years of urolith removal. Unless there are other indications for removing the kidney, the authors recommend nephrotomy rather than nephrectomy for renoliths.

Hematuria of Renal Origin

Nephrotomy may be useful in determining a specific cause for persistent renal hematuria (see *CVT IX,* p. 1130). A ventral cystotomy incision is made so that the ureteral openings can be inspected and the ureters catheterized. Urine is collected from each ureter and examined microscopically, if necessary, to determine which kidney is bleeding. With bilateral renal hematuria, biopsy specimens are taken. With unilateral hematuria from a kidney of normal size and shape, a nephrotomy is performed to identify potentially correctable causes of hemorrhage (e.g., vascular abnormalities, nephroliths, renal parasites, benign tumors). If the source of the bleeding can be identified and corrected, the nephrotomy incision is closed. Otherwise, a nephrectomy is performed as long as the opposite kidney has sufficient function.

References and Suggested Reading

Finco DR, Brown SA, Crowell WA, et al: Effects of aging and dietary protein intake on uninephrectomized geriatric dogs. Am J Vet Res 55:1282, 1994.

An experimental study evaluating the function of the remaining kidney for up to 2 years after nephrectomy.

Gookin JL, Stone EA, Spaulding KA, Berry CR: Unilateral nephrectomy in dogs with renal disease: 30 cases (1985–1994). J Am Vet Med Assoc 208:2020, 1996.
A retrospective evaluation of indications for and complications, efficacy, and effects on renal function of unilateral nephrectomy in dogs with renal disease.

Lirtzman RA, Gregory CR: Long-term renal and hematologic effects of uninephrectomy in healthy feline kidney donors. J Am Vet Med Assoc 20:1044, 1995.
A comparison of renal function and health in cats that had been renal donors with cats in an age- and sex-matched comparison group.

Stone EA, Barsanti JA, eds: Urologic surgery of the dog and cat. Philadelphia: Lea & Febiger, 1992, p 161.
A detailed description, with illustrations of the surgical technique, for nephrectomy and nephrotomy; also includes preoperative and perioperative management of urolithiasis.

Diagnosis and Management of Ureteral Obstruction

ELIZABETH ARNOLD STONE
Raleigh, North Carolina

ANDREW E. KYLES
Davis, California

Acquired ureteral obstruction has numerous causes but most frequently results from nephroliths migrating into the ureter (Table 1). Congenital ureteral obstruction is rarely recognized, although it can occur with an ectopic ureter. Usually, ureteral obstruction is unilateral, unless the source of the obstruction is within the bladder. Reduction in renal function in the affected kidney is a common sequela to ureteral obstruction. Urinary tract infection (UTI) may precede or follow ureteral obstruction and can be difficult to eradicate until the primary disease is removed. The risk of UTI is exacerbated by catheterization, instrumentation, and surgery for obstruction.

CLINICAL SIGNS OF URETERAL OBSTRUCTION

Pain may occur with acute obstruction and is thought to be caused by stretching of the renal capsule or collecting system. The severity of the pain correlates with the rate of distention, rather than the degree of obstruction or distention. Acute obstruction is associated with severe pain, whereas a massive hydronephrosis caused by gradual stricture of the ureter may be asymptomatic. Pain may be manifested by anorexia, restlessness, and gastrointestinal signs and may be alleviated when the obstruction is removed. Signs of uremia are not apparent unless bilateral ureteral obstruction is present or the opposite kidney has subnormal function.

The case history should identify any previous urinary tract infections, history of uroliths, recent surgery, and diet. Abdominal palpation may reveal changes in the shape or size of the kidney. Abnormal findings on urinalysis in animals with ureteral obstruction are nonspecific. Microscopic hematuria is a common finding. Crystals in a freshly voided urine sample may give a clue as to the type of ureterolith, if present, but crystals may also occur in normal animals. During chronic obstruction, a concentrating defect develops, leading to dilute urine production by the affected kidney. With unilateral obstruction, urine retrieved from the bladder may still be in the concentrated range because the other kidney retains concentrating ability. Likewise, serum urea nitrogen and creatinine concentrations may be within normal ranges.

Usually, ureteroliths can be identified on survey abdominal radiographs. When obstruction is suspected, ultrasonography is particularly helpful in diagnosing hydronephrosis and hydroureter. Renal size, dilatation of the renal pelvis and ureter, renal cortical thinning, and intraureteral uroliths may be apparent. In cats, it may be difficult to follow an individual ureter using ultrasonography because the ureters lie fairly close together in the midureteral region, and the ultrasound probe may detect one ureter and then the other within a short distance. Although ultrasonographic findings may suggest the presence of obstruction, excretory urography helps confirm and locate the obstruction. Unfortunately, if the kidney has a low glomerular filtration, the kidney may not be visualized on the excretory urogram because of poor excretion of the contrast agent. In addition, with complete obstruction, the kidney may not excrete enough contrast material to locate the obstruction. Nuclear

TABLE 1. Causes of Acquired Ureteral Obstruction

Intraluminal	*Extraureteral*
Ureteroliths	Accidental ligation of ureter during
Intramural	ovariohysterectomy (OHE)
Ureteral stricture	Extensive retroperitoneal fibrosis
Ureteral tumors	Braided nonabsorbable suture used during
Urinary bladder tumors	OHE
	Migrating plant awn
	Retroperitoneal tumors

scintigraphy, available in some referral centers, may give an indication of total and individual kidney function at the time of obstruction.

POTENTIAL FOR RECOVERY OF RENAL FUNCTION

Partial obstruction of the ureter results in reduced renal blood flow, reduced glomerular filtration rate, and eventual irreversible damage to the kidney. Obstruction and infection may lead to permanent impairment of ureteral peristalsis, which might predispose to vesicoureteral reflux or repeated infection.

Estimating the amount of functional damage to the obstructed kidney helps the clinician decide whether to preserve or remove the affected kidney and ureter. However, determining the potential for recovery is problematic because the degree of dilatation does not correlate with the degree of functional damage. The potential for recovery of renal function depends on the duration and completeness of the obstruction as well as the presence of UTI. In experimental studies in dogs, 7 days of complete unilateral ureteral obstruction resulted in a variable and permanent reduction in renal blood flow. No return of renal function was observed after 40 days of unilateral ligation. However, case reports in humans demonstrated some recovery after 69 days of ureteral obstruction. The degree of recovery after naturally occurring obstruction in dogs and cats has not been established.

Recent information on the management of ureterolithiasis will be discussed in the following sections as a specific example of ureteral obstruction. Detailed discussion on surgically related ureteral obstruction (ureteral surgery, ovariohysterectomy) is presented by Kyles and associates (1998).

URETEROLITHIASIS AND URETERAL OBSTRUCTION

Surgical removal of ureteroliths is indicated when partial or complete obstruction of the ureter occurs, as evidenced by hydronephrosis and hydroureter proximal to the calculus, or with immobility of the ureterolith, as determined by repeated radiographic or ultrasonographic examinations, or both. Small ureteroliths may pass into the bladder, and experimental studies in dogs suggest that the transit time for small, artificial calculi varies from 1 to 24 hours. Although medical dissolution of some types of nephroliths may be successful, ureteroliths are not immersed in undersaturated urine and are unlikely to dissolve. Other factors that influence the decision to remove ureteroliths include the presence of infection, other calculi in the urinary tract, and the degree of renal function in the affected kidney. Chronic renal disease may be exacerbated by the ureteral obstruction. The purpose of surgical removal of the ureterolith is to restore urine flow and to improve or stabilize renal function in the affected kidney. In addition, once the animal recovers from the surgical procedure, ureteral pain may be eliminated.

Although ureteronephrectomy will remove pain and hematuria in animals with unilateral ureteroliths, it also eliminates any contribution to total renal function by the excised kidney. Renal function is then solely dependent on the remaining kidney, which may be diseased and could subsequently develop nephroliths or ureteroliths.

Ureteroliths in Cats

The frequency of ureteroliths in cats is increasing. At North Carolina State University, ureteroliths were first diagnosed in a cat in August, 1993. Since then, more than 15 cats have been diagnosed with ureteroliths (Kyles et al, 1998). All the retrieved ureteroliths were calcium oxalate. Cats with ureteroliths may have nonspecific signs, including weight loss, lethargy, hematuria, pollakiuria, recurrent UTI, or a combination of these conditions. Cats may demonstrate pain by vocalization and restlessness.

In addition to the general criteria described, the decision to remove ureteroliths in cats surgically is also based on the availability of and experience with microsurgical instruments, using either magnifying loupes or, preferably, an operating microscope. The lumen of a normal cat ureter is small, approximately the size of 2–0 suture material. Minimal inflammation and edema can cause acute ureteral obstruction. In a dog, a stent catheter can be used to divert the urine from the ureter. However, in cats, the normal-sized ureter is too small for catheterization.

The specific procedure used to repair the ureteral obstruction depends on the location of the ureterolith (Kyles et al, 1998; Stone, 1997). For ureteroliths in the *middle and distal ureter,* the affected portion of the ureter is excised and the more proximal healthy ureter is reimplanted into the bladder (ureteroneocystostomy). If necessary to relieve tension on the ureter, the bladder dome can be positioned more cranially (psoas cystopexy) and the kidney and proximal ureter can be positioned more caudally (renal descensus). The ureteroneocystostomy technique is similar to the one described for renal transplantation. A urethral catheter is placed to monitor urine output and keep the bladder decompressed.

The proximal ureter will not extend to the bladder, thus when ureteroliths are in the *proximal ureter,* ureteroneocystostomy is not possible. With ureteroliths in this location, ureteral dilatation extends from the level of the ureteroliths proximally into the renal pelvis. After the ureteroliths are removed through a ureterotomy incision, the dilated proximal ureter can be catheterized, which allows placement of a nephrostomy catheter to drain the urine.

After surgery, cats need intensive care to manage fluid therapy, monitor urine output, and ensure the patency of nephrostomy or urethral catheters, or both. Serum biochemistry values and complete blood counts are repeated to assess resolution of azotemia and anemia.

Dietary considerations for prevention of recurrence of calcium oxalate uroliths have been described, but definitive recommendations have not been established (see *CVT XII,* p. 989). Cats that have had ureteral calculi removed should undergo radiography or have an ultrasonographic examination every 3 to 4 months to monitor for recurrence. Also, since many of these cats have renal disease, periodic assessment of renal function and appropriate medical management of renal disease is recommended.

Ureteroliths in Dogs

Ureteral calculi in dogs most often are composed of calcium oxalate or struvite. A detailed study of canine ureteroliths has not been performed, but surgical decision-making is similar to that described in cats. Since the canine ureter (except in miniature breeds) is large enough to catheterize, ureteral stenting can be used to drain urine from the ureterotomy site.

References and Suggested Reading

Curhan GC, Zeidel ML: Urinary Tract Obstruction. In: Brenner BM, ed: Brenner & Rector's The Kidney. Philadelphia: WB Saunders, 1996, p 1936.
This article presents a review of pathophysiology and management of urinary tract obstruction in humans, with a good summary of applicable experimental studies in animals.
Kyles AE, Stone EA, Gookin JL, et al: Diagnosis and surgical management of obstructive ureteral calculi in cats: 11 cases (1993–1996). J Am Vet Med Assoc 213:1150, 1998.
This article discusses a clinical study of calcium oxalate ureteroliths in cats, including preoperative diagnostics, surgical procedure, and postoperative complications.
Stone EA: Surgical management of urinary tract disease: Ureteral calculi in cats and urinary bladder neoplasia in dogs. Suppl Compend Contin Educ Pract Vet 19:62, 1997.
This is a review of the diagnosis and management of cats with ureteroliths.
Stone EA, Barsanti JA: Urologic surgery of the dog and cat. Philadelphia: Lea & Febiger, 1992.
This article provides descriptions of pathophysiology, diagnostic methods, and surgical treatments, with extensive line drawings.

Urine Diversion by Tube Cystostomy

DON R. WALDRON
Blacksburg, Virginia

Urine is normally expelled intermittently from the urinary bladder via the urethra; however, anatomic or neurologic disease may cause disruption of this function. Lower urinary tract obstruction occurs commonly in both the dog and the cat and may be caused by calculi or mucus plugs within the urethra; neoplasia of the urinary bladder, urethra, or prostate; and inflammatory disease of the urethra. Trauma to the lower urinary tract may cause partial or complete disruption of the urethra or urinary bladder, requiring urine diversion before definitive repair. In addition, urine diversion from the bladder aids uncomplicated healing of the urethra after surgical repair. Finally, urethral stricture secondary to naturally occurring disease or to surgical procedures may necessitate urine diversion over the short term.

Obstruction of the lower urinary tract, if prolonged and complete, causes profound metabolic changes, including azotemia, uremia, and acidosis. In many cases, relief of lower urinary tract obstruction may be obtained by urethral catheterization techniques or cystocentesis, or both. If catheterization is not possible, placement of a cystostomy tube may allow urine diversion until the animal is metabolically stable, at which time definitive surgery or medical therapy may be instituted. Tube cystostomy has been used as both a short- and long-term urinary diversion procedure that allows patient stabilization in an emergency setting or as palliative therapy for lower urinary tract neoplasia or other lower urinary tract obstructive disease. Placement of a cystostomy tube may be performed via a minilaparotomy or percutaneously; however, operative placement is easiest and most predictable. The only specific equipment needed is a Foley or Pezzar tipped catheter for minilaparotomy or a Stamey catheter for percutaneous placement. Maintenance of cystostomy catheters is easier than that of urethral catheters.

TECHNIQUE

For operative placement, the animal is anesthetized and placed in dorsal recumbency. If the patient is uremic, administration of opiates and use of local blocks with lidocaine is an alternative to general anesthesia. A 2-cm skin and abdominal wall incision is made on the caudal midline in the female and just lateral to the prepuce in the male. The urinary bladder is located and partially exteriorized, and two "stay" sutures are placed in the cranial ventral bladder wall. Nylon or polypropylene suture material is used to place a pursestring suture between the two "stay" sutures, and a stab incision is made in the middle of the pursestring suture into the bladder lumen. A second paramedian stab skin incision is made lateral to the first incision. An 8F to a 12F Foley or Pezzar (mushroom-tipped catheter) is advanced through the second incision and into the bladder lumen through the pursestring suture. Saline is used to inflate the bulb if a Foley catheter is used, and the pursestring suture is tightened and tied, securing the catheter tip within the urinary bladder. A cystopexy is performed by placing several interrupted sutures between the bladder and ventral abdominal wall. The abdominal wall and skin incisions are closed, and the catheter is connected to a closed drainage system or capped with an infusion plug and three-way stopcock. The catheter may be bandaged or sutured to the body wall or placed under a stockinette cover.

Percutaneous placement of a 10F to 14F Stamey catheter has also been described as a method for cystostomy catheter placement (Botte, 1983; Bellah, 1990). This technique requires that the bladder be palpable; thus, a full urinary bladder is desirable. Local anesthesia is used and a small skin incision is made over the distended bladder. The catheter is advanced through the skin incision and abdominal wall and thrust into the bladder lumen. Fixation and maintenance of the catheter are as described for the operative procedure. A disadvantage of the Stamey catheter is possible difficult placement owing to the freely movable nature of the canine and feline bladders. In addition, long-term maintenance of the polyethylene catheter with its collapsible flanges is more problematic than with the Foley or mushroom-tipped catheter.

MAINTENANCE

Initially, a bandage is applied to minimize fluid discharge from the catheter stoma. Once healing has occurred at 3 to 5 days, the catheter may be maintained under a light body wrap or stockinette. An Elizabethan collar may be necessary to prevent inadvertent catheter removal by the animal; however, most animals tolerate the tube well. If the tube is not connected to a closed system or the tube is intended for long-term maintenance, the bladder should be emptied using a syringe three to four times daily.

The catheter can be removed 5 to 7 days after placement by deflating the bulb on the Foley catheter; alternatively, if definitive abdominal surgery is performed subsequent to catheter placement, the cystopexy can be taken down and the bladder closed primarily. If long-term maintenance of the catheter is desired, the mushroom-tipped catheter may be preferred, as early deterioration of the bulb on the Foley catheter may predispose it to inadvertent early removal (Smith et al, 1995).

Urinary tract infection is a common sequela to cystostomy tube maintenance. Periodic urinalysis and urine culture (2 to 4 weeks) are recommended in animals with long-term cystostomy tubes. Prophylactic use of antibiotics is not advised because of the risk for selecting resistant organisms.

It appears that long-term maintenance of the catheter is possible. In a recent series of six cases of dogs with transitional cell carcinoma, the median time for catheter maintenance before death was 106 days (Smith et al, 1995). The author has maintained catheters in animals with similar disease up to 6 months after diagnosis.

SUMMARY

Cystostomy tube placement is an easy and effective method of urine diversion for both short- and long-term use. Tube cystostomy is valuable in the short term for animals that cannot be catheterized transurethrally either because of obstructive disease or because of urethral trauma in which the urethra is totally disrupted.

Tube cystostomy after urethral anastomosis is an excellent means of providing urine diversion in the postoperative period, and its ease of maintenance makes this technique preferable to indwelling urethral catheters in the dog.

As a palliative technique, tube cystostomy is useful for animals with lower urinary tract obstruction caused by neoplasia or inflammatory disease. The technique may allow time for definitive therapy to be effective or may be used long term as palliative therapy when owners do not desire aggressive surgical therapy.

References and Suggested Reading

Bellah JR: Problems of the urethra, surgical approaches. In: Bradley RL, ed. Problems in Veterinary Medicine. Philadelphia: JB Lippincott, 1990, pp 17–35.
A review of treatment options for clinical disease of the urethra.

Botte RJ: Percutaneous prepubic urinary drainage in normal cats. Vet Surg 12:202, 1983.
An experimental study detailing placement of Stamey urinary catheters in six cats.

Smith JD, Stone EA, Gilson SD: Placement of a permanent cystostomy catheter to relieve urine outflow obstruction in dogs with transitional cell carcinoma. J Am Vet Med Assoc 206:496, 1995.
Original clinical study describing the results of urinary diversion via tube cystostomy in animals with transitional cell carcinoma of the urinary bladder or urethra.

Ammonium Urate Uroliths in Dogs With Portosystemic Shunts

Joseph W. Bartges
Knoxville, TN

Larry M. Cornelius
Athens, Georgia

Carl A. Osborne
St. Paul, Minnesota

Portosystemic shunts (PSSs) are vascular communications linking the portal vein directly to the systemic circulation so that substances in portal blood derived from the intestinal tract bypass the liver without undergoing hepatic metabolism. Dogs with PSSs are at high risk for the development of ammonium urate uroliths. These uroliths occur in both males and females and usually, but not always, are detected in animals before the age of 3 years. The predisposition of dogs with PSSs to urate urolithiasis is associated with concomitant hyperuricemia, hyperammonemia, hyperuricuria, and hyperammonuria. However, not all dogs with PSS acquire ammonium urate uroliths.

ETIOPATHOGENESIS

Uric acid is one of several biodegradation products of purine metabolism. In most dogs, it is converted by hepatic uricase to allantoin (Bartges et al, 1992). However, with PSSs, uric acid produced during purine metabolism does not circulate efficiently through the liver. Therefore, it is incompletely converted to allantoin, resulting in abnormally elevated serum uric acid concentrations. Such concentrations in 15 dogs with portovascular anomalies evaluated at the University of Minnesota Veterinary Teaching Hospital were found to be increased: values ranged from 1.2 to 4.0 mg/dl; values in normal dogs ranged from 0.2 to 0.4 mg/dl (Lulich et al, 1995). Uric acid is freely filtered through the glomerulus, reabsorbed in the early proximal tubule, and secreted into tubular lumina in distal proximal nephrons. Thus, the urine concentration of uric acid is, in part, determined by the serum concentration. Because portosystemic shunting of blood results in elevated concentrations of uric acid in serum, increased concentrations of uric acid are excreted in urine. Uroliths that form in association with PSSs are usually composed of ammonium urate. Ammonium urate uroliths form because urine becomes oversaturated with ammonia and uric acid as a consequence of shunting of blood from the portal system directly into the systemic circulation.

Ammonia is produced primarily by colonic bacteria and is absorbed into the portal circulation. In normal animals, ammonia is extracted from the portal circulation by the liver and is converted to urea. In dogs with PSSs, ammonia is inefficiently converted to urea, and thus ammonia concentrations in the systemic circulation increase. Elevated concentrations of circulating ammonia result in increased excretion of ammonia in urine. The result of portal blood bypassing liver metabolism is elevated systemic concentrations of uric acid and ammonia, which are excreted in urine. If the saturation of urine with ammonia and uric acid exceeds the solubility product of ammonium urate, it will precipitate. If the precipitates are retained in oversaturated urine, ammonium urate uroliths will form.

CLINICAL SIGNS

Urate uroliths associated with PSSs usually form in the urinary bladder; therefore, signs of lower urinary tract disease including hematuria, dysuria, pollakiuria, and inappropriate urination may develop in affected animals. If urethral obstruction results, anuria and signs of postrenal azotemia will occur. Some dogs with urocystoliths do not show signs of lower urinary tract disease. Although it is possible for ammonium urate uroliths to form in the renal pelvis, they are uncommonly recognized. Dogs with PSSs may also have signs of hepatoencephalopathy, including trembling, hypersalivation, seizures, bleeding disorders, and stunted growth.

DIAGNOSIS

Laboratory Evaluation

Dogs with PSSs often have ammonium urate crystalluria (Fig. 1), indicating an increased risk for urolith formation. The urine specific gravity may be low because of decreased renal medullary concentration of urea. Another common laboratory abnormality in dogs with PSSs is microcytic anemia. Routine biochemical analysis of serum is often normal in dogs with PSSs, with the exception of a low blood urea nitrogen concentration caused by inefficient conversion of ammonia to urea. Occasionally, alkaline phosphatase and alanine aminotransferase activities may be increased, and concentrations of albumin and glucose may be low. Serum uric acid concentrations are elevated; however, caution should be used in interpreting values because spectrophotometric methods of uric acid analysis are unreliable (Felice et al, 1990). In dogs with PSSs, liver function tests are abnormal and include elevated concentrations of serum bile acids before and after feeding, elevated concen-

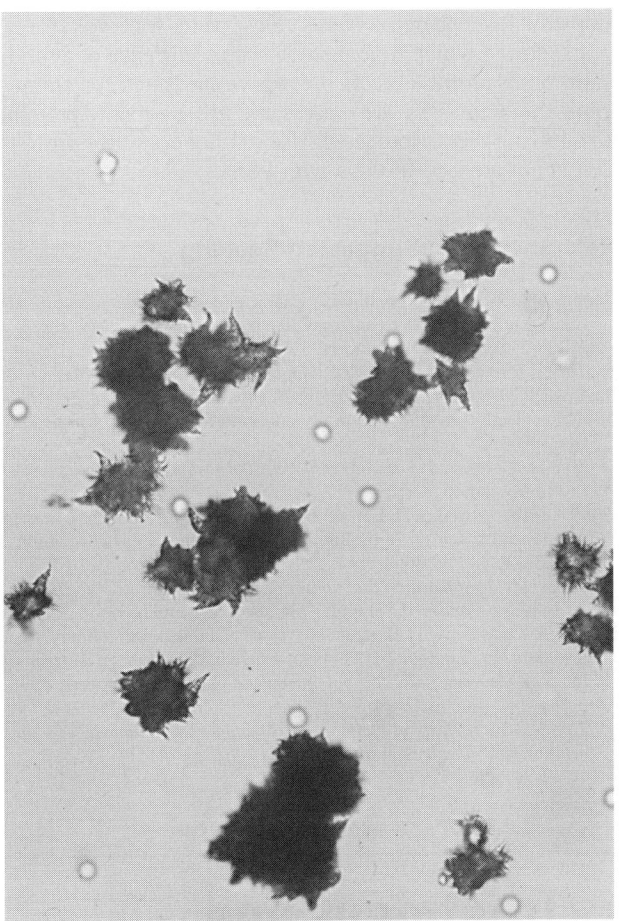

Figure 1. Photomicrograph of urine sediment from a 6-month-old, male Miniature Schnauzer containing ammonium urate crystals (unstained, original magnification, ×100).

trations of plasma or blood ammonia before and after administration of ammonium chloride, and increased retention of Bromsulphalein.

Radiographic Evaluation

Ammonium urate uroliths may be radiolucent; if so, they cannot be detected by survey radiography. However, survey abdominal radiographs may reveal microhepatica associated with hepatic atrophy resulting from portosystemic shunting of blood. Occasionally, renomegaly is observed with PSSs; the significance is unknown. Urate uroliths in the bladder may be visualized by double-contrast cystography (Fig. 2) or by ultrasonography. If uroliths are present in the urethra, contrast urethrography should be performed to evaluate their size, number, and location. Double-contrast cystography and retrograde contrast urethrography have several advantages over abdominal ultrasonography in the evaluation of the lower urinary tract. The urinary bladder and urethra are visualized with contrast radiography, whereas the urinary bladder, but not the urethra, is visualized by ultrasonography. In addition, the number and size of uroliths may be determined during contrast cystography, and small uroliths may be retrieved during the procedure. However, a disadvantage of retrograde contrast

radiography of the lower urinary tract is that it is an invasive procedure that may require sedation or anesthesia. Although the kidneys may be evaluated for the presence of urate uroliths in the renal pelvis, excretory urography provides the most reliable method for examining the kidneys and ureters.

THERAPY

Although ammonium urate uroliths in dogs without PSSs may be dissolved medically using a low-purine, alkalinizing diet in combination with allopurinol, medical therapy has not been consistently effective in inducing urolith dissolution in dogs with PSSs. The efficacy of allopurinol may be altered in these animals because biotransformation of the drug, which has a short half-life, to oxypurinol, which has a longer half-life, requires adequate hepatic function (Bartges et al, 1997). In addition, medical dissolution may not be effective if uroliths contain other minerals besides ammonium urate. Xanthine may form in association with allopurinol administration, which may also impair dissolution.

Urate urocystoliths—which tend to be small, round, and smooth—may be removed nonsurgically using voiding urohydropropulsion. However, the success of this procedure is dependent on the urocystoliths being smaller in diameter than the narrowest part of the urethra. Therefore, dogs with PSSs and urethral obstruction due to uroliths are not candidates for this procedure.

Because medical dissolution is not consistently effective, surgical removal of uroliths that are clinically active is warranted. When possible, uroliths should be removed at the time of surgical correction of PSSs. If uroliths are not removed at the time of PSS ligation, we hypothesize that elimination of hyperuricuria and reduction of urine ammonium concentration after surgical correction of the PSS will dissolve uroliths composed primarily of ammonium urate. Appropriate clinical studies are needed to prove or disprove this hypothesis. Also, use of a low-purine, alkalinizing diet may prevent growth of existing uroliths

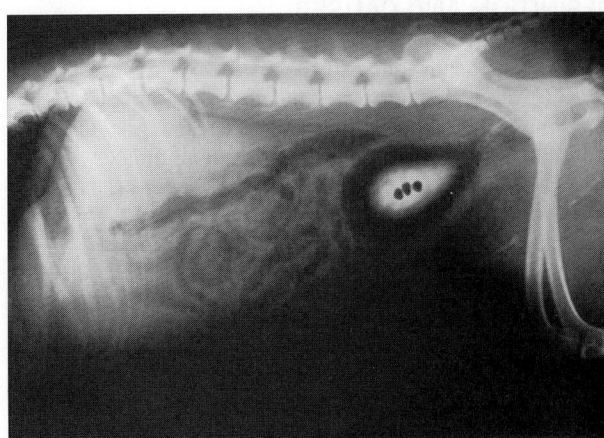

Figure 2. Double-contrast cystogram of a 2-year-old, male Lhasa apso with a PSS, illustrating three radiolucent uroliths and microhepatica. Analysis of surgically removed uroliths revealed that they were composed of 100% ammonium urate.

or promote dissolution of uroliths that are not removed in dogs that undergo PSS ligation.

PREVENTION

After ligation of the PSS, ammonium urate precipitates should not continue to form if adequate blood flow has been returned to the liver. However, in animals in which PSS ligation is not possible or in which partial ligation was performed, the risk of ammonium urate urolith formation still exists. These animals should be monitored by urinalysis for the development of ammonium urate crystals. If crystalluria is present, additional preventive measures should be undertaken. Monitoring of postprandial plasma ammonium concentration may also reveal abnormal levels despite apparent lack of clinical signs. Measurement of serum uric acid concentrations may reveal elevated concentrations. Therefore, urine concentrations of uric acid and ammonia may be elevated in these animals, which increases the risk of ammonium urate uroliths forming. In studies performed at the University of Minnesota, use of a purine-restricted, alkalinizing diet (Prescription Diet Canine u/d, Hill's Pet Products, Topeka, KS) in four dogs with inoperable PSSs resulted in decreasing urine saturation with ammonium urate to a level below which ammonium urate precipitates. In addition, signs of hepatoenceph-

alopathy disappeared. These dogs were followed for 3 years, during which time there was no recurrence of ammonium urate urolithiasis. If preventive measures for ammonium urate uroliths are necessary, use of a low-protein, alkalinizing diet is indicated. Use of allopurinol for prevention is not advised in dogs with PSSs.

References and Suggested Reading

Bartges JW, Osborne CA, Felice LJ: Canine acquired xanthine urocystolithiasis. In: Kirk RW, Bonagura JD, eds: Current Veterinary Therapy XI. Philadelphia: WB Saunders, 1992, p 901.
This is a review of urolithiasis composed of purine metabolites.
Bartges JW, Osborne CA, Felice LJ, et al: Bioavailability and pharmacokinetics of intravenously and orally administered allopurinol in healthy beagles. Am J Vet Res 58:504, 1997.
This is a prospective study evaluating the metabolism of allopurinol in healthy dogs.
Felice LJ, Dombrovskis D, Lafond E, et al: Determination of uric acid in canine serum and urine by high-performance liquid chromatography. Vet Clin Pathol 19:86, 1990.
This study demonstrated that conventional methods of uric acid analysis in plasma and urine samples from dogs are unreliable.
Lulich JP, Osborne CA, Bartges JW, et al: Canine lower urinary tract disorders. In: Ettinger SJ, Feldman EC, eds: Textbook of Veterinary Internal Medicine, 4th ed., vol 2. Philadelphia: WB Saunders, 1995, p 1833.
This volume reviews etiopathogenesis, diagnosis, treatment, and prevention of urolithiasis in dogs.

Compound Uroliths: Treatment and Prevention

JODY P. LULICH
CARL A. OSBORNE
St. Paul, Minnesota

DEFINITION AND CAUSES

Most canine uroliths are composed of a predominant (>70%) mineral, with lesser quantities of other minerals. If a single mineral does not constitute at least 70% of a urolith, and two or more minerals are intimately mixed with each other, it is designated as a *mixed urolith*. Sometimes minerals are separated into distinct bands or layers that may be detected by radiography (Fig. 1) or by bisecting the urolith. If the core or center of a urolith is at least 70% one mineral type, and is surrounded by a different mineral, it is called a *compound urolith*.

Compound uroliths composed approximately 6.5% of 64,000 canine urolith submissions received between 1981 and 1996 at the Minnesota Urolith Center. Compound uroliths form because factors initially promoting precipitation of one type of mineral have been superseded by factors promoting precipitation of a different mineral. For example,

antibiotics and urine acidifiers are used to manage magnesium ammonium phosphate (MAP) uroliths. The antibiotics may eradicate or suppress microbial urease, reducing precipitation of MAP. However, acidemia associated with urine acidifiers may promote hypercalciuria, resulting in a surrounding shell of calcium oxalate (CaOx) or calcium phosphate. Likewise, we have observed shells of sulfadiazine surrounding various types of uroliths (e.g., CaOx, ammonium urate) after empirical administration of sulfonamide antibiotics to animals with lower urinary tract disease.

Some mineral types may serve as a template for deposition of other minerals. This phenomenon may explain why CaOx uroliths occasionally have a nidus of silica and vice versa. All uroliths predispose the animal to bacterial urinary tract infection. If urinary tract infections by microorganisms that produce urease persist, there is increased risk that MAP will precipitate over existing metabolic uroliths (e.g., CaOx, calcium phosphate, urate).

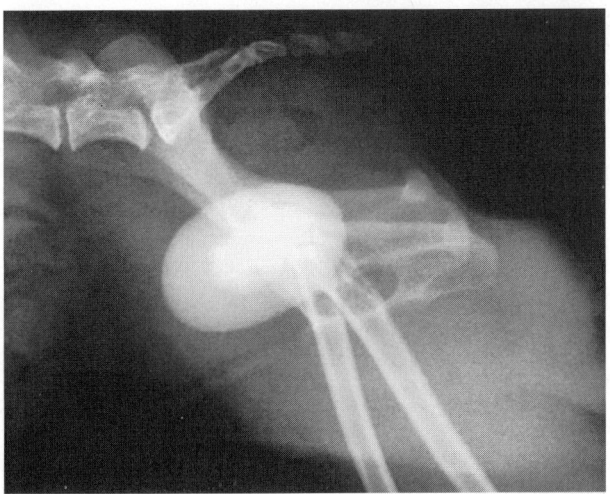

Figure 1. Lateral survey radiograph of a 5-year-old, female Yorkshire terrier with a compound urolith. The core was composed of 100% CaOx monohydrate and the outer layer was composed of 95% phosphate and 5% calcium phosphate.

GENERAL THERAPEUTIC GUIDELINES

Dissolution and Removal of Compound Uroliths

Because risk factors that predispose to precipitation of different minerals in compound uroliths often vary, designing effective medical protocols is a challenge. One strategy is to design protocols to dissolve the outer layer first. Serial survey radiographs may be helpful in monitoring the effectiveness of attempts to dissolve outer layers of uroliths. Once the outer layer of different radiographic density disappears, and there is no further reduction in urolith size, medical therapy can be altered to dissolve different minerals in the inner layers.

In some cases, we have reduced the size of compound uroliths by dissolving their outer layers, followed by removing the remaining portions by voiding urohydropropulsion (see *CVT XII*, p. 1003). Symptomatic compound uroliths that are refractory to medical protocols should be removed surgically. However, in some patients with asymptomatic uroliths, we have chosen a nonsurgical "wait and watch" strategy.

Prevention of Recurring Compound Uroliths

What steps should be followed once compound uroliths have been removed? In the absence of clinical evidence to the contrary, we recommend prevention protocols principally designed to minimize recurrence of the minerals that composed the nucleus, rather than the shell, of compound uroliths. This involves the concept of heterogeneous nucleation. In brief, greater concentrations of lithogenic minerals are required for uroliths to form in the absence of solids in the lumen of the urinary tract (homogeneous nucleation) than are required for uroliths to precipitate around a pre-existing solid (e.g., suture material, catheters, and even pre-existing uroliths of a different mineral type). In the context of compound uroliths, logic suggests that the initial core composed of one mineral type and formed by homogeneous nucleation contributed to the formation of outer layers of a different mineral type by heterogeneous nucleation. Therefore, minimizing risk factors for precipitation of minerals found in the core would eliminate heterogeneous nucleation and thus minimize precipitation of minerals found in the outer layers of the urolith.

Since excessive concentration of minerals in urine is a prerequisite for urolith formation, increased water intake would logically lead to reduction in urine concentration, and thus minimize recurrence of all types of uroliths. In addition to reducing the concentration of lithogenic minerals, production of larger volumes of less concentrated urine decreases the risk of urolithiasis by increasing the frequency of micturition and thus the frequency that crystals would be voided. To minimize formation of concentrated urine, we recommend feeding high-moisture canned foods. Alternatively, water can be added to dry diets with a goal of achieving a urine specific gravity less than 1.020. Although some specific diuretics may be of value in managing certain types of uroliths, in general we avoid indiscriminate use of diuretics because of their propensity for adverse effects (e.g., dehydration, hypokalemia, hypercalcemia, and increased urinary excretion of some lithogenic minerals). Likewise, addition of sodium chloride to food to promote polydipsia and polyuria is no longer recommended because it may promote hypercalciuria. Varying quantities of calcium are commonly found in uroliths.

SPECIFIC THERAPEUTIC GUIDELINES

Compound Uroliths With a Magnesium Ammonium Phosphate Core

The most common type of compound urolith identified at the Minnesota Urolith Center during 1996 contained a core of MAP (Table 1). As is typical of infection-induced MAP uroliths, the majority of this type of compound urolith occurred in female dogs (88%). Other mineral salts surrounding MAP included ammonium urate (5%), silica (3%), and Newberyite (1%). One urolith had a shell of a sulfadiazine metabolite. The animal had been given a drug containing sulfadiazine to treat lower urinary tract disease.

Calcium phosphate (primarily carbonate apatite) was the most common mineral found in the outer layers surrounding cores of MAP (72%). This is not unexpected because MAP and calcium phosphate uroliths share common risk factors. For example, the solubility of both salts is reduced in alkaline urine. Also, increasing urine phosphate concentration increases the risk of formation for both. Precipitation of MAP and calcium phosphate are promoted by urinary tract infections with microorganisms that hydrolyze urea into ammonia and carbonate; ammonia is a component of MAP uroliths and carbonate is a component of calcium phosphate (carbonate apatite) uroliths. What is not yet completely understood is why these salts sometimes form distinct layers in some compound uroliths but become mixed throughout other uroliths without forming distinct layers (i.e., mixed uroliths).

Fortunately, current recommendations to minimize MAP urolith recurrence also minimize calcium phosphate. Eradication or control of urinary tract infections with urease-producing microbes with appropriate antimicrobial agents

TABLE 1. **Distribution of 726 Canine Compound Uroliths**

Core Mineral	Magnesium Ammonium Phosphate	Calcium Oxalate	Silica	Calcium Phosphate	Ammonium Acid Urate	Newberyite	Xanthine	Cystine	Sulfur Metabolite	Mixed
					Mineral Composition of Outer Layer					
Magnesium ammonium phosphate (n = 320)	NA	35	10	229	17	3	0	0	1	25
Calcium oxalate (n = 297)	259	NA	11	12	6	0	2	1	0	6
Silica (n = 34)	4	28	NA	0	2	0	0	0	0	0
Calcium phosphate (n = 23)	14	9	0	NA	0	0	0	0	0	0
Ammonium acid urate (n = 14)	13	0	0	0	NA	0	0	0	0	1
Mixed (n = 38)	35	0	0	1	1	0	1	0	0	NA
Total	325	72	21	242	26	3	3	1	1	32

is fundamental. Reducing dietary protein to reduce the urine concentration of urea will minimize the quantity of ammonia generated by microbial urease. In addition, reduction of dietary protein also minimizes renal medullary urea and thus promotes polyuria. What about diets designed to acidify urine? On the one hand, acidification of urine would minimize the quantity of ionic phosphate available to form MAP and calcium phosphate. On the other hand, however, chronic acidification would promote urine calcium excretion and thus increase the risk for formation of uroliths containing calcium. Attempts to acidify urine of dogs with pre-existing MAP uroliths may be one factor explaining why 11% of uroliths with a core of MAP were surrounded by CaOx (see following section for management of compound uroliths with a CaOx core).

Compound Uroliths With a Calcium Oxalate Core

Forty-one percent of compound uroliths had a core of CaOx monohydrate or CaOx dihydrate, or both. Unlike uroliths predominantly composed of CaOx, which occur more often in males, the majority (87%) of compound uroliths with a CaOx core and a MAP shell occurred in female dogs. The paradox in managing patients forming compound uroliths with CaOx and MAP is that attempts to minimize risk factors for MAP urolith formation (such as pH, magnesium, and phosphorus) increase the risk for CaOx urolith formation. In this situation, we recommend that emphasis be placed on minimizing the recurrence of CaOx uroliths (Lulich et al, 1992), since CaOx uroliths cannot be dissolved medically. In contrast, MAP uroliths that form secondary to infections with urease-producing bacteria can often be dissolved by medical protocols. For uroliths containing both CaOx and infection-induced MAP, it is logical to assume that an initial episode of CaOx uroliths predisposed the animal to infection-induced MAP uroliths. Therefore, preventive management should include eradication or control of recurrent urinary tract infections.

In 12 dogs, a core of CaOx was surrounded by a shell of calcium phosphate. We hypothesize that excessive calcium excretion was a primary abnormality in these dogs. Since control of urine calcium excretion is emphasized in the management of CaOx uroliths, we use the same principles designed for uroliths composed entirely of CaOx to treat these dogs. Some compound uroliths contain a core of CaOx and a shell of urate salts. Consumption of diets

moderately reduced in protein that promote formation of alkaline urine commonly recommended to manage CaOx uroliths (Prescription Diet u/d) are also recommended for prevention of urate uroliths. Therefore, CaOx and urate can be managed simultaneously without apparent adverse effects.

The formation of xanthine surrounding CaOx in two dogs was probably iatrogenic, since both dogs were receiving allopurinol. Xanthine is most likely to form when allopurinol is given without reducing purine precursors in the diet.

Compound Uroliths With a Silica Core

Compound uroliths with a core of silica were primarily retrieved from male dogs (82%). The most common mineral associated with silica was CaOx (82%). Perhaps the common denominator linking these two minerals is consumption of plant-based foods that tend to contain more silica and oxalate than animal-based foods. One mineral may also serve as a template for precipitation of the other.

On the basis of logic, protocols to minimize silica urolith recurrence have been devised (Osborne et al, 1995). Since diets containing substantial quantities of corn gluten feed or soybean and rice hulls, or both, have been associated with silica uroliths and also have increased quantities of oxalate, we recommend that diets containing substantial plant proteins be avoided. When a core of silica is surrounded by CaOx or urate, strategies for prevention of the outer CaOx layer are usually compatible with a reduction in silica. When compound uroliths with a core of silica have an outer layer of MAP, urinary tract infection should also be controlled.

Compound Uroliths With a Calcium Phosphate Core

In our compound urolith series, cores of calcium phosphate were surrounded only by shells of MAP or CaOx. We managed these uroliths in a fashion similar to uroliths with cores of MAP or CaOx and outer layers of calcium phosphate.

Compound Uroliths With a Urate Core

Only 2% of compound uroliths contained a core of urate; all had a shell of MAP, except one (which had a mixture of minerals, including MAP). It is logical to assume that the original urate urolith predisposed the animal to urinary tract infection with urease-producing bacteria, which, in turn, promoted formation of MAP. In addition to protocols designed to prevent recurrence of urate uroliths, urinary tract infections should be controlled to prevent recurrence of MAP.

In our 1996 urolith series, compound uroliths with a core of urate and an outer layer of xanthine were not observed. However, we have observed this type of urolith at the Minnesota Urolith Center in the past. Xanthine precipitation commonly occurs after allopurinol administration to manage urate uroliths (Bartges et al, 1992). Unfortunately, as the urine concentration of uric acid declines in response to allopurinol therapy, the concentration of xanthine increases. Hyperxanthinuria develops because allopurinol minimizes conversion of xanthine to uric acid. The magnitude of xanthinuria increases in proportion to the quantity of purines in the diet and the frequency and dosage of allopurinol administration.

To dissolve compound uroliths containing a core of urate and a shell of xanthine, allopurinol is discontinued while a low-purine diet is continued. In our experience, diet therapy alone (canned Prescription Diet u/d) has often been successful in dissolving outer layers of drug-induced xanthine. After approximately 8 weeks of dietary management, allopurinol can again be added to the purine-restricted diet to dissolve the remaining urate core.

To prevent ammonium urate urolith recurrence, we first consider dietary therapy without giving xanthine oxidase inhibitors (i.e., allopurinol). If xanthine oxidase inhibitors are needed, we administer the smallest dose for the shortest duration. It has been suggested that allopurinol therapy that results in a 24-hour urine excretion of 300 mg of uric acid maintains uric acid and xanthine concentrations in solution (Ling et al, 1991). If the daily uric acid excretion is greater than 300 mg, the dosage of allopurinol should be increased to prevent precipitation of urate salts. When daily uric acid excretion is less than 300 mg, the dosage of allopurinol should be reduced to prevent precipitation of xanthine.

MONITORING RESPONSE

The treatment of compound uroliths often necessitates combining several unrelated treatment regimens. Therefore, it is essential to monitor the efficacy and safety of therapy. Controlling urolith-forming risk factors should reduce urine concentration (e.g., specific gravity) and eliminate crystalluria. We recommend that urinalyses be repeated every 2 to 4 weeks to determine if modifications in therapy achieve desired goals.

Because diet modification and drug therapy usually do not eliminate all underlying risk factors, it is unrealistic to expect complete elimination of all urolith recurrences. In our experience, therapy eliminates urolith recurrence in some dogs and delays urolith recurrence in others. However, the fact that uroliths recur does not always mean that additional surgery is required. The key to eliminating additional surgery is the detection of uroliths when they are small enough to pass easily through the urethral lumen. Small urocystoliths can be quickly and effectively removed by voiding urohydropropulsion (see *CVT XII*, p. 1003). Therefore, we recommend radiographic imaging of the urinary tract at least every 3 to 6 months even if animals are asymptomatic. If animals are re-evaluated only at the time they have clinical signs associated with uroliths, the uroliths are often too large to pass through the urethra.

Scheduled re-examinations may motivate clients to comply with long-term preventive therapy. By continually re-educating clients about the purpose and the expected outcomes of therapy, they are more likely to be motivated to achieve these goals.

References and Suggested Reading

Bartges JW, Osborne CA, Felice LJ: Canine xanthine uroliths: Risk factor management. In: Kirk RW, Bonagura JD, eds: Current Veterinary Therapy XI: Small Animal Practice. Philadelphia: WB Saunders, 1992, pp 900–905.
  Therapy to prevent urate and xanthine urolith recurrence is described.
Ling GV, Ruby AL, Harrold DR, et al: Xanthine-containing urinary calculi in dogs given allopurinol. J Vet Med Assoc 198:1935, 1991.
  Clinical cases of canine xanthine uroliths are described.
Lulich JP, Osborne CA, Smith CL: Canine calcium oxalate urolithiasis: Risk factor management. In: Kirk RW, Bonagura JD, eds: Current Veterinary Therapy XI: Small Animal Practice. Philadelphia: WB Saunders, 1992, pp 892–899.
  Therapy to prevent calcium oxalate urolith recurrence is described.
Osborne CA, Lulich JP, Bartges JW, et al: Canine and feline urolithiasis: Relationship of etiopathogenesis to treatment and prevention. In: Osborne CA, Finco DR, eds: Canine and Feline Nephrology and Urology. Baltimore: Williams & Wilkins, 1995, pp 798–888.
  Therapy to prevent silica urolith recurrence is described.

Urinary Tract Infections Associated With Endocrine Disorders in Dogs

S. Dru Forrester

Gregory C. Troy

Blacksburg, Virginia

The prevalence of urinary tract infection (UTI) in dogs with diabetes mellitus (DM) or hyperadrenocorticism (HAC), or both, is higher than in other dogs presented for veterinary evaluation. Approximately 15% of dogs experience UTI in their lifetime compared with 40 to 50% of dogs with DM or HAC, or both. In addition, the prevalence of UTI in dogs treated with chronic administration of glucocorticosteroids is approximately 50%.

PATHOGENESIS OF URINARY TRACT INFECTION

It is difficult for UTI to develop in normal animals because of intrinsic mechanisms that protect against bacterial colonization of the urinary tract. Except for the distal urethra, the urinary tract of normal dogs is sterile. Organisms that colonize the lower genital tract and distal urethra help prevent UTI by inhibiting adherence of pathogenic bacteria and possibly their growth. Frequent and complete voiding physically removes bacteria from the urinary tract. Anatomic factors that cause unidirectional movement of urine and prevent UTI include ureteral peristalsis, ureterovesical flap valves, prostatic secretions, surface characteristics of urothelium, urethral length, urethral peristalsis, and urethral sphincter pressure. Mucosal defenses, including production of antibody, intrinsic antimicrobial properties, and a surface layer of glycosaminoglycans, help prevent bacterial colonization of the urinary tract. Urine also has intrinsic antimicrobial properties, which include very alkaline or acidic pH, hyperosmolality, and high urea concentration. Lastly, systemic humoral and cellular immunity also play a role in the prevention of UTI in normal animals.

Most UTIs result from organisms that ascend from the distal urogenital tract and establish infection in the urethra and urinary bladder and possibly the ureters and kidneys. Organisms that cause UTI are also the same as those that colonize the lower urogenital tract and perineal area of normal dogs. Any disorder that interferes with host defenses or causes urinary tract dysfunction (e.g., production of dilute urine or the presence of uroliths) predisposes the animal to UTI. Females have a higher incidence of UTIs, possibly because of a relatively shorter urethra and a lack of prostatic secretions.

Several mechanisms have been suggested to explain the predisposition to UTI in dogs with DM or HAC. Both disorders cause polyuria and decreased urine osmolality, which may increase the likelihood of lower UTI. Excessive production of cortisol in dogs with HAC may cause immunosuppression or decrease the normal inflammatory response to infection. In addition to dogs with spontaneous HAC, those treated with long-term prednisone have a high occurrence of UTI. Glucosuria associated with DM may cause dysfunction of neutrophils, which predisposes to infections, including those of the urinary tract.

Organisms that cause UTI in dogs with DM or HAC, or both, are similar to those in dogs with UTI from other causes. *Escherichia coli* is isolated in 65% of dogs; other organisms include *Klebsiella* sp. (15%), *Streptococcus* sp. (14%), *Enterobacter* sp. (7%), *Staphylococcus* spp. (7%), *Enterococcus* spp. (7%), and *Proteus* spp. (7%). Approximately 80% of dogs with UTI and DM or HAC have infection with a single organism, and 20% have two or more infecting organisms.

CLINICAL FINDINGS

Most dogs with DM or HAC and UTI are older, with a median age of 9 years. Miniature Schnauzers, Cocker spaniels, and Poodles appear predisposed to the development of UTI, whereas Golden retrievers, Labrador retrievers, and mixed breeds are underrepresented.

Clinical signs of UTI, including stranguria, dysuria, hematuria, and pollakiuria, are observed in less than 10% of dogs with HAC or DM. This may be due to the anti-inflammatory effects of excessive cortisol in dogs with HAC. It also is possible that owners are more likely to notice polyuria, which is common in dogs with either DM or HAC. Lack of stranguria, dysuria, and pollakiuria may indicate that dogs with DM or HAC have upper UTI (i.e., renal-ureteral infection), which may not cause signs of lower UTI. Physical examination reveals findings typical of DM or HAC, including cataracts, dermatologic abnormalities (pyoderma, thin skin, alopecia, calcinosis cutis), hepatomegaly, and abdominal distention.

DIAGNOSTIC EVALUATION

Routine laboratory evaluation reveals findings characteristic of DM or HAC, including a stress leukogram, hyperglycemia, increased hepatic enzyme activity, hypercholesterolemia, and glucosuria. Urine specific gravity is variable, but most dogs have values less than 1.020. Urine pH is normal and in most dogs ranges from 6 to 7. Proteinuria occurs in two thirds of dogs with HAC or DM, whether UTI exists or not. Urine sediment evaluation reveals hematuria in 45%, pyuria in 60%, and bacteriuria in 65% of dogs with UTI and HAC or DM. Therefore, UTI cannot be ruled out if the urine sediment examination is normal.

Because of the prevalence of UTI in dogs with either

TABLE 1. Antimicrobial Agents for Treatment of Urinary Tract Infections in Dogs With Hyperadrenocorticism or Diabetes Mellitus, or Both, Based on Minimal Inhibitory Concentrations: Results in Clinical Cases

Organism	Recommended Drugs	Alternative Drugs
Escherichia coli	Enrofloxacin or norfloxacin Trimethoprim-sulfa Amoxicillin–clavulanic acid	Nitrofurantoin Chloramphenicol
Klebsiella spp.	Enrofloxacin or norfloxacin	Amoxicillin–clavulanic acid Trimethoprim-sulfa Cephalexin or cefadroxil
Streptococcus spp.	Ampicillin or amoxicillin Amoxicillin–clavulanic acid	Cephalexin or cefadroxil Chloramphenicol Erythromycin
Staphylococcus spp.	Ampicillin or amoxicillin Cephalexin or cefadroxil	Trimethoprim-sulfa Chloramphenicol Erythromycin
Enterobacter spp.	Enrofloxacin or norfloxacin	Trimethoprim-sulfa
Enterococcus spp.	Enrofloxacin or norfloxacin Trimethoprim-sulfa	Chloramphenicol Tetracycline
Proteus spp.	Ampicillin or amoxicillin Enrofloxacin or norfloxacin	Amoxicillin–clavulanic acid Cephalexin or cefadroxil

HAC or DM and a lack of clinical signs, a urine culture should be performed routinely. Urine collected by cystocentesis should be submitted for quantitative culture to determine the number of bacterial organisms per milliliter of urine because small numbers of bacteria (<100 colony-forming units/ml) may indicate contamination during collection or transfer of urine samples. However, if a patient with UTI has received antimicrobial agents within 3 to 7 days of urine collection for culture, bacterial numbers may be lower than expected. Results of culture also should be interpreted together with clinical signs and urine sediment findings. Animals with stranguria, pollakiuria, pyuria, bacteriuria, or hematuria and growth of small numbers of bacteria probably have UTI.

TREATMENT

Antimicrobial treatment is indicated if the urine culture reveals significant bacterial growth. Because UTI in animals with DM or HAC is considered complicated and may interfere with appropriate management of the endocrine disorder, selection of an antimicrobial agent should be based on results of urine culture and susceptibility. While awaiting results of culture, an antimicrobial that is likely to be effective against organisms causing UTI may be administered (Table 1). Unless the patient has received antimicrobial agents recently, the susceptibility of most bacteria that cause UTI is predictable. However, there is enough variation that long-term treatment of UTI in patients with HAC or DM should be based on culture and susceptibility results.

Selection of an appropriate antimicrobial agent for each patient is based on several factors. First, one should consider the drug's minimal inhibitory concentration for the infecting organism (also see p. 33). Antimicrobial agents whose urine concentrations are at least four times the minimal inhibitory concentration generally are effective for treatment of UTI (Table 2). Although the quinolones,

including enrofloxacin (Baytril, Haver; see p. 41) and norfloxacin (Noroxin, Merck), are effective for treatment of most UTIs, they should not be used indiscriminately because this may select for growth of resistant organisms for which there is no effective treatment. If a patient has a polymicrobial infection, an antimicrobial that is effective for all organisms should be selected. If this is not possible, it usually is best to treat each organism sequentially instead of administering a combination of drugs. Although bacteriostatic drugs (e.g., chloramphenicol, erythromycin, nitrofurantoin, tetracycline) may be effective for the treatment of UTI, it is preferable to administer bactericidal antimicrobial agents to patients with DM or HAC because of their impaired host defenses. In intact male dogs, prostatic infection is likely, and an antimicrobial agent that reaches adequate concentrations within the prostate gland is preferred (e.g., chloramphenicol, erythromycin, quinolones, tetracycline, trimethoprim-sulfa).

Except for the quinolones and trimethoprim-sulfa, which are effective when administered twice daily, all antimicrobial agents used to treat animals with UTI should be

TABLE 2. Guidelines for Antimicrobial Treatment of Urinary Tract Infections in Dogs

Drug	MIC Cutoff	Dosage Regimen
Ampicillin	≤ 64 µg/ml	25 mg/kg PO q8hr
Amoxicillin	≤ 32 µg/ml	11 mg/kg PO q8hr
Amoxicillin– clavulanic acid	≤ 32 µg/ml	16.5 mg/kg PO q8hr
Cefadroxil	≤ 32 µg/ml	10–20 mg/kg PO q8hr
Cephalexin	≤ 32 µg/ml	30–40 mg/kg PO q8hr
Chloramphenicol	≤ 16 µg/ml	33 mg/kg PO q8hr
Enrofloxacin	≤ 8 µg/ml	2.5 mg/kg PO q12hr
Nitrofurantoin	≤ 16 µg/ml	5 mg/kg PO q8hr
Tetracycline	≤ 32 µg/ml	18 mg/kg PO q8hr
Trimethoprim (sulfa)	≤ 2 µg/ml (≤ 16 µg/ml)	15 mg/kg PO q12hr

administered three times daily. To help maintain adequate urine concentrations of antimicrobial agents, owners should administer drugs immediately after the animal urinates and just before expected periods of confinement (e.g., bedtime). Ideal duration of treatment for patients with HAC or DM is unknown, although it seems reasonable to administer antimicrobial agents until the underlying endocrine disorder is well controlled. A minimum of 4 to 6 weeks is recommended, although some patients may require longer treatment to eradicate infection.

It is important to monitor patients to determine efficacy and detect relapsing or recurrent infections. Because most patients with HAC or DM and UTI show no clinical signs, and many do not have urine sediment abnormalities, quantitative and qualitative urine culture must be used to monitor treatment. A urine culture should be performed 3 to 5 days after treatment begins and again 7 days after the antimicrobial agents are discontinued. If either culture reveals bacterial growth, treatment is adjusted on the basis of susceptibility results and repeat cultures to ensure the new antimicrobial agent has eradicated the UTI. Because the ideal duration of treatment is unknown, it is recommended that urine culture be performed every month until three consecutive negative cultures are obtained. It is common for animals with DM or HAC to have recurrent UTI throughout life; therefore, urine cultures should be performed routinely whenever these patients are evaluated (e.g., every 3 to 6 months).

References and Suggested Reading

Ihrke PJ, Norton AL, Ling GV, et al: Urinary tract infection associated with long-term corticosteroid administration in dogs with chronic skin diseases. J Am Vet Med Assoc 186:43, 1985.
This retrospective study describes clinical signs and results of urine culture in 71 dogs receiving prednisone for the treatment of dermatologic disorders.
Ling GV, Biberstein EL, Hirsh DC: Bacterial pathogens associated with urinary tract infections. Vet Clin North Am 9:617, 1978.
This is a review of organisms that cause UTI in dogs, including techniques for performing quantitative urine culture.
Ling GV, Stabenfeldt GH, Comer KM, et al: Canine hyperadrenocorticism: Pretreatment clinical and laboratory evaluation of 117 cases. J Am Vet Med Assoc 174:1211, 1977.
This article presents a retrospective study of clinical findings and results of laboratory findings in dogs with hyperadrenocorticism.
Lorenz MD: Diagnosis and medical management of canine Cushing's syndrome: A study of 57 consecutive cases. J Am Anim Hosp Assoc 18:707, 1982.
This article discusses a retrospective study of dogs with HAC, including clinical findings and results of laboratory evaluation and urine culture.
Osborne CA, Lees GE: Bacterial infections of the canine and feline urinary tract. In: Osborne CA, Finco DR, eds: Canine and Feline Nephrology and Urology. Baltimore: Williams & Wilkins, 1995, p 759.
This article presents a thorough review of UTIs, including host defense mechanisms, the pathogenesis of UTI, diagnostic findings, and treatment.

Bacterial Urinary Tract Infection in Cats

JOSEPH W. BARTGES
Knoxville, Tennessee

JEANNE A. BARSANTI
Athens, Georgia

INCIDENCE

A bacterial urinary tract infection exists when bacteria adhere, multiply, and persist in a portion of the urinary tract that is normally sterile. The infection may or may not produce clinical signs. The reported incidence of bacterial urinary tract infections in cats is variable. In prospective studies that have evaluated lower urinary tract disease in young cats, bacterial urinary tract infections were diagnosed in less than 5% of cases (Kruger et al, 1991; Lees, 1996; Buffington et al, 1997). These findings indicate that bacterial urinary tract infection is rarely the cause of lower urinary tract disease in young adult cats. In a number of studies, however, bacterial urinary tract infections were found in 15 to 43% of cats evaluated (Lees, 1996). In one study, urinary tract infections were present in 25% of 1,380 urine cultures performed at a university hospital over a 12-year period (Davidson et al, 1992). The average age of cats with bacterial urinary tract infection was 8.2 years, with the average age of infected males being 6.3 years, and the average age of infected females being 10.6 years. In a retrospective study performed at the University of Georgia, bacterial urinary tract infection was diagnosed in 45% of cats older than 10 years with signs of lower urinary tract disease (Bartges, 1996). Two thirds of these cats also were diagnosed with renal failure, whereas the remaining cats were diagnosed with hyperthyroidism; feline immunodeficiency or feline leukemia virus infection, or both; incontinence; or neoplasia or they were undergoing corticosteroid and diuretic treatment. Only one cat had no identifiable predisposing cause.

Findings from these studies indicate that bacterial urinary tract infection is uncommon in young cats with lower urinary tract disease, but bacterial urinary tract infection is an important problem in geriatric cats (Table 1). Older cats may be at increased risk for the development of bacterial urinary tract infection, because of diminished urinary tract defenses. Whether impaired defenses are intrinsic to the aging process or secondary to disorders that are more common in geriatric cats is unknown. We hypothesize that some conditions that are more common in older cats, such as renal failure, diabetes mellitus, and hyperthyroidism, impair the normal defense mechanisms of older cats.

TABLE 1. Diagnostic and Therapeutic Caveats

Bacterial urinary tract infections are uncommon in young cats (occurring in <5% of cats with lower urinary tract disease) but are common in older cats (occurring in >40% of cats with lower urinary tract disease).

In cats older than 10 yr, bacterial cystitis is often associated with a predisposing cause that alters the body's defense mechanisms; approximately two thirds of affected cats have renal failure that not only predisposes to bacterial infection but also may result from bacterial pyelonephritis.

Because bacterial urinary tract infections are uncommon in young cats, routine use of antibiotics is not indicated in those with lower urinary tract disease. In older cats, use of antibiotics may be indicated once a bacterial infection is confirmed and appropriate testing is performed to determine the type of bacterium and its antibiotic sensitivity pattern.

In older cats, administration of antibiotics for longer than 10 to 14 days may be indicated because bacterial infections are often associated with renal failure, and eradication of bacteria from the upper urinary tract may be difficult.

Follow-up evaluations of cats with urinary tract infections are recommended because bacterial urinary tract infections in cats are often associated with predisposing diseases that may or may not be treatable.

When performing diagnostic or therapeutic procedures that involve insertion of a catheter or endoscope into the lower urinary tract, periprocedural antibiotic therapy for 24 hr before the procedure and continuing for 2 to 3 days after the procedure is indicated. In addition, evaluation of a urine sample collected 5 to 7 days after discontinuing antibiotic therapy is recommended to ensure that bacterial infection of the lower urinary tract has not occurred.

Cats have many defense mechanisms that aid in the prevention of bacterial invasion of the urinary tract (Lulich and Osborne, 1995). Anatomically, the length of the urethra, presence of high-pressure zones within the urethra, urethral and ureteral peristalsis, vesicoureteral flaps to prevent reflux of urine from the bladder into the ureters, and extensive renal blood supply and flow are protective. Mucosal defense barriers that prevent migration of bacteria and subsequent colonization include the presence of a glycosaminoglycan layer, antibody production, intrinsic mucosal antimicrobial properties, exfoliation of cells, and bacterial interference by commensal microbes of the distal urethra and distal genital tract. The composition of the urine also aids in the prevention of bacterial urinary tract infection. Urine produced by cats is normally concentrated, often having a specific gravity greater than 1.045 with an associated high osmolality. Urine also contains substances that are inhibitory to bacterial colonization, including a high urea concentration and the presence of organic acids, low molecular weight carbohydrates, and Tamm-Horsfall mucoproteins. Cell-mediated and humorally mediated immunity present within the urine or urinary tract also impart protection. Although cats void only once or twice a day, they usually empty their bladder completely, and there is a normal turnover of mucosal cells of the urinary tract that helps wash out bacteria that have migrated into the bladder, ureters, and kidneys.

PHYSICAL EXAMINATION FINDINGS AND CLINICAL SIGNS

Clinically, bacterial urinary tract infections may be symptomatic or asymptomatic. Bacterial infection of the lower urinary tract is usually associated with clinical signs that are similar to other diseases of the lower urinary tract. These signs include, but are not limited to, pollakiuria, dysuria, stranguria, hematuria, and inappropriate urination. Bacterial urinary tract infection of the kidneys may be associated with hematuria, or if septicemia develops, the cat may be systemically ill. In addition, upper urinary tract infections may cause recurrent lower urinary tract infections.

DIAGNOSIS

Urinalysis and Urine Culture

Evaluating results of a complete urinalysis of a sample collected by cystocentesis is the best way to screen for bacterial urinary tract infection. Presence of pyuria (>5 white blood cells/high-power field) is important because other causes of lower urinary tract disease in cats are associated with hematuria and proteinuria but minimal pyuria. Identification of bacteria on urine sediment examination is helpful; however, it should not be relied on to rule in or rule out bacterial urinary tract infections. Urine specific gravity may be normal; however, in one study, cats with bacterial urinary tract infection also had dilute urine associated with renal failure, hyperthyroidism, and diuretic therapy (Bartges, 1996).

A urine culture is the most definitive means of diagnosing bacterial urinary tract infections. Care must be taken to collect, preserve, and transport the urine sample to avoid contamination or proliferation or death of bacteria. Urine specimens for aerobic bacterial culture should be transported and stored in sealed, sterilized containers, and processing should begin as soon as possible. If laboratory processing is delayed by more than 30 minutes, the specimen should be refrigerated (4°C). Blood agar plates may be inoculated and incubated for 24 hours. If bacteria are present on the plate after 24 hours, the plate may be submitted for identification and determination of antibiotic sensitivities.

Bacteria that commonly cause urinary tract infections in cats are the same types that frequently cause urinary tract infections in dogs. Infections caused by *Escherichia coli* are the most common, accounting for one third to one half of all organisms isolated from the urine of infected cats. Gram-positive cocci are the second major group of organisms. Staphylococci and streptococci account for one fourth to one third of the isolates recovered. Bacteria that cause the remaining one fourth to one third of urinary tract infections in cats include *Proteus* spp., *Klebsiella* spp., *Pasteurella* spp., *Enterobacter* spp., *Pseudomonas* spp., *Corynebacterium* spp., and *Mycoplasma* spp.; however, each of these types of bacteria has been found in only a few of the infected cats (Lees, 1996).

Unless septicemia is present, results of a complete blood count should be normal. If septicemia is present, leukocytosis and a left shift may be present. Bacterial infection of the lower urinary tract does not cause changes in serum biochemical analysis. In cats with bacterial infection of the kidneys, serum biochemical analysis may be normal if only one kidney is infected or if minimal damage has occurred, or it may reveal biochemical changes consistent with renal failure. Hyperthyroidism has also been associated with inducing a diuresis and bacterial urinary tract infections in cats. Additional laboratory evaluation may include testing for feline leukemia virus and feline immunodeficiency virus, which may compromise the immune system.

Radiography, Ultrasonography, and Endoscopy

In many cats with bacterial urinary tract infections, radiographic results will be normal. However, survey radiography may reveal uroliths, renomegaly, or other defects that may predispose to the development of bacterial urinary tract infection. Uroliths were present in approximately 20% of young cats evaluated for lower urinary tract disease (Kruger et al, 1991; Buffington et al, 1997). In another study, uroliths were present in approximately 10% of cats older than the age of 10 years with signs of lower urinary tract disease (Bartges, 1996). If no abnormalities are found by survey abdominal radiography, ultrasonography or contrast radiography should be performed. The upper urinary tract may be evaluated by excretory urography; whereas the lower urinary tract may be evaluated by contrast cystography and urethrography and double-contrast cystography. A disadvantage of performing contrast radiography of the lower urinary tract is the risk of inducing bacterial urinary tract infections during catheterization. Ultrasonography is a noninvasive technique and can evaluate the kidneys and bladder; however, its use is limited for evaluating the ureters and the majority of the urethra.

Endoscopy of the lower urinary tract may be useful in identifying mucosal and intraluminal lesions of the urinary tract that may predispose to bacterial infection. In one study, a urolith not visible by survey radiography was visualized during cystoscopy (Buffington et al, 1997). Disadvantages of cystourethroscopy include requiring anesthesia to perform the procedure; invasion of the lower urinary tract, which may compromise host defense mechanisms; and the difficulty of performing the procedure in male cats without perineal urethrostomies.

TREATMENT

Treatment of bacterial urinary tract infections in cats is dependent on whether the infection results from a temporary breech in the body's defense mechanisms (uncomplicated) or whether there is an irreversible breech in the defense mechanisms (complicated). Eradication of bacterial urinary tract infection is dependent on selection of the appropriate antibiotic, administering it at the proper dosage and duration, and appropriate follow-up.

Because bacterial urinary tract infection is uncommon in cats less than 10 years of age, routine use of antibiotics in young cats with lower urinary tract disease is not recommended. However, because bacterial urinary tract infection is common in cats older than 10 years, and when present

is often associated with renal failure, infectious disease, or other systemic disease, aggressive antibiotic therapy is recommended. Treatment with antibiotics for longer than the routine 10 to 14 days may be indicated. Furthermore, in older cats, serial evaluations are indicated. Use of once-daily antibiotic treatment may be necessary in order to control bacterial urinary tract infections that are difficult to eradicate.

PREVENTION

Bacterial urinary tract infections in cats can be prevented by minimizing bacterial contamination of the urinary tract and by avoiding or minimizing conditions that impair host defenses. Catheterization and endoscopy of the urinary tract always carries a risk of inducing an infection. The magnitude of the risk increases with the degree of pre-existing urinary tract abnormality, the amount of any additional injury caused by the procedure, and the duration of the procedure. These risks of infection can be minimized by being careful to perform invasive procedures only when necessary, by performing the procedure as atraumatically as possible, and by removing the catheter or endoscope as soon as possible. Cats with perineal urethrostomies are also at higher risk for the development of bacterial urinary tract infections compared with cats without perineal urethrostomies (Lees, 1996; Lulich and Osborne, 1995); thus, other therapeutic interventions should be tried before resorting to this procedure.

References and Suggested Reading

Bartges JW: Lower urinary tract disease in geriatric cats: What's common, what's not. In: Proceedings of a Symposium on Health and Nutrition of Geriatric Cats and Dogs. Orlando, FL, 1996, p 39.
This is a review of lower urinary tract disease in cats older than 10 years.
Buffington CA, Chew DJ, Kendall MS, et al: Clinical evaluation of cats with nonobstructive urinary tract diseases. J Am Vet Med Assoc 210:46, 1997.
This article describes a prospective study of 109 cats with nonobstructive lower urinary tract disease.
Davidson AP, Ling GV, Stevens E, et al: Urinary tract infection in cats: A retrospective study, 1977–1989. California Vet 46:32, 1992.
This is a retrospective study of bacterial urinary tract infections in cats.
Kruger JM, Osborne CA, Goyal SM, et al: Clinical evaluation of cats with lower urinary tract disease. J Am Vet Med Assoc 199:211, 1991.
This article presents a prospective study of lower urinary tract disease in 143 cats.
Lees GE: Bacterial urinary tract infections. Vet Clin North Am Small Anim Pract 26:297, 1996.
This article reviews the incidence, diagnosis, treatment, and prevention of bacterial urinary tract infections in cats.
Lulich JP, Osborne CA: Bacterial urinary tract infections. In: Ettinger SJ, Feldman EC, eds: Textbook of Veterinary Internal Medicine. 4th ed, Philadelphia: WB Saunders, 1995, p 1775.
This is a review of the incidence, diagnosis, treatment, and prevention of bacterial urinary tract infections in cats and dogs.

Management of Difficult Urinary Tract Infections

DAVID F. SENIOR

Baton Rouge, Louisiana

A TYPICAL APPROACH

The usual work-up of an animal with "difficult" urinary tract infection (UTI) includes an evaluation to determine whether appropriate antimicrobial drugs, based on culture and sensitivity tests, were given for appropriate periods. If so, consideration of impaired host defenses requires another urinalysis and culture on urine collected by cystocentesis, evaluation of bladder urine volume at the end of urination, and imaging of the urinary tract to include plain and contrast radiographs and ultrasonography. Underlying conditions that disrupt normal host defenses should be treated and eliminated when possible (Table 1). Antimicrobial treatment should be based on culture and sensitivity test results with consideration given to tissue penetration and duration of treatment. Follow-up bacterial culture of urine is necessary for documenting the success of treatment. If infections tend to recur despite no obvious underlying condition that would lead to disruption of host defenses, long-term low-dose treatment can be given for 6 months. When an untreatable underlying condition is present (e.g.,

neoplasia), treatment with antimicrobials can lead to infection with progressively more resistant bacteria. Under these circumstances, provided that there is no evidence of renal involvement, it may be better to leave the animal untreated.

BACTERIAL VIRULENCE VERSUS HOST DEFENSES

In managing animals with UTI, clinicians must remember the mechanisms by which the urinary tract remains free of infection. Openings to the body—for example, mouth, anus, urethra, and vulva—are colonized by normal flora. Yet the bladder and proximal urethra are normally sterile. Clearly, there are innate defense mechanisms that prevent the development of UTI.

The presence or absence of infection depends on the balance between bacterial virulence and host defenses. If host defenses are normal, only very virulent organisms are capable of invading and colonizing the urinary tract. If host defenses are compromised, relatively avirulent opportunistic organisms can colonize successfully and maintain an infection.

In "simple" infections, a relatively virulent organism has invaded and colonized an otherwise normal urinary tract or a tract that has suffered a temporary reduction in host defenses, for example, temporary placement of an indwelling urinary catheter. Virulent organisms attach avidly to the uroepithelial surface by specific binding mechanisms and trigger a rapid and intense immunologic response. With gram-negative bacteria, the most common isolates in UTI of dogs and cats, the immunologic response is triggered by lipid A (endotoxin) emanating from the surface of the bacterial cell wall. The subsequent inflammatory cascade contributes to the signs of hematuria, dysuria, pollakiuria, and stranguria. Such signs are readily observed by owners who then present their animals for veterinary care. Antimicrobial agents are administered; the invading microorganism is destroyed by a combination of direct antimicrobial effects and the animal's immune system; and all necessary natural defense mechanisms are reestablished. After the cessation of treatment, the animal remains free of infection.

Difficult to treat UTIs are those caused by colonization of the urinary tract by resistant organisms (e.g., *Pseudomonas* spp.), deep-seated infections in difficult to penetrate locations, and infections due to a prolonged breakdown in the natural defense mechanisms so that colonization and subsequent bacterial tissue invasion recur soon after cessation of antimicrobial treatment. When natural host defense mechanisms are depleted, the urinary tract is at risk for colonization by relatively avirulent, opportunistic microor-

TABLE 1. Established and Hypothesized Host Defense Mechanisms in the Urinary Tract

Host Defenses	Disrupting Factors
Normal Micturation	
Adequate urine flow	Urethral obstruction
Frequent voiding	Disc disease
Complete voiding	Atonic bladder
Anatomic Structures	
Urethral high-pressure zone	Perineal urethrostomy
Characteristics of urothelium	Urethral catheterization
Urethral peristalsis	Ureteral obstruction
Prostatic antibacterial fraction	?
Length of urethra	Perineal urethrostomy
Ureterovesical flap valves	Ectopic ureter
Ureteral peristalsis	Ureteral obstruction
Mucosal Defense Barriers	
Antibody production	Hyperadrenocorticoidism
Surface glycosaminoglycan layer	Polyps, neoplasia
Mucosal antimicrobial properties	?
Bacterial interference	Antibiotic-induced yeast Infections
Exfoliation of cells	?
Antimicrobial Properties of Urine	
Extremes of urine pH	Funguria inhibited in high pH
Hyperosmolality	Hyperadrenocorticism
High concentration of urea	Same
Organic acids	?
Renal Defenses	
Glomerular mesangial cells	?
High renal blood flow	Dehydration

883

ganisms. Such microorganisms often do not attach to the uroepithelial surface avidly, do not present endotoxin to the epithelial wall effectively, and do not induce an intense inflammatory response. Infected animals can have few if any clinical signs, except for a pungent urine odor, and the infection can persist almost indefinitely.

Differentiation between persistence of the same infection and reinfection with another infection is possible if the animal becomes infected with an entirely new species of bacteria, for example, reinfection with *Escherichia coli* after initial infection with a *Proteus* sp. However, if the animal becomes reinfected with the same species of bacteria, definitive diagnosis of persistent infection is difficult because analysis of the serotype and biotype of the original and new strains would be necessary to differentiate between them—not a practical proposition in a clinical setting. Factors that may lead to the persistence of infection are shown in Table 2. However, an infection can never be assumed to be persistent; thus, even if it appears to be caused by the same strain as that isolated before treatment, factors that cause both persistent infection and reinfection should always be considered in the evaluation of animals with difficult UTI.

Once it is recognized that infections are persisting or recurring, it is necessary to identify and then eliminate conditions that have compromised host defenses (see Table 1). Clearly, some conditions are easily identified and treated, others are identifiable but not easily treated, and others are beyond the realm of our current diagnostic armamentarium. In all surveys of the infecting organisms in UTI of dogs and cats, *E. coli* is the most common isolate with *Staphylococcus intermedius*, *Streptococcus* spp., and *Proteus* spp. making up most of the other isolates. On occasion, *Klebsiella pneumoniae* may also be included in this number. Certain strains of these species constitute the most common "primary" pathogens causing UTI. However, many strains of *E. coli* and *Klebsiella* spp. are relatively avirulent and can live almost in a commensal relationship in a poorly defended urinary tract. Thus, when urinalysis reveals bacteria but few leukocytes and erythrocytes in the urine sediment, or when known opportunists such as *Pseudomonas aeruginosa*, *Enterobacter cloacae*, and *Acinetobacter* spp. are isolated from a urine culture, the infecting bacteria are relatively avirulent and the host defenses are probably compromised. These circumstances indicate the need for a more extensive diagnostic evaluation.

The difference between virulence and antimicrobial resistance should be recognized. Virulent organisms can invade and colonize a normal urinary tract and induce an intense inflammatory reaction; however, they may be sensi-tive to a wide array of the drugs commonly used to treat UTI. Avirulent organisms are opportunists, capable only of invading a compromised urinary tract, but they may be exceedingly resistant to antimicrobial agents. The obvious example is *P. aeruginosa,* which is an opportunistic infection in the urinary tract but tends to be resistant to antimicrobial action.

MANAGEMENT

Drug Selection

In difficult cases of UTI, urine culture and sensitivity testing should be performed. Accurate documentation of the presence of an infection and accurate determination of the most likely drugs to be successful take much of the conjecture and guesswork out of the management process. To avoid confusion because of contamination from the external genitals and distal urethra, only urine collected by cystocentesis should be used for culture and sensitivity testing. Sensitivity tests are designed to predict the likelihood of successful treatment based on achievable antimicrobial levels in plasma and urine. If four times the minimal inhibitory concentration (MIC) (see p. 33) of the microorganism can be achieved at the site of infection, the likelihood of success in the treatment of UTI is high. In some instances, when four times the MIC cannot be achieved, successful treatment can result with drugs that achieve only twice the MIC. In lower UTIs of female dogs, achievable concentrations of the antimicrobial in urine are applicable (Table 3).

Antimicrobials diffuse into both the prostatic and the renal parenchyma from the blood. Success can be expected in the treatment of infections involving either of these organs only if four times the MIC for the antimicrobial agent can be achieved at the tissue site of infection.

In intact male dogs with UTI, the prostate is almost always a concurrent site of infection. Failure to eliminate infection from the prostate can leave a focus of infection from which the rest of the urinary tract can be recolonized once antimicrobial treatment is discontinued. In addition, a residual focus of infection in the prostate can lead to relatively rare but usually devastating prostatic abscessation. Three factors affect antimicrobial diffusion into the prostate gland: pKa, lipid solubility, and the degree of protein binding in plasma. Based on these criteria, enrofloxacin, trimethoprim, doxycycline, and tetracycline all are good choices, although of these, enrofloxacin and trimethoprim have the broadest spectrum of activity. Recent experimental evidence suggests that castration can enhance resolution of prostatic infections.

Client compliance is enhanced if the medication regimen is relatively inexpensive, easy to administer, and can be readily followed within the owner's schedule. Dividing the total daily dose into two convenient subdoses rather than a more frequent regimen leads to better compliance. Palatable liquids or tablets wrapped in treats may be easier for the client to administer, depending on the nature of the pet. Clinicians are wise to inquire in this regard. Owners appreciate both the thoughtfulness and the higher probability of success compared with a difficult or perhaps impossible medication schedule.

TABLE 2. Factors Causing Persistence of Urinary Tract Infection

Wrong medication
Poor owner compliance
   Inadequate plasma and urine drug levels
   Duration of treatment too short
Impaired absorption of the antimicrobial from the gastrointestinal tract
Persistence of infection in difficult to penetrate locations
   Prostate, kidney, thickened bladder wall, polyps

TABLE 3. Dosage and Mean Urinary Concentration of the Drugs Commonly Used to Treat Urinary Tract Infection

Agent	Dose	Route	Mean Urine Concentration (±S.D.) μg/ml (U/ml)*	BREAKPOINT* μg/ml (U/ml)*
Ampicillin	12 mg/lb t.i.d.	PO	309 (±55)	77
Amoxicillin	5 mg/lb t.i.d.	PO	202 (±93)	50
Tetracycline	8 mg/lb t.i.d.	PO	138 (±65)	35
Chloramphenicol	15 mg/lb t.i.d.	PO	124 (±40)	31
Cephalexin	15 mg/lb t.i.d.	PO	500 (—)	125
Trimethoprim-sulfa	5 mg/lb b.i.d.	PO	246 (±150)	62
	1 mg/lb b.i.d.		55 (±19)	14
Enrofloxacin	2.5 mg/kg b.i.d.	PO	40	10–12
Gentamicin	1 mg/lb t.i.d.	SC	107 (±33)	27
Amikacin	2.3 mg/lb t.i.d.	SC	342 (±143)	85
	(10 mg/kg b.i.d.)	(SC or IM)		

*Organisms are considered sensitive if the MIC is less than the breakpoint.
PO, by mouth; SC, subcutaneously; IM, intramuscularly; t.i.d., three times daily; b.i.d., twice daily.
Courtesy of Dr. G. Ling, UC Davis.

Duration of Treatment

Although the duration of treatment in dogs and cats has not been studied closely, infections of the lower urinary tract in female dogs are usually treated for 7 to 10 days. For infections in male dogs in which the prostate is most likely involved and for infection of the upper urinary tract, treatment for 30 to 40 days is recommended.

More and more frequently, clinicians are confronted with infections caused by multiresistant organisms. Extended sensitivity testing should be performed to identify possible drugs that might be successful. For resistant *Klebsiella* spp., the cephalosporins tend to be relatively successful.

For *P. aeruginosa*, the fluoroquinolones and aminoglycosides are usually successful, although extreme care should be taken when treating with aminoglycosides because of their tendency to induce acute renal failure. Although the toxicity of gentamicin can be reduced by giving the drug only once daily, extended treatment for longer than 7 to 10 days is risky.

The only reliable indicator of successful treatment is a negative urine culture. Owners should be advised that the medication should be continued until the prescription is finished even if clinical signs disappear. The effectiveness of a particular treatment may be established by culturing the urine 3 to 5 days after the beginning of treatment. With effective treatment, a negative urine culture will be obtained. A culture performed at the end of treatment allows detection of superinfections—those that develop during treatment despite the administration of antimicrobial agents. Certainly, cultures should be obtained 10 to 14 days after the cessation of treatment to determine if the infection has recurred. In all instances, urine should be collected by cystocentesis to obtain unequivocal results. Under no circumstances should the bladder be catheterized once treatment has commenced because the catheter will introduce microorganisms into the bladder, and disruption of the urethral mucosa provides easy access for ascending infection.

Special Problems

Animals with hyperadrenocorticism are prone to UTI. The cause of this predisposition is not clear, but it may be due to reduced immunologic response or reduced urine concentration associated with high levels of plasma cortisol. Control of hyperadrenocorticism or withdrawal of glucocorticoid treatment tends to prevent recurrence of infection.

Vulval involution can lead to vulval fold pyoderma. Some animals so affected tend to have a variety of signs, including dysuria and pollakiuria. Passage of urine over the inflamed skin of the vulval fold causes pain; dogs tend to stop urine flow midstream, cry out, and retain a high bladder urine volume. Urine retention and bacterial overgrowth in the perivulval region tends to induce recurrent UTI. Vulvoplasty to surgically correct the conformation defect and prevent skin lesions is indicated to prevent recurrent UTI.

Fungal infections of the urinary tract are often associated with the glucosuria of diabetes mellitus, but nondiabetic animals may also be affected. Resolution of funguria in diabetes may be difficult, but tight control of blood glucose levels to control glucosuria is indicated. Antifungal drugs that undergo renal excretion in the active form must be used. Fluconazole is a good choice in this respect; however, as with most fungal infections, long-term treatment is usually necessary and the drug is expensive. Because fungal growth is inhibited in an alkaline medium, additional nonspecific treatment includes food additives to cause production of alkaline urine.

Animals with atonic bladder or a tendency to empty the bladder incompletely are at risk for the development of UTI. The most obvious example is the animal with convalescent thoracolumbar disc disease. Diagnosis of atonic bladder and urine retention is best achieved by measuring residual bladder volume after the dog has urinated by either ultrasonography or direct catheterization to empty the bladder. Normal dogs should only have 1 to 2 ml of urine remaining in the bladder at the end of urination. In male dogs, determining when the dog has completed urination is more difficult, but the principle is the same.

When catheterization of the bladder is required to allow urine drainage (e.g., spinal injury and atonic bladder), experience in human medicine suggests that intermittent catheterization is preferable to an indwelling catheter. Even with a closed collection system, a biofilm soon develops on the outside of the catheter and the bladder becomes infected. The simultaneous administration of antimicrobial agents delays the onset of UTI by 24 to 48 hours, but UTI is inevitable. Continuous use of antimicrobial agents to control UTI in an animal with an indwelling catheter is not effective. Infection will still occur and the use of the antimicrobial agent guarantees that the infectious agent will be resistant to the drug or drugs used.

Tumors of the bladder in dogs (usually transitional cell carcinoma) induce signs of lower urinary tract inflammation, including hematuria, dysuria, pollakiuria, and stranguria. The disrupted glycosaminoglycan layer renders the bladder prone to secondary bacterial infection, causing the clinical signs to intensify. Antimicrobial treatment often results in dramatic improvement in clinical signs as the inflammation induced by the infection subsides. Subsequent reinfection after antimicrobial treatment is discontinued leads to exacerbation of signs. Veterinarians often believe that the signs of inflammation are solely due to UTI, and repeated treatment with antimicrobial agents is attempted without establishing the underlying cause of the problem. Resolution of the tumor is often the only way of stopping recurrent infection. Many cases are impossible to resolve. Long-term treatment with antimicrobial agents in this circumstance usually leads to the development of infection with multiresistant bacteria.

Sometimes an animal has recurrent UTI and a thorough evaluation fails to reveal any functional or anatomic defect that would explain the loss of normal host defenses. Under these circumstances, long-term low-dose treatment can render the animal free of infection. Antimicrobial agents chosen on the basis of sensitivity tests are given at a full treatment level, initially for a period of 2 to 4 weeks depending on the location of infection. The antimicrobial dose is then reduced to one half to one third of the normal total daily dose given once daily at bedtime after the animal

has urinated. The bladder then fills with urine containing therapeutic levels of antimicrobial agents and remains so overnight. This regimen is usually continued for 6 months, and many animals remain free of infection after the cessation of treatment. Surprisingly few animals acquire resistant infection.

When an anatomic defect or major change in host defenses is apparent, the situation is quite different. Long-term treatment in such instances leads to the development of infection with multidrug-resistant strains. Provided that there is no evidence of renal involvement (dilute urine, white blood cell casts, fever, back pain, and systemic signs), it may be better to leave the animal untreated. The bacteria are secondary opportunists rather than primary pathogens and they seem to act more as commensal agents with mild effects on the host. Not treating such infections avoids contamination of the owner's environment with highly resistant strains.

References and Suggested Reading

Ihrke P, Norton A, Ling G, et al: Urinary tract infection associated with long-term corticosteroid administration. J Am Vet Med Assoc 186:43, 1985.
   The link between corticosteroid administration and chronic low-grade urinary tact infection is described.
Osborne CA: Three steps to the management of bacterial urinary tract infections: Diagnosis, diagnosis, diagnosis. Compend Contin Educ Pract Vet 17:1233, 1995.
   The role of diagnosis in the management of difficult cases of urinary tract infection is discussed.
Prescott J, Baggot J: Antimicrobial Therapy in Veterinary Medicine. Ames, IA: Iowa State University Press, 1993, p 349.
   This is a review of antimicrobial use in urinary tract infections.
Senior DF: Urinary tract infection: Bacterial invasion, host defenses, and new approaches to prevention. Compend Contin Educ Pract Vet 7:334, 1985.
   The relationship between bacterial virulence and host defenses in the development of urinary tract infections is described.

Forceps Biopsy of the Lower Urinary Tract

JODY P. LULICH
CARL A. OSBORNE
St. Paul, Minnesota

Differentiation of potentially reversible disease from progressive irreversible disease is the single most important factor in the management of persistent or recurrent lower urinary tract signs. Biopsy of the urinary bladder and urethra is helpful to make this distinction in the living patient. Many options are available to obtain tissue for microscopic evaluation. If structures to be biopsied can be palpated, they are accessible for aspiration with a needle and syringe. If larger, architecturally intact samples are desired, they can be obtained by catheter biopsy (Osborne and Lulich, 1995), cystoscopy and pinch biopsy (Senior and Sundstrom, 1995), or celiotomy and core resection. A practical

alternative to these procedures is the use of flexible endoscopy forceps to retrieve tissue samples from the lower urinary tract.

MATERIALS NEEDED FOR BIOPSY

A flexible endoscope forceps (not the endoscope) is inserted into the urethra to obtain tissue samples. Several types of grasping units on the end of the forceps are available. We have had the best results using forceps with a fenestrated oval cup and central needle. The fenestrated

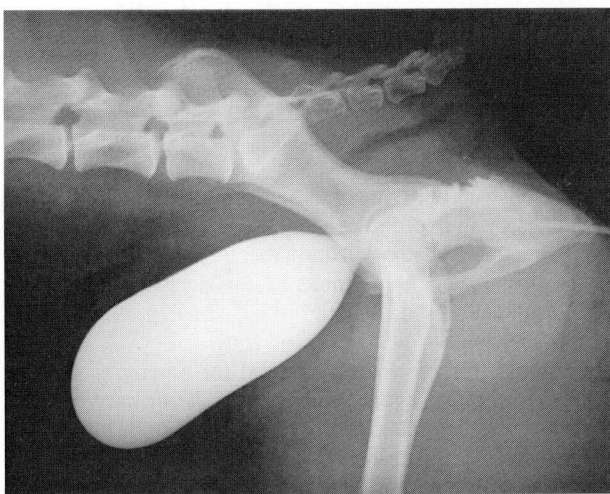

Figure 1. Retrograde urethrocystogram in a 9-year-old Golden Retriever with a proliferative mass in the pelvic urethra.

cup minimizes tissue crushing and the central needle helps anchor the grasping unit to the mucosa that is to be sampled.

No other special equipment is required. However, additional routine supplies would include those needed to assist catheterization in the female dog (e.g., otoscope) and the desired fixative for histologic processing of the sample (e.g., 10% buffered formalin).

PERFORMING FORCEPS BIOPSY

The method used to obtain tissue samples using the endoscopy forceps is similar to methods used to obtain gastrointestinal mucosa with an endoscope. Since the endoscope is not inserted into the urethra, other methods, such as palpation or radiography, are needed to localize the lesion and direct the biopsy forceps. The technique for performing forceps biopsy follows:

- Allow the animal to void urine before biopsy. If micturition is difficult because of partial or complete obstruction, urine can be removed by transurethral catheterization or decompressive cystocentesis. An empty bladder facilitates patient comfort and cooperation.
- Sedate or anesthetize the animal. For many dogs, general anesthesia is not needed. However, tranquilization may facilitate urethral catheterization and palpation of the urethra and bladder and minimizes patient discomfort and anxiety. In lieu of generalized sedation, local anesthesia can be achieved by applying water-soluble lubricants containing lidocaine to the vaginal mucosa or urethra, or both (Anestacon, Polymedica Industries, Division of Alcon Labs, Inc., Woburn, MA). To anesthetize urethral mucosa, the same lubricant can be applied to the biopsy forceps before insertion into the urethra, or it can be diluted and injected into the urethral lumen through a catheter. It has been our experience that most cats usually require general anesthesia to manipulate and catheterize the urethra.

- Identify the site for biopsy by palpation, catheterization, radiography, or a combination of these techniques (Fig. 1).
- With the grasping unit at the end of the forceps closed, insert the flexible endoscopy forceps (not the endoscope) into the urethra.
- Advance the forceps until the grasping unit is near the area to be biopsied (Fig. 2). The tip of the grasping unit can be positioned by abdominal palpation, rectal palpation, radiography, or ultrasonography. For most urethral lesions, the biopsy site is easily determined during insertion, and advancement of the forceps through the urethral lumen; increased friction and force is often required to advance the forceps at the biopsy site. The biopsy site can also be located by using previous radiographs to determine how far the forceps must be inserted into the urethral lumen to reach the lesion. For diffuse urothelial lesions, the apex of the bladder can be sampled by advancing the forceps to the most cranial portion of the bladder. Positioning the forceps fluoroscopically, immediately after contrast urethrocystography, is also an effective method of positioning the biopsy instrument adjacent to the lesion.
- After the biopsy forceps is properly positioned, open the grasping unit and slightly advance the forceps against the lesion.
- Close the grasping unit. With the grasping unit closed, the forceps and tissue sample are retracted from the urinary tract.
- The biopsy sample can be removed from the forceps by lifting the sample from the cup of the grasping unit with a 22- or 25-gauge needle. The sample should then be transferred to formalin for histologic processing.
- Impression smears for immediate cytologic evaluation can be made before placing the sample in formalin. Tissue samples are first lightly blotted on filter paper or dry gauze pads to remove surface blood. Impressions are then made on glass slides and stained before microscopic evaluation.

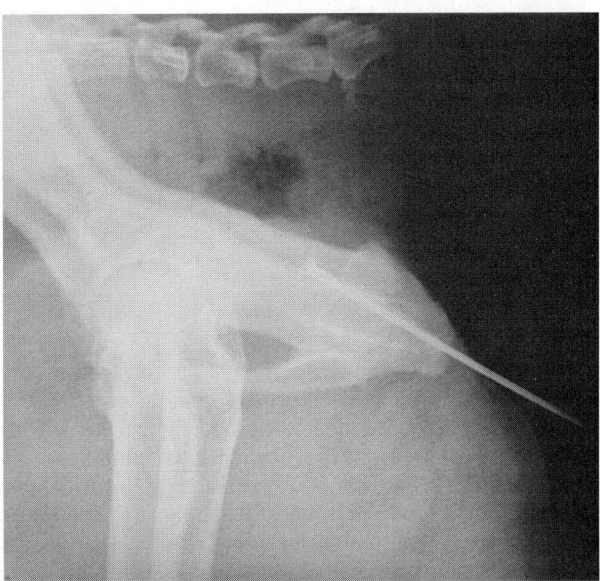

Figure 2. Endoscopy forceps were used to obtain a biopsy of the mass. Microscopic evaluation confirmed a transitional carcinoma.

• Several samples should be retrieved to ensure complete representation of the area in question.

PATIENT CARE AFTER BIOPSY

After bladder biopsy, hematuria and dysuria may be more pronounced. In most cases, bleeding quickly stabilizes (hours to a day) without treatment.

Administration of antibiotics is indicated because the integrity of the mucosal surface of the lower urinary tract is damaged by this procedure, further altering normal host defenses. Infections diagnosed during initial evaluation should be eradicated before biopsy. Eliminating infection before biopsy minimizes hematuria and dysuria associated with sampling of inflamed tissues as well as the potential of extending the infection into the biopsy site and adjacent tissues. In the absence of prior infection, we routinely administer antibiotics orally for the next 3 to 5 days.

LIMITATIONS OF FORCEPS BIOPSY

Standard flexible biopsy forceps are no larger in diameter than an 8F catheter. As a general rule, one should be able to insert the biopsy forceps into the urethral lumen of most male dogs weighing more than 4 kg and into the urethral lumen of most, if not all, female cats and dogs. The lumen of the penile urethra of male cats is usually too small to accommodate insertion of standard flexible biopsy forceps. However, the urethra of male cats after perineal urethrostomy usually is large enough to accommodate insertion of standard biopsy forceps.

It is possible that a thin or weakened bladder wall could be perforated by this procedure. For this reason, we do not recommend biopsy of the lower urinary tract at sites proximal to partial or complete obstruction because increases in intravesicular pressure may result in extravasation of urine into the abdominal cavity. If a tissue sample proximal to a urinary obstruction is desired, constant bladder evacuation by means of indwelling urethral catheterization or antepubic percutaneous catheterization (Stone and Barsanti, 1992) of the urinary bladder should be considered. Minimizing intravesicular pressure should allow small perforations of the bladder wall to heal spontaneously.

Although forceps biopsy is ideal for obtaining samples from the urethra, trigone, and apex of the urinary bladder, directing the flexible forceps to obtain samples from the lateral wall of the urinary bladder requires patience and skill. Use of biopsy forceps with a central needle may help secure samples from this location.

References and Suggested Reading

Osborne CA, Lulich JP: Catheter and forceps biopsy of the urethra, urinary bladder, and prostate. In: Osborne CA, Finco DR, eds: Canine and Feline Nephrology and Urology. Baltimore: Williams & Wilkins, 1995, pp 329–332.
  Biopsy techniques of the urinary bladder are described in this chapter.
Senior DF, Sundstrom DA: Cystoscopy in female dogs. Compend Contin Educ Pract Vet 10:890, 1988.
  Cystoscopic techniques are described.
Stone EA, Barsanti SA: Urologic Surgery of the Dog and Cat. Malvern, PA: Lea & Febiger, 1992.
  Methods of urinary diversion are discussed.

Nonobstructive Idiopathic Feline Lower Urinary Tract Disease: Therapeutic Rights and Wrongs

JOHN M. KRUGER
East Lansing, Michigan

CARL A. OSBORNE

JODY P. LULICH
St. Paul, Minnesota

Since the 1980s, knowledge of the specific causes and natural course of feline lower urinary tract disease (LUTD) has increased, allowing diagnostic and therapeutic efforts to be directed toward identification and elimination of specific underlying causes. However, there is considerable controversy about symptomatic treatment of idiopathic forms of LUTD in male and female cats. This is not surprising because clinical signs associated with this form of the disease are frequently self-limiting and of short duration. In this setting, any form of therapy might appear to be beneficial, as long as it is not harmful. The self-limiting nature of clinical signs in many cats with idiopathic LUTD underscores the need for controlled prospective double-blind clinical studies to prove the efficacy of various forms of therapy.

BIOLOGIC BEHAVIOR

The biologic behavior of nonobstructive idiopathic LUTD has not been evaluated by prospective studies of

TABLE 1. Drugs Commonly Used for Feline Lower Urinary Tract Disorders

Drug	Desired Action	Commonly Used Dose
Amitriptyline (Elavil)	Antidepressant, anticholinergic, anti-inflammatory, analgesic	2.5–12.5 mg/cat PO q24hr
Ammonium chloride (Uroeze)	Urine acidifier	150–300 mg/kg q24hr—to effect
Bethanacol (Urecholine)	Cholinergic agonist	1.25–7.5 mg/cat PO q8hr
Buspirone (Buspar)	Nonbenzodiazepine anxiolytic	2.5–7.5 mg/cat PO q12hr
Dantrolene (Dantrium)	Skeletal muscle relaxant	0.5–2 mg/kg q8hr
Diazepam (Valium)	Skeletal muscle relaxant	1–2.5 mg/cat PO q8–12hr
Dimethylsulfoxide (DMSO; Rimso-50)	Anti-inflammatory	10–20 ml 10% DMSO intravesicularly
Hydrochlorothiazide (Hydrodiuril)	Diuretic—decreases urine calcium	2–4 mg/kg PO q12hr
Methionine-dl (Methiogel; Methioform)	Urine acidifier	1–1.25 g/cat PO q24hr—to effect
2-MPG (Thiola)	Anticystinuric	15 mg/kg PO q12hr
Oxybutin (Ditropan)	Anticholinergic, antispasmodic	0.5–1.25 mg/cat PO q8–12hr
Pentosan polysulfate (Elmiron)	Glycosaminoglycan	2–10 mg/kg PO q12hr
Phenoxybenzamine (Dibenzyline)	Alpha-adrenergic antagonist	2.5–7.5 mg/cat PO q12–24hr
Phenylpropanolamine (Propagest; Dexatrim)	Alpha-adrenergic agonist	1.5–2.2 mg/kg PO q8–12hr
Piroxicam (Feldene)	Anti-inflammatory	0.3 mg/kg PO q24hr
Potassium citrate (Polycitra-K; Urocit-K)	Urine alkalinizing agent	40–75 mg/kg PO q12hr
Prazosin (Minipress)	Alpha-adrenergic antagonist	0.03 mg/kg IV
Prednisolone	Anti-inflammatory	0.5–1.0 mg/kg q12hr
Propantheline (Pro-Banthine)	Anticholinergic	Not established (0.25–0.5 mg/kg PO q12–24hr)

large populations of untreated male and female cats. However, our observations and those of others suggest that clinical signs of hematuria, dysuria, and pollakiuria in many untreated nonobstructed male and female cats with acute idiopathic LUTD frequently subside within 3 to 7 days. These signs may recur after variable periods and again rapidly subside without therapy. It is also our impression that recurrent episodes of acute idiopathic LUTD tend to decrease with frequency and severity over time.

It is commonly assumed that recurrent clinical signs in patients with idiopathic LUTD signal a recurrence of the original disease. However, recurrent LUTD may also be the result of a delayed manifestation of the original disease (e.g., spontaneous or iatrogenic urethral stricture), onset of a different disease associated with clinical manifestations similar to the original disorder (e.g., urolithiasis), or combinations of these factors.

Occasionally, we have encountered cats with signs of hematuria, dysuria, and pollakiuria that have persisted for weeks to months and for which a specific cause cannot be identified. It is unknown whether this chronic form of idiopathic LUTD represents the opposite extreme in the spectrum of clinical manifestations associated with acute self-limiting idiopathic disease caused by similar causative factors, or whether it represents an entirely different mechanism of disease.

MANAGEMENT

Overview

The following generalities recommended for the treatment of nonobstructive forms of idiopathic feline LUTD have not all been substantiated by experimental or clinical investigations, or both. Because some of our recommendations are based on our uncontrolled clinical observations and personal opinion, we are the subject of our own criticism. Therefore, they should be considered with appropriate caution. See Table 1 for desired action and dosages of drugs commonly used to manage feline lower urinary tract disease.

Antibacterial Agents

Antibiotics have commonly been used for decades as empirical therapy for idiopathic LUTD. However, the infrequency (1 to 3%) with which bacteria have been identified at the onset of clinical signs of lower urinary tract disorders in young to middle-aged cats has been well established. The uselessness of antimicrobial agents in the treatment of abacteriuric cats with LUTD has been documented (Table 2). Indiscriminate use of antimicrobial agents has been responsible, at least in part, for the emergence of the resistant strains of microbes that populate veterinary hospitals. We do not recommend routine use of antibiotics to treat cats that do not have confirmed bacterial urinary tract infection (UTI).

Urinary Tract Antiseptics

Urinary tract antiseptics such as methenamine are sometimes used as adjunctive agents for treatment, control, and

TABLE 2. Specific, Supportive, and Symptomatic Therapy Proved to Be Ineffective for the Management of Nonobstructive Idiopathic Lower Urinary Tract Disease

Therapy	Controlled Study?	Efficacy*
Antibiotics†	Yes	Not significant
Antispasmodics‡	Yes	Not significant
Lactated Ringer's solution§	Yes	Not significant
Corticosteroids‖	Yes	Not significant

*Degree of reduction in severity or duration of clinical signs in affected cats treated with a therapeutic agent compared with placebo-treated or untreated controls.

†Chloramphenicol, 100 mg PO q8hr for 5 days.

‡Propantheline bromide, 7.5 mg PO once.

§Lactated Ringer's solution, 100 ml subcutaneously once.

‖Prednisolone, 1.0 mg/kg PO q12hr for 10 days.

TABLE 3. **Specific, Supportive, and Symptomatic Therapy of Uncertain Value for the Management of Nonobstructive Idiopathic Lower Urinary Tract Disease**

Therapy	Rationale	Route	Controlled Study?	Efficacy?*	Our Forecast†
Acepromazine	Antispasmodic	PO, IV, IM, SC	No	ND	Unlikely
Amitriptyline	Anticholinergic Anti-inflammatory Analgesic	PO	No	ND	Probable in some cases
Ammonium chloride	Acidifier	PO	No	ND	Effective for MAP
Butorphanol	Analgesic	PO, IV, IM, SC	No	ND	Possible
Copper coils	Unknown	Intravesicular	No	ND	Contraindicated
Cosequine‡	GAG	PO	No	ND	Probable in some cases
Curcal-feline§	Chelator	PO	No	ND	Very unlikely
Dantrolene	Antispasmodic	PO, IV	No	ND	Unlikely
Debridement	Unknown	Intravesicular	No	ND	Contraindicated
Diazepam	Antispasmodic	PO, IV	No	ND	Unlikely
Diet					
acidifying	Acidifier	PO	No	ND	Effective for MAP
low magnesium	Reduce urine Mg	PO	No	ND	Effective for MAP
moist	Reduce USG	PO	No	ND	Possibly
DMSO	Anti-inflammatory	Intravesicular	No	ND	Unlikely
FCV vaccine	Immunogen	SC	No	ND	Unlikely
Furosemide	Diuretic	PO, IV, IM, SC	No	ND	Unlikely
Glucocorticoids	Anti-inflammatory	PO, IV, IM, SC	No	ND	Unlikely‖
Hydrodistention	Analgesic	Intravesicular	No	ND	Unlikely
Hydroxyzine	Antihistamine	PO	No	ND	Unlikely
Hyaluronidase	Enzyme	SC	No	ND	Unlikely
Interferon alpha-2a	Immunomodulator Antifibrotic Antiviral	PO Intravesicular	No	ND	Possibly
Lugol's solution	Cautery	Intravesicular	No	ND	Contraindicated
Megesterol acetate	Hormone	PO	No	ND	Unlikely
Methenamine	Antiseptic	PO	No	ND	Unlikely
Methionine	Acidifier	PO	No	ND	Effective for MAP
Methylene blue	Antiseptic	PO	No	ND	Contraindicated
Oxybutynin	Antispasmodic	PO	No	ND	May reduce pollakiuria
Pentosan polysulfate	GAG	PO Intravesicular	No	ND	Probable in some cases
Phenazopyridine	Analgesic	PO	No	ND	Contraindicated
Phenol	Cautery	Intravesicular	No	ND	Contraindicated
Phenoxybenzamine	Antispasmodic	PO	No	ND	Unlikely
Piroxicam	Anti-inflammatory	PO	No	ND	Unknown
Potassium chloride	Reduce USG	PO	No	ND	Unlikely
Prazosin	Antispasmodic	PO	No	ND	Unlikely
Propantheline	Antispasmodic	PO	No	ND	May reduce pollakiuria
Prostaglandin E$_1$	Cytoprotective	Intravesicular	No	ND	Unlikely
Sodium chloride	Reduce USG	PO	No	ND	Unlikely
Testosterone	Hormone	IM	No	ND	Unlikely
Vitamin A	Vitamin	PO	No	ND	Unlikely

*Degree of reduction in severity or duration of clinical signs in affected cats treated with a therapeutic agent compared with placebo-treated or untreated controls.
†Our prediction of efficacy if evaluated by a controlled clinical trial.
‡Glucosamine, chondroitin sulfate, and magnesium ascorbate.
§Tetrasodium ethylenediamine tetra-acetic acid, 0.085%, and sodium tripolyphosphate, 0.06%.
‖Ineffective in controlled trial.
DMSO, dimethylsulfoxide; FCV, feline calicivirus; GAG, glycosaminoglycan; IV, intravenous; IM, intramuscular; MAP, magnesium ammonium phosphate; Mg, magnesium; ND, not determined; SC, subcutaneous, USG, urine specific gravity; PO, by mouth; SC, subcutaneous.

prevention of bacterial UTI in humans. Although their use is frequently acknowledged in the treatment of bacterial UTI in dogs, and is occasionally mentioned for treatment of LUTDs in cats, there have been no studies to substantiate their effectiveness in these species (Table 3).

In an acid environment (pH <6.0) methenamine hydrolyzes to form formaldehyde, an essential component of its antimicrobial activity. Because of the necessity of acid urine for the formation of formaldehyde, methenamine is usually given in combination with acidifiers such as mandelic acid (methenamine mandelate) or hippuric acid (methenamine hippurate). Methenamine must remain in the urinary tract for a sufficient period to allow generation of effective concentrations of formaldehyde. However, once generated in sufficient concentration, formaldehyde is capable of killing bacteria, mycoplasma, and viruses at any urine pH.

In light of the hypothesis that some forms of LUTD in cats are caused by viruses, the unproved suggestion that methenamine may have virucidal action in urine is of interest. However, the intracellular location of viruses poses the problem of access of formaldehyde to this location. The lack of definitive proof that viruses are a cause of naturally occurring LUTD in cats and the lack of studies of the efficacy of methenamine in such animals with LUTD are additional problems. At this time, the use of methenamine to treat cats with feline urinary tract disorders represents no more than an idea. We do not recommend methenamine to treat idiopathic LUTD.

Methylene blue (tetramethylthionine chloride) is a weak antiseptic agent that at one time was used in combination products designed to treat lower urinary tract symptoms (see Table 3). Medications containing methylene blue are contraindicated in cats because this agent has the potential to cause Heinz bodies and severe anemia (see *CVT XII*, p. 443).

Urinary Tract Analgesics

Phenazopyridine, an azo dye that is commonly used as a urinary tract analgesic in humans, has recently become available as an over-the-counter preparation. The use of phenazopyridine, alone or in combination with sulfa drugs, is contraindicated in cats because they are susceptible to dose-related methemoglobinemia and irreversible oxidative changes in hemoglobin, resulting in the formation of Heinz bodies and anemia.

Urine Acidifiers

Acidification of urine is of value in helping to dissolve or prevent sterile struvite uroliths, but it is of unlikely value in the treatment of idiopathic LUTD. Many commercially manufactured diets are designed to acidify urine. Systemic overacidification with acidifiers is most likely to occur in cats with pre-existing renal failure, cats consuming acidifying diets, and immature cats. Long-term overacidification may contribute to hypokalemia, renal dysfunction, demineralization of bones, and calcium oxalate urolithiasis. In addition, high doses of methionine may result in Heinz body anemia and methemoglobinemia.

Smooth and Skeletal Muscle Antispasmodics

Cats with inflammation of the lower urinary tract characteristically acquire pollakiuria (frequent voiding of small volumes of urine) or urge incontinence (an uncontrollable desire to void that results in involuntary loss of urine). In both cases, inappropriate voiding of urine usually occurs at low volumes of bladder filling and may be associated with sensations of pain, bladder fullness, and urgency.

Because the exact mechanisms of pollakiuria and urge incontinence are unknown, details about specific therapy are unavailable. Presumably, pollakiuria and urge incontinence are the result of inflammation-induced stimulation of urinary bladder sacral sensory afferents. Sensations of pain and perceptions of fullness and urgency induce a premature micturition reflex and subsequent inappropriate or involuntary voiding of small quantities of urine. Since cholinergic parasympathetic efferents are largely responsible for detrusor contraction, it is logical to consider anticholinergic agents as symptomatic treatment of pollakiuria and urge incontinence. However, the efficacy of these agents in cats with nonobstructive idiopathic LUTD has not been established by properly controlled clinical trials.

The anticholinergic agent propantheline minimizes the force and frequency of uncontrolled detrusor contractions, but has negligible effects on urethral sphincter pressure. In a controlled clinical study of the efficacy of propantheline (7.5 mg given orally on one occasion) in the treatment of naturally occurring hematuria and dysuria in nonobstructed male and female cats, no difference in the rate of recovery was observed between cats treated with propantheline and control groups (see Tables 2 and 4). This is not an unexpected finding because propantheline represents a symptomatic form of therapy. It is possible that therapy with propantheline of longer duration may have reduced the severity of dysuria. We consider propantheline to reduce the severity and frequency of urge incontinence in nonobstructed male and female cats. It has a rapid onset of action. However, care must be used to prevent urinary retention as a result of excessive dosages. Other potential adverse effects include tachycardia, vomiting, and constipation. Because the smallest tablet is 7.5 mg, an empirical dose of 0.25 to 0.5 mg/kg PO every 12 to 24 hours has been suggested. Further studies using appropriate dosages and maintenance intervals are required to substantiate a beneficial symptomatic effect of propantheline in cats with urge incontinence.

Other smooth (oxybutin [0.5 to 1.25 mg/cat PO every 8 to 12 hours], prazosin [0.03 mg/kg IV], phenoxybenzamine [2.5 to 7.5 mg/cat PO every 12 to 24 hours], acepromazine) and skeletal (dantrolene [0.5 to 2.0 mg/kg PO every 8 hours, diazepam [1.0 to 2.5 mg/cat PO every 8 to 12 hours]) muscle antispasmodics have been recommended for symptomatic management of urethrospasm associated with LUTD. Although some of these pharmacologic agents produce significant decreases in intraurethral pressure in normal male cats and cats with naturally occurring urethral obstruction, the role of urethral smooth or skeletal muscle spasm in producing clinical signs associated with idiopathic forms of feline LUTD is unknown. In a limited study of six male cats with urethral obstruction due to unspecified causes, intraurethral pressures before administration of antispasmodics were not significantly different from those of normal nonobstructed male cats. Similar studies in cats with idiopathic forms of LUTD have not been performed. On the basis of available data, we are unable to recommend smooth and skeletal muscle antispasmodics routinely to treat cats with idiopathic LUTD.

Anti-inflammatory Agents

It is reasonable to assume that most cats with idiopathic LUTD have an inflammatory lesion of the lower urinary tract. Hematuria is indicative of (but not pathognomonic of) inflammation; dysuria indicates involvement of the lower urinary tract. The specific cause or causes of inflammation in cats with idiopathic disease is unknown.

Lack of specific therapy for cats with idiopathic causes of hematuria and dysuria has stimulated many to question the value of anti-inflammatory agents to reduce the severity of clinical signs. Success in minimizing the frequency of voiding would not only be beneficial to affected cats but also would eliminate owner frustration associated with the socially unacceptable problem of frequent voiding on floors, carpets, and furniture. Unfortunately, there have been few controlled clinical trials to study the short- and long-term effectiveness of anti-inflammatory agents in the

TABLE 4. Specific, Supportive, and Symptomatic Therapy of Proved Value for Management of Nonobstructive Idiopathic Lower Urinary Tract Disease

Therapy	Controlled Study?	Efficacy?*
Placebo (lactose)	Yes	>70%
Placebo (wheat flour)	Yes	>70%

*Degree of reduction in severity or duration of clinical signs in affected cats.

symptomatic treatment of dysuria and hematuria in cats. Recall that hematuria and dysuria in cats with idiopathic LUTD is often self-limited.

Glucocorticoids. Use of glucocorticoids to minimize dysuria and hematuria associated with inflammation in cats with idiopathic LUTD is logical. To test this logic, we conducted a small double-blind, controlled therapeutic trial using male and female adult cats with previously untreated idiopathic LUTD. Briefly, six symptomatic cats selected randomly were given 1.0 mg/kg of prednisolone orally, twice each day, and six symptomatic cats were given a placebo (Table 4). In both groups, clinical signs subsided in a mean of 1 to 2 days, and in both groups hematuria and pyuria subsided in approximately 2 to 5 days. In one cat with recurrent idiopathic LUTD, one episode was treated with prednisolone. The other episode, which recurred 6 months later, was treated with a placebo. There was no detectable difference in lengths of time before clinical signs subsided after treatment with glucocorticoids or a placebo.

Piroxicam. Piroxicam, a nonsteroidal anti-inflammatory drug, has been empirically suggested to reduce dysuria and pollakiuria in cats with idiopathic LUTD. The empirical dose is 0.3 mg/kg PO every 24 hours. Pending double-blind controlled clinical trials, it is not possible to make recommendations about the safety and efficacy of this drug.

Dimethylsulfoxide. Dimethylsulfoxide (DMSO) is an analgesic anti-inflammatory agent with weak antibacterial, antifungal, and antiviral activity. It has been reported effective in the treatment of a variety of genitourinary disorders in humans, including interstitial cystitis, radiation cystitis, chronic prostatitis, and female chronic trigonitis. Retrograde infusion of 50% solutions of pyrogen-free DMSO into the bladder lumens of humans with interstitial cystitis has been reported to minimize associated clinical signs in some patients.

DMSO has been used to treat LUTD in cats, presumably on the basis of its reported efficacy in humans with interstitial cystitis. Dosages and frequency of administration of DMSO have been entirely empirical. In one uncontrolled study, intravesicular instillation of 10 to 20 ml of 10% DMSO was associated with amelioration of clinical signs in three cats with chronic LUTD. However, appropriately controlled clinical trials designed to evaluate the effectiveness of local instillation of DMSO into the urinary bladder of cats with signs of LUTD have not been reported. In one controlled study of cats with induced cystitis, intravesicular administration of 45% DMSO for 3 days was of no detect-

able benefit in minimizing bacterial infection or inflammation.

Local instillation of varying quantities (up to 25 ml) of solutions containing 25 to 50% DMSO into the urinary bladders of dogs weighing 15 to 40 kg every other week for up to 6 months revealed no detectable side effects. Use of solutions containing 100% DMSO caused mucosal edema and hemorrhage. Licensed products available to veterinarians contain 90% DMSO and are not pyrogen-free; licensed products available to physicians contain 50% DMSO and are pyrogen-free. Side effects of DMSO in cats have apparently not been evaluated. Pending further studies, we discourage its use to treat idiopathic LUTD.

Amitriptyline

Amitriptyline (Elavil), a tricyclic antidepressant and anxiolytic drug with anticholinergic, antihistaminic, anti–alpha-adrenergic, anti-inflammatory, and analgesic properties, has been used extensively for the treatment of interstitial cystitis in humans. Despite amitriptyline's popularity, its exact mechanism of action and its therapeutic value in managing patients with interstitial cystitis is unknown (see p. 894). In an uncontrolled study of 28 human patients with refractory interstitial cystitis, 18 (64%) patients experienced remission of clinical signs, 5 (18%) patients had unacceptable side effects, and 5 (18%) patients had no clinical benefit.

Amitriptyline has recently been advocated for symptomatic therapy of idiopathic feline LUTD. The empirical dose is 2.5 to 12.5 mg/cat PO every 24 hours. Anecdotal reports and limited data suggest that administration of amitriptyline to some cats with chronic idiopathic forms of LUTD was associated with amelioration of clinical signs. Consequently, amitriptyline has gained popularity as an agent for symptomatic therapy for idiopathic feline LUTD. However, appropriately controlled clinical studies designed to evaluate the effectiveness of amitriptyline in controlling signs in cats with idiopathic forms of LUTD have not been reported.

Dose, frequency, and duration of amitriptyline therapy are entirely empirical. Adverse reactions reported in humans treated with antidepressant doses of amitriptyline include urinary retention, dry mucous membranes, blurred vision, hypotension, tachycardia, arrhythmias, sedation, weakness, lethargy, thrombocytopenia, agranulocytosis, elevations in liver enzyme activity, and hypersensitivity reactions. Sedation, urine retention, neutropenia, thrombocytopenia, weight gain, and an unkempt hair coat have been observed in cats treated with amitriptyline. Pending further safety and efficacy studies, we urge caution in the use of amitriptyline to treat idiopathic LUTD.

Glycosaminoglycans

Transitional epithelium of the urinary tract is covered by a thin layer of hydrated extracellular macromolecules called *glycosaminoglycans* (GAGs). Major classes of biologically important GAGs include hyaluronic acid, heparan sulfate, heparin, chondroitin 4-sulfate, chondroitin 6-sulfate, dermatan sulfate, and keratan sulfate. Urothelial

GAGs (1) prevent adherence of microorganisms and crystals to the bladder urothelium and (2) limit transepithelial movement of urine proteins and other ionic and nonionic solutes. Quantitative or qualitative defects in surface GAGs and subsequent increased urothelial permeability have been hypothesized to be a causative factor in the pathogenesis of feline idiopathic LUTD and human interstitial cystitis.

Oral or intravesicular administration of pentosan polysulfate sodium (Elmiron), a semisynthetic low molecular weight heparin GAG analogue, is often used to manage human interstitial cystitis. Pentosan polysulfate reinforced urothelial GAGs and reduced transitional cell injury. Remission of symptoms was observed in 28 to 40% of human interstitial cystitis patients treated with oral or intravesicular pentosan polysulfate compared with only 13 to 20% remission in patients treated with a placebo. Adverse events uncommonly recognized in humans treated with pentosan polysulfate include prolongation of prothrombin time, epistaxis, gingival bleeding, alopecia, abdominal pain, diarrhea, and nausea. The empirical dose extrapolated from human studies is 2 to 10 mg/kg PO every 12 hours. However, evaluation of the safety and efficacy of pentosan polysulfate, or other GAG preparations, for the treatment of feline idiopathic LUTD by controlled clinical trials has not yet been reported. Although treatment with drugs designed to restore the GAG lining of the urinary tract is logical, it is not possible to make recommendations at this time.

Urohydrodistention

Approximately 30% of human interstitial cystitis patients experience substantial, although temporary, relief of signs after controlled distention of the urinary bladder during anesthesia (therapeutic urohydrodistention). Although exact mechanisms of action of urohydrodistention are unknown, possibilities include (1) increased urothelial GAG production, (2) depletion of bladder sensory nerve neuropeptides, or (3) ischemic degeneration of sensory nerve endings within the bladder wall.

Controlled distention of the urinary bladder during cystoscopy has been reported to alleviate clinical signs in some cats with idiopathic LUTD. However, the efficacy of urohydrodistention has not been evaluated by appropriately controlled clinical trials. If retrograde contrast radiography or cystoscopy, or both, are used to diagnose idiopathic LUTD, caution must be exercised in interpreting response to any form of therapy because both techniques distend the urinary bladder. Until other, more specific markers of idiopathic LUTD are identified, it will be difficult to differentiate the effects of bladder distention for diagnostic purposes versus those induced by any form of therapy.

Urothelial Debridement

Cystotomy to lavage and debride the bladder mucosa has been recommended by some to treat animals with chronic cystitis, urethritis, or urethral obstruction, or a combination of these conditions. Although this procedure is still used by some veterinarians, there are no controlled experimental or clinical studies to indicate efficacy for the procedure. In fact, reports of clinical experiences suggest that the technique is of little benefit. This is not surprising because both the urethra and urinary bladder are affected. If one assumes (and we do not) that debridement of the urothelium is of some therapeutic benefit, removal of the bladder mucosa would have no obvious beneficial effect on the urethra. This form of therapy is contraindicated.

Other Agents

A variety of other agents have been advocated by various authors to treat and prevent feline lower urinary tract disorders (see Table 3). None has been evaluated by appropriate selection of patients for study or by controlled clinical trials. Recommendations for testosterone, castor oil, garlic, megestrol acetate, feline calicivirus–feline herpesvirus type 1 vaccines, Lugol's solution, Curcal-feline, vitamin A, hyaluronidase, and various homeopathic preparations appear to be based on supposition rather than fact. We do not recommend them.

References and Suggested Reading

Barsanti JA, Finco DR, Scotts EB, et al: Feline urologic syndrome: Further investigation into therapy. J Am Anim Hosp Assoc 18:387, 1982.
  This article discusses a controlled clinical trial of chloramphenicol, lactated Ringer's solution, and propantheline for the management of idiopathic LUTD.
Buffington CA, Chew DJ, Kendall MS, et al: Clinical evaluation of cats with nonobstructive urinary tract diseases. J Am Vet Med Assoc 210:46, 1997.
  A prospective study of the causes of hematuria, dysuria, pollakiuria, and inappropriate urination in nonobstructed male and female cats is discussed.
Kruger JM, Osborne CA: Recurrent, nonobstructive, idiopathic feline lower urinary tract disease: An illustrative case report. J Am Anim Hosp Assoc 31:312, 1995.
  This is a case report illustrating the natural biologic behavior of untreated feline idiopathic LUTD.
Kruger JM, Osborne CA, Goyal SM, et al: Clinical evaluation of cats with lower urinary tract disease. J Am Vet Med Assoc 199:211, 1991.
  This article describes a prospective study of causes of hematuria, dysuria, pollakiuria, and urethral obstruction in male and female cats.
Kruger JM, Osborne CA, Lulich JP, et al: Management of nonobstructive idiopathic feline lower urinary tract disease. Vet Clin North Am Small Anim Pract 26:571, 1996.
  This is a review of clinical features, potential causes, and management of feline idiopathic LUTD.
Osborne CA, Kruger JM, Lulich JP, et al: Disorders of the feline lower urinary tract disorders. In: Osborne CA, Finco DR, eds: Canine and Feline Nephrology and Urology. Baltimore: Williams & Wilkins, 1995, pp 625–680.
  This is a comprehensive review of etiopathogenesis, clinical features, diagnosis, and management of feline lower urinary tract diseases.
Osborne CA, Kruger JM, Lulich JP, et al: Prednisolone therapy of idiopathic feline lower urinary tract disease: A double-blind clinical study. Vet Clin North Am Small Anim Pract 26:563, 1996.
  This article describes a controlled clinical trial of prednisolone for the management of feline idiopathic LUTD.

CVT Update: Idiopathic (Interstitial) Cystitis in Cats

C. A. TONY BUFFINGTON

D. J. CHEW

Columbus, Ohio

The terms *feline urologic syndrome* and *feline lower urinary tract disease* have become outmoded by the current ability to diagnose at least six distinct causes of the signs of irritative voiding (dysuria, pollakiuria), hematuria, and inappropriate urination in cats. We recently reported our experience with 132 cats examined (Fig. 1) by our urology service for signs of irritative voiding (Buffington et al, 1997). The percentage of cats (61%) with idiopathic (interstitial) cystitis (IC) was similar to that previously reported by others, suggesting that the relative frequency of this problem has been fairly stable during the past four decades. Interstitial cystitis in cats has been discussed previously (see *CVT XII,* p. 1009).

DIAGNOSIS

The evaluation of urinalysis results in cats with signs of irritative voiding is complex (see Fig. 1), because false-negative as well as false-positive results occur. For example, urine pH measured by dipstick and by pH meter do not agree well; a dipstick reading of 6.5 can occur with a meter reading of 5.8 to 7.0. Moreover, increased urine pH may not only be caused by diet or urinary tract infection; urine pH may be greater than 7.0 as a result of the stress of travel and examination by a veterinarian. Hematuria and proteinuria also have been found to wax and wane unpredictably in cats with IC and may occur in cats with urolithiasis or urinary tract infections. Even the presence or absence of crystals can be confusing. Many cats with bladder stones do not have crystalluria (indeed, some cats do not show any signs of the presence of the stone), and many apparently healthy cats have crystals in their urine. Thus, none of these parameters is diagnostic of any particular disease. Radiography can be used to identify radiodense (struvite and calcium oxalate) uroliths, anatomic defects,

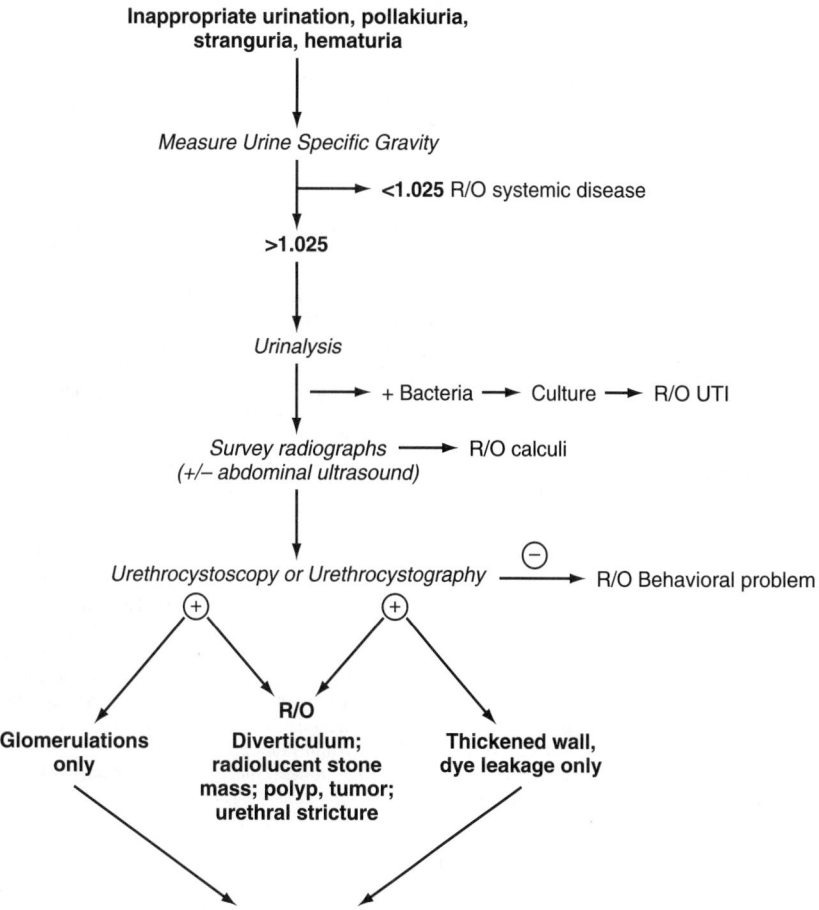

Figure 1. Diagnostic evaluation of lower urinary tract signs in cats.

and neoplasia. A positive urine culture identifies the presence of a urinary tract infection, which should be treated with appropriate antibiotic therapy

Cystoscopy is required for diagnosis of interstitial cystitis to demonstrate the typical findings of prominent vascularity and submucosal petechial hemorrhages. Increased vascularity and glomerulations also result from other bladder diseases, but these conditions have other distinguishing findings (e.g., presence of tumor, stone, bacterial infection). Contrast radiographic studies of cats are more feasible because of the limited availability of cystoscopy in veterinary medicine. Focal or diffuse wall thickening, irregular mucosa, and vesicoureteral reflux are the most commonly found abnormalities in a recent series of cats evaluated at The Ohio State University. Unfortunately, contrast cystography was normal in 80% of cats with IC in this series. When no abnormality can be found after repeated diagnostic investigations, a behavioral problem is presumed.

TREATMENT

Signs related to acute, nonobstructive IC often resolve spontaneously within a few days regardless of treatment, which prevents accurate assessment of the success of treatments given during this time. No treatment is known to be effective in preventing recurrence of clinical signs.

Diet may play multiple roles in the treatment of IC. Most cats with IC already produce acidic (<6.5 pH) urine that contains few crystals. In the presence of macroscopic crystalluria, changing the diet to dilute the urine without increasing the pH is indicated. Although crystalluria is usually benign, severe crystalluria may aggravate an already inflamed bladder. In our most recent study, we found that nearly 60% of cats ate 100% dry cat food; an additional 17% ate 75% or more dry food as their total daily intake (Buffington et al, 1997). This does not mean that dry food consumption causes IC, but it could mean that dry food consumption unmasks or aggravates the disorder in cats that are predisposed to it (making it a nutrient-sensitive rather than a diet-induced disease). Consequently, we recommend either adding water to the dry food or changing to canned foods if this is feasible for the owner and the cat. Because of the risk of urethral obstruction in male cats, we recommend that they be fed a canned diet designed to decrease urine pH. Although a dry diet similarly formulated should inhibit struvite formation, we have found dry foods to be less efficacious than canned foods. Benefits of increased water intake could include dilution of any noxious substances in urine, more frequent urination to decrease bladder contact time with urine, and removal of any excess crystals. We also recommend that the same diet be fed for extended periods to reduce the stress that some cats seem to experience during frequent diet changes.

We believe that stress is important in the development of recurrence of signs in cats with IC and may be important in precipitating the first episode of signs in susceptible animals. Unfortunately, stress is difficult to quantitate. A detailed history is necessary to expose "stressors" in a cat's life, which may include changes in the environment, weather, activity, diet, feeding schedule, use of the litter pan, owner's schedule, additions or subtractions from the household population of humans or animals, and other factors. Regimens to reduce stress may prove essential in the management of cats with IC. To reduce environmental stress, we recommend that the cat be provided places to hide and opportunities to express the natural predatory behavior of cats. These opportunities can include climbing posts and toys that can be chased and caught. The newly available cat pheromones also may prove to be useful to decrease "environmental anxiety" in cats with IC, although to our knowledge they have not yet been tested for this use.

In severe recurrent cases we also treat for pain. Animal behaviorists have prescribed amitriptyline for some time to help treat inappropriate urination in cats. Amitriptyline possesses several potential therapeutic benefits for cats with IC, including analgesia, stabilization of mast cell membranes, norepinephrine reuptake inhibition (that results in down-regulation of noradrenergic transmission) and anticholinergic effects, and antagonism of both glutamate receptors and sodium channels. Preliminary findings in a series of cats with IC at OSU Veterinary Hospital suggest that the clinical signs of some cats are remarkably reduced during amitriptyline treatment. Improvement in clinical signs is, however, not always accompanied by improvement in the cystoscopic appearance of the bladder. Controlled studies of the safety of amitriptyline in cats with IC are not yet available. We prescribe the drug to be given orally once daily before the owner retires for the night. The dosage is adjusted between 2.5 and 12.5 mg to produce a barely perceptible calming effect on the cat. The reduction in severity of clinical signs can be dramatic in some cats; however, in others little or no beneficial effect is observed. Because the long-term safety of amitriptyline in cats has not been well established, we recommend that serum liver enzyme activity (e.g., alanine aminotransferase, alkaline phosphatase, aspartate aminotransferase) be evaluated before and 1 month after institution of therapy and at least yearly thereafter to assure that the drug has not adversely affected liver function. In our experience, however, amitriptyline given at the dosage given is safe for at least 2 years. Potential side effects include excessive urine retention (anticholinergic effects) and increased concentrations of liver enzymes. Other tricyclic drugs, such as desipramine or nortriptyline, may produce fewer side effects, but these also have not yet been tested. We also have used butorphanol to relieve bladder pain with apparent success in a small number of cats with chronic idiopathic cystitis. Longer term studies on the effect of chronic pain relief as therapy for IC are needed.

Experimental justification for many of these recommendations is currently lacking, which is similar to the situation for most therapies for IC in humans. A glycosaminoglycan replacer (pentosan polysulfate [Elmiron]) was approved for use in humans with IC; its safety and efficacy for cats with IC is currently under investigation. We hope that the interest and controversy generated by the demonstration of the occurrence of IC in more than one species will stimulate further research into the causes and treatments for this painful, debilitating disease.

Successful treatment of lower urinary tract disorders

depends on accurate diagnosis of the causes of the signs that prompted the owner to seek veterinary care for the pet. Idiopathic cystitis is the most common cause of these signs, and initial episodes usually are self-limiting. Patients with chronic recurrent disease should be investigated by urinalysis and imaging to identify recognized causes of signs. Once diagnosed, the disorder should be treated appropriately. Variable combinations of diet, "environmental therapy," and analgesic drugs (in severe recurrent cases) may be prescribed, depending on the diagnosis. Until properly controlled clinical trials result in better approaches to treatment, patients should be followed to avoid recurrence of treatable problems.

References and Suggested Reading

Buffington CAT, Chew DJ, Kendall MS, et al: Clinical evaluation of cats with nonobstructive urinary tract diseases. J Am Vet Med Assoc 210:46, 1997.
Presentation of data from 1993 to 1995 showing that the majority of cases of lower urinary tract disease still are idiopathic.

Sant GR, ed: Interstitial Cystitis. New York: Lippincott-Raven, 1997.
This book presents a comprehensive review of IC, including a detailed comparison of the features of IC in cats and in humans.

Scrivani PV, Chew DJ, Buffington CAT, et al: Results of retrograde urethrography in cats with idiopathic, non-obstructive lower urinary tract disease and their association with pathogenesis: 53 cases (1993–1995). J Am Vet Med Assoc 211:741, 1997.
This article presents a detailed examination of the role of anatomy in urethral obstruction of male cats with IC.

Urethral Sphincter Mechanism Incompetence in Male Dogs

SUSI ARNOLD
Zurich, Switzerland

URS WEBER
Tenniken, Switzerland

At rest, the urinary bladder acts as a reservoir for urine, and its closure is maintained by the urethra. Urinary continence is sustained as long as the urethral closure pressure exceeds bladder pressure. If urethral closure pressure cannot exceed bladder pressure, the term *urethral sphincter mechanism incompetence* (USMI) is used. In this situation, the animal is incontinent.

In the dog, urethral pressure is not achieved by a distinct anatomic sphincter but is dependent on the interaction of several physiologic mechanisms. In particular, the smooth urethral musculature, which is controlled by the autonomic nervous system, plays an important role, in concert with the submucosal vascular plexus and fibrous tissue. In bitches, the whole urethra seems to be important for the generation of urethral closure. In male dogs, only the proximal quarter of the urethra—namely, the pars membranacea and the pars prostatica—is important for urethral closure. Therefore, patients suffering from urolithiasis keep voluntary control of micturition after a permanent urethrostomy in a prepubic, scrotal, or perineal location of the pars spongiosa (Stone and Barsanti, 1992). Even surgery at the junction of the pars membranacea and the pars spongiosa can be performed without the risk of incontinence. A transient incontinence can occur after operations on the pars membranacea (Yoshioka and Carb, 1982). However, after surgery in the proximal part of the urethra, such as the surgical removal of abnormal prostatic tissue, urinary incontinence is a common complication (Basinger et al, 1989).

ETIOLOGY

Urethral surgery is not the only cause of USMI-related urinary incontinence in the male dog. Urethral closure can spontaneously deteriorate, thus leading to incontinence. In bitches, this problem occurs especially after spaying (Arnold et al, 1989). Urinary incontinence in the male occurs less often than in the bitch and of these cases, USMI is seen as a minor cause. Holt (1985) reports that in 38 incontinent males, only 5 had a diagnosis of USMI against 60 out of 136 incontinent bitches.

In male dogs, there is also no obvious relationship between castration and urinary incontinence due to USMI. From 1990 to 1996, 22 male dogs with USMI were presented at the Clinic of Zurich; 7 of these animals were intact. Two other dogs were incontinent before castration, but deteriorated further after surgery.

CLINICAL SIGNS

There is also a difference in clinical signs between bitches and male dogs (Table 1). Bitches are mainly incontinent while asleep (Arnold et al, 1989), but male dogs are often permanently incontinent (Weber et al, 1997). Affected dogs urinate normally and are otherwise healthy.

DIAGNOSIS

Even though the history may indicate USMI, affected animals need a thorough work-up. If, by history or physical

TABLE 1. Urethral Closure and Occurrence of Incontinence Due to Urethral Sphincter Mechanism Incompetence: Differences Between Female and Male Dogs

	Females	Males
Urethral zone responsible for continence	Entire urethra	Pars prostatica and pars membranacea
Type of incontinence in dogs with USMI	Urinary leakage mainly during sleep	Constant loss of urine
Occurrence of incontinence in correlation with desexing	Occurs mainly after spaying	More than 30% of the males with USMI are sexually intact
Good response to alpha-adrenergic drugs	In 90% of cases	In <50% of cases

USMI, urethral sphincter mechanism incompetence.

examination, a neurologic problem is suspected, a complete neurologic examination should be performed. If incontinence has been present since birth, an intravenous contrast study should be performed in order to rule out congenital malformations, such as ectopic ureters. In older animals, radiography or ultrasonography of the urinary tract is recommended to exclude neoplasia. Diseases that cause polydipsia and polyuria can be the cause of "urge urination" at night. Using a biochemical profile and urinalysis, diseases causing polydipsia and polyuria can usually be diagnosed. Urinary tract infection can be excluded with a negative bacterial culture of a urine sample collected by cystocentesis. Prostatic diseases are ruled out by rectal palpation and sonography.

If all these examinations and tests are within normal limits, urinary incontinence is most likely caused by USMI, and therapy can be initiated. In the bitch, a urethral pressure profilometry is a suitable tool to confirm the diagnosis. This examination is made either by means of the perfusion method (Rosin et al, 1980) or by the microtranducer method (Holt, 1989). However, urethral pressure profilometry is not a definitely established method for male dogs.

ROLE OF URETHRAL PRESSURE PROFILOMETRY

There are only a few publications on urethral pressure profilometry (Fig. 1) in incontinent male dogs by the perfusion method (Richter and Ling, 1985; Rosin and Barsanti, 1981); however, these studies did not prove the results were reproducible.

In one study, the short- and long-term reproducibility of urethral pressure profiles measured by the microtransducer method was examined in healthy male dogs. In the same study, the tonometric parameters were compared with those of male dogs that were incontinent because of USMI (Kupper, 1995). The maximal urethral closure pressure of the pars prostatica was significantly lower in male dogs with USMI (13.9 ± 5.7 cm H_2O, n = 14) when compared with healthy male dogs (20.0 ± 10.3 cm H_2O, n = 5); in the membranacea region there was no difference in maximal urethral closure pressures (7.4 ± 3.4 cm H_2O versus 7.5 ± 3.8 cm H_2O). These findings agree with the clinical observations that it is mainly the prostatic region of the urethra that is responsible for maintaining urinary continence. However, the microtransducer method does not appear to be suitable as a diagnostic tool because the maximal urethral closure pressures of the proximal urethra varied considerably in repeated measurements. This was attributed to the colliculus seminalis, a permanent fold, which is situated in the dorsomedian aspect along the whole prostatic urethra. This structure gives the urethra a V-shaped cross section (Fig. 2). During measurements, the size of the peak depends on the orientation of the sensor site. If the sensor site touches this rigid tissue structure, a distinct peak results, whereas even a slight rotation of the catheter leads to a different amplitude.

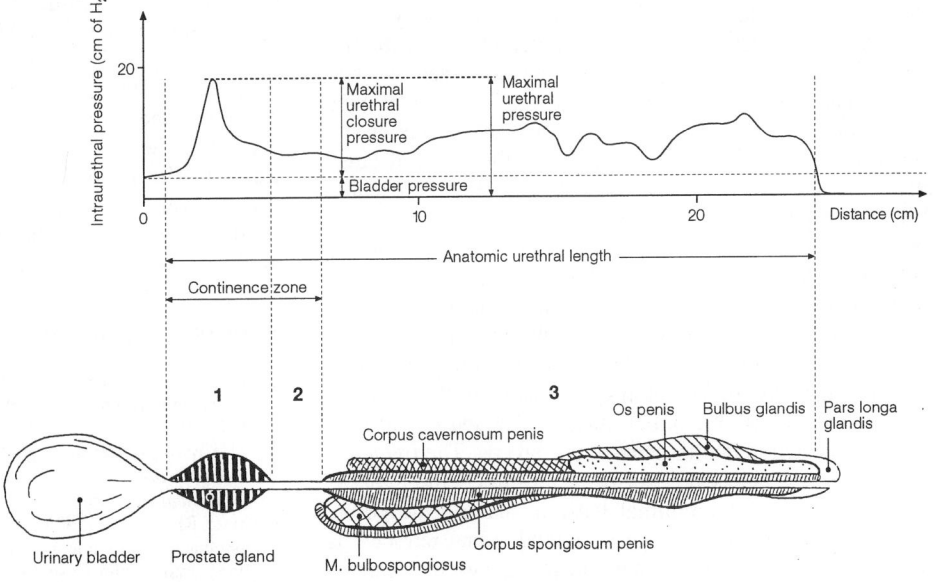

Figure 1. Typical urethral pressure profile of a healthy male Beagle dog recorded by the microtransducer technique: Correlation of function and morphologic characteristics. 1 = pars prostatica; 2 = pars membranacea; 3 = pars spongiosa. (From Weber UTH, Arnold S, Hubler M, et al: Surgical treatment of male dogs with urinary incontinence due to urethral sphincter mechanism incompetence. Vet Surg 26:51–56, 1997, with permission.)

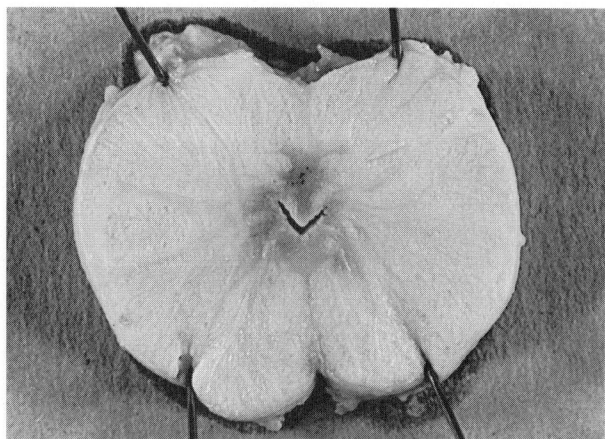

Figure 2. Cross section of the prostatic urethra: V-shaped urethral lumen due to the prominent colliculus seminalis. (From Weber UT, Arnold S, Hubler M, et al: Surgical treatment of male dogs with urinary incontinence due to urethral sphincter mechanism incompetence. Vet Surg 26:51–56, 1997, with permission.)

MEDICAL THERAPY

The recommended medical treatment for USMI is alpha-adrenergic agonist drugs, which stimulate the alpha-receptors of the urethral wall, thereby increasing the urethral closure pressure (Richter and Ling, 1985). Bitches with USMI usually respond well to this therapy. In 90% of cases, urinary continence can be achieved with alpha-adrenergic drugs, but this therapy is less successful in males (see Table 1). Phenylpropanolamine was found to have no effect on more than 50% of male dogs with USMI (Kupper, 1995). In such cases surgery is recommended. Caution should be taken in using these drugs in dogs with pre-existent hypertension or advanced cardiac disease, as blood pressure may increase.

SURGICAL THERAPY

The surgical procedure is similar to the vasopexy that is used as prevention of bladder retroflexion in dogs with perineal hernias (Weber et al, 1997). The patient is anesthetized and positioned in dorsal recumbency. Sexually intact dogs are first castrated by separately ligating the testicular vessels and the ductus deferens. The abdomen is then approached by a caudal median incision. The caudal ends of the deferent ducts are brought into the abdomen by gentle traction. Both deferent ducts are then moved laterally until an angle of 60 degrees to the midline is reached. The cross point of the deferent ducts with the lateral abdominal wall serves as reference for the level of the pexy site. The precise position of the pexy site at this level is perpendicular to the celiotomy and one third of the distance between the midline and the lateral border of the vertebral column (Fig. 3). A 4- to 5-mm incision, perpendicular to the celiotomy, is made in the external sheet of the rectus abdominal muscle. The abdominal wall is bluntly penetrated with hemostatic forceps. The free ends of the deferent ducts are grasped and pulled through the abdominal wall with minimal tension, leaving the pelvic urethra in its original position. The abdominal retractor is then removed in order to obtain normal anatomic relation-

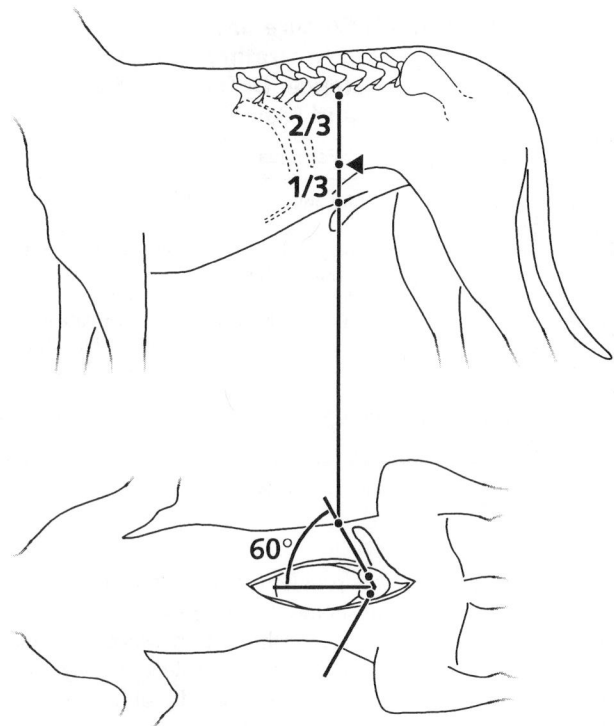

Figure 3. Vasopexy for surgical treatment of male dogs with urethral sphincter mechanism incompetence: Location of the pexy site. (From Weber UT, Arnold S, Hubler M, et al: Surgical treatment of male dogs with urinary incontinence due to urethral sphincter mechanism incompetence. Vet Surg 26:51–56, 1997, with permission.)

ships. Slight tension is applied to the deferent ducts until the prostate gland is moved about 1 cm cranially under digital control. The deferent ducts are anchored to the body wall with 2–0 PDS using a simple interrupted pattern. The ducts are aditionally secured to a double sheet of a PDS band (0.7 × 1.0 cm) with 2–0 PDS sutures. The PDS band is then sutured to the external rectus fascia with 2–0 PDS simple interrupted sutures. Finally, a routine closure of the ventral midline incision is performed.

Immediately before and after surgery, a contrast urethrocystogram is recommended as a control for the result of the operation. The bladder is emptied by catheterization and 5 ml/kg body weight of a diluted contrast medium is instilled into the bladder. Ideally, in the lateral view of the abdomen, the proximal urethra is elongated between 2 and 3 cm and the bladder neck is slightly displaced cranioventrally in the abdomen. This procedure was successful in six of seven incontinent male dogs with USMI, but in three of these cases additional medical therapy was needed to achieve complete continence (Weber et al, 1997).

References and Suggested Reading

Arnold S, Arnold P, Hubler M, et al: Incontinentia urinae bei der kastrierten Hündin: Häufigkeit und Rassedisposition. Schweiz Arch Tierheilkd 131:259, 1989.
This retrospective study of 412 bitches 3 to 10 years after spaying discusses the occurrence, extent of urinary incontinence, and response to medical treatment.
Basinger RR, Rawlings CA, Barsanti JA, et al: Urodynamic alterations associated with clinical prostatic diseases and prostatic surgery in 23 dogs. J Am Anim Hosp Assoc 25:385, 1989.

The urodynamic alterations associated with clinical prostatic disease and prostatic surgery in 23 dogs are described.

Holt PE: Urinary incontinence in the bitch due to sphincter mechanism incompetence: Prevalence in referred dogs and retrospective analysis of sixty cases. J Small Anim Pract 26:181, 1985.
A retrospective analysis of 174 cases of canine incontinence (136 females and 38 males) was made to determine the incidence of sphincter mechanism incompetence.

Holt PE: Simultaneous urethral pressure profilometry in the bitch: Methodology and reproducibility of the technique. Res Vet Sci 47:110, 1989.
The microtransducer technique for urethral pressure profilometry in the bitch is described.

Kupper JR: Urethradruckprofile bei gesunden und harninkontinenten Rüden. Doctoral Thesis, Veterinary Medical Faculty, University of Zurich, 1995.
The microtransducer method was used to examine five normal healthy male dogs. The results were investigated for short- and long-term reproducibility and compared with the results of 14 incontinent male dogs with urethral sphincter mechanism incompetence.

Richter KP, Ling GV: Clinical response and urethral pressure profile changes after phenylpropanolamine in dogs with primary sphincter incompetence. J Am Vet Med Assoc 187:605, 1985.
Urethral pressure profiles were recorded in 11 female and 8 male dogs with urinary incontinence due to USMI before and after treatment with phenylpropanolamine.

Rosin AE, Barsanti JA: Diagnosis of urinary incontinence in dogs: Role of the urethral pressure profile. J Am Vet Med Assoc 178:814, 1981.
Urethral pressure profiles were recorded in six male and three female dogs with urinary incontinence.

Rosin A, Rosin E, Oliver J: Canine urethral pressure profile. Am J Vet Res 41:1113, 1980.
Urethral pressure profiles were recorded in seven females and six male healthy adult dogs; the perfusion technique is described.

Stone EA, Barsanti JA, eds: Postoperative management and surgical complications of canine urethral obstruction. In: Stone EA, Barsanti JA, eds: Urologic Surgery of the Dog and Cat. Philadelphia: Lea & Febiger, 1992, p 157.

Weber UTH, Arnold S, Hubler M, et al: Surgical treatment of male dogs with urinary incontinence due to urethral sphincter mechanism incompetence. Vet Surg 26:51, 1997.
The surgical procedure and follow-up in seven male dogs is described.

Yoshioka MM, Carb A: Antepubic urethrostomy in the dog. J Am Anim Hosp Assoc 18:290, 1982.
The surgical technique and clinical application of the antepubic urethrostomy in three dogs is described.

Use of Anticholinergic Agents in Lower Urinary Tract Disease

INDIA F. LANE

Charlottetown, Prince Edward Island, Canada

Anticholinergic agents are occasionally considered in the management of urinary tract disorders associated with urinary frequency, urgency, incontinence, and pain. The basis for their recommendation extends from the influence of cholinergic transmission in urinary bladder contractility. If a hypercontractile urinary bladder can be "turned off," improved urine storage and continence may be expected. This article summarizes cholinergic pharmacology, as well as the indications, effects, side effects, and veterinary experience with anticholinergic agents.

NEUROPHYSIOLOGY

Anticholinergic agents compete with the action of acetylcholine where preganglionic fibers terminate in the adrenal medulla and the sympathetic and parasympathetic autonomic ganglia (nicotinic receptors) and where postganglionic fibers of the parasympathetic autonomic nervous system (muscarinic receptors) innervate end-organs. Acetylcholine also is the primary neurotransmitter at the somatic neuromuscular junction and in some parts of the central nervous system (nicotinic receptors). At usual doses, anticholinergic agents act primarily as competitive inhibitors at *muscarinic* receptors and are more appropriately termed *antimuscarinic agents* (Fig. 1). Thus, their predominant impact is on effector cells of the parasympathetic nervous system, but additional physiologic effects can be observed because of interference with cholinergic transmission elsewhere.

In the lower urinary tract, parasympathetic impulses are transmitted via the pelvic nerve to ganglia in the urinary bladder wall and to muscarinic receptors in the detrusor smooth muscle (see Fig. 1). During normal urine storage, parasympathetic input is inhibited while the urinary bladder distends and accommodates slow urine filling. Minimal changes in intravesicular pressure or sensory activity develop until threshold volumes are approached. At that time, voiding may be initiated voluntarily or inhibited until appropriate. Intact central nervous system control, adequate distensibility and accommodation of the detrusor muscle, and adequate outlet resistance must coexist for effective urine storage to occur. Antimuscarinic agents, many of which also possess antispasmodic or analgesic properties, have been employed to facilitate urine storage by blocking contractile responses to acetylcholine and facilitating detrusor muscle relaxation.

INDICATIONS

The indication for antimuscarinic administration is the presence of inappropriate, involuntary detrusor contractions, in which detrusor reflexes are triggered at low urinary bladder volume or pressure. Causes of the hypercontractile urinary bladder include neuropathic disorders (*detrusor*

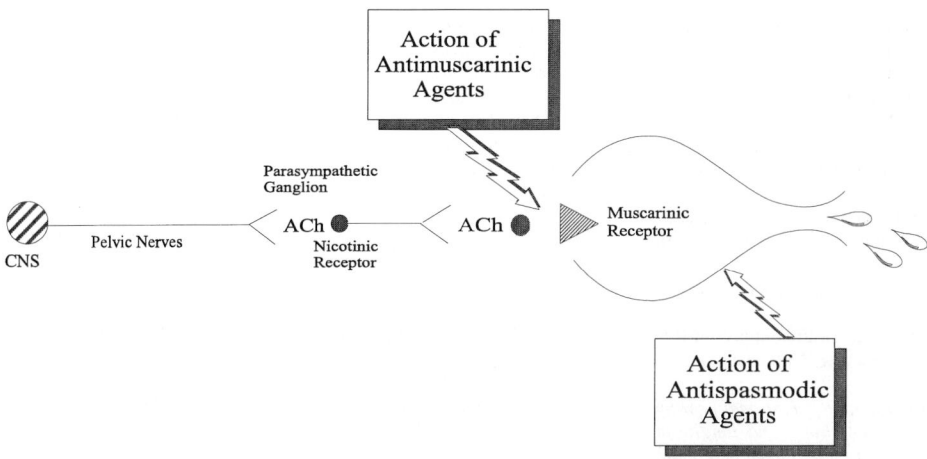

Figure 1. Schematic illustration of parasympathetic innervation to the urinary bladder and the sites of action of antimuscarinic and antispasmodic agents. Ach, acetylcholine.

hyperreflexia), inflammatory or irritative disorders (*sensory hyperreflexia*), and idiopathic disorders (*detrusor instability*). With an overactive detrusor, involuntary contractions cannot be inhibited and lead to a sensation of urgency and leakage of small amounts of urine. Clinically, bladder hypercontractility is manifested by urinary incontinence and pollakiuria. Urinary incontinence may appear similar to the resting intermittent incontinence observed with urethral incompetence or may be associated with positional change such as standing, walking, barking, or jumping. Often, it is difficult to determine whether voiding is voluntary or involuntary. Unstable detrusor contractions or reduced threshold volumes can be documented by cystometric studies, in which intravesicular pressure is measured during bladder filling. A syndrome of reduced bladder storage function, in which urinary bladder capacity and accommodation are reduced but involuntary contractions cannot be documented, may be an additional clinical entity leading to intermittent urinary incontinence.

Antimuscarinic and antispasmodic agents also are advocated for the symptomatic relief of painful and irritating conditions of the urinary bladder, including urinary tract infection, urinary tract neoplasia, urinary bladder fibrosis, and idiopathic feline lower urinary tract disease. For most of these disorders, treatment of the underlying disease process is of primary importance, and antimuscarinic agents are minimally effective.

ANTIMUSCARINIC AGENTS

The prototypical antimuscarinic agents are the naturally occurring belladonna alkaloids, such as atropine, scopolamine, and hyoscyamine. The diffuse cholinergic antagonism and short half-lives of these agents have prompted the development of synthetic antimuscarinics with more specific receptor subtype affinities, minimal adverse effects, and prolonged duration of action. Antimuscarinic agents used in veterinary medicine are summarized in Table 1.

Propantheline (Pro-Banthine, Roberts) is a readily available synthetic quaternary ammonium compound that has been widely used for urinary bladder relaxation. Similar to atropine in potency, this agent increases bladder capacity and abolishes the micturition reflex in healthy humans, and results in increased volume to first contraction, increased total bladder capacity, and decreased amplitude of involuntary bladder contractions in humans with neurogenic bladder dysfunction. In veterinary medicine, propantheline has been recommended in the management of urge incontinence characterized by inappropriate voiding, pollakiuria, and incontinence in dogs. Propantheline administration (7.5 mg PO every 8 hours) was effective in a collie with urethral incompetence and idiopathic detrusor instability in one report; the agent was only partially effective in another dog in the same report (Lappin and Barsanti, 1987). Recommended starting doses in dogs are 7.5 to 15 mg PO

TABLE 1. Recommended Dosing Regimens for Antimuscarinic Agents

Generic Name	Trade Name	Major Actions	Recommended Dosage	Comments
Propantheline	Pro-Banthine	Antimuscarinic	Dog: 7.5–30 mg PO q8–24hr 0.25–0.5 mg/kg PO q8hr Cat: 5–7.5 mg PO q24–72hr	Oral absorption variable; tailor dosage to individual
Oxybutynin	Ditropan	Antispasmodic Antimuscarinic Local anesthetic	Dog: 0.2 mg/kg PO q8–12hr 1.25–3.75 mg PO q12hr (most dogs) Cat: 0.5 mg–1.0 mg PO q8–12hr	
Dicyclomine	Bentyl Bentylol	Antispasmodic Antimuscarinic	Dog: 10 mg PO q6–8hr	
Imipramine	Tofranil	Antimuscarinic Adrenergic agonist Muscle relaxant	Dog: 5–15 mg PO q12hr Cat: 2.5–5 mg PO q12hr	Tremors, sedation possible
Flavoxate	Urispas	Muscle relaxant	Dog and cat: 100–200 mg PO q6–8hr	

every 12 hours; total dosages up to 30 mg every 8 hours are occasionally required.

Propantheline bromide also has been recommended in the symptomatic treatment of nonobstructive feline lower urinary tract disease. In one small controlled study, however, administration of propantheline (7.5 mg per cat given once PO) did not enhance resolution of clinical signs when compared with placebo (Barsanti et al, 1982). Propantheline (5 to 7.5 mg per cat PO) may have a prolonged duration of action in cats, and additional doses may not be required for 2 to 3 days.

Oxybutynin chloride (Ditropan, ALZA Corporation) and *dicyclomine hydrochloride* (Bentyl or Bentylol, Marion Merrell Dow) are antimuscarinic and antispasmodic compounds structurally related to propantheline. These agents exhibit less antimuscarinic activity than do atropine and propantheline, but effect a potent paparavine-like muscle relaxation on smooth muscle cells of the gastrointestinal and genitourinary tract. Oxybutynin also possesses local anesthetic and antihistaminic activity in the lower urinary tract, and has efficacy similar to propantheline in humans. Intravesicular administration has proved efficacious in dog models and in selected human patients refractory to or intolerant of orally administered drug. This route of administration is associated with minimal adverse effects but is unlikely to be routinely practical in small animals. A long-acting preparation of oxybutynin (Ditropan XL, ALZA Corporation) and a more urinary-selective muscarinic receptor antagonist, *tolterodine* tartrate (Detrol, Pharmacia and Upjohn) have recently been introduced for human patients.

Oxybutynin (0.5 mg PO every 12 hours) resulted in resolution of incontinence attributed to feline leukemia–associated detrusor instability in a cat. Improved threshold volume and threshold pressure were documented by follow-up cystometry (Lappin and Barsanti, 1987). Resolution of incontinence and urodynamic improvement also were documented in two dogs with idiopathic detrusor instability. In one dog, previous treatment with propantheline was only partially effective (Lappin and Barsanti, 1987). The author has found oxybutynin administration helpful in the management of documented or suspected detrusor instability, in refractory urinary incontinence, and in juvenile dogs with congenital urogenital abnormalities and compromised urinary bladder capacity. Oxybutynin is available in a 5-mg tablet as well as a 1 mg/ml syrup. Total dosages of 0.5 to 1.0 mg PO every 8 to 12 hours are effective in cats and small dogs; dosages of 1.25 to 3.75 mg/dog PO every 8 to 12 hours are usually effective in medium to large dogs. A prolonged dosing interval is recommended in juvenile animals. Higher doses published elsewhere are unnecessary and may be dangerous.

Imipramine (Tofranil, Geigy) is a tricyclic antidepressant with a variety of potential actions in the lower urinary tract. Tricyclic antidepressants possess anticholinergic, antihistaminic, and adrenergic activities, along with some muscle relaxant, sedative, and analgesic properties. Both the anticholinergic effects and mild stimulatory effects on alpha- and beta-adrenergic receptors in the lower urinary tract may facilitate urine storage. A strong direct inhibitory effect is exerted on the detrusor muscle, which may be mediated by calcium channel antagonism, blockade of nor-epinephrine reuptake, or local anesthetic actions. Tricyclic antidepressants are recommended in the treatment of women with both urge and stress incontinence. Imipramine also has been useful in children with functional enuresis (bedwetting) and in some patients with fibrotic, poorly compliant bladders. Anecdotally, the agent has been effective in the treatment of urinary incontinence in dogs. Recommended dosages are 5 to 20 mg PO every 12 hours in dogs and 2.5 to 5 mg PO every 12 hours in cats. Although clinical experience with imipramine has not been well documented, trial administration is probably worthwhile if other agents fail.

In a study completed by the author, oxybutynin (2.5 mg PO every 8 hours), dicyclomine (10 mg PO every 8 hours), and imipramine (10 mg PO every 8 hours) were administered to 12 healthy Beagles (body weights 9 to 12 kg). Cystometrographic and urethral pressure profile variables obtained after treatment with each agent were compared with pretreatment measurements. With saline cystometry, the mean threshold volume and threshold volume per kilogram of body weight were slightly higher after dicyclomine administration than were pretreatment measurements and measurements after oxybutynin or imipramine administration (mean and median threshold volume 5.3 and 5.4 ml/kg versus 4.2 and 3.7 ml/kg in pretreatment measurements). Similarly, the slope of the filling phase (a measure of bladder compliance and elasticity) was lower after dicyclomine administration (mean 31.1 cm and median 22.5 cm H_2O/dl versus 53.9 and 54.9 cm H_2O/dl in pretreatment measurements). A comparable but blunted effect was observed with carbon dioxide cystometry. At the doses studied, no remarkable differences in cystometric variables were observed for oxybutynin or imipramine when compared with pretreatment measurements. Maximal urethral closure pressure measurements were slightly decreased after oxybutynin and imipramine administration in female Beagles, whereas urethral pressures were slightly increased after treatment with these agents in male dogs. No consistent urethral response was observed after dicyclomine administration. Considerable variability within treatment groups limited the statistical significance of these findings, however, and the cystometric testing method appears limited in detecting subtle effects of antimuscarinic agents in normal dogs. A more demonstrable effect may be observed in clinically affected dogs. Further investigation of dicyclomine appears warranted, however, especially since this drug may be obtained at one-quarter to one-half the cost of oxybutynin.

Emepronium bromide (Cetiprin, Kabi-Vitrum) is an anticholinergic agent with activity at both ganglionic and effector cell sites. The agent is unavailable in North America but may be found in Europe. Emepronium bromide was given to 21 incontinent female dogs that were unresponsive to reproductive hormone supplementation. Overall, only 6 of the 21 dogs exhibited significant improvement with treatment, and the observed improvement was transient in 3 dogs. Sustained improvement was observed in two dogs with signs consistent with detrusor instability and in one dog with suspected urethral incompetence (Holt, 1984).

Flavoxate (Urispar, SmithKline Beecham) is another smooth muscle relaxant with some analgesic and local anesthetic properties similar to those of oxybutynin and dicyclomine. Flavoxate is considered less effective than other muscle relaxants in the urinary tract, however, and has minimal antimuscarinic activity. The agent is used mostly for symptomatic relief of disorders associated with pain and dysuria.

ADVERSE EFFECTS OF ANTIMUSCARINIC AGENTS

Potential adverse effects of anticholinergic agents include sedation, ileus, vomiting, constipation, and urine retention. Dry mouth, dry eye, mydriasis, and tachycardia are problematic complications of anticholinergic administration in humans; the potential exacerbation of closed-angle glaucoma also is a concern. In dogs and cats, vomiting is the most common side effect of anticholinergic agents and usually can be minimized by decreasing the dose or frequency of administration. Hypersalivation is observed in some cats after oral administration of anticholinergic agents and may be minimized by administering the drug in a gelatin capsule. In healthy Beagles studied by the author, no overt adverse effects were observed after administration of oxybutynin, imipramine, and dicyclomine, although mild weight loss was observed. Antimuscarinic agents should be avoided or used cautiously in animals with cardiac disease, hyperthyroidism, arrhythmias, hypertension, or obstructive urinary disease. Pre-existing glaucoma is an absolute contraindication. Imipramine should be avoided in animals with pre-existing hepatic or renal disease, seizures, or hematologic disorders.

Given the potential adverse effects of antimuscarinic agents, the most appropriate indication for their use in small animals remains suspected or documented detrusor instability. When administration of an anticholinergic agent seems warranted, treatment should be initiated with low starting dosages that are titrated slowly to achieve the desired effect without significant adverse effects. Sensory or correctable neurogenic disorders that contribute to the dysfunction should be identified and addressed, if possible. Additional investigation of antimuscarinic agents in dogs and cats affected with disorders of bladder contractility will help define the role of these agents in urologic therapy.

References and Suggested Reading

Barsanti JA, Finco DR, Shotts EB, et al: Feline urologic syndrome: Further investigation into therapy. J Am Anim Hosp Assoc 18:387, 1982.
This article describes a prospective study of cats with nonobstructive feline lower urinary tract disease in which resolution of clinical signs did not differ after propantheline administration, antibiotic administration, fluid diuresis, or no therapy.

Holt PE: Efficacy of emepronium bromide in the treatment of physiological incontinence in the bitch. Vet Rec 114:355, 1984.
This article summarizes the clinical response to emepronium bromide in 21 female dogs with refractory urinary incontinence.

Lane IF, Lappin MR: Urinary incontinence and congenital urogenital anomalies in small animals. In: Bonagura JD, ed: Kirk's Current Veterinary Therapy XII. Philadelphia: WB Saunders, 1992, p 1022.
Included in this article is a summary of urinary bladder storage dysfunction in juvenile dogs and the potential role of anticholinergic agents in their management.

Lappin MR, Barsanti JA: Urinary incontinence secondary to idiopathic detrusor instability: Cystometrographic diagnosis and pharmacologic management in two dogs and a cat. J Am Vet Med Assoc 191:1439, 1987.
This article provides an initial description of idiopathic detrusor instability in small animals, along with a brief review of the disorder and its pharmacologic management.

Levin RM, Wein AJ: Direct measurement of the anticholinergic activity of a series of pharmacological compounds on the canine and rabbit urinary bladder. J Urol 128:396, 1982.
This is a report of a study comparing the relative potency of numerous anticholinergic agents at muscarinic receptors in isolated canine bladder preparations.

Moreau PM, Lappin MR: Pharmacologic management of urinary incontinence. In Kirk RW, ed: Current Veterinary Therapy X. Philadelphia: WB Saunders, 1989, p 1214.
This article reviews the major classes and pharmacologic agents available for treatment of micturition disorders in small animals.

Wein AJ: Pharmacology of incontinence. Urol Clin North Am 22:557, 1995.
This is a comprehensive review of agents that are used to facilitate urine storage in human patients.

Reproductive Disorders

Vicki N. Meyers-Wallen

Consulting Editor

***Still Current Information Found in* Current Veterinary Therapy XII:**

CVT Update: Inherited Disorders of the Reproductive Tract in Dogs and Cats

Vicki N. Meyers-Wallen

Ithaca, New York

NORMAL SEXUAL DEVELOPMENT

Normal sexual development depends on successful completion of three consecutive steps: (1) establishment of chromosomal sex, (2) development of gonadal sex, and (3) development of phenotypic sex. *Chromosomal sex*, which corresponds to genetic sex in normal animals, is established at fertilization. The zygote receives either two X chromosomes or an X and a Y chromosome and maintains this chromosomal constitution in all cells by mitotic division. Morphology of early XX and XY embryos is sexually indifferent. Both have a genital ridge, from which the testis or ovary will develop. They also have müllerian and wolffian ducts, a urogenital sinus, a genital tubercle, and genital swellings, from which the internal and external genitalia will arise (Fig. 1). Differentiation of the genital ridge into a testis or an ovary defines gonadal sex and marks the end of the sexually indifferent stage. Although several genes undoubtedly are necessary for normal development through the sexually indifferent stage, genes that determine gonadal sex have a pivotal role in sexual development.

Gonadal sex is normally determined by sex chromosome constitution: presence of the Y chromosome results in testis development, whereas its absence results in ovarian development. The sex-determining region Y gene, *Sry*, is normally located on the Y chromosome. This gene encodes the testis-determining factor and is the genetic signal for initiating testis differentiation in the genital ridge (reviewed in Goodfellow and Lovell-Badge, 1993). *Sry* is distinctly different from the gene for H-Y antigen, which is no longer thought to have a role in testis induction. Transgenic experiments in mice have demonstrated that *Sry* is the only Y-linked gene needed for testis induction (Koopman et al, 1991), and other evidence supports this theory (reviewed in Goodfellow and Lovell-Badge, 1993). In the absence of the Y chromosome and *Sry*, the genital ridge normally becomes an ovary. The *Dax1* gene, normally located on each X chromosome, is present in double dose in females and may have a role in suppressing male-specific genes during ovarian differentiation (Swain et al, 1996).

Phenotypic sex is normally controlled by gonadal sex. If the genital ridges are removed from XX or XY embryos before gonadal differentiation occurs, a female phenotype develops. This indicates that the embryo is programmed to develop as a female and must be diverted from this pathway to develop as a male. The critical diverting step is testis development. The testis secretes two substances that act within an embryonic critical period to induce masculinization: (1) müllerian inhibiting substance (MIS), which causes the müllerian ducts to regress, and (2) testosterone, which stimulates formation of the vasa deferentia and epididymides from the wolffian ducts (see Fig. 1). In the external genitalia, testosterone (T) is converted to dihydrotestosterone (DHT) by the enzyme 5α-reductase. Dihydrotestosterone stimulates formation of the prostate and male urethra, penis, and scrotum from the urogenital sinus, genital tubercle, and genital swellings, respectively (see Fig. 1). Descent of the testes into the scrotum completes the male external genitalia, but the genetic and hormonal control of this process is incompletely understood. In the absence of a testis and its masculinizing hormones, female genitalia develop (see Fig. 1).

DIAGNOSIS OF DISORDERS OF SEXUAL DEVELOPMENT

Intersex is a general term used to describe an animal with ambiguous genitalia. However, it is nonspecific, in that ambiguous genitalia can arise from an abnormality at any step in sexual development. Disorders in sexual differentiation can be classified by the initial step at which development differs from normal, thus falling into three general categories: abnormalities of chromosomal sex, gonadal sex, and phenotypic sex (Table 1). A more precise diagnosis, which defines the disorder according to its etiol-

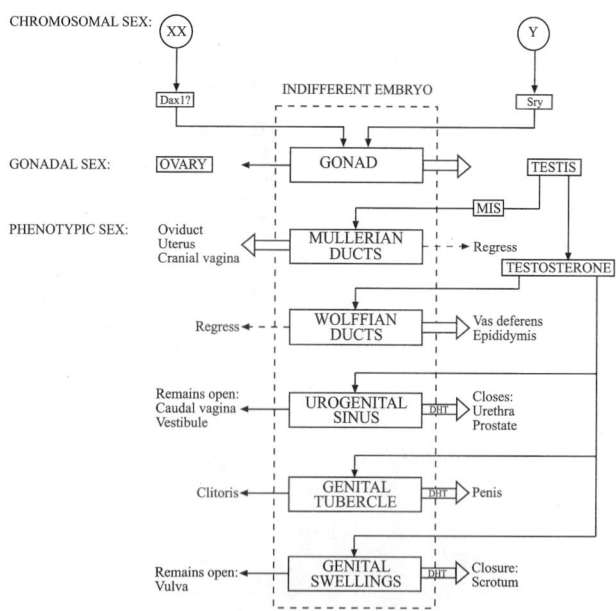

Figure 1. Normal sexual development. (Adapted from Morrow DA: Current Therapy in Theriogenology 2. Philadelphia: WB Saunders, 1986, with permission.)

TABLE 1. **Main Features of Selected Disorders of Sexual Development***

Abnormality Of	Karyotype	Gonad	Müllerian Duct Derivatives	Wolffian Duct Derivatives	External Genitalia	Diagnosis
Chromosomal sex	XXY	Testis	None	Epididymis, vas deferens	Male	XXY syndrome
	XO	Streak gonad	Uterus, oviduct, vagina	None	Female	XO syndrome
	XX/XY	Ovary or ovotestis or testis	Varies depending on amount of functional testis		Female or ambiguous or male	Chimera
Gonadal sex	XX	Testis	Uterus	Epididymis, ± vas deferens	Cryptorchid, hypospadias, displaced prepuce	XX sex reversal (Sry-negative): XX male
		Ovotestis	Uterus, ± oviduct	± epididymis	Female or enlarged clitoris	XX true hermaphrodite
Phenotypic sex Female pseudohermaphrodite	XX	Ovary	Uterus, oviduct	± epididymis	Ambiguous or male	Exogenous androgen/progestagen
Male pseudohermaphrodite	XY	Testis	Uterus, oviduct	Epididymis, vas deferens	Male ± cryptorchid	Persistent müllerian duct syndrome
	XY	Testis	None	None	Female	Complete Tfm
	XY	Testis	None	± epididymis, ± vas deferens	Ambiguous or female	Incomplete Tfm

*Examples are disorders reported in dogs or cats.

ogy, should be made when such information can be obtained. In the near future, for example, these disorders are likely to be defined by the specific gene mutation that is responsible for the defect.

The diagnostic plan should include investigation of chromosomal sex by direct examination of the chromosomes and construction of a karyotype. The presence or absence of the *Sry* gene in dogs can also be examined by molecular assays, such as polymerase chain reaction (see XX sex reversal later). Gonadal sex is best determined by histology and may require serial gonadal sections for identification of the ovotestes. A concise description of the internal and external genitalia is necessary for defining phenotypic sex. Assays of peripheral hormones may be helpful, but gonadotropin-releasing hormone (GnRH) or human chorionic gonadotropin (hCG) stimulation tests are necessary in many cases, particularly those in which peripheral androgen concentrations are of concern (Shille and Olson, 1989; see *CVT X*, pp. 1286–1288).

Abnormalities of Chromosomal Sex

Many disorders of sexual differentiation have been reported in which the primary cause was an abnormality in the number or structure of the sex chromosomes (e.g., see *CVT X*, pp. 1262–1265). To summarize, animals with abnormalities in sex chromosome number, such as those with XXY and XO syndromes, generally have underdeveloped genitalia and are sterile but are unambiguously male or female in phenotype (see Table 1). The gonadal sex of chimeras and mosaics depends on the distribution of XX and XY cells within the genital ridge. Phenotypic sex is then determined by the presence and amount of functional testicular tissue in the gonad. Abnormalities in chromosomal sex are usually due to chance events, such as errors in chromosome segregation or fusion of zygotes. Therefore, familial aggregation of affected individuals is not expected.

Abnormalities of Gonadal Sex

In this category, there is disagreement between the chromosomal sex and the gonadal sex of the individual. These animals are termed *sex-reversed*. In XX sex reversal, the chromosome constitution is XX but the individual develops testicular tissue in the gonad (testis or ovotestis). This has been reported in dogs, but not in cats.

XX Sex Reversal

Dogs affected with XX sex reversal have a 78,XX chromosome constitution and varying amounts of testicular tissue in the gonad. Affected dogs are termed either *XX true hermaphrodites*, which have at least one ovotestis, or *XX males*, which have bilateral testes (see Table 1). Both phenotypes can appear in the same family. Phenotypic masculinization is dependent on the amount of testicular tissue in the affected individual. Thus, XX true hermaphrodites may have normal female external genitalia or have an enlarged clitoris with an os clitoris that resembles a penis or have any phenotype in between. XX males generally have a caudally displaced prepuce and a penis with hypospadias and are bilaterally cryptorchid. XX sex reversal has been reported as a familial disorder in the English Cocker spaniel, Beagle, Weimaraner, Kerry blue terrier, Chinese Pug (see *CVT X*, pp. 1264–1265), and German shorthaired pointer (Meyers-Wallen et al, 1995b). It is likely to be inherited in all of these breeds, but the mode of inheritance has not been determined. In the American Cocker spaniel, XX sex reversal is inherited as an autosomal recessive trait (Meyers-Wallen and Patterson, 1988). The author has also observed individual cases of XX sex reversal in the Soft-Coated Wheaten terrier, Pomeranian, and Doberman pinscher.

Diagnosis of XX sex reversal classically depends on confirmation of a 78,XX chromosome constitution and the presence of at least one ovotestis or testis. Whereas elevation in peripheral T concentrations in response to GnRH or hCG stimulation strongly suggests that testicular tissue is present, it is not diagnostic (see *CVT X*, pp. 1286–1288). The inability to provoke T elevation by a stimulation test does rule out the diagnosis of XX sex reversal. Histologic demonstration of testicular tissue in at least one gonad in a 78,XX dog is necessary for a definitive diagnosis. To define the etiology of XX sex reversal more precisely and aid in genetic counseling, the diagnostic work-up should include a molecular test for the presence or absence of *Sry*. For example, in most humans with XX sex reversal, a Y chromosome is not detectable in the karyotype yet the *Sry* gene is present, as demonstrated by molecular techniques such as PCR. These *Sry*-positive XX individuals have received an *Sry translocation* from the parent. That is, the *Sry* gene has been transferred from the Y to another chromosome through abnormal crossing over, probably during gamete formation. Therefore, only one affected individual with *Sry*-positive XX sex reversal usually occurs within a family. *Sry*-positive XX sex reversal has not been reported in the dog but probably occurs sporadically as it does in humans.

Sry-negative XX sex reversal has been reported in American Cocker spaniels and German shorthaired pointers (Meyers-Wallen et al, 1995a, 1995b), as well as in pigs, goats, and humans. There is no *Sry* translocation detectable in these individuals, because the *Sry* gene is truly absent. The appearance of several affected individuals within a family is common. This form of XX sex reversal is inherited as an autosomal recessive trait in the American Cocker spaniel (Meyers-Wallen and Patterson, 1988). It is currently unclear whether the same autosomal gene is responsible for XX sex reversal in other breeds. However, it is likely to be the same gene in American and English Cocker spaniels because they share recent common ancestry.

XX males are sterile, as are most XX true hermaphrodites. Treatment of XX true hermaphrodite and XX male dogs is limited to surgical removal of the gonads and uterus and, if the dog is uncomfortable, excision of the enlarged clitoris and os clitoris. During breeding studies in the American Cocker spaniel, some XX true hermaphrodites had estrous cycles and a few produced offspring. Nevertheless, the mating of affected dogs of any breed is strongly discouraged. Affected American Cocker spaniels are homozygous for the sex reversal trait, will transmit this gene to all of their offspring, and produce only carrier or affected dogs. Carriers will transmit the gene to half their offspring, on average. Matings of affected or carrier dogs will increase the frequency of the sex reversal gene in the breed. In genetic counseling, it is important to note that both parents of an affected American Cocker spaniel are carriers. Additionally, at least two thirds of the male and female siblings of the affected dog, on average, are expected to be carriers. At present, a laboratory test for detecting carriers and affected dogs is not available.

Abnormalities of Phenotypic Sex

The chromosomal and gonadal sex are in agreement in these animals, yet the internal or external genitalia are ambiguous. Affected individuals are generally termed either *male* or *female pseudohermaphrodites* (see Table 1).

Female Pseudohermaphroditism

Female pseudohermaphrodites have an XX chromosome constitution and bilateral ovaries. Development of ambiguous genitalia is due to the presence of exogenous or endogenous androgens during development (e.g., see *CVT X*, p. 1266). The canine cases were XX individuals with bilateral ovaries and phenotypic masculinization ranging from mild clitoral enlargement to nearly normal male external genitalia with an internal prostate. An iatrogenic cause was known in some cases: either an androgen or a progestagen had been administered during gestation. The presenting signs were related to bleeding at the onset of proestrus, urinary incontinence, or uterine infection. This has not been reported in cats.

Diagnosis of female pseudohermaphrodites depends on confirmation of an XX chromosome constitution and ovaries. Before the gonads are removed, the diagnostic work-up could include tests for investigating endogenous androgen production (see *CVT X*, pp. 1286–1288). Elevation of serum T in response to GnRH or hCG would suggest testicular androgen production. Along with an XX chromosome constitution, this result would suggest a diagnosis of XX sex reversal (see earlier), and not female pseudohermaphroditism. Gonadal histology is necessary for distinguishing the difference. Abnormal elevation of serum androgens in response to adrenocorticotropic hormone stimulation would suggest adrenal androgen production, such as in the human adrenogenital syndromes. If no evidence of endogenous androgen production is found, historical confirmation of exogenous androgen exposure should be sought.

Ovariohysterectomy, with gonadal histopathology, is recommended for female pseudohermaphrodites. However, when urinary abnormalities are present, contrast studies are recommended before surgery to determine whether additional surgical treatment is necessary. Prevention may be best achieved by avoidance of steroid administration, such as androgens or progestagens, during gestation. Because the canine internal and external genitalia normally develop between gestational days 34 and 46, counting from the serum luteinizing hormone peak of the dam (Meyers-Wallen et al, 1991, 1993), it would be prudent to avoid steroid administration during this period.

Male Pseudohermaphroditism

A male pseudohermaphrodite has an XY chromosome constitution and has testes yet has female internal or external genitalia to some degree (see Table 1). Obviously this definition excludes XX males, in which chromosomal and gonadal sex do not agree (see XX sex reversal earlier). Two etiologically distinct categories of male pseudohermaphroditism are recognized: (1) failure of müllerian duct regression (as in persistent müllerian duct syndrome) and (2) failure of androgen-dependent masculinization (including defects in androgen synthesis, 5α reductase, or the androgen receptor).

Persistent Müllerian Duct Syndrome

Persistent müllerian duct syndrome (PMDS) has been reported in the Miniature Schnauzer in the United States and the Basset hound in the Netherlands and may also occur in the Persian cat (reviewed in Meyers-Wallen and Patterson, 1989a). Affected Miniature Schnauzers are XY males with bilateral testes and normal androgen-dependent masculinization of the internal and external genitalia. However, they also have bilateral oviducts, a complete uterus with cervix, and the cranial portion of the vagina. Approximately half of affected dogs have unilateral or bilateral cryptorchidism, while the remaining half have normally descended testes. Therefore, affected males may not be detected by physical examination alone. Affected males are frequently detected when clinical signs related to pyometra, urinary tract infection, or prostate infection arise.

Diagnosis of PMDS depends on confirmation of an XY chromosome constitution, bilateral testes, and the presence of all müllerian duct derivatives (see Table 1). Treatment is limited to castration and hysterectomy. The uterine body terminates in a small cervix and cranial vagina at the craniodorsal aspect of the prostate gland. In some cases, there is a short, small-diameter communication between the cranial vaginal portion and the prostatic urethra, which may allow ascending infection of the uterus. During hysterectomy, care should be taken to remove as much of the vaginal portion as possible.

Prevention is limited to removing affected and carrier dogs from the breeding population. In the Miniature Schnauzer, PMDS is inherited as an autosomal recessive trait (Meyers-Wallen et al, 1989c). Although both females and males can be carriers, only homozygous males express the affected phenotype. Affected dogs with scrotal testes are usually fertile, but breeding of such dogs is strongly discouraged. Affected dogs will transmit the PMDS trait to all of their offspring, producing only carriers or affected dogs. The etiology of this defect is unknown. Affected dogs produce biologically active MIS during the embryonic critical period for müllerian duct regression (Meyers-Wallen et al, 1989c, 1993). Therefore, it is suspected that the müllerian ducts are insensitive to MIS, possibly because of a receptor defect.

Defects in Androgen-Dependent Masculinization

Affected animals in this category are XY males that have bilateral testes and normal regression of the müllerian duct system. However, genitalia that require androgens for masculinization fail to develop normally (see Table 1). Inherited defects of this type generally affect both prenatal and postnatal male development. Failure of androgen-dependent masculinization can range from mild (incomplete failure) to severe (complete failure). The primary defect causing these phenotypes may lie in (1) androgen production, (2) conversion of T to DHT, or (3) androgen reception at the target organ level. Defects in androgen production have not been documented in the dog or cat. The terms *androgen resistance* and *androgen insensitivity* refer to syndromes in which androgen production is normal but there is still failure of masculinization. These include defects in the 5α-reductase enzyme and the androgen receptor. Defects in 5α-reductase affect conversion of T to DHT and have not been reported in dogs and cats. The term *testicular feminization* is reserved for androgen receptor

defects. In the testicular feminization syndromes, both T- and DHT-dependent masculinization can be affected, resulting in either complete or partial failure of masculinization (see Table 1). Defects of this type have been reported in dogs and cats.

Hypospadias. This is an abnormality in location of the urinary orifice, owing to incomplete masculinization of the urogenital sinus during formation of the male urethra. As a result, the urethral opening may be located anywhere along the embryologic course of the urogenital sinus to the genital tubercle. Hypospadias has been reported as a familial defect in some dog breeds, whereas teratogen-induced hypospadias has been reported in other species (see *CVT X*, p. 1267, reviewed in Meyers-Wallen and Patterson, 1989a). The initial differential diagnosis may include inherited defects such as XX sex reversal, particularly when hypospadias is accompanied by scrotal abnormalities or a uterus. A diagnostic plan that includes investigation of chromosomal and gonadal sex will lead to appropriate diagnosis and genetic counseling. Surgical correction of this defect is usually unnecessary, because hypospadias does not usually cause urinary difficulties. Affected dogs with mild hypospadias may be able to breed normally. However, when the etiology of hypospadias is unknown, it is recommended that affected dogs be removed from the breeding program to prevent further dissemination of familial hypospadias.

Testicular Feminization Syndromes. These syndromes are caused by mutations in the X-linked androgen receptor gene. Affected individuals are XY males with bilateral testes (see Table 1). Müllerian duct derivatives are absent, as expected for a male. However, there is either complete or partial failure of androgen-dependent masculinization, depending on whether the androgen receptor is nonfunctional or partially functional. Although T production and conversion to DHT are normal, the target organs are unable to respond appropriately.

In complete testicular feminization, the androgen receptor is completely nonfunctional and androgen-dependent masculinization is entirely absent. Affected males often present as females that fail to cycle and are sterile. A defect of this type has been reported in a domestic shorthaired cat (Meyers-Wallen et al, 1989b). Bilateral abdominal testes were present, but there were no epididymides nor vasa deferentia. The uterus was absent as expected, because MIS production and response is unaffected. The external genitalia were phenotypically female. High-affinity binding of DHT was virtually undetectable in cultured genital fibroblasts, confirming receptor malfunction.

In humans, incomplete testicular feminization syndromes are caused by different mutations of the androgen receptor gene that produce varying degrees of masculinization. The spectrum caused by these defects ranges from individuals with ambiguous genitalia to phenotypic males that are infertile. The author has observed a number of cats that probably have incomplete testicular feminization syndromes. They were XY and had bilateral testes within a bifid scrotum. The external genitalia resemble that of a female, in that there is a vulva-like genital opening with a female urethral orifice and a blind-ending vagina. There is severe perineal hypospadias, and the penis resembles a clitoris yet develops spines. Studies in one cat indicated that neither T nor DHT was deficient (see *CVT X*, p. 1267). Although androgen receptor assays were not performed, this suggests that the partial masculinization was due to an androgen receptor defect where the receptor was partially functional.

A similar case has been described in a mixed breed dog (Peter et al, 1993). In this XY male with bilateral testes in a bifid scrotum the testes appeared as swellings on each side of a vulva that opened into a blind vaginal pouch. Peripheral T and DHT concentrations were normal after hCG stimulation. Epididymides were present adjacent to the testes, indicating that T-dependent masculinization was unimpaired during embryonic development. High-affinity binding of DHT was undetectable in cultured genital fibroblasts. These data suggest that DHT binding was abnormal but T binding was not. Both T and DHT bind to the same androgen receptor, which is encoded by a single gene. Nevertheless, there is pharmacologic evidence that the androgen receptor can exhibit different binding affinity preference for DHT relative to T in adult canine tissues (Summerfield et al, 1995). Therefore, it is possible that a mutation in the androgen receptor could affect DHT-dependent masculinization but not T-dependent masculinization, as the findings in this case would suggest.

Diagnosis of a testicular feminization syndrome is dependent on demonstration of an XY chromosome constitution, bilateral testes, and abnormal androgen binding in androgen-responsive tissues. GnRH/hCG stimulation tests in the intact animal will confirm that peripheral androgens are present (see *CVT X*, pp.1286–1288), providing further evidence for androgen resistance. In the future, when the range of canine and feline androgen receptor mutations has been documented as in humans, it should be possible to diagnose these defects at the level of the androgen receptor gene. Castration is the recommended treatment for affected dogs and cats. Prevention is limited to genetic counseling regarding the X-linked inheritance of this disorder. Carrier females are fertile. Of their offspring, 50% of the males are expected to be affected, whereas 50% of the females are expected to be carriers. However 50% of the male offspring will not receive the X chromosome bearing the testicular feminization mutation. These males should have normal genitalia and can be used in a breeding program.

Cryptorchidism. This disorder is included here somewhat arbitrarily because the underlying mechanisms for abnormal testis descent are incompletely understood. Cryptorchidism is associated with other defects in sexual development, as mentioned earlier, but can also appear as the only defect of the reproductive system, which is referred to here as isolated cryptorchidism. As previously reviewed (see *CVT X*, p. 1268), isolated cryptorchidism is the most common disorder of the reproductive tract reported in dogs. A diagnosis of cryptorchidism is warranted if both testes are not palpable within the scrotum at 8 weeks of age because the testes normally descend by 10 days after birth.

Dogs with bilateral cryptorchidism are sterile, whereas those with unilateral cryptorchidism can be fertile. However, the recommended treatment for both is bilateral castration. First, there is an increased risk of Sertoli cell tumor in cryptorchid testes. Second, isolated cryptorchidism is clearly a familial trait in several breeds and is likely to be inherited in dogs, as it is in other mammals. Although the genetics of this disorder in dogs are incompletely characterized, there are enough data to allow genetic counseling. Inheritance of isolated cryptorchidism as a sex-limited recessive trait is consistent with available data. Using this model, the first recommendation is that affected dogs be removed from the breeding population. The second recommendation is that both the father and mother of affected dogs should be considered to be carriers. Some full siblings of the affected dog will also be carriers. In other species in which cryptorchidism occurs as a simple (single gene) recessive trait, a reduction in the frequency of affected animals was obtained in a few generations by removing carrier parents and affected males from the breeding population. This is probably the minimum program that should be pursued in dogs. It may also be necessary to remove siblings of affected dogs from the breeding program. Although medical regimens have been suggested to induce testicular descent in cryptorchid dogs, there are no published reports to confirm that these are more successful than no treatment. Furthermore, even if the testes descend within a few months, the genes responsible for cryptorchidism remain unchanged and will be transmitted to the offspring. It is recommended that cryptorchid dogs and those with late testicular descent be removed from the breeding program to reduce the gene frequency of these disorders in the breed.

References and Suggested Reading

Goodfellow PN, Lovell-Badge R: *SRY* and sex determination in mammals. Annu Rev Genet 27:71–92, 1993.
This article reviews current medical and experimental evidence supporting the pivotal role of Sry in sex determination.

Koopman P, Gubbay J, Vivian N, et al: Male development of chromosomally female mice transgenic for *Sry*. Nature (London) 351:117, 1991.
This landmark transgenic study demonstrates that Sry is the only gene necessary for testis induction.

Meyers-Wallen VN, Patterson DF: XX sex reversal in the American cocker spaniel dog: Phenotypic expression and inheritance. Hum Genet 80:23, 1988.
This article contains the breeding experiments that defined the mode of inheritance of this disorder and describes the range of phenotypic abnormalities.

Meyers-Wallen VN, Patterson DF: Disorders of sexual development in the dog. In: Kirk RW, Bonagura JD, eds: Current Veterinary Therapy X. 1989a, pp 1261–1269. WB Saunders, Philadelphia:
This is the first review of this subject in dogs, which is updated by the present article.

Meyers-Wallen VN, Wilson JD, Griffin JE, et al: Testicular feminization in a cat. J Am Vet Med Assoc 195:631, 1989b.
This is the only report of complete testicular feminization syndrome in the cat.

Meyers-Wallen VN, Donahoe PK, Ueno S, et al: Mullerian inhibiting substance is present in testes of dogs with persistent mullerian duct syndrome. Biol Reprod 41:881, 1989c.
These experiments demonstrate that bioactive MIS is produced by dogs affected with inherited PMDS.

Meyers-Wallen VN, Manganaro TF, Kuroda T, et al: The critical period for mullerian duct regression in the dog embryo. Biol Reprod 45:626, 1991.
This study defines the gestational ages during which canine mullerian and wolffian development normally occur.

Meyers-Wallen VN, Lee MM, Manganaro TF, et al: Mullerian inhibiting substance is present in embryonic testes of dogs with persistent mullerian duct syndrome. Biol Reprod 48:141, 1993.

This study refines the gestational age at which canine genitalia develop and demonstrates that MIS is produced in embryos affected with PMDS.

Meyers-Wallen VN, Palmer VL, Acland GM, et al: *Sry*-negative XX sex reversal in the American cocker spaniel dog. Mol Reprod Dev 41:300, 1995a.

This study demonstrates that Sry is absent in American cocker spaniels affected with inherited XX sex reversal.

Meyers-Wallen VN, Bowman L, Acland GM, et al: *Sry*- negative XX sex reversal in the German shorthaired pointer dog. J Hered 86:369, 1995b.

This study demonstrates that Sry is absent in German shorthaired pointers affected with XX sex reversal.

Peter AT, Markwelder, Asem EK: Phenotypic feminization in a genetic male dog caused by nonfunctional androgen receptors. Theriogenology 40:1093, 1993.

This is the only report of incomplete testicular feminization in the dog.

Shille VM, Olson PN: Dynamic testing in reproductive endocrinology. In: Kirk RW, Bonagura JD, eds: Current Veterinary Therapy X. 1989, pp 1282–1288. WB Saunders Philadelphia:

This review describes the protocol for canine and feline gonadotropin-releasing hormone and human chorionic gonadotropin stimulation tests.

Summerfield AE, Cruz PJD, Dolenga MP, et al: Tissue-specific pharmacology of testosterone and 5-alpha-dihydrotestosterone analogues: Characterization of a novel canine liver androgen-binding protein. Mol Pharmacol 47:1080, 1995.

This study indicates that the canine androgen receptor can exhibit different binding affinity preference for DHT relative to T.

Swain A, Zanaria E, Hacker A, et al: Mouse *Dax1* expression is consistent with a role in sex determination as well as in adrenal and hypothalamus function. Nat Genet 12:404, 1996.

This study describes embryonic Dax1 expression, providing support for a role in ovarian differentiation.

DNA Testing for Inherited Canine Diseases

GUSTAVO D. AGUIRRE

Ithaca, New York

Recent progress in human genome research, and its application to the understanding and diagnosis of inherited diseases, has had a parallel in canine genetics. This is an area of interest that is shared by both the veterinary profession and the owners and breeders of purebred dogs. At present, over 300 inherited disorders have been identified in dogs, and these are being catalogued in a readily accessible computer database that, when available, will permit the rapid access to canine genetic disease information that is constantly updated (D. Patterson, unpublished). Along with the recognition of new genetic diseases has been the identification of the molecular defects causing some of them. The rapid growth of this area of research will have a major impact not only for the diagnosis of dogs affected with specific inherited diseases but also in genetic counseling in order to produce dogs that are free of these diseases, and to reduce and eventually eliminate the mutant alleles within the susceptible population. This chapter reviews the uses and limitations of DNA testing.

MOLECULARLY DEFINED CANINE DISEASES

Of the recognized genetic diseases in the dog, most of those in which the mode of inheritance is known are autosomal recessive, with fewer being inherited as dominant or X-linked. The reasons for the high proportion of recessively inherited disorders in dogs are complex. In general they are attributed to (1) the difficulty in identification of carrier dogs for some diseases whose age of onset is late and that are difficult to diagnose accurately early in life, and (2) the use of breeding practices where highly desirable individuals, particularly males, are overused. This results in the disproportionate representation of certain bloodlines within the population. When deleterious mutations are present in these individuals, there is the likelihood that the prevalence of the recessive disease will increase.

Autosomal Dominant Inheritance

There are no autosomal dominant diseases that have been identified at the molecular level. When fully penetrant, these diseases do not pose a serious threat to the breeding population because disease control is possible by the elimination of affected dogs. It is only when the diseases are not fully penetrant, e.g., the ocular-skeletal disorder of Labrador retrievers or the posterior cortical cataracts of Golden and Labrador retrievers, that reduction of the disease frequency is more difficult, and the prevalence of the disease remains unchanged or increases.

X-Linked Inheritance

Some of the genes located in the canine X-chromosome, and their corresponding diseases, were the first ones identified in the dog. This is not surprising because the X has been one of the most studied of all human chromosomes, and it is conserved across all placental mammals. There are five molecularly identified X-linked disorders in dogs (Table 1). Because control measures based on breeding practices have been effective, the disease prevalence is usually low.

Autosomal Recessive Inheritance

This mode of inheritance represents the majority of diseases caused by single gene defects; of these, the mutation has been identified in 10 diseases (Table 2). With the advances in human molecular genetics research, and the

TABLE 1. Molecularly Defined Canine Diseases: X-Linked Inheritance

Disease	Gene	Breeds	Contact Person/Institution	Reference
Hemophilia B	Factor IX	Labrador retriever, Lhasa apso, others	M. Brooks, Cornell University	Brooks, 1994; Mauser et al, 1996
X-linked severe combined immunodeficiency (XSCID)	IL-2Rγ	Basset hound, Cardigan Welsh corgi	P. Henthorn, Univ. of Penna.	Henthorn et al, 1994; Somberg et al, 1995
Hereditary nephropathy	α5 (Col. IV)	Samoyed	P. Thorner, Hosp. for Sick Children, Toronto	Zheng et al, 1994
Shaking pup syndrome (hereditary hypomyelination)	Proteolipid protein	English Springer spaniel	I. Duncan, Univ. of Wisconsin	Nadon et al, 1990
Muscular dystrophy	Dystrophin	Golden retriever, Rottweiler	B. Cooper/N. Winand, Cornell Univ.	Winand, 1994

identification of diseases in dogs that are putatively homologous to human disorders, the likelihood is that, in the near future, many of the recessively inherited disorders of dogs will be defined at the molecular level. Because some of these have a relative high disease prevalence or carrier rate, they are the ones in which the use of DNA-based testing for diagnosis of affected individuals or identification of carriers has the greatest potential.

Markers Linked to Disease Loci

It is possible to establish linkage of a genetic disease locus to a DNA marker so that the linked marker is used to identify animals that are affected, normal, or carriers. Linkage can be established without knowledge of the specific gene involved or of the mutation causing the disease. Such a test is now available for *copper toxicosis* in the Bedlington terrier (Yuzbasiyan-Gurkan et al, 1997).

PREVALENCE AND SIGNIFICANCE OF THE DISEASES

Finding a molecular basis for a disease does not mean that a DNA test will be useful in a clinical setting. In several cases, the diseases represent biologic curiosities that are studied because of their potential use to biomedical research rather than because the diseases have a major impact in purebred dogs. With the exception of *hemophilia B*, and possibly *muscular dystrophy*, most of the X-linked diseases are of limited prevalence in the dog population. In contrast, most of the autosomal recessive disorders have a relatively high prevalence for the disease and/or the carrier state, the possible exceptions being *elliptocytosis* and *mucopolysaccharidosis I and VII*.

Mutation Prevalence

Very few studies have been carried out to date to establish the prevalence of a mutation in dog populations, particularly within specific breeds. In testing Irish setters for the mutation in the phosphodiesterase beta (PDEB) gene responsible for the *rcd1* form of progressive retinal atrophy (PRA) (Ray et al, 1994), we have found no affected dogs in a 2.5-year period, but have established that 7.5% of over 300 samples analyzed are from carriers of the disease. Similar high carrier rates have been found in *globoid cell leukodystrophy* in West Highland White terriers (~20%), *phosphofructokinase deficiency* in English Springer spaniels (~10%) and *von Willebrand's disease* in Scottish terriers (~23%) (personal communication from D. Wenger, U. Giger, and P. Venta, respectively). These carrier rates, however, are artificially high. Because the identification of disease-causing mutations and the development of DNA-based testing is very new to canine medicine, it is not surprising that many of the dogs tested initially have a high probability of being carriers, either because they are closely related to obligate heterozygotes, or because of suspected carrier state based on inconclusive biochemical analysis. A

TABLE 2. Molecularly Defined or Linked Canine Diseases: Autosomal Recessive Inheritance

Disease	Gene	Breeds	Contact Person/Institution	Reference
Pyruvate kinase deficiency	PK, R-type	Basenji	C. Lothrop, Jr., Auburn Univ.	Whitney and Lothrop, 1995
Progressive retinal atrophy (*rcd1* form)	PDEB	Irish setter	G. Aguirre, Cornell Univ.	Ray et al, 1994
MPS I	IDUA	Plott hound	R. Shull, Univ. of Tennessee	Menon et al, 1992
MPS VII	GUSB	Mixed breed	P Henthorn, Univ. Penna./J. Ray, Cornell Univ.	Ray et al, 1996
Elliptocytosis 1	protein 4.1	Mixed breed	J. Conboy, Univ. California Berkeley	Conboy et al, 1991
Globoid cell leukodystrophy	GALC	West Highland White and Cairn terriers	D. Wenger, Jefferson Medical College	Victoria et al, 1996
Phosphofructokinase deficiency	PFK, M-type	English Springer spaniel, American Cocker spaniel	U. Giger, Univ. of Penna.	Smith et al, 1996
Copper toxicosis	Linked marker	Bedlington terrier	G. Brewer, Univ. of Mich.	Yuzbasiyan-Gurkan et al, 1997
von Willebrand's disease	vWF	Scottish terrier	P. Venta, Mich. State Univ.	Venta et al., submitted
Fucosidosis	FUCA1	English Springer spaniel	D. Sargan, Univ. of Cambridge	Skelly et al, 1996

MPS, mucopolysaccharidosis.

more accurate determination of carrier rates will be established in the future with the testing of a larger and more random population within each susceptible breed.

Founder Effect Versus Allelic Heterogeneity

The limited studies of mutation prevalence in autosomal recessive diseases in dogs have shown that, *within a breed*, the same disease-causing defect is present. In this case, both alleles of a gene are affected by the same mutation. Such uniformity of mutations within a population suggests a "founder effect" whereby the same genetic defect has increased in prevalence in a population by selection of progeny from the mutant-bearing founder animal over several generations.

In the case of phosphofructokinase deficiency, the same mutation that is present extensively in the English Springer spaniel has been found in the American Cocker spaniel (Smith et al, 1996). Because the probability that the same mutation arose sporadically in two related breeds is extremely low, finding the same mutation in both spaniel breeds would support a founder effect, or would indicate the intentional or inadvertent intercrossing of two breeds.

If more than one mutation exists in the same gene (allelic heterogeneity), it is possible that affected individuals will have a different mutation in each allele; this is a common finding in human autosomal recessive diseases. The issue of allelic heterogeneity is most important when testing for carriers of recessive genes because a heterozygote will be misdiagnosed if it has a mutation different from the one being tested. This area will need to be addressed in the future as research expands our understanding of the molecular basis of inherited diseases within and between dog breeds.

The same situation occurs in X-linked inherited disorders. Although different mutations have been identified in the dystrophin gene that cause *muscular dystrophy*, these are breed-specific in the Golden retriever and Rottweiler (Winand, 1994). Similarly, three different breed-specific mutations have been identified in the Factor IX gene responsible for *hemophilia B* in the Labrador retriever, Lhasa apso, and other breeds (Brooks, 1994; Mauser et al, 1996), and two different mutations in the interleukin-2 receptor γ chain gene have been identified in Basset hounds and Cardigan Welsh corgis affected with *X-linked severe combined immunodeficiency* (XSCID; Henthorn et al, 1994; Somberg et al, 1995). The important point to remember is that the high specificity of mutation-based tests requires that they be used selectively, i.e., to rule out a specific mutation, and that negative results indicate the absence of the specific disease-causing mutation tested, not the absence of a mutation in the gene or one of the alleles when testing carriers.

SPECIFICITY, LIMITATIONS, AND ACCURACY OF DNA TESTS

Linkage-Based Tests

These tests rely on the close physical proximity of a DNA marker (e.g., microsatellite, polymorphic gene, RAPD marker, other) to the disease locus of interest. Such tests usually depend on pedigree analysis in which there is a dog of known disease status, and the linked marker used has to be sufficiently polymorphic in order that genetic variation can be detected among pedigree members; lack of polymorphism prevents the use of the test. The accuracy of the test depends on the distance between the linked marker and the gene locus; this distance is established by determining the number of recombinations that occur between the disease locus and the marker when analyzing a pedigree. Thus a higher recombination fraction means a greater separation between the two, and a lower reliability of the test. Some of these limitations can be overcome by using several linked markers, particularly if they are physically located on either side of the disease gene. A linkage-based test is available for *copper toxicosis* in Bedlington terriers (Yuzbasiyan-Gurkan et al, 1997), and will soon be used in testing for the *prcd* form of PRA in several different dog breeds.

Mutation-Based Tests

Most DNA tests currently used in dogs are directed at identifying a single specific mutation responsible for the disease. The application of a test with such specificity relies on prior knowledge that the mutation being tested is the only one present in the disease, and this information must be known and preferably published before the test is commercially available. Mutation-based tests should not be used in a general screening of dogs in which there is not a high level of suspicion of the specific disease, nor should the test be used in breeds having the same disease, but in which the causative mutation has not been identified. In many cases, diseases that are clinically similar may differ, either because they are the result of mutations of different genes, or different mutations in the same gene (genetic and allelic heterogeneity, respectively).

Comparison of Biochemical and Mutation-Based Tests

Specific biochemical or immunochemical tests are available for the diagnosis of *hemophilia B*, and 7 of the 10 autosomal recessive disorders (exceptions are *rcd1, elliptocytosis,* and *copper toxicosis*) described in Tables 1 and 2. In general, the tests measure the abnormal function of the defective protein in a biochemical reaction. As long as the protein is absent or abnormal in size or function, the test results are reasonably accurate, and the affected sample can be reliably distinguished from the normal. Although carriers for the autosomal recessive diseases have intermediate levels of enzyme activity, the range of values is usually large, and there is some overlap between the normal and affected values at the high and low ends of the range.

Additionally, in some cases such as *pyruvate kinase deficiency* in the Basenji, a compensatory increase in the expression of a related isozyme makes it difficult to identify carriers with a high degree of reliability (Whitney and Lothrop, 1995). This limits the usefulness and accuracy of some biochemical tests for carrier detection. Another limitation is the need to concurrently run normal control samples in some of the assays, as well as the need to pay strict attention to guidelines for collecting and shipping the samples so that the enzyme activity is not lost during transit.

Because of their greater specificity and accuracy, and the need to test only a single animal, mutation-based tests are preferable when testing for specific diseases where the gene and defect are known, and the tests specifically examine the known mutation or mutations present in the population. Biochemical tests are better as a general screening for a suspected disorder in which the abnormal gene has not been identified or the molecular defect defined.

USE OF DNA TESTING

Disease Diagnosis

Because allelic or genetic heterogeneity within the same breed for a specific disease class is not a problem in dogs to date, DNA tests in general, and mutation-based tests in particular, are extremely useful to identify dogs affected with specific inherited disorders. There is no age limitation for the test, which can be run as early as the appropriate DNA-containing sample can be collected (see below).

Genetic Counseling and Breeding

The greatest future potential for DNA testing, particularly for autosomal recessive and some of the X-linked diseases, is in breeding. The specificity and accuracy of mutation-based tests permits the determination at a very young age of dogs who are affected or are carriers for a disease, well before they are used for breeding. For disorders where the disease prevalence and carrier rate are low (e.g., *fucosidosis* in the English Springer spaniel in the *United States* [note that the carrier rate is high in Great Britain and Australia]), the identified carriers can be removed from the breeding population without affecting the genetic diversity of the breed.

On the other hand, for those diseases with a high prevalence of affected individuals and/or carriers (see section on Mutation Prevalence), the test is used to identify carriers that are to be retained within the breeding population as long as they are bred to dogs that are genetically normal by the DNA test. Efforts are made in each subsequent generation to select for breeding genetically normal dogs of superior quality. In this manner, the genetic diversity of a breed can be maintained while gradually reducing or eliminating the prevalence of the mutation, and avoiding producing affected dogs.

DNA TESTING RESOURCES

At present, it is not possible to perform DNA tests in a private veterinary practice setting. The tests require the use of several high-cost instruments that need technical expertise to operate and to interpret the results. Because most of the tests have been developed as a by-product of the specific research interests of university-based scientists, the tests are run as a service by these individuals. In some cases, the mutation and the DNA test have been patented, thus requiring agreement on licensing fees or royalties when used in a commercial basis. More recently, several companies have been started whose aim is to provide a wide spectrum of DNA tests and genetic counseling for a variety of different breeds and diseases. Because of their recent appearance, it has not been possible to evaluate the reliability of the services, or the accuracy of the tests provided. Tables 1 and 2 provide the names and institution of the individuals who have identified the specific molecular defects and/or who have developed the currently available DNA tests; additional details are presented at the end of the article.

SOURCE OF DNA AND SUBMISSION OF THE SAMPLE

Theoretically, any source of DNA (blood, semen, hair bulb, buccal swab, etc.) can be used to carry out the DNA test. In practice, however, most tests have been developed using one specific source of DNA and, for that reason, it is best to submit the appropriate sample to the testing laboratory because this minimizes the costs and increases the reliability of the test. For example, we use citrated whole blood for the PRA test (*rcd1* form) in Irish setters, whereas the *phosphofructokinase* test uses drops of dried blood placed on a modified filter paper (Guthrie card), and the *von Willebrand's disease* test uses buccal smears collected with a small brush as a source of DNA. Regardless of the method in which the sample is collected, it must be remembered that *there must be no contamination* with samples from a different dog. That is, every needle, syringe, brush, etc., must be discarded after a single use, and previously used syringes, even if sterilized, can not be used. The reason for these precautions is that most DNA tests are based on the use of the polymerase chain reaction (PCR) in which a very small quantity of DNA is amplified many times (p. 246). Contaminating DNA from a different animal would be similarly amplified, causing potentially incorrect results in the test.

REFERENCE LABORATORIES FOR DNA TESTING

Aguirre GD, Center for Canine Genetics and Reproduction, James A. Baker Institute for Animal Health, College of Veterinary Medicine, Cornell University, Ithaca, NY 14853.

Brooks M, Comparative Coagulation Section, Diagnostic Laboratory, College of Veterinary Medicine, Cornell University, Ithaca, NY 14853.

Conboy JG, Cell and Molecular Biology, University of California, Berkeley, CA 94720

Cooper B or Winand N, Department of Pathology, College of Veterinary Medicine, Cornell University, Ithaca, NY 14853.

Duncan I, School of Veterinary Medicine, University of Wisconsin, Madison, WI 53706.

Henthorn P, Section of Medical Genetics, School of Veterinary Medicine, University of Pennsylvania, Philadelphia, PA 19104-6010.

Lothrop Jr CD, Scott-Ritchey Research Center, College of Veterinary Medicine, Auburn University, Auburn, AL 36849-5525.

Ray J, James A. Baker Institute for Animal Health, College of Veterinary Medicine, Cornell University, Ithaca, NY 14853.

Sargan D, Department of Clinical Veterinary Medicine, University of Cambridge, Cambridge CB3 OES, UK.

Thorner PS, Department of Pathology, The Hospital for Sick Children and Research Institute, 555 University Ave., Toronto, Ontario, Canada.

Venta P, Department of Small Animal Sciences, College of Veterinary Medicine, Michigan State University, East Lansing, MI 48824-1314.

Wenger DA, Division of Medical Genetics, Jefferson Medical College, Philadelphia, PA 19107.

References and Suggested Reading

Brooks M: Canine hemophilia B: Affected dogs show phenotypic and molecular genetic heterogeneity. AKC Molecular and Canine Health Conference, 1994. (Abstract.)
Description of complete deletion of factor IX gene in affected Labrador retrievers.

Conboy JG, Shitamoto R, Parra M, et al: Hereditary elliptocytosis due to both qualitative and quantitative defects in membrane skeletal protein 4.1. Blood 78:2438, 1991.
Disease-causing mutation presented.

Henthorn PS, Somberg RL, Fimiani VM, et al: IL-2Rγ gene microdeletion demonstrates that canine X-linked severe combined immunodeficiency is a homologue of the human disease. Genomics 23:69, 1994.
Molecular basis of X-linked severe combined immunodeficiency in the Basset hound presented.

Mauser AE, Whitlark J, Whitney KM, et al: A deletion mutation causes hemophilia B in Lhasa apso dogs. Blood 88:3451, 1996.
New disease-causing mutation in factor IX gene.

Menon KP, Tieu PT, Neufeld EF: Architecture of the canine IDUA gene and mutation underlying canine mucopolysaccharidosis I. Genomics 12:763, 1992.
Description of mutation in IDUA gene that causes MPS I in the Plott hound.

Nadon NL, Duncan, ID, Hudson LD: A point mutation in the proteolipid protein gene of the 'shaking pup' interrupts oligodendrocyte development. Development 110:529, 1990.
Description of the mutation of the proteolipid protein gene that causes "shaking pup" syndrome.

Ray K, Baldwin VJ, Acland GM, et al: Cosegregation of codon 807 mutation of the canine rod cGMP phosphodiesterase β gene and *rcd1*. Invest Ophthalmol Vis Sci 35:4291, 1994.
Demonstration that this is the only mutation causing PRA in the Irish setter breed.

Ray J, DeSanto C, Sun W, et al: Studies on the molecular basis of β-glucuronidase deficiency in mucopolysaccharidosis VII (MPS VII) in the retinal pigment epithelium. Suppl Invest Ophthalmol Vis Sci 37:S379, 1996.
Description of mutation in GUSB gene in this rare canine storage disease.

Skelly BJ, Sargan DR, Herrtage ME, et al: The molecular defect underlying canine fucosidosis. J Med Genet 33:284, 1996.
DNA defect responsible for fucosidosis.

Smith BF, Stedman H, Rajpurohit Y, et al: Molecular basis of canine muscle type phosphofructokinase deficiency. J Biol Chem 271:20070, 1996.
Identification of the mutation in English Springer spaniels and one American Cocker spaniel.

Somberg RL, Pullen RP, Casal ML, et al: A single nucleotide insertion in the canine interleukin-2 receptor gamma chain results in X-linked severe combined immunodeficiency disease. Vet Immunol Immunopathol 47:203, 1995.
Mutation causing XSCID in Cardigan Welsh corgi.

Victoria T, Rafi MA, Wenger DA: Cloning of the canine GALC cDNA and identification of the mutation causing globoid cell leukodystrophy in west highland white and cairn terriers. Genomics 33:457, 1996.
Mutation and DNA test for Krabbe disease described.

Whitney KM, Lothrop CD: Genetic test for pyruvate kinase deficiency of basenjis. J Am Vet Med Assoc 207:918, 1995.
DNA test for PK deficiency described and compared to biochemical test.

Winand, NJ: Molecular genetic characterization of spontaneously occurring animal models of Duchenne muscular dystrophy. Ph.D. Thesis, Cornell University, 1994.
Identification of molecular defects causing muscular dystrophy in the dog and cat.

Yuzbasiyan-Gurkan V, Halloran Blanton S, Cao Y, et al: Linkage of a microsatellite to the canine copper toxicosis gene in the Bedlington terrier. Am J Vet Res 58:23, 1997.
First use of linkage-based test to identify an inherited defect of dogs.

Zheng K, Thorner PS, Marrano P, et al: Canine X chromosome-linked hereditary nephritis: A genetic model for human X-linked hereditary nephritis resulting from a single base mutation in the gene encoding the α5 chain of collagen type IV. Proc Natl Acad Sci USA 91:3989, 1994.
Description of mutation causing this rare inherited defect of Samoyed dogs.

Use of Serum Progesterone for Ovulation Timing in the Bitch

MARGARET V. ROOT KUSTRITZ
St. Paul, Minnesota

SHIRLEY D. JOHNSTON
Pomona, California

Traditional breeding management of the bitch is natural service around the bitch's ninth, eleventh, and thirteenth days after proestrus onset, with day 1 defined as the first day of serosanguineous discharge from a swollen vulva. Although the average bitch ovulates on the twelfth day after proestrus onset, many normal bitches ovulate as early as 5 or as late as 25 days after proestrus onset. These will be deemed infertile if they are bred on days 9, 11, and 13 and do not become pregnant. Measurement of serum progesterone concentrations can be used to determine time of ovulation accurately in estrous bitches, and therefore to optimize breeding management.

As the normal bitch enters proestrus, she will exhibit vulvar swelling and transudation of variable amounts of serosanguineous vulvar discharge. Follicle-stimulating hormone (FSH), released from the pituitary, promotes recruitment of a variable number of follicles on the ovary. As the follicles mature, the granulosa cells lining them secrete increasing amounts of estradiol-17β. Estradiol-17β stimulates a gradual cornification of the vaginal epithelial cells. As dogs progress through proestrus, exfoliated vaginal epithelial cells will change from a population of noncornified cells (parabasal and intermediate cells), which are round with healthy nuclei, to a population of cornified cells (superficial and anuclear squame cells), which are large and angular with pyknotic or faded nuclei. Polymorphonuclear leukocytes (PMNs) are abundant in vaginal cytology specimens collected in early proestrus and are absent in late proestrus. Male dogs are attracted to a proestrous female, but most females will not exhibit receptive behaviors for breeding such as standing to be mounted, or lateral deviation of the tail and elevation of the vulva. Proestrus lasts an average of 9 days, with a range of 0 to 17 days in normal bitches.

Late in proestrus or early in estrus, serum concentration of estradiol-17β will drop abruptly, coincident with onset of the luteinizing hormone (LH) surge. Serum progesterone concentration increases above 1 ng/ml on the day of the LH surge, or 2 days prior to ovulation as the ovarian follicles undergo preovulatory luteinization. This decline in the estrogen:progesterone ratio signals the onset of receptive behaviors for breeding.

Estrus, or standing heat, is defined by the bitch's behavior. She will stand to be mounted and bred. The vulva may soften but will still be enlarged. The vulvar discharge will vary in color from serosanguineous to straw-colored and will vary in volume. The exfoliated vaginal epithelial cells will be cornified throughout estrus, with estrus defined cytologically as more than 50% of the cells being anuclear squames. Bacteria may be present in the vaginal smear, and PMNs are absent. Estrus lasts an average of 9 days, with a range of 0 to 21 days in normal dogs.

The LH surge occurs from 3 days before to 5 days after estrus onset (Concannon et al, 1977; Concannon et al, 1989). Because the LH surge, and therefore ovulation, is poorly correlated with estrus onset, defined by breeding behavior or cytologic changes, observation of receptive behaviors for breeding or vaginal cytology alone, or both, are poor prospective predictors of ovulation date for a given bitch.

Conception rate is best if bitches are bred from 4 days before to 2 days after ovulation, and maximal litter size is achieved if the bitch is bred 2 days after ovulation. Bitches can achieve pregnancy with a single insemination 2 to 3 days after ovulation (Holst and Phemister, 1974). The bitch ovulates a primary oocyte that must undergo two meiotic divisions before it can be fertilized. This maturation process takes 48 to 72 hours. The mature egg remains viable for 2 to 3 days. Normal spermatozoa of male dogs may remain viable in the reproductive tract of a female bred by natural service for at least 5 to 6 days.

Measurement of serum LH concentration has been considered for prediction of ovulation day within the canine estrous cycle. A radioimmunoassay (RIA) for canine LH is available through commercial laboratories, but turn-around time is too long to make it a practical test for breeding management in clinical practice. Because LH is a glycoprotein hormone with a unique structure for each species, an assay specific to the canine must be used. An enzyme-linked immunosorbent assay (ELISA) for canine LH is commercially available (Status-LH, Synbiotics, Malvern, PA). The advantage of the canine LH ELISA test is that of time, since it can be run in-house. However, no published reports are available that critically evaluate the accuracy of the test that is currently available, and the short duration of the peak in serum LH concentration in the dog necessitates daily blood testing, which is often impractical and expensive for dog owners.

Measurement of serum progesterone concentrations can be used to predict ovulation day prospectively. In a retrospective study of 49 bitches with serum progesterone concentrations measured during proestrus or estrus, and successful breeding and pregnancy, the following guidelines were reported (Johnston and Root, 1995). Serum progesterone begins to rise concurrently with the LH surge, reaching 1.0 to 1.9 ng/ml (3.1 to 5.9 nmol/L) on that day. The day after the LH surge, 1 day before ovulation, serum progesterone concentration is 2.0 to 3.9 ng/ml (6.2 to 12.1 nmol/L). On the day of ovulation, serum progesterone concentration is 4.0 to 10.0 ng/ml (12.4 to 31.0 nmol/L). After ovulation, a corpus luteum (CL) forms at the site of each ruptured follicle, and serum progesterone concentration will rise rapidly and unpredictably as these corpora lutea begin to produce progesterone; serum progesterone concentrations remain elevated until parturition, peaking at concentrations of 15 to 90 ng/ml in mid-diestrus.

RIAs for serum progesterone are commercially available. Because progesterone is a steroid hormone with a structure common to all species, the assay need not be specific to the canine. RIAs yield a quantitative result. Because serum progesterone rises in a predictable way over the time of the LH surge and ovulation, and remains elevated afterward, daily blood samples to predict ovulation time are not necessary; practical breeding management decisions for insemination with fresh semen can be made with assays run twice each week. The commercial laboratory used should be consulted for particulars of sample submission, and phone or fax results requested.

Several ELISA test kits are available for in-house assay of canine serum progesterone concentrations (Status-Pro, Synbiotics, Malvern, PA; PreMate, Camelot Farms, College Station, TX). ELISA tests yield a qualitative result; i.e., the color change produced is indicative of a range of values. Critical evaluation of ELISA kits, comparing them to RIA, has shown poor correlation between the two techniques, with overall reported inaccuracy of 9.0 to 47.1% of the ELISA. Greatest inaccuracy is in the range of 1.5–3.0 to 5.0–10.0 ng/ml (4.7–9.3 to 15.5–31.0 nmol/L), the range of interest for breeding management. ELISA kits are most accurate in the high range, greater than 5.0 to 10.0 ng/ml (greater than 15.5 to 31.0 nmol/L), with a reported accuracy of 87.3 to 96.0% in that range.

The stage of the canine estrous cycle after estrus is diestrus. In the bitch, corpora lutea are maintained and progesterone is produced for the entire 2 months of diestrus, regardless of whether the animal was bred or conceived. Diestrus onset is defined cytologically by an abrupt decline in percentage of cornified cells. This abrupt change to 50% or less superficial and anuclear squame cells and reappearance of PMNs occurs 6 days after ovulation in the bitch (Holst and Phemister, 1974). Ninety-five percent of pregnant dogs will whelp 61 to 65 days after ovulation. Therefore, determination of the onset of diestrus and knowledge of whelping date, or both, allow one to retrospectively determine ovulation date in a given cycle.

General recommendations for breeding management in clinical practice follow:

- Begin collection of vaginal cytology specimens 4 or 5 days after proestrus onset.

- Once exfoliated vaginal epithelial cell cornification is greater than or equal to 80%, suggesting late proestrus, begin drawing blood samples for measurement of serum progesterone concentration.
- Draw a sample for serum progesterone measurement every 2 to 3 days, until a value is reached that is indicative of the LH peak or ovulation, allowing you to predict optimal fertilizable period for that bitch. If you are measuring serum progesterone concentrations by ELISA, samples should be drawn daily until a "high-range" value (5.0 to 10.0 ng/ml; 15.5 to 31.0 nmol/L) is achieved.
- Conception rate is best if bitches are bred from 4 days before to 2 days after ovulation, and maximal litter size is achieved if the bitch is bred 2 days after ovulation.

References and Suggested Reading

Bouchard GF, Malugani N, Youngquist RS, et al: Determination of ovulation in the bitch with a qualitative progesterone enzyme immunoassay in serum, plasma, and whole blood. J Reprod Fertil Suppl 47:517, 1993.
An accuracy study of an ELISA progesterone assay, using comparison to values predicted by RIA measurement of LH in 180 samples.
Concannon P, Hansel W, McEntee K: Changes in LH, progesterone and sexual behavior associated with preovulatory luteinization in the bitch. Biol Reprod 17:604, 1977.
A study demonstrating the correlation between changes in serum progesterone concentration and occurrence of the LH peak.
Concannon PW, Hansel W, Visek WJ: The ovarian cycle of the bitch: Plasma estrogen, LH and progesterone. Biol Reprod 13:112, 1975.
A description of correlation of LH peak, changes in serum estrogen and progesterone, and onset of sexual receptivity in 20 bitches.
Concannon PW, McCann JP, Temple M: Biology and endocrinology of ovulation, pregnancy and parturition in the dog. J Reprod Fertil Suppl 39:3, 1989.
An excellent review of the reproductive endocrinology of the bitch.
Holst PA, Phemister RD: Onset of diestrus in the beagle bitch: Definition and significance. Am J Vet Res 35:401, 1974.
A prospective study of 400 bitches demonstrating consistent onset of diestrus 6 days after ovulation, and rigorously defining the fertilizable period of the bitch.
Johnston SD, Root MV: Serum progesterone timing of ovulation in the bitch. Proceedings of the Annual Meeting of the Society for Theriogenology, San Antonio, TX, 1995, p 195.
A retrospective study of 49 bitches defining serum progesterone concentrations through the time of ovulation.
Manothaiudom K, Johnston SD, Hegstad RL, et al: Evaluation of the Icagen-Target canine ovulation timing diagnostic test in detecting canine plasma progesterone concentrations. J Am Anim Hosp Assoc 31:57, 1995.
A comparison of measured values of serum progesterone in 166 samples assayed by RIA and ELISA.
Wildt DE, Chakraborty PH, Panko WB, et al: Relationship of reproductive behavior, serum luteinizing hormone and time of ovulation in the bitch. Biol Reprod 18:561, 1978.
A prospective study of 15 bitches correlating measurement of serum LH to laparoscopic observation of ovulation and corpus luteum formation.

Artificial Insemination in the Bitch

Margaret V. Root Kustritz
St. Paul, Minnesota
Shirley D. Johnston
Pomona, California

Artificial insemination (AI) of dogs may be indicated because of abnormal vulvar or vaginal anatomy (vaginal strictures or hyperplasia), narrowing of the vulva or vagina in a virgin bitch, or dominant or aggressive temperament precluding exhibition of normal breeding behaviors. Indications in the male include poor libido, weakness or pain when mounting or ejaculating because of disease of the spine, hindlimbs, or prostate, and either submissive or aggressive temperament. AI also is indicated when chilled extended or frozen semen is sent to a bitch that is geographically or temporally distant from the dog.

In dogs, semen is routinely collected by manual stimulation using a rubber collecting cone attached to a plastic centrifuge tube (Nasco, Fort Atkinson, WI). Presence of a teaser bitch, especially a bitch in estrus or one treated with a topical pheromone preparation (Eau d'Estrus, Synbiotics, Malvern, PA) may improve the quality of the semen sample collected. Nonslip flooring should be present, and the teaser bitch muzzled or well controlled by a handler to prevent injury to the stud dog.

The male dog is allowed to sniff at the hindquarters of the teaser bitch and to mount if he desires. The penis is massaged, briskly and enthusiastically, through the prepuce over the area of the bulbus glandis. As the penis becomes erect, the prepuce is pushed caudal to the enlarging bulbus glandis and the rubber collecting cone with attached centrifuge tube introduced over the engorging penis. The rubber collecting cone is advanced to just proximal to the bulbus glandis, and the penis and collecting cone are tightly encircled with the fingers, simulating the presence of the constricting vulvar lips of the bitch during the copulatory lock of natural service.

Canine semen is ejaculated in three fractions. The first is a small volume of clear fluid, the presperm fraction. The second, or sperm-rich, fraction is cloudy and varies in volume from 0.5 to 3.0 ml. The dog often thrusts vigorously while ejaculating this fraction. The dog may pause and may attempt to step over the operator's arm before ejaculating the final fraction, which consists of clear prostatic fluid. Urethral pulses and concomitant rhythmic anal contractions are evident as pulses of prostatic fluid are ejaculated.

The volume of prostatic fluid collected varies with the intended use of the semen. Because incubation of spermatozoa with autologous prostatic fluid has been shown to decrease progressive motility of those spermatozoa, it is generally recommended that a minimal amount of prostatic fluid be collected in ejaculates that are to be stored. For samples that are to be inseminated immediately, prostatic fluid may be collected so as to yield a final semen volume adequate for insemination. Estimates of these amounts are 1.5 to 3.0 ml for bitches weighing 10 pounds (4.5 kg) or less, 3.0 to 5.0 ml for bitches weighing 10 to 50 pounds (4.5 to 22.7 kg), and 5.0 to 8.0 ml for bitches weighing 50 pounds (22.7 kg) or more.

When semen collection is complete, the rubber collecting cone is gently peeled from the erect penis. The penis should undergo complete detumescence and normal replacement within the prepuce before the male dog is returned to the kennel.

Semen should be evaluated for quality. Assessment of progressive motility (normal >70%) and an objective count or subjective estimate of total number of spermatozoa (normal = 300 million to 2 billion) should be performed. Poorquality samples do not warrant storage or insemination. Complete semen evaluation has been described elsewhere (Root and Johnston, 1994). It is recommended that at least 150 to 200 million normal motile spermatozoa be inseminated.

Semen may be used immediately (fresh semen AI), diluted with an extender that nourishes and protects the spermatozoa, chilled, and shipped for insemination within 24 hours (chilled extended semen AI), or extended with a cryoprotectant, frozen, and stored in liquid nitrogen (frozen semen AI). Extender and shipment materials for chilled extended AI are commercially available (Fresh Express, Synbiotics, Malvern, PA; International Canine Semen Bank, North Ridgeville, OH; Fresh Kooled Canine Semen, Camelot Farms, College Station, TX).

Proper timing of ovulation and insemination is important to achieve best performance with minimal cost (See "Use of Serum Progesterone for Ovulation Timing in the Bitch," *CVT XIII*). For fresh and chilled extended semen AI, at least one breeding 2 days after ovulation is recommended. For frozen semen AI, at least one insemination 3 days after ovulation is recommended. This later time of insemination is recommended with frozen semen because frozen-thawed spermatozoa live within the reproductive tract of the female for only hours after insemination compared with 5 days for chilled extended spermatozoa and at least 6 days for fresh spermatozoa. Mature ova must be present at the time of insemination with frozen semen for conception to occur. Because of the longer viability of the fresh and chilled extended spermatozoa, the fertilizable period of bitches inseminated with these samples is not so narrow.

Insemination can be performed in the cranial vagina or the uterus. For intravaginal insemination, pipettes marketed specifically for bitches are available (Synbiotics, Malvern, PA), but these are too short to reach the cranial vagina of large breeds. Longer pipettes, such as those used for bovine uterine infusions (Nasco, Fort Atkinson, WI), may be trimmed to an appropriate length for a given bitch; the length from the vulvar lips to the cranial vagina can be estimated as half the length from the vulvar lips to the costal arch. Balloon catheters, which help stimulate vaginal muscular contractions and prevent reflux of semen after insemination, also have been described (Osiris probe, I.M.V. Ltd., l'Aigle, France).

The bitch is restrained standing on a table or the floor in such a way that no upward pressure is placed on her caudal abdomen. The semen is drawn into a sterile syringe and the pipette attached. A gloved finger, lubricated with water or scant aqueous lubricant, is inserted into the vagina. The pipette is introduced at the dorsal commissure of the vulva, directed dorsocranially over the gloved finger, and passed as far cranially as possible. The semen sample is injected through the pipette, followed by a bolus of air to clear the pipette of all semen. The pipette is withdrawn. The gloved finger is used to gently stimulate ("feather") the vagina for several minutes, which induces contractions of the vaginal musculature. The gloved finger is withdrawn and the bitch's hindquarters are elevated for 5 to 10 minutes to promote pooling of the semen at the external cervical os. The bitch is restrained by holding her hindlimbs at the stifle or supporting her hindlimbs on an elevated platform. After 5 to 10 minutes, she should be taken to the owner's vehicle and crated or put in a kennel. She should not be allowed to squat and urinate, or to jump up into a vehicle or cage for 30 to 60 minutes.

Intravaginal insemination is appropriate for fresh and chilled extended semen AI. Frozen-thawed spermatozoa should be inseminated into the uterine body because frozen-thawed spermatozoa are usually unable to traverse the cervix. Success with intravaginal insemination of frozen-thawed spermatozoa may occur if a large volume of semen is used.

Intrauterine insemination may be performed surgically, with introduction of the semen sample into the uterine body through a small-gauge needle via laparotomy or laparoscopy, or via transcervical catheterization. Two methods of transcervical catheterization have been described. One involves the use of a rigid catheter that is passed blindly through the vagina and cervix after digital fixation of the cervix through the abdominal wall (Linde-Forsberg and Forsberg, 1989, 1993). The other involves passage of an 8F polypropylene catheter through the cervix after endoscopic visualization of the external cervical os (Wilson, 1993).

Litter size is reported to decrease by 23.3 to 30.5% in frozen semen AI compared with fresh semen AI (Linde-Forsberg and Forsberg, 1989, 1993). Pregnancy rates vary with the type of semen used and the site of insemination. Reported values follow:

Natural service = 80–95%
Fresh AI, intravaginal insemination = 62.3 to 100%
Chilled extended AI, intravaginal insemination = 59 to 80%
Frozen AI, intravaginal insemination = 52.6% to 60%
Frozen AI, intrauterine insemination = 0 to 80%

References and Suggested Reading

Fontbonne A, Badinand F: Canine artificial insemination with frozen semen: Comparison of intravaginal and intrauterine deposition of semen. J Reprod Fert Suppl 47:325, 1993.
This article describes a comparison of intravaginal and intrauterine insemination with frozen semen in 57 bitches.

Gill HP, Kaufman CF, Foote RH, et al: Artificial insemination of Beagle bitches with freshly collected, liquid-stored, and frozen-stored semen. Am J Vet Res 31:1807, 1970.
This is a prospective study comparing insemination with fresh, chilled extended, and frozen semen in Beagle bitches.

Linde-Forsberg C, Forsberg M: Fertility in dogs in relation to semen quality and the time and site of insemination with fresh and frozen semen. J Reprod Fert Suppl 39:299, 1989.
This article describes a retrospective study of 470 bitches inseminated with fresh or frozen semen, with a description of the use of the rigid transcervical catheter.

Linde-Forsberg C, Forsberg M: Results of 527 controlled artificial inseminations in dogs. J Reprod Fert Suppl 47:313, 1993.
This was a retrospective study of 527 bitches inseminated with fresh or frozen semen, with a description of the use of the rigid transcervical catheter.

Root MV, Johnston SD: Basics for a complete reproductive examination of the male dog. Semin Vet Med Surg (Small Anim) 9:41, 1994.
This is a complete description of semen collection and evaluation in the dog.

Silva LDM, Onclin K, Lejeune B, et al: Comparison of intravaginal and intrauterine insemination of bitches with fresh and frozen semen. Vet Rec 138:154, 1996.
This article describes a comparison of intravaginal and intrauterine insemination with fresh or frozen semen in 30 bitches.

Wilson MS: Non-surgical intrauterine artificial insemination in bitches using frozen semen. J Reprod Fert Suppl 47:307, 1993.
This is a comparison of intrauterine insemination of frozen semen with the rigid transcervical catheter or endoscopic visualization of the cervix and passage of a polypropylene catheter in 46 bitches.

Pregnancy Diagnosis in the Bitch

Carlos M. Gradil

Amy E. Yeager

Patrick W. Concannon
Ithaca, New York

Pregnancy diagnosis in the bitch is most commonly done by palpation. This technique is easy and inexpensive. Ultrasonography is becoming more accessible and is the preferred choice for detection or confirmation of pregnancy. Ultrasonography provides the earliest detection of pregnancy (day 20 to 25). Radiography can be used after day 45 to count fetal skeletons, evaluate fetal size, visualize signs of fetal death, and monitor fetal positioning.

The apparent variation in the length of gestation among bitches depends on the event used as the reference point. Counting from the first breeding date, a normal gestation can range from 57 to 72 days. This variation may be influenced by the time between mating and ovulation, the longevity of dog sperm (up to 6 to 7 days), oocyte maturation time (2 to 3 days after ovulation) and the actual time at which the tubo-uterine junction opens (approximately on day 10 after the LH surge) and allows passage of the blastocyst to the uterus. Fertile mating can occur as early as 5 days before ovulation or as late as 7 days after ovulation.

Various methods are used to calculate gestation length more accurately. Commonly, one determines the day of preovulatory serum LH peak, which occurs 48 hours prior to ovulation. The day of LH peak is designated by convention as day 0, and days in the cycle or days of gestation are counted from this reference event; there is little variability between bitches in gestation length if one counts from either day 0 or from the day of ovulation. Thus, gestation length based on determination of day 0 is 65 ± 1 days from the LH peak. The number of laboratories that offer tests for detecting LH levels is limited. Owing to the fact that there is a preovulatory luteinization of follicles, the progesterone rise coincides with the preovulatory LH peak, allowing for the determination of the day of the LH surge based on the increase in plasma progesterone. The designation of day numbers in this article is from day 0 based on the LH peak unless otherwise noted.

When the day of the LH peak is not estimated by progesterone assays, vaginal cytology may be used as a resource. The landmarks obtained from vaginal cytology rely on the determination of the first day of diestrus (diestrus day 1); that is, the first day that the percentage of superficial epithelial cells declines to 50% or less. Diestrus day 1 occurs, on average, on day 8 of gestation or day 8 of the cycle (day 7, 8, or 9 in most bitches). Counting from diestrus day 1, approximately 80% of the bitches will whelp at diestrus day 57. Most bitches can be expected to whelp 57 ± 3 days after diestrus day 1.

Assumption of premonitory signs of an impending whelping, for example, nesting behavior and anorexia, as diagnostic of pregnancy can be problematic. These signs should only be considered as accompanying signs in bitches known to be pregnant using other tests, because pseudopregnant bitches may present similar signs.

PALPATION

Migration of blastocysts between uterine horns occurs on days 12 to 16. Implantation sites are established by day 18 to 19 (Yeager et al, 1992). Implantation occurs on day 20 (Thatcher et al, 1994). Discrete chorioallantoic ovoid swellings (1 to 2 cm) at placental sites along the uterine horns can be detected easily by abdominal palpation, in particular the most caudal swellings (Whitney, 1936), at day 22 to 24 (diestrus days 14 to 16), or 20 to 26 days from the first of multiple breedings. The uterus is quite firm at this stage and should be first palpated at its body (i.e., between the bladder and rectum, immediately cranial to the vagina and cervix) and followed cranially between the palpator's thumb and fingers. Distinction of a pregnant uterus from a stool-filled colon should be a consideration. Uterine swellings are readily palpable for only 10 to 15 days (days 20 to 35). As a rule, palpation for pregnancy should be scheduled for 26 to 28 days after the first breeding if progesterone and vaginal cytology are not known. If no detectable signs of pregnancy can be palpated during this first examination, a second evaluation should be done a week later. In small litters the conceptuses may be engaged too cranially under the ribs to be discernible by palpation. By day 28, uterine swellings have a diameter of 3 to 5 cm for a middle-sized dog and at this time, these structures are most easily and accurately identified. After day 30 of gestation, the uterus enlarges rapidly and occupies a more cranioventral position and it becomes more difficult to palpate discrete swellings. Uterine horns drop to the ventral floor and the anterior portion of the horns are pushed cranially under the rib cage, making it difficult to palpate with certainty. By day 35 the swellings become elongated, almost confluent, and are more pliable and more difficult to palpate as distinct entities, and a diffuse distention of the uterus can make palpation for pregnancy unrewarding. After day 45 to 50 of gestation the individual fetuses are palpable and easily identified. Temperament, body condition, size of the bitch, and number of fetuses can affect ease of palpation. False-positive results may be due to pyometra, particularly forms that present sacculations similar to the ones palpated in normal pregnancies.

Other signs such as mammary gland development are unreliable because overtly pseudopregnant bitches may have enlarged mammary glands. It appears that overt pseu-

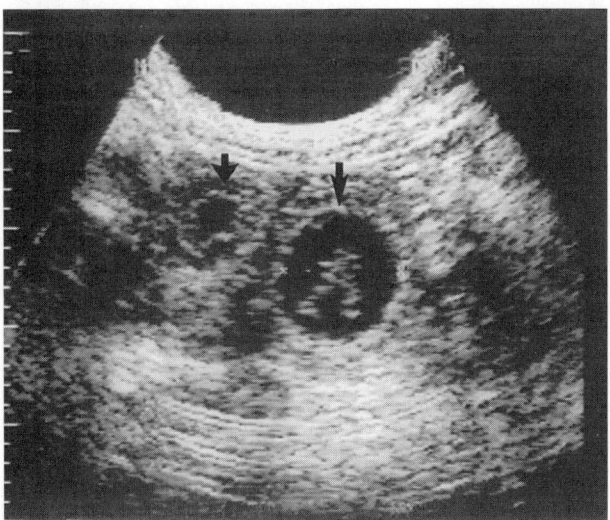

Figure 1. Transverse 7.5-MHz sonograms of two gestational sacs day 26 of gestation. The size and anatomy of a viable gestational sac *(short arrow)* is appropriate for this gestational age. The nonviable gestational sac *(long arrow)* is abnormally small and does not contain embryonic echoes.

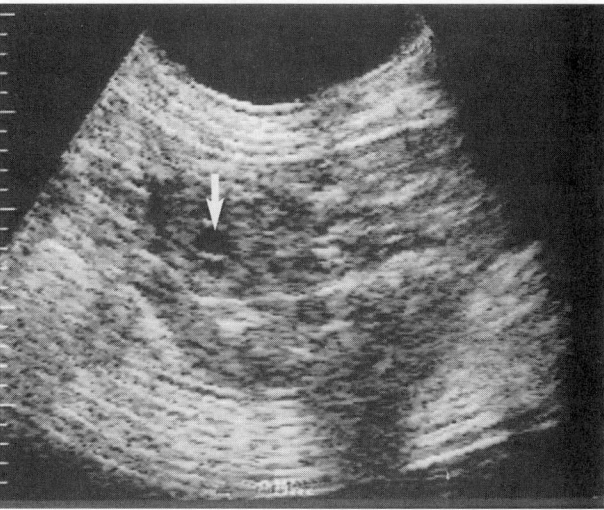

Figure 2. Transverse sonogram of an anechoic 3-mm gestational sac *(arrow)* at day 20 of gestation. At this time, the fetus and membranes are not detectable.

dopregnancy occurs in some nonpregnant bitches in late diestrus due to a sudden or premature drop in progesterone, causing an elevation in prolactin similar to that which occurs in pregnant bitches just prior to parturition (Okkens et al, 1997).

ULTRASONOGRAPHIC DIAGNOSIS OF CANINE PREGNANCY

Transabdominal ultrasonography represents the ideal means of detecting pregnancy in dogs and is becoming a routine diagnostic modality for early pregnancy detection and for determining fetal viability or resorption after day 25 of gestation (Fig. 1; Bondestam et al, 1983). When one is using ultrasonography for pregnancy evaluation in the bitch, the equipment, skill of the operator, and temperament of the bitch should be taken into consideration (Yeager et al, 1992). In some bitches, abdominal hair must be shaved for a thorough examination and permission of the owner must first be granted. Dogs are generally examined in dorsal recumbency but, with some nervous dogs, a standing position may provide adequate imaging. The choice of probes depends on gestational age, size of the bitch, and obesity. A 5.0-MHz transducer is recommended for all-purpose pregnancy detection. In addition, a 7.5-MHz probe is useful for pregnancy detection before day 30 and for any gestational period in smaller dogs (less than 7 kg).

Embryonic vesicles can be visualized as early as day 19 (Yeager and Concannon, 1990; see *CVT XII*, p. 1040), approximately 11 days after diestrus day 1 (Fig. 2). This requires expertise and excellent equipment. The embryo proper can be imaged by day 24, about 16 days after onset of diestrus (Fig. 3). At around day 35 of gestation the fetal head and body are the same size and appearance (Fig. 4). The heart beat can be detected by day 24 or 25 and fetal movement at day 34 to 36. In bitches with small litters, ultrasound gives a good indication of litter size. However, as litter size increases, the estimation of fetal number

becomes more difficult (Fig. 5). Stage of pregnancy can be estimated by measuring the biparietal diameter (longitudinal plane of the head aligned with the rest of the fetal body) and the trunk diameter (transverse plane at the level of the stomach) for one or more pups (Fig. 6). Consider measuring at least two to three fetuses due to differences in fetal size within a litter. Biparietal and trunk diameter are correlated with fetal age (England et al, 1990). The times at which various structures can be detected have been studied (Yeager et al, 1992). Times of first ultrasonographic detection of selected features of canine pregnancy are shown in Table 1. Fetal well-being is often based on fetal heart rate. Normal rates have been reported as 200 to 255 heart beats per minute, from before day 30 throughout pregnancy (Verstegen et al, 1993). Further studies are needed to relate deceleration of fetal heart beat (e.g., to less than 200 heart beats per minute) to fetal distress.

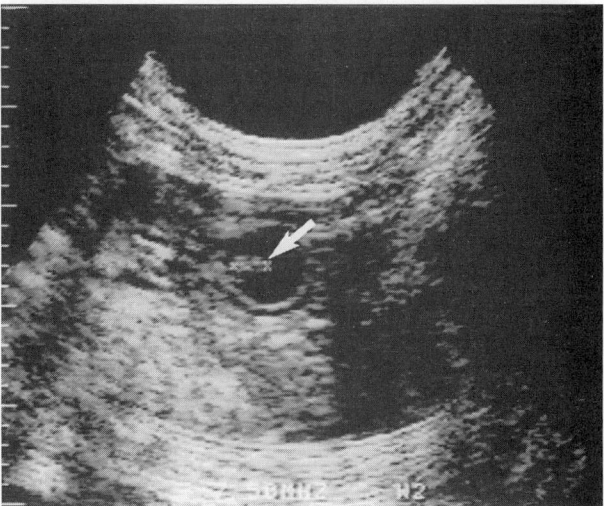

Figure 3. Transverse sonogram of an anechoic 7-mm spherical gestational sac at day 25 of gestation. At this time the fetus *(arrow)* is 4 mm long, and marked by calipers *(x)*. It is "apposed" to the placenta, and fetal membranes are not detectable.

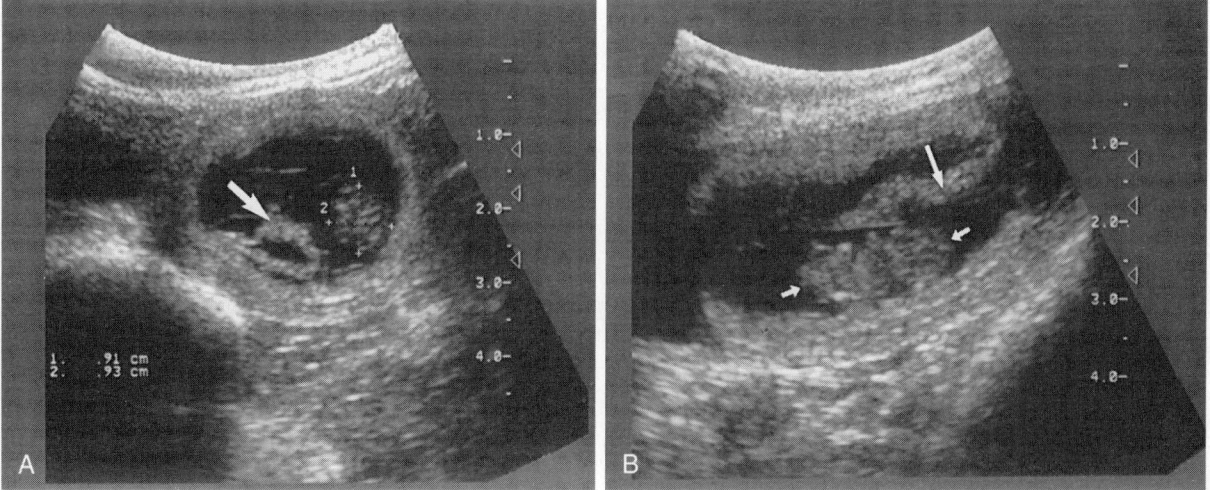

Figure 4. Transverse *(A)* and sagittal *(B)* sonograms of a gestational sac at approximately day 35 of gestation. *A,* The fetal pole is 9 mm in diameter (calipers 1 and 2). The yolk sac *(arrow)* has a prominent hyperechoic folded ring shape. *B,* Short arrows mark the fetal crown-rump length of 2 cm. At this time, the fetal head and body have about the same size and yield a bipolar appearance. The yolk sac *(long arrow)* is the cord-like membrane. The 2-cm fetus is shorter than the 5-cm wide (and 0.7-cm thick) zonary placenta, which appears as an echogenic band just below the fetus in the sonogram. The other side of the placenta is the band to which the yolk sac membrane is attached.

Ultrasound is a valuable tool for ruling out pregnancy in nonpregnant bitches with pyometra that may have been falsely identified as being pregnant by palpation (Fig. 7).

RADIOGRAPHIC DIAGNOSIS OF CANINE PREGNANCY

The most common use of radiographs is for prepartum determination of litter size, or for postpartum determination that all pups have been whelped. In nonpregnant bitches, the uterus very often cannot be identified radiographically.

In pregnant bitches, uterine enlargement is not detect-able until after 21 days of pregnancy. Between 21 and 42 days, enlarged fluid-filled horns may be visualized. Fetal skeletons become radiopaque at about days 44 to 47 or diestrus days 35 to 40, with skull and vertebrae visible before the long bones and digits. An additional 2 days are often required until an unequivocal diagnosis of pregnancy can be made (Concannon and Rendano, 1983). Fetal teeth become detectable only at day 58 to 63. Based on breeding dates, the time of first detection of skeletal mineralization may range from 42 to 52 days after mating.

Radiography is useful to determine litter size from 47 days onward, when ossification of the fetal skeleton has

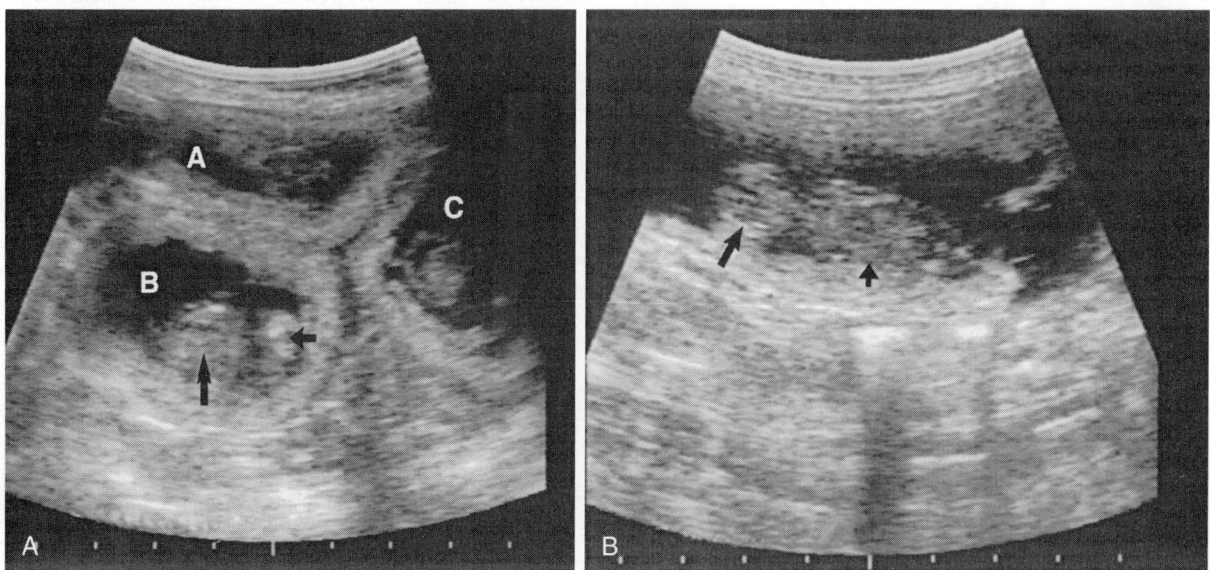

Figure 5. Transverse *(A)* and sagittal *(B)* 5-MHz sonograms of gestational sacs at day 40 of gestation. *A,* Three confluent gestational sacs (A, B, and C) are depicted. One gestational sac shows a fetal body *(long arrow)* and fetal head *(short arrow)*. *B,* The shape and size of the fetal head *(long arrow)* are now obviously different from those of the fetal body *(short arrow)*. Other anatomic structures are faintly visible, such as the hypoechoic heart surrounded by hyperechoic lung; anechoic lateral ventricles in the brain; and hyperechoic ribs that do not cast discrete acoustic shadows at this gestational age.

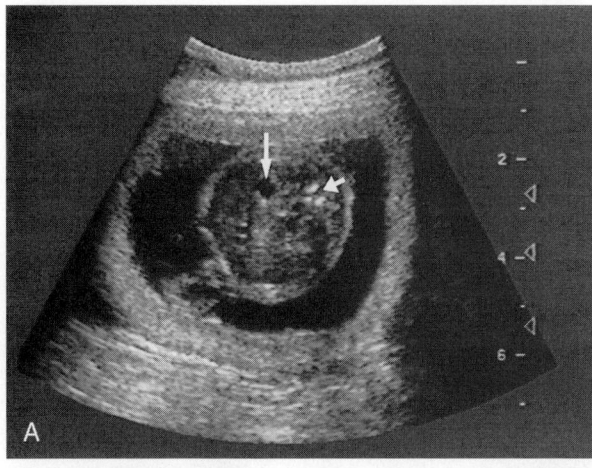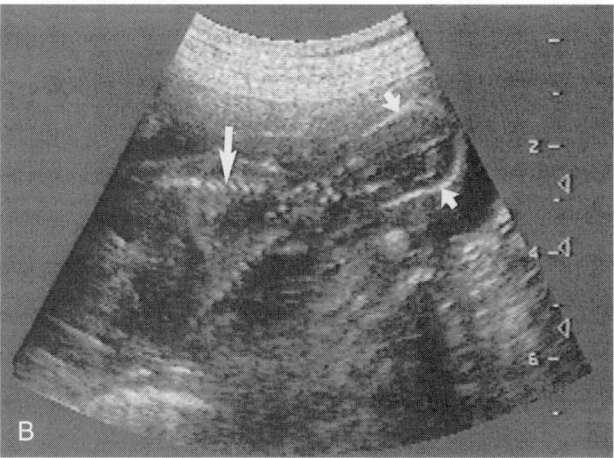

Figure 6. Transverse *(A)* and sagittal *(B)* 7-MHz sonograms of a fetus day 50 of gestation. *A,* The 3.7-cm diameter fetus is shown inside the 6-cm diameter anechoic chorionic structure. The body of the fetus shows distinct anatomic features. The vertebrae *(short arrow)* are hyperechoic structures that cast a faint acoustic shadow below (vertical anechoic area). The stomach lumen *(long arrow)* is an anechoic structure surrounded by hypoechoic liver. The cross-sectional area of the fetus fills approximately half of the gestational sac. *B,* The hyperechoic fetal skeleton including the skull *(short arrows,* depicting biparietal diameter of 1.8 cm) and ribs *(long arrow)* are distinct. The liver is hypoechoic compared with the lung, and the heart is located in the center of the lung. Crown-rump length is much greater than the length of the placenta.

occurred to a threshold as to become radiopaque. Litter size depends on many factors but in general, small-sized breeds have 2 to 4 pups, medium-sized breeds 4 to 7, and large-sized breeds 6 to 10. Radiography allows for the visualization of the minimal number of fetuses present, but despite being more accurate than ultrasonography in determining litter size, it does not always allow all fetuses to be counted. Enumerating skulls or vertebral columns is the easiest method for estimating litter size (Figs. 8 and 9).

Radiology is also useful for the determination of fetal viability based on the absence of intrauterine gas pockets and deformed or excessively flexed skeletal elements that occur as a consequence of fetal death (Fig. 10). Radiology may be a useful tool for determining size of fetal skulls in relation to maternal pelvic canal. Concerned owners may request radiography of the abdomen to predict difficulty of the approaching whelping. However, unless there is an obviously oversized fetus, as may occur in litters of one to two pups, measurement of fetal skeletal elements for radiographic prediction of dystocia is of debatable merit. Radiographs can also be used to determine whether one or more fetuses have been retained following completion of spontaneous parturition.

ENDOCRINOLOGIC AND BIOCHEMICAL DIAGNOSIS OF CANINE PREGNANCY

Pregnancy Hormones

Pregnancy-specific gonadotropins similar to equine or human chorionic gonadotropin have not been reported in the dog, and plasma progesterone concentrations are not

TABLE 1. Times of Ultrasonographic Detection of Selected Features of Canine Pregnancy

Gestational Age (Days)	Ultrasound Feature
20–24	Small anechoic gestational sac ≤ 7 mm. No fetus(es) or membranes.
25–27	Echogenic fetal mass and heart beat became detectable.
28–33	Head and body of the fetus are similar in size and appearance although the beating heart is obviously located in the body. Fetal membranes and zonary placenta are prominent.
34–39	The fetus has motion. Shape and size of the fetal head is distinctively different from the body. Fetal anatomy starts to be detectable (limbs, stomach, bladder, liver, lung, and skeleton). Fetal membrane and zonary placenta are prominent.
≥42	The fetus is longer than the zonary placenta. Anechoic fetal fluid surrounds the fetus.
≥55	Fetal anatomy is obvious. Only scant amounts of fetal fluid are detected between fetus and uterus.

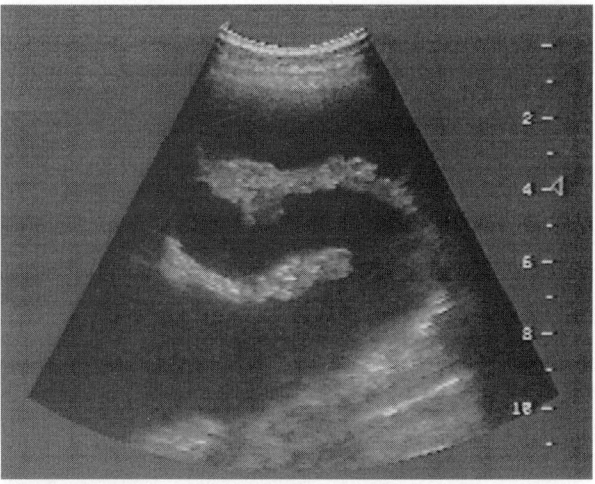

Figure 7. Sagittal 7-MHz sonogram of a pyometra. The lumen of the uterus is the serpentine, anechoic fluid-distended structure. There is no evidence of fetal structures, fetal membranes, or placenta, which rules out pregnancy.

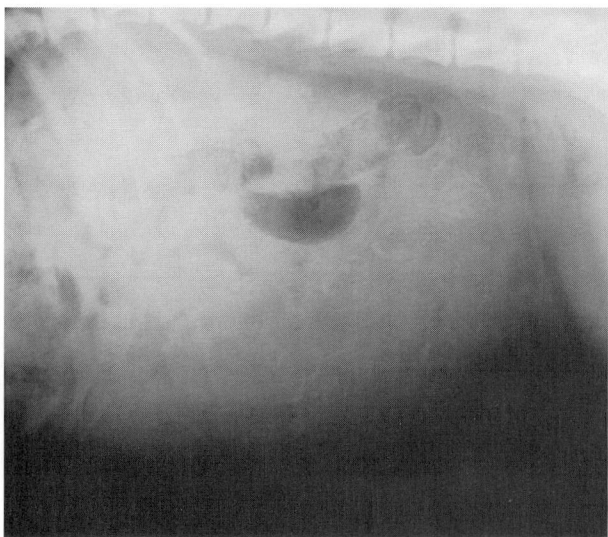

Figure 8. Lateral abdominal radiograph of a pregnant dog, approximately day 55 of gestation, with a normal large litter.

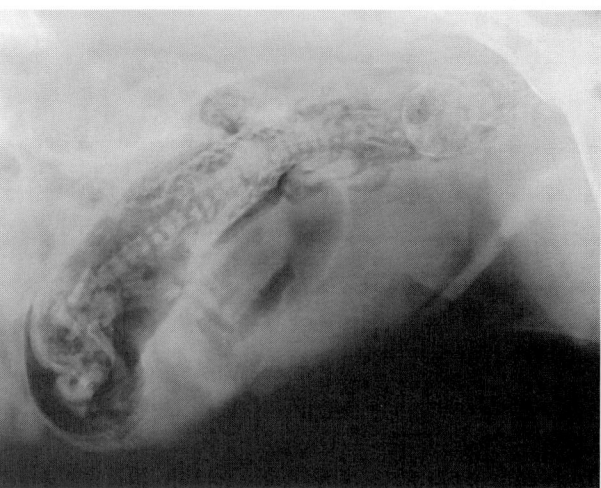

Figure 10. Lateral abdominal radiograph of a pregnant dog with a large single dead fetus. Note the collapsed thorax, overlapping pelvic limbs, and the presence of gas. (Courtesy of Dr. V. Rendano, Radiology Department, Cornell University, Ithaca, NY.)

significantly enough different in pregnant and nonpregnant bitches as to identify pregnancy.

Progesterone in late proestrus is less than 1 ng/ml, peaks around day 30 at 15 to 80 ng/ml, and then slowly declines to 4 to 5 ng/ml by day 62, with a sharp decline to less than 2 ng/ml in the 48 to 24 hours preceding parturition. Progesterone secretion by the corpus luteum is necessary for supporting canine pregnancy throughout gestation. Progesterone tends to be slightly higher in the pregnant dog than in the nonpregnant dog, but not enough to be of diagnostic value.

Relaxin (Rlx) is the only known pregnancy-specific hormone in dogs. Serum Rlx concentration increases during gestation but is not detectable at any time in nonpregnant bitches. In pregnant bitches, serum Rlx is detectable as early as day 28 to 30, and reaches peak levels by 40 to 50 days of gestation. Rlx levels decrease dramatically after parturition, but may remain detectable at low levels for up to 50 days during lactation. Evidence suggests that Rlx is

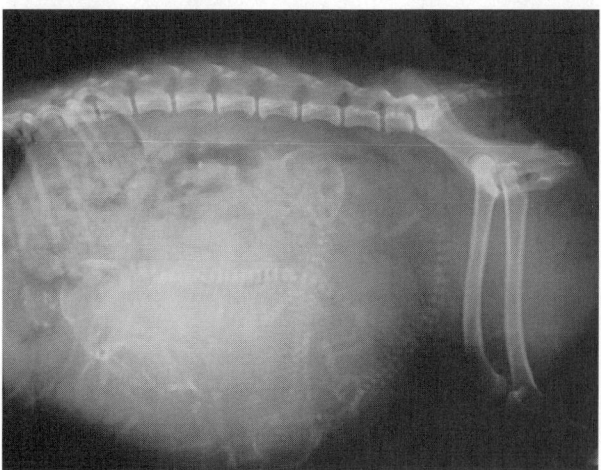

Figure 9. Lateral abdominal radiograph of a pregnant dog, day 63 of a normal gestation, with a small litter with four skulls/vertebral columns evident.

produced primarily by the placenta with smaller amounts probably produced by the ovary (Steinetz et al, 1989). Rlx is detectable by immunoassays that have been proposed for pregnancy diagnosis. However, Rlx assay is not commercially available as a canine pregnancy test (p. 924).

Plasma Proteins

Commercial pregnancy testing services currently available in North America and Europe are based on the assay of acute-phase protein concentration in submitted serum or plasma samples. Whether such measurements include fibrinogen, C-reactive protein (CRP), or both, is unclear, although one such test (Serono Diagnostic, United Kingdom) is reportedly based on fibrinogen measurement (Eckersall et al, 1993). Concentrations of fibrinogen are typically elevated by day 25 to 30, and appear to be diagnostic of pregnancy between days 30 and 50, and then decline near term (Concannon et al, 1996; Günzel-Apel et al, 1997). With an homologous canine CRP assay, CRP levels are also observed to be sufficiently elevated between days 30 and 50 as to be nearly diagnostic of pregnancy (Eckersall et al, 1993), but a commercially available human-CRP assay was only marginally effective as a diagnostic in dogs (Concannon et al, 1996). The incidence of false-positive diagnosis is likely to be high with the use of assays of acute-phase proteins to test for pregnancy in dogs because these proteins are elevated during nonspecific inflammatory states and in inflammatory disease states such as pyometra. Furthermore, their use would depend on a reasonable estimate of the physiologic day of gestation. The elevation in these proteins during pregnancy is presumably due to an inflammatory-like response initiated in the uterus in response to placentation.

In summary, there are no fully reliable blood tests available for pregnancy diagnosis in dogs; assay of relaxin as a reliable diagnostic is likely to become available in the future; and ultrasonography of fetal heart beats after day 25 remains the only reliable means of confirming and monitoring a viable pregnancy in the bitch.

References and Suggested Reading

Bondestam S, Alitalo I, Kurkkainen M: Real-time ultrasound pregnancy diagnosis in the bitch. J Small Anim Pract 24:145, 1983.
Reports on the use of ultrasound for pregnancy diagnosis in eight bitches as a safe, rapid and easy method of investigation.

Concannon PW, Gimpel T, Newton L, et al: Postimplantation increase in plasma fibrinogen concentration with increase in relaxin concentration in pregnant dogs. Am J Vet Res 57:1382, 1996.
Reports the nearly simultaneous increases in fibrinogen and relaxin beginning between days 26 and 30 in 24 Beagle dogs and the potential to use fibrinogen assay as a pregnancy test between days 30 and 50.

Concannon P, Rendano V: Radiographic diagnosis of canine pregnancy: Onset of fetal skeletal opacity in relation to times of breeding, preovulatory luteinizing hormone release, and parturition. Am J Vet Res 44:1506, 1983.
Reports on a radiographic study for pregnancy diagnosis in 6 pregnant Beagle bitches providing basic information for timing and evaluating radiographs during the last trimester of canine pregnancy.

Eckersall PD, Harvey MJA, Ferguson JM, et al: Acute phase proteins in canine pregnancy (Canis familiaris). J Reprod Fertil Suppl 47:159, 1993.
Reports on the development and use of an homologous canine C-reactive protein radioimmunoassay and its application to pregnancy testing in dogs, including large increases in 7 dogs during mid-gestation and again after parturition in 3 of the dogs.

England GCW, Allen WE, Porter DJ, et al: Studies on canine pregnancy using B-mode ultrasound: Development of the conceptus and determination of gestational age. J Small Anim Pract 31:324, 1990.
Reports on events of pregnancy development (biparietal diameter and trunk diameter) to characterize growth of the conceptus and gestational age in 50 Labrador retrievers, Golden Retrievers and their crosses.

Günzel-Apel A-R, Hayer M, Mischke R, et al: Dynamics of haemostasis during the oestrous cycle and pregnancy in bitches. J Reprod Fertil Suppl 51:185, 1997.
Reports on increases in fibrinogen, fibrinogen degradation products, and platelet number at days 30 and 60 of pregnancy in dogs.

Okkens AC, Dieleman SJ, Kooistra HS, et al: Plasma concentrations of prolactin in overtly pseudopregnant Afghan hounds and the effect of metergoline. J Reprod Fertil Suppl 51:295, 1997.
Reports on the high plasma concentrations of prolactin and its associ-ation with the development and maintenance of pseudopregnancy and the use of metergoline, a serotonin antagonist, to decrease the clinical signs of pseudopregnancy.

Steinetz BG, Goldsmith LT, Harvey HJ, et al: Serum relaxin and proges-terone concentrations in pregnant, pseudopregnant, and ovariecto-mized, progestin treated pregnant bitches: Detection of relaxin as a marker of pregnancy. Am J Vet Res 50:68, 1989.
In this report it is proposed that in bitches both the ovary and placenta secrete relaxin during pregnancy based on hormone sampling of 18 Labrador retrievers.

Thatcher M-J, Shille VM, Buhi WC, et al: Canine conceptus appearance and de novo protein synthesis in relation to the time of implantation. Theriogenology 41:1679, 1994.
Report on secretory proteins: canine protein 1 (cP1), cP2, cP4, and cP6 synthesized by the endometrium and de novo by the conceptus. Canine conceptus protein 7 was found to be secreted prior to implan-tation, only by the blastocyst.

Verstegen JP, Silva LDM, Onclin K, et al: Echocardiographic study of heart rate in dog and cat fetuses in utero. J Reprod Fertil 47:175, 1993.
Reports on the heart rates of dog fetuses in utero in 15 bitches monitored from day 19 using real-time B- and M-mode ultrasonogra-phy.

Whitney LF: The diagnosis of pregnancy in the bitch by palpation. Vet Med 31:216, 1936.
Descriptive and diagrammatic report of cumulative data on palpation findings from about 20 days after fertilization in different breeds of dogs.

Yeager AE, Concannon PW: Association between the preovulatory lutein-izing hormone surge and the early ultrasonographic detection of preg-nancy and fetal heart beats in Beagle dogs. Theriogenology 34:655, 1990.
Report on the size of the gestational sac and embryonic mass, and the embryonic heart beat examined by ultrasound from day 16 to 25 of pregnancy in 15 Beagle bitches.

Yeager AE, Mohammed HO, Meyers-Wallen V, et al: Ultrasonographic appearance of the uterus, placenta, fetus, and fetal membranes throughout accurately timed pregnancy in Beagles. Am J Vet Res 53:342, 1992.
Reports on the serial ultrasonographic examinations performed on 8 Beagle bitches from 20 to 60 days pregnant to determine time of first detection, appearance and sizes of selected features (gestational sac, uterine wall, embryo position, fetal membranes, embryo and fetal characteristics, and relative size and relationships) of pregnancy.

Use of Serum Relaxin for Pregnancy Diagnosis in the Bitch

BERNARD G. STEINETZ
Tuxedo, New York

LAURA T. GOLDSMITH
Newark, New Jersey

MICHAEL C. BROWN
Malvern, Pennsylvania

GEORGE LUST
Ithaca, New York

There are currently no inexpensive and reliable methods available for early detection of pregnancy in the bitch following mating or artificial insemination. The patterns of the reproductive hormones, estrogen, progesterone, and pituitary gonadotropins are virtually the same in true pregnancy and in false (pseudo) pregnancy in dogs. Bitches do not produce a placental gonadotropin such as the chorionic gonadotropin (hCG) used to determine human pregnancy. Owners of valuable bitches have therefore had to resort to expensive procedures such as ultrasonic imaging to determine if a pregnancy has actually ensued following a planned insemination or an unwanted exposure to a mongrel; alternatively, they have had to wait until the conceptuses could be felt by manual palpation of the uterus. These methods are not useful until about the fourth and fifth weeks, respectively, of a 9-week pregnancy (see previous article).

We have found that the 6-kD polypeptide hormone relaxin is a specific marker of pregnancy in the bitch (Steinetz et al, 1987, 1989). Relaxin can be detected by radioimmunoassay (RIA) or enzyme immunoassay (EIA) in the blood soon after implantation of the fertilized egg, which occurs about 19 to 21 days after mating (Holst and Phemister, 1971). This is consonant with our finding that relaxin is secreted primarily by the placenta (Steinetz et al, 1990). Relaxin never appears in the blood of pseudopregnant bitches, providing a reliable means of discriminating between true and false pregnancy (Steinetz et al, 1987, 1989).

There is as yet no commercially available immunoassay kit for the determination of canine relaxin; however, we shall describe our results in pregnancy detection using our assay. Materials and methods have been described elsewhere (Büllesbach and Schwabe, 1991; Rodbard, 1974; Sherwood, 1994; Steinetz et al, 1996).

Currently, an RIA and EIA are available for measuring relaxin in research laboratories. The EIA is under further development to offer a rapid, in-office canine pregnancy test in the near future. To estimate the earliest time of pregnancy that relaxin could be detected, seven bitches of three different breeds underwent carefully timed matings. Serial blood samples (1 to 2 ml) were drawn from the bitches every other day, starting in proestrus and continuing through pregnancy until whelping. After clot formation and centrifugation, serum was collected and stored frozen until time of assay. The luteinizing hormone (LH) peak was identified by specific EIA (ICG Status-LH Kit or quantitative ICG LH EIA) and the progesterone rise by specific RIA (International Canine Genetics Biomedicals), signaling that ovulation had occurred. The bitches were artificially inseminated from the time of the progesterone rise. The relaxin data were plotted as days from the LH peak and days from whelping. For routine pregnancy testing, blood samples (1 to 2 ml) should be obtained from bitches 25 days after observed copulation or suspected exposure. For timed matings, the LH peak and progesterone rise should be determined by EIA or RIA, and blood samples (1 to 2 ml) for relaxin assay should be drawn on days 23 to 26 after the LH peak. We routinely use serum for the pregnancy test, but plasma is also suitable (see p. 914).

RESULTS

Serum relaxin concentrations were determined by RIA in sequential blood samples of seven bitches from proestrus throughout pregnancy up to the day of whelping (Fig. 1). The data are plotted on a $\log_{10}$ scale in order to show the earliest detection of relaxin, 42 to 38 days before whelping. Relaxin was first detected in serum between 22 and 27 days after the LH surge in all seven bitches by RIA, and 1 or 2 days earlier by the EIA in 3 of the bitches (Table 1).

TABLE 1. Time From Luteinizing Hormone (LH) Surge Until First Detection of Relaxin in Serum Following Timed Matings

Dog I.D.	Days From LH Surge Until First Relaxin by RIA*	Days From LH Surge Until Whelping
C948	26	67
Poly	27	67
A33	24	64
A53	24–27	63–65
A14	23–25	66
B62	22–25	65
Anubis	24–26	66

*Where daily samples were not available at the time of the LH surge or first detection of relaxin, the days are given as a range. Relaxin was detected at least 1 day earlier by EIA in Poly, A33, and A53, and the same day as the RIA in the remaining bitches.

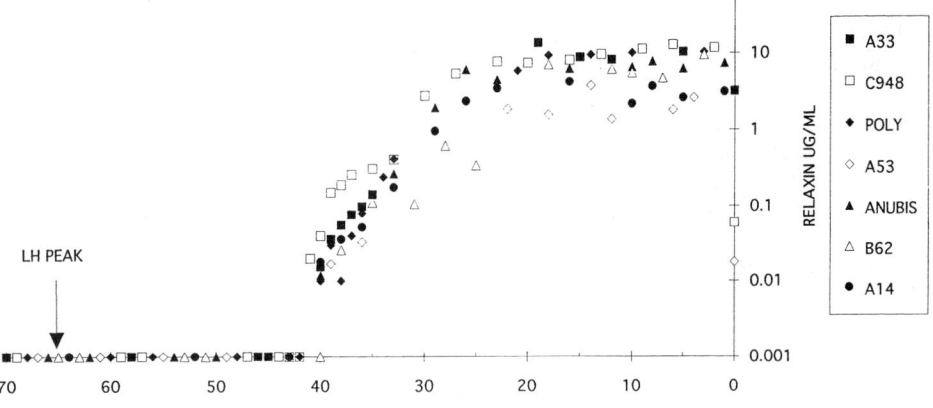

Figure 1. Plot of the serum relaxin concentrations of seven bitches from proestrus through pregnancy following timed matings. The average luteinizing hormone (LH) peak is shown by the arrow. All bitches whelped between 63 and 67 days after the LH surge.

The method has been sensitive, specific, and reproducible in tests of over 300 serum samples obtained from various breeds of dogs, without a single false-positive, even when large sample volumes (300 to 400 μl) were used. Relaxin has never been detected in the serum of male dogs or of pseudopregnant bitches. Relaxin is present in serum and milk during lactation (Goldsmith et al, 1994) for variable periods, but that physiologic state is readily distinguishable from early pregnancy. A sudden loss of serum relaxin is also a useful indicator that spontaneous abortion has occurred (Steinetz et al, 1996).

The relaxin test for pregnancy offers an early, inexpensive and reliable means of determining the success or failure of a planned mating or an unwanted exposure, and thus should soon be a welcome addition to the armamentarium of the veterinarian.

References and Suggested Reading

Büllesbach EE, Schwabe C: Total synthesis of human relaxin and human relaxin derivatives by solid-phase peptide synthesis and site-directed chain combination. J Biol Chem 266:10754, 1991.
First practical synthesis of relaxin molecule.
Goldsmith LT, Lust G, Steinetz BG: Transmission of relaxin from lactating bitches to their offspring via suckling. Biol Reprod 50:258, 1994.
Shows presence of relaxin in serum and milk of lactating bitches and transmission of relaxin to suckling pups.

Holst PA, Phemister RD: The prenatal development of the dog: Preimplantation events. Biol Reprod 5:194, 1971.
Establishes the time of implantation of fertilized eggs in bitches.
Rodbard D: Statistical quality control and routine data processing for radioimmunoassays and immunoradiometric assays. Clin Chem 20:1255, 1974.
Classic paper on data analysis for radioimmunoassays.
Sherwood OD: Relaxin. In: Knobil E, Neill JD, eds: The Physiology of Reproduction, 2nd ed. New York: Raven Press, 1994, p 861.
Contains excellent review of methods for extraction and purification of relaxin, including yields to be expected.
Steinetz BG, Büllesbach EE, Goldsmith LT, et al: Use of synthetic canine relaxin to develop a rapid homologous radioimmunoassay. Biol Reprod 54:1252, 1996.
Describes and validates the homologous canine relaxin radioimmunoassay.
Steinetz BG, Goldsmith LT, Harvey HJ, et al: Serum relaxin and progesterone concentrations in pregnant, pseudopregnant, and ovariectomized, progestin-treated pregnant bitches: Detection of relaxin as a marker of pregnancy. Am J Vet Res 50:68, 1989.
Establishes sources of secretion of relaxin in pregnant bitches.
Steinetz BG, Goldsmith L, Hasan S, et al: Diurnal variation of serum progesterone, but not relaxin, prolactin, or estradiol-17β in the pregnant bitch. Endocrinology 127:1057, 1990.
Shows that the placenta is the primary source of relaxin during pregnancy in bitches.
Steinetz BG, Goldsmith LT, Lust G: Plasma relaxin levels in pregnant and lactating dogs. Biol Reprod 37:719, 1987.
Relaxin is present in the serum of pregnant, but not pseudopregnant, bitches.

CVT Update: Infertility in the Bitch

JANICE L. CAIN
San Ramon, California

A complete reference regarding infertility in the bitch can be found in *CVT XI: Infertility in the bitch* by Johnston (Johnston, 1992). That article is organized by categorizing a bitch's reproductive history as (1) persistent anestrus; (2) abnormal estrous cycles; (3) failure to naturally breed; and (4) apparent conception failure. This *CVT update* is de-signed to provide recommendations for evaluating a bitch presented at any stage of the estrous cycle. Evaluating infertility in the bitch is similar to management for optimal fertility. After the initial evaluation, subsequent phases of the estrous cycle can be further managed to assist an owner in obtaining optimal reproductive performance from a bitch.

PRESENTATION DURING ANESTRUS

Ideally, a bitch with a history of infertility or breeding difficulty is presented for evaluation during anestrus. This will allow time to complete diagnostic procedures and plan breeding management. A prebreeding examination of a previously unbred (maiden) bitch is also recommended. If recommended procedures fail in the subsequent estrous cycle, the bitch is again examined during anestrus. At that time, further diagnostic evaluation is performed and management of future estrous cycles can be planned.

Examination of the Bitch

A complete medical history and physical examination are necessary to ascertain the general health of the bitch. Any underlying illness can cause reproductive failure. The bitch's interestrous interval is determined. Interestrous intervals shorter than 4.5 or longer than 10 months are considered abnormal. Short interestrous intervals theoretically fail to allow sufficient time for endometrial involution after the trophic influence of progesterone during diestrus. Long interestrous intervals can occur in bitches with an underlying illness, although some bitches with long or irregular interestrous intervals are fertile. Anestrus is also the time to review events of prior breedings and assess breeding management. The fertility of stud dogs used for breedings can be investigated retrospectively.

Vaginal Examination

As part of a complete physical examination, and essential to determining the reproductive health of the bitch, the veterinarian must be proficient in digital vaginal palpation of the bitch and have knowledge of normal anatomy. Vulvar and vestibulovaginal stenosis and vaginal septa are common anomalies that can be surgically corrected, ideally during anestrus (Wykes and Soderberg, 1983). Vaginoscopy is well tolerated in nonsedated bitches and is performed to verify normal anatomy. Vaginoscopy can also detect vaginal neoplasia and is essential for an evaluation of vaginitis. The use of a rigid pediatric proctoscope with insufflation is necessary in all but toy breeds; an otoscope will suffice in bitches weighing less than 5 to 8 kg.

Genetic Screening and Population Management

Breed-dependent genetic screening tests are necessary to help the owner determine whether a bitch should be bred. As well, mindful of the pet overpopulation problem, dog owners should be responsible for offspring produced by their bitches.

Laboratory Evaluation

A minimal database (complete blood count, serum biochemistry profile, and urinalysis) should be obtained from any bitch intended for breeding. Many owners will request this standard evaluation annually for their brood bitches. Serum is screened for antibodies to *Brucella canis* prior to each breeding. Owners often request culture from the bitch's vaginal canal prior to natural breedings. Because the differentiation of normal flora from potential pathogens, including those from the cranial vagina, is generally not possible in the bitch, the benefit of this procedure is questionable (Bjurstrom and Linde-Forsberg 1992).

Ultrasonography

Abdominal ultrasonography to evaluate the ovaries and uterus is recommended during anestrus for bitches with undiagnosed infertility. This procedure is also recommended if clinical signs referable to ovarian or uterine disease occurred during the previous estrous cycle. The healthy reproductive tract of the bitch is difficult to image, but abnormalities such as ovarian cysts or hydrometra can be detected (see *CVT XII*, p. 1040).

Surgical Uterine Biopsy and Culture

This invasive procedure is considered for bitches when successful pregnancy has not occurred despite adequate evaluation throughout all phases of the estrous cycle. Anestrus is the best phase to evaluate the endometrium for pathologic abnormalities. Trophic influences of progesterone during diestrus can interfere with interpretation of endometrial biopsies. Direct culture of the uterine lumen for bacteria (aerobic ± anaerobic) and *Mycoplasma sp.* is obtained via the uterine biopsy site. Subclinical bacterial infection of the uterus can be treated with appropriate antimicrobial therapy prior to the next proestrus. The finding of severe cystic endometrial hyperplasia indicates a poor prognosis. Ovaries are usually palpated during laparotomy because the fatty ovarian bursa typically obscures visual inspection. Biopsy or unilateral ovariectomy can be performed if unilateral ovarian disease (e.g., cyst or mass) is found.

Planning the Breeding

Anestrus is the time to help the owner plan the upcoming breeding and consider male selection. *Bitches with a history of questionable fertility are not suitable candidates for breeding with chilled or frozen semen.* Ideally, a known fertile stud dog is chosen that will be available at the time of this bitch's cycle, and one that will not be bred concurrently to other bitches. Bitches with a history of infertility should not be shipped for breeding in order to avoid potential stress of shipping. Either shipping the stud dog to the bitch's locale or choosing a local stud dog should be considered. The owner is advised of ovulation timing procedures and instructed to return the bitch for evaluation at the beginning of proestrus.

PRESENTATION DURING PROESTRUS AND ESTRUS

Initial Evaluation

A bitch may be presented in proestrus or estrus for the beginning of a reproductive evaluation. It is possible to obtain a partial diagnostic evaluation at this time. Procedures performed that are similar to a bitch presented originally in anestrus include medical history; physical examination including digital vaginal palpation; *Brucella canis* screening; and minimal database. Vaginoscopy is performed as an adjunct to ovulation timing, but vaginal mucosal edema at this time will hinder a thorough visual evaluation.

Ovulation Timing

Ovulation timing is recommended for each estrous cycle in which the bitch is to be bred, rather than relying on information from a previous estrus. Variations can occur and bitches ovulate too infrequently (i.e., 1 to 2 times per year) for a breeding to fail because of poor breeding management. Breeding management error is the most common, and most correctable, cause of apparent infertility in the bitch. Typically, two to three breedings are planned to occur during days 9 through 13 (day 1 = first day of sanguineous vaginal discharge). Owners commonly request artificial insemination for the bitch when natural breeding has not occurred by day 12 to 14. Although the average durations of proestrus and estrus are each 7 to 9 days, considerable variation can occur. Ovulation can occur relatively early (i.e., day 3) or late (i.e., day 19). The observation of breeding behavior of the bitch or stud dog can be erroneous when used as the only factor to determine breeding management method. Bitches can begin behavioral estrus from 4 days before to 5 days after the surge of luteinizing hormone (LH) release that triggers ovulation (Concannon, 1986). When a limited number of breedings are allowed, a bitch can be bred too far in advance of ovulation. Estimating when a bitch ovulates, by performing ovulation timing, is used to ensure that breeding occurs during the period of peak fertility (Table 1).

Ovulation timing is performed by evaluating several parameters sequentially during proestrus and estrus (Table 2; Concannon, 1986; Cain, 1992; Goodman, 1992). Serial evaluation of serum progesterone by radioimmunoassay (RIA) or LH concentrations by an in-house semiquantitative assay is an essential service that the veterinarian can provide. Evaluation of serum progesterone concentration

TABLE 1. Physiologic Principles of Ovulation Timing in the Bitch

Folliculogenesis: Follicular growth causes estrogen production, which causes cornification of vaginal epithelium.

Preovulatory LH peak: A spontaneous release of luteinizing hormone (LH) from the pituitary causes ovulation to occur approximately 48 hours later.

Peak fertile period: Approximately 4–6 days after the preovulatory LH peak, mature ova are within the oviducts and are available for fertilization.

Estrus: Behavioral sexual receptivity is usually over a longer duration than the peak fertile period.

Serum progesterone concentration: Increases from <1.0 ng/ml to 1.0–2.5 ng/ml at the time of the preovulatory LH peak. At the time of ovulation, serum progesterone concentration is 4–10 ng/ml.

Vaginal mucosal crenulation: High serum estrogen concentration causes edema of the vaginal mucosa. As the edema recedes, the mucosa appears characteristically wrinkled or crenulated.

TABLE 2. Ovulation Timing Parameters

Vaginal cytology: Used to determine when to begin serum assays for progesterone or luteinizing hormone (LH). Also used to define onset of cytologic diestrus (i.e., increase in parabasal cells after a period of full cornification), which coincides with the end of the fertile period.

Serum progesterone concentration: Begin evaluation when 50–70% of vaginal cells are the superfical type (i.e., 50–70% cornified). Determine every 24–48 hours to detect a first rise in concentration above basal level of <1.0 ng/ml, which correlates with the preovulatory serum LH peak.

Serum LH assay: Determined daily when ≥50% of vaginal cells are the superficial type (i.e., 50% cornified). Values return to baseline after the preovulatory LH peak. False LH peaks can occur prior to the preovulatory LH peak but will not be associated with a progesterone rise. Serum progesterone concentration will rise 1–3 days after the preovulatory LH peak and is measured to confirm the LH peak.

Vaginal mucosal crenulation: Changes seen in the vaginal mucosa during the estrous cycle are as follows:

Anestrus: Mucosa is flat and smooth.

Proestrus/estrus prior to preovulatory LH peak: Mucosa is edematous; vaginal folds are distended and rounded, causing obliteration of the vaginal canal.

Preovulatory LH peak ±24 hours: Initial crenulation is a fine wrinkling in mucosa as vaginal edema begins to recede.

Post–LH peak/period of peak fertility: Crenulation continues with angulated appearance of mucosa with sharp-appearing profiles. Vaginal lumen easy to observe without insufflation.

Diestrus: Mucosa is irregularly flattened, and blotchy red and white.

every 24 to 48 hours, or serum LH concentration every 24 hours (Status-LH; ICG—A Synbiotics Company), is combined with evaluation of exfoliative vaginal cytology. Serial evaluation of vaginal mucosa by vaginoscopy for evidence of crenulation (wrinkling) is another method to estimate ovulation timing and is an excellent adjunct to hormonal assays and vaginal cytology (Lindsay, 1990).

Breeding Assistance

After ovulation timing, breedings are planned to occur on days 2, 4, and 6 (day 0 = day of estimated preovulatory serum LH surge); or if only two breedings are possible, on days 3 and 5. If natural breeding does not occur on the prescribed dates, artificial insemination (AI) is performed. An AI also provides an opportunity to evaluate the stud dog's semen prior to insemination. A complete semen analysis including parameters of motility, total sperm count, and morphology is performed (Olson, 1992; see *CVT XII*, p. 1060). If the first breeding is by AI, the owner will have the option of selecting an alternate male if the semen is of poor quality.

Planning the Diestrus Evaluation

Owners are advised to return the bitch for pregnancy diagnosis via ultrasonography. If the bitch is not pregnant, evaluation in early to mid-diestrus is important to determine other possible causes of infertility.

PRESENTATION DURING DIESTRUS

Initial Evaluation

Owners commonly present their bitch to a veterinarian for pregnancy diagnosis. If she is not pregnant, it may be the first indication to the owner that the bitch has a reproductive problem. A complete medical history and physical examination are essential to help rule out occult disease. The veterinarian can also retrospectively determine if ovulation timing was performed accurately, or if breeding management error could be a problem. Obtaining a minimal database is also indicated for a nonpregnant bitch, if she was not evaluated earlier in the estrous cycle.

Ultrasonography

The only method to correctly diagnose pregnancy early in gestation, and assess fetal viability, is by abdominal ultrasonography (see p. 918). Pregnancy can be detected, and litter size estimated, as early as 21 days after the last breeding. Early pregnancy diagnosis is important to document fetal resorption. Litter resorption can be erroneously diagnosed in pseudopregnant bitches when pregnancy is assessed by abdominal palpation. Ultrasonography is repeated every 2 to 3 weeks for bitches suspected of litter resorption.

Bitches that are not pregnant benefit from ultrasonographic examination during diestrus to detect subclinical pyometra or other uterine disease. Unless severe, cystic endometrial hyperplasia may escape detection by ultrasonography, however.

Serum Progesterone Concentration

After ovulation, progesterone concentrations reach 5 to 80 ng/ml by mid-diestrus, and then slowly return to basal values (<1 ng/ml) by the end of pregnancy. This pattern of progesterone secretion is the same during diestrus of the nonpregnant bitch. Serum progesterone concentration cannot be used to detect pregnancy or assess fetal viability. It is an indicator, however, of luteal function, which is required to sustain pregnancy. Serum progesterone concentration below 1 to 2 ng/ml in early diestrus indicates either ovulatory failure or luteal insufficiency. If pregnancy is documented and serum progesterone concentration is detected below 5 ng/ml prior to day 50 of gestation, luteal insufficiency is possible. This condition is extremely rare in the bitch, and inappropriate supplementation with progesterone can cause masculinization of female fetuses. Supplementation with progesterone in oil (3 mg/kg IM every 24 hours) can maintain serum progesterone concentration of a bitch at 10 ng/ml (Scott-Moncreiff et al, 1990). Supplementation with progesterone must be discontinued for spontaneous parturition to occur; the duration for withdrawal has not been documented for the bitch.

Evaluation of Fetal Resorption or Abortion

The first step to evaluating fetal resorption or abortion is to assess the bitch for underlying illness. Any infectious, metabolic, or endocrinologic disease can prevent the completion of normal pregnancy. To diagnose canine herpesvirus as a cause, viral isolation from a vaginal swab and serum viral antibody titer from the bitch are performed. Uterine bacterial infection may also cause fetal death. Vaginal cultures of aerobic bacteria and *Mycoplasma* sp. are

obtained (see *CVT XII*, p. 1090), but are probably an indication only of uterine disease at the time of abortion and cervical patency. Aborted fetuses are necropsied and cultures are obtained as indicated. Serum progesterone concentration of the bitch is measured to assess luteal function. If the progesterone concentration is low, it is possibly a result and not a cause of the resorption or abortion. It is not uncommon to find that results of all tests are normal. Factors including developmental defects in the fetuses and local uterine abnormalities may cause resorption or abortion. Some bitches with historical litter resorption or abortion do not have problems with future litters.

Whelping Assistance and Cesarean Section

Loss of fetuses or neonates due to lack of veterinary intervention during whelping is common. Cesarean section can prevent fetal loss when whelping does not progress normally. Owners need help deciding when intervention is necessary, and veterinary care must be available at all times.

Evaluating Continued Infertility

Bitches that either failed to conceive or carry a litter to term should be evaluated again during anestrus. At that time, management of the entire estrous cycle can be reviewed. Plans can be made for future breedings if a correctable problem can be isolated. Additional diagnostic testing may be indicated (see section on anestrus evaluation). Fertility can be achieved in some cases by repeating the breeding during another estrous cycle. Some bitches, however, have idiopathic infertility for which no correctable causes can be found.

References and Suggested Reading

Bjurstrom L, Linde-Forsberg C: Long-term study of aerobic bacteria of the genital tract in breeding bitches. Am J Vet Res 53:665, 1992.
    A description of the normal bacterial flora obtained from daily vaginal cultures from bitches.
Cain JL: Introduction to reproduction section. In: Morgan RV, ed: Handbook of Small Animal Practice, 2nd ed. New York: Churchill Livingstone, 1992, p 637.
    Ovulation timing techniques, including evaluation of serum progesterone concentrations and vaginoscopy.
Concannon PW: Clinical and endocrine correlates of canine ovarian cycles and pregnancy. In: Kirk RW, ed: Current Veterinary Therapy IX. Small Animal Practice. Philadelphia: WB Saunders, 1986, p 1214.
    A description of the reproductive physiology of the bitch pertaining to ovulation and measured parameters.
Goodman MF: Canine ovulation timing. In: Problems in Veterinary Medicine: Canine Reproduction. Philadelphia: JB Lippincott, 1992, p 433.
    A review of reproductive physiology and ovulation timing techniques emphasizing the use of serum progesterone assays.
Johnston SD: Infertility in the bitch. In: Kirk RW, Bonagura JD, eds: Current Veterinary Therapy XI. Small Animal Practice. Philadelphia: WB Saunders, 1992, p 954.
    A well-organized discussion describing the causes of infertility in the bitch.
Lindsay FEF: Postuterine endoscopy in the bitch. In: Tams TR, ed: Small Animal Endoscopy. St. Louis: CV Mosby, 1990, p 327.
    Excellent description of the visual changes that occur to the vaginal mucosa during proestrus and estrus, including color photographs.
Olson PN: Collection and evaluation of canine semen. In: Kirk RW, Bonagura JD, eds: Current Veterinary Therapy XI. Small Animal Practice. Philadelphia: WB Saunders, 1992, p 938.

A guide to semen analysis that can be performed in a veterinary hospital, including normal values and a sample evaluation form.

Scott-Moncrieff JC, Nelson RW, Bill RL, et al: Serum deposition of exogenous progesterone after intramuscular administration in bitches. Am J Vet Res 51:893, 1990.

Injections of progesterone in oil (3 mg/kg IM q24hr) will maintain serum progesterone concentration at 10 ng/ml.

Wykes PM, Soderberg SF: Congenital abnormalities of the canine vagina and vulva. J Am Anim Hosp Assoc 19:995, 1983.

A description of the types of anomalies of the vagina and vulva that can occur in bitches.

Yeager AE, Concannon PW: Ultrasonography of the reproductive tract of the female dog and cat. In: Bonagura JD, ed: Current Veterinary Therapy XII. Small Animal Practice. Philadelphia: WB Saunders, 1995, p 1040.

A discussion of normal ultrasonographic findings and examples of some disease conditions, including ultrasonographic photographs.

CVT Update: Infertility in the Queen

Autumn P. Davidson

Davis, California

Evaluation of the queen presented for infertility is an infrequent and challenging event in most small animal practices. Valuable queens from purebred catteries are most commonly presented for a complete failure to reproduce or deterioration in their reproductive performance. An efficient, thorough method of addressing infertility in the queen is necessary, with realistic expectations concerning outcome.

A thorough history reviewing cattery husbandry (feeding, housing, infectious disease control) and reproductive management (lighting, social interaction, breeding methods) should be taken. The queen's health and reproductive (puberty, frequency of cycles, known matings, pregnancies, abortions, litters) histories should also be reviewed. The reproductive status of relatives and other queens in the cattery can be of interest. A complete physical examination and clinicopathologic database (hemogram, serum chemistry profile, urinalysis and urine culture, feline leukemia virus/feline immunodeficiency virus/feline infectious peritonitis [FELV/FIV/FIP] serologies) should be performed initially to rule out any underlying health problems in the queen presented for infertility (Wolf, 1992).

DEFINITION OF INFERTILITY

Infertility in the queen is defined as a failure to produce an expected number of live kittens successfully, due to a failure to breed and conceive, carry fetuses to term, or reproduce. True infertility needs to be differentiated from the failure to reproduce as a consequence of cattery management problems. The prognosis for fertility is better when management problems are discovered and corrected, inasmuch as queens with reproductive pathology generally have a poor prognosis for return to fertility.

Cattery Management Issues

Optimal reproductive performance depends on good husbandry. Catteries should not be overcrowded because social stresses can negatively impact fertility. Travel stress should also be minimized. Cattery sanitation should be optimal. Adequate nutrition resulting from the use of high-quality approved commercial feeds is essential. Prevention of endemic infectious diseases based on judicious immunization, quarantine of new individuals, and appropriate test and removal procedures is important for reproductive success (Stabenfeldt, 1991).

Cattery owners should have a working knowledge of feline reproductive physiology and successful breeding techniques, including the ability to detect estrous cycles in queens, and organize and observe successful copulations. The feline estrous cycle is characterized by variability, and is best monitored by behavioral changes, because the queen shows minimal external physical evidence of estrus. Vaginal cytology is useful for confirming estrus in queens with vague behavioral changes, most enlightening during estrus, when superficial (cornified) vaginal epithelial cells are predominant, and vaginal mucus diminishes. Ideally, breedings should begin on the third day of estrus. Although the queen initiates mating by displaying lordosis, the tom must be in a territory he has adequately established by urine marking in order for him to willingly participate. The past use of a proven (fertile) tom cat with a queen presented for infertility should be ascertained. Toms should not be used excessively or outside of the cattery. Breeding queens should ideally be between 1 and 6 years of age, although they can remain fertile until 8 to 10, but with diminished litter size and an increased incidence of stillbirths (Shille and Sojka, 1995).

Reproductive Failure

When no physical or health abnormalities are found and cattery breeding management is adequate, the queen should be further categorized based on her reproductive status. Vaginoscopy utilizing anesthesia and a vaginoscope with insufflation, vaginography, and ultrasound evaluation of the uterus and ovaries can provide additional information. Laparotomy or laparoscopy with visualization of the ovaries and biopsy and culture of the uterus can be performed.

Whether or not the owner believes the queen cycles, evidence for ovarian activity should be obtained. During appropriate photoperiod or adequate light exposure, queens with cyclical ovarian follicular activity will have estrogen levels of over 12 to 50 pg/ml. Several serum samples should be acquired to assure that sampling did not occur during the interfollicular phase. Failure to cycle under appropriate photoperiod or light exposure is categorized as prolonged anestrus. Prior ovariohysterectomy must be ruled out. Prepubescent and geriatric queens require no further work-up. Queens of appropriate age with prolonged anestrus should be evaluated for socially induced estrus suppression. Housing separate from dominant queens, near a compatible male, can be effective. Estrus induction can be attempted. If no ovarian response occurs, a congenital error in the hypothalamic pituitary ovarian axis or an error in sexual differentiation is probable (Shille and Sojka, 1995).

Queens with regular cycles and breeding behavior should be evaluated for ovulation and conception. Successful ovulation depends on the presence of mature follicles and an adequate luteinizing hormone (LH) surge, which in turn is dependent on an adequate frequency and number of copulations. Ovulation and luteinization of the follicle can be documented by measuring serum progesterone levels 48 hours after breedings. Progesterone levels greater than 2 ng/ml (often above 20 ng/ml) indicate ovulation occurred. Failure to ovulate indicates that copulations were incomplete, too infrequent, too late, or too early during estrus. Breeding management needs to be revised, or artificial insemination and ovulation induction performed.

Documented ovulation should be followed up with an ultrasound evaluation in 14 to 21 days, looking for evidence of conception and implantation. Serial ultrasound evaluations can document fetal resorption versus a failure to conceive (Davidson et al, 1986). Fetal resorption occurs most commonly with congenital defects (chromosomal anomalies, teratogens) and infectious disorders, most commonly feline panleukopenia virus, feline leukemia virus, feline corona virus, and the feline respiratory complex viruses. Toxoplasma and mycoplasma have been detected in infertile cats but have not yet been definitively shown to cause infertility. Bacterial infection of the fetuses is likely to result in abortion. Nutritional disorders (taurine deficiency) have been implicated in abortion.

Maintenance of pregnancy depends upon the presence of functional corpora lutea through the fortieth day of gestation. Placental production of progesterone begins after 40 gestational days. The fetoplacental unit produces prostaglandin $F_{2\alpha}$ ($PGF_{2\alpha}$) and relaxin. Relaxin softens pelvic connective tissues, facilitating delivery, and acts in concert with progesterone to maintain the endometrium in a quiescent state. Hypoluteoidism has not been documented as a cause for infertility in the queen (Feldman and Nelson, 1995).

Ovulation followed by a failure to conceive can occur with the cystic endometrial hyperplasia complex. Cystic endometrial hyperplasia occurs in queens as a consequence of chronic exposure of the endometrium to estrogen. Hydrometra, the accumulation of noninflammatory fluid within the uterus, can occur in the absence of bacterial infection, and causes infertility. Endometritis or pyometra occurs as a consequence of bacterial contamination and colonization of the uterus, associated with progesterone-induced increases in uterine glandular secretions, inhibition of leukocyte function, and decreased myometrial activity. Pyometra is commonly associated with the luteal phase of the estrous cycle, when progesterone is elaborated. Hydrometra is characterized by uterine enlargement and mucinous vaginal discharge with no other clinical signs of disease. Endometritis and pyometra cause systemic illness. Queens are frequently febrile, lethargic, and anorexic and can have a purulent/hemorrhagic vaginal discharge, if the cervix is open. Closed cervix pyometra causes serious, fulminant illness. Ultrasound examination shows uterine distention with flocculation. An inflammatory leukogram, evidence of sepsis, and polyuria secondary to endotoxin-mediated nephrogenic diabetes insipidus can be present. Ovariohysterectomy is curative and indicated when the queen is stabilized. Medical management of open cervix pyometra with $PGF_{2\alpha}$, 0.10 to 0.20 mg/kg per day, with concurrent bactericidal antibiotics can be successful in queens intended for future breeding. Hydrometra can be treated with $PGF_{2\alpha}$ or ovariohysterectomy (Potter et al, 1991; Davidson et al, 1992).

Queens exhibiting prolonged periods of estrus behavior (up to 45 days) during the breeding season, caused by overlapping waves of folliculogenesis, can fail to conceive although fertile, because correct timing of breedings is difficult. Prolonged estrus behavior outside of the breeding season is associated with cystic follicular degeneration of the ovary. Follicles are morphologically abnormal and oocytes not viable. Ovariohysterectomy is indicated because these queens are at risk for endometrial hyperplasia. A functional granulosa cell tumor of the ovary is another cause of persistent nonseasonal estrus in the queen (Stabenfeldt and Pederson, 1991).

The failure to deliver viable fetuses at term results in infertility. $PGF_{2\alpha}$ produced by the fetoplacental unit and the endometrium initiates parturition by causing regression of term corpora lutea and inducing uterine contractions. Fetal adrenal cortisol synthesis at term induces placental estrogen secretion, which subsequently increases $PGF_{2\alpha}$ production. Delivery of fetuses between 61 and 63 days of gestation results in reduced fetal viability, and delivery of fetuses at less than 61 gestational days usually results in neonatal death. Complete histopathologic evaluation of aborted or stillborn kittens and any associated placental tissues, including bacterial and viral evaluation, can be informative. Careful monitoring of labor with intervention as indicated by fetal or maternal distress can prevent late-term fetal death as a consequence of dystocia.

References and Suggested Reading

Davidson AP, Feldman EC, Nelson RW: Treatment of pyometra in cats, using prostaglandin $F_{2\alpha}$: 21 cases (1982–1990). J Am Vet Med Assoc 200:825, 1992.
  Outlines the pathophysiology, diagnosis, and treatment options for feline pyometra.
Davidson AP, Nyland TG, Tsutsui T: Pregnancy diagnosis with ultrasound in the domestic cat. Vet Radiol 27:109, 1986.
  Describes and illustrates the progression of ultrasonographic findings in early pregnancy diagnosis in the queen.
Feldman EC, Nelson RW: Feline reproduction. In: Canine and Feline Endocrinology and Reproduction. Philadelphia: WB Saunders, 1995, p 741.
  Reviews feline reproductive physiology and pathology.
Potter K, Hancock DH, Gallina AM: Clinical and pathologic features of

endometrial hyperplasia, pyometra, and endometritis in cats: 79 cases (1980–1985). J Am Vet Med Assoc 198:1427, 1991.
Summarizes the records of 79 cats with endometrial hyperplasia, endometritis, and pyometra.

Root MV, Johnston SD, Olson PN: Estrous length, pregnancy rate, gestation and parturition lengths, litter size, and juvenile mortality in the domestic cat. J Am Anim Hosp Assoc 31:429, 1995.
Reviews reproductive performance in a research colony of 14 queens.

Shille VM, Sojka NJ: Feline reproduction. In: Ettinger SJ, Feldman EC, ed: Textbook of Veterinary Internal Medicine, 4th ed. Philadelphia: WB Saunders, 1995, p 1690.

Complete review of feline reproductive physiology.

Stabenfeldt GH, Pederson NC: Reproduction and reproductive disorders. In: Pederson NC, ed: Feline Husbandry: Diseases and Management in the Multiple Cat Environment. Goleta, CA: American Veterinary Publications, 1991, p 129.
Complete review of feline clinical reproduction.

Wolf AM: Infertility in the queen. In: Kirk RW, Bonagura JD, eds: Current Veterinary Therapy. Philadelphia: WB Saunders, 1992, p 947.
Summarizes the approach to infertility in the queen, including a review of reproductive physiology.

Current Therapeutic Recommendations for Pregnant Dogs

JONI L. FRESHMAN
Colorado Springs, Colorado

The time a fetus spends in the intrauterine environment can have lasting effects that influence the puppy throughout its life. For this reason the pregnant bitch needs special attention in several areas. Diet, exercise, preventative medicine, and medical care combine to maximize our ability to produce healthy offspring.

DIET

During the first 3 weeks of gestation the well-conditioned bitch may undergo little or no weight gain. The consumption of a good-quality maintenance dog food is sufficient unless the bitch is underweight. Bitches who enter pregnancy excessively thin should eat a growth or performance food to rapidly correct their condition. At about 3 weeks' gestation many bitches suffer a loss of appetite that persists for about a week. Nausea and mild vomiting occasionally accompany the anorexia. Appetite typically will return at about week 4.

Pregnant bitches do require increased protein and carbohydrate over their maintenance state, but this is usually provided by their increased intake of a high-quality maintenance ration. Some texts recommend changing the pregnant bitch to a growth formula; however, this should not be necessary with a well-conditioned bitch, and alteration of diet may lead to gastroenteric distress. Obese bitches should undergo weight reduction prior to breeding, to improve the chances of conception and decrease risks of dystocia and poor lactation. Pregnancy is not a good time to pursue weight loss. The amount of food required by a pregnant bitch in later gestation increases in proportion with litter size and growth. A 40% average increase in food counsumption accompanies the 20 to 55% increase in body weight. Because of the increased intra-abdominal pressure from the enlarging uterus, multiple smaller meals are easier for the bitch to consume than two larger meals. Bitches carrying large litters may have extreme discomfort

the last week of gestation and suffer a decreased appetite again at this time. Many, but not all, bitches will stop eating 24 to 48 hours before parturition.

The administration of vitamins and supplements to pregnant bitches should be discouraged. Calcium supplementation, though unfortunately still common, is contraindicated. Although calcium requirements increase in the pregnant bitch, they are met by the increased amount of food ingested. Excess calcium above the amount provided by a high-quality diet suppresses parathyroid hormone production and increases the bitch's risk of puerperal hypocalcemia. Breeders should be cautioned not to add calcium in any form to the pregnant bitch's diet. Supplementation of fat-soluble vitamins can also be problematic. Excess vitamin A has been associated with congenital defects, including cleft palate. Folate deficiency has been associated with fetal defects in infants. Although premium dog foods should contain enough folate, supplementation of B vitamins is not harmful. Dogs produce sufficient vitamin C of their own and do not require supplementation. Excess vitamin D may complicate the calcium mobilization ability of the bitch. My recommendation is to feed a premium-quality, balanced ration with no supplements.

ROUTINE CONDITIONING

Exercise

Fit, well-conditioned bitches are less likely to suffer dystocia. Regular exercise during pregnancy is important in maintaining condition. Brisk walking is the safest exercise for this purpose. In late gestation, bitches carrying large litters may need to limit this to short walks. Performance bitches should stop heavy work during pregnancy; herding, agility, field, and advanced obedience work are discouraged because of the risk of abdominal trauma and the potential stress to fetuses. Studies performed on pregnant bitches revealed that even relatively mild stress, such as restraint in a harness, can permanently reset the hypothalamic-pituitary-adrenal axis of the fetuses (Nathanielsz, 1996). This results in excess and protracted production of cortisol in response to stress in the resultant puppies. Therefore, it behooves us to keep the pregnant bitch's life as tranquil as possible. Shows, classes, and performance events should be discouraged.

Vaccinations

Vaccinations for rabies, canine distemper, hepatitis, coronavirus parainfluenza, and leptospirosis should be current prior to breeding. The puppies' early immunity is dependent upon consumption of colostrum containing high levels of antibodies and therefore upon the bitch's immune status. Modified live vaccinations should not be given during pregnancy.

Parasites

Toxocara canis larvae encysted in muscle tissue of the pregnant bitch are reactivated during the last trimester and migrate transplacentally to the pups. It is important to realize that routine deworming of the bitch will not affect this process. The infestation of pups can be interrupted by administration of fenbendazole at 50 mg/kg PO from day 40 of gestation to day 14 after whelping. *Ancylostoma caninum* can also be transmitted transplacentally and is responsive to the above treatment.

Microfilariae of *Dirofilaria immitis* can cross the placenta. Although they will not create a patent infestation, they can result in a pup that is a reservoir for spreading heartworm disease and may put the puppy at risk for adverse reactions to routine heartworm preventive medication. Pregnant bitches should be routinely tested for heartworms and maintained on heartworm preventative in areas at-risk. Both ivermectin and milbemycin oxime monthly preventives are safe in pregnant bitches.

MEDICAL CONSIDERATIONS

Parameter Changes

Certain blood values are altered by the pregnant state. The most notable is packed cell volume (PCV), which decreases to approximately 40% by day 35 of gestation. At term, the PCV is often below 35%. The anemia is normocytic and normochromic and is caused by hemodilution. Creatinine decreases by 25 to 35% as well. Fibrinogen increases during pregnancy. Diagnostic testing and medical treatment in the pregnant bitch should be performed with these alterations in mind.

Hypoglycemia

Also known as pregnancy toxemia, this serious illness is most common in thin, poorly conditioned bitches. These bitches have inadequate fat stores, muscle mass, and dietary carbohydrate. They may present with nonspecific signs of illness or seizures. Ketonemia and ketonuria without

glucosuria often accompany the hypoglycemia. Because hypocalcemia presents with similar signs and can occur in term bitches, serum calcium level should also be evaluated. Hypoglycemia should be treated with intravenous administration of dextrose-containing fluids. Nutritional supplementation will be needed in bitches who do not eat voluntarily. Termination of pregnancy may be necessary in severe cases.

Hyperglycemia

Pre-existing subclinical diabetes mellitus may be aggravated by the pregnant state. Insulin should be given if indicated by carefully monitored blood glucose levels. Insulin resistance is usually present. The varying demands and hormonal alterations during pregnancy and parturition make glucose control challenging. Cross-fostering of pups and retirement from breeding should be encouraged.

Hypoluteodism

Although rare, failure to maintain appropriate serum progesterone levels throughout pregnancy is a treatable cause of fetal loss. Monitoring of serum progesterone levels allows accurate diagnosis of this problem (see p. 914). Serum progesterone levels greater than 2 ng/ml are required to maintain pregnancy. In a normal pregnancy, progesterone reaches peak levels of 15 to 90 ng/ml by 15 to 30 days after the luteinizing hormone peak. During the last trimester, progesterone decreases to 4 to 16 ng/ml before dropping below 2 ng/ml approximately 1 day before parturition. Monitoring of serum progesterone level can be performed weekly if the levels are 20 to 50 ng/ml or daily if they are 5 to 10 ng/ml. Hypoluteodism can be treated with injections of progesterone in oil 2 to 3 mg/kg IM every 24 hours. Alternatively, ally-trenbolone (Regumate, Hoechst-Roussel Agri-Vet Co) at 0.088 mg/kg PO daily can be given (Eilts, 1992). Ultrasonographic monitoring of fetuses can be helpful in assessing fetal viability. Fetal heart rates less than twice that of the dam indicate fetal distress, as does decreased fetal movement. Exact timing of ovulation and therefore parturition date is necessary so that progesterone supplementation can be stopped about 72 hours prior to the expected parturition date, allowing an approximation of normal decline of progesterone. Milk production by the bitch may not be adequate, so supplementation of milk for pups may be necessary. Providing progesterone or ally-trenbolone supplementation for too long or short of a time will result in stillborn pups.

Canine Herpesvirus (CHV)

The fatal form of this disease results from exposure of the pups during the last 3 weeks of gestation and the first

TABLE 1. Drugs Considered Safe in Pregnancy

Cephalosporins	Fenbendazole
Penicillins	Ivermectin
Amoxicillin with clavulanic acid	Milbemycin oxime
Clindamycin	Praziquantel
Pyrantel pamoate	

TABLE 2. Some Drugs To Be Avoided in Pregnancy

Aminoglycosides	Griseofulvin	Diethylstilbestrol
Tetracyclines	Fluoroquinolones	Organophosphates
Trimethoprim	Enalapril	Omeprazole
Chloramphenicol	Theophylline	Mitotane
Metronidazole	Misoprostol	

3 weeks of life. Canine herpesvirus is most commonly spread as a mild respiratory infection between adult dogs. Because no vaccination is currently available, prevention is the most effective approach. Complete isolation of the pregnant bitch and her pups for this 6-week danger period is effective in preventing infection. Unfortunately, no successful treatment is available if the pups become infected.

Drug Administration

Administration of any medication is best avoided in the pregnant bitch, especially during days 13 to 30 of gestation. Some drugs have proven relatively safe, whereas others are definitely dangerous to the developing fetus (Tables 1 and 2). Many other drugs carry potential risks that have not been researched or established. The safest course is to avoid any medication of questionable safety and to administer medication only if absolutely necessary.

References and Suggested Reading

Bebiak DM, Lawler DF, Reutzel LF, et al: Nutrition and management of the dog. Vet Clin North Am 17:3:505, 1987.
Review includes biochemical changes during pregnancy and feeding recommendations.

Concannon PW: Physiology and endocrinology of canine pregnancy. In: Morrow DA, ed: Current Therapy in Theriogenology 2. Philadelphia: WB Saunders, 1986, p 491.
An extensive review of hormonal events during pregnancy.

Eilts BE: Pregnancy maintenance in the bitch using Regumate. Proc Soc Therio Annu Meeting (Texas), 1992, p 144.
Review of hypoluteodism and research results on use of ally-trenbolone.

Evermann JF: Comparative clinical and diagnostic aspects of herpesvirus infections of companion animals with primary emphasis on the dog. Proc Soc Therio Annu Meeting (Idaho), 1989, p 335.
A comprehensive review of canine herpesvirus.

Feldman EC, Nelson RW: Breeding, pregnancy and parturition. In: Canine and Feline Endocrinology and Reproduction. Philadelphia: WB Saunders, 1996, p 547.
A review of events preceding, following, and occurring during gestation.

Nathanielsz PW: Long-term effects of the uterine environment. Proc Soc Therio Annu Meeting (Missouri), 1996, p 11.
Discussion of the effects of the intrauterine environment on later life.

Papich M: Pharmacological considerations during pregnancy in small animals. Proc Soc Therio Annu Meeting (Ontario), 1990, p 224.
Thorough review of pharmacology in pregnancy, including an exhaustive list of medications.

Medical Management of Dystocia and Indications for Cesarean Section in the Bitch

Christine M. Schweizer
Vicki N. Meyers-Wallen
Ithaca, New York

Minutes count when a dystocia presents. It is imperative that the clinician work through each case quickly, thoroughly, and calmly in order to maximize the chances of a successful outcome for the dam and each of her pups. Not only may the bitch have emotional value for the client, but also a valuable brood bitch and her offspring may represent a considerable investment in time and capital by the breeder-owner.

EVALUATION OF THE DAM AND FETUSES

History

A dystocia may present in a variety of ways. The most common in our experience are the following:

1. The bitch with no signs of labor perceived as *overdue* by the owner.

2. The bitch that has had a significant decrease in rectal temperature within the last 24 hours yet shows no signs of first- or second-stage labor.

3. The bitch that has been actively straining for more than 20 minutes without producing a pup, and that may or may not have fetal membranes protruding from the vulva.

4. The bitch that has produced one or more pups, but now labor has ceased, even though more pups are present in utero.

Typically, the history is gathered over the phone and/or during the physical examination by thorough and succinct questioning. Factors such as the bitch's age, breed, reproductive history, and previous or chronic medical conditions and their treatments are important pieces of information. For example, older bitches may have an increased risk of primary uterine inertia, and certain breeds have a high incidence of relative fetal oversize. Breeding dates, vaginal cytology information, and, most important, the date of the bitch's preovulatory serum progesterone rise/luteinizing hormone (LH) peak aid in determining whether a pregnancy is full term. Parturition occurs at 57 to 72 days from any one breeding date, or approximately 57 ± 3 days from the first day of diestrus as determined by serial vaginal cytology, or 65 ± 1 days from the preovulatory serum progesterone rise/LH peak.

Establishing a *timeline* of the bitch's labor is also important. Many, but not all, normal bitches exhibit a decrease in rectal temperature 24 to 48 hours prior to delivery that is 1° to 3°F below their normal baseline temperature (commonly below 99°F). This temperature drop is related to the abrupt decrease in serum progesterone concentrations at the end of gestation. Typically, the *average* bitch that is progressing normally into first-stage labor* will show outward signs of panting, restlessness, and intensified nesting behavior within 6 to 18 hours of the temperature drop. She will then progress to second-stage labor,† typified by abdominal press, usually within 24 hours after the temperature drop. Once the bitch enters second-stage labor, pups will be produced every ½ to 1 hour on average, but patterns can vary markedly between litters. A bitch may produce two or more pups in rapid succession and then rest for 1 or more hours between pups before continuing labor. In general, we like to examine a bitch if any of the following circumstances exist:

1. She has reached her expected due date without any sign of a temperature drop or labor.
2. There are no signs of first-stage labor within 12 to 18 hours of a temperature drop.
3. The bitch has failed to progress to second-stage labor after 6 to 8 hours of first-stage labor.
4. The bitch has been actively straining for more than 20 minutes or has had weak, intermittent abdominal contractions for 1 hour and has not expelled a pup or has only presented membranes.
5. It has been more than 1 hour between delivery of pups with no further signs of active labor.

These guidelines may be more stringent than previous recommendations. However, they are designed to increase pup survival by allowing early problem identification and resolution. It is also important that the clinician investigate when an experienced owner suspects that something is wrong. It has been our experience that the owner is often correct.

The clinician needs to ask other specific questions. When did the bitch last eat or drink? Not all bitches are anorexic before parturition. It is a concern particularly if anesthesia is anticipated. Has she vomited? Some bitches vomit as a matter of course, but in others it may be a sign of toxicity. Excessive vomiting can cause dehydration and electrolyte imbalance. Has she urinated or defecated recently? A full bladder or rectum may hinder a laboring bitch by causing discomfort and/or by obstructing the pelvic canal. Sometimes behavior associated with labor may be attributed to a need to defecate, so defecation and urination should be supervised. More than once has an owner found a pup when asked to check the lawn!

The clinician should inquire whether the owner has tried vaginal manipulations or administered medications to the bitch because some breeders use oxytocin. Information on character and amount of vulvar discharge should be obtained. Passage of clear or white mucus can indicate that the cervix has dilated. Thick, black-green discharge *prior* to the delivery of any pups indicates placental separation and a potential emergency for unborn pups. A heavy persistent flow of fresh blood may indicate injury with hemorrhage in the dam and requires evaluation. It is also useful to know when rupture of the chorioallantois (breaking water) occurred, inasmuch as it indicates that the cervix has dilated. If a pup is not expelled soon afterward, it may be lodged in the birth canal.

When it is determined from the history that the bitch should be examined, we recommend that the owner bring any pups already born along with the dam. To ensure that the pups are warm and not inadvertently stepped on during transport, they are placed in a box separate from the dam with a towel and a warm (not hot!) water bottle. Ideally, a second person should accompany the driver to monitor the dam in case more pups are delivered in transit and assistance is required.

Physical Examination of the Dam

Care is taken to examine the whole patient by performing a quick but thorough physical examination before focusing on the reproductive tract. Rapidly assess the bitch's attitude and gait as she enters the room. A quick check of the vulvar area will determine whether fetal membranes or a pup are present. If in doubt, a digital examination, using sterile gloves, will determine whether the priority should shift first to assist delivery of a live pup. If no immediate delivery assistance is needed, physical examination should be continued. While obtaining temperature, pulse, and respirations (TPR), auscultate the heart and lungs, and assess pulse quality, mucous membrane color, capillary refill time, and hydration. Quickly check the sclera and pupillary light responses. Hypocalcemic bitches may have sluggish pupillary responses. If the bitch is trembling, differentiate between tetanic muscle tremors due to hypocalcemia and trembling due to pain or anxiety. Palpate the abdomen and first assess whether she is guarding her abdomen or it is painful. Abdominal pain can be a sign of uterine rupture or torsion, especially if signs of shock are also observed. While palpating the uterus, determine whether pups are present, their relative positions, and whether fetal movement or uterine contractions are present. If pups are near the pelvic inlet, determine whether they are aligned properly for normal delivery. Determine whether there are strong contractions of the abdominal muscles because active abdominal press is a response to stimulation by the fetus or its membranes engaging the cervix and the vaginal canal. Quickly examine the mammary glands for degree of development and attempt to express milk. Milk may be first expressible as early as a week before parturition or as late as a few days postpartum.

---

*Defined as the period when uterine contractions become more synchronous and intensified and the cervix dilates.

†Active expulsion of the pups.

A lack of milk does not necessarily indicate that the bitch is not full term, but it does imply that milk supplementation or replacement will be needed. Determine whether there are signs of mastitis, such as palpably firm glands in a febrile bitch. Typically the examination described above can be accomplished in less than 5 minutes.

A digital vaginal examination is indicated in every dystocia case, with the possible exception of the bitch that has shown no signs of impending labor but is presented as *overdue*. In this case, first determine that the pregnancy is full term or the bitch is in labor, and evaluate fetal well-being before proceeding. In cases of dystocia, examine the vulva for any bruising, vulval tears, or discharge before cleaning. After the vulva has been clipped and cleaned, the bitch is restrained in a standing position or lateral recumbency, and the tail is held to the side. Most bitches do not require a muzzle restraint, but care should be taken to ensure safety. If the bitch is extremely agitated, sedation can be used (meperidine [Demerol] 1 mg/lb SC), but this will also sedate the fetuses and should be avoided if possible. Sterile gloves are recommended for vaginal examination. Depending on the size of the bitch, one or more fingers are introduced dorsally through the vulvar lips into the vestibule, then horizontally over the pelvic brim. This constitutes a cranial 90-degree turn at the vestibulovaginal junction into the vagina. Except in very small bitches, the finger will reach only the caudal vagina. Manual assessment of cervical dilation is usually not possible because the canine vagina is very long, and the cervix is located cranial to the pelvic brim. Assess the diameter of the birth canal. Most bitches need a minimum of 1.5 inches × 1.5 inches in diameter to deliver the fetal head (S. Johnston, personal communication). Check for the presence of soft tissue strictures, tissue bands, or septa, particularly at the vulvar lips and the vestibulovaginal junction, and for vaginal obstructions such as a misshapen bony pelvis, vaginal neoplasm, or prolapse. Determine whether fetal membranes or a pup is present in the vagina, and whether strong abdominal contractions can be elicited in response to digital stimulation (feathering). If abdominal contractions can be elicited, it is a good sign that medical management may still be feasible. If a pup is in the vagina, it is important to determine its presentation, position, and posture within the birth canal. If position allows and the pup is alive, or it is not clear that it is dead, endeavor to deliver the pup by manipulation and eliciting abdominal effort by the dam (see Medical Management of Dystocia below).

Laboratory Values

Blood samples should be quickly drawn and submitted for testing by a technician (where possible) during the physical examination. Quick assessment tests (packed cell volume [PCV], total protein, blood glucose, and AZO Stick) should be performed on every bitch. The bitch with dystocia may be dehydrated, hypoglycemic, or hemorrhaging. Anemia caused by hemorrhage should be differentiated from normal physiologic anemia of pregnancy. These values aid in decisions regarding supportive therapy, such as IV fluids. Early assessment by laboratory tests also aids in efficient management of cases that have no complications but require cesarean section.

When serum calcium can be tested on site, it should be measured. If results can be obtained only after the case has been treated, they can provide valuable information and testing before specific treatment is still recommended. Although hypocalcemia usually occurs postpartum, signs such as muscle spasms, tetany, or convulsions can appear prepartum or at parturition. A nonionized serum calcium concentration below 7 mg/dl confirms the diagnosis. Marginally low calcium concentrations may contribute to ineffective myometrial contractions and slow the progression of labor without causing any other outward clinical signs. Heavy panting in a bitch may produce a respiratory alkalosis, and alkalosis will decrease blood levels of the biologically important ionized calcium (Kaufman, 1986). Serum calcium concentrations above 7 mg/dl but below 9.8 mg/dl, the low normal level in our laboratory, may also justify supplementation.

In the bitch, serum progesterone concentrations remain elevated (more than 2 ng/ml) throughout diestrus. In the normal pregnancy, serum progesterone concentrations decrease abruptly below 2 ng/ml at approximately 63 to 64 days following the LH peak, which is approximately 24 to 48 hours prior to parturition. The due date is accurately predicted as day 65 ± 1 from the preovulatory serum progesterone rise/LH peak, and other methods are much less accurate (see *CVT XII*, p. 1085). In the absence of an accurate estimate of due date, a recorded rectal temperature drop, or active signs of labor, a serum progesterone concentration less than 2 ng/ml will confirm that gestation is full term and that parturition should be imminent. Surgical delivery of premature pups is undesirable; therefore it is important that serum progesterone concentrations be measured accurately. In our experience, interpretation of progesterone enzyme-linked immunosorbent assay (ELISA) tests can be subjective; thus, serum progesterone results using this method can be inaccurate. Confirmation of the serum progesterone concentrations by radioimmunoassay (RIA) is preferable when results can be obtained within 12 to 24 hours. In most cases when a bitch is presented as *overdue* based on breeding dates or vaginal cytology but shows no sign of labor, an emergency cesarean section is rarely warranted. In most cases, there is time to wait for RIA results, unless ultrasound results indicate that fetal well-being is compromised (see below). In the latter case, measurement of serum progesterone by an ELISA test is preferable to no progesterone measurement. Note that bitches supplemented beyond their due date with exogenous progesterone will not have low serum progesterone concentrations and should not exhibit a rectal temperature drop. Fetal death will occur if pregnancy is maintained just 1 to 2 days past term by exogenous progesterone administration. Therefore when progesterone supplementation is indicated for treatment of luteal insufficiency, an accurate due date based on the preovulatory LH peak/ serum progesterone rise is essential. Timely progesterone withdrawal is necessary for the initiation of parturition.

Fetal Monitoring

Direct observation of fetal well-being via transabdominal, two-dimensional ultrasound is invaluable in accurately assessing whether immediate, emergency cesarean section is warranted (*CVT XII*, p. 1085). That is, from the standpoint of pup survival, is there *time* to do the following:

1. Pursue further diagnostics
2. Allow the bitch more time to progress in labor
3. Intervene with medical management before proceeding directly to a cesarean section

Outward detection of fetal motion and assessment of vaginal discharge are helpful in indirectly assessing fetal well-being, but are not precise in predicting fetal well-being. In its simplest application, an ultrasound examination quickly determines whether pups are alive or dead by detecting the presence or absence of cardiac motion. A thorough assessment of live pups determines whether they are so compromised that immediate surgical intervention is warranted. In our experience, this is best determined by measuring fetal heart rates.

In human fetuses, bradycardia with a lack of rate accelerations indicates fetal distress related to anoxia/placental insufficiency. In our clinical experience this principle can be applied to the dog. Our observations of ultrasound examinations performed in full-term and laboring bitches indicate that fetal heart rates greater than 150 bpm (and ideally near 200 bpm) indicate that pups are not compromised. Heart rates lower than 150 bpm are a cause for concern, particularly when upward rate excursions are not observed during fetal movement or several minutes of repeated observation. On occasion we have observed pups with temporary decelerations below our estimated *normal range,* which have then rapidly recovered. This could be related to fetal stress associated with a uterine contraction, but is unconfirmed at this time. A fetal heart rate of 100 bpm or lower is a clear indication of fetal distress. Rapid action is needed if the pup is to survive. Our experience has been that severely bradycardic pups identified in this manner have been meconium stained or difficult to resuscitate upon delivery by cesarean section.

Fetal assessment via transabdominal ultrasound should be performed as soon as physical examination of the dam is completed, that is, within the first 10 minutes after presentation. Most bitches tolerate this examination, and we usually perform it with the bitch standing or in lateral recumbency. The abdomen is clipped as needed, and alcohol is used as a connector for the probe (unless it will damage the transducer). Full-term pups and their chest cavities are easily identified. Heart rates are determined by visually counting the number of beats in a 15-second period and multiplying that count by 4. The upward limit for accurate counting by this method is 200 bpm. M-mode can be utilized to count but it is usually unavailable in private practice, and is not necessary. Pups with decreased heart rates should be observed for at least 2 to 3 minutes and/or repeatedly during a single examination to check for possible rate accelerations. The surface of the entire abdomen should be carefully explored with the probe in order to observe all pups. If no distressed pups are observed during the first examination, examinations are repeated at 1-hour intervals throughout first-stage labor. Our experience has been that this examination interval is adequate to detect deterioration of the fetuses while still being practical, and is well tolerated by the bitch. After the bitch begins delivery, repeated ultrasound and vaginal examinations are per-formed only as needed to update the pups' condition when the interval between deliveries is more than 1 hour. A superior ultrasound machine is not required to perform these examinations. In our opinion ultrasound is indicated in every case because it eliminates guesswork and facilitates decision-making. Where ultrasound is unavailable, simple auscultation with a stethoscope on the bitch's abdomen may identify fetal heartbeats. However, fetal heartbeats cannot always be assessed by this method, and it provides little information regarding the number of pups already dead.

Radiographs

Abdominal films are indicated once evaluation of both dam and pups demonstrates there is time to perform radiography without compromising pup survival. Two views (a lateral and dorsoventral [DV] or ventrodorsal [VD], depending on which is more comfortable for the bitch) should be obtained. Most bitches cooperate if calmly and gently handled, so chemical sedation should be avoided. From the radiograph one can determine the number of fetuses, skeletal size relative to the width of the dam's bony pelvis, signs of fetal death (skeletal collapse), and relative position of the fetuses at the pelvic inlet, such as two pups presenting at once, or transverse presentation. There are limitations regarding the interpretation of these findings because fetal or maternal soft tissue impediments to a vaginal delivery may be present but radiographically undetectable. However, the information is usually helpful in efficient management of dystocia.

MEDICAL MANAGEMENT OF DYSTOCIA

Obstetrical Mutation

If a pup is encountered in the birth canal during a vaginal examination, it is best from the standpoint of pup survival to make manual delivery attempts immediately unless there is a clear indication of a superior alternative. For example, it would be better to proceed directly to a cesarean section if an incorrigible vaginal obstruction, fetal malposition, or blatantly oversized dead pup is lodged in the birth canal. For the pup that appears to be a good candidate for vaginal delivery, manipulation should be performed cleanly and gently using an excess of sterile lubrication. It is our preference to use only fingers and not forceps or snare devices because one can easily damage the bitch and/or fetus when working blindly in this tight space. To assist delivery of a pup in posterior presentation, which is a normal presentation in the dog that occurs in approximately 40% of canine births, one snares both hocks with the fingers, or grasps the pup just in front of its pelvis. To assist delivery of a pup in anterior presentation, initially hook a finger under the mandible if that is all that can be reached. When there is room to do so, place the hand on the pup's dorsum, placing the fingers on either side of the head and around the shoulders. It is important to apply steady, firm, but gentle traction when the bitch strains, and to maintain gentle tension when she rests. Otherwise the pup tends to slip back to its former position. The line of traction should follow the birth canal; that is, horizontally through the vagina and then, as the pup enters the vestibule, pull down at a 90-degree angle from the horizontal vagina, aiming toward the dam's hocks. When the pup is palpable only with the fingertips but is otherwise out of reach, it may help to stroke the dorsal vaginal wall or gently use two fingers to stretch the vaginal walls apart. This may stimulate the bitch to push the pup caudally. A short walk may also help. Elevating the bitch's forelegs and chest will sometimes help move a pup within reach. Conversely, if the problem is the malposition of one pup, or two pups presenting at the same time, then elevating the hindquarters may move the pup cranially into the uterus, providing room for repositioning. At all times it is important to avoid forceful or rushed manipulations because the pup or dam may be injured. Allow time for the birth canal to stretch, particularly with passage of the first pup. One can aid this by gently stretching the tissues in front of the pup as it moves through the canal. If the vulvar opening is narrow and will not stretch sufficiently to permit delivery, an episiotomy should be performed.

Throughout all manipulations, it is important to make steady progress toward vaginal delivery of the pup. Do not waste time on a protracted or impossible delivery. If no progress is made after 10 minutes, it is best to stop and check for fetal death or distress (heart rates). Reassess whether a vaginal delivery is possible and likely with reasonable effort. If the fetuses are not compromised, there is time to try vaginal delivery again. If not, cesarean section is recommended.

Oxytocin

Judicious use of exogenous oxytocin is a proven method to stimulate uterine contractions and facilitate labor. However, each dystocia should be carefully evaluated prior to its use. Evidence that the cervix has dilated is necessary prior to oxytocin administration. Presence of any obstructive lesion (fetal or maternal) absolutely contraindicates the use of oxytocin. Therefore, each bitch should be evaluated by abdominal and vaginal palpation and abdominal radiographs. Bitches demonstrating strong uterine/abdominal contractions are unlikely to benefit from oxytocin treatment. The reason for their failure to deliver should be identified. Depressed fetal heart rates indicate that there is not enough time to try oxytocin. In such a case, oxytocin therapy may actually induce further fetal compromise or death by promoting placental separation. Cesarean section would be the preferred treatment in such a case. On the other hand, if there is a single unobstructed pup in utero, oxytocin therapy may allow the pup to be delivered vaginally, and in some cases, more quickly than could be expected by cesarean section. If the dam is already exhausted but is still a good anesthetic candidate, and there are multiple pups in utero, cesarean section is the preferred treatment.

If the cervix is dilated, there are no vaginal obstructions, the dam and pups are stable, but labor is failing to progress owing to ineffective contractions, then treatment with oxytocin is indicated, and manual assistance should be anticipated. We use a dosage of 5 to 20 IU oxytocin IM, given 20 to 30 minutes apart p.r.n., for a total of three injections. Our initial dose is subjectively dependent on the dam's

body weight. (For example, we start with a single dose of 5 to 10 IU oxytocin IM for a 20- to 40-pound bitch). If second or third injections are required, the dose is increased, again subjectively, depending upon the effect of the previous injection. It is our preference to use the lowest dose possible to achieve delivery of a puppy. Bitches that do not respond after the second injection probably have uterine inertia and are unlikely to respond to further oxytocin treatment. The abdomen can be clipped and cleaned for cesarean section while awaiting a response from the third and final injection.

After a pup is successfully delivered, the reason for the original failure in progression of labor should be reassessed. Repeated oxytocin treatments, using the three-dose rule to effect per pup, should be used only if the bitch fails to deliver any remaining pups spontaneously. Excessive, repeated oxytocin injections in our clinical experience can lead to secondary uterine inertia. It may help to allow the delivered pups to suckle while a cooperative dam rests between labor, inasmuch as a continual release of endogenous oxytocin may be reflexly induced by suckling.

Once a bitch presents with a dystocia, it is unwise to discharge the bitch until delivery of all pups is completed, even if the initial problem has been corrected. In our experience bitches that leave during parturition are often presented again before all pups are delivered. Repeated trips back and forth to the clinic waste valuable time and are likely to be more disruptive to labor than a quiet hospital experience.

Calcium and Intravenous Fluids

Adequate blood calcium levels are necessary for effective uterine contractions, and calcium may need to be supplemented in some patients. A serum calcium concentration of less than 9 mg/dl in a bitch with dystocia probably indicates supplementation is needed. In general, 10% calcium gluconate (5 to 10 ml) may be given to a 10- to 20-lb bitch. Higher doses (5 to 25 ml) *may* be given *as needed* in larger dogs. Calcium may be given as a *slow* IV bolus, or as a slow IV drip when diluted in balanced IV fluids, or be given diluted in sterile, balanced fluids subcutaneously. However, the label of the preparation should be followed *precisely* because some preparations will cause skin sloughing if given by an inappropriate route. Only bitches exhibiting clinical signs of hypocalcemia (muscle spasms, tetany, seizures), or that have serum calcium concentrations below 7 mg/dl should be given calcium by the bolus IV route. We recommend that it be given as a slow IV bolus, and then only while heart rate and rhythm are closely monitored via auscultation and/or preferably by electrocardiogram (ECG). Cardiac arrhythmias and sudden death can result when IV calcium is administered too rapidly. All other bitches in need of supplementation should receive calcium subcutaneously or diluted in a slow drip of IV fluids, taking care to follow the label of the preparation being used. The subcutaneous delivery route may be used initially routinely when tests for serum calcium are unavailable and low serum calcium is suspected to be contributing to poor uterine contractility, or abnormal progression of labor. However, it is recommended that a blood sample be drawn prior to treatment to confirm the diagnosis later.

Intravenous fluids are not indicated for every dystocia case, but they are recommended for dehydrated or hypovolemic bitches, regardless of the cause. Dehydration is deleterious to the dam, but may also cause poor uterine perfusion, reducing placental exchange of oxygen and nutrients. Therefore, dehydration should be corrected with balanced polyionic (.9% NaCl, lactated Ringer's solution) or dextrose solutions (D_5W, .45% NaCl + 2.5% dextrose). Maternal hypotension before, during, or after surgical delivery is frequently encountered. Therefore, intravenous fluids are strongly recommended for any bitch undergoing a cesarean section.

Other Supportive Measures for the Bitch

A bitch that is anxious or frightened may actively inhibit labor. It is imperative that she be kept comfortable in a quiet, calm environment. Thus veterinary examinations and procedures should be performed in as gentle a manner and as calmly as possible. Most bitches will contentedly whelp away from home if they are made comfortable. We prefer to let them whelp on a pile of clean blankets in a small, clean, quiet room where they can be alone with only one or two observers. Some bitches are comfortable in a cage, but these are usually too small for a large or giant breed bitch and her litter. We prefer to use a whelping room where the clinician may remain or enter and leave this room quietly as needed. All necessary equipment is kept in the room for the duration of the medical management of dystocia, and pediatric support such as a heat source for the pups should also be provided. It can also be used as a recovery area after cesarean section, where the bitch and pups can be monitored in a quiet environment. Such a room also allows the owner to be present to support the bitch. However, a nervous or disruptive owner is counterproductive and is best replaced by a calm, trained observer.

Throughout first-stage labor, in particular, the bitch should be permitted short, closely attended walks outside so she may urinate and defecate. During second-stage labor, if all is progressing well, the bitch can be offered small amounts of water or ice cubes, Karo syrup, or Nutrical between delivery of pups. Bitches are particularly eager to accept Karo syrup, which may provide energy for labor and gives the attendant useful employment while monitoring the progress of labor. However, we are careful not to allow the bitch to ingest too much per os, in case anesthesia is required later on. For this reason we usually allow the bitch to eat only one afterbirth if she is inclined and anxious to do so.

INDICATIONS FOR CESAREAN SECTION

To maximize the number of live pups delivered, an emergency cesarean section is indicated in every case in which multiple pups are retained and fetal heart rates are depressed (below 150 bpm). Sometimes this is the situation found at presentation. In other cases the initial ultrasound examination may indicate that all pups seem normal (heart rate > 150 bpm, and usually approximately 200 bpm).

Then fetal well-being is found to deteriorate over the course of hourly ultrasound monitoring. The most common pattern we have observed is that heart rates in the whole litter decrease from 200 bpm to 150 bpm over the course of an hour. One hour later, heart rates of one or two pups are observed to abruptly decrease (less than 100 bpm), indicating that those pups are seriously compromised.

Even if heart rates are normal initially, there are other clear indications that a cesarean section is immediately warranted. These include the following:

1. Primary or secondary uterine inertia that is unresponsive to oxytocin and calcium administration
2. Relative fetal oversize due to one or more large pups, anasarca, fetal monsters, etc.
3. Soft tissue or bony obstructions of the birth canal
4. Incorrigible malposition that precludes vaginal delivery
5. Uterine torsion or rupture

To reduce the likelihood of further fetal compromise, the bitch should be stabilized as soon as possible prior to anesthesia, and emergency cesarean section should be pursued.

If the need for a cesarean section can be identified preterm, such as at the time of proestrus or estrus, arrangements can be made for an elective surgery when the bitch is full term (see *CVT XII*, p. 1085). Scheduling surgery ahead of time allows personnel to be readily available and prevents the dam and fetuses from undergoing an arduous labor prior to surgical delivery. An elective cesarean section can be considered if there is (1) a history of uterine inertia, dystocia, or surgical delivery; (2) a history of pelvic trauma or congenital malformation that has narrowed the pelvic canal; (3) a high breed or family incidence of dystocia due to relative fetal oversize; or (4) if radiographs taken in the last week of pregnancy indicate relative fetal oversize in one or more pups. Ideally, for elective cesarean section, preovulatory serum progesterone rise/LH peak data should be available to determine an accurate due date (i.e., day 65 ± 1 from LH peak). Therefore, breeding management using ovulation timing is strongly recommended for all bitches that have a history suggesting that cesarean section is a possible outcome. When the date of the serum LH peak is unknown, daily serial serum progesterone concentrations may be measured and/or the bitch's daily temperature should be monitored. This regimen is begun 3 to 5 days before the earliest possible due date, as estimated from breeding dates or vaginal cytology. In this manner, the clinician can determine when the pregnancy has reached full term and cesarean section is timely.

The dam should be given IV fluids and inhalant oxygen prior to anesthesia in an effort to maximize fetal oxygen levels. Anesthetic and surgical protocols have been discussed elsewhere in great detail (Grandy, 1989; Gilson, 1993), but in all cases the lightest possible surgical plane of anesthesia should be maintained and the surgeon should work quickly. Several personnel should be available to assist with surgery, monitor the dam's condition during anesthesia, and revive pups. When pups are severely compromised, one person per pup may be necessary to successfully resuscitate them. Each pup should be manually stimulated by vigorous but gentle rubbing and pinching. We routinely use inhalant anesthetics that are rapidly eliminated by respiration. Once pups are gasping or breathing, we find that oxygen supplied via a face mask is invaluable in improving color, respiration, and general pup activity. It is also important to dry pups well and keep them on a warm surface during and after resuscitation. Airways should be cleared of any aspirated fluid via careful swinging of pups and suction. Dopram (doxapram HCl), 1 to 2 drops sublingually, and epinephrine, 0.02 to 0.2 mg/kg lingually or intratracheally (personal communication with Dr. Paula Moon), can be given as needed as respiratory and cardiac stimulants, respectively. These neonatal resuscitation techniques should also be used to resuscitate compromised pups that have been delivered vaginally.

MEDICAL MANAGEMENT OF RETAINED DEAD FETUSES AND RETAINED FETAL MEMBRANES

There are cases in which surgical delivery may not be an option even when indicated. It is the clinician's responsibility to ensure that the owner fully understands that delaying surgery when it is indicated increases the likelihood of losing one or all pups and endangers the dam. The clinician may be presented with a bitch with retained dead fetuses where the options are limited to medical treatment or euthanasia. This dilemma could arise when the bitch is in poor health or the range of treatment is limited by an owner. In such cases, we recommend broad-spectrum antibiotic therapy and subcutaneous fluid administration in an attempt to save the bitch. If metritis and peritonitis can be prevented, decomposing fetal debris may be delivered without serious effects in the bitch. However, it may be wise for the owner to sign a treatment consent form that states that the owner understands that the bitch may well develop life-threatening complications such as metritis or peritonitis. If the bitch becomes febrile or develops signs of shock or painful abdomen, metritis or peritonitis is likely and the treatment course should be altered accordingly. Good nursing care of the bitch and/or orphan care of the remaining litter is likely to be necessary.

While many bitches show no clinical signs when fetal membranes are retained and require no treatment, others may develop complications. Oxytocin treatment soon after parturition may prevent complications in some bitches, but for most bitches it is unnecessary. If it is to be used, oxytocin should be administered in the first 24 hours postpartum to induce expulsion of retained membranes. It should be first determined, by palpation, ultrasound, or radiographs, that the bitch has completed whelping. Then one to two injections (each 5 to 20 IU oxytocin IM), 4 to 6 hours apart, can be given, with the dosage being dependent upon body weight. Owners should be cautioned that

the bitch may expel the membranes and consume them, and this may not be observed by the owner. Lochia discharge will be heavier than normal, and close monitoring of the character of the discharge (i.e., purulent, foul-smelling, or sanguineous), along with monitoring of rectal temperature, attitude, and appetite is required, because postpartum metritis can be a sequela. Treatment does not always need to be initiated immediately after parturition if retained placenta is suspected. However, if the owner is concerned, if the whelping area is contaminated, or if manual manipulation was performed during vaginal delivery, it is prudent to prescribe antibiotics for 7 to 10 days while the bitch is monitored for signs of metritis. Our first antibiotic choice is oral cephalosporin (cefadroxil, 22 mg/kg PO b.i.d.) because it is effective against a broad spectrum of bacteria and has not been observed to adversely affect nursing pups.

References and Suggested Reading

Concannon PW: Physiology and endocrinology of canine pregnancy. In: Morrow DA, ed: Current Therapy in Theriogenology 2. Philadelphia: WB Saunders, 1986, p 491.
   A thorough review of the physiology and endocrinology of canine pregnancy.
Duncan JR, Prasse KW: Veterinary Laboratory Medicine, 2nd ed. Ames: Iowa State University Press, 1986, pp 182, 231.
   A description of serum calcium concentrations and their interpretation.
Ellington J, Surman V: Whelping emergencies. AKC Gazette (August) 110(8):6a, 1993.
   A review of whelping and dystocia management.
Gilson SD: Cesarean section. In: Slatter DS, ed: Textbook of Small Animal Surgery, 2nd ed, vol 2. Philadelphia: WB Saunders, 1993, pp 1322–1325.
   A review of cesarean section of the dog.
Grandy JL: Anesthetic considerations for cesarean section. In: Kirk RW, ed: Current Veterinary Therapy X: Small Animal Practice. Philadelphia: WB Saunders, 1989, p 1321.
   A review of anesthetic protocols of the dog.
Johnson CA: Review of small animal reproductive disorders. In: The North American Veterinary Conference Proceedings Jan 14–18, 1995. Gainesville: Eastern States Veterinary Association, 1995, p 370.
   A review of the endocrinology and physiology of canine and feline reproduction, and the diagnosis and management of a variety of reproductive disorders.
Kaufman J: Eclampsia in the Bitch. In: Morrow DA, ed: Current Therapy in Theriogenology 2. Philadelphia: WB Saunders, 1986, p 511.
   A description of the physiology and treatment of puerperal hypocalcemia in the bitch.
Schott II HC: Assessment of fetal well-being. In: McKinnon AO, Voss JL, eds: Equine Reproduction. Philadelphia: Lea & Febiger, 1993, p 964.
   A presentation of fetal assessment techniques in the horse.
Schweizer CM, Meyers-Wallen V, Yeager A: Previously unpublished clinical observations and interpretations of canine fetal heart rates, 1992–1996, SAC NYSCVM Cornell University.
Varney HP: Nurse-Midwifery. Boston: Blackwell Scientific Publications, 1987, p 325.
   A description of abnormal human fetal heart rate patterns and their interpretation.

Effects of Hypothyroidism on Canine Male Infertility

CHERI A. JOHNSON

East Lansing, Michigan

Hypothyroidism has been cited as a cause of subfertility, diminished libido, poor semen quality, and/or diminished ejaculate volume in male dogs, goats, and human beings (Johnson, 1999). The citations are usually based on the observation of one or more of these abnormalities in individual patients being evaluated for reproductive dysfunction in whom thyroid hormone concentrations are subsequently found to be low. In clinical settings, reproductive function is commonly evaluated by reviewing the reproductive history for breeding behavior and conception rates, and by collecting and analyzing a single semen sample. When reproductive abnormalities are identified and the patient is simultaneously found to have low serum concentrations of thyroid hormones, a diagnosis of infertility due to hypothyroidism is often made, but such a diagnosis may not be justified.

Normal male fertility requires the physical ability to mate, normal libido, and normal semen quality. The physical ability to mate is dependent upon normal musculoskeletal and neurologic function for mounting and intromission. Additionally, the mechanisms for erection and ejaculation must be intact. Canine mating ability is usually assessed by physical examination of the orthopedic, neurologic, and genital systems, and by evaluating historic information (Meyers-Wallen, 1991) about ability to mount, achieve intromission, and the presence or absence of a postcoital tie. The postcoital tie is not necessarily a requisite for canine fertility, but its presence indicates that mounting, intromission, and erection did occur. The absence of a history of a postcoital tie raises questions about mating ability (or opportunity), and the possibility that ejaculation, if it occurred, may not have been intravaginal. Ability to achieve erection and ejaculation can be further assessed during attempts to collect semen. Ability or willingness to achieve erection and ejaculation may be a reflection of libido as well as mating ability.

Normal libido and semen production are dependent upon proper endocrine interactions of the hypothalamus, pituitary, and gonad, all of which ultimately support spermatogenesis and gonadal hormone production, the most significant of which is testosterone. Testosterone serves as the prohormone for dihydrotestosterone, which together with testosterone, supports all aspects of spermatogenesis, maturation of the genitalia and prostate, the development of secondary sexual characteristics, libido, and other types of typical "masculine" behavior such as urine marking of territory. The behavioral manifestations of libido can be influenced by painful conditions, psychologic factors such as the presence of a more dominant male or female, and environmental conditions such as slippery floors, noise, or other distractions. The presence of an estrual bitch and the technique of the person collecting the semen can affect the degree of arousal.

Once collected, semen is analyzed for the number, motility, and morphology of spermatozoa, and the presence of other material such as blood cells or urine. The number of spermatozoa in an ejaculate reflects the daily sperm production within the testes, and the number of spermatozoa present in the extragonadal sperm reserves of the epididymides and ductus deferentia (Olar, 1983). Sperm production in the testes is directly related to testicular size, with larger testes capable of greater sperm production. Testicular size, and therefore daily sperm production, is positively correlated with total scrotal width in dogs. The number of sperm stored in the extragonadal sperm reserves of the epididymis and ductus deferens is influenced by the frequency of ejaculation and by the time interval between ejaculations. The extragonadal sperm reserves of dogs can reportedly be depleted by once-daily ejaculation for 5 to 7 days. Once the sperm reserves are depleted, the daily sperm output in an ejaculate approximates the daily sperm production in the testes. Because of the variable, but substantial, contribution of the sperm reserves to the total number of sperm in an ejaculate, conclusions about the spermatogenic capacity of a male being evaluated for subfertility based on the results of a single, random specimen, can be misleading. Serial semen analyses, or actual determination of daily testicular sperm production, has been recommended (Meyers-Wallen, 1991).

The estimation of spermatozoal motility is known to be imprecise and lacking reproducibility (Johnston, 1991). Nevertheless, the estimation of motility remains an important part of semen analysis because it demonstrates one functional aspect of spermatozoa, movement. Motility is easily affected by external factors such as environmental temperature, exposure to lubricants, and chemicals found in latex and plastic containers, such as artificial vaginas and collection vials. Motility and morphology can be adversely affected by bacterial prostatitis (Meyers-Wallen, 1991), a relatively common problem in dogs as they age, and one that has no known relationship with hypothyroidism. Secondary morphologic abnormalities may be artifacts of semen collection and preparation.

It is well known that serum concentrations of thyroid hormones can be suppressed by nonthyroidal illness and certain medications, and that age and breed affect serum concentrations of thyroid hormones as well (Ferguson, 1994). Therefore, it is recommended that the diagnosis of hypothyroidism be based upon the finding of serum concentrations of thyroxine below the reference range, in a patient with clinical signs typical of hypothyroidism, and confirmed by demonstrating inadequate response to exogenous thyroid stimulating hormone (TSH) or elevated concentrations of endogenous cTSH (also see p. 321). Because the quality of an ejaculate is likewise affected by many factors, such as degree of arousal, frequency of ejaculation, collection technique, and sample handling, it is very difficult to control these confounding variables and establish a cause-and-effect relationship, if one exists, between hypothyroidism and reproductive dysfunction in a clinical patient.

When the reproductive function of dogs made hypothyroid by the administration of ^{131}I was compared with that of age- and breed-matched euthyroid dogs over a 2-year period, no differences were found (Johnson, 1999). Daily testicular sperm production was assessed by determining daily sperm output (i.e., depleting the extragonadal sperm reserves) and by determining total scrotal width. Pituitary and gonadal endocrine function was assessed by determination of serum concentrations of luteinizing hormone (LH) and testosterone, respectively, before and after the administration of gonadotropin releasing hormone. Libido was subjectively assessed by the ease with which semen could be collected. No differences in these parameters of reproductive function were found between the hypothyroid and euthyroid dogs. An aspect of reproductive performance not evaluated in that study was the physical ability to mount and achieve intromission. Because the hypothyroid dogs were profoundly obese and lethargic, it is possible that they might have had difficulty with copulation. However, despite their overt hypothyroidism, they continued to ejaculate readily, and their semen quality and serum concentrations of LH and testosterone were normal. When evaluating male dogs for subfertility, explanations other than hypothyroidism should be sought because a cause-and-effect relationship between hypothyroidism and poor reproductive performance has not been identified in dogs.

References and Suggested Reading

Ferguson DC: Update on diagnosis of canine hypothyroidism. Vet Clin North Am 24:515, 1994.
A review of the diagnostic tests, and their interpretation, for the diagnosis of canine hypothyroidism.
Johnson CA, Olivier NB, Nachreiner RF, Mullaney TP: Effect of ^{131}I-induced hypothyroidism on indices of reproductive function in adult male dogs. J Vet Intern Med 13:104, 1999.
A comparison of semen quality, libido and endocrine function in hypothyroid and age- and breed-matched euthyroid male dogs over a 2-year time period.
Johnston SD: Performing a complete semen evaluation in a small animal hospital. Vet Clin North Am 21:545, 1991.
A practical review of indications and techniques for, and interpretation of results of, semen collection and evaluation in dogs.
Meyers-Wallen VN: Clinical approach to infertile male dogs with sperm in the ejaculate. Vet Clin North Am 21:609, 1991.
An in-depth, yet very practical, discussion of the diagnostic and therapeutic approaches to canine male infertility.
Olar TT, Amann RP, Pickett BW: Relationships among testicular size, daily sperm production and output of spermatozoa, and extragonadal spermatozoal reserves of the dog. Biol Reprod 29:1114, 1983.
The classic study of the dog's ability to produce and ejaculate spermatozoa.

Diseases of the Canine Testes

JAMES A. FLANDERS
DONALD H. SCHLAFER
AMY E. YEAGER
Ithaca, New York

Testicular disease in the dog is manifested by a change in the size or shape of the testes and/or by decreased fertility. Therefore, two very important tools for recognition of testicular disease are palpation and semen evaluation. Normal testicular size is related to body size. Careful palpation can help a clinician to discern between unilateral or bilateral disease or differentiate between focal and diffuse testicular swelling, and can localize the testes to a scrotal, subcutaneous, or abdominal location. Abnormal testicular size is characteristic of many diseases (Table 1). Semen evaluation (see *CVT XII,* p. 1060; see p. 321) quantifies the effect of testicular disease on sperm motility and number. It also provides information about the causes of oligospermia, such as inflammation or infection.

Ultrasonic evaluation of the testes has become a commonly used means of assessing testicular disease. Both scrotal and abdominal testes can be studied noninvasively. Ultrasonic studies can reveal abnormalities in parenchyma density, distinguish focal from diffuse involvement, and help differentiate testicular from epididymal disease.

To reach a definitive diagnosis concerning testicular disease, histopathologic evaluation of testicular tissue is necessary. Tissue samples are often composed of an entire excised testis, but in cases where fertility is to be main-

TABLE 1. **Diseases That Cause Change in Testicular Size**

Large Testes	Small Testes
Neoplasia	Hypoplasia
Acute infection	Chronic inflammation
Testicular torsion	Cryptorchidism
Inguinoscrotal hernia	Degeneration
Sperm granuloma	Intersex

TABLE 2. Relationship Between Body Weight, Testis Size, and Sperm Count in Adult Dogs

Body weight(lb)	10–34	35–39	60–84
Total scrotal testes width (mm)	36 ± 2	50 ± 1	56 ± 1
Semen volume per ejaculate (ml)	2.4 ± 0.3	3.9 ± 0.5	5.4 ± 1.3
After Sexual Rest			
Semen concentration (10^6/ml)	209 ± 42	359 ± 72	228 ± 58
Total sperm (10^9)	0.4 ± 0.11	1.12 ± 0.13	1.43 ± 0.46

The investigator used a thumb and forefinger to force the testes down into the scrotum. Testicular width was measured with calipers placed across both testes at the widest point. Modified from Amann RA: Reproductive physiology and endocrinology of the dog. In: Morrow DA, ed: Current Therapy in Theriogenology, 2nd ed. Philadelphia: WB Saunders, 1986, pp 532–541.

tained, a small portion of testicular tissue is excised and evaluated.

NORMAL TESTICULAR ANATOMY AND PHYSIOLOGY

The testes of the dog are paired, ovoid organs located within the scrotum in the ventral perineal region. The testes are separated within the scrotum by a median raphe of connective tissue. The size of the testes in the mature dog is roughly proportional to body size (Table 2). The testes range from approximately 1 to 5 cm long and 1 to 3 cm in transverse diameter.

The body of each testis is surrounded by a layer of dense connective tissue, the tunica albuginea. Spermatogenic cells and Sertoli cells, which support the development of spermatozoa, are located on the walls of seminiferous tubules within the testicular parenchyma. The testicular parenchyma is partitioned into wedge-shaped sections by connective tissue that contains testosterone-secreting interstitial or Leydig cells. After spermatozoa mature under the influence of testosterone and pituitary gonadotrophs, they migrate out of the testicular parenchyma and are stored in the epididymis, which is attached to the craniomedial surface of each testis. The head of the epididymis is the widest portion. The epididymis gradually tapers as it passes around the cranial pole of the testis. The tail of the epididymis is attached to the caudal pole of the testis, where it gives rise to the ductus deferens, which ascends cranially out of the scrotum and through the inguinal ring. The ductus deferens terminates in the prostatic urethra at the seminal colliculus.

The testicular arteries originate from the abdominal aorta caudal to the renal arteries. The testicular veins form the pampiniform plexus, a complex network of venules that wrap around the testicular artery from the cranial pole of the testicle to the inguinal rings. This venous plexus, along with the cremaster muscle and muscular tissue within the scrotum, maintains the temperature of the blood in the testicular artery below body temperature to promote optimal spermatogenesis. The vessels of the testicle are innervated by sympathetic nerve fibers. The testes have a rich lymphatic system that drains into the lumbar lymph nodes.

The testes, epididymides, vessels, and nerves distal to the inguinal rings are surrounded by the vaginal tunic, which is continuous with the abdominal peritoneum. The spermatic cord is an extra-abdominal neurovascular complex that consists of the testicular vessels, nerves, lymphatics and the ductus deferens surrounded by the vaginal tunic.

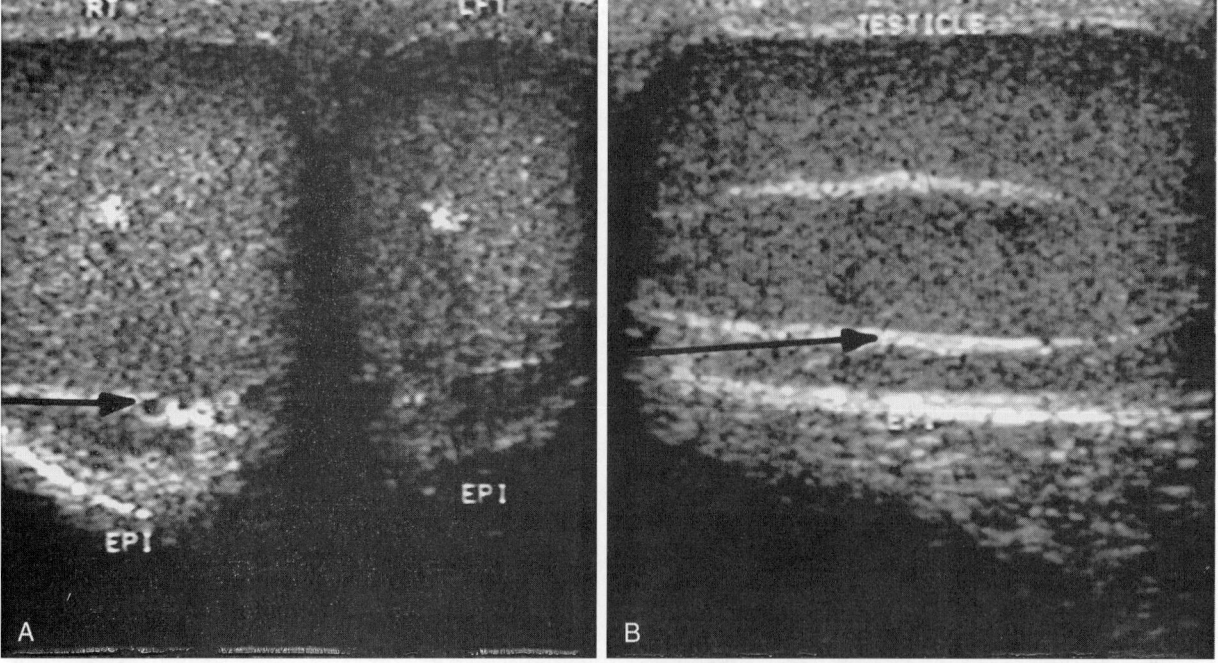

Figure 1. Ultrasonograms of normal canine testes. *A,* Transverse scan plane showing cross section of testes. The bright spot in the center of the testicular parenchyma is the mediastinum testis. The long black arrow indicates the tunica albuginea between the testis *(above)* and the body of the epididymis *(below)*. *B,* Longitudinal scan plane. The arrow indicates the tunica albuginea between the testicular parenchyma *(above)* and the body of the epididymis *(below)*. The mediastinum testis appears as a long echodense line in the center of the testicular parenchyma.

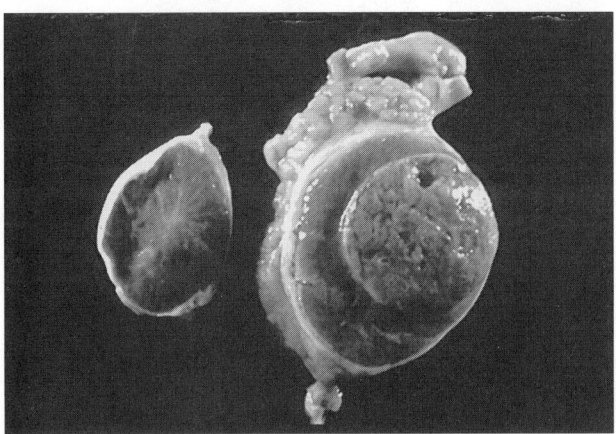

Figure 2. Cross-sectioned canine testis with a large compressing interstitial cell tumor in the right testis. The left testis is small.

Ultrasonographic Appearance of Normal Testes

The parenchyma of the normal testis has a medium-coarse, homogeneous ultrasonographic appearance surrounded by a hyperechoic tunic albuginea (Fig. 1A and B). The connective tissue making up the median raphe can be seen as an echodense line if the testis is scanned along the longitudinal axis, and as a dot in a cross-sectional view. The tail of the epididymis appears as an echolucent mass attached to the caudal pole of the testis. The head of the epididymis is smaller but has a similar ultrasonographic appearance.

DISEASES THAT CAUSE TESTICULAR ENLARGEMENT

Testicular Neoplasia

There are three common types of testicular tumors in dogs, Sertoli cell tumor, seminoma, and interstitial cell tumor. The overall incidence is approximately equal. However, in descended testes, Sertoli cell tumors are only half as common as the other two types. During the period from 1990 to 1996, there were 109 Sertoli cell tumors, 143 seminomas, and 143 interstitial cell tumors diagnosed from 446 canine testes that contained gross or microscopic lesions submitted to the Department of Pathology at Cornell University. Clinical signs usually consist of a palpable enlargement in a scrotal or an abdominal testis. Small testicular tumors may not be palpable but may interfere with sperm passage into the epididymis.

Sertoli cell tumors have the greatest potential for malignancy of all the testicular tumors that occur in dogs. Approximately 10 to 20% metastasize. Sertoli cell tumors are derived from the Sertoli cells within the seminiferous tubules. They are the most commonly diagnosed tumor in cryptorchid testes. Precancerous changes have been found in the mitochondria of Sertoli cells in young cryptorchid dogs. Sertoli cell tumors involving abdominal testes can achieve large size (10 to 15 cm) before diagnosis. They may be nodular and firm on palpation. Signs of hyperestrogenism are often associated with Sertoli cell tumors. The paraneoplastic syndrome associated with hyperestrogenism

consists of some or all of the following: aplastic anemia, bilaterally symmetrical alopecia, gynecomastia, and attraction of male dogs.

Seminomas are typically benign (5 to 10% metastasize) testicular tumors that present as a soft mass within the testes. Most seminomas are small (1 to 2 cm in diameter), but they may occasionally present as a large mass affecting an abdominal testis. The tissue of origin is the spermatogenic tissue within the seminiferous tubules. Seminomas can be functional and secrete estrogen or, more commonly, androgens. Hyperandrogenism may result in prostatic enlargement or promote the development of perianal adenomas.

Interstitial cell tumors are derived from Leydig cells of the testicle. They are almost always benign and usually present as a small, soft mass within the testicular parenchyma (Figs. 2 and 3). Many are found as an incidental finding at necropsy. Interstitial cell tumors are rarely found in abdominal testes.

It is not possible to reliably differentiate between the three tumor types with the use of ultrasound examination. Each type produces a change in echogenicity within the testicular parenchyma (see Fig. 3). Large tumors tend to have an increased blood supply, which may become more tortuous in malignant neoplasms. Histopathologic examination remains the only way of diagnosing tumor type with certainty.

Testicular tumors are best treated with orchiectomy. Clinically, the cancer can be staged by examination of thoracic radiographs and abdominal ultrasound. If an abdominal testis is suspected of containing a neoplasm, thorough exploration of the abdomen is done during abdominal

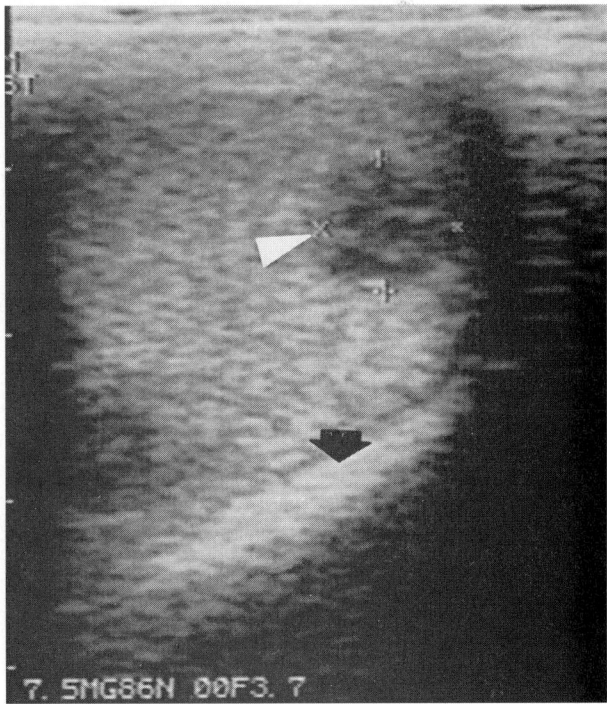

Figure 3. Ultrasonogram of canine testis with interstitial cell tumor within the testicular parenchyma. The tumor *(white arrowhead)* appears as an echolucent sphere within the testis. The body of the epididymis is indicated by the black arrow.

orchiectomy. Metastases are most commonly found in the lumbar lymph nodes, spleen, and liver. Testicular tumor metastases responded with a greater than 50% tumor reduction in dogs treated with combination chemotherapy consisting of vinblastine, cyclophosphamide, and methotrexate (Madewell and Theilen, 1987). Canine seminoma metastases are responsive to radiation therapy (McDonald et al, 1988). However, in the vast majority of cases, there are no metastases at the time of diagnosis and orchiectomy is curative.

Testicular Infection

The testes and/or epididymides may become infected by direct penetrating wounds or by hematogenous or lymphatic spread from distant sites. It is also possible for infection to spread from the urinary tract or prostate gland to the testes via the ductus deferens. Acute orchiepididymitis causes scrotal swelling and pain. Chronic infection may result in sterility owing to destruction of the spermatogenic tissue. There were 28 testes with orchitis diagnosed from 446 canine testes that contained gross or microscopic lesions submitted to the Department of Pathology at Cornell University during the period from 1990 to 1996.

Orchiepididymitis is associated with many microorganisms, including *Staphylococcus, Streptococcus,* coliforms, *Mycoplasma, Ureaplasma,* and *Brucella canis.* In particular, the diagnosis of *B. canis* should be pursued, since it can be transmitted to other dogs and to humans. Male dogs are most commonly infected with *B. canis* through an oronasal route or through sexual transmission. *B. canis* is harbored in the prostate and epididymis and is shed in semen and urine. *B. canis* usually does not cause orchitis; it localizes in the tail of the epididymis, where local inflammation causes sperm leakage (Fig. 4). The immune response to sperm, sperm granuloma, contributes to swelling and inflammation within the epididymis.

Diagnosis of orchiepididymitis is made from the physical findings of scrotal swelling, pain, and fever. Ultrasonographic evaluation of the testes helps define whether the infection is unilateral or bilateral and aids in the differentia-

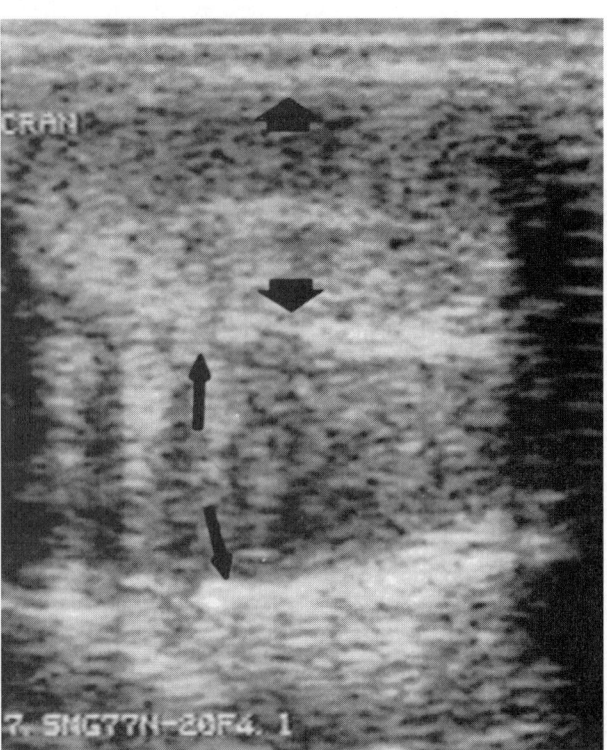

Figure 5. Ultrasonogram of canine testis with severe epididymitis associated with *Brucella canis* infection. The body of the epididymis *(long arrows)* is equal in diameter to the testis *(short arrows).* Compare this to the ultrasonographic appearance of the normal epididymis in Figure 1*B.*

tion of orchiepididymitis from other causes of testicular enlargement. Brucellosis should be considered if ultrasound examination indicates that the inflammation primarily affects the epididymides (Fig. 5).

If brucellosis is suspected, serologic testing by the rapid slide agglutination test, and possibly other follow-up tests, should be performed. The merits of these tests have been discussed elsewhere (see *CVT XII,* p. 1094). Bacterial culture of the ejaculate is helpful in detecting other microorganisms that cause orchiepididymitis, since they are usually present in high numbers. The sample should be placed in Amies medium, as it allows *Ureaplasma, Mycoplasma,* and aerobic bacteria to be isolated from the sample.

Antibiotic and anti-inflammatory agents are recommended for eliminating bacterial infection and minimizing the associated inflammation. Castration is recommended in addition for the dog that has no reasonable potential as a stud dog. Dogs with orchiepididymitis due to *B. canis* have no reproductive future, since chronic carrier states are common and are difficult to diagnose (see *CVT XII,* p. 1094). For dogs that have an established record as a valuable stud dog, castration may be postponed while medical treatment is attempted. Cool compresses applied to the scrotum may alleviate local heat due to inflammation, and may be of benefit in sparing spermatogenesis. If the infection is arrested, castration may not be required. However, even if infection is arrested, effects due to inflammation are likely to have a permanent effect on spermatogenesis. The merits of semen evaluation and testis biopsy for evalu-

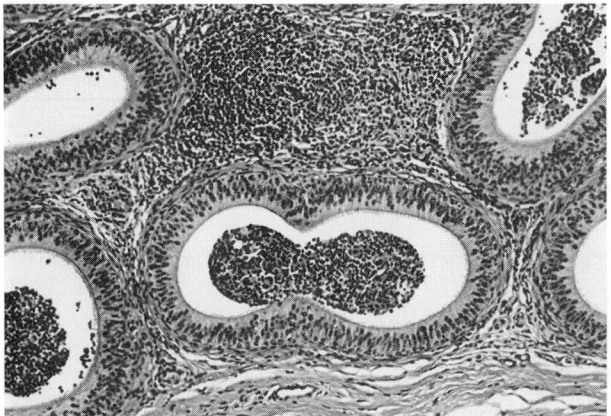

Figure 4. Photomicrograph of the epididymis of a dog with canine brucellosis. Note the severe inflammatory infiltrate within the epididymal parenchyma and within the lumen of multiple sections of the epididymal duct.

ating spermatogenesis is discussed elsewhere in this section.

Testicular Torsion and Inguinoscrotal Hernia

Testicular torsion is a twisting of the testis around the vascular pedicle. Venous return from the testis is severely compromised and the testis becomes engorged with blood. The acute enlargement of the testis is extremely painful and affected dogs may present in a state of shock. Severely affected dogs should be treated for shock before further diagnostics are done. Testicular torsion of abdominal testes is more common than in scrotal testes and should be included in the list of differential diagnoses for painful abdomen in a cryptorchid dog. Abdominal palpation reveals a large, turgid mass in the abdomen or scrotum. A large, echolucent mass is seen around the testes with ultrasound examination. Treatment includes shock therapy and castration. Derotation of the testis is usually not possible. Severe damage to the testis due to vascular compromise prevents any possibility of salvaging a torsed, previously fertile scrotal testis.

Spontaneous inguinoscrotal hernias are uncommon in dogs. Trauma or rare congenital abnormalities may cause a weakening or widening of the inguinal canal in male dogs and allow passage of intestinal loops or omentum into the vaginal process, separating the testis from the scrotal wall. Affected dogs present for acute enlargement of the scrotum. Even less frequently, abdominal contents may herniate through the inguinal ring adjacent to the vaginal process. This is an inguinal hernia and usually appears as an acute swelling adjacent to the prepuce.

Inguinoscrotal hernias are usually not painful, but if a herniated intestinal loop becomes twisted or the intestinal vasculature becomes compromised, hypovolemic shock may ensue. Palpation of the scrotum may reveal a movable, soft, extratesticular mass within the scrotum. Herniated intestine may appear as a tubular mass adjacent to the testis during ultrasound examination. Treatment of shock is first priority, followed by surgical reduction of the hernia. The inguinal ring in the area of the hernia is surgically enlarged to allow safe reduction of the hernia. Any herniated bowel is examined for signs of vascular compromise. Unhealthy bowel is resected. The inguinal incision is closed with a nonabsorbable suture material and care is taken to reduce the size of the inguinal ring without compromising the external pudendal artery and vein and the spermatic cord within the inguinal canal.

Sperm Granuloma

Obstruction of the epididymis secondary to trauma or inflammation may result in accumulation of sperm proximal to the obstruction. Initially there is a dilation of the epididymis (spermatocele) proximal to the obstruction. Subsequent rupture of the epididymis induces an inflammatory response and a sperm granuloma can form. The granuloma may be small and the epididymal swelling may be nonpalpable. Dogs with sperm granulomas are most often presented for evaluation of infertility rather than for evaluation of gross testicular changes. Ultrasonographic examination of a sperm granuloma may show epididymal enlargement in the early stages and an increased echogenicity at the site of the granuloma later in the course of the disease. Surgical correction of the obstruction is usually not possible. Orchiectomy is the recommended treatment.

DISEASES THAT CAUSE DECREASED TESTICULAR SIZE

Testicular Hypoplasia

Idiopathic testicular hypoplasia is an uncommon condition in dogs caused by a lack or severe reduction of spermatic tissue in one or both testes. Testicular hypoplasia is diagnosed by the presence of uni-or bilateral small testes in young adult dogs. Since 50 to 70% of testicular size is due to seminiferous tubules and spermatogonia, the absence of this tissue results in palpably small testes. Ultrasonic examination usually shows a decrease in the size of the testicular parenchyma with a normal-sized epididymis. The diagnosis is confirmed by testicular biopsy. Histologic evaluation shows markedly decreased or absent seminiferous tubules and spermatogonia. Leydig cells can be present in normal numbers, however, so testosterone levels and libido may be normal. Bilaterally affected dogs are usually sterile.

The cause of testicular hypoplasia is unknown. There may be a failure of germinal cells to migrate to the fetal testes or early destruction of spermatic germinal cells within the fetus. Treatment with gonadotropins in an attempt to stimulate proliferation of germinal cells has been unsuccessful.

Chronic Inflammation

Testicular inflammation that persists for more than 2 to 4 weeks may shift from an acute to a more chronic form. Chronic testicular inflammation is characterized by a decreased number of inflammatory cells and increased fibrosis. Elevated temperature and presence of inflammatory mediators within the testicular parenchyma associated with acute inflammation may cause the destruction of the spermatic tissue. As a result, chronically inflamed testes may become small and fibrotic. Ultrasound examination shows small, diffusely echodense testicular parenchyma.

Cryptorchidism

During gestation and the first 14 days of postnatal development, the normal canine testes migrate from a perinephric fetal location, across the abdominal cavity, through the inguinal canal, through the parapreputial subcutaneous tissue, and into the scrotum. There is some variation in the duration of complete testicular descent. At least two studies have documented that canine testes are abdominally located at birth, and descend completely (into the scrotum) within 10 to 14 days after birth. Most authorities agree that in a clear majority of dogs, both testes are in the scrotum by 8 weeks of age (Nelson, 1996). Although other studies have reported testis descent as late as 6 months after birth in a minority of dogs (Cox, 1986), it would be questionable to

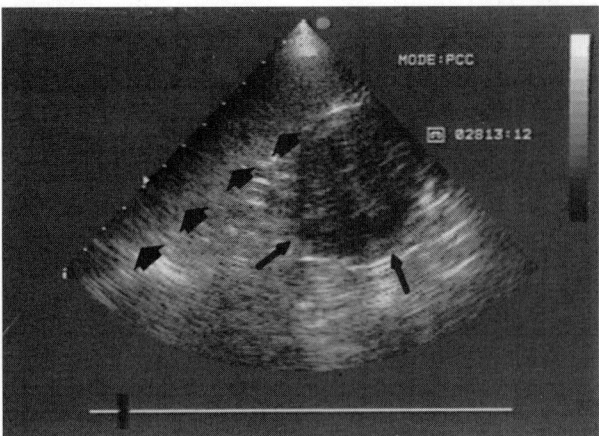

Figure 6. Ultrasonogram of a cryptorchid, neoplastic testis within a dog's abdomen. The enlarged (4 cm in diameter) testis *(long arrows)* has nonuniform echogenicity. The spleen *(wide arrows)* is adjacent to the testis. The testis contained an interstitial cell tumor.

conclude that this is a normal variation in testis descent rather than an abnormal delay in testis descent. Cryptorchid testes may remain in the abdomen (Fig. 6) or migrate through the inguinal ring and remain in the subcutaneous, parapreputial tissue.

The incidence of cryptorchidism has been reported to be 1 to 15% of adult dogs. Approximately 75% of dogs are unilaterally cryptorchid, with the right testicle being retained almost twice as often as the left. The cryptorchid testis is smaller than the scrotal testis, owing to the loss of spermatogonia. However, Sertoli cells and Leydig cells remain, and androgen synthesis is unimpaired.

Cryptorchidism is reported to be inherited as a sex-limited autosomal recessive trait (see p. 904). The American Veterinary Medical Association Principles of Veterinary Ethics indicates that, "Performance of surgical procedures for the purpose of concealing genetic defects in animals to be shown, raced, bred, or sold as breeding animals is unethical. However, should the health or welfare of the individual patient require correction of such genetic defects, it is recommended that the patient be rendered incapable of reproduction." (Principles of Veterinary Medical Ethics, 1997, In: AVMA Directory and Resource Manual, AVMA, Schaumburg, IL, p 45.) Nevertheless, medical therapy to induce testis descent in dogs has been described in a previous review (Nelson, 1996). The author indicates, "Results are variable and unpredictable and may be coincidental with spontaneous descent of mobile testes." In that report, testes were observed to descend in 21 of 25 cryptorchid dogs (less than 16 weeks of age) treated with 100 to 1,000 IU of human chorionic gonadotropin, four times, in a 2-week period.

Cryptorchid testes have an increased risk of developing a Sertoli cell tumor, which is 6- to 13-fold over that of scrotal testes. They also have an increased risk of testicular torsion. Because of these health risks and the likelihood that offspring will carry the genes for this genetic disorder, castration is highly recommended for cryptorchid dogs.

Testicular Degeneration

Testicular degeneration is a loss of seminiferous tubules, germinal cells. interstitial cells, and spermatogonia secon-

dary to an inflammatory or noninflammatory process within the testes. Typical primary testicular diseases that result in degeneration include vascular compromise due to thrombosis, trauma, or inguinoscrotal hernia. Idiopathic testicular degeneration is not associated with an obvious primary disease and most commonly affects middle-aged dogs. During the period from 1990 to 1996 there were 139 testes with degenerative changes diagnosed from 446 canine testes that contained gross or microscopic lesions submitted to the Department of Pathology at Cornell University. Early testicular degeneration may not cause obvious changes in testicular morphology. As the degeneration progresses, the testes may become small and soft. Dogs with testicular degeneration often have normal libido because the Leydig cells are spared from the degenerative process. There is no effective treatment for testicular degeneration except in those few cases where prompt treatment of the primary problem is possible.

Testicular Biopsy

In order to definitively diagnose testicular disease, it is necessary to perform histologic analysis of a representative portion of the testis that has been appropriately fixed. Bouin's fixative, NOT formalin, is essential if an evaluation of spermatogenesis is expected. If orchiectomy was done, then the entire testis is submitted for histology. If it is desirable to attempt to maintain fertility, then a testicular biopsy can be done. A needle aspirate may be sufficient for the diagnosis of inflammation, infection, or neoplasia, but to determine the effect of a disease on the structural elements of the testis, it is necessary to examine a larger sample of tissue.

A wedge of testicular parenchyma can be safely excised from the testis through a standard prescrotal approach. The testis is pushed out of the scrotum into a midline prescrotal location ventral to the penis. The skin and subcutaneous tissue over the testis are incised. The spermatic fascia over the testis is dissected, and a wedge of testicular tissue including the tunica albuginea is excised. The defect in the testis is closed by apposing the tunica albuginea with fine absorbable suture material. The subcutaneous tissue and skin are closed routinely.

References and Suggested Reading

Cox VS: Cryptorchidism in the dog. In: Morrow DA, ed: Current Therapy in Theriogenology, 2nd ed. Philadelphia: WB Saunders, 1986, pp 541–543.
    A thorough review of canine cryptorchidism.
Johnson CA, Walker RD: Clinical signs and diagnosis of *Brucella canis* infection. Compend Contin Educ Pract Vet 14:763, 1992.
    Well-written recent discussion of B. canis diagnosis and treatment.
Madewell BR, Theilen GH: Tumors of the urogenital tract. In: Theilen GH, Madewell BR, eds: Veterinary Cancer Medicine, 2nd ed. Philadelphia, Lea & Febiger, 1987, pp 583–600.
    A good review of neoplasia of the urinary and genital tract in many species of animals.
McDonald RK, Walker M, Legendre AM, et al: Radiotherapy of metastatic seminoma in the dog. J Vet Intern Med 2:103, 1988.
    One of the few published reports of radiotherapy for treatment of testicular neoplasia in dogs.
Meyers-Wallen VN, Patterson DF: Disorders of sexual development in dogs and cats. In: Kirk RW, ed: Current Veterinary Therapy X. Philadelphia: WB Saunders, 1989, pp 1261–1265.
    A detailed review of the pathogenesis of sexual development disorders in dogs and cats.

Nelson RW: Disorders of the testes and epididymides. In: Feldman EC, Nelson RW, eds: Canine and Feline Endocrinology and Reproduction, 2nd ed. Philadelphia: WB Saunders, 1996, pp 697–710.
Well-written discussion of male genital tract disorders including current treatment modalities.

Pugh CR, Kinde LJ: Sonographic evaluation of canine testicular and scrotal abnormalities: A review of 26 case histories. Vet Radiol 32:243, 1991.
Good description of sonographic appearance of various testicular and scrotal disorders in dogs.

Overview of Mismating Regimens for the Bitch

JOHN PAUL L. VERSTEGEN
Liège, Belgium

Methods for postcoital contraception and induction of abortion in dogs are needed to prevent the birth of unwanted litters. Many reasons may be at the base of the decision to induce abortion or prevent implantation in the bitch: mismating, first estrous mating in young bitch; reproduction management; and actual health problems or expected problems at birth related to the mother, such as pelvis abnormalities or disproportionate size between male and female. Abortion induction is a frequent reason for clients to consult. Indeed, mismating in small animals is frequently observed in such countries as France and the United Kingdom, where a mean of around 100,000 canine abortions are induced each year.

The objectives when planning such treatment should be: (1) to induce abortion only if the bitch is pregnant (accurate diagnosis); (2) to use a product that is safe in the short and long term both for the animal's health and her fertility, and (3) to use a drug that is reliable and easy to administer and can be controlled by the veterinarian. Finally, the treatment should be atraumatic for the owner. In the last decades, several experimental or clinical methods for termination of pregnancy following unwanted mating have been demonstrated to be effective and reliable. Prostaglandin and dopamine agonist induction of luteolysis have been incorporated into veterinary practice, slowly replacing the problematic estrogen treatments. However, these protocols are still often associated with many side effects. Some problems are related to the high dosages of drugs used, which cause emesis, diarrhea, prostration, or other undesirable and unpleasant clinical features. Newer protocols and drugs are increasingly proposed that overcome these inconveniences. These protocols are mainly based on: (1) available new drugs such as aglepristone, an inhibitor of progesterone action (antiprogesterone); (2) new derivatives of existing drugs such as cloprostenol, synthetic derivatives of prostaglandins that are more potent and have fewer side effects than natural prostaglandins; or (3) re-evaluation of old treatments such as glucocorticoids. Finally, the use of drug combinations to induce what we can call *balanced luteolysis* has been proposed, in the same sense that pre-emptive analgesia and balanced anesthesia have been proposed. The objective of this new concept in small animal reproduction, which has already been abundantly described and used in other veterinary fields, is to combine different pharmaceutical classes of molecules at low doses to minimize side effects yet obtain supra-additive or synergistic clinical effects that are not observed with single-drug use. These methods are reviewed herein. The essential mechanism of action of the treatments presented is the removal of progesterone support essential to the maintenance of the uteroplacental unit.

ENDOCRINE BIOLOGY OF PREGNANCY IN THE BITCH

A better understanding of endocrine factors regulating pregnancy and of their mode of action in the bitch should lead to efficacious and safe use of abortive drugs now available (Concannon et al, 1989). Progesterone is required for initiation and maintenance of pregnancy. In dogs a plasma progesterone level of 2 ng/ml is required to maintain pregnancy. Progesterone induces the differentiation of the endometrium and endometrial gland secretion and maintains endometrial integrity and placental attachment. Prior to the plasma luteinizing hormone (LH) peak, uterotonic contractions are stimulated by high plasma estrogen concentrations. These are no longer present by 5 days post–LH peak when rising plasma progesterone concentrations suppress uterotonic contractions. For those reasons, changes in the estrogen progesterone ratio or corpus luteum (CL) progesterone secretion will induce uterine changes that can lead to abnormal glandular secretion, myometrial contractility, and impaired implantation or abortion.

No placental or embryonic steroids or luteotrophins have been demonstrated in this species. Both pituitary LH and prolactin appear to be luteotropic in dogs and exogenous prostaglandins are luteolytic, as is endogenous prostaglandin at the end of pregnancy.

- Prolactin appears to be the main pituitary hormone sustaining corpus luteum steroidogenesis. Prolactin removal by dopamine agonists or other mechanisms inhibits prolactin secretion, leading to functional luteal arrest and luteolysis, a blockage of progesterone secretion and abortion.

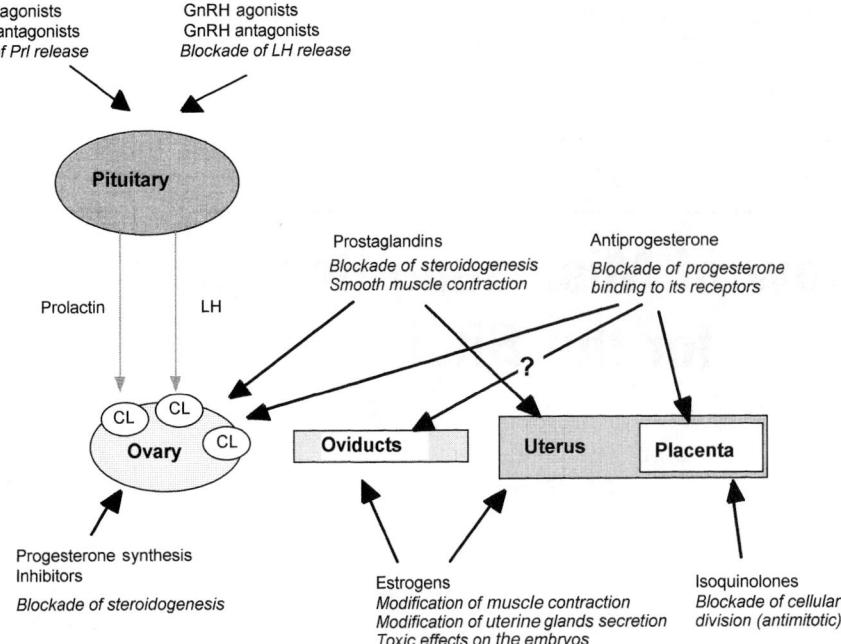

Figure 1. Mechanisms for induction of abortion in the bitch.

- The role of pituitary LH is still controversial, and if it is required, it appears to be more luteotropic than luteotrophic. Indeed, recent studies indicate that LH does not appear to be necessary for pregnancy maintenance but does stimulate progesterone secretion when injected into pregnant animals.

Prostaglandins are the natural inhibiting factors causing luteal functional arrest prior to parturition. The binding of prostaglandin to its receptors is thought to reduce CL blood supply by vasoconstriction and to directly suppress luteal steroidogenesis.

All abortion induction treatments available have the objective of preventing progesterone secretion, or of modifying, blocking, or counteracting progesterone effects on the reproductive tract (Fig. 1). Abortion induction methods involve for this reason:

1. Modification of the estrogen-progesterone ratio by administration of estrogen or synthetic estrogen derivatives or glucocorticoids.
2. Induction of functional luteal arrest or luteolysis by substances that act directly (prostaglandins) or indirectly on the CL by inhibiting luteotrophic or luteotropic support. For example, dopamine agonists suppress prolactin secretion whereas GnRH antagonists deplete LH.
3. Blockage of progesterone secretion by inhibiting steroidogenesis (epostane).
4. Blockage of progesterone action at the receptor level (antiprogesterone—mefiprestone or aglepristone).

PERIODS OF TREATMENT AND CLINICAL INTERESTS

Pregnancy in the bitch can be divided into three periods. The first begins at fertilization and ends at implantation (days 20 to 22 from the plasma LH peak). The second begins at implantation and ends at the time of fetal ossifi-

cation (40 to 42 days). This corresponds to the period of embryogenesis and the beginning of fetal development. The last period begins at fetal ossification and ends at parturition. Methods to induce abortion are available for all three periods; however, only the second period is of practical clinical interest.

First Third of Pregnancy

During this first term of gestation, positive pregnancy diagnosis is difficult to confirm (see p. 924) and abortion induction at this time may simply represent treatment of a nonpregnant bitch. Furthermore, abortion induction during this period is often difficult to achieve due to the apparent refractoriness of the CL to exogenous treatment. This refractoriness may be due to a relative CL autonomy or to a complex interplay of regulatory mechanisms that allow resistance to the withdrawal of one or more supporting elements. Three types of molecules could be used during this first period of pregnancy:

1. Estrogens, which inhibit oocyte transport in the uterine horns or have a direct embryotoxic effect, and have no direct effect on the CL.
2. Prostaglandins, which must be used at high doses to induce functional luteal arrest and concurrently produce undesirable side effects.
3. Inhibitors of progesterone secretion (epostane) or progesterone action (antiprogesterone: mifeprestone or aglepristone). However these drugs are not yet available in most countries.

Second Third of Pregnancy

During this second period, positive pregnancy diagnosis can be obtained and abortion induced if necessary. Abortion induction during this period is mainly associated with embryonic/fetal resorption, which, in the author's experience, is the best, safest, and most reliable method by which to induce abortion in bitches. Abortion can be induced by prostaglandins (natural or synthetic), antiprolactinic agents such as dopamine agonists (bromocryptine, cabergoline) or antiserotoninergic agents (methergoline), the combination of prostaglandins and dopamine agonists, and the inhibitors of progesterone secretion (epostane) or progesterone action (antiprogesterone: mifeprestone or aglepristone). Antagonists of gonadotropin releasing harmone (GnRH) have also been proposed, but are not yet available, and their efficacy remains to be confirmed because the luteotropic role of LH during pregnancy in bitches is still controversial. Finally, new evidence has demonstrated that glucocorticoid treatment might be useful in some instances.

Last Third of Pregnancy

During the last third of pregnancy, fetuses are well developed and ossified, and their body weight dramatically and exponentially increases. Abortion induction during this term is always associated with fetal expulsion. The author does not recommend abortion during this period because it may be traumatic to the animal or the owner. Due to the wide variation in duration of pregnancy (when calculated from the breeding date), abortion induced after day 50 to 55 from first mating might induce premature parturition with delivery of live pups (see *CVT XII,* pp. 1075 and 1080). For this reason, abortion induction during the last third of pregnancy is not advocated.

ABORTION INDUCTION TREATMENTS

In this article, only available therapeutic methods useful for inducing abortion in bitches are presented. Future treatments, such as GnRH antagonists or progesterone synthesis inhibitors, have been promising in experimental trials, but are not available commercially in many countries. A short summary of these future treatments is given at the end of this article.

Treatment of Bitches Not Intended for Reproduction

For the majority of bitches, the most appropriate method to prevent the birth of an unwanted litter is to perform a sterilization by ovariohysterectomy before implantation or following pregnancy diagnosis by ultrasound or palpation around 3 to 4 weeks after mating.

Treatment of Bitches Intended for Reproduction

Abortion Induction Before Implantation

Two types of treatment are available in most countries. The first type is based on the use of estrogens and prevents implantation by modifying tubo-uterine mobility and secretion, thereby inducing embryonic death. The second type is based on the prevention or neutralization of progesterone secretion and can be attained using prostaglandins. However the CL is relatively independent of all hormonal control until at least days 20 to 25 post–LH peak. Therefore, induction of functional luteal arrest before this period can only be obtained with high doses of prostaglandins, which can have undesirable side effects.

Estrogens

Large doses of estrogen have been used for many years to prevent implantation following an undesirable mating in dogs as in cats. However, currently, estrogens are to be avoided because of their toxic side effects.

Fertilization and the first 10 days of embryonic canine development occur in the oviduct. Embryos then migrate to the uterus for another 5 to 10 days before implantation. During this period, important relationships are established between embryos and the oviduct or uterus. Any changes in these relationships lead to embryonic death or prevent implantation. Estrogens exert their actions in at least two ways:

1. When given before the migration of embryos from the oviducts to the uterus, the uterotubal junction remains closed, migration is prevented, and the embryos degenerate.
2. When given after the embryos migrate into the uterus, development of the uterine glands is perturbed and the nutritive requirements of the embryos are no longer satisfied. This prevents embryonic development and increases uterine motility, which prevents implantation. Due to estrogens, embryonic death occurs following transport disturbances and/or direct toxic effects.

Abortion Induction Protocols With Estrogens. Numerous protocols are available and clearly reflect the absence of clear, well-constructed studies to define the minimal effective dose of estrogens necessary for inducing canine abortion. Furthermore, the biologic side effects vary depending on the preparation used, the dose, and the route of administration. Whatever the drug or dose, the use of these drugs is no longer advisable, owing to serious side effects. If used, however, these precautions must be kept in mind:

1. Use of estrogens in a bitch intended for reproduction is *not* recommended. Indeed, estrogens often induce uterine disease or hypothalamo-pituitary blockade leading to irreversible sterility.
2. Estrogen should never be used when progesterone levels are already high. The combination of high estrogen with progesterone often leads to uterine pathologies (cystic endometrial hyperplasia and pyometra).
3. Repeated low doses of estrogen are less toxic than the same cumulative dose given once.
4. Always advise the owners of the serious risks of this treatment, and try to convince them to choose an alternative therapy.
5. Don't forget that the probability of the bitch to become pregnant after a single mating is less than 40% (Feldman et al, 1993). Treating with this method before positive pregnancy diagnosis can be obtained exposes the bitch to serious risk when the bitch may not be pregnant.

The two main estrogen drugs available for abortion induction are estradiol benzoate (Intervet, The Netherlands) in

Europe, and estradiol cypionate (ECP) in the United States. ECP is more potent, has a longer duration of action, and is apparently more toxic than estradiol benzoate. Injectable DES (diethylstilbestrol) is no longer available in Europe or the United States, and oral DES has proven to be ineffective in inducing abortion (Bowen et al, 1985). With the precautions outlined above in mind, the recommended protocols are:

- estradiol benzoate (Estradiol benzoate): Calculate the dose based on 5 to 10 µg/kg with a maximum of 1 mg per dog. Divide this into two or three subcutaneous injections to be given at 48-hour intervals, beginning on day 2 to 4 after mating.
- estradiol cypionate (ECP, Upjohn): Doses vary widely among authors (from 5 to 44 µg/kg). The highest dosage is injected once IM between the fourth day of estrus and the second day of diestrus, as determined by vaginal cytology.
- It is often difficult to determine when treatment should be initiated. Some bitches may accept mating as early as 4 to 5 days before the LH surge or as late as 5 to 6 after the LH surge. Estrogens have to be administered during estrus, and not in proestrus or diestrus, as determined by vaginal cytolog (see p. 925). The efficacy of the protocol described is considered good, but toxic side effects have been reported.

Side Effects and Toxicity of the Estrogens. Numerous side effects are associated with the use of estrogens, particularly when high doses are used. The most important side effect is related to the toxic effects of estrogens on the bone marrow, inducing medullary aplasia resulting in thrombocytopenia, leukopenia, severe anemia, and death. The toxicity is clearly dose dependent. The first hematologic signs could be observed from 5 to 10 days after treatment at a dose of ECP as low as 100 µg/kg. At doses over 500 µg/kg, death was always observed. This bone marrow sensitivity to estrogen is not well understood but is clearly associated with the estrogen treatment (Verstegen et al, 1981; Bowen et al, 1985).

The second complication in terms of frequency and importance is the development of metritis and pyometra related to the abnormal increase in estrogen:progesterone ratio, cystic hyperplasia of the uterine glands, abnormal epithelial secretion, relaxation of the cervix, and ascending infection. In some studies, 25 to 50% of bitches presented with metritis had received estrogen for abortion induction within the previous 6 months.

A less important complication is the observation a few days after injection of the development of an estrus-like behavior associated with vulva swelling, metrorrhagia, vaginal keratinization, male attraction, and sometimes mating. This behavioral estrus is never associated with ovulation and is only due to the exogenous estrogens injected in a bitch already in diestrus. Hypothalamic or pituitary irreversible infertility has also been described.

Prostaglandins

Repeated multiple doses of prostaglandin have been demonstrated to prevent pregnancy in mated bitches by inhibition of CL progesterone synthesis and release. The treatment is efficacious if initiated after the end of cytologic estrus, from day 5 of diestrus, which is approximately day 13 to 15 post-LH surge. There is no evidence indicating that prostaglandin is effective prior to this time. The efficacy is dependent on dose, frequency, and the stage of pregnancy. In general, treatment early in this period requires a longer course of therapy.

Use of Natural and Synthetic Analogues of Prostaglandins. Abortion by natural prostaglandins is induced in three different ways: (1) by inducing vasoconstriction, reducing blood flow to the corpora lutea and causing cellular degeneration; (2) by interfering with steroidogenesis through binding to specific receptors and reducing progesterone production; and (3) by acting directly on the myometrium to cause smooth muscle contractions. Such uterine effects, in addition to luteolysis, play a role particularly in late pregnancy abortion and fetal expulsion.

Prostaglandin analogues have been developed to improve the efficacy over natural prostaglandins and at the same time reduce the side effects associated with their use. The side effects are essentially related to the muscle stimulant properties of natural prostaglandins. The objectives in developing synthetic analogues were have been to reduce muscle contraction side effects and increase the duration of action so that luteolysis can be obtained at relatively low doses.

When inducing abortion during early or mid-pregnancy, the objective is to arrest CL function, and thereby eliminate progesterone support that is necessary to pregnancy maintenance. The myometrial contraction effects of prostaglandins are clear side effects that are not directly related to the treatment objective. Because pregnancy termination by resorption is most desirable, there is clearly no need for the myocontracting effects. Therefore there is interest in synthetic analogues that are devoid of those side effects. Finally, a prolonged duration of action that will reduce the frequency of injections provides more convenient protocols for clinical situations. Cloprostenol (Estrumate, Mallinckrodt Veterinary) has at least 12 to 24 hours of action in comparison to 4 to 8 hours for dynoprostum (prostaglandin F2α THAM [Lutalyse, Upjohn, United States, or Dinolytic, Upjohn, Europe]). In Europe, several authors have used synthetic analogues under clinical conditions to induce abortion and have tried to define the minimal dose that will induce abortion with minimal side effects (see discussions of side effects and protocols).

Side Effect of Prostaglandins. The side effects of natural prostaglandins are mainly related to smooth muscle stimulation. These unwanted effects appear within minutes after injection, are clearly dose and preparation dependent, and are more important at equimolar levels for natural than for synthetic analogues. Adaptation also seems to occur after repeated treatment inasmuch as side effects diminish considerably after several injections. Maximum side effects occur between 20 and 60 minutes after injection, then slowly decrease, with a return to normal in approximately 2 to 3 hours. The return to normal is drug and dose dependent, and is subject to considerable individual variation. Clinical reactions include excessive salivation, vom-

TABLE 1. **Effective Methods Reported for Termination of Pregnancy in Dogs Following Unwanted Matings**

Drug*	Day of Cycle (After LH Surge)	Dose	Duration of Treatment (Days)	Efficacy (%)
Natural PgF$_{2\alpha}$	From 13 to 49	10–250 μg/kg (from b.i.d. to f.i.d.—IM or SC—the lower the dose, the higher the number of injections per day)	3–11 (the lower the dose or earlier the treatment, the longer the treatment)	80–100
Synthetic PgF$_{2\alpha}$ (cloprostenol)	Between 30 and 40	2.5 μg/kg SC once every day	4–5	100
Dopamine Agonists				
Bromocriptine	From 35 to 45	50–100 μg/kg b.i.d. IM or PO	4–7	50–100
Cabergoline	Beginning at day:			
	30/40/50	5 μg/kg PO once/day	5	25/100/100
	25/30/40	1.65 μg/kg SC once/day	5	25/66/100
Combination of cabergoline and cloprostenol	Beginning at day 25	5 μg/kg PO daily and 1 μg/kg SC q48hr	7 for cabergoline/3 for cloprostenol	100

*The majority of the medications listed are not registered for use in small animal reproduction in all countries.

iting, diarrhea, defecation, hyperpnea, ataxia, urination, anxiety, and pupil dilatation followed by constriction. Parasympatholytic agents such as atropine (0.025 mg/kg) or prifinium bromide (0.75 mg/kg) and butylscopolamine (4 to 8 mg/dog) given IM have been reported to reduce severity of side effects, particularly salivation, emesis, diarrhea, and respiratory distress. However, in experimental and clinical trials, we have observed that doses of natural prostaglandins of 10 μg/kg or less and doses of cloprostenol of 1 μg/kg or less are not associated with side effects yet still have an effect on the CL. We have shown that 1 μg/kg of cloprostenol once a day for 5 days can induce functional luteal arrest. This is characterized by a decrease in serum progesterone secretion below 2 ng/ml for more than 24 hours, which is considered to be the minimal concentration necessary for pregnancy maintenance. Similar results could be obtained with 10 μg/kg of dinoprost. However, due to the short life of this molecule, it must be injected at least five times a day, which renders this protocol impractical for clinical use. Table 1 summarizes the different protocols available.

Antiprogestin Therapy

Administration of a progesterone antagonist at effective doses will prevent establishment of pregnancy or terminate pregnancy in several species if administered before implantation. The most extensively studied antiprogestin, mifepristone (RU 486, Roussel Uclaff, not registered for animal use) has been shown to bind to the progesterone receptor with high affinity and to prevent progesterone induced changes in DNA transcription. More recently, a new antiprogestin aglepristone (Alizine, Hoechst Roussel Vet, France), has been marketed in several European countries for use in dogs. Aglepristone was administered at a dose of 10 mg/kg, twice at 24-hour intervals, in a study involving 367 bitches from 0 to 45 days of pregnancy. Treatment was effective in 94.8% of animals confirmed pregnant on the first day of treatment, and in 100% of those dogs in which a positive pregnancy diagnosis could not be obtained on the first day of treatment (Fieni, 1995). No general or local side effects were observed except for mammary

development and lactation. Whether this kind of drug will be available in all countries is still a controversial question, mainly due to issues surrounding the potential use of such compounds (e.g., RU 486) for human contraception. However, due to their efficacy, safety margin, and absence of side effects, they would be of great advantage in abortion induction in small animals and are certainly needed.

Abortion Induction After Implanation

Prostaglandins

Because abortion is more easily induced after implantation, lower doses of prostaglandin can be given over a short duration to induce abortion during this period. The advantage is that pregnancy can be confirmed prior to treatment, and nonpregnant animals are not treated, unnecessarily. Second because a lower dose can be used, fewer side effects are observed. Table 1 describes different natural or synthetic prostaglandins analogue protocols that are available to induce abortion after implantation. The author's preference is cloprostenol, 1 to 2 μg/kg SC given once a day for 5 to 7 days, beginning at least 30 days after mating. Recommendations below concerning the monitoring of abortion must be followed.

Dopamine Agonist Agents

Because prolactin is the main luteotrophic hormone in dogs, inhibition of its synthesis and release causes functional luteal arrest and a decrease in progesterone secretion. If treatment is applied long enough during the second part of pregnancy, luteolysis occurs. Prolactin secretion is a complex phenomenon but is essentially controlled by direct inhibition at the pituitary level by dopamine, and by indirect stimulatory tone at the hypothalamic level by serotonin, which inhibits dopamine secretion. During pregnancy, prolactin has been shown to significantly increase from day 25 to 30 post–LH surge. During this period, dopamine agonists can be given orally or systemically to induce abortion. Bromocriptine and cabergoline belong to the dopamine agonist class, inhibiting prolactin secretion by direct action on D-2 pituitary receptors. Methergoline belongs to the class of serotonin antagonist agents that increase dopamine-inhibiting tone at the hypothalamic level.

Bromocriptine (Parlodel, Sandoz, Switzerland, not approved for animal use except in Italy) was the first inhibitor for which an effective dose was established. However, its use was not extensive because of the high incidence of emesis observed with doses of 50 to 100 μg/kg given once or twice a day. The lowest dose was not consistently effective in inducing abortion in some dogs. The highest dose has to be given for at least 5 days, and ideally should be given to effect, which could require more than 7 days. In fact, oral bromocriptine is not 100% effective in inducing abortion in dogs before day 40 of gestation. This is due to its relatively short duration of action (±8 hours). Emesis associated with inappetence is likely when used at this dose level. Peripherally acting emesis inhibitors could be given at least 30 minutes before administration to prevent emesis. However, as described earlier, inducing abortion after day 40 might be considered undesirable because it is likely to result in fetal expulsion rather than resorption.

Cabergoline (Galastop, Vetem Centralvet, Italy) is a more specific dopamine agonist that is approved and available in Europe but not in the United States. It has been developed explicitly as an antiprolactin drug for use in dogs and cats and is being considered for human applications such as pathologic hyperprolactinemia. It is safe, effective, and easy to administer, being available in a syrup form. It is long acting because it binds to pituitary dopamine receptors for more than 48 hours. Emetic side effects are mild or rarely observed and are of short duration. Oral cabergoline (5 μg/kg/day for 5 days) has been demonstrated to induce abortion in 100% of bitches treated from 40 days after the LH surge, but only in 25% of bitches when given from day 30 (Verstegen et al, 1993). As described earlier, after 40 days of gestation it is probably not advisable to induce abortion. Injections of 1.65 μg/kg SC, administered on alternate days over 5 days, was more effective, with abortions induced in 100%, 66%, and 25% of bitches, when treatments were started at 40, 30, and 25 days post–LH surge, respectively (Onclin et al, 1995). However, the injectable formulation is not available commercially. Due to the relative inefficiency of oral dopamine agonists used in early or mid-pregnancy, it appears that there is a need for injectable, long-acting formulations. Once available, they could be used as the sole agent to induce abortion. Table 1 summarizes the different protocols available.

Combination Therapy of Low Dose of Prostaglandins and Dopamine Agonists

The simultaneous administration of low doses of prostaglandins and a dopamine agonist to induce abortion has recently been described. The objective of this combination is to reduce CL function and progesterone release by a double mechanism of action: (1) direct local effects of prostaglandins on CL steroidogenesis and (2) an indirect effect due to withdrawal of pituitary prolactin support. In this way an additive, if not synergistic, effect is obtained, which allows a lower dose to be used and consequently reduces the side effects known to occur when prostaglan-

dins are used alone at higher doses. This protocol induces abortion in 100% of dogs treated from day 25 post–LH surge (20 to 28 days after first mating) with a combination of cloprostenol (1 μg/kg, three injections on every alternate day SC) and oral cabergoline (5 μg/kg/day for 7 days). The abortion induced was always by resorption and occurred 5 to 8 days after the beginning of treatment. No serious side effects were recorded. As in all abortion induction treatments, some sanguinous vaginal discharge was observed. This was noted 5 to 10 days after the beginning of treatment and was coincident with sonographic evidence of resorption (Onclin and Verstegen, 1996). Finally, recent results have confirmed the safety of this protocol, in the short and long term and in subsequent fertility. The day on which the treatment is initiated is important. Indeed, treatment after day 40 is still efficacious, but abortion is more often observed by fetal expulsion rather than by resorption. Before day 25, the CL is refractory to luteolysis and positive pregnancy diagnosis can be difficult. However, in practice the day of mating is known more often than the LH surge. For these reasons, it is recommended that the treatment be started as soon as pregnancy diagnosis is confirmed by palpation or sonography because this corresponds to approximately 25 days after the LH surge (Yeager et al, 1992).

Instead of cloprostenol, we have used alphaprostol (Gabbrostim, Vetem, Italy) in combination with cabergoline (Onclin et al, 1995). This treatment was effective but was associated with local reactions (granuloma, abscess, pain) and was thus discontinued. Recent data have demonstrated the efficacy of not only cloprostenol associated with cabergoline but also of dinoprostum combined with bromocriptine to induce abortion in the bitch. Bromocriptine was given twice a day for 7 to 8 days at 25 μg/kg instead of cabergoline.

Similarly, abortion could be induced using only two doses of prostaglandin administered at days 1 and 5 (1 μg/kg) combined with cabergoline at 5 μg/kg per day for 7 to 8 days.

It is expected that once the correct dose and protocols are defined using the different dopamine agonists in combination with prostaglandins, similar results could be obtained with many different combinations based on this principle of "balanced polypharmaceutic treatments." Thus for the first time, treatments are available that can induce abortion as soon as a positive pregnancy diagnosis can be obtained by sonography, as early as 25 days post–LH surge. Then the treatment is used only if the animal is pregnant. These treatments are not associated with any side effects and fertility is conserved. Finally, this kind of treatment does not require hospitalization or multiple treatments at the veterinary office. It ensures the necessary veterinary control over the procedure because the animal is seen on alternate days for injections, but at the same time involves the owner in the therapy. Table 1 summarizes the different protocols available.

Antiprogestin Therapy

The antiprogesterone drugs described here can also be used once pregnancy diagnosis has been established. However the results were not as impressive and pseudopregnancy has been described as a side effect after aglepristone treatment.

Corticosteroid Treatments

Administration of dexamethasone has been demonstrated to induce abortion in cattle and sheep. Several injections terminated pregnancy in dogs when doses of 5 mg/kg were administered IM every 12 hours for 10 days, starting at day 30 or 45 of pregnancy. More recently, dexamethasone was demonstrated to terminate pregnancy in 20 bitches when administered from day 35 of pregnancy. Oral dexamethasone (0.2 mg/kg) was given two to three times a day for 5 days, then the dose was progressively reduced to zero in the following 3 to 5 days. Abortion was observed in all animals within a few days of the end of treatment. The exact mode of action is not yet understood, but progesterone was observed to be consistently less than 2 ng/ml at the end of treatment. Therefore, it is likely that abortion is mediated by a direct or indirect luteolytic effect of dexamethasone. This kind of treatment has certain advantages over the use of estrogens given during estrus, in that the side effects are of short term and are unlikely to be life threatening. The efficacy of this treatment is surprising and might be useful. However obvious corticoid-induced side effects (anorexia, polydipsia, and polyuria) were observed and additional information is certainly necessary to determine: (1) the exact mode of action; (2) the effects on future fertility; and (3) if dexamethasone treatment should be recommended as an alternative method of pregnancy termination in cases where other alternatives or veterinary care are not easily available, or hospitalization or surgery is not possible. Therefore the use of corticoids to terminate pregnancy cannot be recommended until further information on efficacy and side effects is documented (Zone et al, 1995).

Medications in the Near Future

Epostane is a steroid molecule that inhibits steroid synthesis at the level of the hydroxysteroid-dehydrogenase-isomerase enzyme system, which converts pregnenolone to progesterone. Epostane has been shown to terminate pregnancy when given orally at 50 mg/kg/day for 7 days, starting on the first day of diestrus. It will also terminate pregnancy when administered later. No adverse side effects have been described. This interesting compound is unfortunately not available for use in small animal practice.

Antagonists of GnRH act by competitive binding to GnRH receptors and rapidly suppress pituitary secretion of LH and follicle-stimulating hormone (FSH). Because LH is a luteotropic support for CL function, its withdrawal is supposed to impair steroidogenesis and then to decrease progesterone secretion. A single high-dose injection of a potent GnRH antagonist was demonstrated to suppress luteal function and terminate pregnancy when administered at midpregnancy. These preliminary results were promising but controversial, and remain to be confirmed. Finally, this preparation is not available in clinical practice.

MONITORING OF ABORTION AND ASSOCIATED THERAPEUTICS

Abortion induction must be carefully monitored to confirm success and prevent complications. If abortion has to be induced, the flow chart (Fig. 2) can be followed to determine which is the best treatment to use. Treatment success can be confirmed by sonography around day 20 to 25 when early luteal phase abortion is induced. Although pregnancy diagnosis is not obtained before treatment, the integrity of the uterus should be assessed by sonography because pyometra is often a complication of estrogen treatment.

If pregnancy termination is begun after implantation,

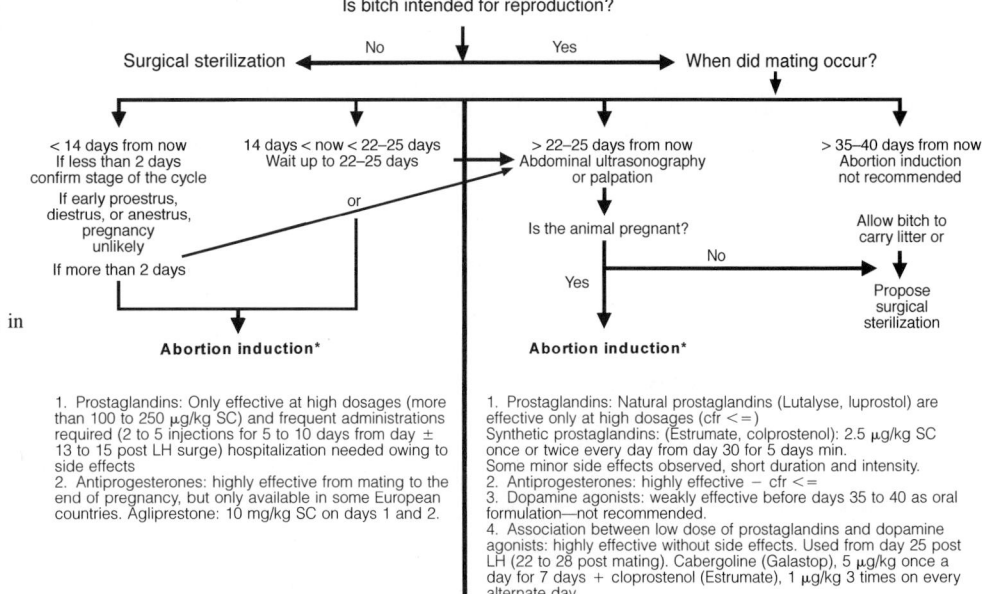

Figure 2. Induction of abortion in the bitch.

post-treatment sonography will confirm treatment efficacy as well as the absence of uterine side effects. It is recommended that a sonographic examination to confirm treatment efficacy be done at 5 to 7 days after treatment initiation. If abortion is not observed, as characterized by changes in fetal anatomy and images of placental detachment and fetal decomposition and resportion (compact dense masses in the gestational sacs), then prolongation of the treatment for another 2 to 5 days is recommended. It is important to know that at sonography pregnancy termination is always sudden, without any preceding ultrasonographic signs such as altered fetal heart rate. In all cases followed by the author, the fetus appeared normal, with a normal heart rate, and then 24 hours later there was no cardiac activity. Ultrasonographic monitoring is highly recommended to monitor treatment success and in abortion induction mediated by inhibition of progesterone synthesis (prostaglandins, antiprolactinic, glucocorticoids, etc). However, practitioners who do not have access to ultrasonography could monitor treatment efficacy by monitoring the decrease in plasma progesterone. Basal plasma progesterone concentrations below 1 ng for more than 2 days would indicate pregnancy termination.

References and Suggested Reading

Bowen RA, Olson PN, Behrendt MD, et al: Efficacy and toxicity of estrogens commonly used to terminate canine pregnancy. J Am Vet Med Assoc 186:783, 1985.
  A dose-titration study of the effects of estrogens in pregnancy termination in bitches.
Concannon PW, McCann JP, Temple M: Biology and endocrinology of ovulation, pregnancy and parturition in the dog. J Reprod Fertil Suppl 39:3, 1989.
  A review of endocrine regulation of pregnancy in the bitch.
Feldman EC, Davidson AP, Nelson RW, et al: Prostaglandin induction of abortion in pregnant bitches after misalliance. JAVMA 202:1855, 1993.
Fieni F: An original molecule to induce abortion in bitches: Aglepristone. A clinical study defining efficacy and absence of side effects. Proc 1995 CNVSA meeting, Paris, November 1995, p 279.
  A clinical study in French describing the efficacy of a progesterone antagonist commercialized in some European countries to induce abortion in bitches. More than 95% efficacy without major side effects is described.
Fieni F: Fuhrer M, Tainturier D, et al: Use of cloprostenol for pregnancy termination in dogs J Reprod Fertil Suppl 39:323, 1989.
Onclin K, Verstegen J: Practical use of a combination of a dopamine agonist and synthetic prostaglandin analogue to terminate unwanted pregnancy in dogs. J Small Anim Pract 37:211, 1966.
Onclin K, Verstegen J: Comparisons of different combinations of PGF2 alpha analogues and dopamine agonists to induce termination of unwanted pregnancy in dogs. Vet Rec 1999 (accepted for publication).
Onclin K, Silva LDM, Verstegen J: Termination of unwanted pregnancy in dogs with the dopamine agonist cabergoline in combination with a synthetic analog of PgF2 alpha either cloprostenol or alphaprostol. Theriogenology 43:813, 1995.
  Description of the clinical efficacy of two dopamine agonists–prostaglandins to induce abortion in bitches. A practical description of a efficacious abortion induction treatment devoid of side effects to be used in bitches after implantation.
Verstegen J, Decoster R, Brasseur M: Influence of estrogens on blood parameters in bitches. Ann Med Vet 125:397, 1981.
  A dose-titration characterization of the toxic effects of ECP on hematologic parameters in bitches.
Verstegen J, Onclin K, Silva LDM, et al: Abortion induction in queens and bitches using cabergoline, a specific dopamine agonist. Ann Med Vet 137:251, 1993.
  Reports on pregnancy termination in dogs and cats using oral or injectable dopamine agonist administration from day 25 to 50 after LH surge.
Yeager AE, Mohammed HO, Meyers-Wallen, et al: Ultrasonic appearance of the uterus, placenta, fetus and fetal membranes throughout accurately timed pregnancy in beagles. Am J Vet Res 53:342, 1992.
  A review of pregnancy diagnostic and follow-up using ultrasonography.
Zone M, Wanke M, Rebuelto, et al: Termination of pregnancy in dogs by oral administration of dexamethasone. Theriogenology 43:487, 1995.
  A clinical study describing the efficacy of dexamethasone treatment to induce abortion in bitches.

Neurologic and Musculoskeletal Disorders

STEVEN C. SCHRADER
KYLE G. BRAUND

Consulting Editors

Still Current Information Found in Current Veterinary Therapy XII:

Diagnosis and Management of Dysautonomia in Dogs

DENNIS P. O'BRIEN
Columbia, Missouri

RANDALL C. LONGSHORE
Phoenix, Arizona

Dysautonomia is characterized by degeneration of neurons in the autonomic ganglia with associated failure of sympathetic and parasympathetic functions. The cause is unknown. Equine dysautonomia (grass sickness) was first described in England around the turn of the century. Dysautonomia was recognized in cats in England in the early 1980s, and the feline disease reached epidemic proportions before subsiding (Edney et al, 1987). During the feline dysautonomia outbreak, a handful of cases of dysautonomia in dogs were recognized in England and Europe (Wise and Lappin, 1990). More recently an increasing number of cases of canine dysautonomia have been diagnosed in the midwestern United States (Longshore et al, 1996). This article describes the diagnostic and therapeutic approaches applied to these cases at the University of Missouri, Veterinary Medical Teaching Hospital.

HISTORY AND CLINICAL SIGNS

Dysautonomia has been diagnosed primarily in young adult dogs (median age 14 months with a range from 8 weeks to 10 years of age). Although Labrador retrievers were slightly overrepresented, a wide variety of breeds have been affected. The most common presenting complaints in affected dogs have been dysuria, regurgitation, purulent nasal discharge, photophobia, anorexia, and weight loss (Table 1). The duration of clinical signs averaged about 2 weeks.

Physical examination findings reflected primarily loss of parasympathetic functions, although sympathetic dysfunction was also present. Pupillary light responses were absent with normal vision, and the pupils varied from maximally dilated to midrange (Fig. 1). Ocular and oral mucous membranes lacked normal secretion. The dogs would frequently posture to urinate, but they produced little urine. On abdominal palpation, the bladder was distended and pain was occasionally noted.

Sympathetic dysfunction was often less obvious. Loss of sympathetic as well as parasympathetic innervation of the iris may have contributed to the midrange pupils seen in some dogs. Other signs of Horner's syndrome such as elevated third eyelids, ptosis, and enophthalmos were often present. The distended bladder was easily expressed, suggesting diminished sphincter tone. Heart rate and blood pressure were generally in the low end of the normal range but did not increase with stress or excitement.

The only sign of somatic motor system involvement was decreased anal sphincter tone; this was present in most dogs. Myotatic and withdrawal reflexes, sensory perception, and postural reactions were normal. Secondary effects of the autonomic dysfunction such as aspiration pneumonia and lethargy soon developed. Rhinitis secondary to dry mucous membranes and/or regurgitation was a common finding. Weight loss was often dramatic, with many of the dogs presenting cachexic. No consistent changes were observed in the complete blood cell counts, urinalyses, serum chemistries, or cerebrospinal fluid analyses.

DIAGNOSTIC TESTS

Confirming a diagnosis of dysautonomia depends on documenting diffuse sympathetic and parasympathetic dysfunction without significant somatic nervous system involvement or sensory loss. A complete neurologic examination will be necessary to rule out somatic involvement. For example, a dog with a sacral cord lesion due to canine distemper may have urinary retention and loss of anal tone, but it should also have other signs such as loss of sensation to the perineum and loss of tail movements. In cases with limited signs initially (e.g., dysuria or photophobia alone),

TABLE 1. Historical and Physical Examination Findings in 11 Dogs with Necropsy-Confirmed Dysautonomia

Historical and/or Physical Finding	Number of Dogs Affected/Number in Which Evaluation was Recorded
Dysuria	11/11
Distended urinary bladder	10/10
Mydriasis	11/11
Absent pupillary light reflex	11/11
Dry mucous membranes	10/11
Weight loss	8/10
Decreased Schirmer tear test (< 15 mm/min)	8/10
Lethargy	7/11
Decreased appetite	7/10
Decreased anal reflex	7/9
Vomiting/regurgitation	6/9
Elevated third eyelid	5/11
Constipation	3/9
Dysphagia	3/9
Diarrhea	3/9
Weakness	2/9
Abdominal pain	1/10

From Longshore RC, O'Brien DP, Johnson GC, et al: Dysautonomia in dogs: A retrospective study. J Vet Intern Med 10:103–109, 1996, with permission.

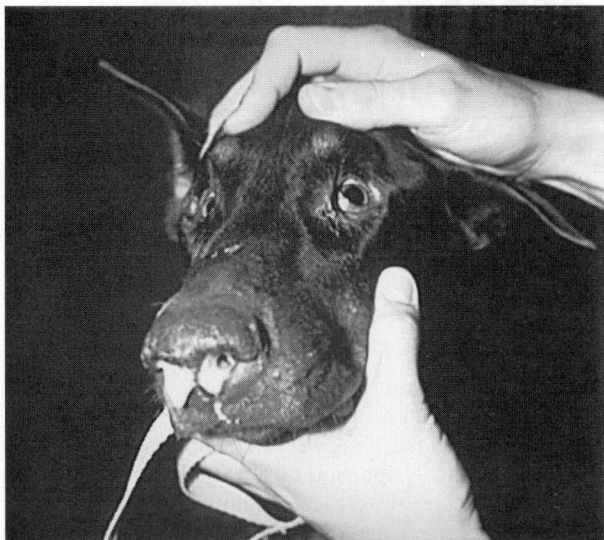

Figure 1. Typical facial appearance of a dog with dysautonomia showing mydriasis, elevated third eyelids, ptosis, and purulent nasal discharge. (From Longshore RC, O'Brien DP, Johnson GC, et al: Dysautonomia in dogs: A retrospective study. J Vet Intern Med 10:103–109, 1996, with permission.)

more common causes of the signs (e.g., cystitis or corneal ulcer respectively) must be ruled out. Because parasympathetic signs predominate in dysautonomia, cholinergic blockade with toxins or drugs (e.g., atropine) must be ruled out. Necropsy confirmation of autonomic ganglia degeneration without inflammation provides the definitive diagnosis, but a variety of tests can be used to support an antemortem diagnosis of dysautonomia.

Pharmacologic testing of the pupils is probably the best single test for confirming the diagnosis. Pilocarpine ophthalmic solution (Isopto Carpine 1%, Alcon) is diluted to 0.05% with normal saline and 1 to 2 drops placed in one eye. Pupil size is then observed every 15 minutes. Dogs with dysautonomia generally show a rapid constriction of the pupils. Even at the 0.05% dilution, some normal dogs may show some constriction of the pupils, but it will take 45 to 60 minutes. If no response is seen 90 minutes after instilling the 0.05% solution, the test is repeated with full strength (1 to 2%) pilocarpine. Because drugs such as atropine produce their effects by blocking cholinergic receptors, dogs who have parasympathetic signs due to such drugs or toxins should not respond to even the full-strength pilocarpine solutions.

Thoracic radiographs can confirm the presence of megaesophagus and detect secondary aspiration pneumonia. Abdominal radiographs may demonstrate a distended urinary bladder and occasionally ileus. Alternatively, ultrasound can be used to document the distended bladder, ileus, and lack of normal gastrointestinal motility. Attempts to urinate will have little effect on bladder volume. The dog can then be tested with a low dose (0.04 mg/kg SC) of bethanechol (Urecholine, Merck Sharp & Dohme) and bladder volume re-evaluated with ultrasound. Emptying of the bladder with low-dose bethanechol would suggest denervation supersensitivity. Some affected dogs have not responded to bethanechol, presumably because of secondary detrusor atony.

Confirming sympathetic involvement is more problematic. Orthostatic hypotension can be documented by measuring blood pressure in the thoracic and pelvic limbs with the dog first in lateral recumbency and then tilted at a 30- to 45-degree angle. In normal dogs this has little effect on blood pressure. In the dogs with dysautonomia, blood pressure drops in the elevated limbs and increases in the down limbs. Heart rate is usually within normal limits but does not increase as expected when the blood pressure drops. Provocative challenges with drugs that affect heart rate and blood pressure are not recommended owing to the risk of deleterious effects. The wheal and flare response to histamine depends on normal sympathetic innervation of the blood vessels. Thus, dogs with dysautonomia should not respond normally to intradermal histamine, but this has not been evaluated systematically.

THERAPY

Because the cause of dysautonomia is still unknown, we are limited to symptomatic therapy. Cholinergic drugs can help relieve some of the signs of parasympathetic dysfunction. Bethanechol (1.25 to 5 mg q12hr) given orally provided some improvement in secretion and urination, but better results have been seen with subcutaneous administration (started at 0.04 mg/kg q12hr and slowly increased as necessary). Frequent expressing of the bladder will be necessary if the bladder does not empty adequately with the bethanechol. Pilocarpine eye drops will stimulate tear production and relieve photophobia. Use of artificial tears is also beneficial. Gastrointestinal motility can be improved by the use of prokinetic drugs such as metaclopramide (Sidmack Laboratories). Humidifying the air can help relieve some of the dryness to the oral and nasal mucous membranes. Parenteral nutrition may be necessary to prevent the development of cachexia.

The prognosis in dysautonomia is grave. In the feline epidemic, mortality was about 70% (Edney et al, 1987), and our experience with the canine disease suggests a similar high mortality. Animals who survived have been largely left with permanent dysfunction and require intensive nursing care. One dog recovered after 3 months with only dilated pupils and occasional regurgitation as residual signs. He died 2½ years later of unrelated causes. Dysautonomia was confirmed at necropsy. Fortunately, the disease appears to still be uncommon, but the increasing number of cases seen in the Midwest raises the concern that an epidemic such as occurred in cats in England could be on the horizon.

References and Suggested Reading

Bannister R: Autonomic Failure. New York: Oxford Medical Publications, 1988.
    Textbook of clinical disorders of the autonomic nervous system in humans.
Edney ATB, Gaskell CJ, Sharp NJH, eds: Feline dysautonomia—an emerging disease. J Small Anim Pract 28:333, 1987.
    Symposium reviewing the emergence of the feline disease as well as background on the equine and human disease.
Longshore RC, O'Brien DP, Johnson GC, et al: Dysautonomia in dogs—a retrospective study. J Vet Intern Med 10:103, 1996
    Report of the first 11 necropsy-confirmed cases in the midwest United States.

O'Brien DP, ed: The autonomic nervous system: Functions and dysfunctions. Semin Vet Med Surg (Small Anim) 5:1, 1990.
  Reviews of the anatomy, physiology and diseases of the autonomic nervous system. Note that the recommendations for evaluation of the pupils have changed, as outlined in this article.

Wise LA, Lappin MR: Canine dysautonomia. Semin Vet Med Surg (Small Anim) 5:72, 1990.
  Review of the early cases of canine dysautonomia.

Seizure Management in Dogs

MICHAEL PODELL
Columbus, Ohio

Epilepsy is the most common neurologic problem seen in the dog. Any dog has the potential to undergo a seizure, and it is often very difficult to predict when, why, or how often the seizures will occur. To complicate matters, many dogs that have experienced a seizure appear completely normal in the examination room. Thus, the clinician must often formulate a diagnostic and therapeutic plan based on a normal examination and unpredictable occurrence of signs. This article has been designed to present 15 guiding principles in the management of seizures in dogs as a means for the clinician to develop a sound foundation in canine epilepsy treatment. Although the specific therapy for seizure disorders may change with time, gaining the fundamental knowledge about this condition will allow veterinarians to adapt future therapeutic advances to their clinical practice.

THE BRAIN IS SIMILAR TO OTHER ORGANS IN THE BODY

The brain is an organ that can get sick and recover, similar to other body systems. The brain is a remarkably resilient organ, with a tremendous capacity to overcome serious pathophysiologic insults. In particular, the large number of neurons in the cerebral cortex affords a greater relative plasticity compared with other parts of the central nervous system. Overlapping and underutilized cerebral cortical function in the dog also allows function to return after significant loss has occurred. Conversely, significant pathologic alterations may be present in the cerebral cortex (e.g., tumors) of dogs, with minimal neurologic deficits.

Epileptic seizures are a sign of a sick brain. The outcome of the illness may vary from the benign (no treatment necessary), to the managed situation (treatment with one drug), to the unmanaged situation (requiring treatment with multiple drugs), to death. Each of these scenarios can occur without any evidence of structural pathology of the brain. Thus, all epileptic seizures in the dog should be taken seriously, and are best approached in a similar fashion.

BE CERTAIN THAT EPILEPTIC SEIZURES HAVE OCCURRED

In making the diagnosis, it is essential to ascertain that an epileptic seizure has occurred. A *seizure* is defined as a nonspecific, "sudden, often catastrophic event." An *epileptic seizure* is the clinical manifestation of excessive and/or hypersynchronous abnormal neuronal activity in the cerebral cortex. Thus, an epileptic seizure has a specific neural origin, which is not true of all seizures. Many events may mimic epileptic seizures. Distinguishing nonepileptic seizures is just as important, inasmuch as an incorrect diagnosis could lead to failure to identify another serious medical condition, administering unnecessary medication to the dog, and undue emotional and financial strain on the owner. More common causes of non-neurologic, nonepileptic seizures are syncope of cardiovascular origin, metabolic disturbances (e.g., transient hypoglycemia, endocrine diseases), and toxicities. The major neurologic causes of nonepileptic seizures are acute vestibular attacks (often peripheral in nature), narcolepsy, and a myasthenia gravis crisis. In practically all instances, dogs with nonepileptic seizures will not exhibit postictal effects. Possible exceptions are dogs that demonstrate autonomic release phenomena (e.g., urination) after a syncopal episode, and dogs with vestibular disease that continue to appear disoriented from their vertigo.

IDENTIFY THE SEIZURE ETIOLOGY

The most important aspect of seizure management is knowing the underlying cause. The etiology of epileptic seizures (ES) in dogs generally falls into one of three basic categories of diagnosis: primary (PES; idiopathic), secondary (SES; structural pathology in the brain), and reactive (RES; a normal brain reacting to an abnormal metabolic problem). Dogs with recurring PES or SES are classified as having epilepsy. The differential diagnoses in terms of prevalence of diagnosis differs according the age at onset of the seizure. Overall, dogs that present at less than 1 or greater than 5 years of age, have an initial interictal interval of less than 4 weeks, or have a partial seizure as the first observed seizure should carry a high suspicion for an underlying identifiable etiology for their seizures with appropriate diagnostic tests done (Podell, 1995).

ALWAYS TREAT THE UNDERLYING DISEASE

Secondary or RES can be viewed as a sign of the underlying disease. This sign can potentially be eliminated or greatly reduced by directing specific therapy to the primary diagnosis. For RES, antiepileptic drug (AED) therapy is often not needed, or only for a short duration. An example is hepatic encephalopathy from a congenital portosystemic shunt (see *CVT XII*, p. 1153). Neoplastic, inflammatory, or vascular accidents of the brain may be treated successfully to reduce or even eliminate seizures.

START AED TREATMENT EARLY IN THE COURSE OF DISEASE

The earlier AED therapy is started, the better the potential outcome may be for seizure control. The decision to initiate AED therapy is based on the underlying etiology, seizure type and frequency, and diagnostic evaluation. Indications to begin phenobarbital are listed in Table 1. A log should be maintained by the owner to document observed seizures and record problems in order to provide an objective method of deciding when to start therapy, or determine the benefit of therapy.

START WITH THE APPROPRIATE AED

Limiting total AED dosage is advantageous and a goal in treating epileptic dogs. With any AED drug, there is a balance between seizure control and quality of life afforded. As such, monotherapy is recommended to reduce adverse effects, allow better owner compliance, and reduce overall costs. Unfortunately, the dog cannot be treated safely or effectively with the majority of available, nonsedating AEDs due to potential hepatotoxicity or rapid drug metabolism. As a result, phenobarbital and bromide are the most widely used initial AEDs. Unfortunately, both drugs have the potential adverse effects of sedation and/or a less active lifestyle for the dog. Phenobarbital is a relatively inexpensive, well-tolerated drug that can be administered two to three times per day with well-documented success to prevent seizures in animals. Oral and IV dosing instructions are listed in Table 1.

Bromide monotherapy has yet to be proved effective as a first-line AED. One potential problem is that it may take upward of 4 months to achieve a steady concentration of bromide in the brain. Dogs may suffer from "unprotected" serum concentrations during this period.

MONITOR TROUGH SERUM CONCENTRATIONS

The objectives of monitoring trough serum concentrations of an AED are to:

1. Determine whether a therapeutic value is present at the time when the lowest serum concentration is present, inasmuch as dogs will be most susceptible to seizure at this time.
2. Document that serum concentration fluctuates within the established therapeutic range for that drug when chronically administered (steady-state concentration).
3. Prevent toxic effects from occurring.
4. Individualize therapy.

Serum trough concentrations of phenobarbital should be measured at 14, 45, 90, 180, and 360 days after the initiation of treatment, at 6-month intervals thereafter, if at any point a dog has more than two seizure events between these scheduled times, or 2 weeks after a dosage change. Blood samples are best taken in the early morning, prior to dosing, in a fasted dog. This increases consistency in comparison to published information and removes diurnal fluctuation of absorption. To avoid factitious decreases in drug concentration, blood samples should not be submitted in serum separation tubes (Booth, 1996; also see p. 26).

KNOW HOW AND WHEN TO ADJUST THE DOSAGE: TO SEDATE OR TOO SEDATE

Adjustments in AED dosages are done either to enhance the effect or to reduce the adverse effects. The most effective trough therapeutic phenobarbital range for the dog is 20 to 40 μg/ml. An optimal starting level is between 20 to 25 μg/ml. Increasing concentration in 5 μg/ml increments is beneficial if seizures are occurring at an equal frequency or worsening after 30 days of therapy. Some dogs may take 30 to 60 days to stabilize the metabolic tolerance associated with autoinduction of the hepatic p450 system. Adjustments of the trough phenobarbital concentration can be calculated with the following formula:

$$\left(\frac{DC}{AC}\right) \times \text{mg PB} = \text{Total mg PB}$$

This new value can then be divided either b.i.d. or t.i.d. The only advantage of t.i.d. administration is less fluctuation between the peak and trough serum concentrations, which may be important in animals requiring tighter therapeutic windows. Note that no adjustment is made according to weight and no upper limit dosage is present. Peak levels are taken 4 to 6 hours after dosing if toxic effects are anticipated. Remember that serum drug concentrations are only a guide and that each dog must be individually managed.

MAKE SURE THERE IS GOOD OWNER COMPLIANCE IN DOSING AND MONITORING

Owners should be sent home with a specialized calendar to record seizure events, adverse effects, and changes in drug dosing. A 20% or greater drop in the trough serum concentration is often an indicator of poor administration compliance. Ensure that the owner is giving the drugs at regular intervals, and that the dog is not managing to spit out pills (behind couches and backyards are favorite hiding places). Plan future re-evaluations on this calendar at the time the first prescription is written.

KNOW WHEN AND HOW TO ADD OR CHANGE MEDICATIONS

Antiepileptic drug therapy should be changed when either no improvement in seizure control is seen despite maximal trough therapeutic serum concentration and/or

TABLE 1. Summary of Antiepileptic Drug Therapy in the Dog

Drug	Indications	Administration	Monitoring	Potential Adverse Effects
Phenobarbital	Identification of a structural lesion Status epilepticus Two or more isolated seizures within an 8-wk period Two or more cluster seizures episodes within a 12-wk period The first observed seizure is within a week of head trauma Prolonged, severe, or unusual postictal periods	Initial oral dose: 2.5 mg/kg PO b.i.d. IV loading dose: Total mg IV = (Body weight [kg]) × (0.8 L/kg) × (25 µg/ml)	Measure trough serum phenobarbital Therapeutic range is between 20 and 40 µg/ml Evaluate serum chemistry panel at 45 days and every 6 months	Transient: lethargy, behavior change Persistent: polyuria, polydipsia, polyphagia, weight gain, excessive sedation Severe: hepatotoxicity
Potassium bromide	Persistent seizure activity with steady state trough serum phenobarbital concentration > 30 µg/ml for at least 1 month Hepatotoxicity from phenobarbital or primary hepatic disease (e.g., portosystemic shunt) Severe cluster seizures	Potassium bromide dissolved in double-distilled water as 200 mg/ml solution Dose: 20–30 mg/kg/day orally in food as initial dose	Measure trough serum concentrations 30 days, 120 days, and every 6 months after initiation. Therapeutic range is 100–200 mg/dl (1.0–2.0 mg/ml) with concurrent phenobarbital (25–30 µg/ml)	Lethargy Polydipsia, polyuria Pancreatitis Ataxia Stupor
Felbamate	Complex partial seizures Refractory to phenobarbital and bromide therapy	Initial dose: 20 mg/kg PO t.i.d. Maximum dose: 1,200 mg PO t.i.d.	Therapeutic range is 20–100 mg/L (expensive) Monitor complete blood counts every 6–12 weeks to check for bone marrow suppression Monitor liver enzymes every 6–12 weeks to check for hepatotoxicity	Hepatotoxicity (people) Aplastic anemia (people) Gastrointestinal upset
Gabapentin	Complex partial seizures Refractory to phenobarbital and bromide therapy	Initial dose: 300 mg PO b.i.d. Increase: Up to 1,200 mg PO t.i.d. over 4 weeks	No benefit of drug monitoring	Sedation No organ toxicity reported
Diazepam per rectum	Generalized cluster epileptic seizures Status epilepticus	On phenobarbital: 2 mg/kg per rectum of diazepam parenteral solution (5 mg/ml) Administer at the onset of a seizure up to three times in 24 hours	Instruct owners to stay with pet for 1 hour after administration	Sedation

when toxic effects are developing. The potential for hepatotoxicity for the dog increases when the trough serum phenobarbital concentration is greater than 35 μg/ml (Dayrell-Hart, 1991). Furthermore, dogs will rarely benefit in seizure control from increases in dosage at this level. At this time, the epileptic dog can be labeled refractory to phenobarbital.

The recommended add-on AED of choice in the dog is bromide (Podell and Fenner, 1993). Bromide is administered as the inorganic salt, potassium bromide, as a 200 mg/ml solution dissolved in double-distilled water. Bromide can be started at 20 to 30 mg/kg/day divided every 12 hours given in food. This protocol allows for a gradual adaptation to the cumulative sedative effects of bromide and phenobarbital. Dosages are then adjusted based on trough serum concentrations (see Table 1). When bromide approaches a steady-state serum concentration in the therapeutic range, the clinician can attempt to decrease the total daily phenobarbital dose. My ultimate goal is to achieve steady-state trough serum concentrations of 25 μg/ml and 150 to 200 mg/dl for phenobarbital and bromide, respectively. Further reductions in phenobarbital can be attempted if a seizure-free period is maintained for 6 months. Some dogs can be successfully weaned off of phenobarbital when steady-state bromide serum concentrations are obtained. Higher concentrations may be needed for bromide monotherapy (200 to 300 mg/dl).

Several new AEDs have recently been introduced. Efficacy in the dog has not been documented for any of these drugs. Felbamate (Felbatol) is believed to increase seizure threshold and prevent seizure spreading by reducing excitatory neurotransmission in the brain. Several dogs with complex partial and generalized seizures have been successfully managed with felbamate at The Ohio State University Veterinary Teaching Hospital. In dogs with partial seizures, immediate and long-term resolution of all seizures can be achieved. Dosing recommendations based on this experience are listed in Table 1. Recently, a higher incidence of aplastic anemia and liver toxicity was found in people treated with felbamate compared with the general population. As such, concurrent phenobarbital therapy is not recommended. Overall, felbamate may prove to be a beneficial AED in dogs after controlled clinical trials have been completed.

Gabapentin (Neurontin) is an interesting new AED whose mechanism of action is still not fully understood. Initially designed to mimic GABA (the major inhibitory neurotransmitter) in the brain, gabapentin does not have the same pharmacologic properties of GABA nor does it bind to GABA receptors. A major benefit of the drug is that it is not metabolized by the liver; thus it can be used in conjunction with drugs with hepatic elimination, such as phenobarbital. Gabapentin may be tried with phenobarbital at doses listed in Table 1. Potential adverse effects include excessive sedation and gastrointestinal upset.

KNOW WHEN AN EMERGENCY SITUATION IS PRESENT

Dogs should be considered to require emergency therapy if:

1. A single generalized seizure persists for greater than 5 minutes.

2. Status epilepticus occurs. This is defined as a state of continuous seizure activity lasting longer than 30 minutes or repeated seizures with impaired consciousness if the recurrence rate does permit a return of consciousness.

3. A dog has more than one seizure per hour for 3 consecutive hours, regardless of seizure length.

4. A dog has more than three seizures per day, regardless of seizure length.

Two main components are essential in treating seizures in the emergency situation: restoring homeostatic conditions and providing specific seizure treatment. Specific seizure treatment can be divided into successive phases. Initial phases involve the initiation of both a short-acting AED to stop immediate seizure activity and a long-acting AED to prevent further seizures. Diazepam is the drug of choice in treating prolonged convulsions, including status epilepticus and cluster seizures, at a dose of 0.5 mg/kg IV (up to 3 times in a 24 hour period). A loading dose of phenobarbital is then administered, followed by initiation of maintenance phenobarbital (see above). Further treatment can involve either continuous diazepam intravenous drip (0.1 to 0.3/mg/kg per hour), parenteral pentobarbital, or inhalation gas anesthesia (isoflurane) to stop seizures. To implement this protocol, it is important for a clinician to have access to injectable AEDs and a 24-hour monitoring facility (Podell, 1996).

PRESCRIBE AT-HOME DIAZEPAM THERAPY FOR DOGS WITH CLUSTER SEIZURES

A safe, affordable home treatment for cluster seizures is available to reduce owner cost, decrease patient morbidity, and contribute positively to the overall AED therapy. A study at The Ohio State University demonstrated that home therapy of dogs with idiopathic epilepsy and generalized cluster seizures using diazepam, per rectum, at a dose at 0.5 mg/kg, was associated with a significant decrease in the number of cluster seizure events in a 24-hour period, a decrease in the total number of seizure events when compared with an identical time period without such therapy, and a significant decrease in the total cost in emergency care per dog, as compared with a similar time period prior to the onset of use of diazepam per rectum (Podell, 1995).

Recent pharmacokinetic studies of diazepam per rectum from our laboratory in nontreated dogs found that chronic phenobarbital dosing significantly reduced total benzodiazepine plasma levels in the dog (Wagner et al, 1998). As a result, dogs on phenobarbital can receive up to 2 mg/kg diazepam, per rectum, up to 3 times in a 24-hour period without significant adverse effects (but not within 15 minutes of each other) to stop cluster seizures (see Table 1). The parenteral solution of diazepam (5 mg/ml) is injected through a plastic teat cannula with a water-soluble lubricant. The diazepam should be stored in the glass dispenser vial because the plastic syringe will adsorb the drug.

KNOW WHEN TO DISCONTINUE MEDICATIONS

Stopping AED therapy is always a gamble. Dogs that are seizure-free for 1 year or longer are candidates for phenobarbital withdrawal. Certain breeds with proven or highly suspected inherited epilepsy (e.g., German shepherds, Siberian huskies, Keeshonds) probably should not have their phenobarbital stopped due to the high likelihood that seizures will recur in these dogs. Phenobarbital withdrawal must be gradual because withdrawal seizures may occur. A 25% reduction every 2 weeks until the trough serum concentration is less than 15 μg/ml can help to prevent this withdrawal reaction. At this time, phenobarbital can be stopped. Reintroduction of therapy is recommended if three or more seizures occur within the ensuing first year.

CALL THE CLIENT BEFORE THE CLIENT CALLS YOU

Seizure prevention is better than intervention. It is important to stay in regular contact with the owners. Because seizures may occur randomly, owners may "lose" track of time or be unaware of a pattern suggesting a change in seizure type or severity. Owners should be contacted every 3 to 6 months, at a minimum. The most important time is the first year after starting therapy. Achieving good seizure control during this time in a first-time treated idiopathic epileptic dog can lead to a rewarding relationship between the client and veterinarian.

CONSULT A SPECIALIST IF YOUR PLAN IS NOT WORKING

Not every epileptic dog can be managed successfully with the above guidelines. Individualized therapy beyond what can be described in a short review article may still be needed. Moreover, newer therapeutic protocols may be available to offer to your patients. A specialist can often provide important insights to help the common goal of improving your patient's quality of life.

References and Suggested Reading

Booth DM, Simpson G, Foster T: Effects of serum separation tubes on serum benzodiazepine and phenobarbital concentrations in clinically normal and epileptic dogs. Am J Vet Res 57:1299, 1996.

Dayrell-Hart B, Steinberg SA, Van Winkle TJ, et al: Hepatotoxicity of phenobarbital in dogs: 18 cases (1985–1989). J Am Vet Med Assoc 199:1060, 1991.

Podell M: The use of diazepam per rectum at home for the acute management of cluster seizures in dogs. J Vet Intern Med 8:68, 1995.

Podell M: Seizures in dogs. Vet Clin North Am Small Anim Pract 26:779, 1996.

Podell M, Fenner WR: Bromide therapy in refractory canine idiopathic epilepsy. J Vet Intern Med 7:318, 1993.

Podell M, Fenner WR, Powers JD: Seizure classification in dogs from a nonreferral-based population. J Am Vet Med Assoc 206:1721, 1995.

Theodore WH, Porter RJ: Epilepsy: 100 Elementary Principles, 3rd ed. Philadelphia: WB Saunders, 1995.

Wagner SO, Sams R, Podell M: Chronic phenobarbital therapy reduces plasma benzodiazepine concentrations after intravenous and rectal administration of diazepam in the dog. J Vet Pharmacol Therap 21:335, 1998.

Feline Seizure Disorders

LINDA G. SHELL
Blacksburg, Virginia

GENERAL INFORMATION

Types of Seizures

A seizure is an episode of abnormal brain wave activity that commonly causes a loss or change in consciousness. Signs often include chewing, involuntary limb movements and twitching of muscles, salivation, urination, defecation, and dilation of pupils. Changes usually last seconds to 1 or 2 minutes. Such seizures are classified as generalized motor seizures ("grand mal"). The partial motor seizure, manifested by involuntary movements only on one side of the body, is frequently associated with structural brain damage (e.g., trauma, infection, neoplasia) on the side opposite the involuntary movement. A partial seizure can become generalized (the left limbs begin moving, followed by movement of all limbs).

Postictal Signs

After a seizure, the cat may appear normal or may have postictal ataxia, confusion, aggression, or other behavioral changes. Postictal changes last minutes to several hours and are more likely to be present and prolonged after a series of severe generalized seizures.

Epilepsy

A seizure is one episode of abnormal brain wave activity, whereas epilepsy is seizure activity that recurs weeks or months apart and sometimes days apart. Many cases of epilepsy have normal mentation and gait in between the seizure activity. Epilepsy is divided into two types: primary and secondary (Shell, 1993).

Primary Epilepsy

Primary epilepsy refers to recurrent seizures that have no underlying disease; a physiologic or biochemical genetic basis for the seizures is suspected. The emphasis is on "suspected" because primary epilepsy is impossible to confirm without study of the family tree and exclusion of secondary epilepsy in family members with recurrent seizures. Thus, the diagnosis of primary epilepsy is difficult to prove; the closest that we can usually get is to exclude all other possible causes for recurrent seizures. In dogs, primary epilepsy usually develops between 1 and 4 years of age. We assume this same age range applies to cats. However, not enough cats with primary epilepsy have been studied to know for sure.

In general, primary epilepsy should cause generalized seizure activity; the neurologic examination should be normal in between the seizure episodes. All ancillary tests should have normal or nonsignificant results, including routine laboratory work, spinal fluid analysis, and specialized imaging (computed tomography [CT] or magnetic resonance imaging [MRI] scans). In my experience, primary epilepsy is uncommon in cats in the United States. It appears more common in Europe (Schwartz-Porsche and Kaiser, 1989).

Secondary Epilepsy

Secondary epilepsy refers to seizures for which there is an underlying structural lesion such as trauma, neoplasia, hypoxia, infection, and ischemia. Partial seizures or partial seizures with secondary generalization may be more commonly found with secondary epilepsy. In my experience, secondary epilepsy is more common than primary epilepsy in cats.

The treatment for both types of recurrent seizures or epilepsy is anticonvulsants. However, with secondary epilepsy, underlying causes of the recurrent seizures should be treated if possible. An example is congenital hydrocephalus, in which seizure control may be improved if spinal fluid production is decreased with corticosteroid usage.

CAUSES OF SEIZURES

I approach the numerous causes of seizures with a mnemonic device: DAMNNIITT-VP. These letters stand for the following disease processes: Degenerative, Anomalous, Metabolic, Neoplastic, Nutritional, Inflammatory, Idiopathic, Traumatic, Toxic, Vascular, and Parasitic. Table 1 lists potential causes of seizures in cats (Shell, 1991).

DIAGNOSTIC APPROACH

Minimum Database

If a seizure is described or suspected, a minimum feline database, consisting of a complete blood count, chemistry profile, urinalysis, and testing for feline leukemia and immunodeficiency viruses, is recommended. Middle-aged (5+ years) and older cats should also be evaluated for hyperthyroidism. The reason for such tests is twofold. First, because most seizures in cats are from acquired diseases, there is a small chance that disease will be reflected in routine blood work, which is less invasive and less expensive than a spinal tap or CT or MRI scans. An example is the cat who has seizures due to polycythemia or erythrocytosis. Second, it is wise to make sure the cat does not have another concurrent disease that may limit the neurologic work-up.

TABLE 1. Possible Causes of Seizures in Cats

Anomalous:	Congenital hydrocephalus, lissencephaly, lysosomal storage disease
Metabolic:	Hepatic encephalopathy, uremia, hypoglycemia, hypocalcemia, polycythemia
Neoplastic:	Primary brain tumors, metastatic brain tumors
Nutritional:	Thiamine deficiency
Inflammatory:	Feline infectious peritonitis virus, feline immunodeficiency virus, systemic fungal infections, toxoplasmosis, bacterial infections, pseudorabies virus, rabies virus, polioencephalomyelitis
Idiopathic:	Feline hyperesthesia syndrome, primary epilepsy
Traumatic:	Head trauma
Toxic:	Lead, organophosphates, ethylene glycol, others
Vascular:	Ischemic encephalopathy
Parasitic:	Aberrant migration of *Cuterebra* larvae or adult *Dirofilaria immitis*

From Shell LG: Seizures in cats. Proc Sheba Feline Med Symposium 1991, p 25, with permission.

An example is the older cat that may not have historical or clinical signs of renal failure but is obviously in chronic renal failure when the laboratory work is examined; owners may not wish to pursue a neurologic work-up for seizures and there is the outside possibility that the renal disease is contributing to the seizures. Another example is the cat that is feline leukemia virus–positive. Until I can determine whether the infection is transient or permanent, it may not be wise to pursue the seizure problem unless seizures are frequent enough to warrant anticonvulsants.

Neurologic Database

A neurologic examination should be performed. If the cat is abnormal in-between the seizures and has a normal minimum database, one should suspect intracranial disease. Other tests include spinal fluid analysis, (see *CVT XII*, p. 1121), electroencephalography, or CT or MRI scans of the brain.

TREATMENT APPROACH

Stopping a Seizure

If a cat is having a seizure, administer diazepam at a dose of 0.5 to 1 mg/kg IV unless there is a history of insulin therapy (in which case glucose may be more beneficial) or exposure to chlorpyrifos. Diazepam may potentiate the signs of acute organophosphate activity in cats exposed to chlorpyrifos (Jaggy and Oliver, 1990).

Ideally, a hemogram and blood chemistry profile should be evaluated for abnormalities that might precipitate seizures, especially if this is the first seizure. If complete laboratory work is unavailable in an emergency situation, a blood glucose level should be evaluated because hypoglycemic-induced seizures occasionally occur and can be treated immediately. Prolonged seizure activity can also deplete glucose stores and result in hypoglycemia. If hypoglycemia is suspected or documented, administer 1 to 2 ml/kg of 50% dextrose IV. Because this solution is extremely hypertonic and may irritate endothelial cells of peripheral blood vessels, dilute with sterile water or administer via a central vein. Alternatively, one can rub Karo syrup or honey on the cat's buccal mucosa.

Stopping Multiple Seizures

Because diazepam is eliminated more slowly in cats than dogs, one dose is usually sufficient. If necessary it can be administered up to three times per hour; however, respiratory depression may occur. If it is administered more than four times within an 8-hour period, I recommend beginning maintenance phenobarbital to prevent further seizure activity. Phenobarbital (2 mg/kg) can be administered IV or IM every 6 to 8 hours if the cat is unable to swallow the pill or elixir form.

TREATMENT APPROACH TO MAINTENANCE THERAPY

Keep a Record

One episode of seizure activity does not warrant long-term anticonvulsant medication in the majority of cases. Owners should, however, keep a concise record, including dates, description, and duration of all future episodes. Future episodes should be communicated to the veterinarian and owners should be made aware that repeat physical and neurologic examinations or blood work may be necessary.

When to Start Maintenance Anticonvulsants

As a guideline, anticonvulsants are recommended if the cat has more than three to four seizure episodes within a year. Any time there is enough evidence that the cat is having repeated seizures without an obvious reason, anticonvulsants should be considered. Prior to prescribing long-term anticonvulsants, a hemogram and blood chemistry profile should be evaluated. It is also wise to rule out extracranial diseases such as portosystemic shunts, arrhythmias, and metabolic diseases (hypoglycemia, electrolyte disturbances, polycythemia) because anticonvulsants are not likely to effectively treat clinical signs associated with these disorders.

Phenobarbital

Phenobarbital, my drug of choice, has an elimination half-life of 34 to 43 hours in cats. The recommended dosage is 1 to 2 mg/kg PO every 12 hours. Although feline therapeutic serum concentrations have not been determined, recommended concentrations should be between 10 and 30 μg/ml (Dyer and Shell, 1993). Some clinicians recommend checking a serum phenobarbital level 2 weeks after beginning therapy to make sure the dose is within therapeutic range. I evaluate serum phenobarbital levels annually or whenever seizure control is inadequate. Common side effects of phenobarbital can include ataxia, lethargy, and excessive thirst, appetite, or urination. Bone marrow hypoplasia and immune-mediated reactions are rare.

Diazepam

Diazepam appears to be an effective anticonvulsant in cats because unlike dogs, cats do not appear to develop a tolerance to the anticonvulsive effects of diazepam. Unpublished studies suggest that the half-life is 15 to 20 hours (Dyer and Shell, 1993). The recommended dose is 0.25 to 0.5 mg/kg PO every 8 to 12 hours. However, hepatotoxicosis has been reported as an adverse reaction with clinical signs beginning 5 to 11 days after beginning oral administration at recommended doses (Center et al, 1996). Thus, baseline serum biochemical screening is recommended prior to beginning diazepam. Diazepam should be discontinued and serum biochemical profile performed if emesis, lethargy, decreased appetite, or ataxia develops.

Other Anticonvulsants

I rarely use primidone in cats because phenobarbital or diazepam usually works well. In one study, normal cats that were administered primidone at a dose of 40 mg/kg divided three times daily for 3 months had no hematologic, serum chemical, electroencephalographic, or hepatic histologic changes (Sawchuk et al, 1985). The half-life of 7 hours did not change during the study. More reports concerning its effectiveness in clinical cases are needed. It has been recommended as one possible treatment for feline hyperesthesia syndrome.

Bromide (30 mg/kg per day PO) has been used by the author in a few cats that have not responded adequately to phenobarbital or have had a toxic reaction to phenobarbital. A recent study found that steady-state levels were reached at 7 to 8 weeks in normal cats and the mean elimination half-life was 1.5 weeks (Boothe et al, 1996). It is likely that the dosage range for dogs (20 to 40 mg/kg per day PO) will apply to cats, but longer term studies in more cats are needed before we can conclude that cats are exempt from any side effects.

Phenytoin is not used as an anticonvulsant in cats because its long half-life of 41.5 hours in this species makes toxicity more likely to occur. Signs of toxicity in the cat include sedation, ataxia, and decreased appetite.

ADEQUATE AND INADEQUATE CONTROL

Adequate Control

If the owner keeps a record or diary of seizures, it will be rather easy to determine if anticonvulsants are working or not. If the seizures are less frequent and/or less severe in nature, the anticonvulsant is working. Ideally, seizures should not occur more than three or four times per year, but in difficult cases, less than one seizure per month is acceptable.

Inadequate Control

If seizure control has not improved after 1 month of phenobarbital or diazepam, then a serum blood level should be evaluated. If the level is within the low end of the therapeutic range, the dose can be increased by one fourth to one half for 1 month. If seizure control is still unacceptable, consider performing more tests (if not done already) to rule in progressive or active diseases. If further testing is not feasible, increase the dose again and take a serum level 2 weeks later. If the level is at the high end of normal or above normal, then one should consider using another anticonvulsant (e.g., bromide) and/or looking for underlying progressive brain disease. If active brain disease and metabolic disorders have already been eliminated or the owner does not wish to pursue other testing, then the only alternative is to increase the dose of anticonvulsant, switch to another anticonvulsant, or try nonconventional therapy (e.g., acupuncture, all-natural diet, taurine supplementation).

WEANING CATS FROM ANTICONVULSANTS

If a cat is free from seizures for a year or more, you can try weaning it *slowly* from the anticonvulsant. The rule of thumb is to decrease the anticonvulsant dose by one eighth every 2 weeks, which can be difficult given some pill sizes. Using an elixir or having a pharmacy compound the pills into the right dosage may work. If you wean too rapidly, a withdrawal seizure could develop not necessarily as a result of the epilepsy, but as a result of addiction to the anticonvulsant. If the cat has a seizure during the weaning phase or anytime thereafter, it should be maintained on the anticonvulsant indefinitely. Weaning is not a common occurrence in either cats or dogs.

References and Suggested Reading

Boothe D, Nguyen J, Legrange S: Disposition of bromide in cats following oral administration of the potassium salt. Proceedings of the 14th ACVIM Forum, 1996. p 757.
    An abstract concerning the pharmacokinetics of bromide in cats.
Center SA, Elston TH, Rowland PH, et al: Fulminant hepatic failure associated with oral administration of diazepam in 11 cats. J Am Vet Med Assoc 209:618, 1996.
    Case reports describing the clinical signs, hematologic changes, and liver histopathologic changes associated with diazepam-induced liver failure.
Dyer KR, Shell LG: Anticonvulsant therapy: A practical guide to medical management of epilepsy in pets. Vet Med 88:647, 1993.
    A review of the anticonvulsants used in cats and dogs, with emphasis on phenobarbital and bromide.
Jaggy A, Oliver JE: Chlorpyrifos toxicosis in two cats. J Vet Intern Med 4:135, 1990.
    Case report describing the clinical signs and treatment of chlorpyrifos toxicosis.
Sawchuk SA, Parker AJ, Neff-Davis C, et al: Primidone in the cat. J Am Anim Hosp Assoc 21:647, 1985.
    A study of the hematologic, biochemical, and histopathologic changes in normal cats administered primidone for 3 months.
Schwartz-Porsche D, Kaiser E: Feline epilepsy. Prob Vet Med 1:628, 1989.
    A review of seizures, epilepsy, and treatment in cats.
Shell LG: Seizures in cats. Proc Sheba Feline Med Symposium 1991, p 25.
    A review of the causes of seizures in cats.
Shell LG: Understanding the fundamentals of seizures. Vet Med 88:622, 1993.
    A review of how seizures are generated, seizure types, and types of epilepsy.

Vestibular Disease of Dogs and Cats

RODNEY S. BAGLEY
Pullman, Washington

Disease of the vestibular system results in some of the most dramatic clinical presentations seen in clinical neurology. The vestibular system is largely responsible for keeping the animal oriented with respect to gravity. Vestibular dysfunction, therefore, is reflected in malpositioning of the body including the head, limbs, and eyes. Falling, incoordination, head tilting, nystagmus, and ataxia result. This article will review the more common disease processes affecting the vestibular system of dogs and cats.

ANATOMY

The anatomic components of the vestibular system have been reviewed (deLahunta, 1983). Simplistically, the vestibular system is made up of receptor organs within the ear. These receptor organs sense the static position and movement of the head in relation to the ground (gravity). For integration of static posture, small, weighted bodies (statconia) of the vestibular receptors (macula utriculi and sacculi) within the inner ear are acted upon by gravity. Statconia lie within a gelatinous covering. Cilia from the vestibular receptor cells protrude into this gelatinous covering. The force exerted on these statconia results in deflection of the ciliated receptor, thus providing positional information that is integrated centrally.

For detection of head motion, movement of fluid (endolymph) in small tubular structures (semicircular canals) results in motion of cilia on additional receptor cells within terminal dilations (crista ampullaris). This movement of cilia excites the receptor cell which conveys this information, through the vestibular nerve, to the central components of the vestibular system. Thus, the vestibular receptors collect information regarding the movement of the head in space.

Nerve fibers coursing from these peripheral receptors form the vestibular nerve proper. The nerve itself is relatively short. Nerve fibers can then terminate in the vestibular nuclei or within parts of the cerebellum (flocculonodular lobe) associated with vestibular functions, providing the anatomic reason that vestibular-type signs can be seen with cerebellar diseases.

CLINICAL SIGNS OF VESTIBULAR DISEASE

Clinical signs of vestibular dysfunction reflect abnormal orientation of the head, limbs, and eyes. A head tilt, nystagmus, and ataxia are common, regardless of whether the disease involves the peripheral receptors (peripheral vestibular disease) or the central nuclei, cerebellum, or projection pathways (central vestibular disease). The head is usually tilted in the direction of the lesion. With lesions of the caudal cerebellar peduncle, however, the head is tilted away from the side of the lesion. An associated ipsilateral hemiparesis is often helpful in lesion localization as to the side of the lesion.

Nystagmus, a characteristic eye movement with a quick and slow phase, is often associated with vestibular dysfunction. Nystagmus can be induced normally (oculovestibular response) by turning the head from side to side. The fast phase of eye movement is in the direction that the head is moved. This slow drift and quick reset during sideways movement of the head is normal. In animals with bilateral vestibular disease, the oculovestibular response is absent. When the vestibular system is dysfunctional, the eyes have a tendency to spontaneously drift in the direction of the lesion (slow phase), and, through a brain stem reset mechanism, the eyes are quickly returned to their initial location (fast phase).

Abnormal nystagmus can occur spontaneously (present at rest) or with abnormal head positions (i.e., positional nystagmus). This latter nystagmus is only present when the head is forced in an abnormal orientation by the examiner. A positional nystagmus is most easily elicited by placing the animal upside down on its back. The direction of the nystagmus is described in relation to the horizontal axis through the palpebral fissure. With a horizontal nystagmus, eye movement is in the direction of this axis. A vertical nystagmus is in the direction perpendicular to this axis. With a rotatory nystagmus, the eye moves around the axis in either a clockwise or counterclockwise direction.

By convention, the direction of the nystagmus is described according to the direction of its fast phase. This can be confusing because the lesion is present on the side of the slow phase of the nystagmus. With peripheral lesions, the fast phase of the nystagmus is directed away from the side of lesion. With central lesions, the direction of the slow phase in relation to the side of the lesion can vary.

The vestibular system affects limb movement, normally being facilitatory to ipsilateral limb extension. A lack of vestibular input can result in ataxia or falling, and rolling. The laterally recumbent animal will prefer to lie on the side of the body with the lesion. The ipsilateral limb often will have decreased extensor tone, with the opposite side limbs having increased extensor tone. The animal may circle, usually towards the side of the lesion. Central lesions that affect the vestibular system often involve ascending and descending motor and sensory pathways to the limb. Paresis, therefore, is common. Because the vestibular influence over limb function is ipsilateral, a brain stem lesion will affect the limbs on the same side of the body as the lesion.

Normal vestibular control is also important for maintenance of the eye in a normal position within the orbit. Vestibular information is projected through the medial longitudinal fasciculus to cranial nerves III, IV, and VI. If the vestibular input is abnormal, an abnormal eye position (strabismus) may be seen when the examiner moves the head into an aberrant position. This is most readily seen as the animal's head is extended dorsally. When viewed from above, a ventral or ventrolateral strabismus is present in the eye on the affected side. The dorsal sclera of this affected eye is more exposed than in the unaffected eye.

Vomiting and nausea are common in human beings with vestibular disease and are more often associated with peripheral vestibular disease. Vomiting is also recognized in animals, more often with acute vestibular dysfunction. Nausea is difficult to assess in animals but may contribute to the anorexia often seen with acute vestibular dysfunction.

NEUROANATOMIC LOCALIZATION

Differentiation as to whether the lesion is central (within the brain stem) or peripheral (within CN VIII proper or its peripheral receptors) is important for selection of appropriate diagnostic tests (Table 1). The presence of certain clinical signs is associated with a central vestibular lesion. If these signs are not present, however, a central lesion cannot be excluded. A head tilt, horizontal or rotatory nystagmus, and ataxia can occur with both peripheral and central vestibular disease. A positional vertical nystagmus and limb paresis are the most consistent signs of central vestibular disease. With unilateral central vestibular lesions, hemiparesis may be seen ipsilateral to the lesion. Occasionally, a hemiparesis is present on the side of the body opposite to the direction of the head tilt (paradoxical vestibular syndrome). In this situation, the lesion occurs on the side of the body ipsilateral to the hemiparesis.

In dogs with bilateral peripheral vestibular abnormalities, no oculovestibular response is elicited upon head movement. The animal often has a wide-based stance. The head is held closer to the ground and may be swung in wide excursions from side to side.

TABLE 1. Differentiation of Peripheral Versus Central Vestibular Disease

Clinical Sign	Central	Peripheral
Nystagmus		
Spontaneous	Horizontal Rotatory *Vertical*	Horizontal Rotatory
Positional	*Changing*	Constant
Head tilt	Present	Present
Cranial nerve deficits	*Any other than VII*	VII
Horner's syndrome	+/−	+/−
Conscious proprioceptive abnormalities	*Present*	Absent

Once the lesion has been localized, appropriate differential diagnoses can be formulated. Unfortunately, intracranial lesions occasionally result in signs indicative of a peripheral lesion. Conversely, animals with acute, severe peripheral vestibular dysfunction may be so incapacitated that accurate interpretation of neurologic examination findings may not be possible. Because of these nuances, if the examiner is unsure of location of the lesion, an evaluation for central vestibular disease should occur concurrently with an evaluation for peripheral disease.

PERIPHERAL VESTIBULAR DISEASES

Idiopathic peripheral vestibular disease occurs in both dogs and cats (Schunk, 1990). Older dogs (canine geriatric vestibular disease) and young to middle-aged cats are most commonly affected. Cats in the Northeast are commonly affected in late summer and early fall. No cause is defined. In the Southeast, a similar syndrome is suspected to be caused in cats by eating of the tail of the blue tail lizard.

Clinical signs are of an acute peripheral vestibular disorder with nystagmus (horizontal or rotary), head tilt (toward the side of the lesion), rolling, and falling. No other neurologic signs are seen. Clinical signs are initially severe. If Horner's syndrome or facial nerve paresis is also present, other differentials should be considered. Differential diagnosis of peripheral vestibular disease include otitis interna in dogs and cats, middle ear polyps in cats, and neoplasia (squamous cell carcinoma of the middle ear) in both species. Otoscopic examination, bulla radiographs, and other advanced imaging studies (computed tomography [CT], magnetic resonance [MR] imaging) are normal.

Clinical signs of idiopathic vestibular disease usually improve dramatically in 1 to 2 weeks. The nystagmus usually resolves quickly (within the first few days). Improvements in posture and walking occur within 5 to 7 days, whereas a mild head tilt may remain persistent. Although most animals compensate well, some may have episodic ataxia when performing tasks such as jumping up on furniture. No treatment has proved beneficial and recurrence is possible.

Otitis media/interna is a common cause of vestibular dysfunction (see *CVT XII*, p. 1128). Most often this is due to a bacteria infection, either from inward extension from the external ear or migration from the pharynx via the auditory tube. Less commonly, infection stems from hematogenous spread. Foreign bodies such as grass awn migration may predispose to severe ear infections.

Clinical signs may reflect either primary ear, vestibular, or auditory dysfunction. A painful external ear and/or pain on opening the mouth is often present. It has been suggested that up to 50% of animals with otitis media/interna have associated facial nerve involvement. Otoscopic examination should be used to examine the tympanic membrane. This may be difficult in animals with severe otitis externa prior to cleansing. The tympanic membrane is often discolored (hyperemic), opaque, and bulging outward with middle ear disease. Clear to yellow fluid may be seen behind the membrane. Diagnosis may also be supported by bulla radiographs or advanced imaging studies (Remedios et al, 1991) (Fig. 1). Definitive diagnosis is made through culture

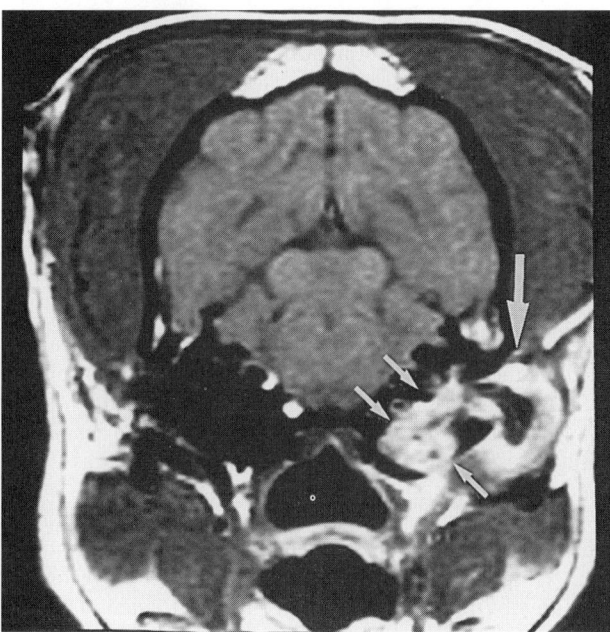

Figure 1. Transaxial, contrast-enhanced T_1-weighted magnetic resonance image of a dog with otitis externa. Note the contrast enhancing lesion within the right bulla *(small arrows)*. The external ear canal is also enhanced *(large arrow)*. Histologic diagnosis was chronic infection due to grass awn foreign body migration.

of the organism via a myringotomy or at surgical exploration.

Tumors of the ear more often occur in older animals. Squamous cell carcinoma and adenocarcinoma are most common. Inflammatory polyps occur in cats. Tumors that extend through the tympanic membrane may be seen during otoscopic examination (Fig. 2). Skull radiographs or advanced imaging is necessary to assess the middle and inner ear. Abnormalities seen with these studies, however, are not always definitive for neoplasia, and tissue diagnosis at surgery is often necessary for accurate assessment. Destruction (lysis) of the bone of the bulla is more often associated with neoplasia as compared to inflammation. Treatment options include surgical resection/debulking, radiation, and chemotherapies.

Congenital peripheral vestibular disease is seen in German shepherds, Doberman pinschers, English Cocker spaniels, Siamese and Burmese cats. While often this is an idiopathic condition, congenital peripheral vestibular disease has been associated with lymphocytic labyrinthitis in young Doberman pinschers (Forbes and Cook, 1991). Bilateral congenital vestibular disease is seen in Beagles and Akitas. Clinical signs include head tilt, ataxia, and, in some, deafness. Signs may remain persistent throughout life or may improve spontaneously. There is no treatment.

Toxicity with metronidazole may result in central vestibular signs in both dogs and cats (Dow et al, 1989; Saxon and Magne, 1993). Usually, this is associated with high doses of the drug. As metronidazole is metabolized by the liver, however, toxic serum levels can occur with appropriate doses in animals with liver dysfunction. Ataxia is usually the initial clinical sign, progressing to nystagmus and more severe vestibular dysfunction. Clinical signs often reflect central vestibular dysfunction and morphologic le-

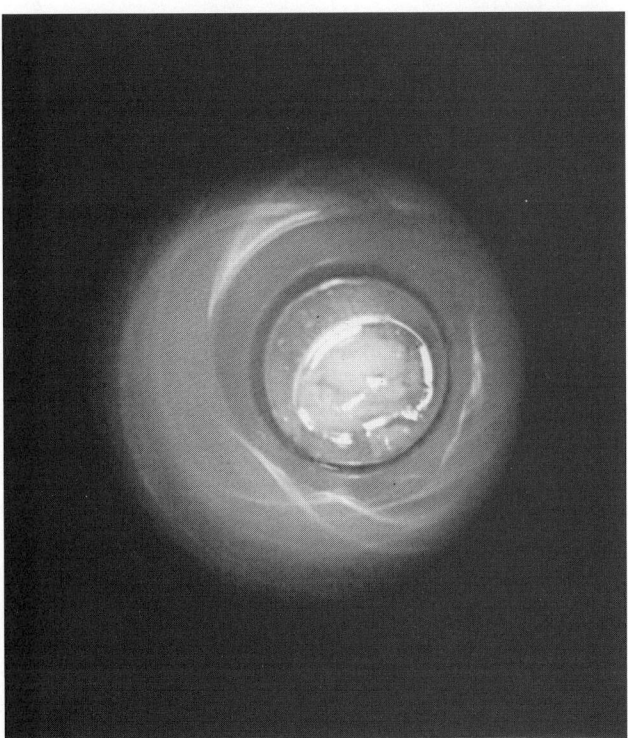

Figure 2. Otoscopic view of the external ear of a dog with a head tilt. A clear fluid is overlying a mass. Histologic diagnosis was inflammatory polyp.

sions have been found in the brain stem of affected dogs. Serum concentrations of metronidazole will be in the toxic range if measured soon after clinical signs begin. If there is a delay in collecting blood for drug concentrations after the initiation of clinical signs, serum concentrations of metronidazole may be decreased into the normal range even as the clinical signs remain persistent.

There is no specific treatment for metronidazole toxicity. Discontinuation of the drug is imperative. If clinical signs are initially severe, some dogs may die. Other dogs will recovery completely, usually over 1 to 2 weeks.

Aminoglycosides, administered either systemically or topically, may cause deafness and vestibular signs. Streptomycin and gentamicin have the most pronounced effects on the vestibular receptors, whereas neomycin, kanamycin, and amikacin preferentially damage auditory receptors. Chlorhexidine solution used to clean the external ear may result in vestibular abnormalities.

Other *idiopathic or inflammatory neuropathies* may affect the vestibular nerve. Overall, these diseases are poorly described and difficult to definitively diagnose. Similarly, a possible relationship exists between some metabolic diseases such as hypothyroidism and a vestibular neuropathy. A cause-and-effect relationship, however, is not always established.

CENTRAL VESTIBULAR DISEASES

Tumors of the infratentorial space such as meningiomas and choroid plexus tumors may cause vestibular signs due to infiltration or compression of the vestibular nerve (Fig. 3). Meningiomas may form a mass or grow in a sheet-like configuration ("en plaque"). Choroid plexus tumors arise around the fourth ventricle, often at the level of the lateral apertures. Diagnosis of a intracranial mass is made with advanced imaging studies. Lesions and associated brain structures are often better seen with MR imaging as compared with CT because beam-hardening artifact with the latter commonly obscures structural detail in this area. Surgical debulking or resection of these tumors is ideal, but is often hindered by lack of surgical exposure and intimate association with vital brain structures. Irradiation may provide some benefit by slowing tumor growth. Choroid plexus tumors, however, are relatively radiation-resistant.

Thiamine deficiency is the most common nutritional deficiency affecting the central nervous system. This deficiency most often affects cats and results in lesions in the oculomotor and vestibular nuclei, the caudal colliculus, and lateral geniculate. The earliest clinical sign is vestibular ataxia, progressing to seizures with ventral neck flexion

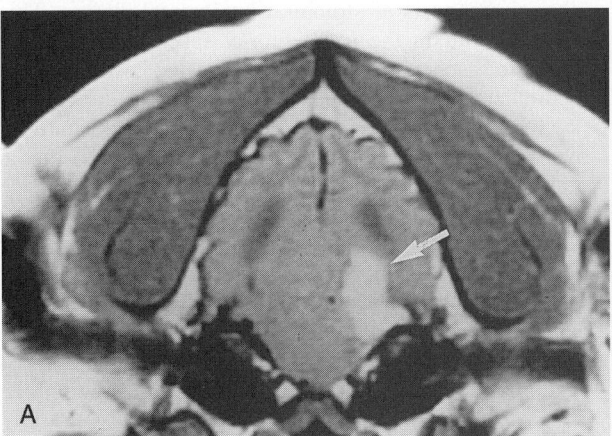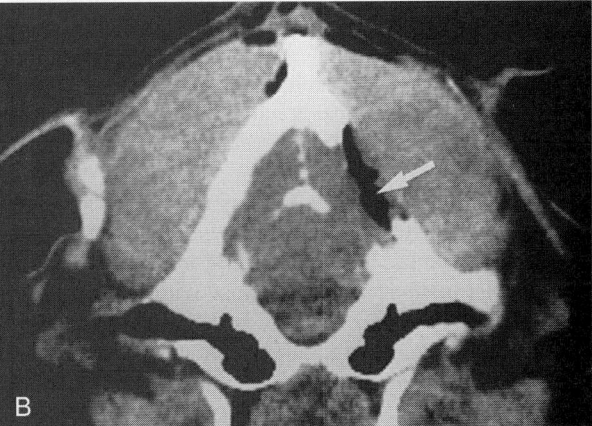

Figure 3. Preoperative, T₁-weighted contrast-enhanced magnetic resonance image *(A)* of a dog with a right head tilt. There is a contrast-enhancing mass in the right cerebellopontine angle *(arrow)*. *B*, Postoperative, contrast-enhanced computed tomography image (3B) at approximately the same level showing resection of the mass *(arrow)*. Histologic diagnosis was a meningioma.

and dilated, nonresponsive pupils. Treatment is administration of thiamine, either parenterally or intravenously.

Inflammatory disease can affect the brain stem as well as other areas of the nervous system. These include both infectious and noninfectious etiologies. The incidence of infectious diseases associated with meningitis varies with geographic location. Most meningitis syndromes (60%) in small animals do not have a definable infectious cause. Infectious agents causing brain disease include *viruses* (distemper, parvovirus, parainfluenza, herpes, feline infectious peritonitis, pseudorabies, rabies), *bacteria, rickettsia* (Rocky Mountain spotted fever, *Ehrlichia*), *spirochetes* (Lyme disease, leptospirosis), *fungi* (blastomycosis, histoplasmosis, cryptococcosis, coccidioidomycosis, aspergillosis), *protozoa* (toxoplasmosis, neosporosis), and *unclassified organisms* (prototheccosis).

Specifically, the rickettsia associated with Rocky Mountain spotted fever commonly involves the brain stem, particularly the vestibular system (Greene et al, 1985). Usually there is a history of systemic illness (usually with thrombocytopenia) 5 to 10 days prior to development of neurologic signs. As the animal's fever is decreasing, neurologic signs appear. There is no mass lesion present on intracranial advanced imaging studies. Occasionally, increased contrast enhancement is noted in the choroid plexus area in affected dogs. This must be differentiated from the degree of contrast enhancement normally seen in these structures. Cerebrospinal fluid usually contains milder increases in nucleated cells (<50 nucleated cells/μl; normal <5 nucleated cells/μl) and milder increases in protein concentration (<50 mg/dl; normal <25 mg/dl). Diagnosis is supported by increasing serum titers to the organism, but results often are available after the disease has progressed. Prognosis is dependent primarily on the severity of clinical signs prior to treatment. Dogs that are severely obtunded prior to treatment are less likely to recover. Therefore, dogs with clinical features of vestibular disease after a systemic febrile illness associated with thrombocytopenia should be treated with tetracycline or doxycycline prior to establishing a definitive diagnosis with titers.

Brain stem trauma usually occurs secondary to being hit by a car. Brain stem function can be assessed by evaluation of cranial nerve function, particularly the oculovestibular response. Occasionally, dogs have brain stem signs with cranial cervical lesions; therefore, manipulation for the oculovestibular response should be made only after assessing for unstable cervical fracture or luxations. Also, an otoscopic examination may reveal hemorrhage in the ear canals.

Diagnosis is supported by a history of a witnessed traumatic event. Skull fractures may be seen with skull radiography. Advanced imaging studies are used to assess for intracranial hemorrhage and edema. With acute trauma (within the first 12 hours), CT may be better at delineating intracranial hemorrhage. Treatments center around recognizing and treating the pathophysiologic sequelae to brain trauma such as brain edema. Surgical removal of debris or hemorrhage is occasionally necessary to stabilize intracranial pressure.

Vascular diseases that involve the central vestibular areas and associated cerebellum are uncommon. With the advent of advanced imaging studies, however, antemortem diagnosis should be improved.

DIAGNOSTIC TESTING

If a lesion is suspected to involve the central vestibular structures (forebrain, brain stem, or cerebellum) in small animals, an advanced imaging study such as CT or MR imaging is used to assess the structural integrity of these areas. These studies are noninvasive but do require anesthesia in all but the comatose animal. Survey radiographs of the skull are useful in instances of skull fracture or middle ear (bulla) disease; however, they do not allow for assessment of nervous system parenchyma. If peripheral disease is suspected, a thorough otoscopic examination, preferably while the animal is anesthetized, is mandatory.

Cerebrospinal fluid (CSF) analysis is helpful primarily to determine the presence of inflammatory diseases. In general, collection of spinal fluid caudal to the level of the lesion is most accurate for diagnosis. Fluid is analyzed for cellularity, protein content, and cell morphology. Although CSF analysis is often helpful in determining the presence of nervous system disease, used alone, it does not often lead toward a specific etiologic diagnosis. Titers to specific infectious agents can be measured in CSF to assess for intrathecal production of antibody. In the presence of blood-brain barrier breakdown, however, antibodies may nonspecifically cross into the CSF from the systemic circulation. In this instance, correlation of the CSF to serum titer may be necessary. An increased antibody titer in the CSF relative to the serum antibody titer suggests local production of antibodies within the central nervous system (CNS) suggestive of actual CNS infection. Protein electrophoresis on CSF can give additional information concerning integrity of the blood-brain barrier and local production of immunoglobulins.

Recording the brain stem auditory potential (BAEP or BAER; see next chapter) may be helpful in determining the presence of intact hearing pathways and may also provide some information about the integrity of central (brain stem) projection pathways associated with hearing (Steiss et al, 1994, Fischer and Obermaier, 1994).

Surgical biopsy is often necessary for definitive antemortem diagnosis of structural intracranial disease. This is more difficult in the infratentorial space because surgical exposure, especially of ventrally located lesions, is often incomplete. Surgical exposure of lesions at the cerebellopontine angle area may be increased by occlusion of the overlying transverse sinus. The limited access to this area often hinders complete lesion resection.

For lesions of the ear canal and bulla, lateral ear canal resection and bulla osteotomy, respectively or in combination are useful for biopsy, lesion resection, and drainage of infected tissue. If these procedures are performed for ear exploration in animals without vestibular signs, then head tilts, ataxia, and nystagmus may result from damage of the vestibular structures during the surgical procedure itself.

TREATMENT

Specific treatments can best be recommended after a definitive diagnosis is made. If intracranial tumors are diagnosed, specific treatments such as surgical debulking/resection and radiation therapy may be helpful. With primary inflammatory diseases, the etiologic organism should be determined, if possible, and specific treatments directed toward killing the organism. With Rocky Mountain spotted fever, tetracycline and doxocycline can eliminate the vestibular signs (*CVT XII,* p. 293). With toxoplasmosis, a combination of clindamycin and trimethoprim/sulfadiazine will often improve or eliminate clinical signs. Noninfectious, inflammatory CNS disease will initially be responsive to corticosteroids. Granulomatous meningoencephalitis has also been treated with irradiation.

Nonspecific treatments include protecting the eyes from damage, especially if there is an associated facial nerve deficit or if the animal is lateral recumbent and rolling into the ground. Antihistamines (p. 48), such as diphenhydramine (1 to 2 mg/kg PO or IV every 12 to 24 hours), have been useful in decreasing anxiety and anorexia and, in some instances, the severity of the associated head tilt and nystagmus.

References and Suggested Reading

deLahunta A: In: Veterinary Neuroanatomy and Clinical Neurology, 2nd ed. Philadelphia: WB Saunders, 1983.
  A review of the pertinent anatomy of the vestibular system in animals.
Dow SW, LeCouteur RA, Poss ML, et al: Central nervous system toxicosis associated with metronidazole treatment of dogs: Five cases (1984–1987). J Am Vet Med Assoc 3:365 1989.
  Description of metronidazole toxicity in dogs.
Fischer A, Obermaier G: Brainstem auditory-evoked potentials and neuropathologic correlates in 26 dogs with brain tumor. J Vet Int Med 8:363, 1994.
  Brain stem auditory evoked potential abnormalities in dogs with brain tumor.
Forbes S, Cook JR Jr: Congenital peripheral vestibular disease attributed to lymphocytic labyrinthitis in two related litters of Doberman Pinscher pups. J Am Vet Med Assoc 198:447, 1991.
  A description of cause for congenital vestibular disease.
Greene CE, Burgdorfer W, Cavagnolo R, et al: Rocky Mountain spotted fever in dogs and its differentiation from canine ehrlichiosis. J Am Vet Med Assoc 186:465, 1985.
  A description of the central nervous system effects associated with Rocky Mountain spotted fever.
Mansfield PD: Ototoxicity in dogs and cats. Comp Contin Ed 12:331, 1990.
  A review of neurotoxic products that affect the ear.
Remedios AM, Fowler JD, Pharr JW: A comparison of radiographic versus surgical diagnosis of otitis media. J Am Anim Hosp Assoc 27:183, 1991.
  A description of diagnostic tests for middle/inner ear disease.
Saxon B, Magne ML: Reversible central nervous system toxicosis associated with metronidazole therapy in three cats. Prog Vet Neuro 4:25, 1993.
  Description of metronidazole toxicity in cats.
Schunk KL: Disease of the vestibular system. Prog Vet Neurol 1:247–254, 1990.
  A general review of vestibular diseases of dogs and cats.
Steiss JE, Cox NR, Hathcock JT: Brain stem auditory-evoked response abnormalities in 14 dogs with confirmed central nervous system lesions. J Vet Int Med 8:293, 1994.
  Brain stem auditory evoked potential abnormalities in dogs with CNS lesions.

CVT Update: Deafness in Dogs and Cats

KIM KNOWLES
North Grafton, Massachusetts

Evaluation of dogs and cats with a hearing loss is no longer a topic of limited interest. During the past decade there has been an increase in basic—and clinical—research reports concerning deafness. This increased interest has resulted in part from attention to the importance of congenital deafness; considerations that arise from this problem are of concern to breeders and owners of congenitally deaf animals. In a recent study of 1,031 Dalmatians, the incidence of congenital deafness, assessed by the brain stem auditory evoked response (BAER), was 29.7% (Strain et al, 1992). The prevalence of congenital deafness in other breeds also appears to be high. Another area of expanding interest is hearing loss associated with advancing age. Owners of older pets often seek advice when loss of this sense appears to exclude the animal from much of what is going on around them. Hence an understanding of the different types of hearing loss, their causes, treatment, and prevention is an important concern for the clinician.

ANATOMY AND PHYSIOLOGY OF THE AUDITORY SYSTEM

The auditory system can be subdivided into the external, middle, and inner ear and central auditory pathways. Sound is collected via the external ear and mechanically transmitted through the tympanic membrane and ossicular chain to the fluid system of the cochlea. The cochlea houses the receptor for hearing, the organ of Corti. It consists of rows of hair cells resting on the basilar membrane. Projecting from each hair cell are stereocilia, which are embedded in the tectorial membrane, a gelatinous structure overlying the organ of Corti. Acoustic vibrations cause the basilar membrane to vibrate; the upward displacement of the basilar membrane bends the stereocilia of the organ of Corti. This displacement results in mechanical deformation of the hair cells, which, in turn, alters the electrical conductance of the cell and provides the adequate stimulus for activating them. Hair cell activation generates neural activity in the cochlear nerve. The cell bodies of the cochlear nerve lie in the spiral ganglion. Central fibers from spiral ganglion cells enter the cranial cavity through the internal acoustic meatus (accompanied by the facial and vestibular nerves). On entering the brain stem, the cochlear nerve terminates in the cochlear nuclei which ultimately project to the auditory cortex of the temporal lobe.

CLASSIFICATION OF DEAFNESS

Impairments in hearing can occur anywhere along the auditory pathway and are classified according to the anatomic site of pathologic change. Deafness or hearing loss may be divided into two types: conductive and sensorineural. Conductive deafness is secondary to pathologic changes of the external or middle ear; this results in a defect in mechanical transmission of sound to the cochlea. Diseases causing external ear canal occlusion, rigidity or rupture of the tympanum, damage to the ossicular chain or effusion into the middle ear, can result in conductive hearing loss. Sensorineural deafness (also called nerve deafness) results from cochlea or cochlear nerve dysfunction and is caused by conditions that cause degeneration of the organ of Corti or cochlear nerve. Hearing disorders secondary to lesions of the cochlear nuclei or ascending auditory pathways are rarely recognized because an extensive lesion (resulting in severe neurologic deficits) is required to interrupt these central projections.

COMMON CAUSES OF HEARING LOSS

Conductive Hearing Loss

External Ear

Obstruction of the external ear canal can be caused by impacted cerumen, otitis externa with stenosis of the ear canal, and neoplasia. Dogs with atopy often have persistent otitis externa and perforation of the tympanum, and, in chronic cases, may result in spread of inflammation to the middle ear. Aural foreign bodies and trauma secondary to head injury or penetrating wounds may cause effusion in the ear canal and subsequent conductive hearing loss.

Middle Ear

Otitis media with effusion is a common cause of conductive hearing loss. Infection or inflammation reaches the middle ear cavity by three main routes: by direct spread across a diseased or ruptured eardrum; by extension through the eustachian tube; or by hematogenous dissemination. Middle ear effusions may be caused by bacterial, viral, or mycotic agents. Obstruction of the eustachian tube secondary to chronic inflammation or tumors can result in an effusion of the middle ear. Inflammatory polyps in cats often originate in the middle ear or eustachian tube and produce a serous or suppurative inflammatory response. Irradiation of the head and neck region may cause osteoradionecrosis of the bulla or disturbed lymphatic drainage of the nasopharynx, resulting in middle ear effusion.

Sensorineural Hearing Loss

Inner Ear

The majority of conditions causing sensorineural hearing loss cause degeneration of the hair cells of the organ of Corti or the cochlear nerve. Although there are many causes, genetic and congenital disorders and hearing loss associated with aging are the most common types.

Congenital/hereditary sensorineural deafness produces a total hearing loss in the affected ear and may be unilateral or bilateral. The overall incidence of congenital/hereditary deafness is unknown, but it is clearly a major, if not the main cause of sensorineural deafness in young animals. At least 48 breeds of dogs (Table 1) are affected with congenital/inherited deafness. Dalmatians, Bull terriers, and English setters have the highest prevalence. Congenital/hereditary deafness is usually found in conjunction with pigmentation anomalies. Affected breeds of dogs either carry the merle or piebald genes, and the incidence of deafness is often higher with increasing white in the hair coat. Inherited deafness is transmitted as a autosomal dominant trait in some white cats with blue irises. In almost every dog and cat with congenital/hereditary deafness the histopathologic lesion is a cochleosaccular degeneration. It is characterized by loss of the vascular supply to the cochlea (stria vascularis) followed by degeneration of the hair cells of the organ of Corti. In Dalmatians and white cats with blue irises, the pathology is at an advanced stage by 3 weeks of age; secondary loss of spiral ganglion cells occurs before 1 year of age and degeneration of neurons of the central auditory pathway has been reported in older animals. An absence or reduction of melanocytes in the stria vascularis of the Dalmatian has been reported and may be related to the initial strial degeneration.

Congenital peripheral vestibular disease, associated with deafness secondary to degeneration of the organ of Corti, has been described in young Doberman pinschers. Congen-

TABLE 1. Breeds of Dogs With Congenital or Hereditary Deafness

Akita	Jack Russell terrier
American Staffordshire terrier	Kuvasz
Australian cattle dog	Maltese
Australian shepherd	Miniature pinscher
Beagle	Miniature poodle
Border collie	Mixed breed
Boston terrier	Norwegian dunkerhound
Boxer	Old English sheepdog
Bulldog	Papillon
Bull terrier	Pit bull terrier
Catahoula leopard dog	Pointer
American Cocker spaniel	Rhodesian ridgeback
Collie	Rottweiler
Dalmatian	Saint Bernard
Dappled dachshund	Schnauzer
Doberman pinscher	Scottish terrier
Dogo Argentino	Sealyham terrier
English setter	Shetland sheepdog
Foxhound	Shropshire terrier
Fox terrier	Siberian husky
German shepherd	English Springer spaniel
Great Dane	Toy Poodle
Great Pyrenees	American Walker foxhound
Ibizan hound	West Highland White terrier

ital peripheral vestibular disease has been described in the English cocker spaniel, beagle, German shepherd dog, Akita, and Siamese and Burmese cats. Although deafness has occasionally been reported in this syndrome, valid tests of auditory function have been performed in a minority of the cases, and the true incidence of concomitant deafness may have been underestimated.

Acquired sensorineural hearing loss, secondary to dysfunction of membranous structures within the cochlea, can be seen in hypothyroidism, infectious labyrinthitis, trauma, and neoplasia of the temporal bone. Ototoxicity from systemic and topical aminoglycosides can result in severe cochlear and hair cell degeneration. Other documented ototoxic agents in dogs and cats are loop diuretics and topical otic antiseptic agents. Age-related hearing loss and deafness in dogs is degenerative and associated with atrophy and loss of spiral ganglion cells in the cochlea; this loss is probably secondary to degenerative changes of the hair cells of the organ of Corti.

CLINICAL SIGNS OF DEAFNESS

The clinical diagnosis of deafness poses a problem in cases of incomplete bilateral or complete unilateral involvement of an affected ear. In cases of complete bilateral deafness, the animal usually startles easily when approached without visual cues, sleeps soundly in noisy environments, and cannot be aroused with loud noises. When awake, a bilaterally deaf animal fails to respond to sounds of different intensities, is difficult to train without hand signals and can be anxious or aggressive. The only clinical sign a unilaterally deaf animal may show is defective sound localization.

DIAGNOSTIC APPROACHES

Given the many possible causes of hearing loss, a thorough history is essential for diagnosis. The age of onset, course of the hearing loss, and history of previous ear disease or exposure to ototoxic agents should be explored. If the onset is less than 5 weeks of age, breed predisposition for congenital deafness as well as familial history of deafness are important considerations. As conductive losses are likely to improve with treatment, the primary emphasis of a diagnostic work-up is to rule out all possible causes of external and middle ear disease. The physical examination should not only include a complete otoscopic examination, but also a complete head and neck and cranial nerve examination. The presence of head shaking, aural pain or discharge, or other cranial nerve deficits (Horner's syndrome, keratoconjunctivitis sicca, head tilt, nystagmus), will help direct the subsequent evaluation. Cytology, culture, and sensitivity of the external or middle ear may be indicated in cases of suppurative otitis media/interna. Radiographs of the bullae and petrous temporal bone or computed tomography of the bullae may be indicated in cases of infectious labyrinthitis or suspected neoplasia.

AUDITORY TESTING

The most widely used electrodiagnostic test for assessing the integrity of the auditory system is the BAER.

It has proven to be particularly useful in the evaluation of uncooperative and young animals in which behavioral responses may be difficult to assess. This test does not require conscious participation on the part of the animal, and therefore provides an objective assessment of auditory function. In this test, neural responses to auditory stimuli can be detected during electroencephalography by signal averaging techniques. Electrical activity resulting from a series of auditory clicks, delivered first to one ear and then to the other, is recorded through scalp electrodes. Because each ear is tested individually, unilateral deafness may be diagnosed. A BAER tracing consists of a series of four to seven waves, at approximately 1.0-msec intervals after presentation of sound stimuli; these waves reflect electrical activity in the cochlear nerve and central auditory pathways. As the organ of Corti and cochlear nerve must be functional to record a BAER, complete deafness results in absence of waveforms from the affected ear. By varying the intensity of acoustic stimuli, a threshold approximating the behavioral threshold can be determined. Recordings, using different intensities of sound, may show an elevated threshold, which can be seen in a conductive or sensorineural hearing loss. Impedance audiometry (tympanometry, acoustic reflex) can be used to investigate the integrity of the middle ear, cochlea, seventh and eighth cranial nerves, and brain stem pathways. These tests are useful when combined with the BAER and clinical judgments. Impedance audiometry is still in varying stages of development and is of limited availability.

TREATMENT, PROGNOSIS, AND MANAGEMENT

Many patients with conductive hearing loss, due to otitis media, will improve or their hearing loss will resolve with long-term antibiotic therapy. Sensorineural deafness due to congenital/hereditary causes or from aging is not reversible. Some recovery of auditory function may occur following treatment of infectious labyrinthitis or discontinuation of ototoxic agents. Hearing aids, which essentially amplify sound, would be beneficial in cases of conductive hearing loss not amenable to medical and surgical management. Hearing aids also appear to help some cases of age-related sensorineural hearing loss. However, animals do not tolerate the currently available model.

In breeds at high risk for congenital deafness, sire, dam, and littermate BAER testing is highly recommended. Owners of animals with congenital deafness should be discouraged from breeding them. Although there is some breed variation, bilateral congenitally deaf animals generally do not make good pets because they are often anxious, aggressive, and prone to vehicular trauma. Unilaterally congenitally deaf animals still make excellent pets.

References and Suggested Reading

Delack JB: Hereditary deafness in the white cat. Compend Contin Educ Pract Vet 6:609, 1984.
This article reviews the genetics of coat and eye color, histologic features and pathogenesis of cochleosaccular degeneration, and the incidence of hereditary deafness in the white cat.
Knowles K, Blauch B, Leipold H, et al: Reduction of spiral ganglion

neurons in the aging canine with hearing loss. J Vet Med (Series A) 36:188, 1989.
Quantification of spiral ganglion neurons in a series of dogs of different ages and hearing abilities revealed an age-associated reduction and atrophy of ganglion cells in dogs that appeared to be deaf and lacked brain stem auditory evoked responses.

Knowles K: Diseases of the middle and inner ear. In: Morgan RV: Handbook of Small Animal Practice, 3rd ed. Philadelphhia: WB Saunders (in press).

A review of the causes, pathophysiology, clinical signs, diagnosis, and treatment of diseases of the middle and inner ear.

Strain GB, Kearney MT, Gignac IJ, et al: Brainstem auditory-evoked potential assessment of congenital deafness in Dalmatians: Association with phenotypic markers. J Vet Intern Med 3:175, 1992.
A study of the relationship between deafness, assessed using the brain stem auditory evoked response, and phenotypic markers in 1,031 Dalmatians from three geographically separate areas of the United States.

Neurologic Manifestations of Canine Hypothyroidism

ANDRÉ JAGGY
Bern, Switzerland

Primary hypothyroidism due to lymphocytic thyroiditis or idiopathic atrophy of the thyroid gland is a relatively common endocrine disorder with characteristic symptoms (Peterson and Ferguson, 1989). The most consistent clinical signs result from the effects on the dog's mental status and activity. Most often the skin is affected by the thyroid hormone deficiency. Recently, a neurologic form of hypothyroidism has been described in dogs (Jaggy et al, 1994b). These cases and five additional dogs with seizures studied at the University of Georgia and Institute of Animal Neurology in Bern are the basis of this report.

CASE SIGNALMENT

Neurologic signs with primary hypothyroidism occur mainly in older large-breed dogs with neither sex predilection nor breed predisposition. The onset of the clinical signs is in most cases acute and nonprogressive; however, the course of the disease may be chronic progressive in a few cases.

CLINICAL SIGNS

Characteristic signs of systemic involvement of hypothyroidism may include weight gain, dry hair coat, hyperpigmentation, cold intolerance, anestrus, and bradycardia (Jaggy et al, 1994b). However, neurologic signs predominate and include either focal or generalized lower motor neuronal dysfunction with laryngeal paralysis and/or megaesophagus, peripheral vestibular involvement, and seizures (Jaggy et al, 1994a).

Neuromuscular Signs

Most dogs are initially depressed and may show weakness with generalized mild muscle atrophy, although myalgia is not common. Generalized ataxia is usually characterized by knuckling of the toes, wearing of the nails, and stumbling. In a few cases tetraparesis or tetraplegia with proprioceptive positioning deficits and decreased segmental spinal reflexes may be observed. Other signs of lower motor neuronal dysfunction, including unilateral or bilateral facial nerve paralysis and/or laryngeal paralysis, as well as megaesophagus, may develop over time or be seen as a sole neurologic involvement (Jaggy et al, 1994a).

Peripheral Vestibular Signs

Neurologic signs of peripheral vestibular disease are evident and include head tilt, vestibular strabismus, drifting and/or circling and generalized ataxia. In addition, a more generalized form of hypothyroidism with abnormal proprioceptive positioning and decreased segmental spinal reflexes may be seen.

Seizures

Generalized seizures ("grand mal" type), typically characterized by loss of consciousness, opisthotonus, limb rigidity, and tonic-clonic muscle activity, followed by paddling movements, have been reported in a few dogs with hypothyroidism (Jaggy, 1990). Duration of clinical signs before confirmed diagnosis ranged from months to years. Some of them have been treated unsuccessfully with antiepileptic medication for several months. On neurologic examination no significant abnormalities were noted (Jaggy, 1990).

DIAGNOSIS

The most common abnormalities on clinicopathology are nonregenerative, normocytic, and normochromic anemia, elevated creatine kinase activity, hyperlipidemia (i.e., hypertriglyceridemia), and hypercholesterolemia (Jaggy et al, 1994b; Feldman and Nelson, 1996). These findings should serve as marker for possible thyroid dysfunction;

however, the diagnosis has to be confirmed by low T_4 levels before and after TSH stimulation or by low T_4 and high TSH levels (see p. 321 and *CVT XII*, pp. 360 and 364).

Diagnostic tests of the neuromuscular system should reveal abnormal electromyographic findings characterized by either fibrillation potentials and positive sharp waves and/or complex repetitive discharges (Jaggy and Oliver, 1994).

In addition, dogs with peripheral vestibular signs have abnormal brain stem auditory evoked responses (BAER; see previous chapter) including decreased amplitudes and increased latencies that are suggestive of impaired peripheral acoustic perception. Selective electromyographic abnormalities are not only seen in dogs with peripheral vestibular signs and concurrent diffuse lower motor neuronal disease, but also in cases with vestibular deficits alone. Therefore, vestibular signs in dogs frequently may be only one clinical sign of an underlying, more generalized polyneuropathy and clinical expression. The exact pathogenesis of vestibular and facial nerve paralysis that can develop is not known, but such neuropathies are likely to result from compression by mucinous deposits in and around the affected nerves as they pass through the internal acoustic meatus of the temporal bone.

The histologic muscular changes, in our experience, are mainly degenerative and characterized by type II myofiber atrophy and focal aggregation and accumulation of some substances in type I myofibers (Braund, 1986). Additional histopathologic findings on teased nerve preparations may show segmental demyelination/remyelination, and biopsies of the thyroid gland may show lymphocytic thyroiditis (Jaggy et al, 1994a).

TREATMENT

Thyroxine supplementation (e.g., levothyroxine 0.02 mg/kg PO every 12 hours) is indicated for confirmed hyperthyroidism. Confirmation of the diagnosis will depend on history, neurologic signs, clinicopathologic results including abnormal low T_4 levels after TSH stimulation, and characteristic electrodiagnostic findings, whereas successful treatment is based on adequate response of thyroxine supplementation. The initial dosage of levothyroxine may need to be modified in dogs with concurrent illness in which thyroid hormone–induced alterations in cellular metabolic functions may have a deleterious effect. The dosage may then be gradually increased over 3 to 4 weeks. Serum T_4 levels should be maintained above 2.5 μg/dl. Thyroid supplementation should be continued for a minimum of 1 month before beginning to critically evaluate the effectiveness of treatment. With appropriate therapy, all of the clinical signs and clinicopathologic abnormalities are reversible. An increase in mental alertness, activity, and muscle strength are the initial signs of improvement within the first days of treatment. The neurologic deficits are less pronounced within the first month, complete recovery may take several months.

In severe cases of spinal neuromuscular involvement and concomitant laryngeal paralysis, additional surgical treatment is indicated (Gaber et al, 1985). Different surgical methods have been described including arytenoidectomy and vocal fold removal, arytenoid lateralization, and castellated laryngofissure (Harvey et al, 1983). Dogs with concurrent hypothyroidism—in some cases with additional focal muscle atrophy of the shoulder, neck, and head—may show dramatic improvement with thyroid supplement therapy, even when minimal surgery is performed.

Some animals with megaesophagus may develop permanent neurologic disabilities (Boudrieau and Rogers, 1985). Although they may improve somewhat with thyroxine supplementation, prognosis is poor (Jaggy et al, 1994b).

Hypothyroidism is not always a simple diagnosis. In many cases either vestibular or lower motor neuron signs, megaesophagus, and laryngeal paralysis may be the only clinical sign of an underlying, more generalized polyneuropathy associated with hypothyroidism. Recently, thyroxine-responsive unilateral forelimb lameness has been reported in dogs with normal neurologic examinations but electromyographic findings suggestive of generalized neuromyopathy (Budsberg et al, 1993). Therefore, electrodiagnostic abnormalities may be seen sometimes in advance of clinical disease and are supportive in confirming the diagnosis of hypothyroidism in dogs.

References and Suggested Reading

Boudrieau RJ, Rogers WA: Megaesophagus in the dog: A review of 50 cases. J Am Anim Hosp Assoc 21:33, 1985.

Braund KG: Myopathies in dogs and cats: Recognizing endogenous causes. Pet Pract 23:803, 1986.

Budsberg SC, Moore GE, Klappenbach K: Thyroxine-responsive unilateral forelimb lameness and generalized neuromuscular disease in four hypothyroid dogs. J Am Vet Med Assoc 202:1859, 1993.

Feldman EC, Nelson RW: Hypothyroidism. In: Feldman EC, Nelson RW, eds: Canine and Feline Endocrinology and Reproduction, 2nd ed. Philadelphia: WB Saunders, 1996, p 67.

Gaber CE, Amis TC, LeCouteur A: Laryngeal paralysis in dogs: A review of 23 cases. J Am Vet Med Assoc 186:377, 1985.

Harvey HJ, Irby NL, Waltrous BJ: Laryngeal paralysis in hypothyroid dogs. In: Kirk RW, ed: Current Veterinary Therapy VIII. Philadelphia: WB Saunders, 1983, p 694.

Jaggy A: Seizures in hypothyroid dogs. Proc ESVN, Berne, 1990, p 51 (abstract).

Jaggy A, Glaus T, Tipold A: Neurologische Ausfallserscheinungen im Zusammenhang mit Hypothyreose beim Hund: Literaturübersicht und Fallbeschreibung. Schweiz Arch Tierheil 136:257, 1994a.

Jaggy A, Oliver JE: Neurologic manifestations of thyroid disease. Vet Clin North Am Small Anim Pract 24:487, 1994.

Jaggy A, Oliver JE, Ferguson DC, et al: Neurological manifestations of hypothyroidism. J Vet Intern Med 8:328, 1994b.

Peterson ME, Ferguson DC: Thyroid disease. In: Ettinger SJ, ed: Textbook of Veterinary Internal Medicine, 3rd ed. Philadelphia: WB Saunders, 1989, p 1632.

Borna Disease in Cats

ANNA-LENA BERG

Uppsala, Sweden

Since the early 1950s, cases of nonsuppurative encephalomyelitis in domestic cats and large *Felidae* have been reported from different parts of the world. Although viral infection has been presumed to be the cause of this poorly defined disease complex, several attempts to isolate a virus have failed. In Sweden and Austria, a feline neurologic disorder apparently belonging to the same group of idiopathic encephalitides has been described (Kronevi et al, 1974; Nowotny and Weissenböck, 1995). After exclusion of various other plausible infectious pathogens, an association between this so-called staggering disease in Swedish cats and Borna disease virus (BDV) was found. Diseased cats were shown to carry serum antibodies against BDV. Furthermore, a feline variant of BDV was isolated from brain and spinal cord material from cats with "staggering disease" (Lundgren et al, 1995). When inoculated intracerebrally into specific pathogen free (SPF) cats, this feline BDV induced neurologic signs and inflammatory brain lesions (Lundgren et al, 1997). Since no other infectious agent has been identified in the central nervous system of cats with "staggering disease," BDV appears to be the most likely cause of the disease. Although BDV so far has been isolated only from Swedish cats, BDV-specific antibodies have been detected in German, Austrian, and Japanese cats. Accordingly, the possibility of BDV infection ought to be considered in cases of feline encephalomyelitis of unknown etiology, also in countries outside Scandinavia.

BORNA DISEASE VIRUS

Originally described in horses in southern Germany, Borna disease (BD) also affects sheep, cattle, and ostriches (Ludwig et al, 1988; Rott and Becht, 1995). The causative agent, BDV, is a nonsegmented negative-stranded (NNS) RNA virus with a genome of 8.9 kb, containing five major open reading frames (Briese et al, 1994; Cubitt et al, 1994). Transcription and replication of BDV take place in the nucleus of the infected cell. This property, which is unique among animal viruses of the NNS RNA order, suggests that BDV may represent a new class of virus. BDV was recently assigned its own family, *Bornaviridae*, within the *Mononegavirales* order.

In naturally infected animals, BDV causes a nonsuppurative encephalomyelitis clinically manifested as a subacute neurologic disorder with behavioral and motor disturbances. Experimentally, a wide range of animals (e.g., rats, rabbits, monkeys, chickens) are susceptible to BDV infection. However, not all of these experimentally infected animals develop neurologic disease. For instance, newborn rats inoculated intracerebrally have high BDV titers in the brain but no encephalitis and show only subtle signs of altered behavior. In adult hamsters, mice, and black-hooded rats the infection frequently runs a subclinical course (Rott and Becht, 1995). Therefore, it seems that the severity of disease is dependent on factors related to the age, immune status, and genetic background of the host.

Serologic findings of BDV-specific antibodies in human neuropsychiatric patients in Europe, Japan, and the United States have raised the question of a possible relationship between BDV and certain mental disorders in man (Bode, 1995). Further evidence for the existence of human BDV infections was obtained recently, with the isolation of infectious BDV from human peripheral blood mononuclear cells (Bode et al, 1996). The natural reservoir of human BDV infections is unknown. So far, there are no indications of a transmission from animals to humans. However, considering the wide host spectrum of BDV, it is important to further investigate the epidemiology of the agent.

CLINICAL SIGNS IN CATS

The majority of cats with BD belong to the rural cat population, accustomed to hunting birds and rodents. Males are more frequently affected than females. There is no age predisposition; however, no case of feline BD has been observed in cats younger than 6 months. Following a few days of unspecific illness (fever, apathy, reduced appetite), neurologic signs appear. The most common clinical manifestation of the disease is hindleg ataxia (Fig. 1). Affected cats move about with a stiff, staggering gait, unable to jump up and down normally. In some cases, the animals lose their ability to retract the claws. In addition to these motor disturbances, many cats show mental changes. Cats that have previously been shy become sociable and affectionate, mewing more than usual, whereas cats that are customarily cheerful become introverted and shy. Aggressive behavior is rare. Less frequent signs include pruritus, hypersensitivity to sound and light, increased salivation,

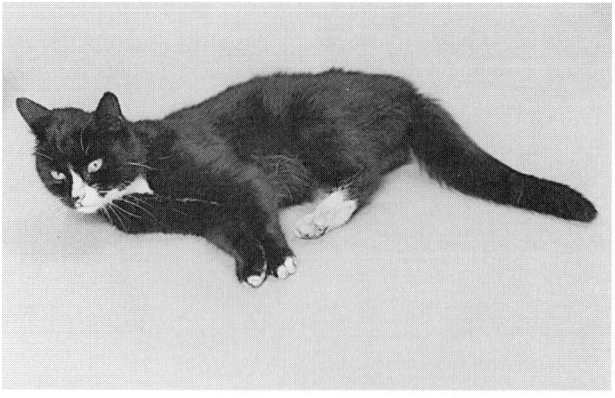

Figure 1. A cat with staggering disease, showing hindleg paresis.

impaired vision, staring gaze, hyperesthesia, constipation, tremor, circling, and seizures.

The progress of the disease is usually subacute to chronic, lasting 1 to 4 weeks until the clinical condition either deteriorates to complete paralysis of the hindlegs and death or stabilizes, leaving most cats permanently afflicted with ataxia and/or personality changes. In a few cases, following recovery from the acute stage of disease, the cats later on develop a ravenous appetite and quickly become obese.

PATHOLOGY OF FELINE BORNA DISEASE

Macroscopically, the brain and spinal cord as well as the internal organs usually appear normal. In severe cases, a slight internal hydrocephalus may be noted. Histopathologic examination reveals a nonsuppurative meningoencephalomyelitis, predominantly located in the gray matter of the central nervous system. The inflammatory reaction is characterized by extensive adventitial mononuclear cell cuffing, neuronophagia, and the presence of inflammatory nodules consisting of lymphoid cells and macrophages/microglial cells within the neural parenchyma. The cells of the adventitial cuffs have been immunohistochemically characterized as CD4$^+$ T cells, CD8$^+$ T cells, B cells, plasma cells, and monocytes/macrophages. Although the adventitial cell infiltrates sometimes seem to compress the lumen of vessels, vasculitis is not present. Intranuclear inclusion bodies, although prominent in horses with BD, are rarely observed in cats. Axonal degeneration and loss of myelin are observed both in the brain and in the ventrolateral tracts of the spinal cord.

The inflammatory lesions in the brain show a certain localization pattern, the most pronounced inflammatory changes being observed in the brain stem (thalamus, mesencephalon, caudal colliculus), basal ganglia, hippocampus, and the olfactory bulb. The cerebral cortex is moderately affected. In the cerebellum, lesions in the neural parenchyma are minimal. However, cerebellar meningitis is usually a prominent feature of the disease.

Outside the central nervous system, lesions are either nonexistent or minimal. Some cats show degeneration and depletion of lymphoid cells in the follicles of the spleen. In the kidneys, small accumulations of mononuclear cells are sometimes observed in the cortex.

DIFFERENTIAL DIAGNOSES

The clinical picture of feline BD reflects multifocal involvement of the central nervous system. The major differential diagnosis is feline infectious peritonitis (FIP). Although cats with the central nervous system form of FIP tend to be younger and more severely affected (usually emaciated) than cats with BD, differentiation between these two diseases based solely upon the clinical picture is not possible. A serologic test for coronavirus antibodies may be helpful. Other plausible agents that should be kept in mind are feline leukemia virus and feline immunodeficiency virus. Both of these agents have the potential to cause multifocal neurologic signs and encephalitis. Aujeszky's disease and rabies both present different clinical

pictures than feline BD. Cerebral neoplasms should be considered in older cats.

At present, there is no single diagnostic test available that can establish an in vivo diagnosis of feline BD. Only about 45% of diseased cats have been shown to carry BDV-specific antibodies. Whether this reflects an inability of the present test systems to detect low titers or a true absence of antibodies in some animals is unknown. Viral RNA can be extracted from white blood cells and used for reverse transcriptase–polymerase chain reaction with BDV-specific primers in order to detect BDV nucleic acid in the blood. Although this technique has been used successfully in horses with BD, preliminary results in cats indicate that the presence of BDV in white blood cells is rare.

Laboratory findings in feline BD usually include a moderate leukopenia (2.6 to 4.1 $\times$ 10^9 cells per L). The cerebrospinal fluid often shows a moderate elevation in protein content, and a slightly increased white blood cell count (mainly mononuclear cells).

A definitive diagnosis of feline BD can presently only be made by postmortem examination. The characteristic distribution pattern of lesions in the brain, together with immunohistochemical detection of BDV antigen in the neural parenchyma, provides the criteria necessary for diagnosis.

TREATMENT AND PROGNOSIS

There is no specific drug available for treatment of feline BD. Besides supportive care, corticosteroids may substantially relieve clinical signs, especially when given at an early stage of disease. Prednisolone is the drug of choice, initially at a dose of 1 to 2 mg/kg PO divided in two doses for 7 days or until a satisfactory clinical response is achieved. The dose is then gradually reduced over 6 to 8 weeks to 0.125 mg/kg on alternate days. In some instances, cats treated with corticosteroids for several months seem to have recovered almost completely. However, the long-term prognosis must be regarded with caution. Presumably, BDV remains in the brain as a persistent infection that may be reactivated during periods of immunosuppression. The cat owner should be informed about the possibility of a later relapse, as well as the risk for permanent motor disturbances and personality changes. It is the author's experience that the majority of cats with BD are euthanized within a year after the onset of disease. Currently, no vaccine against feline BD is available.

References and Suggested Reading

Bode L: Human infections with Borna disease virus and potential pathogenic implications. In: Koprowski H, Lipkin WI, eds: Borna Disease. (Curr Topics Microbiol Immun vol 190). Berlin: Springer-Verlag, 1995, p 103.
A review of human BDV infections.

Bode L, Dürrwald R, Rantam FA, et al: First isolates of infectious human Borna disease virus from patients with mood disorders. Molecular Psychiatry 1:200, 1996.
Describes how BDV was isolated from peripheral blood mononuclear cells of human patients and propagated in tissue culture as well as in rabbits.

Briese T, Schneemann A, Lewis AJ, et al: Genomic organization of Borna disease virus. Proc Natl Acad Sci USA 91:4362, 1994.

Molecular characterization of BDV, including the complete genomic sequence.

Cubitt B, Oldstone C, de la Torre JC: Sequence and genome organization of Borna disease virus. J Virol 68:1382, 1994.
Contains information similar to the paper by Briese and colleagues.

Kronevi T, Nordström M, Moreno W, et al: Feline ataxia due to nonsuppurative meningoencephalomyelitis of unknown aetiology. Nord Veterinärmed 26:720, 1973.
The original report on Swedish cats with staggering disease. Outlines the clinical picture and the histopathology of the brain lesions.

Ludwig H, Bode L, Gosztonyi G: Borna disease: A persistent virus infection of the central nervous system. Progr Med Virol 35:107, 1988.
A review of BDV infections in naturally and experimentally infected animals.

Lundgren A-L, Zimmermann W, Bode L, et al: Staggering disease in cats: Isolation and characterization of the feline Borna disease virus. J Gen Virol 76:2215, 1995.

The first report on isolation of BDV from cats with staggering disease.

Lundgren A-L, Johannisson A, Zimmermann W, et al: Neurological disease and encephalitis in cats experimentally infected with Borna disease virus. Acta Neuropath 93:391, 1997.
Experimental infection of SPF cats with the feline BDV isolate.

Nowotny N, Weissenböck H: Description of feline nonsuppurative meningoencephalomyelitis ("Staggering disease") and studies on its etiology. J Clin Microbiol 33:1668, 1995.
Clinical picture and pathology of staggering disease in Austrian cats.

Rott R, Becht H: Natural and experimental Borna disease in animals. In: Koprowski H, Lipkin WI, eds: Borna Disease. (Curr Topics Microbiol Immun vol 190). Berlin: Springer-Verlag, 1995, p 17.
Provides an overview of Borna disease in a wide range of animal species.

Steroid-Responsive Meningitis-Arteritis in Dogs

ANDREA TIPOLD
Bern, Switzerland

Since the first description about 15 years ago, the so-called steroid responsive meningitis-arteritis (SRMA) in dogs has become a well-known disease in small animal practice (Meric et al, 1985; Presthus, 1991; Tipold and Jaggy, 1994). Before that time a similar condition was already mentioned and a vasculitis of the central nervous system (CNS) described histopathologically. Recently, another similar disease has been published under the name of *corticosteroid-responsive meningomyelitis,* describing the additional involvement of spinal cord tissue (Irving and Chrisman, 1990). A similar condition is known in laboratory dog colonies under various names such as *Beagle pain syndrome* (Hayes et al, 1989), *necrotizing vasculitis* (Scott-Moncrieff et al, 1992), *polyarteritis, canine pain syndrome,* and *canine juvenile polyarteritis syndrome* (Felsburg et al, 1992). This variety of different names not only shows that little is known about this disease but also reflects the most important clinical signs such as pain, improvement after corticosteroid treatment, and involvement of the meninges and blood vessels.

NOMENCLATURE AND PATHOLOGY

Two different forms of SRMA may be distinguished. The typical or acute form is characterized by clinical symptoms such as cervical rigidity and pain, fever, and pleocytosis with polymorphonuclear cells in the cerebrospinal fluid (CSF). In an atypical, more protracted form additional neurologic deficits consistent with a spinal cord or a multifocal lesion, and lack of suppurative inflammation in the CSF, are found. Post mortem examinations in our cases rarely reveal extraneural lesions, with the exception of mild arteritis in the heart and the mediastinum, myocarditis,

mild focal hepatitis and interstitial nephritis and infiltration of plasma cells in the jejunum (Tipold et al, 1995). In another report on Beagles, extraneural lesions were found more frequently (Snyder et al, 1995). Macroscopic lesions are also rarely found in the CNS and consist of dilated lateral ventricles. In the protracted form of the disease, enlarged and thickened vessels in the leptomeninges of the cervical spinal cord may be seen. In the acute stage of the disease the histopathologic examination reveals a marked meningitis with invasion of macrophages, plasma cells, lymphocytes, and varying numbers of polymorphonuclear cells. The meninges of all regions of the CNS are affected with the most marked effect in the cervical region. Lesions of the meningeal arteries consist of swelling of the nuclei of the tunica muscularis, hyaline degeneration, and periarteritis. Focal suppurative inflammation with vascular changes and hemorrhage may also occur in the epidural fat, the outer layers of the dura mater, and the epineurium of the spinal roots. In the protracted form of the disease, the infiltration of the meninges with inflammatory cells is milder. However, marked fibrous thickening and focal mineralization of the leptomeninges are present. The walls of many arteries are thickened with considerable stenosis due to cellular proliferation of the intima and fibrosis (Tipold et al, 1995). Some arterial walls have infiltration with polymorphonuclear cells, macrophages, and lymphocytes, and the vessels may be thrombosed or even recanalized or mineralized (Figs. 1 and 2).

ETIOLOGY AND PATHOGENESIS

The etiology of SRMA is unknown. Epidemiologic data suggest that SRMA may be triggered by an environmental

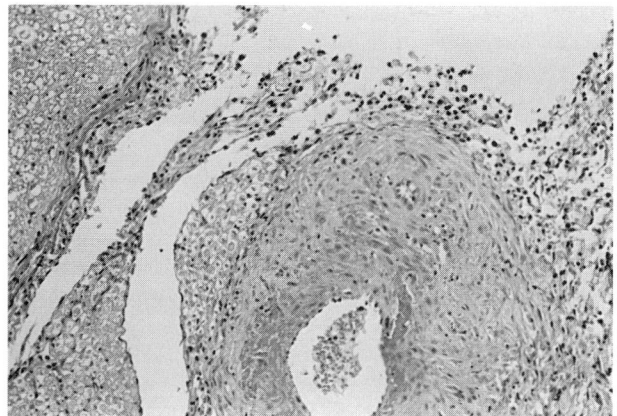

Figure 1. Histopathologic examination: spinal cord section, acute stage of SRMA, arteritis with fibrinoid necrosis, periarteritis, and meningitis with predominantly mononuclear cells.

factor, possibly of infectious nature. However, bacterial and virus isolation attempts so far have been unsuccessful. Activated T cells are found, which means that these cells had contact with an antigen that has not yet been further characterized and might even be a self-antigen. The marked response to steroids as well as pathologic and laboratory observations suggests that immunopathologic mechanisms are involved in SRMA. Morphologic features of the vascular changes bear some similarity to immune complex–mediated vascular injury. However, so far, it has not been possible to demonstrate unequivocally the deposition of immunoglobulins in blood vessels. It has been concluded that the meningeal lesions in SRMA are a primary event rather than the result of a generalized immune complex disease. The dogs synthesize IgG intrathecally, indicating that the immune response in SRMA is in part specifically directed towards the CNS. In this intrathecal humoral immune response, IgA appears to play a central role and to be important in the pathogenesis of the disease (Tipold et al, 1995). Besides elevated intrathecal IgA production, IgA levels are also elevated in serum. Thus, in addition to being an important factor for the pathogenesis, combined intrathecal and systemic high IgA levels are very useful for the clinical diagnosis because this phenomenon is not found in other inflammatory and infectious CNS diseases. This is particularly helpful in the protracted form of the disease, in which the typical neutrophilic pleocytosis in the CSF is lacking.

INCIDENCE

SRMA occurs worldwide in companion dogs and, next to canine distemper encephalitis, granulomatous meningo-encephalitis (GME), and protozoal infections, represents one of the most important inflammatory diseases of the canine CNS. About 10% of dogs of our caseload have inflammatory and infectious diseases, and 15% of these have steroid-responsive meningitis-arteritis (Tipold, 1995). Epidemiologic studies in Beagle colonies revealed that SRMA is mostly found in springtime and has an increased frequency approximately every 5 years (Felsburg et al, 1992). Our study and studies in Beagle kennels probably underestimated the true frequency of occurrence of SRMA.

There is a breed predisposition for Beagles, and Bernese mountain dogs and boxers are over-represented, but every breed can be affected. Genetic factors may play a role, as suspected in Beagle colonies. The disease mostly affects young adult dogs with an age range from 8 to 18 months. However, SRMA can occur in younger animals (up to 4 months) and in older ones (up to 7 years). There is no sex predilection.

CLINICAL COURSE

SRMA mostly has an acute onset, and the clinical signs are recurrent after a short period of improvement. After several relapses without adequate therapy the dogs may develop the more protracted form with continuous worsening of the neurologic dysfunction.

CLINICAL SIGNS

The most important extraneural sign is an elevated body temperature of up to 42°C in the acute stage of the disease. The "classic" signs found during the neurologic examination are hyperesthesia, cervical rigidity, and stiff gait (Fig. 3). With the exception of a decreased menace reaction or slight deficits in postural reactions in some animals, the neurologic examination is normal in the acute stage of SRMA. In the more protracted course of the disease, clinical signs are dominated by further neurologic deficits, usually reflecting a spinal cord or multifocal lesion. Gait abnormalities include hypermetria and generalized ataxia, pacing, tetraparesis, and paraparesis. Postural reactions are affected. Spinal reflexes are either exaggerated or in rare cases diminished. In rare cases cranial nerve deficits are observed, such as decreased menace reaction and vestibular strabismus. An occasional finding is myoclonus.

DIAGNOSIS

The clinical diagnosis is based on a combination of clinical findings, laboratory tests, and ancillary studies, which are performed to exclude other causes of the symptoms, especially in the protracted form of the disease. The

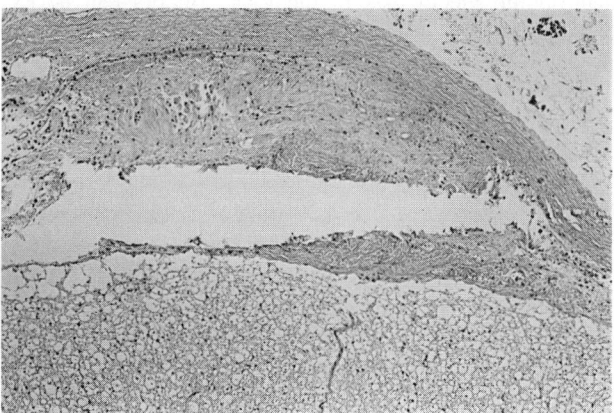

Figure 2. Histopathologic examination: spinal cord section, protracted stage of SRMA, meningitis with massive fibrous thickening.

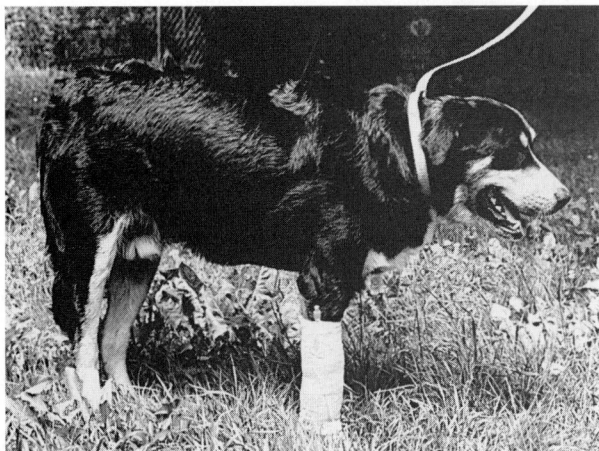

Figure 3. Bernese mountain dog, male, 1 year; SRMA: note the cervical rigidity.

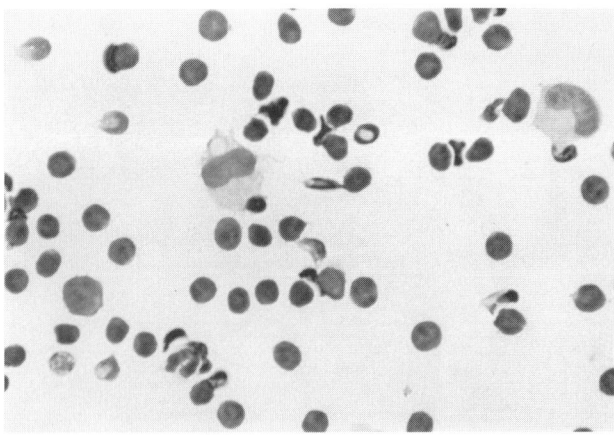

Figure 5. CSF: cytospin preparation, protracted stage of SRMA with predominantly mononuclear cells (lymphocytes, monocytes, macrophages, a few neutrophils). A mild erythrocyte contamination is frequently seen in combination with arteritis.

most important findings in blood profiles of the acute form of SRMA are leukocytosis with a left shift and an increased erythrocyte sedimentation rate. Electrophoresis might reveal elevated alpha$_2$-globulins, which is considered to be an unspecific finding. In the protracted stage the blood examination is frequently inconspicuous. The urinalysis is generally normal, with the exception of protein elevation in a few cases. In protracted cases of SRMA, other causes for the neurologic deficits have to be excluded with the help of imaging and electrodiagnostic techniques.

Cerebrospinal fluid should be collected by cisternal puncture under general anesthesia. In the classic form of the disease there is a mild to clear elevation of the protein content (Pandy reaction + + up to + + + + positive) and a pleocytosis with several hundreds to thousands of leukocytes, predominantly polymorphonuclear cells (Fig. 4). The bacteriologic examination has been negative in all known cases. In protracted cases, the protein content is normal or only slightly elevated, with a mild to moderate pleocytosis with a mixed cell population or even with a predominance of mononuclear cells (Fig. 5).

The acute form of the disease does not produce problems in the clinical diagnosis, but in more protracted cases a clinical diagnosis is not always possible. However, in the

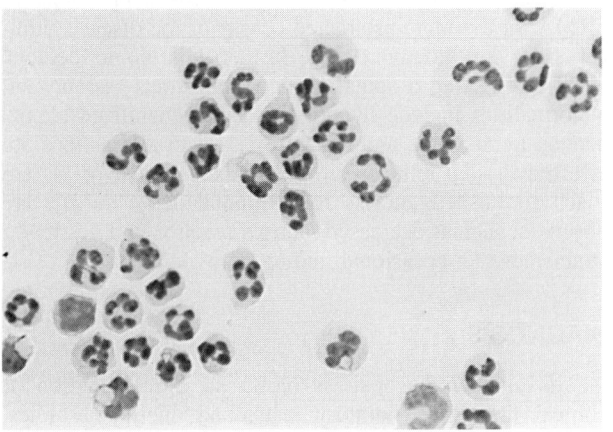

Figure 4. CSF: cytospin preparation, neutrophilic pleocytosis in the acute "classic" form of SRMA.

vast majority of cases with SRMA a combination of *elevated IgA levels* in the CSF and serum is found and strongly supportive of the diagnosis (Tipold and Jaggy, 1994). This finding is typical for SRMA and is not found in other inflammatory and infectious diseases of the CNS, with the exception of tumors of the hematopoietic system (lymphoma, myeloma, histiocytosis).

DIFFERENTIAL DIAGNOSIS

SRMA is the most frequently occurring meningitis with neutrophilic pleocytosis in the dog. However, an important differential diagnosis is a bacterial meningitis that is not treatable with corticosteroids. Bacterial meningitis occurs in young dogs after trauma or biting injuries or by extension of discospondylitis. Other bacterial infections of the CNS are mostly hematogenous and affected dogs may have extensive neurologic deficits (e.g., forebrain or brain stem lesions). In addition to the history, a search for skin lesions or extraneural bacterial infections such as endocarditis, pyelonephritis, pleuritis, and otitis should be performed. Other encephalitides with neutrophilia in the CSF such as protozoal diseases and GME have more profound neurologic deficits due to invasive lesions and are not limited to the meninges. Some meningiomas can produce a marked neutrophilic pleocytosis in the CSF. Tumors can be excluded by appropriate imaging techniques.

Chronic SRMA is more difficult to diagnose. A larger list of possible differential diagnoses must be considered such as all viral encephalitides, GME, protozoal infections, and neoplasms. GME especially can be mistaken for SRMA because this disease also improves after corticosteroid treatment. Besides specific examinations to exclude other inflammatory and infectious diseases and imaging techniques, the determination of IgA in serum and CSF is helpful because values are elevated in a high percentage of cases.

PROGNOSIS AND TREATMENT

The prognosis is relatively good in young dogs in the acute stage of the disease and treated aggressively. In more protracted cases, relapses are frequent, and the prognosis is guarded. Therapy in these dogs becomes more complicated and time consuming. In our experience, about 60% of the dogs have been cured after immunosuppressive treatment. Others were either euthanized on request of the owners because of continuous deterioration of the signs, or required continuous therapy to control clinical signs.

Therapy is anti-inflammatory and immunosuppressive. If initial signs are mild and neutrophilic pleocytosis is not higher than 200 cells/μl in CSF, nonsteroidal anti-inflammatory drugs might be used with careful monitoring of the animal. After the first relapse, or when symptoms become worse and are combined with massive pleocytosis in the CSF, long-term treatment with prednisolone for at least 6 months must be initiated. The dosage is individually adjusted. Prednisolone is given at an initial dose of 4 mg/kg every 24 hours PO or IV. After 2 days, the steroid dosage is reduced to 2 mg/kg every 24 hours for about 1 to 2 weeks followed by 1 mg/kg every 24 hours. The dogs are re-examined including a CSF tap and blood profile every 4 to 6 weeks after the beginning of therapy. As soon as the neurologic examination and CSF are found to be normal, the steroid dose can be reduced to half of the previous dosage until a dosage of 0.5 mg/kg every 48 hours or every 72 hours is reached. If pleocytosis persists, the same dosage should be continued. After about 6 months, when the dogs are clinically normal and present a normal CSF tap and blood profile in the last two examinations, the treatment is stopped. In protracted cases the same regimen is used from the beginning. If the dogs do not respond well to therapy with prednisolone alone, immunosuppressive drugs such as purine analogues like azathioprine may be used in combination with steroids. There are no controlled studies. In my experience, it appears useful to alternate azathioprine treatment every other day with prednisolone. Purine analogues are effective because they affect both T- and B-cell responses and even inhibit the production of macrophages, which are also involved in SRMA. Azathioprine may be given in a dosage of 1.5 mg/kg PO every 48 hours. Since neutrophils are an important cell population in SRMA, prednisolone is still a useful drug because of its "broad-spectrum" ability to suppress inflammation. Corticosteroids do not deplete lymphocytes in dogs at the beginning of a treatment schedule. Perhaps treatment advantages might be expected in protracted cases using drugs that affect lymphocytes. Antibiotics can be given at the beginning of the treatment schedule, if a bacterial infection cannot be excluded. Furthermore, protection against ulceration in the gastrointestinal tract should always be considered with long-term corticosteroid treatment. Treatment with high doses of corticosteroids can lead to serious complications in addition to non-life-threatening side effects such as polyuria, polydipsia, polyphagia, and weight gain. Treatment is not tolerated in about 5% of the dogs.

References and Suggested Reading

Felsburg PJ, Hogenesch H, Somberg RL, et al: Immunologic abnormalities in canine juvenile polyarteritis syndrome: A naturally occurring animal model of Kawasaki disease. Clin Immunol Immunopathol 65:110, 1992.
Immunologic abnormalities in three Beagles with CJPS are described.

Hayes TJ, Roberts GKS, Halliwell WH: An idiopathic febrile necrotizing arteritis syndrome in the dog: Beagle pain syndrome. Toxicologic Pathology 17:129, 1989.
Clinical, laboratory, and pathologic features of the Beagle pain syndrome are described.

Irving G, Chrisman C: Long-term outcome of five cases of corticosteroid-responsive meningomyelitis. J Am Anim Hosp Assoc 26:324, 1990.
Clinical description of five dogs presented with hyperesthesia and spastic paraparesis or quadriparesis and mixed pleocytosis in the CSF.

Meric SM, Perman V, Hardy RM: Corticosteroid-responsive meningitis in ten dogs. J Am Anim Hosp Assoc 21:677, 1985.
Ten cases of SRMA in young dogs seen during a 6-year period are described. Corticosteroid therapy was effective in all cases.

Presthus J: Aseptic suppurative meningitis in Bernese mountain dogs. Eur J Companion Anim Pract 1:24, 1991.
A review of the clinical symptoms of assumed SRMA in 11 Bernese mountain dogs is given.

Scott-Moncrieff JC, Snyder PW, Glickman LT, et al: Systemic necrotizing vasculitis in nine young beagles. J Am Vet Med Assoc 201:1553, 1992.
Nine young Beagles with JPS are studied. If untreated, clinical signs and laboratory abnormalities had a remitting and relapsing course in most dogs.

Snyder PW, Kazacos EA, Scott-Moncrieff JC, et al: Pathological features of naturally-occurring juvenile polyarteritis in beagle dogs. Vet Pathol 32:337, 1995.
In 18 young Beagle dogs with canine juvenile polyarteritis syndrome, the major histopathologic alterations were a systemic vasculitis and perivasculitis.

Tipold A: Diagnosis of inflammatory and infectious-diseases of the central-nervous-system in dogs: A retrospective study. J Vet Intern Med 9:304, 1995.
The medical records of 220 dogs with inflammatory and infectious diseases of the CNS were retrospectively examined.

Tipold A, Jaggy A: Steroid-responsive meningitis-arteritis in dogs: Long-term study of 32 cases. J Small Anim Pract 35:311, 1994.
Clinical symptoms and long-term treatment of 32 dogs with steroid-responsive meningitis-arteritis are studied.

Tipold A, Vandevelde M, Zurbriggen A: Neuroimmunological studies in steroid-responsive meningitis-arteritis in dogs. Res Vet Sci 58:103, 1995.
The present study is concerned with the intrathecal humoral immune response of 13 dogs suffering from SRMA.

Chronic Inflammatory Demyelinating Polyneuropathy in Dogs

KYLE G. BRAUND

Auburn, Alabama

The classification of peripheral nerve (PN) disease in domestic animals continues to evolve in veterinary medicine. The majority of PN disorders in small domestic animals are degenerative, usually breed-related, and hereditary or congenital. Inflammatory or infectious neuropathies in dogs and cats also are well recognized. This present review documents clinical and pathologic findings on an unusual demyelinating inflammatory neuropathy that has previously been limited to single case reports.

CLINICAL FINDINGS

This article summarizes this condition in 20 animals—12 dogs (5 males, 7 females; mean age, 6.3 years; range, 1.5 to 13 years; Table 1) and 8 cats (3 males, 5 females; mean age, 7.1 years; range, 1 to 14 years; Table 2). Muscle and nerve biopsy specimens from affected animals were processed in the Neuromuscular Laboratory, Scott-Ritchey Research Center, Auburn University, for routine histology, histochemistry, single nerve fiber teasing, semithin and ultrathin sections, and peripheral nerve immunocytochemistry.

Onset of clinical signs in our dogs and cats was typically insidious and the course chronic, sometimes relapsing, and often slowly progressive. Clinical signs were usually first noticed in the pelvic limbs and, in most animals, progressed to involve the thoracic limbs. Signs included paraparesis, tetraparesis, stumbling gait, hyporeflexia, sometimes tetraplegia, and variable muscle wasting. Additional signs included muscle trembling when standing in dogs 2 and 7; intermittent shifting limb lameness characterized by a plantigrade stance in cat 1; and ventroflexion of the neck in cat 8. Possible cranial nerve involvement was suggested by voice alteration in dog 4, right facial paresis in dog 7, and prior history of laryngeal paralysis in dog 12 that was surgically treated. A prior history of regurgitation was recorded in cat 6, and there was radiographic evidence of megaesophagus in cat 5. No clinical sensory deficits were observed in any animal.

LABORATORY FINDINGS

With the exception of an IgG monoclonal gammopathy found in cat 8, results of routine hematologic and blood biochemical analyses, cortisol and thyrotropin response testing, blood lead concentration, serum cholinesterase activity, immunologic function, serologic testing for infectious disease, and chemical testing for myasthenia gravis were normal. Analysis of cerebrospinal fluid (CSF) collected from the cerebellomedullary cistern was normal in all animals except for moderately elevated protein content in dog 5 (106 mg/dl) and cat 5 (58 mg/dl). Motor nerve conduction velocity (MNCV) in the sciatic-tibial nerves was slow in all animals tested, ranging from 13 to 45 meters per second (m/sec) in dogs and 20 to 55 m/sec in cats (established normal MNCV values for sciatic-tibial nerves in dogs and cats are 60 to 70 m/sec and 70 to 80 m/sec, respectively). Temporal dispersion, decreased amplitudes, and prolonged latencies of the compound muscle action potentials were also present. Sensory nerve conduction velocities were slow in 1 of 2 dogs tested. Electromyographic testing revealed no abnormal spontaneous

TABLE 1. Clinical Features in 12 dogs With Chronic Inflammatory Demyelinating Neuropathy

Dog No.	Age (Years)	Breed	Sex	Chronic Course	Relapsing Course	Steroid-Responsive	Slowed Motor NCV
1	1.5	Alaskan malamute	F	yes	yes	yes	37
2	1.5	English Springer	F	yes	yes	yes	32
3	2.5	Rottweiler	F	yes	yes	yes	42
4	3	Cocker spaniel	M	yes		yes	45
5	5	Labrador retriever-X	F	yes	yes	yes	17
6	5.5	Great Dane	M	yes	no	yes	39
7	6	Cocker spaniel	M	yes	yes	yes	13
8	10	Mixed-breed	F	yes	no	unknown	34
9	10.5	Mastiff	F	yes	yes	no	25
10	11	Old English sheepdog	M	yes	no	yes	36
11	12	Mixed-breed	F	yes	yes	yes	27
12	13	Brittany spaniel	M	yes	no	yes	14

NCV = nerve conduction velocity.

Adapted from Braund KG, Vallat JM, Steiss JE, et al: Chronic inflammatory demyelinating polyneuropathy in dogs and cats. J Periph Nerv Syst 1(2):149–155, 1996, with permission.

982

TABLE 2. Clinical Features in 8 Cats With Chronic Inflammatory Demyelinating Neuropathy

Cat No.	Age (Years)	Breed	Sex	Chronic Course	Relapsing Course	Steroid-Responsive	Slowed Motor NCV
1	1.0	Abyssinian	F	yes	yes	yes	not tested
2	1.4	DSH	M	yes	no	yes	35
3	1.5	DSH	F	yes	yes	yes	34
4	8	DSH	M	yes	no	yes	25
5	8	DLH	F	yes	no	no	40
6	10	DSH	M	yes	yes	yes	22
7	13	DSH	F	yes	yes	yes	unavailable
8	14	DSH	F	yes	no	yes	63

NCV = nerve conduction velocity; DSH = domestic shorthair; DLH = domestic longhair.

From Braund KG, Vallat JM, Steiss JE, et al: Chronic inflammatory demyelinating polyneuropathy in dogs and cats. J Periph Nerv Syst 1(2):149–155, 1996, with permission.

activity in dogs 7, 9, and 10, or in cats 1, 2, 5, and 8. In the other animals, a mild, patchy pattern of fibrillation potentials and positive sharp waves was recorded in some limb muscles. There was no preferential involvement of proximal or distal muscles.

PATHOLOGIC FINDINGS

Nerve changes were most readily appreciated using teased nerve fiber preparations, the results of which are quantitatively shown in Tables 3 and 4. The dominant abnormality in nerves from all animals was demyelination, usually paranodal, sometimes segmental, and occurring alone (grade C) or in combination with remyelinating intercalated internodes (grade D) on the same fiber. Other changes included remyelination (grade F) and variable numbers of fibers with internodal globules (grade G). Axonal degeneration, characterized by linear rows of myelin ovoids and balls (grade E), was infrequently observed.

In cross-sectional semithin preparations of nerves from affected animals, abnormal findings were typically mild and included variable numbers of fibers with inappropriately thin myelin sheaths and scattered presence of myelin-ated fibers with voluminous Schwann cell cytoplasm, sometimes containing one or more macrophages and myelin debris. The most severe changes seen in semithin sections were those from dog 7, with a 3-year history of chronic relapsing signs. These were characterized by prominent loss of myelinated fibers and apparent onion-bulbs and/or cluster formations.

Ultrastructural studies of nerves from affected dogs and cats revealed frequent presence of one or more macrophages within Schwann cells of myelinated fibers, often separating and stripping myelin sheaths, scattered naked and remyelinating axons, and multifocal presence of endo-neurial mononuclear cells, including lymphocytes, rare plasma cells, macrophages with myelin debris, and vacuo-lated fibroblasts. Axons of myelinated fibers appeared normal.

Indirect immunofluorescence revealed positive IgG staining in peripheral nerve myelin sheaths from two dogs (4, 5). Mild fiber size variation was seen in appendicular skeletal muscle. Antimuscle antibodies were not detected and there was no evidence of necrosis, phagocytosis, or inflammation in any muscle.

No abnormalities have been observed in the brain or

TABLE 3. Incidence (Percentage) of Abnormalities in Teased Nerve Fibers From Dogs With Idiopathic Demyelinating Neuropathy

Dog No.	Age (Years)	Nerve	Histological Classification*					Percentage of Abnormal Fibers
			C	D	E	F	G	
1	1.5	Sciatic	16	6	0	2	0	24 (0)†
2	1.5	CPN	40	0	0	0	0	40 (0)
3	2.5	Tibial	8	0	0	0	0	8 (0)
4	3	CPN	26	0	0	0	0	26 (0)
5	5	Tibial	29	8	2	3	2	44 (0–3)
6	5.5	Tibial	7	5	0	10	2	22 (0–3)
8	10	CPN	15	20	5	20	2	62 (0–7)
9	10.5	Tibial	3	40	1	3	10	57 (0–7)
10	11	CPN	21	1	1	2	2	27 (0–10)
11	12	Tibial	15	10	2	8	0	35 (0–10)
12	13	UN	20	30	2	8	2	62 (0–15)

*A = normal appearance; B = excessive irregularity of myelin not attributable to preparative artifacts; C = single or multiple regions of nodal lengthening or internodal myelin absence; D = single or multiple C and F abnormalities combined; E = linear rows of myelin ovoids and balls; F = 50% or more difference in myelin thickness between internodes; G = thickening or reduplication of myelin to form globules within internodes.

†Figures in parentheses refer to range of abnormalities in comparable nerves from age-matched control dogs.

CPN = common peroneal nerve; UN = ulnar nerve.

From Braund KG, Vallat JM, Steiss JE, et al: Chronic inflammatory demyelinating polyneuropathy in dogs and cats. J Periph Nerv Syst 1(2):149–155, 1966, with permission.

TABLE 4. Incidence (Percentage) of Abnormalities in Teased Nerve Fibers From Cats With Idiopathic Demyelinating Neuropathy

Cat No.	Age (Years)	Nerve	Histological Classification*					Percentage of Abnormal Fibers
			C	D	E	F	G	
1	1	CPN	30	0	0	0	0	30 (0)†
2	1.4	CPN	40	0	0	7	0	47 (0)
3	1.5	CPN	7	14	0	10	0	31 (0)
4	8	CPN	47	0	0	1	0	48 (0–3)
5	8	CPN	18	5	1	10	1	35 (0–3)
6	10	Sciatic	9	0	0	30	0	39 (0–7)
7	13	CPN	12	1	0	5	0	18 (0–13)
8	14	UN	15	0	0	7	0	23 (0–12)

*A = normal appearance; B = excessive irregularity of myelin not attributable to preparative artifacts; C = single or multiple regions of nodal lengthening or internodal myelin absence; D = single or multiple C and F abnormalities combined; E = linear rows of myelin ovoids and balls; F = 50% or more difference in myelin thickness between internodes; G = thickening or reduplication of myelin to form globules within internodes.

†Figures in parentheses refer to range of abnormalities in comparable nerves from age-matched control cats.

CPN = common peroneal nerve; UN = ulnar nerve.

Adapted from Braund KG, Vallat JM, Steiss JE, et al: Chronic inflammatory demyelinating polyneuropathy in dogs and cats. J Periph Nerv Syst 1(2):149–155, 1966, with permission.

spinal cord, and no evidence of polyradiculoneuritis has been seen in nerve roots. In the cat with the monoclonal gammopathy, lymphosarcoma was present in the stomach and intestinal tract.

ETIOLOGY

In absence of metabolic, endocrine, infectious, or storage disease, it is possible that the demyelinating neuropathy in our animals has an underlying immune-mediated pathogenesis, based on presence of endoneurial mononuclear cell infiltrates, macrophage stripping of myelin sheaths, high initial clinical response to corticosteroids, and observation of anti-IgG antibody on the myelin lamellae in two dogs. We suggest this condition be termed *chronic inflammatory demyelinating polyneuropathy* (CIDP) because of its clinical and pathologic similarity to CIDP in people, a probable immune-mediated disease based on pathologic findings, and response to various therapeutic agents, including corticosteroids, immune-modulating agents, plasma exchange, and human immune globulin. Immunocytochemical evidence of IgG antibody staining of myelin lamellae seen in two of our dogs is also occasionally observed in human CIDP patients.

DIFFERENTIAL DIAGNOSIS

The dominant pathologic feature of the peripheral neuropathy in our animals was demyelination, primarily paranodal, which makes this neuropathy pathologically different from the breed-related axonopathies, and from those neuropathies in dogs and cats characterized by mixed axonal degeneration, demyelination, and remyelination as seen in infectious, metabolic, and paraneoplastic neuropathies, and in several generalized, probable immune-mediated inflammatory neuropathies including coonhound paralysis, idiopathic polyradiculoneuritis, chronic relapsing polyradiculoneuritis, cauda equina polyradiculoneuritis, and brachial plexus neuropathy. Furthermore, the insidious onset and slow, often relapsing clinical course seen in our animals differs from the acute onset of coonhound paralysis,

brachial plexus neuropathy, and idiopathic polyradiculoneuritis. There is a single report of a cat with chronic relapsing polyradiculoneuritis in which there was prominent mononuclear inflammatory cell infiltration in nerve roots, ganglia, and cranial and peripheral nerves. Findings comparable to those in our cats included chronic relapsing course, segmental demyelination, remyelination, and onion-bulb formation. However, clinical differences from our cases included presence of a fine, whole-body tremor, biting and excessive grooming of the hind feet, loss of superficial sensation, tendency to fall over when walking, high-stepping gait, and exaggerated patellar reflexes. This cat was not steroid-responsive. Another condition in a cat, termed *chronic relapsing polyneuropathy*, appears quite similar to our cases in every respect; however, one biopsy specimen also contained prominent axonal degeneration, a finding that was not a feature in our cases.

Currently, well-defined demyelinating neuropathies in dogs and cats are restricted to two conditions—inherited chronic hypertrophic neuropathy in Tibetan Mastiff puppies and inherited sphingomyelinosis in Siamese kittens, both of which are clinically, genetically and pathologically different to our cases. The demyelinating condition in our animals is also clinically and pathologically distinct from congenital hypomyelinating neuropathy in Golden retriever puppies.

TREATMENT/PROGNOSIS

The majority of dogs and cats were clinically steroid-responsive, although to varying degrees. In dogs and cats, prednisone may be used at a dosage of 1.0 to 2.0 mg/kg PO bid. The dose is reduced after remission of signs and is gradually withdrawn with alternate-day therapy. Among the dogs of our study, 90% were initially responsive. Six dogs showed a strong and immediate response (dogs 1, 3, 4, 5, 7, and 11) with a return to normality. Dog 11 continued to show a strong response for 18 months, at which time she became steroid-resistant and deteriorated clinically. Five dogs showed a moderate but incomplete clinical response to steroids (dogs 2, 6, 8, 10, and 12). Dog 9 was not steroid-responsive. There is historical evidence that at least four dogs relapsed when the dose of corticosteroids was reduced (dogs 1, 3, 6, 7).

Approximately 88% of cats were initially clinically steroid-responsive. Three cats were strongly responsive (cats 1, 6, and 7) with a return to normality. Four cats showed a moderate but incomplete clinical response to steroids (cats 2, 3, 4, and 8). Cat 5 was not steroid-responsive. Three cats relapsed when the dose of steroids was reduced (cats 1, 3, and 6). In addition, cat 7 had four clinical episodes that were steroid-responsive with a return to normality before she became nonresponsive.

Acknowledgments

I wish to thank the following clinicians for providing clinical data and/or tissue specimens for this study: Drs. Jaggy; Laterza, Lowrie, Shores, Plummer, Shell, Simpson, Katherman, Coates, Sorjonen, Steinberg (HS and SA); McVey, de Carlo, Joseph, Matz, Hardie, and Hohenhaus.

References and Suggested Reading

Braund KG: Clinical Syndromes in Veterinary Neurology, 2nd ed. St. Louis: Mosby–YearBook, 1994.
A clinical textbook that relates to neurologic syndromes in dogs and cats, including the neuropathic syndromes and their associated signs and diseases, as well as a detailed description of nerve biopsy techniques, nerve handling and processing, and illustrated nerve pathology.
Braund KG: Peripheral nerve disorders. In: Ettinger SJ, Feldman EC, eds: Textbook of Veterinary Internal Medicine, 4th ed. Philadelphia: WB Saunders, 1995, pp 701–728.
A comprehensive review of peripheral neuropathies seen in dogs and cats, including inherited, metabolic, infectious, traumatic, and vascular causes.

Hypokalemic Myopathy in Cats

BOYD R. JONES
Dublin, Ireland

Hypokalemia results from one of the following: reduced potassium intake, increased potassium entry into the cells, or increased potassium loss from the body. Of these causes in cats, renal potassium loss is the most important, especially if such loss is associated with inadequate intake. In healthy cats the daily potassium intake should equal daily loss. Potassium maintains the intracellular fluid volume and normal membrane potential. If the ratio between intra- and extracellular potassium is significantly altered, the muscle membrane potential of excitatory tissue such as nerve and muscle is affected. Hypokalemia significantly affects muscle membrane activity and muscle function and can, if severe, result in rhabdomyolysis. As potassium is depleted, a progressive increase in the muscle cell resting transmembrane potential (hyperpolarization) results so that the myocyte becomes increasingly refractory to electrical stimulation. Eventually, however, the muscle cell membrane suddenly becomes permeable to sodium ions and the resulting sudden membrane hypopolarization induces rapid, severe weakness. If the potassium deficit is not corrected, the muscular dysfunction may progress to paralysis. The increase in intracellular sodium (and chloride) often exceeds the degree of potassium depletion that predisposes to rhabdomyolysis by osmotic expansion of the cell (Fettman, 1989). Additional factors that may contribute to the myopathy and rhabdomyolysis are a reduction in muscle blood flow that occurs with exercise, and altered muscle carbohydrate metabolism (Fettman, 1989).

There have been numerous reports of polymyopathy in cats associated with a variety of different causes of hypokalemia (Table 1). Of these causes, cats with chronic renal failure and Burmese kittens that develop hypokalemia associated with disturbances in the intracellular and extracellular balance of potassium show the most severe myopathic signs. The syndrome in Burmese kittens (2 to 6 months of age) bears many similarities to hypokalemic periodic paralysis in humans, a condition that is thought to be related to a calcium channel disorder. The condition has a familial and inherited basis (putative autosomal recessive), with affected kittens being produced in specific lines of this breed.

In the acquired disease, dietary factors appear to contribute significantly to the development of hypokalemia and subsequent myopathy: Potassium-depleted diets, acidifying

TABLE 1. Some Conditions Associated With Hypokalemia in Cats

Hyperaldosteronisim (Conn's syndrome) caused by an
    adrenocortical tumor
Renal tubular acidosis
Thyrotoxicosis
Chronic renal failure
Metabolic acidosis
Dietary
    Potassium deficient
    Acidified diets
Insulin overdose
Diuretic therapy (furosemide)
Metabolic alkalosis
Chronic vomiting/diarrhea
Fluid administration (plasma dilution and volume-induced diuresis)
Idiopathic (Burmese breed)
Systemic diseases
    Hepatic disease
    Infectious disease

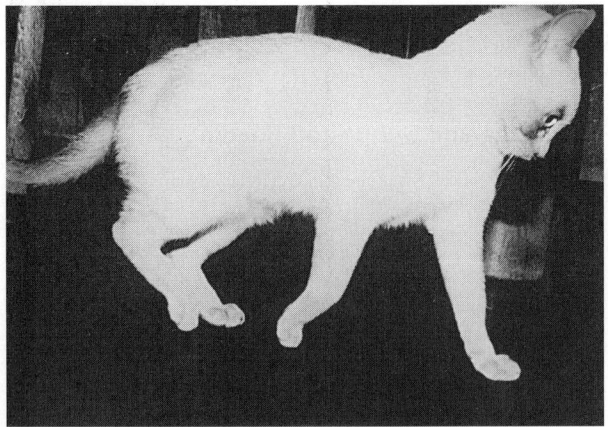

Figure 1. A 9-month-old Burmese cat with hypokalemia and ventroflexion of the head.

diets, magnesium-restricted diets, and high-protein diets have been incriminated. Pet food manufacturers have in recent years ensured that appropriate concentrations of minerals are added and that the formulation of diets for cats is not overacidifying.

CLINICAL SIGNS

Whatever the cause of hypokalemia, the clinical signs shown by the affected cats are similar. The clinical signs may be transient or persistent. The earliest sign of severe potassium depletion is muscle dysfunction. There is generalized muscle weakness with persistent ventroflexion of the neck, with the head being tucked into the sternum (Fig. 1). The cats are intolerant of exercise and some walk with an awkward, stiff, stilted gait. There may be exertional muscle tremor followed by sudden fatigue and collapse. Severely affected cats are reluctant to move, and some owners report that their cat showed lethargy and tiredness for some months before a severe episode occurred. Some cats show pain when their muscles are palpated. The clinical course in Burmese kittens is much more transient, with moderate to severe episodes followed by improvement (with or without treatment) and relapse. Postural reactions and spinal reflexes are normal.

Cats with advanced potassium depletion may show other signs, including poor body condition with weight loss; a poor, unkempt hair coat; and polydipsia and polyuria. These latter signs are mostly present in cats where concurrent chronic renal failure is present.

DIAGNOSIS

The history, clinical findings, and breed (Burmese) provide a high index of suspicion of hypokalemia and the likely cause of potassium depletion.

The presence of a low serum potassium, usually less than 3.0 mmol/L, will confirm the diagnosis of hypokalemia; however, clinical signs can occasionally develop in cats with higher serum potassium values. Furthermore, serum potassium concentrations can increase after cage confinement or hospitalization because the myopathy and clinical signs are frequently precipitated or exacerbated by exercise. The low serum potassium concentration is frequently accompanied by increased serum activity (5,000–10,000 IU/L) of serum creatine kinase (CK). The CK is released only when the concentration of potassium in muscle is very low. In affected Burmese kittens, serum CK values can be very elevated (>50,000 IU/L).

Other biochemical abnormalities that have been observed in hypokalemic cats include azotemia, hypercholesterolemia, hyperchloridemia, hyperglycemia, and elevated serum creatinine. Such findings are frequently associated with concurrent renal dysfunction.

Determination of the fractional excretion of potassium as ascertained by the formula below may help differentiate renal and nonrenal sources of potassium loss. The FE_{K^+} should be less than 5% in a healthy cat with normal renal function and a potassium-depleted cat with normal renal function, for example, in Burmese kittens with idiopathic hypokalemia. An FE_{K^+} of greater than 10 to 15% indicates significant renal potassium loss. Urinary loss may be determined more accurately by measuring the 24-hour urinary potassium loss.

$$FE_{K^+} (\%) = \frac{UK^+}{PK^+} \times \frac{PCr}{UCr} \times 100$$

(where P = plasma, U = urine, Cr = creatinine, and K = potassium).

The differential diagnosis of hypokalemic myopathy includes polyneuropathy, myasthenia gravis, organophosphate toxicity, thiamine deficiency, other electrolyte abnormalities, primary myopathies, tick paralysis, and snake bite.

Diffuse electromyographic abnormalities are sometimes present (e.g., positive sharp waves may be recorded). Muscle biopsy specimens are mostly normal on light microscopy, but mild myofiber necrosis is occasionally observed.

TREATMENT

The goal of treatment of the cat with hypokalemia and myopathic signs is to restore the serum potassium concentration to and maintain it in the reference range without causing the toxic side effects of potassium therapy. The clinical signs of muscle weakness are reversible, and the response to potassium supplementation is rapid. If potassium depletion is severe, potassium supplementation should be administered both orally and intravenously ac-

TABLE 2. IV Potassium Administration*

Serum Potassium (mmol/L)	Potassium Chloride Added to Fluids†	Maximum Volume Infusion Rate ml/kg/hr‡
3.6–5.0	20	25
3.1–3.5	30	17
2.6–3.0	40	12
2.1–2.5	60	8
<2.0	80	6

*Includes quantity and rate of administration so as not to exceed 0.5 mmol/L potassium per hour.
†mmol (mEq) of potassium per liter of crystalloid fluid; sufficient KCl should be added to achieve this concentration per liter.
‡Infusion rate of crystalloid (e.g., lactated Ringer's solution) containing supplemental KCl.
Note: Never inject KCl solution IV.

cording to the dose and administration rates detailed in Table 2. Intravenous potassium supplementation should not exceed 0.5 mmol(mEq)/kg per hour; otherwise cardiac dysrhythmias or asystole may occur. Electrocardiographic monitoring during therapy should be considered and administration stopped if dysrhythmias occur. It should be noted that in some cats the serum potassium may actually decline with IV fluid therapy, and frequent determinations should be made.

Once acute potassium depletion is corrected, oral treatment should be continued (see below). If the cat is not severely affected, oral potassium supplementation is safe and effective for correcting clinical signs.

Potassium gluconate solution (Kaon Elixir, Adria Laboratories), tablets, or powder (Tumil K, Daniels Pharmaceuticals) can be administered in food. Potassium chloride is not an appropriate oral form of potassium because it can contribute to metabolic acidosis. A dose rate of 2 to 4 mmol/cat PO per day is a safe and usually effective starting dose. The serum potassium concentration should be rechecked every 10 to 14 days until serum values are stable in the reference range.

The link between renal disease and potassium depletion is well established and, importantly, there is evidence that oral potassium supplementation will improve or stabilize the remaining renal function. Potassium depletion can contribute to ongoing renal damage; therefore, cats with chronic renal failure should receive daily oral potassium supplementation (2 to 4 mmol/cat PO per day). Burmese kittens with transient periodic hypokalemia also benefit from daily oral supplementation.

If a diagnosis of hypokalemia is correct, the response to intravenous or oral potassium therapy is usually favorable and rapid (2 to 5 days). However, complete recovery of normal muscle strength in cats with myopathy can take up to several weeks. The prognosis is favorable with most affected cats, especially Burmese kittens, but the severity of the renal disease may alter that prognosis in some cats. In cats with Conn's syndrome, the prognosis depends on identification and effective surgical treatment of the adrenal tumor (see p. 368).

References and Suggested Reading

Dow SW, Fettman MJ, Le Couteur RA, et al: Hypokalemia in cats: 186 cases (1984–87). J Am Vet Med Assoc 194:1604, 1989.
   A retrospective survey of hypokalemia in cats in the United States.
Edwards CM, Belford CJ: Hypokalaemic polymyopathy in Burmese cats. Aust Vet Practit 25:58, 1995.
   A report of five cases of hypokalemic myopathy in Burmese cats.
Fettman MJ: Feline kaliopenic polymyopathy/nephropathy syndrome. Vet Clin North Am Small Anim Pract 19:415, 1989.
   A review of hypokalemia and polymyopathy in the cat.
MacIntire DK: Disorders of potassium, phosphorus and magnesium in critical illness. Compend Contin Educ Pract Vet 19:41, 1997.
   A summary of electrolyte disturbances in severe illness and their correction.

Congenital Myotonia in the Cat

FIONA H. HICKFORD
Palmerston North, New Zealand

BOYD R. JONES
Dublin, Ireland

Myotonia is a disorder of skeletal muscle resulting in continued active contraction of a muscle after cessation of voluntary effort or stimulation. Myotonia has been reported in several breeds of dogs, most notably the Chow Chow, and in goats, horses, and humans. A myotonic condition in four related domestic shorthaired kittens similar to human myotonia congenita has recently been discovered and investigated (Hickford et al, 1998; Toll et al, 1998).

The four affected kittens reported by Hickford (1998) were from separate litters, of two related queens, and with an unknown father or fathers. Two males and two females were affected. Their problem was detected after the owner noticed that the kittens walked awkwardly with a stiff gait, and their claws became trapped in the carpet. Two kittens also had difficulty in grasping food with their claws and chewing it.

CLINICAL SIGNS

Affected kittens walk with a stiff, stilted gait, with the hind limbs being more severely affected. The stiffness is worse in cold weather and usually improves with exercise. The limbs are abducted when walking owing to reduced ability to flex the proximal limb joints. When the kittens are startled all four limbs become hyperextended, and they fall into lateral recumbency, often lying in this position for up to 10 seconds before being able to rise. On other occasions when they are startled there is prolapse of the nictitating membranes, spasm of the orbicularis oculi muscle, retraction of the lips, and flattening of the ears (Fig. 1).

Muscle hypertrophy is present with hypertrophy of the gastrocnemius muscle being consistent, and more diffuse muscle hypertrophy involving the triceps, biceps, quadriceps femoris and tongue being present in some kittens.

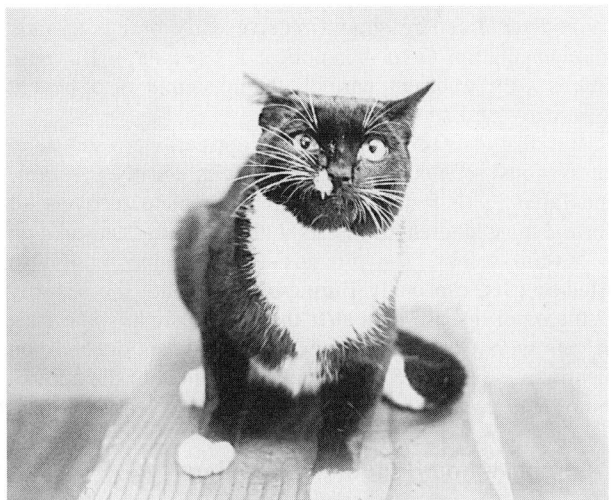

Figure 1. An affected kitten showing flattening of the ears and retraction of the lip after receiving a fright.

Their mouths can be difficult to open fully owing to increased tone of the masticatory muscles. Dysphagia may be present because of difficulty in opening the mouth and chewing. Sometimes a hoarse meow and quiet purr can be heard.

DIAGNOSIS

Muscle Percussion

In anesthetized kittens, percussion of the tongue with the handle of artery forceps results in sustained dimpling of the muscle. This finding is similar to that reported in dogs, and percussion of other muscles can also result in a dimple (Griffiths and Duncan, 1973), but this response is difficult to demonstrate in the kittens without shaving the haircoat. Care should be taken when anesthetizing affected animals because endotracheal intubation can be difficult owing to difficulty in opening the mouth widely and narrowing of the glottis. The latter has been described in other species and is thought to be due to spasm of the muscles controlling the arytenoid cartilage movement (Farrow and Malik, 1981).

Clinical Pathology

Serum chemistry and complete blood counts from all affected kittens showed no abnormalities. The serum creatine kinase (CK) concentrations were within the reference range. Serum CK may be elevated in canine myotonia but is usually normal in humans with myotonia congenita (Farrow and Malik, 1981).

Electromyography

The unique electromyographic changes characteristic of myotonia are present in the kittens. Spontaneous waxing and waning bizarre high-frequency discharges are seen following needle electrode insertion and movement (Fig. 2). Audioprojection of the electromyogram recordings pro-

duces noises like a revving motorcycle or dive-bomber airplane. These electromyographic changes are similar to those described in myotonic humans and dogs (Jones et al, 1977). Percussion of the muscle while the needle is in place will also induce myotonic discharges.

Muscle Biopsy

Histology of muscle tissue from the kittens shows mild nonspecific changes, including occasional hypertrophied myofibers, central nuclei, and degenerate fibers. The severity of histopathologic change varies among affected kittens. The histopathologic abnormalities seen are similar to those described in dogs, and in this species individual variation also occurs (Kortz, 1989).

Histochemical staining with myosin adenosine triphosphatase, oil red O, periodic acid–Schiff, modified Gomori trichrome, and reduced nicotinamide adenine dinucleotide tetrazolium reductase has detected no abnormalities.

PATHOPHYSIOLOGY

Bryant (1973) showed reduced chloride conductance of the muscle fiber membrane from myotonic goats, and this has subsequently been described in humans with myotonia congenita. It is now known than human myotonia congenita is caused by a mutation of the gene encoding the muscle chloride channel (Koch et al, 1992). The chloride channel is responsible for the high resting membrane potential of skeletal muscle cells. Loss of function of the chloride channel leads to reduced chloride conductance and hyperexcitability of cells, and results in uncontrolled bursts of spontaneous action potentials. This causes muscle spasm and stiffness (Hoffman et al, 1995). A similar defect is suspected to be the cause of the myotonia in the kittens, but attempts to determine the muscle chloride conductance have not yet been made.

DIFFERENTIAL DIAGNOSES

Feline myopathies that may cause muscle stiffness and an awkward gait include feline X-linked muscular dystrophy, nemaline myopathy, ossifying myositis, hypokalemic polymyopathy, and immune-mediated and protozoal polymyositis (Cuddon, 1994). These can be differentiated by serum chemistry, serology, muscle biopsy, and electromyography (EMG). The most important to differentiate is

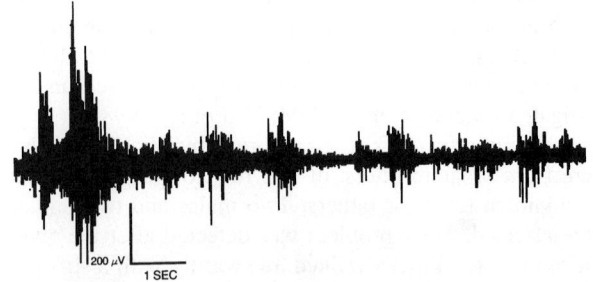

Figure 2. Electromyographic recording from the triceps muscle of an affected kitten showing waxing and waning high-frequency discharges following needle insertion.

feline X-linked muscular dystrophy, which is due to a lack of dystrophin. Affected cats have more marked muscle hypertrophy than kittens with congenital myotonia, and large elevations in serum CK concentration are seen. Histopathologic changes in muscle include marked dystrophic changes such as myofiber necrosis, phagocytosis, mineralization, and muscle splitting, and EMG reveals high-frequency discharges that do not wax and wane (pseudomyotonic discharges). Histochemistry reveals a lack of dystrophin in muscle (Blot and Fuhrer, 1995).

TREATMENT

Treatment has not been necessary for the kittens. They live without distress but do require enhanced supervision to avoid misadventure. Owners should be advised to avoid exposing the kittens to cold weather and shag pile carpets! The disease does not appear to be progressive. It is suspected to be inherited, and although the mode of inheritance is not yet known, affected cats certainly should not be bred.

In dogs, therapy is aimed at stabilizing the muscle membrane using sodium channel blockers such as procainamide, phenytoin, and quinidine. These drugs are associated with a high risk of side effects and toxicity in cats, and extreme caution is warranted. Phenytoin and quinidine are not recommended for use in cats owing to drug accumulation and toxic signs such as ataxia, sedation, seizures, anorexia, vomiting, and diarrhea. Procainamide can cause gastrointestinal side effects and hypotension (Plumb, 1995).

References and Suggested Reading

Blot S, Fuhrer L: Les myopathies des carnivores domestiques. Prat Med Chir Anim Comp 30:27, 1995.
A review (in French) of feline and canine myopathies.
Bryant SH: The electrophysiology of myotonia, with a review of congenital myotonia of goats. In: Desmedt JE, ed: New Developments in Electromyography and Clinical Neurophysiology. Basel: Karger, 1973, p 420.
A review of myotonia in goats and the current knowledge of the electrophysiology of the disorder.
Cuddon PA: Feline neuromuscular disease. Feline Pract 22:7, 1990.
A review of feline neuromuscular diseases and their diagnosis.
Farrow BRH, Malik R: Hereditary myotonia in the chow chow. J Small Anim Pract 22:451, 1981.
A description of the clinical features, diagnosis, and treatment of hereditary myotonia in four Chow Chow dogs.
Griffiths IR, Duncan ID: Myotonia in the dog: A report of four cases. Vet Rec 93:184, 1973.
The first report of myotonia in dogs.
Hickford FH, Jones BR, Gethine MA, et al: Congenital myotonia in related kittens. J Small Anim Pract 39:281, 1998.
A report of the investigation of myotonia in four related kittens.
Hoffman EP, Lehmann-Horn F, Rudel R: Overexcited or inactive: Ion channels in muscle disease. Cell 80:681, 1995.
A review of muscle disease resulting from abnormalities in muscle sodium, chloride, and calcium channels.
Jones BR, Anderson LJ, Barnes GRG, et al: Myotonia in related chow chow dogs. NZ Vet J 25:217, 1977.
The first report of myotonia in related Chow Chow dogs in New Zealand.
Koch MC, Steinmeyer K, Ricker K, et al: Tight linkage of recessive and dominant forms of human myotonia to skeletal muscle chloride channel gene. Science 257:797, 1992.
This details the discovery of a genetic mutation in the chloride channel gene linked to Thomsen and Becker myotonia (myotonia congenita) in humans.
Kortz G: Canine myotonia. Semin Vet Med Surg 4:141, 1989.
A review of canine myotonia and comparison with human myotonic conditions.
Plumb DC: Veterinary Drug Handbook. Ames: Iowa State University Press, 1995, p 548.
Veterinary clinical pharmacology textbook.
Toll J, Cooper B, Altschul M: Congenital myotonia in two domestic cats. J Vet Intern Med 12:116, 1998.
A report of the investigation of myotonia in two cats.

Gracilis-Semitendinosus Myopathy

DANIEL D. LEWIS
Gainesville, Florida

Myopathy of the gracilis and semitendinosus muscles has been reported as an infrequent cause of hindlimb lameness in dogs. This syndrome has been described as gracilis-semitendinosus muscle complex, myopathy, contracture, and fibrotic myopathy. Gracilis-semitendinosus myopathy has been reported in dogs from the United Kingdom, throughout Europe, and from Australia and North America. A review of the literature reveals that gracilis-semitendinosus myopathy has been reported in 48 dogs (Vaughan, 1979; Moore et al, 1981; Thoren, 1981; Clarke, 1989; Capello et al, 1993; Lewis et al, 1997). Eighty-eight percent of the affected dogs have been German (39/48) or Belgian (3/48) shepherds. Other breeds of dogs reported with this condition include Doberman pinscher, Bobtail, St. Bernard,

Boxer, and Old English sheepdog. Young adult (range 8 months to 9 years; mean and median 5 years) male (81%) dogs are most often affected. Bilateral involvement has been reported in 26% of affected dogs; however, the onset of lameness is not always synchronous and the severity of lameness is not always symmetrical between the hindlimbs. Although the gracilis muscle was affected in 86% of affected dogs, the semitendinosus muscle can also be affected. Occasionally, both muscles can be affected in the same dog. Ipsilateral gracilis and semitendinosus muscle involvement has been reported in two dogs and contralateral involvement of the gracilis and semitendinosus muscles in another dog (Moore et al, 1981; Capello et al, 1993).

Several theories have been proposed regarding the etiopathogenesis of this condition. It has been suggested the gracilis-semitendinosus myopathy may result from: (1) a single traumatic event; (2) repeated microtrauma; (3) an autoimmune process; (4) a primary neuropathy; and, (5) vascular compromise. Histologic examination of muscle specimens from affected dogs have not unequivocally substantiated any of these etiologies (Vaughan, 1979; Moore et al, 1981; Capello et al, 1993; Lewis et al, 1997).

DIAGNOSIS

Although some owners perceived that their dog's lameness had a distinct, acute onset and that the onset of lameness was associated with a specific traumatic episode, in one study the majority of owners reported that their dog's lameness had an insidious onset and the severity of lameness gradually progressed over a period of weeks to months before reaching a static state (Lewis et al, 1997). The lameness associated with myopathy of either the gracilis or the semitendinosus muscle is distinctive and is characterized by a shortened stride with a rapid, elastic, internal rotation of the paw, external rotation of the calcaneal tuber, and internal rotation of the stifle during the middle-to-late swing phase of the stride. The lameness typically is more pronounced at a trot or when running and can be best appreciated when watching the dog from behind. This gait abnormality has been described as "goose stepping" or a "jerky gait" (Fig. 1). The lameness is similar in appearance regardless of which muscle is affected because both muscles have similar insertions and functions. The gracilis muscle arises from the pelvic symphysis, while the origin of the semitendinosus muscle is located more lateral on the caudoventral portion of the ischiatic tuberosity. In the caudomedial stifle region, both muscles have broad flat

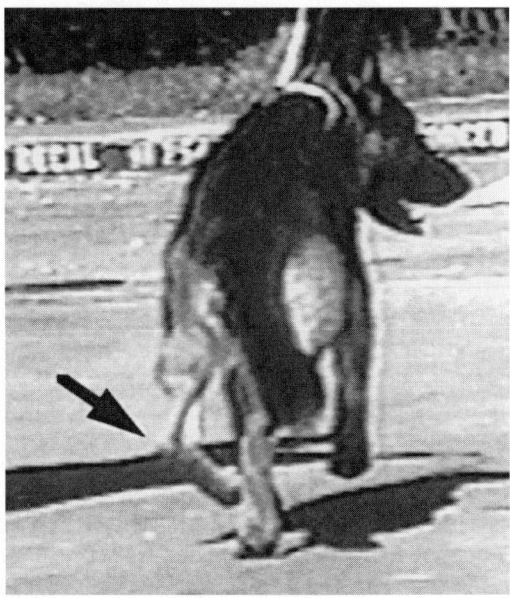

Figure 1. A German shepherd dog with gracilis myopathy walking. The arrow points to the left calcaneal tuber, which is undergoing rapid, elastic external rotation during the mid-swing phase of the stride. Characteristic medial rotation of the paw and internal rotation of the stifle are also present. (From Lewis DD, Packer RB, Bloomberg MS [eds]: Self-assessment Colour Review of Small Animal Orthopaedics. London: Manson Publishing, 1998, p 53, with permission.)

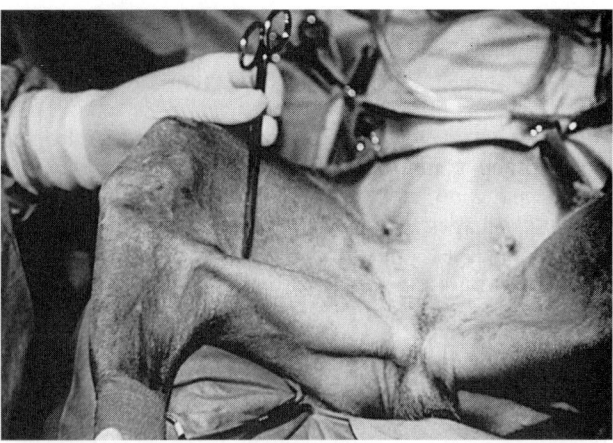

Figure 2. A German shepherd dog with bilateral gracilis myopathy that has been prepared for surgery. The scissors point to the enlarged, firm distal myotendinous portion of the muscle. Visual identification of the remainder of the affected muscle, which originates on the pelvic symphysis, is readily apparent.

tendons that pass over the head of the medial gastrocnemius muscle in the popliteal space and insert on the cranial border of the tibia. Both muscles also have distal aponeuroses that extend from their caudal borders, blending with the crural fascia and contributing a well-developed reinforcing band to the calcaneal tendon. The gait abnormality is the result of a tethering effect by the affected muscle that restricts abduction of the coxofemoral joint and extension of the stifle and hock.

On physical examination the distal myotendinous portion of the affected muscle is palpably firm and enlarged. Increase in the cross-sectional area of the distal myotendinous portion of the affected muscle can also be apparent on radiographs and ultrasound (Lewis et al, 1997). If the dog is positioned in dorsal recumbency, abduction of the affected coxofemoral joint or joints as well as extension of the affected stifle or stifles and hock joint or joints will be limited. Visual identification of the involved muscle or muscles is usually possible (Fig. 2). It is possible to determine whether the gracilis or semitendinosus muscle is affected by carefully palpating the proximal location of the taut muscle band: The semitendinosus muscle originates laterally on the ischiatic tuberosity, whereas the origin of the gracilis muscle is located near midline on the pelvic symphysis.

The lameness associated with this condition would appear to be primarily mechanical. Whether affected dogs experience pain or discomfort is an issue that has not been clarified. Owners of affected dogs often note that their dog's activity level decreased as the lameness progressed and increased following surgery, suggesting that the lameness may, at least in some dogs, have some associated pain. This is supported by the observation that digital pressure exerted on the affected muscle or muscles and abduction of the ipsilateral coxofemoral joint elicited a pain response in the majority of dogs in one study (Lewis et al, 1997).

Abnormal laboratory values have not been consistently associated with this condition. When obtained, results of serum creatine phosphokinase and lactate dehydrogenase have been normal or only marginally elevated (Moore et

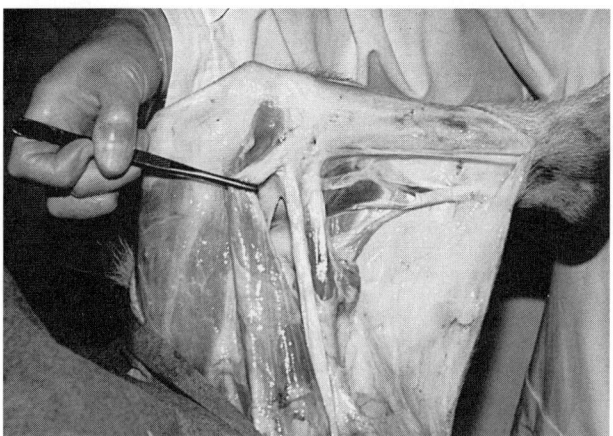

Figure 3. Photograph taken at necropsy of the left hind limb of a German shepherd dog with gracilis myopathy. The atrophic portion of the gracilis muscle has been elevated, revealing an isolated fibrous band associated with the caudolateral border of the muscle. (Courtesy of A. Paris, Collecchio, Italy.)

al, 1981; Capello et al, 1993; Lewis et al, 1997). Electromyographic abnormalities have not been a consistent finding in affected dogs. Some dogs evaluated have had normal electromyographic evaluations (Moore et al, 1981; Lewis et al, 1997). Abnormal electrical activity, consisting of a 2- to 3-second myotonic discharge of waxing and waning high-frequency, high-amplitude potential was reported after electrostimulation of the affected muscle or muscles in one study (Capello et al, 1993). Fibrillation potentials were reported in one other dog (Moore et al, 1981). A lack of insertional activity was found in one dog when electrodes were placed in that portion of the muscle replaced by dense fibrous connective tissue (Moore et al, 1981).

PATHOLOGY

Definition of the gross pathologic abnormalities associated with this condition has often been limited by the sporadic occurrence of this condition and the limited extent of the muscle exposed at surgery. The distal myotendinous portion of the affected muscle or muscles has been consistently observed to be thickened and fibrotic. When the entire length of the affected gracilis muscle has been examined at surgery or necropsy, a thick fibrous band has been observed associated with the caudolateral border of the muscle having its origin on the pubic symphysis and merging with the thickened tendon of insertion of the gracilis muscle proximal to the stifle. This fibrous band has a gross appearance similar to a tendon. Necropsies of several normal dogs have failed to reveal an analogous structure. The band is likely a fibrous remnant of the caudal portion of the gracilis muscle (Lewis et al, 1997). The remaining cranial portion of the gracilis muscle can have a normal or slightly mottled appearance (Fig. 3). Reports detailing the pathology involving the semitendinosus muscle describe a similar thick fibrous band within the muscle belly extending from the tuber ischii to the distal myotendinous junction (Moore et al, 1981).

The most consistent histologic abnormality observed associated with this condition has been variable replacement of muscle fibers with fibrous connective tissue. In some dogs there was complete replacement of muscle fibers with mature collagen oriented parallel to the muscle's long axis in affected regions. Some collagen bundles were surrounded by fat and loosely arranged fibrous tissue. In other dogs, the replacement of muscle fibers was less complete and the collagen bundles were less organized and more variable in size. Myofibers on the periphery of the fibrotic process were often in varying stages of degeneration. Other pathologic changes observed less consistently include mild multifocal nonsuppurative inflammation, focal hemorrhage or hemosiderin deposits, and focal mineralization. Histologic abnormalities are not uniformly distributed throughout the affected muscle or muscles and may not be present in regions of the muscle that appeared grossly normal (Moore et al, 1981; Capello et al, 1993; Lewis et al, 1997).

TREATMENT

Medical treatments (systemic, topical, or intralesional glucocorticoid administration; nonsteroidal anti-inflammatory drugs; acupuncture) have been ineffective in resolving lameness. Any procedure that disrupts the continuity of the affected muscle (simple transection, partial excision, and complete resection) results in immediate improvement in abduction of the coxofemoral joint, as well as increased extension of the stifle and hock (Fig. 4). Lameness is typically resolved the day following surgery unless seroma formation or inflammation of the surgical wound develops. Recurrence of lameness, however, has been reported 1.5 to 5 months following surgery in all dogs with adequate follow-up evaluations. Recurrence of lameness is the result of fibroplasia in the wound reuniting the severed ends of the affected muscle. This occurs irrespective of the extent of the affected muscle that is removed. Adjunctive surgical procedures (inverting the incised margins of the muscle or tendon, or implanting free autogenous fat grafts in an attempt to prevent scar tissue from reuniting the severed segments) and administration of glucocorticoids, nonsteroidal anti-inflammatory drugs, or lathyrogenic agents (D-penicillamine and colchicine) following surgery have not

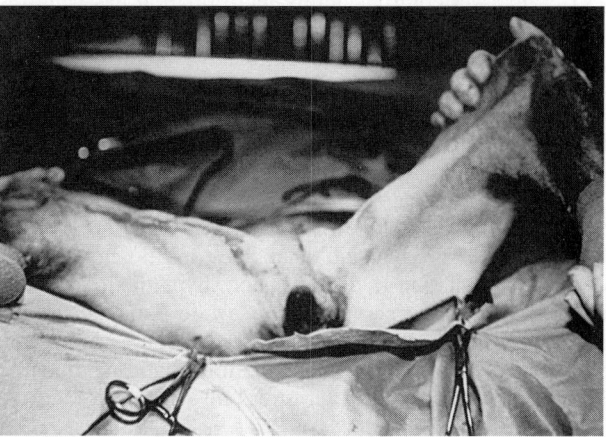

Figure 4. Photograph taken at surgery of a German shepherd dog with bilateral gracilis myopathy. A segment of the distal myotendinous portion of the right gracilis muscle has been excised. Note how abduction of the right coxofemoral joint (from 60 to 85 degrees), and extension of the right stifle (from 160 to 175 degrees) and right hock (from 145 to 155 degrees), are increased following transection of the gracilis muscle.

prevented lameness from recurring (Moore et al, 1981; Thoren et al, 1981; Capello et al, 1993; Lewis et al, 1997).

It is likely that an effective treatment for this condition will not be established until the etiopathogenesis of the condition is known. Affected dogs that are not treated, or have recurrence of lameness following surgical intervention, continue to remain active despite the persistence of lameness (Vaughan, 1979).

References and Suggested Reading

Capello V, Mortellaro CM, Fonda D: Myopathy of the "gracilis semitendinosus muscle complex" in the dog. Eur J Comp Anim Pract 3:57, 1993.
Review of the literature concerning gracilis and semitendinosus myopathy with a report of an additional 13 cases.
Clarke R: Fibrosis and contracture of the semitendinosus muscle in a dog. Aust Vet J 66:259, 261, 1989.
Case report of a dog with semitendinosus myopathy.
Lewis DD, Shelton GD, Paris A, et al: Gracilis or semitendinosus myopathy in 18 dogs. J Am Anim Hosp Assoc 33:177, 1997.
Case summaries of 18 dogs with gracilis or semitendinosus myopathy and literature review of the condition.
Moore RW, Rouse SP, Piermatte DL, et al: Fibrotic myopathy of the semitendinosus muscle in four dogs. Vet Surg 10:169, 1981.
Contains case summaries of four dogs with semitendinosus myopathy.
Thoren L: Kontrakturar m. gracilis och m. semitendinosus som haltorsak hos hund. Sevensk Verterinaertidning 33:319, 1981.
Contains case summaries of four dogs with gracilis or semitendinosus myopathy.
Vaughan LC: Muscle and tendon injuries in dogs. J Small Anim Pract 20:711, 1979.
Contains case summaries of eight dogs with gracilis myopathy.

Diagnosis and Treatment of Cervical Vertebral Instability-Malformation Syndromes

HOWARD B. SEIM III
Fort Collins, Colorado

Cervical vertebral instability-malformation syndromes include disorders of the caudal cervical vertebrae and intervertebral discs of large breed dogs (spondylopathy) resulting in spinal cord compression (myelopathy). Terms commonly used to describe these syndromes include wobbler syndrome, cervical vertebral instability, cervical spondylomyelopathy, cervical malformation-malarticulation, cervical spondylolisthesis, and cervical spondylopathy.

GENERAL CONSIDERATIONS

Cervical vertebral instability-malformation has been reported as a relatively common disorder in Doberman pinschers, Great Danes, and other large breed dogs. The etiology is unknown but is felt to be nutritional, traumatic, hereditary, or acquired. It is a "syndrome" that probably has multiple etiologies. It has been divided into five relatively distinct classifications. Each classification is distinguished by the location and/or nature of the compressive lesion with respect to the spinal canal (Table 1). Lesions may be static or dynamic. Static lesions do not change during manipulation (hyperextension, hyperflexion, or linear traction) of the cervical spine, while dynamic lesions may cause increased compression or decompression of the spinal cord during spinal manipulation. Static or dynamic lesions are documented using stress myelography.

PATHOPHYSIOLOGY
Chronic Degenerative Disc Disease

Chronic degenerative disc disease may originate from either vertebral instability (i.e., stress) or primary degenera-tion of the intervertebral disc (Hansen type II disc protrusion). Regardless of the cause, the degenerate anulus fibrosus undergoes hypertrophy and/or hyperplasia resulting in collapse of the intervertebral disc space and subsequent redundancy of the anulus fibrosus. Spinal cord compression results when the disc space collapses and buckles the redundant anulus fibrosus dorsally. Spinal cord compression in chronic degenerative disc disease is a dynamic compression in that flexion and extension of the neck may vary the degree of spinal cord compression. Generally, dorsal extension of the neck results in an increased spinal cord compression whereas ventral flexion and linear traction result in decreased spinal cord compression.

Congenital Osseous Malformations

Congenital osseous malformations may occur in one or usually multiple vertebrae anywhere along the cervical spine. There is narrowing of the spinal canal due to stenosis of the cranial vertebral canal orifice, articular facet deformities, malformation of vertebral pedicles, and/or deformation of vertebral arches.

Vertebral Tipping

Vertebral tipping is characterized by displacement (tipping) of the cranial, dorsal surface of the vertebral body (generally C6 or C7) into the spinal canal causing spinal cord compression. It is thought that instability secondary

TABLE 1. Classification of Cervical Vertebral Instability-Malformation

Classification	Age/Breed	Lesion Location	Cause of Compression	General Prognosis*
Chronic degenerative disc disease	Adult/male Doberman pinscher	Compresses ventral aspect of spinal cord C5 to C7	Disc degeneration and subsequent hypertrophy of dorsal anulus fibrosus	Favorable
Congenital osseous malformation	Young/Great Dane and Doberman pinscher	Compresses spinal cord laterally or dorsoventrally C3 to C7	Congenital malformation of vertebral bodies and articular facets	Unfavorable
Vertebral tipping	Adult/male Doberman pinscher	Compresses ventral aspect of spinal cord C5 to C7	Dorsal malposition of the affected vertebral body	Favorable
Hypertrophied ligamentum flavum/ vertebral arch malformation	Young/Great Dane	Compresses dorsal aspect of spinal cord C4 to C7	Hypertrophy and hyperplasia of the ligamentum flavum; vertebral arch malformation	Favorable
Hourglass compression	Young/Great Dane	Compresses spinal cord on all sides C2 to C7	Hypertrophy of ligamentum flavum and anulus fibrosus, and malformation or DJD of articular facets	Favorable to guarded

*Prognosis is also influenced by severity of neurologic deficits and number of lesions (see Table 4).
DJD, degenerative joint disease.

to chronic degenerative disc disease (or vice versa) may be the predisposing factor that allows the vertebral body to assume its malposition. Vertebral tipping is not always associated with spinal cord compression.

Hypertrophied Ligamentum Flavum–Vertebral Arch Malformation

The compressive lesion in hypertrophied ligamentum flavum–vertebral arch malformation occurs on the dorsal aspect of the spinal cord. Patients with ligamentum flavum disease only most likely develop hypertrophy or hyperplasia secondary to instability. Patients with vertebral arch malformation are thought to have either a genetic predisposition or nutritional etiology or both. Whatever the cause, the vertebral arch and articular facets become deformed and asymmetrical. Spinal cord compression is not due solely to deformation, but to a combination of static deformation and dynamic compression. In dorsal extension, the cranial tip of the deformed vertebral arch of one vertebra is brought closer to the caudodorsal rim of the body of the adjacent cranial vertebra, increasing spinal cord compression. When the neck is flexed ventrally, the cranial tip of the elongated vertebral arch is retracted, decreasing spinal cord compression.

"Hourglass" Compression

"Hourglass" compression, as detected by myelography, is derived from spinal cord compression that occurs dorsally, ventrally, and laterally. Hypertrophy or hyperplasia of the anulus fibrosus results in ventral spinal cord compression; hypertrophy or hyperplasia of the ligamentum flavum results in dorsal spinal cord compression; and degenerative joint disease or malformation or malarticulation of the articular facets results in lateral spinal cord compression. "Hourglass" lesions may occur at any level of the cervical spine and may be dynamic.

DIAGNOSIS

Signalment

Information concerning age, sex, and breed may assist in determining the specific classification of cervical vertebral instability-malformation syndrome (see Table 1). About 80% of cases are seen in the Doberman pinscher and Great Dane (Bruecker et al, 1989). Chronic degenerative disc disease has a 2:1 male to female ratio.

History

Animals affected with cervical vertebral instability-malformation syndrome generally present with a history of progressive incoordination over a period of months to years. All four limbs are affected, but signs are generally more pronounced and begin in the rear limbs. Occasionally, an acute exacerbation, precipitated by minor trauma, may be the owner's principal complaint. A history of neck pain is seen in approximately 40% of cases.

Neurologic Examination

General physical examination findings are normal in the majority of patients with cervical vertebral instability-malformation syndrome. On neurologic examination, the general pattern of pelvic limb reflex changes is that of upper motor neuron signs; there is often a crossed extensor reflex in dogs with chronic disease. A broad-based stance is often noted in the rear legs. Thoracic limb reflex changes are generally mild. A stiff, straight-legged gait and atrophy of the supraspinatus and infraspinatus muscles are commonly seen in chronic cases. The neck is often carried in ventral flexion. Due to the dynamic nature of most lesions, this position results in the least amount of spinal cord and nerve root compression. Dorsal extension of the neck may cause pain or, more importantly, accentuate spinal cord compression resulting in increased motor signs. One should be careful to avoid excessive manipulation of the head and neck during physical examination of affected animals. Tetraparetic dogs with cervical vertebral instability-malformation may be strongly ambulatory, weakly ambulatory, or nonambulatory.

Imaging

There may be no abnormalities evident on survey radiographs of the affected cervical spine. Abnormalities seen on plain radiographs typical of each classification of cervical vertebral instability-malformation syndrome are summarized in Table 2. Although survey radiography may suggest the presence of cervical vertebral instability-malformation syndrome, myelography is essential in *all* cases to determine (1) location and number of affected vertebrae and intervertebral spaces; (2) location of the lesion within the spinal canal (i.e., dorsal, ventral, or lateral); (3) degree of spinal cord compression; and (4) presence or absence of dynamic compression (Seim and Withrow, 1982). Typical myelographic changes expected with each classification of cervical vertebral instability-malformation syndrome are given in Table 2.

Stress myelography is defined as radiographic imaging of the cervical spine in various positions (ventral flexion, dorsal extension, and linear traction) during myelography. Stress myelography is essential to determine the presence or absence of a dynamic component to a compressive lesion. Classically, compression seen on the ventral aspect of the spinal cord (ventral compression) with chronic degenerative disc disease is worsened with the neck in dorsal extension and improved in ventral flexion and linear traction. Similarly, dorsal compression associated with a dorsal dynamic lesion may be improved by ventral flexion (hypertrophied ligamentum flavum–vertebral arch malformation). Dorsal extension is *not* recommended in routine radiographic evaluation of patients with cervical vertebral instability-malformation syndrome because this may increase spinal cord compression. A complete myelographic examination including lateral and ventrodorsal views plus ventral flexion and linear traction lateral views should allow the clinician to accurately classify each case and formulate a rational therapeutic approach.

DIFFERENTIAL DIAGNOSIS

Any disorder causing neck pain, paraparesis, or tetraparesis in large breed dogs (especially Doberman pinschers and Great Danes) should be considered in the differential diagnosis of cervical vertebral instability-malformation syndrome. Potential differential diagnoses of diseases that mimic cervical vertebral instability-malformation syndrome include cervical disc extrusion, neoplasia, atlantoaxial instability, discospondylitis, fracture or luxation, and fibrocartilaginous embolism. Diagnostic differentials can usually be eliminated by considering signalment, neurologic examination, serum chemistry, cerebrospinal fluid analysis, and radiography. Diagnosis of cervical vertebral instability-malformation syndrome is confirmed by plain and stress myelography.

TREATMENT

Cervical vertebral instability-malformation syndrome is considered to be a chronic progressive disorder characterized by subtle weakness in the hind limbs and often progressing to nonambulatory tetraparesis. Medical therapy may improve a dog's neurologic status (nonambulatory to ambulatory) for a period of time; however, signs often progress to an unacceptable ambulatory to nonambulatory neurologic status. Whether a patient is treated medically depends upon classification of the disorder, degree of neurologic dysfunction at presentation, and number of affected vertebrae or intervertebral spaces. Generally, patients that present with pain, paraparesis, or ambulatory tetraparesis are treated medically and assessed with serial neurologic examinations. If the neurologic status deteriorates or remains unacceptably static, surgery should be considered. Dogs that present weak or nonambulatory, with tetraparesis, should be treated surgically. Patients considered for surgical therapy should have a preoperative myelogram to determine the number of affected intervertebral spaces. Generally, patients with multiple lesions have a guarded to unfavorable prognosis.

Medical Management

The most important aspect of medical management is strict confinement for 3 to 4 weeks; it is recommended that

---

TABLE 2. **Survey Radiographic and Myelographic Findings Seen in Cervical Vertebral Instability-Malformation**

Classification	Possible Survey Radiographic Changes	Typical Myelographic Changes
Chronic degenerative disc disease	None, collapse of the intervertebral space, spondylosis, sclerotic end-plates, calcified disc	Extradural mass compressing the ventral surface of the spinal cord; lesions are generally dynamic
Congenital osseous malformation	Various osseous malformations	Extradural mass compressing the lateral, ventral, and/or dorsal surface of the spinal cord; lesions are generally static
Vertebral tipping	Tipping of the cranial dorsal end of a vertebra into the spinal canal and loss of continuity of the interspace	Extradural mass compressing the ventral aspect of the spinal cord; lesion may be static or dynamic
Ligamentum flavum hypertrophy	None	Extradural mass compressing the dorsal surface of the spinal cord (soft tissue); lesions are generally static
Vertebral arch malformation	None, sclerosis and malformation of affected laminae	Extradural mass compressing the dorsal surface of the spinal cord (malformed laminae); lesions often have a static and dynamic component
Hourglass compression	None	Extradural mass compressing the lateral, ventral and dorsal surfaces of the spinal cord (soft tissue and osseous); lesions are generally dynamic

TABLE 3. Anti-inflammatory Drug Dosages and Regimens Used in Treatment of Cervical Vertebral Instability-Malformation

CORTICOSTEROIDS	
Dexamethasone	0.2 mg/kg twice daily for 3 days; then once daily for 3 days; re-evaluate patient; may repeat treatment one or two more times; if no response, consider surgery.
Prednisolone	0.5 to 1.0 mg/kg twice daily for 3 days; then once daily for 3 days; re-evaluate patient; may repeat treatment one or two more times; if no response, consider surgery.
Methylprednisolone sodium succinate	30 mg/kg given once at anesthetic induction prior to surgery; this corticosteroid is given only preoperatively and discontinued after one dose.

Comments: The dosage for corticosteroids varies dramatically among clinicians. A general rule to follow is to begin with the above dosage schedule, taper the patient over a 6-day period, follow the patient with serial neurologic examinations, and consider repeat corticosteroid therapy or surgery if no response is seen.

NONSTEROIDAL ANTI-INFLAMMATORY DRUGS	
Aspirin	10 mg/kg twice daily for 7 days; re-evaluate patient; if no response, consider alternate medical therapy or surgery.
Phenylbutazone	10 mg *or* 22 mg/kg three times daily (not to exceed 800 mg/day) for 7 days; re-evaluate patient; if no response, consider corticosteroid therapy or surgery.
Flunixin meglumine	0.5 mg/kg twice daily for 2 days maximum; re-evaluate patient; if no response, consider corticosteroid therapy or surgery.

Comments: Nonsteroidal anti-inflammatory drugs may cause severe gastric irritation and ulceration if given above the recommended dose, for too long duration, or in combination with corticosteroids. A general rule to follow is *never* treat a patient with a nonsteroidal anti-inflammatory drug in combination with corticosteroids. In general, nonsteroidal anti-inflammatory drugs are not as effective as corticosteroids for relief of pain and paresis.

patients be fitted with a neck brace if tolerated by the day. During the next 3 to 4 weeks, a gradual return to normal activity is recommended. Collars encircling the neck should be avoided. Although this duration of forced rest allows resolution of spinal cord inflammation, the long-term beneficial effect on cervical spinal stabilization, malformations, disc degeneration, and tissue hypertrophy and hyperplasia is unknown. Strict confinement, use of a neck brace, and exercise control are accompanied by anti-inflammatory therapy. Client education as to the potential euphoric effects of anti-inflammatory drugs is an important consideration. If strict confinement is not maintained during drug therapy, the patient could potentially become more paretic due to acute spinal cord contusion. Commonly used anti-inflammatory and muscle relaxant drugs (and dosages) are listed in Table 3. Patients treated with anti-inflammatory drugs should be monitored for gastrointestinal disorders (i.e., vomiting fresh or digested blood, bloody diarrhea, or melena). At the first sign of a gastrointestinal lesion, anti-inflammatory medication should be discontinued and the patient treated with an H_2 receptor blocker (cimetidine at 5 to 10 mg/kg PO, IV, SC t.i.d. to q.i.d., ranitidine at 1 to 2 mg/kg PO, IV, SC b.i.d. to t.i.d., or famotidine at 0.5 mg/kg PO s.i.d. to b.i.d.) and gastrointestinal protectant (sucralfate, 0.5 to 1.0 gm PO, t.i.d. to q.i.d.). If medical treatment is successful, spinal cord edema resolves, remyelination may occur, and neurologic recovery results. If no improvement is noted by 3 to 4 weeks, or if neurologic deterioration occurs, surgical intervention should be considered.

Surgical Management

Preoperative Preparation

The dog is given intravenous methylprednisolone sodium succinate at 30 mg/kg. Intravenous fluids are administered throughout the procedure. Prophylactic antibiotics are generally administered at the time of anesthetic induction (cefazolin, 20 mg/kg IV) and may be repeated at 4- to 6-hour intervals for 24 hours.

Patient Positioning

Patients requiring a ventral approach (Table 4) are placed in dorsal recumbency, in a V-trough, and carefully secured to the table to prevent lateral motion. Patients with a dynamic lesion (chronic degenerative disc disease, hourglass compression, vertebral arch malformation, redundant ligamentum flavum) are secured to the table with the neck in linear traction (Fig. 1). Linear traction results in spinal cord decompression during surgical manipulation.

Patients requiring a dorsal approach (see Table 4) are placed in sternal recumbency. The use of dynamic positioning is based on patient classification and results of stress myelography (see Table 4). As a general rule, patients

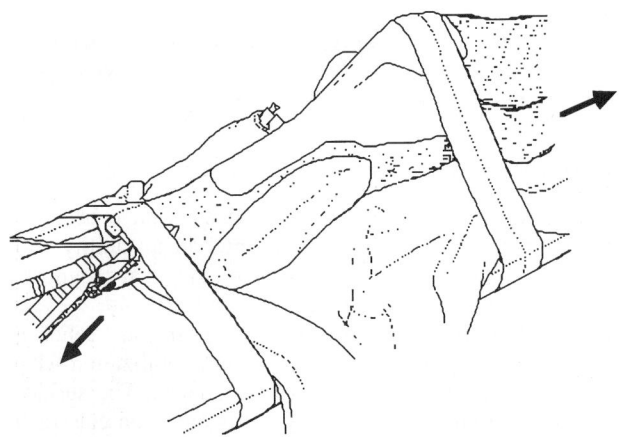

Figure 1. Proper position for ventral approach to the cervical spine. Note that the head and front limbs are pulled to place the neck in linear traction.

TABLE 4. Surgical Techniques for Treatment of Cervical Vertebral Instability-Malformation

Classification	Clinical Presentation	Number of Sites Affected	Dynamic or Static Lesion	Surgical Technique Recommended	Prognosis*
Chronic degenerative disc disease/vertebral tipping	Pain alone	Single or 2 adjacent	Dynamic	Ventral slot or traction-stabilization	Excellent
			Static	Ventral slot	Excellent
	Paraparetic	Single	Dynamic	Ventral slot or traction-stabilization	Excellent to favorable
			Static	Ventral slot ± stabilization	Excellent to favorable
		2 adjacent	Dynamic	Ventral traction-stabilization	Favorable
			Static	Ventral slot and stabilization	Favorable
	Ambulatory tetraparetic	Single	Dynamic	Ventral traction-stabilization	Favorable
			Static	Ventral slot and stabilization	Favorable
		2 adjacent	Dynamic/static	Ventral traction-stabilization	Guarded to favorable
		More than 2 lesions	Dynamic/static	Dorsal laminectomy	Guarded to favorable
	Weakly ambulatory tetraparetic	Single	Dynamic	Ventral traction-stabilization	Guarded to favorable
			Static	Ventral slot and stabilization	Guarded to favorable
		2 adjacent	Dynamic/static	Ventral traction-stabilization	Guarded
		More than 2 lesions	Dynamic/static	Dorsal laminectomy	Guarded
	Nonambulatory tetraparetic	Single	Dynamic	Ventral traction-stabilization	Guarded
			Static	Ventral slot and stabilization	Guarded
		2 adjacent	Dynamic/static	Ventral traction-stabilization	Guarded to unfavorable
		More than 2 lesions	Dynamic/static	Dorsal laminectomy	Guarded to unfavorable
Congenital osseous malformation	Paraparesis to tetraparesis	Single lesion (rare)	Static	Dorsal laminectomy	Favorable
		Multiple lesions	Static	Dorsal laminectomy	Unfavorable
Ligamentum flavum hypertrophy	Paraparesis to tetraparesis	Single lesion	Dynamic	Dorsal laminectomy Ventral traction-stabilization	Favorable
			Static	Dorsal laminectomy	Favorable
		Multiple lesions	Dynamic/static	Dorsal laminectomy	Guarded
Ventral arch malformation	Paraparesis to tetraparesis	Single lesion	Dynamic	Dorsal laminectomy Ventral traction-stabilization	Favorable
			Static	Dorsal laminectomy	Favorable
		Multiple lesions (rare)	Dynamic/static	Dorsal laminectomy	Guarded
Hourglass compression	Paraparesis to tetraparesis	Single lesion	Dynamic	Ventral traction-stabilization Dorsal laminectomy	Favorable
			Static	Dorsal laminectomy	Favorable
		Two lesions	Dynamic/static	Ventral traction-stabilization Dorsal laminectomy	Guarded
		Multiple lesions	Dynamic/static	Dorsal laminectomy	Guarded

*The definition of each prognosis is given below:
   Excellent: patient will return to a normal neurologic status.
   Favorable: patient will return to a near-normal neurologic status (minor deficits will remain).
   Guarded: patient may or may not return to an acceptable neurologic status.
   Unfavorable: patient most likely will not return to an acceptable neurologic status.
   Grave: patient will not return to an acceptable neurologic status.

requiring dorsal decompression are positioned with the neck elevated and gently flexed over a rolled fleece or rigid vacuum-type apparatus.

Surgical Techniques

Although numerous surgical techniques have been described for treatment of cervical vertebral instability-malformation syndrome, only a few have long-term prognostic merit. The objectives of surgery in patients with cervical vertebral instability-malformation syndrome are relief of spinal cord compression, cervical spinal stabilization when indicated, and reversal of neurologic deficits. The surgical technique of choice for each patient is based on classification, clinical presentation, vertebral body or interspace affected, number of lesions present, location of lesion within the spinal canal, and presence or absence of a dynamic lesion. This information for each classification is presented in Table 4. Surgical techniques currently used to treat patients with cervical vertebral instability-malformation syndrome include ventral decompression (i.e., ventral slot), ventral traction-stabilization (i.e., Steinmann pins and methylmethacrylate or interbody methylmethacrylate plug), and dorsal decompression (i.e., dorsal laminectomy).

Ventral Decompression via Ventral Slot

A ventral slot is used to gain entrance and visualization of the ventral cervical spinal canal and limited access to the intervertebral foramen. A ventral midline cervical approach is performed to expose the longus colli muscles. Lateral subperiosteal elevation of the longus colli muscle from the ventral aspect of the vertebral bodies adjacent to the affected interspace or interspaces allows adequate visualization necessary for adequate exposure to the intervertebral disc space. A rectangular defect is created over the affected intervertebral space with a pneumatic drill. In order to center the bony defect over the intervertebral space at the level of the spinal canal, the slot should be centered slightly cranial to the interspace. The depth of the defect is gauged by visualizing three distinct layers of bone while drilling. First, the hard outer cortical layer of the vertebral body is penetrated. Second, the softer, more hemorrhagic marrow layer is visualized and drilled. Finally, the inner cortical layer of the vertebral body is seen. Once this layer is visualized, care is taken to remove it using 000 curette and dental spatula. The dorsal anulus fibrosus and dorsal longitudinal ligament are identified, tented with ophthalmic forceps, and carefully excised with a No. 11 Bard Parker scalpel blade. Care is taken to remove as much redundant ligament as possible. Full decompression is reached when the dura mater is visualized.

Advantages of the ventral slot procedure include minimal dissection through normal tissue planes, minimal disruption of normal anatomic structures, adequate visualization of the spinal canal, minimal manipulation of spinal cord, quick recovery, few complications, and relatively rapid operating time. Disadvantages of ventral slot decompression include difficulty in adequately removing the entire compressive lesion, iatrogenic laceration of vertebral venous sinus, and possible instability caused by the slot.

Ventral Traction and Stabilization

Techniques that employ spinal traction and stabilization have significantly improved the outcome of patients with a dynamic lesion. Based on pathophysiology of the compressive lesion, techniques utilizing linear traction stretch the anulus fibrosus, thus relieving spinal cord compression. Once the spine is stabilized in traction, the spinal cord remains decompressed. Later, atrophy of the anulus fibrosus occurs, further improving decompression. Several ventral traction-stabilization techniques have been successfully used to treat patients with cervical vertebral instability-malformation syndrome, particularly chronic degenerative disc disease. The two recommended by the author are Steinmann pins and methylmethacrylate bone cement, and interbody methylmethacrylate plug. The initial approach in both techniques is as previously described for ventral slot; however, once the affected intervertebral space is located, the intervertebral spaces *and* vertebral bodies cranial and caudal to the affected interspace must also be exposed. This increased exposure is necessary for placement of vertebral spreaders and/or the stabilizing device chosen.

Steinmann Pins and Methylmethacrylate Bone Cement. This method (Bruecker et al, 1989) is the author's technique of choice for patients requiring dynamic ventral traction-stabilization. A ventral slot is performed at the affected intervertebral space or spaces, to the level of the inner cortical layer (75% transdiscal slot) (Fig. 2). The maximal width of the slot is no more than one half the width of the vertebral body. Slot length is determined by the thickness of the vertebral endplates. Drilling is discontinued once the cortical end-plate of each vertebral body is removed. A Gelpi retractor is modified by blunting

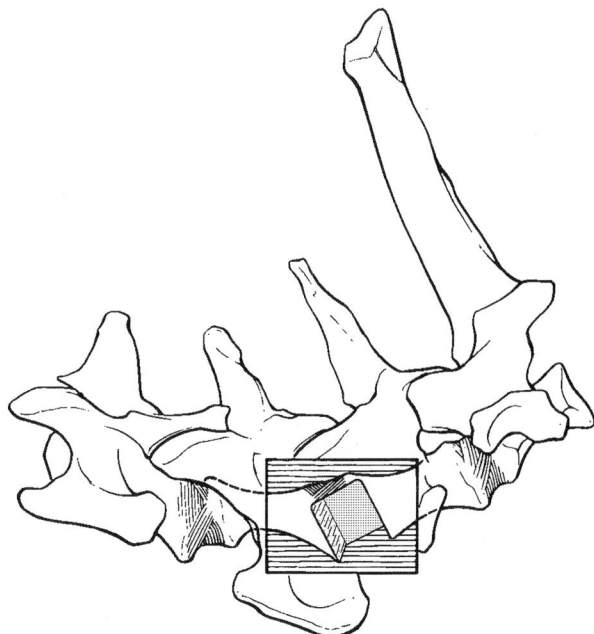

Figure 2. A 75% transdiscal slot is required when one uses traction-stabilization techniques.

the tips and then placed in holes burred in the vertebral bodies cranial and caudal to the affected vertebral bodies (Fig. 3). The holes are burred just large enough to accept the blunted tips of the modified Gelpi retractor. The Gelpi retractor is engaged and the affected intervertebral space placed in approximately 2 to 3 mm of linear traction. Autogenous cancellous bone is harvested from the greater tubercles of the humeri and placed into the distracted slot. Two 7/64- or 1/8-inch Steinmann pins are placed into the ventral surface of the vertebral body cranial to the affected intervertebral space, and two similar size pins are placed into the vertebral body caudal to the affected intervertebral space. Pins are inserted on the ventral midline of the vertebral body and directed 30 to 35 degrees dorsolateral to avoid entering the spinal canal (Fig. 4). It is important to engage two cortices with each pin. Pins are cut leaving approximately 1.5 to 2 cm exposed. The exposed portion of each pin is notched with pin cutters to allow bone cement to grip the pin and prevent migration. Sterile methylmethacrylate bone cement powder is mixed with liquid monomer until it reaches a doughy consistency and can be handled without sticking to surgical gloves. The cement is molded around each pin, making sure each pin is completely surrounded and covered with bone cement (see Fig. 4). The bone cement is irrigated with sterile saline solution for 5 to 10 minutes to dissipate the heat of polymerization. The vertebral spreaders are removed after the cement has hardened. The paired longus colli muscles are sutured cranial and caudal to the cement mass. The remainder of the closure is routine.

This technique can be used to distract and stabilize up to two affected intervertebral spaces. Advantages of this technique over ventral slot decompression alone include complete spinal cord decompression without entering the spinal canal, reduced risk of iatrogenic cord trauma, no requirement for a neck brace, and a expected favorable to

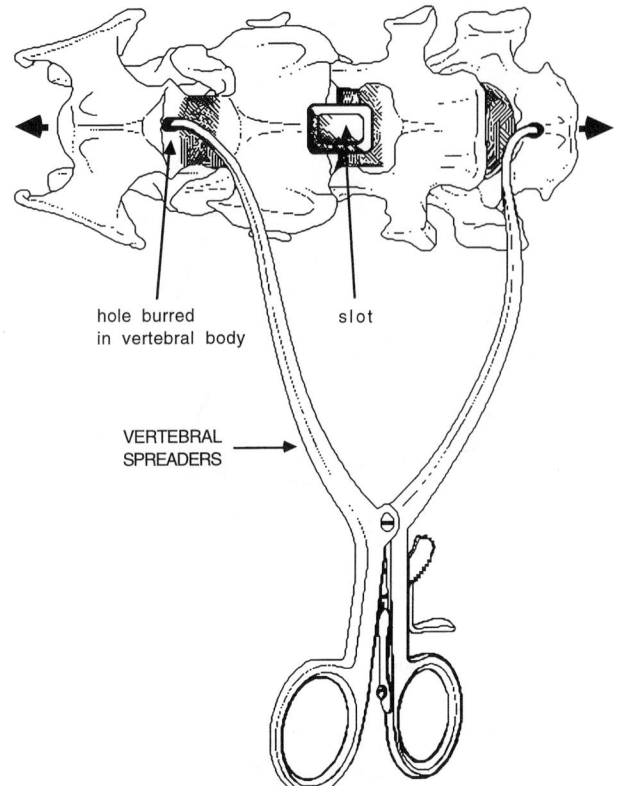

Figure 3. Ventral traction and stabilization technique. Holes are drilled in the vertebral body cranial and caudal to the involved interspace to allow placement of vertebral spreaders. Activating the spreaders results in spinal traction spreading the affected disc space 2 to 4 mm.

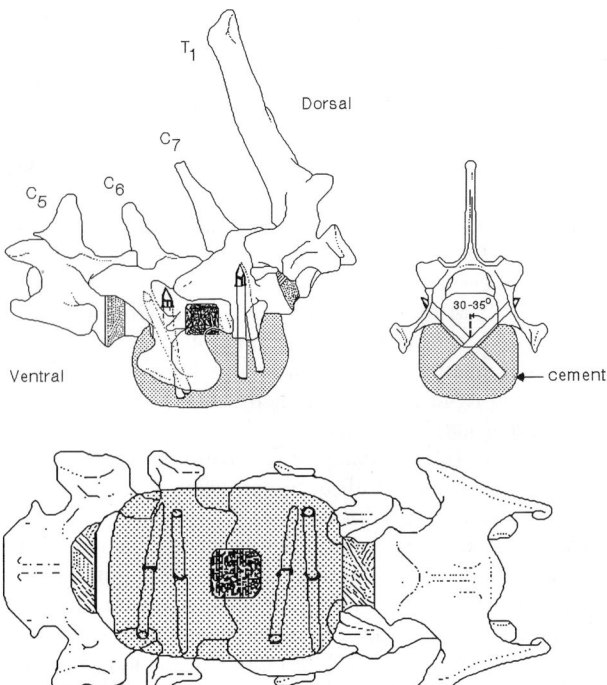

Figure 4. Ventral traction and stabilization technique. Ventral decompression with Steinmann pins and methylmethacrylate stabilization. The pins are placed at a 30- to 35-degree angle to the midline to allow penetration of two cortices without entering the vertebral canal. Methylmethacrylate is placed over all four protruding pins to accomplish stabilization.

excellent prognosis in most patients. The major disadvantage is the technical ability necessary to properly place the Steinmann pins.

Interbody Methylmethacrylate Plug. The affected intervertebral space or spaces are exposed as described for ventral slot in this procedure (Dixon et al, 1996). A fenestration window is made in the ventral anulus fibrosus of the affected interspace one half to two thirds the width of the vertebral body with a No. 11 scalpel blade. Linear traction is applied using the method described for Steinmann pins and methylmethacrylate traction-stabilization. Approximately 4 to 5 mm of linear traction is placed on the affected intervertebral space. Traction facilitates complete removal of the nucleus pulposus and a portion of the lateral and dorsal anulus fibrosus using a high-speed pneumatic drill and Lempert rongeurs. It is important to remove as much disc material and end-plate cartilage as possible without entering the vertebral canal. Approximately 3 to 5 mm of dorsal anulus fibrosus and the bony end-plates corresponding to each affected disc space are left intact. A pneumatic drill is then used to create an undercut in each vertebral body to provide an anchor hole for the methylmethacrylate (Fig. 5). Liquid methylmethacrylate is then injected in the slot with a catheter-tipped syringe; digital pressure is applied to ensure complete filling of the anchor holes. As the cement begins to harden, the area is irrigated with room-temperature 0.9% NaCl solution to dissipate the heat of polymerization. Cancellous

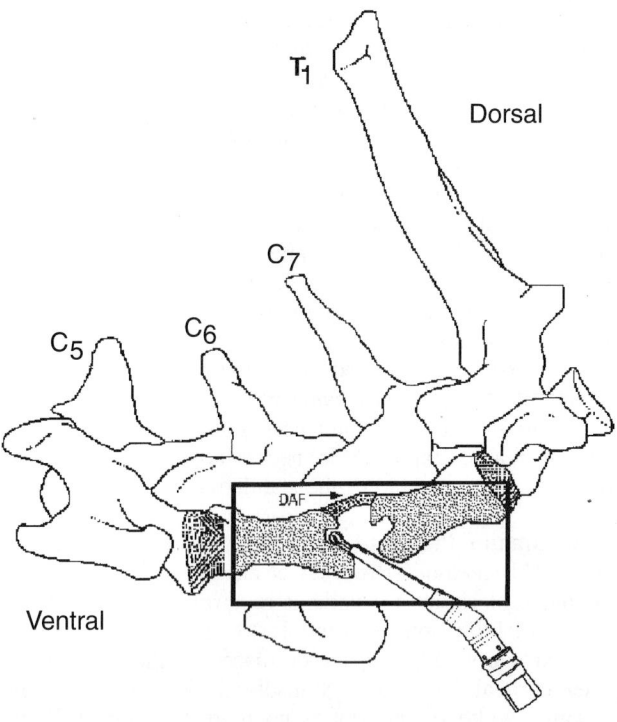

Figure 5. Interbody methylmethacrylate plug technique. The affected interspace is placed in 4 to 5 mm linear traction. Disc material and endplate cartilage are removed with a pneumatic drill. Anchor holes are then drilled to accommodate methylmethacrylate. Care is taken to leave 3 to 4 mm of dorsal anulus fibrosus (DAF) intact.

bone is harvested from the greater tubercles of the humeri and placed on the ventral surface of the exposed vertebrae (Fig. 6). Routine closure of the longus colli muscles holds the graft in place.

Advantages of this technique include the following: (1) There is no need to enter the spinal canal to achieve adequate decompression; drilling the slot and anchor holes is not technically demanding; and multiple spaces can be successfully operated. A possible disadvantage is the need for a neck brace postoperatively, particularly if the patient does not tolerate it.

Dorsal Laminectomy. Prior to laminectomy (Lyman, 1987), affected vertebrae are identified by palpating the prominent dorsal spinous process of C2 and counting caudad. The dorsal aspect of affected cervical vertebrae are exposed and dorsal spinous processes and laminae are removed with rongeurs and a high speed surgical bur, respectively. The laminectomy may be from three fourths of the length of each adjacent vertebrae, to a continuous laminectomy extending from C4 to C7, depending upon the extent of the compressive lesion. The width of the laminectomy is limited by staying between the articular facets of the cranial vertebra. The lamina is burred to the level of the periosteum of the inner cortical layer. A dental or iris spatula is used to carefully penetrate the periosteal layer and enter the spinal canal. Ophthalmic forceps and No. 11 scalpel blade are used to gently excise and remove the ligamentum flavum en bloc. An autogenous fat graft is placed over the laminectomy site to help prevent formation of a fibrous laminectomy membrane that could result in spinal cord compression. Paraspinal muscles and fascia are approximated and remaining tissues closed routinely.

Advantages include decompression of multiple sites and

excellent visualization of dorsal and dorsolateral lesions. Disadvantages include severe disruption of hard and soft tissues, prolonged operating time, poor visualization of ventral and ventrolateral lesions, excessive manipulation of spinal cord necessary to approach the floor of the spinal canal, and prolonged morbidity postoperatively.

POSTOPERATIVE CARE

Patients are assessed initially by immediate postoperative radiographs of the cervical spine to evaluate implants and by neurologic examination 48 hours after surgery to determine neurologic status. Immediate postoperative care includes intravenous fluids, pain control with appropriate analgesics (butorphanol at 0.2 to 0.4 mg/kg IV, IM every 4 hours as needed; oxymorphone at 0.05 to 0.1 mg/kg IV, IM every 4 hours as needed; buprenorphine at 5 to 15 µg/kg IV, IM every 6 hours as needed), discontinue corticosteroids, monitor respiration, measure abdominal girth every 4 hours for 24 hours (gastric dilatation volvulus alert), and monitor for possible seizure activity (particularly if the patient had immediate preoperative myelography). The neck collar should be replaced with a body harness in all patients.

Postoperative management of ambulatory patients includes strict confinement with leash walks two to three times daily for the first 2 to 3 weeks, then a gradual increase in exercise over the next 6 to 8 weeks. Slippery surfaces should be avoided.

Postoperative management of nonambulatory patients includes physiotherapy (passive range of motion exercises), hydrotherapy (swimming, whirlpool), and use of a supporting cart until the dog has regained the ability to walk. Neoprene, nylon, or leather harnesses provide a useful means of assisting weakly ambulatory tetraparetic patients. Special attention to good nursing care of recumbent patients is necessary to avoid decubital ulcers, urinary tract infections, and pneumonia. Heavily padded, dry, soft bedding or waterbeds are useful to prevent decubital ulcers.

Long-term assessment includes radiographic evaluation at 3, 6, 9, and 12 months postoperatively and neurologic examinations as needed depending on status (generally daily until ambulatory, then 1, 2, 3, 6, 9, and 12 months postoperatively).

COMPLICATIONS OF SURGERY

Short-term complications (immediate postoperative to 1 month) generally vary depending upon the surgical procedure chosen but are generally related to implant failure or technical difficulty during surgery.

Complications associated with Steinmann pins and bone cement include pin migration, pin fracture, iatrogenic spinal cord injury, or implant loosening, and are generally related to improper technique. These complications occur in less than 10% of patients. Complications associated with methylmethacrylate plugs were rare and included one case of implant loosening and one case of discospondylitis. The major complication associated with dorsal laminectomy is iatrogenic spinal cord injury.

The most common long-term complication (longer than

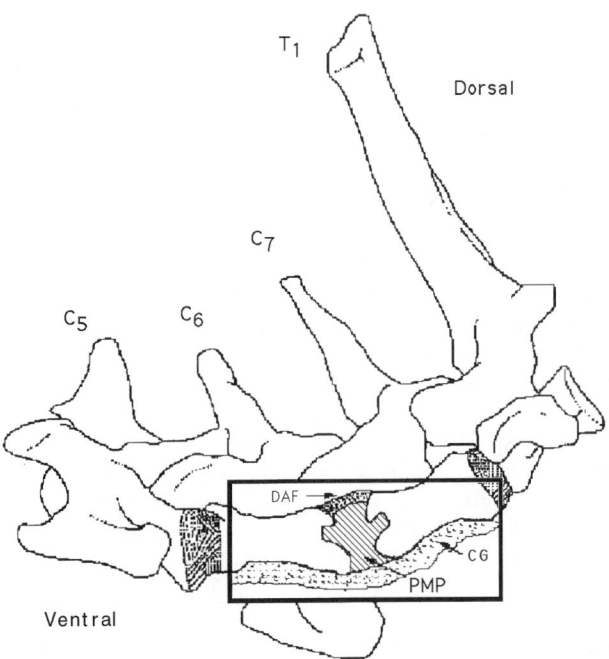

Figure 6. Interbody methylmethacrylate plug technique. Methylmethacrylate (PMP) is placed in the slot and anchor holes; cancellous bone graft (CG) is packed along the ventral surfaces of the affected vertebrae.

1 month postoperative) in patients treated with ventral slot or ventral traction-stabilization for chronic degenerative disc disease, vertebral tipping, or hourglass compression is development of a second compressive lesion at the interspace adjacent to the previously affected interspace. It is presumed that once an intervertebral space is fused, stress at the adjacent interspaces is increased. It is possible that in some patients this increased stress encourages development of spinal instability and subsequent spinal cord compression or that some patients have a predisposition to disc degeneration in the lower cervical spine thus encouraging development of a second lesion. Whatever the cause, this phenomenon is referred to as the *domino effect* and has been reported to occur in 25% of patients at 5 to 60 months postoperatively treated with Steinmann pins and methylmethacrylate stabilization. The domino effect was identified in only one case of methylmethacrylate plugs.

PROGNOSIS

Prognosis for patients treated medically is generally guarded to unfavorable, and is somewhat dependent upon classification, severity of neurologic signs, and number of lesions. Prognosis for surgically treated patients is dependent on disease classification, severity of neurologic deficit, number of lesions, method of therapy available, and quality of aftercare (see Tables 1 and 4).

References and Suggested Reading

Bruecker KA, Seim HB, Blass CE: Caudal cervical spondylomyelopathy: Decompression by linear traction and stabilization with Steinmann pins and polymethyl methacrylate. J Am Anim Hosp Assoc 25:677, 1989.

Bruecker KA, Seim HB, Withrow SJ: Clinical evaluation of three surgical methods for treatment of caudal cervical spondylomyelopathy of dogs. Vet Surg 18:197, 1989.

Dixon BC, Tomlinson JL, Kraus KH: Modified distraction-stabilization technique using an interbody polymethyl methacrylate plug in dogs with caudal cervical spondylomyelopathy. J Am Vet Med Assoc 208:61, 1996.

Lyman R: Continuous dorsal laminectomy for treatment of Doberman pinschers with caudal cervical vertebral instability and malformation. Proceedings of the 5th Annual Veterinary Medical Forum, San Diego, 1987.

Seim HB, Withrow SJ: Pathophysiology and diagnosis of caudal cervical spondylomyelopathy with emphasis on the Doberman pinscher. J Am Vet Med Assoc 18:241, 1982.

Incomplete Ossification of the Humeral Condyle in Dogs

DENIS J. MARCELLIN-LITTLE
Raleigh, North Carolina

Incomplete ossification of the humeral condyle (IOHC) has been recently described in 28 skeletally mature spaniels (Marcellin-Little et al, 1994). The presence of IOHC may explain the findings of others (Vannini et al, 1988; Kaderly and Lamothe, 1992) that suggest that spaniels are predisposed to humeral condylar fractures (HCF) and that such fractures may develop after minor trauma in these breeds.

The cause of IOHC remains unknown. The disease appears to be polygenic, with a recessive mode of inheritance (Marcellin-Little et al, 1994). Little is known about the pathogenesis of the disease. In the pup, normal ossification of the humeral condyle starts at 2 weeks of age and is complete between 8 and 12 weeks of age. The two major centers of ossification, on the medial and lateral sides of the condyle, fail to fuse in affected dogs. The two sides of the condyle remain separated by fibrous tissue. The fibrous tissue is the weakest part of the humeral condyle, and makes it more prone to a HCF. The extent of the IOHC is variable, ranging from a nearly complete ossification of the humeral condyle to a complete fibrous union of the medial and lateral sides of the condyle.

CLINICAL PRESENTATION

Signalment

IOHC has been documented in Cocker spaniels, Brittany spaniels, Boykin spaniels, a Rottweiler, and a mixed-breed dog having a Cocker spaniel dam. IOHC has recently been documented in a dog crossbred between an English setter and a pointer. IOHC is likely present, based on reports of HCFs secondary to minor trauma in skeletally mature dogs, in Springer spaniels, Cavalier King Charles spaniels, and Clumber spaniels. The affected Cocker spaniels generally are indoor dogs with a sedentary lifestyle. The affected Brittany spaniels and Boykin spaniels generally are active hunting dogs. IOHC should be suspected in any adult dog with an HCF secondary to a minor or unknown trauma, especially in spaniels and other working dogs.

Classically, dogs with IOHC present with lameness or HCF at a mean age of 6 years (range: 2 to 12 years). Male Cocker spaniels are 3 to 5 times more likely to have IOHC than female Cocker spaniels (Marcellin-Little et al, 1994). Affected Cocker spaniels originally did not appear overweight when compared with a control population of Cocker spaniels (Marcellin-Little et al, 1994), but a recent report has shown otherwise (Brown et al, 1996).

Clinical Signs

Dogs with IOHC may present with or without an apparent HCF. The history often includes a mild intermittent weightbearing lameness lasting a few days to a few months. This lameness is unresponsive to anti-inflammatory drugs. Most dogs with this history have IOHC without HCF, though some of these dogs may have a chronic HCF. An acute non-weightbearing episode may develop after seemingly normal activities, such as jumping, running, and walking up or down stairs. Most dogs with an acute non-weightbearing forelimb lameness have an HCF, but some of these dogs have no radiographically visible fracture (Kaderly and Lamothe, 1992; Marcellin-Little et al, 1996).

In dogs with IOHC without HCFs, the findings on palpation are similar to the findings associated with degenerative joint disease (DJD) of the elbow joint. They include mild crepitus, a 20- to 30-degree loss of range of motion in flexion, and a pain response in hyperextension or in hyperflexion with pronation of the paw. In dogs with acute HCFs, the clinical signs include focal swelling over the elbow joint, gross malalignment and edema of the forearm, and pain response and crepitus on manipulation. Dogs with chronic HCFs may have severe crepitus and abnormal joint laxity, a 60- to 90-degree loss of range of motion in flexion,

and minimal or no apparent pain response during palpation. In our experience, all dogs with IOHC have been affected *bilaterally.* IOHC is suspected at the time of a unilateral HCF, and confirmed by diagnosing the incomplete ossification of the nonfractured, contralateral condyle. It is critical to perform a complete examination of both elbow joints when examining potentially affected dogs.

DIAGNOSIS

Radiography

A careful radiographic evaluation of both humeral condyles is critical to diagnose IOHC. The radiographic views include a flexed mediolateral, hyperflexed mediolateral, and craniocaudal view with 15 degrees of external rotation (cranial 15 degrees medial-caudolateral oblique). The latter view can be obtained using a horizontal or vertical radiographic beam. This specific positioning is best achieved in sedated dogs (oxymorphone, 0.05 mg/kg IV and acepromazine, 0.025 mg/kg IV).

In nonfractured humeri, the fibrous plane present between the medial and the lateral side of the condyle is visible as a radiolucent line on the craniocaudal view, i.e., when the radiographic beam strikes the bone parallel to the fibrous plane (Fig. 1). On this view, the radiolucent line extends from the midpoint of the trochlea proximally. Sometimes, it may only be 1 or 2 millimeters long (partial radiolucent line). More often, it reaches the level of the

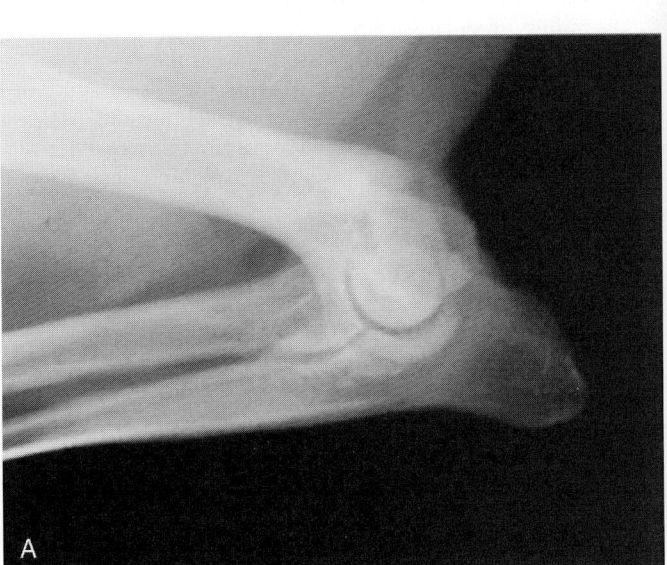
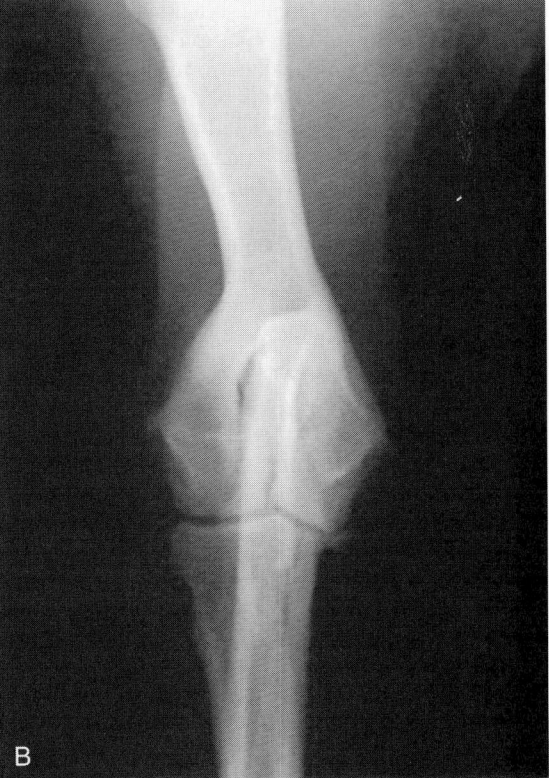

Figure 1. Hyperflexed mediolateral *(A)* and cranial 15-degree medial-caudolateral oblique *(B)* radiographic views of the elbow of a 7-year-old female Cocker spaniel having IOHC. Osteophytes are present on the anconeal process, radial head, and medial coronoid process. On *B*, the midpoint of the trochlea is equidistant from the medial and lateral ulnar cortices. A radiolucent line is visible across the humeral condyle.

physeal scar or the supratrochlear foramen (complete radiolucent line). Because the radiolucent line is only 0.5 to 1 mm wide, it is necessary to use high-detail film and to maintain optimal film exposure. Also, with 5 degrees of internal or external rotation from the reference positioning, the bone of the humeral condyle will be superimposed on the fibrous cleavage plane and prevent its visualization. Surprisingly, most dogs with IOHC (92%, Marcellin-Little et al, 1994) have mild to severe DJD, and 25% of the dogs with IOHC have a displaced fragmented medial coronoid process visible on radiographs. It is important to differentiate IOHC and fragmented medial coronoid process as causes of DJD. In spaniel breeds, fragmented medial coronoid process in the absence of IOHC is rare. Therefore, IOHC should be suspected in spaniels with DJD or with fragmented medial coronoid process. A periosteal reaction on the supratrochlear ridge is visible in half of the dogs with IOHC, and is suggestive of a fracture or stress remodeling in the supracondylar region.

With acute HCF in adult dogs, "Y", lateral, and medial fractures are present. DJD is also common (88%), and fragmented medial coronoid process can be seen in 56% of the dogs. Periosteal proliferation is present on the supratrochlear ridge in 16% of the fractures.

Chronic HCFs are lateral fractures. This may be because Y fractures are diagnosed immediately because the associated mechanical impairment precludes any use of the leg. Also, chronic HCFs may develop over time without a major initiating event. Lateral fractures develop more commonly than medial fractures because the radial head articulates with the lateral aspect of the condyle. In dogs with chronic HCFs, the radiographic abnormalities include demineralization of the affected portion of the condyle, periosteal proliferation, and callus formation. Other causes of pathologic fractures should be included in the initial differential diagnosis of a skeletally mature dog with HCF occurring after a minor or unknown trauma. In these dogs, IOHC can be confirmed by finding radiographic changes in the contralateral humeral condyle.

In immature dogs with acute HCFs, IOHC cannot be confirmed because the ossification of the distal part of the fractured and contralateral humeri is incomplete. The contralateral condyle should be evaluated radiographically for IOHC when the dog reaches 1 year of age.

Computed Tomography

Computed tomography (CT) is useful because the radiolucent line may be difficult to visualize on radiographs. CT is more sensitive and specific than radiographs. The dogs are anesthetized and placed in dorsal recumbency with forelimbs extended. One- to two-millimeter cross-sectional images of the distal humerus, proximal ulna, and proximal radius are made. The fibrous plane is visible as an area of hypoattenuation, either limited to the caudal aspect of the trochlea (Marcellin-Little et al, 1994) or separating the medial and lateral side of the condyle (Fig. 2). Sclerosis of the adjacent bone is usually present, and is seen as an area of hyperattenuation. The presence of a fragmented medial coronoid process can be confirmed using CT.

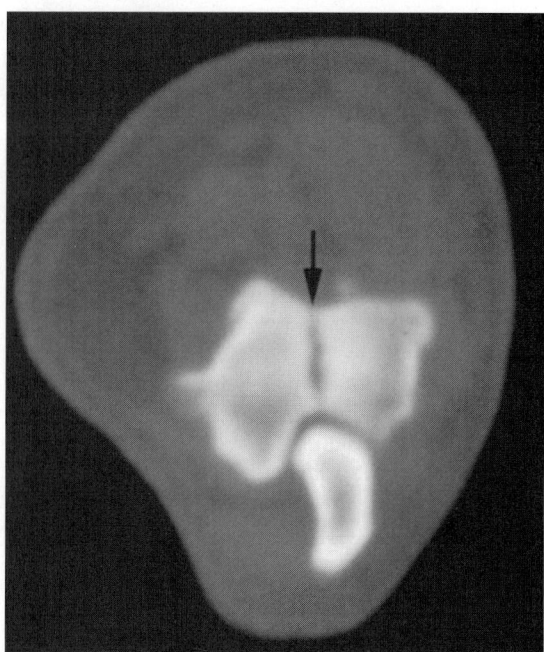

Figure 2. Computed tomographic image of the elbow shown in Figure 1, sectioning the humeral condyle and anconeal process. Incomplete ossification of the condyle (*arrow*) and adjacent sclerosis are present.

Nuclear Scintigraphy

Nuclear scintigraphy can be used to evaluate the soft tissue and bone metabolic activity in dogs with chronic lameness, without specific abnormalities on orthopedic examination. Increased radiotracer uptake in the distal humerus is present in dogs with IOHC.

Intraoperative Evaluation

In the dogs with HCF secondary to IOHC, the fractured surface of the condyle resembles flat cortical bone, with a mildly irregular surface, covered by a 1-mm–thick layer of fibrous tissue. Articular cartilage wear may be present near the fractured edges. Little bleeding follows scraping of the fractured surfaces with a periosteal elevator. When the humeral condyle is drilled prior to transcondylar screw placement, the bone resembles solid cortical bone and bleeding is often absent.

TREATMENT

Humeral Condylar Fracture

Thirty-nine of 42 (93%) dogs presenting with IOHC had an HCF. Nine dogs (21%) had bilateral fractures. Twenty-five of 47 HCFs (53%) were Y fractures, 17 of 47 (36%) were lateral HCFs, 5 of 47 (11%) were medial HCFs, and 1 fracture was of unknown type. Surgery, with open reduction and internal fixation, is the treatment of choice for HCFs. The Y HCFs were repaired using a caudal approach to the distal humerus combined with an osteotomy of the olecranon. A transcondylar bone screw, and one or two bone plates were placed on the caudomedial and caudolateral aspects of the distal part of the humerus. Lateral HCFs were repaired using a lateral approach to the distal part of the humerus. A transcondylar screw was placed and one to three additional bone screws or Kirschner wires were placed in the supracondylar portion of the fractured fragment. All bone screws were used in lag fashion. Medial HCFs were repaired using a medial approach to the distal part of the humerus, and internal fixation similar to that of lateral HCFs. With all types of HCFs combined, the failure rate after internal fixation (23%) tends to be higher in dogs with IOHC than in other dogs (4.6%). Affected condyles may not heal after reconstruction, because of the presence of fibrous tissue at the site of incomplete ossification or because of the sclerosis of the condyle. This may increase implant micromotion and fatigue of the implant. Even though we do not know what primary force or combination of forces is present at the site of fibrous union, larger implants are stronger and stiffer and should probably be used in such cases. Placement of a 4.5 mm cortical screw (Synthes, Inc., Paoli, PA) is recommended whenever possible; 3.5 mm screws (Synthes, Inc., Paoli, PA) are used in smaller dogs. A soft padded bandage can be placed around the limb to prevent swelling, and left in place for 3 to 5 days. The use of a splint is not necessary after fracture repair. The dog's activity is limited to leash walks for 6 to 8 weeks after surgery.

With chronic HCFs and when implant failure occurs following repair of acute HCFs, periarticular fibrosis, bone remodeling, and callus formation are inevitable. The chronic fractures are lateral HCFs that may remain undiagnosed for several weeks. The displacement of the fractured lateral part of the humeral condyle can range from 2 millimeters to 2 centimeters. A nonsurgical approach, including weight control, supervision of the activity, and intermittent nonsteroidal anti-inflammatory therapy, generally gives satisfactory results, even with a large amount of fragment displacement. It is unlikely that anatomic reduction could be achieved in these cases by surgical intervention.

Incomplete Ossification Without Condylar Fracture

The optimal treatment of dogs with documented IOHC but without HCF is unknown. Seven partial radiolucent lines and twelve complete radiolucent lines have been diagnosed radiographically in 19 condyles with IOHC. Three of seven condyles (43%) with a partial radiolucent line and one of 12 condyles (8%) with a complete radiolucent line fractured 11 days to 18 months after diagnosis. Based on the above numbers, approximately one dog with IOHC in five will have an HCF within 18 months of initial diagnosis.

A bone screw can be placed across the humeral condyle with IOHC, in order to reinforce the bone (Fig. 3). The long-term effects of prophylactic transcondylar screw placement have not been evaluated in a prospective, randomized study. A transcondylar bone screw has been placed in 10 nonfractured humeral condyles affected by IOHC. None of the condyles fractured after surgery. Four dogs, with five operated condyles, have been reevaluated 6

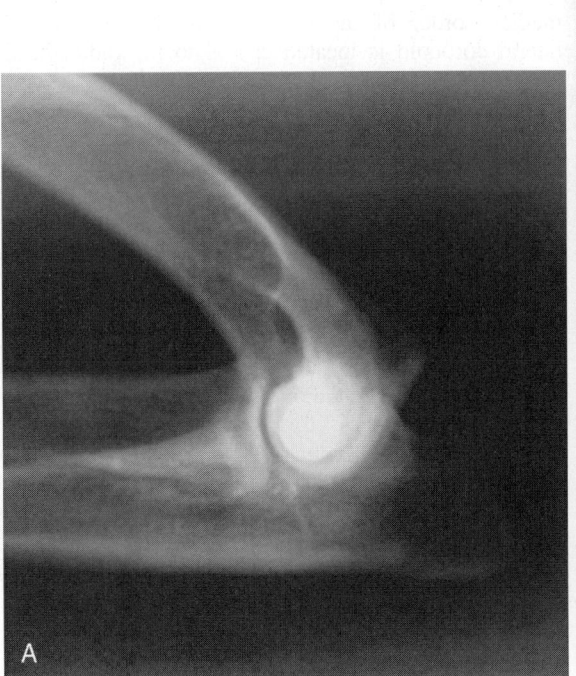
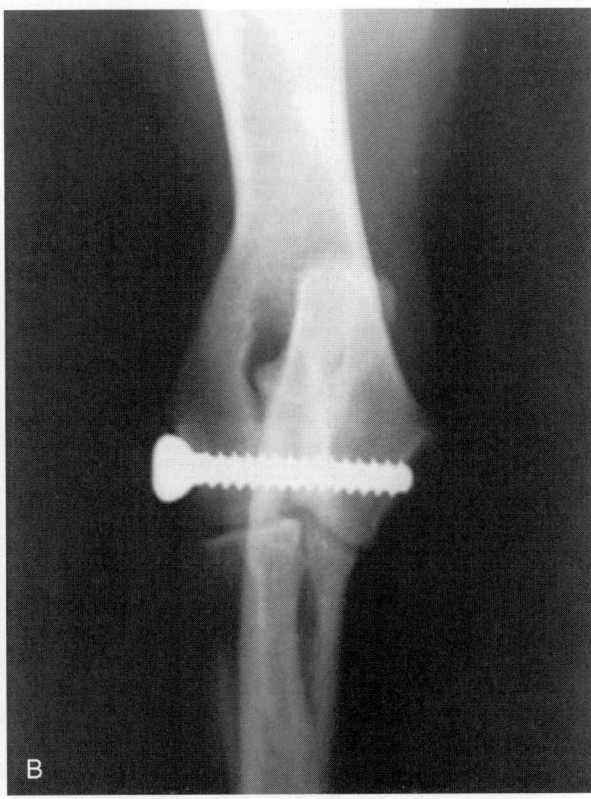

Figure 3. Hyperflexed mediolateral (A) and cranial 15-degree medial-caudolateral oblique (B) radiographic views of the elbow of a 2-year-old male Brittany spaniel having IOHC, immediately after placement of a 4.5-mm cortical transcondylar screw. A radiolucent line is visible across the humeral condyle. Radiographic signs of degenerative joint disease are absent.

to 23 months (mean: 18 months) after screw placement, and are free of lameness. However, on craniocaudal radiograph, the radiolucent lines remain visible across the humeral condyle, suggesting that incompletely ossified condyles do not heal after transcondylar screw placement. Currently, in light of the high fracture rate in dogs with IOHC, we recommend prophylactic use of a transcondylar screw in all dogs with a radiolucent line across the humeral condyle.

PREVENTION

Because of the genetic nature of the disease, we recommend avoiding breeding affected dogs. However, because the mean age at the time of diagnosis of IOHC is 6 years of age, those affected may already have been bred several times. We recommend screening the sire and dam, siblings, and offspring of affected dogs for a history of chronic forelimb lameness, restricted range of motion of the elbow joint, or a history of HCF after an unknown or minor trauma.

References and Suggested Reading

Brown DC, Conzemius MG, Shofer FS: Body weight as a predisposing factor for humeral condylar fractures, cranial cruciate rupture and intervertebral disc disease in cocker spaniels. Vet Comp Orthop Traumatol 9:75, 1996.
Cocker spaniels with humeral condylar fractures weighed significantly more (P < 0.05) than Cocker spaniels without humeral condylar fractures.
Kaderly RE, Lamothe M: Incomplete humeral condylar fracture due to minor trauma in a mature cocker spaniel. J Am Anim Hosp Assoc 28:361, 1992.
Spaniel breeds (P = 0.001), and Cocker spaniels (P = 0.03) are predisposed to humeral condylar fractures.
Marcellin-Little DJ, DeYoung DJ, Ferris KK, Berry CM: Incomplete ossification of the humeral condyle in spaniels. Vet Surg 23:475, 1994.
Retrospective study of 157 dogs with humeral fractures and prospective study of 18 skeletally mature spaniels with humeral condylar fractures caused by a minor or unknown trauma.
Marcellin-Little DJ, Roe SC, DeYoung DJ: What is your diagnosis? J Am Vet Med Assoc 209:727, 1996.
Radiographic and computed tomographic images of incomplete ossification of the humeral condyle in a Brittany spaniel.
Vannini R, Olmstead ML, Smeak DD: Humeral condylar fracture caused by minor trauma in 20 adult dogs. J Am Anim Hosp Assoc 24:355, 1988.
Cocker spaniels over 2 years of age are predisposed (P < 0.01) to humeral condylar fractures caused by a minor trauma.

Canine Elbow Dysplasia

PETER D. SCHWARZ
Albuquerque, New Mexico

In young growing dogs, developmental disorders of the elbow joint are one of the most common causes of forelimb lameness. Veterinary clinicians frequently refer to these disorders as *elbow dysplasia*. Elbow dysplasia is a general term that describes a series of four developmental abnormalities that lead to malformation and degeneration of the elbow joint. Three well-recognized forms of elbow dysplasia include: ununited anconeal process (UAP); fragmented medial coronoid process (FMCP); and osteochondritis dissecans (OCD) of the medial portion of the humeral condyle. A fourth type of elbow dysplasia currently recognized is incongruity (IC), which is manifested by malalignment and malformation of the elbow joint. Incongruity may be present by itself or more commonly in conjunction with UAP, FMCP, and OCD.

ANATOMY OF THE ELBOW JOINT

The radial head provides 75 to 80% of the weightbearing surface of the combined radial and ulnar joint surfaces of the elbow joint, whereas the medial and lateral coronoid processes of the ulna provide 20 to 25%. The coronoid processes are articular eminences of the ulna located distal to the trochlear notch and partially surround the medial and caudal aspect of the radial head (Fig. 1). The larger and more prominent medial coronoid process forms the medial border of the elbow joint, whereas the smaller lateral coronoid is located caudal to the radial head. The radial head lies on the same plane as the lateral coronoid and lateral aspect of the medial coronoid process. The medial coronoid process slopes distally approximately 30 to 35 degrees, laterally to medially. In order to maintain congruity of the radioulnar joint surfaces, the single distal ulnar physis must grow at a rate equal to that of the combined rates of the proximal and distal radial physes.

The humeroulnar joint is a tight-fitting, congruent joint that is formed by the articulation of the trochlea of the humeral condyle with the trochlear (semilunar) notch of the ulna. This joint's main role is to restrict motion in the sagittal plane and to add overall stability to the elbow joint. The anconeal process forms the proximal extent of the trochlear notch, and it fits into the olecranon fossa during extension of the elbow joint. The anconeal process helps to prevent lateral and rotatory instability of the joint during weightbearing. The normal range of motion of the elbow joint is from 30 to 40 degrees flexion to 170 to 180 degrees extension.

ETIOLOGY AND PATHOPHYSIOLOGY
General Considerations

Controversy surrounds the cause of canine elbow dysplasia. One must first realize that there is probably no

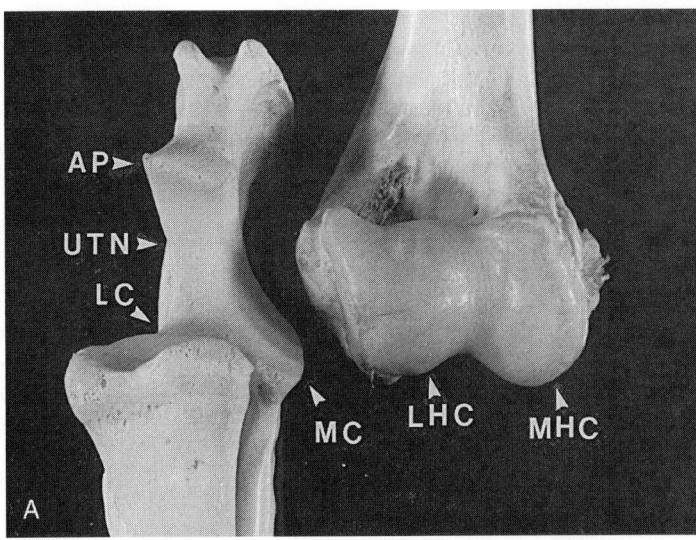

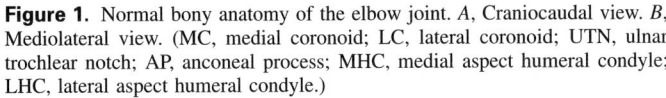

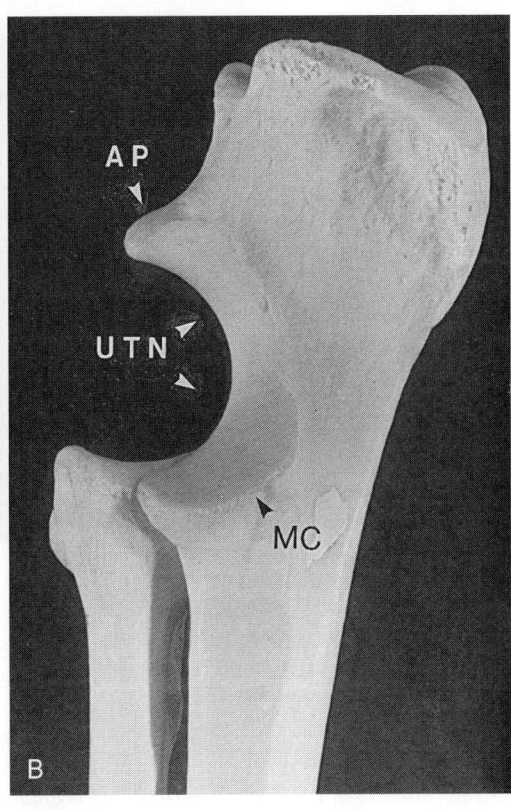

Figure 1. Normal bony anatomy of the elbow joint. *A*, Craniocaudal view. *B*, Mediolateral view. (MC, medial coronoid; LC, lateral coronoid; UTN, ulnar trochlear notch; AP, anconeal process; MHC, medial aspect humeral condyle; LHC, lateral aspect humeral condyle.)

single cause for the various forms of elbow dysplasia presently recognized. Also, the four recognized conditions may occur alone or concurrently with other forms of elbow dysplasia.

Many believe that elbow dysplasia in its various forms is a manifestation of the more general condition known as osteochondrosis (Olsson, 1993). Osteochondrosis (OC) is a pathologic process in growing cartilage. Several etiologic factors have been implicated in causing canine OC, including nutrition, rapid growth, joint conformation, and genetic transmission. The main feature of OC is a disturbance of endochondral ossification that leads to excessive retention of cartilage. In articular cartilage, necrosis and mechanical stress can lead to fissuring of the thickened cartilage and result in a flap lesion. In growth plates (physes), retention of cartilage may make the physes more susceptible to slippage and asymmetrical growth.

The role of nutrition in developmental skeletal disorders, such as elbow dysplasia, is controversial and complex. Rate of growth, excessive energy (calories) and calcium, level of food consumption, and feeding methods have all been shown to increase the likelihood of developing skeletal disease. Nutrition's main role appears to be in modulating the frequency and severity of disease, especially during the early, high-growth-rate period. The greatest harm is caused by overnutrition from excess consumption of energy-rich foods and oversupplementation of calcium. Nutritional management alone will not completely eliminate or prevent developmental skeletal disease.

A polygenic basis for developmental skeletal disease of the elbow joint has been shown for the Labrador retriever, Bernese Mountain dog, Rottweiler, German shepherd dog, and Bassett hound. Heritability estimates indicate a range

of 0.27 to 0.77, which strongly suggests that controlled breeding is required to limit the occurrence of elbow dysplasia. Dogs diagnosed with elbow dysplasia should not be bred. Dam and sire breedings that result in offspring with documented elbow dysplasia should be prevented from breeding again. Breeders and owners alike should be educated as to the hereditary transmission of these disorders.

As a result of OC, genetics, nutritional factors, trauma, or other unknown causes, the development of a growth imbalance between the radius and ulna or within the ulnar trochlear notch can result in conformational changes within the elbow joint (Wind, 1993). As a result of accelerated growth rates, large and giant breeds seem to be most susceptible to developmental skeletal disease such as elbow dysplasia. Abnormalities associated with incongruity include widening of the humeroradial and humeroulnar joint spaces, asymmetrical longitudinal growth between the radius and ulna, cranial displacement of the humeral condyle, and failure of the trochlear notch to form a congruent arc with the trochlea of the humeral condyle. These malformation changes lead to abnormal mechanical stresses and wear within the elbow joint.

Ununited Anconeal Process

Ununited anconeal process has been described as a failure of the anconeal ossification center to unite with the proximal ulnar metaphysis. Normally, bony union should be complete at 16 to 20 weeks of age in dogs. If the anconeal process is not radiographically united at 20 weeks, a disease state exists and spontaneous union will not occur. In most instances, a fibrous tissue or fibrocartilaginous bridge connects the anconeal process to the ulnar metaphysis.

Asynchronous growth between the radius and ulna has been proposed as the cause of UAP (Olsson, 1993; Sjöstrom et al, 1995). Proximally, if the radius becomes relatively longer than the ulna at the level of the elbow joint, the radial head will exert a proximally directed pressure on the humeral trochlea. This pressure, transferred via the trochlea of the humerus to the anconeal process, may cause plastic deformation of the anconeal process and/or prevent bony union of the secondary ossification center of the anconeal process.

Failure of the ulnar trochlear notch to develop a sufficient arc of curvature to congruently fit and accommodate the humeral trochlea may also be a predisposing malformation that leads to development of UAP. As a consequence of this malarticulation, micromotion may occur between the ossification center of the anconeal process and the ulnar metaphysis preventing bony union.

UAP has been documented primarily in large-breed dogs: German shepherd dog, St. Bernard, Great Dane, Labrador retriever, Irish wolfhound, pointers, Bloodhound, Great Pyrenees, Weimaraner, and Newfoundland. The highest incidence has been reported in German shepherd dogs. UAP has also been reported in the chondrodystrophoid breeds: Basset hound, French bulldog, and Dachshund. In about one third of the cases, the condition is bilateral. A genetic predisposition is thought to lead to the development of UAP. No sex predisposition has been demonstrated for UAP.

Fragmented Medial Coronoid Process

FMCP is the chondral or osteochondral fragmentation or fissure of the medial coronoid process. It is considered a manifestation of osteochondrosis of the coronoid process (Olsson, 1993). The pathophysiology is different from that of UAP because the coronoid process does not have a separate ossification center. In the immature dog, the medial coronoid process is composed entirely of cartilage that tends to undergo a delayed endochondral ossification process when compared with other regions of the articular surface. This delay in ossification of the medial coronoid process may predispose it to fragmentation when mechanical stresses are applied.

Another proposed cause of FMCP is joint incongruity due to asynchronous growth between the radius and ulna (Wind, 1993). If the radius becomes relatively shorter than the ulna at the level of the elbow joint, the coronoid will exert a proximally directed pressure on the humeral trochlea. Instead of the radius providing the major weightbearing surface of the forelimb, the coronoid process would now assume the role. The resulting abnormal mechanical stress could disturb development of the coronoid process, leading to fragmentation or abnormal ossification. This type of growth disturbance would result in widening of the humeroradial joint and a step discrepancy of the radioulnar joint surface. Osteochondrosis of the growth plates may be responsible for causing asynchronous growth between the radius and ulna.

FMCP is a developmental condition most commonly observed in large-breed dogs, usually Labrador retrievers,

Rottweilers, Golden retrievers, Bernese Mountain dogs, German shepherd dogs, Chow Chows, Bearded Collies, and Newfoundlands. Males are more often affected than females and the condition is commonly bilateral (30 to 80%). A genetic predisposition is thought to lead to the development of FMCP.

Osteochondritis Dissecans (OCD) of the Humeral Condyle

The pathophysiology of OCD of the medial aspect of the humeral condyle is similar to that of OCD found in the shoulder joint (Olsson, 1993). In animals with OC, the cells of the growth plates and of the immature articular cartilage do not differentiate normally. The process of endochondral ossification is retarded while cartilage continues to grow, resulting in abnormally thick regions that are less resistant to mechanical stress. In immature articular cartilage where nutrition is maintained by diffusion of nutrients from the synovial fluid, increased cartilage thickness results in impaired metabolism with degeneration and necrosis of the poorly nourished cartilage cells. Due to mechanical stress, fissures can result within this thickened cartilage that eventually lead to the formation of a cartilage flap, i.e., osteochondritis dissecans (OCD).

OCD of the humeral condyle is a developmental condition most commonly observed in large-breed dogs, usually Labrador retrievers, Rottweilers, Golden retrievers, German shepherds, and Newfoundlands. There is no established sex predilection and the condition is commonly bilateral (30 to 80%). A genetic predisposition is thought to lead to the development of OCD.

Incongruity (IC) of the Elbow Joint

Incongruity is the manifestation of malalignment and malformation of the elbow joint (Wind, 1993). There are at least two forms of elbow incongruity that may be present alone or concurrently in the same or opposite elbow joints of a dog. One form of IC is due to asynchronous growth between the radius and ulna leading to proximal overgrowth of the coronoid process relative to the radial articular surface. This type of IC would lead to abnormal load and wear, erosion of cartilage in the humeroulnar compartment of the elbow joint, a widened humeroradial joint and a step discrepancy between the coronoids and radial head. An FMCP may be associated with this form of IC.

Incongruity may also be the result of malformation of the trochlear notch of the ulna. A slightly elliptical trochlear notch with a decreased arc of curvature would be too small to articulate congruently with the humeral trochlea. This would result in major points of contact in areas of the anconeal process, coronoid process, and medial aspect of the humeral condyle and little or no contact in other areas of the trochlea. Abnormal mechanical stress on the anconeal process, medial coronoid, and medial humeral condyle may predispose to UAP, FMCP, and OCD, respectively. This form of incongruity would result in a malformed humeroulnar joint space.

Incongruity is most commonly seen in the same breeds where UAP, FMCP, and OCD develop. To date, no sex predisposition has been demonstrated for IC. Until proven otherwise, a genetic predisposition should be considered a contributing factor.

CLINICAL SIGNS AND PHYSICAL FINDINGS

It is virtually impossible to distinguish the various manifestations of elbow dysplasia by clinical signs and physical findings. The clinical signs of elbow dysplasia are often first noticed at 4 to 6 months of age but may not be obvious until 8 months of age or older. Initial lameness may range from intermittent to persistent and from mild to severe. Dogs are often presented with a history of being stiff when rising from rest as well as following vigorous exercise. Many owners claim that their dogs are mildly lame and that this lameness is exacerbated by activity. The elbow is often held abducted and the limb supinated. A gait disturbance characterized by limited range of motion (extension and flexion) of the affected elbow joint is often present.

Joint effusion and swelling may be present. Joint effusion is appreciated most commonly on the lateral aspect between the lateral epicondyle of the humerus and olecranon. Pain can often be elicited on hyperextension and flexion of the elbow joint. Sensitivity and pain, as determined by application of digital pressure on the medial side of the joint, around the medial collateral ligament may be present. Holding the elbow and carpal joints at 90 degrees of flexion and then pronating and supinating the carpus will often elicit a painful response in dogs having elbow dysplasia. Crepitus may or may not be palpable; crepitus is most prevalent with advanced osteoarthritic changes. Physical findings in dogs with chronic elbow dysplasia include crepitus, muscle atrophy, limited range of motion, periarticular thickening, joint effusion, and the palpation of osteophytes. Osteophytes are most readily palpated as a "string-of-pearls" on the lateral aspect of the ulna in the region of the trochlear notch. Chronic elbow dysplasia results in severe damage to the joint surfaces and the periarticular soft tissues. Advanced osteophytosis, partial to full cartilage erosion, and ligament and periarticular ossification may ensue.

Careful historical and physical examination will usually allow the veterinarian to differentiate elbow dysplasia from other common causes of forelimb lameness in young, growing dogs, i.e., panosteitis, shoulder OCD, trauma, septic arthritis, and avulsion or calcification of the flexor tendons of the medial epicondyle.

RADIOGRAPHIC EXAMINATION

Four radiographic views are necessary for adequate evaluation of an elbow joint for dysplasia. The views are mediolateral; mediolateral hyperflexed; 15 degrees craniolateral-caudomedial oblique (extended and supinated mediolateral); and craniocaudal (Fig. 2). It is strongly advised that radiographs of both elbow joints be taken because of the high incidence of bilateral disease. Radiographic evidence of osteoarthritis is a common finding with all of the various manifestations of elbow dysplasia; however, the presence of osteophytes, periarticular lipping, subchondral sclerosis, and cysts are not pathognomonic.

Ununited Anconeal Process

The definitive diagnosis of UAP is readily made from well-positioned plain-film radiographs (Fig. 3). UAP is easiest to see on the hyperflexed mediolateral view. Non-flexed mediolateral views tend to obscure the anconeal process by the overlying medial humeral epicondylar ridge. If the dog is older than 5 to 6 months of age, the presence of a radiolucent line between the anconeal process and the proximal ulnar metaphysis is diagnostic. Separation and displacement of the anconeal process is more common in older aged dogs.

Fragmented Medial Coronoid Process

A fragmented medial coronoid process is rarely visualized on plain-film radiographs. Fragments from the medial coronoid process involving only cartilage or small bone fragments are of insufficient density to allow direct visualization on radiographs, and superimposition of the radial head over the medial coronoid process contributes to poor direct radiographic visualization. The presumptive diagnosis of FMCP is made by finding abnormalities that indicate secondary osteoarthritis and excluding other more radiographically visible causes (UAP, OCD). All four radiographic views are mandatory to diagnose probable FMCP within an elbow joint (see Fig. 2).

The most consistent location to observe developing osteophytes is on the proximal border of the anconeal process when viewing the hyperflexed mediolateral radiograph. These osteophytes can be very subtle and are generally obscured in other radiographic views. The standard mediolateral view often demonstrates sclerosis of the trochlear notch and of the ulna caudal to the base of the coronoid process, osteophyte production on the cranial margin of the radial head, and a step discrepancy between the lateral coronoid process and radial head. Periarticular lipping, in addition to osteophyte formation on the medial coronoid process (often mistaken as an FMCP) and the medial and lateral epicondyles, is best visualized on the craniocaudal and oblique views. These changes are not unique to FMCP and will occur with UAP, OCD, and IC. Occasionally, a fragmented coronoid process may be seen on one of these four radiographic views.

Specialized diagnostic techniques such as linear tomography, contrast arthrography, xeroradiography, computed tomography (CT), and magnetic resonance imaging (MRI) have been evaluated as to their sensitivity, accuracy, and negative predictive value in the diagnosis of FMCP (Carpenter et al, 1993). CT and MRI have been shown to be the most sensitive and specific diagnostic techniques (>90%) in identifying the presence or absence of FMCP and coronoid disease. These techniques enable the veterinarian to diagnose nondisplaced "in-situ" fragments, nondisplaced nonmineralized coronoid processes, and nondisplaced abnormally mineralized coronoid processes when radiography as well as gross visualization is nondiagnostic or equivocal. Arthroscopic exploration of the medial elbow joint compartment is an excellent alternative diagnostic modality to arthrotomy when trying to identify and confirm the presence of FMCP.

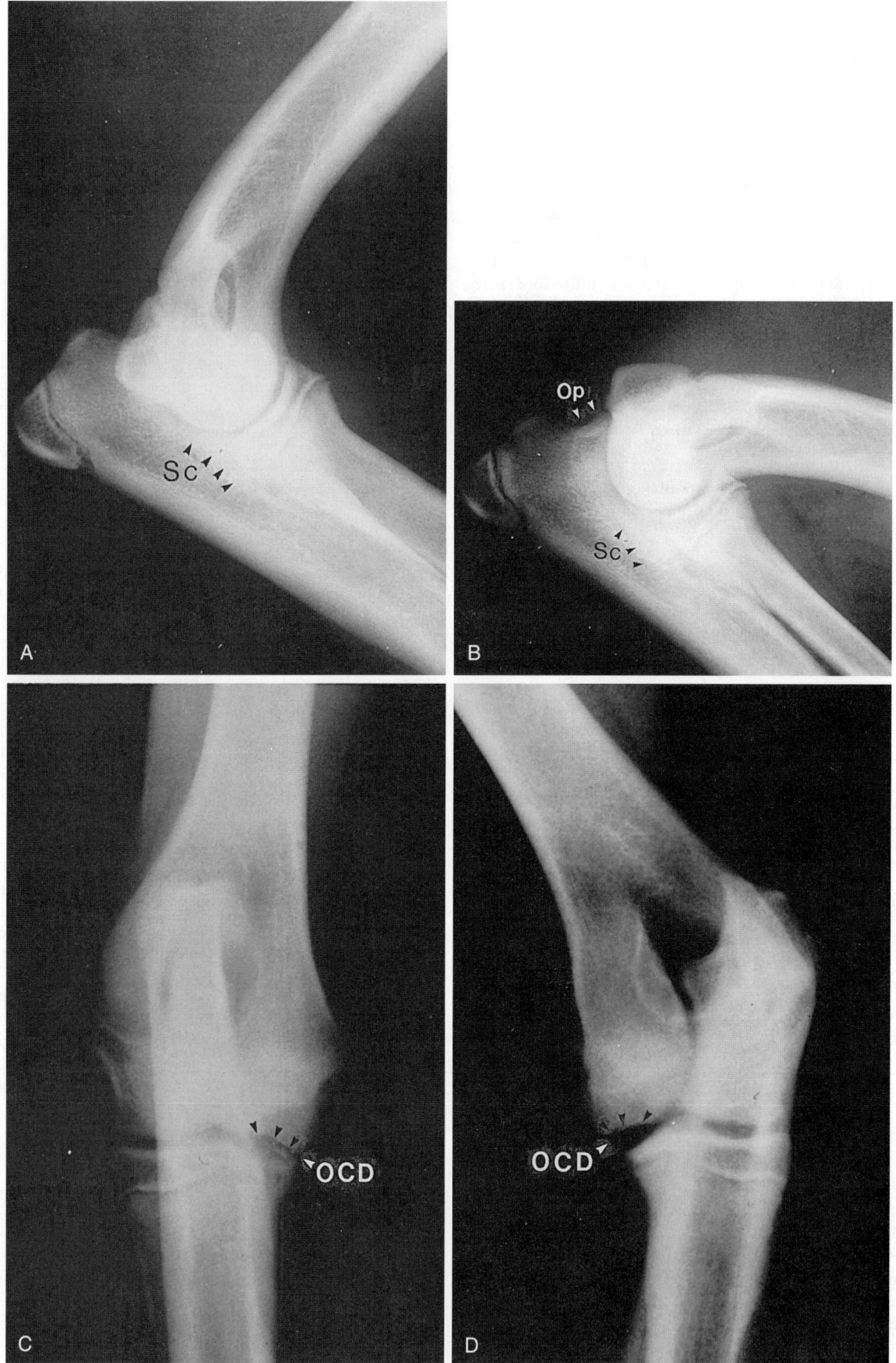

Figure 2. Radiographs of an 8-month-old Labrador retriever with fragmented medial coronoid process (FMCP) and OCD demonstrating the four views recommended for assessing elbow dysplasia. *A*, Mediolateral; *B*, mediolateral hyperflexed; *C*, craniocaudal; and *D*, 15-degree craniolateral-caudomedial oblique views. (Op, osteophytes; Sc, subchondral sclerosis; OCD, osteochondritis dissecans lesion.) The FMCP was discovered during exploratory surgery.

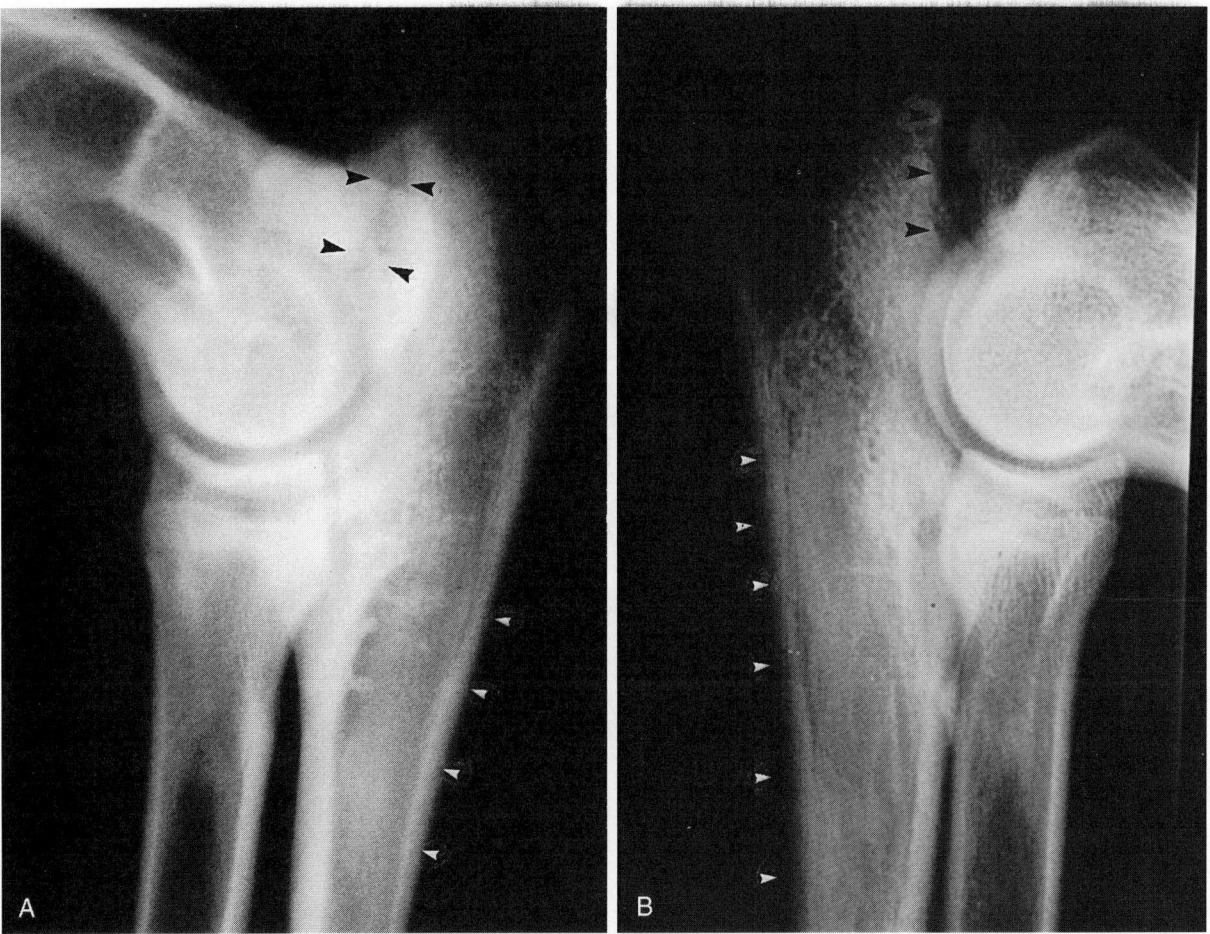

Figure 3. Radiographs of a 9-month-old German shepherd dog with ununited anconeal process (UAP; *black arrowheads*) and panosteitis *(white arrowheads).* A, Mediolateral; and B, mediolateral hyperflexed views. Notice that is is difficult to identify the UAP on the standard mediolateral view.

Osteochondritis Dissecans

OCD of the humeral condyle is most reliably diagnosed on the craniocaudal and oblique radiographic views. The initial radiographic sign is a dome-shaped to triangular radiolucent defect in the subchondral bone of the medial aspect of the humeral condyle directly apposing the medial coronoid process. Generally, this radiolucent region is bordered by a sclerotic margin. As the disease progresses, osteoarthritic changes, similar to those associated with FMCP, develop. Arthroscopy is an excellent diagnostic tool to use in confirming the presence of OCD. Medial portals are used when exploring the medial elbow joint compartment.

Incongruity of the Elbow Joint

It is difficult to accurately and consistently diagnose IC by conventional radiography. Several measurement techniques comparing overall length of the radius to that of the ulna have been reported that can indicate asymmetrical growth between the two bones. However, subtle joint surface discrepancies of less than 1 mm are poorly visualized and appreciated. The sensitivity, accuracy, and positive and negative predictive abilities of plain-film radiographs

versus CT or MRI in detecting IC have not been documented, but it seems likely that the latter are more accurate in demonstrating joint surface discrepancies than that visible on routine radiography. CT and MRI are the preferred diagnostic modalities for fully appreciating the joint irregularities and incongruence associated with this type of elbow dysplasia (Fig. 4). These diagnostic techniques also have the ability to accurately diagnose the presence of concurrent disease such as FMCP, OCD, and UAP. Diagnostic criteria for IC includes widening of the humeroradial and humeroulnar joint spaces, step discrepancy between the radial head and lateral coronoid process, failure of the trochlear notch to form a congruent arc matching the trochlea of the humeral condyle, and sclerotic subchondral bone changes of the coronoid and apposing medial aspect of the humeral condyle.

TREATMENT OPTIONS

There are no proven "best" methods of treating the various forms of elbow dysplasia. Nonsurgical therapies (weight control, exercise limitation, nonsteroidal anti-inflammation drugs, and chondroprotective drugs) have been reported to be as effective as surgical treatment of elbow dysplasia. Unfortunately, most of the studies, both surgical

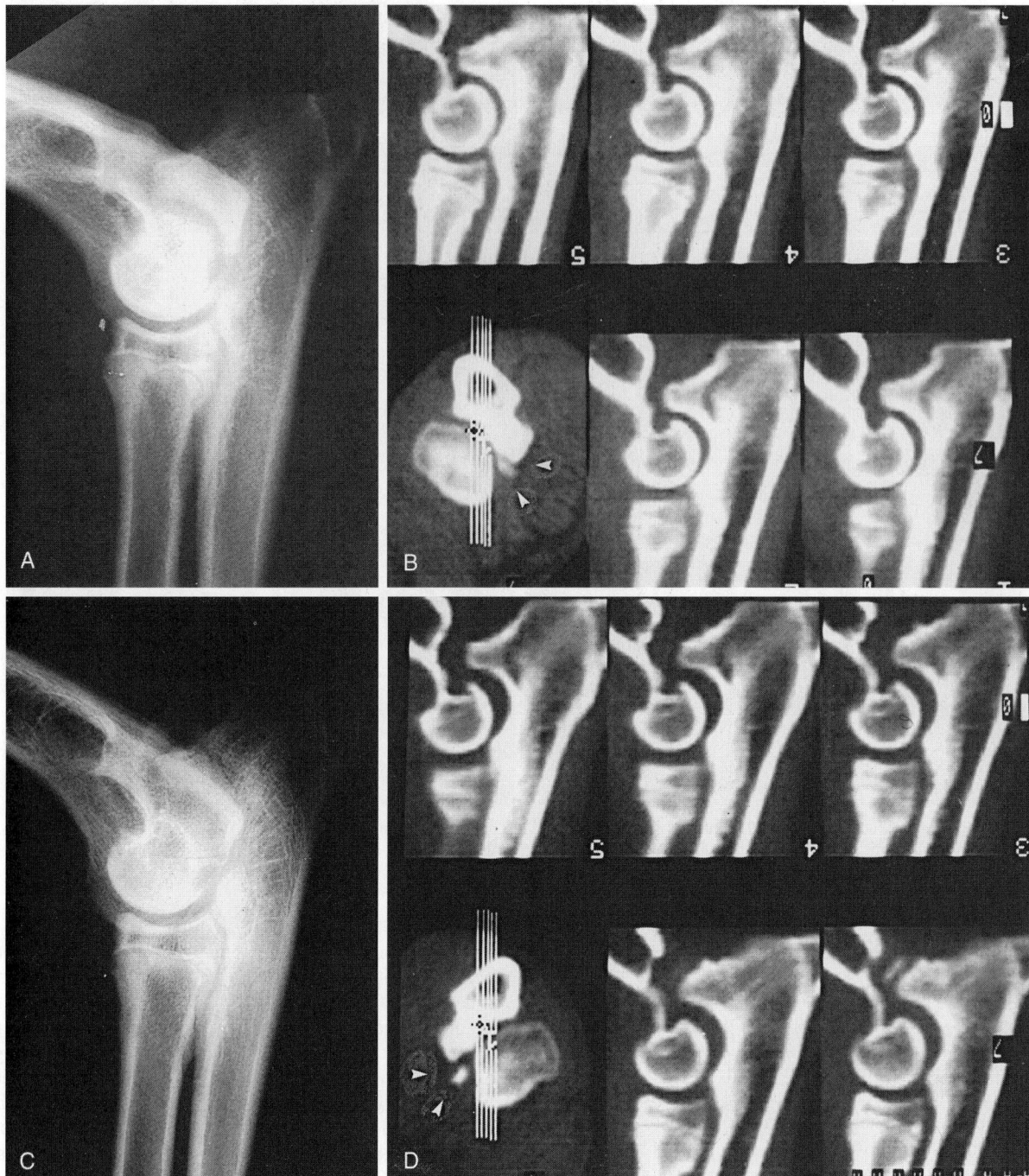

Figure 4. Radiographs and computed tomograms of an 8-month-old Bernese Mountain dog diagnosed with bilateral FMCP and IC. *A*, Mediolateral radiograph of right elbow. *B*, Sagittal and transverse computed tomograms of the right elbow. *C*, Mediolateral radiograph of left elbow. *D*, Sagittal and transverse computed tomograms of the left elbow. The FMCP is indicated by the arrows. The computed tomograms clearly demonstrate incongruity. The right elbow has both ulnar trochlear notch malformation and asymmetrical growth between the radius and the ulna, whereas the left elbow has only the latter.

and nonsurgical, have had relatively short follow-up periods; as such, they may not accurately represent the long-term outcome of their respective treatment approach. Dogs surgically treated before 1 year of age that do not have advanced osteoarthritis have the best clinical results. Surgery has been shown to reduce the time interval from onset of clinical signs and diagnosis to time of best improvement, lessen the severity of lameness, and improve the activity level of dogs when compared with dogs not treated surgi-

cally. Until more studies document long-term outcome, surgery should be considered the primary treatment for UAP, FMCP, and OCD. Regardless of the treatment method chosen, osteoarthritis tends to progress. In all cases, the dog's owner must be informed that progression of osteoarthritis will occur and that medical therapy is likely in the future. Corticosteroids should be avoided because of the potential side effects and the articular cartilage damage associated with long-term usage. Chondroprotective drugs such as polysulfated glycosaminoglycans, and glucosamine and chondroitin sulfates may be of benefit in limiting cartilage damage and degeneration. They may also help alleviate pain and inflammation.

Ununited Anconeal Process

Surgery is the treatment of choice for UAP. Three different surgical procedures have been used. Removal of the UAP is the most commonly performed procedure. Although removal has been recommended only after the dog has neared completion of growth (>9 months), most surgeons recommend removal as soon as the definitive diagnosis has been made. A loose anconeal process may induce inflammation within the joint and exacerbate the development of degenerative joint disease. Early removal may minimize the progression of arthritis (Roy et al, 1994). Surgically, the UAP is most accessible through a lateral approach to elbow joint (Piermattei, 1993).

An alternative to the more frequent practice of removing the anconeal process is lag-screw fixation. The premise of saving the anconeal process is that the process inherently provides stability to the elbow joint and its removal may induce joint instability. With lag-screw fixation, the bone screw can be inserted either in a caudal-to-cranial or cranial-to-caudal direction. The former screw orientation may be easier to perform and requires a less extensive surgical approach. Although a limited number of cases have been documented in the literature, lag-screw fixation for treating UAP has yielded encouraging results (Fox et al, 1996). Severe remodeling and degeneration of the anconeal process precludes lag-screw fixation. In such cases, removal is warranted.

Performing a proximal ulnar osteotomy is another surgical option to consider when treating UAP (Gilson et al, 1989; Sjöstrom et al, 1995). The main goal of this procedure is to realign the humeroulnar joint space. This procedure is relatively simple to perform; it does not require arthrotomy. The proximal ulnar shaft is exposed by a caudal approach (Piermattei, 1993). An oblique osteotomy of the ulna is made just distal to the elbow joint using an oscillating saw or Gigli wire. Use of an osteotome is not recommended because it tends to fragment the bone. A small nonthreaded intramedullary pin or Kirschner wire 0.062 to 3/32 inches diameter (1.6 to 2.4 mm) is driven from the olecranon across the osteotomy site and seated into the midshaft region of the bone. The oblique osteotomy and the pin protect against angular displacement of the proximal ulna from triceps muscle forces. Some widening of the gap will be seen postoperatively as realignment of the humeroulnar joint occurs, especially in severe cases. Ulnar osteotomy distal to the level of the elbow joint does not have the potential to change the configuration of the ulnar trochlear notch but conceivably alters the relative positions of the radial and ulnar joint surfaces within the elbow joint. In a recent report, bony union of the UAP and improved clinical function were observed in 95% (21/22) of the elbows treated. Proximal ulnar osteotomy can be performed either as an alternative treatment option to UAP removal or as a concurrent treatment with either UAP removal or lag-screw fixation.

Fragmented Medial Coronoid Process

Controversy exists concerning the treatment of FMCP. Several published reports have demonstrated no distinct advantage of surgical removal of loose fragments versus nonsurgical or medical treatment (Huibregtse et al, 1994; Bouck et al, 1995). Unfortunately most studies do not include long-term results and most do not evaluate medical versus surgical plus medical treatment. There is much interest in the benefits of using chondroprotective drugs in the early postoperative period, but their efficacy has yet to be documented. Controlled clinical studies are required to establish the true benefits of this type of medical therapy. Until further studies are conducted, early surgical treatment of this condition, involving an exploratory arthrotomy (or via arthroscopy) and removal of loose fragments in addition to medical treatment is advocated. Medical treatment should consist of rest, weight reduction, low-impact exercise, and nonsteroidal anti-inflammatory drugs (NSAIDs) or chondroprotective drugs. Medical therapy instead of surgery should be recommended in older dogs with advanced osteoarthritis and in dogs whose owners are reluctant to pursue surgery.

Surgery should be considered an exploratory procedure. Clients should be forewarned about the possibility of finding no overtly loose osteochondral fragments within the joint. In one study of 30 consecutive elbows that were radiographically suspected of having an FMCP and surgically explored, only 57% (17/30) had a grossly visible fragmented coronoid process (Carpenter et al, 1993).

Several surgical approaches have been described to gain access to the medial coronoid process including osteotomy of the medial epicondyle; tenotomy of the pronator teres alone or in combination with tenotomy of the flexor carpi radialis with or without desmotomy of the medial collateral ligament; intermuscular separation between the pronator teres and flexor carpi radialis or between the flexor carpi radialis and digital flexor muscles; and proximal ulnar diaphyseal osteotomy (Piermattei, 1993). For ease, speed, adequate exposure, and minimal morbidity, the intermuscular separation techniques are preferred. Limited exposure, as compared with the other techniques, is the primary drawback to these approaches. Regardless of which of the surgical approaches is used, it is imperative to adequately identify the entire articular surface of the medial coronoid process once access to the joint is obtained. The area of the medial coronoid most frequently involved is either the cranial tip or the lateral margin that articulates with the radial head. False-negative results can readily be obtained if only the medial aspect of the coronoid is observed. False-positive results can occur when the radioulnar (coronoid) articulation is mistaken for the edge of a bone fragment. Inducing motion within the joint during visual inspection prevents misdiagnosis. Stabilizing the proximal ulna in one hand while pronating and supinating the carpus with the other hand allows the surgeon to differentiate normal from abnormal structures. With this manipulation, the radial head is seen to rotate whereas the ulna and coronoid fragment will not. The entire articular surface should be probed with a blunt-tipped instrument to define the presence and extent of an osteochondral fragment. Following fragment removal, the coronoid stump should be curetted to remove all residual loose or diseased bone and the joint generously lavaged before closure. Surgical findings vary from large, loose fragments within the joint to cartilaginous fissures to mild discoloration of the cartilage. In some reports, FMCP and OCD have been associated with each other as "kissing" lesions. Although these two lesions may occur together, their concurrent presence is uncommon and a direct cause-and-effect has not been demonstrated. More typically, "kissing" lesions are wear lesions indicating abnormal articulation between apposing articular surfaces. Fragment removal using arthroscopically guided instruments is an excellent alternative treatment option to open arthrotomy. Diagnosis and treatment can be performed successfully using medial portals for both scope and instruments.

Osteochondritis Dissecans

Early surgical treatment of this condition, involving an exploratory arthrotomy and removal of loose fragments is advocated. A medial approach to the elbow joint by an intermuscular incision that does not require an osteotomy or desmotomy is strongly recommended (Piermattei, 1993). All loose and undermined cartilage should be removed and the subchondral defect curetted to healthy bleeding bone. Arthroscopy is an excellent alternative treatment option to open arthrotomy. Diagnosis and treatment can be performed successfully using medial portals for both scope and instruments.

Incongruity of the Elbow Joint

Plain-film radiography is unable to adequately define the type and degree of incongruity and therefore the basis for surgery. Also, a malformed ulnar trochlear notch and asynchronous growth between the radius and ulna are not readily apparent during open arthrotomy or arthroscopic exploration. Without the preoperative diagnostic benefits of CT or MRI, it is difficult to know which surgical treatment method or methods are indicated to treat IC in a particular elbow joint. Until comparative studies are conducted, caution should be exercised when recommending surgical treatment for IC.

At surgery, IC will grossly appear as wear lesions on the coronoid and medial aspect of the humeral condyle, in which deep erosions, furrows, and streaking of the articular cartilage are apparent. The objective of surgical treatment of IC in which the ulna is relatively long when compared with the radius is to re-establish normal articulation of the humeroradial joint. This could be accomplished by a lengthening osteotomy of the radius using rigid fixation (bone plate or external skeletal fixator). The difficulty with this is knowing when the radius is in perfect alignment with the humeral condyle. A very small residual malalignment could lead to continued incongruity, cartilage abrasion, and osteoarthritis.

Two other surgical options should be considered when trying to treat IC: coronoidectomy or dynamic ulnar ostectomy, in which part of the medial coronoid or a section of the proximal ulna is removed, respectively. If enough bone is removed (coronoid or proximal ulnar diaphysis) to allow the radial head to contact the lateral portion of the humeral

condyle, muscular forces and weightbearing will seat the head anatomically, and the humeroradial joint will be re-established. Coronoidectomy can be accomplished with either a high speed bur or osteotome in which the articular cartilage and underlying subchondral bone of the medial coronoid process is removed. The level of bone removed should equal the suspected gap present between the radial head and humeral condyle. Coronoidectomies can be done through a medial approach to the elbow joint similar to that performed for FMCP and OCD. Conversely, elbow joint congruity can be achieved by shortening the ulna by performing a proximal ulnar ostectomy (Gilson et al, 1989). The ulna is exposed by a caudal approach to the proximal shaft of the ulna and an oblique ostectomy of the ulna performed distal to the trochlear notch. The width of the removed bone must be at least equal to the gap present between the humeral condyle and radial head and sufficient to allow the radius and distal ulna to move proximally until the radial head articulates normally with the lateral portion of the humeral condyle. A small nonthreaded intramedullary pin or Kirschner wire is driven from the olecranon across the osteotomy site and seated into the midshaft region of the bone. The oblique osteotomy and the pin protect against angular displacement of the proximal ulna from triceps muscle forces. Some narrowing of the gap will be seen postoperatively as realignment occurs. A recent report advocates against using an intramedullary alignment pin, suggesting that the resultant angular malalignment induced by triceps muscle forces is beneficial to re-establishing joint congruity (Thomson et al, 1995). Further investigation is required to substantiate this claim. Arthroscopy is an excellent alternative treatment option. Arthroscopic visualization of the medial elbow compartment allows excellent assessment of the articular surface of the coronoid process. Wear lesions are readily visualized and coronoidectomies can be performed arthroscopically.

RECOMMENDATIONS

Diagnosis

There is a lack of correlation between the degree of clinical, radiographic, and pathologic findings in this disease complex. Dogs with minimal radiographic changes can have significant clinical signs of pain and lameness while dogs with advanced radiographic evidence of osteoarthritis can be relatively asymptomatic. The astute clinician should always consider elbow dysplasia, especially FMCP and IC, when presented with a medium- to large-breed dog with a forelimb lameness.

When findings on radiography are equivocal, but the elbow joint is the suspected origin of lameness, a repeat examination 4 to 8 weeks later is warranted. During this observation period, further progression of osteoarthritis allows a diagnosis to be made with greater confidence. Unfortunately, this waiting period may be detrimental to affected dogs, because early diagnosis and surgical intervention appear to offer the best hope for a favorable outcome.

Joint tap with analysis of synovial fluid is useful to confirm the presence of pathology within the elbow joint but is not diagnostic for elbow dysplasia. Grossly, the synovial fluid should be straw colored with normal to decreased viscosity. Cytologic evaluation demonstrates fewer than 10,000 nucleated cells/μl, with more than 90% being mononuclear cells.

Bone scans, using radiolabeled markers, can be useful in isolating the location of a particular lameness. Although bone scans do not definitively diagnose the cause of a particular lameness, they can assist the clinician in identifying the location (bone, joint, soft tissue). Once the elbow joint is identified as the source of lameness, CT, MRI, or exploratory surgery can be offered to the client. With appropriate client counseling, surgical exploration (arthrotomy/arthroscopy) may be warranted when advanced diagnostic modalities are not available or affordable.

It is not uncommon for more than one type of elbow dysplasia to be present in the same elbow or opposite elbow. Each condition can develop independently or may coexist with other lesions. Unless demonstrated not to be present by CT or MRI, IC should be considered present in all elbows with clinical symptoms associated with dysplasia. Elbow incongruity may be a predisposing cause of UAP, FMCP, and OCD, and removal of bone and cartilage fragments without correction of IC is treating only part of the pathologic problem. Although not always readily available, CT and MRI should be offered to clients who desire complete assessment of their dog's elbow joint prior to initiating treatment. Lack of a simple and cost-effective method of diagnosis that is always accurate (high positive and negative predictive values) continues to be a major clinical dilemma.

Arthroscopy is an excellent surgical modality to asses the medial elbow joint compartment. Structures readily visualized include the medial coronoid process, lateral coronoid process, medial and lateral aspect of the humeral condyle, medial aspect of the radial head, trochlear notch of the ulna, and caudal aspect of the anconeal process. Wear lesions on the humeral condyles and coronoid process (IC) are strikingly apparent as well as FMCP and OCD chondral and osteochondral lesions. Arthroscopy offers minimal soft tissue morbidity concerns and improved postoperative recovery, though these potential benefits have not yet been validated in dogs.

Treatment

The following treatment protocols are based on my personal experiences and beliefs. I prefer arthroscopy as the method of joint exploration and treatment for FMCP, IC (coronoidectomy), and OCD and feel that the use of chondroprotective drugs should be considered in the treatment of all elbow dysplastic dogs.

Ununited Anconeal Process

Once the diagnosis of UAP is made, surgery is recommended. Based on radiographic evidence of osteoarthritis and the appearance of the anconeal process, perform either a proximal ulnar osteotomy alone or in combination with removal of the UAP. If there is significant radiographic evidence of osteoarthritis and the UAP appears misshapen or deformed, preserving the process is not warranted. This assertion is based on histologic evaluation of removed anconeal processes in long-standing cases that have demonstrated fibrous tissue infiltration and chondroid metaplasia of the UAP. In such cases, attempting osteosynthesis is neither justified nor likely to occur. The ulnar osteotomy will realign the proximal ulna in relation to the radius, minimizing IC that is a result of asymmetrical growth between these two bones. An underdeveloped ulnar trochlear notch will not benefit from this procedure. One can always recommend the ulnar osteotomy first, and if spontaneous osteosynthesis between the anconeal process and ulnar metaphysis does not occur within 8 to 12 weeks and clinical signs do not improve, the UAP can be removed during a second surgery.

Fragmented Medial Coronoid Process

Removal via arthroscopy or arthrotomy is the recommended treatment for suspected FMCP. Without a preoperative CT or MRI, surgery should be presented to the client as an "exploratory" surgery. Up to 43% of the joints explored may not have obvious fragmentation or fissuring of the coronoid process. These joints may appear grossly normal or have evidence of wear lesions on the articular surfaces of the coronoid and medial aspect of the humeral condyle. These joints are probably incongruent.

Young to middle-aged dogs with mild to moderate osteoarthritis are considered good surgical candidates. Dogs with advanced osteoarthritis are generally treated medically prior to considering surgery. If an arthrotomy is performed, an intermuscular approach to the medial elbow is used. The intermuscular incision is generally made between the flexor carpi radialis and the deep digital flexor muscles. There appear to be fewer neurovascular branches at this site, and the medial collateral ligament is better protected than with the incision between the pronator teres and flexor carpi radialis muscles. Joint capsule and muscle retraction using small Gelpi retractors is recommended. It is imperative that the antebrachium be strongly pronated and abducted to adequately open the medial joint compartment. In cases of FMCP with a fragmented or fissured coronoid without obvious wear lesions adjacent to the fragment or on the apposing humeral condylar articular surface, simple fragment removal is performed. If the presence of an FMCP is combined with deep erosions of the adjacent coronoid or medial humeral condyle, fragment removal is combined with coronoidectomy.

Osteochondritis Dissecans

Similar to FMCP, a medial muscle separation approach to the elbow is recommended if arthroscopy is not available. The differentiation between OCD and FMCP before surgery is not essential, because a medial approach to the joint is warranted in either case. Often the subchondral bone following fragment removal is sclerotic and difficult to curet. In these cases, drilling numerous small holes (forage) using a drill bit or Kirschner wire that penetrate into the underlying trabecular bone is recommended to encourage revascularization of the region. The articular surface of the coronoid should be closely inspected for wear lesions or a concurrent FMCP lesion.

Incongruity of the Elbow Joint

Most typically, IC is diagnosed during an otherwise negative surgical exploratory of the medial elbow compartment for FMCP. Wear lesions combined with FMCP and OCD or in their absence is probably indicative of IC. The value of CT and MRI becomes apparent when faced with this dilemma. If there is extensive erosion and significant furrowing or streaking of the medial coronoid articular surface, coronoidectomy should be performed. Routinely recommending a proximal ulnar ostectomy is probably not warranted at this time without the aid of more accurate diagnostic tests (CT or MRI) and further comparative studies. If a preoperative CT or MRI is available, a coronoidectomy and/or proximal ulnar ostectomy can be planned to best correct the malalignment. Based on personal experience, not every dog having IC will benefit from one of these two procedures.

PROGNOSIS

It is very difficult to accurately predict the long-term outlook for a particular dog. The overall prognosis for dogs with elbow dysplasia is generally considered fair to good. Most dogs have mild to moderate osteoarthritis already at the time of diagnosis and progression of disease is likely even following treatment. Moderately affected dogs, treated conservatively or surgically, tend to be quite functional although they naturally are inclined to limit their exercise to accommodate elbow discomfort. Working and hunting dogs are frequently limited in their performance, especially over time. In severely affected dogs, secondary degenerative joint disease is often a debilitating disease.

References and Suggested Reading

Bouck GR, Miller CW, Taves CL: A comparison of surgical and medical treatment of fragmented coronoid process and osteochondritis dissecans of the canine elbow. Vet Comp Orthop Traum 8:177, 1995.
A prospective clinical study comparing surgical versus medical treatment of FMCP and OCD of the elbow joint over a 9-month follow-up.
Carpenter LG, Schwarz PD, Lowry JE, et al: Comparison of radiologic imaging techniques for diagnosis of fragmented medial coronoid process of the cubital joint in dogs. J Am Vet Med Assoc 203:78, 1993.
A prospective study in which 30 canine elbow joints suspected of having an FMCP were evaluated, comparing the accuracy of diagnosis of five imaging techniques (plain film radiography, xeroradiography, linear tomography, arthrography, and computed tomography) to surgical observation.
Fox SM, Burbidge HM, Bray JC, et al: Ununited anconeal process: Lagscrew fixation. J Am Anim Hosp Assoc 32:52, 1996.
The description of a new technique for lag-screw fixation of UAP and the clinical results in eight dogs (10 elbow joints).
Gilson SD, Piermattei DL, Schwarz PD: Treatment of humeroulnar subluxation with a dynamic proximal ulnar osteotomy. Vet Surg 18:114, 1989.
The clinical results of surgically treating humeroulnar subluxation in 13 dogs with 18 affected elbows by proximal ulnar osteotomy.
Huibregtse BA, Johnson AL, Muhlbauer MC, et al: The effect of treatment of fragmented coronoid process on the development of osteoarthritis of the elbow. J Am Anim Hosp Assoc 30:190, 1994.
A retrospective clinical study comparing surgical versus medical treatment of FMCP of the elbow joint during evaluation of clinical function and the development of osteoarthritis.
Olsson SE: Pathophysiology, morphology, and clinical signs of osteochondrosis in the dog. In: Bojrab MJ, ed: Disease Mechanisms in Small Animal Surgery. Philadelphia: Lea & Febiger, 1993, p 777.
An in-depth review of the pathophysiology, diagnosis, and treatment of canine elbow dysplasia with an emphasis on osteochondrosis as the underlying cause.
Piermattei DL: An Atlas of Surgical Approaches to the Bones and Joints of the Dog and Cat, 3rd ed. Philadelphia: WB Saunders, 1993.
A comprehensive atlas, descriptions and illustrations, of surgical approaches to the bones and joints of the dog and cat.
Roy RG, Wallace LJ, Johnston GR: A retrospective long-term evaluation of ununited anconeal process excision on the canine elbow. Vet Comp Orthop Traum 7:94, 1994.
Seven dogs were clinically evaluated at a mean of 65 months following surgical removal of a UAP.
Sjöstrom L, Kasstrom H, Kallberg M: Ununited anconeal process in the dog: Pathogenesis and treatment by osteotomy of the ulna. Vet Comp Orthop Traum 8:170, 1995.
A prospective study of UAP in 22 canine elbow joints (20 dogs) treated with proximal ulnar osteotomy.
Thomson MJ, Robins GM: Osteochondrosis of the elbow: A review of the pathogenesis and a new approach to treatment. Aust Vet J 72:375, 1995.
A review of the causes of elbow dysplasia and the case presentation of 7 dogs treated with proximal ulnar osteotomy.
Wind AP: Elbow dysplasia. In: Slatter D, ed: Textbook of Small Animal Surgery, 2nd ed. Philadelphia: WB Saunders, 1993, p 1966.
An in-depth review of the pathophysiology, diagnosis and treatment of canine elbow dysplasia with an emphasis on asynchronous growth of the radius and ulna and insufficient development of the ulnar trochlear notch as the underlying causes.

Bicipital Tenosynovitis in Dogs

DANIEL STOBIE

Tinton Falls, New Jersey

Bicipital tenosynovitis is an inflammatory condition affecting the biceps brachii tendon and its surrounding synovial sheath. The disease produces a chronic, mild to marked, weightbearing lameness in affected dogs that can impair normal activity. It is a common cause for forelimb lameness in the mature dog (Brinker et al, 1990).

ANATOMY

The biceps brachii muscle originates from the supraglenoid tubercle of the scapula by means of a long tendon that crosses the shoulder joint and continues distally along the humerus through the intertubercular groove. The tendon is held in place within the intertubercular groove by the transverse humeral ligament. The tendon invaginates the joint capsule in this region so that the joint capsule surrounds the tendon, forming its synovial sheath. There is no true bursa between the biceps tendon and the humerus in the dog. It is this intracapsular, extrasynovial region of the biceps tendon that becomes diseased in bicipital tenosynovitis (Lincoln et al, 1984; Stobie et al, 1995).

ETIOLOGY

In the majority of cases, no underlying cause is found. Canine bicipital tenosynovitis has been reported to occur secondary to acute trauma to the tendon, tendon strain or rupture, and entrapment of joint mice within the tendon sheath (Lincoln et al, 1984). It may result from activities that cause overuse and chronic repetitive trauma to the tendon. Damage to the tendon from high biomechanical stress and repetitive trauma incites an inflammatory response leading to lameness.

SIGNALMENT, HISTORY, AND CLINICAL FINDINGS

Although any dog can become affected, bicipital tenosynovitis develops in predominantly middle-aged to older, medium- and large-breed dogs. No breed or sex predilection is noted. Dogs can be affected unilaterally or bilaterally. Affected dogs tend to be either active, athletic, sporting dogs; or overweight, sedentary dogs in poor physical condition. Strenuous activities performed by athletic dogs probably traumatize the tendon, thereby inciting the disease. Why dogs in poor physical condition become affected is less clear.

Affected dogs have a history of intermittent or progressive, weightbearing lameness that becomes worse after exercise. The lameness typically improves with rest. Because pain occurs only when the tendon is gliding along the bone, dogs are not reluctant to bear weight when standing. However, when walking or running, affected dogs guard against flexion and extension of the shoulder, which limits the swing phase of the gait. In general, the lameness is refractory to oral medications such as nonsteroidal anti-inflammatory medications, corticosteroids, and polysulfated glycosaminoglycans and nutriceuticals.

Pain on digital pressure on the biceps tendon in the intertubercular groove, especially while flexing and extending the shoulder, is a classic clinical feature of bicipital tenosynovitis. A small number of dogs will also have disuse atrophy of the supraspinatus and infraspinatus muscles.

DIAGNOSIS

Bicipital tenosynovitis is often frustrating and difficult to definitively diagnose due to the subtle nature of the clinical and radiographic findings. Combining findings from history, physical examination, radiography, and synovial fluid analysis will allow other conditions of the shoulder joint to be excluded and a presumptive diagnosis of bicipital tenosynovitis to be made. It is important to evaluate affected dogs carefully to rule out other disease. In one study, several dogs that were originally diagnosed with bicipital tenosynovitis were subsequently found to have other disease such as osteosarcoma of the proximal humerus, cervical vertebral osteosarcoma, cervical intervertebral disc disease with nerve root compression, brachial plexus neoplasia, polyarthritis, and axillary sarcoma (Stobie et al, 1995).

In acute cases of bicipital tenosynovitis radiography is often unremarkable. As the disease becomes more chronic, osteophytes in the intertubercular groove and dystrophic mineralization of the biceps tendon can be visualized (Fig. 1). Many dogs will also often have mild evidence of degenerative joint disease of the shoulder characterized by periarticular osteophytes about the caudal humeral head or the caudal aspect of the glenoid rim. Because radiographic changes can be subtle even in chronic cases, radiographic sensitivity can be increased by obtaining a craniodistal-cranioproximal (skyline) view of the intertubercular groove in addition to standard craniocaudal and mediolateral views of the shoulder. The skyline view is obtained by positioning the dog in dorsal recumbency with the affected shoulder joint hyperflexed and the limb rotated externally approximately 30 degrees (Fig. 2). This view isolates the intertubercular groove, allowing subtle irregularities in the groove and mineralization of the tendon to be identified (Fig. 3). These abnormalities may not be detected on standard radiographic views due to superimposition of the intertubercular groove and proximal end of the humerus.

In cases where plain film radiography is normal, positive contrast arthrography is useful for identifying abnormalities associated with bicipital tenosynovitis. Arthrography will demonstrate filling defects and irregularities along the biceps tendon in a high percentage of affected dogs (Fig. 4). In one study of dogs with chronic bicipital tenosynovitis, arthrograms were abnormal in 92% of the cases (Stobie et al, 1995). Filling defects along the tendon correspond to proliferative synovium, adhesions between the tendon sheath and tendon, or joint mice.

Ultrasonography has been used to diagnose bicipital tenosynovitis and other disorders of the biceps tendon in horses and human beings. Ultrasonography may detect effusion surrounding the biceps tendon, and irregularities between the biceps tendon and the intertubercular groove. However, results of a recent prospective study indicate that ultrasonography is not as sensitive as arthrography for diagnosing bicipital tenosynovitis in dogs (Rivers et al, 1992).

Arthrocentesis and cytologic examination of synovial fluid is a useful ancillary diagnostic test to help support a diagnosis of bicipital tenosynovitis. Because the synovial sheath surrounding the biceps tendon is continuous with the shoulder joint capsule, inflammatory changes are frequently seen in the synovial fluid of the associated scapulohumeral joint. Cytology generally reveals increased numbers of mononuclear cells (consistent with degenerative joint disease) with cell counts ranging from 1500 to 4800 cells/μl. The mucin content and viscosity of the fluid are usually normal. Observing increased numbers of mononuclear cells in the synovial fluid allows the clinician to rule out other arthropathies such as sepsis or immune-mediated disease.

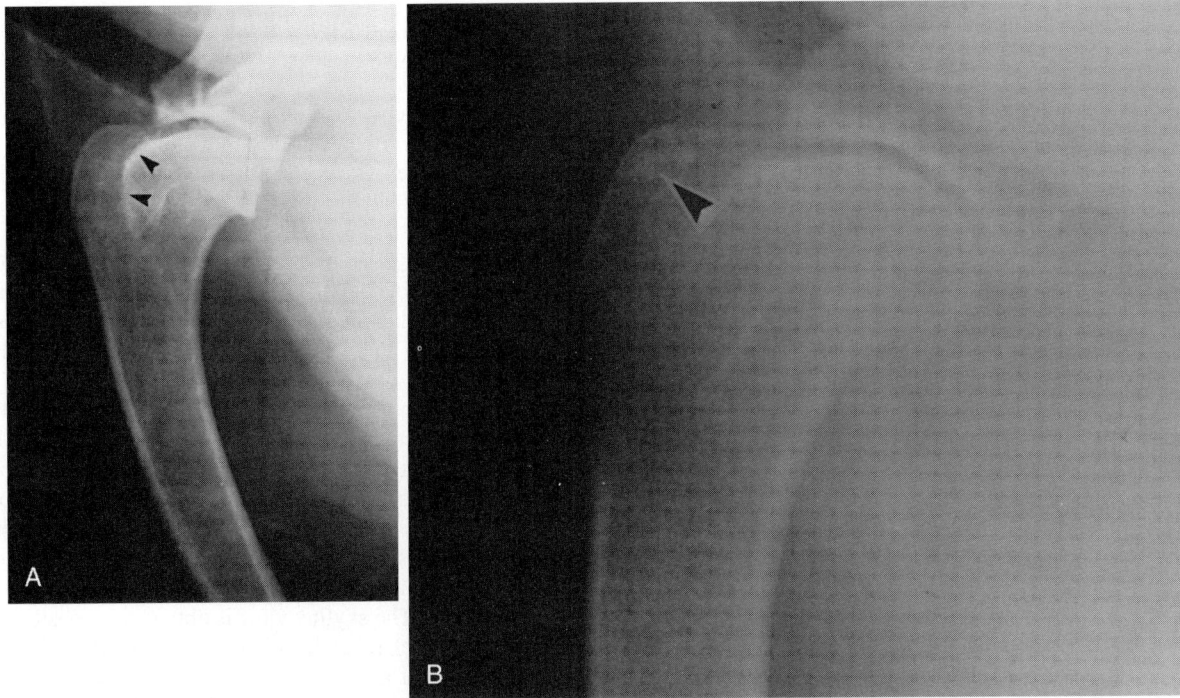

Figure 1. Mediolateral radiographic views of the shoulder joints of two dogs with chronic bicipital tenosynovitis. *A,* Osteophytes can be seen in the intertubercular groove *(arrows). B,* Focal mineralization of the biceps tendon is evident *(arrow).* (From Stobie D, Wallace LJ, Lipowitz AJ, et al: Chronic bicipital tenosynovitis in dogs: 29 cases (1985–1992). J Am Vet Med Assoc 207:201, 1995, with permission.)

TREATMENT

Acute Cases

Treatment of bicipital tenosynovitis is aimed at reducing and preventing inflammation of the biceps tendon and synovial sheath. Medical therapy consists of aseptically injecting methylprednisolone acetate (Depo-Medrol, Upjohn) 1 mg/kg (generally 20 to 40 mg) into the tendon and tendon sheath and restricting all activity for 2 to 3 weeks.

Injection of the tendon and tendon sheath can be performed by palpating the tendon percutaneously and infiltrating the methylprednisolone directly into the tendon itself. Conversely, arthrocentesis of the scapulohumeral joint can be performed. Once synovial fluid is aspirated, confirming an intra-articular injection, the methylprednisolone is injected directly into the joint. As the scapulohumeral joint capsule is continuous with the tendon sheath, intra-articular injection allows delivery of corticosteroids to the affected tissues.

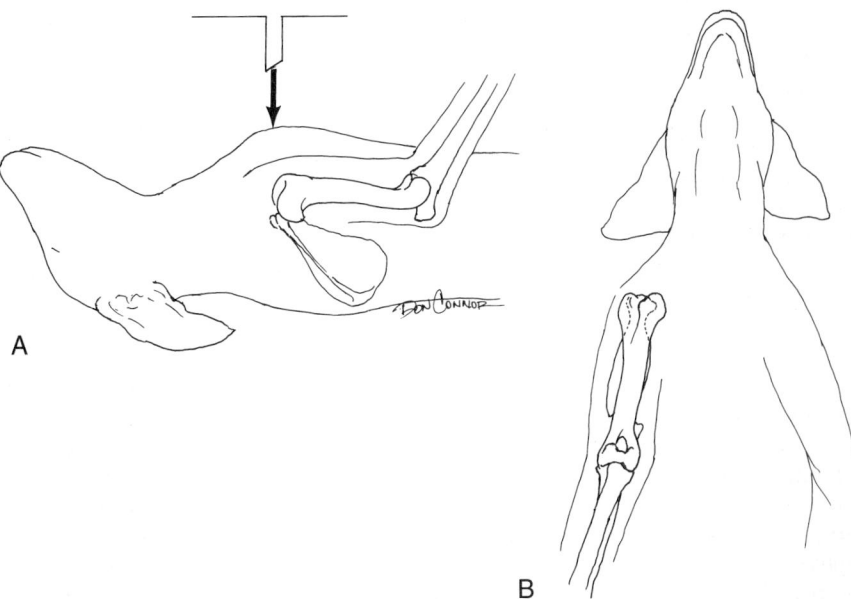

Figure 2. *A* and *B,* Schematic drawings of positioning used to obtain a craniodistal-cranioproximal (skyline) radiographic view of the shoulder joint. The dog is placed in dorsal recumbency with the shoulder joint hyperflexed and the limb rotated externally approximately 30 degrees. (From Stobie D, Wallace LJ, Lipowitz AJ, et al: Chronic bicipital tenosynovitis in dogs: 29 cases (1985–1992). J Am Vet Med Assoc 207:201, 1995, with permission.)

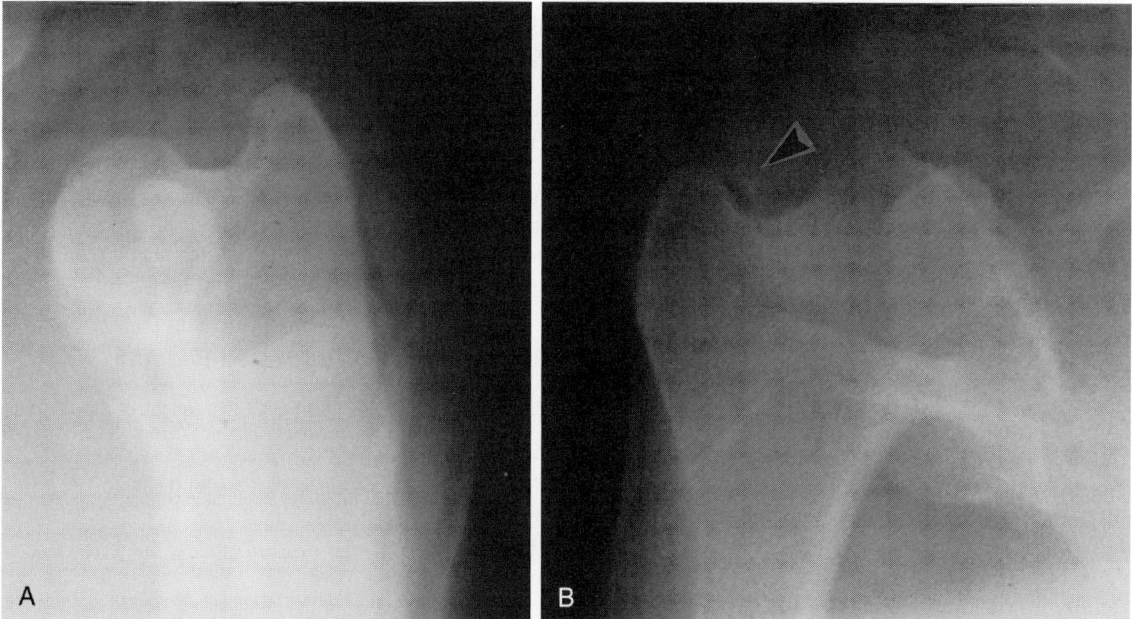

Figure 3. Craniodistal-cranioproximal (skyline) radiographic views of two different shoulder joints. *A,* A normal dog. *B,* A dog with chronic bicipital tenosynovitis. Notice how this view highlights areas of mineralization within the intertubercular groove *(arrow).* (From Stobie D, Wallace LJ, Lipowitz AJ, et al: Chronic bicipital tenosynovitis in dogs: 29 cases (1985–1992). J Am Vet Med Assoc 207:201, 1995, with permission.)

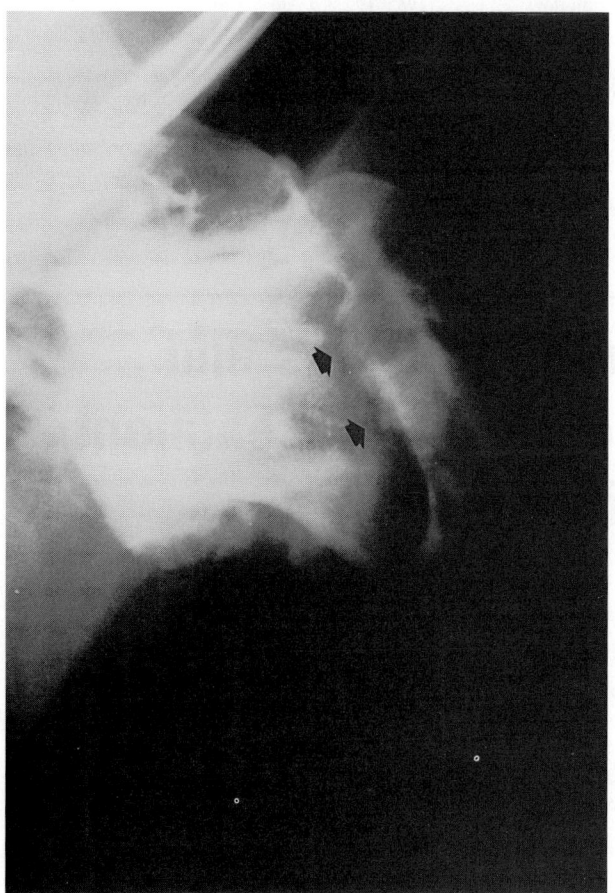

Figure 4. Positive contrast arthrogram of the shoulder joint of a dog with chronic bicipital tenosynovitis. Notice the filling defects and irregularities along the biceps tendon *(arrows).* (From Stobie D, Wallace LJ, Lipowitz AJ, et al: Chronic bicipital tenosynovitis in dogs: 29 cases (1985–1992). J Am Vet Med Assoc 207:201, 1995, with permission.)

If minimal or no response is seen following the initial injection and rest period, a second injection should be performed followed again by absolute exercise restriction. Most acute cases of bicipital tenosynovitis will respond favorably to this treatment, and a poor response should prompt referral to an orthopedic surgeon. Some dogs will have recurrence of lameness several months or even years later. These cases can be treated in a similar fashion.

Chronic Cases

Dogs with chronic bicipital tenosynovitis and radiographic evidence of the disease are less likely to respond to medical therapy. Medical therapy (see above) should be attempted first; however, less than 50% of the dogs will respond favorably. In a recent study, all dogs that responded to medical therapy did so after one or two injections of methylprednisolone acetate (Stobie et al, 1995). Although no complications associated with medical therapy have been reported, repeated injections of corticosteroids should be avoided because they can impair the biomechanical properties and metabolic activities of articular cartilage and long-term use can lead to collagen necrosis and tendon rupture. Surgery should be considered in dogs that do not improve following one or two doses of corticosteroids.

The goal of surgical treatment in dogs with bicipital tenosynovitis is to eliminate pain caused by contact of the biceps tendon with the inflamed tendon sheath, adhesions to the tendon sheath, or osteophytes in the intertubercular groove. This is accomplished by relocating the tendon via a tenodesis procedure. A cranial approach to the shoulder joint is performed. The transverse humeral ligament and joint capsule are opened to expose the tendon and intertubercular groove. Gross abnormalities visible at surgery include osteophytes along the edges of the intertubercular groove, mineralization of the tendon, proliferative synovium, and fibrous adhesions between the tendon and its sheath. Observing these changes confirms a diagnosis of bicipital tenosynovitis. In cases that are unclear, biopsy of affected tissues should be performed to confirm disease. Histologic findings are characterized by synovial proliferation, edema, fibrosis, and lymphocytic-plasmacytic infiltration of the tendon and synovium. Some biopsies may also reveal dystrophic mineralization or chondroid metaplasia secondary to chronic inflammation.

Tenodesis of the biceps tendon can be achieved by one of two methods. In the first procedure the origin of the biceps tendon is transected from the supraglenoid tubercle and the tendon is passed in a medial to lateral direction through a hole drilled in the greater tubercle. The free end of the tendon is then secured to the humerus by suturing it to the supraspinatus muscle, joint capsule, and/or periosteum with nonabsorbable suture, or by using a bone screw and spiked washer. In the second procedure the tendon remains attached to the supraglenoid tubercle and is transposed laterally following osteotomy of the greater tubercle. The greater tubercle is then replaced and secured to the humerus with two small Kirschner wires (Brinker et al, 1990). No external coaptation is required postoperatively, but exercise restriction should be enforced for 6 to 8 weeks following surgery.

In a study of 29 cases of chronic bicipital tenosynovitis, good or excellent results were achieved in all dogs undergoing surgery, compared with only 48% of the dogs that were treated medically. All performance dogs were able to return to work following surgery (Stobie et al, 1995). Surgical transposition of the biceps tendon does not alter shoulder joint stability or function of the biceps tendon (Vasseur et al, 1983). Both tenodesis procedures are highly effective in resolving the lameness associated with the tenosynovitis, but laterally transposing the biceps tendon through a hole in the greater tubercle avoids complications related to implant migration that can occur following greater tubercle osteotomy.

Although the prognosis is favorable in dogs undergoing surgery, time to full return to function may be prolonged in some dogs. Recovery time required until dogs are clinically normal following tenodesis of the biceps tendon for tenosynovitis averages between 3 and 4 months.

References and Suggested Reading

Brinker WO, Piermattei DL, Flo GL: Handbook of Small Animal Orthopedics and Fracture Management, 2nd ed. Philadelphia: WB Saunders, 1990, p 472.
A brief overview of bicipital tenosynovitis as well as diagrams and descriptions of the anatomy and surgical procedures for tenodesis of the biceps tendon.

Lincoln JD, Potter K: Tenosynovitis of the biceps brachii tendon in dogs. J Am Anim Hosp Assoc 20:385, 1984.
Description of the pathophysiology and treatment options for bicipital tenosynovitis as well as six case reports of the disease.

Rivers B, Wallace L, Johnston GR: Biceps tenosynovitis in the dog: Radiographic and sonographic findings. Vet Comp Orthop Trauma 5:51, 1992.
A prospective study comparing the accuracy of arthrography and ultrasonography for diagnosing bicipital tenosynovitis in dogs.

Stobie D, Wallace LJ, Lipowitz AJ, et al: Chronic bicipital tenosynovitis in dogs: 29 cases (1985–1992). J Am Vet Med Assoc 207:201, 1995.
This paper reports the clinical features and diagnostic findings in a large series of cases of canine bicipital tenosynovitis and compares the outcomes of medical and surgical therapy for this condition.

Vasseur PB, Pool RR, Klein K: Effects of tendon transfer on the canine scapulohumeral joint. Am J Vet Res 44:811, 1983.
Scientific biomechanical study demonstrating the effects of transposing the biceps tendon on the stability and function of the scapulohumeral joint.

Use of Chondromodulating Drugs and Substances in the Prevention and Treatment of Osteoarthritis in Dogs

STEVEN C. BUDSBERG
Athens, Georgia

RORY J. TODHUNTER
Ithaca, New York

PAUL S. MCNAMARA, Jr.
Pattersonville, New York

The use of the term *chondroprotective compounds* provokes strong opinions within the medical research community. Rather than spending time debating the merits of this terminology, this article reviews cartilage pathology in osteoarthritis (degenerative joint disease), ideas on slowing this process, and pragmatic expectations for compounds introduced into this field for treatment. An admirable goal of any therapy prescribed for this disease would be the inhibition of abnormal enzymatic and degenerative processes within cartilage. To this end, alternate terminology has been created to classify therapeutic agents in this area. The agents are collectively defined as slow-acting drugs in osteoarthritis (SADOA). The SADOA products can be subdivided into symptomatic slow-acting drugs (SYSA-DOA) and disease-modifying osteoarthritis drugs (DMOADs). SYSADOA are agents that claim to improve pain or function with a delay (weeks to months) but may have persistent benefits after treatment discontinuation. DMOADs are products that claim to prevent, reduce, or reverse the cartilaginous lesions of osteoarthritis (OA). Agents that have been previously called chondroprotective are now considered DMOADs (Theiler et al, 1994).

OSTEOARTHRITIS

At a cellular level, OA is characterized by the progressive depletion of articular cartilage matrix macromolecules. The failure of the chondrocytes in injured articular cartilage to restore a functional matrix despite high metabolic activity is a hallmark of OA. Data suggest that in OA joints, matrix loss is related to overactivity of proteolytic enzymes (metalloproteinases), which degrade matrix macromolecules such as the different collagen types and proteoglycans (Caron et al, 1996). A large group of molecules act as soluble mediators of inflammation and repair within the joint; these are collectively called cytokines. Cytokines, like interleukin-1, and growth factors, may be produced by both chondrocytes and synovial lining cells. These cytokines and other mediators have been implicated as key factors in the synthesis and release of neutral matrix metalloproteinases (Caron et al, 1996).

Within the local environment of the joint, interdependent interactions among chondrocytes, matrix macromolecules, metalloproteinases, and cytokines exist. Disruption during osteoarthritis causes biochemical and pathologic changes accompanied by clinical signs. Disease progression is a slow insidious event; thus, by the time clinical signs occur there may be significant cartilage structural damage. Currently, there is no evidence that such structural damage can be reversed; that is, there are *no current data* to suggest OA can be reversed and the condition "cured."

TREATMENT OF OSTEOARTHRITIS

It is safe to assume that by the time the diagnosis of OA is made, there is structural alteration in the cartilage matrix. Therefore, current recommendations for treatment of OA are primarily ameliorating and palliative. Weight loss, exercise modification, and drug therapy for analgesia and anti-inflammatory effects are often successful in alleviating clinical signs. However, this management doesn't attempt to alter the pathologic process within the diarthrodial joint surface and supporting tissues. Several classes of therapeutic agents have been used to treat OA. Many of these products may protect the metabolism of chondrocytes or cartilage matrix in some fashion. The following discussion will examine these major therapeutic classes.

Nonsteroidal Anti-Inflammatory Drugs (NSAIDs)

NSAIDs are used for their analgesic and anti-inflammatory properties (also see p. 214). Clinically, NSAIDs are fast-acting symptomatic drugs; however, they also have effects on cartilage metabolism. Although one might not initially think of NSAIDs as potential cartilage-modifying agents, their often long-term use can have important effects on cartilage metabolism. Depending on the specific NSAID, there are primarily in vitro data that support the claim of both articular cartilage–sparing effects or potentiation of damage to the articular cartilage. Cartilage damage may be caused by suppression of proteoglycan or collagen synthesis. Conversely, certain NSAIDs may slow the progression of cartilage damage by decreasing metalloproteinase synthesis partially through reduced prostaglandin and interleukin-1 (IL-1) synthesis (Ghosh, 1993). The degree of damage to the cartilage may play a very important role in rendering it vulnerable to the metabolic effects of these drugs. It must also be reiterated that effects of pharmaceuticals on cartilage metabolism in vitro are not necessarily of significance in vivo (Ghosh, 1993).

Buffered aspirin is still a common NSAID currently used in small animal practice. Although dosage recommendations vary, 10 to 20 mg/kg every 12 hours is a widely used starting dose in the dog. Aspirin has been implicated to be damaging to both normal and arthritic cartilage. However, it is our opinion that there is not enough evidence to justify clinicians stopping the use of buffered aspirin in short-term treatment situations. In contrast, there are at least two NSAIDs that may not damage cartilage and may even have some ability to prevent detrimental effects of mediators on cartilage. These two products are carprofen (Rimadyl, Pfizer) and etodolac (Etogesic, Fort Dodge). Carprofen is a recently approved NSAID for use in the treatment of osteoarthritis in dogs. It is a member of the aryl propionic acid class and the dose recommendation is 2.2 mg/kg every 12 hours. Etodolac is also a recently approved NSAID for the treatment of osteoarthritis in dogs. It is a member of the pyranocarboxylic acid class of NSAIDs and has been shown to improve rear limb function in dogs with chronic hip OA at 10 to 15 mg/kg every 24 hours (Budsberg et al, 1999). Finally, piroxicam (Pfizer) is an example of a product that has had conflicting data on its effects on cartilage, making it difficult to draw any conclusions regarding the use of this drug. Piroxicam is a member of the oxicam family of NSAIDS, is a reversible inhibitor of cyclooxygenase, and is often mentioned as a therapeutic agent for use in dogs with osteoarthritis.

Complex Sugars

Polysulfated Glycosaminoglycan

Polysulfated glycosaminoglycan (PSGAG) (Adequan, Luitpold Pharmaceuticals) is a DMOAD (Todhunter and Lust, 1994). Adequan has recently been approved for use in dogs in the US. Polysulfated glycosaminoglycan (Arteparon, Luitpold, Germany) has been available in Europe since the mid-1960s. The interested reader is referred to a recent review on PSGAG (Todhunter et al, 1994). PSGAG is a mixture of highly sulfated glycosaminoglycans, the major component of which, chondroitin sulfate (CS), is extracted from bovine trachea and lungs. It is licensed for intra-articular and for intramuscular use in horses, but is not licensed for use in dogs.

Biochemical and autoradiographic evidence showed incorporation of some components of PSGAG into the articular cartilage and meniscus following injection of PSGAG either intra-articularly, intramuscularly, or subcutaneously in a variety of species. Concentrations of PSGAG achieved in cartilage appear to be high enough to inhibit proteinase activity. Anabolic effects of PSGAG have been demonstrated on articular cartilage explants and isolated chondrocytes and synovial fibroblasts, but results have not been consistent. Hyaluronan (a polymer of n-acetyl glucosamine and glucuronic acid) is a major constituent of synovial fluid and is the boundary lubricant of synovial membrane. An increase in the concentration of hyaluronan in synovial fluid has been reported as a result of treatment with PSGAG in humans (Verbruggen and Veys, 1979).

PSGAG decreases cartilage catabolism. PSGAG ameliorates the effects of degradative enzymes on articular cartilage in vitro (Ghosh et al, 1993). In the Pond-Nuki model of canine OA in which the cranial cruciate ligament is transected surgically, concentrations of active and latent collagenase in the cartilage of PSGAG-treated dogs were lower than those in control cartilage (Altman et al, 1989). Treatment with PSGAG was associated with decreased concentrations of active neutral metalloproteinases in cartilage in a partial medial meniscectomy model of OA in rabbits (Howell et al, 1986) but not in partial or full-thickness articular defects in horses (Yovich et al, 1987). When PSGAG is used intra-articularly immediately postoperatively, it may be detrimental (Todhunter et al, 1993). Therefore, the authors usually begin treatment with PSGAG for joints with osteochondral defects at 7 to 10 days following surgery.

PSGAG generally had a protective effect on cartilage homeostasis in models of OA based on decreased microscopic structural alteration, retention of proteoglycan in cartilage, and decreased proteinase activity when compared with activity in control joints (Ghosh et al, 1993). When PSGAG (5 mg/kg IM twice weekly) was given to groups of very young dogs predisposed to hip dysplasia, the treated dogs had significantly better radiographic hip conformation than did untreated control dogs (Lust et al, 1992). On the basis of a total score for gross pathologic and biochemical measurements of OA, there was a disease-modifying effect of the drug. However, a multicenter, clinical, dose-response study in dogs with hip dysplasia and OA failed to show a significant beneficial effect of treatment with PSGAG (de-Hann et al, 1994).

A variety of dosages have been used experimentally in in vivo models of canine OA. Based on Lust and colleagues' (1992) work in a small group of very young dogs predisposed to hip dysplasia, we currently use PSGAG at a dose of 5 mg/kg twice weekly in dogs with OA. The label dose is 4.4 mg/kg twice weekly for 4 weeks, then as needed. There are, however, no clinical data proving efficacy of any treatment protocol using PSGAG for either symptomatic relief or disease modification. Prior to the establishment of any therapeutic regimens for PSGAG, controlled clinical trials must be performed. Until that time, all recommendations are personal impressions and extrapolation of experimental data. Also, it should be remembered that Lust et al injected hip dysplasia–prone dogs from 6 weeks until 8 months of age, so that the drug was administered in the incipient stages of the development of OA. It is not our intention to recommend a similar dosage regimen for all young dysplastic dogs. Thus, candidates for treatment with PSGAG may include dogs with developmental joint disease (osteochondrosis, fragmented medial coronoid process, ununited anconeal process, and hip dysplasia) and postoperatively following stifle stabilization for cruciate injuries. Administration of PSGAG is an adjunctive treatment for OA in animals; it is not a panacea. We believe, and data support that the earlier the drug is administered, the more likely it will decrease synovitis and protect against cartilage degradation in OA.

PSGAG increased the activated partial thromboplastin, prothrombin, activated clotting, and bleeding times when administered to dogs (Beale et al, 1990; Lust et al, 1992). Administration of PSGAG to animals with a history of hypersensitivity, in shock, or with bleeding tendencies is contraindicated, and complications (including thrombocytopenia) in humans have been reported.

Pentosan Polysulfate

Pentosan polysulfate (PPS) is another DMOAD that can be given by injection or per os. The molecular "backbone" of PPS is isolated from beechwood hemicellulose and consists of repeating units of xylanopyranoses that are sulfated synthetically. Because PPS is not readily available or approved for use in dogs in the United States, we provide only a brief summary of its effects on the OA process. Most of the effects of PPS on articular cartilage and synovial joints that are attributed to PSGAG apply also to PPS. It modulates cytokine action and preserves proteoglycan content of articular cartilage in animal models of OA (Rogachefsky et al, 1993).

In research models of OA in dogs, PPS administered at 2 mg/kg intramuscularly once weekly for 3 weeks resulted in significantly decreased articular cartilage damage based on gross and histologic evaluation and maintained normal articular cartilage proteoglycan content (Rogachefsky et al, 1993). Dogs with fragmented medial coronoid process or osteochondritis dissecans of the elbow were treated in a prospective randomized study with either 3 mg/kg PPS intramuscularly or standard surgical intervention (Bouck et al, 1995). Based on force plate evaluation, a more rapid return to function was observed in the PPS treated group and at 9 months there was no difference between groups in the gait parameters measured. It should be noted that there was no placebo control group in this study and thus no comparison of PPS to conservative therapy can be made. It remains unknown if the drug-treated group would remain the same clinically as the surgically treated group over a life span. Few complications of its use have been reported. It will increase clotting profile times, prolong the action of antithrombin III, and may cause thrombocytopenia presumably through interaction with platelet receptors.

Nutraceuticals

Unlike the parenterally administered complex sugars, which are at least partially purified and modified drugs, oral products are considered nutritional supplements and do not require FDA approval. These DMOADs are touted to have the same effects as parenterally available DMOADs such as PSGAG, namely a positive effect on cartilage matrix synthesis and hyaluronan synthesis by the synovial membrane, and an inhibitory effect on catabolic enzymes. Neutraceuticals contain precursors for synthesis of hyaline cartilage matrix and are reported to provide these precursors in supraphysiologic quantities to diarthrodial joints. Well-controlled studies investigating their efficacy for the treatment of OA in companion animals are unavailable.

The majority of nutritional supplements contain glucosamine and CS in either purified, extracted, or complexed form. Two commonly used products are Glycoflex (Vetriscience Laboratories) and Cosequin (Nutramax Laboratories). Glycoflex is an extract from the *Perna canaliculus* mollusk exoskeleton that contains glucosamine and CS. Cosequin contains purified glucosamine, CS, and manganese ascorbate. Glucosamine is a ubiquitous aminomonosaccharide used in the synthesis of disaccharide units of glycosaminoglycans. Glycosaminoglycans form the side chains of the core proteins of aggrecan (the large aggregating proteoglycan) and the small nonaggregating proteoglycans found in hyaline cartilage. A variety of glucosamine-based complexes are available, including glucosamine sulfate, glucosamine hydroiodide, and glucosamine hydrochloride. Chondroitin sulfates are glycosaminoglycans found in hyaline cartilage. Manganese is a trace element necessary as a cofactor in the biosynthesis of glycosaminoglycans.

The bioavailability of orally administered amino sugars and glycosaminoglycans has been debated when considering the potential efficacy of DMOADs. Questions arise regarding the ability of glucosamine and chondroitin sulfate polymers to traverse the gastrointestinal-blood barrier intact or as active subunits. Approximately 54% of glucosamine is nonionized in the small intestine, yet most of the glucosamine is ionized in the acidic environment of the stomach (Setnikar et al, 1991). This creates a favorable condition for absorption from the small intestine but not the stomach. In fact, based upon fecal excretions of radioactivity after oral administration, approximately 87% of the administered dose of radiolabeled glucosamine was absorbed (Setnikar et al, 1991). The amount of glucosamine absorbed intact is unknown. Oral absorption of CS has been reported in the rat, dog, and human, as determined by significant increases in serum levels of CS moieties after oral administration of ^{35}S-labeled CS. High-molecular-weight CS was detected in the blood, suggesting that some of the CS is absorbed intact (Morrison and Schjeide, 1974).

It is hypothesized that in OA, the demand for hyaline cartilage precursors, or "building blocks," is greater than the body's natural synthetic capability. The authors are unaware of any data to support that this occurs in vivo in OA. By providing these building blocks exogenously, the rate-limiting step of cartilage synthesis may be bypassed; allowing the body to counteract the degradative processes more efficiently and re-establish cartilage homeostasis (Hansen, 1996). Additionally, the individual components of these products may have direct inhibitory effects on the degradation in the OA joint. Orally administered glucosamine has been shown to stimulate glycosaminoglycan, proteoglycan, and collagen synthesis by chondrocytes and fibroblasts (Karzel and Domenjoz, 1971).

Although there are numerous anecdotal reports claiming improvement in mobility and reduction in pain in dogs receiving oral nutraceuticals, there is no scientific evidence that these products, in fact, are DMOADs in the companion animal. To date, most of the evidence of efficacy used by manufacturers to support their products comes from human clinical trials performed in Europe and South America. Numerous studies are reported in which oral glucosamine was used in the treatment of OA. Many report subjective improvement or reductions in pain and mobility scores in response to therapy. Several studies involving individual components of Cosequin have demonstrated no significant toxic or detrimental side effects. In the veterinary literature, one report assessed clinically normal dogs given Cosequin over a 30-day period and showed statistically significant, but clinically irrelevant, changes in hematologic and hemostatic effects, most notably platelet-function tests (McNamara et al, 1996). The product appeared safe, at least in the short term. In dogs and mice, no adverse effects were noted, even with chronic (greater than 1 year) oral administration (Setnikar et al, 1991). Likewise, CS appears well tolerated. No LD_{50} could be established in mice, even when given saturated solutions of CS, and no adverse effects were seen in dogs given 500 mg of chondroitin sulfate. Orally protective agents appear safe; however, additional long-term studies are warranted. The authors (RT, PM) use Cosequin at the manufacturer's recommended dose for most of the OA conditions included in the section on PSGAG. As for PSGAG, some improvement in clinical signs should be apparent by 4 to 6 weeks of treatment; otherwise, it is difficult to justify its continued use to companion animal owners.

Hyaluronan

Hyaluronan (HA), which is also known as hyaluronic acid and sodium hyaluronate, is a linear polydisaccharide. It is a polyanionic, nonsulfated glycosaminoglycan consisting of repeating disaccharide units of D-glucuronic acid and N-acetylglucosamine linked by (1 to 3) glycosidic bonds. HA can be considered a SYSADOA intra-articular drug. Although there is research and clinical experience regarding the use of hyaluronan in equine OA, there is a paucity of information relating to its use in the companion animal. Most of the literature on the use of hyaluronan in the dog arises from its use in animal models of OA for human applications, rather than clinical trials. Anecdotal evidence suggests some efficacy in the dog; however, the lack of extensive scientific evaluation obviates a thorough discussion.

References and Suggested Reading

Altman RD, Dean DD, Muniz OE, et al: Prophylactic treatment of canine osteoarthritis with glycosaminoglycan polysulfuric acid ester. Arthritis Rheum 32:759, 1989.
An experimental study evaluating whether pretreatment with a glycosaminoglycan product can prevent formation of experimentally induced OA.
Beale BS, Goring, RL, Clemmons RM, et al: The effect of semi-synthetic

polysulfated glycosaminoglycan on the hemostatic mechanism in the dog. Vet Surg 19:57, 1990.
A paper evaluating the effects of polysulfated glycosaminoglycan on both the intrinsic and the extrinsic hemostatic systems in healthy dogs.

Bouck GR, Miller CW, Taves CL: A comparison of surgical and medical treatment of fragmented coronoid process and osteochondritis dissecans of the canine elbow. Vet Comp Orthop Traumatol 1:105, 1995.
A prospective trial that examined ground reaction forces in dogs with clinical lameness attributable to either fragmented coronoid process or OCD lesions. Dogs were treated with either PPS or surgery. The study period was limited to 9 months.

Budsberg SC, Johnston S, Schwarz P, et al: Efficacy of etodolac for the treatment of osteoarthritis of hip joints in dogs. J Am Vet Med 214:1, 1999.
A paper discussing the results of a well-controlled blinded clinical trial evaluating the efficacy of etodolac in dogs with OA in the hip.

Caron JP, Fernandes JC, Martel-Pelletier J, et al: Chondroprotective effect of intraarticular injections of interleukin-1 receptor antagonist in experimental osteoarthritis. Arthritis Rheum 39:1535, 1996.
An experimental project examining the ability of an IL-1 receptor agonist to reduce the amount of induced OA that forms in dogs.

deHann JJ, Goring RL, Beale BS: Evaluation of polysulfated glycosaminoglycan for the treatment of hip dysplasia in dogs. Vet Surg 23:177, 1994.
A prospective clinical trial examining the efficacy of polysulfated gylcosaminoglycan in eliminating the clinical signs in dogs with chronic hip OA.

Ghosh P: Nonsteroidal anti-inflammatory drugs and chondroprotection: A review of the evidence. Drugs 46:834, 1993.
Review of the data involving NSAIDs and cartilage metabolism.

Ghosh P, Smith M, Wells C: Second-line agents in osteoarthritis. In: Dixon JS, Furst DE, eds: Second-Line Agents in the Treatment of Rheumatic Diseases. New York: Marcel Dekker, 1993, pp 363–427.
A review of the therapeutic options currently used in human medicine for the treatment of rheumatic diseases.

Hansen R: Mode of action of oral chondroprotective agents: Round table discussion of degenerative joint disease in dogs. Canine Pract 21:9, 1996.
Transcripts of an informal discussion of veterinarians, detailing their personal views on the potential uses of products claiming chondroprotective effects.

Howell DS, Carreno MR, Pelletier JP, et al: Articular cartilage breakdown in a lapine model of osteoarthritis: Action of glycosaminoglycan polysulfate ester (GAGPS) on proteoglycan enzyme activity, hexuronate, and cell counts. Clin Orthop Rel Res 213:69, 1986.
Experimental study evaluating the effect of a glycosaminoglycan compound's ability to modulate certain aspects of articular cartilage damage in induced OA.

Karzel K, Domenjoz R: Effects of hexosamine derivatives and uronic acid derivatives on glycosaminoglycan metabolism of fibroblast cultures. Pharmacology 5:337, 1971.
In vitro study examining the effects of certain hexosamine and uronic acid derivatives on metabolism of fibroblasts.

Lust G, Williams AJ, Burton-Wurster N, et al: Effects of intramuscular injections of glycosaminoglycan polysulfates on signs of incipient hip dysplasia in growing dogs. Am J Vet Res 53:1836, 1992.
A prospective study looking at the use of glycosaminoglycan polysulfates prophylactically on the development of OA in young growing dogs who were prone to the formation of hip dysplasia.

McNamara P, Barr S, Erb H: Hematologic, hemostatic and biochemical effects in dogs receiving an oral chondroprotective agent for thirty days. Am J Vet Res 57:1390, 1996.
A study examining the effects of Cosequin on standard hematologic, hemostatic, and platelet function test in healthy dogs.

Morrison L, Schjeide O: Absorption, distribution, metabolism, and excretion of acid mucopolysaccharides administered to animals and humans. In: Coronary Heart Disease and the Mucopolysaccharides (Glycosaminoglycans). Springfield, IL: Charles C Thomas, 1974, pp 109–127.
Review of data collected on the pharmacodynamics of mucopolysaccharides in different species.

Rogachefsky RA, Dean DD, Howell DS, et al: Treatment of canine osteoarthritis with insulin like growth factors-1 (IGF-1) and sodium pentosan polysulfate. Osteoarthritis Cartilage 1:105, 1993.
Experimental study evaluating the effects of IGF-1 and PPS ability to modulate certain aspects of articular cartilage damage in induced OA.

Setnikar I, Giaccheti C, Zanolo G: Pharmacokinetics of glucosamine in the dog and in man. Arzneim Forschung 36:729, 1991.
A review of the pharmacokinetics and pharmacodynamics of glucosamine in dogs and humans.

Setnikar I, Pacini M, Revel L: Antiarthritic effects of glucosamine sulfate studied in animal models. Arzneim Forschung 41:542, 1991.
Review of data collected on the potential beneficial effects of glucosamine in different animal models.

Theiler R, Ghosh P, Brooks P: Clinical, biochemical and imaging methods of assessing osteoarthritis and clinical trials with agents claiming "chondromodulating" activity. Osteoarthritis Cartilage 2:1, 1994.
A review of methods for clinically assessing the outcome efficacy of products claiming chondrocyte modification.

Todhunter RJ, Lust G: Polysulfated glycosaminoglycan in the treatment of osteoarthritis. Am J Vet Med Assoc 204:1245, 1994.
An excellent review of the scientific data currently available on polysulfated glycosaminoglycan and its potential usage in the treatment of OA.

Todhunter RJ, Minor RR, Wootton JAM, et al: Effects of exercise and polysulfated glycosaminoglycan on the repair of articular cartilage defects in the equine carpus. J Orthop Res 11:782, 1993.
An experimental study evaluating the effects of intra-articular polysulfated glycosaminoglycan and exercise on healing of full-thickness defects in ponies.

Verbruggen G, Veys EM: Influence of an oversulphated heparinoid upon hyaluronate metabolism of the human synovial cell in vivo. J Rheumatol 6:554, 1979.
An experimental study evaluating the effects of oversulphated heparinoid on hyaluronate metabolism.

Yovich J, Trotter GW, McIlwraith CW: Effects of polysulphated glycosaminoglycan on chemical and physical defects in equine articular cartilage. Am J Vet Res 48:1407, 1987.
An experimental study evaluating the effects of polysulphated glycosaminoglycan on histologic healing of full and partial articular cartilage defects in horses.

Sacral Fractures and Sacrococcygeal Injuries in Dogs and Cats

Charles A. Kuntz

Fort Collins, Colorado

Sacral fractures and sacrococcygeal injuries are uncommon but not rare injuries in dogs and cats. Reports of these potentially devastating fractures have been relatively underrepresented in the veterinary literature. Sacral fractures and sacrococcygeal injuries are often missed on conventional radiography; accurate diagnosis requires an increased level of suspicion at initial evaluation of patients with pelvic trauma. Diagnosis is often made based on the presence of characteristic neurologic signs that are due to damage to nervous structures present within or adjacent to the vertebrae. An understanding of the anatomy of the sacrum and related nerves and of the physiology associated with normal micturition and defecation is imperative when attempting diagnosis and prognostication.

ANATOMY AND PHYSIOLOGY

The sacrum is made up of the fused bodies and processes of the three sacral vertebrae. Sacralization of the first coccygeal vertebral body is a common anatomic variation. The first sacral vertebral body and the cranial portion of the second lie between and articulate with the ilial wings through a partially fibrous and partially synovial joint. The dorsal and ventral sacral foramina lie just lateral to the fused sacral bodies. Lateral to the sacral foramina are the fused transverse processes. Cranially, the transverse processes of S1 and S2 make up the sacral wing. The three fused dorsal spinous processes make up the median sacral crest. The ventral aspect of the sacrum is smooth and is the cranial part of the dorsal boundary of the pelvic canal. The sacrum is the weight-transmitting structure between the hind limbs and the lumbar vertebrae. The sacrum houses a portion of the cauda equina, that is, the sacral and coccygeal nerves. The three sacral nerves exit their respective foramina at S1-2, S2-3, and S3-Cd1.

Innervation of the viscera (urinary bladder, terminal colon, and rectum) is critical for normal voiding of urine and feces. Normal micturition and defecation rely on somatic and autonomic innervation. The spinal cord ends at the level of L6 in dogs and L7 in cats. Caudal to the termination of the spinal cord, the distal continuation of the nerve fibers is the cauda equina. Somatic innervation of the pelvic viscera is through the pudendal nerve, which usually arises from the three sacral nerves. It is directly responsible for voluntary contraction and relaxation of the external urethral sphincter and indirectly responsible for the voluntary contraction and relaxation of the external anal sphincter via the caudal rectal nerve. The perineal nerve, a branch of the pudendal nerve, allows cutaneous sensation in the perineal region. Parasympathetic innervation of the bladder and rectum is via the pelvic nerve,

which receives contribution via the three sacral nerves. Parasympathetic innervation is responsible for reflex voiding of urine and feces following stimulation of parasympathetic nerve fibers within the urinary bladder and rectum, respectively. Sympathetic innervation of the pelvic viscera is via the hypogastric nerve, which joins the pelvic nerve to form the pelvic plexus. The hypogastric nerves represent the postganglionic connections between the caudal mesenteric ganglion, which lies just cranial to the bifurcation of the terminal aorta, and the pelvic plexus. Sympathetic stimulation allows bladder filling. S1 and S2 also contribute to the formation of the sciatic nerve.

Normal bladder function can be divided into filling and emptying phases. Filling is facilitated by sympathetic stimulation of the bladder and the internal urethral sphincter. Efferent beta-adrenergic fibers within the bladder wall are inhibitory and result in relaxation of smooth muscle cells allowing storage of urine. Efferent beta-adrenergic fibers present in the internal urethral sphincter are excitatory and prevent emptying. Emptying occurs when, at a threshold, afferent parasympathetic fibers that are stimulated by filling carry nerve impulses back to the terminal spinal cord, where they stimulate efferent parasympathetic nerve fibers, resulting in a detrusor contraction of the urinary bladder. At this point, if urination is inappropriate, voluntary contraction of the external urethral sphincter can prevent voiding. This requires cerebral input and an intact spinal cord. An analogous reflex system is present in the terminal rectum, colon, and internal and external anal sphincters, and is responsible for storage and voiding of feces. Sacral fracture or sacrococcygeal injuries may injure the neurologic structures that control these processes.

PATIENT EVALUATION

Sacral fractures and sacrococcygeal injuries in dogs and cats almost always result from trauma, which is most often automobile related. Pelvic fractures in dogs and cats are among the most common orthopedic injuries resulting from automobile-related trauma (Kolata et al, 1974). In one study, 20% of cats with pelvic fractures had concurrent sacral fractures. The need for careful physical examination is underscored by the fact that greater than 70% of animals sustaining orthopedic injury have injury of the thoracic structures including pneumothorax, hydrothorax, pulmonary contusion, rib fracture, and traumatic myocarditis. Urinary integrity should be assessed by patient observation, abdominal palpation, and abdominal radiography. Animals should urinate within several hours of fluid administration following trauma. Of 100 dogs sustaining blunt injury resulting in pelvic fractures, 39 had concurrent urinary tract injury including ureteral avulsion, urinary bladder rupture, urethral tear, urinary bladder mucosal irregularities, urinary bladder displacement or herniation, hydroureter, and hydronephrosis (Selcer, 1982). At least three of these dogs with urinary tract injury had documented sacral fractures, and several more had sacroiliac luxations.

Rectal examination should be performed as an initial assessment of the bony integrity of the pelvis. Anal tone can be simultaneously evaluated. A complete *neurologic examination* should then be performed to evaluate the extent of injury, and to aid in prognostication. This should include an assessment of ambulation, myotactic reflexes, perineal sensation, bladder tone, tail voluntary motor ability and sensation, and bladder palpation. The ability to initiate and complete urination should be assessed. If manual expression of the bladder is required, residual urine volume should be measured. Abnormal rectal palpation, the presence of neurologic deficits of the pelvic viscera, and inability to ambulate should increase suspicion of pelvic and sacral fractures.

Dogs and cats with sacral fractures and denervation of the tail almost always have some denervation of the pelvic viscera. Dogs and cats that have intact perineal reflex, anal tone, and perineal sensation but large residual urinary volume likely have intact pudendal nerve fibers, but have damage to the pelvic nerve fibers. This is possible because the pelvic nerve fibers are thought to be more fragile than pudendal nerve fibers. These patients' bladders are usually easily expressible. The inability of the patient to void completely after initiating urination may be due to the lack of a detrusor reflex. These animals may have a better chance of recovery than those who also have diminished perineal sensation and anal tone. Dogs and cats with no anal tone; large, flaccid, and easily expressed urinary bladders; and perineal hypalgesia have severe damage to both pelvic and pudendal nerve fibers, and are less likely to recover function.

In some animals, urinary bladder function may be impossible to evaluate directly because of concurrent urinary tract injury, that is, urinary bladder rupture or urethral injury. However, there is a high degree of correlation between urinary continence and fecal continence because of the common dependence on pudendal and pelvic nerve function. Therefore, if a decrease in anal tone is present, it can be assumed that urinary incontinence will also be present.

Some dogs and cats with sacral fractures have sciatic nerve deficits characterized by conscious proprioceptive deficits and knuckling of the hind limb, and diminished cranial tibial, and gastrocnemius and withdrawal reflexes (Kuntz et al, 1995). It is possible that these deficits may result from injury of the sacral components of the sciatic nerve or be the result of peripheral sciatic nerve injury associated with ipsilateral pelvic fractures that frequently coexist in animals with sacral or sacrococcygeal injuries.

RADIOLOGIC EVALUATION

Pelvic radiography should be performed whenever physical or neurologic examinations suggest that sacral or sacrococcygeal injuries have occurred. Care should be taken to prevent further damage to neurologic structures during pel-

vic radiography by careful patient handling and light sedation if necessary. The sensitivity of radiography in the assessment of patients with sacral fractures in dogs and cats has not been adequately evaluated, but, in the author's experience, many patients initially diagnosed with pelvic fractures had sacral fractures that had been missed on initial examination. The most common is the misdiagnosis of a sacroiliac luxation when a sacral fracture is actually present. Conventional radiographs are generally sufficient to make a diagnosis, especially when neurologic deficits are present that would increase one's level of suspicion that these injuries exist. Plain radiography has been shown to be insensitive in the diagnosis of sacral fractures in humans, and computed tomography has greatly improved diagnostic accuracy. Other diagnostic modalities that have been helpful in elucidating the diagnosis of sacral fractures include linear tomography, nuclear scintigraphy, and oblique conventional radiographic views.

A scheme for classification of sacral fractures in dogs has been devised that may be helpful in prognostication. Fractures that are lateral to the sacral foramina are called abaxial (Fig. 1), whereas those which are medial to the sacral foramina are called axial (Fig. 2). Abaxial fractures are similar to sacroiliac fracture-separations relative to clinical signs, prognosis, and surgical treatment. They are unlikely to be associated with urinary or fecal incontinence, and often carry a good prognosis. Axial fractures are almost always associated with neurologic deficits of the pelvic viscera (tail, perineum), and carry a less favorable prognosis. A similar classification scheme, independently devised in humans, has been useful in predicting the incidence

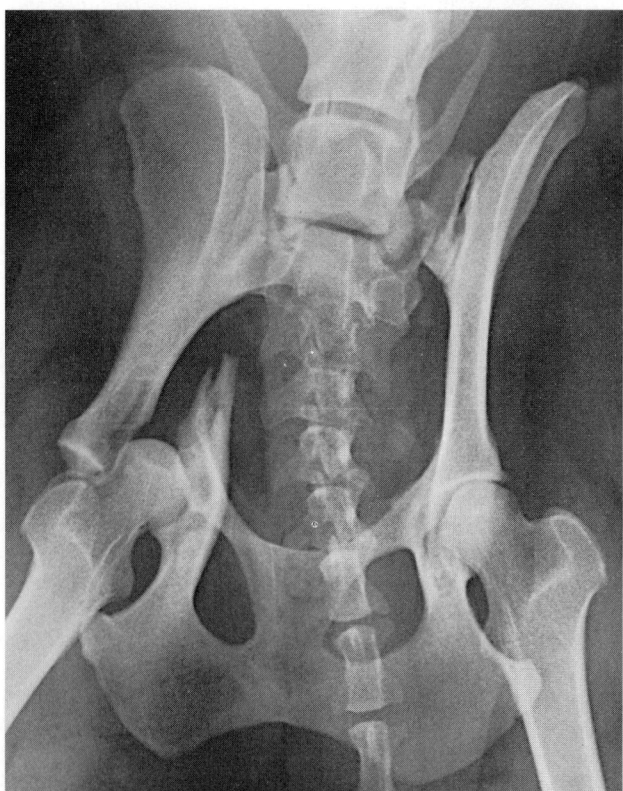

Figure 1. Radiograph showing an abaxial sacral fracture in a dog.

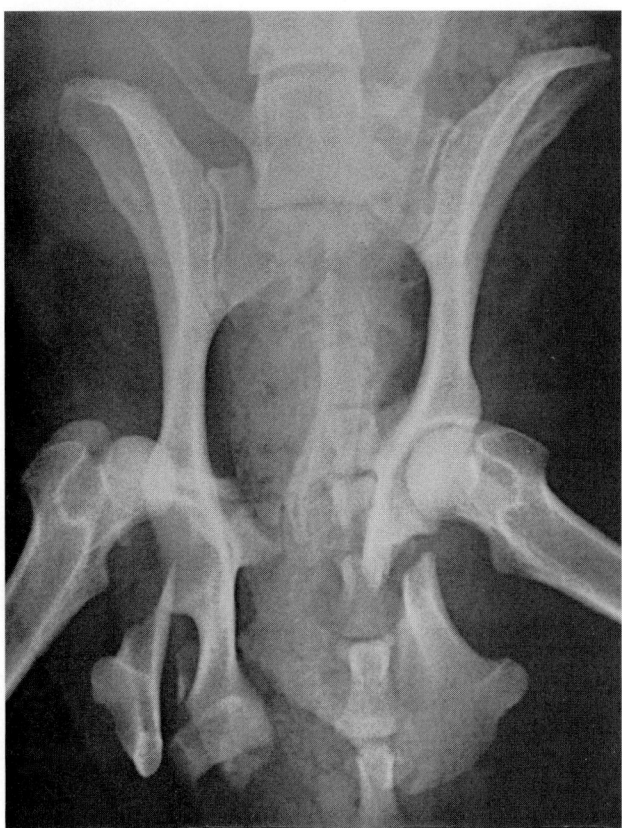

Figure 2. Radiograph showing an axial sacral fracture in a dog.

and severity of neurologic deficits in people with sacral fractures.

MEDICAL AND SUPPORTIVE CARE

If a patient has urine retention, the bladder must be intermittently emptied to prevent the development of an atonic bladder through excessive or persistent stretching of tight junctions. This may be done manually or by use of a urinary catheter. Use of an indwelling closed urinary catheter system is often beneficial in a recumbent patient in that it allows complete urine evacuation, avoids painful bladder expression, and helps prevent urine scalding. Urine scalding can result in patient discomfort, infection of surgical sites, progression of pressure sores, and owner dissatisfaction. Urine scalding must be avoided at all costs even if daily bathing is required. This is usually well tolerated and can be performed with minimal assistance. Petrolatum in the perivulvar or preputial region can also be used to help prevent minor urine scalding. The use of antibiotic therapy in patients with indwelling urinary catheters is controversial, but is generally not recommended because it can result in the development of resistant bacterial strains. Patients should be closely monitored for the development of urinary tract infection by frequent urinalysis and culture. If systemic illness or pyelonephritis develops, appropriate antibiotic therapy based on sensitivity should be administered. Pyelonephritis may be initially characterized by fever, pain, and leukocytosis, but signs are often limited to those of recurrent lower urinary tract infection. Pyelone-

phritis is diagnosed by urine sediment examination and culture. Confirmation is made with contrast dye studies of the renal pelvis or ultrasonography. Urinary culture and sensitivity should be performed 1 week after removal of urinary catheters.

Urethral spasm due to unopposed alpha-adrenergic innervation may be alleviated by the use of phenoxybenzamine, an alpha-antagonist (Dibenzyline, Smith, Kline and French) (1 mg/kg t.i.d.). This should not be used in hypotensive patients because it can cause further hypotension. Complete bladder emptying may be assisted by the use of bethanechol (Urecholine, Merck, Sharpe and Dohme) (1 to 2 mg/kg orally b.i.d. or t.i.d.), a parasympathomimetic. Bethanecol should not be used in patients with markedly increased urethral tone because urinary bladder rupture may result. These drugs may take several days to begin working, so early administration should be attempted when the need is anticipated. Striated muscle relaxants (diazepam, 1.25 to 2.5 mg/kg) can also be used to reduce external urethral sphincter spasm, and may have the advantage of a more rapid onset of effect. Diazepam should not be used in cats for this purpose due to the recent recognition of fatal hepatocellular necrosis in some cats receiving this drug (p. 241). Fecal retention in patients with neurologic injuries does not frequently occur. If associated pelvic fractures are causing fecal retention, stool softeners may be used.

TREATMENT OF SACRAL FRACTURES

Surgical decompression of sacral nerve roots using dorsal laminectomy of the sacrum has been recommended in dogs and cats with axial sacral fractures (Taylor, 1981). Results were similar to those seen in the author's study, where no decompression of nerve roots was performed (Kuntz et al, 1995). The primary difficulty is in identifying which patients have nerve root compression. Animals that have evidence of excessive pain without neurologic deficits may warrant the use of decompressive and exploratory surgery. Surgical stabilization of abaxial fractures resembling sacroiliac fracture-separations is recommended following guidelines used for the repair of the other pelvic fractures. Indications for pelvic fracture repair include presence of articular fractures, disruption of major weightbearing structures, evidence of nerve compression and marked displacement of fracture fragments resulting in collapse of the pelvic canal. Surgical repair is similar to that of sacroiliac fracture-separations using one or two screws placed in lag fashion from the lateral aspect of the ilial wing to the sacral body using previously described guidelines (DeCamp and Braden, 1985). Surgical anatomy is disrupted, and screw placement can be difficult.

In dogs with abaxial sacral fractures, the prognosis for complete return to function is excellent. The prognosis in dogs with axial sacral fractures is good, in that most dogs that are not euthanized during the immediate post-trauma period make nearly complete recoveries even though they may have significant neurologic dysfunction (Kuntz et al, 1995). It is important to note that dogs made significant neurologic recovery only after release from the hospital, and that many dogs with complete urinary and fecal incontinence later become continent. Dogs should not be euthanized during the initial hospital stay despite a lack of early neurologic recovery. A prolonged opportunity for recovery should be allowed, and owners should be warned that although complete neurologic recovery frequently occurs, in some cases, it does not.

SACROCOCCYGEAL INJURIES IN CATS

Sacrococcygeal (SC) separations in cats comprise a distinct clinical syndrome that is markedly different from sacral fractures in dogs and cats (Smeak and Olmstead, 1985). Sacrococcygeal separations result when the tail of a cat is forcefully and abruptly pulled away from the body, whereas sacral fractures result from blunt trauma to the pelvis. Sacrococcygeal separations can occur when the tail is caught under the tire of a moving vehicle or in a closing door. Denervation of the tail, pelvic viscera, and hind limbs results from "tethering" of the cauda equina and laceration of nerve roots or their avulsion from the distal tip of the spinal cord. The salient anatomy is similar to that of the dog.

Clinical signs are related to the degree of the neurologic injury and to the presence of other orthopedic and soft tissue trauma. Hyperesthesia at the base of the tail is common. Some cats may have paraparesis; this almost always resolves during the weeks following the initial injury. Most cats with SC separations have some degree of analgesia and diminished motor function of the tail. This may, in some cats, be the only deficit (group 1). Some cats have residual urine and tail denervation with normal anal tone, perineal sensation, and a maintained ability to posture to urinate (group 2). Cats with decreased anal tone and decreased perineal sensation who do not posture to urinate have damage to both pudendal and pelvic nerve fibers or segmental damage to the spinal cord (group 3). Cats with no anal tone and no perineal sensation have complete urinary and fecal incontinence (group 4). The prognosis for cats in groups 1 and 2 is excellent. All cats will recover tail function, and most cats in group 2 will recover urinary function. Cats in group 3 have a reasonably good prognosis with appropriate medical management. Approximately 75% of these cats will recover completely. Cats in group 4 have a guarded prognosis, but as many as 50% of these cats may make a complete recovery. It is generally accepted that most of the neurologic recovery will occur within the first month after the initial trauma, and that if recovery does not occur by this point, it is unlikely to occur at all. Surgical decompression of nerve roots in cats with sacrococcygeal separations is controversial, but is generally not recommended because injury is generally not compressive but avulsive. Tail amputation should not be performed at initial diagnosis. Indications for tail amputation include ischemic necrosis, frequent soiling with feces and urine, and persistent pain.

References and Suggested Reading

DeCamp CE, Braden TD: The surgical anatomy of the canine sacrum for lag screw fixation of the sacroiliac joint. Vet Surg 14:131, 1985.
  Describes salient surgical anatomy relative to the placement of lag screws used to repair sacroiliac luxations.
Kolata RJ, Kraut NH, Johnston DE: Patterns of trauma in urban dogs and cats: A study of 1000 cases. J Am Vet Med Assoc 164:499, 1974.
  Describes clinical findings in dogs and cats sustaining trauma in urban areas.
Kuntz CA, Waldron D, Martin RA, et al: Sacral fractures in dogs: A review of 32 cases. J Am Anim Hosp Assoc 31:142, 1995.
  Describes clinical findings and classification scheme for dogs with sacral fractures.
Selcer BA: Urinary tract trauma associated with pelvic trauma. J Am Anim Hosp Assoc 19:785, 1982.
  Evaluates urinary tract trauma in 100 dogs with pelvic fractures.
Smeak DD, Olmstead ML: Fracture/luxations of the sacrococcygeal area in the cat. Vet Surg 14:319, 1985.
  Describes neurologic deficits and other clinical signs seen with sacrococcygeal separations in cats.
Taylor RA: Treatment of fractures of the sacrum and sacrococcygeal region. Vet Surg 10:119, 1981.
  Describes decompression of sacral nerve roots in eleven dogs and cats with sacrococcygeal fractures.

Diagnosis and Management of Pelvic Fractures and Dislocation of the Sacroiliac Joint

STEVEN C. SCHRADER
Columbus, Ohio

Pelvic fractures and sacroiliac dislocation are common injuries in dogs and cats; pelvic fractures account for 20 to 30% of fractures diagnosed in dogs and cats (Brinker et al, 1990). Pelvic fractures and sacroiliac dislocation are frequently found concurrently and are almost always the result of blunt trauma.

There are several issues concerning treatment that should be considered once the diagnosis has been made. Because the incidence of injuries to adjacent soft tissues (abdominal wall, urinary bladder, urethra, lumbosacral trunk, or sciatic nerve) and bony structures (lumbar, sacral, coccygeal vertebrae) is quite high, successful management

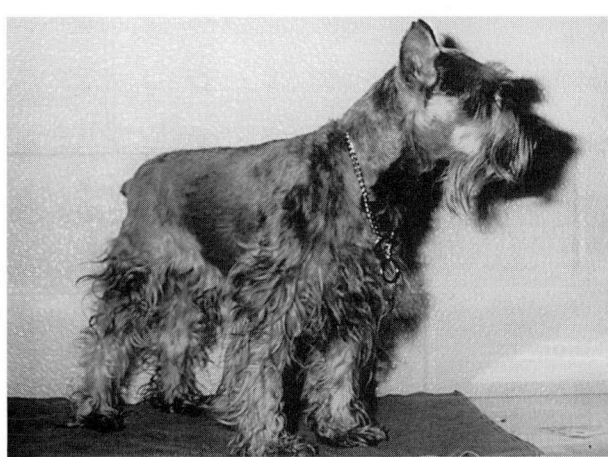

Figure 1. A male Schnauzer 5 months following blunt trauma that caused multiple pelvic fractures, right sacroiliac dislocation, and ventral abdominal hernia. Only the hernia had been repaired. The dog had no detectable alteration of gait or signs of constipation and little external evidence of previous injury at the time this photograph was taken.

of the patient with pelvic fractures and sacroiliac dislocation often depends on timely identification and appropriate management of these injuries as well (see also the previous article, "Sacral Fractures and Sacrococcygeal Injuries in Dogs and Cats"). A significant degree of malalignment of the pelvis can be present without long-term functional disability (gait disturbance, constipation) or altering the outward appearance of the animal (Figs. 1 and 2). Most

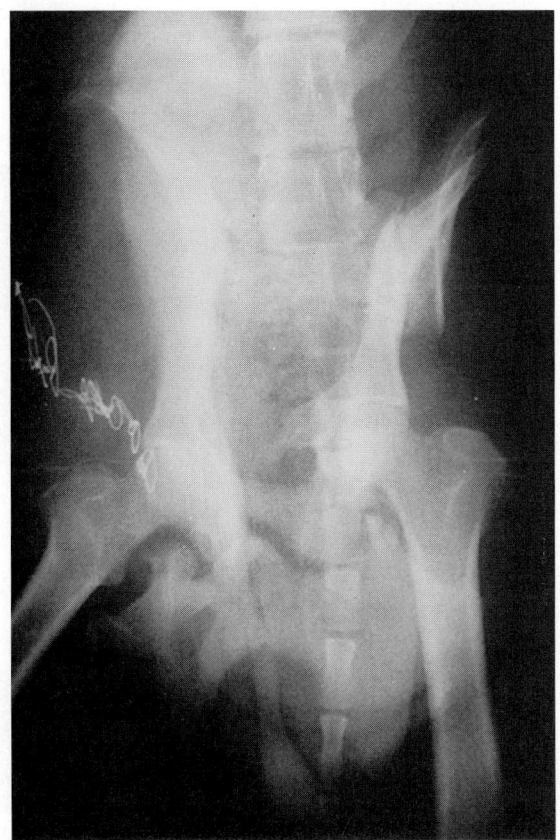

Figure 2. Ventrodorsal radiograph of the pelvis of the dog in Figure 1.

pelvic fractures will heal without reduction or fixation. However, even a small degree of malalignment of acetabular fractures will lead to degenerative joint disease and perhaps to its clinical sequelae; a large degree of medial displacement of the ilium or acetabulum may interfere with defecation or parturition. Narrowing of the pelvic canal is of greatest clinical significance in cats and very small dogs.

DIAGNOSIS

Physical Examination

The high incidence of concurrent injuries in animals that have sustained pelvic fractures and sacroiliac dislocation underscores the importance of a complete physical examination. Careful examination of the caudal abdominal wall for hernias and the urinary bladder and urethra for rupture is imperative. Urethral trauma associated with pelvic fractures is much more common in males than in females. The sensory status of the tail, anus, and perineum should be determined. Anal tone and the status of the anal reflex should be evaluated. Fractures of the lumbar, sacral, and caudal (coccygeal) vertebrae may alter sensory and motor function of these structures; in such cases, a painful response can usually be elicited by manipulation of the base of the tail or by application of digital pressure at the level of the fracture (see also the previous article "Sacral Fractures and Sacrococcygeal Injuries in Dogs and Cats").

The neurologic status of the limbs should be evaluated in all animals that have sustained trauma to the pelvic region. The intimate relationship between the lumbosacral trunk-sciatic nerve and adjacent bony structures (sacrum, sacroiliac joint, and ilium) predispose them to injury. In one study, approximately 11% of dogs and cats with pelvic fractures and sacroiliac dislocation had evidence of peripheral nerve injury (Jacobson and Schrader, 1987). Injury to the lumbosacral trunk or sciatic nerve may result in various degrees of proprioceptive deficit (knuckling of the paw) and diminished sensory status over the dorsal, lateral, and plantar aspects of the paw. Accurate assessment of proprioceptive, sensory, and motor status can sometimes be difficult. Animals with pelvic fractures and sacroiliac injuries may be unwilling to bear weight on the limb, may be less willing to respond to a noxious stimulus because movement of the limb is painful, and may have soft tissue bruising and swelling that alters voluntary movement or sensory perception. Severe avulsive, crushing, or lacerative injuries of the lumbosacral trunk and sciatic nerve will result in diminished or absent withdrawal reflex, loss of voluntary motor function distal to the stifle region, and slight to moderate hyperflexion of the tarsus with weightbearing. Complete denervation of the muscles that extend the tarsus does not result in marked tarsal hyperflexion and a plantigrade stance because the animal's ability to extend the stifle will reciprocally extend the tarsus. There may be hyperextension of the stifle and exaggerated patellar tendon reflexes with denervation of the biceps femoris, semitendinosus, and semimembranosus muscles (loss of antagonists). Entrapment of peripheral nerves often evokes a painful response; entrapment of the lumbosacral trunk or sciatic nerve must be considered whenever the animal appears to have intractable pain or has a marked response to manipu-

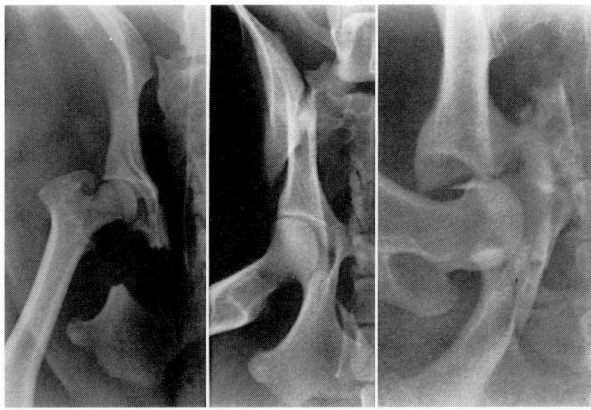

Figure 3. Ventrodorsal radiographs of common pelvic injuries. Craniodorsal displacement of the ilium is commonly associated with disruption of the sacroiliac joint *(left)*. Fractures of the ilium *(center)* and acetabulum *(right)* usually result in medial displacement of bone fragments and the femur. Lumbosacral trunk or sciatic nerve injuries are most commonly associated with sacroiliac dislocation *(left)* or ilial fractures that allow craniomedial displacement of the ilium *(center)*.

lation of the limb. It is common for animals with pelvic fractures to allow manipulation without marked painful response.

The physical findings associated with pelvic fractures and sacroiliac dislocation can be predicted with knowledge of the pathology created by the trauma. Bone is usually displaced away from the site of direct impact. Cranial displacement of the ilium occurs with sacroiliac dislocation, and bone is usually displaced in a medial direction with ilial and acetabular fractures (Fig. 3). The sacrum, sacroiliac joint, ilium, ischium, pubis, and pelvic symphysis form a continuous structure ("pelvic ring"). Disruption of one portion of this structure is almost always accompanied by disruption at another site. Therefore, isolated (single) fracture of the pelvis or sacroiliac dislocation is highly unlikely. Although gross inspection would lead one to believe that the pelvis is somewhat fragile, its shape and the protection afforded by surrounding muscles make it less vulnerable to fracture. A significant amount of kinetic energy is needed to disrupt the "pelvic ring." This would explain the prevalence of associated bony and soft tissue injuries. Soft tissue disruption may be severe; the extent of soft tissue injury, as defined by swelling and bruising, is often not fully apparent until 3 to 4 days have elapsed.

Animals with pelvic fractures and sacroiliac dislocation have a variable degree of functional disability. Some animals are unable or unwilling to rise and walk on the affected limb; others can rise and walk with little or no assistance. Functional abilities often improve, sometimes dramatically, during the first 48 to 72 hours.

Crepitus can usually be detected in the pelvic region when the limb (hip) is manipulated. Doing a rectal examination at the time of such manipulation may facilitate detection of crepitus or movement of bone fragments. Rectal examination allows simultaneous evaluation of anal tone and reflex, the rectum, and the size and shape of the pelvic canal. Rectal examination is much more accurate than radiographic evaluation for determining the extent of narrowing or adequacy of the pelvic canal. The intrapelvic

portions of the sciatic nerve and urethra can sometimes be identified by rectal examination.

In animals having craniodorsal dislocation of the sacroiliac joint (see Fig. 3), the area about the iliac crest may appear swollen or the iliac crest will be more prominent or easier to palpate than on the unaffected side. The greater trochanter may seem less prominent or be more difficult to palpate in animals having medially displaced fractures of the ilium or acetabulum (see Fig. 3).

Radiographic Examination

Standard ventrodorsal and lateral views of the pelvis usually suffice for the diagnosis of pelvic fractures and sacroiliac dislocation. Animals with these injuries seem to tolerate positioning for the dorsoventral "frog-leg" view (Fig. 4) better than ventrodorsal "hip-extended" view (Fig. 5); however, dorsoventral views are generally more difficult to evaluate (compare Fig. 4 and Fig. 5). The ventrodorsal view is particularly helpful in the diagnosis of sacral fracture and sacroiliac injuries. Because even slight rotational malpositioning may cause the width of the two sacroiliac joints to appear different, sacroiliac dislocation is not usually diagnosed unless there is unequivocal widening of the joint or cranial displacement of the ilium (Fig. 6).

Making standard ventrodorsal and lateral views of the pelvis also allows radiographic evaluation of the proximal portion of the femur, the last 2 to 3 lumbar vertebrae, the sacral and caudal vertebrae, and the caudal abdomen (urinary bladder, abdominal wall). Each of the above structures should be carefully examined when evaluating radiographs of animals that have sustained pelvic trauma. Thoracic radiography is recommended in all animals that have sustained blunt trauma; concurrent thoracic injuries are com-

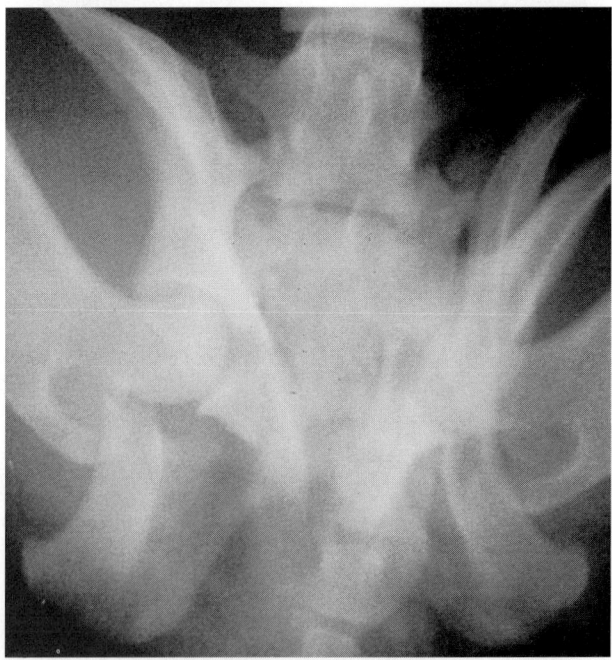

Figure 4. Dorsoventral "frog-leg" radiograph of the pelvis of a dog having multiple pelvic fractures and right sacroiliac dislocation.

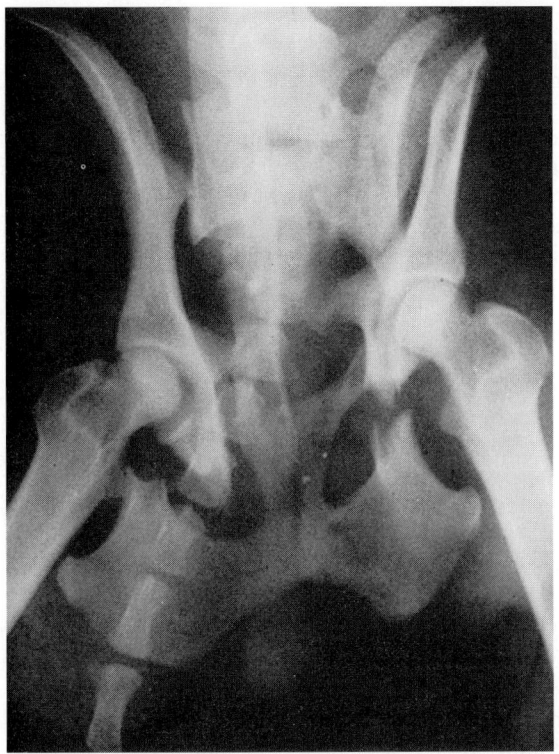

Figure 5. Ventrodorsal "hip-extended" radiograph of the pelvis of the dog in Figure 4. Although dogs and cats are more likely to resist or struggle during positioning for this view, it is preferred over dorsoventral views because the bony injuries are more clearly defined.

mon and such injuries may not be detected by physical examination methods.

The radiographic findings associated with pelvic fracture and sacroiliac dislocation are limited predictors of concurrent soft tissue injury, severity of limb dysfunction, and degree of pelvic narrowing. As such, therapeutic decisions

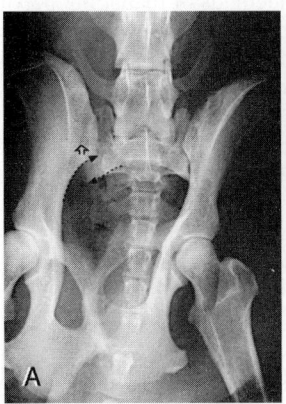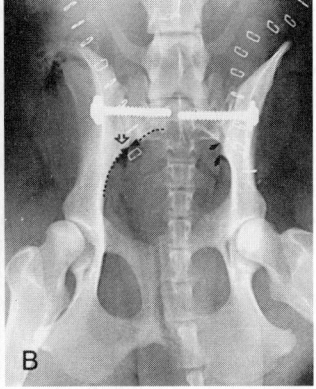

Figure 6. Preoperative *(A)* and postoperative *(B)* ventrodorsal radiographs of the pelvis of a dog having bilateral sacroiliac dislocation and fracture of the pelvic symphysis. The normally confluent bony margin created by union of the medial portion of the ilium and the sacral body has been disrupted on both sides *(dotted line arrows, right joint)*; this disruption confirms that sacroiliac dislocation has occurred. Following reduction *(B)*, confluence has been re-established on the right side *(dotted line arrows)*. The left dislocation has been slightly over-reduced; that is, the ilium has been moved slightly caudal to its normal position *(solid arrowheads)*.

concerning such injuries should be based on both radiographic and physical findings with emphasis on the latter.

INDICATIONS FOR SURGICAL INTERVENTION

Concurrent Soft Tissue Injuries

The presence of an abdominal hernia, a ruptured bladder or urethra, or suspected peripheral nerve injury warrants serious consideration. Management of these injuries usually takes precedence over treatment of the associated fracture or dislocation.

In the case of peripheral nerve injury, surgical treatment usually includes reduction and repair of the bone or joint injury. Injury to the lumbosacral trunk or sciatic nerve is most commonly associated with craniodorsal sacroiliac dislocation and with fractures of the ilium where there is medial or craniomedial displacement of the caudal fragment (see Fig. 3). Surgical exploration is usually warranted when the animal has neurologic deficits, appears especially painful, or is experiencing intractable pain concurrent with radiographic evidence that bone fragments may be causing persistent attenuation of the lumbosacral trunk or the sciatic nerve (see earlier). Exploration may be warranted even when the neurologic examination suggests that nerve injury is severe or complete. In one study (Jacobson and Schrader, 1987), limb function was regained in six of eight dogs and cats that were found to have moderate to severe attenuation, fraying, or stretching of the lumbosacral trunk or sciatic nerve at the time of surgical exploration. Surgery should be performed as soon as possible so that nerve entrapment can be relieved, further nerve damage can be avoided, and prognosis can be determined. If the peripheral nerve is partially intact, the ilial fracture or sacroiliac dislocation should be reduced and fixed. Amputation or tendon relocation techniques (Lesser, 1990) are surgical options when laceration is complete. Nerve anastomosis is impractical because the nerve ends are often badly damaged, adequate exposure is difficult to achieve, and, even under ideal circumstances, reinnervation of the limb will be prolonged or incomplete.

Limb Dysfunction (Pain)

There is a variable degree of limb dysfunction associated with all pelvic fractures and sacroiliac dislocations. Limb dysfunction is the result of soft tissue disruption, bone instability, and the pain associated with each. The degree of dysfunction helps the veterinarian decide whether or not reduction and fixation are warranted.

Regardless of radiographic findings, dogs and cats with pelvic fractures and sacroiliac dislocation that are able or willing to rise and walk without assistance do not usually require surgery (see exceptions below). These animals will recover more slowly than those having open reduction and internal fixation but the end or long-term result is often the same. Although animals with fracture of the acetabulum are often willing to bear weight on the affected limb, early open reduction and internal fixation is recommended because persistent joint incongruence and instability will lead to degenerative joint disease (see Acetabular Fractures).

Assuming that there are no other injuries that require immediate surgical intervention, serial evaluation over a 2- to 3-day period is the best way to evaluate the degree of limb dysfunction. Many animals that initially are unwilling or unable to walk, that is, appear to be surgical candidates, will be able to walk by the third day. Conversely, the decision to surgically intervene should not be delayed too long (more than 3 to 4 days) because, as time passes, reduction becomes more difficult.

Excessively Narrowed Pelvic Canal

Excessive narrowing of the pelvic canal may interfere with defecation and parturition. Excessive narrowing is usually the aftermath of medial displacement of bone following fracture of the ilium or acetabulum. Less commonly, bilateral craniodorsal sacroiliac dislocation allows craniodorsal displacement of the pubic bones and symphysis which decreases the dorsoventral dimension of the pelvic inlet.

The extent of pelvic canal narrowing is best determined by careful rectal examination. Even severe distortion (30 to 40% narrowing) of the pelvic canal is rarely sufficient to cause persistent signs of constipation or obstipation in dogs weighing more than 10 kg. However, a relatively small degree of pelvic narrowing (15 to 25%) may lead to these signs in cats. Attempting to widen the pelvic canal by per-rectum digital manipulation is potentially dangerous and rarely successful. In cats, signs of constipation or obstipation may not become evident until weeks or months have passed, that is, after the fractures have healed. Chronic partial rectal obstruction leads to chronic distention of the colon (megacolon). In cats, widening the pelvic canal via pelvic osteotomy or ostectomy is usually ineffective in diminishing signs of obstruction once megacolon has developed (Schrader, 1992). Subtotal colectomy, with or without a widening procedure, is often helpful in such situations (Matthiesen et al, 1991). It would seem prudent that open reduction and internal fixation be employed whenever there is doubt about the adequacy of the pelvic canal or as soon as there is any sign of obstruction in those cats having pelvic narrowing associated with pelvic fractures. Likewise, surgery should be performed whenever there is narrowing of the canal in a breeding female of either species, especially if the individual is prone to dystocia (brachycephalic breeds).

Acetabular Fractures

Physical examination findings are the primary basis for determining if there is peripheral nerve entrapment, significant limb dysfunction (pain), or excessive narrowing of the pelvic canal in animals with pelvic fractures or sacroiliac dislocation. Although physical examination is useful in the diagnosis of acetabular fracture, radiographic examination is required to confirm the diagnosis and provide an insight to the method of treatment and prognosis.

Surgical intervention is usually recommended in dogs and cats with acetabular fractures. Anatomic reduction and rigid fixation help to avoid the sequelae of joint incongruity and instability (degenerative joint disease) and any restriction of motion associated with medial displacement. Careful evaluation of the radiographs allows the veterinarian to determine the shape, size, number, and location of fragments, that is, whether anatomic reconstruction and fixation are possible. Comminuted fractures of the acetabulum are especially difficult to repair.

Femoral head and neck excisional arthroplasty is warranted when satisfactory reduction and fixation of acetabular fragments cannot be achieved. In addition, excisional arthroplasty should be considered a reasonable alternative to acetabular reconstruction in light-weight (less than 15 kg) dogs and in cats because a good functional outcome can be expected in these animals. Regardless of whether reconstruction or excisional arthroplasty is planned, surgery should not be delayed in animals having acetabular fractures. Acetabular reconstruction will be more difficult after just a few days and the outcome of excisional arthroplasty becomes progressively less favorable as muscle atrophy and restricted hip motion become more pronounced.

Surgical intervention may not be necessary when the acetabular fracture is nondisplaced, especially in skeletally immature animals that have a high capacity to heal and remodel. Fractures that involve the caudal one fourth to one third of the acetabulum do not usually need to be repaired if the hip is stable and noncrepitant, that is, the bone fragments are not interfering with motion. In such cases, the status of the hip is most accurately determined by palpation of the hip with the dog under general anesthesia. There is evidence to suggest that most dogs with fractures of the caudal acetabulum will have restricted range of pain-free motion and develop degenerative joint disease when nonsurgical methods of management are employed (Boudrieau and Kleine, 1988).

Presence of Factors That Adversely Influence Convalescence Following Nonsurgical Methods of Treatment

Compared with nonsurgical methods of managing pelvic fractures and sacroiliac dislocation, convalescence is generally shorter and the degree of limb dysfunction is initially milder with open reduction and internal fixation. In many situations, this alone is reason enough to warrant surgical intervention. It may be especially helpful to repair pelvic fractures and sacroiliac dislocation when there are injuries in other limbs. Rigid fixation of the pelvic injuries may hasten return to ambulatory status, thus reducing the likelihood of complications associated with recumbency (pneumonia, decubital sores, urine or fecal soiling). Repair of pelvic fractures or sacroiliac dislocation has a sparing effect on the repair of fractures in other limbs. Convalescence may be significantly reduced by internal fixation in very large, obese, or debilitated animals or animals with preexisting conditions, such as arthritis in other joints, that adversely affect their ability to walk. Some owners may not be willing or able to provide the nursing care that may be necessary when nonsurgical methods are employed.

SURGICAL CONSIDERATIONS

Specific methods of reduction and internal fixation are described in most surgical textbooks (see References and

Suggested Reading). Although a detailed description of these methods is beyond the scope of this discussion, several points should be considered:

1. Isolated disruption of the "pelvic ring" is uncommon, i.e., if there is one fracture, there is usually another (Fig. 7).
2. Reduction and fixation of one disrupted segment of the "pelvic ring" will often realign or stabilize other disrupted segments as well. Thus, many animals do not need more than one (unilateral) surgery (Fig. 8; see Fig. 7).
3. Fractures involving the pubis, ischium, and pelvic symphysis do not generally need to be repaired; reduction and fixation is usually reserved for acetabular or ilial fractures and sacroiliac dislocation, i.e., to re-establish the bony connection between the hip and the spine (see Figs. 7 and 8).
4. Anatomic reduction of ilial fractures and sacroiliac dislocation is not necessary as long as fixation is stable and the other goals of surgery, such as decompression of nerves and enlargement of the pelvic canal, are achieved.
5. Most ilial fractures can be repaired via a lateral incision (Piermattei and Greeley, 1979); fixation with plate and screws is the most common method but a variety of methods are useful.
6. The cranial ilium and sacroiliac joint can be visualized

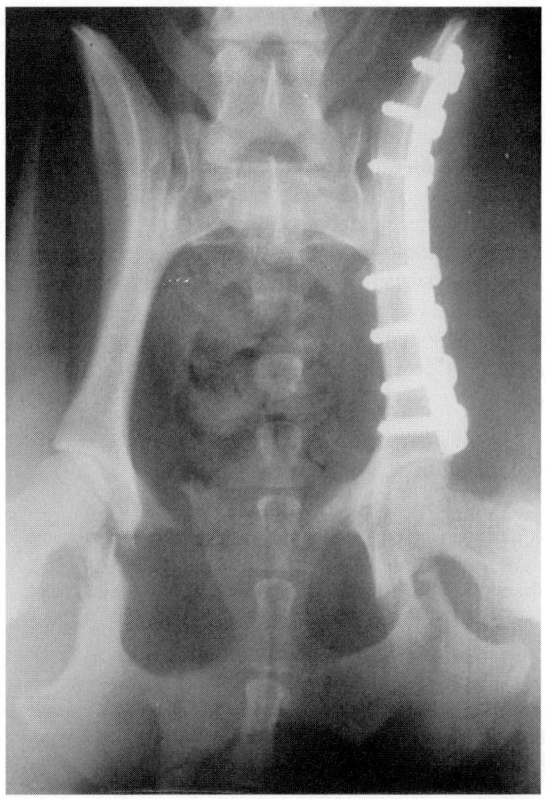

Figure 8. Ventrodorsal radiograph of the pelvis of the dog in Figure 7 following reduction and fixation of the left ilial fracture. Repair of the left ilium has re-established a stable connection between the left limb and the spine, re-established the width of the pelvic canal, and realigned the pubic and ischial fractures. Open reduction and internal fixation of pubic and ischial fractures is rarely necessary.

via a craniodorsal incision (Piermattei and Greeley, 1979); a screw or screws is most commonly employed for fixation of the sacroiliac joint (see Fig. 6); care must be taken to avoid screw placement in the spinal or pelvic canal and the lumbar vertebrae or lumbosacral joint.
7. Gaining exposure to the acetabulum without excessive disruption of the periarticular soft tissues is difficult; widest exposure is usually obtained via trochanteric osteotomy (Piermattei and Greeley, 1979).
8. It is difficult to preserve joint stability, achieve anatomic reduction, and effect rigid fixation of fragments in animals having fracture of the acetabulum; repair of these fractures should be delegated to those having experience with such surgery.

NONSURGICAL TREATMENT

Nonsurgical treatment of pelvic fractures and sacroiliac dislocation consists of rest, controlled exercise, and use of analgesic medications. Rest and controlled exercise may be the primary treatment or follow open reduction and internal fixation. The animals should be confined to a small space; the floor or sleeping area should be clean, dry, and well padded. No running, jumping, or climbing stairs should be allowed for 3 to 4 weeks; thereafter, restrictions on physical activities are generally not necessary. During the first 10 to 14 days, the animal may seem reluctant to

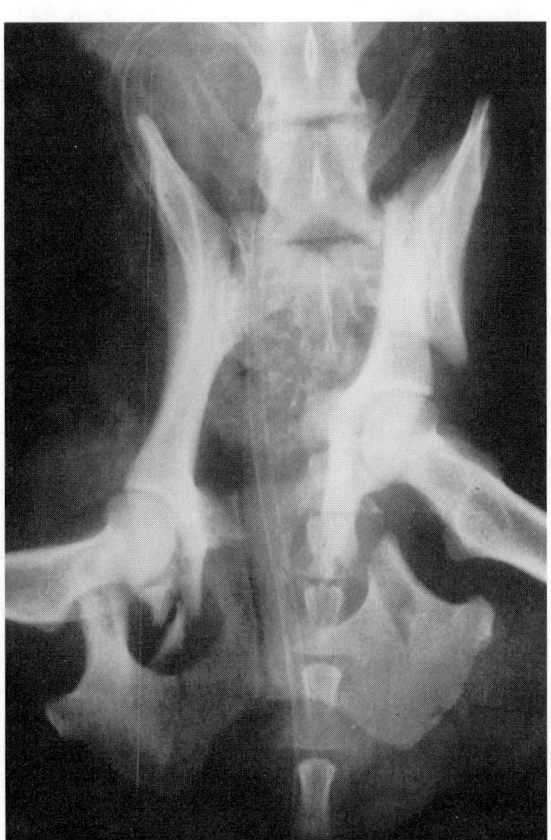

Figure 7. Ventrodorsal radiograph of the pelvis of a dog having multiple pelvic fractures. Disruption of the "pelvic ring" at one site almost invariably is accompanied by disruption elsewhere. The linear radiopacity represents a urinary catheter; the dog had a ruptured urethra.

rise and walk; however, it is important to encourage this in order to prevent muscle atrophy and joint stiffness as well as reduce the likelihood of decubital sores and urine or fecal soiling. Limb function seems to improve more rapidly if the animal has been encouraged to rise and walk numerous times during each day. The owner can help the animal rise and walk as well as prevent falls by placing a towel under the caudal abdomen and using it as a sling. The animal should be re-evaluated by a veterinarian at 10- to 14-day intervals to confirm that limb function is improving, to monitor neurologic status, and to reassess the size of the pelvic canal by rectal examination. Radiographic re-evaluation is warranted whenever internal fixation has been employed.

References and Suggested Reading

Betts CW: Pelvic fractures. In: Slatter D, ed: Textbook of Small Animal Surgery, 2nd ed. Philadelphia: WB Saunders, 1993, p 1769.
An overview of surgical and nonsurgical treatments of pelvic fractures.
Boudrieau RJ, Kleine LJ: Nonsurgically managed caudal acetabular fractures in dogs: 15 cases (1979–1984). J Am Vet Med Assoc 193:701, 1988.
Found that degenerative joint disease and hip pain developed in dogs having caudal acetabular fractures that were not surgically repaired.
Brinker WO, Piermattei DL, Flo GL: Handbook of Small Animal Orthopedics and Fracture Treatment. Philadelphia: WB Saunders, 1990, p 76.
Describes various methods of open reduction and internal fixation of pelvic fractures and sacroiliac dislocation.
Jacobson A, Schrader SC: Peripheral nerve injury associated with fracture or fracture-dislocation of the pelvis in dogs and cats: 34 cases (1978–1982). J Am Vet Med Assoc 190:569, 1987.
Describes the diagnosis, treatment, and outcome of treatment in 34 animals having peripheral nerve injury due to pelvic trauma.
Lesser AS: Tendon transfer for treatment of sciatic paralysis. In: Bojrab MJ, ed: Current Techniques in Small Animal Surgery, 3rd ed. Philadelphia: Lea & Febiger, 1990, p 59.
Describes a method of salvaging limb function following severe sciatic nerve injury.
Matthiesen DT, Scavelli TD, Whitney WO: Subtotal colectomy for the treatment of obstipation secondary to pelvic fracture malunion in cats. Vet Surg 20:113, 1991.
Found that subtotal colectomy helped alleviate signs of constipation and obstipation in cats having pelvic narrowing due to pelvic fracture.
Olmstead ML: Surgical repair of acetabular fractures. In: Bojrab MJ, ed: Current Techniques in Small Animal Surgery, 3rd ed. Philadelphia: Lea & Febiger, 1990, p 656.
Describes surgical methods for open reduction and internal fixation of acetabular fractures.
Piermattei DL, Greeley RG: An Atlas of Surgical Approaches to the Bones of the Dog and Cat, 2nd ed. Philadelphia: WB Saunders, 1979.
Comprehensive guide to the surgical exposure of the bones and joints of dogs and cats.
Schrader SC: Pelvic osteotomy as a treatment for obstipation in cats with acquired stenosis of the pelvic canal: Six cases (1978–1989). J Am Vet Med Assoc 200:208, 1992.
Found that procedures used to widen the pelvic canal of cats having signs of constipation and obstipation were not effective in alleviating signs once megacolon had developed (5 to 6 months).
Tarvin GB, Lenehan TM: Management of sacroiliac dislocations and ilial fractures. In: Bojrab MJ, ed: Current Techniques in Small Animal Surgery, 3rd ed. Philadelphia: Lea & Febiger, 1990, p 649.
Description of the management of sacroiliac dislocations and ilial fractures, including specific methods of open reduction and internal fixation.

Shearing and Degloving Wounds on the Extremities of Dogs and Cats

STEPHANIE L. BEARDSLEY
Austin, Texas

Traumatic injuries of the limbs are common in dogs and cats. These injuries are usually the result of automobile-induced trauma and occur most often in young animals of many breeds. The injuries range in severity from simple lacerations to degloving wounds with loss of skin and underlying soft tissues and associated bone and joint injuries. Shearing and degloving wounds are often highly contaminated because bone, joints, and supportive structures are frequently exposed. Disruption of blood supply, direct tissue damage, and contamination may result in infection. Loss of supportive tissues may lead to joint instability, causing gait or conformational abnormalities. Shearing wounds occur most frequently on the distal portions of the limb, the most common site being the medial aspect of the tarsometatarsal region.

INITIAL ASSESSMENT

Dogs and cats with life-threatening injuries should be stabilized prior to the management of degloving injuries.

A thorough physical examination should be performed because as many as 70% of dogs with shearing and degloving injuries have been reported to have concurrent injuries such as skin laceration, fractures, and cardiopulmonary problems (Beardsley and Schrader, 1995). If definitive management of the wound needs to be delayed, the wound should be cleansed as well as possible and a sterile bandage should be applied to prevent further contamination and to provide support. In most cases, sedation or anesthesia is needed to fully assess and manage the wound. The general physical condition of the animal, along with the degree of injury, dictates the degree and form of anesthesia or analgesia necessary. Neuroleptanalgesics such as acepromazine maleate (Acepromazine, Fermenta Animal Health Co.) and butorphanol tartrate (Torbugesic, Fort Dodge Laboratories Inc.) or oxymorphone (Numorphan, DuPont Merck Pharma) with or without local anesthetics typically provide enough pain relief to allow management of the wounds (see p. 57). In more severe wounds and with a stable animal, a neuroleptanalgesic may be followed by a combination of ketamine (Ketaset, Fort Dodge Laboratories) and diazepam (Valium, Steris Laboratories Inc.) or inhalation anesthesia. Once proper restraint and pain relief have been provided, initial treatment may be performed.

INITIAL WOUND MANAGEMENT

Cleansing and Lavage

The primary focus of treatment is early removal of contaminants and devitalized or contaminated tissues. First, the hair surrounding the wound should be closely and widely clipped. To prevent further contamination by the loose hair, sterile water-soluble jelly (K-Y Jelly, Johnson & Johnson) or sterile gauze sponges should be placed in the wound. The surrounding skin is then aseptically prepared with an effort to minimize the amount of surgical scrub that enters the wound.

Next, the wound should be copiously lavaged to remove foreign material and exudates and to reduce the number of microorganisms. There is controversy about which type of lavage solution is the best. Irrigants that can be used range from tap water to sterile physiologic solutions such as 0.09% NaCl or lactated Ringer's solution with or without the addition of an antiseptic such as chlorhexidine or Betadine. Solutions of 0.05% chlorhexidine and 1.0% Betadine have been recommended. Although researchers have reported on the relative merits and detriments of various solutions used for wound lavage, one study showed there was no relationship between the solutions used and the healing time or outcome (Beardsley and Schrader, 1995). The amount of lavage and the pressure at which it is delivered to the tissues might be more important factors in wound healing. Copious amounts of lavage solution can remove foreign material such as grass and soil and can significantly decrease the bacterial count. Objects such as grass and soils contain infection-potentiating factors (IPFs) that impair the tissue's ability to resist infection by interacting with leukocyte phagocytosis and other humoral factors. For the reasons listed above, the wound should be lavaged before and after surgical debridement until no further necrotic tissue or foreign debris is evident. The lavage solution should be applied under moderate pressure (7 to 8 psi) which can be obtained using an 18-gauge hypodermic needle and a 35-ml syringe. Moderate pressure has been shown to reduce the number of IPFs and bacteria with minimal tissue trauma. Low pressure does not decrease bacterial contamination significantly and high pressure may drive bacteria into the wound and further traumatize the tissues. I use tap water delivered at a moderate pressure before, during, and after surgical debridement. A final rinse with a physiologic solution is used because tap water is hypotonic and the tissues will become edematous if tap water is left in contact with them.

Surgical and Enzymatic Debridement

The next step is debridement of the wound, which can be accomplished by surgery, enzymes, or adherent bandages. Various enzymatic debriding agents containing agents such as *Bacillus subtilis* protease or trypsin are available (Granulex, Beecham Inc). The enzymes aid in the breakdown of necrotic tissue and also cause liquefaction of the bacteria-containing coagulum that forms on the wound surface, thus allowing antibiotics to reach the sequestered bacteria. Enzymatic debriding agents are expensive, are slower than surgical debridement, and thus are rarely used. Surgical debridement of necrotic tissues is a practical and successful method of treatment. All tissues that are unquestionably necrotic or nonviable should be excised, remembering that it is important to leave as much viable tissue as possible for healing or reconstruction. The color and ability to bleed are not reliable indicators of tissue viability. If viability is questioned, the tissue should remain and be reassessed at the next bandage change. Usually tissue that is going to become necrotic has done so by 48 hours after trauma. Several surgical debridements may be necessary when there is severe soft tissue injury and contamination. The use of adherent dressing materials facilitates debridement at each dressing change (see Dressings and Contact Layer).

Closure

The degree of contamination, extent of soft tissue injury, and the degree of skin loss determine whether a wound can be closed primarily. Only degloving injuries with minimal damage to the underlying tissues that can be converted to clean wounds by lavage and debridement should be considered candidates for primary wound closure (Swaim, 1988). Generally, wounds should be left completely or at least partially open when there is any doubt about the efficacy of debridement or the viability of the exposed tissues. Less than 10% of shearing wounds could be closed primarily in one large study (Beardsley, 1995). If sufficient skin is present, but the wound is contaminated, it is best to treat it as an open wound until the degree of contamination is reduced and then close it primarily. This is considered delayed primary closure and is usually done 3 to 5 days after trauma. When compared with primary closure this technique will decrease infection and dehiscence rates while providing a more rapid healing time.

If severed nerves and tendons have identifiable ends they may be anastomosed; however, repair should be delayed until the wound is free from necrotic tissue and infection. When tendon repair is delayed, the cut ends can be tagged with suture or loosely anastomosed to make identification easier when definitive repair is attempted. The limb should be immobilized to reduce tension on the anastomotic sites (Swaim, 1990).

Dressings and Contact Layer

Once lavage and debridement have been performed, the wound should be covered with dry or moistened wide-meshed gauze sponges. Removal of these sponges during bandage changes provides further removal of exudate, foreign material, and necrotic tissue. Dry-to-dry bandages help with debridement of wounds with a copious low-viscosity exudate. The fluid is wicked into the dry contact layer and, as it dries, loose debris and necrotic tissue becomes entrapped in the gauze mesh. When the bandage is removed, so are the debris and necrotic tissue. Similarly, wet-to-dry bandages are advantageous when the exudate is viscous. The moisture in the gauze sponges dilutes the exudate, thus allowing it and debris to be wicked into the gauze mesh. The contact layer of gauze sponges should be sterile, and if moistened, sterile 0.9% NaCl or lactated Ringer's solution used. Bandages should be changed daily until a complete bed of healthy granulation tissue is evident and the degree of drainage is minimal. In practice, dry-to-dry and wet-to-dry are misnomers because the bandage frequently will not have time to dry out before the bandage is changed. A layer of absorbent material such as cast padding or rolled cotton should be applied on top of the contact layer. The quantity needed is dictated by the amount of drainage from the wound. The drainage should not soak through the bandage completely before the next changing because this will allow bacteria to be wicked into the wound. Rolled gauze is applied next and then a final protective layer of loose white tape or self-adherent materials such as Vetrap (Johnson & Johnson) or Co-Flex (Andover).

Typically a neuroleptanalgesic or general anesthesia is needed to change the bandage for the first several days after trauma. Surgical debridement and lavage should be performed at the time of bandage change if necessary. One study showed an average of 1.7 anesthetic or surgical procedures per dog with a mean hospitalization of 4.6 days (Beardsley and Schrader, 1995).

Antimicrobials

Systemic antibiotics should be used in the majority of animals with degloving injuries due to the severe tissue trauma and high contamination rate. A broad-spectrum antibiotic with efficacy against the most common wound contaminants (*Staphylococcus* spp., coliforms, and *Pseudomonas* spp.) such as a cephalosporin (cephalexin [Keflex, Biocraft Laboratories Inc.]), potentiated sulfonamide (sulfamethoxazole trimethoprim [SMZ-TMP, Goldline Laboratories]), or amoxicillin clavulanate acid (Clavamox, SmithKline Beecham Animal Health) is recommended. If topical antibiotics or antiseptics are used, they should be in a water-soluble form. Oil-based topical preparations make it more difficult to cleanse the wounds and can trap debris in the tissues. No improvement in healing rate or outcome has been reported with the use of topical antimicrobial preparations. It has been suggested that healthy granulation tissue is resistant to infection and that neither topical nor systemic antibiotics are necessary once a healthy bed of granulation tissue has developed.

LONG-TERM MANAGEMENT

Nonadherent dressings that do not damage granulation tissue should be applied once a healthy bed of granulation tissue is established and the need for further debridement has diminished. The tissue will appear red and granular, and will bleed easily when disrupted. I prefer to use a semiocclusive petroleum-impregnated gauze (Adaptic, Johnson & Johnson) that promotes granulation tissue production and enhances wound contraction while allowing for

drainage. Perforated polyethylenes with a layer of cotton interposed between (Telfa-Pads, Kendall Healthcare Products, or Melolite, Smith & Nephew Inc.) are other semiocclusive dressings commonly used. These do not wick the discharge well, and therefore should be avoided if the wound is still productive. Two occlusive dressings—hydrogel (Curity Conforma Gel, Kendall Canada Inc.) and hydrocolloid (Comfeel Systems, Smith & Nephew Inc.)—have been used more recently by some to treat open wounds. The advantage of these dressings is that they prevent absorption of fluid from the wound surface, thus providing more nutrients for wound healing. The disadvantages are increased bacterial counts in the wound and possible maceration due to the moist environment. One study of full-thickness wounds showed decreased wound healing with the hydrocolloid and no difference in wound healing time with the hydrogel and perforated polyethylene (Morgan et al, 1994). More studies need to be performed to fully evaluate these dressings. They should be avoided in wounds with excessive granulation tissue because they do promote exuberant granulation tissue.

Once there is no need for further debridement and healthy granulation tissue is present, bandages should be changed every few days or weekly depending on the condition of the bandage and the amount of drainage from the wound. If the secondary layer is soaked with discharge or the outer layer has strike-through, the bandage needs to be changed. Infection increases the amount of drainage and, therefore, the frequency of bandage changes should increase accordingly. Infection should be considered to be present whenever drainage from the wound is excessive, persists, or is purulent in nature; when granulation tissue is discolored or exuberant; and when wound healing is progressing at a slow rate. If a wound appears infected, thorough wound lavage, debridement of necrotic or infected tissues, daily bandage changes, and a change in systemic antibiotics is recommended until the wound appears healthy. Do not depend on a change of antibiotics to clear the infection. Changing the method of the wound care is more important and productive in treating the infection.

The limb should be kept in a protective bandage until the wound is completely healed. The bandage protects against further contamination, self-trauma (licking, chewing), and desiccation of the wound. Bandages provide a collection depot for exudates and may reduce tension forces along suture lines or wound margins, especially with wounds located near joints. Counteracting tensile forces may reduce the likelihood of dehiscence and deforming contractures as well as reduce pain. Problems associated with prolonged immobilization (joint stiffness, muscle atrophy) are not uncommon, but are usually mild or temporary, especially if there is no joint involvement. A mild degree of joint stiffness may be desirable in dogs that had initial joint instability. Prevention of deformities and bandage-associated complications requires proper construction and application of coapting devices and proper care by the owner.

Joint instability secondary to disruption of the supportive ligaments occurs in about 60% of animals with shearing and degloving injuries (Beardsley and Shrader, 1995). Careful palpation of the involved joints is essential to fully assess the extent of the injury. Shearing injuries that result in unstable joints need to have some form of stabilization. A splint or external fixator can provide support while allowing for continued wound therapy. I prefer to use lateral splints constructed of aluminum rods on animals with joint instability. There are benefits of aluminum rod splints over preformed plastic splints (Mason-Meta; Quik-Splint). Rod splints can be formed to fit each animal regardless of the size, the splint can be bent in such a way that the limb is placed in valgus or varus to help correct ligamentous laxities, the joints can be held in a normal flexed position unlike with a straight splint, and the metal rod splints are significantly less expensive. The animal may need to have the splint or external fixator on for 6 to 10 weeks to allow for proper healing of the periarticular tissues. In the majority of animals with unstable joints, adequate healing and stabilization occurs with external coaptation alone. One study showed that 85% of animals with joint instability secondary to a shearing injury had an excellent or good outcome when treated with a splint only (Beardsley and Schrader, 1995). If a joint is still relatively unstable after 3 to 4 weeks of coaptation, surgical intervention with a prosthetic ligament(s) or arthrodesis may be necessary. Internal fixation or external fixators may be indicated when shearing and degloving wounds are associated with fractures. The type and location of the fracture will dictate the form of treatment.

The length of time for healing of a degloving injury depends on the extent of contamination and injury and the type of wound closure if any. For minor injuries with minimal skin defects that are left open, an average of 3 weeks is needed for healing whereas 6 to 8 weeks are needed if there is bone or joint exposure. The wounds with joint instability take an average of 7 to 9 weeks to heal. Although the extent of injury and degree of contamination ultimately dictate the time for wound healing, I have found that even severe degloving and shearing injuries can heal if these methods of treatment are followed. Very few animals require amputation of a limb, arthrodesis of a joint, or reconstructive skin surgeries. In one large study of animals with shearing and degloving injuries treated with the above mentioned methods, 91% had a good or excellent outcome (Beardsley and Schrader, 1995).

References and Suggested Readings

Beardsley SL, Schrader SC: Treatment of dogs with wounds of the limbs caused by shearing forces: 98 cases (1975–1993). J Am Vet Med Assoc 207:1071, 1995.
   A retrospective study of the overall treatment and outcome of 98 dogs with shearing injuries to the extremities.
Johnston DE: Care of accidental wounds. Vet Clin North Am Small Anim Pract 20:27, 1990.
   A review of wound management from the initial presentation to healing.
Morgan PW, Binnington AG, Miller CW, et al: The effect of occlusive and semi-occlusive dressings on the healing of acute full-thickness wounds on the forelimbs of dogs. Vet Surg 23:494, 1994.
   Compares the use of hydrogel, hydrocolloid, and semi-occlusive dressings on full-thickness wounds.
Swaim SF: Bandages and topical agents. Vet Clin North Am Small Anim Pract 20:47, 1990.
   A guide for wound management and selection of bandage materials for various types of wounds.
Swaim SF, Pope ER: Early management of limb degloving injuries. Semin Vet Med 3:274, 1988.
   A useful discussion and review of how to treat shearing and degloving injuries.

Ophthalmologic Diseases

THOMAS J. KERN
MARK P. NASISSE

Consulting Editors

Still Current Information Found in Current Veterinary Therapy XII:

Diagnosis of Blindness

HOLLY L. HAMILTON
Baton Rouge, Louisiana

SUSAN A. MCLAUGHLIN
Auburn, Alabama

Numerous diseases can cause the bilateral loss of vision. Blindness can result from lesions that interfere with the formation of the image by the retina, transmission of the image to the visual cortex, or interpretation of the image by the visual cortex.

CONFIRMATION OF BLINDNESS

The first diagnostic step in a case of possible blindness is confirmation of blindness. This can be achieved by watching the animal walk around the examination room, or by setting up an obstacle course. Evaluation should be performed in both bright and dim lighting. Some animals, particularly cats, will not attempt to walk in an unfamiliar environment. Observing the animal's response to noiseless objects, like cotton balls, dropped through its visual field works well with animals that will not ambulate. The menace response (a menacing gesture such as a hand moving towards one eye) can be used to assess vision and should elicit rapid eyelid closure, provided that the facial nerve (VII) is intact. Care must be taken when testing the menace response not to stimulate the trigeminal nerve by touching the animal, its vibrissae, or by creating air currents. Such stimuli can induce a palpebral reflex (CN V and VII). A Plexiglas shield or vertical hand movements prevent air currents. Vision can also be assessed by the visual placing reaction. The animal is held just in front of a table, then advanced towards the table. If the table is seen, the animal will reach out and place its front feet on the table.

In this chapter the causes of blindness will be grouped by the anatomic segment of the affected visual pathway. Disorders will be discussed in an order typically encountered during an ophthalmic examination. Blindness can occur in a normal-appearing eye, and in these cases, additional diagnostic tests are required. Most ophthalmic lesions are not pathognomonic for an etiologic agent. Even if the structure causing blindness is identified, additional diagnostic tests are required to identify the etiology.

Pupillary Light Reflex

The pupillary light reflex (PLR) should be evaluated in a darkened room with a bright, focal light source. The direct (constriction of the stimulated pupil) and consensual (constriction of the unstimulated pupil) PLR should be evaluated. Absence of a direct and consensual PLR in a blind animal is consistent with a lesion in the retina, optic nerve, optic chiasm, or optic tracts. Abnormal direct and consensual responses can occur without blindness with the following bilateral abnormalities: synechia (iris adhered to lens or cornea), iris atrophy, topical mydriatic application, or oculomotor nerve (CN III) deficits. A frightened or nervous animal may have no PLR owing to stimulation of the sympathetic nervous system. If the PLR is reduced or absent, it should be reassessed later in the examination to determine if it returns to normal as the animal becomes accustomed to its surroundings. Bilateral lesions in the lateral geniculate nucleus, optic radiation, or visual cortex, often referred to as *central or intracranial blindness*, cause loss of sight without affecting the PLR. The presence of a PLR does not always exclude blindness secondary to retinal disease because some retinal degenerations and detachments may be severe enough to cause blindness but a PLR may persist. In most of these cases the PLR is not completely normal.

OPACITY OF THE OCULAR MEDIA

Opacification of the normally clear ocular media (cornea, aqueous, lens, and vitreous) can prevent formation of the image by the retina.

Corneal Opacification

Blindness secondary to corneal disease occurs only with bilateral, severe, diffuse corneal lesions that prevent evaluation of intraocular structures. Causes include corneal pigmentation from chronic exposure, eyelid abnormalities (entropion, ectropion, lagophthalmos, facial nerve paralysis), keratoconjunctivitis sicca, and chronic superficial keratitis (pannus). Diffuse, severe corneal edema due to endothelial dystrophy, endothelial degeneration, or endotheliitis can result in blindness. Diffuse corneal edema can also occur with glaucoma or anterior uveitis. Infiltration by blood vessels or cells, scarring, symblepharon (conjunctiva adhered to cornea), and inherited corneal dystrophy can opacify the cornea.

Aqueous Humor Opacification

Blindness caused by opacification of the aqueous humor results from blood aqueous barrier disruption (uveitis). The underlying cause should be investigated. Red blood cells (hyphema), white blood cells (hypopyon), lipid, or fibrin clots can cause opacification. The cellular exudates typically gravitate ventrally, but if the anterior chamber is diffusely and severely affected to the extent that the iris and other intraocular structures are not visible, blindness may result. Hypopyon can occur secondary to immune-mediated, neoplastic (lymphosarcoma), or infectious diseases (blastomycosis, cryptococcosis, histoplasmosis, coccidioidomycosis, toxoplasmosis, feline infectious peritonitis, prototheclosis, brucellosis, bacterial septicemia). Hyphema can result from coagulopathies (factor deficiencies, warfarin toxicosis, immune-mediated thrombocytopenia), infectious diseases (ehrlichiosis, rickettsiosis), trauma, neoplasia, or retinal detachments. Lipemic aqueous can occur in patients with lipemia (increased blood triglycerides) and concurrent blood aqueous barrier disruption. Hypertriglyceridemia can be primary (see *CVT XII*, p. 430) or secondary to diabetes mellitus, hyperadrenocorticism, or hypothyroidism. Ocular ultrasonography is useful for evaluation of posterior ocular structures, which could be concurrently affected, particularly for the presence of retinal detachment. A complete physical examination also is indicated in these patients. Enlarged lymph nodes, subcutaneous masses, and draining skin tracts, if present, should be aspirated for cytologic evaluation. Diagnostics include a laboratory database (complete blood count, chemistry profile, urinalysis), and chest radiographs. Serology for infectious diseases and a coagulation profile may be beneficial.

Lens Opacification

Cataracts are a frequent cause of blindness in dogs, and the majority are inherited. Cataracts also can occur secondary to diabetes mellitus, retinal degeneration, hypocalcemia, trauma, nutritional deficiencies, electric shock, uveitis, or lens luxation. Cataracts are uncommon in cats, but when they occur, they are most commonly the result of uveitis or lens luxation. For a cataract to be the cause of blindness, the entire lens must be involved and the cataract must be dense enough to prevent evaluation of the ocular fundus. Cataracts do not interfere with the PLR. If the PLR is abnormal, a retinal, optic nerve, or optic tract lesion may be present concurrently, which would preclude cataract removal for improvement of vision. Cataracts must be differentiated from senile nuclear (lenticular) sclerosis, a normal aging change of the lens. The cloudy appearance of the lens in nuclear sclerosis is due to an increased density of the nuclear lens fibers causing partial reflection of light. The ocular fundus is visible by direct or indirect ophthalmoscopy in cases of nuclear sclerosis. Dilation of the pupil with tropicamide facilitates the differentiation between cataracts and nuclear sclerosis.

Vitreous Opacification

Blindness due to opacification of the vitreous can occur secondary to congenital defects such as persistent hyperplastic primary vitreous (PHPV), a developmental abnormality caused by failure of the hyaloid vessel in the primary vitreous to regress, with proliferation of the posterior portion of the tunica vasculosa lentis surrounding the developing lens. Leukocoria ("white pupil") results from fibrovascular plaque formation adjacent to the posterior lens capsule. PHPV is inherited in the Doberman pinscher and Staffordshire bull terrier and occurs sporadically in other breeds.

Severe, diffuse hemorrhage or cellular infiltrate into the vitreous can also cause blindness. The vitreous is avascular and contains very few cells, so inflammation and hemorrhage result from disease in adjacent tissues. Vitreous hemorrhage can occur with systemic hypertension, retinal detachment, blood dyscrasias, neoplasia, and trauma (see hyphema and retinal detachment). Vitreous centesis for cytology and bacterial and fungal culture are indicated in cases of inflammatory cell infiltrate (see chorioretinitis).

RETINAL DISEASE

Chorioretinitis

The retina is thin and in close approximation to the underlying choroid; thus, inflammation of the retina is frequently accompanied by inflammation of the choroid and is referred to as chorioretinitis. Bilateral, diffuse, severe chorioretinitis causes blindness with a significantly reduced or absent PLR. Chorioretinitis is characterized by the presence of hazy, hyporeflective lesions, or if more severely affected, grayish-white infiltrative lesions in the tapetal or nontapetal fundus. In severe cases there may be partial retinal elevation or complete retinal detachment. Differential diagnoses include fungi (*Blastomyces dermatitidis, Cryptococcus neoformans, Histoplasma capsulatum, Coccidioides immitis, Aspergillus* sp., *Fusarium* sp.), *Ehrlichia canis, Rickettsia rickettsii*, canine distemper virus, *Toxoplasma gondii*, feline infectious peritonitis virus, prototheclosis, *Brucella canis*, bacterial septicemia, intraocular larval migrans, and neoplasia. There may be concurrent anterior uveitis. Diagnostic measures include those discussed for uveitis. Vitreous centesis for cytology and bacterial and fungal culture is indicated if detection of the etiologic agent is not possible by less invasive methods.

Retinal Detachment

Retinal detachment typically occurs between the retinal pigmented epithelium (RPE) and the photoreceptors (rods and cones) and must be bilateral and complete to cause blindness. Retinal detachment can be caused by retinal tears (rhegmatogenous retinal detachment), which can occur secondary to cataracts, lens luxation, glaucoma, and endophthalmitis. Nonrhegmatogenous retinal detachment occurs owing to fluid exudation separating the RPE from the rods and cones. Retinal detachment secondary to inflammatory exudate, typically white to tan in color, is often due to infectious causes (see chorioretinitis).

Retinal detachment with serous retinal exudate can occur owing to systemic hypertension or hyperviscosity syndrome, and is frequently accompanied by hemorrhage. Secondary hypertension is more common than primary hypertension, and causes include renal disease, cardiac disease, hyperthyroidism in cats, and hypothyroidism in dogs (see p. 327). Diagnostics should include blood pressure measurement, a thorough physical examination with careful attention to palpation of the cervical area and thoracic inlet for an enlarged thyroid gland, a laboratory database, and serum thyroid concentrations.

Retinal detachment can occur secondary to immune-mediated diseases such as uveodermatologic syndrome (Vogt-Koyanagi-Harada syndrome) and systemic lupus erythematosus. Uveodermatologic syndrome is caused by an immune-mediated response to pigment. Other clinical signs include depigmentation of the skin and hair around the nose, eyes, and lips. In addition to the retinal detachment, there is frequently anterior uveitis and secondary glaucoma.

Inherited congenital diseases such as collie eye anomaly and retinal dysplasia can lead to retinal detachment in severely affected individuals. Idiopathic retinal detachments also occur, and this diagnosis is made after ruling out other causes of retinal detachment.

Retinal Degeneration

Retinal degeneration is a common cause of blindness in dogs. The typical ophthalmoscopic appearance is vascular attenuation, diffuse tapetal hyper-reflectivity, optic nerve pallor, and mottling of the nontapetal fundus. If the retina is not diffusely affected, but has focal or multifocal hyper-reflective tapetal or depigmented nontapetal lesions, there may be another cause for the blindness and further evaluation is needed. Animals with blindness due to retinal degeneration have a diminished or extinguished electroretinogram (ERG).

Progressive retinal atrophy (PRA) is a group of inherited retinal diseases including photoreceptor dysplasias and later onset photoreceptor degenerations. PRA is much more common in dogs than in cats. Because the rods are affected first, the first clinical sign is decreased night vision. The disease progresses to complete blindness as the cones become affected. The age of onset and rate of progression of PRA varies by breed. The progression of vision loss can be very gradual such that the pet compensates extremely well, and the owners may not detect vision loss until the animal is taken to a strange environment. As a result, these cases occasionally present as an acute blindness.

Central progressive retinal atrophy (CPRA) is an uncommon disorder in dogs in the United States. CPRA is a retinal pigment epithelium dystrophy with secondary retinal degeneration. Other causes of retinal degeneration include taurine deficiency in cats, vitamin E deficiency, and glaucoma. Glaucoma causes diffuse retinal degeneration with end-stage disease, and there is usually concurrent optic nerve cupping and buphthalmos.

Sudden acquired retinal degeneration (SARD) causes blindness overnight, or in some cases, within a few weeks. In most cases the PLR is absent or severely reduced at the onset of blindness, but the retina and optic nerve appear normal. SARD is confirmed by ERG, which is extinguished. The cause of SARD is unknown. Typically, overweight female dogs of any breed (or mixed breeds) are affected. Some SARD dogs also have a history of polyuria, polydipsia, and increased appetite. Over several weeks to months after the onset of blindness, the retinal degenerative changes (diffuse hyper-reflectivity of the tapetum, vascular attenuation, and optic nerve pallor) develop and are indistinguishable from other causes of end-stage retinal degeneration. Histologically, the photoreceptors show severe damage immediately after the onset of blindness, and rods and cones are equally affected.

OPTIC NERVE DISEASE

Bilateral lesions of the optic nerves interfere with transmission of the image to the visual cortex and result in blindness and an absent PLR.

Optic Neuritis

Inflammation of the optic nerves (optic neuritis) can be due to infectious agents (canine distemper virus, T. gondii, B. dermatitidis, C. neoformans, H. capsulatum, feline infectious peritonitis virus), granulomatous meningoencephalitis (GME), neoplasia, trauma, and idiopathic causes. A swollen, out of focus optic disc with or without hemorrhage is consistent with optic neuritis. The peripapillary retina may also be involved with inflammation, hemorrhage, and detachment. Optic neuritis must be differentiated from papilledema which is optic nerve swelling without inflammation, blindness, or PLR deficits. Optic neuritis posterior to the globes (retrobulbar optic neuritis) results in blindness with a normal fundic examination. These cases must be differentiated from SARD by an ERG which will be normal with optic nerve disease. The diagnostic plan includes a laboratory database, thorough physical examination, aspiration of lymph nodes if enlarged, chest radiographs, and a cerebrospinal fluid aspirate for cytology, culture, and serology.

Optic Nerve Atrophy

Optic nerve atrophy can be diagnosed by the small, pale to pigmented, depressed, avascular appearance of the optic disk with peripapillary tapetal hyper-reflectivity and a severely diminished or absent PLR. Causes of optic nerve atrophy include previous optic neuritis, trauma, retrobulbar inflammation or compression, glaucoma, and end-stage retinal degeneration.

Congenital Optic Nerve Anomalies

Optic nerve atrophy must be differentiated from optic nerve hypoplasia, a congenital cause of blindness, with small optic nerves and an otherwise normal fundus. Another congenital cause of blindness, optic nerve colobomas, are notch-like defects of the optic nerve. Extensive colobomas can cause blindness and are a predisposition to retinal detachment. Optic nerve colobomas can be a component of collie eye anomaly and are also frequently found in animals with microphthalmos and excessive merling of the coat.

INTRACRANIAL BLINDNESS

There is a long intracranial course of the visual pathway. Lesions in the optic chiasm, optic tracts, and optic radiations result in failure of transmission of the visual image. Visual cortex lesions result in failure of interpretation of the image. Bilateral lesions of the optic chiasm or optic tracts result in blindness with an abnormal PLR. Lesions located posterior to the site where pupillary light fibers branch from the visual pathway (lateral geniculate nucleus, optic radiation, or visual cortex) result in blindness with a normal PLR. Animals with intracranial blindness typically have a normal fundic examination unless there is retrograde degeneration of the optic nerves. They will also have a normal ERG. Causes of intracranial blindness include neoplasia, GME, infectious agents (canine distemper virus, systemic mycoses, T. gondii, feline infectious peritonitis virus), trauma, feline cerebral infarction, obstructive hydrocephalus, various storage diseases, and hypoxemia. These animals may or may not show additional central nervous system (CNS) signs. In a recent report, the majority of dogs with blindness secondary to neoplasia of the optic chiasm did not have other CNS signs (Davidson et al, 1991).

DIAGNOSTICS

Diagnostics for intracranial blindness include a laboratory database, physical and neurologic examinations, cerebrospinal fluid analysis, and computed tomography (CT) or magnetic resonance imaging (MRI).

Cerebrospinal fluid (CSF) analysis (see *CVT XII*, p. 1121) is indicated for patients with optic neuritis and intracranial blindness. The CSF should be cultured and evaluated cytologically, and may be submitted for serology. General anesthesia is required to avoid movement while placing the needle for cisternal puncture.

ERG demonstrates a mass retinal response to light stimuli. The ERG primarily evaluates the outer retinal layers and is severely diminished or absent with blindness due to SARD, or end-stage retinal degeneration. The ERG may be normal in early glaucoma because glaucoma affects the ganglion cell and nerve fiber layers of the inner retina before the outer retinal layers (photoreceptors). An ERG can be performed in an awake or anesthetized animal, but does require special equipment and is thus only available at referral centers. The ERG waveform and amplitude is affected by anesthetics, breed, age, equipment, and technique.

Magnetic resonance imaging or computed tomography may be indicated for evaluation of intracranial and optic nerve lesions. These are highly reliable, noninvasive diagnostic modalities requiring general anesthesia; their use may be limited by availability or expense.

Ocular ultrasound is useful for evaluation of the globe in cases of opacification of the ocular media and may aid in identification of retinal detachment or intraocular mass lesions. In most animals, this can be performed awake with topical anesthesia. Ultrasound is also used for evaluation of orbital contents such as optic nerves, but CT or MRI provides superior information.

Vitreous centesis is performed under general anesthesia. A 23-gauge needle is inserted 6 to 8 mm posterior to the limbus and is directed towards the posterior pole. Aspiration is performed in a slow, controlled manner and 0.1 to 0.2 ml of vitreous may be aspirated for cytology and bacterial and fungal culture. There is some risk of hemorrhage and retinal detachment. In young, normal animals, the vitreous is gel-like and difficult to aspirate. In cases of inflammatory posterior segment disease, the vitreous becomes liquefied and is easier to aspirate. Aqueous can be similarly evaluated by culture and cytology, but it is less frequently diagnostic. Aqueous centesis is most likely to yield positive results with cytologic evaluation in cases of suspected intraocular lymphosarcoma or in evaluation for intraocular antibody production against infectious agents such as *T. gondii*. A 25-to 30-gauge needle is inserted at the limbus, and 0.1 ml of fluid can be slowly aspirated for analysis.

Visual evoked potential (VEP) evaluates postretinal visual pathways and the visual cortex. The VEP is produced by electrical activity in the visual cortex in response to light stimulation of the eye, which is recorded by scalp electrodes. The VEP is not as frequently used or as standardized as the ERG, but can be useful in cases of blindness due to lesions in the optic nerve, visual tracts, or visual cortex.

References and Supplemental Reading

Davidson MG, Nasisse MP, Breitschwerdt EB, et al: Acute blindness associated with intracranial tumors in dogs and cats: Eight cases (1984–1989). J Am Vet Med Assoc 199:755, 1991.
   A retrospective study of 7 dogs and 1 cat with optic chiasm tumors causing acute blindness and no other neurologic deficits.
Hendrix DV, Nasisse MP, Cowen P, Davidson MG: Clinical signs, concurrent diseases, and risk factors associated with retinal detachment in dogs. Prog Vet Comp Ophthalmol 3:87, 1993.
   A retrospective study of 46 dogs with retinal detachment to identify cause and type of detachment and prognosis for reattachment with comparisons to 1,847 cases of retinal detachment from the Veterinary Medical Data Base.
McLaughlin SA, Hamilton HL: Acute vision loss. In Ettinger SJ, Feldman EC, ed: Textbook of Veterinary Internal Medicine, 4th ed. Philadelphia: WB Saunders, 1995, p 208.
   A review of the diagnosis and causes of acute vision loss.
Millichamp NJ: Retinal degeneration in the dog and cat. Vet Clin North Am [Small Anim Pract] 20:799, 1990.
   A review of retinal anatomy, physiology, and inherited and acquired causes of retinal degenerations in dogs and cats.
van der Woerdt A, Nasisse MP, Davidson MG: Sudden acquired retinal degeneration in the dog: Clinical and laboratory findings in 36 cases. Prog Vet Comp Ophthalmol 1:11, 1991.
   A retrospective analysis of 36 dogs with blindness due to SARD including history, signalment, ophthalmoscopy, ERG, and laboratory data.

Differential Diagnosis of the Red Eye

DIANE V. H. HENDRIX

Knoxville, Tennessee

A "red eye" is the most common ocular clinical sign noticed by pet owners. The clinical sign of a red eye does not give any specifics as to severity of disease, type of disease, or prognosis. Localization of the redness must be the first step undertaken when a patient presents with a red eye. Ocular redness may be focal or generalized. It may involve the exterior globe and adnexa or the interior of the globe. External redness may involve the conjunctiva, the nictitans, the episcleral region, or the cornea. Redness from within the globe is usually caused by hemorrhage in the anterior chamber or vitreous. Redness may be the only obvious sign that a blinding disease such as glaucoma or anterior uveitis is present. The purpose of this chapter is to introduce causes of a red eye. Please refer to the other chapters on ocular and infectious diseases for specific information about the diseases and their treatments.

DETERMINATION OF THE ORIGIN OF THE REDNESS (Fig. 1)

When an animal has a red eye, it is imperative that the precise anatomic location of the redness be determined. The redness may be focal or generalized. Focal redness may represent hemorrhage or a mass. Generalized redness is usually caused by conjunctivitis, corneal disease, or intraocular disease. The most important and difficult aspect of localizing ocular redness is in the differentiation of vessels associated with the conjunctival and episcleral regions. Actual conjunctivitis itself poses little threat to vision, but some of the diseases that cause conjunctival/episcleral hyperemia may lead to rapid blindness. If an eye with a blinding disease such as glaucoma or anterior uveitis

were treated as if only conjunctivitis were present, disastrous results can occur. The redness associated with conjunctivitis generally involves the capillaries of the conjunctiva. These superficial blood vessels are more rapidly blanched with topical phenylephrine or epinephrine than deeper episcleral vessels. Conjunctival vessels are also mobile in comparison to the episcleral vessels. One can either try to wiggle the bulbar conjunctiva by sliding the eyelid over the globe while gentle digital pressure is placed on the lids, or a moistened cotton-tipped applicator can be used to slide the conjunctiva over the sclera after topical anesthetic has been instilled. If the engorged vessels are easily moved, they are conjunctival vessels.

The surface redness associated with intraocular disease tends to involve the episcleral vessels. The episcleral vessels are large and immobile. These vessels do not blanch quickly with topical epinephrine or phenylephrine. They may radiate caudally from the limbus as is seen frequently with glaucoma or they may primarily involve the perilimbal region as is seen commonly with anterior uveitis.

Chronic corneal disease may lead to corneal vascularization with or without the development of corneal granulation tissue. Hyphema may fill the entire chamber, making the cornea appear red and completely hide the iris and pupillary aperture. Vitreal hemorrhage can cause the eye to appear red (this must be distinguished from the normal red fundic reflections in dogs and cats with albinotic fundi). A retinal detachment may be visible as blood vessels against the caudal aspect of the lens.

Once the location of the redness has been determined, a complete ocular examination should be performed to diagnose the current disease process, evaluate for prognosis,

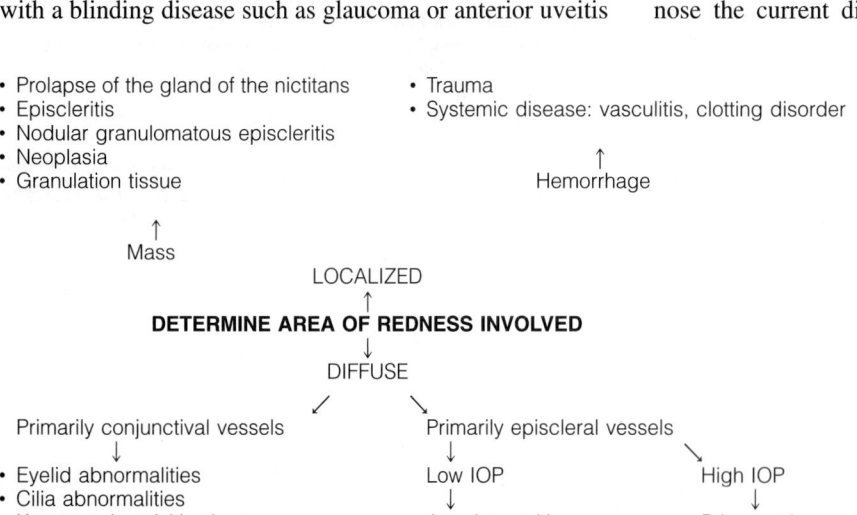

- Prolapse of the gland of the nictitans
- Episcleritis
- Nodular granulomatous episcleritis
- Neoplasia
- Granulation tissue

↑
Mass

- Trauma
- Systemic disease: vasculitis, clotting disorder

↑
Hemorrhage

LOCALIZED
↑
DETERMINE AREA OF REDNESS INVOLVED
↓
DIFFUSE

Primarily conjunctival vessels
↓
- Eyelid abnormalities
- Cilia abnormalities
- Keratoconjunctivitis sicca
- Corneal ulceration
- Allergic conjunctivitis
- Bacterial/fungal conjunctivitis
- Dacryocystitis
- Orbital disease

Primarily episcleral vessels
↓
Low IOP
↓
- Anterior uveitis

High IOP
↓
- Primary glaucoma
- Secondary glaucoma

Figure 1. Algorithm for determining the cause of a red eye in the dog or cat. IOP, intraocular pressure.

and determine the proper treatment. Pupillary light reflexes, menace response, Schirmer tear test, intraocular pressures, examination for aqueous flare, fluorescein staining of the cornea, and complete examination of the eyelids, cornea, iris, lens, vitreous, and fundus should be performed.

FOCAL REDNESS

Focal redness is usually due to hemorrhage or the presence of a mass. Trauma is the most common cause of subconjunctival hemorrhage. Although the hemorrhage may appear severe, no treatment is necessary provided that findings during the remainder of the examination are normal. If there is no trauma in the history, the possibility of a systemic bleeding disorder should be investigated. Prolapse of the gland of the nictitans (cherry eye) is the most common cause of a red mass on the eye. The prolapsed gland should be replaced by either tacking the gland to the orbit or burying the gland using the pocket technique. Neoplasia of the conjunctiva is rare but does occur; biopsy of any questionable mass is indicated. Episcleritis and nodular granulomatous episcleritis are inflammatory diseases that commonly affect the lateral limbus and may respond to treatment with topical and/or systemic prednisone or azathioprine.

GENERALIZED REDNESS

Conjunctival Redness

Localization of the redness to the conjunctiva leads to a diagnosis of conjunctivitis. Even this diagnosis is not final because there are many differential diagnoses that should be explored. One must also keep in mind that dogs with painful intraocular disease such as anterior uveitis and glaucoma often have conjunctival hyperemia as well as episcleral injection; therefore, a diagnosis of conjunctival hyperemia or episcleral injection is not mutually exclusive. In this case the intraocular disease is the primary threat, and with treatment the conjunctival disease will resolve. Complete ophthalmic examination of a dog or cat with isolated conjunctivitis should reveal negative retention of fluorescein stain, normal intraocular pressures, and normal pupillary light responses.

Causes of Conjunctival Hyperemia

Keratoconjunctivitis sicca is a common cause of bacterial conjunctivitis in the dog. Clinically, a mucoid to mucopurulent discharge and a dull cornea that may be ulcerated, pigmented, or vascularized are present. Because of the high incidence of this disease in dogs, a Schirmer tear test should be done on all dogs with conjunctivitis. A result below 8 mm/min of wetting is diagnostic for keratoconjunctivitis sicca. A result of 8 to 14 mm/min of wetting is suggestive of keratoconjunctivitis sicca and treatment should be based on clinical signs or the results of a retest at a later date. Treatment for keratoconjunctivitis sicca includes replacing the tears with an artificial tear ointment, resolving secondary bacterial infections with a broad-spectrum antibiotic (bacitracin-neomycin-polymyxin B [TriOptic P, Smith Kline Beecham Animal Health]) and increasing

tear production with topical cyclosporine used twice daily (Optimmune [Schering Plough Animal Health]) (see p. 1061).

Mechanical irritation is one of the more common causes of conjunctival hyperemia in the dog. Distichia, ectopic cilia, trichiasis, entropion, and ectropion are all commonly incriminated. Clinically, conjunctival hyperemia, epiphora, or a mucoid discharge and corneal disease may be evident. A complete ocular examination is warranted with these cases because occasionally the most apparent abnormality such as distichia, trichiasis, or ectropion may not be the culprit. When it has been determined that the eyelid abnormality is causing the ocular signs, the appropriate surgical therapy should be undertaken.

Allergic conjunctivitis associated with atopy is often seasonal. These dogs and cats have conjunctival hyperemia and epiphora. Another type of conjunctivitis that is thought to be caused by local antigen exposure is follicular conjunctivitis. These dogs are usually young large breed dogs. Ocular examination reveals an abundance of lymphoid follicle formation, conjunctival hyperemia and epiphora. The follicles most commonly occur on the bulbar side of the nictitans but may also occur on the palpebral side or anywhere on the conjunctiva. Cytologic examination of scrapings of the follicles reveals numerous lymphocytes. A mild topical steroid such as hydrocortisone will frequently bring relief. If follicles are present, they may require mechanical disruption. After several doses of topical anesthetic have been instilled in the conjunctival sac, a 4 × 4 gauze wrapped around the end of a cotton-tipped applicator can be used to gently disrupt the follicles. Treating with topical hydrocortisone following debridement is often effective.

Canine distemper virus frequently causes conjunctivitis with epiphora or a mucoid to purulent discharge. Keratoconjunctivitis sicca, corneal ulceration, chorioretinitis, and optic neuritis may also be present in association with systemic signs. Cytologic evaluations of conjunctival scrapings from the nictitans gland may reveal cytoplasmic inclusion bodies. Direct or indirect immunofluorescent antibody testing done on the conjunctival scrapings may also be beneficial. Treatment with topical antibiotics to prevent secondary bacterial infections and treatment with tear replacement ointments may be indicated.

Primary bacterial conjunctivitis is very rare in the dog and cat. *Staphylococcus* spp. are usually the offending bacteria. These dogs present with a purulent ocular discharge with or without swollen eyelid margins. Cytology, culture, and a nasolacrimal duct flush (to rule out dacryocystitis) should be done. Pending culture and sensitivity, try ophthalmic bacitracin, neomycin, polymyxin B for grampositive infections and try ophthalmic bacitracin, neomycin, polymyxin B, gentamicin, or tobramycin for gramnegative infections. Systemic antibiotics will be necessary if the eyelids are involved or dacryocystitis is present. The choice of antibiotic should be based on culture and sensitivity results. If a complete and rapid response does not occur with treatment, re-evaluate.

Occasionally a dog or cat will be presented with a history of exposure to a chemical irritant. In these cases corneal ulceration should be ruled out with fluorescein stain. The cornea and conjunctiva (including the fornices) should be flushed copiously with sterile saline. Often I will treat with a broad-spectrum antibiotic ointment for lubrication and to prevent bacterial infection of any ulcerated surfaces.

Clinical signs of corneal ulceration include blepharospasm, conjunctival hyperemia, photophobia, an uneven corneal surface, vascularization of the cornea, aqueous flare, and miosis. Fluorescein stain retention is diagnostic. One should try to identify the primary cause of the corneal ulcer by doing a complete ophthalmic examination. If the ulcer is deep or rapidly progressing, a bacterial culture should be done. Most corneal ulcers will heal rapidly when treated with a topical broad-spectrum antibiotic and a parasympatholytic drug such as ophthalmic atropine. Occasionally conjunctival graft placement will be required if the ulcer is deep or has perforated.

Feline herpesvirus I (FHV-1) or feline rhinotracheitis virus is a common cause of conjunctivitis in cats. FHV-1 infection is characterized by sneezing and ocular and nasal discharge in neonatal and adolescent cats. Usually the conjunctivitis associated with FHV-1 is characterized by bilateral conjunctival hyperemia and a serous ocular discharge. A mucoid to mucopurulent discharge with conjunctival swelling may develop. Most cases will resolve in 10 to 14 days. Many cats become latently infected. Often adult cats will show unilateral disease without signs of an upper respiratory infection. In adults the disease is more likely to be chronic or recurrent. Fluorescent antibody techniques, virus isolation, and polymerase chain reaction may aid in diagnosis in acute infections. Because the conjunctival form is often self-limiting, antivirals are not used routinely. Topical antibiotics such as tetracycline or chloramphenicol are used to prevent secondary bacterial infections.

Infection with *Chlamydia* is a common cause of conjunctivitis in cats. Clinically the disease is initially unilateral and becomes bilateral. Chemosis and a serous ocular discharge occur. The discharge may become purulent. Cytology revealing intracytoplasmic inclusions or fluorescent antibody testing may be diagnostic. Ophthalmic tetracycline should be used four times daily with the treatment duration extending for two weeks after complete resolution of signs.

Mycoplasma has been associated with conjunctivitis in cats. The clinical signs include unilateral or bilateral epiphora, papillary hypertrophy of the conjunctiva, chemosis, and pseudomembrane formation. Treatment with ophthalmic tetracycline administered four times daily is generally effective. The role of mycoplasma in feline conjunctivitis is questionable because it is frequently cultured from normal cats.

Orbital disease causes secondary conjunctival hyperemia due to inflammation and exposure. If exophthalmos is present or the affected globe is difficult to retropulse, orbital disease should be suspected.

Episcleral Redness

Anterior Uveitis

The clinical signs of anterior uveitis include aqueous flare/hypopyon/hyphema, miosis, resistance to pupillary dilation with mydriatics, anterior or posterior synechia, a darkened iris, and decreased intraocular pressure (if secondary glaucoma is present, the intraocular pressure will be elevated). Aqueous flare, the presence of protein and/or cells in the aqueous humor, is pathognomonic for anterior uveitis. To detect aqueous flare, the smallest white light spot on the direct ophthalmoscope is focused on the cornea. If aqueous flare is present, the light will be scattered and a continuous beam of light will extend from the cornea to the lens. Low levels of aqueous flare are best detected in a completely dark room. Detection of a slightly miotic pupil will be easier in a darkened room as well.

Anterior uveitis has a multitude of etiologies (see *CVT XII*, p. 1248). The goals of treatment of anterior uveitis are to decrease the inflammation and prevent its sequelae. Inflammation may lead to synechia, cataract formation, iris bombé, secondary glaucoma, and blindness. Pending the etiologic diagnosis, the eye should be treated locally using ophthalmic drops. Parasympatholytic drugs, such as atropine (1% ophthalmic solution or ointment) and tropicamide (1% ophthalmic solution), decrease pain by paralyzing the ciliary body muscle and dilate the pupil, thereby decreasing the amount of iris lens contact to prevent or decrease the severity of synechia formation. Corticosteroids, such as prednisone acetate (Econopred Plus 1% suspension, Alcon, Humacao, Puerto Rico), are used to decrease the inflammation. Corticosteroids are contraindicated when a corneal ulcer is present. Topical ophthalmic nonsteroidal anti-inflammatory drugs may also be used; however, they are not as efficacious. The advantage of the topical ophthalmic nonsteroidal anti-inflammatory drugs is that they may be used in the presence of a corneal ulcer.

Hyphema

Hyphema may be noticed by clients. Because hyphema is a form of anterior uveitis, these patients often have episcleral injection as well as the redness in the anterior chamber. There are many causes of hyphema, probably the most common of which is trauma. A one-time episode of hemorrhage generally will resolve quickly. Recurrent bleeding such as that seen secondary to a retinal detachment may lead to secondary glaucoma or synechia. If evaluation of the retina is not possible because of the hyphema, ocular ultrasonography is helpful in determining the presence of a retinal detachment. The primary disease should be diagnosed and treated as well as local ocular treatment for anterior uveitis. If the hemorrhage is recurrent, the intraocular pressure should be evaluated periodically and treated appropriately if secondary glaucoma develops.

Glaucoma

Early glaucoma is the most overlooked cause of a red eye. Early glaucoma (intraocular pressure < 35 mm Hg) often causes a red eye with or without epiphora, with no other clinical signs. These dogs are frequently treated for "conjunctivitis" when they actually have episcleral injection. Later in glaucoma when the pressures are extremely elevated, many other clinical signs are also often present such as pain, corneal edema, mydriasis, blindness, optic nerve cupping, retinal degeneration, buphthalmos, and lens luxation. Schiøtz tonometry should be performed on all dogs and cats that present with a red eye unless corneal ulceration is severe or the globe is ruptured. Breed predisposition should also lead one to suspect glaucoma.

References and Suggested Reading

Gelatt KN, ed: Veterinary Ophthalmology, 2nd ed. Philadelphia: Lea & Febiger, 1991.
An in-depth review of all of the diseases that can cause a red eye.
Kaswan RL, Martin CL: Surgical correction of third eyelid prolapse in dogs. J Am Vet Med Assoc 186:83, 1983.
A description of the surgical technique for repairing prolapse of the gland of the third eyelid by tacking the gland to the ventral orbital rim.
Morgan RM, Duddy JM, McClurg K: Prolapse of the gland of the third eyelid in dogs: A retrospective study of 89 cases (1980–1990). J Am Anim Hosp Assoc 29:56, 1993.
A description of the pocket technique of surgical replacement of prolapse of the gland of the third eyelid.

Differential Diagnosis of Anisocoria

NANCY B. COTTRILL
Metairie, Louisiana

Anisocoria, or different size pupils, is abnormal. The clinician's role is to first determine which pupil is abnormal, and then to determine the underlying cause—be it ophthalmic, neurologic, or otherwise—by using his or her powers of observation and deduction to solve the mystery. The purpose of this article is to guide the reader toward a diagnosis by first examining the normal pupil and pupillary light reflexes and then determining the cause of the abnormality. Once the cause is known, a prognosis can be given. And, after all, these are the essential elements that the client wants to know: What is wrong? What caused it? How is it treated? Will it get better? (And how much will it cost?)

There are two types of anisocoria: dynamic and static. Dynamic anisocoria is present when the pupils are of different sizes depending on which pupil is stimulated. It is normal for the pupil receiving direct stimulation to be more miotic than the fellow pupil because of the decussation of fibers at two locations, the optic chiasm and the pretectal nucleus, yielding more input to the stimulated eye. At the first site, the optic chiasm, the fibers are crossing to the contralateral side, and at the second site, the pretectal nucleus, the fibers are crossing back to the ipsilateral side. Static anisocoria refers to unequal pupils when both eyes are receiving equal illumination, in either ambient room light or dim light.

A thorough medical history, not restricted to ophthalmologic or neurologic queries, is essential. Standard questions should be posed regarding past medical history, current medications, current medical conditions, and physical signs. The owner should be asked about any trauma, or an absence of the pet from its environment for a period of time. The practitioner should ask about prior treatment, by either the owner or a previous veterinarian. Occasionally, a veterinarian will use atropine in the examination room as a diagnostic tool, instead of the appropriate, short-acting, mydriatic-cycloplegic tropicamide. Unfortunately, atropine effects may last 2 weeks in the uninflamed eye, confounding diagnostic efforts. Owners may try home remedies which can include medications used for a previous condition that may alter the pupil size.

A complete ophthalmic examination should be done. This examination must include tonometry; other ophthalmic diagnostic tests (fluorescein stain, Schirmer tear test, etc.) should be done as indicated. Finally, a physical examination is done.

Recording the examination findings is encouraged. This activity is helpful in that it commits the examiner to a decision about the observations. It is also invaluable in compiling the information for review before making a decision regarding the etiology of the anisocoria.

THE PUPIL

Anatomy

The afferent arm of the pupillary light reflex (PLR) consists of the retina, optic nerve, optic chiasm, and optic tract. Nerve fibers in the nasal retina decussate to the opposite optic tract. In the dog, approximately 75% of the optic nerve fibers decussate to the contralateral optic tract, with the remaining fibers remaining ipsilateral. In the cat, approximately 65% of the optic nerve fibers decussate. The optic tract includes both sensory visual fibers and pupillomotor fibers. The destinations of these two fiber types differ and aid in localizing lesions by noting the presence or absence of vision in each eye. The pupillomotor fibers progress to the pretectal nucleus and from there the majority of these fibers decussate to the parasympathetic nucleus of the oculomotor nerve on the contralateral side. This second decussation marks a return to the originating side of the impulse. The visual fibers proceed sequentially to the lateral geniculate nucleus, the optic radiation, and the occipital cortex. Therefore, lesions causing anisocoria affecting both pupillary light reflexes *and* vision are limited to the retina, optic nerve, optic chiasm, and optic tract. Lesions affecting vision, but not PLRs, are located in the lateral geniculate, optic radiation, or occipital

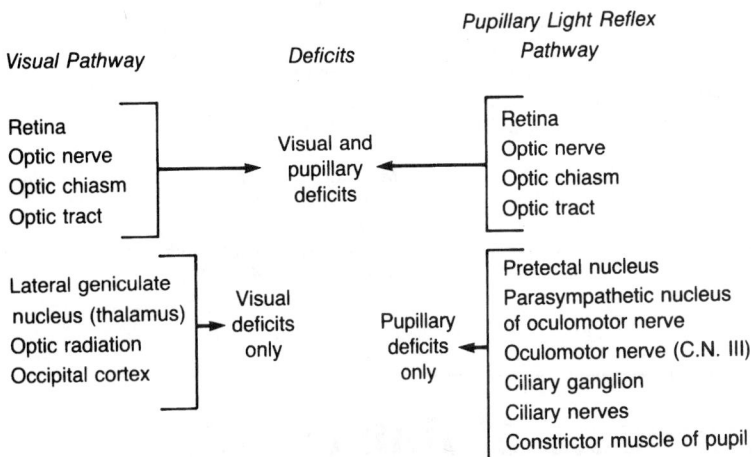

Figure 1. Deficits from lesions of the visual and pupillary light reflex pathways. (From Oliver JE, Lorenz MD, Kornegay JN, eds: Blindness, anisocoria, and abnormal eye movements. In: Handbook of Veterinary Neurology, 3rd ed. Philadelphia: WB Saunders, 1997, p 274, with permission.)

cortex. Lesions affecting the optic chiasm and parasympathetic nucleus of CN III usually are bilateral (Fig. 1).

The efferent arm of the PLR consists of the parasympathetic fibers in the oculomotor nerve that travel to the ciliary ganglion, ciliary nerves, and finally the iris constrictor muscle (see Fig. 3). There are distinct differences in the composition of the canine and feline postganglionic fibers (ciliary nerves). In the dog, there are five to eight short ciliary nerves that have both sympathetic and parasympathetic efferent fibers. Therefore, the canine short ciliary nerves are considered "mixed." A lesion of the ciliary nerve in the dog results in a midrange pupil because both autonomic fibers are lost. The cat, in contrast, has two short ciliary nerves that are solely parasympathetic. These nerves are the nasal and malar (temporal) nerves. In the right eye, a lesion of the nasal nerve will result in a D-shaped pupil. A lesion of the malar nerve will result in a reverse D-pupil in the right eye.

The efferent sympathetic arm affects the iris dilator muscle. The path that the sympathetic axons traverse is as follows: hypothalamus, preganglionic cell bodies in spinal cord segments T1 to T3, spinal nerve ventral roots, thoracic and cervical sympathetic trunk, cranial cervical ganglion, middle ear, cavernous sinus, into the periorbita, nasociliary nerve, long ciliary nerve, ciliary body and finally the iris dilator muscle (see Fig. 3).

Normal Pupillary Light Reflexes

A direct PLR is elicited by directing a *bright* light source into the pupil. Ideally, this is a focused, 3.5-volt halogen light source such as a Finoff transilluminator (Welch-Allyn). The Finoff head can be attached to the battery handle used for a direct ophthalmoscope or otoscope. A penlight's illumination is too diffuse and often dim. A weak light source decreases the amplitude of contraction, the length of time before contraction, and the duration of the contraction. The light source should be of a consistent illumination to allow the examiner to be familiar with the expected response in the examination room. Pupillary constriction upon direct light stimulation is known as the direct PLR. The constriction in the fellow eye is known as the consensual response, is usually not quite as complete as the direct response, and is the result

of the decussation of fibers at the optic chiasm to the contralateral side. If the PLR is not complete, the light should be redirected to another part of the fundus. Areas of the retina have different sensitivities; the "area centralis" in the dorsotemporal region near the optic disc is the most sensitive when measuring pupillary contraction. It is easiest to see the direct and consensual reflexes by gently retracting both upper eyelids and directing the light into the eye being tested, while an assistant is holding the pet. The clinician can easily look at the consensual pupil while still directing the light into the other eye. Normal pupillary responses include physiologic anisocoria, equal pupils in diffuse light, and pupils that are dilated maximally and equally after dark adaptation.

THE OPHTHALMIC EXAMINATION

Visual Status

It is important to determine the visual status of each eye *before* checking the PLRs. The strongest menace reflex is usually obtained in the initial part of the examination, before the pet has been subjected to having bright lights shone in its eyes numerous times, but after it is relatively calm on the table. A properly done menace test, done without creating air currents or noise, is often the most helpful test for vision. Tracking, usually done with cotton balls dropped in front of the patient while shielding one eye, is also helpful. Brightly colored soft balls used for kitten toys provide better contrast against the background of the clinician's white coat than a white cotton ball when determining tracking ability. Maze tests and visual placing are other vision tests. Findings should be recorded (Fig. 2).

Pupillary Light Reflexes

The PLRs should be assessed in ambient light first, with findings recorded as normal, absent, incomplete, or minimal (see Fig. 2). Committing to a response and some qualifying information about the response is valuable.

Swinging Flashlight Test

The swinging flashlight test is used to assess and compare the function of the retina and optic nerve in one eye

	OD	OS
Vision	−	+
Pupillary Light Reflexes		
Direct	−	+
Consensual	+	−

Figure 2. Grid to record visual status and pupillary light reflexes (PLRs). Entry variables include " + " = normal, " − " = absent, "I" = incomplete, "M" = minimal. The latter two variables are used to designate degrees of constriction in the PLRs. The "incomplete" designation may be used in cases of iris atrophy, for example. The example in the chart above depicts the responses of a lesion of the right retina or prechiasmal optic nerve.

versus the other. The bright light is directed into one pupil for a few seconds, and then redirected into the fellow eye. The normal response is for the first pupil to fully constrict. A slight redilation can occur after the constriction in a normal eye. This redilation is a normal response to adaptation of the retina to the light stimulus and is known as *pupillary escape*. The abnormal response is for the second eye to continue to dilate as the light is directed into it. This is known as a *positive swinging flashlight test* (or Marcus Gunn sign) and is a hallmark of an afferent lesion in the retina or prechiasmal optic nerve. A negative swinging flashlight test will be discussed later.

Dark Adaptation Test

Once these initial tests are completed, the lights should be turned off to allow the pet's eyes (and the examiner's) to adapt to the darkness for approximately two minutes. With the light source set at a bright illumination and centered between *the examiner's* eyes, a tapetal reflex should be obtained simultaneously from both of the patient's eyes. Are the pupils now equal and maximally dilated? Or is the anisocoria still present? The findings should be recorded. The examiner should repeat the swinging flashlight test in the dark because differences are more marked after dark adaptation.

Balance of the Ophthalmic Examination

After vision testing and pupillary light reflexes are assessed, a thorough ocular examination is in order. The only lesions that you will miss are the ones that you do not look for. This part of the examination will allow the examiner to rule out, or in, ophthalmic causes of anisocoria.

NON-NEUROLOGIC CAUSES OF ANISOCORIA

Ophthalmic Causes of Anisocoria

Ophthalmic causes of anisocoria can be divided into conditions that cause miosis (a constricted pupil) or those that cause mydriasis (a dilated pupil).

Conditions That Cause Miosis

Anterior uveitis is recognized by miosis, generalized corneal edema, "cloudiness" of the anterior chamber due to an increase in the protein content of the aqueous humor, hyperemic conjunctiva, and low intraocular pressure (as measured by tonometry). PLRs may be sluggish, or they may be difficult to see in cases of extreme miosis.

Posterior synechiae, which are the result of anterior uveitis, are the adhesion of the iris to the anterior lens capsule. The posterior synechiae often create an irregular pupil. PLRs may be slow or absent, depending on the extent of the adhesions. Please note that in some cases, posterior synechiae may form in the position of a dilated pupil.

Corneal ulcers and corneal lacerations cause a reflex miosis mediated by the trigeminal nerve, called the axonal reflex. These conditions are easily recognized by focal corneal edema, plus or minus a corneal stromal defect, and the retention of fluorescein dye.

Conditions That Cause Mydriasis

Iris atrophy is recognized by an irregular or scalloped-edge pupil, and transillumination defects in the iris. When a light is directed toward the fundus, the tapetum reflects light back through the pupil. In the presence of iris atrophy, light can be seen through the body of the iris. Initial constriction may be normal or minimal, and is often best seen with magnification. The constriction is incomplete. Iris atrophy is more common in older patients, particularly poodles, and in Siamese cats.

Iris hypoplasia, a congenital defect, is seen as an irregular area of pigmentation where iris stroma is absent. The darker pigmentation seen in these areas is due to the posterior pigmented epithelium of the iris. The pupil margin is irregular and scalloped, and transillumination defects may be seen. The constriction characteristics are similar to those of iris atrophy.

Posterior synechiae may form when the pupil is dilated, as often occurs in cases of glaucoma that are preceded by anterior uveitis. Chow chows and Bassett hounds are particularly prone to this sequence of events. PLRs are slow or absent.

Other conditions may cause mydriasis. Iridoplegia may result from severe blunt trauma to the eye that damages the constrictor fibers. Glaucoma features episcleral congestion, generalized corneal edema, and intraocular pressure above normal (as measured by tonometry). PLRs are slow or absent. Visual deficits are usually present. Retinal detachment has the appearance of a veil containing blood vessels coming toward the observer. The "veil" is often undulating. Retinal detachment may predispose to glaucoma; the intraocular pressure should be measured, as in all cases of anisocoria. PLRs are slow or absent. Visual deficits are usually present.

Severe chorioretinitis, active or inactive, that affects one eye more than the other, can cause mydriasis unilaterally. Areas of active chorioretinitis have a dull tapetal reflex, are often gray, and have indistinct edges. Areas of inactive chorioretinitis have a brighter than normal tapetal reflex (due to retinal atrophy) and distinct edges. There are usually visual deficits.

Pharmacologic Causes of Anisocoria

Pharmacologic causes of anisocoria can also be divided into drugs that produce miosis and those that produce mydriasis. Miosis is most often caused by pilocarpine administration. Mydriasis can be caused by atropine administration, ocular contact with jimsonweed or other toxic plants, or topical administration of collyria or ocular decongestants containing phenylephrine. Exposure to pharmacologic agents that alter the pupil size should be revealed when the patient history is obtained.

NEUROLOGIC CAUSES OF ANISOCORIA

Afferent Versus Efferent PLR Defects

Two rules of thumb are of great service. The first is that the pupils in afferent lesions dilate maximally and equally in the dark. The second is that in efferent lesions, pupils remain unequal after dark adaptation.

Afferent Lesion Characteristics

Anisocoria due to an afferent arm lesion is replaced with equal, maximally dilated pupils in the dark since the stimulus (light) for the abnormal response (mydriasis) is eliminated. Thus, another distinguishing feature of afferent lesions is that anisocoria is more prominent in the light. If the pupils remain unequal, or do not dilate completely in the dark, the lesion must be in the efferent (parasympathetic) arm of the PLR, in the sympathetic efferent arm, or be ophthalmic or pharmacologic in origin. Afferent lesions cause abnormal PLRs in *both* the abnormal and the normal pupil (Table 1; Fig. 3).

Efferent Lesion Characteristics

An efferent lesion causes persistent anisocoria after dark adaptation. This is true except for lesions in the efferent arm of the PLR in cats. Efferent lesions also cause the pupil on the affected side to have diminished, or absent, responses to both direct and indirect light. The pupil on the unaffected side will have normal direct and consensual PLRs. Efferent lesions of the parasympathetic system will cause an anisocoria that increases in light because the

deficit in constriction will be more apparent. The abnormal pupil will be the mydriatic one. Efferent lesions of the sympathetic system will cause an anisocoria that increases in the dark because the deficit in dilation, and unopposed constriction by the parasympathetic system, will be more apparent. The abnormal pupil will be the miotic one. Efferent lesions do not cause visual deficits (see Table 1 and Fig. 3).

Afferent Lesions

Unilateral Retinal or Prechiasmal Optic Nerve

These lesions feature mydriasis on the affected side, a slow or absent direct PLR but a normal consensual PLR, visual deficits, and a positive swinging flashlight test. The last feature is pathognomonic for lesions in these sites. The fundus is examined to determine which of these sites contains the lesion. If the fundic examination is normal, an electroretinogram (ERG) can be done to localize the lesion. If the ERG is normal (the retina is functioning), then the retrobulbar (prechiasmal) optic nerve is affected.

Unilateral Optic Tract

These lesions feature a consistently miotic pupil on the side of the lesion regardless of which eye is receiving the light stimulus, visual deficits, and a *negative* swinging flashlight test. The pupil is consistently miotic because of the lack of input to the pretectal nucleus on the side of the lesion. Because the majority (75% in dogs, 65% in cats) of the nerve fibers in each optic tract decussated from the *contralateral* optic nerve, the pretectal nucleus no longer receives that input, so no impulses progress from there to decussate a second time to the contralateral parasympathetic nucleus of CN III, which would then deliver the impulse to the oculomotor nerve. A different way to phrase this is to describe the contralateral pupil as being slightly mydriatic regardless of which eye is being stimulated. The eye opposite the lesion will have a partial visual deficit

TABLE 1. **Signs of Lesions in the Visual Pathways**

Complete Lesion on Right Side	Vision		Resting Pupil		Pupillary Light Reflex	
	Right Eye	Left Eye	Right Eye	Left Eye	Light in Right Eye	Light in Left Eye
1. Retina or optic nerve	Absent	Normal	Slightly dilated	Normal	No response	Both constrict
2. Orbit (CN II, III)	Absent	Normal	Dilated	Normal	No response	Left constricts
3. Optic chiasm (bilateral)*	Absent	Absent	Dilated	Dilated	No response	No response
4. Optic tract	Normal	Absent†	Normal or slightly miotic	Normal or slightly dilated	Both constrict	Both constrict
5. Lateral geniculate nucleus	Normal	Absent†	Normal	Normal	Both constrict	Both constrict
6. Optic radiation	Normal	Absent†	Normal	Normal	Both constrict	Both constrict
7. Occipital cortex	Normal	Absent†	Normal	Normal	Both constrict	Both constrict
8. Parasympathetic nucleus of CN III (bilateral)*	Normal	Normal	Dilated	Dilated	No response	No response
9. Oculomotor nerve	Normal	Normal	Dilated	Normal	Left constricts	Left constricts
10. Sympathetic nerve	Normal	Normal	Constricted	Normal	Both constrict	Both constrict

*Unilateral lesions of these structures are rare.
†Possibly loss of sight in left visual field with partial sparing of right visual field.
Modified from Oliver JE, Lorenz MD: Blindness, anisocoria, and abnormal eye movements. In: Oliver JE, Lorenz MD: Handbook of Veterinary Neurology. Philadelphia: WB Saunders, 1994, p 261, with permission.

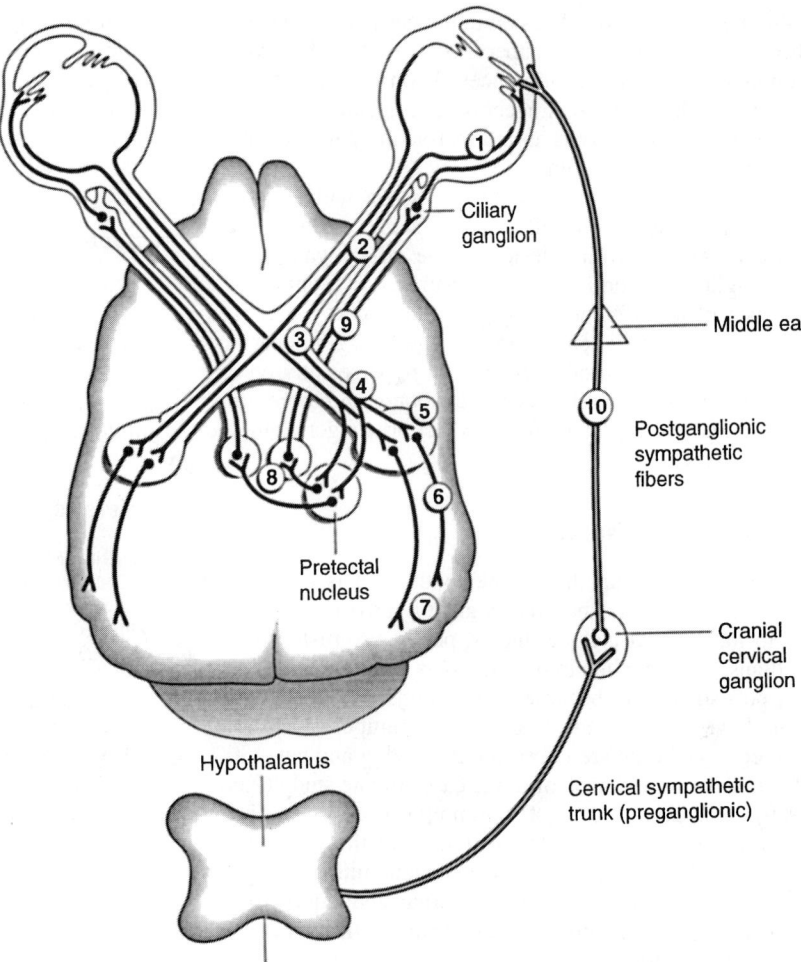

Figure 3. Pathways for vision, the pupillary light reflex, and the sympathetic pathway affecting the eye. Numbers correspond to structures, as lesion sites, in Table 1. (Modified and redrawn from Oliver JE, Lorenz MD, Kornegay JN: Blindness, anisocoria, and abnormal eye movements. In: Oliver JE, Lorenz MD, Kornegay JN, eds: Handbook of Veterinary Neurology, 3rd ed. Philadelphia: WB Saunders, 1997, p 275, with permission.)

because the majority of the optic tract is composed of the nasal retinal fibers of the fellow eye.

Optic Chiasm

Chiasm lesions rarely cause anisocoria because a lesion in this site usually causes bilateral mydriatic pupils, PLR absence, and vision loss.

Efferent Lesions

Parasympathetic Efferent

Lesions of the nucleus of CN III and the preganglionic fibers cause similar signs, previously described (see "Efferent Lesion Characteristics"), in dogs and cats. Unilateral lesions of CN III, preganglionic fibers, ciliary ganglion, or short ciliary nerves *in the cat* produce the same signs because only parasympathetic fibers are affected. In the cat, a lesion of the nasal nerve causes a "D" pupil in the right eye because only the temporal half of the iris can constrict, and a "reverse D" pupil if the malar (temporal) nerve is diseased because only the nasal half can constrict. Efferent arm lesions in the cat produce symmetrical, maximally dilated pupils after dark adaptation. The short ciliary nerves *in the dog* are mixed, containing both parasympa-

thetic and sympathetic fibers; lesions of the ciliary ganglion or ciliary nerves will affect the ability of the iris to constrict *and* to dilate. Therefore, in the dog, anisocoria will persist after dark adaptation; the pupil on the affected side will not match the dilation of the normal side.

Internal ophthalmoplegia, which is not a result of pharmacologic blockade, usually results from impairment of either the iris sphincter muscle or the parasympathetic innervation to the muscle. Internal ophthalmoplegia may be due to trauma from proptosis or retrobulbar disease (retrobulbar abscess/cellulitis/hemorrhage/neoplasm), midbrain lesions, or it may be idiopathic. The parasympathetic fibers are superficial and medial to the oculomotor fibers of CN III; they are more susceptible to trauma and can be affected without the oculomotor fibers being affected. If the oculomotor fibers are impaired, this is referred to as external ophthalmoplegia, and ptosis and lateral strabismus are present.

Pharmacologic Localization of Parasympathetic Lesions

Pharmacologic testing confirms the presence of a lesion in the efferent arm of the PLR, and rules out pharmacologic blockade and iridal disease. It also serves to localize the lesion as preganglionic or postganglionic related to denervation hypersensitivity. A lesion in the ganglion or postganglionic fibers will cause supersensitivity to what would normally be an ineffective concentration of a parasympathomimetic drug. The first agent used in localizing a lesion in the efferent pathway is an indirect-acting parasympathomimetic, 0.5% physostigmine.

The desired response is miosis. An eye with a central or preganglionic lesion will constrict sooner than the normal eye. An eye with a lesion in the ciliary ganglion or postganglionic fibers will not constrict. To confirm the presence of an efferent arm lesion, but not its location, a direct-acting parasympathomimetic agent, 2% pilocarpine (Isopto Carpine) is used. Denervation hypersensitivity will cause the affected pupil to constrict sooner and more completely, and to maintain the constriction longer than the normal eye.

Sympathetic Efferent

The loss of sympathetic tone to the eye is commonly known as Horner's syndrome. Signs of Horner's syndrome are ipsilateral and include miosis, ptosis, protrusion of the nictitans, and enophthalmos. Miosis is the most consistent and persistent sign, because it may remain after the other signs have disappeared. A significant number of cases of Horner's syndrome are idiopathic in the dog and cat—50% of canine cases and 42% of feline cases in one study (Kern, 1989). However, the most common causes of Horner's syndrome in small animals are trauma to the head, neck, and chest; brachial plexus root avulsion; intracranial and thoracic neoplasia; otitis media/interna; and injury to the external ear canal incurred during cleaning. In my practice, the most common cause is chronic otitis.

Pharmacologic Localization of Sympathetic Efferent Lesions

Mydriasis is the desired response in this test. The same principles for denervation hypersensitivity apply to sympathetic lesions. The first step is to instill an indirect-acting sympathomimetic, 1% hydroxyamphetamine (Paredrine), into both eyes. The affected pupil will dilate if the lesion is central or preganglionic. No or little dilation will occur if the lesion is postganglionic. The second step, to confirm a postganglionic lesion, is to instill a direct-acting sympathomimetic, 10% phenylephrine, into each eye. The denervated pupil reacts by dilating; this concentration is too weak to cause dilation in a normal pupil.

Spastic Pupil Syndrome

This syndrome occurs only in cats and is characterized by a static anisocoria, a failure to dilate after dark adaptation, a fluctuating anisocoria that can change from day to day, no visual deficits or iris deficits, and a positive feline leukemia virus status. There may be intervals where the pupils are normal.

References and Suggested Reading

Bercovitch M, Krohne S, Lindley D: A diagnostic approach to anisocoria. Compendium 17:661, 1995.
  A review of anisocoria with a step-by-step approach to diagnosis.
Collins BK: Disorders of the pupil. In: August JR, ed: Consultations in Feline Internal Medicine 2. Philadelphia: WB Saunders, 1994, p 421.
  A review of the neuroanatomy of pupillary function and disorders of the pupil in the cat with differential diagnoses, and an easy-to-understand discussion of pharmacologic testing of efferent lesions.
Kern TJ, Aromando MS, Erb HN: Horner's syndrome in dogs and cats: 100 cases (1975-1985). J Am Vet Med Assoc 195:369, 1989.
  Retrospective study of Horner's syndrome with an emphasis on etiology.
Morgan RV, Zanotti SW: Horner's syndrome in dogs and cats: 49 cases (1980-1986). J Am Vet Med Assoc 194:1096, 1989.
  Retrospective study examining etiology, pharmacologic testing, recovery rates, resolution time, treatment and prognosis.
Neer TM, Carter JD: Anisocoria in dogs and cats: Ocular and neurologic causes. Compend Contin Educ Pract Vet 9:817, 1987.
  Review of anisocoria and other pupillary disorders (feline dysautonomia, tonic pupils) with somewhat more emphasis on neurology than ophthalmology.
Oliver JE, Lorenz MD: Blindness, anisocoria, and abnormal eye movements. In: Oliver JE, Lorenz MD: Handbook of Veterinary Neurology. Philadephia: WB Saunders, 1994, p 261.
  Practical guide to establishing a diagnosis in anisocoria with helpful tables and diagrams.
Scagliotti R: Current concepts in veterinary neuro-ophthalmology. Vet Clin North Am 10:417, 1980.
  The classic reference for veterinary neuro-ophthalmology.

Eyelid Diseases

Erin S. Champagne
Columbia, Missouri

EYELID DISEASES

Normal eyelid anatomy and function are essential to ocular health. The following is a discussion of some of the more commonly seen medical conditions that affect the lids of dogs and cats. Therapy of eyelid disorders that are considered surgical conditions (entropion, ectropion, lash disorders, eyelid agenesis, dermoids, etc.) are described in appropriate textbooks of surgery, and are not included here.

Infectious and Inflammatory Diseases

Hordeolum and Chalazion

A hordeolum is a focal abscess of a sebaceous gland of the lid usually due to a staphylococcal infection. An external hordeolum involves the glands of Zeis and Moll, whereas an internal hordeolum involves the meibomian glands and is the type more commonly seen in the dog. Treatment includes warm compresses, manual expression of the glands to remove retained secretions and appropriate topical antibiotic therapy. When retained meibomian secretions elicit a foreign-body response and granuloma formation occurs, this is termed a chalazion. A chalazion appears as a firm, yellow mass on the conjunctival surface of the lid margin, and may not require treatment. Curettage may aid resolution, and is performed by applying topical anesthetic, everting the lid, and removing the material with a chalazion curet or other appropriate instrument. Topical antibiotics and corticosteroids for several days may be indicated.

Bacterial Blepharitis

Inflammation of the eyelids is termed blepharitis. *Staphylococcus,* the most commonly incriminated organism, may cause blepharitis as a result of simple infection or a hypersensitivity response. A condition most often seen in puppies is a hypersensitivity reaction characterized by multifocal, often large, abscesses along the lid margin with marked edema. The abscesses can be cultured by aspiration with a fine-gauge needle following topical anesthesia, or by lancing an abscess with a larger gauge needle. Treatment should consist of warm compresses several times a day and appropriate topical and systemic antibiotic therapy (e.g., cephalosporins). Concurrent oral corticosteroid therapy is often necessary beginning with 1.1 mg/kg prednisolone b.i.d. for 10 to 14 days and then tapered to effect. If clinical signs do not resolve or improve dramatically following 3 to 4 weeks of therapy, or if recurrence is a problem, then the use of staphage lysate (Delmont Laboratories) should be considered. Bacterial blepharitis in older dogs is often associated with other conditions such as keratoconjunctivitis sicca, atopy, seborrhea, and hypothyroidism. Lid scrubs (commercially prepared or dilute baby shampoo), topical and systemic antibiotics, and prevention of self-trauma with an Elizabethan collar are indicated. Staphage lysate may be beneficial.

Parasitic Blepharitis

In young dogs, localized *Demodex* infestation may involve the lids and periocular areas. Clinical signs may include alopecia, crusting, and secondary pyoderma. Diagnosis is made with routine skin scrapings. The condition may be self-limiting, and treating any secondary bacterial involvement may be all that is indicated. Topical therapy with rotenone ointment (Goodwinol) may be beneficial. When treating localized or generalized demodicosis, one should take care to avoid corneal contact with acaricides, and a protective ointment should be placed in the eye before treatment.

Feline scabies, caused by *Notoedres cati*, may involve the eyelids as well as the pinna, face, and neck. The condition causes alopecia and is very pruritic, leading to excoriation. Diagnosis is by skin scraping. Treatment consists of six to eight weekly lime sulfur dips. Because the condition is highly contagious, isolation and treatment of all affected animals is recommended.

Mycotic Blepharitis

Crusting and alopecia of the lids may also be caused by fungal infections. Skin scrapings, fungal cultures, and Wood's lamp examination should be performed. Dermatophytosis is more common in cats, but may also be seen in dogs. Following application of a protective lubricant ointment, topical therapy using miconazole (Conofite, Pitman-Moore) or thiabendazole (Tresaderm, MSD AgVet) may be used. If the condition is generalized, or is nonresponsive to topical therapy, systemic antifungals may be needed. Ketoconazole (Nizoral, Jannsen) at a dose of 10 to 20 mg/kg every 24 hours or griseofulvin (Fulvicin, Schering) at a dose of 50 mg/kg every 24 hours has been recommended. Isolation of affected animals is recommended. Recently, it has been suggested that the chronic use of oily ophthalmic preparations (such as homemade cyclosporin solutions containing corn oil or olive oil) may predispose some dogs to Malassezia dermatitis. This condition may be diagnosed by skin-scraping (see p. 574) and is treated by discontinuation of the oil-containing product and, if needed, by using one of the antifungal medications listed above.

Immune-Mediated and Autoimmune Diseases

Allergic Blepharitis

Atopy is frequently manifested as periocular pruritus. Secondary alopecia, excoriation, and pyoderma may be seen. Medical therapy consisting of topical and/or systemic corticosteroids or antihistamines may be used; however, hyposensitization following intradermal skin testing is recommended. A number of topical ophthalmic preparations, most notably the aminoglycosides, are commonly incriminated as a cause for allergic blepharoconjunctivitis. However, if worsening of the condition occurs while on a medication, any topical drug should be suspected as a possible culprit, and a trial withdrawal period considered.

Uveodermatologic Syndrome

Uveodermatologic syndrome, also called Vogt-Koyanagi-Harada (VKH)-like syndrome, is believed to be an autoimmune disease where melanocytes are the target cells. Along with an often severe bilateral anterior uveitis, posterior uveitis, or panuveitis, poliosis and vitiligo of the lids, periocular, and perioral skin are seen. The skin lesions are often intensely pruritic, with crusting, ulceration, and excoriation common. Although the condition may occur in any number of breeds of dogs, the Akita is predisposed. Initial treatment consists of immunosuppressive doses of oral corticosteroids, tapering to the lowest dose that will control the condition. The disease is often difficult to manage, and high doses are frequently needed, leading to significant side effects. The addition of azathioprine (Imuran, Buroughs-Wellcome) is often necessary. If the condition is controlled, the poliosis and vitiligo may resolve. Autoimmune dermatoses (pemphigus foliaceus, pemphigus erythematosus, systemic lupus erythematosus, discoid lupus) may involve the lids and periocular region before more generalized signs are present. Lesions involve the surface and mucocutaneous junctions of the eyelid margins, and may manifest as vesicles or bullae, ulcers, crusts, and alopecia. Skin biopsies should be performed to confirm the diagnosis, and treatment using immunosuppressive doses of oral corticosteroids is frequently necessary. Refractory cases may require azathioprine (see *CVT XII,* pp. 636 to 638).

Neoplasia

The most common lid neoplasms in dogs (adenomas, papillomas, melanomas) are benign and can be treated by sharp resection, cryosurgery, or laser ablation. All tissue removed should be submitted for histopathologic examination because malignant masses do occur. Squamous cell carcinoma, basal cell carcinoma, adenocarcinoma, mast cell tumor, malignant melanoma, hemangiosarcoma, and myoblastoma have been reported. Further treatment, including radiation therapy, repeat cryosurgery or laser surgery, or wide excision followed by a skin flap may be needed following histopathologic results. The lids may be involved in cases of multicentric lymphoma, and appropriate medical therapy is indicated (see *CVT XII,* pp. 494 to 497). Feline lid neoplasms are most commonly malignant and often life-threatening. Squamous cell carcinoma is the most common tumor, and tends to be locally invasive, with frequent recurrences and occasional metastasis. Treatment options include wide surgical excision (often not possible without extensive undermining and the use of skin flaps), cryosurgery, laser ablation, radiation therapy, or a combination of these. Other reported tumors include fibrosarcomas, basal cell carcinomas, and mast cell tumors.

Miscellaneous Conditions

Zinc-Responsive Dermatosis

An uncommon skin condition may be seen in young adult Siberian huskies, Alaskan malamutes and Bull terriers. Even when fed a diet adequate in zinc, these dogs develop zinc deficiencies probably related to decreased absorption (see p. 519). The condition may also be seen in dogs, especially rapidly growing puppies fed a zinc-deficient diet and in dogs on diets high in phytates (high-calcium or high-cereal diet), which bind zinc. Signs are often most pronounced in the periocular skin and lids and consist of alopecia, erythema, crusts, and variable pruritus. Diagnosis is made via history, physical examination, and skin biopsy. Treatment consists of correcting any underlying dietary deficiency, or by lifelong supplementation of zinc when poor absorption is suspected.

Sterile Pyogranulomas

Sterile pyogranulomas of unknown etiology may involve the eyelids. These simulate neoplasms, can be quite extensive and multiple, and may ulcerate. Recurrence may be seen. On histopathologic examination, the lesions appear as nodular to diffuse granulomatous or pyogranulomatous inflammation. No evidence of neoplasia is seen, and no etiologic agents are identified. Bacterial and fungal cultures are negative. In the majority of dogs, no response is seen to systemic antibiotics; however, a good response is noted to immunosuppressive doses of oral corticosteroids.

References and Suggested Reading

Angarano DW: Dermatologic disorders of the eyelid and periocular region. In: Kirk RW, ed: Current Veterinary Therapy X. Philadelphia: WB Saunders, 1989, pp 678–681.

Barrie KP, Parshall CJ: Eyelid pyogranulomas in four dogs. J Am Anim Hosp Assoc 15:433, 1979.

Chambers ED, Severin GA: Staphylococcal bacterin for treatment of chronic staphylococcal blepharitis in the dog. J Am Vet Med Assoc 185:422, 1984.

Gelatt KN: The canine eyelids. In: Gelatt KN, ed: Veterinary Ophthalmology, 2nd ed. Philadelphia: Lea & Febiger, 1991, pp 256–275.

Johnson BW, Campbell KL: Dermatoses of the canine eyelid. Compend Contin Educ Pract Vet 11:385, 1989.

Kirschner SE: Diseases of the eyelids and conjunctiva. In: Kirk RW, Bonagura JD, eds: Current Veterinary Therapy XI. Philadelphia: WB Saunders, 1992, pp 1085–1092.

Nasisse MP: Feline ophthalmology. In: Gelatt KN, ed: Veterinary Ophthalmology, 2nd ed. Philadelphia: Lea & Febiger, 1991, pp 529–575.

Panich R, Scott DW, Miller WH: Canine cutaneous sterile pyogranuloma/granuloma syndrome: A retrospective analysis of 29 cases (1979–1988). J Am Anim Hosp Assoc 27:519, 1991.

Roberts SM, Severin GA, Lavach JD: Prevalence and treatment of palpebral neoplasms in the dog: 200 cases (1975–1983). J Am Vet Med Assoc 189:1355, 1986.

Scott DW, Miller WH, Griffin CE: Muller and Kirk's Small Animal Dermatology, 5th ed. Philadelphia: WB Saunders, 1995, pp 956–960.

Diagnosis and Treatment of Canine Conjunctivitis

BRIAN C. GILGER

Raleigh, North Carolina

Canine conjunctivitis, or inflammation of the conjunctiva, is rarely primary; it is almost always secondary to another ocular, periocular, or systemic cause. When presented with a dog that has an inflamed conjunctiva, it is important that the clinician search for the underlying cause or causes of the conjunctivitis and treat it specifically, and avoid nonspecific therapy.

CONJUNCTIVITIS: RESPONSE TO INJURY

An injured conjunctiva responds by developing hyperemia, chemosis, ocular discharge, and possibly forming follicles. Hyperemic, or reddened, conjunctival vasculature may appear similar to deeper episcleral vascular hyperemia. It is important to differentiate conjunctival from episcleral vascular hyperemia because the latter typically is in response to intraocular inflammation such as uveitis or glaucoma. To differentiate between conjunctival and episcleral vessels, the clinician can place 1 drop of 0.5% proparacaine on the affected eye and, using a cotton-tipped applicator, gently attempt to move the conjunctiva. If the hyperemic vessels move with the conjunctiva, the dog most likely has conjunctivitis. If the conjunctiva moves freely over the vessels, the dog probably has intraocular inflammation. Conjunctival vessels also blanch quickly in response to topically applied diluted epinephrine or phenylephrine; episcleral vessels blanch very slowly, if at all. If intraocular inflammation is suspected, measurement of intraocular pressure is indicated. High intraocular pressures would suggest glaucoma as the cause of the episcleral hyperemia; low intraocular pressures would suggest uveitis. Conjunctival hyperemia also tends to be bright red and intense at the conjunctival fornix. Chemosis is swelling or edema of the conjunctiva. Lymphoid follicles can also develop and, like chemosis, are a nonspecific finding associated with chronic irritation.

OCULAR DISEASES MASQUERADING AS CONJUNCTIVITIS

Five ocular conditions may initially appear as mild to moderate conjunctivitis, and these conditions should always be ruled out by the clinician when a dog presents with a hyperemic conjunctiva. These five ocular conditions are keratitis (ulcerative or nonulcerative), keratoconjunctivitis sicca (dry eye), scleritis, uveitis, and glaucoma. As mentioned previously, intraocular pressure should be measured in all cases of suspected conjunctivitis. Schirmer tear test values should also be measured to rule out keratoconjunctivitis sicca. Schirmer tear test values of less than 10 mm of wetting per minute suggests dry eye. Fluorescein

dye should be applied to the cornea to determine whether a corneal ulcer is present.

CAUSES OF CANINE CONJUNCTIVITIS

Dogs typically develop noninfectious conjunctivitis (in contrast to cats). There are several common causes for canine conjunctivitis (Table 1). Follicular conjunctivitis is a nonspecific inflammation of the conjunctiva that is commonly seen in young, large, active breeds of dogs. The conjunctiva is hyperemic with characteristic multiple follicle formation; these follicles are most prominent on the bulbar surface of the nictitans. Follicular conjunctivitis is thought to be immune mediated or a result of chronic irritation. Some dogs have accompanying eyelid abnormalities such as ectropion. Treatment consists of correcting eyelid abnormalities and use of topical corticosteroids (Table 2) until signs abate. Rupturing the follicles is not necessary and may lead to increased conjunctival inflammation and damage. Follicular conjunctivitis is typically recurrent but will usually resolve as the dog ages, unless the eyelid abnormalities remain uncorrected.

Allergic conjunctivitis is usually associated with atopy or food allergies. Occasionally, however, conjunctivitis is the only manifestation of the allergic condition. Allergic conjunctivitis may be seasonal. It is associated with hyperemic conjunctiva with serous discharge, and also possible periocular hyperemia, alopecia, or blepharitis. Conjunctival cytology may be helpful in diagnosing allergic conjunctivitis. A cytology sample can be obtained by gently scraping the conjunctival surface with a small spatula after use of a topical anesthetic. Presence of eosinophils in the cytology sample help confirm allergic conjunctivitis. Presence of other signs of atopy, seasonal occurrence, and lack of response to recurrence after other treatment suggest allergic conjunctivitis. Treatment consists of removing or avoiding the allergen, desensitization, topical antihistamines, or corticosteroids (see Table 2).

Bacterial infection is not a primary cause of conjunctivitis in the dog. Instead, bacterial conjunctivitis occurs when a predisposing insult alters the normal bacterial flora ho-

TABLE 1. Causes of Canine Conjunctivitis

Follicular
Allergic
Anatomic (eyelid) abnormality
Parasitic (*Thelazia*)
Bacterial
Systemic disease (distemper, rickettsial diseases)
Iatrogenic (hypersensitivity)

TABLE 2. Ocular Medication for Treatment of Canine Conjunctivitis

Medication (Trade Name)	Frequency	Indication
Antibiotics	b.i.d.–q.i.d.	
Neomycin/bacitracin/ polymyxin B		Most cases of conjunctivitis
Gentamycin		Bacterial conjunctivitis
Corticosteroids	b.i.d.–q.i.d.	
Dexamethasone 0.1%		Follicular conjunctivitis
Nonsteroidal Anti-Inflammatory Medications	q.i.d.	
Ketorolac tromethamine 0.5%		Allergic conjunctivitis
Lodoxamide tromethamine 0.1%		Allergic conjunctivitis

meostasis, allowing bacteria to proliferate. Insults to the conjunctiva that may allow this to occur include eyelid abnormalities (ectropion, entropion, lagophthalmos, trichiasis, etc.), trauma, foreign body, and possibly chronic skin disease (blepharitis, pyoderma, seborrhea). Keratoconjunctivitis sicca is another major cause of conjunctival bacterial overgrowth in dogs. A thorough ocular examination will rule out most predisposing causes of bacterial conjunctivitis. Examination of conjunctival cytology will reveal neutrophils and bacteria. Aerobic bacterial culture and sensitivity is indicated in chronic or recurrent cases; however, rarely are resistant bacteria a cause for lingering conjunctivitis. Instead, a predisposing or underlying cause is usually missed in chronic and/or recurrent conjunctivitis in dogs. Treatment for bacterial conjunctivitis in dogs involves resolving the underlying cause and use of topical broad-spectrum antibiotics (see Table 2 and *CVT XII*, p. 1211).

Parasitic conjunctivitis is uncommon, but can be caused by *Thelazia* spp. This is sometimes seen in the western United States.

SYSTEMIC DISEASE

Several infectious systemic illnesses may cause conjunctivitis. Canine distemper and Rocky Mountain spotted fever are two examples.

IATROGENIC/TOPICAL OCULAR MEDICATION HYPERSENSITIVITY

Several topical ocular medications may cause a hypersensitivity conjunctivitis. Medications that are particularly sensitizing include neomycin, trifluridine, acetylcysteine, and fortified antibiotics, among others. Dogs developing ocular medication hypersensitivity typically have conjunctivitis that clears up somewhat initially, then worsens and intensifies to severe painful conjunctivitis. Cessation of the medication allows improvement of the conjunctivitis, usually within 12 to 24 hours.

SPECIAL CONSIDERATIONS IN TREATMENT OF CANINE CONJUNCTIVITIS

As mentioned frequently above, the primary goal when treating canine conjunctivitis is to resolve the underlying or anatomic defects. Antibiotics (without hydrocortisone) should be the mainstay of treatment (see Table 2) in most cases of canine conjunctivitis. Topical corticosteroids should be avoided because they may mask underlying disorders such as uveitis or glaucoma. An exception to this is the use of corticosteroids for immune-mediated follicular conjunctivitis and in cases of allergic conjunctivitis in which topical antihistamines or desensitization have not been effective. Topical corticosteroids should be used with caution in cases with a bacterial component and should be strictly avoided in eyes that have corneal ulcers (corneal fluorescein dye retention). If the conjunctivitis does not resolve in 5 to 7 days, the underlying cause was probably missed or not treated appropriately and the dog will need to be re-evaluated. If the conjunctivitis recurs after cessation of treatment, the underlying cause was missed and the dog will need further examination and diagnostic testing.

References and Suggested Reading

Brooks DE: Canine conjunctiva and nictitating membrane. In: Gelatt KN, ed: Veterinary Ophthalmology, 2nd ed. Philadelphia: Lea & Febiger, 1991, pp 290–306.
This is a good comprehensive review of diagnosis and treatment of disorders affecting the canine conjunctiva.
Slatter D: Conjunctiva. In: Slatter D, ed: Fundamentals of Veterinary Ophthalmology, 2nd ed. Philadelphia: WB Saunders, 1990, pp 204–225.
This chapter is well illustrated and has many tables, which is good for quick reference.

Epiphora

CHARLOTTE B. KELLER
Guelph, Ontario, Canada

Epiphora originates from the Greek word *epipher(esthai)* (to rush upon) and is defined as an overflow of tears from the conjunctival sac, as may occur with faulty function of the lacrimal drainage system or from excessive lacrimation. Excessive lacrimation is always a result of ocular pain or irritation. To find the cause of the pain, a thorough and systematic eye examination is performed. Conditions that lead to excessive lacrimation ought to be ruled out first before making the diagnosis of a faulty drainage system. The patency of the nasolacrimal drainage system can be evaluated by applying topical fluorescein and observing it exiting at the nares, by flushing the duct and by dacryocystorhinography. The results of these tests have to be interpreted carefully. In some animals the nasolacrimal duct opens into the pharynx, allowing the dye to exit before it reaches the nares. Also, while the duct is being flushed, the lid is everted and therefore the normal position of the lid is altered. A positive result, therefore, indicates a patent duct but does prove that tears can drain under normal physiologic conditions. The causes of epiphora are listed in Table 1. Chronic epiphora usually leads to staining of the facial hair and moist facial dermatitis, which results in a noncosmetic appearance and an unpleasant odor.

EPIPHORA IN SMALL BREEDS

Shallow orbits, as seen in brachycephalic dogs and cats, cause prominent globe positions and, as a result, very tight fitting lids with very small lacrimal lakes. Subsequently, the tears spill over onto the face instead of remaining in the lake and draining through the nasolacrimal duct. Many of these animals also have long hairs coming from the caruncle and the medial canthal area that act as a wick and facilitate drainage of the tears onto the face (Fig. 1). In many animals the punctum, although normally developed and in the correct location, is occluded due to entropion of the medial lower lid or the entire medial canthus region. When the lid rolls in, it closes the punctum, preventing normal tear drainage. Each of these conditions alone or in combination can lead to epiphora. A careful examination of the medial canthus region and the nasolacrimal system is necessary for identifying these abnormalities.

Treatment consists of surgically correcting the abnormal lid position. A Hotz-Celsus procedure is used to correct lower medial entropion, and a medial canthoplasty with removal of the caruncle is performed in cases of medial canthal entropion (Peiffer et al, 1987). This allows better drainage through the puncta and reduces epiphora. Cryoepilation of the caruncular hair can also be helpful if surgery is not an option. The shallow orbit, the actual underlying problem, cannot be corrected.

Medical palliative treatments with oral tetracycline (50 mg/dog per day) or metronidazole (100 to 200 mg/dog per day) have been used with variable success in dogs with epiphora to reduce staining of the facial hair. They may alter tear secretion and reduce bacterial growth. Keeping the facial hair short and clean is beneficial in most cases, especially if the problem is minor. Removal of the membrana nictitans gland is a poor choice of therapy because of the risk of keratoconjunctivitis sicca in predisposed animals.

IMPERFORATE PUNCTUM

This anomaly is congenital, or acquired secondarily to scarring after trauma or severe inflammation. Atresia of the punctum mostly occurs alone but may be associated with atresia of the canaliculus or the nasolacrimal duct. Sometimes the punctum exists but is abnormally small. Epiphora is the predominant sign if the lower punctum is abnormally developed. Imperforate puncta are commonly seen in Cocker spaniels and poodles but can occur in any breed. A slight indentation in the conjunctiva is often seen in the area of the missing punctum. Flushing through the other (upper) punctum using a lacrimal cannula results in ballooning of the mucous membrane over the canaliculus. Treatment consists of surgically removing the mucous membrane over the canaliculus. The ballooning mucous membrane is held with fine forceps and excised using scissors. The opening is enlarged along the canaliculus. An antibiotic/steroid combination drug is used topically postoperatively every 8 hours for 7 to 10 days to prevent infection and reduce scarring.

OBSTRUCTED PUNCTUM

The punctum can be obstructed by inflammatory cells, debris, plant material or other foreign bodies. Usually the lower punctum is affected, causing epiphora and possibly mucopurulent discharge and conjunctivitis. Sometimes the medial canthal area is swollen. Flushing of the nasolacrimal duct through the upper punctum can dislodge debris or foreign material. This may have to be performed under

TABLE 1. Causes of Epiphora

Shallow orbits and prominent globes with tight-fitting lids and small lacrimal lakes
Aberrant hair at medial canthus and caruncle acting as a wick
Medial lower lid entropion or medial canthal entropion with punctum closure
Imperforate or obstructed punctum or canaliculus
Dacryocystitis
Obstruction of nasolacrimal duct
Irritation or pain due to distichiasis, trichiasis, ectopic cilia, entropion, conjunctival or corneal disease, uveitis, glaucoma

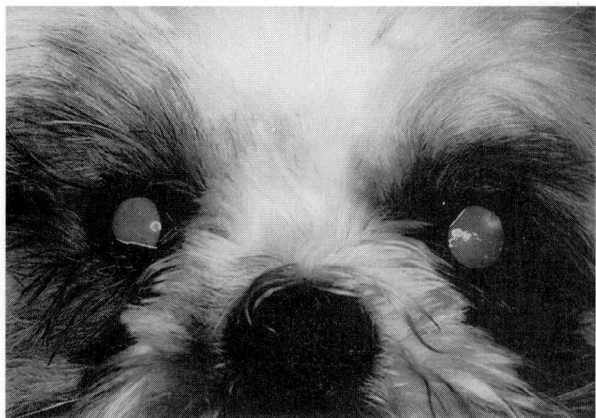

Figure 1. Bilateral epiphora in a 4-month-old Shih tzu with distichiasis, trichiasis, and ectopic cilia. Chronic epiphora leads to tear-staining of the facial hair.

sedation or general anesthesia, especially in cats. Foreign bodies may be grasped with forceps if protruding through the punctum or the punctum may need to be enlarged surgically. After the obstructing material has been removed, topical treatment with an antibiotic solution every 8 hours for 10 days is initiated.

IMPERFORATE CANALICULUS

This anomaly is relatively uncommon and usually concurrent with atresia of the punctum. Flushing of the nasolacrimal duct through the other punctum does not result in ballooning of the conjunctiva. Dacryocystorhinography may confirm the diagnosis. Treatment ideally consists of creating a new drainage pathway; however, this may be difficult to achieve. If one punctum and canaliculus exist, it may be possible to surgically create the other canaliculus and punctum. A metal cannula is placed in the existing canaliculus to define its location while a new punctum and canaliculus are created in the appropriate position using an 18-gauge needle. A size 0 monofilament suture or small polyethylene (PE50 or 90) tubing is placed in the duct and left for 2 to 3 weeks (Severin, 1982). Topical antibiotic/steroid therapy every 6 hours is maintained for the same duration. Other options include a conjunctivorhinostomy or a conjunctivobuccostomy (conjunctivoralostomy) to create a new drainage pathway into the nose or mouth, respectively (Covitz et al, 1977).

OBSTRUCTED CANALICULUS

Foreign bodies, such as plant seeds or cellular debris, can occlude the canaliculus, and in rare cases a cyst (canaliculops) can press onto the canaliculus. Clinical signs include epiphora, possibly mucopurulent discharge and swelling of the medial canthus area. Although flushing through the lower punctum is often not successful, flushing through the upper punctum may dislodge the obstructing material. Foreign bodies can sometimes be pulled out through the punctum after flushing. Surgical enlargement of the punctum and/or canaliculus may be necessary. Surgical removal of a canaliculops is performed after a dacryocystorhinogra-

phy study. Postoperative treatment with a topical antibiotic/steroid solution every 8 hours is recommended for 10 days. A large suture or small polyethylene tubing may be placed in the nasolacrimal duct after surgery for 2 to 3 weeks to prevent scarring.

LACERATION OF THE CANALICULUS

Medial canthus trauma is uncommon; however, it often results in laceration of the canaliculus. Hemorrhage and edema make recognition of the tissues difficult. Cannulation of the duct through the punctum will identify the proximal portion of the canaliculus. Finding the distal part is more challenging but may be achieved by flushing or cannulating the opposite punctum. A size 0 monofilament synthetic suture or small polyethylene tubing is placed in the nasolacrimal duct. The canaliculus may be sutured with 8-0 absorbable suture material. After the lid laceration is closed in two or more layers, the ends of the suture or tubing are sutured to the skin outside the nares and near the medial canthus. This catheter is left in place for 2 to 3 weeks. Treatment consists of systemic and topical (every 6 hours) antibiotics until the catheter is removed.

DACRYOCYSTITIS

Inflammation of the lacrimal sac is relatively uncommon. Clinical signs may include epiphora, mucopurulent discharge, conjunctivitis, and swelling of the medial canthal region just below the lower eyelid. Pain may be felt at palpation, and discharge may be forced out of the punctum. Abscessation can occur with fistulation medioventral to the lower eyelid. Cellular debris, foreign material, and swelling of the mucosa lead to obstruction of the nasolacrimal drainage system. Dacryocystorhinography may be helpful in making a diagnosis. Vigorous flushing, under sedation or general anesthesia, may dislodge obstructing material through the punctum, the fistula, or the nose. It is recommended to collect material for bacterial cultures and sensitivity testing before and/or after flushing. *Staphylococcus*, *Streptococcus*, and *E. coli* bacteria are found most commonly (Lavach et al, 1984). A nasolacrimal catheter is placed after the flushing and left in place for 2 to 3 weeks if signs improve. Topical and systemic antibiotic therapy is indicated. The choice of antibiotics may be guided by the sensitivity results. Anti-inflammatory drugs are used only if severe swelling is present. Fistulas usually heal if infection is controlled and patency restored. If clinical signs persist, repeated flushing is indicated. If the material cannot be dislodged, or if the position becomes chronic, surgical exploration of the nasolacrimal sac (dacryocystotomy) is performed. The sac is flushed through an opening made in the lacrimal bone (Laing et al, 1988).

OBSTRUCTION OF NASOLACRIMAL SYSTEM

Foreign material, inflammation, scarring from trauma, and neoplasm can cause obstruction of the nasolacrimal duct. Epiphora, mucopurulent discharge from eye and nose, and conjunctivitis may be seen. Dacryocystorhinography is necessary to make a diagnosis and localize the obstruction. Nasal endoscopy may also be helpful. Foreign material such as inflammatory debris and foreign bodies may be dislodged through vigorous flushing, restoring patency of the duct. Topical antibiotic solution is applied every 6 hours for 10 days. Repeated flushing may be necessary.

Facial trauma with bony fractures can lead to laceration and scarring of the nasolacrimal duct with secondary epiphora. Creation of a new drainage pathway into the nose (conjunctivorhinostomy) or into the mouth (conjunctivobuccostomy) is necessary to improve the clinical signs.

Nasal and paranasal tumors as well as osteomyelitis of the orbital and nasal bones may lead to deviation, occlusion, or invasion of the duct.

CILIA DISORDERS

Facial hair (trichiasis) or cilia originating from the meibomian glands (distichiasis/districhiasis) cause ocular irritation if they rub against the cornea. Clinical signs include epiphora and slight blepharospasm (see Fig. 1). Not all extra eyelashes cause irritation because they do not always touch the cornea.

Treatment of trichiasis includes shortening of the facial hair or surgical removal of the facial fold or the skin containing the cilia. Treatment of distichiasis consists of destruction of the hair follicle by heat or cold. This can be achieved using electro-, cryo- or thermo(coagulation)epilation. Hairs should not be pulled because they grow back, causing more irritation due to being short and bristly. Postoperative treatment consists of a topical antibiotic solution every 8 hours for 7 to 10 days. Postoperative ice compresses may prevent some of the swelling seen after cryoepilation.

Ectopic cilia, hairs originating from the meibomian glands but exiting through the palpebral conjunctiva, cause severe irritation often accompanied by a linear or oval corneal ulcer. The underside of the lids, mostly the upper lid, needs to be examined carefully with magnification to see the tiny hair. Often the conjunctiva around the hair is slightly elevated. After staining with fluorescein, a small positive dot may be seen in the location of the ectopic cilia.

Treatment of ectopic cilia consists of surgically removing a rectangular wedge-shaped piece of palpebral conjunctiva and meibomian gland containing the ectopic cilia. Postoperative treatment consists of a topical antibiotic solution every 8 hours for 7 to 10 days.

OTHER IRRITATING CONDITIONS

Entropion, corneal ulceration, anterior uveitis, and glaucoma are irritating and painful conditions often leading to epiphora. Diagnosis and therapy are described elsewhere in this section.

References and Suggested Reading

Covitz D, Hunziker J, Koch SA: Conjunctivorhinostomy: A surgical method for the control of epiphora in the dog and cat. J Am Vet Med Assoc 171:251, 1977.
A report on the surgical technique of conjunctivorhinostomy and the outcome of this method of therapy in 21 dogs.
Laing EJ, Spiess B, Binnington AG: Dacryocystotomy: A treatment for chronic dacryocystitis in the dog. J Am Anim Hosp Assoc 24:223, 1988.
A description of the surgical technique of dacryocystotomy and a review of three dogs receiving this therapy.
Lavach JD, Severin GA, Roberts SM: Dacryocystitis in dogs: A review of twenty-two cases. J Am Anim Hosp Assoc 20:463, 1984.
A retrospective study of dacryocystitis in dogs, describing diagnosis and therapy.
Peiffer RL, Nasisse MP, Cook CS, Harling DE: Surgery of the canine and feline orbit, adnexa and globe. Part 2: Congenital abnormalities of the eyelid and cilial abnormalities. Companion Animal Practice 27, 1987.
The second part of a nine-part series of ophthalmic surgeries in dogs and cats focusing on eyelid abnormalities including medial canthus entropion.
Severin GA: Nasolacrimal duct catheterization in the dog. J Am Anim Hosp Assoc 18:13, 1982.
A report on the technique of placing a nasolacrimal catheter in the dog.

Ocular Feline Herpesvirus-1 Infection

MARK P. NASISSE
Greensboro, North Carolina

PATHOPHYSIOLOGIC CONSIDERATIONS

Feline herpesvirus-1 (FHV-1) is probably the most common viral pathogen of domestic cats. FHV-1 is a typical alpha-herpesvirus in that it replicates in epithelial tissues during primary infection and subsequently establishes latency in the trigeminal ganglia. In response to stress, latent virus reactivates and spreads along the sensory axons to cause recrudescent disease. Because primary infection is nearly always self-limiting, specific therapy is generally reserved for recrudescent infections. The following discussion summarizes the clinical features of FHV-1 infection and provides treatment guidelines for its various clinical manifestations.

DIAGNOSIS OF FHV-1 INFECTIONS

Clinical Signs

Primary Infection

Primary infection typically occurs in young or neonatal cats and is characterized by bilateral conjunctivitis and signs of upper respiratory infection. An initially serous ocular discharge becomes purulent as the disease progresses, and the conjunctiva is severely hyperemic and moderately swollen. Although corneal lesions are usually not noticed during primary infection, close inspection after the application of rose bengal stain may reveal small, branching epithelial lesions (microdendrites). All lesions induced during primary infection are the result of direct viral cytolysis. If infection is atypically severe, symblepharon may result.

Recrudescent Infection

The clinical signs seen during recrudescent FHV-1 infection may be quite diverse. In contrast to primary infection, respiratory disease is usually absent and ocular involvement may be either unilateral or bilateral. Chronic and/or recurrent conjunctivitis is the most common manifestation of recrudescent infection (Stiles, 1995). The most consistent clinical signs are mild blepharospasm and persistent ocular discharge. For unknown reasons, chronic FHV-1 infection in cats is often associated with accumulation of a dark brown material in the medial canthus. Keratitis caused by FHV-1 occurs in two general forms; infection may be limited to the epithelium or it may involve the corneal stroma. Similar to conjunctival disease, epithelial lesions are the direct result of viral cytolysis. Although dendritic lesions are considered pathognomonic for FHV-1 infection, the majority of cases are characterized by random patterns of corneal ulceration and superficial vascularization. Stromal keratitis is usually the sequela to chronic or recurrent episodes of epithelial keratitis. In contrast to epithelial keratitis, however, stromal inflammation is thought not to be the direct result of virus infection, but presumably occurs as CD4+ T lymphocytes mount a specific immune response to viral proteins (Nasisse et al, 1995).

Interestingly, recent studies using polymerase chain reaction (PCR) technology have found that many keratectomy specimens from cats with corneal sequestration and eosinophilic keratitis are positive for FHV-1 DNA. It appears, therefore, that some or many cases of these diseases are caused by, or at least associated with, FHV-1 infection. The implications of these findings must be considered when treating these diseases.

Laboratory Methods

Virus Isolation

Although virus isolation has long been considered the gold standard for the diagnosis of viral disease, the logistics of transporting labile culture specimens makes this approach to diagnosing FHV-1 infections impractical. Furthermore, the greater sensitivity provided by PCR testing essentially makes virus isolation obsolete for clinical diagnosis.

Immunofluorescence

For more than 30 years immunofluorescence testing of conjunctival scrapings has been the laboratory method most commonly used to diagnose FHV-1 infections. Despite the low cost and simplicity of the procedure, immunofluorescence is inherently insensitive (Nasisse et al, 1993). As a consequence, like virus isolation, this procedure has largely been supplanted by PCR testing for the diagnosis of FHV-1 infections in clinical patients.

Serology

Neutralizing antibody titers from paired serum samples are commonly compared as a means of diagnosing viral infections. Because clinically relevant FHV-1 infections are usually recrudescent rather than primary, the titer to FHV-1 may not rise predictably during convalescence. Furthermore, most adult cats have been vaccinated for FHV-1, and serologic assays cannot distinguish antibodies produced by natural exposure from those produced by vaccination. Serology, therefore, is of little value in the diagnosis of this disease.

Polymerase Chain Reaction

Due to its high sensitivity and specificity, and short processing time, PCR technology has largely replaced all other methods as the procedure of choice for diagnosing FHV-1 infections (Weigler et al, 1997). In PCR it is viral DNA rather than viral proteins that are detected. For FHV-1 diagnosis we use PCR to detect a short sequence (322 base pairs) in the thymidine kinase gene of the virus. This is accomplished by mixing the clinical sample with short (approximately 20 bases) primers that are complementary to each end of the target sequence in the presence of excess deoxynucleotides and DNA polymerase. The sample is then processed in a thermal cycler where numerous temperature fluctuations cause the target DNA to sequentially denature, bind to the primer sequence, and produce new copies of the DNA. Thus, theoretically at least, a diagnosis can be made if there is as little as one copy of FHV-1 DNA in the sample.

Any clinical sample can be used to search for FHV-1 DNA using PCR (Nasisse and Weigler, 1997). Conjunctival swabs, and conjunctival or corneal scrapings are most commonly submitted. Because FHV-1 is found predominantly within epithelial cells, the test will be more reliable if many cells are present in the sample. Therefore, samples should be aggressively collected. Samples should be immediately placed in a small volume (1 ml) of sterile saline, frozen, and express-mailed on ice to the laboratory.

TREATMENT OF FHV-1 INFECTIONS

Antiviral Therapy

Topical Antiviral Agents

Ocular FHV-1 infections have historically been treated with either idoxuridine (Herplex, Allergan), vidarabine (Vira-A, Parke-Davis) or trifluorothymidine (Viroptic, Glaxo Wellcome). Each of these drugs functions by acting as a competitive nucleoside analogue or by inhibiting DNA polymerase (Nasisse, 1990). At least in vitro, Viroptic is the most effective of these drugs (Nasisse et al, 1989).

Unfortunately, however, Viroptic is also the most expensive and the most likely of these agents to cause conjunctival irritation. As a consequence, I recommend using idoxuridine initially (1 drop 5 times daily) and switching to Viroptic if improvement is not seen after 1 week. Despite the fact that Stoxil was removed from the market in 1996, a 0.1% ophthalmic solution can be obtained from pharmacies specializing in compounding preparations. It must be kept in mind that topical antiviral agents are virostatic, and must be frequently and regularly applied to be effective.

Systemic Antiviral Agents

Because viruses rely on host cell genetic machinery to produce their DNA and proteins, it has been difficult to find antiviral agents that interrupt viral synthesis without affecting host cell function. As a consequence, those antiviral agents that are used topically are too toxic for routine systemic use. Without question the most important breakthrough in anti-herpesvirus pharmacology was the development of acyclovir (Zovirax, GlaxoWellcome). Acyclovir is an acyclic nucleotide that must be phosphorylated in order to exert its antiviral effects. Because phosphorylation of acyclovir requires exposure to the thymidine kinase enzyme produced by herpesviruses, the drug is largely nontoxic in noninfected cells. Acyclovir, therefore, has become the most commonly used drug to treat herpes simplex virus infections of humans. Unfortunately, FHV-1 is considerably less susceptible to acyclovir than many other herpesviruses. Furthermore, it is very difficult to produce theoretically effective blood concentrations of this drug even after large oral dosing. It is for these reasons that acyclovir is not routinely used in cats. Nonetheless, despite the theoretical limitations of this therapeutic approach, acyclovir therapy in cats is still attempted when other forms of therapy fail. I normally recommend a starting dose of 30 to 40 mg/kg PO b.i.d. Acyclovir is available as 200-mg tablets and as a pediatric suspension (40 mg/ml). It must be emphasized that this drug is not approved for use in cats, and previous studies have shown that prolonged high blood levels can cause bone marrow depression (Nasisse et al, 1987). Acyclovir therapy, therefore, should be used only when other forms of therapy fail, and only after owners have been informed of the potential risks. I recommend keeping the course of therapy to less than 3 weeks and performing a weekly complete blood count (CBC) while on acyclovir to monitor leukocyte levels.

Immunotherapy

Interferon

Human, recombinant alpha-interferon has been used by many veterinarians to treat ocular FHV-1 infections (Intron A, Schering Corporation). Interferon therapy is highly effective only if initiated prior to exposure to the virus, and clinical efficacy studies involving herpes simplex infections of humans have produced conflicting results. Nonetheless, due to the frustrating nature of chronic FHV-1 infections, interferon therapy is often attempted, and some ophthalmologists recommend a solution containing 10^3 to 10^6 units/ml be applied topically b.i.d. to q.i.d. In a recent preliminary study, we found that very low oral doses (25 units) of alpha-interferon were partially effective at minimizing the clinical signs of FHV-1 infection even when administered after exposure. It is important to emphasize that this recommendation has been derived entirely empirically and has little scientific basis. Interestingly, at least in tissue culture, the concentration of acyclovir required to inhibit FHV-1 was reduced by a factor of 8 in the presence of alpha-interferon. Consequently, there may be some value in using these drugs concurrently in FHV-1 infected cats.

Vaccination

It has historically been recommended that cats be vaccinated with modified live, parenterally administered FHV-1 vaccines. Vaccination does produce a humoral immune response to FHV-1, and vaccination has been shown to lessen the severity of disease upon subsequent exposure. Vaccination, however, does not prevent infection, nor does it prevent establishment of latency. Because it is the interaction of the virus with the immune system at the level of the exposed mucosal surfaces that subsequently dictates what type of disease is to be produced, stimulating humoral immunity is at best an ineffective strategy for dealing with FHV-1 infections. In fact, high titers are typically found in those animals with the most severe recrudescent FHV-1 infections. Therefore, giving a parenteral vaccine to a cat with a chronic or persistent FHV-1 infection is probably a waste of time. Topical vaccination, however, may have considerably more merit as modified live topical vaccines undoubtedly stimulate a mucosal immune response and local antibody production. Although the reasons for this have yet to be determined, improvement is often noted if cats with chronic, low-grade FHV-1 conjunctivitis are vaccinated with modified live, intranasal-intraocular vaccine.

Lysine Therapy

The replication of FHV-1 is highly dependent on the amino acid arginine. At least in tissue culture, high concentrations of lysine appear to competitively inhibit the incorporation of arginine into the virus and thus suppress virus replication. We commonly use dietary lysine supplementation in an attempt to suppress virus reactivation and recrudescence in chronic FHV-1 infections. The currently recommended dosage is 250 mg per day mixed in the food. Lysine is inexpensive and is provided in 500-mg capsules as a nutritional supplement. Although the efficacy of oral lysine supplementation has yet to be proven, this form of therapy appears to be of little or no risk to the patient. It is important to use lysine for at least 4 weeks before drawing conclusions about its efficacy.

General Treatment Recommendations

Acute Conjunctivitis

Because most acute FHV-1 infections are primary infections, antiviral therapy is generally not indicated. Antibiotics that are effective against the other common feline conjunctival pathogen *Chlamydia psittaci* are applied topically 3 to 4 times daily. My preference is either tetracycline, erythromycin, or chloramphenicol ointment. Systemic antibiotics are not used unless there is conspicuous respiratory involvement.

Chronic Conjunctivitis

Provided the diagnosis has been confirmed by laboratory means, topical antibiotics are not indicated in chronic or recurrent FHV-1 conjunctivitis. My first choice for mild but persistent cases is oral lysine supplementation. If after 4 weeks there is no improvement, or if the condition is severe, topical antiviral therapy is initiated. If this fails to result in improvement, a different topical antiviral drug is selected and/or systemic acyclovir therapy is initiated. In severe cases acyclovir therapy can be combined with interferon treatment. Alternatively, the animal can be vaccinated with modified live topical vaccine.

Epithelial Keratitis

Epithelial keratitis is a clear indication for topical antiviral therapy. As stated previously, idoxuridine solution is my first choice at a frequency of five times daily. If no improvement is seen after 1 week, the animal is switched to Viroptic. If there still is no improvement, consider the recommendations described for chronic conjunctivitis.

Stromal Keratitis

Stromal keratitis is the most difficult manifestation of FHV-1 infection to treat. Because the corneal disease is perpetuated by an immune response to viral antigen, some type of anti-inflammatory therapy is indicated. However, because corticosteroids suppress viral clearance and can exacerbate epithelial infection, concurrent topical antiviral therapy should also be used. My first preference is to combine 0.2% cyclosporine ointment (Optimune, Schering Corporation)(b.i.d.) with 0.1% idoxuridine solution (t.i.d.). In more severe cases corticosteroids (0.1% dexamethasone) may be required. Concurrent lysine therapy is also indicated, and acyclovir and interferon should be tried in refractory cases.

In contrast to chronic conjunctival infections, stimulating the local immune response to FHV-1 via vaccination may be a poor therapeutic choice in cases of stromal keratitis. Because the clinical signs in stromal keratitis result from an immune response to viral antigens within the corneal stroma, it is conceivable that further sensitizing the local environment to FHV-1 antigens via vaccination may actually exacerbate the condition. As a result, I do not recommend vaccination in cats with stromal disease.

It is assumed that chronic stromal keratitis occurs because viral antigens persist within the cornea rather than being cleared. This is presumably attributable to the cornea's so-called "immune privilege" status that is created by the lack of stromal blood vessels and lymphatics, and the lack of turnover of normal stromal cells. Several therapeutic strategies can be employed to circumvent these unique corneal features. Lamellar keratectomy may be done with the rationale of physically ridding the cornea of the offending antigen. In addition, covering the keratectomy site with a pedicle conjunctival flap appears to prevent recurrences.

References and Suggested Reading

Nasisse MP: Feline herpesvirus ocular disease. Vet Clin North Am 20:667, 1990.
A thorough review of the pathophysiology, clinical signs, and treatment of FHV-1 infection.

Nasisse MP, Dorman DC, Jamison KC, et al: Effects of valaciclovir in cats infected with feline herpesvirus 1. Am J Vet Res 58:1141, 1987.
A research study describing the potential toxic effects of acyclovir treatment in cats.

Nasisse MP, English RV, Tompkins MB, et al: Immunologic, histologic, and virologic features of herpesvirus-induced stromal keratitis in cats. Am J Vet Res 56:51, 1995.
An original research article describing the immune responses in chronic stromal infection.

Nasisse MP, Guy JS, Davidson MG, et al: In vitro susceptibility of feline herpesvirus-1 to vidarabine, idoxuridine, trifluridine, acyclovir and bromovinyldeoxyuridine. Am J Vet Res 50:158, 1989.
An experimental study describing the relative potencies of topical antiviral drugs.

Nasisse MP, Guy JS, Stevens JB, et al: Clinical laboratory findings in chronic conjunctivitis in cats: 91 cases (1983–1991). J Am Vet Med Assoc 203:834, 1993.
A retrospective study describing the relative value of laboratory testing procedures for determining the cause of chronic conjunctivitis in cats.

Nasisse MP, Weigler BJ: The diagnosis of ocular feline herpesvirus infection. Vet Comp Ophthalmol 7:44, 1997.
A review that discusses in detail the comparative value of diagnostic tests for FHV-1 infection.

Stiles J: Treatment of cats with ocular disease attributable to herpesvirus infection: 17 cases. J Am Vet Med Assoc 207:599, 1995.
A review of the clinical signs and treatment outcomes of 17 cats with presumed FHV-1 ocular infections.

Weigler BJ, Babineau CA, Sherry B, Nasisse MP: High sensitivity polymerase chain reaction assay for active and latent feline herpesvirus-1 infections in domestic cats. Vet Rec 140:335, 1997.
An original research study describing the sensitivity of PCR for the diagnosis of FHV-1 infection.

Keratoconjunctivitis Sicca

CECIL P. MOORE
Columbia, Missouri

PATHOPHYSIOLOGY

Keratoconjunctivitis sicca (KCS) is a common clinical condition of dogs, characterized by ocular discharge, discomfort, redness, and corneal opacities, that may lead to blindness. KCS results primarily from deficiency of aqueous tear, the fluid comprising over 95% of the total tear volume, and, therefore, is sometimes referred to as a quantitative tear deficiency. Deficiency of the other primary tear components (mucin and lipid) has been referred to as qualitative tear deficiencies (Moore, 1990). In dogs, aqueous tears are normally secreted by orbital and third eyelid lacrimal glands and consist of water, inorganic salts, proteins, glucose, urea, and surface active polymers composed primarily of glycoproteins. Tears meet the metabolic needs of the avascular cornea by providing this tissue with glucose, electrolytes, oxygen, and water. In addition, metabolic products such as CO_2 and lactic acid are removed from the ocular surface by tears. Basal and reflex tears also lubricate the surface tissues and flush away bacteria and particulate debris from the cornea and conjunctiva. Direct antibacterial activity is provided by antibodies and lysozyme present in tears.

Deficiency of aqueous tears may result in inflammation, metaplasia, and necrosis of surface cells by several mechanisms. Tear deficiency results in hypertonicity and dehydration of the conjunctiva and cornea, hypoxia of corneal epithelium and subepithelial corneal stroma, increased susceptibility to ocular infections, frictional irritation by the eyelids and third eyelid, and accumulation of potentially toxic tissue metabolites such as lactic acid, desquamated cells, denatured mucus, and other "micro" debris.

CAUSES

Absence or loss of lacrimal secretions may result from a single disease process or a combination of conditions affecting the orbital and third eyelid glands. Recognized infectious causes of lacrimal adenitis in dogs include canine distemper virus and bacterial blepharoconjunctivitis resulting from chronic staphylococcal infection. Although KCS is relatively uncommon in cats, herpesvirus infection may result in feline dry eye. Congenital acinar hypoplasia is recognized as a breed-related cause in some canine breeds, for example, Yorkshire terriers. Drug-induced KCS may occur in dogs with either systemic sulfonamides or repeated topical administration of topical atropine. Preanesthetic and anesthetic agents are known to reduce tear secretion, although the reduction noted is usually only transient. An important iatrogenic cause is removal of the third eyelid gland. Other events associated with KCS in dogs include uncorrected third eyelid gland prolapse, traumatic and inflammatory orbital diseases, loss of parasympathetic innervation to the lacrimal glands (CN VII), or loss of sensory innervation to the ocular surface (CN V). Decreased aqueous tear production may occur with systemic metabolic diseases such as hypothyroidism, diabetes mellitus, and Cushing's disease.

Although the list of possible causes of KCS is extensive, in most cases the cause is not determined. Histologic studies of lacrimal tissue of dogs affected with idiopathic KCS have revealed varying degrees of mononuclear cell (lymphocytic-plasmacytic) infiltrates and acinar atrophy, suggesting an immunologic basis for the disease (Kaswan et al, 1984). Immune-mediated KCS appears to constitute the largest group of clinical cases. Although KCS may occasionally be associated with systemic autoimmune conditions (Kaswan et al, 1985), KCS more commonly occurs as a tissue-specific immune-mediated disorder. West Highland terriers, miniature schnauzers, and American Cocker spaniels appear to be disproportionately affected by immune-mediated KCS, suggesting a genetic predisposition in these breeds.

CLINICAL SIGNS

Early in the disease, affected eyes appear red and inflamed with intermittent mucoid or mucopurulent discharge. Because clinical signs are nonspecific in the early stages, KCS is often misdiagnosed as an irritant or primary bacterial conjunctivitis. As the KCS becomes subacute or chronic, the ocular surface becomes lackluster, the conjunctiva appears extremely hyperemic, and tenacious mucopurulent ocular discharge is observed. As the KCS progresses, keratitis develops, characterized by corneal vascularization and pigmentation with or without ulceration. Blepharitis with periocular dermatitis often appears simultaneously with accumulation of exudates along the eyelids. As the condition progresses, the level of discomfort intensifies and affected eyes are often squinted partially or completely closed.

DIAGNOSIS

Diagnosis of KCS is based on the presence of typical clinical signs, positive ocular staining using vital stains, and reduced quantitative tear readings. Rose bengal stain will detect devitalized cells and subtle epithelial defects on either conjunctival or corneal surfaces. Fluorescein stain is used primarily to detect concurrent corneal ulceration but may also be used to evaluate tear breakup, or the ability of the corneal surface to retain a homogeneous tear covering. Normal tear breakup times in dogs are reported to be 30 seconds or greater (Moore et al, 1987). The Schirmer tear test (STT) remains the standard for quantifying aqueous tear production. Any dog with a red irritated eye, ocular discharge, and/or corneal disease of undetermined cause should have STTs performed.

STTs may be done either with topical anesthetic (Schirmer I) or without topical anesthetic (Schirmer II) (Gelatt et al, 1975). Testing without anesthetic measures the ability of the eye to produce reflex tears and is most commonly performed. Schirmer II tear test readings *in dogs* are generally interpreted as follows: $\geq$ 15 mm/min = normal production; 11 to 14 mm/min = early or subclinical KCS; 6 to 10 mm/min = moderate or mild KCS; $\leq$ 5 mm/min = severe KCS. Some tear test strips are impregnated with a dye that marks the test strip at the level of tear fluid migration, allowing easier reading of the results (Wyman et al, 1995). Repeating STT measurements is advised in dogs stressed by examination or receiving medical therapy for ulcerative corneal disease because either of these factors, that is, sympathetic stimulation or current topical treatments (specifically atropine administration), may reduce tear secretions.

Evaluation of KCS patients should also include examination for possible associated systemic disease conditions, assessment of eyelid function and blink reflexes, and cultures and cytology in selected cases. Secondary bacterial conjunctivitis is common in KCS cases, and resistant organisms may develop if previous treatment has included a number of different antibiotic preparations.

TREATMENT

Medical Therapy

Medical therapy is the mainstay of KCS management whereby specific treatment regimens are tailored to individual patients and are influenced by the client's ability to comply with recommended treatment schedules. Depending on the severity of KCS, medical treatment generally consists of some combination of the following: (1) tear stimulation; (2) tear replacement; (3) topical antimicrobial drugs; (4) mucinolytic therapy; and (5) anti-inflammatory agents.

Lacrimostimulants

Lacrimostimulants, drugs administered to promote tear secretion, include two categories of therapeutic agents.

Cholinergic Agents

Because lacrimal glands are parasympathetically innervated, cholinergic drugs have historically been used to stimulate tearing. Ophthalmic pilocarpine solution may be administered either topically or orally as a tear stimulant (Rubin and Aguirre, 1967; Smith et al, 1994). Oral administration consists of applying 1 to 2% ophthalmic solution to the food. A safe initial oral dosage is one drop of 2% topical pilocarpine per 10 kg body weight in food twice daily. The dose may be gradually increased by one-drop increments at each dosage until signs of systemic reaction develop, i.e., salivation, vomiting, bradycardia, or diarrhea. Alternatively, topical dilute pilocarpine may be applied directly to the eyes. Concentrations of 0.125% or 0.25% have generally been applied after being diluted as follows: add 1 ml of 2% solution to 15 ml of artificial tears to make 0.125%, or add 2 ml of 2% solution to 14 ml of artificial tears to make 0.25% solution. Topical pilocarpine may

cause conjunctival hyperemia and miosis and, in some cases, sufficient irritation to necessitate discontinuing topical treatments. The route of pilocarpine administration may be determined by the individual patient's tolerance for one method over the other. Results of a recent study where topically applied pilocarpine did not significantly increase tear production in normal dogs have cast doubt on the efficacy of this method of administration (Smith et al, 1994).

Immunomodulation

The ability of the immunosuppressive agent cyclosporine A (CsA) to stimulate tear production in dogs is well documented (Salisbury et al, 1990; Morgan and Abrams, 1991; Olivero et al, 1991; Fullard and Kaswan, 1994; Bounous et al, 1995). Although the specific mechanisms of action of CsA on tear production are not completely understood, both immunomodulating and tear-stimulating properties appear to account for the dramatic responses observed in many affected dogs after topical application of this agent. An important mechanism of action of CsA is the inhibition of T-helper lymphocytes. In laboratory animal models of immune-mediated lacrimal disease, the ratio of T-suppressor to T-helper cells plays an important role in lacrimal gland regulation. Although T-suppressor cells normally predominate, in immune-mediated KCS, T-helper cells become the prevalent T lymphocytes. Therefore, by suppressing T-helper cells, CsA allows the T-suppressor cells to sustain normal lacrimal function.

Because of the probable immune-mediated pathogenesis of many cases of KCS and the marked improvement in tear production observed following its topical use, CsA has now become the primary treatment for canine KCS. Prior to the commercial availability of CsA for ophthalmic use, 1 to 2% oil-based solutions were compounded from 10% oral CsA solution and vegetable oil (either olive or corn oil; see *CVT XII*, p. 1231). Currently, the 0.2% commercial ointment (Optimmune, Schering-Plough) is prescribed. The vehicle used for the commercial product reportedly increases bioavailability by providing sustained release (Fullard et al, 1995) and, thereby, results in efficacy equivalent to higher concentrations of the compounded solutions.

To stimulate tear production, topical CsA is generally recommended for initial application every 12 hours to affected eyes; however, in severe cases treatments every 8 hours may be initiated. Several weeks of continuous treatment is usually needed before substantial increases in tear production are observed. Alternatively, in cases where treatments have been administered every 12 hours, if STT values remain at or below 10 mm/min after 3 weeks of topical therapy, the topical frequency may then be increased to every 8 hours. To provide the most accurate assessment of response to CsA, measuring tear production 3 hours after topical administration is recommended. When a favorable response to treatment every 12 hours restores tears to physiologic levels, that is, STT at or above 15 mm/min, topical CsA therapy may often be reduced to once-daily maintenance therapy.

Dogs with STT values of 0 to 1 mm/min have roughly a 50% chance of responding with increased tear secretion to topical CsA, whereas dogs with 2 mm/min or higher pretreatment values have greater than an 80% chance of improved tear production (Kaswan and Salisbury, 1990). Most dogs will show clinical improvement even in the absence of increased tear production, including those with STT values below 2 mm/min.

Tear Substitutes (Lacrimomimetics)

Tear substitutes contain ingredients or combinations of ingredients to replace deficiencies of one or more of the three primary tear components, that is, aqueous, mucin, and lipid. Many ophthalmic solutions and ointments are commercially available for tear replacement therapy (Table 1). Selection of a particular agent is influenced by availability, costs, clinician preference, patient compatibility, and owner acceptance. Aqueous tear replacement agents are usually initially applied four to six times daily to affected eyes. These agents are generally used concurrently with other topical therapeutic agents.

Methylcellulose and hydroxyethylcellulose are semisynthetic cellulose colloids that are water soluble, viscous, and virtually inert. Because cellulose derivatives are nonirritating to the eye and are compatible with most drugs, they are commonly used as aqueous tear substitutes and as aqueous vehicles for other ophthalmic preparations. These agents do not significantly delay healing of corneal epithelial wounds. Sustained-release artificial tear inserts containing 5 gm hydroxypropyl methylcellulose have been developed for treatment of human KCS patients. Although these small rod-like inserts offer prolonged release of viscous material, that is, for 6 to 12 hours, they have not been used extensively in dogs with KCS largely because owners seem to prefer conventional topical preparations. A newer ocular lubricant (AquaSite, Ciba) consists of a viscous droplet that is placed in the inferior cul-del-sac to serve as a reservoir for sustained tear delivery. This product appears promising for canine use.

Polyvinyl alcohol (PVA) is a synthetic hydrophilic resin that is less viscous than methylcellulose but has good corneal adhesive properties. Available usually as a 1.4% solution, PVA is the primary ingredient in a number of artificial tear products. Because nonviscous polymers are better tolerated by many human patients, many products containing PVA have been formulated and marketed commercially. One product (HypoTears, Ciba) is formulated as a hypotonic fluid to counter the hypertonic tears of KCS patients. A newer artificial tear preparation (Bion Tears, Alcon) employs an electrolyte-based formulation that has been shown to be beneficial to the ocular surface in an animal model of KCS (Gilbard and Rossi, 1992).

Linear polymers, such as dextran and polyvinylpyrrolidone (povidone), have mucinomimetic properties. Patented polymers are often combined with buffered solutions of substituted cellulose esters to form preparations for treating both deficiencies of aqueous and mucin components of the preocular tear film. Among tear substitutes advocated for both their lubricating and hydrating properties, solutions containing linear polymers remain on the eye for longer periods than solutions without these derivatives.

Viscoelastic substances have mucinomimetic properties and include sodium hyaluronate, chondroitin sulfate, and higher concentrations of methylcellulose. Sodium hyaluronate is a naturally occurring, high-molecular-weight glycosaminoglycan that has excellent viscoelastic and lubricating properties. Sodium hyaluronate veterinary products have been diluted with artificial tears to make a 0.04% solution (0.2 ml 1% sodium hyaluronate [Healon, Pharmacia] added to 5 ml of tear substitute) to increase viscosity, prolong retention, and enhance lubrication of dry eyes. This artificial tear/viscoelastic combination has been advocated for topical use every 4 hours initially, then reduced to 2 to 4 times daily for treating eyes of KCS patients. In clinical studies, treated eyes markedly improved, although STT values did not increase with this treatment (Schadler, 1987). A hyaluron derivative viscoelastic tear supplement is available commercially in Canada (Hylashield, I-med) as either a 0.15% or 0.40% drop. Anecdotal reports indicate that this product has been quite helpful in managing dogs with very low or persistently low STT values.

Chondroitin sulfate, which is a glycosaminoglycan polymer made up of disaccharide units, is not as viscous as sodium hyaluronate. High-viscosity methylcellulose (hydroxypropyl methylcellulose) in concentrations of 1 to 2% has been proposed as a less expensive substitute for sodium hyaluronate or chondroitin sulfate. One such product has recently been introduced commercially (Celluvisc, Allergan). An ocular gel has been used in Europe for a number of years as a sustained contact product, and similar products are under investigation in the United States.

Lanolin, petrolatum, and mineral oil are commonly used as bases for ophthalmic lubricant ointments. These ingredients mimic the function of naturally occurring meibomian lipids by preventing evaporation and preserving existing tears. Because ointments may cause blurring of vision in human patients, the use of these products is primarily limited to bedtime and as an adjunct to artificial tears used throughout the day. Because duration of lubrication is usually of greater concern than transient blurring in animals, ointments are used extensively in veterinary patients. Nonmedicated ophthalmic ointments containing one or more of these ingredients are used to lubricate and protect eyes in instances where corneal exposure is a problem, that is, during anesthesia and surgery, or in cases of eyelid paresis or eyelid swelling. Lanolin, petrolatum, and mineral oil vehicles prolong corneal and conjunctival contact for agents such as corticosteroids and antibiotics. Ointment bases may also provide a sustained-release mechanism for delivery of lipophilic agents such as cyclosporine.

Antibiotic ointments may be more economical and as effective as straight lubricants with the additional advantage of having antibacterial effects. Triple antibiotic ointment is often prescribed for use two to three times daily in cases of canine KCS. Although ophthalmic ointments remain on the eye longer, they may be more difficult than drops for some clients to apply.

Antibacterials

Antibiotics with broad-spectrum activity, such as triple antibiotic ointment or solution, are commonly administered to control secondary bacterial infections, which frequently occur with inadequate cleansing of the ocular surface. Frequency of treatment is usually three to four times daily initially, reduced to twice daily as mucopurulent discharge

TABLE 1. Tear Substitutes*

Product	Viscosity Agents/Concentration(s)	Preservative	Source
Polyvinyl Alcohol Solutions			
Akwa Tears	PVA 1.40%	BAC, EDTA	Akorn
Artificial Tears	PVA 1.40%	BAC, EDTA	Generic (many)
Dry Eyes	PVA 1.40%	BAC, EDTA	Bausch & Lomb
Liquifilm Forte	PVA 3%	Thimerosal, EDTA	Allergan
Liquifilm Tears	PVA 1.40%	Chlorobutanol	Allergan
Ocutears PF	PVA 0.10%	None	Ocumed
Cellulose-Based Solutions			
Cellufresh	CMC 0.50%	None	Allergan
Celluvisc	CMC 1%	None	Allergan
Comfort Tears	HEC	BAC, EDTA	Barnes-Hinds
Isopto Alkaline	HPMC 1%	BAC, EDTA	Alcon
Isopto Tears Plain	HPMC 0.50%	BAC, EDTA	Alcon
Murocel	MC 1%	Methylparaben Propylparaben	Bausch & Lomb
Refresh Plus	CMC 0.50%	None	Allergan
TearGard	HPMC 0.50%	Sorbic acid, EDTA	Med Tech
Tearisol	HPMC 0.50%	BAC, EDTA	Iolab
Polymer Combinations			
Adsorbotear	HEC 0.40%, Povidone 1.67%, Adsorbobase	Thimerosal, EDTA	Alcon
AquaSite	PEG-400 0.20%, DEX 0.10%	EDTA	Ciba
Bion Tears	DEX 0.10%, HPMC 0.30%	None	Alcon
HypoTears	PVA 1%, HEC, DEX	BAC, EDTA	Iolab
HypoTears PF	PVA 1%, HEC, DEX 3.30%	EDTA	Iolab
Lacril	HPMC 0.50%, GEL 0.01%, PSB	Chlorobutanol	Allergan
Lubrifair Solution	DEX-70, HPMC	None	Pharmafair
LubriTears	HPMC 0.50%, DEX 0.10%	BAC, EDTA	Bausch & Lomb
Murine Eye Lubricant	PVA 1.40%, Povidone 0.60%	BAC, EDTA	Ross
Moisture Drops	HPMC 0.50%, DEX 0.10%, Povidone 0.10%, Glycerin 0.20%	BAC, EDTA	Bausch & Lomb
Nature's Tears	HPMC 0.40%, DEX	BAC, EDTA	Rugby
Refresh	PVA 1.40%, Povidone 0.60%	None	Allergan
Tears Naturale	HPMC 0.30%, DEX 0.10%	BAC, EDTA	Alcon
Tears Naturale II	HPMC 0.30%, DEX-70 0.10%	POLYQUAD, EDTA	Alcon
Tears Naturale Free	HPMC 0.30%, DEX 0.10%	None	Alcon
Tears Plus	PVA 1.40%, Povidone 0.60%	Chlorobutanol	Allergan
Tears Renewed	HPMC 0.30%, DEX-70 0.10%	BAC, EDTA	Akorn
Vasoclastic Products			
Hylashield	Hylan 0.15%	None	I-Med
Hylashield Nite	Hylan 0.40%	None	I-Med
Glycerin Products			
Dry Eye Therapy	Glycerin 0.30%	None	Bausch & Lomb
Eye-Lube-A	Glycerin 0.25%	BAC, EDTA	Optoptics
Ointments			
Akwa Tears Ointment	White petrolatum, MO	None	Akorn
Dry Eyes	White petrolatum, MO	None	Bausch & Lomb
Duolube	White petrolatum 80%, MO 20%	None	Bausch & Lomb
Duratears Naturale	White petrolatum, lanolin, MO	None	Alcon
Hypo Tears	White petrolatum 85%, lanolin, MO 15%	None	Iolab
Lacri-Lube	White petrolatum 55%, lanolin, MO 41.50%	Chlorobutanol	Allergan
Lacri-Lube NP	White petrolatum 55%, lanolin, MO 42.50%	None	Allergan
Lacri-Lube S.O.P.	White petrolatum 55%, MO 41.50%, 2% nonionic lanolin derivatives	Chlorobutanol	Allergan
Lipo-Tears	White petrolatum, MO	None	Coopervision
LubriTears	White petrolatum, lanolin, MO	Chlorobutanol	Bausch & Lomb
Ocutube	White petrolatum	Methylparaben	Ocumed
Paralube	White petrolatum, lanolin 2%, MO	None	Fougera
Refresh PM	White petrolatum 56.80%, lanolin, MO 41.50%	None	Allergan

BAC, benzalkonium chloride; CMC, carboxymethyl cellulose; DEX, dextran; EDTA, ethylenediaminetetraacetic acid; GEL, gelatin; HEC, hydroxyethyl cellulose; HPMC, hydroxypropyl methylcellulose; MC, methylcellulose; MO, mineral oil; PEG, polyethylene glycol; POLYQUAD, polyquaternium-1; PSB, polysorbate 80; PVA, polyvinyl alcohol.

*Percentage composition given where information available

decreases, and eventually discontinued when signs of infection have abated. In cases of persistent mucopurulent discharge, bacterial culture and sensitivity testing should be performed.

Mucinolytic/Anticollagenase Agents

Good ocular hygiene, that is, frequent cleansing of discharges, is essential to minimize accumulation of degradative enzymes that contribute to ocular surface inflammation and ulceration. A 5 to 10% solution of acetylcysteine may be applied topically 2 to 4 times daily to facilitate removal of copious exudates and mucoid debris that accompany KCS. In addition, acetylcysteine's anticollagenase properties may aid in preventing enzymatic degradation of surface tissues and may be useful in the treatment of corneal ulceration. Acetylcysteine solution has been advocated as one component of a combination solution for treating dry eye, for example, Severin's KCS solution containing artificial tears, pilocarpine, antibiotic, and acetylcysteine (Severin, 1996).

Anti-inflammatory Therapy

Anti-inflammatory therapy may be a valuable adjunct to other medical therapy in improving clinical signs in cases of KCS. Topical corticosteroids are commonly administered to minimize conjunctivitis, alleviate discomfort, and reduce corneal opacities associated with chronic keratitis. Triple antibiotic ointment in combination with hydrocortisone is beneficial to many KCS patients. However, caution must be exercised when administering topical corticosteroids because their use will complicate healing of an ulcerated cornea, and, therefore, they are contraindicated when the cornea retains fluorescein stain. Chronic administration of topical corticosteroids can also cause local immunosuppression and predispose the eye to secondary infections.

Besides its marked lacrimostimulant effects, topical CsA also has beneficial anti-inflammatory properties such as reducing corneal vascularization. Cyclosporine use appears to be safe in the presence of corneal ulceration, and it does not alter ocular surface flora (Salisbury et al, 1995). Cyclosporine may also be beneficial in reducing corneal pigmentation in animals with chronic pigmentary keratitis associated with KCS.

Additional Considerations

Cases of acute KCS may present with corneal stromal ulceration, which requires aggressive medical and/or surgical therapy. Because opportunistic infections may contribute to rapid degradation of ulcerated cornea, bacterial culture of the ulcer margins with subsequent sensitivity testing is indicated. When corneal ulceration occurs as a sequela to KCS, *local atropine administration is contraindicated*, because surface drying will be exacerbated by its application. In cases of deep stromal ulceration or descemetocele formation, reconstructive corneal surgery, that is, conjunctival grafting, may be necessary for stabilizing the cornea and stimulate fibrovascular resolution of the ulceration.

Surgical Therapy

Surgical procedures that may be indicated in the management of selected cases of KCS are parotid duct transposition (saliva as a substitute for tear) and permanent partial tarsorrhaphy (reduces exposure, enhances blinking). Occlusion of the nasolacrimal puncta is used in human patients as a tear-conserving procedure by blocking tear drainage. Replacement of the third eye gland (versus gland removal) is regarded as a preventative surgical procedure for canine KCS.

Parotid Duct Transposition

Because saliva may serve as a substitute for tears, parotid duct transposition (PDT) surgery is performed to provide symptomatic relief in KCS patients refractory to medical therapy. Surgery is delayed until the KCS has proven to be unresponsive to at least 8 weeks of conventional medical therapy. Even if only a minimal response is noted to medical treatment during this period, treatment should probably be extended for an additional 4 weeks before recommending PDT. Rarely, dogs with KCS have concurrent xerostomia and, therefore, are not candidates for PDT surgery. Testing of salivary flow from the parotid papilla can be done by administering a bitter substance, for example, one drop of ophthalmic atropine, to the tongue and observing for salivary flow. The reader is referred to other sources for detailed description of the PDT surgery (Gelatt, 1991; Severin, 1996).

Following PDT surgery, multiple daily feedings are administered to stimulate parotid secretions. Clients should be alerted that because salivary secretions differ from lacrimal secretions, mineral precipitates often form on the ocular surface. The abundance of salivary secretions may result in facial wetting and discoloration that may be objectionable, especially in light-coated dogs. A chelating solution containing 1 to 2% ethylenediaminetetraacetic acid (EDTA) in artificial tears may be applied topically 1 to 3 times daily to help control mineral precipitates. Continued use of topical cyclosporine also appears helpful in reducing irritation from gritty mineral deposits, probably by virtue of both its lubricant and anti-inflammatory properties.

Partial Tarsorrhaphy

Partial permanent tarsorrhaphy surgery may be beneficial in brachycephalic breeds with KCS to afford greater corneal protection and to conserve existing tears. Although lateral canthoplasty is easier to perform, medial canthoplasty provides additional protection from nasal trichiasis, nasal fold hairs, and medial canthal entropion. When performing medial canthoplasty, the surgeon must take care not to sever the lacrimal canaliculi.

Replacement of Prolapsed Third Eyelid Gland

Either removing a prolapsed third eyelid gland or allowing chronic prolapse without treatment predisposes the affected eye to KCS. Repair of a prolapsed third eyelid gland with an appropriate replacement procedure will usually prevent the sequela of KCS. A number of third eyelid gland replacement techniques have been described, and the reader is referred to another source for a review of available techniques (Moore and Constantinescu, 1997).

References and Suggested Reading

Bounous DI, Carmichael KP, Kaswan RL, et al: Effects of ophthalmic cyclosporine on lacrimal gland pathology and function in dogs with keratoconjunctivitis sicca. Vet Comp Ophthalmol 5:5, 1995.
Increased tear values and regeneration of atrophied lacrimal glands were noted in KCS-affected dogs treated with topical cyclosporine.

Fullard RJ, Kaswan RL: Effect of cyclosporine on tear protein profiles of dogs with KCS. Invest Ophthalmol Vis Sci 35:1693, 1994.
Topical cyclosporine returned tear profile to normal in KCS-affected dogs.

Fullard RJ, Kaswan RL, Keller DA, et al: Comparison of vehicles used in topical cyclosporine treatment of canine KCS. Invest Ophthalmol Vis Sci 36:S994, 1995.
A topical 0.2% cyclosporine emulsion decreased inflammation and increased tear production in dogs with KCS.

Gelatt KN, Peiffer RL, Erickson JL, et al: Evaluation of tear function in the dog using a modification of the Schirmer tear test. J Am Vet Med Assoc 166:368, 1975.
Normal canine tear values and effects of lacrimal gland removal and systemic atropine administration on tear production are reported.

Gilbard JP, Rossi SR: An electrolyte-based solution that increases corneal glycogen and conjunctival goblet-cell density in a rabbit model for keratoconjunctivitis sicca. Ophthalmology 99:600, 1992.
An electrolyte-based solution reduced tear osmolarity and increased corneal glycogen and conjunctival goblet cells when applied topically in a rabbit model of KCS.

Kaswan RL, Martin CL, Chapman WL: Keratoconjunctivitis sicca: Histopathologic study of nictitating membrane and lacrimal glands from 28 dogs. Am J Vet Res 45:112, 1984.
Histologic examination of lacrimal tissue from 28 dogs diagnosed with KCS.

Kaswan RL, Martin CL, Dawe DL: Keratoconjunctivitis sicca: Immunological evaluation of 62 canine cases. Am J Vet Res 46:376, 1985.
Report indicating that canine KCS is an immunologic disorder targeting lacrimal tissue.

Kaswan RL, Salisbury MA: A new perspective on canine keratoconjunctivitis sicca. Treatment with ophthalmic cyclosporine. Vet Clin North Am Small Anim Pract 20:583, 1990.
A review of canine KCS, its causes, and treatments.

Moore CP: Qualitative tear film disease. Vet Clin North Am Small Anim Pract 20:583, 1990.
A review of mucin- and lipid-deficient canine tear deficiencies.

Moore CP: Diseases and surgery of the lacrimal secretory system. In: Gelatt KN, ed: Veterinary Ophthalmology, 3rd ed. Media, PA: Williams & Wilkins (in press).
A general review of KCS in the latest edition of this comprehensive text.

Moore CP, Constantinescu GM: Surgery of the adnexa. Vet Clin North Am Small Anim Pract 27:1011, 1997.
Review of surgical procedures of the ocular adnexa including repair of third eyelid gland prolapse.

Moore CP, Wilsman NJ, Nordheim EV, et al: Density and distribution of canine conjunctival goblet cells. Invest Ophthalmol Vis Sci 28:1925, 1987.
A histologic description of goblet cell location within normal canine conjunctiva.

Morgan RV, Abrams KL: Topical administration of cyclosporine for treatment of keratoconjunctivitis sicca in dogs. J Am Vet Med Assoc 199:1043, 1991.
A study evaluating cyclosporine's ability to increase tear production in canine KCS.

Morgan RV, Duddy JM, McClug K: Prolapse of the gland of the third eyelid in dogs: A retrospective study of 89 cases (1980–1990). J Am Anim Hosp Assoc 29:56, 1993.
Retrospective study evaluating outcomes of different surgical techniques versus no surgery for third eyelid gland prolapse.

Olivero DK, Davidson MG, English RV, et al: Clinical evaluation of 1% cyclosporine for topical treatment of keratoconjunctivitis sicca in dogs. J Am Vet Med Assoc 199:1039, 1991.
Topical 1% cyclosporine is reported to be effective in increasing tear production in dogs with KCS.

Rubin LF, Aguirre G: Clinical use of pilocarpine for keratoconjunctivitis sicca in dogs and cats. J Am Vet Med Assoc 151:313, 1967.
Oral pilocarpine stimulated tear production in 6 dogs and 1 cat affected with KCS, with salivation noted as a frequent side effect.

Salisbury MR, Kaswan RL, Brown J: Microorganisms isolated from the corneal surface before and during topical cyclosporine treatment in dogs with keratoconjunctivitis sicca. Am J Vet Res 56:880, 1995.
A 12-month study of corneal cultures taken before and during 2% cyclosporine therapy for KCS in dogs indicating no significant effect on ocular surface microflora.

Salisbury MA, Kaswan RL, Ward DA, et al: Topical application of cyclosporine in the management of keratoconjunctivitis sicca in dogs. J Am Anim Hosp Assoc 26:269, 1990.
An early report on topical 2% cyclosporine treatment for idiopathic canine KCS.

Schadler HJ: An alternative treatment for keratoconjunctivitis sicca. Vet Med 71:1145, 1987.
Topical sodium hyaluronate solution relieved signs of KCS in dogs and cats.

Severin GA: Keratoconjunctivitis sicca. In: Severin's Veterinary Ophthalmology Notes, 3rd ed. Ft. Collins, CO: Veterinary Ophthalmology Notes, 1996, p 230–233.
Discussion of formulation and use of Severin's KCS solution.

Smith EM, Buyukmihci NC, Farver TB: Effect of topical pilocarpine treatment on tear production in dogs. J Am Vet Med Assoc 205:1286, 1994.
Topical application of 0.25, 1.0 or 2.0% pilocarpine had little effect on tear production in normal dogs.

Wyman M, Gilger B, Mueller P, et al: Clinical evaluation of a new Schirmer tear test in the dog. Vet Comp Ophthalmol 5:211, 1995.
Schirmer test strips with a millimeter scale and dye impregnation for ease of reading were compared with standard STTs in normal dogs.

Nonulcerative Corneal Disease

VICTORIA L. GREVAN
West Palm Beach, Florida

Although nonulcerative corneal disease has numerous causes, the cornea has only a limited number of ways in which it may respond. The cornea is normally transparent because of its nonkeratinized epithelium, precise organization of small-diameter collagen fibrils, endothelial pump function, and absence of blood vessels and pigment. The pathologic responses of the cornea may include various combinations of edema, vascularization, pigmentation, accumulation of cellular or metabolic (e.g., lipid or mineral) infiltrates, fibrosis, and ulceration. Due to the requirement for corneal transparency, these changes may produce corneal opacification and loss of vision.

The main differential diagnoses for nonulcerative corneal disease include keratoconjunctivitis sicca (see p. 1061), chronic superficial keratitis, pigmentary keratitis, corneal dystrophy, corneal degeneration, lipid keratopathy, nodular granulomatous episclerokeratitis, corneal sequestration, eosinophilic keratitis, and stromal keratitis associated with herpesvirus infection. Keratoconjunctivitis sicca and herpesvirus stromal keratitis will be covered in separate articles.

CHRONIC SUPERFICIAL KERATITIS (PANNUS)

Chronic superficial keratitis (CSK) or pannus is a bilateral, progressive, vision-threatening, generally nonulcerative, inflammatory disease that typically begins in the lateral or ventrolateral cornea. The third eyelid may be involved simultaneously or exclusively (atypical pannus). Chronic superficial keratitis is characterized by superficial corneal vascularization, pigmentation, and infiltration by lymphocytes and plasma cells. If inadequately controlled, permanent blindness may result from severe corneal pigmentation. Chronic superficial keratitis is most common in the German shepherd dog but any breed may be affected. An increased prevalence of CSK has also been documented in Belgian tervurens, Border collies, Greyhounds, Siberian huskies, and Australian shepherds. Middle-aged dogs are most likely to be affected. Although the exact etiology is unknown, immune-mediated mechanisms are suspected and ultraviolet radiation is known to play a role in the pathogenesis. Exposure to high altitudes with increased ultraviolet light exposure increases the incidence and severity of pannus.

A presumptive diagnosis of CSK may be made based on the suggestive clinical signs. However, corneal vascularization and pigmentation secondary to chronic irritation from other causes (such as keratoconjunctivitis sicca, entropion, lagophthalmos) must be ruled out. Tear production should be evaluated and a complete eye examination, with particular attention focused on eyelid conformation, should be performed. The diagnosis of CSK may be facilitated by

cytologic examination of ocular lesions, which should consist primarily of lymphocytes and plasma cells.

The goal of treatment is to control, rather than cure, the disease. Lifelong therapy should be expected; however, less aggressive therapy may be required in the winter months. The main agents utilized in medical therapy are topical corticosteroids and/or cyclosporine (Optimmune, Schering-Plough Animal Health). The severity of the disease varies markedly; therefore, therapy needs to be tailored to the individual patient. In severe cases (assuming the corneas are negative for fluorescein stain retention), a subconjunctival injection of 4 to 6 mg triamcinolone (Vetalog, Solvay Animal Health) or 1 mg dexamethasone (Azium, Schering-Plough Animal Health) may be given at the time of diagnosis and periodically as necessary. The cases I see are generally mild to moderate (midwestern United States) in severity, and I generally initiate treatment with a combination of cyclosporine ointment every 12 hours and 1% prednisolone acetate suspension (Econopred Plus, Alcon,) every 6 to 12 hours. Alternatively, 0.1% dexamethasone (Maxidex, Alcon,) may be used instead of prednisolone acetate. I do prefer one of these two corticosteroids because they are more potent and penetrate the cornea better than other corticosteroids. The goals of therapy are to reduce corneal inflammatory cell infiltrates and vascularization and prevent progressive corneal pigmentation. Corneal opacification should decrease during therapy and vision should improve as a result. Once the clinical signs are controlled with medical therapy, medications are tapered to the minimum required to control the disease. Follow-up on CSK patients is crucial because the requirement for medical therapy may vary as the disease progresses.

Cases refractory to medical therapy or with severe corneal pigmentation may benefit from either a superficial keratectomy or beta-irradiation, however, ongoing medical therapy will be necessary. Beta-irradiation is noninvasive and reduces much of the superficial pigmentation within 3 to 6 weeks. Cryosurgery of the cornea, with liquid nitrogen or nitrous oxide, will also reduce the superficial corneal pigmentation within several weeks and thus improve vision.

PIGMENTARY KERATITIS

Pigmentary keratitis is characterized by pigmentation of the corneal epithelium and subepithelial stroma. It may be accompanied by varying degrees of superficial corneal vascularization. Corneal pigmentation is a nonspecific response to chronic irritation, which may result from a variety of causes including keratoconjunctivitis sicca and conformational abnormalities. Critical to the management of this condition is determination of the underlying cause.

Keratoconjunctivitis sicca may be diagnosed by determination of subnormal tear production (see p. 1061). The pigmentary keratitis discussed in this section is that which occurs secondary to chronic irritation from a structural abnormality such as entropion, distichiasis, nasal fold trichiasis, and lagophthalmos (incomplete blink). Some of the most severe cases occur in dogs with large palpebral fissures, lagophthalmos, medial lower lid entropion, and nasal trichiasis (e.g., Pug and Pekingese). Pigmentary keratitis is most common in brachycephalic breeds of dogs. They may suffer severe visual compromise due to severe, diffuse corneal pigmentation.

The key to managing cases of pigmentary keratitis is early detection of corneal pigmentation and recognition of precipitating causes. The disease is best managed by prevention through elimination of the underlying cause. Surgical correction of any structural abnormalities is imperative and may include nasal fold resection, entropion correction, or medial canthoplasty. Many of the brachycephalic dogs will benefit from medial canthoplasties, which may eliminate both the lagophthalmos and medial lower lid entropion. Medial canthoplasty (or medial *and* lateral canthoplasty) is oftentimes more effective than lateral canthoplasty in ameliorating the clinical signs, due to the frequent presence of nasal trichiasis.

Many cases already have some degree of corneal pigmentation by the time of examination. Elimination of pre-existing pigmentation is an unrealistic goal of therapy. The goal is to prevent progressive, blinding corneal pigmentation. In addition to correcting the underlying problem, cyclosporine every 12 hours may be tried in an attempt to reduce the density of corneal pigmentation. If corneal pigmentation is severe, surgical options may be considered *if* the underlying cause has been eliminated (otherwise the pigmentation will just recur). Surgeries that may be performed in an attempt to reduce the severity of corneal pigmentation are beta-irradiation, lamellar keratectomy, and cryosurgery.

CORNEAL DYSTROPHY

Corneal dystrophy is exceedingly more common in the dog than in the cat. Corneal dystrophy in the dog is categorized according to the anatomic location of the lesion as epithelial, stromal, or endothelial. Feline corneal dystrophy has been described in the Manx and the domestic shorthair. The few reported cases had disease of the corneal stroma and/or endothelium and severe stromal edema was the consequence.

Epithelial Dystrophy

The most common form of corneal epithelial dystrophy is actually a dystrophy of the epithelial basement membrane, which occurs most commonly in boxers but may occur in any breed. Indolent ulcers are the manifestation of this disorder, which are discussed elsewhere in this book.

Stromal Dystrophy

Corneal stromal dystrophy refers to a primary, usually bilateral, presumably inherited condition of the cornea that is not due to an underlying systemic or inflammatory disease. Corneal stromal dystrophy most commonly begins in young to middle-aged dogs. The clinical appearance is that of a white, crystalline, corneal opacity that frequently resembles "ground glass." The lesions are typically well-delineated, in a central to paracentral location in the cornea, and may assume an oval, circular, or ring shape.

The corneal opacities consist of extracellular and intracellular deposits of phospholipids, neutral fats, and cholesterol in the superficial or deep corneal stroma, which will vary depending upon the breed affected. Lipid deposits are most common in a subepithelial location, and the overlying epithelium is usually uninvolved; therefore, the lesions are typically negative for fluorescein stain retention. Although corneal dystrophy may occur in any breed or mixed breed, several forms of corneal dystrophy have been described in specific breeds of dogs such as the Siberian husky, Beagle, Shetland sheepdog, Bichon frise, and Cavalier King Charles spaniel.

A tentative diagnosis is based on the characteristic features previously described. The primary differential diagnosis is corneal lipid deposition secondary to systemic hyperlipidemia; therefore, the diagnostic work-up may include a serum biochemical profile (including cholesterol and triglycerides), particularly in atypical cases.

Although there is no effective medical therapy for corneal dystrophy, the lesions are usually nonpainful and stationary. The corneal opacities may be resected by superficial keratectomy, particularly if they are compromising vision. Some degree of corneal scarring will result, and the potential for recurrence of the lesions exists. Requirements for performing a keratectomy are magnification, possession of several small and delicate instruments designed for corneal surgery, and a certain level of surgical expertise because the cornea is less than 1 mm in thickness (to avoid inadvertent full-thickness corneal penetration).

Endothelial Dystrophy

Endothelial dystrophy is most common in middle-aged to older Boston terriers, Chihuahuas, and Dachshunds but may occur in any breed. It is more common in females than in males. Endothelial dystrophy results in decreased numbers of functional endothelial cells. Because the most important function of the corneal endothelium is to actively pump fluid out of the cornea to maintain a state of relative deturgescence, the clinical effect of endothelial dysfunction is corneal edema (initially stromal, eventually epithelial). The corneal edema in cases of endothelial dystrophy tends to be diffuse (homogeneous, bluish-white color), bilateral (not necessarily symmetrical initially), progressive, and eventually severe and potentially blinding. The corneal edema may begin temporally with subsequent axial progression. With severe corneal edema, epithelial and subepithelial bullae may develop, which may rupture and cause corneal ulcers. In advanced cases of endothelial dystrophy, especially when corneal ulcers are present, corneal vascularization may develop. These types of corneal ulcers are often slow to heal due to persistence of the underlying cause, and a grid keratotomy may be necessary to promote healing.

There is no highly effective medical therapy available

for endothelial dystrophy. If corneal ulcers develop secondary to rupture of bullae, they should be treated with topical antibiotics. Refractory corneal ulcers may be treated by placement of a soft contact lens or a grid keratotomy. Some veterinarians favor treatment of the corneal edema with topical hyperosmotic agents such as 5% sodium chloride ointment (Muro 128, Bausch & Lomb). Theoretically, it should create an osmotic gradient across the cornea and facilitate movement of fluid out of the cornea to reduce corneal edema and bullae. However, resolution of the edema is at best minimal, and some animals are irritated by its topical application.

In patients with severe corneal edema due to endothelial dystrophy or recurrent corneal ulcers from rupture of epithelial and subepithelial bullae, surgical options should be considered. Penetrating keratoplasty ("corneal transplant") is an option, but graft rejection leads to opacification of the donor cornea; thus, restoration of vision may not result. Thermokeratoplasty is the cautious, controlled application of thermal cautery to the cornea in an attempt to induce formation of a superficial layer of fibrous tissue. The idea is that this may reduce or eliminate the egress of edema fluid into the corneal epithelium, which may prevent the development of corneal bullae and resultant corneal ulcers.

CORNEAL DEGENERATION

Corneal degeneration consists of the stromal deposition of lipids (sometimes referred to as lipid keratopathy), cholesterol, or calcium, and it may be accompanied by vascularization. The degenerative lesions are typically white and crystalline in appearance. The most common location is in the central cornea, but they may occur anywhere depending upon the cause. Occasionally, ulceration of the overlying corneal epithelium may occur with these lesions.

Corneal degeneration may occur as a sequela to corneal trauma, ulceration, chronic irritation, uveitis, or topical corticosteroid therapy. Degenerations may also be secondary to hyperlipidemia or hypercalcemia. Corneal degeneration may be unilateral (more commonly) or bilateral, in contrast to corneal dystrophies, which are typically bilateral.

Calcium degeneration (band keratopathy) may occur secondary to derangements in systemic calcium and phosphorus metabolism and has been reported in dogs with hyperadrenocorticism. Corneal lipid infiltration may be associated with systemic hyperlipidemia due to hypothyroidism, diabetes mellitus, hyperadrenocorticism, pancreatitis, nephrotic syndrome, hepatic disease, or primary hyperlipoproteinemia (e.g., Miniature Schnauzers). Diagnostic evaluation should include a serum biochemical profile including cholesterol and triglycerides, and possibly thyroid testing.

Treatment of corneal degeneration is not necessarily required if the eye is visual and comfortable; however, any underlying problems must be controlled. In the case of calcium degeneration, medical therapy may be attempted to try to reduce the amount of mineral infiltrating the cornea. Topical disodium ethylenediaminetetraacetic acid (EDTA) solution (0.4 to 1.38%) may be used every 6 to 8 hours in an attempt to chelate calcium from the degenerative lesions and reduce the density of the lesion. In cases

of corneal cholesterol and lipid deposition, a fat-restricted diet has been recommended. Although the response is unpredictable, particularly in the absence of hyperlipidemia, cases have been reported with improvement in the corneal lesions despite a lack of reduction of the serum cholesterol and triglyceride levels.

In cases that are problematic due either to compromised vision, corneal ulceration, or ocular irritation, the corneal degenerative lesion may be surgically removed by a keratectomy. The corneal sample should be submitted for histopathologic examination, including special stains for calcium and lipid. This would be advisable only if the underlying condition has been controlled; otherwise the lesion is likely to recur.

ARCUS LIPOIDES CORNEAE

Arcus lipoides corneae refers to the bilateral condition of peripheral, corneal stromal lipid deposition in a characteristic band that encircles the limbus. The lipid deposition begins in the deeper stromal layers and eventually involves the superficial layers. There may be a thin, clear zone between the limbus and the outer edge of the arcus. Arcus lipoides corneae has been most commonly associated with hypothyroidism but may result from any disease that elevates cholesterol and triglyceride levels. Treatment should be directed at the underlying cause (e.g., thyroid supplementation in the case of hypothyroidism).

NODULAR GRANULOMATOUS EPISCLEROKERATITIS

Nodular granulomatous episclerokeratitis (NGE) refers to an inflammatory, nodular lesion of the corneoscleral limbus. Other descriptive terms that have been commonly used in referring to these types of lesions include fibrous histiocytoma, nodular fasciitis, pseudotumor, and collie granuloma. Although the issue is somewhat controversial, many feel that these all refer to the same basic disease with variable histologic manifestations. Histologically, the limbal nodules vary primarily in the proportions of lymphocytes, plasma cells, histiocytes, and fibroblasts.

Nodular granulomatous episclerokeratitis may be unilateral but is commonly bilateral, and there may be more than one nodule on a particular eye. Young to middle-aged dogs are most commonly affected. The exact etiology is unknown, but immune-mediated mechanisms are considered likely. The lesions most commonly develop at the lateral limbus, tend to be slowly progressive if untreated, and may gradually invade the corneal stroma (and thus eventually interfere with vision if untreated). They are characterized by a high incidence of local recurrence in the absence of ongoing therapy. The characteristic appearance is of a raised, smooth, pink ("fleshy") nodule arising at the limbus. Concurrent involvement of the third eyelid (or eyelids) may occur. The breeds reported to be affected most commonly are the Collie, and to a lesser extent the Shetland sheepdog, but they develop in other dog breeds and mixed breeds as well.

A diagnosis may be made based on cytologic examination of a fine-needle aspirate of the mass or a biopsy of the lesion. A keratectomy may be performed for diagnostic and therapeutic purposes, but additional medical therapy will be required. Ideally, histologic confirmation of the presumptive diagnosis is made at the onset of the disease or in cases that do not respond predictably to medical therapy. Less likely differential diagnoses include neoplastic or infectious disease.

Medical therapy for this condition generally relies on either corticosteroids alone or in conjunction with azathioprine (Imuran, Burroughs Wellcome Co.). In the mildest of cases, therapy may be initiated with topical 1% prednisolone acetate or 0.1% dexamethasone every 6 hours. Subconjunctival or intralesional injections of corticosteroids may also be administered. A potential role of topical corticosteroid therapy is as a maintenance treatment, once remission has been induced with azathioprine.

In more severe cases or cases that are not responding markedly by recheck examination, I treat concurrently with an initial dosage of 2 mg/kg of azathioprine, which is gradually tapered over 1 to 2 months. Prior to initiating azathioprine therapy, baseline complete blood count (CBC) and serum biochemical profile values should be determined (see p. 509). The hematologic parameters should be periodically monitored, especially during the first few months of therapy, due to the potential side effects of hepatotoxicity and myelosuppression, in addition to gastrointestinal toxicosis. The lowest possible maintenance dose of topical corticosteroids and/or azathioprine should be determined in each individual patient. Recurrences are still possible, at which time therapy is resumed at a more aggressive level until remission occurs.

In addition to lamellar keratectomy, surgical therapies which have shown some success in the treatment of NGE are beta-irradiation and cryosurgery. However, these are not routinely used due to the high rate of success with noninvasive medical therapy.

CORNEAL SEQUESTRATION

Corneal sequestration is a unique disorder of cats. The appearance is pathognomonic and consists of stromal necrosis and variable pigmentation. The lesion is a brown to black plaque, which may be accompanied by varying degrees of corneal vascularization and edema. The sequestrum may be slightly raised from the surface, and the overlying epithelium is frequently absent. Corneal sequestra are frequently associated with herpesvirus infection but may develop secondary to any source of chronic irritation, such as entropion. Testing for feline herpesvirus is advisable in cats affected by corneal sequestration (see p. 1057).

The ideal treatment for corneal sequestra is somewhat controversial. As the lesion may eventually slough spontaneously, some elect the conservative approach of monitoring the lesions. Because affected cats commonly exhibit signs of ocular pain, including epiphora and blepharospasm, I usually recommend surgical excision by a keratectomy (with or without a conjunctival flap) inasmuch as this is generally associated with a reduced healing time. Concurrent antiviral therapy may be indicated in those cats that test positive for feline herpesvirus.

EOSINOPHILIC KERATITIS

Eosinophilic keratitis is a disease that affects cats and is characterized by a proliferative, pink to white, vascularized, edematous lesion most commonly arising near the lateral or medial limbus, unilaterally or bilaterally. Diagnosis is achieved by biopsy or cytologic examination and identification of eosinophils. The pathogenesis of eosinophilic keratitis is not completely understood, but a large percentage of affected corneas are positive for feline herpesvirus.

Eosinophilic keratitis usually responds very well to medical therapy; however, recurrences are common in the absence of maintenance therapy. Medical therapy consists of topical corticosteroids or systemic megestrol acetate (Ovaban, Schering-Plough Animal Health). Treatment every 6 hours with either topical 0.1% dexamethasone or 1% prednisolone acetate suspension is usually effective at controlling lesions. However, corticosteroids may exacerbate herpesvirus infections, so I concurrently treat herpesvirus-positive cats with antiviral therapy such as trifluridine (Viroptic, Burroughs Wellcome Co.). Alternatively, I more commonly treat affected cats with megestrol acetate at a dose of 5 mg daily for 5 days, reduced to 5 mg every other day for 7 days, then 5 mg weekly for maintenance. Cats usually respond dramatically to this protocol. The disadvantage is that megestrol acetate has been associated with side effects including pyometra and diabetes mellitus, but these appear to be uncommon.

"FLORIDA SPOTS"

"Florida spots" ("acid-fast keratopathy") are corneal lesions that may occur in dogs or cats living in tropical or subtropical climates. The clinical appearance is that of multifocal, gray-white, nonulcerative, circular lesions in the corneal stroma. The lesions tend to have a dense center and less dense periphery. Signs of inflammation and irritation are generally absent. The etiology has not been determined but infection by an acid-fast organism has been proposed as the cause. The condition tends to be self-limiting and there is no known effective therapy; therefore, no treatment is necessary.

References and Suggested Reading

Chavkin MJ, Roberts SM, Salman MD, et al: Risk factors for development of chronic superficial keratitis in dogs. J Am Vet Med Assoc 10:1630, 1994.
   A retrospective, statistical analysis of demographic and environmental risk factors for CSK.
Cooley PL, Dice PF: Corneal dystrophy in the dog and cat. Vet Clin North Am 20:681, 1990.
   A discussion including the characteristics of corneal dystrophy according to breed.
Crispin SM: Lipid keratopathy in the dog. Vet Ann 27:196, 1987.
   A review of the clinical signs, pathogenic mechanisms, and treatment of this disorder.
Holmberg DL, Scheifer HB, Parent J: The cryosurgical treatment of pigmentary keratitis in dogs. Vet Surg 15:1, 1986.
   A description of the technique, potential complications, and clinical outcome of corneal cryosurgery.
Jackson PA, Kaswan RL, Merideth RE, et al: Chronic superficial keratitis in dogs: A placebo controlled trial of topical cyclosporine treatment. Prog Vet Comp Ophthalmol 1:269, 1991.
   A prospective study evaluating the clinical effect of twice daily cyclosporine therapy for CSK.

Linton LL, Moore CP, Collier LL: Bilateral lipid keratopathy in a Boxer dog: Cholesterol analyses and dietary management. Prog Vet Comp Ophthalmol 3:9, 1993.
A description of the clinical manifestations, diagnostic evaluation, surgical, and medical treatment of lipid keratopathy.
Morgan RV: Feline corneal sequestration: A retrospective study of 42 cases (1987–1991). J Am Anim Hosp Assoc 30:24, 1994.
A retrospective analysis of the clinical features, diagnostic testing, and treatments of corneal sequestration.
Morgan RV, Abrams KL, Kern TJ: Feline eosinophilic keratitis: A retrospective study of 54 cases: (1989–1994). Vet Comp Ophthalmol 6:131, 1996.
A review of eosinophilic keratitis with a discussion of diagnostic testing and treatment.
Paulsen ME, Lavach JD, Snyder SP, et al: Nodular granulomatous episclerokeratitis in dogs: 19 cases (1973–1985). J Am Vet Med Assoc 190:1581, 1987.
A retrospective study evaluating the success, remission duration, and complications associated with various medical therapies for NGE.
Whitley RD: Canine cornea. In: Gelatt KN, ed: Veterinary Ophthalmology. Philadelphia: Lea & Febiger, 1991, p 307.
A review of the various forms of nonulcerative corneal disease, including numerous photographs.

Ulcerative Keratitis

RUTH MARRION
North Andover, Massachusetts

The cornea is composed of four layers: the epithelium, stroma, Descemet's membrane, and endothelium. The epithelium provides an effective barrier to entry of bacteria and other organisms into the corneal stroma. A corneal ulcer is a full-thickness loss of corneal epithelium, exposing the underlying stroma.

There are no organisms that are documented to invade a canine cornea in the absence of a corneal ulcer. Causes of ulceration include damage due to conformational abnormalities, foreign objects, trauma, chemicals, inability to blink completely, and the presence of a diseased cornea due to conditions such as keratoconjunctivitis sicca. (Feline herpesvirus, which is capable of causing corneal ulceration in cats, is discussed on p. 1057.)

DIAGNOSIS

Patients presenting with corneal ulcers will generally have some degree of pain, manifested as blepharospasm and epiphora, and often conjunctival hyperemia. Diagnosis of corneal ulceration is straightforward and is based on the principle that fluorescein is unable to penetrate the hydrophobic corneal epithelium, but is absorbed well by the hydrophilic stroma. Application of fluorescein dye to an ulcerated cornea and excitation of the fluorescein using a light source fitted with a cobalt blue filter will reveal a green stain in the ulcerated area. A corneal ulcer may extend through the full thickness of the stroma to Descemet's membrane, forming a descemetocele. Fluorescein staining of a descemetocele results in a ring of green stain in the stroma with a clear center where Descemet's membrane, which does not absorb fluorescein, is exposed.

The corneal epithelium heals rapidly by a combination of mitosis and cellular migration. By contrast, the relatively hypocellular corneal stroma heals much more slowly. As a result of this discrepancy in growth, the epithelial component of an ulcer may heal and cover a relatively thin stroma, leaving an obvious depression in the cornea known as a corneal facet. Although a depression is clearly present,

the area will not absorb fluorescein stain because it is completely covered with corneal epithelium.

A secondary uveitis may be seen concurrently with corneal ulceration; signs of uveitis include aqueous flare, miosis, and low intraocular pressure.

UNCOMPLICATED ULCERS

These are defined as epithelial ulcers that are not infected or otherwise impaired from healing (see below). Patients generally exhibit mild to moderate pain and often no evidence of secondary uveitis.

Treatment (Table 1)

Topical Antibiotics

Topical antibiotic ointment or solution every 6 hours is indicated because the cornea is devoid of a blood supply and therefore susceptible to infection. A good choice for a first-line antibiotic is a broad-spectrum agent such as a triple antibiotic (Tri-Optic P, SmithKline Beecham) or chloramphenicol (Chloramphenicol solution, Rugby) solution or ointment (also see *CVT XII*, p. 1211). Antibiotics such as tobramycin, amikacin, and fluoroquinolones are appropriately used to treat infected corneal ulcers but are *not* indicated for uncomplicated ulcers.

Cycloplegics and Analgesics

Pain in corneal ulceration is the result of stimulation of corneal sensory nerves, which also results in a secondary uveitis. The treatment for uveitis in the absence of corneal ulceration is topical corticosteroid treatment; however, this is *contraindicated* in corneal ulceration. If the patient appears painful, topical atropine ointment (Atropine sulfate ophthalmic 1%, Fougera) or solution (Atropine sulfate 1% solution, Bausch and Lomb) may be prescribed and oral aspirin may be given. For an uncomplicated ulcer, one

TABLE 1. Treatment of Corneal Ulcers

Treatment	Uncomplicated Ulcers	Infected Ulcers	Indolent Ulcers
Antibiotics	Topical antibiotics q6h—triple antibiotic	Topical antibiotics >q6h—consider ciprofloxacin, tobramycin	Topical antibiotics q6h—triple antibiotic
Cycloplegics	± Atropine—one dose may be adequate	Atropine to effect q6–12h	Atropine to effect q12–24h
Analgesics	± Aspirin	Aspirin q12h	Aspirin q12h
Anticollagenases	Not indicated	Serum q2–6h	Not indicated
Surgery	Not indicated	Conjunctival graft may be indicated	Debride loose epithelium Superficial keratotomy ± contact lens, nictitans flap
Observation	Recheck within a week	Hospitalize	Recheck within a week

application of atropine given in the examination room may be sufficient to control pain because atropine is absorbed by uveal melanocytes and is released over a period of days. Atropine solution is bitter and often causes profuse salivation in cats when it enters the mouth following passage down the nasolacrimal duct; atropine ointment is better tolerated in feline patients.

Protective Therapies

If excessive exposure of the cornea is a concern, a third eyelid flap or a partial temporary tarsorrhaphy can be used to increase coverage of the cornea and thereby help correct the problem of exposure. Of these two options, a temporary tarsorrhaphy is preferable because the cornea may be left exposed medially for regular inspection. Furthermore, medications may be directly applied to the cornea if a partial tarsorrhaphy is in place, whereas the presence of a third eyelid flap may hinder access of medications to the cornea.

In most cases, corneal ulcers heal within several days. If the ulcer appears infected at initial presentation (see below), it will need to be treated more aggressively and the patient observed more closely. If an apparently uncomplicated ulcer is not healing when rechecked within a week after the initial visit, an underlying or exacerbating factor should be suspected.

EXACERBATING FACTORS

Chronic Irritation

Conformational Abnormalities

Several types of hairs can rub on the cornea and cause corneal ulceration. Unless this underlying cause is removed, the cornea will not heal. In some cases, the underlying cause is readily apparent, but some such as ectopic cilia may be difficult to find even with magnification.

Distichiasis is the presence of hairs that emanate from the meibomian gland margins and may rub on the cornea. Some distichiasis hairs are long and soft and rarely cause a problem, whereas others are thick and stiff and are able to cause corneal ulceration. These hairs may be removed by electroepilation or cryoepilation (see p. 1051).

It is important to realize that not all animals exhibiting distichiasis need to have distichiasis hairs removed. The great majority of Cocker spaniels have multiple rows of such hairs and no associated problems.

Ectopic cilia exit the conjunctival surface, most commonly in the middle of the upper lid, and cause corneal ulceration associated with a moderate amount of pain. The blinking of the upper eyelid often results in a vertically oriented ulcer in the superior cornea. A high degree of suspicion must be present to detect these hairs because they are often not easily visible even with magnification. Ectopic cilia are best removed by surgical dissection.

Trichiasis hairs are normal hairs that rub on the cornea due to a conformational problem. Prominent nasal folds and entropion are examples of situations that result in trichiasis. Most cases of trichiasis may be successfully treated surgically. Medial canthoplasty surgery generally alleviates irritation caused by nasal folds and medial lower lid entropion. Standard procedures such as the Hotz-Celsus procedure offer relief from trichiasis due to entropion affecting the central portions of the lid.

Lagophthalmos (literally rabbit-like eye), seen in a number of brachycephalic breeds, may result in an incomplete blink. As a result, the horizontal axial cornea becomes dry and prone to ulceration. If the condition is mild, application of lubricant ointment several times daily and at bedtime may supply relief. Permanent correction may be achieved by medial canthoplasty, which alleviates both lagophthalmos and nasal trichiasis.

Neurotrophic keratitis may result from a decreased to absent blink due to damage to either the corneal sensory nerves or facial nerve. In severe cases tarsorrhaphy, sometimes permanent, may be indicated to prevent corneal desiccation.

Other Causes of Chronic Irritation

Ocular foreign bodies may become lodged underneath the third eyelid and cause deep corneal ulcers. This condition is most often seen in the fall of the year in dogs that spend time in woods and fields. Foreign bodies may be found by gently grasping the nictitans (nictitating membrane) with serrated nonlocking forceps following application of topical anesthetic to the ocular surface. The nictitans is gently lifted and the fornix of the nictitans-globe junction inspected. It is never wrong to "look behind the third eyelid" on initial presentation of a patient with a corneal ulcer, but this procedure is certainly indicated if the ulcer has not healed on recheck examination.

Other Ocular Disease

Keratoconjunctivitis Sicca

Keratoconjunctivitis sicca (KCS, "dry eye") is commonly seen in breeds including Cocker spaniels, English bulldogs, and a variety of brachycephalic breeds (see p. 1061). Patients present with varying amounts of ocular pain and often have mucoid ocular discharge. The deficiency in the aqueous portion of tears that occurs in this disease results in poor corneal health in affected animals.

Tear production may be measured using the Schirmer tear test. Normal tear production in an unanesthetized eye is over 15 mm wetting/minute. Diagnosis of KCS is made on the basis of low tear production in the presence of clinical signs such as conjunctival hyperemia, mucoid ocular discharge, and often superficial corneal pigmentation and vascularization. The majority of patients respond well to application of topical cyclosporine ointment (Optimmune, Schering-Plough) every 8 to 12 hours, which stimulates tear production. Cyclosporine ointment may be supplemented with a topical artificial tear ointment or solution as needed. If a secondary bacterial infection is present, an antibiotic ointment or solution may be applied every 6 hours. In cases in which copious mucoid discharge is present, the above medications may be more effective when applied after rinsing the ocular surface with a commercial eye wash. In the minority of cases that are refractory to cyclosporine treatment, parotid duct transposition surgery may be considered.

INFECTED ULCERS

The loss of corneal epithelium deprives the stroma of its main barrier to infection with the bacteria that are normally found in the conjunctival sac. (Fungal organisms are rarely found in infected corneal ulcers in small animals.) Infection results in deepening of the ulcer, due to the action of bacterial and host enzymes that destroy corneal stroma. If a corneal infection goes untreated, it may progress to perforation of the eye.

Diagnosis

Infection of a corneal ulcer should be suspected if an ulcer does not heal within the expected time frame, especially if it enlarges. A white to yellow appearance to the cornea is suggestive of leukocyte infiltration, which is indicative of infection. An edematous or gelatinous appearance is consistent with collagenase activity causing stromal digestion, characteristic but not diagnostic of a *Pseudomonas* infection. An animal diagnosed with an infected ulcer should be hospitalized and examined frequently until the infection is controlled or surgery is performed.

If infection is suspected, a spatula is used to gently collect samples from the affected cornea for culture, sensitivity, and cytology. Slides may be stained with a Wright-Giemsa stain for identification on the basis of morphology—the majority of gram-positive organisms are cocci and gram-negative organisms are rods. Organisms commonly found in infected canine corneal ulcers include *Staphylococcus, Streptococcus,* and *Pseudomonas* spp. Of these, *Pseudomonas* is most likely to be resistant to commonly used antibiotics.

Treatment (see Table 1)

Medical Treatment

Antibiotic Treatment. Antibiotic treatment of a suspected infected corneal ulcer should be based on the results of initial diagnostic testing. If cytology indicates the presence of gram-negative bacteria, the use of agents known to be effective against resistant *Pseudomonas* species, such as topical Ciloxan solution (ciprofloxacin 0.3% solution, Alcon) or tobramycin (tobramycin 0.3% solution, Bausch and Lomb) is indicated. If cocci are seen, triple antibiotic solution (neomycin/polymyxin/gramicidin) would be an appropriate choice. Application of more than one antimicrobial may be performed sequentially, allowing 2 to 3 minutes between application of different solutions. An infected ulcer should be treated more frequently than every 6 hours; treatment every 2 hours is desirable in order to sterilize the ulcer.

Cycloplegics and Analgesics. Animals will also be in considerably more pain than patients with uninfected ulcers and may benefit from topical atropine of an adequate frequency to maintain mydriasis (generally every 8 to 12 hours). Oral aspirin is also useful to relieve discomfort.

Topical Serum. The melting in a corneal ulcer is due to the action of host and bacterial proteases that degrade collagen. Serum contains a number of protease inhibitors; therefore application of serum to an ulcer may be used to slow degradation of collagen. Application of serum may be done at a similar frequency to topical antibiotic treatment.

Surgical Treatment

Surgical intervention is indicated when an ulcer extends greater than one half to two thirds of stromal depth or when the ulcer is progressive despite aggressive medical therapy.

Conjunctival grafts are the surgical treatment of choice because they supply a source of fibrovascular infiltrate to the thinned, compromised cornea. Additional benefits from a conjunctival flap include the antimicrobial and anticollagenase effects of leukocytes and plasma. Intensive antibacterial therapy is indicated prior to placement of a conjunctival flap because if the graft site is heavily infected, the cornea underneath the graft may slough, resulting in loss of the graft. Correct placement of a conjunctival flap is technically demanding and should be performed by veterinarians with experience in corneal surgery, ideally by an ophthalmologist.

Corneoscleral transposition surgery is another alternative procedure used to repair corneal defects. In this procedure normal cornea and sclera adjacent to the diseased tissue are mobilized and transposed to cover the corneal defect. This procedure has no advantages over conjunctival graft surgery. Experience and correct instrumentation are required in order to perform this procedure satisfactorily.

Ophthalmic cyanoacrylate is another alternative for therapy of a deep corneal ulcer. Cyanoacrylate adhesives are reported to have antibacterial effects but do not supply healthy tissue to a corneal defect as conjunctival grafts or corneoscleral transposition does. If cyanoacrylate is used, it is important to dry the ulcer prior to application and to apply a small amount of adhesive to the wound. Application of glue should be considered for a deep corneal ulcer if a competent corneal surgeon is not available, or if finances prohibit conjunctival graft surgery.

There is no rational basis for placing a third eyelid flap

over an infected ulcer, because the most likely result of this procedure is to prevent topically applied medications from reaching the ulcer. If a veterinarian desires to cover a corneal ulcer, a partial temporary tarsorrhaphy offers advantages over a third eyelid flap. Medication may be applied at the medial canthus and is not inhibited from reaching the ulcer. Furthermore, a partial tarsorrhaphy often allows some visualization of the ulcer, which would be completely obscured from view by a third eyelid flap. A mattress suture may be placed over a stent and tied with a bow, allowing the veterinarian to untie the suture, examine the ulcer, and retie the suture if desired.

INDOLENT ULCERS

Also known as nonhealing ulcers or Boxer ulcers, these corneal ulcers do not heal following weeks of therapy. Their superficial nature correctly indicates a lack of infection, and often no exacerbating cause can be found. In some long-standing cases, exuberant granulation tissue may be present in the adjacent cornea, especially in Boxers. Some affected patients have an abnormal corneal epithelial basement membrane and a decrease in the amount of hemidesmosomes that participate in adhesion between the epithelium and basement membrane. As a result of the underlying abnormalities, the epithelium at the edge of the wound is loosely adherent and is unable to migrate over the denuded stroma.

Diagnosis

Diagnosis is based on the history as well as detection of loose epithelium at the margin of the ulcer. Loose epithelium may be detected by inspection of the cornea with magnification, and fluorescein applied to the cornea may be seen migrating underneath epithelium. If loose epithelium is not detected but the history suggests an indolent ulcer, a dry cotton swab can be used to debride the cornea following administration of topical anesthetic. If epithelium can be removed with a cotton swab, it is nonadherent; healthy corneal epithelium is resistant to debridement.

Treatment (see Table 1)

Several types of treatment are used for indolent ulcers, including application of contact lenses, collagen shields, third eyelid flaps, superficial punctate and grid keratotomy, and topical treatments such as aprotinin and epidermal growth factor. In a large clinical study, superficial keratotomy was found to be the most effective treatment, resulting in a 72% resolution rate by 2 weeks.

Superficial Keratotomy

I routinely perform a superficial grid keratotomy for persistent corneal ulcers. The first step is debridement of all loose epithelium using a dry cotton swab. (The owner should be advised that the ulcer is going to be larger when the patient leaves than when it was presented!) A superficial keratotomy is then performed using a 25-gauge needle in a grid pattern. The keratotomy should start in normal cornea, traverse the ulcer and end in normal cornea. To avoid corneal penetration I hold the needle nearly parallel to the surface of the cornea and stabilize my hand on the patient's head. The keratotomy need only be of sufficient depth that a grid pattern is visible following the procedure. Following the keratotomy a contact lens may be placed to further encourage adhesion between the epithelium and stroma. The debridement and keratotomy result in increased pain in affected animals that can be treated by application of topical atropine every 12 to 24 hours for 2 to 3 days and oral aspirin for several days. Application of topical antibiotics is also indicated, as for any ulcer.

Keratotomy may be performed in the examination room with a cooperative patient. If a patient is nervous or objects to restraint the procedure may require sedation. If sedation is used and a contact lens is placed, a temporary tarsorrhaphy may be performed to prolong the retention time of the contact lens. If a contact lens is not available, a third eyelid flap may be performed. In my opinion, an indolent ulcer is one of the few indications for placement of a third eyelid flap. The owner should be advised of the prolonged time for resolution of the disease, as well as the possibility that the condition may recur because of an underlying abnormality.

FELINE HERPESVIRUS–ASSOCIATED DISEASE

Feline herpesvirus is a common respiratory and ocular pathogen of cats. This virus replicates in and is pathogenic for conjunctival epithelium and, to a lesser extent, corneal epithelium.

In my experience the majority of corneal ulcers in cats are caused by feline herpesvirus. The conformational abnormalities seen commonly in canine patients are observed less often in cats, with the exception of brachycephalic cats. Diagnosis and treatment of herpesvirus-associated disease in cats is covered elsewhere in this section. Two of the relevant sequelae to herpesvirus infection are symblepharon and deep corneal ulcers.

Symblepharon is adhesion of conjunctiva to itself or to cornea. Prerequisite to symblepharon formation is extensive damage to the epithelial surface of cornea and conjunctiva such as may occur with feline herpesvirus infection. If extensive areas of cornea are involved in symblepharon, performance of a keratectomy may be considered to achieve a clear visual axis.

As is the case with corneal ulcers in dogs, corneal ulcers in cats may become infected. Medical and surgical treatment considerations of deep corneal ulcers are the same as for dogs.

References and Suggested Reading

Hakanson NE, Merideth RE: Conjunctival pedicle grafting in the treatment of corneal ulcers in the dog and cat. J Am Anim Hosp Assoc 23:641, 1987.
Describes instrumentation required and surgical technique used in conjunctival pedicle grafting for corneal ulceration, as well as results in 35 cases.

Kern TJ: Ulcerative keratitis. Vet Clin North Am Small Anim Pract 20:643, 1990.
Covers the same subject discussed in this chapter in more depth.

Kirschner SE, Niyo Y, Betts DM: Idiopathic persistent corneal erosions: Clinical and pathological findings in 18 dogs. J Am Anim Hosp Assoc 25:84, 1989.
Clinical and histologic study of nonhealing ulcers in dogs with discussion of the pathogenesis of the condition.

Leahey AB, Gottsch JD, Stark WJ: Clinical experience with N-butyl cyanoacrylate (Nexacryl) tissue adhesive. Ophthalmology 100:173, 1993.
A study of the outcomes of use of cyanoacrylate glue in people with deep corneal ulcers.

Morgan RV, Abrams KL: A comparison of six different therapies for

persistent corneal erosions in dogs and cats. Vet Comp Ophthalmol 4:38, 1994.
A study of the success rate of treatment of persistent corneal erosions with third eyelid flaps, contact lenses, collagen shields, aprotinin application and punctate keratotomy.

Nasisse MP: Feline ophthalmology. In: Gelatt KN, ed: Veterinary Ophthalmology. Philadelphia: Lea & Febiger, 1991, p 529.
An in-depth discussion of the pathogenesis and treatment of feline herpesvirus–associated disease.

Whitley RD: Canine cornea. In: Gelatt KN, ed: Veterinary Ophthalmology. Philadelphia: Lea & Febiger, 1991, p 307.
Extensive discussion of the pathophysiology and treatment of corneal ulceration.

Canine Glaucoma

JAMES GAARDER

Ithaca, New York

Glaucoma occurs when elevated intraocular pressure (IOP) impairs normal function of the eye. With a reported incidence of 0.5%, it is one of the common vision-threatening diseases diagnosed in dogs. In canine glaucoma, intraocular pressure is elevated because the egress of aqueous from the anterior chamber is reduced or absent. Glaucoma destroys vision because it kills ganglion cells by the direct effects of increased pressure and by the indirect effects of impaired intraocular circulation. Normal ganglion cell function is essential for normal vision. In most cases the diagnosis of glaucoma in dogs is not complicated: An intraocular pressure measured by indentation (Schiøtz) or applanation tonometry that is over 30 mm Hg is pathologic and diagnostic. That is the easy part. The challenge presented by glaucoma lies not in its diagnosis but in its treatment. *Before appropriate therapy can be implemented, the clinician must distinguish primary glaucoma from secondary glaucoma and assess the potential for vision of the affected eye.* The following discussion is designed to facilitate the critical evaluation of glaucomatous eyes and to guide the therapeutic decision-making process based on this assessment.

CLASSIFICATION OF GLAUCOMA

Canine glaucoma can be divided into primary and secondary forms. It is important to recognize primary glaucoma because it is, by definition, ultimately *bilateral* and the normal fellow eye is *at risk.* In at least 50% of cases, the initially normotensive fellow eye becomes overtly glaucomatous within 6 to 12 months after the onset of disease in the first eye. Primary glaucoma is due to an inherited defect of the iridocorneal angle or trabecular meshwork that eventually impairs aqueous outflow. Primary glaucoma is diagnosed when IOP is elevated in the absence of signs of concurrent ocular disease. Females, middle-aged dogs, and certain breeds are at increased risk (Slater and Erb, 1986). There are two subtypes of primary glaucoma. Primary open angle glaucoma (POAG), the most common type of glaucoma in humans, is an unusual form of canine glaucoma and is seen almost exclusively in the Beagle. Closed or narrow angle glaucoma (CAG) is by far the more common form in the dog and affects several breeds, including Cocker spaniels, Basset hounds, Miniature Poodles, Boston terriers, Dalmatians, and Arctic breeds. This form of glaucoma is much more resistant to conventional medical therapy alone than POAG and is usually best managed by surgery. It should be emphasized that both types of primary glaucoma in the dog are *incurable* disorders that, at best, can be effectively *managed* for variable periods of time. Canine primary glaucoma is an *inherited* disease: Affected dogs should not be used for breeding.

Secondary glaucoma is *usually* a unilateral disease and can sometimes be successfully treated with preservation of vision if the underlying cause can be identified and corrected. Secondary glaucoma is associated with concurrent ocular disease such as inflammation, neoplasia, or hemorrhage. Careful examination of the anterior and posterior segments with a focal light source, magnification, and indirect or direct ophthalmoscopy will usually identify these underlying disorders. Glaucoma secondary to uveitis results from decreased aqueous outflow because of peripheral anterior synechia, posterior synechia, or iridocorneal angle occlusion with inflammatory debris. Intraocular tumors cause glaucoma when they grow anteriorly to a size that impedes aqueous outflow or when exfoliated tumor cells obstruct the iridocorneal angle. Hyphema can result in secondary glaucoma; IOP must be carefully monitored in eyes with anterior chamber hemorrhage because red blood cells can obstruct the drainage apparatus. Intraocular neoplasia should always be considered as an underlying cause of hyphema.

Glaucoma often occurs in association with luxation or subluxation of the lens, especially in predisposed breeds (e.g., terriers, Norwegian elkhounds, Brittany spaniels, Welsh Springer spaniels, Poodles, Beagles). Although this form of glaucoma is often considered secondary to lens luxation, several characteristics of this disorder resemble primary glaucoma. First, although the diagnosis of glaucoma in these breeds often coincides with lens luxation, removing the luxated lens does *not* cure glaucoma in most cases and glaucoma often *precedes* overt anterior lens luxation. Second, this is an inherited disease. Third and most important, this is a *bilateral* disease and the normal, unaffected eye is *at risk*. It should be noted that in most nonterrier breeds, lens luxation is *secondary* to zonular disinsertion in a buphthalmic globe with chronic glaucoma. In dogs predisposed to lens luxation, however, the lens luxates early in the course of disease when vision is still present and often must be removed as an adjunct in treating the disease.

DIAGNOSIS

Glaucoma is a disease that simply *cannot* be accurately diagnosed or effectively treated without a precise and objective method of estimating intraocular pressure. Digital tonometry is notoriously imprecise and inaccurate. Instrumental tonometry is essential for diagnosis and management of the glaucomatous eye. The Schiøtz tonometer is an inexpensive and reliable indentation tonometer and should be owned by all small animal practices. When used and maintained properly, it provides a level of accuracy similar to that of the much more expensive applanation tonometers. When using the Schiøtz tonometer, scale readings must be converted to estimates of IOP using a conversion table. The human (Friedenwald) conversion table provided with the tonometer is preferred (Miller, 1995). Normal canine IOP is 15 to 25 mm Hg with less than 5 mm Hg difference between eyes. Tonometry is also useful for diagnosing uveitis. It should be performed in all red eyes without obvious corneal defects. Ocular hypotony (IOP less than 10 mm Hg) is suggestive of active anterior uveitis. Severe corneal edema may falsely decrease the tonometer reading, and an anteriorly luxated lens may falsely elevate the reading. NOTE: *Schiøtz tonometry is contraindicated in the presence of deep corneal ulcers, penetrating ocular wounds, or recent corneal incisions.*

Gonioscopy facilitates examination of the iridocorneal angle. A special lens is required to overcome the internal reflection of light in the canine eye. Although gonioscopy is helpful in further classifying certain types of glaucoma, the gonioscopic appearance of the canine iridocorneal angle is of little benefit in predicting which eyes will develop glaucoma. Although commonly performed by veterinary ophthalmologists, gonioscopy is not essential for the management of most clinical cases.

CLINICAL SIGNS OF GLAUCOMA

After establishing a diagnosis of glaucoma with objective tonometric measurements, one must determine the vision potential of the affected eye before appropriate therapy can be employed. There are some important clinical signs that can aid the clinician in accurately making this assessment. The following discussion emphasizes those signs as they pertain to acute and chronic disease. Eyes afflicted with *chronic* glaucoma are usually irreversibly blind and uncomfortable. Blind eyes with *acute* glaucoma may still have *potential* for vision provided the IOP can be normalized in a timely manner and the disease is still in its early stages. Because greatly elevated IOP can cause irreversible damage to the visual potential of the eye within hours, acute glaucoma is *truly an ocular emergency.* By the time the signs of chronic glaucoma are evident, the vision potential of the eye is usually lost.

Acute Glaucoma

Early in its course, glaucoma causes acute *blindness*, ocular *pain*, conjunctival and *episcleral* vascular congestion, and *diffuse corneal edema.* The pupil is usually *dilated* and unresponsive or sluggishly responsive to bright light stimulation. Blindness occurs early in glaucoma because of impaired axoplasmic transport within the ganglion cell axons and compromised circulation to the optic nerve. If glaucoma is diagnosed early and the pressure is lowered to normal levels (15 to 25 mm Hg), blindness may be partially reversible. The pain associated with glaucoma is often a referred pain. Humans with angle-closure glaucoma often complain of a migraine-like headache. Many dogs do not show classic signs of ocular pain such as blepharospasm, epiphora, or photophobia. Episcleral congestion is very suggestive of glaucoma and appears as a uniform vascular engorgement of the deep episcleral veins that parallel each other and radiate perpendicular to the limbus. The corneal edema associated with acute glaucoma is usually diffuse, affects the entire cornea, and gives the eye a bluish discoloration. The edema occurs because of impaired endothelial pump activity secondary to increased IOP and often disappears within hours after the IOP has been normalized. Mydriasis occurs because of impaired retinal function secondary to pressure-related obstruction of axoplasmic flow of ganglion cells and iridal paralysis secondary to pressure inhibition of the iris sphincter muscle and oculomotor neuropraxia. The pupil, like the cornea, may return to normal size and motility on IOP reduction. Careful assessment of the *consensual pupillary light response* (from the affected eye to the normal eye) with bright focal light stimulation is very helpful in deciding whether or not the eye has *potential* for vision. The dazzle reflex can be helpful in evaluating the optic nerve. A very strong light source (e.g., a fiberoptic or Finhoff transilluminator) when directed into the eye at close range should produce a rapid blink referred to as the dazzle reflex. These tests should be performed initially and repeated when IOP is normalized. Sometimes a simple test such as blindfolding the normal fellow eye and assessing functional vision using an obstacle course can be helpful. The fundus, when it can be seen, is usually *normal*. Routine electroretinography assesses the photoreceptor cells, bipolar cells, and retinal pigment epithelium but not the ganglion cells, so this diagnostic test is not helpful in early glaucoma. Favorable prognostic clinical signs for a sighted or potentially sighted eye include: (1) normal direct and consensual pupillary light responses (PLRs); (2) normal dazzle reflex; and (3) normal menace or functional vision tests. Unfavorable signs include: (1) absent direct and consensual PLRs; (2) absent dazzle reflex;

and (3) lack of detectable functional vision or history of blindness for more than 3 to 5 days.

Although the aforementioned clinical signs are very suggestive, *there are no pathognomonic signs of acute glaucoma* (in contrast to chronic glaucoma). Because any or all of these signs can be seen in other ocular disorders, *tonometry is essential for accurate diagnosis*. When in doubt as to the visual potential of the eye, institute emergency therapy to reduce the IOP. If the eye is irreversibly blind, this will become evident soon enough.

Chronic Glaucoma

The classic and *pathognomonic* clinical signs of chronic glaucoma are *buphthalmia, corneal striae*, and *optic disk cupping*. Buphthalmia occurs owing to stretching and thinning of the collagen fibers that compose the cornea and sclera. This change occurs over a period of chronic IOP elevation of weeks to months. It should be emphasized that by the time IOP has been elevated for long enough to cause stretching of the cornea and sclera, irreversible damage has been done to the retina and optic nerve. In other words, the buphthalmic eye is almost always a blind eye. An exception to this rule is occasionally seen in puppies. In the juvenile dog buphthalmia can occur within days because of the marked elasticity of the cornea and sclera in young animals. In puppies this elasticity may protect the retina as the eye enlarges with even moderate increases in IOP and makes IOP alone an unreliable indicator of glaucoma in young animals. Buphthalmia in puppies may be reversible if IOP is normalized. Another exception is occasionally seen in Chinese Shar peis, Chow Chows, and Beagles that present with corneal striae and buphthalmia in sighted eyes. This preservation of vision in enlarged eyes may be due to mucinosis of collagen fibrils in the former two breeds increasing the elasticity of the sclera and cornea and the insidious nature of primary open angle glaucoma, which almost exclusively affects the last breed.

With buphthalmia, the cornea stretches and linear tears occur in Descemet's membrane, allowing aqueous to enter the corneal stroma. These linear breaks or tears in Descemet's membrane are referred to as corneal striae, Descemet's striae, or Haab's striae. They are pathognomonic for chronic glaucoma and are usually seen only in blind eyes. These linear striae are permanent changes and do not disappear even if IOP is normalized.

Optic nerve head "cupping" appears as a darker than normal and depressed or recessed optic disk due to axonal degeneration and posterior displacement of the lamina cribrosa. The change is best appreciated with indirect ophthalmoscopy, comparing the normal eye with the affected eye. By the time cupping of the optic nerve head is visible ophthalmoscopically, IOP has usually been elevated for weeks or even months. Most canine eyes that have obvious cupping of the optic nerve head are blind or at least have severe visual impairment. Other signs consistently seen with chronic glaucoma include corneal neovascularization secondary to buphthalmia-related exposure keratitis, lens luxation or subluxation, cataract, vitreal degeneration, and generalized retinal degeneration evidenced by tapetal hyper-reflectivity and retinal vascular attenuation.

GLAUCOMA THERAPY

Choosing the proper therapy depends on proper and thorough diagnostic evaluation. What may be appropriate therapy for the sighted eye is often entirely inappropriate for the blind painful eye. The client should be aware of both the short- and the long-term prognosis when informed of the diagnosis and all of its implications. The goal of therapy depends on the prognosis for vision of the eye. For the sighted or potentially sighted eye acutely affected by glaucoma, the goal of therapy is to maintain vision and comfort as long as possible using any or all appropriate medical and surgical therapy. In acute cases IOP must be reduced as rapidly, effectively, and safely as possible. The clinician and client should realize, however, that eyes affected with primary glaucoma have a *poor* long-term prognosis for vision, regardless of the therapeutic modality employed. When the eye becomes irreversibly blind, the goal of therapy changes. The most important thing the clinician can do for the blind glaucomatous eye is make it *comfortable*. There is little doubt that severely hypertensive eyes are **painful**. This pain is often manifested as subtle lethargy, depression, or withdrawal that many owners overlook until the pain is alleviated. Although POAG in humans is usually manifested as a painless progressive form of vision loss, most forms of canine glaucoma are more analogous to human angle-closure glaucoma in which affected individuals describe severe and intense pain around the eye accompanied by nausea and vomiting.

Because primary glaucoma is bilateral, sadly, most affected dogs ultimately become totally blind in both eyes. Dogs are not nearly as dependent on their vision as are people. Their other senses (smell, hearing, touch) are much more acute than in humans; thus, complete vision loss is not nearly as debilitating as for people if the eyes are **comfortable**. Blind but comfortable animals can continue to be active, enjoyable companions.

THERAPY FOR SIGHTED OR POTENTIALLY SIGHTED EYES

Medical Therapy

The goal of medical therapy is to decrease intraocular pressure by shrinking the intraocular volume, decreasing the production of aqueous, and/or increasing the outflow of aqueous (Table 1). Osmotic agents are useful in the emergency treatment of acute glaucoma because they dehydrate the vitreous and decrease the intraocular volume. Carbonic anhydrase inhibitors, beta-blockers, and sympathomimetic agents decrease the production of aqueous. Miotics, sympathomimetic agents, and prostaglandin analogues increase the outflow of aqueous.

Osmotic Agents

Hyperosmotic agents (e.g., intravenous mannitol, oral glycerol) should be used in acute severe elevations of IOP in sighted or potentially sighted eyes. Hyperosmotic agents increase plasma osmolality, which produces an osmotic gradient between the ocular vasculature and intraocular fluids (primarily the vitreous). The hyperosmotics are the

TABLE 1. Commonly Used Drugs for the Treatment of Canine Glaucoma

Hyperosmotics

Mannitol (25%)—1–2 gm/kg IV; administer over 20 min; withhold water for 4 hours after administration; repeat in 4 to 6 hr if necessary. Useful for emergency therapy for acute glaucoma in potentially sighted eyes.

Glycerol (50%)—1–2 gm/kg PO. May cause vomiting. Do not use in diabetic dogs.

Systemic Carbonic Anhydrase Inhibitors

Dichlorphenamide (Daranide, Merck & Co.)—2–4 mg/kg q8–12hr; most potent CAI with fewest side effects in dogs.

Methazolamide (Neptazane, Lederle)—2–4 mg/kg q8–12hr; available in 25-mg tablets, which facilitates accurate dosing for small dogs.

Acetazolamide (Diamox, Lederle)—4–8 mg/kg q8–12hr; is the least expensive CAI but produces the highest incidence of side effects.

Topical Carbonic Anhydrase Inhibitors

Dorzolamide (Trusopt, Merck & Co.)—q8hr (in humans); unproven efficacy in dogs; not as potent as the oral CAIs.

Miotic Agents (Parasympathomimetics)

Pilocarpine solution (2%)—q6–12hr; should not be used if uveitis is present; topically irritating.

Pilocarpine gel (Pilopine HS, Alcon)—4% q24hr.

Echothiophate iodide (Phospholine Iodide, Wyeth-Ayerst)—0.06%, 0.125% q12–24hr; do not use in conjunction with organophosphate flea products.

Demecarium bromide (Humorsol, Merck & Co.—0.125%, 0.25% q12–24hr; do not use in conjunction with organophosphate flea products.

Beta-Adrenergic Antagonists (Topical)

Timolol maleate (Timoptic, Merck & Co.)—0.5% q12hr; also available in a 0.25% solution that is ineffective in dogs; a nonselective beta-blocker; may cause bronchoconstriction.

Betaxolol HCl (Betoptic, Alcon)—0.5% q12hr; a selective beta-blocker; has fewer side effects than timolol but is not as potent.

Sympathomimetics

Dipivefrin HCl (Propine, Allergan)—0.1% q12hr.

Prostaglandin Analogues

Latanoprost (Xalatan, Pharmacia & Upjohn)—q24hr (in humans); unproven efficacy in dogs; in humans, administration at bedtime is recommended.

Potassium Supplementation

Potassium chloride (Slow-K, Summit)—600 mg tablet/25 kg PO q24hr. Recommended to use in conjunction with oral CAIs.

CAI, carbonic anhydrase inhibitor.

most potent medical therapy available in terms of reducing severe IOP elevations and usually produce ocular hypotension that lasts 5 or more hours within 30 minutes after administration. The hyperosmotics are useful only in emergency situations because they lose their effectiveness after the second or third administration, making osmotherapy ineffective for chronic therapy. Mannitol should be administered intravenously at a dosage of 1 to 2 gm/kg over 20 minutes. High concentrations of mannitol (over 20%) may crystallize at room temperature, so warming to dissolve the crystals and administering the solution through a blood filtration set are indicated. Water should be withheld for a minimum of 4 hours after mannitol administration to maintain intraocular dehydration. Mannitol is never the sole agent used for treatment of glaucoma. An oral carbonic anhydrase inhibitor (see below) should be given during or before mannitol administration along with one or more topical agents. Glycerol (50%) is an oral osmotic diuretic and also produces ocular hypotension. It is not as potent as mannitol and often produces vomiting. The dose is 1.4 gm/kg but should not be used in diabetics because it can produce hyperglycemia. After the IOP is normalized and maintained, referral to a veterinary ophthalmologist should be discussed with the client. If IOP does not normalize within 6 to 8 hours after instituting therapy, emergency referral to a veterinary ophthalmologist should be considered.

Carbonic Anhydrase Inhibitors

The oral carbonic anhydrase inhibitors (CAIs) are the mainstay of veterinary medical therapy for glaucoma and

are the only systemic agents used in the long-term management of patients with glaucoma. Carbonic anhydrase catalyzes the combination of carbon dioxide and water to form carbonic acid. The CAIs decrease the production of aqueous by blocking this process. Because CAIs reduce the production of aqueous, they are useful in all forms of glaucoma. The onset of action of orally administered CAIs is 2 to 3 hours after administration, the maximum effect occurs in 4 to 8 hours, and the IOP is usually reduced by 20 to 30%. The oral carbonic anhydrase inhibitors are the most potent medical agent available for long-term control of IOP. The carbonic anhydrase enzyme is present in many nonocular tissues, including the kidney, pancreas, central nervous system, red blood cells, and lungs. Because of the ubiquitous nature of carbonic anhydrase, side effects to CAIs are expected and include polyuria/polydipsia, metabolic acidosis, depression, confusion, anorexia, vomiting, diarrhea, and rarely blood dyscrasias. In humans, these side effects are severe enough in 40 to 50% of patients to require discontinuation of therapy. Potassium excretion is increased by oral administration of CAIs, and hypokalemia is a potential sequela of chronic use. Supplementation with oral potassium is recommended. Although dogs appear more tolerant than humans to systemic CAI therapy, side effects are still common in the canine patient. Like the pain of glaucoma, these side effects may be subtle and not easily appreciated by the owner or veterinarian until discontinuation of therapy produces notable change in the dog's attitude, activity level, and appetite. When severe side effects are noted, reducing the dosage, substituting another oral CAI, or discontinuing oral CAI therapy is recommended. Most dogs seem to tolerate dichlorphena-mide and methazolamide better than acetazolamide. Some human patients that are intolerant of one CAI can better tolerate an alternative drug in the same class (Derick et al, 1994). Regardless of the dose or type of systemic CAI used, at least 50% of dogs probably experience some side effects. If the side effects are mild and the dog remains sighted, continued CAI administration is warranted. If the side effects are severe or the dog is permanently blind and in pain, better options are available.

Recently, a new *topical* CAI, dorzolamide (Trusopt, Merck & Co.), has become available. Dorzolamide is ad-ministered three times daily in humans and appears very effective in reducing IOP while minimizing the side effects of the systemic CAIs. To date there are mainly anecdotal reports of its use in dogs. It appears to be beneficial in some cases of canine glaucoma but is not nearly as effective in reducing IOP as oral CAIs. A recent study in humans found that adding oral acetazolamide to topically administered dorzolamide increased the ocular hypotensive effect, but adding dorzolamide to oral acetazolamide did not produce an additional reduction in IOP (Maus et al, 1997).

Miotic Agents

Topical miotic agents produce pupillary constriction, contraction of the ciliary musculature, and increased out-flow of aqueous through a configurational change in the trabecular meshwork. Pilocarpine is a direct-acting cholin-ergic miotic that is available in several concentrations: 2% appears most effective in the dog. Theoretically pilocarpine is most effective in treating POAG, the least common form in dogs. Most forms of canine glaucoma are due to narrowing or closure of the iridocorneal angle, not the trabecular meshwork, making the effectiveness of pilocar-pine questionable for CAG. Advantages of pilocarpine are that it is fairly effective for some forms of glaucoma and relatively inexpensive. Disadvantages are that it is topically irritating and often must be administered 3 to 4 times daily to be effective, reducing owner compliance. A 4% pilocarpine gel (Pilopine HS, Alcon Laboratories) is avail-able and has the advantage of once-daily administration. Because it potentiates breakdown of the blood aqueous barrier, pilocarpine should *not* be used when *uveitis* is present or when treating *secondary* glaucoma. The indirect-acting miotics include echothiophate iodide (Phospholine Iodide, Wyeth-Ayerst) and demecarium bromide (Hu-morsol, Merck) and act by inhibiting cholinesterase, thus increasing endogenous acetylcholine. These agents are less irritating and longer acting than pilocarpine but are more expensive. As with pilocarpine, they can activate latent uveitis and intensify concurrent uveitis. Thus they are most useful in primary glaucoma and are especially useful in primary glaucoma with early lens luxation or subluxation because they can produce miosis and discourage a luxated lens from gaining access to the anterior chamber, resulting in acute pupillary block glaucoma, which necessitates sur-gical intervention.

Beta-Blockers

Although topical beta-blockers are the most frequently prescribed agents for treating glaucoma in man, their effec-tiveness in dogs is controversial. Beta-blockers reduce IOP by decreasing aqueous production. The most commonly used drug is 0.5% timolol maleate (Timoptic, Merck). Timolol is useful in both primary and secondary glaucoma because it reduces aqueous production and does not po-tentiate uveitis as do the topical miotic agents. Because beta-blockers decrease aqueous production by a different mechanism than the CAIs, their ocular hypotensive effect when used together is additive. Timolol is most commonly used as an adjunctive therapy and combined with oral CAIs. Although it is not useful as the sole agent when treating a glaucomatous eye, it may be useful in prophylac-tic therapy for the fellow eye in primary glaucoma.

Sympathomimetic Agents

Adrenergic compounds decrease IOP by stimulating alpha-receptors and increasing aqueous outflow and stimu-lating beta-receptors and decreasing production. As with beta-blockers, they are minimally effective when used as sole agents but can be useful adjuncts when combined with other classes of drugs. Topical epinephrine and epineph-rine-pilocarpine combinations are available, as is dipivefrin hydrochloride (Propine, Allergan, Inc.), an epinephrine pro-drug that is converted to epinephrine in the anterior cham-ber. Dipivefrin hydrochloride is the drug of choice in this group because it has better penetration into ocular tissues, is less irritating, and has more potency and less toxicity. It is more expensive than epinephrine or epinephrine-pilocar-pine combinations.

Prostaglandin Analogues

Latanoprost (Xalatan, Pharmacia & Upjohn) is a re-cently released commercial prostaglandin analogue devel-oped to reduce intraocular pressure in humans. Early re-ports indicate that it is as effective as 0.5% timolol maleate in reducing IOP in humans affected with POAG (Watson et al, 1996). It reduces IOP by increasing aqueous outflow by the unconventional or uveoscleral route. In humans the recommended dosage is one drop once daily at bedtime. This particular prostaglandin analogue has not been exten-sively evaluated for effectiveness in animals, although topi-cal application of $PGF_{2\alpha}$ and similar drugs was shown to cause a significant IOP reduction in rabbits, cats, dogs, and monkeys. In humans the most common side effect is an iris color change with long-term use. The use of latanoprost has not been extensively evaluated in humans or animals with angle-closure glaucoma. It is very expensive but may offer yet another medical alternative.

Surgical Therapy

Glaucoma surgical procedures can be divided into two categories: those that decrease aqueous production by de-stroying part of the ciliary body (cyclodestructive proce-dures) and those that increase aqueous outflow by surgi-cally creating an alternative outflow mechanism (filtering procedures). Both types of surgeries have inherent advan-tages and disadvantages. When surgery is elected, the method employed is dependent on the individual situation and the preferences and experiences of the veterinary ophthalmologist.

Cyclodestructive procedures include trans-scleral cryosurgery and laser cyclophotocoagulation. Cryosurgery can be effective in reducing IOP but is associated with many complications including cataract formation, severe uveitis, and hypotony. The most important complication is a transient but severe postoperative IOP elevation that is very difficult to control and often results in permanent blindness. Cyclophotocoagulation (CPC) using the Nd:YAG or diode laser has shown promise recently in decreasing IOP in both visual and blind eyes. Although a transient IOP rise often occurs as in cryosurgery, it is more amenable to control with antiglaucoma medications. Cyclophotocoagulation is a noninvasive surgery but requires a brief period of general anesthesia. Diode laser CPC has been shown to be effective in reducing IOP about 80% of the time and in preserving vision in medically unresponsive eyes about 50% of the time. It is a relatively new procedure and long-term results are unknown. The primary indication for laser CPC is as adjunctive therapy for sighted or potentially sighted eyes in which the IOP cannot be controlled with medical therapy alone. Laser CPC is proving helpful in preserving vision in glaucomatous eyes for longer periods of time than with medical therapy alone. It has also been used to prophylactically treat the normal fellow eye in cases of primary glaucoma, but there is risk involved because some sighted eyes are blinded by postoperative pressure elevations and uveitis.

Several filtering surgical procedures are available including sclerotomy with iridencleisis and gonioimplant devices. In the past, these procedures rarely offered long-term success because the alternative outflow channels created soon became obstructed with fibrin and eventually closed because of scar tissue. Recent improvements in microsurgical technique and the use of antiproliferative agents such as mitomycin-C (Bristol-Meyers Oncology) and 5-fluorouracil (Roche) have improved the outcome and effectiveness of these procedures, and their use has found a renewed enthusiasm among some veterinary ophthalmologists. Because filtering surgeries are expensive and may generate complications, their use should be reserved for visual or potentially visual eyes.

The surgical management of sighted or potentially sighted eyes with early lens luxation/subluxation requires discussion. There is little doubt that acute anterior luxation of the lens into the anterior chamber in a sighted eye requires emergency therapy consisting of medications to reduce IOP and intracapsular lensectomy to relieve the associated pupillary block glaucoma. There is disagreement among veterinary ophthalmologists, however, regarding the management of the subluxated lens that remains in the patellar fossa posterior to the iris. I believe that intracapsular lensectomy in these eyes has an unacceptably high complication rate, including vitreous presentation due to adhesion of the anterior vitreous to the posterior lens capsule and secondary retinal detachment. In my experience, these eyes remain sighted for longer periods of time with conservative medical treatment including miotics to decrease the access of the lens to the anterior chamber and other antiglaucoma medications. Despite medical therapy,

many of these lenses eventually luxate into the anterior chamber and must be surgically removed.

THERAPY FOR BLIND, PAINFUL EYES

Medical Therapy

Medical therapy has no place in the long-term management of blind painful glaucomatous eyes. Most antiglaucoma medications are expensive and generally ineffective in the long run. More importantly, all antiglaucoma medications, including topical drugs, have potential for systemic toxicity and side effects. The oral CAIs are the most effective antiglaucoma drugs but also have the greatest potential for severe side effects. Many humans receiving pilocarpine therapy complain of a brow-ache and blurred vision. Topical beta-blockers can cause cardiovascular and respiratory compromise. In my opinion, the expense and potential for side effects of antiglaucoma medications are warranted as long as there is vision or at least potential for vision. But if the eye is irreversibly blind and painful, the animal and the client are better served by a salvage procedure to make the eye comfortable and eliminate the need for chronic medication.

Surgical Therapy

Salvage procedures for the blind glaucomatous eye include enucleation, intraocular evisceration-implantation, and pharmacologic ciliary body ablation using intravitreal gentamicin. Intraocular evisceration-implantation is my therapy of choice for treating eyes blinded by primary glaucoma. This procedure offers a high success rate and results in a relatively cosmetic and very comfortable globe that usually requires no further therapy. In my experience, the evisceration-implant procedure can be a potentially lifesaving procedure for dogs with primary glaucoma because nearly all owners can adjust to the idea of caring for a blind dog, but a dog without eyes is cosmetically unacceptable for most people. The implant procedure produces a high rate of client satisfaction and complications are rare.

Another option is intravitreal injection of gentamicin. Gentamicin is toxic to the ciliary body epithelium that produces aqueous but it is also toxic to the retina, so it *must only be used in eyes that are already blind*. It should be used with caution in eyes that have active inflammation because it can potentiate uveitis. It should never be used in eyes with intraocular tumors or eyes with glaucoma of an undetermined cause. Advantages are that the procedure can be performed with sedation and local anesthesia, precluding the need for general anesthesia, and it is inexpensive to perform. Complications are *common*, and include failure to reduce IOP, chronic persistent uveitis that can leave an eye hypotonic but still painful, recurrent hemophthalmos, and phthisis bulbi. These complications should be discussed with the owner before the injection because they occur in 30 to 40% of procedures. Despite these complications, pharmacologic ciliary ablation is a viable treatment option in certain situations. Intravitreal gentamicin injection is indicated only when a definitive diagnosis of end-stage primary glaucoma has been made and confirmed with tonometry. It is contraindicated in sighted eyes or eyes with intraocular tumors or infection.

THERAPEUTIC APPROACH

The clinician must realize and communicate to clients that primary glaucoma in dogs is *not a curable disorder*. The goals of therapy are to maintain vision for as long as possible using medical and/or surgical therapy and, if unilateral, to prevent or delay occurrence in the fellow eye. Multiple drug therapy is often required. Oral carbonic anhydrase inhibitors are the most potent ocular hypotensive drugs for long-term use. For topical therapy alone to be effective the IOP must be less than 35 to 40 mm Hg. Most patients are best managed with an oral CAI and one or more topical agents of different classes. I prefer the combination of an oral CAI and timolol. Most antiglaucoma drugs lose their efficacy over time. When the pressure begins to rise despite medical therapy, surgical intervention is indicated. When the eye becomes irreversibly blind and painful, a salvage procedure is indicated. Glaucomatous eyes require frequent monitoring and tonometry should be performed at least every 3 months. More important, the owners should be educated regarding the early clinical signs of glaucoma and instructed to contact their veterinarian if any redness, pain, cloudiness, or change in vision is noted in affected or unaffected fellow eyes. In dogs with primary glaucoma, it appears that prophylactic therapy, using a topical beta-blocker, sympathomimetic agent, or miotic drug is effective in prolonging the period of time until the fellow eye becomes affected, but does not necessarily prevent glaucoma.

Despite many recent advances in veterinary ophthalmology, glaucoma remains one of the most frustrating ocular conditions for both the clinician and the owner. Although there are more antiglaucoma drugs available to veterinarians than ever before, one should recognize that most of the pharmacologic testing for efficacy of these drugs is performed in humans or dogs with POAG, and the effectiveness of many of these agents for closed or narrow angle glaucoma, the most intractable form, in dogs remains speculative. Consultation with a veterinary ophthalmologist is advised early in the management of all cases of canine glaucoma.

References and Suggested Reading

Bingaman DP, Lindley DM, Glickman NW, et al: Intraocular gentamicin and glaucoma: A retrospective study of 60 dog and cat eyes (1985–1993). Vet Comp Ophthal 4:113, 1994.
A discussion of the indications, dosages, and complications of pharmacologic ciliary body ablation using gentamicin.

Brooks DE: Canine and feline glaucomas. In: Kirk RW, ed: Current Veterinary Therapy, 9th ed. Philadelphia: WB Saunders, 1986, pp 656–659.
A discussion of the pathologic features and treatment of canine and feline glaucoma.

Cook C, Brinkmann M, Priehs D, et al: Diode laser transcleral cyclophotocoagulation for glaucoma in dogs. 25th Sci Prog Am Coll Vet Ophthalmol 4:113, 1995.
A description of the early results and outcome of diode laser CPC.

Derick RJ, Craig EL, Weber PA: Glaucoma therapy. In: Mauger TF, Craig EL, eds: Havener's Ocular Pharmacology, 6th ed. St. Louis: Mosby, 1994, pp 172–200.
A discussion of the pharmacokinetics, uses, indications, and side effects of systemic and topical antiglaucoma therapy in humans.

Glover TL, Nasisse MP, Davidson MG: Effects of topically applied mitomycin-C on intraocular pressure, facility of outflow, and fibrosis after glaucoma filtration surgery in clinically normal dogs. Vet Comp Ophthal 56:936, 1995.
This study showed that mitomycin suppresses fibrosis around silicone filtering implants.

Kural E, Lindley D, Krohne S: Canine glaucoma—Part I. Compend Contin Educ 17:1017, 1995.
A thorough discussion of the pathophysiology, clinical signs, and diagnosis of canine glaucoma.

Kural E, Lindley D, Krohne S: Canine glaucoma—Part II. Compend Contin Educ 17:1253, 1995.
A thorough discussion of the goals of therapy for glaucoma and the medical and surgical therapy available for canine glaucoma.

Martin CL, Ward DA: Medical therapy for glaucoma. In: Kirk RW, Bonagura JD, eds: Kirk's Current Veterinary Therapy, 10th ed. Philadelphia: WB Saunders, 1989, pp 647–651.
A discussion of the medical agents used in the treatment of canine and feline glaucoma.

Maus TL, Larsson LI, McLaren JW, et al: Comparison of dorzolamide and acetazolamide as suppressors of aqueous humor flow in humans. Arch Ophthalmol 115:45, 1997.
This study found that 2% dorzolamide was not as effective as systemically administered acetazolamide in reducing IOP in humans.

Miller PE: Glaucoma. In: Kirk RW, Bonagura JD, eds: Kirk's Current Veterinary Therapy, 12th ed. Philadelphia: WB Saunders, 1995, pp 1265–1272.
A discussion of the pathogenesis, diagnosis, and therapy for glaucoma.

Quinn RF, Parkinson K, Wilcock BP, et al: The effects of continuous wave Nd:YAG and semiconductor diode laser energy on the canine ciliary body: In vitro thermographic analysis. Vet Comp Ophthal 6:45, 1996.
Comparison of the effects of the Nd:YAG and diode lasers on the canine ciliary body.

Scherlie JPH: Glaucoma. In: Kirk RW, Bonagura JD, eds: Kirk's Current Veterinary Therapy, 11th ed. Philadelphia: WB Saunders, 1992, pp 1125–1132.
A discussion of aqueous humor dynamics, glaucoma classification, and treatment.

Slater MR, Erb HN: Effects of risk factors and prophylactic treatment on primary glaucoma in the dog. J Am Vet Med Assoc 188:1028, 1986.
An epidemiologic survey and discussion of the potential benefit of antiglaucoma prophylaxis in primary glaucoma of dogs.

Watson P, Stjernschantz J: Latanoprost Study Group: A six-month, randomized, double-masked study comparing latanoprost with timolol in open-angle glaucoma and ocular hypertension. Ophthalmology 103:126, 1996.
This study found that latanoprost administered once daily reduced IOP as well as timolol administered twice daily in human patients with POAG.

Hypertensive Retinopathy

Patricia J. Smith
Fremont, California

Hypertensive retinopathy occurs in association with systemic vascular hypertension in cats and dogs. Hypertension is an organ-destructive and self-perpetuating disease. Without early diagnosis and treatment, hypertensive retinopathy often results in visual impairment in companion animals. Typical ocular findings include retinal hemorrhages, retinal edema, vitreal hemorrhages, hyphema, and partial to complete retinal detachment. Blindness or hyphema often prompts owners to seek veterinary care. Results of the ocular examination may lead the clinician to suspect, and subsequently diagnose, systemic hypertension. The treatment of hypertension can often result in restoration of some vision.

INCIDENCE AND CLINICAL FINDINGS

The causes and pathogenesis of systemic hypertension have been reviewed elsewhere (see *CVT IX,* p. 360; Dukes, 1992; Labato and Ross, 1996; Snyder, 1991). Systemic hypertension may be primary (essential) or secondary. In contrast to humans, in whom essential hypertension constitutes more than 90% of cases, essential or primary hypertension is considered rare in small animals, with a reported incidence of 0.5 to 2% in dogs (Paulsen et al, 1989). Essential hypertension in cats has not been reported, although certain cases may have actually had primary hypertension (Morgan, 1986; Labato and Ross, 1996). Secondary hypertension is much more common in companion animals. Causes of secondary hypertension include renal disease; hyperthyroidism; hypothyroidism; hyperadrenocorticism; diabetes mellitus; coarctation of the aorta; acromegaly; polycythemia; and pheochromocytoma. An isolated case of hypertension in a cat resulting from high dietary salt is also in the literature. Several studies have shown that 50 to 93% of dogs (Snyder, 1991; Paulsen et al, 1989) and 61% of cats (Kobayashi et al, 1990) with renal disease have systemic hypertension. In a group of cats with hyperthyroidism, 87% had elevated blood pressure (Kobayashi et al, 1990).

Animals with systemic hypertension are often presented because of visual deficits or sudden blindness, dilated pupils, or hyphema (Lane et al, 1993; Sansom et al, 1994). It is not uncommon for animals to compensate amazingly well for significant visual deficits, with blindness ensuing only after complete vision loss, that is, with bilateral retinal detachment. Often, an animal will compensate for a slow onset of blindness or severe visual deficit but may manifest "blindness" on movement to a new, unfamiliar environment. In cats and dogs, early ophthalmic findings include retinal edema, foci of intraretinal exudates, and shallow small to segmental retinal detachments. Large intraretinal or preretinal (vitreal) hemorrhage and large areas of complete bullous retinal detachments are present in advanced hypertensive retinopathy (Lane et al, 1993; Sansom et al, 1994; Stiles et al, 1994). Hyphema may occur at any time if larger retinal blood vessels hemorrhage.

In a study of 24 cats with systemic hypertension, all cats had hypertensive retinopathy and 20 of 24 (83.3%) presented for blindness (Littman, 1994). In another study of 36 cats, the incidence of hypertensive retinopathy in cats with renal failure or hyperthyroidism was found to be 80% and 33%, respectively (Stiles et al, 1994). Hypertensive retinopathy may be present at the time of the diagnosis of hypertension but may also appear several months later (Stiles et al, 1994).

The incidence of hypertensive retinopathy in dogs with systemic hypertension has not been determined but is probably much lower than in cats. Over a 22-month period in one study, five dogs were presented for blindness due to intraocular hemorrhage or retinal detachment, and all these animals had systemic hypertension. Four of these dogs had renal insufficiency, and one was diagnosed with essential hypertension (Littman et al, 1988). Isolated reports of systemic hypertension in dogs with ocular abnormalities are in the literature and these abnormalities often prompted referral.

PATHOGENESIS

In experimental canine hypertension, hypertensive retinopathy was characterized by increased vessel tortuosity, preretinal and retinal hemorrhages, retinal and optic disc edema, retinal detachment, and occasionally diffuse intraocular hemorrhage with eventual secondary glaucoma and phthisis bulbi (Paulsen et al, 1989). Three main posterior segment manifestations associated with systemic hypertension are found in hypertensive human patients: optic retinopathy, hypertensive retinopathy, and hypertensive choroidopathy (Hayreh, 1989). All three may occur in animals, but the author believes hypertensive retinopathy and choroidopathy with their respective ocular manifestations of retinal hemorrhage–edema and retinal detachment, are most prevalent in small animals. This terminology—*hypertensive retinopathy, choroidopathy, and optic neuropathy*—has emerged because the vascular systems that supply these three tissues are different in their anatomic and physiologic properties. Specifically, in retinal arterioles, vascular autoregulation is present, and retinal capillaries are nonfenestrated with tight interendothelial junctions. The optic nerve head vasculature has a similar autoregulatory capability. In the choroid (the huge vascular bed within the uvea), choroidal capillaries are fenestrated and the blood-ocular barrier is present at the level of the retinal pigment epithelium. The choroidal vascular bed is under autonomic control (primarily sympathetic) and does not have autoregulatory capabilities.

The hallmark of hypertensive retinopathy is retinal vessel change, including tortuosity, focal intraretinal periarteriolar transudates (FIPTs) or areas of retinal edema, and hemorrhages (Hayreh, 1989). The exudation is believed to represent a breakthrough of autoregulation. The object of autoregulation is to keep the blood flow in a tissue constant; during increases or decreases in perfusion pressure, blood vessels will constrict or dilate, respectively. With chronic hypertension, autoregulatory vasoconstriction will compensate for higher pressures but with chronic or very high blood pressures, or both, breakthrough will occur and result in vasodilatation. These dilated arterioles are exposed to high transmural pressure and exhibit endothelial cell loss and discontinuity, both of which result in breakdown of the blood retinal barrier and increased permeability (Hayreh, 1989). Clinically, FIPTs and retinal edema occur. FIPTs appear clinically as pinpoint- to pinhead-sized, round or oval, dull white lesions adjacent to the major retinal arteries (Stiles et al, 1994), and these may correspond to the foci of intraretinal fluid accumulation seen in cats and dogs. With persistent hypertension, plasma macromolecules leak into the arteriole walls eventually to cause fibrinoid necrosis and thrombosis. *Fibrinoid necrosis* is the term used to denote artery and arteriolar thickening, hyalinization, and fibrin deposition in vessel walls. Retinal hemorrhages may appear "flame-shaped" when small but may break through the internal limiting membrane to form large intravitreal (preretinal) hemorrhages.

Hypertensive choroidopathy results from several changes in the choroidal vascular bed. Hypertensive choroidopathy is primarily due to choroidal ischemia, which produces ischemic damage of the overlying RPE, resulting in the development of the subretinal exudation and retinal detachment. Choroidal arteriolar constriction occurs first, resulting in ischemia with subsequent focal necrosis of the choriocapillaris (CC) and of the adjacent overlying retinal pigment epithelium (RPE), which relies on the CC for nutrition. Subretinal exudation and retinal detachment are observed clinically. Arterioles and CC vessels then become occluded with thrombi, and fibrinoid necrosis may occur. Serous retinal detachment is believed to be a primary manifestation of the choroidopathy.

Pathologically, choroidal arteries and arterioles show marked hyperplastic changes with narrowed or occluded lumina, fibrin deposition in arterial walls, and proliferation of intimal cells with elastic membrane layering, giving vessels an onion skin appearance. Leakage of plasma macromolecules into the vascular smooth muscle results in hyalinization of arterioles. In the nonhuman primate model, there was a significant correlation between the choroidal circulatory disturbances and the blood pressure level. In the few small animal cases that have been examined histologically, retinal and choroidal vascular changes similar to those described earlier have been observed (Paulsen et al, 1989).

Thus hemorrhage and edema in the inner retinal layers results primarily from a retinal vascular pathologic condition or hypertensive retinopathy, and retinal detachment probably is associated with choroidal vascular damage, that is, hypertensive choroidopathy. Retinal degeneration is associated with retinal and choroidal vascular abnormalities that cause ischemia, necrosis, and exudation with retinal

detachment. When one considers how diffuse and bullous retinal detachment often is in hypertension in small animals, it would be logical to presume that diffuse choroidal vascular bed abnormalities with diffuse breakdown of the RPE blood-retinal barrier is the underlying cause for these detachments.

DIAGNOSIS

Diagnosis of hypertensive retinopathy requires a complete ophthalmic examination and documentation of elevated blood pressure. In general hypertension is considered present in dogs and cats if systolic blood pressure is greater than 160 to 180 mm Hg and if diastolic pressure is greater than 100 mm Hg (Dukes, 1992; Snyder, 1991; Littman, 1994). Several articles review the various methods of blood pressure measurement and their reliability (Labato and Ross, 1996; Dukes, 1992; also see p. 835).

A complete ophthalmic examination should be performed, including determination of intraocular pressure (IOP) and mydriasis. In animals with hyphema, uveitis is also present with low IOP, but sometimes high IOP may be present, which is indicative of a secondary glaucoma. Pupils are often dilated and poorly responsive when retinal detachment has been present for sometime. However, depending on the duration and degree of retinal detachment, (i.e., if of short duration) pupillary light reflexes may still be present. If light reflexes are present and glaucoma is absent, pupils should be dilated with 1% tropicamide to facilitate thorough posterior segment examination. The examiner may note the presence of blood vessels, with or without veil-like tissue (the retina), visible just behind the lens. This is suggestive of a highly elevated, bullous retinal detachment.

Posterior segment examination ideally should be performed by direct and indirect ophthalmoscopy. Indirect ophthalmoscopy performed with a light source and 20-D lens allows better screening of a large area of the fundus, because of less magnification, and stereopsis. Common findings include retinal hemorrhages, retinal edema, foci of intraretinal serous exudates, and flat to bullous retinal detachments. Arterial tortuosity may be observed but is not always a prominent feature. Vitreal or preretinal hemorrhage may also be present. Lesions may be asymmetric in distribution; however, in many feline cases, ocular changes are similar in both eyes. In cats, it is typical to have older animals present with sudden blindness caused by bilateral serous retinal detachments. Several owners referred to this ophthalmologist have been told that the bilateral detachments are due to trauma. However, it is unlikely that trauma would cause such significant ocular changes. Hypertensive retinopathy occurs much less frequently in dogs, but there are reports in the literature (Snyder, 1991; Paulsen et al, 1989). Ocular manifestations are similar to those found in the cat, with the additional occasional finding of papilledema. The latter may occur in the cat as well, but because the cat's optic nerve is not myelinated and vessels do not anastomose on the surface of the nerve head, it may be more difficult to recognize. If hyphema is present and precludes posterior segment examination, ocular ultrasonography may help rule out the presence of intraocular neoplasia and may diagnose vitreal hemorrhage or retinal detachment, or both.

If ocular examination is suggestive of hypertensive retinopathy, documentation of elevated blood pressure should follow. All animals in which arterial hypertension is documented should be given a thorough clinical evaluation and physical examination to determine if hypertension is primary or secondary. The diagnostic plan should include a complete history, physical examination (include cardiac auscultation and kidney and thyroid palpation), determination of thyroid hormone level (especially in cats), complete blood count, biochemical profile, and urinalysis. If the most common underlying causes, renal disease or hyperthyroidism, are not identified, additional diagnostic techniques might include abdominal and thoracic radiography and ultrasonography, renal biopsy, coagulation profile, serologic studies for infectious agents that might cause vasculitis or hemorrhage (i.e., ehrlichiosis or Rocky Mountain spotted fever), and testing for other endocrine causes of hypertension such as hyperadrenocorticism, pheochromocytoma, diabetes mellitus, or primary hyperaldosteronism. Because secondary left ventricular hypertrophy is often induced by hypertension, cardiac ultrasonography may be indicated in hypertensive patients. A more detailed discussion of an appropriate diagnostic work-up for systemic hypertension can be found elsewhere (see *CVT IX*, p. 360; *CVT XI* p. 309; Labato and Ross, 1996).

The differential diagnosis of retinal hemorrhage includes clotting disorders, immune-mediated thrombocytopenia, myelophthisic neoplasia, multiple myeloma, coumarin toxicity, estrogen-induced bone marrow suppression, infectious causes of vasculitis or coagulopathy such as ehrlichiosis or rickettsial diseases, hyperviscosity, lymphosarcoma, polycythemia, and systemic lupus erythematosus. Severe anemia in cats, that is, from haemobartonellosis, can also cause retinal hemorrhages because of ischemic damage to vasculature. The differential diagnosis of serous retinal detachment in cats includes hypertension, hyperviscosity, infectious diseases (histoplasmosis, toxoplasmosis), lymphosarcoma, multiple myeloma, or any disease that might cause exudation into the subretinal space. The differential diagnosis for serous retinal detachment in dogs is similar to that of cats but should also include hyperlipidemia, idiopathic immune-mediated (steroid-responsive) retinal detachment, and uveodermatologic syndrome. Differential diagnoses will be ruled out upon recognition of hypertension and during the search for an underlying cause.

TREATMENT

The goal of therapy in hypertensive retinopathy and choroidopathy is to lower the arterial blood pressure. Therapy should be directed against the underlying disease or mechanism of hypertension. Several articles have described therapeutic strategies for hypertension (see *CVT IX*, p. 360; *CVT XI*, p. 309; Snyder, 1991; Labato and Ross, 1996; Dukes, 1992). The basic strategies of therapy are to restrict sodium intake to 0.1 to 0.3% of diet. Dietary therapy alone will not be effective. Medical therapy includes the use of diuretics to alleviate sodium and water retention, sympatholytic agents to reduce cardiac output and renin release, and vasodilators to lower blood pressure.

Uveitis associated with hyphema without glaucoma should be treated with topical steroids (0.1% dexamethasone every 6 to 8 hours or 1% prednisolone acetate every 6 to 8 hours) and mydriatic cycloplegics (1% atropine) as needed to achieve and maintain pupillary dilatation. Secondary glaucoma (from hyphema) should be treated with topical steroids as described, the topical beta-blocker 0.5% timolol maleate every 12 hours and, if needed, systemic carbonic anhydrase inhibitors (i.e., dichlorphenamide or methazolamide, 2 to 5 mg/kg every 8 to 12 hours PO). IOP should be monitored continually and if low, judicious use of short-acting mydriatics (1% tropicamide) may prevent posterior synechiae formation that can later impair vision. (Refer to p. 1090 for details of treating secondary glaucoma.) Topical or systemic steroids should be used with caution, especially if hyperadrenocorticism is suspected, as steroids may theoretically contribute to hypertension by increasing the production of angiotensinogen and increasing the cardiovascular system's sensitivity to catecholamines (see *CVT XI*, p. 309).

Treatment of hypertension and hypertensive retinopathy in companion animals has met with variable success using a variety of treatments. Each case must be handled on an individual basis. The dihydropyridine calcium channel blocker, amlodipine besylate (Norvasc, Pfizer Inc., NY, NY) is often effective at a dose of 0.625 mg every 24 hours per cat as a once-daily single agent. There are minimal side effects (Snyder and Henik, 1994). In refractory cases, 1.25 mg has also been administered every 24 hours with success and without side effects. We have seen lowering of blood pressure and retinal reattachment within 1 week of instituting therapy but have also seen retinal detachments persist for several weeks despite the lowering of blood pressure. Treatment of hypertensive retinopathy in dogs uses a similar approach. Other treatments for hypertension are discussed on page 838. The author has also used amlodipine (0.625 to 1.25 mg/10 pounds) as a single agent in dogs with hypertensive retinopathy with good success at achieving blood pressure control. Urgent control of blood pressure may be attained with sodium nitroprusside (see p. 194)

The addition of diuretics or a systemic carbonic anhydrase inhibitor theoretically may facilitate retinal reattachment, but this has not been substantiated in experimental or clinical studies. Both thiazide and loop diuretics (furosemide) have been used in dogs and cats (Labato and Ross, 1996; Snyder, 1991). Theoretically, diuretics may accelerate resorption of the subretinal fluid in animals with severe bullous detachment.

With these therapies, the author has seen restoration of some vision in several cats; however, underlying renal failure may worsen. In all cases, frequent monitoring of blood pressure, clinical status, and serum biochemistry profiles is imperative. Weekly to bimonthly monitoring of blood pressure is recommended, with long-term evaluations every 2 to 4 months. If the single antihypertensive therapy fails, additional agents can be added and response to therapy reassessed.

PROGNOSIS

The prognosis for return of vision with hypertensive retinopathy depends on the severity of the retinal and vitreal changes as well as of any secondary ocular disease, that is, hyphema and glaucoma. Restoration of vision after retinal reattachment is influenced by the duration of the detachment and how elevated the retina was from the RPE. Both of these findings are probably influenced by the severity and duration of the systemic hypertension. The intraretinal vasculature supplies the inner retina, whereas the outer retina relies primarily on the choroid. Thus with retinal detachment, retinal degeneration occurs, and with higher detachments, (i.e., very bullous retinal detachment, which is typical for cats with hypertensive retinopathy) retinal degeneration is more severe and occurs more rapidly. Retinal damage also occurs in association with intraretinal vascular damage, ischemia, and secondary retinal degeneration. Underlying renal or cardiac disease could further compromise retinal vascular supply, and uremia may cause toxic changes within retinal tissues. Lastly, if hyphema induces a secondary glaucoma that cannot be controlled medically, vision is seriously threatened.

In the author's opinion, the prognosis for maintaining vision with hypertensive retinopathy is guarded to good. Although reports in the literature often indicate a poor prognosis for return of vision, in most of these cases, sufficient antihypertensive therapy was not used or onset of treatment was delayed. If blood pressure as well as the underlying disease can be controlled, the prognosis for vision can be considered guarded to good. If medical intervention occurs in early hypertensive retinopathy, that is, before bullous retinal detachment is present, the prognosis is better. However, even with severe bilateral bullous retinal detachment, the author has seen several cats regain limited vision after retinal reattachment. The prognosis for life may also be guarded to good depending on the underlying cause of the hypertension, that is, hyperthyroidism versus chronic renal failure.

References and Suggested Reading

Dukes J: Hypertension: A review of the mechanisms, manifestations and management. J Small Anim Pract 33:119, 1992.
This is a good review of the causes of hypertension, equipment choices for blood pressure measurement, and treatment of hypertension.
Hayreh SS: Classification of hypertensive fundus changes and their order of appearance. Ophthalmologica 198:247, 1989.
This article reviews lesions found in the fundus of a hypertensive monkey model, many of which are found in domestic species.

Kobayashi DL, Peterson ME, Graves TK, et al: Hypertension in cats with chronic renal failure or hyperthyroidism. J Vet Intern Med 4:58, 1990.
The incidence of hypertension in cats that is associated with renal failure or hyperthyroidism is examined.
Labato MA, Ross LA: Diagnosis and management of hypertension. In: August JR, ed: Consultations in Feline Internal Medicine. Philadelphia: WB Saunders, 1996, p 301.
This article presents a broad review of blood pressure control and measurement, diseases associated with systemic hypertension, clinical signs of hypertension, and dietary and medical management of hypertension in cats.
Lane I, Roberts S, Lappin M: Ocular manifestations of vascular disease: hypertension, hyperviscosity, and hyperlipidemia. J Am Anim Hosp Assoc 29:28, 1993.
This article discusses pathophysiology and ophthalmic clinical signs associated with hypertension and contains good fundus photographs of retinal lesions.
Littman M, Robertson J, Bovee K: Spontaneous systemic hypertension in dogs: Five cases (1981–1983). J Am Vet Med Assoc 193:486, 1988.
This article discusses five dogs that presented for blindness and ocular manifestations secondary to hypertension and the various strategies used to treat them.
Littman MP: Spontaneous systemic hypertension in 24 cats. J Vet Intern Med 8:79, 1994.
Twenty-four cases of feline hypertension are reviewed, with discussion of common clinical findings, underlying causes, and choice of and response to medical treatment of hypertension.
Morgan R: Systemic hypertension in four cats: Ocular and medical findings. J Am Anim Hosp Assoc 22:615, 1986.
A series of feline cases, all with renal failure and secondary hypertension, is presented, along with good-quality photographs of hemorrhagic ocular changes.
Paulsen M, Allen T, Jaenke R, et al: Arterial hypertension in two canine siblings: Ocular and systemic manifestations. J Am Anim Hosp Assoc 25:287, 1989.
This article presents clinical photographs of ocular changes associated with hypertension in two dogs along with a discussion and photomicrographs of histopathologic changes.
Sansom J, Barnett KC, Dunn KA, et al: Ocular disease associated with hypertension in 16 cats. J Small Anim Pract 35:604, 1994.
This is a review of ocular disease associated with hypertension in cats, with good clinical photographs of retinal changes.
Snyder P: Canine Hypertensive Disease. Compend Contin Educ Pract Vet [Small Anim Pract] 13:1785, 1991.
This article reviews the incidence, pathophysiology, causes, diagnosis, and treatment of systemic hypertension in dogs.
Snyder PS, Henik RA: Feline Systemic Hypertension. San Francisco: Proceedings of the 12th American College of Veterinary Internal Medicine Forum, 1994, p 126.
This is a brief review of diagnosis and treatment of hypertension with discussion of use of amlodipine.
Stiles J, Polzin D, Bistner S: The prevalence of retinopathy in cats with systemic hypertension and chronic renal failure or hyperthyroidism. J Am Anim Hosp Assoc 30:564, 1994.
This review discusses the signs and prevalence of hypertensive retinopathy in renal failure or hyperthyroidism in cats and has good photographs of retinal changes.

Exophthalmos

DAVID T. RAMSEY

East Lansing, Michigan

Exophthalmos is defined as abnormal protrusion of the globe. It is the most common clinical sign of orbital disease in dogs and cats and is usually attributable to the mass effect of space-occupying orbital disease. However, the presence of exophthalmos does not invariably imply orbital disease. Extreme variability in the conformation of the orbit and skull of different canine and feline breeds results in large differences in orbital volume. Dogs and cats with a brachycephalic skull conformation have shallow orbits that result in a more conspicuous exophthalmic globe compared with those with mesaticephalic or dolichocephalic skull conformation that have a less prominent or enophthalmic globe.

Exophthalmos must be differentiated from pseudoexophthalmos (simulation of an abnormally prominent globe) and from buphthalmos (absolute enlargement of the globe—a complication of chronic glaucoma) (see p. 1075). Pseudoexophthalmos may be caused by enophthalmos or phthisis bulbi of the contralateral globe, or by asymmetrical eyelid (including nictitating membrane) position. Retraction of the ipsilateral upper eyelid or dilatation of the pupil simulates exophthalmos of the ipsilateral globe. Intraocular pressure and horizontal corneal diameter should always be measured and the optic nerve assessed and compared with the fellow eye when buphthalmos is suspected.

CHARACTERIZING EXOPHTHALMOS

Orbital disorders are characterized by clinical signs that alter the appearance, function, or position of the globe, eyelids, or ocular adnexal structures. When orbital disease is suspected, a thorough history should be acquired and a complete ophthalmic and physical examination performed. Exophthalmos may be unilateral or bilateral and congenital or acquired. The direction of displacement of the globe in relation to the orbital rim is useful in localizing a mass effect and is usually opposite that of the mass effect. When exophthalmos is evident, it is usually attributable to orbital diseases of infectious, inflammatory, neoplastic, or cystic origin that arise from orbital tissues or extend into the orbit from surrounding tissues. Exophthalmos occurs less frequently from trauma, vascular anomalies of the orbit, aberrant parasite migration, bleeding and clotting disorders, craniofacial and orbital malformation (associated with hydrocephalus), and proliferative bone diseases affecting the flat bones of the orbit or vertical ramus of the mandible (craniomandibular osteopathy). Inflammatory and cystic orbital diseases have a favorable prognosis for cure, whereas neoplastic orbital disease bears a poor to grave prognosis.

Rapid onset or progression of exophthalmos and clinical signs of severe pain are typical of acute inflammatory, traumatic, hemorrhagic, or septic-infectious orbital disease. Slowly progressive or static exophthalmos and absence of clinical signs of pain are more typical of cystic, vascular, or structural abnormalities of the orbit. Gradual induction of exophthalmos and minimal or absent clinical signs of pain are most frequently associated with chronic inflammatory or neoplastic orbital disease. Dynamic, intermittent exophthalmos that is dependent (when the head is lowered) is diagnostic of an orbital vascular anomaly with primarily a venous component. Pulsatile, static exophthalmos with or without an audible bruit over the orbit is consistent with a vascular orbital anomaly with a predominant arterial component.

GENERAL APPROACH TO THE EXOPHTHALMIC ANIMAL

A thorough ophthalmic examination is indicated whenever orbital disease is suspected. Vision, pupillomotor function, ocular movements, and eyelid function and position should be assessed whenever exophthalmos is evident. The bony orbital rim and rostral orbital tissues should be palpated for excessive warmth, differences in tissue texture or consistency, or solitary or infiltrative masses and compared with the fellow eye. Increased resistance to digital retropulsion of the globe through the closed upper eyelid is evidence of nonspecific orbital mass effect, which may obstruct venous drainage of the orbit and result in vascular congestion of periorbital tissues. Conjunctival hyperemia, chemosis, and blepharoedema may be dramatic. Mild episcleral injection and intraocular pressure just above the normal reference range may occur from obstruction to episcleral and orbital venous drainage. Funduscopic examination may reveal posterior scleral indentation, overlying choroidal folds, and a flat retinal detachment when exophthalmos is caused by a focal neoplastic or cystic orbital mass. Compressive optic neuropathy attributable to orbital disease may be evident as papilledema.

A complete oral examination should be performed whenever orbital disease is suspected and may require heavy sedation or general anesthesia. The papillae of the zygomatic salivary gland should be examined for erythema or evidence of zygomatic sialoadenitis. Areas of induration of the oral mucosa caudal and medial to the maxillary second molar tooth are infrequently detected but are suggestive of orbital cellulitis or abscess formation. Examination of the caudal maxillary teeth using a periodontal probe and dental explorer may reveal periodontal disease related to or complicating orbital sepsis. Grossly visible abnormalities of the caudal maxillary teeth are not prerequisites for necrosis of the pulp canal, development of a periapical abscess, and orbital cellulitis or abscess. When results of oral examination fail to reveal an abnormality related to orbital disease, orbital echography should be performed and radiographs made of the caudal maxillary teeth. When a lesion is detected, ultrasonographically guided fine-needle aspiration and biopsy may be performed for cytologic examination and bacterial culture and susceptibility testing. Orbital imaging modalities (echography, magnetic resonance imaging or computed tomography) are frequently used to delineate and determine the extent of orbital disease before attempting treatment.

Inflammatory Orbital Disease

The most common causes of inflammatory orbital disease in dogs (and less frequently in cats) include orbital cellulitis and orbital abscess associated with orbital foreign bodies, bacterial organisms, dental disease, dacryoadenitis, or fungal or aberrant parasitic organisms. Masticatory myositis, extraocular polymyositis, and zygomatic sialoadenitis are also common causes of exophthalmos in dogs but have not been reported in cats.

Orbital Cellulitis and Orbital Abscess

Orbital cellulitis is diffuse inflammation of the soft tissues of the orbit and is most frequently attributable to aerobic or anaerobic bacterial infection. An exudate of low viscosity tends to spread through cleavage planes of interstitial and tissue spaces. Infection and inflammation of the extraconal space may result in destruction of tissue planes and involvement of the intraconal space. Orbital cellulitis may develop from infectious or nonseptic inflammatory disease of contiguous periorbital structures or spaces (periodontal or endodontic disease, sinusitis, dacryoadenitis, sialoadenitis, panophthalmitis); from transconjunctival, transpalpebral, or transoral origin; from orbital foreign bodies; or secondary to septicemia. Clinical signs include exophthalmos, erythema, edema of the eyelids, chemosis, conjunctival hyperemia, protrusion of the nictitating membrane, and signs of pain during retropulsion of the globe or when the mouth is opened. Cellulitis may jeopardize vision or cause decreased ocular movements, afferent pupillary defect, rising intraocular pressure, and decreased eyelid and periorbital sensation, and may result in exposure keratitis. Areas of induration or fistulization of the oral mucosa caudal and medial to the maxillary second molar tooth are infrequently observed in this author's experience. Comparison of B-mode orbital ultrasonographic images of the normal and affected orbit may show irregular or poorly defined lesions or echolucent areas within orbital soft tissues. Ultrasonographically guided fine-needle aspiration may be performed for aerobic and anaerobic bacterial culture and susceptibility testing.

Treatment of orbital cellulitis depends on the severity of clinical signs. Cellulitis may ultimately result in formation of an orbital abscess if left untreated. Initial medical treatment requires oral or parenteral administration of a broad-spectrum antibiotic (e.g., amoxicillin-clavulanate). Anti-inflammatory doses of corticosteroids or nonsteroidal anti-inflammatory drugs may be administered, but vigilant monitoring (every 2 hours) for signs of functional deterioration is critical during the first 24 to 48 hours. In the opinion of this author, surgical treatment of orbital cellulitis (described further on) is indicated only when response to

medical treatment is not evident during the first 12 to 24 hours or when progressive deterioration and a threat to ocular function is evident. If ultrasonographic signs of orbital abscess are evident, surgical intervention is indicated. If dental radiographs show evidence of periodontal or endodontic disease of the caudal maxillary teeth, transalveolar drainage should be established by extraction of the affected tooth; establishing transmucosal drainage caudal to the maxillary second molar tooth is not necessary. If dental radiographs appear normal and an orbital abscess is evident ultrasonographically, transmucosal drainage should be established under general anesthesia. The oral mucosa is prepared for aseptic surgery and a 1-cm mucosal incision is created caudal and medial to the maxillary second molar tooth. Care should be used not to incise deeper than the mucosa. A sterile, blunt-tipped probe is inserted into the mucosal incision and gently forced through the medial pterygoid muscle into the extraconal space. Whether or not drainage of purulent material from the wound occurs, a sterile, premoistened culture swab should be inserted into the orbital space for aerobic and anaerobic bacterial culture and susceptibility testing, Gram staining, and cytologic examination. The orbital space may be flushed with 0.9% saline solution or chlorhexidine gluconate solution that has been diluted to 0.05% in sterile water. Exposure keratitis should be prevented by administering a topical ophthalmic ointment that does not contain a corticosteroid. Placement of a temporary tarsorrhaphy or external pressure bandages should be avoided because they can increase intraorbital pressure and compromise delicate neurovascular structures. Frequent and vigilant postoperative monitoring (vision, ocular movements, pupillomotor function, intraocular pressure) is necessary to detect signs of functional deterioration.

Masticatory Myositis

Masticatory myositis is an immune-mediated disorder affecting muscles derived from the first branchial arch, innervated by the mandibular branch of the trigeminal nerve, and containing type 2M myofibers. Myositis is attributable to cellular and humoral responses selectively directed against type 2M myofibers. Three of these muscles form the medial, caudolateral, and ventral soft tissue boundaries of the orbit and often result in exophthalmos (bilateral most common) and diplopia when these muscles are swollen. Masticatory muscles encroaching on the orbital space also cause passive elevation of the nictitating membrane. Blindness has been reported but is considered uncommon. Trismus is often evident, and signs of pain are elicited when attempting to open the mouth or when pressure is applied over the temporalis or masseter muscles. Several case reports have suggested a predisposition for the German shepherd dog and Weimaraner, but the two largest studies (representing 48 dogs) did not detect a breed or gender predilection. The predominant cell types in most muscle biopsy samples are lymphocytes and plasma cells, not eosinophils; hence, the designation eosinophilic myositis is inappropriate for this disorder. Presumptive diagnosis of masticatory myositis is based on typical clinical signs, elevated serum creatine kinase levels, and absence of clinical or laboratory evidence of other systemic or muscular disease (e.g., toxoplasmosis, polymyositis). The diagnosis is supported by histologic examination of frozen masticatory muscle sections demonstrating autoantibodies against type 2M myofibers or circulating in serum. Immunosuppressive doses of corticosteroids (1 to 1.5 mg/kg PO every 12 hours) should be administered for a minimum of 21 days before decreasing the dosage (0.5 mg/kg PO every 12 hours) for 21 days and then gradually decreasing it to an alternate-day dosage. A favorable response to initial treatment is usually evident during the first week, but recrudescence is common if the initial dosage is decreased before 21 days of treatment (see *CVT X,* p. 816).

Extraocular Polymyositis

Bilateral extraocular polymyositis (BEP) is an inflammatory myopathy that is restricted to the extraocular muscles in dogs. A retrospective study of 35 dogs with BEP determined the common clinical signs and course of disease, identified demographic trends and risk factors for the development of BEP, and histochemically characterized the mononuclear inflammatory cell infiltrate of extraocular muscles in a large group of dogs with BEP (Ramsey et al, 1995). The median age of affected dogs was 8 months. Twenty-two female dogs (63%) and 12 male dogs (34%) were affected. Twenty-three of the 35 dogs were Golden retrievers (66%). Other breeds included the Doberman pinscher (4 dogs, 11%), German shorthair pointer (3 dogs, 9%), Labrador retriever (1 dog, 3%), and mixed breeds (4 dogs, 11%). An antecedent "stressor" (ovariohysterectomy, estrous cycle, castration, boarding at a kennel) was historically present in 15 of 35 dogs (43%) and occurred within 14 days of the onset of clinical signs of BEP.

Chemosis of the bulbar conjunctiva, the earliest observed clinical sign, was present 2 to 8 days before the onset of bilateral exophthalmos. The exophthalmos was always bilateral but not symmetrical. Retraction of the upper eyelid and 360-degree scleral show were noted in 12 of 35 dogs (34%). Elevation of the nictitating membrane and clinical signs of pain during retropulsion of the globe or oral examination were not clinical features of BEP. Eight of 35 dogs (23%) exhibited clinical signs suggestive of diplopia, loss of depth perception, or blindness. Funduscopic abnormalities consisted of compressive optic neuropathy, tortuosity of retinal venules, or focal retinitis in five dogs and were reversible after treatment in all instances. Intraocular pressure was minimally elevated to greater than the normal reference range in 10 dogs and was attributable to increased episcleral pressure from obstruction of orbital venous drainage.

A study on normal extraocular muscles of dogs detected unique myofibers of extraocular muscles that differ significantly from limb and masticatory muscle. Three types of myofibers (fine, coarse, granular) predominate in extraocular muscle based on histochemical and immunohistochemical staining characteristics. Examination of extraocular muscle biopsy samples by immunohistochemical staining from eight dogs with BEP compared with samples from normal control dogs revealed a mononuclear cell infiltrate composed primarily of CD3+ T lymphocytes and myeloid histiocyte macrophages. The monoclonal cellular infiltrate of the retractor bulbi muscle was inconspicuous and was limited to the peripheral layer of the muscle containing fine myofibers, suggesting a cellular immune response against fine extraocular myofiber proteins. Tissues did not stain with monoclonal antibodies for IgM, IgG, or IgA. Diffuse, mild muscle fibrosis, discoid degeneration, and regeneration of myofibers were evident in all tissues examined. Extraocular muscle tendons and orbital connective tissues were devoid of inflammatory cells. None of the dogs had autoantibodies against type 2M myofibers, or serologic evidence of elevated creatine kinase levels, dysthyroidism, or toxoplasmosis.

Treatment with immunosuppressive doses of corticosteroids (1 to 2.2 mg/kg PO every 12 hours) resulted in rapid resolution of exophthalmos, but recrudescence was common when the initial dosage was decreased before 21 days or when the dosage interval was increased to every 24 hours (20 dogs, 57%). Twenty-one of 26 dogs (81%) that were available for follow-up evaluation had recurrences of exophthalmos. Recurrences correlated repeatedly with estrous cycle or boarding at kennels in 6 of 26 dogs (23%).

Although the fundamental mechanisms have not been thoroughly defined, BEP appears to be a unique and separate form of orbital myositis from masticatory myositis of dogs and is similar in many respects to idiopathic inflammatory orbital disease in humans. Serum from affected dogs is being evaluated for evidence of circulating autoantibodies against extraocular muscle fine fibers.

Cystic Orbital Disease

Exophthalmos may occur from cystic orbital structures that develop from the orbital lacrimal gland, gland of the nictitating membrane, zygomatic salivary gland, or epithelium of the conjunctiva, nasal cavity, or paranasal sinuses. Developmental ocular anomalies and neoplasms of glandular orbital tissue may also form cystic orbital structures. Cysts may protrude into the conjunctival fornix and may appear pale blue-gray when transilluminated and viewed through the conjunctival surface. Cystic orbital disease is usually painless unless concurrent adenitis or cellulitis is present. An orbital cyst appears anechoic or hypoechoic by orbital echography. Fine-needle aspiration usually reveals a clear or rust-colored viscous or serous fluid. Marsupialization to the conjunctival surface may be curative for cysts of lacrimal gland or conjunctival tissue origin. Surgical excision by limited orbitotomy is usually indicated for cysts of salivary tissue origin or from epithelium of the nasal cavity or paranasal sinus origin. Blunt surgical dissection of the cyst should be done before aspiration of cyst contents. Excised tissues should always be examined histologically.

Orbital Neoplasia

Orbital neoplasms are characterized as primary if they arise directly from orbital structures or tissues, secondary if they occur by local extension or via metastasis or multicentric disease. Primary orbital neoplasms are most frequently reported in dogs and are classified as malignant based on histologic criteria. Secondary orbital neoplasia attributable to infiltration of the orbit by local extension from adjacent tissues constitutes the majority of orbital neoplasms in cats. The median age of dogs and cats diagnosed with orbital neoplasia is 8 and 9 years, respectively. Unilateral exophthalmos is the most common clinical sign of orbital neoplasia and is characterized by insidious onset and gradual progression. Clinical signs of pain are usually absent. Strabismus, nonaxial displacement of the globe, and protrusion of the nictitating membrane are common. Radiographs of the skull and thorax should be obtained to determine if osteolysis or metastases are evident. Treatment is dependent on the type and extent of orbital neoplasm present. Ultrasonographically or computed tomographically guided fine-needle aspiration and biopsy for cytologic examination should be performed and tissues examined histologically to determine the type of neoplasm present before considering treatment options. Ideally magnetic resonance imaging or computed tomographic images should be obtained to determine the extent of the lesion and facilitate development of a surgical treatment plan. Well-delineated malignant orbital masses and solitary, noninfiltrative benign masses occur infrequently but may be excised by orbitotomy. Exenteration is indicated for invasive or infiltrative orbital masses that do not extend beyond the confines of the orbit. When a mass extends beyond the confines of the orbit, subtotal or partial orbitectomy is indicated. Adjuvant radiation or chemotherapy is planned based on the results of histologic examination of excised tissues. Local recurrence or metastasis is common after exenteration and orbitectomy, but a disease-free interval is greater after orbitectomy.

Traumatic Proptosis

Proptosis occurs when the globe is displaced rostrally from the orbit. Marginal eyelid entrapment at the orbital rim is exacerbated by spasm of the orbicularis oculi muscle and compromises vascular circulation to the globe. Dogs with a brachycephalic skull conformation, shallow orbits, and macropalpebral fissures are most frequently affected. Substantial traumatic force is necessary to induce proptosis in cats and nonbrachycephalic dogs, and concurrent and severe intraocular, craniofacial, and central nervous system trauma is common. Strabismus, chemosis, exposure keratitis, corneal ulceration, and hyphema are the most common complications associated with proptosis in dogs. In cats, common complications include facial bone fractures, hyphema, and corneal perforation. All globes that have undergone proptosis and do not have obvious optic nerve transection or catastrophic and irremediable perforation should be replaced; dogs with eyes blinded by proptosis that have been surgically replaced have a better cosmetic appearance compared with dogs that have had enucleation surgery. Favorable prognostic indicators for vision in globes undergoing surgical replacement include proptosis in a brachycephalic dog, sight in a globe that has undergone proptosis, positive direct and consensual pupillary light reflexes, and a normal-appearing posterior segment. Pupil size does not correlate with a visual outcome and should not be used as a prognostic indicator for vision. Unfavorable prognostic indicators for vision before replacement include proptosis in a cat or nonbrachycephalic dog, optic nerve transection, avulsion of three or more extraocular muscles, extensive hyphema, no visible pupil, and facial fractures. Regaining vision after replacement of an eye that has undergone proptosis is uncommon in cats.

Traumatic proptosis constitutes a true ocular emergency that requires timely replacement of the globe, but stability of the animal (physical and neurologic status) must be ensured (also see the next article). Blood and debris should be removed from the periorbital skin and a lateral canthotomy performed using blunt-tipped scissors after induction of general anesthesia if the animal is stable, or after infiltrative local anesthesia if the animal's condition is unstable. A globe that has undergone proptosis should *never* be forced back into the orbit. The eyelid margins are elevated to relieve entrapment while gentle counter pressure is used to replace the globe. The lateral canthotomy incision is then closed in two layers, and temporary tarsorrhaphy sutures are placed over stints, leaving the medial canthus open to expedite administration of topical medication. Since ulcerative keratitis develops in many eyes, use of topical corticosteroid ointment should be discouraged. A broad-spectrum antibiotic ointment should be applied every 6 hours. Atropine should be administered every 12 hours to treat traumatic iridocyclitis. Optic neuropathy, iridocyclitis, and orbital inflammation should be treated by oral administration of prednisone (dog, 1 mg/kg of body weight, every 12 hours; cat, 2 mg/kg every 12 hours) for 7 days and then the dosage should be decreased over the subsequent 14 days. Retrobulbar injection of substances (including corticosteroids) should *never* be performed because they increase orbital pressure and may compromise delicate neurovascular structures. Oral administration of a broad-spectrum antibiotic is also recommended. Tarsorrhaphy sutures are removed 10 to 28 days after placement and may be removed sequentially. Lagophthalmos, keratoconjunctivitis sicca, neurotrophic keratitis, strabismus, corneal ulceration, permanent blindness, and phthisis bulbi are frequent complications of proptosis.

References and Suggested Reading

Gilger BC, Hamilton HL, Wilkie DA, et al: Traumatic ocular proptosis in dogs and cats: 84 cases (1980–1993). J Am Vet Med Assoc 206:1186, 1995.
Risk factors for traumatic proptosis and results of treatment outcome are reviewed.
Gilger BC, McLaughlin SA, Whitley RD, et al: Orbital neoplasms in cats: 21 cases (1974–1990). J Am Vet Med Assoc 201:1083, 1992.
A retrospective report of the clinical signs and course of orbital disease in cats is reported.
Ramsey DT, Gerding PA, Hamor RE, et al: Histochemical and morphometric analysis of fiber types in extraocular muscles of dogs. Proc Am Coll Vet Ophthalmol 26:129, 1995.
This article describes histochemical staining characteristics and myofiber morphologic features of normal extraocular muscle of dogs.
Ramsey DT, Hamor RE, Gerding PA, et al: Clinical and immunohistochemical characteristics of bilateral extraocular polymyositis of dogs. Proc Am Coll Vet Ophthalmol 26:130, 1995.
This is a review of bilateral extraocular polymyositis of dogs.
Ramsey DT, Manfra Marretta S, Hamor RE, et al: Ophthalmic manifestations and complications of dental disease in dogs and cats. J Am Anim Hosp Assoc 32:215, 1996.
Common ophthalmic manifestations of dental disease and treatment recommendations are described.
Shelton GD, Cardinet GH III: Canine masticatory muscle disorders. In: Kirk RW, Bonagura JD, eds: Current Veterinary Therapy X. Philadelphia: WB Saunders, 1989, p 816.
A clinical description of masticatory myopathy, results of histochemical staining of affected masticatory muscle, and recommendations for treatment are given.

Ocular Emergencies

TONY GLOVER

Charlotte, North Carolina

An ocular emergency is often a matter of perspective. What an owner considers to be an emergency usually is not. What a veterinarian considers to be an emergency usually is, but the owner often fails to recognize the problem in time to obtain effective treatment. In this article, ocular emergencies include conditions that, if left undiagnosed and untreated for a matter of hours, can result in permanent loss of structure or function. Also included are conditions that may have an acute onset but are not an immediate threat to vision.

ORBIT

Proptosis

The orbit represents a cavity encased by bone (except the floor) that contains the eyeball, its muscles, blood supply, nerve supply, and fat. By convention, exophthalmos represents a condition in which the globe protrudes, or bulges, outward from its normal position (see previous article). It is most often associated with retrobulbar disease such as abscessation or neoplasia. In comparison, proptosis refers to an acute condition in which the globe has been forced anteriorly beyond the rim of the orbit and eyelids, where it often becomes entrapped. Proptosis can be unilateral or bilateral and is invariably secondary to trauma. Brachycephalic breeds are predisposed because of their prominent globes, shallow orbits, and large eyelid openings.

Globes that have undergone proptosis often present with blindness, strabismus from torn extraocular muscles, chemosis, corneal ulceration, scleral blowout, pupillary abnormalities, uveitis, glaucoma or hypotony, hyphema, or facial injuries such as lacerations or fractures. The presence or absence of any of these clinical signs does not provide a reliable predictor of outcome. The prognosis for vision of any globe that has undergone proptosis is poor in dogs and grave in cats. (Cats have a limited amount of retrobulbar space when compared with dogs). Vision loss usually results from optic nerve damage sustained at the time of trauma. The prognosis for cosmesis is guarded and is dependent on the degree of orbital and adnexal injury.

When the globe has sustained extensive damage and cannot be salvaged (i.e., avulsion of all the extraocular muscles), enucleation is indicated. In all other cases, attempts to reposition the globe should be considered. If surgery fails, the eye can be removed at a later time. Replacing the globe is typically performed with the patient under general anesthesia or intravenous sedation. In most cases, it is difficult to reduce the globe because of secondary swelling of adnexal and orbital tissues. Coating the globe and surrounding tissues with a lubricating ointment (Lacrilube, Allergan) may be helpful, but more often a lateral canthotomy is indicated to increase the eyelid opening and lessen the applied force needed to reduce the globe. After the eye has been repositioned and the lateral canthotomy closed, the eyelid margins should be temporarily sutured together with 5–0 or 6–0 suture material to keep the globe in place while orbital tissue swelling subsides. In most cases, the medial aspect of the temporary tarsorrhaphy should be left open so that topical medication can be applied. Generally, the temporary sutures should be kept in place for 2 to 3 weeks.

Medical treatment consists of a broad-spectrum topical antibiotic ointment (neomycin, polymyxin B sulfates, and gramicidin ophthalmic solution, Bausch & Lomb, every 8 hours) and 1% atropine ointment (atropine sulfate, Fougora, every 8 hours to effect). High-dose systemic corticosteroid therapy (prednisone, Schein Pharmaceutical, 0.25 mg/kg PO every 12 hours, then tapered and discontinued over 14 days) is recommended in an attempt to reduce inflammation, especially in the optic nerve. Systemic antibiotics may be indicated in some cases.

Extraocular Polymyositis

Extraocular polymyositis is a rare condition that refers to the acute onset of profound bilateral exophthalmia due to severe inflammation of the extraocular muscles. The pathogenesis is poorly understood. As the extraocular muscles swell, the globe is displaced anteriorly. There is no apparent discomfort or vision loss, and the intraocular pressure (IOP) is normal or mildly elevated. Young retriever-type dogs appear predisposed. Treatment involves an extended course of high-dose oral corticosteroids. Recurrence is likely once therapy is decreased and may necessitate the use of more potent immunosuppressant drugs such as azathioprine or systemic cyclosporine. For further details, see p. 509).

EYELIDS

Lacerations

Proper apposition of the eyelid to the eyeball is of critical importance, and even seemingly minor eyelid defects can result in marked discomfort and secondary corneal disease. The eyelids are extremely vascular, and the inflammatory response to injury can be dramatic; however, because of the rich blood supply, eyelids tend to heal remarkably well.

When one repairs any eyelid defect, a few basic principles should be considered:

1. Priority should be given to restoration of the eyelid margin. Minimal debridement should be used and as much tissue as possible should be preserved. The function of the upper eyelid is more important than that of

the lower eyelid (during blinking, the upper eyelid moves to meet a relatively stationary lower eyelid).

2. If tissue loss to the eyelid and eyelid margin involves approximately 30% or less, the defect can be closed directly without loss of function or cosmesis. If tissue loss is greater than 30%, some blepharoplastic procedure (i.e., sliding skin graft) is usually recommended.

3. When one closes eyelid defects, 5–0 or 6–0 suture material should be used in a simple interrupted pattern. A two-layered closure (tarsoconjunctival and skin) is desired. If possible, the tarsus should be incorporated because of its strength. In most cases, the conjunctival layer need not be closed.

4. When working around the medial canthus, the clinician should identify and preserve the lower puncta and canaliculi—or postoperative epiphora may result. In the event that the lower canaliculus is severed, patency can be maintained by implantation of retention catheters and direct suturing of the free ductal ends.

CORNEA

Ulceration and Laceration

Corneal ulcers seldom remain static. Typically, they either heal or worsen in a matter of a few days. *There are three fundamental reasons why a corneal ulcer will not heal: (1) it is infected, (2) it is indolent, or (3) the underlying cause is still present.* Every corneal ulcer has a cause, and it is vital that this cause be determined. Delayed wound healing or recurrence may result if the underlying cause is allowed to persist. *Simply switching topical antibiotics is rarely helpful in treating nonhealing ulcers.*

Superficial Corneal Ulcers

Uninfected superficial ulcers are managed by prophylactic treatment with a topical broad-spectrum antibiotic (every 8 hours) until the cornea is fluorescein-negative. Topical 1% atropine (Atrosulf-1, Optopics, every 8 hours to effect) is routinely used to block painful secondary ciliary body spasms. Oral antibiotics are of no value in treating any nonperforating corneal ulcer because of the low concentration of drug in the tear film. The prognosis for vision is excellent, provided that the underlying cause is no longer present.

Deep Corneal Ulcers

Once a corneal ulcer becomes infected, tissue destruction results from proteases and collagenases produced by host cells (i.e., polymorphonuclear leukocytes, fibroblasts) and some bacteria (i.e., *Pseudomonas*). This process has been termed *melting*. In these cases, initiation of prompt medical therapy is imperative and is largely based on clinical impression alone. Currently, the drug of choice in rapidly progressive corneal ulcers is topical ciprofloxacin (Ciloxan, Alcon, every 1 to 2 hours for 2 days and then tapered with improvement) and topical atropine (every 8 hours to effect). The prognosis for infected corneal ulcers involving 50% stromal depth or less is good provided that

appropriate therapy is initiated early. Some residual corneal scarring can be expected.

Corneal ulcers that have progressed to about 60% stromal depth or greater may benefit from a conjunctival grafting procedure (i.e., rotational pedicle graft) or a corneal transplant. A descemetocele occurs when the overlying corneal stoma has eroded, exposing a clear, thin, and fragile Descemet's membrane. This membrane will not stain with fluorescein. Perforation is imminent, and surgery is indicated. When the conjunctiva is sutured directly to the cornea with 7–0 to 9–0 absorbable suture, the underlying corneal defect is provided immediate structural and vascular support. In comparison, deep and uncomplicated corneal lacerations can often be sutured directly without a conjunctival graft. Partial-thickness, rather than full-thickness, sutures should be placed perpendicular to the corneal wound and placed 1 to 1.5 mm apart. Overall, the prognosis for vision and cosmesis in an eye with a nonperforating corneal ulcer treated with a conjunctival graft and appropriate topical antibiotic therapy is fair to good.

In contrast to popular opinion, *third eyelid flaps are contraindicated in almost every corneal ulcer.* A third eyelid flap impedes medical therapy, prevents critical assessment of progress, and provides absolutely no structural or vascular support. Subjectively, any corneal ulcer that heals with a third eyelid flap will heal without one. Tissue adhesives, soft hydrophilic contact lenses, and collagen shields also offer little or no benefit in the emergency treatment of corneal ulcers.

Perforating Corneal Ulcers

Eyes with corneal perforation from full-thickness ulceration or lacerations typically present with a formed anterior chamber because the defect is plugged with fibrin and an anteriorly displaced iris. Surgery is indicated, and attempts are made to reduce or, in some cases, amputate the prolapsed iris before closing the cornea directly or covering the affected area with a conjunctival graft or transplanted cornea. After the full-thickness defect has been sealed, the globe can be inflated with balanced salt solution. Although less desirable, a small amount of sterile saline solution or a small air bubble, or both, will suffice. Medication consists of topical antibiotics, oral antibiotics (cephalexin, Biocraft, 22 mg/kg every 8 hours PO for 7 days), and topical atropine. The prognosis for vision and cosmesis is guarded but is dependent on the nature of the injury.

In any full-thickness corneal injury, especially lacerations, it is important to assess the lens critically. Lens capsule rupture can result in a particularly severe form of uveitis that may not become evident until several days after injury. Phacoclastic uveitis often responds poorly to anti-inflammatory therapy and commonly progresses to secondary glaucoma. Eyes sustaining extensive damage to the lens often benefit from lens extraction at the time of corneal repair. Evaluation of the lens is especially important in cats because they are predisposed to formation of a particularly aggressive intraocular tumor after ocular trauma severe enough to rupture the lens capsule.

Foreign Bodies

Corneal foreign bodies such as plant material or metal flecks can easily become embedded in the corneal epithelium so that the eyelids cannot dislodge them. Under topical anesthesia, superficial foreign bodies can usually be removed by aggressive flushing with a sterile eye wash or direct removal with a moistened cotton-tipped applicator. Removal of foreign bodies embedded deeper in the corneal stroma may benefit from the use of intravenous sedation and a 25- or 26-gauge hypodermic needle to remove the embedded material. Another alternative in removal of deeper implanted objects is to use a fine surgical blade to make a small, deliberate corneal incision over the long axis of the foreign body. When using this method, caution must be used to avoid corneal perforation. After complete removal, therapy should include a topical broad-spectrum antibiotic (every 8 hours) and topical atropine (every 8 hours to effect) because contamination with bacteria or fungus is likely. The prognosis is generally good.

Alkali Burns

In veterinary medicine, alkali burns to the cornea are rare and result in rapid dissolution of the corneal stroma. Typically, this rapidly advances to severe corneal ulceration and anterior uveitis. Initial treatment includes aggressive, copious irrigation with 500 to 1000 ml of sterile solution and a topical collagenase inhibitor such as acetylcysteine (Mucomyst, Apothecon). Symptomatic therapy is indicated for the secondary conditions that often arise. The prognosis for vision is poor to grave, and in many cases surgery may be required to salvage the globe.

Feline Acute Spontaneous Bullous Keratopathy

Acute spontaneous bullous keratopathy represents a rare syndrome unique to cats in which the cornea becomes profoundly edematous, usually over the course of several hours. The condition can affect one or both eyes and either heals spontaneously or progresses to perforation. The underlying cause is not known. A conjunctival graft is often needed to prevent perforation while the underlying stroma remodels. The long-term prognosis is guarded because recurrence is likely.

UVEITIS

Penetrating and Blunt Trauma

Focal puncture wounds to the globe may cause minimal damage to the cornea and sclera and may seal spontaneously. In such cases, the resulting anterior uveitis should be treated with oral corticosteroids (0.25 mg PO every 12 hours and then tapered and discontinued over 10 to 14 days) and topical atropine (every 8 hours to effect). Topical prednisolone acetate (Pred Forte, Allergan, every 4 to 6 hours initially and then tapered with improvement) is indicated, provided that there is no active corneal ulceration. In addition, oral antibiotics are indicated because of the potential for intraocular contamination after penetrating trauma. The prognosis is dependent on the extent of injury. Frequent complications include lens capsule rupture and secondary phacoclastic uveitis, cataracts, secondary glaucoma, and infectious endophthalmitis. More extensive penetrating injuries that rupture the fibrous tunic of the eye generally require surgical repair and have a much poorer prognosis.

Blunt trauma to the globe can cause extensive intraocular injury without apparent damage to the cornea or sclera. If trauma is limited to the anterior segment, signs of anterior uveitis (conjunctival and episcleral hyperemia, corneal edema, iris swelling, miosis, hypotony, aqueous flare, and hyphema) can be expected. Treatment includes topical prednisolone acetate (every 4 to 6 hours and then tapered with improvement) and topical atropine (every 8 hours to effect). The prognosis is good to excellent. However, if the blunt force delivered to the globe is great enough to displace (cave in) the anterior aspect of the globe posteriorly instantaneously, the force rebounds off the back wall of the eye and is reflected forward. This frequently results in retinal detachment or a blowout lesion at the limbus, or both. Therefore, blunt trauma can easily cause as much damage to an eye as sharp, penetrating trauma. Treatment includes aggressive topical prednisolone acetate (every 4 to 6 hours and then tapered with improvement), oral corticosteroid therapy (0.125 mg/kg every 12 hours PO and then tapered and discontinued over 10 to 14 days) and topical atropine (every 8 hours to effect). The prognosis for vision is poor. Phthisis bulbi is a common sequela.

GLAUCOMA

Since the eyeball represents a relatively closed container, if IOP is to remain constant it is necessary that aqueous humor exit the eye at a rate similar to that at which it is produced. If more aqueous exits than is produced, hypotony results. Conversely, if more aqueous is produced than exits the eye, glaucoma results. If acute glaucoma goes undetected and untreated, blindness from damage to the optic nerve and retina can occur in a matter of hours.

There are three fundamental concepts important in managing any case of glaucoma: (1) Is glaucoma present? (2) Is the glaucoma primary or secondary? and *(3) At what stage is the glaucoma?* (Also see p. 1075 for a detailed discussion of glaucoma).

Is Glaucoma Present?

The presence of glaucoma can be ascertained only by obtaining an accurate IOP. Clinical signs and digital palpation are crude indicators at best. The clinical signs associated with glaucoma are nonspecific and frequently occur with other ocular diseases in which the IOP can be normal or even low. Normal canine and feline IOP ranges from 12 to 22 mm Hg with little variation between eyes. Generally, IOP greater than 30 mm Hg is considered diagnostic for glaucoma. The most readily available and commonly used method to measure IOP is Schiotz tonometry. Although somewhat cumbersome, when used properly, this instrument is accurate. When converting Schiotz tonometer readings to IOP in millimeters of mercury, human conversion tables are considered more accurate than canine conversion tables.

Is the Glaucoma Primary or Secondary?

By convention, glaucoma is classified as either primary or secondary. Primary glaucoma is an inherited defect in which the drainage angle closes, impairing aqueous outflow. Since aqueous is still produced, IOP rises. Many purebred dogs (i.e., Cocker spaniel, Basset hound, Chow Chow) are predisposed. Glaucoma eventually affects both eyes, but seldom does it occur simultaneously. Typically, glaucoma affects one eye and then affects the other eye within 1 year. Once glaucoma has occurred in one eye, prophylactic medical therapy appears to delay the onset of glaucoma in the second eye only a few months. The diagnosis of primary glaucoma is based on history, signalment, clinical presentation, and lack of other ocular diseases that could cause an increase in IOP. Gonioscopy, which allows direct examination of drainage angle morphologic characteristics, provides a further basis for classification. In secondary glaucoma, the aqueous outflow system is impaired because of some other disease process (neoplasia, uveitis, lens luxation). Proper management of secondary glaucoma is dependent on identifying and treating the underlying cause. Cats are rarely affected with primary glaucoma but are susceptible to secondary glaucoma because of their high rate of aqueous production.

At What Stage Is the Glaucoma?

The stage of glaucoma determines treatment. There are two major phases of primary glaucoma, acute and chronic. In acute glaucoma, IOP can rapidly increase from normal to pressures of 60 mm Hg or higher. When pressures are this elevated, permanent optic nerve damage occurs in a matter of hours. There are a wide variety of glaucoma medications and treatment protocols used to reduce IOP rapidly in emergency situations. One such protocol is presented here. The prognosis for temporarily lowering IOP with this protocol is good to excellent.

- *Latanoprost* (Xalatan, 0.005%, 1 drop every 24 hours). Latanoprost is a prostaglandin receptor agonist that apparently reduces intraocular pressure by facilitating aqueous outflow. A single dose is recommended because more frequent administration may decrease the desired effect. The topical application of a single dose of Xalatan may preclude the need for IV mannitol therapy.
- *Intravenous mannitol* (Abbott), 1 to 1.5 gm/kg intravenously slowly over 10 to 15 minutes). Mannitol reduces IOP by creating an osmotic imbalance between the ocular vasculature, the aqueous humor, and the vitreous body. Its onset of action is about 30 minutes and its effects last up to 6 hours. It should not be used more than twice in a 24-hour period. Water should be withheld for approximately 5 to 6 hours. Mannitol is contraindicated with concurrent congestive heart disease.
- *Oral dichlorphenamide* (Daranide, Merck & Co., 10 to 15 mg/kg every 8 hours PO). Dichlorphenamide, a carbonic anhydrase inhibitor, reduces IOP by reducing aqueous humor formation. The onset of action is typically within 4 to 8 hours after oral administration.
- *Topical pilocarpine* (Pilocarpine, Steris, 2%, every 6 hours). Pilocarpine, a miotic agent, reduces IOP primarily

by increasing aqueous outflow. Its onset of action occurs within 15 minutes after instillation, and its effects last up to 6 to 8 hours. There is no added benefit in using concentrations greater then 2%. Pilocarpine is contraindicated with significant uveitis.

If effective, the preceding protocol should be considered a short reprieve from elevated IOP. In primary glaucoma, medical therapy can be expected to fail in every case, usually warranting surgical intervention. One treatment option uses laser energy to destroy the ciliary body epithelium selectively, reducing aqueous production and lowering IOP. Another option is filtration surgery, which shunts aqueous from the anterior chamber around a defective drainage angle and to the subconjunctival space, where it can be absorbed by the systemic circulation. Unfortunately, to date, the long-term prognosis for vision and control of IOP is guarded, regardless of treatment.

In chronic glaucoma, sustained elevated IOP results in permanent blindness. Typically, these eyes have buphthalmos and are painful. Treatment objectives include comfort and cosmesis. Common treatment recommendations include enucleation, evisceration with intrascleral prosthesis or, less commonly, laser treatment. Some authors advocate chemical ablation of the ciliary body (Gentocin, Schering-Plough, 25 mg intravitreally) as an alternative to surgery (see p. 1075). It is important to note that this drug destroys not only the ciliary body epithelium but also the retina. If a dog is not totally blind before injection, it will be soon thereafter.

RETINA

Sudden Acquired Retinal Degeneration

Sudden loss of vision (24 hours to 1 week), mydriasis, and no ocular abnormalities to account for bilateral blindness characterize sudden acquired retinal degeneration. The retina appears clinically normal in the initial stages of the disease. Adult dogs are usually affected, and no one breed of dog appears to be predisposed, with the possible exception of dachshunds. Definitive diagnosis is made through electroretinography, which distinguishes vision loss from optic neuritis or central nervous system disorders. After several months, the retina shows signs of generalized atrophy. Some animals with sudden acquired retinal degeneration may have a recent history of obesity, polyuria, polydipsia, polyphagia, and other signs of hyperadrenocorticism. Cortisol levels may be elevated in some cases. Most of these clinical signs resolve over a 2-month period. There is no apparent discomfort, and vision loss is total and permanent. There is no treatment.

Retinal Detachment

Retinal detachment involves separation of the neural retina from the retinal pigment epithelium. Vision loss is related to the extent of the detachment. The mechanisms of retinal detachment include (1) retinal tears in which vitreous gains access to the subretinal space (i.e., trauma); (2) uveitis, which allows exudate from the underlying choroidal vasculature into the subretinal space; and (3) traction forces that tear the retina as hemorrhage and fibrin attached to the retina contracts (i.e., resolving vitritis). Exudative retinal detachment carries the most favorable prognosis after treatment with high-dose systemic corticosteroids (0.25 mg/kg every 12 hours and then tapered over 14 days). Segmental retinal tears are the most amenable to reattachment surgery and have been associated with advanced cataracts.

OPTIC NERVE

Optic Neuritis

Inflammation of any portion of the optic nerve is referred to as *optic neuritis*. Clinically, optic neuritis most often presents as acute bilateral blindness. Funduscopic abnormalities include a swollen (raised) optic disc, vascular congestion, hemorrhage, and peripapillary retinal edema. Although most cases are considered idiopathic, optic neuritis has been associated with canine distemper, granulomatous meningoencephalomyelitis, neoplasia, systemic mycosis, and trauma. Idiopathic optic neuritis is treated with high doses of systemic corticosteroids (0.25 mg every 12 hours PO and then tapered over 14 days). Vision may initially improve while the animal is receiving steroids, but relapse and gradual vision loss often occurs even while maintenance doses are being administered.

References and Suggested Reading

Gelatt KN: Veterinary Ophthalmology. Philadelphia: Lea & Febiger, 1991.
  The most comprehensive reference text pertaining to veterinary ophthalmology.
Millichamp NJ, Dziezyc J: Vet Clin North Am 20:136, 1990.
  A concise text pertaining to major ophthalmic disorders for the general practitioner.
Roberts SM: Assessment and management of the ophthalmic emergency. Comp Cont Ed 7:739, 1985.
  A good review of management of common ocular emergencies.
Severin GA: Severin's Veterinary Ophthalmology Notes. Colorado: Severin, 1995.
  Although some concepts may be outdated, probably the best overall reference text for the general practitioner.

Ocular Neoplasia

RALPH E. HAMOR

KARIN M. HINKLE
Urbana, Illinois

Although ocular tumors are not frequently encountered in dogs and cats, they are potentially blinding and may carry significant risk to the animal's life. The biologic behavior of ocular tumors depends on the tumor type, tumor location, and the species of animal. Accurate histologic identification of the tumor type is crucial to case management and prognosis. Systemic spread of an intraocular neoplasm is much more common in cats.

When confronted with an ocular neoplasm, one must first determine whether the tumor is primary (with or without metastasis) or secondary to systemic neoplasia. This determination is based on clinical signs (Table 1), systemic signs (if any), and tumor type. Ocular neoplasia can masquerade initially as chronic uveitis or glaucoma, so neoplasia must be considered when these clinical signs are present, especially in older animals. For example, one of the most common causes of spontaneous intraocular hemorrhage in an older animal, especially in dogs, is an intraocular neoplasm.

PRIMARY NEOPLASMS OF THE CANINE GLOBE

Anterior Uveal Melanoma

Anterior uveal melanoma (AUM) is the most common primary neoplasm in the dog. Iridal melanomas usually present as focal, dark, raised lesions on the anterior surface of the iris in young dogs. These neoplasms grow slowly, cause little intraocular disease, are benign histologically, and rarely metastasize.

Canine AUMs most commonly occur in dogs greater than 7 years of age and are usually benign both histologically and behaviorally. The clinical presentation is based on the primary site of origin of the neoplasm. Frequently, the patient exhibits changes in the color, shape, and texture of the iris or ciliary body. In dogs, the neoplasm is more discrete than in feline AUM, in which it is most often

TABLE 1. Clinical Signs of Intraocular Neoplasia

Change in texture, color, thickness, or surface of the iris
Uveitis (anterior or posterior, or both)
  Aqueous flare
  Iritis
  Chorioretinitis
  Vitreal inflammation
  Optic neuritis (rare)
Glaucoma
  Corneal edema
  Scleral injection
Hyphema
Blindness
Retinal hemorrhage
Retinal detachment

diffuse. Typically, a smooth, raised, pigmented lesion is seen growing from the iris or ciliary body. Pigmentation of the mass does not confirm the presence of melanoma because some melanomas are nonpigmented. It is also possible for a nonpigmented ciliary body neoplasm to push the anterior surface of the iris forward and mimic an AUM. Other clinical signs typical of any intraocular neoplasm may be identified. As with any primary ocular tumor, this neoplasm progressively enlarges and causes secondary uveitis and glaucoma if not treated. Uveal cysts may mimic the appearance of an AUM. Transillumination usually allows one to differentiate between the two masses. Uveal cysts usually transilluminate, whereas AUMs do not.

Diagnosis can be attempted by fine-needle aspiration or incisional biopsy. Fine-needle aspiration of an anterior uveal neoplasm usually has limited side effects, especially if the mass is located within the anterior chamber. An incisional biopsy does require intraocular surgery and may be best referred to a veterinary ophthalmologist. Ocular ultrasonography can provide more accurate information as to the extent or site of origin of the neoplasm, especially if the ocular media is not clear. Enucleation can also provide a diagnosis but is usually reserved for painful or blind globes, or both.

Forms of treatment include resection, cryosurgery, enucleation, or laser photocoagulation. Of all these, laser photocoagulation has demonstrated the most promise for causing remission, shrinking, or slowing the growth rate of primary intraocular neoplasms in dogs. The benefit of laser photocoagulation is that it is possible to save vision and treat the neoplasm with minimal side effects. Because laser energy is preferentially absorbed by pigmented tissues, one would expect that pigmented neoplasms would be treated more successfully than nonpigmented ones. In fact, laser photocoagulation has shown efficacy in nonpigmented ocular neoplasms in dogs as well. Potential side effects from laser photocoagulation include hyphema, vitreal hemorrhage, corneal edema, mild anterior uveitis, corneal scarring, and cataract formation (if the mass is adjacent to the lens). Aside from scarring and potential cataract formation, side effects are transient and usually resolve with treatment within 2 weeks. Neoplasms confined to the ciliary body have responded the most favorably to this method of treatment. Because most primary ocular neoplasms in dogs have an extremely low metastatic potential, we think that the use of laser photocoagulation provides a safe and effective alternative to enucleation. If there are signs of severe secondary uveitis or glaucoma, we recommend enucleation and histopathologic examination. Before any treatment, the patient should undergo a thorough evaluation for any evidence of systemic metastasis, including a complete physical examination, complete blood work, thoracic radiographs, and abdominal ultrasonography. When canine AUMs do metastasize, the lungs, liver, kidney, spleen, adrenal gland, and heart can be affected. It is also possible for a systemic melanoma to spread to the eye from a distant site.

Canine Epibulbar Melanoma

Canine epibulbar melanomas arise in the sclera adjacent to the cornea and typically present as smooth, raised, pigmented masses at the scleral limbus that may encroach onto the cornea. Systemic metastasis from this neoplasm has not been reported but these lesions can be locally invasive. If allowed to grow, they can invade the globe, cause uveitis and secondary glaucoma, and necessitate enucleation. Proposed methods of treatment include full-thickness resection with homologous or synthetic grafting, partial resection, cryosurgery, or laser photocoagulation. Because of the complications associated with full-thickness resection and the difficulty in finding replacement tissue, we think that laser photocoagulation or cryosurgery is the optimal treatment. The earlier these procedures are performed, the more efficacious and safe the treatment will be.

Choroidal Melanoma

Choroidal melanomas also tend to occur in older dogs. In contrast to their occurrence in humans, in dogs, these neoplasms exhibit benign characteristics histologically and behaviorally. They occur rarely and usually demonstrate slow, expansive growth that eventually necessitates enucleation. As they enlarge, they can cause retinal atrophy and detachment. Clinically, ophthalmic evaluation reveals a well-delineated, raised, subretinal, pigmented mass. Again, ocular ultrasonography may aide the diagnosis when the ocular media is not clear.

Anterior Uveal Epithelial Neoplasms

Epithelial tumors of the anterior uvea consist most commonly of adenomas and adenocarcinomas of the ciliary body and are the second most common primary intraocular neoplasm in dogs. They are usually nonpigmented, white to pink, and slow growing and occupy the posterior chamber. They typically do not cause profound secondary ocular disease until they are rather large. The difference between adenomas and adenocarcinomas is a histopathologic differentiation and does not generally affect the prognosis. Both types can invade local tissues, but metastasis is rare. As with canine AUMs, laser photocoagulation may provide the best option for maintaining vision and providing effective treatment if severe secondary uveitis or secondary glaucoma is not present.

Medulloepithelioma

Medulloepithelioma has been reported rarely in the dog and arises from embryonal neuroepithelium. These neoplasms tend to occur in young dogs but can be slow growing and may not be evident for a few years. The clinical appearance of this neoplasm is similar to a ciliary body adenoma or adenocarcinoma. Regional extraocular extension or metastasis has not been reported in dogs.

PRIMARY NEOPLASMS OF THE FELINE GLOBE

Feline Anterior Uveal Melanoma

Melanoma is the most common primary ocular neoplasm in cats. Feline AUM often presents as a diffuse pigmentation and thickening of the anterior iris surface. As the disease progresses, the neoplastic cells cause thickening and distortion of the iris as well as obstruction of the filtration angle, which leads to secondary glaucoma. This must be differentiated from diffuse iris melanosis, which causes diffuse iridal pigmentation without thickening and distortion of the anterior iris surface. This clinical differentiation can be difficult. Whenever the anterior surface of the iris is raised, or if the normal iridal architecture is obscured, melanoma must be suspected. Cytologic or histologic examination often provides the most accurate diagnosis. Cells for cytologic examination can be obtained by aspiration or "vacuuming" pigmented cells from the anterior surface of the iris. This is performed with a 25-gauge needle connected to a 3-ml syringe. The anterior iris surface is approached in a manner similar to that in an aqueous centesis. With the needle bevel down, the surface of the mass is "vacuumed" to collect cells. One must try not to obtain aqueous, only cells. The aspirated cells are placed on a slide and the slide is air-dried and submitted for evaluation. Histologic samples can be obtained by performing an iridectomy; they provide more accurate information about cell structure and invasion. Because 50 to 60% of feline AUMs are reported to metastasize, it is crucial to evaluate the cat for metastasis at the time of diagnosis. Metastatic disease can occur several months to 2 to 3 years after diagnosis and may not be affected by enucleation. The liver and lung tend to be primary sites of initial metastasis. The presence of secondary uveitis or, especially, secondary glaucoma is associated more frequently with metastasis. Histologically, a large number of mitotic figures is also associated with metastasis.

It can be difficult, perhaps impossible, to differentiate melanoma from melanosis clinically. We find that cytologic studies and, more often, histopathologic studies provide much better information to inform accurately and make recommendations to the owner. Depending on the location of the lesion, a small iridectomy is relatively easy to obtain and is well tolerated by the globe. This procedure is best performed by a veterinary ophthalmologist. Again, before iridectomy or enucleation, we evaluate the thorax (radiographically) and the abdomen (ultrasonographically) for metastasis. If metastasis is present or strongly suspected, we recommend consultation with an oncologist. If ocular malignant melanoma is found or is strongly suspected, we recommend early enucleation and histopathology. The presence of melanoma cells within the scleral vessels is closely associated with distant metastasis. We also recommend re-evaluation for metastasis every 2 months for a year if histopathologic examination of the globe demonstrates malignant AUM. If the mass is small, localized to a small portion of the iris, and not invading the drainage angle, we have performed an iridectomy to remove the entire iridal mass. In this situation, it is crucial to perform histopathologic studies to determine if the entire mass has been removed, and we are more comfortable if the histopathologic examination demonstrates a benign lesion. If iridectomy demonstrates diffuse iris melanosis or a benign melanoma, we observe the patient closely for any signs of malignancy but do not routinely perform enucleation. If, at any time, the globe develops secondary uveitis or glaucoma, we recommend enucleation and histopatho-

logic examination. Because malignant AUM is frequently associated with metastasis that is life-threatening, we would rather remove a visual globe than risk an animal's life. This has to be balanced against not removing a visual globe unnecessarily. If the diagnosis is not clear, we recommend referral to a veterinary ophthalmologist.

Feline Post-traumatic Sarcoma

Numerous cases of intraocular sarcoma have been reported in cats with a history of ocular trauma. The period between the initial trauma and the development of an intraocular sarcoma can be several months to many years. If examined histologically, almost all cases exhibit severe lenticular disease, and it has been suggested that the sarcomas may have originated from lens epithelial cells. These sarcomas often demonstrate malignant behavior with extension to the optic nerve, orbit, and brain, and metastasis to distant sites has been reported. Because of this behavior, early enucleation is recommended. If there are any signs of orbital extension such as exophthalmos or third eyelid elevation, or both, the extent of tumor invasion should be evaluated before enucleation by orbital ultrasonography, computed tomography, or magnetic resonance imaging. In our experience, computed tomography or magnetic resonance imaging provides better information about the extent of orbital and brain invasion than does orbital ultrasonography.

Feline Limbal Melanoma

Feline limbal melanoma is clinically similar to canine epibulbar melanoma and is also typically benign. In cats, however, it is more important to be sure that the mass is scleral in origin and has not grown through the sclera from the anterior uveal tract. Thorough intraocular examination and gonioscopy can aid in this determination. Treatment is as with canine epibulbar melanoma.

SECONDARY NEOPLASMS OF THE CANINE AND FELINE GLOBES

Secondary neoplasms of the eye of dogs and cats (Table 2) are not common but are seen with some regularity in a referral ophthalmology practice. Hematogenous spread of systemic neoplasia can occur, as the ciliary body and choroid have a significant blood supply and are, in fact, one of the most vascular organs in the body. The clinical signs associated with secondary neoplasia are dependent on the amount and location of the affected ocular tissues. Secondary neoplasms can occur as solitary masses but more commonly manifest as diffuse lesions because the spread occurs through vascular tissues. In the posterior segment (retina and choroid), secondary neoplasms may appear as diffuse or multifocal hyporeflective lesions in the retina and choroid. They may even appear as intraretinal or subretinal hemorrhages. In the anterior segment (iris and ciliary body), secondary neoplasms tend to mimic diffuse anterior uveitis with iridal hyperemia, iridal thickening, aqueous flare, and hyphema. As signs of anterior uveitis worsen, the incidence of secondary glaucoma increases. Secondary glaucoma occurs because of blockage of aqueous outflow by posterior or peripheral anterior synechiae, or both, or by physical clogging of the drainage angle with inflammatory or neoplastic cells. One might expect secondary neoplasms to affect both eyes if the eyes are involved; however, any or all of these ocular signs can occur unilaterally or bilaterally.

If ocular spread of a systemic neoplasm is suspected, a thorough systemic evaluation of the animal should be instituted. This includes a physical examination and blood work, including a complete blood count, biochemical profile, and urinalysis. We also recommend thoracic radiography and abdominal ultrasonography to determine the location of the primary neoplasm and the presence of other metastasis. As with primary neoplasia, ocular ultrasonography may be of benefit, especially if the ocular media is not clear.

Lymphosarcoma (LSA) is the most common secondary neoplasm to affect the eye of both dogs and cats. The ocular clinical signs are usually diffuse and mimic anterior uveitis. Choroidal lesions and optic neuritis can also be present. If optic neuritis is present, one must consider that the central nervous system is affected and institute additional appropriate therapy. In dogs and cats with ocular lesions from LSA, one can usually identify systemic involvement without too much difficulty. In both dogs and cats, ocular LSA carries a worse prognosis than if ocular lesions were not present.

About one third of dogs with LSA exhibit ocular signs, with diffuse anterior uveitis being the most common ocular clinical sign. The presence of ocular lesions and lymphadenopathy is associated with stage V disease (using the World Health Organization protocol) and suggests that the patient has hematologic cell involvement. This stage usually represents a poorer prognosis for life expectancy.

In cats with LSA, anterior uveitis or panuveitis is the most common clinical sign of ocular disease. Cats are more likely than dogs to present with unilateral signs and may appear systemically healthy at the time of initial examination. The association of LSA and feline leukemia virus (FeLV) remains, so routine testing for FeLV should be performed in all suspected cases. Because of the strong association of FeLV and LSA, we recommend that an indirect fluorescent antibody test of a blood smear or bone marrow be performed on all negative enzyme-linked immunosorbent assay FeLV screening tests.

Adenocarcinomas are the second most commonly reported secondary neoplasms in dogs and cats. They are more commonly seen in dogs than in cats. Many types of adenocarcinomas have been reported to spread to the eye in both dogs and cats. These secondary neoplasms tend to be more solitary or discrete and are more often unilateral than bilateral.

Other secondary neoplasms can be found in both dogs and cats but are less commonly seen, especially in cats. A thorough ocular examination should be part of any evaluation of an animal with systemic neoplasia. It is often impossible to differentiate secondary neoplasms simply by a clinical ophthalmic evaluation. Many of the ocular signs

TABLE 2. Types of Intraocular Neoplasms

Canine
Primary
  Melanomas
    Anterior uveal
    Epibulbar
    Choroidal
  Adenoma, adenocarcinoma
  Medulloepithelioma (teratoid, nonteratoid)
  Astrocytoma
  Hemangioma
  Others
Secondary
  Lymphosarcoma
  Adenocarcinoma
  Hemangiosarcoma
  Melanoma
  Meningioma
  Others
Feline
Primary
  Melanomas
    Anterior uveal
    Limbal
  Post-traumatic sarcoma
  Others
Secondary
  Lymphosarcoma
  Adenocarcinoma
  Others

are similar, and the exact identification can be determined only by histopathologic examination.

References and Suggested Reading

Cocoran KA, Peiffer RL Jr, Koch SA: Histopathologic features of feline ocular lymphosarcoma: 49 cases (1978–1992). Vet Comp Ophthalmol 5:35, 1995.
This article presents a complete review of the histologic, serologic, and clinical data of 49 feline cases.

Dubielzig RR, Everitt J, Shadduck JA, et al: Clinical and morphologic features of post-traumatic ocular sarcomas in cats. Vet Pathol 27:62, 1990.
This article reviews 13 cases with clinical and histologic data.

Dubielzig RR, Hawkins KL, Toy KA, et al: Morphologic features of feline ocular sarcomas in 10 cats: Light microscopic, ultrastructure, and immunohistochemistry. Vet Comp Ophthalmol 4:7, 1994.
This is a complete review of 10 cases, with data supporting a cell of origin for this neoplasm.

Duncan DE, Peiffer RL: Morphology and prognostic indicators of anterior uveal melanomas in cats. Vet Comp Ophthalmol 1:25, 1991.
This article presents a complete review of 38 feline primary anterior uveal melanomas, with clinical, histologic, and prognostic data.

Krohne SG, Henderson NM, Richardson RC, et al: Prevalence of ocular involvement in dogs with multicentric lymphoma: Prospective evaluation of 94 cases. Vet Comp Ophthalmol 4:127, 1994.
This is a complete review of the ocular signs, hematologic data, clinical signs, and prognosis of 94 canine cases of lymphosarcoma.

Nasisse MP, Davidson MG, Olivero DK, et al: Neodymium:YAG laser treatment of primary canine intraocular tumors. Vet Comp Ophthalmol 3:152, 1993.
This article describes the methods, treatment, complications, and follow-up of 15 cases.

Sullivan TC, Nasisse MP, Davidson MG, et al: Photocoagulation of limbal melanoma in dogs and cats: 15 cases (1989–1993). J Am Vet Med Assoc 208:891, 1996.
This review describes the methods, treatment, complications, and follow-up of 15 canine and feline cases.

Diseases of Birds and Exotic Pets

Nancy L. Anderson

R. Eric Miller

Consulting Editors

***Still Current Information Found in* Current Veterinary Therapy XII:**

Nonsurgical Means of Sex Determination in Psittacine Birds, p. 1275
Antimicrobials in Pet Birds, p. 1278

Care of Orphan Birds

JANETTE ACKERMANN
Molalla, Oregon

In recent years, with the advent of new environmental awareness and conservation attitudes, there has been a growing demand for veterinarians to provide advice about and medical care for sick and injured or orphaned wildlife. Although the impact of releasing rehabilitated animals to the wild, at the population level, is minimal, the care of these animals does benefit the individual person by increasing his or her education and sensitivity toward nature. Thus, that person is more inclined to contribute to more aggressive conservation efforts, such as decreasing pollution, recycling, conserving energy, and so forth. On a more economic level, the treatment of wildlife is a community service and a good client builder.

There are many state and federal laws that protect wildlife, of which veterinarians and the general public should be aware. Most birds are protected under the Migratory Bird Act. The possession of any wild birds, their bodies, parts, feathers, nests, or eggs requires a state or federal permit, or both. These animals may not be kept as pets, killed, trapped, harassed, bought or sold, transported, or held in captivity by private citizens. Domestic waterfowl, turkeys, pigeons, starlings, sparrows, doves, and other non-native species are not included under this law. If a citizen is acting in good faith to rescue an animal and transports it immediately to an appropriate care facility, he or she is allowed temporary custody of the animal. Although government agencies such as the Department of Conservation, the Department of Natural Resources, and the United States Fish and Wildlife Agency have done much to help preserve native bird populations, they have done little to create standards for the proper care of sick, injured, or orphaned wildlife. The National Wildlife Rehabilitators Association and the International Wildlife Rehabilitation Council, although having no legal authority, have done much to improve the professionalism in the field of wildlife rehabilitation through publications and national meetings (Carpenter et al, 1992).

INITIAL PATIENT EVALUATION

Many of the problems found in sick, injured, or orphaned wildlife are similar to those found in their domestic counterparts, and much of what veterinarians need to know can be extrapolated from this knowledge. When an animal is admitted, the veterinarian should first consider two questions:

1. What is medically wrong with the animal, and can it be treated?
2. If treated, can the animal be released back into the wild?

If the answers to these questions are "yes," the next critical fact to determine is if the bird is actually orphaned. It is natural for some species to leave their young for extended periods while foraging for food. In many cases, with good questioning of the client, it can be determined that the baby may just have fallen from the nest and has not truly been abandoned by the parents. In this case, if the baby is not injured, it is best to return it to the nest. It is an unfounded myth that human handling of the chick will drive the parents away. During the history-taking process, it is important to find out when and where the baby was found. This gives the veterinarian an idea as to the duration of the injury or time the baby has been without parental care. It also gives one a good release site for the baby when it is finished being hand reared. The last question that should be asked of the person bringing an orphan bird to the clinic is what medical or supportive care has already been given to the bird so that overdosing can be avoided.

When it has been determined that the baby bird is truly injured or orphaned, its species and age must be determined. A field guide to nestlings is commercially available to help with the identification (Harrison, 1978). Categorization of size, bill structure and color, and down and feather pattern are characteristics that will help in identification.

At hatching, most birds are either precocial (chick covered with down, eyes open, well developed, and soon able to feed itself) or altricial (chick is naked, blind, unable to support itself, and relies on food supplied by parents). Precocial birds include the Galliformes (pheasants, quail, grouse, and turkeys), Anseriformes (ducks, geese), and Gruiformes (coots, gallinules, rails, and cranes). Altricial birds include the Passeriformes (most songbirds), Piciformes (woodpeckers, flickers), Apodiformes (swifts, hummingbirds), Caprimulgiformes (nighthawks, poor-wills), and Columbiformes (doves, pigeons). There are some semiprecocial birds (eyes open, downy, can walk but stay in the nest and are fed by their parents) such as Charadriiformes (gulls, terns), and semialtricial (downy, unable to leave the nest, and are fed by parents) such as Ciconiiformes (herons, egrets, bitterns), Falconiformes (hawks), and Strigiformes (owls).

INITIAL TREATMENT

When an orphan bird is brought to the veterinarian, a physical examination is conducted using procedures similar to those used with domestic animals, although the examination frequently is more cursory until the animal has been rehydrated and warmed. Fluids can be administered in a variety of ways depending on the patient's hydration status and concomitant injury or disease. Different routes include subcutaneous, intravenous, intraosseous, or oral (which is the most common route). Warmed, lactated Ringer's solution or a multielectrolyte solution is used at a dose of 40 to 50 ml/kg body weight divided into three or four treatments in a 24-hour period until rehydration has occurred.

Neonatal animals are not able to thermoregulate and have a tremendous surface area for heat loss. Hypothermia may result in an impaired gaping (feeding) reflex and gastrointestinal hypomotility and maldigestion. Hypothermia decreases the immune system and makes the animal susceptible to secondary bacterial and yeast infections (*Candida* being most common). Supplemental heat can be provided with heat lamps, incubators, heating pads, hot water bottles, or incandescent light bulbs. Care must be taken to insulate the baby so that burns and overheating are avoided. The initial temperature should be between 80 and 95°F, depending on the age and species of bird. A hypothermic, dehydrated baby bird should not be fed until it has been warmed to nearly normal temperature and rehydrated. During this rewarming, energy can be met with a 10 to 20% dextrose solution or a commercial product such as Emeraid I (Lefeber).

In addition to heat and fluids, initial therapy should include antibiotics, vitamin supplements, and other medications as indicated by physical findings. Once the bird is stabilized, it can be placed in an appropriate-sized artificial nest (to avoid splay-legged abnormal growth) and fed. Housing should be clean, have nonslip surfaces, and be quiet to avoid stress. It is important to have an idea of the natural history of a species to provide adequate nesting and housing.

HAND-FEEDING ORPHAN BIRDS

Most baby birds can be hand-fed readily; however, there are a few species that need to be gavaged either into the crop or directly into the stomach. Feeding tube sizes can be found in Table 1. Examples of species that need the latter are doves and nighthawks. A comment must be made regarding feeding problems that can be encountered when hand-rearing orphan birds. One problem is underfeeding birds, causing malnutrition and runting. The opposite extreme is overfeeding baby birds, causing aspiration pneumonia, stress, crop stasis, enteropathies, and secondary diseases. Most orphan birds eat 10 to 20% of their body weight in a 24-hour period. Birds should be weighed daily to monitor weight gain and, therefore, the adequacy of the diet. As stated earlier, although hand-feeding of baby birds generally is not difficult, it requires a tremendous commitment of time and appropriate selection of diet (discussed further on). Forceps, toothpicks, syringes, or plastic coffee stirrers (with the edges rounded) can be used to deliver small bits of food. Whenever possible, one should avoid prying the mouth open to feed baby birds. The food-begging reflex can be elicited by tapping the bill (the yellow or orange flanges at the base of the bill in passerines) or feathers around the bill, which will stimulate the bird to gape for food. Chicks should not continue to be fed until the begging ceases, as they will beg well beyond the point of fullness. The proper amount to feed an orphan bird depends on the rate of growth and development of the species. If the species of bird being reared has a crop (e.g., owls do not), it should be full after each feeding but not stuffed to impaction. After a bite of food is given, a small amount of water should follow to help the passage of food and keep the bird hydrated. The bill and surrounding skin should be cleaned after each feeding. The food should be fresh and warmed to room temperature. Care must be taken, especially with the unequal heating of a microwave, to avoid crop burns. Orphan birds should be encouraged to eat on their own as quickly as possible. Offer a wide variety of foods while following the natural diet for the species as much as possible. Color contrasts may stimulate self-feeding (Hickman and Guy, 1973).

The final problem with hand-rearing is imprinting. Imprinting is an innate response to sight, sound, smell, and other stimuli that teach the orphan bird what species it is. If the bird imprints onto the wrong species, including humans, the bird may become unable to function in the wild. Even if the bird survives, it still will be unable to breed or associate in an appropriate manner to conspecifics. There have been reports of humans being injured by improperly hand-raised animals because the animals lack the fear of humans normally exhibited by their wild counterparts. Even if they are not imprinted, tameness makes them easy prey. It is important to minimize human contact during the hand-rearing process and to keep them with conspecifics, especially during their critical imprinting stage, which is usually the first 24 to 48 hours of life in most species. Some individuals play natural adult bird calls and songs to the orphans. It would be beneficial to place them in aviaries with adults as soon as they are self-thermoregulating and mobile. This works even if they are not finished with the hand-feeding process. Care must be taken if species are mixed in the aviary to avoid injuries to the babies from the adults or from other species of birds. For example, many raptors can be safely placed in a flight pen with adults; however, some species, such as great horned owls, will often kill the juveniles. Orphans in this setting should be carefully monitored (Fowler, 1979; Weber, 1978).

SPECIFIC DIETS AND INFANT CARE

Raptors

Raptor chicks usually start begging within a few hours of pipping (hatching). There is no need to force-feed these babies before this reflex occurs because a yolk sac is present, providing them with nutrients for the first 12 to 24 hours. Ground muscle, liver, and organ meat, excluding the stomach and intestines, should be fed every 2 to 3 hours until the begging has stopped or the crop is full. The meat should be from natural prey species as much as possible, for example, mice for buteos and quail for falcons. Do not

TABLE 1. Feeding Tube Sizes

Weight of Animal	French Size
Less than 50 gm	3–5
50–100 gm	5–10
100–500 gm	10–14
500–1000 gm	15–18
1–2 kg	18–20
2–5 kg	20–24
5–10 kg	28–30
10–20 kg	32–34

From Evans, RH: Care and feeding of orphan mammals and birds. In: Kirk RW, ed: Current Veterinary Therapy IX. Philadelphia: WB Saunders, 1986, p 785, with permission.

TABLE 2. Nesting Diets

Species	Diet
Insectivores	5 ounces canned dog food, 1 ounce turkey starter, 2 drops vitamin supplement, 1 brewer's yeast tablet (Hayes; 1980). Mealworms, waxworms and live insects are added to the diet at 2–3 wk of age.
Omniviores Frugivores	High-protein baby cereal, strained beef baby food, hard-boiled egg yolks, cooked rice, applesauce, vitamin and mineral supplement (Hayes, 1980). Mixed berries are added to the diet (20%).
Seed eating and granivores	Egg yolk, turkey starter, 2 drops vitamin supplement, 1 brewer's yeast tablet, water, to mix to a soupy consistency (Hayes, 1980). For galliformes, add insects and for waterfowl, add aquatic vegetables and water.
Raptors	Chopped muscle, organ (other than stomach and intestines), and bone of skinned rodents or plucked quail.
Fish eating	Insectivorous diet with the addition of slivers of fish, aquatic and terrestrial invertebrates, and insects. Ground or minced rodents and insects can be added to the diet.

use day-old chicks because they provide little nutritional value. After the first 2 to 3 days, small bits of bone can be added to the diet for a calcium source. The amount of food and time interval between feedings can be increased gradually as the bird grows. Whole food usually is not fed until orphans are almost full adult size, at about 8 weeks of age.

Insectivores

General guidelines for hand-rearing orphan insectivorous species are presented in Table 2. The natural diet should be included as much and as quickly as possible. Obviously, many of the insectivorous species eat varieties of insects as well as fruits, berries, and seeds. More information on the natural food sources can be found in *American Wildlife Plants: A Guide to Wildlife Food Habits* (Martin et al, 1951). Nestling songbirds should be fed initially every 15 minutes (1- to 4-day-old birds), for 12 hours of the day. This expands to every 30 to 60 minutes for 5 to 10 days after hatching, and eventually extends to every 2 to 3 hours at 2 weeks after hatching. Self-feeding should be started as early as possible. This usually occurs once the bird becomes a fledgling, leaving the nest.

Age determination in altricial birds is important. The egg teeth at the tip of the bill in these babies are lost after 3 days. Nestlings, up to 1 week, are naked except for pin feathers. By 2 weeks of age, they have feathers covering most of the body. By 3 weeks, they should be completely covered with feathers and starting to fledge. In 4 to 6 weeks, the birds should be able to fly.

Omnivores and Frugivores

A good frugivorous nestling formula can be found on Table 2. The feeding schedule closely follows that which was described previously for insectivorous birds. Again, the sooner the natural diet can be added to the formula, the better is the chance of successful normal growth in the nestling.

Seed Eaters–Granivores

An appropriate diet for nestling seed- and grain-eating chicks is found in Table 2. The same feeding schedule given for the insectivorous chicks is followed, adding the natural diet as soon as possible to the formula and weaning them as quickly as possible. Many waterfowl such as ducks and geese are grain eaters and can be raised on the seed-eater formula with some supplementation. Shredded carrots and lettuce may elicit earlier self-feeding behavior in waterfowl, as they are attracted to the yellow and green. Many shorebirds can be fed on the preceding diet, but it is advisable to add live mealworms and waxworms or other insects on top of the food to stimulate feeding. Keeping waterfowl's food very wet, almost submerged, stimulates appetite, even in the adult. Depending on the grain source fed to the chicks, a calcium and phosphorus supplement should be given. Many waterfowl are gregarious, and housing them together in groups keeps them happier and encourages feeding. For example, wood duck chicks are notorious for not eating, and mallard chicks eat well right from the start. Housing them together may help stimulate feeding. Nestlings housed together should be of similar size or they will outcompete the smaller birds.

Encouraging foster parenting, either by the addition of orphans to wild bird nests or by obtaining surrogate parents in the captive situation, can significantly decrease the labor of hand-rearing and decrease the behavioral abnormalities of the chicks. Foster hens can be obtained from local pigeon breeders and chicken and duck farms. Cross-fostering can also be carried out where wild gallinaceous chicks can be fostered onto domestic chickens, and wild ducklings of many different species can be cross-fostered onto domestic ducks.

Fish Eaters

The same starter diet that is used for the insectivorous birds can be used for these chicks. Small slivers of fish, aquatic and terrestrial insects, and crustaceans are added to the diet within a couple of days of hatching. If fresh fish cannot be found and frozen is used, a thiamine supplement of 25 mg/kg of fish should be used. If these birds will not eat, force-feeding them fish is necessary, or a fish purée can be administered by stomach tube to get them started.

HOUSING YOUNG BIRDS

In general, it is better to house young birds outside if the weather permits. It decreases the nestlings' exposure to humans and decreases stress. Enclosures that are predator-resistant are a must so that the the babies do not fill the belly of a raccoon, weasel, hawk, or other predator. The enclosures should be in as natural a setting as possible for the fledglings. Perches of varying sizes and textures should be offered to all perching birds. Nonslip flooring should be used and it should be easy to clean. There should be adequate shade and water. Many waterfowl and shorebirds like small pools. The perches should be situated to avoid feather damage and should be appropriate for the particular species of bird. For example, most hawks like round perches, whereas falcons like flat, block perches.

Many species of birds can be housed in groups; however, supervision is necessary and this approach does not work with all species. Gamebirds and many raptor species have severe conspecific aggression. It may be helpful to obtain advice on new introductions from someone who has had experience with the species. Food and water dishes should be situated so that they can be removed daily and cleaned without having to enter the enclosure. This decreases stress and minimizes tameness in the young birds. For many of the raptor species, it is important to train the young birds with live prey to ensure that they can hunt successfully before being released. This is where housing with conspecifics, either in the same or the next cage and within visual range of more experienced hunters, can be helpful. Prevention of damage to feathers is important. Once feather damage occurs, the rehabilitator must either "imp" new feathers in or wait for the bird to molt naturally (Arent and Martel, 1996). This can take 6 months to a year, although fledglings undergo a couple of molts just to reach juvenile and adult plumage. Thyroid supplementation has been used to cause a premature molt. Use of this hormone supplement is recommended only under the supervision of an experienced veterinarian because incorrect dosing can cause serious illness, and this hormone does not work consistently in all species. It is much better to prevent feather damage in advance and avoid these headaches.

Hand-rearing of orphan birds can be rewarding; however, before it is attempted, one must consider the time and energy needed to commit to this endeavor. It is important to have a good working knowledge of the individual species'

natural history in order to raise these orphans successfully. Success is defined not only in terms of a living juvenile or adult but also in terms of the development of a physically and behaviorally normal adult bird that is capable of fending for itself once released back into the wild. It may be wise to limit the number of species one offers to hand-raise at first so that this expertise can be developed gradually, after which one can grow and diversify. It is hard to turn down orphans, but it is even harder to see inadequately raised babies being released into the wild only to die of starvation or predation. Starting small and working one's way up is always a wise decision.

References and Suggested Reading

Arent LR, Martel M: Care and Management of Captive Raptors. The Raptor Center, St. Paul, University of Minnesota, 1996.
Carpenter JW, Ackermann J, Mashima T: Medical and Supportive Care of Orphaned Wildlife. Second Mid-western Exotic Animal Medicine Conference Proceedings. Manhattan, Kansas State University College of Veterinary Medicine, 1992.
Evans RH: Care and feeding of orphan mammals and birds. In: Kirk's Current Veterinary Therapy IX. Philadelphia: WB Saunders, 1986.
Fowler ME: Care of Orphaned Wild Animals. Vet Clin North Am 9:447, 1979.
Harrison CA: Field Guide to the Nests, Eggs, and Nestlings of North American Birds. Glasgow, William Collins, 1978.
Hayes MB: Rehabilitation Guidebook for Birds and Mammals. Troy, Ohio: Brukner Nature Center, 1980.
Hickman M, Guy M: Care of the Wild, Feathered, and Furred. Santa Cruz, CA: Unity Press, 1973.
Martin AC, Zim HS, Nelson AL: American Wildlife and Plants: A Guide to Wildlife Food Habits. New York: Dover Publications, 1951.
Weber WJ: Wild Orphaned Babies: Mammals and Birds, Caring for Them and Setting Them Free. New York: Holt, Rinehart, and Winston, 1978.

Psittacine Behavior and Training

BARBARA L. OGLESBEE
Columbus, Ohio

Because of the rise in popularity of psittacine birds as pets, veterinarians are now frequently consulted to assess problems related to abnormal or misunderstood behaviors in these animals. Familiarity with normal psittacine behaviors may help bird-owning clients to better understand their pets and thus learn to prevent or correct unacceptable behavioral problems.

In order to understand parrot behavior, several unique characteristics of these animal should be considered. First, one must recognize the extremely gregarious nature of these birds. Parrots are social flock animals and in the wild will spend their entire lives in the company of their flock. Paired animals will usually spend 24 hours a day with their mate. The flock has a specific social hierarchy and is essential in providing protection from predators. Second, birds, unlike most traditional mammalian pets, are prey animals whose reactions to their owners are often quite different from those of predatory animals such as dogs and

cats. Parrots are also much more intelligent than many people realize. Studies performed on African Grey parrots have shown their cognitive abilities to be similar to the great apes. They are capable of complex behaviors such as using tools, numeric competency, and problem solving. A fourth unique feature of parrots as pets is that they are not truly domesticated animals. Most parrots available to the pet trade today have been bred in captivity, but they are only one, or at most, two generations removed from the wild. They will therefore retain most of their wild characteristics. They have not had generations of breeding to adapt to life with humans.

The combination of all these factors makes life in a home, rather than a forest, a difficult adjustment for birds, even when born in captivity. If proper preventive measures are taken, however, many common behavioral problems may be avoided, and bird and client may form a mutually rewarding relationship.

FLOCK AND MATE BEHAVIOR

Before purchasing a parrot, one should take into consideration his or her daily schedule and determine if it will be possible to be an acceptable mate or flock substitute. This does not preclude bird ownership if the average 8-hour work day is routine, as long as the bird is provided with adequate stimulation during the hours in which the owners are away. However, if the bird will be left alone for prolonged periods or will be faced with a very irregular schedule, behavioral problems are much more likely to occur. The owner may wish to reconsider whether a bird is an appropriate pet in this situation. In some cases, it may be helpful to provide the bird with a psittacine companion when long or irregular schedules are unavoidable.

Many behavioral problems may be avoided by providing the bird with activities during the hours it is alone. The bird should be given a large cage area, with toys and other items for chewing, swinging, and preening. Many birds appear to comforted by noise from a radio or television left turned on while the owners are away. Although a large living space is desired, pet birds should never be allowed to remain uncaged without supervision because of the potential for serious injury. Freedom from the cage is necessary, however, when the owners are home. Most birds become accustomed to an established routine, such as getting out of the cage in the morning, staying with their owners during the breakfast routine, and then returning to the cage for the day. Evenings are again spent outside the cage, interacting with the owners. Disruptions in this routine may result in problem behaviors, such as excessive screaming or feather plucking. Birds should also be introduced to new situations, environments, and people from an early age. A bird that is accustomed to only one room, area, or person becomes fearful of new situations.

DOMINANCE BEHAVIORS

Within a flock and within a bonded pair of parrots, a hierarchy of dominance is established. It is important for bird owners to establish who is the dominant "bird" early in the relationship. Parrots generally accept humans as part of the flock or as a mate, but despite the large differences in size, may not willingly accept the human as the dominant animal. There are several ways in which a bird attempts to establish dominance. One is by protecting what it views as its territory. This may be the cage, the perch, or a favorite area of the house. It also attempts to protect what it views as its possessions, which may be a favorite toy or person. It attempts to drive away an intruder which it considers to be subordinate. These attempts, usually characterized by vocalizing, threatening displays, charging, and biting, must be prohibited immediately. Problems most frequently arise when the person being protected tolerates or even encourages this behavior.

There are two methods often used to curtail this behavior. First, all members of the family must establish themselves as dominant members of the flock. The owners should define what is and is not the bird's territory, including the cage. The owners, not the bird, should control the bird's movement so that whenever the bird is removed from the cage or perch, it should be given the "up"

command (see further on), picked up by the owners, and placed in a desired location. The bird should not be allowed to leave its cage or perch of its own volition and walk or fly freely in the house. Another more subtle way in which a bird establishes dominance is by placing itself in a position where it is physically at eye level or higher than its owner. Most birds become significantly more aggressive (and vocal) when placed on a high perch. To help establish the human as the dominant animal, birds should not be placed on a perch or on the owner's body at eye level or higher. This means that the bird should not be allowed to perch on shoulders but be trained to perch on the hand, with the elbow bent, keeping it at chest level.

Second, negative reinforcement should be used to inhibit any dominance or territorial behaviors, such as screaming, biting, or charging. The most effective negative reinforcement method is to physically remove the bird from its flock substitute, human companionship. As soon as the first sign of threatening behavior begins, a firm "No!" command should be given and the bird removed from the area or person that it is attempting to protect. In mild cases, just placing the bird on the floor is sufficient. If this does not stop the behavior, the bird should be removed from the room and placed in a "time out" area, such as a small cage or sturdy box. The time out area should not be the bird's regular cage or travel carrier. In some cases, a water sprayer has been used as a negative reinforcer, as a sharp stream of water will usually startle a bird. This method should not be used, however, if the bird is regularly misted with a water bottle for grooming purposes.

A bird should never be struck. The chance for serious injury is far too great. Even gentler physical reprimands, such as flicking the bird on the beak, generally do not discourage aggressive behaviors. On the contrary, most birds do not back down when struck on the beak but instead become even more aggressive.

DOMINANCE AND SEXUAL BEHAVIOR

Dominance problems encountered in pet birds usually intensify as the bird reaches sexual maturity. These behaviors may become severe during the "breeding season," which is generally late winter through summer. During this time, many dominant birds become highly protective of their territories and their chosen mate. Aggression may be directed both against intruders and against the person whom the bird has chosen as his "mate." The latter is usually due to displaced aggression, as the bird tries to drive its perceived mate to safety (such as a nestbox) by charging or striking at its mate when faced with a potential threat. Owners often perceive these attacks as being unprovoked and claim that the bird would suddenly bite them and then return to its more docile temperament just a few moments after the attack. These bites can be severe and often draw blood. Obviously, this behavior cannot be tolerated in an acceptable pet, and steps can be taken to temper this aggression.

First, the client should be taught to recognize when the bird is becoming sexually active. A bird may make sexual displays toward the client. These displays may consist of attempting to lure the owner to a chosen nest site (often a confined space such as under a couch or in a closet) and preening the client with the beak. These behaviors may then progress to regurgitating food from the crop toward the client or performing a mating "dance" on the client. In male birds, this is manifested by a squealing noise accompanied by fluffing feathers, bobbing motion, and raising a leg in a mock mounting attempt; females may fan the tail and back into the client. These behaviors are often accompanied by the severe aggression described earlier, especially if the bird perceives an outside threat. Biting incidents are usually triggered by another person walking into the room, other pets, or even humans or animals seen through a window or on television.

To help curtail these problems, *all* sexually motivated behavior toward the client or an object should be completely discouraged. (Many clients find mating behaviors endearing.) At the first sign of courting behavior, the bird should be reprimanded and removed from its perceived mate. Bear in mind that this is a strong instinct in birds and may be difficult to suppress. In some cases, the drive to reproduce is so strong that discouraging dominance behavior and negative reinforcement is insufficient. In this case, it may be prudent to allow the bird an opportunity to go to nest with a mate of the same species and not be handled by humans during this period. There is currently no safe and effective method of castrating parrots.

BASIC TRAINING

Pet birds should be trained to obey a few basic commands, such as "up," "stay," and "potty." The verbal commands may vary according to owner preference but should be short and clear in order to identify them as commands. Training is most successful when begun at weaning before unwanted behaviors have been established as habit. Positive reinforcement works well with parrots. A food or favorite toy may be used as the reinforcement, but in most cases, the strongest reward is owner companionship.

"Step" or "Up" Command

As discussed previously, every time the bird is let out of the cage or off a perch, it should be removed by the owner and not allowed to exit on its own in order to establish owner dominance. The bird must consistently be given the verbal "step" or "up" command every time it is picked up. A bare hand is placed in front of the bird's feet and the command is given. A gentle push up into the abdomen may be necessary at first to encourage the bird to step. Once it is on the hand, the thumb is placed over the dorsal surface of the feet to secure them. With the feet secure, the bird will have less of a tendency to dig its nails in when the owner is moving. No reward is necessary, as being with the client is the reinforcement.

Housebreaking

One of the most common complaints about bird ownership is the mess that unhousebroken birds create. With a little work and knowledge about the natural habits of parrots, housebreaking is attainable. There are some important differences between birds and cats or dogs. In most instances, the client must take the bird to the designated toilet area periodically. The time interval between defecations is shorter than that for dogs or cats and may range from 15 minutes to 3 hours, depending on the size of the bird. To begin training, the client should observe the bird over a period of days to determine the time interval between defecations.

The first training session should last about 3 hours and begin in the morning or after the bird is awakened from a nap. At this time, the bird has an immediate need to defecate. Before the bird is removed from the cage with the "step" command, the "potty" command is given as the bird defecates. The owner must then return the bird to the designated area (e.g., a T-stand) at the interval in which the bird would naturally need to defecate. For larger birds, such as parrots, macaws, and cockatoos, this is usually every 30 minutes. For smaller birds, the interval will be much shorter. The client then waits until the bird is about to defecate, and the command is given as soon as the bird begins to squat. A reward, such as food or a toy may be given along with praise; however, in most cases, just being picked up again is sufficient reward. This process should be repeated at least three to four times during the first session. Most birds catch on fairly quickly. If an "accident" occurs in the beginning, the bird should not be reprimanded, as it usually indicates that the bird was not returned to the designated area quickly enough. Eventually, if this method is followed every time the bird is with the owner, it will learn to defecate only on command or in the designated area. With time, large parrots can learn to control their defecation for up to 3 hours.

Screaming

Most pet birds go through a period each day, usually at dawn and dusk, when they would naturally become very vocal. This is an important flock behavior, and attempting to override this instinct can be difficult and frustrating. When possible, an attempt should be made to avoid the behavior entirely by planning an activity, such as playing or a training session during these periods. If the bird insists on being vocal during these periods, the owner can provide a less irritating and quieter substitute for screaming. If the bird is able to talk or mimic, he or she may be taught some quiet vocalizations, songs, or whistles to be encouraged at these times. If the bird starts to become loud and agitated, the client should sing, speak, or whisper the mimicry the bird knows, since birds in a flock would be trading vocalizations at this time. If the bird still has trouble remaining calm, negative reinforcers, such as the time out area, should be used. The client should never scream at the bird, as this will only encourage further screaming. It is important to emphasize that whenever possible the bird should be given a substitute behavior. Parrots have an instinctual need to be vocal at these times. Constant negative reinforcement or solitary confinement at these times will only serve to frustrate both the bird and the owner. If the substitute behavior begins to deteriorate into screaming, a combination of positive and negative reinforcement should be used to redirect the behavior, not to stifle the bird completely.

With some understanding of the natural behavior of

parrots, and the key differences between bird and mammalian behavior, detrimental behaviors such as screaming, biting, and feather plucking may be curtailed. The owner must understand, however, that although born in captivity, parrots are not domesticated animals. Often, the best one can hope for is a peaceful compromise between human and flock behavior.

References and Suggested Reading

Athan M-S: Guide to a Well-Behaved Parrot. Hauppauge, NY: Barron's Educational Series, Inc., 1993.
This is a client-oriented book detailing normal behavior and avoidance of behavior problems.

Davis C: Behavior. In: Altman RB, Clubb SL, Dorrestein GM, et al, eds: Avian Medicine and Surgery. Philadelphia: WB Saunders, 1996, p 96.
This is a thorough review of the behavior of psittacine birds in captivity.

Davis C: Behavioral Problems. In: Altman RB, Clubb SL, Dorrestein GM, et al, eds: Avian Medicine and Surgery. Philadelphia: WB Saunders, 1996, p 653.
This is a detailed review of commonly encountered behavioral problems in captive psittacine birds.

Harrison GJ: Perspective on parrot behavior. In: Ritchie BW, Harrison GJ, Harrison LR, eds: Avian Medicine: Principles and Application. Lake Worth: Wingers, 1994, p 96.
This is a comprehensive review of wild psittacine bird behavior, training, common behavioral problems, and behavioral modification techniques.

Diagnostic Use of Protein Electrophoresis in Birds

CAROLYN CRAY
Miami, Florida

Serum protein fractionation has been a valuable tool in mammalian diagnostics for more than 30 years. Originated in studies of human serum proteins and immunoglobulins, the techniques of protein fractionation matured to assist in the diagnosis of hepatic disease, autoimmunity, and multiple myeloma. Laborious research-based technologies were improved to facilitate its wider use in human diagnostics.

Small animal diagnostics have made serum protein electrophoresis (EPH) commonplace in most veterinary diagnostic laboratories, where it has been a widely accepted tool in the diagnosis of feline infectious peritonitis (FIP), ehrlichiosis, multiple myeloma, and immune deficiencies (Kaneko, 1989). Only recently has protein EPH been applied to avian diagnostics (Quesenberry and Moroff, 1991; Cray, et al, 1995; Cray and Tatum, 1998). Using plasma samples, EPH has been a valuable aid for diagnosing chlamydiosis, aspergillosis, hepatitis, and nephritis, among other infectious and noninfectious diseases. More recently, high-resolution EPH has been employed at the research level to refine the plasma proteins and better define diagnostic exclusions (Cray et al, 1996a).

TECHNIQUE OF PROTEIN ELECTROPHORESIS

There are many techniques for performing fractionation of plasma or serum proteins, but the one most commonly used in diagnostic laboratories involves EPH. Commercial diagnostic systems by Beckman and Helena Laboratories have led to major improvements in this technique, in addition to cost-saving and timesaving advantages.

The principle of EPH is simple. Plasma is overlayed on a thin agarose gel, which is exposed to an electric field. The way in which proteins migrate is dependent on their charge. The gel is then fixed and stained for the protein bands. Interpretation can be performed visually, or protein fractions can be quantified using a laser tracing by a densitometer. The percentage of proteins can be evaluated, or absolute concentrations of the fractions can be generated if the concentration of total protein has been determined through other means. Using a more advanced electrophoretic technique called *high-resolution EPH,* individual globulin protein components can be defined to monitor specific changes in these fractions.

AVIAN PLASMA PROTEINS

Generally six protein fractions are resolved in psittacine plasma using EPH. These fractions include prealbumin, albumin, alpha₁, alpha₂, beta, and gamma (Fig. 1). The latter four fractions represent the globulin families. Using high-resolution EPH, the globulins can be further defined into more than 10 additional components.

Prealbumin is generally negligible or absent in most mammalian species. It likely serves as a carrier or transporter protein like albumin, the protein that composes the major portion of plasma protein in healthy birds. Alpha-globulins are divided into two fractions by EPH (alpha₁ and alpha₂). These fractions include the acute-phase proteins alpha-lipoprotein, alpha₁-antitrypsin, and haptoglobin. Alpha₂-macroglobulin is also a member of the alpha-globulin class but often migrates in the beta fraction range in EPH of avian specimens. For the most part, alpha₁ globulins are difficult to resolve in psittacine species, but are more easily observed in specimens from raptors and ratites. Beta-globulins are generally reported as one fraction, al-

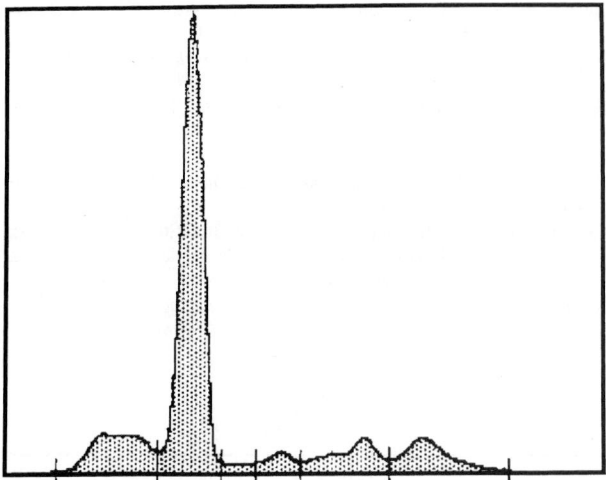

Figure 1. Normal electrophoretogram from an adult macaw. Six fractions are defined (from the left): prealbumin, albumin, alpha$_1$, alpha$_2$, beta, and gamma. The A:G ratio is 2.9.

though two fractions (beta$_1$ and beta$_2$) are observed in psittacines. The latter is especially true with African Grey parrots. These fractions include the acute-phase proteins such as alpha$_2$-macroglobulin, fibronectin, transferrin, and beta-lipoprotein. Gamma globulins can be subdivided into two fractions (gamma$_1$ and gamma$_2$) in mammals. In healthy avians, only one fraction is generally observed. The fractions represent circulating immunoglobulins. In addition, acute-phase proteins, including complement and complement degradation products, migrate in this region.

NORMAL ELECTROPHORETOGRAMS

In psittacines, the normal electrophoretogram is composed of minimal concentrations of the globulins and a predominance of albumin. This is reflected in a normal A:G ratio that can be produced by EPH. Veterinarians should inquire about how the A:G ratio is generated in their diagnostic laboratory. For best results, the formula that should be used is (prealbumin + albumin)/(alpha- + beta- + gamma globulins). Normal values range from 1.6 to 4.5 in psittacine species. The inclusion of prealbumin is important. In some psittacine species, such as cockatiels, lovebirds, and parakeets, prealbumin is also a major fraction, composing up to 40% of the total plasma protein. In most other psittacine species, the prealbumin is present in either negligible amounts or up to 20% of the total plasma protein. The significance of these differences is unknown. The albumin fraction should represent 45 to 70% of plasma protein in psittacines. Lower amounts of albumin are observed in healthy psittacines that have normally higher levels of prealbumin (e.g., cockatiels). In these species, a prealbumin:albumin ratio can also be produced from the EPH data, where the ratio should not exceed 0.80 in normal samples. The globulin fractions generally range from 2 to 8% of plasma protein in psittacine species. Beta-globulins can be higher in healthy African Grey parrots, Amazon parrots, and cockatoo species and may represent up to 13% of plasma protein. Understandably, for proper interpreta-

tion, protein fractions should be compared with laboratory-established species-specific reference ranges.

ABNORMAL ELECTROPHORETOGRAMS

Abnormal electrophoretograms are punctuated by changes in the A:G ratio. EPH results show changes in the major globulin fractions, and high-resolution EPH defines specific acute-phase protein increases or decreases. Through studies of clinical cases, these changes have been categorized to provide the practitioner a more defined list of clinical exclusions (Quesenberry and Moroff, 1991; Cray et al, 1995; Cray et al, 1996a). Together with other clinical data, a diagnosis can be made.

A typical EPH is observed in cases of *acute chlamydiosis* (Fig. 2). Changes include a moderate to marked decrease in albumin, a mild to moderate increase in beta-globulins, and a moderate to marked increase in gamma globulins. Chronic cases of chlamydiosis often have normal EPH patterns or demonstrate mild increases in beta-globulins. Aspergillosis and other mycotic diseases often result in moderate increases in beta-globulins, especially if the disease is chronic in nature. Conversely, immune responsive (e.g., seropositive) cases of *aspergillosis* exhibit mild to moderate increases in gamma globulins in the absence of beta-globulin changes (Fig. 3).

Hepatitis and nephritis are detected through decreases in albumin, which may be mild to moderate. In addition, mild to moderate beta-globulin increases (generally in alpha$_2$-macroglobulin) are seen with acute nephritis. This protein has a large molecular weight and often increases as the other plasma proteins are lost through the disease process. Chronic active hepatitis often results in a mild to moderate beta-globulin increase, with a similar increase in gamma globulins. Many acute-phase proteins that migrate in these fractions increase in concentration so that the EPH tracing demonstrates beta-gamma bridging where the definition between these two fractions becomes ill-defined.

Other EPH abnormalities can also be observed, but the definition of clinical exclusions becomes more variable.

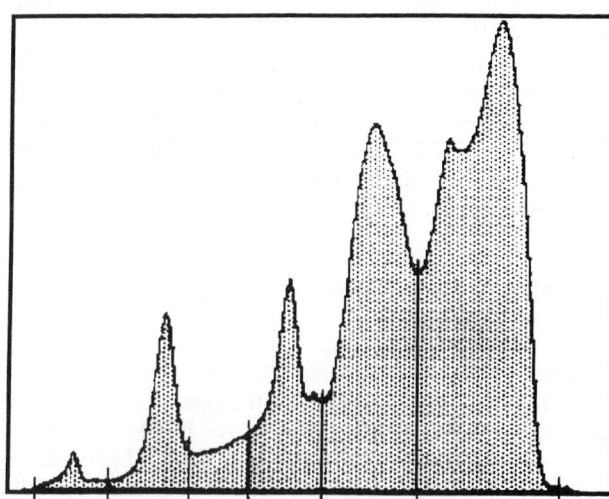

Figure 2. Abnormal electrophoretogram from an adult macaw with confirmed chlamydiosis. Note the large increases in beta- and gamma globulins and the decrease in albumin. The A:G ratio is 0.1.

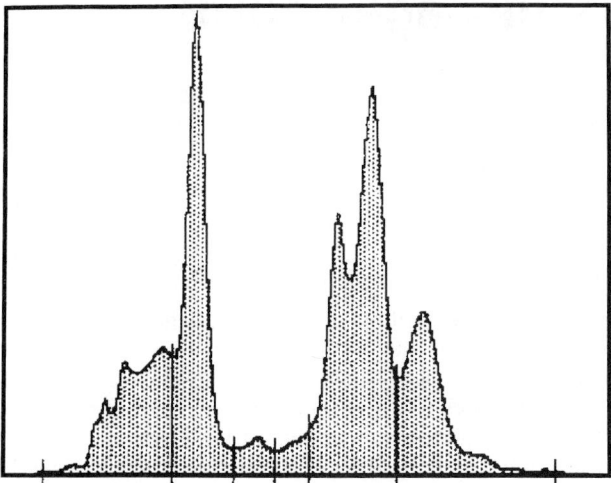

Figure 3. Abnormal electrophoretogram from an adult cockatiel with confirmed aspergillosis. Note the large increase in beta-globulins. The A:G ratio is 0.7.

Parasitism has been observed to result in mild decreases in albumin and mild increases in alpha$_1$-globulins. Malnutrition is typified by decreased albumin and gamma globulins (Romagnano, et al, 1996). This EPH pattern is often characterized by mild to moderate changes in these fractions. Albumin decreases are also observed in young psittacines (through 8 months of age), but gamma globulin decreases are generally normalized by 2 months of age. Infection with *Sarcocystis* spp. has been observed to result in mild to moderate increases in beta and gamma globulins (Cray et al, 1996b). Mycobacteriosis demonstrates similar changes, although most chronic cases are typified by predominately beta-globulin changes (Hoefer et al, 1996). This fraction is also subject to mild to moderate elevations with other diseases that result in an acute or chronic inflammatory response. These include nonspecific feather-plucking cases, mild bacterial infections, and heavy metal toxicities. No defined EPH changes have been reproducibly observed in cases of psittacine beak and feather disease or polyomavirus.

USES OF ELECTROPHORESIS BY THE VETERINARIAN

EPH is now commonly used as an accessory test in the new or well bird examination. As a complement to a complete blood count and chemistry panel, EPH provides not only an accurate quantitation of albumin and globulin (versus chemistry analyzers) but also a different view of the liver, kidney, and immune system. EPH abnormalities are observed in approximately 30% of apparently healthy birds that demonstrate normal or mild changes in the routine chemistry and hematologic analyses.

EPH is also a useful accessory tool to delineate complicating results in chlamydiosis and aspergillosis. Positive serologic results by the *Chlamydia* immunofluorescent antibody test may be interpreted as acute, chronic, or previously resolved infection. Abnormal EPH patterns can thus define these categories for the clinician. Serologic testing for aspergillosis is still difficult because infected birds do not produce high titers of antifungal antibodies. Abnormal beta-globulin increases can thus assist in maintaining this as a possible diagnosis. In addition, the aforementioned changes in beta- and gamma globulins provide useful diagnostic information in conjunction with traditional chemistry analyses such as uric acid, aspartate aminotransferase, and bile acid determinations.

EPH is also a valuable prognostic indicator. Changes in acute-phase plasma proteins can often occur before changes in traditional chemistry and hematologic analyses and thus can reflect positive changes in the patient status. EPH patterns can be examined for normalization with successful treatment regimens. Mild changes or continued elevations in the globulin fractions can thus uncover chronic infection that may not otherwise be detected in the treated bird.

References and Suggested Reading

Cray C, Tatum LM: Applications of protein electrophoresis in avian diagnostics. J Avian Med Surg 12:4, 1998.

Cray C, Bossart G, Harris D: Plasma protein electrophoresis: Principles and diagnosis of infectious disease. Proc Annu Conf Assoc Avian Vet 55, 1995.
This is a general review of the application of EPH to avian diagnostics, with specific abnormal electrophoretograms from clinical cases.

Cray C, Bossart G, Harris D: Plasma protein electrophoresis: An update. Proc Annu Conf Assoc Avian Vet 97, 1996a.
This article reports the investigations with lactate dehydrogenase and creatine phosphokinase isoenzymes in psittacines and the application of high-resolution EPH in avian diagnostics.

Cray C, Greiner E, Zielzienski K: Serological diagnosis of Sarcocystis. Proc Annu Conf Assoc Avian Vet 202, 1996b.
This article reports on a serologic test for Sarcocystis infection in cowbirds and psittacines, with EPH as an accessory test.

Hoefer HL, Kiehn TE, Friedan TR: Systemic *Mycobacterium tuberculosis* in a green winged macaw. Proc Annu Conf Assoc Avian Vet 167, 1996.
This is a clinical case presentation involving the use of EPH in diagnosis.

Kaneko JJ: Serum proteins and the dysproteinemias. In: Kaneko JJ, ed: Clinical Biochemistry of Domestic Animals. New York: Academic Press, 1989, p 142.
This is a review of the technique of protein EPH, the serum proteins, and applications to small animal diagnostics.

Quesenberry K, Moroff S: Plasma protein electrophoresis in psittacine birds. Proc Annu Conf Assoc Avian Vet 112, 1991.
This is an initial report on the application of EPH to avian diagnostics, with an extensive review of chicken and pigeon plasma proteins.

Romagnano A, Wolf C, Schubot S, et al: Maldigestion and hypoproteinemia in palm cockatoo chicks. Proc Annu Conf Assoc Avian Vet 89, 1996.
This article discusses chemistry analyses of malnutrition in young birds, with EPH as an accessory test.

Egg Laying Problems in Caged Birds

Brian L. Speer
Oakley, California

Many cases of advanced, moderate, and early stage oviposition-related disease are encountered in veterinary practice. These problems develop both in companion birds and in those kept for breeding. This article discusses some of the most common of these disorders. Differences between individual pet bird medicine and avicultural medicine are also considered.

EGG BINDING AND DYSTOCIA

Egg binding is defined as the failure of an egg to pass through the oviduct at a normal rate. Binding may or may not be associated with dystocia, which involves the mechanical obstruction of oviposition. Dystocia is a more advanced clinical sign than is egg binding alone and is more likely to require therapeutic intervention.

Reasons for egg binding and dystocia are multifactorial. Causes may include, but are not limited to, oviductal contraction deficits (hypocalcemia, mechanical tears or damage, infections), systemic disease, nutritional imbalances, obesity, inadequate exercise, genetic predisposition, hypothermia, hyperthermia, oviposition in primiparous hens, and breeding stressors. Many of these predisposing factors are difficult to ascertain clearly at the time of diagnosis and treatment.

Clinical signs of egg binding and dystocia vary according to the severity and duration of the incident, the degree of secondary complications, and the size and species of the bird affected. An egg lodged in the pelvic canal may compress the pelvic vessels and kidneys, causing circulatory disorders and shock. The obstruction may cause severe metabolic disturbances related to gastrointestinal ileus and obstructive renal disease. Metabolic derangements progress more quickly in small species such as finches, canaries, budgerigars, lovebirds, and cockatiels. Common clinical signs, particularly in small avian species, include acute onset of depression, tenesmus, abdominal distention, and sudden death. Other signs may include lameness (most frequently of the left leg in larger birds) and bilateral leg paralysis or paresis. Some birds with egg binding or dystocia may have concurrent egg yolk peritonitis.

The diagnosis of egg binding or dystocia is based on the combination of history, clinical signs, physical examination and supportive diagnostic methods, including ultrasonography and radiography. Care should be taken to expedite the physical examination and diagnostic tests to minimize stress that may be detrimental to the patient. Careful abdominal palpation is frequently diagnostic because the egg often is detected as a hard ovoid mass. Soft-shelled eggs, eggs without shells, or eggs in the proximal oviduct may be difficult to palpate and may not be easily identified by radiography. Ultrasonography with a 7.5-MHz

(or greater) sector scanner is a valuable diagnostic tool in these situations.

Calcium malnutrition or aberrant calcium metabolism, or both, are frequent contributors to egg binding and dystocia. High-fat diets, such as a seed-exclusive diet, can exacerbate calcium malnutrition. Some caged bird species (cockatiel or budgerigar) present in fairly advanced stages of calcium metabolic disease in addition to their obstetric crisis and, as a result, are prone to higher mortality.

Treatment is dictated by the severity of the clinical signs and the bird's stability. The primary cause of the egg binding or dystocia should be addressed if possible. Some passerine species and small psittacine species may die during examination or shortly afterward unless careful but aggressive supportive care is delivered.

For minimally depressed birds, fluid therapy is provided (lactated Ringer's solution, 50 to 75 ml/kg per day). The state of the bird's hydration determines the route of administration. Parenteral calcium (5 to 10 mg/kg of calcium glycerophosphate and calcium lactate [Calphosan, Glenwood Pharmaceuticals Inc., Tenafly NJ]), administered subcutaneously or intramuscularly. This therapy combined with heat (approximately 85°F) is usually adequate to address the problem. Most hens in this condition respond favorably within a few hours and pass the egg on their own. Manual "delivery" of the egg can be accomplished with careful side-to-side digital pressure, but care must be taken not to induce additional respiratory difficulty or prolapse the oviduct or cloaca in the process. Isoflurane may be helpful to increase relaxation and decrease pain. If prolapsed tissues are present, they are carefully cleaned and replaced after removal of the egg. Dilute chlorhexidine or Betadine solution has been recommended for cleaning prolapsed cloacal or reproductive tracts. Two vertical sutures may be placed in the cloacal sphincter to prevent further prolapse if indicated. During restraint of the hen, particular care must be taken to monitor stress levels and respiratory quality, and rest periods may be allowed if indicated.

Oxytocin (5 to 10 IU/kg IM, single dose) has traditionally been used in dystocia when no physical obstruction to oviposition is suspected. In some cases, multiple injections are recommended. It is believed that oxytocin exerts its effects on oviductal contractility by stimulating prostaglandin release. Endogenous prostaglandins, which contribute to the contractility of the smooth muscle of the oviduct and vagina, also influence egg transport and expulsion. Prostaglandins have been shown to induce powerful oviductal contractions and help expel retained eggs.

Exogenous prostaglandins should be administered only when there is no significant concern about the possibility of obstruction because oviductal rupture, most frequently at the uterovaginal junction, may be encountered. The relative risk of rupture at the uterovaginal sphincter is believed to be greater with the use of prostaglandin F_2-alpha (Dinoprost tromethamine; Lutalyse, The Upjohn Company, Animal Health Division, Kalamazoo, MI) than with PGE_2 (Prepidil Gel, The Upjohn Company). The recommended dose of prostaglandin E_2 is 0.2 mg/kg applied on the uterovaginal sphincter. This gel can be preserved by freezing it in small aliquots, which makes it economically feasible to keep in stock for cases of egg binding or dystocia. If there are no adhesions or obstructions between the egg and the oviduct, the egg is usually laid within 5 to 10 minutes after prostaglandin E_2 administration.

In more critical cases, in addition to the basic supportive care already mentioned, ovocentesis and implosion of the egg may be a less stressful and safer approach to consider over manual "delivery." Ovocentesis can be accomplished through visualization and access to the egg shell from the cloaca or, most commonly, through transabdominal aspiration with a syringe and needle. Soft-shelled eggs, once their contents have been removed, implode easily, and are much easier for the hen to pass. Normal or hard-shelled eggs may not implode easily and fracture through cloacal access may be required before the egg can be passed. Lacerations of the oviduct by the fractured shell walls seem to be uncommon. In caged birds, surgical removal of a retained egg is most frequently indicated when there are adhesions between oviduct and egg that prohibit oviposition or when the egg is ectopic. At the time the oviduct is entered surgically, care should be taken to seek potential infectious causes. Normograde flushing of the oviduct is recommended before closure.

After removal of the bound egg, appropriate follow-up is indicated. Cloacal prolapse, scarring or damage to the oviduct, and secondary salpingitis can occur, and these complications may be identified early by recurrence of binding or dystocia. Medroxyprogesterone has been recommended in the past to inhibit further ovulation; however, its use is no longer endorsed because of side effects that include obesity, hepatic lipidosis, lethargy, and polyuria and polydipsia. Human chorionic gonadotropin (HCG) (1,000 mg/kg IM, in a single dose or repeated in 3 to 7 days) has been shown to have merit as a means of inhibiting further ovulation in some hens and has no known adverse side effects at present time. Some birds must be repeatedly dosed with HCG, and recommended intervals range, depending on individual clinician's preferences and specifics pertinent to the individual case. Complications that may occur after egg binding may include egg yolk peritonitis, ruptured or traumatized oviducts, cloacal paralysis, ascending infectious salpingitis, and abdominal hernias. These sequelae should be kept in mind after resolution of the binding incident.

Perhaps most importantly, the underlying cause of the incident should be investigated and ultimately eliminated. Nutritional deficits, environmental stressors, and excessive sexual drive issues in pet birds must be discussed with their owners and hopefully eliminated. Pet birds with recurrent histories of egg binding or dystocia may be best served by presenting salpingohysterectomy as a preventive option for further problems. Regardless, unless the underlying cause of the incident is removed, it is entirely likely that egg binding will recur.

EXCESSIVE OR CHRONIC EGG LAYING

Excessive or chronic egg laying occurs when a hen lays eggs in a larger than normal clutch or has repeated clutches regardless of the presence of a suitable mate or appropriate breeding season. Twenty or more eggs have been laid by some cockatiel hens in as short as 1 month's time. Some of the more commonly predisposed pet bird species include the budgerigar, lovebird, and cockatiel. It is theorized that imprinting on humans or possibly even a genetic lack of hormonal balance in controlling egg laying may be involved as predisposing factors.

Careful and detailed education of the pet bird owner is important in preventing complications due to chronic or excessive egg laying. The key to success in chronic egg laying problems is preventive education and early owner recognition, rather than treatment of advanced secondary problems and nutritional depletion, conditions that carry a more guarded prognosis.

If excessive egg laying is not addressed, a depletion of the hen's body stores occurs, ultimately predisposing the bird to egg binding, osteoporosis, and malnutrition. Weight loss, muscle weakness, pathologic fractures of long bones, and calcium metabolic disturbances are all seen. Preventive management includes behavioral modification techniques as well as medical and surgical options.

The dietary plan of the hen should be improved to decrease the severity of the nutritional and metabolic drain. Overall, a more appropriate balance of protein, carbohydrates, fat, vitamins, and minerals should be recommended (pellets, cooked beans, dark leafy greens). When there may be actual clinical signs of malnutrition, nutritional or vitamin and mineral supplementation should be considered. This may include parenteral administration as well as oral supplementation. Eggs should not be removed from the hen's laying site, as this is a stimulus to lay more eggs. The presence of a "nest" is a powerful reproductive trigger in many species. Therefore, it is prudent to remove any designated nesting sites that the hen prefers. On a similar note, the owner should remove toys or other cage items toward which the bird has a sexual affinity. It may be appropriate to consider changing cages and location in the home to a different or "new" environment. Photoperiod manipulation may prove to be of benefit in some of these birds, and there has been a standard recommendation to decrease the photoperiod of the hen to a maximum of 8 to 10 hours per day. Clinical benefit from this approach is poor in many cases.

Leuprolide acetate (Lupron, TAP Pharmaceuticals, Deerfield, IL; 52 or 156 μg/kg per day—dosed in a single intermuscular injection calculated for a 28-day slow release) may be used to prevent egg laying reversibly in cockatiels. HCG has been used to inhibit ovarian activity and has shown favorable results with no obvious adverse effects.

Salpingohysterectomy may provide a definitive solution to the problem of overproduction of eggs in a companion bird kept with no breeding intent. This option is viewed as the definitive treatment for chronic egg laying hens, although it is not generally recommended as a preventive measure in healthy hens.

AVICULTURAL OR FLOCK MEDICINE

The entire aviary is the defined patient in flock medicine. This "patient" differs dramatically from the single bird encountered in companion bird medicine. The building, cages, breeding management, and production records all can play significant roles in veterinary detection of early reproductive disease. Reproductive "disease" in the flock is defined not only as the types of clinical disease processes mentioned earlier in this article but also as subclinical disease and management flaws that are capable of resulting in suboptimal production performance. In avicultural medicine, the attending veterinarian's role is to provide professional input to assist the aviculturist in attaining desired production goals.

Suboptimal breeding performance is best detected initially by regular record review of the collection. It is the records that are kept at a facility that allow an independent veterinary analysis of production and efficiency. Mortality rates, patterns of disease, or production deficits can be identified through careful review of the data collected in all areas of the facility.

Annual reminders for record review and analysis should become a routine part of the private practice setting in the same manner that reminders for annual examinations are sent for pet birds. Clients who identify themselves as aviculturists or designate specific birds or pairs for breeding intent should have an additional file initiated—the *flock file*. This file is where patterns of infectious disease are summarized, reminders for review or medical action are maintained, and production goals for the client are recorded and maintained. Practitioners should keep sample record systems for aviculturists to maintain about breeder production, pediatrics, and incubation.

Production goals of the aviculturist must be stated clearly. Often, these goals are poorly clarified by the aviculturist and poorly understood by the attending veterinarian. Veterinarians should ask their clients key questions about their goals to avoid the "trap" of assuming what the client wants and failing to meet their expectations and goals. Why do they keep these birds? What do they want to accomplish with this collection? Over what time frame is this collection to achieve their goal? Do they need a specific income per annum from the sale of chicks? What are key overhead expenses?

Veterinary analysis of production records is best done away from the aviary and flock. The primary intent of this analysis is to determine if there is an indication to investigate production deficit trends. Deficits in production are best identified in the absence of distracters such as the birds, their owners, or the facility. After overall aviary production statistics have been calculated, activities of individual breeding pairs, species, or birds should be similarly analyzed by the attending veterinarian.

The economic efficiency of the breeding population can be calculated based on sale values for the species and chicks produced per total pairs in the population. Key overhead expenses can be subtracted from this figure to approximate the profitability of the facility. Awareness of these issues allows the veterinarian to be more sensitive to the economics of operating the facility and, as a result, guarantee that they do no economic harm. A large veterinary expense, without compensatory income in chick sales, can be prohibitory to maintaining a successful flock health relationship.

References and Suggested Reading

Bennett RA, Harrison GJ: Soft tissue surgery. In: Ritchie BW, Harrison GJ, Harrison LR, eds: Avian Medicine: Principles and Application. Lake Worth, FL: Wingers Publishing, 1994, pp 1096–1136.

Echols MS, Speer BL: A comprehensive approach for the management of flock reproductive performance. Semin Avian Exotic Pet Med, 1996.

Farner DS, Wingfield JC: Reproductive endocrinology in birds. Annu Rev Physiol 42:457, 1980.

Harrison GJ: Reproductive medicine. In: Harrison GJ, Harrison LR, eds: Clinical Avian Medicine and Surgery. Philadelphia: WB Saunders, 1986.

Harrison GJ: Progesterone implants in cases of chronic egg laying. Proc Assoc Avian Vet, 1989, pp 6–10.

Hasholt J: Disease of the female reproductive organs of pet birds. J Small Anim Pract 32:313, 1966.

Hicks KD: Ratite Reproduction. Proc Assoc Avian Vet, 1992, pp 318–325.

Hochleithner M: Biochemistries. In: Ritchie BW, Harrison GJ, Harrison LR, eds: Avian Medicine: Principles and Application. Lake Worth, FL: Wingers Publishing, 1994, pp 223–245.

Hudelson S, Hudelson P: Egg binding, hormonal control and therapeutic considerations. Compend Contin Educ 15:427, 1993.

Hudelson KS, Hudelson MA: A brief review of the female avian reproductive cycle with special emphasis on the role of prostaglandins and clinical applications. J Avian Med Surg 10:67, 1996.

Jochim L, Millam JR: Behavior of orange-winged amazon parrots before and after nest box presentation. Proc Assoc Avian Vet, 1994, p 435.

Johnson AL: Reproduction in the female. In: Sturkie PD, ed: Avian Physiology. New York: Springer-Verlag, 1986, pp 403–431.

Joyner KL: Theriogenology. In: Ritchie BW, Harrison GJ, Harrison LR, eds: Avian Medicine: Principles and Application. Lake Worth, FL: Wingers Publishing, 1994, pp 748–804.

Kenton B, Milam JR: Photostimulation and serum steroids of orange-winged Amazon parrots. Proc Assoc Avian Vet, 1994, p 437.

Keymer IF: Disorders of the avian female reproductive system. Avian Pathol 9:405, 1980.

Lowenstine LJ: Avian anatomy and its relation to disease processes. Proc Assoc Avian Vet, 1983, pp 1–9.

Millam JR: Environmental enrichment stimulates egg laying in native orange-winged Amazon parrots. Proc Assoc Avian Vet, 1994, p 436.

Millam JR, Finney H: Leuprolide acetate can reversibly prevent egg laying in cockatiels. Proc Assoc Avian Vet, 1993, p 46.

Olsen JH: Anseriformes. In: Ritchie BW, Harrison GJ, Harrison LR, eds: Avian Medicine: Principles and Application. Lake Worth, FL: Wingers Publishing, 1994, pp 1237–1275.

Reece RL: Reproductive diseases. In: Burr E, ed: Companion Bird Medicine. Ames, IA: Iowa State University Press, 1987, pp 89–100.

Ritchie BW, Harrison GJ: Formulary. In: Ritchie BW, Harrison GJ, Harrison, LR eds: Avian Medicine: Principles and Application. Lake Worth, FL: Wingers Publishing, 1994, pp 457–478.

Rosskopf WJ, Woerpel RW: Egg binding in cage and aviary birds. Mod Vet Pract 65:437, 1985.

Rosskopf WJ, Woerpel RW: Pet Avian Obstetrics. Proceedings of the First International Conference of Zoology and Avian Medicine, 1987, pp 213–231.

Rzasa J: The Effect of arginine vasotocin on prostaglandin in production of the hen uterus. Gen Comp Endocrinol 53:260, 1984.

Sharma DN, Singh CM: Studies on pathology of the female genital tract of poultry with special reference to egg peritonitis incidence, pathoanatomy and experimental study. Indian J Poult Sci 8:81, 1973.

Shimada K, Asai I: Effects of prostaglandin E_2 alpha and indomethacin on uterine contraction in hens. Biol Reprod 21:523, 1979.

Singh MP: Studies on the incidence of egg peritonitis, salpingitis and oophoritis in laying hens. Indian J Vet Med 1:38, 1977.

Speer BL: Avicultural medical management: An introduction to basic principles of flock medicine and the closed aviary concept. Vet Clin North Am Small Anim Pract 21:1393, 1991a.

Speer BL: A Clinical Approach to Psittacine Infertility. Proceedings of the Association of Avian Veterinarians, Chicago, 1991b, pp 173–187.

Speer BL, Abramson J: Management and Maintenance of a Macaw Breeding Facility. Proceedings of the Association of Avian Veterinarians, 1992, pp AM2-1–AM2-17.

Stewart JS: Ratites. In: Ritchie BW, Harrison GJ, Harrison LR, eds: Avian Medicine: Principles and Application. Lake Worth, FL: Wingers Publishing, pp 1284–1326.

Zoonotic Diseases of Pet Birds

PATRICK J. MORRIS
San Diego, California

INTRODUCTION

In the modern world, zoonotic diseases are increasingly being recognized as significant threats to human health. While many factors have been associated with this trend (Morse, 1995), the author believes that the following four are especially noteworthy causes of the increased zoonotic potential of avian species:

- Modern transportation technology, which has removed geographic barriers that once separated novel hosts (humans) from animals and their pathogens.
- Immunodeficiency states, which have increased human susceptibility to, and the severity of, infectious diseases. These conditions include acquired immunodeficiency syndrome (AIDS), due primarily to human immunodeficiency virus (HIV) infection; ionizing radiation and immunosuppressive therapy used to treat cancer and organ transplant patients; and the effects of certain pollutants on the immune system.
- Poor preventive medicine practices among some of those who come into contact with animals.
- Increasing associations between humans and animals, and among animals from different geographic areas (nontraditional agriculture, owner-pet relationships, conservation-rehabilitation efforts).

Birds represent one of the most diverse groups of vertebrates kept as pets. Dealing with this tremendous diversity is part of the significant challenge of avian medicine, as more and more birds become the focus of interaction with humans. Many view the veterinarian as a key authority on the health risks associated the human-avian relationship (pet owners—those with and without birds—farmers, conservation project employees, veterinary support staff, and physicians). It is especially important for veterinarians engaged in the practice of avian medicine to have ready access to information on zoonoses.

One consistent feature of a review of this type involves potential zoonoses versus documented zoonoses (Ritchie and Dreesen, 1988; Carpenter and Gentz, 1997). Diseases like psittacosis and salmonellosis can be traced directly to avian hosts. However, other diseases remain listed as potential zoonoses. As our technology grows, and our ability to clearly identify pathogens increases, it is logical to assume that some of the pathogens listed as potential human zoonoses will become documented human zoonoses. The following two examples demonstrate this trend. In the first example, a bird fancier was plagued with chronic keratoconjunctivitis. The lesion had been treated without success, and when treatment failed, conjunctival bacterial and chlamydial cultures failed to reveal the etiology. Ultimately, polymerase chain reaction (PCR) and immunofluorescent technologies identified the causative agent as chlamydial, most likely *Chlamydia psittaci*. Treatment with doxycycline resolved the condition. Recently, human mycobacteriosis has been described due to *Mycobacterium genavense* in AIDS patients. *Mycobacterium genavense* has also recently been reported in canaries (Ramis et al, 1996) and other birds (Hoop et al, 1995) with mycobacterial disease (see p. 1116). In one study, *M. genavense* was the major mycobacterial pathogen isolated (34 of 204 birds necropsied), followed by *M. avium* (8 of 204) (Hoop et al, 1995). Although the relationship, if any, between birds, humans, and *M. genavense* infection remains to be documented, this information cannot be found in any of the existing references on general avian medicine. These two examples demonstrate the dynamics of zoonotic disease investigation, and why supplemental sources should be used when one investigates the zoonotic potential of avian pathogens.

There are two recent reviews in the avian medical literature relating to avian zoonoses in general (Ritchie and Dreesen, 1988; Carpenter and Gentz, 1997), and chlamydiosis specifically (Vanrompay et al, 1995). In both of the general references, the authors have attempted to categorize each avian pathogen in terms of significance to the pet owner. Another major reference on diseases common to humans and animals that should be part of the practitioner's review of zoonotic diseases is the one by Beran (1994). Guidelines have also been developed to help veterinarians better understand their role in dealing with human immunodeficiencies and animal diseases (Gill and Stone, 1992). Although these guidelines were written with cat owners in mind, the general principles apply to avian species as well. Together, these references should be used by the clinician as a starting point for any in-depth review of avian zoonoses, rather than the final word. The last step involves updating one's understanding of avian zoonotic diseases. One significant development in the field of informatics has been the World Wide Web. With this resource, clinicians can quickly locate the most recent information on zoonotic diseases. Table 1 lists readily accessible web sites pertaining to zoonotic diseases.

TABLE 1. World Wide Web Information Sites

Home Page Name/URL	Comment
Centers for Disease Control and Prevention Home Page (CDC) http://www.cdc.gov/	Main page for CDC, Atlanta, GA USA. Contains general information about human health hazards, links to related sites.
Morbidity/Mortality Weekly Report (CDC) http://www.cdc.gov/mmwr/mmwr.html	On-line downloads of MMWR/EID journal articles.
Emerging Infectious Diseases (CDC) http://www.cdc.gov/ncidod/EID/eid.htm	
Emerging/Reemerging Infections—EIIN Network http://info.med.yale.edu/EIINet/infections.html	Network dedicated to providing researchers, interested professionals, public information about emerging infectious diseases.
The World-Wide Web Virtual Library: Veterinary Medicine http://netvet.wustl.edu/Vetmed.htm	General veterinary information geared toward a veterinary audience. Links to related sites.
National Foundation for Infectious Diseases http://www.medscape.com/Affiliates/NFID/	Bibliographic information, links to related sites.
Zoonosis References http://med-med1.bu.edu/dshapiro/zooref.htm	Bibliographic information, links to related sites.
Association of Avian Veterinarians http://www.upatsix.com/aav/	International veterinary organization dedicated to the advancement of avian medicine and surgery. Links to related sites.
U.S. Dept. of Labor, Occupational Health and Safety Administration (OSHA) http://www.osha-scl.gov/	National administrative organization responsible for enforcing job safety standards. Federal code of regulations

TABLE 2. Significant Zoonoses of Pet Birds

Disease	Species of Concern	Signs in Birds	Signs in Humans	Comment
Allergic alveolitis	All species, most reports in budgies, pigeons	Not applicable	R, Vr, F, M	Allergic reaction to birds. Also called bronchiolitis, hypersensitivity pneumonitis, allergic interstitial pneumonitis, pigeon lung disease, parakeet dander pneumoconiosis. Type IV cell-mediated immune reaction typified by IgG and IgA, rather than IgE. Skin test often useful for diagnosis. Acute, subacute, chronic forms documented. Easily overlooked as common, nonzoonotic human respiratory illness. Chronic form is irreversible, often leading to fibrosis. Life-long prevention of exposure to antigen is necessary in these cases. Chronic form is most commonly associated with pet birds.
Campylobacteriosis	Wild birds, passerines, especially poultry	**S**, D, L, Dh	Ap, D, V, F, M, L,	Epizootiology can be complicated. Multiple sources of organisms, including eggs and meat. Wild birds are significant sources of organisms. Sometimes difficult diagnosis in humans, requiring special stains, serologic methods, advanced diagnostic techniques.
Mycobacteriosis	All species, canaries, psittacines, columbiformes	**W**, L, D, R, S, G	**W**, R, Ln, Vr	Sources of mycobacteria infecting humans is not fully documented, although the body of knowledge is rapidly advancing. Treatment often successful, immunodeficiency is a key risk factor for human disease.
Newcastle viral conjunctivitis	Psittacines, ostrich, pigeons, domestic poultry, many other species	Cn, C, U, W, L	C, F, H, M, Cn, Vr	Reportable disease (USDA only). Virus is fairly resistant to sunlight and pH changes. Only 37 cases of human infection were reported over a 28-year period. Live NDV vaccines are a zoonotic source for humans.
Psittacosis	Psittacines, columbiformes especially	R, D, G, C, U, L, W, Cn	F, M, H, L, V, V, R, A	Reportable human zoonosis in 47 of 50 states. Aerosol and fecal-oral transmission most common routes of transmission. Often difficult diagnosis frequently requiring novel diagnostic techniques (e.g., PCR) to document etiology. Chlortetracycline, oxytetracycline, doxycycline, fluoroquinolones most frequently employed in therapy.
Salmonellosis	Very wide species range	**S**, D, W, L, Vr	**G, D, L, Dh,** F, V, M, H, Vr	Frequently source does not appear ill. *S. enteritidis* phage type IV is reportable (USDA). Multitude of sources often cloud epidemiology. More than 2,000 serotypes known. Most infections in humans can be traced to food or water sources.
Yersiniosis	Mainly passerines, especially canaries; turkeys also	L, D, R, Cn	Ln, Ap	Wild birds are significant source of organism. Acute appendicitis is the most common form in humans, while diarrhea is rare. Variable signs in humans from chronic disease.

Key to disease signs: A, arthropathy, polyarthritis; Ap, abdominal pain; C, conjunctivitis; Cn, CNS signs; Ln, lymphadenopathy; M, myalgia; P, pleuritis; R, respiratory tract disease; D, diarrhea; Dh, dehydration; F, fever, chills, G, gastrointestinal disease; H, headache; L, lethargy/debility; S, subclinical; U, upper respiratory signs; V, vomiting; Vr, variable signs or multiple organ involvement; W, weight loss. **Bold** indicates primary sign, or otherwise of special significance.

1115

SIGNIFICANT ZOONOSES OF AVIAN SPECIES

It is important for a veterinarian to understand that different human-animal relationships will change the significance of zoonotic diseases. Even though psittacosis is considered the most significant zoonotic disease of birds (Ritchie and Dreesen, 1988; Carpenter and Gentz, 1997), it may not always be the most important disease of concern when one advises a client. Additionally, a zoonosis of significance in one country may not be of the same importance in another. This suggests that clinicians should regionalize their knowledge for the benefit of the communities they serve. In addition, it is important for the veterinarian to remember that today more avian patients fall into categories other than that of the traditional pet (e.g., zoologic parks, rehabilitation centers). In these cases, the veterinarian must recognize that there are significant differences in the zoonoses of concern (Beran, 1994).

It is also important to recognize that some zoonoses indirectly involve birds as reservoirs or hosts or in other contributing ways (trematodiasis, encephalitides, influenza A, systemic mycoses). Zoonoses result from avian meat products from commercial poultry and exotic meat producers (toxoplasmosis, bacterial toxicoses, cestodiasis, and others). Still other pathogens await identification as bona fide human pathogens (especially cryptosporidiosis). Finally, birds can act as vectors for zoonotic diseases (Lyme borrelliosis, salmonellosis, shigellosis). Within the scope of a normal human-pet relationship, the pet bird should not be considered as a significant source for these latter zoono-ses. In reality, the greatest zoonotic exposure potential from pets resides in the veterinary hospital, especially in the necropsy room. Table 2 lists avian pathogens that are currently considered to be of significance to the pet owner (Ritchie and Dreesen, 1988; Carpenter and Gentz, 1997).

References and Suggested Reading

Beran GW, ed: CRC Series Handbook of Zoonoses. Boca Raton: CRC Press, 1994.

Carpenter JW, Gentz EJ: Zoonotic diseases of avian origin. In: Altman RB, Clubb SL, Dorrestein GM, et al, eds: Avian Medicine and Surgery. Philadelphia: WB Saunders, 1997, p 350.

Dean D, Shama A, Schachter J, et al: Molecular identification of an avian strain of *Chlamydia psittaci* causing severe keratoconjunctivitis in a bird fancier. Clin Infect Dis 20:1179, 1995.

Gill DM, Stone DM: Special Commentary: The veterinarian's role in the AIDS crisis. J Am Vet Med Assoc 201:1683, 1992.

Hoop RK, Bottger EC, Pfyffer GE: Etiological agents of mycobacterioses in pet birds between 1986 and 1995. J Clin Microbiol 34:991, 1996.

Morse SS: Perspectives: Factors in the emergence of infectious diseases. Emerging Infect Dis 1:7, 1995.

Ramis A, Ferrer L, Aranaz A, et al: *Mycobacterium genavense* infection in canaries. Avian Dis 40:246, 1996.

Ritchie BW, Dreesen DW: Avian Zoonoses: Proven and potential diseases part II. Viral, fungal, and miscellaneous diseases. Compend Contin Educ Pract Vet 10:688, 1988.

Ritchie BW, Dreesen DW: Avian Zoonoses: Proven and potential diseases part I. Bacterial and parasitic diseases. Compend Contin Educ Pract Vet 10:484, 1988.

Tortoli E, Simoneti MT, Dionisio D, et al: Cultural studies on two isolates of *Mycobacterium genavense* from patients with acquired immunodeficiency syndrome. Diagn Microbiol Infect Dis 18:7, 1994.

Vanrompay D, Ducatelle R, Haesebrouck F: *Chlamydia psittaci* infections: a review with emphasis on avian chlamydiosis. Vet Microbiol 45:93, 1995.

Avian Mycobacteriosis

DAVID N. PHALEN
College Station, Texas

Mycobacterial infections occur sporadically in a wide range of wild, domestic, and captive birds. Epizootic diseases may occur in collections of captive waterfowl, zoo birds, gray-cheeked (*Brotogeris pyrrhopterus*) and canary-winged parakeets (*B. versicolorus*), certain species of tropical doves, and Australian finches. *Mycobacterium avium* (MA), serotypes 1, 2, 3, and 8, *Mycobacterium genavense* (MGE), and *Mycobacterium tuberculosis* (MTB) are most common causes of mycobacteriosis in birds.

EPIZOOTIOLOGY AND PATHOGENESIS

Ingestion of MA and MGE is the primary route of infection in birds. Birds contract MTB directly from humans by inhalation of aerosolized bacteria. MA appears to be ubiquitous in the environment, yet only certain species and individuals within species appear susceptible to these low concentrations. In closely confined populations, the grounds may become heavily contaminated, resulting in high infection rates. Iatrogenic transmission has also occurred with contaminated tattoo ink and inadequately disinfected surgical sexing instruments.

On rare occasions, mycobacterial infections are focal, causing isolated lesions on the face, skin, or leg. In most cases, the disease is generalized. After ingestion, MA and MGE are believed to colonize the intestinal tract. Histologically, histocytes containing acid-fast organisms are found in the lamina propria of the intestinal villa. The extent of these lesions can vary from scattered foci to diffuse lesions in which the villi are massively distended with sheets of histiocytes. When lesions are extensive, the intestines are grossly thickened. From the lamina propria, the bacteria are believed to disseminate via macrophages to other organs. Mycobacterial organisms and associated lesions have been identified in nearly every tissue, but the liver, spleen, lung, air sac, skin, and bone marrow are most commonly involved. Clinical signs depend on the affected organ systems and the severity of the disease within the organ system.

Grossly, mycobacterial granulomas are of variable size, yellow to gray tan, soft nodules. They may be singular, widely scattered, or coalescing. When organs are diffusely infiltrated with histiocytes, especially the liver, generalized enlargement or a diffuse change in color may be the only indication that the organ is affected. Amyloidosis of the kidney and liver is a common complication of MA infections and may contribute to the clinical signs. Histologically, mycobacterial infections exhibit two primary forms but may contain elements of both. In the first, classic tubercles form that contain a central necrotic area surrounded by macrophages, multinucleated giant cells, histiocytes, and plasma cells. Bacteria may be scarce in these lesions. At the other extreme, lesions are composed of extensive sheets of histiocytes. In these lesions, bacteria are generally abundant. The specific organism, the species of the host infected, the host's immune response, and the stage of infection all contribute to the nature of the lesion (Montali et al, 1976).

HISTORICAL AND PHYSICAL FINDINGS

The clinical picture caused by mycobacterial infections is extremely diverse. Most commonly, however, birds present with a chronic, slowly progressive disease. Owners may report gradual weight loss, reduced vocalization, inappetence, weakness, lethargy, and feather ruffling. Birds may show decreased exercise tolerance or overt dyspnea. When musculoskeletal lesions of the leg are present, birds may be lame. Infrequently, cutaneous masses are the first noticeable sign of disease. Poor-quality feathering, an abnormal molt, polyuria, and diarrhea may all be presenting complaints. Mycobacteriosis should always be suspected in birds that have proved highly susceptible to infection, in birds originating from flocks in which mycobacterial infections have been previously identified, and in birds that fail to respond adequately to routine antibiotic therapy. Mycobacteriosis occurs predominantly in birds 2 to 5 years of age but can occur at any age.

On physical examination, some degree of weight loss and pectoral muscle atrophy is generally expected. Feather quality may be poor. Cutaneous masses may occur around the head and neck and on the body and legs. Lesions may also involve the joints. Periocular swelling, buphthalmia, upper respiratory signs, and oral masses are all suggestive of mycobacterial granulomas. Lesions of the skin and head are especially common with MTB infections. Abdominal distention, caused by organ enlargement, celomic granulomas, or perihepatic effusion may also be evident. Lower airway sounds may reflect pulmonary and air sac disease. Soiling of the tail feathers is indicative of diarrhea.

DIAGNOSIS

Historical and physical findings are rarely specific for mycobacteriosis, and these diseases must be differentiated from other chronic granulomatous diseases such as psittacosis and aspergillosis, as well as neoplasia, visceral gout, and internal parasites. A minimal database for birds presenting with these signs includes a complete blood count, chemistry profile (uric acid, aspartate aminotransferase, creatinine kinase, albumin, and gamma globulin levels), parasitologic examination of the feces, fecal Gram and acid-fast stains, and radiographs. Assessable masses should be aspirated or biopsied.

Significant changes in the hemogram are common but not universal. Leukocyte counts ranging from 20,000 cells/μl to as high as 200,000 cells/μl with heterophilia, left shift, and heterophils evidencing toxic changes have been reported. A monocytosis ($\geq 1,500$ cells/μl) is also common. Anemia is variably present. Serum chemistry changes are generally nonspecific and include elevations in the aspartate aminotransferase and often the creatinine kinase levels. In some stages of the disease, there may be hypoalbuminemia and significant elevation in the globulin fraction. Changes in the serum electrophoretogram may also be suggestive of a mycobacterial infection.

Radiographically, hepatomegaly and splenomegaly are common but nonspecific findings. Thickening of the small intestines is not commonly seen but is a significant finding if present. One or more soft tissue masses in the air sacs or lungs are suggestive of mycobacterial granulomas. Intramedullary lesions of the long bones occur infrequently but are highly suggestive of mycobacterial infections. These lesions are characterized by an increase in the soft tissue density of the medullary canal that is interrupted by circular lucent areas. Soft tissue masses may be identified in the skull. Ultrasonography may be used to define celomic masses, evaluate intestinal thickening, and differentiate among causes of widened liver shadows.

Fecal stains for acid-fast organisms are not sensitive tests, but the presence of acid-fast organisms in clusters in several areas of the slide is diagnostic. Aspirates or biopsy specimens of cutaneous or oral lesions are generally more definitive; however, in some infections, organisms are few and they may be missed. Bone marrow aspirates, either from the ulna or the tibia, provide an easy but only intermediately sensitive assay. Endoscopy with biopsy of the liver, spleen, or celomic masses, or aspiration of thickened intestinal loops is most likely to result in a diagnosis.

Intradermal skin testing has been useful in poultry but is unsatisfactory in most other species. Serologic examination has been used in selected cases as an early indicator of mycobacterial infection. A complement fixation assay has been developed for general use (Phalen et al, 1995). Preliminary evidence suggests that the presence of antibody is specific for infection; however, a negative antibody response has no predictive value (Phalen et al, 1995).

Polymerase chain reaction (PCR) technology appears to have considerable potential in the diagnosis of mycobacterial disease. PCR primers have been developed that can detect all the mycobacterial organisms known to infect birds. These assays are extremely sensitive and would be expected to detect even low concentrations of organisms in feces and biopsy specimens. Humans with MA infections are generally bacteremic. If the same is true for birds with MA or MGE infections, PCR of processed blood samples may prove a powerful diagnostic tool.

Culturing the organism is a complex and often unrewarding process. Mycobacteria are grown on special media and take weeks to months to be identified. Complicating

TABLE 1. Treatment Protocols for *Mycobacterium avium* Infections in Cage Birds

Drugs*	I	II	III	IV
Protocol 1†	Ciprofloxacin 20 mg/kg PO q12 hr *or* enrofloxacin 15 mg/kg PO or IM‡ q12hr for 10 days	Clofazimine 1.5 mg/kg PO q24hr	Cycloserine 5 mg/kg PO q12hr	Ethambutol 20 mg/kg PO q12hr
Protocol 2§	Clofazimine 6 mg/kg PO q24hr	Ethambutol 30 mg/kg PO q24hr	Rifampin 45 mg/kg PO q24hr	
Protocol 3§	Ciprofloxacin 80 mg/kg PO q24 hr *or* enrofloxacin 30 mg/kg PO q24hr	Ethambutol 30 mg/kg PO q24hr	Rifampin 45 mg/kg PO q24hr *or* rifabutin 15 mg/kg PO q24hr	

*All treatments are for a minimum of 6 months unless otherwise noted.
†Data from Rosskopf WJ, Woepel RW: Successful treatment of avian tuberculosis in pet psittacines. Proceedings of the Association of Avian Veterinarians, Chicago, IL, 1991.
‡Repeated intramuscular injections lead to muscle necrosis.
§Data from van Der Heyden N: Update on avian mycobacteriosis. Proceedings of the Association of Avian Veterinarians, Nashville, TN, 1994.

the issue further, many mycobacteria cannot be routinely isolated by standard methods.

ZOONOTIC IMPLICATIONS

MTB, MGE, and the MA serotypes infecting birds are all potential human pathogens. MTB is of greatest concern, as the bird probably contracted this organism from one of its owners and MTB readily infects healthy humans. MA infections are common in patients with acquired immunodeficiency syndrome and are generally a complication of the advanced and near-terminal stages of this disease (Masur, 1993). Children may also be at increased risk for MA infections. The source of MA for humans has not been conclusively defined but probably represents low-level environmental exposure and not direct bird-to-human transmission. MGE, like MA, is a disease of the immunosuppressed, although it is far less common than MA in humans. Both MA and MGE infections in pet birds appear to pose little risk to the healthy general population. However, when a mycobacterial infection is diagnosed in a pet bird, the owners should be warned of the potential zoonotic nature of the disease and should be asked to consult with a physician before a decision is made for treatment or euthanasia of the pet bird. It should also be emphasized to the owner that infected birds pose a significant risk to other birds in the home. The author *does not recommend* treating birds with MTB.

TREATMENT

Controlled clinical trials optimizing treatment protocols for mycobacterial infections in birds have not been performed. Case reports, however, suggest that treatment can be successful in many cases. Successful treatment of any mycobacterial infection requires a combination drug therapy to prevent the development of resistance, prolonged therapy (6 to 12 months), and an adequate immune response from the host. Originally, most protocols were modeled after the treatment protocols used for MTB infections in humans and combined treatment with ethambutol (Myambutol, Lederle, Wayne, NJ), rifampin (Rifadin, Hoechst-Marion Roussel, Kansas City, MO), and isoniazid (Dura-med Pharmaceuticals, Cincinnati, OH) was used. Even though MA is resistant to isoniazid and has variable resistance to ethambutol and rifampin, these protocols were often effective. Combination treatment protocols using ciprofloxacin (Cipro, Bayer, West Haven, CT), enrofloxacin (Baytril, Bayer, Shawnee Mission, KS), clofazimine (Lamprene, Novartis, Summit, NJ), ethambutol, rifampin, and rifabutin (Mycobutin, Pharmacia & Upjohn, Columbus, OH) are shown in Table 1. These protocols have had limited use; therefore, treated birds must be monitored carefully and adjustments made in the regimens as needed. Clarithromycin (Biaxin, Abbott, North Chicago, IL) is used routinely in combination with other drugs for MA infections in humans. There is no information on the efficacy or dosage of this drug in birds. Even with treatment, bacterial shedding may persist for some time. Additionally, a cure can never be guaranteed, even with the resolution of clinical signs and extended treatment.

Environmental contamination poses a major problem for the reintroduction of animals into a facility where *Mycobacterium*-infected birds have previously been held. Extensive cleaning of indoor facilities and cages and disinfection with inorganic chlorine solutions may be effective. It is questionable if pastures and outdoor enclosures with dirt floors can ever be properly sanitized.

References and Suggested Reading

Masur H: Recommendations on prophylaxis and therapy for disseminated *Mycobacterium avium* complex disease in patients infected with the human immunodeficiency virus. N Engl J Med 329:898, 1993.
This article summarizes the role MA plays in acquired immunodeficiency syndrome and discusses current therapies.

Montali RJ, Bush M, Thoen CO, et al: Tuberculosis in captive exotic birds. J Am Vet Med Assoc 169:920, 1976.
This article provides a detailed look at the clinical and pathologic presentation of mycobacterial infections in zoo birds.

Phalen DN, Grimes JE, Phalen SW, et al: Serologic diagnosis of mycobacterial infections in birds (a preliminary report). Proceedings of the Association of Avian Veterinarians, Philadelphia, PA, 1995, p 67.
The complex nature of the host immune response in mycobacterial infections is discussed.

Rosskopf WJ, Woerpel RW: Successful treatment of avian tuberculosis in pet psittacines. Proceedings of the Association of Avian Veterinarians, Chicago, IL, 1991, p 238.
This article describes mycobacteriosis in pet birds and details various treatment protocols.

Van Der Heyden N: Update on avian mycobacteriosis. Proceedings of the Association of Avian Veterinarians, Nashville, TN, 1994, p 53.
This article summarizes the disease presentation and reviews current therapeutic regimens.

Diagnosis and Treatment of Common Diseases of Finches

LANI A. STEINOHRT
Columbus, Ohio

Finches (order Passeriformes) are popular and relatively hardy birds. The main families kept for breeding and as pets include the Fingillidae (European goldfinch, greenfinch, chaffinches, and bramblings) and, most important, the Estrildidae, which includes the Australian finches (i.e., Zebra and Lady Gouldian), African finches (i.e., Cordon Bleu, St. Helena, and orange-cheeked waxbills), and the Bengalese (Society) finches.

ANATOMY AND PHYSIOLOGY

The right and left paranasal sinuses do not communicate. Separate samples should be taken if bilateral nasal discharge is present. The highly efficient lungs of Passeriforme species result in an increased susceptibility to airborne toxins. The basal metabolic rate of passerine birds is approximately 65% greater than that of nonpasserines. In general, most small finches may drink from 250 to 300 ml/kg per day of water. Zebra finches, however, have been known to survive months without drinking any water. This results in erratic blood levels in finches when drugs are administered in drinking water.

HOUSING

Finches may be kept as individual pets or as flocks in aviaries. Depending on the climate, many finches may be maintained in outdoor aviaries. Indoor, temperature-controlled rooms work well in harsher climates. Plenty of space should be provided: multiple, clean, nontoxic perches of varying diameters should be long enough to provide a minimum of 4 inches per bird. Perches should be placed to prevent fecal contamination of food, water dishes, or cage mates. Corn cob, pine, cedar, or walnut shells should be avoided as substrates. Noncolored newspaper, brown paper, and paper towels are ideal. Concrete, gravel, or grass is recommended for outdoor aviaries.

DIET AND HUSBANDRY

Diet requirements for finches are diverse. Most are granivorous or seed eating. Some, however, are insectivorous, omnivorous, carnivorous, nectivorous, or fructivorous. Finches may consume up to 30% of their body weight daily in food: therefore, overdosage of vitamins and minerals may occur if diets other than those specifically formulated for finches are used. Granivorous finches should eat three parts of a good seed mixture to one part of a "soft food" (Protein 25, Higgens Group Corp., Miami, FL). Many species readily adapt to commercially available pel-leted diets (Pretty Bird, Stacy, MN). Fresh fruits and vegetables chopped into fine pieces should be offered but removed before they spoil.

Birds with health problems or poor diets may consume excessive grit and acquire gastrointestinal obstruction; therefore, spontaneous feeding of insoluble grit should be avoided. Providing small amounts of soluble grit such as oyster shell or cuttle bone provides a rich mineral source (Taylor, 1996) and is not associated with obstructions.

PHYSICAL EXAMINATION

The small size of finches can limit diagnostic and treatment options. Veterinary care is often directed toward appropriate preventive husbandry measures and approaching medical problems from a flock perspective. A diagnostic necropsy is often necessary to prevent further losses. A thorough history is essential.

The client should be encouraged to transport the bird in its own uncleaned cage. Special attention should be directed to the droppings, feed and water dishes, cage floor, and substrate. During this time, the bird's activity level, balance, and breathing should be noted.

Before performing the physical examination, all necessary supplies should be placed within reach. A strong light source and magnification device facilitates the examination. In the critically ill bird, the physical examination and diagnostic tests must be done in steps. A "lights out" and "perches out" approach aids in capture. One should ensure that windows and doors are closed. Once captured, the bird can be gently restrained by placing the head between the index and middle fingers with the bill pointing away from the palm. The body should rest in the palm of the hand. Care must be used not to put pressure on the sternum. If the bird becomes stressed or weak, it should be placed in its cage immediately to recover. Physical examination is performed as with other birds (see "References and Suggested Reading").

DIAGNOSTIC PROCEDURES

A complete fecal examination, including flotation, direct wet preparation and Gram stain, should be performed. Finches normally do not have large numbers of resident gut or respiratory flora, but a few gram-positive bacteria may be seen in stained fecal smears. Routine microbiologic aerobic cultures are usually negative.

A direct wet preparation of crop contents can be obtained via crop lavage or by directly inserting a small cotton-tipped swab (Calgiswab, Spectrum Laboratories, Inc., Houston, TX) into the crop.

Small blood samples may be obtained by clipping a toenail or puncturing peripheral veins with a 27-gauge needle, allowing blood to be collected directly into a microhematocrit tube. The right jugular vein is the best site for large-sample blood collection. A preheparinized (thoroughly flushed) 0.5- or 1-ml insulin syringe with a 27-gauge needle is used. A volume of 1% of the bird's body weight in grams (e.g., 0.19 ml from a 19-gm finch) must not be exceeded.

CLINICAL MANAGEMENT

The right jugular vein (intravenous) or the tibia or ulna (intraosseous) can be used for fluid administration in the critical bird. Subcutaneous fluids placed in the lateral flank area may be used for maintenance fluid therapy.

Hemorrhage is often a problem after intramuscular injections into the pectoral muscles. To decrease the risk of hemorrhage, the caudal one third of the chest muscles and a 27-gauge needle placed at an acute angle are used. A cotton-tipped applicator can be used to place pressure on the injection site.

Direct oral administration of drugs is preferred; however, treatment frequency and stress often preclude this route. Drugs may also be administered into "soft" foods. Administering drugs via the bird's drinking water often results in a subtherapeutic drug blood level, disappointing clinical response, and development of resistant organisms.

DIAGNOSIS AND TREATMENT

Nutritional deficiencies and poor husbandry practices are usually the primary causes of many disease processes in finches. The goal of the practitioner is to identify and treat specific disease (Table 1) and prevent further disease through improvement of diet, strict aviary hygiene, proper quarantine procedures, and insect and rodent vector control.

Viral Disease

Avian pox may occur in Society finches but is uncommon (Bauck, 1989). Eastern equine encephalitis has caused deaths in Lady Gouldian finches (Curtis-Velasco, 1992). Mosquito control is imperative in the control of both these viruses. Papillomavirus causes slow-growing, wart-like proliferations on the skin of the feet and legs. Diagnosis is based on histopathologic examination. Treatment includes surgical excision. An autogenous vaccine may be tried. Differential diagnosis should include Knemidokoptes pilae, pox virus, chronic malnutrition, and aging. Polyomavirus infections have been associated with high morbidity and mortality in finches (especially Lady Gouldian). Asymptomatic adults may produce persistently infected young or neonates that acquire clinical signs and die in an acute condition. Fledglings that survive usually fledge late and have poor feather development and long tubular mandibles. Gross postmortem lesions include perirenal or intestinal hemorrhage and hepatosplenomegaly. Fluorescent antibody staining or DNA probe analysis of affected tissues or feces is available (Research Associates, Milford, OH). There is no effective treatment for polyomavirus. Birds shedding the virus as well as their offspring should be depopulated, separated from the collection, or rested from breeding. An inactivated vaccine is currently available for use in psittacines but use in passerines has not been reported. Paramyxovirus infection is common in African silver bills, Lady Gouldian, and zebra finches and is associated with variable degrees of wasting and neurologic signs. Diagnosis must be confirmed by serologic testing and virus isolation. No current treatment is available. Aviary fecal contamination by feral birds should be avoided.

BACTERIAL INFECTIONS

Gram-Positive Bacteria

Staphylococcus aureus and S. epidermidis have been isolated in finches with gastrointestinal and respiratory disease as well as conjunctivitis, arthritis, omphalitis, and embryonic mortality.

Acid-Fast Organisms

Atypical Mycobacterium avium is not uncommon in Lady Gouldian finches. Most birds are presented dead from an acute condition. Other nonspecific signs include polyurea, diarrhea, chronic wasting, anemia, and dull plumage. Leukocytosis is often present. Definitive antemortem diagnosis is difficult because fecal acid-fast stains are often negative. Culture is unrewarding because atypical M. avium are difficult to isolate. Acid-fast stains on tissue specimens may be diagnostic. Culling of affected birds is recommended because M. avium is shed in urine and feces and is highly resistant in the environment and potentially zoonotic (Gerlach, 1994).

Listeria monocytogenes can cause torticollis, tremors, stupor, paralysis, and paresis in canaries and more rarely in finches. Marked monocytosis may occur. Tetracyclines are used for treatment. If central nervous system signs are already present, treatment is usually unrewarding.

Gram-Negative Bacteria

Enterobacteriaceae are generally secondary pathogens that cause diarrhea, metritis, and septicemia. Oral antibiotics treat infections of the intestinal mucosa, but parenteral antibiotics are necessary in cases of septicemia. Salmonella typhimurium var copenhagen is associated with granulomatous ingluvitis in finches that is similar in appearance to crop candidiasis or capillariasis. Antibiotic choice is based on culture and sensitivity results. Vector control should be instituted.

Yersinia pseudotuberculosis is a common cause of peracute mortality in finches in rodent-infested environments. Enteritis and liver abscesses are characteristic. Birds are often unresponsive to therapy. Treating exposed birds with antibiotics based on culture and sensitivity testing may stop an outbreak. Vector control is essential.

Campylobacter fetus var jejuni is associated with pale, voluminous feces. Adding animal protein, vitamins, and minerals to the diet may be helpful in preventing recurrent infections. Erythromycin and tetracyclines are effective treatments.

TABLE 1. Commonly Used Drugs for Finches*

Drug	Route	Dosage
Antimicrobials		
Chlortetracycline (Pfichlor, Pfizer, Lee's Summit, MO)	Drinking water	1000–1500 mg/L
	Soft food	1500 mg/kg
Doxycycline (Vibramycin, Pfizer, Lee's Summit, MO)	Drinking water	250 mg/L
	Soft food	1000 mg/kg
Enrofloxacin (Baytril, Miles, Shawnee Missions, KS)	Drinking water	200 mg/mL
	Soft food	200 mg/kg
	Oral	10–15 mg/kg b.i.d.
	IM	10–15 mg/kg b.i.d.
Erythromycin (E-Mycin, Upjohn, Kalamazoo, MI)	Drinking water	125 mg/L
	Soft food	200 mg/kg
Spectinomycin (Spectam, Syntex, W. Des Moines, IA)	Drinking water	200–400 mg/L
	Soft food	400 mg/kg
Trimethoprim and sulfamethoxazole (Tribrissen Paste, Mundelein, IL)	Drinking water	50–100 mg/L
	Soft food	100 mg/kg
Tylosin (Tylan, Butler, Dublin, OH)	Drinking water	250–400 mg/L
	Soft food	400 mg/kg
Antifungals		
Amphotercin B (Fungizone, Squibb, Princeton, NJ)	Nebulize	1 mg/ml saline for 15 min b.i.d.
Chlorhexidine† (Nolvasan, Fort Dodge, IA)	Oral	10–30 ml/gallon drinking water
	Topical	0.5% as a wound cleanser
Fluconazole (Diflucan, Roerig, New York, NY)	Oral	2–5 mg/kg s.i.d.
Itraconazole (Sporanox, Janssen, Piscataway, NJ)	Oral	5–10 mg/kg b.i.d. for 4 to 5 wk
Ketoconazole (Nizoral, Janssen, Piscataway, NJ)	Oral	20–30 mg/kg b.i.d.
	Drinking water	200 mg/L
	Soft food	10–20 mg/kg
Nystatin (Mycozo, Squibb, Princeton, NJ)	Oral	0.1 ml/30 gm
Antiparasitics		
Amprolium (Corid, Amprol plus, Ag Vet, Rahway, NJ)	Drinking water	2–4 ml/gallon for 5–7 days
Carbaryl (Sevin, Meijer, Inc, Grand Rapids, MI)	Topical	Light dusting on feathers
Carnidazole (Spartrix, Janssen, Piscataway, NJ)	Oral	20–30 mg/kg single dose
Febendazole (Panacur, Hoechst-Roussel, Somerville, NJ)‡	Oral	10–50 mg/kg s.i.d. for 3–5 days
Ivermectin (Ivomec, Merck Rahway, NJ)§	Topical	200 µg/kg, repeat in 14 days
Levamisole (Levasole, Pitman-Moore, Mundlein, IL)‖	Drinking water	5–15 ml/gallon for 1–3 days
Metronidazole (Searle, Chicago, IL)**	Drinking water	100 mg/L
Oxfendazole (Syanthic, Syntex W. Des Moines, IA)	Oral	10–40 mg/kg single dose
Piperazine (Agri-labs, St. Joseph, MO)	Drinking water	300 mg/gal
Praziquantel (Droncit, Bayer, Shawnee Missions, KS)††	Oral	10–20 mg/kg, repeat in 10–14 days
	IM	9 mg/kg, repeat in 10 days
Pyrantel pamoate (Strongid T, Pfizer, Lee's Summit, MO)	Oral	4.5 mg/kg, repeat in 10–14 days
Pyrethrins (Km, Des Moines, IA)	Topical	Lightly mist (Vet-feathers)
Ronidazole (Ridzol-S, AUV, Cuijik, Holland)	Oral	6–10 mg/kg orally for 10 days
	Drinking water	400 mg of 10% powder/L for 10 days
Sulfachlorpyridazine (Vetisulid, Solvay, Mendota Hts, MN)	Drinking water	0.25–1 tsp/gal
Miscellaneous		
Dinoprost Tromethamine (Prosin E2, Upjohn, Kalamazoo, MI)	Topical	1 drop to cloacal region
Furosemide (Lasix, Hoescht-Roussel, Somerville, NJ)	IM, SC, oral	0.15 mg/kg s.i.d. to b.i.d.
Lactobacillus Powder (Benebac, Pet Ag Elgin, IL)	Oral	1 pinch per bird per day

*Not all drug doses are based on pharmocokinetic data; values represent the author's clinical experience and a review of the literature.
†When added to drinking water, it may prevent finches from drinking, resulting in dehydration and death. Topically, it is irritating and may be toxic to finches.
‡Has a low therapeutic index in finches. Use low dose range.
§Toxic in bullfinches and goldfinches when used topically at 0.4 mg/kg (Macwhirter, 1994). Propylene glycol (used as the carrier) may also be toxic in large doses.
‖ Low therapeutic index. Do not use in debilitated finches.
**Contraindicated in finches.
††Injectable form is toxic in finches.
b.i.d., twice daily; IM, intramuscular; SC, subcutaneous; s.i.d., once a day.

MYCOTIC INFECTIONS

Many finches are fed bread products that contain non-budding yeast. Zero to two budding yeast per high power field may be considered normal. Candidiasis may be related to nutritional disease, poor hygiene, and overuse of antibiotics. Clinical signs are vomiting, anorexia, weight loss, and crop stasis. Diarrhea and poor molting are frequent symptoms in adults. Diagnosis is based on cytologic or histopathologic examination. Localized infections are treated with nystatin. Ketoconazole is used for systemic or resistant infections.

Immunosuppression and poor nutrition, sanitation, and ventilation predispose birds to aspergillosis. Postmortem findings include granulomatous nodules in the liver, lung, air sacs, and kidney. Antemortem clinical signs include weight loss, anorexia, vomiting, diarrhea, or respiratory distress. A presumptive diagnosis may be based on history and severe leukocytosis (>25,000 white blood cells/μl). Lesions or feces may be cultured on Sabouraud's dextrose agar. Treatment is expensive and protracted; it includes nebulization with amphotericin B and oral ketoconazole for 4 to 6 weeks. Prognosis is poor to grave.

Dermatomycosis (*Microsporum gallinae*) and *Trichophyton* spp) occasionally causes alopecia (especially of head and neck) or hyperkeratosis of the skin. Diagnosis is made by culturing on dermatophyte test media. Treatment includes topical baths with dilute chlorhexadine or systemic ketoconazole and fluconazole. Underlying immunocompromise is often present. Differential diagnoses of alopecia of head and neck include mite infestation and cage mate aggression.

EXTERNAL PARASITES

Scaly mites (*Knemidokoptes pilae*) cause hyperkeratotic lesions of the feet. Differential diagnoses include chronic malnutrition and papillomavirus. Treatment consists of a small drop of 0.01% ivermectin diluted in propylene glycol placed on the skin over the jugular vein; treatment is repeated 2 weeks later. Some finches have had toxic reactions to ivermectin. Cage mates are treated and the environment is cleaned.

INTERNAL PARASITES

Air Sac Mites

Air sac mites (*Sternostoma tracheacolum*) may inhabit the respiratory tract of passerines. Lady Gouldian finches and finches housed with canaries primarily are affected. Clinical signs include wheezing, squeaking, clicking, coughing, and voice change. Tracheal transillumination may reveal the mites. Secondary bacterial infections often complicate pulmonary acariasis. Ivermectin and antibiotics are used as necessary.

Cestodes

Zebra and parrot finches, and Diamond Firetails are prone to cestodiasis. Clinical signs include diarrhea, emaciation with increased appetite, and occasionally death from intestinal obstruction. Diagnosis is made by identifying proglottids or hexacanth larvae in fecal droppings. Serial fecal flotations may be necessary. Treatment includes praziquantel or oxfendazole and limiting access to intermediate hosts.

Nematodes

The round worms, *Ascaridia* spp and *Porrocaecum* spp, are rare but may cause signs of general debilitation, diarrhea, weight loss, and occasional neurologic symptoms. Diagnosis is based on fecal flotation. Treatment consists of ivermectin, fenbendazole, piperazine, or levamisole.

Capillaria may be subclinical or cause general debilitation, weight loss, diarrhea, and death. These worms often are associated with white to gray plaques in the pharynx or buccal cavity. Diagnosis is made by finding bioperculate eggs in swabs of lesions or in fecal flotations. Capillaria may be resistant, so preventive measures, including strict aviary hygiene and removal of earthworms, is imperative. Levamisole, fenbendazole, and oxfendazole are the treatment choices.

The spiruroid nematodes (*Acuaria skrjavi, Dispharynx nasuta,* and *Spiropter incerta*) inhabit the proventriculus and under the koilin lining of the ventriculus in passerines. Clinical signs include mechanical blockage of food. Resistance is common. Oxfendazole is used for treatment.

Protozoa

Society finches can be asymptomatic carriers of *Cochlosoma* spp. When used as foster parents, they may infect 6- to 12-week-old nestlings, causing high mortality. Clinical signs include dehydration and passing of whole seeds. At necropsy, the intestines are filled with yellow fluid containing whole seeds. Direct wet preparation of fresh, warm droppings or of intestinal contents at necropsy is diagnostic. Treatment is with ronidazole. Metronidazole causes toxicity in some finches and should not be used. *Giardia* is occasionally seen in finches and is associated with gastrointestinal disease. Diagnosis and treatment are as for cochlosomiasis.

Trichomonas infections cause symptoms such as respiratory distress, nasal discharge, regurgitation, green diarrhea, and emaciation. Lesions seen post mortem include caseous material lining the esophagus and crop. Microscopic examination of fresh fecal samples or swabs of lesions may reveal the flagellate. Birds may be treated with ronidazole.

Numerous genera of coccidia in the family Eimeriidae have been associated with hemorrhagic diarrheal syndrome and emaciation. Finding the oocysts in fresh fecal samples is diagnostic. Therapy consists of strict hygiene and medicating with coccidiostatic drugs.

NONINFECTIOUS DISEASE

Trauma

Finches can be very territorial. Feather plucking, head trauma, and other injuries may occur to individuals attacked by a companion. Injuries are treated as with other birds. Aggression is prevented by avoiding overcrowding and providing extra vegetation or visual barriers. Aggression is reduced when all birds are introduced simultaneously into a new environment.

Digit, wing, or foot necrosis frequently occurs because of entanglement of the fine synthetic fibers used as nesting material or constricting leg bands. Use of burlap and coconut fiber may reduce these incidences. Magnification is needed to identify the fibers, which may be gently cut using a 27- to 30-gauge needle. Bands should be removed. Marginal tissue is treated with warm water soaks and antibiotics. Amputation of the affected appendage is often necessary.

Miscellaneous

Hepatic lipidosis is occasionally seen in the family Estrildidae. Obesity, inadequate exercise, and overfeeding of high-energy diets predispose birds to the condition. At necropsy, the liver is yellow and swollen and may float in formalin. Antemortem diagnosis of liver disease is based on history, elevated aspartate aminotransferase levels with normal creatine kinase levels, or elevated bile acids. Liver biopsy is diagnostic. Treatment is directed toward supportive therapy and prevention of recurrence.

Amyloidosis is common in Gouldian finches. A hereditary predisposition is suspected. Most birds have a history of chronic nonspecific illnesses or suffer from concurrent diseases. Histopathologic examination of the kidneys and liver is diagnostic. No treatment is successful at this time.

Egg binding is common in malnourished, prolific egg layers.

References and Suggested Reading

Bauck L: Diseases of the finch as seen in a common commercial import station. Proc Assoc Avian Vet, 1989, pp 196–201.
Curtis-Velasco M: Eastern equine encephalomyelitis in a Lady Gouldian finch. J Assoc Avian Vet 6:227–228, 1992.
Dorrenstein GM: Passerines. In: Altman RB, Clubb SL, Dorrenstein GM, Quesenberry K, eds: Avian Medicine and Surgery. Philadelphia: WB Saunders, 1997, p 867.
    This is a detailed review of passerines.
Macwhirter P: Passeriformes. In: Ritchie BW, Harrison GJ, Harrison LR, eds: Avian Medicine: Principles and Applications. Lake Worth, FL: Wingers Publishing, 1994, p 1172.
    This is an excellent detailed overview of passerines.
Massey JG: Clinical medicine in small passerines. Proceedings of the Association of Avian Veterinarians, Tampa, FL, 1996, p 49.
    This is a good general discussion of passerine clincal medicine.
Scott JR: Passerine aviary diseases: Diagnosis and treatment. Proceedings of the Association of Avian Veterinarians, Tampa, FL, 1996, p 39.
    This article discusses common diseases of passeriformes and includes an excellent reference list.
Taylor EJ: An evaluation of the importance of insoluble versus soluble grit in the diet of canaries. J Avian Med Surg 10:248, 1996.
    This article discusses original research.

Salmonellosis in Birds

NADINE LAMBERSKI
Columbia, South Carolina

The term *avian salmonellosis* refers to a large group of acute or chronic diseases of birds caused by organisms from the bacterial genus *Salmonella*, family Enterobacteriaceae. Salmonellae are usually motile (flagellated), non–spore-forming, gram-negative bacilli. These organisms are ubiquitous and may survive and multiply in the environment. They are naturally found in and capable of infecting a wide variety of vertebrate hosts. They occur primarily in the intestinal tract and can cause localized as well as systemic disease. Salmonellae are distributed worldwide and have public health significance, causing mild to severe gastroenteritis in humans.

Subclinical carriers, such as rodents and some free-living birds, exist and may serve as reservoirs of infection for aviary birds and birds held in zoologic collections. Host susceptibility and development of carrier states vary among species of birds. Birds lacking well-developed ceca (e.g., psittacines, passerines, and columbines) may be more susceptible to salmonella infections than birds with functioning ceca. It is thought that the cecal flora, particularly the anaerobic flora, is a natural antagonist for *Salmonella* spp.

ETIOLOGY AND EPIDEMIOLOGY

This genus includes approximately 2000 species that have been classified based on both biochemical and serologic differences. Serotype, biotype, phage type, antibiotic resistance patterns, and analysis of plasmic profiles are used for epidemiologic studies of the organism but are not useful in predicting virulence. The species considered to be of major pathogenic significance in human and veterinary medicine include *S. arizonae, S. choleraesuis, S. enteritidis,* and *S. typhimurium*. The incidence of *Salmonella* spp. may vary with geographic location as well as the type of diet consumed. Some salmonella strains are host-adapted such as *S. gallinarum* and *S. pullorum* in chickens. *S. typhimurium* is commonly isolated from diseased children and animals. *S. typhimurium* is the most common isolate from wild and companion birds.

The most common modes of transmission are ingestion of contaminated food or water and direct contact with carrier species. Aerogenous spread via contaminated fecal or feather dust can also occur. Egg transmission also occurs and is most common with host-adapted strains. Poultry and pigeons can be asymptomatic carriers of *Salmonella* and contaminate their eggs during oviposition when they enter the egg through pores in the shell. Studies have shown that embryos can become infected with fewer than ten organisms and that more than ten organisms may result in the death of the embryo. The organism can become host-adapted during the egg incubation period, making the chick a subclinical carrier. If the chick hatches, *Salmonella* can colonize the intestines, thus facilitating the spread of *Salmonella* by direct contact. If the environmental conditions are poor, *Salmonella* can cause septicemia and death in some chicks after they hatch. Vertical infections also occur when infected hens feed contaminated crop contents to their young.

PATHOGENESIS

Enterobacteriaceae produce endotoxins; however, death due to ingestion of endotoxin-contaminated food is rare in birds. Most clinical cases are the result of direct infection. Nonvirulent and virulent strains of salmonella can exist in a single host. Nonvirulent strains colonize the intestinal tract, resulting in asymptomatic infections and intermittent shedding. Nonvirulent strains require a break in the mucosal barrier for entry, whereas virulent strains are able to penetrate intact mucosa. Septicemia can occur once virulent or nonvirulent strains have passed the mucosal barrier. Colonization of other tissues can result, leading to death if an appropriate immune response does not ensue. *Salmonella* spp. can also produce chronic infections characterized by acute intermittent septicemic episodes and clinical signs. Recurrent infections usually result in progressive organ involvement, with the central nervous and musculoskeletal systems frequently affected in terminal cases.

CLINICAL FINDINGS

The time from exposure to expression of disease varies with the strain of salmonella, the route of infection, and the immune status of the host. Incubation periods are usually 3 to 5 days in acute cases and can be prolonged in subclinical carriers. The incubation period with egg transmission is usually 1 to 2 days.

Clinical signs can range from mild enteritis to acute death. Nonspecific clinical signs such as anorexia, lethargy, crop stasis, diarrhea, polydipsia, and polyuria characterize acute forms of salmonellosis. Neurologic signs, arthritis, dyspnea, and evidence of liver, spleen, and heart involvement can be seen with subacute and chronic infections. Ocular lesions such as conjunctivitis, iridocyclitis, and panophthalmitis occur in some cases. Granulomatous dermatitis induced by biting insects has been reported in several avian species.

Species-Specific Presentations

Signs of avian salmonellosis vary among various species. Examples of clinical presentations include peracute disease with high flock mortality in lories and penguins; chronic disease characterized by granulomatous dermatitis, arthritis, cellulitis, and tenosynovitis in African Grey par-

rots; neurologic disease in geese and ducks; ocular lesions in turkeys, ducks, parrots, and canaries; septicemia in thick-billed parrots; and dyspnea and myocardial disease in quetzels, red-headed barbets, terns, and house sparrows. Additionally, pigeons can have localized infections such as meningitis, arthritis, tenosynovitis, or osteomyelitis. Finches in Europe are susceptible to a subacute form of the disease characterized by granulomatous ingluvitis caused by *S. typhimurium* var *copenhagen*. *S. pullorum* causes oophoritis in domestic fowl, whereas *S. pullorum* and *S. enteritidis* can also cause embryonic and neonatal mortality in these species. Neonatal anseriforms can acquire necrotizing colitis and omphalitis. Ratites 3 to 6 weeks of age can present with acute weight loss, lethargy, and bilaterally symmetrical distal leg edema resulting from *Salmonella* infection.

Clinical Laboratory Findings and Diagnosis

Depending on the severity and duration of infection, leukocytosis or leukopenia characterized by an absolute heterophilia or heteropenia may occur. Toxic leukocytes may be present in cases of septicemia. An increased hematocrit and total protein often reflect dehydration. Increases in serum enzyme levels indicate specific organ involvement. Septicemic birds may show increased aspartate aminotransferase, lactate dehydrogenase, and creatine phosphokinase levels.

Isolation and identification of the *Salmonella* species is necessary to confirm the diagnosis. However, isolation of the organism does not confirm that the organism is causing clinical disease unless the sample is cultured from blood or a lesion.

Serologic evaluation is of value only if the exact species of *Salmonella* is known. The development of a serologic response requires penetration of the mucosal barrier; therefore, most chronically infected subclinical and carrier birds have negative serological test results because infections are limited to the intestinal lumen.

PATHOLOGIC FINDINGS

Post mortem findings are consistent with the clinical presentation and can include muscle degeneration or necrosis, gastroenteritis, hepatomegaly, splenomegaly, air sacculitis, bile congestion, or nephropathy, or a combination of these conditions. Purulent leptomeningitis and exudate formation in the subarachnoid space has been noted in birds with central nervous system signs. Pericarditis, epicarditis, oophoritis, or orchitis may be seen with chronic infections. Multifocal yellow foci are often present in organs that may demonstrate gram-negative bacilli cytologically. Positive cultures confirm the diagnosis of *Salmonella*. Histopathologic changes are nonspecific and are characterized by purulent inflammation in the affected organs. Granulomas are seen more commonly with chronic infections.

TREATMENT, PREVENTION, AND CONTROL

The treatment of salmonella infections in many mammalian species is controversial. The same is true for avian species. Elimination of infection is difficult, and carrier states can develop. Antibiotics are frequently used in human and veterinary medicine to treat cases of salmonellosis involving prolonged fever or septicemia. Their use is often contraindicated in mild cases because of the possibility of prolonging the carrier period and causing antibiotic-resistant strains to emerge.

Because of the potential for septicemia and death, clincally ill birds should be treated. Therapy includes appropriate antibiotics based on sensitivity testing as well as supportive care, including fluid therapy (see *CVT XI,* p. 1154–1163), nutritional support (see *CVT XI,* p. 1160–1163), and supplemental heat. While waiting for sensitivity results, it is useful to initiate antimicrobial therapy. *Salmonella* strains are usually susceptible to commonly available antibiotics such as trimethoprim-sulfa (Septra, Burroughs Wellcome, Research Triangle Park, NC) (50 to 100 mg/kg every 12 hours dependent upon species) or enrofloxacin (Baytril, Bayer Corp, Shawnee Mission, Kansas) (5 to 15 mg/kg every 12 hours dependent upon species) (see *CVT XII,* p. 1278–1283). In some cases, it may be necessary to extend antibiotic therapy for up to 3 weeks; however, chronic infections and those involving the central nervous system can be refractory to treatment. Concurrent disease due to viral infections or *Aspergillus* infection can also complicate treatment.

Flock management should focus on prevention of egg transmission by identifying and removing subclinically infected breeders and housing birds in an environment where exposure to salmonellae is minimal. Eggs that are artificially incubated should be kept clean. Cleaning eggs with cold water or wiping with a damp cloth can facilitate bacterial penetration and thus transfer the infection. Dry sanding is a better way to remove dirt and dried feces from eggs. Egg-dipping and -spraying procedures have been used in poultry to destroy salmonellae on the surface of hatching eggs before the organisms can penetrate through the shell and shell membranes. To be effective, dipping and spraying must be carried out immediately after egg collection. Care must be taken, as wash solutions can become contaminated with organic material and bacteria and may do more harm than good. For these reasons, egg-dipping and -spraying are not routinely recommended for prevention of egg-borne salmonellosis. Fumigation of eggs with formaldehyde within 2 hours after laying has been found to be effective in preventing salmonellae infections but, again, care must be taken because improper fumigation can kill the embryo. Valuable eggs from known carriers of *Salmonella* can be injected with antibiotics in an attempt to protect the embryo.

Good hygiene is the best way to prevent salmonella outbreaks. Control of possible vectors such as insects, rats, mice, rabbits, other vermin, and free-flying birds is essential. These species should be restricted from the enclosure as well as from food and water pans. Insect control is also important. Humans can be mechanical vectors by carrying the organism on footwear and clothing. Proper food storage is important as is the use of potable water. Regular cleaning and disinfection of the enclosure, aviary, nursery, and feeding utensils is necessary. Phenolic compounds, quaternary ammonium compounds, or household bleach (diluted 1:32 or 4 ounces per gallon of water) are effective disinfectants for salmonella.

Vaccines have been evaluated experimentally and may be beneficial to populations at risk; however, none have proved effective for general use. Vaccination in addition to antibiotics and culling clinically affected birds has been recommended for pigeon flocks after an outbreak (Uyttebroek et al, 1990).

PUBLIC HEALTH CONSIDERATIONS

Strains of *Salmonella* isolated from birds may be of public health significance in infants, geriatric patients, or immunocompromised persons. *S. enteriditis* is commonly isolated from companion birds and is a known enteric pathogen for humans. *S. enteriditis* has been associated with egg consumption. *S. typhimurium* can also cause human disease. Conversely, humans with salmonellosis can infect companion birds.

References and Suggested Reading

Dorrestein GM: Bacteriology. In: Altman RB, Clubb SL, Dorrestein GM, et al, eds: Avian Medicine and Surgery. Philadelphia: WB Saunders, 1997, p 255.
This is a review of salmonellosis in birds.
Gerlach H: Bacteria. In: Ritchie BW, Harrison GJ, Harrison LR, eds: Avian Medicine: Principles and Application. Lake Worth, FL: Wingers Publishing, 1994, p 949.
This chapter is also a review of salmonellosis in birds.
Greene CE: Salmonellosis. In: Greene CE, ed: Infectious Diseases of the Dog and Cat. Philadelphia: WB Saunders, 1990, p 542.
This is a review of salmonellosis in dogs and cats.
Rupiper DJ, Briggs KT, Ehrenberg M: Management of trichomoniasis, paramyxovirus-1, and salmonellosis in the pigeon loft. Proceedings of the annual conference of the Association of Avian Veterinarians, Reno, NV, 1994, p 241.
Husbandry practices used to manage multiple infectious diseases in a pigeon loft are discussed.
Snoeyenbos GH, Williams JE: Salmonellosis. In: Calnek BW, ed: Diseases of Poultry. Ames, IA: Iowa State University Press, 1991, p 72.
Salmonellosis in poultry is reviewed, including recommendations for hatchery and egg sanitation.
Tudor DC: Bacterial diseases. In: Pigeon Health and Disease. Ames, IA: Iowa State University Press, 1991, pp 54–60.
This is a review of salmonellosis in pigeons.
Tully TN: Acute salmonellosis in a breeding facility of eclectus parrots. Proceedings of the annual conference of the Association of Avian Veterinarians, Phoenix, AZ, 1990, p 119.
The clinical aspects of a salmonella outbreak in an aviary are presented.
Uyttebroek E, Devriese LA, Goevaert D, et al: The protective effects of vaccines against experimental salmonellosis in racing pigeons. Vet Rec 128:152, 1991.

Avian Analgesia

VICTORIA L. CLYDE
Milwaukee, Wisconsin

JOANNE PAUL-MURPHY
Madison, Wisconsin

Avian analgesia is in its infancy. Limited information is available regarding avian pain perception and analgesia. The studies that have been performed suggest that pain perception in birds is mediated by neural pathways and neurotransmitters that are similar to those in mammals. Clinical experience also indicates that pain perception in birds differs little from that in mammals, and that many analgesics used in mammalian medicine can be utilized in birds. Unfortunately, specific dosages, drug effects, and species differences are poorly described in birds.

RECOGNITION OF PAIN IN BIRDS

Pain is a subjective experience, generally assessed in human patients by their verbal statement of pain. In animals, the assessment of pain is based on observed behaviors. Active behaviors stimulated by acute pain, such as writhing or vocalizations, are easily interpreted. However, these overt behaviors may be stimulated only by severe or acute pain. The assessment of pain based solely on readily observed behaviors consistently underestimates many instances of pain. Therefore, careful observation of subtle behaviors, behavioral changes, and the absence of normal behaviors is necessary for assessing pain in animals.

Birds react to pain in many ways. Pain often evokes avoidance behavior in which the bird attempts to remove itself from the stimulus. If effective retreat is not possible, the bird may become anxious, display restless behaviors, vocalize, struggle, or become aggressive. A painful area may be guarded, resulting in a decreased interest or active avoidance of social interactions. Abnormal, stiff, or crouched postures may be observed. A site of irritation may be overgroomed, resulting in feather loss, feather picking, or self-mutilation.

Birds may respond to a strong pain stimulus with tonic immobility. This dramatic lack of reaction should not be interpreted as a lack of pain, as it represents just the opposite. Low-grade or chronic pain in birds may produce withdrawal behaviors such as decreased appetite, irritability, lethargy, dyspnea, constipation, weight loss, or poor grooming. The bird may appear preoccupied, becoming less interested in external stimuli as it focuses on an internal source of pain or discomfort.

Accurate assessment of the behavioral changes indicative of pain requires the veterinarian to be familiar with the normal behavior of both the individual bird and its species, as well as being open to the concept that the observed changes in behavior are the result of pain. If the lesion would be painful in a human patient, if tissue damage is induced, or if the bird is displaying aversive responses such as changes in temperament, posture, or nor-mal behaviors, the veterinarian should assume that the bird is perceiving pain, and an analgesic plan should be instituted.

ANALGESIC AGENTS

Analgesics are substances that decrease or eliminate the perception of pain without the loss of consciousness. Analgesics work by a variety of methods, including modulation of the inflammatory process, blockade of nociceptor activation, or the elevation of the activation threshold of a nociceptor. The quality of analgesia induced by different mechanisms may vary, and the combination analgesia obtained by simultaneous administration of different classes of analgesic agents may produce a superior result.

The dosages listed here are a compilation of doses reported in the literature and from personal communications from avian, exotic animal, and zoo veterinarians. Many are extrapolations of mammalian dosages that appear to be clinically effective in limited case numbers. Numerous additional studies are needed to clarify species differences, optimal drugs, and dosages, and to elucidate possible complications of analgesic medications in birds.

Opioids

Opioids are a diverse group of natural and synthetic drugs with morphine-like action that combine reversibly with specific receptors in the central nervous system. Although these drugs are considered the most effective class of centrally acting analgesics for sharp or acute pain, marked species differences in required dosages and clinical effects have been noted. These differences may be due to variations in the subclasses of opioid receptors present in the forebrain of different species. Birds possess opioid receptors and are able to recognize and respond to a variety of opioids. Autoradiographic studies show a marked predominance of kappa receptors in the forebrain of pigeons, in comparison to the mammalian species studied (Mansour et al, 1988).

If other species of birds have an increased percentage of kappa receptors in the forebrain similar to pigeons, mixed agonist-antagonists with kappa activity, such as butorphanol (Torbugesic, Fort Dodge), pentazocine (Talwin, Sanofi Winthrop), and nalbuphine (Nubain, DuPont Merck), should be effective analgesics in birds. Only butorphanol has been investigated in birds to date. The recommendation for dosage range in psittacines is 2 to 4 mg/kg IM. Butorphanol has a short duration of action, and frequent redosing at intervals of 2 to 4 hours is needed to maintain analgesia. Initial anecdotal reports of analgesia of longer duration with buprenorphine (Buprenex, Reckitt & Colman) have not been substantiated. In experimental trials, analgesia was not observed in birds given this mu agonist, even at high dosages (Paul-Murphy, unpublished data).

Possible adverse effects of opioids include respiratory and cardiovascular depression, increased intracranial pressure, behavioral changes, and development of tolerance. Minimal respiratory and cardiovascular changes are observed after the administration of butorphanol to psittacines and other birds. The opioid antagonist naloxone (Astra Pharmaceutical Products, Inc.) should be effective in birds at the standard mammalian dosage (0.05 to 0.25 mg/kg IM or slow IV). Tolerance to opioid analgesia following several days of treatment has been noted in mammals, but no information is available for birds.

Alpha₂-Adrenergic Agonists

Alpha₂-adrenergic agonists induce sedation, analgesia, anxiolysis, and muscle relaxation in mammals, although these effects vary considerably between species. Limited data suggest that these drugs have similar effects in birds. Xylazine (Fermenta Animal Health Co.), 1 to 4 mg/kg IM, provides sedation for ketamine (Ketaset, Fort Dodge Laboratories) anesthesia and has been used at doses up to 10 mg/kg for sedation in small psittacines. Detomidine (Dormosedan, Pfizer Animal Health), 0.3 mg/kg IM, or medetomidine (Domitor, Farmos Group Ltd.), 0.1 mg/kg IM, provides marked sedation in chickens, ostriches, and other birds, but data on duration, cardiopulmonary effects, or complications have not been published. While analgesia has not been assessed directly, this class of drugs should be able to provide analgesia and warrants further investigation.

The possible complications of alpha₂-adrenergic agonists include a short duration of analgesia, hypotension, bradycardia, and hypothermia. Reversal agents for alpha₂-adrenergic agonists appear to be effective in birds at the following doses: yohimbine (Yobine, Lloyd Laboratories) 0.1 mg/kg IV, tolazoline (Priscoline, Novartis) 15 mg/kg IV, or atipamezole (Antisedan, Farmos Group Ltd.) 0.5 mg/kg IM.

Anti-inflammatory Drugs

Anti-inflammatory drugs are indicated for the relief of pain induced by inflammation. While not adequate as a single agent for sharp or acute pain, anti-inflammatory drugs are synergistic with other classes of analgesic agents and can be used effectively in combined analgesic regimens. Preoperative use of anti-inflammatory drugs may lessen the need for postoperative opioids. Two classes of anti-inflammatory agents, corticosteroids, and nonsteroidal anti-inflammatory drugs (NSAIDs), are recognized. Dexamethasone (Steris Laboratories), 1 to 2 mg/kg IM, betamethasone (Betameth, Kay Pharmacal Co.), 0.1 mg/kg IM, and methylprednisolone acetate (Depo-Medrol, Upjohn Co.), 0.5 to 1.0 mg/kg, have been used in a variety of species. Possible immunosuppression and other complica-

tions of steroids make nonsteroidal anti-inflammatory drugs preferable to corticosteroids in many situations.

Nonsteroidal anti-inflammatory drugs act by inhibiting cyclooxygenase and the subsequent production of prostaglandins. Clinical doses include flunixin meglumine (Banamine, Schering-Plough Animal Health), 1.0 to 10.0 mg/kg IM every 24 hours, meclofenamic acid (Meclofenamate, Rugby Labs), 2.2 mg/kg PO every 24 hours, ketoprofen (Ketofen, Fort Dodge) 2 mg/kg IM every 8 to 24 hours, and carprofen (Rimadyl, Pfizer Animal Health) 2 mg/kg PO every 8 to 24 hours. Acetylsalicylic acid (Aspirin, Rugby Labs), 5.0 mg/kg PO t.i.d., can be used but appears less effective than other agents. Gastrointestinal side effects are not frequently recognized following the use of these agents in birds. Renal ischemia with resultant damage may be the greatest complication with the use of NSAIDs in birds. Daily administration of flunixin meglumine to northern bobwhite quail for 7 days produced renal disease in birds even at dosages as low as 0.1 mg/kg IM (Klein et al, 1994). Renal disease and death occur occasionally in psittacines after repeat doses of flunixin meglumine. Use of the lowest possible therapeutic dose for the shortest duration along with supplemental hydration is advisable.

Local Anesthetics

Local anesthetics block ion channels, stopping the transmission of pain impulses. This blockade interferes with nociceptor sensitization and prevents central changes that occur secondary to activation of pain pathways. The use of a local nerve block prior to tissue trauma significantly reduces postoperative pain, and blockade prior to nerve transection in amputation decreases the incidence of "phantom pain" in humans. Lidocaine (Phoenix Pharmaceutical) can be used for local anesthesia in birds, as long as the dose does not exceed 4 mg/kg. Administration of this dose to small birds requires dilution of the commercially available solutions. Overdosage can result in seizures and possible cardiac arrest. Little information is available on the use of longer-acting local anesthetics, such as bupivacaine (Marcaine, Sanofi Winthrop), in birds. Intravenous, epidural, and intrathecal routes of administration of local anesthetics, often in combination with opioids or alpha₂-agonists, have provided superior analgesia in mammals, but these routes have not been investigated in birds.

Adjunctive Medications

While sedatives and tranquilizing agents do not provide analgesia, the induced behavioral changes and reduction in limbic activity can decrease pain perception and allow for improved efficacy of concurrent analgesics. Diazepam (Valium, Roche), 0.5 to 2.0 mg/kg IV or IM, and midazolam (Versed, Roche), 1.0 to 2.0 mg/kg IM or IV, have been used in birds. Additionally, both drugs provide skeletal muscle relaxation, which affords pain reduction in appropriate cases.

TREATMENT OF PAIN IN BIRDS

When evidence of pain is noted in an avian patient, or when tissue trauma has occurred, an analgesic plan should be designed and instituted. The analgesic plan should incorporate multiple methods of pain reduction, including simple, nonchemical methods of analgesia. The source of pain should be identified and treated. The removal of fear and anxiety reduces muscle tension and central nervous system activation. Anxiolytics, tranquilizers, and muscle relaxants should be used judiciously along with environmental modifications. A dry, warm, quiet, comfortable, and nonstressful environment is essential.

Mechanical forms of analgesia provided by good nursing care are important. The first mechanical consideration should be rest for the traumatized area. The affected area should be bandaged or splinted, if necessary, to provide protection and support. Perches should provide easy and comfortable footing without the need for excess gripping. Food and water should be readily available to the bird without excess movement. Other mechanical methods of analgesia (alternating heat and cold, massage, physical therapy, controlled exercise, and transcutaneous electrical nerve stimulation) should be considered, although they may not be applicable to all patients.

The chemical forms of analgesia selected should be appropriate for the type of pain. Acute, sharp pain is best treated by opioids or alpha$_2$-adrenergic agonists. Kappa agonists, such as butorphanol, appear beneficial in birds, although the short duration of action requires multiple redosing. Inflammatory or chronic pain is usually treated with NSAIDs. In chronic situations, a gradual increase in dosage is recommended until pain control is achieved. Corticosteroids can provide pain relief and temporary euphoria, which may stimulate appetite.

The basic principles of analgesia should be reviewed when one formulates an analgesic plan. The earliest possible disruption of the pain pathway is beneficial in reducing sensitization of pain pathways. Pre-emptive analgesia prior to the onset of pain stimulation should be implemented, when possible. Nerve blockade with infiltration of a local anesthetic is recommended prior to nerve transection. Combination analgesia utilizing drugs that interrupt the pain pathway at different steps may improve the level of analgesia afforded to the patient.

References and Suggested Reading

Bauck L: Analgesics in avian medicine. Proceedings of the 1990 Annual Conference of the Association of Avian Veterinarians, 1990, vol 239.
A clinical investigation of the effects of butorphanol or flunixin meglumine on healthy parakeets.

Clyde V, Paul-Murphy J: Avian Analgesia. In: Fowler ME, ed: Zoo and Wild Animal Medicine, Current Therapy 4. Philadelphia: WB Saunders, 1999, pp 309–314.
A review of pain perception and analgesia in multiple species of birds.

Curro TG, Brunson D, Paul-Murphy J: Determination of the ED$_{50}$ of isoflurane and evaluation of the analgesic properties of butorphanol in cockatoo (*Cacatua* spp.). Vet Surg 23:429, 1994.
An experimental study investigating the analgesic effect of butorphanol on cockatoos by determination of its "isoflurane-sparing" effect.

Klein PN, Charmatz K, Langenberg J: The effect of flunixin meglumine (banamine) on the renal function in northern bobwhite (*Colinus virginianus*): An avian model. Proceedings of the Association of Reptilian and Amphibian Veterinarians and American Association of Zoo Veterinarians, vol 128, 1994.
An experimental study detailing the renal damage induced by administration of flunixin meglumine to bobwhite quail.

Livingston A: Physiological basis for pain perception in animals. 5th International Congress of Veterinary Anesthesia, August 21–25, 1994.
A review of pain pathophysiology, with discussion of the role of analgesic agents in pain management for veterinary medicine.

Mansour A, Khachaturian H, Lewis ME, et al: Anatomy of CNS opioid receptors. Trends Neurosci 11:308, 1988.
A review of the anatomical distribution of opioid receptor subtypes in the central nervous system.

Sackman JE: Pain, Part I. The physiology of pain. Compend Small Anim 13:71, 1991.
A succinct review of the pathophysiology of pain.

Sackman JE: Pain, Part II. Control of pain in animals. Compend Small Anim 13:181, 1991.
A review of analgesic agents commonly used in veterinary medicine with suggested dosages for small animals.

General Husbandry and Medical Care of Hedgehogs

ANTHONY J. SMITH
San Jose, California

Hedgehogs have recently gained popularity as household pets. They are fairly easy to care for and can be friendly if provided with proper socialization. There are many different species of hedgehogs, but the majority now kept as pets are of two species. The African pygmy, four-toed, and white-bellied hedgehog all are common names for the single species *Atelerix albiventris*. The natural habitat of this animal extends throughout the central African continent. The European species, *Erinaceus europaeus*, may be found throughout Europe, including Great Britain.

In the United States, the African species is more commonly kept as a pet.

Hedgehogs are crepuscular, or nocturnal, in habit. In the wild, hedgehogs hibernate or sleep for much of the year. They are omnivores, but primarily insectivorous. Because of their classification in the order Insectivora, many wildlife management authorities consider hedgehogs as injurious or detrimental species. Therefore, in certain locales, owners may need to get special permits to keep these animals.

ANATOMY

The most obvious unique feature of the hedgehog is its collection of spines, which range in size from 0.5 to 2 cm in length. The spines are not barbed and do not usually cause serious injury to handlers. Most hedgehogs have spines that are ticked brown and white, but color variants including animals with all white spines (snowflake) have been bred. The spines are arranged dorsally and overlie a layer of loose fat and subcutaneous tissue. Beneath this layer is a powerful orbicular muscle that allows the skin to be pulled around the animal, similar to a pursestring. In some species, particularly the African hedgehog, the spines are absent from a small area over the head in a cranial caudal tract approximately 2 cm long by 0.5 cm wide. The legs and ventral surface of the animal are covered with sparse, light-colored hair. The teeth are similar to those of other insectivores, numbering 36 with the formula: I-3/2, C-1/1, P-3/2, M-3/3. The penis and prepuce are external and located on the midventral abdomen. The testicles, however, are normally raised within the abdominal cavity and are not easily palpable. In females, the vagina is located near the anus, as in other small animals.

BEHAVIOR

Although hedgehogs are now routinely bred in captivity, they have not been domesticated and retain many "wild" behavior patterns. For example, when hedgehogs encounter new items or smells in their environment, they may begin to salivate profusely and rub this frothy saliva onto the spines. This self-anointing behavior is called "anting."

Hedgehogs make a wide variety of vocalizations, including grunts, squeals, snuffling, and sneezing. It is important not to confuse these sounds with respiratory tract abnormalities that might require treatment. Vocalizations are usually made only when an animal is disturbed or encounters another animal. In contrast, respiratory abnormalities may be heard when the animal is at rest.

Many hedgehogs bred in captivity and handled as youngsters can be quite docile. Wild-caught and some captive-born animals can be irritable, especially if they are not accustomed to being handled. Young animals and females tend to be more easily handled than are adult males. Males are also more likely to hiss and struggle when they are handled. When threatened, hedgehogs roll into a tight ball, exposing only their spines. This position makes the animal difficult to handle, examine, and treat.

HUSBANDRY

Hedgehogs can be housed singly or in groups; however, no more than one male should be kept in any group. Males, and occasionally females, may fight, inflicting serious damage on one another with their teeth and spines. Hedgehogs prefer quiet, dimly lit environments and may react poorly to loud noises and bright sunlight. If possible, it is best to maintain hedgehogs on a reverse day-night light cycle, which allows the caretaker to observe the animal more closely.

The ideal temperature range is 22 to 30°C (70 to 85°F). If the temperature falls below this level, activity levels will decrease and animals become more susceptible to respiratory and other opportunistic infections. If the ambient temperature falls below 18°C (65°F), hedgehogs may go into a state of induced torpor, further compromising the animal.

Several types of cages are suitable for housing hedgehogs, including large aquariums and airline carriers. In general, the walls and floor of the enclosure should be smooth, nonclimbable, and easily cleaned. Wire should be avoided because animals may catch toes or limbs in the wire, resulting in trauma and possible fractures. Ample floor space (at least 8 ft^2 per animal) encourages hedgehogs to exercise and prevents obesity. A variety of devices, such as exercise wheels and balls, are commercially available or may be fashioned to encourage exercise. Exercise wheels should have a solid running surface to avoid limb entrapment.

Bedding must be clean, nontoxic, absorbent, and relatively free from dust. Shredded newspaper, pelleted bedding, and wood shavings all are appropriate. Cedar chips or scented shavings should be avoided, since these materials have been associated with respiratory and liver disease. Bedding should be spot-cleaned daily and changed frequently to avoid irritation and infection of sensitive skin.

Many hedgehogs learn to use a litter box. If litter is provided, use only the nonclumping, clay varieties and make sure that it is changed frequently. Use extreme care when preparing litter for males, since the particles may cling to the preputial opening and cause urinary blockage.

Hedgehogs prefer to sleep in hide boxes, and at least one should be provided at all times. The hide box should be slightly larger than the animal, with an access hole cut into one side. Plastic flowerpots, food containers, or polyvinyl chloride (PVC) tubes work well for this purpose. Cages and hide and litter boxes should be cleaned and disinfected at least weekly.

Nutrition

The exact nutrient requirements for hedgehogs are unknown; however, commercially produced hedgehog diets are now available. In the wild, hedgehogs feed on a wide variety of insects, small animals, fruits, and vegetables. Diets consisting of dry cat food, mixed fresh or thawed frozen vegetables, and occasional live insect treats have proved successful in maintaining healthy adult animals over many generations.

Many other food items, such as hard-boiled eggs, evaporated milk, powdered cottage cheese, waxworms, small mice, and vegetable or beef baby food may be provided as treats. When homemade diets are provided, it is important that the diet provide adequate protein, be balanced for calcium and phosphorus levels, and provide adequate vitamins and other minerals. In the absence of definitive nutrient requirements, a variety of high-quality food items should be provided—the owner should not rely on a single food source. Animals with increased metabolic requirements (e.g., growing, pregnant, or lactating animals) should receive appropriate nutrient-dense diets. Commercial vitamin and mineral supplements intended for small animals may also be added when necessary.

Live insects provide variety and behavioral enrichment

for hedgehogs. Dry food and hard-bodied insects also help to keep the teeth clean and free from tartar. However, animals that are maintained solely on insects may not obtain adequate calcium and risk metabolic bone disease.

Hedgehogs can easily become overweight. It is important to monitor the animal's weight frequently and adjust the amount fed appropriately. Feeding adults a light or reduced-calorie cat food helps maintain the animal's weight without compromising the nutritional quality of the diet. Kitten food, waxworms, and ferret foods are very high in fat and calories. If fed in large amounts, these foods can contribute to obesity.

Since hedgehogs are active mainly at night, it is best to provide freshly prepared food early in the evening, with uneaten food removed in the morning to prevent spoilage. This practice is particularly important when one uses foods such as uncooked fresh or frozen meat products, which are susceptible to bacterial overgrowth. Some hedgehogs are resistant to changes in diet. When dietary items are changed, it is wise to introduce new foods gradually and mix the diet thoroughly. Keeping the size and consistency of new food items similar to the old diet tends to improve acceptance. Water may be provided in water bottles equipped with sipper tubes or shallow, heavy dishes. Some hedgehogs never learn to drink from sipper tubes and must have water provided in a dish. In either case, water containers should be emptied, cleaned, and refilled daily.

Handling

Many even-tempered pet hedgehogs can be handled with bare hands. A pair of latex examination or light leather work gloves can be worn when one handles more apprehensive animals. When picking a hedgehog up, cup it gently in both hands. When a hedgehog rolls up into a ball, there are several methods for coaxing it to unroll. The most effective one is to leave the animal alone for several minutes, until it feels comfortable. Other methods include heavy backward stroking of the spines over the rump, holding the hedgehog head downward over a flat surface and then waiting for it to unroll and reach for the surface, or placing the hedgehog in a shallow (less than 2 cm deep) container of water. As a last resort, inhalation anesthesia with isoflurane may be needed.

REPRODUCTION

Reproductive data are summarized in Table 1. Hedgehogs may be bred in pairs or by placing multiple females together with a single male. Pregnancy detection in the hedgehog can be difficult. The most common method for identifying pregnant animals is to compare weights obtained on a weekly basis. Females that gain more than 50 gm within 3 weeks of having access to a male are usually pregnant. Prior to the female giving birth, she should be isolated to avoid cannibalism of the young.

Caring for Orphans

The use of a milk-replacing formula should be initiated for weak pups and in situations of maternal neglect. Com-

TABLE 1. Hedgehog Biologic and Reproductive Data

	African	European
Life span	3–8 yr	6–10 yr
Adult body weight (male)	500–600 gm	800–1,200 gm
(female)	250–400 gm	400–800 gm
Rectal temperature	36.1–37.2°C (97–99°F)	35.1°C (95.2°F)
Cage temperature range	22–30°C (70–85°F)	22–27°C (70–80°F)
Breeding age (female)	2–6 mo	9–10 mo
(male)	6–8 mo	9–10 mo
Gestation period	32 days	34–37 days
Litter size	1–7 young	3–8 young
Birth weight	8–13 gm	8–15 gm
Eyes open	13–16 days	13–16 days
Weaning age	4–5 wk	5–6 wk

mercial canine or feline milk-replacing formula (Esbilac, KMR, Pet-Ag), at the manufacturer's recommended dilutions can be used to raise orphans. A small amount of lactase enzyme (Lactaid, Lactaid, Inc.) should be added to milk-replacing formulas to prevent excessive gas build-up and bloating. Very small animals should be fed every 3 to 4 hours with a medicine dropper, small syringe, or feeding tube, as needed. Weight should be monitored at least daily, and the anus should be massaged gently after each feeding, to promote defecation.

MEDICAL CARE

If the hedgehog is tame or can be picked up by the scruff of the neck before it can roll into a ball, a brief physical examination or short treatment can be performed. However, to carry out most in-depth examinations or procedures, the animal must usually be sedated or anesthetized (see later).

Diagnostics and Therapeutics

Small amounts (up to 0.5 ml) of blood may be obtained from a variety of superficial veins. The lateral saphenous vein, located on the lateral aspect of the rear leg, can be visualized as it crosses the stifle. The cephalic vein of the forelimb can also be utilized. If larger amounts of blood are required, the jugular veins, femoral veins, or cranial vena cavae may be used. Clipping a nail may also provide sufficient blood for minimal testing. Standard reference values are available in Johnson-Delaney (1996). Urine may be collected via catheterization of the bladder with a small-gauge flexible catheter or by cystocentesis through a ventral percutaneous approach. Respiratory samples for microbiologic or cytologic analysis may be obtained with a sterile small-gauge needle or catheter inserted percutaneously through the trachea.

Subcutaneous fluids and other medications injected dorsally into the loose tissue beneath the spines are absorbed slowly over several hours; however, a very large volume may be administered. Volumes of more than 100 ml/kg are possible with a single treatment divided into two or three injection sites.

Anesthesia and Analgesia

The most effective means of inducing and maintaining anesthesia in the hedgehog is through the use of isoflurane (AErrane, Ohmeda). Animals may be induced in an induction chamber with the use of isoflurane at 3 to 5% in 100% oxygen. Maintenance is accomplished via either mask or endotracheal tube at a concentration of 0.5 to 3%. For smaller animals, endotracheal tubes may be fashioned from feeding tubes or intravenous catheters.

Injectable agents can be used, but recovery may be prolonged and occasionally rough. The combination-drug tiletamine HCl/zolazepam (Telazol, Fort Dodge) may be used at a dosage of 1.0 to 5.0 mg/kg (of the combined drug) IM. Analgesia may be provided with buprenorphine (Buprenex, Reckitt & Colman) at 0.01 mg/kg SC or IM or butorphanol (Torbugesic, Fort Dodge) at 0.2 to 0.4 mg/kg SC or IM every 6 to 8 hours (either drug) as needed.

DISEASES AND CONDITIONS

Dermatitis

Dermatitis may be caused by parasitism, bacterial, viral, and fungal infections, neoplasia, immune-mediated diseases, or trauma. Hedgehogs are susceptible to a large number of external parasites, and wild-caught animals are nearly always afflicted. Commonly encountered parasites include fleas, a wide variety of ticks, and several species of mites, especially *Chorioptes* spp. Ticks may be seen with the naked eye and are easily removed manually. Mite infestations may be subclinical or result in severe skin scaling and/or otitis. Mite infestation may be diagnosed with standard skin-scraping techniques. Ivermectin (Ivomec, Merck AgVet) at 0.2 to 0.4 mg/kg PO or SC 2 weeks apart for a total of three treatments is generally effective. It is important to remember to treat and/or thoroughly clean the environment when one treats for any ectoparasite. Follow-up skin scrapings several months after treatment should be performed to ensure complete eradication of the parasite.

Fungal infections of the skin are also commonly encountered in hedgehogs, particularly in animals recently taken from the wild. The clinical signs include crusting of the skin, particularly around the base of the spines, spine loss, and pruritus. Infections may also be subclinical. Commonly isolated fungi include *Trichophyton* and *Microsporum* spp. Dermatomycoses may be found secondary to bacterial infections, mite infestations, or traumatic wounds. Diagnosis is made with standard Dermatophyte Test Medium and/or microscopic examination of the affected spines. Reported treatments include griseofulvin (Grifulvin V, Ortho Pharmaceuticals) at 50 mg/kg PO or ketoconazole (Nizoral, Janssen Pharmaceutical, Titusville, NJ 08560-0200) 10 mg/kg PO once daily for 6 to 8 weeks.

Trauma

Male-male or interspecific interactions may result in moderate to severe wounds. Topical and systemic antibiotics should be used where appropriate and according to culture and sensitivity results. Hedgehogs typically tolerate a variety of bandages and splints without a problem; however, anesthesia may be required in the application and changing of bandages. When needed, animals may be soaked in dilute topical disinfectants, such as chlorhexidine (Nolvasan, Fort Dodge), by placing them in a bucket and pouring properly diluted disinfectant over the animal to a depth of 2 to 4 cm (taking care to avoid the face and eyes). This therapy can be a useful adjunct in wound treatments.

Otitis

The clinical signs of otitis include scratching, aural discharge, head shaking, and, rarely, disturbances of balance. Otitis in the hedgehog is similar to that described in other small animals. There may be a discharge ranging from ceruminal to hemorrhagic. Occasionally, plugs of caseous material completely occlude the otic canal. Microscopic examination of ear exudate should always be performed with Gram's or cytology stains. Culture and sensitivity should be performed when indicated. In cases of otitis media or interna, radiographs of the skull are indicated. If generalized pruritus or dermatitis is present, investigate for underlying systemic disease, such as mites or ticks, bacterial or fungal agents, hypothyroidism, or allergies.

Diet-Related Illnesses

Obesity is the most commonly encountered diet-related illness in pet hedgehogs and may be caused by overfeeding, lack of adequate exercise, or feeding an excessively high-fat diet. Obesity may result in poor skin condition, fatty liver, respiratory and immune system compromise, and dermatitis secondary to excessive skin folds. Other diet-related illnesses include hepatic lipidosis, rickets, dental tartar or periodontitis, hyper- or hypovitaminosis (vitamins A and D), poor integumentary spine growth, and other growth abnormalities. Treatment is aimed at correcting the diet and providing appropriate supplementation when necessary. Owners should frequently monitor the weight of pet hedgehogs and adjust the amounts fed appropriately. Exercise should be encouraged by provision of adequate cage space, exercise wheels, or other equipment.

Dental Disease

Fractured and/or abscessed teeth are a relatively common cause of anorexia, weight loss, and salivation in hedgehogs. Periodontal disease is also frequently observed. Hedgehogs presenting with dental disease frequently have a history of poor diet and/or of being fed only soft foods. Diagnosis may be made by observation of dental tartar accumulation, inflamed gingiva, deep periodontal pockets, mobile teeth, or facial abcessation. The use of a dental probe to determine the depth of gingival sulci aids in the evaluation of periodontal disease. Radiography may be helpful in selected cases.

The progression of disease is similar to that found in other small animals. Early forms of periodontitis respond well to traditional therapies. Once teeth have become mobile, they must usually be extracted. Animals thrive on a soft diet even when all teeth have been extracted. In mild cases of periodontal disease, extraction of mobile teeth and systemic antibiotic therapy is usually curative. Dental disease may be prevented by providing a sound diet that includes firm foods (e.g., dry commercial cat food, hard-bodied insects, and raw vegetables). If the hedgehog is a pet that tolerates tooth brushing, the teeth may be brushed with either a soft-bristled cat toothbrush or gauze sponges wrapped around a finger. Commercial dentifrices made for cats work well for hedgehogs.

Endoparasites

A variety of nematode, cestode, and protozoal internal parasites have been identified in the hedgehog. The incidence of infestation is greatest in wild-caught animals. Animals may be asymptomatic or exhibit clinical signs, such as diarrhea or weight loss. Nematode infestations are treated with either ivermectin at 0.2 mg/kg PO or SC or fenbendazole (Panacur, Hoechst Roussel) at 10 to 15 mg/kg PO. Cestodiasis may be treated with praziquantel (Droncit, Bayer) at 7 mg/kg SC or PO. Each of these should be repeated in 2 or 3 weeks. Metronidazole (Flagyl, Searle) at 25 mg/kg PO b.i.d. for 5 days is generally effective for most protozoal infections.

Diarrhea

Diarrhea is a common clinical condition in hedgehogs with etiologies similar to those found in other small mammals. Clues to diagnosis are provided by complete physical examination, radiography, complete blood count (CBC) and serum chemistry panels, fecal culture and sensitivity, fecal smear and flotation, and ultrasonography. Whenever possible, treatment should be directed at the primary cause. Supportive care includes administration of a bland, hypoallergenic diet (e.g., low-fat cottage cheese and boiled lamb), parenteral electrolyte fluids, and antibiotics when indicated.

Salmonellosis has been reported in several species of hedgehogs. Its incidence and course are similar to that in most other animals. In addition to animals with obvious signs of diarrhea, *Salmonella* may be shed by asymptomatic carriers. Owners should be warned of the zoonotic potential and the possibility of the development of a carrier state. As with other animals, strict hygiene is important for people handling hedgehogs.

Anorexia and Weight Loss

Anorexia is another common clinical presentation in hedgehogs. The common etiologies include dental or gastrointestinal disease, parasites, hepatic lipidosis, neoplasia, pneumonia, chilling, systemic disease, pain, and behavioral factors (competition, diet, or husbandry change). Treatment should be aimed at the specific etiology and instituted as rapidly as possible, since extended periods of anorexia may predispose animals to the development of hepatic lipidosis. Supportive care may include force-feeding or tube feeding (with the use of a commercial feline tube-feeding formula and narrow-gauge soft catheter), parenteral administration of balanced electrolyte solutions, and increasing the environmental temperature to 28 to 30°C (80 to 85°F).

TABLE 2. Antibiotics and Antifungals

Amoxicillin	15 mg/kg IM PO q12hr
Ampicillin	10 mg/kg IM PO q24hr
Chloramphenicol	50 mg/kg PO q12hr
	30–50 mg/kg SC, IM, IV, IO q12hr
Enrofloxacin	5.0–10 mg/kg PO, SC q12hr
Griseofulvin	50 mg/kg PO
Penicillin G	40,000 IU/kg IM s.i.d.
SMZ/TMP	30 mg/kg IM PO q12hr
Sulfadimethoxine	2–20 mg/day IM, SC, PO

SMZ, sulfamethazine; TMP, trimethoprim.

Neoplasia

A wide variety of tumors and disseminated neoplastic processes have been described, affecting virtually every body system. Animals more than 3 years of age are particularly susceptible. Diagnosis is based on biopsy or necropsy and histopathology. A report demonstrated the presence of a retrovirus that may contribute to the pathogenesis of tumors in these animals. Treatments other than surgical excision have not been reported. Prognosis and management depend on the type and stage of the neoplastic process.

Respiratory Infections

As mentioned previously, animals that are kept at low environmental temperatures are particularly susceptible to respiratory infections, including rhinitis, laryngitis, tracheitis, and pneumonia. Typical clinical signs include nasal discharge, sneezing, wheezing, dyspnea, and anorexia and weight loss. Reported etiologies include *Bordetella bronchiseptica*, *Pasteurella*, and cytomegalovirus. Respiratory tract nematodes (common in wild animals), such as *Crenosoma striatum* and *Capillaria aerophila,* may contribute to the development or pathogenesis of pneumonia. Common differential diagnoses for snuffling, sneezing, and/or nasal discharge include normal vocalizations, allergies, and foreign body inhalation. Standard techniques such as hematology, radiology, fecal examinations, and tracheal washes may be employed to aid in the diagnosis. Ideally, antibiotic treatment should be based on the results of appropriate culture and sensitivity studies (Table 2). Useful adjunct therapy includes parenteral fluids, supplemental heat and oxygen, and nebulization.

Other Conditions

Other diseases that have been reported in the literature, but are seen less frequently include papillomas, foot-and-mouth disease, Q fever, pseudotuberculosis (*Yersinia pseudotuberculosis*), mycobacterial infections, and rabies.

References and Suggested Reading

Done LB, Dietze M, Cranfield M, et al: Necropsy Lesions by Body Systems in African Hedgehogs (*Atelerix albiventris*): Clues to Clinical Diagnosis. Proceedings of the American Association of Zoo Veterinarians, 1992, pp 110–112.
  A systematic review of postmortem lesions found in a large collection of hedgehogs at a zoologic institution.
Hoefer HL: Hedgehogs. Vet Clin North Am Small Anim Pract 24:113, 1994.

A guide to the care and treatment of captive hedgehogs.

Isenbugel E, Baumgartner RA: Diseases of the hedgehog. In: Fowler ML, ed: Zoo and Wild Animal Medicine Current Therapy 3. Philadelphia: WB Saunders, 1993, pp 294–301.
A thorough review of diseases and conditions in European hedgehogs, including a complete formulary.

Johnson-Delaney CA: Hedgehogs. In: Exotic Companion Medicine Handbook. Lake Worth, FL: Wingers Publishing, 1996, pp 2–14.
A concise guide to the diagnosis and treatment of common pet hedgehog conditions, including formulary and blood reference values.

Keymer IF, Gibson EA, Reynolds DJ: Zoonoses and other findings in hedgehogs (*Erinaceus europaeus*): A survey of mortality and review of the literature. Vet Record 128:245, 1991.
A review of zoonotic and infectious diseases previously reported in European hedgehogs.

Smith AJ: Neonatology of the hedgehog (*Atelerix albiventris*). J Small Exotic Anim Med 3:15, 1995.
A review of hedgehog reproduction, neonatal care, and pediatric therapeutics.

Dental Disease in Lagomorphs and Rodents

DAVID A. CROSSLEY

Chorlton, United Kingdom

INTRODUCTION

Before one can recognize the abnormal, it is necessary to have an idea of what is normal. When the clinician is unsure about a potentially abnormal finding, it is usually accurate to extrapolate from closely related species. If there is still uncertainty, the clinician should contact a more experienced colleague. Access to a good library or reliable sources on the Internet is also useful.

Lagomorphs. The most likely lagomorph to be presented in general practice is the domesticated rabbit (*Oryctolagus cuniculus*). All lagomorphs are principally grazers, feeding on grasses and other low-growing plants. Their dentition has evolved to provide an effective mechanism for slicing off vegetation and then grinding it sufficiently for digestion. Lagomorphs are distinguished from rodents by having two incisor teeth on each side of the maxilla—rodents have only one. The second maxillary incisor of lagomorphs is small and peg shaped. This "peg tooth" is positioned palatal to the substantial main incisor. Congenital absence of the peg teeth occurs in some lines of domestic rabbits. The first maxillary and the mandibular incisors normally wear in a chisel pattern (Fig. 1) because the enamel is much thicker on the labial surface. The three maxillary and two mandibular premolars have large ridged occlusal surfaces and are similar in structure to all but the most caudal molars. The third molars tend to be small or, in dwarf breeds, absent. The cheek teeth are arranged in almost parallel rows on either side of the mouth. The width between the mandibular cheek tooth arcades is less than that of the maxillary teeth, the jaw pattern being similar to that seen in horses. In lagomorphs, the entire dentition grows and erupts throughout life without the formation of anatomic tooth roots.

Unlike rodents, lagomorphs do not regularly gnaw. During feeding, the animal gathers vegetation into the mouth, using the tongue and lips, where the slicing action of the incisors cuts it into manageable pieces. The cheek teeth grind food with a lateral chewing action. The anatomy of the rabbit's temporomandibular joint is such that the incisors and cheek teeth are not normally in occlusion at the same time (see Fig. 1). Considerable tooth wear occurs from food abrasion while the animal chews natural foods. Under normal circumstances, the rate of tooth growth and eruption matches the rate of wear.

Rodents. Rodents have four continuously growing incisor teeth, one in each quadrant of the mouth. These teeth are used for gnawing, using a dorsoventral-rostrocaudal chewing action. Considerable variation exists in the cheek tooth dentition. For simplicity, it is easiest to consider the cheek tooth dentition as falling into one of two functional groups that affect the dental problems to which they are susceptible. These two groups correspond with the type of diet the animals naturally eat. Species such as the rat (*Rattus* spp.), mouse (*Mus* spp.), and hamster (*Mesocricetus* spp.) have reduced numbers of small brachyodont (short-crowned) cheek teeth, which develop roots, stop growing, and stop erupting once they are in occlusion. Rodents with brachyodont cheek teeth tend to have a small

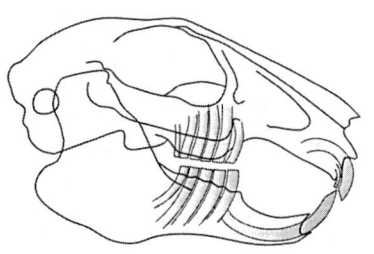
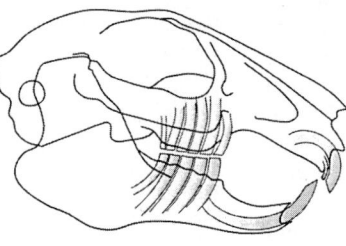

Figure 1. Normal occlusion in the European rabbit *Oryctolagus cuniculus.* Note the chisel form of the principal incisor teeth. *Left,* At rest, the incisor teeth are held in occlusion. In this position, the cheek teeth are separated a little so that they do not interfere with incisor function. *Right,* Cheek tooth occlusion. When the molars and premolars are brought into occlusion, the incisors are separated.

TABLE 1. Signs Associated With Dental Disease

Weight loss
Emaciation
Death
Poor coat condition
Matting of feces around anus
Other digestive disturbances
Fly strike (myiasis)
Noticeable reduction in food intake
Epiphora
Excessive salivation (slobbers)
Purulent ocular or nasal discharge
Dysphagia
Inability to fully close jaw
Reduced range of jaw movement
Discomfort on palpation over cheek teeth
Discomfort on manipulating jaw
Palpable bony swelling of ventral mandible
Mandibular prognathism
Visible incisor malocclusion or overgrowth
Facial abscessation
Mandibular abscessation
Submandibular or cervical lymphadenopathy
Exophthalmos
Systemic disease
Opportunistic infections

chewing surface area. These animals are adapted to a minimally abrasive diet that has a high energy concentration and requires little chewing. Species such as the guinea pig (*Cavia porcellus*) and chinchilla (*Chinchilla laniger*) have minimally reduced numbers of aradicular hypsodont (long-crowned, rootless) cheek teeth that continue growing and erupting throughout life and have a relatively large occlusal surface area. These animals eat large quantities of tough, low-energy, abrasive food. As with rabbits, cheek tooth growth and eruption match the rate of wear under normal circumstances.

Recognition of Dental Problems. Dental disease is common in pet rabbits and rodents and is a potential cause of many other problems. One of the earliest signs, frequently missed by owners, is reduction in food intake and resultant weight loss. An animal that is having difficulty eating will lose condition, will become susceptible to secondary infections, and may develop metabolic problems such as hepatic lipidosis. The author recommends accurate weighing of small pets during clinical examination and suggests that owners do this at home on a weekly basis, with the results being recorded in a "health logbook." Table 1 lists other signs of dental problems.

CLINICAL EXAMINATION

A good clinical history provides a database from which to work. The next stage is an initial clinical examination. If the clinician recognizes a significant level of debility, he or she should start supportive therapy before completing all necessary investigations. A thorough oral examination is essential. Examination of the conscious patient's oral cavity is restricted in many species by small size, a long diastema, and a limited oral aperture. An exception to this is the Syrian hamster (*Mesocricetus auratus*), because the highly elastic cheeks can be drawn back to open the mouth

for a thorough examination, which should include the cheek pouches.

A bright light source and magnification are necessary for visualization of oral lesions. In many species, an otoscope can be used as an oral endoscope. Many oral lesions can be recognized in conscious patients, *but* negative findings do not rule out a dental problem. Approximately 50% of visible oral lesions are missed when this technique is used. Chemical immobilization facilitates oral examination because it permits the use of mouth gags and cheek dilators to improve access and visibility within the oral cavity. The use of a small dental mirror is also helpful. The tongue and cheeks are highly sensitive and are easily irritated by minor tooth irregularities. Periodontal probing (with a standard human instrument that has been shortened) helps detect periodontal lesions and mobile teeth. Caries and other coronal lesions can be detected by running the tip of a sharp dental explorer over exposed tooth surfaces. When possible, a finger should be inserted into the mouth for direct palpation of structures. This is the most sensitive technique for detecting sharp edges on teeth. Grossly visible spikes on the teeth represent an advanced stage of disease. Even with the use of anesthesia, approximately 25% of visible lesions are still missed by experienced observers, as revealed by postmortem examination in unsuccessful cases. Table 2 lists common oral lesions.

Obviously, tooth root and bone pathology are not usually visible, so radiography is routinely indicated. In rabbits and the larger rodents, high-definition screen-film combinations may be of use when one uses radiography purely as a screening method, but to obtain adequate definition for dental investigations it is necessary to use nonscreen or dental film. Films should be examined with the use of magnification. Common radiographic lesions are listed in Table 3.

TREATMENT OF DENTAL PROBLEMS

Once a dental problem has been recognized, the prognosis must be assessed and an appropriate treatment regimen started. An important aspect of treatment is ensuring the welfare of the patient. If the disease is advanced, it may

TABLE 2. Probable Findings on Oral and Dental Examination

Perioral saliva staining, erythema, alopecia, pyoderma
Pain on palpation of maxillary zygomatic process
Swellings on ventral surface of mandible
Ocular and/or nasal discharge
Lip scarring, ulceration, laceration, perforation
Cheek pouch inflammation, impaction, etc.
Incisor tooth overgrowth, damage, dysplasia, deformity, or absence
Gingivitis, periodontitis, pyorrhea of incisor teeth
Mucosal ulceration: tongue, cheek, palate, lip
Fibrous scarring of cheeks and sides of tongue
Deep laceration to tongue and/or cheek
Sharp "spikes" on cheek teeth (may not be visible—test by palpation)
Cheek tooth overgrowth, damage, dysplasia, deformity, caries, or absence
Gingivitis, periodontitis, pyorrhea, food impaction between cheek teeth
Mass lesions, abscesses, and occasionally tumors
Foreign bodies
Jaundice, petechiae

TABLE 3. Dental- and Jaw-Related Lesions Detectable on Radiography

Coronal overgrowth of incisors and/or cheek teeth
Coronal deformities
Tooth and jaw fractures
Irregularity of occlusal plane
Relative mandibular prognathism
Temporomandibular joint abnormalities
Tooth root elongation and deformities
Apical perforation of alveolar bone
Increased lacrimal canal radiodensity
Periodontal bone destruction
Tooth root abscesses
Facial and some retrobulbar abscesses
Bone tumors

be necessary to recommend euthanasia on humane grounds. A high proportion of affected animals have severe pain that can, at best, be only temporarily relieved by treatment. It is unfair to subject such animals to a continued life of misery. Certain dental problems can be easily cured, and some others successfully managed in the longer term. Whichever the case may be, adequate follow-up is required in monitoring for recurrence or other problems.

Fractured Incisors. A common traumatic injury is fracture of an incisor tooth. Treatment is undertaken in three stages. First, treat visible injuries. Second, administer antibiotics and analgesics. Once the condition of the animal is stabilized, smooth sharp edges on the fractured teeth with a dental bur. Treat pulp exposures under aseptic conditions by partial pulpectomy and pulp capping by application of a hard-setting calcium hydroxide cement. The teeth will be expected to wear once they have grown back; thus, it is important *not* to use a hard or toxic restorative material in these teeth. The opposing teeth need trimming at regular intervals to compensate for the lack of wear until the damaged teeth regrow and return to function. The affected teeth may fail to regrow or they may develop a deformity if the periapical tissues were seriously damaged. In this situation, there are two options: regular trimming or extraction of the affected and the opposing teeth.

Methods of Tooth Trimming. Traditionally, tooth trimming in rabbits and rodents has been performed while the animal is conscious and with the use of nail clippers or wire cutters. This method is unacceptable for several reasons. Excessive force is applied to the tooth crown, and this force damages the periapical germinal tissues and periodontal ligament, affecting future tooth growth. Longitudinal splits often occur in the teeth, extending subgingivally or exposing the pulp cavity. The procedure is painful even if pulp exposure is avoided. The teeth are not returned to their natural chisel shape. Accurate tooth trimming requires the use of a high-speed dental drill, which cuts while applying minimal force to the tooth. A fine-taper fissure bur in a low-speed dental handpiece is also acceptable. The pulp cavity usually does not extend beyond the tooth's normal occlusal height, often reaching only just above the level of the gingiva, so exposure should not occur when the teeth are simply returned to normal shape and length. While sedation or anesthesia is preferred, the reshaping can

be humanely performed in conscious animals with minimal restraint, provided that they are accustomed to handling. In unconscious animals, a bur in a straight, low-speed handpiece is also the best instrument for removing spikes and adjusting the occlusal planes in species with continuously growing cheek teeth. The common method of rasping rabbit and rodent cheek teeth is both inefficient and damaging to the periodontal tissues.

Abscesses. Facial abscessation in rabbits and rodents is usually associated with dental disease, foreign bodies, or wounds from fighting. Preoperative radiography is essential in forming a surgical plan. Surgical excision of the abscess is preferred whenever feasible. Any tracts of infection should be traced back to their origin. The wound is usually left open to granulate. Recurrence of abscessation should be anticipated if the underlying cause was not found and removed.

Extractions. Preoperative radiography allows the identification of abnormal root morphology that can complicate extraction. When brachyodont teeth are affected, extractions are usually straightforward. Gentle progressive elevation and luxation can be achieved with the use of fine instruments. When necessary, hypodermic needles can be bent to create custom-made instruments. Rarely, supereruption of an opposing tooth occurs following extraction of a brachyodont tooth. Extraction of hypsodont teeth is not as simple. Careful elevation, with sectioning and removal of successive portions, is generally effective when the root is too long to remove in one piece. An extraoral approach via the ventral mandible can also be used for mandibular cheek teeth. The affected tooth is elevated and either repulsed into the oral cavity or removed via the surgical access. Access to the maxillary cheek teeth may be improved by performing a buccotomy. This is a traumatic procedure and should be avoided if possible. Follow-up must be maintained if hypsodont teeth are extracted, as the opposing teeth will need occasional occlusal adjustment to prevent overgrowth.

Extraction of incisor teeth is quite straightforward once the anatomy is accurately identified. Radiography is routinely required for assessing root length and morphology. The crowns should be shortened, preferably with the use of a high-speed dental bur, so that there is just enough remaining to accommodate a mouth gag. Once any intraoral work has been completed (it is difficult to hold the mouth open following extraction of the incisors), the area is cleansed with a dilute oral disinfectant solution. A No. 11 scalpel blade is used to cut the gingival epithelial attachment within the gingival sulcus around each incisor tooth, and the incision is extended as far down the periodontal ligaments as possible. At this stage, the fairly straight-rooted peg teeth of rabbits are extracted with a small carnivore elevator, like that used for cats' teeth. Extraction of these teeth at this stage avoids the risk of their fracture during extraction of the larger incisor teeth. By repeatedly inserting a purpose-designed curved luxator or, if that is not available, a fine-tipped feline dental elevator lateral and medial to each large incisor and holding the tooth under lateral pressure for 20 seconds in each position, the fibers of the periodontal ligament are stretched and

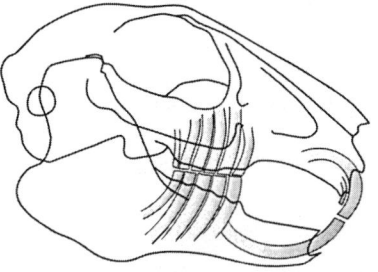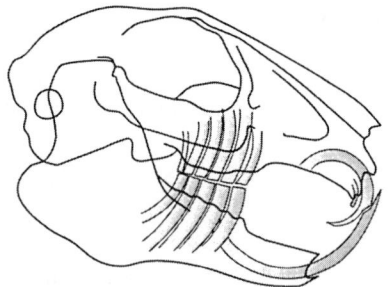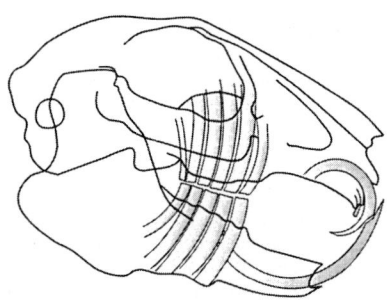

Figure 2. Development of incisor and cheek tooth overgrowth in dwarf-breed rabbits. Compare the tooth alignment with the normal occlusion shown in Figure 1. *Left,* Many dwarf rabbits have a relative mandibular prognathism that leads to the incisors and cheek teeth being in occlusion at the same time. Incisor wear abnormalities may be recognized early in life. *Center,* Over a period of time, the reduced wear leads to coronal elongation of all the teeth. As the mouth is forced open, the resting angle between the palate and the rostral mandible becomes almost parallel. *Right,* Increased resting occlusal pressure prevents normal tooth eruption. Root elongation occurs as a result of continued apical growth. The affected teeth are now more susceptible to periodontal and endodontic disease.

torn. After a few minutes, patience will be rewarded by loosening of the teeth. Once a tooth loosens sufficiently, it can be extracted with the fingers or gentle use of forceps by applying rotational tension along the path of eruption. The extracted tooth should be examined to ensure that it is intact and the pulpal tissue has also been removed from the alveolus. Hemorrhage is usually minimal. If the gingiva has been torn or hemorrhage persists, suturing is advised with the use of a fine absorbable material with a swaged-on cutting needle, otherwise the gingiva is just squeezed together across the sockets. Antibiotics are indicated only if there is evidence of alveolar infection. The normal reason for extraction is nonfunctional incisors; thus, most patients will already have adapted to eating without the use of these teeth. Incisor extraction is an excellent means of managing incisor overgrowth in rabbits when repeated trimmings are undesirable to the owner. This situation most frequently arises in dwarf-breed rabbits with congenital relative mandibular prognathism (Fig. 2). These animals often have cheek tooth problems (crown and root) in addition to the obvious overgrowth of the incisors, so a full assessment should be performed prior to treatment.

Potential Complications. Extractions in rabbits and rodents require a gentle technique to avoid root or jaw fracture. Iatrogenic folding fractures of the lower jaw are a potentially serious complication in rabbits and rodents, resulting in secondary cheek tooth malocclusion. As rabbit and rodent incisor teeth grow continually, when a root fractures, the remaining portion may continue growing. In the author's experience, rabbits' small peg teeth are the most likely to break, but the fractured roots are also quite easy to extract, unlike any remaining portions of the strongly curved larger first incisors. When the clinician discusses cases prior to treatment, clients are routinely advised that a second anesthetic may be required at a later date to complete the procedure. If root fragments are left, the owners are advised accordingly and arrangements are made to assess the patient for their regrowth.

Provided that the teeth are extracted in their entirety, aradicular hypsodont teeth do not normally regrow and have never done so in the author's experience; however, two cases have been reported to him in which the veterinar-

ian performing the procedure was certain that the teeth were extracted intact. It is suspected that in these two cases the operative technique was so gentle that the periapical tissues were not traumatized by the extractions. To reduce this possibility, it is now recommended that the clinician ensure that the pulp is removed along with the tooth. If it is not, a pair of curved mosquito forceps are inserted into the alveolus to grasp this tissue and remove it.

PREVENTION OF DENTAL DISEASE

More important than the treatment of disease is its prevention. In the wild, each species has evolved to cope with its natural environment and diet. Careful management of an animal's environment and diet to mimic what would be found in the wild provides the best way of preventing dental and other health problems from developing. Many species of rodent spend much of their spare time gnawing. Providing a suitable medium is essential for preventing incisor malocclusion. In contrast, rabbits do not require materials to gnaw, as this is not a normal behavior in lagomorphs.

Rabbits and rodents are selective feeders. If they are provided with a choice, they will eat more concentrated energy sources first. Other dietary components containing essential vitamins and mineral supplements may remain uneaten, with resulting dietary imbalances and deficiencies. Also, preferred items generally require less chewing and are less abrasive than natural foods. In species with continuously growing teeth, this results in tooth overgrowth and root elongation. In hypsodont rodents and lagomorphs, limiting concentrates and providing a source of grass or hay reduce the incidence of oral disease. Exposure to sunlight can also help improve bone and tooth structure, as increased vitamin D activation helps promote calcium metabolism.

References and Suggested Reading

Brown SA: Incisor removal in the rabbit. Proceedings of the North American Veterinary Conference, 1993: Orlando, 791–792.
Burling K, Murphy CJ, Silva PA, et al: Anatomy of the rabbit nasolacrimal

duct and its clinical implications. Prog Vet Comp Ophthalmol 1:33, 1991.

Crossley DA: Dental Disease in Rabbits and Herbivorous Rodents. In: Proceedings of British Veterinary Dental Association, Birmingham, April 1995.

Crossley DA: Clinical aspects of lagomorph dental anatomy: The rabbit (Oryctolagus cuniculus). J Vet Dent 12:131, 1995.

Crossley DA: Clinical aspects of rodent dental anatomy. J Vet Dent 12:137, 1995.

Harcourt-Brown FM: A review of clinical conditions in pet rabbits associated with their teeth. Vet Rec 137:34, 1995.

Harcourt-Brown FM: Calcium deficiency, diet and dental disease in pet rabbits. Vet Rec 139:567, 1996.

Harkness JE, Wagner JE: The Biology and Medicine of Rabbits and Rodents, 3rd ed. Philadelphia: Lea & Febiger, 1983, pp 23, 27–28, 34, 48, 68–71, 86, 90–91, 97, 101, 142–143, 145–146.

Kennedy AH: Chinchilla Diseases and Ailments. Bewdley, Ontario: Clay Publishing, 1970, pp 60–74.

Lobprise HB, Wiggs RB: Dental and oral disease in lagomorphs. J Vet Dent 8:11, 1991.

Okerman L: Diseases of Domestic Rabbits. Oxford: Blackwell Scientific Publications, 1988, pp 9–12, 22–36, 40–41, 74, 86–87.

Remeeus PGK: The use of calcium hydroxide in the treatment of abscesses in the cheek of the rabbit resulting from a dental periapical disorder. J Vet Dent 12:1, 1995.

Richardson VCG: Diseases of Domestic Guinea Pigs. Oxford: Blackwell Scientific Publications, 1992, pp 74–78.

Wiggs RB, Lobprise HB: Dental disease in rodents. J Vet Dent 7:5, 1990.

Wiggs RB, Lobprise HB: Dentistry in pet lagomorphs and rodents. In: Crossley DA, Penman S, eds: BSAVA Manual of Small Animal Dentistry, 2nd ed. Cheltenham, UK: BSAVA, 1995, pp 67–91.

Neutering of Rabbits and Rodents

SUSAN A. BROWN
Westchester, Illinois

REASONS FOR NEUTERING

The primary reason clients request castration of rabbits and rodents is to prevent certain behaviors or to prevent pregnancy in cage mates. Primary testicular disease is uncommon in these species. Mature male rabbits spray urine to mark their territory in a manner similar to that of tomcats, and the odor of the urine can be very strong. Some male rodents also mark their territory with urine and develop a strong unpleasant urine odor. Male rabbits and rodents can become aggressive when they are sexually mature and may be difficult to handle.

The primary reasons an ovariohysterectomy (OVH) is requested in rabbits and rodents are to prevent disease and to prevent pregnancy. The most common neoplasia of female rabbits is uterine adenocarcinoma (Hillyer and Quesenberry, 1997; Harkness and Wagner, 1995). This malignancy occurs with such frequency that routine spaying of female rabbits is recommended as a preventive measure. In addition, spaying female rabbits prevents aggression, spraying of urine, and false pregnancies. Rodents have a lower incidence of uterine disease than do rabbits; however, they are more prone to ovarian and mammary gland disease. There is some evidence that ovariectomized rats may have a lower incidence of mammary and pituitary tumors (Hillyer and Quesenberry, 1997).

RECOMMENDED AGE FOR NEUTERING

Rabbits and rodents should be neutered after they reach sexual maturity. This age varies for each species and, as in the case of rabbits, for different breeds. It is unknown whether neutering prior to sexual maturity is detrimental to the long-term health of these animals; however, there is speculation that early neutering may cause a disruption in the maturation of the endocrine system, leading to later disease. In addition, it is more difficult to identify and locate the sexual organs in immature animals.

PRESURGICAL CONSIDERATIONS

A thorough presurgical examination is a necessity in all cases. Do not perform elective neutering procedures on animals that are overweight or are exhibiting other signs of disease. It may be useful, particularly in older patients, to obtain a presurgical complete blood cell count and serum biochemistry for surgical evaluation.

ANESTHESIA

This article does not include a detailed discussion of anesthesia in these species. There is a wealth of information on anesthetic protocols in all of the references listed (see *CVT XII*, p. 1322). The author uses isoflurane anesthesia by mask or endotracheal intubation for neutering procedures in rabbits and rodents. Preanesthetics are rarely necessary in small rodents; they can be anesthetized effectively in an anesthetic chamber or by anesthetic mask. It may be advantageous to use preanesthetic medications in rabbits and the larger rodents, such as guinea pigs, chinchillas, and prairie dogs, particularly if the patient is difficult to handle. Anesthetic monitoring is particularly important in these small species. Preanesthetic or intraoperative analgesia is very useful in both rabbits and rodents in minimizing stress due to pain. The use of analgesics improves the surgical success rate. Common analgesics include butorphanol (0.1 to 0.5 mg/kg SC or IV every 2 to 4 hours), buprenorphine (0.01 to 0.05 mg/kg SC, IM, or IV every 8 to 12 hours), flunixin (0.3 to 2.0 mg/kg PO or deep IM every 12 to 24 hours for no more than 3 consecutive days), and carprofen (1 mg/kg PO every 12 to 24 hours).

GENERAL SURGICAL CONSIDERATIONS

Prolonged presurgical fasting is not necessary because these species do not have the ability to vomit. Withholding food and water for periods longer than 6 hours presurgically can lead to a delay in the return to normal food consumption after surgery. Withhold food for a short period of time (2 to 3 hours) in large rodents, such as guinea pigs, chinchillas, and prairie dogs, to empty the cheek pouches of food material. In addition, clean the cheek pouches carefully with cotton-tipped applicators once the patient is anesthetized to prevent inhalation of this material.

One of the most important surgical considerations is keeping the patient warm during and after the surgical procedure. Avoid the excessive use of alcohol and water during surgical preparation because a wet patient's body temperature will drop precipitously. Use a surgical heating pad that covers as much of the patient's surface area as possible. An overhead heat lamp can be used for additional warmth. Clear plastic adhesive drapes are very useful because they not only allow visualization of the patient for anesthetic monitoring but also retain body heat more effectively than paper or cloth drapes. Monitor the patient's temperature during surgery. After surgery, provide a warm environment until the patient is fully conscious and observe the patient closely to prevent overheating.

It is important to elevate the patient's head slightly during the surgical procedure to prevent unnecessary and potentially life-threatening pressure on the diaphragm and small thoracic cavity. Gently express the bladder prior to abdominal procedures. Rabbits have a large vaginal vault, which can fill with urine cranially if the bladder is expressed while the patient is in dorsal recumbency. Excessive urine in the cranial vaginal vault may interfere with an OVH. Therefore, express the rabbit's bladder with the caudal aspect of the abdomen lowered.

Handle rabbit and rodent tissues, including the skin, with great care because they are more friable than tissues in the canine and feline patient. Keep the skin flat, avoid clipping over the nipples, and use a fine clipper blade when preparing the surgical site. Use monofilament synthetic absorbable suture material for neutering rabbits and rodents. The use of chromic gut has been associated with granulomas and a higher rate of wound dehiscence, in the author's experience. Stainless steel and tantalum surgical clips can also be used for vessel and small pedicle ligation. Since rabbits and rodents can and often will effectively remove skin sutures with their sharp incisors, use a subcuticular layer to close the skin. Apply a thin layer of surgical glue to completely oppose the skin edges as needed. Alternatively, skin staples can be used in some species. The disadvantage to skin staples is that they may not hold well in animals with thin skin and they can occasionally be removed and ingested. Avoid restraint apparatuses, such as Elizabethan collars, unless absolutely necessary because they are poorly tolerated by most rabbit and rodent patients and may interfere with postsurgical recovery.

Antibiotics are not necessary for routine, uncomplicated neutering procedures. Postsurgical adhesions can be seen, particularly in rabbit OVHs. Wash any powder from surgical gloves, and handle the abdominal viscera as little as possible. If postsurgical adhesions are anticipated, verap-amil (Calan, Searle Pharmaceuticals, Gadsden, AL) can be used at 200 µg/kg slowly IV or PO immediately after surgery and every 8 hours for a total of nine doses (Hillyer and Quesenberry, 1997).

Postsurgical analgesia should be used, particularly in patients that have had abdominal procedures. There are excellent and extensive discussions on analgesia in all of the references listed (see *CVT XII*, p. 1322).

ORCHIECTOMY

Rabbits

Sexually mature male rabbits have readily identifiable scrotal sacs, and retained testicles are uncommon. The rabbit can pull its testes into the inguinal canal; however, they can be easily pushed back into the scrotal sacs by applying caudoventral pressure to the prepubic area. Although male rabbits have an open inguinal canal, herniation of viscera rarely takes place even with an open castration; however, it is still advisable to functionally close the inguinal canal to prevent any potential problems. The techniques described for rabbit castration include open and closed techniques with prescrotal or scrotal approaches (Laber-Laird et al, 1996; Harkness and Wagner, 1995; Brown and Rosenthal, 1997; Hillyer and Quesenberry, 1997). Two techniques are described here that have been used successfully by the author. Both methods effectively close the superficial inguinal canal and prevent herniation.

The first technique described is for a closed castration. Place the rabbit in dorsal recumbency and carefully clip or pluck the hair on the scrotal sacs and disinfect the area. Make a 1 cm to 1.5 cm vertical incision midway along the length of the scrotum without incising the tunic. Remove the tunic intact, and pull off the proper ligament attaching the tunic to the scrotum. Strip away the facial attachments of the tunic with a dry gauze sponge and retract the testis caudally. Apply one or two clamps to the narrow portion of the tunic containing the spermatic vessels and vas deferens. Double-ligate the cord and tunic with 3-0 or 4-0 suture material. Alternatively, transfix the cord and tunic with suture material, taking care to avoid puncturing the spermatic vein or artery. Remove the tunic and associated structures caudal to the ligature. Appose the scrotal skin edges with your fingers, and leave the incisions open or alternatively apply a small amount of surgical glue to close the wound. The disadvantage of this technique in older animals is that the increased amount of fat associated with the cord may predispose it to slippage within the tunic after ligation.

The second technique described is for an open castration. The preparation and approach to the patient are the same as those for the closed technique; however, the initial incision should be made all the way through the tunic. Pull the testis away from its attachment to the tunic with the use of a dry gauze sponge. Retract the testis caudally until resistance is encountered. Clamp and double-ligate the spermatic cord and vas deferens, and remove the testis and cord caudal to the ligation. Allow the pedicle to slip back into the abdomen. Grasp the now empty tunic and retract it caudally while stripping its facial attachments with a dry gauze sponge. Clamp the tunic at the narrow cranial portion close to the body wall and double-ligate it. Remove the tunic caudal to the ligation. The scrotal incision is closed in the same manner as that described for the closed technique.

It is very important to keep recently castrated male rabbits away from intact females for 3 to 4 weeks postsurgically to prevent pregnancy due to the possibility of viable sperm being present in the remaining portion of the vas deferens.

Rodents

Rodents are castrated with the same techniques as those described for rabbits. Rodents are prone to herniation of viscera through the open inguinal canal after surgery; therefore, it is critical to functionally close this area. Guinea pigs, chinchillas, and prairie dogs do not have dependent scrotums, and it may be more difficult to identify the testis externally. Rodents can retract the testes into the inguinal canal; however as in the rabbit, the testes can be moved back out of the canal with ventrocaudal pressure. Retained testicles are uncommon in these species. Rodents have a larger epididymal fat pad than rabbits, and in some species it may be up to four times the size of the testicle. For this reason, the author finds the open castration technique, as described for the rabbit, the easiest method to use in order to be able to identify and ligate the proper structures. Close scrotal incisions in rodents with either surgical glue or subcuticular suture using 5-0 or smaller suture material. Keep recently castrated rodents away from intact females of the species for at least 3 weeks after surgery.

OVARIOHYSTERECTOMY

Rabbits

The technique for rabbit OVH has been described in a number of references (Hillyer and Quesenberry, 1997; Brown and Rosenthal, 1997; Laber-Laird et al, 1996). Rabbits have a bicornuate uterus, with each uterine cornua ending in a cervix and the absence of a uterine body. The uterus lies cranial and dorsal to the urinary bladder in a coiled position. The suspensory ligaments are loose, allowing the ovaries to be easily exteriorized. The mature female may have a large amount of fat in the mesovarium, mesosalpinx, and mesometrium. Handle this tissue with care because this fat is very friable.

Place the patient in dorsal recumbency, and clip the hair and surgically prepare the abdomen from the sternum to the pubis. Make a 2- to 3-cm midline incision approximately halfway between the umbilicus and the pubis. Identify the scant linea alba, grasp it with forceps, and lift it prior to making a shallow stab incision in order to avoid puncturing the cecum or bladder, which lie directly below. Carefully extend the incision with scissors. The uterus in sexually mature females is found dorsal to the cranial pole of the bladder. Grasp one horn with forceps. If a spay hook is used to exteriorize the horn, take great care to avoid tearing the delicate cecum. Retract the horn and locate the ovary and its associated oviduct, which is coiled around the ovary in the periovarian fat pad. It is important to remove all ovarian tissue and its associated structures. Handle the friable ovary as little as possible to avoid detaching pieces of ovarian tissue that may later reattach in the abdomen and become functional. It is not necessary to tear the suspensory ligament. The ovarian vessels in all but obese or pregnant animals are small but should be identified, clamped, and single- or double-ligated with 4-0 suture material. Bluntly dissect the broad ligament to allow visualization of the large uterine vessels lateral to the uterine horns and vagina. Double-ligate the uterine vessels just caudal to the cervices. Ligate the uterus just caudal to the cervices with 3-0 or 4-0 suture material to ensure that all uterine tissue is removed. Oversew the stump of the vagina as an additional barrier to urine contamination. If urine is present in the vaginal vault prior to ligation, carefully milk it out caudally and place a clamp at the area to be ligated to prevent leakage. Close the abdominal wall with 4-0 suture material. Place a continuous subcuticular suture layer, along with surgical glue, to appose the edges or use skin staples. Skin staples are removed in 7 to 10 days.

Rodents

Rodents have a bicornuate uterus with a short uterine body and one cervix. The suspensory ligaments are not significant and do not need to be ruptured in order to exteriorize the ovaries. The broad ligament is a fat storage site; in overweight animals, it can be difficult to readily identify blood vessels, and some dissection may be necessary. In chinchillas, guinea pigs, and prairie dogs, the gastrointestinal (GI) tract, particularly the cecum, can interfere with visualization of the ovaries. Handle the GI tract as little and as gently as possible to avoid postsurgical adhesions, rupturing delicate mesenteric blood vessels, and postsurgical ileus. If ovarian disease is diagnosed without uterine disease, it may be easier to perform an ovariectomy than an OVH.

The technique for OVH in rodents is similar to that described for rabbits. With the patient in dorsal recumbency and the abdomen surgically prepared, an incision is made halfway between the umbilicus and the pubis. The uterus is identified at the cranial pole of the kidney and exteriorized with forceps. Do not use a spay hook in rodents. As in the rabbit, retract the ovary and its associated fat pad and oviduct. Bluntly dissect through the fat, and identify and single- or double-ligate the ovarian vessels. In some species, it is necessary to ligate vessels in the fat of the broad ligament as it is dissected down to the body of the uterus. Ligate the large uterine vessels either separately or transfix them to the body of the uterus. Ligate and remove the uterus just cranial to the cervix. It is not necessary to oversew this area if the cervix is left intact. Close as described for the rabbit.

OVARIECTOMY

In rodents, ovariectomy is an option for treating primary ovarian disease or for preventing pregnancy. Techniques for ovariectomies have been described in several references (Harkness and Wagner, 1995; Laber-Laird et al, 1996; Brown and Rosenthal, 1997).

Place the patient in ventral recumbency, and clip the

hair and surgically prepare the dorsal abdominal area from approximately T13 to L6. In small rodents make either a midline incision from L2 to L5 or two transverse incisions on either side of L3. If a midline incision is made, the skin can be shifted to each side to make the approach through the muscle into the abdominal cavity. In rats and guinea pigs, make two transverse incisions just caudal to the last rib and lateral and ventral to the paralumbar muscles. Bluntly dissect through the muscles of the flank lateral to the paralumbar muscles, and incise the peritoneum. Each ovary is located near the caudal pole of the kidney within the periovarian fat pad. Paralumbar fat can be mistaken for periovarian fat, the difference being that the periovarian fat is freely movable. Identify the ovary and associated oviduct, and ligate the ovarian vessels. Handle the periovarian fat, rather than the ovary, to avoid producing ovarian remnants that may be released into the abdomen and later reattach and become functional. One source recommends—in addition to removing the ovaries—locating the cranial tip of the uterine horn and ligating this area (Brown and Rosenthal, 1997). Some rodents have remnants of ovarian tissue associated with each uterine tube, and removal of the cranial tip of the uterine horn removes this tissue. Close the abdomen with 4-0 or smaller suture material and the skin with subcuticular sutures or skin staples.

References and Suggested Reading

Brown SA, Rosenthal KL: Self-Assessment Color Review of Small Mammals. Ames: Iowa State University Press, 1997.
A self-assessment book containing detailed information on the medical and surgical care of rabbits, rodents, hedgehogs, and primates.
Harkness JE, Wagner JE: The Biology and Medicine of Rabbits and Rodents. Media, PA: Williams & Wilkins, 1995.
A comprehensive textbook covering the medical and surgical care of rabbits, guinea pigs, rats, hamsters, gerbils, and mice.
Hillyer EV, Quesenberry KE: Ferrets, Rabbits and Rodents: Clinical Medicine and Surgery. Philadelphia: WB Saunders, 1997.
A comprehensive textbook covering the medical and surgical care of rabbits, guinea pigs, chinchillas, rats, hamster, gerbils, and mice.
Laber-Laird K, Swindle MM, Flecknell P: Handbook of Rodent and Rabbit Medicine. Oxford, UK: Elsevier Science Ltd., 1996.
A comprehensive textbook covering all aspects of the medical and surgical care of rabbits, guinea pigs, chinchillas, rats, hamsters, gerbils, and mice.

Trichobezoars and Gastric Stasis in Rabbits

JAMES W. CARPENTER

Manhattan, Kansas

INTRODUCTION

Trichobezoars (hairballs, fur balls, "wool block") are masses of hair that occur commonly in the stomachs of mature rabbits. The prevalence of masses of hair retained within rabbits' stomachs is unknown, but hairballs are common in the stomachs of healthy rabbits. Although trichobezoar is the common term used to describe these cases, some authors prefer the terms *gastric stasis* or *gastrointestinal hypomotility* to better reflect the clinical condition. These terms are probably appropriate, because this syndrome can occur in rabbits that have not ingested large amounts of hair, but have developed gastric retention of ingested foods.

Multiple factors lead to hairball formation; however, the major contributing factor in rabbits appears to be a low-fiber diet. Contributing factors include the following: the small, relatively nondistensible, but well-developed and muscular lapine pyloric sphincter; an inability to vomit; and the common habit of consuming hair during grooming. Another clinically relevant feature of the rabbit gastrointestinal system is the myoelectrical initiation of peristalsis that occurs in the distal duodenum or jejunum, rather than in the stomach. These factors allow hair to accumulate in the lapine stomach, which may account for the common occurrence of trichobezoars in rabbits. Additional factors, including the animal's physiologic state (i.e., pregnancy and obesity, boredom, and stress), may contribute to the formation of trichobezoars.

NUTRITION

Rabbits require large amounts of fiber in the diet (approximately 15 to 16% crude fiber) to promote intestinal motility and minimize intestinal disease. Diets low in fiber increase the incidence of intestinal hypomotility, prolong cecal retention time, reduce feed intake, and predispose to diarrhea. Coarse, nondigestible particles stimulate normal gastrointestinal processes, including secretion, digestion, absorption, peristalsis, and excretion. Normal peristalsis occurs with the ingestion of a high-fiber diet that provides a large particle size and that results in a lattice-like food ball for effective gastric acid penetration. Incomplete gastric acid penetration of foods consisting of small particles may result in the production of hard-packed food balls, especially in rabbits consuming marginal amounts of water (Brooks, 1997).

The preferred diet for the pet rabbit is a high-quality, high-fiber (15 to 16% crude fiber) pelleted diet containing 13 to 18% crude protein, at the rate of one-quarter cup of pellets per 2.3 kg body weight divided into two meals per day. Some rabbits do well when pellets are offered ad libitum, provided that overeating and obesity are avoided and the rabbit consumes adequate amounts of loose hay.

Pellets must be supplemented with loose hay (mixed grass hay, timothy hay, or high-quality dried grass clippings), provided ad libitum. Alfalfa hay can be offered throughout the growth stages, but should then be discontinued because of its high protein content. The diet can be supplemented with a small amount (up to one cup) of dark fibrous, leafy greens (kale, mustard greens, carrot tops, parsley, or dandelion greens) and fresh vegetables (carrots, broccoli, green peppers, cauliflower, or cabbage) per 2.3 kg body weight daily or several times per week. In addition, rabbits can receive a small amount (up to one tablespoon per 2.3 kg body weight) of fresh fruit (strawberries, other berries, apples) daily or several times per week.

HISTORY AND CLINICAL SIGNS

Trichobezoars and gastric stasis are most commonly characterized by anorexia (frequently of 2 to 7 days' duration) and oligodipsia (hypodipsia). The volume and number of fecal pellets produced are decreased, they may contain hair, and in some cases there is a lack of fecal production. The rabbit may be alert or depressed. There may be weight loss, depending on the chronicity of the problem and the hydration status. In some cases of trichobezoars and gastric stasis, diarrhea may be present. The history may also reveal the following: a high-carbohydrate, low-fiber diet; excessive grooming and ingestion of hair (especially during the shedding season); boredom; or a stressful environment.

In acute pyloric obstruction, severe depression, lethargy, bloating, dehydration, hypothermia, and shock may occur (Quesenberry, 1994). Death can result from prolonged anorexia and metabolic imbalance if the obstruction is not removed or the stasis is not corrected. Hepatic lipidosis is a lesion commonly associated with this syndrome.

DIAGNOSIS

Although the diagnosis of trichobezoars and gastric stasis in rabbits is generally made on the basis of the history, clinical signs, physical examination, and results of abdominal radiographs, a definitive diagnosis can be difficult in some cases. Generally, a complete blood count and serum chemistry analysis are obtained to assess the overall condi-

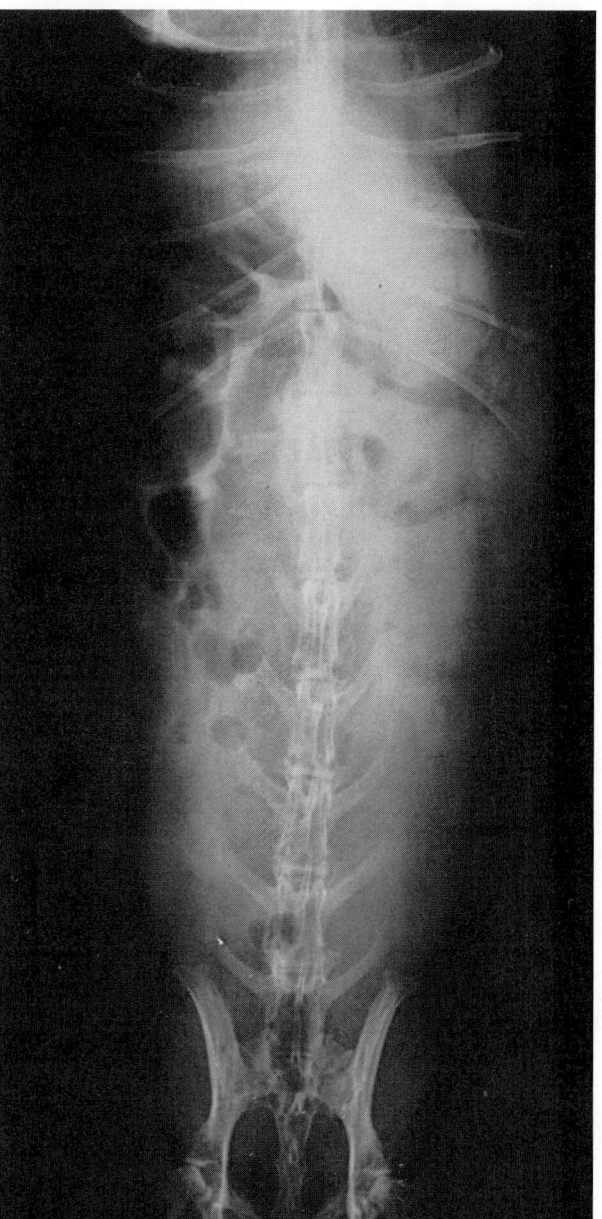

Figure 2. A ventrodorsal radiograph of the abdomen of a rabbit with a trichobezoar and gastric stasis. Note the tubular distention of the stomach. (From Gentz EJ, Harrenstien LA, Carpenter JW: Dealing with gastrointestinal, genitourinary, and musculoskeletal problems in rabbits. Vet Med [April]:365–372, 1995, with permission.)

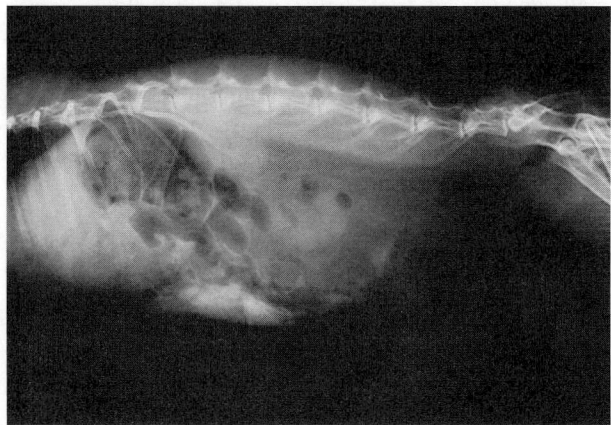

Figure 1. A lateral radiograph of the abdomen of a rabbit with a trichobezoar and gastric stasis. Note the gas-distended stomach and intestines.

tion of the rabbit and to help rule out other causes of the generally nonspecific clinical signs.

The antemortem diagnosis is frequently confirmed by palpation. The stomach can be palpated in the cranial abdomen as a large, doughy mass, although in some cases the mass may feel rather firm. However, it should be noted that the size of the mass does not always correlate with the incidence of clinical illness, because small, nonpalpable trichobezoars at the pylorus can be clinically significant. Gas also may be palpable in the gastrointestinal tract, supporting the diagnosis of gastrointestinal stasis.

Radiographically, distention of the stomach with ingesta and displacement of the intestines is suggestive of a gastric trichobezoar (Figs. 1 and 2), although delayed emptying from other causes results in the same radiographic appearance. In some cases, the radiographic appearance may be very similar to normal ingesta, so it cannot be relied on to differentiate gastric hairballs from normal gastric contents (Gillett et al, 1983). Gas-filled bowel loops or a gas-filled stomach may be seen. Gas in the gastrointestinal tract is generally caused by bacterial fermentation secondary to hypomotility or stasis. Contrast radiography, with the use of barium at 10 to 14 ml/kg PO, may aid in the diagnosis but is often nondiagnostic (Fig. 3).

Often, a definitive diagnosis of trichobezoar and gastric stasis can be made only following exploratory laparotomy (Fig. 4).

TREATMENT

Most rabbits with trichobezoars and gastric stasis respond to aggressive medical management consisting of parenteral fluids, force-feeding, and rehydration of the stomach contents, and stimulation of gastric motility by administering a high-fiber diet with metoclopramide or cisapride (Table 1).

Subcutaneous administration of isotonic fluids (i.e., lactated Ringer's solution) helps to improve and maintain hydration. Although the daily fluid requirements of a rabbit is approximately 100 to 120 ml/kg, administering 50 to 60

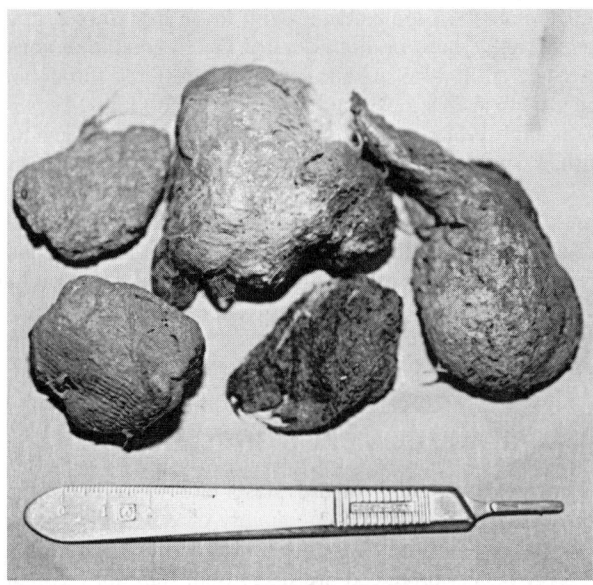

Figure 4. The gastric trichobezoar removed in pieces from the rabbit in Figures 2 and 3 weighed a total of 107 gm. Trichobezoars and gastric stasis are most commonly associated with a low-fiber diet. (From Gentz EJ, Harrenstien LA, Carpenter JW: Dealing with gastrointestinal, genitourinary, and musculoskeletal problems in rabbits. Vet Med [April]:365–372, 1995, with permission.)

ml/kg per day may be adequate in mild or moderately ill rabbits in conjunction with per os fluids. Although seldom needed, the placement of an intravenous catheter in the cephalic vein or an intraosseous catheter in the proximal femur or tibia can also be used to hydrate the patient (see *CVT XII,* p. 1331).

Rehydrating both the rabbit and the hairball may improve the passage of excess hair through the gastrointestinal tract. This can be accomplished with force-fed, blenderized alfalfa pellets with mixed-vegetables or fruit baby food mixed in water or an electrolyte solution (i.e., Pedialyte, Ross, Columbus, OH). Some practitioners use a human enteric feeding formula or juice in the slurry. Anorectic rabbits can be syringe-fed a slurry at a rate of approximately 10 to 15 ml/kg (or as much food as they will comfortably take) every 8 to 12 hours. In addition, always provide the patient with access to fresh greens (e.g., parsley, romaine lettuce, carrot tops, kale), vegetables, small amounts of fruit, hay (i.e., timothy, clover, grass, or alfalfa), pellets, and fresh water. Vitamin supplements (especially vitamin B) also can be administered.

Proteolytic enzymes such as bromelain (present in fresh pineapple juice), papain (papaya juice), or Viokase-V Powder (Fort Dodge Laboratories, Fort Dodge, IA) have also been used empirically in cases of trichobezoars. Although these enzymes do not dissolve the hair, they may aid in the breakdown of trichobezoars by dissolving the proteinaceous matrix that binds them together, helping to rehydrate the gastric mass. Although the value of such therapy is unresolved, enzymes may be of some value, even if just part of the rehydrating strategy. In general, however, proteolytic enzymes are becoming less commonly used in the treatment regimen for trichobezoars.

The value of broad-spectrum antibiotics, oral cat laxatives (Laxatone, Evsco, Buena, NJ), feline hairball prepara-

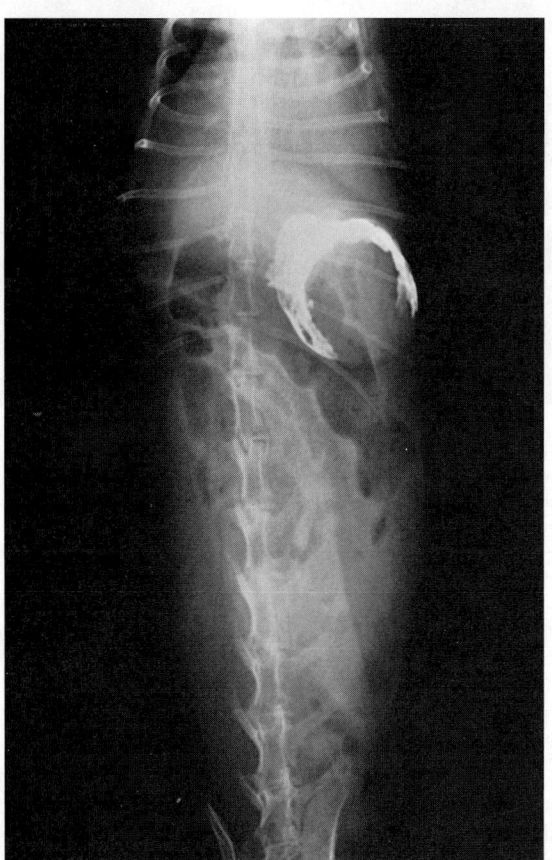

Figure 3. A ventrodorsal radiograph of the abdomen of the rabbit in Figure 2 following a barium swallow. The contrast outlines the mass filling the gastric lumen. (From Gentz EJ, Harrenstien LA, Carpenter JW: Dealing with gastrointestinal, genitourinary, and musculoskeletal problems in rabbits. Vet Med [April]:365–372, 1995, with permission.)

TABLE 1. **Medical Treatment for Trichobezoars in Rabbits**

Treatment	Comments
Fluid therapy	Rehydration is essential May be administered PO, SC, IV Maintenance fluid rate is $\approx$100–120 ml/kg/day
Nutritional support	Important in the anorectic rabbit; helps prevent hepatic lipidosis Force-feed $\approx$10–15 ml/kg (or as much food as they will comfortably take) q8–12h (see text) Offer fresh greens (parsley, romaine lettuce, carrot tops, kale, etc.), vegetables, small amounts of fruit, hay, pellets, and fresh water ad libitum Vitamin supplements (especially vitamin B) as needed
Stimulate gastric motility	Feed a high-fiber diet Metoclopramide (Reglan [AH Robins, Richmond, VA] 0.5 mg/kg PO, SC, q8h) or cisapride (Propulsid [Janssen, Titusville, NJ] 0.5 mg/kg PO q8–12h for 3–5 days) Avoid use in cases of gastrointestinal obstruction or other signs of an acute abdomen

Enzyme supplements	Response to treatment is equivocal
	Pineapple juice, fresh (contains the proteolytic enzyme bromelain)
	  1 ml/0.5 kg PO q12h until the condition is resolved
	  10 ml PO q24h for 3–5 days q2–3 months for the prevention of trichobezoars (questionable efficacy)
	Papaya enzymes (papain)
	  Viokase-V Powder (Fort Dodge Labs, Fort Dodge, IA)

Additional adjuncts to therapy	Antibiotics (broad-spectrum)
	  Use when indicated (i.e., prophylactically in debilitated patients or in cases of concurrent infections); trimethoprim-sulfa or enrofloxacin are generally the drugs of choice; use parenterally until stools are passed
	Grooming
	  Brushing the hair
	Laxatives (feline Laxatone, *Evsco*, Buena, NJ)
	  1–2 ml PO q24h for 3–5 days
	Response to treatment is equivocal
	Exercise
	Analgesics (for abdominal discomfort)
	  Flunixin meglumine (Banamine [Schering, Kenilworth, NJ]) 1 mg/kg SC, IM q12h)
	Supplemental heat
	  May be required in cases of hypothermia

tions, dioctyl sodium sulfosuccinate, modest exercise, and analgesics (in case of abdominal discomfort) is difficult to assess. Brushing the hair may prevent exacerbation of the problem. Supplemental heat may be required in cases of hypothermia.

On rare occasions, the mass of material in the stomach is so dessicated that the rabbit fails to respond to medical treatment, and surgical intervention is necessary (Jenkins, 1997a). All of the ingesta must be removed from the stomach to ensure that potential obstructing masses are removed. This includes less discrete aggregates of hair located in the pyloric opening. The prognosis for a successful outcome is greatly reduced in patients requiring a gastrotomy, especially when the surgery occurs in the later stages of gastric stasis. Complications of hepatic lipidosis are a common cause of death in these patients (Jenkins, 1997a).

Treatment strategies and adjunctive therapy for the medical treatment of trichobezoars and gastric stasis in rabbits are summarized in Table 1.

PREVENTION

The prevention of trichobezoars and gastric stasis in rabbits is best accomplished by feeding high-fiber, high-quality diets because the increased fiber component stimulates gastrointestinal motility, thereby decreasing hair accumulation. Avoiding stress and obesity and reducing boredom through environmental enrichment are reasonable recommendations for prevention. The prophylactic use of juices containing proteolytic enzymes, such as fresh pineapple juice or papaya juice, has also been advocated by some clinicians. Owners should be encouraged to brush their rabbits frequently to remove excess hair. Brushing may help prevent, but will not eliminate, trichobezoar formation in both long- and short-haired rabbits. Access to blankets and carpets, which may be ingested, should also be eliminated.

References and Suggested Reading

Brooks D: Nutrition and gastrointestinal physiology. In: Hillyer EV, Quesenberry KE, eds: Ferrets, Rabbits, and Rodents: Clinical Medicine and Surgery. Philadelphia: WB Saunders, 1997, pp 169–175.

Carpenter JW, Mashima TY, Gentz EJ: Caring for rabbits: An overview and formulary. Vet Med (April): 340–364, 1995.

Carpenter JW, Mashima TY, Rupiper DJ: Exotic Animal Formulary. Manhattan, KS: Greystone Publications, 1996, pp 209–229.

Cheeke PR: Nutrition and nutritional diseases. In: Manning PJ, Ringler DH, Newcomer CE, eds: The Biology of the Laboratory Rabbit, 2nd ed. San Diego: Academic Press, 1994, pp 321–333.

Cheeke PR: Rabbits. In: Pond WG, Church DC, Pond KR, eds: Basic Animal Nutrition and Feeding. New York: John Wiley & Sons, 1995, pp 451–459.

Gentz EJ, Harrenstien LA, Carpenter JW: Dealing with gastrointestinal, genitourinary, and musculoskeletal problems in rabbits. Vet Med (April): 365–372, 1995.

Gillett NA, Brooks DA, Tillman PC: Medical and surgical management of gastric obstruction from a hairball in the rabbit. J Am Vet Med Assoc 183:1176, 1983.

Harkness JE, Wagner JE: The Biology and Medicine of Rabbits and
    Rodents, 4th ed. Baltimore: Williams & Wilkins, 1995, pp 305–
    307.
Jenkins JR: Gastrointestinal diseases. In: Hillyer EV, Quesenberry KE,
    eds: Ferrets, Rabbits, and Rodents: Clinical Medicine and Surgery.
    Philadelphia: WB Saunders, 1997a, pp 176–188.

Jenkins JR: Soft tissue surgery and dental procedures. In: Hillyer EV,
    Quesenberry KE, eds: Ferrets, Rabbits, and Rodents: Clinical Medi-
    cine and Surgery. Philadelphia: WB Saunders, 1997b, pp 227–239.
Quesenberry KE: Rabbits. In: Birchard SJ, Sherding RG, eds: Saunders
    Manual of Small Animal Practice. Philadelphia: WB Saunders, 1994,
    pp 1345–1362.

Heart Disease in Ferrets

HEIDI L. HOEFER
New York, New York

Heart disease is common in middle-aged and geriatric domestic ferrets (*Mustela putorius furo*). The average life span of the normal ferret is 6 to 8 years. Cardiac disease is first evident at about 3 to 4 years of age, and the incidence increases as the ferret ages. Ferrets most typically suffer from acquired cardiac diseases. While dilated cardiomyopathy is the most common heart disorder of ferrets, hypertrophic cardiomyopathy, valvular disease, and dirofilariasis also occur. There have been no reports of congenital cardiac defects in ferrets. The clinical signs can be variable; ferrets may present asymptomatic or in heart failure. Geriatric ferrets often have multiple disease processes; for example, cardiomyopathy, insulinoma, and hyperadrenocorticism (see pp. 357 and 372).

CLINICAL SIGNS

Ferrets often present in congestive heart failure (CHF). The clinical signs are similar to those seen in canine and feline patients: weakness, lethargy, inappetence or anorexia, and tachypnea. Abdominal enlargement from ascites may be present. Some ferrets have difficulty in walking because of the rear legs; this may be from weakness, poor cardiac output, or the mechanical interference of a greatly enlarged abdomen. Coughing or emesis is rare. Some ferrets with heart disease are asymptomatic and present for an unrelated illness or routine check-up.

PHYSICAL EXAMINATION

Affected ferrets can be weak and nonambulatory, or normal in activity. The physical examination in ferrets with CHF reveals poor capillary refill time, weak pulses, and hypothermia (body temperature less than 38°C [100°F]). Tachypnea can be mild or severe, with abdominal respirations and open-mouth breathing. There may be tense ascites on abdominal palpation or a cranial organomegaly from congestion (hepatomegaly, splenomegaly). Auscultation of the thorax often reveals a holosystolic murmur with the point of maximal intensity (PMI) along the left sternal border. The ferret is a "tubular" animal with an elongated thorax. The PMI of the mitral valve lies farther caudal in the thorax than one would expect, given the anatomic location in the dog and cat. Murmurs can be focal and are often best heard along the sternum on the left side caudal aspect of the thorax. Right-sided murmurs are unusual. In some cases, a murmur is not auscultated. Pleural effusion may be present and muffle the heart sounds. Crackles (rales) may be auscultable in any or all lung fields. The normal ferret has a respiratory sinus arrhythmia that can be quite pronounced at times. Ferrets with heart disease may have other arrythmias, or a gallop may be heard.

DIAGNOSTIC TESTING

Several diagnostics tests should be performed on a ferret with suspected heart disease. Thoracic and abdominal radiographs, cardiac ultrasonography, and occult heartworm testing in endemic areas provide the framework for evaluation of the heart. Electrocardiography should be performed if there is a cardiac arrhythmia. A high incidence of concurrent disease is found in the ferret, especially insulinoma, adrenal disease, or lymphosarcoma; thus, a complete blood count and serum biochemistry testing should be performed in all cases. Adjunct tests can be added as necessary; for example, serum or plasma insulin concentrations. Any ferret that presents weak or has collapsed should have a quick, in-house, blood glucose level obtained.

Radiography

Thoracic and abdominal radiographs are essential. Whole body radiographs are often taken on initial presentation to evaluate both body cavities. Thoracic films can be taken as needed for increased radiographic detail. The ferret has a long, narrow, and compliant thorax with a trachea and bronchi that are of relatively large diameter. The normal cardiac apex lies 10 cm cranial to the diaphragm and is easy to assess on the lateral thoracic radiographic view (Fig. 1). It is also important to include the entire mediastinum in the radiograph to evaluate for the presence of a cranial mediastinal mass. Ferrets with cardiac disease often have an enlarged, globoid heart and tracheal elevation (Fig. 2). While there is not an established "rule of thumb" for assessing normal cardiac size in the ferret,

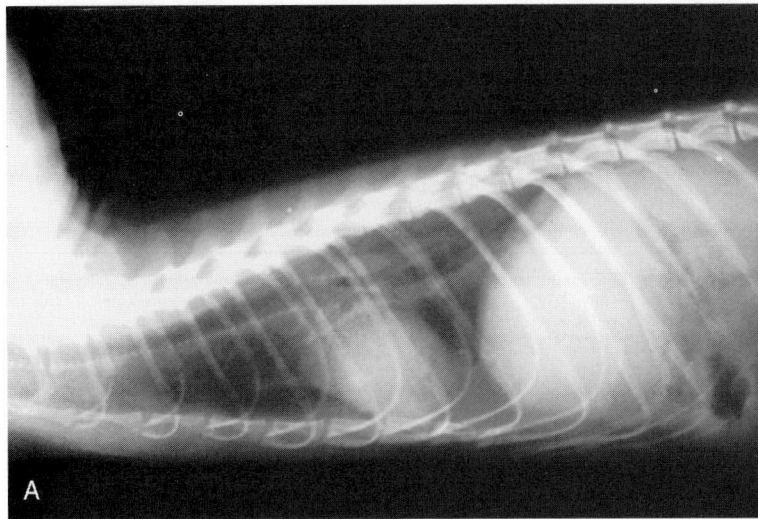

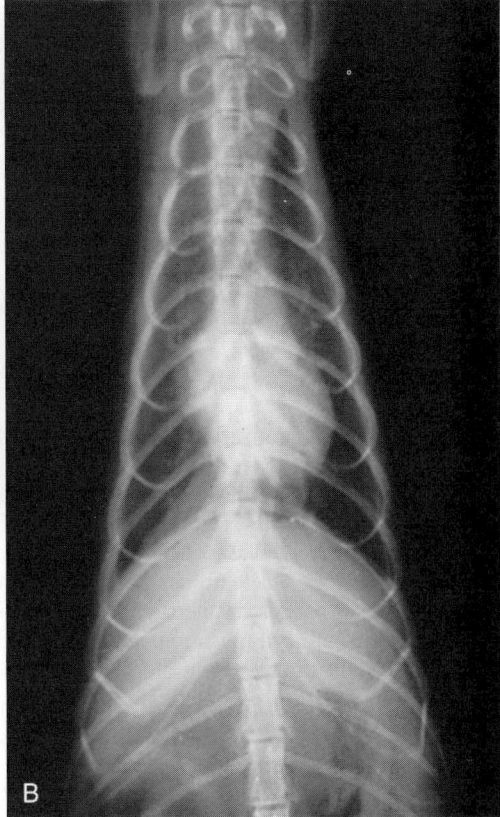

Figure 1. Normal ferret thoracic radiographs. *A,* Lateral; *B,* ventrodorsal.

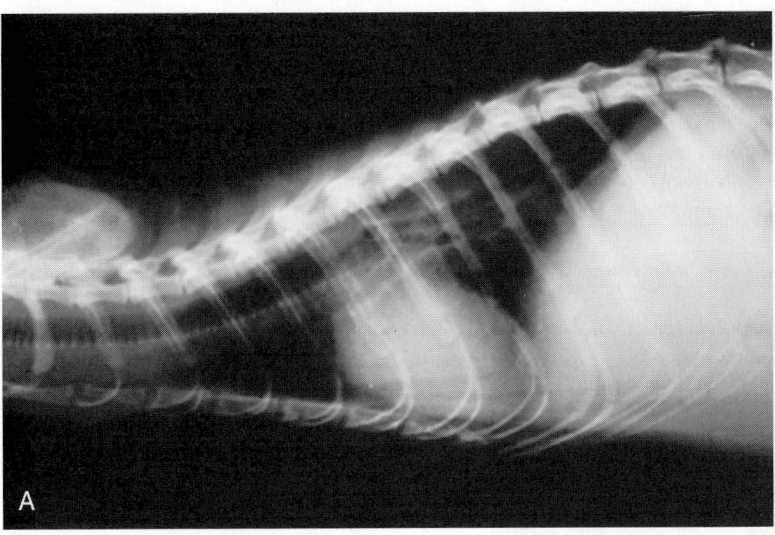

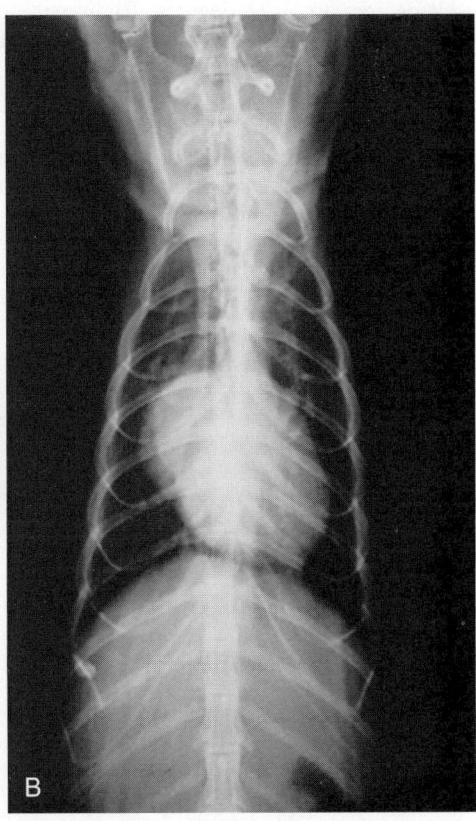

Figure 2. *A* and *B,* Thoracic radiographs of a ferret with dilated cardiomyopathy. The lateral view *(A)* demonstrates increased sternal contact and elevation of the trachea at the hilus. There is an overall increase in the cardiac silhouette, and the apex of the heart makes contact with the diaphragm in both views.

it is helpful to check the distance of the apex from the diaphragm. Respirations do not seem to greatly affect this distance in the normal ferret.

Pleural effusion may be present and, in some cases, is so extensive that the heart cannot be visualized. Differential diagnosis in cases of severe effusion should include an imperceptible mediastinal or heart-base mass. Lymphoma is relatively common in ferrets. Varying degrees of pulmonary edema can also be visualized in many cases of CHF. The liver and spleen are usually enlarged from passive congestion. Ascites can be mild to severe in some cases.

Electrocardiography

The electrocardiogram (ECG) provides important information about conduction disturbances and arrhythmias. Electrocardiographic testing can be difficult to perform in most ferrets because they rigorously reject the ECG clips and the application of alcohol. To reduce stress and facilitate testing, soft ECG electrodes can be used with ECG gel, or the metal prongs on the standard ECG clips can be hammered flat before application. Isoflurane sedation can also be used, but it is safer and more accurate to obtain an ECG without sedation. A practical alternative to sedation is to "scruff" the ferret and syringe-feed Nutri-Cal (Evsco Pharmaceuticals, Buena, NJ) as a distraction while applying the clips or electrodes and running the ECG strip. The normal heart rate for the unanesthetized pet ferret is 180 to 250 beats/min. In limb lead II, normal ferrets have very tall R waves, similar to dogs (Fig. 3). The normal R-wave amplitude can range from 1.4 to 3.0 mV. P waves tend to be small, as in cats. ST-segment elevation is often seen in normal ferrets. Mean electrical axis ranges from +69 degrees to +97 degrees. Right-axis deviation was not observed in one study with experimentally induced right-sided ventricular hypertrophy in 20 adult male ferrets (Smith and Bishop, 1985).

Ferrets with cardiac disease may have a sinus rhythm or a sinus tachycardia. Atrial or ventricular premature complexes may be noted, and second- or third-degree atrioventricular block is common. The most common ECG abnor-

TABLE 1. Mean Echocardiographic Values for 34 Normal Adult Ferrets

Parameter	Mean Value
Left ventricle, end-diastolic	11.0 mm
Left ventricle, end-systolic	6.4 mm
Left ventricular posterior or free wall	3.3 mm
Fractional shortening	42%
End-point septal separation	None

From Stamoulis ME, Miller MS, Hillyer EV: Cardiovascular diseases. In: Hillyer EV, Quesenberry KE, eds: Ferrets, Rabbits, and Rodents: Clinical Medicine and Surgery. Philadelphia: WB Saunders, 1996, pp 63–76, with permission.

mality recorded in ferrets at CardioPet (Little Falls, NJ) is second-degree atrioventricular block. The genesis of the conduction disturbance is unknown but could represent cardiomyopathy or intercurrent conduction system degeneration.

Echocardiography

Echocardiography is the most important part of the cardiac work-up in the ferret. Two-dimensional sonography provides information on the size, shape, and function of the chambers. It can also determine whether a thoracic mass is present. Pleural and pericardial effusions are readily seen. M-mode echocardiography provides indices of systolic function and allows measurement of chamber and wall thickness. Color-flow Doppler imaging can be used to visualize the direction of blood flow. Pulsed-wave or continuous-wave Doppler imaging can then be applied to assess blood flow velocity and verify valvular regurgitation. The author currently uses values obtained from an unpublished study at the Animal Medical Center as guidelines (Table 1).

THERAPY

In general, the treatment of heart disease in ferrets follows the same therapeutic guidelines as those used in

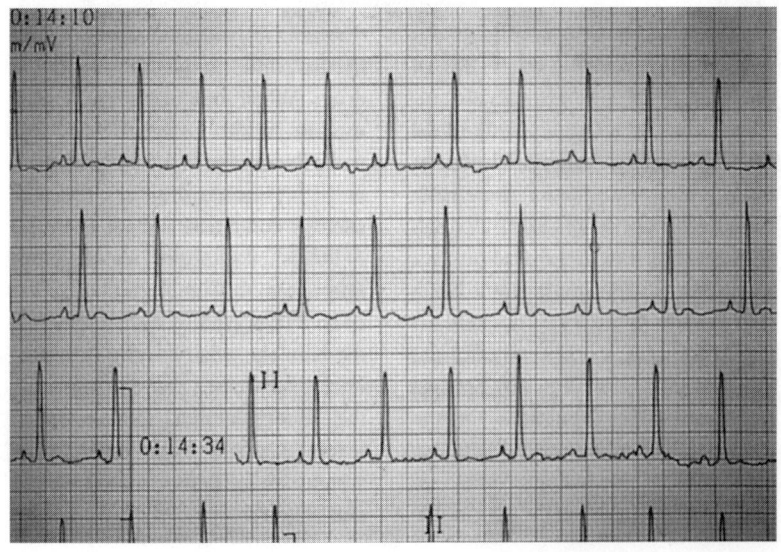

Figure 3. ECG (lead II) of a normal ferret. Note the large R waves.

dogs and cats. Pharmacokinetic studies have not been done for cardiovascular drugs in ferrets; scaling down doses already in use for cats works well clinically.

Furosemide (Lasix, Hoechst Marion Roussel) at 2 to 3 mg/kg IM or IV every 8 to 12 hours is used initially for ferrets in fulminant CHF; 1 to 2 mg/kg PO every 12 hours is used for long-term maintenance therapy. Ferrets tolerate the higher doses of furosemide relatively well. Generic furosemide is readily available in a elixir (10 mg/ml).

Nitroglycerin 2% cream (Nitrol, Adria, Columbus, OH) is a venous dilator that reduces preload to the heart. It is used just for the first 24 hours of therapy for cardiac failure and is used at ⅛-inch strip applied to the inside of the pinna every 12 hours. Enalapril (Enacard, Merck AgVet, Rahway, NJ) and captopril (Capoten, Bristol-Myers Squibb, Princeton, NJ) are angiotensin-converting enzyme (ACE) inhibitors. Enalapril is prescribed at 0.5 mg/kg PO every 48 hours initially and can be increased to once-daily dosing if tolerated well. Captopril was useful prior to the availability of the veterinary formulation of enalapril and was used at ⅛ of a 12.5-mg tablet every 48 hours in the ferret. Ferrets seem to be very sensitive to these vasodilators and can become quite lethargic if hypotensive. Inappetence is also a possible side effect of enalapril or captopril. Renal function (blood urea nitrogen and creatinine levels) must be monitored when one uses ACE inhibitors. A blood chemistry assay should be performed prior to the initiation of therapy, and then again during a recheck examination 1 or 2 weeks later. Guidelines for the management of azotemia during the use of enalapril are outlined in the package insert. Enalapril is only available in tablet form; thus, a suspension can be made to facilitate administration to ferrets. The author dissolves the tablet or tablets in distilled water with equal amounts of a methylcellulose-suspending agent (OraPlus, Paddock Laboratories, Minneapolis, MN) and cherry syrup for flavor. Compounding pharmacies routinely make suspensions for use in small mammals (Island Pharmaceutical Services, Woodruff, WI) and are very convenient to use.

Digoxin is a positive inotropic drug that stimulates the myocardium and depresses the atrioventricular node during supraventricular tachyarrhythmias. It is commercially available in a pediatric elixir (Lanoxin, Glaxo Wellcome). Ferrets with dilated cardiomyopathy are given at 0.01 mg/kg every 24 hours for the initial dose. The digoxin dose can be gradually increased to twice daily if needed. Care should be taken to prevent digoxin toxicity, although this is rarely seen clinically. Guidelines for monitoring digoxin levels in canine and feline patients are used (see p. 748).

Thoracentesis is beneficial in dyspneic animals with pleural effusion. Fluid samples should be submitted for cytologic examination because mediastinal lymphosarcoma is an important possibility in the differential diagnosis for pleural effusion. Thoracic radiographs can be repeated following thoracentesis and diuretic therapy. Oxygen therapy is usually indicated for ferrets in heart failure. Hypothermia must be monitored and controlled. Ferrets have a relatively large surface area and can lose heat quickly in an unheated oxygen cage.

Dilated Cardiomyopathy

Dilated (congestive) cardiomyopathy is the most common heart disease in the ferret. The etiology is unknown.

Most affected ferrets are older than 3 years of age at the time of diagnosis. In the author's practice, most of the cases that present with overt signs of heart failure have dilated cardiomyopathy. Radiographs reveal cardiomegaly and varying degrees of pulmonary edema and pleural effusion. Ascites is possible. Diagnosis cannot be made based on radiographs alone. Echocardiography usually shows left atrial enlargement and right ventricular dilation, similar to the disease in cats. Contractility is reduced and may be very low in advanced cases, resulting in a decrease in fractional shortening (see Table 1). Mitral regurgitation is common, and tricuspid regurgitation is seen occasionally by Doppler studies.

Treatment is similar to the protocol used in cats: furosemide, enalapril, and digoxin (see earlier). Ferret owners should be instructed to use only a commercial ferret formulation or a high-quality kitten diet (The Iams Co., Dayton, OH; or Science Diet, Hill's Pet Nutrition, Topeka, KS) and to avoid table food treats that may be high in salt. Taurine is considered ineffective but can be supplemented if the ferret has been on an inappropriate diet.

The long-term prognosis for ferrets with dilated cardiomyopathy is guarded. With early diagnosis and proper therapy, many of these ferrets can have a good quality of life for many months.

Hypertrophic Cardiomyopathy

Hypertrophic cardiomyopathy (HCM) is not as frequently diagnosed as is the dilated form of the disease. The clinical signs are often vague; the ferret may be asymptomatic or may experience varying degrees of lethargy. Sudden death is possible. Acute thromboembolic disease has not been reported in the ferret. Thoracic radiographs may show an enlarged heart. Cardiac auscultation may reveal an arrhythmia or a murmur. Tachycardia is not a consistent feature. Some ferrets do not have auscultable cardiac abnormalities or abnormal radiographs. The author has had at least three cases in which the cardiomyopathy was subclinical until 24 hours following abdominal surgery. The ferrets then became tachycardiac and weak and went into irreversible cardiac arrest.

Diagnosis is best achieved with echocardiography. The etiology of hypertrophic cardiomyopathy or left ventricular hypertrophy is unknown in ferrets. It is not related to hyperthyroidism.

The treatment of HCM is similar to that used in feline patients. Furosemide and enalapril are used to treat CHF. Nitroglycerin 2% cream can be applied to the inner ear during the initial 24-hour period if the ferret presents in heart failure. Beta-adrenergic blocking drugs, such as atenolol 6.25 mg PO every 24 hours, or calcium channel blockers, such as diltiazem (Cardizem, Hoechst Marion Roussel) 1 mg to 2 mg/kg PO every 12 hours can be considered to reduce heart rate or improve diastolic function.

Valvular Disease

Valvular heart disease is seen occasionally in the ferret and is best detected using two-dimensional imaging with

Doppler technology. Mitral regurgitation (with or without tricuspid regurgitation) is a common finding on Doppler echocardiograms. Varying degrees of aortic valvular insufficiency can be seen in some ferrets, but the significance is unclear. Affected ferrets usually have an auscultable murmur along the left sternal border. Treatment of CHF consists of furosemide and enalapril initially. Digoxin can be added later if systolic function becomes impaired. The prognosis depends on the severity of the cardiac disease at the time of diagnosis.

Heartworm Disease

Ferrets in heartworm-endemic areas are susceptible to filariasis. *Dirofilaria immitis* infection can result in severe cardiac disease in the ferret. Because of the relatively small heart and pulmonary arteries of the ferret, even a very low parasite burden (one or two worms) can have serious consequences. The clinical signs include dyspnea, lethargy, and ascites. Sudden death is possible. The heart may be muffled on auscultation, and radiographs show an enlarged heart, pleural effusion, and ascites. There is nothing pathognomonic about the clinical presentation; any ferret in an endemic area that presents with thoracic disease must be considered suspect. Other possibilities in the differential diagnosis include cardiomyopathy and lymphosarcoma.

Diagnosis. Ferrets with natural infections are not microfilaremic. Heartworm testing kits utilizing the enzyme-linked immunosorbent assay (ELISA) antigen test should be used. One ELISA test (Snap heartworm antigen test kit, Idexx Laboratories, Westbrook, ME) has proved successful in the detection of even very low worm numbers in ferrets (Dr. Deborah Kemmerer, Gainesville, FL, personal communication). Ultrasonography may show the nematodes within the right ventricle, vena cava, or pulmonary artery, but this may not be a reliable diagnostic test for dirofilariasis.

Treatment. Treatment of dirofilariasis in ferrets is possible but carries a guarded prognosis. Successful treatment depends on early diagnosis and long-term antithrombotic therapy following adulticide treatment. One practitioner (Dr. Deborah Kemmerer, personal communication) has treated more than 30 ferrets with heartworm disease with a greater than 70% success rate. Her protocol consists of placing an intravenous catheter (24-gauge) in the cephalic vein. Thiarcetarsemide (Carparsolate, Rhone Merieux, Athens, GA) is administered at 2.2 mg/kg IV every 12 hours for 2 days. Oral prednisolone is started immediately at 1.0 mg/kg every 24 hours and continued for 4 months or until the ferret has a negative occult heartworm test. Post-therapy heartworm testing (ELISA) should be performed at 3 months and, if positive, repeated at 4 months. The successfully treated ferret should be negative at 4 months. Treatment with melarsomine hydrochloride (Immiticide, Rhone-Merieux, Athens, GA) has shown promise and has been used successfully in several ferrets. The protocol for canine intramuscular use is followed, except the injection is given in the thigh muscles instead of the often atrophied lumbar muscle mass. Prednisolone is used, as described earlier, to prevent thromboembolic disease.

Prevention. Prevention is best achieved with the use of ivermectin at 0.02 mg/kg PO monthly to prevent maturation of the third stage of larval development. The smallest tablet (68 µg) of oral ivermectin (Heartgard-30, Merck AgVet, Rahway, NJ) can be dosed at ¼ tablet PO monthly. These tablets cannot be reused once they are removed from the wrapper and broken into quarters. An oral suspension is easier to dose. The 1% bovine preparation (Ivomec, Merck AgVet, Rahway, NJ) can be used orally following dilution with propylene glycol as follows: 0.3 ml of 1% ivermectin injectable is mixed into 1 ounce (30 ml) of propylene glycol to achieve a 0.1 mg/ml solution. The ferret is then dosed at 0.2 ml/kg PO monthly. The suspension should maintain potency until the expiration date of the ivermectin *if kept in an amber bottle and protected from light.*

References and Suggested Reading

Bone L, Battles AH, Goldfarb RD, et al: Electrocardiographic values from clinically normal, anesthetized ferrets (*Mustela putorius furo*). Am J Vet Res 49:1884, 1988.
A detailed study of ECG parameters.
Fox JG: Normal clinical and biologic parameters. In: Fox JG, ed: Biology and Diseases of the Ferret. Philadelphia: Lea & Febiger, 1988, pp 159–173.
A basic overview of the normal ferret.
Lipman N, Fox JG: Clinical, functional, and pathologic changes associated with a case of dilatative cardiomyopathy in a ferret. Lab Anim Sci 37:210, 1987.
Reviews one case of cardiomyopathy in detail, including histopathology.
Parrot TY, Greiner EC, Parott JD: *Dirofilaria immitis* infection in three ferrets. J Am Vet Med Assoc 184:582, 1984.
An early report of naturally occurring heartworm disease in the ferret.
Smith SH, Bishop SP: The electrocardiogram of normal ferrets and ferrets with right ventricular hypertrophy. Lab Anim Sci 35:268, 1985.
Experimentally induced cardiac disease and its effects on the ECG.
Stamoulis ME, Miller MS, Hillyer EV: Cardiovascular diseases. In: Hillyer EV, Quesenberry KE, eds: Ferrets, Rabbits, and Rodents: Clinical Medicine and Surgery. Philadelphia: WB Saunders, 1996, pp 63–76.
A practical overview of cardiac diseases with echocardiogram photographs.

Neoplasia in Ferrets

NATALIE ANTINOFF
Houston, Texas

As ferrets increase in popularity, our knowledge of neoplastic disease in this species also grows. Ferrets are unusually predisposed to the development of one or multiple neoplasms, often concurrently, during their lifetime. This may be attributed to genetic influences, diet or environment, age of altering, or a combination of factors still unidentified. The intent of this discussion is to present the clinical signs, diagnostic tests, and treatments of the most commonly identified neoplasms in ferrets (also see pp. 357 and 368).

ENDOCRINE NEOPLASIA

Endocrine neoplasias appear to be the most frequently encountered group of tumors in ferrets; most middle-aged and older ferrets are likely to acquire one or more of these tumors. It is common for endocrine neoplasias to be present concurrently and for one type to be identified as an asymptomatic incidental finding at the time of surgery for another. In such cases, treatment for all the tumor types present is indicated, as one endocrinopathy may mask clinical signs by providing negative feedback for another.

Insulinoma

Although insulinomas are most commonly diagnosed in ferrets 3 to 5 years of age, they have been reported in ferrets as young as 2 years of age. These are insulin-secreting, pancreatic beta-cell tumors, and clinical signs are associated with hypoglycemia. Ferrets with insulinoma frequently are presented with lethargy, depression, weakness, posterior paresis, ptyalism, "star gazing," bruxism, and collapse. Less common findings include inappetance, twitching, and seizures. In some ferrets, pawing at the mouth may be present, probably attributed to nausea. This pawing may be violent, often causing owners to believe a foreign body has been ingested. Hypoglycemic episodes are cyclic in many ferrets and may be exacerbated by exercise, a prolonged fast, or feeding, particularly of high-carbohydrate treats. The severity of clinical signs varies with both the rate of development and the severity of hypoglycemia. Many ferrets are asymptomatic and the insulinoma is either diagnosed during exploratory surgery for another procedure or by routine biochemical evaluation.

Diagnosis of insulinoma is based on clinical signs and documentation of hypoglycemia. Blood glucose levels should be measured immediately after collection, using a glucometer to avoid artifactual decreases associated with routine biochemical sample processing. Blood glucose levels less than 60 mg/dl (3.3 mmol/L) are highly suggestive of insulinoma. Measurement of insulin levels is recommended in hypoglycemic ferrets. Although not always present, hyperinsulinemia greater than 250 pmol/L (35 uU/ml)

accompanying hypoglycemia further supports the diagnosis of insulinoma. Insulin assays should be validated for ferrets. Because of the cyclic secretion of insulin, controlled fasting (3 to 6 hours) may be required to document hypoglycemic episodes.

Complete blood counts and biochemical panels on most affected ferrets are normal, although some may demonstrate leukocytosis characterized by neutrophilia or monocytosis. Elevations in alanine aminotransferase and alkaline phosphatase may be present. Splenomegaly and hepatomegaly are sometimes detected by palpation or radiography but are not specific indicators of insulinoma. Although of limited value in most cases, ultrasonography may aid in the identification of larger pancreatic masses. Histologically, these masses may be carcinomas, adenomas, or hyperplasia of islet cells. Local recurrence and metastasis is frequent, most commonly affecting the regional lymph nodes and liver.

Therapy is directed at maintaining euglycemia and controlling clinical signs. Frequent modification is required as the disease progresses. Insulinomas may be treated either medically or surgically, and often a combination of both is required. Surgical treatment is strongly recommended for ferrets with insulinomas. Although not evaluated as an independent parameter, in one recent study survival time of ferrets with medical management alone was 6 to 8.9 months, whereas ferrets treated with surgery or combined surgical and medical therapy had a median survival time of 17 months. These latter results were accompanied by disease-free postoperative intervals in some patients (Caplan et al, 1996).

Ferrets should fast 3 to 6 hours before surgery, and intravenous dextrose (2.5 to 5.0%) is recommended to prevent hypoglycemia during the preoperative and intraoperative period. In addition to visual inspection of the pancreas during laparotomy, gentle palpation frequently reveals multiple nodules. When few nodules are found, nodulectomy can be performed. When multiple nodules are present, partial pancreatectomy of the most severely affected area is preferable, with removal of additional nodules as required. Liver biopsy is recommended to evaluate for metastasis. Blood glucose levels should be monitored at least every 12 hours for 48 hours postoperatively and rechecked 1 to 2 weeks after surgery. Some ferrets will still require medical therapy but, in most cases, at decreased dosages; others may remain euglycemic for several months after surgery. Postoperative complications such as pancreatitis and diabetes are extremely rare in ferrets. No difference has been found between the survival times of ferrets who are euglycemic and those that are hypoglycemic postoperatively or between ferrets with benign neoplasms and those with malignant neoplasms (Caplan et al, 1996) (Ehrhart et al, 1996).

Medical management includes frequent feedings, along

with glucocorticoids and diazoxide. Either drug may be chosen as initial therapy. Prednisone increases hepatic gluconeogenesis and decreases peripheral tissue uptake of glucose. Therapy should begin with 0.5 mg/kg every 12 hours and may be increased to 2.0 mg/kg every 12 hours. A pediatric oral elixir (Pediapred, Fisons Pharmaceuticals, Rochester, NY) is readily accepted by most ferrets. As clinical signs progress, diazoxide can be added, which may enable a reduction in the dose of prednisone. Diazoxide acts on pancreatic beta cells to inhibit insulin secretion, increase hepatic gluconeogenesis, and decrease uptake of glucose by peripheral tissues. Therapy with diazoxide should begin at 5 to 10 mg/kg every 12 hours and can be increased to a total of 60 mg/kg per day. Proglycem (Baker Norton Pharmaceuticals, Inc., Miami, FL) is a commercially available formulation of diazoxide, but its cost may be prohibitive for some owners. Commercial compounding pharmacies are a less costly alternative. Resistance to both drugs may develop but is more common with diazoxide. Food should be available at all times. High-carbohydrate treats and supplements, including dextrose and fruit, should be avoided, as these will stimulate insulin release and may precipitate a hypoglycemic crisis.

Adrenal Gland Neoplasia

The average age of ferrets with adrenal cortical neoplasias is 3.5 years, although these neoplasias have been identified in ferrets as young as 18 months. Clinical signs are variable and are attributed to excess androgen production. The most common presentation is bilaterally symmetrical endocrine alopecia, usually beginning with the tail base or tail tip and progressing cranially. On occasion, hair may regrow after a few months, but alopecia recurs within 1 year without subsequent regrowth. Pruritus is the second most common clinical sign, usually occurring in the dorsal scapular region. Vulvar enlargement, frequently accompanied by mild discharge, is present in most affected females. Males may have paraprostatic cysts as a result of excessive androgen production, resulting in urethral obstruction. These males may be presented with owner observations of stranguria or dribbling, or complete urinary obstruction may be the only clinical sign. Less commonly occurring signs include polyuria and polydipsia and lethargy.

Unlike Cushing's syndrome, ferrets with hyperadrenocorticism do not have elevations of circulating cortisol levels (Rosenthal et al, 1993). Clinical signs associated with cortisol excess in other species are typically absent in ferrets (also see p. 372). Hematologic and biochemical parameters are usually normal, although mild elevations in ALT are occasionally present. Anemia and thrombocytopenia are rare but have been reported, probably as a sequela to estrogen-induced bone marrow suppression (Rosenthal et al., 1993). Radiographs are normal in most cases, but may infrequently reveal calcification of the adrenal gland. Ultrasonography is useful in confirming the presence of an enlarged adrenal gland, but the detection rate in one study was only 50% and varies with the resolution of the equipment and the experience of the sonographer (Rosenthal et al, 1993). The most accurate means of establishing a diagnosis is an androgen panel, which is currently validated for ferrets at the University of Tennessee. Elevations of one or more hormones (17-hydroxyprogesterone, androstenedione, dehydroepiandrosterone sulfate, and estradiol) are consistent with the presence of an adrenal tumor (Rosenthal and Peterson, 1996). Urine cortisol: creatinine ratios have been evaluated; however, since serum cortisol is not elevated, the predictive value of this test is limited.

Treatment for adrenal cortical neoplasia is adrenalectomy. A complete abdominal exploratory procedure should be performed before adrenalectomy. It is essential to palpate both adrenal glands for changes in size and consistency before removal. In many cases, both adrenal glands are affected; in these instances the larger should be removed and the smaller debulked, leaving some adrenal tissue to prevent iatrogenic hypoadrenocorticism. Although left adrenalectomies are generally uncomplicated, the enlarged right adrenal gland may surround or invade the vena cava, and attempts at removal may lead to life-threatening complications. Referral to a veterinary surgeon is recommended because bilateral involvement is often detected intraoperatively. If prostatic enlargement or paraprostatic cysts are present, it is not necessary to remove these, although biopsy is recommended. Prostatic enlargement begins to resolve almost immediately after the surgical removal of the tumors. Vulvar swelling begins to decrease within 1 week, and hair regrowth typically occurs within 3 months. Biopsy may reveal hyperplasia, adenoma, or adenocarcinoma. On rare occasions, the opposite adrenal gland may become affected after removal of the first, necessitating a second surgery to debulk the remaining tumor tissue. Mitotane (Lysodren, Bristol-Myers Squibb, Princeton, NJ) has been used in some cases at a dose of 50 mg/kg PO for 7 days and then every 72 hours with limited success. Ketoconazole has not been found to have any effect on this disease. The use of leuprolide acetate (Leupron, Tap Pharmaceuticals), 100 μg/kg IM every 4 to 8 weeks, may show some benefit; however, no formal studies are available to date.

LYMPHOMA

Lymphoma is the most common hematopoetic neoplasia of ferrets. Lymphoma has been described in all age groups; however, acute onset, multicentric lymphoma, and mediastinal masses are more common features in ferrets less than 2 years of age. A more insidious onset with nonspecific, episodic clinical signs seems to predominate in older ferrets. Cluster outbreaks of lymphoma have prompted investigation of an infectious cause. A ferret-specific retrovirus has been proposed; an association with feline leukemia virus and Aleutian disease virus has been suggested, but recent studies have disproven the association of either virus with the development of lymphoma in ferrets (Erdman et al, 1996b).

Clinical signs in younger ferrets typically include lethargy, weight loss, anorexia, dyspnea, extreme weakness and, occasionally, collapse. Physical examination and diagnostic evaluation may reveal dyspnea and pleural effusion, often associated with a mediastinal mass; splenomegaly; a palpable abdominal mass; and peripheral or visceral lymphadenopathy. Lymphocytosis (>8,000 cells/μl) is often a feature of lymphoma in younger ferrets, although the presence of lymphocyte atypia is variable.

Clinical features of lymphoma in ferrets greater than 2 years of age are typically nonspecific and may be cyclic in nature. Signs include lethargy, weight loss, intermittent diarrhea, weakness, and inappetence. Anemia and lymphopenia or leukopenia are more frequently present in older ferrets, but hematologic parameters may also remain normal. Splenomegaly, hepatomegaly, abdominal masses, and peripheral or visceral lymphadenopathy are variable, but multiple site involvement is common. Hypercalcemia is a rare feature of lymphoma in ferrets.

Lymph node aspirates are often inaccurate or nondiagnostic because ferret lymph nodes are often surrounded by a large amount of adipose tissue. Therefore, biopsy is recommended if lymphoma is suspected. Cytologic studies of bone marrow are essential if hematologic abnormalities are present. The marrow is easily collected from the femur using a 20- or 22-gauge spinal needle. Splenic aspirates are often diagnostic and can be obtained with a 25-gauge needle and 3-ml syringe in a properly restrained ferret without sedation. Ultrasonographically guided liver aspiration may be performed; abdominal exploratory surgery may be required to obtain biopsy specimens of affected lymph nodes or organs. Cytologic studies of pleural effusion or mediastinal masses frequently aid in diagnosis.

Several chemotherapy protocols have been proposed for ferrets; however, a controlled study evaluating remission and survival times is lacking (Table 1). When there are severe splenic infiltrates, splenectomy decreases tumor load and may aid in achieving remission. In one study, young ferrets with multicentric lymphoma were unlikely to survive more than 2 months from the time of diagnosis, and the mean survival time of older ferrets ranged from 6 to 8 months (Erdman et al, 1996a). Survival times of older ferrets are variable, and treatment may not prolong survival; however, chemotherapy may provide partial remission and improvement in clinical signs. Many older ferrets have concurrent disease that complicates their chances for remission. Ferrets receiving prednisone for the treatment of insulinoma acquire multiple drug resistance and are less likely to achieve benefit from chemotherapy. An indwelling intravenous catheter (or vascular access port) should always be used in ferrets receiving chemotherapeutic agents, and isofluorane sedation is recommended during drug administration to prevent catheter movement and extravasation. A complete blood count must be evaluated before each treatment; if the patient becomes leukopenic (<1500 cells/μl) or anemic, therapy must be discontinued. Side effects in ferrets are similar to those reported in dogs and cats (see p. 465).

CUTANEOUS NEOPLASMS

Cutaneous neoplasms are the third most commonly reported form of neoplasia in ferrets (Parker and Picut, 1993). Although the early literature suggests a high degree of malignancy in cutaneous neoplasms of ferrets, more recent studies have demonstrated that most skin tumors of ferrets are benign. One study reported that 58% of cutaneous neoplasms were basal cell tumors and 16% were mastocytomas (Parker and Picut, 1993). Another survey identified 30% of cutaneous masses as mastocytomas, 13% as hemangiomas, and 9% as benign cystic adenomas (Brown, 1997). Basal cell tumors are well-demarcated, pedunculated, minimally invasive cutaneous masses that may become ulcerated. Mast cell tumors in ferrets are generally benign, beginning as small discolored areas that may be pruritic, and developing into ulcerated masses. Systemic mastocytosis is rare in ferrets. These tumors respond well to surgical excision. Premedication with antihistamines and wide surgical margins are not necessary in ferrets. Other reported cutaneous neoplasms include fibroma, fibrosarcoma, adenocarcinoma, polyp, squamous cell carcinoma, and lymphosarcoma. Although malignancy is rare, surgical excision of any cutaneous neoplasm is recommended.

CHORDOMA AND CHONDROSARCOMA

Chordomas are tumors arising from notochordal remnants and are typically located at the most distal aspect of the tail. These tumors appear as firm, nonencapsulated ulcerated masses. Chondrosarcomas of the tail have also been reported. Histologically, these two tumor types must be differentiated based on immunohistochemistry. Amputation of the tail several vertebrae proximal to the tumor is curative for both tumor types.

OTHER NEOPLASMS

Many other neoplasms can be present in ferrets. Endocrine neoplasias, including pancreatic exocrine adenocarcinoma, glucagonoma, and pheochromocytoma have been reported. Sporadic cases of hepatic and urogenital neoplasms have been identified. Reproductive neoplasias, such as leiomyosarcoma, are prevalent in breeding colonies but rarely present in domestic pets unless they are unaltered. Gastrointestinal neoplasia, although rare, may be mistaken for a foreign body. As in any patient, a complete work-up is essential to the diagnosis, treatment, and prognosis of any neoplastic disease.

TABLE 1. Chemotherapy Protocol for Lymphosarcoma

Week	Drug	Dose
1	Vincristine	0.07 mg/kg, IV
	Asparaginase	400 IU/kg, IP
	Prednisone	1 mg/kg PO, SID, continued throughout therapy
2	Cyclophosphamide	10 mg/kg, SQ
3	Doxorubicin	1 mg/kg, IV
4–6	Repeat weeks 1–3 but discontinue asparaginase	
8	Vincristine	0.07 mg/kg, IV
10	Cyclophosphamide	10 mg/kg, SQ
12	Vincristine	0.07 mg/kg, IV
14	Methotrexate	0.5 mg/kg, IV
Continue protocol at biweekly intervals after week 14.		

IV, intravenous; IP, intraperitoneal; PO, orally; SID, once a day; SQ, subcutaneous.

From Rosenthal KE: Ferrets. Vet Clin North Am 24:19–20, 1994, with permission.

References and Suggested Reading

Brown SA: Neoplasia. In: Hillyer EV, Quesenberry KE, eds: Ferrets, Rabbits, and Rodents: Clinical Medicine and Surgery. Philadelphia, WB Saunders, 1997, p 99.
This is a comprehensive review of neoplastic diseases in the ferret.

Caplan ER, Peterson ME, Mullen HS, et al: Diagnosis and treatment of insulin-secreting pancreatic islet cell tumors in ferrets: 57 cases. J Am Vet Med Assoc 209:1741, 1996.
This article evaluates clinical, diagnostic, surgical, and histologic findings, as well as long-term outcome in 57 ferrets with insulinomas.

Ehrhart N, Withrow SJ, Ehrhart EJ, et al: Pancreatic beta cell tumor in ferrets: 20 cases. J Am Vet Med Assoc 209:1727, 1996.
A comparison of survival times, disease free intervals, and prognostic factors in ferrets with insulinomas.

Erdman SE, Brown SA, Kawasaki TA, et al: Clinical and pathologic findings in ferrets with lymphoma: 60 cases. J Am Vet Med Assoc 208:1285, 1996a.
This is a retrospective evaluation of clinical and pathologic findings in ferrets with lymphoma, as well as an analysis of prognostic variables.

Erdman SE, Kanki PJ, Moore FM, et al: Clusters of lymphoma in ferrets. Cancer Invest 14:225, 1996b.
This study described epidemiologic, clinical, and pathologic features of cluster outbreaks of lymphoma.

Parker GA, Picut CA: Histopathologic features and post-surgical sequelae of 57 cutaneous neoplasms in ferrets. Vet Pathol 30:499, 1993.
This article describes a survey of signalment, histologic features, and post-surgical sequelae of cutaneous neoplasms in ferrets.

Rosenthal KL, Peterson ME, Quesenberry KE, et al: Hyperadrenocorticism associated with adrenocortical tumor or nodular hyperplasia of the adrenal gland in ferrets: 50 cases. J Am Vet Med Assoc 203:271, 1993.
This article describes a survey of clinical, laboratory, surgical, and histologic findings and surgical outcomes in ferrets with hyperadrenocorticism.

Rosenthal KL, Peterson ME: Evaluation of plasma androgen and estrogen concentrations in ferrets with hyperadrenocorticism. J Am Vet Med Assoc 209:1097, 1996.
This study measured pre- and postoperative concentrations of estrogens and androgens in ferrets with hyperadrenocorticism and evaluated their diagnostic value.

Diseases of Chinchillas

PILAR M. HAYES
Oklahoma City, Oklahoma

HISTORY

The chinchilla (*Chinchilla lanigera*) is classified as a hystricomorph rodent and is closely related to the guinea pig. Chinchillas originate from the cold, rocky slopes of the high Andes Mountains in Peru and Chile. Historically, they have been used in the fur industry and in medical research for hearing studies and the study of Chagas' disease. Recently, chinchillas have become popular as pets because they are generally clean, docile, and inquisitive. Chinchillas are nocturnal, but can occasionally be active during the day. Table 1 contains biologic and physiologic values useful for physical examinations and reproductive cases.

TABLE 1. Biologic and Physiologic Data of Chinchillas

Temperature °C (°F)	36.1–37.8 (97.0–100.0)
Heart rate (BPM)	40–100
Respiratory rate/min	40–80
Ave. wt. (g) male/female	450–600/550–800
Life span (yr)	8–10
Age at puberty (days)	240–540
Estrus length (days)	30–50
Gestation (days)	105–115
Litter size	2–3
Birth weight (g)	30–50
Age eyes open (days)	Birth
Weaning age (days)	36–48

Modified from Carpenter JW, Mashima TY, Rupiper DJ: Exotic Animal Formulary. Manhattan, KS: Greystone Publications, 1996, pp 191–206, with permission.

PHYSICAL RESTRAINT

Chinchillas rarely bite and respond better to minimal physical restraint. It is recommended to handle them by gently holding the base of the tail and hind legs in one hand, while holding the ventral thorax or shoulders with the other hand.

If chinchillas are frightened and handled roughly, they can release a portion of hair, leaving a bald spot. This defense mechanism is called fur-slip, and it can take 3 to 5 months for the fur to regrow. Another defensive behavior is spraying urine at the handler.

CHEMICAL RESTRAINT

Isoflurane is the anesthetic of choice because of its rapid induction and recovery, and high margin of safety. It is recommended to administer isoflurane through a face mask or an induction chamber. A small face mask can be made from a syringe case to fit over a chinchilla's muzzle. Cover the open end of the case with part of a rubber glove and cut a slit in it to insert the muzzle and form a tight seal. A small induction chamber can be made with a 2-L plastic bottle. Secure part of a rubber glove over the cut bottom of the bottle as an entrance. Intubation of chinchillas is very difficult. The oral cavity is long and narrow, and the tongue fills a large portion of it, obscuring visualization of the epiglottis. Blind intubation is not recommended because it can lead to epiglottal edema and dyspnea.

Injectable anesthetics can be used for short procedures, but gas anesthesia is recommended for longer ones. Table 2 lists the dosages for chemical restraint, anesthesia, and analgesics used in chinchillas.

TABLE 2. Chemical Restraint, Anesthetic, and Analgesic Agents Used in Chinchillas

Agent	Dosage
Acepromazine	0.5–1.0 mg/kg IM, preanesthetic
Acetaminophen	1–2 mg/ml drinking water, analgesia
Butorphanol	0.2 mg/kg IM, analgesia
Isoflurane	2–5%, induction: 0.25–4.0%, maintenance (anesthetic of choice)
Ketamine	40 mg/kg IM, light sedation
Ketamine (K)/acepromazine (A)	(K) 40 mg/kg/(A) 0.5 mg/kg IM, anesthesia
Ketamine (K)/diazepam (D)	(K) 20–40 mg/kg/(D) 1–2 mg/kg IM, anesthesia
Ketamine (K)/xylazine (X)	(K) 35–40 mg/kg(X) 4–8 mg/kg IM, anesthesia

Modified from Carpenter JW, Mashima TY, Rupiper DJ: Exotic Animal Formulary. Manhattan, KS: Greystone Publications, 1996, pp 191–206, with permission.

VENIPUNCTURE

The lateral saphenous and cephalic veins are the recommended sites for venipuncture. The ear vein can be pricked to collect a small sample, but repeated use can lead to thrombosis. A toenail clip is not recommended because chinchilla toenails are almost rudimentary and there may be a problem with pain and hemostasis. Table 3 lists hematologic and serum biochemical values.

DIET

Chinchillas are hind gut fermenters and coprophagic. A recommended diet consists of hay, supplemented with pellets. Several commercial chinchilla pellets are available, such as Mazuri Chinchilla Diet (Purina Mills, Inc., St. Louis, MO) and Kaytee Forti-Diet Chinchilla (Kaytee Products, Inc., Chilton, WI). Feeding a pelleted diet without hay does not provide enough fiber and can lead to enteritis. Hay, such as timothy or prairie, should be offered

TABLE 3. Hematologic and Serum Biochemical Values of Chinchillas

PCV (%)	27–54
RBC (10⁶/ml)	5.6–8.4
Hgb (g%)	11.8–14.6
WBC (10³/ml)	5.4–15.6
Neutrophils (%)	39–54
Lymphocytes (%)	45–60
Monocytes (%)	0–5
Eosinophils (%)	0–5
Basophils (%)	0–1
ALT (IU/L)	10–35
AP (IU/L)	6–72
AST (IU/L)	96
Bilirubin, total (mg/dl)	0.6–1.28
Calcium (mg/dl)	5.6–12.1
Chloride (mEq/L)	108–129
Cholesterol (mg/dl)	50–302
Creatinine (mg/dl)	0.4–1.3
Glucose (mg/dl)	109–193
Phosphorus (mg/dl)	4–8
Potassium (mEq/L)	3.3–5.7
Protein, total (g/dl)	3.8–5.6
Albumin (g/dl)	2.3–4.1
Globulin (g/dl)	0.9–2.2
Sodium (mEq/L)	142–166
Urea nitrogen (mg/dl)	17–45

Modified from Carpenter JW, Mashima TY, Rupiper DJ: Exotic Animal Formulary. Manhattan, KS: Greystone Publications, 1996, pp 191–206, with permission.

daily ad libitum. It is important to monitor hay quality, since aflatoxicosis has been reported in chinchillas. Treats can be offered in small amounts a few times a week. Recommended treats are fresh fruits, vegetables, seeds, and grains.

INTEGUMENT

Chinchilla fur is very thick, with as many as 90 hairs growing from each follicle. In the wild, chinchillas keep their fur clean by bathing in fine volcanic dust. A similar dust is available commercially and consists of a mixture of silver sand and Fuller's earth at a ratio of 9:1. It is recommended to offer dust baths daily in a pan deep enough to allow the animal to roll over. The pan should be removed after use to keep it free from feces and prevent excessive bathing.

INTEGUMENTARY DISEASES

Dermatophytosis

Outbreaks of ringworm have been reported in the chinchilla fur industry owing to poor husbandry practices, but ringworm is rarely seen in pet chinchillas. *Trichophyton mentagrophytes* is usually isolated from chinchillas, but *Microsporum canis* is occasionally found. The clinical signs are alopecia, scaling, and inflammation of the nose, ears, and forefeet. Treatment is with oral griseofulvin (Fulvicin-U/F, Schering-Plough, Kenilworth, NJ) or lime sulfur dips (Lymdyp, DVM Pharmaceuticals, Inc., Miami, FL). Also, Captan (Orthocide, Chevron) or Desenex antifungal powder (Ciba Self-Medication, Inc., Woodbridge, NJ) can be mixed in the dust bath to help prevent the spread to cagemates. See Table 4 for dosages.

Bite Wounds and Traumatic Injuries

Chinchillas housed in groups rarely fight, but occasionally bite wound abscesses occur during breeding. Females are larger than males and can be aggressive when selecting a mate. *Streptococcus* spp. and *Staphylococcus* spp. are usually isolated from abscesses. Surgical excision of abscesses yields better results than surgical incision and debridement (Jenkins, 1992). Collecting samples for culture and sensitivity is recommended for selecting an appropriate antibiotic (see the section on drug therapy and Table 4 for treatment options). To avoid aggressive behavior, a large

TABLE 4. Antimicrobial and Antifungal Agents Used in Chinchillas

Agent	Dosage
Amikacin	2–5 mg/kg SC, IM q8–12h
Captan powder	1 tsp/2 cups dust
Chloramphenicol	30–50 mg/kg PO, SC, IM q12h
Chlortetracycline	50 mk/kg PO q12h
Enrofloxacin	5–10 mg/kg PO, IM q12h
Gentamicin	2–4 mg/kg SC, IM q8–24h
Griseofulvin	25 mg/kg PO q24h × 30–60 days
Lime sulfur dip	Dip q7d × 6 wk
Metronidazole	10–40 mg/kg PO q24h
Oxytetracycline	50 mg/kg PO q12h
Tetracycline	50 mg/kg PO q8–12h
Trimethoprim-sulfa	30 mg/kg PO, SC, IM q12h

Modified from Carpenter JW, Mashima TY, Rupiper DJ: Exotic Animal Formulary. Manhattan, KS: Greystone Publications, 1996, pp 191–206, with permission.

cage is needed with several hiding areas, such as boxes or PVC pipes. A male can be housed with a pregnant female, since male aggression toward neonates is rare.

Cage injuries usually result from inadequate housing. Chinchillas are very active and need cages with ample vertical space and multiple levels to climb and jump. Wire mesh should be of a small gauge, such as 15 mm by 15 mm or ½ inch by ½ inch, to avoid limb injuries. Foot pad lesions can be prevented by making a portion of the floor solid, providing a place for the animals to get off the wire.

Tibial fractures commonly occur from cage injuries or accidents during restraint. The tibia is a long, thin bone with minimal muscle padding; therefore, it is prone to fracture. Transverse and short spiral fractures with fragments usually occur. Surgical repair with cerclage wires or external fixators is reported to have greater success than external coaptation. Postoperative complications, such as malunion, can result because it is difficult to restrict a chinchilla's activity. It is strongly recommended to confine the chinchilla to a small cage during recovery.

Fur Chewing

Fur chewing or barbering occurs when a chinchilla chews off most of its fur or another animal's fur, leaving a moth-eaten appearance to the coat. The cause is unknown but believed to be a behavioral response to boredom or stress. Taking a detailed history about husbandry is important, including questions about cage size and levels, hide areas, chewing objects, and dust baths. Suggesting improvements in husbandry practices may alleviate boredom or stress and help resolve fur chewing. For example, chinchillas are nocturnal and become stressed if kept in a busy room during the day. Moving the chinchillas' cage into a quiet room can allow them to sleep undisturbed. Other factors implicated in causing fur chewing are hereditary, hormonal, and dietary imbalances.

Fur Ring

Adult male chinchillas can develop paraphimosis if a ring of fur accumulates around the penis, inside the pre-puce. The clinical signs are excessive grooming, pollakiuria, or dysuria. In chronic, severe cases, the urethra may become constricted and completely obstructed. Treatment includes manually withdrawing the penis from the prepuce and lubricating it to gently remove the fur ring. Examination for a developing fur ring should be done at least every 3 months. Owners can be shown how to exteriorize the penis and examine it. Breeding can lead to a fur ring; therefore, males should be examined every few days during breeding.

DENTITION

The dental formula of chinchillas is 1/1 incisors, 0/0 canines, 1/1 premolars, and 3/3 molars. All of the teeth are open-rooted. The incisors are yellowish and grow at a rate of 6.4 cm to 7.6 cm (2.5 to 3 inches) a year. Chinchillas gnaw often and should be provided daily with branches, wood blocks, pumice stones, and other hard objects to wear their teeth down.

DENTAL DISEASE

Malocclusion

Malocclusion, or slobbers, is a common problem in chinchillas. Early clinical signs are drooling, pawing at the mouth, anorexia, weight loss, and selecting finer food particles over coarser. As the cheek teeth (premolars and molars) overgrow, ulcers of the buccal mucosa and tongue can result. Advanced cases have involved periodontitis, alveolar abscesses, and periostitis. A reported complication of severely maloccluded molars is invasion of the orbit by tooth roots.

Examination of the narrow oral cavity can be facilitated by using an otoscope to visualize the cheek teeth. Treatment for malocclusion consists of trimming the teeth. A Dremel Rotary Tool (Dremel, Racine, WI) with its cutting wheel is useful in cutting the incisors without shattering them. A tongue depressor should be placed behind the incisors while cutting to protect the soft tissues. Bone rongeurs can be used to clip the spurs of overgrown cheek teeth. Malocclusion is caused by hereditary factors or husbandry problems, such as a lack of hard objects to gnaw. Since grossly misaligned teeth can be genetic, it is recommended that these animals not be bred. Owners should be informed that routine trimmings may be necessary.

CONJUNCTIVITIS

Conjunctivitis is often caused by irritation from dust baths. Excessive dust bathing can be limited by offering dust for only 30 minutes a day. The type of bedding used in a cage can also lead to conjunctivitis. The resins of pine and cedar chips are irritating to mucous membranes. Hardwood chips, such as aspen, or shredded paper are recommended for bedding. Other causes of conjunctivitis are soiled bedding and inadequate ventilation. Treatment includes ophthalmic antibiotic ointment, plus a steroid if no corneal ulcer is present. Dust baths should be discontinued during treatment.

RESPIRATORY DISEASE

Pneumonia has been associated with husbandry problems, such as overcrowding, poor ventilation, and high humidity. These problems are more common in the fur industry than with pet chinchillas. Infections with *Bordetella* spp., *Pasteurella* spp., *Pseudomonas* spp., and *Streptococcus* spp. have been isolated from chronic respiratory infections in chinchillas. The clinical signs of pneumonia are nasal discharge, dyspnea, anorexia, depression, and lymphadenitis. Diagnosis is by auscultation, cultures, and radiographs. Treatment consists of antibiotics and nebulization, if possible.

GASTROINTESTINAL DISEASES

Esophageal Choke

There have been cases of chinchillas with objects, such as treats, bedding, or placentas, lodged in the esophagus. Like rabbits and rats, chinchillas cannot vomit, and esophageal choke can result after the ingestion of a large object. The clinical signs are drooling, retching, dyspnea, and anorexia. Diagnosis is by palpation and plain and contrast-enhanced radiographs. Treatment is routine therapy for the removal of an esophageal foreign body.

Gastric Bloat

A history commonly associated with gastric bloat is a lactating female that eats excessive clover, has a sudden addition of fresh greens or fruits in the diet, or has gastroenteritis. The clinical signs are a distended, painful abdomen, dyspnea, and the reluctance to move. Treatment is routine, by decompression with a stomach tube or a transabdominal trocar.

Gastric Trichobezoars

Trichobezoars can result from excessive fur chewing. Patients usually present with a history of anorexia and lethargy. Diagnosis is by palpation and plain and contrast-enhanced radiographs. Treatment is similar to that in rabbits, including fluid therapy, proteolytic enzymes (fresh pineapple juice and papaya tablets), cat laxatives (Felaxin, Schering-Plough, Kenilworth, NJ), increased dietary fiber, and force-feeding a gruel if the animal is anorectic.

Enteritis

A frequently occurring and potentially fatal disease in chinchillas is enteritis. The most common cause of enteritis is an improper diet, such as excessive fat or protein, low fiber, or an abrupt diet change. A history that may reveal this includes feeding excessive pellets, excessive fresh green vegetables, damp or young hay, or no hay. These dietary problems change the normal gastrointestinal bacterial flora, fermentative processes, and motility, allowing pathogenic bacteria to overgrow and potentially leading to enterotoxemia. Bacteria associated with enterotoxemia in chinchillas are *Pseudomonas* spp., *Salmonella* spp., *E. coli*, and *Clostridium* spp. Clostridial enterotoxemia has been reported to cause severe diarrhea and acute death in young chinchillas, 2 to 4 months old.

Less common causes of enteritis are inappropriate or prolonged antibiotic use, nematodes, coccidia, *Cryptosporidium* spp., *Sarcocystis* spp., *Listeria monocytogenes*, and *Yersinia pseudotuberculosis*. *Giardia* can be present in chinchillas without causing clinical disease and is suggested to be a normal gastrointestinal inhabitant. However, stress and poor husbandry can cause an increase in the number of *Giardia*, inducing clinical disease. With cases of diarrhea, examine fresh fecal smears for *Giardia*. If giardiasis is suspected, it can be treated with metronidazole; however, metronidazole toxicity has been anecdotally reported in chinchillas, involving liver failure. Alternative treatments are with albendazole or fenbendazole at a dose of 50 to 100 mg/kg PO or 25 mg/kg PO daily for 3 days. Giardiasis in chinchillas appears to occur more often on the West Coast of the United States than the East Coast. The pathogenicity of *Giardia* in chinchillas remains controversial until further research is performed or cases reported.

Diagnosing an etiologic agent of enteritis can be difficult. Fecal parasite examinations, cultures, and radiographs should be performed as indicated. Treatment is symptomatic with fluids, antiparasitics, and antibiotics as needed. The clinical problems associated with enteritis are diarrhea, anorexia, bloating, and grinding teeth. Conditions resulting from chronic enteritis are impactions, intussusceptions, and rectal prolapses.

Constipation

In chinchillas, constipation may be more common than diarrhea, but goes unnoticed by owners until it progresses. The main cause of constipation is feeding a diet excessive in pellets, which are high in calories and protein, and deficient in hay as a fiber source. Other causes of constipation are obesity, lack of exercise, and pregnancy. The clinical signs are straining to defecate, decreased fecal production, and abnormal pellets, such as small, hard, blood-stained pellets. Constipation is treated by increasing dietary fiber by slowly adding small amounts of hay or fresh vegetables. A cat laxative, such as Felaxin, can be given daily. In unresponsive cases, cisapride (Propulsid, Janssen Pharmaceuticals, Inc., Titusville, NJ) can used to increase motility at a dose of 0.5 mg/kg PO every 8 hours and enemas if indicated. Conditions associated with chronic constipation are rectal prolapses, ileus, impactions, and intussusceptions.

NEUROLOGIC DISEASES

Lead poisoning has occurred in chinchillas allowed to roam free in houses and chew lead-based paint. The clinical signs are convulsions and blindness. Blood lead levels of 25 µg/ml or above are considered indicative of lead poisoning. Nucleated red blood cells and basophilic stippling of red blood cells have not been seen in chinchillas with lead poisoning. Treatment is with calcium EDTA at 30 mg/kg SC every 12 hours.

Cerebrospinal nematodiasis from *Baylisascaris procyonis* has been reported. The chinchillas were infected by eating feed and hay contaminated with raccoon feces. Neurologic signs include torticollis, ataxia, and paralysis. There is no treatment, and a zoonotic potential exists from handling the contaminated feed.

Chinchillas have been reported to be highly susceptible to infection with *Listeria monocytogenes*. Outbreaks in the fur industry were associated with contaminated feed and poor sanitation, but cases have not been reported in pet chinchillas. The clinical signs include ataxia, circling, convulsions, and peracute death. Infections are treated with chloramphenicol or oxytetracycline, but they are usually ineffective once clinical signs appear.

NEOPLASIA

Reports of neoplasias in chinchillas are rare, despite their long life span of 8 to 10 years. In the 1950s, there were reports of neoplasias, such as neuroblastoma, carcinoma, lipoma, hemangioma, and lymphoma. The lack of recorded information on neoplasias since then is probably due to the lack of geriatric chinchillas used in the fur industry and research. With the recent increase in pet chinchillas, there may be an increase in reports of tumors as they become geriatric.

HEATSTROKE

Chinchillas are well adapted to colder, dry climates and do not tolerate temperatures above 25.1°C (80°F). If the ambient temperature is above 80°F and the humidity is high, heatstroke can result. A method for predicting heatstroke is to add the unit values of temperature and humidity (Donnelly and Schaeffer, 1996). Any value greater than 150 is dangerous, such as 85°F + 65% humidity = 150. The clinical signs of heatstroke are panting, drooling, elevated rectal temperatures (>103°F), bloody diarrhea, reddened ears and mucous membranes, and prostration. Prolonged heat stress can lead to hemoptysis, cyanosis, and acute death. Treatment consists of cool water baths and fluid therapy. Heatstroke is prevented by moving cages out of sunny windows and away from heaters, and maintaining a room temperature of 60 to 70°F and humidity of 40 to 50%. The relevance of heatstroke to the veterinarian is to monitor the stress level and body temperature during physical examinations or procedures. Also, the clinician should avoid using heating pads during anesthesia unless hypothermia develops.

REPRODUCTION

Sex Determination

Sexing can be difficult, especially in young chinchillas. The clitoris is a large, cone-shaped papilla ventral to the vagina and is similar in appearance to the penis. Males do not have a true scrotum, and the testes are inguinal. Sex can be determined by comparing the length of the perineum, which is longer in males than in females.

Castrations

The male chinchilla can be placed in dorsal recumbency for a castration. A clear, adhesive drape, such as that sold by Veterinary Specialty Products, Inc. (Boca Raton, FL), can be used to allow visualization of respirations during anesthesia. The testes can be manipulated out of the inguinal canal, and an incision made over each one. If the testes are difficult to exteriorize, elevating the cranial portion of the animal and applying gentle caudoventral pressure to the abdomen can help. A closed castration is recommended, but if the tunic is incised, the incision should be extended cranially to close the inguinal ring and prevent herniation. The skin incisions can be left open to heal by second intention, closed with 5-0 absorbable suture, or tissue adhesive.

Dystocia

A dystocia can result from large feti, a small pelvis, poor nutrition, or uterine inertia. The clinical signs are excessive restlessness, crying, and genital grooming. The initial treatment includes giving oxytocin at 0.2 to 3.0 IU/kg SC, IM, or IV. If there is no response to repeated oxytocin therapy and the chinchilla is in labor more than 4 hours, surgery is indicated. A cesarean section or an ovariohysterectomy of the gravid uterus can be performed. The main advantage of an ovariohysterectomy over a C-section is to avoid possible abdominal contamination by uterine contents. The viability of the neonates is not affected by an ovariohysterectomy. However, an ovariohysterectomy should not be performed if the uterus is exceptionally large or engorged with blood, or the animal is anemic. An alternative procedure is to perform a C-section first to allow the uterus to involute and blood to return to the peripheral circulation, then to perform an ovariohysterectomy.

The procedure for performing an ovariohysterectomy or a C-section is routine, with a ventral midline approach. The subcutaneous tissue is thin in chinchillas, and the linea alba is wide and easily identified. The two uterine horns open separately into the cervix. After the neonates are delivered, 3-0 or 4-0 absorbable suture material can be used to close routinely.

DRUG THERAPY

Antibiotics that have a selective gram-positive spectrum, such as macrolides and beta-lactam antibiotics, *should be avoided* because of the potential for gram-negative overgrowth and endotoxemia. The use of oral *Lactobacillus*

TABLE 5. Antiparasitic Agents Used in Chinchillas

Agent	Dosage
Carbaryl powder 5%	Topically q7d × 3 wk
Ivermectin	0.2 mg/kg PO, SC q7d × 3 wk
Metronidazole	50–60 mg/kg PO q12h × 5 days
Praziquantel	6–10 mg/kg PO
Pyrethrin powder	Topically q7d × 3 wk
Sulfamerazine, sulfamethazine	1 mg/ml drinking water

Modified from Carpenter JW, Mashima TY, Rupiper DJ: Exotic Animal Formulary. Manhattan, KS: Greystone Publications, 1996, pp 191–206, with permission.

spp. to repopulate the gastrointestinal flora during antibiotic therapy is controversial. Its use has not been reported in chinchillas, but it has been used safely in other rodents. A suggested dose is to give a small amount of yogurt with live cultures or a lactobacillus product such as Probios Ruminant Gel (Micobial Genetics, West Des Moines, IA) orally, 2 hours prior to antibiotic treatment and continue for 5 to 7 days beyond the cessation of antibiotics. Table 4 lists the antimicrobial and antifungal dosages used in chinchillas. Table 5 contains antiparasitic dosages.

References and Suggested Reading

Carpenter JW, Mashima TY, Rupiper DJ: Exotic Animal Formulary. Manhattan, KS: Greystone Publications, 1996, pp 191–206.
A thorough, informative book containing an extensive formulary and user-friendly tables of common medical problems of and treatments in many exotic pets.

Donnelly TM, Schaeffer DO: Disease problems of guinea pigs and chinchillas. In: Hillyer EV, Quesenberry KE, eds: Ferrets, Rabbits, and Rodents: Clinical Medicine and Surgery. Philadelphia: WB Saunders, 1996, pp 270–281.
An extensive review of chinchilla medicine and surgery with an emphasis on clinical application.

Hoefer HL: Chinchillas. Vet Clin North Am Small Anim Pract 24:1, 103, 1994.
A complete review of chinchilla biology, husbandry, and medicine, focused for clinical use.

Jenkins JR: Husbandry and common diseases of the chinchilla (*Chinchilla laniger*). J Small Exotic Anim Med 2:15, 1992.
A journal review of common chinchilla diseases and treatments.

Webb RA: Chinchillas. In: Beyen PH, Cooper JE, eds: British Small Animal Veterinary Association: Manual of Exotic Pets. Ames: Iowa State University Press, 1991, pp 15–22.
A general review of chinchilla biology and medicine.

General Husbandry and Medical Care of Sugar Gliders

ROSEMARY J. BOOTH

Currumbin, Queensland, Australia

The sugar glider, *Petaurus breviceps,* is a small pugnacious, arboreal marsupial native to Australia and New Guinea. Sugar gliders can glide (volplane) at least 50 m between trees by extending a patagium (gliding membrane) that stretches from the fifth finger to the first toe on each side. They are gregarious and sexually dimorphic. Males generally weigh 115 to 160 gm, and females weigh 95 to 135 gm. Body length ranges from 160 to 210 mm, and tail length from 165 to 210 mm (Suckling, 1995). Adult sugar gliders are differentiated from the larger and rarer squirrel glider, *Petaurus norfolcensis,* by having a tail shorter than 210 mm that often has a white tip, and weighing less than 200 gm. Chromosome numbers are identical in both species (2N = 22), and fertile hybrids have occurred in captivity.

Sugar gliders and the nonvolant equivalent, the Leadbeaters possum *(Gymnobelideus leadbeateri),* are of similar size and ecology, both eat primarily exudates from trees and insects, both are nocturnal, and both nest communally in well-insulated tree trunks. However, sugar gliders expend 169 kJ/day, compared with 226 kJ/day in the Leadbeaters possum, suggesting that gliding may be an efficient way of conserving energy where food resources are scarce (Nagy and Suckling, 1985). During extreme cold or food shortage, sugar gliders can conserve energy by going into a torpor for periods of up to 16 hr/day (Fleming, 1980). Colonies of 2 to 12 individuals occupy a territory of up to 1 hectare in forest habitat that ranges from cold temperate to tropical climates. Dominant males mark their territory and group members with secretions from androgen-sensitive frontal (forehead), gular (throat), and paracloacal scent glands.

REPRODUCTION

Sugar gliders are seasonally polyestrous (June to November in Australia) and polygynous, with most young born in the spring, coinciding with increased insect availability. Litter size is usually two (81%) or one (19%), although there are four teats. A second litter is commonly produced in one breeding season. The estrus cycle is 29 days, and gestation is 15 to 17 days (Tyndale-Biscoe and Renfree, 1987). Young are born at 0.2 gm and are carried in the pouch for 70 to 74 days. When the young are too large to remain in the pouch, they are left in the nest hollow until they are weaned at 110 to 120 days. The young are usually forcibly dispersed at 7 to 10 months of age. Longevity in the wild is usually 4 to 5 years, but individuals may survive up to 9 years in the wild or 12 years in captivity.

Familiarity with normal reproductive anatomy is important in order to recognize pathology. Female sugar gliders have two uteri and two long, thin lateral vaginae that open proximally into a central vaginal cul-de-sac divided by a septum. Both sexes possess anterior, dorsal, and ventral paracloacal glands that are more developed in males. Males have a large, carrot-shaped prostate just distal to the bladder with a constriction at the anterior third. They possess two pairs of Cowper's glands in addition to the paracloacal glands. The penis is bifid. The testes are permanently descended in the prepenile scrotum, as is characteristic of marsupials (Smith, 1984).

HUSBANDRY

Housing

The essential requirements are an aviary, a nest box, and branches for climbing. The ideal enclosure is an aviary as large as possible, but at least 1,800 mm long × 1,800 mm high × 1,200 mm wide with wire mesh 1 cm × 2.5 cm. Rat walls or mesh floors should be used to prevent rodent access. The cage should be furnished with runways of branches or ropes set high off the ground. Freshly cut branches from nontoxic species should be added two or three times per week for bark stripping and to provide leaves for nest lining.

Sugar gliders need permanent access to a nest box for sleeping and hiding, and daytime disturbances should be minimized. Nest box size depends on colony size but should be at least 15 cm³; the box should have a hinged lid and a circular opening on the front with a sliding closure. Bird nest boxes or small hollow logs are suitable. Nesting material should consist of shredded bark and dried leaves, or equivalent. Shredded paper is unsuitable, as it can entrap the animals' limbs. Nest boxes should be cleaned and bedding material changed every 1 or 2 weeks. If nest box closures are secure, the nest box can be relocated into the house for interaction each evening and then returned to the aviary to allow ad libitum nocturnal activity. If hospitalization is required, a nest box should be placed in the hospital cage, and the cage front covered during the day.

Food and water should be provided in an elevated position. Nectar mixes must be offered in enclosed feeders (e.g., bird or mouse drinkers) that do not allow the animals to get nectar on their fur. Feeding stations should be sheltered from predator access with solid walls. Owls, in particular, can kill small animals through wire.

Captive Colony Size

A "typical" wild colony contains one dominant male, two subordinate males, and four adult females. This is the most natural situation for a captive group, but any number greater than two is acceptable if animals are compatible. Young should be removed at or soon after weaning, or they may be killed because they cannot disperse in captivity. New adults must be introduced to an established group with care. Introduction of new members can sometimes be achieved by locking up established animals in a small cage within the aviary and allowing new animals to establish themselves in the main aviary for a few weeks before allowing animals to interact directly. Fighting will occur, so animals should be examined daily to check for injuries. If animals are to be kept as pets, a pair is the *minimum number*.

Nutrition

Sugar gliders are omnivores with a number of specialized features that the captive diet should aim to utilize. They possess enlarged lower incisors for chewing into the bark of trees, a lengthened fourth digit on the manus that may aid in the extraction of insects from crevices, and an enlarged cecum whose principal function is probably microbial fermentation of the complex associations of polysaccharides in gum. Observations of wild sugar gliders averaged over all seasons show that approximately 40% of foraging time is spent obtaining acacia gum, 30% is spent foraging for arthropods, and 11% is spent obtaining sap from eucalyptus trees (Smith, 1982). Examination of feces and stomach contents, however, suggests that 49% arthropods and 48% gum are actually ingested (Nagy and Suckling, 1985). Manna, pollen, nectar, and honeydew are minor components of the natural diet in all seasons. See Table 1 for a description of these components.

Field energetics studies have demonstrated that wild sugar gliders consume 10.1 to 12.7 gm/day of dry food, which provides 182 to 229 kJ/day (Nagy and Suckling, 1985). This is equivalent to approximately 9% of body weight in dry matter per day or about 17% of body weight in fresh food (Nagy and Suckling, 1985). The captive glider expends less energy in exercise and is generally offered more assimilable foods than the wild glider, so the total energy offered in captivity should be less than or equal to this. Table 2 shows a suitable menu for captive sugar gliders.

TABLE 1. Definition and Composition of Dietary Components of Wild Sugar Gliders[1,3,7]

Component	Definition	Composition
Gum	Exuded on trunks and branches by some species of Acacia to bind sites of damage, particularly those made by boring insects	Complex associations of polysaccharides (cellulose, starch, and sugars), low in protein (1.3–3.1%)
Arthropods	Moths, scarab beetles, caterpillars, weevils and small spiders	Vary in composition but contain in the region of 50–75% protein, and 5–20% fat on a dry weight basis
Sap	Liquid obtained by biting through the bark of some eucalyptus trees into the phloem	1.4% or less protein, predominantly carbohydrate of which 70–85% is sucrose
Manna	Sugary exudate produced at sites of insect damage on the leaves and branches of certain eucalyptus and angophoras	Composition of sugars slightly changed from phloem sap by the action of insects' salivary enzymes
Honeydew	Sap-sucking insects ingest large quantities of sap to obtain sufficient protein and then excrete surplus carbohydrates as honeydew	About 79% mono- and oligosaccharides and 9% polysaccharides
Nectar	Produced in usable quantities by larger eucalyptus flowers (>5 mm in diameter)	Mainly simple sugars

TABLE 2. Suitable Diet for Captive Sugar Gliders*

Group 1	Insects	75% Moths, Crickets, Beetles; 25% Fly Pupae, Mealworms
	Meat Mix	Commercial small carnivore or insectivore mix (e.g., Mazuri, PMI Feeds, St. Louis, MO; Wombaroo Glen Osmond, Australia); or coarse ground low-fat dry cat food (e.g., Iams) blended with fresh mince with balanced multivitamin and mineral supplement added according to weight of mince component.
Group 2	Nectar mix	1.5 cups fructose, 1.5 cups sucrose (brown sugar), 0.5 cup glucose made up to 2 L with warm water. Commercially available mixes from Roudybush, Australia (Hamilton, NSW), Nekton-Produkte (Pfurzheim, Germany), or Wombaroo have the advantage of balanced vitamin and mineral additives.
	Dry Lorikeet Mix	4 cups rolled oats, 1 cup wheat germ, 1 cup brown sugar, 0.5 cup glucose, 0.5 cup raisins or sultanas.
Group 3	Fruit and vegetables	Select from diced apple, nectarine, melons, grapes, raisins, sultanas, figs, tomato, sweet corn, sweet potato, beans, and butternut pumpkin.
	Greens	Mixed sprouts; shredded carrot, lettuce, broccoli, and parsley; corn kernels, sultanas. Vitamin-mineral supplement at manufacturer's directions.

*Offer a total of 15–20% of body weight daily. Select one diet from each group each day. Animals will benefit from a major effort to provide a regular supply of vitamin-mineral–enriched insects.

Live food can provide behavioral enrichment as well as nutrition. Insect-attracting lights just outside the aviary help to provide ad libitum live food. Larval insects (e.g., mealworms and fly pupae) contain more fat than adult insects, so they should be limited. Fruits and vegetables are a useful source of carbohydrates, but soft sugary foods do not promote dental health and should be limited. Many fruits are low in calcium, and individuals may consistently select low-calcium components from a mixture.

The suitability of the captive diet can be judged by monitoring body weight, body condition, coat condition, and fecal consistency. Obesity is a common problem in captivity. Captive animals are often fed an excess quantity of food, excess simple sugars, and excess fat, combined with insufficient exercise. The quantity of food provided should be limited to 15 to 20% of body weight, depending on energy requirements associated with age, ambient temperature, breeding condition, and enclosure size. Body weight should be monitored regularly, and the quantity fed adjusted accordingly. Body condition can be assessed by palpation of the gliding membrane, which should be thin and flexible, not rounded with fat. Normal feces are elongated, firm ellipses 12 mm × 4 mm and dark-brown to black, and are sometimes joined by hairs ingested when the animal grooms.

In groups, some individuals may emerge early to consume more than their share of the food. Multiple feeding stations in the enclosure should be provided, or obese dominant animals can be locked in the nest box until subordinate animals have fed.

Hand Rearing

Orphaning due to cat trauma is common in Australia. Hand rearing should be carried out by one individual so that there is consistency in technique and an opportunity for bonding with the foster parent. Success rates approach 0% for furless young, but experienced hand raisers may wish to try. Once the young are furred, success rates approach 100%. A substitute pouch is required for providing security and warmth. A cotton sock or the sleeve of a fleecy sweat shirt can be easily modified. Pouch-dependent marsupials cannot efficiently thermoregulate, and so they require a stable artificial heat source until they are ready to leave the nest. Just-furred young require a temperature in the range of 30 to 34°C. As they develop, the temperature can be reduced gradually, until they are left at ambient temperature by about 100 days of age. Figures 1 to 4 show some stages in the development of mother-reared sugar gliders.

Unfurred young should be fed every 1 to 2 hours. Recently furred young should be fed every four hours, and then the frequency of feeding should gradually be reduced to once or twice daily prior to weaning. Feed a low-lactose milk formula (e.g., Di-Vetalact, Sharpe Laboratories, Birmington, NSW, Australia; Wombaroo Food Products, Glen Osmond, South Australia; Biolac Universal Milk Products, Bonnyrigg, NSW, Australia). Guidelines for volume of milk to feed per day are shown in Table 3, along with milestones and body weight with respect to age. Juvenile sugar gliders usually lap readily from the tip of a syringe,

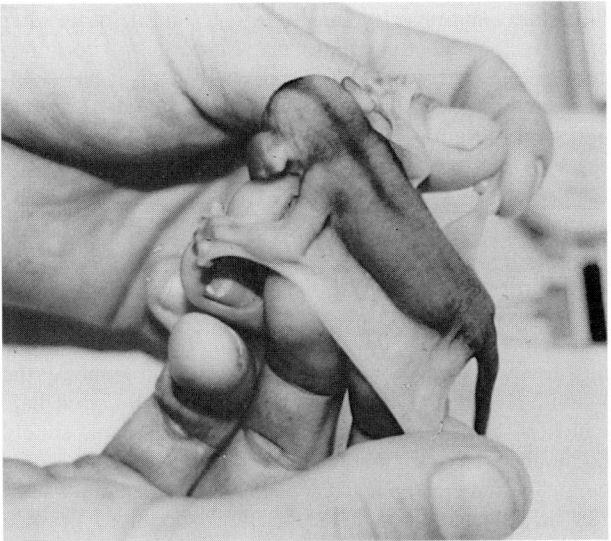

Figure 1. Mother-reared young sugar glider at 65 days and 13 gm. Young are now intermittently detached from the teat, the fur is beginning, the body and tail become pigmented, the dorsal stripe develops on the head and shoulders, and the gliding membrane becomes prominent.

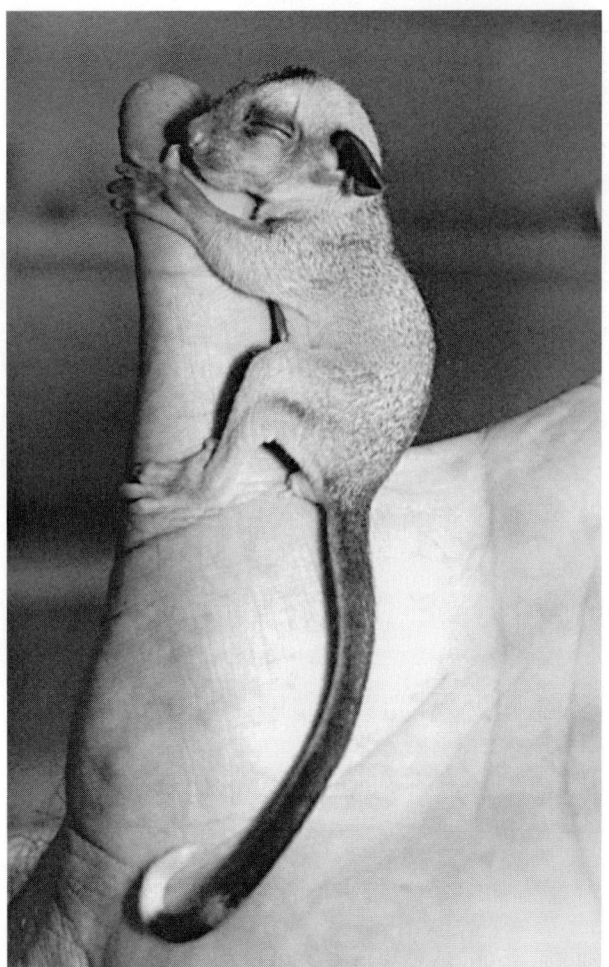

Figure 2. At 72 days and weighing 20 gm; the eyes are still closed and the body is now covered in short fur.

TABLE 3. Growth and Development of Young Sugar Gliders, *Petaurus breviceps breviceps*, from South East Queensland

Age (d)	Weight (g)	Feed (ml/d)	Milestones
1	0.2		Mouth and forelimbs most developed feature
20	0.8		Ears free from head, papillae of mystacial vibrissae visible
35	2.0	1.0	Mystacial vibrissae (whiskers) erupt, ears pigmented
40	3.0	1.5	Pigmentation starts on shoulders, eyeslits present
60	12	3	Detaching from teat, fur emerging, dorsal stripe developing
70	20	4	Eyes open, fully furred, left in nest
80	35	6	Fur lengthens
90	44	7	
100	54	8	Emerging from nest, starting to eat solid foods
130	78		Weaned

Sedation and Anesthesia

Tiletamine-zolazepam has been associated with the mortality of three apparently healthy squirrel gliders when used at a dose of 10 mg/kg IM (Holz, 1992). Therefore, this drug combination is not recommended for use in sugar gliders, although it is a very useful anesthetic agent in possum species.

Isoflurane administered with oxygen via vaporizer and T-piece is the anesthetic of choice. Induction is achieved by application of a small face mask and inhalation of 5% isoflurane. Intubation is possible with the use of a 1-mm endotracheal tube with stylet (Cook's). The tongue is extended, and a fine-bladed laryngoscope is used to visualize the larynx, with the head gently extended maximally to

or they can be taught to lap from a small plastic lid. Food intake should be measured and recorded at each feed. Stimulate hand-raised young to urinate and defecate after each feed by gently wiping the cloaca with moistened cotton wool. Measure body weight daily until it has stabilized, and then weekly. Start offering solid foods at around 100 days (50 gm). Wean by 130 days (80 gm).

MEDICINE

Handling and Restraint

Capture is best achieved by blocking the entrance to the nest box and then opening the hinged lid and grabbing the individual with the hand protected by a small cotton bag, which is then inverted over the glider. Bag seams should be double-sewn so that no frayed threads can become tangled around the animal's appendages. The animal's head can be palpated through the bag and should be grasped firmly behind the ears, with the rest of the animal's body cupped in the hand. Peel the bag back to expose the face for examination or to apply a face mask for induction of anesthesia.

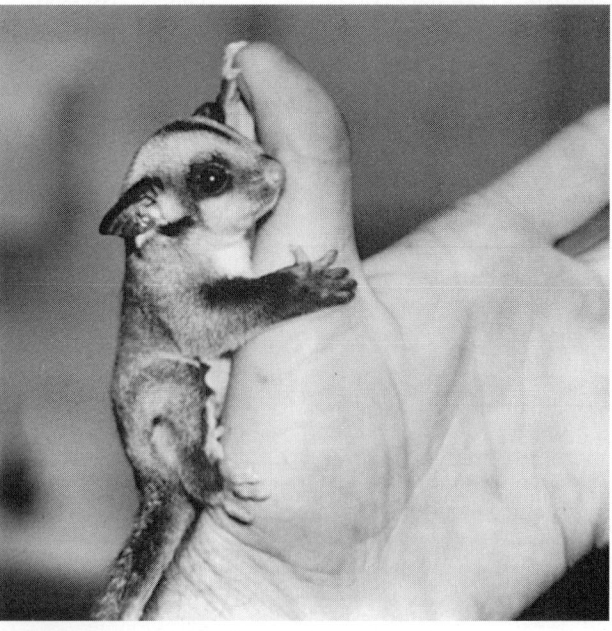

Figure 3. At 87 days and weighing 38 gm; the eyes are now open and juveniles are well furred.

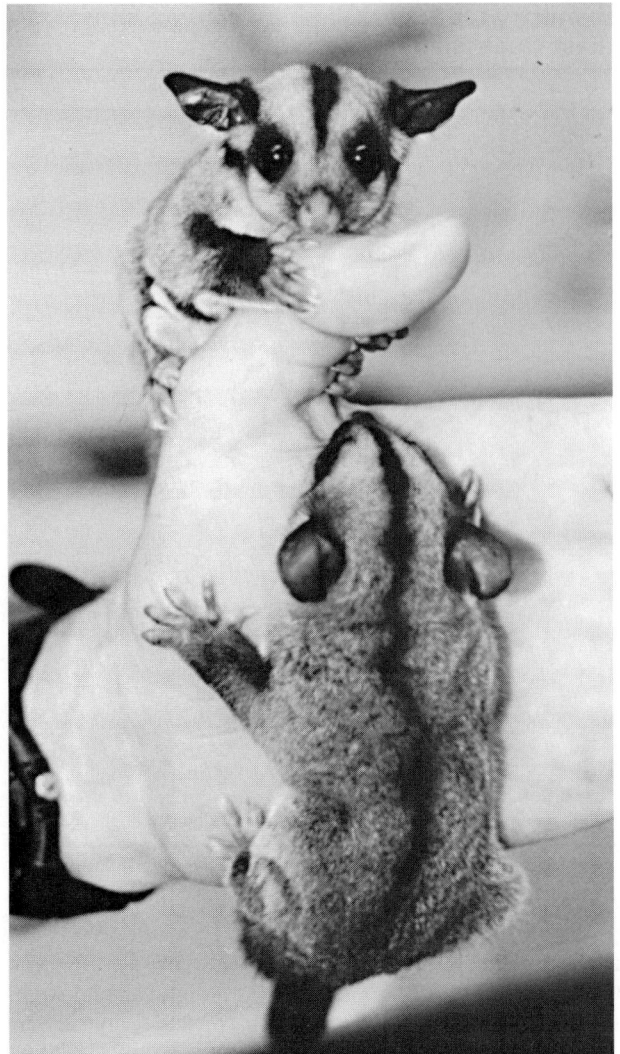

Figure 4. At 94 days, weighing 42 gm, young start to emerge from the nest and eat solid foods.

marsupials of less than 300 gm have been bled from this vessel without harmful sequelae.

Jugular Vein. The jugular cannot be visualized because the neck is short, the skin is loose, and subcutaneous fat is prominent in this region. Clip the hair. Identify the thoracic inlet and the angle of the jaw to determine the direction of the jugular groove.

Lateral Tail Vein. There is a vein running down each side of the tail. If the hair is clipped and a rubber band tourniquet applied, the vein can be visualized and pricked with a 25-gauge needle to obtain a drop of blood, which can be collected into hematocrit tubes. Alcohol interferes with blood droplet formation on the skin surface by reducing the surface tension, so use an aqueous antiseptic.

Femoral Vein. This site is not usually successful for obtaining useful quantities.

Cardiac Puncture. This procedure is not recommended except in nonsurvival procedures.

Orbital Bleeding. Orbital bleeding is not recommended for exophthalmic species.

Reference Ranges

Table 4 shows reference ranges for hematology and biochemistry for *Petaurus breviceps breviceps* from South East Queensland. These ranges differ from reference ranges from up to 17 captive animals from North America recorded on the International Species Inventory System (ISIS) database in that there are significantly higher lymphocyte counts in the Queensland animals. The reason for this finding is uncertain, but it could be the result of population-specific genetic variation or may reflect a difference between arterial blood and venous blood. Queensland animals were bled from the medial tibial artery. Table 5 lists some physiologic data for sugar gliders.

Common Diseases

Parasites. There are no reported diseases caused by parasites in sugar gliders. Parasites that have been identified in sugar gliders include the trematode *Athesmia* sp. found in the liver, and nematodes *Parastrongyloides* sp., *Paraustrostrongylus* sp., and tentatively identified *Paraustroxyuris* sp. (Spratt et al, 1991) from the gut. Ectoparasites include the Trombiculid mite *Guntheria kowanyama*, the Astigmatid mite *Petauralges rackae,* and an Atopomelid mite. Anthelmintics used without apparent side effects in possums and gliders include fenbendazole at a dose of 20 to 50 mg/kg PO s.i.d. for 3 days, oxfendazole at a dose of 5 mg/kg PO once only, and ivermectin at a dose of 0.2 mg/kg PO or SC once only. Carbaryl powder (50 gm/kg) has been used topically and in the nest box to control mites.

Infectious Diseases. Sugar gliders have no recorded susceptibility to specific pathogens, but the following infectious agents are significant pathogens in possum species:

lift the soft palate clear. Maintenance is generally achieved with 2% isoflurane. See Table 5 for normal body temperature, heart rate, and respiratory rates with the animal under isoflurane anesthesia. Transient apnea during induction is common and, if the heart rate is stable, can generally be overcome with gentle pressure to the thorax.

Blood Collection

General anesthesia is required for achieving adequate restraint for blood collection. The volume of blood that can be safely collected is up to 1% of the body weight.

Medial Tibial Artery. There is an artery running medially and very superficially from just above the stifle to the tarsus. It is possible to insert a 29-gauge needle attached to a tuberculin syringe into this artery. It is quite mobile but easiest to enter just distal to the stifle. As much as 0.5 ml of blood can usually be drawn from each side. Care must be taken to minimize hematoma formation. Many

TABLE 4. Reference Ranges for Hematology and Biochemistry for Sugar Gliders, *Petaurus breviceps breviceps,* from South East Queensland

Parameter	Units	n	Mean	Range
Erythrocytes	$\times 10^{12}$/L	7	7.5	6.5–8.3
Hemoglobin	gm/L	7	151	128–162
Packed cell volume	%	7	47.6	40–51
MCH	$\mu\mu$g	7	20.2	18.5–21.9
MCHC	gm/L	7	318	310–338
MCV	fl	7	63.7	57.8–69.6
Leukocytes	$\times 10^9$/L	7	16.3	9.1–22.8
Segmented Neutrophils	$\times 10^9$/L	7	1.01	0.45–1.75
Lymphocytes	$\times 10^9$/L	7	14.99	8.28–21.2
Monocytes	$\times 10^9$/L	7	0.05	0–0.23
Eosinophils	$\times 10^9$/L	7	0.23	0–0.99
Basophils	$\times 10^9$/L	7	0	0
Nucleated RBC	/100 WBC	7	0	0
Glucose	mmol/L	2	4.0	1.1–6.88
Urea	mmol/L	7	6.39	3.61–9.71
Creatinine	μmol/L	5	48.0	20–70
Calcium	mmol/L	1	2.4	2.4
Phosphorus	mmol/L	1	2.6	2.6
Sodium	mmol/L	5	144.2	138–158
Potassium	mmol/L	3	5.4	4.4–6.3
Chloride	mmol/L	5	105.2	101–109
Bicarbonate	mmol/L	2	21.1	20.8–21.3
Cholesterol	mmol/L	3	5.17	3.3–6.4
Total protein	gm/L	6	62.5	56–69
Albumin	gm/L	6	33.3	30–35
Globulin	gm/L	6	29.2	22–36
Alanine aminotransferase	U/L	3	36	28–44
Alkaline phosphatase	U/L	1	188	188
Aspartate aminotransferase	U/L	3	49.7	20–70
Creatine phosphokinase	U/L	1	224	224

MCH, mean cell hemoglobin; MCHC, mean cell hemoglobin concentration; MCV, mean cell volume.

Cryptococcus neoformans, Yersinia pseudotuberculosis, Salmonella spp., *Mycobacterium* spp., *Toxoplasma gondii,* and *Leptospira* spp. Bacterial meningitis was the cause of death in 2 of 14 (14%) of squirrel gliders in one captive institution. Organisms were not identified.

Noninfectious Diseases. Nutritional osteodystrophy, or hindlimb paresis-paralysis, is a commonly reported disease of pet sugar gliders, but it has never been reported in zoo collections. From unpublished reports, the condition closely resembles the nutritional osteodystrophy seen in calcium-deficient lizards. The clinical manifestation is sudden onset of hindlimb paresis or paralysis. Radiography may demonstrate vertebral, pelvic, and long bone osteoporosis. Spinal trauma is a differential diagnosis for nutritional osteodystrophy. Many pet gliders are maintained on a potentially

TABLE 5. Selected Physiologic Data for Sugar Gliders, *Petaurus breviceps*

Parameter	Reference Range/Mean
Heart rate	200–300/min*
Respiratory rate	16–40/min*
Body temperature†	36.3°C
Body temperature in torpor†	≥15°C
Thermoneutral zone†	27–31°C
Basal metabolic rate†	2.54 W kg$^{0.75}$

*Under isoflurane anesthesia.
†Fleming MR: Thermoregulation and torpor

calcium-deficient diet of 75% fruit and 25% muscle meat. Cases identified early may respond to a high-calcium, high-vitamin D_3 diet and strict cage rest. Nocturnal animals are presumed to rely on gut absorption of vitamin D_3, rather than skin absorption of ultraviolet light, to convert vitamin D_1 to D_3. Diets should contain approximately 1% calcium, 0.5% phosphorus, and 1,500 IU/kg of vitamin D_3 on a dry weight basis. Insects fed to gliders should be supplemented with calcium. Dusting insects with calcium powder is less reliable than feeding (gut loading) insects a high-calcium diet (e.g., Mazuri, PMI Feeds, St. Louis, MO) 48 hours before they are fed out.

Neoplasia. Neoplasia, particularly lymphoid neoplasia (50% of reported neoplasms), is relatively common in captive gliders. A review of mortalities in one captive institution revealed that 3 of 14 (21%) squirrel gliders died with neoplasia, specifically one malignant lymphoma in spleen, liver, and kidney; one basal cell tumor of the pouch; and one bronchogenic carcinoma. Two of three mortalities in the greater glider, *Petauroides volans,* were due to neoplasia, with one chondrosarcoma in the jaw with metastases to the liver, and one malignant lymphoma in lymph nodes and spleen. There is also a published report of cutaneous lymphosarcoma in a sugar glider (Hough et al, 1992).

Severe Allergic Dermatitis. Severe allergic dermatitis from Seleen shampoo (selenium sulfide 1% in a detergent base) has occurred in a squirrel glider.

Obesity. This condition has been associated with fatal coronary artherosclerosis in a Leadbeaters possum. Abdominal fat necrosis was the only pathology identified in an obese 300-gm, 3½-year-old sugar glider at death.

Dental Problems. Periodontal disease and tartar accumulation is common in captive sugar gliders, particularly those fed soft, carbohydrate-rich diets. Removal of tartar with the animal under general anesthesia, followed by broad-spectrum antibiotic treatment, is indicated. The diet should also be modified to include as much live food as possible, particularly insects with coarse exoskeletons.

Exposed root canals may occur secondary to tooth decay or traumatic fracture of incisors. The diameter of the root canals is too small to allow root canal filling, and it is almost impossible to remove a lower incisor without fracturing the mandibular symphysis. Animals have tolerated exposed root canals without intervention but may select soft components of the diet and therefore should be monitored regularly for tartar accumulation.

Eye Problems. Sugar gliders are exophthalmic and frequently sustain traumatic injury to the cornea during fighting. Corneal ulcers are relatively common and usually respond well to temporary tarsorrhaphy and application of antibiotic eye ointment. Bite wounds to the face may result in retrobulbar abscessation, which may need to be differentiated from molar root abscessation. Drain and flush the wounds with the patient under general anesthesia, culture the discharge for aerobes, anaerobes, and *Cryptococcus*, and treat as indicated.

Traumatic Injuries. The most common cause of presentation of wild sugar gliders to wildlife rehabilitation facilities in Australia is cat predation. Typical injuries include pneumothorax, hemothorax, and spinal trauma with paralysis; the prognosis is guarded. The skin is usually intact. Owl predation typically involves subcutaneous and muscular hemorrhage to the dorsal neck and thorax. Conspecific trauma can vary from minor puncture wounds to fatal injury.

Acknowledgments

I would like to express my appreciation to Jeff McKee for editorial assistance, Jim Phelan for providing autopsy data, and Wes Caton for husbandry advice and growth rate data, and to Geoff Pye, Katie Reid, and Sue Whyte for assistance with determining reference ranges.

References and Suggested Reading

Basden R: The occurrence and composition of manna in eucalyptus and angophora. The Proceedings of the Linnean Society of NSW, 90:152, 1965.

Fleming MR: Thermoregulation and torpor in the sugar glider *Petaurus breviceps* (Marsupialia: Petauridae). Aust J Zool 28:521, 1980.

Henry SR, Suckling GC: A review of the ecology of the sugar glider *Petaurus breviceps*. In: Smith A, Hume I, eds: Possums and Gliders. Chipping Norton, NSW: Surrey Beatty and Sons Pty Ltd, 1984, pp 355–358.

Holz P: Immobilisation of marsupials with tiletamine and zolazepam. J Zoo Wild Med 23:426, 1992.

Hough I, Reuter RE, Rahaley RS, et al: Cutaneous lymphosarcoma in a sugar glider. Aust Vet J 69:93, 1992.

Nagy KA, Suckling GC: Field energetics and water balance of sugar gliders, *Petaurus breviceps* (Marsupialia: Petauridae). Aust J Zool 33:683, 1985.

Smith AP: Diet and feeding strategies of the marsupial sugar glider in temperate Australia. J Anim Ecol 51:149, 1982.

Smith MJ: Observations on growth of *Petaurus breviceps* and *P. norfolcensis* (Petauridae: Marsupialia) in captivity. Aust J Wild Res 6:141, 1979.

Smith MJ: The reproductive system and paracloacal glands of *Petaurus breviceps* and *Gymnobelideus leadbeateri* (Marsupialia: Petauridae) In: Smith A, Hume I, eds: Possums and Gliders. Chipping Norton, NSW: Surrey Beatty and Sons Pty Ltd, 1984, pp 321–330.

Spratt DM, Beveridge I, Walter EL: A catalogue of Australasian monotremes and marsupials and their recorded helminth parasites. Rec. S. Aust. Mus., Monogr. Ser. No. 1:30, 1990.

Suckling GC: Sugar glider *Petaurus breviceps* Waterhouse 1839. In: Strahan R, ed: The Mammals of Australia. Chatswood, NSW: Reed Books, 1995, pp 229–231.

Tyndale-Biscoe H, Renfree M: Reproductive Physiology of Marsupials. Cambridge: Cambridge University Press, 1987, pp 18, 19, 22, 59, and 123.

Diagnostic Imaging of Reptiles

MARK D. STETTER

Lake Buena Vista, Florida

Even for experienced practitioners, reptilian diseases can be difficult to diagnose. Ill reptiles commonly exhibit nonspecific clinical signs, or sometimes none at all. Our limited knowledge and understanding of normal reptilian anatomy and physiology may confound the interpretation of physical examination and laboratory findings. Diagnostic imaging can provide important clues about the diagnosis of certain diseases and can help document and monitor the animal's response to therapy. Radiography and ultrasonography are readily available and provide excellent images of normal and abnormal anatomy (Fig. 1*A* to *B*). Computed tomography (CT) scan and magnetic resonance imaging (MRI) can produce higher-quality images but are less available to the practitioner (see Fig. 1*C* to *D*).

RESTRAINT AND POSITIONING

Based on an animal's size and demeanor, the experience of the personnel, and the procedure being performed, either manual or chemical restraint can be used when one works

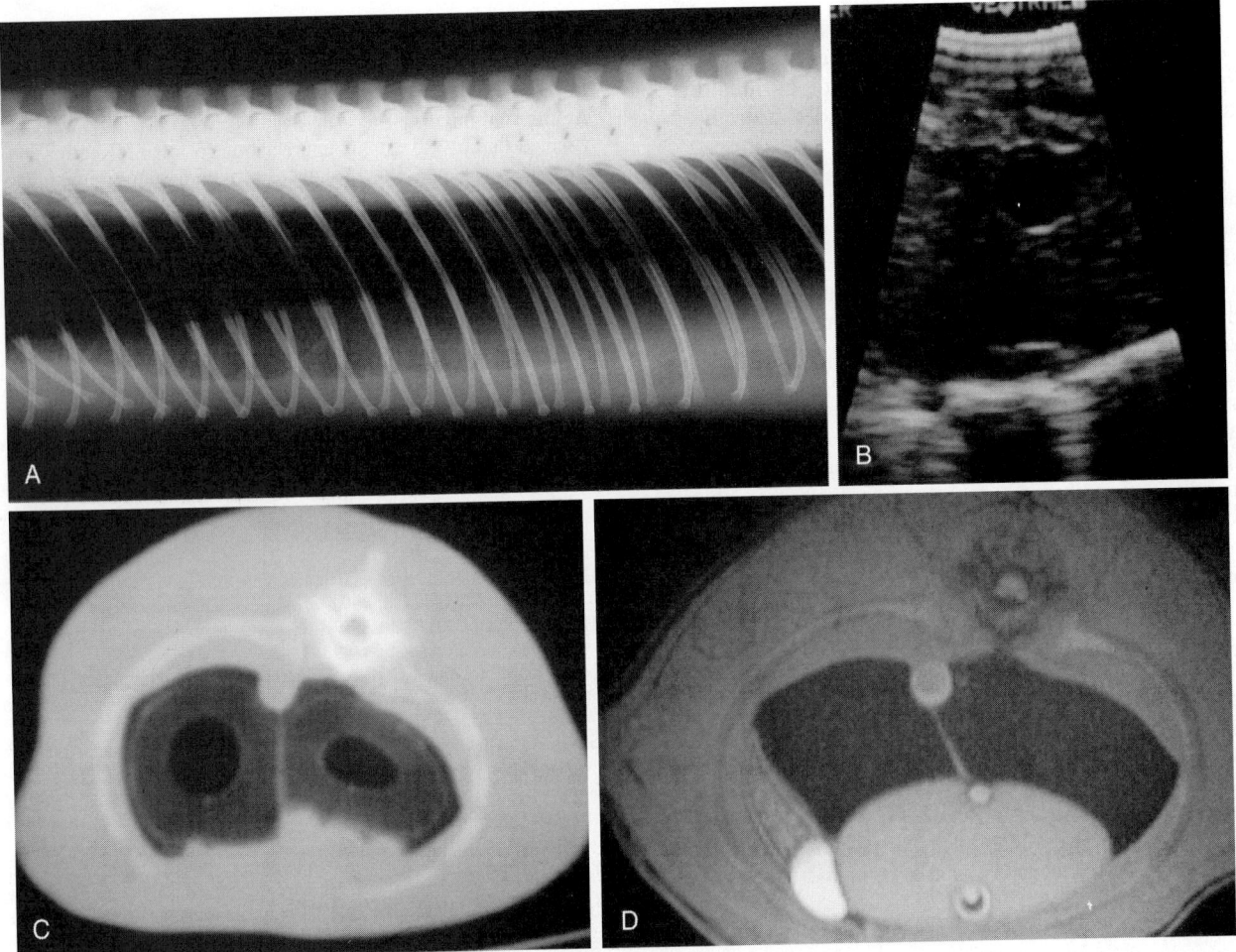

Figure 1. *A* to *D*, Comparison of four methods of diagnostic imaging in the cranial third of a clinically normal Burmese python *(Python molurus bivittatus)*. *A*, Lateral radiograph demonstrates the decreasing size of the lungs and corresponding enlargement of the liver. Note the good contrast between bone, air, and soft tissue but the general lack of contrast between the soft tissue structures. *B*, Ultrasound image of the liver taken at the same location as the radiograph. Note the normal hepatic parenchyma and the large portal vessel. Ultrasound is unable to image the adjacent air-filled lungs or skeletal structures. Note the detailed imaging of bone and pulmonary anatomy but poor contrast of the soft tissue structures. *D*, Magnetic resonance image demonstrates the spinal cord, dorsal aorta, lung spaces, liver, portal vessel, fat body, and esophagus. Note the excellent soft tissue contrast and detail that MRI can provide.

with reptiles. For radiography, snakes can be placed in long, clear acrylic tubes than can be placed directly on the x-ray cassette. Smaller reptiles can be placed in a sealable plastic bag that has been vented for air exchange. Turtles can be taped directly to the cassette or elevated on a small box that keeps their feet from touching the ground. Dorsoventral positioning is the most useful view (Figs. 2 and 3) but should always be complemented with a horizontal view (either lateral or anteroposterior). Lateral views can be acquired by rotating the unit 90 degrees into a horizontal x-ray beam direction. If this is not possible, the animal can be "sandwiched" between two foam blocks and placed onto its side. Another useful view in chelonians is the anteroposterior view. Pneumonia in chelonians is best visualized with the anteroposterior view because it highlights the radiodensity of the right and left lung fields (Fig. 4).

Ultrasonography is commonly performed with manual restraint. Reptiles can be imaged in either dorsal or sternal recumbency. If sternal, the patient can be placed on a cut-out platform with the visceral area of interest placed over the open section. To improve imaging, small animals can be immersed in a water bath (keeping the head out). Many reptiles have very thick scales that may interfere with ultrasound imaging. Commonly, the thickest scales are located ventrally; and in these species, placement of the transducer laterally may produce a better image. In chelonians, the transducer is placed in the inguinal area just cranial to the rear legs on the soft skin between the femur and bridge of the shell. For cardiac imaging, the transducer can be placed between the left or right front leg and the neck.

REPTILE RADIOGRAPHY

Rare earth radiographic film and screens provide excellent images of reptile species. The principles and techniques of domestic animal radiography also apply to reptiles. However, owing to a lack of visceral fat in reptiles, individual organs (e.g., kidney, spleen, liver) are poorly differentiated and often cannot be specifically identified.

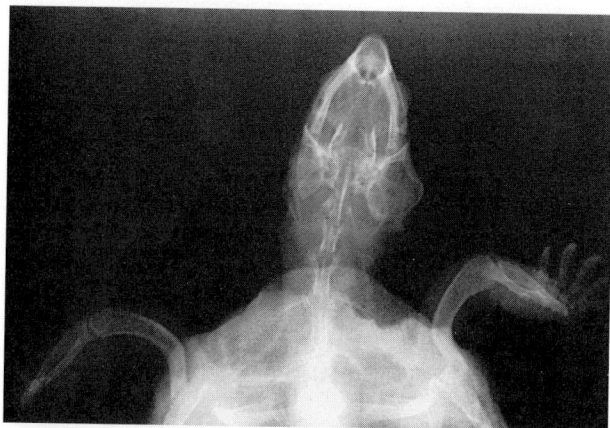

Figure 2. Dorsoventral radiograph of an Eastern box turtle *(Terrapene carolina)* with a chronic severe otitis. Note the soft tissue enlargement and capsular calcification of this right ear granuloma.

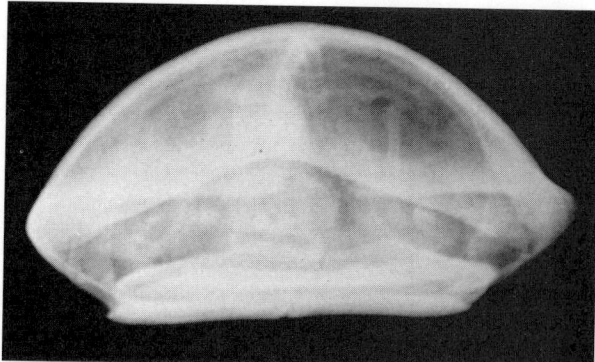

Figure 4. Anteroposterior radiograph of a spotted pond turtle *(Geoclemmys hamiltoni)* with pneumonia. Note the increased radiodensity of the right lung field as compared with the left.

Knowledge of normal reptilian anatomy and availability of comparison films of other reptiles are useful when interpreting films. Radiography is commonly used to determine if a reptile is gravid. Eggs can be easily seen in oviparous species (Fig. 5), and skeletal structures can be seen in viviparous species (Fig. 6). The presence of calcified hemibaculum in certain monitor species can be used for sex determination (Fig. 7). Gastrointestinal contrast studies can be performed to help identify organomegaly or masses. Nonionic, iodinated contrast media at 10 to 15 ml/kg is commonly used by the author. Reptiles (Fig. 8) have much longer gastrointestinal transit times than mammals, and contrast media may take several days or longer to reach the colon.

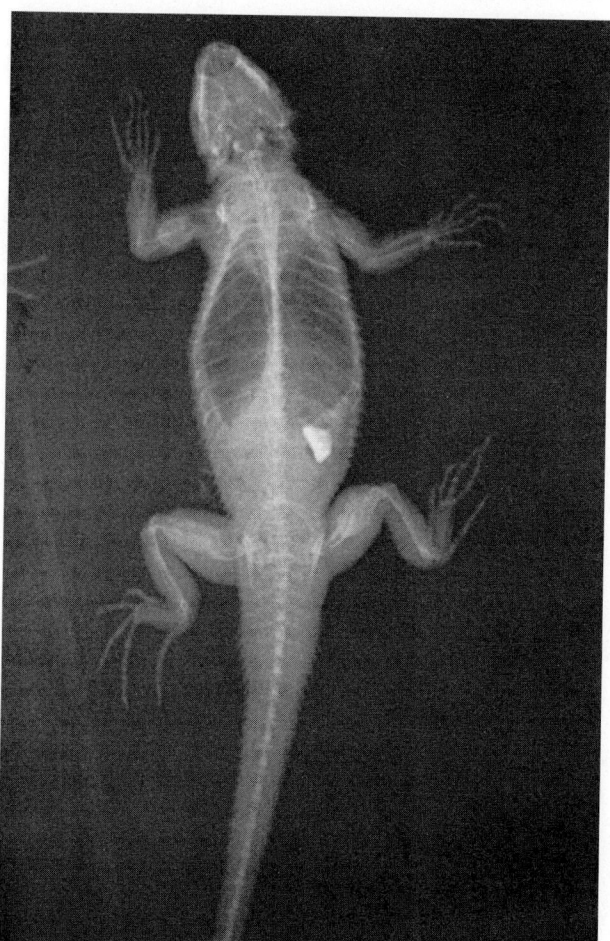

Figure 3. Dorsoventral radiograph of a granite spiney lizard *(Sceloporas orcutti)* demonstrating severe metabolic bone disease. Note the pathologic fractures and poor bone calcification in both humerus and femurs.

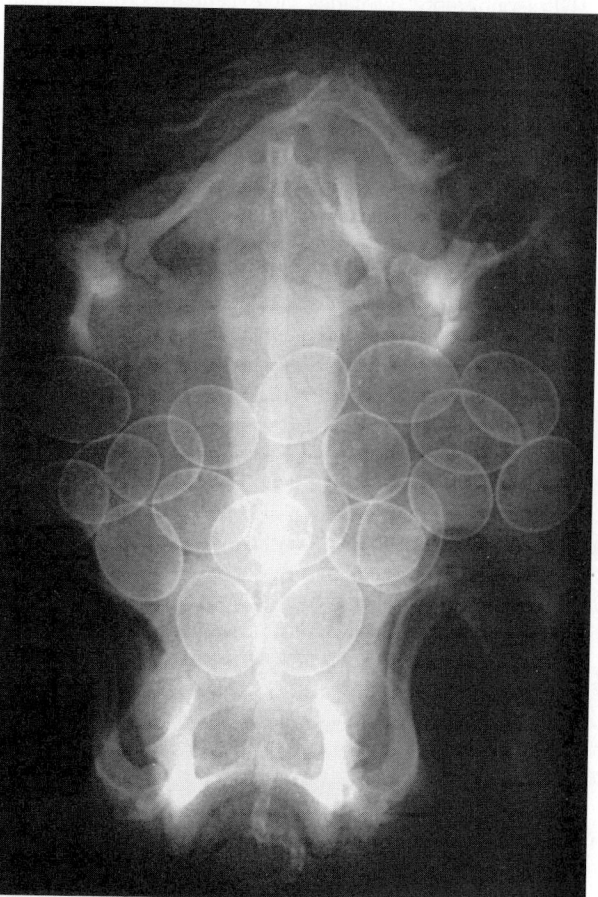

Figure 5. A gravid giant side-necked turtle *(Chelodina expansa)*. This dorsoventral radiograph demonstrates normal calcified ova.

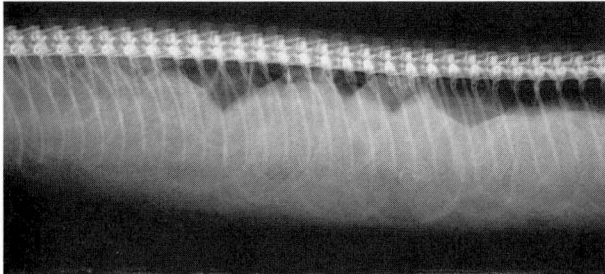

Figure 6. Lateral radiograph of the caudal portion of an emerald tree boa *(Corallus caninus)*. Note the numerous calcified spines that represent fetuses in this gravid viviparous snake.

Another radiographic technique that has been rapidly gaining popularity is the use of mammography film (Fig. 9) This film not only provides outstanding contrast and detail when imaging reptiles but also can be used with either specialized mammography units or with conventional x-ray machines. The advantage of using mammography machines is that they have a sensor that can determine the animal's density and automatically adjust the appropriate MAS. Mammography film must be used with corresponding cassettes and with a shorter focal film distance of 66 cm.

REPTILE ULTRASONOGRAPHY

Ultrasonography provides an excellent complement to radiography. Unlike radiography, ultrasound imaging can differentiate various soft tissue structures and provide information regarding organ location and pathologic changes. The basic principles of mammalian ultrasound should be used when working with reptiles. This modality provides excellent images of the heart, liver, gallbladder, and female reproductive organs. Depending on the ultrasound equip-

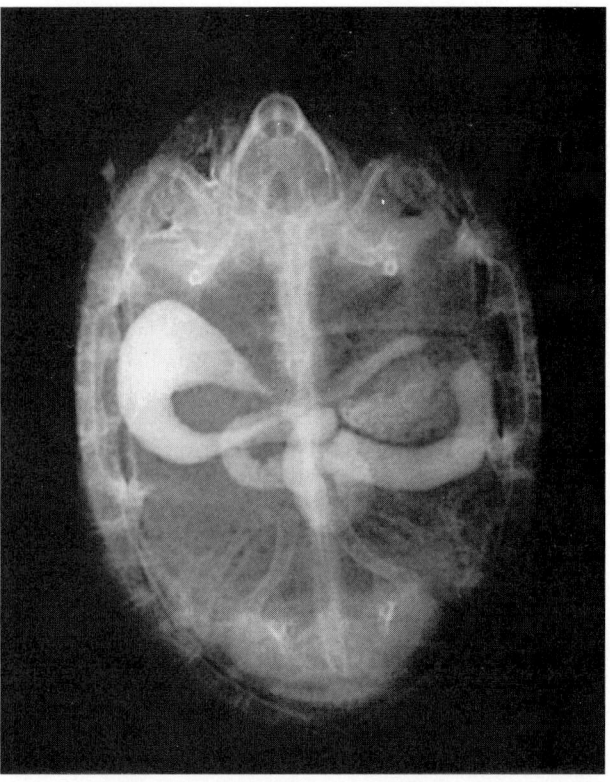

Figure 8. Dorsoventral radiograph of an Indochinese box turtle *(Cistoclemmys galbinifrons)* that is undergoing a gastrointestinal series with barium sulfate. Note the large amount of barium within the stomach and its normal passage through the small intestines.

ment, the operator's experience, and the animal's size, ultrasonography may be useful in evaluating the gastrointestinal tract, kidneys, or testes. Ultrasound has been particularly useful for reproductive studies of female reptiles

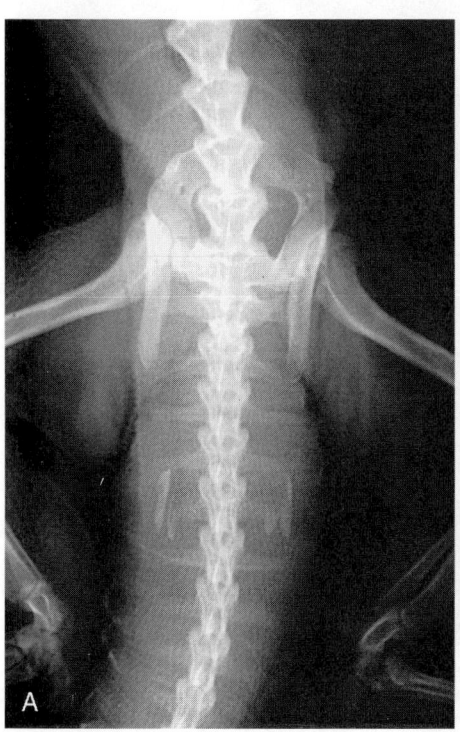

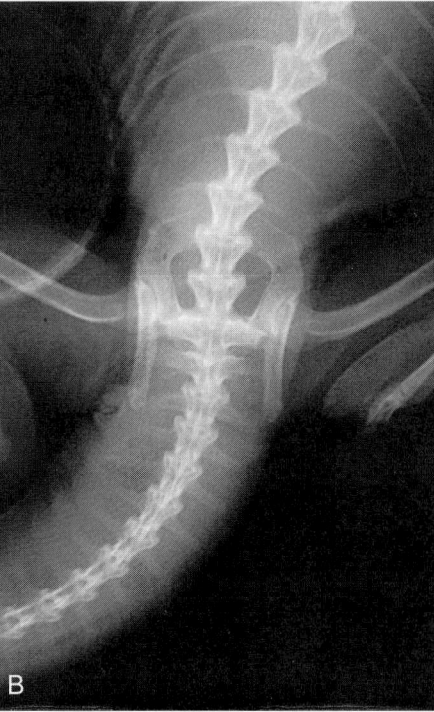

Figure 7. *A* and *B*, Dorsoventral radiographs of male and female monitor lizards demonstrating the normal calcified hemibaculum in certain male monitor species that can be used for sex determination.

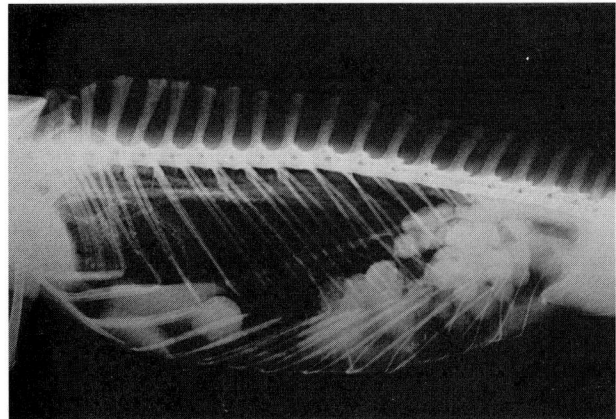

Figure 9. Lateral radiograph of a Meller's chameleon *(Chamaeleo melleri)* using mammography film. Note the excellent skeletal detail and contrast between the air-filled lungs and the other visceral organs. A large number of uncalcified ova can be seen as a grapelike cluster in the caudal abdomen. The large gallbladder, liver, heart, and lungs can also be visualized.

(Fig. 10). Ovarian activity can be monitored, and the presence of ova within the reproductive tract can be easily determined (Fig. 11). Some species of lizards (Varanus spp. and Heloderma spp.) are not sexually dimorphic, and ultrasound has been useful in sex determination of immature animals. Ultrasound is of no value when attempting to image the skeletal or respiratory systems.

B-mode real-time ultrasound machines are most commonly used. Smaller patients are best imaged using a 7.5- or 10-MHz transducer. Larger reptiles may require the use of a 5.0-MHz transducer. Many veterinary and pediatric transducers are made with a smaller contact area than

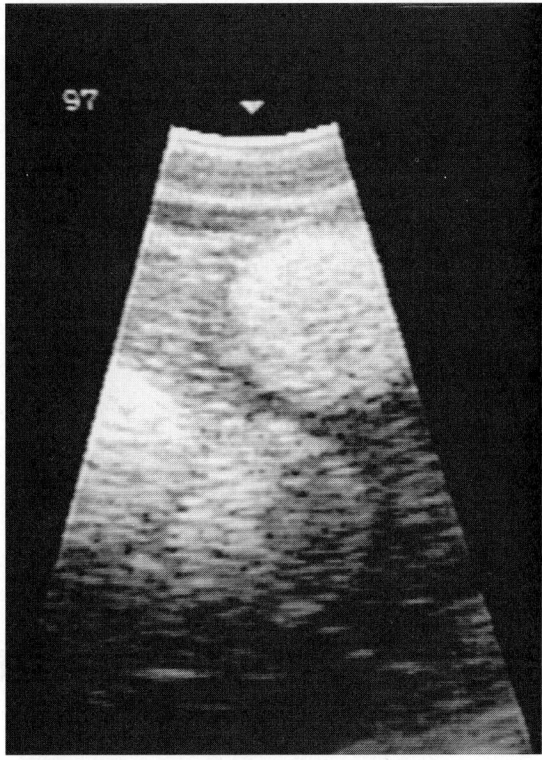

Figure 11. Ultrasound image of the ova of the animal in Figure 8, using a 7.5-MHz transducer placed just cranial to the hindleg.

transducers used for adult humans and are better suited for use with reptiles. Acoustic coupling gel should be applied freely to remove the air interface between the patient and the probe.

Unlike many other diagnostic imaging modalities, ultrasound imaging and interpretation is greatly limited by the experience of the operator. Practitioners are encouraged to enhance their ultrasound diagnostic capabilities by taking every opportunity to correlate surgical and postmortem anatomy with ultrasound findings.

REPTILE COMPUTED TOMOGRAPHY AND MAGNETIC RESONANCE IMAGING

The hard external scales of reptiles usually cause various degrees of artifact and interference when imaging with either radiography or ultrasonography. CT and MRI both offer superior detail of internal anatomy without interference from external scales. CT can be used for examining skeletal structures and imaging of the respiratory tract (see Fig. 1C), whereas MRI provides unparalleled detail of soft tissue structures and visceral anatomy (see Fig. 1D). Unlike the large scanning image that radiographs provide, CT and MRI create images of thin anatomical slices that are better suited for evaluation of a specific organ or lesion. CT and MRI require that the patient be immobile for relatively long periods and typically require manual restraint devices or sedation.

References and Suggested Reading

DeShaw B, Schoenfeld A, Cook RA, et al: Imaging of reptiles: A comparison study of various radiographic techniques. J Zoo Wildl Med 27:364, 1996.

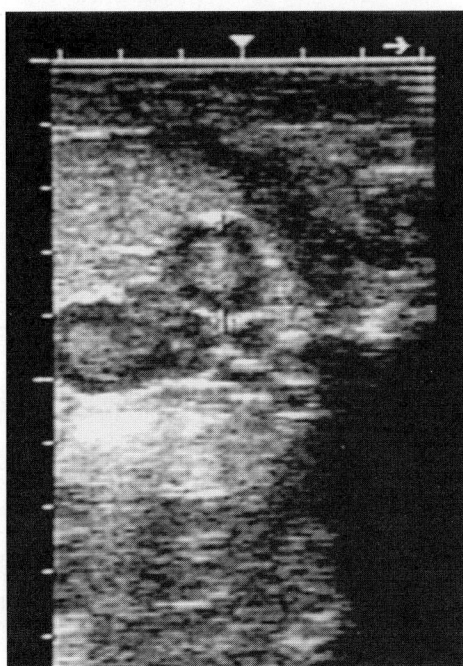

Figure 10. Ultrasound image of a female blood python *(Python curtus)*. Note numerous ovarian follicles with measurements being taken with the machine's electric calipers.

An in-depth discussion of mammography and its use with reptiles as compared with conventional radiography.

Robeck TR, Rostal DC, Burchfield PM, et al: Ultrasound imaging of reproductive organs and eggs in Galapagos tortoises (Geochelone elephantopus spp.). Zoo Biol 9:349, 1990.
A prospective study using ultrasonography to document and monitor reproductive physiology in giant tortoises.

Rubel GA, Isenbugel E, Wolverkamp P: Atlas of Diagnostic Radiology of Exotic Pets. Philadelphia: WB Saunders, 1991.
A radiology text of exotic animals that includes a section on reptile radiology.

Rubel GA, Kuoni W, Augustiny N: Emerging techniques: CT scan and MRI in reptile medicine. Semin Avian Exot Pet Med 3:156, 1994.
A prospective study introducing the use of CT and MRI with reptiles.

Rubel GA, Kuoni W, Frye FL: Radiology and imaging. In: Frye FL, ed: Biomedical and Surgical Aspects of Captive Reptile Husbandry. Malabar, FL: Krieger Publishing, 1991, p 185.
A book chapter that uses illustrations to introduce normal and abnormal diagnostic images of reptiles.

Sainsbury AW, Gili C: Ultrasonographic anatomy and scanning technique of the coelomic organs of the bosc monitor (*Varanus exanthematicus*). J Zoo Wildl Med 22:421, 1991.

A prospective study documenting the normal ultrasonographic anatomy of monitor lizards.

Schildger BJ, Casares M, Kramer M, et al: Technique of ultrasonography in lizards, snakes, and chelonians. Semin Avian Exot Pet Med 3:147, 1994.
A prospective study introducing the use of ultrasonography in reptiles.

Silverman S: Advances in avian and reptilian imaging. In Kirk RW, ed: Current Veterinary Therapy X: Small Animal Practice. Philadelphia: WB Saunders, 1989, p 786.
A review chapter that presents imaging techniques in birds and reptiles.

Silverman S, Janssen DL: Diagnostic imaging. In Mader RM, ed: Reptile Medicine and Surgery. Philadelphia: WB Saunders, 1996, p 258.
A book chapter that describes and illustrates basic imaging techniques in reptiles.

Stetter MD, Raphael BL, Cook RA, et al: Comparison of magnetic resonance imaging, computerized axial tomography, ultrasonography and radiology for reptilian diagnostic imaging. Proceedings of the American Association of Zoo Veterinarians. 1996, p 450.
A prospective study comparing the use of MRI, CT, ultrasound, and radiology for imaging various organ systems in snakes.

Antibiotic Therapy for Reptiles

ELLIOT JACOBSON

Gainesville, Florida

TABLE 1. Antimicrobial Drug Doses in Chelonians (Turtles and Tortoises) and Crocodilians (Alligators, Crocodiles)

Order	Drug	Species	Dose	Dose Interval	Route of Administration	Reference
Chelonia	Carbenicillin	Greek tortoise	400 mg/kg	48 hr	IM	Lawrence et al, 1986
	Ampicillin	Hermann's tortoise	50 mg/kg	12 hr	IM	Spörle et al., 1991
	Doxycycline	Hermann's tortoise	50 mg/kg	Loading dose	IM	Spörle et al, 1991
			25 mg/kg	72 hr		
	Gentamicin	Painted turtle	10 mg/kg	48 hr	IM	Bush et al, 1977
		Red-Eared slider	6 mg/kg	72–96 hr	IM	Raphael et al, 1985
		Gopher tortoise	5 mg/kg	48 hr	IM	Caligiuri et al, 1990
	Enrofloxacin	Box turtle	2.5 mg/kg	96–120 hr	IM	Aucoin, pers. comm., 1994
		Hermann's tortoise	10 mg/kg	24 hr	IM	Spörle et al, 1991
		Gopher tortoise	5 mg/kg	24–48 hr	IM	Prezant et al, 1994
		Indian Star tortoise	10 mg/kg	12–24 hr	IM	Raphael et al, 1994
	Ketoconazole	Gopher tortoise	15–30 mg/kg	24 hr	Oral	Page et al, 1991
Crocodilia	Gentamicin	American alligator	1.75 mg/kg	72–96 hr	IM	Jacobson et al, 1988
	Amikacin	American alligator	2.25 mg/kg	72–96 hr	IM	Jacobson et al, 1988

TABLE 2. Antimicrobial Drug Doses in Squamates (Lizards and Snakes)

Suborder	Drug	Species	Dose	Dose Interval	Route of Administration	Reference
Lacertilia (lizards)	Cefoperazone	Tegu	125 mg/kg	24 hr	IM	Speroni et al; cited in Klingenberg, 1996
Ophidia (snakes)	Carbenicillin	Mangrove snake King snake Reticulated python Great Plains rat snake Yellow rat snake Black rat snake	400 mg/kg	24 hr	IM	Lawrence et al, 1984

TABLE 2. Antimicrobial Drug Doses in Squamates (Lizards and Snakes) *Continued*

Suborder	Drug	Species	Dose	Dose Interval	Route of Administration	Reference
	Piperacillin	Blood python	100 mg/kg	48 hr	IM	Hilf et al, 1991
	Cefoperazone	False water cobra	100 mg/kg	96 hr	IM	Speroni et al; cited in Klingenberg, 1996
	Ceftazidime	Mangrove snake Boa constrictor Reticulated python Burmese python Yellow rat snake	20 mg/kg	72 hr	IM	Lawrence, 1984
	Chloramphenicol	Bull snake	40 mg/kg	24 hr	SC	Bush et al, 1976a
		Red-bellied water snake Midland water snake Gray rat snake Corn snake Eastern king snake Eastern indigo snake Black racer Hog-nose snake Copperhead Cottonmouth Timber rattlesnake Eastern diamondback rattlesnake Reticulated python Indian rock python Burmese python Boa constrictor	50 mg/kg	12–72 hr	SC	Clark et al, 1985
	Gentamicin	Bull snake	2.5 mg/kg	24 hr	SC	Bush et al, 1976b
		Blood python	2.5 mg/kg 1.5 mg/kg	Loading dose 96 hr	IM	Hilf et al, 1989
	Amikacin	Bull snake	5 mg/kg 2.5 mg/kg	Loading dose 72 hr	IM	Mader et al, 1985
	Ciprofloxacin	Reticulated python	2.5 mg/kg	48–72 hr	Oral	Klingenberg and Backner, 1991
	Enrofloxacin	Burmese python	10 mg/kg 5 mg/kg	Loading dose 48 hr	IM IM	Young et al, 1997

References and Suggested Reading

Bush M, Smeller JM, Charache P, et al: Preliminary study of antibiotics in snakes. American Association of Zoo Veterinarians Annual Proceedings, St. Louis, 1976a, pp 50–54.

Bush M, Smeller JM, Charache P, et al: Biological half-life of gentamicin in gopher snakes. Am J Veterinarians Res 39:171, 1976b.

Bush M, Custer R, Smeller JM, et al: Preliminary study of gentamicin in turtles. American Association Zoo Veterinarians Annual Proceedings, Honolulu, 1977, pp 71–73.

Caligiuri RL, Kollias GV, Jacobson ER, et al: The effects of ambient temperature on amikacin pharmacokinetics in gopher tortoises. Vet Pharmacol Ther 13:287, 1990.

Clark CH, Rogers ED, Milton SL: Plasma concentrations of chloramphenicol in snakes. Am J Vet Res 46:2654, 1985.

Hilf M, Swanson D, Wagner R, et al: Pharmacokinetics of gentamicin and piperacillin in blood pythons: New dosing regimen. In: Proceedings of the 13th International Symposium for the Propagation and Husbandry of Reptiles, Phoenix, Arizona, 1989, pp 87–90.

Hilf M, Swanson D, Wagner R, et al: Pharmacokinetics of piperacillin in blood pythons (Python curtis) and in vitro evaluation of efficacy against aerobic gram-negative bacteria. J Zoo Wildlf Med 22:199, 1991.

Jacobson ER, Brown MP, Chung M, et al: Serum concentration and disposition kinetics of gentamicin and amikacin in juvenile American alligators. J Zoo Anim Med 19:188, 1988.

Klingenberg RJ, Backner B: The use of ciprofloxacin, a new antibiotic, in snakes. In: Proceeding of the 15th International Symposium on Captive Propagation and Husbandry of Reptiles and Amphibians, Seattle, Washington, 1991, pp 127–140.

Klingenberg RJ: Therapeutics. In: Mader DR, ed: Reptile Medicine and Surgery. Philadelphia, WB Saunders, 1996, pp 299–321.

Lawrence K: Preliminary study on the use of ceftazidime, a broad-spectrum cephalosporin antibiotic, in snakes. Res Vet Sci 36:16, 1984.

Lawrence K, Needham JR, Palmer GH, et al: A preliminary study on the use of carbenicillin in snakes. J Vet Pharmacol Ther 7:119, 1984.

Lawrence K, Palmer GH, Needham JR: Use of carbenicillin in 2 species of tortoise (Testudo graeca and T. hermanni). Res Vet Sci 40:413, 1986.

Mader DR, Conzelman GM, Baggot JD: Effects of ambient temperature on the half-life and dosage regimen of amikacin in the gopher snake. J. Am Vet Med Assoc 187:1134, 1985.

Page CD, Mautino M, Derendorf H, et al: Multiple-dose pharmacokinetics of ketoconazole administered to gopher tortoises (Gopherus polyphemus). J Zoo Wildlf Med 22:191, 1991.

Prezant RM, Isaza I, Jacobson ER: Plasma concentrations and disposition kinetics of enrofloxacin in gopher tortoises (Gopherus polyphemus). J Zoo Wildlf Med 25:82, 1994.

Raphael BL, Clark CH, Hudson R: Plasma concentrations of gentamicin in turtles. J Zoo Anim Med 16:138, 1985.

Raphael BL, Papich M, Cook RA: Pharmacokinetics of enrofloxacin after a single intramuscular injection in Indian star tortoises (Geochelone elegans). J Zoo Wildlf Med 25:88, 1994.

Spörle H, Göbel T, Schildger B: Blood-levels of some anti-infectives in the Hermann's tortoise (Testudo hermanni). In: 4th International Colloquium on Pathology and Medicine of Reptiles and Amphibians. Abstract, 1991.

Young LA, Schumacher J, Papich MG, Jacobson ER: Disposition of enrofloxacin and its metabolite ciprofloxacin after intramuscular injection in juvenile Burmese pythons (Python molurus bivittatus). J Zoo Wildlf Med 28:71,1997.

Fluid Therapy in Reptiles

Juergen Schumacher

Knoxville, Tennessee

Often, dehydrated reptiles are presented to the veterinary practitioner. Severe dehydration (15 to 20% of body weight) can cause a moribund state. Abnormalities in fluid status should be diagnosed and treated before anesthesia, surgery, or other invasive procedures are performed. Although species, size, age, season, physical condition of the reptile, and the nature of the disease influence fluid and electrolyte imbalances, the general guidelines of fluid therapy known from domestic animals do apply in reptiles.

All reptiles are ectothermic animals. It has been shown that each reptile species has a preferred body temperature. Reptilian body functions depend on an adequate temperature and to ensure optimal response to therapy, it is necessary to maintain the patient within the appropriate preferred body temperature for the species. Reptiles have a renal portal system that is of clinical significance in respect to various drugs, their pharmacokinetics, and the administration of fluids. Drugs that are eliminated by renal excretion may not enter the systemic circulation at a therapeutic level if injected into areas that are drained by branches of the renal portal vein. Drugs with potential nephrotoxic potential may enter the kidneys in high concentrations. It is recommended that the renal portal system be avoided when using these compounds. Fluid therapy can be crucial to the maintenance of renal function, especially in the setting of nephrotoxic drug administration.

FLUID THERAPY

Before fluid therapy, it is essential to determine the degree of dehydration and the nature of the electrolyte imbalance accurately. This includes a thorough history from the owner and information on the type of fluids lost as well as the duration and estimated volume of fluids. This should be followed by a thorough physical examination. In many cases, the nature of the disease gives information about the type of imbalance present. A blood sample, to determine hematologic and plasma biochemical parameters, should be collected before the institution of therapy.

The goal of fluid therapy is to restore homeostasis and maintain organ function. If the patient is dehydrated and if electrolyte and acid-base imbalances have been determined, it is essential that these imbalances are corrected before any invasive procedures are performed. In emergency cases, it may become necessary to initiate and continue fluid therapy with the onset of anesthesia and into the recovery period. If the patient is chronically dehydrated, fluid therapy should be performed over a longer period to avoid rapid dilution of plasma proteins and electrolytes and loss of fluids by the kidneys. Anemic reptiles require transfusion of blood, whereas hypoproteinemic reptiles require plasma or colloids.

Blood Sampling Sites

In chelonians, the jugular vein is the most accessible vein and does not carry the risk of lymph contamination that can affect hematologic and plasma biochemical determinations. The anticoagulant of choice is lithium heparin because ethylenediaminetetraacetic acid has been shown to hemolyze chelonian red blood cells (Jacobson, 1992). Another sample site in chelonians is the brachial vein or plexus; however, it is surrounded by lymphatic vessels. In both fresh water and marine turtles, blood samples may be collected from the occipital sinus, located lateral to the cervical vertebrae cranial to the carapace. The dorsal tail vein is also commonly used in chelonians. In some chelonians, sedation may be required to obtain a blood sample.

In snakes, blood samples may be obtained via cardiocentesis or from the ventral tail vein. In lizards, samples can be obtained from the ventral tail vein, the abdominal vein or, in larger species, from the cephalic vein. In crocodilians, the occipital sinus can be used. (For more information see *CVT XII,* p. 1344 and Jacobson, 1992.)

Fluid Requirements and Selection

Reptiles have a higher percentage of total body water (63.0 to 74.4%) per unit body weight than do mammals. A higher percentage (45.8 to 58.0%) of fluid is also found in the intracellular space, whereas interstitial fluid volume, plasma volume, and extracellular fluid volume are lower in reptiles (Thorson, 1968). Therefore, it has been recommended that hypotonic fluids be administered in cases of severe dehydration to reduce extracellular fluid osmolality and achieve osmotic movement of water in the intracellular compartment (Jarchow, 1988). Hypotonic and dextrose-containing solutions provide sodium-free water. Administration of isotonic solutions will not change the osmolality of the extracellular fluid, and therefore only the volume of the extracellular fluid compartment is expanded.

Hypertonic solutions should be given with caution because they cause a shift of fluids from the intracellular space to the extracellular compartment. The recommendation for the volume to be administered varies among authors and ranges from 2 to 5% of the reptile's body weight (Jackson, 1981; Jarchow, 1988). It is advisable not to exceed 3% of the animal's body weight in fluids because too large a volume may cause signs of overhydration (Pokras et al, 1992; Jarchow, 1988). For maintenance purposes, the daily water requirement is 30 ml/kg per day and should be given, if possible, over 24 hours to avoid electrolyte abnormalities. Before therapy, the reptile should be acclimated to its preferred body temperature to ensure maximal function of all organ systems, and fluids should be warmed to the preferred body temperature to avoid hypothermia or shock.

Lactated Ringer's solution is often used when large volumes need to be given rapidly. It expands the extracellular volume without causing fluid shifts between the intracellular and extracellular space. However, long-term administration of lactated Ringer's solution results in hypokalemia and should be supplemented with potassium chloride. Physiologic saline can also be given for rapid expansion of the circulatory volume and for correction of hyponatremia and alkalemia. Dextrose solutions provide the body with free water and are indicated in cases of severe dehydration. However, they will not expand the circulatory volume because the water enters all fluid compartments. Lactated Ringer's solution containing 2.5% dextrose expands the circulatory volume without causing fluid shifts between fluid compartments. Dextran, hydroxyl starch, and plasma are not routinely used at present in reptilian fluid therapy (Seeler, 1996; Miller et al, 1992).

Routes of Fluid Therapy

Intravenous access is not as easily accomplished in reptiles as in mammalian species because of their size and anatomy. In chelonians, intravenous catheters can be placed in the jugular vein. In lizards, an appropriately sized catheter can be inserted in the ventral abdominal vein and can be sutured and taped in place. In larger specimens, the cephalic vein can be visualized after a cutdown procedure, and a catheter can be inserted and taped in place. In snakes, the jugular vein is the only accessible vein for catheterization and requires a cutdown procedure.

Intraosseous placement of a catheter can be accomplished in almost all lizards and chelonians, with the reptile's size being the limiting factor (see *CVT XII,* p. 1331). In lizards, the tibia is most commonly used and, depending on the size of the reptile, a spinal needle (20-gauge or 22-gauge) or small-gauge hypodermic needle can be inserted. In chelonians, the femur and the tibia may be used for intraosseous catheter placement. Studies in mammals and avian species have shown that intraosseous administration of fluids and drugs is comparable to intravenous administration. Fluids and blood products are generally given at the same rate and dose as by the intravenous route. The effects of various drugs on the bone has not been studied intensively. Hypertonic solutions cause mild necrosis. The advantages of intraosseous catheters over intravenous catheters include easier access and maintainance. Complications include the potential of osteomyelitis and a limited flow rate, especially in small patients. In reptiles with metabolic bone disease, special care has to be taken when placing the intraosseous catheter to avoid creating a hole in the tibia that is too large, which will result in leakage or even fractures. Drugs with established bone marrow toxicity should not be administered via an intraosseous catheter. Correct placement of the needle is ensured with aspiration of bone marrow or, if necessary, by radiography of the tibia. In the reptile with severe dehydration or shock, intravenous or intraosseous routes are the most effective and rapidly expand the circulatory volume and perfuse the kidneys. Intracoelomic administration of fluids is commonly used in reptiles. Care has to be taken to avoid visceral organs and not to administer volumes that are too large and cannot be absorbed adequately. Subcutaneous fluid administration is indicated in cases of mild dehydration or for maintenance purposes.

Oral administration of fluids is indicated in cases of mild dehydration. This can be accomplished via stomach tube in most reptiles. This route is contraindicated with gastrointestinal stasis (common in reptiles), and seizures, and after head trauma. In some instances, oral fluid administration may promote and activate gastrointestinal motility.

Disturbances of Hydration Status

The priority of fluid therapy is to maintain an effective circulating blood volume. In most cases, administration of a balanced electrolyte solution is required to achieve this goal. If electrolyte imbalances are determined, every effort should be made to identify the underlying problem and initiate corrective measures. Normal electrolyte levels in reptiles are species-dependent and a wide range of values has been published (Campbell, 1996). Interpretation of values is difficult because of differences in season, sex, temperature, and underlying disease as well as differences in sample collection and handling. It is often best to establish a blood sampling protocol and rely on reference values from the veterinarians's own laboratory.

Evaluation of hematologic and plasma biochemical parameters helps one assess the need for fluid therapy, the kind of fluids needed, and electrolyte imbalances. A packed cell volume higher than 50% should be considered a sign of dehydration, as should elevated plasma proteins (normal 3 to 8 gm/dl), elevated uric acid levels (normal 0 to 10 mg/dl), and high creatinine (>1 mg/dl) values.

Hyponatremia

Plasma sodium (Na) concentration normally ranges between 120 and 170 mEq/L in reptiles. Therapy is indicated if Na is less than 130 mEq/L. Chronic hyponatremia can be caused by water retention, edema, and a ruptured urinary bladder. Therapy includes treatment of the underlying disease, administration of Na-containing solutions, and diuretics. Severe hyponatremia should be treated immediately with hypertonic saline to change plasma concentration by 1 mEq/l per hour. The amount of sodium to be administered in millimoles (mEq) can be calculated using the formula:

$$\text{mmol } Na^+ = 0.2 \, BW_{kg} \, (\text{Normal } [Na^+] - \text{Patient's } [Na^+])$$

In mild to moderate cases, administration of normal (0.9%) saline ($Na^+ = 154$ mEq/L) is adequate to change plasma Na concentration by 0.5 mEq/L per hour.

Hypernatremia

Hypernatremia is most often seen as a result of dehydration, gastrointestinal disease, and renal failure. Therapy is indicated if serum Na is more than 170 mEq/L. Hypernatremia causes hyperosmolality, resulting in the shift of water from the intercellular space to the intravascular space, causing tissue dehydration. Clinical signs are often associated with central nervous system disease such as depression, seizures, coma, and stupor. Acute hypernatremia should be treated with intravenous 5% dextrose in water or 2.5% dextrose with lactated Ringer's solution. In hypovolemic reptiles, it is necessary first to administer balanced electrolyte solutions to expand the circulating fluid volume, followed by appropriate therapy as mentioned earlier. Chronic hypernatremia, often seen in reptiles as a result of inadequate fluid intake and renal failure should be corrected gradually to prevent cerebral edema. The plasma volume must be expanded slowly, and the Na level should not be lowered more than 1 mEq/L per hour.

Hypokalemia

Serum potassium (K) concentrations of less than 2.5 mEq/L require therapy. These low levels are caused by gastrointestinal loss of K, administration of K-poor fluids, or inadequate intake of K with the diet. Clinically, muscle weakness and intestinal ileus are associated with hypokalemia. K replacement therapy should include administration of 1 mEq/kg of KCl per day or 20 to 40 mEq/L of fluid. Replacement therapy should be slow and in acute cases no more than 0.5 mEq/kg per hour of KCl should be given.

Hyperkalemia

If plasma K concentration is more than 7 mEq/L treatment is required. Causes of hyperkalemia in reptiles include renal failure, ruptured urinary bladder, tissue trauma, acidosis, and administration of K-rich fluids. Clinical signs include lethargy, weakness, vomiting in some reptiles, anorexia, and arrhythmias. In mild cases, administration of normal saline is adequate, whereas in moderate to severe cases, dextrose or bicarbonate should be administered in addition to appropriate fluid therapy. Dextrose solutions promote cellular uptake of potassium. In severe cases, glucose at a dose of 1.0 gm/kg significantly increases uptake of potassium by the cells. The success of treatment should be monitored frequently. If severe electrocardiographic disturbances are present, calcium gluconate (10%) should be given at a rate of 1.0 ml/kg intravenously over 15 to 20 minutes.

Metabolic Acidosis

The most common causes of metabolic acidosis are renal failure, hypovolemia, and diarrhea. Treatment, such as volume replacement therapy in cases of hypovolemia, should eliminate the underlying problem. In severe cases, administration of sodium bicarbonate is indicated. The dose of sodium bicarbonate can be calculated using the formula:

$$\text{Base deficit} \times 0.3 \times \text{BW in kg} = \text{mEq of NaHCO}_3$$

Metabolic Alkalosis

Lethargy, seizures, and general weakness are often seen in cases of metabolic alkalosis. In addition, hypokalemia and hypochloremia (normal = 100 to 150 mEq/L) are often present. Treatment includes correction of the underlying problem, expansion of the fluid volume, and electrolyte replacement therapy. For most cases, normal saline supplemented with KCl is indicated.

Monitoring

The most reliable way to determine the extent of dehydration is comparison of the current weight with a weight obtained before the onset of illness. In acute cases of weight loss caused by fluid loss, this will allow the clinician to estimate the degree of dehydration. Unfortunately, in most cases a previous weight is not available. Clinical signs of dehydration include eyes sunken into the orbit, decreased skin turgor, dry mucous membranes, and decreased heart rate. In combination with a proper diagnosis and understanding of reptilian pathophysiology, these findings lead to a rough estimate of dehydration. Care has to be taken not to apply these criteria to chronically sick reptiles because emaciated reptiles may show similar symptoms. Before initiating fluid therapy, the degree of dehydration must be estimated, and samples for hematologic, serologic, and plasma biochemical determinations should be collected to obtain baseline values. Frequent measurement of body weight and essential electrolyte determinations can be used to monitor the success of fluid therapy. More invasive monitoring devices such as determination of arterial blood pressure and central venous pressure are not routinely used in reptile medicine.

TRANSFUSION MEDICINE

Little information has been made available on transfusion medicine in reptiles. In some instances, one-time transfusions, which minimize the risk of acute immunologic complications, have been used and may have been successful. For the practitioner specializing in reptile medicine, it may be advisable to keep blood donors representing the most common reptile species for emergency cases.

Before transfusion therapy, it is essential to evaluate the patient's status critically and diagnose the primary disease. Blood samples must be collected before transfusion therapy. Transfusion of blood is only a temporary option and does not replace the need to treat underlying disorders (Brooks, 1992). The need for transfusion therapy is dictated by the clinical status of the patient and laboratory test results, indicating anemia by a significant decrease in packed cell volume. Minimally, the packed cell volume and total protein should be determined before initiating transfusion of blood. The packed cell volume for most reptiles ranges between 20 and 40% (Campbell, 1996). Total protein for normal healthy reptiles ranges between 3 and 8 gm/dl (Campbell, 1996).

Indications

The decision for transfusion therapy in most cases is aimed at increasing red blood cells, thus increasing the oxygen carrying capacity of the blood. The best determinant of when to transfuse are clinical signs, including tachypnea, tachycardia, tissue hypoxia, and hypovolemia, which are sometimes difficult to determine in reptiles. Except for trauma cases or reptiles undergoing surgery with blood loss, most reptiles are presented in a stage of chronic illness. It is advisable to transfuse reptiles with acute anemia sooner than those with chronic anemia. Packed cell volume and total protein help support the need for therapy.

Hypoproteinemia is most often found in cachectic reptiles but can also be seen in cases of chronic liver and kidney disease as well as with chronic parasitism and malabsorption-maldigestion symptoms. Hyperproteinemia is most often associated with chronic infections and severe dehydration. The type of anemia (blood loss anemia, nonregenerative anemia, or hemolytic anemia) should be diagnosed before transfusion therapy is started. In acute cases, a blood loss of 20% or more of the total blood volume indicates the need for transfusion of whole blood.

Collection and Handling of Blood

In reptile transfusions, the commonly used anticoagulant is heparin (5 to 10 units per 1 ml of blood). Heparin does not contain preservatives, so the blood must be used within 2 days of collection. Additionally, since the viability of red blood cells decreases with the length of storage, it is advisable to transfuse only freshly collected blood. For most purposes, blood is collected from the donor animal just before its administration, for example, surgeries with anticipated blood loss. Since only small volumes of blood are usually collected from donor reptiles, blood may be collected in a plastic syringe containing the anticoagulant. Reptiles kept as blood donors should be in excellent health and free of parasites and infectious or noninfectious diseases. For most reptile species, the total blood volume accounts for approximately 5 to 8% of their body weight and 10% of the total blood volume can safely be withdrawn at a time (Jacobson, 1992). Frequency of blood collection should not exceed more than once every 1 to 2 months. After collection, whole blood should be kept in a cool place and should be administered warmed within 6 hours to maintain red blood cell viability.

Administration

It is recommended by the author not to exceed 20 ml/kg per hour in reptiles in shock. It is more advisable to transfuse 10 to 15 ml/kg every 24 hours at a rate of 5 to 10 ml/kg per hour. To prevent red cell hemolysis, blood should ideally be administered through a large intravenous catheter. If catheter placement is not possible, a butterfly catheter can be used for short-term venous access. When venous access is not possible, placement of an intraosseous catheter is recommended. Intraperitoneal administration is recommended only when venous or intraosseous access is not possible, as with snakes.

Whole blood should be administered warmed to a temperature of 25 to 30°C. Inline filters should be used in administration sets to avoid transfusion of blood clots and cellular debris. In most reptiles, transfusions are given with a syringe, and it is recommended that syringe filters with a pore size of 80 μm be used.

Transfusions appear to be safe, and although blood groups have been described in some reptile species, crossmatching is not routinely performed. However, several immunologic or nonimmunologic responses can complicate the success of transfusion, and most occur shortly after transfusion has been initiated. Clinical signs include, hypotension, edema, and intravascular or extravascular hemolysis. In these cases, discontinuation of the transfusion and administration of an immunosuppressive dose of a short-acting corticosteroid may be indicated. Acute reactions are visible shortly after the transfusion has been started and include tremors, collapse, shock, or vomiting, which is rarely seen in reptiles. This most often occurs in reptiles sensitized by previous transfusions. A variety of reasons are responsible for nonimmunologic reactions, such as improper storage, processing and administration of the blood, contamination, or circulatory overload. Therefore, strict aseptic technique has to be followed in the handling of the blood to be transfused. Overloading the recipient with too much blood too quickly results in clinical signs that include vomiting, dyspnea, tachycardia, and death.

Monitoring

Constant monitoring of the transfused reptile is essential to avoid complications and ensure success in transfusion medicine. If transfusion of whole blood is successful, the onset of response is usually rapid and should occur within hours of administration. Although more difficult to assess in reptiles than in mammals, respiratory rate, overall strength, mucous membrane color, and pulse quality should all improve. The hematocrit should be monitored and determined 2 hours after the transfusion has been terminated. If there is no improvement or there is a further decline in hematocrit, the causes may be continued blood loss, hemolysis, or decreased hematopoiesis.

References and Suggested Reading

Brooks M: Transfusion medicine. In: Murtaugh RJ, Kaplan PM, eds: Veterinary Emergency and Critical Care Medicine. St. Louis: Mosby–Year Book, 1992, pp 536–546.

Campbell TW: Clinical pathology. In: Mader DR, ed: Reptile Medicine and Surgery. Philadelphia: WB Saunders, 1996, p 248.

Jackson OF: Clinical aspects of diagnosis and treatment. In: Cooper JE, Jackson OF, eds: Diseases of the Reptilia. London: Academic Press, 1981, p 507.

Jacobson ER: Laboratory investigations. In: Beynon PH, ed: Manual of Reptiles. British Small Animal Veterinary Association, Ames, Iowa: Iowa State University Press, 1992, p 50.

Jarchow JL: Hospital care of the reptile patient. In: Jacobson ER, Kollias GV, eds: Exotic Animals. New York: Churchill Livingstone, 1988, p 19.

Miller MW, Schertel ER, DiBartola SP: Conventional and hypertonic fluid therapy: Concepts and applications. In: Murtaugh RJ, Kaplan PM, eds: Veterinary Emergency and Critical Care Medicine. St. Louis: Mosby–Year Book, 1992, p 618.

Pokras MA, Sedgwick CJ, Kaufman GE: Therapeutics. In: Beynon PH, ed: Manual of Reptiles. British Small Animal Veterinary Association. Ames, Iowa: Iowa State University Press, 1992, p 194.

Seeler DC: Fluid and electrolyte therapy. In: Thurmon JC, Tranquilli WJ, Benson GJ, eds: Lumb & Jones' Veterinary Anesthesia, 3rd ed. Baltimore: Williams & Wilkins, 1996, p 572.

Thorson TB: Body fluid partitioning in the Reptilia. Copeia 3:592, 1968.

Viral Diseases of Reptiles

JUERGEN SCHUMACHER
Knoxville, Tennessee

A variety of DNA and RNA viruses has been detected in reptiles, but few are associated with clinical disease. Viruses with established pathogenicity include paramyxovirus infection of viperid and nonviperid snakes, inclusion body disease (IBD) in boid snakes, and herpesvirus infection of tortoises and turtles.

This article describes pathology, clinical signs, and treatment options for the most significant viral diseases affecting private and zoologic collections of reptiles. Detailed information on the pathologic and viral characteristics can be obtained from original reports and review articles (Jacobson, 1986, 1993; Schumacher, 1996).

GENERAL PRINCIPLES OF SAMPLE COLLECTION

Proper collection, handling, and processing of tissue samples is necessary to confirm a viral cause. Tissue samples may be collected for histopathologic, electron microscopic, and viral isolation attempts. Biopsy specimens (e.g., from liver, kidney and skin) collected from sick reptiles or at postmortem examination are placed in 10% neutral buffered formalin for histologic examination. For electron microscopy, samples should be transferred into an appropriate fixative such as Trump's solution. For direct viral detection, samples of fluids (e.g., from vesicles) can also be collected and processed for negative staining electron microscopy. (See Jacobson [1992] for detailed information on collection and handling of various diagnostic samples.)

Post mortem, all organ systems should be examined carefully and gross changes noted. Samples from all major organ systems should be collected and placed in 10% formalin for histopathologic evaluation. Samples from representative organs should also be placed in an electron microscopic fixative. For viral isolation attempts, it is necessary to collect tissues aseptically from all major organs (liver, kidney, spleen, heart, lung). Tissue samples should be stored frozen at −70°C. Several reptilian cell lines are commercially available and are used by specialized laboratories. Not all viruses will grow in these cell lines, and it may become necessary to establish other primary cell cultures. For the practitioner seeing a high number of reptiles, it is recommended that a laboratory be contacted to establish a protocol for tissue collection and handling.

DIAGNOSIS AND TREATMENT

Clinically, a viral infection is often suspected on the basis of characteristic clinical and histopathologic findings. Biopsy specimens from major organs (liver, stomach, skin) can be collected (with ultrasonographic guidance, if indicated) from a live reptile and submitted for histologic and electron microscopic evaluation. Body fluids, for example, urine, saliva, and fluid from vesicles, can be submitted for negative staining electron microscopy and direct demonstration of viral particles. As of yet, few laboratories have the expertise and capability to work with reptilian cell cultures, and relatively few viruses have been isolated.

Few serologic tests have been developed in reptiles. For paramyxovirus infection in viperid snakes, a hemagglutination inhibition test has been developed (Jacobson, 1993).

A viral cause should be suspected if an infectious cause for disease has been established, but clinical symptoms do not resolve, or only temporarily resolve, after the proper use of antibiotics or antifungal agents.

Unfortunately, there are no specific treatments for most viral diseases in reptiles. In most cases, treatment is limited to supportive measures, including prevention of secondary bacterial or fungal infections, or both, by the use of appropriate antimicrobial and antifungal agents. Vaccines that protect reptiles from viral infections have not yet been developed. Paramyxovirus vaccines have been evaluated in western diamondback rattlesnakes; however, the response to these vaccines was not reliable.

PREVENTION

Strict hygienic measures, such as regular disinfection of cages and equipment, and a strict quarantine protocol should be followed to prevent introduction of a viral agent into a collection. During quarantine, each animal should be examined thoroughly. Blood and fecal samples should be collected at the beginning and the end of the quarantine period. Underlying diseases should be diagnosed and treated before introduction of the animal into the collection. Sick animals should never be introduced into an established collection and should be kept in isolation. Every animal in the collection that dies during quarantine should be examined and appropriate postmortem samples collected.

HERPESVIRUS INFECTION OF CHELONIANS

Herpesviruses have been identified in marine and fresh water turtles and in tortoises. Herpesviruses have caused clinically significant disease and have contributed to high morbidity and mortality of infected animals. In many cases, affected animals are kept under stressful conditions resulting from overcrowding, transport, and unfavorable environmental conditions, Such poor conditions may impair immune function. Significant diseases in marine turtles include lung, eye, and trachea disease in green sea turtles *(Chelonia mydas)*. Gray-patch disease and fibropapillomatosis have also been associated with herpesvirus infection.

Fresh water turtles, including Pacific pond turtles *(Clemmys marmorata),* painted turtles *(Chrysemys picta),* and map turtles *(Graptemys* spp.) have also been diagnosed with herpesvirus infections. Herpesviruses have been detected in a variety of tortoise species, including Argentine tortoises *(Geochelone chilensis),* a desert tortoise *(Gopherus agassizii),* and spur-thighed tortoises *(Testudo graeca),* and in Europe many imported Mediterranean tortoises have been diagnosed with herpesvirus infection. The route of transmission is unknown but is most likely oral. Infected tortoises often exhibit nasal and ocular discharge, anorexia, and lethargy. Secondary bacterial infections often complicate clinical signs and conjunctivitis. Dyspnea and edema within the oral and nasal cavity may be seen. In addition, necrotizing lesions and abscesses in the oral cavity can also be present and can lead to open mouth breathing. In fresh water turtles, no specific clinical symptoms were observed before death (Jacobson, 1986).

Necropsy findings in many cases include hepatomegaly, fatty degeneration of the liver, and necrotizing lesions of the oral and pharyngeal cavities and upper airway. Histologically, intranuclear inclusions may be found in hepatocytes, spleen, lung, kidneys, and degenerating epithelial cells. Areas of necrosis and infiltrates of mixed inflammatory cells are often present.

A diagnosis can be made only by critical evaluation of clinical signs, collection of biopsy specimens from the oral cavity, and ultimately by histopathologic detection of intranuclear inclusions and electron microscopic demonstration of viral particles in epithelial cells of the oral mucosa.

Treatment should attempt to prevent or treat secondary bacterial infections. Local and systemic antibiotics do not alter the course of the viral infection. Application of 5% acyclovir ointment produced some improvement in spur-thighed tortoises with oral lesions. Prophylactic measures and strict quarantine protocols should be established before introducing new animals into a collection. In addition, husbandry factors contributing to impaired immune function should be eliminated.

ADENOVIRUS INFECTION

Adenovirus infections have been detected in a variety of reptile species, including snakes, lizards, and crocodiles, and may contribute to high morbidity in private and zoologic collections of reptiles. Under conditions suppressing immune function, including stress from shipping, overcrowding, improper husbandry, and underlying infectious diseases, adenovirus infections are likely to develop. In some cases, an oral route of transmission has been suggested.

Clinical signs of infection may be absent; infected rosy boas, crocodiles, and a Savannah monitor have died without prior signs of illness. In most cases, however, symptoms of gastrointestinal disease are present and include regurgitation and anorexia. In addition, lethargy, limb paresis, and opisthotonus have been reported, especially shortly before death.

Although in some cases, no gross changes were noted at necropsy, necropsy findings generally include signs of gastrointestinal disease with multifocal areas of hemorrhage on the serosa of the gastrointestinal tract. The small intestine may be edematous and may contain large amounts of mucus in its lumen. Hemorrhagic areas may also be seen on the surface of a typically enlarged, pale liver, which often shows swollen borders. By light microscopy, a necrotizing enteritis and hepatic necrosis with large, basophilic intranuclear inclusion bodies in hepatocytes, renal epithelial cells, and epithelial cells of the gastrointestinal tract are most commonly seen.

A diagnosis in most cases is made by postmortem histologic examination of multiple organs and demonstration of typical intranuclear inclusion bodies. An ultimate diagnosis can be made only by electron microscopy and detection of viral particles. Clinically, a thorough history and evaluation of biologic samples aids in the diagnosis. In suspected cases, biopsies may be obtained from the liver, esophagus, and stomach for histopathologic evaluation and demonstration of intranuclear inclusions. Using commercially available viper heart cells and inoculation with suspensions from the liver of suspected specimens, viral isolation attempts should be made whenever possible.

Treatment should include antimicrobial therapy to prevent and treat secondary bacterial infections and supportive measures, including fluid therapy in dehydration and nutritional support. Routine fecal examinations should be performed to diagnose and treat parasitic infections. Treatment of underlying disease processes helps prevent the virus from causing clinical disease.

PARAMYXOVIRUS IN SNAKES

Paramyxoviruses have been isolated most often from viperid snakes, but the disease has also been identified in nonviperid snakes (Jacobson et al, 1980, 1981, 1992). The route of transmission is horizontal, and viral particles are transmitted by secretions from the respiratory tract.

Clinically, signs of respiratory disease include increased respiratory sounds, nasal discharge, and open mouth breathing. Secondary bacterial infections can cause stomatitis. In the final stages of the disease, neurologic symptoms are often evident.

At necropsy, caseous material is found in the nasal passageways and trachea. Lungs often are edematous and are sometimes filled with caseous material from secondary bacterial infections. Histologically, hypertrophy of lining epithelial cells and eosinophilic intracytoplasmic inclusions may be present. In addition, interstitial pneumonia with predominantly gram-negative bacterial organisms is commonly seen.

A clinical diagnosis of paramyxovirus infection can be made by evaluation of clinical symptoms, unresponsiveness to antibiotic treatment, and serologic tests. A hemagglutination inhibition test has been developed and is used at the Veterinary Medical Teaching Hospital, University of Florida, to measure antibodies against ophidian paramyxovirus (OPMV) in private and zoologic collections of snakes (Jacobson, 1993). Postmortem, histologic, and electron microscopic evaluation of lung tissue of infected snakes helps confirm a diagnosis. Paramyxovirus of viperid snakes grows in cell cultures established from commercially available viper heart cells, and viral isolation can be attempted by specialized laboratories.

No specific treatment has been recommended. Antimicrobial therapy is indicated for secondary gram-negative bacterial infections. If an outbreak of OPMV is suspected, separation of sick animals and strict hygiene procedures are recommended to prevent the virus from spreading through a collection. Although in most cases, only a few species are affected when an outbreak occurs, potentially all snakes are at risk for becoming infected. A vaccine has been tested in western diamondback rattlesnakes, but the antibody response was variable (Jacobson et al, 1991). Ultimately, the development of a vaccine may protect valuable private and zoologic collections of snakes against OPMV infections.

INCLUSION BODY DISEASE OF BOID SNAKES

IBD has been detected in almost all members of the family Boidae and is a major cause of morbidity and mortality in private and zoologic collections of boids (Schumacher et al, 1994). The agent is most likely a member of the family Retroviridae. The exact route of transmission has not been determined, but it has been suggested that arthropods, for example, the snake mite *Ophionyssus natricis,* may play a role in transmitting the virus. Although *Boa* spp. may be a natural host for this virus, viral particles and inclusions typical of IBD have been identified in nonboid snakes. In several cases, *Python* spp. acquired IBD after introduction of boa constrictors into the collection. Once present in a collection, this infection spreads rapidly, especially among *Python* spp.

The most common clinical symptom in *Boa* spp. during the initial phase of infection is regurgitation; however, this has not been observed in *Python* spp. In boas, neurologic symptoms, including head tremor, disorientation, and stargazing, develop during the several months it takes the disease to progress. Secondary bacterial infections causing pneumonia or stomatitis are often seen in chronically sick snakes. In pythons, severe neurologic disorders such as head tremor, disorientation, an inability to right itself, opisthotonus, and flaccid paralysis have been noted soon after exposure to the agent. Eventually, affected snakes become anorectic and die. A nonsuppurative meningoencephalitis is commonly seen on histologic examination of the brain of infected snakes, especially pythons.

Characteristic of this infection is the presence of eosinophilic intracytoplasmic inclusions in epithelial cells of all major organs, especially in kidneys, pancreas, and brain. Detection of typical inclusions in biopsy specimens, together with a thorough history and clinical examination, including hematologic and plasma biochemical determinations, help make a diagnosis. In live snakes, collection of liver and kidney biopsy specimens and histologic demonstration of inclusions is currently the best method to diagnose the disease in boas. In addition, biopsy specimens may be obtained from the stomach and esophagus for histologic evaluation. A serologic test is currently being developed.

No treatment is available, and it is recommended that strict quarantine procedures be followed when introducing newly acquired snakes (especially boas) into an established collection. Once the disease has been diagnosed within a collection, isolation and euthanasia of infected snakes is recommended to prevent further spread.

References and Suggested Reading

Jacobson ER: Viruses and viral associated diseases of reptiles. In: Bels VL, Van den Sande AP (eds): Acta zoologica et pathologica antverpiensia. Maintenance and reproduction of reptiles in captivity. Belgium, 1986.

Jacobson ER: Laboratory investigations. In: Beynon PH, ed: Manual of Reptiles. British Small Animal Veterinary Association. Ames, Iowa: Iowa State University Press, 1992, p 50.

Jacobson ER: Viral diseases of reptiles. In: Fowler ME, ed: Zoo and Wild Animal Medicine. Philadelphia: WB Saunders, 1993, p 153.

Jacobson ER, Gaskin JM, Flanagan JP, et al: Antibody responses of western diamondback rattlesnakes (*Crotalus atrox*) to inactivated ophidian paramyxovirus vaccines. J Zoo Wildl Med 22:184, 1991.

Jacobson ER, Gaskin JM, Page D, et al.: Paramyxo-like virus associated illness in a zoologic collection of snakes. J Am Vet Med Assoc 179:1227, 1981.

Jacobson ER, Gaskin JM, Simpson CF, et al: Paramyxo-like virus infection in a rock rattlesnake. J Am Vet Med Assoc 177:796, 1980.

Jacobson ER, Gaskin JM, Wells S, et al: Epizootic of ophidian paramyxovirus in a zoological collection: Pathological, microbiological and serological findings. J Zoo Wildl Med 23:318, 1992.

Schumacher J: Viral diseases of reptiles. In: Mader DR: Reptile Medicine and Surgery. Philadelphia: WB Saunders, 1996, p 224.

Schumacher J, Jacobson ER, Homer BL, et al: Inclusion body disease in boid snakes. J Zoo Wildl Med 25:511, 1994.

Dysecdysis (Abnormal Skin Shedding) in Reptiles

NOHA ABOU-MADI

Ithaca, New York

Veterinarians who treat reptiles are often confronted with snakes that have difficulty shedding. Dysecdysis in reptiles is a complete or partial failure of the skin to molt and is the most common skin condition observed in captive snakes. Although often associated with poor husbandry techniques, dysecdysis can also reflect disease in the animal. The sequence of events associated with ecdysis (normal shedding) in snakes is reviewed, followed by a discussion of causes and treatments for dysecdysis.

ECDYSIS

The skin of reptiles is dry and scaly, forming a highly effective protective barrier against the environment, as in mammals. Normal skin shedding occurs continuously in crocodilians and chelonians. Squamates (snakes and lizards) renew the epidermis periodically, and ecdysis is a more complex process. During this cyclic event, the entire skin is shed in one piece (snakes) or in large patches (most lizards). Ecdysis is highly dependent on environmental and physiologic conditions.

As a snake enters a shedding cycle, it becomes anorectic. In the wild, it will seek sheltered areas. The scales covering its body become increasingly dull over 5 to 7 days, after which the spectacles (transparent scales covering the eyes and formed by the fusion of the lids) turn opaque with a milky blue coloration. The scales clear within 3 to 4 days, and 3 to 6 days later the snake sheds. Rubbing the rostrum and chin against an abrasive surface initiates the separation between the old epidermis and the new one. As the scales around the mouth loosen, the snake is able to reflect the old epidermis and crawl out of it. In a normal shed, both spectacles come away attached to the old skin. A normal skin is shed as a single piece. In an adequate environment and with an appropriate diet, a snake adapted to captivity sheds regularly. The frequency of shedding, however, varies considerably with age, species, size, nutritional status, abundance of food, endocrine balance, and environmental factors. The period between sheds may vary from a few days to a few months.

Each shedding cycle is characterized by two major phases. During the renewal phase (approximately 14 days in most reptiles), the new epidermis is produced and the old one is shed. It is characterized clinically by the changes in the scale appearance and ends with the molt. The second phase is the resting phase, which is further divided into a postshedding resting phase, a perfect resting phase, and a late resting phase. Individual or species-related variation in the total resting phase can occur with the perfect resting phase, lasting from 2 days to many months. Some snakes and lizards are known to eat their shed skin. This is a normal behavior, and the skin is a good source of protein.

Histologically, the epidermis of snakes is composed of six different cell types (the clear layer cells, the lacunar cells, the alpha cells, the meso cells, the beta cells, and the most superficial layer of Oberhautchen) overlaying the basal stratum germinativum. These cells are organized into two epidermal generations (old or outer epidermis, new or inner epidermis). All epidermal cells originate from the stratum germinativum, migrate, and undergo a sequence of changes until they acquire their specific mature characteristics. Germinal proliferation and cell differentiation are synchronized over the entire body of the snake. After a shed, the epidermis is composed of three cell types: the Oberhautchen, beta, and immature alpha cells. During the postshedding resting phase, proliferation of germinal cells occurs, and mature alpha cells are produced. During the perfect resting phase, little or no cellular activity occurs. Toward the end of the late resting phase and the renewal phase, proliferation of the stratum germinativum generates cells that will complete the outer epidermis (six cell types) and form the new epidermis (three cell types). The deepest cell layer (clear cell) of the old epidermis is attached to the most superficial cell layer (Oberhautchen) of the new epidermis. Shedding results from the separation of these two layers (Maderson, 1985). Premature separation of the epidermis from traumatic handling or restraint during the renewal phase results in exposure of immature epithelium and potentially serious damage to the skin.

The presence of lipid-rich granules located within the meso layer provides the reptile skin effective protection against the environment. These granules form intercellular junctional complexes that are thought to maintain the osmotic gradient and prevent cutaneous water loss. The structural and physiologic characteristics of the epidermis and the dynamic changes associated with ecdysis are actively involved in protecting the snake from dehydration (Maderson, 1985).

Extensive studies have attempted to identify the mechanism that controls shedding; the role of endogenous hormones has been confirmed and narrowed to the "pituitary-thyroid axis." However, the specific hormone or hormones still remain to be identified. The thyroid gland of snakes plays an important role in the frequency of shedding; however, contradictory results are described in the literature. In one study, thyroidectomy in snakes initially increased the shedding frequency (three to six cycles were observed), but the animals were unable to complete the molts successfully after the first shed. Death occurred within 10 weeks of the surgery. Histologic examination of the skin revealed that the meso cells were particularly affected and the intercellular junctional complexes were disorganized. It is postulated that with the thyroid gland controlling the lipid metabolism, the high turnover of the granules would lead to the synthesis of deficient granules and a loss of integrity of the skin as a physical barrier. In another study, thyroidectomy in lizards slowed the shedding frequency and did not affect the synthesis of the epidermal cells. These paradoxical results are still unexplained (Maderson, 1985).

DYSECDYSIS

Dysecdysis is a difficult or impaired molt, with complete or partial failure to shed the outer epidermis. Dysecdysis is also reported in lizards and less frequently in chelonians. The clinician encounters varying clinical signs, including failure of the reptile to come out of the old skin, large patches of old epidermis still attached to the body, increased frequency of shedding cycles (sometimes with several old sheds adhering), dermatitis, retained spectacles, loss of physical condition, and underlying infectious diseases. Multiple causes may be involved. The work-up should include a thorough history with emphasis on captive management techniques and biologic characteristics of the species, physical examination, and analysis of the lesions identified.

Environmental stress and inadequate husbandry are the most frequent causes of dysecdysis. Ambient temperature and humidity should be emphasized. Snakes rely on ambient temperature for maintaining their own body temperature. Species-specific ranges of temperature have been established. Through thermoregulation, reptiles can maintain their preferred body temperature to ensure optimal enzymatic activity and immunologic function. Direct correlation between ambient temperature and rate of shedding has been established. With a rapid rise in temperature, the shedding frequency increases until the snake is acclimated to the new condition. At lower temperature, shedding frequency is decreased. Immunosuppression usually occurs and the snake is more susceptible to disease. The rate of skin wound healing has also been correlated with ambient temperature, with optimal healing occurring at or around the snake's preferred body temperature (Smith et al, 1988). A low humidity level in the cage is detrimental and predisposes the snake to chronic dehydration. This is frequently seen during the winter months. Depending on the species, the environmental humidity should range between 35 and 70% (i.e., desert to tropical species). Misting of the animal or the foliage of the cage provides additional humidity. Proper ventilation must be maintained to avoid excessive moisture, even in desirable high-humidity conditions. Vesicular lesions or blisters (subcutaneous, fluid-filled lesions) can result from an environment that is too damp and where the snake has no dry substrate. Secondary bacterial or fungal infection can invade the untreated wounds and cause septicemia. In chelonians, an inability to shed scutes may be due to a poor diet (nutritional osteodystrophy) or an inadequate basking area.

As mentioned previously, restraint of a snake that has just entered a cycle of ecdysis can cause severe damage to the fragile skin. Conversely, if no suitable rough surfaces are provided in the cage, the snake may have difficulty separating the new and old epidermis. Large rocks or branches can be used. The importance of providing a proper diet is again emphasized. Either from a lack of food intake or from an inappropriate diet, malnourished snakes are not able to sustain the energy or protein demand necessary for cellular proliferation and shedding. "Scale rot," or necrotizing dermatitis, can result from prolonged starvation.

The presence of wounds and old scars from bites, thermal or chemical burns, dermatitis, or trauma interferes with the normal eversion of the old epidermis by creating areas of abnormal adhesion. Scabs over the chin or rostrum (created by excessive rubbing on the cage walls or roof from increased activity, stress, failure to adapt to captivity, improper housing) may cause delays in the separation of the skin. Wounds along the body may retain successive patches of unshed skin and become a nidus for bacterial or fungal proliferation. Traumatic wounds or surgical wounds stimulate an ecdysis cycle that accelerates the rate of healing of the integument.

Systemic disease often results in secondary skin disease (red discoloration, necrosis and ulceration of the scales, cellulitis, or granuloma formation). These secondary conditions and the primary bacterial and mycotic necrotizing dermatitis are associated with abnormal shedding (Rossi, 1996). Neurologic disorders may prevent a snake from shedding normally because of incoordinated behavior. Heavy loads of ectoparasites (mites or ticks) can also cause ulcerative lesions, contributing to dysecdysis. They may also be vectors of disease transmission (Jacobson, 1977; Mader, 1996).

Endocrine dysfunction has been documented in cases of dysecdysis, but treatments are still unresolved. Frye (1991) reported successful treatment of pathologically increased shedding frequency in snakes with antithyroid drugs; however, the author strongly recommended thyroid function determination before these treatments to confirm thyroid dysfunction.

THERAPY

The treatment of a completely retained shed consists in soaking the snake for 30 to 60 minutes in warm water. If skin wounds are present, a diluted solution of a disinfectant solution may be used, for example, chlorhexidine, 2% solution (Nolvasan, Fort Dodge Laboratories, Inc.) should be diluted 1:100. Since snakes can drown, the water level should be low and the animal closely supervised. Working from the head to the tail with a damp towel, the clinician gently rubs away the slough. An alternative method consists of placing the snake in a small container between heavy damp towels. In many cases, the weight of the towels creates enough friction to remove the retained shed. In cases of partial skin retention, the affected areas can be soaked for 15 to 20 minutes in warm water and worked away with a moist towel (Frye, 1991).

Retained spectacles result when one or both fails to come off with the shed. They are soaked for 15 minutes and, using a wet cotton-tipped applicator, the spectacle can be rubbed away from the medial canthus to the lateral canthus. Some authors have advised using a blunt instrument to work away the edges (Frye, 1991). If performed, this procedure should be done carefully. Occasionally, several layers of unshed spectacles are observed. Careful removal of the ones that will peel off is carried out, and further attempts are performed after subsequent sheds. Permanent injuries to the eye have resulted from aggressive manipulation of the spectacle or the use of sharp or pointed instruments. These injuries include premature separation of the old epidermis, subspectacular abscess, exposure of the cornea from complete removal of the new and old epidermis, perforation of the cornea, and destruction of the globe.

In the presence of any skin lesion, biopsy specimens of the affected scales and skin should be submitted for histologic evaluation and bacterial and fungal culture and sensitivity. Appropriate topical and systemic antibiotic or antifungal drugs, or both, should be prescribed (Klingenberg, 1996).

In conclusion, for a successful correction of dysecdysis, the clinician must investigate and address all underlying causes. Precise record keeping of periodic weights and lengths of each animal, as well as dates of feeding, voiding, and shedding, greatly enhances the health management of reptiles.

References and Suggested Reading

Frye FL: Biomedical and Surgical Aspects of Captive Reptile Husbandry. Malabar: Krieger, 1991, p 173–177.
   The causes of dysecdysis in reptiles are reviewed and the clinical approach using antithyroid drugs is discussed.
Jacobson ER: Histology, endocrinology, and husbandry of ecdysis in snakes (a review). Vet Med Small Anim Clin 72:275, 1977.
   The clinical approach to dysecdysis is reviewed.

Klingenberg RJ: Therapeutics. In: Mader DR, ed: Reptile Medicine and Surgery. Philadelphia: WB Saunders, 1996, p 299.
The principles of antimicrobial use, treatment techniques, and dosages in reptiles are discussed.

Mader DR: Dysecdysis: Abnormal shedding and retained eye caps. In: Mader DR, ed: Reptile Medicine and Surgery. Philadelphia: WB Saunders, 1996, p 368.
The different treatments for dysecdysis are reviewed.

Maderson PFA: Some developmental problems of the reptilian integument. In: Gans C, ed: Biology of the Reptilia, vol 14. New York: Wiley-Interscience Publications, 1985, p 523.

This is an extensive review of the reptilian integument, the healing process, and mechanism of control of ecdysis.

Rossi JV: Dermatology. In: Mader DR, ed: Reptile Medicine and Surgery. Philadelphia: WB Saunders, 1996, p 104.
The dermatologic problems encountered in reptiles are reviewed.

Smith DA, Barker IK, Allen OB: The effect of ambient temperature and the type of wound on healing of cutaneous wounds in the common garter snake (*Thamnophis sirtalis*). Can J Vet Res 52: 120, 1988.
The effect of the type of wound and various ambient temperatures on skin healing is discussed.

Nutritional Secondary Hyperparathyroidism in Green Iguanas

DOUGLAS R. MADER

Long Beach, California

Metabolic bone disease (MBD) is a complicated, but also very common finding in captive herpetofauna (Boyer, 1991, 1996). *MBD* is a term that describes a variety of medical disorders affecting the integrity and function of the bony skeleton. Nutritional secondary hyperparathyroidism (NSHP) is the most common MBD diagnosed in captive herpetofauna. NSHP occurs as a result of dietary or husbandry mismanagement. The most commonly implicated factors are a prolonged deficiency of dietary calcium and/or vitamin D_3, an imbalance of the calcium-to-phosphorus ratio in the diet (usually an excess of phosphorus), or inadequate exposure to ultraviolet radiation in diurnal animals. Although diets of the green iguana have been studied in the wild (Troyer, 1984), nutritionally balanced diets in captivity have yet to be fully elucidated.

In NSHP there is an excessive production of parathyroid hormone from the parathyroid gland in response to hypocalcemia induced by diet or management practices (McCance and Huether, 1990). Calcium is resorbed from the bones to compensate for the deficiency. The resulting osteopenia weakens the integrity of the bones. If this occurs in a young, growing animal it is called rickets. If it occurs in an adult it is referred to as osteomalacia (McCance and Huether, 1990).

NSHP can potentially affect all reptilian and amphibian species, but it is most commonly described in lizards and aquatic turtles (Frye, 1991). Young animals experiencing active bone growth are the most often affected. There are no typical presentations of the disease. Affected animals may show any or all of the following: thickening of the long bones and mandibles, pathologic fractures of the long bones and spine (Fig. 1), horizontal (rather than the normal vertical) rotation of the scapulae, tetany, muscle fasciculations, hyper-reflexivity, prolapsed rectum or cloaca, anorexia, inability to ambulate, and stunted growth. The severity of presenting signs depends on a number of factors, including extent of the disease, the age and type of patient,

and the experience of the owner at recognizing early signs of disease.

There have been numerous reviews and suggested treatments of NSHP in the recent literature (Boyer, 1996). Therapy for NSHP generally centers around the treatment of life-threatening disorders (e.g., hypocalcemic tetany),

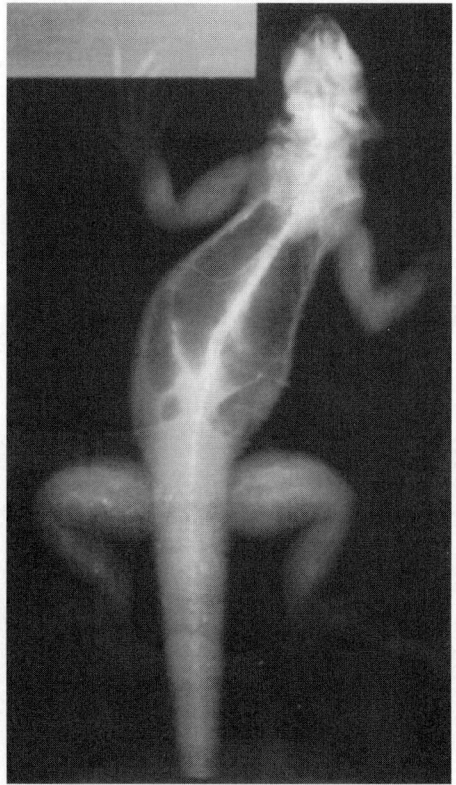

Figure 1. Radiograph of a juvenile green iguana (*Iguana iguana*) with severe MBD due to NSHP.

repairing and splinting pathologic fractures, and correcting any management or nutritional deficiencies. Vitamin and mineral supplements are routinely included as part of the follow-up care.

Most of the information available regarding NSHP and vitamin D₃ is derived from the mammalian literature. Very little research has been done in reptiles and recommended treatments are empirical.

Calcium deficits cause partial depolarization of nerves and muscle because of an increase in the threshold potential (Ganong, 1981; McCance and Huether, 1990). Resultant symptoms (in humans) include confusion, paresthesias around the mouth and in the digits, carpopedal spasms, and hyper-reflexia (McCance and Huether, 1990). An increase in neuromuscular excitability, caused by hypocalcemia, can account for the patient's spastic tremors when stimulated with a pinch of a limb. Intestinal cramping and bloating result from the effects of the hypocalcemia on the smooth muscle of the gastrointestinal tract (McCance and Huether, 1990). Rectal prolapse is a common finding in the young iguana.

As the blood calcium levels drop, parathyroid hormone (PTH) is released that increases blood calcium levels by increasing bone resorption and increasing renal tubular reabsorption of calcium while simultaneously increasing phosphate excretion in the urine. PTH also stimulates formation of 1,25-dihydroxycholecalciferol, which increases absorption of intestinal calcium.

In conditions in which calcium levels are chronically low, such as renal disease and rickets, feedback stimulation of the parathyroid glands causes a compensatory parathyroid hypertrophy and secondary hyperparathyroidism (McCance and Huether, 1990). This situation results in a myriad of detrimental effects on the body, including demineralization of the bones. Of particular significance with this parathyroid hypertrophy is the loss of the negative feedback influence by increasing levels of serum calcium or the production of parathyroid hormone from the parathyroid gland.

Reptiles with NSHP that present with pathologic fractures carry a guarded prognosis. When the fractures affect the vertebral column the prognosis changes from guarded to grave.

TREATMENT

Until recently, the focus on treatment for NSHP has been to correct husbandry problems and provide supple-

mental nutrients and exposure to natural sunlight. However, this is often not enough, especially in severe cases of NSHP. The intended goal of treatment for NSHP is not only to correct and replace the nutritional and mineral deficiencies but also to reverse the bone loss and promote new bone production.

Blood calcium concentration is mediated by a feedback system primarily involving two hormones. Low blood calcium stimulates PTH secretion. When the blood calcium concentration is above normal, PTH secretion is halted and calcitonin, which is produced from the ultimobranchial bodies, increases.

Calcitonin lowers circulating calcium and phosphorus levels by inhibiting bone resorption. There is a decrease in osteoclast activity and number, as well as a stimulatory effect on osteoblast bone formation. Calcitonin also decreases blood calcium concentration by increasing urinary calcium excretion (Riggs, 1991).

A synthetic form, called salmon calcitonin (SCT), has been used successfully to treat osteoporosis in post-menopausal women (Riggs, 1991; Wallach, 1992). SCT, which has been approved by the Food and Drug Administration for the treatment of MBDs since 1975, is modeled after the salmon calcitonin molecule, and is 40 to 50 times more potent than human calcitonin (Wallach, 1992).

Based on the value of calcitonin in the therapy for osteoporosis in women, similar applications have been utilized with success in the green iguana for the treatment of NSHP. The dose of SCT for the iguana is 50 IU, given once per week for 2 weeks (Figs. 2 and 3). Based on the clinical response to treatment and radiographic changes in over 400 animals in a clinical setting, this dose appears to be adequate. On occasion an animal may require a third dose, but this is not common. See Table 1 for guidelines for the treatment of NSHP.

The side effects of SCT in humans include anorexia, nausea, vomiting, skin flushing, nonspecific rash, urticaria, polyuria, pruritus, and edema (Wallach, 1992). The amino acid sequence of SCT is not the same as that in human calcitonin. As a result, it is not uncommon to see an antibody response (as evidenced by a type I hypersensitivity reaction) to SCT after chronic administration lasting longer than 6 months (Wallach, 1992). Because the duration of treatment using SCT for NSHP in iguanas is substantially shorter than it is for osteoporosis, an antibody response is unlikely and to date has not been reported.

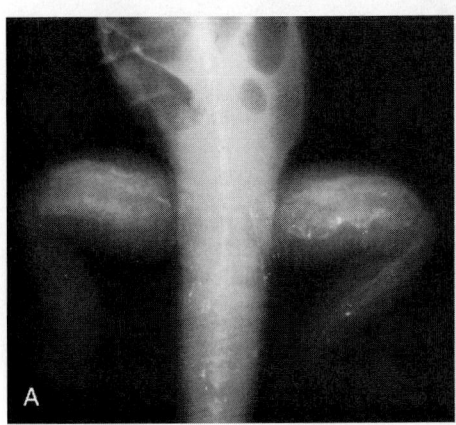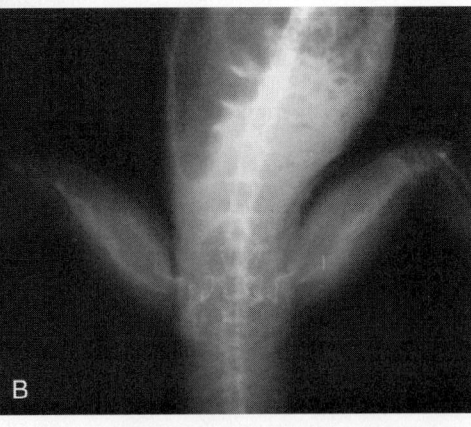

Figure 2. *A*, The pelvis and femurs of the patient in Figure 1. *B*, Follow-up radiograph taken 3 weeks after therapy that included SCT.

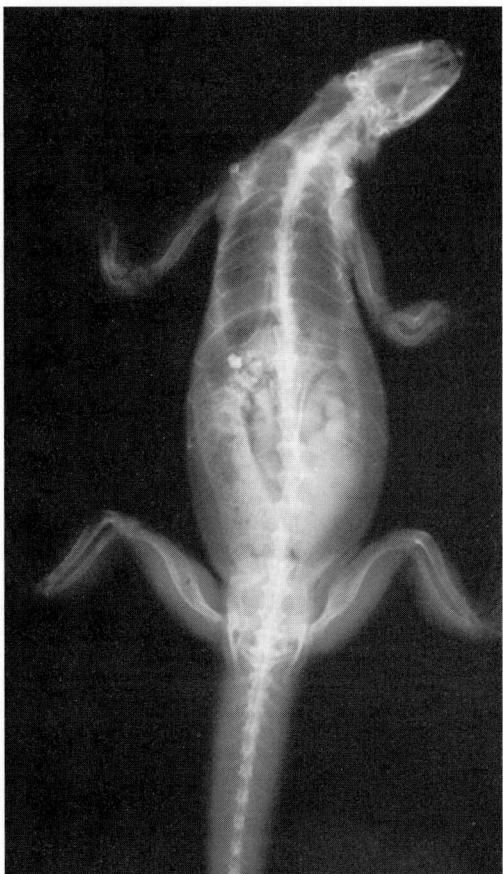

Figure 3. Radiograph from recheck 1 year after treatment.

SCT is also reported to have an analgesic effect against skeletal pain in human medicine. This results from SCT's ability to stabilize or augment bone mass, change the skeletal blood flow, stimulate endogenous endorphin production and directly affect the pain centers in the brain (Wallach, 1992). This is a potential benefit when using SCT in the treatment of MBD in reptiles.

TABLE 1. Protocol for Treatment With Calcitonin

Initial visit
    Evaluate patient (radiographs).
    Determine plasma calcium.
    0.1 ml/kg Injacom* 100, IM
    1.0 ml/kg Neocalglucon,† PO, b.i.d.
    Support patient (tube feeding, etc.).
One-week follow-up
    Second Injacom injection (0.1 ml/kg).
    First calcitonin‡ injection (50 IU/kg).§
    Continue with Neocalglucon.
    Continue with supportive care.
Two-week follow-up
    Second calcitonin injection (50 IU/kg).
    Supportive care as needed.

*Injacom 100, Roche, Nutley, NJ, 07110.
  †Neocalglucon, Sandoz Pharmaceuticals, Inc., East Hanover, NJ 07936.
  ‡Calcitonin, Calcimar, Rhone-Poulenc Rorer Pharmaceuticals, Inc., Fort Washington, PA 19034.
  §Hypocalcemic animals with low normal plasma calcium should not receive calcitonin until after their calcium level has been stabilized. Calcitonin can cause acute death if administered in patients with marginal calcium values! Never give calcitonin to an animal that has not had its calcium stabilized.

The administration of calcitonin has the potential of causing life-threatening hypocalcemic tetany, although no cases have been reported in the human literature. Because of this liability, SCT should not be given to an animal with unknown or suspected low blood calcium levels. If owner compliance prevents proper preadministration screening (plasma calcium, normal range 9.0–25.1 mg/dl), then it is wise to start the animal on appropriate supplements. Vitamin D₃ and supplemental calcium, preferably administered orally, should be given for at least 3 days before dosing with SCT (see Table 1 for specific instructions).

Animals presenting with hypocalcemic tetany should be treated for their life-threatening condition before addressing their bone pathology. Animals in tetany should be treated with appropriate fluid therapy, warmth, calorie replacement, and a calcium supplement. If tetany is present, calcium gluconate 10% (American Regent Laboratories, Inc., Shirley, NY) can be administered at 100 mg/kg IM q6hr until the tetany ceases. Once the tetany stops, the animal should be switched to oral calcium supplementation with calcium glubionate (Neocalglucon, Sandoz Pharmaceuticals, Inc., East Hanover, NJ).

There is never any justification to treat bone involvement with injectable calcium. Aside from being a dangerous practice, calcium injections have been demonstrated to be painful and, most importantly, at high doses can cause permanent damage to the kidneys. Long-term therapy for NSHP should only be conducted using appropriate oral calcium supplementation.

SCT should not be used in cases of hypocalcemia. Its best use will be in animals with NSHP that have clinically apparent bone involvement, such as softening or swelling of the long bones and/or the mandible. Animals that were requiring 4 to 6 months of intensive supportive care to recover from NSHP are now responding, with the addition of SCT in the treatment regimen, in 4 to 6 weeks. SCT should not be used alone but as an adjunct to proper medical care and, most importantly, coinciding with necessary corrections in the animal's husbandry and diet (Table 2).

Until the nutritional requirements of the many different reptile species are established, NSHP will continue to be a problem. In the meantime, SCT, with its ability to reverse the destructive processes of NSHP and its apparent analgesic effect on the skeleton is an asset to current treatment protocols.

TABLE 2. Suggested Convalescent Care for the Iguana With Nutritional Secondary Hyperparathyroidism (NSHP)

Temperature: 88°–95° F
Humidity: Approximately 100%
UV light: As much exposure to natural sunlight as possible
Artificial UV light: Vita-lite (Duro Test), Chroma 50 (General Electric), Reptisun UVB (Zoo Med)
Enteral supplement: Blend 1 can of Ensure, 1 banana and 1 multivitamin (feed 1–3% of body weight every 24 hours)
Normal diet: Dark, leafy green vegetables, no animal protein
Cage rest: Remove climbing items from cage
Minimize handling

For further information refer to Barten SL: Lizards. In: Mader DR, ed: Reptile Medicine and Surgery. Philadelphia, WB Saunders, 1997, pp 47–61.

References and Suggested Reading

Anderson NL: Diseases of *Iguana iguana*. Compend Contin Educ Prac Vet 14:1335, 1992.

Bernard JB, Oftedal OT, Barboza PS, et al: The response of vitamin D–deficient green iguanas *(Iguana iguana)* to artificial ultraviolet light. In: Proceedings of the American Association of Zoo Veterinarians, 1991, p 147.

Boyer TH: Common problems and treatment of the green iguana *(Iguana iguana)*. Bull Assoc Rept Amphib Vet 1:8, 1991.

Boyer TH: Metabolic bone disease. In: Mader DR, ed: Reptile Medicine and Surgery. Philadelphia: WB Saunders, 1996, p 385.

Frye FL: Biomedical and Surgical Aspects of Captive Reptile Husbandry, 2nd ed. Malabar, FL: Krieger Publishing, 1991, p 47.

McCance KL, Huether SE: Pathophysiology: The Biological Basis of Disease in Adults and Children. St Louis: CV Mosby, 1990, p 97.

Riggs BL: Overview of osteoporosis. West J Med 154:63, 1991.

Scott PW: Nutritional diseases. In: Beynon PH ed: Manual of Reptiles. Gloucestershire, Brittish Small Animal Veterinary Association, 1992, p 133.

Troyer K: Diet selection and digestion in *Iguana iguana*, the importance of age and nutrient requirements. Oecologia 61:201, 1984.

Wallach S: Calcitonin treatment in osteoporosis. The Female Patient 17:35, 1992.

Egg Laying Problems in Green Iguanas, *Iguana iguana*

STEPHEN L. BARTEN

Mundelein, Illinois

Green iguanas, *Iguana iguana*, are oviparous, with a complex reproductive biology that is controlled by a variety of environmental, behavioral, and social stimuli. Because captive conditions inevitably differ from the natural conditions that influence reproduction, and females can produce eggs without the presence of a male, egg laying problems among adult, female iguanas is a common clinical complaint.

REPRODUCTIVE BIOLOGY

Iguanas begin producing eggs at the end of their second year of life and reproduce every year thereafter. Breeding cycles vary with the rainy season rather than the length of daylight. Follicular growth and deposition of yolk, or vitellogenesis, begins in mid-October as the rainy season ends. Courtship and mating coincide with the onset of the dry season in December and January. Courtship lasting 2 to 4 weeks precedes copulation, and females undergo multiple copulations with multiple partners. Ovulation occurs throughout January when ova reach 20 mm in diameter, 5 weeks after the first copulations. Nesting follows 3 to 4 weeks after ovulation, in February and March (Dugan, 1982). Well-drained, thermally favorable nesting sites are scarce, so females migrate long distances to use them, traveling up to 3.0 km and even swimming to offshore islands. Communal nesting is common (Wiewandt, 1982). Nests tend to be a complex series of tunnels and chambers, often a meter underground, with egg chambers dug into the side walls of the tunnels. Clutches vary from 14 to 76 eggs with average measurements of 39 × 26 mm and weights of 9 to 14 g (Wiewandt, 1982). There are anecdotal reports of clutches numbering up to 100 eggs in captive iguanas. Eggs hatch in April and May.

CLINICAL PRESENTATION OF GRAVID CAPTIVE IGUANAS

Variable environmental conditions cause captive iguanas to exhibit breeding behavior at almost any time of year. Behavior may mimic the pattern of wild populations, exhibit two short seasons in the spring and fall, or one longer season lasting from fall through spring or spring through summer. Female iguanas greater than 260 mm in snout to vent length (SVL) can produce eggs, as maturity is determined by size rather than age. As vitellogenesis progresses, the presence of two to five dozen or more ova measuring 20 mm each fill the coelom and cause decreased appetite or complete anorexia. The coelomic cavity may or may not be visibly distended.

In some captive lizards, the process stops before ovulation and is termed *preovulatory egg retention* or *follicular stasis*. The cause is unknown but probably relates to missing environmental or social cues. One of several sequelae may result. Most commonly, the iguana continues to refuse food, loses fat and muscle mass, and may eventually die of dehydration, starvation, and hypocalcemia unless treatment is instituted. Often the fragile ova rupture when lizards jump or fall, or rupture occurs iatrogenically during palpation, resulting in yolk peritonitis. Sometimes the ova inspissate and remain, causing prolonged hypophagia. In a few, rare cases the ova may resorb, being demonstrable on one visit and absent a month later. Egg resorption requires no treatment but is rare and should not be counted on as a likely outcome. Furthermore, egg resorption is not possible after ovulation and shell deposition.

In other cases, ovulation ensues. The ova pass through the fimbria into the oviducts or shell glands, where shell deposition occurs. Some iguanas pause at this stage and fail to oviposit. This is termed *postovulatory egg retention* and may be caused by the lack of a suitable nest site, poor muscle tone from lack of exercise, any physical obstruction of the pelvic canal (sequelae of metabolic bone disease, nephromegaly, urolith, or misshapen eggs), metabolic imbalances such as hypocalcemia, and infections of the reproductive tract or cloaca (Barten, 1993; Divers, 1996). Affected lizards continue to refuse food; become dehydrated, cachectic, and often hypocalcemic; and may die without treatment. Other females drop eggs anywhere in their environment without digging a nest, whereas some seem to hold the eggs until an enclosed nest chamber is provided and then oviposit normally. Many lizards are hyperactive and dig frantically before laying.

When an iguana is found to be gravid, it is not necessarily retaining eggs but may be progressing normally through its reproductive cycle. Precise timing of these cycles is problematic, as there is no set gestation period. Oviposition in captive lizards does not occur within an exact number of days after any measurable behavior—mating displays, copulation, or onset of anorexia.

Sex Determination

The sex of iguanas with SVL greater than 260 mm may be determined by external characteristics. Mature male iguanas have taller dorsal spines, larger dewlap, larger operculum scales, and a bigger head than females. A more accurate means of sexing iguanas greater than 200 mm SVL is to examine the row of femoral pores on the ventral aspect of the thighs. In males, these pores are usually large and well developed but remain small in adult females. Although there is some overlap (small males may have smaller femoral pores than large females), in general males have pores greater than 1 mm in diameter, and females' pores are less than 1 mm. Mathematical comparison of femoral pore diameter, dorsal crest height, SVL, and sex has been reported (Rodda, 1991). The presence of bilateral hemipenal bulges in the ventral base of the tail is an indisputable sign of maleness. Measuring the depth of the inverted hemipenes with a blunt probe is an accurate method for sexing adult iguanas, but the visual methods already described make this exercise unnecessary. In juveniles, probing and eversion of the hemipenes are not reliable sexing methods.

Patient Evaluation

Clinically, iguanas may be found to be gravid as a presenting complaint or an incidental finding. The owner may report any, all, or none of the following: decreased appetite or anorexia, decreased level of activity, distended abdomen, frantic digging behavior, and laying of one or more eggs. A comprehensive history and physical examination are in order. The attitude of the lizard is important—gravid lizards in good condition remain bright, alert, and responsive with good muscle tone. They stand high on their toes and actively inspect their surroundings. Lizards that sprawl and are depressed usually are debilitated. Eye position and skin turgor should be assessed for signs of dehydration. Care must be taken not to mistake a coelom distended with eggs for adequate body mass; condition is assessed by the muscle mass around the pelvis, limbs, and tail base. Coelomic palpation must be performed

with extreme care, as thin-walled, preovulatory ova are easily ruptured, leading to potentially fatal yolk peritonitis. Ova are usually apparent on palpation as multiple, soft, round coelomic masses approximately 20 mm in diameter. It is impossible to differentiate between pre- and postovulatory ova on palpation alone.

A minimal database includes a complete blood count; serum calcium, phosphorus, and uric acid determinations; and radiographs. Blood is taken from the ventral caudal vein. Dehydration, infection, hypocalcemia, and renal disease often accompany egg retention and must be addressed before treating retained ova. The serum calcium in gravid iguanas should measure 20 to 25 mg/dl, which is higher than the 8 to 12 mg/dl normal values for nongravid lizards (Campbell, 1996). Hyperphosphatemia and calcium:phosphorus ratios less than 1 indicate renal disease, and these changes usually precede elevations in uric acid (Campbell, 1996). Radiographs should be evaluated for the presence of various metabolic bone diseases, misshapen or narrowed pelvic canal, nephromegaly, fused or misshapen eggs, uroliths, or anything that might hinder the passage of eggs. In general, preovulatory ova are round, whereas postovulatory eggs tend to be oval. The ova may fill the coelomic cavity in both cases. The presence of shells indicates that eggs are in the oviducts. Lizard egg shells are poorly calcified and more radiolucent than are those of birds and chelonians. If shells are not visible, ova may still be in the oviducts but at a stage before the shells are laid down. Negative contrast radiographs using 5 to 10 cc of room air injected into the coelomic cavity, with care taken to avoid damaging the ova with the needle, allows better visualization when plain radiographs are inconclusive (Divers, 1996). Ultrasonography also may be used to differentiate between pre- and postovulatory ova.

TREATMENT

A gravid iguana with normal physical examination and laboratory parameters may not have egg retention and should be sent home with instructions to optimize temperatures, ultraviolet light, and diet and to provide an enclosed nest box. This can be two kitty litter pans placed rim to rim and taped together with duct tape, with an access hole cut in one end of the upper pan, or a square plastic garbage can on its side, with the lid taped on and an access hole cut in the upper side of the lid. A ramp or other means to reach the access hole is necessary. The box should be filled with a moist, but not drenched, mixture of potting soil and sand, such as 14 quarts of sterile peat potting soil and one quart of sterile sand mixed with 9 cups of warm water (Kaplan, 1994). The box should be in a warm and quiet area and the lizard introduced to the access hole. Iguanas often block the access hole with soil when digging and spend hours laying eggs, after which they emerge with a sunken, emaciated appearance.

The duration of decreased appetite or anorexia should be followed. Normally iguanas lay their eggs after approximately 4 weeks of decreased appetite. The lizard should be re-evaluated if no eggs have appeared after 4 weeks of anorexia, or sooner if the iguana becomes depressed or debilitated. If the lizard is still in good shape and the ova are preovulatory, ovariectomy is performed. If radiographs reveal shelled ova and blood parameters are normal, induction of oviposition is attempted with calcium gluconate, 100 mg/kg IM every 6 hours, followed by oxytocin 10 IU/kg IM every 6 hours, 1 hour after each calcium injection and provision of a nest box (Mader, 1996a). Alternatively, oxytocin may be given at 5 to 10 IU/kg as a slow intraosseous or IV drip (Divers, 1996). If no eggs are passed after 24 hours, salpingotomy or ovariosalpingectomy is performed.

Depressed or debilitated gravid iguanas must be stabilized for 1 to 3 days before surgery. When egg retention causes symptoms, lizards go downhill rapidly when compared with snakes or turtles, and treatment should not be delayed. Ambient temperatures of 35°C are essential. Warmed Ringer's solution or normal saline at 10 to 40 ml/kg is given through an intraosseous catheter in the proximal tibia, cephalic vein catheter, or intracoelomically (Divers, 1996; Jenkins, 1996; Mader, 1996a). The latter route is less favorable because of a lack of space in the gravid coelomic cavity and risk of iatrogenic damage to the ova. Infusion pumps allow accurate dosing of small volumes. Hypocalcemia is treated with calcium gluconate at 100 mg/kg IM every 6 hours or calcium glubionate (NeoCalglucon; Novartis, East Hanover, NJ) at 1 ml/kg PO b.i.d., and a single injection of vitamin D at 100 IU/kg IM (Mader 1996a). Tube feeding should be used cautiously, if at all, as the full coelom may cause regurgitation and aspiration. Enteral nutrition (liquid, nutritionally complete diets for humans) at doses of 5 ml/kg per day or less are recommended (Mader, 1996a). Antibiotics, allopurinol, and other medications may be used when indicated. One to three days of support significantly decreases surgical risk, and normal serum calcium levels should be achieved before performing surgery.

Surgery

Anesthesia and surgical techniques have been described in the literature (Mader, 1996b). The patient is anesthetized using 2 to 3% isoflurane with or without premedication and is prepared for surgery. Perioperative antibiotics are indicated because it is difficult to disinfect reptile skin adequately. Ceftazidime, 20 mg/kg IM every 72 hours, or cephalexin, 20 mg/kg PO every 24 hours for 7 days has been recommended (Divers, 1996; Mader, 1996a). Standard electrocardiographic or pulse oximeter monitors are employed. Adhesive plastic drapes offer better visualization than do opaque, disposable ones. The lizard should be kept at 32 to 35°C before, during, and after the procedure.

Traditionally, a paramedian celiotomy has been recommended to avoid the large ventral abdominal vein on the midline. However, this vein lies in a suspensory ligament and is easily avoided if care is taken during a standard midline approach. This reduces hemorrhage and postoperative pain compared with a paramedian incision. If the vein is accidentally cut, collateral circulation allows ligation without ill effect (Mader, 1996a). The incision is centered between the xiphoid and the pubis. The thin-walled bladder is often distended and must be avoided.

In preovulatory egg retention, the ovaries fill the coelomic cavity. One ovary at a time is elevated through the incision, and caution is exercised to avoid tearing the fragile membranes and spilling yolk into the coelom. Excessive traction also can avulse the ovarian blood vessels from the vena cava, causing hemorrhage that is difficult to control. The left ovary is attached by an ovarian ligament to the renal vein. The left adrenal gland—a white, oblong gland—lies within the ligament between these two structures. The right ovary is connected in a similar fashion to the vena cava, but the right adrenal gland is on the opposite side of the vena cava from the ovary (Fig. 1). Several ovarian vessels in the ovarian ligaments must be ligated with 3–0 to 5–0 monofilament synthetic absorbable suture, taking care to preserve the adrenal glands. Hemostatic clips (Hemoclips, Fort Dodge Animal Health, Fort Dodge, IA) facilitate this task and are preferred. After the first ovary is removed, the procedure is repeated for the contralateral side. It is not necessary to remove the oviducts in these cases, as postovariectomy pyosalpinx has not been reported (Mader, 1996a).

In postovulatory egg retention, it is theoretically possible to perform salpingotomy and remove the eggs, leaving the reproductive tract intact. In reality, the dozens of eggs and the fragility of the shell glands makes the practice impractical. Multiple oviductal incisions are necessary, and the fragile tissue tears easily during manipulation. It is difficult, if not impossible, to suture oviductal tissue. In addition, egg retention would likely recur the following year. Ovariosalpingectomy is the preferred technique. One oviduct is exteriorized. There are multiple vessels in the mesosalpinx or broad ligament, and each must be ligated with 3–0 to 5–0 monofilament synthetic absorbable suture or hemostatic clips. The latter greatly reduce operative time and are highly recommended. The oviduct is ligated and

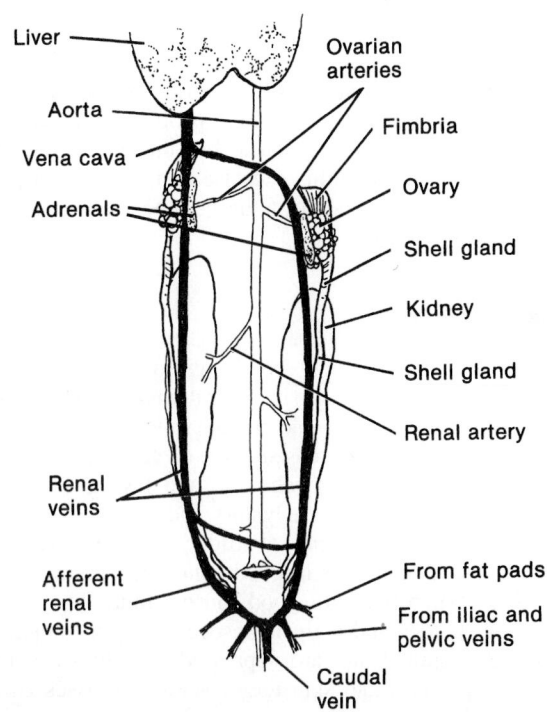

Figure 1. Vascular supply to the female iguana reproductive tract. (Modified from Bennett RA, Mader DR: Soft tissue surgery. In: Mader DR, ed: Reptile Medicine and Surgery. Philadelphia: WB Saunders, 1996, p 295, with permission.)

transected near its attachment to the cloaca. Care must be taken to reflect the bladder and follow the oviduct to its end. Failure to do so could result in ligation of the oviduct too far cranially, leaving one or more eggs behind. The procedure is repeated for the contralateral oviduct. The ovaries are now located and removed as described previously, otherwise future ova could be released into the coelomic cavity. The ovarian ligament is shorter and the ovarian vessels smaller than in preovulatory cases, making ligation more difficult.

If possible, the thin and friable muscle layer is closed with 3–0 to 5–0 monofilament synthetic absorbable suture with care to avoid the ventral abdominal vein. The skin is the strength layer and is sutured in an interrupted horizontal mattress everting pattern using nonabsorbable suture. Cyanoacrylate tissue adhesive or a light bandage is used to protect the incision. Flunixin meglumine, 2 mg/kg IM every 24 hours, or butorphenol, 0.05 mg/kg IM every 24 hours, may be used during the first 48 hours to control pain (Mader, 1996a). Sutures are removed after 4 weeks but may come out before then during ecdysis.

References and Suggested Reading

Barten SL: The medical care of iguanas and other common pet lizards. Vet Clin North Am Small Anim Pract 23:1213, 1993.
A broad overview of the clinically significant aspects of husbandry, disease syndromes, and medical care of iguanas and other common pet lizards.

Campbell TW: Clinical pathology. In: Mader DR, ed: Reptile Medicine and Surgery. Philadelphia: WB Saunders, 1996, p 248.
A thorough review of blood collection, hematology, blood chemistries, and cytodiagnostics in reptiles.

Divers SJ: Medical and surgical treatment of pre-ovulatory and post-ovulatory egg stasis in oviparous lizards. Proceedings of the Association of Amphibian and Reptilian Veterinarians, Tampa, FL, 1996, p 119.
A review of egg retention in lizards, stressing patient evaluation, medical treatments, and surgical techniques.

Dugan B: The mating behavior of the green iguana, *Iguana iguana*. In: Burghardt GM, Rand AS, eds: Iguanas of the World: Their Behavior, Ecology, and Conservation. Park Ridge, NJ: Noyes Publications, 1982, p 320.
A broad description of the mechanisms and adaptive strategies of mate acquisition in the green iguana, based on studies of a wild population on Flamenco Island, Panama.

Jenkins JR: Diagnostic and clinical techniques. In: Mader DR, ed: Reptile Medicine and Surgery. Philadelphia: WB Saunders, 1996, p 264.
Techniques for physical restraint, administration of parenteral medication, venipuncture, intravenous and intraosseous catheterization, sample collection, and endoscopy and laparoscopy.

Kaplan M: Preparing for egg-laying and incubation of potentially fertile eggs. [On-Line]. Available http://www.sonic.net/melissk/index.html. 1994.
A guide for iguana owners on the behavior of the gravid iguana, setting up the egg laying box, and incubation of iguana eggs.

Mader DR: Reproductive surgery in the green iguana. Seminars in Avian and Exotic Pet Medicine 5:214, 1996a.
A practical review of surgical procedures for the reproductive tracts of both male and female iguanas.

Mader DR, ed: Reptile Medicine and Surgery. Philadelphia: WB Saunders, 1996b.
A comprehensive, practical text geared for the practitioner. Sections include normal biology, special techniques and procedures, differential diagnosis by symptoms, and specific diseases and conditions.

Rodda GH: Sexing *Iguana iguana*. Bull Chicago Herp Soc 26:173, 1991.
A simple table was developed from measurements of road-killed iguanas to identify gender based on snout-vent length, dorsal crest height, and femoral pore diameter.

Wiewandt TA: Evolution of nesting patterns in Iguanine lizards. In: Burghardt GM, Rand AS, eds: Iguanas of the World: Their Behavior, Ecology, and Conservation. Park Ridge, NJ: Noyes Publications, 1982, p 119.
A qualitative study of iguanine lizard nesting behavior, including size and age of first nesting; egg, clutch, and hatchling sizes; nesting phenology; nest site selection; and communal nesting.

Salmonella in Reptiles

RICHARD C. CAMBRE
Washington, D.C.

MICHAEL W. MCGUILL
Boston, Massachusetts

Reptiles commonly are carriers of *Salmonella*. All the major types of reptiles have been implicated, including lizards, snakes, tortoises, turtles, and crocodilians. In most instances, the organisms are merely commensal in the intestinal tract, causing no harm to their hosts. Salmonellae may, in fact, be part of the normal intestinal microflora of reptiles. Opinion varies as to whether some *Salmonella* serotypes can act as primary pathogens in reptiles. Generally, opportunistic infection is thought to be the pathophysiologic mechanism at work when a *Salmonella* isolate is implicated in disease in these animals.

Public health officials consider all *Salmonella* isolates to have zoonotic potential. Because of the increasing popularity of reptiles as pets, the risk of transmission to humans has risen correspondingly. Legal importation of iguanas, for example, rose 29-fold from 1986 (22,806) to 1993 (798,405) (Anonymous, 1995). A study in New York state estimated that more than 700 cases of reptile-associated human salmonellosis (gastrointestinal infection with *Salmonella*) occurred there in 1993 (Ackerman, 1995). Although it is a self-limiting disease in most humans, salmonellosis in certain populations—such as infants and young children, immunosuppressed persons, and the elderly—and certainly the sequelae of invasive illness with *Salmonella*, can be life-threatening. Recent human cases have demonstrated that direct handling of the animal is not necessary for zoonotic transmission of the organism. Ingestion of the bacterium through contact with fomites or infected persons (secondary transmission) is common.

THE AGENT

The genus *Salmonella* belongs to the family Enterobacteriaceae: non–spore-forming, motile, facultatively anaerobic, gram-negative, rod-shaped bacteria. Numerous classification schemes have been proposed through the years, and the application of molecular genetics techniques to bacteriology will likely result in further taxonomic revision. The former "Ewing" scheme listed three species within the genus *Salmonella*: *S. typhi*, *S. choleraesuis*, and *S. enteritidis*, with greater than 2,000 serotypes (serovars) contained within the latter species. A newer scheme, adopted by the Centers for Disease Control and Prevention (CDC, United States Public Health Service), divides the genus into only two species: *S. bongori*, with 18 rare serotypes, and *S. enterica* (formerly *choleraesuis*), containing six subspecies with more than 2,300 serotypes (McWhorter-Murlin and Hickman-Brenner, 1994). In either of these schemes, the species name is dropped in common usage and replaced with the serotype name, or subspecies name and numeric code, in cases of unnamed serotypes. For example, *Salmonella enterica* serotype Poona becomes *Salmonella* Poona. The common reptile isolate formerly known as *Arizona hinshawii* is now classified as *Salmonella enterica* subsp. *arizonae*.

According to the CDC, close to 1,000 different serotypes have now been isolated from reptiles, many of which have been associated with zoonotic disease in humans. Although all serotypes of *Salmonella* are considered potentially pathogenic for humans, virulence factors within serotypes may dictate infectivity and severity.

The ways that reptiles acquire *Salmonella* include fecal-oral transmission, ingestion of contaminated food, and transovarial or percloacal contamination of eggs. The young of herbivorous species such as iguanas and other lizards are known to eat feces of adults, possibly to establish normal intestinal flora. *Salmonella* can remain viable in the environment for a considerable time, particularly in moist areas such as many reptile enclosures, rendering these areas and the objects therein potential sources of infection for long periods.

CLINICAL DISEASE IN REPTILES

Healthy reptiles generally do not become ill from the commensal salmonellae that inhabit their digestive tracts. However, certain serotypes have been recovered in pure culture or as the predominant organism from cases of abscessation, spinal osteomyelitis, infectious stomatitis, pneumonia, hepatitis, splenitis, nephritis, gastritis, enteritis, coelomitis, epicarditis, myocarditis, and septicemia. It is unclear whether any of these disease conditions represent cases of *Salmonella* acting as a primary pathogen. More likely, they are manifestations of secondary invasion by the opportunistic bacteria. The true underlying disease condition may or may not be identified clinically or at necropsy. Clinical signs are nonspecific. In some cases, anorexia, regurgitation, and diarrhea occur, but in others, no premonitory signs accompany the sudden death of an affected animal.

DIAGNOSIS

Isolation of a *Salmonella* serotype from diseased tissue, correlated with the finding of gram-negative organisms in histologic lesions, provides evidence of the agent as pathogen. In contrast, isolation of a *Salmonella* serotype from a stool or cloacal swab culture of a sick reptile offers little understanding of the agent's role in the disease because fecal carriage rates even in healthy animals may be greater than 90%.

Veterinarians are sometimes asked to "screen" an individual or group of reptiles for carriage of *Salmonella*. Such requests might come from physicians or public health departments in cases of potential zoonotic exposure, pet store owners or breeders seeking to certify their animals as "*Salmonella*-free," or zoos, wildlife rehabilitators, or other entities wishing to use reptiles in public contact displays or in educational outreach programs at schools or hospitals. The practitioner should be aware that attempting to culture *Salmonella* from specimens obtained from reptiles may harbor many pitfalls, from the taking of the sample through the laboratory technique and interpretation of results.

First, cloacal swabs are less reliable than feces for bacterial culture. A negative result on a single culture sample from either source should *not* be taken as proof that the animal is free of *Salmonella*. A succession of three cultures, at 2-week intervals, has historically been considered a more reliable screening protocol, but even this does not free the animal from suspicion because of the recognized phenomenon of intermittent shedding in reptiles. Finally, the laboratory culture technique may markedly influence the rate of recovery of *Salmonella* organisms. In a 1992 study of morbid chickens and poultry house environmental samples, a greatly increased recovery rate of *Salmonella* (98% versus 55%) was realized with a combination of 24-hour incubation and 5-day delayed secondary enrichment in tetrathionate broth versus plating after 24-hour enrichment in tetrathionate alone (Waltman et al, 1993). In a survey of veterinary diagnostic and independent laboratories in the United States, reported in the same study, 51% of the more than 50 respondents incubated their enrichment cultures for 24 hours only before plating. This would mean that more than half of the laboratories are failing to isolate between 40 and 50% of the potential salmonellae in their samples.

Intermittent shedding and inadequate culture technique are two of probably a number of reasons why a *Salmonella* screening program for reptiles might fail. Perhaps both contributed to the failure of a U.S. Food and Drug Administration–approved screening protocol for pet turtles in the early 1970s, leading to several cases of human illness and recovery of *Salmonella* from animals that had been "certified" as "free" of the bacterium. Unless and until controlled studies elucidate a foolproof screening method, it is better to assume that all reptiles are potentially positive for *Salmonella* and to refuse requests to certify animals as "*Salmonella*-free" by screening.

THERAPY

In general, therapy is not recommended for clinically healthy pet reptiles found to be shedding *Salmonella* in their feces. Antibiotic therapy is known to promote the development of resistant strains and at best might only suppress the organism, creating a carrier state, with resumption of shedding within days, weeks, or even months of cessation of treatment. In ill animals with gastroenteritis, supportive care with fluids and appropriate drugs such as intestinal protectants is indicated, much as it is in humans and other mammals. Occasionally, with valuable individual reptiles, such as with endangered species in a zoo collection, antibiotic therapy might be administered when the clinician suspects disease due to *Salmonella*, when no other causative agent can be identified, and stool cultures are consistently positive. The choice of antibiotic would be based on sensitivity testing.

PUBLIC HEALTH RISKS

In the 1960s and 1970s, the correlation between ownership of pet turtles and human salmonellosis became clear. In 1970, the (then) Centers for Disease Control found that 30% of human *Salmonella* cases in the United States were associated with reptiles in a nationwide case control study (Cohen et al, 1980). Based on concerns over the high incidence of turtle-associated salmonellosis at the time, and following the lead of some state health departments, the U.S. Food and Drug Administration ruled it illegal in 1975 to sell viable turtle eggs or live turtles with carapace length of less than 10.2 cm (4 inches). In the years after these state and federal laws went into effect, the incidence of turtle-associated cases of human salmonellosis decreased by 77%.

In 1996, the CDC estimated that, of the 2 to 6 million human salmonellosis cases each year, 3 to 5% may be attributed to reptiles. Food-associated cases, by contrast, account for as much as 80% of human cases. Most such cases are acquired by eating undercooked poultry and eggs (Miller et al, 1996), and outbreaks attributed to these sources have heightened public awareness of the disease, resulting in improved regulatory controls over the processing and sale of poultry by the U.S. Department of Agriculture.

Recent individual cases and outbreaks illustrate the seriousness of the risk of acquiring *Salmonella* from reptiles. In October 1995, a 3-week-old boy died in Rochester, Indiana, of infection with *S. Poona*. The same serotype was isolated from the family's pet iguana, and transmission was thought to have occurred indirectly because the baby had not touched the animal. In January 1996, an outbreak occurred among people visiting a special exhibit of Komodo dragons at the Denver Zoological Gardens. Although touching the animals was not allowed, 33 children and 1 adult acquired culture-confirmed infection with *S. enteritidis*. The two youngest cases (5 and 7 months) were hospitalized. Phage typing of an isolate from a cloacal swab culture of one of the lizards produced an exact match with the serotype affecting the humans. Swabs of the skin of the animal were culture-negative, whereas environmental swabs of the exhibit barrier used during the demonstration yielded the *Salmonella* organism 2 weeks after it had been placed in storage. Health officials concluded that children acquired the infection by touching the barrier, on which the lizards had climbed, and then had eaten or put unwashed fingers into their mouths.

Young children appear to be at the greatest risk for acquiring reptile-associated *Salmonella* infections, particularly those causing invasive disease. Anyone who is immunocompromised is also at special risk. This includes persons with congenital or acquired immune deficiency diseases, such as acquired immune deficiency syndrome (AIDS), cancer, kidney failure, chronic liver disease, pregnancy, or anyone taking immonosuppressive drugs. Elderly persons, whose immune systems may be weak, may also be at increased risk. Cases of reptile-associated salmonellosis have been documented in persons with AIDS. In fact, recurrent bacteremia caused by *Salmonella* is an AIDS-defining illness, and *Salmonella* infections in persons with AIDS may be 60 times more common than in the general population.

PREVENTION AND CONTROL

There is no known effective way of preventing exposure to or carriage of *Salmonella* by reptiles, and it should be assumed that all reptiles may be carriers. Strict adherence to good hygiene, including the use of disinfectants after thorough cleaning of cages and implements, might reduce the numbers of organisms in the animal's immediate envi-

---

TABLE 1. Ways of Helping to Prevent Humans from Getting *Salmonella* Infections from Reptiles

Always wash hands after handling a reptile, the reptile's cage, or anything in the cage.

Always wash hands before eating, smoking, or doing anything that involves putting the hands in or near the mouth.

Make sure that children wash their hands immediately after touching a reptile or its cage.

To wash hands properly, use soap and warm running water. Rub the hands back and forth, washing all parts of the hands, including the back of the hands, the wrists, between fingers, and under fingernails. Rinse the hands with water and dry with a paper towel. Turn off the water with a paper towel instead of using the hands.

Keep reptiles out of places where food is stored, prepared, or eaten.

Do not use kitchen sinks to clean reptiles or reptile cages and be sure to clean and disinfect any other sinks or tubs that you might use.

Always wear rubber gloves to clean reptile cages and equipment, and even to handle your animals if you have cuts or scratches on your hands.

Do not keep reptiles in places where there are children less than 5 years old.

The following persons should avoid *all* contact with reptiles:
    Infants and children up to 5 years old
    Anyone with HIV/AIDS or a weakened immune system
    Anyone receiving radiation therapy
    Anyone on any drug that suppresses the immune system (such as chemotherapy)
    Pregnant women
    Elderly, frail, or sick individuals

HIV, human immunodeficiency virus; AIDS, acquired immunodeficiency syndrome.

ronment, with possible health implications for the animal, its cage mates, and handlers.

Educating reptile buyers, owners, and handlers about public health risks is the key to minimizing zoonotic transmission. By far, the single most important preventive measure in the home is handwashing after handling of animals or objects in their enclosures. Health officials recommend washing hands with warm water and soap for at least 30 seconds in many circumstances to eliminate bacteria that might be on the hands. This precaution would apply to *Salmonella* from reptiles as well. Other measures recommended include keeping reptiles out of kitchens and away from other surfaces where human food is stored, prepared, or served and not using kitchen sinks to clean reptile accessories or caging materials. Table 1, written for the layperson, lists a number of precautions to prevent human infection from reptiles.

Persons at increased risk of infection should avoid contact with reptiles (pregnant women, children younger than 5 years of age, immunocompromised persons). Reptiles should not be kept in child care centers or taken to children's hospitals or wards for educational or entertainment programs. The American Zoo and Aquarium Association has issued guidelines to member institutions recommending that if reptiles and other zoo animals are used in public contact situations, handwashing stations be available in the immediate vicinity and patrons required to use them on the spot (Miller, 1997).

Veterinarians who see clients with reptile pets are in an excellent position to educate them and their families and friends on the dangers of *Salmonella* transmission from their animals and ways to prevent it. Providing a brochure or one-page handout on the subject at the time of the first visit to the clinic is a recognized and appreciated client education tool used routinely in several animal hospitals. Documenting in the patient record that the client was provided with this written information is highly recommended as protection for the veterinarian and staff against possible litigation in cases of human exposure.

References and Suggested Reading

Ackerman DM, Drabkin P, Birkhead G, et al: Reptile-associated salmonellosis in New York State. Pediatr Infect Dis J 14:955, 1995.
   This retrospective case-control study of New York cases of salmonellosis looks at reptile ownership or contact before the onset of illness.
Anonymous: Reptile-associated salmonellosis—selected states, 1994–1995. MMWR 44:347, 1995.
   This is a description of select, serious cases of reptile-associated salmonellosis in humans, with a discussion of epidemiology, risks, and precautions.
Cohen ML, Potter M, Pollard R, et al: Turtle-associated salmonellosis in the United States: Effect of public health action, 1970 to 1976. J Am Med Assoc 243:1247, 1980.
   This is a review of the effect of state and federal legislative actions on the incidence of turtle-associated salmonellosis in humans in the United States.
Johnson-Delaney CA: Reptile zoonoses and threats to public health. In: Mader DR, ed: Reptile Medicine and Surgery. Philadelphia, WB Saunders, 1996, p 20.
   This chapter presents a historical and epidemiologic summary of reptile-associated salmonellosis in humans.
McWhorter-Murlin AC, Hickman-Brenner FW: Identification and serotyping of *Salmonella* and an update of the Kauffmann-White Scheme. Atlanta, Centers for Disease Control and Prevention, 1994, pp 5–24.
   This is a review of Salmonella classification schemes and nomenclature, with a focus on current CDC, national, and international classification schemes.
Miller RE: AZA guidelines for animal contact with the general public. Wheeling, WV: American Zoo and Aquarium Association, 1997.
   This is a concise zoo industry review of potential zoonotic concerns about contact between the visiting public and a wide variety of zoo animals, with recommendations for prevention.
Miller SI, Hohmann EL, Pegues DA: *Salmonella* (including *Salmonella typhi*). In: Mandell GL, Bennett JE, Dolin R, eds: Principles and Practice of Infectious Diseases, 4th ed. New York: Churchill Livingstone, 1996, p 2013.
   This is a physician's comprehensive guide to epidemiology and treatment of salmonellosis in humans.
Waltman WD, Horne AM, Pirkle C: Influence of enrichment incubation time on the isolation of *Salmonella*. Avian Dis 37:884, 1993.
   This 1992 study compares recovery rates of Salmonella using various incubation enrichment protocols, and presents a survey of current procedures at more than 50 U.S. laboratories.

Cryptosporidia in Reptiles

MICHAEL R. CRANFIELD
THADDEUS K. GRACZYK
Baltimore, Maryland

Cryptosporidia are spore-forming, monogenous life cycle apicomplexan protozoans that, in reptiles, inhabit epithelial cells of the gastric region. The first complete report on infection with *Cryptosporidium* species in snakes was provided by the Baltimore Zoo in 1977 (Brownstein et al, 1977). The name *C. serpentis* was assigned to reptiles in 1980, and since then multiple studies have described pathologic changes associated with cryptosporidiosis in snakes (Cranfield and Graczyk, 1995). *Cryptosporidium* also has been reported in lacertas, chameleons, iguanas, tortoises, and turtles; however, these reports are occasional and fragmentary (Cranfield and Graczyk, 1995).

CLINICAL SIGNS AND PATHOLOGY

There appear to be two manifestations of *Cryptosporidium* infections in reptiles: (1) subclinical (carrier state) and (2) clinical (gastritis) (Cranfield and Graczyk, 1995).

Clinically healthy reptiles are able to intermittently pass oocysts for years. They oscillate between periods of shedding high numbers of *Cryptosporidium* oocysts to producing fecal specimens that are oocyst negative by acid-fast stain (Cranfield and Graczyk, 1995). The prevalence of subclinically infected shedders can be high in a reptile collection with relatively low mortality. Clinical signs in snakes and tortoises are associated with gastric hyperplasia of the mucus-secreting cells. Snakes often display foul-smelling diarrhea and midbody swelling and may live from a few days up to 2 years after the appearance of the clinical signs (Cranfield and Graczyk, 1995). Weight loss often occurs with persistent or periodical postprandial regurgitation 3 to 4 days after ingestion of mice in snakes and of plant material in tortoises. *Cryptosporidium* infections in lizards has been associated with acute bacterial gastritis.

Lesions due to *Cryptosporidium* are limited to the stomach area. They vary from no visible pathology in chronic shedders with no history of clinical signs to increased stomach diameter with a reduction in the diameter of the gastric lumen in clinical cases (Cranfield and Graczyk, 1995). The gastric mucosa of affected snakes is edematous with mucosal thickening and exaggerated longitudinal rugae that have copious amounts of adherent mucus (Brownstein et al, 1977; Cranfield and Graczyk, 1995). In reptiles other than snakes, the lesions are usually limited to histopathologic changes or incidental histopathologic findings.

DIAGNOSIS

Barium Study

In clinical cases with postprandial regurgitation and midbody swelling, a barium study is useful to differentiate between gastric occlusion due to mucosal swelling and nongastrointestinal mass (Cranfield and Graczyk, 1995).

Fecal Examination

Historically, cryptosporidial oocysts have been found in reptile fecal specimens by examination of direct unstained smears or acid-fast stained smears. Recently, it has been found (Graczyk et al, 1995) that the epitopes of *C. serpentis* oocyst wall antigens produce positive reactions with fluorescein-labeled monoclonal antibodies (mAb) of the MER-*IFLUOR* test kit for detection of *C. parvum* oocysts and *Giardia* cysts in human fecal samples (Fig. 1). Studies have found that the MER*IFLUOR* test is over 16 times more sensitive than acid-fast stain for detection of *C. serpentis* oocysts (Graczyk et al, 1995). However, even with the increased sensitivity of the immunofluorescent antibody multiple negative fecal tests must be performed to raise the confidence level of a snake's negativity for *Cryptosporidium* (Cranfield and Graczyk, 1995).

Endoscopy

The procedure requires expensive equipment, and the results of visualization of the gastric rugae are difficult to interpret (Cranfield and Graczyk, 1995).

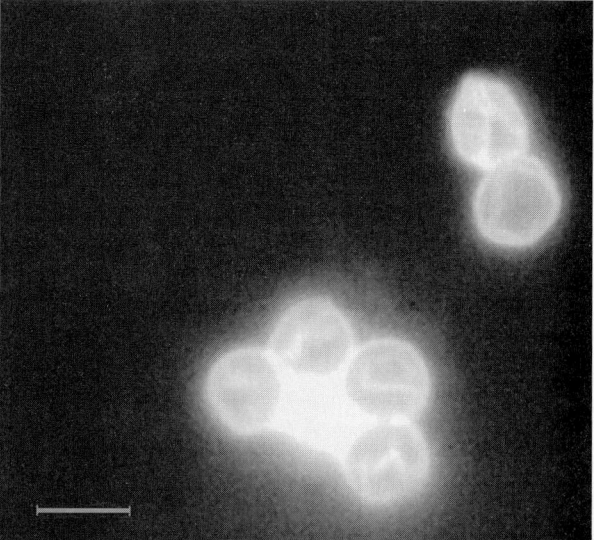

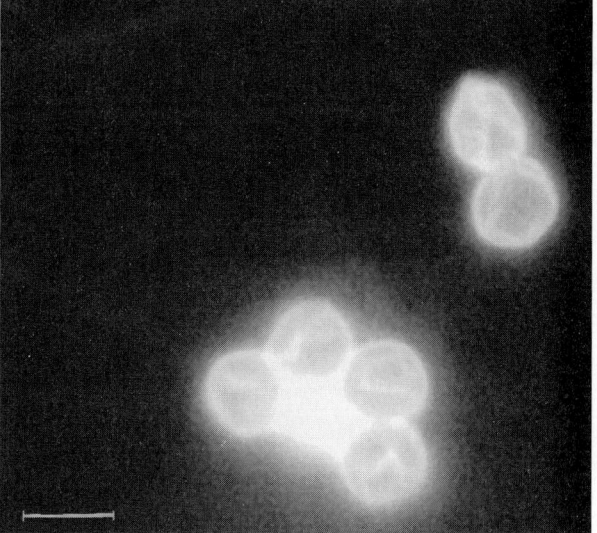

Figure 1. *Cryptosporidium serpentis* oocysts extracted from feces of clinically infected black rat snake *(Elaphe obsoleta obsoleta)* and purified by cesium chloride gradient centrifugation. The oocysts were detected by fluorescein-labeled monoclonal antibody of MER*IFLUOR Cryptosporidium/Giardia* test kit for direct immunofluorescence. Scale bar, 5 μm.

Gastric Lavage and Cloacal Swabs

The advantage of these methods is that they can be performed on anorectic and nondefecating reptiles (Graczyk et al, 1997). Cloacal swab smears were demonstrated to be far less effective than gastric lavage smears. Because the pathogen resides in the stomach area, it is expected that in nondefecating reptiles, *Cryptosporidium* oocysts will be present in higher concentrations in stomach aspirates than in cloacal swabs. Gastric lavage is performed by passing a stomach tube into the stomach located at the midpoint between the head and the cloaca of a snake (Graczyk et al, 1997). Two percent of the animal's body weight of phosphate buffered saline is passed through the tube into the stomach and then aspirated back while the snake is being held head downward. Approximately 50% of the administered fluid is retrieved. The aspirate is centrifuged and a smear prepared from the pellet. Stomach eluants contain little particulate matter, and, therefore, acid-fast stain detection of the oocysts is just about as sensitive as the MER-*IFLUOR* test (Graczyk et al, 1997). Additionally, it was noted that the test was more sensitive if performed within 3 days of eating (Graczyk et al, 1997). Because the metabolic rate of the gastric mucosal tissue increases over 22 times after a meal, it is proposed that the *Cryptosporidium* reproductive cycle increases with the metabolic increases occurring in the gastric mucosa (Graczyk et al, 1997). It may be beneficial to administer an appropriate baby food in a stomach tube meal to an anorectic reptile 3 days before the stomach lavage.

Regurgitated Material

Examination of smears of the parasite-rich mucus surrounding a regurgitated meal utilizing either the acid-fast stain or MER*IFLUOR* test kit can provide a definitive diagnosis (Cranfield and Graczyk, 1995).

Gastric Biopsies

This is a relatively safe procedure that can aid in the prognosis of a case when developmental stages of *Cryptosporidium* are found in the biopsy material. However, the nonuniform distribution of the pathogen on the gastric mucosa makes a negative outcome difficult to interpret (Cranfield and Graczyk, 1995).

Serum Antibody Test

A recently developed serum antibody enzyme-linked immunosorbent assay (ELISA) utilizing *C. serpentis* oocyst wall antigen has shown great sensitivity and specificity in surveys of reptile collections and in blind studies (Graczyk and Cranfield, 1997). The test diagnoses exposure of a snake to *Cryptosporidium* and allows for identification of truly *Cryptosporidium*-negative snakes. The test is expected to help assemble the pathogen-free colonies and select negative snakes for *Cryptosporidium* research.

Postmortem Examinations

Several stomach tissue sections should be trimmed for histologic examination. On a rare occasions, *Cryptosporidium*-positive snakes diagnosed on fecal samples were found to be negative on postmortem examination when limited samples of gastric tissue were collected (Cranfield and Graczyk, 1995).

TREATMENT

The treatment of *Cryptosporidium* infections in reptiles is similar to the situation in humans with human immunodeficiency virus infection who developed cryptosporidiosis, because in both cases the disease is not self limiting. Treatment regimens for reptiles have mainly originated from the experiences of human and domestic animal treatment. The human literature includes more than 100 prophylactic and therapeutic compounds tested in patients with the acquired immunodeficiency syndrome with no consistent

positive outcome. For reptiles, a regimen of trimethoprim-sulfamethoxazole (TMP-SMZ, Biocraft Laboratories), 30 mg/kg once a day for 14 days and then one to three times weekly for several months (Cranfield and Graczyk, 1995), spiramycin, 160 mg/kg for 10 days, and paromomycin, 100 mg/kg for 7 days and then twice a week for 3 months, has been used (Cranfield and Graczyk, 1995). These compounds were all effective for reducing the magnitude of clinical signs of cryptosporidiosis and decreasing or eliminating shedding of the oocysts. Postmortem examination revealed that the spiramycin and paromomycin-treated snakes still had high numbers of *Cryptosporidium* developmental stages in the gastric region (Graczyk et al, 1996a). Biopsies of TMP-SMZ–treated snakes were *Cryptosporidium* negative; however, postmortem results were not available. Halofuginone, which is effective in some domestic animal species, was both ineffective and toxic to the snakes (Graczyk et al, 1996a). Studies are being conducted in which hyperimmune enhanced bovine colostrum is administered orally to snakes clinically and subclinically infected with *Cryptosporidium*. Supportive treatments, such as high temperatures ($\geq$80°F), subcutaneous fluids, regular stomach tubing of highly digestible foods, and the elimination of any concurrent disease problems, appear to act synergistically with treatment aimed at *Cryptosporidium* (Cranfield and Graczyk, 1995).

PREVENTION, CONTROL, AND ZOONOTIC POTENTIAL

All *Cryptosporidium* infections are contracted by the ingestion of oocysts; therefore, effective prevention and control measures must aim to reduce contamination. *Cryptosporidium* can be transmitted directly via the fecal-oral route or indirectly by contamination of food or water (e.g., utensils, feeding bottles, and cages) (Granfield and Graczyk, 1995). The oocysts, which are fully sporulated and infectious when excreted, are resistant to environmental stressors and to a wide range of commonly used disinfectants (Cranfield and Graczyk, 1995). Ammonia (5%) and formal saline (10%) were the most effective in altering oocysts infectivity after 18 hours at greater than or equal to 4°C (Cranfield and Graczyk, 1995). Strict high-standard hygiene, good management, and isolation of infected animals are essential in prevention of spreading of *Cryptosporidium* within captive reptiles (Cranfield and Graczyk, 1995).

Of eight valid *Cryptosporidium* species infecting all vertebrate groups: *C. nasorum* (fish), *C. serpentis* (reptiles), *C. baileyi* and *C. meleagridis* (birds), *C. felis, C. muris, C. wrairi,* and *C. parvum* (mammals), only one, *C. parvum,* is readily cross-transmissible to humans and, therefore, represents zoonotic potential (Fayer et al, 1997). *Cryptosporidium* species from a lizard *(Varanus exanthematicus)* failed to establish infections in mammals (Upton, 1990). Multiple heterogeneous isolates of *C. serpentis* from seven snake species were noninfectious to mammals (e.g., neonatal BALB/c mice) (Fayer et al., 1995) and to birds (e.g., Peking ducks, *Anas platyrhynchos*). Thus, it is unlikely that snake infections are generated by *C. muris,* which is infectious to rodents, and that *C. serpentis* represents a zoonotic potential. A series of cross-transmission experiments in which human/bovine *C. parvum* isolates were used excluded any potentially successful cross-transmission of *C. parvum* to lower vertebrates (e.g., fish, amphibia, or reptiles) (Graczyk et al, 1996b).

References and Suggested Reading

Brownstein DG, Strandberg JD, Montali RJ, et al: *Cryptosporidium* in snakes with hypertrophic gastritis. Vet Pathol 14:606, 1977.

Cranfield MR, Graczyk TK: Cryptosporidiosis. In Mader DR, ed: Manual of Reptile Medicine and Surgery. Philadelphia: WB Saunders, 1995, p 369.

Fayer R, Graczyk TK, Cranfield MR: Multiple heterogenous isolates of *Cryptosporidium serpentis* from captive snakes are not transmissible to neonatal BALB/c mice *(Mus musculus)*. J Parasitol 81:482, 1995.

Fayer R, Speer CA, Dubey JP: The general biology of *Cryptosporidium*. In Fayer R, ed: *Cryptosporidium* and Cryptosporidiosis. Boca Raton, FL: CRC Press, 1997.

Graczyk TK, Cranfield MR: Detection of *Cryptosporidium*-specific immunoglobulins in captive snakes by a polyclonal antibody in the indirect ELISA. Vet Res 28:131, 1997.

Graczyk TK, Cranfield MR, Fayer R: A comparative assessment of direct fluorescence antibody, modified acid-fast stain, and sucrose flotation techniques for detection of *Cryptosporidium serpentis* in snake fecal specimens. J Zoo Wildl Med 26:396, 1995.

Graczyk TK, Cranfield MR, Hill SL: Therapeutic efficacy of halofuginone and spiramycin treatment against *Cryptosporidium serpentis* (Apicomplexa: Cryptosporidiidae) infections in captive snakes. Parasitol Res 82:143, 1996a.

Graczyk TK, Fayer R, Cranfield MR: *Cryptosporidium parvum* is not transmissible to fish, amphibians, or reptiles. J Parasitol 82:748, 1996b.

Graczyk TK, Owens R, Cranfield MR: Diagnosis of subclinical cryptosporidiosis in captive snakes based on stomach lavage and cloacal sampling. Vet Parasitol 50:67:143, 1996.

Upton SJ: *Cryptosporidium* spp. in lower vertebrates. In Dubey JP, Speer CA, Fayer R, eds: Cryptosporidiosis in Man and Animals. Boca Raton, FL: CRC Press, 1990, p 147.

Nutrition of Ornamental Fish

RICHARD T. LOVELL

Auburn University, Alabama

In a natural environment, fish seldom show signs of nutritional disease. Although the quantity of food may be limited, their natural foods are generally balanced in essential nutrients and meet the nutritional needs of the fish for normal health and function. It is usually when fish are confined to an artificial environment, where natural food is absent or limited, that nutritional problems occur. Such a situation can arise if all essential nutrients, pigments, and other diet components essential for growth and development are not provided.

Like warm-blooded animals, fish need dietary sources of energy, protein, vitamins, minerals, and lipids for normal growth, health, and function. Nutrient requirements of fish are similar to those of warm-blooded animals, although there are a few exceptions. For example, fish have lower energy requirements than do terrestrial animals (discussed later); fish can absorb nutrients, namely certain minerals, from water through the gills; many fish require more highly unsaturated fatty acids than do land animals; and most fish require vitamin C in their diet, whereas most warm-blooded animals can synthesize vitamin C.

Because of the commercial aquaculture that has evolved since the 1970s, a great amount of information has been generated on fish nutrition. This is because least-cost, nutritionally balanced feeds are important to successful aquaculture. All the essential nutrient requirements for several species of commercially important fish have been determined, and recommended allowances are provided by the National Research Council (NRC). According to the NRC, nutrient requirements among fishes do not vary greatly; slight differences may be found between warm and cold water species, carnivores and herbivores, or marine and freshwater fish. Thus, when nutrient requirements for a certain species of fish are not available, a prudent analogy from known requirements of a similar species will usually suffice. This indicates that although nutrient requirements specifically for ornamental species have not received much attention, enough information is available from a variety of "food" fishes that reasonable estimates of nutrient requirements of ornamentals can also be made.

NUTRIENT REQUIREMENTS

The minimal dietary requirements for energy and essential nutrients for channel catfish (*Ictalurus punctatus*), rainbow trout (*Oncarhynchus mykiss*), Pacific salmon (*Oncarhynchus* spp.), common carp (*Cyprinus carpio*), and Nile tilapia (*Oreschronus nilotia*), are presented in Table 1 (National Research Council/National Academy of Sciences, 1993). These values were determined with small fish fed highly purified diets under laboratory conditions where there was no natural food. The table shows considerable similarity in nutrient requirements among the species. Diets for several ornamental species have been successfully prepared based on the nutrient requirements in this table.

ENERGY

One of the striking differences in nutrition between fish and farm animals is that the amount of energy required for protein synthesis is less for fish than for warm-blooded food animals. Because fish do not regulate body temperature and expend less energy than terrestrial animals in maintaining posture, their maintenance requirement is

TABLE 1. Nutrient Requirements of Fish Diets (As Fed Basis)

Energy Base* (kcal DE/kg diet)	Channel Catfish 3,000	Rainbow Trout 3,600	Pacific Salmon 3,600	Common Carp 3,200	Tilapia 3,000
Protein, crude (digestible), percent	32 (28)	38 (34)	38 (34)	35 (30.5)	32 (28)
Amino acids					
Arginine, %	1.20	1.5	2.04	1.31	1.18
Histidine, %	0.42	0.7	0.61	0.64	0.48
Isoleucine, %	0.73	0.9	0.75	0.76	0.87
Leucine, %	0.98	1.4	1.33	1.00	0.95
Lysine, %	1.43	1.8	1.70	1.74	1.43
Methionine + cystine, %	0.64	1.0	1.36	0.94	0.90
Phenylalanine + tyrosine, %	1.40	1.8	1.73	1.98	1.55
Threonine, %	0.56	0.8	0.75	1.19	1.05
Tryptophan, %	0.14	0.2	0.17	0.24	0.28
Valine, %	0.84	1.2	1.09	1.10	0.78
n-3 fatty acids, %	0.5–1	1	1–2	1	—
n-6 fatty acids, %	—	1	—	1	0.5–1
Macrominerals					
Calcium, %	R	1E	NT	NT	R
Phosphorus, %	0.45	0.6	0.6	0.6	0.5
Sodium, %	R	0.6E	NT	NT	NT
Potassium, %	R	0.7	0.8	NT	NT
Chlorine, %	R	0.9E	NT	NT	NT
Magnesium, mg/kg	400	500	NT	500	600
Microminerals					
Manganese, mg/kg	2.4	13	R	13	R
Zinc, mg/kg	20	30	R	30	20
Iron, mg/kg	30	60	NT	150	NT
Copper, mg/kg	5	3	NT	3	R
Selenium, mg/kg	0.25	0.3	R	NT	NT
Iodine, mg/kg	1.1E	1.1	0.6–1.1	NT	NT
Fat-soluble vitamins					
Vitamin A, IU/kg	1,000–2,000	2,500	2,500	4,000	NT
Vitamin D, IU/kg	500	2,400	NT	NT	NT
Vitamin E, IU/kg	50	50	50	100	50
Vitamin K, mg/kg	R	R	R	NT	NT
Water-soluble vitamins					
Riboflavin, mg/kg	9	4	7	7	6
Pantothenic acid, mg/kg	15	20	20	30	10
Niacin, mg/kg	14	10	R	28	NT
Vitamin B_{12}, mg/kg	R	0.01E	R	NR	NR
Choline, mg/kg	400	1,000	800	500	NT
Biotin, mg/kg	R	0.15	R	1	NT
Folate, mg/kg	1.5	1.0	2	NR	NT
Thiamine, mg/kg	1	1	R	0.5	NT
Vitamin B_6, mg/kg	3	3	6	6	NT
myo-Insitol, mg/kg	NR	300	300	440	NT
Vitamin C, mg/kg	25–50	50	50	R	50

*Typical energy concentrations in practical diets.

These requirements have been determined with highly purified ingredients in which the nutrients are highly digestible: therefore, the values presented represent near 100% bioavailability.

R, required in diet but quantity not determined; NR, no dietary requirement demonstrated under experimental conditions; NT, not tested; E, estimated.

Reprinted with permission from Nutritional Requirements of Fish. Copyright 1993 by the National Academy of Sciences. Courtesy of the National Academy Press, Washington, DC.

lower. Cho and Kaushik (1990) measured oxygen consumption of fasting rainbow trout and calculated their fasting heat production, in kcal per fish per day, to be 8.85 $W^{0.82}$ where W = body weight in kilograms. When compared with 70 $W^{0.73}$ for mammals and 83 $W^{0.75}$ for birds (Brody, 1945), it is apparent that the fasting heat production of fish is markedly lower.

Another reason that fish have a lower dietary energy requirement is that heat increment, or rise in heat production after eating food, is lower in fish than in warm-blooded animals. This is primarily because the energy expenditure for nitrogen excretion is much lower in fish, which excrete

ammonia, than in mammals and birds, which excrete urea or uric acid. Synthesis of urea and uric acid requires significant energy, whereas excretion of ammonia requires negligible energy. Smith (1989) reported the heat increment for rainbow trout to be 3 to 5% of the metabolizable energy (ME), whereas in mammals it may account for as much as 30% of ME (Brody, 1945).

Because fish evolved in an aqueous environment where carbohydrates were scarce, their digestive and metabolic systems are often better adapted to the utilization of protein and lipids for energy than to carbohydrates. However, warm water herbivores or omnivores, like channel catfish, tilapia, and carp, can digest and metabolize carbohydrates relatively well, whereas carnivores, like rainbow trout, utilize carbohydrates relatively poorly and require fat and protein as energy sources. Nile tilapia and channel catfish may digest more than 70% of the gross energy in cornstarch, whereas rainbow trout digest less than 50% (National Research Council, 1993).

PROTEIN AND AMINO ACIDS

Because commercial fish feeds contain a higher percentage of protein, the perception is common that fish have a higher protein requirement for growth than do livestock. The reason for this higher protein:energy ratio is not because fish have a higher protein requirement; fish, in fact, convert dietary protein into tissue protein with about the same efficiency as warm-blooded animals. Rather, it is because fish require less energy for maintenance and excretion of nitrogen. Because of the lower energy requirement in relation to protein requirement by fish, practical diets with higher concentrations of protein can be more profitably fed to fish than to farm animals. For example, catfish feeds contain approximately 32% protein and 2.9 kcal of ME/g; this provides a protein energy ratio of 110 g/kcal. Pig feeds contain approximately 16% and 3.0 kcal of ME/g, with a protein:energy ratio of 53 g/kcal.

Protein requirements, meaning the minimal amount needed to meet amino acid requirements and to achieve maximal weight gain, have been measured in juvenile fish of many species. Crude protein requirements ranging from 25 to 55% of the diet for various species are presented in the NRC publication.

An absolute requirement for 10 amino acids has been demonstrated in all fish species examined thus far. These are the same amino acids that are required by warm-blooded animals. Quantitative requirements for the 10 essential amino acids for five fish species are presented in Table 1.

ESSENTIAL FATTY ACIDS

Fish have dietary requirements for certain fatty acids. Some species require n-3 or n-6, or both types of fatty acids. Some can convert 18-carbon unsaturated fatty acids to longer chain, more highly unsaturated fatty acids, whereas other species cannot and must consume the metabolically active long-chain highly unsaturated fatty acids in the diet. Tropical species, such as some tilapias, require n-6 series fatty acids, as do humans and other warm-blooded animals, and can utilize linolenic acid, 18:2(n-6), which is commonly found in plant oils. Cold water species such as rainbow trout require n-3 series fatty acids and can convert linolenic acid, 18:3(n-3) to eicosapentaenoic acid, 20:5(n-5) or docosahexaenoic acid, 22:5(n-3), whereas marine species such as red sea bream and yellow tail, require eicosapentaenoic acid or docosahexaenoic acid preformed in the diet. Freshwater species indigenous to temperate zones, such as common carp and channel catfish, have shown benefit from the simultaneous inclusion of n-6 and n-3 fatty acids in the diet.

MINERALS

Although most mineral elements known to be essential for terrestrial animals are also considered important for fish, quantitative requirements for only nine have been reported: calcium, phosphorus, copper, iodine, iron, magnesium, manganese, selenium, and zinc. Fish can obtain minerals from the water by absorbing dissolved minerals directly across the gill membrane or, in the case of marine fish that drink water, across the intestinal wall. Most of the calcium requirements for freshwater and marine fish come from the water. In seawater, significant amounts of copper, iron, magnesium, selenium, potassium, sodium, and zinc are also obtained from the water. However, fish usually require a dietary source of phosphorus to meet their high metabolic requirements because levels of dissolved phosphorus in natural waters are relatively low.

Fish feeds that contain large amounts of fish meal are generally sufficient in all essential minerals, and mineral supplementation is unnecessary. A rule of thumb is that fish feeds containing more than 10% animal byproducts do not need mineral supplementation. Fish meal with high ash content (>20%) should be avoided for fish feeds because it can form complexes with other minerals, such as zinc, and cause deficiency problems.

VITAMINS

Most fish studied have a dietary requirement for all the 15 recognized vitamins. There are some exceptions: channel catfish can synthesize myoinositol de novo and do not show a dietary requirement (Burtle and Lovell, 1989); warm-water fish like Nile tilapia (Limsuwan and Lovell, 1981) and common carp (Kashiwada et al, 1970) show a high rate of intestinal synthesis of several of the B-complex vitamins and do not respond to dietary supplementation of the vitamins. Intestinal microorganisms do not appear to be a significant source of vitamins in cold water carnivorous fish (Hepher, 1988).

Vitamin requirements of fish have been determined by feeding chemically defined diets deficient in a specific vitamin in a controlled environment. Deficiency signs have been described in several species (Table 2). The quantitative requirements for most of the vitamins have been established for Pacific salmon, rainbow trout, common carp, channel catfish, and yellowtail (Seriola lalandi), whereas only some of the requirements are known for other species. The requirements are affected by fish size, feeding rates, environmental factors, and nutrient interrelationships. Also, the response criterion measured influences the requirement for various vitamins. For example, it has been demonstrated in several fish species that maximal resistance to bacterial infection is affected by higher dietary concentrations of vitamin C than maximal weight gain. Requirement data based on subclinical measurements, like enzyme activity or histologic assay, are often lower than determinations based on weight gain or absence of overt deficiency signs. Values presented in Table 1 generally represent requirements for maximal weight gain, determined with young, nonstressed fish.

An important difference in nutritional requirements between fish and land animals is that most warm-blooded

TABLE 2. Major Vitamin Deficiency Signs Reported in Fish

Vitamin	Salmonids	Channel Catfish	Common Carp
A	Skin depigmentation, exophthalmia, corneal thinning, retinal degeneration edema, ascites	Exophthalmia, edema, skin depigmentation	Skin depigmentation, exophthalmia, twisted opercula, hemorrhagic areas
D	Impaired calcium homeostasis, tetany of skeletal muscle	Low bone ash, potassium, and calcium contents	Not tested
E	Skin depigmentation, ascites, fragile erythrocytes, muscular dystrophy	Skin depigmentation, exudative diathesis, muscular dystrophy, fatty liver	Exophthalmia, lordosis, muscular dystrophy, pancreatic degeneration
K	Prolonged blood clotting, hemorrhagic gills and eyes	Hemorrhagic skin	Not tested
Thiamine	Nervous disorders, loss of equilibrium, hyperirritability, convulsions	Dark skin coloration, loss of equilibrium, nervousness	Nervousness, skin depigmentation, subcutaneous hemorrhage
Riboflavin	Dark pigmentation, spinal deformities, photophobia, fin and eye hemorrhage	Short-body dwarfism	Photophobia, dermatitis, fin and abdominal hemorrhage
Pyroxidine	Epileptiform convulsions, hyperirritability, erratic spiral swimming	Nervous disorders, tetany, erratic swimming, greenish coloration	Nervous disorders, low hepatopancreatic transferase
Pantothenic acid	Clubbed gills, distended operculum, atrophied pancreatic acinar cells	Clubbed gills, eroded epidermis	Clubbed gills, exophthalmia, skin hemorrhage
Niacin	Skin, fin, and colon lesions; photosensitivity; sunburn; ascites	Skin and fin lesions, exophthalmia, deformed jaws	Skin hemorrhage, mortality
Biotin	Degenerative gill lamellae, skin lesions, muscle atrophy, reduced hepatic acetyl CoA and pyruvate carboxylase degeneration of pancreatic acinar cells	Skin depigmentation, reduced hepatic pyruvate carboxylase	Lethargy, increased number of dermal mucous cells
Folate	Serious anemia, bilobed erythrocytes, dark skin coloration	Mild anemia, bilobed erythrocytes, increased sensitivity to bacterial infection	None detected
Vitamin B_{12}	Microcytic hypochromic anemia, fragmented erythrocytes	Reduced growth, low hematocrit	None detected
Choline	Fatty liver, exophthalmia, extended abdomen, hemorrhagic kidney and intestine	Enlarged liver, hemorrhagic kidney and intestine	Fatty liver, vacuolization of hepatic cells
Inositol	Dark skin coloration, distended abdomen, reduced activity of cholinesterase and transaminase	None detected	Loss of skin mucosa
Ascorbic acid	Hemorrhagic tissues, hemorrhagic exophthalmia, distorted gill filaments, lordosis and scoliosis, ascites	Hemorrhagic areas, reduced bone collagen, lordosis and scoliosis	Poor growth

Major deficiency signs include anorexia, mild anemia, and poor growth; they are not listed unless those are the only signs observed. Mortality means high and rapid mortality and thus might be useful for distinguishing some vitamin deficiencies.

Reprinted with permission from Nutritional Requirements of Fish. Copyright 1993 by the National Academy of Sciences. Courtesy of the National Academy Press, Washington, DC.

animals can readily synthesize vitamin C (L-ascorbic acid) from glucose, but most fish do not have this ability. Fish are deficient in the enzyme L-gulonolactone oxidase, which is necessary in the conversion, and therefore must obtain vitamin C from the diet. Dietary deficiency of vitamin C in fish readily causes overt deformities (see Table 2). Ingredients commonly used in feeds are devoid of vitamin C, so supplementation of prepared diets is necessary. L-Ascorbic acid, the traditional source of vitamin C, is sensitive to oxidation. Fifty to 100% of the supplemental vitamin is usually destroyed in processing, especially when extreme heat is used, as in flaked feeds. Also, L-ascorbic acid deteriorates with time in feeds (half-life is about 4 weeks). A stable source of vitamin C is now available in the form of L-ascorbyl-2-phosphate, commonly called ascorbic acid phosphate, and should be used in all ornamental fish feeds. Most other vitamins used in fish feeds are fairly stable. Fresh feed should be purchased for ornamental fish about every 3 months to ensure that all nutrients are present and in active form.

DIETARY ENHANCEMENT OF COLOR IN ORNAMENTAL FISH

The commercial value of ornamental fish is dependent on good coloration. Carotenoids are the primary source of pigmentation in the skin of fishes. Yellow, red, and blue colors are caused by various carotenoids or carotenoid-protein complexes. Because carotenoids are synthesized only by plants (although they can be modified in animal tissues), fish must get them from their diet.

Fish in a pond or a natural environment get the carotenoids by ingesting aquatic plants or through the aquatic food chain. Many pigmented carotenoids have been identified in the aquatic environment. The most common are usually lutein and zeaxanthin (yellow and deep orange), found in aquatic plants and animals, and astaxanthin (red), found in micro- and macrocrustaceans. Fish that are grown or held in tanks, recirculating systems, or some type of environment where natural food is absent lose or fail to develop desired coloration unless pigments are supplemented in the prepared diets. Also, if natural food is limiting, such as an infertile pond or dense culture where artificial feed makes up most of the diet, the fish may not have optimal pigmentation.

A trend in ornamental fish farming is to grow the fish in a closed recirculating culture system. Claimed advantages are management convenience, fewer disease problems, and temperature control. The fish must be fed commercial feeds. Feeds made from traditional ingredients are nutritionally sufficient, but unless a satisfactory pigment source is added, the fish will grow well but not color adequately.

Commercial feeds that are rich in certain carotenoids include yellow corn, corn gluten meal, and alfalfa meal. These feedstuffs are sources of zeaxanthin and lutein, which are yellow-orange. Marigold (the flower) meal or extract is a highly concentrated source of lutein and is used in the United States in poultry feeds to enhance yellow in chicken egg and flesh. An extract from red peppers (*Capsicum* spp.), which contains the orange-red carotenoid, capxanthin, is also used commercially. Astaxanthin is a natural pigment in krill or crustacean meal and enhances red in salmon flesh. Spirulina (algae) meal contains a group of yellow-red xanthophylls and is often a component of aquarium feeds. Synthetic astaxanthin and canthaxanthin have been developed but are restricted-use compounds for food fish feed in the United States and are generally unavailable.

Studies were conducted at Auburn University to evaluate supplementation of feeds with various pigment sources on color development in cherry barbs (*Barbus titteya*) and tiger barbs (*B. tetrazona*) grown in recirculating aquaria. In the first test, cherry barbs, which desirably have deep red color of skin and fins, were fed a commercial salmon diet supplemented with 0, 100, or 400 ppm of carotenoids from *Capsicum* extract (primarily capxanthin) or 100 ppm of synthetic canthaxanthin. The carotenoid supplements were mixed with menhaden fish oil, (3 gm of the oil mixture was added per 100 gm of feed), and fish were fed the diets for 8 weeks. In a second study, tiger barbs were fed the salmon starter alone or supplemented with 200 ppm of capxanthin carotenoid from the *Capsicum* extract or from a marigold flower extract (primarily lutein), or a combination of the two pigment sources. The fish were fed the same as those in the first study. All fish were evaluated against pond-grown fish for color development.

The cherry barbs in the recirculating aquaria that were fed the salmon feed with no pigment source were almost devoid of color. Those fed the *Capsicum* extract at 100 ppm had a desirable red color, whereas those fed the same concentration of canthaxanthin had only a faint pink color. Increasing the concentration of carotenoids from *Capsicum* to 400 ppm increased color intensity. Coloration was consistent among fish fed the *Capsicum* extract in the aquaria, but coloration varied among the pond fish from intense to light pigmentation. The tiger barbs that were fed the salmon feed with no pigment supplement were almost devoid of color. Those from the pond varied in color intensity, whereas those fed the pigment supplements in the tanks were uniform. The combination of *Capsicum* and marigold extracts produced the best coloration; the fins were deep red, whereas the body had a yellow sheen that accented the dark stripes. *Capsicum* extract alone produced deep red

fin tips but less body coloration. The marigold extract alone produced yellow to orange coloration that was less intense.

These results indicate that the carotenoids lutein and capxanthin, from natural extracts that are used in commercial poultry feeds, can satisfactorily produce the commercially desirable yellow to deep red colors in ornamental fish.

FOOD PREPARATION FOR ORNAMENTAL FISH

Newly Hatched Fry

Many ornamentals are hatched from small eggs and thus the nutriment from the yolk sac is used up quickly. In such cases, the digestive tract is usually not fully developed when the fry need an exogenous source of nutrients. Because of this, the fry are unable to use artificial diets and must have live foods. This is in contrast to fish like channel catfish and rainbow trout, which hatch from large eggs that nourish the hatchling for a long period, and the digestive tract is fairly well developed when the fish begins consuming food. These species can use artificial (prepared) feeds as their first food.

When ornamentals are spawned and hatched in earthen ponds, natural pond organisms (phytoplankton and zooplankton) are abundant for nourishment. If hatched indoors in tanks or aquaria, live foods must be provided. This is assuming that the fry require live food. (The author knows of no documentation of which ornamental species require live foods and which do not. Most hatchery managers provide some live food even though the fry are able to assimilate prepared diets.) The most common live foods for larval fish are algae, rotifers, and brine shrimp (artemia) nauplii, in increasing order of size. These organisms are cultured in the hatchery and added periodically to the container where the larvae are reared. Brine shrimp eggs (cysts) are widely available in sealed metal cans and can be reconstituted (hatched into nauplii) in saline water. Brine shrimp vary in size of nauplii (the first posthatch stage), hatchability of cysts, and nutritional quality.

Generally, within a week the fry begin accepting dry diets and a combination of live and dry foods are offered. Within 2 to 3 weeks, the fry can usually use dry diet alone provided that the nutritional, physical, and palatability characteristics of the prepared dry diet are satisfactory.

Prepared Diets

For small or newly hatched fish, a powder or meal is usually fed. The primary ingredient is usually good quality fish meal, which is highly nutritious and palatable. A powdered diet must be liberally supplemented with a vitamin mixture because many of the water-soluble nutrients will be lost when the feed is put into the water. Addition of oil to the diet mixture will reduce the loss of nutrients into the water.

If fish are large enough to consume particles as large as 2 mm (based on mouth size), a pelleted feed should be used because pellets may be consumed more efficiently by the fish and there is less fouling of the water. As fish increase in size, the pellet size can be increased. Commercial trout or salmon starter diets can be fed to most fish. These feeds are nutritionally complete, palatable, and available in a range of pellet sizes. Some are available as floating pellets. Trout and salmon feeds do not contain pigment sources, however, so they must be added.

Some fish do not accept dry feeds or their feeding habits are not suited to infrequent offering (once or twice daily) of dry diets. A soft, gelatin-type food that remains in the water for long periods while the fish feed intermittently is sometimes used. This type of food is prepared by mixing a variety of ingredients—wet or dry, finely ground—plus a complete vitamin mixture in a warm gelatin solution and pouring the mixture into a mold to solidify. The hardened mixture, in suitable size, can be suspended in the rearing container, and the fish will nibble on the soft but insoluble chunks.

Flaked diets are popular for aquarium feeding because they stay on the surface and do not dissolve quickly and foul the water. These diets are processed on a drum dryer. The diet ingredients are mixed into an aqueous slurry that is poured onto the surface of a steam heated, rotating cylinder (drum). The moisture is immediately evaporated off, and the dry film is scraped off the drum surface as flakes. Intense heat is involved, so the vitamin supplement should be increased by at least 100% and the vitamins should be in the most stable forms available.

Vitamin C (ascorbic acid) is the vitamin (or nutrient) most sensitive to oxidative deterioration. Some of the ascorbic acid in a diet mix will be lost (about 25%) in steam pelleting, a large amount (>50%) will be lost in extrusion processing (floating feeds), and nearly all will be lost in the flaking process. Ascorbic acid will also deteriorate in feed during storage (half-life is about 2 months). As mentioned earlier, a stable form of vitamin C, ascorbic acid polyphosphate, is now available, and most feed manufacturers use it. Anyone purchasing fish feeds should read the label to determine if the feed contains the stabilized form of vitamin C. The other vitamins are relatively insensitive to deterioration during storage.

References and Suggested Reading

Brody S: Bioenergetics and Growth. New York: Hofner, 1945.
Burtle GJ, Lovell RT: Lack of response of channel catfish (*Ictalurus punctatus*) to dietary myoinositol. Can J Fish Aquat Sci 46:218, 1989.
Cho CY, Kaushik SJ: Nutritional energetics in fish: Energy and protein utilization in rainbow trout (*Oncarhynchus mykiss*). World Rev Nutr Diet 61:132, 1990.
Hepher B: Vitamins. In: Nutrition of Pond Fishes. New York: Cambridge University Press, 1988, p 224.
Kashiwada K, Teshima D, Kanazawa A: Studies on the production of B vitamins by intestinal bacteria of fish. 5. Evidence of the production of Vitamin B_{12} by microorganisms in the intestinal canal of carp, *Cyprinus carpio*. Bull Jpn Soc Sci Fish 36:421, 1970.
Limsuwan T, Lovell RT: Intestinal synthesis and absorption of Vitamin B_{12} in channel catfish. J Nutr 111:2125, 1981.
National Research Council/National Academy of Sciences: Nutritional Requirements of Fish. Washington, DC: National Academy Press, 1993.
Smith RR: Nutritional energetics. In: Halver JE, ed: Fish Nutrition. San Diego: Academic Press, 1989, p 2.

CVT Update: Antibiotic Treatment of Aquarium Fish

GREGORY A. LEWBART
Raleigh, North Carolina

Certainly one of the most commonly asked questions concerning the practice of pet fish veterinary medicine is, "What antibiotic should I use and what is the dose?" This is a straightforward and uncomplicated question with a complex and frequently ambiguous answer. The problem lies in the lack of sound pharmacokinetic data available and the overwhelming number of species involved. When environmental differences such as temperature, pH, and water hardness are tossed into the equation, selecting a drug and dosing regimen becomes even less objective.

Historically, most treatment of aquarium fish diseases has been performed by nonveterinarians using empirical dosing regimens of a variety of chemotherapeutics. The U.S. Food and Drug Administration is currently examining the wide availability of prescription drugs, especially antibiotics, and will possibly restrict their availability to the lay public within the next few years. Such measures will necessitate sound pharmacokinetics studies to support clinical use of antimicrobials in pet fishes by licensed veterinarians. Little research related to pharmacology has been reported in aquarium fishes and few pharmacokinetic data are available. What scant information exists is based on clinical efficacy and in vitro trials using a number of different antimicrobial agents.

The purpose of this article is to familiarize the reader with the most current pet fish pharmacokinetic information, provide a list of frequently used antibiotics, and discuss the variables that influence antibiotic dosing regimens in pet fish.

DOSING ROUTES

Because of their aquatic nature, generally small size, and frequently large numbers, a variety of atypical methods

TABLE 1. **Routes of Antibiotic Administration for Aquarium Fish**

Bath
Usually refers to a treatment in which the drug is dissolved in the water in which the fish are swimming. The treatment usually lasts at least 15 minutes and less than 24 hours. Dosage is usually based on volume of water and not on fish biomass.

Dip
Refers to a treatment in which the fish is submerged in a particular solution for 1 second to 15 minutes. Water volumes are usually smaller than those of bath treatments and drug concentrations are frequently higher.

Flush or flow through
Requires constant water flow. Most frequently used in raceways or narrow vats. Medicine is added to inflow area and fish are exposed to drug as it passes over them with the water current. Similar to dip procedure except fish may not have to be removed from their normal holding area.

Indefinite bath
Medication is added to aquarium and usually there is no water change or immediate retreatment.

Injection
The antibiotic is given by injection with the aid of a hypodermic needle and syringe. Routes may be subcutaneous, intradermal, intramuscular, intravenous, or intraperitoneal.

Oral
Medication is mixed with the food in order to treat the fish. Usually carried out by incorporating drug into a gelatinized food mixture. For larger fish, medication ban be placed in a chunk of food and then fed or force fed to the fish.

Topical
The antibiotic is applied directly to the lesion.

Before using any drug in the water, discontinue chemical (e.g., carbon) filtration during treatment as this will inactivate the medication. Adequate aeration is also important during any water treatment.

When antibiotics are used as bath treatments, they should ideally be used daily for 5 to 7 days. Water changes (at least 50%) should take place between treatments. This protocol is much easier to follow in a home or hospital aquarium than in a pet store or wholesale facility.

are used to deliver antibiotics to aquarium fish. Standard parenteral methods can and commonly are used to dose aquarium fish with antibiotics, but the clinician must also be familiar with the terminology applied to waterborne treatments. Table 1 contains these important definitions.

DRUGS AND DOSAGES

The majority of the current information on antibiotics used in aquarium fish has been extrapolated from the finfish aquaculture literature. There are a number of reasons for this, most of which revolve around the availability of funding for pharmacokinetic research. A recently published review article summarizes the entire body of literature on this subject (Stoffregen et al, 1996). There are currently only two antibiotics (Romet-30 and Terramycin) approved for use in fish intended for human consumption. Most of the literature dealing with antibiotic use in aquarium fish is empirical and anecdotal. Two studies (Lewbart et al,

TABLE 2. **Antibiotics for Aquarium Fish**

Drug	Dose and Route	Comments
Aztreonam	100 mg/kg IM or IP q48hr for 15 days	Used primarily by koi hobbyists. Effective against *Aeromonas salmonicida.**
Enrofloxacin	5 mg/kg given IM or IP q48hr for 15 days: 5 mg/kg PO for 10–14 days or 0.1% (10 mg/10 gm) in food and feed fish for 10–14 days; 2.5–5 mg/L as a 5-hr bath, repeated q24hr for 5–7 days, 50–75% water change between treatments	Injectable or oral form can be used in oral and bath routes
Erythromycin	50–100 mg/kg PO q24hr for 10 days	Bath formulations also available
Florfenicol	20–30 mg/kg IM or IP q48hr for 15 days	
Kanamycin sulfate	50–100 mg/L as a 5-hr bath, repeated q72hr for three treatments, 50–75% water change between treatments	Available through pet products suppliers
Metronidazole	10 mg/L as a 5- to 12-hr bath, repeated q24hr for 3 consecutive days; 0.2% (20 mg/20 gm) in food and feed for 10 days	Good for anaerobes and some flagellates
Nitrofurazone	20 mg/L as a 5-hr bath, repeated q24hr for 5–7 days, 50–75% water change between treatments	Obtain a water-soluble form
Oxytetracycline	20–50 mg/L as a 5- to 24-hr bath, repeated q24hr for 5–7 days, 50–75% water change between treatments; 10 mg/kg given IM or IP q24hr for 5–7 days; 20 mg/kg PO q24hr for 10 days	Many resistant bacteria
Silver sulfadiazine cream	Apply cream directly to wound q12hr; allow affected area to remain out of water for 30–60 sec while medication is absorbed	
Triple antibiotic ointment	Apply ointment directly to wound q12hr; allow affected area to remain out of water for 30–60 seconds while medication is absorbed	
Trimethoprim/ sulfamethoxazole	30 mg/kg PO q24hr for 10–14 days; 0.2% (20 mg/10 gm) in food and feed to fish for 10–14 days; 20 mg/L as a 5- to 12-hr bath, repeated q24hr for 5–7 days, 50–75% water change between treatments	Effective as a bath treatment

*Dosage information courtesy of J Spangenberg and R Hedrick, UC Davis (1996).
IM, intramuscularly; IP, intraperitoneally; PO, orally.

1997; Doi et al, 1998) report on the pharmacokinetics of antimicrobials in the red pacu, a tropical aquarium fish closely related to important species such as the tetras, hatchetfishes, silver dollars, and headstanders. Fortunately, the veterinarian treating aquarium fish can apply current extralabel drug use regulations when selecting and initiating antibiotic therapy.

Whenever possible, appropriate microbiologic culture and sensitivity results should be applied when selecting an antibiotic course of treatment. The majority of aquarium fish pathogens are gram-negative bacteria that are susceptible to a number of antibiotics. Efforts to follow a complete treatment course are encouraged to help reduce antibiotic-resistant organisms. Indiscriminate use of antibiotics in the aquarium fish industry both in the United States and abroad has made antibiotic resistance a significant problem (Dixon et al, 1990). At times, appropriate microbiologic diagnostics are financially or logistically unavailable. In such cases, selecting an antibiotic that has good activity against gram-negative organisms may be the clinician's only recourse.

Table 2 lists a number of antibiotics that are available to the private practitioner and are clinically effective for treating bacterial disease in aquarium fish, including pond koi. This information must be tempered with caution, and the clinician must understand that the routes and dosages are only guidelines. A biotest (or bioassay; i.e., testing of the dosing regimen with one or two fish first) is in order when dealing with an unfamiliar drug, fish species, or particular aquatic environment, or all of these factors.

References and Suggested Reading

Dixon BA, Yanashita J, Evelyn F: Antibiotic resistance of *Aeromonas* spp. isolated from tropical fish imported from Singapore. J Aquatic Anim Health 2:295, 1990.
  This paper describes the important problem of bacterial antibiotic resistance in aquarium fishes.
Doi AM, Stoshopf MK, Lewbart GA: Pharmacokinetics of oxytetracycline in the red pacu (*Colossoma brachypomum*) following different routes of administration. J Vet Pharmacol Ther 21:364, 1998.
  This paper reports on intramuscular and intravenous administration of oxytetracycline in an important aquarium fish model.
Gratzek JB: Aquariology: The Science of Fish Health Management. Morris Plains, NJ: Tetra Press, 1992.
  This is a general up-to-date reference with an emphasis on the health and maintenance of freshwater pet fishes.
Lewbart G, Vaden S, Deen J, et al: Pharmacokinetics of enrofloxacin in the red pacu (*Colossoma brachypomum*). J Vet Pharmacol Ther 20:124, 1997.
  This paper explores and reports on oral, intramuscular, and bath administration of enrofloxacin in an important aquarium fish model.
Noga EJ: Fish Disease: Diagnosis and Treatment. St. Louis: Mosby–Year Book, 1996.
  This fish medicine text presents a problem-based approach to fish medicine and includes a formulary on antibiotics.
Stoffregen DA, Bowser PR, Babish JG: Antibacterial chemotherapeutants for finfish aquaculture: A synopsis of laboratory and field efficacy and safety studies. J Aquatic Anim Health 8:181, 1996.
  This is a comprehensive review article on finfish antibacterial pharmacology.
Stoskopf MK: Fish Medicine. Philadelphia: WB Saunders, 1993.
  This comprehensive reference text on all aspects of ornamental and food fish medicine was written with the veterinarian in mind.

Necropsy Techniques in Aquarium Fish

RENATE REIMSCHUESSEL
Baltimore, Maryland

Fish are becoming an increasingly significant part of pet practice. It is therefore important for companion animal practitioners to become familiar with routine diagnostic procedures in these animals. As in poultry practice, necropsy examination can be an extremely valuable management tool for evaluating the health of fish populations. This is especially true when working with owners of pet shops or avid aquaculturists. In addition, owners of just a few fish may seek professional advice when their pet dies. The clinician can provide valuable insights into the problem by conducting a thorough necropsy examination. With an appropriate diagnosis, the remaining fish can be treated appropriately. Conversely, unwarranted treatments can be avoided.

HISTORY

Once the clinician has decided to provide clinical and necropsy examinations, it is important to let potential cli-

ents know about the availability of these services. The owners' observations before the death of the animals and the length of time after death can significantly affect the amount of information obtained from the post mortem examination. One easy way to let clients know that the practice welcomes fish cases is to place an aquarium in the waiting room. Adjacent to the aquarium, one can provide tips on aquatic animal care, including *what to do when a fish dies*. If fish are moribund, encourage owners to bring them in for euthanasia and necropsy. Dead fish should be removed from the tank immediately and placed in plastic bags. The bodies are refrigerated and taken to the clinic as rapidly as possible. A water sample is brought in a separate container.

When the owner drops off the body for examination, it is important to obtain as much history about the case as possible. If the client does not see the practitioner at this time, it may be useful to have a questionnaire for the receptionist to give to the owner. A sample is provided in Table 1.

TABLE 1. History

Describe the tank that this fish came from:
    Number of gallons
    Temperature and heater type
    Filter type
    Fresh or saltwater
    Number of air pumps
    How long has the tank been set up?
    Are there any living plants?
    Describe any decorations
Did the fish show any signs before dying?
    Irregular feeding
    Aberrant swimming
    Hanging at the bottom or top
    Gulping
    Color changes
    Scale loss
    Spots
How long have you had this fish?
How many other fish are there and what type are in the tank?
Have any other fish shown signs or died?
Have any new fish been introduced into the tank?
How often and how much are the fish fed?
Have any environmental changes occurred?
    High or low temperature
    Filter pump failures
    Air pump failures
How was the water quality before this and have you made any
    water changes recently?
Have any treatments been given to the fish or the water?

EXTERNAL EXAMINATION

Preparation

Sample Media and Fixatives. The appropriate containers should be easily available for microbiologic, virologic, and histologic samples. Since identification of fish pathogens is not a routine procedure in most clinical laboratories, it is best to contact a reference laboratory familiar with fish diseases for the appropriate media in which to submit samples. Culturettes used for mammalian pathogens kept at room temperature will suffice for many aquatic pathogens, but some pathogens require specialized media. Identification of viral pathogens is performed by only a few reference laboratories. The best samples are obtained from live fish, but dead fish can be shipped overnight on ice. Frozen samples can be submitted, but some viruses do not survive the freezing process. Histopathologic examination can often reveal many lesions not evident during the gross necropsy. Tissues for histopathologic examination can be preserved in 10% phosphate buffered formalin. Once samples have been preserved in fixative, the tissues can be stored for prolonged periods. It is therefore a good idea to collect samples of all organs during the necropsy routinely. Later on, the client may or may not elect to submit them for processing. An adequate amount of fixative for the size of the tissues submitted should be used and they should be packaged appropriately for shipping.

Instruments. It is helpful to have a pack of sterile, dedicated necropsy instruments. In addition, a flame and a beaker of alcohol can be used to sterilize the instruments before use or during the necropsy if they become contaminated.

Euthanasia

The external examination is conducted in a manner similar to that of a routine physical examination of living fish. If the owner has submitted a living sample, the animal's clinical condition should be observed before euthanasia. The fish is placed in an aerated container and is examined for increased respiratory rate, equilibrium problems, and other behavioral abnormalities. Also noted are any physical abnormalities, scale loss, or lesions that should be sampled. After an initial clinical evaluation, the fish can be euthanized. Tricane methane sulfonate (MS-222-Finquel, Argent Laboratories, Redmond, WA; www.argent-labs.com/argent.htm) or Crescent Research Chemicals, Phoenix, AZ) is a rapidly acting fish anesthetic that can be used to euthanize fish. A solution of 100 to 200 mg/L (twice the anesthetic dose) induces rapid anesthesia in most species. The fish is left in the solution long enough to ensure that they are dead. Fish may also be killed by severing the cervical spine, but blood samples should be obtained before this procedure (also see *CVT XII, Euthanasia of Poikilotherms*).

Bleeding

Blood samples can be obtained from the caudal tail vein (Fig. 1). For most aquarium fish, a tuberculin syringe and needle are used. The skin is entered at approximately a 45-degree angle below the lateral line on the caudal peduncle. The needle is inserted through the muscles and directed dorsally toward the vertebral column (Fig. 2). Once the vertebrae are felt, the syringe is gently aspirated and the needle directed slightly ventral to the bone. The needle may need to be rotated slightly before obtaining blood. In general, fish blood pressure is low; one must aspirate gently and slowly to avoid collapsing the vein. In small fish, blood may be obtained by cutting off the tail at the caudal peduncle and placing a capillary tube under the spine adjacent to the dorsal aorta to catch the blood. This should be performed only with fish that have been anesthetized. Cardiac punctures can be performed by inserting the needle into the pericardial cavity through the opercular membrane, but usually the caudal vein puncture produces more blood. A few drops of blood can also be obtained by clipping the gills. Blood smears are made as with mammalian smears. Serum or plasma should be separated rapidly from the red cells. Blood cultures are useful indicators of sepsis in fish.

Cultures and Wet Mounts

Cultures. The skin, fins, and eyes are examined for any lesions that should be cultured. Excess water is blotted from around the lesion with sterile gauze and a specimen of the lesion is obtained for culture using a small swab. Sterile thin wooden applicator sticks can also be used to culture samples from small lesions.

Skin Scrape. A skin scrape is prepared using a small coverslip or blade to scrape mucus from the lateral body wall (Fig. 3). The sample is placed on a slide that has a drop of tank water on it. The wet mount is examined as soon as possible because many protozoa die soon after

Necropsy Work Sheet

SAMPLES:

- ☐ Blood Sample
- ☐ Culture Surface Lesions
- ☐ Skin Scrape _____
- ☐ Gill Biopsy _____

General Body Condition Checklist:

- ☐ 1. Body shape
- ☐ 2. Fins
- ☐ 3. Eyes
- ☐ 4. Nares
- ☐ 5. Oral Cavity
- ☐ 6. Anus/Urogenital Pore
- ☐ 7. Weight _____
- ☐ 8. Length _____

Organ Evaluation and Sampling Checklist:

- ☐ 1. Sample Surface Lesions
- ☐ 2. Operculum
- ☐ 3. Gills
- ☐ 4. Eyes
- ☐ 5. Open body cavities
- ☐ 6. Heart
- ☐ 7. Abdominal Body Block
- ☐ 8. Liver
- ☐ 9. Spleen
- ☐ 10 Gonads
- ☐ 11. Swimbladder
- ☐ 12. Cranial and Caudal Kidneys
- ☐ 13. Muscle, Vertebra, Spinal Cord
- ☐ 14. Skin, Lateral Line, Nares
- ☐ 15. Brain
- ☐ 16. Stomach and Intestine

Figure 1. Necropsy work sheet.

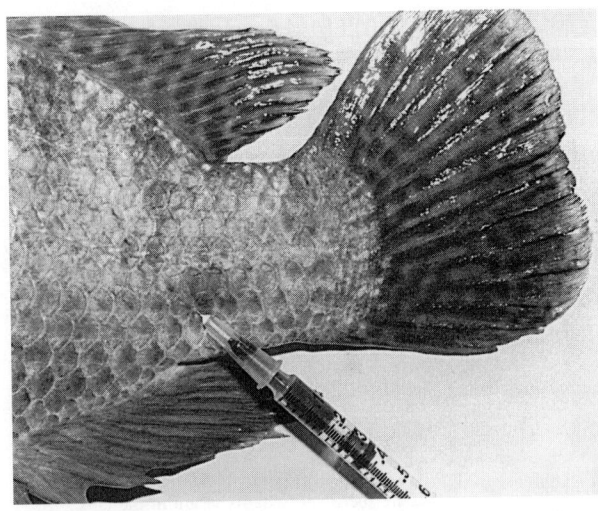

Figure 2. Taking blood from the caudal peduncle. The needle is inserted below the lateral line and directed toward the vertebral column. The needle is retracted slightly after contacting bone and aspiration takes place gently.

tion. A small section of gill is removed using small scissors such as iridectomy scissors. One can use the scissors to hold open the operculum while cutting the gill filaments. Only a small piece is removed, avoiding the cartilage. The filaments are placed on a wet slide and the lamellae are evaluated for the presence of parasites, fusion of secondary lamellae, excess mucus, and hemorrhage or thrombosis in the secondary lamellae.

General Condition

Once cultures and wet mounts have been obtained, the general body condition of the fish is examined.

Body Shape. The body is palpated to determine if the muscles are soft or if the animal is thin. Freshwater fish experiencing osmoregulatory failure retain fluid and have soft, mushy-feeling muscles. Fish that are malnourished lose muscle mass, which is especially evident in the epaxial

leaving the host. Fin clips can also be viewed as wet mounts by snipping off a small piece of fin and placing it on a slide. Lesions may be scraped, but only one side of the lesion is sampled so that the remaining side can be sampled for histopathologic examination.

Gill Biopsy. The gills are examined. Most species of fish have four gill arches. The gill filaments are attached to a white cartilaginous arch, which may have long gill rakers in filter-feeding fish. Healthy gill filaments should be a bright, blood red color. If the gills are pale pink, the fish may be anemic. Thickened gill filaments and gills with excess mucus indicate possible exposure to irritants, parasites, or toxic substances in the water. Brownish or tan gills could indicate nitrite toxicity, which induces methemoglobinemia. Gills rapidly change from red to pale pink and eventually to white after death. These are post mortem changes. Fish with white gills frequently have become autolytic and are not suitable for histopathologic examina-

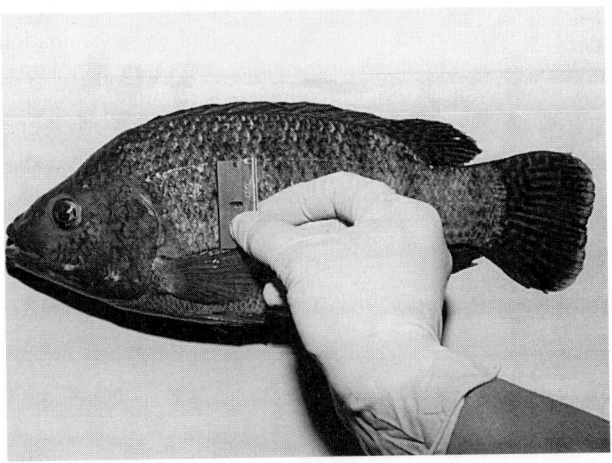

Figure 3. Taking a mucus sample from the lateral body wall. A coverslip or blade is scraped gently along the skin, removing mucus and scales.

muscles to either side of the spine. The spine is examined for lateral or dorsoventral deviations, and the body is examined for other skeletal deformities.

Fins. The condition of all the fins is noted. Ragged edges may indicate aggression from tank mates or bacterial infection. Fluffy white material may indicate fungal infection. Discolored spots on the fins could be parasites. All abnormalities should be examined microscopically.

Eyes. The eyes are examined for corneal opacities, ulcers, hemorrhage, or exophthalmia. The anterior chamber should be examined for exudates or presence of blood. Lenses should be clear.

Nares. Nares are rather small openings in most species but should be examined for any exudates or ulceration.

Oral Cavity. The mouth is opened by gently squeezing the fish in a dorsoventral direction. Some fish have grossly apparent teeth. The oral cavity is examined for any ulcerative lesions or raised foci. Thyroid adenomas are not uncommon and may present as a dark raised lesion at the base of the oral cavity. These neoplasms sometimes extend into the gill arches and the opercular cavity.

Anus–Urogenital Pore. The anus is examined for swelling, redness, or ulceration. The urogenital pore may or may not be grossly apparent. In gravid females, the pore becomes moderately swollen and can have a pinkish color. Feces may be obtained by gently compressing the abdomen from an anterior to a posterior direction. Fecal samples can be examined as a direct smear or by using routine mammalian flotation procedures.

Weight and Length. Weight and length are especially important for fish when monitoring breeding populations. Living fish can be weighed using a water-filled container or by rapidly placing them in a moist container. Length may be measured from the snout to either the tip of the caudal fin margin (total length) or the tail fork (fork length). Fork length is less affected by fin injuries.

INTERNAL EXAMINATION

Disinfection

Disinfection. The body is placed on a nonslip surface such as wood or a disposable drape. The abdominal wall is rinsed with 70% ethanol (a squeeze bottle is convenient for this).

Surface Lesions. Before dissecting the individual organs, samples are obtained for histopathologic examination of any surface lesions noted during the external examination.

Dissection

Operculum and Pseudobranch. The operculum is lifted and cut through its anterior margin. A grossly visible pseudobranch is present in many fish species. It should be

bright red and look similar to gill lamellae. In small fish, it is preserved while still attached to the operculum.

Gills. The second and third gill arches are removed (assuming the first was used for the gill biopsy). One must be sure to handle only the cartilaginous arch with forceps. Note any discoloration, excess mucus, or parasites.

Eye. The eye is removed and the orbit is examined for hemorrhage, exudates, or masses. If one of the eyes has any gross lesions, both eyes are submitted for histopathologic examination.

Body Cavity. The body cavity is opened by tenting the abdomen anterior to the anus; using sterile technique, a small incision is made. Small blunt scissors work well for most small aquarium fish. The incision is extended in a dorsoanterior direction, following the curvature of the abdominal cavity to the pectoral girdle and flaming the scissors after each cut. One then returns to the initial incision and extends the incision forward to the pelvic girdle. Finally, one cuts through the bones of both girdles and removes the flap of skin and muscle (Fig. 4).

The contents of the abdominal cavity and the pericardial cavity should be completely exposed (Fig. 5). A specimen should be obtained of any fluid in the cavities for culture, noting its color and consistency. The organs are then examined in situ. The amount of peritoneal adipose tissue present between the organs is noted. A specimen should be obtained for culture of any organs that appear abnormal. Each organ is then removed (described in the following sections) and its color, size, and any lesions are noted. Areas of necrosis, parasites, and granulomas all can appear as small white foci. Impression smears and wet mounts of small sections can be evaluated microscopically for cytologic characteristics and parasites. Sections from all organs are preserved. Small fish (1 cm or less) may be preserved with the organs in situ.

The Heart. The bulbus arteriosus—an elastic, white portion of the ventral aorta attached to the heart—is located and the connection to the ventral aorta is severed. The

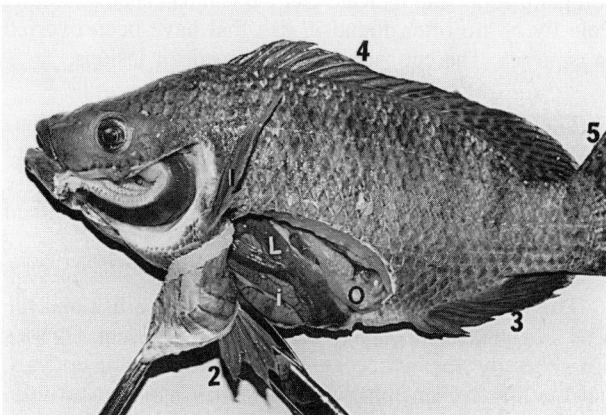

Figure 4. Opening the body cavities. After making a small cut anterior to the anus, the incision is extended both in a craniodorsal direction and cranially along the midline. L, liver; i, intestine; O, ovary with developing oocytes. Fins: 1, pectoral; 2, pelvic; 3, anal; 4, dorsal; 5, tail.

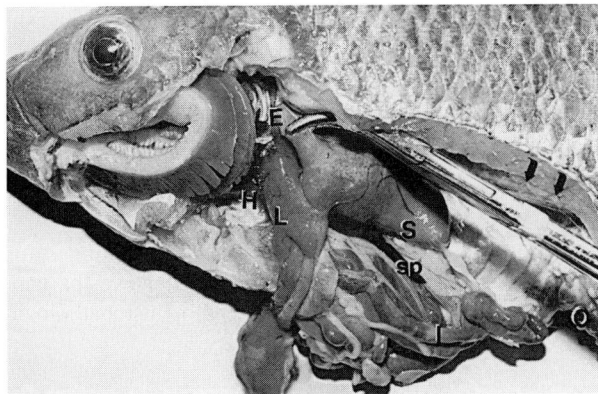

Figure 5. The organs in the body cavities. The ovary has been retracted and the esophagus is being elevated by the hemostats. Arrows on the cut muscles indicate the thin white gas-filled swimbladder located adjacent to the spinal column. Although there is considerable variation in gross anatomy of the swimbladder among different fish species, it is readily identified as a gas-filled sac. In this tilapia, the swimbladder extends along the length of the entire abdominal cavity. E, esophagus; S, stomach; I, intestines; L, liver; Sp, spleen; O, ovary; H, heart.

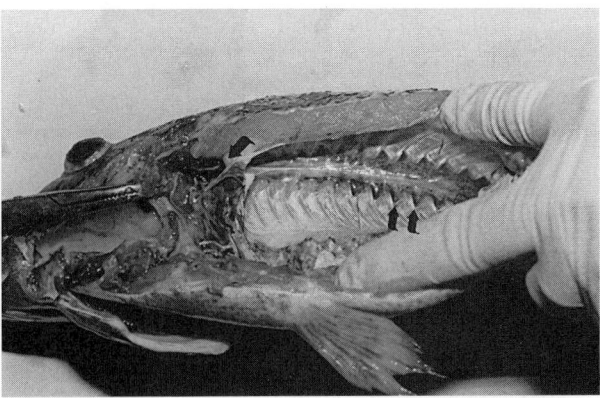

Figure 6. Cranial and caudal kidney. The cranial kidney (dark tissue by the hemostat and *large arrow*) is located approximately at the level of the dorsal margin of the operculum, just anterior to the swimbladder (removed here). The cranial kidney is entirely separate from the caudal kidney in this species. Small wedges of the retroperitoneal caudal kidney extend outward between the vertebra *(small arrows)* along the length of the abdomen.

bulbus is then retracted caudally to pull the heart out of the pericardial cavity. The sinus venous is severed and the heart examined. Small hearts can be preserved whole; larger hearts should be sectioned.

Abdominal Body Block. The contents of the abdominal cavity can usually be removed as a unit by grasping the esophagus and gently retracting caudally. Once adequately exposed, the esophagus is transected and pulling continues caudally until the organs lift out of the abdominal cavity. Usually, the gastrointestinal tract, liver, spleen, and possibly the swimbladder and gonads are removed by this procedure.

The Liver. The liver is dissected free from the surrounding tissue. In some species, the liver has well-defined lobes that can easily be removed. In other fish, the liver consists of small sections that are interlaced between the intestinal loops. The color of the liver is noted. Dark tan livers indicate little glycogen or fat storage, which with a full gallbladder can indicate that the fish has been anorexic. Pale livers are often found in fish that have been overfed in captivity. The cut surface is examined for lesions.

The Spleen. The spleen is dark red and has various shapes in different species, ranging from long and thin to a small oval. In small fish with a large amount of adipose tissue, it may be difficult to find. The spleen is examined for discoloration or swollen edges.

The Gonads. Depending on the age of the fish and the season, gonads may or may not be grossly evident. Ovaries are generally obvious because of the presence of oocytes, but the inactive or immature ovary may appear as a thin, translucent, pale peach structure. Testes are usually white and may at first glance appear to be a large piece of peritoneal fat. Wet mounts of the testes should demonstrate the presence of sperm.

The Swimbladder. The presence, shape, and size of swimbladders vary greatly among fish species (Fig. 6). Some fish have a firm, muscular swimbladder; some have multiple lobes; and some have a prominent red gas-secreting organ. The swimbladder is carefully opened and samples of any exudates or hemorrhage are obtained for culture.

The Kidney. Since bacteria often localize in the kidney during sepsis and because it is a relatively easy organ to approach using sterile technique, the kidney is an ideal organ to culture. With the abdominal body block and swimbladder removed, the kidneys are examined. Depending on the species, cranial and caudal kidneys can be one organ extending the length of the spinal column, or they can be completely separate organs (see Fig. 6). Specimens for culture can be taken by piercing through the thin peritoneal lining with a small culturette, wooden applicator, or wire loop. One must remember to take sections of both cranial and caudal kidneys for histologic examination. An easy way to take a section of tissues containing kidney, spinal cord, muscle, and skin is by cutting a wedge from the abdomen through the dorsal body of the fish.

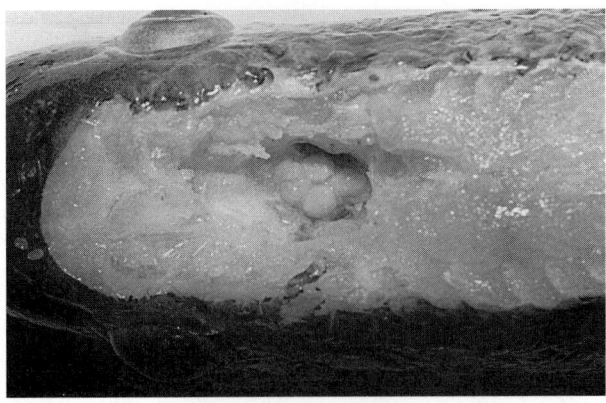

Figure 7. Brain. The brain is located midline, just caudal to the eyes in most fish species.

The Skin, Lateral Line, and Nares. Samples for culture and skin scrapes are obtained in the beginning of the necropsy examination to reduce contamination and loss of parasites during subsequent steps. Samples of skin, lateral line, and nares are, however, important to include for histologic evaluation. One must be sure to sample a piece of skin that was *not* scraped earlier.

The Brain. Depending on the size of the animal, heavy scissors or bone cutters are used to remove the bone overlying the brain. The brain is usually located midline, posterior to the eyes but anterior to the caudal margin of the operculum (Fig. 7). Any hemorrhage or discoloration of the cerebrospinal fluid or the brain itself is noted.

The Gastrointestinal Tract. Any discoloration or lesions on the surface of the stomach and intestines are noted. One must determine if any food is present in the stomach or intestines. The intestines are cut open, and a wet mount of the contents is examined for parasites.

References and Suggested Reading

Gratzek JB: Aquariology, the Science of Fish Health Management. Morris Plains, NJ: Tetra Press, 1992, p 330.
  This is a general reference of fish health, especially as related to pet fish.
Noga EJ: Fish Disease: Diagnosis and Treatment. St. Louis: Mosby 1996, p 367.
  This text uses a case base approach to diagnosing fish diseases. Many photographs detailing procedures and disease agents are included.
Reimschuessel R: Postmortem examination. In: Stoskopf MK, ed: Fish Medicine. Philadelphia: WB Saunders, 1993, p 882.
  This chapter discusses necropsy examination of fish in a comprehensive reference of fish medicine.
Roberts RJ: Fish Pathology, 2nd ed. London: Bailliere Tindall, 1989, p 467.
  This is a comprehensive reference on all aspects of fish pathology.
Tucker CS: Water analysis. In: Stoskopf MK, ed: Fish Medicine. Philadelphia: WB Saunders 1993, p 882.
  This chapter discusses methods of water analysis for aquarium fish.

Appendices

ROBERT M. JACOBS

MARK G. PAPICH

Consulting Editors

Canine and Feline Reference Values

ROBERT M. JACOBS

JOHN H. LUMSDEN

JUDITH A. TAYLOR

Guelph, Ontario, Canada

We provide the following tables as general guidelines for the interpretation of laboratory data in dogs and cats. There is wide variation in test results and reference values between laboratories for several reasons, including the use of different reagents, instruments, and selection of reference animals. We have tried to specify methodologies in most instances, so that other laboratories and users may more directly compare test results. Despite interlaboratory variation, laboratory data can be interpreted correctly if appropriately determined reference values* are supplied with the test results. Laboratory users should demand species' reference values developed in the laboratory to which the samples were submitted.

Laboratories strive to limit intralaboratory variation by careful attention to quality control practices. The performance of a laboratory in quality control programs determines the laboratory users' confidence in test results from that laboratory. Conscientious users should not hesitate to ask for details of quality assurance in their laboratory and for expected within-run and between-run analytic variation. This information is necessary for the laboratory user attempting to separate analytic from animal variation on sequential samples.

The tables show either ranges that include 95% of the population, ranges that extend from the minimum to maximum (min-max) observation, mean ± one or two standard deviations (1 or 2 SD), or mean ± one standard error of the mean (SE). These measurements of error or variation about the mean are specified where appropriate (see *CVT X*, p 8). Reference values should never be presented as simple means without some indication of error or variation or upper and lower limits for 95% of the population when provided for individual animal application. We have used mean values only to demonstrate simple trends in laboratory data with age.

A number of reference sources and scientific journals use Système International (SI) units. In the major tables, we have given reference values in both the traditional and the SI units in the hopes of easing some of the confusion. Tables showing the interconversion of traditional and SI units for most analytes are given.†

For ease of access, literature sources are provided as footnotes to each table. In an attempt to be concise, we did not always cite the primary sources of the data, but these are available in the footnoted articles. Along with the references, we have occasionally given short comments that indicate some aspect important in data interpretation.

Patient variables and sample quality also affect test results and their interpretation. We have attempted to address some patient variables by the inclusion of tables showing the effects of age, gender, pregnancy, and body weight. Unless specified otherwise, all data are for adult animals and include different genders and breeds. In some cases, we have given literature sources so the reader may further explore these effects.

To address problems of sample quality, we have included graphs showing the effects of bilirubinemia, hemolysis, and lipemia on the determination of most serum analytes.‡ Many instrument manufacturers provide interference data for human sera, but generally not for animal sera. If nothing else, these graphs serve to remind laboratory users that interferences do occur and sometimes in a species-specific manner. The interferences due to drugs have not been adequately studied in animals, but such interferences must always be considered.§

Laboratory data should be used to support diagnoses. Laboratory data that are inconsistent with the clinical diagnosis should be interpreted with caution. In these instances, the laboratory user should request that the laboratory reanalyze the same sample. If the result is similar, the laboratory user must consider alternatives to the initial clinical diagnosis or eliminate sample collection and handling or drug-related interferences, where possible, by resubmitting another sample. Samples taken at different times or analyzed in different laboratories are not comparable. Sequential laboratory data are often essential for rendering a prognosis and for determining response to therapy.

---

*Lumsden JH, Mullen K: On establishing reference values. Can J Comp Med 42:293, 1978; Solberg HE: Establishment and use of reference values. In: Burtis CA, Ashwood ER, eds: Tietz Textbook of Clinical Chemistry, 2nd ed. London, WB Saunders, 1994, pp 454–484; Solberg HE: RefVal: A program implementing the recommendations of the International Federation of Clinical Chemistry on the statistical treatment of reference values. Comp Methods Programs Biomed 48:247–256, 1995; Lumsden JH: "Normal" or "reference" values: Questions and comments. J Vet Clin Pathol 27:102, 1998.

†For further information about SI units, refer to Young DS: Implementation of SI units for clinical laboratory data. Ann Intern Med 106:114–129, 1987, which was reprinted in J Nutr 120:20, 1990; and Beeler MF: SI units and the AJCP. Am J Clin Pathol 87:140, 1987.

‡Jacobs RM, Lumsden JH, Taylor JA, Grift E: Effects of interferents on the kinetic Jaffé reaction and an enzymatic colorimetric test for serum creatinine concentration determination in cats, cows, dogs, and horses. Can J Vet Res 55:150, 1991; Jacobs RM, Lumsden JH, Grift E: Effects of bilirubinemia, hemolysis, and lipemia on clinical chemistry analytes in bovine, canine, equine, and feline sera. Can Vet J 333:605, 1992.

§An extensive review of drug interferences in human sera is found in Young DS, Pestaner LC, Gibberman V: Effects of drugs on clinical laboratory tests. Clin Chem 21:1D, 1975.

Hematology—Coulter S Plus IV* with Manual Differential Counts†

	Unit		Canine		Feline	
	Traditional	*SI‡*	*Traditional*	*SI*	*Traditional*	*SI*
Hemoglobin (Hgb)	gm/dl	gm/L	13.2–19.2	132–193	8.0–15.0	80–150
Hematocrit (Hct)	%	L/L	38–57	0.38–0.57	24–45	0.24–0.45
Erythrocytes	$\times 10^6/\mu l$	$\times 10^{12}/L$	5.6–8.5	5.6–8.5	5.0–10.0	5.0–10.0
Mean corpuscular volume (MCV)	μ^3 or mm^3	fl	62–71	62–71	39–50	39–50
Mean corpuscular Hgb (MCH)	$\mu\mu g$ or pg	pg	22–25	22–25	13–17	13–17
Mean corpuscular Hgb concentration (MCHC)	%	gm/L	33.7–36.5	337–365	32.0–36.0	320–360
Red cell distribution width (RDW)	%	%	12–15	12–15	13–17	13–17
Reticulocytes	$\times 10^3/\mu l$	$\times 10^9/L$	20–80	20–80	20–60	20–60
Platelets	$\times 10^3/\mu l$	$\times 10^9/L$	145–440	145–440	190–400	190–400
Mean platelet volume (MPV)	μ^3 or mm^3	fl	7.0–10.3	7.0–10.3	—	—
Platelet distribution width (PDW)	%	%	15.5–17.5	15.5–17.5	—	—
Total nucleated cell count	$\times 10^3/\mu l$	$\times 10^9/L$	6.1–17.4	6.1–17.4	5.5–15.4	5.5–15.4
Segmented neutrophils	$\times 10^3/\mu l$	$\times 10^9/L$	3.9–12.0	3.9–12.0	2.5–12.5	2.5–12.5
Band neutrophils	$\times 10^3/\mu l$	$\times 10^9/L$	0.0–1.0	0.0–1.0	0.0–0.3	0.0–0.3
Lymphocytes	$\times 10^3/\mu l$	$\times 10^9/L$	0.8–3.6	0.8–3.6	1.5–7.0	1.5–7.0
Monocytes	$\times 10^3/\mu l$	$\times 10^9/L$	0.1–1.8	0.1–1.8	0.0–0.85	0.0–0.85
Eosinophils	$\times 10^3/\mu l$	$\times 10^9/L$	0.0–1.9	0.0–1.9	0.0–0.75	0.0–0.75
Basophils	$\times 10^3/\mu l$	$\times 10^9/L$	0.0–0.2	0.0–0.2	0.0–0.2	0.0–0.2

*This automated cell counter was configured using Isoton III and Lyse S III DIFF. The mean nucleated cell aperature voltage was 94.2 and the mean red cell/platelet aperature voltage was 165.5.

†From Clinical Pathology Laboratory, Animal Health Laboratory, Laboratory Services Division, University of Guelph. Feline leukocyte differential count is modified from Jain NC: Schalm's Veterinary Hematology, 4th ed. Philadelphia: Lea & Febiger, 1986, p 127.

‡Systéme International.

Hematology—Technicon H-1 Hematology Analyzer*

	Unit	Canine	Feline
Hemoglobin	gm/dl	14.1–20.0	9.0–15.6
Hematocrit	%	43.3–59.3	29.3–49.8
Erythrocytes	$\times 10^6/\mu l$	6.15–8.70	6.12–11.86
Mean corpuscular volume	fl	63.0–77.1	41.9–54.8
Mean corpuscular hemoglobin	pg	21.1–24.8	12.5–17.6
Mean corpuscular hemoglobin concentration	gm/dl	29.9–35.6	28.1–32.0
Red cell distribution width	%	11.9–14.9	14.0–18.1
Hemoglobin distribution width	gm/dl	1.49–2.17	1.89–2.73
Platelets	$\times 10^3/\mu l$	164–510	26†–470
Mean platelet volume	fl	3.9–6.1	4.1–8.3
White blood cell count	$\times 10^3/\mu l$	6.02–16.02	4.87–20.10
Neutrophils	$\times 10^3/\mu l$	3.23–10.85	—
Lymphocytes	$\times 10^3/\mu l$	0.53–3.44	—
Monocytes	$\times 10^3/\mu l$	0.00–0.43	—
Eosinophils	$\times 10^3/\mu l$	0.00–1.82	—
Basophils	$\times 10^3/\mu l$	0.01–0.54	—
Large unstained cells (LUC)	$\times 10^3/\mu l$	0.26–2.09	—
Lobularity index (LI)‡	—	1.88–3.15	1.3–2.68
Mean peroxidase index (MPXI)‡	—	−19 to −7	−47 to −16

*From Tvedten H: Reference values for the veterinary clinical center laboratory, Michigan State University, May 1991. These data were derived from approximately 120 dogs and 40 cats. Canine reference values include 95% of the population, whereas the feline values represent the minimum to maximum.

†The lower limit of feline platelets is falsely decreased owing to clumping.

‡Interpretation of these determinations is undetermined in canine and feline blood.

Système International (SI) Units in Hematology

Analyte	Example Values		Conversion Factors	
	SI	Traditional	Traditional to SI	SI to Traditional
Hemoglobin (Hgb)	15.0 gm/dl	150 gm/L	10	0.1
Hematocrit (Hct) or packed cell volume (PCV)	45%	0.45 L/L	0.01	100
Erythrocytes	$6.0 \times 10^6/mm^3$	$6.0 \times 10^{12}/L$	10^6	10^{-6}
Mean corpuscular volume (MCV)	$75 \mu^3$	75 fl	No change	No change
Mean corpuscular Hgb (MCH)	$25 \mu\mu g$	25 pg	No change	No change
Mean corpuscular Hgb concentration (MCHC)	33 gm/dl	33 gm/L	10	0.1
White blood cell count	$15.0 \times 10^3/mm^3$	$15.0 \times 10^9/L$	10^6	10^{-6}
Platelets	$250 \times 10^3/mm^3$	$250 \times 10^9/L$	10^6	10^{-6}

Hematology—Manual or Semiautomated Methods*

	Adult Dog		Adult Cat	
	Range	Mean	Range	Mean
Red Cell Determinations				
Erythrocytes (millions/dl)	5.5–8.5	6.8	5.5–10.0	7.5
Hemoglobin (gm/dl)	12.0–18.0	14.9	8.0–14.0	12.0
Packed cell volume (%)	37.0–55.0	45.5	24.0–45.0	37.0
Mean corpuscular volume (fl)	66.0–77.0	69.8	40.0–55.0	45.0
Mean corpuscular hemoglobin (pg)	19.9–24.5	22.8	13.0–17.0	15.0
Mean corpuscular hemoglobin concentration (gm/dl)				
Wintrobe	31.0–34.0	33.0	31.0–35.0	33.0
Microhematocrit	32.0–36.0	34.0	30.0–36.0	33.2
Reticulocytes (%, excluding punctate reticulocytes)	0.0–1.5	0.8	0.2–1.6	0.6
Resistance to hypotonic saline (% saline solution)				
Minimum (initial hemolysis)	0.40–0.50	0.46	0.66–0.72	0.69
Maximum (complete hemolysis)	0.32–0.42	0.33	0.46–0.54	0.50
Erythrocyte life span (days)	100–120		66–78	
White Blood Cell Determinations				
Leukocytes (cells/μl)	6,000–17,000	11,500	5,500–19,500	12,500
Neutrophils—bands (%)	0–3	0.8	0–3	0.5
Neutrophils—mature (%)	60–77	70.0	35–75	59.0
Lymphocytes (%)	12–30	20.0	20–55	32.0
Monocytes (%)	3–10	5.2	1–4	3.0
Eosinophils (%)	2–10	4.0	2–12	5.5
Basophils (%)	Rare	0.0	Rare	0.0
Neutrophils—bands (cells/μl)	0–300	70	0–300	100
Neutrophils—mature (cells/μl)	3,000–11,500	7,000	2,500–12,500	7,500
Lymphocytes (cells/μl)	1,000–4,800	2,800	1,500–7,000	4,000
Monocytes (cells/μl)	150–1,350	750	0–850	350
Eosinophils (cells/μl)	100–1,250	550	0–1,500	650
Basophils (cells/μl)	Rare	0	Rare	0

*From Jain NC: Schalm's Veterinary Hematology, 4th ed. Philadelphia: Lea & Febiger, 1986.

Canine Hematology (Means) at Different Ages—Manual or Semiautomated Methods*

Age	RBC (millions/μl)	Retic. (%)†	Nucl. RBC per 100 WBC†	Hgb (gm/dl)	PCV (%)	WBC/μl	Neut./μl	Bands/μl	Lymph./μl	Eos./μl
Birth	5.75	7.1	1.8	16.70	50	16,500	1,300	400	2,500	600
2 weeks	3.92	7.1	1.8	9.76	32	11,000	6,500	100	3,000	300
4 weeks	4.20	7.1	1.8	9.60	33	13,000	8,600	0	4,000	40
6 weeks	4.91	3.6	1.8	9.59	34	15,000	10,000	0	4,500	100
8 weeks	5.13	3.9	0.3	11.00	37	18,000	11,000	234	6,000	270
12 weeks	5.27	3.9	Rare	11.60	36	15,300	9,400	115	4,600	322

*From Andersen AC, Gee W: Normal values in the beagle. Vet Med 53:135, 156, 1958.
†From Ewing GO, Schalm OW, Smith RS: Hematologic values of normal Basenji dogs. J Am Vet Med Assoc 161:1661, 1972.
Also see *CVT XI*, p 981.

Canine Hematology (Means and Ranges) With Different Ages and Genders—Manual or Semiautomated Methods*

	Sex	Birth to 12 Months		1–7 Years		7 Years and Older	
		Range	*Mean*	*Range*	*Mean*	*Range*	*Mean*
Erythrocytes (millions/µl)	Male	2.99–8.52	5.09	5.26–6.57	5.92	3.33–7.76	5.28
	Female	2.76–8.42	5.06	5.13–8.6	6.47	3.34–9.19	5.17
Hemoglobin (gm/dl)	Male	6.9–16.5	10.7	12.7–16.3	15.5	14.7–21.2	17.9
	Female	6.4–18.9	11.2	11.5–17.9	14.7	11.0–22.5	16.1
Packed cell volume (%)	Male	22.0–45.0	33.9	35.2–52.8	44.0	44.2–62.8	52.3
	Female	25.8–55.2	36.0	34.8–52.4	43.6	35.8–67.0	49.8
Leukocytes (thousands/µl)	Male	9.9–27.7	17.1	8.3–19.5	11.9	7.9–35.3	15.5
	Female	8.8–26.8	15.9	7.5–17.5	11.5	5.2–34.0	13.4
Mature neutrophils (%)	Male	63–73	68	65–73	69	55–80	66
	Female	64–74	69	58–76	67	40–80	64
Lymphocytes (%)	Male	18–30	24	9–26	18	15–40	29
	Female	13–28	21	11–29	20	13–45	29
Monocytes (%)	Male	1–10	6	2–10	6	0–4	1
	Female	1–10	7	0–10	5	0–4	1
Eosinophils (%)	Male	2–11	3	1–8	4	1–11	4
	Female	1–9	5	1–10	6	0–19	6

*From Normal Blood Values for Dogs, Ralston Purina Co. Professional Marketing Services, Checkerboard Square, St. Louis, 1975.
Also see *CVT XI*, p 981.

Canine Hematology (Means ± SD) at Different Ages*

Age	RBC (millions/µl)	Hgb (gm/dl)	PCV (%)	MCV (fl)	MCH (pg)	MCHC (gm/dl)	WBC/µl
0–3 days	4.8 ± 0.8	15.8 ± 2.9	46.3 ± 8.5	94.2 ± 5.9	32.7 ± 1.8	34.6 ± 1.4	16,800 ± 5,700
14–17 days	3.5 ± 0.3	9.9 ± 1.1	28.7 ± 2.9	81.5 ± 3.3	28.0 ± 2.0	34.3 ± 1.6	13,600 ± 4,400
28–31 days	3.9 ± 0.4	9.6 ± 0.9	28.4 ± 2.5	71.7 ± 3.5	24.3 ± 1.6	33.5 ± 1.4	13,900 ± 3,300
40–45 days	4.1 ± 0.4	9.3 ± 0.7	28.3 ± 2.3	68.2 ± 2.6	22.4 ± 1.0	32.4 ± 1.7	15,300 ± 3,700
56–59 days	4.7 ± 0.4	10.3 ± 0.9	31.4 ± 2.4	65.8 ± 2.3	21.8 ± 1.2	32.6 ± 1.8	15,700 ± 4,400

*From Jain NC: Schalm's Veterinary Hematology, 4th ed. Philadelphia: Lea & Febiger, 1986; derived from between 42 and 48 dogs at each time interval.

Effects of Pregnancy and Lactation on Canine Hematology (Means)*

	Gestation				Term	Lactation		
	2 Weeks	*4 Weeks*	*6 Weeks*	*8 Weeks*	*0 Weeks*	*2 Weeks*	*4 Weeks*	*6 Weeks*
RBC (millions/µl)	8.85	7.48	6.73	6.26	4.53	5.13	5.65	6.15
PCV (%)	53	47	44	37	32	34	38	43
Hgb (gm/dl)	19.6	16.4	14.7	13.8	11.0	11.7	12.8	13.4
WBC (thousands/µl)	12.0	12.2	15.7	19.0	18.9	16.9	17.1	15.9

*From Andersen AC, Gee W: Normal values in the beagle. Vet Med 53:135, 156, 1958.

Relative Distribution of Cell Types in Canine Bone Marrow*

Cell Type	Range (%)	Mean (%)
Myeloid (granulocytic) series		
Myeloblasts	0.7–1.1	0.9
Promyelocytes	1.7–2.5	2.1
Neutrophil myelocytes	5.3–7.3	6.3
Neutrophil bands	9.1–13.5	11.3
Neutrophil segmenters	22.2–24.8	23.5
Eosinophil myelocytes	0.4–0.8	0.6
Eosinophil metamyelocytes	0.4–1.0	0.7
Eosinophil bands	0.8–1.6	1.2
Eosinphil segmenters	0.3–1.3	0.8
Basophil series	0.0–0.06	0.02
Total myeloid series	49.3–61.1	55.2
Erythrocytic series		
Rubriblasts and prorubricytes	6.1–6.9	6.5
Rubricytes and metarubricytes	23.2–32.0	27.6
Total erythroid series	29.4–38.8	34.1
Myeloid/erythroid (M/E) ratio	1.3–2.1	1.7
Other cells		
Lymphocytes	5.5–10.9	8.2
Plasma cells	0.4–1.0	0.7
Monocytes	0.2–5.2	1.2
Macrophages	0.2–0.6	0.4
Mitotic figures	1.1–1.7	1.4

*From Latimer KS, Meyer DJ: Leukocytes in health and disease. In: Ettinger SJ, ed: Textbook of Veterinary Internal Medicine, Diseases of the Dog and Cat, 3rd ed. Philadelphia: WB Saunders, 1989, pp 2185–2186. These data are based on the following citations: Prasse KW, Mahaffey EA: Hematology of normal cats and characteristic responses to disease. In: Holzworth J, ed: Diseases of the Cat: Medicine and Surgery. Philadelphia: WB Saunders, 1987, p 739; Duncan JR, Prasse KW: Veterinary Laboratory Medicine: Clinical Pathology, 2nd ed. Ames: Iowa State University Press, 1986; Melveger BE, et al: Sternal bone marrow biopsy in the dog. Lab Anim Care 19:866, 1969; Bloom F, Meyer LM: The morphology of the bone marrow cells in normal dogs. Cornell Vet 34:13, 1944. For a comprehensive review of peripheral blood and bone marrow changes with illness, see Hoff B, Lumsden JH, Valli VEO: An appraisal of bone marrow biopsy in assessment of sick dogs. Can J Comp Med 49:34, 1985.

Feline Hematology (Means and Ranges) With Different Ages and Genders—Manual or Semiautomated Methods*

	Sex	Birth to 12 Months		1–7 Years		7 Years and Older	
		Range	Average	Range	Average	Range	Average
Erythrocytes (millions/μl)	Male	5.43–10.22	6.96	4.48–10.27	7.34	5.26–8.89	6.79
	Female	4.46–11.34	6.90	4.45–9.42	6.17	4.10–7.38	5.84
Hemoglobin (gm/dl)	Male	6.0–12.9	9.9	8.9–17.0	12.9	9.0–14.5	11.8
	Female	6.0–15.0	9.9	7.9–15.5	10.3	7.5–13.7	10.3
Packed cell volume (%)	Male	24.0–37.5	31	26.9–48.2	37.6	28.0–43.8	34.6
	Female	23.0–46.8	31.5	25.3–37.5	31.4	22.5–40.5	30.8
Leukocytes (thousands/μl)	Male	7.8–25.0	15.8	9.1–28.2	15.1	6.4–30.4	17.6
	Female	11.0–26.9	17.7	13.7–23.7	19.9	5.2–30.1	14.8
Neutrophils—mature (%)	Male	16–75	60	37–92	65	33–75	61
	Female	51–83	69	42–93	69	25–89	71
Lymphocytes (%)	Male	10–81	30	7–48	23	16–54	30
	Female	8–37	23	12–58	30	9–63	22
Monocytes (%)	Male	1–5	2	1–5	2	0–2	1
	Female	0–7	2	0–5	2	0–4	1
Eosinophils (%)	Male	2–21	8	1–22	7	1–15	8
	Female	0–15	6	0–13	5	0–15	6

From Normal Blood Values for Cats, Ralston Purina Co., Professional Marketing Services, Checkerboard Square, St. Louis, 1975. Also see *CVT XI,* p 981.

Feline Hematology (Means) at Different Ages*

Age	RBC (millions/μl)	Hgb (gm/dl)	PCV (%)	MCV (fl)	MCH (pg)	MCHC (gm/dl)	WBC/μl
0–6 hr	4.95	12.2	44.7	90.3	24.6	27.3	7,550
12–48 hr	5.11	11.3	41.7	81.6	22.1	27.1	10,180
7 days	5.19	10.9	35.7	68.8	21.0	30.5	7,830
21 days	4.99	9.3	31.3	62.7	18.6	29.7	8,820
42 days	6.75	9.0	35.4	52.4	13.3	25.4	8,420
80 days	7.69	10.3	39.0	50.7	13.4	26.4	9,120
Adult male	9.02	12.2	40.6	45.0	13.5	30.0	12,400
Adult female	8.39	12.0	41.3	49.2	14.3	29.1	10,500

*From Jain NC: Schalm's Veterinary Hematology, 4th ed. Philadelphia: Lea & Febiger, 1986; data derived from between 18 and 26 cats at each time interval. Also see *CVT XI,* p 981.

Effects of Pregnancy and Lactation on Feline Hematology (Means)*

| | Gestation | | | | | Term | Lactation | |
	1 Day Past Conception	2 Weeks	4 Weeks	6 Weeks	8 Weeks	0 Weeks	2 Weeks	4 Weeks
RBC (millions/μl)	8.0	7.9	7.1	6.7	6.2	6.2	7.4	7.4
PCV (%)	36.1	37.0	33.0	32.0	28.0	29.0	33.0	33.0
Hgb (gm/dl)	12.5	12.0	11.0	10.8	9.5	10.0	11.5	11.2
Reticulocytes (%, includes punctate reticulocytes)	9	11	9	10	20.1	15	9	6

*From Berman E: Hemogram of the cat during pregnancy and lactation and after lactation. Am J Vet Res 35:457, 1974.

Relative Distribution of Cell Types in Feline Bone Marrow*

Cell Type	Range (%)	Mean (%)
Myeloid (granulocytic) series		
Myeloblasts	0.0–1.8	0.4
Promyelocytes	0.6–3.8	1.2
Neutrophil myelocytes	0.4–5.4	2.2
Neutrophil metamyelocytes	0.6–9.6	4.2
Neutrophil bands	5.0–19.4	11.0
Neutrophil segmenters	17.8–38.6	27.8
Eosinophil series	0.6–7.2	3.0
Basophil series	0.0–0.4	0.2
Total myeloid cells	39.4–64.4	52.0
Erythrocytic series		
Rubriblasts	0.0–1.6	0.6
Prorubricytes and rubricytes	—	12.4
Metarubricytes	15.6–32.2	23.6
Total erythroid cells	24.0–48.8	36.6
Myeloid/erythroid (M/E) ratio	0.9–2.5	1.5
Other cells		
Lymphocytes	3.2–22.6	11.4
Plasma cells	0.0–1.2	0.2
Mitotic cells	0.0–2.0	1.0

*From Latimer KS, Meyer DJ: Leukocytes in health and disease. In: Ettinger SJ, ed: Textbook of Veterinary Internal Medicine, Diseases of the Dog and Cat, 3rd ed. Philadelphia: WB Saunders, 1989, pp 2185–2186. These data are based on the following citations: Prasse KW, Mahaffey EA: Hematology of normal cats and characteristic responses to disease. In: Holzworth J, ed: Diseases of the Cat: Medicine and Surgery. Philadelphia: WB Saunders, 1987, p 739; Duncan JR, Prasse KW: Veterinary Laboratory Medicine: Clinical Pathology, 2nd ed. Ames: Iowa State University Press, 1986; Melveger BE, et al: Sternal bone marrow biopsy in the dog. Lab Anim Care 19:866, 1969; Bloom F, Meyer LM: The morphology of the bone marrow cells in normal dogs. Cornell Vet 34:13, 1944.

Clinical Chemistry—Hitachi 911*

	Unit		Canine		Feline	
	Traditional	*SI†*	*Traditional*	*SI*	*Traditional*	*SI*
Alanine aminotransferase	IU/L	U/L	15–90	15–90	20–85	20–85
Albumin	gm/dl	gm/L	2.8–3.9	28–39	2.4–3.5	24–35
Albumin/globulin	—	—	0.5–1.2	0.5–1.2	0.5–1.4	0.5–1.4
Alkaline phosphatase	IU/L	U/L	18–94	18–94	13–116	13–116
Amylase	IU/L	U/L	190–1,350	190–1,350	570–1,320	570–1,320
Anion gap	mEq/L	mmol/L	10–32	10–32	13–28	13–28
Asparate aminotransferase	IU/L	U/L	10–50	10–50	10–35	10–35
Bilirubin, conjugated	mg/dl	μmol/L	0–0.18	0–3	0–0.06	0–1
Bilirubin, unconjugated	mg/dl	μmol/L	0–0.23	0–4	0–0.18	0–3
Bilirubin, total	mg/dl	μmol/L	0–0.23	0–4	0–0.23	0–4
Calcium	mg/dl	mmol/L	9.42–11.74	2.35–2.93	8.74–11.94	2.18–2.98
Carbon dioxide, total	mEq/L	mmol/L	11–27	11–27	10–21	10–21
Chloride	mEq/L	mmol/L	108–131	108–131	115–125	115–125
Cholesterol	mg/dl	mmol/L	106.2–368.2	2.74–9.50	69.8–197.7	1.8–5.1
Creatine kinase	IU/L	U/L	0–460	0–460	0–820	0–820
Creatinine	mg/dl	μmol/L	0.68–1.45	60–128	0.68–1.84	60–163
Globulins	gm/dl	gm/L	2.6–4.4	26–44	2.9–5.5	29–55
Glucose	mg/dl	mmol/L	63.1–109.9	3.5–6.1	46.8–151.3	2.6–8.4
γ-Glutamyl transferase	IU/L	U/L	0–6	0–6	0–7	0–7
Iron‡	μg/dl	μmol/L	72.6–189.8	13–34	78.2–111.7	14–20
Iron-binding capacity, total	μg/dl	μmol/L	363–475	65–85	296–318	53–57
Transferrin saturation	%	%	16–40	16–40	27–35	27–35
Lipase	IU/L	U/L	0–680	0–680	50–700	50–700
Phosphorus	mg/dl	mmol/L	2.8–6.2	0.9–2.0	3.7–9.3	1.2–3.0
Potassium	mEq/L	mmol/L	4.1–5.4	4.1–5.4	4.3–6.1	4.3–6.1
Protein, total serum	gm/dl	gm/L	5.7–7.6	57–76	5.3–8.5	53–85
Sodium	mEq/L	mmol/L	143–168	143–168	147–161	147–161
Urea	mg/dl	mmol/L	8.7–30.5	3.1–10.9	13.4–32.5	4.8–11.6

*Tentative ranges prepared with the assistance of Dr. B. Hoff and the Clinical Pathology Laboratory, Animal Health Laboratory, Laboratory Services Division, University of Guelph (for most analytes: dogs, n = 55; cats, n = 45). Trends in serum chemistry values with age and original citations concerning this topic are found in Lowseth LA, Gillett NA, Gerlach RF, Muggenburg BA: The effects of aging on hematology and serum chemistry values in the Beagle dog. Vet Clin Pathol 19:13, 1990. For temperature stability of enzymes see Kaneko JJ: Stability of serum enzymes under various storage conditions. In: Kaneko JJ, ed: Clinical Biochemistry of Domestic Animals, 4th ed. San Diego: Academic Press, 1989, p 883.

†Système International.

‡Feline values derived from Fulton R, Weiser MG, Freshman JL, Gasper PW, Fettman MJ: Electronic and morphologic characterization of erythrocytes of an adult cat with iron deficiency anemia. Vet Pathol 25:521, 1988.

Also see *CVT XI*, p 981, for pediatric values.

Clinical Chemistry—Selected Manual Procedures*

Analyte	Unit	Canine	Feline
Ammonia (bromophenol blue, Kodak Ektachem, Rochester, NY)			
Resting	μmol/L	20–80	—†
30 min after provocation	μmol/L	≤140	—
Anion gap	mmol/L	15–25	—
Bile acids (colorimetric, Enzabile, Nycomed, Oslo, Norway)			
Fasting	μmol/L	0–9	≤2.2‡
2 hr postprandial	μmol/L	0–30	≤12.6
Sulfobromophthalein retention	% at 30 min	≤5	≤3§
Indocyanine green retention§	% at 30 min	7.7–15.6	4.7–14.0
Osmolality (freezing point depression)	mmol/kg	295–315	301–314

*Data are from the Clinical Pathology Laboratory, Animal Health Laboratory, Laboratory Services Division, University of Guelph unless indicated otherwise. Methods and reagent sources given in brackets where appropriate.

†Data for four cats with portosystemic shunts are reported in Center SA, Baldwin BH, de Lahunta A, et al: Evaluation of serum bile acid concentrations for the diagnosis of portosystemic venous anomalies in the dog and cat. J Am Vet Med Assoc 186:1090, 1985.

‡From Center SA, Baldwin BH, Erb H, et al: Bile acid concentrations in the diagnosis of hepatobiliary disease in the cat. J Am Vet Med Assoc 189:891, 1986.

§From Center SA, Bunch SE, Baldwin BH, et al: Comparison of sulfobromophthalein and indocyanine green clearances in the cat. Am J Vet Res 44:727, 1983; Center SA, Bunch SE, Baldwin BH, et al: Comparison of sulfobromophthalein and indocyanine green clearances in the dog. Am J Vet Res 44:722, 1983.

Système International (SI) Units in Clinical Chemistry

Analyte	Traditional Unit (with examples)	Conversion Factor	SI Unit (with examples)
Alanine aminotransferase	0–40 U/L	1.00	0–40 U/L
Albumin	2.8–4.0 gm/dl	10.0	28–40 gm/L
Alkaline phosphatase	30–150 U/L	1.00	30–150 U/L
Ammonia	10–80 μg/dl	0.5871	5.9–47.0 μmol/L
Amylase	200–800 U/L	1.00	200–800 U/L
Aspartate aminotransferase	0–40 U/L	1.00	0–40 U/L
Bile acids (total)	0.3–2.3 μg/ml	2.45	0.75–5.64 μmol/L
Bilirubin	0.1–0.2 mg/dl	17.10	2–4 μmol/L
Calcium	8.8–10.3 mg/dl	0.2495	2.20–2.58 mmol/L
Carbon dioxide	22–28 mEq/L	1.00	22–28 mmol/L
Chloride	95–100 mEq/L	1.00	95–100 mmol/L
Cholesterol	100–265 mg/dl	0.0258	2.58–5.85 mmol/L
Copper	70–140 μg/dl	0.1574	11.0–22.0 μmol/L
Cortisol	2–10 μg/dl	27.59	55–280 nmol/L
Creatine kinase	0–130 U/L	1.00	0–130 U/L
Creatinine	0.6–1.2 mg/dl	88.40	50–110 μmol/L
Fibrinogen	200–400 mg/dl	0.01	2.0–4.0 gm/L
Folic acid	3.5–11.0 μg/L	2.265	7.93–24.92 nmol/L
Glucose	70–110 mg/dl	0.05551	3.9–6.1 mmol/L
Iron	80–180 μg/dl	0.1791	14–32 μmol/L
Lactate	5–20 mg/dl	0.1110	0.5–2.0 mmol/L
Lead	150 μg/dl	0.04826	7.2 μmol/L
Lipase Sigma Tietz (37°C)	≤1 ST U/dl	280	≤280 U/L
Lipase Cherry Crandall (30°C)	0–160 U/L	1.00	0–160 U/L
Lipids (total)	400–850 mg/dl	0.01	4.0–8.5 gm/L
Magnesium	1.8–3.0 mg/dl	0.4114	0.80–1.20 mmol/L
Mercury	≤1.0 μg/dl	49.85	≤50 nmol/L
Osmolality	280–300 mOsm/kg	1.00	280–300 mmol/kg
Phosphorus	2.5–5.0 mg/dl	0.3229	0.80–1.6 mmol/L
Potassium	3.5–5.0 mEq/L	1.0	3.5–5.0 mmol/L
Protein (total)	5–8 gm/dl	10.0	50–80 gm/L
Sodium	135–147 mEq/L	1.00	135–147 mmol/L
Testosterone	4.0–8.0 mg/ml	3.467	14.0–28.0 nmol/L
Thyroxine	1–4 μg/dl	12.87	13–51 nmol/L
Triglyceride	10–500 mg/dl	0.0113	0.11–5.65 mmol/L
Urea	10–20 mg/dl	0.3570	3.6–7.1 nmol/L
Uric acid	3.6–7.7 mg/dl	59.44	214–458 μmol/L
Urobilinogen	0–4.0 mg/dl	16.9	0.0–6.8 μmol/L
Vitamin A	90 μg/dl	0.03491	3.1 μmol/L
Vitamin B$_{12}$	300–700 ng/L	0.738	221–516 pmol/L
Vitamin E	5.0–20.0 mg/L	2.32	11.6–46.4 μmol/L
D-Xylose	30–40 mg/dl	0.06666	2.0–2.17 mmol/L
Zinc	75–120 μg/dl	0.1530	11.5–18.5 μmol/L

Clinical Chemistry—Test Characteristics for Analytes Determined on the Hitachi 911*

Analyte	Methodology
Alanine aminotransferase	Modified IFCC† (L-alanine and α-oxoglutarate substrate)
Albumin	Modified Doumas (bromcresol green)
Alkaline phosphatase	Modified Bowers and McComb (p-nitrophenyl phosphate substrate)
Amylase	Modified Wallenfels (p-nitrophenylmaltohexaoside substrate)
Bilirubin, total	Modified Walters and Gerarde (diazo)
Bilirubin, conjugated	Modified Jendrassik and Grof (diazotized sulfonilic acid)
Calcium	Modified Connerty and Briggs (O-cresolphthalein complexone)
Total carbon dioxide	Enzymatic phosphoenol-pyruvate carboxylase
Chloride	Ion selective electrode
Cholesterol	Enzymatic (cholesterol esterase/oxidase)
Creatine kinase	Modified Oliver-Rosalki (creatine phosphate substrate)
Creatinine‡	Enzymatic creatinine deiminase
Glucose	Modified hexokinase/glucose-6-phosphate dehydrogenase
γ-Glutamyl transferase	Modified Szasz (L-γ-glutamyl-p-nitroanilide and glycylglycine substrate)
Lipase	Triolein substrate
Phosphorus	Modified Daly and Ertingshausen (molybdate)
Potassium	Ion-selective electrode
Protein, total serum	Modified biuret (cupric sulfate)
Sodium	Ion-selective electrode
Urea	Modified Talke and Schubert (urease)

*From Clinical Pathology Laboratory, Animal Health Laboratory, Laboratory Services Division, University of Guelph. Unless indicated otherwise all reagents are from Bochringer Mannheim, Dorval, Quebec.
†International Federation of Clinical Chemistry.
‡Randox Laboratories Canada Ltd., Mississauga, Ontario.

Interferences Caused by Lipid, Bilirubin, and Hemoglobin for Analytes Determined on the Hitachi 911

The following series of graphs are termed *interferograms*. The protocols for preparing these data are described in Glick MR, Ryder KW, Jackson SA: Graphical comparisons of interferences in clinical chemistry instrumentation. Clin Chem 32:470, 1986. These interferograms show the effects of common interferents on the concentrations or activities of analytes determined on the Hitachi 911 (methods given in previous table) in canine (▼) and feline (▽) sera. See *CVT XII* for the effect of these interferences on the Coulter DACOS. The X axes show increasing amounts of lipid, bilirubin, or hemoglobin, while the Y axes show the percentage change (final/original × 100%) in any particular analyte. In instances in which the concentration or activity of a particular analyte was numerically small, the absolute values are given on the Y axes. These data are provided by the Clinical Pathology Laboratory, Animal Health Laboratory, Laboratory Services Division, University of Guelph and were prepared with the assistance of B. Jefferson, E. Grift, and Dr. B. Hoff. For a more complete discussion of interferences on creatinine, refer to Jacobs RM, Lumsden JH, Taylor JA, et al: Effects of interferents on the kinetic Jaffé reaction and an enzymatic colorimetric test for serum creatinine concentration determination in cats, cows, dogs, and horses. Can J Vet Res 55:150, 1991; and Jacobs RM, Lumsden JH, Grift E: Effects of bilirubinemia, hemolysis, and lipemia on clinical chemistry analytes in bovine, canine, equine, and feline sera. Can Vet J 33:605, 1992. Also see *CVT XII*, pp. 14 and 20.

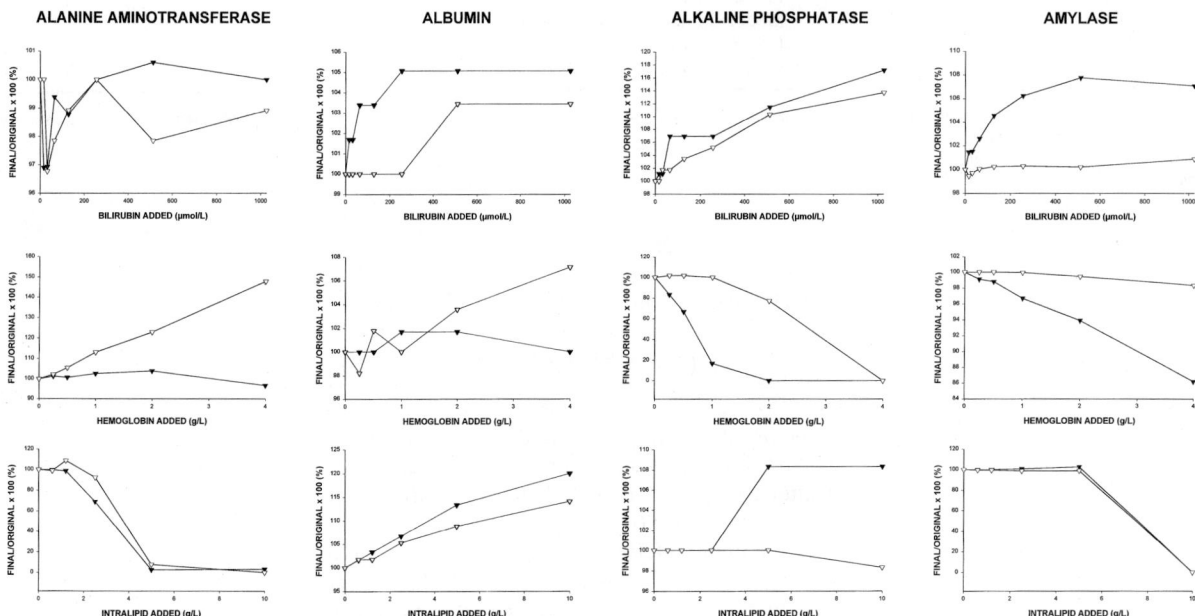

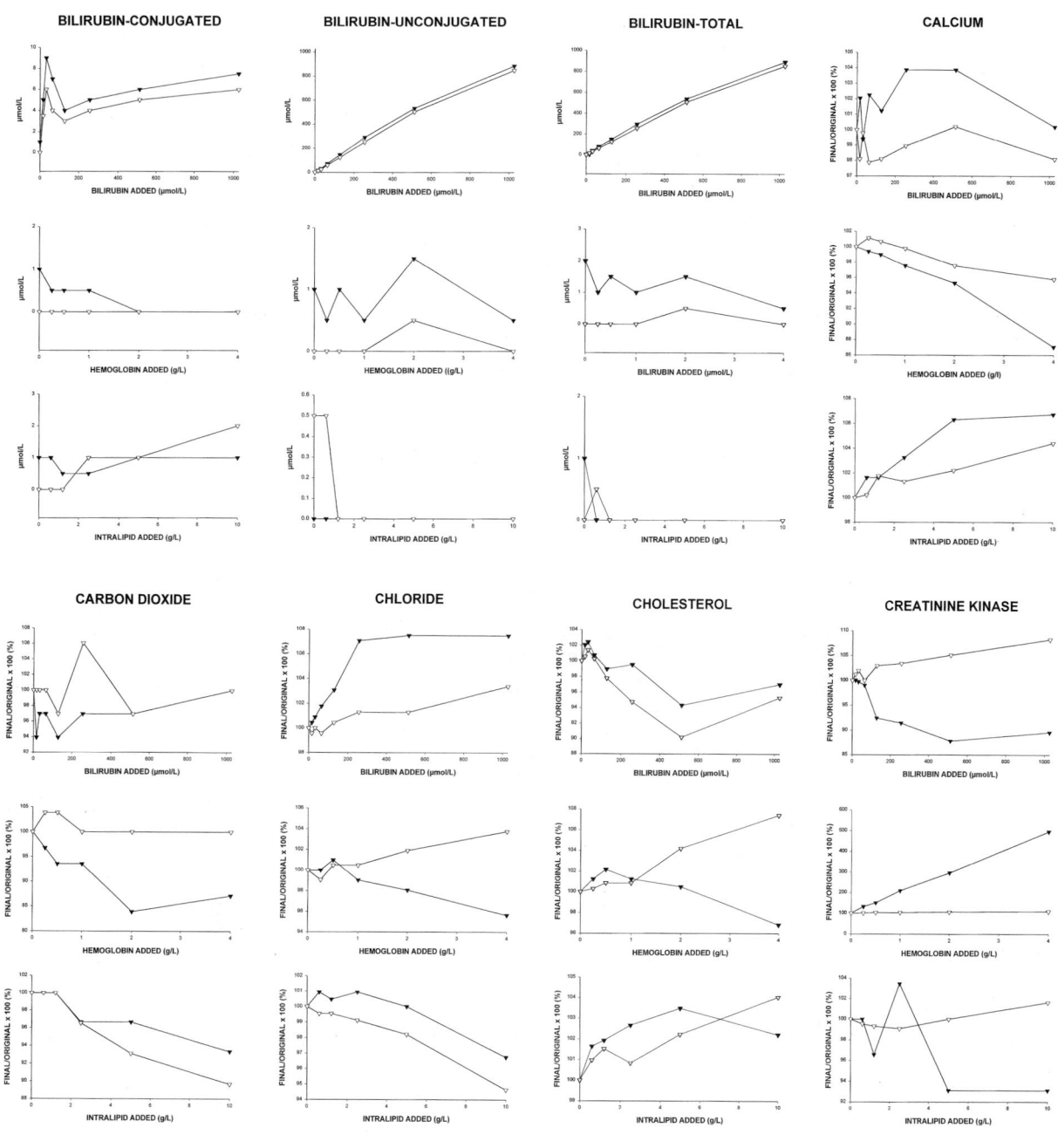

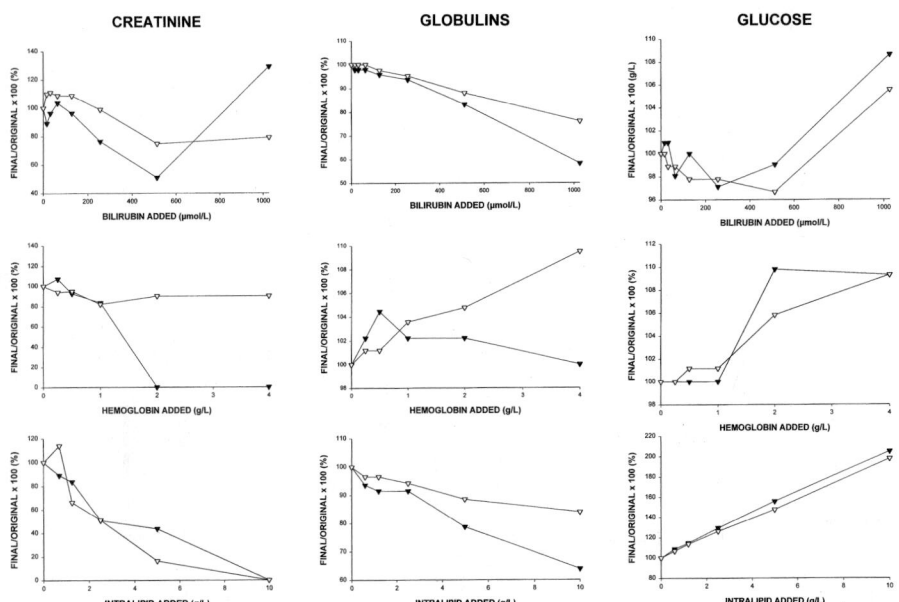

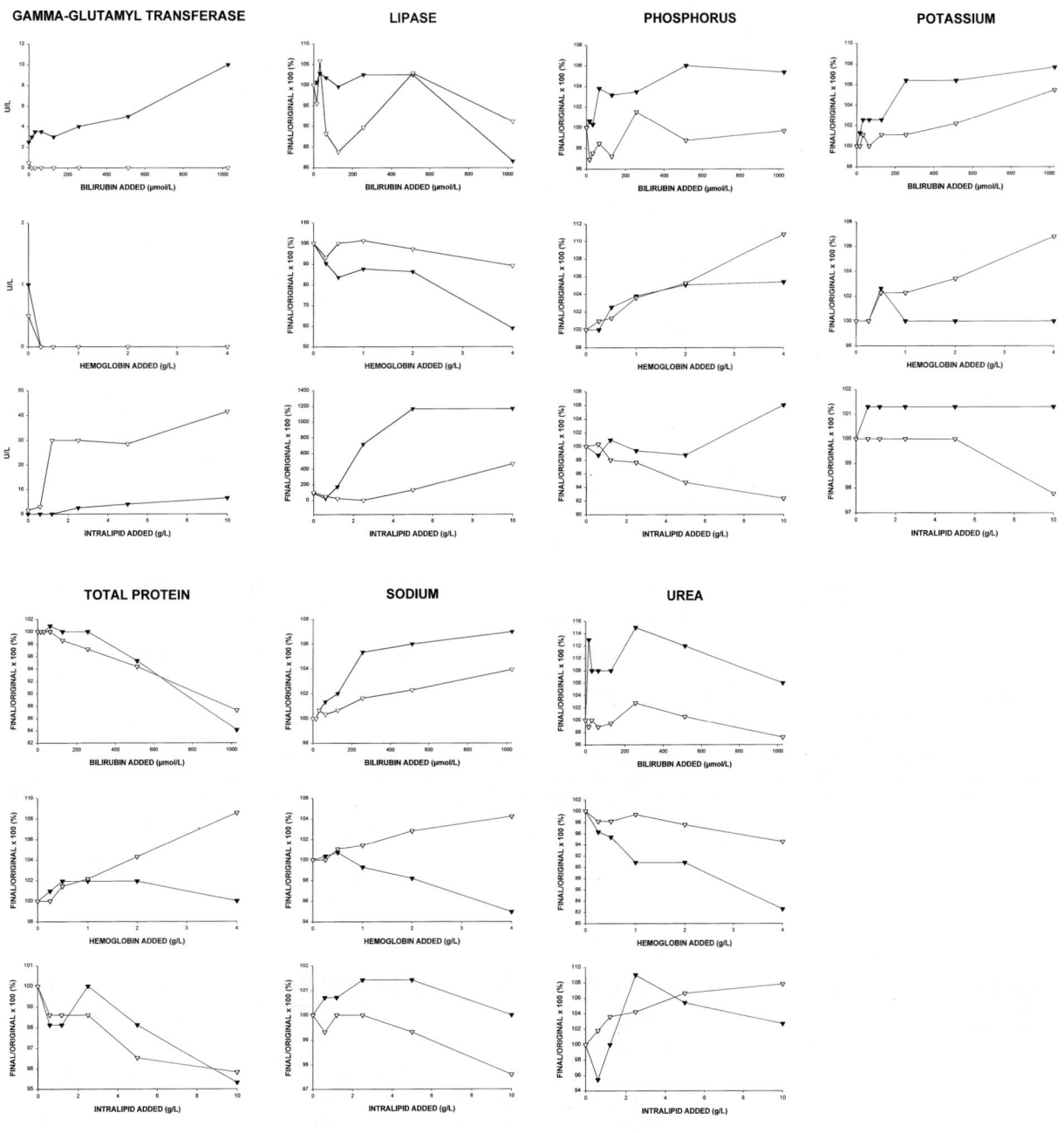

Serum Protein Fractions*

	Unit	Canine	Feline
Plasma protein	gm/L	58–76	60–80
Serum protein	gm/L	50–75	60–82
Albumin	gm/L	22–35	25–39
Globulins	gm/L	22–45	26–50
A/G ratio	—	0.50–1.20	0.53–1.36
IgA	gm/L	0.40–1.6	0.10–0.58
IgM	gm/L	1.0–2.0	0.06–0.39
IgG	gm/L	10.0–20.0	11.7–22.6
Agarose gel electrophoresis:			
α_1	gm/L	5–8	2–5
α_2	gm/L	5–8	8–11
β_1	gm/L	5–11	3–5
β_2	gm/L	3–7	3–6
γ	gm/L	5–18	12–32

*From Clinical Pathology Laboratory, Animal Health Laboratory, Laboratory Services Division, University of Guelph. Immunoglobulin concentrations from Schultz RD, Adams LS: Immunologic methods for the detection of humoral and cellular immunity. Vet Clin North Am 8:721, 1978; Schultz RD, Scott FW, Duncan JR, et al.: Feline immunoglobulins. Infect Immun 9:391, 1974; and Barlough JE, Jacobson RH, Scott FW: The immunoglobulins of the cat. Cornell Vet 71:397, 1981.

Serum Iron and Iron-Binding Capacities in Iron-Deficient and Normal Dogs*

		Iron-Deficient Dogs		Normal Dogs	
Analyte	Unit	Mean	Range (min-max)	Mean	Range (min-max)
Serum iron	μmol/L	5	1–11	27	15–42
Total iron-binding capacity	μmol/L	69	42–118	70	51–102
Saturation	%	8	2–19	39	19–59

*Derived from Harvey JW, French TW, Meyer DJ: Chronic iron deficiency in dogs. J Am Animal Hosp Assoc 18:946, 1982. For a review of similar data from dogs with various hematologic changes, see Hoff B, Lumsden JH, Valli VEO: An appraisal of bone marrow biopsy in assessment of sick dogs. Can J Comp Med 49:34, 1985.

Serum Immunoglobulin Concentrations (mg/ml, Mean ± SD) of Normal Beagle Dogs at Various Ages*

Immunoglobulin Type	6–12 Months ($n = 10$)	1–2 Years ($n = 10$)	2–3 Years ($n = 10$)	3–5 Years ($n = 10$)	5–7 Years ($n = 10$)	7 Years ($n - 6$)
IgM	1.24 ± 1.69	1.34 ± 1.43	1.3 ± 1.8	1.52 ± 0.33	1.67 ± 1.1	1.84 ± 0.35
IgA	0.64 ± 0.34	1.13 ± 0.42	1.04 ± 0.53	1.29 ± 0.39	1.77 ± 0.56	1.62 ± 0.61
IgG$_1$	3.74 ± 1.44	3.97 ± 0.87	2.09 ± 0.68	3.16 ± 0.69	3.34 ± 1.3	2.24 ± 1.71
IgG$_{2a + 2b}$	5.0 ± 1.58	5.94 ± 1.16	6.13 ± 0.88	6.97 ± 0.92	9.05 ± 1.82	7.47 ± 1.68
IgG$_{2c}$	1.25 ± 0.36	1.43 ± 0.21	1.49 ± 0.39	1.6 ± 0.27	1.88 ± 0.51	1.77 ± 0.58

*From Gorman NT, Halliwell REW: Immunoglobulin quantitation and clinical interpretation. In: Halliwell REW, Gorman NT, eds: Veterinary Clinical Immunology. Philadelphia: WB Saunders, 1989, p 61.

Acid-Base and Blood Gases (Mean ± SD)*

Analyte	Unit	Canine		Feline	
		Arterial	*Venous*	*Arterial*	*Venous*
pH	—	7.407 ± 0.0097	7.405 ± 0.0097	7.386 ± 0.038	7.300 ± 0.087
P_{CO_2}	mm Hg	36.8 ± 3.0	36.6 ± 1.21	31.0 ± 2.9	41.8 ± 9.12
P_{O_2}	mm Hg	92.1 ± 5.6	52.1 ± 2.11	106.8 ± 5.7	38.6 ± 11.44
HCO_3	mmol/L	22.2 ± 1.7	22.3 ± 0.43	18.0 ± 1.8	19.4 ± 4.0

*From Senior DF: Fluid therapy, electrolyte and acid-base control. In: Ettinger SJ, ed: Textbook of Veterinary Internal Medicine, Diseases of the Dog and Cat, 3rd ed. Philadelphia: WB Saunders, 1989, p 440. These data are based on the following original citations: Haskins SC: Blood gases and acid-base balance: Clinical interpretation and therapeutic implications. In: Kirk RW, ed: Current Veterinary Therapy VIII. Philadelphia: WB Saunders, 1980, p 201; Rodkey WG, et al: Arterialized capillary blood used to determine the acid-base and blood gas status of dogs. Am J Vet Res 39:459, 1978; Middleton DJ, et al: Arterial and venous blood gas tensions in clinically healthy cats. Am J Vet Res 42:1609, 1981.

Coagulation Screening Tests*

		Unit	Canine	Feline
Buccal mucosal bleeding time (BMBT)†	Lip	Min	1.7–4.2	1.0–3.2
(Simplate, Organon Teknika)		Min	2.62 ± 0.49 (mean ± SD)	—
Cuticle bleeding time (CBT)‡	Nail bed	Min	6.0 ± 3.7 (mean ± SD)	—
		Min	4.3 ± 0.3 (mean ± SEM)	—
Activated coagulation time (ACT)§	37°C	Sec	64–95	≤65
	Room temperature	Sec	60–125	—
		Sec	83–129	—
Tests using a mechanical end point‖				
Prothrombin time (PT, Thromboplastin·C, Dade)		Sec	9–14	—
Activated partial thromboplastin time (APTT, Actin Activated Cephaloplastin, Dade)		Sec	≤20	—
Tests using an electro-optical end point¶				
Prothrombin time (PT, Permaplastin, Dade)		Sec	13.2–22.0	15.5–25.9
Activated partial thromboplastin time (APTT, Actin Activated Cephaloplastin, Dade)		Sec	21.0–35.0	22.8–38.0
Thrombin clotting time (TCT, Thrombostat, Parke-Davis)		Sec	8.3–13.8	8.9–14.9
Russell's viper venom time (RVVT)		Sec	10–15	—

*Prepared with the assistance of **Dr. I.B. Johnstone**, Hemostasis Laboratory, Department of Biomedical Sciences, University of Guelph. Abbreviations, methods, names, and sources of reagents are given in parentheses. These reference values are provided only as general guidelines. Reference values for PT, APTT, TCT, and other coagulation tests differ between laboratories depending on the type and concentration of reagents used and on the type of end-point detection (visual, mechanical, electro-optical). In interpreting patient test results, comparisons must always be made with reference values for that particular laboratory. Some laboratories may elect to run a species-specific reference plasma concurrent with patient plasma and report patient/control time. In such cases, the patient/control (P/C) ratio may be used to determine the significance of the test results. P/C ratios <0.75 or >1.25 in the PT, PTT, and TCT tests should be considered questionable or abnormal and worthy of further investigation (Johnstone IB: Classical haemophilia [haemophilia 'A'] in German shepherd dogs: Different expressions of the disease. Aust Vet Pract 17:71, 1987).

†From Parker MT, Collier LL, Kier AB, Johnson GS: Oral mucosa bleeding times of normal cats and cats with Chediak-Higashi syndrome or Hageman trait (factor XII deficiency). Vet Clin Pathol 17:9, 1988; Jergens AE, Turrentine MA, Kraus KH, et al: Buccal mucosa bleeding times of healthy dogs and of dogs in various pathologic states, including thrombocytopenia, uremia, and von Willebrand's disease. Am J Vet Res 48:1337, 1987.

‡From Giles AR, Tinlin S, Greenwood R: A canine model of hemophilic (factor VIII:C deficiency) bleeding. Blood 60:727, 1982; Pijnappels MIM, Briët E, van der Zwet GTh, et al: Evaluation of the cuticle bleeding time in canine haemophilia A. Thromb Haemost 55:70, 1986.

§From Byars TD, Ling GV, Ferris NA, et al: Activated coagulation time (ACT) of whole blood in normal dogs. Am J Vet Res 37:1359, 1976; Middleton DJ, Watson ADJ: Activated coagulation times of whole blood in normal dogs and dogs with coagulopathies. J Small Anim Pract 19:417, 1978.

‖Fibrometer, reference values from Clinical Pathology Laboratory, Department of Pathology, University of Guelph. This APTT test uses ellagic acid and kaolin as activators.

¶BioData PC8, reference values from **Dr. I.B. Johnstone**, Hemostasis Laboratory, Department of Biomedical Sciences, University of Guelph. This APTT test uses ellagic acid as an activator.

Specific Coagulation Tests*

	Unit	Canine	Feline
Fibrinogen (fibrometer, thrombin time, TT, Thrombostat, Parke-Davis)	gm/L	1.6–4.5	—
Fibrinogen (heat precipitation)	gm/L	1.3–4.4	0.8–2.9
Platelets (manual, phase contrast)	× 10⁹/L	200–600	190–750
Fibrinogen degradation products (FDP, latex agglutination, Burroughs Wellcome)	µg/ml	≤20	—
Factor VIII coagulant (FVIII:C, one-stage differential PTT)	% of normal	55–135	—
von Willebrand factor antigen (vWF:Ag, Laurell Electroimmunoassay)†	% of normal	50–178	—
vWF:Ag (enzyme-linked immunosorbent assay, Diagnostica Stago)‡	% of normal	60–152	—
Antithrombin III (AT III, chromogenic substrate, Diagnostica Stago)§	% of normal	80–136	—

*Prepared with the assistance of **Dr. I.B. Johnstone**, Hemostasis Laboratory, Department of Biomedical Sciences, University of Guelph. Abbreviations, methods, names, and sources of reagents are given in parentheses. Specific hemostatic factors are generally assayed by comparing test plasma to a species-specific reference plasma. The reference plasma is arbitrarily designated as having 100% activity and the activity in the patient plasma is expressed as a percentage of the "normal" plasma.

†From Johnstone IB, Crane S: Determination of canine factor VIII–related antigen using commercial antihuman factor VIII serum. Vet Clin Pathol 9:31, 1980.

‡From Johnstone IB, Crane S: Quantitation of canine plasma von Willebrand factor antigen using a commercial enzyme-linked immunosorbent assay. Can J Vet Res 55:11, 1991.

§Johnstone IB, Petersen D, Crane S: Antithrombin III (AT III) activity in plasmas from normal and diseased horses, and in normal canine, bovine, and human plasmas. Vet Clin Pathol 16:14, 1987.

Quantitative Tests of Gastrointestinal Function*

Fecal determinations

Fecal output (gm feces/kg body weight/day, mean ± SEM)

Canine

Normal (*n* = 14)	8.5 ± 1.1
Malabsorption (*n* = 6)	42.3 ± 8.0
Colitis (*n* = 10)	11.9 ± 1.1
Nonsteatorrheal small intestinal diarrheal disease (*n* = 17)	13.9 ± 2
Exocrine pancreatic insufficiency (EPI) (*n* = 20)	34.4 ± 4.5

Fecal fat output (g fecal fat/kg body weight/day, mean ± SEM)

Canine

		Feline	
Normal (*n* = 14)	0.24 ± 0.01	Normal	0.35 ± 0.23 (mean ± SD)
Malabsorption (*n* = 6)	1.14 ± 0.11	Steatorrhea	>3.5 gm fecal fat/day
EPI (*n* = 20)	2.08 ± 0.36		

Note: Values greater than 0.3 indicate steatorrhea. Fat balance in dogs with colitis and other nonmalabsorptive intestinal diseases is indistinguishable from normal dogs.

Fecal proteolytic activity (FPA) (mean of 3 samples)†

Canine   **Feline**

Radial enzyme diffusion (mm)

		Feline	
Normal	7–15	Normal	6–17
EPI	≤5	EPI	≤5

Azocasein digestion (ACU/gm feces)

Normal	19–122	Normal	29–207
EPI	≤10	EPI	≤10

Serum concentrations of orally administered or naturally occurring substances

Xylose (0.5 gm/kg body weight)

Canine   **Feline**

Peak at 60 min of 65 mg/dl ± 6 (mean ± SEM, *n* = 13), decreasing to 48 ± 5 at 90 min. Only 10% of dogs have 45 to 50 mg/dl at 60 min. All dogs with concentrations greater than 50 mg/dl at 60 min or 45 mg/dl at 90 min are considered normal.

Feline: Peaks between 12 and 42 mg/dl

Note: This test has poor sensitivity for detecting malabsorption in the dog and cat.

N-Benzoyl-L-tyrosyl-*para*-aminobenzoic acid (BT-PABA)

Canine (50 mg/kg body weight)
>400 μg/dl at 60 to 90 min

Feline
Peaks at 386 ± 134 μg/dl (mean ± SD, *n* = 17, 16.7 mg/kg body weight). At 50 mg/kg body weight, the peak occurred at 90 min and the range (min-max) was approximately 400–1,100 μg/dl.

Vitamin E (mg/L)

Canine	>5	**Feline**	>5

Vitamin B₁₂ (ng/L)

Canine	225–661	**Feline**	200–1,680

Folic acid (μg/L)

Canine	6.7–17.4	**Feline**	13.4–38.0

Trypsin-like immunoreactivity (TLI) (μg/L)

Canine

		Feline	
Normal	5.0–35		17–49
EPI	≤2.5		

*Prepared with the assistance of **Dr. D.A. Williams**. Review and original citations in Jacobs RM, Norris AM, Lumsden JH, et al: Laboratory Diagnosis of Malassimilation. Vet Clin North Am [Small Anim Pract] 19:951, 1989.

†From Williams DA, Reed SD, Perry L: Fecal proteolytic activity in clinically normal cats and in a cat with exocrine pancreatic insufficiency. J Am Vet Med Assoc 197:210, 1990; Williams DA, Reed SD: Comparison of methods for assay of fecal proteolytic activity. J Vet Clin Pathol 19:20, 1990.

Tests of the Endocrine System*

Hormone	Unit	Canine	Feline
Adrenocorticotrophic hormone, basal (ACTH, plasma)	pmol/L	2–15	1–20
Aldosterone† (plasma)			
Basal	pmol/L	14–957	194–388
Post-ACTH	pmol/L	197–2,103	277–721
Cortisol (serum or plasma, urine)			
Basal	nmol/L	25–125	15–150
Post-ACTH	nmol/L	200–550	130–450
Post–**low**-dose dexamethasone (0.01 or 0.015 mg/kg)	nmol/L	≤40	≤40
Post–**high**-dose dexamethasone (0.1 or 1.0 mg/kg)‡	nmol/L	≤40	≤40
Urinary cortisol/creatinine ratio	× 10⁻⁶	8–24†, 10§	—
Insulin, basal (serum)	pmol/L	35–200	35–200
Intact parathormone† (serum)	pmol/L	2–13	0–4
Progesterone (serum or plasma, female)	mmol/L	≤3.0 in anestrus, proestrus 50–220 in diestrus, pregnancy	≤3.0 in anestrus, proestrus 50–220 in diestrus, pregnancy
Testosterone (serum or plasma, male)	nmol/L	1–20	1–20
Thyroxine (T₄, serum)			
Basal	nmol/L	12–50	10–50
Post–thyroxine-stimulating hormone (TSH)	nmol/L	>45	>45
Triiodothyronine (T₃) suppression‖	nmol/L	—	≤20
Triiodothyronine, basal (T₃, serum)	nmol/L	0.7–2.3	0.5–2.0

*Prepared with the assistance of **Dr. M.E. Peterson**, The Animal Medical Center, New York, NY. Unless indicated otherwise, values in this table are adapted from Kemppainen RJ, Zerbe CA: Common endocrine diagnostic tests: Normal values and interpretations. In: Kirk RW, ed: Current Veterinary Therapy X. Philadelphia, WB Saunders, 1989, p 961. Hormone determinations are variable between laboratories. The laboratory performing the analysis should provide reference values. Before submitting samples for hormone determinations, consult the laboratory for sample specifications, use of anticoagulants, and sample preservation. General sampling conditions are discussed in Reimers TJ: Guidelines for collection, storage, and transport of samples for hormone assay. In: Kirk RW, ed: Current Veterinary Therapy X. Philadelphia: WB Saunders, 1989, p 968. The effects of age, gender, and size on canine serum thyroid and adrenocortical hormone concentrations are discussed in Reimers TJ, Lawler DFG, Sutaria PM, et al: Effects of age, sex, and body size on serum concentrations of thyroid and adrenocortical hormones in dogs. Am J Vet Res 51:454, 1990.

†Provided by **Dr. R.F. Nachreiner**, Animal Health Diagnostic Laboratory, Endocrine Diagnostic Section, Michigan State University.

‡This test is used after adrenocortical hyperfunction has been confirmed. It is used to differentiate adrenal tumor (where no suppression is seen) from pituitary-dependent cases (where suppression occurs, but is variable).

§From Stolp R, Rijnberk A, Meiher JC, et al: Urinary corticoids in the diagnosis of canine hyperadrenocorticism. Res Vet Sci 34:141, 1983; Rijnberk A, van Wees A, Mol JA: Assessment of two tests for the diagnosis of canine hyperadrenocorticism. Vet Rec 122:178, 1988.

‖From Peterson ME, Ferguson DC: Thyroid diseases. In: Ettinger SJ, ed: Textbook of Veterinary Internal Medicine: Diseases of the Dog and Cat, 3rd ed. Philadelphia: WB Saunders, 1989, pp 1632–1675.

There are many potential drug-induced physiologic changes that can affect the results of endocrine testing; see *CVT XII*, pp 341–345.

Système International (SI) Units for Hormone Assays*

Hormone	Unit		Conversion Factors	
	Traditional	*SI*	*Traditional → SI*	*SI → Traditional*
Aldosterone	ng/dl	pmol/L	27.7	0.036
Corticotrophin (ACTH)	pg/ml	pmol/L	0.22	4.51
Cortisol	µg/dl	mmol/L	27.59	0.36
β-Endorphin	pg/ml	pmol/L	0.289	3.43
Epinephrine	pg/ml	pmol/L	5.46	0.183
Estrogen (estradiol)	pg/ml	pmol/L	3.67	0.273
Gastrin	pg/ml	ng/L	1.00	1.00
Glucagon	pg/ml	ng/L	1.00	1.00
Growth hormone (GH)	ng/ml	µg/L	1.00	1.00
Insulin	µU/ml	pmol/L	7.18	0.139
α-Melanocyte–stimulating hormone (α-MSH)	pg/ml	pmol/L	0.601	1.66
Norepinephrine	pg/ml	nmol/L	0.006	169
Pancreatic polypeptide (PP)	mg/dl	mmol/L	0.239	4.18
Progesterone	ng/ml	mmol/L	3.18	0.315
Prolactin	ng/ml	µg/L	1.00	1.00
Renin	ng/ml/hr	ng/L/s	0.278	3.60
Somatostatin	pg/ml	pmol/L	0.611	1.64
Testosterone	ng/ml	nmol/L	3.47	0.288
Thyroxine (T₄)	µg/dl	nmol/L	12.87	0.078
Triiodothyronine (T₃)	ng/dl	nmol/L	0.0154	64.9
Vasoactive intestinal polypeptide (VIP)	pg/ml	pmol/L	0.301	3.33

*Contributed by **Dr. M.E. Peterson**, The Animal Medical Center, New York, NY.

Urinary and Renal Function Tests*

	Unit	Canine	Feline
Random specific gravity (SG)	—	1.001–1.070	1.001–1.080
SG after 5% dehydration	—	1.050–1.076	1.047–1.087
Random osmolality	mmol/kg	50–2,500	50–3,000 +
Osmolality after 5% dehydration	mmol/kg	1,787–2,791	1,581–2,984
Urine/plasma osmolality after 5% dehydration	—	5.7–8.9	—
Volume output	ml/kg body weight/day	24–41	22–30
Protein—sulfosalicylic acid†	0.1, 0.2. 0.3, 0.4, 0.5, 0.75, and 1.0 gm/L stds.	<0.1	
Protein—dipstick‡	Negative, trace, 0.3, 1.0, 3.0, and 20+ gm/L stds.	Negative when SG <1.035 Trace when SG >1.035	
Blood—dipstick	Negative, +, ++, and +++ stds.	Negative	
Glucose—dipstick	Negative, 6, 14, 28, 56, and 111+ mmol/L stds.	Negative	
Ketones—dipstick	Negative, 0.5, 1.5, 4, 8, and 16 mmol/L stds.	Negative	
Bilirubin—dipstick	Negative, +, ++, and +++ stds.	+ when SG > 1.035	Negative
Protein output§	mg/kg body weight/day	<22	<30
	mg/day	<200 or <600	<115
Protein/creatinine ratio‖			
Normal	—	<0.2	<0.6
Questionable	—	0.2–1.0	0.6–1.0
Abnormal	—	>1.0	>1.0
Effective renal plasma flow by clearance of	ml/min/m² body surface	266±66	—
$para$-aminohippurate or [131I]iodohippurate¶	ml/min/kg body weight	13.5±3.3	14.1±5.75 or 10.6±1.7
Glomerular filtration rate (GFR) by clearance	ml/min/m² body surface	84.4±19	—
of [14C]inulin, [125I]iothalamate, or other	ml/min/kg body weight	4.2±1.8 or 3.6±0.1	51.±1.5
labelled chemicals#			3.5±0.6
GFR by sodium sulfanilate clearance**—$t_{0.5}$	Min	58±13 or 66.1±10.8	44.7±5.7
GFR by exogenous creatinine clearance††	ml/min/kg body weight	4.0±0.5	2.9±0.3
GFR by endogenous creatinine clearance‡‡	ml/min/m² body surface	60±22	—
	ml/min/kg body weight 20 min	3.0±1.0	2.7±1.1
	24 hr	3.7±0.8	2.3±0.5
Fractional clearances§§			
Sodium	%	0–0.7	0.24–0.96
Chloride	%	0–0.8	0.41–1.33
Potassium	%	0–20	6.7–23.9
Calcium	%	0–0.4	—
Phosphorus	%	3–39	17–73

*Prepared with the assistance of **Dr. J. Barsanti**, University of Georgia. Data are given in mean ± SD rounded to one decimal place. In a few instances, alternative reference values are listed. An extensive bibliography and a review of these tests can be found in Chew DJ, Dibartola SP: Diagnosis and pathophysiology of renal disease. In: Ettinger SJ, ed: Textbook of Veterinary Internal Medicine: Diseases of the Dog and Cat, 3rd ed. Philadelphia: WB Saunders, 1989, pp 1893–1961.

†Albumin in Urine Test Set, Harleco, Gibbstown, NJ.

‡Multistix, Miles Canada Inc, Etobicoke, Ontario. Also applies for the semiquantitative analysis of blood, glucose, ketones, and bilirubin. Refer to the discussion in the package insert entitled "Ames Reagent Strips for Urinalysis" for potential interferents.

§From DiBartola SP, Chew DJ, Jacobs G: Quantitative urinalysis including 24-hour protein excretion in the dog. J Am Anim Hosp Assoc 16:537, 1980; Russo EA, Lees GE, Hightower D: Evaluation of renal function tests in cats, using quantitative urinalysis. Am J Vet Res 47:1308, 1986; Barsanti JA, Finco DR: Protein concentration in urine of normal dogs. Am J Vet Res 40:1583, 1979. Applies to urine samples with no hemorrhage or inflammation. Some differences in test results occur with different quantitative methods.

‖From White JV, Olivier B, Reimann K, et al: Use of protein-to-creatinine ratio in a single urine specimen for quantitative estimation of canine proteinuria. J Am Vet Med Assoc 185:882, 1984; Grauer GF, Thomas CB, and Eicker SW: Estimation of quantitative proteinuria in the dog, using the protein-to-creatinine ratio from a random, voided sample. Am J Vet Res 46:2116, 1985; Center SA, Wilkinson E, Smith CA, et al: 24-hour urine protein/creatinine ratio in dogs with protein-losing nephropathies. J Am Vet Med Assoc 187:820, 1985; McCaw DL, Knapp DW, Hewett JE: Effect of collection time and exercise restriction on the prediction of urine protein excretion, using urine protein/creatinine ratio in dogs. Am J Vet Res 46:166, 1985; Jergens AE, McCaw DL, Hewett JE: Effects of collection time and food consumption on the urine protein/creatinine ratio in dogs. Am J Vet Res 48:1106, 1987. Applies to urine samples with no hemorrhage or inflammation.

¶From Mercer HC, Garg RC, Powers JD, et al: Bioavailability and pharmacokinetics of several dosage forms of ampicillin in the cat. Am J Vet Res 38:1353, 1977; Ross LA, Finco DR: Relationship of selected clinical renal function tests to glomerular filtration rate and renal blood flow in cats. Am J Vet Res 42: 1704, 1981.

#From Ross LA, Finco DR, 1981; Carlson GP, Kaneko JJ: Simultaneous estimation of renal function in dogs using sodium sulfanilate and sodium iodohippurate-131I. J Am Vet Med Assoc 158:1229, 1971; Maddison JE, Pascoe PJ, Jansen BS: Clinical evaluation of sodium sulfanilate clearance for the diagnosis of renal disease in dogs. J Am Vet Med Assoc 185:961, 1984; Mercer HC, et al, 1977.

**From Ross LA, Finco DR, 1981; Osborne CA, Low DG, Finco DR: Canine and Feline Urology. Philadelphia: WB Saunders, 1972; Finco DR, Coulter DB, Barsanti JA: Simple, accurate method for clinical estimation of glomerular filtration rate in the dog. Am J Vet Res 42:1874, 1981; Fettman MJ, Allen TA, Wilke WL, et al: Single-injection method for evaluation of renal function with 14C-inulin and 3H-tetraethylammonium bromide in dogs and cats. Am J Vet Res 46:482, 1985; Powers TE, Powers JD, Garg RC: Study of the double-isotope single-injection methods for estimating renal function in purebred beagle dogs. Am J Vet Res 38:1933, 1977.

††From Ross LA, Finco DR, 1981; Finco DR, et al, 1981. Creatinine given subcutaneously in dog and intravenously in cat.

‡‡From Russo EA, et al, 1986; Osborne CA, et al, 1972; Bovee KC, Joyce T: Clinical evaluation of glomerular function: 24 hour creatinine hippurate, and phenolsulphothalein in the cat. Can J Comp Med 24:138, 1970.

§§From Dibartola SP, et al, 1980; Russo EA, et al, 1986. Values vary markedly with diet.

Bronchoalveolar Lavage Fluid Cell Populations*

	Canine (n = 6)	Feline (n = 11)
Total nucleated cells/μl	≤500	≤400
Cell types (mean %)		
Macrophages	70 ± 11 (49–93)	70.6 ± 9.8
Lymphocytes	7 ± 5 (1–19)	4.6 ± 3.2
Neutrophils	5 ± 5 (1–27)	6.7 ± 4.0
Eosinophils	6 ± 5 (1–19)	16.1 ± 6.8
Mast cells	1 ± 1 (0–5)	NR†
Epithelial cells	1 ± 1 (0–12)	NR

*Canine data given as mean % ± SD (range). Feline data given as mean % ± SE. Data derived from and original citations listed in Hawkins EC, DeNicola DB, Kuehn NF: Bronchoalveololar lavage in the evaluation of pulmonary disease in the dog and cat. J Vet Intern Med 4:267, 1990.
†Not reported.

Cerebrospinal Fluid (CSF)*

	Canine		Feline	
Protein (gm/L)†	0.10–0.30		0.04–0.32	
Total nucleated cells (× 10⁹/L)‡	0–0.002		0–0.002	
	Sediment (n = 40)	Cytospin (n = 50)	Sediment (n = 20)	Cytospin (n = 22)
Cell types (mean %, [range])				
Large foamy mononuclear	3 (0–32)	6 (0–46)	—	—
Monocytoid	—	17 (0–50)	87 (69–100)	77 (25–100)
Small mononuclear	26 (3–52)	37 (0–73)	—	—
Large mononuclear	38 (9–74)	33 (0–68)	—	—
Small lymphocyte	5 (0–76)	4 (0–61)	9 (0–27)§	14 (0–50)
Neutrophil	1 (0–10)	3 (0–7)	1 (0–9)	2 (0–25)
Eosinophil	0	0.3 (0–13)	0	0
Macrophage	0	0	0 (0–3)	3 (0–33)

*Canine data adapted from Jamison EM, Lumsden JH: Cerebrospinal fluid analysis in the dog: Methodology and interpretation. Semin Vet Med Surg (Small Anim) 3:122, 1988, and other unpublished data describing the CSF characteristics of histologically normal dogs. Feline data adapted from Rand JS, Parent J, Jacobs RM, et al: Reference intervals for feline cerebrospinal fluid: Cell counts and cytologic features. Am J Vet Res 51:1044, 1990, describing CSF characteristics in histologically normal cats. All feline CSFs had red blood cell counts between 0 and 0.030 × 10⁹/L. All data are for cerebellomedullary CSF. There are significant differences between lumbar and cerebellomedullary CSF (Bailey CS, Higgins RJ: Comparison of total white blood cell count and total protein content of lumbar and cisternal cerebrospinal fluid of healthy dogs. Am J Vet Res 46:1162, 1985); Thomson CE, Kornegay JN, Stevens JB: Analysis of cerebrospinal fluid from the cerebellomedullary and lumbar cisterns of dogs with focal neurologic disease: 145 cases (1985–1987). J Am Vet Med Assoc 196:1841–1844, 1990.

†The protein concentrations here are for the Ponceau S method and the reference interval represents the range. For a comparison of Ponceau S and urine dipstick methods, see Jacobs RM, Cochrane SM, Lumsden JH, et al: Relationship of cerebrospinal fluid protein concentration determined by dye-binding and urinary dipstick methodologies. Can Vet J 31:587, 1990.

‡Range for hemocytometer cell counts.
§Includes all sizes of lymphocytes.

Cerebrospinal Fluid Biochemical Analytes in Histologically Normal Cats*

Analyte	Unit	Mean	Range (min–max)
Glucose	mmol/L	4.1	0.5–8.1
Creatine kinase	U/L	47	2–236
Lactate dehydrogenase	U/L	12	4–30
Aspartate aminotransferase	U/L	17	0–39
IgG	gm/L	0.015	0.005–0.56
[CSF IgG]/[serum IgG]	—	0.8	0.3–2.1

*Adapted from Rand JS, Parent J, Jacobs RM, et al: Reference intervals for feline cerebrospinal fluid: Biochemical and serologic variables, IgG concentration, and electrophoretic fractionation. Am J Vet Res 51:1049, 1990. All feline CSFs had red blood cell counts between 0 and 0.030 × 10⁹/L. See also CVT XII, p 1121.

Characteristics of Body Cavity Fluids in Healthy Dogs and Cats*

Volume	0–15 ml for peritoneal cavity
	Approximately 3 ml in pleural cavity
	Approximately 0.3 ml in pericardial sac
Color	Colorless to slight yellow
Odor	None
Transparency	Clear, with no tissue fragments
Protein†	≤2.5 gm/dl (≤25 gm/L)
	Does not coagulate
Specific gravity	≤1.014
Electrolytes and pH	As for plasma
Total nucleated cell count	≤3,000/μl (≤3.0 × 10⁹/L)
Cell types	Mesothelial cells
	Occasional well-preserved neutrophils
	Occasional lymphocytes and monocytes
	Occasional erythrocytes

*From O'Brien PJ, Lumsden JH: The cytologic examination of body cavity fluids. Semin Vet Med Surg (Small Anim) 3:140, 1988. The original citations are listed in this review.

†For the Goldberg refractometer (Fisher Scientific, Toronto, Ontario), 2.5 gm protein/dl corresponds to a specific gravity of 1.014 on he plasma/serum scale. The serum/plasma specific gravity scale should be used for the estimation of protein concentration in body cavity fluids. If the urine specific gravity scale is used erroneously or unknowingly, the corresponding specific gravity is 1.020 for a protein concentration of 2.5 gm/dl.

Cytologic Findings in Normal and Abnormal Canine Synovial Fluids*

	Clarity	Color	Mucin Clot	Fibrin	Cell Count (× 10⁹/L)	Mononuclear Cells (%)	Neutrophils (%)
Normal	Clear	None to light yellow	Good	—	0.0–3.0	90–100	0–10
Nonsuppurative inflammation							
Degenerative	Clear	None to light yellow	Good to fair	—	0.0–3.5	90–100	0–10
Traumatic	Clear to turbid	Normal to bloody	Good	±	2.5–3.0	90–100	0–10
Chronic hemarthrosis	Turbid	Bloody	Fair to poor	—†	Variably increased	Predominate	Occasional
Suppurative inflammation							
Rheumatoid-like	Turbid	Yellow to bloody	Fair to poor	+	3.0–38	20–80	20–80
SLE‡-like	Turbid	Yellow to bloody	Good to poor	+	4.4–370	5–85	15–95
Bacterial	Turbid	Gray to bloody	Poor to very poor	+	110–267	1–10	90–99

*From Ellison RS: The cytologic examination of synovial fluid. Semin Vet Med Surg (Small Anim) 3:133, 1988. The original citations are listed in this review. The protein concentration in normal joint fluid is ≤30 gm/L.

†In acute hemarthrosis, fibrin clots may be present.

‡Systemic lupus erythematosus.

Also see *CVT XII*, p. 1166.

Canine Semen (Mean ± SEM)*

Semen Characteristics After Sexual Rest	Unit	Body Weight (pounds)		
		10–34	*35–59*	*60–84*
Volume†	ml	2.4 ± 0.3	3.9 ± 0.5	5.4 ± 1.3
Sperm concentration	× 10⁶/ml	209 ± 42	359 ± 72	228 ± 58
Total sperm	× 10⁶/ml	400 ± 110	1,120 ± 130	1,430 ± 460

*Data derived from Amann RP: Reproductive physiology and endocrinology of the dog. In: Morrow DA, ed: Current Therapy in Theriogenology 2. Philadelphia: WB Saunders, 1986, p 536. In one study, inseminations with greater than 200 × 10⁶ morphologically normal sperm resulted in a pregnancy rate of 81% (22 of 27 bitches). As the total number of morphologically normal sperm declined, so did the pregnancy rate and litter size (Michelsen WD, Society for Theriogenology, Orlando, FL, September, 1988, p 387).

†The presperm and sperm-rich fractions were collected together, but ejaculation was terminated when ejaculation of the postsperm prostatic fluid was started.

Canine Prostatic Fluid (Third Fraction)*

Volume	Variable, depending on length of ejaculation
pH	6.1–7.2
Appearance	Clear
Sediment	Acellular

*From Bartlett DJ: Studies on dog semen II. Biochemical characteristics. J Reprod Fertil 3:190, 1962.

Electrocardiography*

It is recognized that normal and abnormal electrocardiographic measurements overlap and that the criteria for the normal electrocardiogram serve only as a guide for the clinician. Deviations from normal in an individual electrocardiogram suggest, but are not always diagnostic of, heart disease. As additional statistical data become available for the electrocardiograms of dogs of each breed, body type, age, and sex, the data herein may require revision and "normal" may be more precisely defined. The value of serial electrocardiograms from an individual cannot be overemphasized, since serial changes best demonstrate electrocardiographic abnormalities.

Criteria for the Normal Canine Electrocardiogram†

Heart rate—60 to 160 bpm for adult dogs, up to 180 bpm in toy breeds, and 220 bpm for puppies.
Heart rhythm—Normal sinus rhythm; sinus arrhythmia; and wandering sinoatrial pacemaker.
P wave—Up to 0.4 mV in amplitude; up to 0.04 sec in duration (may be longer in giant breeds); always positive in leads II and aVF; positive or isoelectric in lead I.
P-R interval—0.06- to 0.14-sec duration.
QRS complex—Mean electric axis, frontal plane, 40 to 100 degrees.
Amplitude—Maximum amplitude of R wave 2.5 to 3.0 mV in leads II, III, and aVF. Complex positive in leads II, III, and aVF; negative in lead V_{10}.
Duration—To 0.05 sec (0.06/sec in dogs over 40 lb).
Q-T segment—0.15- to 0.22-sec duration.
ST segment and T wave—ST segment free of marked coving (repolarization changes).
ST segment depression not greater than 0.2 mV.
ST segment elevation not greater than 0.15 mV.
T wave negative in lead V_{10}.
T wave amplitude no greater than 25% of amplitude of R wave.

Criteria for the Normal Feline Electrocardiogram†

Heart rate—240 bpm maximum.
Heart rhythm—Normal sinus rhythm or, infrequently, sinus arrhythmia.
P wave—Positive in leads II and aVF; may be isoelectric or positive in lead I; should not exceed 0.03 sec in duration.
P-R interval—0.04- to 0.08-sec duration (inversely related to the heart rate).
QRS complex—More variable than in the canine; the mean electric axis in the frontal plane is often insignificant. Often the QRS complex is nearly isoelectric in all frontal plane limb leads (so-called horizontal heart).
QRS amplitude—The amplitude of the R wave is usually low; marked amplitude of R wave (>0.8 mV) in the frontal plane leads may suggest ventricular hypertrophy.
QRS duration—<0.04 sec.
Q-T segment—0.16- to 0.18-sec duration.
ST segment and T wave—ST segment and T wave should be small and free of repolarization changes as well as marked depression or elevation.

*From Ettinger SJ, Suter PF: Canine Cardiology. Philadelphia: WB Saunders, 1970, pp 102–169.
†From Ettinger SJ: Textbook of Veterinary Internal Medicine, Diseases of the Dog and Cat, 3rd ed, vol 1. Philadelphia: WB Saunders, 1989, p 1055.

AAFCO Dog and Cat Food Nutrient Profiles

David A. Dzanis

Santa Clarita, California

The Association of American Feed Control Officials (AAFCO) is an advisory body composed of representatives from individual states and territories, the U.S. Food and Drug Administration, and Canada. A primary function of AAFCO is the publication of a model feed bill, animal feed regulations, and ingredient definitions, all of which a state may adopt as a part of its own feed laws and regulations. A pet food that bears a "complete and balanced" label claim that does not, in fact, offer adequate nutrition is both misbranded and unsafe. To address this concern, included in the model pet food regulations are means of substantiating nutritional adequacy for complete and balanced dog and cat foods.

One method of substantiating nutritional adequacy requires that the product be formulated so that essential nutrient levels meet a prescribed profile. Historically, AAFCO relied on the publications of the National Research Council (NRC) as its authority with respect to the levels of nutrients that constituted a complete and balanced dog or cat food. However, to address several technical concerns regarding the applicability of the NRC recommendations to the practical formulation of pet foods, they were replaced by the AAFCO Dog and Cat Food Nutrient Profiles (Tables 1 and 2) in the early 1990s.

The profiles are the product of the AAFCO Canine Nutrition Expert (CNE) and Feline Nutrition Expert (FNE) Subcommittees, which met in 1990 and 1991, respectively. Nationally recognized experts from both academia and industry were convened to establish practical profiles based on commonly used ingredients. In addition to this author, members of the CNE included Dr. Jim Corbin, University of Illinois; Dr. Gail Czarnecki-Maulden, Westreco, Inc.; Dr. Diane Hirakawa, The Iams Company; Dr. Francis Kallfelz, Cornell University; Dr. Mark Morris, Mark Morris Associates; and Dr. Ben Sheffy, Cornell University. Added to the original members of the CNE were two new members on the FNE to bring additional expertise in the field of cat nutrition: Dr. Quinton Rogers, University of California-Davis; and Dr. Angele Thompson, Kal Kan Foods. Mr. Wendell Kerr of Westreco, Inc., also participated to provide statistical support to both subcommittees. The CNE and FNE met once again in 1995 to review and update both the dog and the cat food profiles.

Nutrient levels in the AAFCO Dog and Cat Food Nutrient Profiles are based on the CNE and FNE members' knowledge of published and unpublished research, as well as their personal expertise and experiences in practical formulation. Much of the scientific data on nutrient requirements are based on studies using purified diets and the presumption of 100% bioavailability. However, since commercial products are composed of nonpurified, complex ingredients, allowances to account for the effects of ingredients, ingredient interactions, and processing on bioavailability were also considered in establishing nutrient levels.

Comments on the bioavailability or the effect of processing and ingredient interaction on some nutrients are also added in the footnotes to the tables.

In addition to minimum nutrient levels, the AAFCO Dog and Cat Food Nutrient Profiles also set maximum levels of intake of some nutrients. This was done out of concern that the risk of nutrient excess, rather than deficiency, was a concern with some pet foods. Thus, maximum limits on the amounts of calcium, phosphorus, magnesium, fat-soluble vitamins, and most trace minerals in dog foods are established. While the list of maximum levels for cat foods is not as extensive as that for dog foods, it should not imply that cats are more tolerant of nutrient excesses than dogs. Rather, it reflects the paucity of information on the toxic effects of nutrients in cats. Establishing maximum levels arbitrarily might prove worse than no maximum at all. Setting a maximum level implies safety below that level, which the subcommittees could not reasonably ensure.

Replacing the previous "meets or exceeds the NRC recommendations" verbiage, the required label wording for reference to the nutrient profiles is that the product is "...formulated to meet the AAFCO Dog (or Cat) Food Nutrient Profile for..." a given life stage. For both dog and cat foods, there are two separate AAFCO profiles: one for growth and reproduction (gestation and lactation), and one for adult maintenance. This allows foods formulated for adult dogs or cats to contain lower amounts of some nutrients, eliminating unnecessary excesses. Products that meet only the adult maintenance profile should include "maintenance" as its given life stage. Since products suitable for the more stringent nutrient requirements of growth and reproduction are also presumed to be adequate for adult maintenance, products meeting the growth and reproduction profile can list their intended use for either maintenance, growth, gestation and lactation, or "all life stages."

Nutrient levels in the tables are expressed on a dry matter (DM) basis. To accurately compare levels for a pet food as given in the guaranteed analysis portion of a label or elsewhere on an "as fed" basis, the values must first be corrected for moisture content. For most dry pet foods (10% moisture), "as fed" values should be multiplied by 1.1. For a 75% moisture canned product, values should be multiplied by 4.0. The profiles are also set at presumed energy densities (3.5 kcal ME/gm DM for dog foods, 4.0 kcal ME/gm DM for cat foods). Since a dog or cat is presumed to eat less of a high-calorie food, the levels of the nutrients must be proportionally higher in order for the animal to meet its needs with the lower food intake. Thus, products very high in caloric density should also be corrected for energy content before comparisons with the profiles are made.

The AAFCO Dog and Cat Food Nutrient Profiles and accompanying information on using the tables are published annually in the AAFCO Official Publication. Information on AAFCO and how to obtain a copy of the AAFCO Official Publication can be found on its web site (http://www.aafco.org) or by writing to: Ms. Sharon Senesac, AAFCO Assistant Treasurer, P.O. Box 478, Oxford, IN 47971.

TABLE 1. **AAFCO Dog Food Nutrient Profiles***

Nutrient	Units DM Basis	Growth & Reproduction Minimum	Adult Maintenance Minimum	Maximum
Protein	%	22.0	18.0	
Arginine	%	0.62	0.51	
Histidine	%	0.22	0.18	
Isoleucine	%	0.45	0.37	
Leucine	%	0.72	0.59	
Lysine	%	0.77	0.63	
Methionine-cystine	%	0.53	0.43	
Phenylalanine-tyrosine	%	0.89	0.73	
Threonine	%	0.58	0.48	
Tryptophan	%	0.20	0.16	
Valine	%	0.48	0.39	
Fat†	%	8.0	5.0	
Linoleic acid	%	1.0	1.0	
Minerals				
Calcium	%	1.0	0.6	2.5
Phosphorus	%	0.8	0.5	1.6
Ca:P ratio		1:1	1:1	2:1
Potassium	%	0.6	0.6	
Sodium	%	0.3	0.06	
Chloride	%	0.45	0.09	
Magnesium	%	0.04	0.04	0.3
Iron‡	mg/kg	80	80	3,000
Copper§	mg/kg	7.3	7.3	250
Manganese	mg/kg	5.0	5.0	
Zinc	mg/kg	120	120	1,000
Iodine	mg/kg	1.5	1.5	50
Selenium	mg/kg	0.11	0.11	2
Vitamins and others				
Vitamin A	IU/kg	5,000	5,000	250,000
Vitamin D	IU/kg	500	500	5,000
Vitamin E	IU/kg	50	50	1,000
Thiamine¶	mg/kg	1.0	1.0	
Riboflavin	mg/kg	2.2	2.2	
Pantothenic acid	mg/kg	10	10	
Niacin	mg/kg	11.4	11.4	
Pyridoxine	mg/kg	1.0	1.0	
Folic acid	mg/kg	0.18	0.18	
Vitamin B$_{12}$	mg/kg	0.022	0.022	
Choline	mg/kg	1,200	1,200	

*Presumes an energy density of 3.5 kcal ME/gm DM, based on the "modified Atwater" values of 3.5, 8.5, and 3.5 kcal/gm for protein, fat, and carbohydrate (nitrogen-free extract, NFE), respectively. Rations greater than 4.0 kcal/gm should be corrected for energy density; rations less than 3.5 kcal/gm should *not* be corrected for energy.

†Although a true requirement for fat per se has not been established, the minimum level was based on recognition of fat as a source of essential fatty acids, as a carrier of fat-soluble vitamins, and on the amount needed to enhance palatability and to supply an adequate caloric density.

‡Because of very poor bioavailability, iron from carbonate or oxide sources that are added to the diet should not be considered in determining the minimum nutrient level.

§Because of very poor bioavailability, copper from oxide sources that are added to the diet should not be considered in determining the minimum nutrient level.

¶Because processing may destroy up to 90% of the thiamine in the diet, allowances in formulation should be made to ensure that the minimum nutrient level is met after processing.

TABLE 2. AAFCO Cat Food Nutrient Profiles*

Nutrient	Units DM Basis	Growth and Reproduction Minimum	Adult Maintenance Minimum	Maximum
Protein	%	30.0	26.0	
Arginine	%	1.25	1.04	
Histidine	%	0.31	0.31	
Isoleucine	%	0.52	0.52	
Leucine	%	1.25	1.25	
Lysine	%	1.10	0.83	
Methionine-cystine	%	1.10	1.10	
Methionine	%	0.62	0.62	1.5
Phenylalanine-tyrosine	%	0.88	0.88	
Phenylalanine	%	0.42	0.42	
Threonine	%	0.73	0.73	
Tryptophan	%	0.25	0.16	
Valine	%	0.62	0.62	
Fat†	%	9.0	9.0	
Linoleic acid	%	0.5	0.5	
Arachidonic acid	%	0.02	0.02	
Minerals				
Calcium	%	1.0	0.6	
Phosphorus	%	0.8	0.5	
Potassium	%	0.6	0.6	
Sodium	%	0.2	0.2	
Chloride	%	0.3	0.3	
Magnesium‡	%	0.08	0.04	
Iron§	mg/kg	80	80	
Copper (extruded)¶	mg/kg	15	5	
Copper (canned)¶	mg/kg	5	5	
Manganese	mg/kg	7.5	7.5	
Zinc	mg/kg	75	75	2,000
Iodine	mg/kg	0.35	0.35	
Selenium	mg/kg	0.1	0.1	
Vitamins and others				
Vitamin A	IU/kg	9,000	5,000	750,000
Vitamin D	IU/kg	750	500	10,000
Vitamin E‖	IU/kg	30	30	
Vitamin K**	mg/kg	0.1	0.1	
Thiamine††	mg/kg	5.0	5.0	
Riboflavin	mg/kg	4.0	4.0	
Pantothenic acid	mg/kg	5.0	5.0	
Niacin	mg/kg	60	60	
Pyridoxine	mg/kg	4.0	4.0	
Folic acid	mg/kg	0.8	0.8	
Biotin‡‡	mg/kg	0.07	0.07	
Vitamin B_{12}	mg/kg	0.02	0.02	
Choline§§	mg/kg	2,400	2,400	
Taurine (extruded)	%	0.10	0.10	
Taurine (canned)	%	0.20	0.20	

*Presumes an energy density of 4.0 kcal ME/gm DM, based on the "modified Atwater" values of 3.5, 8.5, and 3.5 kcal/gm for protein, fat, and carbohydrate (nitrogen-free extract, NFE), respectively. Rations greater than 4.5 kcal/gm should be corrected for energy density; rations less than 4.0 kcal/gm should *not* be corrected for energy.

†Although a true requirement for fat per se has not been established, the minimum level was based on recognition of fat as a source of essential fatty acids, as a carrier of fat-soluble vitamins, to enhance palatability, and to supply an adequate caloric density.

‡If the mean urine pH of cats fed ad libitum is not below 6.4, the risk of struvite urolithiasis increases as the magnesium content of the diet increases.

§Because of very poor bioavailability, iron from carbonate or oxide sources that are added to the diet should not be considered in determining the minimum nutrient level.

¶Because of very poor bioavailability, copper from oxide sources that are added to the diet should not be considered in determining the minimum nutrient level.

‖Add 10 IU of vitamin E above minimum level per gram of fish oil per kilogram of diet.

**Vitamin K does not need to be added unless diet contains more than 25% fish on a dry matter basis.

††Because processing may destroy up to 90% of the thiamine in the diet, allowances in formulation should be made to ensure that the minimum nutrient level is met after processing.

‡‡Biotin does not need to be added unless diet contains antimicrobial or antivitamin compounds.

§§Methionine may be used to substitute for choline as a methyl donor at a rate of 3.75 parts for 1 part choline by weight when methionine exceeds 0.62%.

Compendium of Animal Rabies Control, 1999*
National Association of State Public Health Veterinarians, Inc.

The purpose of this Compendium is to provide rabies information to veterinarians, public health officials, and others concerned with rabies control. These recommendations serve as the basis for animal rabies control programs throughout the United States and facilitate standardization of procedures among jurisdictions, thereby contributing to an effective national rabies control program. This document is reviewed annually and revised as necessary. Immunization procedure recommendations are contained in Part I; all animal rabies vaccines licensed by the United States Department of Agriculture (USDA) and marketed in the United States are listed in Part II; Part III details the principles of rabies control.

Part I: Recommendations for Parenteral Immunization Procedures

A.　**VACCINE ADMINISTRATION:** All animal rabies vaccines should be restricted to use by, or under the direct supervision of, a veterinarian.

B.　**VACCINE SELECTION:** In comprehensive rabies control programs, only vaccines with a 3-year duration of immunity should be used. This constitutes the most effective method of increasing the proportion of immunized dogs and cats in any population. (See Part II.)

C.　**ROUTE OF INOCULATION:** All vaccines must be administered in accordance with the specifications of the product label or package insert. If administered intramuscularly, it must be at one site in the thigh.

D.　**WILDLIFE AND HYBRID ANIMAL VACCINATION:** The efficacy of parenteral rabies vaccination of wildlife and hybrids (the offspring of wild animals crossbred to domestic dogs and cats) has not been established, and no such vaccine is licensed for these animals. Zoos or research institutions may establish vaccination programs which attempt to protect valuable animals, but these should not replace appropriate public health activities that protect humans.

E.　**ACCIDENTAL HUMAN EXPOSURE TO VACCINE:** Accidental inoculation may occur during administration of animal rabies vaccine. Such exposure to inactivated vaccines constitutes no rabies hazard.

F.　**IDENTIFICATION OF VACCINATED ANIMALS:** All agencies and veterinarians should adopt the standard tag system. This practice will aid the administration of local, state, national, and international control procedures. Animal license tags should be distinguishable in shape and color from rabies tags. Anodized aluminum rabies tags should be no less than 0.064 inches in thickness.

1.　**RABIES TAGS**

YEAR	COLOR	SHAPE
1999	Green	Bell
2000	Red	Heart
2001	Blue	Rosette
2002	Orange	Oval

2.　**RABIES CERTIFICATE:** All agencies and veterinarians should use the NASPHV form #51, "Rabies Vaccination Certificate," which can be obtained from vaccine manufacturers. Computer-generated forms containing the same information are acceptable.

THE NASPHV COMMITTEE
Suzanne R. Jenkins, VMD, MPH, Chair
Michael Auslander, DVM, MSPH
Robert H. Johnson, DVM
Mira J. Leslie, DVM
F. T. Satalowich, DVM, MSPH
Faye E. Sorhage, VMD, MPH

*Address all correspondence to:
Suzanne R. Jenkins, VMD, MPH
Virginia Department of Health
Office of Epidemiology
Post Office Box 2448, Room 113
Richmond, VA 23218

CONSULTANTS TO THE COMMITTEE
Deborah J. Briggs, PhD; Kansas State University Rabies
　Laboratory
James E. Childs, ScD; Centers for Disease Control
　and Prevention (CDC)
Mary Currier, MD, MPH; CSTE
David W. Dreesen, DVM, MPVM; private consultant
Nancy Frank, DVM, MPH; AVMA Council on Public Health and
　Regulatory Veterinary Medicine
Jim McCord, DVM; Animal Health Institute
Robert B. Miller, DVM, MPH; Animal and Plant Health
　Inspection Service, USDA
Charles E. Rupprecht, VMD, PhD; CDC
Charles V. Trimarchi, MS; New York State Rabies Laboratory

ENDORSED BY:
American Veterinary Medical Association (AVMA)
Council of State and Territorial Epidemiologists (CSTE)

Part II: Rabies Vaccines Licensed in U.S. and NASPHV Recommendations, 1999

Product Name	Produced by	Marketed by	For Use In	Dosage	Age at Primary Vaccination[1]	Booster Recommended	Route of Inoculation
A) MONOVALENT (Inactivated)							
TRIMUNE	Fort Dodge Animal Health License No. 112	Fort Dodge Animal Health	Dogs Cats	1 ml 1 ml	3 months & 1 year later 3 months & 1 year later	Triennially Triennially	IM[2] IM
ANNUMUNE	Fort Dodge Animal Health License No. 112	Fort Dodge Animal Health	Dogs Cats	1 ml 1 ml	3 months 3 months	Annually Annually	IM IM
DEFENSOR 1	Pfizer, Incorporated License No. 189	Pfizer, Incorporated	Dogs Cats	1 ml 1 ml	3 months 3 months	Annually Annually	IM or SC[3] SC
DEFENSOR 3	Pfizer, Incorporated License No. 189	Pfizer, Incorporated	Dogs Cats Sheep Cattle	1 ml 1 ml 2 ml 2 ml	3 months & 1 year later 3 months & 1 year later 3 months 3 months	Triennially Triennially Annually Annually	IM or SC SC IM IM
RABDOMUN	Pfizer, Incorporated License No. 189	Schering-Plough	Dogs Cats Sheep Cattle	1 ml 1 ml 2 ml 2 ml	3 months & 1 year later 3 months & 1 year later 3 months 3 months	Triennially Triennially Annually Annually	IM or SC SC IM IM
RABDOMUN 1	Pfizer, Incorporated License No. 189	Schering-Plough	Dogs Cats	1 ml 1 ml	3 months 3 months	Annually Annually	IM or SC SC
RABVAC 1	Fort Dodge Animal Health License No. 112	Fort Dodge Animal Health	Dogs Cats	1 ml 1 ml	3 months 3 months	Annually Annually	IM or SC IM or SC
RABVAC 3	Fort Dodge Animal Health License No. 112	Fort Dodge Animal Health	Dogs Cats Horses	1 ml 1 ml 2 ml	3 months & 1 year later 3 months & 1 year later 3 months	Triennially Triennially Annually	IM or SC IM or SC IM
PRORAB-1	Intervet, Incorporated License No. 286	Intervet, Incorporated	Dogs Cats Sheep	1 ml 1 ml 2 ml	3 months 3 months 3 months	Annually Annually Annually	IM or SC IM or SC IM
PRORAB-3F	Intervet, Incorporated License No. 286	Intervet, Incorporated	Cats	1 ml	3 months & 1 year later	Triennially	IM or SC
IMRAB 3	Merial License No. 298	Merial	Dogs Cats Sheep Cattle Horses Ferrets	1 ml 1 ml 2 ml 2 ml 2 ml 1 ml	3 months & 1 year later 3 months & 1 year later 3 months & 1 year later 3 months 3 months 3 months	Triennially Triennially Triennially Annually Annually Annually	IM or SC IM or SC IM or SC IM or SC IM or SC SC
IMRAB BOVINE PLUS	Merial License No. 298	Merial	Cattle Horses Sheep	2 ml 2 ml 2 ml	3 months 3 months 3 months & 1 year later	Annually Annually Triennially	IM or SC IM or SC IM or SC
IMRAB 1	Merial License No. 298	Merial	Dogs Cats	1 ml 1 ml	3 months 3 months	Annually Annually	IM or SC IM or SC
B) COMBINATION (Inactivated rabies)							
ECLIPSE 3 + FeLV/R	Fort Dodge Animal Health License No. 112	Schering-Plough	Cats	1 ml	3 months	Annually	IM or SC
ECLIPSE 4 + FeLV/R	Fort Dodge Animal Health License No. 112	Schering-Plough	Cats	1 ml	3 months	Annually	IM or SC
Fel-O-Guard 3 + FeLV/R	Fort Dodge Animal Health License No. 112	Fort Dodge Animal Health	Cats	1 ml	3 months	Annually	IM or SC
Fel-O-Guard 4 + FeLV/R	Fort Dodge Animal Health License No. 112	Fort Dodge Animal Health	Cats	1 ml	3 months	Annually	IM or SC
Fel-O-Vax PCT-R	Fort Dodge Animal Health License No. 112	Fort Dodge Animal Health	Cats	1 ml	3 months & 1 year later	Triennially	IM
FELINE 4 + IMRAB	Merial License No. 298	Merial.	Cats	1 ml	3 months & 1 year later	Triennially	SC
FELINE 3 + IMRAB	Merial License No. 298	Merial	Cats	1 ml	3 months & 1 year later	Triennially	SC
EQUINE POTOMAVAC + IMRAB	Merial License No. 298	Merial	Horses	1 ml	3 months	Annually	IM
MYSTIQUE II	Bayer Corporation License No. 52	Bayer Corporation	Horses	1 ml	3 months	Annually	IM
C) ORAL (Rabies glycoprotein, live vaccinia vector) - RESTRICTED TO USE IN STATE AND FEDERAL RABIES CONTROL PROGRAMS							
RABORAL V-RG	Merial License No. 298	Merial	Raccoons	N/A	N/A	determined by state authorities	Oral

* Formerly Rhone Merieux.
1 Three months of age (or older) and revaccinated one year later.
2 Intramuscularly.
3 Subcutaneously.

Part III: Rabies Control

A. PRINCIPLES OF RABIES CONTROL

1. **RABIES EXPOSURE:** Rabies is transmitted only when the virus is introduced into bite wounds, open cuts in skin, or onto mucous membranes.

2. **HUMAN RABIES PREVENTION:** Rabies in humans can be prevented either by eliminating exposures to rabid animals or by providing exposed persons with prompt local treatment of wounds combined with appropriate passive and active immunization. The rationale for recommending preexposure and postexposure rabies prophylaxis and details of their administration can be found in the current recommendations of the Immunization Practices Advisory Committee (ACIP), of the Public Health Service (PHS). These recommendations, along with information concerning the current local and regional status of animal rabies and the availability of human rabies biologics, are available from state health departments.

3. **DOMESTIC ANIMALS:** Local governments should initiate and maintain effective programs to ensure vaccination of all dogs, cats, and ferrets and to remove strays and unwanted animals. Such procedures in the United States have reduced laboratory confirmed cases in dogs from 6,949 in 1947 to 126 in 1997. Since more rabies cases are reported annually involving cats (300 in 1997) than dogs, vaccination of cats should be required. The recommended vaccination procedures and the licensed animal vaccines are specified in Parts I and II of the Compendium.

4. **RABIES IN WILDLIFE:** The control of rabies among wildlife reservoirs is difficult. Vaccination of free-ranging wildlife or selective population reduction may be useful in some situations, but the success of such procedures depends on the circumstances surrounding each rabies outbreak. (See Part C. Control Methods in Wildlife.)

B. CONTROL METHODS IN DOMESTIC AND CONFINED ANIMALS

1. **PREEXPOSURE VACCINATION AND MANAGEMENT**
   Parenteral animal rabies vaccines should be administered only by, or under the direct supervision of, a veterinarian. This is the only way to ensure that a responsible person can be held accountable to assure the public that the animal has been properly vaccinated. Within 1 month after primary vaccination, a peak rabies antibody titer is reached and the animal can be considered immunized. An animal is currently vaccinated and is considered immunized if it was vaccinated at least 30 days previously, and all vaccinations have been administered in accordance with this Compendium. Regardless of the age at initial vaccination, a second vaccination should be given one year later. (See Parts I and II for recommended vaccines and procedures.)

   (a) DOGS, CATS, AND FERRETS
   All dogs, cats and ferrets should be vaccinated against rabies at 3 months of age and revaccinated in accordance with Part II of this Compendium. If a previously vaccinated animal is overdue for a booster, it should be revaccinated with a single dose of vaccine and placed on an annual or triennial schedule depending on the type of vaccine used.

   (b) LIVESTOCK
   It is neither economically feasible nor justified from a public health standpoint to vaccinate all livestock against rabies. However, consideration should be given to vaccination of livestock which are particularly valuable and/or may have frequent contact with humans.

   (c) OTHER ANIMALS
      (1) WILD
      No parenteral rabies vaccine is licensed for use in wild animals. Because of the risk of rabies in wild animals (especially raccoons, skunks, coyotes, foxes, and bats), the AVMA, the NASPHV, and the CSTE strongly recommend the enactment of state laws prohibiting the importation, distribution, relocation, or keeping of wild animals or hybrids as pets.

      (2) MAINTAINED IN EXHIBITS AND IN ZOOLOGICAL PARKS
      Captive animals not completely excluded from all contact with rabies vectors can become infected. Moreover, wild animals may be incubating rabies when initially captured; therefore, wild-caught animals susceptible to rabies should be quarantined for a minimum of 180 days before exhibition. Employees who work with animals at such facilities should receive preexposure rabies immunization. The use of pre- or postexposure rabies immunizations of employees who work with animals at such facilities may reduce the need for euthanasia of captive animals.

2. **STRAY ANIMALS**
   Stray dogs, cats, or ferrets should be removed from the community. Local health departments and animal control officials can enforce the removal of strays more effectively if owned animals are confined or kept on leash. Strays should be impounded for at least 3 days to give owners sufficient time to reclaim animals and to determine if human exposure has occurred.

3. **IMPORTATION AND INTERSTATE MOVEMENT of ANIMALS**

(a) INTERNATIONAL

CDC regulates the importation of dogs and cats into the United States, but present PHS regulations (42 CFR No. 71.51) governing the importation of such animals are insufficient to prevent the introduction of rabid animals into the country. All dogs and cats imported from countries with endemic rabies should be currently vaccinated against rabies as recommended in this Compendium. The appropriate public health official of the state of destination should be notified within 72 hours of any unvaccinated dog or cat imported into his or her jurisdiction. The conditional admission of such animals into the United States is subject to state and local laws governing rabies. Failure to comply with these requirements should be promptly reported to the Division of Quarantine, CDC, 404-639-8107.

(b) INTERSTATE

Prior to interstate movement, dogs, cats, and ferrets should be currently vaccinated against rabies in accordance with the Compendium's recommendations (See Part III, B.1. Preexposure Vaccination and Management). Animals in transit should be accompanied by a currently valid NASPHV Form #51, Rabies Vaccination Certificate.

4. **ADJUNCT PROCEDURES**

Methods or procedures which enhance rabies control include:

(a) LICENSURE. Registration or licensure of all dogs, cats, and ferrets may be used to aid in rabies control. A fee is frequently charged for such licensure and revenues collected are used to maintain rabies or animal control programs. Vaccination is an essential prerequisite to licensure.

(b) CANVASSING OF AREA. House-to-house canvassing by animal control personnel facilitates enforcement of vaccination and licensure requirements.

(c) CITATIONS. Citations are legal summonses issued to owners for violations, including the failure to vaccinate or license their animals. The authority for officers to issue citations should be an integral part of each animal control program.

(d) ANIMAL CONTROL. All communities should incorporate stray animal control, leash laws, and training of personnel in their programs.

5. **POSTEXPOSURE MANAGEMENT**

ANY ANIMAL POTENTIALLY EXPOSED TO RABIES VIRUS (See Part III, A. 1. Rabies Exposure) BY A WILD, CARNIVOROUS MAMMAL OR A BAT THAT IS NOT AVAILABLE FOR TESTING SHOULD BE REGARDED AS HAVING BEEN EXPOSED TO RABIES.

(a) DOGS, CATS, AND FERRETS

Unvaccinated dogs, cats, and ferrets exposed to a rabid animal should be euthanized immediately. If the owner is unwilling to have this done, the animal should be placed in strict isolation for 6 months and vaccinated 1 month before being released. Animals with expired vaccinations need to be evaluated on a case by case basis. Dogs, cats, and ferrets that are currently vaccinated should be revaccinated immediately, kept under the owner's control, and observed for 45 days.

(b) LIVESTOCK

All species of livestock are susceptible to rabies; cattle and horses are among the most frequently infected. Livestock exposed to a rabid animal and currently vaccinated with a vaccine approved by USDA for that species should be revaccinated immediately and observed for 45 days. Unvaccinated livestock should be slaughtered immediately. If the owner is unwilling to have this done, the animal should be kept under very close observation for 6 months.

The following are recommendations for owners of unvaccinated livestock exposed to rabid animals:

(1) If the animal is slaughtered within 7 days of being bitten, its tissues may be eaten without risk of infection, provided liberal portions of the exposed area are discarded. Federal meat inspectors must reject for slaughter any animal known to have been exposed to rabies within 8 months.

(2) Neither tissues nor milk from a rabid animal should be used for human or animal consumption. However, since pasteurization temperatures will inactivate rabies virus, drinking pasteurized milk or eating cooked meat does not constitute a rabies exposure.

(3) It is rare to have more than one rabid animal in a herd, or herbivore to herbivore transmission; therefore, it may not be

necessary to restrict the rest of the herd if a single animal has been exposed to or infected by rabies.

(c) OTHER ANIMALS

Other animals bitten by a rabid animal should be euthanized immediately. Animals maintained in USDA licensed research facilities or accredited zoological parks should be evaluated on a case by case basis.

6. **MANAGEMENT OF ANIMALS THAT BITE HUMANS**

A healthy dog, cat, or ferret that bites a person should be confined and observed for 10 days; it is recommended that rabies vaccine not be administered during the observation period. Such animals should be evaluated by a veterinarian at the first sign of illness during confinement. Any illness in the animal should be reported immediately to the local health department. If signs suggestive of rabies develop, the animal should be euthanized, its head removed, and the head shipped under refrigeration (not frozen) for examination of the brain by a qualified laboratory designated by the local or state health department. Any stray or unwanted dog, cat, or ferret that bites a person may be euthanized immediately and the head submitted as described above for rabies examination. Other biting animals which might have exposed a person to rabies should be reported immediately to the local health department. Prior vaccination of an animal may not preclude the necessity for euthanasia and testing if the period of virus shedding is unknown for that species. Management of animals other than dogs, cats, and ferrets depends on the species, the circumstances of the bite, the epidemiology of rabies in the area, and the biting animal's history, current health status, and potential for exposure to rabies.

C. CONTROL METHODS IN WILDLIFE

The public should be warned not to handle wildlife. Wild mammals and hybrids that bite or otherwise expose people, pets or livestock should be considered for euthanasia and rabies examination. A person bitten by any wild mammal should immediately report the incident to a physician who can evaluate the need for antirabies treatment. (See current rabies prophylaxis recommendations of the ACIP.)

1. **TERRESTRIAL MAMMALS**

The use of licensed oral vaccines for the mass immunization of free-ranging wildlife should be considered in selected situations, with the approval of the state agency responsible for animal rabies control. Continuous and persistent government-funded programs for trapping or poisoning wildlife are not cost effective in reducing wildlife rabies reservoirs on a statewide basis. However, limited control in high-contact areas (picnic grounds, camps, suburban areas) may be indicated for the removal of selected high-risk species of wildlife. The state wildlife agency and state health department should be consulted for coordination of any proposed vaccination or population reduction programs.

2. **BATS**

(a) Indigenous rabid bats have been reported from every state except Hawaii, and have caused rabies in at least 32 humans in the United States. It is neither feasible nor desirable, however, to control rabies in bats by programs to reduce bat populations.

(b) Bats should be excluded from houses and adjacent structures to prevent direct association with humans. Such structures should then be made bat-proof by sealing entrances used by bats.

Immunization of Wild Mammal Species Against Common Diseases

R. Eric Miller
St. Louis, Missouri

Nancy L. Anderson
Columbus, Ohio

Susceptibility to disease is variable among exotic animals, sometimes even among species of the same family. Often, because thoroughly tested vaccination regimens and subsequent challenge studies are lacking, vaccination schedules for nondomestic species must be considered as recommendations. Given that, it is always important to weigh the risk of disease versus the risks associated with vaccination, particularly in many of these exotic species for which side effects can be more common and/or severe. Obviously, any vaccination program should also be based on a knowledge of the local prevalence of the diseases in question.

The following information focuses on vaccination recommendations for the species that a veterinary practitioner is likely to see in nondomestic animal practice and is based, in part, on vaccination schedules found to be effective for related domestic species (see *CVT X*, p. 727, for more information and a discussion of immunization of exotic carnivores). Whenever possible, inactivated or recombinant vaccines should be used in preference to modified live virus (MLV) products. The use of MLV vaccines in nonapproved species carries the risk of vaccine-induced disease, possible immunosuppression, and the risk that vaccinated animals may shed virus to unvaccinated individuals. No rabies vaccine is licensed for use in wild animal species, but if it is used, it must contain only inactivated virus. Before administering any rabies vaccine to *any* nondomestic species, always contact your local and state veterinary authorities regarding the legal aspects of rabies vaccination in their jurisdiction.

Further information on vaccinations may be obtained by contacting the veterinarian at your local zoo or a member of the American College of Zoological Medicine (members listed in the board specialty section of the *AVMA Directory*).

Additionally, it should be noted that private ownership of wild animal species is strongly discouraged and, in many localities, is restricted by law. Be aware that in most states, ownership of native nondomestic species requires special permission, and threatened and endangered species can only be held subject to the regulations of the Endangered Species Act.

FAMILY CANIDAE (e.g., Wolf, fox)

Canine Distemper. Commercial canine vaccines are currently available only as MLV preparations. In nondomestic canids, it appears that the avian-origin MLV vaccine (Fromm D, Solvay Veterinary) was the safest vaccine for the widest variety of species (Montali et al, 1983). However, this formulation is no longer commercially available. Current choices for safe vaccination of nondomestic canids are limited. The Species Survival Plan (SSP) Committees of the American Zoo and Aquarium Association (AZA) recommend vaccination of wolves and maned wolves with a univalent CD product (Galaxy-D, Fort Dodge). In most other species, especially gray wolves and kit foxes, LMV canine distemper vaccines of canine cell origin should be carefully avoided because they are associated with a high incidence of vaccine-induced distemper (Halbrooks et al, 1981). Currently, Merial manufactures a multivalent vaccination for dogs that includes a canary pox vectored recombinant DNA univalent CD vaccine. The recombinant CD portion of the vaccine, when manufactured as a univalent product, appears to provide safe protection against CD for many nondomestic canids. Unfortunately, the univalent vaccine is not commercially available, and the multivalent vaccine cannot be recommended for vaccination in nondomestic canids owing to the MLV components for adenovirus and parvovirus. Considering the high incidence of vaccine-induced disease associated with commercially available products, in some cases strict isolation from sources of CD virus may be preferable to vaccination until safer products are available.

Infectious Canine Hepatitis. Inactivated vaccines are not commercially available. If performed, vaccination is recommended with canine adenovirus-2 products to reduce the risk of corneal opacity.

Canine Parvovirus. Infection with canine parvovirus has been reported in numerous wild canid species, particularly those from South America (maned wolf, raccoon dogs, bush dogs); (Mann et al, 1980). Vaccination with an inactivated vaccine is warranted.

Leptospirosis. Vaccination with a multivalent commercial bacterin is recommended.

FAMILY FELIDAE (e.g., Tiger, lion, ocelot, margay, bobcat).

Feline Panleukopenia. Exotic felids appear to be particularly sensitive to this virus, so vaccination is required. Vaccination should be performed only with an inactivated virus (see later) according to the manufacturer's recommendation or the following schedule: vaccination every 2 weeks from 8 to 16 weeks of age, then boostered at 6 months, then annually.

Feline Rhinotracheitis and Calicivirus. Infection with feline rhinotracheitis and calicivirus has been reported in exotic felids, often with devastating consequences. All exotic felids should be vaccinated for these diseases with an inactivated vaccine (commercially available in combination with inactivated feline panleukopenia as Fel-O-Vax, Fort Dodge; Bush et al, 1981). Humoral titers with these vaccines are generally short-lived and boosters every 3 months may be warranted in high-risk situations (Wack et al, 1993).

Feline Leukemia. Reports of infection with feline leukemia virus (FeLV) in exotic felids are uncommon; however it is advisable to test all felids for exposure. A present, FeLV vaccination is not commonly practiced in zoological parks (Citino, 1988), although some institutions do so when there is close contact with feral cats.

Feline Infectious Peritonitis. Although feline infectious peritonitis can occur in exotic felid species, vaccination for this disease is not generally practiced.

Canine Distemper. Canine distemper has been reported in large nondomestic felids both in Africa and in North America. However, at the present time, most nondomestic cats that are in zoological institutions or are privately owned are not vaccinated for this disease.

FAMILY PROCYONIDAE (Raccoons, coatimundi, kinkajou)

Canine Distemper. Members of this family are extremely susceptible to disease caused by the canine distemper virus (Mehren, 1986). Vaccinate with caution, as for the canid family. Kinkajous have exhibited a particular sensitivity to CD vaccines. Only inactivated vaccines are safe in red pandas (Montali et al, 1983).

Feline Panleukopenia. Although reports of infection with feline panleukopenia virus are less common than those with canine distemper, most facilities currently vaccinate procyonids for this disease. Use an inactivated vaccine without components for the feline respiratory viruses (Phillips, 1989).

FAMILY MUSTELIDAE (Ferrets, skunks)

Canine Distemper. Vaccination of all mustelids for canine distemper is recommended, as for the canids. Ferravac (United Vaccines) is specifically made for ferrets; however, anaphylaxis is still seen more commonly than in dogs, and postvaccinal signs of vague malaise are relatively common. Otters are particularly sensitive to vaccine-induced distemper. Additionally, particular caution should be exercised with black-footed ferrets (an endangered species); they have developed vaccine-induced disease with MLV vaccines (They are currently vaccinated with a killed CD vaccine that is not commercially available.)

Feline Panleukopenia. All mustelids except ferrets (Parrish et al, 1987) are considered susceptible to feline panleukopenia. However, because of the uncommon reports of the disease in skunks kept as pets, there are regional differences in the frequency of vaccination for this disease. If practiced for skunks and for other mustelids, vaccination for members of this family should be as for felids, but without the feline respiratory component. Mink can be vaccinated with either feline panleukopenia or mink viral enteritis vaccines.

Botulism. Mink and ferrets are susceptible to botulism induced by *Clostridium botulinum* type C toxin. Commercial mink are routinely vaccinated with the appropriate toxoid, but owing to different management conditions (unless they are fed a commercial mink diet), vaccination is not routinely practiced in pet ferrets.

Rabies. An inactivated rabies vaccine (Imrab, Rhone Poulenc, Athens, GA) has been approved for use in ferrets; however, local veterinary authorities should be contacted regarding the legal aspects of vaccination in each community.

FAMILY VIVERRIDAE (Binturong, civet, fossa)

Canine Distemper. Canine distemper has been reported in binturongs and civets. It is generally recommended that all captive viverrids be vacccinated (Phillips, 1989).

Feline Panleukopenia. Although cases of feline panleukopenia are not well documented, it is generally recommended that captive viverrids be vaccinated as for procyonids.

FAMILY URSIDAE (Bears)

Canine Distemper and Feline Panleukopenia. Bears are not generally considered to be susceptible to either of these diseases, and no vaccinations are routinely administered.

Infectious Canine Hepatitis. Infectious canine hepatitis has been reported from a colony of American black bears (Whetstone et al, 1988). However, vaccination of captive bears for canine adenovirus is not generally recommended.

ORDER MARSUPIALIA, FAMILY DIDELPHIDAE (opossums), and FAMILY PETAURIDAE (sugar gliders)

Routine vaccination of these species is not practiced.

ORDER PRIMATES

Tetanus. Primates are susceptible to tetanus and should be vaccinated with tetanus toxoid products. After two initial doses, vaccination can be practiced at more prolonged intervals (2 to 3 years) or in the interim if an injury occurs.

Measles, Yellow Fever, Rabies, Hepatitis A and B, Poliomyelitis. Vaccination for all are used in certain or all primate species when circumstances warrant. Inoculation for poliomyelitis is advisable for great apes. Advice for these and other primate preventive medicine techniques should be sought from a primate research center. The CDC immunization recommendations for humans is also another valuable information resource.

ORDER RODENTIA

Mice, rats, hamsters, gerbils, guinea pigs, squirrels. No routine vaccines are recommended for these animals when they are kept as caged pets.

ORDER LAGOMORPHA (Rabbits, hares)

No routine vaccinations are recommended for these animals when they are kept as caged pets.

ORDER ARTIODACTYLA, FAMILY CAMELIDAE (Llama)

Tetanus. Llamas are routinely vaccinated for tetanus with a commercial toxoid (Fowler, 1989).

Enterotoxemia. Llamas are susceptible to enterotoxemia produced by *Clostridium perfringens* types C and D, particularly in the first 3 weeks of life. Adults should be vaccinated annually, and vaccination of pregnant dams 8 and 5 weeks prior to parturition confers immunity on the neonate until it can respond to its own vaccination regimen (Fowler, 1989).

ORDER ARTIODACTYLA, FAMILY CERVIDAE
(Deer, moose)

Clostridial Diseases. Deer can be affected by enterotoxemia caused by *Clostridium perfringens* types C and D.

Vaccination can be practiced with the appropriate bacterin. Owing to the occurrence of blackleg (*Clostridium chauveoi*) in moose, many vaccinate moose species with a multivalent clostridial bacterin.

Rabies. In endemic areas, killed rabies vaccines have been used.

References and Suggested Reading

Bush M, Povey RC, Koonse H: Antibody response to inactivated vaccine for rhinotracheitis, caliciviral disease, and panleukopenia in non-domestic felids. J Am Vet Med Assoc 179:1203, 1981.

Citino SB: Use of a subunit feline leukemia virus vaccine in exotic cats. J Am Vet Med Assoc 192:957, 1988.

Fowler ME: Llama basics. In: Kirk RW, ed: Current Veterinary Therapy X. Philadelphia: WB Saunders, 1989, p 736.

Halbrooks RD, Swango LJ, Schnurrenberger PR, et al: Response of gray foxes to modified live virus canine distemper vaccines. J Am Vet Med Assoc 179:1170, 1981.

Mann PC, Bush M, Appel MJG, et al: Canine parvovirus infection in South American canids. J Am Vet Med Assoc 177:779, 1980.

Mehren KG: Procyonidae. In: Fowler ME, ed: Zoo and Wild Animal Medicine. Philadelphia: WB Saunders, 1986, p 820.

Montali RJ, Barty CR, Teare JA, et al: Clinical trials with canine distemper vaccines in exotic carnivores. J Am Vet Med Assoc 183:1163, 1983.

Parrish CR, Leathers CW, Pearson R: Comparisons of feline panleukopenia virus, canine parvovirus, raccoon parvovirus and mink enteritis and their pathogenicity for mink and ferrets. Am J Vet Res 48:1429, 1987.

Phillips LG: Preventive medicine in nondomestic carnivores. In: Kirk RW, ed: Current Veterinary Therapy X. Philadelphia: WB Saunders, 1989, pp 728–729.

Wack RF, Kramer LW, Cupps WL: The response of cheetahs (*Acinonyx jubatus*) to routine vaccination. J Zoo Wildlife Dis 24:109, 1993.

Whetstone CA, Draayer H, Collins JE: Characterization of canine adenovirus type I isolated from American black bears. Am J Vet Res 47:778, 1988.

Treatment of Parasites

CRAIG R. REINEMEYER

Knoxville, Tennessee

TABLE 1. Anthelmintics for Nematode Parasites of Dogs and Cats*

Drug	Nematode Spectrum	Species	Dosage
Dichlorvos (Task Tabs, TechAmerica)	Ascarids, hookworms	Canine, feline	11 mg/kg PO
Dichlorvos (Task Dog Anthelmintic, TechAmerica)	Ascarids, hookworms, whipworms	Canine	33 mg/kg PO
Diethylcarbamazine (DEC) + oxibendazole (Filaribits Plus, Pfizer)	Ascarids, hookworms, whipworms	Canine	6.6 mg/kg DEC and 5 mg/kg oxibendazole PO q24h
Febantel (Rintal, Bayer)	Ascarids, hookworms, whipworms	Canine, feline	10 mg/kg PO q24h for 3 days
Febantel + praziquantel (Vercom, Bayer)	Ascarids, hookworms, whipworms	Canine, feline	Febantel 10 mg/kg, and praziquantel 1 mg/kg PO q24h for 3 days; 15 mg/kg and 1.5 mg/kg for animals <6 months
Febantel + pyrantel pamoate + praziquantel (Drontal Plus, Bayer)	Ascarids, hookworms, whipworms	Canine	Febantel 25 mg/kg PO, and pyrantel 5 mg/kg PO, and praziquantel 5 mg/kg PO
Fenbendazole (Panacur, Hoechst)	Ascarids, hookworms, whipworms	Canine	50 mg/kg PO q24h for 3 days
Mebendazole (Telmintic, Schering Animal Health)	Ascarids, hookworms, whipworms	Canine	22 mg/kg PO q24h for 3 days
Milbemycin (Interceptor, Novartis)	Ascarids, hookworms, whipworms	Canine	0.5 mg/kg PO once monthly
Piperazine (generic, various sources)	Ascarids	Canine, feline	44–66 mg/kg PO
Pyrantel pamoate (Nemex, Pfizer)	Ascarids, hookworms	Canine, feline†	Dogs: 5 mg/kg PO Cats: 20 mg/kg PO
Pyrantel pamoate + ivermectin (Heartgard Plus, Merck)	Ascarids, hookworms	Canine	>5 mg/kg pyrantel, and ivermectin >6 µg/kg PO once monthly
Pyrantel pamoate + praziquantel (Drontal, Bayer)	Ascarids, hookworms	Feline	Pyrantel 20 mg/kg, and praziquantel 5 mg/kg PO

*For more complete information on treatment and control of internal parasites, see Reinemeyer CR: Canine gastrointestinal parasites. In: Bonagura JD, Kirk RW, eds: Current Veterinary Therapy XII. Philadelphia: WB Saunders, 1995, p 711; Reinemeyer CR: Feline gastrointestinal parasites. In: Kirk RW, Bonagura JD, eds: Current Veterinary Therapy XI. Philadelphia: WB Saunders, 1992, p 626.

†Extra-label application.

Ascarids (i.e., *Toxocara canis, Toxocara cati, Toxascaris leonina*); hookworms (i.e., *Ancylostoma caninum, Ancylostoma tubaeforme, Uncinaria stenocephala*); whipworms (i.e., *Trichuris vulpis*).

TABLE 2. Anthelmintics for Cestode Parasites of Dogs and Cats*

Drug	Cestode Spectrum	Species	Dosage
Epsiprantel (Cestex, Pfizer)	*Dipylidium caninum, Taenia pisiformis, T. taeniaeformis*	Canine, feline	Dogs: 5.5 mg/kg PO Cats: 2.75 mg/kg PO
Praziquantel (Droncit, Bayer)	*D. caninum, Echinococcus granulosus, E. multilocularis, T. pisiformis, T. taeniaeformis*	Canine, feline	5–12.5 mg/kg PO, IM, SC
Praziquantel + febantel	*D. caninum, T. pisiformis, T. taeniaeformis*	Canine, feline	See Vercom, Table 1
Praziquantel + pyrantel pamoate	*D. caninum, T. taeniaeformis*	Feline	See Drontal, Table 1
Praziquantel + pyrantel pamoate + febantel	*D. caninum, E. granulosus E. multilocularis, T. pisiformis*	Canine	See Drontal Plus, Table 1
Fenbendazole (Panacur, Hoechst Roussel Vet)	*T. pisiformis*	Canine	50 mg/kg PO q24h 3 days
Mebendazole (Telmintic, Schering Animal Health)	*T. pisiformis*	Canine	22 mg/kg PO q24h 3 days

*See footnote, Table 1.

TABLE 3. **Compounds for Protozoal Parasites of Dogs and Cats***

Drug	Protozoal Spectrum	Species	Dosage
Albendazole (Valbazen, Pfizer)	*Giardia*	Canine,† feline†	Dogs: 25 mg/kg PO q12h for 2 days; Cats: 25 mg/kg PO q12h for 5 days
Amprolium (Amprovine, Merial)	*Isospora* spp	Canine†	0.75% solution as sole source of drinking water
Fenbendazole (Panacur, Hoechst Roussel Vet)	*Giardia*	Canine,† feline†	50 mg/kg PO q24h for 3 days
Metronidazole (Flagyl, Searle)	*Giardia*	Canine,† feline†	25 mg/kg PO q12h for 5 days
Sulfadiazine + trimethoprim (Tribrissen, Schering Animal Health; Di-Trim, Fort Dodge)	*Isospora*	Canine,† feline†	30 mg/kg PO q24h for 10 days
Sulfadimethoxine (Albon, Pfizer; Bactrovet, Schering Animal Health)	*Isospora*	Canine, feline	50 mg/kg q24h once; 25 mg/kg PO q24h for 4–9 days

*See footnote, Table 1.
†Extra-label application.

Table of Common Drugs: Approximate Dosages

MARK G. PAPICH

Consulting Editor

Drug Name	Other Names	Formulations Available	Dosage
Acemannan	Acemannan Immunostimulant	10-mg vial reconstituted to 1 mg/ml	Dog: intraperitoneal (1 mg/kg) and intralesional injection (2 mg) every week for 6 treatments Cat: 2 mg/kg intraperitoneal or SC per week for 6 weeks
Acepromazine	PromAce and many generic brands	5-, 10-, and 25-mg tablets and 10-mg/ml injection	Dog: 0.56–1.13 mg/kg IM, SC, IV; 0.56–2.25 mg/kg PO q6–8hr Cat: 1.13–2.25 mg/kg IM, SC, IV
Acetaminophen	Tylenol and many generic brands	120-, 160-, 325-, and 500-mg tablets	Dog: 15 mg/kg PO q8hr Cat: not recommended
Acetaminophen with codeine	Tylenol with codeine and many generic brands	Oral solution and tablets. Many forms (e.g., 300 mg acetaminophen plus either 15, 30, or 60 mg codeine)	Follow dosing recommendations for codeine
Acetazolamide	Diamox	125- and 250-mg tablets	5–10 mg/kg PO q8–12hr Glaucoma: 4–8 mg/kg PO q8–12hr
Acetylcysteine	Mucomyst	20% solution	Antidote: 140 mg/kg (loading dose) then 70 mg/kg IV or PO q4hr for five doses Eye: 2% solution topically q2hr
Acetylsalicylic acid	*See* Aspirin		
ACTH	*See* Corticotropin		
Actinomycin D	Cosmegen	Powder for IV injection	0.5 to 0.9 mg/m² IV (consult anti-cancer protocol for intervals)
Activated charcoal	*See* Charcoal, activated		
Adequan	*See* Polysulfated glycosaminoglycan (PSGAG)		
Albendazole	Valbazen	113.6-mg/ml suspension and 300-mg/ml paste	25–50 mg/kg PO q12hr × 3 days For *Giardia* use 25 mg/kg q12hr × 2 days
Albuterol	Proventil or Ventolin	2-, 4-, and 5-mg tablets; 2 mg/5 ml syrup	20–50 μg/kg four times/day; up to maximum of 100 μg/kg four times daily
Allopurinol	Lopurin, Zyloprim	100- and 300-mg tablets	10 mg/kg q8hr, then reduce to 10 mg/kg q24hr
Aluminum carbonate gel	Basalgel	Capsule (equivalent to 500 mg aluminum hydroxide)	10–30 mg/kg PO q8hr (with meals)
Aluminum hydroxide gel	Amphojel	64-mg/ml oral suspension; 600-mg tablet	10–30 mg/kg PO q8hr (with meals)
Amikacin	Amiglyde-V (veterinary) and Amikin (human)	50- and 250-mg/ml injection	Dog, cat: 6.5 mg/kg IV, IM, SC q8hr or 20 mg/kg IV, IM, SC q24hr
Aminopentamide	Centrine	0.2-mg tablet; 0.5-mg/ml injection	Dog: 0.01–0.03 mg/kg IM, SC, PO q8–12 hr Cat: 0.1 mg/cat IM, SC, PO q8–12 hr
Aminophylline	Many (generic)	100- and 200-mg tablets: 25-mg/ml injection	Dog: 10 mg/kg PO, IM, IV q8hr Cat: 6.6 mg/kg PO q12hr
6-Aminosalicylic acid	*See* Mesalamine, Olsalazine		

Table continued on following page

Drug Name	Other Names	Formulations Available	Dosage
Amitraz	Mitaban	10.6-ml concentrated dip (19.9%)	10.6 ml per 7.5 L water (0.025% solution). Apply three to six topical treatments q2 wk. For refractory cases, this dose has been exceeded to produce increased efficacy. Doses that have been used include 0.025, 0.05, and 0.1% concentration applied twice a week and 0.125% solution applied to one-half body every day for 4 weeks to 5 months.
Amitriptyline	Elavil	10-, 25-, 50-, 75-, 100-, and 150-mg tablets; 10-mg/ml injection	Dog: 1–2 mg/kg PO q12–24hr (range: 0.25–4 mg/kg q12–24hr) Cat: 2 mg/kg or approx. 5–10 mg per cat per day PO
Amlodipine besylate	Norvasc	2.5-, 5-, and 10-mg tablets	Dog: 2.5 mg/dog or 0.1 mg/kg PO once daily Cat: 0.625 mg/cat/day PO initially and increase if needed to 1.25 mg/cat/day (average is 0.18 mg/kg)
Ammonium chloride	Generic	Available as crystals	Dog: 100 mg/kg PO q12hr Cat: 800 mg/cat (approximately ⅓ to ¼ tsp) mixed with food daily
Amoxicillin trihydrate	Amoxi-Tabs, Amoxi-drops, Amoxil, and others	50-, 100-, 200-, and 400-mg tablets; 50-mg/ml oral suspension	6–20 mg/kg PO q8–12hr
Amoxicillin/clavulanic acid	Clavamox	62.5-, 125-, 250-, and 375-mg tablets; 62.5-mg/ml suspension	Dog: 12.5–25 mg/kg PO q12hr Cat: 62.5 mg/cat PO q12hr; consider administering these doses q8hr for gram-negative infections
Amphotericin B	Fungizone	50-mg injectable vial	0.5 mg/kg IV (slow infusion) q48hr, to a cumulative dose of 4–8 mg/kg
Amphotericin B	Other forms include amphotericin B cholesteryl sulfate complex (Amphotec); amphotericin B lipid complex (Abelcet); and amphotericin B liposomal complex (AmBisome). Use in dogs has been limited for these products.		
Ampicillin	Omnipen, Principen, others	250- and 500-mg capsules; 125-, 250-, and 500-mg vials of ampicillin sodium	10–20 mg/kg IV, IM, SC q6–8hr (ampicillin sodium) 20–40 mg/kg PO q8hr
Ampicillin + sulbactam	Unasyn	1.5 and 3 gm vials in 2:1 combination for injection	10–20 mg/kg IV, IM q8hr
Ampicillin trihydrate	Polyflex	10- and 25-mg vials for injection	6.5–10 mg/kg IM, SC q12hr
Amprolium	Amprol, Corid	9.6% (9.6 gm/dl) oral solution; soluble powder	1.25 gm of 20% amprolium powder to daily feed, or 30 ml of 9.6% amprolium solution to 3.8 L of drinking water for 7 days
Antacid drugs	*See* Aluminum hydroxide gel, Magnesium hydroxide, and Calcium carbonate		
Apomorphine hydrochloride	Generic	6-mg tablet	0.02–0.04 mg/kg IV, IM, 0.1 mg/kg SC, or instill 0.25 mg in conjunctiva of eye (dissolve 6-mg tablet in 1–2 ml of saline)
Ascorbic acid	Vitamin C	Various forms	100–500 mg/animal/day (diet supplement) or 100 mg/animal q8hr (urine acidification)
L-Asparaginase	Elspar	10,000 U per vial for injection	400 U/kg IV, IP, IM weekly
Aspirin	Many generic and brand names (Bufferin, Ascriptin)	81-mg and 325-mg tablets	Dog: Mild analgesia: 10 mg/kg q12hr; anti-inflammatory: 20–25 mg/kg q12hr; antiplatelet: 5–10 mg/kg q24–48hr Cat: 10–20 mg/kg q48hr; antiplatelet: 80 mg q48hr
Astemizole	Hismanal	10-mg tablet	Dog: 0.2 mg/kg q24hr, up to 1.0 mg/kg PO q12hr
Atenolol	Tenormin	25-, 50-, and 100-mg tablets; 25-mg/ml oral suspension; and 0.5-mg/ml ampule for injection	Dog: 6.25–12.5 mg/dog q12hr (or 0.25–1.0 mg/kg q12–24hr) Cat: 6.25–12.5 mg/cat q12hr (approx. 3 mg/kg)

Drug Name	Other Names	Formulations Available	Dosage
Atipamezole	Antisedan	5-mg/ml injection	Inject same volume as used for medetomidine
Atracurium	Tracrium	10-mg/ml injection	0.2 mg/kg IV initially, then 0.15 mg/kg q30min (or IV infusion at 3–8 μg/kg/min)
Atropine	Many generic brands	400-, 500-, and 540 μg/ml injection; 15-mg/ml injection	0.02–0.04 mg/kg IV, IM, SC q6–8hr 0.2–0.5 mg/kg (as needed) for organophosphate and carbamate toxicosis
Auranofin (triethylphosphine gold)	Ridaura	3-mg capsule	0.1–0.2 mg/kg PO q12hr
Aurothioglucose	Solganol	50-mg/ml injection	Dog < 10 kg: 1 mg IM first week, 2 mg IM second week, 1 mg/kg/week maintenance Dog > 10 kg: 5 mg IM first week, 10 mg IM second week, 1 mg/kg/week maintenance Cat: 0.5–1 mg/cat IM q7days
Azathioprine	Imuran	50-mg tablet; 10-mg/ml for injection	Dog: 2 mg/kg PO q24hr initially then 0.5–1 mg/kg q48hr Cat (use cautiously): 1 mg/kg PO q48hr
Azithromycin	Zithromax	250-mg capsule; and 250- and 600-mg tablets; 20 mg/ml oral suspension	Dog: 10 mg/kg PO once every 5 days or 3.3 mg/kg once daily for 3 days Cat: 5 mg/kg PO every other day
AZT (azidothymidine)	*See* Zidovudine		
Bactrim (sulfamethoxazole + trimethoprim)	*See* Trimethoprim-sulfonamide combinations		
BAL	*See* Dimercaprol		
Benazepril	Lotensin	5-, 10-, 20-, and 40-mg tablets	Dog: 0.25–0.5 mg/kg PO q24hr Cat: Same
Betamethasone	Celestone	600-μg (0.6-mg) tablet; 3-mg/ml sodium phosphate injection	0.1–0.2 mg/kg PO q12–24hr
Bethanechol	Urecholine	5-, 10-, 25-, and 50-mg tablets; 5-mg/ml injection	Dog: 5–15 mg/dog PO q8hr Cat: 1.25–5 mg/cat PO q8hr
Bisacodyl	Dulcolax	5-mg tablet	5 mg/animal PO q8–24hr
Bismuth subcarbonate			0.3–3.0 gm PO q4hr
Bismuth subsalicylate	Pepto Bismol	Oral suspension; 262 mg/15 ml or 525 mg/ml in extrastrength formulation; 262-mg tablet	1–3 ml/kg/day (in divided doses) PO
Bleomycin	Blenoxane	15-U vials for injection	10 U/m^2 IV or SC for 3 days, then 10 U/m^2 weekly (maximum cumulative dose 200 U/m^2)
Bromide	*See* Potassium bromide		
BSP (Bromsulphalein); *see* Sulfobromophthalein (BSP)			
Bunamidine hydrochloride	Scolaban	400-mg tablet	20–50 mg/kg PO
Bupivacaine	Marcaine and generic	2.5- and 5-mg/ml solution injection	1 ml of 0.5% solution per 10 cm for an epidural
Buprenorphine	Temgesic (Vetergesic in the UK)	0.3-mg/ml solution	Dog: 0.006–0.02 mg/kg IV, IM, SC q4–8hr Cat: 0.005–0.01 mg/kg IV, IM q4–8hr
Buspirone	BuSpar	5- and 10-mg tablets	Cat: 2.5–5 mg/cat PO q24hr (may be increased to twice daily for some cats)
Busulfan	Myleran	2-mg tablet	3–4 mg/m^2 PO q24hr

Table continued on following page

Drug Name	Other Names	Formulations Available	Dosage
Butorphanol	Torbutrol Torbugesic	1-, 5-, and 10-mg tablets; 0.5- or 10-mg/ml injection	Dog: antitussive: 0.055 mg/kg SC q6–12hr or 0.55 mg/kg PO; preanesthetic: 0.2–0.4 mg/kg IV, IM, SC (with acepromazine); analgesic: 0.2–0.4 mg/kg IV, IM, SC q2–4hr or 0.55–1.1 mg/kg PO q6–12hr Cat: analgesic: 0.2–0.8 mg/kg IV, SC q2–6hr, or 1.5 mg/kg PO q4–8hr
Calcitriol	Rocaltrol, Calcijex	Available as injection (Calcijex) and capsules (Rocaltrol): 0.25- and 0.5-μg capsules; 1- or 2-μg/ml injection	Dog (renal failure): 0.25 to 0.5 μg/dog/day PO Cat (hypocalcemia): 0.01 to 0.04 μg/kg/day PO (or 0.25 μg/cat every other day)
Calcium carbonate	Many brands available: Titralac, Tums, generic	Many tablets or oral suspension (e.g., 650-mg tablet (contains 260 mg calcium ion)	5–10 ml of oral solution PO q4–6hr For phosphate binder: 60–100 mg/kg/day in divided doses PO
Calcium chloride	Generic	10% (100 mg/ml) solution	0.1–0.3 ml/kg IV (slowly)
Calcium citrate	Citracal (OTC)	950-mg tablet (contains 200 mg calcium ion)	Cat: 10–30 mg/kg PO q8hr (with meals)
Calcium disodium EDTA	*See* Edetate calcium disodium		
Calcium gluconate	Kalcinate and generic	10% (100 mg/ml) injection	0.5–1.5 ml/kg IV (slowly)
Calcium lactate	Generic	OTC tablet	Dog: 0.5–2.0 gm/dog/day PO (in divided doses) Cat: 0.2–0.5 gm/cat/day PO (in divided doses)
Captopril	Capoten	25-mg tablet	Dog: 0.5–2 mg/kg PO q8–12hr Cat: 3.12–6.25 mg/cat PO q8hr
Carbenicillin	Geopen, Pyopen	1-, 2-, 5-, 10-, and 30-gm vials for injection	40–50 mg/kg and up to 100 mg/kg IV, IM, SC q6–8hr
Carbenicillin indanyl sodium	Geocillin	500-mg tablet	10 mg/kg PO q8hr
Carbimazole	Neo-mercazole	Available in Europe	Cat: 5 mg/cat PO q8hr (induction), followed by 5 mg/cat PO q12hr
Carboplatin	Paraplatin	50- and 150-mg vial for injection	Dog: 300 mg/m² IV q3–4 wk Cat: 200 mg/m² IV q4wk
Carprofen	Rimadyl (Zinecarp in the UK)	25-, 75-, and 100-mg tablets	Dog: 2.2 mg/kg PO q12hr Cat: doses not available
Cascara sagrada	Many brands (e.g., Nature's Remedy)	100- and 325-mg tablets	Dog: 1–5 mg/kg day PO Cat: 1–2 mg/cat/day
Castor oil	Generic	Oral liquid (100%)	Dog: 8–30 ml/day PO Cat: 4–10 ml/day PO
Cefaclor	Ceclor	250- and 500-mg capsules and 25-mg/ml oral suspension	4–20 mg/kg PO q8hr
Cefadroxil	Cefa-Tabs, Cefa-Drops	50-mg/ml oral suspension; 50-, 100-, 200-, and 1,000-mg tablets	Dog: 22–30 mg/kg PO q12hr Cat: 22 mg/kg PO q24hr
Cefazolin sodium	Ancef, Kefzol, and generic	50 and 100 mg/50 ml for injection	20–35 mg/kg IV, IM q8hr For perisurgical use: 22 mg/kg q2hr during surgery
Cefdinir	Omnicef	300-mg capsules; 25-mg/ml oral suspension	Dose not established (human dose is 7 mg/kg PO q12hr)
Cefixime	Suprax	20-mg/ml oral suspension and 200- and 400-mg tablets	10 mg/kg PO q12hr For cystitis: 5 mg/kg PO q12–24hr
Cefotaxime	Claforan	500-mg and 1-, 2-, and 10-gm vials for injection	Dog: 50 mg/kg IV, IM, SC q12hr Cat: 20–80 mg/kg IV, IM q6hr
Cefotetan	Cefotan	1-, 2-, and 10-gm vials for injection	30 mg/kg IV, SC q8hr
Cefoxitin sodium	Mefoxin	1-, 2-, and 10-gm vials for injection	30 mg/kg IV q6–8hr
Ceftazidime	Fortaz, Ceptaz, Tazicef	0.5-, 1-, 2- and 6-gm vials reconstituted to 280 mg/ml	30 mg/kg IV, IM q6hr
Ceftiofur	Naxcel (ceftiofur sodium); Excenel (ceftiofur HCL)	50-mg/ml injection	2.2–4.4 mg/kg SC q24hr (for urinary tract infections)

Drug Name	Other Names	Formulations Available	Dosage
Cephalexin	Keflex and generic forms	250- and 500-mg capsules; 250- and 500-mg tablets; 100-mg/ml or 125- and 250-mg/5-ml oral suspension	10–30 mg/kg PO q6–12hr; for pyoderma, 22–35 mg/kg PO q12hr
Cephalothin sodium	Keflin	1- and 2-gm vials for injection	10–30 mg/kg IV, IM q4–8hr
Cephapirin	Cefadyl	500-mg and 1-, 2-, and 4-gm vials for injection	10–30 mg/kg IV, IM q4–8hr
Cephradine	Velosef	250- and 500-mg capsules; 250- and 500-mg and 1- and 2-gm vials for injection	10–25 mg/kg PO q6–8hr
Charcoal, activated	ActaChar, Charcodote, Toxiban, generic	Oral suspension	1–4 gm/kg PO (granules) 6–12 ml/kg (suspension)
Chlorambucil	Leukeran	2-mg tablet	2–6 mg/m² *or* 0.1–0.2 mg/kg PO q24hr initially, then q48hr
Chloramphenicol and chloramphenicol palmitate	Chloromycetin, generic forms	30-mg/ml oral suspension (palmitate); 250-mg capsule; and 100-, 250-, and 500-mg tablets	Dog: 40–50 mg/kg PO q8hr Cat: 12.5–20 mg/kg PO q12hr
Chloramphenicol sodium succinate	Chloromycetin, generic	100-mg/ml injection	Dog: 40–50 mg/kg IV, IM q6–8hr Cat: 12.5–20 mg/cat IV, IM q12hr
Chlorothiazide	Diuril	250- and 500-mg tablets; 50-mg/ml oral suspension and injection	20–40 mg/kg PO q12hr
Chlorpheniramine maleate	Chlor-Trimeton, Phenetron, and others	4- and 8-mg tablets	Dog: 4–8 mg/dog PO q12hr (up to a maximum of 0.5 mg/kg q12hr) Cat: 2 mg/cat PO q12hr
Chlorpromazine	Thorazine	25-mg/ml injection solution	0.5 mg/kg IM, SC q6–8hr (before cancer chemotherapy administer 2 mg/kg SC q3hr)
Chlortetracycline	Generic	Powdered feed additive	25 mg/kg PO q6–8hr
Chorionic gonadotropin	*See* Gonadotropin		
Cimetidine	Tagamet (OTC and prescription)	100-, 150-, 200-, and 300-mg tablets and 60-mg/ml injection	10 mg/kg IV, IM, PO q6–8hr (in renal failure administer 2.5–5 mg/kg IV, PO q12hr)
Ciprofloxacin	Cipro	250-, 500-, and 750-mg tablets; 2-mg/ml injection	5–15 mg/kg PO, IV q12hr
Cisapride	Propulsid (Prepulsid in Canada)	10-mg tablet	Dog: 0.1–0.5 mg/kg PO q8–12hr (doses as high as 0.5–1.0 mg/kg have been used in some dogs) Cat: 2.5–5 mg/cat PO q8–12hr (as high as 1 mg/kg q8hr has been administered to cats)
Cisplatin	Platinol	1-mg/ml injection; 50-mg vials	Dog: 60–70 mg/m² IV q3–4wk (administer fluid for diuresis with therapy) Cat: not recommended
Clavamox	*See* Amoxicillin-clavulanic acid combination		
Clavulanic acid	*See* Amoxicillin-clavulanic acid combination		
Clemastine	Tavist, Contac 12-hr allergy, and generic	1.34-mg tablet (OTC); 2.64-mg tablet (Rx); 0.134-mg/ml syrup	Dog: 0.05–0.1 mg/kg PO q12hr
Clindamycin	Antirobe, Cleocin	Oral liquid 25-mg/ml; 25-, 75-, and 150-mg capsule; and 150-mg/ml injection (Cleocin)	Dog: 11 mg/kg PO q12hr or 22 mg/kg PO q24hr Cat: 5.5 mg/kg q12hr, or 11 mg/kg q24hr (staphylococcal infections); 11 mg/kg q12hr or 22 mg/kg q24hr (anaerobic infections) PO Toxoplasmosis: 12.5 mg/kg PO q12hr for 4 weeks
Clofazimine	Lamprene	50- and 100-mg capsules	Cat: 1 mg/kg PO up to a maximum of 4 mg/kg/day
Clomipramine	Anafranil (human label); Clomicalm (veterinary label)	10-, 25-, and 50-mg tablets (human) 5-, 20-, and 80-mg tablets (veterinary)	Dog: 1–2 mg/kg PO q12hr up to a maximum of 3 mg/kg PO q12hr Cat: 1–5 mg/cat PO q12–24hr

Table continued on following page

Drug Name	Other Names	Formulations Available	Dosage
Clonazepam	Klonopin	0.5-, 1-, and 2-mg tablets	0.5 mg/kg PO q8–12hr
Clorazepate	Tranxene	3.75-, 7.5-, 11.25-, 15-, and 22.5-mg tablets	2 mg/kg PO q12hr
Cloxacillin	Cloxapen, Orbenin, Tegopen	250- and 500-mg capsules; 25-mg/ml oral solution	20–40 mg/kg PO q8hr
Codeine	Generic	15, 30-, and 60-mg tablets; 5-mg/ml syrup; 3-mg/ml oral solution	Analgesia: 0.5–1 mg/kg PO q4–6hr Antitussive: 0.1–0.3 mg/kg PO q4–6hr
Colchicine	Generic	500- and 600-μg tablets; 500-μg/ml ampule injection	0.01–0.03 mg/kg PO q24hr
Colony-stimulating factor	Amgen		2.5 μg/kg SC q12hr
Corticotropin (ACTH)	Acthar	Gel 80 U/ml	Response test: collect pre-ACTH sample and inject 2.2 IU/kg IM; collect post-ACTH sample in 2 hr in dogs and at 1 and 2 hr in cats
Cosequin	See Glucosamine chondroitin sulfate		
Cosyntropin	Cortrosyn	250 μg per vial (can be stored in freezer for 6 months)	Response test: collect pre-ACTH sample and inject 5 μg/kg IV in dogs and 0.125 mg IV in cats; collect post sample at 1 hr
Cyanocobalamin (vitamin B_{12})	Many	100 μg/ml injection	Dog: 100–200 μg/day PO Cat: 50–100 μg/day PO
Cyclophosphamide	Cytoxan, Neosar	25-mg/ml injection; 25- and 50-mg tablets	Anticancer: 50 mg/m² PO once daily 4 days/wk or 150–300 mg/m² IV and repeat in 21 days Immunosuppressive therapy: 50 mg/m² (approx. 2.2 mg/kg) PO q48hr or 2.2 mg/kg once daily for 4 days/wk Cat: 6.25–12.5 mg/cat once daily 4 days/wk
Cyclosporine (cyclosporin A)	Neoral; Sandimmune, Optimmune (ophthalmic)	Neoral: 25-mg and 100-mg microemulsion capsules; 100-mg/ml oral solution (for microemulsion) Sandimmune: 100-mg/ml oral solution; 25- and 100-mg capsules. Optimmune: 0.2% ointment	Dog: 3–7 mg/kg PO q12hr (adjust dose by monitoring blood concentrations) Cat: 4–6 mg/kg PO q12hr
Cyropheptadine	Periactin	4-mg tablet; 2-mg/5 ml syrup	Antihistamine: 1.1 mg/kg PO q8–12hr Appetite stimulant: 2 mg/cat PO
Cytarabine (cytosine arabinoside)	Cytosar-U	100-mg vial	Dog (lymphoma): 100 mg/m² IV, SC once daily or 50 mg/m² twice daily for 4 days Cat: 100 mg/m² once daily for 2 days
Dacarbazine	DTIC	200-mg vial for injection	200 mg/m² IV for 5 days q3wk; or 800–1,000 mg/m² IV q3wk
Danazol	Danocrine	50-, 100-, and 200-mg capsules	5–10 mg/kg PO q12hr
Dantrolene	Dantrium	100-mg capsule and 0.33-mg/ml injection	For prevention of malignant hyperthermia: 2–3 mg/kg IV Dog: 1–5 mg/kg PO q8hr Cat: 0.5–2 mg/kg PO q12hr
Dapsone	Generic	25- and 100-mg tablets	1.1 mg/kg PO q8–12hr
Darbazine (prochlorperazine + isopropamide)	Darbazine	No. 1, 2, and 3 capsules	Dog and cat: 0.14–0.2 ml/kg SC q12hr Dog 2–7 kg: 1-#1 capsule PO q12hr Dog 7–14 kg: 1-#2 capsule PO q12hr Dog > 14 kg: 1-#3 capsule PO q12hr
Deferoxamine	Desferal	500-mg vial for injection	10 mg/kg IV, IM q2hr for two doses; then 10 mg/kg q8hr for 24 hr

Drug Name	Other Names	Formulations Available	Dosage
Deprenyl (L-deprenyl)	*See* Selegiline (Anipryl)		
Desmopressin acetate	DDAVP	100-μg/ml injection and desmopressin acetate nasal solution (0.01% metered spray); 0.1- and 0.2-mg tablets	Diabetes insipidus: 2–4 drops (2 μg) q12–24hr intranasally or in eye. Animal oral dose not established, but dose extrapolated from humans is 0.05 mg/animal, q12hr PO, and increase to 0.1 or 0.2 mg/animal as needed. von Willebrand's disease treatment: 1 μg/kg (0.01 ml/kg) SC, IV, diluted in 20 ml of saline administered over 10 minutes
Desoxycorticosterone pivalate	Percorten-V, DOCP, or DOCA pivalate	Injection	1.5–2.2 mg/kg IM q25days
Detomidine	Dormosedan	10-mg/ml injection	Doses not established for small animals
Dexamethasone (dexamethasone solution and dexamethasone sodium phosphate)	Azium solution in polyethylene glycol. Sodium phosphate forms include Dexaject SP, Dexavet, and Dexasone. Tablets include Decadron and generic	Azium solution, 2 mg/ml. Sodium phosphate forms are 3.33 mg/ml; 0.25-, 0.5-, 0.75-, 1-, 1.5-, 2-, 4-, and 6-mg tablets	Anti-inflammatory: 0.07–0.15 mg/kg IV, IM, PO q12–24hr. For shock, spinal injury: 2.2–4.4 mg/kg IV (of sodium phosphate form) Dexamethasone suppression test: Dog: 0.01 mg/kg IV Cat: 0.1 mg/kg IV Collect sample at 0, 4 and 8 hours
Dextran	Dextran 70 Gentran-70	Injectable solution: 250, 500, and 1,000 ml	10–20 ml/kg IV to effect
Dextromethorphan	Benylin and others	Available in syrup, capsule, and tablet; many OTC products	0.5–2 mg/kg PO q6–8hr
Dextrose solution 5%	D5W	Fluid solution for IV administration	40–50 ml/kg IV q24hr
Diazepam	Valium and generic	2- and 5-mg tablets; 5-mg/ml solution for injection	Preanesthetic: 0.5 mg/kg IV Status epilepticus: 0.5 mg/kg IV, 1.0 mg/kg rectal; repeat if necessary Appetite stimulant (cat): 0.2 mg/kg IV
Dichlorophen	Vermiplex (*See* Toluene)		
Dichlorphenamide	Daranide	50-mg tablet	3–5 mg/kg PO q8–12hr
Dichlorvos	Task	10- and 25-mg tablets	Dog: 26.4–33 mg/kg PO Cat: 11 mg/kg PO
Dicloxacillin	Dynapen	125-, 250-, and 500-mg capsules; 12.5-mg/ml oral suspension	25 mg/kg IM q6hr Oral doses not absorbed
Diethylcarbamazine (DEC)	Caricide, Filaribits	Chewable tablets; 50-, 60-, 180-, 200-, and 400-mg tablets	Heartworm prophylaxis: 6.6 mg/kg PO q24hr
Diethylstilbestrol (DES)	DES, generic (no longer manufactured in US)	1- and 5-mg tablet; 50-mg/ml injection	Dog: 0.1–1.0 mg/dog PO q24hr Cat: 0.05–0.1 mg/cat PO q24hr
Difloxacin	Dicural	11.4-, 45.4-, and 136-mg tablets	5–10 mg/kg/day PO
Digitoxin	Crystodigin	0.05- and 0.1-mg tablets	0.02–0.03 mg/kg PO q8hr
Digoxin	Lanoxin, Cardoxin	0.0625-, 0.125-, 0.25-mg tablets; 0.05- and 0.15-mg/ml elixir	Dog: < 20 kg body weight: 0.01 mg/kg q12hr; >20 kg use 0.22 mg/m^2 PO q12hr (subtract 10% for elixir) Dog (rapid digitalization): 0.0055–0.011 mg/kg IV q1hr to effect Cat: 0.008–0.01 mg/kg PO q48hr (approximately ¼ of a 0.125-mg tablet/cat)
Dihydrotachysterol (vitamin D)	Hytakerol, DHT	0.125-mg tablet; 0.5 mg/ml oral liquid	0.01 mg/kg/day PO; for acute treatment administer 0.02 mg/kg initially, then 0.01–0.02 mg/kg PO q24–48hr thereafter

Table continued on following page

Drug Name	Other Names	Formulations Available	Dosage
Diltiazem	Cardizem, Dilacor	30-, 60-, 90-, and 120-mg tablets; 50-mg/ml injection	Dog: 0.5–1.5 mg/kg PO q8hr, 0.25 mg/kg over 2 min IV (repeat if necessary) Cat: 1.75–2.4 mg/kg PO q8hr For Dilacor XR or Cardizem CD dose is 10 mg/kg PO once daily
Dimenhydrinate	Dramamine (Gravol in Canada)	50-mg tablets; 50-mg/ml injection	Dog: 4–8 mg/kg PO, IM, IV q8hr Cat: 12.5 mg/cat IV, IM, PO q8hr
Dimercaprol (BAL)	BAL in oil	Injection	4 mg/kg IM q4hr
Dinoprost tromethamine	*See* Prostaglandin F$_{2\alpha}$ 5-mg/ml injection		
Dioctyl calcium sulfosuccinate	*See* Docusate calcium		
Dioctyl sodium sulfosuccinate	*See* Docusate sodium		
Diphenhydramine	Benadryl	Available OTC: 2.5-mg/ml elixir; 25- and 50-mg capsules and tablets; 50-mg/ml injection	2–4 mg/kg PO q6–8hr or 1 mg/kg IM, IV (for dogs, administer 25–50 mg/dog IV, IM, PO q8hr)
Diphenoxylate	Lomotil	2.5 mg	Dog: 0.1–0.2 mg/kg PO q8–12hr Cat: 0.05–0.1 mg/kg PO q12hr
Diphenylhydantoin	*See* Phenytoin		
Diphosphonate disodium etidronate	*See* Etidronate disodium		
Dipyridamole	Persantine	25-, 50-, 75-mg tablets; 5-mg/ml injection	4–10 mg/kg PO q24hr
Dipyrone		No longer available	
Disophenol	DNP	No longer available	10 mg/kg (0.22 ml/kg) SC, once
Disopyramide	Norpace (Rhythmodan in Canada)	100- and 150-mg capsules (10-mg/ml injection in Canada only)	6–15 mg/kg PO q8hr
Dithiazanine iodide	Dizan	10-, 50-, 100-, and 200-mg tablets	Heartworm: 6.6–11 mg/kg PO q24hr for 7–10 days For other parasites: 22 mg/kg PO
Divalproex sodium	*See* Valproic acid		
Dobutamine	Dobutrex	250 mg/20 ml vial for injection (12.5 mg/ml)	Dog: 5–20 μg/kg/min IV infusion Cat: 0.5–2 μg/kg/min IV infusion
Docusate calcium	Surfak, Doxidan	60-mg tablet (and many others)	Dog: 50–100 mg/dog PO q12–24hr Cat: 50 mg/cat PO q12–24 hr
Docusate sodium	Colace, Doxan, Doss, many OTC brands	50- and 100-mg capsules; 10-mg/ml liquid	Dog: 50–200 mg/dog PO q8–12hr Cat: 50 mg/cat PO q12–24hr
Domperidone	Motilium	Not available in US	2–5 mg/animal PO
Dopamine	Intropin	40-, 80-, or 160-mg/ml	Dog, cat: 2–10 μg/kg/min IV infusion
Doxapram	Dopram No longer available in US	20-mg/ml injection	5–10 mg/kg IV Neonate: 1–5 mg SC, sublingual, or via umbilical vein
Doxorubicin	Adriamycin	2-mg/ml injection	30 mg/m^2 IV q21 days or >20 kg use 30 mg/m^2 and <20 kg use 1 mg/kg Cat: 1 mg/kg IV q3wk
Doxycycline	Vibramycin and generic forms	10-mg/ml oral suspension; 100-mg tablet; 100-mg injection vial	3–5 mg/kg PO, IV q12hr or 10 mg/kg PO q24hr For *Rickettsia* in dogs: 5 mg/kg q12hr
Edetate calcium disodium (CaNa$_2$EDTA)	Calcium disodium versenate	20-mg/ml injection	25 mg/kg SC, IM, IV q6hr for 2–5 days
Edrophonium	Tensilon and others	10-mg/ml injection	Dog: 0.11–0.22 mg/kg IV Cat: 2.5 mg/cat IV
Enalapril	Enacard, Vasotec	2.5-, 5-, 10-, and 20-mg tablets	Dog: 0.5 mg/kg PO q12–24 hr Cat: 0.25–0.5 mg/kg PO q12–24hr
Enflurane	Ethrane	Available as solution for inhalation	Induction: 2–3% Maintenance: 1.5–3%

Drug Name	Other Names	Formulations Available	Dosage
Enilconazole	Imaverol, Clina-Farm-EC	10% or 13.8% emulsion	Nasal aspergillosis: 10 mg/kg q12hr instilled into nasal sinus for 14 days (10% solution diluted 50/50 with water) Dermatophytes: dilute 10% solution to 0.2% and wash lesion with solution four times at 3- to 4-day intervals
Enrofloxacin	Baytril	68-, 22.7-mg, and 5.7-mg tablets. Taste Tabs are 22.7 and 68 mg; 22.7-mg/ml injection	5–20 mg/kg/day PO, IM
Ephedrine	Many, generic	25- and 50-mg/ml injection	Urinary incontinence: 4 mg/kg, or 12.5–50 mg/dog PO q8–12hr (2–4 mg/kg for cats) Vasopressor: 0.75 mg/kg, IM, SC; repeat as needed
Epinephrine	Adrenaline and generic forms	1-mg/ml (1:1,000) injection solution	Cardiac arrest: 10–20 µg/kg IV or 200 µg/kg intratracheal (may be diluted in saline before administration) Anaphylactic shock: 2.5–5 µg/kg IV or 50 µg/kg intratracheal (may be diluted in saline)
Epsiprantel	Cestex	Coated tablet	Dog: 5.5 mg/kg PO Cat: 2.75 mg/kg PO
Ergocalciferol (vitamin D_2)	Calciferol, Drisdol	400-U tablet (OTC); 50,000-U tablet (1.25 mg); 500,000-U/ml (12.5 mg/ml) injection	500–2,000 U/kg/day PO
Erythromycin	Many brands and generic	250-mg capsule or tablet	Antibacterial dose: 10–20 mg/kg PO q8–12hr Prokinetic dose: 0.5–1.0 mg/kg PO q8hr
Erythropoietin (r-HuEPO)	Epogen, epoetin alfa (r-HuEPO)	2,000-U/ml injection	Doses range from 35 or 50 U/kg three times/wk to 400 U/kg/wk IV, SC (adjust dose to hematocrit of 0.30–0.34)
Esmolol	Brevibloc	10-mg/ml injection	500 µg/kg IV, which may be given as 0.05–0.1 mg/kg slowly every 5 minutes or 50–200 µg/kg/min infusion
Estradiol cypionate (ECP)	ECP, Depo-Estradiol, generic	2-mg/ml injection	Dog: 22–44 µg/kg IM (total dose not to exceed 1.0 mg) Cat: 250 µg/cat IM between 40 hr and 5 days of mating
Etidronate disodium	Didronel	200- and 400-mg tablets; 50-mg/ml injection	Dog: 5 mg/kg/day PO Cat: 10 mg/kg/day PO
Etodolac	EtoGesic, veterinary; Lodine, human	150- and 300-mg tablets	Dog: 10–15 mg/kg PO once daily Cat: Dose not established
Etretinate	Tegison	10- and 25-mg capsules	Dog: 1 mg/kg PO, with food/day or for <15 kg 10 mg/dog PO q24hr; >15 kg 10 mg/dog PO q12hr Cat: 2 mg/kg/day
Famotidine	Pepcid	10-mg tablet; 10-mg/ml injection	0.25 mg/kg IM, SC, PO, IV q12hr; or 0.5 mg/kg IM, SC, PO, IV q24hr
Felbamate	Felbatol	400- and 600-mg tablets; 120-mg/ml oral flavored suspension	Dog: Start with 15 mg/kg PO q8hr and increase gradually to maximum of 65 mg/kg q8hr
Fenbendazole	Panacur, Safe-Guard	Panacur granules 22.2% (222 mg/gm); 100-mg/ml liquid	50 mg/kg/day PO for 3 days
Fentanyl	Sublimaze, generic	250-mg/5 ml injection	0.02–0.04 mg/kg IV, IM, SC q2hr or 0.01 mg/kg IV, IM, SC (with acetylpromazine or diazepam) For analgesia: 0.01 mg/kg IV, IM, SC q2hr

Table continued on following page

Drug Name	Other Names	Formulations Available	Dosage
Fentanyl transdermal	Duragesic	25-, 50-, 75-, and 100-μg/hr patch	Dog: 10–20 kg, 50 μg/hr patch q72hr Cat: 25 μg patch every 118 hr
Ferrous sulfate	Many OTC brands	Many	Dog: 100–300 mg/dog PO q24hr Cat: 50–100 mg/cat PO q24hr
Finasteride	Proscar	5-mg tablets	Dog (BPH): 5-mg tablet/dog PO q24hr
Florfenical	Nuflor	300 mg/ml (cattle)	Dog: 20 mg/kg q6hr PO, IM Cat: 22 mg/kg q12hr IM, PO
Fluconazole	Diflucan	50-, 100-, 150-, and 200-mg tablets; 10- or 40-mg/ml oral suspension; 2-mg/ml IV injection	Dog: 10–12 mg/kg day PO Cat: 50 mg/cat PO q12hr or 50 mg/cat/day PO
Flucytosine	Ancobon	250-mg capsule; 75-mg/ml oral suspension	25–50 mg/kg PO q6–8hr (up to a maximal dose of 100 mg/kg PO q12hr)
Fludrocortisone	Florinef	100-μg (0.1 mg) tablet	Dog: 0.2–0.8 mg/dog or 0.02 mg/kg PO q24hr (13–23 μg/kg) Cat: 0.1–0.2 mg/cat PO q24hr
Flumazenil	Romazicon	100-μg/ml (0.1 mg/ml) injection	0.2 mg (total dose) IV as needed
Flumethasone	Flucort	0.5-mg/ml injection	Dog: 0.0625–0.25 mg/day IV, IM, SC Cat: 0.03–0.125 mg/day IV, IM, SC Anti-inflammatory: 0.15–0.3 mg/kg IV, IM, SC q12–24hr
Flunixin meglumine	Banamine	250-mg packet granules; 10- and 50-mg/ml injection	1.1 mg/kg IV, IM, SC once or 1.1 mg/kg/day PO 3 days/wk Ophthalmic: 0.5 mg/kg IV once
5-Fluorouracil	Fluorouracil	50-mg/ml vial	Dog: 150 mg/m² IV once/week Cat: do not use
Fluoxetine	Prozac	10- and 20-mg capsules; 4-mg/ml oral solution	Dog: 0.5 mg/kg day initially PO then increase to 1 mg/kg/day PO (10–20 mg/dog) Cat: 0.5–4 mg/cat PO q24hr
Follicle-stimulating hormone (FSH)	*See* Urofollitropin		
Fomepizole	*See* 4-Methylpyrazole		
Furazolidone	Furoxone	100-mg tablet	4 mg/kg PO q12hr for 7–10 days
Furosemide	Lasix, generic	12.5-, 20-, and 50-mg tablets; 10-mg/ml oral solution; 50-mg/ml injection	Dog: 2–6 mg/kg IV, IM, SC, PO q8–12hr (or as needed) Cat: 1–4 mg/kg IV, IM, SC, PO q8–24hr
Gemfibrozil	Lopid	300-mg capsules; 600-mg tablets	7.5 mg/kg PO q12hr
Gentamicin	Gentocin	50- and 100-mg/ml solution for injection	Dog: 2–4 mg/kg q6–8hr or 6–10 mg/kg IV, IM, SC q24hr Cat: 3 mg/kg q8hr or 9 mg/kg IV, IM, SC q24hr
Glipizide	Glucotrol	5- and 10-mg tablets	2.5–7.5 mg/cat PO q12hr. Usual dose is 2.5 mg/cat initially, then increase to 5 mg/cat q12hr
Glucosamine chondroitin sulfate	Cosequin and others	Regular (RS) and double-strength (DS) capsules	Dog: 1–2 RS capsules per day (2–4 capsules of DS for large dogs) Cat: 1 RS capsule daily
Glyburide	Diabeta, Micronase, Glynase	1.25-, 2.5-, and 5-mg tablets	0.2 mg/kg/day PO
Glycerin	Generic	Oral solution	1–2 ml/kg, up to PO q8hr
Glycopyrrolate	Robinul-V	0.2-mg/ml injection	0.005–0.01 mg/kg IV, IM, SC
Gold sodium thiomalate	Myochrysine	Injection	1–5 mg IM on first week, then 2–10 mg IM on second week, then 1 mg/kg once/wk IM maintenance
Gold therapy	*See* Aurothioglucose, Gold sodium thiomalate, or Auranofin		
GoLYTELY	*See* Polyethylene glycol electrolyte solution		

Drug Name	Other Names	Formulations Available	Dosage
Gonadorelin (GnRH, LHRH)	Factrel	50-μg/ml injection	Dog: 50–100 μg/dog/day IM q24–48hr Cat: 25 μg/cat IM once
Gonadotropn, chorionic (HCG)	Profasi, Pregnyl, generic, A.P.L.	Injection sizes of 5,000, 10,000 and 20,000 U	Dog: 22 U/kg IM q24–48hr or 44 U IM once Cat: 250 U/cat IM once
Gonadotropin-releasing hormone	*See* Gonadorelin		
Granisetron	Kytril	1-mg/ml injection; 1-mg tablets	0.01 mg/kg (10μg/kg) IV
Griseofulvin (microsize)	Fulvicin U/F	125-, 250-, and 500-mg tablets; 25-mg/ml oral suspension; 125-mg/ml oral syrup	50 mg/kg PO q24hr (up to a maximum dose of 110–132 mg/kg/day in divided treatments)
Griseofulvin (ultramicrosize)	Fulvicin P/G, GrisPEG	100-, 125-, 165-, 250-, and 330-mg tablets	30 mg/kg/day in divided treatments PO
Growth hormone (hGH, somatrem, somatropin)	Protropin, Humatrope, Nutropin	5- and 10-mg/vial	0.1 U/kg SC, IM three times per week for 4–6 weeks (Usual human pediatric dose is 0.18–0.3 mg/kg/wk)
Halothane	Fluothane	250-ml bottle	Induction: 3% Maintenance: 0.5–1.5%
Heparin sodium	Liquaemin (US); Hepalean (Canada)	1,000- and 10,000-U/ml injection	100–200 units/kg IV loading dose; then 100–300 units/kg SC q6–8hr Low-dose prophylaxis (dog and cat): 70 U/kg SC q8–12hr
Hetastarch	*See* Hydroxyethyl starch (HES)		
Hycodan	*See* Hydrocodone bitartrate		
Hydralazine	Apresoline	10-mg tablet; 20-mg/ml injection	Dog: 0.5 mg/kg (initial dose); titrate to 0.5–2 mg/kg PO q12hr Cat: 2.5 mg/cat PO q12–24hr
Hydrochlorothiazide	HydroDIURIL, and generic	10- and 100-mg/ml oral solution and 25-, 50-, and 100-mg tablets	2–4 mg/kg PO q12hr
Hydrocodone bitartrate	Hycodan	5-mg tablet	Dog: 0.22 mg/kg PO q4–8hr Cat: no dose available
Hydrocortisone	Cortef, and generic	5-, 10-, 20-mg tablets	Replacement therapy: 1–2 mg/kg PO q12hr Anti-inflammatory: 2.5–5 mg/kg PO q12hr
Hydrocortisone sodium succinate	Solu-Cortef	Various size vials for injection	Shock: 50–150 mg/kg IV Anti-inflammatory: 5 mg/kg IV q12hr
Hydroxyethyl starch (HES)	HES, Hetastarch	Injection	10–20 ml/kg IV to effect
Hydroxyurea	Hydrea	500-mg capsule	Dog: 50 mg/kg PO once daily, 3 days/wk Cat: 25 mg/kg PO once daily, 3 days/wk
Hydroxyzine	Atarax	10-, 25-, and 50-mg tablets; 2-mg/ml oral solution	Dog: 1–2 mg/kg q6–8hr IM, PO Cat: safe dose not established
Ibuprofen	Motrin, Advil, Nuprin	200-, 400-, 600-, and 800-mg tablets	Safe dose not established
Imipenem	Primaxin	250- or 500-mg vials for injection	3–10 mg/kg IV, IM q6–8hr
Imipramine	Tofranil	10-, 25-, and 50-mg tablets	2–4 mg/kg PO q12–24hr
Indomethacin	Indocin		Safe dose has not been established
Insulin, regular crystalline		100-U/ml injection	Ketoacidosis: animals <3 kg, 1 U/animal initially, then 1 U/animal q1hr; animals 3–10 kg, 2 U/animal initially, then 1 U/animal q1hr; animals >10 kg, 0.25 U/kg initially, then 0.1 U/kg IM q1hr *Table continued on following page*

Drug Name	Other Names	Formulations Available	Dosage
Insulin, NPH isophane		100-U/ml injection	Dog <15 kg: 1 U/kg SC q24hr (to effect) Dog >25 kg: 0.5 U/kg SC q24hr (to effect) Cat: NPH not recommended for cats
Interferon (interferon alpha, HuIFN-alpha)	Roferon	3-million U/vial	Cat: 15–30 U per cat IM or SC once daily for 7 days and repeated every other week
Iodide	*See* Potassium iodide		
Ipecac syrup	Ipecac	Oral solution: 30-ml bottle	Dog: 3–6 ml/dog PO Cat: 2–6 ml/cat PO
Iron	*See* Ferrous sulfate		
Isoflurane	AErrane	100-ml bottle	Induction: 5% Maintenance: 1.5–2.5%
Isoproterenol	Isuprel	0.2-mg/ml ampules for injection	10 μg/kg IM, SC q6hr; or dilute 1 mg in 500 ml of 5% dextrose or Ringer's solution and infuse IV 0.5–1 ml/min (1–2 μg/min) or to effect
Isosorbide dinitrate	Isordil, Isorbid, Sorbitrate	2.5-, 5-, 10-, 20-, 30-, and 40-mg tablets; 40-mg capsules	2.5–5 mg/animal PO q12hr (or 0.22–1.1 mg/kg PO q12hr)
Isosorbide mononitrate	Monoket	10- and 20-mg tablets	5 mg/dog PO two doses per day 7 hours apart
Isotretinoin	Accutane	10-, 20-, and 40-mg capsules	1–3 mg/kg/day (up to a maximum recommended dose of 3–4 mg/kg/day PO)
Itraconazole	Sporanox	100-mg capsules	Dog: 2.5 mg/kg PO q12hr or 5 mg/kg PO q24hr Cat: 1.5–3.0 mg/kg PO up to 5 mg/kg PO q24hr
Ivermectin	Heartguard, Ivomec, Eqvalan liquid	1% (10 mg/ml) injectable solution; 10-mg/ml oral solution; 18.7-mg/ml oral paste; 68-, 136-, and 272-μg tablets	Heartworm preventative: dog: 6 μg/kg PO q30days; cat: 24 μg/kg PO q30days Microfilaricide: 50 μg/kg PO 2 weeks after adulticide therapy Ectoparasite therapy (dog and cat): 200–300 μg/kg IM, SC, PO Endoparasites (dog and cat): 200–400 μg/kg SC, PO weekly Demodex therapy: 600 μg/kg/day PO for 60–120 days
Kanamycin	Kantrim	200- and 500-mg/ml injection	10 mg/kg IV, IM, SC q6–8hr
Kaopectate (kaolin + pectin)	Kaopectate	Oral suspension 12 oz	1–2 ml/kg PO q2–6hr
Ketamine	Ketalar, Ketavet, Vetalar	100-mg/ml injection solution	Dog: 5.5–22 mg/kg IV, IM (recommend adjunctive sedative or tranquilizer treatment) Cat: 2–25 mg/kg IV, IM (recommend adjunctive sedative or tranquilizer treatment)
Ketoconazole	Nizoral	200-mg tablet; 100-mg/ml oral suspension (only available in Canada)	Dog: 10–15 mg/kg PO q8–12hr (for *Malassezia canis* infection use 10 mg/kg PO q24hr or 5 mg/kg PO q12hr); Hyperadrenocorticism: 15 mg/kg PO q12hr Cat: 5–10 mg/kg PO q8–12hr
Ketoprofen	Orudis-KT (human OTC tablet); Ketofen (veterinary injection)	12.5-mg tablet (OTC); 100-mg/ml injection	Dog and cat: 1 mg/kg PO q24hr for up to 5 days or 2.0 mg/kg IV, IM, SC for one dose
Ketorolac tromethamine	Toradol	10-mg tablet; 15- and 30-mg/ml injection in 10% alcohol	Dog: 0.5 mg/kg PO, IM, IV q12hr for not more than 2 doses
L-Dopa	*See* Levodopa		

Drug Name	Other Names	Formulations Available	Dosage
Lactated Ringer's solution	Generic	250-, 500-, and 1,000-ml bags	Maintenance: 40–50 ml/kg/day IV Shock therapy dog: 90 ml/kg IV; cat: 60–70 ml/kg IV
Lactulose	Chronulac, generic	10 gm/15 ml	Constipation: 1 ml/4.5 kg PO q8hr (to effect) Hepatic encephalopathy: dog: 0.5 ml/kg PO q8hr; cat: 2.5–5 ml/cat PO q8hr
Leucovorin (folinic acid)	Wellcovorin and generic	5-, 10-, 15-, and 25-mg tablets; 3- and 5-mg/ml injection	With methotrexate administration: 3 mg/m² IV, IM, PO Antidote for pyrimethamine toxicosis: 1 mg/kg PO q24hr
Levamisole	Levasole, Tamisol, Ergamisol	0.184-gm bolus; 11.7 gm/13-gm packet; 50-mg tablet (Ergamisol)	Dog (hookworms): 5–8 mg/kg PO once (up to 10 mg/kg PO for 2 days) Microfilaricide: 10 mg/kg PO q24hr for 6–10 days Immunostimulant: 0.5–2 mg/kg PO 3 times/wk Cat: 4.4 mg/kg once PO (for lungworms: 20–40 mg/kg PO q48hr for five treatments)
Levodopa (L-dopa)	Larodopa, L-dopa	100-, 250-, and 500-mg tablets or capsules	Hepatic encephalopathy: 6.8 mg/kg initially then 1.4 mg/kg q6hr
Levothyroxine sodium (T₄)	Soloxine, Thyro-Tabs, Synthroid	0.1- to 0.8-mg tablets (in 0.1-mg increments)	Dog: 22 µg/kg PO q12hr (adjust dose via monitoring) Cat: 10–20 µg/kg/day PO (adjust dose via monitoring)
Lidocaine	Xylocaine and generic brands	5-, 10-, 15-, and 20-mg/ml injection	Dog (antiarrhythmic): 2–4 mg/kg IV (to a maximum dose of 8 mg/kg over 10-minute period); 25–75 µg/kg/min IV infusion; 6 mg/kg IM q1.5hr Cat (antiarrhythmic): 0.25–0.75 mg/kg IV slowly For epidural (dog and cat): 4.4 mg/kg of 2% solution
Lincomycin	Lincocin	100-, 200-, and 500-mg tablets	15–25 mg/kg PO q12hr For pyoderma: doses as low as 10 mg/kg q12hr have been used
Liothyronine (T₃)	Cytomel	60-µg tablet	4.4 µg/kg PO q8hr For T₃ suppression test (cats): collect presample for T₄ and T₃; administer 25 µg q8hr for 7 doses, then collect post samples for T₃ and T₄ after last dose
Lisinopril	Prinivil, Zestril	2.5-, 5-, 10-, 20-, and 40-mg tablets	Dog: 0.5 mg/kg PO q24hr Cat: no dose established
Lithium carbonate	Lithotabs	150-, 300-, and 600-mg capsules; 300-mg tablet; 300-mg/5 ml syrup	Dog: 10 mg/kg PO q12hr Cat: not recommended
Lomotil	*See* Diphenoxylate		
Loperamide	Imodium and generic	2-mg tablet; 0.2-mg/ml oral liquid	Dog: 0.1 mg/kg PO q8–12hr Cat: 0.08–0.16 mg/kg PO q12hr
Lufenuron	Program	45-, 90-, 135-, 204.9-, and 409.8-mg tablets; 135- and 270-mg suspension per unit pack	Dog: 10 mg/kg PO q30days Cat: 30 mg/kg PO q30days, 10 mg/kg SC q6mo
Lufenuron + milbemycin oxime	Sentinel tablets and Flavor Tabs	Milbemycin/lufenuron ratio is as follows: 2.3/46-mg tablets; 5.75/115, 11.5/230, and 23/460-mg Flavor Tabs	Administer 1 tablet q30days. Each tablet formulated for size of dog
Luteinizing hormone	*See* Gonadorelin		
Magnesium citrate	Citroma, Citro-Nesia (Citro-Mag in Canada)	Oral solution	2–4 ml/kg PO

Table continued on following page

Drug Name	Other Names	Formulations Available	Dosage
Magnesium hydroxide	Milk of Magnesia	Oral liquid	Antacid: 5–10 ml/kg PO q4–6hr Cathartic: dog: 15–50 PO ml/kg; cat: 2–6 ml/cat PO q24hr
Magnesium sulfate	Epsom salts	Crystals, many generic preparations	Dog: 8–25 gm/dog PO q24hr Cat: 2–5 gm/cat PO q24hr
Mannitol	Osmitrol	5–25% solution for injection	Diuretic: 1 gm/kg of 5–25% solution IV to maintain urine flow Glaucoma or central nervous system edema: 0.25–2 gm/kg of 15–25% solution IV over 30–60 min (repeat in 6 hr if necessary)
Marbofloxacin	Marbocyl, Zeniquin	25-, 50-, 100-, and 200-mg tablets	Dog: 2.75–5.55 mg/kg PO q24hr Cat: Dose not established
MCT oil	MCT oil (many sources)	Oral liquid	1–2 ml/kg/day in food
Mebendazole	Telmintic	Each gram of powder contains 40 mg	22 mg/kg (with food) q24hr for 3 days
Meclizine	Antivert, generic	12.5-, 25-, and 50-mg tablets	Dog: 25 mg PO q24hr (for motion sickness, administer 1 hr before traveling) Cat: 12.5 mg PO q24hr
Meclofenamic acid (meclofenamate sodium)	Arquel, Meclomen	50- and 100-mg capsules	Dog: 1 mg/kg/day PO for up to 5 days
Medetomidine	Domitor	1.0-mg/ml injection	750 μg/m² IV or 1,000 μg/m² IM
Medium-chain triglycerides	*See* MCT oil		
Medroxyprogesterone acetate	Depo-Provera (injection); Provera (tablets)	150- and 400-mg/ml suspension injection; 2.5-, 5-, and 10-mg tablets	1.1–2.2 mg/kg IM q7days; for behavioral use 10–20 mg/kg SC; for prostate 3–5 mg/kg SC, IM
Megestrol acetate	Ovaban	5-mg tablet	Dog: proestrus: 2 mg/kg PO q24hr for 8 days; anestrus: 0.5 mg/kg PO q24hr for 30 days; behavior: 2–4 mg/kg q24hr for 8 days (reduce dose for maintenance) Cat: dermatologic therapy or urine spraying: 2.5–5 mg/cat PO q24hr for 1 wk, then reduce to 5 mg once or twice/wk; suppress estrus: 5 mg/cat/day for 3 days, then 2.5–5 mg once/wk for 10 wk
Melarsomine	Immiticide	25-mg/ml injection; after reconstitution retains potency for 24 hr	Administer via deep IM injection. Class 1–2 dogs: 2.5 mg/kg/day for 2 consecutive days. Class 3 dogs: 2.5 mg/kg once, then in 1 mo two additional doses 24 hr apart
Melphalan	Alkeran	2-mg tablet	1.5 mg/m² (or 0.1–0.2 mg/kg) PO q24hr for 7–10 days (repeat every 3 wk)
Meperidine	Demerol	50- and 100-mg tablets; 10-mg/ml syrup; 25-, 50-, 75-, and 100-mg/ml injection	Dog: 5–10 mg/kg IV, IM as often as q2–3hr (or as needed) Cat: 3–5 mg/kg IV, IM q2–4hr (or as needed)
Mepivacaine	Carbocaine-V	2% (20 mg/ml) injection	Variable dose for local infiltration. For epidural, 0.5 ml of 2% solution q30sec until reflexes are absent
6-Mercaptopurine	Purinethol	50-mg tablet	50 mg/m² PO q24hr
Meropenem	Merrem	500 mg in 20-ml vial, or 1-gm vial in 30-ml vial for injection	20 mg/kg IV q8hr; for meningitis 40 mg/kg IV q8hr
Mesalamine	Asacol, Mesasal, Pentasa	400-mg tablet; 250-mg capsule	Veterinary dose has not been established. The usual human dose is 400–500 mg q6–8hr (also see Sulfasalazine, Olsalazine)

Drug Name	Other Names	Formulations Available	Dosage
Metamucil	*See* Psyllium (bulk-forming laxative)		
Metaproterenol	Alupent, Metaprel	10- and 20-mg tablets; 5-mg/ml syrup; inhalers	0.325–0.65 mg/kg PO q4–6hr
Methazolamide	Neptazane	25- and 50-mg tablets	2–4 mg/kg (to a maximum dose of 4–6 mg/kg) PO q8–12hr
Methenamine hippurate	Hiprex, Urex	1-gm tablet	Dog: 500 mg/dog PO q12hr Cat: 250 mg/cat PO q12hr
Methenamine mandelate	Mandelamine and generic	1-gm tablet; granules for oral solution; 50- and 100-mg/ml oral suspension	10–20 mg/kg PO q8–12hr
Methimazole	Tapazole	5- and 10-mg tablets	Cat: 2.5 mg/cat q12hr PO for 7–14 days then 5–10 mg/cat PO q12hr and adjust by monitoring T_4
DL-Methionine	*See* Racemethionine		
Methocarbamol	Robaxin-V	500- and 750-mg tablets; 100-mg/ml injection	44 mg/kg PO q8hr on the first day then 22–44 mg/kg PO q8hr
Methohexital	Brevital	0.5-, 2.5-, and 5-gm vials for injection	3–6 mg/kg IV (give slowly to effect)
Methotrexate	MTX, Mexate, Folex, Rheumatrex, generic	2.5-mg tablet; 2.5- or 25-mg/ml injection	2.5–5 mg/m² PO q48hr (dose depends on specific protocol) or Dog: 0.3–0.5 mg/kg IV once/wk Cat: 0.8 mg/kg IV q2–3wk
Methoxamine	Vasoxyl	20-mg/ml injection	200–250 µg/kg IM or 40–80 µg/kg IV
Methoxyflurane	Metofane	4-oz bottle for inhalation	Induction: 3%; maintenance: 0.5–1.5%
Methylene Blue 0.1%	Generic, also called New Methylene Blue	1% solution (10 mg/ml)	1.5 mg/kg IV, slowly
Methylprednisolone	Medrol	1-, 2-, 4-, 8-, 18-, and 32-mg tablets	0.22–0.44 mg/kg PO q12–24hr Compared to prednisolone, methylprednisolone is 1.25 times more potent.
Methylprednisolone acetate	Depo-Medrol	20- or 40-mg/ml suspension for injection	Dog: 1 mg/kg (or 20–40 mg/dog) IM q1–3wk Cat: 10–20 mg/cat IM q1–3wk
Methylprednisolone sodium succinate	Solu-Medrol	1- and 2-gm and 125- and 500-mg vials for injection	For emergency use: 30 mg/kg IV and repeat at 15 mg/kg IV in 2–6 hr For replacement or anti-inflammatory therapy, see Prednisolone
4-Methylpyrazole (fomepizole)	5% solution	Antizol-Vet (Fomepizole)	20 mg/kg initially IV, then 15 mg/kg at 12- and 24-hr intervals, then 5 mg at 36 hr
Methyltestosterone	Android, generic	10- and 25-mg tablets	Dog: 5–25 mg/dog PO q24–48h Cat: 2.5–5 mg/cat PO q24–48h
Metoclopramide	Reglan, Clopra, and others	5- and 10-mg tablets; 1-mg/ml oral solution; 5- mg/ml injection	0.2–0.5 mg/kg IV, IM, PO q6–8hr (or 1–2 mg/kg/day via continuous IV infusion—approximately 0.1–0.2 mg/kg/hr)
Metoprolol tartrate	Lopressor	50- and 100-mg tablets; 1 mg/ml injection	Dog: 5–50 mg/dog (0.5–1.0 mg/kg) PO q8hr Cat: 2–15 mg/cat PO q8hr
Metronidazole	Flagyl and generic	250- and 500-mg tablets; 50-mg/ml suspension; 5-mg/ml injection	For anaerobes: dog: 15 mg/kg PO q12hr or 12 mg/kg q8hr; cat: 10–25 mg/kg PO q24hr For *Giardia:* dog: 12–15 mg/kg PO q12hr for 8 days; cat: 17 mg/kg (⅓ tablet per cat) q24hr for 8 days
Mexiletine	Mexitil	150-, 200-, and 250-mg capsules	Dog: 5–8 mg/kg PO q8–12hr (use cautiously) *Table continued on following page*

Drug Name	Other Names	Formulations Available	Dosage
Mibolerone	Cheque-drops	55-μg/ml oral solution	Dog: 0.45–11.3 kg, 30 μg; 11.8–22.7 kg, 60 μg; 23–45.3 kg, 120 μg; >45.8 kg, 180 μg or approximately 2.6–5 μg/kg/day PO Cat: safe dose not established
Midazolam	Versed	5-mg/ml injection	0.1–0.25 mg/kg IV, IM (or 0.1–0.3 mg/kg/hr IV infusion)
Milbemycin oxime	Interceptor and Interceptor Flavor Tabs	23-, 11.5-, 5.75, and 2.3-mg tablets	Dog: microfilaricide; 0.5 mg/kg; demodex: 2 mg/kg PO q24hr for 60–120 days; heartworm prevention: 0.5 mg/kg PO q30days
Milk of Magnesia	*See* Magnesium hydroxide		
Mineral oil	Generic	Oral liquid	Dog: 10–50 ml/dog PO q12hr Cat: 10–25 ml/cat PO q12hr
Minocycline	Minocin	50- and 100-mg tablets; 10-mg/ml oral suspension	5–12.5 mg/kg PO q12hr
Misoprostol	Cytotec	0.1-mg (100 μg), 0.2-mg (200 μg) tablets	Dog: 2–5 μg/kg PO q6–8hr Cat: dose not established
Mithramycin	*See* Plicamycin (Mithracin)		
Mitotane (*o,p'*-DDD)	Lysodren	500-mg tablet	Dog: for pituitary-dependent hypercorticism: 50 mg/kg/day (in divided doses) PO for 5–10 days, then 50–70 mg/kg/week PO; for adrenal tumor: 50–75 mg/kg day for 10 days, then 75–100 mg/kg/wk PO
Mitoxantrone	Novantrone	2-mg/ml injection	Dog: 6 mg/m² IV q21days Cat: 6.5 mg/m² IV q21days
Morphine	Generic	1- and 15-mg/ml injection; 30- and 60-mg delayed-release tablets	Dog: 0.1–1 mg/kg IV, IM, SC (dose is escalated as needed for pain relief) q4–6hr; epidural: 0.1 mg/kg Cat: 0.1 mg/kg q3–6hr IM, SC (or as needed)
Moxidectin	Cydectin	Injection	Dog: heartworm prevention: 3 μg/kg; endoparasites: 25–300 μg/kg
Myochrysine	*See* Gold sodium thiomalate		
Naloxone	Narcan	20- or 400-μg/ml injection	0.01–0.04 mg/kg IV, IM, SC as needed to reverse opiate
Naltrexone	Trexan	50-mg tablet	For behavior problems: 2.2 mg/kg PO q12hr
Nandrolone decanoate	Deca-Durabolin	Nandrolone decanoate injection: 50, 100, and 200 mg/ml	Dog: 1–1.5 mg/kg/wk IM Cat: 1 mg/cat/wk IM
Naproxen	Naprosyn, Naxen, Aleve (naproxen sodium)	220-mg tablet (OTC); 25-mg/ml suspension liquid; 250-, 375-, and 500-mg tablets (Rx)	5 mg initially, then 2 mg/kg q48hr
Neomycin	Biosol	500-mg bolus; 200-mg/ml oral liquid	10–20 mg/kg PO q6–12hr
Neostigmine bromide and neostigmine methylsulfate	Prostigmin; Stiglyn	15-mg tablet (neostigmine bromide); 0.25- and 0.5-mg/ml injection (neostigmine methylsufate)	2 mg/kg/day PO (in divided doses, to effect) Injection: antimyasthenic: 10 μg/kg IM, SC, as needed; antidote for nondepolarizing neuromuscular block: 40 μg/kg IM, SC; diagnostic aid for myasthenia gravis: 40 μg/kg IM or 20 μg/kg IV
Nifedipine	Adalat, Procardia	10- and 20-mg capsules	Dose not established. In humans, the dose is 10 mg/human three times a day and increased in 10-mg increments to effect
Nitrates	*See* Nitroglycerin, Isosorbide dinitrate, or Nitroprusside		

Drug Name	Other Names	Formulations Available	Dosage
Nitrofurantoin	Macrodantin, Furalan, Furatoin, Furadantin, or generic	Macrodantin and generic 25-, 50-, and 100-mg capsules; Furalan, Furatoin, and generic 50- and 100-mg tablets; Furadantin 5-mg/ml oral suspension	10 mg/kg/day divided into four daily treatments, then 1 mg/kg PO at night
Nitroglycerin ointment	Nitrol, Nitro-Bid, Nitrostat	0.5-, 0.8-, 1-, 5-, and 10-mg/ml injection; 2% ointment; transdermal systems (0.2 mg/hr patch)	Dog: 4–12 mg (up to 15 mg) topically q12hr Cat: 2–4 mg topically q12hr (or ¼ inch of ointment per cat)
Nitroprusside	Nitropress	50-mg vial for injection	1–5, up to a maximum of 10 μg/kg/min IV infusion
Nizatidine	Axid	150- and 300-mg capsules	Dog: 5 mg/kg PO q24hr
Norfloxacin	Noroxin	400-mg tablet	22 mg/kg PO q12hr
o,p'-DDD	See Mitotane (Lysodren)		
Olsalazine	Dipentum	500-mg tablet	Dose not established (usual human dose is 500 mg or 5–10 mg/kg PO twice daily)
Omeprazole	Prilosec (formerly Losec), Gastrogard (equine paste)	20-mg capsule	Dog: 20 mg/dog PO once daily (or 0.7 mg/kg q24hr) Cat: not recommended
Ondansetron	Zofran	4- and 8-mg tablets; 2-mg/ml injection	0.5 to 1.0 mg/kg IV, PO 30 minutes before administration of cancer drugs
Orbifloxacin	Orbax	5.7-, 22.7-, and 68-mg tablets	2.5 to 7.5 mg/kg PO once daily
Ormetoprim	See Primor (ormetoprim-sulfadimethoxine)		
Oxacillin	Prostaphlin and generic	250- and 500-mg capsules; 50-mg/ml oral solution	22–40 mg/kg PO q8hr
Oxazepam	Serax	15-mg tablet	Cat: appetite stimulant: 2.5 mg/cat PO
Oxtriphylline	Choledyl-SA	400- and 600-mg tablet (oral solutions and syrup available in Canada but not US)	Dog: 47 mg/kg (equivalent to 30 mg/kg theophylline) PO q12hr
Oxybutynin chloride	Ditropan	5-mg tablet	Dog: 5 mg/dog PO q6–8hr
Oxymetholone	Anadrol	50-mg tablet	1–5 mg/kg/day PO
Oxymorphone	Numorphan	1.5- and 1-mg/ml injection	Dog, cat: analgesia: 0.1–0.2 mg/kg IV, SC, IM (as needed), redose with 0.05–0.1 mg/kg q1–2hr; preanesthetic: 0.025–0.05 mg/kg IM, SC
Oxytetracycline	Terramycin	250-mg tablets; 100- and 200-mg/ml injection	7.5–10 mg/kg IV q12hr; 20 mg/kg PO q12hr
Oxytocin	Pitocin and Syntocinon (nasal solution) and generic	10- and 20-U/ml injection; 40-U/ml nasal solution	Dog: 5–20 U/dog SC, IM (repeat every 30 min for primary inertia) Cat: 3–5 U/cat SC, IM (repeat every 30 min)
2-PAM	See Pralidoxime chloride		
Pancreatic enzyme	See Pancrelipase		
Pancrelipase	Viokase	16,800 U of lipase, 70,000 U of protease, and 70,000 U of amylase per 0.7 gm; also capsules and tablets	Mix 2 tsp powder with food per 20 kg body weight or 1–3 tsp/0.45 kg of food 20 min before feeding
Pancuronium bromide	Pavulon	1- and 2-mg/ml injection	0.1 mg/kg IV or start with 0.01 mg/kg and additional 0.01-mg/kg doses every 30 min
Paregoric	Corrective Mixture	2 mg morphine per 5 ml of paregoric	0.05–0.06 mg/kg PO q12hr
Paroxetine	Paxil	10-, 20-, 30-, and 40-mg tablets	Cat: ⅛ to ¼ of a 10-mg tablet daily PO
D-Penicillamine	Cuprimine, Depen	125- and 250-mg capsules and 250-mg tablets	10–15 mg/kg PO q12hr

Table continued on following page

Drug Name	Other Names	Formulations Available	Dosage
Penicillin G benzathine	Benza-Pen and other names	150,000 U/ml, combined with 150,000 U/ml of procaine penicillin G	24,000 U/kg IM q48hr
Penicillin G potassium; penicillin G sodium	Many brands	5- to 20-million unit vials	20,000–40,00 U/kg IV, IM q6–8hr
Penicillin G procaine	Generic	300,000 U/ml suspension	20,000–40,000 U/kg IM q12–24hr
Penicillin V	Pen-Vee	250- and 500-mg tablets	10 mg/kg PO q8hr
Pentazocine	Talwin-V	30-mg/ml injection	Dog: 1.65–3.3 mg/kg IM q4hr Cat: 2.2–3.3 mg/kg IV, IM, SC
Pentobarbital	Nembutal and generic	50 mg/ml	25–30 mg/kg IV
Pentoxifylline	Trental	400-mg tablet	Dog: For use in canine dermatology and for vasculitis, 10 mg/kg PO q12hr Cat: ¼ of 400-mg tab PO, q8–12hr
Pepto Bismol	*See* Bismuth subsalicylate		
Phenobarbital	Luminal and generic	15-, 30-, 60-, and 100-mg tablets; 30-, 60-, 65-, and 130-mg/ml injection; 4-mg/ml oral elixir solution	Dog: 2–8 mg/kg PO q12hr Cat: 2–4 mg/kg PO q12hr Dog and cat: adjust dose by monitoring plasma concentration Status epilepticus: administer in increments of 10–20 mg/kg IV (to effect)
Phenoxybenzamine	Dibenzyline	10-mg capsule	Dog: 0.25 mg/kg PO q8–12hr or 0.5 mg/kg q24hr Cat: 2.5 mg/cat q8–12hr or 0.5 mg/cat PO q12hr. (In cats, doses as high as 0.5 mg/kg IV have been used to relax urethral smooth muscle)
Phentolamine	Regitine (Rogitine in Canada)	5-mg vial for injection	0.02–0.1 mg/kg IV
Phenylbutazone	Butazolidin and generic	100-, 200-, 400-mg and 1-gm tablets; 200-mg/ml injection	Dog: 15–22 mg/kg PO, IV q8–12hr (44 mg/kg/day) (800 mg/dog maximum) Cat: 6–8 mg/kg IV, PO q12hr
Phenylephrine	Neo-Synephrine	10-mg/ml injection; 1% nasal solution	0.01 mg/kg IV q15min 0.1 mg/kg IM, SC q15min
Phenylpropanolamine	Dexatrim, Propagest and others	15-, 25-, 30-, and 50-mg tablets	1.5–2 mg/kg PO q12hr
Phenytoin	Dilantin	30- and 125-mg/ml oral suspension; 30- and 100-mg capsules; 50-mg/ml injection	Antiepileptic dog: 20–35 mg/kg q8hr Antiarrhythmic: 30 mg/kg PO q8hr or 10 mg/kg IV over 5 min
Physostigmine	Antilirium	1-mg/ml injection	0.02 mg/kg IV q12hr
Phytomenadione	*See* Vitamin K₁		
Phytonadione	*See* Vitamin K₁		
Piperacillin	Pipracil	2-, 3-, 4-, and 40-gm vials for injection	40 mg/kg IV or IM q6hr
Piperazine	Many	860-mg powder; 140-mg capsule, 170-, 340- and 800-mg/ml oral solution	44–66 mg/kg PO administered once
Piroxicam	Feldene and generic	10-mg capsule	Dog: 0.3 mg/kg PO q48hr Cat: dose not established
Pitressin (ADH)	*See* Vasopressin, Desmopressin acetate		
Plicamycin (old name is mithramycin)	Mithracin	2.5-mg injection	Dog: Antineoplastic: 25–30 μg/kg/day IV (slow infusion) for 8–10 days Antihypercalcemic: 25 μg/kg/day IV (slow infusion) over 4 hours Cat: Not recommended
Polyethylene glycol electrolyte solution	GoLYTELY	Oral solution	25 ml/kg PO repeat in 2–4 hr PO
Polysulfated glycosaminoglycan (PSGAG)	Adequan Canine	100-mg/ml injection in 5-ml vial (for horses vials are 250 mg/ml)	4.4 mg/kg IM twice weekly for up to 4 weeks

Drug Name	Other Names	Formulations Available	Dosage
Potassium bromide (KBr)	No commercial formulation	Usually prepared as oral solution	Dog and cat: 30–40 mg/kg PO q24hr If administered without phenobarbital higher doses of up to 40–50 mg/kg may be needed. Adjust doses by monitoring plasma concentrations. Loading doses of 400 mg/kg divided over 3 days have been administered.
Potassium chloride (KCl)	Generic	Various concentrations for injection (usually 2 mEq/ml); oral suspension and oral solution	0.5 mEq potassium/kg/day; or supplement 10–40 mEq/500 ml of fluids, depending on serum potassium
Potassium citrate	Generic, Urocit-K	5-mEq tablet; some forms are in combination with potassium chloride	2.2 mEq/100 kcal of energy/day PO or 40–75 mg/kg PO q12hr
Potassium gluconate	Kaon, Tumil-K, generic	2-mEq tablet; 500-mg tablet; Kaon elixir is 20-mg/15 ml elixir	Dog: 0.5 mEq/kg PO q12–24hr Cat: 2–8 mEq/day PO divided twice daily
Potassium iodide			30–100 mg/cat daily (in single or divided doses) for 10–14 days
Pralidoxime chloride (2-PAM)	2-PAM, Protopam Chloride	50-mg/ml injection	20 mg/kg q8–12hr (initial dose) IV slow or IM
Praziquantel	Droncit	23- and 34-mg tablets; 56.8-mg/ml injection	Dog (PO): <6.8 kg, 7.5 mg/kg, once; >6.8 kg, 5 mg/kg, once; (IM, SC): <2.3 kg, 7.5 mg/kg, once; 2.7–4.5 kg, 6.3 mg/kg, once; >5 kg, 5 mg/kg, once Cat (PO): <1.8 kg, 6.3 mg/kg, once; >1.8 kg, 5 mg/kg, once (for *Paragonimus* use 25 mg/kg q8hr for 2–3 days); (IM, SC): 5 mg/kg
Prazosin	Minipress	1-, 2-, and 5-mg capsules	0.5- and 2-mg/animal (1 mg/15 kg) PO q8–12hr
Prednisolone	Delta-Cortef and many others	5- and 20-mg tablets	Dog (cat often requires 2× dog dose) Anti-inflammatory: 0.5–1 mg/kg IV, IM, PO q12–24hr initially, then taper to q48hr Immunosuppressive: 2.2–6.6 mg/kg/day IV, IM, PO initially, then taper to 2–4 mg/kg q48hr Replacement therapy: 0.2–0.3 mg/kg/day PO Shock, spinal trauma: see Prednisolone sodium succinate
Prednisolone sodium succinate	Solu-Delta-Cortef	100- and 200-mg vials for injection (10 and 50 mg/ml)	Shock: 15–30 mg/kg IV (repeat in 4–6 hr) Central nervous system trauma: 15–30 mg/kg IV, taper to 1–2 mg/kg q12hr
Prednisone	Deltasone and generic; Meticorten for injection	1-, 2.5-, 5-, 10-, 20-, 25-, and 50-mg tablets; 1 mg/ml syrup (LiquidPred in 5% alcohol) and 1 mg/ml oral solution (in 5% alcohol); 10- and 40-mg/ml prednisone suspension for injection	Same as prednisolone
Primidone	Mylepsin, Neurosyn (Mysoline in Canada)	50- and 250-mg tablets	8–10 mg/kg PO q8–12hr as initial dose, then is adjusted via monitoring to 10–15 mg/kg q8hr
Primor (ormetoprim + sulfadimethoxine)	Primor	Combination tablet (ormetoprim + sulfadimethoxine)	27 mg/kg on first day, followed by 13.5 mg/kg PO q24hr *Table continued on following page*

Drug Name	Other Names	Formulations Available	Dosage
Procainamide	Pronestyl, generic	250-, 375-, 500-mg tablets or capsules; 100- and 500-mg/ml injection	Dog: 10–30 mg/kg PO q6hr (to a maximum dose of 40 mg/kg), 8–20 mg/kg IV, IM; 25–50 μg/kg/min IV infusion Cat: 3–8 mg/kg IM, PO q6–8hr
Prochlorperazine	Compazine	5-, 10-, and 25-mg tablets (prochlorperazine maleate); 5-mg/ml injection (prochlorperazine edisylate)	0.1–0.5 mg/kg IM, SC q6–8hr
Progesterone, repositol	*See* Medroxyprogesterone acetate		
Promethazine	Phenergan	6.25- and 25-mg/5 ml syrup; 12.5-, 25-, 50-mg tablets; 25- and 50-mg/ml injection	0.2–0.4 mg/kg IV, IM, PO q6–8hr (up to a maximum dose of 1 mg/kg)
Propantheline bromide	Pro-Banthine	7.5- and 15-mg tablet	0.25–0.5 mg/kg PO q8–12hr
Propiomazine	Tranvet, Largon	20-mg/ml injection	1.1–4.4 mg/kg q12–24hr
Propofol	Rapinovet and PropoFlo (veterinary); Diprivan (human)	1% (10 mg/ml) injection in 20-ml ampules	6.6 mg/kg IV slowly over 60 seconds. Constant-rate IV infusions have been used at 2 mg/kg/hr
Propranolol	Inderal	10-, 20-, 40-, 60-, 80-, and 90-mg tablets; 1-mg/ml injection; 4- and 8-mg/ml oral solution	Dog: 20–60 μg/kg over 5–10 min IV; 0.2–1 mg/kg PO q8hr (titrate dose to effect) Cat: 0.4–1.2 mg/kg (2.5–5 mg/cat) PO q8hr
Propylthiouracil (PTU)	Generic, Propyl-Thyracil	50- and 100-mg tablets	11 mg/kg PO q12hr
Prostaglandin F2 alpha (dinoprost)	Lutalyse	5-mg/ml solution for injection	Pyometra: dog: 0.1–0.2 mg/kg SC once daily for 5 days; cat: 0.1–0.25 mg/kg SC once daily for 5 days Abortion: dog: 0.025–0.05 mg (25–50 μg)/kg IM q12hr; cat: 0.5–1 mg/kg IM for 2 injections
Pseudoephedrine	Sudafed and many others (some formulations have other ingredients)	30- and 60-mg tablets; 120-mg capsule; 6-mg/ml syrup	0.2–0.4 mg/kg (or 15–60 mg/dog) PO q8–12hr
Psyllium	Metamucil and others	Available as powder	1 tsp/5–10 kg (added to each meal)
Pyrantel pamoate	Nemex, Strongid	180-mg/ml paste and 50-mg/ml suspension	Dog: 5 mg/kg PO once and repeat in 7–10 days Cat: 20 mg/kg PO once
Pyridostigmine bromide	Mestinon, Regonol	12-mg/ml oral syrup; 60-mg tablet; 5-mg/ml injection	Antimyasthenic: 0.02–0.04 mg/kg IV q2hr or 0.5–3 mg/kg PO q8–12hr Antidote (nondepolarizing muscle relaxant): 0.15–0.3 mg/kg IM, IV
Pyrimethamine	Daraprim	25-mg tablet	Dog: 1 mg/kg PO q24hr for 14–21 days (5 days for *Neosporum caninum*) Cat: 0.5–1 mg/kg PO q24hr for 14–28 days
Quibron	*See* Theophylline		
Quinacrine	Atabrine (no longer available in US)	100-mg tablet	Dog: 6.6 mg/kg PO q12hr for 5 days Cat: 11 mg/kg PO q24hr for 5 days
Quinidine gluconate	Quiniglute, Duraquin	324-mg tablets; 80-mg/ml injection	Dog: 6–20 mg/kg IM q6hr; 6–20 mg/kg PO q6–8hr (of base)
Quinidine sulfate	Cin-Quin, Quinora	100-, 200-, and 300-mg tablets; 200- and 300-mg capsules; 20-mg/ml injection	Dog: 6–20 mg/kg PO q6–8hr (of base); 5–10 mg/kg IV
Quinidine polygalacturonate	Cardioquin	275-mg tablet	Dog: 6–20 mg/kg PO q6hr (of base) (275 mg quinidine polygalacturonate = 167 mg quinidine base)
Racemethionine (DL-methionine)	Uroeze, MethioForm, and generic. Human forms include Pedameth, Uracid, and generic	500-mg tablets and powders added to animal's food; 75-mg/5 ml pediatric oral solution; 200-mg capsule	Dog: 150–300 mg/kg/day PO Cat: 1–1.5 gm/cat PO (added to food each day)

Drug Name	Other Names	Formulations Available	Dosage
Ranitidine	Zantac	75-, 150-, and 300-mg tablets; 150- and 300-mg capsules; 25-mg/ml injection	Dog: 2 mg/kg IV, PO q8hr Cat: 2.5 mg/kg IV q12hr, 3.5 mg/kg PO q12hr
Retinoids	*See* Isotretinoin (Accutane), Retinol (Aquasol-A), or Etretinate (Tegison)		
Retinol	*See* Vitamin A (Aquasol-A)		
Riboflavin (vitamin B₂)	*See* Vitamin B₂		
Rifampin	Rifadin	150- and 300-mg capsules	10–20 mg/kg PO q24hr
Ringer's solution	Generic	250-, 500-, and 1000-ml bags for infusion	40–50 mg/kg/day IV, SC, IP
Salicylate	*See* Aspirin, acetylsalicylic acid		
Selegiline (deprenyl)	Anipryl (also known as deprenyl, and *l*-deprenyl); human dose form is Eldepryl	2-, 5-, 10-, 15-, and 30-mg tablets	Dog: begin with 1 mg/kg PO q24hr. If there is no response within 2 months, increase dose to maximum of 2 mg/kg PO q24hr Cat: dose not established
Senna	Senokot	Granules in concentrate, or syrup	Cat: syrup: 5 ml/cat q24hr; granules: ½ teaspoon/cat q24hr (with food)
Septra (sulfamethoxazole + trimethoprim)	*See* Trimethoprim/sulfonamides		
Sodium bicarbonate (NaHCO₃)	Generic, Baking Soda, Soda Mint	325-, 520-, and 650-mg tablets; injection of various strengths (4.2% to 8.4%), and 1 mEq/ml	Acidosis: 0.5–1 mEq/kg IV Renal failure: 10 mg/kg PO q8–12hr Alkalization of urine: 50 mg/kg PO q8–12hr (1 tsp is approximately 2 gm)
Sodium chloride 0.9%	Generic	500- and 1,000-ml infusion	40–50 ml/kg/day IV, SC, IP
Sodium chloride 7.5%	Generic	Infusion	2–8 ml/kg IV
Sodium iodide 20%	Iodopen, generic	100 μg elemental iodide (118 μg sodium iodide) per ml injection	20–40 mg/kg PO q8–12hr
Sodium thiomalate	*See* Gold sodium thiomalate		
Somatrem, Somatropin	*See* Growth hormone		
Sotalol	Betapace	80-, 160-, 240-mg tablets	Dog: 1–2 mg/kg PO q12hr. (One can start with 40 mg/dog q12hr, then increase to 80 mg if no response) Cat: 1–2 mg/kg PO q12hr
Spironolactone	Aldactone	25-, 50-, and 100-mg tablets	2–4 mg/kg/day (or 1–2 mg/kg PO q12hr)
Stanozolol	Winstrol-V	50-mg/ml injection; 2-mg tablet	Dog: 2 mg/dog (or range of 1–4 mg/dog) PO q12hr; 25–50 mg/dog/wk IM Cat: 1 mg/cat PO q12hr; 25 mg/cat/wk IM
Succimer	Chemet	100-mg capsule	10 mg/kg PO q8hr for 5 days, then 10 mg/kg PO q12hr for 2 more weeks
Sucralfate	Carafate (Sulcrate in Canada)	1-gm tablet; 200-mg/ml oral suspension	Dog: 0.5–1 gm/dog PO q8–12hr Cat: 0.25 gm/cat PO q8–12hr
Sufentanil citrate	Sufenta	50-μg/ml injection	2 μg/kg IV, up to a maximum dose of 5 μg/kg
Sulfadiazine	Generic, combined with trimethoprim in Tribrissen	500-mg tablet	100 mg/kg IV, PO (loading dose), followed by 50 mg/kg IV, PO q12hr (see also Trimethoprim)
Sulfadimethoxine	Albon, Bactrovet, and generic	125-, 250-, and 500-mg tablets; 400-mg/ml injection; 50-mg/ml suspension	55 mg/kg PO (loading dose), followed by 27.5 mg/kg PO q12hr (see also Primor)
Sulfamethazine	Many brands (e.g., Sulmet)	30-gm bolus	100 mg/kg PO (loading dose), followed by 50 mg/kg PO q12hr

Table continued on following page

Drug Name	Other Names	Formulations Available	Dosage
Sulfamethoxazole	Gantanol	50-mg tablet	100 mg/kg PO (loading dose), followed by 50 mg/kg PO q12hr (see also Bactrim, Septra)
Sulfasalazine (sulfapyridine + mesalamine)	Azulfidine (Salazopyrin in Canada)	500-mg tablet	10–30 mg/kg PO q8–12hr (see also Mesalamine, Olsalazine)
Sulfisoxazole	Gantrisin	500-mg tablet; 500-mg/5 ml syrup	50 mg/kg PO q8hr (urinary tract infections)
Sulfobromophthalein sodium	Bromsulphalein (BSP) (this drug's availability is limited)		5 mg/kg IV, collect plasma or serum 30 min after BSP injection
Tamoxifen	Nolvadex	10- and 20-mg tablets (tamoxifen citrate)	Veterinary dose not established. 10 mg PO q12hr is human dose
Taurine	Generic	Available in powder	Dog: 500 mg PO q12hr Cat: 250 mg/cat PO q12hr
Telezol	*See* Tiletamine-Zolazepam		
Terbutaline	Brethine, Bricanyl	2.5- and 5-mg tablets; 1-mg/ml injection (equivalent to 0.82 mg/ml)	Dog: 1.25–5 mg/dog PO q8hr Cat: 0.1–0.2 mg/kg PO q12hr (or 0.625 mg/cat, ¼ of 2.5-mg tablet)
Terfenadine	No longer available (Seldane)		
Testosterone cypionate ester	Andro-Cyp, Andronate, Depo-Testosterone and other forms	100- and 200-mg/ml injection	1–2 mg/kg IM q2–4wk (see also Methyltestosterone)
Testosterone propionate ester	Testex (Malogen in Canada)	100-mg/ml injection	0.5–1 mg/kg 2–3 times/wk IM
Tetracycline	Panmycin	250- and 500-mg capsules; 100-mg/ml suspension	15–20 mg/kg PO q8hr; or 4.4–11 mg/kg IV, IM q8hr
Thenium closylate	Canopar	500-mg tablet	Dog: >4.5 kg: 500 mg PO once, repeat in 2–3 weeks; 2.5–4.5 kg: 250 mg q12hr for 1 day, repeat in 2–3 weeks
Theophylline	Many brands and generic	100-, 125-, 200-, 250-, and 300-mg tablets; 27-mg/5 ml oral solution or elixir; injection in 5% dextrose	Dog: 9 mg/kg PO q6–8hr Cat: 4 mg/kg PO q8–12hr (see also Aminophylline)
Theophylline sustained-release	Theo-Dur, Slo-bid Gyrocaps	100-, 200-, 300-, and 450-mg tablets (Theo-Dur); 50- to 200-mg capsules (Slo-bid)	Dog: 20 mg/kg PO q12hr (Theo-Dur); 30 mg/kg q12hr (Slo-bid) Cat: 25 mg/kg PO q24hr (at night) for Theo-Dur and Slo-bid
Thiabendazole	Omnizole, Equizole	2 or 4 gm per oz (30 ml) suspension or liquid	Dog: 50 mg/kg q24hr for 3 days, repeat in 1 mo; respiratory parasites: 30–70 mg/kg PO q12hr Cat: *Strongyloides:* 125 mg/kg q24hr for 3 days
Thiacetarsamide sodium	Caparsolate	10 mg/ml	Dog: 2.2 mg/kg IV twice daily for 2 days Cat: not recommended
Thiamine (vitamin B₁)	Bewon and others	250-µg/5 ml elixir; tablets of various size from 5 mg to 500 mg; 100- and 500-mg/ml injection	Dog: 10–100 mg/dog/day PO Cat: 5–30 mg/cat/day PO (up to a maximum dose of 50 mg/cat/day)
Thiamylal sodium	No longer available. Substitute Thiopental		
Thioguanine (6-TG)	Generic	40-mg tablet	40 mg/m² PO q24hr
Thiomalate sodium	*See* Gold sodium thiomalate		
Thiopental sodium	Pentothal	Various size vials from 250 mg to 10 gm (mix to desired concentration)	Dog: 10–25 mg/kg IV (to effect) Cat: 5–10 mg/kg IV (to effect)
Thiotepa	Generic	15-mg injection (usually in solution of 10 mg/ml)	0.2–0.5 mg/m² weekly, or daily for 5–10 days IM, intracavitary, or intratumor
Thyroid hormone	*See* Levothyroxine sodium (T₄), or Liothyronine		

Drug Name	Other Names	Formulations Available	Dosage
Thyrotropin, thyroid-stimulating hormone (TSH)	Thytropar	10-U vial	Dog: collect baseline sample, followed by 0.1 U/kg IV (maximum dose is 5 U); collect post-TSH sample at 6 hr Cat: collect baseline sample, followed by 2.5 U/cat IM and collect a post-TSH sample at 8–12 hr
Ticarcillin	Ticar, Ticillin	6-gm/50 ml vial; vials containing 1, 3, 6, 20, and 30 gm	33–50 mg/kg IV, IM q4–6hr
Ticarcillin + clavulanate	Timentin	3-gm/vial for injection	Dose according to rate for ticarcillin
Tiletamine + zolazepam	Telazol, Zoletil	50 mg of each component per milliliter	5–7 mg/kg IM
Tobramycin	Nebcin	40-mg/ml injection	2–4 mg/kg IV, IM, SC q8hr
Tocainide	Tonocard	400- and 600-mg tablets	Dog: 15–20 mg/kg PO q8hr Cat: no dose established
Toluene	Vermiplex		267 mg/kg PO (of toluene), repeat in 2–4 wk
Trandolapril	Mavik	1-, 2-, and 4-mg tablets	Not established for dogs. Human dose is 1 mg/person/day to start, then increase to 2–4 mg/day
Triamcinolone	Vetalog, Trimtabs, Aristocort, generic	Veterinary (Vetalog) 0.5- and 1.5-mg tablets. Human form: 1-, 2-, 4-, 8-, and 16-mg tablets; 10-mg/ml injection	Anti-inflammatory: 0.5–1 mg/kg PO q12–24hr, then taper dose to 0.5–1 PO mg/kg q48hr (however, manufacturer recommends doses of 0.11 to 0.22 mg/kg/day)
Triamcinolone acetonide	Vetalog	2- or 6-mg/ml suspension injection; 0.5- and 1.5-mg tablets	0.1–0.2 mg/kg IM, SC, repeat in 7–10 days Intralesional: 1.2–1.8 mg, or 1 mg for every cm diameter of tumor q2wk
Triamterene	Dyrenium	50- and 100-mg capsules	1–2 mg/kg PO q12hr
Tribrissen	*See* Trimethoprim-sulfadimethoxine combination		
Trientine hydrochloride	Syprine	250-mg capsule	10–15 mg/kg PO q12hr
Trifluoperazine	Stelazine	10-mg/ml oral solution; 1-, 2-, 5-, and 10-mg tablets; 2-mg/ml injection	0.03 mg/kg IM q12hr
Triflupromazine	Vesprin	10- and 20-mg/ml injection	0.1–0.3 mg/kg IM, PO q8–12hr
Tri-iodothyronine	*See* Liothyronine		
Trimeprazine tartrate	Temaril (Panectyl in Canada)	2.5-mg/5 ml syrup; 2.5-mg tablet	0.5 mg/kg PO q12hr
Trimethobenzamide	Tigan and others	100-mg/ml injection; 100- and 250-mg capsules	Dog: 3 mg/kg IM, PO q8hr Cat: not recommended
Trimethoprim + sulfonamides (sulfadiazine or sulfamethoxazole)	Tribrissen and others	30-, 120-, 240-, 480-, and 960-mg tablets	15 mg/kg PO q12hr, or 30 mg/kg PO q12–24hr (for *Toxoplasma*: 30 mg/kg PO q12hr)
Tripelennamine	Pelamine, PBZ	25- and 50-mg tablets; 20-mg/ml injection	1 mg/kg PO q12hr
TSH (thyroid-stimulating hormone)	*See* Thyrotropin		
Tylosin	Tylocine, Tylan, Tylosin tartrate	Available as soluble powder 2.2 gm tylosin per tsp (tablets for dogs in Canada)	Dog and cat: 7–15 mg/kg PO q12–24hr Dog: for colitis: 11 mg/kg q8hr with food
Urofollitropin (FSH)	Metrodin	75-U/vial for injection	Doses not established
Ursodiol (ursodeoxycholate)	Actigall	300-mg capsule	10–15 mg/kg PO q24hr
Valproic acid, divalproex	Depakene (valproic acid); Depakote (divalproex)	125-, 250-, and 500-mg tablets (Depakote); 250-mg capsule; 50-mg/ml syrup (Depakene)	Dog: 60–200 mg/kg PO q8hr; or 25–105 mg/kg/day PO when administered with phenobarbital

Table continued on following page

Drug Name	Other Names	Formulations Available	Dosage
Vancomycin	Vancocin, Vancoled	Vials for injection (0.5 to 10 gm)	Dog: 15 mg/kg q6–8hr IV infusion Cat: 12–15 mg/kg q8hr IV infusion
Vasopressin (ADH)	Pitressin	20 U/ml (aqueous)	10 U IV, IM
Verapamil	Calan, Isoptin	40-, 80-, and 120-mg tablet; 2.5-mg/ml injection	Dog: 0.05 mg/kg IV q10–30min (maximum cumulative dose is 0.15 mg/kg) Cat: 1.1–2.9 mg/kg PO q8hr
Vinblastine	Velban	1-mg/ml injection	2 mg/m² IV (slow infusion) once/week
Vincristine	Oncovin, Vincasar, generic	1-mg/ml injection	Antitumor: 0.5–0.7 mg/m² IV (or 0.025–0.05 mg/kg) once/wk For thrombocytopenia: 0.02 mg/kg IV once/wk
Viokase	*See* Pancrelipase		
Vitamin A (retinoids)	Aquasol A	Oral solution: 5,000 U (1,500 RE) per 0.1 ml 10,000-, 25,000- and 50,000-U tablets	625–800 U/kg PO q24hr
Vitamin B₁	*See* Thiamine		
Vitamin B₂ (riboflavin)	Riboflavin	Various-size tablets in increments from 10 to 250 mg	Dog: 10–20 mg/day PO Cat: 5–10 mg/day PO
Vitamin B₁₂ (cyanocobalamin)	Cyanocobalamin	Various-size tablets in increments from 25 to 100 µg and injections	Dog: 100–200 µg/day PO Cat: 50–100 µg/day PO
Vitamin C (ascorbic acid)	See Ascorbic acid	Tablets of various sizes and injection	100–500 mg/day
Vitamin D	*See* Dihdyrotachysterol or Ergocalciferol		
Vitamin E (alpha-tocopherol)	Aquasol E, and generic	Wide variety of capsules, tablets, oral solution available (e.g., 1,000 units per capsule)	100–400 units PO q12hr (or 400–600 U PO q12hr for immune-mediated skin disease)
Vitamin K₁ (phytonadione, phytomenadione)	AquaMEPHYTON (injection), Mephyton (tablets); Veta-K1 (capsules)	2- or 10-mg/ml injection; 5-mg tablet (Mephyton) 25-mg capsule (Veta-K1)	Short-acting rodenticides: 1 mg/kg/day IV, IM, SC, PO for 10–14 days Long-acting rodenticides: 2.5–5 mg/kg/day IV, IM, SC, PO for 3–4 wk Birds: 2.5–5 mg/kg q24hr
Warfarin	Coumadin, generic	1-, 2-, 2.5-, 4-, 5-, 7.5-, and 10-mg tablets	Dog: 0.1–0.2 mg/kg PO q24hr Cat: (thromboembolism) start with 0.5 mg/cat/day and adjust dose based on clotting time assessment
Xylazine	Rompun and generic	20- and 100-mg/ml injection	Dog: 1.1 mg/kg IV, 2.2 mg/kg IM Cat: 1.1 mg/kg IM (emetic dose is 0.4–0.5 mg/kg IV)
Yohimbine	Yobine	2-mg/ml injection	0.11 mg/kg IV or 0.25–0.5 mg/kg SC, IM
Zidovudine (AZT)	Retrovir	10-mg/ml syrup; 10-mg/ml injection	Cat: 15 mg/kg PO q12hr to 20 mg/kg q8hr (doses as high as 30 mg/kg/day also have been used)
Zolazepam	*See* Tiletamine-zolazepam combination		

Note: Doses listed are for dogs *and* cats, unless otherwise listed. Many of the doses listed are extra-label or are human drugs used in an off-label or extra-label manner. Doses listed are based on best available evidence at the time of table preparation; however the author cannot ensure efficacy of drugs used according to recommendations in this table. Adverse effects may be possible from drugs listed in this table of which author was not aware at the time of table preparation. Veterinarians using these tables are encouraged to check current literature, product label, and the manufacturer's disclosure for information regarding efficacy and any known adverse effects or contraindications not identified at the time of preparation of these tables.

IM, intramuscular; IV, intravenous; OTC, over-the-counter (without prescription); Rx, prescription only; PO, per os (oral); SC, subcutaneous; U, units.

INDEX

Note: Page numbers followed by the letter f refer to figures; those followed by the letter t refer to tables. Page numbers following roman numeral XII refer to pages in the previous edition.

ISBN 0-7216-5523-8

Conversion Table (Weight to Body Surface in Square Meters) For Dogs*

kg	m²	kg	m²	kg	m²	kg	m²
0.5	0.06	26.0	0.88	13.0	0.55	39.0	1.15
1.0	0.10	27.0	0.90	14.0	0.58	40.0	1.17
2.0	0.15	28.0	0.92	15.0	0.60	41.0	1.19
3.0	0.20	29.0	0.94	16.0	0.63	42.0	1.21
4.0	0.25	30.0	0.96	17.0	0.66	43.0	1.23
5.0	0.29	31.0	0.99	18.0	0.69	44.0	1.25
6.0	0.33	32.0	1.01	19.0	0.71	45.0	1.26
7.0	0.36	33.0	1.03	20.0	0.74	46.0	1.28
8.0	0.40	34.0	1.05	21.0	0.76	47.0	1.30
9.0	0.43	35.0	1.07	22.0	0.78	48.0	1.32
10.0	0.46	36.0	1.09	23.0	0.81	49.0	1.34
11.0	0.49	37.0	1.11	24.0	0.83	50.0	1.36
12.0	0.52	38.0	1.13	25.0	0.85		

*From Ettinger SJ: *Textbook of Veterinary Internal Medicine, Diseases of the Dog and Cat,* 2nd edition. Philadelphia, WB Saunders Co, 1975, p 146.

Although the above chart was compiled for dogs, it can also be used for cats. A formula for more precise values follows: BSA in $m^2 = (K \times W^{2/3}) \times 10^{-4}$ where m^2 = square meters, BSA = body surface area, W = weight in gm, and K = constant of 10.1 in dogs and 10.0 in cats.

Système International (SI) Units in Clinical Chemistry

Analyte	Traditional Unit (with examples)	Conversion Factor	SI Unit (with examples)
Alanine aminotransferase	0–40 U/L	1.00	0–40 U/L
Albumin	2.8–4.0 gm/dl	10.0	28–40 gm/L
Alkaline phosphatase	30–150 U/L	1.00	30–150 U/L
Ammonia	10–80 µg/dl	0.5871	5.9–47.0 µmol/L
Amylase	200–800 U/L	1.00	200–800 U/L
Aspartate aminotransferase	0–40 U/L	1.00	0–40 U/L
Bile acids (total)	0.3–2.3 µg/ml	2.45	0.74–5.64 µmol/L
Bilirubin	0.1–0.2 mg/dl	17.10	2–4 µmol/L
Calcium	8.8–10.3 mg/dl	0.2495	2.20–2.58 mmol/L
Carbon dioxide	22–28 mEq/L	1.00	22–28 mmol/L
Chloride	95–100 mEq/L	1.00	95–100 mmol/L
Cholesterol	100–265 mg/dl	0.0258	2.58–5.85 mmol/L
Copper	70–140 µg/dl	0.1574	11.0–22.0 µmol/L
Cortisol	2–10 µg/dl	27.59	55–280 nmol/L
Creatine kinase	0–130 U/L	1.00	0–130 U/L
Creatinine	0.6–1.2 mg/dl	88.40	50–110 µmol/L
Fibrinogen	200–400 mg/dl	0.01	2.0–4.0 gm/L
Folic acid	3.5–11.0 µg/L	2.265	7.93–24.92 nmol/L
Glucose	70–110 mg/dl	0.05551	3.9–6.1 mmol/L
Iron	80–180 µg/dl	0.1791	14–32 µmol/L
Lactate	5–20 mg/dl	0.1110	0.5–2.0 mmol/L
Lead	150 µg/dl	0.04826	7.2 µmol/L
Lipase Sigma Tietz (37°C)	≤1 ST U/dl	280	≤280 U/L
Lipase Cherry Crandall (30°C)	0–160 U/L	1.00	0–160 U/L
Lipids (total)	400–850 mg/dl	0.01	4.0–8.5 gm/L
Magnesium	1.8–3.0 mg/dl	0.4114	0.80–1.20 mmol/L
Mercury	≤1.0 µg/dl	49.85	≤50 nmol/L
Osmolality	280–300 mOsm/kg	1.00	280–300 mmol/kg
Phosphorus	2.5–5.0 mg/dl	0.3229	0.80–1.6 mmol/L
Potassium	3.5–5.0 mEq/L	1.0	3.5–5.0 mmol/L
Protein (total)	5–8 gm/dl	10.0	50–80 gm/L
Sodium	135–147 mEq/L	1.00	135–147 mmol/L
Testosterone	4.0–8.0 mg/ml	3.467	14.0–28.0 nmol/L
Thyroxine	1–4 µg/dl	12.87	13–51 nmol/L
Triglyceride	10–500 mg/dl	0.0113	0.11–5.65 mmol/L
Urea nitrogen	10–20 mg/dl	0.3570	3.6–7.1 nmol/L
Uric acid	3.6–7.7 mg/dl	59.44	214–458 µmol/L
Urobilinogen	0–4.0 mg/dl	16.9	0.0–6.8 µmol/L
Vitamin A	90 µg/dl	0.03491	3.1 µmol/L
Vitamin B_{12}	300–700 ng/L	0.738	221–516 pmol/L
Vitamin E	5.0–20.0 mg/L	2.32	11.6–46.4 µmol/L
D-Xylose	30–40 mg/dl	0.06666	2.0–2.71 mmol/L
Zinc	75–120 µg/dl	0.1530	11.5–18.5 µmol/L